DISEASES OF THE KIDNEY

DISEASES OF THE KIDNEY

FIFTH EDITION

VOLUME II

EDITED BY

ROBERT W. SCHRIER, M.D.
Professor and Chairman, Department of Medicine,
University of Colorado School of Medicine,
Denver, Colorado

CARL W. GOTTSCHALK, M.D.
Career Investigator, American Heart Association;
Kenan Professor of Medicine and Physiology,
University of North Carolina School of Medicine,
Chapel Hill, North Carolina

LITTLE, BROWN and COMPANY
BOSTON/TORONTO/LONDON

Fifth Edition

Library of Congress Cataloging-in-Publication Data

Diseases of the kidney—5th ed. / edited by
Robert W. Schrier, Carl W. Gottschalk.
p. cm.
Includes bibliographical references and index.
ISBN 0-316-77501-0
1. Kidneys—Diseases. I. Schrier, Robert W.
II. Gottschalk, Carl W.
[DNLM: 1. Kidney Diseases. WJ 300 D611]
RC902.D57 1992
616.6'1—dc20
DNLM/DLC
for Library of Congress 92-15282
CIP

Printed in the United States of America

MV-NY

Contents

Preface xv
Contributing Authors xvii
Acknowledgment xxix

VOLUME I

I
Biochemical, Structural, and Functional Correlations in the Kidney

1. Structural–Functional Relationships in the Kidney 3
   Steven C. Hebert
   Wilhelm Kriz
2. Renal Circulation and Glomerular Hemodynamics 65
   William J. Arendshorst
   L. Gabriel Navar
3. Regulation of Water Balance: Urine Concentration and Dilution 119
   William E. Lassiter
   Carl W. Gottschalk
4. Tubular Sodium Transport 139
   W. Brian Reeves
   Thomas E. Andreoli
5. Tubular Potassium Transport 181
   Heino Velàzquez
   Fred S. Wright
6. Renal Acid-Base Transport 207
   Michael F. Flessner
   Mark A. Knepper
7. Renal Metabolism 233
   Anton C. Schoolwerth
   Krystyna Drewnowska
8. Renal Transport of Organic Anions and Cations 261
   T. Dwight McKinney
9. Hormones and the Kidney 283
   Ralph Rabkin
   David C. Dahl

II
Clinical Evaluation of the Kidney

10. Urinalysis 335
    Kenneth F. Fairley
11. Laboratory Evaluation of Renal Function 361
    Jeanine A. Carlson
    John T. Harrington
12. Intravenous Urography, Ultrasonography, and Radionuclide Studies 407
    Judith A. W. Webb
    Keith E. Britton
13. Computed Tomography and Magnetic Resonance Imaging 449
    Barbara E. Demas
    Hedvig Hricak
14. Diagnostic and Therapeutic Angiography of the Renal Circulation 465
    Mark H. Knelson
    N. Reed Dunnick
15. Indications for and Interpretation of the Renal Biopsy: Evaluation by Light, Electron, and Immunofluorescence Microscopy 485
    C. Craig Tisher
    Byron P. Croker

III
Hereditary Diseases of the Kidney

16. Medullary and Miscellaneous Renal Cystic Disorders 513
    Kenneth D. Gardner, Jr.
17. Medullary Sponge Kidney 525
    Edmund R. Yendt
18. Polycystic Kidney Disease 535
    Patricia A. Gabow
    Jared J. Grantham
19. Alport Syndrome 571
    Martin C. Gregory
    Curtis L. Atkin
20. Fabry's Disease and Nail-Patella Syndrome 593
    Karen A. Douek
    William M. Bennett
21. Isolated Renal Tubular Disorders 611
    Aaron L. Friedman
    Russell W. Chesney

IV
Urologic Diseases of the Genitourinary Tract

22. Congenital Urologic Anomalies 637
    William A. Cook
    F. Douglas Stephens
23. Urinary Tract Obstruction 657
    Douglas R. Wilson
    Saulo Klahr
24. Vesicoureteric Reflux and Reflux Nephropathy 689
    Ross R. Bailey
    Thomas M. J. Maling
    Charles P. Swainson

25. Urolithiasis 729
Charles Y. C. Pak

26. Prostatitis, Orchitis, and Epididymitis—Acute and Chronic 743
Edwin M. Meares, Jr.

27. Disorders of Micturition 759
M. Susan Tucker
Steven J. Stafford

V
Neoplasms of the Genitourinary Tract

28. Molecular Mechanisms of Malignancy 777
Harry A. Drabkin
York E. Miller

29. Primary Neoplasms of the Kidney and Renal Pelvis 785
Marc B. Garnick
Jerome P. Richie

30. Bladder Carcinoma and Uroepithelial Carcinomas 811
Harold A. Frazier, II
David F. Paulson

31. Prostatic Carcinoma 835
L. Michael Glode

32. Testicular Carcinoma 851
John N. Wettlaufer
Paul H. Lange

VI
Infections of Urinary Tract and Kidney

33. Host Defense Mechanisms in Urinary Tract Infections 885
Jack D. Sobel
Donald Kaye
Harald Reinhart

34. Urinary Tract Tuberculosis 909
Mark S. Pasternack
Robert H. Rubin

35. Fungal Infections of the Kidney and Urinary Tract 929
David J. Drutz

36. Renal and Perirenal Abscesses 959
Vincent T. Andriole

37. Infections of the Upper Urinary Tract 973
Allan R. Ronald
Lindsay E. Nicolle

38. Cystitis and Urethritis 1007
Walter E. Stamm

Index [3]

VOLUME II

VII
Nephrotoxin-Induced Diseases of the Kidney

39. The Cellular Basis of Nephrotoxicity 1031
Joel M. Weinberg

40. Lithium-Induced and Analgesic-Induced Renal Diseases 1099
Priscilla Kincaid-Smith
Ranjit S. Nanra

41. Aminoglycoside Nephrotoxicity 1131
George J. Kaloyanides

42. Renal Diseases Induced by Antineoplastic Agents 1165
Richard E. Rieselbach
Marc B. Garnick

43. Radiocontrast Media-Induced Acute Renal Failure 1187
Robert E. Cronin

44. Nephrotoxicity of Nonsteroidal Antiinflammatory Agents 1203
William L. Henrich

45. Drug Abuse with Narcotics and Other Agents 1219
David S. Baldwin
Gloria R. Gallo
Joel Neugarten

46. Heavy Metals 1237
Richard P. Wedeen

VIII
Acute Renal Failure

47. Pathophysiology of Cell Ischemia 1257
Thomas J. Burke
Robert W. Schrier

48. Acute Tubular Necrosis 1287
Robert J. Anderson
Robert W. Schrier

49. Acute Renal Vein Thrombosis 1319
Francisco Llach
Bijan Nikakhtar

50. Acute Interstitial Nephritis 1331
Jean-Pierre Grünfeld
Dieter Kleinknecht
Dominique Droz

51. The Hepatorenal Syndrome 1355
Ori S. Better
Robert W. Schrier

52. Treatment of Acute Renal Failure 1371
Carl M. Kjellstrand
Kim Solez

IX
Hypertension

53. Blood Pressure and the Kidney 1407
Hugh E. de Wardener
Graham A. MacGregor

54. Nephrosclerosis 1433
Robert G. Luke
John J. Curtis

55. Renovascular Hypertension 1451
Thomas G. Pickering
John H. Laragh
Thomas A. Sos

56. The Syndrome of Primary Aldosteronism and Pheochromocytoma 1475
Emmanuel L. Bravo

57. Hypertension and Pregnancy 1505
John M. Davison
Marshall D. Lindheimer

58. Hypertension in Cushing's Syndrome 1541
Bruce A. Scoggins
Judith A. Whitworth

59. Malignant Hypertension and Other Hypertensive Crises 1555
Charles R. Nolan III
Stuart L. Linas

X
Chronic Glomerulonephritis and Chronic Interstitial Nephritis

60. Immunopathology of Glomerular and Interstitial Disease 1647
Charles D. Pusey
D. Keith Peters

61. Glomerulonephritis with Bacterial Endocarditis, Ventriculovascular Shunts, and Visceral Infections 1681
Sharon G. Adler
Arthur H. Cohen

62. Rapidly Progressive Glomerulonephritis 1689
Robert C. Atkins
Napier M. Thomson

63. Acute Poststreptococcal Glomerulonephritis 1715
Bernardo Rodríguez-Iturbe

64. Nephrotic Syndrome: Minimal Change Disease, Focal Glomerulosclerosis, and Related Disorders 1731
H. William Schnaper
Alan M. Robson

65. Membranous Nephropathy 1785
Cecil H. Coggins

66. Membranoproliferative Glomerulonephritis 1815
James V. Donadio, Jr.

67. IgA Nephropathy and Henoch-Schönlein Purpura 1839
Anthony R. Clarkson
Andrew J. Woodroffe
Ian Aarons

68. Antiglomerular Basement Membrane Antibody-Mediated Nephritis 1865
Neil Turner
C. Martin Lockwood
Andrew J. Rees

69. The Long-Term Outcome of Glomerular Diseases 1895
J. Stewart Cameron

70. Chronic Tubulointerstitial Nephropathies 1959
Garabed Eknoyan

XI
Collagen, Vascular, Hematologic, and Vasculitis-Related Renal Disease

71. Mechanisms of Vascular Injury 1993
John Savill
Leopoldo Raij
Andrew J. Rees

72. Nephropathy of Systemic Lupus Erythematosus 2019
John P. Hayslett
Michael Kashgarian

73. Renal Involvement in Systemic Sclerosis 2039
Alvin P. Shapiro
Thomas A. Medsger, Jr.
Virginia D. Steen

74. Rheumatoid Arthritis, Sjögren's Syndrome, and Dermatomyositis-Polymyositis 2049
Woodruff Emlen
James C. Steigerwald
William P. Arend

75. Thrombotic Thrombocytopenic Purpura, Hemolytic-Uremic Syndrome, and Acute Cortical Necrosis 2063
Giuseppe Remuzzi
Arrigo Schieppati
Piero Ruggenenti
Tullio Bertani

76. Vasculitic Diseases of the Kidney: Polyarteritis, Wegener's Granulomatosis, Necrotizing and Crescentic Granulomatosis, and Other Disorders 2095
James E. Balow
Anthony S. Fauci

77. Renal Thromboembolism, Atheroembolism, and Other Acute Diseases of the Renal Arteries 2119
Jack W. Coburn
Keith L. Agre

78. Essential Mixed Cryoglobulinemia 2137
Claudio Ponticelli
Giuseppe D'Amico

Index [3]

VOLUME III

XII
Systemic Diseases of the Kidney

79. Diabetic Nephropathy 2153
S. Michael Mauer
Carl E. Mogensen
Carl M. Kjellstrand

80. Dysproteinemias: Multiple Myeloma, Amyloidosis, and Related Disorders 2189
Carlos A. Vaamonde
Guido O. Pérez
Victoriano Pardo

81. Hyperuricemia, Gout, and the Kidney 2239
Bryan T. Emmerson

82. Nonrenal Neoplasms and the Kidney 2265
Manuel Martínez-Maldonado
Julio E. Benabe

83. Pregnancy and Renal Disease 2287
M. Roy First
Victor E. Pollak

84. Sickle Cell Disease 2311
L. W. Statius van Eps
Paul E. de Jong

85. Tropical Nephrology 2331
Asghar Rastegar
Visith Sitprija
Heonir Rocha

86. Renal Diseases Associated with Human Immunodeficiency Virus (HIV) Infection (HIV-Associated Nephropathy) 2361
Mark H. Gardenswartz
T. K. Sreepada Rao

87. Kidney Disease in Children 2379
Cyril Chantler

88. Aging and the Kidney 2405
Moshe Levi
John W. Rowe

XIII
Clinical Disorders of Fluid, Electrolyte, and Acid-Base

89. Mechanisms of Diuretic Action 2435
Mark A. Dillingham
Robert W. Schrier
Rainer Greger

90. Cardiac Failure, Liver Disease, and Nephrotic Syndrome 2453
Daniel G. Bichet
Robert W. Schrier

91. Idiopathic Edema 2493
Graham A. MacGregor
Hugh E. de Wardener

92. Diabetes Insipidus and the Syndrome of Inappropriate Antidiuretic Hormone Secretion 2503
Isaac Teitelbaum
Stephen P. Kelleher
Tomas Berl

93. Disorders of Sodium and Water Balance Associated with Adrenal, Thyroid, and Pituitary Disease 2539
Alan G. Robinson
Frederick R. DeRubertis

94. Fluid-Electrolyte and Acid-Base Disorders Complicating Diabetes Mellitus 2563
Robert G. Narins
G. Gopal Krishna
Nelson P. Kopyt

95. Disorders of Phosphorus, Calcium, and Magnesium Metabolism 2599
Eduardo Slatopolsky
Keith Hruska
Saulo Klahr

96. Disorders of Potassium Metabolism Associated with Renal Disease 2645
Asghar Rastegar
Ralph A. DeFronzo

97. Acid-Base Disorders in Association with Renal Disease 2669
Nicolaos E. Madias
Ronald D. Perrone

XIV
Uremic Syndrome

98. Pathophysiology and Nephron Adaptation in Chronic Renal Failure 2703
Leon G. Fine
Ira Kurtz
Adrian S. Woolf
Gabriel M. Danovitch
Cheryl Emmons
Dean A. Kujubu
Jill T. Norman

99. Anemia in Renal Disease 2743
Joseph W. Eschbach
John W. Adamson

100. The Osteodystrophy of Chronic Renal Failure 2759
Dennis L. Andress
Donald J. Sherrard

101. Nervous System Manifestations of Renal Failure 2789
Cosmo L. Fraser
Allen I. Arieff

102. Cardiovascular Complications of End-Stage Renal Disease 2817
Kwan Eun Kim
Charles Swartz

103. Metabolic and Endocrine Dysfunctions in Uremia 2845
Franz Schaefer
Eberhard Ritz
Franciszek Kokot
Shaul G. Massry

XV
Management of End-Stage Renal Failure

104. Immunobiology and Immunopharmacology of Graft Rejection 2879
Terry B. Strom
Nicholas L. Tilney

105. Outcome and Complications of Renal Transplantation 2911
Laurence Chan
Igal Kam
Everett K. Spees

106. Peritoneal Dialysis 2969
Ramesh Khanna
Dimitrios G. Oreopoulos

107. Center and Home Chronic Hemodialysis 3031
Suhail Ahmad
Christopher R. Blagg
Belding H. Scribner

108. Outcome and Complications of Chronic Hemodialysis 3069
Eli A. Friedman
Andrew Peter Lundin, III

109. Ethical Considerations in End-Stage Renal Disease 3097
Nancy Boucot Cummings
with contributions by
Patricia Schoenfeld
Ronald Baker Miller

XVI
Nutrition, Drugs, and the Kidney

110. Protein Intake and Prevention of Chronic Renal Disease 3131
Thomas Heard Hostetter
William Evans Mitch

111. Phosphate, Aluminum, and Other Elements in Chronic Renal Disease 3153
Allen C. Alfrey

112. Dietary Considerations in Patients with Advanced Chronic Renal Failure, Acute Renal Failure, and Transplantation 3167
Joel D. Kopple

113. Use of Drugs in Patients with Renal Failure 3211
John G. Gambertoglio
Francesca T. Aweeka
William B. Blythe

Index [3]

VII

Nephrotoxin-Induced Diseases of the Kidney

Notice

The indications and dosages of all drugs in this book have been recommended in the medical literature and conform to the practices of the general medical community. The medications described do not necessarily have specific approval by the Food and Drug Administration for use in the diseases and dosages for which they are recommended. The package insert for each drug should be consulted for use and dosage as approved by the FDA. Because standards for usage change, it is advisable to keep abreast of revised recommendations, particularly those concerning new drugs.

The Cellular Basis of Nephrotoxicity

Joel M. Weinberg

The structural heterogeneity of the kidney and the complex interplay between tubule cell injury and alterations of nephronal function have posed substantial challenges to the elucidation of the pathogenesis of nephrotoxic renal failure. However, an increasing amount of information is becoming available about the cellular mechanisms for tubule injury and serves to highlight the primary role of tubule cell injury in most types of nephrotoxic renal failure.

In considering the nephrotoxic potential of various agents, it is important to keep in mind that their intrinsic toxicity may be only moderate, but the functional properties of the kidneys to concentrate or metabolize the agent result in nephrotoxicity while other tissues are spared. Factors that make the kidney particularly prone to the actions of nephrotoxins have generally been considered to include (1) high levels of toxin delivery secondary to the kidney's large blood supply; (2) the large surface area of the renal tubular epithelium providing sites for toxin interaction and uptake; (3) the availability of specific transport mechanisms that mediate cellular uptake; (4) the normal concentrating mechanisms of the kidney, which can act to increase the urinary and interstitial concentrations of nonreabsorbed agents; (5) the presence of metabolic processes within renal tubular cells which release toxic components of agents or produce toxic by-products of metabolism; and (6) the high metabolic rates of tubule cells required for normal function.

Damage by nephrotoxins may result from their direct reactivity with cellular macromolecules and membrane components or from metabolism within tubular cells to toxic products. Among agents with structural characteristics that impart direct toxicity are the heavy metals because of their affinities for macromolecular sulfhydryl groups [628], the organic cations, such as spermine [393], cationic amino acids [508] and aminoglycosides [357], which interact with anionic membrane phospholipids [357], and the polyene antibiotics, such as amphotericin B [156], which interact with membrane cholesterol. Metabolic activation of nephrotoxins may release well-defined metabolites with nephrotoxic activity, such as the fluoride and oxalate produced by hepatic metabolism of methoxyflurane [433] or may involve complex, as yet incompletely identified, intermediates, such as cisplatin [210, 691], cysteine conjugates [17, 568], the haloalkanes [422], cephaloridine [443], and acetominophen [215]. Of these intermediates resulting from intracellular toxic activation, toxic metabolites, including free radicals producing membrane damage by means of covalent binding and peroxidation, are the most important [215, 422].

Nephrotoxins generally damage specific segments of the nephron to a much greater degree than others (Fig. 39-1). The proximal tubule is most commonly affected and, within the proximal tubule, effects of individual nephrotoxins tend to be more prominent in either S1 and S2 segments or in S3 segments. S1 and S2 segments are major sites of damage produced by aminoglycosides [357], cephaloridine [756], chromate [230], and citrinin [486]. S3 segments are the most prominent site of tubule cell injury produced by Hg^{++} [284], uranyl nitrate [303], cisplatin [211], many of the haloalkanes [246, 422, 423, 458], cysteine conjugates [389], and maleic acid [864]. Theoretically, a number of factors may contribute to selective sensitivity of various nephronal segments to toxins: (1) degree of exposure resulting from the amount of toxin delivery, (2) presence of transport and uptake mechanisms facilitating intracellular access of toxin, (3) presence of intracellular sites particularly susceptible to toxin, and (4) availability of metabolic pathways that produce toxic metabolites or by-products. The proximal straight tubule, which is prominently affected by a number of nephrotoxins, is the richest in the inducible type of microsomal mixed-function oxidases, which have been implicated in the toxic activation of various agents [223, 247, 289, 422]. The same segment has the highest concentration of glutathione and glutathione-metabolizing enzymes [105, 289, 559] and glucosyltransferase and sulfotransferase activities [335].

The time frame over which nephrotoxicity becomes manifest depends on both how acutely tubular cells are injured and how widespread such injury is. The extent of injury, in turn, reflects the abundance of susceptible cells and the quantity of toxin administered. Agents that injure tubule cells rapidly, so that cell necrosis and renal failure appear during the first 24 hours after exposure, include heavy metals, such as Hg^{++} [284] and uranyl [303], many of the haloalkanes [246, 422, 458], cephaloridine [756], methoxyflurane [433], and maleic acid [864]. Agents whose pattern of injury develops during several days or which may require several doses of drug include the aminoglycosides [357], cisplatin [211], and the mycotoxin, citrinin [486]. Delayed manifestation of injury over periods of weeks to months may result from low levels of acute direct cellular toxicity or from toxicity to only limited numbers of cells during individual episodes of drug exposure, but with cumulative effects over long periods. Lead clearly accumulates within renal tubular cells but, in the amounts delivered during usual exposure, appears to have only a relatively low-grade chronic toxicity at the cellular level [887]. Limited information is available about the acute effects of mithramycin [412] and the nitrosoureas [585] but both appear to damage tubular cells and can eventuate, after repeated courses, in clinically significant chronic renal failure. The observations that acute episodes of renal failure are occasionally seen with mithramycin and that mice treated with methyl-CCNU develop renal tubule cell necrosis over several days [202] make it likely that, for these drugs,

Preparation of this chapter and the author's work in it were supported by NIH grants DK-01337, DK-34275, and DK-39255.

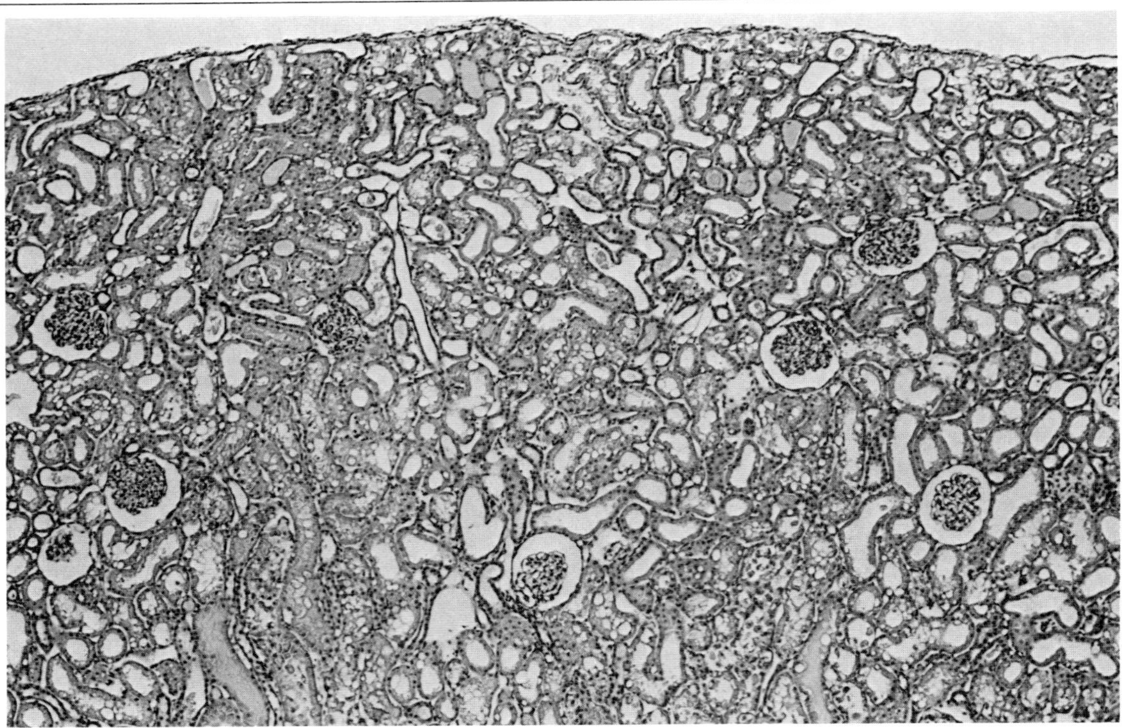

Fig. 39-1. Photograph of renal cortex from rat treated with $HgCl_2$, illustrating the heterogeneity of response of proximal tubule segments to toxic injury. S3 and S2 segments in the medullary rays show severe damage with many exfoliating necrotic cells. Although cells of S1 segments are injured, integrity of the epithelium is preserved.

each insult involves relatively few nephrons, but the effects are cumulative over long periods. Combined insults from multiple nephrotoxins or nephrotoxins in combination with ischemia can induce accelerated patterns of damage and are frequently implicated as causes of acute renal failure in the clinical setting [31, 62, 104, 120, 224, 329, 390, 543, 752, 783, 822, 848, 956, 957].

Functional manifestations of nephrotoxicity may occur at several levels. Tubular function abnormalities, such as K^+ wasting and failure of acidification during amphotericin treatment [215], Mg^{++}, K^+, and Na^+ wasting and concentrating defects after cisplatin [85, 358], and concentrating defects and Mg^{++} wasting after aminoglycosides [357] may be detected. However, these are not always ideal clues to the occurrence or localization of tubular cell injury because effects in the proximal tubule tend to be masked by retained distal transport mechanisms, thus blunting the final net manifestations of any disorder. Any associated reductions of glomerular filtration also act to obscure the full extent of nephrotoxin-induced tubular function abnormalities.

Nephrotoxin-induced changes in tubule cell integrity may be sublethal or lethal. Extensive sublethal changes can occur even during drug exposure not otherwise considered to be nephrotoxic. Such prelethal changes include development of abnormally enlarged lysosomes and myeloid bodies, loss of brush-border membranes, and vacuolization and dilatation of the endoplasmic reticulum. Enzymuria resulting from loss of some of these damaged membranes in the urine has been used to gauge the occurrence of renal tubule cell injury and to follow it serially. Brush-border and lysosomal enzymes have received the most study [566, 927]. Ultrastructural studies of urine sediment may also reveal subcellular structures from injured cells [512, 567].

The relationships between tubular cell injury and significant loss of renal clearance function during nephrotoxicity are complex. Since nephrons function as units in series, injury localized to limited nephron segments may lead to substantial end-organ failure if the degree of obstruction, back-leak, or secondary alterations in glomerular hemodynamics are sufficient to compromise function of the whole nephron. Sublethally injured cells may exhibit functional abnormalities for prolonged periods. As previously noted, the presence of tubular functional defects prior to the occurrence of cell necrosis in acute renal failure is well documented [175, 771, 855]. Loss of brush borders of proximal tubular cells is a common feature of many types of injury and may be sustained for relatively long periods without the development of further loss of cell integrity [346, 776, 960]. Such loss of a major portion of the luminal surface has the potential to alter markedly the transport capacity of affected tubules. Decreases of basolateral membrane surface area have also been described (Fig. 39-2). Additionally, loss of cell polarity with redistribution of Na^+-K^+-ATPase from the basolateral to the apical surface can contribute to functional deficits [564]. On the other hand, lethal tubule cell

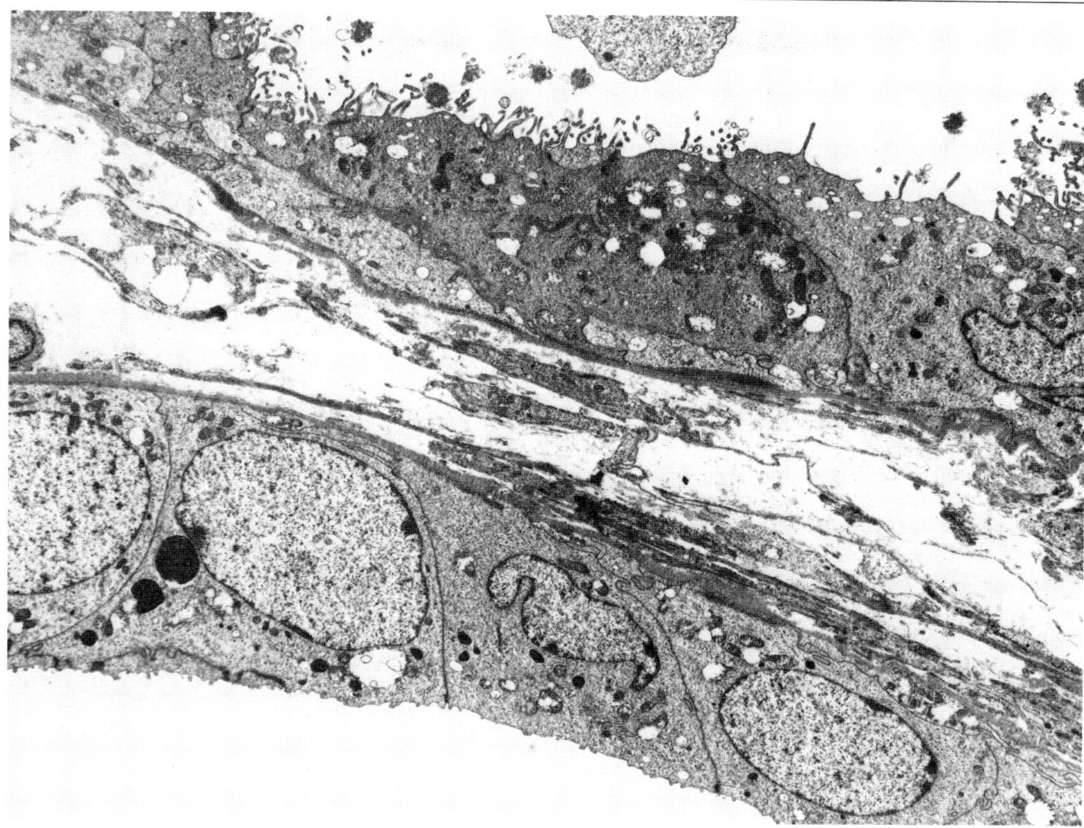

Fig. 39-2. Loss of plasma membrane surface areas in remodeled renal tubular cells in a case of human acute renal failure. (Photograph from D. B. Jones, Ultrastructure of human acute renal failure. *Lab. Invest.* 46:254, 1982, with permission.)

injury of limited extent may be associated with no detectable changes in overall clearance [439], presumably due to the plasticity of function of the remaining less-injured or uninjured nephrons. This type of observation has led to substantial controversy about the existence of a necessary relationship between lethal renal tubular cell injury and acute renal failure. It is now generally agreed, however, that (1) the presence and extent of lethal cell injury must be considered in such an analysis; (2) in animal models, a reasonably good correlation between the extent of lethal cell injury and loss of function exists; and (3) sustained acute loss of renal clearance function that is unresponsive to volume expansion is virtually always accompanied by extensive lethal renal tubule cell injury [208, 777, 915]. Furthermore, despite concomitant decrements of renal blood flow that may develop in the presence of extensive lethal renal tubule cell injury, agents with vascular effects to increase renal blood flow in this setting generally have been ineffective in reversing the loss of clearance [448, 523, 773].

Interactions of Toxins with Tubule Cells Associated with Their Uptake

The combination of high renal blood flow to the kidney and large surface area of tubule cell membranes, which is instrumental for its normal function, results in exposure of renal tubular cells to higher levels of toxins than cells in other organs. Toxins can interact directly with the plasma membrane to produce damage there, irrespective of their uptake. This is true for amphotericin B, which has well-documented acute membrane effects to increase membrane monovalent cation permeability due to its interaction with plasma membrane cholesterol to form aqueous channels appropriate in size for Na^+ and K^+ [156]. More common are mechanisms by which toxins either bind to the surface of tubular cells and are internalized, such as seen with the aminoglycosides [357], or utilize existing transport systems, such as seen with the cephalosporins [842] and cysteine conjugates [451, 967]. Toxins also may be internalized into renal tubular cells bound to other molecules. This is well illustrated by studies of the interactions of cadmium and cadmium plus metallothionein with the kidney [147, 610, 885] and may also be true for Hg^{++} [352, 416, 912, 962]. Lipophilic agents, such as halogenated hydrocarbons and cyclosporine, may simply partition in the lipophilic regions of the plasma membrane and thereby rapidly gain access to the intracellular space and other organelles.

Renal tubule cells accumulate high levels of aminoglycosides that, if they were free, would be 50- to 100-fold greater than serum concentrations [232, 493]. The net accumulation process is energy dependent [424, 694].

Aminoglycoside renal membrane interactions that account for uptake are well understood. Autoradiographic studies had shown that tracer doses of labeled aminoglycosides transiently localized to the apical surface of the cell and are then internalized over 30 minutes, largely to lysosomes [396, 757] (Fig. 39-3). The membrane recycling involved in internalization requires energy; the initial binding does not and can be analyzed using isolated membranes. Studies of the binding of gentamicin to isolated brush-border membranes demonstrated that this binding could be characterized using Scatchard analysis to have K_ds in the range of 20 to 125 μM and n_{max}, ranging from 2 to 18 nmol/mg protein [397, 477, 700] (Fig. 39-4). Binding with similar affinities but with two- to threefold greater capacity to basolateral membrane vesicles has also been reported [392, 931–933] and tissue slices with collapsed lumina concentrate the drug [68, 424], suggesting the occurrence of basolateral uptake. However, most autoradiographic [396, 757, 888], micropuncture [629, 736], and whole kidney clearance [168] data favor luminal uptake by means of the brush-border membrane as the most important route. Whether differences in the perimembrane microenvironment, membrane turnover, or fluid fluxes primarily account for the preferential apical uptake by the intact proximal tubule cells is not known.

Based on observations that the aminoglycosides are cationic at physiological pH [357] and that neomycin had been shown to have a particularly high affinity for binding to polyphosphoinositides [487], it was proposed that aminoglycoside binding to renal plasma membranes was to anionic membrane sites comprised of membrane acidic phospholipids [700]. In support of this possibility, it was found that the in vitro affinities for gentamicin binding to individual phospholipids in a simple partitioning system were in the same range as its affinity for binding to renal brush-border membranes. Gentamicin had relatively high affinities for most acidic phospholipids, not just the polyphosphoinositides, and, in contrast, showed no binding to nonacidic phospholipids. Treatment of isolated renal brush-border membranes with phospholipases to specifically reduce their acidic phospholipid content reduced gentamicin binding while increasing brush-border membrane content of the acidic phospholipid, phosphatidylinositol, increased gentamicin binding [700].

Other aminoglycosides as well as other organic polycations [477] were effective competitive inhibitors of gentamicin binding to the brush-border membranes according to their degree of cationicity [432, 700, 932]. Both Ca^{++} and Mg^{++} competitively inhibit gentamicin binding to renal brush-border membranes, with Ca^{++} being the more effective of these two divalent cations [355]. Gentamicin-induced aggregation of brush-border membranes is antagonized by Ca^{++} and Mg^{++} [415]. Aminoglycosides exhibit competitive interactions with Ca^{++} binding to liposomes, lipid monolayers, red cell ghosts, and cardiac sarcolemma [101, 152, 415, 497, 880]. These latter observations are consistent with well-established effects of divalent cations to antagonize aminoglycoside bacterial uptake [968] and neurological effects [639]. The polycations, spermine and polylysine, inhibited renal cortical uptake of gentamicin in vivo [393]. Thus strong evidence favors binding of aminoglycosides as a result of their cationic properties to plasma membrane acidic phospholipids as the initial and major step in their renal tubular cell uptake. It is well established that, ultimately, the major site of aminoglycoside localization within renal tubular cells is in lysosomes, and autoradiographic studies indicated a direct transition of labeled aminoglycosides from the plasma membrane to lysosomes [396, 757]. However, using different tissue fixation techniques, evidence for a phase of cytosolic localization prior to lysosomal uptake has been described [888] and studies of gentamicin binding, using subcellular fractionation techniques, have revealed substantial binding

Fig. 39-3. Autoradiographic studies of gentamicin uptake by mouse proximal tubule cells. Initially, following I.V. injection of ^{3}H-gentamicin, both brush-border and basolateral membrane surfaces are labeled (*left panel*). After 20 minutes, most label is found in apical lysosomes (*right panel*). (From M. Just, G. Erdmann, and T. Habermann. The renal handling of polybasic drugs. I. Gentamicin and aprotinin in intact animals. *Naunyn Schmiedebergs Arch. Pharmacol.* 300:57, 1977, with permission.)

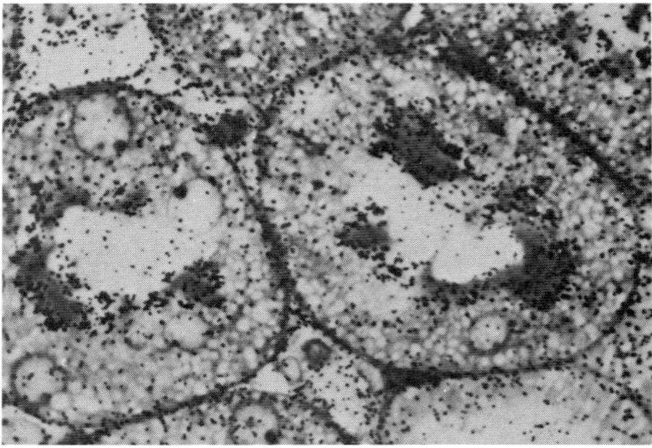

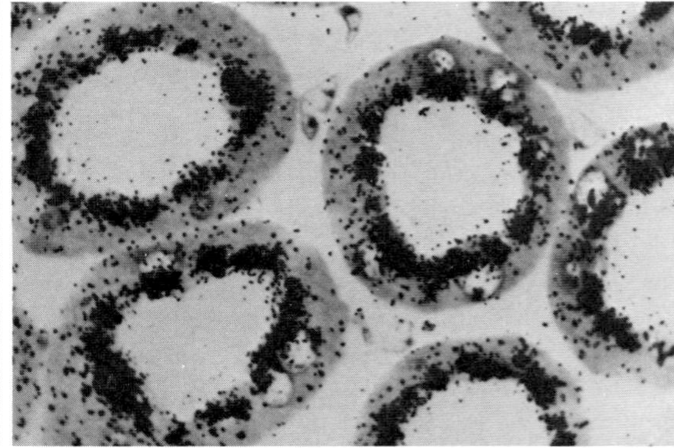

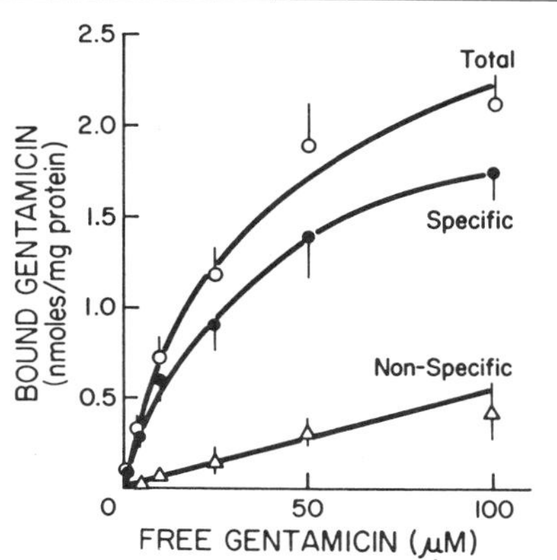

Fig. 39-4. Binding of ³H-gentamicin to isolated renal brush-border membranes. (From M. Sastrasinh, T. C. Knauss, J. M. Weinberg, and H. D. Humes. Identification of the aminoglycoside receptor of renal brush border membranes. *J. Pharmacol. Exp. Ther.* 222:350, 1982, with permission.)

to multiple subcellular membranes, with potential for redistribution among them [35, 594].

The relevance of the saturable mechanism delineated for brush-border membrane uptake of aminoglycosides to interactions of aminoglycosides and renal tubular cells in vivo is suggested by observations that frequent or continuous dose regimens are more toxic than drug administration at higher doses but at prolonged intervals [69, 557]. The latter type of regimen would be expected to favor drug excretion because of greater delivery of antibiotic at times when binding sites are relatively saturated [700]. This has been confirmed experimentally [267, 869, 944].

Amelioration of toxicity by competitive inhibition of uptake has been assessed. Organic polycations, i.e., other aminoglycosides, spermine, and polylysine, have yielded mixed results because of their intrinsic potential for direct toxicity [393, 508, 932]. Important, recently described actions of neutral and polyanionic amino acids to strongly antagonize aminoglycoside nephrotoxicity appear to relate primarily to actions to complex with the aminoglycosides intracellularly rather than to effects on the initial uptake or accumulation [55, 417, 418, 932]. The inorganic cations Ca^{++} and Mg^{++} do provide significant protection from toxicity [65, 355, 652, 943], but again this does not appear to be a result of inhibition of uptake or accumulation. The modulating effects of polyamino acids and divalent cations on aminoglycoside toxicity are detailed below. Alterations of membrane anionic phospholipid-binding sites for aminoglycosides did not explain the modulatory effects of parathyroidectomy [339] or streptozotocin-induced diabetes [392] on aminoglycoside toxicity. Protective effects of thyroid hormone were associated with decreased gentamicin accumulation [174], but the full mechanism for this effect has not been established.

Tubular cell uptake of nephrotoxins in complexed form is typified by the renal handling and nephrotoxicity of Cd^{++}. Available data on the short-term effects of this heavy metal on renal structure and function are not extensive but do suggest that it has substantially less acute toxicity than other heavy metals, such as Hg^{++}, and less than would be predicted from its high level of direct membrane reactivity in vivo [371, 435, 942]. This finding, in large part, appears due to the nature of cadmium handling by the kidney. Highest levels of Cd^{++} after acute administration were found in liver, the earliest site of toxic manifestations [435]. Within 2 weeks following administration of Cd^{++}, levels in most tissues except for liver and kidney dropped substantially. Liver levels decreased minimally during this time, while renal levels increased fourfold, with much of the increase accounted for by Cd^{++} bound to metallothionein [435]. Cd^{++} is a potent inducer of both hepatic and renal metallothionein. Within hours of its administration, most intracellular Cd^{++} is bound to this low-molecular-weight intracellular protein [883]. It has been found that, in contrast to ionized Cd^{++}, cadmium-thionein administered systemically is a potent acute nephrotoxin, producing substantial morphological changes in proximal tubule cells, including loss of brush border, cytoplasmic blebbing, large increases in numbers of intracellular vacuoles, and mitochondrial swelling within 4 hours after its administration. Over 12 to 24 hours, widespread necrosis of proximal tubule cells develops [147, 610, 884, 885]. This acute toxicity of cadmium-thionein is associated with a major shift in distribution of Cd^{++} to the kidney as compared to when Cd^{++} alone is administered. Acute renal Cd^{++} levels were 20 times greater after administration of cadmium-thionein than after an equimolar amount of Cd^{++} as $CdCl_2$ [147]. The distribution of Cd^{++} between cytosol and particulate fractions was not different with the two modes of administration; however, after $CdCl_2$, most cytosolic Cd^{++} was bound to high-molecular-weight proteins, while after Cd-thionein, most was initially present in the tissue as Cd-thionein [147]. The Cd-thionein is degraded since, if the thionein is labeled with ^{35}S or ^{3}H, most of the label is recovered in other proteins after 48 hours [885]. This finding suggests that the toxicity of Cd-thionein is that of Cd^{++} rather than that of the complex or of the metallothionein. Consistent with this interpretation, Cd-thionein does not appear to have substantial direct membrane toxicity of its own [883], Zn-thionein is relatively nontoxic [885], and other low-molecular-weight Cd^{++} complexes, such as Cd-cysteine and Cd-penicillamine, are highly nephrotoxic [293, 412].

Toxin uptake in complexed form, with subsequent intracellular release of the active toxin due to metabolic degradation of the complex, is not limited to cadmium, although no other agent has been subjected to such extensive study with regard to this issue. Hg^{++}, for example, circulates virtually completely in protein-bound form [352, 416], and this probably influences the nature of its uptake by tubules, although details of the process remain to be delineated [962].

The toxicity of the cephalosporins is importantly related to their uptake and subsequent excretion [844,

845]. Uptake is by means of the organic anion transport system and can be inhibited by probenecid or *p*-aminohippurate (PAH) [842]. Most cephalosporins do not substantially accumulate within tubular cells due to luminal membrane secretion and do not exhibit high degrees of toxicity. Luminal secretion, however, is apparently much lower for cephaloridine than for the other cephalosporins, possibly due to the presence of a fixed cationic charge on its pyridyl side ring. This results in substantial intracellular accumulation of cephaloridine, which likely contributes to its higher degree of nephrotoxicity [844, 845]. Glutamate has also been recently shown to potently inhibit tubule cell cephaloridine uptake and toxicity [687].

Cis-platinum is concentrated by renal cortical slices in an energy- and temperature-dependent fashion. Uptake is inhibited by probenecid and a number of the organic bases, including mepiperphenidol, tetraethylammonium, and tolazoline, but not by the organic anions *p*-aminohippurate and pyrazinoate [691]. Cisplatin also inhibits organic cation transport but not organic anion transport in isolated brush-border and basolateral membrane vesicles [660]. In vivo, probenecid decreases apparent cisplatin clearance in the human [370], but increases it in the rat [188]. Circulating cisplatin is highly protein bound [231]. Substantial differences in both protein binding and renal uptake and distribution have been noted between cisplatin and the less nephrotoxic platinum derivatives, carboplatin and iproplatin [188, 231]. These observations indicate a complex mode of handling for platinum compounds that importantly contributes to the pattern of nephrotoxicity and remains to be more fully defined.

Mechanisms and Sites of Toxin-Induced Damage

TOXIC ACTIVATION AND FREE-RADICAL PRODUCTION

General Mechanisms. Metabolism of toxic agents intracellularly by the endoplasmic reticulum (ER) mixed-function oxidases, with resulting formation of reactive metabolites, many of which are free radicals, has long been implicated in the pathogenesis of toxic cell injury caused by haloalkanes [422, 667, 688, 954]. Reactions catalyzed by these cytochrome P450-dependent enzymes include hydroxylation of both aromatic and aliphatic structures, O-, N-, and S-dealkylation, sulfoxidation, N-oxidation, and epoxidation. This phase 1 metabolism may be followed by detoxification reactions, such as sulfation or glucuronidation, producing more readily excreted water-soluble metabolites, or it may result in damage to cellular macromolecules through arylation or alkylation or by the initiation of free-radical metabolic events [688, 938].

It is now being appreciated that many more toxic cell insults as well as cell damage due to inflammatory processes and oxygen-deprivation–induced cell injury are mediated, at least in part, by reactive metabolites generated by several mechanisms, including the mixed-function oxidases [686, 825, 938], metabolism by xanthine oxidase of hypoxanthine and xanthine to uric acid with production of superoxide [277, 525], autoxidation of ubiquinone and NADH dehydrogenase during electron transport by damaged mitochondria [95, 374, 854], infiltrating inflammatory cells [277, 678], arachidonic acid metabolism by prostaglandin endoperoxide synthetase [723, 963], and conjugation with glutathione at a number of subcellular sites [303, 688] (Fig. 39-5). In this section, the general processes will be reviewed and available information about their applicability to individual nephrotoxins will be detailed. Distinctly separate processes—lipid peroxidation produced by radicals, covalent binding of reactive metabolites, and depletion of low-molecular-weight and protein thiols—are involved in the formation of reactive oxygen metabolites and toxic derivatives of various agents, but the frequent related occurrence of several of these events in multiple models makes it most informative to consider them together. The injury they produce often involves perturbation of cellular energy and calcium metabolism. Those events are considered in separate sections.

Free radicals may be defined simply as atoms or groups of atoms having an unpaired number of electrons that may enter into covalent bond formation. These unpaired electrons are chemically unstable, highly reactive, and may induce chemical chain reactions in susceptible compounds [136, 250]. Any aromatic compound can be involved in free-radical formation [519]. Biologically important free radicals include metabolic products of chemicals and drugs, such as CCl_4 and free radicals formed during oxidative metabolic reactions, including superoxide, hydroxyl radical, and singlet oxygen, a high-energy state of oxygen [519].

Superoxide ion is formed during natural oxidation reactions. These include the action of endoplasmic reticulum mixed-function oxidases, other NADPH oxidases, such as those in leukocyte plasma membranes, the mitochondrial electron transport system, and xanthine oxidase. Superoxide dismutase catalyzes the conversion of superoxide ions to hydrogen peroxide and molecular oxygen [303]. Superoxide is far more reactive in nonaqueous environments than in aqueous solution [708]. Thus, when generated within membranes, the toxicity of superoxide may arise from its direct reactivity, but when generated in solution, as has usually been the case in most studies of its toxicity, additional mediators are involved [303]. To explain the toxicity of superoxide in aqueous solutions, it was proposed that hydroxyl radicals were formed by the Haber-Weiss reaction [244], in which hydrogen peroxide combines with superoxide to form oxygen, hydroxyl radical, and hydroxyl anion. Because of the slow rate of this reaction in aqueous solution, it is more likely that, to the extent it occurs in biological systems, the reaction is catalyzed by transition metal ions, a process termed the *Fenton reaction* [303].

Fe^{++} appears to be the major physiological intracellular mediator of the Fenton reaction, and the effectiveness of deferoxamine to inhibit hydroxyl radical formation supports this concept [32, 235, 298]. Although Fe^{++} is kept extremely low within cells, sufficient amounts are available to participate in the Fenton reaction [140, 303]. Cu^{++} may also be important. Cu^{++} is substantially more active than Fe^{++} in promoting hy-

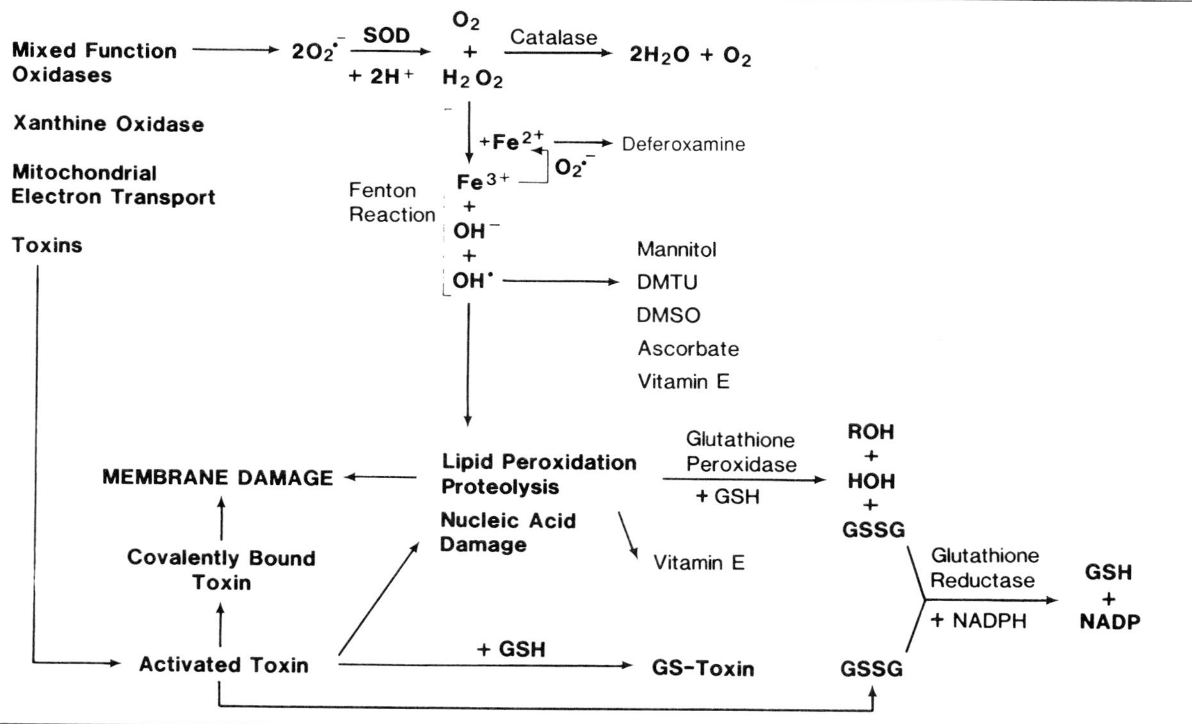

Fig. 39-5. Some major pathways for cell damage produced by intracellular toxic activation and free-radical generation. Important protective mechanisms and agents are also diagrammed. As detailed in the text, additional pathways and interactions have been identified for various cell types, and most of the illustrated pathways are still under study. Processes that have been identified to date only in neutrophils, such as formation of hypohalus acids by myeloperoxidase [925], are not included.

droxyl radical formation from H_2O_2 in vitro [303]. Intracellular free Cu^{++} availability is limited, but bound Cu^{++} may be capable of generating hydroxyl radical [699].

The hydroxyl radical is highly reactive. In considering the potential for various oxygen metabolites to exert toxicity, it is important that hydroxyl radicals react rapidly with adjacent molecules and will not, as a result, cross membranes. Superoxide and H_2O_2, because they are less reactive, can diffuse away from the sites of their production, thus exposing remote cellular structures to the potential for hydroxyl radical generation from interaction with these metabolites. H_2O_2 readily crosses cell membranes; superoxide does not [303]. All aspects of how various oxygen metabolites induce lipid peroxidation have not been resolved. In some systems, hydroxyl radical generation is readily detected, but radical scavengers have no effect on the degree of lipid peroxidation that occurs, suggesting the involvement of other factors, such as ferryl radicals [296, 303].

Oxidative metabolism of arachidonate by cyclooxygenase in the presence of hydroperoxides can result in formation of hydroxyl radical as a by-product. Prostaglandin endoperoxide synthetase (PES), consisting of cyclooxygenase that converts arachidonic acid to PGG2 and a hydroperoxidase that converts PGG2 to PGH2, can mediate metabolic activation of drugs by co-oxidation [517, 556]. The hydroperoxidase component of the enzyme complex appears most important in the co-oxidation process [964], which has been shown to affect a variety of agents, including acetaminophen, oxyphenbutazone, benzidine, and benzo(a)pyrene [517, 964]. The involvement of free-radical mechanisms in the co-oxidation process is strongly suggested by observations that free-radical scavengers, such as ethoxyquin, vitamin E, and butylated hydroxytoluene inhibit co-oxidation [516]. Highest levels of PES in the kidney are found in the medulla [963, 966]. Activity there is present in tubular, vascular, and interstitial cells [963, 966].

Leukocytes are major sources of reactive oxygen metabolites due to the presence of a membrane NADPH oxidase, which produces superoxide anion, and as a result of arachidonic acid metabolism with production of hydroxyl radical [34].

Metabolism by xanthine oxidase of hypoxanthine and xanthine to uric acid with production of superoxide [277, 525] is a potentially important mechanism by which degradation of endogenous purines can contribute to the production of damaging reactive oxygen metabolites. It has received considerable attention in studies of the pathogenesis of ischemic tissue damage where the combination of extensive purine nucleotide catabolism and Ca^{++}-induced proteolytic conversion of the non–radical-producing xanthine dehydrogenase to xanthine oxidase could produce a potent radical-generating system

[474, 804, 827]. However, there are major species differences regarding the availability of xanthine oxidase. Isolated tubules and whole kidney in the rat show higher levels of xanthine oxidase activity than those found in the rabbit [25, 212, 959]. Neither rabbit kidney nor isolated rabbit tubules appreciably metabolize nucleosides beyond hypoxanthine [122, 514, 897]. Human kidney also appears to have relatively low xanthine oxidase activity [780]. Consistent with this and similar to results from the studies with isolated rabbit tubules, very little degradation beyond hypoxanthine was seen in human kidneys stored in preservation solutions containing high concentrations of adenosine [780]. An unusually high susceptibility to oxidant damage of rat tissues as compared to human tissues is also indicated by work showing a 30-fold greater rate of spontaneous autooxidation in homogenates of rat kidney as compared to human kidney [185]. It is also of note that the activities of nonmitochondrial oxidases such as xanthine oxidase may be limited at physiological tissue PO_2s [266, 385]. This may be particularly relevant in view of the relatively low PO_2 present in normally perfused kidneys [107, 727, 742].

Conjugation with glutathione (GSH) can result in production of reactive intermediates as well as in detoxification, and the former process may be particularly prominent in the kidney given its high levels of GSH metabolism [18, 568, 688]. There are several mechanisms by which GSH metabolism may be involved in the formation of damaging reactive intermediates. Mutagenic effects of glutathione derivatives of dihaloalkanes have been related to the propensity for these compounds to form episulfonium ions nonenzymatically [332, 484, 858]. A number of quinone-linked, glutathione conjugates are highly nephrotoxic via a mechanism dependent on metabolism of the compounds by gamma-glutamyl transpeptidase [456, 457, 568–572]. Promotion of toxicity by gamma-glutamyl transpeptidase may be due to facilitated cellular uptake of the cysteine and cysteinylglycine derivatives or greater oxidative activity of the quinone moiety in the latter form [456, 457, 568–572]. Of note, N-acetylation of the the compounds can either diminish [571] or enhance [457] toxicity.

Another, even better characterized pathway for toxicity of multiple haloalkenes involves cleavage of cysteine conjugates by cysteine conjugate beta-lyase to reactive thiol intermediates (plus ammonia and pyruvate) [18, 21, 80, 568]. Both a cytosolic and a mitochondrial glutamine transaminase have cysteine conjugate beta-lyase activity which, along with toxicity, can be inhibited by aminooxyacetic acid [449, 452, 501, 792–794]. All enzymes present for toxicity by this pathway, including glutathione-S-transferase for initial conjugation with glutathione, are present in the renal tubules [316]. However, in vivo, glutathione conjugates are predominantly formed in the liver by glutathione-S-transferase–catalyzed reactions [638] and are excreted into the bile. They are metabolized by gamma-glutamyl transpeptidases on biliary tract and intestinal epithelium to cysteine conjugates, which are reabsorbed and can reach the kidney unchanged or after further hepatic metabolism to N-acetyl derivatives [365, 366, 593]. Any glutathione conjugates directly reaching the kidney can also be metabolized to cysteine conjugates by the action of renal gamma-glutamyl transpeptidase and dipeptidase [199]. Uptake of cysteine conjugates occurs by more than one amino acid transporter [451, 967]; uptake of the N-acetyl derivatives is by the probenecid-sensitive anion transporter [92, 967]. Uptake of intact glutathione conjugates can also potentially occur [453], but is probably not significant for the beta-lyase pathway of injury. The N-acetyl cysteine conjugates are deacetylated to cysteine conjugates by acetylases present within tubule cells [485, 648, 967].

Compounds for which beta-lyase metabolism of cysteine conjugates has been strongly implicated in nephrotoxicity include hexachloro-1,3-butadiene, trichloroethylene, chlorotrifluoroethylene, tetrachloroethylene, tetrafluoroethylene, dichloroacetylene, perfluoropropene, and a number of others [258, 568, 613]. Toxic intracellular processes subsequent to activation by beta-lyase have been studied in detail for the cysteine conjugates of several of these compounds. That information is reviewed in detail below and in the sections on alterations of energy and calcium metabolism.

Lipid peroxidation, a major deleterious effect of intracellular free-radical generation, is the oxidative deterioration of polyunsaturated lipids and is equivalent to the process by which fats become rancid. Peroxidation of unsaturated lipids has far greater biochemical effects than mere deterioration of lipids, especially when lipid peroxidation occurs in membrane lipids. Dramatic alterations in membrane structure and function can be ultimate consequences of this process due to disruptive effects of loss of membrane lipids, production of toxic lipid breakdown products, and peroxidative damage to nearby membrane proteins [136, 250].

Peroxidation of lipids usually involves the reaction of free radicals and polyunsaturated lipids to form free-radical intermediates and semistable hydroperoxides. Polyunsaturated fatty acids are especially prone to become involved in free-radical metabolism, because the presence of the double bond weakens the carbon-hydrogen bond on the carbon atom adjacent to the unsaturated carbon-carbon bond. These allylic hydrogens are less tightly bound and are susceptible to abstraction by free radicals so as to initiate lipid peroxidation.

Lipid hydroperoxides are relatively stable, but their decomposition is catalyzed by metals in forms that are present in vivo. This includes both heme and nonheme iron proteins as well as complexes of iron salts with phosphate or phosphorylated compounds, such as ADP. The alkoxy and peroxy radicals produced by the interaction of reduced iron compounds and lipid hydroperoxides then propagate the reaction [303]. Membranes of mitochondria and endoplasmic reticulum contain large amounts of unsaturated fatty acids [288], making them important sites of lipid peroxidation damage. Some of the most potent initiators of free-radical formation, including iron and hemoproteins, are found in mitochondria and endoplasmic reticulum. It is of interest that some degree of hypoxia may favor the occurrence of microsomal toxic activation and resulting lipid peroxidation [198, 608].

Although lipid peroxidation has received the most attention as a process by which intracellular free-radical metabolism produces injury, proteins and nucleic acids are also subject to free-radical metabolite-induced damage [27, 190, 191, 243, 250, 304, 404, 674, 721]. Even minimal oxidant damage can denature proteins, resulting in a loss of function or increased susceptibility to proteolysis [190, 191]. Oxidants can also inappropriately activate proteins, with damaging effects as shown for neutrophil collagenase [924]. Oxidant damage to nucleic acids limits cell repair and proliferation [27, 722]. The other major process by which toxic activation of xenobiotics to radical intermediates is involved in the pathogenesis of cell injury is covalent binding of activated metabolites of toxins to cellular macromolecules, with resulting functional changes and damage to membranes [686].

The highly reactive, transient nature of oxygen free radicals and the reactive intermediates they produce in target molecules makes their direct measurement impractical by current techniques. Instead, a variety of more stable and measurable markers have been used. These include spin trap behavior using electron paramagnetic resonance; oxidation of benzoic acid, phenol, salicylate, or methionine; lipid peroxidation–induced polyunsaturated fatty acid products such as malondialdehyde and 4-hydroxnonenal; lipid hydroperoxides; volatile hydrocarbons such as ethane; conjugated dienes; nonmitochondrial oxygen consumption; oxidized products of proteins and nucleic acids; levels of endogenous antioxidant compounds such as glutathione, ascorbate, and alpha-tocopherol; and behavior of the fluorescent probe, dichlorofluorescein [297, 650]. No single approach is applicable to all systems. Most data on lipid peroxidation during nephrotoxic renal injury pertain to malondialdehyde, a by-product of enzymatic oxygenation of polyunsaturated fatty acids and of nonenzymatic fatty peroxide formation and decomposition [375]. Although more direct methods are available, usually malondialdehyde has been assayed by the thiobarbituric acid test. The validities of both malondialdehyde as an index of lipid peroxidation and of the thiobarbituric acid test as a measure of malondialdehyde have been seriously questioned on multiple grounds [375]. Consequently, the results of malondialdehyde determinations are mentioned below because they are the only available information on a parameter potentially related to lipid peroxidation, but with the understanding that they must be cautiously interpreted. The situation with regard to studies of acute renal failure in vivo is further complicated by the vascular congestion that commonly occurs in that setting. The absorption spectrum of hemoglobin and other tissue chromogens overlaps with that of the thiobarbituric acid product measured during the usual thiobarbituric acid assay [257] and can confound measurement of the thiobarbituric acid product unless appropriate corrections are employed [257]. Detailed consideration of the merits of the various other methods for measuring malondialdehyde is beyond the scope of this chapter and is available elsewhere [297, 650].

Multiple intrinsic mechanisms modulate intracellular free-radical metabolism. They affect processes involved in both the generation of free-radical metabolites and other toxic intermediates and the disposition of these compounds when formed. Superoxide dismutase metabolizes superoxide but produces hydrogen peroxide [136, 250, 688]. Catalase enhances the metabolism of hydrogen peroxide to water and molecular oxygen, reducing the availability of hydrogen peroxide to participate in the Fenton reaction [136, 250, 688].

Glutathione (GSH) is a tripeptide with the amino acid sequence, gamma-glutamylcysteinylglycine. It is the most abundant cellular peptide and the major nonprotein thiol of most cells [529, 538, 539]. Roles for glutathione as an intracellular antioxidant and participant in detoxification reactions in the kidney and other tissues are well documented [26, 60, 123, 169, 299, 301, 539, 544, 627, 788], and it is a widely held view that a critical, minimal level of cellular glutathione is necessary for the prevention of oxidant damage to cellular lipids and proteins [546, 617, 627]. Glutathione acts to limit oxidant injury by serving as a substrate for glutathione peroxidase in the metabolism of hydrogen peroxide and lipid hydroperoxides [142, 483], is involved in the antioxidant effects of vitamin E [50, 627, 826, 891], and can interact directly with free-radical metabolites [681, 890]. It also plays an important role in maintaining protein sulfhydryl groups in the reduced state, by reducing oxidant availability through the latter mechanisms as well as by direct enzymatic reduction [60, 84]. Conjugation of glutathione mediated by glutathione-S-transferases or direct interactions with reactive compounds is an important detoxification mechanism and, as previously discussed, can also contribute to toxic activation of some compounds [539, 638, 688, 792].

Vitamin E, alpha-tocopherol, is a scavenger largely localized within membranes because of its high lipid solubility and thus plays a special role at the critical membrane lipid targets of free radicals [171, 627]. Tocopheryl radicals formed during reduction of lipid peroxyl radicals to lipid hydroperoxides by vitamin E are converted back to alpha-tocopherol by GSH with the participation of a labile membrane factor [123, 299, 627, 826]. Ascorbic acid can also scavenge free radicals [16] and act cooperatively with vitamin E [48, 627]. Whether glutathione predominantly acts to directly scavenge lipid peroxides or to maintain alpha-tocopherol and trap initiators of lipid peroxidation remains under investigation [627].

Because of its involvement in metabolizing oxygen radicals and other toxic metabolites, depletion of GSH, particularly when accompanied by accumulation of its oxidized disulfide form, GSSG, has been used as an index of "oxidant stress" [527, 627]. When applied to the kidney, this interpretation is complicated by the normal rapid turnover of glutathione in proximal tubule cells [539, 560, 735]. Glutathione constantly cycles out of the cell as both GSH and GSSG, is catabolized to its component amino acids via the sequential action of gamma-glutamyl transpeptidase and dipeptidase [437, 530, 539], and is then resynthesized after uptake of the precursors [43, 281, 282, 328, 539]. The purpose of this cycling has not been established, but it has been suggested to be involved in amino acid transport and in the protection of membranes from oxidant damage [539]. Since both uptake of precursor amino acids and intracellular resynthesis of glutathione are ATP-dependent processes [539, 710, 902, 903, 920], any injurious process that reduces ATP can substantially affect glutathione levels, irrespective of whether oxidants or toxic metabolites are involved.

The role of glutathione in the tubule response to injury is further complicated by recent observations that one of its component amino acids, glycine, has a critical, independent action to preserve the structural integrity of tubule cells against a variety of insults. This phenomenon was initially recognized in studies of hypoxic tubules [898, 899, 904, 922], but has since been demonstrated with chemical inhibitors of mitochondrial oxidative phosphorylation [903, 907], iodoacetate [900], ouabain [905], and, importantly, the calcium ionophore, ionomycin [907]. In the latter model, glycine protected tubule cells even though it did not prevent large increases of cytosolic free calcium [907]. Protection occurs at physiological amino acid levels [920], is not mediated by preservation of cell ATP or glutathione [513, 902, 903], and does not require metabolism of the amino acid [900, 904, 920, 922]. It is not limited to the proximal tubule, since it is expressed strongly with respect to hypoxic damage of the medullary thick ascending limb in the isolated perfused rat kidney [39, 755]. At present, information on glycine modulation of additional forms of toxic injury is limited. Glycine did not substantially protect against $HgCl_2$ toxicity [192]. It was not protective in one study using *tert*-butyl hydroperoxide [301], but in another study that tested *tert*-butyl hydroperoxide as well as menadione and hydrogen peroxide, protective effects of glutathione that required catabolism of the glutathione were suggestive of glycine involvement [454]. The mechanism for glycine's effects remains to be established [898, 900, 902–904, 907].

A number of agents with major effects on metabolic activation and free-radical metabolites have been widely used as probes for testing the contribution of these processes to various forms of injury. Phenobarbitol induces a group of mixed-function oxidases that participate in the metabolism of a variety of agents. Benzamphetamine-*N*-demethylase, one of these enzymes, has been widely used as a marker for the response [649]. SKF 525A inhibits the mixed-function oxidases produced by phenobarbital [262].

Another group of mixed-function oxidases is induced by polycyclic aromatic hydrocarbons, such as 3-methylcholanthrene. The spectrum of agents metabolized by this group of P450-dependent enzymes is narrower than that induced in response to phenobarbital. Ethoxyresofulin-*O*-deethylase may be used as a marker for this response [125]. Beta-naphthoflavone inhibits the mixed-function oxidases induced by methylcholanthrene [262]. Exposure to polybrominated or polychlorinated biphenyls increases levels of renal and hepatic microsomal enzymes [342].

Piperonyl butoxide inhibits both renal and hepatocyte microsomal enzyme activity [445]. Cobalt chloride decreases cytochrome P450 synthesis [531] and increases GSH levels [699]. Methionine sulfoximine inhibits gamma-glutamyl cysteine synthetase and markedly reduces glutathione levels throughout the proximal tubule [105]. Buthionine sulfoximine acts similarly [283]. Diethyl maleate decreases tissue GSH [688]. 1,3-Bis (2-chloroethyl)-1-nitrosourea (BCNU) inhibits glutathione reductase [237]. Cysteine can increase GSH levels. L-2-oxothiazolidine-4-carboxylate facilitates intracellular delivery of cysteine and, as a result, increases glutathione levels [935]. Alternatively, glutathione monoesters can be used to facilitate cellular uptake of intact glutathione [20, 709].

DMSO, mannitol, and dimethylthiourea are hydroxyl radical scavengers [248, 270, 732]. Deferoxamine chelates the Fe^{++} required for the Fenton reaction [298] and can also scavenge peroxyl and alkoxyl radicals at higher concentrations [313]. *N,N'*-diphenyl-*p*-phenylenediamine (DPPD) has been widely used as an antioxidant but also can inhibit microsomal cytochrome P450 bioactivation reactions [379].

Interpreting the effects of agents altering intracellular toxic activation and free-radical metabolism is complex because of several factors. (1) Differential effects in liver and kidney may alter drug distribution. For example, increased hepatic metabolism may decrease delivery to the kidney, thus reducing toxicity on that basis. This occurs with cyclosporine [180]. (2) Within a given tissue, competing metabolic pathways may be evoked to various degrees so that both toxin activation and inactivation are simultaneously increased, and the net effect is a balance of the two processes. (3) The agents used may affect the nature of toxicity by means of processes that are independent of toxic activation or free-radical production, e.g., alterations of cellular toxin transport.

The processes by which toxic activation and free-radical production ultimately lead to cell death remain under study. Considerable data are available on two major processes implicated in the general pathogenesis of cell injury—abnormal calcium metabolism and phospholipase activation. Lipid peroxidation decreases microsomal enzyme activity in general [263, 336, 338, 644], and microsomal calcium sequestration has been shown to be inhibited by CCl_4 [578], bromotrichloromethane [492], and 1,1-dichloroethylene [577, 664]. The loss of microsomal calcium transport activity resulting from treatment with CCl_4 is very rapid. It occurs within 10 to 15 minutes of intragastric administration and is substantial—85 percent [491]. Microsomal calcium sequestration can be compromised either by covalent binding or by lipid peroxidation [878].

Lipid peroxidation of lysosomes enhanced phospholipid degradation and production of lysophospholipids, suggesting an action of lipid peroxidation to enhance susceptibility of membrane phospholipids to phospholipases [892]. Synthetic peroxidized lipids are more sensitive to phospholipases [737]. Lipid peroxidation increases the mitochondrial membrane sensitivity to phospholipases [950]. Decreased intramitochondrial GSH/GSSG ratios have been implicated in the promotion of Ca^{++}-dependent membrane phospholipase-mediated injury to the inner mitochondrial membrane, possibly by means of reduction of lysophospholipid acyltransferase activity induced by the decreased GSH/GSSG ratios [54].

A major question about the pathogenesis of injury produced by intracellular free-radical generation is how metabolites are distributed in cells so as to cause damage at sites that are distant from where they are generated initially. CCl_4 hepatotoxicity has been an important model system for study. Lipid peroxidation in CCl_4 toxicity is largely locally confined to the ER [667]. It has been proposed that aldehyde products, such as 4-hydroxynonenal, may result from lipid peroxidation and cause injury to membranes both locally and remotely [63, 64, 207, 229]. However, the role of 4-hydroxyalkenals in mediating injury has been disputed based on the fact that the concentration of Fe^{++} required for injury to be mediated by this mechanism is far above that likely to be present in vivo [667]. Additionally, the amounts of 4-hydroxyalkenals needed for production of injury are unlikely to result from the degree of lipid peroxidation that can be measured. If high levels of 4-hydroxyethanols developed, they would likely decrease hepatic glutathione levels. Such changes in glutathione levels are not prominent features of CCl_4 toxicity [667].

In considering the role of toxic activation and free-radical production in injury, it is important to distinguish between causes and effects of injury. CCl_4-induced cell damage is present prior to measurable lipid peroxidation [785]. In isolated hepatocytes, blebbing of the plasma membrane occurs within 5 minutes after CCl_4 exposure, prior to morphological alterations of the ER associated with CCl_4 toxicity there [632]. Lipid peroxidation may occur consequent to cell damage [768] or as a coincident process that is not actually involved in the determination of cell viability. Treatment with iodoacetamide, diethyl maleate, or vanadate decreased viability of isolated hepatocytes and was accompanied by lipid peroxidation. DPPD, in each case, effectively prevented lipid peroxidation but did not have as consistent an effect on the losses of viability [787]. Lipid peroxidation can occur without cell damage [419, 785, 786, 953]. In a coordinated series of studies, it was possible to demonstrate (1) lipid peroxidation without inhibition of microsomal Ca^{++} sequestration or lethal cell injury after cumene hydroperoxide treatment, (2) lipid peroxidation with lethal cell injury and inhibition of microsomal Ca^{++} sequestration after CCl_4, and (3) inhibition of microsomal calcium sequestration and lethal cell injury without lipid peroxidation after thioacetamide [953].

Covalent binding of toxic metabolites need not necessarily result in cell injury. In studies of acetaminophen (APAP)-treated hepatocytes, CaEDTA, by unclear mechanisms, exerted a marked protective effect after transient toxin exposure without altering covalent binding but did reduce lipid peroxidation. CaEDTA was not protective against the toxicity of prolonged APAP exposure, and this toxicity was not associated with lipid peroxidation [51]. Hepatic necrosis secondary to bromobenzene occurred when glutathione levels dropped to 2.5 to 3.5 nmol/mg protein and was accompanied at that time by lipid peroxidation. Covalent binding was also observed; however, the correlation between its occurrence and cell injury was weaker. Treatment with a vitamin E analogue was highly protective against lipid peroxidation and cell injury but did not alter the extent of covalent binding [139]. APAP sensitivity of cultured hepatocytes induced by methylcholanthrene was further potentiated by BCNU, an inactivator of glutathione reductase, without any increases in covalent binding. Deferoxamine ameliorated sensitivity to injury, while ferric chloride restored sensitivity. No concomitant changes in covalent binding were observed during any of these maneuvers, suggesting a more important role for oxygen metabolites than for covalent binding in APAP toxicity [262].

Several processes may interact in complex fashion. It is well established that vitamin E deficiency can enhance membrane damage [124, 300, 327, 815] due to various oxidative stresses. Removal of medium Ca^{++} accelerated loss of membrane vitamin E and increased the toxic effects of treating isolated hepatocytes with doxorubicin (Adriamycin) and BCNU or with the alkylating agent, ethylmethanesulfonate. Replacement of vitamin E reduced toxicity in the Ca^{++}-free medium. In a vitamin E replete medium, raising medium Ca^{++} enhanced toxicity. Thus the effects of modulating medium Ca^{++} were dependent on membrane vitamin E levels, which, in turn, were sensitive to modulation of medium Ca^{++} [237].

The specific activities of drug-metabolizing enzymes in the kidney, particularly the cytochrome P450–dependent mixed-function oxidases, are substantially less than those in the liver [251, 481, 831]. To some extent, this is due to the functional heterogeneity of the renal tubule, with higher levels of enzymes found in particular nephron segments. Cytochrome P450 is present throughout the proximal tubule; however, S3 segments appear to be the most prominent sites of inducible mixed-function oxidases [197, 686, 688]. The degree of inducibility varies from one species to another. In rabbit kidney, both phenobarbital and polycyclic aromatic hydrocarbons are effective inducers. In rat, only the polycyclic aromatic hydrocarbons are effective [444, 831, 965].

FREE-RADICAL AND TOXIC ACTIVATION INJURY WITH SPECIFIC NEPHROTOXINS

Chloroform. Chloroform produces proximal tubule cell injury to various degrees, depending on species and sex, with a prominent reproducible lesion that is amenable to study in male mice and is dependent on the presence of testosterone [363, 688]. The hepatic metabolism of chloroform proceeds by means of phenobarbital-inducible cytochrome P450–dependent mixed-function oxidases to trichloromethanol and then to phosgene, a highly electrophilic compound [643, 688], which reacts with cellular macromolecules, or with water to form HCl and CO_2 (the major pathway), or can be conjugated with glutathione or cysteine [119, 642, 688]. Covalent binding of ^{14}C after administration of $^{14}CHCl_3$ was found in both liver and kidney and was concentrated in areas of greatest injury, suggesting a role for covalent binding of a reactive metabolite in the pathogenesis of injury [363]. An important detoxification role for glutathione during chloroform nephrotoxicity is suggested by the early occurrence of renal glutathione depletion during developing nephrotoxicity and the potentiation of chloroform toxicity by pretreatment with diethyl maleate to decrease available glutathione [421].

Studies of the effects of inducers and inhibitors of mixed-function oxidase activity on chloroform nephrotoxicity have been complicated by the variable and different effects of these agents in liver and kidney and the difficulty of determining whether renal effects were independent or were secondary to metabolites produced in liver [688]. However, recent studies using renal slices have demonstrated that injury requiring metabolism of $CHCl_3$ occurs preferentially in slices from male mice [766]. Chloroform is metabolized by renal microsomes by a mechanism typical of mixed-function oxidases, which can be induced by phenobarbital pretreatment [766, 767]. This metabolism results in covalent binding, which can be ameliorated by glutathione or cysteine [767], and a cysteine conjugate of phosgene is identifiable after kidney-slice metabolism of chloroform [767].

Acetaminophen. Several mechanisms involving toxic metabolites have been proposed for acetaminophen (APAP). These mechanisms include (1) activation of APAP itself by mixed-function oxidases to an electrophilic metabolite, which covalently binds to cellular macromolecules [532]; (2) deacetylation of APAP to paraminophenol (PAP) [261, 772], which, in turn, is metabolized to a free-radical product, which covalently binds to cellular macromolecules [261, 596]; and (3) activation of APAP to an arylating metabolite by the prostaglandin endoperoxide synthetase system [97, 138, 558]. The first two mechanisms could contribute to injury of cortical tubules, while the third would be limited to medullary structures where the required enzymes are concentrated. GSH depletion has been postulated to play a major role in the development of APAP toxicity by allowing for binding of reactive metabolites to cellular macromolecules rather than detoxification by means of conjugation with GSH [532]. Studies comparing the relative importance of covalent binding and oxygen metabolites, such as done for hepatic APAP toxicity [262], have not been reported for renal APAP toxicity.

Cephalosporins. As detailed previously, uptake of cephaloridine by means of the organic acid transport system and achievement of relatively high intracellular levels because of a slow efflux process have been proposed by major factors in the pathogenesis of cephaloridine-induced renal tubular cell injury [150, 842, 843, 853, 926]. Toxic activation of intracellular cephaloridine may mediate its intracellular toxicity. In support of this possibility, it was observed that phenobarbital potentiated cephaloridine toxicity [531] while piperonyl butoxide protected against it [215, 441, 531]. However, phenobarbital also increased tissue cephaloridine, while piperonyl butoxide decreased drug levels [441] so that primary effects on drug handling rather than on metabolism probably explain the actions of these agents.

Cephaloridine may promote lipid peroxidation as a result of a one-electron reduction of the pyridine ring of the antibiotic (structurally similar to paraquat) to a free radical, which is then oxidized by O_2 with the formation of superoxide ions [443]. Isolated rat kidney microsomes incubated with NADPH produced superoxide anion and malondialdehyde [163]. Malondialdehyde production could be inhibited by superoxide dismutase plus catalase, as well as by the hydroxyl radical scavengers, mannitol and (+)-cyanidanol-3, and by the singlet oxygen scavenger, histidine [163]. Involvement of lipid peroxidation in the pathogenesis of cephaloridine toxicity was supported by the finding of increased levels of conjugated dienes in the kidney during cephaloridine toxicity and the observation that vitamin E– or selenium-deficient diets potentiated toxicity [443]. Isolated kidney slices showed increases of malondialdehyde with cephaloridine, but not with cefotaxime [165]. The cephaloridine-induced increases of malondialdehyde and associated impairment of slice tetraethylammonium accumulation were blocked by DPPD and alpha-tocopherol [165]. Tissue GSH depletion was observed during cephaloridine toxicity and diethylmaleate-enhanced toxicity [442], suggesting an important role for GSH. Since no GSH conjugates of cephaloridine metabolites were detectable and the loss of GSH could be completely accounted for as GSSG, it was proposed that GSH was being depleted as a result of its activity to reduce lipid hydroperoxides [443].

Although these observations support a role for lipid peroxidation in cephaloridine nephrotoxicity, other reports indicate that it may not be the critical factor. When cephaloridine was compared to another highly nephrotoxic cephalosporin, cephaloglycin, both agents sharply reduced renal cortical GSH, but only cephaloridine led to increases in GSSG and malondialdehyde [847]. However, cephaloridine and cephaloglycin had equivalent effects on mitochondrial function, suggesting that this effect was more closely related to injury [847]. In isolated rabbit proximal tubules treated with cephaloridine, GSH depletion, ATP depletion, and malondialdehyde formation preceded lethal cell injury. The presence of DPPD during the first 3 hours of cephaloridine exposure protected the tubules and blocked the malondialdehyde formation and ATP depletion but not the GSH depletion. During 5 additional hours of incubation, however, the protective effect of DPPD was lost, even though malondialdehyde continued to be suppressed [687].

Carbon Tetrachloride. Carbon tetrachloride has been implicated in cases of human acute renal failure [290, 595, 762] but has proved to be elusive as a nephrotoxin in animal models, where effects on tubular cells, although present, were relatively mild [499, 798]. Striking structural alterations of the ER after CCl_4, such as those seen in liver [665], were not seen in kidney [798]. Although still subject to investigation, lipid peroxidation as a result of CCl_4 metabolism by mixed-function oxidases to trichloromethyl free radical can be identified readily in the liver during CCl_4 toxicity [665]. No such evidence of lipid peroxidation has been found in studies of kidney [154, 784, 871].

Mercuric Chloride. Treatment of cultured Chinese hamster ovary cells with $HgCl_2$ resulted in increased leakage of superoxide radicals [132]. Evidence for free-radical formation and lipid peroxidation during in vivo mercuric chloride nephrotoxicity, based on increased levels of conjugated dienes, increased malondialdehyde, and decreased glutathione peroxidase activity was obtained following two daily doses of mercuric chloride [951]. A recent study has assessed this issue using a common model of acute toxicity, a single subcutaneous dose of 4 mg/kg. The study also evaluated maleate nephrotoxicity. At 12 hours after mercuric chloride, renal cortical levels of superoxide dismutase and catalase were unchanged from controls, while both glutathione peroxidase and glutathione reductase were significantly reduced. At 24 hours after mercuric chloride, all four enzymes were reduced. Two hours after maleate, only glutathione peroxidase was reduced. Total glutathione (GSH + GSSG) was normal at 6 hours after mercuric chloride but was severely reduced at 24 hours and at 2 hours after maleate. Malondialdehyde levels were not altered in mercuric chloride or maleate-treated kidneys; however, in vitro formation of malondialdehyde by renal cortical homogenates in response to cumene hydroperoxide was enhanced after both toxins [287]. After subcutaneous Hg^{++} administration, tissue Hg^{++} levels peak within the first 3 to 4 hours; subcellular effects of Hg^{++} are detectable over that time frame [912]; and cell necrosis becomes evident after about 6 hours [210]. The absence of more striking changes in the free-radical metabolism parameters measured during the first 6 hours after mercuric chloride suggests a minor role, if any, for them in the pathogenesis of mercuric chloride nephrotoxicity. Consistent with this, infusion of superoxide dismutase had no effects to alter the course of mercuric chloride toxicity in vivo [622]. In studies of the effects of mercuric chloride on isolated hepatocytes, malondialdehyde levels and ethane, another lipid peroxidation product, increased along with losses of viability as assessed by enzyme leakage, and GSH levels fell. However, treatment with antioxidants inhibited lipid peroxidation without substantially affecting cell viability [786]. These observations argue against a major role for lipid peroxidation in the toxicity of mercuric chloride and suggest that it may occur as a secondary process. Decreasing cellular glutathione with buthionine sulfoximine aggravates $HgCl_2$ nephrotoxicity while augmenting glutathione ameliorates nephrotoxicity [72, 589]. Glutathione probably acts mainly by producing sulfhydryl binding sites for Hg^{++}, alternative to those on important cellular macromolecules, and by favoring excretion of the metal in the urine [911, 912, 962]. Similar considerations apply to models where cadmium is acutely nephrotoxic [761, 806, 807].

Gentamicin. Gentamicin-induced alterations of mitochondrial electron transport have been shown to increase mitochondrial hydrogen peroxide production in vitro [876]. Gentamicin treatment in vivo increased renal cortical malondialdehyde levels [659, 660, 877], decreased total glutathione [659, 660], increased the GSSG/GSH ratio [659, 660], sharply reduced levels of esterified arachidonic acid, and induced a generalized shift from polyunsaturated to saturated fatty acids [368, 660]. All of these changes are consistent with an oxidative insult. Gentamicin also decreased activities of catalase and superoxide dismutase [660]. Several different hydroxyl radical scavengers, dimethylthiourea, dimethyl sulfoxide, and sodium benzoate, and two iron chelators, deferoxamine and 2,3-dihydrobenzoic acid, strongly ameliorated nephrotoxicity [877]. The effect of dimethylthiourea was accompanied by suppression of malondialdehyde formation [877]. However, neither DPPD [659] nor alpha-tocopherol [660] ameliorated nephrotoxicity, even though DPPD prevented increases of malondialdehyde and oxidation of glutathione [659] and pretreatment with alpha-tocopherol prevented those effects as well as the shift from polyunsaturated to saturated fatty acids [660]. Depletion of cellular glutathione with buthionine sulfoximine did not aggravate gentamicin nephrotoxicity [946]. Primary cultures of rat proximal tubule cells were not suitable for further assessing radical mechanisms in gentamicin toxicity because the antibiotic did not induce either malondialdehyde formation or increased fluorescence of intracellular dichlorofluorescein, which would have been suggestive of radical formation [810]. Thus, there is evidence for oxidant stress, lipid peroxidation, and Fe^{++}-mediated damage during gentamicin nephrotoxicity in vivo, but lipid peroxidation per se does not appear to play a necessary role in toxicity.

Cisplatin. Nephrotoxicity of cisplatin is importantly modulated as a result of biotransformation, but the complete mechanisms for toxic activation and detoxification have not been defined. Substitution of the chlorides on cisplatin with water, a process favored by the relatively low intracellular Cl^- concentration, produces a positively charged, more reactive compound that has been suggested to mediate both antitumor efficacy and nephrotoxicity [383, 480, 482]. Unbound platinum in ultrafiltrates of cytosol from kidney had a different chromatographic migration pattern than the parent compound and was substantially less mutagenic, suggesting metabolism within renal tubular cells to a less toxic form [691]. The elution pattern of this derivative suggested that the compound was a neutral one formed by nucleophilic substitution for chloride [691]. In contrast to the rapid development of lethal cell injury seen with other heavy-metal acute nephrotoxins such as Hg^{++} [284] and uranyl [405], lethal cell injury produced by cisplatin is delayed until 48 to 72 hours after administration [211]. Whether this is due to the time required for transformation or to a unique nature of the target sites injured is not known.

Lipid peroxidation, generally assessed as increases of malondialdehyde levels, accompanied cisplatin-induced tissue damage both in vivo and in vitro [88, 307, 308, 573, 801, 802]. In a study of isolated rat proximal tubules and inner medullary collecting duct cells, both cell types exhibited effects on mitochondrial respiration, but only the proximal tubules had increases of malondialdehyde and lytic plasma membrane damage indicated by release of ^{51}Cr [291].

DPPD and alpha-tocopherol have been reported to at least partially ameliorate cisplatin toxicity [307, 800–802]. These reports did not fully exclude effects on drug uptake or metabolism. In a study using rabbit renal cortical slices, DPPD did ameliorate cisplatin-induced depression of organic cation and anion concentrative capacity without altering cisplatin accumulation; however, the effect was relatively small [308]. Transplatin, a stereoisomer of cisplatin that lacks both antitumor properties and nephrotoxic effects in vivo [468] despite accumulation in the kidney in amounts equivalent to cisplatin [337], induced greater malondialdehyde production and impairment of concentrative capacity in the renal cortical slices than did cisplatin [308]. The effects of transplatin on the slices were associated with severalfold higher levels of accumulation than those of cisplatin in the slices. Carboplatin, an effective antitumor agent considered to have reduced nephrotoxic potential [310, 609, 764], was accumulated the least, did not impair concentrative capacity, and produced little increase of malondialdehyde [308]. Firmer conclusions about a pathogenetic role for lipid peroxidation after cisplatin will require an assessment of the degree to which antioxidants can modify progression to lytic cell damage. In this regard, it is relevant that cisplatin, transplatin, and hydrolysis products of cisplatin inhibited lactate dehydrogenase, a widely applied marker for lytic cell damage [165], so that alternative parameters are more appropriate for studies of platinum compounds.

Unlike most other forms of nephrotoxicity where it has been assessed, glutathione depletion is not a prominent feature of cisplatin nephrotoxicity. The majority of studies have described either normal or elevated glutathione levels after cisplatin [470, 473, 574], suggesting that glutathione turnover is retarded. Consistent with this, glutathione reductase, glutathione peroxidase, and glutathione-S-transferase were all inhibited after cisplatin treatment [88, 89]. Cisplatin can complex with glutathione [194, 482] and these complexes are less nephrotoxic, at least when formed extracellularly [574]. Depletion of cellular glutathione in most studies has enhanced cisplatin nephrotoxicity [19, 368, 574]. Systemic infusion of glutathione is protective [19, 971, 972] and glutathione monoisopropyl ester, which has a greater effect on intracellular glutathione content than glutathione itself, is more potent [19]. These observations taken together with the efficacy of other sulfhydryl reagents, diethyldithiocarbamate and thiosulfate [93, 94, 348, 574], favor the concept that cellular nonprotein sulfhydryl compounds trap toxic platinum derivatives and protect critical protein sulfhydryl groups [93, 94, 470]. Glutathione may also protect by acting as a source of glycine, since glycine alone was recently shown to afford a similar degree of protection [330]. Whether this effect of glycine is related to an interaction of the amino with cisplatin [194, 699] or to the recently identified, general cytoprotective action of glycine for kidney tubules [898, 904] has not been fully clarified.

Cyclosporine. Treatment with Aroclor 1254, a polychlorinated biphenyl, or phenobarbital, but not 3-methylcholanthrene, protected against cyclosporine-induced nephrotoxicity as a result of induction by these agents of hepatic mixed-function oxidases [180]. However, reported changes of ER morphology in renal tubular cells after cyclosporine suggest that some events in the cellular handling of the drug in the kidney may occur at that subcellular level [895].

Cysteine Conjugates. Roles for depletion of glutathione and lipid peroxidation in toxicity of cysteine conjugates activated by beta-lyase have been assessed in several systems. Mice treated with either trichloroethylene [161] or its active cysteine conjugate, dichlorovinylcysteine (DCVC) [79], had decreases of renal cortical glutathione and increases of ethane exhalation and cortical malondialdehyde, but the timing of these changes relative to the appearance of necrosis was not precisely established. Isolated rabbit proximal tubules had 50 percent decreases of GSH content within 15 minutes of exposure that were associated with inhibition of organic anion and cation transport; supplementation with exogenous GSH maintained cellular GSH levels and prevented the transport effects, but development of lethal cell injury was not assessed [315].

Depletion of nonprotein sulfhydryls (predominantly GSH) and accumulation of malondialdehyde clearly preceded lethal cell injury in LLC-PK_1 cells treated with DCVC [145]. Deferoxamine as well as several phenolic antioxidants including DPPD, butylated hydroxytoluene, propyl gallate, and butylated hydroxyquinone decreased the extent of lethal cell damage in this system. DPPD, the most effective of the antioxidants, and deferoxamine markedly suppressed malondialdehyde formation without altering metabolism of DCVC, covalent binding of its products, or depletion of nonprotein sulfhydryls. The sulfhydryl-reducing agent, dithiothreitol (DTT), also prevented cell death and lipid peroxidation despite metabolism and covalent binding of DCVC [145]. DPPD also protected primary cultures of rat proximal tubule cells against DCVC, but was effective only against a relatively low concentration of DCVC (25 μM) in suspensions of freshly isolated proximal tubule cells [145].

In suspensions of isolated rabbit proximal tubules, butylated hydroxytoluene and DPPD delayed lethal cell injury produced by 25 μM DCVC, but the effect was largely lost by 6 hours despite continued suppression of DCVC-induced malondialdehyde formation [286]. Deferoxamine acted similarly to DPPD and butylated hydroxytoluene in providing limited protection against lethal cell injury while completely suppressing malondialdehyde formation. Comparable effects of DPPD, butylated hydroxytoluene, and deferoxamine were also found in this system for several other nephrotoxic cysteine conjugates including pentachlorobutadienylcysteine, chlorotrifluoroethylcysteine, and tetrafluoroethylcysteine except that, for tetrafluoroethylcysteine, suppression of malondialdehyde production by deferoxamine and butylated hydroxytoluene was not associated with a significant reduction in cell killing [286]. Of note, chlorpromazine was also tested in this study. It suppressed malondialdehyde production and provided greater and more consistent protection than any butylated hydroxytoluene, DPPD, or deferoxamine [286].

These recent comprehensive studies with isolated cell systems [145, 286] have thus provided evidence for involvement of iron-dependent lipid peroxidation in the pathogenesis of cysteine conjugate–induced tubule cell damage, but it is only one of a number of factors involved and its role varies with different degrees of insult and stages of injury. The mechanisms by which it occurs and its relationship and importance to the other factors implicated in damage—covalent binding of reactive metabolites, soluble and nonsoluble thiol depletion, inhibition of mitochondrial ATP production, and disturbances of intracellular Ca^{++} homeostasis—remain to be determined.

Thus, toxic activation and free-radical production are central processes in the pathophysiology of the cellular toxicity of multiple agents and play an important role in several nephrotoxic lesions. Additional studies are needed to more precisely define their occurrence and contribution to injury produced by the commonly studied nephrotoxins, with particular reference to whether the phenomena observed are primary events leading to loss of cell integrity.

Disturbances of Tubule Cell Energy Metabolism

Renal tubule cells are abundantly supplied with mitochondria, which provide the controlled oxidative metabolism to produce the ATP required to drive transport and other energy-consuming processes. Mitochondria comprise about 30 percent of the protein and volume of renal proximal tubule cells [356, 634]. The surface area of the inner mitochondrial membrane, the site of oxidative phosphorylation, exceeds the sum of the basolateral and brush-border membrane surface areas [356, 634]. Kidney tubules normally respire at rates that are only about one-third maximal, suggesting the availability of redundant functional capacity [311, 894].

Renal cortex ATP levels are reduced by a number of nephrotoxins prior to the appearance of lethal cell injury. Total ATP levels are depressed in kidney during the early stages of nephrotoxicity induced by gentamicin and *cis*-platinum when mitochondrial dysfunction is demonstrable [758, 759]. These events occur well before loss of cellular integrity. Sequential studies of adenine nucleotide and lactate levels in a standard rat model of nephrotoxicity, produced by subcutaneous injection of $HgCl_2$ (4 mg/kg), have demonstrated falls in ATP to 80 percent of control levels in the first hour, 60 to 70 percent at 6 hours, 57 percent at 24 hours, and 42 percent at 48 hours. Total adenine nucleotides showed a parallel but slightly less marked decrease. Lactate increased to three times control levels at 6 hours and remained elevated through 48 hours [633, 834]. Renal cortical ATP levels fell rapidly after maleic acid treatment and at 1 hour were 60 percent of control [22, 712, 812]. Total adenine nucleotides were reduced to 80 percent of control [22]. Further decreases of ATP to 20 percent of control and of total adenine nucleotides to 40 percent of control were seen at 3 hours [677]. While these alterations of adenine nucleotide metabolism could be due to decreases in oxygen supply as a result of changes in renal blood flow or of increases in ATP consumption due to various cellular effects of nephrotoxins on ATP consuming processes, such changes in ATP levels have been associated in several models with simultaneous impairment of functional properties of isolated renal cortical mitochondria [356], suggesting a primary role for mitochondrial damage in early nephrotoxic renal cell injury.

The complex balance of transport functions at the inner mitochondrial membrane, requiring maintenance and precise regulation of its selective permeability properties, makes it highly sensitive to perturbation by toxins [356]. All nephrotoxins that have been evaluated have direct effects on mitochondrial function in vitro, and these are usually highly specific in nature. However, several factors dictate caution in comparing the changes in mitochondrial function after in vivo exposure with those after in vitro exposure.

1. Assessment of a limited number of mitochondrial functional parameters can be misleading. Changes in state 4 and state 3 rates and acceptor control ratios (ACRs) are, in and of themselves, nonspecific in the absence of additional information, since similar rate alterations may result from different mechanisms. Simply showing that a particular toxin produces the same effects on one of these parameters in vivo and in vitro does not imply an identical mechanism for the effects.
2. The precise degree of exposure of mitochondria to toxins in situ is unknown for most toxins and, with present methods, may be difficult to determine. Aminoglycosides are a good example. As detailed in the following discussion, the in vitro conditions for their maximal activity include the absence of added Mg^{++}, a condition unlikely to be present within cells. Furthermore, the concentration of aminoglycoside associated with mitochondria after in vivo treatment, sufficient to produce nephrotoxicity, is unknown and is very difficult to assess; large amounts of gentamicin are concentrated in lysosomes, which contaminate other organelle fractions obtained by subcellular fractionation procedures.
3. Redistribution of toxins during mitochondrial isolation may occur. Of necessity, mitochondria must be isolated from disrupted tissues, which results in a mixing of the intracellular and extracellular compartments, albeit under metabolically quiescent conditions at relatively high dilutions. Nonetheless, the po-

tential exists for toxins that were associated with mitochondria in situ to be lost as well as for toxins not associated with mitochondria in situ to gain access to them. The actual extent to which this redistribution occurs depends on the unique properties and compartmentalization of the agent in question and must be determined empirically for each agent studied.

4. Mitochondrial function may be altered during isolation as a result of the exposure of mitochondria from undamaged cells to toxic products that have accumulated in damaged cells. The increased levels of calcium present in injured tissue may further damage mitochondria during the isolation unless a Ca^{++} chelator is present [916]. Free esterified fatty acids present at increased levels in injured tissues could be redistributed with damaging effects on mitochondria [103, 406]. Mitochondria from injured tissues also could be nonspecifically more sensitive to the physical forces involved in the isolation and the components of the isolation medium.
5. Toxins may induce early cellular metabolic alterations, such as free-radical production and perturbation of phospholipid metabolism, which produce mitochondrial effects to a greater degree in vivo than direct toxin-mitochondria interactions in vitro.

Used in conjunction with studies of isolated mitochondria, studies of oxygen consumption of intact samples of renal tissue potentially offer the opportunity to determine whether the changes in bioenergetics of the isolated mitochondria are actually expressed in situ. However, results of studies with tissue slices have been inconclusive and, at times, contradictory. One problem has been that, by and large, most investigators have only measured total O_2 consumption. In the absence of additional manipulations, this single measurement provides only limited information. No determination of how efficiently O_2 consumption is coupled to ATP production and how the measured values relate to the maximal capacity of the tissue can be obtained. Furthermore, it has been demonstrated that the state of oxygenation of tissue slices is relatively poor and their work of transport is relatively low compared to the in vivo situation, adding to the difficulty of interpreting the data [41]. Preparations of isolated tubules [41] can overcome many of the problems with tissue slices and information using this approach is available for acute effects of some nephrotoxins, as detailed below. Since many agents have time courses of action extending over hours to days, it would be desirable to isolate tubules after toxin treatment in vivo. Whether such already damaged tubules will tolerate the isolation procedure without further damage that obscures the underlying in vivo effects remains to be determined but success with postischemic tubules [259] supports the feasibility of this approach.

Mitochondria isolated from kidneys of rats treated with gentamicin exhibit functional abnormalities prior to the occurrence of renal tubule cell necrosis and calcium overload, and renal cortex ATP levels are reduced, findings consistent with the actions of aminoglycosides to alter mitochondrial function in vivo during the developmental stages of cell injury [758, 913]. Whether the in vivo changes seen are direct or indirect effects of the aminoglycosides remains uncertain. Although sufficient total cell gentamicin is present to affect mitochondria, much of this is compartmentalized within lysosomes and is not available for direct interaction [918]. The high levels of intracellular Mg^{++} would be expected to blunt the specific interactions of aminoglycosides with Mg^{++}-sensitive sites, which are demonstrable in vitro [910, 914]. In fact, the pattern of respiratory effects observed in the isolated mitochondria, inhibition of state 3 and uncoupled respiratory rates, differs from the main effect, stimulation of state 4 rates, seen with the lowest effective levels of gentamicin in vitro [758, 913]. This finding suggests that gentamicin exposure in vitro during mitochondrial isolation is not altering respiratory rates but indicates either that direct interaction of gentamicin with mitochondria in vivo leads to further functional alterations than are manifested during short-term in vitro experiments or that the mitochondrial functional changes are secondary to other gentamicin-induced subcellular effects. In this regard, mitochondria isolated from kidneys during gentamicin treatment had decreased levels of cytochrome oxidase and cytochrome *c*, suggesting that reduced synthesis of respiratory chain enzymes coated outside the mitochondrion played a role in the decreases of respiratory chain activity seen [540]. Studies of renal slices taken early during the course of gentamicin toxicity have revealed diminished respiration, gluconeogenesis, and ammoniagenesis consistent with the presence of altered mitochondrial function [425].

Small amounts of reactive oxygen metabolites are normally produced during electron transport [95, 854]. This production is greater with increased rates of electron transport and in the presence of partial blocks at any of several points in the electron transport chain [95, 854]. Both of these latter conditions occur during exposure of mitochondria to gentamicin [61, 758, 910, 914], and isolated renal cortical mitochondria treated with gentamicin showed increased rates of hydrogen peroxide production [876] that have been implicated in development of toxicity in vivo [877].

The potency of Hg^{++} to alter the normal integrated function of the inner mitochondrial membrane is well recognized [114, 447, 734, 779, 781]. Its interactions with biological macromolecules have been generally associated with its high affinity for sulfhydryl groups [155, 628]. Renal cortical mitochondria exposed to Hg^{++} in vitro exhibited stimulation of state 4 respiration at 2 nmol Hg^{++}/mg mitochondrial protein. Increasing Hg^{++} to 10 nmol/mg mitochondrial protein resulted in generalized respiratory inhibition. Sulfhydryl reagents and albumin, as well as the mix of other subcellular organelles and cytosolic proteins present in renal cortical homogenates, provided alternative Hg^{++} binding sites that could ameliorate its mitochondrial effects [912]. Renal cortical mitochondria isolated from rats within 1 to 3 hours after treatment with 5 mg/kg $HgCl_2$ subcutaneously showed depressed state 3 and dinitrophenol (DNP) uncoupled rates and adenine nucleotide translocase activity. Hg^{++} levels were 0.72 nmol/mg protein, and this Hg^{++} was more tightly bound than that present after acute in vitro Hg^{++} exposure. The data thus implicate mitochondria as an early intracellular site of Hg^{++} action during the development of $HgCl_2$ toxicity but suggest, as was the case for the aminoglycosides, that the response to Hg^{++} is conditioned by intracellular factors more complex than conditions present in studies of isolated mitochondria [912]. Isolated tubules treated with $HgCl_2$ show alterations in plasma membrane permeability before changes of mitochondrial respiration occur [106], but, as discussed in the calcium section, these may be due to differences in the mode of delivery.

Cephalosporins, including cephaloridine, cephaloglycin, and cephalexin (nontoxic), inhibit state 3 mitochondrial respiratory rates in vitro [844, 845, 852]. Renal cortical mitochondria isolated 2 hours after cephaloridine or cephaloglycin treatment also had inhibited respiratory rates, but mitochondria isolated after cephalexin were unaffected [844]. These effects have been shown to predominantly result from inhibition by cephalosporins of the mitochondrial anion transporter [849, 851]. All cephalosporins tested have this action in vitro, but it is only found after treatment in vivo with the nephrotoxic cephalosporins. This difference between nephrotoxic and nonnephrotoxic compounds has been attributed to higher cellular levels and affinity for the transport site of the toxic agents and to an ability of the toxic agents to acylate the transporter [842, 844, 845, 849, 851]. The thienamycin, imipenem, behaves like the toxic cephalosporins [846].

As detailed in the section on reactive metabolite–induced injury, oxidative damage has been proposed as a major mechanism for cephalosporin nephrotoxicity [163, 443, 687]. The relative importance of primary mitochondrial effects of cephalosporins versus oxidative damage remains under study [687, 847]. Cephaloridine and cephaloglycin, which are highly nephrotoxic, had similar strong effects on mitochondrial function, but only cephaloridine altered the cellular parameters of oxidant damage [847]. In studies that directly assessed cephalosporin effects on energetics in situ, the respiratory rates of intact tubules isolated 2 hours after cephaloridine exposure in vivo were inhibited, as were the rates of normal isolated tubules exposed to cephaloridine in vitro for 2 hours [845]. However, in detailed serial time course studies that followed respiration, ATP levels, and lactate dehydrogenase release as a measure of cytotoxicity, a causal relationship between mitochondrial dysfunction and cell injury was not clear. In the presence of 5 mM cephaloridine, respiratory inhibition and substantial ATP depletion clearly preceded lactate dehydrogenase release. But, with 0.5 mM cephaloridine, which also ultimately produced lethal cell injury, respiratory inhibition was not evident and decreases of ATP seemed to be only a reflection of loss of cell viability [687].

Mitochondria isolated from kidney prior to the development of overt cell necrosis during *cis*-platinum nephrotoxicity are functionally compromised [273, 759, 921]. Direct acute toxicity of the agent in vitro is variable [356], but intracellular metabolism could readily produce more active derivatives [691] and recent studies of both isolated proximal tubules [99] and medullary collecting ducts [100] have provided evidence for early mitochondrial functional effects of cisplatin in the intact tubule, as indicated by decreases of both ouabain-sensitive and -insensitive respiration and by loss of cell K^+ despite preservation of Na^+-K^+-ATPase activity in isolated cell membranes. Similar effects on cell K^+ had previously been demonstrated in renal slices that were precision-cut to improve their stability [636]. In this latter study, these K^+ losses were accompanied by a reduction of cell ATP, and both events considerably preceded leakage of lactate dehydrogenase to the medium. However, the nontoxic isomer, transplatin, also depressed ATP levels somewhat [636], thus complicating assignment of a critical pathogenetic role to that event. Also of importance for interpreting studies of cisplatin-induced lethal cell injury is that cisplatin, transplatin, and cisplatin hydrolysis products have been reported to directly inhibit lactate dehydrogenase [306]. The proximal tubule mitochondrial effects of cisplatin were associated with increased mitochondrial generation of reactive oxygen metabolites, lipid peroxidation, and progression to lethal cell injury as indicated by ^{51}Cr release; the mitochondrial effects in the inner medullary collecting ducts were not associated with an increase in reactive oxygen metabolites, lipid peroxidation, or lethal cell injury [291].

Other metals with defined tubule toxicity that have distinct mitochondrial functional effects include arsenic [102, 279], uranyl [136], cadmium [371], tin [113, 581, 795], copper [359, 671], silver [201, 673], and gold [844]. Treatment of isolated proximal tubules with Ag^{++} initially produced plasma membrane permeability changes with preserved mitochondrial function [429], but as discussed in the calcium section with regard to sites of Hg^{++} action, the mode of delivery and balance between sites of toxicity may be different in vivo. Isolated proximal tubules treated with uranyl nitrate showed respiratory inhibition before a loss of cell K^+, suggesting mitochondria as a very early target of toxicity [98].

Recent studies have provided evidence for early mitochondrial dysfunction during tubule cell injury secondary to several organic toxins. Cysteine conjugate beta-lyase activity is present in tubule cell glutaminases that are found in both cytosol and mitochondria [452, 501, 792–794]. Isolated rat renal cortical mitochondria treated with *S*-(1,2-dichlorovinyl)-L-cysteine (DCVC) showed inhibition of state 3 respiration and matrix enzymes, loss of membrane potential, and impaired ability to retain Ca^{++}, followed by leakage of matrix protein and increased permeability to polyethylene glycol [450]. These effects were associated with covalent binding of ^{35}S-labeled conjugates and both binding and functional effects were blocked by treatment with the beta-lyase inhibitor aminooxyacetic acid [321]. Isolated rat proximal tubule cells treated with DCVC had substantial decreases of oxygen consumption rates and ATP levels that preceded lytic plasma membrane damage [449].

S-(1,2,3,4,4,-pentachloro-1,3-butadienyl)-L-cysteine (PCBC), a toxic metabolite of hexachlorobutadiene, initially stimulated basal and ouabain-insensitive respiration of isolated rabbit proximal tubules and then inhibited respiration before resulting in lactate dehydrogenase release [720]. Like the classic uncouplers, PCBC acted to dissipate the proton gradient across the inner mitochondrial membrane [718]. Although stimulation of respiration followed by inhibition is consistent with a primary uncoupling action, since a similar pattern is seen even with classic uncouplers such as carbonyl cyanide-*m*-chlorophenylhydrazone [903], PCBC likely affected multiple targets. The uncoupling effect was not blocked by inhibiting cysteine conjugate beta-lyase with aminooxyacetic acid, but inhibition of state 3 respiration and binding of ^{35}S-labeled conjugates were prevented [321], suggesting that the uncoupling effect was a direct action of PCBC while the inhibition of state 3 was secondary to covalent binding of a toxic species resulting from metabolism by the beta-lyase. Consistent with these actions on inner mitochondrial membrane permeability and electron transport, PCBC treatment collapsed the mitochondrial membrane potential and impaired ability of the mitochondria to retain Ca^{++} [605]. A slow nonenzymatic loss of mitochondrial glutathione was also found [605]. A study using isolated rat proximal tubule cells identified only a severe inhibitory effect on respiration by pentachlorobutadienyl-glutathione, the parent compound of PCBC, but it was accompanied by profound ATP depletion and clearly preceded lytic plasma membrane damage [879]. 2-Bromohydroquinone, the nephrotoxic metabolite of bromobenzene, inhibited both ouabain-sensitive and -insensitive respiration well before the development of lethal cell injury and this was associated with a substantial drop in ATP content [719].

In isolated rabbit tubules treated with *tert*-butyl hydroperoxide, mitochondrial function and cell ATP levels were initially well preserved in the face of extensive K^+ losses that were apparently due to a primary plasma membrane lesion [544, 717]. Mitochondrial function then went on to deteriorate ahead of lytic plasma membrane damage, as indicated by lactate dehydrogenase release [717]. Mitochondrial injury during *tert*-butyl hydroperoxide injury was related to the oxidant actions of the compound, since the damage could be prevented by a variety of antioxidants as well as by chelation of iron [98, 544]. *N*-(3,5-dichlorophenyl)maleimide, a potential toxic metabolite of the nephrotoxin, *N*-(3,5-dichlorophenyl)succinimide, inhibited respiration of isolated rat tubules and mitochondria, apparently by means of action at site I of the electron transport chain [6]. Two mycotoxins with well-defined tubule toxicity, ochratoxin [7] and citrinin [8], had early actions on mitochondrial respiration with apparently different mechanisms. Ochratoxin inhibited respiration by effects on electron transport or carrier proteins that were not distinguished [7]. Citrinin appeared to have at least a partial uncoupling action [8].

In addition to affecting mitochondrial function by means of actions at the inner mitochondrial membrane, toxins may act by altering enzyme function required for normal operation of the citric acid cycle. Agents that likely act, at least in part, by this general mechanism include maleic acid and fluoroacetate [356, 528, 945]. The glycolytic enzyme, glyceraldehyde-3-phosphate dehydrogenase, has been suggested to be a relatively specific target during oxidant cell injury [360], but there is no information on its behavior in the kidney. The limited role for glycolytic metabolism in proximal tubules compared to other tubule segments and cell types [289] makes it less likely to be a central target of injury.

Aside from the direct actions of nephrotoxins and their reactive metabolites, damage to mitochondria during nephrotoxic injury can develop as a result of disturbances of cellular Ca^{++} metabolism. Mitochondria from all tissues have a ruthenium red–sensitive inner membrane uniporter for calcium, which can utilize either the electrochemical gradient derived from electron transport or intramitochondrial ATP to drive calcium uptake [135, 294]. Depending on the conditions of study, the K_m for mitochondrial calcium uptake has been estimated to be in a range from 1 to 100 μM [135]. More relevant to the way they function in both normal and injured cells is the observation that, as long as an energy source is available, mitochondria take up calcium added to their medium so as to attain medium concentrations of about 0.2 to 0.5 μM, depending on the presence of polyamines [57, 598]. The calcium uptake process is so avid and so preferentially utilizes available energy supplies that it readily occurs under conditions of mitochondrial isolation done at 4°C [159, 916] and even occurs at subzero temperatures if precautions are taken to prevent the formation of ice crystals [141]. The utilization of the electrochemical gradient across the mitochondrial membrane for calcium transport makes that electrochemical gradient unavailable for ATP production while calcium uptake is occurring [465, 860]. Of even greater importance to the deleterious effects of calcium on mitochondrial function are the alterations that calcium uptake produces in the permeability properties of the inner mitochondrial membrane [294]. Normal mitochondrial function depends on the maintenance of limited, highly selective permeability properties of the inner mitochondrial membrane, so that the translocation of H^+ across this membrane can be used in a controlled fashion to drive the proton ATPase of the membrane to effect ATP production. Unregulated movement of cations other than H^+, such as Na^+ and K^+, or movement of H^+ through abnormal channels alternative to the proton ATPase, so that the electrochemical gradient across the membrane cannot be maintained, compromises mitochondrial capacity for oxidative phosphorylation. Additionally, losses of intramitochondrial enzymes and adenine nucleotides, because of abnormal inner mitochondrial membrane permeability properties, can further contribute to sustained loss of mitochondrial functional capacity [356].

Mitochondria are capable of the uptake and retention of calcium without any sustained deleterious effects up to certain levels; however, above these calcium levels, mitochondrial calcium uptake is followed by a spontaneous release of a large fraction of the calcium that had been taken up. This release occurs through both ruthenium red–sensitive and –insensitive pathways and is accompanied by loss of intramitochondrial K^+, Mg^{++}, and adenine nucleotides, loss of the ability of mitochondria to generate and maintain a membrane potential, and large amplitude mitochondrial swelling [52, 53, 294, 318, 356]. Studies using polyethylene glycols of various sizes have elegantly quantitated the marked changes of membrane permeability responsible for these effects in cardiac mitochondria [318].

The precise amounts of calcium uptake required for such changes of inner mitochondrial membrane permeability to develop differ between mitochondria from different tissues. Renal cortical mitochondria are notably sensitive to the effects of calcium [916]. The sequence in which various inner mitochondrial membrane permeability properties are lost also varies depending on the source of the mitochondria and the experimental conditions, and it has been argued that the permeability alterations related to calcium uptake are not uniformly manifestations of membrane damage but, instead, are due to changes in the regulation of normal membrane permeability pathways [576, 832]. Most data, however, favor the hypothesis that permeability changes evoked by calcium mainly represent an abnormal process at the inner mitochondrial membrane [52, 53, 118, 294, 916, 969]. Calcium-induced inner mitochondrial membrane permeability alterations occur at substantially lower calcium levels than would otherwise be required to evoke them when calcium uptake occurs in the presence of several other agents, including phosphate, oxalacetate, thyroxin, *N*-ethylmaleimide, and *tert*-butyl hydroperoxide [52, 53, 118, 294]. The action of phosphate to promote calcium-induced mitochondrial membrane alterations is of particular interest with regard to their role during in vivo injury because of the ready availability of phosphate to mitochondria in vivo and the increases in phosphate levels that may occur during certain states of injury, e.g., hydrolysis of adenine nucleotides during ischemia. It is also of particular relevance to toxic mitochondrial damage that this process may be regulated by intramitochondrial glutathione, in that the Ca^{++}-induced membrane alterations were prevented so long as the mitochondrial GSH/GSSG ratio remained high [54].

The development of calcium-induced mitochondrial membrane permeability alterations can be prevented by blocking the initial calcium uptake with ruthenium red. It can be ameliorated, in spite of calcium uptake to levels that would otherwise evoke permeability changes, by the presence of extra medium Mg^{++}, adenine nucleotides, agents with activity to inhibit membrane phospholipases, such as dibucaine, verapamil, promethazine, and trifluoperazine, and, to a striking degree, by the presence of fatty acid free albumin [52, 53, 118, 242, 318, 394, 916, 970]. The sensitivity of the calcium-induced mitochondrial membrane alterations to moderation by agents affecting phospholipases and the actions of the resulting lipid degradation products, as well as the documented presence of a calcium-dependent phospholipase A_2 in the inner mitochondrial membrane have led to the hypothesis that the effects of calcium on mitochondrial membrane permeability are due mainly to activation of this phospholipase A_2 along with inhibition of lysophospholipid-acyltransferase [52, 53, 118]. It has been proposed that lysophospholipids are mediators of the permeability changes [52, 53] and that maintenance of a high GSH/GSSG ratio by keeping critical sulfhydryl groups reduced preserves lysophospholipid-acyltransferase activity [54, 294]. Additionally, alterations in regulation of a specific protein pore may be involved [117, 318, 319]. The results of studies of mitochondrial aging suggest that this process is similarly mediated by calcium-induced activation of mitochondrial membrane phospholipases and occurs at "normal" levels of endogenous mitochondrial calcium [143, 144, 624, 625]. Most recently, it has been shown for renal cortical mitochondria that mild Ca^{++} loading potentiates damage produced by a free-radical generating system consisting of hypoxanthine and xanthine oxidase [507]. The mitochondrial alterations included a site I specific inhibition of electron transport and decreases of ATPase and adenine nucleotide translocase activity [507]. Consistent with activation of phospholipase A_2, these functional changes were accompanied by release of polyunsaturated fatty acids [509] and both the functional changes and fatty acid release were ameliorated by dibucaine [507, 509]. These findings are of particular relevance to in vivo injury because they occur in the presence of the moderate levels of mitochondrial Ca^{++} loading that could conceivably occur prelethally, and they provide a link to the damaging actions of reactive oxygen metabolites that have been found to occur in both toxic and ischemic insults due to disordered mitochondrial electron transport, degradation of purines by xanthine oxidase, and toxic activation.

The potential for interactions between nephrotoxic and ischemic or hypoxic damage is also of considerable importance to the role of abnormal energetics in nephrotoxicity. Although blood flow in the kidney is high, oxygenation of large areas is potentially marginal, even under normal conditions. As a result of preglomerular shunting which is likely due to countercurrent exchange between the lobular arteries and veins, PO_2s in superficial glomeruli averaged only 46 mm Hg [728]. A further sharp drop to around 10 mm Hg takes place in the outer medulla, largely as a result of countercurrent diffusion between arteries and veins in the vasa recta (reviewed in [107]) and contributes to the high susceptibility of medullary thick ascending limb cells to injury [107]. The decreased O_2-carrying capacity that results from the absence of erythrocytes in standard isolated perfused kidney preparations [108] exaggerates expression of this medullary thick ascending limb injury [107, 108, 727] and has made that system a very useful one for studying the process. Studies in the isolated perfused kidney have established the importance of transport and work-related damage in that reduction of transport activity by ouabain suppressed cell damage even when membrane permeability was increased by treatment with the polyene antibiotics, amphotericin and nystatin [109]. Comparable effects were also seen in S3 segment proximal tubules [741]. The simplest explanation for these findings is that the restrictions of ATP production capacity produced by limited oxygenation were aggravated by nephrotoxin (polyene antibiotic)-induced increases of plasma membrane permeability and ATP consumption so that a more severe state of ATP depletion and resulting cell injury was achieved. However, this cannot be the sole mechanism, at least not for the medullary thick ascending limb cells, because the characteristic injury they sustain is *suppressed* by inhibition of electron transport or mitochondrial substrate metabolism [111, 112]. The notable exception to this pattern among electron transport inhibitors was cyanide [112] which also inhibits catalase [614]. Taken together, these observations suggest a role for mitochondrial oxidant generation in the medullary thick ascending limb lesion, although this remains to be firmly established.

Decreases of total renal blood flow occur commonly after treatment with nephrotoxins [345, 351, 523, 941]. Although their role in sustaining reductions of glomerular filtration rate remains controversial, the decreases of oxygen delivery could contribute to a hypoxic component of injury if falls in glomerular filtration do not commensurately decrease reabsorptive workload or other toxin actions, such as mitochondrial uncoupling activity or induction of increased plasma membrane cation permeability, promote ATP consumption. Aside from the information available for the isolated perfused kidney, these interactions have not been experimentally defined for any nephrotoxin. It is well established, however, that mild ischemia and gentamicin have synergistic damaging effects that show a morphological pattern of injury similar to that produced by severe ischemia alone [783, 956]. Ischemia also aggravates cephaloridine nephrotoxicity [120], and endotoxemia, which can have potent effects to selectively reduce renal perfusion, aggravates both gentamicin [31, 960] and cephaloridine [848, 850] toxicity. It is not clear, however, whether these interactions relate primarily to additive inhibitory effects on the energetic process or simply to enhancement of the cellular toxin uptake due to increased contact time of toxin and tubule cell resulting from lower rates of perfusion and urine flow. Synergistic damage between radiocontrast and hypoxia, however, occurs in isolated tubule preparations where contact time is not a variable [543].

Thus, there is substantial evidence that disturbances of cellular energy metabolism arising from both direct and indirect effects of nephrotoxins play an important role in nephrotoxic tubule cell damage. They may cause functional changes or contribute to the development of lethal cell injury. Ideally, before assigning mitochondria a primary role as a target for a particular nephrotoxin in the development of lethal cell injury, a number of criteria should be met:

1. Direct effects of the agent or a likely metabolite should be present in isolated mitochondria.
2. Either uncoupling of respiration (suggested but not proven by increases of the ouabain-insensitive component) or suppression of maximally stimulated respiration should be seen in intact tubules well before loss of plasma membrane integrity (lactate dehydrogenase release).
3 Intact tubules should show a degree of ATP depletion similar to that sufficient for production of injury under similar conditions when that degree of ATP depletion is produced by a specific inhibition of mitochondrial and glycolytic ATP synthesis, and the depletion should clearly precede lactate dehydrogenase release.
4. Blocking other effects of the nephrotoxin such as lipid peroxidation, glutathione depletion, and covalent binding should not protect against lethal cell injury unless mitochondrial function is also protected.
5. Differences between modes of delivery and available levels between toxicity in vivo and the isolated test system must be considered.

These criteria have not been fully met for any agent. The levels of ATP required to maintain basic cell structural integrity under various conditions remain under investigation even for relatively "pure" anoxic and related forms of injury produced by metabolic inhibitors [689, 863]. However, sufficient progress has been made with a variety of nephrotoxins to establish the importance of this aspect of the cellular response to nephrotoxins.

Disrupted Cell Calcium Homeostasis

Disturbances of cellular calcium metabolism have received much attention in studies of the pathophysiology of nephrotoxicity and of cell injury in general [234, 395, 617, 724, 750, 821, 836, 893, 896]. It is now appreciated that, for virtually all cell types, cytosolic free calcium is normally kept at about 100 nM, 1/10,000th of the extracellular level; exchangeable intramitochondrial Ca^{++} is extremely low; an inositol trisphosphate-sensitive pool sufficient to substantially raise cytosolic free calcium is present in microsomes; and considerable additional Ca^{++} can be bound to cellular macromolecules [135, 778, 936]. Recent studies of isolated proximal tubules with fluorescent Ca^{++} indicators [372, 907] and by electron probe microanalysis [430, 462] have shown this to be true for tubule cells. The endoplasmic reticulum Ca-ATPase and plasma membrane Ca-ATPase and Ca^{++}-Na^{+} exchange regulate free cytosolic Ca^{++} at physiological resting levels [135, 936]. Mitochondrial uptake and retention of Ca^{++} becomes substantial only when cytosolic levels exceed 400 to 500 nM [25, 57], although the presence of physiological levels of polyamines can lower this value to about 200 nM [526, 598].

Disturbances of cellular calcium homeostasis are damaging in large part due to exaggerated and uncoordinated expression of processes that are normally regulated by Ca^{++}. Virtually every cellular structure is a potential site of damage including the plasma membrane, mitochondria, the endoplasmic reticulum, the cytoskeleton, and the nucleus. Mechanisms of action include activation of membrane-bound and free phospholipases, alterations of membrane permeability properties as a result of both direct effects on permeability pathways and activation of membrane phospholipases, effects on intracellular contractile and cytoskeletal structures, and activation of proteases and nucleases [10, 23, 53, 234, 541, 809, 837, 838, 947].

Calcium overload is characteristic of tissues with lethally injured cells because loss of the plasma membrane barrier to calcium allows unrestricted uptake by mitochondria (Fig. 39-6). Even damaged mitochondria can sustain high intramitochondrial Ca^{++} levels [682, 893, 916]. This has been shown for both toxic and ischemic injury to the kidney, where mitochondria exhibit the morphological features of Ca^{++} overload [302, 837] and very high Ca^{++} levels are measured in isolated mitochondria [24, 724, 893, 913] and using electron probe microanalysis [837]. Even when it occurs after lethal cell injury, mitochondrial Ca^{++} uptake is an active process utilizing any available ATP as well as electron transport. This is illustrated by the behavior of isolated proximal tubules in suspension. During hypoxic injury, the cells gain substantial amounts of calcium, which is predominantly localized in mitochondria [813, 894, 909]. During complete anoxia, which produces an apparently similar amount of injury, no such Ca^{++} uptake is observed [782, 813], presumably because mitochondrial electron transport is not available to drive it.

More relevant to the question of a pathophysiological role for Ca^{++} is whether either cytosolic free calcium or mitochondrial calcium increase *prior* to lethal cell injury as a result of enhanced membrane permeability, reversal of the normal outward direction of Ca^{++} movement by Na-Ca exchange [774], diminished ATP to drive active Ca^{++} extrusion and nonmitochondrial sequestration, or damage to extrusion and sequestration enzymes [714].

Since cytosolic free calcium cannot be readily measured in vivo, evidence for prelethal disturbances of cellular calcium homeostasis during nephrotoxic injury overload was sought during serial studies of mercuric chloride and gentamicin nephrotoxicity that systematically correlated tissue and mitochondrial cation levels, mitochondrial functional changes, and morphologic alterations [913]. Three hours after 5 mg/kg mercuric chloride, cells in all proximal tubule segments remained intact, although ultrastructural changes consisting of increased numbers of small vesicles and microbodies and occasional loss of brush-border membranes were seen. Isolated mitochondria had mild but consistent altera-

Fig. 39-6. Severely damaged Ca^{++} overloaded mitochondria in lethally injured renal tubular cell. The dark granular deposits in the mitochondria are composed largely of calcium phosphate.

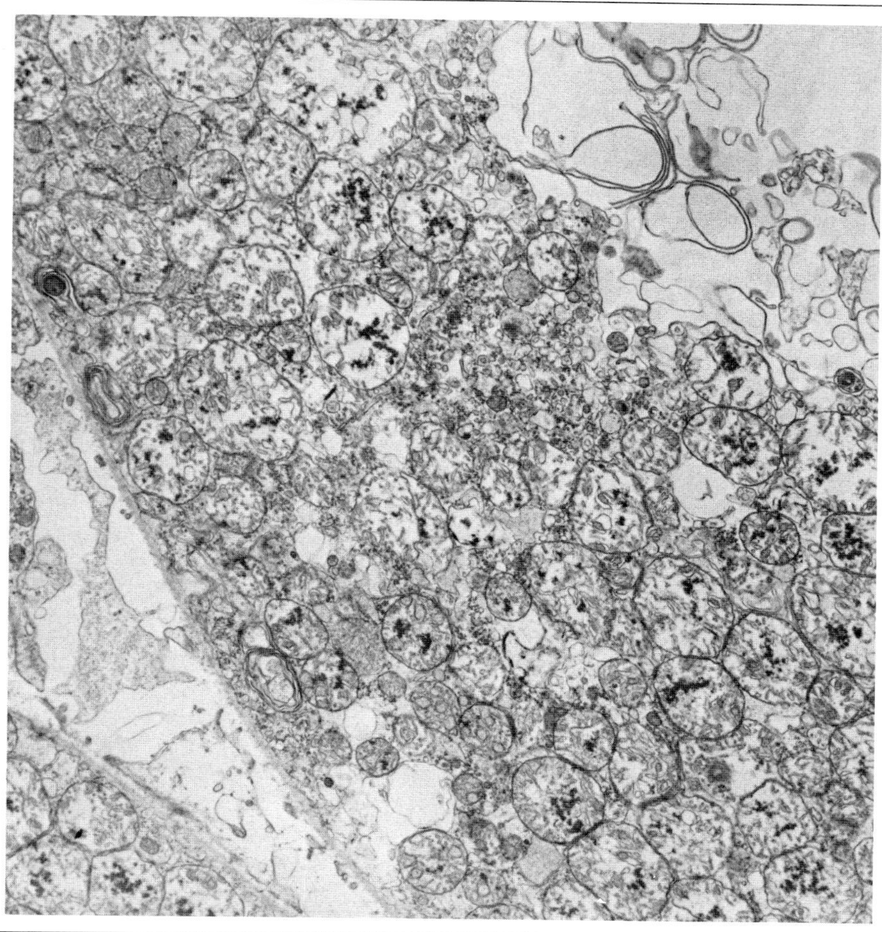

tions of a number of bioenergetic parameters of this point and showed small decreases in their potassium and magnesium levels. However, mitochondria isolated using techniques to minimize artifactual in vitro redistribution of Ca^{++} [896, 916] did not show increases of their calcium content relative to similarly isolated mitochondria from control rats. Measurements of whole cortex water, sodium, potassium, and magnesium also did not differ from control values at this time interval [913].

Detailed morphologic studies have demonstrated that cell necrosis appears between 6 and 12 hours after mercuric chloride exposure in this model [44]. At 12 hours, S3 segments in both medullary rays and outer medulla showed widespread cell necrosis, renal cortex water and sodium were elevated, and calcium was markedly increased. Mitochondria isolated at this point showed severe functional abnormalities, reduced potassium content, and markedly elevated levels of calcium [913]. The correlation between severity of renal functional loss and level of tissue calcium was high [915].

Four single daily 100-mg/kg doses of gentamicin in the Sprague-Dawley rat produced extensive morphological changes throughout S1 and S2 segments of the proximal tubule, characterized by marked increases in the size of lysosomes, formation of myeloid bodies, and moderate but widespread focal losses of brush-border membranes. Progressive rises in BUN were not seen up to this point. Isolated mitochondria showed mild but consistent functional abnormalities. Tissue potassium was slightly reduced [913]. Tissue magnesium was more markedly decreased and this magnesium depletion appeared to be selective for kidney [913]. Cortex sodium and water were unaffected and neither tissue nor mitochondrial calcium levels differed from controls. With continued daily gentamicin, tubular cell necrosis is apparent after 6 doses and becomes widespread to involve virtually all S1 and S2 segments after 10 doses [775, 913]. The appearance of tubule cell necrosis correlated with progressive rises in BUN and with parallel and marked increases in tissue and mitochondrial calcium levels. After 10 doses, there was a high correlation between BUN and tissue calcium [355]. Elevated renal cortex calcium levels at approximately this stage of injury have also been reported in other experimental models of gentamicin nephrotoxicity [177, 178] (Fig. 39-7).

Increases of tissue and mitochondrial Ca^{++} have also been reported during the first 48 hours of cisplatin-induced nephrotoxicity [206, 273] and, in this setting, have been attributed to enhanced microsomal sequestration resulting from stimulation of the endoplasmic reticulum calcium pump [206]. However, in each of these studies, an element of necrosis sufficient to account for the increases of Ca^{++} was present at the time points sampled.

Nephrotoxins can act to reduce mitochondrial Ca^{++} uptake by means of specific competitive effects as well as by induction of generalized mitochondrial damage [260, 701]. The Ca^{++} accumulation that occurs in the presence of lethal cell injury, however, indicates that inhibition of uptake cannot account for the absence of prelethal increases of mitochondrial and tissue Ca^{++}.

Taken together, the failure of these in vivo studies to provide evidence for the accumulation of Ca^{++} that

Fig. 39-7. Calcium levels of renal cortex and isolated renal cortical mitochondria during $HgCl_2$ and gentamicin-induced nephrotoxicity. The data are from Weinberg et al. [913].

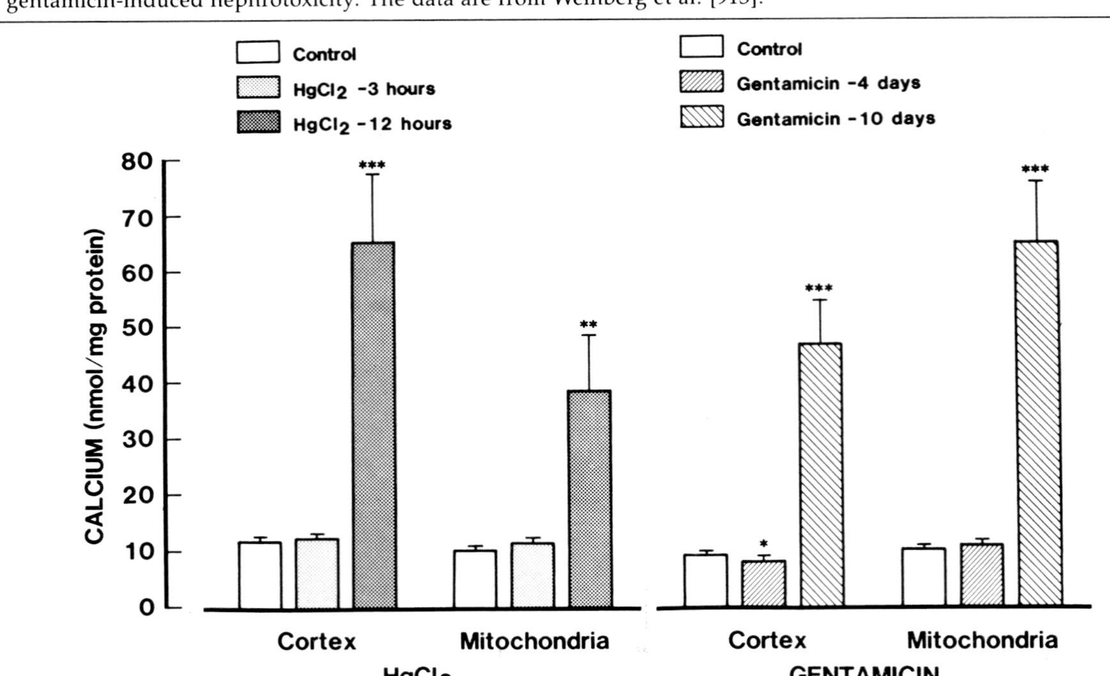

would have resulted from action of mitochondrial and other active sequestering mechanisms to compensate for elevations of cytosolic free Ca^{++} argues strongly against the occurrence of a prolonged state of elevated cytosolic free Ca^{++} during the development of nephrotoxic injury secondary to the agents studied. But the work does not exclude the possibility that Ca^{++} can play a pivotal role during an accelerated phase of membrane damage that immediately precedes lethal cell injury. Recent studies using fluorescent probes for cytosolic free Ca^{++} (Ca_f) have begun to provide information about its behavior during rapidly evolving forms of proximal tubule cell injury, although data on fresh fully differentiated tubules, which are most relevant to understanding nephrotoxin behavior in vivo, remain limited.

In freshly isolated rabbit proximal tubules (predominantly S2 segments), the Ca^{++} ionophore, ionomycin, increased Ca_f to micromolar levels and rapidly produced lethal cell injury, as indicated by a loss of lactate dehydrogenase to the medium by suspended tubules and an accelerated leak of fura and failure to exclude trypan blue by superfused tubules (Fig. 39-8). Decreasing medium Ca^{++} to 100 nM prevented the ionomycin-induced increases of Ca_f and the injury. In contrast, cells treated with 1799, an uncoupler of oxidative phosphorylation that produced severe ATP depletion, did not develop increases of Ca_f until just before loss of viability. Preventing these increases of Ca_f with 100 nM Ca^{++} medium did not protect 1799-treated cells [907] (Fig. 39-9).

Data on Ca_f during injury secondary to common nephrotoxins are presently limited to cultured tubule cells. Initial reports that gentamicin could produce acute [340] and chronic [33] increases of Ca_f in LLC-PK_1 cells were not confirmed in detailed studies of both primary cultures of rat proximal tubules and LLC-PK_1 cells [811]. Hg^{++} at concentrations ranging from 2.5 to 100.0 μM unequivocally produces large increases of Ca_f due to release from intracellular stores followed by massive influx, both of which preceded blebbing and lethal cell injury [637, 769, 770, 811]. Reducing medium Ca^{++} to less than 5 μM substantially blunted the increases of Ca_f and delayed blebbing and loss of the ability to exclude trypan blue [769]. Similar effects of low medium Ca^{++} to reduce blebbing and delay cell death have been found during treatment of LLC-PK_1 cells with several membrane active toxins: the polycation, polylysine; the phospholipase activator, mellitin; and the heavy metal, mercuric chloride [835].

A recent study of $HgCl_2$ effects on isolated hepatocytes using digital imaging identified only the second component of increased Ca_f due to influx of medium Ca^{++} and showed that blebs were hot spots of increased Ca_f. However, blebbing *preceded* the increases of Ca_f, and reducing medium Ca^{++} to 2.6 μM did not delay either

Fig. 39-8. Measurements of cytosolic free Ca^{++} (Ca_f) in fura-2–loaded superfused proximal tubules. Studies were done in the presence of probenecid to block fura-2 secretion as detailed elsewhere [907]. The top set of panels (*A1, B1,* and *C1*) are the ratio values plotted against calculated Ca_f. The bottom set of panels (*A2, B2,* and *C2*) are the raw 340- and 380-nm signals. In panels A1 and A2, the tubule is observed under control conditions for 1,000 seconds followed by calibration employing 15 μM ionomycin plus 2.5 mM EGTA in Ca^{2+}-free medium (labeled as EGTA), then 15 μM ionomycin in 3.5 mM Ca^{2+} medium (labeled ION). In panels B1 and B2, 10 μM ionomycin was introduced at 175 seconds of perfusion. An accelerated leak of fura began at the point indicated by the arrow in B2. The experiment ended with the same calibration procedure as in panels A1 and A2. In panels C1 and C2, the tubule was perfused with 100 nM Ca^{2+} medium at 100 seconds followed by 15 μM ionomycin in 100 nM Ca^{2+} medium followed by the calibration procedure. (Adapted from J. M. Weinberg, J. A. Davis, N. F. Roeser, et al. Role of increased cytosolic free calcium in the pathogenesis of rabbit proximal tubule cell injury and protection by glycine or acidosis. *J. Clin. Invest.* 87:581, 1991.)

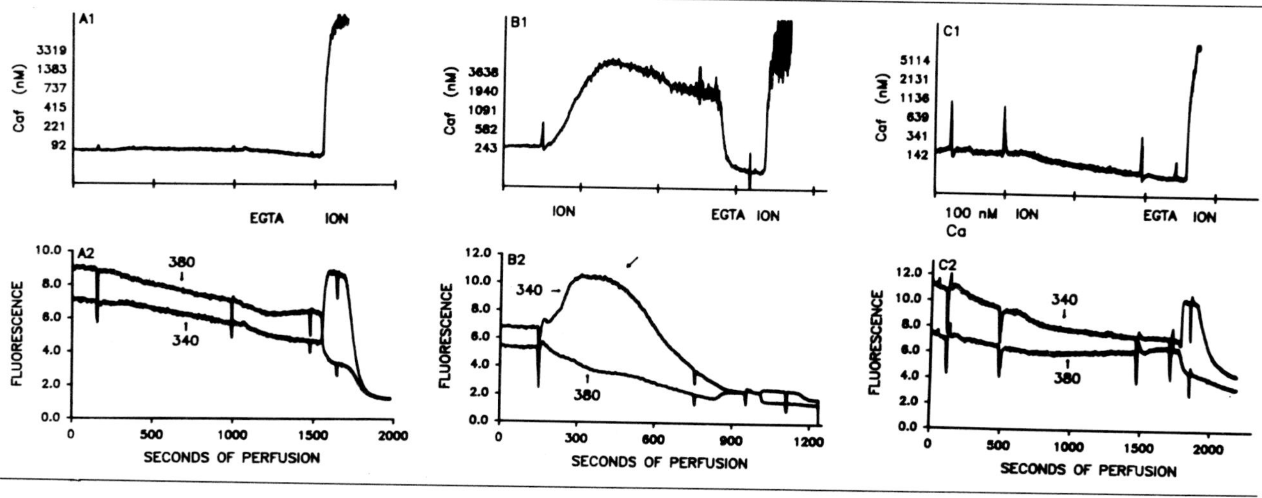

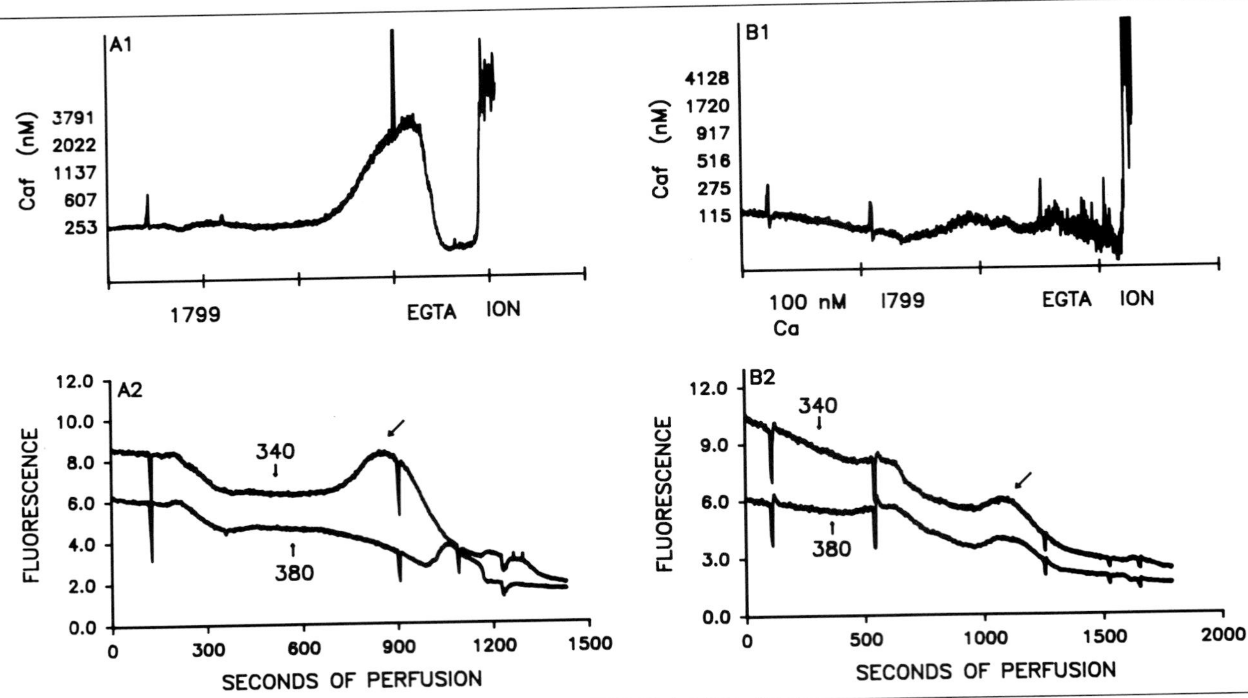

Fig. 39-9. Measurements of cytosolic free Ca^{2+} in fura-2–loaded superfused proximal tubules treated with 20 μM 1799. The experimental design and figure format are the same as in Fig. 39-8. The tubule in panels A1 and A2 was treated with 20 μM 1799 during the experimental period, and the tubule in panels B1 and B2 was treated with 100 nM Ca^{2+} medium followed by 20 μM 1799 in 100 nM Ca^{2+} medium. (Adapted from J. M. Weinberg, J. A. Davis, N. F. Roeser, et al. Role of increased cytosolic free calcium in the pathogenesis of rabbit proximal tubule cell injury and protection by glycine or acidosis. *J. Clin. Invest.* 87:581, 1991.)

blebbing or cell death even though it prevented the increases of Ca_f [602]. In this system the most prominent event that preceded blebbing and cell death was a collapse of the mitochondrial membrane potential [602].

These studies unequivocally demonstrate substantial changes of Ca_f after $HgCl_2$ in vitro, but indicate that the role of Ca_f as a necessary mediator of injury varies with cell type. They contrast with the lack of evidence for early changes of cell Ca^{++} during in vivo damage [913]. The differences may be explained by the fact that Hg^{++} delivery to the kidney in vivo is likely in a form complexed to protein [352] so that the plasma membrane is never directly exposed to the levels of Hg^{++} achieved by direct treatment of isolated cells with $HgCl_2$ in protein-free media.

With regard to the oxidant damage potentially involved in several types of nephrotoxic tubule cell injury, studies in a number of nonrenal cell types have shown that early oxidation of glutathione and sulfhydryl groups impairs cellular mechanisms for sequestering and extruding Ca^{++} [59, 378, 386, 599]. The release of sequestered Ca^{++} initially produces a loss of total cell Ca^{++} [59, 361, 378] and an increase of Ca_f that may be either transient [695, 865] or sustained [249, 334, 361]. Influx of medium Ca^{++} also contributes to the increase of Ca_f [249, 695]. Later, larger and uniformly sustained increases of Ca_f secondary to influx precede lytic plasma membrane damage [334, 361, 695]. To the extent it has been studied, blunting both types of increases of Ca_f by lowering medium Ca^{++} delays but does not prevent lethal cell damage [695, 746]. Protection against lytic plasma membrane damage by deferoxamine, DPPD or catechol did not prevent the early Ca_f transient, but blocked the later sustained increase in one model using *tert*-butyl hydroperoxide in hepatocytes [695]. The nephrotoxic glutathione conjugate, pentachlorobutadienyl-glutathione [879], its metabolite, PCBC [285], and another nephrotoxic haloalkane cysteine conjugate, *S*-(1,1,2,2-tetrafluoroethyl)-L-cysteine, induced increases of Ca_f of isolated rat proximal tubule cells within the first several minutes of exposure. The precise role of these changes of Ca_f in the injury response and their mechanisms remain to be more fully defined.

Although the accumulation of Ca^{++} after cell death is not important for understanding the early pathogenesis of cell injury, it can contribute to the ultimate tissue response if it results in locally high Ca^{++} concentrations that promote damage to neighboring cells, serve as foci for the development of nephrocalcinosis, or alter responses to physiological regulators of cytosolic free calcium in neighboring cells. This area of study remains largely unexplored; however, the potential for experimentally manipulating the degree of pathological calcification is suggested by recent work showing that saline loading of animals prior to induction of mercuric chloride nephrotoxicity dramatically lowers tissue Ca^{++} deposition without necessarily reducing the extent of lethal tubule cell injury [919].

The role of calcium in renal tubule cell injury produced by aminoglycosides may be particularly complex. As detailed previously there is substantial evidence that these drugs, because of their cationic properties, interact at cell membranes with divalent cations and with binding sites that would normally be occupied by divalent cations [357]. The initial observation [65] that a high-calcium diet (4%) as calcium carbonate, which results in hypercalciuria with little or no rise in serum calcium, produces striking protection from the progression of experimental gentamicin nephrotoxicity has been amply confirmed based on studies of renal functional parameters [355, 652], morphology [652], and marked attenuation of increases in tissue and mitochondrial calcium, reflecting the development of lethal cell injury [355].

Calcium at physiological levels was demonstrated to be an effective competitive inhibitor of gentamicin binding to brush-border membranes [355]. In one study, the high-calcium carbonate diet delayed the time of appearance of peak tissue gentamicin levels [65]; however, in another it did not [355], suggesting that cellular sites in addition to brush-border membranes may be involved in any competitive interactions between gentamicin and calcium, which play a role in the protective effects seen.

It has not been reported whether calcium carbonate alters the characteristic phospholipidosis produced by aminoglycosides in vivo [460]. This determination is of considerable interest to understanding the roles of both calcium and the phospholipidosis during aminoglycoside-induced tubule injury, since it would help localize the site of calcium action and provide another test of whether the phospholipidosis is essential for progression of toxicity. An action of calcium most consistent with a necessary role for the phospholipidosis would be to compete with aminoglycosides for membrane sites where they acted to inhibit phospholipase activity [934]. Increasing medium $CaCl_2$ from 1.8 to 5.4 mM did not ameliorate the phospholipidosis induced by gentamicin in cultured LLC-PK_1 cells [731], but it is not clear how well this actually simulates the effects of calcium carbonate in vivo since they do not require increases of serum Ca^{++} [65, 355].

An effect of the high-calcium diet to suppress PTH-mediated increases of membrane phospholipids has been considered [70, 176, 222]. In two studies, parathyroidectomy was protective against gentamicin nephrotoxicity [70, 222], while in another it was not [176]. The high-calcium diet, however, was still protective after parathyroidectomy, suggesting an additional effect of calcium unrelated to PTH status [70]. Parathyroidectomy reduced renal cortical accumulation of gentamicin but did not change either the affinity or the number of binding sites present on isolated brush-border or basolateral membranes [339].

The protective effects of high calcium did not appear to be due to urinary alkalinization resulting from administration of Ca^{++} as calcium carbonate, because urinary alkalinization alone is not protective [221]. Thus the protection produced by the calcium carbonate diet is, indeed, likely to be directly related to the resulting increases of intestinal calcium absorption and urinary excretion. The protective effect of increased dietary calcium appears to be specific for aminoglycoside toxicity, since no protection was seen after a similar feeding protocol prior to mercuric chloride nephrotoxicity [651]. Mg^{++}, which can also compete with gentamicin at both the plasma membrane [355] and subcellular membranes [910, 914], also protects against gentamicin nephrotoxicity when provided orally [943].

Short-term administration of 1-25-$(OH_d)_2$-D_3 to increase renal calcium delivery and hypercalciuria by mechanisms different from dietary calcium carbonate loading did not protect from gentamicin toxicity, but, in fact, markedly exacerbated it [158, 354]. In considering why hypercalcemia and hypercalciuria secondary to vitamin D administration have effects opposite to those produced by increased dietary calcium carbonate, the possibility of a role for concomitant changes in phosphate metabolism arises. Oral calcium and magnesium produce phosphate depletion as a result of intestinal phosphate binding by the cations [218]. No such effect is expected from vitamin D. Hyperphosphatemia has been reported to exacerbate ischemic acute renal failure [955], and the deleterious interactions between calcium and phosphate in mitochondria [916] suggest at least one type of cellular mechanism for such an effect of phosphate. It is thus possible that phosphate depletion plays a role in the protective effects of oral calcium and magnesium loading. In fact, phosphate-depleted rats were reported to be protected from gentamicin toxicity, while phosphate-loaded rats were not, despite the development of similar degrees of hypercalcemia and hypercalciuria in both groups [219, 310a].

Thus information is available to support a role for disordered cell calcium homeostasis in toxic cell injury in the kidney, and evaluation of changes in cellular calcium homeostasis is an essential part of analyzing the pathogenesis of any type of nephrotoxic injury. However, the mechanisms by which calcium mediates cell injury are complex; they vary with different types of injury and act in conjunction with noncalcium-mediated injurious processes. Indeed, there are settings in which calcium may be protective against injury. Simply documenting increases in tissue or mitochondrial calcium at a time when lethal cell injury is already present provides little information on calcium's pathogenetic role. Instead, careful documentation of the time course of alterations in cell calcium metabolism, the subcellular loci involved, and ideally the behavior of cytosolic free calcium are required to evaluate such a role for calcium. Manipulating the availability of calcium or altering its cellular actions, and thereby affecting the development of injury, provides the strongest support for a pathogenetic role.

Alterations of Membrane Phospholipid Metabolism

INCREASED DEGRADATION OF PHOSPHOLIPIDS

Since it occurs in close proximity to the level at which cell viability is ultimately determined, the integrity of cell membranes, disruption of phospholipid metabolism by means of abnormally increased phospholipase activity, decreased normal phospholipid synthetic activity, or combinations of these two events appears to be critically important in the pathogenesis of cell injury. Besides contributing to the structural framework for membranes [760], membrane phospholipids have been shown to play important roles in regulating membrane permeability properties [278] and the activity of membrane-bound enzymes, such as Na-K-ATPase [478]. Additionally, the products of phospholipid metabolism, lysophospholipids and free fatty acids, have toxic detergent properties, which further contribute to ongoing membrane injury unless their activity is limited [278, 356, 406, 522]. Intrinsic membrane phospholipases, present in all subcellular membranes, provide a basis for membrane phospholipid degradation should conditions arise that impair the regulation of their activity or prevent normal compensatory synthetic mechanisms from salvaging phospholipid degradation products and reconstituting membrane phospholipids [149, 281, 522, 635, 870, 874, 875]. Factors that contribute to abnormally high activity of membrane phospholipases and inadequate resynthesis include failure of cell Ca^{++} homeostasis, depletion of cellular high-energy phosphate supplies, effects of agents with high activity at membrane sulfhydryl groups, such as heavy metals and *N*-ethylmaleimide, and lipid peroxidation resulting from free-radical production [149, 281, 377, 522, 635, 751, 892, 893].

Information on the role of phospholipid degradation in the pathogenesis of nephrotoxic renal injury is relatively limited. Accelerated rates of phosphatidylcholine degradation were not found during incubation of prelabeled slices from $HgCl_2$-treated animals [828], and decreases of total cortex levels of the major phospholipids were not seen after $HgCl_2$ treatment [426]. However, isolated mitochondria and basolateral and brush-border membranes had reduced phospholipid levels after $HgCl_2$ [584]. $HgCl_2$ injury to cultured fibroblasts was accompanied by accelerated phospholipid hydrolysis, which was attributed to a Ca^{++} mimetic action of Hg^{++} [751]. Cultured LLCPK$_1$ cells injured by $HgCl_2$ showed significant depletion of phosphatidylethanolamine and phosphatidylcholine accompanied by marked increases of unesterified arachidonic acid and lysophospholipids [835]. Free fatty acids and lysophospholipids added to the medium of control primary cultures of tubule cells were highly damaging [522].

More detailed information pertinent to understanding the role of phospholipid degradation during tubule cell injury is available from a study of ATP depletion–induced damage to cultured tubule cells. LLC-PK$_1$ cells required a combination of glucose deprivation and mitochondrial electron transport inhibition with antimycin to maximally lower ATP levels and induce lethal cell injury, which occurred after several hours [863]. This allowed definition of a relatively early, large increase of both saturated and unsaturated free fatty acids that accompanied the initial rapid drop of ATP levels during the first hour of exposure to antimycin without glucose, well before lethal cell injury. Free fatty acid accumulation continued during 5 hours of incubation, at the end of which time most cells were dead. At 5 hours there were significant decreases of phospholipid content (predominantly of phosphatidylcholine). However, cells exposed for 5 hours to antimycin with a low concentration of glucose (0.55 mM) showed similar decreases of phospholipid content yet did not develop lethal cell injury. The latter group also did not show any increases of free fatty acids. These data implicate prelethal accumulation of fatty acids as a pathogenetic event in this system and suggest that loss of phospholipid mass is less important than fatty acid accumulation [863].

DECREASED PHOSPHOLIPID DEGRADATION

Accumulation of phospholipids due to inhibition of phospholipid degradation is a prominent feature of aminoglycoside nephrotoxicity [402, 460]. As detailed in the section on uptake of nephrotoxins, acidic phospholipids are major cellular sites of aminoglycoside binding. This is due to the cationicity of the molecule and its general configuration [357, 393, 487]. The aminoglycosides accumulate predominantly within renal tubular cell lysosomes and lead to marked changes in their morphology including, though not limited to, the development of a lamellar appearance (myeloid bodies) reflecting the accumulation of undegraded membrane phospholipid [434].

Gentamicin was first reported to induce a marked generalized phospholipidosis in cultured fibroblasts. All measured phospholipids, including phosphatidylethanolamine, phosphatidylcholine, sphingomyelin, and an unresolved area, including the acid phospholipids, were substantially increased. Neutral lipids and cholesterol were unaffected. Furthermore, a substantial amount of a lipid that is normally almost undetectable and was tentatively identified as bis(monoacylglycerol)phosphate was found. Marked increases in this lipid are a unique feature of the phospholipidosis induced by several of the cationic amphiphilic drugs. The activity of 14 intralysosomal enzymes was assessed, and the only one affected was the single tested phospholipase, sphingomyelinase. This was markedly reduced due to a decrease in V_{max} [30].

Subsequently, phospholipidosis was shown to be a prominent feature of aminoglycoside nephrotoxicity in vivo [193, 238, 401, 426, 459] and was also demonstrated in cultured tubule cells treated with aminoglycosides [654, 656, 731] where the predominant effect to inhibit phospholipid degradation as well as increased synthesis were observed [656]. The renal phospholipidosis is demonstrable in measurements of cortical phospholipids within 1 to 2 days after initiation of gentamicin, well before lethal tubule cell injury and at doses of aminoglycosides that do not go on to produce lethal tubule cell injury or acute renal failure [193, 460, 833, 841]. Proportionately, the greatest increases are always found in the acidic phospholipid, phosphatidylinositol; however, substantial increases of phosphatidylcholine have been consistently described, as have increases of phosphatidylethanolamine, phosphatidylserine, and the polyphosphoinositides, depending on the system studied [238, 401, 426, 459, 654, 656, 731].

The major part of this excess phospholipid is generally considered to be intralysosomal secondary to inhibition of lysosomal phospholipases [401, 460]. Aminoglycosides inhibit lysosomal phospholipase A_1, A_2, and C in vitro [137, 344, 459]. Inhibition of lysosomal phospholipase A_1 and sphingomyelinase can be measured after in vivo treatment, including therapeutic doses in humans [193, 266]. In vivo inhibition of sphingomyelinase is believed to be secondary to accumulation of intralysosomal phospholipids [459] rather than to a direct aminoglycoside effect. Aminoglycoside inhibition of phospholipases is not solely due to direct aminoglycoside interaction with the target phospholipid [662] because it clearly affects phospholipids (e.g., phosphatidylcholine and phosphatidylethanolamine) that do not have high affinities for the aminoglycosides. Activity of aminoglycosides in this setting has been attributed to targeting of the aminoglycosides by nearby acidic phospholipid and to a requirement for an acidic phospholipid for phospholipase activity directed against neutral phospholipids [137, 460, 550].

Induction of phospholipidosis is specific for aminoglycosides among acute nephrotoxins. Studies of acute renal injury induced by $HgCl_2$ and glycerol showed that these lesions were also characterized by increases in phosphatidic acid and phosphatidylinositol content; however, in contrast to gentamicin, which produced its effects prior to manifestations of advanced cell injury and at doses that would never go on to advanced cell injury, the effects of $HgCl_2$ and glycerol were only evident at times when extensive renal tubular cell necrosis was present and were not seen with doses that do not produce necrosis [426].

Aminoglycosides also inhibit nonlysosomal phospholipases including cytosolic and plasma membrane–bound phospholipase C [479, 730]. Given the effects of aminoglycosides to inhibit extralysosomal phospholipases, phospholipid alterations of nonlysosomal cellular membranes are also likely during aminoglycoside toxicity. Subcellular fractionation studies have provided evidence for this [426, 655], although definitive assignment of such changes to specific intracellular sites is complicated by possibilities for lysosomal contamination and redistribution of phospholipids among the subcellular membranes. The polyphosphoinositides are potential extralysosomal sites of aminoglycoside action of particular importance, given their role in mediating hormonal effects [73, 555]. Aminoglycosides have been shown to have a particularly high affinity for binding to polyphosphoinositides in vitro [487, 880], they alter phosphoinositide metabolism in red blood cell membranes [515], and they have been used to inhibit polyphosphoinositide hydrolysis in isolated cell and membrane systems [157, 553, 765, 856]. Although an early study failed to detect gentamicin-induced alterations of the turnover of ^{32}P-labeled polyphosphoinositides in vivo [426], more recent work has shown inhibition of hormone-induced inositol phosphate formation and protein kinase C activation in both primary cultures of rabbit proximal tubule cells and rat renal cortex in vivo [655].

The acidic phospholipids have important roles in the regulation of membrane permeability properties, hormone receptor interactions, and enzyme activity [73, 131, 179, 187, 236, 278, 387, 555] so that binding of aminoglycosides to them and alterations in their content in multiple cell membranes could contribute to changes in a variety of cellular processes. Modulation by aminoglycosides of Na^+-K^+-ATPase [478] and Ca-ATPase [553] activity by means of effects on acidic phospholipids necessary for enzyme function has been shown. The aminoglycosides act antagonistically to Ca^{++} to fluidize liposomes composed of phosphatidylinositol bisphosphate [880], increase permeability of polyphosphoinositide-containing liposomes to carboxyfluorescein [29], decrease permeability of phosphatidic acid and phosphatidylinositol-containing liposomes to glycerol [661, 662], and promote membrane aggregation [415, 662].

Which of the multiple consequences of the aminoglycoside acidic–phospholipid interactions that have already been studied and of the many other additional possibilities that remain to be studied is most critically involved in development of nephrotoxicity is unknown. Their importance to toxicity is emphasized by recent observations on the remarkable protective effects against aminoglycoside toxicity of polyaspartic acid and other anionic and neutral polyamino acids [55, 56, 265, 417, 418, 654, 658, 930, 932]. These compounds appear to act predominantly by complexing with the aminoglycosides intracellularly [417, 418]. They do not decrease uptake, but rather promote accumulation of increased amounts of aminoglycoside [265, 658]. Much of this accumulation is in lysosomes, as seen in the absence of polyamino acids [55, 417]. However, the lysosomes differ ultrastructurally in that myeloid body formation is diminished and an osmophilic homogenous material, possibly the complexed polyamino acid, accumulates [55, 418]. This is accompanied by potent amelioration of aminoglycoside-induced phospholipidosis [55, 654] and of aminoglycoside-induced inhibition of polyphosphoinositide-mediated hormonal responsiveness [654]. Polyaspartic acid also blocked the in vitro effects of gentamicin to decrease permeability of liposomes to glycerol and promote aggregation [654]. Although these elegant observations with polyamino acids still do not distinguish which of the processes blocked are most critical to nephrotoxicity, they provide a powerful tool for further studies of this issue.

Disruption of Cell Monovalent Cation, Volume, and pH Regulation

Nephrotoxin-induced disruption of cellular monovalent cation homeostasis can impair the normal reabsorptive function of renal tubules resulting in cation wasting and, when more severe, could disrupt volume regulation, and thereby promote cell injury. Toxins can directly affect membrane permeability as typified by amphotericin

B and the other polyene antibiotics [156]. Hg^{++} and the organic mercurials are known to increase membrane monovalent cation permeability [628, 683, 684]; however, available evidence does not suggest that such effects are expressed early during in vivo nephrotoxicity [913]. As discussed previously, this may relate to the fact that most mercury delivery to the kidney in vivo is in protein-bound form so that concentrations of Hg^{++} available to act directly at the surface of the cell are limited, as compared to those present in experimental systems in vitro where the only available binding sites are on the target cell [913].

Tubular reabsorption of Na^+ and multiple other solutes dependent on secondary active transport as well as tubule cell volume regulation require active Na^+ extrusion and maintenance of a negative intracellular potential to exclude Cl^- [502]. Both processes depend on Na^+-K^+-ATPase activity so that uptake of these extracellular solutes and osmotic swelling would result even without major changes in membrane permeability, from impaired function of Na^+-K^+-ATPase due to limitations of ATP availability, damage to the enzyme itself, or changes in the phospholipid microenvironment surrounding the enzyme and required for optimal function and regulation.

The major cation shifts occurring during oxygen deprivation are attributable to lack of ATP [899]. As previously detailed in the section on abnormalities of cellular energetics, toxic lesions are generally not associated with such severe perturbations of cellular adenine nucleotide metabolism, although recent studies have suggested that the K_m for Na^+-K^+-ATPase is higher in vivo than in vitro so that even moderate decreases of tubule cell ATP levels could potentially affect its activity [15, 312]. Acute, cisplatin-induced K^+ loss from isolated proximal tubules decreased Na^+-K^+-ATPase activity resulting from primary impairment of mitochondrial ATP production [99].

Heavy metals directly affect the activity of numerous enzymes including Na^+-K^+-ATPase [672]. Aminoglycosides, by binding to anionic phospholipids required for optimal Na^+-K^+-ATPase function, inhibit the enzyme [478]. Inhibition of Na^+-K^+-ATPase both acutely and chronically after gentamicin in vivo has been described [176, 933] and restoration of Na^+-K^+-ATPase activity by thyroxine treatment ameliorated toxicity [176]. However, additional effects of thyroxine on gentamicin accumulation [174] and its potential for enhancing regeneration [547] complicate this interpretation. In addition to its effects on Na^+-K^+-ATPase that are secondary to inhibition of mitochondrial function [99], cisplatin can produce direct inhibition of the enzyme [194, 817].

The extent to which these various abnormalities of Na^+-K^+-ATPase activity impact on cellular volume and cation homeostasis in vivo and whether this contributes to injury at the cellular level have not been fully defined. Serial measurements of tissue K^+ and Na^+ during the development of gentamicin and $HgCl_2$ nephrotoxicity showed only small or absent changes prior to necrotic cell damage [913]. Fractional lithium clearance, a marker for proximal tubule Na^+ reabsorption, was increased after cisplatin in vivo [189] over a rapid time frame similar to that for effects on Na^+-K^+-ATPase in isolated tubules [99]. Additional information on the importance of cell volume and monovalent cation alterations in the pathogenesis of injury is available from studies of oxygen deprivation that have been recently reviewed [899]. The available data strongly support a major role for cell swelling in cold injury as seen during tissue preservation, but its contribution is less important relative to other processes during injury at 37°C [899].

Alterations of cell pH during toxic injury have not been well documented; however, studies with both renal tubules and other cell types have demonstrated important modulating effects on cellular susceptibility to injury. Early studies described better preservation of K^+ in hypoxic renal slices at reduced pH [631] as well as protective effects against anoxic injury to myocardial tissue [83], Ehrlich ascites tumor cells [936], and isolated hepatocytes [630]. More recent work detailing behavior of a number of injury-related metabolic parameters in freshly isolated hepatocytes [91] and renal proximal tubules [126, 894] clearly showed the critical pH to be 6.9 to 7.0. In isolated proximal tubules studied in suspension, susceptibility to hypoxic injury increased linearly as the pH was dropped from 7.5 to 7.0 by titrating the Krebs-Ringer bicarbonate-buffered medium with HCl. Between pH 6.4 and 7.0, the cells were highly resistant to injury [894].

The protective effects of reduced pH were not limited to conditions where metabolic acidosis was induced by addition of HCl to tubule suspensions. When tubules were incubated at high density as pellets during oxygen deprivation, they spontaneously lowered the surrounding pH to about 7.0 and showed the same increased resistance to oxygen deprivation–induced injury, as seen in the suspended tubules kept at pH 7.0 or less [894].

Protective effects of reduced pH have subsequently been reported for suspensions of rat proximal tubules [126] and in the isolated perfused rat kidney [744] where reduced pH also decreased sensitivity to damage produced by elevated levels of perfusate calcium [745]. Kidneys flushed with simple phosphate-buffered saline plus sucrose solutions at pH 7.0 prior to warm ischemia had better recovery of function than those flushed with pH 7.4 solution [239]. Isolated rabbit tubules are also protected by reduced pH against damage from ATP-depleting metabolic inhibitors [674, 901] and ouabain [901], but not from damage produced by *tert*-butyl hydroperoxide or ochratoxin A [674].

Although direct measurements of intracellular pH during kidney tubule injury models have not been reported, recent studies with primary cultures of isolated hepatocytes, where similar protective effects occur, are probably relevant. In hepatocytes that were metabolically inhibited by a combination of cyanide and iodoacetate in pH 7.4 medium, intracellular pH dropped to approximately 6.5 and remained there until immediately prior to the apparent time of cell death, when it rose moderately just before abrupt leakage of bis-carboxyethylfluorescein, the fluorescent pH probe. Cells incubated in low pH medium showed the same sequence of changes, except the period of intracellular acidosis and the time to cell death were prolonged. A similar prolongation of the period of intracellular acidosis and protection was produced by treatment with amiloride in pH 7.4 medium, while replacement of medium chloride with gluconate or treatment with a disulfonic stilbene or monensin to ameliorate the metabolic inhibitor–induced intracellular acidosis accelerated injury [274, 275].

The mechanism for protection by reduced pH is unknown. Reduced pH can inhibit H^+-ATPases [685] and could affect Na^+-H^+ exchange, a process that can consume a substantial amount of ATP in the proximal tubule [606]. ATP levels during hypoxia were slightly preserved in the isolated rabbit proximal tubules protected by reduced pH [894]; however, observations that low pH did not markedly decrease respiration by oxygenated tubules [894], that intracellular acidosis with normal medium pH protected hepatocytes [275], and that ATP levels were not preserved during protection of isolated hepatocytes [91, 274] or in the isolated perfused kidney [743] argue against a necessary role for ATP preservation in protection. Maintenance of ATP in some systems could simply reflect better general levels of cellular integrity, as detailed elsewhere in this review to explain improved ATP levels at the end of hypoxia in glycine-protected tubules [902]. Better cellular integrity may also account for the improved preservation of AMP in tubules protected by low pH [894], although this could alternatively be explained by inhibition of 5′-nucleotidase by reduced pH [464].

Reduced pH can decrease transmembrane Ca^{++} fluxes [14, 872] and the affinity of calmodulin for Ca^{++} drops sharply as pH is decreased from 7.5 to 6.5 [128, 827]. Thus, multiple Ca^{++}-calmodulin–regulated processes could be inhibited as pH decreases. Studies of plasma membrane phospholipases A_2 and C and mitochondrial phospholipase A_2 have indicated a pH optima above 7.0, with sharp decreases of activity below pH 7.0 [272, 729, 870, 874]. Inhibition of phospholipase activity by reduced pH by means of direct effects as well as reductions of Ca^{++} availability and Ca^{++}-calmodulin binding could, therefore, contribute to protection. However, the roles of all these events in oxygen deprivation and toxic injury remain to be more completely defined, and numerous other mechanisms for protection are possible, including effects on membrane recycling [697], the cytoskeleton [407], cell-cell junctional permeability [127], and the generation [255] and metabolism [40] of reactive oxygen metabolites.

Alterations of pH could also affect metabolic activation of toxins. Protection of isolated proximal tubules by reduced pH against toxicity of 2-bromohydroquinone has been related to decreased formation of toxic metabolites [675].

Abnormalities of Cell Proteases

Uncontrolled activation of proteases in lysosomes, the cytosol, and associated with the cell membrane [90, 666] could contribute to tissue damage during nephrotoxic renal injury. As detailed in the section on lysosomes, most data do not favor a prelethal pathogenetic role for release of lysosomal proteases and other hydrolases. Involvement of the calcium-activated neutral cysteine protease [541, 809], calpain, is of greater potential relevance. High- and low-affinity (relative to Ca^{++}) forms of the enzyme as well as an autocatalytic effect of Ca^{++} have been characterized [809]. The enzyme is both cytosolic and membrane associated [170, 271, 809] and activity may be regulated by membrane phospholipids as well as by a specific inhibitor protein, calpistatin [586, 809]. Calpain has been implicated in the control of cell membrane fusion, receptor expression, activation of kinases including protein kinase C, cytoskeletal proteins, and membrane channels [58, 500, 541, 809]. Both forms of calpain and calpistatin are found in kidney and have been reported to be present in tubule cells [87, 587, 952]. Renal brush-border membranes are very rich in proteases such as meprin and endopeptidase 24.11 as well as expopeptidases [90]. Their regulation and potential involvement during injury have not been studied. ATP-dependent proteases and ubiquitin, which targets damaged proteins, are widely distributed [90, 666]. As yet there is little information about their role during acute cell injury in the kidney or other tissues.

In a preliminary report [349], primary cultures of S3 segments in the proximal tubule were protected against anoxic injury by L-3-carboxy-*trans*-2,3-epoxypropionyl-leucylamido-(4-guanidino)butane (E64), a cysteine protease inhibitor active against calpain [626]. Inhibitors of lysosomal proteolysis and other nonlysosomal proteases were not effective [349]. Freshly isolated hepatocytes with elevated cytosolic calcium secondary to cystamine, exogenous ATP, or the divalent cation ionophore, A 23187, had accelerated proteolysis associated with blebbing and cell death [600, 601]. The proteolysis, blebbing, and cell death were substantially ameliorated by antipain and leupeptin, two cysteine protease inhibitors active against calpain. Lysomotrophic reagents did not have the same protective effect, suggesting that leupeptin and antipain were not acting by means of effects on lysosomal proteases [600, 601]. In contrast, cultured hepatocytes treated with the same agents did not exhibit injury related to proteolysis [518].

Disruption of the Cytoskeleton

Nephrotoxins can potentially alter cytoskeletal components and cytoskeletal-membrane interactions as a result of interference with cellular energetics, elevation of cytosolic free Ca^{++}, promotion of phospholipid degradation, and production of free radicals. ATP is required for both polymerization and depolymerization of actin and tubulin [76–78] as well as for actin-myosin interactions [797]. GTP is required for polymerization of tubulin [347]. Ca^{++} mediates the interactions of actin and myosin [5] and regulates microtubule formation [923]. It also modulates the effects of actin-binding proteins including gelsolin and profilin, which control the state of actin polymerization, and of alpha-actinin, which plays an important role in actin-membrane interactions [314, 604, 889]. Additionally, activation of calpains could affect interactions among actin and the many other proteins linking it to the plasma membrane, e.g., integral membrane proteins such as uvomorulin and the laminin and fibronectin receptors [292, 604], membrane-associated proteins such as ankyrin, fodrin, alpha-actinin, vinculin, brush-border myosin I, and cross-linking proteins such as villin and fimbrin [172, 292, 564, 579, 604].

Membrane phospholipids interact with and regulate the function of cytoskeletal proteins. Specific interactions of this type include preferential binding of diacylglycerol and palmitic acid to alpha-actinin [604] and inhibition by phosphatidylinositol bisphosphate of gelsolin and profilin activity [376, 455]. Lipid interactions with other membrane-associated proteins such as spectrin, vinculin, and protein 4.1 as well as with intermediate filaments, microtubules [604], and myosin [4] have also been described. Additionally, cytoskeletal proteins can be covalently linked to fatty acids, a posttranslational modification that could occur directly at the membrane. There is good evidence for covalent linkage of fatty acids to ankyrin, vinculin, and protein 4.1 [604]. Oxidants could alter these interactions by lipid peroxidation as well by direct effects on cytoskeletal proteins. Actions of oxidants to cross-link actin and actin-binding protein and to oxidize cytoskeleton protein thiols have been documented [551, 823].

There is relatively little information about expression of these processes during nephrotoxic renal tubule cell injury. Their potential for involvement and interactions is illustrated by a recent study of cytoskeletal changes in platelets treated with menadione, a redox-active quinone frequently used in experimental models of oxidant damage [551]. Multiple cytoskeletal abnormalities were found: proteolysis of actin-binding protein by Ca^{++}-activated proteases; direct effects of increased cytosolic Ca^{++} to dissociate actin, alpha-actinin and actin-binding protein from the Triton X-100–insoluble cytoskeleton; and oxidative modification of actin with cross-linking of actin, alpha-actinin, and actin-binding protein.

Microfilament alterations have been observed during ATP depletion induced by metabolic inhibitors in cultured fibroblasts [78], epithelial cells [698], and endothelial cells [333, 948]. The general pattern consisted of disassembly and shortening of stress fibers with retraction from the membrane and appearance of side-side aggregates by electron microscopy. In all these systems, the changes were rapidly reversed during recovery from the metabolic inhibitor and were not associated with loss of cell viability or adherence.

Plasma membrane blebbing is a common manifestation of both ischemic and toxic injury in a variety of cell types [214, 378, 466, 467, 637, 835, 861]. It has been related to Ca^{++}-mediated activation of phospholipases with production of amphiphilic, membrane disrupting, free fatty acids, lysophospholipids, and diglycerides as well as to intramembrane phase alterations resulting from Ca^{++}-phospholipid interactions [835, 868]. However, the precise mechanism for bleb formation is not known. Given its close interrelationship and dynamic interactions with membrane components, the cytoskeleton probably plays a critical role in these events, but this also is incompletely defined [803].

In primary cultures of rabbit proximal tubule cells treated with a variety of toxins and metabolic inhibitors, cytosolic Ca^{++} increased and the degree and duration of the Ca^{++} increase correlated closely with both the extent of blebbing and the rapidity of development of cell death [637, 770]. Some blebs were hot spots of increased Ca^{++} [770]. These observations support a causal relationship between Ca^{++} and blebbing by means of one or more of the mechanisms detailed above. They are different from results of studies of primary cultures of isolated hepatocytes where blebbing induced by $HgCl_2$ and metabolic inhibitors was not preceded by elevations of cytosolic Ca^{++} [466, 602, 603]. In that system, cell death appeared to be precipitated abruptly by rupture of the plasma membrane in an area of a large or particularly unstable bleb [466, 603]. An important role for this type of membrane instability in areas weakened by blebs has also been suggested in myocardial ischemia where plasmalemma fragmentation was observed primarily in areas of the sarcolemma overlying blebs [791] and was accelerated by osmotic swelling conditions that did not damage oxygenated cells [790, 859]. Anoxic damage was accompanied by loss of vinculin and subplasmalemma microfilament structures [692, 791].

Major structural rearrangements likely involving the cytoskeleton occur in ischemic tubule cells. The proximal tubule brush-border membrane is prominently affected. Ischemia durations as short as 5 minutes produce coalescence and interiorization of a majority of the microvilli. Some microvilli are shed into the lumen, although luminal obstruction does not occur [214, 861]. Reoxygenation allows recovery of apparently normal morphology within several hours due to recycling of the interiorized membranes [862]. With longer durations of ischemia (60 minutes), much more shedding of membranes with extensive obstruction distally secondary to impaction of tubule lumina with blebs is seen [214]. These morphological alterations are also accompanied by a significant sustained loss of polarity with redistribution of Na^{+}-K^{+}-ATPase from the basolateral to the apical surface and decrease of the characteristically high sphingomyelin-phosphatidylcholine ratio of the brush-border membrane [562, 563, 565]. The brush-border sphingomyelin-phosphatidylcholine ratio is also reduced after gentamicin treatment [471, 561] and a recent report has shown redistribution of Na^{+}-K^{+}-ATPase to this membrane during gentamicin treatment [561].

Toxin-induced remodeling of the tubule cell surface, irrespective of the mechanisms, can change the area available for transport processes. Evidence for such alterations has been reported in human acute renal failure [387] and has been quantified in the development of acute renal failure secondary to mercuric chloride [287, 634]. Such losses of plasma membrane surface area may be due to internalization of membranes, to failure of membrane production and replacement of normal losses, or to loss of membranes into the tubule lumen [214, 960].

MDCK cells treated with H_2O_2 showed increases of transepithelial conductance and permeability to mannitol, pulling apart of neighboring cells, fragmentation of cytoplasmic staining for F-actin, and thinning and beading of F-actin staining at cell-cell junctions [929]. Disruption of the cytoskeleton also can impair cell adhesion to the basement membrane [121]. Loss of otherwise viable cells from the tubule epithelium could contribute just as much to backleak as necrosis of those cells. The relevance of this process to acute renal failure in vivo is supported by the finding that urine from patients with acute renal failure contain greatly increased numbers of tubule cells, of which a surprisingly large fraction are viable, based on morphological criteria and ability to be placed into tissue culture [653].

In view of increasing information about reciprocal regulatory interactions between membrane polyphosphoinositides and the cytoskeleton and the high affinity of aminoglycosides for those acidic phospholipids, it is conceivable that these processes will be altered during aminoglycoside nephrotoxicity. This remains to be assessed. It has been suggested that aminoglycosides can cause mistargeting of newly synthesized phospholipids and proteins to the surface membrane [561]. Aminoglycoside abnormalities of endosomal processing are detailed in the section on lysosomes. The extent to which these changes are due to primary membrane effects or effects on the cytoskeletal membrane interactions necessary for these processes [151, 295, 564, 676] has not yet been reported.

In addition to the actions on the sodium pump detailed previously, toxins can affect both activity and adherence of other plasma membrane enzymes. Histochemical studies following mercuric chloride showed widespread but transient loss of cell surface enzyme activity within an hour after toxin administration, well before the manifestations of advanced cell injury [961]. Aminoglycosides impair glucose and phosphate transport and Na^+-H^+ exchange [343, 367, 471]. Since these effects are present in isolated brush-border membranes, they are not explained by sodium pump inhibition and must represent changes either in the number of transporters or in the lipid membrane environment required for optimal transporter function.

Aminoglycosides induce marked early losses of brush-border membrane enzymes, including but not limited to alkaline phosphatase [357, 426, 927]. This phenomenon may be due to effects of aminoglycosides on membrane phosphatidylinositol to which alkaline phosphatase is anchored [490], as well as to the loss of whole membrane fragments [426].

Enzymuria originating from the surfaces of renal tubule cells and from within them is a prominent feature of renal exposure to virtually all toxins, even at toxin levels that otherwise do not produce toxic manifestations [38]. Because of the high sensitivity of this parameter to toxin exposure, its occurrence nonspecifically in other types of renal disease, and the large variation in absolute levels between individuals, measurements of enzymuria have not gained wide application in the clinical assessment of renal disease in individual patients. However, serial assessments in individuals can be a useful noninvasive means of monitoring drug effects under well-controlled experimental conditions [566].

Abnormalities of Protein and Nucleic Acid Synthesis

Although some data are available on the acute effects of Hg^{++} in cell culture models [132, 364], interference with cell nucleic acid metabolism and protein synthesis have not been implicated as major mediators of acute nephrotoxic cell injury. The vigorous proliferative repair responses seen after acute nephrotoxic lesions [181–183] also do not support severe suppression. However, inhibition of protein and nucleic acid synthesis might be expected to play a more important role in lesions that evolve over several days such as aminoglycoside and cisplatin nephrotoxicity. Netilmicin, tobramycin, and neomycin all inhibited protein synthesis by isolated hepatic ribosomes. Neomycin and gentamicin C_2, one of the components of gentamicin, caused misreading [489]. Incorporation of ^{3}H-leucine into protein by renal cortex in vivo [561] and by isolated renal cortical microsomes [67] was inhibited early during the course of gentamicin nephrotoxicity. Cyclosporine added to renal microsomes in vitro did not affect ^{3}H-leucine incorporation, but treatment in vivo for 2 to 10 days had substantial dose-dependent inhibitory effects that were attributed to the presence of a translation inhibitor [129]. During serial measurements, inhibition of protein synthesis occurred a day later than reduction of glomerular filtration rate and renal plasma flow, and also recovered sooner when cyclosporine was withdrawn [66].

Renal DNA, RNA, and protein synthesis were inhibited within 6 hours after cisplatin treatment of rabbits [817]. LLC-PK_1 cells were lethally injured during 72 hours exposure to cisplatin in a dose-dependent fashion [574]. Immediate cisplatin inhibition of protein and RNA but not DNA synthesis was predictive of later loss of viability [574]. Killing of Chinese hamster ovary cells by cisplatin was accompanied by DNA fragmentation and was blocked by cycloheximide [47], characteristic features of apoptotic cell death mediated by activation of endonucleases [11, 23, 947]. Cells with morphological features of apoptosis are seen during acute renal failure [616] and during regression of renal hyperplasia [461]. More remains to be learned about this form of cell damage in the kidney. Activation of polyadenosine diphosphate-ribose polymerase has been implicated in the pathogenesis of oxidant injury [721], but this mechanism has yet been demonstrated in the kidney.

Chronic lead intoxication is accompanied by the development of characteristic intranuclear inclusion bodies in proximal tubule cells [245, 749]. They are comprised primarily of protein and lead and probably serve to sequester the metal.

Lysosomes

Lysosomes can contribute to nephrotoxic tubule cell injury by accumulating toxin, failing to perform their normal degradative functions, and leaking damaging hydrolytic enzymes. Lysosomes are involved in the degradation and turnover of macromolecules both from intracellular and extracellular sources, in the storage of undegradable material, and in turnover of cellular membranes and organelles (autophagy) [195, 524]. They contain multiple hydrolytic enzymes that are active against the full range of cellular macromolecules and generally have acidic pH optima [46]. A lysosomal membrane proton ATP-ase pump maintains the intralysosomal pH at 4 to 5 [668, 669, 715]. Primary lysosomes consist of the membrane-bound aggregation of enzymes as packaged in the Golgi apparatus. Secondary lysosomes are derived from the fusion of primary lysosomes with either autophagic or endocytic vacuoles. Depending on their appearance and presumed derivations, secondary lysosomes have been variously termed *cytosomes, cytosegrosomes,* or *phagosomes* [226, 373]. The lysosomal character of an intracellular membrane-bound body is established by the histochemical localization within it of typical lysosomal enzyme activity, e.g., acid phosphatase. The formation of new autophagic secondary lysosomes is not inhibited by cessation of protein synthesis but is markedly diminished by compromise of the cell's energy supply [748].

Methods for assessing the structural and functional integrity of a lysosome system include a variety of approaches. Their size, number, and intracellular locations may be quantified. Nonmetabolized, intralysosomal material, as in myeloid bodies, may be seen. The presence or absence of enzyme activity may be assessed histochemically. Depending on the tissue and nature of injury, lysosomal preparations of varying purity can be isolated by differential and gradient centrifugation methods. The latency of lysosomal enzyme activity is evaluated on such isolated lysosome preparations. Total enzyme activity is measured by disrupting the lysosomal membrane, which may be done with detergents, such as Triton, thermal stress, sonication, or combinations of more than one treatment. Free enzyme activity is the amount present in the absence of such disruptive treatment and is generally taken as a measure of lysosomal fragility. Unsedimentable free activity represents enzyme that has leaked into solution and is no longer associated with the lysosomal membrane. Sedimentable free activity is enzyme that has remained associated with lysosomal particles but, due to apparent changes in the barrier characteristics of the lysosomal membrane or other factors, has greater effective access to substrate. Agents that "stabilize" lysosomes decrease the ratio of free to total activity while agents that "labilize" lysosomes increase this ratio. Much useful information has been derived from studies with ^{125}I-labeled formaldehyde-treated bovine serum albumin [533]. The tissue uptake of this compound, given adequate controls for delivery, can be used as an index of the effectiveness of phagosome formation. Measurement of the conversion of trichloroacetic acid-insoluble radioactivity to acid-soluble radioactivity during in vitro incubation of lysosomes prelabeled with ^{125}I-albumin is a good index of the effectiveness of intralysosomal proteolysis [533]. Effectiveness of intralysosomal degradative processes in vivo also may be assessed by determining whether there has been abnormal accumulation of a particular macromolecule, e.g., the phospholipids comprising myeloid bodies.

ACCUMULATION OF TOXINS IN LYSOSOMES

Lysosomes are major intracellular storage sites for a number of toxins and drugs. It has been shown that a variety of metals, including Hg^{++}, which can be phagocytized bound to filtered albumin [352, 503, 505, 612], uranium [256], chromium [74], copper [269], beryllium [940], iron [413], and zinc [816], accumulate in lysosomes. The metals, though concentrated in lysosomes relative to other cellular organelles at various stages of treatment, never reach massive levels. Lysosomal processing of complexed toxin (e.g., cadmium-thionein [703]) may, in fact, serve mainly to release toxins for effects elsewhere within the cell. In contrast to the metals, a number of organic agents, including the aminoglycoside antibiotics, accumulate in lysosomes in very large quantities. The brush-border membrane–binding characteristics of the aminoglycosides have been reviewed previously in this chapter. Sequential autoradiographic studies have shown redistribution of labeled aminoglycoside bound to proximal tubular cell plasma membrane into intracellular, apparently lysosomal, vacuoles within minutes after the initial binding [396]. Cell fractionation studies have demonstrated accumulation of tracer quantities of ^{14}C-gentamicin in lysosomes within 6 hours after administration [396, 583]. The subcellular distribution of gentamicin during a longer high-dose protocol, of the type that most consistently produces experimental gentamicin nephrotoxicity, is not as well defined. There is little doubt that predominant intralysosomal localization continues; however, additional subcellular sites may become involved [918]. A more generalized cytosolic distribution of aminoglycosides has also been suggested to occur during the early uptake period [594, 888]. The most striking morphological feature of the early phases of gentamicin nephrotoxicity is the appearance of very large secondary lysosomes, many with myeloid bodies (Fig. 39-10). Such changes are apparent within 12 to 24 hours after a single dose of gentamicin [434] and are evident in human kidneys after brief courses of gentamicin at therapeutic levels [193].

A number of drugs induce striking morphologic changes, with development of numerous myeloid bodies, most commonly in liver but in kidney as well [86, 496]. They include chloroquine [2, 3, 521], chlorpromazine [216], chlorphentermine [216, 398], the tricyclic antidepressants [216, 496, 498, 789], 4,4′-diethylaminoethoxyhexestrol [200, 949], 4,4′-bis(diethylaminoethoxy)-diethyldiphenylethane [521], 2-*N*-methylpiperazinomethyl-1,3-diazafluoranthen 1-oxide (AC3579) [331, 824], and others. Detailed studies on the intracellular accumulation and metabolism of all these agents are not available; however, two that have been assessed, chloroquine and 4-4′-bis(diethylaminoethoxy)-diethyldiphenylethane [521], do preferentially accumulate in lysosomes. Al-

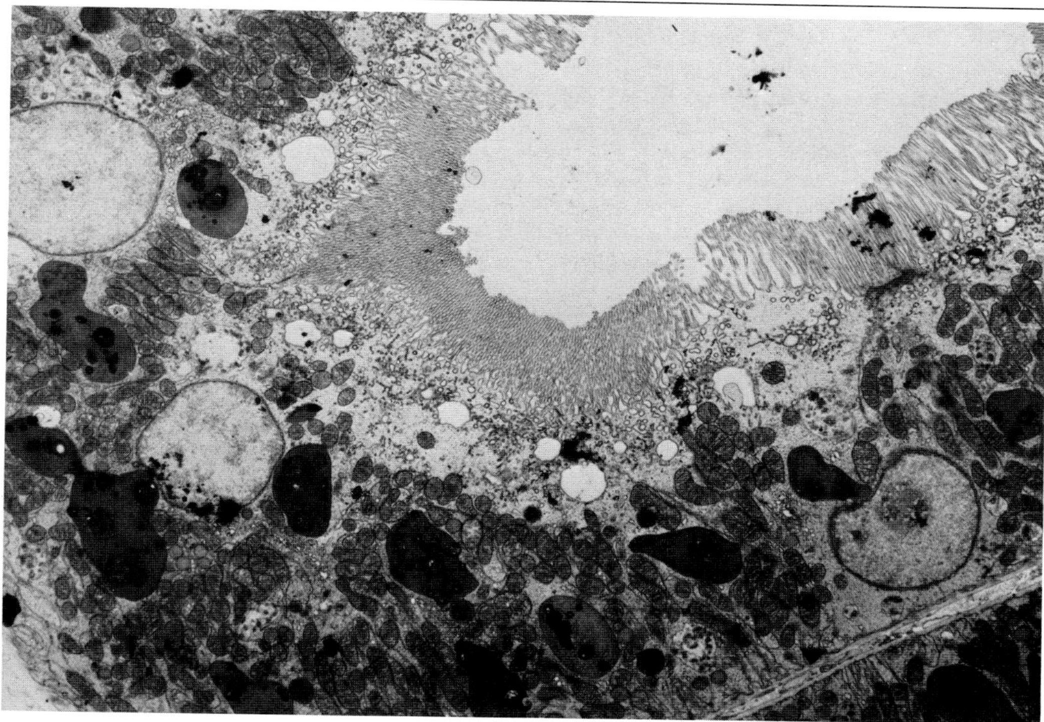

Fig. 39-10. Proximal tubule cells during gentamicin nephrotoxicity, illustrating enlargement of lysosomes and myeloid bodies.

though the major target organ for most of these agents is liver, kidney may also be prominently involved [498] and the effects appear generalized for many types of cells [216]. The common feature of all these agents is that they are cationic amphiphiles, i.e., their molecular structure includes highly hydrophobic and cationic hydrophilic moieties in close proximity. Structural analogues of these agents whose hydrophilic side chains are anionic do not possess similar properties [496].

Myeloid body formation during gentamicin treatment is prevented by polyaspartic acid and other polyamino acids. Large lysosomes still form but, instead of myeloid bodies, they contain an amorphous, osmophilic material that likely consists of polyamino acid–gentamicin complexes [55, 417, 418]. The importance of having an intact polyamino acid is shown by the observation that poly-D-glutamic acid, which is nonmetabolizable by lysosomes, prevented myeloid body formation (and nephrotoxicity). Poly-L-glutamic acid, which was shown to be metabolizable by lysosomes, was not effective [418].

EFFECTS ON LYSOSOMAL FUNCTION

Once nephrotoxins have accumulated in lysosomes, they have the potential to alter lysosomal function. Metal ions inhibit lysosomal cathepsins with K_is in the μM range. Cu^{++} and Zn^{++} were most effective in inhibiting cathepsins B and C, while Hg^{++} and Ag^{++} were most effective with cathepsins A and D [552]. Cu^{++}, Sn^{+++}, Pb^{++}, Hg^{++}, and Zn^{++} all inhibited intralysosomal proteolysis when added to suspensions of phagolysosomes, but the 1 mM levels used to achieve these effects were relatively high compared to levels in situ [534]. Data suggest, however, that, for $HgCl_2$, levels in the range of 3 to 30 nmol/mg lysosomal protein do inhibit intralysosomal proteolysis in vitro [504]. Of more significance regarding in vivo toxicity is the observation that within 2 to 5 hours after administration of acutely toxic doses of $HgCl_2$ and $CdCl_2$, both phagolysosome formation and intralysosomal proteolysis were inhibited in the major target organs—kidney for $HgCl_2$ and liver for $CdCl_2$ [535, 537]. Whether these effects were due to primary lysosomal actions of the metals or are secondary to their other metabolic effects is not clear, since ATP synthesis is potentially already compromised at those intervals with both toxins [834, 912] and ATP may be required for both formation of secondary lysosomes [748] and maintenance of optimal intralysosomal pH [668, 669, 715].

Gentamicin has also been reported to inhibit cathepsins B and L of microdissected S1 and S2 segments. The effect did not increase with 4 days of treatment as compared to 1 day. Although gentamicin inhibited activity of cathepsins B and L in vitro, the in vivo effect was considered more likely to be a result of interference with the synthesis and delivery of cathepsin to lysosomes rather than to a direct interaction in the lysosome [615].

Appearance in the urine of cationic, low-molecular-weight proteins (lysozyme, beta-2-microglobulin) is one of the earliest renal effects of aminoglycoside treatment. This appears to relate in large part to competition between aminoglycoside and the proteins for endocytic uptake [71, 162, 164, 166]. However, there is also evidence for impaired intracellular degradation [166]. This could be due to inhibition of lysosomal protease activity or to abnormal interactions between endosomes and primary lysosomes. With regard to the latter possibility, it has been shown that gentamicin treatment in vivo did not impair total accumulation of horseradish peroxidase, a marker for endocytic uptake, but a decreased fraction of "normal-appearing" lysosomes contained horseradish peroxidase and very few lysosomes with myeloid bodies contained the marker [268]. Results of available studies of cultured tubule cells differ. In LLC-PK_1 cells, endocytic uptake of sucrose and Lucifer yellow was inhibited by growth in a high concentration of gentamicin [410]. During 7 days of gentamicin exposure, cultured human proximal tubule cells did not have substantial decreases of endocytic activity as measured by uptake of fluorescein isothiocyanate–dextran [670]. There were also no major changes in intralysosomal pH [670].

Appearance of lysosomal enzymes in the urine is another early feature of aminoglycoside nephrotoxicity [927, 928]. Myeloid bodies are also found on ultrastructural examination of urine sediments [511]. Whether the lysosomal enzymuria results entirely from such release of whole lysosomes or is also due to exocytosis of lysosomal contents is not known.

The formation of myeloid bodies induced by the cationic amphiphilic drugs is associated with development of phospholipidosis. The type of phospholipids preferentially accumulated vary with the agent and often include some increase in all major phospholipids, i.e., the quantitatively preponderant zwitterionic phospholipids phosphatidylcholine and phosphatidylethanolamine as well as the acidic phospholipids—phosphatidic acid, phosphatidylinositol, and phosphatidylserine [86]. However, frequently, the acidic phospholipids, particularly phosphatidylinositol and a normally rare acidic phospholipid, bis(monoacylglycerophosphate), make up a disproportionate share of the increase [86, 200, 521], although this is not a completely uniform finding [824]. With the drugs in which it has received detailed study, i.e., chloroquine, 4-4′-bis(diethylaminoethoxy)-diethyldiphenylethane [521], and 2,2′-diethylaminoethoxyhexestrol [200], almost all of the increased phospholipid, after chronic drug exposure, could be localized within lysosomes. Several mechanisms for this effect have been proposed. There is little doubt that these drugs can complex with phospholipids by both hydrophobic bonding, utilizing their apolar moiety and electrostatic interactions between their cationic side chain and the polar component of the phospholipid. Indeed, such interactions have been demonstrated directly using NMR techniques [738, 739]. Such an interaction will be strongest with the acidic phospholipids because of their negatively charged head groups. Binding of drug to phospholipid would make it a poor substrate for intralysosomal phospholipases and both drug and lipid would, therefore, accumulate. Support for the operation of such a mechanism derives from the observation that AC3579 induced a marked phospholipidosis, including increased phosphatidylethanolamine without increasing incorporation of ^{14}C ethanolamine into phosphatidylethanolamine or ^{32}P into total phospholipids. On the other hand, degradation of ^{32}P-labeled phospholipids was diminished [331]. Inhibitory effects of the cationic amphiphilic drugs on a variety of phospholipases including those of lysosomal origin have been shown [440, 520] and, at least for some of the agents, the effects occur by a direct drug-enzyme interaction rather than by means of a drug substrate action [440].

However, the actions of these agents are not limited to lysosomal degradative processes. Substantial data are available that another mode of action is to diminish the activity of phosphatidate phosphohydrolase and, thereby, redirect de novo phospholipid synthesis toward additional phosphatidylinositol at the expense of phosphatidylcholine and phosphatidylethanolamine [1, 9, 96, 115, 116, 548, 640]. This mechanism opens the possibility of alterations in the phospholipid composition of multiple cell membranes rather than only lysosomal degradative pools. Such alterations of phospholipid content may have significant functional consequences on such processes as cation transport [357].

Gentamicin, although not amphiphilic, is similar to the cationic amphiphilic drugs in that phospholipids, specifically the acidic phospholipids, are major cellular sites of its binding. This is due to the cationicity of the molecule and its general configuration [357]. As described earlier in this section, gentamicin accumulates within renal tubular cell lysosomes and leads to marked changes in their morphology including, though not limited to, the production of myeloid bodies. This effect of gentamicin has been detailed in the section on alterations of phospholipid metabolism.

The importance of lysosomal phospholipid accumulation in the pathogenesis of nephrotoxicity remains to be clarified. The deleterious consequences of the naturally occurring lysosomal storage diseases, such as Niemann-Pick [716], Tay-Sachs [431, 818], and Fabry's disease [36, 510, 620] are well known and, indeed, they share many morphological features with the drug-induced phospholipidosis. However, the injury produced in these settings, even though it can lead to profound organ dysfunction and failure over prolonged periods, is chronic in nature and does not have many of the features of acute injury. Similarly, cationic amphiphilic drugs may produce chronic organ dsyfunction but, in spite of extensive lysosomal phospholipidosis, general cell integrity and integrity of intracellular organelles remain well preserved [2, 3, 200, 216, 350, 398, 824]. Aminoglycoside nephrotoxicity is quite different in that early progressive injury is evident at multiple cellular sites, with evolution to a classical pattern of cell death. It is clear, however, that a phospholipidosis is a very early tubule cell alteration produced by aminoglycoside treatment. At the time phospholipidosis is first detected, prior to any large or progressive loss of clearance function or direct morphologic evidence of lethal cell injury, a significant increase in the normal turnover of tubule cells can be shown by thymidine labeling [266]. Protection by polyaspartic acid against both this low-level injury and against more widespread, overt tubule cell necrosis is clearly associated with prevention of phospholipidosis despite continued aminoglycoside accumulation. This supports the notion that the phospholipidosis is either a mediator of injury or a closely associated parallel process.

COMPROMISED LYSOSOMAL INTEGRITY

Available data on the in vitro effects of various nephrotoxins on lysosomal fragility are limited and, in some cases, insufficient to determine the significance of the effect. Thus Hg^{++}, at levels down to about 10 μM (the minimal active level was not precisely determined), increased the ratio of free/total activity (i.e., decreased latency) of several lysosomal enzymes; however, the lack of data on whether the increased activity was sedimentable or nonsedimentable makes it difficult to ascertain the degree of disruption of lysosomal integrity [867]. Concentrations of 1 mM Hg^{++} and Cu^{++} increased markedly the unsedimentable activity, but the pathophysiologic significance of observations on the effects of such massive levels is minimal. It is of interest, though, that, in the same system, 1 mM Zn^{++} decreased the amount of unsedimentable activity relative to controls, suggesting a substantial stabilizing effect of even this high level of Zn^{++} [153].

The importance of determining whether an increase in free activity is sedimentable or nonsedimentable is demonstrated by observations on the in vitro effects of gentamicin. During in vitro exposure of normal lysosomes to gentamicin over the range of 5 to 50 μg/ml, a marked increase in free/total lysosomal enzyme activity was seen. Incubation of lysosomes without gentamicin for 60 minutes at 37°C also increased the amount of nonsedimentable enzyme. Addition of gentamicin to lysosomes incubated for 60 minutes at 37°C further increased the free/total enzyme ratio but completely prevented the increase in the amount of nonsedimentable enzyme [582]. Thus gentamicin, at the levels tested, acts to decrease the latency of lysosomal enzymes, but it does not apparently do so by disrupting lysosomal structure and, instead, serves to "stabilize" the lysosomal membrane against other labilizing treatments. Other tested aminoglycosides had similar qualitative effects [582]. Another study of in vitro effects of aminoglycosides on renal cortical lysosomes also found inhibition of NAG release from lysosomes by low concentrations of the antibiotics [646]. The polyamines, spermine and spermidine, had similar effects. As aminoglycoside concentrations were raised above approximately 0.1 mM, their "protective" effect was lost and the degree of NAG release returned toward that seen in untreated lysosomes [646]. At millimolar levels, gentamicin labilized lysosomes, producing loss of multiple hydrolases in amounts substantially greater than those seen in controls [597]. Mepacrine, a cationic amphiphilic drug with effects to inhibit phospholipases, behaved similarly to the aminoglycosides at low and intermediate concentrations [647]. Extrapolating from these observations to in vivo effects of gentamicin is further complicated because, in vivo, lysosomal membranes are exposed to far higher levels of gentamicin from within than from without.

Direct exposure of lysosomes to 0.5 mM or 1 mM cephaloridine, levels in the range of those seen in renal cortex after in vivo treatment and similar to those which produce mitochondrial dysfunction [844, 845], had a stabilizing effect similar to that seen with gentamicin in that it ameliorated the increase in nonsedimentable activity that occurred upon incubation at 37°C. On the other hand, 10 mM cephaloridine rapidly and markedly increased the amount of nonsedimentable enzyme activity, suggesting marked lysosomal disruption by this level of drug. Stabilizing effects were seen with the cationic amphiphilic agents chlorpromazine, chloroquine, triparanol, chlorphentermine, and mepacrine. These agents, as well as cephaloridine, had parallel effects to inhibit the hemolysis of red blood cells produced by a lysosomal phospholipase A_2. From this observation, it was proposed that the lysosomal stabilization was secondary to inhibition of the action of endogenous lysosomal phospholipase A_2 [252, 253].

Information on changes in the integrity of lysosomes isolated after in vivo exposure to nephrotoxins is relatively limited. Lysosomes isolated after treatment of female Sherman rats with 6 to 12 mg/kg of gentamicin for 7 days did not differ from controls, but after 150 mg/kg for 21 days, free/total activity ratios were increased. No intermediate treatment conditions were assessed and determination of sedimentable versus nonsedimentable activity was not reported. Lysosomes from the rats treated for 21 days were resistant to the action of gentamicin added in vitro to increase the amount of free activity [582]. Decreased latency of *N*-acetylglucosaminidase was seen within a day after treatment of male rats with 50 mg/kg of gentamicin. In dose-response studies employing an 8-day course of treatment, daily doses as low as 4 mg/kg reduced latency [583]. Increased fragility of lysosomes from cultured human proximal tubule cells was not found until 10 days of exposure, long after the appearance of myeloid bodies [670].

Lysosomes isolated 24 hours after treatment with 5 mg/kg of $HgCl_2$ showed increased proportions of free/total enzyme activity. Sedimenting properties were not assessed. Total acid phosphatase activity was substantially diminished [866]. The presence of necrosis at the time that lysosomal changes were found makes it difficult to assign the importance of these changes in the sequential pathophysiology of the lesion. Lysosomes isolated after cephaloridine treatment have not been characterized, but shortly after treatment, when injury is otherwise not fully developed, urinary excretion of acid phosphatase is diminished [641]. This observation has been attributed to the "stabilizing" effects of low doses of cephaloridine on lysosomal membranes [252, 253]. Of note, however, even though gentamicin also has "stabilizing" effects, as discussed previously, lysosomal enzyme excretion is increased after in vivo treatment with the antibiotic [494]. More extensive work on associations between fragility of isolated lysosomes and cell injury has been done using hepatocytes, but, as for the studies of renal tubule cells, the results do not conclusively establish a pathogenetic role [196, 200, 205, 280, 369, 536, 763, 789, 896, 973, 974].

Data on altered lysosomal integrity from intact renal tubule cell models are relatively limited but, in combination with several studies on nonrenal cells, are more informative about the pathogenetic role of the organelle. Microscopic observation of isolated flounder tubules developing lethal cell injury secondary to treatment with potassium cyanide or organic mercurials revealed that integrity of lysosomal granules was preserved well into the period of advanced injury [693, 839, 840]. Histochemical studies of acid phosphatase in kidneys of rats during $HgCl_2$ toxicity showed loss of staining 30 minutes after $HgCl_2$ exposure but subsequent spontaneous recovery at 3 hours. Thereafter, a steady loss of staining for the enzyme occurred concomitantly with the development of generalized loss of cellular integrity [961]. Lysosomes in ischemic kidney slices were stable until after necrotic cell damage had occurred [225]. Interpreting negative results of this type is complicated because (1) fixation of the tissue prior to histological study may decrease enzyme activity; (2) enzyme activity that has leaked into the cytoplasm will be substantially diluted; and (3) lysosomes may leak enzyme without severe disruption of their structure [227].

To circumvent these difficulties in assessing enzyme release from lysosomes in situ during tissue injury, marker agents have been used to evaluate more sensitively the timing of the release of lysosomal contents. Lysosomes of Chang liver tumor cells in tissue culture were labeled in situ with the fluorochrome, acridine orange, or horseradish peroxidase, and were then treated with either the combination of potassium cyanide and iodoacetamide to inhibit energy metabolism or the combination of immunoglobulin and complement to primarily damage the plasma membrane. Acridine orange escaped from the lysosomes relatively early during injury that was produced by the metabolic inhibitors but was retained well into the stages of advanced injury produced by immunoglobulin and complement. Ferritin was retained within lysosomes well into stages of advanced injury in both models. The results do not suggest major lysosomal disruption during the early phases of development of either type of injury [317].

In the presence of oxygen and blue light, cells treated with acridine orange sustain rapid damage due to excitation by light of the acridine orange, with production of reactive oxygen metabolites [12] Because acridine orange concentrates in lysosomes, these organelles are major targets in this process. Following exposure to blue light, rapid disappearance of dye and parallel loss of histochemical staining for acid phosphatase in lysosomes occurred. However, carefully timed morphological observations revealed substantial alterations in the morphology of endoplasmic reticulum and mitochondria prior to histochemical evidence of leakage of enzyme and fluorescent dye. Furthermore, lysosomal membranes were morphologically intact when leakage was occurring [520].

Silica taken up by macrophages localizes in lysosomes. This is followed by redistribution of acid phosphatase activity from lysosomes to the cytoplasm [13]. A similar redistribution of horseradish peroxidase is seen if lysosomes are labeled with this marker prior to silica exposure [588]. How this early lysosomal disruption contributes to injury has been assessed [403]. It was confirmed that silica produced lysosomal disruption in situ as measured by redistribution of either acridine orange or horseradish peroxidase. However, cell death occurred only if Ca^{++} was present in the medium despite similar degrees of lysosomal disruption with and without Ca^{++}. This observation might only indicate, however, that the damage caused by release of lysosomal enzymes was present but was not expressed as cell death in the absence of Ca^{++}. However, there was also no evidence for degradation of DNA, RNA, protein, or phospholipid, as might be expected if uncontrolled hydrolase activity were present. Promethazine protected against cell death produced by silica but not against lysosomal rupture. Indomethacin protected against lysosomal rupture produced by silica but not against cell death. The calcium ionophore A23187 itself caused lysosomal rupture irrespective of the presence of extracellular Ca^{++} but caused cell death only when extracellular Ca^{++} was present [403]. Thus in a lesion with high potential to be mediated by lysosomal disruption, alterations in lysosomal integrity could be dissociated in multiple ways from the development of injury.

Taken together, the available information on lysosomal damage in situ argues that lysosomes in the intracellular milieu are relatively stable structures that, even when disrupted, do not predictably contribute to the progression of acute cell injury.

Intrinsic Protective Mechanisms and Protective Maneuvers Offering Insights into the Cellular Basis of Nephrotoxicity

PROTECTIVE MANEUVERS

Several protective maneuvers with actions that have been related to specific cellular processes contributing to nephrotoxicity have already been considered. These include oral calcium loading, polyamino acids, and possibly thyroxine in aminoglycoside toxicity and various approaches for modulating toxic activation and free-radical damage.

In assessing modes of action of protective maneuvers and the information they can provide about mechanisms of nephrotoxic cell damage, changes in tubule cell exposure to nephrotoxins and accumulation of nephrotoxins due to alterations in toxin delivery to the kidney, toxin contact time with the epithelium, and reabsorptive and secretory processes must be carefully considered before attributing effects to specific intracellular mechanisms. This has not always been done.

Mannitol has been reported to ameliorate the severity of amphotericin nephrotoxicity [326], chronic gentamicin nephrotoxicity in the rabbit [488], and the acute fall in GFR produced by intravenous $HgCl_2$ in the dog [323]. Results of studies on the use of mannitol in *cis*-platinum nephrotoxicity have been contradictory [322, 463, 801]. In most of these nephrotoxic models, the data are insufficient to draw firm conclusions about the mechanism for mannitol's effects. Increased toxin excretion and lower urinary toxin concentration, as well as action to promote clearance of intratubular debris, must be considered [204, 937] and differences in effects between studies may be secondary to variation in these processes. Mannitol also has antioxidant properties [409] and this action has frequently been cited to explain its efficacy in various forms of acute renal failure, but has not generally been subject to rigorous experimental testing. A pathogenetic role for hydroxyl radical formation related to the release of Fe from free myoglobin has been described for hemoglobin- and glycerol-induced acute renal failure [621, 740]. Mannitol is protective against acute renal failure induced by glycerol [937] and injection of methemoglobin and ferrocyanide [819], but the protective effect of mannitol appears to relate more to its actions to maintain tubule patency, rather than to prevent tubule cell damage [958]. In this regard, mannitol has also been reported to promote release of atrial natriuretic peptide [264, 446], which has been reported to ameliorate ischemic acute renal failure [592, 747] as well as gentamicin [711, 713], cyclosporine [134], cisplatin [133], uranyl nitrate [324], and other forms of nephrotoxic acute renal failure, by relieving a sustained vasoconstrictive element that contributes to both functional impairment and potentially ameliorating concurrent ischemic damage promoted by this vasoconstriction.

Furosemide has been of interest because of its clinical efficacy and availability as a diuretic as well as for its actions to reduce transport-related medullary thick ascending limb damage [107, 110]. However, its major actions are distal to the proximal tubule sites of damage for most nephrotoxins and its effects to stimulate renin production could aggravate nephrotoxic damage by decreasing renal perfusion. For these reasons, it is not surprising that furosemide did not have clearly beneficial effects in $HgCl_2$ [37, 857] or uranyl nitrate [475] nephrotoxicity. In the latter study of uranyl nitrate nephrotoxicity in the dog, dopamine also did not ameliorate acute renal failure, but the combination of furosemide and dopamine was beneficial. This combination, but not the agents individually, produced a sustained sodium and water diuresis. Thus the protection may have resulted from a modification of tissue uptake of uranyl nitrate, although this was not directly assessed. In support of this theory is the observation that furosemide alone can be protective against $HgCl_2$ if it is simultaneously accompanied by heavy saline loading to induce a large sustained diuresis [820]. Furosemide may worsen the acute renal failure produced by cephaloridine [37, 213] and gentamicin [607]. Most, but not all, studies have reported that furosemide provides some protection against *cis*-platinum nephrotoxicity [186, 463, 881, 882]. A mechanism for the latter effect has not been determined and a large acute saline diuresis in the absence of diuretic drugs is just as beneficial [937].

Chronic saline loading is effective for ameliorating nephrotoxicity, particularly that of heavy metals, such as uranyl nitrate [690] and $HgCl_2$ [45, 209, 241]. Saline loading has received considerable study because of the proposition that its beneficial effects were mediated by its suppression of the renin-angiotensin system [240]. This hypothesis minimized any role for saline loading in altering the interaction of heavy metal and renal tubule cells, because it was emphasized that acute renal failure was ameliorated in spite of the presence of renal tubular cell necrosis in the groups where renal function was protected by chronic saline loading [45, 209]. However, subsequent studies showed that suppression of renin can be dissociated from protection, since both plasma and renal renin levels were elevated by furosemide, but it still effectively protected against $HgCl_2$ toxicity when a constant diuresis similar to that produced by chronic saline loading was maintained [82, 408]. Additionally, the amount of tubule cell damage can be reduced by saline loading. Such protection has been described in the potassium dichromate model [469] and in some reports of protection against $HgCl_2$ toxicity [45, 241]. A close review of the data (Table 4 of [209]) from a $HgCl_2$ study in which morphologic protection originally was not considered to be present indicates that it probably did occur [209].

There is evidence that chronic saline loading reduces renal tissue levels of Hg^{++}. In two studies [416, 618], renal tissue Hg^{++} levels were substantially lower in saline drinking rats than in controls 20 and 24 hours after $HgCl_2$. The decrease in tissue Hg^{++} produced by chronic saline loading was correlated with a fourfold increase in urine Hg^{++} excretion [416]. However, conflicting data showing no effect of saline loading on tissue levels of Hg^{++} also have been reported [203]. A major difficulty that arises in studies of tissue levels of nephrotoxins is the loss of necrotic cells along with their accumulated toxin as injury advances. This can lead to an underestimation of maximal tissue levels contributing to toxicity if sampling is done only relatively late in the course of injury.

Cisplatin nephrotoxicity is clearly reduced by administration of the drug in isotonic saline, and hypertonic saline is more effective than normal saline [480, 619]. As previously detailed, one proposed mechanism for this is that, when dissolved in fluids containing low chloride concentrations, the chlorides of cisplatin (*cis*-diamminedichloroplatinum, II) are replaced by water and form, via an aquation reaction, a compound [680] that may be more reactive with nucleophilic sites than the parent compound, and thus more potent and more toxic. However, saline administration has also been found to lower tissue uptake of cisplatin [320, 554].

Streptozotocin-induced diabetes in the rat is associated with strong protection against aminoglycoside and cisplatin nephrotoxicity [276, 733]. These animals undergo a sustained, heavy osmotic diuresis and protection can be reversed by insulin treatment [733]. It has been argued that the diuresis and associated reductions of toxin uptake cannot fully explain protection [276], but this remains the most tenable explanation [391, 657].

Chelators such as British anti-Lewsinite (BAL), dithiothreitol (DTT), and 2,3-dimercaptosuccinic acid are effective for ameliorating heavy metal toxicity in both clinical and experimental settings [44, 388, 420, 663]. The protection of renal function correlates with protection against morphologic injury. These agents may act both by complexing the agents and promoting elimination and by decreasing toxicity of metal still in the tissue by preventing its interaction with cellular components. Several studies have emphasized the role of glutathione as a preexisting endogenous chelator for Hg^{++} and Cd^{++} [72, 254, 589, 761, 807]. The role of metallothionein as an inducible chelator is considered below. As previously detailed, many thiol-containing compounds including dithiocarbamates, sodium thiosulfate, methionine and its derivatives, glutathione, and 2-mercaptoethanesulfonate have been reported to ameliorate cisplatin nephrotoxicity, probably by complexing the toxin and promoting its clearance or keeping it within cells in a form that it is not reactive with cellular macromolecules [49, 93, 94, 194, 348, 470, 482, 574]. A variety of additional compounds have been reported to substantially ameliorate cisplatin toxicity: prochlorperazine [438], piperacillin [320], fosfomycin [320, 873], procaine [228], acetazolamide [325], bismuth nitrate [590], probenecid [188, 370], glycine [330], and others. Whether the primary actions of these agents are on uptake of cisplatin, elimination, intracellular sequestration, or processes distal to the interaction of cisplatin with cellular macromolecules has not been fully determined for these agents.

Calcium channel blockers are of potential benefit because of actions to relieve renal vasoconstriction and to prevent damage from cellular Ca^{++} overload. Despite much interest, the latter process has not been convincingly demonstrated [148, 724, 893]. However, the vascular effects can have a significant impact on cyclosporine and amphotericin nephrotoxicity [81, 362, 830], probably by antagonizing direct calcium-mediated vasoconstrictive action of these agents [545, 707]. Actions of calcium-channel blockers against other nephrotoxins have been equivocal.

Pyridoxal-5-phosphate has been reported to complex with cyanide, spermine, and gentamicin and to ameliorate their systemic toxicity [411]. Activity of pyridoxal-5-phosphate to block gentamicin-induced phospholipidosis and enzymuria has been described during a 2-week course of 60 mg/kg of gentamicin in association with decreased tissue gentamicin levels. Pyridoxal-5-phosphate was not effective against the changes induced by a higher dose of gentamicin, 100 mg/kg, for 4 days despite an equivalent reduction of tissue levels, although loss of gentamicin from damaged cells complicates interpretation of this change [399].

Beneficial effects of amino acid infusions during $HgCl_2$ nephrotoxicity have been reported [828]. They were attributed to amino acid–induced enhancement of phosphatidylcholine synthesis. Infusion of amino acids in vivo or exposure of renal slices in vitro increased the incorporation of ^{14}C-choline into membrane phosphatidylcholine. The effect was seen in both normal kidneys and after $HgCl_2$ treatment. In the latter case, this enhancement was superimposed on the accelerated rate of ^{14}C-choline phospholipid incorporation produced by the nephrotoxin alone. The amino acids acted to both increase ^{14}C-choline tissue accumulation and to enhance two of the steps in the Kennedy pathway of phosphatidylcholine synthesis [828, 829]. Which specific amino acids are responsible has not been established. It is also not known whether this is primarily a repair mechanism for damaged cells or a process facilitating replacement of the damaged epithelium by regeneration.

Treatment with thyroxine has been found to have a beneficial effect on the course of nephrotoxic acute renal failure secondary to mercuric chloride [725, 726], potassium dichromate [753], gentamicin [176], and ischemia [805]. The protection from dichromate occurred even when thyroxine was started 24 hours after toxin administration [753]. Whether this effect is related to thyroxine-induced changes in Na-K-ATPase [176], cell phospholipid metabolism, regenerative capacity, or toxin handling [174] is presently unclear and it may differ depending on the model. There is increasing interest in the potential to enhance regeneration by manipulation of growth levels. Accelerated recovery resulting from treatment with epidermal growth factor has been reported for both ischemic [353, 611] and $HgCl_2$-induced [160] acute renal failure. Thyroxine, an essential constituent of serum-free culture media for proximal tubule cells, has been shown to upregulate expression of epidermal growth factor receptors in primary cultures of rabbit proximal tubule cells [173], and protection against dichromate-induced acute renal failure was associated with moderate enhancement of thymidine incorporation into DNA [547]. Also potentially related is the observation that administration of ATP-$MgCl_2$ up to 24 hours after the toxin ameliorates the course of acute renal failure [754]. The initial rationale for this approach was to improve cellular energetics and there is some evidence that exogenous purines can help restore depleted intracellular pools in the kidney [514, 796, 906, 917]. However, it has become evident during the past several years that many cell types, including renal tubule cells, have surface receptors for both purine nucleotides and their metabolites [908] and that the resulting intracellular signaling events can modify the cellular proliferation that would figure importantly during regeneration [580, 623]. Whether this latter mode of action best explains the beneficial effects of ATP administration during both ischemic and nephrotoxic injury is being investigated.

Concurrent selenium administration markedly reduces the nephrotoxicity of both acute and chronic mercury administration irrespective of whether the mercury is given in organic or inorganic form [233, 309, 428, 542, 557, 645]. Selenium compounds, possibly by direct interaction with Hg^{++}, appear able to alter markedly the biological activity of Hg^{++} by changing its affinity for tissue components. Thus whole body retention of Hg^{++} given concurrently with selenium is increased, circulating levels of Hg^{++} increase due to increased binding to formed elements of the blood [557], intracellular Hg^{++} binding to metallothionein is largely eliminated [309, 428, 542], and the intracellular distribution of Hg^{++} is further altered in that a larger proportion is recovered in the nuclear fraction at the expense of the cytoplasmic fraction [233]. From the available data, fractional mitochondrial binding does not appear to change markedly. The contribution of these subcellular effects to ameliorating Hg^{++} toxicity, however, has not been intensively investigated in either in vivo or in vitro systems. It is also complicated by the net effect of selenium treatment to markedly decrease total Hg^{++} levels in the kidney [233, 557], despite the greater whole body retention that reflects increases in Hg^{++} in all other tissues studied, particularly liver and spleen. However, the fact that these increases of Hg^{++} induced by selenium in other tissue are not associated with increased extrarenal toxicity and, depending on the mercurial used, may be associated with decreased extrarenal toxicity [645] confirms the importance of the protective effects occurring at the subcellular level.

Several different modes of selenium administration have also shown promise in ameliorating cisplatin nephrotoxicity [42, 75, 704, 706]. The basis for these effects has not been as extensively studied as the action of selenium during $HgCl_2$ toxicity, but it also presumably resides in a nucleophilic interaction between selenium and platinum.

ENDOGENOUS MECHANISMS

The metallothioneins are low-molecular-weight cytoplasmic proteins having a high content of sulfur, mainly as cysteine and with high affinity for Cd^{++}, Zn^{++}, Cu^{++}, and Hg^{++} so that on isolation they contain the metal and, thence, the name metallothionein [146, 400, 883]. Their physiological role may be to provide a reservoir for the essential but highly toxic trace metals Cu^{++} and Zn^{++} [305, 400, 883, 896]. Levels of metallothionein in liver and kidney, as well as other tissues, increase markedly after heavy metal administration due to increased synthesis secondary to an increased rate of transcription from the metallothionein gene within the first several hours after administration of the metal [217, 883]. In fact, metallothionein-bound metal accounts for the largest fraction of intracellular Cd^{++} and Hg^{++} during acute and chronic intoxication [227, 702, 883, 939].

The ability of toxic heavy metals to induce synthesis of metallothioneins that can bind them and prevent their interaction with sensitive cellular macromolecules provides an important protective mechanism for both acute and chronic heavy-metal exposure. Preinduction of metallothionein by either prior metal exposure or other maneuvers has been shown to substantially ameliorate both Cd^{++} and Hg^{++} nephrotoxicity [380–382, 427, 506, 549, 605, 886]. However, as detailed previously, Cd-thionein formed in the liver appears to be more toxic to the kidney than Cd^{++} itself. Whether all Cd^{++} in the kidney during in vivo toxicity arises from leakage of liver Cd-thionein has been controversial [610, 884].

Considerable work has been done to assess whether metallothionein plays a role in cisplatin nephrotoxicity. Cisplatin does not induce either hepatic or renal metallothionein [414]. Although studies from one group have suggested that metallothionein induction can ameliorate cisplatin toxicity [590, 591, 705], this has not been a consistent finding [575, 808].

Brief exposure to heat or a variety of other nonlethal stresses induces production of a group of closely related proteins, usually termed *heat shock proteins*, in virtually all species. Concomitantly there is a generalized inhibition of synthesis of other proteins. The response is associated with enhanced tolerance to a second insult [476]. Although attention has focused on the most prominent heat shock proteins falling into three size classes—70, 83 to 90, and 20 to 30 kd—heat shock proteins number in the dozens, and even the major size classes consist of families of proteins [167, 476, 799]. Additionally, a related and interacting, but distinct stress response is seen during conditions of glucose deprivation [799]. Despite much work, full functional characterization of even the major heat shock proteins remains incomplete. However, most data indicate involvement of heat shock proteins in the regulation of cell protein metabolism to control degradation of damaged proteins [476, 666] and to regulate synthesis of new proteins [167, 679] during adverse conditions or recovery. Interactions with the cytoskeleton [436, 476] and regulation by Ca^{++}-calmodulin [436] have been reported, thus further linking these proteins to structures and cellular mediators involved in the injury process.

Ischemia, anoxia, ATP-depleting metabolic inhibitors, and heavy metals have been shown to induce the heat shock response in various cell types [130, 184, 472, 476, 749, 799]. Induction of the heat shock response with hyperthermia has been reported to ameliorate subsequent ischemic injury in the heart [230]. As yet, there is no published information on the role of the heat shock response of the kidney during nephrotoxic renal injury, but it could play a very important role, especially during subacutely evolving damage.

Enhanced resistance by the kidney to second insults has been found after heavy-metal– and glycerol-induced nephrotoxicity [341, 495, 506, 886]. Prolonged treatment of rats with high doses of gentamicin results in an "acquired" insensitivity without apparent substantial decreases in cortical concentration of the antibiotic [220]. Interpretation of the available data on altered renal susceptibility to second insults is complex because of the potential for altered hemodynamics and solute delivery patterns [341]. Additionally, at the cellular level, recovering cells with decreased surface area and transport capacity [384] as well as different patterns of metabolism (e.g., enhanced glycolysis [28, 814]) may have altered susceptibility on the basis of these effects, rather than due to heat shock protein–related phenomena. As previously detailed, induction of metallothionein will contribute to increased resistance to heavy metals.

References

1. Abdel-Latif, A. A., and Smith, J. P. Effects of DL-propranolol on the synthesis of glycerolipids by rabbit iris muscle. *Biochem. Pharmacol.* 25: 1697, 1976.
2. Abraham, R., and Hendy, R. Effects of chronic chloroquine treatment of lysosomes of rat liver cells. *Exp. Mol. Pathol.* 12: 148, 1970.
3. Abraham, R., Hendy, R., and Grasso, P. Formation of myeloid bodies in rat liver lysosomes after chloroquine administration. *Exp. Mol. Pathol.* 9: 212, 1968.
4. Adams, R. J., and Pollard, T. D. Binding of myosin I to membrane lipids. *Nature* 340: 565, 1989.
5. Adelstein, R. S., and Eisenberg, E. Regulation and kinetics of the actin-myosin-ATP interaction. *Annu. Rev. Biochem.* 49: 921, 1980.
6. Aleo, M. D., Rankin, G. O., Cross, T. J., and Schnellmann, R. G. Toxicity of N-(3,5-dichlorophenyl)-succinimide and metabolites to rat renal proximal tubules and mitochondria. *Chem. Biol. Interact.* 78: 109, 1991.
7. Aleo, M. D., Wyatt, R. D., and Schnellmann, R. G. Mitochondrial dysfunction is an early event in ochratoxin A but not oosporein toxicity to rat renal proximal tubules. *Toxicol. Appl. Pharmacol.* 107: 73, 1991.
8. Aleo, M. D., Wyatt, R. D., and Schnellmann, R. G. The role of altered mitochondrial function in citrinin-induced toxicity to rat renal proximal tubule suspensions. *Toxicol. Appl. Pharmacol.* 109: 155, 1991.
9. Allan, D., and Michell, R. H. Enhanced synthesis de novo of phosphatidylinositol in lymphocytes treated with cationic amphiphilic drugs. *Biochem. J.* 148: 471, 1975.
10. Allbritton, N. L., Verret, C. R., Wolley, R. C., and Eisen, H. N. Calcium ion concentrations and DNA fragmentation in target cell destruction by murine cloned cytotoxic T lymphocytes. *J. Exp. Med.* 167: 514, 1988.
11. Alles, A., Alley, K., Barrett, J. C., et al. Apoptosis: A general comment. *FASEB J.* 5: 2127, 1991.
12. Allison, A. C. Lysosomes and Cancer. In J. T. Dingle and H. B. Fell (eds.), *Lysosomes in Biology and Pathology*, Vol. 2. Amsterdam: North Holland Publishing Co., 1969. P. 178.
13. Allison, A. C., Harrington, J. S., and Berbeck, M. An examination of the cytotoxic effects of silica on macrophages. *J. Exp. Med.* 124: 141, 1966.
14. Altschuld, R. A., Hostetler, J. R., and Brierley, G. P. Response of isolated heart cells to hypoxia, reoxygenation and acidosis. *Circ. Res.* 49: 307, 1981.
15. Ammann, H., Noel, J., Boulanger, Y., and Vinay, P. Relationship between intracellular ATP and the sodium pump activity in dog renal tubules. *Can. J. Physiol. Pharmacol.* 68: 57, 1989.
16. Anbar, M., and Neta, P. A compilation of specific bimolecular rate constants for the reactions of hydrated electrons, hydrogen atoms, and hydroxyl radicals with inorganic and organic compounds in aqueous solution. *Int. J. Appl. Radiat. Isot.* 18: 495, 1967.
17. Anders, M. W., Elfarra, A. A., and Lash, L. H. Cellular effects of reactive intermediates: Nephrotoxicity of S-conjugates of amino acids. *Arch. Toxicol.* 60: 103, 1987.
18. Anders, M. W., Lash, L., Dekant, W., Elfarra, A. A., and Dohn, D. R. Biosynthesis and biotransformation of glutathione S-conjugates to toxic metabolites. *Crit. Rev. Toxicol.* 18: 311, 1988.
19. Anderson, M. E., Naganuma, A., and Meister, A. Protection against cisplatin toxicity by administration of glutathione ester. *FASEB J.* 4: 3251, 1990.
20. Anderson, M. E., Powrie, F., Puri, R. N., and Meister, A. Glutathione monoethyl ester: Preparation, uptake by tissues, and conversion to glutathione. *Arch. Biochem. Biophys.* 239: 538, 1985.
21. Anderson, P. M., and Schultze, M. O. Cleavage of S-(1,2-dichlorovinyl)-L-cysteine by an enzyme of bovine origin. *Arch. Biochem. Biophys.* 111: 593, 1965.
22. Angielski, S., Pempkowiak, L., Gmaj, P., Hoppe, A., and Nowicka, C. The Effect of Maleate and Lithium on Renal Function and Metabolism. In U. Schmidt and U. C. Dubach (eds.), *Renal Metabolism in Relation to Renal Function*. Bern: Huber, 1976. P. 142.
23. Arends, M. J., Morris, R. G., and Wyllie, A. H. Apoptosis. The role of the endonuclease. *Am. J. Pathol.* 136: 593, 1990.
24. Arnold, P. E., Lumlertgul, D., Burke, T. J., and Schrier, R. W. In vitro versus in vivo mitochondrial calcium loading in ischemic acute renal failure. *Am. J. Physiol.* 248: F845, 1985.
25. Arnold, P. E., VanPutten, V. J., Lumlertgul, D., Burke, T. J., and Schrier, R. W. Adenine nucleotide metabolism and mitochondrial Ca^{2+} transport following renal ischemia. *Am. J. Physiol.* 250: F357, 1986.
26. Arrick, B. A., Nathan, C. F., Griffith, O. W., and Cohn, Z. A. Glutathione depletion sensitizes tumor cells to oxidative cytolysis. *J. Biol. Chem.* 257: 1231, 1982.
27. Aruoma, O. I., Halliwell, B., and Dizdaroglu, M. Iron ion-dependent modification of bases in DNA by the superoxide radical-generating system hypoxanthine/xanthine oxidase. *J. Biol. Chem.* 264: 13024, 1989.
28. Ash, S. R., and Cuppage, F. E. Shift toward anaerobic glycolysis in the regenerating rat kidney. *Am. J. Pathol.* 60: 385, 1970.
29. Au, S., Weiner, N. D., and Schacht, J. Aminoglycoside antibiotics preferentially increase permeability in phosphoinositide-containing membranes: A study with carboxyfluorescein in liposomes. *Biochim. Biophys. Acta* 902: 80, 1987.
30. Aubert-Tulkens, G. A., VanHoff, T., and Tulkens, P. Gentamicin-induced lysosomal phospholipidosis in cultured rat fibroblasts. *Lab. Invest.* 40: 481, 1979.
31. Auclair, P., Tardif, D., Beauchamp, D., Gourde, P., and Bergeron, M. G. Prolonged endotoxemia enhances the renal injuries induced by gentamicin in rats. *Antimicrob. Agents Chemother.* 34: 889, 1990.
32. Aust, S. D., Morehouse, L. A., and Thomas, C. E. Role of metals in oxygen radical reactions. *J Free Radic. Biol. Med.* 1: 3, 1985.
33. Aynedjian, H. S., Nguyen, D., Lee, H. Y., Sablay, L. B., and Bank, N. Effects of dietary electrolyte supplementation on gentamicin nephrotoxicity. *Am. J. Med. Sci.* 295: 444, 1988.
34. Babior, B. M. Oxygen-dependent microbial killing by phagocytes. *N. Engl. J. Med.* 298: 659, 1978.
35. Baccino, F. M., Cantino, D., and Zuretti, M. F. Studies on the hepatotoxicity of *Amanita phalloides* in the rat. *Exp. Mol. Pathol.* 24: 159, 1976.
36. Bagdade, J. D., Parker, F. Ways, P. O., Morgan, T. E., Lagunoff, D., and Eidelman, S. Fabry's disease. *Lab. Invest.* 18: 681, 1968.
37. Bailey, R. R., Natale, R., Turnbull, I., and Linton, A. L. Protective effect of furosemide in acute tubular necrosis and acute renal failure. *Clin. Sci. Mol. Med.* 45: 1, 1973.
38. Bailie, M. B., Smith, J. H., Newton, J. F., and Hook, J. B. Mechanism of chloroform nephrotoxicity: IV. Phenobarbital potentiation of in vitro chloroform metabo-

lism and toxicity in rabbit kidneys. *Toxicol. Appl. Pharmacol.* 74: 285, 1984.

39. Baines, A. D., Shaikh, N., and Ho, P. Mechanisms of perfused kidney cytoprotection by alanine and glycine. *Am. J. Physiol.* 259: F80, 1990.
40. Baker, M. S., and Gebicki, J. M. The effect of pH on the conversion of superoxide to hydroxyl free radicals. *Arch. Biochem. Biophys.* 234: 258, 1984.
41. Balaban, R. S., Soltoff, S. P., Storey, J. M., and Mandel, L. J. Improved renal cortical tubule suspension: Spectrophotometric study of O_2 delivery. *Am. J. Physiol.* 238: F50, 1980.
42. Baldew, G. S., McVie, J. G., van der Valk, M. A., Los, G., de Goeij, J. J., and Vermeulen, N. P. Selective reduction of cis-diamminedichloroplatinum(II) nephrotoxicity by ebselen. *Cancer Res.* 50: 7031, 1990.
43. Bannai, S., and Tateishi, N. Role of membrane transport in metabolism and function of glutathione in mammals. *J. Membr. Biol.* 89: 1, 1986.
44. Barnes, J. L., McDowell, E. M., McNeil, J. S., Flamenbaum, W., and Trump, B. F. Studies on the pathophysiology of acute renal failure. IV. Protective effect of dithiothreitol following administration of mercuric chloride in the rat. *Virchows Arch. B [Cell Pathol.]* 32: 201, 1980.
45. Barnes, J. L., McDowell, E. M., McNeil, J. S., Flamenbaum, W., and Trump, B. F. Studies on the pathophysiology of acute renal failure. V. Effect of chronic saline loading on the progression of proximal tubular injury and functional impairment following administration of mercuric chloride in the rat. *Virchows Arch. B [Cell Pathol.]* 32: 233, 1980.
46. Barrett, A. J. Lysosomal Enzymes. In J. T. Dingle (ed.), *Lysosomes. A Laboratory Handbook.* Amsterdam: North Holland Publishing Co., 1972. P. 46.
47. Barry, M. A., Behnke, C. A., and Eastman, A. Activation of programmed cell death (apoptosis) by cisplatin, other anticancer drugs, toxins and hyperthermia. *Biochem. Pharmacol.* 40: 2353, 1990.
48. Bascetta, E., Gunstone, F. D., and Walton, J. C. Electron spin resonance study of the role of vitamin E and vitamin C in the inhibition of fatty acid oxidation in a model membrane. *Chem. Phys. Lipids* 33: 207, 1983.
49. Basinger, M. A., Jones, M. M., and Holscher, M. A. L-Methionine antagonism of cis-platinum nephrotoxicity. *Toxicol. Appl. Pharmacol.* 103: 1, 1990.
50. Bast, A., and Haenen, G. R. M. M. Interplay between lipoic acid and glutathione in the protection against microsomal lipid peroxidation. *Biochim. Biophys. Acta* 963: 558, 1988.
51. Beales, D., Hue, D. P., and McLean, A. E. M. Lipid peroxidation, protein synthesis, and protection by calcium EDTA in paracetamol injury to isolated hepatocytes. *Biochem. Pharmacol.* 34: 19, 1985.
52. Beatrice, M. C., Palmer, J. W., and Pfeiffer, D. R. The relationship between mitochondrial membrane permeability, membrane potential, and the retention of Ca^{2+} by mitochondria. *J. Biol. Chem.* 255: 8663, 1980.
53. Beatrice, M. C., Stiers, D. L., and Pfeiffer, D. R. Increased permeability of mitochondria during Ca^{2+} release induced by t-butyl hydroperoxide or oxalacetate. *J. Biol. Chem.* 257: 7161, 1982.
54. Beatrice, M. C., Stiers, D. L., and Pfeiffer, D. R. The role of glutathione in the retention of Ca^{2+} by liver mitochondria. *J. Biol. Chem.* 259: 1279, 1984.
55. Beauchamp, D., Laurent, G., Maldague, P., Abid, S., Kishore, B. K., and Tulkens, P. M. Protection against gentamicin-induced early renal alterations (phospholipidosis and increased DNA synthesis) by coadministration of poly-L-aspartic acid. *J. Pharmacol. Exp. Ther.* 255: 858, 1990.
56. Beauchamp, D., Laurent, G., Maldague, P., and Tulkens, P. M. Reduction of gentamicin nephrotoxicity by the concomitant administration of poly-l-aspartic acid and poly-l-asparagine in rats. *Arch. Toxicol. Suppl.* 9: 306, 1986.
57. Becker, G. L., Fiskum, G., and Lehninger, A. L. Regulation of free calcium by liver mitochondria and endoplasmic reticulum. *J. Biol. Chem.* 255: 9009, 1980.
58. Belles, B., Hescheler, J., Trautwein, W., Blomgren, K., and Karlsson, J. O. A possible physiological role of the Ca-dependent protease calpain and its inhibitor calpastatin on the Ca current in guinea pig myocytes. *Pflugers Arch.* 412: 554, 1988.
59. Bellomo, G., Jewell, S. A., Thor, H., and Orrenius, S. Regulation of intracellular calcium compartmentation: Studies with isolated hepatocytes and t-butyl hydroperoxide. *Proc. Natl. Acad. Sci. U.S.A.* 79: 6842, 1982.
60. Bellomo, G., Thor, H., and Orrenius, S. Modulation of cellular glutathione and protein thial status during quinone metabolism. *Methods Enzymol.* 181: 627, 1990.
61. Bendirdjian, J. P., Foucher, B., and Fillastre, J. P. Influence des aminoglycosides sur le metabolisme respiratoire des mitochondries isolees de foie et de rein de rat. In J. P. Fillastre (ed.), *Nephrotoxicity: Interaction of Drugs with Membrane Systems Mitochondria-Lysosomes.* New York: Masson, 1978. P. 315.
62. Bendirdjian, J. P., Prime, D. J., Browning, M. C., Hsu, C. Y., and Tune, B. M. Additive nephrotoxicity of cephalosporins and aminoglycosides in the rabbit. *J. Pharmacol. Exp. Ther.* 218: 681, 1981.
63. Benedetti, A., Casini, A. F., Ferrali, M., and Comporti, M. Extraction and partial characterization of dialysable products originating from the peroxidation of liver microsomal lipids and inhibiting microsomal glucose 6-phosphatase activity. *Biochem. Pharmacol.* 28: 2909, 1979.
64. Benedetti, A., Fulceri, R., Ferrali, M., Ciccoli, L., Esterbauer, H., and Comporti, M. Detection of carbonyl functions in phospholipids of liver microsomes in CCl_4- and $BrCCl_3$-poisoned rats. *Biochim. Biophys. Acta* 712: 628, 1982.
65. Bennett, W. M., Elliott, W. C., Houghton, D. C., Gilbert, D. N., DeFehr, J., and McCarron, D. A. Reduction of experimental gentamicin nephrotoxicity in rats by dietary calcium loading. *Antimicrob. Agents Chemother.* 22: 508, 1982.
66. Bennett, W. M., Houghton, D. C., and Buss, W. C. Cyclosporine-induced renal dysfunction: Correlation between cellular events and whole kidney function. *J. Am. Soc. Nephrol.* 1: 1212, 1991.
67. Bennett, W. M., Mela-Riker, L. M., Houghton, D. C., Gilbert, D. N., and Buss, W. C. Microsomal protein synthesis inhibition: An early manifestation of gentamicin nephrotoxicity. *Am. J. Physiol.* 255: F265, 1988.
68. Bennett, W. M., Plamp, C. E., Elliott, W. C., Parker, R. A., and Porter, G. A. Effect of basic amino acids and aminoglycosides on ^{3}H-gentamicin uptake in cortical slices of rat and human kidney. *J. Lab. Clin. Med.* 99: 156, 1982.
69. Bennett, W. M., Plamp, C. E., Gilbert, D. N., Parker, R. A., and Porter, G. A. The influence of dosage regimen on experimental gentamicin nephrotoxicity: Dissociation of peak serum levels from renal failure. *J. Infect. Dis.* 140: 576, 1979.

70. Bennett, W. M., Pulliam, J. P., Porter, G. A., and Houghton, D. C. Modification of experimental gentamicin nephrotoxicity by selective parathyroidectomy. *Am. J. Physiol.* 249: F832, 1985.
71. Bernard, A., Viau, C., Ouled, A., Tulkens, P., and Lauwerys, R. Effects of gentamicin on the renal uptake of endogenous and exogenous protein in conscious rats. *Toxicol. Appl. Pharmacol.* 84: 431, 1986.
72. Berndt, W. O., Baggett, J. M., Blacker, A., and Houser, M. Renal glutathione and mercury uptake by kidney. *Fundam. Appl. Toxicol.* 5: 832, 1985.
73. Berridge, M. J., and Taylor, C. W. Inositol triphosphate and calcium signaling. *Cold Spring Harbor Symp. Quant. Biol.* 53: 927, 1988.
74. Berry, J. P., Hourdry, J., Galle, P., and Lagrue, G. Chromium concentration by proximal renal tubule cells: An ultrastructural, microanalytical and cytochemical study. *J. Histochem. Cytochem.* 26: 651, 1978.
75. Berry, J. P., and Lespinats, G. Cis DDP in combination with selenium and sulfur. Subcellular effect in kidney cells. Electron microprobe study. *J. Submicrosc. Cytol. Pathol.* 20: 59, 1988.
76. Bershadsky, A. D., and Gelfand, V. I. ATP-dependent regulation of cytoplasmic microtubule disassembly. *Proc. Natl. Acad. Sci. U.S.A.* 78: 3610, 1981.
77. Bershadsky, A. D., and Gelfand, V. I. Role of ATP in the regulation of stability of cytoskeletal structures. *Cell Biol. Int. Rep.* 7: 173, 1983.
78. Bershadsky, A. D., Gelfand, V. I., Svitkina, T. M., and Tint, I. S. Destruction of microfilament bundles in mouse embryo fibroblasts treated with inhibitors of energy metabolism. *Exp. Cell Res.* 127: 421, 1980.
79. Beuter, W., Cojocel, C., Muller, W., Donaubauer, H. H., and Mayer, D. Peroxidative damage and nephrotoxicity of dichlorovinylcysteine in mice. *J. Appl. Toxicol.* 9: 181, 1989.
80. Bhattacharya, R. K., and Schultze, M. O. Enzymes from bovine and turkey kidneys which cleave S-(1,2-dichlorovinyl)-L-cysteine. *Comp. Biochem. Physiol.* 22: 723, 1967.
81. Bia, M. J., and Tyler, K. Evidence that calcium channel blockade prevents cyclosporine-induced exacerbation of renal ischemic injury. *Transplantation* 51: 293, 1991.
82. Bidani, A., Churchill, P., and Fleischman, L. Sodium chloride induced protection in nephrotoxic acute renal failure: Independence from renin. *Kidney Int.* 16: 481, 1979.
83. Bing, O. H. L., Brooks, W. W., and Messer, J. V. Heart muscle viability following hypoxia: Protective effect of acidosis. *Science* 180: 1297, 1973.
84. Bjelland, S., Wallevik, K., Kroll, J., Dixon, J. E., Morin, J. E., Freedman, R. B., Lambert, N., Varandani, P. T., and Nafz, M. A. Immunological identity between bovine preparations of thiol:protein-disulphide oxidoreductase, glutathione-insulin transhydrogenase and protein-disulphide isomerase. *Biochim. Biophys. Acta* 747: 197, 1983.
85. Blachley, J. D., and Hill, J. B. Renal and electrolyte disturbances associated with cisplatin. *Ann. Intern. Med.* 95: 628, 1981.
86. Blohm, T. R. Drug-induced lysosomal lipidosis: Biochemical interpretations. *Pharmacol. Rev.* 30: 593, 1978.
87. Blomgren, K., Nilsson, E., and Karlsson, J. O. Calpain and calpastatin levels in different organs of the rabbit. *Comp. Biochem. Physiol.* [*B*] 93: 403, 1989.
88. Bompart, G. Cisplatin-induced changes in cytochrome P-450, lipid peroxidation and drug-metabolizing enzyme activities in rat kidney cortex. *Toxicol. Lett.* 48: 193, 1989.
89. Bompart, G. J., Prevot, D. S., and Bascands, J. L. Rapid automated analysis of glutathione reductase, peroxidase, and S-transferase activity: Application to cisplatin-induced toxicity. *Clin. Biochem.* 23: 501, 1990.
90. Bond, J. S., and Butler, P. E. Intracellular proteases. *Annu. Rev. Biochem.* 56: 333, 1987.
91. Bonventre, J. V., and Cheung, J. Y. Effects of metabolic acidosis on viability of cells exposed to anoxia. *Am. J. Physiol.* 249: C149, 1985.
92. Boogaard, P. J., Commandeur, J. N., Mulder, G. J., Vermeulen, N. P., and Nagelkerke, J. F. Toxicity of the cysteine-S-conjugates and mercapturic acids of four structurally related difluoroethylenes in isolated proximal tubular cells from rat kidney. Uptake of the conjugates and activation to toxic metabolites. *Biochem. Pharmacol.* 38: 3731, 1989.
93. Borch, R. F., Katz, J. C., Lieder, P. H., and Pleasants, M. E. Effect of diethyldithiocarbamate rescue on tumor response to *cis*-platinum in a rat model. *Proc. Natl. Acad. Sci. U.S.A.* 77: 5441, 1980.
94. Borch, R. F., and Pleasants, M. E. Inhibition of *cis*-platinum nephrotoxicity by diethyldithiocarbamate rescue in a rat model. *Proc. Natl. Acad. Sci. U.S.A.* 76: 6611, 1979.
95. Boveris, A., and Chance, B. The mitochondrial generation of hydrogen peroxide. General properties and effect of hyperbaric oxygen. *Biochem. J.* 134: 707, 1973.
96. Bowley, M., Cooling, J., Burditt, S. L., and Brindley, D. N. The effects of amphiphilic cationic drugs and inorganic cations on the activity of phosphatidate phosphohydrolase. *Biochem. J.* 165: 447, 1977.
97. Boyd, J. A., and Eling, T. E. Prostaglandin endoperoxide synthetase-dependent cooxidation of acetaminophen to intermediates which covalently bind in vitro to rabbit renal medullary microsomes. *J. Pharmacol. Exp. Ther.* 219: 659, 1981.
98. Brady, H. R., Kone, B. C., Brenner, R. M., and Gullans, S. R. Early effects of uranyl nitrate on respiration and K^+ transport in rabbit proximal tubule. *Kidney Int.* 36: 27, 1989.
99. Brady, H. R., Kone, B. C., Stromski, M. E., Zeidel, M. L., Giebisch, G., and Gullans, S. R. Mitochondrial injury: An early event in cisplatin toxicity to renal proximal tubules. *Am. J. Physiol. Renal Fluid Electrolyte Physiol.* 258: F1181, 1990.
100. Brady, H. R., Zeidel, M. L., Kone, B. C., Giebisch, G., and Gullans, S. R. Cisplatin (CP) inhibits K^+ transport and oxygen consumption (QO_2) in rabbit inner medullary collecting duct (IMCD) cells. *FASEB J.* 3: A326, 1989. (Abstract.)
101. Brasseur, R., Laurent, G., Ruysschaert, J. M., and Tulkens, P. Interactions of aminoglycoside antibiotics with negatively charged lipid layers. Biochemical and conformational studies. *Biochem. Pharmacol.* 33: 629, 1984.
102. Brazy, P. C., Balaban, R. S., Gullans, S. R., Mandel, L. J., and Dennis, V. W. Inhibition of renal metabolism. Relative effects of arsenate on sodium, phosphate and glucose transport by the rabbit proximal tubule. *J. Clin. Invest.* 66: 1211, 1980.
103. Brecher, P. The interactions of long-chain acyl CoA with membranes. *Mol. Cell. Biochem.* 57: 3, 1983.
104. Bregman, C. L., and Williams, P. D. Comparative nephrotoxicity of carboplatin and cisplatin in combination with tobramycin. *Cancer Chemother. Pharmacol.* 18: 117, 1986.
105. Brehe, J. E., Chan, A. W. K., Alvey, T. R., and Burch, H. B. Effect of methionine sulfoximine on glutathione

and amino acid levels in the nephron. *Am. J. Physiol.* 231: 1536, 1976.
106. Brenner, R. M., Kone, B. C., and Gullans, S. R. Increased plasma membrane K^+ permeability precedes mitochondrial injury by $HgCl_2$ in rabbit proximal tubule (PT) segments. *Kidney Int.* 33: 354, 1988. (Abstract.)
107. Brezis, M., Rosen, S., Silva, P., and Epstein, F. H. Renal ischemia: A new perspective. *Kidney Int.* 26: 375, 1984.
108. Brezis, M., Rosen, S., Silva, P., and Epstein, F. H. Selective vulnerability of the medullary thick ascending limb to anoxia in the isolated perfused kidney. *J. Clin. Invest.* 73: 182, 1984.
109. Brezis, M., Rosen, S., Silva, P., Spokes, K., and Epstein, F. H. Polyene toxicity in renal medulla: Injury mediated by transport activity. *Science* 224: 66, 1984.
110. Brezis, M., Rosen, S., Spokes, K., Silva, P., and Epstein, F. H. Transport-dependent anoxic cell injury in the isolated perfused rat kidney. *Am. J. Pathol.* 116: 327, 1984.
111. Brezis, M., Rosen, S., Spokes, K., Silva, P., and Epstein, F. H. Substrates induce hypoxic injury to medullary thick limbs of isolated rat kidneys. *Am. J. Physiol.* 251: F710, 1986.
112. Brezis, M., Shanley, P., Silva, P., Spokes, K., Lear, S., Epstein, F. H., and Rosen, S. Disparate mechanisms for hypoxic cell injury in different nephron segments. Studies in the isolated perfused rat kidney. *J. Clin. Invest.* 76: 1796, 1985.
113. Brierley, G. P., Jurkowitz, M., and Jung, D. W. Osmotic swelling of heart mitochondria in acetate and chloride salts. *Arch. Biochem. Biophys.* 190: 181, 1978.
114. Brierley, G. P., Scott, K. M., and Jurkowitz, M. Ion transport by heart mitochondria. XXI. Differential effects of mercurial reagents on adenosine triphosphatase activity and on adenosine triphosphate-dependent swelling and contraction. *J. Biol. Chem.* 246: 2241, 1971.
115. Brindley, D. N., Allan, D., and Michell, R. H. The redirection of glyceride and phospholipid synthesis by drugs including chlorpromazine, fenfluramine, imipramine, mepyramine and local anaesthetics. *J. Pharm. Pharmacol.* 27: 462, 1975.
116. Brindley, D. N., and Bowley, M. Drugs affecting the synthesis of glycerides and phospholipids in rat liver. *Biochem. J.* 148: 461, 1975.
117. Broekemeier, K. M., Dempsey, M. E., and Pfeiffer, D. R. Cyclosporin A is a potent inhibitor of the inner membrane permeability transition in liver mitochondria. *J. Biol. Chem.* 264: 7826, 1989.
118. Broekemeier, K. M., Schmid, P. C., Schmid, H. H. O., and Pfeiffer, D. R. Effects of phospholipase A_2 inhibitors on ruthenium red-induced Ca^{2+} release from mitochondria. *J. Biol. Chem.* 260: 105, 1985.
119. Brown, D. M., Langley, P. F., Smith, D., and Taylor, D. C. Metabolism of chloroform. I. The metabolism of ^{14}C chloroform by different species. *Xenobiotica* 4: 151, 1974.
120. Browning, M. C., Hsu, C. Y., Wang, P. L., and Tune, B. M. Interaction of ischemic and antibiotic-induced injury in the rabbit kidney. *J. Infect. Dis.* 147: 341, 1983.
121. Buck, C. A., Shea, E., Duggan, K., and Horwitz, A. F. Integrin (the CSAT antigen): Functionality requires oligomeric integrity. *J. Cell Biol.* 103: 2421, 1986.
122. Buhl, M. R. Purine metabolism in ischaemic kidney tissue. *Dan. Med. Bull.* 29: 1, 1982.
123. Burk, R. F. Glutathione-dependent protection by rat liver microsomal protein against lipid peroxidation. *Biochim. Biophys. Acta* 757: 21, 1983.
124. Burk, R. F., and Lane, J. M. Ethane production and liver necrosis in rats after administration of drugs and other chemicals. *Toxicol. Appl. Pharmacol.* 50: 467, 1979.
125. Burke, M. D., Prough, R. A., and Mayer, R. T. Characteristics of a microsomal cytochrome P-448 mediated reaction: Ethoxyresorufin O-deethylation. *Drug Metab. Dispos.* 5: 1, 1977.
126. Burnier, M., Van Putten, V. J., Schieppati, A., and Schrier, R. W. Effect of extracellular acidosis on ^{45}Ca uptake in isolated hypoxic proximal tubules. *Am. J. Physiol.* 254: C839, 1988.
127. Burt, J. M. Block of intercellular communication: Interaction of intracellular H^+ and Ca^{2+}. *Am. J. Physiol.* 253: C607, 1987.
128. Busa, W. B., and Nuccitelli, R. Metabolic regulation via intracellular pH. *Am. J. Physiol.* 246: R409, 1984.
129. Buss, W. C., Stepanek, J., and Bennett, W. M. A new proposal for the mechanism of cyclosporine A nephrotoxicity. Inhibition of renal microsomal protein chain elongation following *in vivo* cyclosporine A. *Biochem. Pharmacol.* 38: 4085, 1989.
130. Cairo, G., Bardella, L., Schiaffonati, L., and Bernelli-Zazzera, A. Synthesis of heat shock proteins in rat liver after ischemia and hyperthermia. *Hepatology* 5: 357, 1985.
131. Calderon, P., Furnelle, J., and Cristophe, J. Phosphatidylinositol turnover and calcium movement in the rat pancreas. *Am. J. Physiol.* 238: G247, 1980.
132. Cantoni, O., Nelwyn, C. T., Swann, A., Drath, D. B., and Costa, M. Mechanism of $HgCl_2$ cytotoxicity in cultured mammalian cells. *Mol. Pharmacol.* 260: 360, 1984.
133. Capasso, G., Anastasio, P., Giordano, D., Albarano, L., and DeSanto, N. G. Beneficial effects of atrial natriuretic factor on cisplatin-induced acute renal failure in the rat. *Am. J. Nephrol.* 7: 228, 1987.
134. Capasso, G., Rosati, C., Ciani, F., Giordano, D. R., Russo, F., and DeSanto, N. G. The beneficial effect of atrial natriuretic peptide on cyclosporine nephrotoxicity. *Am. J. Hypertens.* 3: 204, 1990.
135. Carafoli, E. Intracellular calcium homeostasis. *Annu. Rev. Biochem.* 56: 395, 1987.
136. Carafoli, E., Tiozzo, R., Pasquali-Ronchetti, I., and Laschi, R. A study of Ca^{2+} metabolism in kidney mitochondria during acute uranium intoxication. *Lab. Invest.* 25: 516, 1971.
137. Carlier, M. B., Laurent, G., Claes, P. J., Vanderhaeghe, H. J., and Tulkens, P. M. Inhibition of lysosomal phospholipases by aminoglycoside antibiotics: In vitro comparative studies. *Antimicrob. Agents Chemother.* 23: 440, 1983.
138. Carpenter, H. M., and Mudge, G. H. Acetaminophen nephrotoxicity: Studies on renal acetylation and deacetylation. *J. Pharmacol. Exp. Ther.* 218: 161, 1981.
139. Casini, A. F., Pompella, A., and Comporti, M. Liver glutathione depletion induced by bromobenzene, iodobenzene, and diethylmaleate poisoning and its relation to lipid peroxidation and necrosis. *Am. J. Pathol.* 118: 225, 1985.
140. Cederbaum, A. I., and Dicker, E. Inhibition of microsomal oxidation of alcohols and of hydroxyl-radical-scavenging agents by the iron-chelating agent desferrioxamine. *Biochem. J.* 210: 107, 1983.
141. Chance, B., Nakase, Y., and Itshak, F. Membrane energization at subzero temperatures: Calcium uptake and oxonol-V responses. *Arch. Biochem. Biophys.* 198: 360, 1979.
142. Chance, B., Sies, H., and Boveris, A. Hydroperoxide

metabolism in mammalian organs. *Physiol. Rev.* 59: 527, 1979.
143. Chefurka, W. Oxidative phosphorylation in in vitro aged mitochondria. I. Factors controlling the loss of the dinitrophenol-stimulated adenosine triphosphatase activity and respiratory control in mouse liver mitochondria. *Biochemistry* 5: 3887, 1966.
144. Chefurka, W., and Dumas, T. Oxidative phosphorylation in in vitro aged mitochondria. II. Dinitrophenol-stimulated adenosine triphosphatase activity and fatty acid content of mouse liver mitochondria. *Biochemistry* 5: 3904, 1966.
145. Chen, Q., Jones, T. W., Brown, P. C., and Stevens, J. L. The mechanism of cysteine conjugate cytotoxicity in renal epithelial cells. Covalent binding leads to thiol depletion and lipid peroxidation. *J. Biol. Chem.* 265: 21603, 1990.
146. Cherian, M. G., and Goyer, R. A. Role of metallothioneins in disease. *Ann. Clin. Lab. Sci.* 8: 91, 1978.
147. Cherian, M. G., Goyer, R. A., and Delaquerriere-Richardson, L. Cadmium-metallothionein-induced nephropathy. *Toxicol. Appl. Pharmacol.* 38: 399, 1976.
148. Cheung, J. Y., Bonventre, J. V., Malis, C. D., and Leaf, A. Calcium and ischemic injury. *N. Engl. J. Med.* 314: 1670, 1986.
149. Chien, K. R., Abrams, J., Serroni, A., Martin, J. T., and Farber, J. L. Accelerated phospholipid degradation and associated membrane dysfunction in irreversible, ischemic liver cell injury. *J. Biol. Chem.* 253: 4809, 1978.
150. Child, K. J., Dodds, M. G., Cullis, P. R., de Krujiff, B., Hope, M. J., Nayar, R., and Schmid, S. L. Mechanism of urinary excretion of cephaloridine and its effects on renal function in animals. *Br. J. Pharmacol.* 26: 108, 1966.
151. Christensen, E. I., and Maunsbach, A. B. Proteinuria induced by sodium maleate in rats: Effects on ultrastructure and protein handling in renal proximal tubule. *Kidney Int.* 17: 771, 1980.
152. Chung, L., Kaloyanides, G., McDaniel, R., McLaughlin, A., and McLaughlin, S. Interaction of gentamicin and spermine with bilayer membranes containing negatively charged phospholipids. *Biochemistry* 24: 442, 1985.
153. Chvapil, M., Ryan, J. N., and Brada, Z. Effects of selected chelating agents and metals on the stability of liver lysosomes. *Biochem. Pharmacol.* 21: 1097, 1972.
154. Ciccoli, L., Casini, A. F., and Benedetti, A. Free radical damage produced by carbon tetrachloride in the lipids of various rat tissues. *Agents Actions* 8: 303, 1978.
155. Clarkson, T. W. The pharmacology of mercury compounds. *Annu. Rev. Pharmacol. Toxicol.* 12: 375, 1972.
156. Clejan, S., and Bittman, R. Rates of amphotericin B and filipin association with sterols. A study of changes in sterol structure and phospholipid composition of vesicles. *J. Biol. Chem.* 260: 2884, 1985.
157. Cockcroft, S., and Stutchfield, J. Effect of pertussis toxin and neomycin on G-protein-regulated polyphosphoinositide phosphodiesterase. A comparison between HL60 membranes and permeabilized HL60 cells. *Biochem. J.* 256: 343, 1988.
158. Cohen, R., Johnson, K., and Humes, H. D. Potentiation of aminoglycoside nephrotoxicity by vitamin-D-induced hypercalcemia. *Miner. Electrolyte Metab.* 14: 121, 1988.
159. Cohn, D. V., Bawdon, R., Newman, R. R., and Hamilton, J. W. Effect of calcium chelation on the ion content of liver mitochondria in carbon tetrachloride poisoned rats. *J. Biol. Chem.* 243: 1089, 1968.
160. Coimbra, T. M., Cieslinski, D. A., and Humes, H. D. Epidermal growth factor accelerates renal repair in mercuric chloride nephrotoxicity. *Am. J. Physiol.* 259: F438, 1990.
161. Cojocel, C., Beuter, W., Muller, W., and Mayer, D. Lipid peroxidation: A possible mechanism of trichloroethylene-induced nephrotoxicity. *Toxicology* 55: 131, 1989.
162. Cojocel, C., Dociu, N., Maita, K., Sleight, S. D., and Hook, J. B. Effects of aminoglycosides on glomerular permeability, tubular reabsorption, and intracellular catabolism of the cationic low-molecular-weight protein lysozyme. *Toxicol. Appl. Pharmacol.* 68: 96, 1983.
163. Cojocel, C., Hannemann, J., and Baumann, K. Cephaloridine-induced lipid peroxidation initiated by reactive oxygen species as a possible mechanism of cephaloridine nephrotoxicity. *Biochim. Biophys. Acta* 834: 402, 1985.
164. Cojocel, C., and Hook, J. B. Effects of acute exposures to gentamicin on renal handling of proteins. *Toxicology* 28: 347, 1983.
165. Cojocel, C., Laeschke, K. H., Inselmann, G., and Baumann, K. Inhibition of cephaloridine-induced lipid peroxidation. *Toxicology* 35: 295, 1985.
166. Cojocel, C., Smith, J. H., Maita, K., Sleight, S. D., and Hook, J. B. Renal protein degradation: A biochemical target of specific nephrotoxicants. *Fundam. Appl. Toxicol.* 3: 278, 1983.
167. Colbert, R. A., Hucul, J. A., Scorsone, K. A., and Young, D. A. Alpha subunit of eukaryotic translational initiation factor-2 is a heat-shock protein. *J. Biol. Chem.* 262: 16763, 1987.
168. Collier, V. U., Lietman, P. S., and Mitch, W. E. Evidence for luminal uptake of gentamicin in the perfused rat kidney. *J. Pharmacol. Exp. Ther.* 210: 247, 1979.
169. Comporti, M. Glutathione depleting agents and lipid peroxidation. *Chem. Phys. Lipids* 45: 143, 1987.
170. Cong, J., Goll, D. E., Peterson, A. M., and Kapprell, H.-P. The role of autolysis in activity of the Ca^{2+}-dependent proteinases (μ-calpain and m-calpain). *J. Biol. Chem.* 264: 10096, 1989.
171. Corwin, L. M. Studies on peroxidation in vitamin E-deficient rat liver homogenates. *Arch. Biochem. Biophys.* 97: 51, 1962.
172. Coudrier, E., Kerjaschki, D., and Louvard, D. Cytoskeleton organization and submembranous interactions in intestinal and renal brush borders. *Kidney Int.* 34: 309, 1988.
173. Cozzaglio, L., Doci, R., Colella, G., Zunino, F., Casciarri, G., Gennari, L., and Colla, G. A feasibility study of high-dose cisplatin and 5-fluorouracil with glutathione protection in the treatment of advanced colorectal cancer [published erratum appears in *Tumori* 77: 93, 1991]. *Tumori* 76: 590, 1990.
174. Cronin, R., Inman, L., Eche, T., Southern, P., and Griggs, M. Effect of thyroid hormone on gentamicin accumulation in rat proximal tubule lysosomes. *Am. J. Physiol.* 257: F86, 1989.
175. Cronin, R. E., Bulger, R., Southern, P., and Henrich, W. Natural history of aminoglycoside nephrotoxicity in the dog. *J. Lab. Clin. Med.* 95: 463, 1980.
176. Cronin, R. E., and Newman, J. A. Protective effect of thyroxine but not parathyroidectomy on gentamicin nephrotoxicity. *Am. J. Physiol.* 248: F332, 1985.
177. Cronin, R. E., Nix, K. L., Ferguson, E., Southern, P. M., and Henrich, W. L. Changes in renal cortex electrolyte content and Na-K-ATPase activity in early gentamicin nephrotoxicity. *Am. J. Physiol.* 242: F477, 1982.

178. Cronin, R. E., Splinter, K. L., Ferguson, E. R., and Henrich, W. L. Gentamicin nephrotoxicity: Protective effect of diabetes on cell injury. *Mineral Electrolyte Metab.* 9: 38, 1983.
179. Cullis, P. R., deKruijff, B., Hope, M. J., Nayar, R., and Schmid, S. L. Phospholipids and membrane transport. *Can. J. Biochem.* 58: 1091, 1980.
180. Cunningham, C., Burke, M. D., Wheatley, D. N., Thomson, A. W., Simpson, J. G., and Whiting, P. H. Amelioration of cyclosporin-induced nephrotoxicity in rats by induction of hepatic drug metabolism. *Biochem. Pharmacol.* 34: 573, 1985.
181. Cuppage, F. E., Chiga, M., Tate, A., and Cunningham, N. Cell cycle studies in the regenerating rat nephron following injury with mercuric chloride. Nucleic acid synthesis in the regenerating nephron following injury with mercuric chloride. *Lab. Invest.* 21: 449, 1969.
182. Cuppage, F. E., Cunningham, N., and Tate, A. Nucleic acid synthesis in the regenerating nephron following injury with mercuric chloride. *Lab. Invest.* 21: 449, 1969.
183. Cuppage, F. E., and Tate, A. Repair of the nephron following injury with mercuric chloride. *Am. J. Pathol.* 51: 405, 1967.
184. Currie, R. W. Effects of ischemia and perfusion temperature on the synthesis of stress-induced (heat shock) proteins in isolated and perfused rat hearts. *J. Mol. Cell. Cardiol.* 19: 795, 1987.
185. Cutler, R. G. Peroxidizing potential of tissues: Inverse correlation with longevity of mammalian species. *Proc. Natl. Acad. Sci. U.S.A.* 82: 4798, 1985.
186. Cvitkovic, E., Spaulding, J., Bethune, V., et al. Improvement of *cis*-dichlorodiammine-platinum therapeutic index in an animal model. *Cancer* 39: 1357, 1977.
187. Dahl, J. L., and Hokin, L. E. The sodium-potassium adenosine triphosphatase. *Annu. Rev. Biochem.* 44: 327, 1974.
188. Daley-Yates, P. T., and McBrien, D. C. The renal fractional clearance of platinum antitumour compounds in relation to nephrotoxicity. *Biochem. Pharmacol.* 34: 1423, 1985.
189. Daugaard, G., Holstein-Rathlou, N.-H., and Leyssac, P. P. Effect of cisplatin on proximal convoluted and straight segments of the rat kidney. *J. Pharmacol. Exp. Ther.* 244: 1081, 1988.
190. Davies, K. J. A. Intracellular proteolytic systems may function as secondary antioxidant defenses: An hypothesis. *J. Free Radic. Biol. Med.* 2: 155, 1986.
191. Davies, K. J. A., Lin, S. W., and Pacifici, R. E. Protein damage and degradation by oxygen radicals. IV. Degradation of denatured protein. *J. Biol. Chem.* 262: 9914, 1987.
192. Davis, J. A., and Weinberg, J. M. Effects of glycine and GSH on toxic maneuvers altering tubule cell plasma membrane cation permeability. *Clin. Res.* 36: 517A, 1988. (Abstract.)
193. DeBroe, M. E., Paulus, G. J., Verpooten, G. A., Roels, F., Buyssens, N., Wedeen, R., VanHoof, F., and Tulkens, P. M. Early effects of gentamicin, tobramycin, and amikacin on the human kidney. *Kidney Int.* 25: 643, 1984.
194. Dedon, P. C., and Borch, R. F. Characterization of the reactions of platinum antitumor agents with biologic and nonbiologic sulfur-containing nucleophiles. *Biochem. Pharmacol.* 36: 1955, 1987.
195. deDuve, C. The Lysosome in Retrospect. In J. T. Dingle and H. B. Fell (eds.), *Lysosomes in Biology and Pathology,* Vol. 1. New York: Wiley, 1969. P. 3.
196. deDuve, C., and Beaufay, H. Tissue fractionation studies. X. Influence of ischaemia on the state of some bound enzymes in rat liver. *Biochem. J.* 73: 610, 1959.
197. Dees, J. H., Masters, B. S. S., Moller-Berhard, U., and Johnson, E. F. Effect of 2,3,7,8-tetrachlorodibenzo-*p*-dioxin and phenobarbital on the occurrence and distribution of four cytochrome P-450 isozymes in rabbit kidney, lung and liver. *Cancer Res.* 42: 1423, 1982.
198. deGroot, H., and Noll, T. The crucial role of hypoxia in halothane-induced lipid peroxidation. *Biochem. Biophys. Res. Commun.* 119: 139, 1984.
199. Dekant, W., Vamvakas, S., and Anders, M. W. Bioactivation of hexachlorobutadiene by glutathione conjugation. *Food Chem. Toxicol.* 28: 285, 1990.
200. de la Iglesia, F., Feuer, G., McGuire, E. J., and Takada, A. Morphological and biochemical changes in the liver of various species in experimental phospholipidosis after diethylaminoethoxyhexestrol treatment. *Toxicol. Appl. Pharmacol.* 34: 28, 1975.
201. Dempsey, E. W., and Wislocki, G. B. The use of silver nitrate as a vital stain, and its distribution in several mammalian tissues as studied with the electron microscope. *J. Cell Biol.* 1: 111, 1955.
202. Denine, E. P., Harrison, S. D., and Peckham, J. C. Qualitative and quantitative toxicity of sublethal doses of methyl-CCNLU in BDFI mice. *Cancer Treat. Rep.* 61: 409, 1977.
203. deRougemont, D., Wunderlich, P. F., Torhorst, J., Keller, M., Peters-Hafeli, L., Thiel, G., and Brumer, F. P. $HgCl_2$ induced acute renal failure in the rat: Effect of water diuresis, saline loading and diuretic drugs. *J. Lab. Clin. Med.* 99: 646, 1982.
204. DeSimone, P. A., Yancy, R. S., Coupal, J. J., Butts, J. D., and Hoeschel, J. D. Effect of a forced diuresis on the distribution and excretion (via urine and bile) of ^{195m}Platinum *cis*-dichlorodiammine platinum (II). *Cancer Treat. Rep.* 63: 951, 1979.
205. Deter, R. L., and deDuve, C. Influence of glucagon, an inducer of cellular autophagy on some physiological properties of rat liver lysosomes. *J. Cell Biol.* 35: 437, 1967.
206. De Witt, L. M., Jones, T. W., and Moore, L. Stimulation of the renal endoplasmic reticulum calcium pump: A possible biomarker for platinate toxicity. *Toxicol. Appl. Pharmacol.* 92: 157, 1988.
207. Dianzani, M. U. Biochemical Effects of Saturated and Unsaturated Aldehydes. In D. C. H. McBrien and T. F. Slater (eds.), *Free Radicals, Lipid Peroxidation and Cancer.* London: Academic Press, 1982. P. 129.
208. DiBona, G. F. Light Microscopic Structural-Functional Correlations in Acute Renal Failure. In K. Solez and A. Whelton (eds.), *Acute Renal Failure—Correlations Between Morphology and Function.* New York and Basel: Marcel Dekker, 1984. P. 43.
209. DiBona, G. F., McDonald, F. D., Flamenbaum, W., Dammen, G. J., and Oken, D. E. Maintenance of renal function in salt loaded rats despite severe tubular necrosis induced by $HgCl_2$. *Nephron* 8: 205, 1971.
210. Dobyan, D. C., Levi, J., Jacobs, L. C., Kosek, J., and Weiner, M. W. Mechanisms of *cis*-platinum nephrotoxicity: II. Morphologic observations. *J. Pharmacol. Exp. Ther.* 213: 551, 1980.
211. Dobyan, D. C., Levi, J., Jacobs, C., and Kosek, J. A. U. W. Mechanism of cis-platinum nephrotoxicity: II. Morphologic observations. *J. Pharmacol. Exp. Ther.* 213: 551, 1980.

212. Doctor, R. B., and Mandel, L. J. Minimal role of xanthine oxidase and oxygen free radicals in rat renal tubular reoxygenation injury. *J. Am. Soc. Nephrol.* 1: 959, 1991.
213. Dodds, M. G., and Foord, R. D. Enhancement by potent diuretic of renal tubular necrosis induced by cephaloridine. *Br. J. Pharmacol.* 40: 227, 1970.
214. Donohoe, J. F., Venkatachalam, M. A., Bernard, D. B., and Levinsky, N. G. Tubular leakage and obstruction after renal ischemia: Structural-functional correlations. *Kidney Int.* 13: 208, 1978.
215. Douglas, J. B., and Healey, J. K. Nephrotoxic effects of amphotericin B including renal tubular acidosis. *Am. J. Med.* 46: 151, 1969.
216. Drenckhahn, D., Kleine, L., and Lullmann-Rauch, R. Lysosomal alterations in cultured macrophages exposed to anorexigenic and psychotropic drugs. *Lab. Invest.* 35: 116, 1976.
217. Durham, D. M., and Palmiter, R. D. Transcriptional regulation of the mouse metallothionein-I gene by heavy metals. *J. Biol. Chem.* 256: 5712, 1981.
218. Eby, B., Hsu, C., and Lau, K. Evidence that PO_4 depletion mediates the antihypertensive effects of dietary Ca supplementation. *Clin. Res.* 31: 328A, 1983.
219. Eknoyan, G., Gentry, L., Bulger, R., and Dobyan, D. Attenuation of gentamicin induced acute renal failure by phosphate depletion. *Kidney Int.* 25: 229, 1984.
220. Elliott, W. C., Houghton, D. C., Gilbert, D. N., Baines-Hunter, J., and Bennett, W. M. Gentamicin nephrotoxicity. I. Degree and permanence of acquired insensitivity. *J. Lab. Clin. Med.* 100: 501, 1982.
221. Elliott, W. C., Parker, R. A., Houghton, D. C., Gilbert, D. N., Porter, G. A., DeFehr, J., and Bennett, W. M. Effect of sodium bicarbonate and ammonium chloride ingestion in experimental nephrotoxicity in rats. *Res. Commun. Chem. Pathol. Pharmacol.* 28: 483, 1980.
222. Elliott, W. C., Patchin, D. S., and Jones, D. B. Effect of parathyroid hormone activity on gentamicin nephrotoxicity. *J. Lab. Clin. Med.* 109: 48, 1987.
223. Endou, H. Cytochrome P-450 monooxygenase system in the rabbit kidney: Its intranephron localization and its induction. *Jpn. J. Pharmacol.* 33: 423, 1983.
224. Engineer, M. S., Bodey, G. P., Newman, R. A., and Ho, D. H. Effects of cisplatin-induced nephrotoxicity on gentamicin pharmacokinetics in rats. *Drug Metab. Dispos.* 15: 329, 1987.
225. Ericsson, J. L., Biberfeld, P., and Seljelid, R. Electron microscopic and cytochemical studies of acid phosphatase and aryl sulfatase during autolysis. *Acta Pathol. Microbiol. Scand.* 70: 215, 1967.
226. Ericsson, J. L. E. Mechanism of Cellular Autophagy. In J. T. Dingle and H. B. Fell (eds.), *Lysosomes in Biology and Pathology,* Vol. 2. New York: Wiley, 1969. P. 345.
227. Ericsson, J. L. E., and Brunk, U. T. Alterations in Lysosomal Membranes as Related to Disease Processes. In B. F. Trump and A. K. Arstila (eds.), *Pathobiology of Cell Membranes,* Vol. 1. New York: Academic Press, 1975. P. 217.
228. Esposito, M., Fulco, R. A., Collecchi, P., Zicca, A., Cadoni, A., Merlo, F., Rosso, R., and Sobrero, A. Improved therapeutic index of cisplatin by procaine hydrochloride. *J. Natl. Cancer Inst.* 82: 677, 1990.
229. Esterbauer, H. Aldehydic Products of Lipid Peroxidation. In D. C. H. McBrien and T. F. Slater (eds.), *Free Radicals, Lipid Peroxidation and Cancer.* London: Academic Press, 1982. P. 101.
230. Evan, A. P., and Dail, W. G. The effects of chromate on the proximal tubules of the rat kidney. *Lab. Invest.* 30: 704, 1974.
231. Ewen, C., Perera, A., Hendry, J. H., McAuliffe, C. A., Sharma, H., and Fox, B. W. An autoradiographic study of the intrarenal localisation and retention of cisplatin, iproplatin and paraplatin. *Cancer Chemother. Pharmacol.* 22: 241, 1988.
232. Fabre, J., Rudhardt, M., Blanchard, P., Regamey, C., and Chauvin, P. Persistence of sisomicin and gentamicin in renal cortex and medulla compared with other organs and serum of rats. *Kidney Int.* 10: 444, 1976.
233. Fang, S. C. Interaction of selenium and mercury in the rat. *Chem. Biol. Interact.* 17: 25, 1977.
234. Farber, J. L. Membrane injury and calcium homeostasis in the pathogenesis of coagulative necrosis. *Lab. Invest.* 47: 114, 1982.
235. Farber, J. L., Kyle, M. E., and Coleman, J. B. Biology of disease. Mechanisms of cell injury by activated oxygen species. *Lab. Invest.* 62: 670, 1990.
236. Farese, R. V., Bidot-Lopez, P., Sabir, A., Smith, J. S., Schinbeckler, B., and Larsen, R. Parathyroid hormone acutely increases polyphosphoinositides of the rabbit kidney cortex by a cyclohexamide-sensitive process. *J. Clin. Invest.* 65: 1523, 1980.
237. Fariss, M. W., Pascoe, G. A., and Reed, D. J. Vitamin E reversal of the effect of extracellular calcium on chemically induced toxicity in hepatocytes. *Science* 227: 751, 1985.
238. Feldman, S., Wang, M., and Kaloyanides, G. J. Aminoglycosides induce a phospholipidosis in the renal cortex of the rat: An early manifestation of nephrotoxicity. *J. Pharmacol. Exp. Ther.* 220: 514, 1982.
239. Ferwana, O. S., Pirie, S. C., and Potts, D. J. Effect of phosphate-buffered sucrose flush solution upon the initial phase of ischaemic acute renal failure in the rat. *Clin. Sci.* 77: 77, 1989.
240. Flamenbaum, W. Pathophysiology of acute renal failure. *Arch. Intern. Med.* 131: 911, 1977.
241. Flamenbaum, W., Kotchen, T. A., Nagle, R., and McNeil, J. S. Effect of potassium on the renin-angiotensin system and $HgCl_2$-induced acute renal failure. *Am. J. Physiol.* 224: 305, 1973.
242. Fleschner, C. R., Pershadsingh, H. A., Vorbeck, M. L., Long, J. W., Jr., and Martin, A. P. Phosphate-dependent, trifluoperazine-sensitive Ca^{2+} efflux from rat liver mitochondria. *FEBS Lett.* 141: 45, 1982.
243. Fligiel, S. E. G., Lee, E. C., McCoy, J. P., Johnson, K. J., and Varani, J. Protein degradation following treatment with hydrogen peroxide. *Am. J. Pathol.* 115: 418, 1984.
244. Foote, C. S. In A. P. Autor (ed.), *Pathology of Oxygen.* New York: Academic Press, 1982. P. 21.
245. Fowler, B. A. Mechanisms of metal-induced renal cell injury: Roles of high-affinity metal-binding proteins. *Contrib. Nephrol.* 64: 83, 1988.
246. Fowler, B. A., and Brooks, R. E. Effects of the herbicide paraquat on the ultrastructure of mouse kidney. *Am. J. Pathol.* 63: 505, 1971.
247. Fowler, B. A., Hook, G. E., and Lucier, G. W. Tetrachlorodibenzo-*p*-dioxin-induction of renal microsomal enzyme systems: Ultrastructural effects on pars recta (S_3) proximal tubule cells of the rat kidney. *J. Pharmacol. Exp. Ther.* 203: 712, 1977.
248. Fox, R. B. Prevention of granulocyte-mediated oxidant lung injury in rats by a hydroxyl radical scavenger, dimethylthiourea. *J. Clin. Invest.* 74: 1456, 1984.
249. Franceschi, D., Graham, D., Sarasua, M., and Zollinger,

R. M., Jr. Mechanisms of oxygen free radical-induced calcium overload in endothelial cells. *Surgery* 108: 292, 1990.

250. Freeman, B. A., and Crapo, J. D. Biology of disease. Free radicals and tissue injury. *Lab. Invest.* 47: 412, 1982.
251. Fry, J. R., Wiebkin, P., Kao, J., Jones, C. A., Gwynn, J., and Bridges, J. W. A comparison of drug-metabolizing capability in isolated viable rat hepatocytes and renal tubule fragments. *Xenobiotica* 8: 113, 1978.
252. Fry, M., and Plummer, D. T. The Stabilization of Renal Lysosomes by Cephaloridine: The Role of a Membrane-Bound Phospholipase A_2. In J. P. Fillastre (ed.), *Nephrotoxicity: Interactions with Drugs with Membrane Systems, Mitochondria, Lysosomes*. New York: Masson, 1978. P. 193.
253. Fry, M., and Plummer, D. T. The interaction of cephaloridine with model membrane systems and rat kidney lysosomes. *Chem. Biol. Interact.* 25: 113, 1979.
254. Fukino, H., Hirai, M., Hsueh, Y. M., Moriyasu, S., and Yamane, Y. Mechanism of protection by zinc against mercuric chloride toxicity in rats: Effects of zinc and mercury on glutathionine metabolism. *J. Toxicol. Environ. Health* 19: 75, 1986.
255. Gabig, T. G., Bearman, S. I., and Babior, B. M. Effects of oxygen tension and pH on the respiratory burst of human neutrophils. *Blood* 53: 1133, 1979.
256. Galle, P. Role des lysosomes et des mitochondries dans les phenomenes de concentration et d'elimination d'elements mineraiux (uranium et or) par le rein. *J. Microsc.* 19: 17, 1974.
257. Gamelin, L. M., and Zager, R. A. Evidence against oxidant injury as a critical mediator of postischemic acute renal failure. *Am. J. Physiol.* 255: F450, 1988.
258. Gandolfi, A. J., Nagle, R. B., Soltis, J. J., and Plescia, F. H. Nephrotoxicity of halogenated vinyl cysteine compounds. *Res. Commun. Chem. Pathol. Pharmacol.* 33: 249, 1981.
259. Gaudio, K. M., Thulin, G., Ardito, T., Kashgarian, M., and Siegel, N. J. Metabolic alterations in proximal tubule suspensions obtained from ischemic kidneys. *Am. J. Physiol.* 257: F383, 1989.
260. Gemba, M., Nakatani, E., Teramoto, M., and Nakano, S. Effect of cisplatin on calcium uptake by rat kidney cortical mitochondria. *Toxicol. Lett.* 38: 291, 1987.
261. Gemborys, M. W., and Mudge, G. H. Formation and disposition of the minor metabolites of acetaminophen in the hamster. *Drug Metab. Dispos.* 9: 340, 1981.
262. Gerson, R. J., Casini, A., Gilfor, D., Serroni, A., and Farber, J. L. Oxygen-mediated cell injury in the killing of cultured hepatocytes by acetaminophen. *Biochem. Biophys. Res. Commun.* 126: 1129, 1985.
263. Ghoshal, A. K., and Recknagel, R. O. On the mechanism of carbon tetrachloride nephrotoxicity: Coincidence of loss of glucose-6-phosphatase activity with peroxidation of microsomal lipid. *Life Sci.* 4: 2195, 1965.
264. Gianello, P., Squifflet, J. P., Carlier, M., Jamart, J., Pirson, Y., Mahy, B., Berbinschi, A., Donckier, J., Ketelslegers, J. M., Lambotte, L., and Alexandre, G. P. J. Evidence that atrial natriuretic factor is the humoral factor by which volume loading or mannitol infusion produces an improved renal function after acute ischemia. *Transplantation* 48: 9, 1989.
265. Gilbert, D. N., Wood, C. A., Kohlhepp, S. J., Kohnen, P. W., Houghton, D. C., Finkbeiner, H. C., Lindsley, J., and Bennett, W. M. Polyaspartic acid prevents experimental aminoglycoside nephrotoxicity. *J. Infect. Dis.* 159: 945, 1989.
266. Giuliano, R. A., Paulus, G. J., Verpooten, G. A., Pattyn, V. M., Pollet, D. E., Nouwen, E. J., Laurent, G., Carlier, M. B., Maldague, P., Tulkens, P. M., and DeBroe, M. E. Recovery of cortical phospholipidosis and necrosis after acute gentamicin loading in rats. *Kidney Int.* 26: 838, 1984.
267. Giuliano, R. A., Verpooten, G. A., and De Broe, M. E. The effect of dosing strategy on kidney cortical accumulation of aminoglycosides in rats. *Am. J. Kidney Dis.* 8: 297, 1986.
268. Giurgea-Marion, L., Toubeau, G., Laurent, G., Heuson-Stiennon, J. A., and Tulkens, P. M. Impairment of lysosome-pinocytic vesicle fusion in rat kidney proximal tubules after treatment with gentamicin at low doses. *Toxicol. Appl. Pharmacol.* 86: 271, 1986.
269. Goldfischer, S., and Moskal, J. Electron probe microanalysis of liver in Wilson's disease. *Am. J. Pathol.* 48: 305, 1966.
270. Goldstein, S., and Czapski, G. Mannitol as an OH^- scavenger in aqueous solutions and in biological systems. *Int. J. Radiat. Biol.* 46: 725, 1984.
271. Gopalakrishna, R., and Anderson, W. B. Ca^{2+}- and phospholipid-independent activation of protein kinase C by selective oxidative modification of the regulatory domain. *Proc. Natl. Acad. Sci. U.S.A.* 86: 6758, 1989.
272. Goracci, G., Porcellati, G., and Woelk, H. Subcellular Localization and Distribution of Phospholipases A in Liver and Brain Tissue. In C. Gali (ed.), *Advances in Prostaglandin and Thromboxane Research,* Vol. 3. New York: Raven Press, 1978. P. 55.
273. Gordon, J. A., and Gattone, V. H. Mitochondrial alterations in cisplatin-induced acute renal failure. *Am. J. Physiol.* 250: F991, 1986.
274. Gores, G. J., Nieminen, A.-L., Fleishman, K. E., Dawson, T. L., Herman, B., and Lemasters, J. J. Extracellular acidosis delays onset of cell death in ATP-depleted hepatocytes. *Am. J. Physiol.* 255: C315, 1988.
275. Gores, G. J., Nieminen, A.-L., Wray, B. E., Herman, B., and Lemasters, J. J. Intracellular pH during "chemical hypoxia" in cultured rat hepatocytes. Protection by intracellular acidosis against the onset of cell death. *J. Clin. Invest.* 83: 386, 1989.
276. Gouvea, W. L., Alpert, H. C., Kelley, J., Pardo, V., and Vaamonde, C. A. Phlorizin-induced glycosuria does not prevent gentamicin nephrotoxicity in rats. *Kidney Int.* 35: 1041, 1989.
277. Granger, D. N. Role of xanthine oxidase and granulocytes in ischemia-reperfusion injury. *Am. J. Physiol.* 255: H1269, 1988.
278. Green, D., Fry, M., and Blondin, G. Phospholipids as the molecular instruments of ion and solute transport in biological membranes. *Proc. Natl. Acad. Sci. U.S.A.* 77: 257, 1980.
279. Gresser, M. J. ADP-arsenate. *J. Biol. Chem.* 256: 5981, 1981.
280. Griffin, C. C., Waravdekar, V. S., Trump, B. F., Goldblatt, P. J., and Stowell, R. E. Studies on necrosis of mouse liver in vitro. *Am. J. Pathol.* 47: 833, 1965.
281. Griffith, O. W. The role of glutathione turnover in the apparent renal secretion of cystine. *J. Biol. Chem.* 256: 12263, 1981.
282. Griffith, O. W., Bridges, R. J., and Meister, A. Evidence that the gamma-glutamyl cycle functions in vivo using intracellular glutathione: Effects of amino acids and selective inhibition of enzymes. *Proc. Natl. Acad. Sci. U.S.A.* 75: 5405, 1978.

283. Griffith, O. W., and Meister, A. Potent and specific inhibition of glutathione synthetase synthesis by buthionine sulfoximine (S-*n*-butyl homocysteine-sulfoximine). *J. Biol. Chem.* 254: 7558, 1979.
284. Gritzka, T. L., and Trump, B. F. Renal tubular lesions caused by mercuric chloride. *Am. J. Pathol.* 52: 1225, 1968.
285. Groves, C. E., Lock, E. A., and Schnellmann, R. G. The effects of haloalkene cysteine conjugates on cytosolic free calcium levels in suspensions of rat renal proximal tubules. *J. Biochem. Toxicol.* 5: 187, 1990.
286. Groves, C. E., Lock, E. A., and Schnellmann, R. G. Role of lipid peroxidation in renal proximal tubule cell death induced by haloalkene cysteine conjugates. *Toxicol. Appl. Pharmacol.* 107: 54, 1991.
287. Gstraunthaler, G., Pfaller, W., and Kotanko, P. Glutathione depletion and in vitro lipid peroxidation in mercury or maleate induced acute renal failure. *Biochem. Pharmacol.* 32: 2969, 1981.
288. Guarnieri, M., Johnson, R. M., and Du, J. T. The unsaturated fatty-acid content of mitochondria in relation to oxidation of exogenous NADH. *Biochim. Biophys. Acta* 254: 28, 1971.
289. Guder, W. G., and Ross, B. D. Enzyme distribution along the nephron. *Kidney Int.* 26: 101, 1984.
290. Guild, W. R., Young, J. V., and Merril, J. P. Anuria due to carbon tetrachloride intoxication. *Ann. Intern. Med.* 48: 1221, 1958.
291. Gullans, S. R., Brady, H. R., Kone, B. C., Giebisch, G., and Zeidel, M. L. Lipid peroxidation: A consequence of cisplatin-induced free radical formation in proximal tubule (PT) but not inner medullary collecting duct cells. *Kidney Int.* 37: 483, 1990. (Abstract.)
292. Gumbiner, B. Structure, biochemistry, and assembly of epithelial tight junctions. *Am. J. Physiol.* 253: C749, 1987.
293. Gunn, S. A., Gould, T. C., and Anderson, W. A. A. Specificity in protection against lethality and testicular toxicity from cadmium. *Proc. Soc. Exp. Biol. Med.* 128: 591, 1968.
294. Gunter, T. E., and Pfeiffer, D. R. Mechanisms by which mitochondria transport calcium. *Am. J. Physiol. Cell Physiol.* 258: C755, 1990.
295. Gutmann, E. J., Niles, J. L., McCluskey, R. T., and Brown, D. Colchicine-induced redistribution of an apical membrane glycoprotein (gp330) in proximal tubules. *Am. J. Physiol.* 257: C397, 1989.
296. Gutteridge, J. M. The role of superoxide and hydroxyl radicals in phospholipid peroxidation catalysed by iron salts. *FEBS Lett.* 150: 454, 1982.
297. Gutteridge, J. M. C., and Halliwell, B. The measurement and mechanism of lipid peroxidation in biological systems. *Trends Biochem. Sci.* 15: 129, 1990.
298. Gutteridge, J. M., Richmond, R., and Halliwell, B. Inhibition of the iron catalyzed formation of hydroxyl radicals from superoxide and of lipid peroxidation by desferrioxamine. *Biochem. J.* 184: 469, 1979.
299. Haenen, G. R. M. M., and Bast, A. Protection against lipid peroxidation by a microsomal glutathione-dependent labile factor. *FEBS Lett.* 159: 24, 1983.
300. Hafeman, D. G., and Hoekstra, W. G. Lipid peroxidation in vivo during vitamin E and selenium deficiency in the rat as monitored by ethane evolution. *J. Nutr.* 107: 666, 1977.
301. Hagen, T. M., Aw, T. Y., and Jones, D. P. Glutathione uptake and protection against oxidative injury in isolated kidney cells. *Kidney Int.* 34: 74, 1988.
302. Hagler, H., Sherwin, L., and Buja, L. Effect of different methods of tissue preparation on mitochondrial inclusions of ischemic and infarcted canine myocardium. *Lab. Invest.* 40: 529, 1979.
303. Halliwell, B., and Gutteridge, J. M. C. Oxygen toxicity, oxygen radicals, transition metals and disease. *Biochem. J.* 219: 1, 1984.
304. Halliwell, B., and Gutteridge, J. M. C. Oxygen radicals in biological systems. Part B: Oxygen radicals and antioxidants. Role of free radicals and catalytic metal ions in human disease: An overview. *Methods Enzymol.* 186: 1, 1990.
305. Hamer, D. H. Metallothionein. *Annu. Rev. Biochem.* 55: 913, 1986.
306. Hannemann, J., and Baumann, K. Inhibition of lactate-dehydrogenase by cisplatin and other platinum-compounds: Enzyme leakage of LDH is not a suitable method to measure platinum-compound-induced kidney cell damage in vitro. *Res. Commun. Chem. Pathol. Pharmacol.* 60: 371, 1988.
307. Hannemann, J., and Baumann, K. Cisplatin-induced lipid peroxidation and decrease of gluconeogenesis in rat kidney cortex: Different effects of antioxidants and radical scavengers. *Toxicology* 51: 119, 1988.
308. Hannemann, J., and Baumann, K. Nephrotoxicity of cisplatin, carboplatin and transplatin. A comparative in vitro study. *Arch. Toxicol.* 64: 393, 1990.
309. Hansen, J. C., and Kristensen, P. On the influence of zinc on mercury/selenium interaction. *Arch. Toxicol.* 46: 273, 1980.
310. Harrap, K. R. Preclinical studies identifying carboplatin as a viable cisplatin alternative. *Cancer Treat. Rev.* 12(Suppl. A): 21, 1985.
310a. Harris, D. C. H., Gabow, P. A., Linas, S. L., Rosendale, D. E., Guggenheim, S., and Schrier, R. W. Prevention of hypercalcemia-induced renal concentrating defect and tissue calcium accumulation by phosphate restriction in the rat. *Am. J. Physiol.* 251: F642, 1986.
311. Harris, S. I., Balaban, R. S., Barrett, L., and Mandel, L. J. Mitochondrial respiratory capacity and Na^+- and K^+-dependent adenosine triphosphatase-mediated on ion transport in the intact renal cell. *J. Biol. Chem.* 256: 10319, 1981.
312. Harris, S. I., Patton, L., Barrett, L., and Mandel, L. J. (Na^+, K^+)-ATPase kinetics within the intact renal cell. The role of oxidative metabolism. *J. Biol. Chem.* 257: 6996, 1982.
313. Hartley, A., Davies, M. J., and Rice-Evans, C. Desferrioxamine and membrane oxidation: Radical scavenger or iron chelator. *Biochem. Soc. Trans.* 17: 1002, 1989.
314. Hartwig, J. H., Chambers, K. A., and Stossel, T. P. Association of gelsolin with actin filaments and cell membranes of macrophages and platelets. *J. Cell Biol.* 108: 467, 1989.
315. Hassall, C. D., Brendel, K., and Gandolfi, A. J. Regulation of a *S*(*trans*-1,2-dichlorovinyl)-L-cysteine-induced renal tubular toxicity by glutathione. *J. Appl. Toxicol.* 3: 321, 1983.
316. Hassall, C. D., Gandolfi, A. J., Duhamel, R. C., and Brendel, K. The formation and biotransformation of cysteine conjugates of halogenated ethylenes by rabbit renal tubules. *Chem. Biol. Interact.* 49: 283, 1984.
317. Hawkins, H. K., Ericsson, J. L. E., Biberfeld, P., and Trump, B. F. Lysosome and phagosome stability in lethal cell injury. *Am. J. Pathol.* 68: 255, 1972.
318. Haworth, R. A., and Hunter, D. R. The Ca^{2+}-induced membrane transition in mitochondria. II. Nature of the Ca^{2+} trigger site. *Arch. Biochem. Biophys.* 195: 460, 1979.

319. Haworth, R. A., and Hunter, D. R. Allosteric inhibition of the Ca^{2+}-activated hydrophilic channel of the mitochondrial inner membrane by nucleotides. *J. Membr. Biol.* 54: 231, 1980.
320. Hayashi, T., Watanabe, Y., Kumano, K., Kitayama, R., Muratani, T., Yasuda, T., Saikawa, I., Katahira, J., Kumada, T., and Shimizu, K. Protective effect of piperacillin against the nephrotoxicity of cisplatin in rats. *Antimicrob. Agents Chemother.* 33: 513, 1989.
321. Hayden, P. J., and Stevens, J. L. Cysteine conjugate toxicity, metabolism, and binding to macromolecules in isolated rat kidney mitochondria. *Mol. Pharmacol.* 37: 468, 1990.
322. Hayes, D. M., Cvitkovic, E., Golbey, R. B., Scheiner, E., Helson, H., and Krakoff, I. H. High dose *cis*-platinum diamine dichloride. Amelioration of renal toxicity by mannitol diuresis. *Cancer* 39: 1372, 1977.
323. Hebert, S. C., and Sun, A. Hypotonic cell volume regulation in mouse medullary thick ascending limb: Effects of ADH. *Am. J. Physiol.* 255: F962, 1988.
324. Heidbreder, E., Schafferhans, K., Heyd, A., Schramm, L., and Heidland, A. Uranyl nitrate-induced acute renal failure in rats: Effect of atrial natriuretic peptide on renal function. *Kidney Int.* 34(Suppl. 25): S79, 1988.
325. Heidemann, H. T., Hoffmann, K., and Inselmann, G. Long-term effects of acetazolamide and sodium chloride loading on cisplatin nephrotoxicity in the rat. *Eur. J. Clin. Invest.* 20: 214, 1990.
326. Hellebusch, A. A., Salama, F., and Eadie, E. The use of mannitol to reduce the nephrotoxicity of amphotericin B. *Surg. Gynecol. Obstet.* 134: 241, 1972.
327. Herschberger, L. A., and Tappel, A. L. Effect of vitamin E on pentane exhaled by rats treated with methyl ethyl ketone peroxide. *Lipids* 17: 686, 1982.
328. Heuner, A., Schwegler, J. S., Silbernagl, S., and Mildenberger, S. Renal tubular transport of glutathione in rat kidney. *Pflugers Arch.* 414: 551, 1989.
329. Heyman, S. N., Brezis, M., Reubinoff, C. A., Greenfeld, Z., Lechene, C., Epstein, F. H., and Rosen, S. Acute renal failure with selective medullary injury in the rat. *J. Clin. Invest.* 82: 401, 1988.
330. Heyman, S. N., Rosen, S., Silva, P., Spokes, K., Egorin, M. J., and Epstein, F. H. Protective action of glycine in cisplatin nephropathy. *Kidney Int.* 40: 273, 1991.
331. Hildebrand, J., Thys, O., and Gerin, Y. Alterations of rat liver lysosomes and smooth endoplasmic reticulum induced by the diazafluoranthen derivative AC-3579. *Lab. Invest.* 28: 83, 1973.
332. Hill, D. L., Shih, T.-W., Johnston, T. P., and Struck, R. F. Macromolecular binding and metabolism of the carcinogen 1,2-dibromoethane. *Cancer Res.* 38: 2438, 1978.
333. Hinshaw, D. B., Armstrong, B. C., Beals, T. F., and Hyslop, P. A. A cellular model of endothelial cell ischemia. *J. Surg. Res.* 44: 527, 1988.
334. Hinshaw, D. B., Burger, J. M., Armstrong, B. C., and Hyslop, P. A. Mechanism of endothelial cell shape change in oxidant injury. *J. Surg. Res.* 46: 339, 1989.
335. Hjelle, J. T., Hazelton, G. A., Klaassen, C. D., and Hjelle, J. J. Glucuronidation and sulfation in rabbit kidney. *J. Pharmacol. Exp. Ther.* 236: 150, 1986.
336. Hochstein, P., and Ernster, L. Microsomal Peroxidation of Lipids and its Possible Role in Cellular Injury. In A. V. S. de Reuck and J. Knight (eds.), *Ciba Foundation Symposium on Cellular Injury.* Boston: Little, Brown, 1964. P. 123.
337. Hoeschele, J. D., and Van Camp, L. Whole body counting and the distribution of cis 195mPt(NH3)2(cl2) in the major organs of swiss white mice. *Adv. Antimicrob. Antineoplast. Chemother.* 2: 241, 1972.
338. Hogberg, J., Bergstand, A., and Jakobsson, S. V. Lipid peroxidation of rat-liver microsomes. Its effect on the microsomal membrane and some membrane-bound microsomal enzymes. *Eur. J. Biochem.* 37: 51, 1973.
339. Holohan, P. D., Elliott, W. C., Grace, E., and Ross, C. R. Effect of parathyroid hormone on gentamicin plasma membrane binding and tissue accumulation. *J. Pharmacol. Exp. Ther.* 243: 893, 1987.
340. Holohan, P. D., Sokol, P. P., Ross, C. R., Coulson, R., Trimble, M. E., Laska, D. A., and Williams, P. D. Gentamicin-induced increases in cytosolic calcium in pig kidney cells ($LLC\text{-}PK_1$). *J. Pharmacol. Exp. Ther.* 247: 349, 1988.
341. Honda, N., Hishida, A., Ikuma, K., and Yonemura, K. Acquired resistance to acute renal failure. *Kidney Int.* 31: 1233, 1987.
342. Hook, J. B., and Serbia, C. Potentiation of the Action of Nephrotoxic Agents by Environmental Contaminants. In G. A. Porter (ed.), *Nephrotoxic Mechanisms of Drugs and Environmental Toxins.* New York: Plenum, 1982. P. 345.
343. Horio, M., Chin, K.-V., Currier, S. J., Goldenberg, S., Williams, C., Pastan, I., Gottesman, M. M., and Handler, J. Transepithelial transport of drugs by the multidrug transporter in cultured Madin-Darby canine kidney cell epithelia. *J. Biol. Chem.* 264: 14880, 1989.
344. Hostetler, K. Y., and Hall, L. B. Inhibition of kidney lysosomal phospholipases A and C by aminoglycoside antibiotics: Possible mechanism of aminoglycoside toxicity. *Proc. Natl. Acad. Sci. U.S.A.* 79: 1663, 1982.
345. Hostetter, T. H., Wilkes, B. M., and Brenner, B. M. *Renal Circulatory and Nephron Function in Experimental Acute Renal Failure.* Philadelphia: Saunders, 1983. P. 99.
346. Houghton, D., Hartnett, M., Campbell-Boswell, M., Porter, G., and Bennett, W. A light and electron microscopic analysis of gentamicin nephrotoxicity in rats. *Am. J. Pathol.* 82: 589, 1976.
347. Howard, W. D., and Timasheff, S. N. Linkages between the effects of taxol, colchicine, and GTP on tubulin polymerization. *J. Biol. Chem.* 263: 1342, 1988.
348. Howell, S. B., and Taetle, R. Effect of sodium thiosulfate on *cis*-dichlorodiammineplatinum(II) toxicity and antitumor activity in L1210 leukemia. *Cancer Treat. Rep.* 64: 611, 1980.
349. Hreniuk, D., Guerra, E., and Wilson, P. D. A common final pathway of renal tubule cell killing by toxins and anoxia (AN): Attenuation by protease inhibition. *Kidney Int.* 408, 1989. (Abstract.)
350. Hruban, Z., Siesers, A., and Hopkins, E. Drug-induced and naturally occurring myeloid bodies. *Lab. Invest.* 27: 62, 1972.
351. Hsu, C.-H., and Kurtz, T. W. Renal hemodynamics in experimental acute renal failure. *Nephron* 27: 204, 1981.
352. Hultman, P., and Enestrom, S. Localization of mercury in the kidney during experimental acute tubular necrosis studied by the cytochemical silver amplification method. *Br. J. Exp. Pathol.* 67: 493, 1986.
353. Humes, H. D., Cieslinski, D. A., Coimbra, T. M., Messana, J. M., and Galvao, C. Epidermal growth factor enhances renal tubule cell regeneration and repair and accelerates the recovery of renal function in postischemic acute renal failure. *J. Clin. Invest.* 84: 1757, 1989.
354. Humes, H. D., Sastrasinh, M., and Weinberg, J. M. Modification of gentamicin-induced renal tubular cell injury and renal excretory failure. *Clin. Res.* 31: 430, 1983.
355. Humes, H. D., Sastrasinh, M., and Weinberg, J. M. Cal-

cium is a competitive inhibitor of the gentamicin-renal membrane binding interaction and dietary calcium supplementation protects against gentamicin nephrotoxicity. *J. Clin. Invest.* 73: 134, 1984.

356. Humes, H. D., and Weinberg, J. M. Cellular Energetics in Acute Renal Failure. In B. M. Brenner and J. M. Lazarus (eds.), *Acute Renal Failure*. Philadelphia: Saunders, 1983. P. 47.
357. Humes, H. D., Weinberg, J. M., and Knauss, T. C. Clinical and pathophysiologic aspects of aminoglycoside nephrotoxicity. *Am. J. Kidney Dis.* 2: 5, 1982.
358. Hutchison, F. N., Perez, E. A., Gandara, D. R., Lawrence, H. J., and Kaysen, G. A. Renal salt wasting in patients treated with cisplatin. *Ann. Intern. Med.* 108: 21, 1988.
359. Hwang, K. M., Scott, K. M., and Brierley, G. P. Ion transport by heart mitochondria. The effect of Cu^{2+} on membrane permeability. *Arch. Biochem. Biophys.* 150: 746, 1972.
360. Hyslop, P. A., Hinshaw, D. B., Halsey, W. A., Jr., Schraufstatter, I. U., Sauerheber, R. D., Spragg, R. G., Jackson, J. H., and Cochrane, C. G. Mechanisms of oxidant-mediated cell injury. The glycolytic and mitochondrial pathways of ADP phosphorylation are major intracellular targets inactivated by hydrogen peroxide. *J. Biol. Chem.* 263: 1665, 1988.
361. Hyslop, P. A., Hinshaw, D. B., Schraufstatter, I. U., Sklar, L. A., Spragg, R. G., and Cochrane, C. G. Intracellular calcium homeostasis during hydrogen peroxide injury to cultured P388D1 cells. *J. Cell. Physiol.* 129: 356, 1986.
362. Iaina, A. D., Herzog, D., Cohen, D., Gavendo, S., Kapuler, S., Serban, I., Schiby, G., and Eliahou, H. E. Calcium entry-blockade with verapamil in cyclosporine A plus ischemia induced acute renal failure in rats. *Clin. Nephrol.* 25: S168, 1986.
363. Ilett, K. F., Reid, W. D., Sipes, I. G., and Krishna, G. Chloroform toxicity in mice: Correlation of renal and hepatic necrosis with covalent binding of metabolites to tissue macromolecules. *Exp. Mol. Pathol.* 19: 215, 1973.
364. Inamoto, H., Ino, Y., Inamoto, N., Wada, T., Kihara, H. K., Watanabe, I., and Asano, G. Effect of $HgCl_2$ on rat kidney cells in primary culture. *Lab. Invest.* 34: 489, 1976.
365. Inoue, M., Okajima, K., and Morino, Y. Hepato-renal cooperation in biotransformation, membrane transport, and elimination of cysteine-S-conjugates of xenobiotics. *J. Biochem. (Tokyo)* 95: 247, 1982.
366. Inoue, M., Okajima, K., and Morino, Y. Metabolic coordination of liver and kidney in mercapturic acid biosynthesis. *Hepatology* 2: 311, 1982.
367. Inui, K., Saito, H., Iwata, T., and Hori, R. Aminoglycoside-induced alterations in apical membranes of kidney epithelial cell line (LLC-PK1). *Am. J. Physiol.* 254: C251, 1988.
368. Ishikawa, M., Takayanagi, Y., and Sasaki, K. The deleterious effect of buthionine sulfoximine, a glutathione-depleting agent, on the cisplatin toxicity in mice. *Jpn. J. Pharmacol.* 52: 652, 1990.
369. Iturriaga, H., Vaisman, S., Pino, E. M., and Pereda, T. Lysosomal injury and hepatic necrosis effects of triton WR-1339 on liver cells in the rat. *Exp. Mol. Pathol.* 14: 350, 1971.
370. Jacobs, C., Coleman, C. N., Rich, L., Hirst, K., and Weiner, M. W. Inhibition of cis-diamminedichloroplatinum secretion by the human kidney with probenecid. *Cancer Res.* 44: 3632, 1984.
371. Jacobs, E. E., Jacob, M., Sanadi, D. R., and Bradley, L. B. Uncoupling of oxidative phosphorylation by cadmium ion. *J. Biol. Chem.* 223: 147, 1956.
372. Jacobs, W. R., Sgambati, M., Gomez, G., Vilaro, P., Higdon, M., Bell, P. D., and Mandel, L. J. Role of cytosolic Ca in renal tubule damage induced by anoxia. *Am. J. Physiol. Cell Physiol.* 260: C545, 1991.
373. Jacques, P. J. Endocytosis. In J. T. Dingle and H. B. Fell (eds.), *Lysosomes in Biology and Pathology*, Vol. 2. New York: Wiley, 1969. P. 395.
374. Jaeschke, H., and Mitchell, J. R. Mitochondria and xanthine oxidase both generate reactive oxygen species in isolated perfused rat liver after hypoxic injury. *Biochem. Biophys. Res. Commun.* 160: 140, 1989.
375. Janero, D. R. Malondialdehyde and thiobarbituric acid-reactivity as diagnostic indices of lipid peroxidation and peroxidative tissue injury. *Free Radic. Biol. Med.* 9: 515, 1990.
376. Janmey, P. A., and Stossel, T. P. Modulation of gelsolin function by phosphatidylinositol 4,5-bisphosphate. *Nature* 325: 362, 1987.
377. Jennings, R. B., and Reimer, K. A. Lethal myocardial ischemic injury. *Am. J. Physiol.* 102: 241, 1981.
378. Jewell, S., Bellomo, G., Thor, H., Orrenius, S., and Smith, M. T. Bleb formation in hepatocytes during drug metabolism is caused by disturbances in thiol and calcium ion homeostasis. *Science* 217: 1257, 1983.
379. Jiang, Q. G., and Moldeus, P. Effect of the antioxidant *N,N*1-diphenyl-*p*-phenylenediamine (DPPD) on bromobenzene metabolism and toxicity in isolated hepatocytes. *Pharmacol. Toxicol.* 62: 104, 1988.
380. Jin, T., and Nordberg, G. F. Cadmium toxicity in kidney cells. Resistance induced by short term pretreatment in vitro and in vivo. *Acta Pharmacol. Toxicol. (Copenh.)* 58: 137, 1986.
381. Jin, T., Nordberg, G. F., and Nordberg, M. Uptake of cadmium in isolated kidney cells—Influence of binding form and in vivo pretreatment. *J. Appl. Toxicol.* 6: 397, 1986.
382. Jin, T., Nordberg, G. F., and Nordberg, M. Influence of cadmium-metallothionein pretreatment on tolerance of rat kidney cortical cells to cadmium toxicity in vitro and in vivo. *Pharmacol. Toxicol.* 60: 345, 1987.
383. Johnson, N. P., Hoeschele, J. D., and Rahn, R. O. Kinetic analysis of the in vitro binding of radioactive cis- and trans-dichlorodiammineplatinum(II) to DNA. *Chem. Biol. Interact.* 30: 151, 1980.
384. Jones, D. B. Ultrastructure of human acute renal failure. *Lab. Invest.* 46: 254, 1982.
385. Jones, D. P. Renal metabolism during normoxia, hypoxia, and ischemic injury. *Annu. Rev. Physiol.* 48: 33, 1986.
386. Jones, D. P., Thor, H., Smith, M. T., Jewell, S. A., and Orrenius, S. Inhibition of ATP-dependent microsomal Ca^{2+} sequestration during oxidative stress and its prevention by glutathione. *J. Biol. Chem.* 258: 6390, 1983.
387. Jones, L. M., Cockcroft, S., and Mitchell, R. H. Stimulation of phosphatidylinositol turnover in various tissues by cholinergic and adrenergic agonists, by histamine and by coerulein. *Biochem. J.* 182: 669, 1979.
388. Jones, M. M., Basinger, M. A., Topping, R. J., Gale, G. R., Jones, S. G., and Holscher, M. A. Meso-2,3-dimercaptosuccinic acid and sodium N-benzyl-N-dithiocarboxy-D-glucamine as antagonists for cadmium intoxication. *Arch. Toxicol.* 62: 29, 1988.
389. Jones, T. W., Qin, C., Schaeffer, V. H., and Stevens,

J. L. Immunohistochemical localization of glutamine transaminase K, a rat kidney cysteine conjugate beta-lyase, and the relationship to the segment specificity of cysteine conjugate nephrotoxicity. *Mol. Pharmacol.* 34: 621, 1988.

390. Jongejan, H. T., Provoost, A. P., and Molenaar, J. C. Potentiation of cis-diamminedichloroplatinum nephrotoxicity by amikacin in rats. *Cancer Chemother. Pharmacol.* 22: 178, 1988.

391. Josepovitz, C., Farruggella, T., Levine, R., Lane, B., and Kaloyanides, G. J. Effect of netilmicin on the phospholipid composition of subcellular fractions of rat renal cortex. *J. Pharmacol. Exp. Ther.* 235: 810, 1985.

392. Josepovitz, C., Levine, R., Farrugella, T., Lane, B., and Kaloyanides, G. J. ^{3}H-netilmicin binding constants and phospholipid composition of renal plasma membranes of normal and diabetic rats. *J. Pharmacol. Exp. Ther.* 233: 298, 1985.

393. Josepovitz, C., Pastoriza-Munoz, E., Timmerman, D., Scott, M., Feldman, S., and Kaloyanides, G. J. Inhibition of gentamicin uptake in rat renal cortex in vivo by aminoglycosides and organic polycations. *J. Pharmacol. Exp. Ther.* 223: 314, 1982.

394. Judah, J. D. The action of antihistamine drugs in vitro. I. Mitochondrial swelling. *Biochim. Biophys. Acta* 53: 375, 1961.

395. Judah, J. D., Ahmed, K., and McLean, A. E. M. Possible Role of Ion Shifts in Liver Injury. In A. V. S. De Reuck and J. Knight (eds.), *Cellular Injury.* Boston: Little, Brown, 1964. P. 187.

396. Just, M., Erdmann, G., and Habermann, E. The renal handling of polybasic drugs. I. Gentamicin and aprotinin in intact animals. *Naunyn Schmiedebergs Arch. Pharmacol.* 300: 57, 1977.

397. Just, M., and Habermann, E. The renal handling of polybasic drugs. II. In vitro studies with brush border and lysosomal preparations. *Naunyn Schmiederbergs Arch. Pharmacol.* 300: 67, 1977.

398. Kacew, S. Cationic amphiphilic drug-induced renal cortical lysosomal phospholipidosis: An in vivo comparative study with gentamicin and chlorphentermine. *Toxicol. Appl. Pharmacol.* 91: 469, 1987.

399. Kacew, S. Inhibition of gentamicin-induced nephrotoxicity by pyridoxal-5′-phosphate in the rat. *J. Pharmacol. Exp. Ther.* 248: 360, 1989.

400. Kagi, J. H. R., and Vallee, B. L. Metallothionein: A cadmium and zinc containing protein from equine renal cortex. *J. Biol. Chem.* 236: 2435, 1961.

401. Kaloyanides, G. J. Aminoglycoside-induced functional and biochemical defects in the renal cortex. *Fund. Appl. Toxicol.* 4: 930, 1984.

402. Kaloyanides, G. J. Metabolic interactions between drugs and renal tubulointerstitial cells: Role in nephrotoxicity. *Kidney Int.* 39: 531, 1991.

403. Kane, A. B., Stanton, R. P., Raymond, E. G., Dobson, M. E., Knafelc, M. E., and Farber, J. L. Dissociation of intracellular lysosomal rupture from the cell death caused by silica. *J. Cell Biol.* 87: 643, 1980.

404. Kappus, H. Oxidative stress in chemical toxicity. *Arch. Toxicol.* 60: 144, 1987.

405. Karmazyn, M. Amiloride enhances postischemic ventricular recovery: Possible role of Na^{+}-H^{+} exchange. *Am. J. Physiol.* 255: H608, 1988.

406. Katz, A. M., and Messineo, F. C. Lipid-membrane interactions and the pathogenesis of ischemic damage in the myocardium. *Circ. Res.* 48: 1, 1981.

407. Katz, J., and Wals, P. A. Studies with digitonin-treated rat hepatocytes (nude cells). *J. Cell. Biochem.* 28: 207, 1985.

408. Kauppinen, R. A., McMahon, H. T., and Nicholls, D. G. Ca^{2+}-dependent and Ca^{2+}-independent glutamate release, energy status and cytosolic free Ca^{2+} concentration in isolated nerve terminals following metabolic inhibition: Possible relevance to hypoglycaemia and anoxia. *Neuroscience* 27: 175, 1988.

409. Kellogg, E. W., III, and Fridovich, I. Liposome oxidation and erythrocyte lysis by enzymically generated superoxide and hydrogen peroxide. *J. Biol. Chem.* 252: 6721, 1977.

410. Kempson, S. A., Ying, A. L., McAteer, J. A., and Murer, H. Endocytosis and Na^{+}/solute cotransport in renal epithelial cells. *J. Biol. Chem.* 264: 18451, 1989.

411. Keniston, R. C., Cabellon, S., Jr., and Yarbrough, K. S. Pyridoxal 5′-phosphate as an antidote for cyanide, spermine, gentamicin, and dopamine toxicity: An in vivo rat study. *Toxicol. Appl. Pharmacol.* 88: 433, 1987.

412. Kennedy, B. J. Metabolic and toxic effects of mithramycin during tumor therapy. *Am. J. Med.* 49: 494, 1970.

413. Kent, G., Volini, E. I., Orfei, E., Minick, O. T., and de la Heurga, J. Effect of hepatic injuries upon iron storage in the liver. *Lab. Invest.* 12: 1094, 1963.

414. Kinsler, S., and Bell, J. U. Failure of cis-platinum to alter metal concentrations in the liver and kidney of the rat. *Biochem. Int.* 10: 847, 1985.

415. Kirschbaum, B. B. Interactions between renal brush border membranes and polyamines. *J. Pharmacol. Exp. Ther.* 229: 409, 1984.

416. Kirschbaum, B., Sprinkle, F., and Oken, D. Renal function and mercury level in rats with mercuric chloride nephrotoxicity. *Nephron* 26: 28, 1980.

417. Kishore, B. K., Kállay, Z., Lambricht, P., Laurent, G., and Tulkens, P. M. Mechanism of protection afforded by polyaspartic acid against gentamicin-induced phospholipidosis. I. Polyaspartic acid binds gentamicin and displaces it from negatively charged phospholipid layers *in vitro. J. Pharmacol. Exp. Ther.* 255: 867, 1990.

418. Kishore, B. K., Lambricht, P., Laurent, G., Maldague, P., Wagner, R., and Tulkens, P. M. Mechanism of protection afforded by polyaspartic acid against gentamicin-induced phospholipidosis. II. Comparative *in vitro* and *in vivo* studies with poly-L-aspartic, poly-L-glutamic and poly-D-glutamic acids. *J. Pharmacol. Exp. Ther.* 255: 875, 1990.

419. Klaassen, C. D. Inhibition of lipid peroxidation without prevention of cellular injury in isolated rat hepatocytes. *Toxicol. Appl. Pharmacol.* 58: 8, 1981.

420. Kleinman, J. G., McNeil, J. S., Schwartz, J. H., Hamburger, R. J., and Flamenbaum, W. Effect of dithiothreitol on mercuric chloride- and uranyl nitrate-induced acute renal failure in the rat. *Kidney Int.* 12: 115, 1977.

421. Kluwe, W. M. Acute toxicity of 1,2-dibromo-3-chloropropane in the F344 male rat. II. Development and repair of the renal, epididymal, testicular and hepatic lesion. *Toxicol. Appl. Pharmacol.* 59: 84, 1981.

422. Kluwe, W. M. The Nephrotoxicity of Low Molecular Weight Halogenated Alkane Solvents, Pesticides and Chemical Intermediates. In J. B. Hook (ed.), *Toxicology of the Kidney.* New York: Raven Press, 1981. P. 179.

423. Kluwe, W. M., Harrington, F. W., and Cooper, S. E. Toxic effects of organohalide compounds on renal tubular cells in vivo and in vitro. *J. Pharmacol. Exp. Ther.* 220: 597, 1982.

424. Kluwe, W. M., and Hook, J. B. Analysis of gentamicin

uptake by rat renal cortical slices. *Toxicol. Appl. Pharmacol.* 45: 531, 1978.

425. Kluwe, W. M., and Hook, J. B. Functional nephrotoxicity of gentamicin in the rat. *Toxicol. Appl. Pharmacol.* 45: 163, 1978.
426. Knauss, T. C., Weinberg, J. M., and Humes, H. D. Alterations in renal cortical phospholipid content induced by gentamicin: Time course, specificity, and subcellular localization. *Am. J. Physiol.* 244: F535, 1983.
427. Koizumi, T., and Yamane, Y. Protective effect of sodium molybdate on the acute toxicity of mercuric chloride. V. Enhancement of renal regeneration after exposure to $HgCl_2$. *Chem. Biol. Interact.* 67: 185, 1988.
428. Komsta-Szumska, E., Chmielnicka, J., and Piotrowski, J. K. Binding of inorganic mercury by subcellular fractions and proteins of rat kidneys. *Arch. Toxicol.* 37: 57, 1976.
429. Kone, B. C., Kaleta, M., and Gullans, S. R. Silver Ion (Ag^+)-induced increases in cell membrane K^+ and Na^+ permeability in the renal proximal tubule: Reversal by thiol reagents. *J. Membr. Biol.* 102: 11, 1988.
430. Kopolovic, J., Brezis, M., Spokes, K., and Rosen, S. Polyethylene glycol effect on the oxygenated and hypoxic isolated perfused rat kidney. *Virchows Arch.* [*A*] 414: 429, 1989.
431. Korey, S. R., Gonatas, J., and Stein, A. Studies in Tay-Sachs disease. III. Biochemistry. *J. Neuropathol. Exp. Neurol.* 22: 56, 1963.
432. Kornguth, M. L., Bayer, W. H., and Kunin, C. M. Binding of gentamicin to subcellular fractions of rabbit kidney: Inhibition by spermine and other polyamines. *J. Antimicrob. Chemother.* 6: 121, 1980.
433. Kosek, J. C., Mazze, R. I., and Cousins, J. M. The morphology and pathogenesis of nephrotoxicity following methoxylurane anesthesia: An experimental model in rats. *Lab. Invest.* 27: 575, 1972.
434. Kosek, J. C., Mazze, R. I., and Cousins, M. J. Nephrotoxicity of gentamicin. *Lab. Invest.* 30: 48, 1974.
435. Kotsonis, F. N., and Klaassen, C. D. Toxicity and distribution of cadmium administered to rats at sublethal doses. *Toxicol. Appl. Pharmacol.* 41: 667, 1977.
436. Koyasu, S., Nishida, E., Miyata, Y., Sakai, H., and Yahara, I. HSP100, a 100-kDa heat shock protein, is a Ca^{2+}-calmodulin-regulated actin-binding protein. *J. Biol. Chem.* 264: 15083, 1989.
437. Kozak, E. M., and Tate, S. S. Glutathione-degrading enzymes of microvillus membranes. *J. Biol. Chem.* 257: 6322, 1982.
438. Kramer, R. A. Protection against cisplatin nephrotoxicity by prochlorperazine. *Cancer Chemother. Pharmacol.* 25: 156, 1989.
439. Kreisberg, J. I., Bulger, R. E., Trump, B. F., and Nagle, R. B. Effect of transient hypotension on the structure and function of rat kidney. *Virchows Arch. B* [*Cell Pathol.*] 22: 121, 1976.
440. Kunze, H., Nahas, N., Traynor, J. R., and Wurl, M. Effects of local anaesthetics on phospholipases. *Biochim. Biophys. Acta* 441: 93, 1976.
441. Kuo, C. H., Braselton, W. E., and Hook, J. B. Effect of phenobarbital on cephaloridine toxicity and accumulation in rabbit and rat kidneys. *Toxicol. Appl. Pharmacol.* 64: 244, 1982.
442. Kuo, C. H., and Hook, J. B. Depletion of renal glutathione content and nephrotoxicity of cephaloridine in rabbits, rats and mice. *Toxicol. Appl. Pharmacol.* 63: 292, 1982.
443. Kuo, C. H., Maita, K., Sleight, S. D., and Hook, J. B. Lipid peroxidation: A possible mechanism of cephaloridine-induced nephrotoxicity. *Toxicol. Appl. Pharmacol.* 67: 78, 1983.
444. Kuo, C. H., Rush, G. F., and Hook, J. B. Renal cortical accumulation of phenobarbital in rats and rabbits: Lack of correlation with induction of renal microsomal monooxygenases. *J. Pharmacol. Exp. Ther.* 220: 547, 1982.
445. Kuo, C. H., Tune, B. M., and Hook, J. B. Effect of piperonyl butoxide on organic anion and cation transport in rabbit kidneys. *Proc. Soc. Exp. Biol. Med.* 174: 165, 1983.
446. Kurnik, B. R. C., Weisberg, L. S., Cuttler, I. M., and Kurnik, P. B. Effects of atrial natriuretic peptide versus mannitol on renal blood flow during radiocontrast infusion in chronic renal failure. *J. Lab. Clin. Med.* 116: 27, 1990.
447. Kurup, C. K., and Sanadi, D. R. Studies on oxidative phosphorylation. XVI. Sulfhydryl involvement in the energy transfer pathway. *Biochemistry* 7: 4483, 1968.
448. Lameire, N., Ringoir, S., and Leusen, I. Effect of variation in dietary NaCl intake on total and fractional renal blood flow in the normal and mercury-intoxicated rat. *Circ. Res.* 39: 506, 1976.
449. Lash, L. H., and Anders, M. W. Cytotoxicity of S-(1,2-dichlorovinyl)glutathione and S-(1,2-dichlorovinyl)-L-cysteine in isolated rat kidney cells. *J. Biol. Chem.* 261: 13076, 1986.
450. Lash, L. H., and Anders, M. W. Mechanism of S-(1,2-dichlorovinyl)-L-cysteine- and S-(1,2-dichlorovinyl)-L-homocysteine-induced renal mitochondrial toxicity. *Mol. Pharmacol.* 32: 549, 1987.
451. Lash, L. H., and Anders, M. W. Uptake of nephrotoxic S-conjugates by isolated rat renal proximal tubular cells. *J. Pharmacol. Exp. Ther.* 248: 531, 1989.
452. Lash, L. H., Elfarra, A. A., and Anders, M. W. Renal cysteine conjugate beta-lyase. Bioactivation of nephrotoxic cysteine S-conjugates in mitochondrial outer membrane. *J. Biol. Chem.* 261: 5930, 1986.
453. Lash, L. H., and Jones, D. P. Uptake of the glutathione conjugate S-(1,2-dichlorovinyl)glutathione by renal basal-lateral membrane vesicles and isolated kidney cells. *Mol. Pharmacol.* 28: 278, 1985.
454. Lash, L. H., and Tokarz, J. J. Oxidative stress in isolated rat renal proximal and distal tubular cells. *Am. J. Physiol.* 259: F338, 1990.
455. Lassing, I., and Lindberg, U. Specific interaction between phosphatidylinositol 4,5-bisphosphate and profilactin. *Nature* 314: 472, 1985.
456. Lau, S. S., Hill, B. A., Highet, R. J., and Monks, T. J. Sequential oxidation and glutathione addition to 1,4-benzoquinone: Correlation of toxicity with increased glutathione substitution. *Mol. Pharmacol.* 34: 829, 1988.
457. Lau, S. S., Jones, T. W., Highet, R. J., Hill, B. A., and Monks, T. J. Differences in the localization and extent of the renal proximal tubular necrosis caused by mercapturic acid and glutathione conjugates of 1,4-naphthoquinone and menadione. *Toxicol. Appl. Pharmacol.* 104: 334, 1990.
458. Lau, S. S., Monks, T. J., and Gillette, J. R. Identification of 2-bromohydroquinone as a metabolite of bromobenzene and O-bromophenol: Implications for bromobenzene-induced nephrotoxicity. *J. Pharmacol. Exp. Ther.* 230: 360, 1984.
459. Laurent, G., Carlier, M. B., Rollman, B., VanHoof, F., and Tulkens, P. Mechanism of aminoglycoside-induced lysosomal phospholipidosis: In vitro and in vivo studies

with gentamicin and amikacin. *Biochem. Pharmacol.* 31: 3861, 1982.

460. Laurent, G., Kishore, B. K., and Tulkens, P. M. Aminoglycoside-induced renal phospholipidosis and nephrotoxicity. *Biochem. Pharmacol.* 40: 2383, 1990.
461. Ledda-Columbano, G. M., Columbano, A., Coni, P., Faa, G., and Pani, P. Cell deletion by apoptosis during regression of renal hyperplasia. *Am. J. Pathol.* 135: 657, 1989.
462. LeFurgey, A., Spencer, A. J., Jacobs, W. R., Ingram, P., and Mandel, L. J. Elemental microanalysis of organelles in proximal tubules: I. Alterations in transport and metabolism. *J. Am. Soc. Nephrol.* 1: 1305, 1991.
463. Lehane, D., Winston, A., Gray, R., and Daskal, Y. The effect of diuretic pretreatment on clinical, morphological and ultrastructural *cis*-platinum induced nephrotoxicity. *Int. J. Radiat. Oncol. Biol. Phys.* 5: 1393, 1979.
464. Le Hir, M., and Dubach, U. C. An ATP-inhibited soluble 5'-nucleotidase of rat kidney. *Am. J. Physiol.* 254: F191, 1988.
465. Lehninger, A. L., Rossi, C. S., and Greenawalt, J. W. Respiration-dependent accumulation of inorganic phosphate and Ca^{++} by rat liver mitochondria. *Biochem. Biophys. Res. Commun.* 10: 444, 1963.
466. Lemasters, J. J., DiGuiseppi, J., Nieminen, A. L., and Herman, B. Blebbing, free Ca^{2+} and mitochondrial membrane potential preceding cell death in hepatocytes. *Nature* 325: 78, 1987.
467. Lemasters, J. L., Stemkowski, C. J., Ji, S., and Thurman, R. G. Cell surface changes and enzyme release during hypoxia and reoxygenation in the isolated perfused liver. *J. Cell Biol.* 97: 778, 1983.
468. Leonard, B. J., Eccleston, E., Jones, D., Todd, P., and Walpole, A. Antileukaemic and nephrotoxic properties of platinum compounds. *Nature* 234: 43, 1971.
469. Lê Quôc, K., and Lê Quôc, D. Involvement of the ADP/ATP carrier in calcium-induced perturbations of the mitochondrial inner membrane permeability: Importance of the orientation of the nucleotide binding site. *Arch. Biochem. Biophys.* 265: 249, 1988.
470. Levi, J., Jacobs, C., Kalman, S. M., McTigue, M., and Weiner, M. W. Mechanism of *cis*-platinum nephrotoxicity: I. Effects of sulfhydryl groups in rat kidneys. *J. Pharmacol. Exp. Ther.* 213: 545, 1980.
471. Levi, M., and Cronin, R. E. Early selective effects of gentamicin on renal brush-border membrane Na-Pi cotransport and Na-H exchange. *Am. J. Physiol.* 258: F1379, 1990.
472. Levinson, W., Oppermann, H., and Jackson, J. Transition series metals and sulfhydryl reagents induce the synthesis of four proteins in eukaryotic cells. *Biochim. Biophys. Acta* 606: 170, 1980.
473. Leyland-Jones, B., Morrow, C., Tate, S., Urmacher, C., Gordon, C., and Young, C. W. *cis*-Diamminedichloroplatinum(II) nephrotoxicity and its relationship to renal gamma-glutamyl transpeptidase and glutathione. *Cancer Res.* 43: 6072, 1983.
474. Linas, S. L., Whittenburg, D., and Repine, J. E. Role of xanthine oxidase in ischemia/reperfusion injury. *Am. J. Physiol. Renal Fluid Electrolyte Physiol.* 258: F711, 1990.
475. Lindner, A., Cutler, R. E., and Goodman, W. G. Synergism of dopamine plus furosemide in preventing acute renal failure in the dog. *Kidney Int.* 16: 158, 1979.
476. Lindquist, S. The heat-shock response. *Annu. Rev. Biochem.* 55: 1151, 1986.
477. Lipsky, J. J., Cheng, L., Sacktor, B., and Lietman, P. S. Gentamicin uptake by renal tubule brush border membrane vesicles. *J. Pharmacol. Exp. Ther.* 215: 390, 1980.
478. Lipsky, J. J., and Lietman, P. S. Neomycin inhibition of adenosine triphosphatase: Evidence for a neomycin-phospholipid interaction. *Antimicrob. Agents Chemother.* 18: 532, 1980.
479. Lipsky, J. J., and Lietman, P. S. Aminoglycoside inhibition of a renal phosphatidylinositol phospholipase C. *J. Pharmacol. Exp. Ther.* 220: 287, 1982.
480. Litterst, C. L. Alterations in the toxicity of cis-dichlorodiammineplatinum-II and in tissue localization of platinum as a function of NaCl concentration in the vehicle of administration. *Toxicol. Appl. Pharmacol.* 61: 99, 1981.
481. Litterst, C. L., Mimnaugh, E. G., Reagan, R. L., and Gram, T. E. Comparison of in vitro drug metabolism by lung, liver, and kidney of several common laboratory species. *Drug Metab. Dispos.* 3: 259, 1975.
482. Litterst, C. L., Tong, S., Hirokata, Y., and Siddik, Z. H. Alterations in hepatic and renal levels of glutathione and activities of glutathione S-transferases from rats treated with *cis*-dichlorodiammine-platinum-II. *Cancer Chemother. Pharmacol.* 8: 67, 1982.
483. Little, C., and O'Brien, P. J. An intracellular GSH-peroxidase with a lipid peroxide substrate. *Biochem. Biophys. Res. Commun.* 31: 145, 1968.
484. Livesey, J. C., and Anders, M. W. In vitro metabolism of 1,2-dihaloethanes to ethylene. *Drug Metab. Dispos.* 7: 199, 1979.
485. Lock, E. A., Odum, J., and Ormond, P. Transport of N-acetyl-S-pentachloro-1,3-butadienylcysteine by rat renal cortex. *Arch. Toxicol.* 59: 12, 1986.
486. Lockard, V. G., Phillips, R. D., Hayes, A. W., Berndt, W. O., and O'Neal, R. M. Citrinin nephrotoxicity in rats: A light and electron microscopic study. *Exp. Mol. Pathol.* 32: 226, 1980.
487. Lodhi, S., Weiner, N. D., and Schacht, J. Interactions of neomycin and calcium in synaptosomal membranes and polyphosphoinositide monolayers. *Biochim. Biophys. Acta* 426: 781, 1976.
488. Louis, B., Gorfein, P., Shani, J., and Lipner, H. Partial protection by mannitol against gentamycin induced acute renal failure in rabbits. *Kidney Int.* 19: 208, 1981.
489. Loveless, M. O., Kohlhepp, S. J., and Gilbert, D. N. The influence of aminoglycoside antibiotics on the in vitro function of rat liver ribosomes. *J. Lab. Clin. Med.* 103: 294, 1984.
490. Low, M. G., and Zilversmit, D. B. Role of phosphatidylinositol in attachment of alkaline phosphatase to membranes. *Biochemistry* 19: 3913, 1980.
491. Lowrey, K., Glende, E. A., Jr., and Recknagel, R. O. Rapid depression of rat liver microsomal calcium pump activity after administration of carbon tetrachloride or bromotrichloromethane and lack of effect after ethanol. *Toxicol. Appl. Pharmacol.* 59: 389, 1981.
492. Lowrey, K., Glende, E. A., Jr., and Recknagel, R. O. Destruction of liver microsomal calcium pump activity by carbon tetrachloride and bromotrichloromethane. *Biochem. Pharmacol.* 30: 135, 1981.
493. Luft, F. C., and Kleit, S. A. Renal parenchymal accumulation of aminoglycoside antibiotics in rats. *J. Infect. Dis.* 656: 659, 1974.
494. Luft, F. C., and Patel, V. Lysosomal Acid Hydrolases as Urinary Markers of Aminoglycoside Nephrotoxicity in the Rat. In J. P. Fillastre (ed.), *Nephrotoxicity: Interactions of Drugs with Membrane Systems, Mitochondria, Lysosomes.* New York: Masson, 1978. P. 127.

495. Luft, F. C., Yum, M. N., and Kleit, S. A. The effect of concomitant mercuric chloride and gentamicin on kidney function and structure in the rat. *J. Lab. Clin. Med.* 89: 622, 1977.
496. Lullman, H., Lullman-Rauch, R., and Wassermann, O. Drug induced phospholipidosis. *CRC Crit. Rev. Toxicol.* 4: 185, 1975.
497. Lullmann, H., and Vollmer, B. An interaction of aminoglycoside antibiotics with Ca binding to lipid monolayers and to biomembranes. *Biochem. Pharmacol.* 31: 3769, 1982.
498. Lullmann-Rauch, R. Lipidosis-like renal changes in rats treated with chlorphentermine or with tricyclic antidepressants. *Virchows Arch. B* [*Cell Pathol.*] 18: 51, 1975.
499. Lundh, H. A. B. Sequence comparison between kidney and liver lesions in the rat following carbon tetrachloride poisoning. *J. Occup. Med.* 6: 123, 1964.
500. Lynch, G., and Baudry, M. The biochemistry of memory: A new and specific hypothesis. *Science* 224: 1057, 1984.
501. MacFarlane, M., Foster, J. R., Gibson, G. G., King, L. J., and Lock, E. A. Cysteine conjugate β-lyase of rat kidney cytosol: Characterization, immunocytochemical localization, and correlation with hexachlorobutadiene nephrotoxicity. *Toxicol. Appl. Pharmacol.* 98: 185, 1989.
502. Macknight, A. D. C., and Leaf, A. Regulation of Cellular Volume. In T. E. Andreoli, J. F. Hoffman, D. D. Fanestil, and S. G. Schultz (eds.), *Physiology of Membrane Disorders*. New York: Plenum, 1986. P. 311.
503. Madsen, K. M. Mercury accumulation in kidney lysosomes of proteinuric rats. *Kidney Int.* 18: 445, 1980.
504. Madsen, K. M., and Christensen, E. I. Effects of mercury on lysosomal protein digestion in the kidney proximal tubule. *Lab. Invest.* 38: 165, 1978.
505. Madsen, K. M., and Hansen, J. L. Subcellular distribution of mercury in the rat kidney cortex after exposure to mercuric chloride. *Toxicol. Appl. Pharmacol.* 54: 443, 1980.
506. Magos, L., Webb, M., and Butler, W. H. The effect of cadmium pretreatment on the nephrotoxic action and kidney uptake of mercury in male and female rats. *Br. J. Exp. Pathol.* 55: 589, 1974.
507. Malis, C. D., and Bonventre, J. V. Mechanism of calcium potentiation of oxygen free radical injury to renal mitochondria. A model for post-ischemic and toxic mitochondrial damage. *J. Biol. Chem.* 261: 14201, 1986.
508. Malis, C. D., Racusen, L. C., Solez, K., and Whelton, A. Nephrotoxicity of a single dose of aminoglycoside in rats given lysine. *J. Lab. Clin. Med.* 103: 660, 1984.
509. Malis, C. D., Weber, P. C., Leaf, A., and Bonventre, J. V. Incorporation of marine lipids into mitochondrial membranes increases susceptibility to damage by calcium and reactive oxygen species: Evidence for enhanced activation of phospholipase A_2 in mitochondria enriched with *n*-3 fatty acids. *Proc. Natl. Acad. Sci. U.S.A.* 87: 8845, 1990.
510. Malmqvist, E., Ivemark, B. I., Lindsten, J., Maunsbach, A. B., and Martensson, E. Pathologic lysosomes and increased urinary glycosylceramide excretion in Fabry's disease. *Lab. Invest.* 25: 1, 1971.
511. Mandal, A. K., and Bennett, W. M. Transmission electron microscopy of urinary sediment in the assessment of aminoglycoside nephrotoxicity in the rat. *Nephron* 49: 67, 1988.
512. Mandal, A. K., Sklar, A. H., and Hudson, J. B. Transmission electron microscopy of urinary sediment in human acute renal failure. *Kidney Int.* 28: 58, 1985.
513. Mandel, L. J., Schnellmann, R. G., and Jacobs, W. R. Intracellular glutathione in the protection from anoxic injury in renal proximal tubules. *J. Clin. Invest.* 85: 316, 1990.
514. Mandel, L. J., Takano, T., Soltoff, S. P., and Murdaugh, S. Mechanisms whereby exogenous nucleotides improvement rabbit renal proximal function during and after anoxia. *J. Clin. Invest.* 81: 1255, 1988.
515. Marche, P., Koutouzov, S., and Girard, A. Impairment of membrane phosphoinositide metabolism by aminoglycoside antibiotics: Streptomycin, amikacin, kanamycin, dibekacin, gentamicin and neomycin. *J. Pharmacol. Exp. Ther.* 227: 415, 1983.
516. Marnett, L. J., Bienkowski, M. J., and Pagels, W. R. Oxygen 18 investigations of the prostaglandin synthetase-dependent co-oxidation of diphenylisobenzofuran. *J. Biol. Chem.* 254: 5077, 1979.
517. Marnett, L., Wlodawer, P., and Samuelsson, B. Co-oxidation of organic substrates by the prostaglandin synthetase of sheep vesicular gland. *J. Biol. Chem.* 250: 8510, 1975.
518. Masaki, N., Sakaida, I., and Farber, J. L. Protease inhibitors do not prevent the killing of cultured hepatocytes by cystamine. *Biochem. Biophys. Res. Commun.* 163: 412, 1989.
519. Mason, R. P. Free-Radical Intermediates in the Metabolism of Toxic Chemicals. In *Free Radicals in Biology*, Vol. V. New York: Academic Press, 1982. P. 161.
520. Matsuzawa, Y., and Hostetler, K. Y. Inhibition of lysosomal phospholipase A and phospholipase C by chloroquine and 4,4'-bis(diethylaminoethoxy)-diethyldiphenylethane. *J. Biol. Chem.* 255: 5190, 1980.
521. Matsuzawa, Y., and Hostetler, K. Y. Studies on drug-induced lipidosis: Subcellular localization of phospholipid and cholesterol in the liver of rats treated with chloroquine or 4,4'-bis(diethylaminoethoxy)-diethyldiphenylethane. *J. Lipid Res.* 21: 202, 1980.
522. Matthys, E., Patel, Y., Kreisberg, J., Stewart, J. H., and Venkatachalam, M. Lipid alterations induced by renal ischemia: Pathogenic factor in membrane damage. *Kidney Int.* 26: 153, 1984.
523. Mauk, R. H., Patak, R. V., Fadem, S. Z., Lifschitz, M. D., and Stein, J. H. Effect of prostaglandin E. Administration in a nephrotoxic and a vasoconstrictor model of acute renal failure. *Kidney Int.* 12: 122, 1971.
524. Maunsbach, A. B. Function of Lysosomes in Kidney Cells. In J. T. Dingle and H. B. Fell (eds.), *Lysosomes*. New York: Wiley, 1969. P. 115.
525. McCord, J. M. Oxygen-derived free radicals in postischemic tissue injury. *N. Engl. J. Med.* 312: 159, 1985.
526. McCormack, J. G. Effects of spermine on mitochondrial Ca^{2+} transport and the ranges of extramitochondrial Ca^{2+} to which the matrix Ca^{2+}-sensitive dehydrogenases respond. *Biochem. J.* 264: 167, 1989.
527. McCoy, R. N., Hill, K. E., Ayon, M. A., Stein, J. H., and Burk, R. F. Oxidant stress following renal ischemia: Changes in the glutathione redox ratio. *Kidney Int.* 33: 812, 1988.
528. McDowell, E. M. Light and electron microscopic studies of the rat kidney after administration of inhibitors of the citric acid cycle in vivo. I. Effects of sodium fluoroacetate on the proximal convoluted tubule. *Am. J. Pathol.* 66: 513, 1972.
529. McIntyre, T. M., and Curthoys, N. P. The interorgan metabolism of glutathione. *Int. J. Biochem.* 12: 515, 1980.
530. McIntyre, T., and Curthoys, N. P. Renal catabolism of

glutathione. Characterization of a particulate rat renal dipeptidase that catalyzes the hydrolysis of cysteinylglycine. *J. Biol. Chem.* 257: 11915, 1982.

531. McMurtry, R. J., and Mitchell, J. R. Renal and hepatic necrosis after metabolic activation of 2-substitute furans and thiophenes, including furosemide and cephaloridine. *Toxicol. Appl. Pharmacol.* 42: 285, 1977.
532. McMurtry, R. J., Snodgrass, W. R., and Mitchell, J. R. Renal necrosis, glutathione depletion and covalent binding after acetaminophen. *Toxicol. Appl. Pharmacol.* 46: 87, 1978.
533. Mego, J. L. A Biochemical Method for the Evaluation of Heterolysosome Formation and Function. In J. T. Dingle (ed.), *Lysosomes in Biology and Pathology,* Vol. 3. New York: Elsevier, 1973. P. 527.
534. Mego, J. L. Inhibition of intralysosomal proteolysis in mouse liver and kidney phagolysosomes by zinc. *Biochem. Pharmacol.* 25: 753, 1976.
535. Mego, J. L., and Barnes, J. Inhibition of heterolysosome formation and function in mouse kidneys by injection of mercuric chloride. *Biochem. Pharmacol.* 22: 373, 1973.
536. Mego, J. L., and Cain, J. A. The effect of carbon tetrachloride on lysosome function in kidneys and livers of mice. *Biochim. Biophys. Acta* 297: 343, 1973.
537. Mego, J. L., and Cain, J. A. An effect of cadmium on heterolysosome formation and function in mice. *Biochem. Pharmacol.* 24: 1227, 1975.
538. Meister, A. Glutathione metabolism and its selective modification. *J. Biol. Chem.* 263: 17205, 1988.
539. Meister, A., and Anderson, M. E. Glutathione. *Annu. Rev. Biochem.* 52: 711, 1983.
540. Mela-Riker, L. M., Widener, L. L., Houghton, D. C., and Bennett, W. M. Renal mitochondrial integrity during continuous gentamicin treatment. *Biochem. Pharmacol.* 35: 979, 1986.
541. Mellgren, R. L. Calcium-dependent proteases: An enzyme system active at cellular membranes. *FASEB J.* 1: 110, 1987.
542. Mengel, H., and Karlog, O. Studies on the interaction and distribution of selenite, mercuric, methoxyethyl mercuric and methyl mercuric chloride in rats. II. Analysis of the soluble proteins and the precipitates of liver and kidney homogenates. *Acta Pharmacol. Toxicol.* 46: 25, 1980.
543. Messana, J. M., Cieslinski, D. A., Nguyen, V. D., and Humes, H. D. Comparison of the toxicity of radiocontrast agents, iopamidol and diatrizoate, to rabbit proximal tubule cells in vitro. *J. Pharmacol. Exp. Ther.* 3: 1139, 1988.
544. Messana, J. M., Cieslinski, D. A., O'Connor, R. P., and Humes, H. D. Glutathione protects against exogenous oxidant injury to rabbit renal proximal tubules. *Am. J. Physiol.* 255: F874, 1988.
545. Meyer-Lehnert, H., and Schrier, R. W. Potential mechanism of cyclosporin A-induced vascular smooth muscle contraction. *Hypertension* 13: 352, 1989.
546. Miccadei, S., Kyle, M. E., Gilfor, D., and Farber, J. L. Toxic consequence of the abrupt depletion of glutathione in cultured rat hepatocytes. *Arch. Biochem. Biophys.* 265: 311, 1988.
547. Michael, U. F., Logan, J. L., and Meeks, L. A. The beneficial effects of thyroxine on nephrotoxic acute renal failure in the rat. *J. Am. Soc. Nephrol.* 1: 1236, 1991.
548. Michell, R. H., Allan, D., Bowley, M., and Brindley, D. N. A possible metabolic explanation for drug-induced phospholipidosis. *J. Pharm. Pharmacol.* 28: 331, 1976.
549. Min, K. S., Hatta, A., Onosaka, S., Ohta, N., Okada, Y., and Tanaka, K. Protective role of renal metallothionein against Cd nephropathy in rats. *Toxicol. Appl. Pharmacol.* 88: 294, 1987.
550. Mingeot-Leclercq, M. P., Laurent, G., and Tulkens, P. M. Biochemical mechanism of aminoglycoside-induced inhibition of phosphatidylcholine hydrolysis by lysosomal phospholipases. *Biochem. Pharmacol.* 37: 591, 1988.
551. Mirabelli, F., Salis, A., Vairetti, M., Bellomo, G., Thor, H., and Orrenius, S. Cytoskeletal alterations in human platelets exposed to oxidative stress are mediated by oxidative and Ca^{2+}-dependent mechanisms. *Arch. Biochem. Biophys.* 270: 478, 1989.
552. Misaka, E., and Tappel, A. L. Inhibition studies of cathepsins A, B, C and D from rat liver lysosomes. *Comp. Biochem. Physiol.* 38B: 651, 1971.
553. Missiaen, L., Wuytack, F., Raeymaekers, L., De Smedt, H., and Casteels, R. Polyamines and neomycin inhibit the purified plasma-membrane Ca^{2+} pump by interacting with associated polyphosphoinositides. *Biochem. J.* 261: 1055, 1989.
554. Mistry, P., Lee, C., and McBrien, D. C. Intracellular metabolites of cisplatin in the rat kidney. *Cancer Chemother. Pharmacol.* 24: 73, 1989.
555. Mitchell, J. R., McMurtry, R. J., Statham, C. N., and Nelson, S. D. Molecular basis for several drug-induced nephropathies. *Am. J. Med.* 62: 618, 1977.
556. Miyamoto, T., Ogino, N., Yamamoto, S., and Hayaishi, O. Purification of prostaglandin endoperoxide synthetase from bovine vesicular gland microsomes. *J. Biol. Chem.* 251: 2629, 1976.
557. Moffitt, A. E., and Clary, J. J. Selenite-induced binding of inorganic mercury in blood and other tissues in the rat. *Res. Commun. Chem. Pathol. Pharmacol.* 7: 593, 1974.
558. Mohandas, J., Duggin, G. G., Horvath, J. S., and Tiller, D. J. Metabolic oxidation of acetaminophen (paracetamol) mediated by cytochrome P-450 mixed function oxidase and prostaglandin endoperoxide synthetase in rabbit kidney. *Toxicol. Appl. Pharmacol.* 61: 252, 1981.
559. Mohandas, J., Marshall, J. J., Duggin, G. G., Hovarth, J. S., and Tiller, D. J. Differential distribution of glutathione and glutathione-related enzymes in rabbit kidney. Possible implications in analgesic nephropathy. *Biochem. Pharmacol.* 33: 1801, 1984.
560. Moldeus, P., Ormstad, K., and Reed, D. J. Turnover of cellular glutathione in isolated rat-kidney cells. Role of cystine and methionine. *Eur. J. Biochem.* 116: 13, 1981.
561. Molitoris, B. A. Gentamicin (G) inhibits protein (P) and phospholipid (PL) synthesis and translocation to the apical membrane. *Kidney Int.* 37: 490, 1990. (Abstract.)
562. Molitoris, B. A., Falk, S. A., and Dahl, R. H. Ischemia-induced loss of epithelial polarity. Role of the tight junction. *J. Clin. Invest.* 84: 1334, 1989.
563. Molitoris, B. A., Hoilien, C. A., Dahl, R., Ahnen, D. J., Wilson, P. D., and Kim, J. Characterization of ischemia-induced loss of epithelial polarity. *J. Membr. Biol.* 106: 233, 1988.
564. Molitoris, B. A., and Nelson, W. J. Alterations in the establishment and maintenance of epithelial cell polarity as a basis for disease processes. *J. Clin. Invest.* 85: 3, 1990.
565. Molitoris, B. A., Wilson, P. D., Schrier, R. W., and Simon, F. R. Ischemia induces partial loss of surface membrane polarity and accumulation of putative calcium ionophores. *J. Clin. Invest.* 76: 2097, 1985.

566. Mondorf, A., Brier, J., Hendus, J., Scherberich, J. D., Mackenrodt, G., Shah, P. M., Stille, W., and Schoeppe, W. Effect of aminoglycosides on proximal tubular membranes of the human kidney. *Eur. J. Clin. Pharmacol.* 13: 133, 1978.
567. Mondorf, A. W., Scherberich, J. E., Falkenberg, F. W., Sachse, H. J., Gauh, C., and Schoeppe, W. Brush Border Enzymes and Drug Nephrotoxicity. In K. Solez and A. Whelton (eds.), *Acute Renal Failure: Correlations Between Morphology and Function*. New York: Marcel Dekker, 1983. P. 179.
568. Monks, T. J., Anders, M. W., Dekant, W., Stevens, J. L., Lau, S. S., and Van Bladeren, P. J. Glutathione conjugate mediated toxicities. *Toxicol. Appl. Pharmacol.* 106: 1, 1990.
569. Monks, T. J., Highet, R. J., and Lau, S. S. 2-Bromo-(diglutathion-S-yl)hydroquinone nephrotoxicity: Physiological, biochemical, and electrochemical determinants. *Mol. Pharmacol.* 34: 492, 1988.
570. Monks, T. J., Highet, R. J., and Lau, S. S. Oxidative cyclization, 1,4-benzothiazine formation and dimerization of 2-bromo-3-(glutathion-S-yl)hydroquinone. *Mol. Pharmacol.* 38: 121, 1990.
571. Monks, T. J., and Lau, S. S. Glutathione, gamma-glutamyl transpeptidase, and the mercapturic acid pathway as modulators of 2-bromohydroquinone oxidation. *Toxicol. Appl. Pharmacol.* 103: 557, 1990.
572. Monks, T. J., Lau, S. S., Highet, R. J., and Gillette, J. R. Glutathione conjugates of 2-bromohydroquinone are nephrotoxic. *Drug Metab. Dispos.* 13: 553, 1985.
573. Monroe, D. M., Sherrill, G. B., and Roberts, H. R. Use of *p*-aminobenzamidine to monitor activation of trypsin-like serine proteases. *Anal. Biochem.* 172: 427, 1988.
574. Montine, T. J., and Borch, R. F. Quiescent LLC-PK_1 cells as a model for *cis*-diamminedichloroplatinum(II) nephrotoxicity and modulation by thiol rescue agents. *Cancer Res.* 48: 6017, 1988.
575. Montine, T. J., and Borch, R. F. Role of endogenous sulfur-containing nucleophiles in an in vitro model of cis-diamminedichloroplatinum(II)-induced nephrotoxicity. *Biochem. Pharmacol.* 39: 1751, 1990.
576. Moore, G. A., Jewell, S. A., Bellomo, G., et al. On the relationship between Ca^{2+} efflux and membrane damage during t-butyl hydroperoxide metabolism by liver mitochondria. *FEBS Lett.* 153: 289, 1983.
577. Moore, L. Inhibition of liver-microsome calcium pump by in vivo administration of CCl_4, $CHCl_3$ and 1,1-dichloroethylene (vinylidene chloride). *Biochem. Pharmacol.* 29: 2505, 1980.
578. Moore, L., Davenport, G. R., and Landon, E. J. Calcium uptake of a rat liver microsomal subcellular fraction in response to in vivo administration of carbon tetrachloride. *J. Biol. Chem.* 251: 1197, 1976.
579. Mooseker, M. S., Conzelman, K. A., Coleman, T. R., Heuser, J. E., and Sheetz, M. P. Characterization of intestinal microvillar membrane disks: Detergent-resistant membrane sheets enriched in associated brush border myosin I (110K-calmodulin). *J. Cell Biol.* 109: 1153, 1989.
580. Morgan, M., Dettmer, R., Liuzzo, J., Johnson, R., Safirstein, R., and Goligorsky, M. S. Mechanisms of oxidative stress-induced proliferative response (PR) in renal tubular cells. *Kidney Int.* 37: 490, 1990. (Abstract.)
581. Mori, Y., Iesato, K., Ueda, S., Wakashin, Y., Wakashin, M., Iwasaki, I., and Okuda, K. [Heavy metal nephropathy induced by tributyltin oxide (author's transl.)]. *Nippon Jinzo Gakkai Shi* 23: 89, 1981.
582. Morin, J. P., Fresel, J., Fillastre, J. P., and Vaillant, R. Aminoglycoside Actions on Rat Kidney Lysosomes "in Vivo" and "in Vitro." In J. P. Fillastre (ed.), *Nephrotoxicity: Interactions of Drugs with Membrane Systems, Mitochondria, Lysosomes*. New York: Masson, 1978. P. 253.
583. Morin, J. P., Viotte, G., Vanderwulle, A., VanHoff, F., Tulkeny, P., and Fillastre, J. P. Gentamicin induced nephrotoxicity: A cell biology approach. *Kidney Int.* 18: 583, 1980.
584. Morrison, A. R., Pascoe, N., Tank, N., and Kennerly, D. Biochemical alterations of membrane lipids associated with renal injury. *Fed. Proc.* 43: 2811, 1984.
585. Morrow, J. S., Cianci, C. D., Ardito, T., Mann, A. S., and Kashgarian, M. Ankyrin links fodrin to the alpha subunit of Na,K-ATPase in Madin-Darby canine kidney cells and in intact renal tubule cells. *J. Cell Biol.* 108: 455, 1989.
586. Murachi, T. Intracellular regulatory system involving calpain and calpistatin. *Biochem. Int.* 18: 263, 1989.
587. Murachi, T., Hatanaka, M., Yasumoto, Y., Nakayama, N., and Tanaka, K. A quantitative distribution study on calpain and calpastatin in rat tissues and cells. *Biochem. Int.* 2: 651, 1981.
588. Nadler, S., and Goldfischer, S. The intracellular release of lysosomal contents in macrophages that have ingested silica. *J. Histochem. Cytochem.* 18: 368, 1970.
589. Naganuma, A., Anderson, M. E., and Meister, A. Cellular glutathione as a determinant of sensitivity to mercuric chloride toxicity: Prevention of toxicity by giving glutathione monoester. *Biochem. Pharmacol.* 40: 693, 1990.
590. Naganuma, A., Satoh, M., and Imura, N. Prevention of lethal and renal toxicity of cis-diamminedichloroplatinum(II) by induction of metallothionein synthesis without compromising its antitumor activity in mice. *Cancer Res.* 47: 983, 1987.
591. Naganuma, A., Satoh, M., Koyama, Y., and Imura, N. Protective effect of metallothionein inducing metals on lethal toxicity of cis-diamminedichloroplatinum in mice. *Toxicol. Lett.* 24: 203, 1985.
592. Nakamoto, M., Shapiro, J. I., Chan, L., Shanley, P., and Schrier, R. W. In vitro and in vivo protective effects of atriopeptin III in ischemic acute renal failure. *J. Clin. Invest.* 80: 698, 1987.
593. Nash, J. A., King, L. J., Lock, E. A., and Green, T. The metabolism and disposition of hexachloro-1:3-butadiene in the rat and its relevance to nephrotoxicity. *Toxicol. Appl. Pharmacol.* 73: 124, 1984.
594. Nassberger, L., Bergstrand, A., and DePierre, J. W. Intracellular distribution of gentamicin within the rat kidney cortex: A cell fractionation study. *Exp. Mol. Pathol.* 52: 212, 1990.
595. New, P. S., Lubash, G. D., Scherr, L., and Rubin, A. L. Acute renal failure associated with carbon tetrachloride intoxication. *J.A.M.A.* 181: 903, 1962.
596. Newton, J. F., Kuo, C. H., Gemborys, M. W., Mudge, G. H., and Hook, J. B. Nephrotoxicity of *p*-aminophenol, a metabolite of acetaminophen, in the Fischer 344 rat. *Toxicol. Appl. Pharmacol.* 65: 336, 1982.
597. Ngaha, E. O., and Ogunleye, I. O. Studies on gentamicin-induced labilization of rat kidney lysosomes in vitro. Possible protection by selenium. *Biochem. Pharmacol.* 32: 2659, 1983.
598. Nicchitta, C. V., and Williamson, J. R. Spermine. A regulator of mitochondrial calcium cycling. *J. Biol. Chem.* 259: 12978, 1984.
599. Nicotera, P., Bellomo, G., and Orrenius, S. The role of Ca^{2+} in cell killing. *Chem. Res. Toxicol.* 3: 484, 1990.
600. Nicotera, P., Hartzell, P., Baldi, C., Svensson, S.-A.,

Bellomo, G., and Orrenius, S. Cystamine induces toxicity in hepatocytes through the elevation of cytosolic Ca^{2+} and the stimulation of a nonlysosomal proteolytic system. *J. Biol. Chem.* 261: 14628, 1986.

601. Nicotera, P., Hartzell, P., Davis, G., and Orrenius, S. The formation of plasma membrane blebs in hepatocytes exposed to agents that increase cytosolic Ca^{2+} is mediated by the activation of a nonlysosomal proteolytic system. *FEBS Lett.* 209: 139, 1986.
602. Nieminen, A.-L., Gores, G. J., Dawson, T. L., Herman, B., and Lemasters, J. J. Toxic injury from mercuric chloride in rat hepatocytes. *J. Biol. Chem.* 265: 2399, 1990.
603. Nieminen, A.-L., Gores, G. J., Wray, B. E., Tanaka, Y., Herman, B., and Lemasters, J. J. Calcium dependence of bleb formation and cell death in hepatocytes. *Cell Calcium* 9: 237, 1988.
604. Niggli, V., and Burger, M. M. Interaction of the cytoskeleton with plasma membrane. *J. Membr. Biol.* 100: 97, 1987.
605. Nishiyama, S., Taguchi, T., and Onosaka, S. Induction of zinc-thionein by estradiol and protective effects on inorganic mercury-induced renal toxicity. *Biochem. Pharmacol.* 36: 3387, 1987.
606. Noel, J., Tejedor, A., Vinay, P., Laprade, R., and Gougoux, A. BBM H^+-ATPase activity in the dog kidney: Modulation by substrate availability. *Kidney Int.* 37: 529, 1990. (Abstract.)
607. Noel, P., and Levy, V. G. Toxicite renale de l'association gentamicin-furosemide. *Nouv. Presse Med.* 7: 351, 1978.
608. Noll, T., and deGroot, H. The critical steady-state hypoxic conditions in carbon tetrachloride-induced lipid peroxidation in rat liver microsomes. *Biochim. Biophys. Acta* 795: 356, 1984.
609. Nonclercq, D., Toubeau, G., Laurent, G., Tulkens, P. M., and Heuson-Stiennon, J. A. Tissue injury and repair in the rat kidney after exposure to cisplatin or carboplatin. *Exp. Mol. Pathol.* 51: 123, 1989.
610. Nordberg, G. F., Goyer, R., and Nordberg, M. Comparative toxicity of cadmium-metallothionein and cadmium chloride on mouse kidney. *Arch. Pathol.* 99: 192, 1975.
611. Norman, J., Tsau, Y.-K., Bacay, A., and Fine, L. G. Epidermal growth factor accelerates functional recovery from ischaemic acute tubular necrosis in the rat: Role of the epidermal growth factor receptor. *Clin. Sci.* 78: 445, 1990.
612. Norseth, T. The intracellular distribution of mercury in rat liver after a single injection of mercuric chloride. *Biochem. Pharmacol.* 17: 581, 1968.
613. Odum, J., and Green, T. The metabolism and nephrotoxicity of tetrafluoroethylene in the rat. *Toxicol. Appl. Pharmacol.* 76: 306, 1984.
614. Ogura, Y., and Yamazaki, I. Steady-state kinetics of the catalase reaction in the presence of cyanide. *J. Biochem. (Tokyo)* 94: 403, 1983.
615. Olbricht, J. C., Fink, M., and Gutjahr, E. Alterations in lysosomal enzymes of the proximal tubule in gentamicin nephrotoxicity. *Kidney Int.* 39: 639, 1991.
616. Olsen, S., Burdick, J. F., Keown, P. A., Wallace, A. C., Racusen, L. C., and Solez, K. Primary acute renal failure ("acute tubular necrosis") in the transplanted kidney: Morphology and pathogenesis. *Medicine (Baltimore)* 68: 173, 1989.
617. Orrenius, S., and Nicotera, P. On the role of calcium in chemical toxicity. *Arch. Toxicol. Suppl.* 11: 11, 1987.
618. Ozaki, H., Satoh, T., Karaki, H., and Ishida, Y. Regulation of metabolism and contraction by cytoplasmic calcium in the intestinal smooth muscle. *J. Biol. Chem.* 263: 14074, 1988.
619. Ozols, R. F., Corden, B. J., Jacob, J., Wesley, M. N., Ostchega, Y., and Young, R. C. High dose cisplatin in hypertonic saline. *Ann. Intern. Med.* 100: 19, 1984.
620. Pabico, R. C., Atanacio, B. C., McKenna, B. A., Pamukcoglu, T., and Yodaiken, R. Renal pathologic lesions and functional alterations in a man with Fabry's disease. *Am. J. Med.* 55: 415, 1973.
621. Paller, M. S. Hemoglobin- and myoglobin-induced acute renal failure in rats: Role of iron in nephrotoxicity. *Am. J. Physiol.* 255: F539, 1988.
622. Paller, M. S., Hoidal, J. R., and Ferris, T. F. Oxygen free radicals in ischemic acute renal failure in the rat. *J. Clin. Invest.* 74: 1156, 1984.
623. Paller, M. S., Schnaith, E. J., and Rosenberg, M. E. ATP enhances recovery from renal ischemia by stimulating cellular proliferation. *J. Am. Soc. Nephrol.* 1: 601, 1990. (Abstract.)
624. Parce, J. W., Cunningham, C. C., and Waite, M. Mitochondrial phospholipase A_2 activity and mitochondrial aging. *Biochemistry* 17: 1634, 1978.
625. Parce, J. W., Spach, P. I., and Cunningham, C. C. Deterioration of rat liver mitochondria under conditions of metabolite deprivation. *Biochem. J.* 188: 817, 1980.
626. Parkes, C., Kembhavi, A. A., and Barrett, A. J. Calpain inhibition by peptide epoxides. *Biochem. J.* 230: 509, 1985.
627. Pascoe, G. A., and Reed, D. J. Cell calcium, vitamin E, and the thiol redox system in cytotoxicity. *Free Radic. Biol. Med.* 6: 209, 1989.
628. Passow, H., Rothstein, A., and Clarkson, T. W. The general pharmacology of the heavy metals. *Pharmacol. Rev.* 13: 185, 1961.
629. Pastoriza-Munoz, E., Bowman, R. L., and Kaloyanides, G. J. Renal tubular transport of gentamicin in the rat. *Kidney Int.* 16: 440, 1979.
630. Penttila, A., Glaumann, H., and Trump, B. F. Studies on the modification of the cellular response to injury. IV. Protective effect of extracellular acidosis against anoxia, thermal, and p-chloromercuribenzene sulfonic acid treatment of isolated rat liver cells. *Life Sci.* 18: 1419, 1976.
631. Penttila, A., and Trump, B. F. Extracellular acidosis protects Ehrlich ascites tumor cells and rat renal cortex against anoxic injury. *Science* 185: 277, 1974.
632. Perrissoud, D., Auderset, G., Reymond, O., and Maignan, M. F. The effect of carbon tetrachloride on isolated rat hepatocytes. *Virchows Arch B [Cell Pathol.]* 35: 83, 1981.
633. Pfaller, W., Gunther, R., and Silbernagl, S. Pathogenesis of $HgCl_2$ and maleate induced acute renal failure. *Pfluegers Arch.* 379: R18, 1979.
634. Pfaller, W., and Rittinger, M. Quantitative morphology of the rat kidney. *Int. J. Biochem.* 12: 17, 1980.
635. Pfeiffer, D. R., Schmid, P. C., Beatrice, M. C., and Schmid, H. H. O. Intramitochondrial phospholipase activity and the effects of Ca^{2+} plus N-ethylmaleimide on mitochondrial function. *J. Biol. Chem.* 254: 11485, 1979.
636. Phelps, J. S., Gandolfi, A. J., Brendel, K., and Dorr, R. T. Cisplatin nephrotoxicity: In vitro studies with precision-cut rabbit renal cortical slices. *Toxicol. Appl. Pharmacol.* 90: 501, 1987.
637. Phelps, P. C., Smith, M. W., and Trump, B. F. Cytosolic ionized calcium and bleb formation after acute cell injury of cultured rabbit renal tubule cells. *Lab. Invest.* 60: 630, 1989.
638. Pickett, C. B., and Lu, A. Y. H. Glutathione S-transfer-

ases: Gene structure, regulation, and biological function. *Annu. Rev. Biochem.* 58: 743, 1989.

639. Pittinger, C., and Adamson, R. Antibiotic blockage of neuromuscular function. *Annu. Rev. Pharmacol.* 12: 169, 1972.
640. Plantavid, M., Chap, H., Lloveras, J., and Douste-Blazy, L. Cationic amphiphilic drugs as a potential tool for modifying phospholipids of tumor cells. An in vitro study of chlorpromazine effects on Krebs II ascites cells. *Biochem. Pharmacol.* 30: 293, 1981.
641. Plummer, D., and Ngaha, E. Urinary Enzymes as an Index of Kidney Damage by Toxic Compounds. In J. P. Fillastre (ed.), *Nephrotoxicity: Interaction of Drugs with Membrane Systems, Mitochondrial, Lysosomes.* New York: Masson, 1978. P. 175.
642. Pohl, L. R., Branchflower, R. V., Highet, R. J., Martin, J. L., Nunn, D. S., Monks, T. J., George, J. W., and Hinson, J. A. The formation of diglutathionyl dithiocarbonate as a metabolite of chloroform, bromotrichloromethane, and carbon tetrachloride. *Drug. Metab. Dispos.* 9: 334, 1981.
643. Pohl, L. R., Martin, J. L., and George, J. W. Mechanism of metabolic activation of chloroform by rat liver microsomes. *Biochem. Pharmacol.* 29: 3271, 1980.
644. Poli, G., and Gravela, E. Lipid Peroxidation in Isolated Hepatocytes. In D. C. H. McBrien and T. F. Slater (eds.), *Free Radicals, Lipid Peroxidation and Cancer.* London: Academic Press, 1982. P. 215.
645. Potter, S., and Matrone, G. Effect of selenite on the toxicity of dietary methyl mercury and mercuric chloride in the rat. *J. Nutr.* 104: 638, 1974.
646. Powell, J. H., and Reidenberg, M. M. In vitro response of rat and human kidney lysosomes to aminoglycosides. *Biochem. Pharmacol.* 31: 3447, 1982.
647. Powell, J. H., and Reidenberg, M. M. Further studies of the response of kidney lysosomes to aminoglycosides and other cations. *Biochem. Pharmacol.* 32: 3213, 1983.
648. Pratt, I. S., and Lock, E. A. Deacetylation and further metabolism of the mercapturic acid of hexachloro-1,3-butadiene by rat kidney cytosol in vitro. *Arch. Toxicol.* 62: 341, 1988.
649. Prough, R. A., and Ziegler, D. M. The relative participation of liver microsomal amine oxidases and cytochrome P-450 in N-demethylation reactions. *Arch. Biochem. Biophys.* 180: 363, 1977.
650. Pryor, W. A. On the detection of lipid hydroperoxides in biological samples. *Free Radic. Biol. Med.* 7: 177, 1989.
651. Pulliam, J. P., Houghton, D. C., and Bennett, W. M. High calcium intake does not protect against mercuric chloride-induced acute renal failure. *Kidney Int.* 25: 236, 1984.
652. Quarum, M. L., Houghton, D. C., Gilbert, D. N., McCarron, D. A., and Bennett, W. M. Increasing dietary calcium moderates experimental gentamicin nephrotoxicity. *J. Lab. Clin. Med.* 103: 104, 1984.
653. Racusen, L. C., Li, Y., Fivush, B., and Solez, K. Shedding of viable tabular cells (TC) into the urine in experimental "acute tabular necrosis" (ATN). *Kidney Int.* 35: 416, 1989. (Abstract.)
654. Ramsammy, L., Josepovitz, C., Lane, B., and Kaloyanides, G. J. Polyaspartic acid inhibits gentamicin-induced perturbations of phospholipid metabolism. *Am. J. Physiol. Cell Physiol.* 258: C1141, 1990.
655. Ramsammy, L. S., Josepovitz, C., Jones, D., Ling, K. Y., Lane, B. P., and Kaloyanides, G. J. Induction of nephrotoxicity by high doses of gentamicin in diabetic rats. *Proc. Soc. Exp. Biol. Med.* 186: 306, 1987.
656. Ramsammy, L. S., Josepovitz, C., and Kaloyanides, G. J. Gentamicin inhibits agonist stimulation of the phosphatidylinositol cascade in primary cultures of rabbit proximal tubular cells and in rat renal cortex. *J. Pharmacol. Exp. Ther.* 247: 989, 1988.
657. Ramsammy, L. S., Josepovitz, C., Lane, B., and Kaloyanides, G. J. Effect of gentamicin on phospholipid metabolism in cultured rabbit proximal tubular cells. *Am. J. Physiol.* 256: C204, 1989.
658. Ramsammy, L. S., Josepovitz, C., Lane, B. P., and Kaloyanides, G. J. Polyaspartic acid protects against gentamicin nephrotoxicity in the rat. *J. Pharmacol. Exp. Ther.* 250: 149, 1989.
659. Ramsammy, L. S., Josepovitz, C., Ling, K. Y., Lane, B. P., and Kaloyanides, G. J. Effects of diphenylphenylenediamine on gentamicin-induced lipid peroxidation and toxicity in rat renal cortex. *J. Pharmacol. Exp. Ther.* 238: 83, 1986.
660. Ramsammy, L. S., Josepovitz, C., Ling, K. Y., Lane, B. P., and Kaloyanides, G. J. Failure of inhibition of lipid peroxidation by vitamin E to protect against gentamicin nephrotoxicity in the rat. *Biochem. Pharmacol.* 36: 2125, 1987.
661. Ramsammy, L. S., and Kaloyanides, G. J. Effect of gentamicin on the transition temperature and permeability to glycerol of phosphatidylinositol-containing liposomes. *Biochem. Pharmacol.* 36: 1179, 1987.
662. Ramsammy, L. S., and Kaloyanides, G. J. The effect of gentamicin on the biophysical properties of phosphatidic acid liposomes is influenced by the O-C=O group of the lipid. *Biochemistry* 27: 8249, 1988.
663. Randall, R. V., and Seeler, A. O. BAL. *N. Engl. J. Med.* 239: 1004, 1948.
664. Ray, P., and Moore, L. 1,1-Dichloroethylene inhibition of liver microsomal calcium pump in vitro. *Arch. Biochem. Biophys.* 218: 26, 1982.
665. Rechsteiner, M. Ubiquitin-mediated pathways for intracellular proteolysis. *Annu. Rev. Cell Biol.* 3: 1, 1987.
666. Recknagel, R. O. A new direction in the study of carbon tetrachloride hepatotoxicity. *Life Sci.* 33: 401, 1983.
667. Recknagel, R. O., and Glende, E. A. Carbon tetrachloride hepatotoxicity: An example of lethal cleavage. *CRC Crit. Rev. Toxicol.* 2: 263, 1973.
668. Reeves, J. P. Accumulation of amino acids by lysosomes incubated with amino acid methyl esters. *J. Biol. Chem.* 254: 8914, 1979.
669. Reeves, J. P., and Reames, T. ATP stimulates amino acid accumulation by lysosomes incubated with amino acids methyl esters. *J. Biol. Chem.* 256: 6047, 1981.
670. Regec, A. L., Trump, B. F., and Trifillis, A. L. Effect of gentamicin on the lysosomal system of cultured human proximal tubular cells. Endocytotic activity, lysosomal pH and membrane fragility. *Biochem. Pharmacol.* 38: 2527, 1989.
671. Reynolds, E. S., Tannen, R. L., and Tyler, H. R. The renal lesion in Wilson's disease. *Am. J. Med.* 40: 518, 1966.
672. Rifkin, R. J. In vitro inhibition of Na^+-K^+ and Mg^{2+} ATPases by mono, di, and trivalent cations. *Proc. Soc. Exp. Biol. Med.* 120: 802, 1965.
673. Riley, M. V., and Lehninger, A. L. Changes in sulfhydryl groups of rat liver mitochondria during swelling and contraction. *J. Biol. Chem.* 239: 2083, 1964.
674. Rodeheaver, D. P., and Schnellmann, R. G. Extracellular acidosis ameliorates metabolic inhibitor-induced and potentiates oxidative-induced cell death in rabbit renal proximal tubules (RPT). *Kidney Int.* 37: 493, 1990. (Abstract.)

675. Rodeheaver, D. P., and Schnellmann, R. G. Mechanism of pH amelioration of 2-bromohydroquinone-induced toxicity to rabbit renal proximal tubules. *J. Pharmacol. Exp. Ther.* 256: 917, 1991.
676. Rodman, J. S., Seidman, L., and Farquhar, M. G. The membrane composition of coated pits, microvilli, endosomes, and lysosomes is distinctive in the rat kidney proximal tubule cell. *J. Cell Biol.* 102: 77, 1986.
677. Rogulski, J., Strzelecki, T., and Pacanis, A. Effects of Maleate on Renal Carbohydrate Metabolism in Vivo and in Vitro. In S. Angielski and V. C. Dubach (eds.), *Biochemical Aspects of Renal Function*. Bern: Huber, 1975. P. 106.
678. Romson, J. L., Hook, B. G., Kunkel, S. L., Abrams, G. D., Schork, M. A., and Lucchesi, B. R. Reduction of the extent of ischemic myocardial injury by neutrophil depletion in the dog. *Circulation* 67: 1016, 1983.
679. Rose, D. W., Welch, W. J., Kramer, G., and Hardesty, B. Possible involvement of the 90-kDa heat shock protein in the regulation of protein synthesis. *J. Biol. Chem.* 264: 6239, 1989.
680. Rosenberg, B. Platinum analysis. *Biochimie* 60: 859, 1978.
681. Ross, D., Cotgreave, I., and Moldeus, P. The interaction of reduced glutathione with active oxygen species generated by xanthine-oxidase-catalyzed metabolism of xanthine. *Biochim. Biophys. Acta* 841: 278, 1985.
682. Rossi, C. S., and Lehninger, A. L. Stoichiometry of respiratory stimulation, accumulation of Ca^{2+} and phosphate, and oxidative phosphorylation in rat liver mitochondria. *J. Biol. Chem.* 239: 3971, 1964.
683. Rothstein, A. Sulfhydryl groups in cell membrane structure and function. *Curr. Top. Membr. Transp.* 1: 135, 1970.
684. Rothstein, A., and Mack, E. Actions of mercurials on cell volume regulation of dissociated MDCK cells. *Am. J. Physiol. Cell Physiol.* 260: C113, 1991.
685. Rouslin, W. Protonic inhibition of the mitochondrial oligomycin-sensitive adenosine 5′-triphosphatase in ischemic and autolyzing cardiac muscle. Possible mechanism for the mitigation of ATP hydrolysis under nonenergizing conditions. *J. Biol. Chem.* 258: 9657, 1983.
686. Rush, G. F., Maita, K., Sleight, S. D., and Hook, J. B. Induction of rabbit renal mixed-function oxidases by phenobarbital: Cell specific ultrastructural changes in the proximal tubule. *Proc. Soc. Exp. Biol. Med.* 172: 430, 1983.
687. Rush, G. F., and Ponsier, G. D. Cephaloridine-induced biochemical changes and cytotoxicity in suspensions of rabbit isolated proximal tubules. *Toxicol. Appl. Pharmacol.* 109: 314, 1991.
688. Rush, G. F., Smith, J. H., Newton, J. F., and Hook, J. B. Chemically induced nephrotoxicity: Role of metabolic activation. *CRC Crit. Rev. Toxicol.* 13: 99, 1984.
689. Russell, J. H., and Dobos, C. B. Mechanisms of immune lysis. II. CTL-induced nuclear disintegration of the target begins within minutes of cell contact. *J. Immunol.* 125: 1256, 1980.
690. Ryan, R., McNeil, J. S., Flamenbaum, W., and Nagle, R. Uranyl nitrate induced acute renal failure in the rat: Effect of varying doses and saline loading. *Proc. Soc. Exp. Biol. Med.* 143: 289, 1973.
691. Safirstein, R., Miller, P., and Guttenplan, J. B. Uptake and metabolism of cisplatin by rat kidney. *Kidney Int.* 25: 753, 1984.
692. Sage, M. D., and Jennings, R. B. Alterations to subplasmalemmal leptomeres in adult canine myocytes during total in vitro ischemia. *Lab. Invest.* 61: 171, 1989.
693. Sahaphong, S., and Trump, B. F. Studies of cellular injury in isolated kidney tubules of the flounder. V. Effects of inhibiting sulfhydryl groups of plasma membrane with the organic mercurials, parachloromercuribenzoate and parachloromercuribenzenesulfonate. *Am. J. Pathol.* 63: 277, 1971.
694. Saito, H., Inui, K., and Hori, R. Mechanisms of gentamicin transport in kidney epithelial cell line (LLC-PK1). *J. Pharmacol. Exp. Ther.* 238: 1071, 1986.
695. Sakaida, I., Thomas, A. P., and Farber, J. L. Increases in cytosolic calcium ion concentration can be dissociated from the killing of cultured hepatocytes by *tert*-butyl hydroperoxide. *J. Biol. Chem.* 266: 717, 1991.
696. Samuni, A., Aronovitch, J., Godinger, D., Chevion, M., and Czapski, G. On the cytotoxicity of vitamin C and metal ions. A site-specific Fenton mechanism. *Eur. J. Biochem.* 137: 119, 1983.
697. Sandvig, K., Oisnes, S., Peterson, O. W., and van Deurs, B. Inhibition of endocytosis from coated pits by acidification of the cytosol. *J. Cell. Biochem.* 36: 73, 1988.
698. Sanger, J. W., and Sanger, J. M. Differential response of three types of actin filament bundles to depletion of cellular ATP levels. *Eur. J. Cell Biol.* 31: 197, 1983.
699. Sasame, H. A., and Boyd, M. R. Paradoxical effects of cobaltous chloride and salts of other divalent metals on tissue levels of reduced glutathione and microsomal mixed-function oxidase components. *J. Pharmacol. Exp. Ther.* 205: 718, 1978.
700. Sastrasinh, M., Knauss, T. C., Weinberg, J. M., and Humes, H. D. Identification of the aminoglycoside receptor of renal brush border membranes. *J. Pharmacol. Exp. Ther.* 222: 350, 1982.
701. Sastrasinh, M., Weinberg, J. M., and Humes, H. D. The effect of gentamicin on calcium uptake by renal mitochondria. *Life Sci.* 30: 2309, 1982.
702. Sato, M., and Nagai, Y. Mode of existence of cadmium in rat liver and kidney after prolonged subcutaneous administration. *Toxicol. Appl. Pharmacol.* 54: 90, 1980.
703. Sato, M., and Nagai, Y. Cadmium in rat kidney subcellular particles after injection of cadmium-metallothionein. *J. Toxicol. Sci.* 11: 29, 1986.
704. Satoh, M., Naganuma, A., and Imura, N. Deficiency of selenium intake enhances manifestation of renal toxicity of cis-diamminedichloroplatinum in mice. *Toxicol. Lett.* 38: 155, 1987.
705. Satoh, M., Naganuma, A., and Imura, N. Metallothionein induction prevents toxic side effects of cisplatin and Adriamycin used in combination. *Cancer Chemother. Pharmacol.* 21: 176, 1988.
706. Satoh, M., Naganuma, A., and Imura, N. Optimum schedule of selenium administration to reduce lethal and renal toxicities of cis-diamminedichloroplatinum in mice. *J. Pharmacobiodyn.* 12: 246, 1989.
707. Sawaya, B. P., Weihprecht, H., Campbell, W. R., Lorenz, J. N., Webb, R. C., Briggs, J. P., and Schnermann, J. Direct vasoconstriction as a possible cause for amphotericin-B-induced nephrotoxicity in rats. *J. Clin. Invest.* 87: 2097, 1991.
708. Sawyer, D. T., and Valentine, J. S. How super is superoxide? *Acc. Chem. Res.* 14: 393, 1981.
709. Scaduto, R. C., Jr., Gattone, V. H., II, Grotyohann, L. W., Wertz, J., and Martin, L. F. Effect of an altered glutathione content on renal ischemic injury. *Am. J. Physiol.* 255: F911, 1988.
710. Schafer, J. A., and Williams, J. C. Transport of metabolic substrates by the proximal nephron. *Annu. Rev. Physiol.* 47: 103, 1985.
711. Schafferhans, K., Heidbreder, E., Sperber, S., Damm-

rich, J., and Heidland, A. Atrial natriuretic peptide in gentamicin-induced acute renal failure. *Kidney Int.* 34: S101, 1988.
712. Scharer, K., Yoshida, T., Voyer, L., Berlow, S., Pietra, G., and Metcalf, J. Impaired renal gluconeogenesis and energy metabolism in maleic acid-induced nephropathy in rats. *Res. Exp. Med.* 157: 136, 1972.
713. Schefferhans, K., Heidbreder, E., Schmatz, R., and Heidland, A. Atrial natriuretic peptide protects against gentamicin-induced acute renal failure in the rat. *Kidney Int.* 33: 366, 1988.
714. Schieppati, A., Wilson, P. D., Burke, T. J., and Schrier, R. W. Effect of renal ischemia on cortical microsomal calcium accumulation. *Am. J. Physiol.* 249: C476, 1985.
715. Schneider, D. L. ATP-dependent acidification of intact and disrupted lysosomes. *J. Biol. Chem.* 256: 3858, 1981.
716. Schneider, P. B., and Kennedy, E. P. Sphingomyelinase in normal human spleens and in spleens from subjects with Niemann-Pick disease. *J. Lipid Res.* 8: 202, 1967.
717. Schnellmann, R. G. Mechanisms of t-butyl hydroperoxide-induced toxicity to rabbit renal proximal tubules. *Am. J. Physiol.* 255: C28, 1988.
718. Schnellmann, R. G., Cross, T. J., and Lock, E. A. Pentachlorobutadienyl-L-cysteine uncouples oxidative phosphorylation by dissipating the proton gradient. *Toxicol. Appl. Pharmacol.* 100: 498, 1989.
719. Schnellmann, R. G., Ewell, F. P., Sgambati, M., and Mandel, L. J. Mitochondrial toxicity of 2-bromohydroquinone in rabbit renal proximal tubules. *Toxicol. Appl. Pharmacol.* 90: 420, 1987.
720. Schnellmann, R. G., Lock, E. A., and Mandel, L. J. A mechanism of S-(1,2,3,4,4-pentachloro-1,3-butadienyl)-L-cysteine toxicity to rabbit renal proximal tubules. *Toxicol. Appl. Pharmacol.* 90: 513, 1987.
721. Schraufstatter, I. U., Hinshaw, D. B., Hyslop, P. A., Spragg, R. G., and Cochrane, C. G. Oxidant injury of cells. DNA strand-breaks activate polyadenosine diphosphate-ribose polymerase and lead to depletion of nicotinamide adenine dinucleotide. *J. Clin. Invest.* 77: 1312, 1986.
722. Schraufstatter, I. U., Hyslop, P. A., Hinshaw, D. B., Spragg, R. G., Sklar, L. A., and Cochrane, C. G. Hydrogen peroxide-induced injury of cells and its prevention by inhibitors of poly(ADP-ribose) polymerase. *Proc. Natl. Acad. Sci. U.S.A.* 83: 4908, 1986.
723. Schreiber, J., Foureman, G. L., Hughes, M. F., Mason, R. P., and Eling, T. E. Detection of glutathione thiyl free radical catalyzed by prostaglandin H synthase present in keratinocytes. Study of cooxidation in a cellular system. *J. Biol. Chem.* 264: 7936, 1989.
724. Schrier, R. W., Arnold, P. E., Van Putten, V. J., and Burke, T. J. Cellular calcium in ischemic acute renal failure: Role of calcium entry blockers. *Kidney Int.* 32: 313, 1987.
725. Schulte-Wissermann, H., Straub, E., and Funke, P. J. Influence of L-thyroxin upon enzymatic activity in the renal tubular epithelium of the rat under normal conditions and in mercury-induced lesions. II. *Virchows Arch. B [Cell Pathol.]* 23: 175, 1977.
726. Schulte-Wissermann, H., Straub, E., and Funke, P. J. Influence of L-thyroxin upon enzymatic activity in the renal tubular epithelium of the rat under normal conditions and in mercury-induced lesions. I. *Virchows Arch. B [Cell Pathol.]* 23: 163, 1977.
727. Schurek, H-J., and Kriz, W. Morphologic and functional evidence for oxygen deficiency in the isolated perfused rat kidney. *Lab. Invest.* 53: 145, 1985.
728. Schurek, H. J., Jost, U., Baumgartl, H., Bertram, H., and Heckmann, U. Evidence for a preglomerular oxygen diffusion shunt in rat renal cortex. *Am. J. Physiol.* 259: F910, 1990.
729. Schwertz, D. W., Kreisberg, J. I., and Venkatachalam, M. A. Characterization of rat kidney proximal tubule brush border membrane associated phosphatidylinositol phosphodiesterase. *Arch. Biochem. Biophys.* 224: 555, 1983.
730. Schwertz, D. W., Kreisberg, J. I., and Venkatachalam, M. A. Effects of aminoglycosides on proximal tubule brush border membrane phosphatidylinositol-specific phospholipase C. *J. Pharmacol. Exp. Ther.* 231: 48, 1984.
731. Schwertz, D. W., Kreisberg, J. I., and Venkatachalam, M. A. Gentamicin-induced alterations in pig kidney epithelial (LLC-PK1) cells in culture. *J. Pharmacol. Exp. Ther.* 236: 254, 1986.
732. Scott, J. A., An Kaw, B., Locke, E., Haber, E., and Homey, C. The role of free radical-mediated processes in oxygen-related damage in cultured murine myocardial cells. *Circ. Res.* 56: 72, 1985.
733. Scott, L. A., Madan, E., and Valentovic, M. A. Attenuation of cisplatin nephrotoxicity by streptozotocin-induced diabetes. *Fundam. Appl. Toxicol.* 12: 530, 1989.
734. Scott, R. L., and Gamble, J. L., Jr. Effect of mercurial compounds on potassium binding by mitochondria. *J. Biol. Chem.* 236: 570, 1961.
735. Sekura, R., and Meister, A. Glutathione turnover in the kidney: Considerations relating to the gamma-glutamyl cycle and the transport of amino acids. *Proc. Natl. Acad. Sci. U.S.A.* 71: 2969, 1974.
736. Senekjian, H. O., Knight, T. F., and Weinman, E. J. Micropuncture study of the handling of gentamicin by the rat kidney. *Kidney Int.* 19: 416, 1981.
737. Sevanian, A., Stein, R. A., and Mead, J. F. Metabolism of epoxidized phosphatidylcholine by phospholipase A_2 and epoxide hydrolase. *Lipids* 16: 781, 1981.
738. Seydel, J. K., and Wasserman, O. NMR studies on the molecular basis of drug induced phospholipidosis, interaction between chlorphentermine and phosphatidylcholine. *Naunyn Schmiedebergs Arch. Pharmacol. Exp. Pathol.* 279: 207, 1973.
739. Seydel, J. K., and Wasserman, O. NMR studies on the molecular basis of drug induced phospholipidosis. II. Interaction between several amphiphilic drugs and phospholipids. *Biochem. Pharmacol.* 25: 2357, 1976.
740. Shah, S. V., and Walker, P. D. Evidence suggesting a role for hydroxyl radical in glycerol-induced acute renal failure. *Am. J. Physiol.* 255: F438, 1988.
741. Shanley, P. F., Brezis, M., Spokes, K., Silva, P., Epstein, F. H., and Rosen, S. Transport-dependent cell injury in the S3 segment of the proximal tubule. *Kidney Int.* 29: 1033, 1986.
742. Shanley, P. F., Brezis, M., Spokes, K., Silva, P., Epstein, F. H., and Rosen, S. Hypoxic injury in the proximal tubule of the isolated perfused rat kidney. *Kidney Int.* 29: 1021, 1986.
743. Shanley, P. F., and Johnson, G. C. Adenine nucleotides, transport activity and hypoxic necrosis in the thick ascending limb of Henle. *Kidney Int.* 36: 823, 1989.
744. Shanley, P. F., Shapiro, J. I., Chan, L., Burke, T. J., and Johnson, G. C. Acidosis and hypoxic medullary injury in the isolated perfused kidney. *Kidney Int.* 34: 791, 1988.
745. Shanley, P. F., Turke, T. J., and Johnson, G. C. Acidosis and calcium in hypoxia. *Kidney Int.* 37: 494, 1990. (Abstract.)
746. Shasby, D. M., Lind, S. E., Shasby, S. S., Goldsmith,

J. C., and Hunninghake, G. W. Reversible oxidant-induced increases in albumin transfer across cultured endothelium: Alterations in cell shape and calcium homeostasis. *Blood* 65: 605, 1985.
747. Shaw, S. G., Weidmann, P., Hodler, J., Zimmerman, A., and Paternostro, A. Atrial natriuretic peptide protects against acute ischemic renal failure in the rat. *J. Clin. Invest.* 80: 1232, 1987.
748. Shelbourne, J. D., Arstila, A. U., and Trump, B. F. Studies on cellular autophagocytosis. The relationship of autophagocytosis to protein synthesis and to energy metabolism in rat liver and flounder kidney tubules in vitro. *Am. J. Pathol.* 73: 641, 1973.
749. Shelton, K. R., Todd, J. M., and Egle, P. M. The induction of stress-related proteins by lead. *J. Biol. Chem.* 261: 1935, 1986.
750. Shen, A. C., and Jennings, R. B. Myocardial calcium and magnesium in acute ischemic injury. *Am. J. Pathol.* 67: 417, 1972.
751. Shier, W. T., and DuBourdieu, D. J. Stimulation of phospholipid hydrolysis and cell death by mercuric chloride: Evidence for mercuric ion acting as a calcium-mimetic agent. *Biochem. Biophys. Res. Commun.* 110: 758, 1983.
752. Shusterman, N., Strom, B. L., Murray, T. G., Morrison, G., West, S. L., and Maislin, G. Risk factors and outcome of hospital-acquired acute renal failure. *Am. J. Med.* 83: 65, 1987.
753. Siegel, N. J., Gaudio, K. M., Katz, L., Reilly, H., Ardito, T. A., Hendler, F. G., and Kashgarian, M. Beneficial effect of thyroxine on recovery from toxic renal failure. *Kidney Int.* 25: 906, 1984.
754. Siegel, N. J., Meade, R., and Kashgarian, M. Amelioration of dichromate-induced acute renal failure by infusion of ATP-$MgCl_2$. *Kidney Int.* 18: 776, 1979.
755. Silva, P., Rosen, S., Spokes, K., and Epstein, F. H. Effect of glycine on medullary thick ascending limb injury in perfused kidneys. *Kidney Int.* 39: 653, 1991.
756. Silverblatt, F., Turck, M., and Bulger, R. Nephrotoxicity due to cephaloridine: A light and electron-microscopic study in rabbits. *J. Infect. Dis.* 122: 33, 1970.
757. Silverblatt, F. J., and Kuehn, C. Autoradiology of gentamicin uptake by the rat proximal tubule cell. *Kidney Int.* 15: 335, 1979.
758. Simmons, C. F., Jr., Bogusky, R. T., and Humes, H. D. Inhibitory effects of gentamicin on renal cortical mitochondrial oxidative phosphorylation. *J. Pharmacol. Exp. Ther.* 214: 709, 1980.
759. Simmons, C. F., Jr., and Humes, H. D. Effects of *cis*-platinum on renal cortical mitochondrial respiration. *Clin. Res.* 27: 602A, 1979.
760. Singer, S., and Nicholson, G. The fluid mosaic model of the structure of cell membranes. *Science* 175: 720, 1972.
761. Singhal, R. K., Anderson, M. E., and Meister, A. Glutathione, a first line of defense against cadmium toxicity. *FASEB J.* 1: 220, 1987.
762. Sirota, J. H. Carbon tetrachloride poisoning in man. I. The mechanisms of renal failure and recovery. *J. Clin. Invest.* 28: 1412, 1949.
763. Slater, T. F., and Greenbaum, A. L. Changes in lysosomal enzymes in acute experimental liver injury. *Biochem. J.* 96: 484, 1965.
764. Sleijfer, D. T., Smit, E. F., Meijer, S., Mulder, N. H., and Postmus, P. E. Acute and cumulative effects of carboplatin on renal function. *Br. J. Cancer* 60: 116, 1989.
765. Slivka, S. R., and Insel, P. A. Phorbol ester and neomycin dissociate bradykinin receptor-mediated arachidonic acid release and polyphosphoinositide hydrolysis in Madin-Darby canine kidney cells. Evidence that bradykinin mediates noninterdependent activation of phospholipases A_2 and C. *J. Biol. Chem.* 263: 14640, 1988.
766. Smith, J. H., and Hook, J. B. Mechanism of chloroform nephrotoxicity. II. In vitro evidence for renal metabolism of chloroform in mice. *Toxicol. Appl. Pharmacol.* 70: 480, 1983.
767. Smith, J. H., and Hook, J. B. Mechanism of chloroform nephrotoxicity. III. Renal and hepatic microsomal metabolism of chloroform in mice. *Toxicol. Appl. Pharmacol.* 73: 511, 1984.
768. Smith, M. T., Thor, H., and Orrenius, S. The role of lipid peroxidation in the toxicity of foreign compounds to liver cells. *Biochem. Pharmacol.* 32: 763, 1983.
769. Smith, M. W., Ambudkar, I. S., Phelps, P. C., Regec, A. L., and Trump, B. F. $HgCl_2$-induced changes in cytosolic Ca^{2+} of cultured rabbit renal tubular cells. *Biochim. Biophys. Acta* 931: 130, 1987.
770. Smith, M. W., Phelps, P. C., and Trump, B. F. Cytosolic Ca^{2+} deregulation and blebbing after $HgCl_2$ injury to cultured rabbit proximal tubule cells as determined by digital imaging microscopy. *Proc. Natl. Acad. Sci. U.S.A.* 88: 1991.
771. Smith, P., Guntupalli, J., Eby, B., and Lau, K. Evidence that gentamicin produces tubular wastage of K^+ and Mg^{++} independent of reduced GFR and aldosterone. *Clin. Res.* 29: 475A, 1981.
772. Smith, T. F., and Griffiths, L. A. Comparative metabolic studies of phenacitin and structurally related compounds in the rat. *Xenobiotica* 176: 217, 1976.
773. Smolens, P., and Stein, J. H. Hemodynamic Factors in Acute Renal Failure: Pathophysiological and Therapeutic Implications. In B. M. Brenner and J. H. Stein (eds.), *Acute Renal Failure.* New York: Churchill-Livingstone, 1980. P. 180.
774. Snowdowne, K. W., Freudenrich, C. C., and Borle, A. B. The effects of anoxia on cytosolic free calcium, calcium fluxes, and cellular ATP levels in cultured kidney cells. *J. Biol. Chem.* 260: 11619, 1985.
775. Soberon, L., Bowman, R. L., Pastoriza-Munoz, E., et al. Comparative nephrotoxicities of gentamicin, netilmicin and tobramycin in the rat. *J. Pharmacol. Exp. Ther.* 210: 334, 1981.
776. Solez, K., Morel-Maroger, L., and Sraer, J. The morphology of acute tubular necrosis in man: Analysis of 57 renal biopsies and a comparison with the glycerol model. *Medicine* 58: 362, 1979.
777. Solez, K., and Whelton, A. Correlation of Structural and Functional Changes in Nephrotoxic and Postischemic Acute Renal Failure (Acute Tubular Necrosis). In P. Periti and G. G. Grassi (eds.), *Current Chemotherapy and Immunotherapy.* Washington, D.C.: American Society of Microbiology, 1982. P. 837.
778. Somlyo, A. P. Calcium content of mitochondria and endoplasmic reticulum in liver frozen rapidly in vivo. *Nature* 314: 622, 1985.
779. Southard, J. H., and Green, D. E. Control of the energy coupling modes in mitochondria by mercurials. *Biochem. Biophys. Res. Commun.* 61: 1310, 1974.
780. Southard, J. H., Marsh, D. C., McAnulty, J. F., and Belzer, F. O. Oxygen-derived free radical damage in organ preservation: Activity of superoxide dismutase and xanthine oxidase. *Surgery* 101: 566, 1987.
781. Southard, J. H., Penniston, J. T., and Green, D. E. Induction of transmembrane proton transfer by mercurials in mitochondria. I. Ion movements accompanying transmembrane proton transfer. *J. Biol. Chem.* 218: 3546, 1973.

782. Spencer, A. J., LeFurgey, A., Mandel, L. J., and Ingram, P. Anoxia-induced changes in elemental compartmentation in renal proximal tubules as studied by high resolution x-ray imaging. *Kidney Int.* 37: 495, 1990.
783. Spiegel, D. M., Shanley, P. F., and Molitoris, B. A. Mild ischemia predisposes the S3 segment to gentamicin toxicity. *Kidney Int.* 38: 459, 1990.
784. Srinivasan, S., and Recknagel, R. O. Ultraviolet spectra of rat kidney lipids after carbon tetrachloride administration. *Exp. Mol. Pathol.* 18: 214, 1973.
785. Stacey, N., and Priestly, B. G. Lipid peroxidation in isolated rat hepatocytes: Relationship to toxicity of CCl4, ADP/Fe^{3+}, and diethyl maleate. *Toxicol. Appl. Pharmacol.* 45: 41, 1978.
786. Stacey, N. H., and Kappus, H. Cellular toxicity and lipid peroxidation in response to mercury. *Toxicol. Appl. Pharmacol.* 63: 29, 1982.
787. Stacey, N. H., and Klaassen, C. D. Inhibition of lipid peroxidation without prevention of cellular injury in isolated rat hepatocytes. *Toxicol. Appl. Pharmacol.* 58: 8, 1981.
788. Starke, P. E., and Farber, J. L. Endogenous defenses against the cytotoxicity of hydrogen peroxide in cultured rat hepatocytes. *J. Biol. Chem.* 260: 86, 1985.
789. Staubli, W., Schweizer, W., and Suter, J. Some properties of myeloid bodies induced in rat liver by an antidepressant drug (Maprotiline). *Exp. Mol. Pathol.* 28: 177, 1978.
790. Steenbergen, C., Hill, M. L., and Jennings, R. B. Volume regulation and plasma membrane injury in aerobic, anaerobic, and ischemic myocardium in vitro. Effects of osmotic cell swelling on plasma membrane integrity. *Circ. Res.* 57: 864, 1985.
791. Steenbergen, C., Hill, M. L., and Jennings, R. B. Cytoskeletal damage during myocardial ischemia: Changes in vinculin immunofluorescence staining during total in vitro ischemia in canine heart. *Circ. Res.* 60: 478, 1987.
792. Stevens, J., Hayden, P., and Taylor, G. The role of glutathione conjugate metabolism and cysteine conjugate B-lyase in the mechanism of S-cysteine conjugate toxicity in LLC-PK1 cells. *J. Biol. Chem.* 261: 3325, 1986.
793. Stevens, J. L., Ayoubi, N., and Robbins, J. D. The role of mitochondrial matrix enzymes in the metabolism and toxicity of cysteine conjugates. *J. Biol. Chem.* 263: 3395, 1988.
794. Stevens, J. L., Robbins, J. D., and Byrd, R. A. A purified cysteine conjugate beta-lyase from rat kidney cytosol. Requirement for an alpha-keto acid or an amino acid oxidase for activity and identity with soluble glutamine transaminase K. *J. Biol. Chem.* 261: 15529, 1986.
795. Stockdale, M., Dawson, A. P., and Selwyn, M. J. Effects of trialkyltin and triphenyltin compounds on mitochondrial respiration. *Eur. J. Biochem.* 15: 342, 1970.
796. Stomski, M. E., Cooper, K., Thulin, G., Avison, M. J., Gaudio, K. M., Shulman, R. G., and Siegel, N. J. Postischemic ATP-$MgCl_2$ provides precursors for resynthesis of cellular ATP in rats. *Am. J. Physiol.* 250: F834, 1986.
797. Straub, F. B., and Feuer, G. Adenosinetriphosphatase: The functional group of actin. *Biochim. Biophys. Acta* 4: 455, 1950.
798. Striker, G. E., Smuckler, E. A., Kohnen, P. W., and Nagle, R. B. Structural and functional changes in rat kidney during CCl_4 intoxication. *Am. J. Pathol.* 53: 769, 1968.
799. Subjeck, J. R., and Shyy, T. T. Stress protein systems of mammalian cells. *Am. J. Physiol.* 250: C1, 1986.
800. Sugihara, K., and Gemba, M. Modification of cisplatin toxicity by antioxidants. *Jpn. J. Pharmacol.* 40: 353, 1986.
801. Sugihara, K., Nakano, S., and Gemba, M. Effect of cisplatin on in vitro production of lipid peroxides in rat kidney cortex. *Jpn. J. Pharmacol.* 44: 71, 1987.
802. Sugihara, K., Nakano, S., Koda, M., Tanaka, K., Fukuishi, N., and Gemba, M. Stimulatory effect of cisplatin on production of lipid peroxidation in renal tissues. *Jpn. J. Pharmacol.* 43: 247, 1987.
803. Sugrue, S. P., and Hay, E. A. Responses of basal epithelial cell surface and cytoskeleton to solubilized extracellular matrix molecules. *J. Cell Biol.* 91: 45, 1981.
804. Sun, A., and Hebert, S. C. Rapid hypertonic cell volume regulation in the perfused inner medullary collecting duct. *Kidney Int.* 36: 831, 1989.
805. Sutter, P. M., Thulin, G., Stromski, M., Ardito, T., Gaudio, K. M., Kasgarian, M., and Siegel, N. J. Beneficial effect of thyroxin in the treatment of ischemic acute renal failure. *Pediatr. Nephrol.* 20: 1, 1988.
806. Suzuki, C. A., and Cherian, M. G. Effects of cadmium-metallothionein on renal organic ion transport and lipid peroxidation in rats. *J. Biochem. Toxicol.* 3: 11, 1988.
807. Suzuki, C. A., and Cherian, M. G. Renal glutathione depletion and nephrotoxicity of cadmium-metallothionein in rats. *Toxicol. Appl. Pharmacol.* 98: 544, 1989.
808. Suzuki, C. A., and Cherian, M. G. The interactions of cis-diamminedichloroplatinum with metallothionein and glutathione in rat liver and kidney. *Toxicology* 64: 113, 1990.
809. Suzuki, K., Imajoh, S., Emori, Y., Kawasaki, H., Minami, Y., and Ohno, S. Calcium-activated neutral protease and its endogenous inhibitor. Activation at the cell membrane and biological function. *FEBS Lett.* 220: 271, 1987.
810. Swann, J. D., and Acosta, D. Failure of gentamicin to elevate cellular malondialdehyde content or increase generation of intracellular reactive oxygen species in primary cultures of renal cortical epithelial cells. *Biochem. Pharmacol.* 40: 1523, 1990.
811. Swann, J. D., Ulrich, R., and Acosta, D. Lack of changes in cytosolic ionized calcium in primary cultures of rat kidney cortical cells exposed to cytotoxic concentrations of gentamicin. *Toxicol. Appl. Pharmacol.* 106: 38, 1990.
812. Szczepanska, M., and Angielski, S. Prevention of maleate-induced tubular dysfunction by acetoacetate. *Am. J. Physiol.* 239: F50, 1980.
813. Takano, T., Soltoff, S. P., Murdaugh, S., and Mandel, L. J. Intracellular respiratory dysfunction and cell injury in short-term anoxia of rabbit renal proximal tubules. *J. Clin. Invest.* 76: 2377, 1985.
814. Tang, M.-J., Suresh, K. R., and Tannen, R. L. Carbohydrate metabolism by primary cultures of rabbit proximal tubules. *Am. J. Physiol.* 256: C532, 1989.
815. Tappel, A. L., and Dillard, C. J. In vivo lipid peroxidation: Measurement via exhaled pentane and protection by vitamin E. *Fed. Proc.* 40: 174, 1981.
816. Tappel, A. L., Shibko, S., Stein, M., and Susz, J. P. Studies on the composition of lysosomes. *J. Food Sci.* 30: 498, 1965.
817. Tay, L. K., Bregman, C. L., Masters, B. A., and Williams, P. D. Effects of cis-diamminedichloroplatinum(II) on rabbit kidney in vivo and on rabbit renal proximal tubule cells in culture. *Cancer Res.* 48: 2538, 1988.
818. Terry, R. D., and Weiss, M. Studies in Tay-Sachs disease. II. Ultrastructure of the cerebrum. *J. Neuropathol. Exp. Neurol.* 22: 18, 1963.
819. Teschan, P. E., and Lawson, N. L. Studies in acute renal failure. *Nephron* 3: 1, 1966.
820. Thiel, G., Brunner, F., Wunderlich, P., Huguenin, M., Bienko, B., Torhorst, J., Peters-Haefeli, L., Kirchertz,

E. J., and Peters, G. Protection of rat kidneys against $HgCl_2$-induced acute renal failure by induction of high urine flow without renin suppression. *Kidney Int.* 10: S191, 1976.
821. Thomas, C. E., and Reed, D. J. Current status of calcium in hepatocellular injury. *Hepatology* 10: 375, 1989.
822. Thomsen, H. S., Skaarup, P., Larsen, S., Golman, K., and Hemmingsen, L. Gentamicin nephropathy and contrast media. A comparison between diatrizoate and iohexol in rats. *Acta Radiol.* 31: 401, 1990.
823. Thor, H., Mirabelli, F., Salis, A., Cohen, G. M., Bellomo, G., and Orrenius, S. Alterations in hepatocyte cytoskeleton caused by redox cycling and alkylating quinones. *Arch. Biochem. Biophys.* 266: 397, 1988.
824. Thys, O., Hildebrand, J., Gerins, Y., and Jacques, P. J. Alterations of rat liver lysosomes and smooth endoplasmic reticulum induced by the diazafluoranthen derivative AC-3579. *Lab. Invest.* 28: 70, 1973.
825. Tien, M., and Aust, S. D. Rabbit liver microsomal lipid peroxidation. The effect of lipid on the rate of peroxidation. *Biochim. Biophys. Acta* 712: 1, 1982.
826. Tirmenstein, M., and Reed, D. J. Effects of glutathione on the α-tocopherol-dependent inhibition of nuclear lipid peroxidation. *J. Lipid Res.* 30: 959, 1989.
827. Tkachuk, V. A., and Menshikov, M. Y. Effect of pH on calcium binding properties of calmodulin and on its interaction with Ca-dependent cyclic nucleotide phosphodiesterase. *Biokhimiia* 46: 965, 1981.
828. Toback, F. G. Amino acid enhancement of renal regeneration after acute tubular necrosis. *Kidney Int.* 12: 193, 1977.
829. Toback, F. G., Teegarden, D. E., and Havener, L. J. Amino acid-mediated stimulation of renal phospholipid biosynthesis after acute tubular necrosis. *Kidney Int.* 15: 542, 1979.
830. Tolins, J. P., and Raij, L. Chronic amphotericin B nephrotoxicity in the rat: Protective effect of calcium channel blockade. *J. Am. Soc. Nephrol.* 2: 98, 1991.
831. Tominaga, T., Katagi, H., and Ohnishi, S. T. Is Ca^{2+}-activated potassium efflux involved in the formation of ischemic brain edema. *Brain Res.* 460: 376, 1988.
832. Toninello, A., Siliprandi, D., and Siliprandi, N. On the mechanism by which Mg^{2+} and adenine nucleotides restore membrane potential in rat liver mitochondria deenergized by Ca^{2+} and phosphate. *Biochem. Biophys. Res. Commun.* 111: 792, 1983.
833. Toubeau, G., Laurent, G., Carlier, M. B., Abid, S., Maldague, P., Heuson-Stiennon, J. A., and Tulkens, P. M. Tissue repair in rat kidney cortex after short treatment with aminoglycosides at low doses. A comparative biochemical and morphometric study. *Lab. Invest.* 54: 385, 1986.
834. Trifillis, A. L., Kahng, M. W., and Trump, B. F. Metabolic studies of $HgCl_2$-induced acute renal failure in the rat. *Exp. Mol. Pathol.* 35: 14, 1981.
835. Troyer, D. A., Kreisberg, J. I., and Venkatachalam, M. A. Lipid alterations in LLC-PK1 cells exposed to mercuric chloride. *Kidney Int.* 29: 530, 1986.
836. Trump, B. F., and Berezesky, I. K. The role of calcium in cell injury and repair: A hypothesis. *Surv. Synth. Pathol. Res.* 4: 248, 1985.
837. Trump, B. F., Berezesky, I. K., Collan, Y., Kahng, M. W., and Mergner, W. J. Recent studies on the pathophysiology of ischemic cell injury. *Beitr. Path. Bd.* 158: 363, 1976.
838. Trump, B. F., Berezesky, I. K., Laiho, K. U., Osornio, A. R., Mergner, W. J., and Smith, M. W. The Role of Calcium in Cell Injury. A Review. In *Scanning Electron Microscopy.* Chicago: SEM Inc., A. M. F. O'Hare, 1980. P. 437.
839. Trump, B. F., and Bulger, R. E. Studies of cellular injury in isolated flounder tubules. III. Light microscopic and functional changes due to cyanide. *Lab. Invest.* 18: 721, 1968.
840. Trump, B. F., and Bulger, R. E. Studies of cellular injury in isolated flounder tubules. IV. Electron microscopic observations of changes during the phase of altered homeostasis in tubules treated with cyanide. *Lab. Invest.* 18: 731, 1968.
841. Tulkens, P. M. Experimental studies on nephrotoxicity of aminoglycosides at low doses. Mechanisms and perspectives. *Am. J. Med.* 80: 105, 1986.
842. Tune, B. M. Effect of organic acid transport inhibitors on renal cortical uptake and proximal tubular toxicity of cephaloridine. *J. Pharmacol. Exp. Ther.* 181: 250, 1972.
843. Tune, B. M., Fernholt, M., and Schwartz, A. Mechanism of cephaloridine transport in the kidney. *J. Pharmacol. Exp. Ther.* 191: 311, 1974.
844. Tune, B. M., and Fravert, D. Cephalosporin nephrotoxicity. Transport, cytotoxicity and mitochondrial toxicity of cephaloglycin. *J. Pharmacol. Exp. Ther.* 215: 186, 1980.
845. Tune, B. M., and Fravert, D. Mechanisms of cephalosporin nephrotoxicity: A comparison of cephaloridine and cephaloglycin. *Kidney Int.* 18: 591, 1980.
846. Tune, B. M., Fravert, D., and Hsu, C.-Y. Thienamycin nephrotoxicity. Mitochondrial injury and oxidative effects of imipenem in the rabbit kidney. *Biochem. Pharmacol.* 38: 3779, 1989.
847. Tune, B. M., Fravert, D., and Hsu, C.-Y. Oxidative and mitochondrial toxic effects of cephalosporin antibiotics in the kidney. A comparative study of cephaloridine and cephaloglycin. *Biochem. Pharmacol.* 38: 795, 1989.
848. Tune, B. M., and Hsu, C.-Y. Augmentation of antibiotic nephrotoxicity by endotoxemia in the rabbit. *J. Pharmacol. Exp. Ther.* 234: 425, 1985.
849. Tune, B. M., and Hsu, C.-Y. The renal mitochondrial toxicity of cephalosporins: Specificity of the effect on anionic substrate uptake. *J. Pharmacol. Exp. Ther.* 252: 65, 1990.
850. Tune, B. M., Hsu, C. Y., and Fravert, D. Mechanisms of the bacterial endotoxin-cephaloridine toxic synergy and the protective effects of saline infusion in the rabbit kidney. *J. Pharmacol. Exp. Ther.* 244: 520, 1988.
851. Tune, B. M., Sibley, R. K., and Hsu, C. Y. The mitochondrial respiratory toxicity of cephalosporin antibiotics. An inhibitory effect on substrate uptake. *J. Pharmacol. Exp. Ther.* 245: 1054, 1988.
852. Tune, B. M., Wu, K. Y., Fravert, D., and Holtzman, D. Effect of cephaloridine on respiration by renal cortical mitochondria. *J. Pharmacol. Exp. Ther.* 210: 98, 1979.
853. Tune, B. M., Wu, K. Y., and Kempson, R. I. Inhibition of transport and prevention of toxicity of cephaloridine in the kidney. Dose-responsiveness of the rabbit and the guinea pig to probenecid. *J. Pharmacol. Exp. Ther.* 202: 466, 1977.
854. Turrens, J. F., and McCord, J. M. Mitochondrial Generation of Reactive Oxygen Species. In G. B. Zelenok (ed.), *Clinical Ischemic Syndromes. Mechanisms and Consequences of Tissue Injury.* St. Louis: Mosby, 1990. P. 203.
855. Tyrakowski, T., Knapowski, J., and Baczyk, K. Disturbances in electrolyte transport before the onset of uranyl acetate induced renal failure. *Kidney Int.* 10: S144, 1976.
856. Tysnes, O.-B., Steen, V. M., and Holmsen, H. Neomycin inhibits platelet functions and inositol phospholipid metabolism upon stimulation with thrombin, but not with

ionomycin or 12-*O*-tetradecanoyl-phorbol 13-acetate. *Eur. J. Biochem.* 177: 219, 1988.

857. Ufferman, R. C., Jaenike, J. R., Freeman, R. B., and Pabico, R. C. Effects of furosemide on low-dose mercuric chloride acute renal failure in the rat. *Kidney Int.* 8: 362, 1975.
858. van Bladeren, P. J., van der Gen, A., Breimer, D. D., and Mohn, G. R. Stereoselective activation of vicinal dihalogen compounds to mutagens by glutathione conjugation. *Biochem. Pharmacol.* 28: 2521, 1979.
859. Vander Heide, R. S., and Ganote, C. E. Increased myocyte fragility following anoxic injury. *J. Mol. Cell. Cardiol.* 19: 1085, 1987.
860. Vasington, F. D., and Murphy, J. V. Ca^{++} uptake by rat kidney mitochondria and its dependence on respiration and phosphorylation. *J. Biol. Chem.* 237: 2670, 1962.
861. Venkatachalam, M. A., Bernard, D. B., Donohoe, J. F., and Levinsky, N. G. Ischemic damage and repair in the rat proximal tubule: Differences among the S_1, S_2, and S_3 segments. *Kidney Int.* 14: 31, 1978.
862. Venkatachalam, M. A., Jones, D. B., Rennke, H. G., Sandstrom, D., and Patel, Y. Mechanism of proximal tubule brush border loss and regeneration following mild renal ischemia. *Lab. Invest.* 45: 355, 1981. (Abstract.)
863. Venkatachalam, M. A., Patel, Y. J., Kreisberg, J. I., and Weinberg, J. M. Energy thresholds that determine membrane integrity and injury in a renal epithelial cell line (LLC-PK1). Relationships to phospholipid degradation and unesterified fatty acid accumulation. *J. Clin. Invest.* 81: 745, 1988.
864. Verani, R. R., Brewer, E. D., Ince, A., Gibson, J., and Bulger, R. E. Proximal tubular necrosis associated with maleic acid administration to the rat. *Lab. Invest.* 46: 79, 1982.
865. Vercellotti, G. M., Severson, S. P., Duane, P., and Moldow, C. F. Hydrogen peroxide alters signal transduction in human endothelial cells. *J. Lab. Clin. Med.* 117: 15, 1991.
866. Verity, M. A., and Brown, W. J. Hg^{2+}-induced kidney necrosis. *Am. J. Pathol.* 61: 57, 1970.
867. Verity, M. A., and Reith, A. Effect of mercurial compounds on structure-linked latency of lysosomal hydrolases. *Biochem. J.* 105: 685, 1967.
868. Verleij, A. J., and Post, J. A. Physico-chemical properties and organization of lipids in membranes: Their possible role in myocardial injury. *Basic Res. Cardiol.* 82: 85, 1987.
869. Verpooten, G. A., Giuliano, R. A., Verbist, L., Eestermans, G., and DeBroe, M. E. Once-daily dosing decreases renal accumulation of gentamicin and netilmicin. *Clin. Pharmacol. Ther.* 45: 22, 1989.
870. Victoria, E. J., Van Golde, L. M. G., Hostetler, K. Y., Scherphof, G. L., and Van Deenen, L. L. M. Some studies on the metabolism of phospholipids in plasma membranes from rat livers. *Biochim. Biophys. Acta* 239: 443, 1971.
871. Villarruel, M. C., de Toranzo, E. G., and Castro, J. A. Carbon tetrachloride activation, lipid peroxidation, and the mixed function oxygenase activity of various rat tissues. *Toxicol. Appl. Pharmacol.* 41: 337, 1977.
872. Vogel, S., and Sperelakis, N. Blockade of myocardial slow inward current at low pH. *Am. J. Physiol.* 233: 99, 1977.
873. Wagner, T., Kreft, B., Bohlmann, G., and Schwieder, G. Effects of fosfomycin, mesna, and sodium thiosulfate on the toxicity and antitumor activity of cisplatin. *J. Cancer Res. Clin. Oncol.* 114: 497, 1988.
874. Waite, J., Scherphof, G. L., Boshouwers, F. M. G., and Van Deenen, L. L. M. Differentiation of phospholipases A in mitochondria and lysosomes of rat liver. *J. Lipid Res.* 10: 411, 1969.
875. Waite, M. Isolation of rat liver mitochondrial membrane fractions and localization of the phospholipase A. *Biochemistry* 8: 2536, 1969.
876. Walker, P. D., and Shah, S. V. Gentamicin enhanced production of hydrogen peroxide by renal cortical mitochondria. *Am. J. Physiol.* 253: C495, 1987.
877. Walker, P. D., and Shah, S. V. Evidence suggesting a role for hydroxyl radical in gentamicin-induced acute renal failure in rats. *J. Clin. Invest.* 81: 334, 1988.
878. Waller, R. L., Glende, E. A., Jr., and Recknagel, R. O. Carbon tetrachloride and bromotrichloromethane toxicity. Dual role of covalent binding of metabolic cleavage products and lipid peroxidation in depression of microsomal calcium sequestration. *Biochem. Pharmacol.* 32: 1613, 1983.
879. Wallin, A., Jones, T. W., Vercesi, A. E., Cotgreave, I., Ormstad, K., and Orrenius, S. Toxicity of S-pentachlorobutadienyl-L-cysteine studied with isolated rat renal cortical mitochondria. *Arch. Biochem. Biophys.* 258: 365, 1987.
880. Wang, B. M., Weiner, N. D., Ganesan, M. G., and Schacht, J. Interaction of calcium and neomycin with anionic phospholipid-lecithin liposomes. A differential scanning calorimetry study. *Biochem. Pharmacol.* 33: 3787, 1984.
881. Ward, J. M., Grabin, M. E., Berline, E., and Young, D. M. Prevention of renal failure in rats receiving *cis*-diamminedichloroplatinum (II) by administration of furosemide. *Cancer Res.* 37: 1238, 1977.
882. Ward, J. M., Grabin, M. E., LeRoy, A. F., and Young, D. M. Modification of the renal toxicity of *cis*-dichlorodiammine-platinum (II) with furosemide in male F344 rats. *Cancer Treat. Rep.* 61: 375, 1977.
883. Webb, M. The Metallothioneins. In M. Webb (ed.), *The Chemistry, Biochemistry and Biology of Cadmium.* Amsterdam: Elsevier, 1979. P. 195.
884. Webb, M. Toxicology of Cadmium-Thionein. In M. Webb (ed.), *The Chemistry, Biochemistry and Biology of Cadmium.* Amsterdam: Elsevier/North-Holland Biomedical Press, 1979. P. 423.
885. Webb, M., and Etienne, A. T. Studies on the toxicity and metabolism of cadmium-thionein. *Biochem. Pharmacol.* 26: 25, 1977.
886. Webb, M., and Magos, L. Cadmium-thionein and the protection by cadmium against the nephrotoxicity of mercury. *Chem. Biol. Interact.* 14: 357, 1976.
887. Wedeen, R. P. Lead Nephrotoxicity. In G. A. Porter (ed.), *Nephrotoxic Mechanisms of Drugs and Environmental Toxins.* New York: Plenum, 1982. P. 255.
888. Wedeen, R. P., Batuman, V., Cheeks, C., Marquet, E., and Sobel, H. Transport of gentamicin in rat proximal tubule. *Lab. Invest.* 48: 212, 1983.
889. Weeds, A. Actin-binding proteins—Regulators of cell architecture and motility. *Nature* 296: 811, 1982.
890. Wefers, H., and Sies, H. Oxidation of glutathione by the superoxide radical to the disulfide and the sulfonate yielding singlet oxygen. *Eur. J. Biochem.* 137: 29, 1983.
891. Wefers, H., and Sies, H. The protection by ascorbate and glutathione against microsomal lipid peroxidation is dependent on vitamin E. *Eur. J. Biochem.* 174: 353, 1988.
892. Weglicki, W. B., Dickens, B. F., and Mak, I. T. Enhanced lysosomal phospholipid degradation and phospholipid

production due to free radicals. *Biochem. Biophys. Res. Commun.* 124: 229, 1984.
893. Weinberg, J. M. Calcium as a mediator of renal tubule cell injury. *Semin. Nephrol.* 4: 174, 1984.
894. Weinberg, J. M. Oxygen deprivation induced injury to isolated rabbit kidney tubules. *J. Clin. Invest.* 76: 1193, 1985.
895. Weinberg, J. M. Issue in the pathophysiology of nephrotoxic renal tubular cell injury pertinent to understanding cyclosporine nephrotoxicity. *Trans. Proc.* 17: 81, 1985.
896. Weinberg, J. M. The Cellular Basis of Nephrotoxicity. In R. W. Schrier and C. W. Gottschalk (eds.), *Diseases of the Kidney*. Boston: Little, Brown, 1988. P. 1137.
897. Weinberg, J. M. Adenine nucleotide metabolism by isolated kidney tubules during oxygen deprivation. *Biochem. Med. Metab. Biol.* 39: 319, 1988.
898. Weinberg, J. M. The effect of amino acids on ischemic and toxic injury to the kidney. *Semin. Nephrol.* 10: 491, 1990.
899. Weinberg, J. M. The cell biology of ischemic renal injury. *Kidney Int.* 39: 476, 1991.
900. Weinberg, J. M., Buchanan, D. N., Davis, J. A., and Abarzua, M. Metabolic aspects of protection by glycine against hypoxic injury to isolated proximal tubules. *J. Am. Soc. Nephrol.* 1: 949, 1991.
901. Weinberg, J. M., and Davis, J. A. A comparison between protection by glycine, acidosis and mannitol against proximal tubule cell injury. *Clin. Res.* 38: 577A, 1990. (Abstract.)
902. Weinberg, J. M., Davis, J. A., Abarzua, M., and Kiani, T. Relationship between cell ATP and glutathione content and protection by glycine against hypoxic proximal tubule cell injury. *J. Lab. Clin. Med.* 113: 612, 1989.
903. Weinberg, J. M., Davis, J. A., Abarzua, M., and Kiani, T. Glycine-dependent protection of proximal tubules against lethal cell injury due to inhibitors of mitochondrial ATP production. *Am. J. Physiol.* 258: C1127, 1990.
904. Weinberg, J. M., Davis, J. A., Abarzua, M., and Rajan, T. Cytoprotective effects of glycine and glutathione against hypoxic injury to renal tubules. *J. Clin. Invest.* 80: 1446, 1987.
905. Weinberg, J. M., Davis, J. A., Abarzua, M., Smith, R. K., and Kunkel, R. Ouabain-induced lethal proximal tubule cell injury is prevented by glycine. *Am. J. Physiol.* 258: F346, 1990.
906. Weinberg, J. M., Davis, J. A., Lawton, A., and Abarzua, M. Modulation of cell nucleotide levels of isolated kidney tubules. *Am. J. Physiol.* 254: F311, 1988.
907. Weinberg, J. M., Davis, J. A., Roeser, N. F., and Venkatachalam, M. A. Role of increased cytosolic free calcium in the pathogenesis of rabbit proximal tubule cell injury and protection by glycine or acidosis. *J. Clin. Invest.* 87: 581, 1991.
908. Weinberg, J. M., Davis, J. A., Shayman, J. A., and Knight, P. R. Alterations of cytosolic calcium in LLC-PK1 cells induced by vasopressin and exogenous purines. *Am. J. Physiol.* 256: C967, 1989.
909. Weinberg, J. M., Davis, J. A., and Trivedi, B. Calcium compartmentation in isolated renal tubules in suspension. *Biochem. Med. Metab. Biol.* 39: 234, 1988.
910. Weinberg, J. M., Harding, P. G., and Humes, H. D. Mechanisms of gentamicin-induced dysfunction of renal cortical mitochondria. II. Effects on mitochondrial monovalent cation transport. *Arch. Biochem. Biophys.* 205: 232, 1980.
911. Weinberg, J. M., Harding, P. G., and Humes, H. D. Mitochondrial bioenergetics during the initiation of mercuric chloride-induced renal injury. I. Direct effects of in vitro mercuric chloride on renal mitochondrial function. *J. Biol. Chem.* 257: 60, 1982.
912. Weinberg, J. M., Harding, P. G., and Humes, H. D. Mitochondrial bioenergetics during the initiation of mercuric chloride-induced renal injury. II. Functional alterations of renal cortical mitochondria isolated after mercuric chloride treatment. *J. Biol. Chem.* 257: 68, 1982.
913. Weinberg, J. M., Harding, P. G., and Humes, H. D. Alterations in renal cortex cation homeostasis during mercuric chloride and gentamicin nephrotoxicity. *Exp. Mol. Pathol.* 39: 43, 1983.
914. Weinberg, J. M., and Humes, H. D. Mechanisms of gentamicin induced dysfunction of renal cortical mitochondria. I. Effects on mitochondrial respiration. *Arch. Biochem. Biophys.* 205: 222, 1980.
915. Weinberg, J. M., and Humes, H. D. Renal Tubular Cell Integrity During Mercuric Chloride and Gentamicin Nephrotoxicity. In K. Solez and A. Whelton (eds.), *Acute Renal Failure: Correlations Between Morphology and Function*. New York: Marcel Dekker, 1983. P. 179.
916. Weinberg, J. M., and Humes, H. D. Calcium transport and inner mitochondrial membrane damage in renal cortical mitochondria. *Am. J. Physiol.* 248: F876, 1985.
917. Weinberg, J. M., and Humes, H. D. Increases of cell ATP produced by exogenous adenine nucleotides in isolated rabbit kidney tubules. *Am. J. Physiol.* 250: F720, 1986.
918. Weinberg, J. M., Hunt, D., and Humes, H. D. Distribution of gentamicin among subcellular fractions from rat renal cortex. *Biochem. Pharmacol.* 34: 1779, 1985.
919. Weinberg, J. M., Johnson, K., De la Iglesia, F., and Allen, E. Acute alterations of tissue Ca^{++} and lethal tubular cell injury during $HgCl_2$ nephrotoxicity in the rat. *Toxicol. Pathol.* 17: 483, 1989.
920. Weinberg, J. M., Nissim, I., Roeser, N. F., Davis, J. A., Schultz, S., and Nissim, I. Relationships between intracellular amino acid levels and protection against injury to isolated proximal tubules. *Am. J. Physiol.* 260: 410, 1991.
921. Weinberg, J. M., Simmons, C. F., Jr., and Humes, H. D. Renal mitochondrial injury is an early pathogenetic event in *cis*-platinum nephrotoxicity. *Clin. Res.* 28: 464A, 1981.
922. Weinberg, J. M., Venkatachalam, M. A., Garza-Quintero, R., Roeser, N. F., and Davis, J. A. Structural requirements for protection by small amino acids against hypoxic injury in kidney proximal tubules. *FASEB J.* 4: 3347, 1990.
923. Weisenberg, R. C. Microtubule formation in vitro in solutions containing low calcium concentrations. *Science* 177: 1104, 1972.
924. Weiss, S. J., Peppen, G., Ortiz, X., Ragsdale, C., and Test, S. T. Oxidative autoactivation of latent collagenase by human neutrophils. *Science* 227: 747, 1985.
925. Weiss, S. J., and Slivka, A. Monocyte and granulocyte-mediated tumor cell destruction. A role for hydrogen peroxide-myeloperoxidase chloride system. *J. Clin. Invest.* 69: 255, 1982.
926. Wells, J. S., Gibson, W. R., Harris, P. N., Small, R. M., and Anderson, R. C. Toxicity, distribution and excretion of cephaloridine in laboratory animals. *Antimicrob. Agents Chemother.* 1965: 863, 1966.
927. Wellwood, J. M., Lovell, D., Thompson, A. E., et al. Renal damage caused by gentamicin: A study of the effects

on renal morphology and urinary enzyme excretion. *J. Pathol.* 118: 171, 1976.

928. Wellwood, J. M., Simpson, P. M., Tighe, J. R., and Thompson, A. E. Evidence of gentamicin nephrotoxicity in patients with renal allografts. *Br. Med. J.* 3: 278, 1975.
929. Welsh, M. J., Shasby, D. M., and Husted, R. M. Oxidants increase paracellular permeability in a cultured epithelial cell line. *J. Clin. Invest.* 76: 1155, 1985.
930. Williams, P. D., and Hottendorf, G. H. Inhibition of renal membrane binding and nephrotoxicity of gentamicin by polyasparagine and polyaspartic acid in the rat. *Res. Commun. Chem. Pathol. Pharmacol.* 47: 317, 1985.
931. Williams, P. D., and Hottendorf, G. H. [^{3}H]gentamicin uptake in brush border and basolateral membrane vesicles from rat kidney cortex. *Biochem. Pharmacol.* 35: 2253, 1986.
932. Williams, P. D., Hottendorf, G. H., and Bennett, D. B. Inhibition of renal membrane binding and nephrotoxicity of aminoglycosides. *J. Pharmacol. Exp. Ther.* 237: 919, 1986.
933. Williams, P. D., Trimble, M. E., Crespo, L., Holohan, P. D., Freedman, J. C., and Ross, C. R. Inhibition of renal Na^+, K^+-adenosine triphosphatase by gentamicin. *J. Pharmacol. Exp. Ther.* 231: 248, 1984.
934. Williams, S. E., and Schacht, J. Binding of neomycin and calcium to phospholipids and other anionic compounds. *J. Antibiot. (Tokyo)* 39: 457, 1986.
935. Williamson, J. M., Boettcher, B., and Meester, A. Intracellular delivery system that protects against toxicity by promoting glutathione synthesis. *Proc. Natl. Acad. Sci. U.S.A.* 79: 6246, 1982.
936. Williamson, J. R., and Monck, J. R. Hormone effects on cellular Ca^{2+} fluxes. *Annu. Rev. Physiol.* 51: 107, 1989.
937. Wilson, D. R., Thiel, G., Arce, M. L., and Oker, D. E. Glycerol induced hemoglobinuric acute renal failure in the rat. III. Micropuncture study of the effects of mannitol and isotonic saline on individual nephron functions. *Nephron* 4: 337, 1967.
938. Wislocki, P. G., Miwa, G. T., and Lu, A. Y. H. Reactions Catalyzed by the Cytochrome P-450 System. In W. B. Jakoby (ed.), *Enzymatic Basis of Detoxification*, Vol. 1. New York: Academic Press, 1980. P. 135.
939. Wisniewska, J. M., Trajanowska, B., Piotrowski, J., and Jakubowski, M. Binding of mercury in the rat kidney by metallothionein. *Toxicol. Appl. Pharmacol.* 16: 754, 1970.
940. Witschi, H. P., and Aldridge, W. N. Uptake distribution and binding of beryllium to organelles of the rat liver cell. *Biochem. J.* 106: 811, 1968.
941. Wolfert, A. I., Laveri, L. A., Reilly, K. M., Oken, K. R., and Oken, D. E. Glomerular hemodynamics in mercury-induced acute renal failure. *Kidney Int.* 32: 246, 1987.
942. Wong, K. L., Cachia, R., and Klaassen, C. D. Comparison of the toxicity and tissue distribution of cadmium in newborn and adult rats after repeated administration. *Toxicol. Appl. Pharmacol.* 56: 317, 1980.
943. Wong, N. L., Magil, A. B., and Dirks, J. H. Effect of magnesium diet in gentamicin-induced acute renal failure in rats. *Nephron* 51: 84, 1989.
944. Wood, C. A., Norton, D. R., Kohlhepp, S. J., Kohnen, P. W., Porter, G. A., Houghton, D. C., Brummett, R. E., Bennett, W. M., and Gilbert, D. N. The influence of tobramycin dosage regimens on nephrotoxicity, ototoxicity, and antibacterial efficacy in a rat model of subcutaneous abscess. *J. Infect. Dis.* 158: 13, 1988.
945. Worthen, H. G. Renal toxicity of maleic acid in the rat: Enzymatic and morphologic observation. *Lab. Invest.* 12: 791, 1963.
946. Wu, D. F., Griffith, O. W., and Reidenberg, M. M. Lack of effect of glutathione depletion by L-buthionine-S,R-sulfoximine on gentamicin nephrotoxicity in rats. *Pharmacology* 40: 250, 1990.
947. Wyllie, A. H., Kerr, J. F. R., and Currie, A. R. Cell death: The significance of apoptosis. *Int. Rev. Cytol.* 68: 251, 1980.
948. Wysolmerski, R. B., and Lagunoff, D. Inhibition of endothelial cell retraction by ATP depletion. *Am. J. Pathol.* 132: 28, 1988.
949. Yamamoto, A., Adachi, S., Ishikawa, K., Yokomura, T., Kitani, T., Nasu, T., Imoto, T., and Nishikawa, M. Studies on drug-induced lipidosis. *J. Biochem.* 70: 775, 1971.
950. Yasuda, M., and Fujita, T. Effect of lipid peroxidation on phospholipase A_2 activity of rat liver mitochondria. *Jpn. J. Pharmacol.* 27: 429, 1977.
951. Yonaha, M., Saito, M., and Sagai, M. Stimulation of lipid peroxidation by methyl mercury in rats. *Life Sci.* 32: 1507, 1983.
952. Yoshimura, N., Hatanaka, M., Kitahara, A., Kawaguchi, N., and Murachi, T. Intracellular localization of two distinct Ca^{2+}-proteases (calpain I and calpain II) as demonstrated by using discriminative antibodies. *J. Biol. Chem.* 259: 9847, 1984.
953. Younes, M., Albrecht, M., and Siegers, C.-P. Interrelationship between in vivo lipid peroxidation, microsomal Ca^{2+}-sequestration activity and hepatotoxicity in rats treated with carbon tetrachloride, cumene hydroperoxide or thioacetamide. *Res. Commun. Chem. Pathol. Pharmacol.* 40: 405, 1983.
954. Younes, M., and Siegers, C. P. Interrelation between lipid peroxidation and other hepatotoxic events. *Biochem. J.* 33: 2001, 1984.
955. Zager, R. A. Hyperphosphatemia: A factor that provokes severe experimental acute renal failure. *J. Lab. Clin. Med.* 100: 230, 1982.
956. Zager, R. A. Gentamicin nephrotoxicity in the setting of acute renal hypoperfusion. *Am. J. Physiol.* 254: F574, 1988.
957. Zager, R. A. A focus of tissue necrosis increases renal susceptibility to gentamicin administration. *Kidney Int.* 33: 84, 1988.
958. Zager, R. A., Foerder, C., and Bredl, C. Mannitol's influence on myoglobinuric acute renal failure: Functional, biochemical, and morphologic assessments. *J. Am. Soc. Nephrol.* 2: 1991.
959. Zager, R. A., and Gmur, D. J. Effects of xanthine oxidase inhibition on ischemic acute renal failure in the rat. *Am. J. Physiol.* 257: F953, 1989.
960. Zager, R. A., and Prior, R. B. Gentamicin and gram-negative bacteremia. A synergism for the development of experimental nephrotoxic acute renal failure. *J. Clin. Invest.* 78: 196, 1986.
961. Zalme, R., McDowell, E., Nagle, R., McNeil, J., Flamenbaum, W., and Trump, B. F. Studies on the pathophysiology of acute renal failure. II. A histochemical study of the proximal tubule of the rat following administration of mercuric chloride. *Virchows Arch. Abt. B. Zellpath.* 22: 197, 1976.
962. Zalups, R. K., Robinson, M. K., and Barfuss, D. W. Factors affecting inorganic mercury transport and toxicity in the isolated perfused proximal tubule. *J. Am. Soc. Nephrol.* 2: 1991.
963. Zenser, T. V., and Davis, B. B. Enzyme systems involved in the formation of reactive metabolites in the renal medulla: Cooxidation via prostaglandin H synthase. *Fund. Appl. Toxicol.* 4: 922, 1984.

964. Zenser, T. V., Mattammal, M. B., Brown, W. W., and Davis, B. B. Cooxygenation by prostaglandin cyclooxygenase from rabbit inner medulla. *Kidney Int.* 16: 688, 1979.
965. Zenser, T. V., Mattammal, M. B., and Davis, B. B. Differential distribution of the mixed function oxidase activities in rabbit kidney. *J. Pharmacol. Exp. Ther.* 207: 719, 1978.
966. Zenser, T. V., Mattammal, M. B., and Davis, B. B. Demonstration of separate pathways for the metabolism of organic compounds in rabbit kidney. *J. Pharmacol. Exp. Ther.* 208: 418, 1979.
967. Zhang, G. H., and Stevens, J. L. Transport and activation of S-(1,2-dichlorovinyl)-L-cysteine and N-acetyl-S-(1,2-dichlorovinyl)-L-cysteine in rat kidney proximal tubules. *Toxicol. Appl. Pharmacol.* 100: 51, 1989.
968. Zimelis, V. M., and Jackson, G. G. Activity of aminoglycoside antibiotics against *Pseudomonas aeruginosa:* specificity and site of calcium and magnesium antagonism. *J. Infect. Dis.* 127: 663, 1973.
969. Zoccarato, F., and Nichols, D. The role of phosphate in the regulation of the independent calcium-efflux pathway of liver mitochondria. *Eur. J. Biochem.* 127: 333, 1982.
970. Zoccarato, F., Rugulo, M., Siliprandi, D., and Siliprandi, N. Correlated effluxes of adenine nucleotides, Mg^{2+} and Ca^{2+} induced in rat-liver mitochondria by external Ca^{2+} and phosphate. *Eur. J. Biochem.* 114: 195, 1981.
971. Zunino, F., Pratesi, G., Micheloni, A., Cavalletti, E., Sala, F., and Tofanetti, O. Protective effect of reduced glutathione against cisplatin-induced renal and systemic toxicity and its influence on the therapeutic activity of the antitumor drug. *Chem. Biol. Interact.* 70: 89, 1989.
972. Zunino, F., Tofanetti, O., Besati, A., Cavalletti, E., and Savi, G. Protective effect of reduced glutathione against cis-dichlorodiammine platinum (II)-induced nephrotoxicity and lethal toxicity. *Tumori* 69: 105, 1983.
973. Zuretti, M. F., and Baccino, F. M. Biochemical and structural changes of rat liver lysosomes by ethionine. *Exp. Mol. Pathol.* 22: 271, 1975.
974. Zuretti, M. F., and Baccino, F. M. Studies on the hepatotoxicity of *Amanita phalloides* in the rat. II. Biochemical analysis of the lysosomal changes. *Exp. Mol. Pathol.* 24: 176, 1976.

Lithium-Induced and Analgesic-Induced Renal Diseases

Priscilla Kincaid-Smith (Section 1)
Ranjit S. Nanra (Section 2)

1

LITHIUM-INDUCED RENAL DISEASE

Historical Background

Lithium was introduced as a pharmacological agent as long ago as 1859 by Alfred Garrod and was featured in the *British Pharmacopoeia* in 1864 as a therapeutic agent for urate stones and gout [29]. Subsequently, Lange [51] and Haig [34] advocated its use for depression. In the 1940s, lithium was used as a salt substitute in low-sodium diets, and it was at this time that acute intoxication was first described [17, 36].

By 1949, lithium had been totally discredited as a therapeutic agent, but in that year Cade reintroduced it for the treatment of acute mania [10]. It proved to be very effective, not only in the treatment of acute mania, but subsequently as a prophylactic agent in recurring unipolar and bipolar mood disorders [1, 40, 47, 68].

Lithium was initially used mainly in Australia, where it was introduced, and in Scandinavia, where psychiatrists began to use it with some enthusiasm. Only during the past 10 to 15 years has it been used widely in other countries, including the United States, where FDA approval for the use of lithium was only given in 1970 [69]. Lithium is now extensively used. Estimates in Scotland [31] and Scandinavia [66] suggest that 1 in 1,000 persons are taking lithium on a long-term basis.

As early as 1876, Garrod noted polyuria as a side effect of lithium, and serious nephrotoxicity, with a fatal outcome, was first reported by Hanlon et al. [36]. Subsequently, reports of acute renal failure appeared from time to time [20, 53, 59], but the whole emphasis was on the renal effects of lithium being acute and reversible. In 1977 [42] there was a suggestion that chronic renal damage may occur as a result of lithium use.

Lithium undoubtedly causes acute functional and histological lesions in renal tubular cells that are usually reversible. It may also cause chronic progressive morphological and functional changes.

Acute Changes Induced by Lithium

ACUTE REVERSIBLE TUBULAR EFFECTS

Within 24 hours of administration of lithium to humans or animals, a sodium diuresis occurs [2] and impairment in the renal concentrating capacity becomes apparent [27, 39]. This functional defect, which may be associated with gross polyuria, is accompanied by other measurable disturbances of distal tubular function, such as inability to acidify the urine [57, 62, 63].

The defective concentrating capacity is caused by a vasopressin-resistant diabetes insipidus [27]. This occurrence is, in part, related to lithium inhibition of adenyl cyclase and impairment of vasopressin-induced generation of cAMP, but it is likely that this is not the only mechanism involved, because the defect is only partially corrected by dibutyryl cyclic AMP [27, 55]. In addition, one group of workers has shown that lithium does not alter the response to vasopressin in isolated perfused rat papillae [12] and suggest that a factor present in plasma from rats treated with lithium interferes with the action of vasopressin at receptor sites in the distal nephron [58]. The exact mechanism(s) involved in lithium-induced functional tubular disturbances is, therefore, not fully resolved.

Acute lithium intoxication in humans and animals can cause acute renal failure. This occurrence is associated with degenerative changes and necrosis of tubular cells [65, 67]. At an ultrastructural level, Evan and Ollerich [26] found mitochondrial swelling, dilatation of the cisternae of the rough endoplasmic reticulum, and swelling of apical cytoplasm. In humans with lithium-induced acute renal failure, biopsies have shown acute tubular necrosis [37, 68].

Biopsies in humans also show a specific histological lesion in the distal tubule and collecting duct [9, 78–80]. On light microscopy, this lesion is shown to consist of swelling and vacuolization in cells associated with considerable accumulation of PAS-positive glycogen (Fig. 40-1). The lesion is present in all renal biopsies from patients taking lithium and appears within days after administration of lithium and disappears when lithium ingestion is ceased [78]. This acute glycogen accumulation, associated with a characteristic appearance in distal tubular and collecting duct cells, is not seen in rats whose tubules do not contain glycogen but does appear in rabbits.

Rabbits, unlike rats, show glycogen reserves [43, 73] in the distal portion of distal convoluted tubules and collecting ducts. Adult rabbits are also known to increase cellular levels of glycogen in distal convoluted tubules and collecting ducts under physiological conditions associated with low intracellular levels of cyclic AMP [18]. Low cyclic AMP levels favor the synthesis of glycogen [28] and inhibit the breakdown of glycogen [50, 61]. The inhibition of vasopressin-sensitive adenyl cyclase in the distal tubule and collecting duct during lithium administration would be associated with low cyclic AMP levels [22]. Lithium has other actions that would favor glycogen synthesis and inhibit breakdown. It inhibits the protein kinase inhibitor of glycogen synthetase [44] and inhibits other enzymes involved in glycogen breakdown [56]. All these mechanisms would favor glycogen accumulation in distal tubule cells and collecting ducts during lithium administration. These acute tubular changes, which consist mainly of glycogen accumulation, are the histological counterpart of the acute changes in renal function.

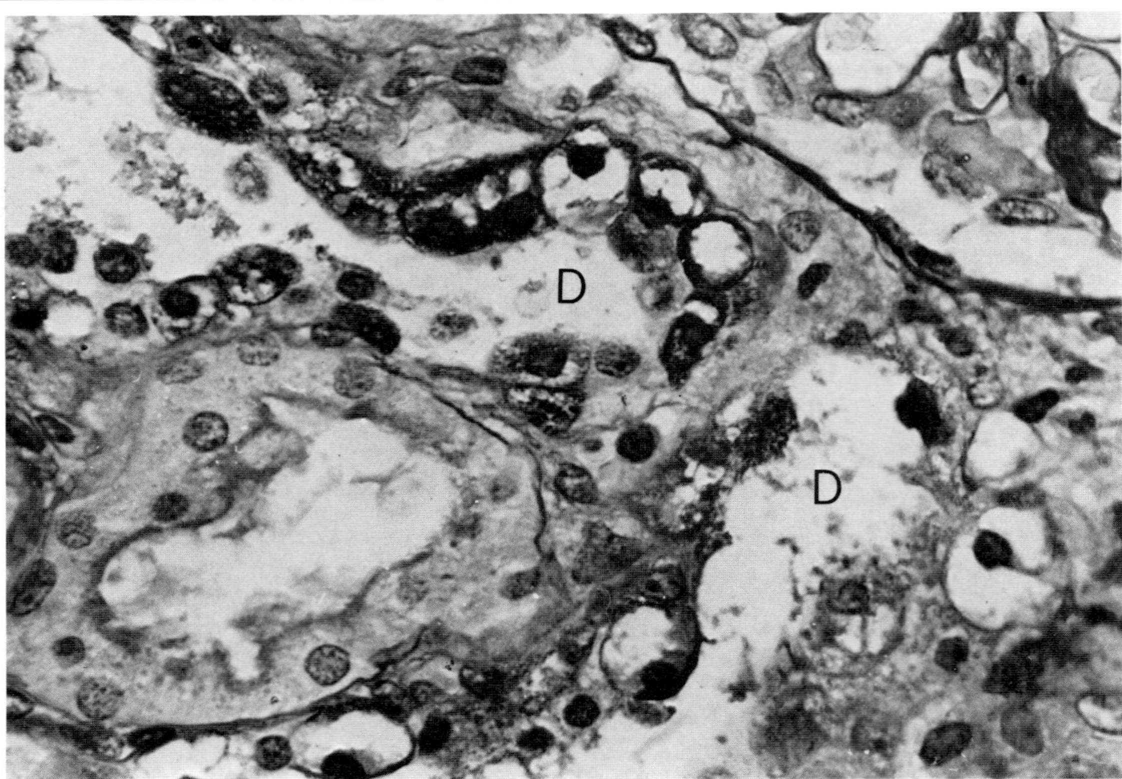

Fig. 40-1. Ballooning, vacuolation, and accumulation of PAS-positive glycogen in epithelial cells in distal tubules (D) in a patient taking lithium. These changes appear within days of starting lithium and disappear soon after lithium is ceased. (PAS, × 900.)

ACUTE RENAL FUNCTIONAL ABNORMALITIES IN PATIENTS TAKING LITHIUM

Renal Handling of Water. Polyuria and polydipsia were first documented with lithium ingestion in 1876 by Garrod and are now recognized as common side effects in patients taking lithium [4, 54, 60, 70, 82]. The incidence of polyuria has varied in different studies from 4 to 50 percent [13, 27, 75, 76]. Ten percent of patients studied by Walker et al. [79] had urine volumes above 3,000 ml in 24 hours. Polydipsia has been less well documented, but Forrest et al. [27] noted polydipsia in 40 percent of 96 patients.

A number of different mechanisms have been suggested to explain the polyuria and polydipsia but, undoubtedly, the major one is a nephrogenic diabetes insipidus. This is a disorder of the distal portion of the distal convoluted tubule and the collecting tubule, characterized by an insensitivity to both endogenous and exogenous vasopressin. The generation of electrolyte-free water during water loading in these patients is intact, but the ability to reabsorb solute-free water under hydropenic conditions is reduced markedly [27].

Patients taking lithium who have polyuria and polydipsia show a reduction in both symptoms after administration of thiazides. These agents produce an antidiuresis in nephrogenic diabetes insipidus by decreasing the delivery of water to the distal nephron. This results from a sodium diuresis, diminished extracellular fluid volume, decreased glomerular filtration rate, and increased fractional reabsorption of sodium and water in proximal tubules [23]. Lithium reabsorption is also increased and this may result in acute lithium intoxication. Amiloride, a potassium-sparing diuretic, may reduce the incidence of polyuria in patients on lithium by inhibiting cellular uptake of lithium in the distal tubule [3]. This is a preferred method of reducing polyuria in patients taking lithium.

Impaired Acidification of Urine. In addition to the defect in urinary concentrating capacity, several groups have documented impairment of distal urinary acidification [57, 63, 79].

Perez et al. [63] noted this defect in most patients; however, Donker et al. [21] found that only 2 of 28 patients ingesting lithium could not acidify their urine to a pH of 5.4 or below after an acid load, and Coppen et al. [16] found no defect in urinary acidification in 16 patients on lithium for 1 to 12.5 years.

Because the fractional excretion of bicarbonate at normal plasma bicarbonate levels was very small [63] and urinary excretion of phosphate and ammonium was normal [46, 63], the defect in acidification with lithium ingestion was attributed to distal rather than proximal tubular abnormalities.

Progressive Renal Damage in Patients Taking Lithium

CONCENTRATING CAPACITY

Bucht and Wahlin [7, 8] showed that impaired concentrating ability may persist for months after discontinuation of lithium, and Rabin [64] reported severe polyuria persisting 18 months after discontinuation of lithium.

In one study, Bucht and Wahlin [8] noted impaired urine concentrating capacity in 17 of 27 patients a year after discontinuation of lithium, and Smigan et al. [71] reported similar results in patients 2 years after stopping lithium. One case has been described in which severe nephrogenic diabetes insipidus, together with two other effects of lithium toxicity, namely hyperparathyroidism and hypothyroidism, all persisted for 2 years after lithium was ceased [11].

Several groups have shown a correlation between the duration of lithium therapy and the degree of impairment of concentrating ability [16, 33, 38, 72, 77, 79]; this observation suggests that progressive damage may occur. A recent longitudinal study supported the view that progressive impairment of the distal tubular responsiveness to arginine vasopressin is common [81]. Contrary evidence came from Coppen et al. [16], who found no difference in maximum urine osmolalities following exogenous vasopressin when 101 patients on maintenance lithium for 12.5 years were compared to a control group that had affective disorders but had not received lithium.

GLOMERULAR FILTRATION RATE

The first suggestion that serious progressive impairment of glomerular filtration rate may occur in patients taking lithium came from Hestbech's group [42]. This observation stimulated a number of cross-sectional studies of patients taking lithium, and most failed to show evidence of impaired renal function [15, 19, 21, 35, 46, 74–76].

Controlled studies have been few [24], but Hullin and colleagues [45] compared 30 patients on lithium with 30 age- and sex-matched patients who had affective disorders but were not on lithium. They observed no difference in serum creatinine, blood urea, or creatinine clearance. Coppen et al. [16] reported similar results, comparing 99 patients on lithium and 52 other patients with affective disorders who had never ingested lithium. On the other hand, Walker et al. [79], comparing 32 age- and sex-matched patients who had affective disorders but had not received lithium with 47 patients who were receiving lithium, found that serum creatinine, ^{51}CrEDTA clearance, and serum β_2-microglobulin levels, all measurements of glomerular function, demonstrated significant impairment in the group on lithium; these results tended to support the view of Hestbech et al. [42].

Thus although the findings in these functional studies are not uniform, there is a suggestion that progressive impairment of both concentrating capacity and glomerular function may occur during long-term lithium treatment.

Fig. 40-2. Cystic dilatation of tubules, or "microcyst," formation, the only hisotological feature suggesting chronic damage, which distinguished biopsies from patients receiving lithium from those of patients with manic-depressive psychosis who had not received lithium. (PAS, × 900.)

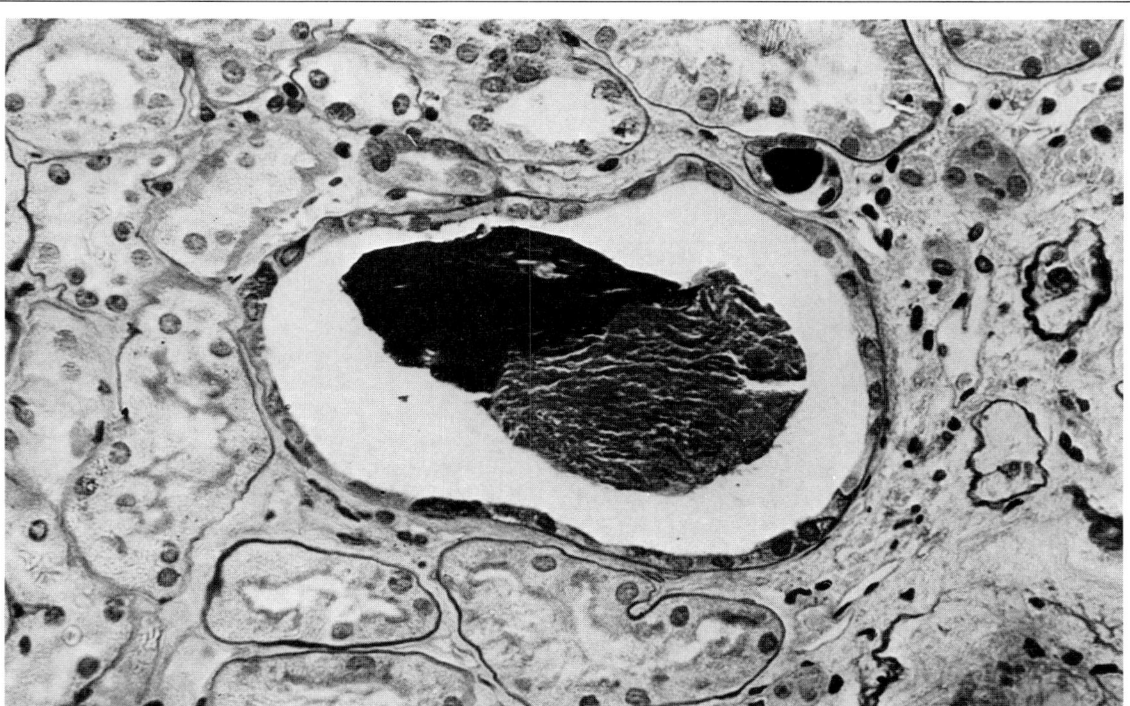

HISTOLOGICAL STUDIES

Hestbech et al. [42] were the first to suggest that progressive chronic interstitial lesions occurred in the kidneys of patients receiving lithium.

The significance of their observations [42] has been questioned because some groups were unable to document a difference in renal function between a control group and patients receiving lithium [16, 47]. Others [13] also failed to find any evidence of a correlation between the duration of lithium therapy and the degree of functional impairment. The only controlled histological study was carried out by Walker et al. [79, 80]. Morphometric analysis failed to show any difference between biopsies from patients taking lithium and those from a group of patients who had affective disorders but were not ingesting lithium. Specifically, there was no difference in the incidence of glomerular sclerosis, interstitial fibrosis, tubular atrophy, cast formation, or interstitial volume. A significant difference was noted, however, in the occurrence of microcyst formation in the lithium-treated patients (Fig. 40-2). Microcysts had also been noted as a significant feature of lithium ingestion, by Hansen et al. [38].

Clinical Features Associated with Lithium-Induced Renal Disease

Polyuria and polydipsia are the major clinical manifestations of lithium-induced renal disease. These symptoms are rarely disturbing to the patient and most tolerate them well. Patients on lithium are almost all aware of considerable benefit in terms of control of their psychiatric illness and, in relation to this benefit, accept polyuria and polydipsia as minor symptoms.

The other functional defect, namely, renal tubular acidosis, is incomplete and does not produce hyperchloremic acidosis in patients, although this can be produced experimentally with high doses of lithium.

Uremia has been described in patients taking lithium [41]; hence the symptoms and signs of uremia may be present. However, the incidence of this complication is very low and lithium's role in the causation of uremia remains controversial.

Other features of lithium toxicity, such as central nervous system (CNS) toxicity and hypothyroidism, may be aggravated by administration of a low-sodium diet or by administration of thiazide diuretics in an attempt to control polyuria. Both these measures will reduce lithium excretion and increase serum lithium concentrations.

Investigations Aimed at Prevention or Detection of Lithium-Induced Renal Disease

SERUM LITHIUM LEVELS

Long before there was any implication that lithium may cause renal disease, psychiatrists recognized the need to monitor serum lithium levels because of the narrow margin of safety between its therapeutic and toxic effects. Since Hestbech [42] raised the possibility of chronic nephrotoxicity resulting from lithium, regular serum lithium levels have assumed greater importance. Whereas previously the aim was to keep the serum lithium level between 0.8 and 1.2 mmol/liter, some groups [45] now recommend that they can be maintained between 0.4 and 0.8 mmol/liter without losing the therapeutic effect in affective disorders.

TEST OF RENAL FUNCTION

Since the first suggestion by Hestbech [42] that lithium may produce serious progressive renal damage, the question of the need to perform renal function tests in patients receiving long-term lithium has been debated.

Hallgren et al. [35] have suggested regular monitoring of the glomerular filtration rate and measurement of albumin and β_2-microglobulin excretion to detect renal damage in patients on lithium. As commented elsewhere [25], this seems rather demanding for psychiatrists dealing with manic-depressive patients, particularly in view of the difficulties of collecting 24-hour urines in such patients.

A simple test, such as estimation of the serum creatinine, is probably all that is necessary. Tests of concentrating capacity and urinary acidification are more troublesome and, even if abnormal, they may not be harbingers of impaired renal function in most patients receiving lithium [81].

Until the question of chronic lithium nephrotoxicity is resolved, an annual serum creatinine estimation is recommended in patients receiving lithium therapy.

Does Lithium Cause Chronic Renal Damage?

There is some skepticism about the suggestion, which has come mainly from Hestbech's group, that lithium may cause a progressive interstitial lesion and progressive impairment of function [32].

Studies from Melbourne [78–80] have generally supported Hestbech's views, although clearly some of the chronic histological changes observed by Hestbech in biopsies from patients taking lithium are not due to the lithium because they appear in biopsies from patients with manic-depressive psychosis who have not taken lithium. Cystic dilatation of tubules (Fig. 40-2) was, however, a feature that clearly distinguished the biopsies of patients receiving lithium from those of other patients with affective disorders [80].

One reason why it has been difficult to answer the question about lithium-induced chronic renal damage has been the lack of a suitable animal model in which lesions similar to those noted in human biopsies can be demonstrated.

In the rat, although tubular dilatation occurs [49], even with prolonged use of lithium at high doses, the major effect is an increase in the size of tubules and of the kidney (Figs. 40-3 and 40-4). No convincing evidence of nephron loss or progressive interstitial lesions has been reported.

When the acute tubular lesion was first described in patients receiving lithium, it seemed likely that this may

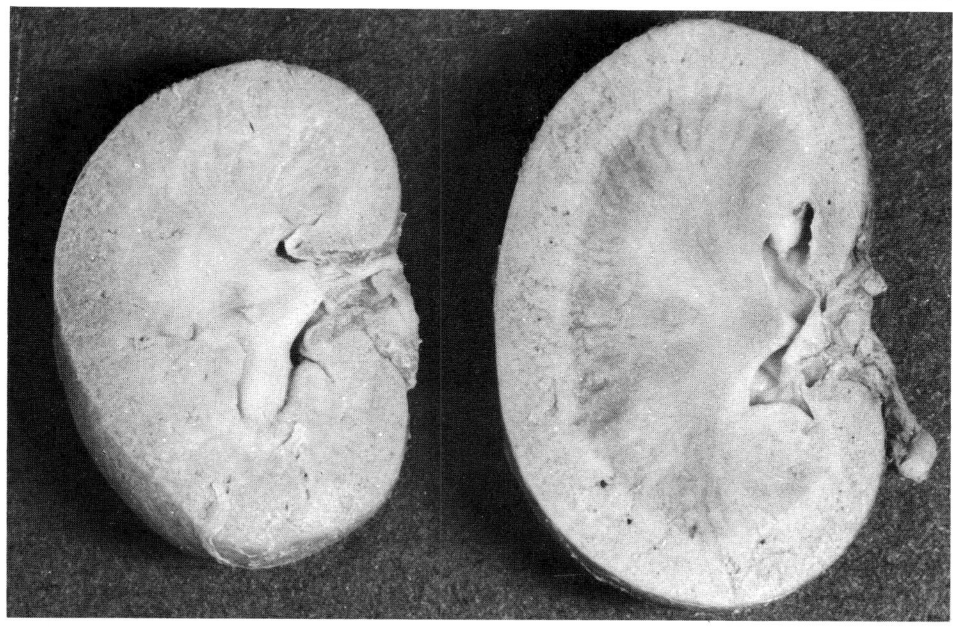

Fig. 40-3. Comparison of rat kidney from a control rat (*left*) and a rat that had received lithium for 18 months (*right*). An increase in size was consistently observed in rats receiving lithium for 12 to 18 months.

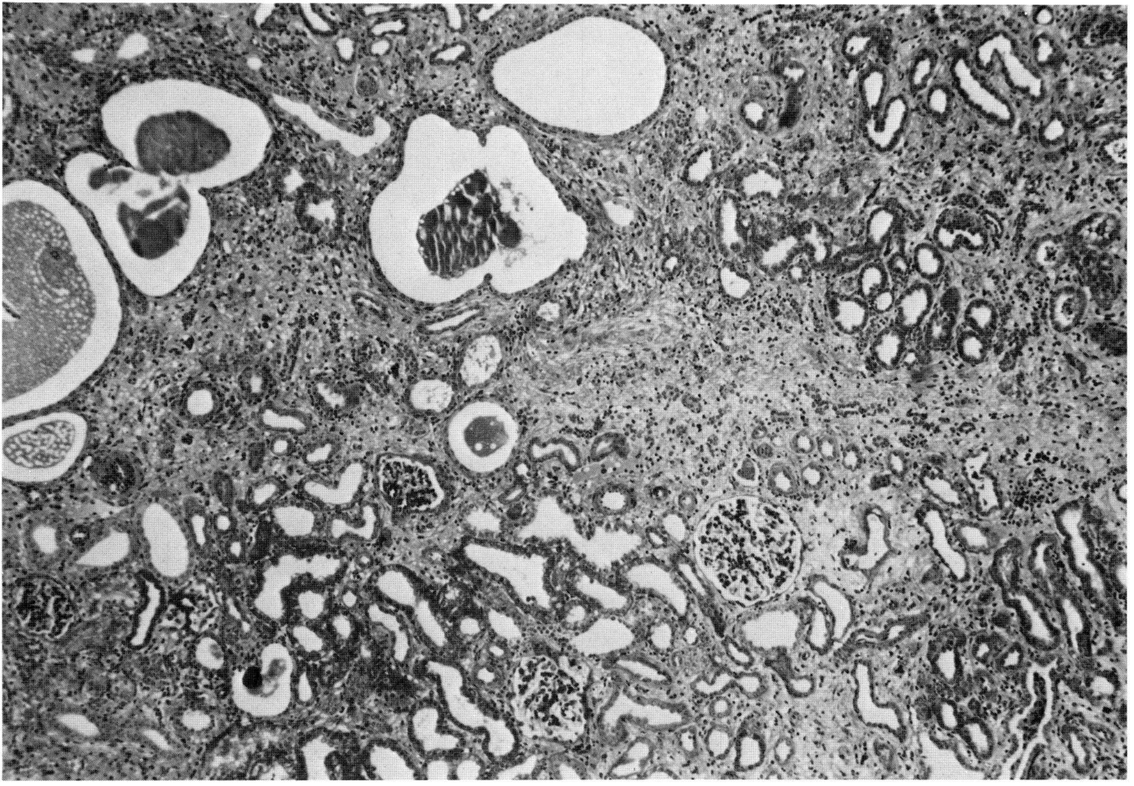

Fig. 40-4. Section of renal cortex of a biopsy taken from an animal that was on lithium supplementation for 12 months. Apart from extensive interstitial fibrosis and atrophic tubules, note the gross dilatation of some distal tubules (microcysts) containing amorphous casts. (Masson trichrome, × 2000.) On PAS stains, casts are strongly PAS-positive.

be responsible for chronic progressive lesions [9]. The acute lesions are seen in tubules within areas of interstitial fibrosis and tubular atrophy, and it was proposed that desquamation of cells and cast formation could cause tubular obstruction and subsequent atrophy.

Because the acute tubular lesion is associated with glycogen accumulation and because glycogen is not seen in the rat tubules—but does occur in the distal and collecting tubules of the rabbit—a study of lithium nephrotoxicity has recently been carried out in the rabbit. This study has shown clear-cut evidence of progressive histological and functional impairment in the rabbit. Rabbits were given lithium chloride, 50 to 250 mmol/kg of food, over 12 months. They developed significant interstitial fibrosis, tubular atrophy, glomerular sclerosis, and cystic tubular lesions. These lesions were quite advanced (Fig. 40-4) and were associated with impaired renal function at 12 months. In this animal model, as in biopsies from patients receiving lithium, microcyst formation is prominent. This is the strongest experimental evidence to date supporting Hestbech's suggestion [42] that lithium causes progressive renal disease.

Management of Lithium-Induced Renal Disease

Polyuria and polydipsia due to nephrogenic diabetes insipidus and other acute manifestations of the effect of lithium on the kidney usually disappear rapidly if lithium is withdrawn. The decision about management, however, usually revolves around the relative benefit of the lithium in controlling and preventing the manifestations of manic-depressive psychosis and the disadvantage to the patient of the major side effect of lithium, namely polyuria. Lithium is so clearly beneficial in most patients that the polyuria is accepted as a side effect and lithium is usually continued.

It is much more difficult to decide appropriate management in a patient who has been on lithium for a number of years and in whom there is some evidence of progressive impairment of glomerular function as well as tubular function. Not all patients develop evidence of progressive impairment of renal function and in some patients, renal function remains normal after 30 years of lithium use [14].

Even where renal function is clearly impaired, both the psychiatrist and the patient will often accept the risks of further deterioration in renal function rather than accept the deterioration in the features of manic-depressive psychosis, which occur if lithium is discontinued.

It is likely that the serum concentration of lithium is important and that renal damage is more likely to occur if the serum concentration is consistently high or if repeated episodes of lithium toxicity occur [48]. The serum lithium concentration should thus be maintained at the lowest level that will provide adequate control of the manic-depressive psychosis, and episodes of toxicity should be avoided by careful monitoring of serum lithium levels.

2

ANALGESIC-INDUCED RENAL DISEASE

Renal papillary necrosis (RPN) complicating chronic urinary tract obstruction was recognized in 1877 [115], and in diabetes mellitus in 1937 [116, 140]. There were, however, numerous reports of RPN where there was no obstruction or diabetes [19, 162, 202, 349, 354]. In 1953, Spuhler and Zollinger [357], in Switzerland, first drew attention to the association between analgesics, chronic interstitial nephritis, and RPN. They believed that this form of new disease had increased in frequency since 1945 [382].

The early reports of analgesic nephropathy appeared almost exclusively from Europe. Publications from English-speaking countries emerged after 1960, and by 1973 at least 3,200 cases of analgesic nephropathy had been reported in the literature [329]; analgesic nephropathy has now been reported from most parts of the world [315].

Analgesic nephropathy appears to be a disease of the twentieth century, and its prevalence appears to be highest in Australia. The abuse of analgesics in the Australian community was recognized as early as 1907 [101]. Between 5 and 45 percent of different subpopulations in the Australian community consumed analgesics daily [54, 69, 112, 127, 128, 155, 178, 206, 319, 374]. Similar patterns of community abuse of analgesic mixtures were reported from many countries; between 2 and 41 percent of populations were found to use analgesics regularly [38, 86, 105, 136, 161, 176, 181, 205, 216, 221, 257, 301, 335, 378].

The per-capita consumption of phenacetin in analgesic mixtures in many countries [123] appeared to correspond to the prevalence of analgesic nephropathy, its contribution to dialysis and transplantation, the incidence of uroepithelial tumors, and to the autopsy incidence of RPN [26–28, 41, 45, 50, 63, 68, 80, 105, 123, 125, 129, 130, 169, 193, 226, 240, 280, 299, 305, 339, 341, 347] (Table 40-1). The abuse of analgesics was also associated with an increase in the autopsy incidence of RPN in several countries as well as an increase in new cases of renal pelvic carcinoma [75, 129, 341]; in Australia, the autopsy incidence of RPN rose from 4 to over 20 percent between 1962 and 1977 [18, 48, 61, 169, 266, 280], and in Switzerland, new cases of renal pelvic carcinoma rose from 2,400 to 2,900 per 100,000 population per year between 1963 and 1977 [239–241].

The geographical distribution of analgesic nephropathy within different countries [20, 43, 135, 260, 322, 366] has been, previously, partly explained on the basis of a hot climate and dehydration [47, 49, 187, 280, 364]. A more likely explanation for the geographical variation is the pattern of analgesic sales and consumption in different areas; in Australia, there was a clear association between analgesic sales and advertisement, and the inci-

Table 40-1. Relationship between consumption of phenacetin and dialysis and transplantation, uroepithelial tumors, and autopsy incidence of renal papillary necrosis

Country	Phenacetin (gm/yr, 1967)	AN (% of Dx/Tx program)	Crude incidence rate of renal pelvic carcinoma/ million population/yr	Autopsy incidence of RPN
Australia	40	18–20 (1979–1983)	0.7–1.6 (Sydney/Newcastle)	3.7–21.4
Scandinavia	25	9.6 (1970) (Sweden) 14.0 (1970) (Denmark)	0.8 (Sweden)	0.2–2.5 (Denmark)
Belgium	25 (Analgesic mixtures)	17.9		
Switzerland	22	16.7 (1970)	High	0.76–1.32
South Africa	12	20 (1978)		
U.S.A.	10	2–10 (1975)	Low	0.23
United Kingdom	8 (Scotland 12)	12	0.3 (England/Wales)	0.16–0.60
Canada	7	2.5 (1976) 5.5	0.4 (British Columbia)	

AN = Analgesic nephropathy; Dx = dialysis; Tx = transplantation; RPN = renal papillary necrosis.

dence of end-stage renal disease in different states [322]; a similar association was noted in Belgium as well [105].

The high morbidity, mortality, and health costs related to analgesic nephropathy led to the introduction of legislation in many countries to restrict analgesic sales and advertisement. In the Scandinavian countries, restriction of phenacetin in 1961 led to prompt reduction in consumption of phenacetin-containing analgesics, a slow decrease in mortality from analgesic nephropathy and chronic interstitial nephritis, and a gradual decline in analgesic nephropathy in dialysis and transplantation programs [42, 126, 136, 137, 160, 180, 183, 193, 221, 295]. Phenacetin was removed from analgesic mixtures in Finland in 1965, in Canada in 1973, and in the United Kingdom in 1975 [125, 316]; in most countries the expected decrease in the incidence of chronic renal failure did not occur. In Switzerland, analgesic sales had not been restricted, and analgesic nephropathy remained a major cause of end-stage renal disease: 17 percent in 1970 and 18 percent in 1979 [42]. In Australia, in 1979, the advertising and sale of analgesic mixtures were restricted, instead of removing phenacetin from analgesic mixtures. There has been a significant change in the use of analgesics in the community [143]; a decrease in the number of new patients with analgesic nephropathy commencing dialysis, from 23 percent in 1977 to 12 percent in 1990 [373]; and a significant reduction in the number of new cases of analgesic nephropathy seen at Royal Newcastle Hospital, Australia, from a mean of 66 per year between 1972 and 1979 to 37 per year between 1984 and 1986 [273, 275].

Definition

Analgesic nephropathy is a form of renal disease characterized by RPN and chronic interstitial nephritis caused by prolonged and excessive consumption of analgesic mixtures; similar disease also results from long-term use or misuse of nonsteroidal antiinflammatory drugs (NSAIDs). The analgesic mixtures in European countries have commonly contained antipyrine, phenacetin, and caffeine, and in Anglo-Saxon countries, aspirin and caffeine or codeine combined with phenacetin, paracetamol (acetaminophen), or salicylamide. Significant analgesic abuse may be defined as an intake of at least 1 to 2 kg of aspirin or phenacetin or paracetamol in the form of an analgesic mixture [266, 269, 290]. Thus this may represent a minimum average consumption of three "powders," containing aspirin + phenacetin + caffeine (900 mg), daily for 5 years or, equally, an intake of one "powder" daily for 15 years; the total quantity of analgesics rather than the duration of abuse has been recently emphasized [20]. Most patients with analgesic nephropathy caused by NSAIDs have used the drugs on a regular basis for over 10 years.

The renal disease associated with analgesic abuse is part of a much wider clinical syndrome—the analgesic syndrome. The other aspects of the analgesic syndrome are neuropsychiatric disorders, cardiovascular and cerebrovascular complications, gastrointestinal disorders (predominantly gastric ulcer and its complications), anemia, gonadal and pregnancy-related problems, pigmentation, and premature aging [20, 24, 67, 76, 94, 123, 125, 150, 209, 260, 264–266, 269, 290, 316, 342] (Table 40-2).

Etiology

In spite of extensive clinical, epidemiological, and experimental evidence that prolonged consumption of analgesics leads to renal disease and renal failure, some authorities have questioned the existence of analgesic nephropathy [208, 356, 378]. The evidence that analgesics cause renal disease is overwhelming. By 1973, more than 3,200 cases of analgesic nephropathy were reported in the literature [290, 329]. There are numerous reports associating analgesic abuse with chronic renal disease and RPN [1, 8, 25, 55, 76, 89, 123, 136, 137, 149, 154, 163, 192, 203, 217, 220, 262–264, 290, 298, 310, 312, 334, 344, 350, 351, 369] and RPN at autopsy, with retrospective estimates of analgesic abuse [50, 129, 130, 139, 169, 239]. These studies emphasized that the incidence of RPN and the extent of renal damage increased with higher abuse of analgesics. The clinical syndrome of analgesic nephropathy [20, 24, 67, 76, 94, 123, 125, 150, 209, 260, 264–266, 269, 290, 316, 342] and the pathological changes of analgesic-induced RPN [46, 47, 49, 129, 130, 341] are characteristic and distinctive. Analgesic nephropathy patients who continue to abuse analgesics have progressive renal failure, and renal function tends to improve or stabilize when patients stop taking analgesics [22, 24, 67, 68, 121, 122, 125, 135, 149, 179, 187, 188, 191, 192, 218, 257, 262, 265, 269, 290, 294, 329, 350, 353, 355, 359]. Experimental RPN is readily produced in laboratory animals by most NSAIDs, and the pathological and functional changes seen are identical to those in clinical analgesic nephropathy (reviewed in [1, 21, 186, 270, 283, 287, 316, 327, 350, 379]). The prospective controlled longitudinal epidemiological studies involving 600 female patients over 11 years reported by Dubach et al. [86–91] clearly demonstrate a significant association between analgesic consumption and renal disease; the studies showed a significant reduction in urine concentration capacity, and an increase in serum creatinine, bacteriuria, and mortality from renal and urinary tract disorders and cardiovascular causes.

Analgesic nephropathy is invariably caused by compound analgesic mixtures containing aspirin or antipyrine in combination with phenacetin, paracetamol, or salicylamide and caffeine or codeine in popular "over-the-counter" proprietary mixtures. Case-control studies related to regular consumption of analgesic mixtures containing phenacetin or paracetamol have suggested a 20-fold risk of RPN, an odds ratio of 5.11 for renal disease, and a relative risk of 2.65 for end-stage renal failure [229, 309, 337, 362]. However, analgesic nephropathy with RPN or chronic interstitial nephritis has also been reported with most individual analgesics and NSAIDs [36, 68, 156, 168, 331, 345] (reviewed in [20, 53, 316]).

Table 40-2. The analgesic syndrome

1. Renal manifestations—analgesic nephropathy
   - Acute/chronic renal failure
   - Hypertension
   - Urinary tract infection
   - Sodium-losing state
   - Renal tubular acidosis
   - Renal artery stenosis/thrombosis
   - Proteinuria—glomerular/tubular
   - Renal calculi
   - Hydronephrosis/pyonephrosis
   - Uroepithelial carcinoma
2. Gastrointestinal manifestations
   - Gastric ulcer—giant
     - Gastrointestinal hemorrhage
     - Perforation
     - Pyloric stenosis
     - Hour-glass stomach
     - Partial gastrectomy and complications
     - Milk–alkali syndrome
   - Abnormal liver function tests
   - Chronic pancreatitis
3. Hematological manifestations
   - Anemia
     - Iron deficiency anemia
     - Anemia of chronic renal failure
     - Hemolytic anemia
     - Refractory sideroblastic anemia
     - Macrocytic and megaloblastic anemia
   - Met- and sulph-hemoglobinemia
   - Splenomegaly
4. Neuropsychiatric manifestations
   - Headaches
   - Migraine
   - Personality inadequacies
     - Introversion
     - Neuroticism
     - External locus of control
   - Addictive syndrome
   - Dementia
   - Psychosis
5. Cardiovascular manifestations
   - Hypertension
   - Generalized atherosclerosis
     - Cerebrovascular disease
     - Renal artery stenosis
     - Abdominal aortic aneurysm
     - Peripheral vascular disease
   - Ischemic heart disease
   - Cardiac valve annulus calcification
6. Pregnancy and gonadal manifestations
   - Toxemia of pregnancy
   - Postmaturity
   - Infertility
   - Teratogenicity ?
   - Congenital malformations
7. Pigmentation
8. Premature aging

In animal studies with the aspirin + phenacetin + caffeine mixture, aspirin appears to be the major nephrotoxic agent, and phenacetin plays a secondary and synergistic role (reviewed in [267, 283–285, 287, 288, 316]). The chronic nephrotoxicity of aspirin is also supported by the significant incidence of RPN and chronic interstitial nephritis (8–100%) in patients with rheumatoid arthritis who are known to take mainly aspirin over many years [20, 40, 48, 51, 64, 82, 119, 133, 207, 225, 283, 285, 286, 302, 380]. However, severe renal failure is rare in rheumatoid arthritis patients; when present, the patient has invariably been abusing compound analgesics [285, 286]. In contrast to aspirin, there are no clinical reports of RPN with phenacetin alone, and all reports of phenacetin-related analgesic nephropathy are due to phenacetin-containing compound analgesic mixtures.

The nephrotoxicity of phenacetin is related to its major immediate metabolite, paracetamol (acetaminophen), and in hydropenic animals, paracetamol and not phenacetin concentrates in the renal medulla [35, 96–99]. The other metabolites of phenacetin and a contaminant in phenacetin, *p*-chloracetanilide, have not been shown to be nephrotoxic but may induce met- and sulph-hemoglobinemia [15, 44, 282, 307, 314, 340, 347, 367]; another minor and inconstant metabolite, *p*-aminophenol, may cause acute proximal tubular necrosis [134], but this is not directly relevant to the chronic nephrotoxicity seen in analgesic nephropathy.

Although the role of caffeine in analgesic nephropathy had been previously discounted and, in fact, postulated to have a protective role [277, 283, 358, 361], a recent study found RPN and hematuria in animals fed caffeine alone [78]. The role of caffeine in analgesic nephropathy should therefore be reconsidered.

In animal studies, RPN has been produced with almost all NSAIDs (Table 40-3) (reviewed in [21, 55, 192, 241, 270, 283, 287, 288, 316, 327, 329, 350, 351, 379]), suggesting that this form of chronic nephrotoxicity associated with RPN and chronic interstitial nephritis is common to all the NSAIDs. Clinical analgesic nephropathy has been reported with a variety of proprietary analgesic mixtures as well most single analgesics (Table 40-4) [36, 68, 156, 168, 186, 274, 275, 331, 345] (reviewed in [20, 53, 283, 316, 350]). NSAID-associated analgesic nephropathy is not uncommon: RPN was found in 23 percent of 230 patients with NSAID-related renal lesions, 88 cases of aspirin-associated RPN were reviewed in 1982, and more cases are being recognized and reported [53, 274, 275, 316].

Pathology

The pathological changes in analgesic nephropathy have been well documented [5, 20, 46, 47, 49, 62, 122, 129, 130, 186, 215, 243, 267, 269, 283, 290, 338].

MACROSCOPIC APPEARANCE

Characteristically, in analgesic nephropathy, the kidneys are reduced in size. The renal capsule is adherent and strips with difficulty. The surface of the kidney is scarred and coarsely granular, and often there are numerous small cortical cysts. In patients who have stopped abusing analgesics, prominent pale tumor-like nodules may be seen and represent hypertrophied columns of Bertin. The cut surface of the kidney reveals marked cortical atrophy. Black necrotic papillae may be seen toward the tip of the medulla (Fig. 40-5). Small, shrunken, streaky, and pale areas of medullary necrosis may be readily missed unless they are specifically looked for by serial coronal cuts through the kidney.

MICROSCOPIC APPEARANCE

RPN is a bland coagulative necrosis, involving the tip of the papilla and extending toward the outer medulla to a variable degree. In total papillary necrosis, all the elements of the medulla, loops of Henle, vasae rectae, collecting tubules, and the interstitium are involved and necrotic. Ghost structures may be identified, particularly with the periodic acid–Schiff stain. There is a striking absence of an inflammatory infiltrate and a clear line of demarcation between necrotic and viable tissue. In partial papillary necrosis, the collecting tubules are spared. In the very early stages of papillary damage, there is patchy necrobiosis, involving the loops of Henle and vasae rectae, and damage to and loss of interstitial cells, usually toward the tip of the papillae. The nuclei in the loops of Henle and vasae rectae are absent and the basement membrane of these structures is thickened and stains prominently. Special stains have also revealed loss of acid mucopolysaccharide staining in the medulla, lipid in necrotic tissue, and needle-shaped cholesterol esters and unsaturated fatty acids [47, 49, 130]. Patchy papillary calcification is common in all stages of RPN with occasional bone formation [49]. Electron microscopic studies have confirmed the necrosis of the loops of Henle and vasae rectae and basement membrane thickening, and in addition reveal the characteristic lesion of capillary sclerosis [122, 238].

The cortex overlying the papilla shows changes of chronic interstitial nephritis, which is characterized by prominent tubular atrophy, interstitial fibrosis, and a nonspecific mononuclear cell infiltrate (Fig. 40-6). The mononuclear cells may represent interference of the normal trafficking of these cells through the interstitium as well as the effect of chemotactic metabolites in the lipooxygenase pathway [20]. Tubular protein casts may be present with occasional areas of "thyroidization." Prominent accumulations of the golden-brown lipofuchsin-like pigment are characteristically seen.

The glomerular changes are varied and range from completely normal or hypertrophied glomeruli to global glomerular sclerosis. The glomerular changes also include periglomerular fibrosis and ischemic changes. In a review of 62 biopsies in analgesic nephropathy patients with proteinuria, chronic interstitial nephritis was seen in all biopsies, focal glomerular sclerosis in 28 percent, focal glomerular hyalinosis in 44 percent, proliferative glomerular lesions in 10 percent, and typical membranous glomerulopathy in 3 percent [236, 269, 272, 290]. The glomeruli with focal and segmental glomerular sclerosis and hyalinosis may show focal deposits of immunoglobulins, especially IgM and C3, albumin, and fibrin; these are likely to be nonspecific deposits that are

Table 40-3. Experimental renal papillary necrosis

Drug	Dose (mg/kg/day)	Duration of feeding (wk)	RPN %	RPN Grade	CIN %	Ca^{2+} %
Compound analgesics						
A + P + C	900	8–30	46–70	+ +		
A + NAPAP + C	900	8–30	38–75	+ +		
A + S + C	900	12–30	54	+ +		
A + P	750	8–20	40	+ +		
AnP + P + C	840	12–30	17–36	+		
MA + C	200	16	62	+ +		
Single analgesics and NSAIDs						
Phenacetin	137–3,000	4–80	8–80	+	+	+
Paracetamol	894–3,000	8–36	43–60	+		
Aspirin	200–500	8–66	33–75	+ – + +	+	+
Aspirin (uninephrectomy)	325	12–15	100	+ +		
Caffeine	100	16	23	+		
Antipyrine	1,000	12–30	13	+	–	38
Amidopyrine	500–1,200	7	83	+		
Phenylbutazone	10	8–20	11	+ +	–	33
Indomethacin	12	12–30	29	+ +	14	43
Flufenamic acid			+			
	50–100	Single dose	+			
Meclofenamic acid			+			
Mefenamic acid	100	8–20	66–67	+ – + +	–	89
Naproxen			+		+	
Sudoxicam	2		+			
Fenoprofen	40–305	78	+		+	
Homozygous Gunn rats						
Phenacetin	320–500	4	7	+		
Phenacetin	1,150	Single dose	33	+		
Paracetamol	268–420	4	37	+		
Paracetamol (uninephrectomy)	3 mmol/kg	Single dose	85	+	+	
Aspirin	200–500	3–4	45–63	+ +		
Aspirin	175–1,150	Single dose	17–100	+ +		
Aspirin (uninephrectomy)	1.25 mmol/kg	Single dose	90	+ +	+	
Sodium salicylate	3 mmol/kg	Single dose	50	+ +		
Antipyrine (uninephrectomy)	2.5 mmol/kg	Single dose	80	+ +	40	
A + P + C	1,190	5–18 days	100	+ +		
A + P + C	238	25–34	70	+ +		
A + NAPAP	4.25 mmol/kg	Single dose	100	+ +	70	
AntiP + NAPAP	5.25 mmol/kg	Single dose	95	+ +	75	

CIN = chronic interstitial nephritis; Ca^{2+} = calcification; A = aspirin; P = phenacetin; C = caffeine; NAPAP = paracetamol; S = salicylamide; AnP = antipyrine; MA = mefenamic acid.

trapped in diseased glomeruli. Arterial changes of benign nephrosclerosis, with thickening of the wall, reduplication of elastic lamina interna, and hyaline sclerosis of the arterioles, were present in 61 percent of biopsy specimens and those of malignant nephrosclerosis in 11 percent.

The walls of capillaries, arterioles, and venules in the renal papilla and the mucosa of the urinary tract, especially in the renal pelvis, ureter, and the bladder mucosa, commonly have a homogeneous thickening, and these changes have been referred to as analgesic microangiopathy or capillary sclerosis [6, 7, 122, 130, 189, 190,

238, 242, 243, 372]. Similar vessels have been described in the skin of analgesic nephropathy patients [3]. Capillary sclerosis occurs in 82 percent of analgesic abusers and its severity correlates with the estimated daily intake of phenacetin. The vessel walls stain heavily with periodic acid–Schiff and fat stains, and these changes are not related to age, blood pressure, or diabetes mellitus. Electron microscopy of these vessels shows irregularities, thickening, and multilayering of the basement membrane, with empty lipid vacuoles and large numbers of highly osmophilic bodies. It is not known whether these changes are primary or secondary, but in histologic studies, capillary sclerosis provides a significant clue to an analgesic etiology.

Table 40-4. Clinical analgesic nephropathy

Analgesic mixtures	Single analgesic compound
A + P + C or codeine	Aspirin
A + paracetamol + C or codeine	Indomethacin
A + salicylamide + C	Paracetamol
Antipyrine + P + C	Phenylbutazone
	Ibuprofen
	Benoxeprofen
	Fenoprofen
	Mefenamic acid
	Naproxen
	Antipyrine
	Alclofenac ?

A = aspirin; P = phenacetin; C = caffeine.

Clinical Features

The clinical syndrome associated with abuse of analgesics is well recognized and has been reviewed extensively. In Australia, with the restriction of sales of analgesic mixtures in 1979, there has been a reduction of analgesic abuse [143] in the community; this has resulted in significant changes in the analgesic syndrome [273, 275]. Three distinct analgesic syndromes can be identified: (1) the syndrome associated with active analgesic abuse, (2) the syndrome following cessation of analgesic abuse, and (3) the NSAID-associated analgesic syndrome [273–275]. The differences between the three syndromes are given in Table 40-5.

ANALGESIC SYNDROME ASSOCIATED WITH ACTIVE ANALGESIC ABUSE

With the exception of one report where there were more males than females [296], analgesic nephropathy is a predominantly female disease, with a female-to-male ratio of 5 to 7:1 [22, 68, 76, 94, 123, 290]. The majority of

Fig. 40-5. Macroscopic appearance of analgesic nephropathy. Note the black necrotic papillae and loss of renal cortical substance. (Reproduced with permission of the author [271].)

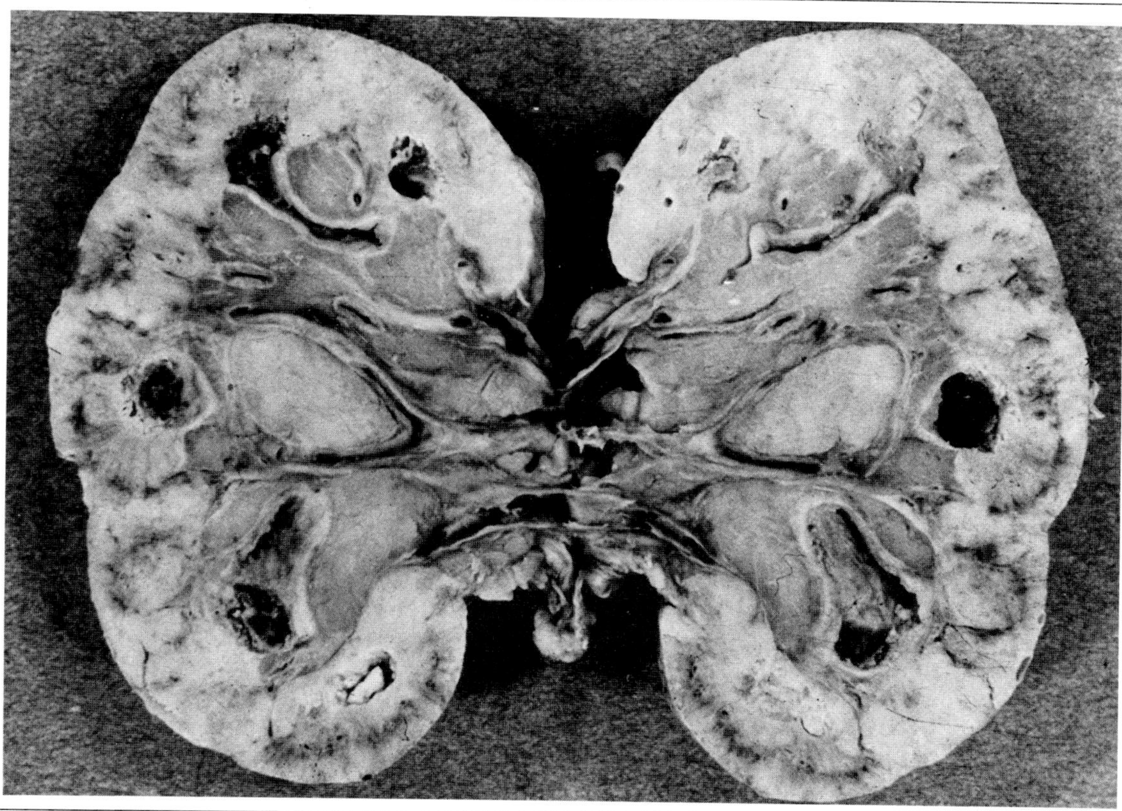

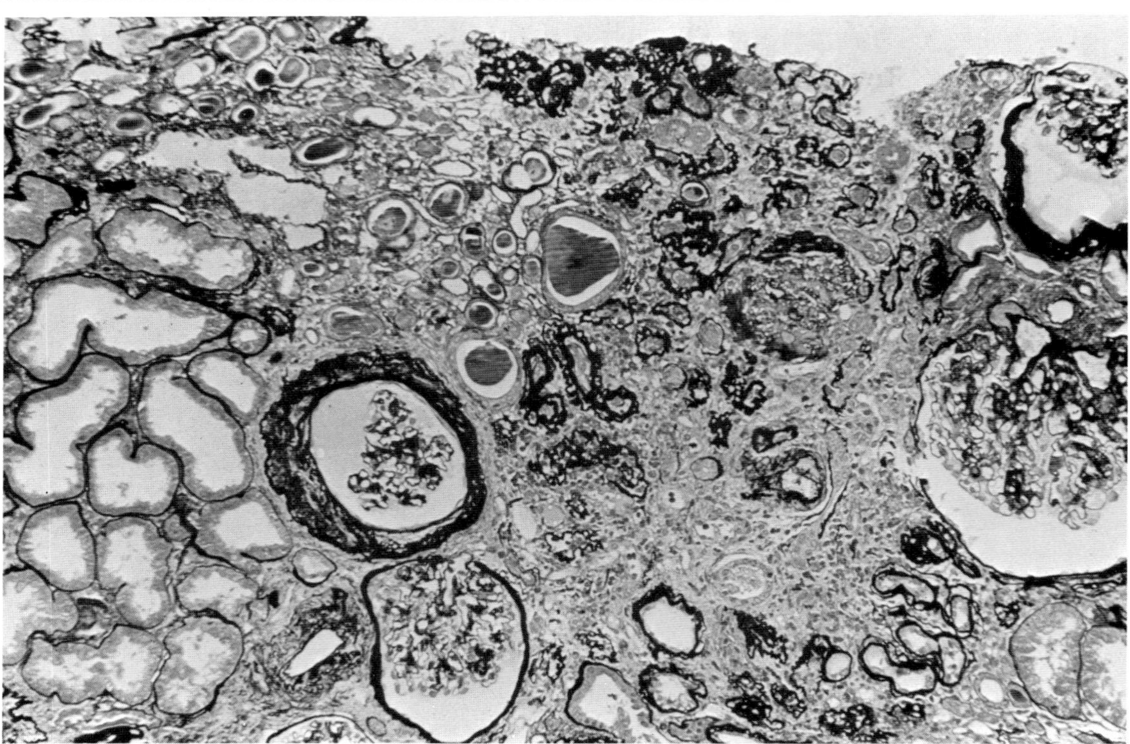

Fig. 40-6. Chronic interstitial nephritis. There is prominent tubular atrophy and interstitial fibrosis, with some mononuclear infiltrate. Periglomerular fibrosis is noted.

Table 40-5. Differences between analgesic syndrome associated with active analgesic abuse, cessation of analgesic abuse, and NSAID-associated analgesic syndrome

Feature	AS—active analgesic abuse	AS—no analgesic abuse	AS—NSAID-associated
No. of patients	100	100	29
NSAID misuse (%)	4	14	100
Smoking (%)	63	36	21
Age (yr)	49 (SD 11)	60 (SD 9)	63 (SD 11)
Female-male ratio	6.1:1	5.7:1	0.9:1
Presenting C_{cr} < 19 ml/min/ 1.73 m² (%)	42	17	0
Sterile pyuria (%)	43	27	41
Hematuria (%)	41	20	28
Urinary tract infections (%)	34	22	0
Proteinuria (gm/day)	1.1 (SD 1.6)	1.2 (SD 2.3)	0.3 (SD 0.6)
Secondary hyperparathyroidism (%)	34	31	0
Malignant hypertension (%)	7	0	0
Renal pelvic carcinoma (%)	0	6	0
Coronary artery disease (%)	31	18	17
Anemia (%)	40	13	10
Cyanosis (%)	5	0	0
Gastric ulcer (%)	12	0	0

AS = analgesic syndrome; C_{cr} = creatinine clearance.
Source: Adapted from Nanra [273–275].

patients present in the fourth and fifth decade of life. The disease is uncommon under the age of 30 years, and an alternative diagnosis should be considered in younger patients [266, 269, 290]. Analgesic nephropathy may have a familial tendency [138, 263, 290, 295], and the increased frequency of HLA antigen B-12 in analgesic nephropathy patients suggests a possible additional genetic factor [222].

NONRENAL MANIFESTATIONS OF THE ANALGESIC SYNDROME

Gastrointestinal Manifestations. Gastrointestinal symptoms are common and peptic ulcer disease has been reported in at least 35 percent of patients [76, 95, 110, 123, 312]. Characteristically, the peptic ulcer is a large gastric ulcer, which is prone to complications, including hemorrhage, perforation, pyloric obstruction, hour-glass stomach, milk-alkali syndrome, and recurrence of anastomotic ulcer and hemorrhage after gastric surgery. Peptic ulcer disease is seen exclusively in patients who abuse aspirin-containing analgesics and, therefore, it is not a feature of the analgesic syndrome in Europe. Single-cell hepatic necrosis [103, 324] with asymptomatic abnormalities in liver function tests and relapsing pancreatitis [12, 142] have been reported in patients with analgesic nephropathy.

Hematological Manifestations. Anemia occurs in 60 to 90 percent of patients with analgesic nephropathy, and the commonest cause of anemia is chronic renal failure. The other causes of anemia include iron deficiency secondary to peptic ulcer and aspirin-related gastrointestinal blood loss, hemolytic anemia, refractory and sideroblastic anemias, macrocytic and megaloblastic anemia, and pancytopenia (reviewed in [71, 76, 92, 110, 113, 218, 298, 316]). Splenomegaly may be seen in 10 percent of patients [92, 113]. Mild cyanosis due to met- and sulphhemoglobinemia is mainly related to *p*-phenetidine, a metabolite of phenacetin, and *p*-chloracetanilide, a contaminant [55, 70, 124, 194, 340, 344]. Cyanosis and hemolysis are more common in Europe, and it is suggested that antipyrine and amidopyrine in the analgesic mixtures in Europe cause induction of microsomal enzymes, which increase the conversion of phenacetin to metabolites that produce methemoglobin [347, 373].

Psychological and Psychiatric Manifestations. Psychological and psychiatric manifestations are seen in over 90 percent of patients, and the frequent associated headaches do not have an organic basis; these are most likely related to caffeine withdrawal [83]. The neuropsychiatric manifestations are reflected in the frequency of associated addictive habits, such as purgative abuse, smoking, alcoholism, and use of psychotropic drugs [59, 61, 110, 195, 258, 374]. Distinct personality traits and inadequacies have been identified and these include introversion, neuroticism, and an external locus of control on the background of disturbed family and social circumstances [259, 326, 328]. Organic features also occur and migraine, dementia, psychosis, hallucinations, and reversible electroencephalographic abnormalities have all been described [84, 182, 261, 376, 381].

Cardiovascular Manifestations. Cardiovascular changes are common and serious complications in patients with analgesic nephropathy. They adversely influence the management of chronic renal failure in these patients. There is premature and often aggressive diffuse atherosclerosis, leading to significant cerebrovascular insufficiency syndromes, coronary artery disease, abdominal aortic aneurysm, peripheral vascular disease, and renal artery stenosis [177, 187, 199, 269, 290]; some patients have associated cardiac valve annulus calcification [255]. Increased mortality from cardiovascular causes has also been reported by Dubach and associates; life table analyses revealed a relative risk of cardiovascular mortality of 2.9, and of cardiovascular disease, fatal or nonfatal myocardial infarction, heart failure, or stroke of 1.8 [66, 90, 91]. In patients with analgesic nephropathy and resistant hypertension, atheromatous renal artery stenosis is common [187, 269, 290]; it is present in 64 percent of cases and is bilateral in 15 percent. Associated renal artery thrombosis is present in 16 percent of cases (R. S. Nanra. Unpublished data, 1991). These features assume greater significance in premenopausal women. The factors that may contribute to severe atherosclerosis are hypertension, the hyperlipidemia and hyperinsulinemia of chronic renal failure, and smoking habits. It has been suggested that, unlike native nonoxidized low-density lipoproteins (LDLs), oxidized LDLs may play a crucial role in atherogenesis [363]. Analgesics, particularly phenacetin, are potent oxidants, and the long-term oxidant effect of these agents in analgesic abusers on LDLs may be an important mechanism in the severe atherogenesis; this hypothesis is supported by the recent epidemiological linkage of phenacetin to hypertension, and cardiovascular morbidity and mortality [91].

Gonadal and Pregnancy-Related Manifestations. These manifestations include infertility, pregnancy-associated hypertension, postmaturity due to reduced uterine prostaglandin, and, possibly, congenital malformations and teratogenicity [9, 39, 102, 107, 213, 266, 325].

Pigmentation. Many patients with analgesic nephropathy appear pigmented and this is accentuated by uremia and a salt-wasting state. The brown-black appearance of necrotic papillae and occasional dark urine in analgesic abusers is related to a breakdown pigment product of phenacetin, 3-amino-7-ethoxyphenazone [244, 318]. A golden-brown lipofuchsin-like pigment is widely distributed throughout the body in the brain, heart, liver, kidney, skin, cartilage (like ochronosis), and the lower urinary tract [33, 129, 209, 254]. Lipofuchsin is a highly oxidized polymer of unsaturated fatty acids [303], and its accumulation in organs is probably related to the oxidant effect of phenacetin.

Premature Aging. Patients with analgesic nephropathy look many years older than their stated age. The presence of severe and aggressive premature atheroma, the reports of presenile dementia, the multiorgan dysfunction, and the widespread distribution of the wear-and-tear lipofuchsin-like pigment in the body all support the notion of premature biologic aging in these patients [123, 266, 269, 290].

RENAL MANIFESTATIONS OF THE ANALGESIC SYNDROME—ANALGESIC NEPHROPATHY

Analgesic nephropathy is a predominantly tubulointerstitial disorder, and the varied clinical manifestations of the renal disease are a reflection of tubulointerstitial dysfunction, varying degrees of renal insufficiency, and complications related to severe atheromatous arterial disease and obstructive uropathy.

Analgesic nephropathy is often asymptomatic, and renal disease is only suspected when reduced renal function, hypertension, or a urine abnormality is detected on routine examination. Up to 14 percent of patients present with terminal renal failure and 80 percent have a reduced glomerular filtration rate (GFR). The possible mechanisms and hypotheses for reduced GFR include (1) blockage of renal tubules by atrophy and interstitial fibrosis; (2) a reduction in postglomerular capillary surface area causing a fall in renal blood flow and GFR; (3) the modified Thurau hypothesis where impaired proximal sodium reabsorption leads to increased tubular flow rate and reduced local renin and angiotensin production; (4) efferent arteriolar vasodilatation; and (5) increased production of the vasoconstrictor thromboxane A_2 by infiltrating mononuclear cells [148, 276, 291]. The renal dysfunction is characterized by a disproportionate reduction in urinary concentrating capacity, systemic acidosis, and a sodium-losing state [24, 25, 67, 68, 122, 198, 269, 276, 288, 290, 313, 323, 360]. All patients with analgesic nephropathy have a urinary concentrating defect, and 26 percent, an acidifying defect; frank renal tubular acidosis, seen in 10 percent of patients, occurs only when the GFR is reduced [198, 276, 290]. These functional abnormalities, which are partly related to reduced medullary synthesis of proteoglycans and glycosaminoglycans [20, 21], contribute to a number of common clinical manifestations, including nocturia, cramps, medullary calcification, renal calculi with hypercalciuria, and renal osteodystrophy [34, 109, 166, 170, 256, 266, 269, 290]. Acute renal failure often occurs with severe life-threatening systemic acidosis and may result from acute RPN, obstruction, surgery, malignant hypertension, hypotension from dehydration, myocardial infarction, gastrointestinal hemorrhage, acute pancreatitis, or septicemia [30, 76, 149, 169, 196, 290, 312, 366].

Patients with analgesic nephropathy have all the usual manifestations of chronic renal failure and uremia. Clinical gout occurs in 5 percent of analgesic patients with normal renal function and in 27 percent in whom the creatinine clearance is less than 60 ml/min/1.73 m^2 surface area; it is more common in males [281, 290]. Renal osteodystrophy tends to be more prevalent and severe, and this may be due partly to the disproportionate systemic acidosis [109, 166, 170].

Urinary tract infections, which may be recurrent and asymptomatic, occur in 15 to 60 percent of patients with analgesic nephropathy and are a late complication [22, 61, 68, 94, 123, 139, 265]. Any associated decline in renal function usually suggests urinary tract obstruction or septicemia. Sterile pyuria is common and may be due to covert urinary tract infection or renal tubular epithelial celluria; the latter can be distinguished from true leukocytes with special staining techniques [317]. It is generally accepted that urinary tract infections do not play a pathogenetic role in the development of RPN. However, an increased susceptibility to urinary tract infections has been suggested in analgesic nephropathy, and this has also been related to reduced medullary synthesis of proteoglycans and glycosaminoglycans [20, 21].

Thirty five to 40 percent of analgesic nephropathy patients may have hematuria [236, 269, 276]. Hematuria may be related to urinary tract infection and cystitis, acute RPN and papillary separation, renal calculus formation, malignant hypertension, or the development of a glomerular lesion or a uroepithelial tumor. Phase contrast microscopy of urine is helpful in differentiating dysmorphic glomerular from nonglomerular hematuria.

Significant proteinuria, greater than 0.3 gm per day, occurs in 40 to 50 percent of analgesic nephropathy patients [236, 276]. The average proteinuria is approximately 1.0 gm per day and nephrotic syndrome is uncommon. In contrast to proteinuria in glomerulonephritis, the incidence and degree of proteinuria in analgesic nephropathy increase as the GFR declines, and this inverse relationship is significant ($p < 0.01$) [236, 276]; more than 90 percent of patients with a creatinine clearance less than 10 ml/min/1.73 m^2 have proteinuria. The proteinuria in analgesic nephropathy is mixed, glomerular and tubular, with large quantities of low- and high-molecular-weight proteins, particularly β_2-microglobulin and albumin; β_2-microglobulinuria occurs in 56 percent of patients and its concentration in urine increases as GFR declines [10, 11, 276, 289]. Persistent proteinuria usually indicates the presence of chronic interstitial nephritis with secondary glomerular lesions and develops at a relatively late stage of RPN; it is an adverse prognostic marker [236, 276].

Fifteen to 70 percent of patients develop hypertension [22, 25, 61, 76, 94, 110, 122, 218, 298], which increases in severity with declining renal function. Up to 15 percent of patients have resistant hypertension and 7 percent develop malignant hypertension [276, 290], a common mechanism of precipitating patients into terminal renal failure. Hypertension may be more common and severe in analgesic abusers with or without RPN, than in glomerulonephritis patients [201] (R. S. Nanra. Unpublished data, 1980). The recent epidemiological report by Dubach and co-workers suggests an association between phenacetin and hypertension, with an odds ratio of 1.6 for the incidence of hypertension; no association was found with aspirin [91]. A significant proportion of patients with presumed essential hypertension may have subclinical analgesic nephropathy [365]. As in other forms of hypertension secondary to renal parenchymal diseases, the hypertension in analgesic nephropathy is related to a fall in GFR, retention of sodium, elevation of angiotensin II, and a distorted relationship between intravascular volume and pressor agents [81]. The pressor agents in analgesic nephropathy are likely to be exaggerated because of potentially higher angiotensin II levels secondary to impaired sodium conservation and loss of vasodilatory medullary substances due to RPN [253, 276]. Thus, some patients with analgesic nephropathy, acute RPN, and marked intravascular volume depletion may have severe hypertension or even malignant hypertension [269, 290]. When there is resistant or brittle hypertension, an atheromatous renal artery stenosis or thrombosis should be suspected (see Cardiovascular Manifestations).

Urinary tract obstruction is a serious complication in analgesic nephropathy and may be due to a necrotic or calcified papilla [25, 163, 216, 366], a renal calculus, a transitional cell renal pelvic or ureteric tumor, or ureteric fibrosis and stricture [29, 111, 212, 223, 269, 290]. Recurrent renal colic, with passage of fragments of papillae, is not uncommon. Urinary tract obstruction may be silent and the only manifestation of this may be an unexplained rise in serum creatinine or blood urea concentration. Concomitant urinary tract infection may lead to septicemia or pyonephrosis, a potentially fatal complication. Renal calculi occur commonly in analgesic nephropathy [34, 202, 266, 269, 290] and should be differentiated from calcified necrotic papillae. The factors contributing to calculus formation are exfoliation of renal tubular epithelial cells or fragments of necrotic papillae, which provide a nidus for precipitation, the secondary renal tubular acidosis, obstruction and stasis, and urinary tract infection, especially with urea-splitting organisms, such as *Proteus* and *Pseudomonas* [290]; reduced medullary synthesis of proteoglycans and glycosaminoglycans may also contribute to microcrystallization and stone formation [20].

NATURAL HISTORY OF THE ANALGESIC SYNDROME

In Australia, in general, the habit of analgesic intake commenced in secondary school and by graduation age analgesic consumption was at an adult level (Fig. 40-7). The obstetric and gastrointestinal manifestations were usually seen between the ages of 20 and 40 years, whereas the renal and other complications tended to occur after the age of 30 years [269].

ANALGESIC SYNDROME FOLLOWING CESSATION OF ANALGESIC ABUSE

Five to 7 years after restriction of analgesic sales in Australia and a significant fall in analgesic abuse in the community [143], there have been significant changes in the analgesic syndrome [273, 275] (Table 40-5). A comparison of 100 analgesic nephropathy patients with active analgesic abuse seen between 1972 and 1974, with 100 patients with no active analgesic abuse seen between 1984 and 1986, showed significant changes in the analgesic syndrome; in the latter group there was a reduction in severe and terminal renal failure, smoking habit, hematuria, sterile pyuria, coronary artery disease, and anemia; a total disappearance of malignant hypertension, gastric ulcer, and cyanosis; and a significant in-

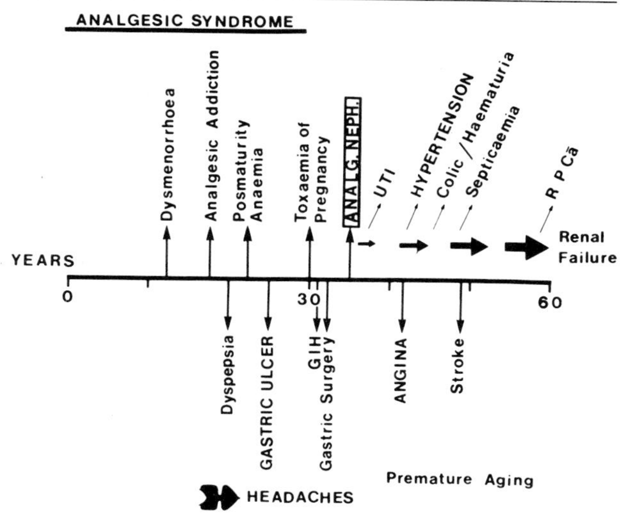

Fig. 40-7. Natural history of a hypothetical case of analgesic syndrome. GIH = gastrointestinal hemorrhage; UTI = urinary tract infection; RPCā = renal pelvic carcinoma. (Reproduced with permission of the author [269].)

crease in age at diagnosis (by 11 years), and renal pelvic carcinoma.

NSAID-ASSOCIATED ANALGESIC SYNDROME

The NSAID-associated analgesic syndrome (Table 40-5) is similar in most respects to the syndrome seen in analgesic nephropathy patients following cessation of analgesic abuse, with a few differences. The usage of NSAIDs is invariably related to rheumatological disorders such as osteoarthritis and rheumatoid arthritis. There is no predominance of females. Severe renal failure, proteinuria, urinary tract infections, and secondary hyperparathyroidism are less common, and renal pelvic carcinoma has not been seen as yet [274, 275].

Pathogenesis of Renal Papillary Necrosis and Analgesic Nephropathy

The primary lesion in analgesic nephropathy is RPN; the cortical change of chronic interstitial nephritis is a secondary lesion, resulting from obstruction to tubules in the necrotic medulla [46, 47, 49, 130, 185, 249, 267, 269].

The pathogenesis of RPN and chronic interstitial nephritis has been studied best in animal experiments with the common analgesic compounds, aspirin, phenacetin, and paracetamol.

In hydropenic animals, aspirin and salicylate develop a corticopapillary gradient of 1:1.9 to 4.5; there is some evidence that aspirin accumulates in the pars recta of proximal tubules [31, 35, 96, 120, 249, 320]. Aspirin and salicylate also have an intracellular distribution, which is augmented by maximal urine acidification [56, 96]. Aspirin has a profound effect on intracellular metabolism and, in large doses, produces massive proximal tubular necrosis [17]; this is related to the formation of a reactive metabolite, which is mediated by a microsomal cytochrome P-450-dependent monooxygenase [245]. Aspirin (1) induces covalent acetylation of cellular proteins, resulting in inhibition of prostaglandin synthetase in both the renal cortex and medulla [57, 151, 332, 348]; (2) reduces renal glutathione probably by inhibition of the hexose-monophosphate shunt [96, 131]; (3) irreversibly blocks fatty acid cyclooxygenase causing reduced lipogenesis in the renal medulla and also leads to reduced glutathione [56, 165, 333]; (4) uncouples cortical oxidative phosphorylation, resulting in decreased intracellular adenosine triphosphate (ATP) [77, 322]; (5) inhibits amino acid incorporation into cellular proteins, an effect that is enhanced by paracetamol [72, 73]; and (6) may induce tissue hypoxia by reducing red cell 2,3-diphosphoglyceride [197].

In hydropenic animals, paracetamol develops a large corticomedullary gradient of 1:10, and the concentration gradient of free paracetamol is 1:16 [35, 56, 96–99]. Paracetamol, and its metabolite, *p*-aminophenol, also undergo P-450-mediated activation to a reactive alkylating intermediate metabolite, probably *N*-acetyl-*p*-benzoquinoneimine [235, 252] as well as peroxidative activation to reactive phenolic and aromatic metabolites [52, 157, 235, 247]. The P-450-mediated activation occurs in the renal cortex, as in the liver, and the covalent binding to proteins in the medulla appears to be different and requires further study [96, 235, 245, 246]. The effects of paracetamol on intermediary metabolism include (1) intracellular depletion of glutathione induced by covalent binding to cellular proteins and nuclei by reactive metabolites in the renal medulla and cortex [252], an effect that is augmented during antidiuresis [235, 252]; and (2) marked depletion of serum sulfate and sulfate clearance, thus limiting its availability for medullary synthesis of proteoglycans and glycosaminoglycans, essential constituents of medullary matrix [214].

Phenacetin does not develop a corticopapillary gradient even under conditions of antidiuresis [99] and as a result of hepatic metabolism [321], systemic and urinary concentrations of phenacetin are extremely low. Paracetamol is the major immediate metabolite of phenacetin; it is paracetamol that concentrates in the renal medulla. However, *p*-phenetidine, the major deacetylated metabolite of phenacetin, also produces biologically active reactive species, with toxic effects similar to those of paracetamol [13].

Most NSAIDs and analgesics interfere with arachidonic acid metabolism resulting in reduced prostaglandin E_2 synthesis by suppression of cyclooxygenase, which leads to vasoconstriction and medullary ischemia [100, 117, 234, 269, 351]. Matsuda et al. [227] have shown that the decreasing rank order of the potency of suppression of prostaglandin synthesis by NSAIDs is flubiprofen, ketoprofen, naproxen, indomethacin, diclofenac, meclofenamic acid, mefenamic acid, and aspirin; this equates with the potency of RPN induction [145]. The NSAIDs also undergo metabolic activation and may generate reactive metabolites via prostaglandin hydroperoxidase or other peroxidase-mediated metabolic pathways (reviewed in [21]). These metabolites have effects similar to those of aspirin, including reduced medullary lipogenesis, reduced tissue levels of glutathione, and medullary ischemia [32].

Thus it may be concluded that (1) aspirin and paracetamol achieve significant medullary concentrations, although the data with aspirin are still debated; (2) aspirin, paracetamol, and the NSAIDs have significant potential for nephrotoxicity; and (3) the nephrotoxicity of phenacetin is likely to be due to its major metabolite, paracetamol, although *p*-phenetidine, the deacetylated metabolite of phenacetin, may contribute to the renal lesion.

The crucial role of the renal concentrating mechanism in the development of RPN has been documented experimentally and clinically (reviewed in [20, 21]) [118, 189, 190, 219, 280, 282–284]. The earliest histological lesions in experimental RPN are toward the tip of the papilla at the site of maximal concentration of analgesics; dehydration increases the incidence and severity of experimental RPN; and a water diuresis or experimental papillectomy protects against the lesion [49, 118, 144, 249, 282–284]. It has been suggested that the renal countercurrent concentration mechanism is responsible for the specific concentration of toxicokinetic factors in target cells in the renal medulla [251]. Dehydration alone may result in significant medullary ischemia [371] and RPN in infants and animals [60, 74, 352].

Medullary ischemia plays a significant role in the pathogenesis of RPN; it has been demonstrated in experimental analgesic nephropathy and correlates with evidence of medullary dysfunction in the form of impaired concentrating ability and sodium conservation [278]. The histological features of analgesic-associated RPN are suggestive of an ischemic infarction, and vasa recta lesions, with endothelial necrosis, vascular obliteration and narrowing, platelet aggregation, and a more generalized microangiopathy or capillary sclerosis have all been demonstrated early in RPN [2, 6, 7, 49, 78, 189, 190, 238, 249, 278, 336]. The medulla is particularly vulnerable to ischemic damage; its blood flow is slow, tissue oxygen tension is low, and ischemic insults, such as renal pedicle or renal vein occlusion or severe shock are sufficient to produce RPN (reviewed in [278]).

The suggested stages in the pathogenesis of RPN and analgesic nephropathy with aspirin and phenacetin are (modified from [288]):

STAGE I. The concentration of analgesics and NSAIDs in the renal medulla by the countercurrent mechanism leads to suppression of prostaglandin synthesis and *reversible* medullary ischemia [308].

STAGE II. The earliest detectable histological lesions in experimental RPN are cytotoxic injury to interstitial cell and medullary matrix, mediated by reactive metabolites, with loss of medullary proteoglycans and glycosaminoglycans [20, 21, 214, 248, 249]. This stage may be associated with a defect in urine concentration, hypertension, papillary calcification, and thickening of the basement membrane in the loops of Henle and vasae rectae [49, 144, 224, 238, 249, 283, 306].

STAGE III. The cytotoxic effects of the reactive metabolites of analgesics and NSAIDs lead to glutathione depletion and necrobiosis of the loops of Henle, endothelial lesions in the vasae rectae, and the characteristic basement membrane change of capillary sclerosis or analgesic microangiopathy. Occlusive changes in the vasae rectae lead to *irreversible* medullary ischemia, with associated impaired urinary concentration capacity and sodium conservation.

STAGE IV. The renal medulla is very vulnerable to ischemic damage, and the combination of irreversible medullary ischemia, cytotoxic cell necrosis, and interstitial damage results in RPN with the histological features of an ischemic infarct.

STAGE V. Obstruction to tubules in the necrotic medulla leads to the nonspecific obstructive change of chronic interstitial nephritis in the cortex.

Analgesic-associated chronic interstitial nephritis also may develop in the absence of RPN, particularly with aspirin [130, 249, 270]. A possible explanation for these findings is a direct cortical toxic effect of aspirin [270]. Aspirin achieves a six-fold concentration in the cortex in hydropenic animals [96] and has significant cortical cytotoxic effects. Prostaglandins have been demonstrated in most cortical structures, glomeruli, arteries, and tubules [308], and suppression of prostaglandin synthesis may lead to cortical ischemia as well.

Transitional Cell Tumors of the Uroepithelium

Since the first description of renal pelvic carcinoma in patients with RPN in 1965 [164], more than 400 cases of transitional cell carcinoma of the uroepithelium had been reported in the literature by 1983 [270]. There appears to be a causal relationship between analgesics and uroepithelial tumors with a relative risk of 5.7 to 13.0 for renal pelvic carcinoma, of 2.6 for bladder carcinoma, and of 2.0 for ureteric carcinoma, related to regular analgesic abuse [106, 228, 231, 232, 330]. The evidence supporting this association is overwhelming and is suggested by a high incidence of these tumors in countries in which analgesic nephropathy is prevalent, including Australia, Sweden, and Switzerland [27, 200, 210, 226, 301] (Table 40-1); an increase in new cases of uroepithelial carcinoma in Switzerland from 2,400 per 100,000 population between 1963 and 1966 to 2,900 per 100,000 population between 1972 and 1977, associated with an increase in RPN [239–241]; a decline in renal papillary carcinoma by 5.1 percent per year, in renal parenchymal carcinoma by 3.4 percent per year, and in bladder carcinoma by 2.1 percent per year following withdrawal of phenacetin-containing analgesics [233]; patients with analgesic-associated tumors being on average 10 years younger than those with nonanalgesic tumors [28, 226, 239–241]; a female-to-male ratio of 2 to 4:1 in an otherwise predominant male disease [27, 28, 132, 164, 226, 239–241, 299]; reversed distribution of tumors in the urinary tract, the ratio of renal pelvic-to-bladder carcinoma being 11:1 instead of the 1:15 in nonanalgesic patients [28, 240]; the presence of renal insufficiency and RPN in 80 to 92 percent of cases [27, 28, 173]; and the induction of uroepithelial hyperplasia, a premalignant change, and tumors in animals fed phenacetin alone or analgesic mixtures containing aspirin, phenacetin, paracetamol, salicylamide, and caffeine [167, 171, 172, 279]. In Australia, the crude incidence rate of renal pelvic carcinoma has been estimated to be 0.7 to 1.6 per million population per year, and this rate is much higher than in other parts of the world [270, 299]. It is suggested that with long-term survival of patients with analgesic nephropathy, uroepithelial tumors may develop in 8 percent of patients [27, 130, 220, 310]. Mihatsch et al. [239–241] have estimated that patients who abuse analgesics experience greater rates of cancer of the ureter (89 times higher), the renal pelvis (77 times higher), and the bladder (7 times higher) than patients who do not abuse these drugs.

The major analgesic-associated tumor is uroepithelial carcinoma (reviewed in [58]). However, hypernephroma, sarcoma, and chorionepithelioma have also been reported in patients with analgesic abuse [16, 41, 200, 220]. The renal pelvic tumors are commonly localized to the calyces, calyceal infundibula, or pelvic ampulla but may also wholly or partly originate from the renal papilla. The tumors tend to be multifocal and in about 5 percent of cases, bilateral simultaneous renal pelvic carcinomas are seen [28]. Both papillary and solid tumors occur, and with increasing tumor size, a lower differentiation of the tumor has been observed. Distant metastases have been reported in 43 percent of cases at autopsy, the predominant sites being lung, liver, and bone [173].

Most investigators have linked phenacetin to the development of uroepithelial tumors, and attention has been focused on the 2-hydroxy and N-hydroxy metabolites of phenacetin [28, 41, 173, 226, 229, 233, 292, 293]; reviewed in [20, 21, 316]. Further evidence in support of the carcinogenicity of phenacetin is the increased relative risk (1.9) of deaths from cancer related to phenacetin and not to aspirin, in a recent epidemiological study [91]. The N-hydroxy metabolites of phenacetin have been shown to inhibit synthesis of DNA and RNA protein, and to alter nuclear chromatin structure [151]. In patients with analgesic-associated tumors, the mean intake of phenacetin has been 9.1 kg; the exposure and latency time, 20 to 30 years; and the induction time, greater than latency time by 5 years [28, 174]. These risks persist even after stopping analgesics for 4 to 8 years [132, 141]. However, definitive proof of carcinogenicity of phenacetin is still lacking and the role of other factors, including cigarettes, caffeine, artificial sweeteners, urinary tract infections, calculi, occupational exposure, and other unknown factors, such as in Balkan nephropathy, which has a strikingly high incidence of uroepithelial carcinoma [104], cannot be ignored [28, 65, 226, 228, 230–232, 330].

Diagnosis

The diagnosis of analgesic nephropathy is based on obtaining a history of significant analgesic abuse or NSAID misuse and the demonstration of renal disease characterized by RPN and chronic interstitial nephritis.

Significant analgesic abuse has been defined previously (see Definition). The actual consumption of analgesics may be as high as 30 kg of aspirin or phenacetin. Precise quantitation of analgesic intake may be difficult, and many patients attempt to conceal or minimize the extent of abuse [61, 110, 112, 123, 258]. Analgesic abuse, seen in 45 percent of patients in the 1970s, has significantly diminished to 5 percent only in the 1980s after the restriction of analgesic sales in Australia [273, 275]. The presence of analgesics and their metabolites in urine is a useful method of detecting analgesic abuse or use [89].

RPN is usually demonstrated by an intravenous urogram. In cases where renal damage is mild and changes in the intravenous urogram are doubtful, the diagnosis of analgesic nephropathy is supported by the biopsy demonstration of chronic interstitial nephritis and disproportionate reduction in concentrating capacity [266, 269, 290]. In renal biopsy specimens, prominent lipofuscin granules are a feature of analgesic abuse, and the golden brown pigment may be seen in renal tubular epithelial cells in 78 percent of specimens [209, 243]. When renal function is significantly reduced and there is poor radiological calyceal definition, retrograde pyelography should be undertaken to confirm RPN; the detection of brown mucosal discoloration during cystoscopy is a valuable diagnostic aid and supports the suspicion of analgesic abuse [49, 55, 114]. Occasionally, RPN may be seen in a renal biopsy, which inadvertently obtains medullary tissue, or it may be confirmed by the demonstration of necrotic papillary tissue voided in urine. Fragments of papillary tissue should always be looked for in urine when a patient has renal colic or macroscopic hematuria; calcified papillae, which may be passed or removed surgically, should be examined histologically for necrotic papillary tissue. The finding of the characteristic capillary sclerosis in urinary mucosal biopsy specimens provides strong evidence for an analgesic etiology [114, 130, 238, 242, 243, 300]. The relationship between renal function, radiological changes, and renal biopsy abnormalities in analgesic nephropathy are shown in Table 40-6 [290].

The radiological features of RPN have been fully described [79, 108, 146, 147, 158, 202, 204, 211, 217, 237, 256, 271, 311]. In acute RPN, the papillae appear swollen. Chronic RPN may be of the medullary or papillary types, and the important features that assist in diagnosis are medullary cavities, papillary calcification, calyceal "horns," ring shadows, and clubbed calyces (Fig. 40-8). In RPN in situ, careful calyceal study, particularly with retrograde pyelography, will often reveal calyceal abnormalities [311]. Papillary calcification may be seen in 30 to 50 percent of patients with analgesic nephropathy [79] and may be readily detected in ultrasound examinations even in end-stage kidneys [159, 250]; 50 percent of end-stage analgesic nephropathy kidneys also show intrarenal cysts [250]. Radiological cortical scarring is not as prominent as that seen in reflux nephropathy, except in patients who have stopped analgesic abuse and compensatory hypertrophy of columns of Bertin has occurred. In serial intravenous urograms, it is common to find a progressive reduction in renal size. Rarely, in patients with

Fig. 40-8. A pyelogram in a patient with analgesic nephropathy. Note (from top to bottom) calyceal "horn," clubbed calyx with medullary cavity, and ring shadow. (Reproduced with permission of the author [269].)

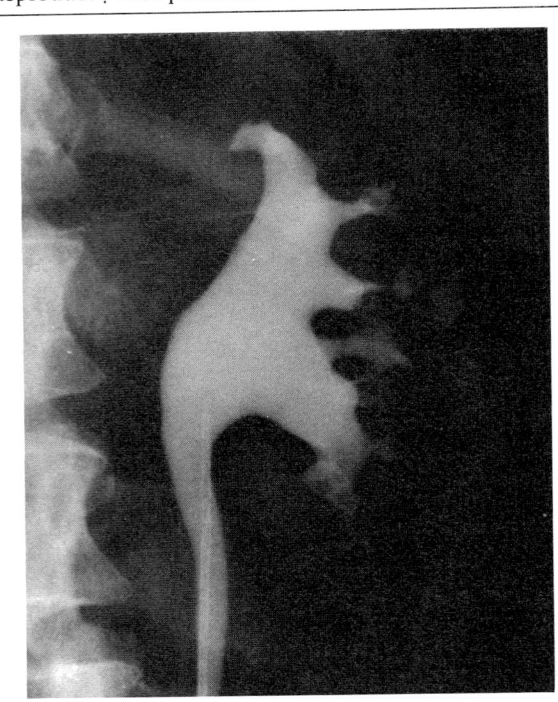

Table 40-6. Relationship between renal function, radiological changes, and renal biopsy abnormalities in analgesic nephropathy

			IVU		
Reduction in GFR	Reduction in concentration capacity	Acidification defect	Renal size	Calyceal abnormality	CIN
−	+	−	−	−	+/−
+	+ +	−/+	−/+	+	+
+ +	+ + +	+	+	+ +	+ +
+ + +	+ + +	+	+ +	+/− (RPN in situ)	+ +

GFR = glomerular filtration rate; CIN = chronic interstitial nephritis; RPN = renal papillary necrosis; (−) = normal; (+) = abnormal; IVU = intravenous urography.

Table 40-7. Differences between analgesic nephropathy and reflux nephropathy

	AN	RN
Clinical		
Age	Rare < 30 yr	Children > adults
Childhood history	–	+/–
Peptic ulcer	+/–	–
Renal colic	+/–	–
Atherosclerosis	+ +	+/–
Radiological		
Radiological changes	Bilateral	Unilateral/bilateral
Medullary calcification	30–50%	Uncommon
Calyceal abnormalities	Most calyceal groups	Usually polar Superior > inferior
Cortical scarring	+	+ + +
Compensatory hypertrophy	+/–	+ +
Reduction in renal size on serial IVUs	+	–
Dilatation lower ⅓ of ureter	–	+/–
Vesicoureteric reflux	–	+/–
Renal calculi	+/–	Uncommon

AN = analgesic nephropathy; RN = reflux nephropathy. (Reproduced with permission of author [271].)

stable analgesic nephropathy, serial intravenous urograms may show some renal hypertrophy [188].

The radiological changes of RPN in analgesic nephropathy cannot be distinguished from those seen in diabetes mellitus or sickle-cell disease. The radiological conditions that need to be considered in differential diagnosis are reflux nephropathy, renal tuberculosis, obstructive uropathies, pyelogenic cysts, medullary sponge kidney, and cortical infarcts with calyceal distortion. Reflux nephropathy is the most important differential diagnosis, and the criteria that may be used to distinguish reflux nephropathy from RPN are summarized in Table 40-7 [271].

Management of Analgesic Nephropathy

The management of analgesic nephropathy patients with severe oliguric acute renal failure associated with urinary tract obstruction and septicemia involves immediate attention to potentially fatal complications, such as hyperkalemia and systemic acidosis, and the use of appropriate broad-spectrum antibiotics, which are active against gram-negative organisms. It is essential to establish adequate urine flow by rapid, but judicious, intravascular volume expansion and the parenteral use of a potent loop diuretic, such as furosemide. Severe hypertension, which may be present, should be managed independently of the negative salt and water balance and responds satisfactorily to standard antihypertensive drugs. Attempts to control hypertension with further sodium restriction may lead to persisting oliguria and terminal renal failure. Early and acute dialysis may be necessary as a life-saving measure. Exclusion of pelvic or ureteric obstruction due to necrotic papillae by renal ultrasound and, if necessary, by ureteric catheterization should be considered early. Recovery from an episode of acute RPN is commonly followed by a severe salt-losing state.

Urological procedures are frequently necessary in the management of analgesic nephropathy patients [37, 152, 153, 174, 175], and in our series of 232 patients [290], 86 procedures were required in 70 patients (30%). The investigative procedures used were cystoscopy, retrograde pyelography, and open renal biopsy. The common indications for these diagnostic procedures were unexplained reduction in renal function, renal colic, macroscopic or microscopic hematuria, and persistent urinary tract infection. Therapeutic urological procedures were necessary in 7 percent of patients and were not associated with any morbidity or mortality. Urinary tract obstruction due to necrotic papillae were managed by cystoscopy and ureteric catheterization, extraction of papillae from ureters, ureterolithotomy, and pyelolithotomy. Endoscopic extraction of papillae were most successful with the Dormia basket, and occasionally ureteric catheter drainage of the renal pelvis was necessary for several days. Contrary to the experience of Johnson [174], pyelolithotomy was not performed for free nonobstructing papillae in the renal pelvis and, on several occasions, large necrotic papillae disintegrated and were passed uneventfully. Transitional cell carcinoma of the pelvis or ureter is treated with nephroureterectomy [164].

In the long-term management of analgesic nephropathy, it is essential to avoid all NSAIDs because of their known acute and chronic nephrotoxicity. Intermittent use of single analgesics by patients with analgesic nephropathy and renal insufficiency has led to progressive deterioration of renal function and fresh RPN [188, 191, 266]. Patients should be regularly monitored for evidence of continuing analgesic abuse by screening for analgesics and their metabolites [85, 89, 95]. All patients are encouraged to maintain a high fluid intake, and there is experimental and clinical evidence that a water diuresis protects the kidney from analgesic nephrotoxicity and reduces the risk of urinary tract infections [14,

282–285]. All manifestations and complications of the analgesic syndrome and analgesic nephropathy, chronic renal failure, and hypertension should be carefully and regularly supervised and managed; particular attention should be paid to evidence of ongoing analgesic abuse.

Many investigators have reported a gloomy outlook, especially in patients with advanced analgesic nephropathy in spite of the withdrawal of phenacetin and other analgesics [22, 24, 68, 121, 149, 179, 192, 249, 265, 294, 353, 355, 359]. However, with total avoidance of all analgesics, including the so-called safe single analgesics, such as aspirin, paracetamol, and NSAIDs, and careful medical management as outlined previously, a better outlook for these patients has been demonstrated [1, 24, 66, 68, 123, 185, 188, 191, 209, 263, 266, 269, 283, 290, 329, 350, 351]. More than 85 percent of patients completely stop analgesic intake and have no evidence of further abuse on the basis of negative blood or urine screening; between 10 and 15 percent take analgesics intermittently and a small minority with very disturbed personalities continue analgesic abuse [268]. The vast majority of patients who take analgesics for headaches completely lose their headaches after stopping analgesic abuse. In a review of 323 consecutive patients with analgesic nephropathy followed for up to 66 months [268, 269, 290], 12 percent presented in terminal renal failure and either died or required maintenance dialysis within 6 months; 17 percent improved, with a significant rise in GFR; 50 percent remained stable; and 23 percent deteriorated. The major factors associated with deterioration were suboptimal blood pressure control or malignant hypertension, persistent proteinuria related to secondary focal glomerular sclerosis, secondary gout and asymptomatic hyperuricemia, and reduced renal size and GFR at the time of presentation. The other factors that contributed to renal decline in individual cases were nephrectomy for pyonephrosis or transitional cell tumors, ischemic heart disease with cardiac failure, atheromatous renal artery thrombosis or bilateral renal artery stenosis (R. S. Nanra. Unpublished data, 1991), and continued analgesic abuse. The 6-year cumulative survival was 72 percent. Overall, 21 percent of patients died and the main causes of mortality were ischemic heart disease (61%), cerebrovascular disease (20%), and septicemia (19%). The finding of a higher mortality from cardiovascular diseases ($p = 0.008$) in the analgesic abuse group compared to the matched control group by Dubach and co-workers [66, 91] in the prospective epidemiological study in Switzerland is, therefore, very significant. In an earlier report involving 43 patients with severe renal insufficiency, the same authors found a 5-year cumulative survival of 74 percent [188, 191]. Other reports, however, have found lower survival rates, with a death rate of 51 percent at 5 years and a mean survival time from diagnosis of 31 months [68, 192].

End-Stage Renal Failure

End-stage renal failure from analgesic nephropathy continues to account for a significant proportion of dialysis patients in many countries, although there has been a decline in terminal renal failure consequent on restriction of analgesic sales, at least in Scandinavia and Australia [42, 126, 136, 137, 160, 180, 183, 193, 221, 295, 370]. Recent reports on end-stage renal failure from analgesic nephropathy show an incidence ranging from 8 percent in Malaysia to 18 percent in Belgium [105, 106, 345]. The relative risk of end-stage renal failure from analgesic abuse has been estimated as 2.65, with an increase in relative risk related to time-dose exposure to analgesics [309, 362]. Anemia, renal osteodystrophy, and dialysis dementia appear to be more prevalent in analgesic nephropathy patients on dialysis treatment, and this has been attributed to the use of aluminum antacids for phosphate control and treatment of peptic ulcer [109, 343]. In Australia, withdrawal of phenacetin-containing analgesics resulted in a fall in the incidence rate of end-stage renal failure of 4.2 percent per year between 1973 and 1983; during the same period, there was an increase in the incidence rate of 1.3 percent for nonanalgesic nephropathy and nondiabetic patients [233].

Analgesic nephropathy adversely affects the outcome of patients treated with dialysis and transplantation [23, 346, 370, 375]. The author had noted a mortality of 51 percent in analgesic nephropathy patients treated with dialysis and transplantation over a 6-year period. More recently, Balle and Schollmeyer [23] also noted a mortality of 47 percent over 57 months, the main causes of death being cardiovascular in 29 percent, hyperkalemia in 19 percent, sepsis in 14 percent, and tumor in 14 percent. The primary cadaver graft survival rate at 12 months in Australia between 1985 and 1989 was 75 percent for analgesic nephropathy and between 81 and 89 percent for glomerulonephritis, polycystic kidney disease, reflux nephropathy, and diabetic nephropathy [370].

Analgesic nephropathy is a major burden on the health resources. In the United States a 2 percent incidence of analgesic nephropathy patients treated with dialysis was estimated to cost $40 million, and this did not take into account the cost of treatment of predialysis chronic renal failure and complications of the analgesic syndrome [66].

References: Lithium-Induced Renal Disease

1. Baastrup, P. C., and Schou, M. Lithium as a prophylactic agent. *Arch. Gen. Psychiatry* 16: 162, 1967.
2. Baer, L., Platman, B. R., Kassir, S., and Fieve, R. R. Mechanisms of renal lithium handling and their relationship to mineralocorticoids: A dissociation between sodium and lithium ions. *J. Psychiatr. Res.* 8: 91, 1971.
3. Batlle, D. C., von Riotte, A. B., Gaviria, M., and Grupp, M. Amelioration of polyuria by amiloride in patients receiving long-term lithium therapy. *N. Engl. J. Med.* 312: 408, 1985.
4. Baylis, P. H., and Heath, D. A. Water disturbances in patients treated with oral lithium carbonate. *Ann. Intern. Med.* 59: 153, 1978.
5. British Pharmacopoeia, 1864.
6. Bucht, G., and Wahlin, A. Impairment of renal concentrating ability by lithium. *Lancet* 1: 778, 1978.
7. Bucht, G., and Wahlin, A. Impairment of renal concentrating ability by lithium. *Lancet* 2: 580, 1978.

8. Bucht, G., and Wahlin, A. Renal concentrating capacity in long-term lithium treatment and after withdrawal of lithium. *Acta Med. Scand.* 207: 309, 1980.
9. Burrows, G. D., Davies, B., and Kincaid-Smith, P. Unique tubular lesion after lithium. *Lancet* 1: 1310, 1978.
10. Cade, J. F. J. Lithium salts in the treatment of psychotic excitement. *Med. J. Aust.* 36: 349, 1949.
11. Cairns, S. R., Wolman, R., Lewis, J. G., and Thakker, R. Persistent nephrogenic diabetes insipidus, hyperparathyroidism and hypothyroidism after lithium treatment. *Br. Med. J.* 290: 516, 1985.
12. Carney, S., Rayson, B., and Morgan, T. The effect of lithium on the permeability response induced in the collecting duct by antidiuretic hormone. *Pfluegers Arch.* 366: 19, 1976.
13. Cattell, W. R., Coppen, A., Bailey, J., and Rama Rao, V. A. Impairment of real concentrating capacity by lithium. *Lancet* 2: 44, 1978.
14. Chiu, E., Davies, B., Walker, R., and Kincaid-Smith, P. Renal findings after 30 years on lithium. *Br. J. Psychiatry* 143: 424, 1983.
15. Colt, E. W. D., Igel, G., Fieve, R. R., and Dunner, D. L. Lithium-associated nephropathy. *Am. J. Psychiatry* 136: 1098, 1979.
16. Coppen, A., Bishop, M. E., Bailey, J. E., Catell, W. R., and Price, R. G. Renal function in lithium and non-lithium treated patients with affective disorders. *Acta Psychiatr. Scand.* 62: 343, 1980.
17. Corcoran, A. C., Taylor, R. D., and Page, R. H. Lithium poisoning from the use of salt substitutes. *J.A.M.A.* 139: 685, 1949.
18. Darnton, S. J. Glycogen metabolism in rabbit kidney under differing physiological states. *Q. J. Exp. Physiol.* 52: 392, 1967.
19. Depaulo, J. R., Jr., Correa, E. I., and Sapir, D. G. Renal glomerular function and long-term lithium therapy. *Am. J. Psychiatry* 138: 324, 1981.
20. Dias, N., and Hocken, A. G. Oliguric renal failure complicating lithium carbonate therapy. *Nephron* 10: 246, 1973.
21. Donker, A. J. M., Prins, E., Meijer, S., Sluiter, W. J., Van Berkestijn, J. W. B. M., and Dols, L. C. W. A renal function study in 30 patients on long-term lithium therapy. *Clin. Nephrol.* 12: 254, 1979.
22. Dousa, T., and Hector, O. The effect of NaCl and LiCl on vasopressin sensitive adenyl cyclase. *Life Sci.* 9: 765, 1970.
23. Earley, L. E., and Orloff, J. The mechanisms of antidiuresis associated with the administration of hydrochlorothiazide to patients with vasopressin-resistant diabetes insipidus. *J. Clin. Invest.* 41: 1988, 1962.
24. Editorial. Lithium nephropathy. *Lancet* 2: 619, 1979.
25. Editorial. Lithium and the kidney: Grounds for cautious optimism. *Lancet* 2: 1056, 1979.
26. Evan, A. P., and Ollerich, D. A. The effect of lithium carbonate on the structure of the rat kidney. *Am. J. Anat.* 134: 97, 1972.
27. Forrest, J. N., Cohen, A. D., Torretti, J., Himmelhoch, I. M., and Epstein, F. M. On the mechanism of lithium-induced diabetes insipidus in man and the rat. *J. Clin. Invest.* 53: 1115, 1974.
28. Friedman, D. L., and Larner, J. Studies in UPDG-a-glucan transglucocyclase. *Biochem. N.Y.* 2: 669, 1963.
29. Garrod, A. B. *The Nature and Treatment of Gout and Rheumatic Gout.* London: Walton and Maberly, 1859.
30. Garrod, A. B. A Treatise on Gout and Rheumatic Gout. In *Rheumatoid Arthritis.* London: Longmans, Green & Co., 1876.
31. Glen, A. I. M. Lithium Regulation of Membrane ATPases. In F. N. Johnson and S. Johnson (eds.), *Lithium in Medical Practice.* Lancaster: MTP Press Ltd., 1978. Chap. 18.
32. Gonick, H. C. Nephropathies of Heavy Metal Intoxication. In S. G. Massry and R. J. Glassock (eds.), *Textbook of Nephrology.* Baltimore: Williams & Wilkins, 1983. P. 6.184.
33. Grof, P., MacCrimmon, D. J., Smith, E. K. M., Daigle, L., Saxena, B., Varma, R., Grof, E., Keitner, G., and Kenny, J. Long term lithium treatment and the kidney. (Interim report on fifty patients). *Can. J. Psychiatry* 25: 534, 1980.
34. Haig, A. Mental depression and the excretion of uric acid. *Practitioner* 41: 342, 1888.
35. Hallgren, R., Alm, P. O., and Hellsing, K. Renal function in patients on lithium treatment. *Br. J. Psychiatry* 135: 22, 1979.
36. Hanlon, L. W., Romaine, M., Gilroy, F. W., and Dietrick, S. E. Lithium chloride as a substitute for sodium chloride in the diet. *J.A.M.A.* 139: 688, 1949.
37. Hansen, H. E., and Amdisen, A. Lithium intoxication (report of 23 cases and review of 100 cases from the literature). *Q. J. Med.* 47: 123, 1978.
38. Hansen, H. E., Hestbech, J., Sorensen, J. L., Norgaard, K., Heilskov, J., and Amdisen, A. Chronic interstitial nephropathy in patients on long-term lithium treatment. *Q. J. Med.* 48: 577, 1979.
39. Harris, C. A., and Jenner, F. A. Some aspects of the inhibition of the action of antidiuretic hormone by lithium ion in the rat kidney and the bladder of the toad, *Bufo marinus. Br. J. Pharmacol.* 44: 223, 1972.
40. Hartigan, G. P. The use of lithium salts in affective disorders. *Br. J. Psychiatry* 109: 810, 1963.
41. Hestbech, J., and Aurrell, M. Lithium induced uremia. *Lancet* 1: 212, 1979.
42. Hestbech, J., Hansen, H. E., Amdisen, A., and Olsen, S. Chronic renal lesions following long-term treatment with lithium. *Kidney Int.* 12: 205, 1977.
43. Hinde, I. T. Glycogen in the collecting tubules of newborn animals. *J. Pathol. Bacteriol.* 61: 451, 1944.
44. Horn, R. S., Walaas, O., and Walaas, E. The influence of sodium, potassium and lithium on the response of glycogen synthetase I to insulin and epinephrine in the isolated rat diagram. *Biochem. Biophys. Acta* 313: 296, 1973.
45. Hullin, R. P., Coley, V. P., Birch, J. N., Thomas, T. H., and Morgan, D. B. Renal function after long-term treatment with lithium. *Br. Med. J.* 1: 1457, 1979.
46. Hwu, H., Ardekani, A. B., and Helzer, J. E. A longitudinal record study of renal function in patients treated with lithium. *J. Affect. Dis.* 3: 101, 1981.
47. Jarrett, D. B., Burrows, G. D., and Davies, B. Lithium as a prophylactic action in recurring affective disorder. *Med. J. Aust.* 1: 325, 1973.
48. Johnson, G. F. A., Hunt, G. E., Duggin, G. G., Horvath, J. S., and Tiller, D. J. Renal function and lithium treatment: Initial and follow-up tests in manic-depressive patients. *J. Affect. Dis.* 6: 249, 1984.
49. Kling, M. S., Fox, J. G., Johnston, S. M., Tolkoff-Rubin, N. E., Rubin, R. H., and Colvin, R. B. Effects of long-term lithium administration on renal structure and function in rats: A distinctive tubular lesion. *Lab. Invest.* 50: 526, 1984.
50. Krebs, E. G., and Fischer, E. H. Molecular properties and transformation of glycogen phosphorylase in animal tissues. *Adv. Enzymol.* 24: 263, 1962.
51. Lange, C. Periodische depressionszustande und ihre pathogenesis auf dem boden der harnsauren diathese. *Mit einer Nachschrift,* Hamburg and Leipzig: Verlag von Leopold Voss, 1896.

52. Lavender, S., Brown, J. N., and Berrill, W. T. Acute renal failure and lithium intoxication. *Postgrad. Med. J.* 49: 277, 1973.
53. Lindop, G. B. M., and Padfield, P. L. The renal pathology in a case of lithium induced diabetes insipidus. *J. Clin. Pathol.* 28: 472, 1975.
54. Marini, J. L., and Sheard, M. H. Sustained-release lithium carbonate in a double-blind study: Serum lithium levels, side-effects and placebo response. *J. Clin. Pharmacol.* 16: 276, 1976.
55. Martinez-Maldonado, M., Stavroulaki-Tsapara, A., Tsaparas, N., Suki, W. N., and Eknoyan, G. Renal effects of lithium administration in rats: Alterations in water and electrolyte metabolism and the response to vasopressin and cyclic-adenosine monophosphate during prolonged administrations. *J. Lab. Clin. Med.* 86: 445, 1975.
56. Mellerup, E. T., and Rafaelson, O. J. In F. N. Johnson and S. Johnson (eds.), *Lithium in Medical Practice.* London: Academic Press, 1975. P. 381.
57. Miller, P. D., Dubovsky, S. L., McDonald, K. M., Katz, F. H., Robertson, G. L., and Schrier, R. W. Central, renal and adrenal effects of lithium in man. *Am. J. Med.* 66: 797, 1979.
58. Myers, J. B., Morgan, T. O., Carney, S. L., and Ray, C. Effects of lithium on the kidney. *Kidney Int.* 18: 601, 1980.
59. Olsen, S. Renal histopathology in various forms of acute anuria in man. *Kidney Int.* 10 (Suppl. 6): S2, 1976.
60. Padfield, P. L., Park, S. J. M., Morton, J. J., and Braidwood, A. E. Plasma levels of antidiuretic hormone in patients receiving prolonged lithium therapy. *Br. J. Psychiatry* 130: 140, 1977.
61. Parmeggiani, A., and Morgan, H. E. The effect of adenine nucleotides and inorganic phosphate on muscle phosphorylase activity. *Biochem. Biophys. Res. Commun.* 9: 252, 1962.
62. Perez, G. O., Oster, J. R., and Vaamonde, C. A. Incomplete syndrome of renal tubular acidosis induced by lithium carbonate. *J. Lab. Clin. Med.* 86: 386, 1975.
63. Perez, G. O., Oster, J. R., Sonneborn, R. E., Magrinat, G., and Vaamonde, C. A. Urinary carbon dioxide tension in lithium carbonate-treated patients. *J. Pharmacol. Exp. Ther.* 201: 456, 1977.
64. Rabin, E. Z., Garston, R. G., Weir, R. V., and Posen, G. A. Persistent nephrogenic diabetes insipidus associated with long term lithium carbonate treatment. *C.M.A.* 121: 194, 1979.
65. Radomski, J. L., Fuyat, H. N., Nelson, A. A., and Smith, P. K. The toxic effects, excretion and distribution of lithium chloride. *J. Pharmacol. Exp. Ther.* 100: 428, 1950.
66. Rafaelson, O. J., Bolwig, T. G., Ladefoged, J., and Brun, C. L. Kidney Function and Morphology in Long-Term Treatment. In T. B. Cooper, S. Gershon, N. Kline, and M. Schou (eds.), *Lithium: Controversies and Unresolved Issues.* Amsterdam: Excerpta Medica, 1979.
67. Schou, M. Lithium studies 1. Toxicity. *Acta Pharmacol. Toxicol.* 15: 70, 1958.
68. Schou, M. Lithium in psychiatric therapy and prophylaxis. *J. Psychiatr. Res.* 6: 67, 1968.
69. Schou, M. Lithium prophylaxis: Is the honeymoon over? *Aust. N.Z. J. Psychiatry* 13: 109, 1979.
70. Schou, M., Baastrup, P. C., Grof, P., Weis, P., and Angst, J. Pharmacological and clinical problems of lithium prophylaxis. *Br. J. Psychiatry* 116: 615, 1970.
71. Smigan, L., Von Knorring, L., Bucht, G., and Wahlin, A. Kidney Function During and After Discontinuation of Lithium Therapy. Presented at IIIrd World Congress of Biological Psychiatry (Stockholm), 1981.
72. Sorensen, J. L., Olsen, S., Norgaard, K., Heilskov, J., and Amdisen, A. Chronic interstitial nephropathy in patients on long-term lithium treatment. *Abstracts of the VIIth International Congress of Nephrology (Montreal)* D-37, 1978.
73. Spicer, S. S. Histological localisation of glycogen in the urinary tract and lung. *J. Histochem. Cytochem.* 6: 52, 1958.
74. Uldall, P. R., Awad, A. G., McCormick, W. O., Carter, L. B., Gonsick, T., Grass, G. L., and Kugelmass, M. I. Renal function in patients receiving long-term lithium therapy. *Can. Med. Assoc. J.* 124: 1471, 1981.
75. Vestergaard, P., Amdisen, A., Hansen, H. E., and Schou, M. Renal Function of Lithium Treated Patients: A Progress Report. In M. Schou and E. Stomgren (eds.), *Origin, Prevention and Treatment of Affective Disorders.* London: Academic Press, 1979. Chap. 9.
76. Vestergaard, P., Amdisen, A., Hansen, H. E., and Schou, M. Lithium treatment and kidney function. A survey of 237 patients in long-term treatment. *Acta Psychiatr. Scand.* 60: 504, 1979.
77. Wahlin, A., Rapp, W., and Jonsson, E. H. Failure of chlorothiazide to improve urinary concentrating capacity in lithium-treated patients. *Acta Med. Scand.* 207: 195, 1980.
78. Walker, R., Dowling, J., Alcorn, D., Ryan, G., and Kincaid-Smith, P. Renal pathology associated with lithium therapy. *Pathology* 15: 403, 1983.
79. Walker, R. G., Bennett, W. M., Davies, B. M., and Kincaid-Smith, P. Structural and functional effects of long-term lithium therapy. *Kidney Int.* 21 (Suppl. 11): S13, 1982.
80. Walker, R. G., Davies, B. M., Holwill, B. J., Dowling, J. P., and Kincaid-Smith, P. A clinicopathological study of lithium nephrotoxicity. *J. Chronic Dis.* 35: 685, 1982.
81. Waller, D. G., Edwards, J. G., Naik, R., and Polak, A. Renal function during lithium treatment. *Q. J. Med.* 211: 369, 1984.
82. Wallin, L., Alling, C., and Aurell, M. Impairment of renal function in patients on long-term lithium treatment. *Clin. Nephrol.* 18: 23, 1982.
83. Williams, W. O., and Gyory, A. Z. Aspects of the use of lithium for the non-psychiatrist. *Aust. N.Z. J. Med.* 6: 233, 1976.

References: Analgesic-Induced Renal Disease

1. Abel, J. A. Analgesic nephropathy—A review of the literature. *Clin. Pharmacol. Ther.* 12: 583, 1971.
2. Abrahams, C. Cause of analgesic-induced RPN. *Lancet* 2: 346, 1976.
3. Abrahams, C., and Levin, N. W. Experimentally induced analgesic nephropathy—Its pathogenesis. *Med. Proc.* 13: 506, 1967.
4. Abrahams, C., Furman, K. I., and Salant, D. Dermal microangiopathy in patients with analgesic nephropathy. *S. Afr. Med. J.* 54: 393, 1978.
5. Abrahams, C., Levin, N. W., Gecelter, L., and Rubenstein, A. H. The diagnosis of analgesic nephropathy by renal biopsy. *Med. Proc.* 13: 501, 1967.
6. Abrahams, C., and Levinson, C. Ultrastructure of the renal papilla in experimentally induced analgesic nephritis in rats. *S. Afr. Med. J.* 44: 63, 1970.
7. Abrahams, C., Van Tonder, H., and Hesse, V. Abnormal vessels in the urinary tract following analgesic abuse in man. *Arch. Pathol. Lab. Med.* 100: 630, 1976.
8. Ager, P. H., Bluth, E. I., Murray, T., and Goldberg, M. Analgesic abuse nephropathy. *Urology* 7: 123, 1976.
9. Aiken, J. W. Aspirin and indomethacin prolong partu-

rition in rats: Evidence that prostaglandins contribute to expulsion of foetus. *Nature* 240: 21, 1972.
10. Alt, J. M., Hacke, H., von der Heyde, D., Janig, H., Junge, P. M., Olbricht, Ch., Schurek, H. J., and Stolte, H. Urinary protein excretion in interstitial and tubular kidney disease as characterised by gradient electrophoresis. *Klin. Wochenschr.* 61: 641, 1983.
11. Alt, J. M., Janig, H., Schurek, H. J., and Stolte, H. Study of renal protein excretion in chronic pyelonephritis. *Contrib. Nephrol.* 16: 37, 1979.
12. Ammann, R. W., Buhler, H., Tuma, J., Schneider, J., Siebenmann, R., and Satz, N. Chronic and relapsing acute pancreatitis associated with chronic renal insufficiency and analgesic (phenacetin) abuse. Observations in 4 patients. *Gastroenterol. Clin. Biol.* 5: 509, 1981.
13. Andersson, B., Larsson, R., Rahimtula, A., and Moldeus, P. Hydroperoxide-dependent activation of p-phenetidine catalyzed by prostaglandin synthase and other peroxidases. *Biochem. Pharmacol.* 32: 1045, 1983.
14. Andriole, V. T., and Epstein, F. H. Prevention of Pyelonephritis by Water Diuresis. Evidence of the Role of Medullary Hypertonicity in Promoting Renal Infection. In E. H. Kass (ed.), *Progress in Pyelonephritis.* Philadelphia: Davis, 1965. Pp. 232–238.
15. Argus, M. F., Newell, M. P., Henderson, J. T., and Ray, F. E. Antipyretic and toxicity studies with acetanilid *o-*, *m-*, and *p*-chloracetanilid. *J. Am. Pharm. Assoc.* 43: 204, 1959.
16. Armstrong, B., Garrod, A., and Doll, R. A retrospective study of renal cancer with special reference to coffee and animal protein consumption. *Br. J. Cancer* 33: 127, 1976.
17. Arnold, L., Collins, C., and Starmer, G. A. The short-term effects of analgesic on the kidney, with special reference to acetylsalicylic acid. *Pathology* 5: 123, 1976.
18. Arnold, L., Collins, C., and Starmer, G. A. Analgesic abuse, RPN and concomitant drug intake. *Aust. N.Z. J. Med.* 7: 253, 1977.
19. Artusi, G. Uber einen Fall von postanginoser Pyamie mit necrotisierender Nephritis papillaris embolica. *Reitr. Path. Anat.* 75: 1, 1926.
20. Bach, P. H., and Bridges, J. W. Chemically induced renal papillary necrosis and upper urothelial carcinoma. Part I. *CRC Crit. Rev. Toxicol.* 15: 216, 1985.
21. Bach, P. H., and Bridges, J. W. Chemically induced renal papillary necrosis and upper urothelial carcinoma. Part II. *CRC Crit. Rev. Toxicol.* 15: 331, 1985.
22. Bailey, R. R., Neale, T. J., and Little, P. J. Analgesic nephropathy. *N.Z. Med. J.* 79: 1053, 1974.
23. Balle, C., and Schollmeyer, P. Morbidity of patients with analgesic-associated nephropathy on regular dialysis treatment and after renal transplantation. *Klin. Wochenschr.* 68: 38, 1990.
24. Bell, D., Kerr, D. N. S., Swinney, J., and Yeates, W. K. Analgesic nephropathy. Clinical course after withdrawal of phenacetin. *Br. Med. J.* 3: 378, 1969.
25. Bengtsson, U. A comparative study of chronic non-obstructive pyelonephritis and RPN. *Acta Med. Scand.* 388(Suppl.), 1962.
26. Bengtsson, U. Prevention of renal disease. *Proc. Eur. Dial. Transplant. Assoc.* 16: 466, 1979.
27. Bengtsson, U., Angervall, L., Ekman, H., and Lehman, L. Transitional cell tumours of the renal pelvis in analgesic abusers. *Scand. J. Urol. Nephrol.* 2: 145, 1968.
28. Bengtsson, U., Johansson, S., and Angervall, L. Malignancies of the urinary tract and their relation to analgesic abuse. *Kidney Int.* 13: 107, 1978.
29. Bergman, S., Forrest, J., Betsill, W., and Gillenwater, J. Acquired upper ureteral stricture in a phenacetin abuser. *J. Urol.* 124: 892, 1980.
30. Berning, H., Orellana, K., and Selberg, W. Nierenpapillennekrosen. *Detsch. Med. Wochenschr.* 99: 1749, 1974.
31. Beyer, K. H., Jr., and Gelanden, R. T. Renal concentration gradients of salicylic acid and its metabolic congeners in the dog. *Arch. Int. Pharmacol. Ther.* 2312: 180, 1978.
32. Beynen, A. C., Buechler, K. F., van der Molen, A. J., and Geelen, M. J. H. Inhibition of hepatic lipogenesis by salicylate. *Toxicology* 24: 33, 1982.
33. Bianchi, L., Berneise, K., and Studer, A. Brown discolouration of cartilage in phenacetin abuse. *Virchows Arch. [Cell Pathol.]* 10: 339, 1972.
34. Blackman, J. E., Gibson, G. R., Lavan, J. N., Learoyd, H. M., and Posen, S. Urinary calculi and the consumption of analgesics. *Br. Med. J.* 2: 800, 1967.
35. Bluemle, L. W., and Goldberg, M. Renal accumulation of salicylate and phenacetin: Possible mechanisms in the nephrotoxicity of analgesic abuse. *J. Clin. Invest.* 47: 2507, 1968.
36. Boletis, J., Williams, A. J., Shortland, J. R., and Brown, C. B. Irreversible renal failure following mefenamic acid. *Nephron* 51: 575, 1989.
37. Bonin, N. Papillary necrosis, pathology and management of the acute attack. *Am. Heart J.* 68: 842, 1964.
38. Boyd, D. H. A. The use and abuse of phenacetin. *Scott. Med. J.* 9: 423, 1964.
39. Boyd, E. M. Sterility from phenacetin. *J. Clin. Pharmacol.* 11: 96, 1971.
40. Brun, C., Olsen, T. S., Raaschau, F., and Sorenson, A. W. S. Renal biopsy in rheumatoid arthritis. *Nephron* 2: 65, 1965.
41. Brunner, F. P., Richtmann, L., Thiel, G., and Dubach, U. C. Tumoren der ableitenden Harnwege und Analgetika-Abusus. *Schweiz. Med. Wochenschr.* 108: 1013, 1978.
42. Brynger, H., Brunner, F. P., Chantler, C., et al. Combined report on regular dialysis and transplantation in Europe. *Proc. Eur. Dial. Transplant. Assoc.* 17: 2, 1980.
43. Buckalew, V. M., Jr., and Schey, H. M. Epidemiology of analgesic-associated nephropathy in North America. N.I.H. Consensus Development Conference, Analgesic-Associated Kidney Disease, 1984. (Abstract) P. 24.
44. Burns, J. J., and Conney, A. H. Biochemical studies with phenacetin and related compounds. *Proc. Eur. Soc. Drug Toxicol.* 6: 76, 1965.
45. Burry, A. F. A profile of renal disease in Queensland: Results of an autopsy survey. *Med. J. Aust.* 1: 826, 1966.
46. Burry, A. F. The evolution of analgesic nephropathy. *Nephron* 5: 185, 1967.
47. Burry, A. F. Pathology of analgesic nephropathy: Australian experience. *Kidney Int.* 13: 34, 1978.
48. Burry, A. F., Axelsen, R. A., and Trolove, P. Analgesic nephropathy: Its present contribution to renal mortality and morbidity profile. *Med. J. Aust.* 1: 31, 1974.
49. Burry, A. F., Cross, R., and Axelsen, R. Analgesic nephropathy and the renal concentrating mechanism. *Pathol. Annu.* (Part 2) 12: 1, 1977.
50. Burry, A. F., de Jersy, P., and Weedon, D. Phenacetin and RPN: Results of a prospective autopsy investigation. *Med. J. Aust.* 1: 873, 1966.
51. Burry, H. C. Renal disorders in rheumatoid arthritis. *Rheumatol. Rehabil.* 11: 2, 1971.
52. Calder, I. C., Yong, A. C., Woods, R. A., Crowe, C. A., Ham, K. N., and Tange, J. D. The nephrotoxicity of p-aminophenol. II. The effect of metabolic inhibitors and inducers. *Chem. Biol. Interact.* 27: 245, 1979.

53. Carmichael, J., and Shankel, S. W. Effects of nonsteroidal anti-inflammatory drugs on prostaglandins and renal function. *Am. J. Med.* 78: 992, 1985.
54. Carrington-Smith, D. Survey of drug use amongst 500 in Hobart, Tasmania. Health Education Council, Health Service Department, Hobart, Tasmania, 1974.
55. Carro-Ciampi, G. Phenacetin abuse: A review. *Toxicology* 10: 311, 1978.
56. Caterson, R. J., and Duggin, G. G. Intrarenal distribution of salicylate. *Proc. Aust. Soc. Med. Res.* 1: 57, 1978.
57. Caterson, R. J., Duggin, G. G., Horvarth, J. S., Mohandas, J., and Tiller, D. J. Aspirin, protein transacetylation and inhibition of prostaglandin synthetase in the kidney. *Br. J. Pharmacol.* 207: 584, 1978.
58. Chasko, S. B., Gray, G. F., and McCarron, J. P. Urothelial neoplasia of the upper urinary tract. *Pathol. Annu.* 16: 127, 1981.
59. Chojnowski, J. R., Adamska-Marcinkowska, H., and Osinska, E. Kidney damage in phenacetin addicts. *Polish Med. J.* 6: 1489, 1967.
60. Chrispin, A. R., Hull, D., Lillie, J. G., and Risdon, R. A. Renal tubular necrosis and papillary necrosis after gastroenteritis in infants. *Br. Med. J.* 1: 410, 1970.
61. Clarkson, A. R., and Lawrence, J. R. The Clinical Features of Analgesic Nephropathy. In P. Kincaid-Smith and K. F. Fairley (eds.), *Renal Infection and Renal Scarring*. Melbourne: Mercedes Press, 1973. Pp. 375–384.
62. Clausen, E., and Jensen, K. Renal biopsies from patients with high analgesic intake. *Acta Pathol. Microbiol. Scand.* 72: 219, 1968.
63. Clausen, E., and Pedersen, J. Stigningen i hyppighed af renal papil-nekrose i et autopsimateriale. *Ugeskr. Laeger.* 123: 620, 1961.
64. Clausen, E., and Pedersen, J. Necrosis of renal papillae in rheumatoid arthritis. *Acta Med. Scand.* 170: 631, 1961.
65. Cole, P. Coffee drinking and cancer of the lower urinary tract. *Lancet* 1: 1335, 1971.
66. Consensus conference. Analgesic kidney disease. *J.A.M.A.* 251: 3123, 1984.
67. Cove-Smith, J. R., and Knapp, M. S. Sodium handling in analgesic nephropathy. *Lancet* 2: 70, 1973.
68. Cove-Smith, J. R., and Knapp, M. S. Analgesic nephropathy: An important cause of chronic renal failure. *Q. J. Med.* 47: 46, 1978.
69. Cullen, K. J., and Woodings, T. Alcohol, tobacco and analgesics; Busselton, 1972. *Med. J. Aust.* 2: 211, 1975.
70. Cumming, R. L. C., and Pollock, A. Drug induced sulphhaemoglominaemia and Heinz body anaemia in pregnancy with involvement of the foetus. *Scott. Med. J.* 12: 320, 1967.
71. Dacie, J. V., and Mollin, D. L. Siderocytes, sideroblasts and sideroblastic anaemia. *Acta Med. Scand.* 445: 237, 1966.
72. Davidson, W., Daffist, L., and Shippey, W. Effect of aspirin and phenacetin metabolites on protein synthesis in dog renal medulla. *Clin. Res.* 21: 683, 1973.
73. Davidson, W., Daffist, L., and Shippey, W. In vitro effects of aspirin and phenacetin metabolites on the metabolism of dog renal medulla. *Clin. Res.* 21: 227, 1973.
74. Davies, D. J., Kennedy, A., and Roberts, C. Renal medullary necrosis in infancy and childhood. *J. Pathol.* 99: 125, 1969.
75. Davies, D. J., Kennedy, A., and Roberts, C. The etiology of renal medullary necrosis: A survey of adult cases in Liverpool. *J. Pathol.* 100: 257, 1970.
76. Dawborn, J. K., Fairley, K. F., Kincaid-Smith, P., and King, W. E. The association of peptic ulceration, chronic renal disease and analgesic abuse. *Q. J. Med.* 35: 69, 1966.
77. Dawson, A. G. Effects of acetylsalicylate on gluconeogenesis in isolated rat tubules. *Biochem. Pharmacol.* 24: 1407, 1975.
78. de Crespigny, P. J. C., Hewitson, Y., Birchall, I., and Kincaid-Smith, P. Caffeine potentiates the nephrotoxicity of mefenamic acid on the rat renal papilla. *Am. J. Nephrol.* 10: 311, 1990.
79. De Leon, A. H., and Nanra, R. S. Radiological changes in analgesic nephropathy and chronic pyelonephritis. *Aust. N.Z. J. Med.* 6: 68, 1976.
80. De Palma, J., Wassanmiller, J., and Abukuran, A. Phenacetin/aspirin nephritis as a cause of chronic renal failure. Presented at Western Dialysis and Transplant Society Meeting, Las Vegas, Nevada, 1975.
81. de Wardener, H. E., and MacGregor, G. A. Blood Pressure and the Kidney. In R. W. Schrier and C. W. Gottschalk (eds.), *Diseases of the Kidney*. Boston: Little, Brown, 1988. Pp. 1543–1572.
82. Doyle, D. V. Renal disease in rheumatoid arthritis—The controversy examined. *Eur. J. Rheum. Inflam.* 3: 91, 1979.
83. Dreisbach, R. H., and Pfeiffer, C. Caffeine-withdrawal headache. *J. Lab. Clin. Med.* 28: 1212, 1943.
84. Drtil, J. Psychotic syndromes after long term use of analgesic pyretics. *Activ. Nerv. Super. (Praha)* 14: 186, 1972.
85. Dubach, U. C. *p*-Aminophenol-Bestimmung in urin als Routinemethode zur Erfassung der Phenacetineinnahme. *Dtsch. Med. Wochenschr.* 92: 211, 1967.
86. Dubach, U. C., Levy, P. S., and Minder, F. Epidemiological study of analgesic intake and its relationship to urinary tract disorders in Switzerland. *Helv. Med. Acta* 34: 297, 1968.
87. Dubach, U. C., Levy, P. S., and Muller, A. Relationships between regular analgesic intake and urorenal disorders in a working female population of Switzerland. I. Initial results. *Am. J. Epidemiol.* 93: 425, 1971.
88. Dubach, U. C., Levy, P. S., Rosner, B., Baumeler, H. R., Muller, A., Peyer, A., and Ehrensperger, T. Relationship between regular intake of phenacetin-containing analgesics and laboratory evidence of urorenal disorders in a working female population of Switzerland. *Lancet* 1: 539, 1975.
89. Dubach, U. H., Rosner, B., Levy, P. S., Baumeler, H. R., Muller, A., Peyer, A., Ehrensperger, T., and Ettlin, C. Epidemiological study in Switzerland. *Kidney Int.* 13: 41, 1978.
90. Dubach, U. H., Rosner, B., and Pfister, E. Epidemiologic study of abuse of analgesics containing phenacetin. Renal morbidity and mortality (1968–1979). *N. Engl. J. Med.* 308: 357, 1983.
91. Dubach, U. H., Rosner, B., and Strumer, T. An epidemiologic study of abuse of analgesic drugs. Effects of phenacetin and salicylate on mortality and cardiovascular morbidity (1968 to 1987). *N. Engl. J. Med.* 324: 155, 1991.
92. Duggan, J. M. Splenomegaly in analgesic takers. *Med. J. Aust.* 2: 580, 1970.
93. Duggan, J. M. The phenestix test in the detection of analgesic abuse. *Med. J. Aust.* 1: 659, 1972.
94. Duggan, J. M. The analgesic syndrome. *Aust. N.Z. J. Med.* 4: 365, 1974.
95. Duggan, J. M. Aspirin in chronic gastric ulcer. An Australian experience. *Gut* 17: 378, 1976.
96. Duggin, G. G. Mechanisms in the development of analgesic nephropathy. *Kidney Int.* 18: 553, 1980.
97. Duggin, G. G., and Mudge, G. H. Renal tubular trans-

port of paracetamol and its conjugates in the dog. *Br. J. Pharmacol.* 54: 359, 1975.
98. Duggin, G. G., and Mudge, G. H. Analgesic nephropathy: Renal distribution of acetaminophen and its conjugates. *J. Pharmacol. Exp. Ther.* 199: 1, 1976.
99. Duggin, G. G., and Mudge, G. H. Phenacetin: Renal tubular transport and intrarenal distribution in the dog. *J. Pharmacol. Exp. Ther.* 199: 10, 1976.
100. Dunn, M. J., and Zambraski, E. J. Renal effects of drugs that inhibit prostaglandin synthesis. *Kidney Int.* 18: 609, 1980.
101. Editorial. Headache cures. *The Lone Hand,* 1907. Pp. 193–195.
102. Editorial. Salicylates and malformations. *Br. Med. J.* 1: 642, 1970.
103. Editorial. Aspirin-induced hepatic injury. *Ann. Intern. Med.* 80: 103, 1974.
104. Editorial. Balkan nephropathy. *Lancet* 1: 683, 1977.
105. Elseviers, M. M., and De Broe, M. E. Is analgesic nephropathy still a problem in Belgium? *Nephrol. Dial. Transplant.* 3: 143, 1988.
106. Elseviers, M. M., and De Broe, M. E. Prevention of analgesic nephropathy. *Arch. Belg.* 47: 77, 1989.
107. Eriksson, M. Salicylate-induced foetal damage late in pregnancy: An experimental study in mice. *Acta Paediatr. Scand. Suppl.* 211: 5, 1971.
108. Fairley, K. F., and Kincaid-Smith, P. Renal papillary necrosis with a normal pyelogram. *Br. Med. J.* 1: 156, 1968.
109. Fassett, R. G., Lien, J. W. K., McClure, J., and Mathew, T. H. Bone disease in analgesic nephropathy. *Clin. Nephrol.* 18: 273, 1982.
110. Fellner, S. K., and Tuttle, E. P. The clinical syndrome of analgesic abuse. *Arch. Intern. Med.* 124: 379, 1969.
111. Finan, B. F., and Finkbeiner, A. E. Renal papillary necrosis and retroperitoneal fibrosis. *J. Urol.* 126: 533, 1981.
112. Finnigan, D., Burry, A. F., and Smith, I. D. B. Analgesic consumption in an antenatal clinic survey. *Med. J. Aust.* 1: 761, 1974.
113. Fordham, C. C., and Huffines, W. D. Splenomegaly, analgesic ingestion and renal disease. *N. Engl. J. Med.* 277: 749, 1967.
114. Fourie, I. J. V. H., Pauw, F. H., and de Bruin, B. Bladder urothelium in analgesic-associated nephropathy—A valuable diagnostic aid. *J. Urol.* 128: 262, 1982.
115. Friedreich, N. Ueber Necrose der Nierenpapillen bei Hydronephrose. *Arch. Pathol. Anat.* 69: 308, 1877.
116. Froboese, C. Uber sequestrierende Marknekrose der Nieren bei Diabetes mellitus. *Vrh. Dtsch. Ges. Path.* 30: 431, 1937.
117. Frolich, J. C., Nies, A. S., and Schrier, R. W. (eds.). Prostaglandins and the kidney. *Kidney Int.* 19: 755, 1981.
118. Fuwa, M., and Waugh, D. Experimental RPN. Effects of diuresis and antidiuresis. *Arch. Pathol.* 85: 404, 1968.
119. Gardner, D. L. In W. S. C. Copeman (ed.), *Textbook of Rheumatic Diseases.* Edinburgh: Livingstone, 1969. P. 122.
120. Gault, M. H. Intrarenal gradients of radioactive acetylsalicylic acid (ASA) and inulin. *Clin. Res.* 19: 808, 1971.
121. Gault, M. H. The clinical course of patients with analgesic nephropathy. *Can. Med. Assoc. J.* 113: 204, 1975.
122. Gault, M. H., Blennerhassett, J., and Muehrcke, R. Analgesic nephropathy—A clinicopathologic study using electron microscopy. *Am. J. Med.* 51: 740, 1971.
123. Gault, M. H., Rudwal, T. C., Engles, W. D., and Dossetor, J. B. Syndrome associated with the abuse of analgesics. *Ann. Intern. Med.* 68: 906, 1968.
124. Gault, M. H., Shahidi, N. T., and Barber, V. E. Methemoglobin formation in analgesic nephropathy. *Clin. Pharmacol. Ther.* 15: 521, 1974.
125. Gault, M. H., and Wilson, D. R. Analgesic nephropathy in Canada: Clinical syndrome, management and outcome. *Kidney Int.* 13: 58, 1978.
126. Geismar, P. The mortality from pyelonephritis in Denmark during the period 1957–67 and its relationship to the use of phenacetin. *Ugeskr. Laeger* 133: 550, 1971.
127. George, A. Survey of drug use in a Sydney suburb. *Med. J. Aust.* 2: 233, 1972.
128. Gillies, M. A., Skyring, A. P., and Livingstone, E. The pattern and prevalence of aspirin ingestion as determined by interview of 2,921 inhabitants of Sydney. *Med. J. Aust.* 1: 974, 1972.
129. Gloor, F. J. Some Morphological Features of Chronic Interstitial Nephritis (Chronic Pyelonephritis) in Patients with Analgesic Abuse. In E. H. Kass (ed.), *Progress in Pyelonephritis.* Philadelphia: Davis, 1965. Pp. 287–296.
130. Gloor, F. J. Changing concepts in pathogenesis and morphology of analgesic nephropathy in Europe. *Kidney Int.* 13: 27, 1978.
131. Goldberg, M., Meyers, C. L., Peshel, W., McCarron, D., and Morrison, A. B. Mechanism of analgesic abuse nephropathy. (Abstract) *J. Clin. Invest.* 50: 37a, 1971.
132. Gonwa, T. A., Corbett, W. T., Schey, H. M., and Buckalew, V. M. Analgesic-associated nephropathy and transitional cell carcinoma of the urinary tract. *Ann. Intern. Med.* 93: 249, 1980.
133. Gradus, D. B., Zuker, N., and Barki, Y. Renal papillary necrosis in a child with rheumatic carditis treated with aspirin. *Isr. J. Med. Sci.* 25: 196, 1989.
134. Green, C. R., Ham, K. N., and Tange, J. D. Kidney lesions induced in rats by *p*-aminophenol. *Br. Med. J.* 1: 162, 1969.
135. Gregg, N. J., Elseviers, M. M., De Broe, M. E., and Bach, P. H. Epidemiology and mechanistic basis of analgesic-associated nephropathy. *Toxicol. Lett.* 46: 141, 1989.
136. Grimlund, K. Phenacetin and renal damage at Swedish factory. *Acta Med. Scand.* 174(Suppl.)405: 1, 1963.
137. Grimlund, K. Fatal injuries from overdosage of phenacetin. *Proc. Eur. Soc. Drug Toxicol.* 6: 90, 1965.
138. Grimlund, K. Phenacetin and Renal Damage. In H. Haschek (ed.), *Problems of Phenacetin Abuse.* Vienna: Facta publication, Verlag M. Egermann, 1973. Pp. 195–201.
139. Gsell, O. Nephropathie durch Analgetica. *Ergeb. Inn. Med. Kinderheilkd.* 35: 67, 1974.
140. Gunther, G. W. Die Papillennekrosen der Niere bei Diabetes. *Munch. Med. Wochenschr.* 84: 1695, 1937.
141. Handa, S. P., and Tewari, H. D. Urinary tract carcinoma in patients with analgesic nephropathy. *Nephron* 28: 62, 1981.
142. Hangartner, P. J., Buhler, H., Munch, R., Zaruba, K., Stamm, B., and Ammann, R. Chronic pancreatitis as a possible result of analgesic abuse. *Schweiz. Med. Wochenschr.* 112: 1347, 1987.
143. Hardes, G., Egger, G., O'Neill, P., Nanra, R. S., and Leeder, S. R. Consequences of legislative restriction on the sale of compound analgesics in Newcastle (N.S.W., Australia). *Aust. N.Z. J. Med.* 11: 654, 1981.
144. Hardy, T. L. Partial renal papillectomy and the study of drug induced RPN in the rat. *Br. J. Exp. Pathol.* 51: 591, 1970.
145. Hardy, T. L. Unpublished data, 1978, quoted by Bach, P. H., and Bridges, J. W. Chemically induced renal papillary necrosis and upper urothelial carcinoma. Part II. *CRC Crit. Rev. Toxicol.* 15: 331, 1985.
146. Hare, W. S. C. The Radiology of Analgesic Nephropa-

thy. In P. Kincaid-Smith and K. F. Fairley (eds.), *Renal Infection and Renal Scarring*. Melbourne: Mercedes Press, 1970. Pp. 409–413.

147. Hare, W. S. C., and Poynter, J. D. The radiology of renal papillary necrosis as seen in analgesic nephropathy. *Clin. Radiol.* 25: 423, 1974.
148. Harris, K. P. G., Schreiner, G. F., and Klahr, S. Effects of leucocyte depletion on the function of the postobstructed kidney in rat. *Kidney Int.* 36: 210, 1989.
149. Harvald, B. Renal papillary necrosis—A clinical survey of sixty six cases. *Am. J. Med.* 35: 481, 1963.
150. Haschek, H. (ed.). *International Symposium on Problems of Phenacetin Abuse*. Vienna: Facta Publications, 1973.
151. Hawkins, D., Pinkard, N., Crawford, I., and Farr, R. Structural changes in human serum albumin induced by ingestion of acetylsalicylic acid. *J. Clin. Invest.* 48: 538, 1969.

151a. Hayward, N. K., and Lavin, M. F. Inhibition of DNA, RNA and protein synthesis and chromatin alteration by *N*-hydroxyphenacetin. *Xenobiotica* 17: 115, 1987.

152. Hellebusch, A. A. Renal papillary necrosis. *J.A.M.A.* 210: 1098, 1969.
153. Hendry, W. F., Harrison, A. R., and Kilpatrick, F. R. Surgical management of renal papillary necrosis. *Proc. R. Soc. Med.* 65: 1023, 1972.
154. Hengstmann, H. Uber Verbreitung und Folgen des Phenazetin-Abusus auf dem Lande. *Munch. Med. Wochenschr.* 108: 1489, 1966.
155. Hennessy, B. L., Bruen, W. J., and Cullen, J. The Canberra mental health survey, preliminary results. *Med. J. Aust.* 1: 721, 1973.
156. Henrich, W. L. Analgesic nephropathy. *Am. J. Med. Sci.* 295: 561, 1988.
157. Hinson, J. A. Reactive metabolites of phenacetin and acetaminophen: A review. *Environ. Health Perspect.* 49: 71, 1983.
158. Hodson, C. J. Differential Diagnosis Between Atrophic Pyelonephritis and Analgesic Nephropathy. In P. Kincaid-Smith and K. F. Fairley (eds.), *Renal Infection and Renal Scarring*. Melbourne: Mercedes Press, 1970. Pp. 415–419.
159. Hoffman, J. C., Schnur, M. J., and Koenisberg, M. Demonstration of renal papillary necrosis by sonography. *Radiology* 145: 785, 1982.
160. Hood, B., Falkheden, T., and Carlsson, M. Trends and present pattern of mortality in chronic uraemia. *Acta Med. Scand.* 181: 561, 1967.
161. Horisberger, B., Grandjean, E., and Lanz, F. Untersuchungen uber den Medicamentenmissbrauch in einem Grossbeittrieb der Schweizerischen Uhrenindustrie. *Schweiz. Med. Wochenschr.* 88: 920, 1958.
162. Hultengren, N. Renal papillary necrosis: A clinical study of 34 cases. *Acta Chir. Scand.* 115: 89, 1958.
163. Hultengren, N. Renal papillary necrosis. A clinical study of 103 cases. *Acta Chir. Scand. Suppl.* 277, 1961.
164. Hultengren, N., Lagergren, C., and Ljungqvist, A. Carcinoma of the renal pelvis in renal papillary necrosis. *Acta Chir. Scand.* 130: 314, 1965.
165. Humes, J. L., Winter, C. A., Sadowski, S. J., and Kuehl, F. A., Jr. Multiple sites on prostaglandin cyclooxygenase are determinants in the action of nonsteroidal anti-inflammatory agents. *Proc. Natl. Acad. Sci. U.S.A.* 78: 2053, 1981.
166. Ingham, J. P., Kleerekoper, M., Stewart, J. H., and Posen, S. Symptomatic skeletal disease in non-terminal renal failure. *Med. J. Aust.* 2: 873, 1974.
167. Isaka, H., Yoshii, H., Otsuji, A., Koike, M., Nagai, Y., Koura, M., Sugiyasu, K., and Kanabayashi, T. Tumours of Sprague-Dawley rats induced by long-term feeding of phenacetin. *Gann* 70: 29, 1979.
168. Itami, N., Akutsu, Y., Yasoshima, K., Tochimaru, H., Takekoshi, Y., and Matsumoto, S. Progressive renal failure despite discontinuation of mefenamic acid. *Nephron* 54: 281, 1990.
169. Jacobs, L. A., and Morris, J. G. Renal papillary necrosis and the abuse of phenacetin. *Med. J. Aust.* 2: 531, 1962.
170. Jaeger, P., Burckhardt, P., Wauters, J. P., Trechsel, U., and Bonjour, J. P. Atteinte particulierement severe du metabolisme calcique dans la nephropathie par abus d'analgesiques. *Schweiz. Med. Wochenschr.* 112: 1791, 1982.
171. Johansson, S., and Angervall, L. Urothelial hyperplasia of the renal papillae in female Sprague-Dawley rats induced by long-term feeding of phenacetin. *Acta Pathol. Microbiol. Scand.* 84: 353, 1976.
172. Johansson, S., and Angervall, L. Urothelial changes of the renal papillae in Sprague-Dawley rats induced by long-term feeding of phenacetin. *Acta Pathol. Microbiol. Scand.* 84: 375, 1976.
173. Johansson, S., Angervall, L., Bengtsson, U., and Wahlqvist, L. Uroepithelial tumours of the renal pelvis associated with abuse of phenacetin-containing analgesics. *Cancer* (Philadelphia) 33: 743, 1974.
174. Johnson, W. Analgesic nephropathy with renal failure: Surgical aspects. *Br. J. Urol.* 44: 723, 1972.
175. Jones, L. W., and Morrow, J. W. Renal papillary necrosis: Management by ureteral catheter drainage. *J. Urol.* 106: 467, 1971.
176. Joubert, P. H., Clark, E. C., Otto, A. C., and Pannall, P. R. Unreliable drug histories, analgesics, and changes in renal function. *S. Afr. Med. J.* 52: 107, 1977.
177. Kaladelfos, G., and Edwards, K. D. G. Increased prevalence of coronary heart disease in analgesic nephropathy: Relationship to hypertension, hypertriglyceridemia and combined hyperlipidemia. *Nephron* 16: 388, 1976.
178. Kamien, M. A survey of drug use in a part-aboriginal community. *Med. J. Aust.* 1: 291, 1975.
179. Kasanen, A. The prognosis of kidney damage and anaemia in the analgesic abuser. *Ann. Med. Int. Fenn.* 56: 93, 1967.
180. Kasanen, A. The effect of restriction of sale of phenacetin on the incidence of papillary necrosis established at autopsy. *Ann. Clin. Res.* 5: 369, 1973.
181. Kasanen, A., and Salmi, H. A. The use of phenacetin and its detrimental effects on a series of hospital patients. *Ann. Med. Int. Fenn.* 50: 195, 1961.
182. Kasanen, A., and Valleala, P. Electroencephalographic findings in chronic phenacetin abusers. *Acta Med. Scand.* 173: 35, 1963.
183. Kassis, V., and Kassis, E. Nyrepapilnekrose og fenacetinforbrug. *Ugeskr. Laeger.* 140: 1406, 1978.
184. Kincaid-Smith, P. The pathogenesis of the renal lesion associated with abuse of analgesics. *Lancet* 1: 859, 1967.
185. Kincaid-Smith, P. Analgesic nephropathy. *Ann. Intern. Med.* 68: 949, 1968.'
186. Kincaid-Smith, P. (ed.). Analgesic nephropathy. *Kidney Int.* 13: 1, 1978.
187. Kincaid-Smith, P. Analgesic nephropathy in Australia. *Contrib. Nephrol.* 16: 57, 1979.
188. Kincaid-Smith, P., Nanra, R. S., and Fairley, K. F. Analgesic Nephropathy: A Recoverable Form of Chronic Renal Failure. In P. Kincaid-Smith and K. F. Fairley

(eds.), *Renal Infection and Renal Scarring*. Melbourne: Mercedes Press, 1970. Pp. 385–400.
189. Kincaid-Smith, P., Saker, B. M., McKenzie, I. F. C., and Muirden, K. D. Lesions in the blood supply of papilla in experimental analgesic nephropathy. *Med. J. Aust.* 1: 203, 1968.
190. Kincaid-Smith, P., Saker, B. M., and McKenzie, I. F. C. Lesions in the vasa recta in experimental analgesic nephropathy. *Lancet* 1: 24, 1968.
191. Kincaid-Smith, P., Whitworth, J., Fairley, K. F., and Nanra, R. S. Clinical Course of Analgesic Nephropathy with Renal Failure. In H. Haschek (ed.), *Problems of Phenacetin Abuse*. Vienna: Facta Publication, Verlag H. Egermann. Pp. 157–184.
192. Kingsley, D. P. E., Goldberg, B., Abrahams, C., Meyers, A. J., Furman, K. I., and Cohen, I. Analgesic nephropathy. *Br. Med. J.* 4: 656, 1972.
193. Kjaerulff, J., and Harvald, B. Incidensen of papillitis necroticans. *Nord. Med.* 80: 1588, 1968.
194. Kneezel, L. D., and Kitchens, C. S. Phenacetin-induced sulfhemoglobinemia: Report of a case and review of literature. *Johns Hopkins Med. J.* 139: 175, 1976.
195. Kolarova-Paneva, D. Syndrome of analgesic abuse and drug addiction. *Nevrol. Psikhiat. Neurokhir. (Sofia)* 14: 200, 1975.
196. Koutsaimanis, K. G., and de Wardener, H. E. Phenacetin nephropathy, with particular reference to the effect of surgery. *Br. Med. J.* 4: 131, 1970.
197. Kravath, R. E., Abel, G., and Colli, A. Salicylate poisoning: Effect on 2,3-diphosphoglycerate levels in the rat. *Biochem. Pharmacol.* 21: 2656, 1972.
198. Krishnaswamy, S., Kuna, K., and Nanra, R. S. Pattern of changes in renal function with analgesic abuse. *Aust. N.Z. J. Med.* 6: 88, 1976.
199. Krishnaswamy, S., Wallace, D. C., and Nanra, R. S. Ischaemic heart disease in analgesic nephropathy. *Aust. N.Z. J. Med.* 4: 426, 1974.
200. Kung, L. G. Hypernephroides Karzinom und Karzinome der ableitenden Harnwege nach Phenacetinabusus. *Schweiz. Med. Wochenschr.* 106: 47, 1976.
201. Kuster, G., and Ritz, E. Analgesic abuse and hypertension. *Lancet* 3: 1105, 1989.
202. Lagergren, C., and Lindvall, N. Renal papillary necrosis. Roentgenologic diagnosis and formation of calculi. *Acta Radiol. [Diagn.] (Stockh.)* 49: 249, 1958.
203. Lakey, W. H. Interstitial nephritis due to chronic phenacetin poisoning. *Can. Med. Assoc. J.* 85: 477, 1961.
204. Lalle, A. F. Renal papillary necrosis. *Am. J. Roentgenol. Rad. Ther. Nucl. Med.* 114: 741, 1972.
205. Larsen, K., and Moller, C. E. A renal lesion caused by abuse of phenacetin. *Acta Med. Scand.* 164: 53, 1959.
206. Lavan, J. M., Benson, W. J., Gatenby, A. H., and Posen, S. The consumption of analgesics by Australian hospital patients. *Med. J. Aust.* 2: 693, 1966.
207. Lawson, A. A. H., and McLean, N. Renal disease and drug therapy in rheumatoid arthritis. *Ann. Rheum. Dis.* 25: 441, 1966.
208. Lawson, D. H. Analgesic consumption and impaired renal function. *J. Chronic Dis.* 26: 39, 1973.
209. Lee, H. A., Davidson, A. R., and Burston, J. Analgesic nephropathy in Wessex: A clinico-pathological survey. *Clin. Nephrol.* 2: 197, 1974.
210. Leistenschneider, W., and Nagel, R. Urotheltumoren und Phenzetinabusus. *Therapiewoche* 27: 4221, 1977.
211. Levine, E., and Bernard, D. Analgesic nephropathy: A clinico-radiological study. *S. Afr. Med. J.* 47: 2439, 1973.
212. Lewis, C. T., Molland, E. A., Marshall, V. F., Tressider, G. C., and Blandy, J. P. Analgesic abuse, ureteric obstruction and retroperitoneal fibrosis. *Br. Med. J.* 2: 76, 1975.
213. Lewis, R. B., and Schulman, J. D. Influence of acetylsalicylic acid, an inhibitor of prostaglandin synthesis, on the duration of human gestation and labour. *Lancet* 2: 1159, 1973.
214. Lin, J. H., and Levy, G. Renal clearance of inorganic sulfate in rats: Effect of acetaminophen-induced depletion of endogenous sulfate. *J. Pharm. Sci.* 72: 213, 1983.
215. Lincke, H. U., Zenker, K., Sickor, H. J., Fischer, H., and Modelmog, D. Biopsiebefunde der Nieren bei Phenacetinabusus. *Dtsch. Ges.* 32: 1228, 1977.
216. Lindholm, T. On RPN with special reference to the diagnostic importance of papillary fragments in urine, therapy (i.e., artificial kidney) and prognosis. *Acta Med. Scand.* 167: 319, 1960.
217. Lindvall, N. Renal papillary necrosis. A roentgenographic study of 155 cases. *Acta Radiol. [Diagn.] (Stockh.)* 192(Suppl.), 1960.
218. Linton, A. L. Renal disease due to analgesics. *Can. Med. Assoc. J.* 107: 749, 1972.
219. Ljungquist, A., and Richardson, J. Studies on the pathogenesis of serum-induced RPN in the rat. *Lab. Invest.* 15: 1395, 1966.
220. Lornoy, W., Morelle, V., Becaus, I., Fonteyne, E., and Vrouwziekenhuis, O. L. Analgesic nephropathy. *N. Engl. J. Med.* 300: 319, 1979.
221. Mabeck, C. E., and Wichmann, B. Mortality from chronic interstitial nephritis and phenacetin consumption in Denmark. *Acta Med. Scand.* 205: 599, 1979.
222. MacDonald, I. M., Dumble, L. J., Doran, T., Bashir, H., Nanra, R. S., and Kincaid-Smith, P. Increased frequency of HLA-B12 in analgesic nephropathy. *Aust. N.Z. J. Med.* 8: 233, 1978.
223. MacGregor, G. A., Jones, N. F., Barraclough, M. A., Wing, A. J., and Cranston, W. I. Ureteric stricture with analgesic nephropathy. *Br. Med. J.* 2: 271, 1973.
224. Macklin, A. W., and Szot, R. J. Eighteen month oral study of aspirin, phenacetin and caffeine in C57BL/6 mice. *Drug Chem. Toxicol.* 3: 135, 1980.
225. Mahallaway, N. M., and Sabour, M. S. Renal lesions in rheumatoid arthritis. *Lancet* 2: 852, 1959.
226. Mahony, J. F., Storey, B. G., Ibanez, R. C., and Stewart, J. H. Analgesic abuse, renal parenchymal disease and carcinoma of the kidney or ureter. *Aust. N.Z. J. Med.* 7: 463, 1977.
227. Matsuda, K., Ohnishi, K., Misaka, E., and Yamazaki, M. Decrease of urinary prostaglandin E_2 and prostaglandin $F_{2'}$ excretion by nonsteroidal anti-inflammatory drugs in the rat. *Biochem. Pharmacol.* 32: 1347, 1983.
228. McCredie, M., Ford, J. M., Taylor, J. S., and Stewart, J. H. Analgesics and cancer of the renal pelvis in New South Wales. *Cancer* 49: 2617, 1982.
229. McCredie, M., and Stewart, J. H. Does paracetamol cause urothelial cancer or renal papillary necrosis? *Nephron* 49: 296, 1988.
230. McCredie, M., Stewart, J. H., and Ford, J. M. Analgesics and tobacco as risk factors of cancer of the ureter and renal pelvis in men. *J. Urol.* 130: 280, 1983.
231. McCredie, M., Stewart, J. H., Ford, J. M., and MacLennan, R. A. Phenacetin-containing analgesics and cancer of the bladder or renal pelvis in women. *Br. J. Urol.* 55: 220, 1983.
232. McCredie, M., Stewart, J. H., and Mahony, J. F. Is phen-

acetin responsible for analgesic nephropathy in New South Wales? *Clin. Nephrol.* 17: 134, 1982.

233. McCredie, M., Stewart, J. H., Mathew, T. H., Disney, A. P., and Ford, J. M. The effect of withdrawal of phenacetin-containing analgesics on the incidence of kidney and urothelial cancer and renal failure. *Clin. Nephrol.* 31: 35, 1989.
234. McGiff, J. C. Prostaglandins, prostacyclin and thromboxanes. *Annu. Rev. Pharmacol. Toxicol.* 21: 479, 1981.
235. McMurtry, M. J., Snodgrass, W. R., and Mitchell, J. R. Renal necrosis, glutathione depletion and covalent binding after acetaminophen. *Toxicol. Appl. Pharmacol.* 46: 87, 1978.
236. Mehta, A. R., White, K. H., and Nanra, R. S. Significance of proteinuria in analgesic nephropathy. *Aust. N.Z. J. Med.* 7: 463, 1977.
237. Mellins, H. Z. Chronic pyelonephritis and renal medullary necrosis. *Semin. Roentgenol.* 6: 292, 1971.
238. Mihatsch, M. J., Hofer, H. O., Gudat, F., Knusli, C., Torhorst, J., and Zollinger, U. Capillary sclerosis of the lower urinary tract and analgesic nephropathy. *Clin. Nephrol.* 20: 285, 1984.
239. Mihatsch, M. J., Hofer, H. O., Gutzwiler, F., Brunner, F. P., and Zollinger, H. U. Phenacetinabusus, 1. Haufigkeit, Pro-Kopf-Verbrauch und Folgefosten. *Schweiz. Med. Wochenschr.* 110: 108, 1980.
240. Mihatsch, M. J., Manz, T., Knusli, C., Hofer, H. O., Rist, M., Guetg, R., Rutishauser, G., and Zollinger, H. U. Phenacetinabusus III. Maligne Harnwegtumoren bei phenacetinabusus in Basel 1963–1977. *Schweiz. Med. Wochenschr.* 110: 255, 1980.
241. Mihatsch, M. J., Schmidlin, P., Brunner, F. P., Hofer, H. O., Six, P., and Zollinger, H. U. Phenacetinabusus. II. Die chronische renale Niereninsuffizienze un Basler Autopsiegut. *Schweiz. Med. Wochenschr.* 110: 116, 1980.
242. Mihatsch, M. J., Torhorst, J., Amsler, B., and Zollinger, H. U. Capillarosclerosis of the lower urinary tract in analgesic (phenacetin) abuse. An electron-microscopy study. *Virchows Arch. A Pathol. Anat. Histopathol.* 381: 41, 1978.
243. Mihatsch, M. J., Torhorst, J., Steinmann, E., Hofer, H., Stickelberger, M., Bianchi, L., Bernies, K., and Zollinger, H. U. The morphologic diagnosis of analgesic (phenacetin) abuse. *Pathol. Res. Pract.* 164: 68, 1979.
244. Miller, A. L., Worsley, L. R., and Chu, P. K. Brown urine as a clue to phenacetin intoxication. *Lancet* 2: 1102, 1970.
245. Mitchell, J. R., McMurtry, R. J., Statham, C. N., and Nelson, S. D. Molecular basis for several drug-induced nephropathies. *Am. J. Med.* 62: 518, 1977.
246. Mohandas, J., Calder, I. C., and Duggin, G. G. Renal oxidative metabolism of drugs in C57BL6J mouse. *Proc. Aust. Soc. Med. Res.* 10: 49, 1977.
247. Mohandas, J., Duggin, G. G., Horvarth, J. S., and Tiller, D. J. Metabolic oxidation of acetaminophen (paracetamol) mediated by cytochrome P-450 mixed function oxidase and prostaglandin endoperoxide synthetase in rabbit kidney. *Toxicol. Appl. Pharmacol.* 61: 252, 1981.
248. Molland, E. A. Aspirin damage in the rat kidney in the intact animal and after unilateral nephrectomy. *J. Pathol.* 120: 43, 1976.
249. Molland, E. A. Experimental renal papillary necrosis. *Kidney Int.* 13: 5, 1978.
250. Mostbeck, G., Derfler, K., Walter, R., Herold, C., Mallek, R., and Tschollakoff, D. Ultrasound in terminal renal failure—Etiologic conclusions? *Ultraschall Med.* 9: 250, 1988.
251. Mudge, G. H. Pathogenesis of Nephrotoxicity; Pharmacological Principles. In P. H. Bach and E. A. Lock (eds.), *Renal Heterogeneity and Target Cell Toxicity*. Chichester, England: John Wiley, 1985. Pp. 1–12.
252. Mudge, G. H., Gembroys, M. W., and Duggin, G. G. Covalent binding of metabolites of acetaminophen to kidney protein and depletion of renal glutathione. *J. Pharmacol. Exp. Ther.* 206: 218, 1978.
253. Muirhead, E. E. The Medullary Antihypertensive System and Its Putative Hormone(s). In J. Genest, P. Kuchel, P. Hamet, and M. Cantin (eds.), *Hypertension* (2nd ed.). London: Academic Press, 1971. Pp. 394–407.
254. Munck, A., Lindlar, F., and Masshoff, W. Die Pigmentierung der Nierenpapillen und der Schleimhaut der ablietenden Harnwege bei der chronischen sklerosierenden interstitiellen Nephritis ("Phenacetinniere"). *Virchows Arch.* [*Path. Anat.*] 349: 323, 1970.
255. Muller, F., and Schneider, J. Complications of calcified annulus fibrosus mitralis of the heart. *Wchweiz. Med. Wochenschr.* 110: 1233, 1980.
256. Murphy, K. J. Calcification of the renal papillae as a sign of analgesic nephropathy. *Clin. Radiol.* 19: 394, 1968.
257. Murray, R. M. The use and abuse of analgesics. *Scott. Med. J.* 17: 393, 1972.
258. Murray, R. M. The origins of analgesic nephropathy. *Br. J. Psychiatry* 123: 99, 1973.
259. Murray, R. M. Personality factors in analgesic nephropathy. *Psychol. Med.* 4: 69, 1974.
260. Murray, R. M. Genesis of analgesic nephropathy in the United Kingdom. *Kidney Int.* 13: 50, 1978.
261. Murray, R. M., Greene, J. G., and Adams, J. H. Analgesic abuse and dementia. *Lancet* 2: 242, 1971.
262. Murray, R. M., Lawson, D. H., and Linton, A. L. Analgesic nephropathy: Clinical syndrome and prognosis. *Br. Med. J.* 1: 479, 1971.
263. Murray, T., and Goldberg, M. Chronic interstitial nephritis: Etiologic factors. *Ann. Intern. Med.* 82: 453, 1975.
264. Murray, T., and Goldberg, M. Analgesic abuse and renal disease. *Annu. Rev. Med.* 26: 537, 1975.
265. Murray, T. G., and Goldberg, M. Analgesic-associated nephropathy in the USA: Epidemiologic, clinical and pathogenetic features. *Kidney Int.* 13: 64, 1978.
266. Nanra, R. S. Analgesic nephropathy. *Med. J. Aust.* 1: 745, 1976.
267. Nanra, R. S. Pathology, etiology and pathogenesis of analgesic nephropathy. *Aust. N.Z. J. Med.* 1 (Suppl.): 33, 1976.
268. Nanra, R. S. Factors which influence the clinical course of analgesic nephropathy. *Proceedings of the VIIth International Congress of Nephrology*, Montreal (Abstract G-20), 1978.
269. Nanra, R. S. Clinical and pathological aspects of analgesic nephropathy. *Br. J. Clin. Pharmacol.* (Suppl. 2)10: 359S, 1980.
270. Nanra, R. S. Renal effects of antipyretic analgesics. *Am. J. Med.* 75: 70, 1983.
271. Nanra, R. S. Analgesic-Associated Nephropathy. In S. G. Massry and R. J. Glassock (eds.), *Textbook of Nephrology*. Baltimore: Williams & Wilkins, 1983. Pp. 6.195–6.201.
272. Nanra, R. S. Renal biopsies in analgesic nephropathy (AN)—A clinicopathological study. *Kidney Int.* 33: 145, 1988.
273. Nanra, R. S. Evolution of the analgesic syndrome (AS) following legislation restricting analgesic sales. *Kidney Int.* 33: 136, 1988.

274. Nanra, R. S. Renal papillary necrosis (RPN) and chronic interstitial nephritis (CIN) with nonsteroidal anti-inflammatory drugs (NSAIDs)—A comparison with the analgesic syndrome. *Annual Scientific Meeting of Australasian Society of Nephrology,* Sydney (Abstract), 1989.
275. Nanra, R. S. The new analgesic syndromes (ASs). *XIth International Congress of Nephrology,* Tokyo (Abstract), 1990. P. 189A.
276. Nanra, R. S. Functional Defects in Analgesic Nephropathy. In J. H. Stewart (ed.), *Kidney Disease due to Analgesics and Anti-inflammatory Drugs.* Oxford: Oxford University Press. (In press.)
277. Nanra, R. S., Chirawong, P., and Kincaid-Smith, P. Renal Papillary Necrosis in Rats Produced by Aspirin, APC and Other Analgesics. In P. Kincaid-Smith and K. F. Fairley (eds.), *Renal Infection and Renal Scarring.* Melbourne: Mercedes Press, 1971. Pp. 347–358.
278. Nanra, R. S., Chirawong, P., and Kincaid-Smith, P. Medullary ischaemia in experimental analgesic nephropathy—The pathogenesis of RPN. *Aust. N.Z. J. Med.* 3: 580, 1973.
279. Nanra, R. S., Daniel, V., Howard, M., Murugasu, R., and White, K. H. Uroepithelial hyperplasia and carcinoma in experimental analgesic nephropathy. *Proceedings of the VIIth International Congress of Nephrology,* Athens (Abstract DK 021), 1981. P. 188.
280. Nanra, R. S., Hicks, J. D., McNamara, J. H., Lie, J. T., Leslie, D. W., Jackson, B., and Kincaid-Smith, P. Seasonal variation in the postmortem incidence of RPN. *Med. J. Aust.* 1: 293, 1970.
281. Nanra, R. S., Howard, M., and Daniel, V. Secondary gout in analgesic nephropathy (AN). *Aust. N.Z. J. Med.* 8: 237, 1978.
282. Nanra, R. S., and Kincaid-Smith, P. Papillary necrosis in rats caused by aspirin and aspirin containing mixtures. *Br. Med. J.* 3: 559, 1970.
283. Nanra, R. S., and Kincaid-Smith, P. Chronic effect of analgesics on the kidney. *Prog. Biochem. Pharmacol.* 7: 285, 1972.
284. Nanra, R. S., and Kincaid-Smith, P. Experimental RPN (RPN) with Nonsteroidal Anti-inflammatory Analgesics. In H. Haschek (ed.), *Problems of Phenacetin Abuse.* Vienna: Facta Publication, Verlag H. Egermann, 1973a. Pp. 67–88.
285. Nanra, R. S., and Kincaid-Smith, P. Experimental and Clinical Analgesic Nephropathy with Aspirin. In H. Haschek (ed.), *Problems of Phenacetin Abuse.* Vienna: Facta Publication, Verlag H. Egermann, 1973. Pp. 89–114.
286. Nanra, R. S., and Kincaid-Smith, P. Renal papillary necrosis in rheumatoid arthritis. *Med. J. Aust.* 1: 194, 1975.
287. Nanra, R. S., and Kincaid-Smith, P. Experimental Effects of Analgesics in Rats. In T. C. Jones (ed.), *Monographs on Pathology of Laboratory Animals.* Berlin-Heidelberg-New York: Springer-Verlag, 1986. Pp. 254–261.
288. Nanra, R. S., and Kincaid-Smith, P. Experimental Evidence for Nephrotoxicity of Analgesics. In J. H. Stewart (ed.), *Kidney Disease due to Analgesics and Anti-inflammatory Drugs.* Oxford: Oxford University Press. (In press.)
289. Nanra, R. S., and Nanra, S. K. The proteinuria in analgesic nephropathy (AN) is glomerular. *Kidney Int.* 33: 141, 1988.
290. Nanra, R. S., Taylor, J. S., de Leon, A. H., and White, K. H. Analgesic nephropathy: Etiology, clinical syndrome and clinico-pathologic correlations in Australia. *Kidney Int.* 13: 79, 1978.
291. Neilson, E. G. Pathogenesis and therapy of interstitial nephritis. *Kidney Int.* 35: 1257, 1989.
292. Nery, R. Some new aspects of metabolism of phenacetin in the rat. *Biochem. J.* 122: 317, 1971.
293. Nery, R. The binding of radioactive label from labelled phenacetin and related compounds to rat tissues in vivo and to nucleic acids and bovine plasma albumin in vitro. *Biochem. J.* 122: 311, 1971.
294. Nitzsche, T., and Bock, K. D. The course of phenacetin-induced nephropathy. *Germ. Med. Mon.* 15: 539, 1970.
295. Nordenfelt, O. Deaths from renal failure in abusers of phenacetin-containing drugs. *Acta Med. Scand.* 191: 11, 1972.
296. Nordenfelt, O., and Ringertz, N. Phenacetin takers dead with renal failure. *Acta Med. Scand.* 170: 385, 1961.
297. Nunn, I. N. Surgical Aspects of Papillary Necrosis. In P. Kincaid-Smith and K. F. Fairley (eds.), *Renal Infection and Renal Scarring.* Melbourne: Mercedes Press, 1970. Pp. 405–408.
298. Olafsson, O., Gudmundsson, K. R., and Brakkan, A. Migraine, gastritis and RPN. A syndrome in chronic non-obstructive pyelonephritis. *Acta Med. Scand.* 121: 128, 1966.
299. Orell, S. R., Nanra, R. S., and Ferguson, N. W. Renal pelvic carcinoma in the Hunter Valley. *Med. J. Aust.* 121: 128, 1966.
300. Palvio, D. H., Andersen, J. C., and Falk, E. Capillary sclerosis in the mucus membrane of the urinary tract; A reliable histological marker for analgesic abuse. *Ugeskr. Laeger.* 149: 2704, 1987.
301. Panzram, C., and Muller, K. H. Amnulante Untersuchungen und Klinische Erfahrungen uber die Haufigkeit des Analgetikamissbrauches; Ergebnis einer Reihenuntersuchung in einem Grossbetrieb. *Dtsch. Ges.* 19: 903, 1964.
302. Pasternack, A., Wegelius, O., and Makisara, P. Renal biopsy in rheumatoid arthritis. *Acta Med. Scand.* 182: 591, 1967.
303. Pearse, A. G. E. *Histochemistry: Theoretical and Applied.* Edinburgh and London: Churchill Livingstone, 1960.
304. Pearson, H. H. Residual renal defects in non-fatal phenacetin nephritis. *Med. J. Aust.* 2: 308, 1967.
305. Pendreigh, D. M., Heasman, M. H., Howitt, L. F., et al. Survey of chronic renal failure in Scotland. *Lancet* 1: 304, 1972.
306. Pinter, G. G. A possible role of mucopolysaccharides in the urinary concentrating process. *Experientia* 23: 100, 1976.
307. Pletscher, A., Studer, A., and Miescher, P. Experimentelle Untersuchungen uber Erythrocyten und Organveranderungen durch N-acetyl-*p*-aminophenol und Phenacetin. *Schweiz. Med. Wochenschr.* 88: 1214, 1958.
308. Plotz, P. L., and Kimberly, R. P. Acute effects of aspirin and acetaminophen on renal function. *Arch. Intern. Med.* 141: 343, 1981.
309. Pommer, W., Bronder, E., Greiser, E., Helmert, U., Jesdinsky, H. J., Klimpel, A., Borner, K., and Molzahn, M. Regular analgesic intake and the risk of end-stage renal failure. *Am. J. Nephrol.* 9: 403, 1989.
310. Porpaczy, P. Ursachen und Folgen langjahriger Einnahme phenacetinhaltiger Analgetike aus der Sicht des Urolgen. *Wien. Klin. Wochenschr.* 91(Suppl. 104): 1, 1979.
311. Poynter, J. D., and Hare, W. S. C. Necrosis in situ: A form of renal papillary necrosis seen in analgesic nephropathy. *Radiology* 111: 69, 1974.

312. Prescott, L. F. Analgesic abuse and renal disease in North-East Scotland. *Lancet* 2: 1143, 1966.
313. Prescott, L. F. The nephrotoxicity of analgesics. *J. Pharm. Pharmacol.* 18: 331, 1966.
314. Prescott, L. F. The Absorption, Metabolism, Excretion and CNS Effects of Phenacetin. In P. Kincaid-Smith and K. F. Fairley (eds.), *Renal Infection and Renal Scarring.* Melbourne: Mercedes Press, 1971. Pp. 359–374.
315. Prescott, L. F. Analgesic nephropathy—The international experience. *Aust. N.Z. J. Med.* 6(Suppl. 1): 44, 1976.
316. Prescott, L. F. Analgesic nephropathy: A reassessment of the role of phenacetin and other analgesics. *Drugs* 23: 75, 1982.
317. Prescott, L. F., and Brodie, D. E. A simple differential stain for urinary sediment. *Lancet* 2: 940, 1964.
318. Prescott, L. F., and Brown, S. S. Brown urine: A clue to phenacetin intoxication. *Lancet* 1: 253, 1970.
319. Purnell, J., and Burry, A. F. Analgesic consumption in a country town. *Med. J. Aust.* 2: 389, 1967.
320. Quantanilla, A., and Kessler, R. H. Direct effect of salicylate on renal function in the dog. *J. Clin. Invest.* 52: 3143, 1973.
321. Raaflaub, J., and Dubach, U. C. Dose-dependent change in the pattern of phenacetin metabolism in man and its possible significance in analgesic nephropathy. *Klin. Wochenschr.* 47: 1286, 1969.
322. Report from Senate Standing Committee on Social Welfare. Drug problems in Australia—An intoxicated society? Canberra: Australian Government Publishing Service, 1977. Pp. 107–126.
323. Reubi, F. Chronische Pyelonephritis mit "salt-losing" syndrome und sekundarem Saridon-abusus. *Wchweiz. Med. Wochenschr.* 88: 294, 1958.
324. Rich, R. R., and Johnson, J. S. Salicylate hepatotoxicity in patients with juvenile rheumatoid arthritis. *Arthritis Rheum.* 16: 1, 1973.
325. Richards, P. D. G. Congenital malformations and environmental influences in pregnancy. *Br. J. Prev. Soc. Med.* 23: 218, 1969.
326. Ricketts, J., and Nanra, R. S. Analgesic abuse in perspective. *Aust. Alcohol/Drug Rev.* 1: 81, 1982.
327. Ringoir, S. Aspects cliniques, epidemiologiques et experimentaux de la nephropathie chronique avec abus d'analgesiques. *Therapie* 29: 483, 1974.
328. Roberts, J. E., and Lawrence, J. R. Personality and the Use and Misuse of Drugs. In H. Haschek (ed.), *Problems on Phenacetin Abuse.* Vienna: Facta Publication, Verlag H. Egermann, 1973. Pp. 299–303.
329. Rosner, I. Experimental analgesic nephropathy. *CRC Crit. Rev. Toxicol.* 4: 331, 1976.
330. Ross, R. K., Paganini-Hill, A., Landolph, J., Gerkins, V., and Henderson, B. E. *Cancer Res.* 49: 1045, 1989.
331. Rossi, E., Menta, R., and Cambi, V. Partially reversible chronic renal failure due to long-term use of non-steroidal anti-inflammatory drugs. *Nephrol. Dial. Transplant.* 3: 469, 1988.
332. Roth, G., and Majerus, P. The mechanism of the effect of aspirin on human platelets: I. Acetylation of platelet particulate protein. *J. Clin. Invest.* 56: 624, 1975.
333. Roth, G. and Soik, C. J. Acetylation of -NH_2 terminal serine of prostaglandin synthetase by aspirin. *J. Biol. Chem.* 253: 3782, 1978.
334. Rubenstein, A. H., Abrahams, C., Stables, D. P., and Levin, N. W. Acetophenitidin nephritis and papillary necrosis. *Arch. Intern. Med.* 113: 378, 1964.
335. Ruikka, I., and Sourander, L. B. Phenacetin consumption, occurrence of urinary tract infection and renal function in a series of aged hospital patients. *Gerontol. Clin.* 9: 99, 1967.
336. Saker, B. M., and Kincaid-Smith, P. Papillary necrosis in experimental analgesic nephropathy. *Br. Med. J.* 1: 161, 1969.
337. Sandler, D. P., Smith, J. C., Weinberg, C. R., Buckalew, V. M., Dennis, V. W., Blythe, W. B., and Burgess, W. P. Analgesic use and chronic renal disease. *N. Engl. J. Med.* 320: 1238, 1989.
338. Sanerkin, N. G. Chronic phenacetin nephropathy with particular reference to the relationship between RPN and "chronic interstitial nephritis." *Br. J. Urol.* 38: 361, 1966.
339. Scheidegger, S. Pathologisch-anatomischer Beitrag zur Frage der chronischen interstitiellen Nephritis im Anschluss an Abusus von phenacetin-haltigen Analgetika. *Bull. Schweiz. Akad. Med. Wis.* 14: 139, 1958.
340. Schnitzer, B., Smith, E. B., and Golden, A. Effects of phenacetin and its contaminant on the kidney of the rat. *Am. J. Pathol.* 46: 917, 1965.
341. Schourup, K. Necrosis of the renal papilla. Post mortem series. *Acta Pathol. Microbiol. Scand.* 41: 462, 1957.
342. Schreiner, G. E., McAnnaly, J. F., and Winchester, J. F. Clinical analgesic nephropathy. *Arch. Intern. Med.* 14: 349, 1981.
343. Schwarz, A., Kraft, D., Keller, F., Gawlik, D., and Offermann, G. Aluminium load in patients with analgesic nephropathy. *Miner. Electrolyte Metab.* 13: 141, 1987.
344. Schweingruber, R. Probleme der chronischen vergiftung mit kombinierten Phenacetinpraparaten. *Schweiz. Med. Wochenschr.* 85: 1162, 1955.
345. Segasothy, M., Suleiman, A. B., Puvaneswary, M., and Rohana, A. Paracetamol: A cause of analgesic nephropathy and end-stage renal disease. *Nephron* 50: 50, 1988.
346. Seventh Report of the Australia and New Zealand Combined Dialysis and Transplant Registry (ANZDATA), 1984.
347. Shahidi, N. T. Acetophenetidin-induced methemoglobinemia. *Ann. N.Y. Acad. Sci.* 151: 82, 1968.
348. Shamsuddin, M. R., Mason, R. G., Ritchey, J. M., Honig, G. R., and Klotz, I. M. Site of acetylation of sickle cell hemoglobin by aspirin. *Proc. Natl. Acad. Sci. U.S.A.* 12: 4693, 1974.
349. Sheehan, H. L. Medullary necrosis of the kidneys. *Lancet* 232: 187, 1937.
350. Shelley, J. H. Phenacetin through the looking glass. *Clin. Pharmacol. Ther.* 8: 427, 1967.
351. Shelley, J. H. Pharmacological mechanisms of analgesic nephropathy. *Kidney Int.* 13: 15, 1978.
352. Shimamura, T., and Trojanowski, S. Effects of repeated deprivation of drinking water on the structure of renal medulla in rats. *Am. J. Pathol.* 84: 87, 1976.
353. Silberbusch, J., Lenstra, J. B., van Es, H. W., and Gerbrandy, J. Follow-study of renal function in patients with a history of phenacetin abuse. *Neth. J. Med.* 16: 58, 1973.
354. Simon, H., Bennett, W., and Emmett, J. Renal papillary necrosis; A clinicopathological study of 42 cases. *J. Urol.* 77: 557, 1957.
355. Smith, J. D., Rabkin, R., Stables, D., Thatcher, G. N., and Eales, L. Analgesic RPN. *S. Afr. Med. J.* 49: 1819, 1975.
356. Sorenson, A. W. S. Is the relationship between analgesics and renal disease coincidental and not causal? *Nephron* 3: 366, 1966.

357. Spuhler, O., and Zollinger, H. U. Die chronische interstitielle Nephritis. *Z. Klin. Med.* 151: 1, 1953.
358. Steele, T. W., and Edwards, K. D. G. Abnormalities of urinary concentrating, acidifying and sodium conserving abilities induced by excess analgesic intake in rats. *Aust. Ann. Med.* 19: 412, 1970.
359. Steele, T. W., and Edwards, K. D. G. Analgesic nephropathy. Changes in various parameters of renal function following cessation of analgesic abuse. *Med. J. Aust.* 1: 181, 1971.
360. Steele, T. W., Gyory, A. Z., and Edwards, K. D. G. Renal function in analgesic nephropathy. *Br. Med. J.* 2: 213, 1969.
361. Steele, T. W., Hung, E. C. Y., and Edwards, K. D. G. Hypercalciuria and reduced daily excretion of citrate, potassium and hydrogen ions induced by excess intake of analgesics in rats. *Med. J. Aust.* 1: 170, 1971.
362. Steenland, N. K., Thun, M. J., Ferguson, C. W., and Port, F. K. Occupational and other exposures associated with male end-stage renal disease: A case/control study. *Am. J. Public Health* 80: 153, 1990.
363. Steinberg, D., Parthasarathy, S., Carew, T. E., Khoo, J. C., and Witztum, J. L. Beyond cholesterol. Modification of low-density lipoprotein that increases its atherogenecity. *N. Engl. J. Med.* 14: 915, 1989.
364. Stewart, J. H. Analgesic abuse and renal failure in Australia. *Kidney Int.* 13: 72, 1978.
365. Stewart, J. H., and Gallery, E. D. M. Analgesic abuse and kidney disease. *Aust. N.Z. J. Med.* 6: 498, 1976.
366. Strimer, R. M., and Morin, L. J. Phenacetin-induced RPN. Pyonephrosis, anuria, and bilateral ureteral obstruction. *Urology* 5: 780, 1975.
367. Studer, A., and Scharer, K. Prolonged phenacetin tolerance test on dogs with consideration of pigmentation of liver and kidney. *Schweiz. Med. Wochenschr.* 95: 933, 1965.
368. Tan, G. H., Rabbino, M. D., and Hopper, J. Is phenacetin a nephrotoxin? *Calif. Med.* 101: 73, 1964.
369. Thiele, K. G., and Berning, H. Nierenpapillennecrosen und Analgetika-Mi (Beta)brauch. *Munch. Med. Wochenschr.* 111: 1673, 1969.
370. Thirteenth Report of the Australia and New Zealand Dialysis and Transplant Registry (ANZDATA), 1990.
371. Thurau, K. Renal haemodynamics. *Am. J. Med.* 36: 698, 1964.
372. Torhorst, J., Rohr, H. P., Zollinger, H. U., Studer, A., and Tranzer, J. P. Ultrastrukturelle Veranderungen der proximalen Tubuluszelle von Rattennieren nach Phenacetinuberbelastung. *Virchows Arch.* [*Pathol. Anat.*] 342: 70, 1967.
373. Uehleke, H. Biochemical Pharmacology and Toxicology of Phenacetin. In H. Haschek (ed.), *Problems of Phenacetin Abuse.* Vienna: Facta Publication, Verlag H. Egermann, 1973. Pp. 31–44.
374. Unisearch Ltd. and School of Applied Psychology, University of N.S.W. A survey of analgesic and sedative consumption in Sydney and Brisbane. Unisearch Ltd., 1968.
375. Veller, M. G., Botha, J. R., Seggie, J., Thomson, P. D., Meyers, A. M., and Myburgh, J. A. Renal transplantation. The Johannesburg Hospital experience. *S. Afr. J. Med.* 71: 752, 1987.
376. Von Zerssen, D., Fliege, K., and Wolff, M. Cerebral atrophy in drug addicts (Letter). *Lancet* 2: 313, 1970.
377. Wainscoat, J. S., and Finn, R. Possible role of laxatives in analgesic nephropathy. *Br. Med. J.* 4: 697, 1974.
378. Waters, W. E., Elwood, P. C., and Asscher, A. W. Community survey of analgesic consumption and kidney function in women. *Lancet* 1: 341, 1973.
379. Wiseman, E. H., and Reinert, H. Anti-inflammatory drugs and RPN. *Agents Actions* 5: 322, 1975.
380. Wortmann, D. W., Kelsch, R. C., Kuhns, L., Sullivan, D. B., and Cassidy, J. T. Renal papillary necrosis in juvenile rheumatoid arthritis. *J. Pediatr.* 97: 37, 1980.
381. Zgirski, L. Fenacetynomania a organiczne uszkodzenie mozgu. *Psychiatr. Pol.* 3: 272, 1976.
382. Zollinger, H. U., and Spuhler, O. Die nichteitrige, chronische interstitielle Nephritis. *Schweiz. Z. Allg. Pathol.* 13: 807, 1950.

Aminoglycoside Nephrotoxicity

George J. Kaloyanides

Nephrotoxic injury is a common complication of aminoglycoside antibiotic therapy. Studies that have used well-defined measures of nephrotoxicity indicate an incidence rate of 7 to 36 percent [21, 68, 75, 85, 86, 102, 152, 154, 163, 225, 274, 280]. A review of multiple studies indicates that the average incidence of gentamicin nephrotoxicity is around 15 percent [126] and that the aminoglycosides at risk of inducing nephrotoxicity are, in decreasing order of relative risk, gentamicin, tobramycin, amikacin, and netilmicin [37, 126]. The pathogenesis of aminoglycoside-induced nephrotoxicity is causally linked to the transport and accumulation in high concentration of these cationic drugs by renal proximal tubular cells that subsequently manifest functional, biochemical, and structural alterations. As a class, few drugs have been studied more extensively with respect to their nephrotoxic potential than have aminoglycoside antibiotics. Consequently an enormous amount of literature has been generated on this subject. This chapter will summarize current concepts about the pathogenesis, treatment, and prevention of this complex and challenging disorder.

Clinical Aspects

The nephrotoxic potential of aminoglycoside antibiotics was recognized shortly after the introduction of streptomycin for use in clinical medicine, when it was appreciated that this agent caused cylinduria and celluria, changes attributed to "chemical irritation" of the kidney [78]. In retrospect, these changes may have reflected the influence of contaminants rather than the parent compound because subsequent studies established that pure streptomycin, even when administered in supranormal doses, has little potential for causing renal injury [173], which reflects the fact that unlike other aminoglycosides, streptomycin is not concentrated within the renal cortex [174]. As each new aminoglycoside was introduced into clinical practice, the potential of this drug class to cause nephrotoxicity and renal failure was rediscovered at the price of considerable patient morbidity and mortality. Today it is widely appreciated that aminoglycoside antibiotics are characterized by a very narrow therapeutic-toxicity ratio such that during a standard course of therapy, most patients will manifest some evidence of renal toxicity [273].

The earliest and most common expression of aminoglycoside nephrotoxicity is increased urinary excretion of low-molecular-weight proteins [88, 256, 261] and of lysosomal and brush-border membrane enzymes [19, 88, 198, 212, 256]. These changes may be detected within 24 hours of initiating drug therapy and the frequency and magnitude of these changes increase as a function of dose and duration of therapy. Unfortunately, these changes do not predict which patients will progress with respect to the development of acute renal failure. This probably reflects the fact that several mechanisms underly the expression of the enzymuria and proteinuria [127]. With repeated dosing, the level of enzymes and low-molecular-weight proteins excreted may increase quite sharply, in which case it usually signifies the onset of proximal tubular cell necrosis [127]. Increased urinary excretion of tubular cell casts, epithelial cells, and white blood cells typically appears as the next expression of nephrotoxicity [256, 258] and generally signifies the presence of more advanced cell injury and necrosis compared to that seen with increased urinary excretion of enzymes and low-molecular-weight protein.

Nonoliguric renal failure is a common expression of aminoglycoside nephrotoxicity [5] and probably reflects in part tubulointerstitial injury resulting in failure to maintain a hypertonic medullary interstitium. In addition, inhibition of adenylate cyclase by aminoglycosides may also contribute to the polyuria [113]. Neither mechanism, however, adequately explains the maintenance of normal to high urine output even in the face of severe depression of whole-kidney glomerular filtration rate (GFR). The slow evolution of acute renal failure, which has been attributed to a variable susceptibility of renal proximal tubular cells to aminoglycoside toxicity [128, 276], may allow for the development of maximal compensatory adaptation by residual intact nephrons. In addition, micropuncture experiments implicate a sharp depression of solute and water transport along the proximal tubule such that the large increase in the fraction of filtrate escaping reabsorption along the proximal tubule may overwhelm the reabsorptive capacity of the distal nephron and contribute to the pattern of nonoliguric renal failure [248]. When oliguria occurs, it usually signifies the influence of one or more complicating factors, e.g., ischemia or another nephrotoxin, especially if the oliguria appears early in the course of aminoglycoside administration. Studies in animals have shown that aminoglycoside therapy sensitizes the kidney to a subsequent ischemic or nephrotoxic insult [15, 105, 175, 278, 315, 316], such that the severity and rapidity of onset of the acute renal failure are substantially greater than those predicted by the sum of the effects of either individual insult.

Deterioration of other proximal tubular transport processes may occur during aminoglycoside toxicity and in rare cases may mimic a Fanconi-like syndrome with glycosuria and aminoaciduria [264]. Hypokalemia and hypomagnesemia secondary to renal potassium and magnesium wasting may also appear [14, 100, 222].

Depression of GFR is a relatively late manifestation of aminoglycoside nephrotoxicity. In humans, depression of GFR typically does not occur before 5 to 7 days of therapy has been completed [165] unless there has been a major complicating factor such as renal ischemia. Enzymuria, proteinuria, decreased urine concentrating capacity, cylindruria, celluria, and altered proximal tubular cell transport processes and plasma membrane enzyme activities are characteristically seen prior to depression of GFR in animal models of aminoglycoside nephrotoxicity [128, 256]. Furthermore, histopathologic lesions of focal proximal tubular cell necrosis may be present in the absence of a measurable decline in whole-kidney GFR [128, 171, 276]. Micropuncture studies have delineated alterations in the determinants of glomerular ultrafiltration in gentamicin nephrotoxicity in the Munich-Wistar rat [17]. A 30 percent decline of GFR in superficial nephrons was identified after 10 days of gentamicin administration at doses of 4 and 40 mg/kg/day and these changes of single-nephron GFR were accompanied by declines of whole-kidney GFR. The primary cause of the reduction of single-nephron GFR was a significant decline of the glomerular capillary ultrafiltration coefficient, K_f. Luft et al. [172] reported dose-dependent decrements in the size, density, and areas of glomerular endothelial fenestrae of rats treated with aminoglycosides. In the study of Baylis et al. [17] no ultrastructural alterations of the glomerular capillaries were detected. Schor et al. [263] reported that the effects of gentamicin on glomerular hemodynamics were almost completely prevented in rats treated with the converting enzyme inhibitor captopril. Although these results are consistent with a role of angiotensin II in the pathogenesis of the altered glomerular hemodynamics, they do not exclude other mechanisms of action. Since both nontoxic and toxic doses of gentamicin produced these glomerular changes, these alterations are likely maximal effects induced by early and mild renal tubular cell injury. In more advanced stages of tubular cell injury and renal failure, Luft et al. [172] detected no beneficial effect of captopril with respect to ameliorating aminoglycoside-induced alterations of renal function or morphology, including ultrastructural alterations at the level of the glomerular capillaries. Thus, this study argues against a dominant role of the renin-angiotensin system in advanced aminoglycoside-induced renal failure. Other investigators have implicated tubular obstruction [208] and increased backleak [248] as pathogenic factors causing depression of GFR in the advanced stages of aminoglycoside nephrotoxicity.

Most patients with aminoglycoside nephrotoxicity recover complete renal function clinically, although the rate of recovery may be prolonged in some [171]. Chronic renal failure is a distinctly uncommon complication of pure aminoglycoside nephrotoxicity. Nevertheless, animal studies indicate that incomplete tubular regeneration with interstitial fibrosis does occur [107].

Morphologic Alterations

Aminoglycosides produce tubular cell necrosis, that is largely confined to the proximal convoluted tubule and pars recta [63, 108, 150, 298]. The earliest lesion, seen by electron microscopy, is an increase in the number and size of secondary lysosomes, also called *cytosegrosomes* or *phagosomes* [63, 108, 150]. Examples of this lesion are shown in Figs. 41-1 and 41-2. Secondary lysosomes are primary lysosomes that have coalesced with endocytic or autophagic vacuoles. Many of these cytosegrosomes contain myeloid bodies, electron-dense lamellar structures of concentrically arranged and densely packed membranes (Fig. 41-2). These lysosomal alterations probably represent autophagic vacuoles arising from sequestration of fragments of membranes and organelles that were damaged in developing toxicity and are undergoing lysosomal processing. In experimental animals receiving single parenteral drug doses or continuous drug infusion, these changes have been observed as early as 6 to 12 hours posttreatment [91]. These morphologic alterations have been convincingly demonstrated by DeBroe and colleagues in a well-controlled manner [66]. Patients about to undergo radical nephrectomy for a renal neoplasm and who had neither impairment of renal function nor proteinuria were randomly allocated to no treatment or to standard daily clinical doses of gentamicin, tobramycin, or amikacin for 4 days. These patients were carefully screened to exclude diabetes mellitus, concurrent infection, or the use of diuretics, antibiotics, nonsteroidal antiinflammatory drugs, or drugs known to affect lipid metabolism. No patient had received an aminoglycoside within 4 months of the study. Morphologic alterations after 4 days of treatment mirrored those observed in the whole animal experimental setting [63, 91, 108, 150]. As in cultured fibroblasts exposed to aminoglycosides [12], histomorphometry showed that lysosomal volume was increased in the proximal tubular epithelial cells of treated patients. Importantly, patients treated with gentamicin or tobramycin had significantly greater accumulations of lamellar material than patients treated with amikacin [66]. It has been shown recently that the development of lysosomal alterations during aminoglycoside administration does not necessitate progression to renal cell necrosis and organ failure [91]. Additionally, these morphologic alterations are not specific for aminoglycoside toxicity and can occur in other tissues after focal cell injury induced by a variety of toxins [82, 110, 125, 177].

Following lysosomal alterations, there occurs a decrease in the density and height of brush-border microvilli, dilatation of the cisternae of rough endoplasmic reticulum, and the appearance of cytoplasmic vacuolization in the tubular epithelial cells [63, 91]. As injury progresses, brush-border membrane fragments and extruded myeloid bodies, membrane vesicles, and cytoplasmic debris begin to be seen within tubular lumina [63, 119] and are excreted in the urine. Later in the course of nephrotoxicity, mitochondrial swelling becomes evident and patchy, but extensive tubular epithelial cell necrosis and desquamation occur. Many tubules, both proximal and distal, are filled with eosinophilic, granular material that according to electron microscopy, is composed of cytoplasmic debris, membrane fragments, and myeloid bodies. Transmission electron microscopy of the urine reveals the presence of myeloid bodies [119, 134, 178] and degrees of brush-border membrane [119]. The degree of renal cortical injury correlates reasonably well with the decline in renal excretory func-

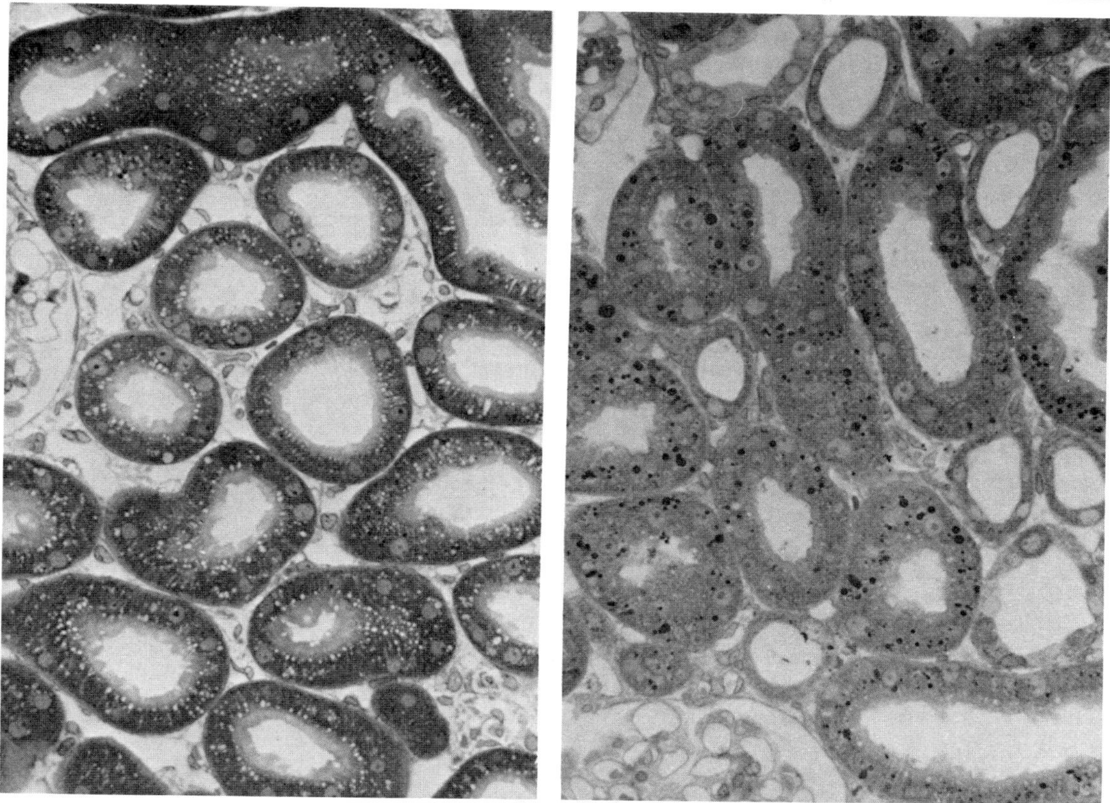

Fig. 41-1. Toluidine blue–stained thin sections (1–2 microns) of outer renal cortex from normal rats or rats with early gentamicin nephrotoxicity (*right*). Increased numbers of secondary lysosomes (*dark circular structures*) are apparent within the renal tubular epithelial cells of gentamicin-treated animals. (Magnification × 400.)

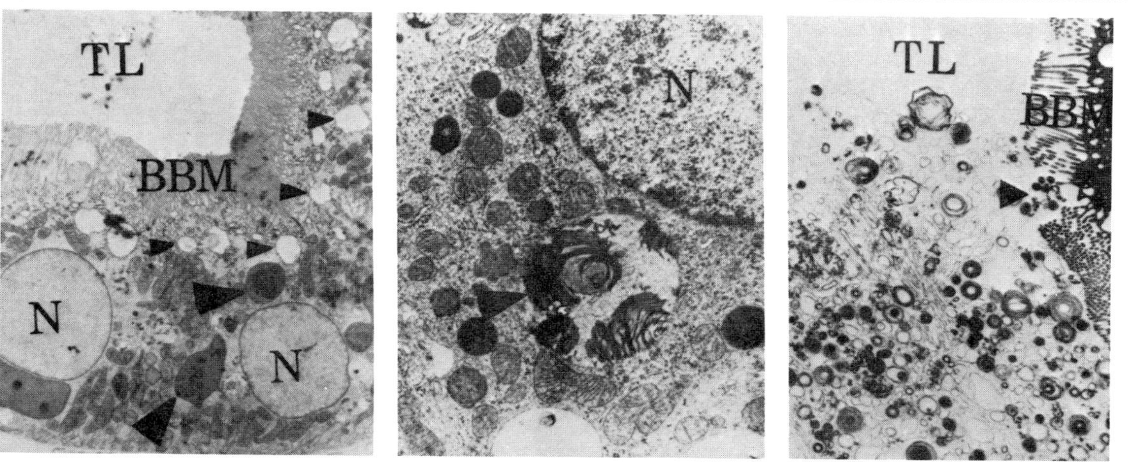

Fig. 41-2. Electron micrographic appearance of representative renal tubular epithelium from rats with established aminoglycoside nephrotoxicity. Increased numbers of apical vesicles (*small arrowheads, left*) and electron-dense lysosomes (*large arrowheads, left*) are apparent, while myeloid bodies are seen within a lysosome (*large arrowhead, center*). Focal loss of brush-border membranes (*small arrowhead, right*) is observed with membrane fragments filling the tubular lumen (*right*). TL, BBM, and N denote tubular lumen, brush-border membrane, and nucleus, respectively. (Magnification × 8000 [*left*]; × 32,000 [*center and right*].)

tion. The pattern of substantial susceptibility of S_2 proximal tubular segments to injury [267] contrasts with heavy-metal nephrotoxicity and ischemia in which a markedly greater susceptibility of S_3 segments is seen [95, 187]. Perhaps this is due to a much higher toxin load presented to the more proximal S_1 and S_2 cells along the tubule. Distal tubules and glomeruli reveal little damage by light and transmission electron microscopy [17, 63]. Scanning electron microscopy, however, has revealed glomerular alterations, including a decrease in the number and size of endothelial fenestrae and endothelial cell swelling [172].

Proximal tubular cells manifest an apparent variable susceptibility to aminoglycoside toxicity evident by the appearance of cell regeneration simultaneously with ongoing cell necrosis [107–109, 159, 276]. Regeneration of proximal tubule cells first appears during the stage of patchy necrosis. The relatively undifferentiated, immature, regenerating cells subsequently begin to regain normal height and structure. Foci of interstitial inflammatory infiltrates appear throughout the cortex during this stage of patchy necrosis and may become more prominent with time [59, 149]. Analysis of functional and morphologic recovery from aminoglycoside nephrotoxicity in vivo is clouded by coexistent and evolving necrosis. In an attempt to temporally dissociate injury from recovery, Giuliano and co-workers [91] used 12-hour, low-, medium-, and high-dose aminoglycoside infusions to achieve rapid and sizable renal cortical drug levels. After 12 hours of aminoglycoside infusion, lysosomal ultrastructural alterations were noted at each dosage level. While lysosomal enlargement, density, and myeloid bodies decreased gradually in size over 2 days in the low-dose group, progressive enlargement of lysosomes and myeloid bodies were noted in the high-dose group. Laurent et al. [158, 159] demonstrated significant increases in [^{3}H]thymidine incorporation into rat renal cortical DNA after low-dose administration (10 mg/kg/day for 4 days). These authors have suggested that stimulation of renal cortical DNA synthesis represents tubular epithelial regeneration following patchy aminoglycoside-induced cell necrosis. Importantly, the absence of identifiable cell necrosis by standard histologic methodologies suggests that this incorporation may be a highly sensitive and quantitative indicator of focal cell necrosis in whole renal cortex. Porter et al. [226] further demonstrated that aminoglycoside-stimulated [^{3}H]thymidine incorporation in vivo is dose related and occurs both in vivo and in vitro. Significantly, labeling is quantitatively similar in tubular epithelial cells and in renal cortical interstitial cells [226]. This finding is of considerable interest because interstitial inflammation is known to develop late in both acute and chronic animal models of aminoglycoside nephrotoxicity [107, 149]. Although tubular regeneration is an attractive explanation for the observed effects of low-dose aminoglycoside administration on [^{3}H]thymidine incorporation into DNA, a direct effect of these cationic drugs on DNA synthesis has not been excluded.

Eventually, most areas of the affected kidney regain normal architecture and function, but residual scarring containing collections of collapsed, atrophic tubules may occur focally in the cortex [59, 63, 109, 149]. Of interest, the regenerative process within the renal cortex continues even in the presence of continued aminoglycoside administration and toxic renal cortical drug levels [69]. Elliott and colleagues [70] demonstrated that protection against gentamicin nephrotoxicity requires prior cell necrosis, and cannot be promoted by other nephrotoxins or mildly nephrotoxic aminoglycosides.

Pathogenesis

The toxic as well as the therapeutic activity of a drug is critically dependent on the concentration of the active moiety reaching sensitive target sites. The susceptibility of the kidney to toxic injury typically derives from the fact that the kidney is the dominant route by which the toxic agent is eliminated from the body. In the case of aminoglycoside antibiotics, the susceptibility of the kidney to toxic injury relates to the fact that the kidney is the sole route by which these drugs are excreted and that during the process of excretion a small fraction of drug is transported by and accumulated in high concentration within proximal tubular cells. Not surprisingly, it is renal proximal tubular cells that manifest functional, biochemical, and structural alterations that frequently progress to extensive cell injury and necrosis. While proximal tubular cell transport and accumulation of aminoglycoside antibiotics are an essential first step in the pathogenesis of their nephrotoxicity, it is well established that the rate of drug transport and accumulation within proximal tubular cells does not predict their relative nephrotoxic potentials. The second step in the pathogenesis of toxicity relates to the potential of these organic polycations to interact with and disrupt the function of a variety of intracellular membranes and organelles. In the following section the renal pharmacology of aminoglycoside antibiotics will be reviewed, followed by an analysis of how these cationic drugs interact with model and cell membranes, disrupt membrane and organellar function, and compromise cell viability.

RENAL PHARMACOLOGY OF AMINOGLYCOSIDE ANTIBIOTICS

Except for streptomycin, the aminoglycoside antibiotics are composed of a central ring structure known as an amino-substituted cyclitol, to which are attached amino-substituted sugars in glycosidic linkage (Fig. 41-3) [204]. Under physiologic pH, these drugs behave as organic polycations and carry a net positive charge that ranges between +2.39 for amikacin to +4.37 for neomycin (Table 41-1) [120]. Being highly polar compounds, aminoglycosides have an infinitesimal lipid solubility and, therefore, are poorly absorbed across the gastrointestinal tract following oral intake [207]. After parenteral administration these drugs are distributed in a volume slightly greater than that of extracellular fluid and are eliminated from the body exclusively by the kidneys without metabolic modification [207].

Ultrafilterability of Aminoglycosides. The first step in the renal excretion of aminoglycosides involves their filtra-

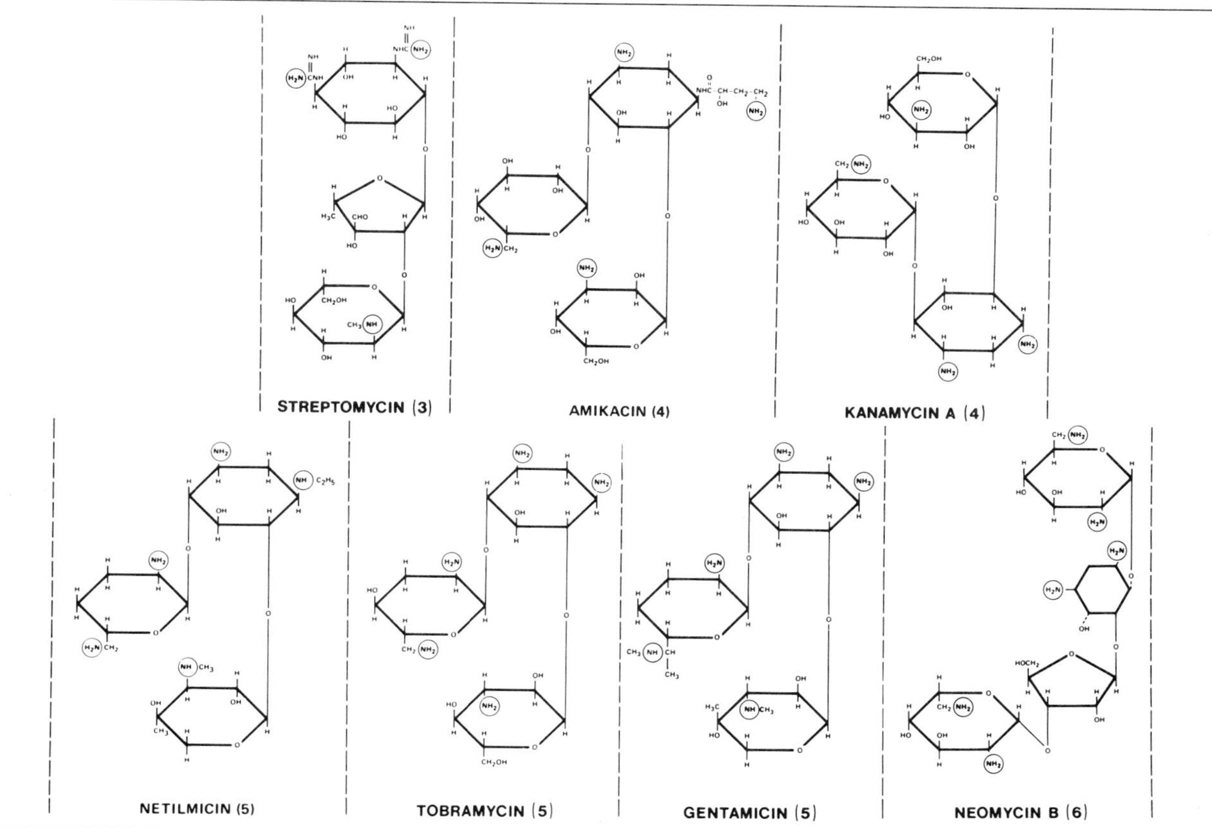

Fig. 41-3. Structures of aminoglycoside antibiotics, depicting ionizable amino groups (*circled*). The total number of ionizable amino groups is indicated in parentheses.

Table 41-1. Ranking of aminoglycoside antibiotics according to net charge

	Maximum charge	Net charge (pH 7.4)
Neomycin	+6.0	+4.37
Netilmicin	+5.0	+3.48
Gentamicin	+5.0	+3.46
Tobramycin	+5.0	+3.10
Amikacin	+4.0	+2.39

tion across the glomerular capillaries. Initial studies had suggested that the ultrafilterable fraction of aminoglycosides was as low as 70 percent due to binding of drug to plasma protein [191]. Subsequently, direct measurements of drug concentration in filtrate collected from Bowman's space of glomeruli located on the kidney surface of Munich-Wistar rats revealed that the ultrafiltrable fraction of gentamicin was 0.86 and that of netilmicin was 0.85 [218]. Given the fact that at pH 7.4 the mean charge of gentamicin is +3.47 and that of netilmicin is +3.48 [120], these ratios closely agree with those predicted by the Donnan equilibrium for the passive distribution of these polycations across a semipermeable membrane and agree with results obtained by in vitro ultrafiltration techniques [218, 266]. Thus, aminoglycosides do not appear to bind appreciably to plasma proteins.

Renal Tubular Transport of Aminoglycosides. Tubular absorption of aminoglycosides was inferred initially from clearance studies in which the urinary excretion of drug was found to be significantly less than the filtered load [46, 206, 259]. Direct evidence of tubular absorption of aminoglycosides was obtained using microinjection [84, 206, 216, 220] and free-flow micropuncture experiments [220, 266, 268]. An absorptive flux of [^{3}H]gentamicin was detected along the proximal convoluted tubule, loop of Henle, and presumably the pars recta, of superficial nephrons, whereas no absorption was detected beyond the early distal tubule [84, 216, 266, 268]. Studies utilizing autoradiography also support the view that the transport and accumulation of gentamicin is confined to the proximal tubule [121, 151, 270, 294, 313]; however, distal tubule uptake has been reported for [^{3}H]tobramycin [206]. Microinjection experiments demonstrate that [^{3}H]netilmicin undergoes a pattern of segmental tubular absorption identical to that of gentamicin, although the rate of absorption appears to be less than that of gentamicin [220]. In agreement with microinjection experiments, free-flow micropuncture experiments provided no evidence of tubular absorption of gentamicin or netilmicin along the distal tubule or the collecting duct [220, 266]. The fractional deliveries of gentamicin and netilmicin to the distal tubule of superficial nephrons were significantly less than the fractional excretion rates of these drugs under all experimental conditions examined [220, 266], a finding consistent with the heterogeneity of nephron function such that deep nephrons excrete a larger fraction of drug than do superficial nephrons [268].

Transtubular secretion of aminoglycosides was initially suggested by clearance studies in which the fractional excretion of gentamicin was reported to be equal to the filtered load calculated without correction for the ultrafilterable fraction of drug [99]. Subsequent micropuncture experiments demonstrated segmental fractional deliveries of gentamicin [268] and netilmicin [220] that exceeded the filtered load, thereby providing unequivocal evidence of tubular secretion.

Transtubular Flux of Aminoglycosides. A transtubular absorptive flux was inferred by Chiu et al. [46] based on the observation that the renal extraction ratio of gentamicin was 0.20, which was significantly less than the simultaneously measured inulin extraction ratio of 0.30. These investigators concluded that the difference in extraction ratios reflected a transtubular absorptive flux of filtered drug. However, this difference largely disappears when the data are corrected for an ultrafilterable fraction of 0.87. Pastoriza-Munoz et al. [216] failed to detect excretion of labeled gentamicin from the contralateral kidney after microinjection of drug into superficial proximal convoluted tubules in the rat. The available evidence suggests that if a transtubular absorptive flux of aminoglycoside antibiotics occurs, it amounts to only a small fraction of the total absorptive flux, most of which is trapped within the cell. Evidence supporting transtubular secretion of gentamicin and netilmicin has been cited above.

Kinetics of Aminoglycoside Accumulation in the Renal Cortex. Virtually all aminoglycosides have been shown to accumulate to some degree within the renal cortex [128, 173], presumably reflecting sequestration within renal proximal tubular cells. The amount of drug present in the renal cortex at a given point in time is determined by the rates of uptake and efflux of drug across the apical and basolateral membranes. While pharmacokinetic studies in humans and experimental animals have provided information about the rate constants for tissue uptake and efflux of these drugs, such studies provide little information about the transport processes involved.

The kinetics of aminoglycoside uptake in rat renal cortex have been examined in vivo [93, 120, 220]. Josepovitz et al. [120], using clearance techniques, examined the accumulation of [^{3}H]gentamicin as a function of increasing plasma concentration of drug. The major finding of this study was that despite achieving pharmacologic concentrations of drug in plasma and extremely high filtered loads, the mechanism mediating the absorption of gentamicin was not saturated. This was reflected by a fractional excretion rate less than the filtered load and a progressive, albeit curvilinear, increase in the renal cortical concentration of drug. The latter finding suggests that the uptake process would eventually reach a plateau but only at a very high plasma concentration and filtered load of drug. A similar pattern of renal cortical accumulation was observed with netilmicin [220]. In the case of netilmicin, however, significantly less drug was accumulated in renal cortex for any given plasma concentration, when compared to gentamicin. This difference most likely reflects the combined influence of a lower absorptive flux and higher secretory flux of netilmicin, which is manifested by a higher fractional excretion rate compared to that of gentamicin [220].

The above data suggest that the transport and accumulation of gentamicin and netilmicin are mediated by a low-affinity, high-capacity system that cannot be readily saturated. Giuliano et al. [93] obtained evidence in support of this concept from measurements of in vivo kinetics of aminoglycoside accumulation in the rat renal cortex. Steady-state elevations of serum concentrations of gentamicin and netilmicin were associated with nonlinear increases of cortical concentrations of drug that followed Michaelis-Menten kinetics suggesting a saturable transport process. The initial rate of gentamicin uptake at serum concentrations below 15 μg/ml was greater than that of netilmicin. The initial rate of tobramycin uptake was less than that of gentamicin and netilmicin and it remained linear over a broad range of serum concentrations. Amikacin uptake exhibited Michaelis-Menten kinetics at low serum concentrations and first-order kinetics at high serum concentrations. These data imply that more than one mechanism mediates the uptake of these drugs. Depending on which mechanism predominates, the kinetics may follow a saturable, linear, or mixed pattern.

The renal cortical accumulation of aminoglycosides measured in the studies cited above reflects the combined influence of apical membrane and basolateral membrane transport. Two lines of evidence suggest that apical membrane transport is the dominant route of uptake. Collier et al. [55] demonstrated that the cortical accumulation of gentamicin in the isolated perfused rat kidney was reduced 80 percent by maneuvers that suppressed glomerular filtration but maintained renal blood flow. Chiu and Long [48] showed that renal cortical accumulation of gentamicin was greatly depressed in rat kidneys subjected to an ischemic insult that depressed GFR but not para-aminohippurate uptake, a basolateral membrane transport function. Based on these two studies, it appears that the low-affinity, high-capacity transport process mediating the renal accumulation of aminoglycosides as defined by clearance studies primarily describes apical membrane transport of these drugs. Recently, Ford et al. [81a] reported that gentamicin is transported at equivalent rates across the apical and basolateral membranes of LLC-PK_1 cells.

Aminoglycosides have been shown to competitively inhibit the renal cortical accumulation of [^{3}H]gentamicin in vivo with the following decreasing order of efficacy:

neomycin, netilmicin, amikacin, and tobramycin [120]. Uptake of [^{3}H]gentamicin in renal cortex can also be inhibited in vivo by simultaneous infusions of organic polycations with the following decreasing order of potency: polylysine, spermine, and tetralysine and cadaverine [120]. The mechanism of inhibition most likely reflects electrostatic interference with drug-membrane binding. Competitive inhibition of membrane transport of gentamicin by aminoglycosides and by other organic polycations has also been demonstrated in microinjection experiments [84, 216] and in renal cortical slices [27, 70, 153]. The findings that aminoglycoside transport exhibits saturation kinetics and is susceptible to competitive inhibition implicate facilitated transport of these drugs, presumably by an active process. Although these observations do not exclude passive transport, in view of the low lipid solubility of these polycationic drugs, simple diffusion is unlikely to contribute significantly to their cellular uptake.

Binding of Aminoglycosides to Apical Membranes. Six groups of investigators have applied the technique of Scatchard analysis to characterize the binding of radiolabeled aminoglycoside to renal brush-border membrane vesicles [118, 133, 166, 251, 303]. Three groups of investigators [118, 122, 251] reported that gentamicin or netilmicin binds to a single class of receptors on rat renal brush-border membrane vesicles with a binding constant ranging between $3 \times 10^4\ M^{-1}$ to $4 \times 10^4\ M^{-1}$. These data signify an intermediate to low binding affinity and are consistent with in vivo data cited above [120, 220]. The maximal drug-binding capacity ranged between 2 and 38 nmol/mg of membrane protein. Amikacin exhibited a very low binding affinity for rat brush-border membrane vesicles [303]. In rabbit brush-border membrane, Lipsky et al. [166] identified two classes of low-affinity receptors, whereas Kardos et al. [133] reported finding a single class of high-affinity receptors that were also present in brush-border membrane vesicles prepared from small intestine. The discrepancy between these two studies remains unexplained. Two groups [7, 166] have reported evidence of intravesicular transport of aminoglycosides.

Recent studies established that the binding of aminoglycosides to artificial membranes containing anionic phospholipids can be described as an electrostatic interaction [50, 87]. If electrostatic binding of aminoglycosides to artificial membranes accurately describes their binding to biologic membranes including brush-border and basolateral membranes, then applying Scatchard analysis is inappropriate, as this technique will generate estimates of apparent binding affinities that are approximately three orders of a magnitude greater than the true binding affinity determined from studies using the technique of microelectrophoresis [50, 87].

Aminoglycoside antibiotics compete for binding to brush-border membrane vesicles with the following decreasing order of affinity as reported by Sastrasinh et al. [251]: neomycin, netilmicin, tobramycin, gentamicin, amikacin, and kanamycin. The decreasing rank order reported by Williams et al. [303] is neomycin, tobramycin, gentamicin, netilmicin, amikacin, and streptomycin. As neither ranking precisely follows the relative nephrotoxicity potentials of these drugs [128], it follows that binding per se is not a sensitive predictor of toxicity potential (vide infra). Gentamicin binding to brush-border membrane vesicles has also been shown to be inhibited by spermine [166, 305] and by polymers of cationic, neutral, and acidic amino acids [305]. Brush-border membrane binding of aprotinin, a cationic low-molecular-weight protein, was competitively inhibited by aminoglycosides with the following decreasing order of potency: neomycin, tobramycin, gentamicin, kanamycin, and streptomycin [122]. This latter observation is consistent with the view that aminoglycosides and low-molecular-weight proteins share a common or closely related transport system, such as endocytosis.

Anionic phospholipids have been implicated as membrane-binding sites for aminoglycoside antibiotics. These polycationic drugs have been shown to bind to acidic phospholipids of model and biologic membranes [10, 34, 50, 139, 156, 176, 240, 251, 255, 291] by an electrostatic interaction [50]. Of the various acidic phospholipids, aminoglycoside antibiotics bind most avidly to phosphatidylinositol 4,5-bisphosphate (PIP_2) [10, 11, 87, 240, 251, 253, 291]. In one study phosphatidylinositol (PI) content of brush-border membrane was found to be insufficient to explain the binding of aminoglycoside observed in vitro [118]. In a second study [87a] a significant correlation between increased binding of gentamicin to the apical membrane and PI content was noted. Although phosphatidylserine (PS) is present in sufficient quantities in brush-border membrane [118], this phospholipid typically is localized to the inner leaflet of the lipid bilayer and, therefore, is unlikely to be accessible for binding aminoglycoside present in tubular fluid. Of interest, little or no binding occurs to anionic nonlipid compounds such as melanin, gangliosides, or chondroitin sulfate [309]. Thus, although the hypothesis that anionic phospholipids serve as apical membrane–binding sites for aminoglycoside remains attractive, it has yet to be unequivocally proved. Recently, Aramaki et al. [6] reported evidence implicating *N*-acetylneuraminic acid as a brush-border membrane binding site for aminoglycosides.

Mechanisms of Apical Membrane Transport of Aminoglycoside. Studies utilizing autoradiographic techniques provide compelling evidence that aminoglycosides are transported across the apical membrane by endocytosis [121, 270]. Ten minutes after a pulse injection, [^{3}H]-gentamicin was found within apical membrane vesicles; 1 hour after a pulse injection, labeled drug was detected within lysosomes [270]. It should be noted that autoradiography is a relatively insensitive technique that provides qualitative rather than quantitative data. As such, the autoradiographic studies cited above do not exclude other modes of transport. Wedeen et al. [294] presented evidence based on immunofluorescent microscopy that drug sequestered in lysosomes may be derived, at least in part, from nonendocytotic uptake. Lipsky et al. [166]

reported that gentamicin is taken up by renal brush-border membrane vesicles. Aramaki et al. [7] reported a similar observation for 3′,4′-dideoxykanamycin. Of interest, no uptake of drug into basolateral membrane vesicles was detected [7]. The fact that aminoglycoside transport can be inhibited by organic polycations and polyamines raises the possibility of a shared transport system. Infusion of L-lysine in quantities sufficient to saturate the amino acid transport system depressed the renal cortical accumulation of gentamicin and tobramycin, whereas saturation of the acidic or neutral amino acid transport system was without effect [299]. An inconsistent effect on gentamicin accumulation has been observed in response to inhibition of the organic base transport system in vivo [115, 300], whereas inhibition of the organic base transport system in renal cortical slices had no effect [143, 216]. Recently, evidence derived from studies of brush-border membrane transport does support the view that a moiety of aminoglycoside uptake may be mediated by the organic base transport system [277]. Inhibition of the organic acid transport system in vitro has no effect on gentamicin uptake [143, 153, 216] whereas depressed uptake was observed in vivo in the rat [84] but not in humans [31]. Although aminoglycosides contain amino-substituted sugars, several studies have failed to detect any evidence that hexose or phlorhizin inhibit aminoglycoside binding or uptake [120, 133, 300]. In LLC-PK_1 cells, gentamicin uptake was depressed by metabolic inhibitors such as rotenone and 2,4-dinitrophenol, findings that implicate an active transport process [249]. That the transport mechanism is dependent on calcium was suggested by the observations that gentamicin transport was stimulated by the calcium ionophore A 23187 and inhibited by EDTA.

Basolateral Membrane Transport of Aminoglycoside. [^{3}H]Netilmicin was shown to bind to a single class of receptors on rat renal cortical basolateral membrane vesicles with an affinity close to that of brush-border membrane vesicles; however, the maximal binding capacity of basolateral membrane was significantly greater than that of brush-border membrane [118]. As in the case of brush-border membrane, the membrane content of PI was insufficient to explain the netilmicin-binding capacity of basolateral membrane. Amikacin, similar to netilmicin, was shown to have a higher binding affinity for rat basolateral than that for brush-border membrane [303]. Evidence for basolateral membrane transport of aminoglycosides includes the demonstration of concentrative uptake of drug in renal cortical slices [111, 128, 143, 153, 216] by a mechanism that is energy dependent [111, 143] and exhibits saturation kinetics and competitive inhibition [216]. Uptake is not inhibited by the organic base, organic acid, or basic amino acid transport system [27, 53, 216]. Basolateral membrane uptake has also been observed in rabbit proximal tubules in suspension [16]. The major evidence for basolateral membrane transport is from the study of Collier et al. [55] which implicates 20 percent of renal cortical accumulation being derived from uptake across the basolateral membrane. Fig. 41-4 illustrates diagrammatically the possible

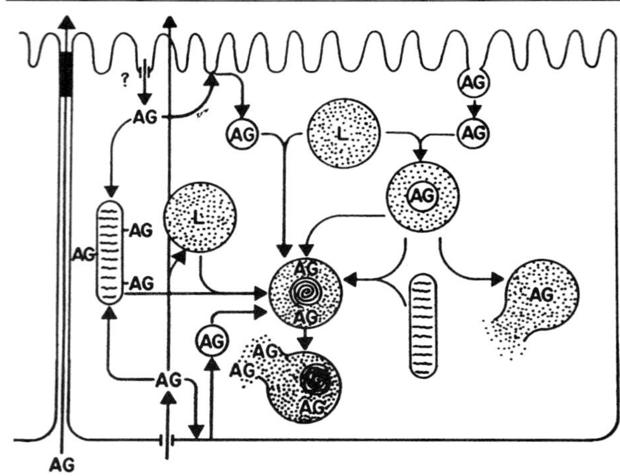

Fig. 41-4. Model of pathways by which aminoglycoside (AG) antibiotics are transported across the plasma membrane, accumulated within the lysosomal (L) compartment, and subsequently released and redistributed within renal proximal tubular cells. The major fraction of aminoglycoside is transported across the brush-border membrane by adsorptive endocytosis and translocated to the lysosomal compartment. Although not shown, a similar transport process occurs at the basolateral membrane. In addition, a small moiety of drug appears to gain access across both membranes by some other transport mechanism. This moiety of drug theoretically is available to interact with intracellular membranes that subsequently are shuttled into the lysosomal compartment. The accumulation of drug in high concentrations within lysosomes impairs phospholipase degradation of phospholipid, which results in the formation of myeloid bodies that congest the lysosomal system. Other lysosomal enzymes may be inhibited as well. Eventually the lysosomal membrane becomes permeable and ruptures, releasing acid hydrolases and high concentrations of drug into the cytoplasm where they interact with other intracellular membranes, disrupting membrane function and structure.

pathways for aminoglycoside transport by renal proximal tubular cells.

Intrarenal Distribution of Aminoglycoside. The concentration of aminoglycoside in renal cortex exceeds that in medulla by a factor of three or greater [77, 216, 276, 301]. Within the renal cortex, drug is localized to proximal tubular cells. The precise location of drug in the medulla has not been established. Micropuncture studies have consistently demonstrated the absence of an absorptive flux beyond the early distal tubule [84, 216, 220]. While it is possible that cells lining the distal nephron accumulate drug across the basolateral membrane, autoradiographic studies suggest that there is little [32, 270] or no uptake [313] beyond the pars recta. It appears likely that drug detected in the medullary portion of the kidney represents drug present in cells lining the pars recta of juxtamedullary nephrons.

Determinants of Aminoglycoside Concentration in Renal Cortex. The nephrotoxicity of aminoglycosides appears to be causally related to the transport and accumulation of these drugs within proximal tubular cells [128, 299]. Although a precise correlation between relative nephrotoxicity potentials and relative accumulation rates in renal cortex of the various aminoglycosides is lacking, it has been shown that for a given aminoglycoside the risk of nephrotoxicity increases as the absolute concentration of drug in renal cortex rises [128, 257, 276, 299]. The dose of drug administered per day and the duration of drug therapy are two obvious determinants of tissue drug level. During the first few days, the drug concentration in renal cortex rises sharply, but then the rate falls off and a plateau is reached, reflecting attainment of an equilibrium between uptake and efflux of drug in proximal tubular cells [260]. Aronoff et al. [8] showed that steady-state tissue levels are attained in rats after 10 to 20 days of daily drug administration. A number of factors have been shown to influence the renal cortical concentration of drug achieved in response to a specific drug regimen. The same daily dose of drug given as two or three divided doses leads to a greater accumulation of drug than when it is given as a single dose [28]. Even greater accumulation occurs when the same amount of drug is administered by continuous intravenous infusion [92]. Male sex [26], older age [182, 188], volume depletion induced by a sodium-deficient diet [24], furosemide [47, 205], water deprivation [160], potassium depletion [35, 142], increased parathyroid hormone activity [73], endotoxemia [211, 284], and obesity [56, 57] are associated with increased accumulation of gentamicin in renal cortex and increased incidence and severity of nephrotoxicity. The contribution of augmented uptake and decreased efflux to the higher tissue drug levels in these conditions has not been assessed.

Depressed renal cortical uptake of aminoglycoside can be induced by the simultaneous administration of organic polycations consequent to decreased apical membrane transport [120]. Sodium bicarbonate loading sufficient to cause alkalinization of the urine has been shown to decrease renal cortical accumulation of gentamicin in the rat [49]. In another study bicarbonate loading plus diamox was protective [13]. One possible mechanism is decreased binding of drug to apical membrane receptors consequent to a reduction in the net cationic charge of the molecule. Thyroid hormone [58], potassium chloride loading [286], and latamoxef [146] have been reported to protect against aminoglycoside nephrotoxicity by decreasing the renal cortical accumulation of drug. A similar claim was made for pyridoxal 5′-phosphate in one study [124] but was not confirmed in an independent study [130]. Rats with streptozotocin-induced diabetes mellitus are resistant to aminoglycoside-induced nephrotoxicity [62, 71, 285]. The mechanism is due to decreased cortical accumulation of drug consequent to decreased apical membrane transport [217]. When an experimental maneuver was introduced to augment the renal cortical content of aminoglycoside, nephrotoxic injury ensued, thereby indicating that the resistance to toxicity was not due to an intrinsic change in susceptibility at the cellular level [231]. Proteinuria was shown to decrease renal accumulation of gentamicin in one study [223] whereas a low-protein diet had a similar effect in another study [302].

INTERACTIONS OF AMINOGLYCOSIDE ANTIBIOTICS WITH MEMBRANES

The second step in the pathogenesis of aminoglycoside nephrotoxicity involves the deleterious interaction between these organic polycationic drugs and membranes of renal proximal tubular cells. Plasma, lysosomal, mitochondrial, and microsomal membranes have been identified as targets of aminoglycoside antibiotics and that the resultant drug-membrane interactions have resulted in a broad array of functional, biochemical, and structural alterations of these organelles. Although these drug-membrane interactions have been described in detail, it has not been possible thus far to establish unequivocally whether such interactions bear a causal relationship to the development of cell injury and necrosis or are a manifestation, i.e., a consequence, of such injury. What does seem incontrovertible, however, is that the toxic potential of individual aminoglycoside antibiotics is directly related to the capacity of these agents to bind to and perturb membrane function.

Aminoglycoside–Model Membrane Interactions. As noted above, the polycationic aminoglycosides bind to anionic [10, 34, 50, 139, 156, 176, 240, 251, 255, 291] but not to neutral phospholipid [50, 139, 156, 251]. Among the anionic phospholipids, aminoglycosides bind most avidly to PIP_2 [11, 87, 251, 253, 291]. Chung et al. [50] demonstrated that the binding of gentamicin to PI and PS of liposomes could be explained by an electrostatic interaction between the cationic amino groups of the polycationic drug and the anionic phosphate groups of the phospholipid. The intrinsic association constant was found to be below 10 M^{-1} for PI and PS [50], whereas Gaver et al. [87] found the intrinsic association constant for PIP_2 to be 10^3 M^{-1}. These data lend support to the hypothesis that anionic phospholipids, especially the phosphoinositides, function as membrane receptors for aminoglycoside antibiotics [251, 255, 309].

Several approaches have been used to gain insight into the geometry of the molecular interaction between aminoglycosides and anionic phospholipids [34, 195, 239, 244]. All models indicate an electrostatic interaction between a protonated amino group and the anionic phosphate head group. Brasseur et al. [34], using the technique of computer-aided conformational analysis, initially proposed a model that involved extension of an amino group of gentamicin into the hydrophobic plane of the lipid bilayer. In a subsequent study [195] this model was modified such that gentamicin interacted only with the hydrophilic region of the membrane. In contrast, Ramsammy and Kaloyanides [239] proposed a model that in addition to an electrostatic interaction between a protonated amino group and the phosphate head group, also involved formation of hydrogen bonds between an amino group of gentamicin and the carbonyl groups of glycerol. This model helped to explain observed changes in the biophysical properties of artificial membranes, i.e., an increase in the transition temperature and a decrease in glycerol permeability of PI-containing liposomes [240]. Both changes signify that gentamicin induces a decrease in membrane fluidity. Several investigators reported that aminoglycosides depress the fluidity of brush-border membrane as assessed by changes in the fluorescence of membrane probes [139] and by electron spin resonance spectroscopy [200].

Aminoglycosides have also been shown to promote membrane aggregation [129]. In order for membrane aggregation to occur, surface charge must be neutralized. In a comparative study of aminoglycoside-induced aggregation of PI-containing liposomes, it was observed that the rank order with respect to efficacy in neutralizing membrane surface charge was: neomycin > gentamicin = tobramycin = netilmicin = spermine; whereas significant differences existed among these polycations with respect to promoting aggregation of liposomes [129]. Of particular interest, the rank order for inducing aggregation of liposomes (neomycin > gentamicin > tobramycin > netilmicin = spermine) was identical to the rank order of these agents with respect to depressing glycerol permeability [129]. This rank order also coincides precisely with the established clinical nephrotoxicity potentials of these aminoglycosides. Since depression of glycerol permeability was shown to be dependent on hydrogen bonding between one or more amino groups of the drug and carbonyl groups of the glycerol backbone [239], these data suggest that the membrane toxicity of aminoglycosides is closely linked to their potentials to engage in hydrogen bonding. Importantly, the rank order in terms of nephrotoxicity potentials does not coincide with the net cationic charge of these agents (see Table 41-1). This observation emphasizes that spatial orientation of charge rather than net charge is a critical determinant of toxicity.

In contrast to the above studies of PI-containing liposomes, Schacht and colleagues utilized a variety of methods for measuring perturbations of PIP_2-containing membranes to assess the ototoxicity potentials of aminoglycosides. Increased fluorescence of 1-anilino-8-naphthalenesulfonate [10], increased permeability to carboxyfluorescein [11], and increased surface tension of monomolecular film of phosphatidylcholine (PC):PIP_2 [139, 292] were shown to correlate precisely with the ototoxicity potentials of aminoglycosides as assessed by the depression of the guinea pig cochlear with aminoglycoside-containing solutions. In contrast, competition for [^{14}C]neomycin binding or $^{45}Ca^{2+}$ binding did not accurately predict the relative toxicities of aminoglycoside antibiotics. Schacht [254] proposed that the ototoxicity of aminoglycosides is causally related to binding of drug to PIP_2 and disruption of this signaling mechanism.

The studies cited above provide strong support for the hypothesis that the toxicity of aminoglycosides is causally related to their capacity to bind to and perturb the function of cell membranes. These studies, however, do not identify whether aminoglycoside toxicity is linked to an interaction with a specific membrane target or multiple membrane targets, nor is it clear whether toxicity results from disruption of a single critical membrane function or multiple membrane functions. In the following sections the effects of aminoglycoside interactions with specific cell membranes will be reviewed and the possible contribution of such interactions to the development of cell injury will be considered.

Aminoglycoside–Plasma Membrane Interactions. The brush-border and basolateral membranes of renal proximal tubular cells are the initial sites of aminoglycoside-cell interactions. Numerous transport and biochemical abnormalities have been identified at the level of the plasma membrane of renal proximal tubular cells early in the course of aminoglycoside administration to experimental animals and to humans (Table 41-2). One of the earliest biochemical abnormalities induced by aminogly-

Table 41-2. Aminoglycoside-induced functional and biochemical alterations of plasma membranes of renal proximal tubular cells

Transport abnormalities		Biochemical abnormalities
	Brush-border membrane (BBM)	
1. ↓ Organic base transport		1. BBM lipiduria
2. ↓ Low-molecular-weight protein transport		2. BBM enzymuria
3. ↓ Glucose transport		3. ↓ BBM enzymes
4. ↓ K^+ transport		a. ↓ γ-Glutamyl transpeptidase
5. ↓ Mg^{2+} transport		b. ↓ Alanine aminopeptidase
6. ↓ Na^+-PO_4^{3-} cotransport		c. ↓ Alkaline phosphatase
7. ↓ Na^+-H^+ exchange		4. Altered phospholipid composition
	Basolateral membrane	
1. ↓ Organic base transport		1. ↓ Na^+-K^+-ATPase
2. ↑ Organic acid transport		2. ↓ Adenylate cyclase
3. ↓ Ca^{2+} transport		3. ↓ Calcium content
4. ↓ Na^+-K^+ transport		4. Altered phospholipid composition
5. ↓ Mg^{2+} transport		

coside antibiotics in experimental animals is phospholipiduria [119]. Within 24 hours of a single injection of gentamicin in rats, the urinary excretion of phospholipid increased threefold; by the third day of gentamicin administration the excretion of phospholipid had increased tenfold above baseline. Of the major phospholipids excreted in the urine, the largest fractional increase (37-fold) was observed with PI, one of the putative membrane receptors for aminoglycoside antibiotics. The phospholipiduria was accompanied by significant increases of alanine aminopeptidase, a brush-border membrane enzyme, and *N*-acetyl-β-glucosaminidase, a lysosomal enzyme, also evident within 24 hours of a single injection of gentamicin. Brush-border membrane and lysosomal enzymuria have been described early in the course of aminoglycoside therapy in humans [19, 88, 198, 219, 256] and in experimental animals [221, 298]. The simultaneous appearance of phospholipiduria, brush-border membrane enzymuria, and lysosomal enzymuria can be explained by several mechanisms. Since aminoglycosides are known to be taken up by endocytosis followed by translocation into lysosomes, the finding of lysosomal enzymes in the urine simultaneously with phospholipid and brush-border membrane enzymes may indicate that components of the brush-border membrane are also shuttled into the lysosomal system and subsequently regurgitated into the lumen by exocytosis. In addition, transmission electron microscopy of rat renal proximal tubule obtained 24 hours after a single dose of gentamicin revealed focal loss of microvillus membrane and the presence of apical blebs that contained organelles including lysosomes [119]. The sloughing of these blebs into the lumen could explain the simultaneous appearance in the urine of phospholipid, brush-border membrane enzymes, and lysosomal enzymes. The formation of apical blebs has been observed with other nephrotoxins [269] and in response to ischemia [95], and implies significant cellular injury. In the rat, apical bleb formation induced by gentamicin remains focal in distribution at 24 and 48 hours [119]. After 6 days of drug, frank proximal tubular cell necrosis is evident by light microscopy [276] and presumably explains the sharp rise in the urinary excretion of brush-border membrane enzymes and lysosomal enzymes that typically occur by days 5 and 6 in this animal model [119]. Sloughing of apical blebs may also explain the increased urinary excretion of ligandin (glutathione S–transferase B), a major organic anion binding protein in the cytosol of proximal tubular cells, observed in rats treated with gentamicin [79] and the decrease in specific activity of several brush-border membrane enzymes [116, 145, 202]. Direct inhibition of the brush-border membrane enzyme alkaline phosphatase by dibekacin has been demonstrated in vitro [281]; however, in view of the high concentrations required, the relevance of this observation to the enzyme changes observed in vivo is uncertain.

Because of the marked phospholipiduria, consideration was given to the possibility that the phospholipid composition of brush-border membrane might be altered. Measurement of the phospholipid composition of brush-border membrane after 2 days of aminoglycoside injections in rats revealed that the only significant change was a slight increase in the content of PI [127]. This finding was confirmed in two other independent studies [116, 118]. The fact that the PI content of brush-border membrane was increased is somewhat surprising considering the urinary losses of this phospholipid, and may signify an adaptive mechanism elicited in response to some stress imposed by gentamicin. This observation lends support to the hypothesis that disturbance of phosphoinositide metabolism is linked to the pathogenesis of aminoglycoside toxicity.

Tubular proteinuria is a prominent manifestation of aminoglycoside nephrotoxicity [88, 136, 261]. An increase in the urinary excretion of β_2-microglobulin, a marker of tubule proteinuria, is usually detectable within 72 hours of aminoglycoside administration. Although aminoglycosides have been shown to compete with low-molecular-weight proteins for binding to and transport across the apical membrane [33, 121, 209], competitive inhibition of transport is not a major factor promoting proteinuria because it persists after the drug has been excreted or discontinued [276]. Cojocel et al. [54] observed that aminoglycosides depressed the fractional absorption of lysozyme in the following decreasing rank order: tobramycin and gentamicin, kanamycin, amikacin, and netilmicin. The decrease in fractional absorption occurred in the face of a depressed filtered load consequent to a reduction of the glomerular sieving coefficient of lysozyme. In addition to decreased tubular transport, these workers presented evidence that indicated decreased lysosomal degradation of the absorbed lysozyme as well. Inhibition of lysosomal proteases as well as impaired lysosome-pinocytic vesicle fusion by aminoglycoside [94] may contribute to the decreased degradation of lysozyme.

Organic base transport in rat brush-border membrane was depressed 30 percent within 90 minutes after a single dose of gentamicin [306]. The mechanism of inhibition is not known nor is it known how long this effect persists. At the time when organic base transport was depressed, para-aminohippurate and glucose uptake in brush-border membrane vesicles was not altered [306]. Glucosuria develops during the course of aminoglycoside nephrotoxicity [59, 90, 144]. Two groups have reported that gentamicin inhibits sodium-dependent D-glucose transport in renal brush-border membrane vesicles [7, 114].

Aminoglycosides induce potassium and magnesium depletion in humans and experimental animals [14, 59, 100, 222]. Perfusion of the isolated kidney with gentamicin promotes kaliuresis attributed to stimulated distal tubular potassium secretion [196]. The observation that gentamicin induces potassium depletion of the renal cortex [61] implies that proximal tubular cell transport of potassium is altered as well. Depression of Na^+-K^+-ATPase activity does not explain this effect [61]. One possibility is that aminoglycosides augment the permeability of the cell membrane to potassium, similar to the effect of other organic polycations [138]. Potassium depletion in turn has been shown to augment the nephrotoxicity of gentamicin [35, 142] by facilitating increased uptake and accumulation of drug in proximal tubular cells. Potassium chloride loading has the opposite effect [286]. In addition to kaliuresis, an acute infusion of gentamicin in the rat stimulates increased urinary excretion of magnesium and calcium [219]. Hypomagnesemia secondary to renal wasting of magnesium has been associated with chronic gentamicin administration in humans [14, 222]. The observation that the renal cortical content of magnesium is depressed early in the course of gentamicin treatment in the dog [61] suggests that impaired proximal tubular cell transport across the apical membrane may contribute to the renal wasting of magnesium. Hypomagnesemia augments gentamicin nephrotoxicity [243, 310] whereas gentamicin nephrotoxicity is ameliorated by a high magnesium intake [202]. The mechanism of protection has not been clearly established but it may involve competitive inhibition of critical aminoglycoside-membrane interactions [112].

Thus, early in the course of aminoglycoside administration, the brush-border membrane of renal proximal tubular cells exhibits significant functional, biochemical, and structural alterations. The precise relationship among these changes, their temporal sequence, and their progression in response to dose and duration of drug treatment remain to be defined, as does their contribution to the propagation of cell injury.

Several lines of evidence implicate the basolateral membrane as another early target for aminoglycoside interaction. It has been shown that aminoglycosides bind to basolateral membrane with an affinity similar to that of brush-border membrane but that the maximum binding capacity of basolateral membrane is greater than that of brush-border membrane [118, 303]. Consistent with this observation is the report of Williams et al. [306] that 90 minutes after the injection of labeled gentamicin, more drug was found associated with basolateral than with brush-border membrane. Furthermore, a number of transport and biochemical abnormalities at the level of the basolateral membrane have been identified early in the course of aminoglycoside treatment in experimental animals (Table 41-3). Williams et al. [306] reported that organic base transport was depressed 32 percent as early as 90 minutes after administration of a single dose of gentamicin in the rat whereas organic acid transport was not affected. This effect was transient, as no change in organic base transport was detected in renal cortical slices 90 minutes after gentamicin administration. Other workers [29, 144] have shown that organic base transport is consistently depressed after 3 or 4 days of gentamicin treatment. In contrast, organic acid transport is stimulated early in the course of gentamicin administration. Cohen et al. [53] found that the uptake of para-aminohippurate in renal cortical slices was significantly increased within 24 hours of administration of a single dose of gentamicin in the rat. With continued daily drug treatment, para-aminohippurate transport eventually declined as progressive cellular injury developed. Stimulation of para-aminohippurate uptake was shown to be due to an increase in the active transport step plus a decrease in the passive permeability of the basolateral membrane to para-aminohippurate [155]. The molecular mechanism and significance of organic acid transport stimulation by aminoglycoside remain unknown. The fact that other proximal tubular cell toxins also augment para-aminohippurate transport [104] raises the possibility that stimulation of this transport system may represent a nonspecific compensatory response to cell injury.

Table 41-3. Effect of gentamicin on degradation rates of labeled phospholipid pools

	t½, days		
Labeled precursor	Control	Gentamicin	*p*
[^{3}H]Myoinositol	1.17 ± 0.08	2.88 ± 0.23	< 0.01
[^{3}H]Choline	1.77 ± 0.16	2.38 ± 0.23	< 0.025
[^{3}H]Ethanolamine	3.14 ± 0.19	4.93 ± 0.34	< 0.01
[^{3}H]Serine	6.30 ± 0.57	8.63 ± 0.65	< 0.05

Rabbit proximal tubular cells grown in primary culture were incubated for 48 h in medium containing labeled precursor followed by 24 h in medium containing 3-fold excess of cold precursors. Then gentamicin (10^{-3} M) was added to half the monolayers and the rate of decline of labeled phospholipid was measured at 2-day intervals for 6 days by assaying the phospholipid extract for radioactivity. Values are means ± SE of 5 experiments. t½ was calculated from regression equation: $A = A_0e^{kt}$ where A_0 equals labeled phospholipid pool expressed as dpm/mg of protein at t_0 and t equals time in days. The data demonstrate that the phosphoinositide-labeled pool has the shortest t½ in control cells and that the t½ is prolonged to 246 percent of control in cells exposed to gentamicin, a change indicative of impaired degradation of [^{3}H]myoinositol-labeled phospholipids.
Source: L. S. Ramsammy, C. Josepovitz, B. Lane, et al. Effect of gentamicin on phospholipid metabolism in cultured rabbit proximal tubular cells. *Am. J. Physiol.* 256:C204, 1989.

Basolateral membrane content and transport of calcium were depressed after a single injection of gentamicin whereas no such changes were evident in the brush-border membrane [306]. Previous studies have shown that aminoglycosides compete with calcium for binding to artificial and biologic membranes [176, 255]. Aminoglycosides have been shown to block a variety of calcium-dependent channels [101, 184, 213, 215]. This action has been implicated in the pathogenesis of aminoglycoside-induced functional alterations of cardiac and vascular smooth muscle [1, 2, 97], in causing neuromuscular blockade [81, 224, 282], and in depressing the microphonic potential of hair cells [255]. The contribution of calcium channel blockade to the observed alterations of basolateral membrane transport and enzyme activities has not been evaluated.

Na^+-K^+-ATPase activity was found to be decreased in basolateral membrane within 30 minutes of administration of a single dose of gentamicin in the rat, with a peak inhibitory effect occurring by 90 minutes [306, 307]. The fact that this key enzyme was depressed so early in the course of aminoglycoside treatment raised the possibility that this effect may be linked to other membrane abnormalities such as depressed solute transport. Enthusiasm for this hypothesis is diminished, however, by the observation that the peak inhibitory effect on Na^+-K^+-ATPase activity was not augmented by increasing the dose of gentamicin. Moreover, within 24 hours Na^+-K^+-ATPase activity had returned to baseline. The mechanism of Na^+-K^+-ATPase inhibition is also uncertain. In a follow-up study, Williams et al. [308] reported that perfusion of the isolated filtering rat kidney with gentamicin inhibited Na^+-K^+-ATPase by 43 percent but that this effect was not observed in the perfused nonfiltering kidney. The inference drawn from this study was that gentamicin induced inhibition of Na^+-K^+-ATPase–required transport of drug across the apical membrane followed by an interaction between the drug and the cytoplasmic face of the enzyme. Other investigators also demonstrated that aminoglycosides inhibit Na^+-K^+-ATPase in vivo [230] and in vitro [4, 7, 45, 167]. Lipsky and Lietman [167] reported that 2×10^{-5} M neomycin inhibited canine renal Na^+-K^+-ATPase by more than 90 percent but that this effect could be blocked by preincubating neomycin with phosphoinositides. The suggestion was made that the inhibitory effect of neomycin may involve binding of drug to the enzyme's phospholipid annulus, similar to the mechanism proposed by Dunst et al. [67] for cationic amphiphilic drugs. Chahwala and Harpur [45] reported that aminoglycosides inhibited Na^+-K^+-ATPase in three in vitro preparations; however, in light of the high concentration of drug (10^{-2} M) required to achieve 50 percent or greater inhibition, these authors questioned whether this effect seen in vitro is relevant to the pathogenesis of toxicity seen in vivo. The question also arises as to whether the 48 percent inhibition of Na^+-K^+-ATPase reported by Williams et al. [306–308] is of physiologic significance. One clue that it might be is the observation that renal cortical slices from gentamicin-treated rats manifested impaired ability to restore sodium and potassium content to normal following exposure to 0°C for 60 minutes. With more prolonged aminoglycoside treatment sufficient to cause elevation of serum creatinine concentration, derangements of intracellular electrolyte composition including increases in sodium and calcium were evident along with depression of renal cortical Na^+-K^+-ATPase activity [61]. At this advanced stage of nephrotoxicity, however, identifying cause-and-effect relationships becomes difficult.

Depression of basal and NaF-stimulated adenylate cyclase activity was also observed in the study of Williams et al. [307]. As to whether the mechanism of inhibition was secondary to displacement of membrane calcium or magnesium or a direct interaction between the drug and the enzyme complex has not been determined. Nor is it known whether this effect is transient or persistent, whether it exhibits dose dependency, and whether it reflects a generalized or selective interaction with specific receptor–adenylate receptor complexes. In contrast to the data of Williams et al., Queener et al. [230] reported that gentamicin treatment of rats stimulated basal and receptor-mediated adenylate cyclase activity of renal cortical plasma membranes.

Altered phospholipid composition of basolateral membrane occurs early in the course of aminoglycoside treatment in the rat. Two doses of gentamicin resulted in significant increases of PC, phosphatidylethanolamine (PE), PI, cardiolipin, and phosphatidic acid (PA), whereas sphingomyelin and PS were unchanged [118, 127]. PI manifested the largest fractional increase above baseline. Phospholipids are known to influence a variety of membrane properties and functions including permeability, fluidity, solute transport, enzyme activity, and agonist receptor interactions [36, 98, 103, 192, 250]. It is possible, therefore, that the functions and biochemical derangements identified at the level of the basolateral membrane are causally related to aminoglycoside alterations of phospholipid metabolism.

Aminoglycoside-Lysosome-Phospholipid Interactions. Morphologic alterations of lysosomes occur early in the course of aminoglycoside administration. Within 12 hours of administration of a single dose of drug, the typical ultrastructural lesion of aminoglycoside toxicity, namely the myeloid body, is evident and is accompanied by an increase in the size of secondary lysosomes [91, 150]. With repeated dosing, the number and size of myeloid bodies and the volume of the cell occupied by secondary lysosomes expand dramatically. Early on, these changes represent prelethal alterations because they are reversible on discontinuation of drug treatment [91]. The myeloid body is not a unique feature of aminoglycoside toxicity. Similar lysosomal ultrastructural lesions have been previously described in association with amphiphilic drugs that are known to accumulate within lysosomes consequent to trapping of the protonated form [110, 125, 177]. Moreover, these drugs induce a lysosomal phospholipidosis due in large measure to impaired degradation consequent to binding of drug to phospholipid, which renders the substrate less susceptible to the action of phospholipases [110, 125, 177, 185, 186]. Because aminoglycosides accumulate in high concentration within lysosomes and induce myeloid bodies that resemble those associated with amphiphilic compounds, it was inferred that myeloid bodies induced by aminoglycosides were also composed of phospholipid [150]. The first clue that this was the case was provided by Aubert-Tulkens et al. [12] who reported that cultured fibroblasts incubated in medium containing gentamicin developed a phospholipidosis that increased in parallel with the increase in the fraction of cell volume occupied by lysosomes engorged with myeloid bodies. Subsequently it was shown in the rat that aminoglycoside antibiotics induce a renal cortical phospholipidosis [80, 91, 116, 117, 156], the magnitude of which correlated with expansion of lysosomes filled with myeloid bodies [91]. Importantly the phospholipidosis was detected within 24 hours of administration of a single dose of aminoglycoside [80, 117]. The phospholipidosis reflected significant increases in the quantities of PC, PE, PI, and PS. Of particular interest, PI demonstrated the greatest fractional increase among the four phospholipids. Subsequently it was shown that the lysosomal fraction prepared from the renal cortex of rats injected with netilmicin was enriched in myeloid bodies (Fig. 41-5), that the phospholipid content of this lysosomal fraction was twice that of control lysosomes lacking myeloid bodies, and that the composition of the lysosomal phospholipidosis was enriched in PI (Fig. 41-6), similar to the pattern observed in the renal cortex [116].

Studies of phospholipid metabolism in primary cultures of rabbit proximal tubular epithelium exposed to gentamicin revealed that the phospholipidosis was due primarily to impaired degradation of phospholipid and that PI manifested the greatest depression of degradation rate (see Table 41-3) [233]. Impaired phospholipid degradation was presumed to be due to the inhibitory effect of high lysosomal concentrations of aminoglycosides on lysosomal phospholipase activity. Administration of low-dose aminoglycosides in the rat was shown to be accompanied by depressed activities of acid sphingomyelinase and phospholipase A [156]. Similar changes were demonstrated in the renal cortex of humans treated with aminoglycosides [66]. Furthermore, in vitro studies have unequivocally established that aminoglycosides can inhibit the activity of lysosomal phospholipases [42, 106, 156]. The mechanism of inhibition of phospholipase A appears to be related to the capacity of aminoglycosides to bind to PI and other acidic phospholipids [42, 156, 193, 194]. The activity of phospholipase A toward PC and PE, neutral phospholipids that do not bind aminoglycosides, could be restored by adding PI to the liposome. These data suggest that PI and possibly other anionic phospholipids serve as membrane-binding sites or anchors for phospholipase A and that membrane binding is an essential first step for the expression of enzyme activity. In the acidic environment of the lysosome, aminoglycoside antibiotics would be maximally protonated and this would greatly enhance the electrostatic interaction with anionic phospholipids. The resulting neutralization of surface charge consequent to the binding of aminoglycoside antibiotics to PI,

Fig. 41-5. Transmission electron micrograph of lysosomal fraction. A. In a control rat, the lysosomal fraction consists primarily of round granules with a homogeneous, moderately electron-dense matrix. No multivesicular or myeloid body–containing lysosomes are seen. Contaminating mitochondria represent 20 percent of the fraction by volume. B. In a netilmicin-injected rat, the lysosomal fraction is comprised largely of irregularly shaped lysosomes containing myeloid bodies. Free-lying myeloid bodies are also seen along with mitochondria. The degree of mitochondrial contamination is similar to that observed in A. (Magnification × 12,000.) (From C. Josepovitz, T. Farruggella, R. Levine, et al. Effect of netilmicin on the phospholipid composition of subcellular fractions of rat renal cortex. *J. Pharmacol. Exp. Ther.* 235:810, 1985. © by the American Society for Pharmacology and Experimental Therapeutics.)

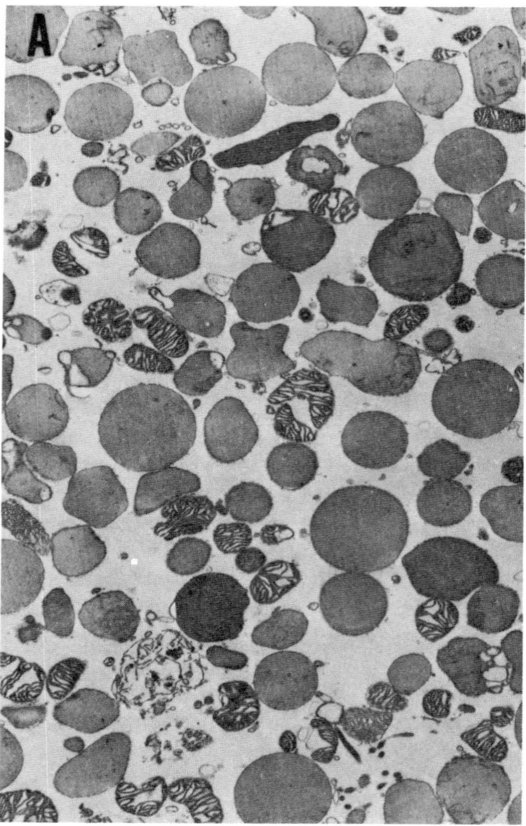

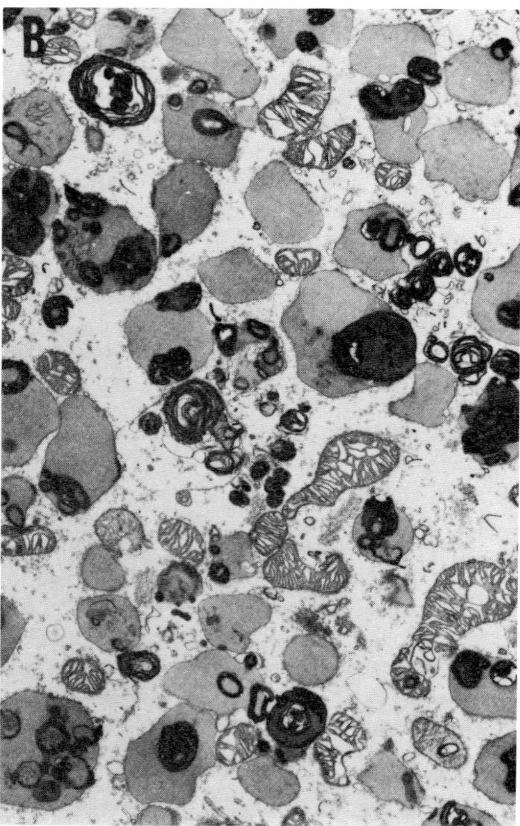

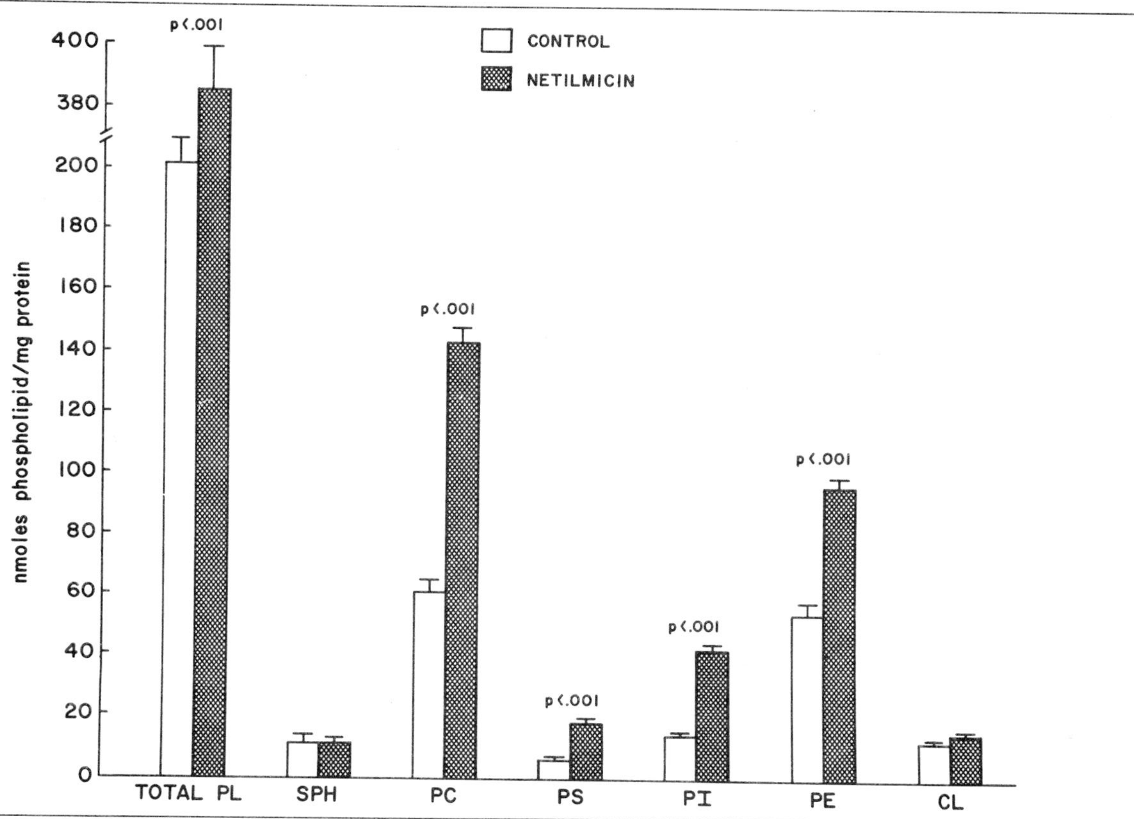

Fig. 41-6. Phospholipid content and composition of renal cortical lysosomal fractions of control and netilmicin-injected rats. The composition of the lysosomal phospholipidosis is identical to that of renal cortical homogenate. PL = phospholipid; SPH = sphingomyelin; PC = phosphatidylcholine; PS = phosphatidylserine; PI = phosphatidylinositol; PE = phosphatidylethanolamine; CL = cardiolipin. (From C. Josepovitz, T. Farruggella, R. Levine, et al. Effect of netilmicin on the phospholipid composition of subcellular fractions of rat renal cortex. *J. Pharmacol. Exp. Ther.* 235:810, 1985. © by the American Society for Pharmacology and Experimental Therapeutics.)

PS, and other negatively charged phospholipids may prevent activation of phospholipases for which PC and PE serve as substrate. This mechanism, however, does not explain the impaired degradation of PI by phospholipase C. Recent studies in our laboratory demonstrated that this inhibition can be overcome by adding increased quantities of PI to the reaction [242]. These observations imply that aminoglycoside-induced inhibition of PI hydrolysis by phospholipase C is due to the formation of a drug-substrate complex that obviates access of phospholipase C to its substrate.

Laurent et al. [157] postulated that the lysosomal phospholipidosis is causally linked to aminoglycoside-induced cell necrosis. These investigators have shown that low-dose aminoglycoside administration, 10 mg/kg/day, in the rat stimulates increased DNA synthesis that correlates with augmented cellular proliferation primarily of proximal tubular cells but also interstitial cells [158, 159, 288]. These changes are presumed to reflect a reparative response to aminoglycoside-induced focal tubular cell necrosis [288]. The decreasing rank order of low-dose aminoglycosides with respect to their effects on DNA synthesis, cell proliferation, and presumably cell necrosis is gentamicin and dibekacin, netilmicin, tobramycin, and amikacin. Although Laurent et al. [157] suggested that this order agrees with the relative potencies of these agents in promoting a lysosomal phospholipidosis, morphometric analysis of cell volume occupied by lysosomes, an indirect measure of aminoglycoside-induced lysosomal phospholipidosis and myeloid body formation revealed no significant differences among these agents. Support for this hypothesis is provided, however, by the report of Josepovitz et al. [117]. These investigators studied a rat model of high-dose-aminoglycoside nephrotoxicity and observed that the potency of four aminoglycoside antibiotics with respect to causing renal cortical phospholipidosis (netilmicin > tobramycin > gentamicin > neomycin) was exactly opposite to their ranking for causing acute renal failure and cell necrosis in the same model (Fig. 41-7) [276]. This apparent discrepancy can be explained by the observation that accompanying the renal cortical phospholipidosis was phospholipiduria, the magnitude of which was exactly opposite to that of the renal cortical phos-

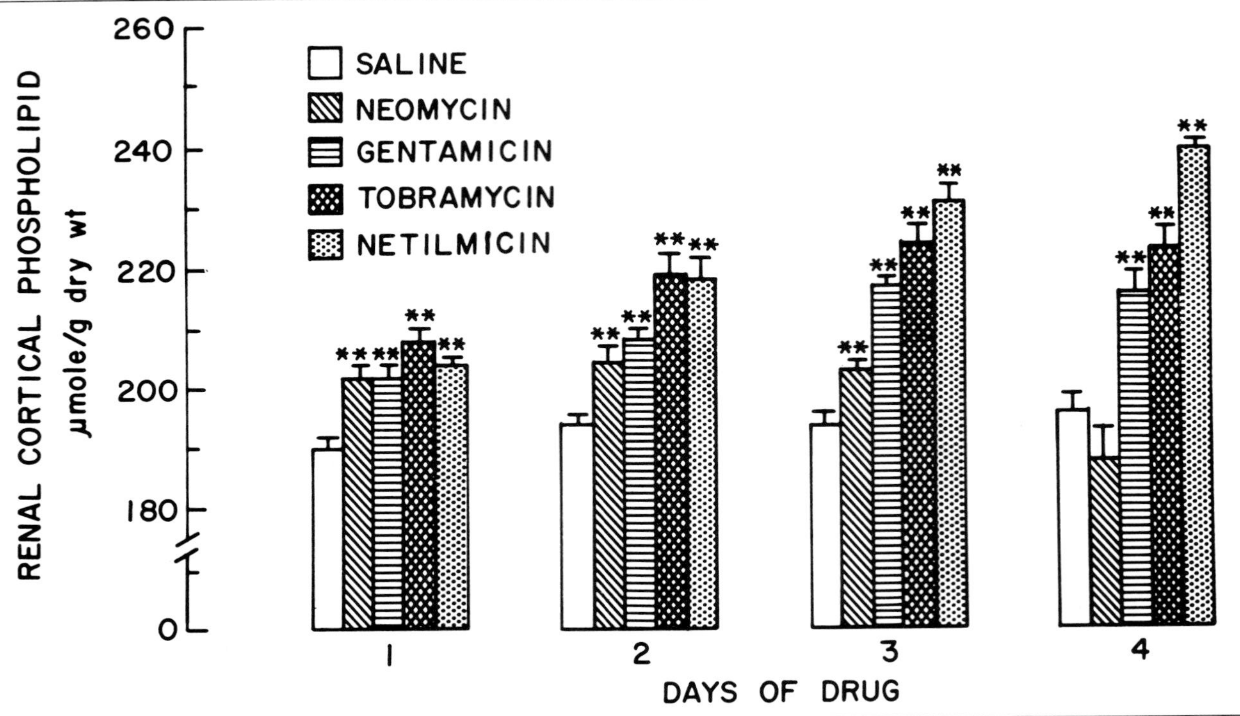

Fig. 41-7. Effect of drug treatment on the phospholipid content of the renal cortex. Rats were injected with drug at 100 mg/kg/day. The data demonstrate an inverse correlation between the magnitude of the renal cortical phospholipidosis and the nephrotoxicity potential of the four aminoglycoside antibiotics. **Significantly different from saline, $p < 0.01$. (From C. Josepovitz, R. Levine, T. Farruggella, et al. Comparative effects of aminoglycosides on renal cortical and urinary phospholipids in the rat. *Proc. Soc. Exp. Biol. Med.* 182:1, 1986. © by the Society for Experimental Biology and Medicine.)

pholipidosis and coincided precisely with the established nephrotoxicity potentials of these agents (Fig. 41-8) [117]. The phospholipiduria, which presumably was derived from cells undergoing necrosis, may explain the lack of correlation between phospholipid accumulation and toxicity.

Although the findings of Josepovitz et al. [117] are consistent with the hypothesis that aminoglycoside-induced cell necrosis is linked to the development of lysosomal phospholipidosis; the mechanism by which lysosomal phospholipidosis progresses to cell necrosis remains uncertain. Two possibilities warrant consideration. Firstly, previous studies suggest that a critical threshold of phospholipid accumulation must be reached before cell death occurs [91]. If this critical value is not exceeded, the cell can survive and fully recover after the drug is withdrawn. This critical value of phospholipid presumably correlates with a critical value of aminoglycoside concentration within the lysosomal compartment. Proximal tubular cells exhibit a high level of endocytotic activity related to the transport of a variety of biologic substances including low-molecular-weight proteins that are normally degraded within this cellular compartment. Aminoglycosides have been shown to inhibit the enzymatic breakdown of transported proteins [54]. The mechanism may be related to an inhibitory effect of aminoglycosides on lysosomal hydrolases or, perhaps more importantly, to inhibition of lysosomal membrane fusion with endocytotic vesicles [94]. If aminoglycosides cause a generalized disturbance of membrane fusion involving lysosomes, it could have far-reaching consequences not only for endocytotic and exocytotic coupled events but also for the process of cell remodeling and repair that is linked to autophagy. Secondly, Powell and Reidenberg [227, 228] have shown that aminoglycosides exert a dual effect on the integrity of the lysosomal membrane in vitro; low doses caused membrane stabilization while higher doses promoted membrane disruption and lysosomal enzyme release. These effects were observed in lysosomes prepared from both human nephrectomy specimens and from rat kidney. Inhibition and promotion of NAG release from lysosomes in vitro was dose related and correlated with the accepted order of nephrotoxicity. Other investigators have also shown that the aminoglycosides cause labilization of lysosomes in vitro and in vivo [189, 201, 202, 210]. In all studies the concentrations of aminoglycosides used were well below the concentrations estimated to be achievable in vivo [12, 106].

Labilization of lysosomes could have two potentially serious consequences. Firstly, increased fragility and permeability of lysosomes might promote the release of potent hydrolases into the cytoplasm where they might

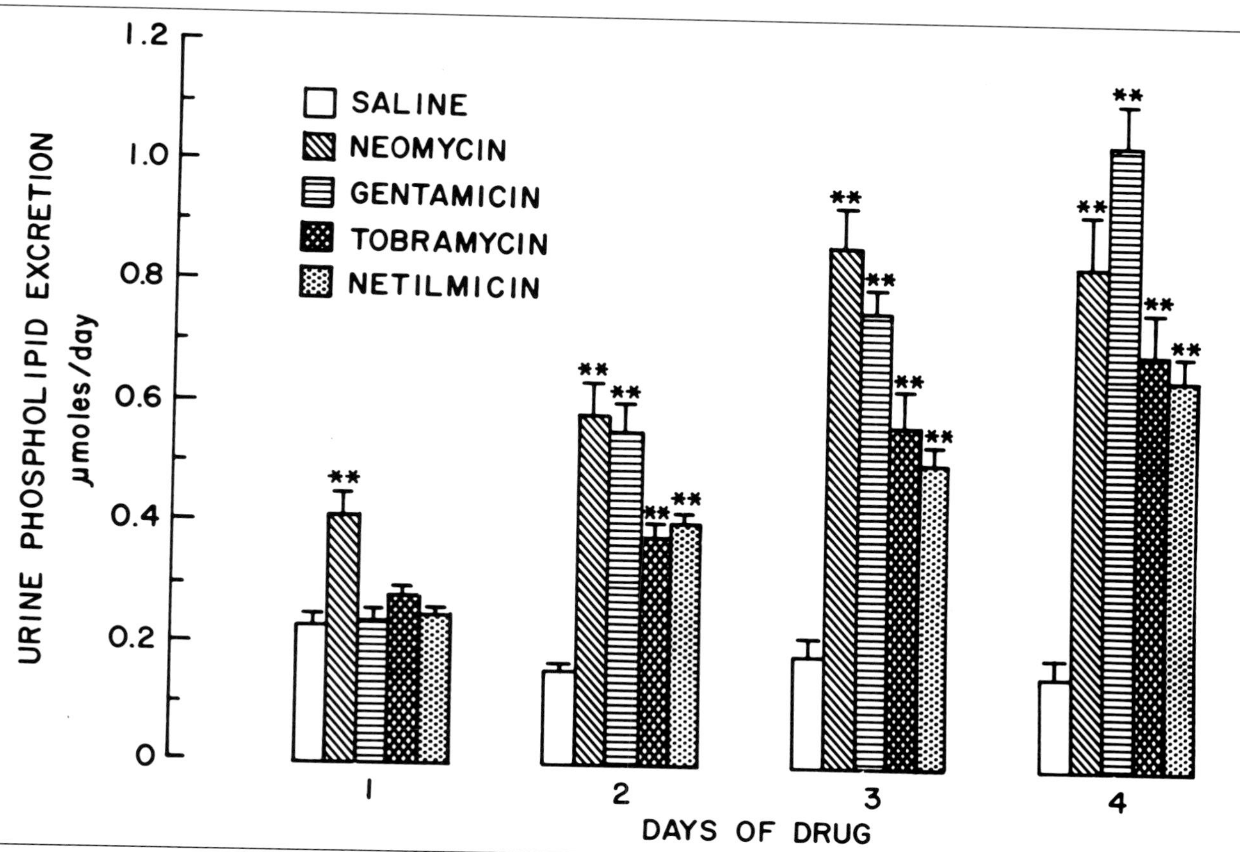

Fig. 41-8. Effect of drug treatment on the urinary excretion of phospholipid. The data demonstrate a direct correlation between the magnitude of the phospholipiduria and the nephrotoxicity potential of the four aminoglycoside antibiotics. **Significantly different from treatment with saline solution, $p < 0.01$. (From C. Josepovitz, R. Levine, T. Farruggella, et al. Comparative effects of aminoglycosides on renal cortical and urinary phospholipids in the rat. *Proc. Soc. Exp. Biol. Med.* 182:1, 1986. © by the Society for Experimental Biology and Medicine.)

begin degrading intracellular organelles. Although a linkage between intracellular release of lysosomal enzymes and cell injury has been suggested in other models of toxin-mediated injury [3, 203, 297], it has been difficult to establish a causal relationship between the two events. In studies designed to assess the issue of causality in injury models where lysosomal disruption appeared to be of primary pathogenic importance, the data suggested that lysosomal disruption in situ does not occur until late during the course of injury, well after the irreversibility of injury has been determined by other factors [132, 272]. Additionally, the pH optima of lysosomal hydrolases are far removed from the ambient intracellular pH. Thus, it is uncertain to what extent these lysosomal enzymes would be activated following their release into the cell interior. Labilization of lysosomes, however, has another and potentially more important consequence with respect to disrupting the functional integrity of the cell than the release of acid hydrolases and that is the release of high concentrations of aminoglycosides. The progressive leakage of aminoglycosides from permeabilized or ruptured lysosomes, their redistribution and interaction with other intracellular membrane targets, and the subsequent disruption of critical metabolic processes including mitochondrial respiration may be the key pathogenic event that initiates the irreversible injury cascade that eventuates in cell death (see Fig. 41-4).

Lysosomal phospholipidosis is a well-described complication of amphiphilic drugs [110, 123, 125, 177, 185, 186]. Despite similar alterations of lysosomal phospholipid metabolism and similar ultrastructural changes of lysosomes, cell injury does not invariably accompany the administration of cationic amphiphilic drugs [110, 123, 125, 177]. The difference between the potentials of aminoglycoside antibiotics and amphiphilic compounds to cause cell injury and necrosis may not reside in their relative effects on lysosomal phospholipid metabolism, which in the case of chlorphentermine and gentamicin are quite similar [123], and labilization of lysosomes but on their relative capacities for interacting with and disrupting other intracellular processes after these drugs are released from the lysosomal compartment.

Aminoglycoside-Phosphoinositide Interactions. If redistribution of aminoglycosides consequent to release from permeabilized or ruptured lysosomes does occur and is of pathogenic significance, then in light of the evidence supporting PIP_2 as the preferred binding site of aminoglycoside [10, 11, 87, 251, 253, 291] one might anticipate that the released drug would interact with this membrane receptor site. Several lines of evidence suggest that one consequence of aminoglycoside binding to PIP_2 would be perturbation of the PI cascade. Aminoglycosides have the capacity to inhibit PI-specific phospholipase C of nonlysosomal origin [123, 168, 265, 314], presumably as a consequence of drug binding to substrate or the formation of a drug-substrate enzyme complex [265]. Neomycin has been shown to block the hydrolysis of PIP_2 and the generation of inositol triphosphate (IP_3) presumably by the same mechanism [43, 52, 279]. Aminoglycosides have been shown to modify the incorporation of phosphorus 32 (^{32}P) into PIP_2 in a variety of tissues, findings that implicate an inhibitory effect of these agents on PIP kinase [179, 180, 181, 214, 252, 262]. Marche et al. [179] observed that the decreasing rank order of potency among the aminoglycosides for this phosphoinositide effect was neomycin, gentamicin, dibekacin, kanamycin, amikacin, and streptomycin and paralleled the nephrotoxicity potentials of these drugs in vivo.

Ramsammy et al. [232] provided direct evidence that gentamicin inhibits agonist stimulation of the PI cascade in a cell culture model of aminoglycoside toxicity. These authors demonstrated that incubation of primary cultures of rabbit proximal tubular cells in medium containing gentamicin at 10^{-3} M completely inhibited the generation of IP_3 (Fig. 41-9) and the redistribution of protein kinase C (Fig. 41-10) in response to stimulation with 10^{-6} M parathyroid hormone, angiotensin II, phenylephrine, and bradykinin. Importantly the generation of cyclic AMP in response to parathyroid hormone was not inhibited. This finding indicated that gentamicin did not interfere with the binding of the agonist to its membrane receptor site but rather implicated an interaction at a more distal site in the cascade. The authors postulated that inhibition of the PI cascade was due to the binding of gentamicin to PIP_2 which prevented the hydrolysis of PIP_2 by phospholipase C and generation of the second messengers IP_3 and diacylglycerol (Fig. 41-11). To establish the relevance of these observations made in cell culture to the in vivo situation, additional experiments were performed in a well-characterized rat model of aminoglycoside nephrotoxicity [232]. Rats were injected with gentamicin at 100 mg/kg/day for 2 days. This dose, if continued for 4 to 6 days causes proximal tubular cell dysfunction and necrosis [276], whereas after 2 days of drug treatment the only significant lesion is the accumulation of phospholipid in association with the appearance of the lysosomal myeloid body in renal proximal tubular cells. Twenty-four hours after the second dose of gentamicin, rats were injected with parathyroid hormone and its effect on the redistribution of protein kinase C, a marker for activation of the PI cascade, was measured in the renal cortex. In control rats, parathyroid hormone had the expected effect on the redistribution of protein kinase C from the cytosolic to the membrane fraction of renal cortex, whereas in rats injected with only two doses of drug this effect was completely abrogated. In contrast, addition of the phorbol ester 12-*O*-tetradecanoylphorbol-13-acetate to renal cortical homogenates activated protein kinase C to the same extent in both groups. This finding eliminated from consideration a direct inhibitory effect of gentamicin on protein kinase C. These data are consistent with the hypothesis that aminoglycosides bind to PIP_2 and prevent its hydrolysis by phospholipase C in response to agonist stimulation. It was suggested that the generalized inhibition of the PI cascade and disruption of critical regu-

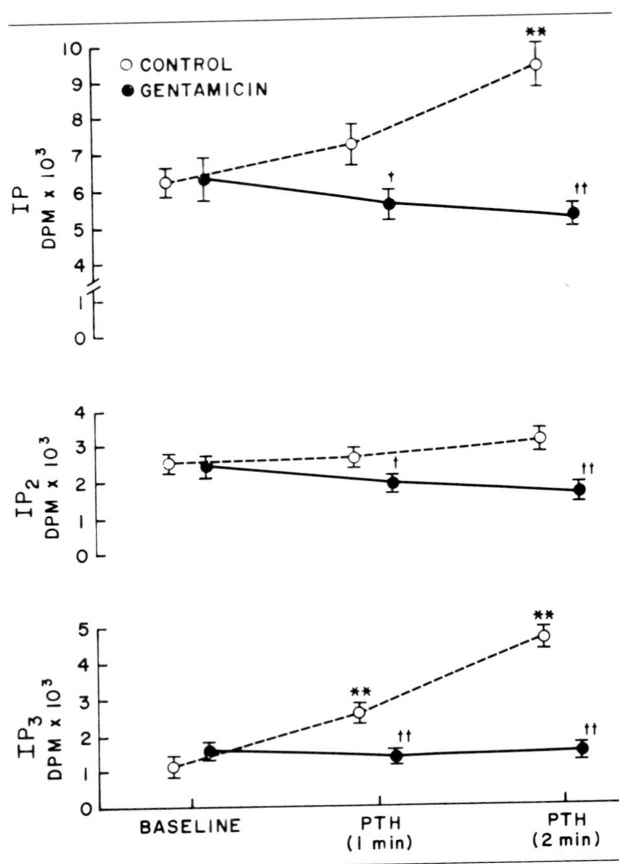

Fig. 41-9. Effect of gentamicin (10^{-3} M) on parathyroid hormone (PTH) (10^{-6} M) stimulation of inositol phosphate (IP), bisphosphate (IP_2), and triphosphate (IP_3) generation in primary cultures of rabbit proximal tubular cells. Exposure of cells to gentamicin for 48 hours resulted in blockade of inositol phosphate generation in response to PTH stimulation. Similar results were obtained after 24 hours of exposure to gentamicin. Data represent mean ± standard error in disintegrations per minute per culture plate; n = 5. **Significantly different from baseline, $p < 0.01$. †,††Significantly different from control, $p < 0.05$ and $p < 0.01$. (From L. S. Ramsammy, C. Josepovitz, and G. J. Kaloyanides. Gentamicin inhibits agonist stimulation of the phosphatidylinositol cascade in primary culture of rabbit proximal tubular cells and in rat renal cortex. *J. Pharmacol. Exp. Ther.* 247:989, 1988. © by the American Society for Pharmacology and Experimental Therapeutics.)

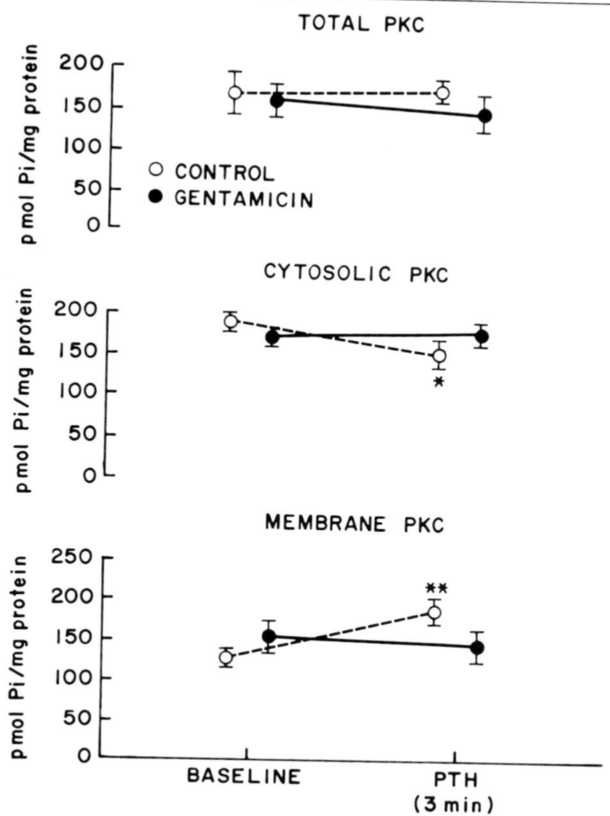

Fig. 41-10. Effect of gentamicin (10^{-3} M) on parathyroid hormone (10^{-6} M)–stimulated redistribution of protein kinase C (PKC) between the cytosolic and membrane fractions of rabbit proximal tubular cells grown in primary culture (1° RPTC). Exposure of cells to gentamicin for 48 hours resulted in blockade of protein kinase C activation in response to parathyroid hormone stimulation. Data represent the mean ± standard error; n = 5. *, **Significantly different from baseline, $p < 0.05$ and $p < 0.01$. (From L. S. Ramsammy, C. Josepovitz, and G. J. Kaloyanides. Gentamicin inhibits agonist stimulation of the phosphatidylinositol cascade in primary culture of rabbit proximal tubular cells and in rat renal cortex. *J. Pharmacol. Exp. Ther.* 247:989, 1988. © by the American Society for Pharmacology and Experimental Therapeutics.)

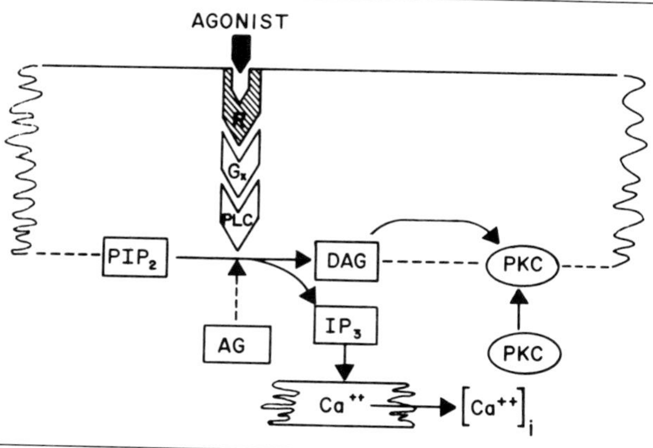

Fig. 41-11. Model depicting aminoglycoside (AG)-induced inhibition of the phosphatidylinositol (PhI) cascade. Aminoglycoside binds electrostatically to phosphatidylinositol bisphosphate (PIP_2) of the cytoplasmic leaflet of the cell membrane, thereby preventing agonist-stimulated phospholipase C–mediated hydrolysis of PIP_2 and generation of second messengers, inositol triphosphate (IP_3) and diacylglycerol (DAG). PLC = phospholipase C; R = receptor; G_x = protein.

latory processes linked to this major signal-transducing mechanism might play a significant role in the pathogenesis of aminoglycoside nephrotoxicity [232]. Particularly noteworthy was the finding that inhibition of the PI cascade was evident very early in the course of drug exposure, both in vitro and in vivo, before other major functional and structural abnormalities had developed. A potentially important implication of this observation is that inhibition of the PI cascade may precede labilization and rupture of phospholipid and drug-ladened lysosomes, in which case serious consideration must be given to the hypothesis that a moiety of drug gains access to the cell by a mechanism other than endocytosis and that this moiety of drug may be responsible for the early functional, biochemical, and structural abnormalities that precede disruption of lysosomal integrity.

Aminoglycoside-Mitochondrial Interactions. Cuppage et al. [63] reported that mitochondria from rats treated with gentamicin for 28 days showed dose-related changes in respiratory rates, but these were not analyzed in detail or at any other treatment interval. The potential of gentamicin and other aminoglycoside antibiotics to interact with the mitochondrial membrane in vitro was initially demonstrated in studies on mitochondria isolated from liver by Bendirdjian and colleagues [20], who suggested that a competitive interaction between gentamicin and Mg^{2+} at the mitochondrial membrane could produce altered mitochondrial respiration and K^+ permeability. They also demonstrated effects of other aminoglycoside antibiotics, the magnitude of which correlated with their nephrotic potential.

Humes and co-workers engaged in a series of investigations to clarify the role of mitochondrial injury in the pathogenesis of aminoglycoside-induced renal injury either as a primary action of gentamicin or as a secondary event arising from an altered intracellular milieu. Renal cortical mitochondria isolated from Sprague-Dawley rats treated with gentamicin, 40 mg/kg/day for 7 days, showed depressed state 3 and DNP uncoupled respiration compared to untreated controls [271]. Of importance, this regimen was not associated with severe gentamicin nephrotoxicity. Ultrastructural studies revealed the characteristic features of early gentamicin treatment, which included secondary lysosomes and myeloid bodies but no signs of substantial loss of cellular integrity. Depression of whole-kidney ATP content suggested that the observed mitochondrial dysfunction constituted a major impact on cellular energetics. These effects appeared to be specific, since liver mitochondria were not affected [271].

In subsequent studies the direct effects of gentamicin at the inner mitochondrial membrane were investigated [296]. The acute in vitro effects of gentamicin on renal cortical mitochondrial function were shown to be due to the competitive displacement of Mg^{2+} at inner mitochondrial membrane sites that regulate monovalent cation permeability. Gentamicin appeared to compete with Mg^{2+} for these sites without itself limiting Na^+ and K^+ permeability to the same degree as Mg^{2+}. Detailed studies showed that exposure to gentamicin also produced increased basal mitochondrial respiration (state 4) secondary to increased monovalent cation permeability. Such stimulation of mitochondrial respiration is suggestive of an uncoupling action of gentamicin on oxidative phosphorylation. However, since gentamicin did not completely release respiratory control or decrease the ADP-oxygen ratio, it differs from classic uncouplers, such as DNP, and fits into the category of agents termed *loose* or *pseudouncouplers* [137]. Additionally, the increased access of Na^+ to inner mitochondrial membrane components, which results from the action of gentamicin, has deleterious effects on maximal rates of electron transport, and these account for the depression of state 3 and DNP uncoupled respiration produced by gentamicin in vitro [296]. The ability of gentamicin to interact with sites normally occupied by Mg^{2+} is consistent with the theory that its membrane interaction is due to the cationic properties of the gentamicin molecule. This similarity of mechanism of action on mitochondrial function of all aminoglycosides was substantiated by the observation that like gentamicin, other aminoglycosides stimulate state 4 and inhibit both state 3 and DNP uncoupled respiration [20]. Of interest, the magnitude of these effects on mitochondrial respiration correlated, in a general way, with the cationicity of the aminoglycosides. These data illustrate the potential for these antibiotics to alter markedly the control of membrane permeability properties.

Mela-Riker et al. [190] examined the effects of chronic gentamicin treatment in the rat on mitochondrial respiratory and calcium transport functions and cytochrome concentrations. During the first 10 days of chronic gentamicin treatment, mitochondrial cytochrome aa_3 and cytochrome c but not cytochrome b concentrations declined significantly along with depression of state 3 respiration and calcium accumulation. The authors concluded that depression of these mitochondrial respiratory chain enzymes and the associated mitochondrial respiratory and transport functions reflected an indirect, extramitochondrial effect of gentamicin, i.e., depressed synthesis of mitochondrial proteins that are regulated by extramitochondrial genes. In contrast to the in vivo study of Simmons et al. [271], these investigators found that state 4 respiration was depressed to an equivalent degree as state 3 respiration so that no change in respiratory control was observed. It is unknown whether this difference is related to a difference in severity of injury, animal species, or both.

Interpretation of the above-mentioned studies is complicated by the fact that neither group of investigators took the necessary precautions to minimize mitochondrial uptake of calcium during the isolation procedure. Weinberg [295] has shown that under conditions where mitochondrial uptake of calcium is inhibited by adding ruthenium red and EGTA to the isolation buffer, mitochondrial respiration is well preserved in rats until late in the course of gentamicin nephrotoxicity.

Other studies have implicated renal mitochondrial injury as an important biochemical pathogenic pathway for renal cell injury secondary to a variety of nephrotoxins besides aminoglycoside antibiotics. Mercurials [295a, 295b], phenacetin [66a], cyclosporin A [213a], and cephaloridine [288a] all inhibit mitochondrial oxidative phosphorylation in vitro, while mercury and cephaloridine cause the same effect in vivo as well [288a, 295b]. Nephrotoxin-related alterations in renal cell bioenergetics, therefore, appear to be a potential common biochemical pathway in the pathogenesis of nephrotoxic acute renal failure. Although this thesis is attractive, current evidence does not assign mitochondrial dysfunction a unique role in the early pathogenesis of aminoglycoside nephrotoxicity. Since rapid and avid intralysosomal sequestration of aminoglycosides has been observed in all models of nephrotoxicity, the amount of aminoglycoside available for significant mitochondrial exposure early in the treatment course has been questioned. Mitochondrial dysfunction may be one component of an irreversible injury cascade initiated by the release of stored aminoglycoside from unstable lysosomes followed by deleterious interactions with other organelles (see Fig. 41-4).

Aminoglycoside-Microsomal Interactions. The concentrations of mitochondrial cytochrome aa_3 and cytochrome c are depressed in the renal cortex of rats treated with gentamicin [190]. Because these proteins are coded by extramitochondrial genes, these data suggest that gentamicin alters the synthesis of these proteins by an extramitochondrial mechanism. Buss et al. [39] demonstrated that gentamicin, kanamycin, and netilmicin, at concentrations readily achievable in vivo, inhibited microsomal protein synthesis in a concentration-dependent manner. In subsequent studies, these investigators demonstrated that injection of gentamicin in rats at a dose used clinically in man significantly depressed protein synthesis in microsomes isolated from the kidney but not from the brain or liver [25, 38]. Importantly, the inhibition of microsomal protein synthesis occurred prior to the appearance of depressed creatinine clearance, organic solute transport, and mitochondrial cytochrome concentrations or the appearance of proximal tubular cell necrosis [25]. The mechanism of microsomal protein synthesis inhibition was not investigated. However, Eustice and Wilhelm [76] have shown that aminoglycosides cause misreading of the eukaryotic code. The fact that depressed microsomal protein synthesis was observed early in the course of aminoglycoside treatment, before other advanced clues of toxicity were seen, raises the possibility that disruption of microsomal function may be a proximal event in the injury cascade of aminoglycoside nephrotoxicity. These data also raise the question as to the mechanism by which aminoglycosides gain access to microsomes at such an early stage.

Role of Free Radicals in Aminoglycoside Nephrotoxicity. Increased lipid peroxides have been identified in the renal cortex of rats injected with gentamicin [9, 241]. Ramsammy et al. [241] observed that by the second dose of gentamicin in rats, a significant decline of arachidonic acid content of renal cortical phospholipids was evident. By the fourth day of gentamicin treatment, arachidonic acid had declined 48 percent below the value of control rats and was accompanied by reciprocal increases of more saturated fatty acids and by a significant increase of malondialdehyde, an end product of lipid peroxidation, in the renal cortex. Catalase activity was depressed as was total and reduced glutathione, whereas oxidized glutathione was increased, a change consistent with glutathione scavenging of free radicals. Superoxide dismustase activity was unaltered. Because these alterations were observed relatively early in the course of aminoglycoside administration, the hypothesis was advanced that accelerated lipid peroxidation secondary to free radical attack may be a proximal cause of aminoglycoside nephrotoxicity [241]. To test this hypothesis, rats were injected with gentamicin plus one of two free radical scavengers, diphenyl-phenylenediamine (DPPD) [237] or vitamin E [238]. Both agents were highly effective in preventing lipid peroxidation and the associated changes involving glutathione. However, neither agent ameliorated gentamicin-induced nephrotoxicity as assessed by no reduction in the magnitude of enzymuria, phospholipiduria, creatininemia, or renal histopathologic changes. Ramsammy et al. [237, 238] concluded that free radical–mediated lipid peroxidation was a consequence and not the cause of gentamicin-induced acute renal failure.

Subsequently, Walker and Shah reported that gentamicin-stimulated mitochondrial production of hydrogen peroxide in vitro [290] and that treatment of rats with a variety of hydroxyl radical scavengers conferred significant protection against gentamicin-induced acute renal failure [289]. Utilizing protocols identical to those described by Walker and Shah [289], Kaloyanides et al. [131] examined the efficacy of three hydroxyl radical scavengers (dimethylthiourea, dimethylsulfoxide, and sodium benzoate) in protecting against gentamicin nephrotoxicity in the rat. Not only did these three hydroxyl radicals not protect rats against gentamicin nephrotoxicity, but in the case of dimethylthiourea and dimethylsulfoxide the severity of the nephrotoxicity was augmented even though these agents inhibited lipid peroxidation. The reason for the different outcomes of the two studies remains unclear. At the present time, the preponderance of the evidence supports the view that free radical–mediated lipid peroxidation is a consequence rather than a cause of aminoglycoside-induced injury.

Interventions for Modifying Experimental Aminoglycoside Nephrotoxicity

Insights into the pathogenesis of aminoglycoside nephrotoxicity have been gleaned from studies of interventions that modify the severity of this disorder in experimental animals.

CALCIUM AND PARATHYROID HORMONE

Because of the fact that aminoglycoside antibiotics have been shown to compete with calcium for membrane binding and to perturb a number of calcium-dependent processes, investigators have examined the influence of increased dietary calcium on the expression of aminoglycoside nephrotoxicity. Bennett et al. [23] have shown that supplementing the diet of rats with $CaCO_3$ so as to augment urinary calcium by 10- to 20-fold significantly ameliorated the severity of gentamicin nephrotoxicity. Decreased rate of accumulation of gentamicin was proposed as the mechanism of protection [229]. Humes et al. [112] extended these observations by demonstrating that oral calcium loading in rats decreased gentamicin-induced depression of renal excretory function and mitochondrial respiratory function and reduced the associated accumulation of calcium by mitochondria. The demonstration that calcium was a competitive inhibitor of gentamicin binding to membranes and to anionic phospholipids in vitro but did not alter the accumulation of gentamicin in renal cortex in vivo led these investigators to postulate that the protective effect of dietary calcium supplementation may be related to competitive antagonism of gentamicin-membrane interactions at a critical intracellular site [112]. The possible role of suppression of parathyroid hormone in the protective action of calcium loading was investigated in several studies. Bennett et al. [30] demonstrated that selective parathyroidectomy ameliorated the severity of gentamicin nephrotoxicity but that the protective effect was enhanced by a high-calcium diet. These data suggested that a high-calcium diet had a beneficial effect independent of suppression of parathyroid hormone. Elliott et al. [73] demonstrated that stimulation of parathyroid hormone augmented gentamicin nephrotoxicity in the rat, whereas parathyroidectomy afforded protection in association with reduced accumulation of drug in the renal cortex. In contrast, Cronin and Newman [60] observed no protection in rats subjected to parathyroidectomy, whereas administration of thyroxine was protective. The reason for the difference among these studies is not known. Other investigators have examined the effect of calcium channel blockers on aminoglycoside nephrotoxicity. Lee and Michael [161] reported that nitrendipine protected rats against gentamicin-induced nephrotoxicity without altering the accumulation of drug. In contrast, no protective effect of calcium channel blockade was observed in two studies involving verapamil [283, 293], whereas in one study involving verapamil [183] and two studies involving diltiazam [96, 183] the severity of gentamicin nephrotoxicity was enhanced.

POLYAMINO ACIDS

Williams and Hottendorf [304] and Williams et al. [305] first reported that polyasparagine and polyaspartic acid (PAA) inhibited binding of [^{3}H]gentamicin to rat renal brush-border membrane in vitro and when injected in vivo, conferred protection against the development of aminoglycoside nephrotoxicity. Because renal cortical accumulation of drug was not depressed, it was concluded that polyamino acids inhibited aminoglycoside-cell interactions at a step distal to the uptake step, and therefore, might serve as a probe for dissecting out drug-membrane interactions of pathogenic importance. Three groups of investigators subsequently confirmed and extended the findings of Williams et al. [305]. Gilbert et al. [89] reported that administration to rats of PAA in a 0.3:1.0 M PAA-gentamicin dosage ratio prevented virtually all AG-induced injury for up to 27 days as assessed by functional (increased urinary NAG excretion, elevated serum creatinine concentration) and histologic (cell necrosis and regeneration) parameters despite the renal cortical accumulation of drug to tenfold that of rats injected with gentamicin alone. Ramsammy et al. [234] reported that the co-administration of PAA and gentamicin at a molar ratio of 0.3:1.0 for 6 days also provided an impressive degree of protection against gentamicin, as indicated by a lower rate of urinary NAG excretion, no elevation of malondialdehyde in the renal cortex, less elevation of phospholipid in the renal cortex, no depression of creatinine clearance, and less evidence of structural injury as assessed by light and electron microscopy. In contrast to the study of Gilbert et al. [89], the renal cortical accumulation of gentamicin was only modestly higher in the rats receiving PAA and gentamicin compared to rats receiving gentamicin alone [234]. Nevertheless, the basic conclusions of the two studies were the same, i.e., that PAA provided dramatic protection against the development of functional and structural lesions of gentamicin nephrotoxicity in the rat by a mechanism that did not involve inhibition of drug uptake and accumulation by renal proximal tubular cells. Ramsammy et al. [236] in a subsequent study demonstrated that injecting rats with PAA 16 hours prior to the injection of gentamicin was also effective in protecting rats against gentamicin nephrotoxicity. Based on the pharmacokinetics of both agents, it was concluded that this injection schedule prevented any appreciable complexation between PAA and gentamicin in the extracellular space so that the protective effect of PAA had to be exerted within renal proximal tubular cells. This concept is strengthened by the observation that PAA induces formation of subapical vesicles suggestive of endocytotic transport and accumulation of this compound [235].

The mechanism by which PAA protects against gentamicin nephrotoxicity was investigated in cultured renal cells [235]. It was demonstrated that co-incubation of cells in medium containing PAA and gentamicin as well as preloading cells with PAA followed by exposure to gentamicin prevented the development of the lysosomal phospholipidosis and myeloid body formation, prevented impaired degradation of lysosomal phospholipids, and prevented disruption of agonist-mediated stimulation of the PI cascade without inhibiting the transport and accumulation of drug. These studies suggested that PAA prevented gentamicin from interacting electrostatically with PIP_2 and other anionic phospholipids. Direct evidence in support of this view was obtained in experiments using PI-containing liposomes [235]. It was demonstrated that PAA prevented gentamicin from depressing glycerol permeability of these liposomes (Fig. 41-12) and from promoting their aggregation (Fig. 41-13), effects previously shown to be dependent on gentamicin binding electrostatically and by hydrogen bonding to PI [239]. Since PAA is a polyanion, these data suggested that the protective effect of this compound might be related to its ability to electrostatically complex gentamicin and, thereby, prevent gentamicin from interacting with anionic phospholipids. In support of this interpretation, it was shown that aggregating complexes of gentamicin and PAA formed in vitro when the molar concentration ratio exceeded 8.25 [235]. Furthermore, an electrostatic interaction between gentamicin and PAA could be demonstrated at molar ratios that did not cause aggregation [235].

Beauchamp et al. [18] also demonstrated that administration of PAA to rats affords protection against the early manifestation of gentamicin-induced nephrotoxicity, including depression of sphingomyelinase activity, increased renal cortical phospholipids, lysosomal enlargement with myeloid bodies, and increased mitoses and [^{3}H]thymidine incorporation into DNA. In other studies, Kishore et al. [140] demonstrated that PAA competitively displaced gentamicin from liposomes containing anionic phospholipids and restored the activity of gentamicin-inhibited lysosomal phospholipase A toward PC. These investigators also presented evidence that the protective effect of different anionic polyamino acids was related to their resistance to hydrolysis by ly-

Fig. 41-12. Effect of polyaspartic acid (PAA), gentamicin (G), and G plus PAA on glycerol permeability of phosphatidylcholine/phosphatidylinositol liposomes. PAA prevented gentamicin-induced depression of glycerol permeability of the liposomes. Data represent mean ± standard error; n = 5. **Significantly different from control (C), $p < 0.01$. $\bar{p}$ = relative permeability coefficient. (From L. Ramsammy, C. Josepovitz, B. Lane, et al. Polyaspartic acid inhibits gentamicin-induced perturbations of phospholipid metabolism. *Am. J. Physiol.* 258:C1141, 1990.)

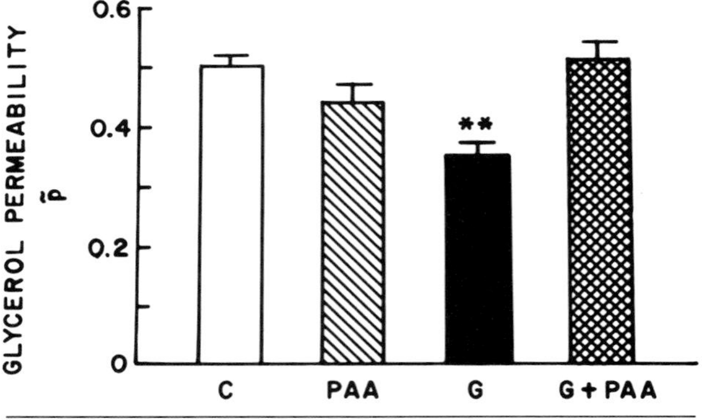

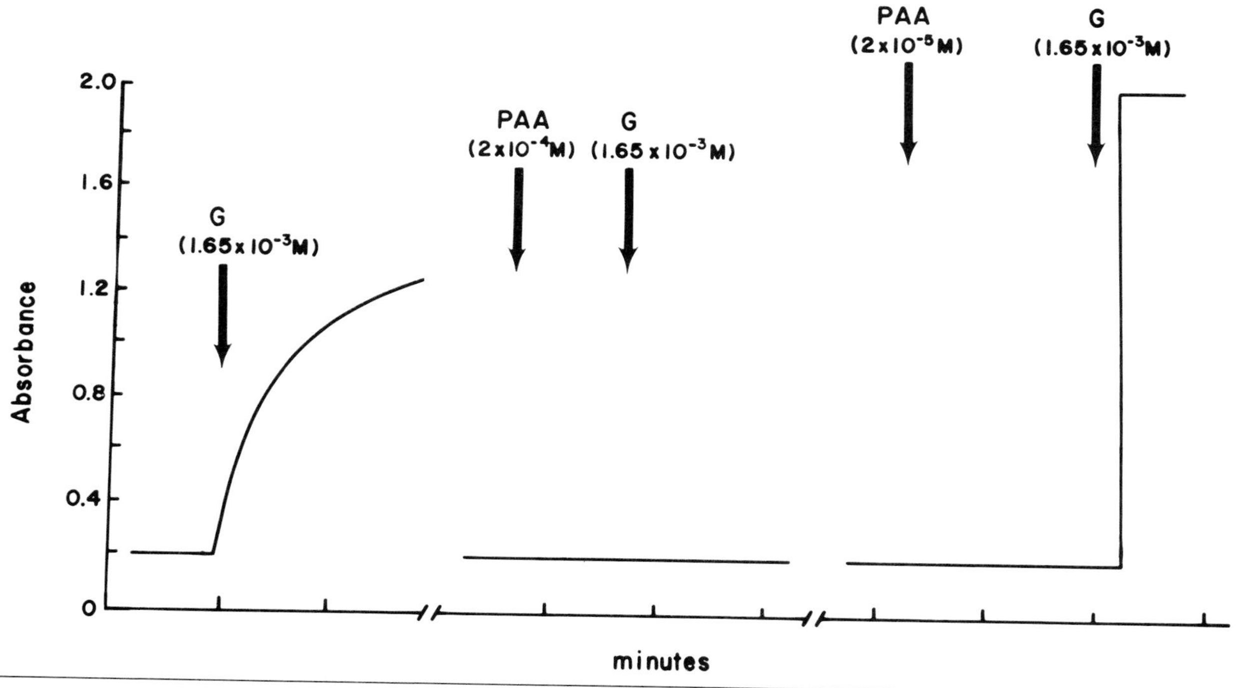

Fig. 41-13. Prior addition of polyaspartic acid (PAA) inhibits gentamicin (G)-induced aggregation of phosphatidylcholine/phosphatidylinositol liposomes. This tracing demonstrates that addition of 1.65×10^{-3} M gentamicin (*left*) caused aggregation of these liposomes, whereas no aggregation was seen when PAA was added to liposomes prior to gentamicin (*middle*). When the concentration of PAA was lowered to 2×10^{-5} M, addition of the same concentration of gentamicin (1.65×10^{-3} M) provoked a maximal rise in absorbance (*right*), a pattern distinctly different from that seen on the left and indicative of formation of PAA and gentamicin electrostatic complexes. (From L. Ramsammy, C. Josepovitz, B. Lane, et al. Polyaspartic acid inhibits gentamicin-induced perturbations of phospholipid metabolism. *Am. J. Physiol.* 258:C1141, 1990.)

sosomal enzymes, thereby indirectly implicating the lysosome in the injury cascade of aminoglycoside nephrotoxicity [141].

A synthesis of the above-mentioned studies indicates that the protective effect of PAA is related to its ability to bind aminoglycoside antibiotics electrostatically, thereby preventing these cationic drugs from binding to anionic constituents of cell membranes. These studies provide strong support for the hypothesis that the toxicity of aminoglycoside antibiotics is causally linked to the electrostatic interaction between these drugs and membrane anionic phospholipids and the resulting disturbances of phospholipid metabolism and membrane function.

PYRIDOXAL 5′-PHOSPHATE

Kacew [124] reported that co-injection of pyridoxal 5′-phosphate protected rats against gentamicin nephrotoxicity as assessed by prevention of enzymuria, depression of renal cortical enzyme activities, and the development of phospholipidosis. The mechanism of protection was attributed to a decreased uptake of drug, presumably consequent to the complexation of pyridoxal 5′-phosphate, a negatively charged compound, with the cationic gentamicin. Pyridoxal 5′-phosphate was also shown to protect against tobramycin nephrotoxicity by a similar mechanism [147], as was inositol hexasulfate [148]. In contrast to the above findings, Kaloyanides et al. [131] observed no reduction of enzymuria or phospholipidosis in rats injected with pyridoxal 5′-phosphate intraperitoneally and gentamicin subcutaneously. However, the elevation of serum creatinine concentration was less marked, as were the depression of creatinine clearance and the severity of proximal tubular cell necrosis. Of interest, the renal cortical concentrations of gentamicin were not different in the two groups. This finding implicates some mechanism other than decreased uptake in the protective effect of pyridoxal 5′-phosphate. Intracellular complexation of gentamicin by pyridoxal 5′-phosphate warrants consideration.

Treatment and Prevention

The treatment of aminoglycoside nephrotoxicity starts with prevention. Prevention requires knowledge of the risk factors, summarized in Table 41-4. These can be categorized into those that are determined by the individual patient and not easily influenced, if at all, and those that are determined by the clinician and potentially controllable.

Table 41-4. Clinical risk factors for aminoglycoside nephrotoxicity

A. Factors not readily modifiable clinically
  1. Age
  2. Sex
  3. Obesity
  4. Preexisting liver disease
  5. Preexisting kidney disease
  6. Underlying disease

B. Factors potentially modifiable clinically
  1. Daily dose, interval, duration
  2. Specific aminoglycoside
  3. Volume depletion
  4. Hypokalemia
  5. Hypomagnesemia
  6. Metabolic acidosis
  7. Concurrent pharmaceutical agents
     a. Amphotericin B
     b. Cephalosporin
     c. Vancomycin
     d. Cisplatin
     e. Furosemide
     f. Calcium channel blockers
     g. Radiocontrast agents

Prominent among the risk factors peculiar to the patient and not modifiable is age. Advanced age had been implicated as a significant risk. Moench and Smith [197] have challenged the assumptions on which this conclusion was based. A subsequent study using stepwise discriminant analysis did demonstrate that age was a significant factor for aminoglycoside nephrotoxicity in humans [199]. The mechanisms underlying the increased risk of advanced age are probably multifactorial and include age-related decline of renal function that, if not appreciated and corrected for, results in excessive dosing [246]. Animal studies suggest that aging is associated with altered renal pharmacokinetics accompanied by increased renal cortical accumulation of drug [182]. In addition, increased susceptibility of the aging kidney to aminoglycoside toxicity has also been suggested [188], possibly on the basis of an age-related, impaired capacity for cellular repair and regeneration [128].

Male gender has been shown to carry increased risk for aminoglycoside nephrotoxicity in the rat [26], whereas female gender has been identified as a risk factor in humans [199]. The reason for this difference has not been established.

Obesity carries increased risk for aminoglycoside nephrotoxicity [57]. Increased toxicity was observed despite dose adjustments for differences in volume of distribution and rate of renal clearance. Experiments in an animal model of obesity suggested that the renal susceptibility to a toxic insult may be heightened in obese subjects [56].

Chronic liver disease has been identified as a risk factor in experimental animals [169, 312] and in human subjects [41, 199]. Increased renal cortical accumulation of gentamicin has been observed in animal models [169, 312]. The mechanism may be related to alterations in renal hemodynamics, volume, and electrolyte metabolism that commonly complicate liver disease.

Preexisting chronic renal insufficiency has been recognized as a major risk factor for developing aminoglycoside nephrotoxicity primarily when the drug dosage is not appropriately adjusted for the decreased excretory capacity of the diseased kidney. However, when appropriate dose adjustments were made, Moench and Smith [197] found no increased risk for aminoglycoside nephrotoxicity associated with chronic renal insufficiency. Animal studies suggest that the influence of chronic renal failure on the susceptibility to aminoglycoside nephrotoxicity is species dependent. In the rat, subtotal nephrectomy was not associated with increased risk [44] whereas in the dog, increased risk for aminoglycoside nephrotoxicity was clearly demonstrable despite careful adjustment in the dose to maintain the serum concentration of drug within normal limits [83]. Increased drug accumulation was identified as the probable cause of the increased risk [83]. Of potential relevance to humans is the observation that administration of gentamicin using the method of reduced dose and fixed interval carries a higher risk of nephrotoxicity in dogs with chronic renal insufficiency than does using the method of fixed dose and prolonged interval [245].

The nature of the underlying disease also influences the risk of nephrotoxicity. Sepsis with hypotension carries a higher risk for nephrotoxicity than does an uncomplicated gram-negative infection [199]. This undoubtedly reflects the fact that sepsis and shock carry an independent risk, as endotoxin was shown to augment the severity of nephrotoxicity in association with increased renal cortical accumulation of drug [211, 284].

Of the risk factors that are potentially modifiable by the clinician, the most important are daily drug dose, interval of dosing, and the duration of therapy. A direct relationship between total dose (daily dose plus duration of therapy) has been consistently found in experimental animals [63, 69, 70, 91, 107, 109, 173, 276] and in humans [22, 37, 40, 68, 102, 275]. More recently, animal studies have shown that the same daily dose of drug given as two or three divided doses leads to greater accumulation of drug and greater nephrotoxicity than if it was given as a single dose [28]. Administration of drug by continuous intravenous infusion carries the highest risk of nephrotoxicity with respect to gentamicin, tobramycin, and netilmicin but not amikacin [65, 92].

Among aminoglycoside antibiotics the risk of developing nephrotoxicity varies and reflects the influence of different rates of drug accumulation by renal proximal tubular cells and different potentials for drug-membrane interactions. Comparative studies in humans suggest that the relative risk for developing nephrotoxicity from gentamicin is greater than that associated with either tobramycin [126, 274], netilmicin [64, 126, 162], or amikacin [126, 275]. Based on such trials, the decreasing rank order for clinical nephrotoxicity potential appears to be gentamicin, tobramycin, amikacin, and netilmicin.

Volume depletion [24, 47, 160, 205], hypomagnesemia

[243, 310], and metabolic acidosis [72] all carry increased risks for nephrotoxicity. In the case of volume depletion and hypokalemia, the increased risk appears to be related to an increased accumulation of drug in the renal cortex. The mechanism underlying the increased risk associated with hypomagnesemia has not been definitively established but may relate to the competition between divalent cations and the cationic aminoglycoside antibiotic for critical membrane-binding sites [112]. In the case of metabolic acidosis, the reduced pH would promote increased protonation of aminoglycoside antibiotics and this would augment the reactivity of these organic polycations.

Finally, the risk of aminoglycoside nephrotoxicity has been shown to be augmented when aminoglycoside antibiotics are administered in conjunction with certain drugs and pharmaceutical agents, some of which have intrinsic nephrotoxicity potential. These include amphotericin [51], cephalosporins [170], vancomycin [247, 274, 311], cisplatin [74, 135], furosemide [47, 205], calcium channel blockers [96, 183], and radiocontrast agents [287]. Many of these synergistic interactions have been identified in animal studies so that the relevance of these observations to humans remains to be established. Nevertheless, prudence dictates that potentially nephrotoxic drugs should be avoided if at all possible in patients who are undergoing or have recently completed therapy with aminoglycoside antibiotics.

The prevention of aminoglycoside nephrotoxicity requires that use of these drugs be limited to appropriate indications. When indicated, these drugs should be used in the appropriate dosage to achieve therapeutic serum concentrations and avoid toxic concentrations. Monitoring of peak and trough serum concentrations generally every 2 to 3 days, but occasionally daily in critically ill patients, is standard practice in pursuing this goal. Finally, these drugs should be continued for the minimum time required to achieve the therapeutic goal. The choice of drug is dictated by the relative sensitivity of the organism to the various aminoglycoside antibiotics. In a patient at increased risk for nephrotoxicity because of advanced age, associated disease, or concomitant drug therapy, the risk may be lessened by selecting an aminoglycoside antibiotic of lower nephrotoxic potential than that of gentamicin. Even when those factors known to influence risk are absent or have been minimized or eliminated, aminoglycoside nephrotoxicity can still occur in a certain percentage of appropriately dosed patients. These patients exhibit excessive renal accumulation of drug or increased sensitivity to a given level of drug accumulation [257]. The clinician must be constantly alert to the possibility of aminoglycoside nephrotoxicity and monitor all patients on aminoglycoside therapy for this potential complication. The intensity of monitoring is dictated in part by the relative risk factors present. At a minimum, frequent measurements of serum creatinine concentration, generally every 2 to 3 days, should be performed. In high-risk patients, daily creatinine clearance measurement and urinalysis may be required in order to detect early signs of toxicity before a rise in serum creatinine concentration or serum trough level of drug becomes evident. If renal injury occurs, then the drug should be stopped if possible or dosage should be reduced to prevent the accumulation of drug in serum and further toxic injury related thereto. Careful attention must be paid to maintaining fluid and electrolyte balance and avoiding potential insults to the kidney related to renal hypoperfusion or exposure to other potential nephrotoxins. Even when nephrotoxicity is recognized and the drug is discontinued early in the course, renal failure may progress over the next 5 to 10 days with a slow rise in the serum creatinine to disturbingly high levels and it may remain there for a number of days before renal function begins to slowly improve. No specific therapy for hastening recovery has been identified to be effective. The prognosis for recovery of renal function is generally good except in those cases where the underlying disease exposes the kidney to persisting or recurrent insults related to sepsis, hypotension, and hypoperfusion.

ACKNOWLEDGMENT. The author expresses his appreciation to Pamela Geller for expert secretarial assistance.

References

1. Adams, H. R., and Durrett, L. R. Gentamicin blockade of slow Ca^{2+} channels in atrial myocardium of guinea pigs. *J. Clin. Invest.* 62: 241, 1978.
2. Adams, H. R., and Goodman, F. R. Differential inhibitory effects of neomycin on contractile responses of various canine arteries. *J. Pharmacol. Exp. Ther.* 193: 393, 1974.
3. Allison, A. C., Harrington, J. S., and Birbeck, M. An examination of the cytotoxic effects of silica on macrophages. *J. Exp. Med.* 124: 141, 1966.
4. Amacher, D. E., and Schomaker, S. J. Selective membrane toxicity of aminoglycoside antibiotics in membrane vesicles isolated from proximal renal tubules of the rat. *Biochem. Pharmacol.* 38: 3872, 1989.
5. Anderson, R. J., Linas, S. L., Berns, A. S., Henrich, W. L., Miller, T. R., Gabow, P. A., and Schrier, R. W. Nonoliguric acute renal failure. *N. Engl. J. Med.* 296: 1134, 1977.
6. Aramaki, Y., Takagi, K., and Tsuchiya, S. Role of N-acetylneuraminic acid in renal brush-border membrane vesicle aggregation by aminoglycosides. *Biochim. Biophys. Acta* 1023: 352, 1990.
7. Aramaki, Y., Takahashi, M., Inabe, A., Ishii, Y., and Tsuchiya, S. Uptake of aminoglycoside antibiotics in brush border membrane vesicles and inhibition of (Na^+,K^+)-ATPase activity of basolateral membrane. *Biochim. Biophys. Acta* 862: 111, 1986.
8. Aronoff, G. R., Pottratz, S. T., Brier, M. E., Walker, N. E., Fineberg, S., Glant, M. D., and Luft, F. C. Aminoglycoside accumulation kinetics in rat renal parenchyma. *Antimicrob. Agents Chemother.* 23: 74, 1983.
9. Aso, Y., Ohtawara, Y., Suzuki, K., Tajima, A., and Fujita, K. The effect of gentamicin and mercuric chloride on cyclic AMP and lipoperoxide in rat kidneys. *Nippon Jinzo Gakkai Shi* 6: 583, 1982.
10. Au, S., Schacht, J., and Weiner, N. Membrane effects of aminoglycoside antibiotics measured in liposomes con-

taining the fluorescent probe, 1-anilino-8-naphthalene sulfonate. *Biochim. Biophys. Acta* 862: 205, 1986.

11. Au, S., Weiner, N. D., and Schacht, J. Aminoglycosides preferentially increase permeability in phosphoinositide-containing membranes: A study with carboxyfluorescein in liposomes. *Biochim. Biophys. Acta* 902: 80, 1987.
12. Aubert-Tulkens, G., Van Hoof, F., and Tulkens, P. Gentamicin-induced lysosomal phospholipidosis in cultured rat fibroblasts: Quantitative ultrastructural and biochemical study. *Lab Invest.* 40: 481, 1979.
13. Aynedjian, H. S., Nguyen, D., Lee, H. Y., et al. Effects of dietary electrolyte supplementation on gentamicin nephrotoxicity. *Am. J. Med. Sci.* 295: 444, 1988.
14. Bar, R. J., Wilson, H. E., and Mazzaferri, E. L. Hypomagnesemic hypocalcemia secondary to renal magnesium wasting: A possible consequence of high dose gentamicin therapy. *Ann. Intern. Med.* 82: 646, 1975.
15. Barr, G. A., Mazze, R. I., Cousins, M. J., and Kosek, J. C. An animal model for combined methoxyflurane and gentamicin nephrotoxicity. *Br. J. Anaesth.* 45: 306, 1973.
16. Barza, M., Murray, T., and Hamburger, R. J. Uptake of gentamicin by separated, viable renal tubules from rabbits. *J. Infect. Dis.* 141: 510, 1980.
17. Baylis, C., Rennke, H., and Brenner, B. M. Mechanisms of the defect in glomerular ultrafiltration associated with gentamicin administration. *Kidney Int.* 12: 344, 1977.
18. Beauchamp, D., Laurent, G., Maldague, P., Abid, S., Kishore, B. K., and Tulkens, P. M. Protection against gentamicin-induced early renal alterations (phospholipidosis and increased DNA synthesis) by coadministration of poly-L-aspartic acid. *J. Pharmacol. Exp. Ther.* 255: 858, 1990.
19. Beck, P. R., Thomson, R. B., and Chaudhuri, A. K. R. Aminoglycoside antibiotics and renal function: Changes in urinary gamma-glutamyl transferase excretion. *J. Clin. Pathol.* 30: 432, 1977.
20. Bendirdjian, J. P., Fillastre, J. P., and Foucher, B. Mitochondria Modifications with the Aminoglycosides. In A. Whelton and H. Neu (eds.), *The Aminoglycosides, Microbiology, Clinical Use and Toxicology.* New York: Marcel Dekker, 1982.
21. Bendush, C. L., Senior, S. L., and Wooller, H. O. Evaluation of nephrotoxic and ototoxic effects of tobramycin in world-wide study. *Med. J. Aust.* 2: 22, 1977.
22. Bendush, C. L., and Weber, R. Tobramycin sulfate: A summary of world-wide experience from clinical trials. *J. Infect. Dis.* 134(Suppl.): S219, 1976.
23. Bennett, W. M., Elliott, W. C., Houghton, D. C., Gilbert, D. N., DeFehr, J., and McCarron, D. A. Reduction of experimental gentamicin nephrotoxicity in rats by dietary calcium loading. *Antimicrob. Agents Chemother.* 22: 508, 1982.
24. Bennett, W. M., Hartnett, M. N., Gilbert, D., Houghton, D., and Porter, G. A. Effect of sodium intake on gentamicin nephrotoxicity in the rat. *Proc. Soc. Exp. Biol. Med.* 151: 736, 1976.
25. Bennett, W. M., Mela-Riker, L. M., Houghton, D. C., Gilbert, D. N., and Buss, W. C. Microsomal protein synthesis inhibition: An early manifestation of gentamicin nephrotoxicity. *Am. J. Physiol.* 255: F265, 1988.
26. Bennett, W. M., Parker, R. A., Elliott, W. C., Gilbert, D. N., and Houghton, D. C. Sex-related differences in the susceptibility of rats to gentamicin nephrotoxicity. *J. Infect. Dis.* 145: 370, 1982.
27. Bennett, W. M., Plamp, E. E., Elliott, W. C., Parker, R. A., and Porter, G. A. Effect of basic amino acids and aminoglycosides on [^{3}H]gentamicin cortical slices of rat and human kidneys. *J. Lab. Clin. Med.* 99: 156, 1982.
28. Bennett, W. M., Plamp, C. E., Gilbert, D. N., Parker, R. A., and Porter, G. A. The influence of dosage regimen on experimental nephrotoxicity: Dissociation of peak serum levels from renal failure. *J. Infect. Dis.* 140: 576, 1979.
29. Bennett, W. M., Plamp, C. E., Parker, R. A., Gilbert, D. N., Houghton, D. C., and Porter, G. A. Alterations in organic ion transport induced by gentamicin nephrotoxicity in the rat. *J. Lab. Clin. Med.* 95: 32, 1980.
30. Bennett, W. M., Pulliam, J. P., Porter, G. A., and Houghton, D. C. Modification of experimental gentamicin nephrotoxicity by selective parathyroidectomy. *Am. J. Physiol.* 249: F832, 1985.
31. Bergant, T., Westlie, L., and Brodwell, E. K. Influence of probenecid on gentamicin pharmacokinetics. *Acta Med. Scand.* 191: 221, 1972.
32. Bergeron, M. G., Marois, Y., Kuehn, C., and Silverblatt, F. J. Autoradiographic study of tobramycin uptake by proximal and distal tubules of normal and pyelonephritic rats. *Antimicrob. Agents Chemother.* 31: 1359, 1987.
33. Bernard, A., Viau, C., Ouled, A., Tulkens, P., and Lauwerys, R. Effects of gentamicin on the renal uptake of endogenous and exogenous proteins in conscious rats. *Toxicol. Appl. Pharmacol.* 84: 431, 1986.
34. Brasseur, R., Laurent, G., Raysschaert, J. M., and Tulkens, P. Interactions of aminoglycoside antibiotics with negatively charged lipid layers: Biochemical and conformational studies. *Biochem. Pharmacol.* 33: 629, 1984.
35. Brinker, K. R., Bulger, R. E., Dobyan, D. C., Stacey, T. R., Southern, P. M., Henrich, W. L., and Cronin, R. E. Effect of potassium depletion or gentamicin nephrotoxicity. *J. Lab. Clin. Med.* 98: 292, 1981.
36. Buldt, G., and Wohlgemuth, R. The head group conformation of phospholipids in membranes. *J. Membr. Biol.* 58: 81, 1981.
37. Buring, J. E., Denis, A. E., Mayrent, S. L., Rosner, B., Colton, T., and Hennekens, C. H. Randomized trials of aminoglycoside antibiotics: quantitative overview. *Rev. Infect. Dis.* 10: 951, 1988.
38. Buss, W. C., and Piatt, M. K. Gentamicin administered in vivo reduces protein synthesis in microsomes subsequently isolated from rat kidneys but not from rat brains. *J. Antimicrob. Chemother.* 15: 715, 1985.
39. Buss, W. C., Piatt, M. K., and Kauten, R. Inhibition of mammalian microsomal protein synthesis by aminoglycoside antibiotics. *J. Antimicrob. Chemother.* 14: 231, 1984.
40. Bygljerg, I. E., and Moller, R. Gentamicin-induced nephropathy. *Scand. J. Infect. Dis.* 8: 203, 1976.
41. Cabrera, J., Arroyo, V., Ballesta, A., Rimola, A., Gual, J., Elena, M., and Rodes, J. Aminoglycoside nephrotoxicity in cirrhosis. Value of urinary B_2-microglobulin to discriminate functional renal failure from acute tubular damage. *Gastroenterology* 82: 97, 1982.
42. Carlier, M. D., Laurent, G., Claes, P. J., Vanderhaeghe, H. J., and Tulkens, P. M. Inhibition of lysosomal phospholipases by aminoglycoside antibiotics: In vitro comparative studies. *Antimicrob. Agents Chemother.* 23: 440, 1983.
43. Carney, D. H., Scott, D. L., Gordon, E. A., and LaBelle, E. F. Phosphoinositides in mitogenesis: Neomycin inhibits thrombin-stimulated phosphoinositide turnover and initiation of cell proliferation. *Cell* 42: 479, 1985.
44. Carver, M. P., Shy-Modjeska, J. S., Brown, T. T., Rogers, R. A., and Riviere, J. E. Dose response studies of gen-

tamicin nephrotoxicity in rats with experimental renal dysfunction. *Toxicol. Appl. Pharmacol.* 80: 251, 1985.

45. Chahwala, S. B., and Harpur, E. S. An investigation of the effects of aminoglycoside antibiotics on Na^+-K^+ ATPase as a possible mechanism of toxicity. *Res. Commun. Chem. Pathol. Pharmacol.* 35: 63, 1982.
46. Chiu, P. J., Brown, A., Miller, G., and Long, J. F. Renal excretion of gentamicin in anesthetized dogs. *Antimicrob. Agents Chemother.* 10: 277, 1976.
47. Chiu, P. J. S., and Long, J. F. Effects of hydration on gentamicin excretion and renal accumulation in furosemide-treated rats. *Antimicrob. Agents Chemother.* 14: 214, 1978.
48. Chiu, P. J. S., and Long, J. F. Urinary excretion and tissue accumulation of gentamicin and para-aminohippurate in post-ischemic kidneys. *Kidney Int.* 15: 618, 1979.
49. Chiu, P. J. S., Miller, G. H., Long, J. F., and Waitz, J. A. Renal uptake and nephrotoxicity of gentamicin during urinary alkalinization in rats. *Clin. Exp. Pharmacol. Physiol.* 6: 317, 1979.
50. Chung, L., Kaloyanides, G., McDaniel, R., McLaughlin, A., and McLaughlin, S. Interaction of gentamicin and spermine with bilayer membranes containing negatively charged phospholipids. *Biochemistry* 24: 442, 1985.
51. Churchill, D. N., and Seeley, J. Nephrotoxicity associated with combined gentamicin-amphotericin B therapy. *Nephron* 19: 176, 1977.
52. Cockcroft, S., and Stutchfield, J. Effect of pertussis toxin and neomycin on G-protein-regulated polyphosphoinositide phosphodiesterase. *Biochem. J.* 256: 343, 1988.
53. Cohen, L., Lapkin, R., and Kaloganides, G. J. Effect of gentamicin on renal function in the rat. *J. Pharmacol. Exp. Ther.* 193: 264, 1975.
54. Cojocel, C., Docin, N., Maita, K., Sleight, S. D., and Hook, J. B. Effects of aminoglycosides on glomerular permeability, tubular reabsorption and intracellular catabolism of the cationic low-molecular-weight protein lysozyme. *Toxicol. Appl. Pharmacol.* 68: 96, 1983.
55. Collier, V. U., Lietman, P. S., and Mitch, W. E. Evidence for luminal uptake of gentamicin in the perfused rat kidney. *J. Pharmacol. Exp. Ther.* 210: 247, 1979.
56. Corcoran, G. B., and Salazar, D. E. Obesity as a risk factor in drug-induced organ injury. IV. Increased gentamicin nephrotoxicity in the obese overfed rat. *J. Pharmacol. Exp. Ther.* 248: 17, 1989.
57. Corcoran, G. B., Salazar, D. E., and Schentag, J. J. Excessive aminoglycoside nephrotoxicity in obese patients. *Am. J. Med.* 85: 279, 1988.
58. Cronin, R., Inman, L., Eche, T., Southern, P., and Griggs, M. Effect of thyroid hormone on gentamicin accumulation in rat proximal tubule lysosomes. *Am. J. Physiol.* 257: F86, 1989.
59. Cronin, R. E., Bulger, R. E., Southern, P., and Henrich, W. C. Natural history of aminoglycoside nephrotoxicity in the dog. *J. Lab. Clin. Med.* 95: 463, 1980.
60. Cronin, R. E., and Newman, J. A. Protective effect of thyroxine but not parathyroidectomy on gentamicin nephrotoxicity. *Am. J. Physiol.* 248: F332, 1985.
61. Cronin, R. E., Nix, K. L., Ferguson, E. R., Southern, P. M., and Henrick, W. L. Renal cortex ion composition and Na-K-ATPase activity in gentamicin nephrotoxicity. *Am. J. Physiol.* 242: F477, 1982.
62. Cronin, R. E., Splinter, K. L., Ferguson, E. R., and Henrich, W. C. Gentamicin nephrotoxicity: Protective effect of diabetes on cell injury. *Mineral Electrolyte Metab.* 9: 38, 1983.
63. Cuppage, F. E., Setter, K., Sullivan, L. P., Reitzes, E., and Melnykovych, A. Gentamicin nephrotoxicity. II. Physiological, biochemical, and morphological effects of prolonged administration to rats. *Virchows Arch. B [Cell Pathol.]* 234: 121, 1977.
64. Daschner, F. D., Just, A. M., Jansen, W., and Lorber, R. Netilmicin versus tobramycin in multicentre studies. *J. Antimicrob. Chemother.* 13(A): 37, 1984.
65. DeBroe, M. E., Giuliano, R. A., and Verpooten, G. A. Choice of drug and dosage regimen. *Am. J. Med.* 80(Suppl. 63): 115, 1986.
66. DeBroe, M. E., Paulus, G. J., Verprooten, G. A., Roels, F., Buyssens, N., Weeden, R., VanHoot, F., and Tulkens, P. M. Early effects of gentamicin, tobramycin and amikacin on the human kidney. *Kidney Int.* 25: 643, 1984.

66a. Druery, C. J., and Dawson, A. G. Inhibition of respiration by phenacetin in isolated tubules and mitochondria of rat kidney. *Biochem. Pharmacol.* 28: 57, 1979.

67. Dunst, J., Lullmann, H., and Mohr, K. Influence of cationic amphiphilic drugs on the characteristics of ouabain-binding to cardiac Na^+/K^+-ATPase. *Biochem. Pharmacol.* 32: 1595, 1983.
68. Eisenberg, J. M., Koffer, H., Glick, H. A., Connell, M. L., Loss, L. E., Talbot, G. H., Shusterman, N. H., and Strom, B. L. What is the cost of nephrotoxicity associated with aminoglycosides? *Ann. Intern. Med.* 107: 900, 1987.
69. Elliott, W. C., Houghton, D. C., Gilbert, D. N., Baines-Hunter, J., and Bennett, W. N. Gentamicin nephrotoxicity. I. Degree and permanence of acquired insensitivity. *J. Lab. Clin. Med.* 100: 501, 1982.
70. Elliott, W. C., Houghton, D. C., Gilbert, D. N., Baines-Hunter, J., and Bennett, W. M. Gentamicin nephrotoxicity. II. Definition of conditions necessary to induce acquired insensitivity. *J. Lab. Clin. Med.* 100: 513, 1982.
71. Elliott, W. C., Houghton, D. C., Gilbert, D. N., Baines-Hunter, J., and Bennett, W. M. Experimental gentamicin nephrotoxicity: Effect of streptozotocin-induced diabetes. *J. Pharmacol. Exp. Ther.* 233: 264, 1985.
72. Elliott, W. C., Parker, R. A., Houghton, D. C., Gilbert, D. N., Porter, G. A., DeFehr, J., and Bennett, W. M. Effect of sodium bicarbonate and ammonium chloride ingestion in experimental gentamicin nephrotoxicity. *Res. Commun. Chem. Pathol. Pharmacol.* 28: 483, 1980.
73. Elliott, W. C., Patchin, D. S., and Jones, D. B. Effect of parathyroid hormone activity on gentamicin nephrotoxicity. *J. Lab. Clin. Med.* 109: 48, 1987.
74. Engineer, M. S., Brown, N. S., Ho, D. H. W., Newman, R. A., and Bulger, R. E. A comparison of the effects of tetraplatin and cisplatin on renal function and gentamicin pharmacology in rats. *Toxicology* 59: 151, 1989.
75. EORTC International Antimicrobial Therapy Project Group. Three antibiotic regimens in the treatment of infection in febrile granulocytopenic patients with cancer. *J. Infect. Dis.* 137: 14, 1978.
76. Eustice, D. C., and Wilhelm, J. M. Fidelity of the eukaryotic codon-anticodon interaction: Interference by aminoglycoside antibiotics. *Biochemistry* 23: 1462, 1984.
77. Fabre, J., Rudhardt, M., Blanchard, P., and Regamey, C. Persistence of sisomicin and gentamicin in renal cortex and medulla compared with other organs and serum of rats. *Kidney Int.* 10: 444, 1976.
78. Farrington, R. F., Hull-Smith, H., Bunn, P. A., and McDermott, W. Streptomycin toxicity. *J.A.M.A.* 134: 679, 1947.
79. Feinfeld, D. A., Fleischner, G. M., and Arias, I. M. Urinary ligandin and glutathione-5-transferase in gentami-

cin-induced nephrotoxicity in the rat. *Clin. Sci.* 61: 123, 1981.

80. Feldman, S., Wang, M., and Kaloyanides, G. J. Aminoglycosides induce a phospholipidosis in the renal cortex of the rat: An early manifestation of nephrotoxicity. *J. Pharmacol. Exp. Ther.* 220: 514, 1982.
81. Fiekers, J. F. Effects of the aminoglycoside antibiotics, streptomycin and neomycin on neuromuscular transmission. I. Presynaptic considerations. *J. Pharmacol. Exp. Ther.* 225: 487, 1983.
81a. Ford, D. M., Dahl, R. H., Weng, C. A., and Molitoris, B. A. Simultaneous apical and basolateral (BLM) aminoglycoside uptake: quantification and localization within the endosomal compartment of LLC-PK_1 cells. *JASN* (In press).
82. Fowler, B. A., and Brooks, R. E. Effects of the herbicide paraquat on the ultrastructure of mouse kidney. *Am. J. Pathol.* 63: 62, 1971.
83. Frazier, D. L., Dix, L. P., Bowman, K. F., Thompson, C., and Riviere, J. E. Increased gentamicin nephrotoxicity in normal and diseased dogs administered identical serum drug concentration profiles: Increased sensitivity in subclinical renal dysfunction. *J. Pharmacol. Exp. Ther.* 239: 946, 1986.
84. Frommer, J. P., Senekjian, H. O., Babino, H., and Weinman, E. J. Intratubular microinjection study of gentamicin transport in the rat. *Mineral Electrolyte Metab.* 9: 108, 1983.
85. Gary, N. E., Buzzeo, L., Salaki, G., and Eisinger, R. P. Gentamicin-associated acute renal failure. *Arch. Intern. Med.* 136: 1101, 1976.
86. Gatell, J. M., San Miguel, J. G., Zamona, L., Araujo, V., Bonet, M., Bohe, M., Jiminez de Anta, M. T., Farre, M., Elena, M., Ballestra, A., and Marin, J. L. Comparison of nephrotoxicity and auditory toxicity of tobramycin and amikacin. *Antimicrob. Agents Chemother.* 23: 897, 1983.
87. Gaver, E., Kasianowicz, J., Abbott, T., and McLaughlin, S. Binding of neomycin to phosphatidylinositol 4,5-bisphosphate (PIP_2). *Biochim. Biophys. Acta* 979: 105, 1989.
87a. Geerdes, A., Dahl, R. H., Meger, C., Weng, C., and Molitoris, B. A. Cellular mechanism of adaptation to long term gentamicin (LTG) administration. *J.A.S.N.*, in press.
88. Gibey, R., Dupond, J.-L., Alber, D., Des Floris, R. L., and Henry, J.-C. Predictive value of urinary N-acetyl-beta-glucosaminidase (NAG), alanine-aminopeptidase (AAP) and beta-2-microglobulin (B_2M) in evaluating nephrotoxicity of gentamicin. *Clin. Chem. Acta* 116: 24, 1981.
89. Gilbert, D. N., Wood, C. A., Kohlhepper, S. J., Kohnen, P. W., Houghton, D. C., Finkbeiner, H. C., Lindsley, J., and Bennett, W. M. Polyaspartic acid prevents experimental aminoglycoside nephrotoxicity. *J. Infect. Dis.* 159: 945, 1989.
90. Ginsburg, D. S., Quintanilla, A. P., and Levin, M. Renal glycosuria due to gentamicin in rabbits. *J. Infect. Dis.* 134: 119, 1976.
91. Giuliano, R. A., Paulus, G. J., Verpooten, G. A., Pattyn, U. M., Pollet, D. E., Nouwen, E. J., Laurent, G., Carlier, M. B., Maldogue, P., Tulkens, P. M., and DeBroe, M. E. Recovery of cortical phospholipidosis and necrosis after acute gentamicin loading in rats. *Kidney Int.* 26: 838, 1984.
92. Giuliano, R. A., Verpooten, G. A., and DeBroe, M. E. The effect of dosing strategy on kidney cortical accumulation of aminoglycosides in rats. *Am. J. Kidney Dis.* 8: 297, 1986.
93. Giuliano, R. A., Verpooten, G. A., Verbist, L., Wedeen, R. P., and DeBroe, M. E. In vivo uptake kinetics of aminoglycosides in the kidney cortex of rats. *J. Pharmacol. Exp. Ther.* 236: 470, 1986.
94. Giurgea-Marion, L., Toubeau, G., Heuson-Stiennon, J. A., and Tulkens, P. M. Impairment of lysosome-pinocytic vesicle fusion in rat kidney proximal tubules after treatment with gentamicin at low doses. *Toxicol. Appl. Pharmacol.* 86: 271, 1986.
95. Glaumann, B., and Trump, B. F. Studies on the pathogenesis of ischemic cell injury. III. Morphological changes of the proximal pars recta tubules of the rat kidney made ischemic in vivo. *Virchows Arch.* [*B*] 19: 303, 1975.
96. Gomez, A., Martos, F., Garcia, R., Perez, B., and de la Cuesta, S. Diltiazem enhances gentamicin nephrotoxicity in rats. *Pharmacol. Toxicol.* 64: 190, 1989.
97. Goodman, F. G., Adams, H. R., and Weiss, G. B. Effects of neomycin on ^{45}Ca binding and distribution in canine arteries. *Blood Vessels* 12: 248, 1975.
98. Green, D. E., Fry, M., and Blondin, G. A. Phospholipids as the molecular instruments of ion and solute transport in biological membranes. *Proc. Natl. Acad. Sci. U.S.A.* 77: 257, 1980.
99. Gyselynck, A. M., Forey, A., and Cutlet, R. Pharmacokinetics of gentamicin: Distribution and plasma and renal clearance. *J. Infect. Dis.* 124: S70, 1971.
100. Hansen, M. M., and Kaaber, K. Nephrotoxicity of combined cephalothin and gentamicin therapy. *Acta Med. Scand.* 201: 463, 1977.
101. Hashimoto, H., Yanagisawa, T., and Taira, N. Differential antagonism of the negative inotropic effect of gentamicin by calcium ions, Bay K 8644 and isoprenaline in canine ventricular muscle: Comparison with cobalt ions. *Br. J. Pharmacol.* 96: 906, 1989.
102. Hewitt, W. L. Reflections on the clinical pharmacology of gentamicin. *Acta Pathol. Microbiol. Immunol. Scand. (B)* 82(Suppl. 241): 151, 1973.
103. Hirota, F., and Axelrod, J. Phospholipid methylation and biological signal transmission. *Science* 209: 1082, 1980.
104. Hirsch, G. H. Differential effects of nephrotoxic agents on renal organic ion transport and metabolism. *J. Pharmacol. Exp. Ther.* 186: 593, 1973.
105. Hirsch, G. H. Enhancement of gentamicin nephrotoxicity by glycerol. *Toxicol. Appl. Pharmacol.* 29: 270, 1974.
106. Hostetler, K. Y., and Hall, L. B. Inhibition of kidney lysosomal phospholipases A and C by aminoglycoside antibiotics: Possible mechanism of aminoglycoside toxicity. *Proc. Natl. Acad. Sci. U.S.A.* 79: 1663, 1982.
107. Houghton, D. C., English, J., and Bennett, W. M. Chronic tubulointerstitial nephritis and renal insufficiency associated with long-term "subtherapeutic" gentamicin. *J. Lab. Clin. Med.* 112: 694, 1988.
108. Houghton, D. C., Hartnett, M., Campbell-Boswell, M., Porter, G., and Bennett, W. A light and electron microscopic analysis of gentamicin nephrotoxicity in rats. *Am. J. Pathol.* 82: 589, 1976.
109. Houghton, D. C., Lee, D., Gilbert, D. M., and Bennett, W. M. Chronic gentamicin nephrotoxicity; Continued tubular injury with preserved glomerular filtrated function. *Am. J. Pathol.* 123: 183, 1986.
110. Hruban, Z., Slessers, A., and Hopkins, E. Drug induced and naturally occurring myeloid bodies. *Lab. Invest.* 27: 62, 1972.
111. Hsu, C. H., Kurtz, T. W., and Weller, J. M. In vitro uptake of gentamicin by rat renal cortical tissue. *Antimicrob. Agents Chemother.* 12: 192, 1977.

112. Humes, H. D., Sastrasinh, M., and Weinberg, J. M. Calcium is a competitive inhibitor of gentamicin-renal membrane binding interactions and dietary calcium supplementation protects against gentamicin nephrotoxicity. *J. Clin. Invest.* 73: 134, 1984.
113. Humes, H. D., and Weinberg, J. M. The effect of gentamicin on antidiuretic hormone-stimulated osmotic water flow in the toad urinary bladder. *J. Lab. Clin. Med.* 101: 472, 1983.
114. Inui, K., Saito, H., Iwata, T., and Hori, R. Aminoglycoside-induced alterations in apical membranes of kidney epithelial cell line. *Am. J. Physiol.* 254: C251, 1988.
115. Jerauld, R., and Silverblatt, F. J. Effect of *N*-methylnicotinamide on the renal accumulation and reabsorption of gentamicin in rats. *Antimicrob. Agents Chemother.* 13: 893, 1978.
116. Josepovitz, C., Farruggella, T., Levine, R., Lane, B., and Kaloyanides, G. J. Effect of netilmicin on the phospholipid composition of subcellular fractions of rat renal cortex. *J. Pharmacol. Exp. Ther.* 235: 810, 1985.
117. Josepovitz, C., Levine, R., Farruggella, T., and Kaloyanides, G. J. Comparative effects of aminoglycosides on renal cortical and urinary phospholipids in the rat. *Proc. Soc. Exp. Biol. Med.* 182: 1, 1986.
118. Josepovitz, C., Levine, R., Farruggella, T., Lane, B., and Kaloyanides, G. J. [^{3}H]Netilmicin binding constants and phospholipid composition of renal plasma membranes of normal and diabetic rats. *J. Pharmacol. Exp. Ther.* 233: 298, 1985.
119. Josepovitz, C., Levine, R., Lane, B., and Kaloyanides, G. J. Contrasting effects of gentamicin and mercuric chloride on urinary excretion of enzymes and phospholipids in the rat. *Lab. Invest.* 52: 275, 1985.
120. Josepovitz, C., Pastoriza-Munoz, E., Timmerman, D., Scott, M., Feldman, S., and Kaloyanides, G. J. Inhibition of gentamicin uptake in rat renal cortex in vivo by aminoglycosides and organic polycations. *J. Pharmacol. Exp. Ther.* 223: 314, 1982.
121. Just, M., Erdmann, G., and Habermann, E. The renal handling of polybasic drugs. 1. Gentamicin and aprotinin in intact animals. *Naunyn Schmiedebergs Arch. Pharmacol.* 300: 57, 1977.
122. Just, M., and Habermann, E. The renal handling of polybasic drugs. 2. In vitro studies with brush border and lysosomal preparation. *Naunyn Schmiedebergs Arch. Pharmacol.* 300: 67, 1977.
123. Kacew, S. Cationic amphiphilic drug induced renal cortical lysosomal phospholipidosis: An in vivo comparative study with gentamicin and chlorphentermine. *Toxicol. Appl. Pharmacol.* 91: 469, 1987.
124. Kacew, S. Inhibition of gentamicin-induced nephrotoxicity by pyridoxal-5′-phosphate in the rat. *J. Pharmacol. Exp. Ther.* 248: 360, 1989.
125. Kacew, S., and Narbaitz, R. The effect of phenobarbitol on chlorphentermine-induced lipidosis-like alterations in renal tissue of adult and newborn rats. *Virchows Arch. B [Cell Pathol.]* 36: 59, 1981.
126. Kahlmeter, G., and Dahlager, J. Aminoglycoside toxicity—A review of clinical studies published between 1975 and 1982. *J. Antimicrob. Chemother.* 13: 9A, 1984.
127. Kaloyanides, G. J. Aminoglycoside-induced functional and biochemical defects in the renal cortex. *Fund. Appl. Toxicol.* 4: 930, 1984.
128. Kaloyanides, G. J., and Pastoriza-Munoz, E. Aminoglycoside nephrotoxicity. *Kidney Int.* 18: 571, 1980.
129. Kaloyanides, G. J., and Ramsammy, L. S. Alterations of Biophysical Properties of Liposomes Predict Aminoglycoside Toxicity: Inhibitory Effect of Polyaspartic Acid. In P. H. Bach, L. Delacrey, N. J. Gregg, and M. F. Wilks (eds.), *Proceedings of the Fourth International Symposium on Nephrotoxicity.* New York: Marcel Dekker, 1990. P. 109.
130. Kaloyanides, G. J., Ramsammy, L., and Josepovitz, C. Assessment of Three Therapeutic Interventions for Modifying Gentamicin Nephrotoxicity in the Rat. In P. H. Bach, L. Delacruz, N. J. Gregg, and M. F. Wilks (eds.), *Proceedings of the Fourth International Symposium of Nephrotoxicity.* New York: Marcel Dekker, 1990. P. 91.
131. Kaloyanides, G. J., Ramsammy, L., and Josepovitz, C. Assessment of Three Therapeutic Interventions for Modifying Gentamicin Nephrotoxicity in the Rat. In P. H. Bach, L. Delacruz, N. J. Gregg, and M. F. Wilks (eds.), *Proceedings of the Fourth International Symposium of Nephrotoxicity.* New York: Marcel Dekker, 1990. P. 103.
132. Kane, A. B., Stanton, R. P., Raymond, E. G., Dobson, M. E., Knafelo, M., and Farber, J. Dissociation of intracellular lysosomal rupture from cell death caused by silica. *J. Cell. Biol.* 87: 643, 1980.
133. Kardos, N., Eicholtz, A., and Schaffner, C. P. Binding of aminocyclitol antibiotics to kidney and intestinal brush border membranes. *J. Antibiot. (Tokyo)* 34: 103, 1981.
134. Katz, S. M., Sufian, S., and Matsumoto, T. Urinary myelin figures in gentamicin nephrotoxicity. *Am. J. Clin. Pathol.* 72: 621, 1979.
135. Kawamura, J., Soedu, A., and Yoshida, O. Nephrotoxicity of cis-diamendichloroplatinum (II) (cis-platinum) and the additive effect of antibiotics: Morphological and functional observations in rats. *Toxicol. Appl. Pharmacol.* 58: 475, 1981.
136. Kaye, W. A., Griffiths, W. C., Camara, P. D., Trebbin, W. M., Solomon, R. J., and Diamond, I. The significance of β-2 microglobulinemia associated with gentamicin therapy. *Ann. Clin. Lab. Sci.* 11: 530, 1981.
137. Kessler, R. J., Tyson, C. A., and Green, D. E. Mechanism of uncoupling in mitochondria: Uncouplers as ionophores for cycling cations and protons. *Proc. Natl. Acad. Sci. U.S.A.* 73: 3141, 1976.
138. Kimmelberg, H. K., and Papahadjopoulos, D. Interactions of basic proteins with phospholipid membranes. *J. Biol. Chem.* 246: 1142, 1971.
139. Kirschbaum, B. B. Interactions between renal brush border membranes and polyamines. *J. Pharmacol. Exp. Ther.* 229: 409, 1984.
140. Kishore, B. K., Kallay, Z., Lambricht, P., Laurent, G., and Tulkens, P. M. Mechanism of protection afforded by polyaspartic acid against gentamicin-induced phospholipidosis. I. Polyaspartic acid binds gentamicin and displaces it from negatively charged phospholipid layers in vitro. *J. Pharmacol. Exp. Ther.* 255: 867, 1990.
141. Kishore, B. K., Lambricht, P., Laurent, B., Maldague, P., Wagner, R., and Tulkens, P. M. Mechanism of protection afforded by polyaspartic acid against gentamicin-induced phospholipidosis. II. Comparative in vitro and in vivo studies with poly-L-glutamic acids. *J. Pharmacol. Exp. Ther.* 255: 875, 1990.
142. Klotman, P. E., Boatman, J. E., Volpp, B. D., Baker, J. D., and Yarger, W. E. Captopril enhances aminoglycoside nephrotoxicity in potassium-depleted rats. *Kidney Int.* 28: 118, 1985.
143. Kluwe, W. M., and Hook, J. B. Analysis of gentamicin uptake by rat renal cortical slices. *Toxicol. Appl. Pharmacol.* 45: 531, 1978.
144. Kluwe, W. M., and Hook, J. B. Functional nephrotoxicity of gentamicin in the rat. *Toxicol. Appl. Pharmacol.* 45: 163, 1978.

145. Knauss, T. C., Weinberg, J. M., and Humes, H. D. Alterations in renal cortical phospholipid content induced by gentamicin: Time course, specificity and subcellular localization. *Am. J. Physiol.* 244: F535, 1983.
146. Kojima, R., Ito, M., and Suzuki, Y. Studies on the nephrotoxicity of aminoglycoside antibiotics and protection from these effects (3): Protective effect of latamoxef against tobramycin nephrotoxicity and its protective mechanism. *Jpn. J. Pharmacol.* 42: 397, 1986.
147. Kojima, R., Ito, M., and Suzuki, Y. Studies on the nephrotoxicity of aminoglycoside antibiotics and protection from these effects (8): Protective effect of pyridoxal-5'-phosphate against tobramycin nephrotoxicity. *Jpn. J. Pharmacol.* 52: 11, 1990.
148. Kojima, R., Ito, M., and Suzuki, Y. Studies on the nephrotoxicity of aminoglycoside antibiotics and protection from these effects (9): Protective effect of inositol hexasulfate against tobramycin-induced nephrotoxicity. *Jpn. J. Pharmacol.* 53: 347, 1990.
149. Kourilsky, O., Solez, K., Morel-Maroger, L., Whelton, A., Duhoux, P., and Sraer, J. D. The pathology of acute renal failure due to interstitial nephritis in man, with comments on the role of interstitial inflammation and sex in gentamicin nephrotoxicity. *Medicine* 61: 258, 1982.
150. Kozek, J. C., Mazze, R. I., and Cousins, M. J. Nephrotoxicity of gentamicin. *Lab. Invest.* 30: 48, 1974.
151. Kuhar, M. J., Mark, L. L., and Lietman, P. S. Autoradiographic localization of [^{3}H]gentamicin in the proximal renal tubules of mice. *Antimicrob. Agents Chemother.* 15: 131, 1979.
152. Kumin, G. D. Clinical nephrotoxicity of tobramycin and gentamicin: A prospective study. *J.A.M.A.* 244: 1808, 1980.
153. Kuo, C. H., and Hook, J. B. Specificity of gentamicin accumulation by rat renal cortex. *Life Sci.* 25: 873, 1979.
154. Lane, A. Z., Wright, G. E., and Blair, D. C. Ototoxicity and nephrotoxicity of amikacin. *Am. J. Med.* 62: 911, 1977.
155. Lapkin, R., Bowman, R., and Kaloyanides, G. J. Effects of gentamicin on PAH metabolism and transport in rat kidney slices. *J. Pharmacol. Exp. Ther.* 201: 233, 1977.
156. Laurent, G., Carlier, M. B., Rollman, B., VanHoop, F., and Tulkens, P. Mechanism of aminoglycoside-induced lysosomal phospholipidosis: In vitro and in vivo studies with gentamicin and amikacin. *Biochem. Pharmacol.* 31: 3861, 1982.
157. Laurent, G., Kishore, B. K., and Tulkens, P. M. Aminoglycoside-induced renal phospholipidosis and nephrotoxicity. *Biochem. Pharmacol.* 40: 2383, 1990.
158. Laurent, G., Maldague, P., Carlier, M. D., and Tulkens, P. M. Increased renal DNA synthesis in vivo after administration of low doses of gentamicin to rats. *Antimicrob. Agents Chemother.* 24: 586, 1983.
159. Laurent, G., Toubeau, G., Heuson-Stiennon, J. A., Tulkens, P., and Maldague, P. Kidney tissue repair after nephrotoxic injury: Biochemical and morphological characterization. *CRC Crit. Rev. Toxicol.* 19: 147, 1988.
160. Lecompte, J., Dumont, L., Hill, J., de Souich, P., and Lelorier, J. Effect of water deprivation and rehydration on gentamicin disposition in the rat. *J. Pharmacol. Exp. Ther.* 218: 231, 1981.
161. Lee, S. M., and Michael, V. F. The protective effect of nitrendipine on gentamicin acute renal failure in rats. *Exp. Mol. Pathol.* 43: 107, 1985.
162. Lerner, A. M., Cone, L. A., Jansen, W., Reyes, M. P., Blair, D. C., Wright, G. E., and Lorber, R. R. Randomized, controlled trial of the comparative efficacy, auditory toxicity and nephrotoxicity of tobramycin and netilmicin. *Lancet* 1: 1123, 1983.
163. Lerner, S. A., Seligsohn, R., and Matz, G. J. Comparative clinical studies of ototoxicity and nephrotoxicity of amikacin and gentamicin. *Am. J. Med.* 62: 919, 1977.
164. Levi, M., and Cronin, R. E. Early selective effects of gentamicin on renal brush-border membrane Na-Pi cotransport and Na-H exchange. *Am. J. Physiol.* 258: F1379, 1990.
165. Lietman, P. S., and Smith, C. R. Aminoglycoside nephrotoxicity in humans. *Rev. Infect. Dis.* 5: S284, 1983.
166. Lipsky, J. J., Cheng, L., Sacktor, B., and Lietman, P. S. Gentamicin uptake by renal tubule brush border membrane vesicles. *J. Pharmacol. Exp. Ther.* 215: 390, 1980.
167. Lipsky, J. J., and Lietman, P. S. Neomycin inhibition of adenosine triphosphatase: Evidence for a neomycin-phospholipid interaction. *Antimicrob. Agents Chemother.* 18: 532, 1980.
168. Lipsky, J. J., and Lietman, P. S. Aminoglycoside inhibition of a renal phosphotidylinositol phospholipase C. *J. Pharmacol. Exp. Ther.* 220: 287, 1982.
169. Lucena, M. I., Gonzalez-Correa, A., Andrade, R. J., Ibanez, J., Torres, D., and Sanchez de la Cuesta, F. Enhanced gentamicin nephrotoxicity after experimental biliary obstruction in rats. *Pharmacol. Toxicol.* 65: 352, 1989.
170. Luft, F. C. Cephalosporin and Aminoglycoside Interactions: Clinical and Toxicological Implications. In A. Whelton and H. C. Neu (eds.), *The Aminoglycosides.* New York: Marcel Dekker, 1982. P. 387.
171. Luft, F. C. Clinical significance of renal changes engendered by aminoglycosides in man. *J. Antimicrob. Chemother.* 13(Suppl. A): 23, 1984.
172. Luft, F. C., Aronoff, G. R., Evan, A. P., Connors, B. A., Weinberger, M. H., and Kleit, S. A. The renin-angiotensin system in aminoglycoside-induced acute renal failure. *J. Pharmacol. Exp. Ther.* 20: 443, 1982.
173. Luft, F. C., Bloch, R., Sloan, R. S., Yum, M. N., Costello, R., and Maxwell, D. R. Comparative nephrotoxicity of aminoglycoside antibiotics in rats. *J. Infect. Dis.* 138: 541, 1978.
174. Luft, F. C., and Kleit, S. A. Renal parenchymal accumulation of aminoglycoside antibiotics in rats. *J. Infect. Dis.* 130: 656, 1974.
175. Luft, F. C., Yum, M. N., and Kleit, S. A. The effect of concomitant mercuric chloride and gentamicin on kidney function and structure in the rat. *J. Lab. Clin. Med.* 89: 622, 1977.
176. Lullmann, H., and Vollmer, B. An interaction of aminoglycoside antibiotics with Ca binding to lipid monolayers and to biomembranes. *Biochem. Pharmacol.* 31: 3769, 1982.
177. Lullmann-Rauch, R. Drug-Induced Lysosomal Storage Disorders. In J. T. Dingle, P. J. Jacques, and I. H. Shaw (eds.), *Lysosomes in Applied Biology and Therapeutics.* Amsterdam: North Holland, 1979. P. 49.
178. Mandel, A. K., and Bennett, W. M. Transmission electron microscopy of urinary sediment in the assessment of aminoglycoside nephrotoxicity in the rat. *Nephron* 49: 67, 1988.
179. Marche, P., Koutouzov, S., and Girard, A. Impairment of membrane phosphoinositide metabolism by aminoglycoside antibiotics: Streptomycin, amikacin, kanamycin, dibekacin, gentamicin and neomycin. *J. Pharmacol. Exp. Ther.* 227: 415, 1983.

180. Marche, P., Koutouzov, S., and Meyer, P. Metabolism of phosphoinositides in the rat erythrocyte membrane. A reappraisal of the effect of magnesium on the ^{32}P incorporation into polyphosphoinositides. *Biochim. Biophys. Acta* 710: 332, 1982.
181. Marche, P., Olier, B., Girard, A., Fillastre, J. P., and Morin, J. P. Aminoglycoside-induced alteration of phosphoinositide metabolism. *Kidney Int.* 31: 59, 1987.
182. Marra, R., Tarara, N., Louton, T., and Sack, K. Age-dependent nephrotoxicity and the pharmacokinetics of gentamicin in rats. *Eur. J. Pediatr.* 133: 25, 1980.
183. Martinez-Molina, J. L., del Ponzo, E., and Baeyens, J. M. Increase by verapamil and diltiazem of gentamicin-induced acute toxicity in mice. *Med. Sci. Res.* 15: 1293, 1987.
184. Martinez-Molina, J. L., del Pozo, E., and Baeyens, J. M. Antagonism by calcium and the calcium channel stimulant Bay K 8644 of gentamicin-induced acute toxicity in mice. *Med. Sci. Res.* 16: 815, 1988.
185. Matsuzawa, Y., and Hostettler, K. Y. Studies on drug-induced lipidosis: Subcellular localization of phospholipid and cholesterol in the liver of rats treated with chloroquine or 4,4′-bis(diethylaminoethoxy)-α,β diethyldiphenylethane. *J. Lipid Res.* 21: 202, 1980.
186. Matsuzawa, Y., and Hostettler, K. Y. Inhibition of lysosomal phospholipase A and phospholipase C by chloroquine and 4,4′-bis(diethylaminoethoxy)-α,β-diethyldiphenylethane. *J. Biol. Chem.* 255: 5190, 1980.
187. McDowell, E. M., Nagle, R. B., Zalme, R. C., McNeil, J. S., Flamenbaum, W., and Trump, B. F. Studies on the pathophysiology of acute renal failure: I. Correlation of ultrastructure and function in the proximal tubule of the rat following administration of mercuric chloride. *Virchows Arch. [B]* 22: 173, 1976.
188. McMartin, D. N., and Engle, S. G. Effect of aging on gentamicin nephrotoxicity and pharmacokinetics in rats. *Res. Commun. Chem. Pathol. Pharmacol.* 38: 193, 1982.
189. Meisner, H. Effect of gentamicin on the subcellular distribution of renal β-A-acetylglucosaminidase activity. *Biochem. Pharmacol.* 30: 2949, 1981.
190. Mela-Riker, L. M., Widener, L. L., Houghton, D. C., and Bennett, W. M. Renal mitochondrial integrity during continuous gentamicin treatment. *Biochem. Pharmacol.* 35: 979, 1986.
191. Meyers, D. R., De Fehr, J., Bennett, W. M., Porter, G. A., and Olsen, G. D. Gentamicin binding to serum and plasma proteins. *Clin. Pharmacol. Ther.* 23: 356, 1978.
192. Michell, R. H. Inositol phospholipids and cell surface receptor function. *Biochim. Biophys. Acta* 415: 81, 1975.
193. Mingeot-Leclercq, M. P., Laurent, G., and Tulkens, P. M. Biochemical mechanism of aminoglycoside-induced inhibition of phosphatidylcholine hydrolysis by lysosomal phospholipases. *Biochem. Pharmacol.* 37: 591, 1988.
194. Mingeot-Leclercq, M. P., Piret, J., Brasseur, R., and Tulkens, P. M. Effect of acidic phospholipids on the activity of lysosomal phospholipases and on their inhibition by aminoglycoside antibiotics—I. *Biochem. Pharmacol.* 40: 489, 1990.
195. Mingeot-Leclercq, M. P., Schanck, A., Ronvaux-Dupal, M. F., Deleers, M., Brasseur, R., Ruys-Schaert, J. M., Laurent, G., and Tulkens, P. M. Ultrastructural physicochemical and conformational study of the interactions of gentamicin and bis (beta-diethylaminoethylether) hexestrol with negatively-charged phospholipid layers. *Biochem. Pharmacol.* 38: 728, 1989.
196. Mitchell, C. J., Bullock, S., and Ross, B. D. Renal handling of gentamicin and other antibiotics by the isolated perfused rat kidney: Mechanism of nephrotoxicity. *J. Antimicrob. Chemother.* 3: 593, 1977.
197. Moench, T. R., and Smith, C. R. Risk Factors for Aminoglycoside Nephrotoxicity. In A. Whelton and H. C. Neu (eds.), *The Aminoglycosides.* New York: Marcel Dekker, 1982. P. 401.
198. Mondorf, A. W., Breier, J., Handus, J., Scherberich, J. E., Mackenrodt, G., Shah, P., Stille, W., and Schieppe, W. Effect of aminoglycosides on proximal tubular membranes of the human kidney. *Eur. J. Clin. Pharmacol.* 13: 133, 1978.
199. Moore, R. D., Smith, C. R., Lipsky, T. J., Mellits, E. D., and Lietman, P. S. Risk factors for nephrotoxicity in patients treated with aminoglycosides. *Ann. Intern. Med.* 100: 352, 1984.
200. Morigama, T., Nakahama, H., Fukahara, Y., Horio, M., Yanase, M., Orita, Y., Ramada, T., Kanashiro, M., and Miyake, Y. Decrease in the fluidity of brush-border membrane vesicles induced by gentamicin. A spin-labelling study. *Biochem. Pharmacol.* 38: 1169, 1989.
201. Morin, J. P., Fresel, J., Fillastre, J.-P. and Vaillant, R. Aminoglycoside actions on rat kidney lysosomes in vivo and in vitro. In J.-P. Fillastre (ed.), *Nephrotoxicity.* New York: Masson, 1978. P. 253.
202. Morin, J. P., Viotte, G., Vandemolle, A., Van Hoot, F., Tulkens, P., and Fillastre, J. P. Gentamicin-induced nephrotoxicity: A cell biology approach. *Kidney Int.* 18: 583, 1980.
203. Nadler, S., and Goldfischer, S. The intracellular release of lysosomal contents in macrophages that have ingested silica. *J. Histochem. Cytochem.* 18: 368, 1970.
204. Nagabhushan, T., Miller, G., and Weinstein, M. Structure-Activity Relationships in Aminocyclitol-Aminoglycoside Antibiotics. In A. Whelton and H. Neu (eds.), *The Aminoglycosides.* New York: Marcel Dekker, 1982.
205. Nakahama, H., Fukahara, Y., Orita, Y., Yamauchi, A., Takama, T., and Kamada, T. Furosemide accelerates gentamicin accumulation in cultured renal cells (LLC-PK_1 cells). *Nephron* 53: 138, 1989.
206. Nedden, R., Fuchs, T., Schroder, K., and Wundt, W. Die renale Ausscheidung von Gentamicin beim Menschen. *Dtsch. Med. Wochenschr.* 97: 1496, 1972.
207. Neu, H. C. Pharmacology of Aminoglycosides. In A. Whelton and H. C. Neu (eds.), *The Aminoglycosides.* New York: Marcel Dekker, 1982.
208. Neugarten, J., Aynedjian, H. S., and Bank, N. Role of tubular obstruction in acute renal failure due to gentamicin. *Kidney Int.* 24: 330, 1983.
209. Neuhaus, O. W. Renal reabsorption of low molecular weight proteins in adult male rats: α_2 μ-Globulin. *Proc. Soc. Exp. Biol. Med.* 182: 531, 1986.
210. Ngaha, E. O., and Ogunleye, J. O. Studies on gentamicin-induced labilization of rat kidney lysosomes in vitro. *Biochem. Pharmacol.* 32: 2659, 1983.
211. Ngeleka, M., Beauchamp, D., Tardif, D., Auclair, P., Gourde, P., and Bergeron, M. G. Endotoxin increases the nephrotoxic potential of gentamicin and vancomycin plus gentamicin. *J. Infect. Dis.* 161: 721, 1990.
212. Nicot, G., Merle, L., Valette, J.-P., Charmes, J.-P., and Lachatre, G. Gentamicin and sisomicin induced renal tubular damage. *Eur. J. Pharmacol.* 23: 161, 1982.
213. Nomura, K., Naruse, K., Watanabe, K., and Sokabe, M. Aminoglycoside blockade of Ca^{2+}-activated K^+ channel from rat brain synaptosomal membranes in-

corporated into planar bilayers. *J. Membr. Biol.* 115: 241, 1990.

213a. O'Connor, R. P., Weinberg, J. M., and Humes, H. D. The effect of cyclosporin A on renal cortical mitochondrial function. *Kidney Int.* 25: 235, 1984.

214. Orsulakova, H., Stockhorst, E., and Schacht, J. Effect of neomycin on phosphoinositide labeling and calcium binding in guinea-pig inner ear tissue in vivo and in vitro. *J. Neurochem.* 26: 285, 1976.

215. Paradelis, A. G., Triantaphyllidis, C. J., Mironidou, M., Crabbaris, L. G., Karachalios, D. N., and Giala, M. M. Interaction of aminoglycoside antibiotics and calcium channel blockers on the neuromuscular functions. *Methods Find. Exp. Clin. Pharmacol.* 10(11): 687, 1988.

216. Pastoriza-Munoz, E., Bowman, R. C., and Kaloyanides, G. J. Renal tubular transport of gentamicin in the rat. *Kidney Int.* 16: 440, 1979.

217. Pastoriza-Munoz, E., Josepovitz, C., Ramsammy, L., and Kaloyanides, G. J. Renal handling of netilmicin in the rat with streptozotocin-induced diabetes mellitus. *J. Pharmacol. Exp. Ther.* 241: 166, 1987.

218. Pastoriza-Munoz, E., Timmerman, D., Feldman, S., and Kaloyanides, G. J. Ultrafiltration of gentamicin and netilmicin in vivo. *J. Pharmacol. Exp. Ther.* 220: 604, 1982.

219. Pastoriza-Munoz, E., Timmerman, D., and Kaloyanides, G. J. Tubular wasting of cations associated with netilmicin infusion. *Clin. Res.* 31: 438A, 1983.

220. Pastoriza-Munoz, E., Timmerman, D., and Kaloyanides, G. J. Renal transport of netilmicin in the rat. *J. Pharmacol. Exp. Ther.* 228: 65, 1984.

221. Patel, V., Luft, F. C., Yum, M. N., Patel, B., Zeman, W., and Kleit, S. A. Enzymuria in gentamicin-induced kidney damage. *Antimicrob. Agents Chemother.* 7: 364, 1975.

222. Patel, R., and Savage, A. Symptomatic hypomagnesemia associated with gentamicin therapy. *Nephron* 23: 50, 1979.

223. Pattyn, V. M., Verpooten, G. A., Giuliano, R. A., Zheng, F., and DeBroe, M. E. Effect of hyperfiltration, proteinuria and diabetes mellitus on the uptake kinetics of gentamicin in the kidney cortex of rats. *J. Pharmacol. Exp. Ther.* 244: 694, 1988.

224. Pittinger, C., and Adamson, R. Antibiotic blockade of neuromuscular function. *Annu. Rev. Pharmacol. Toxicol.* 12: 169, 1972.

225. Plant, M. E., Schentag, J. J., and Jusko, W. J. Aminoglycoside nephrotoxicity: Comparative assessment in critically ill patients. *J. Med.* 10: 257, 1979.

226. Porter, G. A., Laurent, G., Maldague, P., and Tulkens, P. M. Gentamicin-induced stimulation of DNA synthesis in rat kidney. Comparison between in vivo and in vitro models. *Toxicol. Lett.* 23: 205, 1984.

227. Powell, J., and Reidenberg, M. N. In vitro response of rat and human kidney lysosomes to aminoglycosides. *Biochem. Pharmacol.* 31: 3447, 1982.

228. Powell, J. H., and Reidenberg, M. M. Further studies of the response of kidney lysosomes to aminoglycosides and other cations. *Biochem. Pharmacol.* 32: 3213, 1983.

229. Quarum, M. L., Houghton, D. C., Gilbert, D. N., McCarron, D. A., and Bennett, W. M. Increasing dietary calcium moderates experimental gentamicin nephrotoxicity. *J. Lab. Clin. Med.* 103: 104, 1984.

230. Queener, S. F., Luft, F. C., and Hamel, F. G. Effect of gentamicin treatment on adenylate cyclase and Na^+, K^+-ATPase activities in renal tissues of rats. *Antimicrob. Agents Chemother.* 24: 815, 1983.

231. Ramsammy, L. S., Josepovitz, C., Jones, D., Ling, K.-Y., Lane, B. P., and Kaloyanides, G. J. Induction of nephrotoxicity by high doses of gentamicin in diabetic rats. *Proc. Soc. Exp. Biol. Med.* 186: 306, 1987.

232. Ramsammy, L. S., Josepovitz, C., and Kaloyanides, G. J. Gentamicin inhibits agonist stimulation of the phosphatidylinositol cascade in primary cultures of rabbit proximal tubular cells and in rat renal cortex. *J. Pharmacol. Exp. Ther.* 247: 989, 1988.

233. Ramsammy, L. S., Josepovitz, C., Lane, B., and Kaloyanides, G. J. Effect of gentamicin on phospholipid metabolism in cultured rabbit proximal tubular cells. *Am. J. Physiol.* 256: C204, 1989.

234. Ramsammy, L. S., Josepovitz, C., Lane, B. P., and Kaloyanides, G. J. Polyaspartic acid protects against gentamicin nephrotoxicity in the rat. *J. Pharmacol. Exp. Ther.* 250: 149, 1989.

235. Ramsammy, L., Josepovitz, C., Lane, B., and Kaloyanides, G. J. Polyaspartic acid inhibits gentamicin-induced perturbations of phospholipid metabolism. *Am. J. Physiol.* 258: C1141, 1990.

236. Ramsammy, L. S., Josepovitz, C., Lane, B., and Kaloyanides, G. J. Pretreatment of rats with polyaspartic acid protects against gentamicin nephrotoxicity. *Cin. Res.* 39:248A, 1991.

237. Ramsammy, L. S., Josepovitz, C., Ling, K. Y., Lane, B. P., and Kaloyanides, G. J. Effects of diphenyl-phenylenediamine on gentamicin-induced lipid peroxidation and toxicity in rat renal cortex. *J. Pharmacol. Exp. Ther.* 238: 83, 1986.

238. Ramsammy, L. S., Josepovitz, C., Ling, K-Y., Lane, B. P., and Kaloyanides, G. J. Failure of inhibition of lipid peroxidation by vitamin E to protect against gentamicin nephrotoxicity in the rat. *Biochem. Pharmacol.* 36: 2125, 1987.

239. Ramsammy, L. S., and Kaloyanides, G. J. The effect of gentamicin on the biophysical properties of phosphatidic acid liposomes is influenced by the O—C=O group of the lipid. *Biochemistry* 27: 8249, 1988.

240. Ramsammy, L. S., and Kaloyanides, G. J. Effect of gentamicin on the transition temperature and permeability to glycerol of phosphatidylinositol-containing liposomes. *Biochem. Pharmacol.* 36: 1179, 1987.

241. Ramsammy, L., Ling, K.-Y., Josepovitz, C., Levine, R., and Kaloyanides, G. J. Effect of gentamicin on lipid peroxidation in rat renal cortex. *Biochem. Pharmacol.* 34: 3895, 1985.

242. Ramsammy, L. S., Van Cott, C., and Kaloyanides, G. J. Effect of gentamicin on phosphatidylinositol and phosphatidylcholine hydrolysis by phospholipase C in vitro. *FASEB J.* 5: A1406, 1991.

243. Rankin, L. I., Krous, H., Fryer, A. W., and Whang, R. Enhancement of gentamicin nephrotoxicity by magnesium depletion in the rat. *Mineral Electrolyte Metab.* 10: 199, 1984.

244. Reid, D. G., and Gajjar, K. A proton and carbon 13 nuclear magnetic resonance study of neomycin B and its interactions with phosphatidylinositol 4,5-bisphosphate. *J. Biol. Chem.* 262: 7967, 1987.

245. Riviere, J. E., Carver, M. P., Coppoc, G. L., Carlton, W. W., Lantz, G. C., and Shy-Modjeska, J. Pharmacokinetics and comparative nephrotoxicity of fixed-dose versus fixed-interval reduction of gentamicin dosage in subtotal nephrectomized dogs. *Toxicol. Appl. Pharmacol.* 75: 496, 1984.

246. Rowe, J. W. Clinical research on aging: Strategies and directions. *N. Engl. J. Med.* 297: 1332, 1977.

247. Rybak, M. J., Albrecht, L. M., Boike, S. C., and Chandresekar, P. H. Nephrotoxicity of vancomycin, alone and

with an aminoglycoside. *J. Antimicrob. Ther.* 25: 679, 1990.

248. Safirstein, R., Miller, P., and Kahn, T. Cortical and papillary absorptive defects in gentamicin nephrotoxicity. *Kidney Int.* 24: 526, 1983.
249. Saito, H., Inui, K.-I., and Hori, R. Mechanisms of gentamicin transport in kidney epithelial cell line ($LLC-PK_1$). *J. Pharmacol. Exp. Ther.* 238: 1071, 1986.
250. Sandermann, H., Jr. Regulation of membrane enzymes by lipids. *Biochim. Biophys. Acta* 515: 229, 1978.
251. Sastrasinh, M., Knauss, T. C., Weinberg, J. M., and Humes, H. D. Identification of the aminoglycoside binding site in rat renal brush border membranes. *J. Pharmacol. Exp. Ther.* 222: 350, 1982.
252. Schacht, J. Inhibition by neomycin of polyphosphoinositide turnover in subcellular fractions of guinea-pig cerebral cortex in vitro. *J. Neurochem.* 27: 1119, 1976.
253. Schacht, J. Isolation of an aminoglycoside receptor from guinea pig inner ear tissues and kidney. *Arch. Otorhinolaryngol.* 224: 129, 1979.
254. Schacht, J. Molecular mechanisms of drug-induced hearing loss. *Hearing Res.* 22: 297, 1986.
255. Schacht, J., Weiner, N. D., and Lodhi, S. Interaction of Aminocyclitol Antibiotics with Polyphosphoinositides in Mammalian Tissues and Artificial Membranes. In W. W. Wells and F. Eisenberg (eds.), *Cyclitols and Phosphoinositides.* New York: Academic, 1978.
256. Schentag, J. J. Specificity of renal tubular damage criteria for aminoglycoside nephrotoxicity in critically ill patients. *J. Clin. Pharmacol.* 23: 473, 1983.
257. Schentag, J. J., Cumbo, T. J., Jusko, W. J., and Plaut, M. E. Gentamicin tissue accumulation and nephrotoxic reactions. *J.A.M.A.* 240: 2067, 1978.
258. Schentag, J. J., Gengo, F. M., Plaut, M. E., Danner, D., Mangione, A., and Jusko, W. J. Urinary casts as an indication of renal tubular damage in patients receiving aminoglycosides. *Antimicrob. Agents Chemother.* 16: 468, 1979.
259. Schentag, J. J., and Jusko, W. J. Renal clearance and tissue accumulation of gentamicin. *Clin. Pharmacol. Ther.* 22: 364, 1977.
260. Schentag, J. J., Jusko, W. J., Vance, J. W., Cumbo, T., Abrutyn, E., deLattre, M., and Gebracht, L. Gentamicin disposition and tissue accumulation on multiple dosing. *J. Pharmacokinet. Biopharm.* 5: 559, 1977.
261. Schentag, J. J., Sutfin, T. A., Plaut, M. E., and Jusko, W. J. Early detection of aminoglycoside nephrotoxicity with urinary beta-2-microglobulin. *J. Med.* 9: 201, 1978.
262. Schibeci, A., and Schacht, J. Action of neomycin on the metabolism of polyphosphoinositides in the guinea pig kidney. *Biochem. Pharmacol.* 26: 1769, 1977.
263. Schor, N., Ichikawa, I., Rennke, H. G., Troy, J. L., and Brenner, B. M. Pathophysiology of altered glomerular function in aminoglycoside-treated rats. *Kidney Int.* 19: 288, 1981.
264. Schwartz, J. H., and Schein, P. Fanconi syndrome associated with cephalothin and gentamicin therapy. *Cancer* 41: 769, 1978.
265. Schwertz, D. W., Kreisberg, J. I., and Venkatachalam, M. A. Effects of aminoglycosides on proximal tubule brush border membrane phosphatidylinositol-specific phospholipase C. *J. Pharmacol. Exp. Ther.* 231: 48, 1984.
266. Senekjian, H. O., Knight, T. F., and Weinman, E. J. Micropuncture study of the handling of gentamicin by the rat kidney. *Kidney Int.* 19: 416, 1981.
267. Shanley, P. F., and Burke, T. J. Differential susceptibility to gentamicin toxicity within the proximal convoluted tubule. *Ren. Fail.* 12: 83, 1990.
268. Sheth, A. U., Senekjian, H. O., Babino, H., Knight, T. F., and Weinman, E. J. Renal handling of gentamicin by the Munich-Wister rat. *Am. J. Physiol.* 241: F645, 1981.
269. Siegel, F. L., and Bulger, R. E. Scanning and transmission electron microscopy of mercuric chloride-induced acute tubular necrosis in rat kidney. *Virchows Arch. [B]* 18: 243, 1975.
270. Silverblatt, F. S., and Kuehn, C. Autoradiography of gentamicin uptake by the rat proximal tubule cell. *Kidney Int.* 15: 335, 1979.
271. Simmons, C. F., Bogusky, R. T., and Humes, H. D. Inhibitory effects of gentamicin or renal mitochondrial oxidative phosphorylation. *J. Pharmacol. Exp. Ther.* 214: 709, 1980.
272. Slater, T. F., and Greenbaum, A. C. Changes in lysosomal enzymes in acute experimental liver injury. *Biochem. J.* 96: 484, 1965.
273. Smith, C. R. Review of studies evaluating the pathophysiological effects of aminoglycosides in normal human volunteers. Proceedings of the 12th International Congress of Chemotherapy, Florence, July 19–24, 1981. American Society for Microbiology. *Curr. Chemother. Immunother.* 2: 833, 1981.
274. Smith, C. R., Lipsky, J. J., Laskin, O. C., Hellman, D. B., Mellits, E. D., Longstreth, J., and Lietman, P. S. Double-blind comparison of the nephrotoxicity and auditory toxicity of gentamicin and tobramycin. *N. Engl. J. Med.* 302: 1106, 1980.
275. Smith, C. R., Maxwell, R. R., Edwards, C. Q., Rogers, J. F., and Lietman, P. S. Nephrotoxicity induced by gentamicin and amikacin. *Johns Hopkins Med. J.* 142: 85, 1978.
276. Soberon, L., Bowman, R. L., Pastoriza-Munoz, E., and Kaloyanides, G. J. Comparative nephrotoxicities of gentamicin, netilmicin and tobramycin in the rat. *J. Pharmacol. Exp. Ther.* 210: 334, 1979.
277. Sokol, P. P., Huiatt, R., Holohan, P. D., and Ross, C. R. Gentamicin and verapamil compete for a common transport mechanism in renal brush border membrane vesicles. *J. Pharmacol. Exp. Ther.* 251: 937, 1989.
278. Spiegel, D. M., Shanley, P. F., and Molitoris, B. A. Mild ischemia predisposes the S_3 segment to gentamicin toxicity. *Kidney Int.* 38: 459, 1990.
279. Streb, H., Heslop, J. P., Irvine, R. F., Schulz, J., and Berridge, M. J. Relationship between secretagogue-induced Ca^{2+} release and inositol polyphosphate production in permeabilized pancreatinc acinar cells. *J. Biol. Chem.* 260: 7309, 1985.
280. Tablan, O. C., Reyes, M. P., Rintelmann, W. F., and Lerner, A. M. Renal and auditory toxicity of high-dose, prolonged therapy with gentamicin and tobramycin in *Pseudomonas* endocarditis. *J. Infect. Dis.* 149: 257, 1984.
281. Takahashi, M., Aramaki, Y. M., Inaba, A., and Tsuchiya, S. Inhibition of alkaline phosphatase activity and D-glucose uptake in rat renal brush-border membrane vesicles by aminoglycosides. *Biochim. Biophys. Acta* 903: 31, 1987.
282. Talbot, P. A. Potentiation of aminoglycoside-induced neuromuscular blockade by protons in vitro and in vivo. *J. Pharmacol. Exp. Ther.* 241: 686, 1987.
283. Tamir, A., Israeli, B., Aladjem, M., and Bogin, E. The effect of oral calcium load or verapamil on gentamicin-induced nephrotoxicity. *J. Clin. Chem. Clin. Biochem.* 27: 847, 1989.
284. Tardif, D., Beauchamp, D., and Bergeron, M. G. Influence of endotoxin on the intracortical accumulation ki-

netics of gentamicin in rats. *Antimicrob. Agents Chemother.* 34: 576, 1990.
285. Teixeira, R. B., Kelley, J., Alpert, H., Pardo, V., and Vaamonde, C. A. Complete protection from gentamicin-induced acute renal failure in the diabetes mellitus rat. *Kidney Int.* 21: 600, 1982.
286. Thompson, J. R., Simonsen, R., Spindler, M. A., Southern, P. M., and Cronin, R. E. Protective effect of KCl loading in gentamicin nephrotoxicity. *Am. J. Kidney Dis.* 15: 583, 1990.
287. Thomsen, H. S., Skaarup, P., Larsen, S., Golman, K., and Hemmingsen, L. Gentamicin nephropathy and contrast media. *Acta Radiol.* 31: 401, 1990.
288. Toubeau, G., Laurent, G., Carlier, M. B., Abid, S., Maldague, P., Heuson-Stiennon, J. A., and Tulkens, P. M. Tissue repair in rat kidney cortex after short treatment with aminoglycosides at low doses. *Lab. Invest.* 54: 385, 1986.
288a. Tune, B. M., Wu, K. Y., Fravert, D., and Holtzman, D. The effect of cephaloridine on respiration by renal cortical mitochondria. *J. Pharmacol. Exp. Ther.* 210: 98, 1979.
289. Walker, P. D., and Shah, S. V. Evidence suggesting a role for hydroxyl radical in gentamicin-induced acute renal failure in rats. *J. Clin. Invest.* 81: 334, 1988.
290. Walker, P. D., and Shah, S. V. Gentamicin enhanced production of hydrogen peroxide by renal cortical mitochondria. *Am. J. Physiol.* 253: C495, 1987.
291. Wang, B. M., Weiner, N. D., Ganesan, M. G., and Schacht, J. Interaction of calcium and neomycin with anionic phospholipid-lecithin liposomes. *Biochem. Pharmacol.* 33: 3787, 1984.
292. Wang, B. M., Weiner, N. D., Takada, A., and Schacht, J. Characterization of aminoglycoside-lipid interactions and development of a refined model for ototoxicity testing. *Biochem. Pharmacol.* 33: 3257, 1984.
293. Watson, A. J., Giminez, L. F., Klassen, D. K., Stout, R. L., and Whelton, A. Calcium channel blockade in experimental aminoglycoside nephrotoxicity. *Clin. Pharmacol.* 27: 625, 1987.
294. Wedeen, R. P., Batuman, V., Cheeks, C., Marquet, E., and Sobel, H. Transport of gentamicin in rat proximal tubule. *Lab. Invest.* 48: 212, 1983.
295. Weinberg, J. M. Aminoglycoside nephrotoxicity: The role of cell calcium overload in nephrotoxic renal tubular cell injury. *Am. J. Kidney Dis.* 8: 284, 1986.
295a. Weinberg, J. M., Harding, P. G., and Humes, H. D. Mitochondrial bioenergetics during the initiation of mercuric chloride renal injury. I. Direct effects of in vitro mercuric chloride on renal cortical mitochondrial function. *J. Biol. Chem.* 257: 60, 1982.
295b. Weinberg, J. M., Harding, B. G., and Humes, H. D. Mitochondrial bioenergetics during the initiation of mercuric chloride renal injury. II. Functional alterations of renal cortical mitochondria isolated after mercuric chloride treatment. *J. Biol. Chem.* 257: 68, 1982.
296. Weinberg, J. M., and Humes, H. D. Mechanisms of gentamicin-induced dysfunction of renal cortical mitochondria. I. Effects on mitochondrial respiration. *Arch. Biochem. Biophys.* 205: 222, 1980.
297. Weissman, G., Zurier, R. B., Spieler, P. J., and Goldstein, I. M. Mechanisms of lysosomal enzyme release from leukocytes exposed to immune complexes and other particles. *J. Exp. Med.* 134: 149S, 1971.
298. Wellwood, J. M., Lovell, D., Thompson, A. E., and Tighe, J. R. Renal damage caused by gentamicin: A study of the effects on renal morphology and urinary enzyme excretion. *J. Pathol.* 118: 171, 1976.
299. Whelton, A. Renal Tubular Transport and Intrarenal Aminoglycoside Distribution. In A. Whelton and H. Neu (eds.), *The Aminoglycosides.* New York: Marcel Dekker, 1982. P. 191.
300. Whelton, A., and Solez, K. Aminoglycoside nephrotoxicity—A tale of two transports. *J. Lab. Clin. Med.* 99: 148, 1982.
301. Whelton, A., and Walker, W. G. Intrarenal antibiotics distribution in health and disease. *Kidney Int.* 6: 131, 1974. (Editorial.)
302. Whiting, P. H., Powers, D. A., Petersen, J., Innes, A., Simpson, J. G., and Catto, G. R. D. The effect of dietary protein restriction on high dose gentamicin nephrotoxicity in rats. *Br. J. Exp. Pathol.* 69: 35, 1988.
303. Williams, P. D., Bennett, D. B., Gleason, C. R., and Hattendorf, G. H. Correlation between renal membrane binding and nephrotoxicity of aminoglycosides. *Antimicrob. Agents Chemother.* 31: 570, 1987.
304. Williams, P. D., and Hottendorf, G. H. Inhibition of renal membrane binding and nephrotoxicity of gentamicin by polyasparagine and polyaspartic acid in the rat. *Res. Commun. Chem. Pathol. Pharmacol.* 47: 317, 1985.
305. Williams, P. D., Hottendorf, G. H., and Bennett, D. B. Inhibition of renal membrane binding and nephrotoxicity of aminoglycosides. *J. Pharmacol. Exp. Ther.* 237: 919, 1986.
306. Williams, P. D., Holohan, P. D., and Ross, C. R. Gentamicin nephrotoxicity. I. Acute biochemical correlates in the rat. *Toxicol. Appl. Pharmacol.* 61: 234, 1981.
307. Williams, P. D., Holohan, P. D., and Ross, C. R. Gentamicin nephrotoxicity. II. Plasma membrane changes. *Toxicol. Appl. Pharmacol.* 61: 243, 1981.
308. Williams, P. D., Trimble, M. E., Crespo, L., Holohan, P. D., Freedman, J. C., and Ross, C. R. Inhibition of renal Na^+, K^+-adenosine triphosphatase by gentamicin. *J. Pharmacol. Exp. Ther.* 231: 248, 1984.
309. Williams, S. E., and Schacht, J. Binding of neomycin and calcium to phospholipids and other anionic compounds. *J. Antibiot. (Tokyo)* 39: 457, 1986.
310. Wong, N. L. M., Magil, A. B., and Dirks, J. H. Effect of magnesium diet in gentamicin-induced acute renal failure in rats. *Nephron* 51: 84, 1989.
311. Wood, C. A., Kohlhepp, S. J., Kohnen, P. W., Houghton, D. C., and Gilbert, D. N. Vancomycin enhancement of experimental tobramycin nephrotoxicity. *Antimicrob. Agents Chemother.* 30: 20, 1986.
312. Vakil, N., Abu-Alfa, A., and Mujais, S. K. Gentamicin nephrotoxicity in extrahepatic cholestasis: Modulation by dietary calcium. *Hepatology* 9: 519, 1989.
313. Vanderwalle, A., Farman, N., Morin, J. P., Fillastre, J. P., Hatt, P. Y., and Bonvalet, J. P. Gentamicin incorporation along the nephron: Autoradiographic study on isolated tubules. *Kidney Int.* 19: 529, 1981.
314. Van Rooijen, L. A. A., and Agranoff, B. W. Inhibition of polyphosphoinositide phosphodiesterase by aminoglycoside antibiotics. *Neurochem. Res.* 10: 1019, 1985.
315. Zager, R., and Sharma, H. M. Gentamicin increases renal susceptibility to an acute ischemic insult. *J. Lab. Clin. Med.* 101: 670, 1983.
316. Zager, R. A. Gentamicin nephrotoxicity in the setting of acute renal hypoperfusion. *Am. J. Physiol.* 254: F574, 1988.

Renal Diseases Induced by Antineoplastic Agents

Richard E. Rieselbach
Marc B. Garnick

Many types of systemic cancer now are treated either by antineoplastic agents alone or by combining these agents with localized forms of therapy. When curative therapy is not possible, these agents may provide substantial palliative benefit. Thus, many cancer patients receive antineoplastic agents at some time during the course of their illness.

There is a potential for significant nephrotoxicity with many of these agents. Now that cancer patients are surviving for longer periods of time, cumulative and delayed nephrotoxic effects of antineoplastic therapy have been observed with increasing frequency. Also, as increasing numbers of cancer patients have been treated aggressively with a curative goal, nephrotoxicity has increased. Furthermore, some antineoplastic regimens include several agents that have the potential for synergistic nephrotoxicity.

When nephrotoxicity occurs, this may lead to renal insufficiency, ranging from moderate azotemia to advanced uremia. Any significant degree of renal failure may constitute a major problem in the cancer patient. The pharmacokinetics of antineoplastic agents may be altered in renal failure, thus rendering treatment more difficult; furthermore, delayed renal excretion of these agents may enhance their nephrotoxicity. Uremia, with its infectious, hemorrhagic, and metabolic complications, imposes a particularly severe burden on the cancer patient. Thus the importance of avoiding or minimizing the nephrotoxic effects of antineoplastic agents is apparent.

When some antineoplastic agents are administered in the presence of renal failure, their potential for nephrotoxicity is greatly increased. Cancer is frequently associated with renal damage due to the renal infiltrative or obstructive characteristics of the primary cancer, associated metabolic abnormalities, or the nephrotoxicity of various treatment modalities. Because the level of renal function may be an important factor determining nephrotoxicity, we will review briefly the more common causes of renal dysfunction associated with cancer before discussing nephrotoxicity due to various classes of antineoplastic agents. Discussion of these agents will include alkylating drugs, antimetabolites, antitumor antibiotics, and modifiers of biologic response. Finally, we will consider the nephrotoxicity that may occur in the presence of extensive, rapidly proliferating cancer as the result of the metabolic consequences of effective antineoplastic therapy.

Etiology of Renal Failure Associated with Cancer or Its Therapy

The presence of renal failure may increase the cancer patient's vulnerability to the nephrotoxic effect of antineoplastic agents. For example, an excellent correlation has been observed between endogenous creatinine clearance and clearance of methotrexate [102]. Increased plasma levels of this drug contribute to increased nephrotoxicity. Thus an appreciation for the association between cancer and renal dysfunction has relevance when assessing the potential of antineoplastic agents for producing nephrotoxicity in a given clinical setting.

Cancer or its therapy may produce functional impairment of the kidneys through a wide variety of mechanisms, as outlined in Table 42-1. In this section, we shall review briefly the more common settings where cancer produces renal dysfunction. Acute renal failure may be observed in association with cancer or its therapy with some frequency. Chronic renal failure and specific tubular function abnormalities are not as common, but they also may enhance the nephrotoxic potential of antineoplastic agents and thus may limit their effective utilization.

ACUTE RENAL FAILURE

The same clinical spectrum of acute renal failure (ARF) encountered within the general population may be observed in the patient with cancer, who is equally at risk. Moreover, the cancer patient is at additional risk to develop forms of ARF unique to cancer due to primary manifestations of the tumor, its metabolic consequences, or its treatment. Furthermore, the cancer patient has an increased likelihood of developing some other types of ARF with greater frequency than the general population. For example, antibiotic-induced ARF is likely to occur more frequently because the increased incidence of life-threatening infection in association with cancer requires more frequent therapy with potentially nephrotoxic antibiotics. In one large epidemiologic study, cancer was the underlying basic disease in 20 percent of all patients with ARF [52]. The clinical spectrum of ARF in cancer may be classified into three broad categories: prerenal, intrinsic, and postrenal.

Prerenal ARF. Prerenal ARF is frequently encountered in the cancer patient, particularly in association with contraction of the ECF volume. The cause of hypovolemia may be excessive fluid loss from the gastrointestinal tract due to vomiting or diarrhea induced by cancer or its therapy. Also, hypovolemia may occur from internal fluid loss due to translocation of ECF volume, with sequestration in third spaces, as seen in peritonitis, bowel obstruction, and malignant effusion.

A decrease in *effective* intravascular volume may occur due to peripheral vasodilation, as seen in sepsis. A decrease in cardiac output due to cardiac tamponade secondary to malignant pericardial disease also may produce prerenal ARF, as may cardiomyopathy induced by doxorubicin, which usually appears within 2 months of the last dose. In the cancer patient, hepatobiliary disease

Table 42-1. Etiology of renal functional impairment associated with cancer

1. Acute renal failure	
a. *Prerenal*	
Hypovolemia	
Peripheral vasodilation	
Impaired cardiac function	
Functional disorders of intrarenal circulation	
b. *Intrinsic*	
Glomerular abnormalities	Tumor antigen-mediated glomerulopathies
	Disseminated intravascular coagulation
Tubular abnormalities	Ischemic acute tubular necrosis (ATN)
	Exogenous nephrotoxins
	Antineoplastic agents
	Antimicrobials
	Radiocontrast media
	Anesthetic agents
	Endogenous nephrotoxins
	Myoglobin
	Hemoglobin
	Immunoglobulins
	Calcium and phosphorus
	Uric acid and xanthine
Interstitial abnormalities	Drug-induced acute tubulointerstitial nephritis (ATIN)
	Acute pyelonephritis
	Tumor infiltration
	Radiation nephropathy
Abnormalities of intrarenal blood vessels	Disseminated intravascular coagulation
	Acute bilateral renal cortical necrosis
	Malignant hypertension
	Vasculitis
c. *Postrenal*	
Urethral obstruction	Prostatic hypertrophy
Bladder neck obstruction	Prostatic or bladder cancer
	Functional: neuropathy or drugs
	Intraureteral
	Uric acid crystals or stones
	Blood clots
	Pyogenic debris
	Edema
	Necrotizing papillitis
Bilateral obstruction of ureters (or unilateral obstruction of single kidney)	Extraureteral
	Cancer prostate; cervix
	Periureteral fibrosis
	Accidental ureteral ligation during pelvic surgery for cancer
2. Chronic renal failure	
a. *Glomerular abnormalities*	Tumor antigen-mediated
	Lymphokine-mediated
	Immunoglobulins
	Amyloid
	Primary renal cancer
	Antineoplastic agents
b. *Tubulointerstitial abnormalities*	Immunoglobulins
	Radiation nephropathy
	Leukemic infiltration
	Lymphomatous infiltration
	Metastatic infiltration
	Chronic pyelonephritis
	Antineoplastic agents

Table 42-1 (continued)

c. *Renovascular disease*	Hypertension due to malignancy Perirenal vascular involvement by renal or nonrenal cancer Renal vein thrombosis
d. *Obstruction*	Cancer: Prostate Cervix Bladder Retroperitoneal lymphoma Primary renal Uric acid or calcium stones Periureteral fibrosis
3. Specific tubular dysfunction	
a. *Tumor-induced inappropriate hormone concentrations*	PTH-like substances ADH SIADH Diabetes insipidus Adrenocortical excess Adrenal insufficiency
b. *Tumor products or metabolites*	Hypercalcemia Lysozyme Inhibitin Immunoglobulins
c. *Intrinsic*	Nephrogenic diabetes insipidus Multiple myeloma Obstruction
d. *Antineoplastic agents*	SIADH Cyclophosphamide Vincristine Magnesium wasting Cisplatin

may be responsible for the alterations in intrarenal hemodynamics that serve as the basis for the hepatorenal syndrome. In addition, adaptive responses of the intrarenal circulation to potentially deleterious stimuli may be impaired by the administration of nonsteroidal antiinflammatory agents to the cancer patient for analgesia.

Intrinsic ARF. GLOMERULAR ABNORMALITIES. When ARF is caused by a glomerular abnormality, the pathologic process most frequently consists of either diffuse proliferative or crescentic glomerulonephritis. Although immune-complex glomerular disease is not uncommon in patients with cancer [206], glomerular disease causing ARF in the cancer patient has been reported in only a few cases [90].

TUBULAR ABNORMALITIES. ARF may arise either on the basis of ischemia or as a result of exposure to exogenous or endogenous nephrotoxins. Since tubular function is compromised in all cases, all the foregoing are considered as tubular abnormalities for clarity of organization. When intrinsic ARF is not the result of primary anatomic lesions within glomeruli, blood vessels, or the renal interstitium, it has been referred to as *acute tubular necrosis* (ATN). However, since ATN is a renal histologic finding and is not consistently demonstrable in this setting [124], this terminology is not always pathologically accurate. Nevertheless, lacking alternative terminology of any greater etiologic or descriptive accuracy, the term ATN is employed when referring to tubular abnormalities of ischemic origin. The more general term of ARF is utilized when referring to tubular abnormalities secondary to exogenous or endogenous nephrotoxins.

Renal ischemia is usually the initiating factor when ATN follows sepsis or shock or arises as a postsurgical complication. In these settings, which are commonly associated with cancer, an antecedent period of hemodynamic instability may frequently be identified, and renal blood flow is usually depressed out of proportion to any decrease in cardiac output. The pathogenesis, pathology, clinical course, and complications of ATN are discussed in depth in other chapters.

Throughout the last decade, exogenous nephrotoxins have assumed an increasingly prominent role in the etiology of ARF [136]. Some series have indicated a toxic etiology in 25 percent [57] and 21 percent [3] of consecutive patients with ARF. Cancer patients are particularly vulnerable to ARF induced by exogenous nephrotoxins in view of their frequent exposure to a wide variety of nephrotoxic drugs as well as to diagnostic studies utilizing radiocontrast media.

ARF may occur after administration of virtually any intravascular contrast agent and has been reported to follow urography, angiography, computerized tomography, and cholecystography. Although the incidence of this etiology of ARF has been quite low, it is now being recognized more often; the true incidence in the past may have been underestimated. In one review summarizing a number of reports, the incidence was estimated as being between 0.1 and 0.3 percent [26]. The onset of ARF following surgery raises the possibility of nephrotoxicity due to anesthetic agents. Anesthetic administration is a rare cause of ARF, but it has been reported following halothane, methoxyflurane, and enflurane anesthesia [31, 37].

Cancer patients are particularly prone to develop antimicrobial-induced ARF, since they are frequently afflicted with serious infections requiring therapy with potentially nephrotoxic antimicrobials. The nephrotoxicity of these agents is enhanced because sepsis is often associated with hemodynamic alterations, ECF volume contraction, or both, with both leading to renal hypoperfusion. Cancer patients may have additional risk factors that enhance the potential for induction of ARF by these agents: They may be receiving other potential nephrotoxins; they may have preexisting renal disease; they may be of advanced age; or all of these.

Nephrotoxins of endogenous origin are encountered with increased frequency in the cancer patient and may be etiologic factors in producing ARF. Hemoglobin, myoglobin, immunoglobulins, calcium, phosphorus, and uric acid are included in this category. Myoglobin is present in the cytoplasm of striated skeletal and cardiac muscle cells. Thus rhabdomyolysis is required for liberation of this potential nephrotoxin. Nontraumatic rhabdomyolysis may occur in a variety of settings. Those particularly relevant to the cancer patient include (1) profound hypokalemia, as may be seen with severe potassium-losing nephropathy associated with cancer; (2) severe hypophosphatemia, as may occur in association with hyperalimentation in a patient with a previously poor nutritional status; (3) infection with influenza type A viruses, causing myositis, with a degree of muscle damage sufficient to produce myoglobinuria [173]; and (4) prolonged immobilization, such as may be associated with coma or severe weakness. In this setting, interference with local blood supply leads to muscle damage [126]. ARF also may occur in association with hemoglobinuria. In the cancer patient, the usual cause of hemoglobinuria is an incompatible blood transfusion. In this setting, immunologically mediated destruction of erythrocytes results in the liberation of free hemoglobin into the plasma.

Excessive production of immunoglobulins in multiple myeloma may be the basis for ARF, although renal involvement in multiple myeloma usually results in chronic renal failure [176]. When ARF does occur in multiple myeloma, intrinsic tubular pathology produced by immunoglobulins is not necessarily the etiology in that nephrotoxic antibiotics, hyperuricemia, or hypercalcemia may be important factors. Nevertheless, when excessive immunoglobulin production does contribute to the pathogenesis of ARF, factors facilitating intratubular precipitation of Bence Jones protein appear to be important. Thus dehydration, which may be associated with infection, hypercalcemia, or excretory urography, may be of concern. Also, a low urinary pH may contribute to decreased intratubular solubility of these proteins [33].

ARF may occur as a result of the severe hypercalcemia, which may be encountered in the cancer patient [34]. The hypercalcemia-induced reduction in GFR appears to be multifactorial. These factors include a possible direct effect of hypercalcemia on glomerular filtration as well as the natriuretic effect of hypercalcemia, producing ECF volume depletion. Intratubular obstruction by calcium deposition also may be a factor. ARF associated with the acute onset of extreme hyperphosphatemia in cancer patients is discussed in a subsequent section of this chapter, as is ARF produced by acute uric acid nephropathy.

INTERSTITIAL ABNORMALITIES. Acute tubulointerstitial nephritis may be induced in cancer patients by hypersensitivity to various drugs. These patients frequently receive the analgesics and antimicrobials associated with this form of ARF. Also, immunosuppressed cancer patients may be particularly vulnerable to severe, acute bacterial pyelonephritis. ARF may occur in this setting, even in the absence of urinary tract obstruction or other underlying renal disease [8]. Infiltrative and metastatic disease of the kidney may involve the interstitium but rarely causes ARF [118]. Finally, acute radiation nephropathy may occur following radiation therapy for cancer and has been associated with ARF [64].

ABNORMALITIES OF INTRARENAL BLOOD VESSELS. The fourth major anatomic site of intrinsic ARF is the intrarenal vasculature. Disseminated intravascular coagulation may occur in association with sepsis in the cancer patient [111]. This may produce acute bilateral renal cortical necrosis secondary to occlusion of the cortical vasculature. In addition, because the cancer patient is more often in an older age group, atheroembolic disease or malignant hypertension must be considered as possible etiologies of intrarenal vascular occlusion in the presence of ARF. Finally, vasculitis is a consideration, particularly in the presence of hepatitis B antigenemia.

Postrenal ARF. Postrenal ARF is caused by urinary tract obstruction from tumors of the urinary tract or surrounding tissues. Some of the more common causes of bladder-neck obstruction include prostatic hypertrophy [68] and prostatic or bladder cancer [20]. Postrenal ARF also may be produced by bilateral obstruction of both ureters (or unilateral ureteral obstruction in the presence of a single kidney). When obstruction is intraureteral, it is most commonly due to uric acid crystals, blood clots, or stones. The most common basis for extraureteral obstruction is cancer of the prostate, colon, or uterine cervix, although obstruction also may occur with retroperitoneal lymphoma and sarcoma. Obstructive uropathy accounts for 60 to 80 percent of deaths due to cervical cancer [10]. Extraureteral obstruction also may occur due to retroperitoneal fibrosis secondary to malignancy [190].

CHRONIC RENAL FAILURE

Glomerular Abnormalities. Since a report by Lee et al. [105] in 1966 that 11 percent of 105 adults with the nephrotic syndrome also had cancer, many reports concerning a variety of glomerular abnormalities in cancer have appeared; this literature recently has been reviewed in detail [206]. Membranous glomerulopathy is the most frequent glomerular abnormality associated with carcinoma. Granular deposition of immunoglobulins and complement within the glomerular basement membrane has been observed in many cases, suggesting that the lesion is mediated by tumor antigen [106]. By contrast, minimal-change glomerular disease is seen most often when glomerular abnormalities are associated with lymphomas. It has been suggested that lymphokines produced by neoplastic cells may cause glomerular injury in this setting [120]. The most common malignancies associated with glomerular amyloid deposition are multiple myeloma, Hodgkin's disease, and renal carcinoma. Glomeruli are extensively involved, often resulting in severe nephrotic syndrome [197]. Glomerular abnormalities are observed in association with immunoglobulin deposition in multiple myeloma, macroglobulinemia, and cryoglobulinemia [176].

Interstitial Abnormalities. Abnormalities of immunoglobulin production associated with multiple myeloma are a frequent cause of interstitial abnormalities causing chronic renal failure in association with cancer. Renal failure has been reported to develop in up to half of patients with myeloma at some time during their illness and is associated with a significantly worse prognosis [45]. Often renal failure is of multiple etiologies in myeloma, with a variety of specific lesions and metabolic abnormalities contributing to nephron destruction. The most frequently observed renal abnormality in myeloma and the one generally associated with the term *myeloma kidney* is the characteristic change in renal tubules. The typical feature is the presence of amorphous, dense, hyaline, or concentric lamellated casts, associated with tubular atrophy, interstitial fibrosis, and multinucleated giant cells or syncytial cells adjacent to cast-filled tubules. In the majority of myeloma patients, renal pathology is limited to the tubules and interstitium [116].

Radiation nephropathy may produce chronic renal failure due to interstitial abnormalities. This clinical syndrome is characterized by progressive renal failure, proteinuria, hypertension, and profound anemia; it has been described in patients who receive more than 2,300 rads to both kidneys [64]. Chronic radiation nephropathy may not develop until 18 months to many years following therapy. Pathologic examination reveals widespread glomerular sclerosis, tubular atrophy, and arteriolar fibrinoid necrosis. It has been suggested that therapy with antineoplastic agents, such as actinomycin D and vincristine or vinblastine and bleomycin, administered in conjunction with abdominal irradiation, may enhance the potential for development of radiation nephropathy [4, 32].

Metastatic infiltration of the kidneys is a rare cause of functional impairment [118]. Most renal metastases are multiple and bilateral. Glomeruli tend to be spared, possibly because of their lack of lymphatic channels or because of protective humoral factors [204]. Interstitial infiltration by hematologic neoplasms is more frequent but rarely causes renal failure [118]. Infiltration is usually bilateral, diffuse, and more prominent in the cortex [56]. The incidence of lymphomatous infiltration of the kidneys is high. In one series, 33 percent of patients had renal involvement at the time of death [141]. However, kidney failure was the terminal event in only 0.5 percent of these patients. Nevertheless, one report describes a patient with lymphomatous infiltration of the kidneys presenting with uremia of unknown etiology. Renal function markedly improved following chemotherapy [139]. As noted previously with relation to acute bacterial pyelonephritis, the immunosuppressed status of many cancer patients serves to increase their susceptibility to bacterial invasion of the renal interstitium. Thus chronic bacterial pyelonephritis may be a cause of chronic renal failure in the cancer patient, particularly in association with chronic obstruction.

Renovascular Disease. Hypertension due to malignancy may produce renovascular disease. Hypertension may be associated with hypercalcemia of malignancy and is observed frequently in patients with renal carcinoma. Perirenal vascular involvement may be present with primary renal cancer or nonrenal cancer; renal vein thrombosis or occlusion may occur due to external compression by tumor or direct extension of tumor [115].

Obstruction. When obstruction is present at any level of the urinary tract, the continued production of urine results in an increase of volume and pressure proximal to the obstruction. If the obstruction persists, the kidney may be damaged progressively with resultant chronic renal failure. The etiologies for obstruction causing chronic renal failure in association with cancer are similar to those noted in Table 42-1 for acute renal failure.

SPECIFIC TUBULAR DYSFUNCTION

Tumor-Induced Inappropriate Hormone Concentration. Normal renal tubular function is controlled by a delicate balance of humoral mediators. Thus a tumor-induced inappropriate concentration of a hormone that normally contributes to the modulation of this balance may result in a profound disturbance of tubular function, thereby causing impairment of fluid and electrolyte balance as well as other homeostatic defects. Certain mesenchymal tumors may cause renal phosphate loss [41]. The resultant hypophosphatemia appears to be related to some substance or product elaborated by the tumor, since it regresses when the tumor is removed [41]. The substance produced by these tumors appears to act directly on renal phosphate transport; a PTH-like substance could be responsible. Hyponatremia occurs frequently in the patient with cancer; its presence raises the possibility of SIADH as the etiology. Bronchogenic carcinoma is the most frequent cause for this syndrome. Unsuppressed plasma arginine vasopressin in response to water loading has been found in 40 percent of patients with oat cell carcinoma [59]. A number of other tumors also have been reported to be associated with SIADH [174]. Disappearance of SIADH upon removal of the tumor, or improvement following successful chemotherapy, frequently has been observed [174].

Cancer is a common cause of central diabetes insipidus; metastatic lesions have been reported to cause from 5 to 20 percent of all cases. Breast cancer has been the primary malignancy in more than half of the cases reported [77]. Adrenocortical excess may be associated with malignancies and is often manifest by hypokalemia and metabolic alkalosis. Adrenal insufficiency may occur due to metastatic lesions of the adrenal glands. This is uncommon, since extensive destruction of both adrenals or of a solitary adrenal gland is required [25]. Nevertheless, weight loss, anorexia, nausea, vomiting, and fatigue in a hyponatremic, hyperkalemic patient with advancing metastatic disease raises the possibility of adrenal insufficiency.

Tumor Products and Metabolites. Hypercalcemia associated with malignancy may produce profound tubular dysfunction involving impairment of bicarbonate or sodium transport, urinary concentration, hydrogen-ion secretion, or the renal handling of potassium, phosphorus, or magnesium [34].

Massive lysozymuria may be associated with renal damage, leading to kaliuresis and hypokalemia [133]. Elevations of lysozyme are seen with acute myelogenous leukemia. In this setting, proximal tubular defects in urate, phosphate, and amino acid reabsorption also have been noted [165]. The isolation of a sodium transport inhibitory factor, *inhibitin,* from cultured leukemic promyelocytes suggests that this humoral substance may be involved in mediating the natriuresis, which may occur in association with the destruction of leukemic blast cells after chemotherapy [121].

Intrinsic. Cancer may be associated with nephrogenic diabetes insipidus, where the kidney is unresponsive to the action of ADH, with resultant formation of inappropriately dilute urine. This may be seen in multiple myeloma, where causative intrinsic lesions could include intratubular obstruction by myeloma proteins or amyloid deposition in collecting ducts. Also, chronic urinary tract obstruction due to cancer, with associated anatomical disruption of renal medullary structures, may result in nephrogenic diabetes insipidus.

Antineoplastic Agents. The tubular dysfunction produced by antineoplastic agents, such as cyclophosphamide and cisplatin, will be discussed in the specific section devoted to the nephrotoxicity of these agents.

Nephrotoxicity Produced Directly by Antineoplastic Agents

The nephrotoxicity due to antineoplastic agents may be manifest as acute renal failure, chronic renal failure, or specific tubular dysfunction. Nephrotoxicity has been observed with alkylating agents, antimetabolites, antitumor antibiotics, and biologic agents, as outlined in Table 42-2. These antineoplastic agents may induce nephrotoxicity soon after initiation of therapy or only after long-term administration. The risk of nephrotoxicity varies with each agent. Table 42-2 summarizes the risk of nephrotoxicity, time of onset, and type of functional impairment produced by each agent to be discussed in this section.

ALKYLATING AGENTS

Cisplatin. Cisplatin (*cis*-diamminedichloroplatinum, II) is an antineoplastic agent that has a remarkably broad spectrum of clinical activity in the treatment of solid tumors [151]. Administration of this drug has significantly improved the response rate in patients treated for metastatic testicular and ovarian carcinomas [51]. Cisplatin (CP) also is an important component of many treatment programs for the management of bladder carcinoma, squamous cell carcinoma of the head and neck, bronchogenic carcinoma of the lung, cervical and endometrial cancer, and lymphomas [1]. In addition to nephrotoxicity, side effects of CP include myelosuppression, severe nausea and vomiting, peripheral neuropathy, ototoxicity, and acute anaphylaxis. Early preclinical toxicologic studies had predicted renal injury as a major toxicity [161]. As anticipated, nephrotoxicity was a prominent side effect with initial clinical trials [186]. A dose of 50 mg/m^2 of body surface area (BSA), administered either as a single dose or in divided doses over a 5-day period, produced nephrotoxicity in a significant percentage of patients; hydration-diuresis maneuvers were not employed. With higher doses and repeated courses of therapy, nephrotoxicity was severe, frequently irreversible, and a major dose-limiting factor [1].

HISTOPATHOLOGY AND PATHOGENESIS. The kidney accumulates and retains platinum to a greater degree than other organs and is the predominant excretory route for CP [205]. Thus it is not surprising that nephrotoxicity is a major CP side effect and that the primary site of nephrotoxicity is the tubule. Distal tubules and collecting ducts are affected to a greater degree than proximal tubules [61]. In a study of 12 patients who died after receiving CP, coagulative necrosis, interstitial edema, and tubular dilatation were the most prominent findings; glomerular changes were not observed [61]. In another study, electron microscopy revealed swollen, degenerated, and vacuolated mitochondria in tubular cells as well as disruption of brush-border microvilli [150].

After administration of CP in the rat, 50 percent of the administered dose is excreted in the urine within 24 hours [109, 205]; the major portion appears within the first hour [155]. CP is freely filterable at the glomerulus because of its low molecular weight and uncharged character [154]. Thus CP is excreted primarily by glomerular filtration; however, data indicating that free platinum clearance exceeds glomerular filtration rate suggest that tubular secretion also occurs [88]. Thus the drug may gain access to renal tubular cells by means of secretion or reabsorption.

Safirstein et al. have demonstrated that rat kidney slices accumulate CP and a related platinum-containing analogue at concentrations up to five times higher than extracellular concentrations [156]. These studies describe characteristics of the renal accumulation of the drug and reveal that drugs which compete in the kidney

Table 42-2. Antineoplastic agents that produce nephrotoxicity

Alkylating agents	Antimetabolities	Antitumor antibiotics	Biologic agents
1. Cisplatin (1a-I) 2. Carboplatin (3a-I) 3. Cyclophosphamide (3c-I) 4. Nitrosoureas a. Streptozotocin (1a-I) b. Carmustine (BCNU) (3b-L) c. Lomustine (CCNU) (1b-L) d. Semustine (Methyl CCNU) (1b-L)	1. High-dose methotrexate (1a-I) 2. Cytosine arabinoside (3a-I) 3. High-dose 6-thioguanine (3a-I) 4. 5-Fluorouracil (3a-I) 5. 5-Azacytidine (3a-I)	1. Mitomycin (1b-L) 2. Mithramycin (1a-I) 3. Doxorubicin (3a-I)	1. Recombinant interferon alfa and gamma (3a-I) 2. Interleukin-2 (1a-I) 3. *Corynebacterium parvum* (3a-I)

(1) High risk; (2) intermediate risk; (3) low risk; (a) acute renal failure; (b) chronic renal failure; (c) specific tubular dysfunction; I = immediate nephrotoxicity; L = nephrotoxicity from long-term administration.

for transport of organic acids, such as pyrazinamide, have no effect on its transport. However, drugs transported by the organic base system all reduce CP uptake significantly. These studies indicate that CP is biotransformed intracellularly and that in this altered form, it may no longer be toxic. Other work has suggested that the toxic effect of CP appears to occur through its interaction with nucleophilic sites in DNA [145]. In biologic fluids that contain a low chloride concentration (that is, intracellular water in which the chloride concentration is 4 mM), the drug's chloride ligands in the *cis* position are replaced by water molecules, thus forming an aquated compound. This positively charged, aquated species then reacts with nucleophilic sites. In plasma, which has an ambient chloride concentration of 103 mM, CP remains electrically neutral, with the chloride ligands remaining intact on the molecule. Thus the drug may become activated only when present within the cell.

CLINICAL MANIFESTATIONS. A gradual irreversible decline in creatinine clearance may be observed with successive courses of CP therapy, with an associated increase in the BUN and serum creatinine concentrations [16]. Initial cycles of therapy may be associated with only mild reductions in GFR, whereas an apparent cumulative effect occurs with subsequent cycles [193]. Since glomerular injury is not part of the nephrotoxic process, glomerular proteinuria does not occur; tubular proteinuria may be observed as an early indication of toxicity [92]. Cylindruria is a prominent feature only when severe nephrotoxicity is present [74]. Consistent increases in urinary beta-2-microglobulin excretion in the absence of serum creatinine elevations have suggested that most patients sustain some renal tubular damage from CP, even in the presence of hydration [55]. Concomitant administration of potentially nephrotoxic antibiotics with CP may lead to synergistic nephrotoxicity [62]. Recently, renal sodium wasting with associated ECF volume concentration was noted in patients receiving CP [86].

An additional nephrotoxic effect of CP is renal magnesium wasting [22, 163]. The resultant hypomagnesemia may be life-threatening, particularly when accompanied by hypocalcemia and tetany. In one series of 44 patients receiving 70 mg/m^2 of CP every 3 weeks, hypomagnesemia was observed in 52 percent [163]. The median nadir of magnesium concentration in these patients was 0.92 mEq/liter. It usually occurred 21 days following drug administration, after completion of one or two courses of CP. The use of multiple-drug therapy regimens containing CP may lead to a greater incidence of hypomagnesemia than that from CP itself [22]. Also, patients treated with CP often receive antibiotics, such as aminoglycosides or amphotericin, which may induce renal magnesium wasting [9, 129]. The incidence and severity of CP-induced hypomagnesemia have been reported to be dose-related and are reduced when courses are more widely spaced [22]. Although interventions such as calcitriol administration are not effective [184], this complication is readily managed with administration of oral magnesium chloride solution (magnesium, 1 mEq/ml) and usually does not require parenteral magnesium sulfate administration. This tubular defect usually remits spontaneously over a period of weeks if CP therapy is not reinstituted. However, on occasion, it may persist as long as 3 years after CP therapy is discontinued [164]. Hypomagnesemia in these patients may be associated with normal or slightly elevated serum calcium levels which may result from hypocalciuria [117]. The dissociation of renal calcium and magnesium handling resembles that described in Bartter's syndrome [152]. A distal tubular lesion is supported further by the impairment in maximal urinary acidification noted in these patients [185].

PROPHYLACTIC MEASURES. Initial clinical studies with CP indicated its prominent antitumor activity. However, the frequent occurrence of severe nephrotoxicity discouraged interest in this drug. Subsequent development of CP to its present level of clinical effectiveness was facilitated greatly by studies employing hydration-diuresis maneuvers in dogs [40] and, subsequently, in humans [78]. If CP dosage did not exceed 120 mg/m^2 BSA, these maneuvers were extremely effective in preventing or minimizing nephrotoxicity.

Subsequent studies indicated that even higher doses of CP may be tolerated without nephrotoxicity if each dose is administered in 250 ml of 3% saline (over 30 minutes) in association with intravenous infusion of 250 ml/hour of normal saline with potassium chloride added (20 mEq/liter). This infusion is initiated 12 hours before the first dose of CP and continued until 12 hours after the last dose on day 5 of chemotherapy. This regimen allowed administration of 200 mg/m^2 BSA in five divided daily doses without evidence of a decrease in creatinine clearance [127]. These studies are of particular importance because previous studies of CP administration in both ovarian and testicular cancer have not employed CP doses of greater than 100 to 120 mg/m^2 BSA; these data provide evidence in support of a dose-response curve for CP effectiveness. When used with moderate hydration (3 liters per day) and mannitol or furosemide diuresis, doses up to 120 mg/m^2 of CP have produced an acceptable degree of nephrotoxicity. However, previous experience with higher doses of CP has shown that an unacceptable incidence of nephrotoxicity occurs at doses greater than 120 mg/m^2 BSA even with furosemide or mannitol diuresis [14]. Thus the hypertonic saline regimen is highly advantageous, since it allows administration of a higher dose of CP, resulting in a markedly increased antitumor effect in patients with testicular or ovarian cancer. However, the routine use of this regimen must be viewed with some reservations, since severe extrarenal toxicity (including debilitating neuropathy) may occur with these high doses.

Although the mechanism for the apparent protective effect of this saline infusion regimen is unclear, these findings suggest two possible mechanisms of protection. First, this level of ECF volume expansion stimulates a massive natriuresis and diuresis, thereby decreasing the concentration of CP within tubular fluid throughout the nephron and also decreasing contact time with tubular epithelium to a greater degree than most previous hydration-diuresis maneuvers. It is of interest that patients with one kidney who received 60 mg/m^2 BSA of CP in conjunction with an aggressive hydration protocol experienced a significantly lesser decrease in creatinine clearance than patients with two kidneys [85]. Since subjects with one kidney have an increased fractional excretion of sodium and water [19], the foregoing considerations regarding drug concentration and transit time may explain this observation, as well as other data indicating a lack of age-dependent CP-induced nephrotoxicity [85], which otherwise might be expected, considering the progressive decrease in renal excretory capacity for CP associated with nephron loss of advancing age. A second mechanism may relate to the degree of intracellular aquation of CP associated with this saline infusion regimen. A low intracellular concentration of chloride ion favors the formation of the aquated species of CP within renal tubular cells as opposed to a high chloride concentration as accomplished with this regimen, which may decrease the intracellular concentration of the toxic aquated species.

There are other promising approaches to limiting CP nephrotoxicity. Administration of drugs, such as probenecid or tolazoline, may be effective in decreasing the concentration of drug in renal tubular cells by inhibiting its uptake [149, 156]. Also, it is possible that patients who subsequently develop CP nephrotoxicity may be identified on the basis of elevated plasma platinum levels early in the course of an infusion. It is possible that dose attenuation during CP infusion in these patients will lessen the probability of subsequent nephrotoxicity [28]. Extending the duration of CP infusion may have some influence on decreasing the nephrotoxicity, which occurs when the drug is given as a bolus infusion. Toxicity may be related to the high peak plasma levels of CP, whereas continuous infusion therapy avoids this pharmacologic consequence. Regimens have been described for both 1-day and 5-day infusions, which have resulted in decreased nephrotoxicity [87, 158].

When CP is administered intraperitoneally for the therapy of tumors, such as far-advanced ovarian carcinoma, mesothelioma, and malignant carcinoid, a significant incidence of acute renal failure has been noted with the usual intraperitoneal dose of 90 mg/m^2 [113]. In this setting, systemic administration of a neutralizing agent for CP, such as thiosulfate, has been observed to reduce nephrotoxicity [83]. Thiosulfate is thought to react covalently with CP; the resulting complex neither is toxic nor has antitumor activity [84]. In the absence of systemic thiosulfate protection, intraperitoneal doses of 90 mg/m^2 BSA produced approximately the same exposure for the systemic circulation as an intravenous CP dose of 100 mg/m^2 but a fifteenfold greater exposure for the peritoneal cavity. With systemic thiosulfate treatment, protection from CP nephrotoxicity was so effective that the intraperitoneal CP dose could be increased to 270 mg/m^2.

New second-generation platinum compounds have considerable promise [23]. Although they also are excreted by the kidney and require dosage modification in relation to reductions in GFR, they have much less nephrotoxicity than CP, thereby facilitating their administration to ambulatory patients because the CP saline infusion regimen usually is not necessary. The most widely studied of these compounds is carboplatin (*cis*-diamminecyclobutanedicarboxylatoplatinum, II). This compound has established activity against ovarian, small-cell lung, germ cell, and head and neck cancers [23]. Single-agent studies have established that the standard maximum tolerated dose is 400 to 500 mg/m^2 every 4 to 6 weeks [192]. In patients who have been extensively treated with other agents or who have decreased renal function, or in combination with other chemotherapy, a well-tolerated dose has been in the range of 200 to 250 mg/m^2 [49, 50]. The dose-limiting toxicity has been myelosuppression, predominantly thrombocytopenia [49, 50]. This toxicity profile is substantially different from the severe nausea and vomiting and renal, otologic, and neurologic toxicities that accompany therapy with comparably effective CP doses of 60 to 100 mg/m^2. The marked reduction in nonhematologic toxicity establishes carboplatin as a valuable agent in the setting of high-dose chemotherapy, where recovery from myelosuppression can be accomplished by the use of autologous bone marrow transplantation. A recent study in this setting indicated the maximum tolerated dose of carboplatin to be 2,000 mg/m^2 administered with a 4-day continuous infusion. Dose-limiting toxicity consisting of reversible hepatoxicity, renal dysfunction, and moderate to severe ototoxicity was encountered with a dose of 2,400 mg/m^2 [169]. Also, current trials are evaluating carboplatin in combination with the recombinant colony-stimulating factors, where substantial potential exists for modifying chemotherapy-induced white blood cell and red blood cell suppression and possibly platelet suppression.

Thus, carboplatin and similar compounds are expected to assume an increasing role in the practice of oncology over the next decade. Because carboplatin undergoes substantially less protein binding than CP, a much larger percentage is excreted in the urine [42]. This suggests that full doses of carboplatin might produce undue toxicity in patients with reduced renal function. However, that patient population includes those in whom carboplatin might have its greatest clinical efficacy. These include patients who have undergone a decrease in renal function due to previous chemotherapy or the previously described renal complications of cancer such that they could not receive CP, and nevertheless might have tumors with a high probability of platinum responsiveness. Thus, the carboplatin dosage modification described by Van Echo et al. [192], based on the patient's GFR, pretreatment platelet count, desired platelet nadir, and prior chemotherapy status, could be extremely useful [42]. The derived formula provides the ability to calculate a fully therapeutic, but a not unduly toxic dose of carboplatin.

Cyclophosphamide. Cyclophosphamide (CPA) is an antineoplastic agent that has been widely utilized for many years, most frequently in the therapy of hematologic malignancies, lymphomas, multiple myeloma, and a variety of solid tumors. Its toxicity primarily involves bone marrow suppression, gastrointestinal symptoms, alopecia, and hemorrhagic cystitis. CPA has no intrinsic alkylating or cytotoxic activity; conversion to its active metabolites (which are intrinsically toxic to urothelium) requires the action of hepatic microsomal enzymes [114].

The nephrotoxicity of CPA is limited to impairment of water excretion after high-dose therapy (50 mg/kg body weight), as reflected by dilutional hyponatremia and inappropriate concentration of the urine [44, 181]. No other nephrotoxicity has been noted [44]. Impaired water excretion occurs within 12 hours after CPA administration and resolves within 24 hours after drug withdrawal. This time sequence is consistent with the time required for conversion of the drug to its active metabolites and their urinary excretion.

In contrast to the syndrome of "inappropriate ADH secretion," which is an unusual occurrence after administration of vincristine [183] and is associated with elevated plasma vasopressin concentrations [144], CPA-induced water retention occurs commonly and is not accompanied by increased vasopressin concentrations [18]. The origin of CPA-induced water retention appears to be a direct toxic effect of drug metabolite(s) on the renal tubular cells of the distal nephron and collecting duct, facilitating increased water reabsorption. This proposed pathogenesis of CPA nephrotoxicity is consistent with the observed relationship between onset of antidiuresis and the appearance of alkylating metabolites in the urine [43].

CPA nephrotoxicity is usually self-limited and not a serious complication but has resulted in the death of a patient from cerebral edema in one reported case [75]. Its major clinical relevance relates to the need for a sustained diuresis after high-dose CPA therapy in order to avoid hemorrhagic cystitis or acute uric acid nephropathy. In this setting, diuresis should not be induced by water loading because of the potential for severe hyponatremia due to CPA-related water retention. DeFronzo et al. have recommended a regimen of half-normal saline administration prior to high-dose CPA therapy in order to correct preexisting volume deficits and suppress endogenous ADH [44]. This infusion is continued throughout the period of CPA administration. If weight gain is excessive, the infusion volume is reduced. Diuretic therapy is avoided, if possible, in order to eliminate the potential for exacerbating hyponatremia.

Streptozotocin. Streptozotocin (ST) is a nitrosourea compound derived from *Streptomyces acromogenes;* the drug also has been chemically synthesized [66]. ST has well-established roles in the management of patients with metastatic islet cell carcinoma of the pancreas and in carcinoid tumors [201]. Clinical activity also has been reported in Hodgkin's and non-Hodgkin's lymphoma [162]. Nonrenal toxicity includes nausea, vomiting, and febrile reactions. Nephrotoxicity has proved to be the dose-limiting toxicity of this agent. It may cause renal function abnormalities after one dose, and up to 75 percent of patients develop nephrotoxicity to some degree with prolonged administration [201].

The major excretory pathway for ST is the kidney. Animal studies have shown high concentrations of ST in the kidney [15]; up to 73 percent of administered drug and its metabolites are excreted in the urine [94]. Renal histopathology following ST has involved glomerular and tubular cells [112, 122]. Proximal tubules have been affected primarily, with tubular atrophy and interstitial inflammatory infiltrates being a prominent feature [122].

The clinical manifestations of ST nephrotoxicity involve abnormalities of both glomerular and tubular function. In one study, hypophosphatemia due to renal phosphate wasting was the earliest sign of nephrotoxicity and appeared in some cases after one dose of the drug. This study described renal tubular dysfunction in a group of 18 patients treated at a ST dosage of 2 gm/m^2/week [153]. These patients manifest a wide variety of tubular defects and some developed acute renal failure. In two other large series, proteinuria was the initial abnormality noted and was predictive of more severe renal toxicity if ST was continued [21, 162]. It appeared in some patients after only a few doses; the degree of proteinuria usually did not reach nephrotic levels. The onset of renal insufficiency was often delayed and sometimes did not occur despite evidence of other renal dysfunction [162]. If administration of ST was discontinued at the outset of mild renal functional abnormalities, these abnormalities resolved. However, if treatment was continued, progressive nephrotoxicity occurred [162]. Although there are no definitive data relating a cumulative dose with the development of nephrotoxicity, renal damage often has been manifest following a cumulative dose of 4 gm/m^2.

The clinical value of ST would be greatly enhanced if a consistent means of reducing nephrotoxicity were available. In order to minimize nephrotoxicity, it would appear that the optimal dosage schedule may be either 1.5 gm/m^2/week or 0.5 gm/m^2 daily for 5 days, with repeat courses every 3 to 4 weeks. Detection of proteinuria or renal tubular defects is an indication for drug discontinuation until these abnormalities resolve. Utilization of hydration and diuretic regimens or a continuous infusion schedule may possibly reduce nephrotoxicity; however, specific data in this regard are not yet available.

Semustine. Semustine (methyl CCNU) is a lipid-soluble nitrosourea, which is structurally similar to carmustine (BCNU) and lomustine (CCNU). These agents have demonstrated clinical activity in malignant melanoma, brain tumors, and malignant lymphomas [30, 199]. Semustine differs from carmustine by the substitution of a cyclohexyl ring for one chloroethyl group and from lomustine only by the addition of a methyl group on the four position of the cyclohexyl ring. Because of the ease of administration of these agents, their ability to cross the blood-brain barrier because of high lipid solubility, and their broad spectrum of antitumor activity, they have the potential of widespread utilization either alone or in combination with other oncolytic agents. However, to date, their nephrotoxicity has been a factor limiting their more widespread utilization.

All three of these drugs are rapidly metabolized, and the parent compound cannot be detected in the plasma more than 20 minutes after administration [125]. Metabolites are excreted in the urine up to 72 hours after administration [180]. Urinary excretion accounts for approximately 60 percent of the excretion of metabolites; these metabolites are most likely responsible for nephrotoxicity, since none of the parent compound undergoes urinary excretion. Semustine has proved to be the most nephrotoxic of these compounds; the nephrotoxicity of carmustine and lomustine will be discussed subsequently.

Preclinical trials of semustine in mice, dogs, and monkeys led to the prediction of renal toxicity in patients [46]. However, there were no reports of nephrotoxicity during the early years of the drug's utilization in humans [198]. However, long-term observation in patients receiving the drug following the total or partial resection of brain tumors revealed that high-dose therapy may lead to irreversible renal failure [76]. In this study, all six children who received more than 1,500 mg/m^2 BSA of semustine had marked renal damage. Proteinuria, hypertension, and alterations in urine sediment were absent. The degree of toxicity appeared to be dose-dependent. Evidence of renal damage often was not apparent until 18 to 24 months following the completion of semustine therapy. Another extensive series has described nephrotoxicity in children and adults who received semustine for therapy of malignant brain tumors [159]. In these patients, renal failure also developed insidiously, with the initial evidence of renal insufficiency occurring 1 to 6 years after onset of therapy. In 7 patients, clinical evidence of nephrotoxicity did not appear until at least 7 to 28 months after semustine was discontinued. In 4 patients, functional impairment progressed rapidly to advanced uremia despite discontinuation of therapy. The interval between recognition of renal disease and uremia in these patients was 6 months to 1 year after therapy was discontinued. Histologic examination of renal tissue in both of the foregoing studies disclosed glomerulosclerosis, focal tubular atrophy, moderate lymphocyte infiltration, and varying degrees of interstitial fibrosis on light microscopy (Fig. 42-1). Electron microscopy in one patient revealed uniform thickening and wrinkling of the glomerular basement membrane without evidence of immune-complex deposition.

Another study has described the nephrotoxicity of semustine in 45 adult patients with malignant melanoma who received the drug as adjuvant chemotherapy. Abnormalities of renal function were noted in 7 of these patients; all had received more than 1,400 mg/m^2. This represented a nephrotoxicity incidence of 26 percent in patients receiving more than 1,400 mg/m^2 [119]. No clinical signs of renal insufficiency were detected in any patients receiving less than 1,400 mg/m^2 and no changes unequivocally attributable to semustine were seen in 8 patients at autopsy, although 3 of those patients had received greater than 1,900 mg/m^2 of the drug. Thus in adults, the incidence of nephrotoxicity appeared to be significantly lower than that previously reported in children. In those adults who did develop renal failure, there were two distinct patterns. Two patients were observed to develop an increase in serum creatinine concentration while receiving semustine and later progressed to renal failure. Another five patients had normal serum creatinine levels throughout their course of treatment but developed an increased level 1 month to 2 years following the completion of therapy.

Carmustine. Carmustine has not been observed to produce severe nephrotoxicity in humans. DeVita et al. noted an unexplained elevation of BUN in 10 percent of patients treated with this agent, but no reports of severe renal insufficiency have occurred in subsequent studies [47]. Of 89 patients receiving carmustine alone in a report by Schacht et al. [159], only 4 patients experienced renal dysfunction. This consisted of a modest elevation in serum creatinine. One of these patients underwent renal biopsy and only mild interstitial and tubular abnormalities were observed. Unfortunately, the efficacy of this drug is limited because interstitial pneumonitis and fibrosing alveolitis are observed when doses exceed 1,200 to 1,500 mg/m^2 [202].

Lomustine. Lomustine nephrotoxicity has been observed in monkeys at doses exceeding 120 mg/m^2 [160]. Interstitial nephritis was the prominent finding in these acute toxicity studies. Reports of nephrotoxicity from lomus-

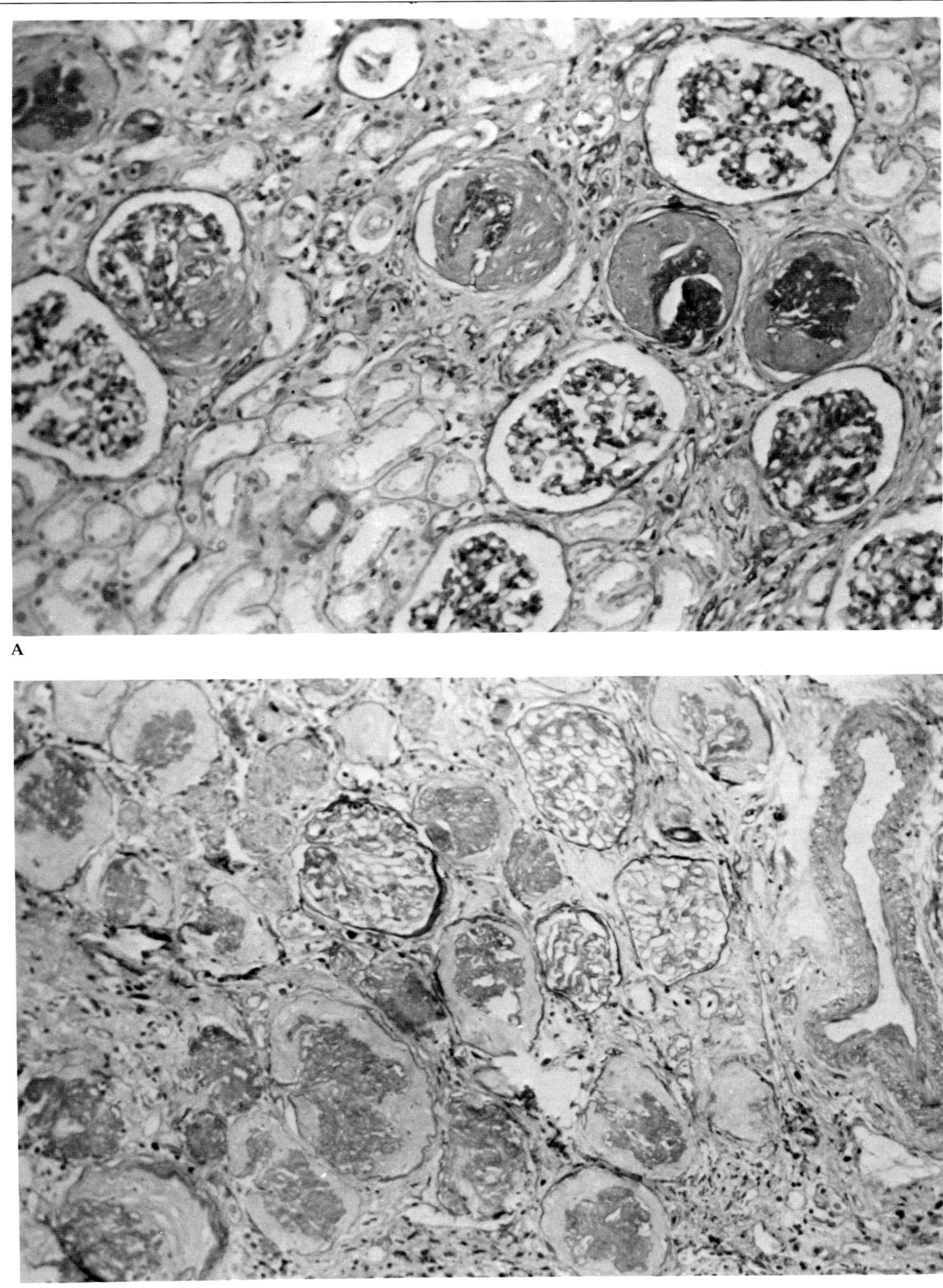

Fig. 42-1. A. Photomicrograph of the late stages of semustine nephrotoxicity from a specimen obtained at autopsy. (Magnification × 125.) B. Photomicrograph of a renal biopsy specimen from a patient with advanced semustine nephrotoxicity. (Magnification × 125.) (From W. E. Harmon et al. [76]; reprinted by permission of the *New England Journal of Medicine*.)

tine in humans have been few and are not well documented. The three cases that have been described received cumulative doses of 3,320, 3,360, and 2,300 mg [13, 63, 172]. In the latter case, azotemia and mild proteinuria were first noted 2 years after initiation of therapy [63]. This patient demonstrated an excellent therapeutic response to lomustine; however, progressive renal failure occurred and, ultimately, hemodialysis was required. Laboratory evaluation revealed minimal proteinuria and a benign urinary sediment; small kidneys were noted at autopsy. Thus it appears that nephrotoxicity is a potential problem only in patients receiving a prolonged course of treatment.

ANTIMETABOLITES

Methotrexate. Methotrexate (MTX), one of the first antineoplastic agents, has proved to be an extremely effective agent when used as a component of combination chemotherapy regimens for gestational trophoblastic choriocarcinoma, acute lymphocytic leukemia, bladder cancer, breast carcinoma, squamous cell carcinoma of the head and neck, osteogenic sarcoma, and non-Hodgkin's lymphoma. The major extrarenal toxicities caused by MTX include myelosuppression, mucositis, diarrhea, dermatitis, and hepatitis. This analogue of folic acid exerts its cytotoxic activity as a consequence of tight binding to dihydrofolate reductase, with subsequent inhibition and depletion of intracellular reduced folate pools.

When administered at conventional dosage, nephrotoxicity is rarely a problem [36]. However, high-dose MTX regimens (50–250 mg/kg to 1–7 gm/m^2) have been associated with a high incidence of nephrotoxicity. Prior to an appreciation of the importance of maintaining a high urinary volume and pH, renal toxicity was noted in approximately 30 percent of treatment courses and was responsible for 20 percent of the drug-related deaths during high-dose MTX-leucovorin rescue therapy [195]. MTX is excreted primarily by the kidneys by means of glomerular filtration and tubular secretion; greater than 90 percent of an intravenous dose appears unchanged in the urine following conventional doses [71, 107]. Thus any change in renal function has an effect on plasma MTX levels and the rate of MTX clearance. If MTX levels are elevated for prolonged periods of time, the organ systems most affected, which are thereby limiting with respect to toxicity, are the bone marrow and gastrointestinal tract [8, 135]. MTX is poorly cleared by hemodialysis [189]; removal by peritoneal dialysis is even less effective [70]. Plasma exchange does not effectively remove MTX because of its extensive volume of distribution and poor binding to serum albumin [182].

The pathogenesis of MTX nephrotoxicity is presently unclear; there are three leading hypotheses. The one most widely accepted is that MTX or a metabolite precipitates within the distal nephron, thereby causing an intrarenal obstructive nephropathy similar to that observed with acute uric acid nephropathy. During high-dose infusions, urinary MTX levels, which may be in excess of 1 mM, exceed the solubility of MTX and promote drug precipitation [71]. At physiologic systemic pH, MTX is completely ionized; however, because the unionized moiety predominates at the more acid pH usually encountered within the distal nephron, solubility is markedly reduced. Thus patients receiving high doses of MTX therapy may be more prone to nephrotoxicity if they are dehydrated and excreting an acid urine; this would promote MTX precipitation in the distal nephron. The 7-OH metabolite of MTX also may precipitate within the kidney. This metabolite may account for as much as 7 to 33 percent of MTX appearing in the urine from 24 to 48 hours after intravenous administration; its solubility is only 25 percent of that observed for MTX [89]. Figure 42-2 represents a renal biopsy specimen from a patient treated with MTX (3 gm/m^2 BSA) followed by leucovorin rescue therapy [58]. This patient became dehydrated and developed acute renal failure. The precipitated material in the renal tubules was demonstrated to be MTX. The incidence of MTX nephrotoxicity has markedly decreased since the institution of prophylactic urinary alkalinization and hydration as part of the treatment regimen associated with high-dose MTX therapy [134]. This observation appears to support the importance of precipitation of intrarenal MTX, its metabolite, or both, as a significant factor in the pathogenesis of nephrotoxicity.

The second proposed mechanism of pathogenesis in-

Fig. 42-2. Renal biopsy specimen from a patient treated with 3 gm/m^2 of methotrexate, with accompanying leucovorin therapy, who became dehydrated and developed acute renal failure. Precipitated material in the renal tubules (*arrow*) strongly reacted with a fluoresceinated rabbit antimethotrexate antibody. (Courtesy of Dr. Susan W. Pitman.) (From M. B. Garnick et al. [58]; reprinted by permission of Grune & Stratton.)

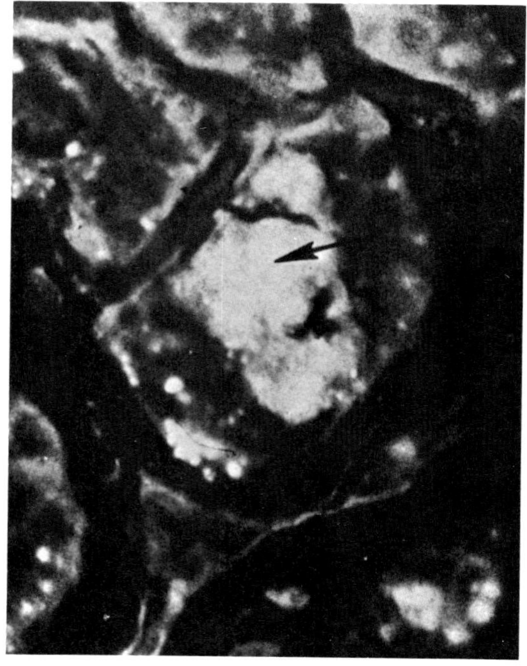

volves direct tubular toxicity. In one report of a patient who developed MTX-induced renal failure following high-dose treatment, postmortem examination revealed evidence of proximal tubular necrosis without demonstration of intraluminal precipitated material [1]. Furthermore, the occurrence of nephrotoxicity following high-dose aminopterin therapy is of great interest in this regard. Aminopterin is a folic acid antagonist, which is ten times more potent than equimolar doses of MTX but has similar solubility characteristics. High-dose aminopterin protocols employ a dosage that is approximately 10 percent of the MTX dosage in similar protocols; nevertheless, nephrotoxicity does occur. The absence of renal tubular precipitates in two patients receiving a high-dose aminopterin protocol, who died with nephrotoxicity, suggests direct tubular toxicity [60].

The third proposed mechanism of MTX nephrotoxicity involves a direct effect on glomerular hemodynamics. The administration of high-dose MTX has uniformly resulted in a decrease in GFR, both in pediatric and adult patients [82, 108]. The consistent and reversible decrease in GFR observed after high-dose MTX therapy suggests that a decrease in renal perfusion due to constriction of afferent arterioles may be a mechanism of toxicity. In this regard, it is of interest that pediatric patients receiving high-dose MTX for treatment of osteogenic sarcoma have been observed to develop hypertension during therapy.

The clinical course of MTX nephrotoxicity often resembles the nonoliguric acute renal failure induced by aminoglycosides. Although serum creatinine may increase progressively, urine output characteristically remains high. Since renal function changes rapidly when nephrotoxicity occurs, alterations in serum creatinine may not reflect accurately the decrease in GFR. Thus serial creatinine clearances are necessary to accurately assess the level of renal function. If renal damage occurs, the excretion of the drug is delayed and leads to systemic toxicity. Plasma MTX levels are essential in confirming the excretion of the drug. MTX levels below 4×10^{-7} M at 48 hours after drug infusion have been associated with a lack of systemic toxicity, while 40 percent of patients with 48-hour levels greater than 5×10^{-7} M had myelosuppression [182]. Parameters for monitoring serum MTX levels and the strategy for both prophylaxis of MTX-induced nephrotoxicity and its management have been reviewed in detail [1].

Cytosine Arabinoside. Cytosine arabinoside (CA) is an analogue of pyrimidine nucleoside and interferes with DNA synthesis by inhibiting DNA polymerase. Free CA is degraded by deaminase to uracil arabinoside, which is excreted in the urine. CA has proved to be an effective agent in the treatment of acute leukemia [101] and has recently been shown to be active against non-Hodgkin's lymphoma [171].

In a study of 33 patients treated with CA in a variety of multidrug regimens, more than half were observed to undergo a greater than 100-percent elevation in serum creatinine concentration or a decrease in creatinine clearance to less than 50 percent of baseline values [177]. Although CA was not the only drug used in these patients, the other drugs employed had not been associated with nephrotoxicity that involved renal insufficiency. The observed renal insufficiency was not dependent on the dose of CA. Renal histology of patients who died with renal failure revealed marked interstitial edema, tubular dilatation, and flattening of epithelial cells. It should be noted that a recent trial employing high-dose CA as a single agent was not associated with significant nephrotoxicity [171].

6-Thioguanine. Administration of high-dose, intravenous 6-thioguanine has been associated with moderate azotemia, which was often reversible within 2 weeks of withdrawing therapy [100, 137]. Nephrotoxicity was dose-related; the highest levels of azotemia occurred at doses in excess of 800 mg/m^2 [137]. Oral 6-thioguanine, when administered at the dosage usually employed in the treatment of acute leukemia, has not been associated with nephrotoxicity.

5-Fluorouracil. 5-Fluorouracil (5-FU) is converted to its active metabolite fluoro-deoxyuridine monophosphate, which inhibits DNA synthesis by blocking the enzyme thymidylate synthetase. Although nephrotoxicity has not been reported with 5-FU alone, renal insufficiency has been observed when this drug has been used in conjunction with mitomycin-C [67, 73, 91]. In one report, 14 of 143 patients with carcinoma of the gastrointestinal tract and pancreas who received combination therapy with these two drugs developed renal insufficiency [73]. Two clinical patterns were recognized. Some patients underwent acute, fulminating renal failure that was rapidly fatal. They manifest microangiopathic hemolytic anemia, with thrombocytopenia and erythrocyte fragmentation. Light and electron microscopy studies of the kidney revealed a primary vascular disease, with intimal hyperplasia of arteries and fibrin thrombi in arterioles. Interstitial fibrosis, tubular atrophy, and widespread glomerular necrosis also were present. These patients died within 3 to 4 weeks. Other patients manifest a more chronic course, with similar but less pronounced pathological findings; microangiopathic anemia was not present. The clinical course of the second group was also fatal but not until 3 to 8 months after the onset of this syndrome. In two patients who were receiving adjuvant therapy with this combination after resection of gastric neoplasms, progressive hemolytic anemia and mild renal impairment were noted [91]. When compatible blood transfusions were administered, exacerbation of the hemolytic process was noted, with evidence of an intravascular coagulopathy, rapidly progressive renal failure, and death. Autopsy revealed microangiopathic changes in the kidneys, with fibrin deposition in the small arterioles. These and the previously noted pathologic findings were distinct from those described when mitomycin-C was administered by itself [39, 110], as will be discussed subsequently.

5-Azacytidine. 5-Azacytidine (5-AZ) is a pyrimidine compound that has been effective in the therapy of patients with refractory acute nonlymphocytic leukemia. Toxicity has involved primarily gastrointestinal side effects and myelosuppression [157]. Preclinical studies indicated the potential for substantial nephrotoxicity [128]; 90 percent of the drug is excreted in the urine in humans [196]. An extensive clinical study revealed no renal toxicity in 745 patients treated with this drug [196]. However, another study has noted a high rate of renal tubular dysfunction in patients being treated with drug combinations that included 5-AZ [130]. In this study of 22 patients who received a total of 33 courses of combination chemotherapy, including 5-AZ, nephrotoxicity was noted in 88 percent of treatment courses. Nephrotoxicity was manifest by abnormalities indicative of tubular transport defects for glucose, bicarbonate, phosphorus, and sodium; polyuria was also a frequent finding. In addition, systemic acidosis without an increased anion gap and a urine pH greater than 7.0 was observed in some patients and was felt to be compatible with renal tubular acidosis. The foregoing defects appeared early in the course of treatment and resolved rapidly following completion of chemotherapy. The mild azotemia that occurred followed the same temporal pattern. It did not appear that other chemotherapy given in conjunction with 5-AZ could be incriminated, since these findings have not been reported on utilization of these agents in the absence of 5-AZ administration. Two reported cases of hypophosphatemia that occurred during therapy with only 5-AZ tend to support this conclusion [80]. While the evidence is not compelling that 5-AZ is nephrotoxic when utilized alone as an antineoplastic agent, at a minimum, it would appear that the drug is potentially nephrotoxic in synergism with other agents when utilized in combination chemotherapy regimens.

ANTITUMOR ANTIBIOTICS

Mitomycin-C. Mitomycin-C (MMC), an antibiotic isolated from the broth of *Streptomyces caespitosis,* has been shown to have clinical activity in the treatment of several solid tumors [29]. It is commonly employed with other agents, particularly 5-FU and doxorubicin, in the treatment of gastric and pancreatic carcinomas. It also has been found useful in the treatment of squamous carcinoma of the cervix and as intravesical therapy for superficial transitional cell carcinoma of the bladder. Major dose-limiting toxicities include cumulative delayed myelosuppression, dermatitis, nausea and vomiting, and pulmonary fibrosis [39]. In preclinical toxicologic investigations, monkeys given a single intravenous dose manifest acute tubular necrosis [132]. Unmetabolized MMC is excreted in the urine of dogs and rodents; recovery varies from 5 to 40 percent of the administered dose [166]. Excretion appears to be entirely by glomerular filtration [166]. The renal excretion of the intact drug in humans is less than in experimental animals, since most of the drug undergoes metabolism by the liver [39]. Although small amounts of the unmetabolized drug are excreted in the urine, the mechanism for nephrotoxicity is unknown.

MMC nephrotoxicity, consisting of azotemia, increased serum creatinine concentration, and proteinuria, was originally described in 3 of 32 patients treated with MMC at a dosage of 0.5 to 1.0 mg/kg, repeated every 4 to 8 weeks [110]. The cumulative dosage in these three cases ranged between 1.5 and 4.0 mg/kg, administered over a 6- to 27-month period. Nephrotoxicity appears to be dose-related and cumulative. Hamner et al. reported renal failure in patients exposed to 10 mg/m^2 of MMC or more; the onset of renal dysfunction followed initiation of MMC therapy by an average of 10 to 11 months [69]. Conflicting results have been reported by another study in which 68 patients were treated at a MMC dosage of 15 to 20 mg/m^2 over 68 weeks, including 29 patients who received greater than a total of 100 mg of MMC; drug-related nephrotoxicity was not demonstrated conclusively [140]. Renal histopathology in MMC nephrotoxicity was described comprehensively in a recently reported case of a 62-year-old man who developed advanced renal failure and microangiopathic hemolytic anemia 12 months after a course of 42 mg/m^2 of MMC was initiated as adjuvant therapy for adenocarcinoma of the colon [138]. Renal biopsy revealed marked glomerular sclerosis, hypocellularity, and necrosis; there was a great deal of interstitial scarring. Immunofluorescence studies were negative for antibody and complement in the 5 to 10 glomeruli studied; IgG deposits were present in the proximal tubular epithelium. On electron microscopy, fibrin was noted within glomeruli and interstitial blood vessels. These findings were interpreted as consistent with a thrombotic microangiopathic process and were thought to be similar to those seen in the hemolytic-uremic syndrome. Of additional interest in this patient was improvement of thrombocytopenia and microangiopathic hemolytic anemia following plasma exchange. At the time this therapy was instituted, renal failure was already far advanced; improvement in renal function did not occur.

In an attempt to establish the true incidence of MMC nephrotoxicity, Ratanatharathorn have reviewed clinical studies with the drug dating back to 1959 and have critically analyzed other potential contributing factors in the development of nephrotoxicity [140]. Of the 1,245 patients treated with MMC, 8 patients (<1%) developed nephrotoxicity, which appeared to be both drug- and dose-related. Thus available data suggest that MMC may occasionally produce nephrotoxicity when given by itself; toxicity appears to be related to the cumulative dosage received. On the other hand, as described previously, when the drug is given with 5-FU, nephrotoxicity occurs frequently and may be severe.

Mithramycin. Mithramycin is an antibiotic produced from the microorganism *Streptomyces tanashiensis.* Although not widely used as an antineoplastic agent at present, this drug has demonstrated activity against testicular carcinomas and glioblastomas [95, 96]. A variety of metabolic and toxic side effects have precluded its widespread use. In one study, the drug was administered in a dosage of 25 or 50 gm/kg daily for 5 days (or until toxicity) or three times weekly, with repeat courses every month [95]. Renal toxicity, reflected by a BUN of >25 mg/dl or a decrease in creatinine clearance, occurred in 22 of 54 (40%) of patients. Toxicity appeared to be cumulative and persistent if mithramycin was given in the presence of a diminished creatine clearance. Proteinuria occurred in 78 percent of the patients; 6 patients had drug-related deaths secondary to renal failure. Histopathologic findings consisted of renal tubular swelling with hydropic degeneration, proximal and distal tubular necrosis, and tubular atrophy; glomeruli were not involved.

Mithramycin is now most frequently utilized in the therapy of malignancy-associated hypercalcemia [97]. A single infusion of 25 μg/kg has been shown to decrease bone absorption and normalize serum calcium in 80 to 85 percent of patients treated. When given as a single injected dose, mithramycin generally has not been associated with renal toxicity [97]. However, recently a patient has been described who manifested renal functional deterioration that was temporally related on two occasions to single-dose mithramycin therapy (25 μg/kg) [12]. Another case of nephrotoxicity with single-dose therapy has been described [175]. Thus constant monitoring of renal function is essential even when this agent is administered in a small, single-dose regimen, particularly in the presence of renal insufficiency.

Doxorubicin. Doxorubicin (Adriamycin), one of the most widely used antineoplastic agents, exerts its antitumor effect by intercalating DNA. The drug is employed in the management of both solid and hematologic neoplasms. Doxorubicin has been shown to be nephrotoxic in animals, with primary involvement of the glomerulus; vacuolization of the tubular epithelium and interstitial fibrosis also have been observed [54, 131]. Nephrotoxicity is dose-dependent and occurs simultaneously with cardiomyopathy [131]. The observed dose dependency and the limitation of dosage in humans because of the risk of cardiomyopathy may explain the lack of nephrotoxicity in clinical studies. In the only published case of nephrotoxicity, the patient developed uremia after two doses of doxorubicin, with a total dose of 180 mg [24]. Renal biopsy revealed interstitial fibrosis and glomerular alterations similar to those observed in animals. The extensive use of this drug without evidence of nephrotoxicity raises doubt as to the significance of this report.

BIOLOGIC AGENTS

Interferons. The interferons are a group of glycoproteins that have been shown to have antitumor activity [81, 104, 187]. The three major types are alfa (leukocyte or lymphoblastoid), beta (fibroblast), and gamma (immune). A patient has been described who developed reversible acute renal insufficiency and the nephrotic syndrome after being treated with interferon alfa [6]. The clinical syndrome and histopathology were consistent with a combination of acute interstitial nephritis and minimal-change nephropathy. Light microscopy revealed unremarkable glomeruli, extensive interstitial edema, and a moderately severe, patchy interstitial infiltrate predominantly composed of lymphocytes, eosinophils, and plasma cells. Tubular dilatation and focal degeneration and necrosis of proximal tubular cells also were observed. Electron microscopy confirmed the tubulointerstitial findings and demonstrated diffuse effacement of glomerular epithelial foot processes. The absence of electron-dense deposits on the glomerular basement membrane was felt to be consistent with the findings of typical minimal-change disease. This latter observation and the absence of circulating immune complexes while the patient had nephrotic-range proteinuria strongly suggested that immune complexes did not play a role in the pathogenesis of the renal lesion. A similar picture has been described in a variety of other patients who received this agent [168]. In addition, nephrotic syndrome due to membranoproliferative glomerulonephritis has been reported recently in a patient with hairy-cell leukemia after treatment with interferon alfa for 1 year [79]. Interferon alfa–induced renal toxicity actually is quite rare, as indicated by a phase I study of interferon in 81 patients with advanced tumors [170]. Two patients developed urinary protein excretion of 1.0 and 2.0 gm per day after treatment three times weekly for a period of 2 weeks. Proteinuria resolved 10 days after discontinuing therapy. A recent case of acute renal failure has been described 19 days after initiating treatment with interferon gamma in a child with acute lymphoblastic leukemia. The renal biopsy specimen revealed acute tubular necrosis, with no evidence of immune complex deposition [5].

Interleukin-2. Interleukin-2 is a glycoprotein with a molecular weight of 15,000 daltons. In vivo, it enhances natural killer cell function, augments alloantigen responsiveness, and improves the recovery of immune function in acquired immunodeficiency states. With the development of recombinant DNA technology, interleukin-2 now can be produced in large quantities. The incubation of human peripheral-blood lymphocytes with interleukin-2 generates lymphokine-activated killer cells. Administration of these cells alone to patients with cancer causes minimal side effects but also mediates no beneficial antitumor effects [146]. However, administration of lymphokine-activated killer cells in conjunction with recombinant interleukin-2 to patients with advanced cancer can induce the regression of metastatic disease in melanoma, renal cell, and colorectal cancer [145]. Unfortunately, the required dosage level in early studies produced severe renal insufficiency. Therefore, nephrotoxicity was one of the major factors limiting the ability of patients to tolerate high doses of this agent [145]. Profound reductions in GFR and sodium excretion have been noted. The rapidity with which these abnormalities develop and resolve suggests that they are largely hemodynamic in origin [188].

Belldegrun et al. studied the effect of a high dose, bolus interleukin-2 regimen on renal function in 99 patients with advanced cancer who received therapy with interleukin-2 alone or in conjunction with lymphokine-activated killer cells. More than 90% of the patients in each group showed some sign of acute renal failure, with rapid improvement after cessation of therapy [11].

However, patients with pretreatment elevations in serum creatinine had significantly prolonged recovery times, and underwent greater decrements of GFR. Therapy with lymphokine-activated killer cells alone was not associated with renal insufficiency, thereby supporting the conclusion that interleukin-2 is the offending agent. The clinical syndrome of hypotension, oliguria, fluid retention, and associated azotemia with extremely high fractional reabsorption of sodium strongly supports prerenal failure as the basis for the observed renal dysfunction. This hypoperfusion state appears to be secondary to translocation of intravascular fluid along with albumin to the extravascular space. This capillary leak syndrome requires management with sufficient ECF volume replacement to reverse hypotension and oliguria.

Both the catabolism of lymphokine-activated killer cells and tumor cells may result in uric acid overproduction and excretion due to accelerated rates of nucleic acid turnover. Since acute uric acid nephropathy is most often seen in patients with uric acid overproduction associated with ECF volume contraction, this etiology has been considered as a possible contributing factor to the renal insufficiency observed due to interleukin-2. However, this possibility has been rendered unlikely by data indicating a urinary uric acid to creatinine ratio substantially less than 1.0 in this setting [11]. A more likely contributing factor to the observed profound prerenal failure is the administration of indomethacin in order to alleviate fever and chills. It is possible that the resultant inhibition of vasodilatory prostaglandins contributes to renal hypoperfusion.

Continuing efforts to modify the nephrotoxicity of interleukin-2 have involved modification of dosage schedules. Constant infusion as opposed to bolus therapy has resulted in maintenance of an antitumor effect with a substantial reduction in toxicity [203]. Repetitive weekly cycles of therapy administered without lymphokine-activated killer cells also has induced antitumor activity with acceptable toxicity [179].

Corynebacterium parvum. Immunotherapy with *Corynebacterium parvum* has been associated with three cases of reversible glomerulonephritis [48]. These patients were oliguric and azotemic in the presence of hypocomplementemia. Examination of tissue from renal biopsies revealed mesangial proliferation with polymorphonuclear aggregates in glomerular capillaries. Immunofluorescent microscopy revealed a finely granular pattern with deposition of IgG, IgA, IgM, and C3 within the mesangium and along the capillary walls. Electron microscopy revealed an increase in mesangial matrix and subendothelial electron-dense deposits.

Nephrotoxicity due to Metabolic Products of Tumor Lysis Produced by Antineoplastic Agents

Treatment with antineoplastic agents may result in the rapid generation of endogenous nephrotoxins, such as uric acid, xanthine, and phosphorus. This complication is of particular concern in patients with rapidly growing tumors that are extremely sensitive to antineoplastic agents. In this setting, intracellular products of malignant cells are released into the circulation as a consequence of massive cytolysis and may produce hyperuricemia, hyperxanthinemia (especially when patients are being treated with allopurinol), hyperphosphatemia, and hyperkalemia. The magnitude of biochemical alterations in this setting is related to tumor burden and is greatly magnified by prior renal insufficiency, since phosphate, potassium, and uric acid homeostasis are particularly dependent on integrity of renal excretory function.

The foregoing metabolic abnormalities have been described as part of the *acute tumor lysis syndrome,* which has been reported as a complication of therapy with antineoplastic agents in patients with acute leukemia, malignant lymphoma, and small-cell bronchogenic carcinoma [27, 35, 53, 191, 194]. Nephrotoxicity due to hyperphosphatemia or hyperxanthinemia occurs only in this setting and thus is a rare occurrence. On the other hand, acute uric acid nephropathy (AUAN) occurs more frequently and thus must be considered prior to initiating therapy for a variety of malignancies.

ACUTE URIC ACID NEPHROPATHY

The sudden onset of renal insufficiency in association with acute hyperuricemia is now a well-recognized occurrence [98, 142]. When a sufficient level of hyperuricosuria can be documented, the diagnosis of acute uric acid nephropathy (AUAN) is established. AUAN is most frequently associated with the therapy of leukemias and lymphomas [98, 103, 200], although it has been reported in a patient with disseminated carcinoma [38]. This form of hyperuricemic nephropathy may occur spontaneously, but most often it is precipitated by or exacerbated by therapy with antineoplastic agents, with a resultant increase in uric acid production by means of the accelerated degradation of nucleoprotein.

The normal renal response to hyperuricemia is an increase in tubular urate secretion [143]. Since urinary concentration of nonionized uric acid approaches saturation under normal physiologic conditions, any significant increase in accession of urate into proximal tubular fluid, with its subsequent acidification and concentration in the distal nephron, provides the potential for uric acid precipitation and associated tubular obstruction [142]. The concentration and physical state of uric acid in tubular fluid are key determinants in the pathogenesis of AUAN. Manipulation of these variables comprises the basis for prophylaxis and therapy. Failure to recognize impending AUAN, or delay in pursuing vigorous therapy, may result in rapidly progressive acute renal failure. The clinical course, pathogenesis, diagnosis, and therapy of AUAN are discussed in detail in Chap. 81.

XANTHINE NEPHROPATHY

Xanthine nephropathy is encountered rarely. Nevertheless, this complication must be considered in patients who develop the acute tumor lysis syndrome and are receiving allopurinol. Although the normal daily excretion of xanthine is approximately 6 mg, patients who experience rapid tumor lysis and who are receiving allopurinol therapy may undergo an increase in urinary xanthine excretion to a level as high as 750 mg/day [72]. The solubility of xanthine in urine at a pH of 5.0 is 50 mg/liter, whereas it is 130 mg/liter at a pH of 7.0 [99]. Hypoxanthine, which is the other immediate precursor of uric acid whose urinary excretion is increased due to allopurinol-induced xanthine oxidase inhibition, is much more soluble than xanthine. Thus hypoxanthine nephropathy is not likely to occur.

Purine excretion was determined following chemotherapy in seven patients with rapidly growing lymphomas who were receiving 300 to 600 mg/day of allopurinol [72]. The peak urinary xanthine excretion postchemotherapy exceeded the solubility of xanthine at pH 7.0 in 4 of 7 patients. Despite intensive hydration, 2 of these 4 patients developed transient renal failure, with creatinine clearances of 28 and 12 ml/min. In another report, xanthine crystalluria, acute renal failure, and a high plasma oxypurine level were observed in a patient with Burkitt's lymphoma who was treated with cyclophosphamide and allopurinol [2].

At a urine pH of 5.0, one would expect that xanthine solubility limits would be exceeded in a significant number of patients receiving high doses of allopurinol and undergoing rapid lysis of tumor cells. Thus it is surprising that more cases of xanthine nephropathy have not been reported in cancer patients who are receiving allopurinol in view of reports of xanthine calculi in 3 of 8 patients with hereditary xanthinuria [167]. Similar reports have appeared in patients with Lesch-Nyhan syndrome treated with allopurinol [65, 178]. Since xanthine solubility is substantially enhanced in an alkaline urine, and since induction of a high urine flow and urinary alkalinization are frequently employed in hyperuricemic cancer patients receiving allopurinol, this may account for the rarity of xanthine nephropathy.

HYPERPHOSPHATEMIC NEPHROPATHY

Profound hyperphosphatemia is frequently observed as part of the acute tumor lysis syndrome, especially when it is associated with lymphoblastic tumors, since lymphoblasts have a higher organic and inorganic phosphorous content than normal cells [27]. Phosphate derived from cell lysis is reutilized by other dividing cells and the excess is excreted by the kidneys [191]. However, in the presence of renal failure, renal phosphate excretion is impaired. Acute hyperphosphatemia may induce a decrease in serum calcium concentrations; this has been ascribed to extraskeletal calcium phosphate deposition [207].

The acute onset of extreme hyperphosphatemia following cancer chemotherapy may result in acute renal failure [27, 53]. Marked hyperphosphatemia, sometimes in excess of 20 mg/dl, may be anticipated after therapy in patients with a large tumor burden associated with renal insufficiency prior to therapy. Intrarenal precipitation of calcium phosphate salts has been suggested as the cause of acute renal failure in this setting [27]. Acute renal failure in response to this "infusion" of phosphate derived from tumor cells undergoing rapid lysis is analogous to reports of acute renal failure observed following the administration of large doses of phosphate [7]. Excessive urinary alkalinization may promote phosphate precipitation in renal tubules and thus should be avoided in the presence of a high urinary phosphate concentration. If the GFR is already substantially reduced in the presence of marked hyperphosphatemia, dialysis may be necessary to prevent further renal damage. Recovery of renal function usually occurs following reduction of the serum phosphate level [53, 93].

Conclusion

Nephrotoxicity due to antineoplastic agents is a frequent cause of acute renal failure and other renal abnormalities in the cancer patient. A decrease in the incidence of this complication can be attained with an increased awareness of (1) the nephrotoxic potential of offending antineoplastic agents, (2) the nephrotoxic dosage of these agents, (3) appropriate prophylactic measures, and (4) the clinical settings that predispose to nephrotoxicity. Additionally, early diagnosis of nephrotoxicity allowing prompt therapy and withdrawal of the offending agent may minimize adverse effects. The foregoing principles have been reviewed and provide an important consideration in the care of the cancer patient.

References

1. Abelson, H. T., and Garnick, M. B. Renal Failure Induced by Cancer Chemotherapy. In R. E. Rieselbach and M. B. Garnick (eds.), *Cancer and the Kidney*. Philadelphia: Lea & Febiger, 1982.
2. Ablin, A., et al. Nephropathy, xanthinuria, and orotic aciduria complicating Burkitt's lymphoma treated with chemotherapy and allopurinol. *Metabolism* 21: 771, 1972.
3. Anderson, R. J., et al. Non-oliguric acute renal failure. *N. Engl. J. Med.* 296: 1134, 1977.
4. Arneil, G. C., et al. Nephritis in two children after irradiation and chemotherapy for nephroblastoma. *Lancet* 1: 960, 1974.
5. Ault, B. H., et al. Acute renal failure during therapy with recombinant human gamma interferon. *N. Engl. J. Med.* 319: 1397, 1988.
6. Averbuch, S. D., et al. Acute interstitial nephritis with the nephrotic syndrome following recombinant leukocyte A interferon therapy for mycosis fungoides. *N. Engl. J. Med.* 310: 32, 1984.
7. Ayala, G., et al. Acute hyperphosphatemia and acute persistent renal insufficiency induced by oral phosphate therapy. *Ann. Intern. Med.* 83: 520, 1975.
8. Baker, L. R. J., et al. Acute renal failure due to bacterial pyelonephritis. *Q. J. Med.* 48: 603, 1979.
9. Barton, C. H., et al. Renal magnesium wasting associated with amphotericin B therapy. *Am. J. Med.* 77: 471, 1984.
10. Beach, E. W. Urologic complications of cancer of the uterine cervix. *J. Urol.* 68: 178, 1952.
11. Belldegrun, A., et al. Effects of interleukin-2 on renal function in patients receiving immunotherapy for advanced cancer. *Ann. Intern. Med.* 106: 817, 1987.
12. Benedetti, R. G., Heilman, J. K., III, and Gabow, P. A. Nephrotoxicity following single dose mithramycin therapy. *Am. J. Nephrol.* 3: 277, 1983.
13. Berglund, J. Progressive renal insufficiency after CCNU therapy. *Lakartidningen* 77: 1760, 1980.

14. Bhuchar, V. K., and Lanzotti, V. J. High-dose cisplatin for lung cancer. *Cancer Treat. Rep.* 66: 375, 1982.
15. Bhuyan, B. K., et al. Tissue distribution of streptozotocin (NSC-85998). *Cancer Chemother. Rep.* 58: 157, 1974.
16. Blachley, J. D., and Hill, J. B. Renal and electrolyte disturbances associated with cisplatin. *Ann. Intern. Med.* 95: 628, 1981.
17. Bleyer, W. A. The clinical pharmacology of methotrexate: New application of an old drug. *Cancer* 41: 36, 1978.
18. Bode, U., Seif, S. M., and Levine, A. S. Studies on the antidiuretic effect of cyclophosphamide: Vasopressin release and sodium excretion. *Med. Pediatr. Oncol.* 8: 295, 1980.
19. Boner, G., Newton, M., and Rieselbach, R. E. Exaggerated carbohydrate-induced calciuria in the remaining kidney of transplant donors. *Kidney Int.* 3: 24, 1973.
20. Boxer, R. J., Garnick, M. B., and Anderson, T. Extrarenal Cancer of the Genitourinary Tract. In R. E. Rieselbach and M. B. Garnick (eds.), *Cancer and the Kidney*. Philadelphia: Lea & Febiger, 1982.
21. Broder, L. E., and Carter, S. K. Pancreatic islet cell carcinoma. *Ann. Intern. Med.* 79: 108, 1973.
22. Buckley, J. E., et al. Hypomagnesemia after cisplatin combination chemotherapy. *Arch. Intern. Med.* 144: 2347, 1984.
23. Bunn, P. A., Jr., et al. *Carboplatin (JM-8): Current Perspectives and Future Directions*. Philadelphia: W. B. Saunders Company, 1990.
24. Burke, J. F., et al. Doxorubicin hydrochloride-associated renal failure. *Arch. Intern. Med.* 137: 385, 1977.
25. Butterly, J. M., et al. Addison's disease secondary to metastatic carcinoma of the adrenal glands. *Ann. Intern. Med.* 37: 930, 1952.
26. Byrd, L., and Sherman, R. L. Radiocontrast-induced acute renal failure. A clinical and pathophysiologic review. *Medicine* 58: 270, 1979.
27. Cadman, E., Lundberg, W., and Bertino, J. Hyperphosphatemia and hypocalcemia accompanying rapid cell lysis in a patient with Burkitt's lymphoma and Burkitt cell leukemia. *Am. J. Med.* 62: 283, 1977.
28. Campbell, A. B., Kalman, S. M., and Jacobs, C. Plasma platinum levels: Relationship to cisplatin dose and nephrotoxicity. *Cancer Treat. Rep.* 67: 169, 1983.
29. Carter, S. K., and Crooke, S. T. (eds.) *Mitomycin C: Current status and new developments*. New York: Academic Press, 1979.
30. Carter, S. K., and Wasserman, T. H. The nitrosoureas—Thoughts for the future. *Cancer Treat. Rep.* 60: 807, 1976.
31. Chapman, A. Etiology of Acute Renal Failure in Adult Patients. In A. Chapman (ed.), *Acute Renal Failure*. New York: Churchill Livingstone, 1980.
32. Churchill, D. N., Hong, K., and Gault, M. H. Radiation nephritis following combined abdominal radiation and chemotherapy (bleomycin-vinblastine). *Cancer* 41: 2162, 1978.
33. Clyne, D. H., Pesce, A. J., and Thompson, R. E. Nephrotoxicity of Bence Jones protein in the rat. Importance of protein isoelectric point. *Kidney Int.* 16: 345, 1979.
34. Coe, F. L. Calcium and Phosphorus Metabolism in Cancer; Hypercalcemic Nephropathy. In R. E. Rieselbach and M. B. Garnick (eds.), *Cancer and the Kidney*. Philadelphia: Lea & Febiger, 1982.
35. Cohen, L., et al. Acute tumor lysis syndrome: A review of 37 patients with Burkitt's lymphoma. *Am. J. Med.* 68: 486, 1980.
36. Condit, P. T., Chanes, R. E., and Joel, W. Renal toxicity of methotrexate. *Cancer* 23: 126, 1969.
37. Cousins, M. J., and Mazze, R. I. Methoxyflurane nephrotoxicity: A study of dose-response in man. *J.A.M.A.* 225: 1611, 1973.
38. Crittenden, D. R., and Ackermann, G. L. Hyperuricemic acute renal failure in disseminated carcinoma. *Arch. Intern. Med.* 137: 97, 1977.
39. Crooke, S. T., and Bradner, W. T. Mitomycin-C—A review. *Cancer Treat. Rev.* 3: 121, 1976.
40. Cvitkovic, E., et al. Improvement of *cis*-dichlorodiammine-platinum (NSC-119875), therapeutic index in an animal model. *Cancer* 39: 1357, 1977.
41. Daniels, R. A., and Weisenfeld, I. Tumorous phosphaturic osteomalacia: Report of a case associated with multiple hemangiomas of bone. *Am. J. Med.* 67: 155, 1979.
42. Deconti, R. C., et al. Clinical and pharmacological studies with cis-diamminedichloroplatinum(II). *Cancer Res.* 33: 1310, 1973.
43. DeFronzo, R. A., et al. Water intoxication in man after cyclophosphamide therapy. *Ann. Intern. Med.* 78: 861, 1973.
44. DeFronzo, R. A., et al. Cyclophosphamide and the kidney. *Cancer* 33: 483, 1974.
45. DeFronzo, R. A., et àl. Renal function in patients with multiple myeloma. *Medicine* 57: 151, 1978.
46. Denine, E. P., Harrison, S. D., Jr., and Peckham, J. C. Qualitative and quantitative toxicity of sublethal doses of methyl-CCNU in BDF_1 in mice. *Cancer Treat. Rep.* 61: 409, 1977.
47. DeVita, V. T., et al. Clinical trials with 1,3-bis(2-chloroethyl)-1-nitrosourea, NSC-409962. *Cancer Res.* 25: 1876, 1965.
48. Dosik, G. M., et al. Nephrotoxicity from cancer immunotherapy. *Ann. Intern. Med.* 89: 41, 1978.
49. Edmonson, J. H., et al. Pilot study of cyclophosphamide plus carboplatin in advanced ovarian carcinoma. *Cancer Treat. Rep.* 71: 199, 1987.
50. Egorin, M. J., et al. Pharmacokinetics and dosage reduction of cis-diammine (1,1-cyclobutanedicarboxylate) platinum in patients with impaired renal function. *Cancer Res.* 44: 5432, 1984.
51. Einhorn, L. H., and Williams, S. D. The role of *cis*-platinum in solid tumor therapy. *N. Engl. J. Med.* 300: 289, 1979.
52. Eliahou, H. E., et al. An epidemiologic study of renal failure. II. Acute renal failure. *Am. J. Epidemiol.* 101: 281, 1975.
53. Ettinger, D., et al. Hyperphosphatemia, hypocalcemia, and transient renal failure: Results of cytotoxic treatment of acute lymphoblastic leukemia. *J.A.M.A.* 239: 2472, 1978.
54. Fajardo, L. F., et al. Adriamycin nephrotoxicity. *Lab Invest.* 43: 242, 1980.
55. Fleming, J. J., Collis, C., and Peckham, M. J. Renal damage after *cis*-platinum. *Lancet* ii: 960, 1979.
56. Frei, E., III, et al. Renal complications of neoplastic disease. *J. Chronic Dis.* 16: 757, 1963.
57. Galpin, J. E., et al. Acute interstitial nephritis due to methicillin. *Am. J. Med.* 65: 756, 1978.
58. Garnick, M. B., and Mayer, R. J. Management of Acute Renal Failure Associated with Neoplastic Disease. In J. Yarboro and R. Bornstein (eds.), *Oncologic Emergencies*. New York: Grune and Stratton, 1981.
59. Gilby, E. D., Rees, L. H., and Bondy, P. K. Ectopic Hormones as Markers of Response to Therapy in Cancer. In C. Maltoni (ed.), *Biological Characterization of Human Tumors*. New York: American Elsevier, 1975.
60. Glode, L. M., et al. A phase I study of high doses of

aminopterin with leucovorin rescue in patients with advanced metastatic tumors. *Cancer Res.* 39: 3707, 1979.
61. Gonzalez-Vitale, J. C., et al. The renal pathology in clinical trials of *cis*-platinum (II) diaminedichloride. *Cancer* 39: 1362, 1977.
62. Gonzalez-Vitale, J. C., et al. Acute renal failure after *cis*-diaminedichloroplatinum (II) and gentamicin cephalothin therapies. *Cancer Treat. Rep.* 62: 693, 1978.
63. Goupil, A., et al. Insuffisance renale chronique apres traitement par le CCNU. *Nouv. Presse Med.* 9: 3069, 1980.
64. Greenberger, J. S., et al. Radiation Nephropathy. In R. E. Rieselbalch and M. Garnick (eds.), *Cancer and the Kidney.* Philadelphia: Lea & Febiger, 1982.
65. Greene, M. L., Fujomoto, W. Y., and Seegmiller, J. E. Urinary xanthine stones; a rare complication of allopurinol therapy. *N. Engl. J. Med.* 280: 426, 1969.
66. Guidelines for the clinical use of streptozotocin (NSC-85998). Prepared by Investigational Drug Branch, Cancer Therapy Evaluation Program Division of Cancer Treatment, National Cancer Institute, Bethesda, Maryland, 1976.
67. Gulati, S. C., et al. Microangiopathic haemolytic anaemia observed after treatment of epidermoid carcinoma with mitomycin C and 5-fluorouracil. *Cancer* 45: 2252, 1980.
68. Gutmann, F. D., and Boxer, R. J. Pathophysiology and Management of Urinary Tract Obstruction. In R. E. Rieselbach and M. B. Garnick (eds.), *Cancer and the Kidney.* Philadelphia: Lea & Febiger, 1982.
69. Hamner, R. W., Verani, R., and Weinman, E. J. Mitomycin-associated renal failure. *Arch. Intern. Med.* 143: 803, 1983.
70. Hande, K. R., Balow, J. E., and Drake, J. C. Methotrexate and hemodialysis. *Ann. Intern. Med.* 87: 495, 1977.
71. Hande, K. R., Donehower, R. C., and Chabner, B. A. Pharmacology and Pharmacokinetics of High Dose Methotrexate in Man. In H. M. Pinedo (ed.), *Clinical Pharmacology of Antineoplastic Drugs.* New York: Elsevier/North Holland, 1978.
72. Hande, K. R., et al. Postchemotherapy hyperxanthinuria in lymphoma patients on allopurinol: A potential cause of nephropathy. (Abstract) *Clin. Res.* 27: 386, 1979.
73. Hanna, W. T., et al. Renal disease after mitomycin C therapy. *Cancer* 48: 2583, 1981.
74. Hardaker, W. T., Stone, R. A., and McCoy, R. Platinum nephrotoxicity. *Cancer* 34: 1030, 1974.
75. Harlow, P. J., et al. A fatal case of inappropriate ADH secretion induced by cyclophosphamide therapy. *Cancer* 44: 896, 1979.
76. Harmon, W. E., et al. Chronic renal failure in children treated with methyl CCNU. *N. Engl. J. Med.* 300(21): 1200, 1979.
77. Hauck, W. A., Olson, K. B., and Horton, J. Clinical features of tumor metastasis to the pituitary. *Cancer* 26: 656, 1970.
78. Hayes, D. M., et al. High-dose *cis*-platinum diammine dichloride: Amelioration of renal toxicity by mannitol diuresis. *Cancer* 39: 1372, 1977.
79. Herrman, J., and Gabriel, F. Membranoproliferative glomerulonephritis in a patient with hairy-cell leukemia treated with alpha-II interferon. (Letter to the editor) *N. Engl. J. Med.* 316: 112, 1987.
80. Ho, M., Bear, R. A., and Garvey, M. B. Symptomatic hypophosphatemia secondary to 5-azacytidine therapy of acute nonlymphocytic leukemia. *Cancer Treat. Rep.* 60: 1400, 1976.
81. Horning, S. J., et al. Clinical and immunologic effects of recombinant leukocyte A interferon in eight patients with advanced cancer. *J.A.M.A.* 247: 1718, 1982.
82. Howell, S. B., and Carmody, J. Changes in glomerular filtration rate associated with high dose methotrexate therapy in adults. *Cancer Treat. Rep.* 61: 1389, 1977.
83. Howell, S. B., et al. Intraperitoneal cisplatin with systemic thiosulfate protection. *Ann. Intern. Med.* 97: 845, 1982.
84. Howell, S. B., and Taetle, R. The effect of sodium thiosulfate on *cis*-dichlorodiammineplatinum (II) toxicity and antitumor activity in the L1210 leukemia. *Cancer Treat. Rep.* 64: 611, 1980.
85. Hrushesky, W. J. M., Shimp, W., and Kennedy, B. J. Lack of age-dependent cisplatin nephrotoxicity. *Am. J. Med.* 76: 579, 1984.
86. Hutchinson, F. N., et al. Renal salt wasting in patients treated with cisplatin. *Ann. Intern. Med.* 108: 21, 1988.
87. Jacobs, C., et al. 24-Hour infusion of *cis*-platinum in head and neck cancers. *Cancer* 42: 2135, 1978.
88. Jacobs, C., et al. Renal handling of *cis*-diaminedichloroplatinum (II). *Cancer Treat. Rep.* 64: 1223, 1980.
89. Jacobs, S. A., et al. 7-Hydroxy methotrexate as a urinary metabolite in human subjects and rhesus monkeys receiving high dose methotrexate. *J. Clin. Invest.* 57: 534, 1976.
90. Jenkins, P. G., and Rieselbach, R. E. Acute Renal Failure: Diagnosis, Clinical Spectrum, and Management. In R. E. Rieselbach and M. B. Garnick (eds.), *Cancer and the Kidney.* Philadelphia: Lea & Febiger, 1982.
91. Jones, B. G., et al. Intravascular haemolysis and renal impairment after blood transfusion in two patients on long-term 5-fluorouracil and mitomycin C. *Lancet* 1: 1275, 1980.
92. Jones, B. R., et al. Comparison of methods of evaluating nephrotoxicity of *cis*-platinum. *Clin. Pharmacol. Ther.* 24: 557, 1980.
93. Kanfer, A., et al. Extreme hyperphosphatemia causing acute anuric nephrocalcinosis in lymphosarcoma. *Br. Med. J.* 1: 1320, 1979.
94. Karunanayake, E. H., Hearse, D. J., and Mellows, G. The metabolite fate and elimination of streptozotocin. *Biochem. Soc. Trans.* 3: 410, 1975.
95. Kennedy, B. J. Metabolic and toxic effects of mithramycin during tumor therapy. *Am. J. Med.* 49: 494, 1970.
96. Kennedy, B. J., Brown, J. H., and Yarbro, J. W. Mithramycin (NSC-24559) therapy for primary glioblastomas. *Cancer Chemother. Rep.* 48: 59, 1965.
97. Kiang, P. T., Loken, M. K., and Kennedy, B. J. Mechanism of the hypocalcemic effect of mithramycin. *J. Clin. Endocrinol. Metab.* 48: 341, 1979.
98. Kjellstrand, C. M., et al. Hyperuricemic acute renal failure. *Arch. Intern. Med.* 133: 349, 1974.
99. Klinenberg, J. R., Goldfinger, S. E., and Seegmiller, J. E. The effectiveness of the xanthine oxidase inhibitor allopurinol in the treatment of gout. *Ann. Intern. Med.* 62: 639, 1965.
100. Konits, P. H., et al. Phase II evaluation of 6-thioguanine in patients with metastatic colorectal carcinoma. *Proc. Am. Assoc. Cancer Res.* 22: 260, 1981.
101. Kremer, W. B. Cytarabine. *Ann. Intern. Med.* 82: 684, 1975.
102. Kristensen, L. O., Weisman, K., and Hutters, L. Renal function and the rate of disappearance of methotrexate. *Eur. J. Clin. Pharmacol.* 8: 439, 1975.
103. Kritzler, R. A. Anuria complicating the treatment of leukemia. *Am. J. Med.* 25: 532, 1958.
104. Krown, S. E. Interferons and interferon inducers in cancer treatment. *Semin. Oncol.* 13: 207, 1986.
105. Lee, J. C., Yamauchi, H., and Hopper, J. The association

of cancer and the nephrotic syndrome. *Ann. Intern. Med.* 64: 41, 1966.
106. Lewis, M. G., Loughridge, L. W., and Phillips, T. M. Immunological studies in nephrotic syndrome associated with extrarenal malignant disease. *Lancet* 2: 134, 1971.
107. Liegler, D. G., et al. The effect of organic acids on renal clearance of methotrexate in man. *Clin. Pharmacol. Ther.* 10: 849, 1969.
108. Link, D. A., Fosburg, M. T., and Ingelfinger, J. R. Renal toxicity of high dose methotrexate. *Pediatr. Res.* 10: 455, 1976.
109. Litterst, L., Torres, I. J., and Guarino, A. M. Plasma levels and organ distribution of platinum in the rat, dog, and dog fish following intravenous administration of *cis*-DDP (II). *J. Clin. Hematol. Oncol.* 7: 169, 1977.
110. Liu, K., Mittelman, A., Sproul, E. E., and Elias, E. G. Renal toxicity in man treated with mitomycin-C. *Cancer* 28: 1314, 1971.
111. Lodish, J. R., and Boxer, R. J. Urinary Tract Hemorrhage. In R. E. Rieselbach and M. B. Garnick (eds.), *Cancer and the Kidney*. Philadelphia: Lea & Febiger, 1982.
112. Loftus, L., Cuppage, F. E., and Hoogstraten, B. Clinical and pathological effects of streptozotocin. *J. Lab. Clin. Med.* 84: 407, 1974.
113. Lucas, W. E., Markman, M., and Howell, S. B. Intraperitoneal chemotherapy for advanced ovarian cancer. *Am. J. Obstet. Gynecol.* 154: 474, 1985.
114. Major, P., Kufe, D., and Frei, E., III. Role of the Kidney in the Pharmacokinetics of Anticancer Agents. In R. E. Rieselbach and M. B. Garnick (eds.), *Cancer and the Kidney*. Philadelphia: Lea & Febiger, 1982.
115. Marks, E. S., and Lee, K. M. Acute renal failure secondary to vascular occlusion by a retroperitoneal plasmacytoma. *Cancer* 53: 1228, 1984.
116. Martinez-Maldonado, M., et al. Renal complications in multiple myeloma; Pathophysiology and some aspects of clinical management. *J. Chronic Dis.* 24: 221, 1971.
117. Mavichak, V., et al. Renal magnesium wasting and hypocalciuria in chronic cis-platinum nephropathy in man. *Clin. Sci.* 75: 203, 1988.
118. Mayer, R. J. Infiltrative and Metastatic Disease of the Kidney. In R. E. Rieselbach and M. B. Garnick (eds.), *Cancer and the Kidney*. Philadelphia: Lea & Febiger, 1982.
119. Micetich, K. C., et al. Nephrotoxicity of semustine (methyl-CCNU) in patients with malignant melanoma receiving adjuvant chemotherapy. *Am. J. Med.* 71: 967, 1981.
120. Moorthy, A. V., Zimmerman, S. W., and Burkholder, P. M. Nephrotic syndrome in Hodgkin's disease. Evidence for pathogenesis alternative to immune complex deposition. *Am. J. Med.* 61: 471, 1976.
121. Morgan, K., and Mir, M. A. Isolation of sodium transport inhibitory factor, inhibitin, from cultured leukemic promyelocytes. *J. Clin. Invest.* 74: 1132, 1984.
122. Mycrowitz, R. L., Sartiano, G. P., and Cavallo, T. Nephrotoxic and cytoproliferative effects of streptozotocin. Report of a patient with a multiple hormone-secreting islet cell carcinoma. *Cancer* 38: 1550, 1976.
123. Narins, R. G., et al. The nephrotoxicity of chemotherapeutic agents. *Semin. Nephrol.* 10: 556, 1990.
124. Oliver, J., MacDowell, M., and Tracy, A. The pathogenesis of acute renal failure associated with traumatic and toxic injury. Renal ischemia, nephrotoxic damage and the ischemuric episode. *J. Clin. Invest.* 30: 1307, 1951.
125. Oliverio, V. T. Toxicology and pharmacology of the nitrosoureas. *Cancer Chemother. Rep.* (Part 3) 4: 13, 1973.
126. Owen, C. A., et al. Intramuscular pressures with limb compression clarification of the pathogenesis of the drug-induced muscle-compartment syndrome. *N. Engl. J. Med.* 30: 1169, 1979.
127. Ozols, R. F., et al. High-dose cisplatin in hypertonic saline. *Ann. Intern. Med.* 100: 19, 1984.
128. Palm, P. E., and Kensler, C. J. Preclinical toxicology of NSC-102816 (5-azacytidine) in mice, hamsters, and dogs. In US Clearing House Fed. Sci. Tech. Inform. P. B. Rep., 194791: 191, 1970.
129. Patel, R., and Savage, A. Symptomatic hypomagnesemia associated with gentamicin therapy. *Nephron* 23: 50, 1979.
130. Peterson, B. A., et al. 5-Azacytidine and renal tubular dysfunction. *Blood* 57: 182, 1981.
131. Philips, F. S., et al. Some observations on the toxicity of adriamycin (NSC-123127). *Cancer Chemother. Rep.* (Part 3) 6: 177, 1975.
132. Philips, F. S., Schwartz, H. S., and Sternberg, S. S. Pharmacology of mitomycin C. I. Toxicity and pathologic effects. *Cancer Res.* 20: 1354, 1960.
133. Pickering, T. G., and Catovsky, D. Hypokalemia and raised lysozyme level in acute myeloid leukemia. *Q. J. Med.* 42: 677, 1973.
134. Pitman, S. W., and Frei, E., III. Weekly methotrexate calcium leukovorin rescue: Effect of alkalinization on nephrotoxicity; pharmacokinetics in the CNS, and use in CNS non-Hodgkin's lymphoma. *Cancer Treat. Rep.* 61: 695, 1977.
135. Pitman, S. W., et al. Clinical trial of high-dose methotrexate (NSC-740) with citrovorum factor (NSC-3590)-toxicologic and therapeutic observations. *Cancer Chemother. Rep.* 6: 43, 1975.
136. Porter, G. A., and Bennett, W. M. Nephrotoxin-Induced Acute Renal Failure. In B. M. Brenner and J. H. Stein (eds.), *Acute Renal Failure*. New York: Churchill Livingstone, 1980.
137. Presant, C. A., et al. Phase I and preliminary phase II observations of high-dose intermittent 6-thioguanine. *Cancer Treat. Rep.* 64: 1109, 1980.
138. Price, T. M., et al. Renal failure and Hemolytic anemia associated with mitomycin C. *Cancer* 55: 51, 1985.
139. Randolph, V. L., Hall, W., and Bromson, W. Renal failure due to lymphomatous infiltration of the kidneys. *Cancer* 52: 1120, 1983.
140. Ratanatharathorn, V. Clinical and Pathologic Study of Mitomycin C Nephrotoxicity. In S. K. Carter and S. T. Crooke (eds.), *Mitomycin C: Current Status and New Developments*. New York: Academic Press, 1979.
141. Richmond, J., et al. Renal lesions associated with malignant lymphomas. *Am. J. Med.* 32: 184, 1962.
142. Rieselbach, R. E., et al. Uric acid excretion and renal function in the acute hyperuricemia of leukemia. *Am. J. Med.* 37: 872, 1964.
143. Rieselbach, R. E., and Steele, T. H. Influence of the kidney upon urate homeostasis in health and disease. *Am. J. Med.* 56: 665, 1974.
144. Robertson, G. L., Bhoopalam, N., and Zelkowitz, L. J. Vincristine neurotoxicity and abnormal secretion of antidiuretic hormone. *Arch. Intern. Med.* 132: 717, 1973.
145. Rosenberg, B. Cisplatin: Its History and Possible Mechanism of Action. In A. W. Prestayko et al. (eds.), *Cisplatin-Current Status and New Development*. New York: Academic Press, 1980.
146. Rosenberg, S. A. Immunotherapy of cancer by systemic administration of lymphoid cells plus interleukin-2. *J. Biol. Response Mod.* 3: 504, 1984.
147. Rosenberg, S. A., et al. Biological activity of recombinant

human interleukin-2 produced in *Escherichia coli*. *Science* 223: 1412, 1984.
148. Rosenberg, S. A., et al. Observations on the systemic administration of autologous lymphokine-activated killer cells and recombinant interleukin-2 to patients with metastatic cancer. *N. Engl. J. Med.* 313: 1485, 1985.
149. Ross, D. A., and Gale, G. R. Reduction of the renal toxicity of *cis*-dichlorodiammineplatinum (II) by probenecid. *Cancer Treat. Rep.* 63: 781, 1979.
150. Rossof, A. H., Slayton, R. E., and Perlia, C. P. Preliminary clinical experience with *cis*-diaminedichloroplatinum (II) (NSC 119875, CACP). *Cancer* 30: 1451, 1972.
151. Rozencweig, M., von Hoff, D. D., Slavik, M., and Muggia, F. M. *Cis*-diamminedichloroplatinum (II), a new anticancer drug. *Ann. Intern. Med.* 86: 803, 1977.
152. Rudin, A., Sjogren, B., and Aurell, M. Low urinary calcium excretion in Bartter's syndrome. *N. Engl. J. Med.* 310: 1190, 1984.
153. Sadoff, L. Nephrotoxicity of streptozotocin (NSC-85998). *Cancer Chemother. Rep.* 54: 457, 1970.
154. Safirstein, R., Daye, M., and Guttenplan, J. Mutagenic activity and identification of excreted platinum in human and rat urine and rat plasma after administration of cisplatin. *Cancer Lett.* 18: 329, 1983.
155. Safirstein, R., et al. Renal disposition and metabolism of liganded platinum: Implications to toxicity. (Abstract) *Fed. Proc.* 40: 651A, 1980.
156. Safirstein, R., Miller, P., and Guttenplan, J. B. Uptake and metabolism of cisplatin by rat kidney. *Kidney Int.* 25: 753, 1984.
157. Saiki, J. H., et al. 5-Azacytidine in acute leukemia. *Cancer* 42: 2111, 1978.
158. Salem, P., et al. *Cis*-diamminedichloroplatinum (II) by 5-day continuous infusion—A new dose schedule with minimal toxicity. *Cancer* 53: 837, 1984.
159. Schacht, R. G., et al. Nephrotoxicity of nitrosoureas. *Cancer* 48: 1328, 1981.
160. Schaeppi, U., et al. (NSC-79037) Preclinical toxicologic evaluation of a single intravenous infusion in dogs and monkeys. *Cancer Chemother. Rep.* (Part 3) 5(1): 53, 1974.
161. Schaeppi, U., et al. *Cis*-dichlorodiamine-platinum (II) (NSC-119875): Preclinical toxicologic evaluation of intravenous injection in dogs, monkeys and mice. *Toxicol. Appl. Pharmacol.* 25: 230, 1973.
162. Schein, P., et al. Clinical antitumor activity and toxicity of streptozotocin (NSC-85998). *Cancer* 34: 993, 1974.
163. Schilsky, R. L., and Anderson, T. Hypomagnesemia and renal magnesium wasting in patients receiving cisplatin. *Ann. Intern. Med.* 90: 929, 1979.
164. Schilsky, R. L., Barlock, A., and Ozols, R. F. Persistent hypomagnesemia following cisplatin chemotherapy for testicular cancer. *Cancer Treat. Rep.* 66: 1767, 1982.
165. Schlosstein, L., Kippen, I., and Bluestone, R. Association between hypouricemia and jaundice. *Ann. Rheum. Dis.* 33: 308, 1974.
166. Schwartz, H. S., and Philips, F. S. Pharmacology of mitomycin C. II. Renal excretion and metabolism by tissue homogenates. *J. Pharmacol. Exp. Ther.* 133: 335, 1961.
167. Seegmiller, J. E. Xanthine stone formation. *Am. J. Med.* 45: 780, 1968.
168. Selby, P., et al. Nephrotic syndrome during treatment with interferon. *Br. Med. J.* 290: 1180, 1985.
169. Shea, T. C., et al. A phase I clinical and pharmacokinetic study of carboplatin and autologous bone marrow support. *J. Clin. Oncol.* 7: 651, 1989.
170. Sherwin, S. A., et al. A multiple-dose phase I trial of recombinant leukocyte A interferon in cancer patients. *J.A.M.A.* 248: 2461, 1982.
171. Shipp, M. A., Takvorian, R. C., and Canellos, G. P. High-dose cytosine arabinoside—Active agent in treatment of non-Hodgkin's lymphoma. *Am. J. Med.* 77: 845, 1984.
172. Silver, H. K. B., and Morton, D. L. CCNU nephrotoxicity following sustained remission in oat cell carcinoma. *Cancer Treat. Rep.* 63: 226, 1979.
173. Simon, N. M., Rovner, R. N., and Berlin, B. S. Acute myoglobinuria associated with type A2 (Hong Kong) influenza. *J.A.M.A.* 212: 1704, 1970.
174. Simpson, D. P., Wen, S. F., and Chesney, R. W. Fluid and Electrolyte Abnormalities Due to Tumors, Their Products, or Metabolites. In R. E. Rieselbach and M. B. Garnick (eds.), *Cancer and the Kidney.* Philadelphia: Lea & Febiger, 1982.
175. Singer, F. R., et al. Mithramycin treatment of intractable hypercalcemia due to parathyroid carcinoma. *N. Engl. J. Med.* 283: 634, 1970.
176. Skarin, A. T., and Canellos, G. P. Nephropathies Due to Excess Production of Immunoglobulins. In R. E. Rieselbach and M. B. Garnick (eds.), *Cancer and the Kidney.* Philadelphia: Lea & Febiger, 1982.
177. Slavin, R. E., Dias, M. A., and Saral, R. Cytosine arabinoside induced gastrointestinal toxic alteration in sequential chemotherapeutic protocols. A clinical pathological study of 33 patients. *Cancer* 42: 1747, 1978.
178. Sorensen, L. B. Discussion of J. E. Seegmiller. Proceedings of the seminars on the Lesch-Nyhan syndrome: management and treatment. *Fed. Proc.* 27: 1097, 1968.
179. Sosman, J. A., et al. Repetitive weekly cycles of recombinant human interleukin-2: Responses of renal carcinoma with acceptable toxicity. *J. Natl. Cancer Inst.* 80: 60, 1988.
180. Sponzo, R. W., DeVita, V. T., and Oliverio, V. T. Physiologic disposition of 1-(2-chloroethyl)-3-cyclohexyl-1-nitrosourea (CCNU) and 1-(2-chloro-ethyl)-3-(4-methylcyclohexyl)-1-nitrosourea (meCCNU) in man. *Cancer* 31: 1154, 1973.
181. Steele, T. H., Serpick, A. A., and Block, J. B. Antidiuretic response to cyclophosphamide in man. *J. Pharmacol. Exp. Ther.* 185(2): 245, 1973.
182. Stoller, R. G., et al. Use of plasma pharmacokinetics to predict and prevent methotrexate toxicity. *N. Engl. J. Med.* 297: 630, 1977.
183. Stuart, M. J., et al. Syndrome of recurrent increased secretion of antidiuretic hormone following multiple doses of vincristine. *Blood* 45: 315, 1975.
184. Sutton, R. A. L., et al. Chronic hypomagnesemia caused by cisplatin: Effect of calcitriol. *J. Lab. Clin. Med.* 117: 40, 1991.
185. Swainson, C. P., Colls, B. M., and Fitzharris, B. M. *Cis*-platinum and distal renal tubular toxicity. *N.Z. Med. J.* 98: 375, 1985.
186. Talley, R. W., et al. Clinical evaluation of toxic effects of *cis*-diaminedichloroplatinum (NSC-119875): Phase I clinical study. *Cancer Chemother. Rep.* 57: 465, 1973.
187. Talpaz, M., et al. Therapy of chronic myelogenous leukemia: chemotherapy and interferons. *Semin. Hematol.* 25: 62, 1988.
188. Textor, S. C., et al. Renal, volume, and hormonal changes during therapeutic administration of recombinant interleukin-2 in man. *Am. J. Med.* 83: 1055, 1987.
189. Thierry, F. X., et al. Acute renal failure after high-dose methotrexate therapy. *Nephron* 51: 416, 1989.
190. Thomas, M. H., and Chisholm, G. C. Retroperitoneal

fibrosis associated with malignant disease. *Br. J. Cancer* 28: 453, 1973.

191. Tsokos, G. C., et al. Renal and metabolic complications of undifferentiated and lymphoblastic lymphomas. *Medicine* 60: 218, 1981.
192. Van Echo, D. A., et al. A phase I clinical and pharmacologic trial of carboplatin daily for 5 days. *Cancer Treat. Rep.* 65: 1103, 1984.
193. Vogelzang, N. Vascular and other complications of chemotherapy for testicular cancer. *World J. Urol.* 2: 32, 1984.
194. Vogelzang, N. J., Nelimark, M. D., and Nath, K. A. Tumor lysis syndrome after induction chemotherapy of small-cell bronchogenic carcinoma. *J.A.M.A.* 249(4): 513, 1983.
195. Von Hoff, D. D., et al. Incidence of drug-related deaths secondary to high-dose methotrexate and citrovorum factor administration. *Cancer Treat. Rep.* 61: 745, 1977.
196. Von Hoff, D. D., and Slavik, M. 5-Azacytidine—A new anticancer drug with significant activity in acute leukemia. *Adv. Pharmacol. Chemother.* 14: 285, 1977.
197. Walker, W. G., Harvey, A. M., and Yardley, J. H. Renal Involvement in Myeloma, Amyloidosis, SLE, and Other Connective Tissue Disorders. In M. D. Strauss and L. G. Welt (eds.), *Diseases of the Kidney*. Boston: Little, Brown, 1971.
198. Wasserman, T. H. The nitrosoureas: An outline of clinical schedules and toxic effects. *Cancer Treat. Rep.* 60: 709, 1976.
199. Wasserman, T. H., Slavik, M., Carter, S. K. Clinical comparisons of the nitrosoureas. *Cancer* 36: 1258, 1975.
200. Weisberger, A. S., and Perksy, L. Renal calculi and uremia as a complication of lymphoma. *Am. J. Med. Sci.* 225: 669, 1953.
201. Weiss, R. B. Streptozocin: A review of its pharmacology, efficacy, and toxicity. *Cancer Treat. Rep.* 66: 427, 1982.
202. Weiss, R. B., Poster, D. S., and Penta, J. S. The nitrosoureas and pulmonary toxicity. *Cancer Treat. Rev.* 8: 111, 1981.
203. West, W. H., et al. Constant-infusion recombinant interleukin-2 in adoptive immunotherapy of advanced cancer. *N. Engl. J. Med.* 316: 898, 1987.
204. Willis, R. A. Secondary Tumors of the Kidneys. In *The Spread of Tumors in the Human Body*, 3rd ed. London: Butterworth, 1973.
205. Wolf, W., and Manaka, R. C. Synthesis and distribution of ^{195m}Pt *cis*-dichlorodiammine platinum (II). *J. Clin. Hematol. Oncol.* 7: 79, 1976.
206. Zimmerman, S. W., et al. Glomerulopathies Associated with Neoplastic Disease. In R. E. Rieselbach and M. B. Garnick (eds.), *Cancer and the Kidney*. Philadelphia: Lea & Febiger, 1982.
207. Zusman, J., Brown, D. M., and Nesbit, M. E. Hyperphosphataemia, hyperphosphaturia and hypocalcaemia in acute lymphoblastic leukemia. *N. Engl. J. Med.* 289: 1335, 1973.

Radiocontrast Media–Induced Acute Renal Failure

Robert E. Cronin

The emergence of radiocontrast material as an important cause of acute renal failure is a relatively recent phenomenon. Isolated case reports of death, anaphylaxis, and renal failure resulting from the use of these agents have not been rare, but it is only in the past 20 years that radiocontrast materials have achieved prominence as a major clinical cause of nephrotoxic acute renal failure. Of 129 consecutive cases of hospital-acquired renal insufficiency, radiocontrast studies were the cause in 16 patients (12%) [80]. In the late 1960s, reports began to appear that several groups of patients were particularly at risk for the development of acute renal failure after exposure to radiocontrast agents, namely, patients with chronic renal failure and patients with diabetes mellitus. Although, initially, acute renal failure was thought to be a rare complication, reports came in rapid succession attesting to the widespread nature of the problem. The appreciation of this association by clinicians and radiologists alike has led to a reappraisal of the use of radiocontrast agents in the diagnosis of renal disease and in the diagnosis of nonrenal disease in patients with impaired renal function. In the presence of renal insufficiency, particularly, there is now a decided trend to avoid radiocontrast studies when alternative imaging procedures are available (e.g., ultrasonography, cystoscopy, or both, and retrograde pyelography to diagnose obstructive uropathy). Additional developments and applications of nuclear magnetic resonance (NMR) also may lead to a lessening of the demand for radiocontrast agents in high-risk patients.

Incidence

A single figure for the incidence of radiocontrast-induced acute renal failure in the entire population at risk cannot be established with certainty since the incidence varies, depending on the population studied and the rigorousness used to diagnose nephrotoxicity.

The recent surge in reports of acute renal failure following the use of radiocontrast agents might suggest that the incidence of this problem is increasing, especially in view of early reports that urographic studies in patients with chronic renal insufficiency were both efficacious and safe [139]. However, a careful reading of such reports suggests that the same risk of renal damage was present then. In recent years, nephrotoxicity or acute renal failure has been defined variously as a rise in serum creatinine concentration of 0.3 mg/dl [33, 113], 0.5 mg/dl [121, 131], 0.6 mg/dl [114], 1.0 mg/dl [32, 37, 69, 93, 149], or 2.0 mg/dl [22, 26] or a 50 percent increase in baseline serum creatinine 1 to 5 days following exposure to radiocontrast material [35, 115]. Byrd and Sherman [22] reported an incidence of acute renal failure of approximately 0.15 percent for urographic and tomographic studies and 0.53 percent for angiographic studies. Two aspects of this report suggest that these incidence figures are low estimates: (1) The study was a retrospective analysis only of cases severe enough to prompt nephrologic consultation by the primary physician, and (2) a rise of 2 mg/dl in serum creatinine was required during the 48 hours following the procedure to make a diagnosis of acute renal failure. These two factors in the study design would not detect mild cases of renal insufficiency. When the criteria for nephrotoxicity are more liberal, the incidence figures are higher. D'Elia et al. [37] found that 0.68 percent of nonazotemic patients and 17.4 percent of azotemic patients had a 1 mg/dl rise in serum creatinine following nonrenal angiography. Swartz et al. [141] reported a 12 percent incidence of acute renal failure in seriously ill, hospitalized patients, using as their criterion a rise in serum creatinine of at least 1 mg/dl within 48 hours of the study. However, believing this to be an overestimate of the true incidence of acute renal failure following radiocontrast studies, Eisenberg et al. [44] prospectively studied 100 consecutive patients undergoing major angiography using criteria similar, but not identical, to that of Swartz et al., and found no episodes of acute renal failure. This study was later extended to include data from 537 consecutive patients and again demonstrated no episodes of acute renal failure [45]. This latter study differed from that of Swartz et al. [141] in that volume expansion with saline solution was done for all patients during angiography, and the criterion for nephrotoxicity was more strict (i.e., a rise in serum creatinine of 1 mg/dl within 24 hours of the study), a point for which the study was criticized [143]. In another study done in response to the report by Swartz et al. [141], Kumar et al. [88] reported a serum creatinine rise of 0.5 mg/dl in only 1 patient during the 48 hours following 100 consecutive angiographic studies. Using even less stringent criteria for nephrotoxicity, Cochran et al. [33] reviewed the records of 800 patients undergoing renal angiography to obtain 266 with preangiography and postangiography serum creatinine values. Using as criteria for nephrotoxicity a rise in serum creatinine of 0.3 mg/dl, or a greater than 20 percent rise of serum creatinine within 5 days of the procedure, they found an incidence of 17 percent (45 of 266). While sensitivity in case detection was improved by these less rigid criteria, the group probably included a number of patients with transient, volume depletion–induced elevations in serum creatinine.

Thus the incidence figures for acute renal failure following radiocontrast administration are dependent on whether the patient has normal or abnormal renal function prior to the procedure and also on what arbitrary change in renal function (usually serum creatinine concentration) is used to make the diagnosis. To group together and equate a transient reversible rise in serum creatinine of 0.3 mg/dl in one patient with a sustained 5.0 mg/dl rise that results in the patient going on to long-term hemodialysis and to classify both as acute renal failure may satisfy the needs of the demographer, but it is of little help to clinicians trying to discern which patients are at the greatest risk of developing acute renal failure.

Risk Factors for Radiocontrast Media–Induced Acute Renal Failure

The list of factors purported to predispose to radiocontrast media–induced acute renal failure is long (Table 43-1) and includes age [5, 22, 26, 33, 82, 96, 141, 150], renal insufficiency [5, 22, 26, 33, 37, 41, 51, 82, 96, 141, 148, 150, 153], diabetes mellitus [5, 9, 14, 22, 26, 32, 41, 51, 69, 82, 116, 132, 141, 150, 153], multiple myeloma [13, 67, 109, 127], anemia [153], proteinuria [26, 33, 118, 141], abnormal liver function [118, 141], volume depletion [89, 96, 153], dehydration [5, 43, 82, 87, 116], hyperuricemia [3, 22, 69], concomitant exposure to other nephrotoxins [3, 9, 14, 43, 116], repeated exposure to radiocontrast media over a few days [3, 33, 87, 113, 118], volume of contrast media [9, 14, 32, 89, 96, 108, 153], injection site (i.e., intraarterial versus intravenous) [22, 153], male sex [33], presence of cardiovascular disease [9, 26, 33, 87, 113, 116, 150, 153], hypertension [3, 26, 33, 87, 113, 148], and renal transplantation [74, 94]. Many of these risk factors may be covariate rather than independent variables. This probably accounts for reports that fail to confirm many of these as risk factors [100]. Harkonen and Kjellstrand [69] were unable to make an association between radiocontrast acute renal failure and volume depletion, the dose of contrast, the use of concomitant nephrotoxic drugs, or hyperuricemia. Volume depletion and dehydration, often the result of purging enemas and restricted food and fluid intake prior to urographic and arteriographic studies, are probably only a contributing factor to radiocontrast-induced acute renal failure. D'Elia et al. [37] studied 378 hospitalized patients undergoing nonrenal angiography and identified the presence of preexisting azotemia as the only risk factor predisposing to nephrotoxicity (defined as a rise in serum creatinine of 1 mg/dl or greater following the procedure). The volume of radiocontrast material injected, the site of injection, a history of prior cardiovascular disease, or diabetes mellitus were not significant factors in the development of acute renal failure. Miller et al. [100] studied prospectively 200 patients requiring intravenous or intraarterial contrast material and found no consistent change in renal function with increasing doses of contrast material. Also, in 10 patients who underwent two procedures with only 1 day between them, there was no tendency toward deterioration of renal function. However, Cigarroa et al. [32] showed that careful limitation of the volume of contrast agent used during cardiac catheterization could limit the incidence of contrast nephropathy. They found that the following formula empirically predicted the amount of radiocontrast material that could be given without impairing renal function:

$$\frac{\text{5 ml of contrast/kg of body weight (maximum, 300 ml)}}{\text{serum creatinine (mg/dl)}}$$

Taliercio et al. [142] have shown that class IV heart failure is an independent risk factor for contrast-induced acute renal failure, particularly when the amount of contrast exceeds 125 ml. They reported a 23 percent incidence of contrast nephropathy (greater than 1 mg/dl rise in serum creatinine) in 139 patients with preexisting abnormal renal function (serum creatinine of 2 mg/dl or higher) who underwent cardiac angiography. The mean increment in serum creatinine was 2.6 mg/dl, the time to peak serum creatinine was 2.8 days, and 9 percent developed anuria or oliguria. Similarly, Gomes et al. [63] showed an increased incidence of contrast-induced acute renal failure in patients receiving digoxin for congestive heart failure or arrhythmias. Cochran et al. [33] studied the interdependency of risk factors in 45 patients who developed a significant elevation of serum creatinine (greater than 0.3 mg/dl) after an angiographic procedure. They found that age, proteinuria, abnormal baseline serum creatinine, use of Renografin 76, and preexisting renal disease were the five independent risk factors. These five clinical factors were those most likely to predict patients who would have an increase in serum creatinine after angiography.

Underlying renal insufficiency is the risk factor most commonly associated with radiocontrast-induced acute renal failure. Factors that may be involved in this predisposition include (1) a reduced glomerular filtration rate that obligates each remaining nephron to excrete a proportionately greater load of contrast material and thus to be exposed to a greater amount of contrast; and (2) with the lack of functional renal reserve in chronic stable renal insufficiency to buffer acute losses in glomerular filtration, any nephron damage or loss is translated immediately into a rise in serum creatinine.

Table 43-1. Risk factors for development of radiocontrast agent–induced acute renal failure

Risk factor
Age
Renal insufficiency
Diabetes mellitus
Multiple myeloma
Anemia
Proteinuria
Abnormal liver function
Volume depletion
Dehydration
Hyperuricemia
Concomitant exposure to other nephrotoxins
Repeated exposure to radiocontrast
Volume of contrast
Injection site, intraarterial vs. intravenous
Male sex
Cardiovascular disease
Hypertension
Renal transplantation

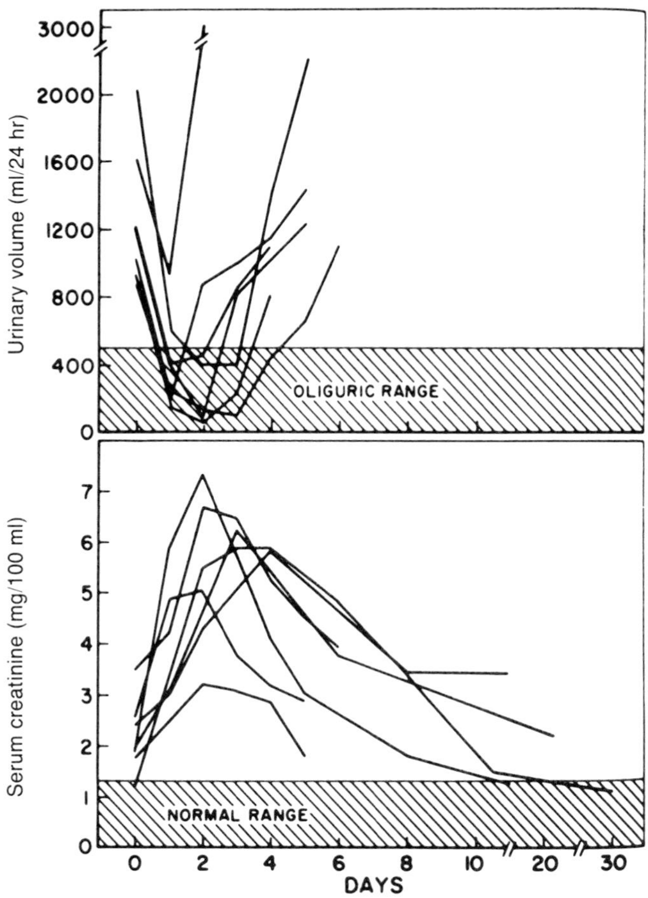

Fig. 43-1. Urinary volume and serum creatinine levels before and after intravenous administration of radiocontrast media in seven diabetic patients. (Reprinted by permission from A. Kamdar, *Diabetes* 26:643, 1977.)

Radiocontrast-Induced Acute Renal Failure and Diabetes

The incidence of radiocontrast-induced acute renal failure in diabetic patients rises sharply as the baseline serum creatinine rises. Diabetic patients with a serum creatinine value greater than 1.5 mg/dl have an approximately 50 percent chance of developing acute renal failure [69, 150]. Harkonen and Kjellstrand [69] reported that 22 of 29, or 76 percent, of all diabetic patients with a serum creatinine greater than 2 mg/dl developed acute renal failure following intravenous pyelography. Diabetic patients with a baseline serum creatinine over 5 mg/dl and those developing diabetes before the age of 40 years had an even greater risk of acute renal failure. In 56 percent of these latter patients, acute renal failure was irreversible. The experience of 13 patients with juvenile-onset diabetes, with advanced diabetic nephropathy (mean serum creatinine of 6.8 mg/dl), undergoing coronary angiography was equally stark, with 12 of 13, or 92 percent, of them developing acute renal failure [153]. The age of onset of diabetes also seems to affect the severity and likelihood of developing radiocontrast-induced acute renal failure. Type II diabetic patients are less likely to develop radiocontrast-induced acute renal failure than type I diabetic patients [69, 134]. Nonetheless, the risk of developing acute renal failure in type II diabetic patients is not trivial. Shieh et al. [134] reported a 6 percent incidence of acute renal failure after excretory urography in 49 type II diabetic patients who, as a group, had only minor renal impairment (mean baseline serum creatinine, 1.3 mg/dl, and mean creatinine clearance of 79.6 ml/min). A recent study by Parfrey et al. [115] supports diabetes as a risk factor for radiocontrast-induced acute renal failure, but only when it occurs in the presence of renal insufficiency. Furthermore, the incidence of acute renal failure of 9 percent in their diabetic patients was lower than previously reported. Why these diabetic patients with near-normal renal function were at a higher risk for acute renal failure is unclear. In addition to the reasons cited previously that may predispose patients with renal insufficiency to further injury, diabetic patients may have as contributing factors increased blood viscosity, postcapillary hypoxia with formation of microthrombi, and altered red-cell deformability [13]. Atherosclerosis, hypertension, and the potential role of glomerulosclerosis induced by hyperfiltration of the nephron, as demonstrated in both human and animal forms of diabetes, also could be involved.

Multiple myeloma has for many years been singled out as a high-risk state for the development of acute renal failure following radiocontrast [13, 67, 109, 127]. Despite numerous case reports documenting this complication, the overall risk of developing acute renal failure is still relatively small. Retrospective studies of the incidence of acute renal failure in multiple myeloma revealed only two cases developing after 376 examinations [106, 109, 152]. In the experimental animal, administration of meglumine diatrizoate further enhances the nephrotoxicity of Bence Jones protein when the latter is given in the presence of an acid urine [76]. Although the results of this animal study may not apply directly to humans, it seems prudent in patients with unexplained renal disease undergoing urography or arteriography, particularly the elderly patient, to screen the urine for Bence Jones proteins with *p*-toluene sulfonic acid (TSA) or, if unavailable, the dipstick and sulfosalicylic acid (SSA) test [34]. A positive TSA test or a negative dipstick (albumin) and positive SSA (all urinary proteins) may be considered presumptive evidence of Bence Jones proteinuria, and radiocontrast studies should then be undertaken only with extreme caution if no alternative imaging procedure is suitable.

CLINICAL FEATURES

Radiocontrast-induced acute renal failure has been reported following virtually every radiographic procedure in which these agents have been used. The list includes excretory urography [22, 26, 41, 132, 148, 150], coronary angiography [5, 22, 32, 118, 142], aortography [5, 22, 37, 63, 95, 118], cerebral angiography [1, 37, 136], pulmonary angiography [22], peripheral angiography [22], computerized tomography of the head [22], percutaneous cholangiography [66, 86], intravenous cholangiography [5], and oral cholecystography [5, 25, 53, 70, 71, 128]. Renal toxicity appears to be favored in the presence of liver disease or excessive dosages [53, 66, 118, 141]. Since the liver and kidney represent major excretory pathways for oral cholecystographic agents, reduced hepatic conjugation and excretion obligate a larger fraction to renal excretion.

Radiocontrast-induced acute renal failure may be oliguric or nonoliguric. Nonoliguric acute renal failure seems to be more common in patients initially having a lower serum creatinine prior to receiving the contrast. In oliguric acute renal failure, the time course of the oliguria and the rise in serum creatinine depends on the baseline serum creatinine prior to receiving the contrast agent. Patients with normal or mild renal functional impairment prior to receiving radiocontrast agents usually have oliguria lasting 2 to 5 days, with recovery to baseline urine volumes and serum creatinine by the seventh day (Fig. 43-1). When more serious impairment of underlying renal function is present, recovery is generally prolonged. Occasionally, renal failure is irreversible and requires long-term hemodialysis [37, 63, 69, 96, 142, 153].

DIAGNOSIS

The diagnosis of radiocontrast-induced acute renal failure is occasionally made when oliguria develops 24 to 48 hours following a radiocontrast study. More often, a subtle, nonoliguric episode of acute renal failure is diagnosed in retrospect by demonstrating a reversible 0.5 to 3.0 mg/dl rise in serum creatinine. One feature that may help to distinguish radiocontrast from other causes of acute renal failure is the paradoxical and, as yet, poorly explained propensity for the urinary sodium concentration and the fractional excretion of sodium to be low [26, 38, 51, 150]. Carvallo et al. [26] observed that 3 of 10 patients developing radiocontrast-induced acute renal failure after drip infusion pyelography had a low urinary sodium concentration (mean 7 mEq/liter). Fang et al. [51] reported 12 patients with radiocontrast-induced acute renal failure that had a low fractional excretion of sodium (mean 0.36%), which persisted for up to 5 days during the oliguric phase. The mechanism of the low fractional excretion of sodium is unknown, but reduced renal perfusion or acute tubular obstruction have been offered as possible explanations [51].

The urinalysis in this disorder may show features compatible with acute renal failure (renal tubular epithelial cell casts or coarsely granular brown casts), but these changes may be absent in the presence of a functional abnormality [37]. In three diabetic patients with angiography-induced acute renal failure, the urinary sediment showed an increase in renal tubular epithelial cells, with epithelial cell casts, muddy brown coarsely granular renal failure casts, or both [153]. Conversely, in the absence of demonstrable nephrotoxicity by functional criteria, radiocontrast agents may still alter the urinary sediment. Gelman et al. [56] demonstrated more formed elements (cells, casts, and debris) in the urine of 12 of 14 patients following angiography, although none of the patients experienced a reduction in glomerular filtration rate. All patients showed amorphous urate crystals and two patients had a heavy shower of calcium oxalate crystals.

A persistent nephrogram 24 to 48 hours after the contrast study is a characteristic but not pathognomonic feature of radiocontrast-induced acute renal failure [37, 53, 114] (Fig. 43-2). In the normal subject given a bolus of radiocontrast material, renal opacification is the most dense immediately after the end of the injection and then fades rapidly with very little nephrogram effect detectable by 6 hours [29]. In most patients with radiocontrast-induced acute renal failure as well as in patients with other forms of acute renal failure, the nephrogram develops quickly but fails to disappear with time. The frequency of this finding was studied by D'Elia et al. [37], who performed a radiographic abdominal flat plate in patients 24 hours following angiography. They found a persistent nephrogram to be a sensitive indicator of the presence of renal failure (83% of patients with renal failure had a positive nephrogram) with high specificity (93% of patients without renal failure lacked the persistent nephrogram). Unfortunately, a high false-positive rate made the predictive accuracy of a persistent nephro-

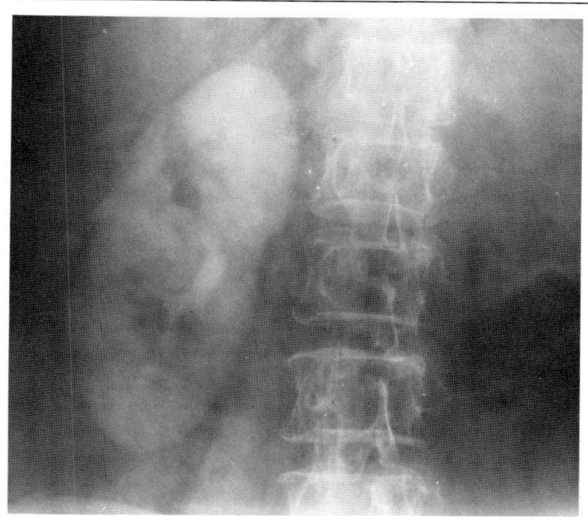

Fig. 43-2. Persistent nephrogram in solitary kidney in a 73-year-old woman 8 hours following excretory urography performed to evaluate hematuria. The contralateral kidney had been removed previously because of nephrolithiasis. Baseline serum creatinine was 1.6 mg/dl. (Courtesy of Dr. Thomas Curry.)

gram a low 19 percent. Thus if a persistent nephrogram is not present, this virtually excludes the presence of radiocontrast-induced acute renal failure, but its presence is of less help in predicting whether renal function will be impaired. For most clinical situations, the serum creatinine will remain the most practical test for diagnosing radiocontrast-induced acute renal failure.

In experimental acute renal failure in the rat, administration of radiocontrast material leads to the same persistent nephrographic pattern that is observed in patients with acute renal failure, but these studies have not provided a plausible mechanism to explain the phenomenon [29, 30].

PATHOLOGY

The characteristic lesion in the kidneys of persons with radiocontrast-induced acute renal failure is an intense vacuolization of proximal tubular cells, often called *osmotic nephrosis* [102, 103]. In 1975, Moreau et al. [103] described their findings from 211 renal biopsies obtained within 10 days of urography or renal arteriography. Osmotic nephrosis was found in 47 of the biopsies; a diffuse form was found in patients with severe preexisting renal disease, while a milder focal form was seen in patients with less severe renal impairment or in patients with previously normal kidneys. However, the presence of the focal or even the diffuse form of osmotic nephrosis did not necessarily predict the presence of renal functional impairment. Conversely, virtually normal proximal tubular cells were found in patients who developed oligoanuric acute renal failure after urography. Hyperosmolality does not seem to be required for the development of these lesions, since even the newer low osmotic contrast media are capable of inducing it [101, 104]. Notably, in 13 patients with histologically normal kidneys, vacuoles were not found in any of the tubular cells, implying that an underlying nephropathy was required to induce this histological lesion. Moreau has suggested that the vacuoles represent molecules of the contrast medium that have entered the cytoplasm by a process of endocytosis. However, Heyman et al. [75] suggested that the origin of the vacuoles is not from endocytosis but from invaginations of membranes of lateral cellular interdigitations. They suggested that the contrast media in the paracellular space may have damaged these membranes, leading to the vesicular outpouchings. The presence of iodine in these vacuoles cannot be demonstrated using several techniques [75, 105].

PATHOGENESIS

In view of the wealth of clinical descriptions of radiocontrast-induced acute renal failure, it is surprising that relatively little is known about the pathogenesis of the renal injury. Unlike other nephrotoxic substances, radiocontrast seems to be nephrotoxic only in humans [75, 105, 151]. The lack of a good experimental model of radiocontrast-induced acute renal failure has slowed the understanding of its pathogenesis. Neither the normal rabbit nor the normal rat is particularly susceptible to renal functional injury, although other properties of radiocontrast agents have been studied successfully in these species [102].

The observations that radiocontrast agents seem to be only nephrotoxic in compromised kidneys suggests that an impaired cell is required for development of acute renal failure [75, 151].

The currently used group of radiocontrast agents was introduced about 35 years ago. They are triiodinated benzoic acid derivatives and are formulated as either the sodium or methylglucamine (meglumine) salts of diatrizoate or iothalamate (Fig. 43-3A). The efficacy of these agents for radiocontrast studies is dependent on their iodine content, which ranges from 28 to 37 percent by weight. The osmolality of the different preparations ranges between 1,400 and 1,700 mOsm/kg.

Generally, there is little biotransformation of the ionic radiocontrast agents. At physiologic pH, they are highly stable and greater than 99.9 percent ionized. Their low pKa, highly ionized form, and polar nature generally do not allow them to cross cell membranes. In humans, the volume of distribution of the triiodinated radiocontrast agents is 20 to 22 percent, which is quite similar to the volume of distribution for inulin [39]. This indicates that following administration, the radiocontrast agents are largely confined to the extracellular fluid compartment. Following injection, radiocontrast agents are generally eliminated in 5 to 6 hours. More than 90 percent of a given dose of currently used urographic and angiographic contrast media is normally excreted through the kidneys. Clearance studies with most of the commonly used radiocontrast agents that are in general use indicate that they are excreted by glomerular filtration and undergo no significant tubular secretion or reabsorption [18, 39, 42]. However, Hypaque may be an exception, with one report indicating that 20 percent of filtered Hy-

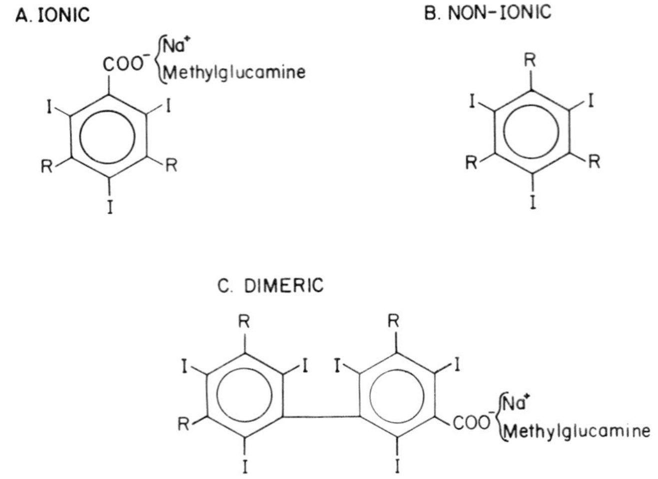

Fig. 43-3. A. Ionic radiocontrast agents are triiodinated benzoic acid derivatives and are formulated as either the sodium or methylglucamine salts of diatrizoate or iothalamate. B. Nonionic radiocontrast agents are also triiodinated benzoic acid derivatives, but they do not dissociate after administration. C. Dimeric radiocontrast agents contain two benzene rings, with a total of six iodine atoms and a cation of either sodium or methylglucamine.

paque is reabsorbed [140]. Studies in humans [60] and dogs [79] of the new nonionic agent metrizamide (Amipaque) indicate substantial reabsorption, with a fractional excretion compared to inulin of 70 percent. The cholecystographic agents, in comparison to the urographic and arteriographic agents, are more completely metabolized and, in addition, are highly protein-bound.

Hemodynamic Changes. There are several reasons to believe that hemodynamic factors may be involved in the pathogenesis of radiocontrast agent–induced acute renal failure. When radiocontrast is injected directly into the renal artery, glomerular filtration rate is reduced, and there is a prolonged vasoconstriction phase [8, 24, 83, 119, 133]. Caldicott et al. [24] demonstrated that intrarenally injected contrast in the dog produced a characteristic biphasic response with an initial vasodilatation, which is common to all vascular beds, followed by vasoconstriction, a characteristic only found in the kidney [22, 57, 130]. Porter et al. [119] demonstrated that when iothalamate was injected into the left ventricle of the dog, cardiac output increased, and renal blood flow decreased by 25 percent. When isosmolar quantities of mannitol were injected, however, the same increase in cardiac output occurred, but renal blood flow increased. In humans, transient decreases in renal plasma flow and glomerular filtration rate occur after large-dose excretory urography [42, 68, 145]. However, this effect is not unique to radiocontrast agents; noncontrast hypertonic solutions also produce it [31]. The response is biphasic, showing initially a transient increase in renal blood flow, followed by a more prolonged 10 to 20 percent decrease that may persist for up to 1 hour. This vasoconstrictor response of the kidney seems to be unique among the vascular beds, since it follows an initial renal vasodilatation, the characteristic and sole response of other vascular beds during the administration of radiocontrast material [22, 57, 130]. The renal vasoconstrictor effect of radiocontrast cannot be blocked with alpha receptor antagonists or by blockade of the renin-angiotensin system [24, 90]. The vasoconstrictor, but not the vasodilator effect, of radiocontrast material appears to be a calcium-dependent phenomenon, since the calcium-channel blockers verapamil and diltiazem and the calcium chelator EGTA all can significantly attenuate the magnitude and duration of radiocontrast-induced intrarenal vasoconstriction as well as attenuate the transient radiocontrast-induced reduction in glomerular filtration rate [8] (Fig. 43-4). Calcium entry blockers block this contrast-induced vasoconstriction. An uncontrolled, retrospective analysis of patients with renal insufficiency who were concomitantly receiving nifedipine at the time they received intravascular radiocontrast did not show a protective effect against the development of acute renal failure when compared to a control group not receiving nifedipine [23]. However, Russo et al. [126a] in a randomized prospective study in essentially healthy patients with normal renal function demonstrated that the addition of nifedipine to a high-osmolar radiocontrast agent (diatrizoate meglumine) prevented the typical transient fall in glomerular filtration rate and renal plasma flow normally seen with this agent. Whether these radiocontrast-induced hemodynamic changes are forerunners of radiocontrast acute renal failure is uncertain and thus the role of calcium entry blockers in protecting against this entity remains unclear.

Byrd and Sherman [22] reported an almost fourfold greater chance of developing acute renal failure after intraarterial administration compared to intravenous administration of radiocontrast. The effect of radiocontrast agents injected intraarterially on renal vascular resistance could be related directly to the osmolality of the

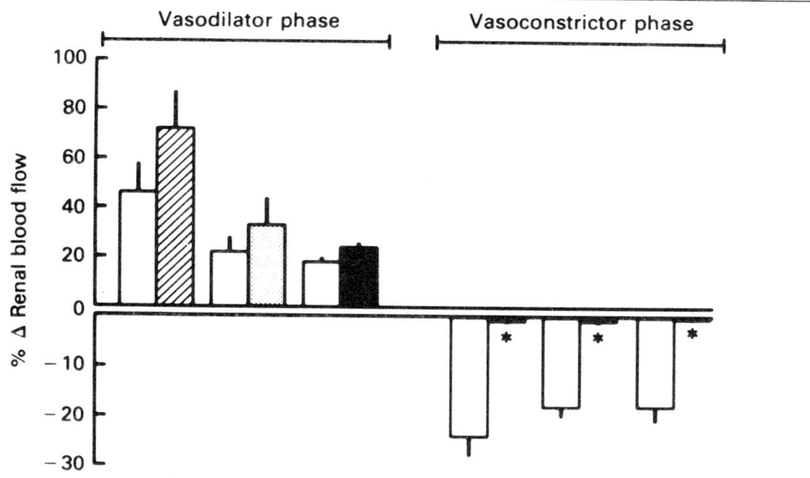

Fig. 43-4. Effects of radiocontrast-medium administration on renal blood flow response in the presence and absence of verapamil, diltiazem, and EGTA in the dog. Symbols are: □, control; ▨, verapamil ($n = 6$); ■, diltiazem ($n = 6$); EGTA ($n = 5$); *, $p < 0.05$. (Reprinted by permission from G. L. Bakris, *Kidney Int.* 27:465, 1985.)

solution. Radiocontrast agents with a high osmolality impair renal blood flow much more than those of lower osmolality [107, 126]. Impaired microcirculatory flow also occurs following injection of contrast material [46, 48, 138]. The mechanism for this decrease in flow may involve blood sludging, resulting from alterations in red cell shape or loss of deformability [16, 94, 129, 138], increased blood viscosity [138], increased platelet aggregation [4, 54, 157], and vascular endothelial injury [48]. These observations, in turn, may partly explain the observations of Fajers and Gelin [50], who showed that hyperosmolar solutions aggregated red blood cells and caused necrosis of proximal tubular cells. However, the osmolality of the radiocontrast agent is not the complete answer, since the newer nonionic contrast agents, which have a much lower osmolality, cause equal degrees of ischemia in the rabbit microcirculation [46]. The interpretation of these data on the microcirculatory effects of radiocontrast material must be tempered by the fact that most of these observations regarding the radiocontrast-induced changes in red blood cells and platelets were made using radiocontrast concentrations far higher than those encountered clinically. Thus the effect of radiocontrast material on these systems may represent minor effects under usual circumstances.

While the hypertonicity of radiocontrast materials injected into the renal artery clearly may have a significant, although temporary, effect on renal vascular resistance, it is less clear that intravenously injected contrast material that is rapidly diluted before it reaches the kidney has an important osmolality-related effect on renal vascular resistance. The importance of the injection site of the radiocontrast agents on the osmolality experienced by renal vasculature was shown by Becker et al. [10], who demonstrated a maximum 2.2 percent increase in plasma osmolality immediately on completion of a high-dose (300-ml) intravenous injection of standard ionic triiodinated radiocontrast agent. Moreover, more than half of the reported cases of radiocontrast-induced acute renal failure have been reported following excretory urography, in which the contrast medium is injected intravenously rather than intraarterially. Thus while theoretically an attractive candidate to explain radiocontrast nephrotoxicity, the hypertonicity of these agents is unlikely to be the sole mediator of renal damage.

Heyman et al. [75] demonstrated selective damage to the medullary thick ascending limbs in uni-nephrectomized, salt-depleted rats injected with indomethacin 24 hours after the administration of sodium iothalamate. The fraction of severely damaged medullary thick ascending limbs correlated with the rise in plasma creatinine. Except for an increase in vacuoles, proximal convoluted tubular cells were not injured. Since medullary thick ascending limbs are a very active, high oxygen–dependent transporting epithelium, these findings suggest that the radiocontrast agent mediated renal failure in some way by causing hypoxia of the renal medulla, an area of the kidney that normally has only a meager blood supply [15, 20]. Supporting this thesis was the further demonstration in isolated perfused kidneys that contrast-induced injury to the medullary thick ascending limbs was almost completely eliminated by inhibiting sodium transport in this segment with ouabain.

Proteinuria. Radiocontrast agents injected intraarterially also have a profound, but short-lived, effect on glomerular permeability to proteins. Nephroangiography is associated with transient but massive proteinuria in humans [147] and dogs [61, 77–79]. Holtas et al. [77–79] found that injection of contrast media into the renal artery produced albuminuria that peaked 45 minutes after injection. Here also, the adverse effect was independent of the osmolality of the agent employed, since both ionic and nonionic compounds caused the same relative increase in albuminuria. This suggested that it was rather a property of the molecule rather than the osmolality of the solution that caused the increase in glomerular permeability. Massive proteinuria only occurs when the glomerulus is directly exposed to high concentrations of the contrast agent during angiography. Only relatively minor proteinuria, 1/300 of that found after angiography, occurred in dogs given intravenous contrast media [78]. The mechanism involved in this transient loss of the glomerular capillary barrier to the movement of large molecular species is unknown, but it may be analogous to the temporary opening of the blood-brain barrier, which occurs following radiocontrast injection into the cerebral circulation [122].

Tubular Obstruction. The pathological hallmark of myeloma kidney is the presence of intratubular casts [73, 123]. The associated renal functional impairment is felt to be at least partly due to tubular obstruction. Such observations have led to the theory that contrast agents may accelerate the precipitation of Bence Jones proteins. Lasser et al. [91] demonstrated that two urographic contrast agents that are no longer in use because of their toxicity—iodopyracet (Diodrast) and sodium acetrizoate (Urokon)—produced in vitro precipitates in the urine of myeloma patients in a pH range of 4.5 to 5.5. However, agents that have been in use for the last 20 to 25 years—meglumine diatrizoate (Renografin) and sodium diatrizoate (Hypaque)—did not produce precipitates in this pH range. Nevertheless, both agents are capable of causing acute renal failure in multiple myeloma [109]. McQueen [98] demonstrated that Bence Jones proteins readily cause Tamm-Horsfall proteins to sludge in vitro. Whether this same phenomenon occurs in vivo and causes tubular obstruction as proposed by Berdon et al. [13] is still unknown.

The uricosuric property of radiocontrast agents prompted the theory that intratubular obstruction might occur from uric acid crystallization in the nephron [108, 120]. The oral cholecystographic agents (Telepaque, Oragrafin, and ChologrAfin) are the agents most often reported to cause uricosuria, but Hypaque, to some degree, also shares this property [120]. A recent clinical study demonstrated a prompt increase in urinary oxalate excretion in normal persons following diatrizoate injection [56]. Whether enhanced oxalate excretion is a factor in tubular obstruction is unknown.

Based on these limited data, it seems unlikely that either acute urate nephropathy or enhanced oxalate excretion is a major factor in the pathogenesis of contrast-induced acute renal failure.

Allergic and Immunologic Radiocontrast Reactions. Radiocontrast agents may cause acute allergic reactions and even anaphylaxis, leading to death [6]. The mechanisms by which this happens are not clear, but radiocontrast agents stimulate histamine release and increase microvascular reactivity, factors that could be participants both in the allergic reactions as well as in the production of acute renal failure. Ring et al. [125] demonstrated that the infusion of radiocontrast material into the rabbit led to a dose-dependent change in systemic arterial pressure, microvascular pressure, and red blood cell volume. In addition, radiocontrast material led to a marked rise in histamine release and a reduction in complement (CH_{50}). Although the initial hemodynamic changes could be mimicked by hypertonic saline, it had only a trivial stimulatory effect on histamine release and had no effect on complement levels. Also, the effects of radiocontrast agents on systemic hemodynamic changes were not as quickly reversible as were those of saline. There are other areas where immunologic and hemodynamic disturbances caused by radiocontrast agents could potentially overlap in producing acute renal failure. Human studies have demonstrated that radiocontrast agents in vitro cause serotonin release [124], impaired platelet function [19], and stimulate the formation of fibrin split products [135].

Radiocontrast material, injected either intravenously or intraarterially, has been implicated in renal transplant rejection [76, 94]. While radiocontrast agents can clearly cause induction of antibodies [19], how these antibodies might lead to acute renal failure is not known. Based on these few reports, it would be premature to suggest that radiocontrast material is capable of triggering acute renal failure through an immunologic reaction in the kidney.

Enzymuria. Radiocontrast agents cause a marked, but short-lived, increase in the urinary excretion of a variety of brush-border enzymes, a finding that is indicative of injury to proximal tubular cells [58, 72]. Peak output of these enzymes usually occurs 24 to 48 hours postangiography, with values then returning quickly to normal. Hartmann et al. [72] angiographically studied 20 patients with benign essential hypertension without evidence of renal insufficiency (endogenous creatinine clearance greater than 80 ml/min). All patients had increases in enzymes, but the magnitude and pattern varied among the individual patients. Despite the enzyme changes, there were no parallel changes in creatinine clearance. The greatest rise in enzyme activity for the group occurred in alkaline phosphatase, which rose 428 percent. Whether this increase in enzyme activity in the urine following angiography, in fact, represented tubular injury was unclear. The suddenness with which enzymuria develops and its rapid reversibility suggest that tubular damage is minimal.

Since hypertonic mannitol and hypertonic saline also produce significant increases in enzymuria (lactic dehydrogenase, glutamic oxaloacetic transaminase, creatine phosphokinase, catalase), it is possible that hypertonicity rather than a direct effect of the contrast agent is the cause of the enzymuria [146]. However, in the dog, the degree of glomerular proteinuria produced by contrast is a hundredfold higher than that resulting from equally hypertonic saline [78]. Clearly, other factors are also important.

Direct Toxicity. A direct nephrotoxic effect of radiocontrast material on tubular cells is the most widely held theory to explain radiocontrast-induced acute renal failure. Diatrizoate and iothalamate alter tubular transport of sodium [36, 119, 156]. Cunningham et al. [36] demonstrated that radiocontrast agents induced more of a diuresis and natriuresis than equiosmolar mannitol and that the diuresis occurred within 3 minutes of injection. Ziegler et al. [156] demonstrated that radiocontrast agents had an inhibitory effect on sodium transport in toad bladders when used in isotonic amounts (Fig. 43-5). Interestingly, the sodium diatrizoate–treated bladder was still responsive to the action of antidiuretic hormone, and the effect on sodium transport was reversible when the contrast agent was washed out. The serosal side of the bladder, analogous to the basolateral or contraluminal aspect of nephronal cells, was more sensitive to the adverse effects. This is of particular interest in view of the histologic observation of osmotic nephrosis in humans, which has focused attention on the abnormalities occurring at the luminal surface of proximal tubular cells. While the mechanism of reduced sodium transport is not clear, an inhibition of Na^+-K^+-ATPase in the basolateral membrane of the toad bladder cells or a direct effect on energy production has been postulated [156]. Although these effects of radiocontrast on sodium transport do not necessarily indicate cellular injury or toxicity, they represent one of the few demonstrations that radiocontrast agents at isotonic concentrations have a direct cellular inhibitory effect apart from hemodynamic effects. Humes et al. [81], using isolated renal proximal tubule cells, showed that diatrizoate sodium and, to a lesser degree, meglumine are directly toxic. When incubated with these tubules for 97 minutes, diatrizoate produced a significant decline in tubule content of K^+ and ATP, a significant decrease in basal and uncoupled tubule respiratory rates, and a significant increase in tubule content of Ca^{2+}. The threshold dose for the diatrizoate effect was between 1 and 10 mM, a concentration range that is achievable in clinical practice [81]. The study also demonstrated that the combination of hypoxia and diatrizoate led to additional injury. When viewed together with the inherent vasoconstrictive properties of radiocontrast agents, these findings may explain why certain clinical states often associated with relative renal ischemia (volume depletion, prior renovascular disease) are more often associated with radiocontrast-induced acute renal failure. The finding that contrast media enhances injury to medullary thick ascending limbs in the isolated perfused kidney, an experimental model that is inherently hypoxic under the best of circumstances, supports this in vitro study [75].

Several observations from clinical and experimental studies suggest that radiocontrast-agent nephrotoxicity is determined by the anionic portion of the molecule. Both sodium acetrizoate and sodium diatrizoate have the same cation and the same number of iodine atoms per molecule, but sodium acetrizoate is now no longer used because of its high incidence of nephrotoxicity. Although the precise reason for the different nephrotoxicities of these two radiocontrast agents is not known, several observations suggest that a difference in access to the interior of proximal tubular cells may explain neph-

Fig. 43-5. Comparison of the effect of the radiocontrast agent sodium diatrizoate and the control impermeant anion methylsulfate on short-circuit current (an index of sodium transport) in the toad urinary bladder. The compounds were added at 78 mM to both mucosal and serosal solutions at time zero. Sodium diatrizoate depressed short-circuit current to about 30 percent of the pretreatment value, while sodium methylsulfate had no significant effect on SCC. The ordinate shows short-circuit current (SCC_t) as a fraction of pretreatment short-circuit current (SCC_o). (Reprinted by permission from T. W. Ziegler, *Kidney Int.* 7:68, 1975.)

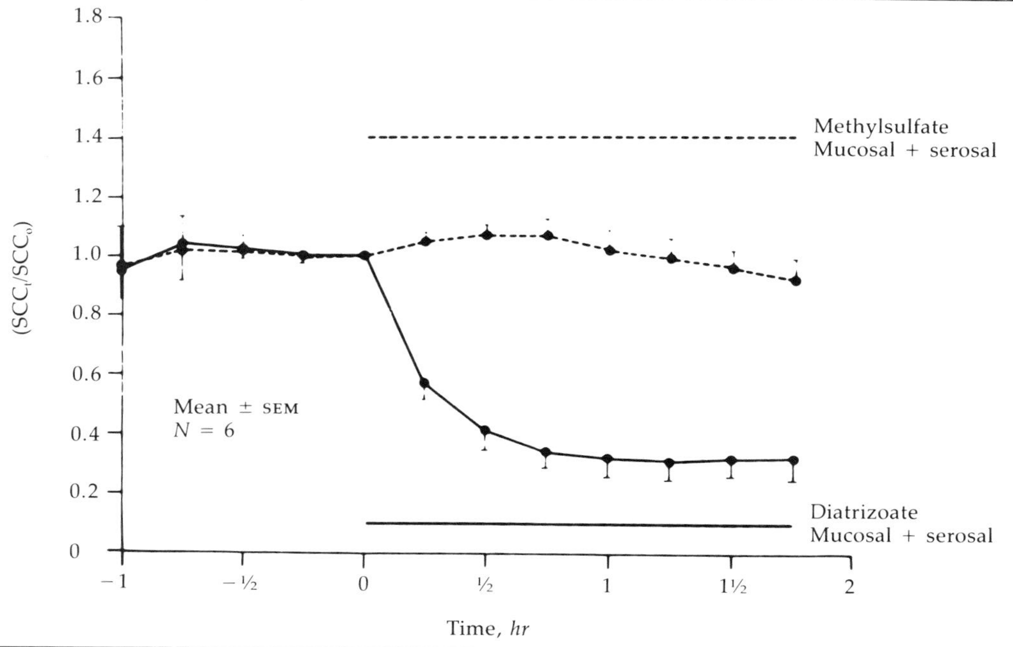

rotoxicity. The renal clearance of acetrizoate in humans is 600 ml/min, indicating a substantial component of tubular secretion [110]. Also, sodium acetrizoate reduces the tubular secretion of *p*-aminohippurate, which is further evidence that this particular radiocontrast agent is transported into the cell along the organic acid secretory pathway [117]. On the other hand, the renal handling of iothalamate, an example of the currently used triiodinate compounds, in humans has a renal clearance that is identical with that of inulin [47], implying neither secretion nor reabsorption. However, another agent from this group, sodium diatrizoate, has been shown to undergo both tubular secretion and tubular reabsorption [42, 140]. For nephrotoxicity to occur with the currently used agents, it is probable that some of the radiocontrast gains access to the cell interior. Lasser et al. [92] studied the histologic effect of several contrast agents injected directly into the dog kidney. The halogen moiety of the molecule appeared to be the toxic portion, since injection of the basic nonhalogenated molecule, constructed with prosthetic groups on all positions on the benzene ring, caused little renal histologic damage. Iodinated contrast agents are usually quite stable at normal body pH, but some deiodination does occur in vivo [97, 144]. Thus after urography or cholecystography, blood iodide may be elevated up to 200-fold for several days [11, 12]. The fractional excretion of ^{131}I is approximately 40 percent, indicating significant tubular reabsorption of the free iodide molecule [21]. Older cholecystographic agents that caused acute renal failure commonly released substantial free iodine into the circulation, and levels remained above normal for up to 5 days [28]. Protein-bound iodine remained high for many months. Also, as much as 5 mg of free iodide per dose may be present as a contaminant in urography dyes [137]. Whether these temporary elevations in iodide levels are nephrotoxic to normal or impaired proximal tubular cells is unclear. Whether renal cortical levels of radiocontrast are high after exposure is also unknown. Moreau et al. [105] were unsuccessful in attempts at demonstrating iodine atoms in renal biopsies of patients with osmotic nephrosis.

In a normal person, the usual contrast load is probably handled with minor impairment of normal cellular function when enzymuria is considered a marker of such transient tubular injury. However, in the presence of chronic disease that is characterized by sublethal cellular dysfunction, the added stress of a contrast load, iodine load, or both might precipitate cellular death. Many questions are left unanswered when examining the problem of radiocontrast-induced acute renal failure. The transient effect of radiocontrast material on renal blood flow and glomerular filtration rate does not suggest that these are primary mechanisms leading to acute renal failure. Toad bladder studies showing impairment of sodium transport raise the possibility that radiocontrast agents may impair sodium transport, possibly by inhibiting the enzyme Na^+-K^+-ATPase [156].

It is even more difficult to correlate the clinical risk factors with the clinical and animal studies described previously. The increased incidence of radiocontrast-induced acute renal failure in older patients may just reflect an increased likelihood for such patients to have vascular disease and renal impairment. Renal insufficiency is also very prevalent in patients with diabetes that develop radiocontrast-induced acute renal failure and is probably the single most important risk factor for this group. Dehydration or volume contraction has been cited as a major risk factor in patients with multiple myeloma or diabetes mellitus. Other factors, such as proteinuria and hyperuricemia, are present in only some patients who develop contrast-induced acute renal failure.

Although several retrospective as well as a few prospective clinical reports of radiocontrast-induced acute renal failure have suggested that renal injury is not a dose-related phenomenon, it seems most prudent to assume that it is. There is no a priori reason to consider that this nephrotoxin is different from others that have been shown to be dose dependent in their toxicities. When appropriate animal models of radiocontrast nephrotoxicity are developed, it is likely that a dose-response relationship will be uncovered. Although not confirmed by controlled studies, the clinical observation that repeated contrast studies over several days' time are associated with a greater risk of nephrotoxicity suggests that total dose is important [3, 33, 87, 113, 118]. Moreover, these observations suggest that radiocontrast-induced acute renal failure is not an all-or-none phenomenon. Rather, mild subclinical or sublethal renal injury only may become clinically detectable after a threshold is reached.

Altered Glomerular Permeability. The experimental model of contrast-induced acute renal failure that most closely approximates the abnormalities seen in humans is that of Vari et al. [151]. These investigators consistently produced reversible acute renal failure in rabbits by placing them on a low-sodium diet for 7 days, using indomethacin (18 mg/kg), and then administering contrast media (7 ml/kg). Glomerular filtration rate was not affected by the contrast material in these rabbits on the low-sodium diet unless indomethacin was also given (Fig. 43-2). Long-term DOCA but not acute saline or acute mannitol infusions prevented acute renal failure. Light microscopy showed no abnormalities of glomeruli or tubules, but micropuncture studies of individual nephrons showed that glomerular hydraulic conductivity, K_f, was significantly reduced during acute renal failure with no significant increase in intratubular pressure or decrease in renal blood flow.

New Radiocontrast Agents

If the hypertonicity of radiocontrast agents ultimately proves to be an important aspect of nephrotoxicity, then the newer nonionic and dimeric radiocontrast agents, although priced 10–20 times higher [49, 52, 154, 155], may prove to be safer than the ionic compounds (see Fig. 43-3). The nonionic agents, unlike for example, sodium diatrizoate, do not dissociate into anionic and cationic components on administration and thus are only moderately hypertonic to blood. The dimeric compounds dissociate into an anion containing two benzene rings that contain six iodine atoms and a cation of either sodium or methylglucamine. Since the iodine content of these dimeric compounds is twice that of either the ionic or the nonionic agents, similar amounts of iodine can be given with only half the osmotic load. The median lethal dose of intravenously administered iohexol, a nonionic agent, is three times greater than that of the ionic contrast agents [64]. Nonionic agents seem to have a particular advantage in myelography, digital subtraction angiography, leg phlebography, and coronary arteriography. Systemic effects, such as a feeling of warmth (especially after intravenous use), that depend on iodine content, osmolality, and sodium ion concentration are less frequent with the nonionic agents [17]. Despite these apparent advantages, there are several problems that will slow their acceptance into general use. The nonionic agents are difficult to manufacture and are unstable in solution. Metrizamide, for example, used for lumbar myelography, is available only as a lyophilized preparation. This factor makes it both difficult and expensive to use. Iohexol and iopamidol are sold as liquids. Unlike the ionic agents that are minimally reabsorbed by the nephron, the nonionic agents are to some extent reabsorbed by the proximal tubule, but there is a species specificity to this property [62]. Like the ionic agents, these nonionic agents also cause proteinuria when injected directly into the renal artery, but the magnitude of this effect is less than with the ionic agents [149]. The nonionic agents also have significantly less cardiac effects, causing less depression of ventricular contractility and less reduction in coronary sinus calcium concentration [17]. The nonionic agents also appear to have less effect on complement consumption, cause fewer hypersensitivity reactions, and have a less disruptive effect on the endothelial wall of blood vessels [111]. Using an in vitro preparation of rabbit renal proximal tubule cells, Messana et al. [99] showed that when these renal tubules were made hypoxic, the nonionic iopamidol caused loss of cellular potassium and impaired basal and uncoupled respiration rates less than diatrizoate under the same conditions.

Prevention of Radiocontrast-Induced Acute Renal Failure

In the absence of a clear understanding of the pathogenesis of radiocontrast-induced acute renal failure, guidelines for preventing this disorder must be based on the best interpretation of published clinical observations. In situations where the renal function is presumed to be normal (e.g., kidney donors), there is little evidence that exposure to radiocontrast agents carries more than a 1 percent incidence of acute renal failure. Since renal insufficiency is indisputably a risk factor, contrast studies should be done on this background only when the results produced by the study outweigh the risk of precipitating acute renal failure. If the patient has a baseline creatinine of 5 mg/dl or greater, the risk of acute renal failure is high and the possibility of irreversible acute renal failure must be considered. Chronic hemodialysis is not an unusual outcome for many of these patients. Although the role of hydration, volume status, dose of contrast, and concomitant nephrotoxins as risk factors is controversial, there are many historical and experimental parallels that suggest that these factors influence what effect radiocontrast agents will have on the kidney. A lack of consistent correlation with renal failure for each of these risk factors is more likely a fault of individual study design.

Mannitol was reported to decrease the incidence of radiocontrast-induced acute renal failure in a small group of patients when given within 1 hour of the radiocontrast [7, 112]. The precise interpretation and weight that should be given to such data are unclear, since in one report only five patients each were studied in the experimental and control groups [112]. Also, since radiocontrast agents promote a vigorous osmotic diuresis, the mechanism by which mannitol traditionally has been credited with protecting man and experimental animals from acute renal failure, it is unclear just how mannitol might afford protection against radiocontrast-induced acute renal failure. Other reports fail to demonstrate a protective effect from mannitol [2, 93]. Nevertheless, unless the patient has an underlying unstable cardiovascular system, volume expansion of every patient prior to receiving radiocontrast seems prudent and warranted. The addition of mannitol and/or furosemide to this regimen would appear to add little in the way of risk and, in experimental forms of acute renal failure, seems to have a beneficial effect.

References

1. Adornato, B., and Winestock, D. Acute renal failure—A complication of cerebral angiography. *Arch. Neurol.* 33: 687, 1976.
2. Agarwal, B. N., Cabebe, E., and McCormick, C. Renal effects of urography in diabetes mellitus. *Ann. Intern. Med.* 83: 902, 1975.
3. Alexander, R. D., Berkes, S. L., and Abuelo, J. G. Contrast media-induced oliguric renal failure. *Arch. Intern. Med.* 138: 381, 1978.
4. Almen, T., Bergentz, S. E., Tornquist, C., and Oystese, B. Selective nephroangiography in the dog causing platelet aggregation and irregular nephrographic phase. *Acta Radiol.* 26: 627, 1985.
5. Ansari, Z., and Baldwin, D. S. Acute renal failure due to radiocontrast agents. *Nephron* 17: 28, 1976.
6. Ansell, G. Adverse reactions to contrast agents. *Invest. Radiol.* 5: 374, 1970.
7. Anto, H. R., Chou, S. Y., Porush, J. G., and Shapiro, W. B. Infusion intravenous pyelography and renal function effects of hypertonic mannitol in patients with chronic renal insufficiency. *Arch. Intern. Med.* 141: 1652, 1981.
8. Bakris, G. L., and Burnett, J. C., Jr. A role for calcium in radiocontrast-induced reductions in renal hemodynamics. *Kidney Int.* 27: 465, 1985.
9. Barshay, M. E., Kaye, J. H., Goldman, R., and Coburn, J. W. Acute renal failure in diabetic patients after intravenous infusion of pyelography. *Clin. Nephrol.* 1: 35, 1973.

10. Becker, J. A., Kimkhabwala, M., and Zolan, S. Urography in renal failure. *Radiology* 105: 505, 1972.
11. Beierwaltes, W. H. The value of radioactive iodine uptake and protein-bound iodine estimations in the diagnosis of thyrotoxicosis. *Ann. Intern. Med.* 44: 40, 1956.
12. Beng, C. G., Welby, M. L., Symons, R. G., Stuart, S., and Marshall, J. The effects of iopodate on the serum iodothyronine pattern in normal subjects. *Acta Endocrinol.* 93: 175, 1980.
13. Berdon, W. E., Schwartz, R. H., Becker, J., and Baker, D. H. Tamm-Horsfall proteinuria: Its relationship to prolonged nephrogram in infants and children and to renal failure following intravenous urography in adults with multiple myeloma. *Radiology* 92: 714, 1969.
14. Bergman, L. A., Ellison, M. R., and Dunea, G. Acute renal failure after drip-infusion pyelography. *N. Engl. J. Med.* 279: 1277, 1968.
15. Berkseth, R. O., and Kjellstrand, C. M. Radiologic contrast-induced nephropathy. *Med. Clin. North Am.* 68: 351, 1984.
16. Bernstein, E. F., Evans, R. L., Blum, J. A., and Avant, R. F. Further experimental observations concerning the protective action of low molecular weight dextran upon intravenous hypaque toxicity. *Radiology* 76: 260, 1961.
17. Bettmann, M. A. Angiographic contrast agents: Conventional and new media compared. *Am. J. Roentgenol.* 139: 787, 1982.
18. Blaufox, M. D., Sanderson, D. R., Tauxe, W. N., Wakim, K. G., Orvis, A. L., and Owen, C. A., Jr. Plasmitic diatrizoate I^{131} and glomerular filtration in the dog. *Am. J. Physiol.* 204: 536, 1963.
19. Brasch, R. C., and Caldwell, J. L. The allergic theory of radiocontrast agent toxicity: Demonstration of antibody activity in sera of patients suffering major radiocontrast reactions. *Invest. Radiol.* 11: 347, 1976.
20. Brezis, M., and Epstein, F. H. A closer look at radiocontrast-induced nephropathy. *N. Engl. J. Med.* 320: 179, 1989.
21. Bricker, N. S., and Hlad, C. J. Observations on the mechanism of the renal clearance of I^{131}. *J. Clin. Invest.* 34: 1057, 1955.
22. Byrd, L., and Sherman, R. L. Radiocontrast-induced acute renal failure: A clinical and pathophysiologic review. *Medicine* 58: 270, 1979.
23. Cacoub, P., Deray, G., Baumelou, A., and Jacobs, C. No evidence for protective effects of nifedipine against radiocontrast-induced acute renal failure. *Clin. Nephrol.* 29: 215, 1988.
24. Caldicott, W. J. H., Hollenberg, N. K., and Abrams, H. L. Characteristics of response of renal vascular bed to contrast media. Evidence of vasoconstriction induced by renin–angiotensin system. *Invest. Radiol.* 5: 539, 1970.
25. Canales, C. O., Smith, G. H., Robinson, J. C., Remmers, A. R., and Sarles, H. E. Acute renal failure after the administration of iopanoic acid as a cholecystographic agent. *N. Engl. J. Med.* 281: 89, 1969.
26. Carvallo, A., Rakowski, T. A., Argy, W. P., and Schreiner, G. E. Acute renal failure following drip infusion pyelography. *Am. J. Med.* 65: 38, 1978.
27. Case records of the Massachusetts General Hospital. *N. Engl. J. Med.* 315: 308, 1986.
28. Cassidy, C. E. The duration of increased serum iodine concentration after ingestion of Bunamoidyl (Orabilex). *J. Clin. Endocrinol. Metab.* 20: 1034, 1960.
29. Cattell, W. R., Sensi, M., Ackrill, P., and Fry, I. K. The functional basis for nephrographic patterns in acute tubular necrosis. *Invest. Radiol.* 15: S79, 1980.
30. Chamberlain, M. J., and Sherwood, T. Intravenous urography in acute renal failure. *Nephron* 4: 65, 1967.
31. Chou, C. C., Hook, J. B., Hsieh, C. P., Burns, T. D., and Dabney, J. M. Effects of radiopaque dyes on renal vascular resistance. *J. Lab. Clin. Med.* 78: 705, 1974.
32. Cigarroa, R. G., Lange, R. A., Williams, R. H., and Hillis, L. D. Dosing of contrast material to prevent contrast nephropathy in patients with renal disease. *Am. J. Med.* 86: 649, 1989.
33. Cochran, S. T., Wong, W. S., and Roe, D. J. Predicting angiography-induced acute renal function impairment: Clinical risk model. *Am. J. Roentgenol.* 14: 1027, 1983.
34. Cohen, E., and Raducha, J. J. Detection of urinary Bence Jones protein by means of *p*-toluene sulfonic acid (TSA). *Am. J. Clin. Pathol.* 37: 660, 1963.
35. Cramer, B. C., Parfrey, P. S., Hutchinson, T. A., et al. Renal function following infusion of radiologic contrast material: A prospective controlled study. *Arch. Intern. Med.* 145: 87, 1985.
36. Cunningham, J. J., Friedland, G. W., and Thurber, B. Immediate diuretic effects of intravenous sodium diatrizoate in injections. *Radiology* 11: 85, 1974.
37. D'Elia, J. A., Gleason, R. E., Alday, M., Malarick, C., Godfey, K., Warram, J., Kaldany, A., and Weinrauch, L. A. Nephrotoxicity from angiographic contrast material. A prospective study. *Am. J. Med.* 72: 719, 1982.
38. D'Elia, J. A., Kaldany, A., Weinbrauch, L. A., and Buchbinder, E. M. Inadequacy of fractional excretion of sodium test. (Letter) *Arch. Intern. Med.* 141: 818, 1981.
39. Denneberg, T. Clinical studies on kidney function with radioactive sodium diatrizoate. *Acta Med. Scand.* [*Suppl.*] 442: 5, 1965.
40. Diaz-Buxo, J. A., Farmer, C. D., Chandler, J. T., and Walker, P. J. Computerized tomography—How safe? (Letter) *Arch. Intern. Med.* 140: 1253, 1980.
41. Diaz-Buxo, J. A., Wagoner, R. D., Hattery, R. R., and Palumbo, P. J. Acute renal failure after excretory urography in diabetic patients. *Ann. Intern. Med.* 83: 155, 1975.
42. Donaldson, I. M. L. Comparison of the renal clearances of inulin and radioactive diatrizoate ("Hypaque") as measures of the glomerular filtration rate in man. *Clin. Sci.* 35: 513, 1968.
43. Dudzinski, P. J., Petrone, A. F., Persoff, M., and Callaghan, E. E. Acute renal failure following high dose excretory urography in dehydrated patients. *J. Urol.* 106: 619, 1971.
44. Eisenberg, R. L., Bank, W. O., and Hedgock, M. W. Renal failure after major angiography can be avoided with hydration. *Am. J. Roentgenol.* 136: 859, 1981.
45. Eisenberg, R. L., Bank, W. O., and Hedgcock, M. W. Renal failure after major angiography. *Am. J. Med.* 68: 43, 1980.
46. Ekeland, A., and Uflacker, R. Effect of meglumine metrizoate and metrizamide on the microcirculation. *Acta Radiol.* [*Diagn.*] *(Stockh.)* 19: 969, 1978.
47. Elwood, C. M., Sigman, E. M., and Treger, C. The measurement of glomerular filtration rate with ^{125}I-sodium lothalamate (Conray). *Br. J. Radiol.* 40: 581, 1967.
48. Endrich, B., Ring, J., and Intaglietta, M. Effects of radiopaque contrast media on the microcirculation of the rabbit omentum. *Radiology* 132: 331, 1979.
49. Evens, R. G. Economic impact of low-osmolality contrast agents on radiology procedures and departments. *Radiology* 162: 267, 1987.
50. Fajers, C. M., and Gelin, L. E. Kidney, liver, and heart damage from trauma and from induced intravascular ag-

gregation of blood cells. *Acta. Pathol. Microbiol. Scand.* 46: 97, 1969.

51. Fang, L. S., Sirota, R. A., Ebert, T. H., and Lichenstein, N. S. Low fractional excretion of sodium with contrast media-induced acute renal failure. *Arch. Intern. Med.* 140: 531, 1980.
52. Fischer, H. W., Spataro, R. F., and Rosenberg, P. M. Medical and economic considerations in using a new contrast medium. *Arch. Intern. Med.* 146: 1717, 1986.
53. Fisher, M. S. Tyropanoate cholecystography and reversible renal failure. *J.A.M.A.* 234: 743, 1975.
54. Gafter, U., Creter, D., Zevin, D., Catz, R., and Djaldetti, M. Inhibition of platelet aggregation by contrast media. *Radiology* 132: 341, 1979.
55. Gale, M. E., Robbins, A. H., Hamburger, R. J., and Widrich, W. C. Renal toxicity of contrast agents: Iopamidol, iothalamate, and diatrizoate. *Am. J. Roentgenol.* 142: 333, 1984.
56. Gelman, M. L., Rowe, J. W., Coggins, C. H., and Athanasoulis, C. Effects of an angiographic contrast agent on renal function. *Cardiovasc. Med.* 4: 313, 1979.
57. Gerber, K. H., Higgins, C. B., Yuh, Y. S., and Koziol, J. A. Regional myocardial hemodynamics and metabolic effects of ionic and nonionic contrast media in normal and ischemic states. *Circulation* 65: 1307, 1982.
58. Goldstein, E. J., Feinfeld, D. A., Fleischner, G. M., and Elkin, M. Enzymatic evidence of renal tubular damage following renal angiography. *Radiology* 121: 617, 1976.
59. Golman, K., and Almen, T. Metrizamide in experimental urography. VI. Effect of renal contrast media on urinary solutes. *Acta Pharmacol. Toxicol.* 38: 120, 1976.
60. Golman, K., Denneberg, T., and Nosslin, B. Metrizamide in urography. II. A comparison of ^{51}Cr EDTA clearance and metrizamide clearance in man. *Invest. Radiol.* 12: 353, 1977.
61. Golman, K., and Holtas, S. Proteinuria produced by urographic contrast media. *Invest. Radiol.* 15: S61, 1980.
62. Golman, G., and Scient, C. Metrizamide in experimental urography. V. Renal excretion mechanism of a non-ionic contrast medium in rabbit and cat. *Invest. Radiol.* 11: 187, 1976.
63. Gomes, A. S., Baker, J. D., Martin-Paredero, V., Dixon, S. M., Takiff, H., Machleder, H. I., and Moore, W. S. Acute renal dysfunction after major arteriography. *Am. J. Roentgenol.* 145: 1249, 1985.
64. Gomes, A. S., Lois, J. F., Baker, J. D., McGlade, C. T., Bunnell, D. H., and Hartzman, S. Acute renal dysfunction in high-risk patients after angiography: Comparison of ionic and nonionic contrast media. *Radiology* 170: 65, 1989.
65. Gornick, C. C., Jr., and Kjellstrand, C. M. Acute renal failure complicating aortic aneurysm surgery. *Nephron* 35: 145, 1983.
66. Gregory, M. C. Acute renal failure after percutaneous cholangiography. *Arch. Intern. Med.* 144: 1288, 1984.
67. Gross, M., McDonald, H., Jr., and Waterhouse, K. Anuria following urography with meglumine diatrizoate (renografin) in multiple myeloma. *Radiology* 90: 780, 1968.
68. Gup, A. K., and Schlegel, J. U. Physiologic effects of high dosage excretory urography. *J. Urol.* 100: 85, 1968.
69. Harkonen, S., and Kjellstrand, C. M. Exacerbation of diabetic renal failure following intravenous pyelography. *Am. J. Med.* 63: 939, 1977.
70. Harrow, B. R., and Sloane, J. A. Acute renal failure following oral cholecystography. *Am. J. Med. Sci.* 249: 26, 1965.
71. Harrow, B. R., and Winslow, O. P. Toxicity following oral cholecystography with oragrafin. *Radiology* 87: 721, 1966.
72. Hartmann, H. G., Braedel, H. E., and Jutzler, G. A. Detection of renal tubular lesions after abdominal aortography and selective renal arteriography by quantitative measurement of brush-border enzymes in the urine. *Nephron* 39: 95, 1985.
73. Healy, J. K. Acute oliguria renal failure associated with multiple myeloma: Report of three cases. *Br. Med. J.* 1: 1126, 1963.
74. Heidemann, M., Claes, G., and Nilson, A. E. The risk of renal allograft rejection following angiography. *Transplantation* 21: 289, 1976.
75. Heyman, S. N., Brezis, M., Reubinoff, C. A., Greenfeld, Z., Lechene, C., Epstein, F. H., and Rosen, S. Acute renal failure with selective medullary injury in the rat. *J. Clin. Invest.* 82: 401, 1988.
76. Holland, M. D., Galla, J. H., Sanders, P. N., and Luke, R. G. Effect of urinary pH and diatrizoate on Bence Jones protein nephrotoxicity in the rat. *Kidney Int.* 46: 50, 1985.
77. Holtas, S., Almen, T., and Tejler, L. Proteinuria following nephroangiography. II. Influence of contrast medium and catheterization in dogs. *Acta Radiol. [Diagn.] (Stockh.)* 19: 33, 1978.
78. Holtas, S., Almen, T., and Tejler, L. Proteinuria following nephroangiography. III. Role of osmolality and concentration of contrast medium in renal arteries in dogs. *Acta Radiol. [Diagn.] (Stockh.)* 19: 401, 1978.
79. Holtas, S., and Tejler, L. Proteinuria following nephroangiography. IV. Comparison in dogs between ionic and nonionic contrast media. *Acta Radiol. [Diagn.] (Stockh.)* 20: 13, 1979.
80. Hou, S. H., Bushinsky, D. A., Wish, J. B., Cohen, J. J., and Harrington, J. T. Hospital acquired renal insufficiency: A prospective study. *Am. J. Med.* 74: 243, 1983.
81. Humes, H. D., Hunt, D. A., and White, M. D. Direct toxic effect of the radiocontrast agent diatrizoate on renal proximal tubule cells. *Am. J. Physiol.* 252: F246, 1987.
82. Kamdar, A., Weidmann, P., Makoff, D. L., and Massry, S. G. Acute renal failure following intravenous use of radiographic contrast dyes in patients with diabetes mellitus. *Diabetes* 26: 643, 1977.
83. Katzberg, R. W., Schulman, G., Meggs, L. G., Caldicott, W. J. H., Damieno, M. M., and Hollenberg, N. K. Mechanism of renal response to contrast medium in dogs. Decrease in renal function due to hypertonicity. *Invest. Radiol.* 18: 74, 1983.
84. Kjellstrand, C. M., Ebben, J., and Davin, T. Time of death, recovery of renal function, development of chronic renal failure and need for chronic hemodialysis in patients with acute tubular necrosis. *Trans. Am. Soc. Artif. Int. Organs* 27: 45, 1981.
85. Kjellstrand, C. M., Gornick, C., and Davin, T. Recovery from acute renal failure. *Clin. Exp. Dial. Apheresis* 5: 143, 1981.
86. Kone, B. C., Watson, A. J., Gimenez, L. F., and Kadir, S. Acute renal failure following percutaneous transhepatic cholangiography. *Arch. Intern. Med.* 146: 1405, 1986.
87. Krumlovsky, F. A., Simon, N., Santhanam, S., del Greco, F., Roxe, D., and Pomaranc, M. M. Acute renal failure: Association with administration of radiographic contrast material. *J.A.M.A.* 239: 125, 1978.
88. Kumar, S., Hull, J. D., Lathi, S., Cohen, A. J., and Pletka, P. G. Low incidence of renal failure after angiography. *Arch. Intern. Med.* 141: 1268, 1981.

89. Lang, E. K., Foreman, J., Schlegel, J. U., Leslie, C., List, A., and McCormick, P. The incidence of contrast medium induced acute tubular necrosis following arteriography: A preliminary report. *Radiology* 138: 203, 1981.
90. Larson, T. S., Hudson, K., Mertz, J. I., Romero, J. C., and Knox, F. G. Renal vasoconstrictive response to contrast medium. The role of sodium balance and the renin-angiotensin system. *J. Lab. Clin. Med.* 101: 385, 1983.
91. Lasser, E. C., Lang, J. H., and Zawadzki, Z. A. Contrast media: Myeloma protein precipitates in urography. *J.A.M.A.* 198: 945, 1966.
92. Lasser, E. C., Lee, S. H., Fisher, E., and Fisher, B. Some further pertinent considerations regarding the comparative toxicity of contrast materials for the dog kidney. *Radiology* 78: 240, 1962.
93. Levitz, C. S., and Friedman, E. A. Failure of protective measures to prevent contrast media-induced renal failure. *Arch. Intern. Med.* 142: 642, 1982.
94. Light, J. A., and Hill, G. S. Acute tubular necrosis in a renal transplant recipient: Complication from drip-infusion excretory urography. *J.A.M.A.* 232: 1267, 1975.
95. Madias, N. E., Kwon, O. J., and Millan, V. G. Percutaneous transluminal renal angioplasty. A potentially effective treatment for preservation of renal function. *Arch. Intern. Med.* 142: 693, 1982.
96. Martin-Paredero, V., Dixon, S. M., Baker, J. D., Takiff, H., Gomes, A. S., Busuttil, R. W., and Moore, W. S. Risk of renal failure after major angiography. *Arch. Surg.* 118: 1417, 1983.
97. McChesney, E. W. The Biotransformation of Iodinated Radiocontrast Agents. In P. D. Knoefel (ed.), *International Encyclopedia of Pharmacology and Therapeutics,* Sect. 76. Oxford: Pergamon Press, 1971. P. 147.
98. McQueen, E. G. The nature of urinary casts. *J. Clin. Pathol.* 15: 367, 1962.
99. Messana, J. M., Cieslinski, D. A., Nguyen, V. D., and Humes, H. D. Comparison of the toxicity of the radiocontrast agents, iopamidol and diatrizoate, to rabbit renal proximal tubule cells *in vitro*. *J. Pharmacol. Exp. Ther.* 244: 1139, 1988.
100. Miller, D. L., Chang, R., Wells, W. T., Dowjat, B. A., Malinosky, R. M., and Doppman, J. L. Intravascular contrast media: Effect of dose on renal function. *Radiology* 167: 607, 1988.
101. Moreau, J. F., Droz, D., and Noel, L. H. Nephrotoxicity of metrizamide in man. (Letter to the editor.) *Lancet* 1: 1201, 1978.
102. Moreau, J. F., Droz, D., Noel, L. H., Leibowitch, J., Jungers, P., and Michel, J. R. Tubular nephrotoxicity of water-soluble iodonated contrast media. *Invest. Radiol.* 15: S54, 1980.
103. Moreau, J. F., Droz, D., Sabto, J., et al. Osmotic nephrosis induced by water-soluble tri-iodinated contrast media in man. *Radiology* 115: 329, 1975.
104. Moreau, J. F., Noel, L. H., Droz, D., and Michel, J. R. Nephrotoxicity of ioxaglic acid (AG 6227 or P286) in humans. (Letter to the editor.) *Invest. Radiol.* 13: 554, 1978.
105. Moreau, J. R. Discussion. Symposium on radiocontrast agents and the kidney. *Invest. Radiol.* 15: S84, 1980.
106. Morgan, C., Jr., and Hammack, W. J. Intravenous urography in multiple myeloma. *N. Engl. J. Med.* 275: 77, 1966.
107. Morris, T. W., Katzberg, R. W., and Fischer, H. W. A comparison of the hemodynamic responses to metrizamide and meglumine/sodium diatrizoate in canine renal angiography. *Invest. Radiol.* 13: 74, 1978.
108. Mudge, G. H. Uricosuric action of cholangiographic agents: A possible factor in nephrotoxicity. *N. Engl. J. Med.* 284: 929, 1971.
109. Myers, G. H., Jr., and Witten, D. M. Acute renal failure after excretory urography in multiple myeloma. *Am. J. Roentgenol.* 113: 583, 1971.
110. Neuhaus, D., Christmann, A. A., and Lewis, H. B. Biochemical studies on Urokon (sodium 2,4,6-triiodo-3-acetylamino-benzoate) a new pyelographic medium. *J. Lab. Clin. Med.* 35: 43, 1950.
111. Nyman, U., and Almen, T. Effects of contrast media on aortic endothelium. *Acta Radiol.* [*Suppl.*] *(Stockh.)* 362: S65, 1980.
112. Old, C. W., and Lehrner, L. M. Prevention of radiocontrast induced acute renal failure with mannitol. *Lancet* 1: 885, 1980.
113. Older, R. A., Korobkin, M., Cleeve, D. M., Schaaf, R., and Thompson, W. Contrast-induced acute renal failure; persistent nephrogram as clue to early detection. *Am. J. Roentgenol.* 134: 339, 1980.
114. Older, R. A., Miller, J. P., Jackson, D. C., Johnsrude, I. S., and Thompson, W. M. Angiographically induced renal failure and its radiographic detection. *Am. J. Roentgenol.* 126: 1039, 1976.
115. Parfrey, P. S., Griffiths, S. M., Barrett, B. J., Paul, M. D., Genge, M., Withers, J., Farid, N., and McManamon, P. J. Contrast material-induced renal failure in patients with diabetes mellitus, renal insufficiency, or both. *N. Engl. J. Med.* 320: 143, 1989.
116. Pillay, V. K. G., Robbins, P. C., Schwartz, F. D., and Kark, R. M. Acute renal failure following intravenous urography in patients with long-standing diabetes mellitus and azotemia. *Radiology* 95: 633, 1970.
117. Porporis, A. A., Elliott, G. V., Fischer, G. L., and Mueller, C. B. The mechanism of urokon excretion. *Am. J. Roentgenol.* 72: 995, 1954.
118. Port, F. K., Wagoner, R. D., and Fulton, R. E. Acute renal failure after angiography. *Am. J. Roentgenol.* 121: 544, 1974.
119. Porter, G. A., Kloster, F. E., and Bristow, J. D. Sequential effect of angiographic contrast agent on canine renal and systemic hemodynamics. *Am. Heart J.* 81: 90, 1971.
120. Postlehwaite, A. E., and Kelley, W. N. Uricosuric effect of radio-contrast agents: Study in man of four commonly used preparations. *Ann. Intern. Med.* 74: 845, 1971.
121. Powe, N. R., Steinberg, E. P., Erickson, J. E., Moore, R. D., Smith, C. R., White, R. I., Jr., Brinker, J. A., Fishman, E. K., Zinreich, S. J., Kinnison, M. L., and Anderson, G. F. Contrast medium-induced adverse reactions: Economic outcome. *Radiology* 169: 163, 1988.
122. Rapoport, S. I., Thompson, H. D., and Bidinger, J. M. Equi-osmolal opening of the blood brain barrier in the rabbit by different contrast media. *Acta Radiol.* 15: 21, 1974.
123. Rees, E. D., and Waugh, W. H. Factors in renal failure in multiple myeloma. *Arch. Intern. Med.* 116: 400, 1965.
124. Ring, J., Arroyave, C. M., Fritzler, M. J., and Tam, E. M. In vitro histamine and serotonin release by radiographic contrast media (RCM). Complement-dependent and -independent release reaction and changes in ultrastructure of human blood cells. *Clin. Exp. Immunol.* 32: 105, 1978.
125. Ring, J., Endrich, B., and Intaglietta, M. Histamine release, complement consumption and microvascular changes after radiographic contrast media infusions in rabbits. *J. Lab. Clin. Med.* 92: 584, 1978.

126. Russel, S. B., and Sherwood, T. Monomer/dimer contrast media in the renal circulation: Experimental angiography. *Br. J. Radiol.* 47: 268, 1974.
126a. Russo, D., Testa, A., Della Volpe, D., and Sansone, G. Randomised prospective study on renal effects of two different contrast media in humans: Protective role of calcium channel blocker. *Nephron* 55: 254, 1990.
127. Sanchez, L. M., and Domz, C. A. Renal patterns in myeloma. *Ann. Intern. Med.* 52: 44, 1960.
128. Sanen, F. J., Myerson, R. M., and Teplick, J. G. Etiology of serious reactions of oral cholecystography. *Arch. Intern. Med.* 113: 241, 1964.
129. Schiantarelli, P., Peroni, F., and Rosati, G. Effects of iodinated contrast media on erythrocytes. *Invest. Radiol.* 8: 199, 1973.
130. Schmidek, H. H., Moreira, D., and Harder, D. R. Diatrizoate meglumine-induced dilation of rat basilar artery. *Neurosurgery* 12: 137, 1983.
131. Schwab, S. J., Hlatky, M. A., Pieper, K. S., Davidson, C. J., Morris, K. G., Skelton, T. N., and Bashore, T. M. Contrast nephrotoxicity: A randomized controlled trial of a nonionic and an ionic radiographic contrast agent. *N. Engl. J. Med.* 320: 149, 1989.
132. Shafi, T., Shyan-Yik Chou, Porush, J. G., and Shapiro, W. B. Infusion intravenous pyelography and renal function. Effects in patients with chronic renal insufficiency. *Arch. Intern. Med.* 138: 1218, 1978.
133. Sherwood, T., and Lavender, J. P. Does renal blood flow rise or fall in response to diatrizoate? *Invest. Radiol.* 4: 327, 1969.
134. Shieh, S. D., Hirsch, S. R., Boshell, B. R., Pino, J. A., Alexander, L. J., Witten, D. M., and Friedman, E. A. Low risk of contrast media-induced acute renal failure in nonazotemic type 2 diabetes mellitus. *Kidney Int.* 21: 739, 1982.
135. Simon, R. A., Schatz, M., Stevenson, D. D., Curry, N., Yamamoto, F., Plow, E., Ring, J., and Arroyave, C. M. Radiographic contrast media infusions: Measurement of mediators and correlation with clinical parameters. *J. Allergy Clin. Immunol.* 61: 145, 1978.
136. Skyhj-Olsen, T., Lund, P., and Praestholm, J. Transient acute renal failure and functional hemispheric depression after cerebral arteriography in diabetic patients. *Acta Neurol. Scand.* 64: 460, 1981.
137. Slingerland, D. W. Effect of an organic iodine compound priodax on tests of thyroid function. *J. Clin. Endocrinol. Metab.* 17: 82, 1957.
138. Sobin, S. S., Frasher, W. G., and Johnson, G. Nature of adverse reactions to radiopaque agents. Preliminary report. *J.A.M.A.* 170: 1546, 1959.
139. Stage, P., Brix, E., Folke, K., and Karie, A. Urography in renal failure. *Acta Radiol. [Diagn.] (Stockh.)* 11: 337, 1970.
140. Stokes, J. M., Conklin, J. W., and Huntley, H. C. Measurements of glomerular filtration rate by contrast media containing I^{131} isotopes. *J. Urol.* 87: 630, 1962.
141. Swartz, R. D., Rubin, J. E., Leeming, B. W., and Silva, P. Renal failure following major angiography. *Am. J. Med.* 65: 31, 1978.
142. Taliercio, C. P., Vlietstra, R. E., Fisher, L. D., and Burnett, J. C. Risks for renal dysfunction with cardiac angiography. *Ann. Intern. Med.* 104: 501, 1986.
143. Talner, L. B. Does hydration prevent contrast material renal injury? (Editorial) *Am. J. Roentgenol.* 136: 1021, 1981.
144. Talner, L. B., Coel, M. N., and Lang, J. H. Salivary secretion of iodine after urography. *Radiology* 106: 263, 1973.
145. Talner, L. B., and Davidson, A. J. Renal hemodynamic effects of contrast media. *Invest. Radiol.* 3: 310, 1968.
146. Talner, L. B., Rushmer, H. N., and Coel, M. N. The effect of renal artery injection of contrast material on urinary enzyme excretion. *Invest. Radiol.* 7: 311, 1972.
147. Tejler, L., Almen, T., and Holtas, S. Proteinuria following nephroangiography. *Acta Radiol. [Diagn.] (Stockh.)* 18: 634, 1977.
148. Teruel, J. L., Marcen, R., Onaindia, J. M., Serrano, A., Quereda, C., and Ortuno, J. Renal function impairment caused by intravenous urography. *Arch. Intern. Med.* 141: 1271, 1981.
149. Tornquist, C., Almen, T., Golman, K., and Hoftas, S. Proteinuria following nephroangiography. VII. Comparison between ionic-monomeric, mono-acidic dimeric and nonionic contrast media in the dog. *Acta Radiol.* 362: S49, 1980.
150. VanZee, B. E., Hoy, W. E., Talley, T. E., and Jaenike, J. R. Renal injury associated with intravenous pyelography in nondiabetic and diabetic patients. *Ann. Intern. Med.* 89: 51, 1978.
151. Vari, R. C., Natarajan, L. A., Whitescarver, S. A., Jackson, B. A., and Ott, C. E. Induction, prevention and mechanisms of contrast media-induced acute renal failure. *Kidney Int.* 33: 699, 1988.
152. Vix, V. A. Intravenous pyelography in multiple myeloma: Review of 52 studies in 40 patients. *Radiology* 87: 896, 1966.
153. Weinrauch, L. A., Healy, R. W., Leland, O. S., Goldstein, H. H., Kassissieh, S. D., Libertino, J. A., Takacs, F. J., and D'Elia, J. A. Coronary angiography and acute renal failure in diabetic azotemic nephropathy. *Ann. Intern. Med.* 86: 56, 1977.
154. White, R. I., and Halden, W. J. Liquid gold: Low osmolality contrast media. *Radiology* 159: 559, 1986.
155. Wolf, G. L. Safer, more expensive iodinated contrast agents: How do we decide? *Radiology* 159: 559, 1986.
156. Ziegler, T. W., Ludens, J. H., Fanestil, D. D., and Talner, L. B. Inhibition of active sodium transport by radiographic contrast media. *Kidney Int.* 7: 68, 1975.
157. Zir, L. M., Carvalho, A. C., Harthorne, J. W., Colman, R. W., and Lees, R. S. Effect of contrast agents on platelet aggregation and ^{14}C-serotonin release. *N. Engl. J. Med.* 291: 134, 1974.

Nephrotoxicity of Nonsteroidal Antiinflammatory Agents

William L. Henrich

Nonsteroidal antiinflammatory drugs (NSAIDs) have come to occupy a preeminent place in modern clinical therapeutics. Although the first NSAID, aspirin, was synthesized and given to patients over 100 years ago, the last decade has brought a profusion of new NSAIDs to market. These drugs have become popular partly because of their accepted efficacy and relative safety and partly because of the wide range of clinical conditions for which they are prescribed: arthritis, traumatic injury, athletic overuse syndromes such as tendonitis and bursitis, headache, and dysmenorrhea, to name a few.

Along with the growing use of these agents has developed an awareness of a number of adverse clinical syndromes associated with them. Among these, a form of acute renal failure, a direct nephrotoxicity, as well as several other clinical problems that primarily involve a derangement in renal homeostasis occur often with highly morbid consequences. The toxicity of NSAIDs in the kidney is inexorably coupled to a disruption in the physiology of renal prostaglandins, substances whose synthesis is inhibited by NSAIDs. Thus in order to clearly understand the mechanism of NSAID-induced renal effects, the renal physiology of prostaglandins is initially discussed briefly. A section on adverse clinical events related to renal functional changes following NSAID administration is then presented.

Renal Effects of Prostaglandins

SYNTHESIS, COMPARTMENTALIZATION, AND INTERACTIONS

Several major pathways for prostaglandin formation in the kidney are outlined in Fig. 44-1. Prostaglandins are derivatives of arachidonic acid, a 20-carbon tetraenoic acid that is acylated to membrane phospholipids. Deacylation of arachidonic acid from the cell membrane is controlled by phospholipases, predominantly phospholipase A_2, an enzyme that is calcium-sensitive and is stimulated by a number of exogenous factors. Vasopressin [36], bradykinin [112], angiotensin [110], and norepinephrine [98] all stimulate arachidonic acid release from membranes, whereas glucocorticoids (via inhibitory proteins called *macrocortin* or *lipomodulin* [172]) inhibit release.

Following release of arachidonic acid from the cell membrane, one of several synthetic pathways may be followed. Molecular oxygen may be added to arachidonic acid via the action of the intracellular endoplasmic reticulum-bound enzyme cyclooxygenase, which leads to the synthesis of the endoperoxide PGG_2. A second endoperoxide (PGH_2) is then formed with the liberation of a superoxide radical. NSAIDs exert their prostaglandin inhibitory effects by primarily inhibiting the cyclooxygenase enzyme. A decrease in prostaglandin biosynthesis follows the use of a NSAID; a decrease in the generation of superoxide and hydroxyl-free radicals into which superoxide is converted also occurs. Part of the effectiveness of NSAIDs in reducing inflammation may be due to a decrease in intracellular substances with oxidizing activity [108, 143]. The degree of the cyclooxygenase inhibition obtained with a NSAID may vary from as much as 90 to 95 percent in in vitro studies to as little as 70 percent in in vivo systems.

The endoperoxide PGH_2 is transformed by a series of enzymes to the dienoic series of prostaglandins (denoted by the suffix 2). It is these prostaglandins that possess biologic activity in the kidney. Prostacyclin synthetase acts to form prostacyclin (PGI_2), thromboxane synthetase forms thromboxane (TXA_2), and isomerases form PGE_2 and PGF_2. PGE_2 may be converted to PGF_2 by 9-keto reductase, an enzyme that may be stimulated by a high-salt diet [163] and inhibited by the loop diuretic furosemide [150]. It should be noted that with the exception of the thromboxane synthetase inhibitors, specific inhibitors of these enzymes are not available.

Prostaglandins exert physiologic effects at the location where they are synthesized; thus they are really autocoids rather than hormones since they are not synthesized to exert effects in distant locations. Prostaglandins that are secreted into renal lymph or into the renal vein, with the exception of PGI_2, are rapidly metabolized into inactive products in the lung. A 15-hydroxyprostaglandin dehydrogenase is responsible for the degradation of biologically active prostaglandins into degradation products.

Prostaglandins synthesized in the renal cortex regulate renal cortical processes (e.g., renal vascular resistance and renin secretion), whereas prostaglandins formed in the medulla modulate medullary physiologic events (e.g., salt and water handling). Table 44-1 lists the anatomic locations in the kidney where the various prostaglandins are synthesized more abundantly. PGE_2 and PGF_2 are synthesized primarily by medullary interstitial cells and less by the papillary collecting tubule and glomeruli. PGI_2 is synthesized in abundance by cortical arterioles and glomeruli, thus accounting for the predominance of PGI_2 located in the renal cortex. PGE_2 and TXA_2 are also produced in the renal cortex by glomeruli [36] and therefore may exert effects in this site.

Despite the rapid growth of interest in the basic physiologic prostaglandin effects, the roles prostaglandins play in renal physiologic processes have been difficult to define with precision. This is true because of the complicated series of counterbalancing effects that are initiated when a physiologic stimulus to prostaglandin synthesis is applied. Two basic concepts have emerged from the prodigious number of recent studies of prostaglandins and renal function: (1) Under baseline, euvolemic circumstances, there is typically a low rate of prostaglandin synthesis, thereby making it difficult to demonstrate that prostaglandins contribute to the normal maintenance of renal function. (2) When prostaglandin synthesis and release are stimulated, it is usually under circumstances in which systemic or renal hemodynamic destabilization has occurred. Under these perturbed cir-

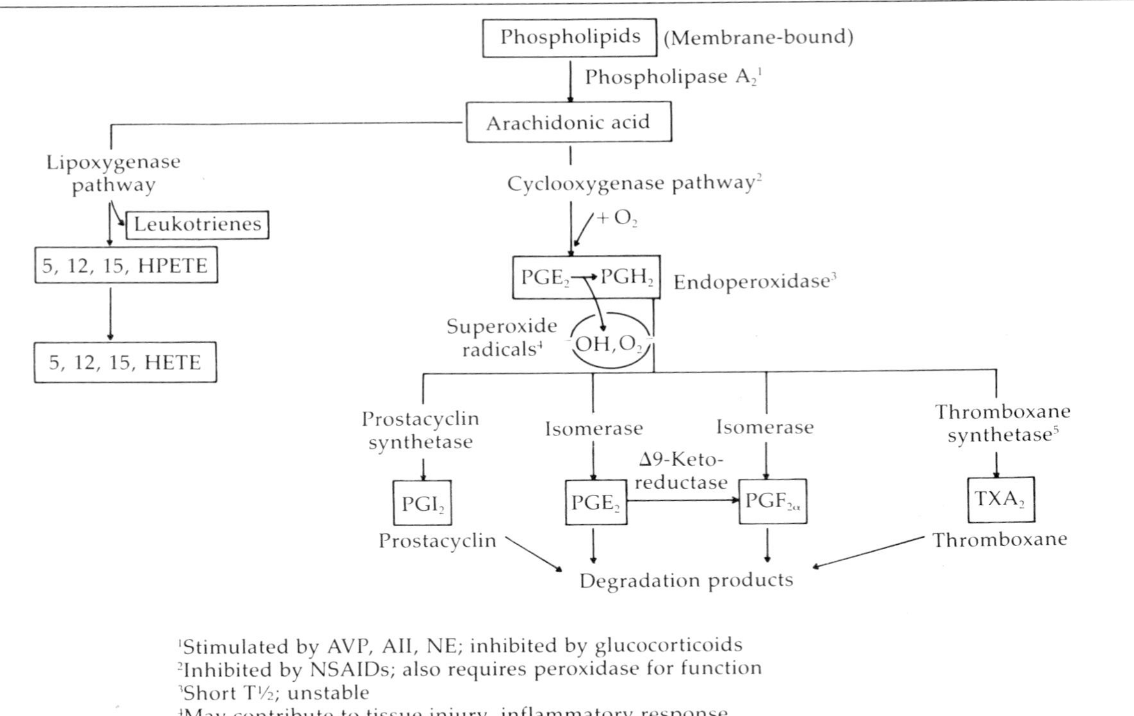

Fig. 44-1. Pathways for prostaglandin formation.

Table 44-1. Location and effects of prostaglandin production in the kidney

Location of synthesis and action	Prostaglandin	Action	Physiologic effects
Arterioles	PGI_2, PGE_2	Vasodilation	Maintain renal blood flow, direct more flow to inner cortical and medullary regions
Glomeruli	PGI_2, PGE_2, TXA_2	Vasodilation (PGE_2 and PGI_2); vasoconstriction (TXA_2)	Modulate glomerular filtration rate
Distal tubules	PGE_2, PGI_2, PGF_2	1. Inhibition of cAMP synthesis	1. Interfere with ADH action
		2. Decreased Na transport	2. Natriuresis
Juxtaglomerular apparatus	PGE_2, PGI_2	Possibly cAMP stimulation	Increase renin release

Source: Adapted from A. Garella and R. A. Matarese. Renal effects of prostaglandins and clinical adverse effects of nonsteroidal anti-inflammatory agents. *Medicine* 63:1655, 1984.

cumstances, prostaglandins may be shown to exert a moderating influence by opposing the stimulus that provoked prostaglandin release. For example, vasopressin stimulates prostaglandin synthesis and release, but prostaglandins antagonize the hydroosmotic effects of vasopressin on collecting tubule epithelium. Similarly, angiotensin II and norepinephrine (both renal vasoconstrictors) are potent stimulators of PGI_2 and PGE_2 formation; PGI_2 and PGE_2 are renal vasodilators that then attenuate any vasoconstrictor response. In the aggregate, then, as will be discussed, prostaglandins promote renal vasodilation, renin secretion, and sodium and water excretion during periods of destabilization or under conditions in which renal function has been compromised. The consequences of inhibiting this moderating, counterbalancing effect of prostaglandins with a NSAID could then be expected to result in exaggerated renal vasoconstrictive, antinatriuretic, antirenin, and antidiuretic effects.

EFFECTS OF PROSTAGLANDINS ON RENAL VASCULAR TONE

The exogenous infusion of the E, D, or I series prostaglandins directly into the kidney induces renal vasodilatation [36, 38, 97, 99]. A postglomerular vasodilatation is most frequently documented, notable because of the fact that the postglomerular circulation is the main target of the vasoconstrictive effect of angiotensin II [6, 7]. Much of the evidence for a postglomerular vasodilatory effect of prostaglandins has been inferred by studies in which administration of a NSAID to anesthetized animals has resulted in relative stability of the glomerular filtration rate (GFR) but a decline in renal blood flow (RBF) coupled with a sharp increase in renal vascular resistance (RVR) [3, 78, 98]. The increase in filtration fraction in such experiments has been attributed to increments in the hydrostatic forces that favor filtration. Studies of RBF distribution with radiolabeled microspheres in anesthetized animals given a NSAID show a predominant reduction in distribution of RBF to the inner cortical nephrons with relative preservation of outer cortical blood flow [86].

These positive studies documenting an effect of prostaglandins or NSAIDs on baseline RBF were performed on anesthetized, surgically prepared animals. As noted previously, it is difficult to demonstrate any major effect of NSAIDs in the conscious, euvolemic state. Thus experiments in the conscious animal typically demonstrate only trivial decrements in RBF after administration of indomethacin and meclofenemate [153, 156, 170]. In fact, one group of investigators attributed the effect of surgery in promoting a response of RBF to a NSAID to secondary increases in angiotensin II [156]. In sodium-replete humans, acute administration of indomethacin does not induce changes in GFR or RBF [30, 32]. Aspirin has been observed to have either no effect on GFR in normal individuals [10, 120] or at best only a modest one [8]. Thus it is clear that in the conscious, unstressed state, both humans and animals have minimal renal dependence on intact prostaglandin synthesis. Synthesis of endogenous prostaglandins is low under these conditions, and inhibition of cyclooxygenase with a NSAID would not be expected to have a deleterious effect.

A sharply different effect of cyclooxygenase inhibition is observed when the systemic hemodynamics are compromised. Under this set of conditions, a series of hormonal and neuronal reflex responses are elicited to protect blood pressure. Angiotensin II, norepinephrine, vasopressin, and sympathetic nerve activity all increase and cause increases in renal vascular resistance. In addition, each of these stimuli is a potent agonist for prostaglandin synthesis [110–112]. If cyclooxygenase inhibition is applied in this physiologic context, renal vascular resistance markedly increases, and both RBF and GFR decline.

That this counterbalancing relationship between vasoconstrictor and vasodilator forces exists in vivo was initially demonstrated by Aiken and Vane [2]. These investigators found that inhibition of prostaglandin synthesis with indomethacin or meclofenamate markedly increased the vasoconstrictor effect of an intrarenal infusion of angiotensin II. This pharmacologic in vivo relationship has also been demonstrated in other models using an angiotensin infusion [48, 136, 153]. Both PGE_2 and PGI_2 antagonize the effects of angiotensin II on the renal vasculature, an effect that has been demonstrated in the renal microcirculation in several species [2, 48, 136]. Furthermore, other renal vasoconstrictors (such as α-adrenergic stimuli and renal nerve stimulation) demonstrate enhanced renal vasoconstriction under conditions in which prostaglandin synthesis is blocked [102, 122, 152].

The physiologic importance of this relationship between vasoconstrictive and vasodilator forces has been demonstrated in several experimental models. Each of these models is characterized by an increase in activity of the renin-angiotensin system, circulating catecholamines, renal sympathetic nerves, and vasopressin. It is under such circumstances that maximum vasoconstrictive input is focused on the kidney and renal prostaglandin (particularly PGI_2 and PGE_2) synthesis is increased. In this setting, inhibition of cyclooxygenase will further reduce GFR and RBF. Hypotensive hemorrhage [69, 70], endotoxemic shock [75], volume depletion [32, 125], heart failure [129], nephrotic syndrome [33], hepatic cirrhosis [17, 171], underlying renal disease [90, 93], and aging [13, 52] are some of the conditions that have been extensively tested (Fig. 44-2). In the hemorrhage studies [69, 70], the degree to which each vasoconstrictive factor

Fig. 44-2. Schematic depiction of relationship between vasodilator and vasoconstrictor input into the kidney. PGI_2 and PGE_2 exert a moderating effect on renal vasoconstrictive stimuli.

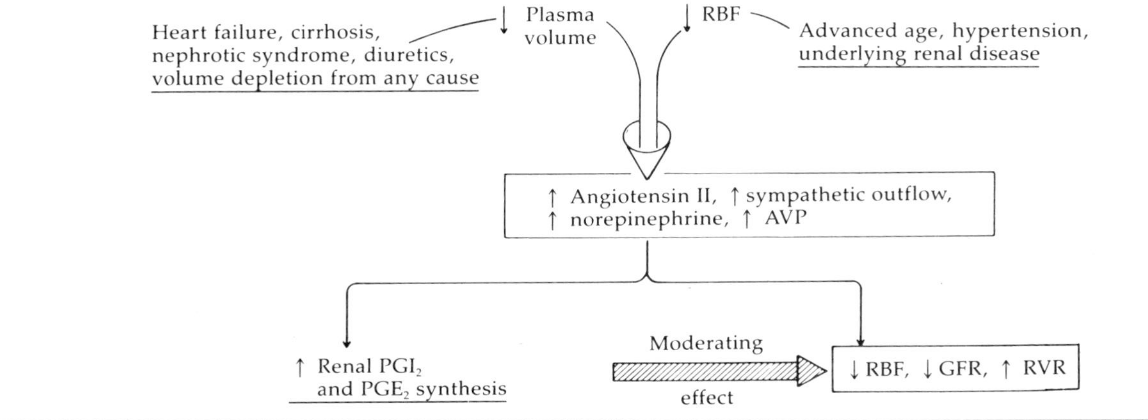

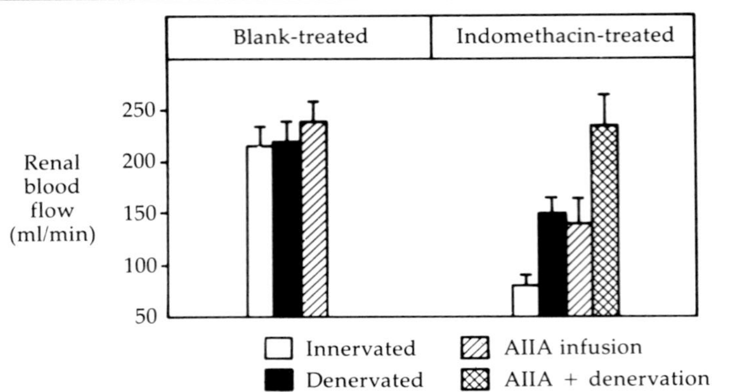

Fig. 44-3. Effects of prostaglandin synthesis inhibition on RBF during hypotensive hemorrhage. These data were obtained during maximum hypotension, at a time when vasoconstriction is greatest. Indomethacin-treated dogs had a significantly lower RBF than blank-treated dogs (open bars). Renal denervation (solid bars) or infusion of an angiotensin II antagonist (AIIA, striped bars) partly blunted the ischemia in the indomethacin-treated animals. The combination of renal denervation and an AIIA infusion improved RBF in the indomethacin-treated dogs to that of the blank-treated dogs. (Adapted from reference [70].)

contributed to renal vasoconstriction was studied by unilateral renal denervation and a unilateral angiotensin-antagonist infusion (Fig. 44-3). Under conditions of documented prostaglandin synthesis inhibition during hemorrhage, RBF was markedly reduced compared to prostaglandin-intact dogs. Renal denervation or an angiotensin-antagonist infusion partly reversed the renal ischemic response. As shown in Fig. 44-3, the combination of renal denervation and an angiotensin-antagonist infusion restored RBF to a level comparable to that in the nonprostaglandin-inhibited animals. This study documented the contribution of the renin-angiotensin system and renal sympathetic nerves to renal ischemia and also demonstrated the interplay of vasoconstrictive and vasodilator factors existing in a dynamic state in vivo.

EFFECTS OF PROSTAGLANDINS ON RENAL SODIUM EXCRETION

Prostaglandins affect sodium excretion both indirectly and directly. Through their activity as renal vasodilators, prostaglandins may cause an increase in the filtered load of sodium [36, 38, 97]. Moreover, prostaglandins preferentially augment blood flow to the inner cortical and medullary regions of the kidney; this effect tends to reduce the hypertonicity of the medullary interstitium and leads to a decrease in water reabsorption in the descending limb of the loop of Henle. Because of this effect, the maximum sodium concentration at the loop is reduced, and the gradient for passive sodium reabsorption along the water-impermeable thin ascending limb is reduced [51, 53, 141]. Finally, since prostaglandins exert their vasodilatory effects more at the efferent arteriolar site, the filtration fraction is thereby reduced, as is the peritubular osmotic pressure; the peritubular hydraulic pressure is increased. The sum of all these changes in Starling forces may cause a decrease in tubular sodium reabsorption [82, 83].

In addition to these hemodynamically mediated changes in renal sodium handling, prostaglandins have direct effects on tubular sodium transport as shown in several recent in vitro investigations. While there is some controversy about this issue [37, 45, 149], a number of in vivo and in vitro studies have demonstrated that prostaglandins have a natriuretic effect via the inhibition of sodium transport in the loop of Henle, distal nephron, and collecting tubule [79, 84, 133, 149, 167]. Recent studies further suggest that prostaglandins may play a key permissive role in the sodium excretion that follows volume expansion and an increase in renal perfusion pressure [23, 166]. Thus the majority of prior investigations have led to the conclusion that prostaglandins (PGE_2 and PGI_2, primarily) promote a natriuresis.

The consequences of NSAID administration for sodium excretion are different depending on the physiologic "set point." In euvolemic circumstances, NSAID administration typically causes little change in sodium excretion. However, in circumstances in which endogenous prostaglandin production is high (such as in the context of reduced renal perfusion), more profound changes in sodium excretion may be expected. The renal vasodilation produced by prostaglandins is muted, and the sodium-retentive effects of an active renin-angiotensin-aldosterone system are then more fully expressed [83, 136]. Positive sodium balance may be expected to ensue in clinical conditions characterized by high renin activity (i.e., in edema-forming states).

Another important practical aspect of the interaction of prostaglandins on renal sodium handling is the prostaglandin dependence of powerful loop diuretics. In particular, a blunting of diuretic effect has been noted in patients with edema-forming states who receive a NSAID [6, 41, 157, 159]. Some studies have suggested that NSAIDs possess a receptor-mediated mineralocorticoid activity analogous to aldosterone [43, 80]. More notable, however, is the fact that the ingestion of indomethacin or aspirin has been shown to result in resistance to the natriuretic action of furosemide [9, 114, 126, 157, 165]. This observation is most pronounced in patients with underlying renal disease or an edema-forming condition. The mechanism of this diuretic resistance was recently examined by Nies et al. [124] in anesthetized dogs on both low and high salt intakes. These investigators demonstrated that renal vasodilation followed furosemide administration in salt-depleted but not in salt-repleted dogs. When indomethacin was given prior to furosemide, this vasodilation was blocked, and a smaller natriuresis occurred. Thus the renal vasodilation accompanying furosemide administration was proposed to be partially responsible for the full natriuretic effect of the drug. When a NSAID is given prior to the diuretic, less vasodilation occurs and the natriuresis that occurs is smaller in magnitude. Examination of these animals in a salt-depleted, high-renin condition was particularly pertinent in view of the fact that this condition more closely resembles the patient group that often requires diuretic therapy. Similar to these findings are the data of Epstein et al. [39], who noted a blunted natriuretic effect of head-out water immersion following indomethacin administration in salt-depleted subjects.

EFFECTS OF PROSTAGLANDINS ON RENAL WATER EXCRETION

In recent years a body of evidence has accumulated that supports the involvement of prostaglandins as modulators of renal water excretion. Prostaglandins impair the ability of the kidney to concentrate the urine maximally, whereas NSAIDs may impair urinary dilution. Several key steps in the excretion of free water are potentially affected by prostaglandins: As suggested above, by increasing renal blood flow to the inner cortical and medullary regions of the kidney, distal delivery may be increased. By increasing medullary blood flow, medullary hypertonicity is reduced, thereby enhancing water excretion. Any action of prostaglandins in blunting sodium reabsorption in the ascending limb of the loop of Henle also further reduces medullary hypertonicity, thus promoting water excretion and reducing maximum urinary concentration. Finally, both in vivo and in vitro experiments have shown that prostaglandins oppose the hydroosmotic effects of vasopressin-induced cyclic AMP synthesis [36, 38, 64, 96, 148]. This effect limits free water reabsorption by the collecting duct. It is of interest that vasopressin stimulates PGE_2 synthesis in epithelial cells; by doing so, vasopressin induces its own antagonist. Hence the system is able to modulate the antidiuretic effect at the end-organ, with PGE_2 playing an important role in opposing the effects of vasopressin. The sum of all these actions of prostaglandins, therefore, is to impair urinary concentrating ability.

Conversely, the inhibition of prostaglandin synthesis by a NSAID would be expected to impair renal diluting ability. Clinically, this could result in water retention and a proclivity toward hyponatremia. In one investigation by Zusman et al. [173], indomethacin reduced urinary volume and impaired free water clearance when given to water-loaded animals treated concomitantly with ACTH. It is possible that NSAIDs may worsen any hyponatremic tendencies in patients taking other drugs known to affect water excretion negatively (e.g., chlorpropamide [90] and thiazide diuretics [92]).

EFFECTS OF PROSTAGLANDINS ON RENIN RELEASE AND CONSEQUENT EFFECTS ON POTASSIUM EXCRETION

Prostaglandins (particularly PGI_2 and PGE_2) are agonists for renin release; this release occurs in a dose-response fashion [73]. Recent evidence obtained in rat renal cortical slices suggests that prostaglandins may stimulate renin release via activation of cyclic AMP and that the final event in the renin release cascade may be a fall in intracellular calcium concentration [72]. In addition to the ability of PGI_2 and PGE_2 to directly elicit renin release, prostaglandins have also been implicated as essential mediators in other powerful pathways to renin release; of these, the renal baroreceptor, macula densa, and the β-adrenergic pathways are the most studied and the most important [68, 89].

Careful studies in the nonfiltering kidney have established a role of the prostaglandins in renin release stimulated by the arterial baroreceptor. Other investigations have confirmed this observation using renal arterial clamping models [12, 14] and hemorrhage [76]. Recently, Gerber and associates [55] provided compelling evidence that the macula densa pathway to renin release also operated in a prostaglandin-dependent manner. In contrast, both in vivo and in vitro studies have established that the β-adrenergic system may stimulate renin release despite prostaglandin synthesis inhibition [12, 68–70, 73, 74]. In summary, prostaglandins are integral to renin release elicited by several pathways (renal baroreceptor and macula densa) and are able to elicit renin release directly, probably by a cyclic AMP-coupled mechanism.

Inhibition of prostaglandin synthesis with NSAID administration would be expected to favor a positive potassium balance in several ways. First, by suppressing endogenous prostaglandin synthesis, hyporeninemia and hypoaldosteronism may occur; this would markedly impair potassium excretion by producing an endogenous hyporenin-hypoaldosterone state. Second, by reducing distal delivery of solute by the mechanisms listed earlier, the distal sodium-potassium exchange sites are deprived of substrate for exchange, thus further limiting potassium excretion. Finally, as discussed earlier, inhibition of prostaglandin synthesis has been shown to decrease angiotensin generation and aldosterone secretion [130]. Obviously, all of these tendencies toward development of a positive potassium balance and hyperkalemia are even more acute in a setting of already reduced ability to excrete potassium—e.g, an underlying reduction in GFR.

Clinical Nephrotoxicity Syndromes Associated with NSAIDs

Table 44-2 provides a list of the more currently used NSAIDs segregated according to derivative chemical structure; the NSAIDs available in the United States are denoted separately. The most widely prescribed group of NSAIDs is the carbocyclic and heterocyclic acetic acid

Table 44-2. Chemical classification of NSAIDS

	Generic name	Proprietary name
I. Carboxylic acids		
A. Proprionic acid derivatives	Ibuprofen[1]	Motrin, Rufen, Advil,[2] Nuprin[2]
	Fenoprofen[1]	Nalfon
	Naproxen[1]	Naprosyn
	Ketoprofen	
	Pirprofen	
	Fenbufen	
	Flurbiprofen	
	Benoxaprofen[3]	Oraflex
	Indoprofen	
B. Acetic acid derivatives (carbocyclic and heterocyclic acids)	Indomethacin[1]	Indocin
	Sulindac[1]	Clinoril
	Tolmetin[1]	Tolectin
	Zomepirac[3]	Zomax
C. Antranilic acid derivatives	Meclofenemate[1]	Meclomen
	Flulenamic	
	Mefenamic acid	Ponstel
D. Salicylic acids and esters	Aspirin[1,2]	
	Diflunisal	Dolobid
II. Enolic acids		
A. Pyrazolone derivatives	Piroxicam[1]	Feldene
	Sudoxicam	
	Isoxicam	

[1]Drugs available in the United States.
[2]Available over the counter.
[3]Removed from market.

derivatives, which include indomethacin (Indocin), sulindac (Clinoril), and tolmetin (Tolectin). The most extensive clinical and laboratory experience exists for indomethacin, which became available in 1972 and possesses antipyretic, antiinflammatory, and analgesic effects. Among the phenylproprionic acids, ibuprofen (Motrin), fenoprofen (Nalfon), and naproxen (Naprosyn) are the most popular. This class of agents was released as antiinflammatory agents in 1974 and 1975. These drugs are highly bound to protein and are slowly excreted in the urine as inactive metabolites. Each is a potent cyclooxygenase inhibitor; they were released with a reported lower incidence of gastrointestinal side effects.

The recognition of nephrotoxicity arising from NSAIDs has grown in recent years for at least two reasons: (1) It has been estimated that up to 40 million people in the United States use a NSAID daily, so the population of patients at risk is quite large. (2) The routine determination of the serum creatinine level in laboratory chemistry profiles has allowed detection of smaller changes in renal function earlier and more reliably than previously [67]. It should be noted that the exact incidence or frequency of nephrotoxicity due to NSAIDs is unknown. This is so because no precise method of detection is in place; the Food and Drug Administration monitors adverse drug reports (ADRs) from physicians, but this methodology seriously underestimates the true incidence rate. The most recent example of an ADR system being useful regards the numerous reports of nephrotoxicity from suprofen, a NSAID on the market for only a brief period of time [66, 135, 144, 149]. The syndrome consisted of flank pain and sudden renal failure, probably from deposition of uric acid crystals in the distal nephron.

Attempts by pharmaceutical companies to devise accurate surveys of renal toxicity based on numbers of prescriptions written have also been flawed. It is clear that in clinical practice nephrologists have come to recognize NSAIDs as a frequent etiologic agent in many patients who experience an acute reduction of renal function. In fact, many nephrologists rank NSAIDs behind only the aminoglycoside antibiotics as a cause of acute renal failure. This awareness among nephrologists is difficult to reconcile with negative surveillance studies showing a low incidence of renal toxicity due to NSAIDs [50]. It seems quite possible that nephrologists are encountering the "numerator" of the problem, while the "denominator" is so vast (i.e., millions of people exposed to NSAIDs daily) that an accurate assessment of incidence is not possible. Thus although the problem of NSAID nephrotoxicity is quite real and important, the overall incidence is probably very low, in part because of the physiologic behavior of prostaglandins discussed earlier. As has been recently pointed out by several authors, improved data bases are needed to accurately determine the scope of the problem [118, 147]. The following discussion of clinical toxicity focuses on the several discrete renal syndromes (listed in Table 44-3) that have emerged in recent years. Awareness of the particular patients at risk of toxicity may serve to further reduce the incidence of adverse side effects of NSAIDs.

Table 44-3. Clinical consequences of NSAID nephrotoxicity

1. Renal failure due to enhanced vasoconstriction: Secondary to prostaglandin synthesis inhibition, which leads to enhanced vasoconstriction; risk factors known
2. Interstitial nephritis: Believed to be a direct form of toxicity
3. Sodium and water retention: Secondary to the antinatriuretic effect of prostaglandin synthesis inhibition; water retention secondary to enhanced ADH effect from prostaglandin synthesis inhibition
4. Hyperkalemia: Secondary to hyporeninemic-hypoaldosteronism as a consequence of prostaglandin synthesis inhibition

RENAL FAILURE DUE TO ENHANCED RENAL VASOCONSTRICTION

This form of toxicity from a NSAID appears to be by far the most commonly encountered type. The clinical features of the disorder are summarized in Table 44-4; indomethacin accounts for the majority of the cases reported in the literature (60 to 70 percent) probably because of its longer availability and continuing popularity. Indomethacin is also one of the most potent cyclooxygenase inhibitors [140]. Typically, the serum creatinine increases sharply within 24 to 48 hours of instituting the drug, urine output declines to oliguric levels (at least initially), and, because this form of toxicity has usually been recognized early in the NSAID course in most patients, recovery of baseline or near-baseline renal function occurs with the discontinuation of the drug. Among the patients carefully reported in the literature [4, 11, 15, 18, 23, 42, 49, 52, 54, 90–93, 101, 107, 109, 127, 154, 171], several other interesting features are noteworthy. In contrast to the usual patient with oliguric acute renal failure, the fractional excretion of sodium (FE_{Na}) was less than 1 percent in 4 of 6 patients in whom it was measured [52]. The urinalysis was unremarkable in the majority of patients during the acute deterioration in function. Obviously, given the reversibility of the renal failure in patients in whom this condition is recognized early, dialysis is not usually required. In one survey of 27 patients with this disorder [54], only 3 of the 27 underwent dialysis. In these 3 patients, 2 had significant underlying renal disease at baseline; 2 of the patients recovered sufficient renal function to not require further dialysis, and only 1 [11] required permanent dialysis. The degree of renal failure was moderate in the group as a whole, with a mean rise of 3.0 mg per deciliter in the serum creatinine, and a peak serum creatinine of 4.8 mg per deciliter. Hyperkalemia out of proportion to the decrement in renal function was a common feature, occurring in approximately 25 percent of cases. In one case [90], a decline in renin and aldosterone concentrations was documented.

This typically reversible form of acute renal failure is most closely related to the inhibition of prostaglandin synthesis in the kidneys of susceptible individuals. Thus the groups at greatest risk for toxicity are those that depend on the counterbalancing vasodilatory properties of prostaglandins for support of RBF and GFR. The patient groups at greatest risk (listed in Table 44-5) are therefore the groups in which the majority of case reports have clustered: the nephrotic syndrome (n = 19 [5]), cirrhosis of the liver and ascites (n = 12 [171]), patients with underlying renal disease [10, 15, 27, 92, 93], patients with congestive heart failure [52, 161, 162], and patients with ineffective circulatory volume [161]. A unifying feature of several of these groups is a high-renin, high-angiotensin state. The most common indication for use of a NSAID in these patients is acute gout, but pericarditis, arthritis, and pseudogout have also been indications. It is under these conditions of a high-renin, high-angiotensin state coupled with enhanced sympathetic outflow that increased vasoconstrictive input to the kidney occurs and prostaglandins can be expected to exert a moderating influence. This balance is similar to the experimental studies previously described in which a clear relationship between prostaglandins and maintenance of renal function was demonstrated under high-angiotensin conditions. While this form of toxicity is usually reversible, progressive renal failure has been reported [6].

A recent demonstration of the relationship between NSAID administration and renal insufficiency was provided by Whelton et al. [164] (Fig. 44-4). These workers gave ibuprofen (800 mg 3 times a day), piroxicam (20 mg every day), and sulindac (200 mg twice a day) to 12 women with moderate renal insufficiency. All three regimens suppressed renal prostaglandin production; 3 pa-

Table 44-4. Clinical features of acute renal failure due to NSAID-induced vasoconstriction

Oliguria (at least initially)
Often occurs in hospitalized patients with other medical problems (e.g., congestive heart failure, cirrhosis)
Usually occurs within a few days of beginning medicine
Usually does not require dialysis (< 10 percent)
Hyperkalemia out of proportion to renal failure
FE_{Na} may be misleading as a diagnostic tool
Usually reversible

Table 44-5. Predisposing factors for developing NSAID-induced vasoconstrictive acute renal failure

Congestive heart failure
Cirrhosis (particularly with ascites)
Underlying renal disease
Advanced age (> 65 years old)
Volume depletion, shock, septicemia
Hypertension
Concomitant diuretic therapy
Postoperative patients with "third space" fluid sequestration

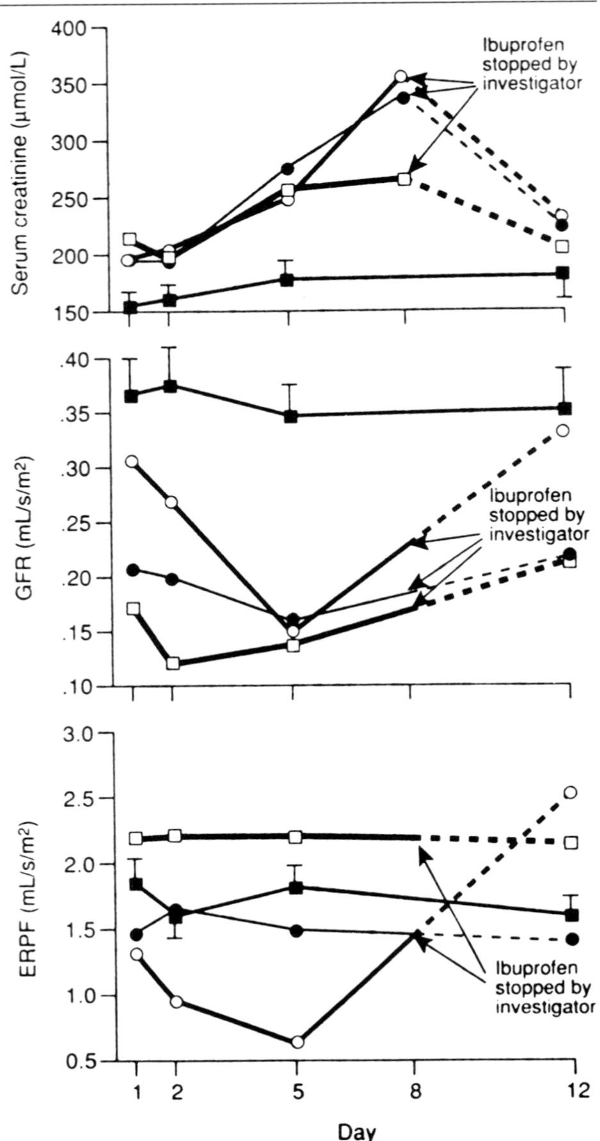

Fig. 44-4. GFR declined after indomethacin therapy (800 mg 3 times a day) in three patients.

tients receiving ibuprofen developed significantly worse renal insufficiency (see Fig. 44-4). Rechallenge of these 3 patients with 400 mg of ibuprofen 3 times a day still resulted in worse renal failure for 2.

Another group of patients at risk is the elderly, as recently emphasized by Blackshear et al. [13]. These observers described 7 patients with a mean age of 70 years who developed reversible acute renal failure on exposure to a NSAID (indomethacin in 4 cases and sulindac, naproxen, and ibuprofen in 1 case each). All of the patients had evidence of atherosclerotic heart disease, and 6 of 7 were taking a diuretic. In 3 of 4 patients in whom it was measured, the FE_{Na} was less than 1 percent at the point of maximum weight gain. Thus the risk factors of age (seventh decade of life and older), underlying renal disease, and diuretic use were emphasized by this report. The relationship between diuretic use and NSAID nephrotoxicity may be secondary to the volume-depleting effect of the diuretic described previously or to a combination of direct toxicities. This direct toxicity issue seems to be particularly true of a combination of triamterene and indomethacin; this combination should be avoided, since it has caused renal insufficiency even in healthy euvolemic normal individuals [41]. Another recent study [119] found that elderly patients were at greater risk for developing renal failure from ibuprofen than were the nonelderly, and recommended closer monitoring of serum creatinine in these patients.

In summary, it is possible to construct a population of patients at risk of this form of nephrotoxicity from the aggregate reports in the literature and from the experimental laboratory experience. The cautious use of NSAIDs with careful monitoring of renal function in such patients (listed in Table 44-5) is mandatory. Hopefully, the advent of prospective monitoring will continue to identify patients in whom renal function deteriorates so that rapid recovery can be effected.

Several additional issues deserve comment. It is obvious from the foregoing discussion that the development of a NSAID that has no effect on renal prostaglandin synthesis would be a major advance. Recently, a series of reports have suggested that sulindac may be "protective" of renal function and still be an effective antiinflammatory agent [22, 25, 26]. Any protective effect of sulindac would be expected to occur because of its unique metabolism [113]: It is administered as a prodrug (sulfoxide), which is then converted in the liver and kidney to the active, prostaglandin-inhibitory drug, sulindac sulfide. The sulfide form is then converted back to the sulfoxide or to an inactive sulfone product by mixed-function oxidases in the kidney. Hence the active drug (the sulfide) does not usually appear in the urine. However, reports of reversible renal failure based on an enhanced renal vasoconstrictive effect due to sulindac do exist [13]. Further, a recent study in dogs with therapeutic plasma levels of sulindac sulfide but without detectable urine levels suggested that sulindac could enhance a renal ischemic insult [71]. Finally, several reports have noted that sulindac may impair furosemide responsiveness in a manner similar to indomethacin and naproxen [19]. Any protection attributed to sulindac may therefore depend on several variables: the rapidity of the need for an increment in prostaglandin synthesis and release, the intrarenal drug distribution, and the metabolism of the drug. Caution should still be used with sulindac, as with all NSAIDs, until this issue of protection is more completely examined. It should be noted that some investigators have used oral prostaglandin therapy to reduce the vasoconstriction from NSAIDs in patients at risk for the syndrome. Misoprostol was used to reduce the effects of indomethacin on renal function in cirrhotic patients [4, 123]. It delayed or blunted the effects of indomethacin on renal function in a short-term study; whether this effect will be sustained is unknown.

A final question relates to the long-term hazards of kidney damage from NSAID use, an issue that has not been adequately addressed. Several NSAIDs have been associated with the development of papillary necrosis either alone [81, 105, 115, 132, 138] or in combination with aspirin [61, 105]. It is difficult to determine the direct contribution of a NSAID to the production of papillary necrosis in several of the cases reported because of the concomitant conditions present (e.g., other medications, urinary tract obstruction). However, the ability of NSAIDs to reduce prostaglandin synthesis and medullary blood flow, thus causing inner medullary ischemia, makes the drugs a likely cofactor in several of these cases [94]. In the clearest examples of NSAID-induced papillary necrosis [40, 81, 115, 132, 138, 168], several different drugs were implicated: phenylbutazone, fenoprofen, tolmetin, aspirin, meclofenamate, ibuprofen, and benoxaprofen. In most reported cases, patients had been treated for a minimum of 3 weeks. Several of the patients had underlying renal disease or reduced renal function. Usually an interstitial infiltrate and some scarring was seen when renal biopsy was performed. In most patients renal function was observed to improve on discontinuation of the NSAID. The only long-term report available on chronic treatment is a preliminary communication [131] in which patients treated with NSAIDs for rheumatoid arthritis and osteoarthritis were prospectively compared to a control arthritis population. Analysis of these groups revealed that NSAID-treated patients had a serum creatinine value of 2.58 mg per deciliter after the NSAID treatment compared to the value of 1.27 mg per deciliter before treatment. Control group values were unchanged. The time to development of a change in serum creatinine was 47.5 months. Thus, while future studies are needed to definitely answer the question of cumulative toxicity, it appears that some chronically treated patients may develop a change in renal function over a long term. Details of the drugs used, dosages, and patient characteristics were not available in this preliminary report.

RENAL FAILURE DUE TO GLOMERULAR AND INTERSTITIAL DISEASE INDUCED BY NSAIDs

A distinct clinical syndrome associated with NSAID exposure has become apparent in the last several years. This disorder is characterized by an interstitial nephritis on renal biopsy but often presents clinically as the nephrotic syndrome. The incidence of this unusual disorder (as with reversible hemodynamically mediated insufficiency) is unknown but is believed to be rare. One estimate for fenoprofen-induced interstitial nephritis was 1 case per 5,300 patient-years of treatment [20]. Another institution reported that a NSAID accounted for 1.3 percent of renal biopsy diagnoses. Abraham and Keene recently extensively reviewed the 36 reported cases in the literature [1]. Of interest is the fact that eight of the NSAIDs were associated with this disorder; the propionic acid derivatives (fenoprofen, ibuprofen, and naproxen) were associated with 27 (75 percent) of 36. Fenoprofen alone was implicated in 22 (61 percent) of the 36 cases [1].

In contrast to hemodynamically mediated NSAID renal failure, there appear to be no clear-cut risk factors for this interstitial nephritis-nephrotic syndrome disorder. The demographics of the 36 patients with an interstitial lesion on biopsy may simply reflect the general population who widely use NSAIDs: The mean age was 65 years, 28 percent were taking a diuretic, 14 percent were also taking aspirin, and 9 percent were diabetic. Unlike the hemodynamic deterioration form of renal failure arising from NSAIDs, the patients with this disorder did not have an underlying renal disease prior to NSAID exposure. Table 44-6 lists several of the differences between hemodynamic NSAID renal failure and NSAID interstitial nephritis.

The clinical features of the 36 patients summarized by Abraham and Keene are detailed in Table 44-7. Three distinct presentations of the interstitial nephritis are described: the nephrotic syndrome with acute renal failure ($n = 26$), the nephrotic syndrome without acute renal failure ($n = 4$), and renal failure without nephrotic syndrome ($n = 6$). Several features of this entity (summarized in Table 44-7) are noteworthy. (1) The time to development is quite variable, with a mean of 5.4 months; (2) only 7 (19 percent) of the 36 patients had a fever, rash, or eosinophilia; and (3) 83 percent (30 of 36) had nephrotic syndrome. Recurrence of the disorder has been described on reexposure to a different NSAID [104].

Renal biopsy findings typically include normal light microscopy with focal interstitial edema and fibrosis. A diffuse or focal monocellular infiltrate is usually present; in 30 percent of the reported cases, eosinophils were seen in the infiltrate. Immunofluorescence studies are usually unremarkable; in some cases weak and variable staining for IgG, IgA, IgM, and C3 were seen in the interstitium or tubular basement membrane. Mesangial electron-dense deposits have been seen in 3 patients [47, 63, 88].

The pathogenesis of the disorder is unknown. Direct tubular toxicity of NSAIDs seems unlikely due to the delayed onset of renal failure. A delayed hypersensitivity response to the NSAID would be compatible with the prolonged drug exposure histories and the predominance of the lymphocytes seen in biopsies [47, 146]. How glomerular damage is inflicted by the interstitial inflammation is unknown. It has been suggested that infiltrating lymphocytes release lymphokines and the vascular permeability factor, recently described as present in nil lesion nephrotic syndrome [145]. NSAIDs could conceivably enhance production of these lymphocyte-derived substances and thus change glomerular permeability [117]. Another possibility is that the inhibition of the cyclooxygenase enzyme shunts arachiodonic acid synthesis to the lipoxygenase pathways to leukotrienes [57, 142]. These leukotrienes mediate inflammation [57, 59, 60], increase vascular permeability [29, 57], and are chemotactic for white blood cells, including T lymphocytes and eosinophils [16, 60, 128].

Table 44-6. Differences in types of NSAID acute renal failure

	Hemodynamic type	Interstitial type
Severity of acute renal failure	Moderate to mild	Severe
Underlying renal disease	Yes	No
Time course to development	Variable, but usually days	Variable, but usually 5 or more months
NSAID involved	All	Fenoprofen over 60 percent; proprionic acid derivatives, 75 percent
Patients in hospital for other acute problems	Yes	No, usually outpatients
Presentation	Volume overload with decreased urine output, increased serum creatinine	Edema or oliguria
Usual symptoms	Insidious	Cramps, edema
Proteinuria	Trivial	Nephrotic syndrome
Recovery time course	Prompt in most patients	Slowly—may take weeks to months. Steroids may help in some cases
Frequency	Common	Unusual

Table 44-7. Clinical presentation of NSAID-induced interstitial and glomerular disease

	Number patients	Age (yr)	Drug exposure (mo)	Peak S_{CR} (mg/dl)	Urinary protein (gm/24h)	Systemic hypersensitivity reactions[1]
Nephrotic syndrome and renal failure	26	65	5.7	6.1	13.2	3
Nephrotic syndrome without renal failure[2]	4	65	11.3	1.1	7.4	0
Renal failure without nephrotic syndrome	6	63	1.2	7.0	0	4

[1]Fever, skin rash, eosinophilia, eosinophiluria.
[2]Documented by renal biopsy [4] or systemic hypersensitivity response [2].
Source: Adapted from P. A. Abraham and W. F. Keane. Glomerular and interstitial disease induced by non-steroidal anti-inflammatory drugs. *Am. J. Nephrol.* 4:1, 1984.

Whether such an effect of leukotrienes would be the result of local (renal) production or infiltrating lymphocytes is unknown [21, 58, 87]. Torres summarized this potential scheme in detail recently [158].

One recent report documented nil disease following ibuprofen exposure without interstitial nephritis [116]; the exact incidence of this syndrome is unknown. Similarly, a spontaneous relapse of the nephrotic syndrome linked to naproxen has been reported [138]. The value of steroids in aiding the resolution of this disorder is unsettled. Prednisone has been used in 75 percent of the cases reported [1]; recovery has generally occurred gradually over several weeks to months. A controlled trial of steroids and/or cytotoxic agents in this disorder has not yet been undertaken. Anecdotal reports of success using prednisone therapy are available [28]. In some patients, NSAID toxicity may appear to be an exacerbation of underlying disease or a rapidly progressive glomerulonephritic syndrome [96, 100].

NSAIDs AND SODIUM BALANCE

Mild sodium retention represents the most commonly encountered side effect of NSAIDs, occurring in as many as 25 percent of patients who use them. Typically, this positive sodium balance is transient and of no major clinical importance. In more tenuous patients with severe congestive heart failure or hypertension, the sodium retention may, however, have serious adverse consequences.

As noted in the previous discussion of sodium excretion with NSAIDs, the amount of sodium retention resulting from NSAID administration depends on the baseline set point of a particular patient. For example, in patients with edema-forming conditions, prostaglandins exert a balancing natriuretic function, which, when ablated, leads to more avid sodium retention and positive balance. Conversely, euvolemic normal individuals with low endogenous prostaglandin production may note either no or trivial accumulations of edema. Massive amounts of sodium retention are rare; the most spectacular case is that of a 70-year-old man who gained 15 kg during a 17-day course of ibuprofen [137].

The issue of diuretic resistance induced by NSAIDs has also been discussed earlier in the physiology section. Clinically this phenomenon could be critically important in sodium-avid individuals taking a NSAID who are found to require larger and larger doses of loop diuretics to maintain weight. Conversely, the administration of a NSAID to a patient already receiving a diuretic may promote sufficient positive sodium balance to cause destabilization. Finally, as noted earlier, the prior use of diuretics increases an individual's risk for a reduction in renal function (GFR and RBF) when a NSAID is added.

EFFECTS OF NSAIDs ON WATER BALANCE

As noted earlier, NSAIDs impair urinary diluting ability by one of several actions. An antidiuresis is maximized by inhibition of endogenous prostaglandin production, which then leads to unopposed vasopressin effect. In addition, if GFR declines as a result of NSAID use, delivery of filtrate to the distal nephron-diluting sites is impaired and water excretion declines. Each of these effects would make patients prone to hyponatremia. Clinically, this problem has not been reported to be common or severe; however, in marginal patients who are already hyponatremic, use of a NSAID should include serial monitoring of the serum sodium concentration. Such a patient has been described by Walshe and Venuto [162]; the diabetic patient receiving chlorpropamide and indomethacin developed worsening hyponatremia, weight gain, and heart failure.

HYPERKALEMIA AND NSAIDs

A tendency toward hyperkalemia in patients receiving a NSAID is to be expected given the known ability of the drugs to suppress the renin-angiotensin-aldosterone system. NSAID administration has resulted in hyperkalemia in patients with both normal and abnormal renal function [44, 62, 95, 154]. The frequency of hyperkalemia clinically is probably quite low in nondiabetic normal individuals. However, patients with diabetes or underlying renal disease and those receiving beta-blocking medication are most at risk of developing hyperkalemia. In virtually all instances of hyperkalemia following NSAID administration, the mechanism invoked has been hyporeninemic hypoaldosteronism. One report suggested a cellular defect in potassium uptake [130], which could be responsible. The opposite of this clinical syndrome of a NSAID-induced hyporeninemic state and hyperkalemia is Bartter's syndrome, which is characterized by hypereninemic hyperaldosteronism, hypokalemia, and exaggerated renal prostaglandin synthesis and release. Of note is the fact that several of the manifestations of Bartter's syndrome are corrected by cyclooxygenase inhibition [34, 56, 65, 160].

References

1. Abraham, P. A., and Keane, W. F. Glomerular and interstitial disease induced by non-steroidal anti-inflammatory drugs. *Am. J. Nephrol.* 4: 1, 1984.
2. Aiken, J. W., and Vane, J. R. Intrarenal prostaglandin release attenuates the renal vasoconstrictor activity of angiotensin. *J. Pharmacol. Exp. Ther.* 184: 678, 1973.
3. Anderson, R. J., Taher, S., Cronin, R. E., et al. Effects of β-adrenergic blockade and inhibitors of angiotensin II and prostaglandins on renal autoregulation. *Am. J. Physiol.* 229: 731, 1975.
4. Antillon, M., Cominelli, F., Lo, S., et al. Effects of oral prostaglandins on indomethacin-induced renal failure in patients with cirrhosis and ascites. *J. Rheumatol.* 20: 46, 1990.
5. Ariz, L., Donker, A. J. M., Brentjens, J. R. H., et al. The effect of indomethacin on proteinuria and kidney function in the nephrotic syndrome. *Acta Med. Scand.* 199: 121, 1976.
6. Attallah, A. A. Interaction of prostaglandins with diuretics. *Prostaglandins* 18: 369, 1979.
7. Baylis, C., and Brenner, B. M. Modulation by prostaglandin synthesis inhibitors of the action of exogenous angiotensin II on glomerular ultrafiltration in the rat. *Cir. Res.* 43: 889, 1978.
8. Beeley, L., and Kendall, M. J. Effect of aspirin on renal clearance on ^{125}I diatrizoate. *Br. Med. J.* 1: 707, 1971.
9. Berg, K. J. Acute effects of acetylsalicylate acid in patients with chronic renal insufficiency. *Eur. J. Clin. Pharmacol.* 11: 111, 1977.
10. Berg, K. J. Acute effects of acetylsalicylate acid on renal function in a normal man. *Eur. J. Clin. Pharmacol.* 11: 117, 1977
11. Berheim, J. L., and Rorzets, Z. Indomethacin-induced renal failure. *Ann. Intern. Med.* 91: 792, 1979.
12. Berl, T., Henrich, W. L., Erickson, A. L., et al. Prostaglandins in the beta-adrenergic and baroreceptor-mediated secretion of renin. *Am. J. Physiol.* 236: F472, 1979.
13. Blackshear, J. L., Davidman, M., and Stillman, M. T. Identification of risk for renal insufficiency from nonsteroidal anti-inflammatory drugs. *Arch. Intern. Med.* 143: 1130, 1983.
14. Blackshear, J. L., Spielman, W. S., Knox, F. G., et al. Dissociation of renin release and renal vasodilatation by prostaglandin synthesis inhibitors. *Am. J. Physiol.* 237: F20, 1979.
15. Blum, M., Bauminger, S., Algueti, A., et al. Urinary prostaglandin E_2 in chronic renal disease. *Clin. Nephrol.* 15: 87, 1981.
16. Bokoch, F., Boeynaems, J., and Hubbard, W. Chemotactic and chemokinetic activity of products of mammalian lipoxygenases. *Pick. Lymphokines* 4: 271, 1981.
17. Boyer, T. D., Zia, P., and Reynolds, T. B. Effect of indomethacin and prostaglandin A_1 on renal function and plasma renin activity in alcoholic liver disease. *Gastroenterology* 77: 215, 1979.
18. Brandstetter, R. D., and Marr, D. D. Reversible oliguric renal failure associated with ibuprofen treatment. *Br. Med. J.* 2: 1194, 1978.
19. Brater, D. C., Anderson, S., Baird, B., et al. Sulindac does not spare the kidney. *Clin. Res.* 31: 868A, 1983.
20. Brezin, J., Katz, S., Schwartz, A., et al. Reversible renal failure and nephrotic syndrome associated with nonsteroidal anti-inflammatory drugs. *N. Engl. J. Med.* 301: 1271, 1979.
21. Brown, D., Gerrard, J., Peller, J., et al. Glomerular prostaglandin metabolism in diabetic rats. *Diabetes* 29: 219, 1980.
22. Bunning, R. D., and Barth, W. F. Sulindac: A potential renal-sparing non-steroidal anti-inflammatory drug. *J.A.M.A.* 248: 2864, 1982.
23. Carmines, P. K., Bell, D. P., Roman, R. J., et al. Prostaglandins in the sodium excretory response to altered renal arterial pressure in dogs. *Am. J. Physiol.* 248 (*Renal Fluid Electrolyte Physiol.* 17): F8, 1985.
24. Chapnick, B. M., Paustian, P. W., Klainer, E., et al. Influence of prostaglandins E, A and F on vasoconstrictor responses to norepinephrine, renal nerve stimulation

and angiotensin in the feline kidney. *J. Pharmacol. Exp. Ther.* 196: 44, 1976.
25. Ciabattoni, G., Cinotti, G. A., Pierucci, A., et al. Effects of sulindac and ibuprofen in patients with chronic glomerular disease. *N. Engl. J. Med.* 310: 279, 1984.
26. Ciabattoni, G., Pugliese, F., Cinotti, G. A., et al. Renal effects of antiinflammatory drugs. *Eur. J. Rheumatol.* 3: 210, 1980.
27. Cinotti, G. A., Manzi, M., Mene, P., et al. Prostaglandin dependence of renal function in chronic glomerular disease, abstract. *Clin. Res.* 30: 445A, 1982.
28. Crespigny, P. J., Becker, G. J., and Ihle, U. Renal failure and nephrotic syndrome associated with sulindac. *Clin. Nephrol.* 30(1): 52, 1988.
29. Dahlen, S., Bjork, J., Hedqvist, P., et al. Leukotrienes promote plasma leakage and leukocyte adhesion in postcapillary venules. In vivo effects with relevance to the acute inflammatory response. *Proc. Nat. Acad. Sci. U.S.A.* 78: 3887, 1981.
30. DeJong, P. E., DeJong-Vandenberg, L., Sewrajsingh, G. S., et al. The influence of indomethacin on renal hemodynamics in sickle cell anemia. *Clin. Sci.* 59: 245, 1976.
31. Donker, A. J. M. The effect of indomethacin on renal function and glomerular protein loss. In M. J. Dunn, C. Patrono, and G. A. Cinotti (eds.), *Prostaglandins and the Kidney: Biochemistry, Physiology, Pharmacology and Clinical Applications.* New York: Plenum, 1900. Pp. 251–262.
32. Donker, A. J. M., Arisz, L., Brentjens, J. R. H., et al. The effect of indomethacin on kidney function and plasma renin activity in man. *Nephron* 17: 288, 1976.
33. Donker, A. J. M., Brentjens, J. R. H., and Van der Hem, G. K. The effect of indomethacin on proteinuria and kidney function in the nephrotic syndrome. *Acta Med. Scand.* 199: 121, 1976.
34. Donker, A. J. M., DeJong, P. E., Statius Van Eps, L. W., et al. Indomethacin in Bartter's syndrome. *Nephron* 19: 200, 1977.
35. Dunn, M. J., Greely, H. P., Valtin, H., et al. Renal excretion of prostaglandins E_2 and F_2 in diabetes insipidus rat. *Am. J. Physiol.* 235: E624, 1978.
36. Dunn, M. J., and Hood, V. L. Prostaglandins and the kidney. *Am. J. Physiol.* 233: F169, 1977.
37. Dunn, M. J., and Howe, D. Prostaglandins lack a direct inhibitory action on electrolyte and water transport in the kidney and the erythrocyte. *Prostaglandins* 13: 417, 1977.
38. Dunn, M. J., and Zambraski, E. Renal effects of drugs that inhibit prostaglandin synthesis. *Kidney Int.* 18: 609, 1980.
39. Epstein, M., Lifschitz, M. D., Hoffman, D. S., et al. Relationship between renal prostaglandin E and renal sodium handling during water immersion in normal man. *Circ. Res.* 45: 71, 1979.
40. Erwin, L., and Jones, J. M. B. Benoxaprofen and papillary necrosis. *Br. Med. J.* 285: 694, 1982.
41. Favre, L., Glasson, P. H., Riondel, A., et al. Interaction of diuretics and non-steroidal antiinflammatory drugs in man. *Clin. Sci.* 64: 407, 1983.
42. Favre, L., Glasson, P., and Vallotton, M. B. Reversible acute renal failure from combined triamterene and indomethacin. A study in healthy subjects. *Ann. Intern. Med.* 96: 317, 1982.
43. Feldman, D., and Couropmitree, C. Intrinsic mineralocorticoid agonist activity of some non-steroidal anti-inflammatory drugs. *J. Clin. Invest.* 57: 1, 1976.
44. Findling, J. W., Beckstrom, D., and Rawsthorne, L. Indomethacin-induced hyperkalemia in three patients with gouty arthritis. *J.A.M.A.* 244: 1127, 1980.
45. Fine, L. G., and Trizna, W. Influence of prostaglandins on sodium transport of isolated medullary nephron segments. *Am. J. Physiol.* 232 (*Renal Fluid Electrolyte Physiol.* 1): F383, 1977.
46. Fink, G. D., Chapnick, B. M., Goldberg, M. R., et al. Influence of prostaglandin E_2, indomethacin and reserpine on renal vascular responses to nerve stimulation, pressor and depressor hormones. *Circ. Res.* 41: 172, 1977.
47. Finklestein, A., Fraley, D., Stachura, I., et al. Fenoprofen nephropathy: Lipoid nephrosis and interstitial nephritis. A possible T-lymphocyte disorder. *Am. J. Med.* 72: 81, 1982.
48. Finn, W., and Arendshorst, W. J. Effect of prostaglandin synthetase inhibitors on renal blood flow in the rat. *Am. J. Physiol.* 231: 1541, 1976.
49. Fong, H. J., and Cohen, A. H. Ibuprofen-induced acute renal failure with acute tubular necrosis. *Am. J. Nephrol.* 2: 28, 1982.
50. Fox, D. R., and Jick, H. Nonsteroidal anti-inflammatory drugs and renal disease. *J.A.M.A.* 251: 1299, 1984.
51. Fulgraff, G., and Meiforth, A. Effects of prostaglandin E_2 on excretion and reabsorption of sodium and fluid in rat kidneys (micropuncture studies) *Plfügers Arch.* 330: 243, 1971.
52. Galler, M., Folkert, V. W., and Schlondorf, D. Reversible acute renal insufficiency and hyperkalemia following indomethacin therapy. *J.A.M.A.* 246: 154, 1981.
53. Ganguli, M., Tobian, L., Azar, S., et al. Evidence that prostaglandin synthesis inhibitors increase the concentration of sodium and chloride in rat renal medulla. *Circ. Res.* 40: 135, 1977.
54. Garella, S., and Matarese, R. A. Renal effects of prostaglandins and clinical adverse effects of nonsteroidal antiinflammatory agents. *Medicine* 63: 165, 1984.
55. Gerber, J. G., Olson, R. D., and Nies, A. S. Control of canine renin release: Macula densa requires prostaglandin synthesis. *J. Physiol.* (Lond.) 319: 419, 1981.
56. Gill, J. R., Jr., Frolich, J. C., Bowden, R. E., et al. Bartter's syndrome: A disorder characterized by high urinary prostaglandins and a dependence of hyperreninemia on prostaglandin synthesis. *Am. J. Med.* 61: 43, 1976.
57. Goetzl, E. Mediators of immediate hypersensitivity derived from arachidonic acid. *N. Engl. J. Med.* 303: 822, 1980.
58. Goetzl, E. Selective feed-back inhibition of the 5 lipoxygenation of the arachidonic acid in human T-lymphocytes. *Biochem. Biophys. Res. Commun.* 101: 344, 1981.
59. Goetzl, E. Oxygenation products of arachidonic acids as mediators of hypersensitivity and inflammation. *Med. Clin. North Am.* 65: 809, 1981.
60. Goetzl, E., Woods, J., and Gorman, R. Stimulation of human eosinophil and neutrophil polymorphonuclear leukocyte chemotaxis and random migration by 12-L-hydroxy-5, 8, 10, 14-eicostetraenoic acid. *J. Clin. Invest.* 59: 179, 1977.
61. Gokal, R., and Matthews, D. R. Renal papillary necrosis after aspirin and alclofenac. *Br. Med. J.* 2: 1517, 1977.
62. Goldzer, R. C., Coodlley, E. L., Rosner, M. J., et al. Hyperkalemia associated with indomethacin. *Arch. Intern. Med.* 141: 802, 1980.
63. Greenstone, M., Hartley, B., and Gabriel, R. Acute nephrotic syndrome with reversible renal failure after phenylbutazone. *Br. Med. J.* 282: 950, 1981.

64. Gross, P. A., Schrier, R. W., and Anderson, R. J. Prostaglandins and water metabolism: A review with emphasis on in vivo studies. *Kidney Int.* 19: 839, 1981.
65. Halushka, P. V., Privatera, P. J., Hurwitz, G., et al. Bartter's syndrome: Urinary prostaglandin E-like material and kallikrein: indomethacin effects. *Ann. Intern. Med.* 87: 281, 1977.
66. Hart, D., Ward, M., and Lifschitz, M. D. Suprofen-related nephrotoxicity. A distinct clinical syndrome. *Ann. Intern. Med.* 106: 235, 1987.
67. Henrich, W. L. Nephrotoxicity of nonsteroidal antiinflammatory agents. *Am. J. Kid. Dis.* 2: 478, 1983.
68. Henrich, W. L. Prostaglandins in renin secretion. *Kidney Int.* 19: 822, 1981.
69. Henrich, W. L., Anderson, R. J., Berl, T., et al. Role of angiotensin II and prostaglandins in renal response to hypotensive hemorrhage. *Am. J. Physiol.* 235: F46, 1978.
70. Henrich, W. L., Anderson, R. J., Berns, A. S., et al. Role of renal nerves and prostaglandins in control of renal hemodynamics and plasma renin activity during hypotensive hemorrhage in the dog. *J. Clin. Invest.* 61: 744, 1978.
71. Henrich, W. L., Brater, D. C., and Campbell, W. B. Sulindac accentuates renal ischemia during hemorrhage. *Kidney Int.* 27: 295, 1985.
72. Henrich, W. L., and Campbell, W. B. Importance of intracellular calcium in tissue renin release. *Clin. Res.* 32: 242A, 1984.
73. Henrich, W. L., and Campbell, W. B. Relationship between prostaglandins and the β-adrenergic pathway to renin secretion. An in vitro study. *Am. J. Physiol.* 247: E343, 1984.
74. Henrich, W. L., and Campbell, W. B. The β-adrenergic pathway to renin release: Relations with the prostaglandin system. *Endocrinology* 113: 2247, 1983.
75. Henrich, W. L., Hamasaki, Y., Said, S. I., et al. Dissociation of systemic and renal effects in endotoxemia: Prostaglandin-inhibition uncovers an important role of renal nerves. *J. Clin. Invest.* 69: 691, 1982.
76. Henrich, W. L., McDonald, K. M., Schrier, R. W., et al. Mechanisms of renin secretion during hemorrhage in the dog. *J. Clin. Invest.* 64: 1, 1979.
77. Henrich, W. L., Pettinger, W. A., and Cronin, R. E. The influence of circulating catecholamine and prostaglandins on canine renal hemodynamics during hemorrhage. *Circ. Res.* 48: 424, 1979.
78. Herbaczynska-Cedro, K., and Vane, J. R. Contribution of intrarenal generation of prostaglandin to autoregulation of renal blood flow in the dog. *Circ. Res.* 33: 428, 1973.
79. Higashihara, E., Stokes, J. B., Kokko, J. P., et al. Cortical and papillary micropuncture examination of chloride transport in segments in the rat kidney during inhibition of prostaglandin production. *J. Clin. Invest.* 64: 1277, 1979.
80. Hofman, L. M., Krupnick, M. I., and Garcia, H. A. Interactions of spironolactone and hydrochlorathiazide with aspirin in the rat and dog. *J. Pharmacol. Exp. Ther.* 180: 1, 1972.
81. Husserl, F. E., Lange, R. K., and Kantrow, C. M., Jr. Renal papillary necrosis and pyelonephritis accompanying fenoprofen therapy. *J.A.M.A.* 242: 1896, 1979.
82. Ichikawa, I., and Brenner, B. M. Mechanism of inhibition of proximal tubule fluid reabsorption after exposure of the rat kidney to the physical effects of expansion of extracellular fluid volume. *J. Clin. Invest.* 64: 1466, 1979.
83. Ichikawa, I., and Brenner, B. M. Importance of efferent arteriolar vascular tone in regulation of proximal tubular fluid reabsorption and glomerulotubular balance in the rat. *J. Clin. Invest.* 65: 1192, 1980.
84. Iino, Y., and Imai, M. Effects of prostaglandins on Na transport in isolated collecting tubules. *Pflügers Arch.* 373: 125, 1978.
85. Itami, N., Akutsu, Y., Yasoshima, K., et al. Progressive renal failure despite discontinuation of mefenamic acid. *Nephron* 54: 281, 1990.
86. Itskovitz, H. D., Stemper, J., Pacholcyzk, D., et al. Renal prostaglandins: Determinants of intrarenal distribution of blood flow in the dog. *Clin. Sci. Mol. Med.* 45: 321s, 1973.
87. Jim, K., Dunn, M., Hassid, A., et al. Lipoxygenase activity in rat renal glomeruli. *Clin. Res.* 30: 571A, 1982.
88. Katz, S., Capaldo, R., Everts, E., et al. Tolmetin: Association with reversible renal failure and acute interstitial nephritis. *J.A.M.A.* 246: 243, 1981.
89. Keeton, T. K., and Campbell, W. B. The pharmacologic alteration of renin release. *Pharmacol. Rev.* 32: 81, 1980.
90. Kimberly, R. P., Bowden, R. E., Keiser, H. R., et al. Reduction of renal function by newer nonsteroidal anti-inflammatory drugs. *Am. J. Med.* 64: 804, 1978.
91. Kimberly, R. P., and Brandstetter, R. D. Exacerbation of phenylbutazone-related renal failure by indomethacin. *Arch. Intern. Med.* 138: 1711, 1978.
92. Kimberly, R. P., Grill, J. R., Bowden, R. E., et al. Elevated urinary prostaglandins and the effects of aspirin on renal function in lupus erythematosus. *Ann. Intern. Med.* 89: 336, 1981.
93. Kimberly, R. P., and Plotz, P. H. Aspirin-induced depression of renal function. *New Engl. J. Med.* 296: 418, 1977.
94. Kincaid-Smith, P., Saker, B. M., McKenzie, J. F. C., et al. Lesions in the blood supply of the papilla in experimental analgesic nephropathy. *Med. J. Aust.* 1: 203, 1968.
95. Kutyrina, J. M., Andosova, S. O., and Tareyeva, I. E. Indomethacin-induced hyporeninaemic hypoaldosteronism. *Lancet* 1: 785, 1979.
96. Laxer, R. M., Silverman, E., Balfe, D., et al. Indomethacin and ibuprofen-induced reversible acute renal failure in a patient with systemic lupus erythematosus. *Neth. J. Med.* 30: 181, 1987.
97. Levenson, D. J., Simmons, C. E., Jr., and Brenner, B. M. Arachidonic acid metabolism, prostaglandins and the kidney. *Am. J. Med.* 72: 354, 1979.
98. Levine, L., and Moskowitz, M. A. Alpha and beta adrenergic stimulation of arachidonic acid metabolism cells in culture. *Proc. Nat. Acad. Sci. U.S.A.* 76: 6632, 1979.
99. Lifschitz, M. D. Prostaglandins and renal blood flow: In vivo studies. *Kidney Int.* 19: 781, 1981.
100. Ling, B. N., Bourke, E., and Campbell, W. G. Naproxen-induced nephropathy in systemic lupus erythematosus. *Nephron* 54: 249, 1990.
101. Lipsett, M. B., and Goldman, R. Phenylbutazone toxicity: Report of a case of acute renal failure. *Ann. Intern. Med.* 41: 1075, 1954.
102. Lonigro, A. J., Itskovitz, H. D., Crowshaw, K., et al. Dependency of renal blood flow on prostaglandin synthesis in the dog. *Circ. Res.* 32: 712, 1973.
103. Lonigro, A. J., Terragno, N. A., Malik, K. U., et al. Differential inhibition by prostaglandins of the renal actions of pressor stimuli. *Prostaglandins* 3: 595, 1973.
104. Lorch, J., Lefavour, G., Davidson, H., et al. Renal effects of fenaprofen. *Ann. Intern. Med.* 93: 509, 1980.

105. Lourie, S. H., Denman, S. J., and Schroeder, E. T. Association of renal papillary necrosis and ankylosing spondylitis. *Arth. Rheum.* 20: 917, 1977.
106. Malik, K. U., and McGiff, J. C. Modulation by prostaglandins of adrenergic transmission in the isolated perfused rabbit and rat kidney. *Circ. Res.* 36: 599, 1975.
107. McCarthy, J. T., Torres, V. E., Romero, J. C., et al. Acute intrinsic renal failure induced by indomethacin. Role of prostaglandin synthetase inhibition. *Mayo Clin. Proc.* 57: 289, 1982.
108. McCord, J. M., and Fridovich, I. The biology and pathology of oxygen radicals. *Ann. Intern. Med.* 89: 122, 1978.
109. McDonald, F. D., Lazarus, G. S., and Campbell, W. L. Phenylbutazone anuria. *South Med. J.* 60: 1318, 1967.
110. McGiff, J. C., Crowshaw, K., Terragno, N. A., et al. Release of a prostaglandin-like substance into renal venous blood in response to angiotensin II. *Circ. Res.* 26/27 (Suppl. I) 1: 121, 1970.
111. McGiff, J. C., Crowshaw, K., Terragno, N. A., et al. Renal prostaglandins: Possible regulators of the renal actions of pressor hormones. *Nature* 227: 1255, 1970.
112. McGiff, J. C., Crowshaw, K., Terragno, N. A., et al. Differential effect of noradrenaline and renal nerve stimulation on vascular resistance in the dog kidney and the release of a prostaglandin E-like substance. *Clin. Sci.* 42: 223, 1972.
113. Miller, M. J. S., Bednar, M. M., and McGiff, J. C. Renal metabolism of sulindac: Functional implications. *J. Pharm. Exp. Ther.* 281: 449, 1984.
114. Mirouze, D., Zisper, R. D., and Reynolds, T. B. Effect of inhibitors of prostaglandin synthesis on induced cirrhosis. *Hepatology* 3: 50, 1983.
115. Morales, A., and Steyn, J. Papillary necrosis following phenylbutazone ingestion. *Arch. Surg.* 103: 420, 1971.
116. Morgenstern, S. J., Burns, F. J., Fraley, D. S., et al. Ibuprofen-associated lipoid nephrosis without interstitial nephritis. *Am. J. Kidney Dis.* 16: 50, 1989.
117. Morley, J. Role of prostaglandins secreted by macrophages in the inflammatory process. *Lymphokines* 4: 377, 1981.
118. Murray, M. D., and Brater, D. C. Adverse effects of nonsteroidal anti-inflammatory drugs on renal function. *Ann. Intern. Med.* 112: 559, 1990.
119. Murray, M. D., Brater, D. C., Tierney, W. M., et al. Ibuprofen-associated renal impairment in a large general internal medicine practice. *Am. J. Med. Sci.* 299: 222, 1990.
120. Muther, R. S., and Bennett, W. M. Effects of aspirin on glomerular filtration rate in normal humans. *Ann. Intern. Med.* 92: 386, 1980.
121. Muther, R. S., Potter, D. M., and Bennett, W. M. Aspirin-induced depression of glomerular filtration rate in normal humans: Role of sodium balance. *Ann. Intern. Med.* 94: 317, 1981.
122. Needleman, P., Marshall, G. R., and Johnson, E. M., Jr. Determinants and modification of adrenergic and vascular resistance in the kidney. *Am. J. Physiol.* 227: 665, 1974.
123. Nicholson, P. A., Klairm, A., and Smith, M. Pharmacokinetics of misoprostol in the elderly, in patients with renal failure and when co-administered with NSAID or antipyrine, propranolol or diazepam. *J. Rheumatol.* 20: 33, 1990.
124. Nies, A. S., Gal, J., Fadul, S., et al. Indomethacin-flurosemide interaction: The importance of renal blood flow. *J. Pharm. Exp. Ther.* 226: 27, 1983.
125. Oliver, J. A., Pinto, J., Sciacca, R. R., et al. Increased renal secretion of norepinephrine and prostaglandin E_2 during sodium depletion in the dog. *J. Clin. Invest.* 66: 748, 1980.
126. Patak, R. V., Moorkejeree, B. K., Bentzel, C. J., et al. Antagonism of the effects of furosemide by indomethacin in normal and hypertensive man. *Prostaglandins* 10: 649, 1975.
127. Pawaz-Estrup, F., and Ho, G., Jr. Reversible acute renal failure induced by indomethacin. *Arch. Intern. Med.* 141: 1670, 1981.
128. Payan, D., and Goetzl, E. The dependence of human T-lymphocyte migration on the 5-lipoxygenation of endogenous arachidonic acid. *J. Clin. Immunol.* 1: 266, 1981.
129. Pethenkamp, S. F., Davis, J. O., DeForrest, J. M., et al. Effects of indomethacin, renal denervation and propranolol on plasma renin activity in conscious dogs with chronic thoracic caval constriction. *Circ. Res.* 49: 492, 1981.
130. Pratt, J. H. Role of angiotensin II in potassium-mediated stimulation of aldosterone secretion in the dog. *J. Clin. Invest.* 70: 667, 1982.
131. Rice, D. *Fed. Proc.* 43: 100, 1984.
132. Robertson, C. E., Van Someren, V., Ford, M. J., et al. Mefenamic acid nephropathy. *Lancet* 2: 232, 1980.
133. Roman, R. J., and Kauker, M. L. Renal effect of prostaglandin synthetase inhibition in rats: Micropuncture studies. *Am. J. Physiol.* 235 (*Renal Fluid Electrolyte Physiol.* 4): F111, 1978.
134. Romero, J. C., Dunlap, C. L., and Strong, C. G. The effect of indomethacin and other anti-inflammatory drugs on the renin-angiotensin system. *J. Clin. Invest.* 58: 282, 1976.
135. Rossi, A. C., Bosco, L., and Faich, G. A. The importance of adverse reaction reporting by physicians. Suprofen and the flank pain syndrome. *J.A.M.A.* 259: 1203, 1988.
136. Satoh, S., and Zimmerman, B. G. Influence of the renin-angiotensin system on the effect of prostaglandin synthesis inhibitors in the renal vasculature. *Circ. Res.* (Suppl. I) 36: 89, 1975.
137. Schooley, R. T., Wagley, P. F., and Lietman, P. S. Edema associated with ibuprofen therapy. *J.A.M.A.* 237: 1716, 1977.
138. Schwartzman, M., and Dagati, V. Spontaneous relapse of naproxen-related nephrotic syndrome. *Am. J. Med.* 82: 329, 1987.
139. Shah, G. M., Muhalwas, K. K., and Winer, R. L. Renal papillary necrosis due to ibuprofen. *Arthr. Rheum.* 24: 1208, 1981.
140. Shelley, J. H. Pharmacological mechanisms of analgesic nephropathy. *Kidney Int.* 13: 15, 1978.
141. Shimizu, K., Kurosawa, T., Maeda, T., et al. Free water excretion and washout of renal medullary urea by prostaglandin E. *Jpn. Heart J.* 10: 437, 1969.
142. Siegl, M., McConnell, R., Porter, N., et al. Arachidonate metabolism via lipoxygenase and 12-L-hydroperoxy-5, 8, 10, 14-eicosatetraenoic acid peroxidase sensitive to anti-inflammatory drugs. *Proc. Nat. Acad. Sci. U.S.A.* 77: 308, 1980.
143. Simon, L. S., and Mills, J. A. Nonsteroidal anti-inflammatory drugs. *N. Engl. J. Med.* 302: 1179, 1980.
144. Snyder, S., and Teehan, B. P. Suprofen and renal failure. *Ann. Intern. Med.* 106: 776, 1987.
145. Sobel, A., Heslan, J. M., Branellec, A., et al. Vascular permeability factor produced by lymphocytes of patients with nephrotic syndrome. *Adv. Nephrol.* 10: 315, 1981.

146. Solez, K., Beschorner, W., Bender, W., et al. The "unique" lesion of fenoprofen nephropathy—an oversimplification? *Am. Soc. Nephrol.* 15: 105A, 1982.
147. Stillman, M. T., and Schlesinger, P. A. Nonsteroidal anti-inflammatory drug nephrotoxicity. Should we be concerned? *Arch. Intern. Med.* 150: 268, 1990.
148. Stokes, J. B. Integrated actions of renal medullary prostaglandins in the control of water excretion. *Am. J. Physiol.* 9: F471, 1981.
149. Stokes, J. B., and Kokko, J. P. Inhibition of sodium transport by prostaglandin E_2 across the isolated, perfused rabbit collecting tubule. *J. Clin. Invest.* 49: 1099, 1977.
150. Stone, K. J., and Hart, M. Inhibition of renal PGE_2 9-ketoreductase in the rabbit kidney. *Prostaglandins* 12: 197, 1976.
151. Strom, B. L., West, S. L., Sim, E., et al. The epidemiology of the acute flank pain syndrome from suprofen. *Clin. Pharmacol. Ther.* 46: 693, 1989.
152. Susic, H., and Malik, K. U. Prostacyclin and prostaglandin E_2 effects on adrenergic transmission in the kidney of the anesthetized dog. *J. Pharmacol. Exp. Ther.* 218: 588, 1981.
153. Swain, J. A., Heyndricks, G. R., Boettcher, D. H., et al. Prostaglandin control of renal circulation in the unanesthetized dog and baboon. *Am. J. Physiol.* 229: 826, 1975.
154. Tan, S. Y., Franco, R., Stockard, H., et al. Indomethacin-induced prostaglandin inhibition with hyperkalemia. A reversible cause of hyporeninemic hypoaldosteronism. *Ann. Intern. Med.* 90: 783, 1979.
155. Tan, S. Y., Shapiro, R., and Kish, M. A. Reversible acute renal failure induced by indomethacin. *J.A.M.A.* 241: 2732, 1979.
156. Terragno, N. A., Terragno, D. A., and McGiff, J. C. Contribution of prostaglandins to the renal circulation in conscious, anesthetized and laparotomized dogs. *Circ. Res.* 40: 590, 1977.
157. Tiggeler, R. G., Koene, R. A., and Wijdeveld, P. G. Inhibition of furosemide-induced natriuresis by indomethacin in patients with nephrotic syndrome. *Clin. Sci. Mol. Med.* 52: 149, 1977.
158. Torres, V. E. Present and future of the nonsteroidal antiinflammatory drugs in nephrology. *Mayo Clin. Proc.* 57: 389, 1982.
159. Tweeddale, M. G., and Ogilve, R. I. Antagonism of spironolactone-induced natriuresis by aspirin in man. *N. Engl. J. Med.* 289: 198, 1973.
160. Veroerckmoes, R., Van Damme, B., Clement, J., et al. Bartter's syndrome with hyperplasia of renomedullary cells: Successful treatment with indomethacin. *Kidney Int.* 9: 302, 1976.
161. Wagoner, R. D. Renal effects of the newer nonsteroidal anti-inflammatory agents. *Mayo Clin. Proc.* 56: 525, 1981.
162. Walshe, J. J., and Venuto, R. C. Acute oliguric renal failure induced by indomethacin: Possible mechanism. *Ann. Intern. Med.* 91: 47, 1979.
163. Weber, P. C., Larsson, C., and Scherer, B. Prostaglandin E_2 9-keto reductase as a mediator of salt-intake related to prostaglandin-renin interaction. *Nature* 266: 65, 1977.
164. Whelton, A., Stout, R. L., Spilman, P. S., et al. Renal effects of ibuprofen, piroxicam, and sulindac in patients with asymptomatic renal failure. *Ann. Intern. Med.* 112: 568, 1990.
165. Williamson, H. E., Bourland, U. A., and Marchand, G. R. Inhibition of furosemide-induced increase in renal blood flow by indomethacin. *Proc. Soc. Exp. Biol. Med.* 148: 164, 1975.
166. Wilson, D. R., Honrath, U., and Sonnenberg, H. Prostaglandin synthesis inhibition during volume expansion: Collecting duct function. *Kidney Int.* 22: 1, 1982.
167. Work, J., Baehler, T. R., Kotchen, A., et al. Effect of prostaglandin inhibition on sodium chloride reabsorption in the diluting segment of the conscious dog. *Kidney Int.* 17: 24, 1980.
168. Wortmann, D. W., Kelsch, R. C., Kuhns, L., et al. Renal papillary necrosis in juvenile rheumatoid arthritis. *J. Pediatr.* 97: 37, 1980.
169. Zambraski, E. J., Chermos, A. N., and Dunn, M. J. Comparison of the effects of sulindac with other cyclooxygenase inhibitors on prostaglandin excretion and renal function in normal and chronic bile duct ligated dogs and swine. *J. Pharm. Exp. Ther.* 228: 560, 1984.
170. Zambraski, E. J., and Dunn, M. J. Renal prostaglandin E_2 secretion and excretion in conscious dogs. *Am. J. Physiol.* 236: F552, 1979.
171. Zisper, R. D., Hoefs, J. C., Speckart, P. F., et al. Prostaglandins: Modulators of renal function and pressor resistance in chronic liver disease. *J. Endocrinol. Metab.* 48: 895, 1979.
172. Zusman, R. M., and Keiser, H. R. Prostaglandin biosynthesis by rabbit renomedullary interstitial cells in tissue culture: Stimulation by angiotensin II, bradykinin, and vasopressin. *J. Clin. Invest.* 60: 215, 1970.
173. Zusman, R. M., Vinci, J. M., Bowden, R. E., et al. Effect of indomethacin and adrenocorticotrophic hormone on renal function in man: An experimental model of inappropriate antidiuresis. *Kidney Int.* 15: 62, 1979.

Drug Abuse with Narcotics and Other Agents

David S. Baldwin
Gloria R. Gallo
Joel Neugarten

Abuse of narcotics, amphetamines, and other illicit substances may be associated with a variety of renal disorders, as listed in Table 45-1. In recent years, the spectrum of renal manifestations of drug abuse has undergone an alarming expansion. In the 1970s and early 1980s, glomerulosclerosis associated with intravenous heroin abuse emerged as a major cause of nephrotic syndrome and end-stage renal disease in urban areas with large addict populations and came to account for approximately 10 percent of patients aged 18 to 45 years undergoing dialysis in these cities [20, 21]. Also, in the early 1980s, a form of secondary amyloidosis was described as an important cause of renal failure in heroin abusers who utilized the subcutaneous route (i.e., "skin poppers") [31, 69, 84, 95]. Most recently, glomerulosclerosis in intravenous drug abusers infected with the human immunodeficiency virus (HIV) has been recognized as an entity distinct from the nephropathy observed in uninfected drug abusers prior to the advent of the HIV epidemic [23]. HIV-associated nephropathy has rapidly supplanted "heroin nephropathy" as the major renal disorder affecting intravenous drug abusers in New York City. Concurrently, the incidence of "heroin nephropathy" and of "skin poppers' amyloidosis" has declined dramatically. In striking contrast, nephropathy in HIV-negative intravenous cocaine users was recently reported as a frequent cause of end-stage renal disease in San Francisco [105].The basis for the geographic variability in the epidemiology of renal disease in drug abusers is unclear and may reflect the relatively high prevalence of HIV infection among drug abusers in New York City, where 50 to 60 percent of intravenous drug users are infected [1]. The presence of HIV infection in such a large proportion of the addict population immediately reduces the number at risk for heroin nephropathy, which by definition necessarily excludes HIV-infected patients. Accordingly, some instances of actual heroin abuse nephropathy could be erroneously classified as HIV-associated nephropathy. Moreover, the early occurrence of HIV infection and associated nephropathy in intravenous heroin abusers would preempt the development of heroin abuse nephropathy, which may require a more prolonged period of heavy drug abuse for its advent. This hypothesis is borne out by epidemiologic data in hospitalized AIDS patients showing that the prevalence of nephropathy (approximately 7–8%) (A. Valeri, personal communication, 1990) far exceeds that of heroin nephropathy (0.1%) [3, 146] as recorded in the era before acquired immune deficiency syndrome (AIDS). Thus, HIV infection in this subgroup of intravenous drug users, many of whom are black with a predisposition to focal glomerulosclerosis (FGS), would selectively reduce those at risk for heroin nephropathy. Finally, one might argue that HIV-associated nephropathy is, in fact, not an entity distinct from FGS as originally described in drug users prior to the advent of AIDS. However, epidemiologic data, particularly the occurrence of FGS in *non*–drug abusers with HIV infection, and distinctive clinical and morphologic features that differentiate the two forms of FGS belie this suggestion (see Chap. 86).

Focal Glomerulosclerosis in Intravenous Heroin Abusers

The occurrence of proteinuria associated with opium addiction was appreciated by nineteenth century clinicians [84]. Albuminuria was observed in 7 to 17 percent of addicts by early investigators [73, 131]. More recent studies have reexamined the nature of renal disease in narcotics abusers [3, 4, 38, 118, 135, 136]. In several cross-sectional studies, investigators attempted to determine the prevalence of glomerular abnormalities in postmortem specimens from heroin addicts and of proteinuria and renal sediment abnormalities in populations of addicts attending drug rehabilitation centers [3, 4, 38, 118, 135, 136]. Markedly disparate data were reported. However, these studies have little relevance to renal disease in heroin addicts as we now understand it.

Heroin-associated FGS is characterized typically by proteinuria progressing to the nephrotic syndrome. The finding of nonspecific urinary abnormalities or "nephritis" in surveys of the addict population cannot be accepted as representative of the incidence of FGS. Moreover, the rarity with which cases would be detected in random prospective studies is readily apparent when one considers that data available from early in the 1980s placed the prevalence of FGS at well below 1 percent [36, 146], with an annual incidence of less than 1 new case per 1000 addicts [3, 146].

In the early 1970s several investigators began to recognize a clinical pathologic entity in heroin addicts characterized by the nephrotic syndrome and glomerulosclerosis. McGinn et al. [82] described seven drug abusers with the nephrotic syndrome and focal glomerular lesions in whom serial renal biopsy specimens showed progressive glomerulosclerosis associated with declining renal function. Similarly, Avram et al. [4] reported on several addicts with end-stage renal disease who presented with the nephrotic syndrome and hyalinized glomeruli. Renal biopsy specimens from seven nephrotic heroin abusers studied by Kilcoyne et al. [60] revealed "focal membranoproliferative glomerulonephritis" with subendothelial electron-dense deposits and granular deposits of predominantly IgM and complement. Similar histologic abnormalities were reported by Thompson et al. [135] in heroin addicts with proteinuria and microscopic hematuria. Rao, Nicastri, and Friedman [106] identified focal and segmental glomerulosclerosis that progressed to global sclerosis as the lesion characteristic of parenteral heroin abuse. These authors described 14 black heroin abusers; the nephrotic syndrome was present in all but one. Renal biopsy specimens showed focal and segmental or global glomerulosclerosis in 11 of 13, associated with focal and segmental glomerular deposition of IgM and complement. This characteristic glomerular sclerosis in intravenous heroin abusers has been confirmed by numerous other investigators [31, 43, 44, 69, 80]. A similar syndrome of glomerulosclerosis associated with the nephrotic syndrome and progressive renal insufficiency has been observed in parenteral abusers of drugs other than heroin, including cocaine and pentazocine with tripelennamine [20, 81, 82].

Table 45-1. Renal disease associated with drug abuse

1. Focal glomerulosclerosis in intravenous heroin abusers
2. Amyloidosis in subcutaneous heroin abusers ("skin poppers' amyloidosis")
3. Endocarditis-associated glomerulonephritis in intravenous drug abusers
4. Acute renal failure due to nontraumatic rhabdomyolysis
5. Systemic necrotizing vasculitis in amphetamine abusers
6. Nephropathy in glue and solvent "sniffers"
7. Hepatitis B–related glomerulonephritis in intravenous drug abusers
8. Focal glomerulosclerosis in intravenous drug abusers with acquired immune deficiency syndrome (AIDS)

PATHOLOGY

Glomerulosclerosis in heroin abusers appears to begin as a focal process in which some glomeruli are affected while others appear normal. At the time of renal biopsy, however, many patients show advanced disease with more than one-half of glomeruli already in stages of sclerosis, so that the process appears diffuse. Within a glomerulus the sclerosis may be segmental, involving only a portion of the tuft (Fig. 45-1), or global, with the whole tuft affected (Fig. 45-2). In some specimens there may be individual glomeruli with early global collapse of tufts as well as segmental obliteration, suggesting a transition between the two types of tuft involvement (Fig. 45-2E).

Stains that delineate the basement membranes, such as periodic acid silver-methenamine or periodic acid–Schiff, show that the pattern of glomerular sclerosis, whether segmental or global, is characterized by col-

Fig. 45-1. Light microscopy of biopsies from nephrotic addicts showing detail of segmental sclerosis (arrows). Most of the glomerular tufts exhibit normal cellularity and have thin capillary walls with smooth basement membrane contours, widely patent capillary lumens, and delicate mesangial regions. A. A segmental sclerosing lesion exhibits a mild increase in matrix of two loops, one of which is adherent to Bowman's capsule. B. One tuft exhibits obliteration of lumens due to collapse and wrinkling of capillary walls associated with proliferation of visceral epithelial cells, which fill adjacent Bowman's space. C. The segmental lesion that is adherent to thickened Bowman's capsule contains amorphous eosinophilic material (hyaline) in capillary lumens. D. There is segmental obliteration of capillary loops due to collapse and retraction of capillary basement membranes that are adherent to Bowman's capsule. Periodic acid-silver methenamine counterstained with H&E. (× 400.)

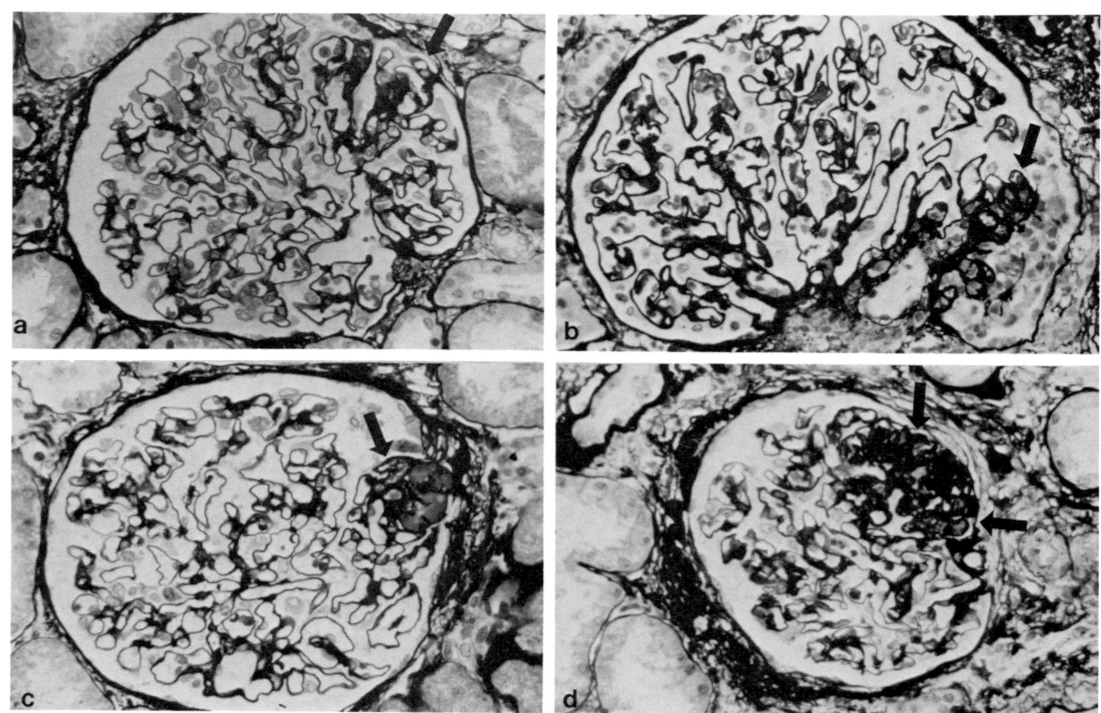

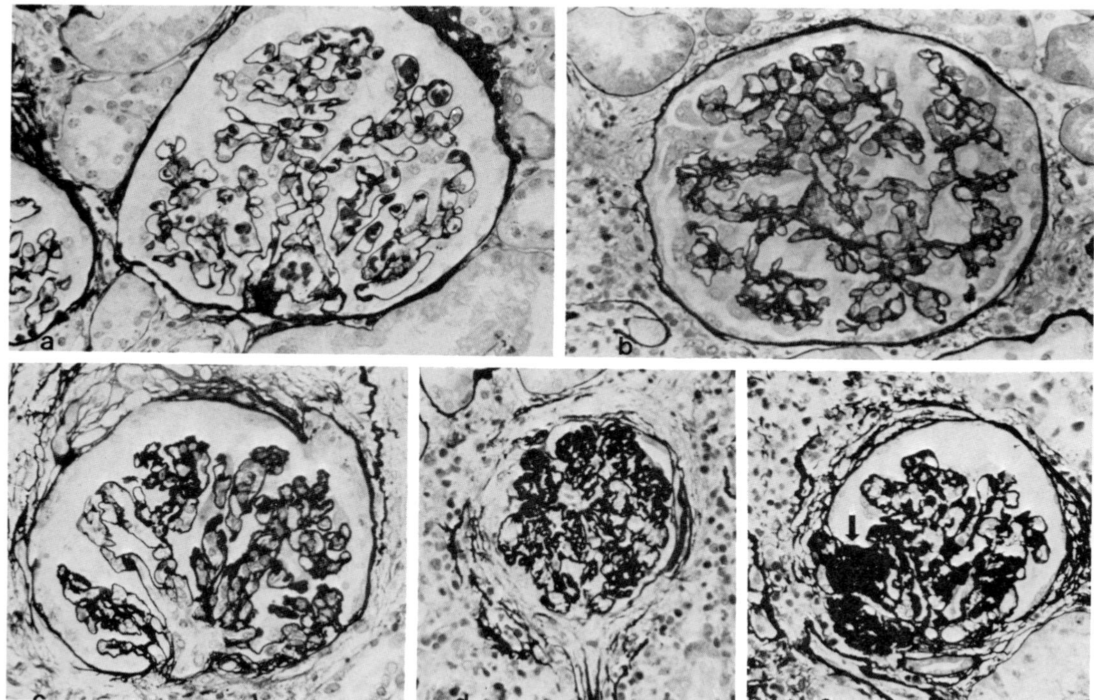

Fig. 45-2. Light microscopy of biopsies from nephrotic addicts showing varying degrees of global sclerosis. A. One of the normal glomeruli in a biopsy with focal glomerular sclerosis exhibits widely patent capillary lumens and thin, delicate smooth capillary walls; the dense silver-stained material in the lower part of the glomerulus is the normal vascular pole, and not segmental sclerosis. B. All capillary tufts exhibit mild thickening and wrinkling of basement membranes, causing narrowing of lumens, and prominent global visceral epithelial cell swelling and proliferation. C, D. Two glomeruli show more advanced stages of global sclerosis as compared to (B), with more exaggerated collapse of tufts, wrinkling of basement membranes, partial to total obliteration of lumens, and, in (D), beginning resorption of Bowman's capsule. E. Global sclerosis with segmental accentuation (arrow). It is uncertain whether the sclerosis began as a segmental or global lesion. Periodic acid silver methenamine, counterstained with H&E. (× 400.) Figs. (C) and (D) from Matalon et al. [80], with permission of the publisher.

lapse, wrinkling, and thickening of the glomerular basement membrane (GBM) such that lumens are narrowed or totally obliterated. Mesangial widening due to increased matrix is seen in some but is inconstant [20, 33]. In the end-stage of sclerosis, portions or all of the glomerular tuft are solidified and acellular but still have detectable shrunken basement membranes that identify the glomerular structure even in stages of partial resorption (Fig. 45-2D). These end-stage structures are often referred to as "obsolescent" glomeruli.

Glomeruli that are undergoing sclerosis may appear hypercellular, especially in hematoxylin and eosin stains. This appearance in most instances is due to a relative increase in glomerular cells because of collapse of tufts and crowding of resident cells. Also contributing to the hypercellular appearance is the prominent swelling and proliferation of visceral epithelial cells, especially in early stages of sclerosis (Fig. 45-2B). Segmental sclerosis may also appear hypercellular due to similar swelling and/or proliferation of visceral epithelial cells and the presence of foam cells in capillary lumens (Fig. 45-1B). Such sclerosing lesions may be difficult to distinguish from the segmental lesions in focal proliferative glomerulonephritis. Usually helpful in this regard are special stains that outline the basement membranes. In FGS the GBM is collapsed, thickened, and wrinkled, with little or no production of new matrix, while in proliferative lesions a fine fibrillar network of increased basement membrane–like material is seen between proliferating cells, or necrosis and interruption of basement membranes are evident. An additional feature that may help to distinguish these two types of segmental lesions is "hyalinosis," which may be found in sclerosing but not proliferative lesions [52]. Such "hyaline" lesions consist of homogeneous eosinophilic material in varying amounts in the lumina of sclerosing capillary tufts, either segmental or global (Fig. 45-1C). Although hyalinosis is common in heroin-associated FGS as well as in idiopathic FGS, it is not unique to these disorders. Similar "hyaline" material may be seen, for example, in diabetic nodular glomerular sclerosis and in other diseases with secondary glomerulosclerosis.

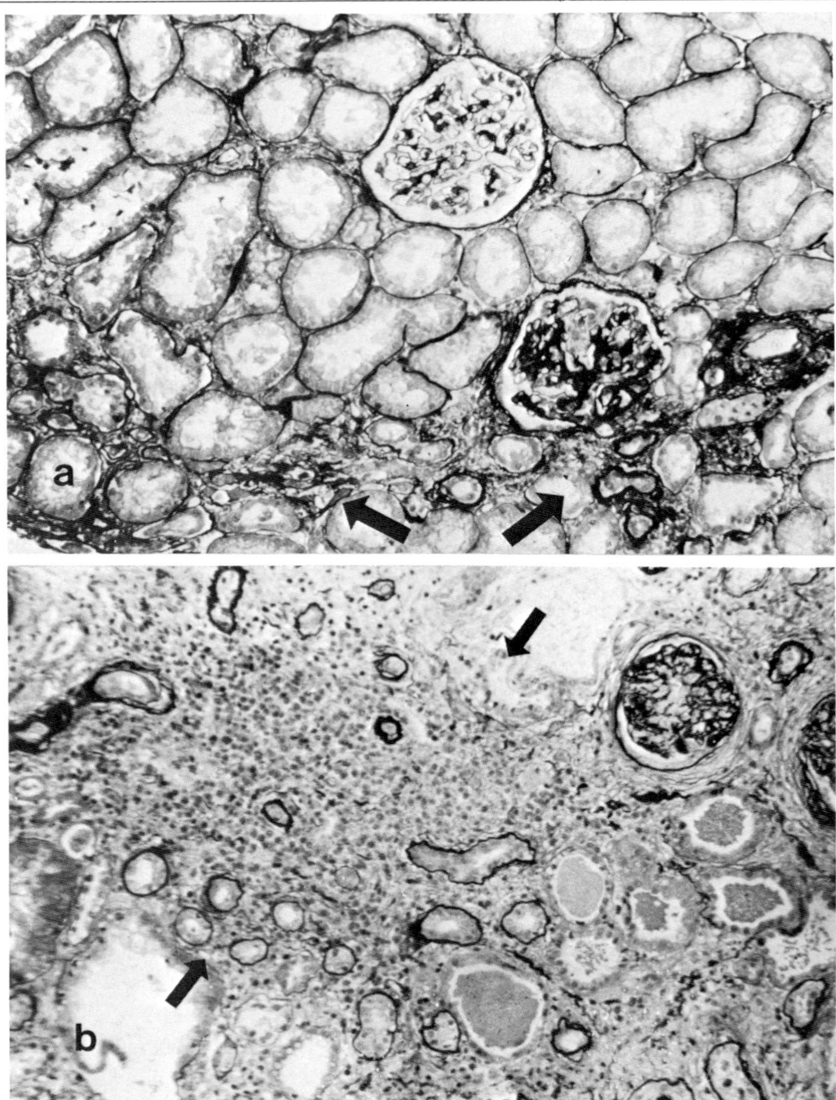

Fig. 45-3. Light microscopy of biopsies from two nephrotic addicts showing focal glomerular sclerosis. A. One normal glomerulus (top) and one sclerosing glomerulus (bottom). The tubulointerstitial abnormalities (arrows) are mild as compared to those in (B), where there is more severe tubular atrophy and dense cellular interstitial infiltration (arrows) as well as sclerotic glomeruli. Periodic acid silver methenamine counterstained with H&E. (× 175.)

Tubular atrophy and interstitial fibrosis, generally accompanied by moderate to severe cellular infiltration, are commonly found [20, 43, 44, 69, 80] (Fig. 45-3). Whether the tubulointerstitial changes represent a primary or secondary process is presently unknown. Several studies have noted that the severity of degenerative tubulointerstitial lesions parallels that of glomerular lesions [20, 44, 80]. Thus interstitial, vascular, and glomerular changes coexist and tend to parallel each other in severity, but their precise interrelationships remain unclear.

Immunofluorescence findings are variable but appear to be of two major types, either granular or linear (Table 45-2). In one study, granular deposits of IgM and complement were most commonly found, predominantly in focal segmental lesions, while other immunoglobulins were infrequent [106]. In our own patients and in those reported by Cunningham et al. [20], linear staining for IgG along the GBM was frequent (Fig. 45-4). The significance of the linear staining pattern is uncertain, but evidence is lacking that it represents binding of anti-GBM antibody [80]. More likely this represents nonspecific trapping of IgG as in other diseases such as diabetic nephropathy. We have also seen focal granular deposits of C3, IgM, and occasionally IgG, usually in sclerotic lesions (Table 45-2).

Table 45-2. Glomerular immunopathology in heroin-associated focal glomerulosclerosis

	Number of specimens positive/number examined		
Reactants and staining patterns observed	NYU	Cunningham et al. [20]	Rao et al. [106]
IgG			
Diffuse linear	28/37	10/16	
Linear and granular	2/37	2/16	
Granular focal	2/37	1/16	1/1
Negative or trace	5/37	3/16	
IgM			
Focal granular	8/32	6/16	8/10
Linear	0/32	1/16	
Negative or trace	24/32	9/16	2/10
IgA			
Focal granular	1/33	1/16	
Linear	0/33	3/16	
Negative or trace	32/33	12/16	
C3			
Focal granular	16/36	9/16	9/12
Negative or trace	20/36	7/16	3/12

Electron microscopic findings include GBM thickening, epithelial podocyte loss, varying degrees of severity of epithelial foot process detachment and loss, degeneration of epithelial cells, and new basement membrane formation [20, 42–44, 80]. In the majority of cases, electron-dense deposits are not seen in peripheral basement membranes; rather, electron-dense material, when present, is usually found along the internal aspects of the capillary wall or in the lumen of collapsed tufts of the sclerosing lesions. The appearance and location of the electron-dense material often corresponded to the hyalinosis lesions, suggesting that these accumulations represent nonspecific trappings of serum proteins in sclerosing lesions rather than deposits of immune complexes.

The sclerosis that typifies the nephrotic heroin abuser closely resembles FGS as it occurs in nonaddicts. In our own experience with 40 heroin addicts and 20 nonaddicts with idiopathic FGS in the pre-AIDS era, biopsy specimens from both groups showed global and segmental sclerosis. The proportions of glomeruli involved by the two types of sclerosis did not differ, and there were no overall differences in the severity of tubulointerstitial and vascular abnormalities. There is disagreement over whether interstitial inflammatory cell infiltration is more prominent in heroin-associated FGS than in the idiopathic form [6, 20, 23, 43, 69, 80]. In our own patients we found both mild and severe degrees of interstitial infiltration in both groups, leading us to conclude that no clear-cut qualitative or quantitative morphologic differences exist between them. It should be noted that the semiquantitative methods used to assess the severity of tubulointerstitial abnormalities may account for variations in observations among different observers.

Progression from focal to diffuse glomerulosclerosis in the absence of proliferation has been amply documented in several studies of heroin-associated FGS, supporting the view that the sclerosis is a primary process rather than a "burned-out" phase of proliferative glomerulonephritis.

The morphologic evolution and natural history of the sclerosing lesions are not clearly defined. In our experience, segmental and global sclerosis are usually found together; 62 percent of the biopsy specimens we have examined had both global and segmental sclerosis, while 38 percent had global sclerosis alone. The frequent coexistence of segmental and global sclerosis suggests a common pathogenesis for both types, but precisely how the lesions evolve is uncertain. Global sclerosis may result from segmental sclerosis by a process that damages portions of the tufts at different times and rates, as suggested by the finding of transition forms in which portions of the tufts are totally obliterated and the remaining ones are in earlier stages of collapse (Fig. 45-2E). Alternatively, damage may be global from onset, leading to sclerosis of all tufts at the same rate and time. The frequent finding in our own cases of glomeruli that exhibit early stages of global sclerosis characterized by contraction and wrinkling of capillary walls with narrowing of capillary lumens favors this hypothesis (Fig. 45-2B and C). Also, the finding of global sclerosis alone in 38 percent of our patients in the absence of segmental lesions lends further support to this view. However, in the Grishman series [44], in which some specimens showed exclusively global sclerosis, segmental lesions were also seen when serial biopsies from the same individual were available.

The etiologic and pathogenetic mechanisms causing glomerular damage and leading to sclerosis remain uncertain. Primary visceral epithelial cell damage, manifested by swelling and vacuolization, as a basis for glomerular sclerosis has been emphasized [42, 43]. In support of this concept, our biopsies have also shown pronounced epithelial cell swelling in both global and segmental distributions (Figs. 45-1B, 45-2B). An immune complex etiology seems unlikely in view of the immunopathologic and ultrastructural evidence reviewed above.

Deposition of talc granules has been observed in arterioles and glomeruli of intravenous drug abusers who inject drugs compounded for oral use [46, 130, 147]. In addition, granulomatous interstitial nephritis in association with interstitial talc deposits has been reported [130].

CLINICAL FEATURES

Detailed descriptions of the course of nephropathy in 90 parenteral drug abusers with biopsy-proven focal glomerulosclerosis are available in the literature [20, 25, 31, 43, 44, 76, 80, 99, 106, 136]; in addition, we have studied 40 patients at our institution. Incomplete information is available in an additional 168 other cited cases [4, 21, 38, 69, 107]. The present discussion gives a composite picture based on the data available from a total of 298 cases (Table 45-3). Only patients with clearly identified focal glomerulosclerosis are included. Seventy-six heroin abusers who have been described with either "focal membranoproliferative glomerulonephritis," focal mesangial proliferation or expansion, focal proliferative glomerulonephritis, membranoproliferative glomerulonephritis, diffuse proliferative glomerulonephritis, nephrotic syndrome and normal glomeruli, or membranous nephropathy are excluded from analysis. The relationship between these various glomerular lesions and heroin abuse is not established.

Where specified, 92 percent of patients were male, and 95 percent were black. Mean age was 29 years. Heroin, often in conjunction with cocaine, was used in all but a few cases in which parenteral cocaine or pentazocine with tripelennamine were the sole drugs abused [20, 81, 82]. The mean duration of drug abuse prior to presentation with renal disease was 6 years, ranging widely from 6 months to 24 years but generally exceeding 1 to 2 years.

Two-thirds of patients presented with edema due to the nephrotic syndrome, one-quarter with an abnormal urinalysis and most of the remainder with uremia. It cannot be stated whether a period of asymptomatic proteinuria existed prior to development of the nephrotic syndrome in the two-thirds who were nephrotic at presentation. Microscopic hematuria is described in one-third and pyuria in half of the cases, but nearly one-fourth had no documented sediment abnormalities. Renal function on presentation varied widely but was reduced in three-fourths of cases. On presentation, the mean BUN was 35 mg per deciliter, and the mean serum creatinine was 3.6 mg per deciliter. Initial serum creatinine was less than 1.3 mg per deciliter in 24 percent of 105 patients, and ranged from 1.2 to 2.0 mg per deciliter in 30 percent, from 2 to 4 mg per deciliter in 22 percent, and 4 to 9 mg per deciliter in 14 percent. Ten percent presented with uremia.

Urinary protein excretion averaged 9.3 gm per 24 hours. Protein excretion was less than 1 gm per 24 hours in only 3 percent of 119 patients and ranged from 1 to 2 gm in another 3 percent, from 2 to 4 gm in 14 percent, and from 4 to 10 gm in 37 percent. Proteinuria exceeded 10 gm in 43 percent. Mean serum albumin was 2.6 gm per deciliter and mean serum cholesterol was 321 mg per deciliter. Serum complement levels were normal and erythrocytosis was a rare finding [80].

In our own patients, hypertension was present in 64 percent on initial presentation. Serum creatinine averaged 4.7 mg per deciliter in hypertensives and 1.4 mg per deciliter in those who were normotensive. Hypertension developed in the remaining patients after serum creatinine had reached an average level of 5.0 mg per deciliter. In the series reported by Cunningham et al. [20] hypertension was found at presentation in 61 percent, developed in all those progressing to uremia.

Table 45-3. Focal glomerulosclerosis in intravenous heroin abusers

Clinical features	
Black	95%
Male sex	92%
Age	29 yr
Duration of drug abuse	6 yr
Hypertension on presentation	64%
Serum creatinine on presentation	3.6 mg/dl
Nephrotic syndrome	80%
Time to uremia	
Initial creatinine clearance >50 ml/min	43 mo
Initial creatinine clearance 20–50 ml/min	23 mo
Initial creatinine clearance <20 ml/min	7 mo

OUTCOME

Follow-up observations demonstrate that heroin-associated FGS typically progresses inexorably to uremia within approximately 4 years. Of 60 patients presenting with a serum creatinine below 2.2 mg per deciliter or creatinine clearance exceeding 50 ml per minute, 77 percent progressed to end-stage renal disease over a mean period of 43 months (range, 6 to 148 months). This group included 4 patients in whom progression occurred despite discontinuation of drug use. Of the remaining 14 patients, serum creatinine rose progressively in all but 5 during a follow-up period that averaged 33 months. Three of those who failed to show progressive functional deterioration had been drug-free for approximately 2 years; data are not available in the remaining 2 patients. Twenty-six of 28 patients who presented with a serum creatinine of 2.2 to 5 mg per deciliter or a creatinine clearance ranging from 20 to 50 ml per minute progressed to end-stage renal disease over a mean of 23 months (range, 2 to 93 months), including 7 patients who had discontinued drug use for periods of 1 to 10 years. The remaining 2 patients showed a progressive rise in serum creatinine over 12 months. Fourteen patients who presented with a creatinine clearance below 20 ml per minute progressed to uremia over a mean period of 7 months.

The effect of abstinence from drug use on the course of established nephropathy is not known. As described above, 11 patients with FGS have been reported who progressed to end-stage renal disease despite discontinuation of drugs. It appears, however, that patients who abstain have followed a somewhat more protracted course to renal failure than those who have continued to use heroin. Moreover, several drug-free former addicts with FGS have been described who underwent sustained remission in proteinuria and/or stabilization or improvement in renal function following abstinence [69, 76, 107]. These isolated observations do not establish an effect of abstinence from further drug use on nephropathy; however, a salutary effect on the course is suggested.

TREATMENT

Corticosteroid and immunosuppressive therapy have generally proved to be ineffective. Despite reputed responses to such therapy, there is no convincing evidence that treatment induces remission of proteinuria or prevents progression to end-stage renal failure. Eight of the 40 patients under our observation received single or multiple courses of corticosteroids, combined in some with immunosuppressive agents. In no patient was there remission of proteinuria. Four of the 5 patients in whom long-term follow-up was available progressed to uremia within 1 year. Davis et al. [25], McGinn et al. [82], and Rao and associates [36, 106] also administered corticosteroids and immunosuppressives to addicts with focal glomerulosclerosis without affecting proteinuria or renal function. Grishman et al. [43] described two patients who experienced a reduction in proteinuria with prednisone and a third patient who experienced a transient remission of the nephrotic syndrome; however, all progressed to renal failure over 2 to 5 years. A fourth patient had no response to therapy.

COMPARISON WITH OTHER FORMS OF FOCAL GLOMERULOSCLEROSIS

Several investigators have suggested that focal glomerulosclerosis as it occurs in heroin abusers is associated with a more aggressive clinical course and more prominent interstitial inflammatory reactions than those encountered in the idiopathic form [43, 69]. However, in our experience with adult patients, the clinical course and morphologic features in these two groups are indistinguishable. In a comparison of renal biopsy specimens from three groups of 13 patients each with either idiopathic FGS, heroin-associated FGS, or HIV-associated FGS, D'Agati et al. [23] found them to be qualitatively similar but noted that the HIV group had more globally "collapsed" glomeruli, less hyalinosis, more severe visceral epithelial cell swelling, more prevalent and severe tubular microcytic dilatation, and more numerous tubuloreticular inclusions. In addition to the above, we have observed more thickening and hyalinosis of small renal vessels (lobular arteries and arterioles) in idiopathic FGS and heroin-associated FGS than in HIV-associated FGS (unpublished observations, 1990).

The clinical course of FGS associated with HIV infection, which is usually characterized by a precipitous loss of renal function over a period of months, contrasts sharply with the less rapid decline generally observed in patients with heroin nephropathy [70]. In studies performed at our institution, we concluded that these two forms of FGS do not differ morphologically on presentation [70]. The appearance of glomerular sclerosis in HIV-infected patients (i.e., varying degrees of obliteration by collapsed and contracted capillary tufts) is similar to the sclerosis we observed in heroin-associated FGS. However, the majority of the patients with HIV nephropathy demonstrated advanced renal failure at the time of renal biopsy, although they lacked histologic evidence of widespread and complete obliteration of glomeruli by sclerosis. In this respect, they differed from the heroin abusers with similar histologic characteristics whose renal function was more in keeping with early stages of obliteration by glomerular sclerosis. An occlusive vascular basis for the rapid progression is ruled out by the absence of significant abnormalities of the arterioles and interlobular arteries; in fact, there is less vascular sclerosis in HIV nephropathy than in heroin nephropathy. Moreover, the fulminant course to renal failure cannot be explained by the severity of tubulointerstitial injury. Moderate to severe interstitial inflammation with a component of epithelial cell necrosis, mild to moderate tubular atrophy, and pronounced visceral epithelial cell swelling and proliferation appeared to be no more severe in the present HIV population than in those with heroin-associated nephropathy. Also contrasting with heroin nephropathy, patients with HIV-associated FGS remained normotensive as they progressed to uremia. In addition, peripheral edema was not observed despite the presence of nephrotic-range proteinuria and hypoalbuminemia, and hypercholesterolemia was generally absent.

EPIDEMIOLOGY

The epidemiology of heroin nephropathy has changed radically in the last 5 years. As discussed above, HIV-associated FGS has reduced the incidence of heroin nephropathy, and has preempted its position as the major cause of end-stage renal disease in the black addict population of urban areas. Nevertheless, epidemiologic studies performed during the 1970s and 1980s are not only of historic interest but also add insight into the pathogenesis of heroin nephropathy. Such epidemiologic studies have not been repeated in the AIDS era.

Cunningham et al. [20] reported on the epidemiology of glomerulosclerosis in the Buffalo metropolitan area from 1967 to 1978, which antedated the AIDS era. The annual incidence of sclerosing glomerular disease in patients aged 18 to 45 years was 41 times greater in addicts than in nonaddicts and 29 times greater in black addicts than in nonaddicted black males. The prevalence and annual incidence rate of end-stage renal disease in black male addicts were at least 10 times greater than those of any other race or sex subcategory [146]. Addicted individuals developed end-stage renal disease 18 times more frequently than nonaddicts. Although representing only 1 percent of the general population, heroin abusers comprised 10 percent of the dialysis population. All patients were black [146]. Ninety percent of drug abusers with end-stage renal disease in their program underwent renal biopsy and all showed FGS. In related studies, the same authors analyzed data obtained by questionnaire from 14 other metropolitan areas [21]. They identified 98 patients with heroin-associated nephropathy, two-thirds with end-stage renal disease. Ninety-four percent were black—79 percent were black males and 15 percent, black females. The prevalence of heroin-related nephropathy in patients 18 to 45 years old with end-stage renal disease was 11 percent. Heroin-related nephropathy was the underlying disease in one-third of black males with end-stage renal failure. Similarly, 95 percent of the 98 patients with heroin-associated FGS followed at Kings County Hospital were black [35].

These data establish the existence of a form of FGS that occurs in intravenous heroin abusers and shows a predisposition to affect young black males. FGS in nonaddicts is likewise more prevalent in blacks than in whites, but this race disparity is more marked in parenteral drug abusers [126]. Cunningham and associates [20, 146] have suggested that parenteral drug abuse may unmask a genetic predisposition in blacks to develop glomerular sclerosis. The emergence of this latent tendency may result from exposure to heroin, adulterants in "street" drugs, bacterial or viral contaminants, or other environmental factors related to heroin abuse. In this regard, Haskell et al. [50] have demonstrated an increased frequency of HLA-BW53 among black intravenous drug abusers with heroin-associated nephropathy. These data suggest a genetic predisposition to the development of FGS in this population [40, 50].

PATHOGENESIS

The presumption had prevailed that FGS in heroin abusers is immunologically mediated [36, 106]. The finding of IgM and C3 in the segmental lesions suggested an immunologic mechanism of damage due to deposition of immune complexes. However, such deposits may represent nonspecific trapping of serum protein in sclerosing lesions analogous to the hyaline lesions found in diabetic glomerulosclerosis. The frequent finding of IgG in a linear global distribution appears to represent nonspecific binding [20, 80]. Also cited in support of an immunopathogenesis is the demonstration of electron-dense deposits in glomeruli by some investigators [36, 106]. However, ultrastructural studies by other investigators, including ourselves, have failed to demonstrate immune complexes.

The multiple antigenic challenges to which parenteral drug abusers are exposed on a daily basis give rise to a wide variety of immunologic disturbances. These immunologic phenomena, though never shown to have any direct pathogenetic role in the development of renal disease, have been cited by numerous authors as indicative of a derangement in immune responsiveness that might favor the development of immune complex nephropathy. Relevant to the issue of pathogenesis is the occurrence of nephropathy in rare parenteral drug abusers who have solely abused drugs other than heroin [20, 81, 82]. The occurrence of idiosyncratic reactions to parenteral administration of heroin has also been cited as evidence that an immunologic response may occur in some addicts [22]. The putative antigen involved in the formation of immune complexes may be self-injected bacterial or viral contaminants, adulterants used to dilute heroin, or the heroin itself [20]. Heroin and morphine, however, lack the chemical configuration to act as antigens but may serve as haptens [22, 117, 140].

In the rabbit, prolonged parenteral administration of morphine has been associated with increased in vitro serum binding of morphine [11, 54, 110]. Administration of morphine to rats by Marchand et al. [77] did not result in glomerular disease but instead caused tubulointerstitial lesions in the cortex, medulla, and papilla consisting of basement membrane thickening, loss of microvilli, and cytoplasmic dense inclusions in proximal, distal, and collecting duct tubules. However, other investigators have demonstrated increased glomerular podocyte microprojections in morphine-treated rats [59]. Clearly, administration of morphine sulfate to rats is not analogous to the nonsterile self-injection of heroin and its adulterants by addicts.

In our studies, electron-dense deposits may be seen in areas of sclerosis but not in uninvolved peripheral capillary walls. Their appearance and location in the lumens of sclerosing tufts suggest that these deposits represent nonspecific trapping of immunoglobulins in segmental lesions rather than immune complexes. Immunofluorescence findings may also be explained by nonspecific trapping of serum proteins rather than by immune-complex deposition. Consequently, no convincing evidence exists to support an immunologic mechanism for FGS in heroin addicts.

Amyloidosis in Subcutaneous Heroin Abusers ("Skin Poppers' Amyloidosis")

In the late 1970s and early 1980s we and others observed the emergence of systemic amyloidosis as a major cause of nephropathy in heroin abusers in the New York metropolitan area [31, 69, 84, 95]. The association was first reported in isolated and small numbers of addicts with proteinuria between 1975 and 1979 [12, 28, 58, 83, 96, 121, 122]. Approximately one-third of heroin abusers who underwent renal biopsy for proteinuria at New York University Medical Center in the late 1970s and early 1980s were found to have amyloidosis [95]. A similar high incidence of amyloid in 40 percent of heroin abusers with proteinuria was observed at Columbia University-affiliated hospitals in New York City between the years 1972 and 1983 [69]. At Beth Israel Hospital in New York City, amyloidosis was found in one-third of renal biopsies from heroin abusers with proteinuria obtained between 1977 and 1980; this percentage rose to 62 percent in the years 1981 to 1983 [31]. However, in the AIDS era, amyloidosis has become an infrequent cause of nephrotic syndrome and renal failure in drug abusers.

PATHOGENESIS

A prospective survey performed in 1983 by Gallo and associates [84] of unselected addicts, predominantly black males who died of accidents or trauma and were examined at necropsy, demonstrated that addicts with suppurative skin infections were at high risk for the development of amyloidosis. Among 150 addicts, 7 (5%) had unsuspected renal amyloidosis; 6 of the 7 had extensive skin infections due to subcutaneous injections. Of 23 addicts with skin infections, 26 percent had renal amyloidosis, indicating a strong association between suppurative skin infections and renal amyloidosis. The skin infections, usually in the extremities, were generally extensive, involving 10 to 20 percent of the body surface area. The amyloid was AA protein–related in all cases as determined by immunofluorescence microscopy as well as by biochemical analysis of amyloid isolated from the kidney in 2 of the subjects. Thus, to the extent examined, amyloid in addicts does not differ from the AA amyloid that characterizes amyloidosis secondary to chronic infections and inflammatory diseases in nonaddicts.

The near universal association of chronic suppurative cutaneous lesions in subcutaneous drug abusers with amyloidosis strongly supports skin infection as important in the pathogenesis [31, 69, 84, 95, 96, 103]. Of note, systemic amyloidosis may occur in nonaddicts in association with chronic cutaneous dermatoses, secondarily infected burns, decubitus ulcers, hydradenitis suppurativa, or dystrophic epidermolysis bullosa [84]. Thus chronic, antigenic stimulation from cutaneous infections appears to be the underlying cause of amyloidosis in addicts.

The average duration of drug abuse in addicts with renal amyloidosis was 18 years, significantly longer than the average 6 years in addicts with focal glomerulosclerosis. The mean age of addicts with amyloidosis was 41 years, while those with focal sclerosis averaged 29 years of age. In general, intravenous abuse antedated the subcutaneous route in those with amyloidosis. The subcutaneous route was initiated due to venous thrombosis and the unavailability of intravenous access. With advancing age and prolonged addiction, intravenous sites for injection of drugs become exhausted, necessitating a shift to the subcutaneous route. Cutaneous ulcerations due to local reactions to the injected heroin or diluent develop and are followed by suppurative complications [88, 122]. Longer survival of addicts in the late 1970s and early 1980s due to improved management of bacterial endocarditis, hepatitis, and other narcotic abuse-related medical illnesses may have allowed the emergence of renal amyloidosis. It is possible that the recent dramatic decline in the incidence of "skin poppers' amyloidosis" in New York City may reflect a shortened life span of intravenous drug users who now succumb at an earlier age due to AIDS.

PATHOLOGY

Deposits of amyloid are typically present in all compartments [i.e., glomeruli, arteries and arterioles, tubular basement membranes, and interstitium (in about one-half of our patients)]. In the majority, glomeruli exhibit prominent mesangial expansion or solidified lobules, which may be misinterpreted as sclerosis on hematoxylin-eosin–stained sections. However, the two processes are readily differentiated by routine stains because amyloid is negative for periodic acid–Schiff and silver, whereas the opposite is true of sclerosis. Peripheral capillary walls are often thickened and have a "spicular" deformity on silver-stained sections produced by the penetration of amyloid fibrils through the GBM. Tubular basement membranes, especially those of the distal segments, are thickened due to deposits of amyloid, and the degree of tubular atrophy appears to parallel the amount of amyloid deposited. While amyloid is seen focally in tubular basement membranes of some proximal tubules, the amount and distribution are far greater in distal segments.

All of the 17 kidneys with skin poppers' amyloidosis that we have examined by immunofluorescence thus far showed predominant staining for amyloid A (AA) protein (Fig. 45-4A). Amyloid that was isolated and biochemically characterized in two instances was AA protein–related and did not differ from AA amyloid secondary to chronic infections and inflammatory diseases [84]. None has been classified as amyloid light chain (AL) amyloid. We have observed several patients with two types of deposits on electron microscopy, both homogeneous electron-dense deposits and fibrils typical of amyloid. Although immunofluorescence microscopy showed predominantly staining for AA protein in the distribution of the amyloid as seen on light microscopy, less prominent small granular deposits of immunoglobulins and/or C3 were also present. By immunoelectron microscopy, amyloid fibrils were labeled with anti-amyloid A protein antibody, while the granular deposits were labeled with antibody to IgG, demonstrating the coexistence of amyloid and immune complex deposits [144].

CLINICAL FEATURES

The following description of the clinical features of skin poppers' amyloidosis is based on data from 57 cases reported in the literature, including 21 cases observed at our own institutions [2, 12, 19, 28, 31, 58, 69, 83, 95, 96, 121, 122] (Table 45-4). The mean age of these patients was 41 years (range, 25 to 57 years). When specified, nearly all patients were black, and all but 8 were male. The reason for this predominance of black males is unclear. Heroin was abused in nearly all cases, often in association with cocaine; however, in 2 patients crushed tablets of pentazocine and tripelennamine were the sole drugs abused. All but 7 patients injected drugs by the subcutaneous route and invariably had multiple and extensive skin ulcerations, usually with active chronic suppuration at the time of presentation. Of the 7 patients without subcutaneous drug use, 6 had chronic skin infections at intravenous injection sites or systemic illnesses associated with systemic amyloidosis. The mean total duration of drug abuse was 18 years, and the time from initiation of the subcutaneous route was 3 years, with a range of 1 to 8 years.

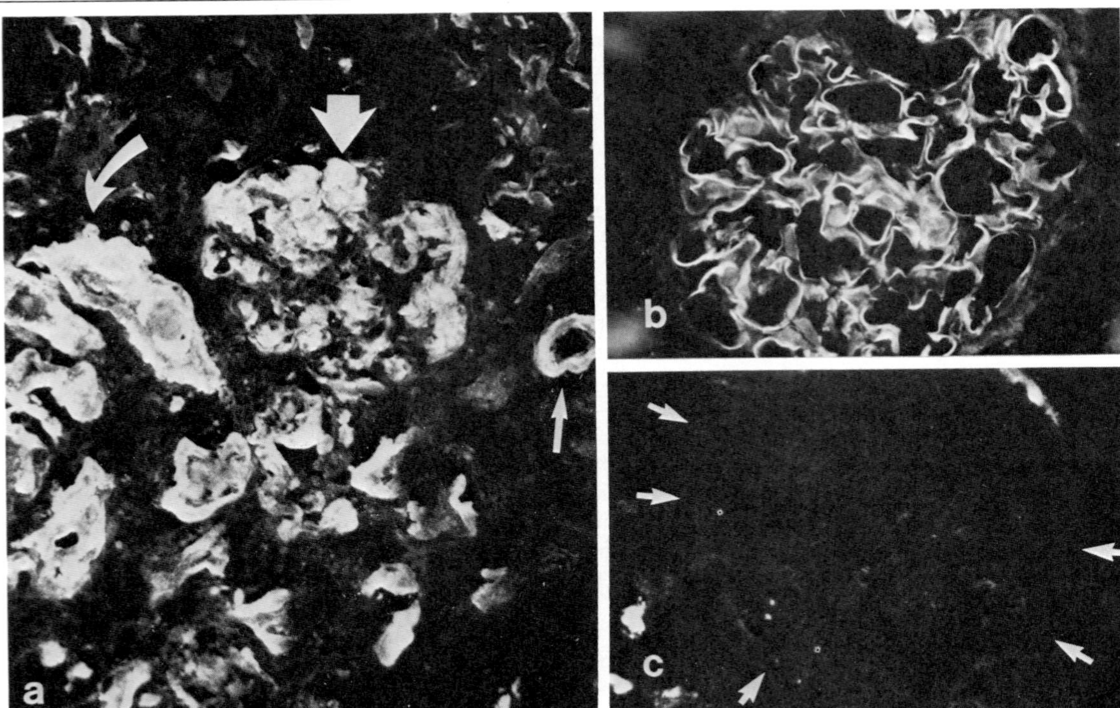

Fig. 45-4. Immunofluorescence microscopy of renal biopsies of addicts with amyloid (A) and focal glomerulosclerosis (B), and of a nonaddict patient with minimal-change nephrotic syndrome (C) A. Frozen section incubated with rabbit anti-AA protein antibody followed by fluoresceinated goat anti-rabbit IgG shows bright fluorescent labeling of amyloid deposits in the glomerulus (large arrowhead), vessel wall (small arrow), and tubular basement membranes (curved arrow). Stains for immunoglobulin (heavy- or light-chain–specific) were negative. (× 200.) B, C. Frozen sections incubated with fluorescein-conjugated anti-human IgG. Note smooth continuous global pattern of localization of IgG in glomerular basement membranes of addict (B), in contrast to negative staining of glomerulus (arrows) from nonaddict (C). (× 400.)

Table 45-4. Amyloidosis in subcutaneous heroin abusers

Clinical features	
Black	98%
Male sex	86%
Age	41 yr
Duration of intravenous route	18 yr
Duration of subcutaneous route	3 yr
Suppurative skin lesions	88%
Nephrotic syndrome on presentation	86%
Hypertension on presentation	17%
Serum creatinine on presentation	2.5 mg/dl

Addicts with amyloidosis typically present with the nephrotic syndrome. Urinary protein excretion exceeded 4 gm per 24 hours in 36 of 42 cases and averaged 13 gm per 24 hours. Mean serum albumin was 2.1 gm per deciliter and mean serum cholesterol was 247 mg per deciliter. Microscopic hematuria and pyuria were uncommon. Hypertension on initial presentation was reported in 17 percent [31]. Average serum creatinine levels did not differ between hypertensive and normotensive patients (2.2 and 2.6 mg/dl, respectively). Dubrow et al. [31] comment on the infrequency of hypertension in heroin abusers with systemic amyloidosis in contrast to its presence at presentation in two-thirds of heroin abusers with focal glomerulosclerosis. Our own experience with systemic amyloidosis differs somewhat; hypertension was observed at presentation in 40 percent. Initial kidney size was normal in 9 and increased in 5 of 14 patients studied. The mean initial BUN and serum creatinine levels were 38 mg per deciliter and 2.5 mg per deciliter, respectively. Initial creatinine clearance averaged 46 ml per minute. On presentation serum creatinine was below 1.2 mg per deciliter in 15 percent of patients, ranged from 1.2 to 2.0 mg per deciliter in 36 percent, from 2 to 4 mg per deciliter in 30 percent, and from 4 to 9 mg per deciliter in 15 percent. The remaining 4 percent were uremic at presentation.

Follow-up data are available in 12 patients. Five progressed to uremia, generally within 2 to 3 years after presenting with serum creatinine levels ranging from 1.5 to 4.7 mg per deciliter. In 5 additional patients, serum creatinine rose from a mean of 1.3 mg per deciliter to 4.8 mg per deciliter over an average period of 9 months. In the remaining 2 patients, renal function stabilized or improved.

One might anticipate that aggressive therapy of skin

infections combined with abstinence would favorably alter the clinical course of systemic amyloidosis in subcutaneous heroin abusers. Two patients have been described in whom abstinence from subcutaneous drug use and clearance of infection were associated with remission of the nephrotic syndrome and improvement or stabilization of renal function [2, 19]. Repeat renal biopsy showed persistent glomerular deposits of AA amyloid in one of the patients [19]. In contrast, nephrotic syndrome and renal amyloid deposits persisted and indolent progression to renal failure occurred in another patient who had discontinued drug use 5 years earlier [122]. We have observed three patients with unremitting nephrotic syndrome and progression to renal failure within 3 years despite clearance of infection and discontinuation of drug use. Postmortem examination of one revealed persistent systemic and renal amyloid deposits.

TUBULAR DISORDERS

We have assessed renal tubular function in 13 addicts with renal amyloidosis [95]. Renal tubular acidosis was found in 8 patients. Five patients complained of polyuria and polydipsia on initial presentation and 4 had urine volumes ranging from 4 to 7 liters per day. Nephrogenic diabetes insipidus that was insensitive to exogenous vasopressin administration was documented in one of these, and postmortem examination revealed amyloid deposits in tubular basement membranes, predominantly involving distal segments. Phosphaturia was demonstrated in 2 cases and glycosuria in 4. Glycosuria has been reported in other series, but since glycosuria may occur in any nephrotic patient, it does not necessarily reflect a specific amyloid-associated tubular defect.

In summary, systemic amyloidosis emerged in the late 1970s and early 1980s as a major cause of nephropathy in drug abusers in New York City, apparently related to use of the subcutaneous route. However, more recently, amyloidosis has disappeared as a major clinical entity in the addict population.

Endocarditis-Associated Glomerulonephritis in Heroin Abusers

We have recently reviewed the epidemiology and clinical features of glomerulonephritis during the course of bacterial endocarditis [92, 93]. Glomerulonephritis, confirmed histologically, occurred frequently in parenteral drug abusers, particularly when the infecting organism was *Staphylococcus aureus,* currently the most common organism causing endocarditis in intravenous drug abusers [14]. Others have reported a similarly high incidence of glomerulonephritis, ranging from 40 to 78 percent, in parenteral drug abusers with bacterial endocarditis due predominantly to *S. aureus* [55, 71, 72, 85, 98]. Not all investigators, however, confirm this frequent occurrence of clinical glomerular involvement in parenteral drug abusers with endocarditis [9, 65]. These discrepancies likely relate to the varying clinical criteria used to define renal involvement. Our data, which are based on postmortem and biopsy material, demonstrate a high incidence of parenteral drug abuse and *S. aureus* etiology in patients with infective endocarditis in whom glomerulonephritis developed. Noteworthy is the occurrence of parenteral drug abuse in 35 of 58 patients reported in the literature since 1969 in whom glomerulonephritis complicating *S. aureus* bacterial endocarditis was confirmed histologically [92]. Predisposition of parenteral drug abusers to develop glomerulonephritis during the course of bacterial endocarditis may be related to preformed serum antibodies to bacterial antigens.

PATHOLOGY

Glomerulonephritis encountered in the course of endocarditis can be classified as diffuse or focal [92]. Diffuse glomerulonephritis, as it occurs often in addicts with acute bacterial endocarditis due to *S. aureus,* is generally indistinguishable from acute poststreptococcal or other postinfectious glomerulonephritis [137]. Proliferation in glomeruli is global and regular, and electron-dense deposits are present in a subepithelial distribution. This contrasts with the morphologic features of diffuse glomerulonephritis formerly seen when a subacute course was more common and infective endocarditis was often due to *Streptococcus viridans.* In this latter setting, deposits were predominantly subendothelial and mesangial rather than subepithelial, and proliferation in glomeruli was irregular with coexistence of segmental and global lesions [92]. Focal glomerulonephritis in infective endocarditis is characterized by varying degrees of segmental glomerular hypercellularity, sclerosis, or capsular adhesions. Epithelial and fibroepithelial crescents, either small or circumferential, may be present.

CLINICAL FEATURES

Clinical manifestations of focal glomerulonephritis are usually mild [93]. Microscopic hematuria, pyuria, or modest proteinuria may be observed; heavy proteinuria and hypertension are rare. Renal functional impairment is uncommon, but when segmental glomerular involvement is severe and extensive, renal insufficiency may supervene [92]. Occasionally, focal glomerulonephritis may be present without clinical evidence of renal involvement.

We have reviewed our experience with the course of diffuse glomerulonephritis during bacterial endocarditis as seen predominantly in heroin abusers [92, 93]. Renal functional impairment was common, ranging from mild effects to advanced. No correlation existed between the duration of symptoms prior to presentation and the initial or peak serum creatinine value. In the majority, serum creatinine reached maximal levels prior to initiation of antibiotic therapy or during the early phase of treatment. Recovery of renal function rarely occurred in those patients with advanced degrees of renal failure. Since failure of antibiotic therapy and death were far more frequent in patients who presented with severe renal insufficiency than in those in whom renal functional impairment was mild or moderate, it is unclear whether the presence of uremia hindered the eradication of infection or whether more "severe" endocarditis gave rise to more severe glomerulonephritis. Thus advanced renal insufficiency on initial presentation was associated with both failure of bacterial cure and failure to recover renal function. By contrast, when antibiotic therapy was effective, recovery of renal function, normalization of the serum complement level, and remission of the clinical features of glomerulonephritis occurred consistently in those patients in whom renal functional impairment was mild or moderate.

Microscopic hematuria and proteinuria are universal in endocarditis-associated diffuse glomerulonephritis with bacterial endocarditis [92]. Gross hematuria may also be observed or may result from renal infarction or concurrent drug-induced interstitial nephritis. It is generally thought that the nephrotic syndrome is a rare feature; however, the nephrotic syndrome has been noted in 14 percent of 126 reported cases of histologically confirmed glomerulonephritis with bacterial endocarditis [92]. This figure may overestimate the true incidence in that patients with heavy proteinuria are more likely to be subjected to renal biopsy. Diffuse glomerulonephritis was present in all but 5 of the 20 patients reported to have the nephrotic syndrome; 56 percent of these were parenteral drug abusers with *S. aureus* bacterial endocarditis [92]. Hypertension is rare despite its frequent occurrence in other forms of postinfectious endocapillary glomerulonephritis [92]. Because of the difficulty in differentiating cardiac, nephrotic, and "nephritic" edema in patients with endocarditis and renal disease, the contribution of primary renal sodium retention cannot be determined with certainty.

OUTCOME

With control of infection by antibiotic therapy, the urinary abnormalities normalize in most patients within several days to several weeks [92]. Occasionally, microscopic hematuria or proteinuria may persist for months to years after bacteriologic cure [92]. In the majority, renal insufficiency of mild to moderate severity resolves promptly with successful antibiotic therapy; infrequently, transient worsening of renal function may occur prior to recovery [92]. Despite the usual fatal outcome in patients who present with uremia, even severe renal failure occasionally resolves with successful antibiotic therapy, sometimes with improvement continuing during weeks or months. Serial renal biopsies may reveal almost complete histologic resolution of glomerulonephritis in association with clinical recovery [92].

Rarely, renal failure requiring dialysis may persist despite bacteriologic cure [92, 93]. This might occur more frequently were it not for the high mortality associated with uremia in bacterial endocarditis due to concomitant failure of antibiotic therapy. Among those cured of endocarditis, later deaths due to chronic renal failure secondary to glomerulonephritis acquired during the active phase of endocarditis have occasionally been reported [92]. Persistent renal insufficiency, nephrotic syndrome, and sediment abnormalities have been described in parenteral drug abusers after bacteriologic cure of *S. aureus* endocarditis [119, 120]. Our own studies demonstrate that glomerulonephritis acquired during the course of endocarditis occasionally may prove to be irreversible after bacteriologic cure and may result in persistent renal insufficiency or sediment abnormalities [93].

Acute Renal Failure due to Nontraumatic Rhabdomyolysis in Drug Abusers

Nontraumatic rhabdomyolysis in drug abusers is a well-recognized clinical syndrome. Although cocaine and parenteral heroin are the agents most frequently responsible, the syndrome has been described as well after intravenous or oral administration of phencyclidine, methadone, barbiturates, or other sedatives singly or in combination. Phencyclidine use has been associated with rhabdomyolysis during periods of involuntary isometric activity against mechanical restraints [8, 17]. Nontraumatic rhabdomyolysis in drug abusers may also arise as a result of tetanus [107] or self-injection of water [33].

Prolonged pressure on dependent muscles by the weight of the patient's own body, with compromise of the regional vascular supply during extended periods of depressed consciousness and immobilization, is generally regarded as the pathogenetic mechanism responsible for heroin-associated rhabdomyolysis [13, 30, 45, 61, 64, 99, 107, 123, 124, 141]. This sequence results in compression myonecrosis and ischemic injury. However, a number of cases of heroin-associated rhabdomyolysis have been reported in which depressed consciousness or muscle compression did not occur [24, 26, 39, 64, 66, 94, 109, 112, 126]. Rhabdomyolysis in these instances has been attributed to a direct toxic effect or an allergic reaction to heroin or a contaminant. Instead of typical localized muscle involvement as seen with pressure myonecrosis, generalized diffuse and symmetric muscle swelling in all extremities may be observed in these cases [109, 126]. Lending further credence to a toxic or allergic pathogenesis in some is the occasional occurrence of swelling of an entire extremity after local injection of heroin [109]. In several cases myocarditis was purported to accompany allergic or toxic nontraumatic rhabdomyolysis due to heroin [66, 126, 138]; however, in only one was myocardial involvement confirmed postmortem [126].

Most heroin abusers with nontraumatic rhabdomyolysis were young men between the ages of 18 and 41 years (mean, 25 years). Prolonged muscle compression during extended periods of stupor and immobilization was present in the vast majority. The degree and duration of stupor usually determined the severity of rhabdomyolysis and the occurrence and severity of acute renal failure [107]. Hypoxia, volume depletion, acidosis, hypotension, and disturbances in temperature regulation, which are frequent concomitants of drug overdose, contribute to the occurrence of rhabdomyolysis in this setting [41, 64, 102]. Clinical evidence of muscle injury such as swelling and tenderness of involved muscles or localized pain and weakness was frequent; however, these findings may be absent or overlooked. Elevation of serum levels of muscle enzymes and myoglobinuria were characteristic features. Acute renal failure occurred in two-thirds of the cases and was frequently oliguric.

Prognosis was excellent, with full recovery in all but three patients who died of uremia during oliguric renal failure [109, 126].

The first reports calling attention to the association between cocaine abuse and nontraumatic rhabdomyolysis appeared in 1987 [86, 89, 125]. Over 60 patients have been described to date [7, 53, 68, 86, 89, 100, 103, 108, 111, 113, 125, 127, 128, 145]. All but 10 were male and their average age was 30 years. The majority of patients experienced complications of cocaine use that may have contributed to the occurrence of rhabdomyolysis or may have been primarily responsible for muscle injury. These complications included hypotension, seizures, hyperpyrexia, and muscle compression after prolonged immobilization. Others abused cocaine together with heroin or alcohol, drugs that are also associated with muscle injury. Myalgia or muscle tenderness accompanied cocaine-induced rhabdomyolysis in one-half of reported cases. Cocaine was administered most frequently by intravenous injection or smoking of the cocaine alkaloid. It has been suggested that the occurrence of renal failure is unrelated to the route of cocaine administration [111]; however, we found the intravenous route to be associated with more severe muscle injury and a greater incidence of renal failure [113, 128].

Urinalyses showed a positive orthotoluidine reaction for heme in 75 percent of reported cases. Proteinuria was detected by dipstick in two-thirds. Renal failure developed in nearly one-half of the patients. Of those who developed renal failure, one-half were oliguric and an equal number required dialysis. Roth et al. [111] described more severe muscle injury as reflected in higher serum levels of creatine kinase, more marked elevation in serum uric acid levels, and more marked decline in serum calcium levels among patients with cocaine-induced rhabdomyolysis who developed renal failure. Mean serum creatine kinase levels in patients with cocaine-induced rhabdomyolysis and renal failure were 150 times the upper limit of normal and twice as high as in the group as a whole [111]. In our own series [128], mean peak serum creatine phosphokinase levels exceeded 90,000 IU per liter in those with renal failure as compared to approximately 1000 IU per liter in nonazotemic patients. Hypotension, hyperpyrexia, volume contraction, diffuse intravascular coagulation, and severe hepatic dysfunction were correlated with the development of renal failure in both series. Of the 13 patients with renal failure reported by Roth et al. [111], 6 died; however, we did not observe so bleak a prognosis [128]. In view of the rapid proliferation of cocaine addiction among young adults, cocaine-induced rhabdomyolysis threatens to become an increasingly frequent cause of acute renal failure in urban areas.

Systemic Necrotizing Vasculitis in Parenteral Amphetamine Abusers

The occurrence of systemic necrotizing vasculitis in parenteral drug abusers, clinically similar to classic polyarteritis nodosa, was initially described by Citron et al. [15], who attributed this syndrome to abuse of amphetamines. Although a variety of drugs were involved, methamphetamine had been abused in all but 2 of their 14 patients and was used exclusively by one of them. In an exploration of the possible pathogenetic role of amphetamines in this disorder, an experimental model of amphetamine-induced cerebral vasculitis was developed in the rhesus monkey [115]. Characterized angiographically by spasm and reduction in cerebral vessel caliber and histologically by generalized cerebral edema, hemorrhage, infarction, and occasional microaneurysms, the validity of these experimentally induced cerebral vascular changes as a model of systemic necrotizing angiitis has been questioned [101]. Further, the severe hypertension that occurs in this model could itself be responsible for the histologic and angiographic features observed [115].

More recently, an association between classic polyarteritis nodosa and hepatitis B surface antigenemia has been described [57]. In addition, hepatitis surface antigen has been found in parenteral drug abusers, in a range varying from 4 to 13 percent [56, 87, 90, 142]. Accordingly, some authors have proposed that systemic necrotizing vasculitis as it occurs in parenteral drug abusers may be related to hepatitis B surface antigenemia, thus discounting a pathogenetic role for amphetamine [63]. When sought, hepatitis B surface antigen has been found in the serum of some, but not all, drug abusers with systemic necrotizing vasculitis [10, 16, 32, 37, 63, 101]. Indeed, in one study, hepatitis B surface antigen was demonstrated in fewer than one-third of 30 drug abusers with this syndrome [16]. However, Koff et al. [63] described one abuser of heroin and amphetamines with systemic necrotizing angiitis in whom hepatitis B surface antigen was documented but antigenemia was transient despite the development of systemic vasculitis. Thus, the roles of methamphetamine and hepatitis B surface antigen in the pathogenesis of systemic necrotizing angiitis in drug abusers are not clear.

The clinical course and angiographic features of systemic necrotizing vasculitis in 39 parenteral drug abusers has been described in varying detail and isolated cerebral angiitis in an additional 20 patients has been described [10, 15, 16, 32, 37, 48, 49, 63, 74, 78, 99, 101, 114, 129, 133]. Patients with widespread vasculitis ranged in age from 18 to 47 years (mean, 24 years); one-half were male. The duration of parenteral drug abuse invariably exceeded 3 months. When specified, amphetamines were among the agents abused in all but two patients, usually in association with multiple other drugs. Hepatitis B surface antigen was demonstrated in the serum of fewer than one-third of the 30 patients evaluated by Citron and Peters [16]. Hepatitis B surface antigen was sought in five additional patients and was present in all [10, 32, 37, 63, 101]. In five asymptomatic patients the diagnosis was made on the basis of typical angiographic findings, which included arterial aneurysms and sacculations involving multiple organs including the kidney, pancreas, liver, and small bowel [15]. In symptomatic cases, the duration of illness prior to presentation ranged widely from several days to 1 year. The severity of hypertension observed in this syndrome and its refractoriness to therapy have been emphasized [10]. Hypertension was present in 13 of 17 patients in whom the level of blood pressure was specified; in 2 of these patients the onset of hypertension followed steroid administration. Malignant hypertension associated with papilledema, encephalopathy, or rapidly progressive renal failure occurred in 6 patients.

Renal manifestations were present in 4 of the 14 patients reported by Citron et al. [15]. Renal failure developed in 2 and hematuria, proteinuria, or azotemia was present in 2 others. Renal involvement has been described in a total of 11 patients in the literature; 7 of these were uremic. Severe or accelerated hypertension was characteristic of all but one of those who developed renal failure. Renal imaging techniques or postmortem examination frequently revealed small kidneys. Renal histopathology was detailed in 6 cases. Small kidneys with segmental ischemic atrophy reflecting old as well as more recent renal infarction were characteristic findings at postmortem examination. Necrotizing arteriolitis often involved the interlobular and arcuate arteries and vascular changes of different ages coexisted. Glomerulonephritis was not observed.

Three patients expired in uremia and four from visceral infarction, cardiovascular complications, or aneurysmal rupture. One patient underwent renal transplantation. Follow-up was not available in the remaining three uremic patients. Four patients responded favorably to therapy with steroids or immunosuppressive agents. In one of these, immunosuppressive therapy induced a remission despite an equivocal response to steroids; relapse occurred with discontinuation of cytotoxic therapy. Two patients expired and a third developed accelerated hypertension and renal failure during corticosteroid therapy.

Nephropathy in Glue and Solvent "Sniffers"

Inhalation of the fumes of toluene or toluene-containing compounds (spray paint, glue, transmission fluid, paint, and lacquer thinners) may be associated with a variety of electrolyte and acid-base disturbances [67, 91, 132, 139]. Taher et al. [134] described hyperchloremic metabolic acidosis with a normal anion gap in association with toluene "sniffing" in two patients, one of whom was studied in detail. Urine pH was inappropriately high, and studies of urinary bicarbonate excretion were indicative of a distal renal tubular acidosis. Azotemia was absent and proximal tubular reabsorption of solutes was unimpaired. The acidifying defect was reversible and recurrent with repeated episodes of toluene abuse. Hypokalemia was associated with renal potassium wasting, which was attributed to hyperaldosteronism accompanying distal renal tubular acidosis. Generalized muscle weakness and flaccid quadriparesis were observed in those with severe hypokalemia. Several other cases of nonanion gap hyperchloremic metabolic acidosis have been reported in association with toluene abuse [34, 67, 91, 139]. Moss et al. [91] described a patient with hyperchloremic metabolic acidosis, hypokalemia, hypouricemia, hypophosphatemia, and hypocalcemia. Proximal reabsorption of uric acid, glucose, phosphate, calcium, and some amino acids was impaired. Fractional excretion of bicarbonate rose to nearly 7 percent with rising serum bicarbonate indicative of a proximal defect, while submaximal urinary acidification during ammonium chloride loading suggested a distal defect as well. Microhematuria and pyuria were additional features. Hyperchloremic metabolic acidosis persisted, whereas other tubular defects reversed with abstinence, only to recur with repeated exposure. Two additional cases with hyperchloremic metabolic acidosis due to proximal bicarbonate wasting are described in this report [91]. Streicher et al. [132] reported 25 cases of toluene abuse associated with hypokalemia in 13, hypophosphatemia in 10, and hyperchloremic metabolic acidosis in 19. Six patients developed nontraumatic rhabdomyolysis, related perhaps to the combined effects on muscle of hypokalemia and hypophosphatemia. These electrolyte disturbances may also have been responsible for muscle weakness, frequently a presenting complaint, which progressed in some to quadriparesis. Rhabdomyolysis in 4 additional patients occurred in the absence of these electrolyte disturbances, and the authors suggested a direct toxic effect of toluene on skeletal and cardiac muscle. Hypokalemia was attributed by these authors to a redistribution of extracellular potassium. Despite normal values at presentation, serum calcium levels declined during fluid repletion and 2 patients developed symptomatic hypocalcemia. Three patients in this series and six described by others [34, 139] presented with an anion gap acidosis that was attributed to the accumulation of products of toluene metabolism (benzoic acid and hippuric acid). It was suggested that these metabolites are more likely to accumulate and cause anion gap acidosis in those with impaired renal function. In contrast, in those with normal renal function, overproduction and urinary excretion of the anions of these organic acids may contribute to the development of nonanion gap hyperchloremic metabolic acidosis [34]. Elevation of serum creatinine, which proved to be reversible, was observed only once in the series of Streicher et al. [132]. Urinary abnormalities were frequent, occurring in 18 of 21 patients, and included hematuria, pyuria, and reversible proteinuria ranging up to 1 gm per 24 hours. One patient underwent renal biopsy, which was unremarkable by light microscopy. By contrast, Voigts and Kaufman [139] found reversible renal insufficiency in 38 percent of 16 episodes. Pyuria was universal in their series, and hematuria and proteinuria each occurred in three-fourths of cases [139].

Among nearly 200 toluene abusers reported in the literature who underwent examination of the urine, pyuria was present in 28 percent, and microscopic hematuria and proteinuria were each present in 16 percent [51, 79, 104, 139]. Several episodes of acute renal failure have been observed in association with toluene inhalation [34, 51, 97, 116, 139, 143]. Reversible renal failure was attributed to hypotension-induced acute tubular necrosis in one patient and was associated with hepatic failure in a second [34, 97]. Serial renal biopsy in one patient with irreversible acute renal failure demonstrated progressive tubulointerstitial injury leading to interstitial fibrosis [116]. Of interest is a report of a long-term regular abuser of toluene who developed recurrent renal calculi related perhaps to toluene-induced distal renal tubular acidosis [67].

Acute renal failure has been observed in inhalation abusers of trichloroethylene, which is contained in cleaning fluid and other solvents ("solvent sniffers") [5, 75]. Oliguric acute renal failure as well as less severe renal functional impairment, with or without associated acute centrilobular necrosis of the liver, has been described in four solvent abusers [5, 75]. Renal injury was reversible in all cases. Modest proteinuria was a universal feature; microscopic hematuria was present in one case. Industrial exposure to trichloroethylene by inhalation has also been associated with reversible acute oliguric renal failure [47], abnormalities of the urinary sediment [18], and fatal combined hepatic and renal failure [27]. Examination of renal tissue in one case of trichloroethylene-induced acute renal failure showed acute tubular necrosis [47].

Hepatitis B–Related Glomerulonephritis in Heroin Abusers

Hepatitis B–related antigen or antibody has been reported in parenteral drug abusers in a range varying between 4 and 13 percent [56, 87, 90, 142]. Glomerular involvement has been described in parenteral drug abusers temporally related to acute viral hepatitis [33, 99] and in association with chronic hepatitis [62]. The relationship between hepatitis B and glomerular disease is discussed in Chap. 65.

HIV-associated Nephropathy in Intravenous Heroin Abusers

This subject is discussed in Chap. 86.

References

1. AIDS and human immunodeficiency virus infection in the United States: 1988 update. *M.M.W.R.* 38(54): 1, 1989.
2. Amigo, J. S., Orriols, J., Modol, J., et al. Resolution of nephrotic syndrome secondary heroin-associated renal amyloidosis. (Letter) *Nephrol. Dial. Transplant.* 5: 158, 1990.
3. Arruda, J. A. L., Kurtzman, N. A., and Pillay, V. K. G. Prevalence of renal disease in asymptomatic heroin addicts. *Arch. Intern. Med.* 135: 535, 1975.
4. Avram, M. M., Iancu, M., and Weiss, S. Heroin usage nephropathy—subclinical to end stage nephrotic syndrome. *Abstr. Am. Soc. Nephrol.* 1971. P. 5.
5. Baerg, R. D., and Kimberg, D. V. Centrilobular hepatic necrosis and acute renal failure in "solvent sniffers." *Ann. Intern. Med.* 73: 713, 1970.
6. Bakir, A. A., Bazilinski, N. G., Rhee, H. L., et al. Focal segmental glomerulosclerosis: A common entity in nephrotic black adults. *Arch. Intern. Med.* 149: 1802, 1989.
7. Barrido, D. T., Joseph, A. J., Rao, T. K. S., et al. Renal disease associated acute and chronic "crack" abuse. (Abstract) *Kidney Int.* 33: 181, 1988.
8. Barton, C. H., Sterling, M. L., and Vaziri, N. D. Rhabdomyolysis and acute renal failure associated with phencyclidine intoxication. *Arch. Intern. Med.* 140: 568, 1980.
9. Bayer, A. S., Theofilopoulos, A. N., Eisenberg, R., et al. Circulating immune complexes in infective endocarditis. *N. Engl. J. Med.* 295: 1500, 1976.
10. Bennett, W. M., Plamp, C., and Porter, G. A. Drug-related syndromes in clinical nephrology. *Ann. Intern. Med.* 87: 582, 1977.
11. Beranek, J. T. Morphine binding by serum globulins from morphine-treated rabbits. *Fed. Proc.* 33: 474, 1974.
12. Brus, I., Steiner, G., Maceda, A., et al. Amyloid fibrils in urinary sediment. Heroin addiction with renal amyloidosis. *N. Y. State J. Med.* 79: 768, 1979.
13. Cadnapaphornchal, P., Taher, S., and McDonald, F. D. Acute drug-associated rhabdomyolysis: An examination of its diverse renal manifestations and complications. *Am. J. Med. Sci.* 280: 66, 1980.
14. Chambers, H. F., Korzeniowski, O. M., and Sande, M. A. *Staphylococcus aureus* endocarditis: Clinical manifestations in addicts and nonaddicts. *Medicine* 62: 170, 1983.
15. Citron, B. P., Halpern, M., McCarron, M., et al. Necrotizing angiitis associated with drug abuse. *N. Engl. J. Med.* 283: 1003, 1970.
16. Citron, B. P., and Peters, R. L. Angiitis in drug abusers. *N. Engl. J. Med.* 284: 112, 1971.
17. Cogen, F. C., Rigg, G., Simmons, J. L., et al. Phencyclidine-associated acute rhabdomyolysis. *Ann. Intern. Med.* 88: 210, 1978.
18. Cotter, L. H. Trichloroethylene poisoning. *Arch. Industr. Hygiene Occup. Med.* 1: 319, 1950.
19. Crowley, S., Feinfeld, D. A., and Janis, R. Resolution of nephrotic syndrome and lack of progression of heroin-associated renal amyloidosis. *Am. J. Kidney Dis.* 13: 333, 1989.
20. Cunningham, E. E., Brentjens, J. R., Zielezny, M. A., et al. Heroin nephropathy—a clinicopathologic and epidemiologic study. *Am. J. Med.* 68: 47, 1980.
21. Cunningham, E. E., Zielezny, M. A., and Venuto, R. C. Heroin-associated nephropathy—a nationwide problem. *J.A.M.A.* 250: 2935, 1983.
22. Cushman, P., and Grieco, M. H. Hyperimmunoglobulinemia associated with narcotic addiction. Effects of methadone maintenance treatment. *Am. J. Med.* 54: 320, 1973.
23. D'Agati, V., Cheng, J. I., Carbone, L., et al. The pathology of HIV-nephropathy: A detailed morphologic and comparative study. *Kidney Int.* 35: 1358, 1989.
24. D'Agostino, R. S., and Arnett, E. N. Acute myoglobinuria and heroin snorting. *J.A.M.A.* 241: 277, 1979.
25. Davis, J. S., and Lie, J. T. Extracellular glomerular microparticles in nephrotic syndrome of heroin users. *Arch. Pathol.* 99: 278, 1975.
26. de Gans, J., Stam, J., and van Wijngaarden, G. K. Rhabdomyolysis and concomitant neurological lesions after intravenous heroin abuse. *J. Neurol. Neurosurg. Psychiatry* 48: 1057, 1985.
27. Defalque, R. J. Pharmacology and toxicology of trichloroethylene. A critical review of the world literature. *Clin. Pharmacol. Ther.* 2: 665, 1961.

28. Derosena, R., Koss, M. N., and Pirani, C. L. Demonstration of amyloid fibrils in urinary sediment. *N. Engl. J. Med.* 293: 1131, 1975.
29. Dikman, S. H., Kahn, T., Gribetz, D., et al. Resolution of renal amyloidosis. *Am. J. Med.* 63: 430, 1977.
30. Dolich, B. H., and Aiache, A. E. Drug-induced coma: a cause of crush syndrome and ischemic contracture. *J. Trauma* 13: 223, 1973.
31. Dubrow, A., Mittman, N., Ghali, V., et al. The changing spectrum of heroin-associated nephropathy. *Am. J. Kidney Dis.* 5: 36, 1985.
32. Duffy, J., Lidsky, M. D., Sharp, J. T., et al. Polyarthritis, polyarteritis and hepatitis B. *Medicine* 55: 19, 1976.
33. Eknoyan, G., Gyorkey, F., Dichoso, C., et al. Renal involvement in drug abuse. *Arch. Intern. Med.* 132: 801, 1973.
34. Fischman, C. M., and Oster, J. R. Toxic effects of toluene—a new cause of high anion gap metabolic acidosis. *J.A.M.A.* 241: 1713, 1979.
35. Friedman, E. A., and Rao, T. S. K. Why does uremia in heroin abusers occur predominantly among blacks. *J.A.M.A.* 250: 2965, 1983.
36. Friedman, E. A., Rao, T. K. S., and Nicastri, A. D. Heroin-associated nephropathy. *Nephron* 13: 421, 1974.
37. Fye, K. H., Becker, M. J., Theofilopoulos, A. N., et al. Immune complexes in hepatitis B antigen-associated periarteritis nodosa. Detection by antibody-dependent cell-mediated cytotoxicity and the Raji cell assay. *Am. J. Med.* 62: 783, 1977.
38. Gardiner, H., Mahajan, S., Briggs, W., et al. Renal disease in heroin addicts. *Abstr. Am. Soc. Nephrol.*, 1977. P. 15A.
39. Gibb, W. R. G., and Shaw, I. C. Myoglobinuria due to heroin abuse. *J. R. Soc. Med.* 78: 862, 1985.
40. Glicklich, D., Haskell, L., Senitzer, D., et al. Possible genetic predisposition to idiopathic focal segmental glomerulosclerosis. *Am. J. Kidney Dis.* 12: 26, 1988.
41. Greenwood, R. J. Lumbar plexitis and rhabdomyolysis following abuse of heroin. *Postgrad. Med. J.* 50: 772, 1974.
42. Grishman, E., and Churg, J. Podocyte degeneration in focal glomerular sclerosis. *Abstr. Am. Soc. Nephrol.*, 1973. P. 44.
43. Grishman, E., and Churg, J. Focal glomerular sclerosis in nephrotic patients: An electron microscopic study of glomerular podocytes. *Kidney Int.* 7: 111, 1975.
44. Grishman, E., Churg, J., and Porush, J. G. Glomerular morphology in nephrotic heroin addicts. *Lab. Invest.* 35: 415, 1976.
45. Grossman, R. A., Hamilton, R. W., Morse, B. M., et al. Nontraumatic rhabdomyolysis and acute renal failure. *N. Engl. J. Med.* 291: 807, 1974.
46. Groth, D. H., Mackay, G. R., Crable, J. V., et al. Intravenous injection of talc in a narcotics addict. *Arch. Pathol. Lab. Med.* 94: 171, 1972.
47. Gutch, C. F., Tomhave, W. G., and Stevens, S. C. Acute renal failure due to inhalation of trichlorethylene. *Ann. Intern. Med.* 63: 128, 1965.
48. Halpern, M. Angiitis in drug abusers. *N. Engl. J. Med.* 284: 113, 1971.
49. Halpern, M., and Citron, B. P. Necrotizing angiitis associated with drug abuse. *Am. J. Roentgenol.* 3: 663, 1971.
50. Haskell, L. P., Glicklich, D., and Senitzer, D. HLA associations in heroin-associated nephropathy. *Am. J. Kidney Dis.* 12: 45, 1988.
51. Hayden, J. W., Peterson, R. G., and Bruckner, J. V. Toxicology of toluene (methylbenzene): Review of current literature. *Clin. Toxicol.* 11: 549, 1977.
52. Heptinstall, R. H. *Pathology of the Kidney*. Boston: Little, Brown, 1983. Pp. 676–696.
53. Herzlich, B. C., Arsura, E. L., Pagala, M., et al. Rhabdomyolysis related to cocaine abuse. *Ann. Intern. Med.* 109: 335, 1988.
54. Hill, J. H., Wainer, B. H., Fitch, F. W., et al. The interaction of ^{14}C-morphine with sera from immunized rabbits and from patients addicted to heroin. *Clin. Exp. Immunol.* 15: 213, 1973.
55. Hurwitz, D., Quismorio, F. P., and Friou, G. J. Cryoglobulinaemia in patients with infectious endocarditis. *Clin. Exp. Immunol.* 19: 131, 1975.
56. Husby, G., Pierce, P. E., and Williams, R. C., Jr. Smooth muscle antibody in heroin addicts. *Ann. Intern. Med.* 83: 801, 1975.
57. Inman, R. D. Rheumatic manifestations of hepatitis B virus infection. *Semin. Arthr. Rheum.* 11: 406, 1982.
58. Jacob, H., Charytan, C., Rascoff, J. H., et al. Amyloidosis secondary to drug abuse and chronic skin suppuration. *Arch. Intern. Med.* 138: 1150, 1978.
59. Johnson, J. E., White, J. J., Walovitch, R. C., et al. Effects of morphine on rat kidney glomerular podocytes: A scanning electron microscopic study. *Drug Alcohol Depend.* 19: 249, 1987.
60. Kilcoyne, M. M., Daly, J. J., Gocke, D. J., et al. Nephrotic syndrome in heroin addicts. *Lancet* 1: 17, 1972.
61. Klock, J. C., and Sexton, M. J. Rhabdomyolysis and acute myoglobinuric renal failure following heroin use. *Calif. Med.* 119: 5, 1973.
62. Knieser, M. R., Jenis, E. H., Lowenthal, D. T., et al. Pathogenesis of renal disease associated with viral hepatitis. *Arch. Pathol.* 97: 193, 1974.
63. Koff, R. S., Widrich, W. C., and Robbins, A. H. Necrotizing angiitis in a methamphetamine user with hepatitis B—Angiographic diagnosis, five-month follow-up results and localization of bleeding site. *N. Engl. J. Med.* 288: 946, 1973.
64. Koffler, A., Friedler, R. M., and Massry, S. G. Acute renal failure due to nontraumatic rhabdomyolysis. *Ann. Intern. Med.* 85: 23, 1976.
65. Korzeniowski, O., and Sande, M. A. Combination antimicrobial therapy for *Staphylococcus aureus* endocarditis in patients addicted to parenteral drugs and in nonaddicts. A prospective study. *Ann. Intern. Med.* 97: 496, 1982.
66. Krige, L. P., Milne, F. J., Margolius, K. A., et al. Rhabdomyolysis and renal failure—unusual complications of drug abuse. A case report. *S. Afr. Med. J.* 64: 253, 1983.
67. Kroeger, R. M., Moore, R. J., Lehman, T. H., et al. Recurrent urinary calculi associated with toluene sniffing. *J. Urol.* 123: 89, 1980.
68. Krohn, K. D., Slowman-Kovacs, S., and Leapman, S. B. Cocaine and rhabdomyolysis. (Letter) *Ann. Intern. Med.* 108: 639, 1988.
69. Kunis, C., Olesnicky, M., Nurse, H., et al. Heroin nephropathy—clinical-pathologic correlations. Proceedings of the 9th International Congress of Nephrology, 1984. P. 102A.
70. Langs, C., Gallo, G. R., Schacht, R. G., et al. Rapid renal failure in AIDS-associated focal glomerulosclerosis. *Arch. Intern. Med.* 150: 287, 1990.
71. Lessin, B. E., and Siegel, L. Endocarditis in drug addicts. *J.A.M.A.* 224: 1650, 1973.

72. Levine, D. P., Cushing, R. D., Jui, J., et al. Community-acquired methicillin-resistant *Staphylococcus aureus* endocarditis in the Detroit Medical Center. *Ann. Intern. Med.* 97: 330, 1982.
73. Light, A. B., and Torrance, E. G. Opium addiction. V. Miscellaneous observations on human addicts during the administration of morphine. *Arch. Intern. Med.* 43: 878, 1929.
74. Lignelli, G. J., and Buchheit, W. A. Angiitis in drug abusers. *N. Engl. J. Med.* 284: 112, 1971.
75. Litt, I. F., and Cohen, M. I. Danger . . . vapor harmful: Spot remover sniffing. *N. Engl. J. Med.* 281: 543, 1969.
76. Llach, F., Descoeudres, C., and Massry, S. G. Heroin associated nephropathy: Clinical and histological studies in 19 patients. *Clin. Nephrol.* 11: 7, 1979.
77. Marchand, C., Cantin, M., and Cote, M. Evidence for the nephrotoxicity of morphine sulfate in rats. *Can. J. Physiol. Pharmacol.* 47: 649, 1969.
78. Margolis, M. T., and Newton, T. H. Methamphetamine ("speed") arteritis. *Neuroradiology* 2: 179, 1971.
79. Massengale, O. N., Glaser, H. H., LeLievre, R. E., et al. Physical and psychologic factors in glue sniffing. *N. Engl. J. Med.* 269: 1340, 1963.
80. Matalon, R., Katz, L., Gallo, G., et al. Glomerular sclerosis in adults with nephrotic syndrome. *Ann. Intern. Med.* 80: 488, 1974.
81. May, D. C., Helderman, H., Eigenbrodt, E. H., et al. Chronic sclerosing glomerulopathy (heroin-associated nephropathy) in intravenous T's and blues abusers. *Am. J. Kidney Dis.* 8: 404, 1986.
82. McGinn, J. T., McGinn, T. G., Cherubin, C. E., et al. Nephrotic syndrome in drug addicts. *N.Y. State J. Med.* 74: 92, 1974.
83. Meador, K. H., Sharon, Z., and Lewis, E. J. Renal amyloidosis and subcutaneous drug abuse. *Ann. Intern. Med.* 91: 565, 1979.
84. Menchel, S., Cohen, D., Gross, E., et al. AA protein-related renal amyloidosis in drug addicts. *Am. J. Pathol.* 112: 195, 1983.
85. Menda, K. B., and Gorbach, S. L. Favorable experience with bacterial endocarditis in heroin addicts. *Ann. Intern. Med.* 78: 25, 1973.
86. Merigian, K. S., and Roberts, J. R. Cocaine intoxication: Hyperpyrexia, rhabdomyolysis and acute renal failure. *Clin. Toxicol.* 25: 135, 1987.
87. Millian, S. J., and Cherubin, C. E. Serologic investigations in narcotic addicts: III. Latex fixation, C-reactive protein, 'monotest,' serum proteins and SH antigen. *Am. J. Clin. Pathol.* 56: 693, 1971.
88. Minkin, W., and Cohen, H. J. Dermatologic complications of heroin addiction—report of a new complication. *N. Engl. J. Med.* 277: 473, 1967.
89. Morrow, J. D. A case of rhabdomyolysis (CPC). *J. Tenn. Med. Assoc.* 80: 613, 1987.
90. Moser, R. H. Heroin addiction. *J.A.M.A.* 230: 728, 1974.
91. Moss, A. H., Gabow, P. A., Kaehny, W. D., et al. Fanconi's syndrome and distal renal tubular acidosis after glue sniffing. *Ann. Intern. Med.* 92: 69, 1980.
92. Neugarten, J., and Baldwin, D. S. Glomerulonephritis in bacterial endocarditis. *Am. J. Med.* 77: 297, 1984.
93. Neugarten, J., Gallo, G. R., and Baldwin, D. S. Glomerulonephritis in bacterial endocarditis. *Am. J. Kidney Dis.* 5: 371, 1984.
94. Neugarten, J., Gallo, G. R., Buxbaum, J., et al. Amyloidosis in subcutaneous heroin abusers. *Am. J. Med.* 81: 635, 1986.
95. Nicholls, K., Niall, J. F., and Moran, J. E. Rhabdomyolysis and renal failure: Complications of narcotic abuse. *Med. J. Aust.* 2: 387, 1982.
96. Novick, D. M., Yancovitz, S. R., and Weinberg, P. G. Amyloidosis in parenteral drug abusers. *Mt. Sinai J. Med.* 46: 163, 1979.
97. O'Brien, E. T., Yeoman, W. B., and Hobby, J. A. E. Hepatorenal damage from toluene in a "glue sniffer." *Br. Med. J.* 2: 29, 1971.
98. O'Connor, D. T., Weisman, M. H., and Fierer, J. Activation of the alternate complement pathway in *Staph. aureus* infective endocarditis and its relationship to thrombocytopenia, coagulation abnormalities, and glomerulonephritis. *Clin. Exp. Immunol.* 34: 179, 1978.
99. Olivero, J., Bacque, F., Carlton, C. E., et al. Renal complications of drug addiction. *Urology* 8: 526, 1976.
100. Parks, J. M., Reed, G., and Knochel, J. P. Cocaine-associated rhabdomyolysis. *Am. J. Med. Sci.* 297: 334, 1989.
101. Pear, B. L. Radiologic recognition of extrahepatic manifestations of hepatitis B antigenemia. *Am. J. Roentgenol.* 137: 135, 1981.
102. Penn, A. S., Rowland, L. P., and Fraser, D. W. Drugs, coma and myoglobinuria. *Arch. Neurol.* 26: 336, 1972.
103. Pogue, V. A., and Nurse, H. M. Cocaine-associated acute myoglobinuric renal failure. *Am. J. Med.* 86: 183, 1989.
104. Press, E., and Done, A. K. Solvent sniffing. Physiologic effects and community control measures for intoxication from the intentional inhalation of organic solvents. II. *Pediatrics* 39: 611, 1967.
105. Qiu, C., Schoenfeld, P., Burnell, M., et al. Impact of the cocaine epidemic on end stage renal disease at San Francisco General Hospital. (Abstract) *J. Am. Soc. Nephrol.* 1: 373, 1990.
106. Rao, T. K. S., Nicastri, A. D., and Friedman, E. A. Natural history of heroin-associated nephropathy. *N. Engl. J. Med.* 290: 19, 1974.
107. Rao, T. K. S., Nicastri, A. D., and Friedman, E. A. Renal Consequences of Narcotic Abuse. In J. Hamburger, J. Crosnier, and M. H. Maxwell (eds.), *Nephrology.* New York: Wiley, 1979. Pp. 843–856.
108. Reinhart, W. H., and Stricker, H. Rhabdomyolysis after intravenous cocaine. *Am. J. Med.* 85: 579, 1988.
109. Richter, R. W., Challenor, Y. B., Pearson, J., et al. Acute myoglobinuria associated with heroin addiction. *J.A.M.A.* 216: 1172, 1971.
110. Ringle, D. A., and Herndon, B. L. In-vitro morphine binding by sera from morphine-treated rabbits. *J. Immunol.* 109: 174, 1972.
111. Roth, D., Alarcon, J. F., Fernandez, J. A., et al. Acute rhabdomyolysis associated with cocaine intoxication. *N. Engl. J. Med.* 319: 673, 1988.
112. Rowland, L. P., and Penn, A. S. Myoglobinuria. *Med. Clin. North Am.* 56: 1233, 1972.
113. Rubin, R., and Neugarten, J. Cocaine-induced rhabdomyolysis masquerading as myocardial ischemia. *Am. J. Med.* 86: 551, 1989.
114. Rumbaugh, C. L., Bergeron, R. T., Fang, H. C. H., et al. Cerebral angiographic changes in the drug abuse patient. *Radiology* 101: 335, 1971.
115. Rumbaugh, C. L., Bergeron, R. T., Scanlan, R. L., et al. Cerebral vascular changes secondary to amphetamine abuse in the experimental animal. *Radiology* 101: 345, 1971.
116. Russ, G., Clarkson, A. R., Woodroffe, A. J., et al. Renal failure from "glue sniffing." *Med. J. Aust.* 2: 121, 1981.

117. Ryan, J. J., Parker, C. W., and Williams, R. C., Jr. Gamma-globulin binding of morphine in heroin addicts. *J. Lab. Clin. Med.* 80: 155, 1972.
118. Sapira, J. D., Ball, J. C., and Penn, H. Causes of death among institutionalized narcotic addicts. *J. Chronic Dis.* 22: 733, 1970.
119. Savin, V. Glomerulonephritis in acute bacterial endocarditis in addicts. *Clin. Res* 22: 208A, 1974.
120. Savin, V., Siegel, L., and Schreiner, G. E. Nephropathy in Heroin Addicts with Staphylococcal Septicemia. In P. Kincaid-Smith, T. H. Mathew, and E. L. Becker (eds.), *Glomerulonephritis, Morphology, Natural History and Treatment.* New York: Wiley, 1973.
121. Scholes, J. V., Derosena, R., Appel, G. B., et al. Amyloidosis and the nephrotic syndrome in chronic heroin addicts. *Proc. 7th Int. Congr. Nephrol.*, 1978. P. L9.
122. Scholes, J., Derosena, R., Appel, G. B., et al. Amyloidosis in chronic heroin addicts with the nephrotic syndrome. *Ann. Intern. Med.* 91: 26, 1979.
123. Schreiber, S. N., Liebowitz, M. R., and Bernstein, L. H. Limb compression and renal impairment (crush syndrome) following narcotic and sedative overdose. *J. Bone Joint Surg.* 54A: 1683, 1972.
124. Schreiber, S. N., Liebowitz, M. R., Bernstein, L. H., et al. Limb compression and renal impairment (crush syndrome) complicating narcotic overdose. *N. Engl. J. Med.* 284: 368, 1971.
125. Schwartz, J. G., and McAfee, R. D. Cocaine and rhabdomyolysis. (Letter) *J. Fam. Pract.* 24: 209, 1987.
126. Schwartzfarb, L., Singh, G., and Marcus, D. Heroin-associated rhabdomyolysis with cardiac involvement. *Arch. Intern. Med.* 137: 1255, 1977.
127. Singhal, P., Horowitz, B., Quinones, M. C., et al. Acute renal failure following cocaine abuse. *Nephron* 52: 76, 1989.
128. Singhal, P., Rubin, R., Santiago, A., et al. Cocaine-induced rhabdomyolysis and acute renal failure. *J. Toxicol. Clin. Toxicol.* 28: 321, 1990.
129. Singleton, E. B., Dunbar, J. S., Fraser, R. G., et al. Film interpretation session. Radiological Society of North America. *Radiology* 13: 853, 1980.
130. Steinmuller, D. R., Kline Bolton, W., Stilmant, M. M., et al. Chronic interstitial nephritis and mixed cryoglobulinemia associated with drug abuse. *Arch. Pathol. Lab. Med.* 103: 63, 1979.
131. Stevens, J. W. Morphinism and kidney disease. *South. Med. J.* 9: 300, 1916.
132. Streicher, H. Z., Gabow, P. A., Moss, A. H., et al. Syndromes of toluene sniffing in adults. *Ann. Intern. Med.* 94: 758, 1981.
133. Streiter, M. L., and Bosniak, M. A. The radiology of drug addiction: Urinary tract complications. *Semin. Roentgenol.* 18: 221, 1983.
134. Taher, S. M., Anderson, R. J., McCartney, R., et al. Renal tubular acidosis associated with toluene "sniffing." *N. Engl. J. Med.* 290: 765, 1974.
135. Thompson, A. M., Anthonovych, T., Lin, R., et al. Focal membranoproliferative glomerulonephritis in heroin users. *Abstr. Am. Soc. Nephrol.*, 1973. P. 105.
136. Treser, G., Cherubin, C., Lonergan, E. T., et al. Renal lesions in narcotic addicts. *Am. J. Med.* 57: 687, 1974.
137. Tu, W. H., Shearn, M. A., and Lee, J. C. Acute diffuse glomerulonephritis in acute staphylococcal endocarditis. *Ann. Intern. Med.* 71: 335, 1969.
138. Tuller, M. A. Acute myoglobinuria with or without drug abuse. *J.A.M.A.* 217: 1868, 1971.
139. Voigts, A., and Kaufman, C. E. Acidosis and other metabolic abnormalities associated with paint sniffing. *South. Med. J.* 76: 443, 1983.
140. Weksler, M. E., Cherubin, C., Kilcoyne, M., et al. Absence of morphine-binding activity in serum from heroin addicts. *Clin. Exp. Immunol.* 13: 613, 1973.
141. Weston, C. F. M., Chalker, J. C., and Heaton, K. W. Multifactorial nature of renal impairment in heroin addicts. (Letter) *J. R. Soc. Med.* 79: 185, 1986.
142. Wetli, C. V., Noto, T. A., and Fernandez-Carol, A. Immunologic abnormalities in heroin addiction. *South. Med. J.* 67: 193, 1974.
143. Will, A. M., and McLaren, E. H. Reversible renal damage due to glue sniffing. *Br. Med. J.* 283: 525, 1981.
144. Yang, G. H., and Gallo, G. R. Protein-A-gold immunoelectron microscopic study of amyloid fibrils, granular deposits, and fibrillar luminal aggregates in renal amyloidosis. *Am. J. Pathol.* 137: 1223, 1990.
145. Zamora-Quezada, J. C., Dinerman, H., Stadecker, M., et al. Muscle and skin infarction after free-basing cocaine (crack). *Ann. Intern. Med.* 108: 564, 1988.
146. Zielezny, M. A., Cunningham, E. E., and Venuto, R. C. The impact of heroin abuse on a regional end-stage renal disease program. *Am. J. Public Health* 70: 829, 1980.
147. Zientara, M., and Moore, S. Fatal talc embolism in a drug addict. *Human Pathol.* 1: 324, 1970.

Heavy Metals

Richard P. Wedeen

More than 45 naturally occurring elements are classified as heavy metals by virtue of their metallic qualities and specific gravities greater than 5. Seven of these metals are generally recognized as nephrotoxic following environmental or occupational exposure: lead, cadmium, mercury, uranium, chromium, copper, and arsenic, although chronic renal failure has been described for only lead, cadmium, uranium, and arsenic. Therapeutic forms of platinum (Chap. 42), gold (Chap. 74), and bismuth may also induce kidney damage. While other heavy metals are potentially damaging to the kidneys, too little evidence of the clinical significance of these renal effects is available to warrant inclusion here. The potentially nephrotoxic heavy metals include cobalt, manganese, nickel, silver, thallium, thorium, tin, and vanadium. The paucity of incriminating evidence against these elements may be more a testimony to our ignorance of the etiologic factors that lead to end-stage renal disease than to the benign nature of the metals. Cause and effect are relatively easy to demonstrate when renal damage is acute. Establishing the contribution of a metal in kidney disease is, however, considerably more difficult if the toxicity is delayed. When renal disease is a consequence of long-term, low-dose, asymptomatic exposure modulated by complex interactions with other metals, nutritional factors, other diseases, and genetic susceptibility, the etiology remains obscure. It has become increasingly clear that metals essential for biologic systems (e.g., calcium, iron, magnesium, and zinc) can ameliorate the nephrotoxicity of other metals. It should also be noted that barium, selenium, molybdenum, lithium (Chap. 40), beryllium, and silicon are nephrotoxic metals with specific gravities less than 5 and are therefore not considered in this chapter.

Occupational exposure to silicon or beryllium is associated with clinical renal disease that is secondary to pulmonary damage. For example, in the accelerated form of silicosis known as silicoproteinosis, silicon dust appears to be indirectly responsible for rapidly progressive, immune complex–mediated, focal glomerulosclerosis [17, 71]. Silica is also believed to induce interstitial nephritis by direct deposition of crystalline material in the renal parenchyma [34, 35, 106]. Inhalation of beryllium can cause sarcoidlike pulmonary interstitial fibrosis sometimes complicated by hypercalcemia-induced interstitial nephritis [132, 146].

Kidney disease arising from exposure to heavy metals plays a special role in nephrology because of the potential for prevention. Disease resulting from relatively intense exposure in the workplace serves as a model for understanding the nephrotoxic effects of the more subtle but ubiquitous environmental exposure [150]. Both the source of exposure and the toxic agents may be multiple in origin. Life-style factors, such as analgesic abuse or consumption of lead-contaminated moonshine (illicit whiskey), and combined exposures to solvents or silica may contribute to the renal damage associated with occupational exposure to heavy metals [130].

Lead Nephropathy

Occupational exposure to lead began over ten thousand years ago in the region of the Aegean Sea. The earliest description of lead poisoning is found in a poem dating from about 200 B.C. by the Greek philosopher Nikander of Colophon [144]. Although possible recognition of renal effects of lead can be traced to the seventeenth century, the first description of lead nephrotoxicity in modern terms was provided by Lancerceaux in 1862. Lancerceaux's patient had saturnine (lead-induced) gout; his kidneys showed interstitial nephritis at postmortem examination. Controversy concerning the renal effects of lead stem from this nineteenth century description and is compounded by the recurrent failure to recognize the late sequelae of chronic absorption of relatively low levels of lead or to distinguish glomerular from extraglomerular renal disease. Additional confusion has been created by the failure to distinguish the transient Fanconi syndrome of acute childhood lead poisoning from the chronic interstitial nephritis characteristic of lead nephropathy in adults. In addition to the difficulty in assigning cause when the effect is delayed in time, identification of the renal effects of lead was further obscured because the late complications of excessive lead absorption, gout and hypertension, can themselves produce renal damage unrelated to lead.

DIAGNOSIS

In the past lead nephropathy was identified in individuals with repeated episodes of acute lead intoxication [144]. The classic symptoms of inorganic lead poisoning (abdominal colic, extensor muscle weakness, encephalopathy, anemia) in patients known to have excessive lead absorption made the diagnosis straightforward. In recent decades the diagnosis was confirmed in the clinical laboratory by finding anemia in association with excessive urinary excretion of lead, coproporphyrins, or δ-aminolevulinic acid. Following the extensive studies of lead metabolism by Kehoe beginning in the 1930s [152], the mainstay of laboratory diagnosis has been the blood lead concentration. Until 1978, a whole blood lead concentration of up to 80 μg per deciliter was considered "acceptable" in occupationally exposed adults. The finding of blood lead levels below 80 μg per deciliter was considered incompatible with the diagnosis of lead poisoning in adults, although levels above 40 μg per deciliter were considered unacceptable in children. The battle over the "safe" blood lead level continues despite a growing consensus that blood levels over 10 μg per deciliter may be associated with lead-induced organ damage [1, 93, 100, 101, 110, 145].

The blood lead concentration is relatively insensitive to cumulative body stores acquired over many years of moderate exposure (i.e., exposure insufficient to produce classic symptoms of acute poisonings). Blood lead concentrations tend to fall markedly within weeks of removal from exposure. Since approximately 95 percent of the body stores of lead is retained in bone with a mean residence time approximating 30 years [6, 113], alternative approaches to the detection of excessive lead absorption have been examined. At present cumulative past lead absorption is best assessed by the $CaNa_2EDTA$ (calcium disodiumtetraacetic acid) lead-mobilization test.

The EDTA test is performed in adults by parenteral administration of 1 to 3 gm of $CaNa_2EDTA$ over 4 to 12 hours with subsequent collection of 24-hour urine samples over 1 to 4 days. A dose of 20 to 30 mg per kilogram is generally used in children. Adults without undue prior lead absorption excrete up to 650 μg of lead-chelate in the urine. Neither the dose (1 to 3 gm) nor the route of administration (intravenous or intramuscular) appears to critically modify the normal response to chelation testing [87, 146], but in the presence of renal failure (serum creatinine greater than 1.5 mg/dl) urine collections should be extended to at least 3 days. The intramuscular administration of 2 gm of $CaNa_2EDTA$ (1 gm of EDTA mixed with local anesthetic in each of two injections, 12 hours apart) may be the preferable method of performing the chelation test because it has been well standardized in both normal subjects and patients with renal failure [7, 8, 156, 157]. In the presence of reduced glomerular filtration rate, urinary excretion of lead-chelate is measured for 3 consecutive days and the adequacy of collection checked by simultaneous measurement of creatinine excretion (1.3 gm of creatinine/day is an acceptable lower limit in normal adult males).

Since lead in bone has a biologic half-life measured in decades, compared to a biologic half-life of lead in blood of only 2 weeks [25], the bone more closely reflects cumulative body lead stores. Chelatable lead correlates well with bone lead [75, 141] (Fig. 46-1). Diagnostic monitoring of the body lead burden can be accomplished by in vivo tibial K x-ray fluorescence, a new, noninvasive technique that is both safe and accurate at bone lead concentrations associated with interstitial nephritis due to lead [127, 128, 148] (Fig. 46-2). The characteristic K x-rays of lead are stimulated by the 88-keV gamma emissions from a ^{109}Cd radioactive source. The fluorescent x-rays are measured with a high-purity, liquid nitrogen–cooled, germanium detector and recorded in a computer equipped with a multichannel pulse height analyzer. The characteristic K x-rays differ from the characteristic L x-rays of lead in that the higher-energy K photons penetrate 2 cm of cortical bone [120]. L x-rays only detect lead within the outermost 0.5 mm of subperiosteal bone. Calibration of the L x-rays is problematic because of major soft tissue absorption. K x-rays, on the other hand, can be accurately calibrated and normalized to the bone calcium content. The K x-ray fluorescence technique records the calcium content of the bone region under study and thus permits measurement of the lead-calcium ratio. This ratio is largely independent of target-source geometry and, therefore, permits calibration by either plaster-of-paris phantoms or absolute physical properties [148]. Whole-body radiation during the ½-hour K x-ray fluorescence test is 0.3 mrem, equivalent to

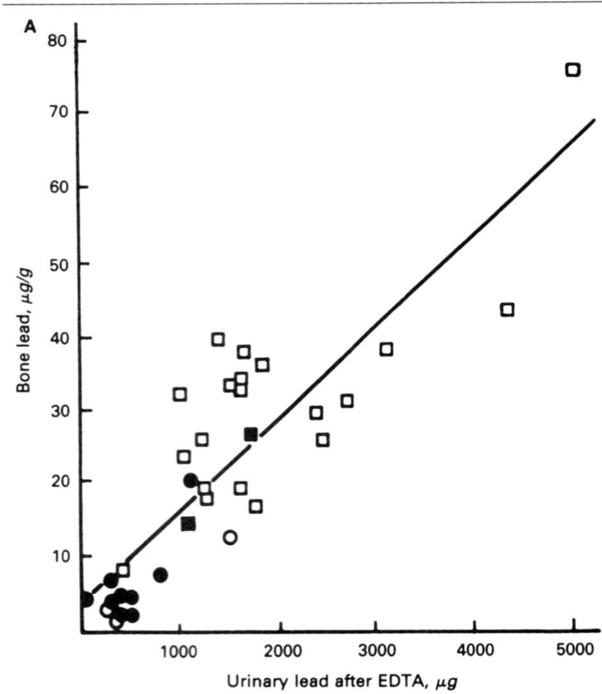

Fig. 46-1. Relationship of bone lead to chelatable lead in 35 Belgians including 22 lead workers (squares). Lead was measured in transiliac bone biopsy specimens by atomic absorption spectroscopy and chelatable lead by the EDTA lead-mobilization test. The linear regression correlation coefficient (r) is 0.87. Open symbols represent subjects with normal glomerular filtration rates; closed symbols, those with reduced glomerular filtration rates. (From F. L. Van de Vyver et al., Bone lead in dialysis patients. *Kidney Int.* 33:601, 1988.)

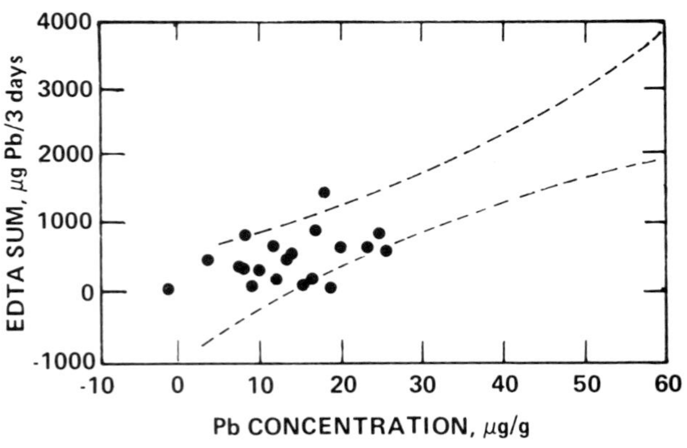

Fig. 46-2. Bone lead determined by in vivo tibial K x-ray fluorescence compared to chelatable lead in American Armed Service veterans without known excessive exposure to lead. Dotted lines represent 95 percent confidence limits of data presented in Fig. 46-1. Transiliac bone lead values in Fig. 46-1 were multiplied by 1.75 to convert to tibial bone values. Pb = lead. (From R. P. Wedeen, Bone lead, hypertension, and lead nephropathy. *Environ. Health Perspect.* 78:57, 1988.)

background radiation absorbed over about 10 hours. Marrow absorption is 0.4 mrem, compared to 0.1 mrem absorbed from an intraoral dental x-ray. In vivo tibial K x-ray fluorescence should prove of value to monitor the loss of lead from bone during prolonged chelation therapy [10]. It is likely that this noninvasive technique for measuring bone lead will largely replace other diagnostic techniques for estimating cumulative lead absorption.

Although the blood lead reflects absorption of both organic and inorganic lead, the clinical symptoms of organic lead are primarily cerebral and acute. DuPont's Chambers Works in Deepwater, New Jersey, became known as the "House of Butterflies" because of the frequency of hallucinations among workers producing tetraethyl lead shortly after discovery of the antiknock gasoline additive in 1923 [152]. Renal disease has not been found following tetraethyl lead absorption [66]. On the other hand, combustion of tetraethyl lead in automobiles is largely responsible for the pervasive background of inorganic lead to which modern industrialized societies are exposed. Environmental inorganic lead from gasoline appears to be responsible for behavioral disorders in children [101] and provides the background on which additional exposure due to accident or occupation causes renal disease in adults.

ACUTE LEAD NEPHROPATHY

In children with lead encephalopathy, a proximal tubule reabsorptive defect characterized by aminoaciduria, phosphaturia, and glycosuria (Fanconi syndrome) has been observed [27, 28]. The Fanconi syndrome is found in the presence of blood lead levels usually in excess of 150 μg per deciliter and appears to be rapidly reversed by chelation therapy designed to treat the far more dangerous encephalopathy [1, 99]. The proximal tubule reabsorptive defect has been induced experimentally in rats fed dietary lead [63]. In both children and experimental animals, acute lead nephropathy is consistently associated with the appearance of acid-fast intranuclear inclusions in proximal tubule epithelial cells [64, 65]. The intranuclear inclusion bodies consist of a lead-protein complex and may be seen in tubular epithelial cells in the urinary sediment during acute poisoning [123]. The inclusions contain about 50 μg of lead per milligram of protein, which is 60 to 100 times the concentration found in the kidney as a whole or in control nuclei [62]. Lead-containing intranuclear inclusions have been observed in liver, neural tissue, and osteoclasts as well as in kidney. Acute poisoning is also associated with morphologic and functional defects in mitochondria.

CHRONIC LEAD NEPHROPATHY

The phrase *chronic lead nephropathy* refers to the slowly progressive interstitial nephritis occurring in adults following prolonged lead exposure. Occupational lead nephropathy has developed after as little as 3 years of intense exposure [156]. Analysis of death certificates of 601 men employed at the Bunker Hill Lead Mine and Smelter in Kellogg, Idaho, up to 1977 indicated a twofold increased risk of dying from chronic renal disease [125]. The increased risk approached fourfold after 20 years of occupational lead exposure. Although most frequently recognized in lead workers after decades of occupational exposure [31, 89, 144], chronic lead nephropathy has also been recognized among young adults in Australia who sustained acute childhood lead poisoning [42, 43] and among illicit whisky ("moonshine") consumers in the southeastern United States. Chronic interstitial nephritis due to lead has also been seen among American workmen whose exposure was never severe enough to produce acute symptoms of lead poisoning [156, 157] and in U.S. Armed Service veterans suffering from renal failure attributed to gout or essential hypertension [7, 8]. In the veterans, exposure to lead had never produced acute symptoms of poisoning, and the source of exposure had never been recognized. The diagnosis was only established by performance of the $CaNa_2EDTA$ lead-mobilization test after renal failure was apparent. Medical histories were often misleading; patient recall frequently contradicted the objective evidence of chelation testing. Sporadic case reports of lead nephropathy arising from unusual accidental exposure such as geophagia [158] or Asian folk remedies and cosmetics continue to appear in the medical literature [144].

"Queensland nephritis" appears to represent the transition from the acute disease of childhood to the chronic nephropathy of adults [43]. This evolution has been observed in experimental animals but has not been reported in American children. The difference between the American and Australian experience may well be due to the fact that the American children with pica who had long-term follow-up received chelation therapy in childhood [28]. In the single American study of untreated childhood lead poisoning, diagnostic criteria for both lead poisoning and renal disease were unacceptably vague [134, 138]. The differences between the American and Australian experience may be more apparent than real, since a number of untreated victims of childhood pica in the United States who have been followed for several decades have developed chronic nephropathy but have not been reported in the medical literature [144].

Chronic lead nephropathy from moonshine came to medical attention because of the dramatic symptoms of acute lead poisoning. As in severely exposed industrial workers, lead colic and anemia were associated with reduced glomerular filtration rates, which often improved following chelation therapy. Transient renal failure, apparently the result of renal vasoconstriction [89], was superimposed on more chronic renal damage that appeared to be less responsive to chelating agents. The chronic lead nephropathy of the moonshiners, more often than not, was accompanied by gout and hypertension, in accord with nineteenth century descriptions of plumbism and contemporary reports from Australia [144]. Recently, a statistically significant odds ratio of 2.4 was reported for moonshine consumption and end-stage renal disease, suggesting a causal association in the absence of acute lead poisoning [130].

Evaluation of renal function in workmen with excessive body lead stores has revealed previously unsuspected reductions in glomerular filtration rates (i.e., less than 90 ml/min/1.73 m^2 body surface area) before renal dysfunction was clinically evident [157]. In these occupationally exposed individuals, minimal (about 30 percent) reductions in glomerular filtration rate were restored to normal by long-term, low-dose chelation therapy (1 gm of $CaNa_2EDTA$ with local anesthetic thrice weekly until the chelation test returned to normal). This therapeutic response in pre-azotemic lead nephropathy may reflect reversal of functional impairment rather than reversal of established interstitial nephritis. Both the renin-angiotensin system and Na^+-K^+-ATPase are inhibited by lead [138, 140, 151], and these effects may have been modified by chelation therapy. Considerable epidemiologic evidence suggests that modest azotemia is significantly more prevalent among lead-exposed workers than among nonexposed counterparts [144], presumably due to both morphologic and functional changes.

Renal biopsies in chronic lead nephropathy show nonspecific tubular atrophy and interstitial fibrosis with minimal inflammatory response as well as mitochondrial swelling, loss of cristae, and increased lysosomal dense bodies within proximal tubule cells [31, 156] (Fig. 46-3). Arteriolar changes indistinguishable from nephrosclerosis are found, often in the absence of clinical hypertension [75, 156]. Intranuclear inclusion bodies are often absent when the renal disease is long standing or following the administration of chelating agents. Clumped chromatin and nuclear invaginations of cytoplasmic contents may be found even in the absence of intranuclear inclusions. Morphologic alterations are minimal in glomeruli until the reduction in glomerular filtration rate is advanced.

The hypothesis derived from acute lead nephropathy—that proximal tubular injury accounts for the pathogenesis of chronic lead nephropathy—has gained little support. The appearance of arteriolar nephrosclerosis before hypertension develops, and the relatively short duration of hypertension before renal failure supervenes, suggest that the initial renal injury from lead may be in the microvascular endothelium [24, 85, 150]. Proximal tubular transport defects have not been convincingly demonstrated in chronic lead nephropathy. The absence of notable low-molecular-weight proteinuria in chronic lead nephropathy suggests a pathogenesis unrelated to the acute proximal tubule injury of acute lead poisoning. The mechanism of such microvascular injury remains speculative. Interference with cation transport is a reasonable hypothesis because the metabolism of lead is similar to that of other cations. The paradox that increased dietary calcium reduces, while increased free intracellular calcium increases, vascular smooth muscle tone could, in part, be explained by lead-calcium interactions [145]. Inhibition of red blood cell Na^+-K^+-ATPase in lead workers correlates with membrane-bound lead [160], and lead increases red blood cell Na-Li countertransport in vitro [9]. Similarly, lead interactions with vasoactive hormones may modulate blood pressure and induce microvascular injury [144].

The functional changes in chronic lead nephropathy appear to be less specific than those observed in acute poisoning. As in other forms of interstitial nephritis, proteinuria and glycosuria are initially absent. In contrast to cadmium nephropathy, the excretion of low-molecular-weight proteins such as lysozyme and β_2-microglobulin [20, 86, 139, 146, 155] is not increased after chronic exposure to lead. *N*-acetyl-β-glucosaminidase excretion is significantly greater among lead-exposed workers than among nonexposed employees [96], but

Fig. 46-3. Renal biopsy obtained from a 28-year-old man who had prepared lead solder for 5 years. His ^{125}I-iothalamate clearance was 52 ml/min/1.73 m^2; hemoglobin, 9.6 gm/dl; uric acid, 13.2 mg/dl; and blood lead, 48 μg/dl when he was initially seen. Lead-chelate excretion following 2 gm of $CaNa_2EDTA$ intramuscularly was 5.2 mg/24 hr. Light microscopy shows periglomerular fibrosis, a sclerotic glomerulus, and tubular atrophy. Trichrome stain; × 304. (From R. P. Wedeen et al., Occupational lead nephropathy. *Am. J. Med.* 59:630, 1975.)

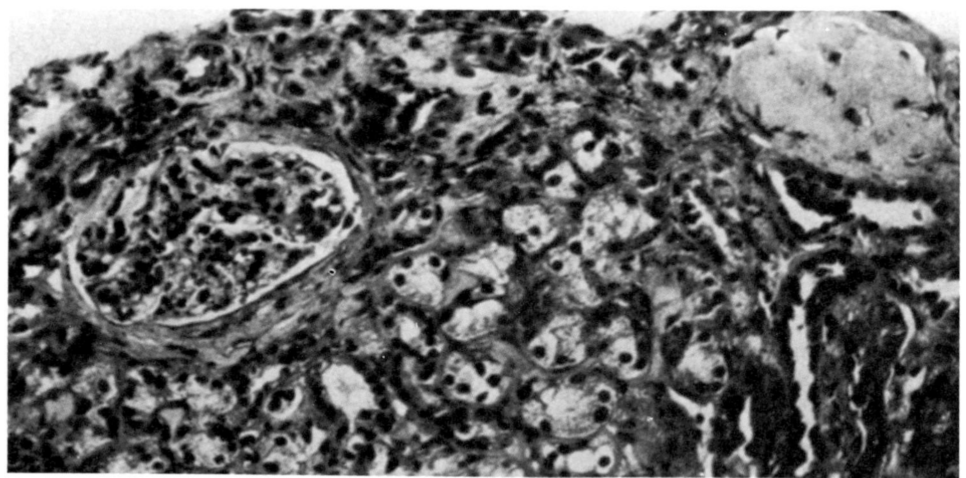

this phenomenon is too nonspecific to be helpful in diagnosis. In contrast to the reabsorptive defect of acute lead nephropathy, saturnine gout is characterized by renal retention of uric acid [144]. The clearance (C_{PAH}) and maximal secretion rate (Tm_{PAH}) for paraaminohippurate (PAH) have been found to be variable in patients with occupational lead nephropathy. A reduced maximal reabsorptive rate for glucose (Tm_G) has been reported, but simultaneous, matched controls were not obtained [72].

The relationship of lead to gout nephropathy has provoked controversy for over a century [11–13, 30, 115, 144]. Hyperuricemia and gout are common among individuals with excessive exposure to lead, apparently the result of decreased excretion and increased production of uric acid. Similarly, although hyperuricemia invariably accompanies azotemia, gout is rare in patients with renal failure except in those with lead nephropathy. Half of uremic patients with lead nephropathy have clinical gout [32, 43], but in the absence of renal failure, gout cannot usually be attributed to lead despite coexisting hypertension [108, 162].

There is substantial evidence that renal failure in gout is sometimes secondary to overt or unsuspected lead poisoning. In Queensland, Australia, as many as 80 percent of gout patients with renal failure have elevated EDTA lead-mobilization tests [43]. In New Jersey, chelatable lead was found to be significantly greater among gout patients with renal failure than among gout patients with normal renal function [7]. Since patients with comparable renal failure due to known causes other than lead show no increase in chelatable lead, the excessive mobilizable lead in these gout patients appears to be the cause rather than consequence of their renal failure. Measurement of lead levels in transiliac biopsy specimens from patients with end-stage renal disease confirm the fact that renal failure per se does not cause increased bone lead levels [141]. Unrecognized lead poisoning may therefore explain the occurrence of renal failure in some gout patients who have neither urinary calculi nor intratubular uric acid deposition disease [21]. Similarly, overt lead poisoning may explain the protean manifestations of gout in past centuries, the so-called irregular gout, as well as the long but almost forgotten association of gout with wine [144]. Sporadic contamination of alcoholic drinks with lead throughout history may have been responsible for gout that terminated in cerebral disease (i.e., uremia, stroke, or encephalopathy).

The association between lead and hypertension has also been a subject of controversy since the first use of the sphygmomanometer. The early view that renal injury induced by lead causes hypertension has gained increasing support. The EDTA lead-mobilization test can sometimes indicate that lead is the most probable cause of hypertension with renal failure, when lead exposure has not been previously suspected. Patients believed to have "essential hypertension with nephrosclerosis" may be identified as having lead nephropathy by the EDTA lead-mobilization test [8]. The duration of hypertension in patients with lead nephropathy tends to be shorter than that in hypertensives without renal failure, suggesting that lead-induced renal injury precedes and therefore causes the hypertension. Lead nephropathy does not account for all renal failure in all hypertensives with renal dysfunction any more than it accounts for renal failure in all gout patients with kidney disease. The heavy metal may, however, contribute to the long and controversial association of gout with hypertension, as well as to the variable incidence of renal failure in each of these conditions. Mortality data show that death from hypertensive cardiovascular disease is more frequent among lead workers than among the general population [44, 125, 126, 146]. In all forms of lead nephropathy (as in other types of interstitial nephritis) proteinuria is meager or absent initially but increases progressively as renal failure advances [7, 8].

A role for lead in hypertension gains further credence from epidemiologic studies of low-level lead exposure (i.e., exposure too low in intensity to produce the classic symptoms of acute lead poisoning). The Second National Health and Nutrition Examination Survey (NHANES II) performed between 1976 and 1980 included blood lead and blood pressure measurements in almost 10,000 noninstitutionalized Americans aged 6 months to 74 years [93, 150]. The correlation between blood lead and blood pressure was robust even when both measurements were within the accepted "normal" range [70, 111]. Similar conclusions have been drawn from studies performed throughout the world [95, 101, 112, 126], although contradictory findings in small studies have also been reported [41, 52, 107]. Although some doubts have been raised about the magnitude of the dose-response relationship, there is a growing consensus that lead contributes to hypertension, particularly in the presence of renal dysfunction, in the general population.

TREATMENT

Lead nephropathy is important because it is one of the few renal diseases that is preventable. Moreover, lead nephropathy can sometimes be reversed or its progression retarded by judicious use of chelation therapy [89, 144, 157]. Lead nephropathy is unusual for a nonsystemic disease involving the kidneys in that an etiologic diagnosis can be established even after renal failure supervenes.

Although chelation therapy effectively reverses acute lead nephropathy [28] and the preclinical renal dysfunction of occupational lead nephropathy [157], there is no evidence that such therapy reverses established interstitial nephritis due to lead. The partial remissions achieved among moonshiners and symptomatic lead workers may represent reversal of acute poisoning superimposed on chronic lead nephropathy. No improvement in renal function can be expected once advanced interstitial nephritis is present and the steady-state serum creatinine concentration exceeds about 3 mg per deciliter [55]. Chronic volume depletion and hyporeninemic hypoaldosteronism may contribute to the reversible component of renal dysfunction [4]. The effect of lead on the renin-angiotensin system, however, remains controversial because increased renin responsiveness has also been observed in lead-exposed experimental animals and humans [18, 19, 22, 140, 150].

Before chelation therapy is undertaken, the diagnosis should be established. It may be necessary to perform the EDTA lead-mobilization test, and other possible causes of renal disease must be rigorously excluded. For the present, attempts of chelation therapy should probably be avoided when the cause of the renal disease is unclear (e.g., in the presence of heavy proteinuria). Moreover, long-term, low-dose EDTA therapy should only be undertaken with a clear end-point in mind, such as reversion of the EDTA test to normal and restoration of renal function. Although the EDTA *test* has been shown to be safe even in the presence of renal failure [153], the cumulative nephrotoxicity of prolonged EDTA *therapy* in patients with markedly reduced glomerular filtration rates is unknown. Reports that $CaNa_2EDTA$ therapy has been followed by deterioration of renal function warrant careful follow-up of treated patients [55, 163]. Despite these caveats, it may be appropriate to perform EDTA lead-mobilization tests in individuals with gout or hypertension and renal failure or interstitial nephritis of unknown etiology since a positive test may provide the best available indication of etiology. Knowledge of etiology may permit identification and removal of the source of lead and prevention of lead nephropathy in others.

Cadmium Nephropathy

Industrial use of cadmium has increased steadily since its discovery by Stromyer in 1817. Cadmium-containing compounds are widely used in the manufacturing of pigments, plastics, glass, metal alloys, and electrical equipment. Acute absorption of as little as 10 mg as dust or fumes may induce severe gastrointestinal symptoms and, after a delay of 8 to 24 hours, fatal pulmonary edema [38, 48–51, 102]. Chronic low-dose exposure, on the other hand, causes slowly progressive emphysema, anosmia, and proximal tubular reabsorptive defects (acquired Fanconi syndrome) characterized by low-molecular-weight proteinuria, aminoaciduria, and renal glycosuria [83, 105]. Hypercalciuria (with normocalcemia), phosphaturia, and distal renal tubular acidosis result in clinically important osteomalacia, pseudofractures, and urinary tract stones [77–79, 81, 82, 84, 124]. Interstitial nephritis resulting from parenteral administration of cadmium to experimental animals was recognized in the nineteenth century [131], but only recently has the progression of early proximal tubular dysfunction to chronic renal failure been documented.

METABOLISM

Nonoccupationally exposed individuals accumulate cadmium throughout their lives through food and cigarettes. The biologic half-life of cadmium in humans exceeds 15 years, and one-third of the total body stores (10 to 20 mg) is retained in the kidneys. No harmful effects are currently recognized from this level of absorption.

Absorbed cadmium is initially sequestered in liver and kidney, where it is bound to a cysteine-rich apoprotein known as metallothionein [39]. Zinc, copper, mercury, and iron, as well as cadmium, induce metallothionein synthesis in these organs. With a molecular mass of 6,500 daltons, the cadmium-thionein complex is filtered at the glomerulus, taken up in the proximal tubule by endocytosis, and transferred to lysosomes, where it is rapidly degraded. Cadmium-thionein is considerably more nephrotoxic than cadmium or metallothionein alone, but cytoplasmic cadmium ions released from lysosomes may be the mediator of tubular cell injury [129]. Although uptake in liver initially exceeds that in kidney, most of the cadmium is eventually bound to protein in the proximal tubules, where it is accumulated until a "critical concentration," approximately 200 μg per gram of renal cortex, is achieved. At this tissue level, renal effects become evident including tubular proteinuria and increased cadmium excretion [75, 78]. Although urinary cadmium excretion is normally less than 2 μg per day, after the critical concentration has been exceeded, urinary cadmium in excess of 10 μg per day is usual. Significant abnormalities of proximal tubular function are associated with urinary cadmium excretion in excess of 30 μg per day [16]. The blood cadmium concentration is less reliable as an indicator of health effects. Although the blood cadmium level rises promptly following occupational exposure, blood is a poor indicator of cumulative absorption. Nevertheless, blood levels greater than 1 μg per deciliter, as well as urine concentrations of over 10 μg per gram of creatinine, are considered evidence of excessive exposure.

Increased urinary excretion of low-molecular-weight proteins such as β_2-microglobulin or retinol-binding protein is an early renal effect of cadmium [40, 50, 51, 83, 116–122, 142]. β_2-Microglobulin has been the most extensively examined urinary protein in cadmium nephropathy. With a molecular mass of approximately 11,000 daltons, β_2-microglobulin is normally filtered at the glomerulus and taken up by endocytosis by proximal tubule cells, where it is metabolized in lysosomes. Screening of cadmium workers for urinary β_2-microglobulin is widely employed for the detection of excessive cadmium absorption in industry. This HLA-associated protein, initially identified in the urine of patients with cadmium nephropathy, is now measured with a commercially available radioimmunoassay kit. Normally, urinary excretion of β_2-microglobulin is less than 1 mg per gram of creatinine. In patients with cadmium nephropathy urinary β_2-microglobulin is increased 50- to 100-fold [83]. Interpretation of β_2-microglobulin excretion is, however, complicated by the fact that it is found in tissues other than kidney, and both blood and urine levels may be increased in the absence of renal disease [69]. Circulating β_2-microglobulin is markedly elevated in systemic amyloidosis and multiple myeloma [57]. Urinary excretion is elevated in the presence of azotemia or proteinuria regardless of etiology. It is unstable in acid urine. Measurement of retinol-binding protein is more reliable [86]. Moreover, β_2-microglobulin is itself nephrotoxic and may be the mediator of both tubular injury and carcinogenesis. Elevated β_2-microglobulin excretion may reflect both increased production and diminished tubular degradation in cadmium nephropathy.

Low-molecular-weight proteinuria in cadmium workers rarely exceeds a few hundred milligrams per day and does not approach nephrotic levels (> 2.5 gm/day). The usual techniques for detecting albuminuria such as Albustix, heat and picric acid, or nitric acid are not sufficiently sensitive or specific to reliably detect tubular proteinuria. Although phosphotungstic, trichloroacetic, and sulfosalicylic acids are more sensitive, immunoelectrophoresis is required for specific protein identification.

There is no convincing evidence that β_2-microglobulin is normally reabsorbed into the circulation; hence, its increase in the urine should not be considered a manifestation of the Fanconi syndrome. Renal tubular lysosomal enzymes such as lysozyme, ribonuclease, alkaline phosphatase, acid phosphatase, transaminases, and *N*-acetyl-β-glucosaminidase are also increased in the urine in cadmium nephropathy, but the excretion of these low-molecular-weight proteins appears to be a nonspecific result of renal tubular injury. Whereas circulating proteins reach the tubular fluid via the glomerular filtrate, urinary lysosomal enzymes are derived primarily from renal tubule cells.

CALCIUM WASTING

Clinical symptoms associated with cadmium nephropathy derive primarily from the increased calcium excretion that accompanies the renal tubular dysfunction. Hypouricemia, hypophosphatemia, intermittent renal glycosuria, or elevated serum alkaline phosphatase (in the absence of renal failure or hyperparathyroidism) may bring acquired Fanconi syndrome to the clinician's attention, but ureteral colic is more likely to be the cadmium worker's chief complaint [51]. Although both osteomalacia and renal failure are distinctly uncommon in cadmium workers [16], urinary calculi have been reported in up to 40 percent of those subjected to industrial exposure [51, 78, 84, 124, 136]. Osteomalacia is associated with diminished renal tubular reabsorption of calcium and phosphate, elevated circulating parathormone levels, and reduced hydroxylation of vitamin D metabolites [103].

ITAI-ITAI DISEASE

In Japan a painful bone disease associated with pseudofractures due to cadmium-induced renal calcium wasting was recognized in the 1950s. Attributed to local contamination of food staples by river water polluted with industrial effluents, particularly cadmium, the syndrome known as "itai-itai" or "ouch-ouch" disease, afflicted postmenopausal, multiparous women [104]. Sustained deficiencies in calcium and vitamin D rendered these women particularly vulnerable to cadmium-induced calcium losses. The women with itai-itai disease tended to have reduced glomerular filtration rates, anemia, lymphopenia, and hypotension as well as osteomalacia. They exhibited a waddling gait, short stature, anemia, glucosuria, and elevated serum alkaline phosphatase levels. Hypertension was absent. β_2-Microglobulin excretion exceeded the normal maximum (1 mg/gram of creatinine) 100-fold, and glomerular filtration rates were substantially reduced in the most severely affected individuals. An increase in mean serum creatinine concentration from 1.19 to 1.68 mg per deciliter in 21 individuals averaging 65 years old who were followed for 9 to 14 years after β_2-microglobulinuria was first detected demonstrated the progression of renal failure [81]. The long-term follow-up demonstrated that β_2-microglobulin predicts the later development of renal failure in patients with itai-itai disease, and that renal damage progresses even after exposure has ceased.

CHRONIC INTERSTITIAL NEPHRITIS

Until recently, the role of cadmium in the induction of chronic interstitial nephritis has been controversial (Fig. 46-4). Whether cadmium contributes to hypertension or prostatic cancer remains subject to debate. Epidemiologic studies do not show a consistent correlation between blood or urine cadmium levels and blood pressure [53]. Mortality studies designed to evaluate the long-term implications of industrial cadmium exposure have yielded conflicting results [2]. Nevertheless, tubulointerstitial nephritis was found in 23 occupationally exposed and in 26 environmentally exposed individuals in whom postmortem tissue or renal biopsy specimens were examined [83]. These findings in conjunction with recent epidemiologic studies in the United States [136] and Belgium [118] and the long-term follow-up of itai-itai disease in Japan [81] leave little room for doubt that cadmium can induce chronic interstitial nephritis [150].

In the United States, Thun et al. [136] examined 45 current and retired nonferrous smelter workers exposed to cadmium for a mean of 19 years. Their blood cadmium levels averaged 7.9 μg per deciliter and urine cadmium levels averaged 9.3 μg per gram of creatinine. Cumulative cadmium dose estimated from air measurements correlated with low-molecular-weight proteinuria, and with decreased fractional calcium and phosphate reabsorption. The cadmium workers had significantly more kidney stones than did controls. Correlations between renal function and cadmium exposure were independent of other diseases in the workmen. A strong association between cumulative cadmium exposure and the later increase in serum creatinine supported the notion that cadmium-induced renal disease progresses slowly after a latent period of several decades. Roels et al. [118] provided further evidence that clinical renal disease results from cadmium. Workers who were exposed to cadmium in a nonferrous smelter in Belgium for up to 5 years and who had low-molecular-weight proteinuria were examined annually for 5 years after exposure had ceased. Cadmium levels in liver ranged from 24 to 158 μg per gram and from 133 to 355 μg per gram in the kidney. Serum creatinine concentrations increased from a mean of 1.2 to 1.5 mg per deciliter over 5 years (Fig. 46-5). The reduction in glomerular filtration rate was accompanied by an increase in mean serum β_2-microglobulin from 0.189 to 0.300 mg per deciliter and an increase in mean urinary β_2-microglobulin excretion from 1.770

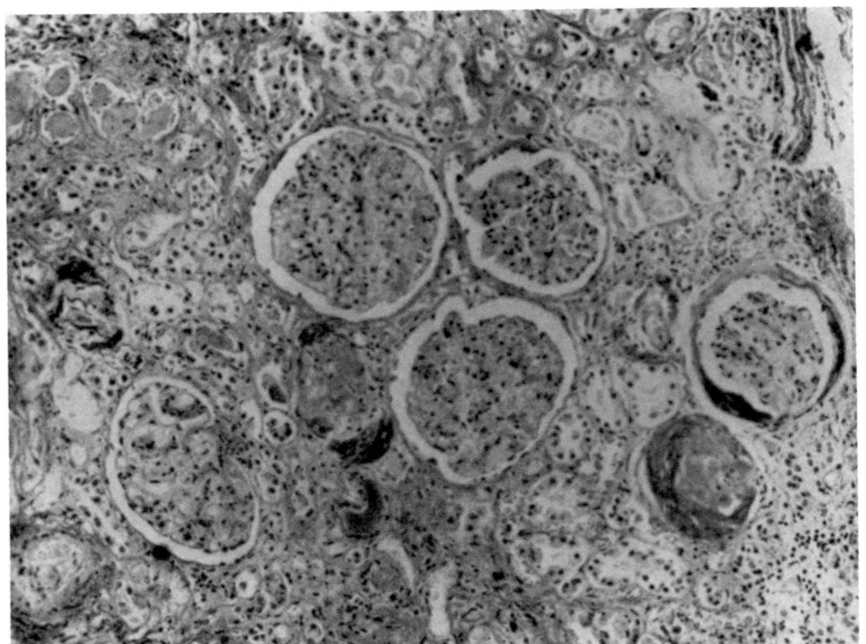

Fig. 46-4. Autopsy section of kidney from a 46-year-old man who had manufactured cadmium pigments for 28 years. He was found to have renal glycosuria, proteinuria, mild hypertension, and severe pulmonary emphysema. Death was attributed to cor pulmonale. His kidneys contained 55 μg Cd/gm wet weight and showed extensive interstitial fibrosis, tubular atrophy, and glomerular sclerosis. (From G. Kazantzis et al., Renal tubular malfunction and pulmonary emphysema in cadmium pigment workers. *Q. J. Med.* 32:165, 1963.)

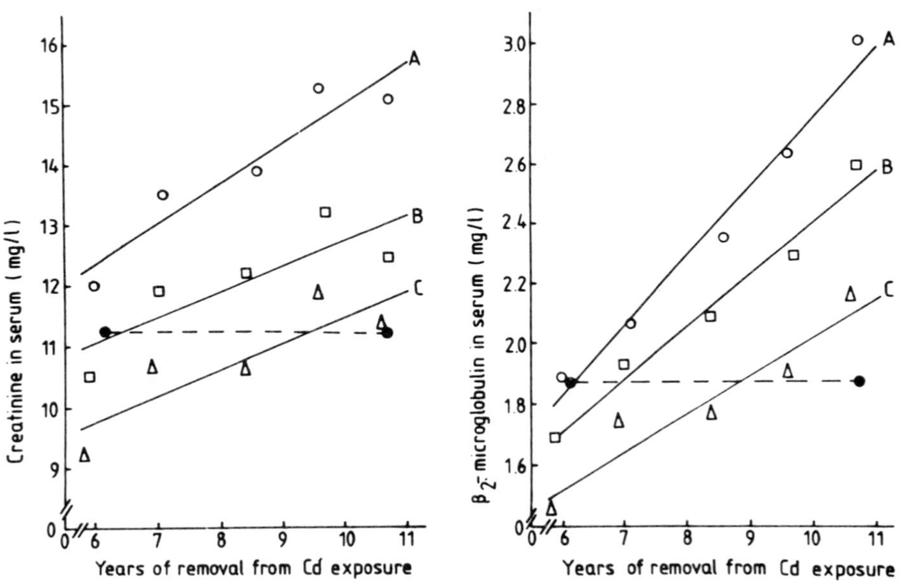

Fig. 46-5. Progression of renal dysfunction in cadmium workers over 5 years after removal from exposure. The mean serum creatinine increased from normal to abnormal levels (1.2 to 1.5 mg/dl). (From H. A. Roels et al., Health significance of cadmium induced renal dysfunction: A five year follow up. *Br. J. Ind. Med.* 46:755, 1989.)

to 2.580 mg per liter. The loss of glomerular filtration over the 5-year period was estimated to be 30 ml per minute; this is 30 times the predicted loss of kidney function for these elderly men.

DIAGNOSIS

Most commonly, the diagnosis of cadmium nephropathy is established by the history of exposure in conjunction with laboratory tests indicative of proximal tubule dysfunction (e.g., low-molecular-weight proteinuria, hypercalciuria, or renal glycosuria). Suspicions are confirmed if the urine cadmium concentration exceeds 10 μg per gram of creatinine.

Renal and hepatic accumulation of cadmium has been exploited for diagnostic purposes by in vivo neutron-activation analysis. This noninvasive technique for assessing organ cadmium content correlates well with tissue and urinary cadmium levels, and β_2-microglobulin excretion. It should prove valuable for monitoring industrial exposure before toxic levels have been attained [118, 119]. In individuals without occupational exposure, renal cadmium content reaches a maximum of about 50 μg per gram of cortex at about 45 years of age and thereafter declines as urinary elimination increases [105]. Renal cadmium concentration tends to fall with the development of renal failure, so that the diagnostic value of neutron-activation analysis of kidney is diminished in azotemic or uremic patients. In vivo neutron-activation studies indicate that when the hepatic cadmium level exceeds about 60 ppm and renal cortical content exceeds 200 ppm (20 mg/kidney), minimal proteinuria is likely to occur [61, 118].

TREATMENT

Although $CaNa_2EDTA$ given to experimental animals simultaneously with cadmium results in prompt excretion of the cadmium chelate and protection from nephrotoxicity, the chelating agent has little effect after cadmium has been complexed with metallothionein [23, 49]. Progression of renal disease has been described despite removal from exposure [81]. While osteomalacia may be arrested by calcium and vitamin D replacement [16], urinary tract stones represent a relative contraindication to such therapy.

Mercury

The toxicity of mercury depends on both its chemical form and the route of absorption. Elemental mercury is virtually harmless when ingested [162], but inhalation of the metallic vapor can produce bronchial damage and later neurologic disease [133, 147]. After in vivo oxidation of metallic mercury to the ionic form, the inhaled vapor readily crosses the blood-brain barrier and is retained in the cerebrum and cerebellum [79]. Although preferentially accumulated in the kidney, neurologic but not nephrologic disease follows exposure to elemental mercury; paresthesias, tremor, ataxia, visual impairment, erythism, and ultimately stupor and death are the clinical course.

Once in the environment, elemental mercury undergoes biotransformation to both organic and inorganic salts that are absorbed by living organisms and thus enter the food chain. Methyl, ethyl, and phenoxyethyl mercury are important organomercurial contaminants arising from industrial and agricultural processes. Methyl and ethyl mercury compounds are widely used as fungicides but also enter the environment as industrial wastes and through biotransformation of less toxic mercurials. Although a diuretic effect of inorganic mercury was documented in the late nineteenth century, diuresis following therapeutic administration of organomercurials was first noted by a medical student in Vienna in 1920 as a side effect of Novasurol used in antisyphilitic therapy [60]. Organomercurials subsequently became the mainstay of diuretic therapy until the advent of ethacrynic acid and furosemide in the 1960s. The inorganic mercurous salt (Hg_2Cl_2, calomel) is relatively nontoxic and was widely used as a medicinal agent until the present century. The mercuric salt ($HgCl_2$, corrosive sublimate), on the other hand, is highly nephrotoxic and continues to be used to create animal models of acute tubular necrosis [154]. Similar nephrotoxicity is produced by phenyl and methoxy methyl mercuric salts [92].

Although all chemical forms of mercury are accumulated in the cells of proximal tubules, the cellular concentration by itself provides little insight into pharmacologic or toxic actions. Inorganic mercury is retained in the kidney with a biologic half-life approximating 2 months [29]. While $HgCl_2$, chlormerodrin, and *p*-chloromercuribenzoate (p-CMB) are each selectively concentrated in the proximal tubule, the inorganic $HgCl_2$ salt produces tubular necrosis, chlormerodrin (Fig. 46-6) is a diuretic, and p-CMB blocks the diuretic effect of chlormerodrin [91, 155]. It has been suggested that the variable effect of different organomercurials on the kidney is due to variability in biotransformation to inorganic mercury within the body [45]. The affinity of mercurials for sulfhydryl groups and the presence of mercury within lysosomes [137, 143, 146] may not, however, reflect specific pharmacologic or toxic mechanisms. Cell injury may result from the interaction of inorganic mercury with phospholipid cell membranes [96]. It has been hypothesized that mercury nephrotoxicity as well as that of other heavy metals may result from stimulation of calmodulin-dependent phosphodiesterase activity [26].

DIAGNOSIS

Although blood mercury levels over 3 μg per deciliter or urine levels above 50 μg per gram of creatinine are considered abnormal, the correlation of blood and urine concentrations with renal disease is poor [78, 117]. Workers exposed to mercury vapors generally excrete more than 200 μg of mercury per liter of urine, but very few have renal dysfunction. Consequently, the diagnosis of mercury-induced renal disease is usually dependent on known exposure in the presence of renal dysfunction. Case reports of acute tubular necrosis or the nephrotic syndrome attributed to occupational, accidental, or intentional exposure to mercury are necessarily limited to situations in which the toxic agent has been identified.

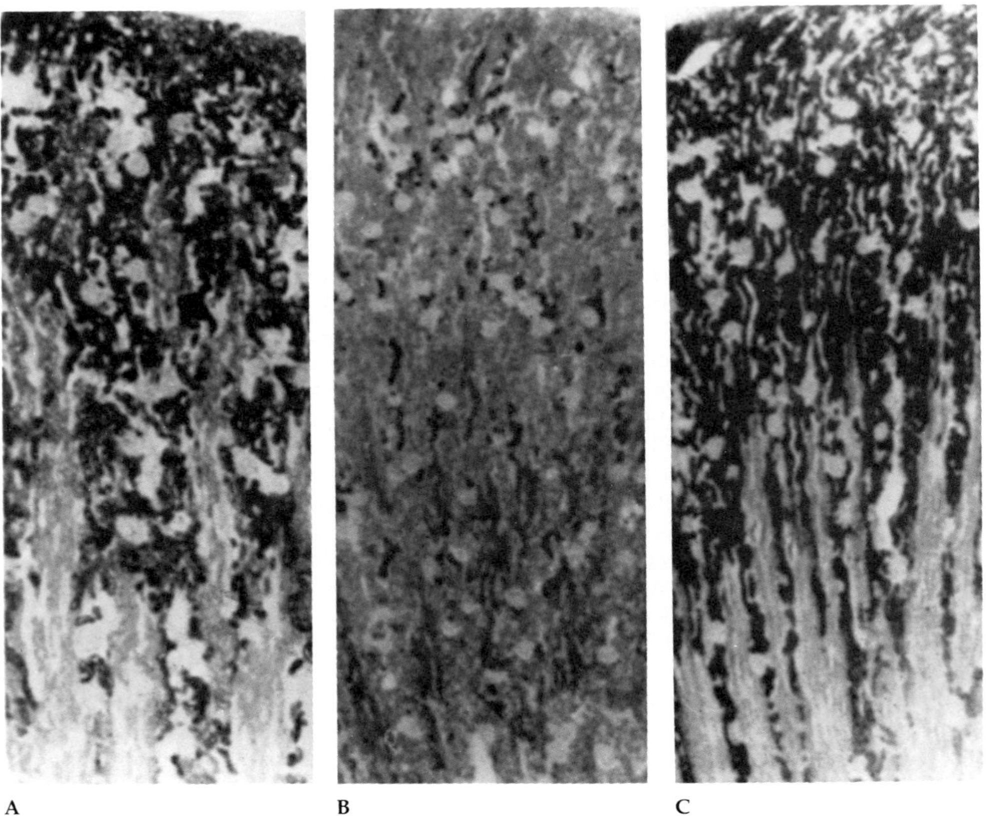

Fig. 46-6. Autoradiograph of ^{203}Hg-chlormerodrin in dog kidney during (A) acidosis, (B) acidosis-BAL, and (C) alkalosis. The proximal tubular accumulation of this organomercurial is comparable under conditions that permit (A) or prevent (C) a diuretic response. × 15. (From E. Littman et al., *J. Pharmacol. Exp. Ther.* 152:130, 1966.)

ACUTE TUBULAR NECROSIS

Ingestion of as little as 0.5 gm of $HgCl_2$ produces acute tubular necrosis in humans. Over the first few days the clinical picture is dominated by gastrointestinal symptoms including errosive gastritis with hematemesis and melena [121]. Before oliguria supervenes, chelation therapy with intravenous BAL (British antilewisite, dimercaprol) may limit renal damage [56]. Initially, oliguria should be treated by volume expansion with close monitoring of central venous or pulmonary wedge pressure. Diuresis induced by hydration, mannitol, and furosemide may not only prevent the development of oliguric acute renal failure, but persisting oliguria in the face of adequate therapy indicates renal parenchymal damage. An elevated urine sodium concentration (> 40 mEq/liter) and diminished concentrating capacity (U_{osm} < 450 mOsm/liter) in association with failure to obtain diuresis in an acutely oliguric patient with adequate circulatory status confirms the diagnosis of acute tubular necrosis. Once oliguria has become established, rigid fluid restriction is mandatory (< 500 ml/day). Acute oliguric renal failure may rapidly lead to death unless dialysis is provided.

Histologic examination of the kidneys reveals necrosis of the proximal tubules, particularly the pars recta. In the experimental model, the tubular basement membrane is spared compared with the damage incurred during ischemic tubular necrosis [15]. Backleak of inulin from the tubular lumen to peritubular capillaries has been observed in experimental animals indicating loss of integrity of the proximal tubule. Such back diffusion contributes to the reduction in inulin or creatinine clearance induced by outer cortical ischemia [73]. In the rat, $HgCl_2$-induced acute tubular necrosis is accompanied by sequestration of mercury sulfide within lysosomes of surviving proximal tubule cells [154]. The extent of damage to individual nephrons is highly variable, although tubular necrosis extends to more proximal segments after larger doses [15].

During the recovery phase, oliguria is replaced by polyuria while the glomerular filtration rate is still low. Urine flow rates may double daily, reaching a maximum of about 5 liters per day while the serum creatinine continues to rise, albeit more slowly than the initial rate of 1 to 2 mg/dl/day. During the diuretic phase, salt and water must be vigorously replaced, but potassium restriction and reduced dosage of toxic drugs normally excreted by the kidneys should be maintained. If death from hypervolemia, hyperkalemia, hemorrhagic complications, uremia, and infection is avoided, spontaneous regeneration of tubular epithelium occurs with subsequent recovery. Dystrophic calcification of necrotic tubules may, however, limit restoration of function [67] and the kidneys may show residual interstitial nephritis. The entire process from acute oliguria through polyuria and recovery may last from a few days to many months.

NEPHROTIC SYNDROME

Sporadic case reports of nephrosis following exposure to elemental or organic mercury have appeared since the middle of the present century [56]. Proteinuria in children with acrodynia ("pink disease") following external use of mercurial ointments or powders has been attributed to allergic reactions. In the occupational setting the causal relationship of mercury exposure to proteinuria and the nephrotic syndrome has been less compelling [60, 76, 117], largely because the dose-response is unpredictable and, in addition, the etiology of nephrotic syndrome unrelated to mercury is rarely known.

Renal biopsies have most often shown deposits within glomerular capillaries consistent with membranous nephropathy [137] (Fig. 46-7), but normal glomeruli (i.e., nil disease) and antiglomerular basement membrane antibody (anti-GBM Ab) deposition have also been described. In most instances proteinuria due to mercury appears to be self-limited and disappears spontaneously when the source of exposure is removed. Although the immunologic mechanisms have not been determined, observations in rats may provide a framework for understanding mercury-induced glomerular disease in humans.

Fig. 46-7. Electron micrograph of kidney from a 24-year-old man exposed to mercury vapor in an industrial electrolysis unit. The urine mercury was 174 μg/24 hr; urine protein, 3.11 gm/24 hr. Creatinine clearance was 116 ml/min/1.73 m^2. Subepithelial electron-dense deposits (arrows), presumably immune complexes, overlie the glomerular basement membrane. Lead citrate and uranyl acetate; × 11,000. (From R. R. Tubbs et al., Membranous glomerulonephritis associated with industrial mercury exposure. *Am. J. Clin. Pathol.* 77:409, 1982.)

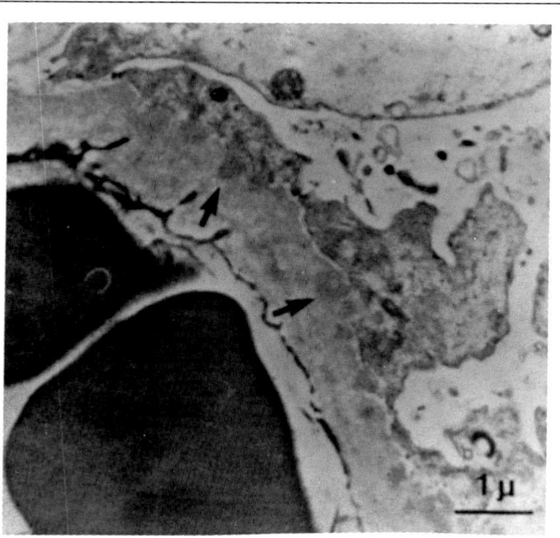

In 1971 Bariety et al. reported that multiple subcutaneous injections of $HgCl_2$ in rats [5], in doses too small to produce acute tubular necrosis, induced membranous nephropathy. Renal disease characterized by glomerular deposition of immune complexes and heavy proteinuria developed in about 2 months. Subsequent studies showed that the immune response is actually biphasic; immune complex deposition is preceded by anti-GBM Ab and complement deposition [59]. The response to mercury in the rat is under precise genetic control [122]. As little as 0.005 mg per 100 gm of body weight will elicit immunologically mediated glomerular disease in selected strains. Similar renal disease has been induced in other rodents and with alternate forms and routes of exposure including organomercurials and inhalation [14, 37]. As in humans, mercury-induced glomerular disease in rats is self-limited. Immunoglobulin localization in the glomeruli is associated with heavy proteinuria, circulating immune complexes, and polyclonal B-cell activation due to antiself Ia autoreactive T cells. The glomerular disease can be transferred to T cell–depleted rats by T cells and helper T cells taken from $HgCl_2$-treated rats of the same strain [109]. Weening et al. found evidence that the autoimmune process is initiated by mercury inhibition of suppressor T-cell functions [159].

MINIMATA DISEASE

In 1956 endemic methyl mercury poisoning was recognized in Japan arising from the contamination of food by industrial effluents in the area of Minimata Bay [104]. Severe neurologic defects including visual, speech, and gait disturbances afflicted several hundred adults whose diet consisted largely of contaminated fish. The mercury pollution had been going on for a decade before the health consequences were recognized. Fish from Minimata Bay contained up to 36 mg of mercury per kilogram [79]. Cerebral palsy was common among the children of affected mothers. Similar clusters of cases were subsequently identified in Nigata, Japan, and in Iraq, where the disease was the result of bread prepared from grain that had been treated with methyl mercury fungicide.

Although methyl mercury is more avidly accumulated by renal than by neural tissue, the kidney manifestations of Minimata disease are minor. Tubular proteinuria occurs [74], but significant albuminuria and azotemia have not been reported. Postmortem examinations have shown minimal nonspecific renal abnormalities, although rats treated with methyl mercury show increased numbers of mercury-containing lysosomes in proximal tubule epithelial cells [45]. In more heavily exposed rats, lysosomal and mitochondrial dysfunction has been observed and may account for the low-molecular-weight proteinuria in patients with Minimata disease [47].

TREATMENT

BAL is an effective chelator for acute inorganic mercury poisoning. Up to 5 mg per kilogram is given initially by the intramuscular route, followed by 2.5 mg per kilogram twice daily for 10 days. In the presence of acute renal failure the mercury chelator can be removed by hemodialysis. BAL is of doubtful value in chronic poisoning, which is effectively treated by removing the patient from the source of exposure. Dimercaptosuccinic acid (DMSA), an oral chelating agent not yet available in the United States, may play an important role in the treatment of mercury toxicity in the future [3].

Other Heavy Metals

As long as the etiology of most end-stage renal disease is unknown, it is not surprising that the contribution of environmental and industrial toxicants to the induction of chronic renal disease remains unclear. Uranium is widely used to induce experimental acute tubular necrosis and, like lead, is stored in bone, but cases of clinical renal failure due to uranium have not been reported. Uranium is selectively accumulated in the proximal tubule with a biologic half-life approximating 1 week for 95 percent of the renal stores [88]. After inhalation, the uranyl ion binds to circulating transferrin, and to proteins and phospholipids in the second and third parts of the proximal tubule. Rats given uranyl nitrate subcutaneously develop intrarenal microcysts 8 weeks after injection [68].

Acute tubular necrosis occurred in men working on the atomic bomb during the Manhattan Project in the 1940s [36], but chronic renal failure due to uranium has not been reported. A workplace hazard evaluation performed by the National Institute of Occupational Safety and Health revealed significantly increased β_2-microglobulin excretion compared to controls in workmen exposed to uranium dust [135]. The significance of this finding is doubtful, however, since the urinary β_2-microglobulin levels were well within the normal range and there was no evidence of reduced renal function. Many of these men had urine uranium levels in excess of the upper acceptable limit of 30 μg per liter.

Acute tubular necrosis has been reported after voluntary ingestion of copper sulfate in young female science students attempting suicide in Delhi, India [33].

Minimal tubular proteinuria in the absence of reduced glomerular filtration has also been reported in chromeplaters, but the implications of this finding for clinically important renal disease also remain speculative [90, 98]. Like other heavy metals, chromium is selectively accumulated in the proximal tubule and induces acute tubular necrosis when absorbed in large doses ($>$ 15 mg/kg) [80, 149]. Chromium has been recognized as an important cause of lung cancer for over 100 years, but chronic renal disease from occupational or environmental exposure has not been reported.

Unequivocal acute tubular necrosis has been produced by bismuth compounds prepared as therapeutic agents. Lower dosage induces the Fanconi syndrome with reduced glomerular filtration and bismuth-containing intranuclear inclusions in proximal tubule cells that are similar to, but distinguishable from, lead inclusions [114].

The acute cardiovascular collapse and hemolysis accompanying arsenic poisoning are associated with renal failure, but whether the mechanism of injury involves

Fig. 46-8. Renal biopsy obtained 2 years after acute renal failure from arsine poisoning in an industrial accident. The patient required peritoneal dialysis and hemodialysis for 6 weeks. The initial renal biopsy showed acute tubular necrosis. At the time of this biopsy the creatinine clearance was 24 ml/min. Left: Light microscopy shows local interstitial fibrosis, tubular atrophy, and sclerosis of 13 out of 17 glomeruli. Hematoxylin and eosin; ×300. Right: Electron microscopy shows normal and damaged proximal tubule cells. In this illustration, normal and distorted mitochondria are present in a single cell adjacent to a normal nucleus. Uranyl acetate and lead citrate; ×9,000. N = nuclei; M = normal mitochondria; m = probably newly formed mitochondria. (From R. O. Muehrcke and C. L. Pinani. Arsine-induced anuria: A correlative clinicopathological study with electron microscopic observations. *Ann. Intern. Med.* 68:853, 1968.)

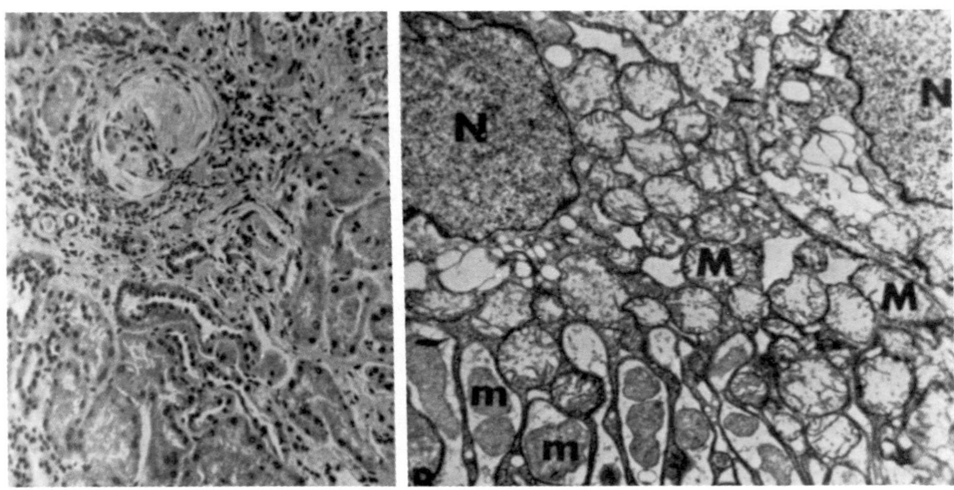

direct cellular toxicity is unclear [58]. Moonshine contaminated with arsenic produces painful polyneuropathy that is distinct from the isolated motor neuropathy of lead poisoning. Patchy cortical necrosis has been reported following consumption of arsenic-contaminated liquor with persistent residual renal failure [54, 97]. When arsenicals react with acid, the deadly, colorless, odorless gas arsine (AsH_3) evolves. Almost invariably the result of an industrial accident, arsine inhalation produces hemolysis, hematuria, and abdominal pain within a few hours, followed by acute oliguric renal failure and jaundice within 2 days [46]. Reticulocytosis, basophilic stippling, bilirubinemia, and free hemoglobin in the plasma may assist diagnosis, which is established by detecting arsenic in the urine. Acute tubular necrosis followed by residual interstitial nephritis 2 years after exposure has been documented (Fig. 46-8). BAL is ineffective once renal failure is present, and, in addition to hemodialysis, exchange transfusion may be necessary to eliminate hemoglobin-bound arsenic from the body.

References

1. Agency for Toxic Substances and Disease Registry. Public Health Service. U.S. Department of Health and Human Services. *The Nature and Extent of Lead Poisoning in Children in the United States. A Report to Congress.* Atlanta: U.S. Department of Health and Human Services, Public Health Service, 1988.
2. Anderson, K., Elinder, C. G., Hogstedt, C., et al. Mortality among cadmium and nickel-exposed workers in a Swedish battery factory. *Toxicol. Environ. Chem.* 9: 53, 1984.
3. Aposhian, H. V. DMSA and DMPS-water soluble antidotes for heavy metal poisoning. *Annu. Rev. Pharmacol. Toxicol.* 23: 193, 1983.
4. Ashouri, O. S. Hyperkalemic distal tubular acidosis and selective aldosterone deficiency: Combination in a patient with lead nephropathy. *Arch. Intern. Med.* 145: 306, 1985.
5. Bariety, J., Druet, P., Laliberte, F., et al. Glomerulonephritis with α and β 1C-globulin deposits induced in rats by mercuric chloride. *Am. J. Pathol.* 65: 293, 1971.
6. Barry, P. S. I. A comparison of concentrations of lead in human tissues. *Br. J. Ind. Med.* 32: 119, 1975.
7. Batuman, V., Landy, E., Maesaka, J. K., et al. Contribution of lead to hypertension with renal impairment. *N. Engl. J. Med.* 309: 17, 1983.
8. Batuman, V., Maesaka, J. K., Haddad, B., et al. The role of lead in gout nephropathy. *N. Engl. J. Med.* 304: 520, 1981.
9. Batuman, V., Dreisbach, A., Chun, E., et al. Lead increases the red cell sodium-lithium countertransport. *Am. J. Kidney Dis.* 14: 200, 1989.
10. Batuman, V., Wedeen, R. P., Bogden, J., et al. Reducing bone lead content by chelation treatment in chronic lead poisoning. An in vivo X-ray fluorescence and bone biopsy study. *Environ. Res.* 48: 70, 1989.
11. Beck, L. H. Requiem for gouty nephropathy. *Kidney Int.* 30: 280, 1986.
12. Behringer, D., Craswell, P., Mohl, C., et al. Urinary lead excretion in uremic patients. *Nephron* 42: 323, 1986.
13. Bennett, W. M. Lead nephropathy. *Kidney Int.* 28: 212, 1985.
14. Bernaudin, J. F., Druet, E., Druet, P., et al. Inhalation or ingestion of organic or inorganic mercurials produces auto-immune disease in rats. *Clin. Immunol. Immunopathol.* 20: 129, 1981.
15. Biber, T. U. L., Mylle, M., Baines, A. D., et al. A study by micropuncture and microdissection of acute renal damage in rats. *Am. J. Med.* 44: 664, 1968.
16. Blainey, J. D., Adams, R. G., Brewer, D. B., et al. Cadmium-induced osteomalacia. *Br. J. Ind. Med.* 37: 278, 1980.
17. Bolton, W. K., Suratt, P. M., and Stingill, A. Rapidly progressive silica nephropathy. *Am. J. Med.* 71: 823, 1981.
18. Boscolo, P., and Carmignani, M. Neurohumoral blood pressure regulation in lead exposure. *Environ. Health Perspect.* 78: 101, 1988.
19. Boscolo, P., Galli, G., Iannaccone, A., et al. Plasma renin activity and urinary kallikrein excretion in lead-exposed workers as related to hypertension and nephropathy. *Life Sci.* 28: 175, 1988.
20. Buchet, J-P., Roels, H., Bernard, A., et al. Assessment of renal function of workers exposed to inorganic lead, cadmium or mercury vapor. *Am. J. Occup. Med.* 22: 741, 1980.
21. Campbell, B. C., Elliott, H. L., and Meredith, P. A. Lead exposure and renal failure: Does renal insufficiency influence lead kinetics? *Toxicol. Lett.* 9: 121, 1981.
22. Campbell, B. C., Meredith, P. A., and Scott, J. J. C. Lead exposure and changes in the renin-angiotensin-aldosterone system in man. *Toxicol. Lett.* 55: 25, 1985.
23. Cantilena, L. R., Jr., and Klaassen, C. D. The effect of repeated administration of several chelators on the distribution and excretion of cadmium. *Toxicol. Appl. Pharmacol.* 66: 361, 1982.
24. Chai, S., and Webb, R. C. Effects of lead on vascular reactivity. *Environ. Health Perspect.* 78: 85, 1988.
25. Chamberlain, A. C. Prediction of response of blood lead to airborne and dietary lead from volunteer experiments with lead isotopes. *Proc. R. Soc. Lond.* [*Biol.*] 244: 149, 1985.
26. Cheung, W. Y. Calmodulin: Its potential role in cell proliferation and heavy metal toxicity. *Fed. Proc.* 43: 2995, 1984.
27. Chisolm, J. J., Harrison, H. C., Eberlern, W. R., et al. Aminoaciduria, hypophosphatemia and rickets in lead poisoning. *Am. J. Dis. Child.* 89: 159, 1955.
28. Chisolm, J. J., Mellits, E. D., and Barrett, M. B. Interrelationships Among Blood Lead Concentration, Quantitative Daily ALA-U and Urinary Lead Output Following Calcium EDTA. In G. F. Nordberg (ed.), *Effects and Dose-Response Relationships of Toxic Metals.* Amsterdam: Elsevier, 1976.
29. Clarkson, T. W., Hursh, J. B., Sager, P. R., et al. Mercury. In T. W. Clarkson, L. Friberg, G. F. Nordberg, et al. (eds.), *Biological Monitoring of Heavy Metals.* New York: Plenum, 1988.
30. Colleoni, N., and D'Amico, G. Chronic lead accumulation as a possible cause of renal failure in gouty patients. *Nephron* 44: 32, 1986.
31. Cramer, K., Goyer, R. A., Jagenburg, R., et al. Renal ultrastructure, renal function, and parameters of lead toxicity in workers with different periods of lead exposure. *Br. J. Ind. Med.* 31: 113, 1974.
32. Craswell, P. W., Price, J., Boyle, P. D., et al. Chronic renal failure with gout: A marker of chronic lead poisoning. *Kidney Int.* 26: 319, 1984.
33. Dash, S. C. Copper sulfate poisoning and acute renal failure. *Int. J. Artif. Organs* 12: 610, 1989.

34. Dobbie, J. W., and Smith, M. J. B. Urinary and serum silicon in normal and uraemic individuals. *Ciba Found. Symp.* 12: 194, 1986.
35. Doll, N. J., Stankus, R. P., Hughes, J., et al. Immune complexes and autoantibodies in silicosis. *J. Allergy Immunol.* 68: 281, 1981.
36. Dounce, A. L. The Mechanism of Action of Uranium Compounds in the Animal Body. In C. Voegtlin and H. C. Hodge (eds.), *Pharmacology and Toxicology of Uranium Compounds.* Div. VI, Vol. 1. New York: McGraw-Hill, 1949. Chap. 15.
37. Druet, P., Druet, E., Potdevin, F., et al. Immune type glomerulonephritis induced by $HgCl_2$ in the Brown Norway rat. *Ann. Immunol.* (Inst. Pasteur). 129: 777, 1978.
38. Elinder, C-G. Other Toxic Effects. In L. Friberg, C-G. Elinder, T. Kjellstrom, et al. (eds.), *Cadmium and Health: A Toxicological and Epidemiological Appraisal.* Vol. II. Boca Raton: CRC Press, 1986.
39. Elinder, C-G., and Nordberg, M. Metallothionein. In L. Friberg, C-G. Elinder, T. Kjellstrom, et al. (eds.), *Cadmium and Health: A Toxicological and Epidemiological Appraisal.* Vol. II. Boca Raton: CRC Press, 1986.
40. Elinder, C-G., Edling, C., Lindberg, E., et al. Beta-2-microglobulinuria among workers previously exposed to cadmium: Follow-up and dose response analysis. *Am. J. Ind. Med.* 8: 553, 1985.
41. Elwood, P. C., Davey-Smith, G., Oldham, P. D., et al. Two Welsh surveys of blood lead and blood pressure. *Environ. Health Perspect.* 78: 119, 1988.
42. Emmerson, B. T. Chronic lead nephropathy: The diagnostic use of calcium EDTA and the association with gout. *Aust. Ann. Med.* 12: 310, 1963.
43. Emmerson, B. T. Chronic lead nephropathy. *Kidney Int.* 4: 1, 1973.
44. Fanning, D. A mortality study of lead workers. 1926–1985. *Arch. Environ. Health* 43: 247, 1988.
45. Fowler, B. A., Hayes, W., Brown, M. S., et al. The effects of chronic oral methyl mercury exposure on the lysosome system of rat kidney. *Lab. Invest.* 32: 313, 1975.
46. Fowler, B. A., and Weissberg, J. B. Arsine poisoning. *N. Engl. J. Med.* 291: 1171, 1974.
47. Fowler, B. A., and Woods, J. S. Ultrastructural and biochemical changes in renal mitochondria during chronic oral methyl mercury exposure. *Exp. Mol. Pathol.* 27: 403, 1977.
48. Friberg, L. Proteinuria and kidney injury among workmen exposed to cadmium and nickel dust. *J. Ind. Hygiene* 30: 32, 1948.
49. Friberg, L. Edathamil calcium-disodium in cadmium poisoning. *Arch. Ind. Health* 13: 18, 1956.
50. Friberg, L. Cadmium and the kidney. *Environ. Health Perspect.* 54: 1, 1984.
51. Friberg, L. Introduction. In L. Friberg, C-G. Elinder, T. Kjellstrom, et al. (eds.), *Cadmium and Health: A Toxicological and Epidemiological Appraisal.* Vol. II. Boca Raton: CRC Press, 1986.
52. Gartside, P. S. The relationship of blood lead levels and blood pressure in NHANES II: Additional calculations. *Environ. Health Perspect.* 78: 31, 1988.
53. Geiger, H., Bahner, U., Anderes, S., et al. Cadmium and renal hypertension. *J. Human Hypertens.* 3: 23, 1989.
54. Gerhardt, R. E., Crecelius, E. A., and Hudson, J. B. Moonshine-related arsenic poisoning. *Arch. Intern. Med.* 140: 211, 1980.
55. Germain, M. J., Braden, G. L., and Fitzgibbons, J. P. Failure of chelation therapy in lead nephropathy. *Arch. Intern. Med.* 144: 2419, 1984.
56. Gerstner, H. B., and Huff, J. E. Selected case histories and epidemiologic examples of human mercury poisoning. *Clin. Toxicol.* 11: 131, 1977.
57. Gertz, M. A., Kyle, R. A., Greipp, P. R., et al. Beta-2-microglobulin predicts survival in primary systemic amyloidosis. *Am. J. Med.* 89: 609, 1990.
58. Gilberson, A., Vaziri, N. D., Mirahamadi, K., et al. Hemodialysis of acute arsenic intoxication with transient renal failure. *Arch. Intern. Med.* 136: 1303, 1976.
59. Goldman, M., Baran, D., and Druet, P. Polyclonal activation and experimental nephropathies. *Kidney Int.* 34: 141, 1988.
60. Goldwater, L. J. Mercury: A History of Quicksilver. Baltimore: York Press, 1972.
61. Gompertz, D., Flecter, J. G., Perkins, J., et al. Renal dysfunction in cadmium smelters: Relation to in-vivo liver and kidney cadmium concentrations. *Lancet* 1: 1185, 1983.
62. Goyer, R. A. Ascorbic acid and EDTA treatment of lead toxicity in rats. *Life* 24: 433, 1979.
63. Goyer, R. A., Leonard, D. L., Bream, P. R., et al. Aminoaciduria in experimental lead poisoning. *Proc. Soc. Exp. Biol. Med.* 135: 767, 1970.
64. Goyer, R. A., and Wilson, M. H. Lead-induced inclusion bodies. Results of ethylenediaminetetraacetic acid treatment. *Lab. Invest.* 32: 149, 1975.
65. Goyer, R. A., Leonard, D. L., Moore, J. F., et al. Lead dosage and the role of the intranuclear inclusion body: An experimental study. *Arch. Environ. Health* 20: 705, 1970.
66. Grandjean, P. *Biological Effects of Organolead Compounds.* Boca Raton, Fla.: CRC Press, 1984.
67. Gritzka, T. L., and Trump, B. F. Renal tubular lesions caused by mercuric chloride. *Am. J. Pathol.* 52: 1225, 1968.
68. Haley, D. P., Bulger, R. E., and Dobyan, D. C. The long-term effects of uranyl nitrate on the structure and function of the rat kidney. *Virchows Arch. B Cell. Pathol.* 41: 181, 1982.
69. Hall, P. W. Endemic Balkan Nephropathy. In G. A. Porter (ed.), *Nephrotoxic Mechanisms of Drugs and Environmental Toxins.* New York: Plenum, 1982.
70. Harlan, W. R. The relationship of blood lead levels to blood pressure in the U.S. population. *Environ. Health Perspect.* 78: 9, 1988.
71. Hauglustaine, D., Van Damme, B., Daenens, P., et al. Silicon nephropathy: A possible occupational hazard. *Nephron* 26: 219, 1980.
72. Hong, C. D., Hanenson, I. G., Lerner, S., et al. Occupational exposure to lead: effects on renal function. *Kidney Int.* 18: 489, 1980.
73. Hsu, C. H., Kurtz, T. W., Rosenzweig, J., et al. Renal hemodynamics in $HgCl_2$-induced acute renal failure. *Nephron.* 18: 326, 1977.
74. Iesato, K., Wakashin, M., Wakashin, Y., et al. Renal tubular dysfunction in Minimata disease. Detection of renal tubular antigen and beta-2-microglobulin in the urine. *Ann. Intern. Med.* 86: 731, 1977.
75. Inglis, J. A., Henderson, D. A., and Emmerson, B. T. The pathology and pathogenesis of chronic lead nephropathy occurring in Queensland. *J. Pathol.* 124: 65, 1978.
76. Joselow, M. M., and Goldwater, L. J. Absorption and excretion of mercury in man. Relationship between uri-

nary mercury and proteinuria. *Arch. Environ. Health* 15: 155, 1967.
77. Kazantzis, G. Cadmium nephropathy. *Contrib. Nephrol.* 16: 161, 1979.
78. Kazantzis, G. Renal tubular dysfunction and abnormalities of calcium metabolism in cadmium workers. *Environ. Health Perspect.* 28: 155, 1979.
79. Kazantzis, G. Mercury. In H. A. Waldron (ed.), *Metals in the Environment*. New York: Academic, 1980.
80. Kaufman, D. B., DiNickola, W., and McIntosh, R. Acute potassium dichromate poisoning. *Am. J. Dis. Child.* 119: 374, 1970.
81. Kido, T., Nogawa, K., Honda, R., et al. The association between renal dysfunction and osteopenia in environmentally cadmium-exposed subjects. *Environ. Res.* 51: 71, 1990.
82. Kido, T., Nogawa, K., Ishizaki, M., et al. Long-term observation of serum creatinine and arterial blood pH in persons with cadmium-induced renal dysfunction. *Arch. Environ. Health* 45: 35, 1990.
83. Kjellstrom, T. Renal Effects. In L. Friberg, C-G. Elinder, T. Kjellstrom, et al. (eds.), *Cadmium and Health: A Toxicological and Epidemiological Appraisal*. Vol. II. Boca Raton: CRC Press, 1986.
84. Kjellstrom, T. Effect on Bone, Vitamin D and Calcium Metabolism. In L. Friberg, C-G. Elinder, T. Kjellstrom, et al. (eds.), *Cadmium and Health: A Toxicological and Epidemiological Appraisal*. Vol. II. Boca Raton: CRC Press, 1986.
85. Kopp, S. J., Barron, J. T., and Tow, J. P. Cardiovascular actions of lead and relationship to hypertension: A review. *Scand. J. Work Environ. Health* 11: 15, 1985.
86. Lauwerys, R. R., and Bernard, A. M. Early detection of the nephrotoxic effects of industrial chemicals: State of the art and future prospects. *Am. J. Ind. Med.* 11: 275, 1987.
87. Leckie, W. J. H., and Tomsett, S. L. The diagnostic and therapeutic use of edathamil calcium disodium (EDTA Versene) in excessive inorganic lead absorption. *Q. J. Med.* 27: 65, 1958.
88. Leggett, R. W. The behavior and chemical toxicity of U in the kidney: A reassessment. *Health Phys.* 57: 365, 1889.
89. Lilis, R., Garilescu, N., Nestoresca, C., et al. Nephropathy in chronic lead poisoning. *Br. J. Ind. Med.* 25: 196, 1968.
90. Lindberg, E. K., and Vesterberg, O. Urinary excretion of proteins in chromeplaters, exchromeplaters and referents. *Scand. J. Work Environ. Health* 9: 505, 1983.
91. Littman, E., Goldstein, M. H., Kasen, L., et al. The relationship of the intrarenal distribution of Hg^{203}-chlormerodrin to the diuretic effect. *J. Pharmacol. Exp. Ther.* 152: 130, 1966.
92. Magos, L., Sparrow, S., and Snowden, R. The comparative renal toxicology of phenylmercury and mercuric chloride. *Arch. Toxicol.* 50: 133, 1982.
93. Mahaffey, K. R., Annest, J. L., Roberts, J., et al. National estimates of blood lead levels: United States, 1976–1980. Association with selected demographic and socioeconomic factors. *N. Engl. J. Med.* 307: 573, 1982.
94. Meyer, B. R., Fischbein, A., Rosenman, K., et al. Increased urinary enzyme excretion in workers exposed to nephrotoxic chemicals. *Am. J. Med.* 76: 989, 1984.
95. Moreau, T., Orsseaud, G., Huet, G., et al. Influence of membrane sodium transport upon the relation between blood lead and blood pressure in a general male population. *Environ. Health Perspect.* 78: 47, 1988.
96. Morrison, A. R., Pascoe, N., Tauk, N., et al. Biochemical alterations of membrane lipids associated with renal injury. *Fed. Proc.* 43: 2811, 1984.
97. Muehrcke, R. C., and Pirani, C. L. Arsine-induced anuria: A correlative clinicopathological study with electron microscopic observations. *Ann. Intern. Med.* 68: 853, 1968.
98. Mutti, A., Lucertini, S., Valcalvi, P., et al. Urinary excretion of brush-border antigen revealed by monoclonal antibody: early indicator of toxic nephropathy. *Lancet* 2: 914, 1985.
99. National Research Council. *Airborne Lead in Perspective*. Washington: National Academy of Sciences, 1972.
100. Needleman, H. L., Schell, A., Bellinger, D., et al. The long-term effects of exposure to low doses of lead in childhood. An 11 year follow-up report. *N. Engl. J. Med.* 322: 83, 1990.
101. Neri, L. C., Hewitt, D., and Orser, B. Blood lead and blood pressure: Analysis of cross-sectional and longitudinal data from Canada. *Environ. Health Perspect.* 78: 123, 1988.
102. Nicaud, P., Lafitte, A., Gros, A., et al. Les lesions osseuses de l'intoxication chronique par le cadmium. Aspects radiologiques a type de syndrome de Milkman. *Bull. Mem. Soc. Med. Hop. Paris* 19: 204, 1942.
103. Nogawa, K., Tsuritani, I., Kido, T., et al. Serum vitamin D metabolites in cadmium-exposed persons with renal damage. *Arch. Environ. Health* 62: 189, 1990.
104. Nomiyama, K. Recent progress and perspectives in cadmium health effects studies. *Sci. Total Environ.* 14: 199, 1980.
105. Nordberg, G. F., Kjellstrom, T., and Nordberg, M. Kinetics and Metabolism. Other Toxic Effects. In L. Friberg, C-G. Elinder, T. Kjellstrom, et al. (eds.), *Cadmium and Health: A Toxicological and Epidemiological Appraisal*. Vol. II. Boca Raton: CRC Press, 1986.
106. Osorio, A. M., Thun, M. J., Novak, R. F., et al. Silica and glomerulonephritis: A case report and review of the literature. *Am. J. Kidney Dis.* 9: 224, 1987.
107. Parkinson, D. K., Hodgson, M. J., Bromet, E. J., et al. Occupational lead exposure and blood pressure. *Br. J. Ind. Med.* 44: 744, 1987.
108. Peitzman, S. J., Bodison, W., and Ellis, I. Moonshine drinking among hypertensive veterans in Philadelphia. *Arch. Intern. Med.* 145: 632, 1985.
109. Pelletier, L., Pasquier, R., Rossert, J., et al. Autoreactive T cells in mercury-induced autoimmunity. Ability to induce the autoimmune disease. *J. Immunol.* 140: 750, 1988.
110. Piomelli, A., Seaman, C., Zullow, D., et al. Threshold for lead damage to heme synthesis in urban children. *Proc. Natl. Acad. Sci.* 79: 3335, 1982.
111. Pirkle, J. L., Schwartz, J., Landis, J. R., et al. The relationship between blood lead levels and blood pressure and its cardiovascular risk implications. *Am. J. Epidemiol.* 121: 246, 1985.
112. Pocock, S. J., Shaper, A. G., Ashby, D., et al. The relationship between blood lead, blood pressure, stroke, and heart attacks in middle-aged British men. *Environ. Health Perspect.* 78: 23, 1988.
113. Rabinowitz, M. B. Kinetic analysis of lead metabolism in healthy humans. *J. Clin. Invest.* 58: 260, 1976.
114. Randall, R. E., Osheroff, R. J., Bakerman, S., et al. Bismuth nephrotoxicity. *Ann. Intern. Med.* 77: 481, 1972.
115. Ritz, E., Mann, J., and Stoeppler, M. Lead and the kidney. *Adv. Nephrol.* 17: 241, 1988.

116. Roels, H., Djubgang, J., Buchet, J. P., et al. Evolution of cadmium-induced renal dysfunction in workers removed from exposure. *Scand. J. Work Environ. Health* 8: 191, 1982.
117. Roels, H. A., Lauwerys, R. R., Buchet, J.-P., et al. Comparison of renal function and psychomotor performance in workers exposed to elemental mercury. *Int. Arch. Occup. Environ. Health* 50: 77, 1982.
118. Roels, H. A., Lauwerys, R. R., Buchet, J. P., et al. Health significance of cadmium-induced renal dysfunction: A five-year follow-up. *Br. J. Ind. Med.* 46: 755, 1989.
119. Roels, H. A., Lauwerys, R. R., Buchet, J.-P., et al. In vivo measurement of liver and kidney cadmium in workers exposed to this metal: Its significance with respect to cadmium in blood and urine. *Environ. Res.* 26: 217, 1981.
120. Rosen, J. F., Markovitz, M. E., Bijur, P. E., et al. L-line x-ray fluorescence of cortical bone lead compared with $CaNa_2EDTA$ test in lead-toxic children: Public health implications. *Proc. Natl. Acad. Sci. U.S.A.* 86: 685, 1989.
121. Sanchez-Sicilia, L., Seto, D. S., Nakamoto, S., et al. Acute mercurial intoxication treated by hemodialysis. *Ann. Intern. Med.* 59: 692, 1963.
122. Sapin, C., Druet, E., and Druet, P. Induction of anti-glomerular basement membrane antibodies in the Brown-Norway rat by mercuric chloride. *Clin. Exp. Immunol.* 28: 173, 1977.
123. Schumann, G. B., Lerner, S. I., Weiss, M. A., et al. Inclusion-bearing cells in industrial workers exposed to lead. *Am. J. Clin. Pathol.* 74: 192, 1980.
124. Scott, R., Cunningham, C., McLelland, A., et al. The importance of cadmium as a factor in calcified upper urinary tract stone disease—a prospective 7 year study. *Br. J. Urol.* 54: 584, 1982.
125. Selevan, S. G., Landrigan, P. J., Stern, F. B., et al. Mortality of lead smelter workers. *Am. J. Epidemiol.* 122: 673, 1985.
126. Sharp, D. S., Becker, C. E., and Smith, A. H. Chronic low-level lead exposure. Its role in the pathogenesis of hypertension. *Med. Toxicol.* 2: 210, 1987.
127. Skerfving, S., Christoffersson, J-O., Schutz, A., et al. Biological monitoring, by in vivo XRF measurements, of occupational exposure to lead, cadmium, and mercury. *Biol. Trace Element Res.* 13: 241, 1987.
128. Somervaille, L. J., Chettle, D. R., Scott, M. C., et al. In vivo tibia lead measurements as an index of cumulative exposure in occupationally exposed subjects. *Br. J. Ind. Med.* 45: 174, 1988.
129. Squibb, K. S., Pritchard, J. B., and Fowler, B. A. Renal Metabolism and Toxicity of Metallothionein. In E. C. Foulkes (ed.), *Biological Roles of Metallothionein.* New York: Elsevier/North Holland Press, 1982.
130. Steenland, N. K., Thun, M. J., Ferguson, C. W., et al. Occupational and other exposures associated with male end-stage renal disease: A case/control study. *Am. J. Public Health* 80: 153, 1990.
131. Stephens, G. A. Cadmium poisoning. *J. Ind. Hygiene* 2: 129, 1920.
132. Stoeckle, J. D., Hardy, H., and Weber, A. L. Chronic beryllium disease. Long-term follow-up of sixty cases and selective review of the literature. *Am. J. Med.* 46: 545, 1969.
133. Stonard, M. D., Chater, B. V., Duffield, D. P., et al. An evaluation of renal function in workers occupationally exposed to mercury vapour. *Int. Arch. Occup. Environ. Health* 52: 177, 1983.
134. Tepper, L. Renal function subsequent to childhood plumbism. *Arch. Environ. Health* 7: 76, 1963.
135. Thun, M. J., Baker, D. B., Streeland, K., et al. Renal toxicity in uranium mill workers. *Scand. J. Work Environ. Health* 11: 83, 1985.
136. Thun, M. J., Osorio, A. M., Schober, S., et al. Nephropathy in cadmium workers—assessment of risk from airborne occupational cadmium exposure. *Br. J. Ind. Med.* 46: 689, 1989.
137. Tubbs, R. R., Gephardt, G. N., McMahon, J. T., et al. Membranous glomerulonephritis associated with industrial mercury exposure. *Am. J. Clin. Pathol.* 77: 409, 1982.
138. United States Environmental Protection Agency. *Air Quality Criteria for Lead.* Final draft. EPA 600/8-83-028dF. Research Triangle Park, N.C.: Environmental Criteria and Assessment Office, 1986.
139. Vacca, C. Heavy metal nephrotoxicity: Lead differentiated from cadmium and mercury. *Am. J. Clin. Pathol.* 73: 308, 1980.
140. Vander, A. J. Chronic effects of lead on the renin-angiotensin system. *Environ. Health Perspect.* 78: 77, 1988.
141. Van de Vyver, F. L., D'Hase, P. C., Visser, W. J., et al. Bone lead in dialysis patients. *Kidney Int.* 33: 601, 1988.
142. Verschoor, M., Herber, R., van Hemmen, J., et al. Renal function of workers with low-level cadmium exposure. *Scand. J. Work Environ. Health* 13: 232, 1987.
143. Wedeen, R. P. Occupational renal diseases. *Am. J. Kidney Dis.* 3: 241, 1984.
144. Wedeen, R. P. *Poison in the Pot: The Legacy of Lead.* Carbondale, Ill: Southern Illinois University Press, 1984.
145. Wedeen, R. P. Blood lead levels, dietary calcium, and hypertension. *Ann. Intern. Med.* 102: 403, 1985.
146. Wedeen, R. P. Occupational and environmental renal diseases. *Curr. Nephrol.* 11: 65, 1988.
147. Wedeen, R. P. Were the hatters of New Jersey "mad?" *Am. J. Ind. Med.* 16: 225, 1989.
148. Wedeen, R. P. *In vivo* tibial XRF measurement of bone lead. *Arch. Environ. Health* 45: 69, 1990.
149. Wedeen, R. P. Chromium-induced kidney disease. *Environ. Health Perspect.* 92: 71, 1991.
150. Wedeen, R. P. Heavy Metals and the Kidney. In J. S. Cameron, A. M. Davison, J.-P. Grunfeld, et al. (eds.), *Oxford Textbook of Clinical Nephrology.* Oxford: Oxford University Press, 1992, pp. 837–852.
151. Wedeen, R. P. Lead, the Kidney, and Hypertension. In H. Needleman (ed.), *Human Lead Exposure.* Boca Raton: CRC Press, 1992, pp. 170–189.
152. Wedeen, R. P. The Politics of Lead. In H. A. Sheehan and R. P. Wedeen (eds.), *Toxic Circles: Workplace to Community.* New Brunswick: Rutgers University Press. (In press.)
153. Wedeen, R. P., Batuman, V., and Landy, E. The safety of the EDTA lead-mobilization test. *Environ. Res.* 30: 58, 1983.
154. Wedeen, R. P., and Cheeks, C. Intrarenal distribution of exchangeable calcium in $HgCl_2$-induced acute tubular necrosis. *J. Histochem. Cytochem.* 36: 1103, 1988.
155. Wedeen, R. P., and Goldstein, M. H. Renal tubular localization of chlormerodrin labelled with mercury-203 by autoradiography. *Science* 141: 438, 1963.
156. Weeden, R. P., Maesaka, J. K., Weiner, B., et al. Occupational lead nephropathy. *Am. J. Med.* 59: 630, 1975.
157. Wedeen, R. P., Mallik, D. K., and Batuman, V. Detection and treatment of occupational lead nephropathy. *Arch. Intern. Med.* 139: 53, 1979.
158. Wedeen, R. P., Mallik, D. F., Batuman, V., et al. Geographic lead nephropathy: A case report. *Environ. Res.* 17: 409, 1978.
159. Weening, J. J., Fleuren, G. J., and Hoedemaeker, P. J.

Demonstration of antinuclear antibodies in mercuric chloride-induced glomerulopathy in the rat. *Lab. Invest.* 39: 405, 1978.

160. Weiler, E., Khalil-Manesh, F., and Gonick, H. Effects of lead and natriuretic hormone on kinetics of sodium-potassium-activated adenosine triphosphatase: Possible relevance to hypertension. *Environ. Health Perspect.* 78: 113, 1988.
161. Wright, L. F., Saylor, R. P., and Cecere, F. A. Occult lead intoxication in patients with gout and kidney disease. *J. Rheumatol.* 11: 517, 1984.
162. Wright, N., Yeoman, W. B., and Carter, G. F. Massive oral ingestion of elemental mercury without poisoning. *Lancet* 206, 1980.
163. Yver, L., Marechaud, R., Picaud, D., et al. Insuffisance renale aigue au cours d'un saturnisme professionel. *Nouvelle Presse Med.* 7: 1541, 1978.

VIII

Acute Renal Failure

Pathophysiology of Cell Ischemia

Thomas J. Burke
Robert W. Schrier

The role of ischemia in causing renal functional injury has been approached both at the whole-kidney and at the cellular level with freshly isolated renal epithelial tissue (tubules) and with tissue culture. Since it has been difficult to obtain reasonably large quantities of renal vascular smooth muscle and renal endothelial cells, these are usually harvested from other vascular areas. Glomerular mesangial cells, which are sensitive to oxygen deprivation and oxidant stress, have, however, been amenable to experimental studies using primary cultures. Several very excellent reviews concerning the pathophysiology of ischemic renal injury have been published, and the reader is referred to these for additional insights and perspectives into various aspects of oxygen deprivation injury [11, 26, 249, 251, 253, 276, 311, 314, 315].

Over the last 5 to 6 years, these complementary studies have permitted investigators to test the relative importance of specific defects in the isolated cellular systems to the overall functional, biochemical, and morphologic injury that accompanies ischemic acute renal failure in vivo. Most of the efforts, however, have been directed at isolated cell systems using freshly prepared tissue, primary tissue culture, or established cell lines, and this chapter highlights the major results from these studies. There are, however, two drawbacks to cultured cell studies: First, both primary and established cultures are quite resistant to the effects of oxygen deprivation, and, second, biochemical diversity appears to be lost with increasing culture time/passage.

It is also apparent that the injury due to complete ischemia induced by, for example, norepinephrine infusion into the renal artery may result in a different pathogenesis of functional injury from that induced by placing a totally occlusive clamp on the renal artery. Furthermore, both of these models of complete renal ischemia apparently induce different degrees of cellular as well as functional injury compared to those that attend less severe reductions in renal blood flow, as may occur, for example, in cyclosporine treatment [68, 340] or ureteral obstruction or hemorrhage [14, 96, 121, 142, 229, 346, 347]. In addition, these latter types of insult often result in either total or regional hypoxia rather than complete anoxia, and studies from several laboratories clearly demonstrate significant differences in cellular metabolism between anoxic and hypoxic injury [1, 24, 107, 134, 150, 158, 292, 317]. It has also been useful to experimentally mimic certain effects of oxygen deprivation in well-oxygenated systems. Thus, chemical hypoxia induced by mitochondrial respiratory inhibitors or proton ionophores, which uncouple oxidation from phosphorylation, provides insight into the mechanism of injury independent from oxygen deprivation itself. Such studies, however, have a propensity to increase oxygen radical–mediated cell damage since buffering or detoxification of reactive oxygen molecules (ROM) is compromised under these conditions.

Finally, it has also become evident that species differences and temperatures, as well as the age of the animal, play significant roles in assessing the mechanisms of, and protection from, cell ischemic injury [7, 8, 30, 56, 77, 80, 139, 221, 348, 350]. Irrespective of these subtle but important experimental differences, it is unquestioned that the first effect of ischemia, hypoxia, or mitochondrial inhibition is on adenine nucleotide metabolism. Decreased production of adenosine triphosphate (ATP) precedes virtually every other mechanism of cell injury during ischemia (Table 47-1).

Adenine Nucleotides

That removal of oxygen from renal cells or whole kidneys results in prompt decreases in the cellular ATP pool is unquestioned. Initially, adenosine diphosphate (ADP) and adenosine monophosphate (AMP) concentrations increase [10], and further catabolism of AMP to hypoxanthine and, in some species, to xanthine occurs as the ischemic period is prolonged [32, 58, 69, 71, 73, 78, 92, 111, 133, 165, 192, 305, 349]. Following the impressive in vivo protective effects resulting from provision of exogenous ATP-$MgCl_2$ to ischemic rat kidneys by Siegel and colleagues [95, 271, 284, 289, 290], several laboratories have sought to define the mechanisms whereby loss of ATP results in cellular injury [12, 66, 83, 84, 118, 120, 179, 188, 259, 280, 287, 302, 306, 310, 323, 327].

It is important to consider the decreases in cellular ATP in response to ischemia first with respect to the regional location of the tissues within the kidney [351]. For example, in the renal cortex, especially in the outer and middle cortex, high rates of blood flow exist and, with this highly efficient delivery of oxygenated blood, proximal convoluted tubules (PT) exhibit substantial oxidative metabolism and little glycolytic capacity [11, 31, 44, 248, 280, 284, 294, 316]. Gluconeogenic pathways are prominent [248], and from the standpoint of studies using freshly isolated PT or primary cultures of PT, this oxidative capacity is quite important. Analysis of individual nephron segments confirms the presence of the appropriate enzymes for these biochemical reactions [31]. In deeper renal locations, especially in the proximal straight tubule (S_3, or pars recta) and in the cortical and medullary thick ascending limb (TAL) [107, 158, 259], regional blood flow is derived from vessels that have already delivered well-oxygenated blood to other tissues [35, 36, 158]. In the medullary rays, cortical labyrinths, and outer medulla, oxygen availability is precariously low [158] and, thus, glycolytic capacity of renal tubules in these regions is higher than that observed in the tubules from the outer cortex. These biochemical observations together with the extensive necrosis that is found in these deeper cortical regions have led to attempts to enhance anaerobic glycolysis by providing certain substrates such as α-ketoglutarate or fumarate. In the perfused rat kidney, such additions improve the functional recovery from ischemia [107], but in the

Table 47-1. Renal biochemical and ionic disturbances during 0 to 60 minutes of ischemia

↓ ATP, ↑ ADP, ↑ AMP
Na^+ entry
K^+ efflux
Membrane depolarization
Ca^{2+} influx
Mitochondrial Ca^{2+} overload (H)
Mg^{2+} efflux
↓ Mitochondrial respiration
↑ Mitochondrial/microsomal PLA_2
↑ Oxygen free radicals
Acidosis (A)
↑ Endothelial-derived relaxing factor via adenosine
Cell swelling
Brush border internalization
↓ Na-K-ATPase
↓ Ca-ATPase
↑ Free fatty acids
Lipid peroxidation
↓ Glutathione (L)
↑ Hypoxanthine/xanthine (L)
Mitochondrial membrane reordering
Lysophospholipid changes (L)
Protease activation
Xanthine oxidase
↓ Glycine concentration
↑ NADH, ↓ NAD
Neutrophil activation
↑ Platelet activating factor
Basement membrane injury
Cytoskeletal changes

(H) = during hypoxia; (A) = during anoxia; (L) = late event; ADP = adenosine diphosphate; AMP = adenosine monophosphate; ATPase = adenosine triphosphatase; NAD, NADH = nicotinamide adenine dinucleotide.

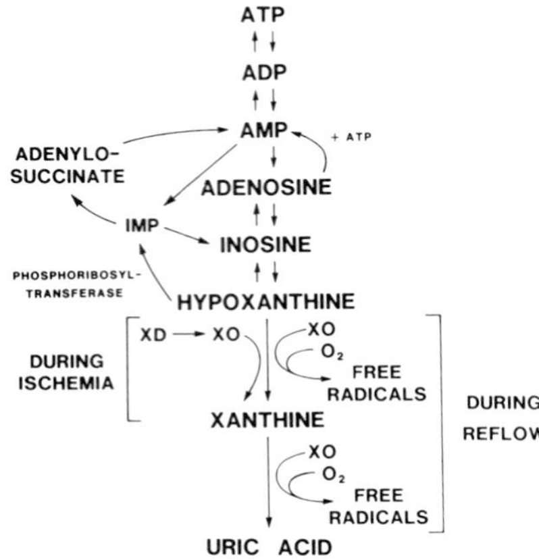

Fig. 47-1. The degradation pathway of ATP to uric acid. During ischemia XD is rapidly converted to XO, which, when reperfusion ensues, can catabolize hypoxanthine and xanthine to uric acid. Free radicals formed during these metabolic steps can be injurious to cell membrane phospholipids. Therefore, during ischemia conditions develop intracellularly that can precipitate renal cell injury during reperfusion.

freshly isolated rabbit proximal tubule preparation, these were not successful [94, 316]. This may represent a species difference or different experimental modeling, or both.

Other approaches that have been employed include those designed to retard the catabolism of adenine nucleotides, with a goal of either preserving ATP levels at nearer to normal values or, at best, delaying the formation of nucleosides, which leak more easily from injured cells [224]. The role of the enzymes critical to these processes and their inhibitors has received significant attention. In general, AMP catabolism can proceed via two pathways: to inosine monophosphate (IMP) or to adenosine (Fig. 47-1). Adenosine is then further catabolized to hypoxanthine (HX). In the rat kidney, but not in the rabbit kidney, further catabolism of HX to xanthine (X) and uric acid occurs [69, 78, 111, 165, 192, 349]. Thus, as mentioned above, experimental studies on the mechanisms of cell injury must consider the species in which experiments are performed. The conversion of HX to X involves the enzyme xanthine oxidase, whose presence is clearly established in rat renal tissue [71, 192]. This enzyme, activated by a calcium (Ca^{2+})-dependent protease, also produces significant amounts of ROM; this contribution to cellular injury during hypoxia or ischemia and reoxygenation is discussed below. It is not surprising, therefore, that, at least in the intact rat, both allopurinol and oxypurinol have been shown to attenuate renal cell injury [219, 305]. The catabolism of AMP to adenosine appears to be the primary pathway for nucleotide degradation since in neither the rat nor the rabbit are appreciable amounts of IMP formed during ischemia [287, 323].

The process of adenine nucleotide regeneration begins with the formation of AMP from adenosine, and therefore maintenance of significant intracellular stores of adenosine should provide for significantly less cell injury. The improved PT viability associated with administration of ATP-$MgCl_2$ in vitro appears to be due to adenosine itself, which is generated during the incubation process from catabolism of AMP [179, 323, 327]. These data are consistent with in vivo results from Siegel's group [286].

Mandel's group has confirmed the importance of adenosine and its role, on entering rabbit proximal tubules, to the subsequent generation of adenine nucleotides [179]. Furthermore, if adenosine is catabolized to inosine extracellularly, cellular protection is lost [179]. The enzyme responsible for this degradation is adenosine deaminase. Studies from Siegel's group support this interpretation and have shown in vivo protection against the ischemic insult in rats if the inhibitor of adenosine deaminase, 2′-deoxycoformycin, is present during ischemia [287]. Adenosine leakage from injured cells, however, is quite rapid, and efforts to minimize AMP degradation (by dephosphorylation) to adenosine have been undertaken. The enzyme responsible, 5′-nucleotidase, has a membrane location in rat tubules and can be inhibited by ATP or ADP as well as by α, β-methylene adenosine-5′-diphosphate (AMP-CP) [153–155]. The cytosolic enzyme is inhibited by low pH such as occurs during ischemia [154, 229]. Thus, two situations develop during in vivo ischemia that tend to offset each other: first, the decreases in ATP and eventually ADP concentrations [10, 306, 310, 323, 327, 347, 351], which would favor activation of the enzyme, and, second, cellular acidosis, which inhibits the enzyme [313, 317, 324]. It appears as if the latter process prevails during ischemia since cellular AMP levels initially become quite high rather than very low, which would be the case if AMP was rapidly degraded to adenosine [10]. Thus, preventing dephosphorylation of AMP retards the formation of nucleosides, which leak from injured renal tissue. Siegel's group has clearly demonstrated the functional and metabolic improvement associated with administration of AMP-CP, as inulin clearance after 24 hours of reflow is more than two times greater than that in untreated, ischemic rats, and ATP recovery rate, measured with nuclear magnetic resonance (NMR), is much swifter [302].

Although it seems quite reasonable that the decrease in ATP during ischemia would place cells at risk for cellular injury and necrosis, this hypothesis has recently been called into question. Shanley and Johnson [258a], using the isolated perfused rat kidney (IPK) as a model, were able to virtually eliminate fragmentation necrosis in the medullary TAL by adding rotenone to the perfusate. This inhibitor blocks mitochondrial electron flow at site I and thus prevents ATP synthesis. The authors, using biopsies of the outer medulla, confirmed profound reductions in ATP equivalent to or greater than those observed during hypoxic injury alone [259], and yet necrosis did not occur [258a]. The interpretation of these studies is that, together with the cessation of mitochondrial ATP synthesis, there was an accompanying cessation of oxygen free radical generation during hypoxia when rotenone was present. Rotenone perfusions differ from hypoxic perfusion conditions in that during hypoxia mitochondrial ATP synthesis is only compromised since ambient oxygen is very low and not totally absent. Under these conditions, however, even though production of ATP is reduced, continued mitochondrial function produces oxygen free radicals or ROM, or both.

These results parallel those reported earlier by our group in which ATP depletion induced by either glycerol or fructose administration did not by itself worsen the functional injury in the IPK that accompanies ischemia [263]. The addition of fructose or glycerol presumably diverts cellular phosphate (PO_4) pools so that phosphorylation of ADP to ATP is retarded. This might be expected, therefore, to also reduce oxidant generation during electron flow through mitochondria. The role of ATP depletion itself, while undoubtedly important, may not be the sole cause of cellular injury during oxygen deprivation, and other events including the capacity of mitochondrial respiratory activity to generate ROM, altered electrolyte transport, cell swelling, and structural changes must also be considered as contributors to the development of cell injury, especially during hypoxia.

Studies on the role of low PO_2 itself have been illuminating in this regard. Galat and associates [91] compared the IPK during exposure to hypoxic gas alone (with continued perfusion) to hypoxia in the presence of a 10- or 30-minute cessation of perfusate flow. These studies therefore extend those of Shanley and Johnson [258a], mentioned previously. Injury was much more extensive when stagnation of flow occurred. The authors suggest that inadequate nutrient delivery or accumulation of metabolic waste products might be critical to this greater propensity toward development of functional and tubular injury.

Low ATP levels at the end of an ischemic interval retard the reestablishment of normal cellular and organ function. Didlake and associates [67] have used fructose 1,6-diphosphate (FDP) to delay utilization, during reperfusion, of newly synthesized ATP for glucose phosphorylation. These authors showed dramatic improvement in rat renal function and histology 24 hours after 30 minutes of renal ischemia when FDP was administered (e.g., beginning 10 minutes after clamp release). These authors also suggested that free radical production by neutrophils was inhibited. Thus, short-term ischemia, although injurious itself, can be largely rendered unimportant if ATP, particularly its synthesis and utilization, is carefully managed during the early reperfusion period. These results suggest that most of the structural or functional changes to cells or mitochondria, or both, are reversible if short-term ischemia is the insult. Linas and co-workers [164] have demonstrated that the major injury induced by short periods of ischemia is due to oxidant generation and that other factors become more important as the time of ischemia is prolonged. A large body of data from several species suggests that the transition period is about 45 minutes; longer periods of ischemia generally result in irreversible cellular and organ damage.

With respect to mitochondrial structure and function, several observations are compatible with this timing. For example, rat kidney mitochondria undergo reversible changes in their membranes as assessed by lipid rotational mobility analysis if the period of ischemia is 45 minutes or less [127]. By 24 hours of reflow, full recovery of mitochondrial membrane integrity [128] as well as ATP synthesis capacity can be demonstrated [128]. However, if the ischemic period is prolonged to 60 minutes, there is a 55 percent irreversible decrease in activity of the ATP/ADP translocator in mitochondria, thus accounting in part for the failure to reestablish either normal synthesis of ATP or cellular respiration [118]. This is a rather unique insult to the mitochondrial ADP translocator since in rat kidney mitochondria the H^+ ion shuttle across the mitochondrial inner membrane is unchanged [15]. The data suggest that ischemia primarily affects electron transport and this is the cause of decreases in coupled (ADP-stimulated) respiration by ischemic mitochondria [9, 292]. Cooling of tissue to 4°C markedly reduced the severity of these changes in mitochondria and prevented the reduction in ATP synthesis, not only in rat kidney but in rat brain and liver as well [15]. Our own work using in vivo ischemia in rats for 50 minutes confirmed that mitochondrial dysfunction is not reversible during reperfusion [9, 10, 335]. Specifically, although mitochondrial respiration transiently increases toward normal with reflow, this recovery pattern becomes arrested and then deteriorates further over 24 hours (Fig. 47-2). This is paralleled by a truncation of ATP recovery as well [10] (Fig. 47-3).

In conclusion, the decrease in ATP synthesis that attends renal ischemia is problematic due to the subsequent loss of purine nucleosides themselves and in some species for the opportunity to generate free radicals especially during reperfusion. However, many other metabolic functions are dependent on adequate ATP levels, and altered metabolic functions, in themselves, may induce renal cell injury. Of particular interest to the question of cell viability is the role(s) played independently by loss of ion gradients, cell swelling, structural and cytoskeletal alterations, and loss of polarization of transport enzymes.

Ion Gradients

Ca^{2+} kinetics across cell membranes determine intracellular K^+ concentrations via effects on K^+ conductance [55]. Takano and associates [292] have measured the abrupt decrease in cellular potassium (K^+) concentration that occurs in rabbit proximal tubules during hypoxia (Fig. 47-4). Most of the decrease in cell K^+ occurs in the first 10 minutes, with more modest decreases seen

Fig. 47-2. Relationship between mitochondrial Ca^{2+} content (•——•) and respiration, as assessed by acceptor control ratio (ACR, ○- - -○) following 50 minutes of renal ischemia. Postischemic reflow is associated with progressive mitochondrial Ca^{2+} accumulation. ACR improves briefly during early reflow, only to deteriorate again progressively as reperfusion continues. Sham mitochondrial Ca^{2+} and ACR are designated by arrows. Basal mitochondrial Ca^{2+} in rats is approximately 13 nmol/mg protein and is virtually unchanged after 50 minutes of total ischemia. (From [9].)

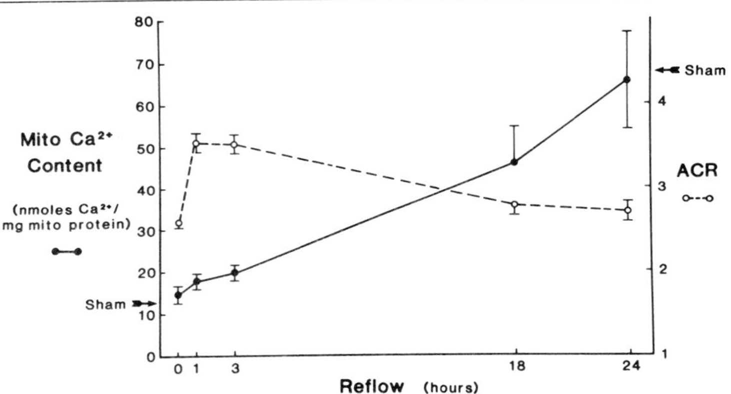

Fig. 47-3. Renal cortical ATP levels during reperfusion following 50-minute ischemia. ATP concentrations fall to 16 percent of control during ischemia and recover to approximately 70 percent of normal after 3 hours of reflow. This recovery is incomplete since ATP levels remain depressed (57 percent) compared to control at 24 hours of postischemic reperfusion. (Adapted from [10].)

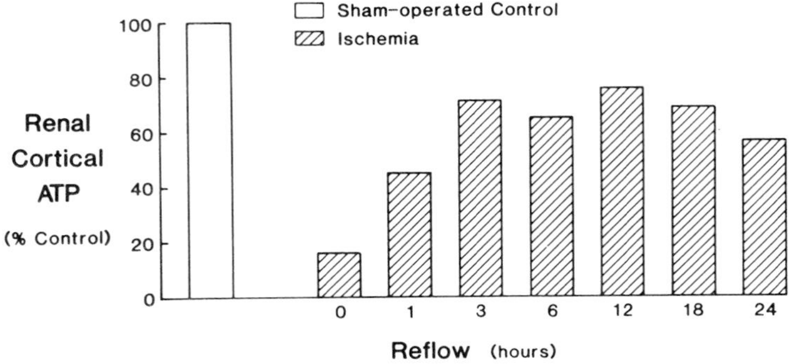

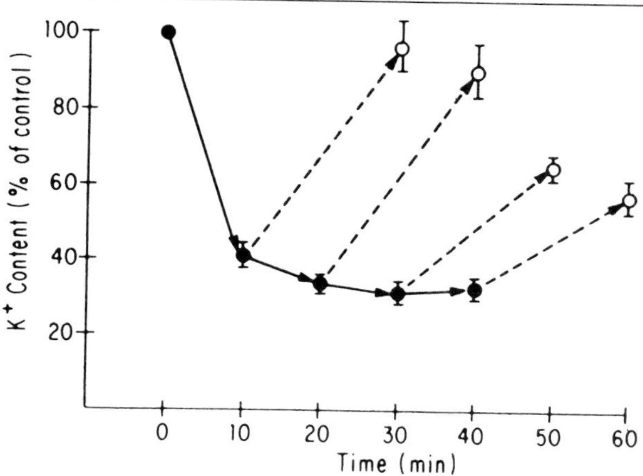

Fig. 47-4. Rabbit proximal tubule potassium (K^+) content (nmol/mg protein) decreases rapidly in the first 10 minutes of anoxia. Only modest further decreases occur over the next 30 minutes [292]. The prompt decrease in K^+ content (and reciprocal increase in Na^+) results in membrane depolarization, which has been associated with increased calcium influx through pathways sensitive to calcium channel blockers. (From [292].)

thereafter. Weinberg and his co-workers have reported similar results [327]. Both groups used atomic absorption spectroscopy to evaluate K^+ content. This technology has not been as useful in evaluating the expected parallel increases of cellular sodium [Na^+] due to the excessive contamination of pelleted tubules by medium Na^+, which obscures the results. Using electron probe analysis, however, Mason and colleagues [181] demonstrated increases in cellular Na^+ in ischemic rat kidneys that were more severe at 60—compared to 20—minutes of complete renal ischemia.

The decrease in extracellular Na^+ has also been confirmed using NMR technology in the guinea pig kidney; as much as one third of the extracellular Na^+ apparently moves intracellularly during ischemia [172]. Therefore, cells gain Na^+ and lose K^+ during ischemia.

SODIUM IONS

The disruption in these ion gradients, in itself, may be important in mediating cell injury. This can best be appreciated, for example, from the results of studies in which rabbit tubules, exposed to normal oxygen levels, suffer substantial cell injury when incubated in the presence of 1 mM ouabain [320]. With ouabain exposure and inhibition of the Na^+-K^+–adenosine triphosphatase (ATPase) enzyme, cell Na^+ increases and cell K^+ decreases, but, unlike in ischemia, ATP is not immediately reduced. This type of study would suggest that ion gradient changes themselves could induce cell injury independent from ATP.

Under normal conditions, a steep gradient for Na^+ exists across the plasma membrane and electrochemical movement of Na^+ into cells is accompanied by Ca^{2+} extrusion: the so-called Na^+-Ca^{2+} exchange process [88, 131, 275, 277]. Renal cortical basolateral membrane vesicles express the Na^+-Ca^{2+} exchanger and this is the cell site where such exchange can be pertubated [131]. With either ouabain treatment or ischemia, this exchanger mechanism does not function well because the transmembrane gradient for Na^+ is reduced as cell Na^+ rises and, thus, the rate of Ca^{2+} extrusion is reduced. The inability to regulate Na^+ transport alone but not sodium co-transport processes occurs within 15 minutes of initiation of renal ischemia [197]. Failure to extrude Ca^{2+} via Na^+-Ca^{2+} exchange or via CaATPase could lead to cellular Ca^{2+} overload, and Takano and associates [292] as well as Weinberg [311, 313] have independently demonstrated progressive increases in total cellular Ca^{2+} during hypoxia.

That the Na^+ gradient may participate in the development of cellular Ca^{2+} overload has been evaluated in other systems in which ATP levels did not decrease. Rat proximal tubules or monkey kidney cells incubated in progressively lower extracellular Na^+ concentrations had increased rates of Ca^{2+} influx and increased Ca^{2+} activated K^+ conductance [55, 151a]. These conditions, therefore, mimic early effects of ouabain treatment in which the transmembrane Na^+ gradient, but not ATP, is reduced and possibly reflect expression of the Na^+-Ca^{2+} exchanger operating in its reverse mode, that is, Na^+ efflux in exchange for extracellular Ca^{2+} [277]. It should be emphasized that Ca^{2+}-ATPase activity may continue to function normally for some time after ouabain administration since ATP levels do not decrease until rather late after drug treatment. Thus, cytosolic-free Ca^{2+} may not rise to as high a level as expected due to the activity of this extrusion mechanism.

Other effects of cellular Na^+ overload include inhibition of transport protein activity, which alters Na^+-dependent glucose and Na^+-PO_4 uptake [196, 200]. The mechanism for cellular Na^+ overload during ischemia includes events other than simply a loss of ATP such as loss of epithelial polarity of enzymes [197, 198, 199, 201] and direct damage to the Na^+-K^+-ATPase [39], possibly due to oxidants [135] and localized at the alpha subunit [173]. Such an ion gradient–mediated mechanism, which itself may drive increased Ca^{2+} entry into renal tubules, resulting in the subsequent development of cell injury during oxygen deprivation, is supported by experimental data. Specifically, reductions in extracellular Ca^{2+} to 2.5 μM markedly reduced lactate dehydrogenase (LDH) release from rabbit proximal tubules during anoxia [291], and these data suggest that the presence of extracellular Ca^{2+} during anoxia is an important contributor to cell injury. Schrier and colleagues [249, 251–253] have recently summarized the possible mechanisms by which Ca^{2+} may initiate cell injury during renal ischemia. The role of cytosolic Ca^{2+} or tissue Ca^{2+}, or both, which should increase as efflux rate decreases and influx rate increases, in mediating oxygen deprivation injury is discussed later; it does appear likely that the cytosolic environment has the potential to be overloaded with Ca^{2+} during ischemia via mechanism(s) related both to the decrease in ATP and to the disrupted transmembrane Na^+ gradient. At least one of these mechanisms may be increased flux of Ca^{2+} into the cells.

POTASSIUM IONS

Accompanying an ischemia-mediated gain in cell Na^+ and loss of cell K^+ is a fall in membrane potential [194, 204]. Upon reperfusion, a large portion of any newly synthesized ATP is presumably used to reestablish these gradients, to effect recovery of transport and reabsorptive processes [148], and to normalize the membrane potential. One method useful in avoiding K^+ depletion and preserving ATP for other functions is to bathe tissues or cells in a buffer or perfusate containing a very high K^+ concentration. As expected, when incubations are conducted, at 37°C in high K^+ medium, injury can be minimized [320]. Weinberg and associates [320] demonstrated that although these maneuvers also partly prevented the ATP depletion of hypoxia, mitochondrial respiration remained inhibited and cell swelling still occurred.

Preliminary results from our laboratory have also demonstrated an important synergistic role for ATP depletion and changes in the transmembrane K^+ gradient. If rat proximal tubules are exposed to low-dose ouabain (10 μM) or to 50 μM amphotericin B or 3 μM valinomycin—each of which decreases cellular K^+—only valinomycin (which markedly reduces cellular ATP) is associated with lethal cell injury [253, 330]. The decreased membrane potential, which is presumably associated with maneuvers that lead to losses of intracellular K^+, can be partially mimicked by increasing extracellular K^+ concentration.

Frindt and co-workers [88] have documented the magnitude of membrane depolarization that accompanies changes in extracellular KCl or NaCl in Necturus proximal tubules. During any of these conditions (i.e., during administration of high-dose ouabain, amphotericin B, or valinomycin, as is the case during hypoxia), the transmembrane K^+ gradient is reduced. We also observed that during incubation of rat proximal tubules in a high KCl buffer, no lethal cell injury occurred and ATP was well maintained [253, 330].

Of potential importance to the mechanism of cell injury, the decreased transmembrane K^+ gradient was attended by an increase in the Ca^{2+} influx rate in each study [253]. These data suggest that, as was the case for a decreased transmembrane Na gradient, an increased influx of Ca^{2+} occurs when the transmembrane K^+ gradient is independently reduced. Under most conditions in which ATP is well maintained, this additional Ca^{2+} burden is either buffered intracellularly and/or returned to the cell exterior by ATP-dependent Ca^{2+} efflux mechanisms; cytosolic and presumably tissue Ca^{2+} overload would not develop under such conditions and cell injury would not occur. These observations therefore contrast with those in in vitro anoxia [1, 134, 278] or very high ouabain [320] or valinomycin [253, 330] treatments, which are all conditions wherein Ca^{2+} influx or tissue Ca^{2+}, or both, are increased in the presence of mitochondrial dysfunction/ATP depletion and cell injury is clearly demonstrable.

The importance of normal transmembrane K^+ gradients to cellular integrity has been explored by Seguro and associates [257], who showed exacerbation of renal ischemic injury in vivo in rats fed a low-K^+ diet for 10 days before renal ischemia, which was reflected in as much as a 50 percent decrease in inulin clearance and higher fractional excretion roles for Na^+, K^+, and water compared to ischemic rats with normal serum K^+ concentrations.

Finally, of additional interest are our observations [330] that the increased Ca^{2+} influx that occurs during high KCl, ouabain, amphotericin B, and valinomycin treatment can be prevented by verapamil, a calcium channel blocker (CCB) (Fig. 47-5). As is the case for CCB protection against hypoxic cell injury [1, 254, 328], verapamil also attenuated cell injury to rat proximal tubules exposed to valinomycin [330] (Fig. 47-6). High ex-

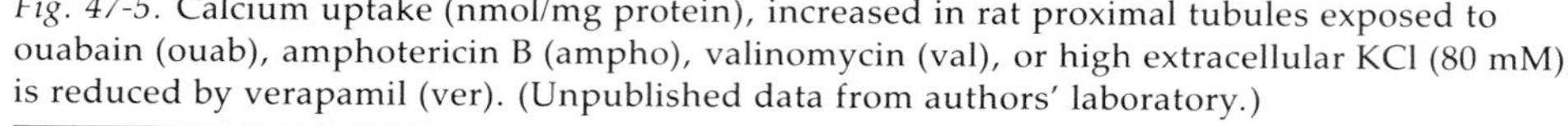
Fig. 47-5. Calcium uptake (nmol/mg protein), increased in rat proximal tubules exposed to ouabain (ouab), amphotericin B (ampho), valinomycin (val), or high extracellular KCl (80 mM), is reduced by verapamil (ver). (Unpublished data from authors' laboratory.)

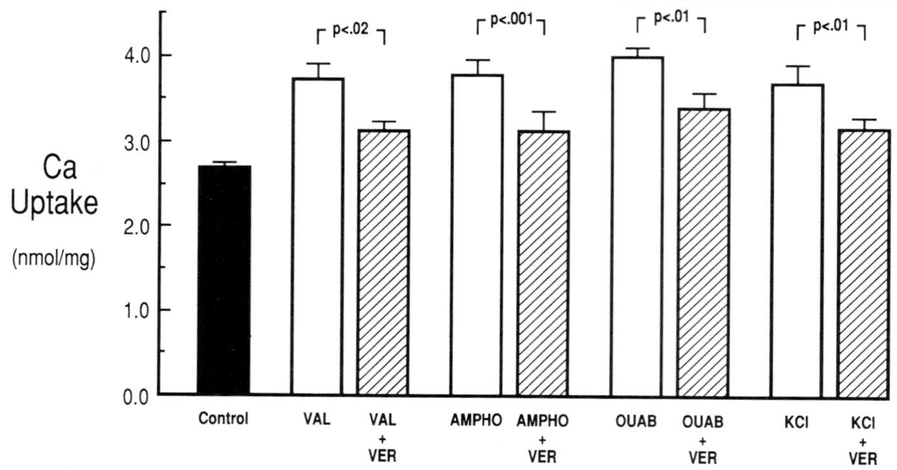

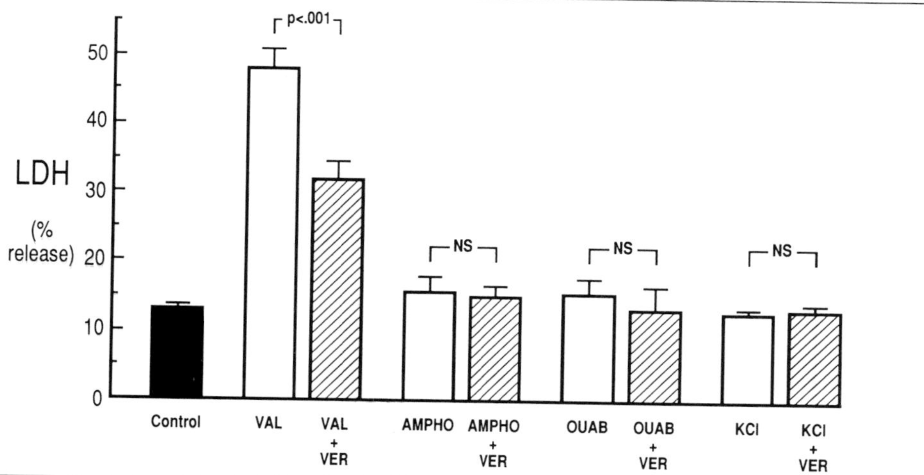

Fig. 47-6. Percent LDH release is increased only in valinomycin (val)-treated rat tubules (and only these tubules had reduced ATP levels). Verapamil (ver) attenuates both Ca^{2+} uptake and LDH release in valinomycin-treated tubules. (Unpublished data from authors' laboratory.)

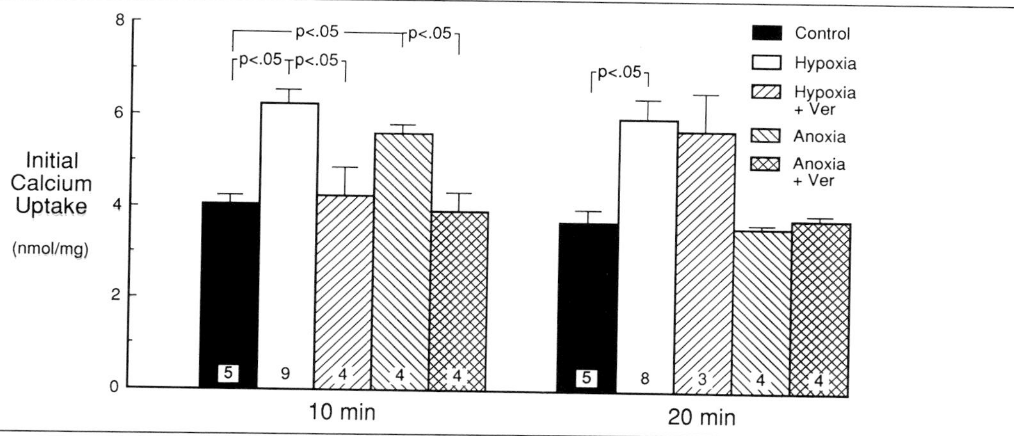

Fig. 47-7. Hypoxia and anoxia induce an early (10 minute) increase in calcium uptake in anoxic and hypoxic rat proximal tubules. Calcium uptake remains increased only in hypoxic tubules at 20 minutes. (From [1].)

tracellular K^+ also enhances renal proximal tubule ammonia production and thus may increase intracellular pH; intracellular alkalosis could contribute to cellular Ca^{2+} overload (see following section) [1a, 2, 48, 206, 308, 313, 324]. Together, these data would appear to support the hypothesis that increased Ca^{2+} influx into ATP-depleted cells is an important contributor to hypoxic cell injury rather than a passive, unimportant marker of cell membrane injury.

CALCIUM IONS

Extracellular Ca^{2+} appears to participate in renal cell injury by virtue of an accelerated Ca^{2+} influx into ischemic cells, which occurs through pathways that are often sensitive to CCB [1, 1a, 9, 37, 53, 62, 66, 87, 103, 121, 136, 137, 156, 222, 249–254, 256, 260, 268, 278, 324, 326, 332, 335, 336]. The experimental conditions must be carefully considered in evaluating this association. In two studies in rats, verapamil in vivo failed to exert cellular or functional protection [24, 175]; both studies used inactin, a drug that inhibits renal autoregulation, as the anesthetic. As was noted previously, a reduction in extracellular Ca^{2+} during the anoxia phase reduces the magnitude of rabbit tubule cell injury assessed by LDH release [292]. Since anoxic rabbit tubules do not accumulate Ca^{2+} over time [292, 313], one possibility is that Ca^{2+} ions are acting at a membrane site and do not in fact enter anoxic cells. This seems unlikely based on the measurable increases in cytosolic Ca^{2+} reported for anoxic, cultured kidney cells [278]. Furthermore, we have measured virtually identical increases in Ca^{2+} influx in rat proximal tubules exposed to 10 minutes of either anoxia or hypoxia [1] (Fig. 47-7). There is probably a generalized, although possibly small, increase in cytosolic calcium in most tissues early in the course of "anoxia," which is really dependent on the degree of oxygen deprivation [24] (Fig. 47-8).

The sensitivity to Ca^{2+} of oxygen-deprived organs

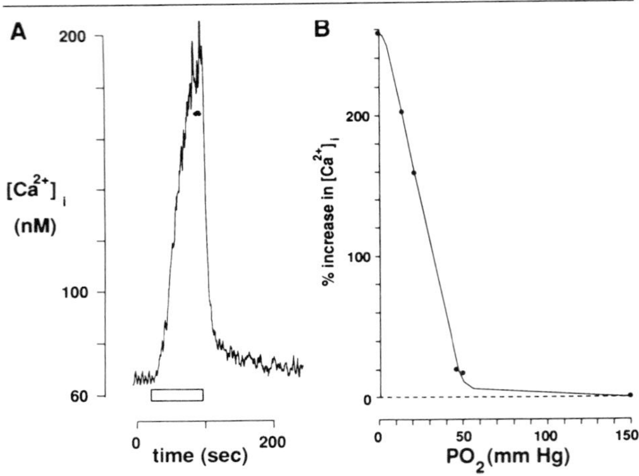

Fig. 47-8. A. Exposure of rabbit cells for 80 seconds to complete anoxia (PO_2 = 0 mm Hg) increases cytosolic-free Ca^{2+} measured with indo-1. B. Steady-state increases in $[Ca^{2+}]_i$ are greatest below PO_2 of 50 mm Hg. (From [24].)

such as kidneys harvested for transplantation can be deduced from the protective effects of adding verapamil to rabbit kidneys flushed and stored for 72 hours [63]. Ca^{2+} added to the flush/storage solution to raise extracellular Ca^{2+} overcomes the protective effects of verapamil, whereas flushing with citrated solutions that bind extracellular Ca^{2+} reduces injury [63]. Since this is not a reperfusion model, it is of interest to note that lipid peroxidation characterizes this organ damage and possibly reflects an increased cytosolic Ca^{2+} during storage [63]. This is supported by the observation that A23187 or ruthenium red, both of which increase cytosolic free Ca^{2+}, exacerbates the injury process [63]. Appropriate to these experimental animal studies, a large patient study recently showed enhanced graft and patient survival if kidneys of the cadaver and the recipient were infused with diltiazem [87]. In addition, intact rats with clamp ischemia suffered less acute tubular necrosis (ATN) if they were given nitrendipine. Direct tubular effects can be deduced from studies in which membrane vesicles obtained from these kidneys showed improvement in sodium-dependent phosphate transport compared to vesicles from untreated ischemic kidneys [273]. Nicardipine has also been shown to prevent the injury due to 60 minutes of warm renal ischemia in dogs [75] and verapamil mimics this protection [74]. Finally, novel, recently developed CCB, including KW-3049 and S-312-d, also show promise in reducing renal ischemic injury, at least in animal models [137, 268].

As was noted previously, anoxic rabbit proximal tubules do not exhibit any increase in total tissue Ca^{2+}, whereas hypoxic tubules exhibit profound time-dependent increases in tissue Ca^{2+} [292, 313], and the mechanism for this difference has been sought [325]. One proposal is that in hypoxic tissues, mitochondrial membrane potential is not totally dissipated; thus, the increased rate of Ca^{2+} influx during hypoxia is accompanied by mitochondrial Ca^{2+} sequestration, which is the cause of the progressive tissue Ca^{2+} overload [292]. Hypoxic and total renal ischemic injury to mitochondria may have different bases [119]. Experimental techniques to prevent mitochondrial and, thus, tissue Ca^{2+} overload during hypoxia are available. Mandel's group has reported that (1) addition of ruthenium red will prevent hypoxic mitochondrial Ca^{2+} accumulation and (2) the calcium burden in these hypoxic rabbit proximal tubules is virtually identical to that seen in anoxia [292]. One interpretation of these results is that Ca^{2+} influx is increased in both anoxia and hypoxia, but that only during hypoxia, in which the mitochondria can accumulate Ca^{2+}, does tissue Ca^{2+} overload occur.

Weinberg advocates another, possibly the primary, cause for the failure of anoxic tissue to accumulate Ca^{2+}. In his hypothesis, it is the more substantive acidosis of anoxia that actually inhibits Ca^{2+} uptake; anoxic acidosis, therefore, prevents tissue Ca^{2+} overload [313]. This reasoning is compatible with the inhibitory effects of acidosis on Ca^{2+} influx in normoxic renal tubules reported some years ago by Studer and Borle [288] and would suggest that reduced intracellular pH lowers Ca^{2+} influx. In a recent study we also observed that the comparable increase in Ca^{2+} influx in anoxic and hypoxic rat proximal tubules is not sustained in the anoxic tubules beyond 10 minutes [1]. Thus, although Ca^{2+} influx is initially quite similar in both states of experimental oxygen deprivation, it remains high only during continued hypoxia, whereas it reverts to nearly normal rates with prolonged anoxia [1]. One could generalize that the progressive development of intracellular acidosis is a protective state during anoxia, that acidosis tends to limit the magnitude of cellular calcium influx, and that this may answer the question as to why tissue Ca^{2+} levels remain virtually unchanged during in vivo ischemia [9, 10, 45, 250, 335], rising only on reperfusion. Finally, it appears as if the rat proximal tubules retain a memory of the acidotic conditions during hypoxia since Ca^{2+} influx and LDH release are markedly reduced during 30 to 60 minutes of reoxygenation [48]. Perhaps this attenuated development of cell injury during reoxygenation reflects the reduced cellular Ca^{2+} overload that occurred during the hypoxic and acidotic conditions. As noted above, Weinberg [313] has clearly demonstrated that there is an attenuation of tissue Ca^{2+} overload during hypoxia if acidosis is maintained. These observations have also been extended to, and confirmed in, the IPK, a more complex model of hypoxic renal injury. Removal of perfusate Ca^{2+} virtually eliminated injury (fragmentation necrosis) in the hypoxic mTAL, and this protection could be mimicked by reducing perfusate pH even in the presence of normal Ca^{2+} levels [260, 261].

There appears to be one additional important role for Ca^{2+} mediating ischemic cell injury, and this may be particularly relevant during hypoxia wherein the ambient oxygen tension is low but not totally absent. Malis and Bonventre [174] have shown in an isolated mitochondria model mimicking hypoxia-induced free radical formation that Ca^{2+} ions enhance the injury caused solely by the free radicals. They further localized the site of mitochondrial damage to pyridine nucleotides, that is, the first step in the oxidation of tricarboxylic acids.

This observation is quite important, for it provides for a relatively intact site II at which generation of ATP from anaerobic conversion of α-ketoglutarate or fumarate to succinate could occur. In fact, the isolated perfused rat kidney demonstrates improved functional capacity when these compounds are provided as metabolic substrates [107]. Hypoxic rabbit tubules, however, show no enhancement of cellular viability with these additions [94, 316]. This may reflect a species difference or alternatively simply a regional (nephron type) difference in the capacity of tissue to carry out anaerobic glycolysis. Thus, the protection seen with α-ketoglutarate or fumarate in the intact rat kidney may be reflective of better cell integrity in S_3 or TAL segments. One cannot rule out the possibility that substrate additions are also exerting protective effects at a vascular or endothelial site in the intact kidney.

In the study by Malis and Bonventre [174], injury to mitochondria via free radicals and Ca^{2+} could be prevented by dibucaine, which inhibits phospholipase activity, and exacerbated by incorporation of marine lipids into mitochondrial membranes [176]. The results suggest that the Ca^{2+} ions activated one or more mitochondrial phospholipases, and, in the presence of increased amounts of fatty acids released in response to free radical injury to mitochondrial membranes, phospholipase activity was increased. An important role for intracellular phospholipases, activated by Ca^{2+} ions, has been proposed by several laboratories. Widener and Mela-Riker [332] have demonstrated attenuation of ischemic mitochondrial damage by verapamil. Schrier's laboratory has quantitated the time-dependent, progressive rise in renal calcium content in dogs and rats [9, 10, 250, 335] and has accumulated preliminary evidence that dibucaine and mepacrine reduce hypoxic injury to rat proximal tubules [43]. Miyahara and associates [195] would suggest that these drugs indeed preserve mitochondrial (and possibly other) membrane structure since ATP levels themselves are not improved. The endoplasmic reticulum in vivo, however, is probably impervious to injury of approximately 50 minutes' duration [245]. Its failure to uptake Ca^{2+} is likely due to the low levels of ATP rather than to structural defects.

MAGNESIUM IONS

Ischemic cells lose magnesium, but the impact of this depletion and its role, if any, in cellular injury has not been explored in depth [332]. Magnesium is, however, important for the activity of Na^+-K^+-ATPase and Ca^{2+}-ATPase; its loss from cells could influence Na^+-H^+ [33, 85, 151, 324] or Na^+-Ca^{2+} [88, 131, 174, 176, 320] exchange and/or Ca^{2+} efflux, thereby leading to cellular Ca^{2+} overload. Furthermore, Mg^{2+} is important in the regulation of mitochondrial Ca^{2+} [332], and Mg^{2+} appears to be important in the protective effects of ATP [179, 271, 285, 289, 290, 310, 322, 327]. It may have a role in generating or maintaining adequate extracellular adenosine for reentry into ischemic cells. Mg^{2+} also has effects similar to those of tetrodotoxin in Purkinje fibers and, thus, like acidosis, Mg^{2+} may alter cellular Ca^{2+} overload via blockade of Na^+ channel activity [138].

In summary, ischemia is attended by an increased flux of Ca^{2+} into renal tubules; this can be attenuated by the development of intracellular acidosis as cells shift toward glycolytic capacity, by reductions in extracellular Ca^{2+} concentration, or through addition of CCB. In these experimental situations, cellular injury is reduced.

Cell Injury

LACTATE DEHYDROGENASE RELEASE

An additional useful parameter that is assessed during the measurement of ATP, cellular ions, and Ca^{2+} flux in hypoxic tubules is the release of LDH into the bathing medium. Generally, it is appreciated that the harvesting conditions, specifically the use of enzymes, including collagenase and hyaluronidase, are more stringent when preparing proximal tubules from the rat than the rabbit [1, 1a, 48, 49, 69, 129, 292, 313, 352]. Mandel and co-workers have performed experiments in very viable suspensions of both rat and rabbit proximal tubules, and their data demonstrate somewhat higher basal levels of LDH release in rat tubules [69, 129, 292]. Furthermore, we and others have shown that LDH release rises quickly to 30 to 40 percent during hypoxic or anoxic incubation of rat proximal tubules, whereas in rabbit tubules, especially during anoxia, LDH release occurs more slowly [1, 292, 352].

Additional studies by Mandel's group have provided an alternative reason to the enzymatic harvesting conditions for this difference in LDH release in rat versus rabbit tubules. They have demonstrated that rat and rabbit tubules contain large amounts of Ca^{2+} in their mitochondria, potentially providing for a releasable pool of Ca^{2+} to the cytosol during oxygen deprivation [69, 129, 202]. The amounts of Ca^{2+} in mitochondria were measured using proton ionophores (that collapse the mitochondrial membrane potential) plus Ca^{2+}-sensitive dyes and are virtually identical (10–15 nmol/mg protein) to those measured by atomic absorption in the rat by our group [9, 170] (see Fig. 47-2). Their studies in rabbit proximal tubules show that, unlike in rat proximal tubules, very little mitochondrial Ca^{2+} was released by ionophores [130]. Thus, at least one additional reason to consider species differences when examining the mechanism of oxygen deprivation injury is the contribution of large-capacity storage sites for Ca^{2+}. In the case of Ca^{2+}, its more rapid release from mitochondria into the cytosol of rat proximal tubules may activate phospholipases, with subsequent deleterious effects on membrane phospholipids. These deleterious effects could express themselves in rat tubules as LDH release that is quicker and more substantial than that found in rabbit tubules, in which it appears that there may be little mitochondrial Ca^{2+} released during oxygen deprivation.

ACIDOSIS

The protective effects of reduced pH demonstrated by Burnier and associates [48], Weinberg [313], and Shanley and co-workers [260, 261] also strongly support a role for Ca^{2+} in the development of ischemic cell injury. However, intracellular pH modulates many other metabolic pathways [50]. Decreased intracellular pH reduces

Ca^{2+}-calmodulin affinity and this may delay the activation of proteases, which have been suggested to be a major cause of cell death [123]. pH also controls the endocytic release of the content of coated pits [242]. This may reduce delivery of substrates to metabolic sites, thereby delaying consumption of energy [242]. A further possible contribution elicited by reduced pH may relate to a decrease in Na^+-H^+ exchange during acidosis. Reduced efflux of H^+ ions from cells in exchange for Na^+ might lessen the cellular Na^+ overload during ischemia and, indirectly, reduce the rate or magnitude of cellular Ca^{2+} overload via reversal of the Na^+/Ca^{2+} exchange process. Since ATP is consumed during Na^+-H^+ exchange [210], acidosis could also preserve cell integrity by reducing ATP consumption in addition to delaying the onset of cellular and mitochondrial Ca^{2+} overload. There are, of course, additional explanations for the protective effects of acidosis.

Recently, Weinberg and associates have provided persuasive evidence in isolated rabbit tubules that acidosis also exerts its protective effect(s) at a site distal to the elevation of cytosolic free Ca^{2+}. Their study, performed in rabbit proximal tubules, involved measuring cell injury during ionomycin exposure. Fura-2 measurable Ca^{2+} rose under both these circumstances (normal pH and acidosis) and yet acidosis greatly attenuated the cell injury.

The increased cytosolic-free Ca^{2+} presumably contributed to the injury process by a mechanism that depended on pH not decreasing to very low levels. One possible mechanism for this response involves phospholipases, whose activity depends on elevated Ca^{2+} in the cytosol and on the ambient intracellular pH. Reduction in either cytosolic Ca^{2+} or pH would lessen the injury normally mediated by phospholipases. Phospholipases and their role in ischemic cell injury are discussed in the following section. Other experiments in rabbit tubules bathed in a Ca^{2+}-free medium and treated with the mitochondrial respiratory inhibitor 1799, which uncouples mitochondrial oxidative phosphorylation and does not interfere with fluorescence measurements, showed virtually no release of Ca^{2+} to the cytosol [324]. These results confirm those of Mandel and associates [130] noted previously and reinforce the observation that very little Ca^{2+} is released from rabbit proximal tubule mitochondria when membrane potential is decreased by either oxygen deprivation or proton ionophores. The usefulness of fura-2 as an index of cytosolic-free Ca^{2+} changes remains problematic, especially where leak of intracellular molecules such as LDH could be accompanied by leak of fura-2 as well. This leak may be the reason why LeFurgey and co-workers [157], using electron microprobe analysis, were unable to detect increases in cytosolic-free Ca^{2+} under conditions in which A23187, another Ca^{2+} ionophore, was administered, but this group has subsequently shown that in anoxia increased cytosolic–free Ca^{2+} is demonstrable [281]. The precise reason for these differences is at present unclear but LDH leak is more prominent during administration of A23187 or ionomycin than during anoxia.

PHOSPHOLIPASES

Phospholipids containing unsaturated fatty acids act as subtrates for phospholipase A_2 (PLA_2). Ordinarily, fatty acids such as arachidonic acid provide substrates for vasodilating prostaglandin synthesis [253]. However, these fatty acids are especially prone to be attacked at the double bonds, with subsequent formation of peroxides and dialdehydes [27, 187, 312]. Phospholipase A_2 activity has been measured directly in normoxic and ischemic renal epithelial tissue and mesangial cells, and there are reports that PLA_2 shifts its activity from cytosolic to membrane sites [206, 228]. Increased PLA_2 activity is observed in mitochondria and microsomal fractions during oxygen deprivation and in the cytosolic fraction as well at 1 hour of reoxygenation [206]. The Ca^{2+} dependency of the enzyme, which may have multiple forms, is between 100 and 1000 nM, that is, physiologic intracellular concentrations [206]. During ischemia itself the development of intracellular acidosis may be responsible for the reduction in the cytosolic activity since the pH optimum for enzyme activity is between 8.5 and 9.5 [206].

One of the earliest effects of PLA_2 activation appears to be a subtle local effect on lipid integrity of the apical membrane, which coincidentally occurs as Na^+-K^+-ATPase moves from its basolateral location to the brush border membrane [198, 201]. Proximal tubule reabsorption of Na^+ is clearly abnormal after ischemia [40]. Furthermore, leucine aminopeptidase moves from a luminal membrane site toward the basolateral membrane and PTH-dependent adenylate cyclase also moves toward the apical membrane [199]. Ischemic rat kidneys have been shown to undergo alterations in membrane composition, which presumably reflect the effects on epithelial tissue primarily [196–201]. In addition, time is an important consideration since the changes in lysophospholipid composition were modest after 60 minutes of ischemia [201]. In concert with these results, Humes' group [126] has demonstrated abrupt increases in free fatty acids (FFA) in hypoxic rabbit tubule suspensions, whereas the lysophospholipid remodeling was not seen until quite late. Taken together, these data suggest that phospholipases are activated quite promptly during hypoxia and the first evidence is a release of fatty acids. However, the degree of ATP depletion modifies the rate of fatty acid release [209]. Our laboratory has also confirmed an early (10–20 minute) increase in fatty acids released from hypoxic rat proximal tubules [331], possibly due to activation of endogenous phospholipases [43].

Fatty acids are thought to participate in cell injury in a number of important ways. First, at least some compounds such as phosphatidic acid (PA) can act as calcium ionophores; rat kidney tissue levels are increased with in vivo ischemia before reflow [201]. Although increased phospholipase activity alone can account for increased levels of FFA during ischemia, there is also a loss over time of the enzymes responsible for oxidation of fatty acids as well as a shift from beta-oxidation, which is favorable for energy production, to the more energy-unfavorable peroxidation of the fatty acids [237]. It has been proposed that lipid peroxidation is one of the earliest pathophysiologic events in experimental acute renal failure (ARF) [132] and prevention of lipid peroxidation in vivo attenuates ischemic ARF in the rat [53]. In addition, methylguanidine, formed from creatinine, is increased in both plasma and urine of ischemic animals and humans, and may provide an additional marker of ischemic injury [38]. Second, FFA are thought to act as membrane detergents, thereby decreasing cell membrane integrity. Lieberthal and co-workers have used albumin to reduce injury to mouse tubule cells in a model of chemical hypoxia [266]. The cellular protection, thought to reside in the scavenging of fatty acids by albumin, could not be duplicated by Humes and colleagues [126], who paradoxically showed enhanced injury during hypoxia to rabbit tubules treated with albumin. Again, the possibility of a species difference must be considered. Kidneys also produce endogenous fatty acid–binding proteins and their role in ischemia has not been fully examined [152].

Finally, if the severity of ATP depletion is only modest, reacylation of fatty acids into membrane phospholipids or esterification of triglycerides would provide for additional reductions of FFA concentrations and presumably less injury. However, in the absence of significant maintenance of ATP, as occurs in hypoxic proximal tubules, we have found, as noted previously, significant, although short-lived, protection against rat renal cell injury with mepacrine and dibucaine, suggesting that phospholipase activation is an early response in rat tubules [43]. Weinberg [315] has reported that he was unable to duplicate such results in rabbit tubules. The reason for this difference may be due, in part, to a more substantial increase in cytosolic Ca^{2+} overload that likely occurs in the rat tubule(s) compared to the rabbit tubule(s) as a consequence of injury to calcium-laden mitochondria [130]. Specifically, Ca_i measured with fluorescent dyes rises from approximately 100 nM to 300 nM in rabbit tubules treated with 1799 and from 100 nM to 600 nM in rat tubules under identical conditions [129, 130, 166, 177, 324]. Phospholipases may be more quickly activated in the rat, accounting therefore for the higher LDH release as well as the protective effects of mepacrine and dibucaine. Canine renal epithelial cells also demonstrate a prompt rise in cytosolic-free Ca^{2+} in response to ATP depletion [190]. Finally, the ability of mitochondria from rat kidneys to "buffer" cytosolic Ca^{2+} is lost during 50 minutes of ischemia [10] (Fig. 47-9).

OXYGEN FREE RADICALS

Since McCord's seminal observations on oxygen free radical–mediated injury during reperfusion following ischemia [189], many investigators utilizing many different types of tissues have contributed to the evaluation and refinement of this theory [51, 58, 63, 69, 81, 89, 93, 106, 133, 191, 219, 256, 283, 284, 301]. With respect to the kidney, two general approaches have been followed: first, treatment either with free radical generating systems to accelerate injury or with scavengers of free radicals to reduce injury [17, 21–23, 30, 32, 104, 108, 110, 111, 140, 149, 162, 178, 193, 247, 262, 305, 307, 309, 318, 339, 349] and, second, evaluation of the contributing effects of activated neutrophils to the cellular injury that occurs in vivo on reperfusion following ischemia [144, 163, 169, 216, 258, 295, 345]. In the last 5 years, however, it has become increasingly evident that the rat model of oxygen radical–mediated damage may not pertain to human ARF. Unlike in the rat, human tissues have been shown to have little xanthine oxidase activity [71], and this is the enzyme that, during reperfusion, would generate superoxide ions during conversion of xanthine to uric acid. In addition, human kidneys apparently do not catabolize hypoxanthine to xanthine; thus, the substrate for xanthine oxidase is also not readily available for superoxide generation. However, oxidants and peroxidation can be produced via other mechanisms [265].

Since many of these experimental studies in animal models involve analysis of whole kidney tissue wherein the renal tubules compose most of the mass, attention has been devoted to specific nephron as well as vascular tissues and endothelial cells in an attempt to discern if specific tissue responses to oxidants or protective agents are masked by analysis of entire organs. For example, human monocytes develop significant superoxide anion levels within 9 seconds after the addition of Ca^{2+} to the media. Both internal redistribution of Ca^{2+} and Ca^{2+} influx into concanavalin-treated monocytes participate in the generation of this ROM [256].

A large body of information concerning the free radical–mediated mechanism of injury has been obtained using in vivo models of ischemia reperfusion. However, even within species genetic differences may temper definitive conclusions. For example, New Zealand white rabbits exhibit greater injury than do French loop rabbits when both are challenged with 60 minutes of renal ischemia followed by reflow for 14 days [110].

Timing of observations is also quite important when assessing oxidant-mediated injury due to ischemia. Following 45 minutes of ischemia in rats, leukotriene B_4 (LTB_4) and thromboxane B_2 (TxB_2) levels are increased only in the first 5 minutes of reperfusion [144]. In agreement with these observations are those showing that malondialdehyde (MDA) levels are increased only in the first 5 minutes of reflow after 45 minutes of renal ischemia [241] and only when PO_2 is between 10 and 50 mm Hg; MDA is not produced when PO_2 is less than 10 mm Hg [241]. Ethane production, a measure of lipid peroxidation, does increase during ischemia [217]. The degree of glutathione (GSH) depletion appears to be critical to whether xanthine dehydrogenase (XD) conversion to xanthine oxidase (XO) has occurred; glutathione must fall to less than 40 percent of normal levels for XO formation to occur [243]. Inhibition of TxA_2 by the synthetase inhibitor DP-1904 results in reduced functional injury compared to the injury induced by ischemia or platelet activating factor (PAF) infusion [186]. Finally, the formation of oxidants can occur through two pathways: one dependent on the presence of iron (and inhibited by deferoxamine) and the other associated with cyclooxygenase activity (and inhibited by indomethacin)

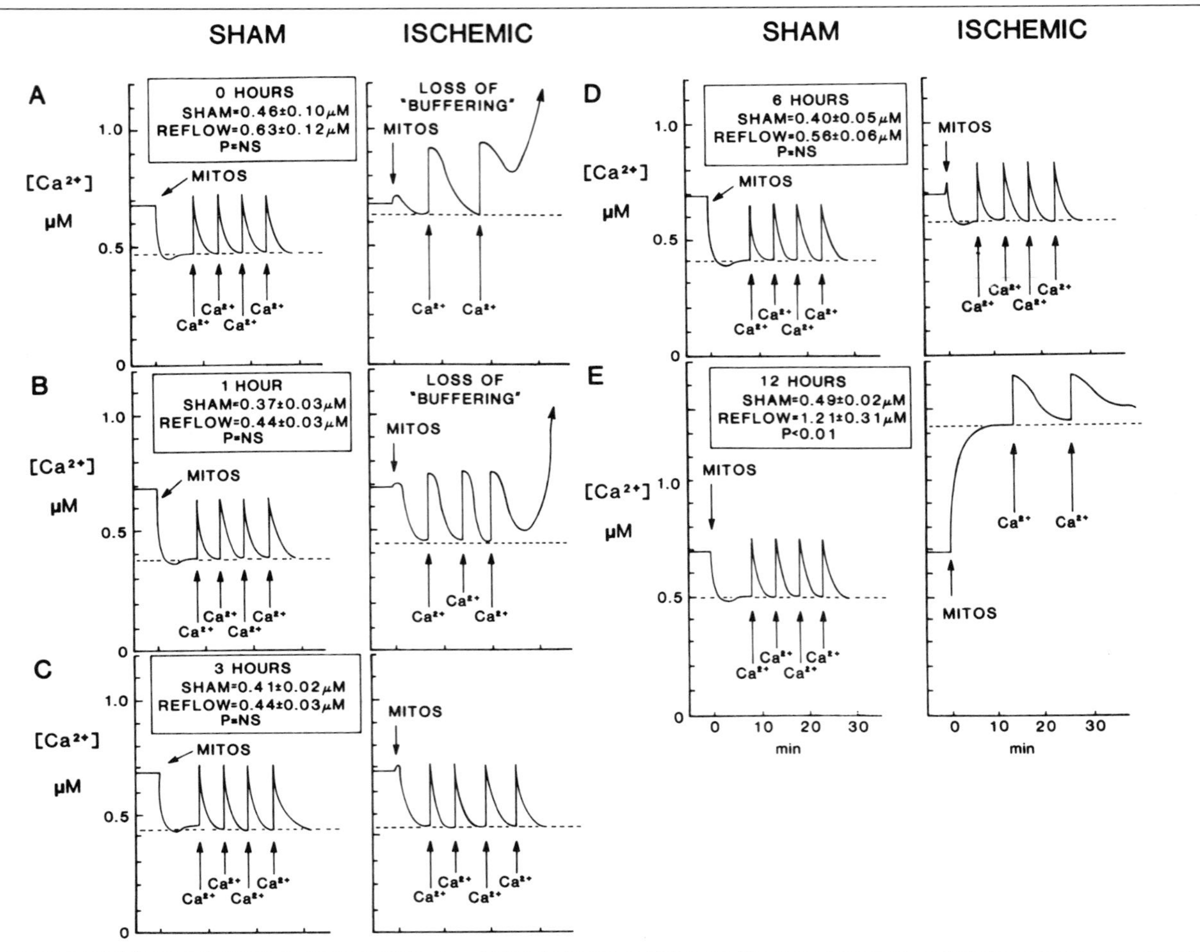

Fig. 47-9. Regulation of extramitochondrial free Ca^{2+} concentration after ischemia. Panels A through E show representative recordings for sham-operated (left) and 50-minute ischemic (right) kidneys after 0 1, 3, 6, and 12 hours' reflow, respectively. (From [10].)

[105]. The iron-mediated injury appears to be directed mainly at the renal cortex whereas indomethacin prevents primarily medullary injury [105]. Storage solutions for organs to be used for eventual transplantation should probably include both deferoxamine and indomethacin [235]. To integrate these observations, it would appear in vivo that ischemia leads to production of TxA_2 in the renal medulla and this vasoconstrictor prolongs the period of oxygen deprivation. This may be a factor as to why medullary tubules exhibit such profound morphologic damage after ischemia [212]. Therefore, even though oxidant-mediated injury may mostly occur early during warm reperfusion, elimination of this process is an important route of cellular protection. An especially fruitful area of investigation presently involves the endothelium and its role in ischemia-reperfusion injury since this tissue also responds to oxygen deprivation and is in intimate contact with both vascular smooth muscle cells and circulating neutrophils. This is discussed later in this chapter.

There are two approaches to the prevention of oxygen radical–mediated ischemic damage. One is to enhance endogenous scavengers and the second is to provide an appropriate and adequate source of exogenous scavengers. The latter is more easily accomplished. Free radicals are generated during normal cellular metabolism, including that performed by the kidney. Superoxide dismutase (SOD), catalase (CAT), and the glutathione peroxidase enzymes all interact to prevent free radical damage during well-oxygenated conditions. Dietary depletion of antioxidants, on the other hand, exacerbates injury to renal tissue [165, 207]. The mechanism of oxidant formation and pathways in which these enzymes function are shown in Fig. 47-10.

Initially, studies in intact rats and in the IPK of the rat have shown that additions of SOD and CAT or allopurinol or dimethylthiourea (DMTU) to the animal or perfusate resulted in attenuation of functional injury, including improved tubular Na^+ transport (T_{Na^+}) [162, 164, 215, 219]. Recently, these data have not been confirmed [93]. In addition DMTU, as well as deferoxamine, which is employed to prevent hydroxyl radical generation via the Haber-Weiss reaction, has been shown to improve renal function and to reduce morphologic injury [135, 162, 218]. Dithiothreitol prevents hydrogen peroxide–induced mitochondrial damage. Finally, inhi-

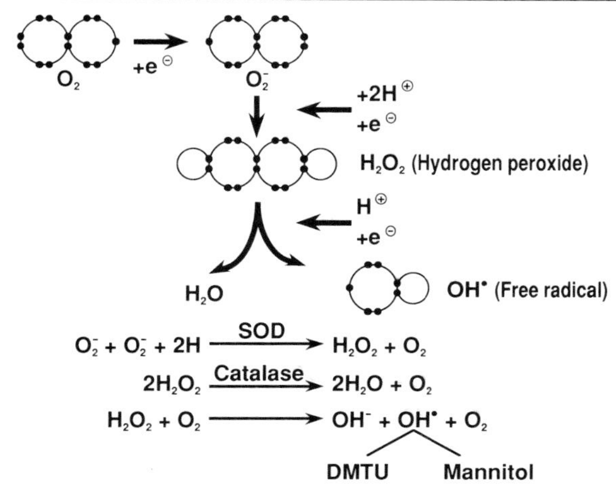

Fig. 47-10. Top panel. Structural changes that result in formation of superoxide (O_2^-), hydrogen peroxide (H_2O_2), and hydroxyl ($OH^\cdot$) ions. Bottom panel. Superoxide dismutase (SOD) decreases oxygen free radical concentration by enhancing H_2O_2, which itself is converted to water and oxygen by catalase. Oxygen plus H_2O_2 yields two molecules of hydroxyl ions. Dimethylthiourea (DMTU) and mannitol scavenge hydroxyl ions. (Adapted from J. Duhault, M. Lonchampt, and L. Alliot. Superoxide dismutase: Pathological and therapeutic implications. *Medicographia* 6:24, 1984.)

bition of the enzyme xanthine oxidase by dietary tungsten feeding also reduces the severity of renal injury in the rat [163]. In the reperfused rabbit kidney, however, oxygen radical scavengers were not protective [337].

Whereas in vivo studies present an additional problem in that neutrophil-mediated postischemic injury would likely occur, this does not happen in tubules or the IPK. During in vivo studies the injurious effects of ROM generation are seen during reperfusion and, thus, they apply primarily to models of total ischemia [189]. A less well-explored area involves in vivo oxygen deprivation in states of hypoperfusion, hemorrhage, or hypoxia, states in which ROM would be generated before reestablishment of normal perfusion. Finally, whole-animal and whole-kidney studies do not identify important nephron or vascular sites of injury, which is why parallel studies of freshly isolated renal tubules, and of cultured vascular smooth muscle cells, mesangial cells, and endothelial cells, have provided important insights into the free radical–mediated processes of cell injury [219a]. By design, however, most of these experimental maneuvers have involved severe hypoxia rather than complete anoxia as the experimental insult.

Although the proximal tubule isolated from rabbit kidney is relatively impervious to ROM injury [42, 310], surprisingly tubular function in the postischemic rabbit kidney is enhanced by oxypurinol [32]. As was noted earlier in this chapter, the absence of xanthine oxidase and xanthine in the rabbit apparently limits generation of free radicals via this mechanism either during in vitro hypoxia or during reoxygenation [42, 310]. It has been observed that in the rabbit tubule preparation hypoxic injury is manifested during hypoxia itself rather than during reoxygenation [313]. Even the addition of extra amounts of hypoxanthine did not exacerbate cell injury [315]. Rat proximal tubules, on the other hand, which exhibit injury during reoxygenation as well as during oxygen deprivation [47, 48], have xanthine oxidase, and although the enzyme could be inhibited by allopurinol the cellular injury persists [28, 69]. These observations suggest, therefore, that other routes of injury to rat proximal tubules occur during in vitro hypoxia.

The protective effects in vivo of scavengers of free radicals in the rat kidney and in the rat IPK can be observed in some but not all isolated tubule preparations [140, 219a]. Because SOD is a large molecular weight enzyme, access to the cell interior, where protection might be more likely, could be problematic. In addition, in plasma the half-life of SOD is rather short. Moreover, in vivo SOD might exert its protective effect by inhibition of neutrophil-mediated free radical production and thus indirectly reduce the severity of postischemic reperfusion injury. Finally, if free radical formation begins with superoxide generation, this might be expected to occur continuously during hypoxic, in vitro injury; thus, the failure of SOD or other scavengers or enzymes to obviate hypoxic injury to isolated proximal tubules may be due to rather large and continuous oxygen free radical production.

It is unquestioned that an index of free radical production in hypoxic isolated rat proximal tubules, namely MDA, can be detected [132, 219, 219a], but in vivo MDA levels increase promptly only in the first 5 minutes of reperfusion. In this period the oxidants formed, which are susceptible to SOD protection, are not due to xanthine oxidase because activity of this enzyme is low at this time [133]. In the IPK, where neutrophils are not present to mediate oxidant injury, their addition can induce cellular injury, which is lessened by SOD and catalase; these data indicate that extracellular production of oxidants is susceptible to SOD or catalase [91]. Conversely, in vivo, neither SOD nor catalase exhibits protection, therefore suggesting that oxidants are likely to be formed intracellularly at sites inaccessible to SOD or catalase [91–93].

There is one additional consideration related to the study of free radical production in hypoxic tissues including renal tubules. For example, especially in the rat proximal tubule, the large stores of mitochondrial Ca^{2+}, some of which could be released to the cytosol, could accelerate a Ca^{2+}-activated, protease-mediated conversion of xanthine dehydrogenase to xanthine oxidase. Furthermore, cellular depletion of glutathione, which decreases rapidly during ischemia and remains low for at least 2 hours of reperfusion [243], also contributes to activation of reversible XO formation [243]. We have observed in the intact rat that the very high levels of HX and X at the end of 50 minutes of in vivo ischemia are catabolized to nearly normal by 1 hour of reperfusion [10]. In complete ischemia, free radical generation in the first hour of reperfusion may be an additional cause of functional and morphologic renal injury. Intermittent reperfusion, which exacerbates renal ischemic injury, may provide for more complete washout of glutathione and more thorough cellular depletion [296]. Thus, in the rat proximal tubule all the necessary components are present to generate substantial cytosolic and mitochondrial free radicals with low oxygen levels (hypoxia), including xanthine, Ca^{2+} ions, and xanthine oxidase. The rabbit kidney, and its proximal tubule in particular, even under similar hypoxic conditions, appears to have much lower levels of both xanthine and free Ca^{2+} ions. It is not surprising then that in the rabbit in vivo ischemia is not prevented by allopurinol [310], and the different degree of free radical–induced cell damage during hypoxia or reoxygenation between rats and rabbits may therefore be related to species differences.

Glutathione is now being used as an additive to perfusion and harvesting solutions of organs for transplantation [7] due to the continued impression that oxidant injury plays an important role in cell/organ dysfunction [30, 51, 106, 110, 149, 232, 274, 307, 318, 319]. The source of at least some of these ROM appears to be the mitochondria [159, 174, 176, 184, 301]. Several years ago Weinberg and his co-workers [319] found that glutathione, added to suspensions of hypoxic rabbit proximal tubules, reduced LDH leakage during hypoxia and permitted almost complete recovery of ATP and intracellular electrolytes after reoxygenation. These investigators also reported that glutathione in the medium was rapidly broken down into its component amino acids, glycine, cysteine, and glutamate, and that only glycine protected hypoxic tubules as well as did intact glutathione [319]. This remarkable protective effect of glycine has yet to be fully explained, but the strongest available evidence suggests that glycine acts before, as well as at some step after, an increase in cytosolic calcium. Specifically, results by Weinberg's group [324] using 1799 in rabbit proximal tubules showed enhanced cell injury and increased cytosolic calcium, but when glycine was present there was less cell injury but no reduction in cytosolic calcium. Glycine also prevents tubule injury during treatment with other mitochondrial inhibitors, including antimycin A, rotenone, cyanide, and oligomycin [318–320, 322]. Recently, glycine has also been shown to enhance organ function after transplantation [246].

The protective effects of glycine are shared in large part by alanine [13, 94, 141]. Alanine is often used in isolated perfused nephron studies [65, 244] and has been incorporated into the isolation media used to harvest renal tubules, rabbit proximal tubules in particular [292]. This addition of alanine may provide an additional degree of protection during harvesting of rabbit tubules, thus explaining their lower baseline level of LDH release.

Glycine is present in significant quantities in renal epithelium, with intracellular levels exceeding extracellular levels by about fourfold [64]. It is postulated that harvesting of tubules for in vitro studies or organs for transplantation leads to a rapid efflux of glycine into the medium and loss, therefore, of its intracellular protective effects [64, 246]. Amino acids also aid in recovery of renal phospholipid regeneration after ischemia [297].

There have been several attempts to prevent in vivo renal injury through administration of glycine: In both a cisplatinum and a uranyl nitrate model of ARF in intact rats, functional improvement with glycine has been shown [79, 90]. Conversely, use of glutathione itself appears to be more protective during complete renal ischemia than during renal hypoperfusion injury [344]. This difference may relate to the greater propensity for cellular calcium overload—and the activation of other injurious processes including phospholipases during hypoxia as compared to complete anoxia [43, 206, 228, 291, 312, 331]. In vitro, renal hypoperfusion experiments or intermittent reperfusion studies are characterized by modest, low levels of blood flow and a loss of glutathione from tissues that would not occur during complete ischemia induced by a mechanical clamp on the renal artery.

We have used a completely phosphate-free medium for incubation of rat proximal tubules to assess the effects of this form of ATP reduction on cellular function. Under these conditions phosphorylation of ADP is compromised and ATP levels fall to 30 percent or lower compared to control during 45 minutes of incubation; in addition, cellular potassium decreases whereas LDH release and calcium influx increase [1a]. Both glycine administration and extracellular acidosis to a level of pH 7.0 prevent the increased calcium uptake and the LDH release [1a]. This model of ATP depletion differs from oxygen deprivation models in the mechanism by which ATP synthesis is impaired. Nevertheless, in both conditions cellular injury and increased fluxes of calcium into the cytosol occur, and each can be arrested by glycine, without any improvement in cellular ATP levels or in cellular potassium stores [1a] (Fig. 47-11). These data suggest that glycine may also limit the severity of cell injury by a mechanism that occurs before, in addition to, or coincidental with increased cytosolic Ca^{2+}. This interpretation may be unique to rat tubules or this particular model of ATP depletion. Finally, low PO_4 conditions and mercuric chloride appear to disrupt disulfide bonds as part of their pathogenic injury process; it has been reported that both glycine and acidosis protect disulfide bonds, which may contribute to their beneficial effects [72]. Disulfide bonds are found throughout the protein structures of ion channels, G-proteins, and receptors, and thus their importance to cell integrity cannot be overlooked.

ENDOTHELIUM

Endothelial cells produce both endothelial-derived relaxing factor (EDRF) and several endothelins [303]. The EDRF appears to be nitric oxide (NO), and maneuvers designed to enhance its production, thereby inducing renal vasodilation, could be a fruitful area of therapy [57]. Adenosine released from injured cells can be a profound stimulator of EDRF [112]. Endothelin is also synthesized by tubule cells in the inner medulla [147]. The absence of renal vasodilatory responses to EDRF-dependent vasodilators such as acetylcholine has confirmed the ischemia-induced derangement in this mechanism [61]. In addition, absence of normal autoregulatory re-

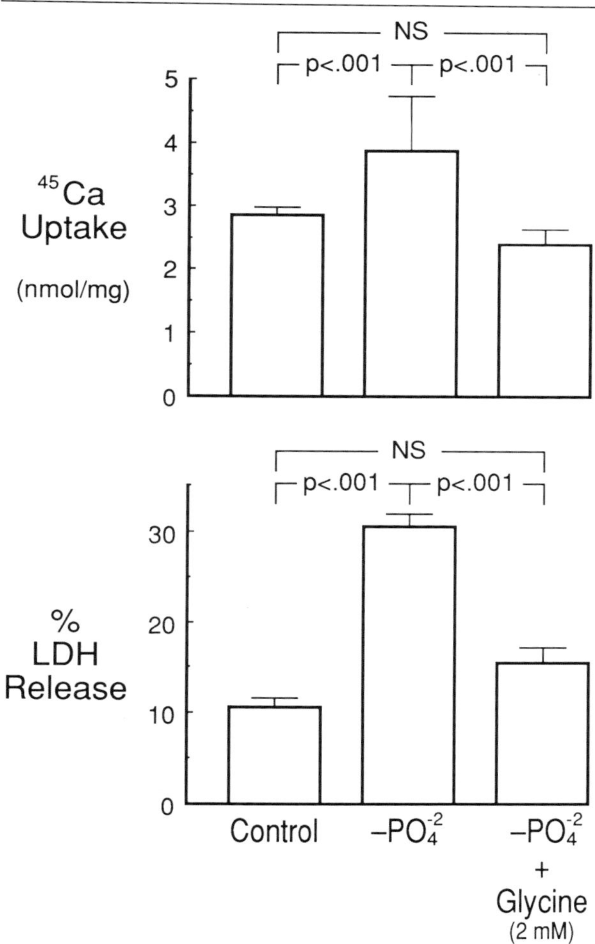

Fig. 47-11. Phosphate depletion increases calcium uptake in rat proximal tubules (upper panel) and LDH release (lower panel). Glycine (2 mM) prevents both increased calcium uptake and increased LDH release. (From [1a].)

sponses—up to one week after renal ischemia—is consistent with very slow endothelial cell recovery from the initial ischemic damage [61]. Oxidants produced during ischemia or reflow may damage endothelial cells [230, 354], resulting in poor recovery of EDRF production or enhanced endothelin release [304]. This slow recovery may also be due in part to the formation of advanced glycosylation products on the collagen that is interspersed between endothelial cells and underlying smooth muscle of the vasculature. These advanced glycosylation products inhibit the vasodilatory effects of nitric oxide [42]. Curiously, hypoxia actually causes release of EDRF while simultaneously releasing endothelin, and this may represent an important difference between hypoxia and complete anoxia [226]. Finally, the paradoxical renal vasoconstriction that accompanies reductions in renal perfusion pressure in postischemic kidneys [142] has provided a new insight into the mechanisms of renal autoregulation in normal kidneys, as is discussed elsewhere in this book (see Chap. 2).

The paradoxical vasoconstriction seen in these rat models of ischemic ARF provides a reasonable physiologic explanation for the fresh ischemic lesions often noted by pathologists who examine kidneys or kidney biopsies, at times well after the initial ischemic or hypotensive event has passed [278]. Taken together, these observations suggest that even modest reductions in renal perfusion pressure in the days following correction of the ischemic insult are not accompanied by either the normal renal vasodilatory response or the maintenance of renal blood flow [114]. Rather, it would appear that proportionate decreases in renal blood flow may ensue and lead to repeated ischemic events. As pointed out earlier these would appear to be most problematic in the outer medulla and cortical rays, where oxygenation is already markedly reduced due to the anatomic arrangement of blood vessels [35]. Endothelin itself may be the cause of this paradoxical vasoconstriction and both antibodies to endothelin and a recently synthesized endothelin antagonist can reduce ischemic functional and morphologic injury as well as decrease the progressive tissue Ca^{2+} overload that occurs during reperfusion [56a, 267]. Moreover, endothelin-dependent contraction of anoxic femoral arteries is blocked by calcium entry blockers and is readily reversible, suggesting a link between Ca^{2+} ions, the endothelium, and vascular smooth muscle. Clearly, endothelin release from injured tissue during reperfusion may exacerbate the severity of tubular cell injury. However, at present, data do not totally support a major effect of endothelin at glomerular sites during ischemia/reperfusion. Wilkes and associates [334] reasoned that if endothelin were to be an important cause of reduced glomerular hemodynamics, there should be either an increase in its receptor number or affinity in postischemic glomerular tissue, but neither of these was observed.

Rather, the outer medullary region of the kidney appears to be highly susceptible to the events that occur during early reperfusion. Specifically, shortly after initiation of reperfusion, red blood cells (RBC) become trapped in the vasa recta [16, 168, 181, 185, 343]. This accumulation of RBC further prolongs the period of oxygen deprivation beyond that of the initial ischemic period, and extended oxygen deprivation is likely the cause of the extensive necrosis seen in the S_3 segments of the proximal tubule and the fragmentation necrosis of the TAL [35–37]. The trapping of these RBC may be the result of underlying endothelial damage initiated by either endogenous free radical generation or by activated neutrophils. Brezis and associates [34] have documented functional and morphologic improvement in vivo and in the IPK when rats are given L-arginine, the precursor of NO. RBC that accumulate in these deeper nephron regions may also compress adjacent tubules, raise intratubular pressure, and reduce effective glomerular filtration pressure [114]. If this is truly a contribution to lower GFR, one would expect its effect to be less important, with more prolonged periods of ischemia when irreversible cell injury becomes the predominate cause of ARF [114]. In addition, one would also expect that hemoconcentration would, for any given period of ischemia, cause greater functional injury, whereas hemodilution would cause less functional injury; this has been experimentally confirmed in the intact rat with an ischemia time of 45 minutes and hematocrits of 31, 46, and 60 percent [113]. Hemodilution, however, reduces the concentration of neutrophils, which could also lessen injury (see below). Curiously, the type of renal cell determines in which direction it will swell when confronted with oxygen deprivation. Mason and her colleagues [182] have demonstrated that proximal tubule cells swell outward from the basolateral side, whereas TAL cells swell inward toward the lumen.

Taken together these data suggest strongly that prevention of medullary congestion should be beneficial to ischemic kidneys. However, there is a potentially detrimental effect of reducing this congestion. Stated simply, improvement in nutrient flow to the outer medulla may cause an enhancement in transport activity in the TAL and S_3 segments of the proximal tubule. Brezis and colleagues [36] noted the precarious balance between oxygen availability in this region and transport-related work, and reported that anything that upset this balance, that is, increased transport alone or decreased oxygen availability, would lead to cellular necrosis. It has recently been shown that addition of SOD to ischemic rat kidneys will reduce the trapping of erythrocytes, which begins within 20 minutes of initiation of reperfusion, but that 1 week or 1 month later functional injury is not decreased [17]. Conversely, although enhancement of RBC trapping is seen during postischemic treatment with hyperosmolar mannitol, renal function is often improved [116]. The beneficial effects of mannitol may be to reduce both cell swelling and mitochondrial Ca^{2+} overload [46, 250]. Thus, the goal of reducing RBC trapping, in an effort to restore reflow to the outer medulla to more normal levels, may be accompanied by cellular injury that develops because of increased transport-related work at a time when, and at nephron sites where, ATP recovery is not yet complete [23, 51]. This reasoning is entirely consistent with the early improvement in nephron function in rats treated with the antioxidant probucol [23].

Trapping of RBC begins quite promptly, within 20 minutes, at least as assessed by increased leakage of plasma from vessels [17]. This leakage is preventable by SOD, by certain steroids, or by use of antineutrophil serum, and in such studies RBC accumulation in the outer medulla is reduced [225]. Thus, in vivo, activated neutrophils release toxic oxygen metabolites whose effects are primarily directed at vessels or endothelial cells, or both, in the outer medulla [17]. Finally, pentoxifylline has been shown to markedly reduce polymorphonuclear leukocyte (PMN)-induced injury in the rat, presumably by inhibiting neutrophil activation. Less medullary congestion was an associated beneficial effect and thus pentoxifylline halts prolongation of ischemia [169]. Neutrophils are clearly responsible for the early extravasation of plasma from capillaries, a process that leads to red blood cell congestion [114].

In the 1970s, it was clearly shown that intact and cultured renal cells underwent massive swelling during experimental oxygen deprivation and that this could be reduced—and cell viability increased—by provision of impermeant solutes such as polyethylene glycol [86]. Shanley and associates [262] have noted endothelial cell swelling in a mouse model of bilateral renal ischemia. These authors suggest that endothelial damage due to swelling or oxygen free radicals exposes the collagen of the basement membrane to platelets, which then become activated. The basement membrane itself is also susceptible to oxidant injury [21], thus further exacerbating the platelet aggregation. The activated platelets aggregate and provide an impediment to vascular flow and eventually result in impaction of RBC within the vessels [262]. Substantial platelet aggregation can be observed as early as 1 hour after reflow begins following 30 minutes of warm ischemia in the mouse [262]. This impediment to flow throughout the outer medulla apparently diverts blood flow from efferent arterioles to the descending vasa recta. Yagil and colleagues have measured a marked increase in papillary flow at both 90 minutes and 24 hours of reperfusion [341, 342]. This increased flow may partly account for the absence of concentrating ability following renal ischemia. Ca^{2+} also plays a predominant role in platelet aggregation [272]. The absence of these same events in the well-oxygenated outer cortex suggests that the poorly oxygenated outer medulla is problematic not only for epithelial tissues, such as TAL and S_3, but for endothelial cells as well. Thus, the series of events in which plasma flow through the outer medulla slows and eventually stops does not simply involve erythrocytes.

Pathologic examination of the outer medulla often reveals large numbers of neutrophils, a phenomenon not seen in the outer cortex. Linas and co-workers [163] have shown that addition of neutrophils enhances injury, which can be prevented by catalase, in the isolated perfused ischemic kidney, and it has been demonstrated that amelioration of renal ischemic injury can be achieved with antisera to neutrophils or neutrophil depletion induced by nitrogen mustard [115, 145, 216]. Thus, sequestration of neutrophils in very small capillaries lined with endothelial cells, which are at risk for oxygen radical–mediated damage, appears to extend the injury process in the kidney beyond the period of oxygen deprivation itself. Neutrophils also damage tubules participating in the back leak that characterizes some models of renal ischemia [117].

Shanley and co-workers [262] have sought to circumvent this problem by use of a unique strain of transgenic (TG) mice, which express the human Cu^{2+}/Zn^{2+} SOD gene at four to six times the normal level. This approach would obviate the problems of intravenous administration of antioxidants such as SOD with short plasma half-lives and poor intracellular accessibility. When subjected to bilateral renal ischemia for 25 to 35 minutes, these TG mice have little or no rise in serum creatinine or BUN after 24 hours of reflow, exhibit only very modest S_3 or TAL necrosis, and have a markedly reduced outer medullary congestion compared to normal mice [262]. Endothelial cell damage also appears to be minimal and platelet aggregation is diminished [262]. These data would support a role for superoxide generation within endothelial cells [303, 354] during reperfusion as a contributing factor in tissue and functional impairment following ischemia. Undoubtedly, coincidental increases in endothelin release or a decrease in EDRF would likely accompany free radical–mediated endothelial injury, and activation of neutrophils could also be facilitated by damaged endothelial cells. In addition to superoxide anion, thromboxane A_2 (TxA_2) is produced by endothelial cells [303]. The injurious effects of vasoconstrictive TxA_2, which can be overcome in vivo, may reflect an imbalance between vasodilatory and vasoconstrictor prostaglandin production and account therefore for the renal dysfunction induced by indomethacin [203].

Andreoli and her colleagues [3–6] have contributed extensively to the interpretation of free radical–mediated injury to endothelial cells, generally concluding that hydrogen peroxide is a major cause of oxidant damage [6]. Using hypoxanthine-xanthine oxidase or glucose-glucose oxidase to generate exogenous free radicals, these workers also noted prompt development of DNA injury and NAD^+ depletion as well as ATP depletion [3]. Their results confirmed that the fall in NAD^+ is due to an attempt to repair DNA via poly-ADP–ribose polymerase, in which NAD^+ is a co-factor. This differs somewhat from the fall in NAD^+ during hypoxia, which occurs in parallel with increases in nicotinamide adenine dinucleotide (NADH). It is possible to measure NAD^+ and NADH using cycling techniques in single cells in real time, and it is anticipated that these techniques will be useful to investigators studying renal hypoxia or anoxia in vitro [3]. Although NAD^+ is an important co-factor in the synthesis of ATP [3] and its depletion could be expected to compromise ATP production, it was found that preservation of NAD^+ did not prevent the fall in cellular ATP that occurred during free radical–mediated injury [3]. The decrease in ATP seen in endothelial cells occurs quickly whereas other indices of cell injury such as LDH release occur much later [3]. Finally, Andreoli's group has shown an important potential role for activated neutrophils in producing direct endothelial cell injury [4]. These data taken together help explain the injurious effects noted by Linas and his group [163] during perfusion of the isolated rat kidney with PMN, since presumably endothelial cell production of superoxide anion or TxA_2 would have been constant.

VASCULAR SMOOTH MUSCLE

The smooth muscle of intact vessels constricts during hypoxia [180], and Rodman and associates [234] have shown that this is due largely to reduced EDRF activity rather than increased endothelin. The degree of hypoxia, the vascular location, and the length of exposure to oxygen deprivation appear to be important variables. For example, very short exposures of the lumen of femoral artery or aorta from rabbits to low PO_2 induce measurable increases in bioassayable EDRF and vasodilation [226]. Thus, low PO_2 in immediate proximity to the endothelia of small vessels may help sustain vasodilation. These data on vessels from areas other than the kidney might be applicable to the outer medulla of the mammalian kidney, where PO_2 is known to be quite low and where surrounding tubules depend on patent arterioles and capillaries to provide oxygen for transport [34, 158].

Although focus has been directed at arteries and capillaries, the conditions in the renal venous circulation have not received much attention. It would seem important to compare responses of renal veins and venules to hypoxia or anoxia to determine if the endothelium that lines them releases vasoconstrictor substances, such as superoxide anion and thromboxane A_2 [303]. Curiously, in some vascular smooth muscle preparations the maximal response to hypoxia is increased two- to threefold for the same dose of endothelin and the response to endothelin-3 exceeds that for endothelin-1 [58a, 70]. There also appears to be a species difference between dog and rabbit vessels with respect to their responses to hypoxia. In dog femoral artery, for example, the endothelium was not crucial for hypoxic vasodilation, but in the rabbit thoracic aorta, the removal of the endothelium lessened the magnitude of relaxation [58a, 76]. Whether species differences are truly responsible for these differences remains to be answered.

As in proximal tubules, hypoxia or high KCl depolarization of vascular smooth muscle increases Ca^{2+} influx and this can be reduced by two-thirds if the temperature is reduced by 10°C [136]. Since temperature changes are often used to evaluate receptor (membrane protein) recycling, the decrease in Ca^{2+} influx at reduced temperature may reflect a decrease in the activity of voltage-gated Ca^{2+} channels, which are themselves proteins, as are receptors [54a, 194, 222]. The IPK of the rat perfused with RBC, as opposed to cell-free perfusate, and exposed to ischemia for 25 minutes at 27°C also exhibits less injury to TAL and coincidentally less vascular congestion is observed [160]. Together, these observations suggest that the protective effects of reduced temperature may lie in the reduction of Ca^{2+} influx into vascular or endothelial cells in the outer medulla. Furthermore, Ca^{2+} itself regulates the epithelial conductance of K^+ and thus membrane potential is dependent on maintenance of appropriate transmembrane Ca^{2+} flux rates [55]. Anoxia and hypoxia also elicit different responses in vascular smooth muscle, as they do in proximal tubules. For example, in porcine pulmonary artery, hypoxia increases the contraction induced by leukotriene D4 (LTD4), but anoxia blunts this effect markedly [220]. At present, one must consider that either LTD4 release is increased more during hypoxia than anoxia or that vascular responsiveness to LTD4 is enhanced with hypoxia. Interleukin-1 also blunts contraction of vascular smooth muscle cells and could provide for a novel route of renal protection [19]. Vascular smooth muscle Ca^{2+} handling is also affected by extracellular Na^+. For example, cell Ca^{2+} is not depleted rapidly from smooth muscle cells stimulated by angiotensin II when extracellular Na^+ is replaced by either KCl or N-methyl-D-glucamine and free Ca^{2+} increases more than twofold under such conditions [275]. Addition of Na^+ to the bathing medium results in rapid Ca^{2+} efflux. Thus,

Ca^{2+} efflux in smooth muscle is dependent on the external Na^+ concentration and occurs by a Na^+-Ca^{2+} exchange in normoxia. This process, like that shown for renal tubules, is probably compromised during hypoxia or anoxia. Genetic disturbances of Na^+-Ca^{2+} exchange appear to be important causes of salt-sensitive hypertension in animals [57]. Recent studies in rats suggest that this is due to altered NO production by endothelial cells and therefore Na^+/Ca^{2+} exchange is important in endothelial cells, as well as in epithelial and smooth muscle cells [57].

Hypoxia or anoxia will also reduce ATP generation by vascular smooth muscle cells and increase calcium influx, an effect that can be prevented by acidosis [211]. Recently, the observation that 1mM ATP will decrease the open probability of the K^+ channel in these cells [282] provides for an additional explanation of the in vivo protective effects of ATP-$MgCl_2$ seen by Siegel and colleagues [271]. These patch clamp studies were made in an attempt to better understand hypertensive phenomena, but the applicability of K^+ channel activity, membrane depolarization, cellular Ca^{2+} regulation, and (renal) vasoconstriction during hypoxia deserves further investigation. At least one additional area in which KCl-induced depolarization has been evaluated involves the effects subsequent to the increase in Ca_i; simultaneously, phosphorylation of myosin light chain is reduced, thereby accounting, in part, for contractile disturbances [101]. Therefore, decreases in the transmembrane K^+ gradient, as occurs in hypoxia, can have multiple effects on both renal epithelial and vascular tissue.

Finally, the absolute importance of low oxygen tension in smooth muscle vasoconstriction has been questioned. Marshall and associates [180] have found that at constant, low-percent oxygen (10% vs. normal 21%), constriction of pulmonary arteries from rat lungs could be enhanced markedly if the ratio of carbon monoxide to oxygen was increased. With carbon monoxide addition, a reduction of the energy state of the vascular smooth muscle cells develops, and thus electron flow or mitochondrial function, or both, may be more important in functional vascular responses than the absolute level of hypoxia.

MESANGIAL CELLS

Mesangial cells exhibit contractile responses to agonists [293], mediated in part by increases in Ca_i^{2+}. In vivo, the administration of phorbol myristate acetate (PMA) results in a 10-fold increase in neutrophil accumulation in, and functional damage to, glomeruli in intact rats [345]. These events can be prevented by scavengers of free radicals or by depletion of PMN. Functional damage from the ROM has been localized to the mesangium (decreased ultrafiltration coefficient) and to the efferent arteriole, at and just downstream from the trapped, activated PMN [345]. Shah and associates [258] have demonstrated an additional effect of activated neutrophils to degrade human glomerular basement membrane. Their results confirm that the basement membrane injury is due to a latent metaloproteinase(s) that becomes activated, likely via hypochlorous acid production; thus, this mechanism may also contribute to acute glomerular injury.

These data, which confirm that mesangial cells, through their effects on single-nephron glomerular filtration rate (SNGFR), do participate in the functional injury associated with ischemia [183], have prompted investigators to seek ways to reverse this damage. The antioxidant, probucol, has been shown to attenuate the decrease in SNGFR [23]. Atrial natriuretic peptide (ANP) is a vasodilatory polypeptide and both the 24 and the 28 amino acid (aa) form are equally beneficial in promoting better glomerular function in dogs and rats [100, 205, 208, 264]. ANP and prostaglandins may work in concert to reduce glomerular dysfunction [97], but ANP must be administered rather promptly after ischemia [99]. ANP exerts these beneficial effects even though hypotension ensues [208, 227], but the beneficial effects of ANP are enhanced if hypotension is avoided by infusions of dopamine [60]. Analogues of ANP are also beneficial [227]. The improvement in GFR can also be seen in the IPK as well, where control of renal perfusion pressure and thus systemic hypotension is not a factor [161, 205]. In this model, mannitol enhances the protective effect of ANP [161]. Since ANP is not bound by glomerular receptors following ischemia, renal venous blood is rich in ANP [333]. It has been suggested that high renal venous levels of ANP, in fact, act as a marker for renal ischemia [333]. Finally, ANP may act as a paracrine rather than endocrine factor since renorenal reflexes are suppressed following unilateral models of renal ischemia [299].

ACTIVATED PLATELETS

Activated platelets may also contribute to glomerular dysfunction during ischemic renal injury [98]. Platelet activating factor infused into intact rats leads to a prompt decrease in glomerular filtration rate (GFR), whereas the administration of two different PAF receptor antagonists before renal ischemia provides for improved postischemic creatinine clearances and a conversion of anuric ARF to polyuric ARF [167]. The activated platelets promote formation of the potent renal vasoconstrictor TxA_2. Inhibition of TxA_2 synthesis with DP-1904 substantially reduces renal injury due to PAF infusion or ischemia [186]. Platelets can be activated by multiple pathways, including Ca^{2+} and oxidants [272]. Once platelets are activated little can be done to reverse the subsequent thrombi formation. However, inhibition of fibrin deposition or fibrinolysis often attenuates reperfusion injury [82].

CYTOSKELETAL CHANGES

The structure and polarity of a cell are intimately related to the energy state and therefore it is not surprising that a hypoxic, an anoxic, or an ischemia-induced decrease in ATP is accompanied by visible and biochemically quantifiable alterations in the structural integrity of cells [171]. Cell swelling is the most pronounced and easily identifiable morphologic alteration that accompanies oxygen deprivation, at least in proximal tubules and endothelial cells. The TAL, which exhibits very low water permeability under normal conditions, thereby contributing to the effectiveness of the countercurrent diluting process, apparently does not swell before the development of fragmentation necrosis, and this is one of the few examples of cellular injury that is not preceded by cell swelling [35, 36].

In addition to cell swelling, a rather prompt internalization of brush border membranes (microvilli) occurs during renal ischemia [306]. Associated with this internalization, approximately 15 minutes after beginning ischemia, there is a disruption of tight junctions (zona adherens) and a redistribution of apical and cytosolic enzymes and possibly receptors to other membrane sites [143, 197, 199, 233]. Redistribution of basolateral enzymes has also been described [197, 201]. Using fluorescent dyes coupled to antibodies to specific cellular proteins and appropriately stained specimens of renal tissue, structural correlates to bleb formation, disruption of cytoskeletal components of tight junction integrity, and apical filament disintegration have been demonstrated morphologically using these cytochemical techniques [143]. In addition, changes in the pattern and quantity of membrane phospholipids, so important to the activity of membrane proteins, have also been described. The apical membrane seems to be at greater risk for these early changes [255]. It has been postulated recently that tight junction and zona adherens breakdown may be protective in ischemia, as this would permit reduced contact between hypoxic and normal cells [49]. It is known especially in smooth muscle that spread of hypoxic damage to neighboring, normoxic cells (1) occurs through such junctions, (2) is enhanced by increased cytosolic Ca^{2+}, and (3) is attenuated by acidosis [49]. This mechanism would tend to isolate the injured cells from more normal, intact cells and provides for focal rather than generalized areas of injury.

Thinning and beading of the subapical and microvilli F-actin network has been demonstrated. This area, known as the terminal web, begins to be disrupted as early as 5 minutes after ischemia begins; this is before, and therefore possibly a cause of, membrane phospholipid alterations and internalization of brush borders [143, 291]. Other structural proteins as well as those destined to direct intracellular proteins toward specific cellular sites are also affected early after ATP depletion due to ischemia. These changes are seen in ankarin, actin, and myosin, among others, and reflect (1) the absence of ATP necessary to remodel (polymerization/depolymerization) cytoskeletal proteins and (2) the aberrant Ca^{2+} metabolism of ischemia [20, 122]. In cultured tubules, an increase in cytosolic free Ca^{2+} precedes bleb formation, which is a sign of cytoskeletal disruption [223]. Finally, the prompt early release of fatty acids from membrane phospholipids due to activation of phospholipases provides for strong covalent bonds between fatty acids and several integral cellular proteins [209a]. Such linkages could disrupt cellular integrity, leading not only to increased permeability of plasma membranes but decreases in transcellular resistance as well. This major new area of investigation is likely to provide, in the future, an extended knowledge of cellular biology, as well as possibly novel methods of delaying or reversing the effects of ischemia, especially in the presence of ATP depletion and cellular Ca^{2+} overload. Until that time, however, the impressive protection against ARF from ischemia seen with use of calcium channel blockers will continue to have an important role in preventing ischemic injury [reviewed in 249, 251–253, 330].

Cell Repair

Beset with the frustration that it is often difficult to anticipate or prevent cell ischemia in vivo, several laboratories have begun to explore the possibility of enhancing the recovery process once reoxygenation and blood flow are normalized. Molecular biology studies designed to detect genes and gene products that could participate in cell recovery are currently providing a strong foundation for future studies [29, 102, 109, 124, 125, 213, 231, 239, 269, 270]. Unmodified cellular Ca^{2+} overload, metabolic derangements (e.g., decreased ATP and GSH), and oxidant formation apparently provide conditions favorable for early gene activation.

Safirstein and colleagues [238] have explored the changes in the preproepidermal growth factor (PPEGF) gene since expression of this gene occurs primarily in renal tissue, where the most extensive cell injury from hypoxic events in the rat IPK is achieved, that is, the TAL. Their work also has identified several promotor elements and has detected significant homology between mouse and rat EGF and PPEGF [240]. The regulation of these promotor elements during or after renal ischemia may eventually provide meaningful approaches to improve cellular recovery.

It is also well known that proximal tubule cells can reline denuded basement membranes after ischemic injury. This observation presupposes that a population of undifferentiated stem cells resides within the proximal tubule mass, and these can be induced to differentiate and grow under postischemic conditions [125]. Humes and co-workers have tested this hypothesis using retinoic acid and EGF on primary cultures of rabbit proximal tubules. These treated cell cultures have been shown to both grow and develop polarized characteristics including lumen formation [124]. Thus, if the period of ischemia is not inordinately prolonged, tubular recovery may occur as stem cells are induced to grow and differentiate, and this may be due to the induction of EGF. EGF is, in fact, one of the earliest genes to be detected following ischemia [213].

Bonventre and associates have directed their studies at the regulation of DNA transcription following ischemia, reasoning that subsequent gene activity or expression must be preceded by transcription [338]. Since proteins with zinc fingers are characteristic of transcription via binding to DNA, these authors have examined adult and neonatal rat kidneys for clones with linkage to zinc finger genes. Adult rat kidneys express a particular clone (14 kb) that is unique (not found in other organs or in neonatal rats), suggesting that its RNA becomes expressed with aging. This clone contains 12 zinc finger regions and appears to be involved in growth regulation and control of ontogeny in adult rat kidneys [338]. Efforts to inhibit this activity might permit a much quicker and more complete return of normal tubular structure and function after ischemia. With all such studies caution must be exercised in attempts to modify gene induction because, if uncontrolled, this can lead to, for example, cystic disease after ischemia [59].

Summary

As noted several times in this chapter, differences in experimental observations may ultimately be related to the degree of oxygen deprivation, the presence of endothelial cells or neutrophils, or the species or cell type used for the experimental model. Although renal tubules from different species and cultured cell lines derived from renal tissue provide the most direct evidence for the pathophysiology of renal epithelial damage, less information is available for renovascular smooth muscle and renal endothelial cells. Although it is likely that the vascular smooth muscle cells and endothelial cells harvested from larger vessels will be found to exhibit the same physiology and pathophysiology as do cells of renal origin, this has not yet been proved to be true. It remains important to continue to describe both the subtle and major differences in experimental results associated with time-related (Fig. 47-12) metabolic derangements in ATP production, in ion regulation including

Fig. 47-12. Time-dependent changes in cellular Ca^{2+} are both a response to decreased oxygen availability and a cause of cellular injury. This schema thus affords a central role to altered calcium homeostasis in the initiation of ischemic cell injury. (From [1].)

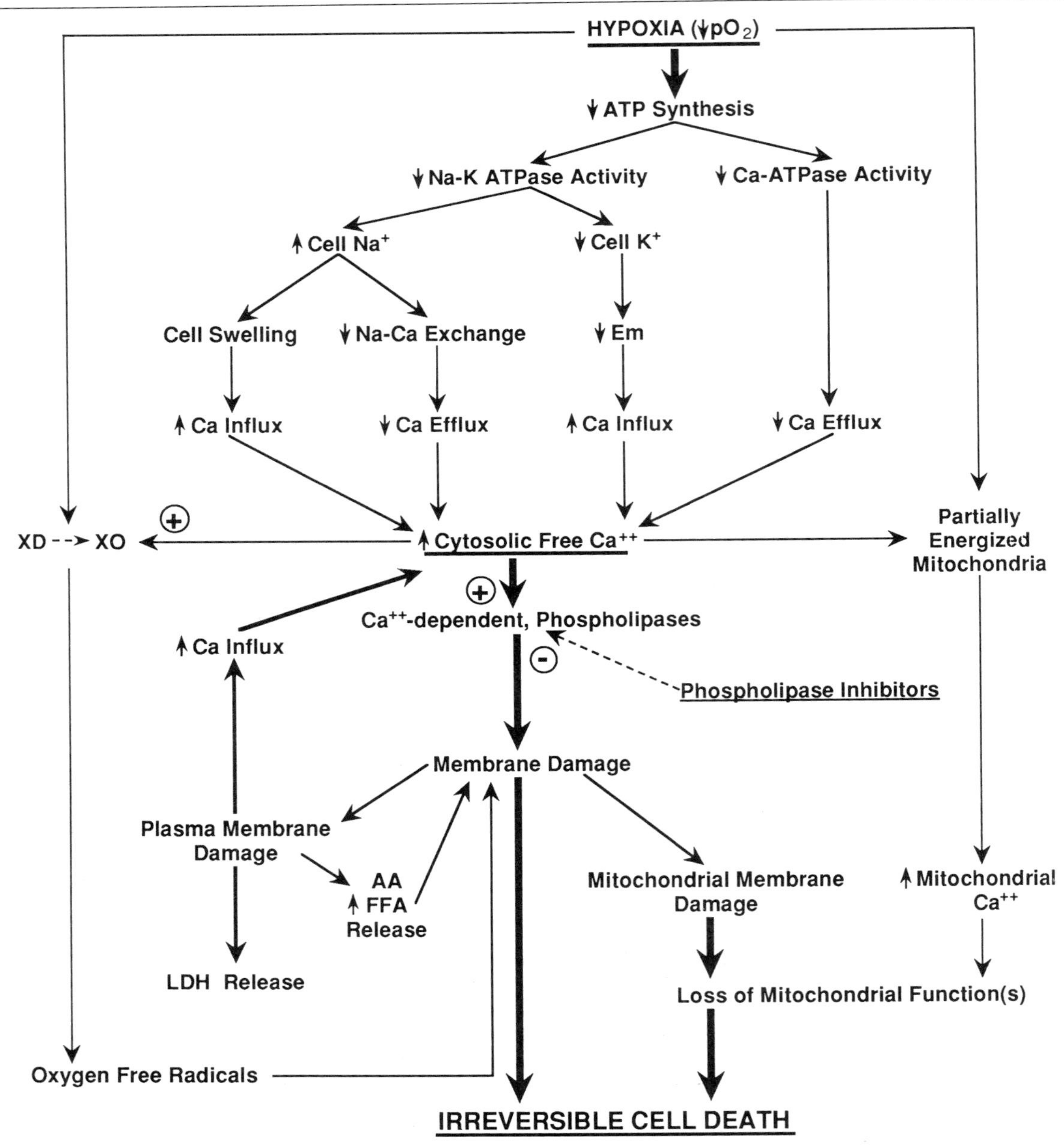

Ca^{2+} and iron, and in oxidant formation in various species and systems as investigators proceed toward the ultimate goal of defining ways to prevent or at the very least salvage the human kidney, with its multiple cell types, from the ravages of an ischemic insult.

References

1. Almeida, A. R. P., Bunnachak, D., Burnier, M., et al. Time-dependent protective effects of calcium channel blockers on anoxia- and hypoxia-induced proximal tubule injury. *J. Pharmacol. Exp. Ther.* 260: 526, 1992.

1a. Almeida, A. R. P., Wetzels, J. F. M., Bunnachak, D., et al. Acute phosphate depletion and in vitro rat proximal tubule injury: Protection by glycine and acidosis. *Kidney Int.* (in press), 1992.

2. Altschuld, R. A., Hostetler, J. R., and Brierley, G. P. Response of isolated heart cells to hypoxia, reoxygenation and acidosis. *Circ. Res.* 49: 307, 1981.
3. Andreoli, S. P. Mechanisms of endothelial cell ATP depletion after oxidant injury. *Pediatr. Res.* 25: 97, 1988.
4. Andreoli, S. P., Baehner, R. L., and Bergstein, J. M. In vitro detection of endothelial cell damage using 2-deoxy-D-^{3}H-glucose: Comparison with chromium 51, ^{3}H-leucine, ^{3}H-adenine, and lactate dehydrogenase. *J. Lab. Clin. Med.* 106: 253, 1985.
5. Andreoli, S. P., Liechty, E. A., Mallett, C., et al. Exogenous adenine nucleotides replete endothelial cell adenosine triphosphate after oxidant injury by adenosine uptake. *J. Lab. Clin. Med.* 115: 304, 1990.
6. Andreoli, S. P., Mallett, C. P., and Bergstein, J. M. Role of glutathione in protecting endothelial cells against hydrogen peroxide oxidant injury. *J. Lab. Clin. Med.* 108: 190, 1986.
7. Andrews, P. M., and Bates, S. B. Improving Euro-Collins flushing solution's ability to protect kidneys from normothermic ischemia. *Miner. Electrol. Metab.* 11: 309, 1985.
8. Andrews, P. M., and Coffey, A. K. Factors that improve the preservation of nephron morphology during cold storage. *Lab. Invest.* 46: 100, 1982.
9. Arnold, P. E., and Lumlertgul, D., Burke, T. J., et al. In vitro versus in vivo mitochondrial calcium loading in ischemic acute renal failure. *Am. J. Physiol.* 248: F845, 1985.
10. Arnold, P. E., Van Putten, V. J., Lumlertgul, D., et al. Adenine nucleotide metabolism and mitochondrial Ca^{2+} transport following renal ischemia. *Am. J. Physiol.* 250: F357, 1986.
11. Avison, M. J., van Waarde, A., Stromski, M. E., et al. Metabolic alterations in the kidney during ischemic acute renal failure. *Semin. Nephrol.* 9: 98, 1989.
12. Avison, M. J., van Waarde, A., Thulin, G., et al. Adenosine transport contributes to the beneficial effect of post-ischemic ATP-$MgCl_2$ (abstract). *Kidney Int.* 37: 476, 1990.
13. Baines, A. D., Shaikh, N., and Ho, P. Mechanisms of perfused kidney cytoprotection by alanine and glycine. *Am. J. Physiol.* 259: F80, 1990.
14. Barber, J. D., and Moss, N. G. Reduced renal perfusion pressure causes prostaglandin-dependent excitation of R2 chemoreceptors in rats. *Am. J. Physiol.* 259: R1243, 1990.
15. Baumann, M., Bender, E., Stommer, G., et al. Effects of warm and cold ischemia on mitochondrial functions in brain, liver and kidney. *Mol. Cell. Biochem.* 87: 137, 1989.
16. Bayati, A., Christofferson, R., Kallskog, O., et al. Mechanism of erythrocyte trapping in ischaemic acute renal failure. *Acta Physiol. Scand.* 138: 13, 1990.
17. Bayati, A., Kallskog, O., and Wolgast, M. The long-term outcome of post-ischaemic acute renal failure in the rat. I. A functional study after treatment with SOD and sucrose. *Acta Physiol. Scand.* 138: 25, 1990.
18. Bayati, A., Nygren, K., Kallskog, O., et al. The effect of loop diuretics on the long-term outcome of post-ischaemic acute renal failure in the rat. *Acta Physiol. Scand.* 139: 271, 1990.
19. Beasley, D., Cohen, R. A., and Levinsky, N. G. Interleukin 1 inhibits contraction of vascular smooth muscle. *J. Clin. Invest.* 83: 331, 1989.
20. Bershadsky, A. D., and Gelfand, V. I. Role of ATP in the regulation of stability of cytoskeletal structures. *Cell. Biol. Int. Rep.* 7: 173, 1983.
21. Betts, W. H., Cleland, L. G., Gee, D. J., et al. Effects of D-penicillamine on a model of oxygen-derived free radical mediated tissue damage. *Agents Actions* 14: 283, 1984.
22. Bird, J. E., Evan, A. P., Peterson, O. W., et al. Early events in ischemic renal failure in the rat: Effects of antioxidant therapy. *Kidney Int.* 35: 1282, 1989.
23. Bird, J. E., Milhoan, K., Wilson, C. B., et al. Ischemic acute renal failure and antioxidant therapy in the rat. The relation between glomerular and tubular dysfunction. *J. Clin. Invest.* 81: 1630, 1988.
24. Biscoe, T. J., and Duchen, M. R. Monitoring pO_2 by the carotid chemoreceptor. *News Physiol. Sci.* 5: 229, 1990.
25. Bock, H. A., Brunner, F. P., Torhorst, J., et al. Failure of verapamil to protect from ischaemic renal damage. *Nephron* 57: 299, 1991.
26. Bonventre, J. V. Mediators of ischemic renal injury. *Ann. Rev. Med.* 39: 531, 1988.
27. Bonventre, J. V., and Nemenoff, R. Renal tubular arachidonic acid metabolism. *Kidney Int.* 39: 438, 1991.
28. Borkan, S. C., and Schwartz, J. H. Role of oxygen free radical species in in vitro models of proximal tubular ischemia. *Am. J. Physiol.* 257: F114, 1989.
29. Bortz, J. D., Rotwein, P., Devol, D., et al. Focal expression of insulin-like growth factor I in rat kidney collecting duct. *J. Cell. Biol.* 107: 811, 1988.
30. Bosco, P. J., and Schweizer, R. T. Use of oxygen radical scavengers on autografted pig kidneys after warm ischemia and 48-hour perfusion preservation. *Arch. Surg.* 123: 601, 1988.
31. Brand, P. H., and Taylor, B. B. Lactate oxidation by three segments of the rabbit proximal tubule. *Proc. Soc. Exp. Biol. Med.* 182: 454, 1986.
32. Bratell, S., Haraldsson, G., Herlitz, H., et al. Protective effects of pretreatment with superoxide dismutase, catalase and oxypurinol on tubular damage caused by transient ischaemia. *Acta Physiol. Scand.* 139: 417, 1990.
33. Breyer, M. D., and Jacobson, H. R. Regulation of rabbit medullary collecting duct cell pH by basolateral Na^+/H^+ and Cl^-/base exchange. *J. Clin. Invest.* 84: 996, 1989.
34. Brezis, M., Heyman, S. N., Dinour, D., et al. Role of nitric oxide in renal medullary oxygenation. *J. Clin. Invest.* 88: 390, 1991.
35. Brezis, M., Rosen, S., Silva, P., et al. Selective vulnerability of the medullary thick ascending limb to anoxia in the isolated perfused rat kidney. *J. Clin. Invest.* 73: 182, 1984.
36. Brezis, M., Rosen, S., Spokes, K., et al. Transport-dependent anoxic cell injury in the isolated perfused rat kidney. *Am. J. Pathol.* 116: 327, 1984.
37. Brezis, M., Shina, A., Kidroni, G., et al. Calcium and

hypoxic injury in the renal medulla of the perfused rat kidney. *Kidney Int.* 34: 186, 1988.
38. Brooks, D. P., Rhodes, G. R., Woodward, P., et al. Production of methylguanidine in dogs with acute and chronic renal failure. *Clin. Sci.* 77: 637, 1989.
39. Brunskill, N., Hayes, C., Morrissey, J., et al. Changes in lipid environment decrease Na,K-ATPase activity in obstructive nephropathy. *Kidney Int.* 39: 843, 1991.
40. Bruun, N. E., Rehling, M., Skott, P., et al. Enhanced fractional sodium reabsorption in the ischaemic kidney revisited with lithium as a probe. *Scand. J. Clin. Lab. Invest.* 50: 579, 1990.
41. Bucala, R., Tracey, K. J., and Cerami, A. Advanced glycosylation products quench nitric oxide and mediate defective endothelium-dependent vasodilation in experimental diabetes. *J. Clin. Invest.* 87: 432, 1991.
42. Buhl, M. R. Purine metabolism in ischaemic kidney tissue. *Dan. Med. Bull.* 29: 1, 1982.
43. Bunnachak, D., Joseph, J., Burke, T. J., et al. Contribution of phospholipases to altered calcium kinetics during hypoxia in isolated rat proximal tubules (abstract). *Kidney Int.* 37: 478, 1990.
44. Burg, M., Patlak, C., Green, N., et al. Organic solutes in fluid absorption by renal proximal convoluted tubules. *Am. J. Physiol.* 231: 627, 1976.
45. Burke, T. J., Arnold, P. A., Gordon, J. A., et al. Protective effect of intrarenal calcium membrane blockers before or after renal ischemia. *J. Clin. Invest.* 74: 1830, 1984.
46. Burke, T. J., Arnold, P. A., Schrier, R. W. Prevention of ischemic acute renal failure with impermeant solutes. *Am. J. Physiol.* 244: F646, 1984.
47. Burke, T. J., Singh, H., and Schrier, R. W. Calcium handling by renal tubules during oxygen deprivation injury to the kidney prior to reoxygenation. *Cardiovasc. Drugs Ther.* 4: 1319, 1990.
48. Burnier, M., Van Putten, V. J., Schieppati, A., et al. Effect of extracellular acidosis on ^{45}Ca uptake in isolated hypoxic proximal tubules. *Am. J. Physiol.* 254: C839, 1988.
49. Burt, J. M. Block of intercellular communication: Interaction of intracellular H^+ and Ca^{2+}. *Am. J. Physiol.* 253: C607, 1987.
50. Busa, W. B., and Nuccitelli, R. Metabolic regulation via intracellular pH. *Am. J. Physiol.* 246: R409, 1984.
51. Canavese, C., Stratta, P., and Vercellone, A. The case for oxygen free radicals in the pathogenesis of ischemic acute renal failure. *Nephron* 49: 9, 1988.
52. Carafoli, E. Intracellular calcium homeostasis. *Ann. Rev. Biochem.* 56: 395, 1987.
53. Catroux, P., Cambar, J., Benchekroun, N., et al. Antilipoperoxydant effect of trimetazidine in post ischaemic acute renal failure in the rat. *Adv. Exp. Med. Biol.* 264: 383, 1990.
54. Catterall, W. A. Functional subunit structure of voltage-gated calcium channels. *Science* 253: 1499, 1991.
55. Chang, H., Yamashita, N., Matsunoga, H., et al. Ca^{2+}-activated K^+ conductance causes membrane hyperpolarizations in a monkey kidney cell line (JTC-12). *J. Membr. Biol.* 103: 263, 1988.
56. Chatson, G., Perdrizet, G., Anderson, C., et al. Heat shock protects kidneys against warm ischemic injury. *Curr. Surg.* 47: 420, 1990.
56a. Chittinandana, A., Chan, L., Suleymanlar, G., et al. Effects of endothelin antagonist on ischemic acute renal failure (abstract). *J. Am. Soc. Nephrol.* 2: 644, 1991.
57. Chen, P. Y., and Sanders, P. W. L-arginine abrogates salt-sensitive hypertension in Dahl/Rapp rats. *J. Clin. Invest.* 88: 1559, 1991.
58. Cighetti, G., Del Puppo, M., Paroni, R., et al. Lack of conversion of xanthine dehydrogenase to xanthine oxidase during warm renal ischemia. *FEBS Lett.* 274: 82, 1990.
58a. Coburn, R. F., Eppinger, R., and Scott, D. P. Oxygen-dependent tension in vascular smooth muscle. Does the endothelium play a role? *Clin. Res.* 58: 341, 1986.
59. Cohen, E. P., and Elliott, W. C., Jr. The role of ischemia in acquired cystic kidney disease. *Am. J. Kidney Dis.* 15: 55, 1990.
60. Conger, J. D., Robinette, J. B., and Schrier, R. W. Smooth muscle calcium and endothelium-derived relaxing factor in the abnormal vascular responses of acute renal failure. *J. Clin. Invest.* 82: 532, 1988.
61. Conger, J. D., Falk, S. A., Yuan, B. H., et al. Atrial natriuretic peptide and dopamine in a rat model of ischemic acute renal failure. *Kidney Int.* 35: 1126, 1989.
62. Cooper, K., Thulin, G., Gaudio, K., et al. Role of intracellular Ca^{2+} overload in the pathogenesis of ischemic renal injury (abstract). *Kidney Int.* 29: 300, 1986.
63. Cotterill, L. A., Gower, J. D., Fuller, B. J., et al. Oxidative damage to kidney membranes during cold ischemia. Evidence of a role for calcium. *Transplantation* 48: 745, 1989.
64. Davis, J. A., Abarzua, M., Laughrey, E., et al. Cellular glycine fluxes during protection by glycine against renal proximal tubule cell injury (abstract). *FASEB J.* 4: A1142, 1990.
65. Dennis, V. W., and Brazy, P. C. Sodium, phosphate, glucose, bicarbonate, and alanine interactions in the isolated proximal convoluted tubule of the rabbit kidney. *J. Clin. Invest.* 62: 387, 1978.
66. Deray, G., Martinez, F., Cacoub, P., et al. A role for adenosine calcium and ischemia in radiocontrast-induced intrarenal vasoconstriction. *Am. J. Nephrol.* 10: 316, 1990.
67. Didlake, R., Kirchner, K. A., Lewin, J., et al. Attenuation of ischemic renal injury with fructose 1,6-diphosphate. *J. Surg. Res.* 47: 220, 1989.
68. Dische, F. E., Neuberger, J., Keating, J., et al. Kidney pathology in liver allograft recipients after long-term treatment with cyclosporin A. *Lab. Invest.* 58: 395, 1988.
69. Doctor, R. B., and Mandel, L. J. Minimal role of xanthine oxidase and oxygen free radicals in rat renal tubule reoxygenation injury. *J. Am. Soc. Nephrol.* 1: 959, 1991.
70. Douglas, S. A., James, S., and Hiley, C. R. Endothelial modulation and changes in endothelin pressor activity during hypoxia in the rat isolated perfused superior mesenteric arterial bed. *Br. J. Pharmacol.* 103: 1441, 1991.
71. Downey, J. M., Hearse, D. J., and Yellon, D. M. The role of xanthine oxidase during myocardial ischemia in several species including man. *J. Mol. Cell. Cardiol.* 20: 55, 1988.
72. Duran, M. A., Spencer, D., Weise, M., et al. Renal epithelial amino acid concentrations in mercury-induced and postischemic acute renal failure. *Toxicol. Appl. Pharmacol.* 105: 183, 1990.
73. Eddy, L. J., Stewart, J. R., Jones, J. P., et al. Free radical-producing enzyme, xanthine oxidase, is undetectable in human hearts. *Am. J. Physiol.* 253: H709, 1987.
74. Eisenger, D. R., Suranyi, M. G., Brocs, P., et al. Effects of verapamil in the prevention of warm ischaemia induced acute renal failure in dogs. *Aust. N.Z. J. Surgery* 55: 391, 1985.
75. Elkadi, H. K., Mardan, A. H., Nghiem, D. D., et al. The

role of calcium antagonists in the management of renal warm ischemia. *J. Urol.* 141: 974, 1989.
76. Elliott, D. A., Ong, B. Y., Bruni, J. E., et al. Role of endothelium in hypoxic contraction of canine basilar artery. *Br. J. Pharmacol.* 96: 949, 1989.
77. Emami, A., Schwartz, J. H., and Borkan, S. C. Transient ischemia or heat stress induces a cytoprotectant protein in rat kidney. *Am. J. Physiol.* 260: F479, 1991.
78. Engerson, T. D., McKelvey, T. G., Thyne, D. B., et al. Conversion of xanthine dehydrogenase to oxidase in ischemic rat tissue. *J. Clin. Invest.* 79: 1564, 1987.
79. Epstein, F., Silva, P., Spokes, K., et al. Prevention with glycine of acute renal failure caused by cis-platinum (abstract). *Kidney Int.* 37: 480, 1990.
80. Evered, D. F. Species differences in amino acid excretion by mammals. *Comp. Biochem. Physiol.* 23: 163, 1967.
81. Fahey, R. C., Newton, G. L., Arrick, B., et al. Entamoeba histolytica: A eukaryate without glutathione metabolism. *Science* 224: 68, 1984.
82. Ferrero, M. E., Marni, A., and Gaja, G. Defibrotide, a profibrinolytic drug, reduced damage due to postischaemic reperfusion in rats. *Biochem. Soc. Trans.* 18: 501, 1990.
83. Ferwana, O. S., Pirie, S. C., and Potts, D. J. Unilateral renal ischaemia in the rat: Effect of contralateral nephrectomy and intrarenal flush with phosphate-buffered sucrose. *Clin. Sci.* 74: 261, 1988.
84. Ferwana, O. S., Pirie, S. C., and Potts, D. J. Effect of phosphate-buffered sucrose flush solution upon the initial phase of ischaemic acute renal failure in the rat. *Clin. Sci.* 77: 77, 1989.
85. Fine, L. G., Holley, R. W., Nasri, H., et al. BSC-1 growth inhibitor transforms a mitogenic stimulus into a hypertrophic stimulus for renal proximal tubular cells: Relationship to Na^+/H^+ antiport activity. *Proc. Natl. Acad. Sci. U.S.A.* 82: 6163, 1985.
86. Flores, J., DiBona, D. R., Beck, C. H., et al. The role of cell swelling in ischemic renal damage and the protective effect of hypertonic solute. *J. Clin. Invest.* 51: 118, 1972.
87. Frei, U., Harms, A., Bakovic-Alt, R., et al. Calcium channel blockers for kidney protection. *J. Cardiovasc. Pharmacol.* 16: S11, 1990.
88. Frindt, G., Lee, C. O., Yang, J. M., et al. Potential role of cytoplasmic calcium ions in the regulation of sodium transport in renal tubules. *Miner. Elect. Metab.* 14: 40, 1988.
89. Fuller, B. J., Gower, J., and Cotterill, L. Reperfusion injury and renal metabolism: The temporal relationship between oxidative stress and functional change. *Adv. Exp. Med. Biol.* 264: 389, 1990.
90. Gabbai, F. B., Peterson, O. W., and Blantz, R. C. Protective effect of glycine (G) infusion in a single nephron model of acute renal failure (ARF) (abstract). *Kidney Int.* 35: 406, 1989.
91. Galat, J. A., Robinson, A. V., and Rhodes, R. S. The contribution of hypoxia to postischemic renal dysfunction. *Surgery* 104: 257, 1988.
92. Galat, J. A., Robinson, A. V., and Rhodes, R. S. Postischemic renal dysfunction: The limited role of xanthine oxidase-generated oxygen free radicals. *J. Surg. Res.* 49: 488, 1990.
93. Gamelin, L. M., and Zager, R. A. Evidence against oxidant injury as a critical mediator of postischemic acute renal failure. *Am. J. Physiol.* 255: F450, 1988.
94. Garza-Quintero, R., Ortega-Lopez, J., Stein, J. H., et al. Alanine protects rabbit proximal tubules against anoxic injury in vitro. *Am. J. Physiol.* 258: F1075, 1990.
95. Gaudio, K. M., Ardito, T. A., Reilly, H. F., et al. Accelerated cellular recovery after an ischemic renal injury. *Am. J. Pathol.* 112: 338, 1983.
96. Gedroyc, W. M., Koffman, G., and Saunders, A. J. Ureteric obstruction in stented renal transplants. *Br. J. Urol.* 62: 123, 1988.
97. Gianello, P., Besse, T., Gustin, T., et al. Atrial natriuretic factor, arachidonic acid metabolites and acute renal ischemia: Experimental protocol in the rat. *Eur. Surg. Res.* 22: 57, 1990.
98. Gianello, P., Janssen, T., Chatzopoulos, C., et al. Beneficial effect of piracetam on renal blood flow in ischemically injured kidneys in the rat. *Transplant. Proc.* 20: 914, 1988.
99. Gianello, P., Poelaert, D., Ramboux, A., et al. Beneficial effect of atrial natriuretic factor on ischemically injured kidneys in the rat. A new approach to improve early renal function. *Transplantation* 45: 860, 1988.
100. Gianello, P., Poelaert, D., Ramboux, A., et al. Beneficial effect of atrial natriuretic factor on ischemically injured kidneys in rats. *Transplant. Proc.* 20: 921, 1988.
101. Gilbert, E. K., Weaver, B. A., and Rembold, C. M. Depolarization decreases the $[Ca^{2+}]_i$ sensitivity of myosin light-chain kinase in arterial smooth muscle: Comparison of aequorin and fura 2 $[Ca^{2+}]_i$ estimates. *FASEB J.* 5: 2593, 1991.
102. Gobe, G. C., Axelsen, R. A., and Searle, J. W. Cellular events in experimental unilateral ischemic renal atrophy and in regeneration after contralateral nephrectomy. *Lab. Invest.* 63: 770, 1990.
103. Goldfarb, D., Iaina, A., and Serban, I. Beneficial effect of verapamil in ischemic acute renal failure in the rat. *Proc. Soc. Exp. Biol. Med.* 172: 389, 1983.
104. Gower, J. D., Fuller, B. J., and Green, C. J. Prevention by antioxidants of oxidative damage to rabbit kidneys subjected to cold ischaemia. *Biochem. Pharmacol.* 38: 213, 1989.
105. Gower, J. D., Healing, G., and Fuller, B. J. Iron redistribution and lipid peroxidation in the cold ischaemic kidney. *Adv. Exp. Med. Biol.* 264: 393, 1990.
106. Gower, J. D., Healing, G., Fuller, B. J., et al. Protection against oxidative damage in cold-stored rabbit kidneys by desferrioxamine and indomethacin. *Cryobiology* 26: 309, 1989.
107. Gronow, G. H. J., and Cohen, J. J. Substrate support for renal functions during hypoxia in the perfused rat kidney. *Am. J. Physiol.* 247: F618, 1984.
108. Hagen, T. M., Aw, T. Y., and Jones, D. P. Glutathione uptake and protection against oxidative injury in isolated kidney cells. *Kidney Int.* 34: 74, 1988.
109. Hammerman, M. R. The renal growth hormone/insulin-like growth factor I axis. *Am. J. Kidney Dis.* 17: 644, 1991.
110. Hansson, R., Bratell, S., Burian, P., et al. Renal function during reperfusion after warm ischaemia in rabbits: An experimental study on the possible protective effects of pretreatment with oxygen radical scavengers or lidoflazine. *Acta Physiol. Scand.* 139: 39, 1990.
111. Hansson, R., Johansson, S., Jonsson, O., et al. Kidney protection by pretreatment with free radical scavengers and allopurinol: Renal function at recirculation after warm ischaemia in rabbits. *Clin. Sci.* 71: 245, 1986.
112. Headrick, J. P., and Berne, R. M. Endothelium-dependent and -independent relaxations to adenosine in guinea pig aorta. *Am. J. Physiol.* 259: H62, 1990.

113. Hellberg, P. O., Bayati, A., Kallskog, T. O., et al. Red cell trapping after ischemia and long-term kidney damage. Influence of hematocrit. *Kidney Int.* 37: 1240, 1990.
114. Hellberg, P. O., Kallskog, T. O., and Wolgast, M. Nephron function in the early phase of ischemic renal failure. Significance of erythrocyte trapping. *Kidney Int.* 38: 432, 1990.
115. Hellberg, P. O., Kallskog, T. O., Ojteg, G., et al. Peritubular capillary permeability and intravascular RBC aggregation after ischemia: Effects of neutrophils. *Am. J. Physiol.* 258: F1018, 1990.
116. Hellberg, P. O., Nygren, A., Hansell, P., et al. Post-ischemic administration of hyperosmolar mannitol enhances erythrocyte trapping in outer medullary vasculature in the rat kidney. *Renal Physiol. Biochem.* 13: 328, 1990.
117. Hellberg, P. O. A., and Kallskog, T. O. K. Neutrophil-mediated postischemic tubular leakage in the rat kidney. *Kidney Int.* 36: 555, 1989.
118. Henke, W., and Jung, K. Ischemia decreases the content of the adenine nucleotide translocator in mitochondria of rat kidney. *Biochim. Biophys. Acta* 1056: 71, 1991.
119. Henke, W., Klotzek, S., Nickel, E., et al. Ischemia-induced alterations of rat kidney mitochondria. *Transplantation* 49: 997, 1990.
120. Henke, W., Nickel, E., and Jung, K. Determination of purine compounds by ion-pair microbore high-performance liquid chromatography: Application to ischemic rat kidney mitochondria. *J. Chromatogr.* 527: 498, 1990.
121. Hess, M. L., and Greenfield, L. J. Calcium entry blockers: Potential applications in shock. *Adv. Shock Res.* 10: 15, 1983.
122. Howard, W. D., and Timasheff, S. N. Linkages between the effects of taxol, colchicine, and GTP on tubulin polymerization. *J. Biol. Chem.* 263: 1342, 1988.
123. Hreniuk, D., Guerra, E., and Wilson, P. D. A common final pathway of renal tubule cell killing by toxins and anoxia (AN): Attenuation by protease inhibition (abstract). *Kidney Int.* 35: 408, 1989.
124. Humes, H. D., and Cieslinski, D. A. Growth selection of renal proximal tubule stem cells in tissue culture (abstract). *J. Am. Soc. Nephrol.* 2: 439, 1991.
125. Humes, H. D., Cieslinski, D. A., Coimbra, T. M., et al. Epidermal growth factor enhances renal tubule cell regeneration and repair and accelerates the recovery of renal function in postischemic acute renal failure. *J. Clin. Invest.* 84: 1757, 1989.
126. Humes, H. D., Nguyen, V. D., Cieslinski, D. A., et al. The role of free fatty acids in hypoxia-induced injury to renal proximal tubule cells. *Am. J. Physiol.* 256: F688, 1989.
127. Irazu, C. E., Rajagopalan, P. R., Orak, J. K., et al. Mitochondrial membrane fluidity changes in renal ischemia. *J. Exp. Pathol.* 5: 1, 1990.
128. Irazu, C. E., Ruidera, E., Singh, I., et al. Effect of ischemia and 24 hour reperfusion on ATP synthesis in the rat kidney. *J. Exp. Pathol.* 4: 29, 1989.
129. Jacobs, W. R., Ferrari, C. M., Brazy, P. C., et al. Cytosolic free calcium regulation in renal tubules from spontaneously hypertensive rats. *Am. J. Physiol.* 258: F175, 1990.
130. Jacobs, W. R., Sgamboli, M., Gomez, G., et al. Role of cytosolic Ca in renal tubule damage induced by anoxia. *Am. J. Physiol.* 260: C545, 1991.
131. Jayakumar, A., Cheng, L., Liang, C. T., et al. Sodium gradient dependent calcium uptake in renal basolateral membrane vesicles. *J. Biol. Chem.* 259: 10827, 1984.
132. Joannidis, M., Bonn, G., and Pfaller, W. Lipid peroxidation—an initial event in experimental acute renal failure. *Renal Physiol. Biochem.* 12: 47, 1989.
133. Joannidis, M., Gstraunthaler, G., and Pfaller, W. Xanthine oxidase: Evidence against a causative role in renal reperfusion injury. *Am. J. Physiol.* 258: F232, 1990.
134. Joseph, J. K., Bunnachak, D., Burke, T. J., et al. A novel method of inducing and assuring total anoxia during in vitro studies of O_2 deprivation injury. *J. Am. Soc. Nephrol.* 1: 837, 1990.
135. Kako, K., Kato, M., Matsuoka, T., et al. Depression of membrane-bound Na^+-K^+-ATPase activity induced by free radicals and by ischemia of kidney. *Am. J. Physiol.* 254: C330, 1988.
136. Karaki, H., and Weiss, G. B. Modification by decreased temperature and hypoxia of ^{45}Ca movements in stimulated smooth muscle of rabbit aorta. *Gen. Pharmacol.* 18: 363, 1987.
137. Karasawa, A., and Kubo, K. Protection by benidipine hydrochloride (KW-3049), a calcium antagonist, of ischemic kidney in rats via inhibitions of Ca-overload, ATP-decline and lipid peroxidation. *Jpn. J. Pharmacol.* 52: 553, 1990.
138. Kaseda, S., Gilmore, R. F., Jr., and Zipes, D. P. Depressant effect of magnesium on early after depolarizations and triggered activity induced by cesium, quinidine and 4-aminopyridine in canine cardiac Purkinje fibers. *Am. Heart J.* 118: 458, 1989.
139. Kasiske, B. L., O'Donnell, M. P., and Keane, W. F. Direct effects of altered temperature on renal structure and function. *Renal Physiol. Biochem.* 11: 80, 1988.
140. Kedar, I., Jacob, E. T., Bar-Natan, N., et al. Dimethyl sulfoxide in acute ischemia of the kidney. *Ann. N.Y. Acad. Sci.* 411: 131, 1983.
141. Kehrer, G., Blech, M., Kallerhoff, M., et al. Contribution of amino acids in protective solutions to postischemic functional recovery of canine kidneys. *Res. Exp. Med. (Berl.)* 189: 381, 1989.
142. Kelleher, S. P., Robinette, J. B., Miller, J. B., et al. Effect of hemorrhagic reduction in blood pressure on recovery from acute renal failure. *Kidney Int.* 31: 725, 1987.
143. Kellerman, P. S., Clark, P. A., Hoilien, C. A., et al. Role of microfilaments in maintenance of proximal tubule structural and functional integrity. *Am. J. Physiol.* 259: F279, 1990.
144. Klausner, J. M., Paterson, I. S., Goldman, G., et al. Postischemic renal injury is mediated by neutrophils and leukotrienes. *Am. J. Physiol.* 256: F794, 1989.
145. Klausner, J. M., Paterson, I. S., Kobzik, L., et al. Vasodilating prostaglandins attenuate ischemic renal injury only if thromboxane is inhibited. *Ann. Surg.* 209: 219, 1989.
146. Klebanoff, S. J., Waltersdorph, A. M., Michel, B. R., et al. Oxygen-based free radical generation by ferrous ions and deferoxamine. *J. Biol. Chem.* 264: 19765, 1989.
147. Kohan, D. E., and Fiedorek, F. T., Jr. Endothelin synthesis by rat inner medullary collecting duct cells. *J. Am. Soc. Nephrol.* 2: 150, 1991.
148. Kokko, J. P. Proximal tubule potential difference. Dependence on glucose, HCO_3, and amino acids. *J. Clin. Invest.* 52: 1362, 1973.
149. Korb, S. M., Albornoz, G., and Light, J. A. Selenium addition to the flush/preservation solution protects kidneys against oxidative stress during warm and cold ischemia. *Transplant. Proc.* 22: 452, 1990.
150. Kotowski, A., Ruhrberg, A., and Kaufmann, P. The influence of hypoxic cell-free perfusion and ischemia on

cell morphology in the proximal tubular S2-segment of the rat kidney. *Virchows Arch. [B]* 59: 329, 1990.

151. Krapf, R. Basolateral membrane H/OH/HCO_3 transport in the rat cortical thick ascending limb. *J. Clin. Invest.* 82: 234, 1988.

151a. Kwon, S., Rothroch, J. K., and Dominguez, J. H. External sodium alters cell calcium homeostasis in rat proximal tubules (abstract). *Kidney Int.* 37: 458, 1990.

152. Lam, K. T., Borkan, S., Claffey, K. P., et al. Properties and differential regulation of two fatty acid binding proteins in the rat kidney. *J. Biol. Chem.* 263: 15762, 1988.

153. Le Hir, M., Angielski, S., and Dubach, U. C. Properties of an ecto-5'-nucleotidase of the renal brush border. *Renal Physiol. (Basel)* 8: 321, 1985.

154. Le Hir, M., and Dubach, U. C. An ATP-inhibited soluble 5'-nucleotidase of rat kidney. *Am. J. Physiol.* 254: F191, 1988.

155. Le Hir, M., and Kaissling, B. Distribution of 5'-nucleotidase in the renal interstitium of the rat. *Cell Tissue Res.* 258: 177, 1989.

156. Leahy, A. L., Fitzpatrick, J. M., and Wait, R. B. Variable results of calcium blockade in post-ischaemic renal failure. *Eur. Urol.* 14: 222, 1988.

157. LeFurgey, A., Ingram, P., Mandel, L. J., et al. Heterogeneity of calcium compartmentation: Electron probe analysis of renal tubules. *J. Membr. Biol.* 94: 191, 1986.

158. Leichtweiss, H.-P., Lubbers, D. W., Weiss, C., et al. The oxygen supply of the rat kidney: Measurements of interrenal pO_2. *Pflugers Arch.* 309: 328, 1969.

159. LeMasters, J. J., DiGuiseppi, J., Nieminen, A.-L., et al. Blebbing, free Ca^{2+} and mitochondrial membrane potential preceding cell death in hepatocytes. *Nature* 325: 78, 1987.

160. Lieberthal, W., Rennke, H. G., Sandock, K. M., et al. Ischemia in the isolated erythrocyte-perfused rat kidney. Protective effect of hypothermia. *Renal Physiol. Biochem.* 11: 60, 1988.

161. Lieberthal, W., Sheridan, A. M., and Valeri, C. R. Protective effect of atrial natriuretic factor and mannitol following renal ischemia. *Am. J. Physiol.* 258: F1266, 1990.

162. Linas, S. L., Shanley, P. F., White, C. W., et al. O_2 metabolite-mediated injury in perfused kidneys is reflected by consumption of DMTU and glutathione. *Am. J. Physiol.* 253: F692, 1987.

163. Linas, S. L., Shanley, P. F., Whittenburg, D., et al. Neutrophils accentuate ischemia-reperfusion injury in isolated perfused rat kidneys. *Am. J. Physiol.* 255: F728, 1988.

164. Linas, S. L. Whittenburg, D., and Repine, J. E. O_2 metabolites cause reperfusion injury after short but not prolonged renal ischemia. *Am. J. Physiol.* 253: F685, 1987.

165. Linas, S. L., Whittenburg, D., and Repine, J. E. Role of xanthine oxidase in ischemia/reperfusion injury. *Am. J. Physiol.* 258: F711, 1990.

166. Llibre, J., LaPointe, M. S., and Batlle, D. C. Free cytosolic calcium in renal proximal tubules from the spontaneously hypertensive rat. *Hypertension* 12: 399, 1988.

167. Lopez-Farre, A., Bernabeu, F., Gomez-Garre, D., et al. Platelet-activating factor antagonists treatment protects against postischemic acute renal failure in rats. *J. Pharmacol. Exp. Ther.* 253: 328, 1990.

168. Losonczy, G. Rheological mechanisms in postischemic acute renal failure. *Contrib. Nephrol.* 67: 22, 1988.

169. Luke, D. R., Berens, K. L., and Verani, R. R. Role of vascular decongestion in ischemic acute renal failure defined by postinsult administration of pentoxifylline. *Renal Fail.* 11: 187, 1989–90.

170. Lumlertgul, D., Harris, D. C. H., Burke, T. J., et al. Detrimental effect of hypophosphatemia on the severity and progression of ischemic acute renal failure. *Miner. Elect. Metab.* 12: 204, 1986.

171. Macknight, A. D. C., and Leaf, A. Regulation of Cellular Volume. In T. E. Andreoli, J. F. Hoffman, D. D. Fanestil, and S. G. Schultz (eds.), *Physiology of Membrane Disorders.* New York: Plenum Medical Book Co., 1986. Pp. 311–328.

172. Maeda, M., Seo, Y., Murakami, M., et al. Sodium-23 MR imaging of the kidney in guinea pig at 2.1 T, following arterial, venous, and ureteral ligation. *Magn. Reson. Med.* 16: 361, 1990.

173. Maixent, J. M., Birkui, P., Fenard, S., et al. Alpha subunits (alpha and alpha+) isoforms of Na^+, K^+-ATPase in dog heart. Alteration of alpha+ in ischemia. *Prog. Clin. Biol. Res.* 268B: 263, 1988.

174. Malis, C. D., and Bonventre, J. V. Mechanisms of calcium potentiation of oxygen free radical injury to renal mitochondria. *J. Biol. Chem.* 261: 14201, 1986.

175. Malis, C. D., Cheung, J. Y., Leaf, A., et al. Effects of verapamil in models of ischemic acute renal failure in the rat. *Am. J. Physiol.* 245: F735, 1983.

176. Malis, C. D., Weber, P. C., Leaf, A., et al. Incorporation of marine lipids into mitochondrial membranes increases susceptibility to damage by calcium and reactive oxygen species: Evidence for activation of phospholipase A_2 in mitochondria enriched in N-3 fatty acids. *Proc. Natl. Acad. Sci.* 87: 8845, 1990.

177. Mandel, L. J., and Murphy, E. Regulation of cytosolic free calcium in rabbit proximal renal tubules. *J. Biol. Chem.* 259: 11188, 1984.

178. Mandel, L. J., Schnellmann, R. G., and Jacobs, W. R. Intracellular glutathione in the protection from anoxic injury in renal proximal tubules. *J. Clin. Invest.* 85: 316, 1990.

179. Mandel, L. J., Takano, T., Soltoff, S. P., et al. Mechanisms whereby exogenous adenine nucleotides improve rabbit renal proximal function during and after anoxia. *J. Clin. Invest.* 81: 1255, 1988.

180. Marshall, C., Cooper, D. Y., and Marshall, B. E. Reduced availability of energy initiates pulmonary vasoconstriction. *Proc. Soc. Exp. Biol. Med.* 187: 282, 1988.

181. Mason, J., Beck, F., Dorge, A., et al. Intracellular electrolyte composition following renal ischemia. *Kidney Int.* 20: 61, 1981.

182. Mason, J., Joeris, B., Welsch, J., et al. Vascular congestion in ischemic renal failure: The role of cell swelling. *Miner. Electrolyte Metab.* 15: 114, 1989.

183. Mason, J., Olbricht, C., Takabotake, T., et al. The early phase of experimental acute renal failure. *Pflugers Arch.* 370: 155, 1977.

184. Mason, J., Torhorst, J., and Welsch, J. Role of the medullary perfusion defect in the pathogenesis of ischemic renal failure. *Kidney Int.* 26: 283, 1984.

185. Mason, J., Welsch, J., and Torhorst, J. The contribution of vascular obstruction to the functional defect that follows renal ischemia. *Kidney Int.* 31: 65, 1987.

186. Masumura, H., Kunitada, S., Irie, K., et al. A thromboxane A2 synthase inhibitor, DP-1904, prevents rat renal injury. *Eur. J. Pharmacol.* 193: 321, 1991.

187. Matthys, E., Patel, Y., Kreisberg, J., et al. Lipid alterations induced by renal ischemia: Pathogenic factor in membrane damage. *Kidney Int.* 26: 153, 1984.

188. Mcanulty, J. F., Southard, J. H., and Belzer, F. O. Comparison of the effects of adenine-ribose with adenosine for maintenance of ATP concentrations in five day hypothermically perfused dog kidneys. *Cryobiology* 25: 409, 1988.
189. McCord, J. M. Oxygen-derived free radicals in postischemic tissue injury. *N. Eng. J. Med.* 312: 159, 1985.
190. McCoy, C. D., Selvaggio, A. M., Alexander, E. A., et al. Adenosine triphosphate depletion induces a rise in cytosolic free calcium in canine renal epithelial cells. *J. Clin. Invest.* 82: 1326, 1988.
191. McCoy, R. N., Hill, K. E., Ayon, M. A., et al. Oxidant stress following renal ischemia: Changes in the glutathione redox ratio. *Kidney Int.* 33: 812, 1988.
192. McKelvey, T. G., Hollwarth, M. E., Granger, D. N., et al. Mechanisms of conversion of xanthine dehydrogenase to xanthine oxidase in ischemic rat liver and kidney. *Am. J. Physiol.* 254: G753, 1988.
193. Messana, J. M., Cieslinski, D. A., O'Connor, R. P., et al. Glutathione protects against exogenous oxidant injury to rabbit renal proximal tubules. *Am. J. Physiol.* 255: F874, 1988.
194. Miller, C. 1990: Annus mirabilis of potassium channels. *Science* 252: 1092, 1991.
195. Miyahara, M., Okimasu, E., Mickasa, H., et al. Improvement of the anoxia-induced mitochondrial dysfunction by membrane modulation. *Arch. Biochem. Biophys.* 233: 139, 1984.
196. Molitoris, B. A., Alfrey, A. C., Harris, R. A., et al. Renal apical membrane cholesterol and fluidity in regulation of phosphate transport. *Am. J. Physiol.* 249: F12, 1985.
197. Molitoris, B. A., Chan, L. K., Shapiro, J. I., et al. Loss of epithelial polarity: A novel hypothesis for reduced proximal tubule Na^+ transport following ischemic injury. *J. Membr. Biol.* 107: 119, 1989.
198. Molitoris, B. A., Falk, S. A., and Dahl, R. H. Ischemia-induced loss of epithelial polarity. Role of the tight injunction. *J. Clin. Invest.* 84: 1334, 1989.
199. Molitoris, B. A., Hoilien, C. A., Dahl, R., et al. Characterization of ischemia-induced loss of epithelial polarity. *J. Membr. Biol.* 106: 233, 1988.
200. Molitoris, B. A., and Kinne, R. Ischemia induces surface membrane dysfunction. Mechanisms of altered Na^+ -dependent glucose transport. *J. Clin. Invest.* 80: 647, 1987.
201. Molitoris, B. A., Wilson, P. D., Schrier, R. W. Ischemia induces partial loss of surface membrane polarity and accumulation of putative calcium ionophores. *J. Clin. Invest.* 76: 2097, 1985.
202. Murphy, E., and Mandel, L. J. Cytosolic free calcium levels in rabbit proximal kidney tubules. *Am. J. Physiol.* 242: C124, 1982.
203. Murray, M. D., and Brater, D. C. Adverse effects of nonsteroidal anti-inflammatory drugs on renal function (editorial). *Ann. Intern. Med.* 112: 559, 1990.
204. Nagami, G. T. Effect of bath and luminal potassium concentration on ammonia production and secretion by mouse proximal tubules perfused in vitro. *J. Clin. Invest.* 86: 32, 1990.
205. Nakamoto, M., Shapiro, J. I., Chan, L., et al. In vitro and in vivo protective effects of atriopeptin III in ischemic acute renal failure. *J. Clin. Invest.* 80: 698, 1987.
206. Nakamura, H., Nemenoff, R. A., Gronich, J. H., et al. Subcellular characteristics of phospholipase A2 activity in the rat kidney. Enhanced cytosolic, mitochondrial, and microsomal phospholipase A2 enzymatic activity after renal ischemia and reperfusion. *J. Clin. Invest.* 87: 1810, 1991.
207. Nath, K. A., and Solatrudeen, A. K. Induction of renal growth and injury in the intact rat kidney by dietary deficiency of oxidants. *J. Clin. Invest.* 86: 1179, 1990.
208. Neumayer, H. H., Seherr-Thohs, U., Blossei, M., et al. Effect of human atrial natriuretic peptide on postischemic acute renal failure in conscious dogs. *Transplant. Proc.* 29: 917, 1988.
209. Nguyen, V. D., Cieslinski, D. A., and Humes, H. D. Importance of adenosine triphosphate in phospholipase A2-induced rabbit renal proximal tubule injury *J. Clin. Invest.* 82: 1098, 1988.
209a. Niggli, V., and Burger, M. M. Interaction of the cytoskeleton with plasma membrane. *J. Membr. Biol.* 100: 97, 1987.
210. Noel, J., Tejedor, A., Vinay, P., et al. BBM H^+-ATPase activity in the dog kidney: Modulation by substrate availability (abstract). *Kidney Int.* 37: 529, 1990.
211. Okada, K., Tsai, P., Briner, V., et al. Effects of extra- and intracellular pH on vascular action of arginine vasopressin. *Am. J. Physiol.* 260: F39, 1991.
212. Olsen, T. S., and Hansen, H. E. Ultrastructure of medullary tubules in ischemic acute tubular necrosis and acute interstitial nephritis in man. *APMIS* 98: 1139, 1990.
213. Ouellette, A. J., Malt, R. A., Sukhatme, V. P., et al. Expression of two "immediate early" genes, Egr-1 and c-fos, in response to renal ischemia and during compensatory renal hypertrophy in mice. *J. Clin. Invest.* 85: 766, 1990.
214. Paller, M. S. Hemoglobin- and myoglobin-induced acute renal failure in rats: Role of iron in nephrotoxicity. *Am. J. Physiol.* 255: F539, 1988.
215. Paller, M. S. Renal work, glutathione and susceptibility to free radical–mediated postischemic injury. *Kidney Int.* 33: 843, 1988.
216. Paller, M. S. Effect of neutrophil depletion on ischemic renal injury in the rat. *J. Lab. Clin. Med.* 113: 379, 1989.
217. Paller, M. S., and Hebbel, R. P. Ethane production as a measure of lipid peroxidation after renal ischemia. *Am. J. Physiol.* 251: F839, 1986.
218. Paller, M. S., and Hedlund, B. E. Role of iron in postischemic renal injury in the rat. *Kidney Int.* 34: 474, 1988.
219. Paller, M. S., Hoidal, J. R., and Ferris, T. F. Oxygen free radicals in ischemic acute renal failure in the rat. *J. Clin. Invest.* 74: 1156, 1984.
219a. Paller, M. S., and Neumann, T. V. Reactive oxygen species and rat renal epithelial cells during hypoxia and reoxygenation. *Kidney Int.* 40: 1041, 1991.
220. Paterson, N. A., Hamilton, J. T., Yaghi, A., et al. Effect of hypoxia on responses of respiratory smooth muscle to histamine and LTD4. *J. Appl. Physiol.* 64: 435, 1988.
221. Perdrizet, G. A., Kaneko, H., Buckley, T. M., et al. Heat shock protects pig kidneys against warm ischemic injury. *Transplant. Proc.* 22: 460, 1990.
222. Peters, T. Calcium in physiological and pathological cell function. *Eur. Neurol.* 25: 27, 1986.
223. Phelps, P. C., Smith, M. W., and Trump, B. F. Cytosolic ionized calcium and bleb formation after acute cell injury of cultured rabbit renal tubule cells. *Lab. Invest.* 60: 630, 1989.
224. Plagemann, P. G. W., Wohlhueter, R. M., and Woffendin, C. Nucleoside and nucleobase transport in animal cells. *Biochim Biophys. Acta* 947: 405, 1988.
225. Podrazik, R. M., Obedian, R. S., Remick, D. G., et al. Attenuation of structural and functional damage from acute renal ischemia by the 21-amino steroid U74006F in rats. *Curr. Surg.* 46: 287, 1989.
226. Pohl, U., and Busse, R. Hypoxia stimulates release of

endothelium-derived relaxant factor. *Am. J. Physiol.* 256: H1595, 1989.
227. Pollock, D. M., and Opgenorth, T. J. Beneficial effect of the atrial natriuretic factor analog A68828 in postischemic acute renal failure. *J. Pharmacol. Exp. Ther.* 255: 1166, 1990.
228. Portilla, D., and Mandel, L. J. Phospholipase A_2 activation during anoxic injury in proximal tubules. *J. Am. Soc. Nephrol.* 1: 602, 1990.
229. Ratcliffe, P. J., Moonen, C. T. W., Holloway, P. A. H., et al. Acute renal failure in hemorrhagic hypotension: Cellular energetics and renal function. *Kidney Int.* 30: 355, 1986.
230. Raytch, R. E., Chuknyiska, R. S., and Bulkley, G. B. The primary localization of free radical generation following anoxia/reoxygenation in isolated endothelial cells. *Surgery* 102: 122, 1987.
231. Reid, I. R., Civitelli, R., Westbrook, S. L., et al. Cytoplasmic pH regulation in canine renal proximal tubule cells. *Kidney Int.* 31: 1113, 1987.
232. Roake, J. A., Toogood, G. J., Cahill, A. P., et al. Reducing renal ischaemia during transplantation (letter; comment). *Br. J. Surg.* 78: 121, 1991.
233. Rocha-Singh, K. J., Hines, D. K., Honbo, N. Y., et al. Concanavalin A amplifies both β-adrenergic and muscarinic cholinergic receptor-adenylate cyclase-linked pathways in cardiac myocytes. *J. Clin. Invest.* 88: 760, 1991.
234. Rodman, D. M., Yamaguchi, T., Hasunuma, K., et al. Effects of hypoxia on endothelium-dependent relaxation of rat pulmonary artery. *Am. J. Physiol.* 258: L207, 1990.
235. Rosenberg, H. G., Martinez, P. S., Vaccarezza, A. S., et al. Morphological findings in 70 kidneys of living donors for renal transplant. *Pathol. Res. Pract.* 186: 619, 1990.
236. Rubanyi, G. M., and Vanhoutte, P. M. Hypoxia releases a vasoconstrictor substance from the canine vascular endothelium. *J. Physiol. (Lond.)* 364: 45, 1985.
237. Ruidera, E., Irazu, C. E., Rajagopalan, P. R., et al. Fatty acid metabolism in renal ischemia. *Lipids* 23: 882, 1988.
238. Safirstein, R., Megyesi, J., Saggi, S. J., et al. Increased KC and JE expression after renal ischemia and inhibition of JE expression by methyl prednisolone (abstract). *J. Am. Soc. Nephrol.* 2: 654, 1991.
239. Safirstein, R., Price, P. M., Saggi, S. J., et al. Changes in gene expression after temporary renal ischemia. *Kidney Int.* 37: 1515, 1990.
240. Safirstein, R., Zelent, A. Z., and Price, P. M. Reduced renal preproepidermal growth factor mRNA and decreased EGF excretion in ARF. *Kidney Int.* 36: 810, 1989.
241. Salaris, S. C., and Babbs, C. F. Effect of oxygen concentration on the formation of malondialdehyde-like material in a model of tissue ischemia and reoxygenation. *Free Radic. Biol. Med.* 7: 603, 1989.
242. Sandvig, K., Oisnes, S., Peterson, O. W., et al. Inhibition of endocytosis from coated pits by acidification of the cytosol. *J. Cell. Biochem.* 36: 73, 1988.
243. Scaduto, R. C., Jr., Gattone, V. H., 2d, Grotyohann, L. W., et al. Effect of an altered glutathione content on renal ischemic injury. *Am. J. Physiol.* 255: F911, 1988.
244. Schafer, J. A., and Williams, J. C. Transport of metabolic substrates by the proximal nephron. *Ann. Rev. Physiol.* 47: 103, 1985.
245. Schieppati, A., Wilson, P. D., Burke, T. J., et al. Effect of renal ischemia on cortical microsomal calcium accumulation. *Am. J. Physiol.* 249: C476, 1985.
246. Schilling, M. K., den Butter, G., Saunder, A., et al. Membrane stabilizing effects of glycine during kidney cold storage and reperfusion. *Transplant. Proc.* 23: 2387, 1991.
247. Schneider, J., Friderichs, E., and Giertz, H. Equieffective protection by human and bovine SOD against renal reperfusion damage in rats. *Basic Life Sci.* 49: 891, 1988.
248. Schoolwerth, A. C., Smith, B. C., and Culpepper, R. M. Renal gluconeogenesis. *Miner. Elect. Metab.* 14: 347, 1988.
249. Schrier, R. W. Role of calcium channel blockers in protection against experimental renal injury. *Am. J. Med.* 90: 21S, 1991.
250. Schrier, R. W., Arnold, P. E., Gordon, J. A., et al. Protection of mitochondrial function by mannitol in ischemic acute renal failure. *Am. J. Physiol.* 247: F365, 1984.
251. Schrier, R. W., Arnold, P. E., Van Putten, V. J., et al. Cellular calcium in ischemic acute renal failure: Role of calcium entry blockers. *Kidney Int.* 32: 313, 1987.
252. Schrier, R. W., and Burke, T. J. Role of calcium channel blockers in preventing acute and chronic renal injury. *J. Cardiovasc. Pharmacol.* 18: 38, 1991.
253. Schrier, R. W., Conger, J. D., and Burke, T. J. Pathogenetic Role of Calcium in Renal Cell Injury. In M. Hatano (ed.), *Nephrology*. Tokyo: Springer-Verlag, 1991. Pp. 648–659.
254. Schwertschlag, U., Schrier, R. W., and Wilson, P. Beneficial effects of calcium channel blockers and calmodulin binding drugs in vitro renal cell anoxia. *J. Pharmacol. Exp. Ther.* 238: 119, 1986.
255. Schwertz, D. W., Kreisberg, J. I., and Venkatachalam, M. A. Characterization of rat kidney proximal tubule brush border membrane associated phosphatidylinositol phosphodiesterase. *Arch. Biochem. Biophys.* 224: 555, 1983.
256. Scully, S. P., Segel, G. B., and Lichtman, M. A. Relationship of superoxide production to cytoplasmic free calcium in human monocytes. *J. Clin. Invest.* 77: 1349, 1986.
257. Seguro, A. C., Shimizu, M. H., Monteiro, J. L., et al. Effect of potassium depletion on ischemic renal failure. *Nephron* 51: 350, 1989.
258. Shah, S. V., Baricos, W. H., and Basci, A. Degradation of human glomerular basement membrane by stimulated neutrophils. *J. Clin. Invest.* 79: 25, 1987.
258a. Shanley, P. F., and Johnson, G. C. Evidence for mitochondrial electron transport dependent necrosis in the thick ascending limb of Henle (abstract). *Kidney Int.* 35: 417, 1989.
259. Shanley, P. F., and Johnson, G. C. Adenine nucleotides, transport activity and hypoxic necrosis in the thick ascending limb of Henle. *Kidney Int.* 36: 823, 1989.
260. Shanley, P. F., and Johnson, G. C. Calcium and acidosis in renal hypoxia. *Lab. Invest.* 65: 298, 1991.
261. Shanley, P. F., Shapiro, J. I., Chan, L., et al. Acidosis and hypoxic medullary injury in the isolated perfused kidney. *Kidney Int.* 34: 791, 1988.
262. Shanley, P. F., White, C. W., Avraham, K. B., et al. Use of transgenic animals to study models of human disease. *Renal Failure* 14: 391, 1992.
263. Shapiro, J. I., Mills, S., Cheung, C., et al. Effect of adenosine triphosphate depletion in vivo on renal function in the rat with and without ischemia. *Miner. Elect. Metab.* 15: 276, 1989.
264. Shaw, S. G., Weidmann, P., Hodler, J., et al. Atrial natriuretic peptide protects against acute ischemic renal failure in the rat. *J. Clin. Invest.* 80: 1232, 1987.
265. Sheng, W. Y., Lysz, T. A., Wyche, A., et al. Kinetic comparison and regulation of the cascade of microsomal en-

zymes involved in renal arachidonate and endoperoxide metabolism. *J. Biol. Chem.* 258: 2188, 1983.

266. Sheridan, A. M., La Raia, J. A., Schwartz, J. H., et al. Resistance of MDCK cells to chemical anoxia and toxic free fatty acids (abstract). *J. Am. Soc. Nephrol.* 1: 604, 1990.
267. Shiboute, Y., Suzuki, N., Shino, A., et al. Pathophysiological role of endothelin in acute renal failure. *Life Sci.* 46: 1611, 1990.
268. Shimizu, T., Kawabata, T., and Nakamura, M. Protective effect of a novel calcium blocker, S-312-d, on ischemic acute renal failure in rat. *J. Pharmacol. Exp. Ther.* 255: 484, 1990.
269. Shoskes, D. A., and Halloran, P. F. Ischemic injury induces altered MHC gene expression in kidney by an interferon-gamma-dependent pathway. *Transplant. Proc.* 23: 599, 1991.
270. Shoskes, D. A., Parfrey, N. A., and Halloran, P. F. Increased major histocompatibility complex antigen expression in unilateral ischemic acute tubular necrosis in the mouse. *Transplantation* 49: 201, 1990.
271. Siegel, N. J., Glazier, W. B., Chaudry, I. H., et al. Enhanced recovery from acute renal failure by the postischemic infusion of adenine nucleotides and magnesium chloride in rats. *Kidney Int.* 17: 338, 1980.
272. Siess, W. Multiple signal-transduction pathways synergize in platelet activation. *News Physiol. Sci.* 6: 51, 1991.
273. Silverman, M., Rose, H., and Puschett, J. B. Modifications in proximal tubular function induced by nitrendipine in a rat model of acute ischemic renal failure. *J. Cardiovasc. Pharmacol.* 14: 799, 1989.
274. Slusser, S. O., Grotyohann, L. W., Martin, L. F., et al. Glutathione catabolism by the ischemic rat kidney. *Am. J. Physiol.* 258: F1546, 1990.
275. Smith, J. B., and Smith, L. Extracellular Na^+ dependence of changes in free Ca^{2+}, $^{45}Ca^{2+}$ efflux and total cell Ca^{2+} produced by angiotensin II in cultured arterial muscle cells. *J. Biol. Chem.* 262: 17455, 1987.
276. Smolens, P., and Stein, J. H. Pathophysiology of acute renal failure. *Am. J. Med.* 70: 479, 1981.
277. Snowdowne, K. W., and Borle, A. B. Effect of low extracellular sodium on cytosolic ionized calcium. *J. Biol. Chem.* 260: 14998, 1985.
278. Snowdowne, K. W., Freudenrich, C. C., and Borle, A. B. The effects of anoxia on cytosolic free calcium, calcium fluxes, and cellular ATP levels in cultured kidney cells. *J. Biol. Chem.* 260: 11619, 1985.
279. Solez, K., Morel-Maroger, L., and Sraaer, J.-D. The morphology of "acute tubular necrosis" in man: Analysis of 57 renal biopsies and a comparison with the glycerol model. *Medicine (Baltimore)* 58: 362, 1979.
280. Southard, J. H., Marsh, D. C., Mcanulty, J. F., et al. Oxygen-derived free radical damage in organ preservation: Activity of superoxide dismutase and xanthine oxidase. *Surgery* 101: 566, 1987.
281. Spencer, A. J., LeFurgey, A., Mandel, L. J., et al. Anoxia-induced changes in elemental compartmentation in renal proximal tubules as studied by high resolution x-ray imaging (abstract). *Kidney Int.* 37: 495, 1990.
282. Standen, N. B., Quayle, J. M., Davies, N. W., et al. Hyperpolarizing vasodilators activate ATP-sensitive K^+ channels in arterial smooth muscle. *Science* 245: 177, 1989.
283. Steiner, M. G., and Babbs, C. F. Hydroxyl radical generation by postischemic rat kidney slices in vitro. *Free Radic. Biol. Med.* 9: 67, 1990.
284. Stratta, P., Canavese, C., Gurioli, L., et al. Oxygen free radicals in mediating tissue damage: Role in nephrological settings. *Contrib. Nephrol.* 77: 132, 1990.
285. Stromski, M. E., Cooper, K., Thulin, G., et al. Postischemic ATP-$MgCl_2$ provides precursors for resynthesis of cellular ATP in rats. *Am. J. Physiol.* 250: F834, 1986.
286. Stromski, M. E., Cooper, K., Thulin, G., et al. Chemical and functional correlates of postischemic renal ATP levels. *Proc. Natl. Acad. Sci. U.S.A.* 83: 6142, 1986.
287. Stromski, M. E., van Waarde, A., Avison, M. J., et al. Metabolic and functional consequences of inhibiting adenosine deaminase during renal ischemia in rats. *J. Clin. Invest.* 82: 1694, 1988.
288. Studer, R. K., and Borle, A. B. Effect of pH on the calcium metabolism of isolated rat kidney cells. *J. Membr. Biol.* 48: 325, 1979.
289. Sumpio, B. E., Chandry, I. H., Clemens, M. G., et al. Accelerated functional recovery of isolated rat kidney with ATP-$MgCl_2$ after warm ischemia. *Am. J. Physiol.* 247: R1047, 1984.
290. Sumpio, B. E., Hull, M. J., Baue, A. E., et al. Effects of ATP-$MgCl_2$ and adenosine-$MgCl_2$ administration on intracellular ATP levels in the kidney. *Biochim. Biophys. Acta* 862: 303, 1986.
291. Tachalam, M. Lipid alterations induced by renal ischemia: Pathogenic factor in membrane damage. *Kidney Int.* 26: 153, 1984.
292. Takano, T., Soltoff, S. P., Murdaugh, S., et al. Intracellular respiratory dysfunction and cell injury in short-term anoxia of rabbit renal proximal tubules. *J. Clin. Invest.* 76: 2377, 1985.
293. Takeda, K., Meyer-Lehnert, H., Kim, J. K., et al. AVP-induced Ca fluxes and contraction of rat glomerular mesangial cells. *Am. J. Physiol.* 255: F142, 1988.
294. Tang, M.-J., Suresh, K. R., and Tannen, R. L. Carbohydrate metabolism by primary cultures of rabbit proximal tubules. *Am. J. Physiol.* 256: C532, 1989.
295. Thornton, M. A., Winn, R., Alpers, C. E., et al. An evaluation of the neutrophil as a mediator of in vivo renal ischemic-reperfusion injury. *Am. J. Pathol.* 135: 509, 1989.
296. Thornton, M. A., and Zager, R. A. Brief intermittent reperfusion during renal ischemia: Effects on adenine nucleotides, oxidant stress, and the severity of renal failure. *J. Lab. Clin. Med.* 115: 564, 1990.
297. Toback, F. G., Teegarden, D. E., and Havener, L. J. Amino acid mediated stimulation of renal phospholipid biosynthesis after acute tubular necrosis. *Kidney Int.* 15: 542, 1979.
298. Tobimatsu, M., Ueda, Y., Saito, S., et al. Effects of a stable prostacyclin analog on experimental ischemic acute renal failure. *Ann. Surg.* 208: 65, 1988.
299. Torikai, S. A renorenal suppression in response to atrial natriuretic peptide in the unilateral ischaemic rat. *Clin. Sci.* 74: 519, 1988.
300. Torsello, G., Schror, K., Szabo, Z., et al. Winner of the ESVS Prize 1988. Effects of prostaglandin E1 (PGE1) on experimental renal ischaemia. *Eur. J. Vasc. Surg.* 3: 5, 1989.
301. Turrens, J. F., and McCord, J. M. Mitochondrial Generation of Reactive Oxygen Species. In G. B. Zelenok (ed.), *Clinical Ischemic Syndromes. Mechanisms and Consequences of Tissue Injury.* St. Louis: Mosby, 1990. Pp. 203–212.
302. van Waarde, A., Stromski, M. E., Thulin, G., et al. Protection of the kidney against ischemic injury by inhibition of 5′-nucleotidase. *Am. J. Physiol.* 256: F298, 1989.

303. Vanhoutte, P. M. Endothelium-derived relaxing and contracting factors. *Adv. Nephrol.* 19: 3, 1990.
304. Vanhoutte, P. M., Auch-Schelk, W., Boulanger, C., et al. Does endothelin-1 mediate endothelium-dependent contractions during anoxia? *J. Cardiovasc. Pharmacol.* 13: S124, 1989.
305. Vasko, K. A., Dewall, R. A., and Riley, A. M. Effect of allopurinol in renal ischemia. *Surgery* 71: 787, 1972.
306. Venkatachalam, M. A., Patel, Y. J., Kreisberg, J. I., et al. Energy thresholds that determine membrane integrity and injury in a renal epithelial cell line (LLC-PK1). Relationships to phospholipid degradation and unesterified fatty acid accumulation. *J. Clin. Invest.* 81: 745, 1988.
307. Vicens, A., Lopez-Boado, M. A., Alcaraz, A., et al. Beneficial effect of superoxide dismutase (SOD) on erythrocyte trapping and 6-keto-PGF1 alpha TxB2 ratio after ischemia-reperfusion in kidney transplantation. *Transplant. Proc.* 22: 2221, 1990.
308. Vogel, S., and Sperelakis, N. Blockade of myocardial slow inward current at low pH. *Am. J. Physiol.* 233: 99, 1977.
309. Wahlberg, J., Jacobsson, J., and Tufveson, G. Relevance of additive components of University of Wisconsin cold-storage solution. An experimental study in the rat. *Transplantation* 48: 400, 1989.
310. Weinberg, J. M. Adenine nucleotide metabolism by isolated kidney tubules during oxygen deprivation. *Biochem. Med. Metab. Biol.* 39: 319, 1988.
311. Weinberg, J. M. Calcium as a mediator of renal tubule cell injury. *Semin. Nephrol.* 4: 179, 1984.
312. Weinberg, J. M. Labeled arachidonate as a probe for membrane damage during oxygen deprivation injury to isolated rabbit tubules (abstract). *Clin. Res.* 33: 501, 1985.
313. Weinberg, J. M. Oxygen deprivation-induced injury to isolated rabbit kidney tubules. *J. Clin. Invest.* 76: 1193, 1985.
314. Weinberg, J. M. The effect of amino acids on ischemic and toxic injury to the kidney. *Semin. Nephrol.* 10: 491, 1990.
315. Weinberg, J. M. The cell biology of ischemic renal injury. *Kidney Int.* 39: 476, 1991.
316. Weinberg, J. M., and Davis, J. A. Protective effects of glycine against hypoxic tubule cell injury are independent of the presence of butyrate (abstract). *Clin. Res.* 35: 559A, 1987.
317. Weinberg, J. M., and Davis, J. A. A comparison between protection by glycine, acidosis and mannitol against proximal tubule cell injury (abstract). *Clin. Res.* 38: 577A, 1990.
318. Weinberg, J. M., Davis, J. A., Abarzua, M., et al. Cytoprotective effects of glycine and glutathione against hypoxic injury to renal tubules. *J. Clin. Invest.* 80: 1446, 1987.
319. Weinberg, J. M., Davis, J. A., Abarzua, M., et al. Relationship between cell ATP and glutathione content and protection by glycine against hypoxic proximal tubule cell injury. *J. Lab. Clin. Med.* 113: 612, 1989.
320. Weinberg, J. M., Davis, J. A., Abarzua, M., et al. Ouabain-induced lethal proximal tubule cell injury is prevented by glycine. *Am. J. Physiol.* 258: F346, 1990.
321. Weinberg, J. M., Davis, J. A., Abarzua, M., et al. Glycine-dependent protection of proximal tubules against lethal cell injury due to inhibitors of mitochondrial ATP production. *Am. J. Physiol.* 258: C1127, 1990.
322. Weinberg, J. M., Davis, J. A., Abarzua, M., et al. Protection by glycine of proximal tubules from injury due to inhibitors of mitochondrial ATP production. *Am. J. Physiol.* 258: C.1127, 1990.
323. Weinberg, J. M., Davis, J. A., Lawton, A., et al. Modulation of cell nucleotide levels of isolated kidney tubules. *Am. J. Physiol.* 254: F311, 1988.
324. Weinberg, J. M., Davis, J. A., Roeser, N. F., et al. Role of increased cytosolic free calcium in the pathogenesis of rabbit proximal tubule cell injury and protection by glycine or acidosis. *J. Clin. Invest.* 87: 581, 1991.
325. Weinberg, J. M., Davis, J. A., and Trivedi, B. Calcium compartmentation in isolated renal tubules in suspension. *Biochem. Med. Metab. Biol.* 39: 234, 1988.
326. Weinberg, J. M., and Humes, H. D. Calcium transport and inner mitochondrial membrane damage in renal cortical mitochondria. *Am. J. Physiol.* 248: F876, 1985.
327. Weinberg, J. M., and Humes, H. D. Increases of cell ATP produced by exogenous adenine nucleotides in isolated rabbit kidney tubules. *Am. J. Physiol.* 250: F720, 1986.
328. Weinberg, J. M., Hunt, D., Humes, H. D. Effects of verapamil on in vitro ischemic injury to isolated rabbit proximal tubules (abstract). *Kidney Int.* 25: 239, 1984.
329. Welsh, M. J., Shasby, D. M., and Husted, R. M. Oxidants increase paracellular permeability in a cultured epithelial cell line. *J. Clin. Invest.* 76: 1155, 1985.
330. Wetzels, J. F. M., Burke, T. J., and Schrier, R. W. Calcium channel blockers: Protective effects in ischemia acute renal failure. *Renal Failure* (in press), 1992.
331. Wetzels, J. F. M., Wang, X.-N., and Arnold, P. E. Glycine protection against hypoxic injury in isolated rat proximal tubules is not mediated by interference with activation or action of phospholipase A_2 (abstract). *J. Am. Soc. Nephrol.* 2: 657, 1991.
332. Widener, L. L., Mela-Riker, L. M. Verapamil pretreatment preserves mitochondrial function and tissue magnesium in the ischemic kidney. *Circ. Shock* 13: 27, 1984.
333. Wiecek, A., Kokot, F., Kuczera, M., et al. Plasma level of atrial natriuretic peptide in renal venous blood—marker of kidney ischemia? *Clin. Nephrol.* 34: 26, 1990.
334. Wilkes, B. M., Pearl, A. R., Mento, P. F., et al. Glomerular endothelin receptors during initiation and maintenance of ischemic acute renal failure in rats. *Am. J. Physiol.* 260: F110, 1991.
335. Wilson, D. R., Arnold, P. E., Burke, T. J., et al. Mitochondrial calcium accumulation and respiration in ischemic acute renal failure in the rat. *Kidney Int.* 25: 519, 1984.
336. Wilson, P. D., and Schrier, R. W. Nephron segment and calcium as determinants of anoxic cell death in renal cultures. *Kidney Int.* 29: 1172, 1986.
337. Winchell, R. J., and Halasz, N. A. Lack of effect of oxygen-radical scavenging systems in the preserved reperfused rabbit kidney. *Transplantation* 48: 393, 1989.
338. Witzgall, R., Guest, S., Ouellette, A. J., et al. Cloning of a developmentally regulated, zinc-finger rich, putative transcription factor from the rat kidney (abstract). *J. Am. Soc. Nephrol.* 2: 447, 1991.
339. Wolgast, M., Bayati, A., Hellberg, O., et al. Prevention of acute renal failure by SOD and sucrose. *Basic Life Sci.* 49: 1053, 1988.
340. Yagil, Y. Acute effect of cyclosporin on inner medullary blood flow in normal and postischemic rat kidney. *Am. J. Physiol.* 258: F1139, 1990.
341. Yagil, Y., Miyamoto, M., and Jamison, R. L. Inner medullary blood flow in postischemic acute renal failure in the rat. *Am. J. Physiol.* 256: F456, 1989.
342. Yagil, Y., Myers, B. D., and Jamison, R. L. Course and

pathogenesis of postischemic acute renal failure in the rat. *Am. J. Physiol.* 255: F257, 1988.
343. Yamamoto, K., Wilson, D. R., and Baumal, R. Outer medullary circulatory defect in ischemic acute renal failure. *Am. J. Pathol.* 116: 253, 1984.
344. Yang, H. C., Gattone, V. H., 2d, Martin, L. F., et al. The effect of glutathione content on renal function following warm ischemia. *J. Surg. Res.* 46: 633, 1989.
345. Yoshioka, T., and Ichikawa, I. Glomerular dysfunction induced by polymorphonuclear leukocyte-derived reactive oxygen species. *Am. J. Physiol.* 257: F53, 1989.
346. Zager, R. A. Hypoperfusion-induced acute renal failure in the rat: An evaluation of oxidant tissue injury. *Circ. Res.* 62: 430, 1988.
347. Zager, R. A. Adenine nucleotide changes in kidney, liver, and small intestine during different forms of ischemic injury. *Circ. Res.* 68: 185, 1991.
348. Zager, R. A., and Alpers, C. E. Effects of aging on expression of ischemic acute renal failure in rats. *Lab. Invest.* 61: 290, 1989.
349. Zager, R. A., and Gmur, D. J. Effects of xanthine oxidase inhibition on ischemic acute renal failure in the rat. *Am. J. Physiol.* 257: F953, 1989.
350. Zager, R. A., Gmur, D. J., Bredl, C. R., et al. Degree and time sequence of hypothermic protection against experimental ischemic acute renal failure. *Circ. Res.* 65: 1263, 1989.
351. Zager, R. A., Gmur, D. J., Bredl, C. R., et al. Regional responses within the kidney to ischemia: Assessment of adenine nucleotide and catabolite profiles. *Biochim. Biophys. Acta* 1035: 29, 1990.
352. Zager, R. A., Gmur, D. J., Bredl, C. R., et al. Temperature effects on ischemic and hypoxic renal proximal tubular injury. *Lab. Invest.* 64: 766, 1991.
353. Zenser, T. V., and Davis, B. B. Enzyme systems involved in the formation of reactive metabolites in the renal medulla: Cooxidation via prostaglandin H synthase. *Fundam. Appl. Toxicol.* 4: 922, 1984.
354. Zweier, J. L., Kuppusamy, P., and Lutty, G. A. Measurement of endothelial cell free radical generation: Evidence for a central mechanism of free radical injury in postischemic tissues. *Proc. Natl. Acad. Sci. U.S.A.* 85: 4046, 1988.

Acute Tubular Necrosis

Robert J. Anderson
Robert W. Schrier

Acute renal failure (ARF) is defined as an abrupt decrease in renal function sufficient to result in retention of nitrogenous waste (e.g., blood urea nitrogen and creatinine) in the body. Recent prospective studies demonstrate that acute renal failure is commonly encountered in the contemporary practice of medicine. For example, 4.9 percent of more than 2200 patients admitted to a general medical-surgical hospital developed an abrupt rise in serum creatinine [147]. In patients undergoing nonemergent surgery, 25 percent will develop either a mild acute rise in serum creatinine or a fall in creatinine clearance in the early postoperative period [57]. In two large intensive care unit studies, 5 to 15 percent of all patients admitted to the units developed an abrupt, significant rise in serum creatinine [157, 242]. A high frequency of occurrence of acute renal failure is encountered in a wide variety of clinical settings [5, 93, 117, 128, 147, 157, 230, 242, 259, 313, 342, 356] (Table 48-1). Not only does acute renal failure occur with high frequency, but it is also associated with significant morbidity and mortality [1, 8, 51, 69, 70, 112, 147, 201, 209, 216, 313, 342, 354] (Fig. 48-1). A recent prospective case control study found that the development of hospital-acquired acute renal failure increased the relative risk of dying by 6.2-fold and the length of stay from 13 to 23 days [313]. Contemporary mortality of patients with oliguric and nonoliguric acute renal failure remains in the 50 to 80 percent and 15 to 40 percent range, respectively [1, 8, 51, 69, 70, 112, 147, 201, 207, 216, 274, 312, 342, 354] (Fig. 48-1). Abrupt and progressive renal failure is the final common pathway for several disease processes (Tables 48-2 through 48-4). The high frequency of occurrence, multiple causes, and significant morbidity demand a logical clinical approach to ARF. In this chapter, we use the term ARF in its most generic sense to describe acute impairment of the kidney function independent of cause and mechanism. We discuss the causes, diagnostic approach, and consequences of such clinically encountered ARF.

Differential Diagnosis

Kidney regulation of the normal volume and composition of body fluids and the process of urine formation begins with ultrafiltration of the blood delivered to the kidney, proceeds through intrarenal processing of the ultrafiltrate by tubular reabsorption and secretion, and ends by elimination of the formed urine through the ureters, bladder, and urethra. It follows that ARF can result from a decrease of renal blood flow (prerenal azotemia, Table 48-2), intrinsic renal parenchymal diseases (renal azotemia, Table 48-3), or obstruction to urine flow (postrenal azotemia, Table 48-4). Since therapy of ARF depends on the underlying cause, the initial step in determining the cause of ARF is to attempt to classify the site of origin of ARF as prerenal, renal, or postrenal. It is also noteworthy that many patients with ARF have more than a single insult to renal function [287]. A number of clinical and laboratory clues may assist in determining the site of ARF (Table 48-5).

PRERENAL AZOTEMIA (TABLE 48-2)

The process of urine formation begins with delivery of blood to the glomerulus. The highly selective permeability of the glomerular capillary combined with the glomerular capillary hydrostatic pressure (which exceeds glomerular capillary oncotic pressure) results in formation of glomerular filtrate. Under unusual clinical circumstances such as mannitol intoxication, high-dose dextran infusion, or marked hyperproteinemia, a "hyperoncotic state" occurs in which glomerular capillary oncotic pressure exceeds hydrostatic pressure [94, 144, 253]. This results in cessation of glomerular filtration and an anuric state. Rapid reversal of this form of acute renal failure occurs with removal (plasmapheresis) of the osmotically active substance from plasma.

The central role of delivery of blood to the glomerulus as the starting point of formation of glomerular filtrate dictates that clinical disorders that decrease renal perfusion are potential causes of acute renal failure. In clinical practice, acute renal failure due to hypoperfusion with a resultant fall in glomerular capillary filtration pressure is one of the most common forms of ARF [93, 112, 128, 147, 287, 313]. A recent prospective study by Hou et al. found prerenal azotemia to be the single most common cause of ARF in a general medical-surgical hospital [287] (Fig. 48-2). In our experience, prerenal forms account for 40 to 80 percent of all cases of ARF. [8, 93, 128, 247]. Shusterman and associates [313] recently found that the elevated odds ratios for development of acute renal failure were increased 9.4-fold and 9.2-fold in the presence of the "prerenal" insults of volume depletion and congestive heart failure, respectively. Prerenal azotemia is not only common but is also potentially often reversible. However, prolonged prerenal azotemia can lead to ischemic acute tubular necrosis (ATN) with significant morbidity (Fig. 48-1). Thus, recognition and prompt therapy of prerenal causes of ARF are important.

Under normal circumstances renal blood flow and glomerular filtration rate are relatively constant over a wide range of renal perfusion pressures, a phenomenon termed autoregulation [65, 169, 293] (Fig. 48-3). Renal autoregulation not only allows constancy of glomerular filtration rate and filtered load of solutes, but also maintains constancy of oxygen delivery in spite of variable renal perfusion pressures. A marked decrease in renal perfusion pressure below the autoregulatory range can lead to an abrupt decrease in glomerular filtration and ARF. Within the autoregulatory range, a reduction in renal perfusion, as occurs with either diminished cardiac output or depletion of extracellular fluid volume, normally results in dilation of the glomerular afferent arte-

Table 48-1. High-risk setting for acute renal failure

Clinical setting	Frequency of acute renal failure (%)
General medical-surgical	3–5
Intensive care unit	5–25
Open heart surgery	5–20
Aminoglycoside therapy	10–30
Severe burns	20–60
Rhabdomyolysis	20–30
Cisplatinum, bleomycin and vinblastine	15–25

Table 48-2. Causes of prerenal acute renal failure

1. *Decreased effective extracellular fluid volume*
   A. Extracellular fluid loss—burns, diarrhea, vomiting, diuretics, salt-wasting renal disease, primary adrenal insufficiency
   B. Extracellular fluid sequestration—pancreatitis, burns, crush injury, nephrotic syndrome, malnutrition, advanced liver disease
2. *Decreased cardiac output*
   A. Myocardial dysfunction—myocardial infarction, arrhythmias, ischemic heart disease, cardiomyopathies, valvular disease, hypertensive disease, severe cor pulmonale
   B. Pericardial tamponade
3. *Peripheral vasodilation*
   A. Drugs—antihypertensive agents
   B. Sepsis
   C. Miscellaneous—adrenal cortical insufficiency, hypermagnesemia, hypercapnia, hypoxemia
4. *Severe renal vasoconstriction*
   A. Sepsis
   B. Drugs—nonsteroidal antiinflammatory agents, α-adrenergic agonists
   C. Hepatorenal syndrome
5. *Mechanical occlusion of renal arteries*
   A. Thrombotic occlusion
   B. Miscellaneous (emboli, trauma [i.e., angioplasty])

riole and constriction of the glomerular efferent arteriole so that glomerular capillary hydrostatic pressure and, thus, glomerular filtration rate remain constant [65, 169, 293]. The afferent dilation is mediated in part by vasodilatory eicosanoids, while efferent constriction can be attributed in part to angiotensin II [16]. It follows that in the setting of compromised cardiac output or intravascular volume depletion, prevention of afferent arteriolar dilation (as occurs following nonsteroidal antiinflammatory agent therapy) and attenuation of efferent arteriolar constriction (as occurs following angiotensin converting enzyme inhibition and perhaps, calcium channel–blocking agents) potentially decrease glomerular capillary filtration pressure and cause an abrupt decline in glomerular filtration.

From a clinical perspective, a potentially reversible "prerenal" form of acute renal failure can be seen when

Table 48-3. Renal causes of acute renal failure

1. *Renal vascular disorders (see Part XI)*
   A. Vasculitis
   B. Malignant hypertension
   C. Scleroderma
   D. Thrombotic thrombocytopenic purpura
   E. Hemolytic-uremic syndrome
   F. Disseminated intravascular coagulation
   G. Mechanical renal artery occlusion (surgery, emboli, thrombotic occlusion)
   H. Renal vein thrombosis
2. *Glomerulonephritis (see Part X)*
   A. Postinfectious
   B. Membranoproliferative
   C. Rapidly progressive glomerulonephritis (idiopathic systemic lupus erythematosus, Wegener's syndrome, Goodpasture's syndrome, polyarteritis, Henoch-Schönlein purpura)
   D. Drugs
3. *Interstitial nephritis (see Part X)*
   A. Drugs (pencillins, sulfonamides, rifampin, phenindiones, cimetidine, azathioprine, phenytoin, captopril, thiazides, furosemide, allopurinol)
   B. Hypercalcemia
   C. Infections
   D. Infiltration (sarcoid, leukemia, lymphoma)
   E. Connective tissue disease
4. *Tubular necrosis*
   A. Renal ischemia (prolonged prerenal; see Table 48-2)
   B. Nephrotoxins (aminolgycosides, radiocontrast agents, heavy metals, organic solvents)
   C. Pigmenturia (myoglobinuria and hemoglobinuria)
   D. Miscellaneous

Table 48-4. Causes of postrenal acute renal failure

1. *Intrarenal (intratubular)*
   A. Crystal deposition—uric acid, oxalic acid, methotrexate, acylovir, triamterene, sulfonamides
   B. Protein deposition—light chains, myoglobin, hemoglobin
2. *Extrarenal*
   A. Ureteral/pelvic
      (1) Intrinsic obstruction—tumor, stone, clot, pus, fungal ball, papilla
      (2) Extrinsic obstruction—retroperitoneal and pelvic malignancy, fibrosis, ligation
   B. Bladder—stones, clots, tumor, neurogenic, prostatic hypertrophy/malignancy
   C. Urethral—stricture, phimosis

nonsteroidal antiinflammatory agents are given to patients with volume depletion, hypoalbuminemia, an edematous disorder, advancing age, underlying chronic renal failure, or recent diuretic (especially triamterene) use [24, 34, 44, 59, 167, 202, 206, 246, 288, 316, 328, 355]. If the nonsteroidal antiinflammatory agent is stopped early, the renal failure readily reverses. With continued administration of the agent, a more severe form of acute renal failure due to ischemic ATN may occur. A similar "prerenal" form of acute renal failure can complicate angiotensin converting enzyme therapy [58, 62, 72, 79,

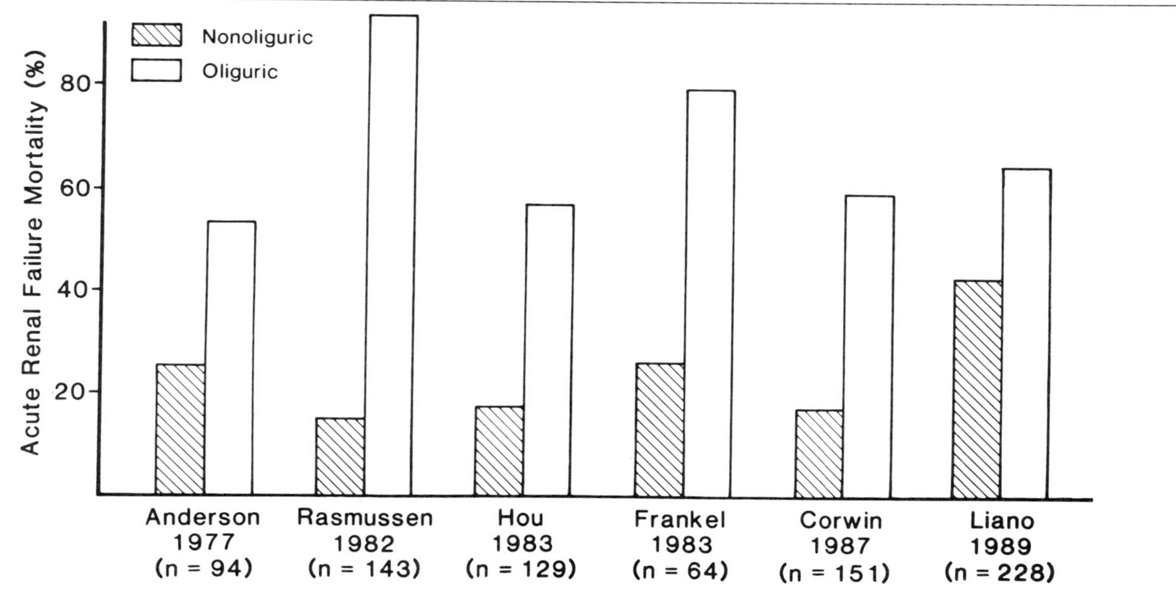

Fig. 48-1. Effect of urine output on acute renal failure mortality. (Data taken from [8], [70], [112], [147], [201], [287].)

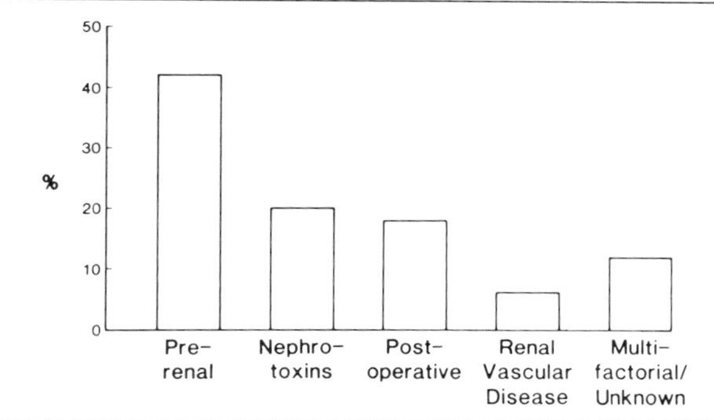

Fig. 48-2. Causes of acute renal failure in a general medical-surgical hospital. (From [147].)

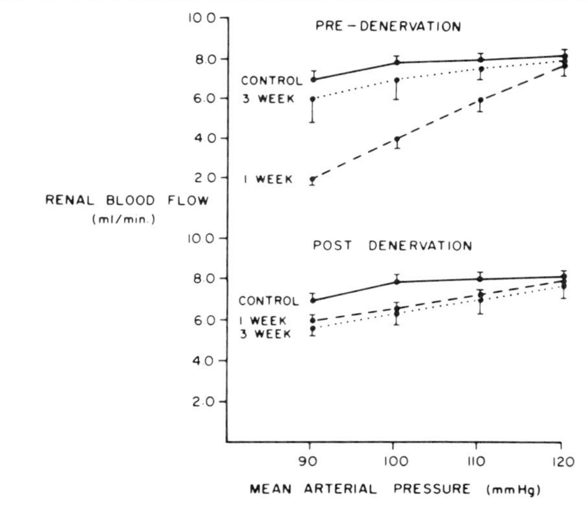

Fig. 48-3. Renal blood flow autoregulation in acute renal failure. (From [169].)

135, 149, 150, 166, 273, 314]. In the presence of a decrease in renal blood flow from severe bilateral renal artery stenosis, renal artery stenosis in a solitary kidney, and other high-renin, high–angiotensin II states (i.e., edematous disorders and volume depletion disorders), angiotensin II converting enzyme inhibition with a resultant decrease in both renal perfusion pressure and efferent arteriolar constriction can precipitously decrease glomerular filtration rate. For example, about one third of patients with severe congestive heart failure will experience an abrupt rise in serum creatinine concentration following angiotensin converting enzyme inhibitor therapy [273]. In the setting of heart failure, this increase in serum creatinine following angiotensin converting enzyme inhibition tends to be mild and readily reversible on discontinuation of the drug. Although the precise cellular mechanisms have not been defined whereby angiotensin-mediated constriction of the efferent arteriole occurs, an increase in cellular calcium uptake appears to be involved. The occasional effect of slow-channel calcium blockers to induce a prerenal form of acute renal failure may be due to a failure of efferent arteriolar constriction [91].

Several clinical conditions can result in enhanced renal afferent arteriolar vasoconstriction, which potentially impairs renal autoregulation. For example, in the setting of hemorrhagic hypotension or gram-negative sepsis, the combined effect of intense renal adrenergic neural traffic, norepinephrine, angiotensin II, endothelin, and endotoxin can all exert potent vasoconstrictor influences on the afferent arteriole of the kidney [137, 138, 159, 215, 301]. Thus, the decrease in systemic and, therefore, renal perfusion pressure that accompanies septic or hemorrhagic shock combines with intense afferent arteriolar constriction, which results in a precipitous fall in glomerular filtration rate and acute renal failure.

It is noteworthy that experimental studies demonstrate that one effect of ischemic ARF (ATN) may be to impair renal autoregulation [65, 169, 293] (Fig 48-3). Some of this impaired autoregulation appears to be due to the effect of enhanced renal adrenergic neural tone and increased action of renal vasoconstrictors such as thromboxane to prevent afferent arteriolar dilation as renal perfusion pressure is reduced [65, 169, 293]. Preliminary studies also suggest that impaired generation of endothelial-derived relaxing factors may be important determinants of abnormal autoregulatory responses under normal and pathologic conditions [65]. Thus, in the setting of ATN it is possible that modest decreases in renal perfusion pressure can serve to maintain a decrease in glomerular filtration rate in the maintenance phase of ARF, thus preventing or prolonging recovery from ATN.

It is also of interest that fixed renal artery stenosis is an important determinant of the renal autoregulatory response. Recent studies by Textor et al. suggest a "critical renal perfusion pressure" in patients with fixed renal artery stenosis [340]. In these studies, 8 patients with unilateral renal artery stenosis tolerated sodium nitroprusside–induced arterial pressure reduction without a change in either glomerular filtration rate (GFR) or estimated renal plasma flow. By contrast, a similar pressure reduction in 8 patients with bilateral renal artery stenosis resulted in marked reductions in GFR and renal plasma flow. Sensitivity of GFR and renal plasma flow to blood pressure reduction was eliminated following revascularization in 4 patients with bilateral renal vascular stenosis [340].

A number of disorders that result in extracellular fluid volume depletion can induce an ARF state [147, 168, 214]. For example, gastrointestinal losses of fluid can precipitate a prerenal state. Prolonged nasogastric and biliary drainage (sodium concentration 150 mEq/liter) of large amounts of fluid can cause ARF [23, 114]. Diarrhea of any cause can induce volume depletion and ARF. Aggressive restoration of extracellular fluid volume has dramatically decreased the frequency of ARF due to prerenal causes that complicate cholera [36, 54, 55, 168, 214]. In recent collected series of 22 patients with villous adenoma (stool sodium 70 to 150 mEq/liter), all had azotemia with BUNs as high as 200 mg per deciliter [15]. Sequestration of extracellular fluid, as occurs with acute pancreatitis, can cause ARF. In recent studies 1 to 5 percent of cases of ARF have occurred in the setting of acute pancreatitis [165, 237]. In series of patients with acute pancreatitis, ARF is occasionally reported. For example, 5 of 78 and 23 of 549 patients with acute pancreatitis developed ARF [152, 155].

Extensive dermal losses of salt and water occur in the setting of burns or heat stroke injury [38, 50, 53, 79, 120, 219, 279, 302, 344]. Early, ARF can often be attributed to volume depletion with prerenal azotemia and rarely ischemic ATN [38, 50, 53, 120, 219, 279, 302, 344]. Later, sepsis and aminoglycoside antimicrobial agents produce a nonoliguric form of ARF in the setting of burns [279]. A less than 15 percent burn rarely leads to either death or ARF [53]. In one study, 22 of 110 patients with a greater than 15 percent area burn developed ARF and 21 died. Half of the cases of ARF were oliguric [53]. Excessive dermal losses with extracellular volume depletion and ARF also occur in heat stroke [302, 344]. In many cases, rhabdomyolysis is also present [302, 323, 344].

ARF resulting from excessive renal loss of extracellular fluid is common [106, 194, 289, 313]. Mild degrees of azotemia are often seen in diabetic ketoacidosis, but ischemic ATN is rare [27, 28]. Of note, ketoacids can interfere with automated serum creatinine assays, producing artifactually high values [251]. Renal loss of salt and water can also lead to ARF in hyperosmolar, nonketotic coma [11, 131].

Hemorrhagic shock, except in rare circumstances or in the obstetric setting, rarely leads to severe ARF. Of 590 patients with serious upper gastrointestinal hemorrhage, only 8 died with ARF [174]. ARF secondary to myocardial infarction is also rare. Only 5 of 500 patients with acute myocardial infarction seen during 2 years developed ARF [189].

POSTRENAL ACUTE RENAL FAILURE (TABLE 48-3)

Obstruction of urine flow is a less common cause of ARF and is encountered in 2 to 10 percent of all cases of ARF (Table 48-4) [98, 128, 147, 178, 235]. However, obstructive uropathy is more common in selected patient populations, such as the very young or older men with prostatic disease and patients with either a single kidney or intraabdominal cancer, particularly pelvic cancer [128, 235, 292]. Moreover, the cause of obstructive uropathy is often amenable to therapy. Thus, obstructive uropathy should be considered in each case of ARF [235, 292].

The cause of obstruction of urine flow can be classified as intrarenal or extrarenal (Table 48-3). Intratubular deposition of either crystalline or proteinaceous material can increase intratubular pressure, thereby decreasing effective glomerular filtration pressure. For example, intratubular precipitation of uric acid can cause tubular obstruction and ARF. Acute uric acid nephropathy is most often seen following chemotherapy for leukemias and lymphomas [176, 224]. In this setting, the liver converts the purine load generated by cytolysis into uric acid. High filtered loads of uric acid and high rates of tubular fluid reabsorption combine to produce high tubular concentrations of soluble urate and uric acid. Acidification of tubular fluid converts urate to uric acid, which can occlude tubular lumens.

Abrupt exposure of the kidneys to high filtered loads of other insoluble crystalline substances can also cause an intrarenal form of obstructive uropathy. For example, ARF associated with calcium oxalate crystalluria can accompany ethylene glycol ingestion, administration of the anesthetic agent methoxyflurane, and small bowel bypass operations [178, 224]. Administration of high doses of methotrexate can be associated with ARF, possibly due to intratubular precipitation of the insoluble 7-hydroxy metabolite of methotrexate [148, 278]. As discussed in Chap. 80, intratubular precipitation of myeloma proteins can lead to ARF. Dehydration with resultant high tubular water reabsorption and radiographic contrast material can also contribute to myeloma protein deposition. Other substances that can potentially precipitate within renal tubules and thereby lead to acute renal failure include acylovir, triamterene, and older sulfonamides [104, 300].

Recognition of intratubular obstruction as a potential cause of ARF has important therapeutic implications. For example, prophylactic therapy with the xanthine oxidase inhibitor allopurinol can prevent accumulation of uric acid in tumor-lysis syndrome [176, 224]. Moreover, forced diuresis decreases tubular salt and water reabsorption, thereby diluting tubular fluid with decreases in crystal and protein concentrations. Finally, manipulation of urinary pH can increase solubility of crystalline substances.

Recent micropuncture and morphologic studies of an animal model of ARF due to uric acid nephropathy illustrate these points [64, 66]. In this model, the underlying pathologic lesion is deposition of uric acid crystals within collecting ducts and deep cortical and medullary vessels [64, 66]. In these studies high rates of urine flow induced by either high-dose furosemide (which produced a solute diuresis) or use of animals with central diabetes insipidus (which resulted in a water diuresis) protected against the development of uric acid–induced ARF [64, 66]. By contrast, either urinary alkalinization or induction of a mild diuresis with a furosemide provided only minimal protection [64, 66]. These observations suggest that maintenance of high urinary flow rates should be a major prophylactic objective in cases of high uric acid loads. It is also noteworthy that clinical experience suggests that maintenance of high urine flow may protect against development of ARF in the setting of high doses of methotrexate infusion and myeloma cases. Finally, in patients with ARF due to uric acid nephropathy, hemodialysis can remove large amounts of uric acid and restore renal function. [176, 224].

Extrarenal causes of postrenal ARF are listed in Table 48-3. Several factors are determinants of renal response to obstruction [292, 298]. The site, degree, and rapidity of onset of obstruction are all important [292]. Without complicating infection, substantial improvement in renal function can follow decompression of the urinary tract after several days of complete obstruction [292]. Obstruction of the upper urinary tract is a less common cause of ARF, since it requires simultaneous obstruction of both ureters or unilateral ureteric obstruction with either absence of or severe disease in the contralateral kidney. Intraureteric obstruction can be due to stone, necrotic papillae, tumor, pus, blood clots, and fungal balls [292, 298]. Papillary necrosis usually occurs in the setting of sickle-cell disorders, diabetes mellitus, chronic urinary tract infections, analgesic abuse, obstructive uropathy, and possibly chronic alcoholism [224, 298]. Extraureteric lesions producing obstruction include retroperitoneal fibrosis and tumors, pelvic tumors, and surgical ligation [292]. Retroperitoneal fibrosis is often idiopathic but may be encountered in the setting of methyldopa and β-blocker therapy, methsergemide, connective tissue disorders, and lymphoma [292, 298]. A high frequency of prostatic carcinoma in males and pelvic carcinoma (predominantly cancer of the cervix) in females causing ARF secondary to ureteric occlusion has been reported. Less commonly encountered causes of extrinsic ureteric obstruction include inflammatory bowel disease (predominantly right-sided obstruction), an inflammatory reaction resulting from a leaking abdominal aortic aneurysm, and the late stages of pregnancy [292, 298, 304].

Ellis and Arnold recently examined their experience with 50 cases of renal failure due to ureteric obstruction experienced over a 5-year interval [98]. The cause of obstruction was malignant disease (cervix, prostate, bladder, bowel, or ovary) in 76 percent of cases. Nonmalignant causes of obstructive uropathy included retroperitoneal fibrosis (16 percent), calculi (4 percent), and ligated ureters (4 percent). Substantial survival time was observed following relief of obstruction (often with percutaneous nephrostomy or ureteral stints) in many of the patients with extensive malignant disease.

Recent reports emphasize that stone-induced obstruction may be a relatively frequent cause of ARF in selected populations [9, 130]. Grundy and collaborators describe urosepsis as the setting of ARF in 5 quadriplegic patients [130]. In 3 of these 5 patients, stone-induced obstructive uropathy played a role in the sepsis. Ansari and co-workers have emphasized that uric acid obstruction of the ureters with anuric acute renal failure can be seen in young male residents of the Near East [9]. From 1978 to 1981, they encountered 8 male patients with ARF, loin pain, and anuria due to ureteral obstruction with uric acid calculi. Retrograde pyelography and either local or systemic alkalinization dissolved the stones, relieved the obstruction, and returned renal function to normal. Pharmacologic agents with anticholinergic activity may impair bladder drainage, resulting in obstructive uropathy. Danziger and Horn have emphasized that the antiarrhythmic agent disopyramide can induce urinary retention with development of renal failure [81].

RENAL AZOTEMIA

A variety of renal disorders can cause ARF (Table 48-4). These diagnoses should be considered when prerenal and postrenal disorders have been excluded. The frequency with which renal causes are encountered in patients with ARF varies between 5 and 50 percent. In series of pediatric patients, as many as 50 percent of all cases of ARF can be attributed to such renal parenchymal disorders as acute glomerulonephritis and hemolytic-uremic syndrome [8, 127, 128]. In hospitalized adults in whom prerenal and postrenal azotemia have been excluded, ARF is often due to ATN. By contrast, in an outpatient setting in which prerenal and postrenal causes have been excluded, ARF is more often due to renal parenchymal diseases. The renal causes of ARF are most systematically categorized as to their anatomic site of origin. Thus, vascular, glomerular, interstitial, and tubular disorders occur. Acute renal failure due to renovascular, glomerular, and interstitial disorders is discussed in detail in Parts VII through XII.

The underlying disorders that usually predispose to ATN are listed in Table 48-3. Recent studies of patients with ATN emphasize that multiple insults to renal function are usually present. For example, in more than 600 well-characterized patients with ATN, about half have more than a single insult to renal function [201, 287].

The most common predisposing factor in the development of ATN appears to be renal ischemia resulting from prolonged prerenal azotemia [5, 6, 8, 112, 128, 147, 287]. Sepsis, and particularly septic shock, has assumed an ever increasing role as a major predisposing factor in the occurrence of ATN [313]. Nephrotoxins (see Part VII) account for about 25 percent of all cases of ATN. Contemporary nephrotoxins commonly encountered include the aminoglycoside antimicrobial agents, radiographic contrast material, nonsteroidal antiinflammatory agents, organic solvents, and heavy metals such as cisplatin and carboplatin [128, 233]. A prospective case control study found that the relative risk for development of acute renal failure was increased five- to sixfold by exposure to either aminoglycoside antimicrobials or radiocontrast agents [313]. The increasing numbers of infections in patients with AIDS has served as a strong reminder of the significant nephrotoxicity that can accompany therapy with pentamidine, sulfamethoxazole-trimethoprim, amphotericin B, and foscarnet [88, 103, 308, 353]. The advent of recombinant cytokine therapy for advanced solid tumors has been associated with nephrotoxicity following gama interferon and interleukin-2 treatment [13, 339]. ATN also can complicate the course of heavy pigment loads such as those in rhabdomyolysis or hemolysis [86, 93]. Finally, in a few cases of ATN, no specific identifiable cause is found.

Frankel and collaborators retrospectively reviewed 64 hospitalized patients with ARF in whom prerenal and postrenal azotemia were excluded [112]. Approximately 75 percent of these cases had ATN. The clinical setting of ATN in these cases included: hypotension 30 percent, nephrotoxins 19 percent, sepsis 15 percent, and rhabdomyolysis 3 percent. Other causes of ARF included interstitial nephritis 9 percent, glomerulonephritis 7 percent, vascular disease 4 percent, and miscellaneous 13 percent. In recent series, 40 to 60 percent of cases of ATN occurred in a postoperative or trauma setting while the remainder were observed in medical settings [127, 128, 237, 248].

Rasmussen and Ibels [287] examined risk factors in the development of ATN. In this study the records of 143 patients who developed an acute increase in serum creatinine of more than 2.2 mg per deciliter and who did not have prerenal or postrenal azotemia, glomerulonephritis, and interstitial nephritis were examined by retrospective multivariate analysis. Approximately 60 percent of these patients were seen in a surgical setting. The following were considered possible acute insults: hypotension (74 percent), sepsis (31 percent), contrast media and aminoglycosides (25 percent), pigmenturia (hemoglobin, myoglobin, 22 percent), and dehydration (35 percent). Nearly two thirds (64 percent) of the 143 patients had more than one acute insult before ATN.

The "graying" of many societies has focused attention on acute renal failure occurring in the elderly. A survey of 4000 patients aged 60 to 97 years old who were admitted to three geriatric units over a 6-month interval revealed that 7 percent had an elevated urea nitrogen and/or creatinine concentration [235]. Most of the renal failure in these elderly patients was prerenal in nature (55%). However, obstructive uropathy was present in 10 percent while the remainder of the patients had chronic renal failure.

In a large longitudinal study, Turney and collaborators [342] found that the mean age of patients with acute renal failure progressively increased from 41 years in the 1950s to 61 years in the 1980s. Pascual and associates [274] compared the cause and clinical course of acute renal failure in 152 patients over 70 years of age with those of 205 concurrently encountered patients less than 70 years old. Prerenal factors and ATN accounted for about 85 percent of all cases of acute renal failure in both age groups. The elderly group of patients tended to recover renal function more slowly and less completely than did younger patients. In this study, patients with advanced age had only a slight increase in acute renal failure mortality relative to younger patients. In contrast, Turney and associates [342] found a striking direct correlation between mortality in acute renal failure and advancing age.

A contemporary study by Preston and associates [281] demonstrates that acute renal failure presenting in selected elderly patients may be caused by an underlying renal parenchymal disorder. In this report, 55 of 363 renal biopsies done on patients aged 65 or over were performed because of acute renal failure. In these elderly biopsied patients with ARF, 42 percent had acute glomerulonephritis, 27 percent had ATN, 16 percent had a renovascular disorder, and 15 percent had acute interstitial nephritis. The results of this study emphasize the need to consider systematically all forms of renal disease in each elderly patient presenting with an acute deterioration in renal function.

ATN occurring in the setting of concomitant respiratory failure has received recent emphasis [29, 188]. Acute renal failure was observed in more than half of patients with acute respiratory distress syndrome [188]. In other studies, Kraman et al. found that 74 of 686 patients with respiratory failure developed ATN [188]. Mortality in these patients with combined acute renal and respiratory failure was 80 percent. By contrast, mortality was only 11 percent in patients without renal failure. The leading predisposing factors in the development of ATN were hypotension (gastrointestinal hemorrhage, sepsis, cardiogenic shock, and hypotension of unknown cause) and aminoglycoside administration.

About half of all currently encountered cases of ATN are seen in patients in the postoperative state [8, 26, 57, 69, 70, 112, 147 201, 209, 342, 354]. Charlson and coworkers [57] prospectively measured daily serum creatinine concentrations and pre- and postoperative (5 day) creatinine clearances in 278 patients undergoing nonemergent, elective surgery. These patients had a mean age of 63 years and many had significant co-morbid conditions, including diabetes mellitus (38%), hypertension (76%), and other cardiovascular disorders (20%). A mild (> 20%) increase in serum creatinine occurred in 23 percent of patients. The increase in serum creatinine tended to occur within 48 hours of operation. In 12 percent of patients, the increase in serum creatinine was transient, lasting 48 hours or less. In 11 percent of patients, the increase in serum creatinine was sustained for more than 48 hours. In these postoperative patients with a sustained increase in serum creatinine, an additional potential renal insult (contrast exposure, reoperation, sepsis, aminoglycoside exposure, or hypotension) occurred in one third and resulted in a further deterioration in renal function. Altogether, 11 percent of patients decreased their creatinine clearance by at least 50 percent from preoperative values. Patients exhibiting such a decrease in creatinine clearance showed an increase in serum creatinine unless they had undergone a limb amputation. This study suggests that a substantial proportion of the contemporary population of patients undergoing elective surgery are at risk for development of acute renal failure. This renal failure appears to be multifactorial in origin.

One clinical situation in which a relationship between renal ischemia and ATN is well established involves surgical procedures on the abdominal aorta [124, 260, 356]. Thus, ATN complicated the course of 10 to 40 percent of patients undergoing abdominal aortic aneurysm surgery [124, 260, 356]. Gornick and Kjellstrand reported their experience with 47 patients with ATN who required dialysis following repair of an abdominal aortic aneurysm [124]. These 47 patients constituted approximately 15 percent of the patient population that required dialysis for ATN over an 11-year interval. Survival in patients with ATN after abdominal aortic aneurysms was low (21 percent), and most patients died of infectious complications. In nine series of 257 patients with acute renal failure occurring after operation for an abdominal aortic aneurysm, survival ranged from 0 to 40 percent and averaged 29 percent [30].

The high mortality of renal failure that accompanies abdominal aortic aneurysm surgery demands that attention be paid to prevention of the renal failure. Hesdorffer and colleagues [140] suggest that meticulous attention to fluid/volume status can preserve renal function in this setting. In their study, 87 patients operated on from 1980 to 1982 were historic control subjects while 61 patients operated on in 1983 to 1984 were the test group. The authors claim that the major difference in treatment between the two groups was a more organized approach to ensure adequate intravascular volume in the more recently operated group of patients. In these patients, a Swan-Ganz catheter was routinely placed and fluids administered to maintain a minimum pulmonary capillary wedge pressure of 10 mm Hg. More recently operated patients with greater attention to intravascular volume had less postoperative hypotension (33% vs. 62%), acute renal failure (10% vs. 33%), and better survival (85% vs. 69%). In patients at highest risk for acute renal failure (those with ruptured aneurysms), greater attention to intravascular volume repletion also was associated with less acute renal failure (33% vs. 58%). Unfortunately, use of historic controls is not optimal and several factors including improved technical skills of the surgical team could account for some of the improved outcome. However, in the absence of evidence that meticulous attention to ensuring adequate intravascular volume is harmful, it seems reasonable to carefully monitor and attempt to ensure adequate volume status in patients undergoing aortic abdominal aneurysm surgery.

Myers and colleagues recently examined renal function early (1 to 2 hours) and later (24 hours) following 15 to 87 minutes of total renal ischemia (suprarenal aortic clamping) in 15 mannitol-treated patients undergoing abdominal aortic surgery [259, 260]. Renal function in these patients was compared with that observed in 15 patients undergoing similar surgery but with infrarenal aortic clamping. Both groups of patients remained nonoliguric throughout the study. Patients with suprarenal aortic clamping had significantly lower GFRs than did patients with infrarenal aortic clamping. The decrease in GFR seen 1 to 2 hours after ischemia was not associated with a decrement in renal blood flow but rather with decreases in urine-to-plasma osmolality and inulin ratios, two indices of renal tubular function. At 24 hours after ischemia, renal blood flow was depressed and transglomerular passage of neutral dextrans of radius 24 to 40 Å was enhanced. Based on a theoretical analysis, the enhanced passage of neutral dextrans could be explained by either the observed decrease in renal blood flow or by an increase in effective glomerular transcapillary ultrafiltration pressure. These studies suggest that the nonoliguric state seen following renal ischemia in humans is characterized by the early onset of renal tubular dysfunction followed by a reduction in renal plasma flow and possibly glomerular capillary filtration pressure.

Several studies confirm that open heart surgery is a high-risk setting for the development of ARF [259, 260]. Corwin and associates [69] found that 7 percent of patients who underwent a cardiac operation developed at least a 50 percent increase in serum creatinine concentration that could not be attributed to a prerenal cause. The frequency of acute renal failure was 6 to 7 percent from either coronary bypass or valve replacement surgery alone and increased to 22 percent for combined coronary bypass and valve surgery. A case control study found that elevated preoperative serum creatinine, advanced age, combined valve and bypass surgery, increased operating room and pump time, and use of vasopressors were significantly associated with the development of acute renal failure. The development of ARF was associated with an increase in mortality (5% to 24%), hospital stay (16 days to 25 days), and frequency of development of one or more significant postoperative complications (21% vs. 60%). This study suggests that three easily obtained presurgery clinical variables (age, type of procedure, and serum creatinine) could be used to risk stratify patients for postoperative acute renal failure and to select patients who might benefit from renal protective maneuvers.

Rhabdomyolysis often occurs following traumatic muscle injury and has also been recognized as predisposing to ARF [109, 117]. Common settings for trauma include seismic and war catastrophes and industrial accidents. An authoritative review [31] highlights five issues relative to traumatic rhabdomyolysis: (1) Hyperkalemia, hyperphosphatemia, hypocalcemia, and metabolic acidosis occur quickly after injury and the hyperkalemia can be life threatening. (2) Early, aggressive alkaline diuresis may protect the kidneys from development of renal failure. (3) Markedly positive fluid balance is often required to sustain a brisk diuresis; much of this positive fluid balance appears to be due to sequestration within injured muscles. (4) The role of fasciotomy to prevent neurovascular entrapment remains unclear; at present a conservative approach with surgery reserved for clinical evidence of neurovascular compromise and/or intracompartmental manometric readings that are increasing or are very high seems to be the best approach. (5) An intensive search for survivors should continue for up to 5 days.

In a recent prospective study, 25 percent of causes of ARF occurred in the setting of nontraumatic rhabdomyolysis [8]. The vast majority of these patients were drug-overdose victims. The mechanism whereby coma predisposes to rhabdomyolysis has been clarified by Owen et al. [272]. These workers found that muscle compression on a hard surface results in intramuscular compartment pressures of 26 to 240 mm Hg. These pressures are sufficient to cause ischemic necrosis of muscle. Other recently appreciated clinical settings of rhabdomyolysis include strenuous exercise, seizures, heat stroke, viral infections (influenza), inflammatory myopathies, drugs (amphetamines, alcohol, phencyclidine, prolonged epsilon aminocaproic acid), and metabolic disorders (hypokalemia and hypophosphatemia) [22, 32, 35, 49, 76, 99, 117, 208, 264]. The occurrence of rhabdomyolysis in association with cocaine use and abuse has recently received attention [296]. In one series, 39 patients were encountered with cocaine intoxication and rhabdomyolysis over an 8 year interval [296]. Of these patients, 13 had acute renal failure. The patients with ARF had lower blood pressures, higher temperatures, and higher serum creatine kinase concentrations than those without renal failure. Of the patients with acute renal failure, 11 had severe hepatic dysfunction, 7 had disseminated intravascular coagulation, and 6 died. Other recent reports demonstrate the occurrence of rhabdomyolysis following Coxsackie viral infection, polymicrobial sepsis, amoxapine overdose, phenylpropanolamine ingestion, extensive trauma, severe exercise, strychnine poisoning, and the "neuroleptic malignant syndrome" [39, 96, 109, 136, 156, 163, 207, 241, 284, 294, 333]. This latter rare syndrome occurs after concomitant use of phenothiazines and haloperidol [96]. It is characterized by hyperpyrexia, muscular rigidity, altered consciousness, and autonomic nervous system dysfunction [96]. In a few patients, recurrent myoglobinuria occurs in the absence of any of these settings. Some of these patients have hereditary defects of muscle glycolytic metabolism (McArdle's syndrome) or an inherited deficiency of muscle carnitine palmityl transferase as a cause of rhabdomyolysis. Although rhabdomyolysis usually results in tender swollen muscles, rhabdomyolysis-induced ARF may be seen with few muscle complaints.

Cadnapaphornchai et al. have provided an overview of rhabdomyolysis following drug overdosage [49]. Thirty patients with rhabdomyolysis occurring after alcohol ingestion or narcotics or sedative-hypnotic usage were observed in an inner-city general hospital population over 4 years. Three clinical courses were observed, including oliguric ARF (N = 10), nonoliguric ARF (N = 10), and no ARF (N = 10). Patients with ARF appeared to have a greater degree of muscle necrosis as determined by serum enzyme levels. Oliguric patients required more dialysis (50 percent) than nonoliguric patients (0 percent). Hypercalcemia complicated the course of 3 patients with oliguric ARF and 1 patient with nonoliguric ARF. Sixteen patients developed nerve entrapment syndromes during the course of their illness.

Gabow and collaborators reported experience with 87 episodes of rhabdomyolysis in 77 patients seen over a 4-year interval [117]. Rhabdomyolysis was defined as an increase of at least sixfold in serum creatinine kinase in the absence of myocardial infarction or cerebrovascular accident and an increase in MM isoenzymes of creatinine kinase. Most patients (66 of 77) were men, with a mean age of 48 years. Causes of rhabdomyolysis included alcoholism (67 percent), muscle compression (39 percent), seizures (24 percent), trauma (17 percent), drugs (5 percent), metabolic (8 percent), and miscellaneous (10 percent). Most (59 percent) of the patients had more than one potential cause of rhabdomyolysis. Muscle pain was noted in half the patients, but muscle swelling was rarely present. In the 87 episodes, 52 (60 percent) were not associated with ARF. Prerenal azotemia was seen in 6 (7 percent), while 29 (33 percent) developed ATN. Of the 29 patients who developed ATN, half had advanced ARF on hospital admission. Nearly one half of the 29 patients with ARF were oliguric, and 13 required dialysis. Rhabdomyolysis following major trauma appeared particularly to predispose to ARF. Six of the twenty-nine ARF patients (21 percent) died. Only 2 patients required fasciotomy for neurovascular compression.

Ward [347] used a multiple logistic regression analysis to determine factors predictive of acute renal failure in 157 patients with traumatic and atraumatic rhabdomyolysis. Rhabdomyolysis was associated with renal failure in 17 percent of these patients and factors predictive of renal failure included the degree of elevation of serum creatine kinase, potassium, and phosphorus; the degree of depression of the serum albumin; the presence of volume depletion on admission; and the presence of sepsis as a cause of rhabdomyolysis. As noted previously, recognition of rhabdomyolysis as a cause of ARF is especially important because recent studies suggest that forced alkaline diuresis can prevent the occurrence of ARF [99, 294].

Renal artery occlusion due to emboli or atherosclerotic plaques and renal artery thrombosis may result in ARF [82, 84, 215, 303, 309, 321]. In this regard, Madias and collaborators recently performed percutaneous transluminal angioplasty on 12 patients with hypertension and decreasing renal function [215]. Ten patients had critical stenosis in a solitary kidney, and 2 had severe bilateral stenosis. In 5 patients, clear-cut improvement in renal function occurred, whereas in 7 patients renal function was either unchanged or worsened. Complications in these 12 patients included three episodes of nonoliguric ARF, occlusion of a renal artery, a femoral arteriotomy, and an episode of gastrointestinal hemorrhage. In studies by Sos et al., 10 renal complications (6 renal artery dissections, 3 cases of ARF, 1 kidney lost) were encountered in 89 patients undergoing percutaneous transluminal angioplasty [321]. Together these studies suggest that transluminal angioplasty may be a reasonable therapeutic modality in patients with decreasing renal function based on arterial stenosis. However, in this setting, the procedure is associated with significant morbidity including ARF. Complications are more frequent in atherosclerotic than fibromuscular disease [321].

Diagnostic Approach

It is important to acknowledge that clinical settings at high risk for ARF (Table 48-1) are often associated with disease states in which all forms of ARF, including prerenal, postrenal, and renal causes should be considered. Determination of the cause of ARF depends on a systematic approach similar to that depicted in Table 48-5 [48].

CHART REVIEW, HISTORY, AND PHYSICAL EXAMINATION

Chart analysis for determination of the underlying disease state and recent clinical events is needed. Careful attention to a history of loss or sequestration of extracellular fluid volume, signs and symptoms of sepsis or heart failure, exposure to nephrotoxins, and symptoms related to the genitourinary tract (urine output, pyuria, dysuria, hematuria, flank or abdominal pain) can provide helpful diagnostic information. Intense thirst, salt craving, orthostatic syncope, and muscle cramps are often symptoms of extracellular fluid volume depletion. Meticulous examination and careful recording in flow sheet fashion of available data on the clinical course of each patient with ARF are necessary. Examination of serial vital signs, hemodynamic data, intake and output, and daily weight can provide important data regarding the cause of ARF. A weight change of greater than 0.25 to 0.50 kg per day indicates gain or loss of salt and/or water. Recording of serial renal functional data and correlation of any deterioration in renal function with clinical events such as those altering systemic hemodynamics (Table 48-2) and use of potential nephrotoxins often are of great diagnostic value. As is discussed subsequently, analysis of the hemogram, routine biochemical data, and special serologic studies can also be of great diagnostic assistance.

Table 48-5. Sequential diagnostic approach to acute renal failure

1. Record review
2. History and physical examination
3. Urinalysis and urinary volume
4. Urinary chemical indices
5. Consideration of urinary tract obstruction
6. Therapeutic trials
7. Miscellaneous
8. Renal biopsy

Physical examination can be of value in determining the presence or absence of prerenal and postrenal cause of ARF as well as the presence of a systemic disorder that could result in a renal cause of ARF. The effect of either loss or sequestration of extracellular fluid volume on systemic hemodynamic responses depends on several variables including the composition and rate of fluid loss and the underlying health state of the patient. For example, a 20 to 40 percent decrease in extracellular fluid volume by sodium depletion over 4 to 5 hours decreases mean arterial pressure by about 35 percent [168]. This decrease in mean arterial pressure is associated with a decline in cardiac output and an increase in total peripheral resistance [168]. By contrast, a 30 percent decrease in extracellular fluid volume by sodium depletion over 11 days causes no decrease in mean arterial pressure [168]. The presence of a significant increase in pulse and a decrease in arterial pressure 2 to 3 minutes following change from supine to either a sitting or standing position is compatible with the presence of extracellular fluid volume depletion. Dry mucous membranes, low jugular venous pressure, absence of axillary moisture, decreased turgor of skin over the forehead and sternum, and absence of skin sheet marks over the back are all findings compatible with either loss or sequestration of extracellular fluid volume [298]. Physical examination can also provide evidence of cardiac dysfunction. Elevated jugular venous pressure, pulsus paradoxus, and the presence of moist pulmonary rales, S_3 sounds, and murmurs are all compatible with prerenal azotemia due to impaired cardiac function. The presence of significant edema is compatible with a number of disorders characterized by a decrease in effective arterial blood volume and prerenal azotemia. These include cardiac failure, hepatic cirrhosis, nephrotic syndrome, and severe hypoalbuminemia. Also, retroperitoneal fibrosis and intraabdominal lymphomas and other extensive cancers as well as acute inferior vena caval or renal vein thrombosis can present as ARF associated with pedal edema.

Physical examination must also include palpation for determining the state of peripheral circulation, renal size, and the possibility of aortic aneurysms. Palpation or percussion of the suprapubic area is necessary to detect bladder distention, and rectal and pelvic examinations are needed to detect prostatic and pelvic disorders. It is beyond the scope of this chapter to detail all of the physical findings that can be associated with causes of ARF other than ATN (Table 48-3). However, the presence of neurologic or pulmonary disease, fever, skin lesions, joint abnormalities, or diffused lymphadenopathy suggests the presence of a systemic disorder associated with ARF.

URINALYSIS AND URINARY FLOW RATE

Chemical and microscopic examination of the urine is critical in assessment of the cause of ARF. Urinalyses in 103 patients with ATN yielded diagnostically useful information in approximately 75 percent of cases [147]. Routine microscopic urinalysis may also provide prognostic information. Hou et al. found that about half of 97 patients with ARF had an abnormal microscopic urinalysis [147]. An abnormal urinalysis (probable "renal" cause of ARF) was associated with a 35 percent mortality, while a normal urinalysis (probable "prerenal" cause of ARF) was associated with a 15 percent mortality [147]. Such a relationship between routine urinalysis and prognosis has not been found in another study of ARF [248]. An entirely normal microscopic urinalysis in the setting of ARF suggests the presence of either prerenal azotemia or obstructive uropathy.

The "dipstick" can provide helpful information in ARF. A positive reaction for "blood" by an ortho-toluidine test indicates the presence of red blood cells (> 5/high-power field). If no red blood cells are present, this reaction will be positive in the presence of either myoglobin or hemoglobin. Because the myoglobin molecule is smaller (17,000 molecular weight) and is not bound to plasma proteins, it is readily filtered and cleared from plasma. By contrast, the larger hemoglobin molecule (65,000 molecular weight), which is bound to hapatoglobin, is less readily cleared from the plasma and thus gives plasma a pink-red color. Definitive differentiation of hemoglobin from myoglobin in the urine is best done by electrophoretic or immunochemical techniques that are not widely available.

The dipstick protein reading reflects the presence of albumin. Urinary protein determination performed by the acid precipitation method (e.g., Exton's reagent) detects the presence of all types of protein in the urine. Thus, a quantitative estimate of proteinuria that is lower with the dipstick method than with Exton's reagent suggests the presence of light chains (globulins) in the urine. Immunoelectrophoretic techniques remain the definitive method for identifying urinary light chains. If heavy proteinuria (2-3 gm/day) is present in ARF, the presence of a vasculitis or glomerular or other renal parenchymal cause of ARF should be sought. It is important to correlate the dipstick proteinuria assessment with the urinary specific gravity. For example, a 1^+ to 2^+ reading in a concentrated specimen may not indicate significant proteinuria. Conversely, a 2^+ reading in a dilute specimen may indicate significant proteinuria. Recent studies indicate that the ratio of a urinary measurement of albumin-to-creatinine concentration in a spot urinary sample provides a reasonable estimate of the grams per day of urinary protein. The ratio approximates the grams of urinary albumin per 24 hours.

Examination of the urinary sediment is of great value in the differential diagnosis of acute impairment of renal function. Sediment containing few formed elements or only hyaline casts strongly suggests prerenal azotemia or obstructive uropathy. With ATN, brownish pigmented cellular casts and many renal tubular epithelial cells are observed in more than 75 percent of patients. Red blood cell casts suggest the presence of glomerular or vascular inflammatory diseases of the kidney and rarely if ever occur with ATN. Red blood cell casts can, however, be seen rarely in acute interstitial nephritis. The presence of large numbers of polymorphonuclear leukocytes, singly or in clumps, suggests acute diffuse pyelonephritis or papillary necrosis. Eosinophilic casts on Hansel's stain of urine sediment supports a diagnosis of acute allergic interstitial nephritis [268]. Other stains that detect the bilobed eosinophil include Hansel's stain and the May-Grünwald-Giemsa stain. These stains are less pH dependent than Wright's stain and often detect eosinophiluria in interstitial nephritis. However, eosinophiluria is also seen in some forms of glomerulonephritis but is rarely encountered in ATN [268]. The combination of brownish pigmented granular casts and positive occult blood tests on urine in the absence of hematuria indicates either hemoglobinuria or myoglobinuria. In ARF the finding in fresh, warm urine of large numbers of football-shaped uric acid crystals may suggest a diagnosis of acute uric acid nephropathy, whereas the finding of large numbers of "back-of-envelope -shaped oxalic acid or needle-shaped hippuric acid crystals suggests ethylene glycol toxicity. The presence of broad casts (defined as > 3 white blood cells in diameter) suggests chronic renal disease.

A recent study has used the technique of transmission electron microscopy (and electron microscopy) to study urinary sediment in the setting of ARF [221]. In this study renal tubular epithelial cells were present in urine sediment only in the presence of ATN [221]. There was a correlation between the severity of cellular damage to urinary renal tubular epithelial cells and clinical course. These observations suggest that transmission electron microscopy may be helpful in determining the cause and severity of ARF.

The urinary flow rate may also provide helpful information about the cause of ARF. *Anuria* should be defined as absence of urine by bladder catheterization. Sustained periods of anuria suggest urinary tract obstruction as the cause of ARF. Other rare causes of anuria include rapidly progressive glomerulonephritis, mechanical occlusion of renal blood flow, and diffuse renal cortical necrosis. Brief intervals of severe oliguria (< 100 ml/24 hr) may be encountered early in the course of some patients with ATN and may be especially common in the setting of ATN and heat stroke [302].

Oliguria (< 400 ml urine/day) has traditionally been considered the cardinal feature of renal failure [331]. However, the first clinical descriptions of progressive azotemia occurring with little or no oliguria were reported in the early 1940s [123]. In the mid-1950s, additional reports suggested that nonoliguric varieties of ARF may be especially common following head injury, military combat casualties, and burns [305, 336–338]. Small series of selected patients in the 1960s and 1970s reemphasized the occurrence of nonoliguric ARF in burned and traumatized patients [25, 119, 153, 345]. More recently, several reports suggest that nonoliguric ARF is more common than generally appreciated. In 1977 in a prospective study we found that the majority (59 percent) of patients with ARF encountered in a general medical-surgical hospital were nonoliguric despite progressive azotemia [8]. The nonoliguric state was seen with all types of ARF including those following surgery, trauma, hypotension, nephrotoxins, and rhabdomyolysis. Additional studies report similar results and demonstrate a frequency of nonoliguric ARF ranging from 25 to 80 percent of all cases of ARF (Fig. 48-1).

Why was the high frequency of occurrence of nonoliguric ARF recognized only relatively recently? Daily biochemical monitoring of renal function in seriously ill patients, regardless of urine output, has contributed to greater recognition of nonoliguric ARF. Aminoglycoside nephrotoxicity, a frequent contemporary cause of hospital-acquired ARF, is often nonoliguric [230]. Prophylactic use of high-dose potent diuretic agents and renal vasodilators may also contribute to a high frequency of nonoliguric ARF, especially after open heart surgery [259, 261, 262]. It is also possible that aggressive resuscitation and improved supportive management of the seriously ill, traumatized patient has altered the natural history of ARF so that nonoliguric varieties are more common. For example, the Maryland Institute of Emergency Medical Services has demonstrated an increasing incidence of nonoliguric and a decreasing incidence of oliguric ARF concomitant with more aggressive fluid resuscitation of traumatized patients [312]. Another influence on the frequency of occurrence of nonoliguric ARF is the means of patient selection. When ARF patients are selected by need for dialytic therapy as the only criterion, few if any nonoliguric patients will be encountered [177]. When all patients with an increasing serum creatinine level are studied [147], the frequency of occurrence of nonoliguric ARF will be very high (Fig. 48-1).

Oliguria with avid renal salt and water retention is the hallmark of reversible prerenal azotemia. Decreasing effective circulating volume results in rising renal vascular resistance (occurring predominantly at the afferent arteriole) and diminishing renal blood flow. A decrease in glomerular capillary hydrostatic pressures decreases glomerular filtration. The resultant decline in peritubular hydrostatic pressure and increase in filtration fraction (with an increased peritubular colloid oncotic pressure) may act to increase proximal tubular fluid reabsorption. Increases in plasma concentration of aldosterone and antidiuretic hormone, decreases in glomerular capillary pressure, and altered peritubular factors combine to result in avid tubular reabsorption of salt and water and decreased urine flow. Thus, urine flow in patients with prerenal azotemia is usually diminished, and the urine is concentrated with a low fractional excretion of sodium.

In 1980 Miller and associates reported on 9 patients with apparent polyuric prerenal failure [245]. These patients ranged from 28 to 76 years of age. No evidence of diabetes insipidus, exposure to nephrotoxins or diuretic drugs, and glycosuria was present. Two patients had mild chronic interstitial renal disease, whereas the other 7 had normal serum creatinine concentrations. Azotemia developed in each patient (mean serum creatinine, 2.5 mg per deciliter), and high urine outputs (ranging from 980 to 2140 ml/day at the time of peak serum creatinine) were present. Prerenal azotemia was suggested by a negative fluid balance, signs of intravascular volume depletion, low urinary sodium concentration (< 22 mEq/liter), and resolution of azotemia with intravenous fluid administration. The authors postulated that a depletion of medullary interstitial solute prevented maximal urinary concentrating ability in the seriously ill patients, allowing the "polyuric" prerenal state to occur. However, since slow recovery of renal function following correction of prerenal factors was seen, some of these patients may have had nonoliguric ATN

Additional support for the concept of nonoliguric prerenal azotemia is found in studies by Myers et al. [259, 261, 262]. These authors studied glomerular dynamics following open heart surgery and noted that postcardiac surgery patients with prerenal azotemia (as determined by renal failure in the presence of a markedly reduced cardiac output and renal blood flow, no tubular back leak of filtered inulin, and low urinary sodium concentration) had a normal urine output. Importantly, these patients had had vasodilation with nitroprusside and had low filtration fractions.

A number of renal causes of ARF may present as nonoliguric ARF. *Acute interstitial nephritis* comprises a group of heterogeneous diseases that involve the tubular and interstitial components of the kidney [92, 118, 205, 285]. In four series the percentage of nonoliguric forms of acute interstitial nephritis has varied from 20 to 60 percent [92, 118, 205, 285]. However, both oliguric and nonoliguric forms of acute interstitial nephritis may require dialysis. The outcome appears good regardless of urine output as long as the offending agent is recognized and promptly withdrawn.

Some glomerular diseases present with acute renal failure [77, 142, 193, 195, 199, 200, 236, 238, 256, 268, 270, 271, 297, 323] (see Part X), and poststreptococcal glomerulonephritis in children is nonoliguric in over 75 percent of cases. Nonoliguric acute glomerulonephritis (poststreptococcal as well as other forms of glomerulonephritis) in symptomatic adults is less common, comprising 40 percent of the patients in the series of Hinglais et al [142]. Rapidly progressive glomerulonephritis presents as nonoliguric ARF in approximately 50 percent of patients from nonselected series [77, 142, 193, 195, 199, 202, 236, 238, 270, 271, 297, 329]. However, the variance is large, ranging from 4 of 4 nonoliguric cases in one series to only 1 of 7 patients in another [49, 271]. The nonoliguric form of rapidly progressive glomerulonephritis may have a significantly better prognosis than oliguric forms. In two series of rapidly progressive glomerulonephritis, 9 of 12 oliguric patients died or developed end-stage renal failure, whereas these events occurred in 4 of 13 nonoliguric patients [270, 329].

Obstructive uropathy can present as anuria, oliguria, fluctuating oliguria, and polyuria, or nonoliguric renal failure [292] (see Chap. 13). Whether oligoanuria or polyuria is the presenting feature of obstructive uropathy depends critically on the underlying etiology and duration and degree of obstruction.

Nephrotoxins account for 11 to 25 percent of all cases of ATN and usually result in a nonoliguric clinical course. Most prominent among them are the aminoglycosides and cisplatin [33, 213, 230]. For example, the recent prospective study by Matzke and colleagues found that 73 percent of ATN attributed to either gentamicin or tobramycin was nonoliguric [230]. Nonoliguric ATN with radiographic contrast exposure, nonsteroidal antiinflammatory agents, aspirin, captopril, methoxyflurane, amphotericin B, heavy metals, and cyclosporin A have all been reported [46, 74, 86, 87, 110, 111, 134, 181, 186, 231, 299, 332].

Heavy metals are potentially nephrotoxic [33, 213]. Cisdichlorodiamine platinum (cisplatin) is being used for treatment of testicular, head and neck, and other tumors. Studies have shown that approximately one third of patients receiving a single moderate dose of cisplatin develop some nephrotoxicity, which is usually manifest as mild, reversible nonoliguric ARF [33, 87, 134, 213]. With increasing dosage and duration of therapy, more severe renal failure with oliguria occurs, possibly leading ultimately to chronic renal failure. Limiting the administered dose and prehydration are the primary prophylactic measures.

Iodinated dye used for radiologic contrast studies is another potential cause of nephrotoxin-induced ARF [4, 10, 47, 86, 249, 332]. In the prospective study by Hou et al. 12 percent of all ARF was due to contrast administration [147]. Early retrospective studies suggested that oliguria commonly complicates the course of contrast-induced ARF [3, 10, 47, 85, 332]. More recently, however, nonoliguric forms of radiocontrast-induced ARF appear to predominate [4, 249]. This may be due to increased awareness leading to increased detection and improved pre- and postprocedure hydration.

Nontraumatic rhabdomyolysis may account for up to 5 to 7 percent of all cases of ARF and one quarter of all cases of ATN [8, 49, 99, 109, 116, 117, 127, 129, 184]. Oliguric ATN was initially reported as the most common presentation for "pigment"-associated ARF. Subsequent studies have revealed that ARF develops in one third to two thirds of episodes of rhabdomyolysis and is nonoliguric 50 to 60 percent of the time [49, 117, 129, 184].

Ischemic ARF due to inadequate renal perfusion such as occurs with cardiac failure, sepsis, or hemorrhagic shock accounts for approximately 50 percent of all cases of ARF [6, 8, 127, 128, 147, 169, 214, 259]. As noted in Table 48-1, many of these patients (postoperative or posttraumatic) present with nonoliguric ARF. In our experience, there is no difference in the prevalence of nonoliguric versus oliguric ARF in postoperative, postsepticemic, or other causes of renal ischemia [8]. Even limited total renal ischemia from a suprarenal aortic clamp during abdominal aortic aneurysm surgery can produce primarily nonoliguric ARF [259, 260]. These latter studies suggest that improved fluid and hemodynamic management with intraoperative mannitol may favor nonoliguric ARF, particularly during controlled elective surgery.

Historically, ARF following severe burns has often been nonoliguric [38, 93, 279, 344]. A recent study suggests that severe burns (second- and third-degree burns over more than 30 percent of the body surface) are associated with about a 40 percent incidence of ARF [38, 279]. The ARF was nonoliguric and associated with a low fractional excretion of sodium in most of these burned patients. A variety of miscellaneous uncommon causes of ARF have been noted to be nonoliguric. These include ARF associated with hypercalcemia, hyperuricemia, and following transfusions (the latter may be a form of pigment nephropathy) [93].

URINARY CHEMICAL INDICES

Urinary concentrations of electrolytes and nitrogenous wastes were first measured in patients with ATN in the late 1940s [42, 315]. These studies found low urine-to-plasma (U/P) creatinine and urea-nitrogen ratios, and high urinary concentrations of sodium (U_{Na}) and chloride (U_{Cl}) in the established phase of ATN. As renal function improved, U/P creatinine and urea-nitrogen ratios increased. These early observations were subsequently confirmed in nearly all studies [6, 18, 19, 41, 101, 102, 123, 132, 141, 154, 161, 204, 211, 247, 262, 275, 276, 295, 322, 334]. In the 1950s Welt and Waugh first suggested that spot urinalysis, specific gravity, and U_{Na} would be helpful in distinguishing between reversible prerenal azotemia and ATN [349, 350]. In 1967 and 1976, Handa et al. and Espinel, respectively, suggested that the diagnostic accuracy of U_{Na} alone in determining the cause of ARF was limited [100, 101, 132]. However, either U_{Na} ÷ U/P creatinine (renal failure index) or the fraction of excretion of sodium (FE_{Na}) was found to have a high degree of accuracy in differentiating between reversible prerenal azotemia and ATN. Several prospective studies have confirmed the utility of selected urinary indices as diagnostic aids in assessing the patient with ARF [247, 259] (Tables 48-6 and 48-7).

In one such prospective study, a urine osmolality (U_{Osm}) of greater than 500 was noted in 15 of 24 patients with prerenal azotemia and only 5 of 48 patients with oliguric and nonoliguric ATN [247]. A U_{Osm} of less than 350 was seen in only 2 of 24 patients with prerenal azotemia compared with 32 of 48 patients with ATN. A large number of patients from both groups had intermediate values (350 to 500). Thus, urine osmolality was only 60 to 70 percent sensitive in differentiating prerenal azotemia from ATN.

Another means of assessing renal tubular function is to examine the ratio of the urine concentration to the plasma concentration of a substance freely filtered by the glomerulus but relatively unaffected by tubular reabsorption or secretion. Much higher ratios might be expected in the setting of intact tubular function, in which a high percentage of filtrate would be reabsorbed, than in the setting of marked tubular dysfunction. In this regard Bull et al. found that the U/P creatinine ratio ranged from 1.4 to 9.6, and Handa and collaborators found a mean U/P creatinine ratio of 11 in 10 patients with ATN

[42, 132]. In our experience a U/P creatinine ratio of > 40 was encountered in 57 percent of patients with prerenal azotemia and 10 percent of patients with ATN [247]. A U/P creatinine ratio of < 20 was present in 70 percent of cases of ATN and 17 percent of patients with prerenal azotemia. Prerenal azotemia was diagnosed by immediate reversibility with correction of the prerenal cause. Nearly 25 percent of all patients had intermediate values. Thus, U/P creatinine ratios are of limited sensitivity and specificity in the clinical setting.

Extremely low values for urinary sodium (U_{Na}) or chloride (U_{Cl}) concentrations appear to be helpful markers for potentially reversible prerenal azotemia. Thus, several studies have demonstrated that in oliguric patients, a U_{Na} of < 20 mEq per liter is a highly specific (> 90 percent) indicator of prerenal azotemia [6, 247]. While low U_{Na} and U_{Cl} values appear to be fairly specific for prerenal azotemia, sensitivity is less because a considerable overlap, especially a U_{Na} in the 20 to 40 mEq per liter range, was present in most studies (Fig. 48-4). Jones and Weil, however, did not find U_{Na} helpful in differentiating who would develop ARF after shock [161].

Handa et al. in 1967 proposed the use of a renal failure index (RFI) (defined by $U_{Na} \div U/P_{Cr}$) to improve on the diagnostic accuracy afforded by either the U/P creatinine ratio or the U_{Na} value [132]. Both the U/P creatinine ratio and the U_{Na} value suffer from a gray zone in the range, coincidentally, of 20 to 40 and 20 to 40 mEq per liter, respectively. In the series of Handa et al. an RFI of < 1 was found in 11 of 13 patients with prerenal azotemia but in no patient with ATN [132]. Espinel in 1976 found that the RFI reliably distinguished ATN from far-advanced prerenal azotemia [100]. We found an FE_{Na} of < 1 percent in 27 of 30 patients with prerenal azotemia compared with 1 of 24 patients with oliguric and 3 of 31 patients with nonoliguric ATN [247]. Thus, the FE_{Na} is about 90 percent sensitive and specific in differentiating potentially reversible prerenal azotemia from ATN. In more recent studies, we have found FE_{Na} of < 1 percent and U_{Cl} of < 20 mEq per liter to be equivalent in sensitivity and specificity for prerenal azotemia [6]. Recent

Table 48-6. Summary of urinary indices in oliguric patients

	Favors prerenal azotemia	Favors acute tubular necrosis
U_{Osm} (mOsm/kg H_2O)	>500	<350
U_{Na} (mEq/liter)	<20	>40
U/P creatinine ratio (mg/dl)	>40	<20
FE_{Na}	<1	>2

U_{Osm} = urine osmolality.

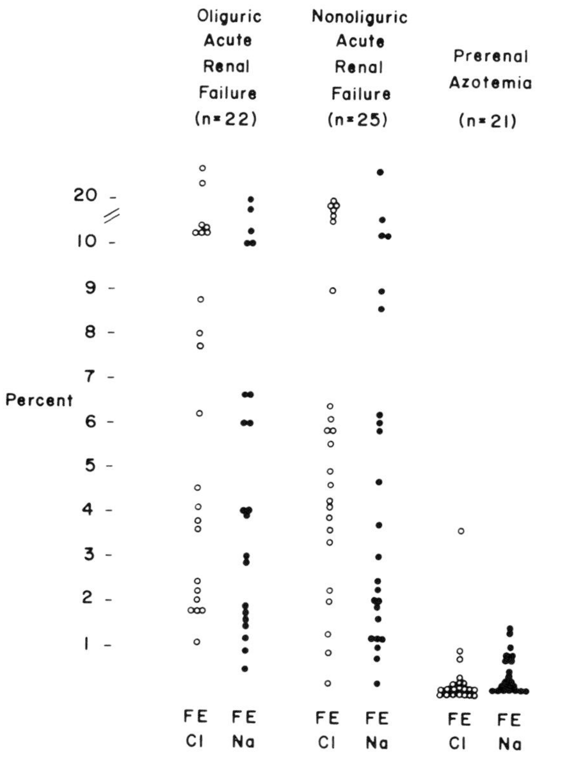

Fig. 48-4. Fractional excretion of sodium (FE_{Na}) and chloride (FE_{Cl}) in acute renal failure. (From [6].)

Table 48-7. FE_{Na} in acute renal failure

FE_{Na} < 1%	FE_{Na} > 1%
1. Prerenal azotemia	1. Diuretic use
A. ECF volume loss or sequestration	2. Nonreabsorbable solute
B. Impaired cardiac output	A. Bicarbonate
2. Severe renal vasoconstriction	B. Glucose
A. Hepatorenal syndrome	C. Mannitol
B. Nonsteroidal antiinflammatory agents	3. Mineralocorticoid deficiency
C. Disease of afferent arteriole (e.g., TTP, scleroderma)	4. Late obstructive uropathy
D. Sepsis	5. Chronic renal failure
E. Early phase of myoglobinuric renal failure	6. Acute tubular necrosis
F. Radiocontrast-induced ARF	
3. Acute glomerulonephritis	
4. Early obstructive uropathy	
5. 10–15% of nonoliguric acute tubular necrosis	

ECF = extracellular fluid; TTP = thrombotic thrombocytopenic purpura studies by Lam and Kaufman provide FE_{Na} data on 8 patients during the maintenance and recovery phases of ARF [191]. The high (> 5 percent) FE_{Na} seen during the maintenance phase persisted for at least 5 days into the recovery phase [191]. Lins and associates [204] have examined standard urinary diagnostic indices in patients with acute renal failure due to acute interstitial nephritis. In these patients, the diagnostic indices were indistinguishable from those found in patients with ATN.

A low FE_{Na} (< 1 percent) suggests the presence of intact renal tubular function and is most often due to extracellular fluid volume loss or sequestration and/or impaired cardiac output [247]. However, the early phase of severe renal vasoconstriction is also associated with a low FE_{Na}. Thus, an FE_{Na} of < 1 percent occurs in the hepatorenal syndrome, in nonsteroidal antiinflammatory agent–induced ARF, after myoglobinuria and radiologic control exposure, in hypotensive septic patients, in acute renovascular diseases such as glomerulonephritis and thrombotic thrombocytopenic purpura, and in early obstructive uropathy [71, 90, 102, 143, 325, 343]. Finally, an FE_{Na} of < 1 percent occurs in approximately 10 to 15 percent of patients with nonoliguric ATN [247] (Table 48-7).

The ratio between urine uric acid and urine creatinine has been used in defining the nature of acute renal failure [171]. In a recent study by Kelton et al., ratios of higher than 1 in patients with renal failure were observed in patients with acute uric acid nephropathy compared with ratios of below 1 in those who had ARF from other causes [171]. For example, the ratio was found to be less than 1 in prerenal azotemia, chronic renal failure, and obstructive uropathy. It was concluded that a ratio of more than 1 in ARF signified a diagnosis of acute uric acid nephropathy. In a more recent study, the urinary uric acid to urinary creatinine ratio was studied in 23 patients with ARF [341]. This ratio was > 1 in 12 patients. These 12 patients had high fever, catabolism, hyperbilirubinemia, and nonoliguric ARF. The 11 patients with ratios of < 1 tended to be less catabolic and oliguric. These results suggest limited diagnostic utility of the urinary uric acid to urine creatinine ratio in determining the cause of ARF [341].

The fractional excretion of uric acid has also been proposed as a reliable marker to differentiate prerenal azotemia from ATN. Fushini and associates [115] found that the fractional excretion of uric acid was 5.9 percent in eight patients with prerenal azotemia and 32.7 percent in seven patients with ATN. The fractional excretion of uric acid was usually > 5.0 percent in patients with chronic renal failure.

Several comments regarding the diagnostic use of urinary indices in ARF are worthwhile. First, as noted in Table 48-7, an FE_{Na} of > 1 percent in the presence of recent diuretic use, bicarbonaturia, glycosuria, mineralocorticoid deficiency, or chronic renal disease does not exclude the possibility of a reversible "prerenal" component to the ARF. Conversely, if these clinical settings are not present, then ATN is the most likely diagnosis with an FE_{Na} of > 1 percent in the setting of ARF. As with any other diagnostic method, urinary indices are really not completely sensitive or specific (Tables 48-6 and 48-7). Moreover, most of the available data were obtained from a single time point, usually relatively late in the course of ARF. Finally, there is no easily obtainable "gold standard" that clearly establishes the presence and degree of ATN. Thus, many studies have defined their patient populations by different criteria. Nevertheless, current data suggest that the criteria outlined in Table 48-6 may be helpful in differentiating prerenal azotemia and ATN.

Eliahou and Bata first suggested that selected urinary diagnostic indices may be a predictor of response to therapy in selected oliguric patients [97]. In a study of 25 oliguric patients, 13 responded to mannitol with sustained diuresis while 12 did not respond. The U/P osmolality and urea nitrogen ratios were significantly higher in patients who responded to mannitol compared with nonresponders. These observations were soon confirmed by Luke et al. [211], who studied 37 patients with oliguria despite correction of deficits in extracellular fluid volume. All patients were given mannitol in an attempt to establish urine flow. Twenty patients responded to mannitol with sustained diuresis. The 20 responders differed from the 17 nonresponders with regard to duration of oliguria (27 hours in responders, 44 hours in nonresponders, $p < 0.05$), U/P osmolality ratio (1.29 in responders, 1:04 in nonresponders, $p < 0.001$), and U/P urea ratio (7.1 in responders, 3.4 in nonresponders, $p < 0.01$).

More recent studies suggest that U_{Na} and FE_{Na} may predict response to therapy [8]. In our experience with 40 furosemide-treated patients who remained oliguric despite correction of deficits in extracellular fluid volume, U_{Na} was lower in furosemide responders (47 ± 6 mEq per liter) than in nonresponders (67 ± 6 mEq per liter, $p < 0.02$) [8]. A recent study by Graziani et al. provides confirmatory data [126]. In this report, combined furosemide and dopamine were administered to 24 oliguric patients in whom mannitol and furosemide failed to produce a diuresis. The 19 patients who responded to combined furosemide and dopamine had ≤ 21 hours of oliguria and a mean U_{Na} value of 45 mEq per liter. By contrast, the 5 nonresponders all had ≥ 28 hours of oliguria and a mean U_{Na} of 70 mEq per liter ($p < 0.05$ versus responders). Together, these studies suggest that the likelihood of a diuretic response to mannitol, furosemide, and/or dopamine is dependent on the duration of oliguria and the integrity of renal tubular function as assessed by selected urinary indices.

Pru and Kjellstrand have suggested that the FE_{Na} provides limited prognostic information in ARF [282]. In their analysis of 45 patients, the FE_{Na} did not differ when the 26 patients who recovered renal function spontaneously (FE_{Na} 4.95 percent) were compared with 19 patients who required dialysis (FE_{Na} 6.28 percent). However, 71 percent of all patients in this study received furosemide before the determination of FE_{Na}. Since it is clear that furosemide increases FE_{Na} [6, 334], the results of this study cannot be applied to patients who have not received furosemide.

We reexamined our prospectively acquired data with regard to FE_{Na} and survival in ARF [307]. In 111 patients with clearly defined categories of ARF [247, 307], mortality in the presence of an $FE_{Na} < 1$ percent was 17.5 percent. When FE_{Na} was > 1 percent, mortality increased to 38 percent ($X^2 = 4.82$, $p < 0.05$). It is also of note that the mortality of nonoliguric ARF was lower with an FE_{Na} of < 1 percent (11 percent) than with an FE_{Na} of > 1 percent (48 percent, $p < 0.05$).

Evidence from other studies also indicates that prognostic information in ARF may be obtained with the use of different urinary indices. In the studies of Eliahou and Bata and Luke et al., survival was 73 percent (24 of 33) in patients with higher U/P osmolality and urea nitrogen ratios and 31 percent (9 of 29) in patients with lower U/P osmolality and urea nitrogen ratios [97, 211]. Moreover, in a study of 36 patients with shock, Jones and Weil [161] demonstrated that the 26 patients who did not develop progressive azotemia had higher U/P osmolality (1.67) than did the 10 patients with progressive azotemia (1.0, $p < 0.05$). Mortality in the nonazotemic group was 46 percent and increased to 80 percent in the azotemic group.

CONSIDER URINARY TRACT OBSTRUCTION

Although a postrenal cause will be encountered in < 10 percent of all cases of ARF, the potential for therapeutic intervention suggests consideration of this diagnosis in each case. The presence of prostatic, pelvic or intraabdominal cancer, a single kidney, anuria, widely fluctuating urinary volumes, recent surgery on the genitourinary tract, or a normal urinalysis demands evaluation for potential obstruction [292].

The best means of excluding obstructive uropathy as cause of ARF remains debatable [292]. Physical examination (suprapubic palpation, pelvic and rectal examinations) and postvoiding bladder catheterization continue to be the best screening methods for bladder neck obstruction. Ultrasonography in experienced hands is an excellent screening tool for the presence of extrarenal obstruction [292, 298]. However, two recent reports suggest that significant obstructive uropathy may occur in the presence of minimal ureteral and renal pelvic dilation [78, 286]. Rascoff and colleagues describe 3 patients with extensive retroperitoneal disease (prostatic cancer in 2, fibrosis in 1) with minimal dilation on either ultrasound or CT scans, in whom renal function improved with nephrostomy drainage [286]. In studies by Curry et al. 27 patients with obstructive uropathy were examined by ultrasound [78]. Three of these twenty-seven (11 percent) were found to have minimal dilation and high-grade obstruction that improved with percutaneous drainage. Two other series of nearly 250 patients reports a somewhat lower frequency (4%) of nondilated obstructive uropathy [217, 265]. Because the majority of patients with acute renal failure and nondilated renal collecting systems do not have either retrograde pyelography or percutaneous nephrostomy, it is likely that the reported frequency of nondilated obstructive uropathy represents a minimal estimate. CT scanning and isotopic methods can also be helpful in the diagnosis of obstructive uropathy, but retrograde pyelography remains the gold standard [292, 298, 311].

Restoration of renal function with extracellular fluid volume expansion and improvement in cardiac output or relief of obstructive uropathy provide evidence for prerenal or postrenal azotemia, respectively.

RENAL BIOPSY

Occasionally, despite a logical sequential approach, the cause of ARF remains unclear. Under such circumstances, renal biopsy may be considered. A renal biopsy is often considered in the setting of ARF when some of the following are present: (1) no obvious cause of ARF; (2) either extrarenal clinical evidence or a history of systemic disease; (3) heavy proteinuria and persistent hematuria; (4) marked hypertension in the absence of volume expansion; (5) prolonged (> 2 to 3 weeks) oliguria; (6) anuria in the absence of obstructive uropathy.

Several studies have examined the clinical utility of renal biopsy in the setting of ARF [257, 318, 357]. Mustonen et al. performed biopsies in 91 of 99 patients and compared biopsy results with the prebiopsy clinical diagnoses [257]. A clinical impression of acute tubular and/or interstitial disease was confirmed by biopsy in 44 of 51 (86 percent) of cases. A clinical impression of acute glomerular disease was confirmed by biopsy in 16 of 23 (70 percent) of cases. In 30 percent of cases, either no clinical diagnosis was obvious or the clinical diagnosis differed from the biopsy diagnosis. Wilson et al. performed a renal biopsy on 84 patients with ARF [357]. All of these patients had undefined "atypical features" for ATN. On biopsy 52 percent had glomerular disease, 30 percent had acute tubulointerstitial disease, and 18 percent had renal vascular disorders [357]. In this study, a clinical diagnosis of an acute tubulointerstitial process was 77 percent sensitive and 86 percent specific. By contrast, a clinical diagnosis of acute glomerulonephritis was less sensitive (56%) and specific (66%). In another prospective study, Cohen and associates [61] found that only one third of the clinical diagnoses of cause of acute renal failure were substantiated by renal biopsy. Moreover, in this small series, the renal biopsy led to a significant change in therapy in more than half of the patients with acute renal failure who were undergoing a biopsy.

Solez et al. reported on their experience with 976 patients with ARF encountered over a 10 year interval [318]. Twenty-two percent of these patients underwent biopsy because the cause of ARF was not apparent. Most of the patients had features atypical of ATN such as gradual onset of ARF, significant hypertension, marked proteinuria, significant hematuria, prolonged (> 3 weeks) oliguria, and underlying systemic disease. Half of the patients who had biopsies had glomerular disease, while the remainder had tubulointerstitial disease. A renal biopsy may thus be warranted when ARF occurs in the setting of some of these features, since some forms of glomerular disease respond to therapy.

Recently Jones studies with light, scanning, and transmission microscopy 19 kidney biopsies of patients with ATN [160]. Kidney specimens were taken several days (range, 11 to 65 days) after onset of ARF. No glomerular changes were seen. In the proximal tubule, abnormal tubular brush border and luminal surface blebs were present. In both proximal and distal tubules, decreased basolateral interdigitations and increased cytosomes were seen. Unfortunately, these tubular findings were not specific for ATN because 2 patients with subacute obstructive uropathy had identical findings [160]. Klingbiel et al. compared light microscopic measurements of renal biopsy samples from oligoanuric and polyuric phases of ATN with 39 controls [180]. Tubular external diameter and lumen width were increased in both oligoanuric and polyuric ATN. Bohle and associates [37], systematically studied renal tissue in several patients with ATN. The primary findings in this study were that while proximal and distal tubular cell swelling was common, cell necrosis was slight and occurred in single cells. Although intratubular casts were frequently seen, the tubules proximal to the casts were not dilated. Clear-cut enlargement of the juxtaglomerular apparatus in oligoanuric ATN was present, but not seen in the nonoliguric phase of ATN. Together, these morphologic observations demonstrate tubular damage in the established phase of ARF.

Complications of Acute Renal Failure

CARDIOVASCULAR SYSTEM

Complications of the cardiovascular system are common in ARF (Table 48-8). Myocardial infarction (7 percent) and arrhythmias (33 percent) were encountered in a series of 276 patients with ATN [237]. In another recent study of 462 patients with ATN, cardiovascular complications (heart failure, arrhythmias, myocardial infarction, and cardiac arrest) occurred in 35 percent of cases [43]. In 64 cases of ATN, Frankel et al. encountered cardiac failure in 34 percent (22 of 64), and Minuth et al. found that 19 of 104 patients with ATN had congestive heart failure [112, 248].

In the oliguric patient with ARF, volume overload with hypertension, edema, and pulmonary congestion is an ever present threat. Early studies of ATN demonstrate that volume overload and congestive heart failure were common causes of death [331]. Therapy with sodium bicarbonate and parenteral nutrition can contribute to volume overload. Volume overload also occurs in nonoliguric patients [8].

Frankel et al. found a direct relationship between pulse rate on initial evaluation and mortality [112]. Mortality was 25 percent with pulse rates from 60 to 69 beats per minute and rose to 100 percent with pulse rate > 100 beats per minute. A similar although inverse relationship was found with systolic blood pressure and mortality [112]. Not only do cardiovascular complications occur frequently during the course of ARF, but they are also associated with increased mortality [43].

ARF frequently occurs in advancing age and often accompanies open heart and abdominal aneurysm surgery. In these populations a number of significant cardiovascular complications are anticipated. McMurray et al. and others found that 7 percent of patients with ARF had a myocardial infarction [237]. The average age of patients with ARF and myocardial infarction was 64 years compared with 51 years for the remaining patients. In patients ages 70 years and older Kumar et al. found that 27 percent of the deaths were due to myocardial infarction [190].

Pericarditis may rarely complicate the course of ARF. Pericarditis occurs at relatively low serum creatinine concentrations in ARF accompanying the hepatorenal syndrome [358]. Pericarditis can lead to tamponade. The presence of hypotension in the setting of ARF suggests volume depletion, gastrointestinal hemorrhage, cardiac/pericardial abnormalities, and sepsis. Hypotension also occurs commonly during acute hemodialysis and can result from hypermagnesemia.

The concomitant presence of significant cardiac dysfunction and ARF may be a manifestation of either systemic disease (i.e., systemic lupus erythematosus, scleroderma) or a complication of cardiac disease (i.e., subacute bacterial endocarditis, atrial fibrillation with emboli). Spontaneous and catheter-induced atheroemboli can cause abdominal and peripheral vascular manifestations as well as ARF. Indwelling arterial and venous catheters can lead to vascular occlusion, inflammation, and infection in the setting of ARF. Cardiac arrest in the setting of ARF should always arouse immediate suspicion of hyperkalemia, a potentially treatable cause of cardiac arrest.

Table 48-8. Frequency (%) of clinical complications in acute renal failure

Study	Neurologic	Gastrointestinal	Cardiovascular	Pulmonary	Infectious
McMurray et al. (N = 276)	—	33	41	—	74
Anderson et al. (N = 92)	38	27	—	28	28
Minuth et al. (N = 104)	—	—	43	—	45
Frankel et al. (N = 64)	—	—	34	36	30
Bullock et al. (N = 462)	—	43	62	54	—
Wheeler et al. (N = 100)	17	40—50	20—30	80	40—50
Maher et al. (N = 90)	—	—	20—30	90	74
Liano et al. (N = 228)	13—26	21	41	38	36

PULMONARY SYSTEM COMPLICATIONS

Pulmonary infiltrates due to edema from volume overload and/or infection are encountered frequently in ARF. In eight series comprising 1900 patients with severe acute renal failure, more than 50 percent had concomitant respiratory failure sufficient to warrant mechanical ventilation [45]. Crosbie and Parsons found hypoxemia ($PaO_2 < 70$ mm Hg) within 2 to 3 days of admission in patients with ATN [75]. This hypoxemia could not be attributed to either decreased alveolar ventilation or cardiac failure. However, extravascular lung water was increased, suggesting the presence of pulmonary edema [75]. Pulmonary function studies by Lee et al. in 55 patients with ATN without clinical or radiologic evidence of pulmonary disease revealed a restrictive and diffusional defect that correlated with the degree of impaired renal function and was also compatible with the presence of pulmonary edema [192].

Pulmonary infiltrates appeared in 26 of 92 (28 percent) patients with ATN in our experience [8]. Pulmonary complications including aspiration pneumonia, respiratory failure, respiratory arrest, and acute respiratory distress syndrome occurred in 54 percent of 462 patients in another recent study [43]. McMurray et al. found 81 episodes of pneumonia in 276 patients with ATN [237]. In the experience of Frankel, endotracheal intubation was required during the course of ATN in 48 percent of oliguric and 10 percent of nonoliguric patients [112]. ARF also appears to be a frequent complication in the respiratory intensive care unit [29, 188]. In the experience of Kraman et al. 74 of 686 patients with respiratory failure developed ARF [188]. The major predisposing factors for ARF in these patients were gastrointestinal bleeding, sepsis, drug nephrotoxicity, and hypotension.

There are several disease processes that can cause simultaneous pulmonary involvement and impairment of renal function [45]. These processes include glomerulonephritis, Goodpasture's syndrome, systemic lupus erythematosus, Wegener's granulomatosis, polyarteritis nodosa, cryoglobulinemia, sarcoidosis, renal vein thrombosis with pulmonary emboli, and bronchogenic carcinoma with immune complex glomerulonephritis [326].

Hypoxemia occurs during acute hemodialysis and can be marked in the presence of underlying pulmonary disease [14, 73]. Some of this hypoxemia results from extrapulmonary shunting due to intravascular sequestration of white blood cells and perhaps platelets; a decrease in alveolar ventilation also contributes to the hypoxemia [14, 73].

The development of pulmonary complications is an adverse prognostic factor in ARF. In a study of prognostic risk factors in 462 patients with ATN, Bullock found the development of pulmonary complications to be the single most significant risk factor for death in ATN, and ARF occurring in the respiratory intensive care unit as associated with an 80 percent mortality [43, 188]. In five series of patients with severe acute renal failure, mortality increased from 49 percent in nonventilated patients to over 80 percent in patients who required mechanical ventilation [45]. Cardiorespiratory failure was the major cause of death in 25 percent of patients with acute renal failure studied by Beaman and associates [26].

GASTROINTESTINAL SYSTEM COMPLICATIONS

The primary gastrointestinal complications of ARF include symptoms of anorexia and nausea, vomiting, and upper-gastrointestinal bleeding. Stress ulcers and gastritis are common. In a recent series of 276 patients with ATN, gastrointestinal bleeding was seen in 90 patients [237]. However, the bleeding was mild and easily controlled in 75 of these patients. Gastrointestinal bleeding did, however, cause deaths in 4 of these 276 ARF patients [237]. In patients with acute renal failure encountered by Beaman and others [26], gastrointestinal hemorrhage accounted for 8 percent of deaths from acute renal failure. Gastrointestinal bleeding may be particularly serious in postoperative and posttraumatic setting of ARF [172]. The effect of gastrointestinal hemorrhage on ARF outcome is unclear. Selected centers reported that gastrointestinal hemorrhage in ARF is associated with high mortality [108, 172, 179, 210]. Other centers find that gastrointestinal hemorrhage is mild and easily controlled and is responsible for only 5 to 8 percent of ARF deaths, especially when encountered in a medical setting [8, 237].

The pathophysiology of gastrointestinal hemorrhage in ARF is not well established [326]. Low acid output and high gastric pH are seen in ARF [326]. This may be due at least in part to high gastric ammonia levels derived from urea nitrogen. Two gastrointestinal hormones that affect acid production and neutralization, gastrin and secretin respectively, are elevated in ARF [133, 306, 335, 351]. In one series about half of the patients with ARF had hypergastrinemia, often in the range seen in Zollinger-Ellison syndrome [133, 306, 335, 351]. Gastrointestinal inhibitory polypeptide and cholecystokinin are also elevated in chronic renal failure [306, 335, 351].

Recent placebo-controlled studies of intensive care unit patients (25 percent of whom had renal failure) demonstrate that cimetidine therapy decreases the frequency of gastroduodenal bleeding and transfusion requirement [63, 283]. Since cimetidine is cleared by the kidney, doses should be reduced to prevent central nervous system toxicity [113]. In other studies cimetidine was superior to infrequent antacid therapy in preventing acute gastrointestinal hemorrhage in the setting of fulminant hepatic failure, a situation often associated with ARF [234]. However, frequent antacid therapy was superior to cimetidine in preventing stress ulceration in other high-risk patients, including several patients with ARF [280]. In regard to antacid prophylaxis after transplantation, gastrointestinal hemorrhage was encountered in 6 of 33 patients not treated with either antacid or cimetidine, while none of 30 patients on cimetidine developed this complication [162]. In a retrospective analysis, Hussy and Belzer found clinical ulcer disease in 3 of 24 patients on cimetidine and in none of 23 patients on antacid [151]. In summary, both cimetidine and frequent antacid therapy offer some protection in several groups of patients with ARF at high risk of acute gastrointestinal hemorrhage. Because of almost exclusive renal elimination of magnesium, extreme caution in utilizing magnesium-containing antacids in the ARF setting is warranted. Furthermore, cimetidine therapy required reduced dosage and careful serial central nervous system monitoring.

Mild hyperamylasemia (two or three times normal) can be seen in ARF [21]. Also noteworthy is the fact that several disease processes such as atheroemboli, vasculitis, and common bile duct stones with bacteremia can present with both acute pancreatitis and ARF. Acute and chronic renal failure can elevate the ratio of the renal clearances of amylase to creatinine [21]. Thus, lipase determinations and clinical assessment are often necessary to assist in the diagnosis of pancreatitis in the setting of ARF. As noted previously, acute pancreatitis can be associated with the development of ATN [152, 155, 165, 237]. It is noteworthy that autopsy studies on patients with shock show a significant direct relationship between the presence of ATN and acute pancreatitis [348].

Jaundice often occurs during the course of ARF. In the experience of Bullock, jaundice occurred in 43 percent of 462 patients with ATN [43]. Jaundice is often multifactorial, with several contributing factors including passive hepatic congestion, blood transfusions, hypotension, medications and toxins, and sepsis. A number of infections (gram-negative sepsis especially in patients with bile duct obstruction, leptospirosis, or hepatitis B) and toxins (hydrocarbons, acetaminophen, *Amanita phalloides* toxin) can cause simultaneous hepatitis and ARF. The development of jaundice in the setting of ARF is an ominous prognostic finding [43].

NEUROLOGIC SYSTEM COMPLICATIONS

Central nervous system disorders have long been recognized as frequent accompaniments of ARF [326]. The frequency of neurologic abnormalities in a recent series of patients with ARF was 38 percent [8]. Beaman and associates [26] found that a cerebrovascular accident was responsible for 7 percent of deaths of patients with acute renal failure. Initially, lethargy, somnolence, lassitude, and fatigue are present. These symptoms may progress to irritability, confusion, disorientation, decreased memory, twitching, asterixis, and myoclonus [326]. In advanced cases generalized tonic-clonic seizures are seen, and marked somnolence and coma can occur. Toxic psychoses with paranoid depression and catatonia may rarely be seen. In rare circumstances in severely encephalopathic patients, transient unilateral facial weakness and hemiparesis can occur [326]. Fluctuating nystagmus and pupillary size, diplopia, and amaurosis have all been reported. Deep tendon reflexes are usually symmetrical and may be either increased or decreased. Myoclonus and "restless legs" syndrome may be present. Clinical evidence of peripheral motor neuropathy attributable solely to ARF is rarely present.

Levitan and collaborators recently examined autonomic nervous system function in patients with ATN [197]. Patients with ARF had significant increases in basal heart rate and arterial pressure and an impaired baroreflex arc as demonstrated by decreases in Valsalva ratio and falls in orthostatic arterial pressure. The defect was reversible on recovery from ARF. Since patients with ARF had decreased heart rate and arterial pressure response to hand grip and a decreased pressor response to norepinephrine infusion, the efferent limb of the autonomic nervous system was abnormal. Control populations with similar critical illnesses but with normal renal function were not studied. Nevertheless, these observations suggest that autonomic nervous system dysfunction occurs in ARF.

The encephalopthy of ARF has not yet been firmly identified as a complication of a single specific identifiable toxin. Thus, the pathophysiology of neurologic complications in ARF remains unclear. Electroencephalographic (EEG) changes correlate to some degree with clinical involvement [326]. Loss of alpha activity with development of nonsymmetrical slow waves is seen early in ARF. Later, more slowing, disorganization, and spiking occur. A systematic examination of the cerebrospinal fluid in ARF is not available.

The neurologic disturbances that complicate ARF have been recently investigated by Cooper et al. [67]. In serial EEGs patients with ARF, the percentage of EEG power less than 5 Hz increased to 41 percent (normal < 2 percent) within 48 hours of onset of ARF. These EEG changes were not influenced by dialysis but normalized on recovery of renal function. To determine the cause of these EEG abnormalities, studies of brain electrolyte content were done in 10 patients who died. Striking increases in cortical gray-matter calcium content were present [67]. This high brain calcium content did not correlate with the calcium $\times$ phosphorus product. In dog studies performed by these and other workers, evidence for parathyroid hormone (PTH) as an important mediator of the increased brain calcium content was found [12, 121, 122]. In patients with ARF, elevated PTH levels are also found. Together, these studies suggest that the central nervous system abnormalities seen in ARF may be mediated by an effect of PTH that increases brain calcium content. In a study performed in dogs, both ARF (induced by bilateral nephrectomy) and exogenous PTH increased peripheral nerve calcium content and diminished motor nerve conduction velocity [122]. These findings were not observed in thyroparathyroidectomized animals. Although these results suggest a role for calcium-PTH in diminishing motor nerve function in experimental ARF, the studies of Cooper et al. [67] did not demonstrate decreased motor nerve conduction in patients with ARF.

There are a number of other causes of neurologic dysfunction in the setting of ARF. Primary neurologic disease, other metabolic disturbances, and the presence of systemic disease (vasculitis, systemic lupus erythematosus, subacute bacterial endocarditis, thrombotic thrombocytopenic purpura, hemolytic-uremic syndrome, malignant hypertension) involve both the kidneys and the nervous system [326]. Recently, pharmacologic agent–induced encephalopathy was found to be a common cause of central nervous system dysfunction in patients with renal failure [290]. Neurologic symptoms appearing after dialytic therapy should arouse suspicion of a dialysis "disequilibrium" syndrome. Development of peripheral neuropathy in the setting of ARF should raise consideration of neurovascular entrapment (rhabdomyolysis), ischemic neuropathy (polyarteritis, emboli), and heavy metal intoxication.

INFECTIOUS COMPLICATIONS

ARF and infections are commonly associated. In the experience of Rasmussen and Ibels, septicemia appeared to be an important factor contributing to the development of ARF in 26 percent of 143 ARF patients [287]. In the studies of McMurray et al. and Frankel et al. 14 percent and 17 percent, respectively, of all cases of ATN occurred in the setting of septicemia, and septicemia accounted for 30 percent of all cases of ATN encountered in a respiratory intensive care unit [112, 237].

Not only is septicemia frequently associated with the onset of ARF, but also infections frequently complicate the course of patients with ARF. McMurray et al. found infections in 74 percent of 276 patients with ATN [237]. In their study the most common sites of infection were pulmonary (29 percent of patients), urinary tract (32 percent of patients), and peritonitis (22 percent of patients). A total of 56 patients had abscesses and 97 patients had documented bacteremia [237]. In a prospective analysis, we found that 11 percent of 92 patients with ARF developed septicemia [8]. Infections from indwelling venous and arterial line and indwelling bladder catheters also occur in ARF. However, urinary tract infections can occur even in patients without indwelling catheters. Pulmonary infections appear to occur later in the course of ARF and are often gram negative in nature.

Because of the frequent presence of infections, many patients with ARF are treated with antibiotics. In the experience of Bullock et al. with 462 ARF patients, 91 percent received an average of three antibiotics for 16 days [43]. In the series of Frankel, 66 percent of ARF patients were treated with antibiotics [112]. Of the patients treated with antibiotics, most (67 percent) received three of more agents [112].

Infectious complications are a leading source of morbidity and mortality in ARF. McMurray et al. found that infectious complications were the cause of death in 54 percent of 102 ATN deaths [237], and Frankel et al. found that infections caused death in 30 percent of 64 patients with ATN [112]. In other series infections have been responsible for 29 to 72 percent of all deaths [107]. It is of interest, however, that septicemia could not be identified as an independent risk factor for death in 462 patients with ATN [43].

ENDOCRINE SYSTEM COMPLICATIONS

Several hormonal abnormalities have been described in ARF. For example, ATN is often associated with disturbances in divalent ion metabolism (hypocalcemia, hyperphosphatemia, and hypermagnesemia). Altered PTH action and vitamin D metabolism may play a pathogenetic role in the hypocalcemia and hyperphosphatemia.

Several studies demonstrate high plasma PTH in ATN [116, 185, 187, 208, 277]. This probably occurs in response to hypocalcemia. The simultaneous presence of hypocalcemia with high PTH levels suggests impaired bone response to PTH. An impaired calcemic response to PTH has been demonstrated in humans, dogs, and rats with ARF [225, 229, 319, 320]. The cause of this impaired calcemic response is debated. In experiments by Massry et al. supplementation with large doses of 1,25-dihydroxyvitamin D_3 (1,25$(OH)_2D_3$) to dogs studied shortly after bilateral nephrectomy only partially restored the calcemic response to PTH. However, the same dose of 1,25$(OH)_3D_3$ given either to dogs with comparable renal failure produced by ureteric caval diversion or to dogs given 24,25$(OH)_3D_3$ completely reverses the calcemic response to PTH [228, 229]. These observations favor a role for diminished 1,25$(OH)_3D_3$ and 24,25$(OH)_2D_3$ in impairing the calcemic response to PTH in ARF. Indeed, low values for 25$(OH)D_3$ have been observed in patients with ARF [277]. However, in rat experiments, no evidence for a role for vitamin D or its metabolites in resistance to the calcemic response to PTH in ARF was found [319, 320].

Calcium homeostasis in ARF related to rhabdomyolysis has recently been investigated by Llach et al. [208]. These workers studied 6 oliguric patients with ARF following rhabdomyolysis. At admission, hypocalcemia, hyperphosphatemia, and low levels of 1,25$(OH)_2D_3$ were present. Hypercalcemia occurred early in the polyuric phase of ARF and was associated with increases in 1,25-dihydroxycholecalciferol and PTH (both amino-terminal and carboxy-terminal). Later in the polyuric phase, serum calcium, vitamin D, and PTH levels returned to normal. A close correlation between serum calcium and vitamin D levels was present. These observations suggest that the hypocalcemia seen during the early phase of ARF is due to hyperphosphatemia and decreased 1,25-dihydroxyvitamin D synthesis. In summary, high PTH, skeletal resistance to PTH, and low 1,25-dihydroxyvitamin D levels occur in ARF.

Recently, data on male gonadal function in ARF have become available. Two groups of investigators found high blood prolactin and low testosterone in males with ARF [185, 198]. The abnormalities in prolactin and testosterone resolved as renal function normalized. In the study of Kokot and Kuska, increased blood concentrations of luteinizing hormone and estradiol were also present [185]. These workers found a negative correlation between plasma prolactin and testosterone but no correlation between PTH and either testosterone or prolactin [185]. By contrast, Levitan et al. found a direct relationship between prolactin and PTH [198]. Together, these observations demonstrate that male gonadal failure frequently occurs in the setting of ARF.

Thyroid function tests have been examined in the setting of ARF [164]. Total T_4 and T_3 were decreased in ARF and returned to normal with recovery of renal function. However, all patients appeared clinically to be euthyroid, and free T_4, T_3 uptake ratios, thyroid-stimulating hormone (TSH), and T_3 concentrations were all normal. Thus, patients with ARF resemble other critically ill patients, and thyroid function is normal.

Kokot and Kuska studied glucogenic insulin release in

patients with ARF [185]. Insulin release from beta cells was studied by intravenous glucose infusions. Fasting insulin concentrations were normal. In response to glucose infusion, insulin concentrations were higher than in controls, and plasma disappearance was prolonged. These findings suggest the presence of insulin resistance such as is commonly seen in chronic renal failure. This conclusion was further documented by finding that insulin (0.1 μ/kg) decreased fasting plasma glucose from 96 to 58 mg per deciliter in patients with ARF and from 90 to 38 mg per deciliter in normal subjects. In acutely uremic rats, insulin resistance appears to be due to skeletal muscle resistance to insulin-mediated glucose uptake [252]. Also, there appears to be impaired hepatic glucose response to glucagon but not to cyclic adenosine monophosphate (cAMP) [252]. Together, these clinical and experimental studies suggest that ARF produces insulin resistance and the resistance occurs at the skeletal muscle level. Also, acute uremia appears to induce a "pre-cAMP" defect in hepatic glucose response to glucagon [252].

High plasma renin activity and angiotensin II often occur in the setting of ARF [183]. In a clinical study, Mitch and Walker found elevated plasma levels of angiotensin II in 13 patients with shock and ARF [250]. Of these 13 patients, 10 had increased plasma renin activity (PRA). However, only slight increases in angiotensin II and PRA levels were frequently found. Furthermore, comparable increases in PRA and angiotensin II were observed in 6 patients undergoing elective drug-induced hypotension who did not develop ARF [250]. The observations confirm that high levels of angiotensin II and PRA are often observed in the clinical setting of ARF. However, similar levels also occur in settings in which renal function is clinically well maintained. Whether the high angiotensin II levels contribute to hypertension that occasionally complicates ARF remains to be determined.

Kokot and Kuska examined growth hormone response to insulin in patients with ARF [185]. Patients with ARF had a threefold greater increase in growth hormone compared with controls. Following hemodialysis, the exaggerated increase in growth hormone response was significantly less but still present. Hyperglucagonemia and increased plasma 17-hydroxycortisol and gastrointestinal inhibitory polypeptide also occur in the setting of ARF [183]. The mechanisms and physiologic importance of these abnormalities have not been determined.

Biochemical Abnormalities in ARF

NITROGEN BALANCE

Since decreased urinary excretion of nitrogenous waste occurs in ARF, plasma urea nitrogen and creatinine increase. The magnitude of increase is dependent on the nitrogen intake, the degree of renal impairment, and the degree of protein catabolism. Urea nitrogen appearance rates ranging from 5 to 30 gm per day can occur depending on the catabolic state of the patient [183]. In the noncatabolic patient with mild renal impairment, daily blood urea nitrogen usually increases < 10 to 15 mg/dl/day and serum creatinine < 1.5 mg/dl/day. Conversely, in the catabolic patient, daily increments of blood urea nitrogen can exceed 50 mg per deciliter (Table 48-9). In 462 patients with ATN, Bullock et al. found that 35 were "catabolic" as defined by an increase of BUN of > 30 mg per deciliter on 2 consecutive days [43]. The degree of renal impairment is also an important determinant of BUN and plasma creatinine in ARF. We found that the duration of BUN of > 50 mg per deciliter in ARF was 18 ± 2 days in oliguric patients and only 8 ± 0.8 days in nonoliguric patients who had a higher glomerular filtration rate [8].

The precise cause of the catabolic state in ARF cannot be stated with certainty. Many patients have necrotic tissue, muscle damage, fever, and sepsis and may be receiving corticosteroids. Several hormonal abnormalities are present in ARF (e.g., elevated levels of glucagon, catecholamines, growth hormone, cortisol, and insulin resistance) that could alter muscle protein metabolism [183, 185]. Several experimental studies suggest that acute uremia per se decreases the release of amino acids from muscle and/or muscle protein synthesis [60]. Enhanced degradation of muscle protein also occurs. Circulating proteases have been found in the blood of catabolic patients with ARF [145, 146]. Finally, diminished nutritional intake can potentially contribute to the depression level of muscle protein synthesis in ARF.

Enhanced muscle breakdown with release of creatinine can lead to a disproportionate increase in serum creatinine relative to BUN in the setting of rhabdomyolysis-induced ARF [109, 117]. For example, Koffler et al. found that about 25 percent of their patients with rhabdomyolysis-induced ARF had disproportionate increases in creatinine relative to BUN [184]. Grossman et al. found daily increments in plasma creatinine varying from 1.6 to 6.6 mg per deciliter [129]. In 15 patients with rhabdomyolysis-related ARF, 9 had daily increments of plasma creatinine of > 3.0 mg per deciliter [129]. However, Gabow et al. did not find any difference in daily increment in plasma creatinine when ARF patients with (1.3 ± 0.7 mg/dl) and without (1.4 ± 0.8 mg/dl) rhabdomyolysis were compared [117].

Clinicians commonly follow daily serum creatinine concentrations to assess whether glomerular filtration rate is increasing, decreasing, or constant in patients with acute renal failure. Unfortunately, the serum creatinine concentration is dependent on creatinine production, volume of distribution, and renal elimination, and all of these variables are subject to wide fluctuations

Table 48-9. Selected biochemical complications in acute renal failure

	Change/day	
	Noncatabolic	Catabolic
BUN (mg/dl)	10–20	>30
Creatinine (mg/dl)	<1.5	>1.5
K^+ (mEq/liter)	<0.5	>0.5
HCO_3^- (mEq/liter)	<2	>2

in patients with acute renal failure [255, 259]. Moran and Myers developed a simple, computerized model of creatinine kinetics in patients with postischemic acute renal failure [255, 259]. This model allows calculation of glomerular filtration rate based on serum creatinine concentration corrected for changes in creatinine volume of distribution and was validated by direct measurements of GFR. Using this model, two clinically noteworthy observations were made. First, in patients with acute renal failure, changes in glomerular filtration rate often correlated poorly with changes in serum creatinine concentration. Second, several patterns (abrupt and large, slow and progressive, and stepwise) of change in glomerular filtration occur during development of and recovery from postischemic acute renal failure and are poorly reflected by daily changes in serum creatinine concentration [255, 259]. These observations suggest that definite conclusions regarding changes in GFR are difficult to make using serum creatinine concentration alone in the setting of acute renal failure.

Disorders of Electrolyte and Uric Acid Metabolism

Hyperkalemia, hyponatremia, metabolic acidosis, and hyperuricemia often occur in ARF. In our experience, a rise in plasma potassium concentrations of > 5.5 mEq per liter was seen in 50 percent of patients with ARF [8]. Minuth et al. found hyperkalemia in 75 percent of 94 patients [248]. Wheeler and associates [354] found that 30 percent of patients with ATN develop an increase in plasma potassium concentration of > 6.0 mEq per liter. The hyperkalemia is due to continued potassium release from cells in spite of impaired renal potassium elimination. For example, the potassium concentration of intracellular water is about 155 mEq per liter in skeletal muscle. Thus, "tumor lysis" syndrome and rhabdomyolysis can induce dangerous levels of hyperkalemia quickly. A recent study of 7 patients with rhabdomyolysis induced by extensive traumatic muscle crush injury revealed plasma potassium concentrations on admission of 4.5 to 8.3 mEq per liter despite rapid evacuation from the site of injury [294]. Three of the seven patients had potassium concentrations of > 6.9 mEq per liter. Gabow et al. found significantly higher peak potassium concentrations in ARF associated with rhabdomyolysis than in other forms of ARF (5.6 ± 0.9 versus 4.7 ± 0.6, respectively, $p < 0.05$) [117]. Other factors including a cellular shift of potassium due to acidemia and hyperosmolality and potassium loads by exogenous sources such as blood, dietary intake, potassium salts (e.g., salt substitutes), or large doses of penicillin G can also contribute to hyperkalemia. Acute renal failure induced by nonsteroidal antiinflammatory agents can also be associated with marked hyperkalemia [34, 232]. An effect of these agents in suppressing renin and aldosterone secretion may in part be responsible.

Metabolic acidosis occurs often in ARF. In 92 patients with ARF, we found metabolic acidosis (plasma bicarbonate of < 15 mEq/liter, pH < 7.40) in 18 (19 percent) [8]. Stable patients without kidney function on chronic hemodialysis usually have a decline of plasma bicarbonate of 2 mEq per day [183]. The metabolic acidosis is often associated with an increased anion gap. Thus, Gabow et al. found an anion gap of 17 ± 6 mEq per liter in ARF; however, when rhabdomyolysis was present, the anion gap increased to 28 ± 14 mEq per liter [117]. The metabolic acidosis results from continued production of nonvolatile acid and decreased renal ability to excrete acid. In severely catabolic states, the usual daily production of 1 mEq per liter of nonvolatile acid can be increased markedly. It is noteworthy that other causes of anion gap metabolic acidosis such as ingestion of ethylene glycol and clinical setting associated with lactic acidosis are often associated with ARF.

Hyponatremia is a common complication of ARF and is due to an absolute or relative increase in free-water intake. In a prospective analysis of hyponatremia, we found that 19 percent of all cases of hyponatremia occur in the setting of excess free-water intake in the presence of renal failure [7]. Hyperuricemia usually occurs in ARF. Peak uric acid was 9.2 ± 3.7 mg per deciliter in 38 patients with ATN [117]. Much higher blood uric acid concentrations occur in cell injury–associated ARF, and peak uric acid concentrations of 14.1 ± 4.4 mg per deciliter were found in patients with ARF and rhabdomyolysis [117]. Uric acid concentrations of greater than 20.0 mg per deciliter were seen in 5 of 21 patients with rhabdomyolysis and ARF in other studies [129, 184]. Striking increases in uric acid concentrations also occur with ARF in the setting of heat stroke and catabolism. Despite high blood uric acid concentrations, there is little evidence of irreversible end-organ disease resulting from hyperuricemia [184, 302, 341].

ION METABOLISM

Hyperphosphatemia in the range of 5 to 8 mg per deciliter usually occurs in ARF [225]. Decreased urinary excretion of phosphorus contributes to hyperphosphatemia. In addition, phosphorus is released from injured tissue in which intracellular phosphate concentrations average 100 mmol per liter. In the presence of tissue destruction as in the "tumor lysis" syndrome and in rhabdomyolysis, extremely high serum phosphorus concentrations are seen. For example, 14 of 34 patients with ARF due to nontraumatic rhabdomyolysis had hyperphosphatemia (> 9 mg/dl) in two studies [129, 184]. In another study peak serum phosphorus in patients with ARF with and without rhabdomyolysis was 7.0 ± 2.7 and 4.5 ± 1.8 mg per deciliter, respectively [117]. Acute acidosis, by decreasing the glycolytic rate and increasing the rate of hydrolysis of sugar phosphates intracellularly, can also contribute to hyperphosphatemia.

Hypocalcemia is also an expected finding in ARF. In the absence of rhabdomyolysis, calcium concentrations usually exceed 6.5 mg per deciliter [225, 226]. In rhabdomyolysis-associated ARF, profound hypocalcemia can be observed. Thus, 8 of 35 patients with rhabdomyolysis and ARF had serum calcium concentrations of < 6.5 mg per deciliter [208]. The cause of the hypocalcemia of ARF is debated. Phosphate retention with calcium-phosphate deposition in soft tissues can cause some degree of hypocalcemia. However, in some studies, no relationship between hyperphosphatemia and hypocalcemia can be demonstrated, suggesting that additional mechanisms are operative [225, 226]. As note previously, skeletal resistance to the calcemic effect of PTH is present in ARF. Evidence that this diminished calcemic response is due to decreased 1,25-dihydroxyvitamin D_3 production has been discussed earlier [227–229]. A contrary view has been proposed by Somerville and Kaye [319, 320]. In these studies, lowering serum phosphorus in urine-reinfused rats resulted in normalization of the calcemic responses to PTH. Moreover, infusion of phosphate produced a significant inverse relationship between the dose of phosphate infused and the calcemic response to PTH. These observations support a role for phosphorus per se in the impaired calcemic response to PTH in this model.

Rarely, hypercalcemia complicates the course of ARF [89, 105, 117, 208]. Although this hypercalcemia usually occurs during the diuretic phase of rhabdomyolysis-induced ARF, it has been reported during the oliguric phase as well [105]. The mechanism of this hypercalcemia is unclear. Both increased and decreased PTH levels are reported [105, 117]. Utilizing electron microscopy and technetium pyrophosphate scanning in 4 patients with rhabdomyolysis, Akmal et al. demonstrated muscular tissue calcification that disappeared during recovery from ARF [2]. Meroney and co-workers administered radiolabled calcium to dogs with experimental muscle trauma [243]. They found that the isotope was deposited in injured skeletal muscle at a rate nine times that observed in control animals. As noted earlier, hypercalcemia occurring in the early polyuric phase of rhabdomyolysis-associated ARF is associated with increases in 1,25-dihydroxyvitamin D_3 and PTH [208]. Two studies demonstrate widespread tissue calcium deposition with calcium-related organ dysfunction in patients becoming hypercalcemic after rhabdomyolysis-associated ARF [89, 105]. These observations emphasize the importance of recognition and control of this complication of ARF.

Hypermagnesemia in the range of 2.5 to 4.0 mg per deciliter occurs frequently in ARF [225, 226]. This range of hypermagnesemia is almost always asymptomatic. However, striking hypermagnesemia can occur if magnesium-containing antacids are administered to patients with ARF.

High plasma aluminum concentrations are traditionally thought to occur exclusively in the setting of chronic renal failure. However, recent reports demonstrate high plasma aluminum concentrations occurring in the setting of ATN [83]. In the majority of these patients with acute renal failure, the source of the aluminum appeared to be untreated water used for dialysis.

Hematologic Status

Anemia is common with ARF. The characteristics, genesis, and treatment of anemia in animals are described in detail in Chap. 99. Of note, a recent report of 10 patients with ATN includes data on serial measurements (radioimmunoassay) of serum erythropoietin [266]. Serum erythropoietin levels were very low in patients with ATN. Moreover, several weeks to months were required before serum erythropoietin levels returned to normal, and the normalization of serum erythropoietin lagged far behind the normalization of the GFR. In one patient with ATN, exogenous recombinant erythropoietin resulted in a brisk reticulocytosis and a progressive increase in hemoglobin, suggesting the lack of any endogenous inhibitor of erythropoiesis. A number of disease states (Table 48-3) resulting in ARF are associated with significant abnormalities of the hemogram. Thus, ARF associated with a microangiopathic hemolytic process suggests a "vascular" form of ARF (Table 48-3). Eosinophilia suggests the possibility of allergic interstitial nephritis, polyarteritis nodosa, and atheroembolic disease [71, 118, 205, 298]. Anemia and rouleaux formation suggest a plasma cell dyscrasia. Leukopenia and thrombocytopenia often occur in systemic lupus erythematosus.

Coagulation disturbances occur frequently in ARF. Acute renal failure associated with traumatic and atraumatic rhabdomyolysis is often accompanied by thrombocytopenia and disseminated intravascular coagulation [294, 296]. A bleeding diathesis complicating the course of acute renal failure occurred in 16 percent of the patients reported by Liano and associates, [201]. Associated liver disease and multiple transfusions are often present in patients with ARF. A functional defect in platelets leading to a prolongation in the bleeding time is seen in ARF. Thus, hemorrhagic complications contributing to hemostatic abnormalities are seen in 5 to 20 percent of patients with ARF [237]. In a clinical study, 19 of 47 patients with intravascular coagulation developed ARF concurrently with or shortly after onset of the coagulopathy [223]. However, the absence of either cortical necrosis or microthrombi in the 11 kidneys examined histologically argues against a role for coagulopathy in directly affecting renal function in these patients. Studies in 3 patients with ARF due to cardiogenic shock also suggest that intravascular coagulation can contribute to ARF [189]. A falling platelet count and a rise in fibrinogen degradation products occurred simultaneously with onset of ARF. A rapid improvement in urine output and renal function was noted after heparin therapy.

Prognostic Factors

The outcome of acute renal failure as reported in the literature is highly dependent on the definition of the disorder and subsequent patient selection [239] (Table 48-10). In many epidemiologic studies, acute renal failure is defined either as a 20 to 50 percent increase or a 0.5 mg/dl increase in basal serum creatinine concentration. Although this appears to be a small degree of renal failure, it likely reflects a 30 to 60 percent decrease in GFR. With a such definition of acute renal failure, a mortality of 20 to 30 percent is seen [57, 239, 242, 313]. This mortality exceeds that for case controls by a factor of six- to eightfold [313]. About 10 to 20 percent of patients who meet this definition of acute renal failure will require dialysis. By contrast, when patients are selected and/or identified as having acute renal failure by either referral to a renal service or by reviewing discharge diagnosis, the selection bias generally produces a much different group of

Table 48-10. Prognostic factors in acute renal failure

1. Clinical setting
   A. Severity and reversibility of underlying disease
   B. APACHE II score
   C. Extremes of age
   D. Cause and reversibility of renal failure
2. Severity of renal failure
   A. Peak serum creatinine
   B. Urine flow rate
   C. Dialysis requirement
   D. Urinalysis/FE_{Na}
3. Development of complications
   A. Number of complications
   B. Presence of multiple organ failure
   C. Development of pulmonary, cardiovascular, hepatic, or neurologic complications
   D. Development of major infection
   E. Development of a second episode of renal failure
   F. Development of disseminated intravascular coagulation
   G. Catabolic state

patients. In such patients, a greater degree of renal failure is present, with 30 to 80 percent of patients requiring dialytic therapy and a reported contemporary mortality of 30 to 60 percent [8, 26, 30, 51, 52, 70, 157, 201, 237, 287, 342, 354]. Finally, many series report outcome and prognostic variables only in patients with acute renal failure who have been dialyzed. In this highly selected population, current mortality ranges from 50 to 90 percent [1, 43, 209, 342].

The causes of death in three recent series of patients with severe ATN are listed in Table 48-11. Infections/sepsis, underlying disease, and cardiopulmonary complications appear to be major causes of death in ATN [26, 43, 201, 237, 342]. The majority of ATN deaths occur within 14 days of onset of the renal failure. Some clinical settings of acute renal failure that have been reported to be associated with an especially high mortality include extensive burn injury, pancreatitis, advanced liver disease, ruptured abdominal aortic aneurysm, and development of a second episode of acute renal failure.

The underlying health of patients in whom acute renal failure develops is a critical outcome determinant. Obviously, a patient in poor general health due to advanced, nonreversible disease will often not fare very well with the development of acute renal failure. Recently, a validated scoring system has been widely utilized in critical care medicine to predict outcome of intensive care unit admissions [216]. The system is based on easily obtainable acute physiologic parameters and chronic health evaluation monitors and is termed APACHE II. This system also appears to be a valid model for assessing prognosis in patients with acute renal failure. When applied to patients with severe ARF who require intensive care unit admission, no patient with a score greater than 40 survived whereas 40 percent with a score of 19 or less survived [216]. The use of this scoring system in future studies will allow patients to be categorized by severity of disease to ensure comparability of groups in interventional studies and to address quality-of-care issues with regard to outcome between hospitals.

Age per se as an outcome factor continues to be debated. In general, advanced age, especially when associated with underlying disease, is a potential marker for a poor outcome. Although much emphasis has been placed in the past on outcome in relationship to the clinical setting in which the acute renal failure occurs (i.e., medical vs. surgical vs. obstetric), the setting appears to have little predictive power when patients are matched for age and underlying disease [239].

A major prognostic factor in patients with ATN is the severity and duration of the resultant renal dysfunction. Hou and collaborators [147], in a large prospective study, found that the presence of urinalysis abnormalities in patients with ARF had a marked influence on outcome. Death occurred in 31 percent of ARF patients with normal urine sediment and in 74 percent of patients with an abnormal urine sediment. These observations have also been reported in other studies and probably reflect outcome differences between prerenal azotemia (normal sediment) and renal azotemia (abnormal sediment). Hou and collaborators also found a direct correlation between mortality and the magnitude of rise in serum creatinine in patients with ARF. The mortality was less than 20 to 30 percent until the increment in serum creatinine exceeded 3 mg/dl, at which time the mortality was 64 percent (Fig. 48-5).

Other indicators of severity of renal insult in patients with ARF are the quantity and quality of urine output. Virtually all contemporary studies of patients with ARF find mortality of nonoliguric patients to be less than half of that of oliguric patients (see Fig. 48-1). Moreover, several studies demonstrate lower mortality in ARF patients with more avid retention of urinary sodium. These results likely also reflect mortality differences in patients with prerenal versus renal forms of azotemia.

Several recent studies have applied numerous statistical analyses (discriminant, univariate, and logistic

Table 48-11. Causes of death in three recent series of patients with severe acute tubular necrosis

Series	Underlying disorder	Sepsis	Pulmonary/ cardiovascular	Gastro-intestinal	CNS	Multiple organ failure
Liano et al. [201]	40%	19%	12%	7%	4%	—
Berisa et al. [30]	—	16%	54%	14%	3%	14%
Beaman et al. [26]	7%	52%	25%	8%	7%	—

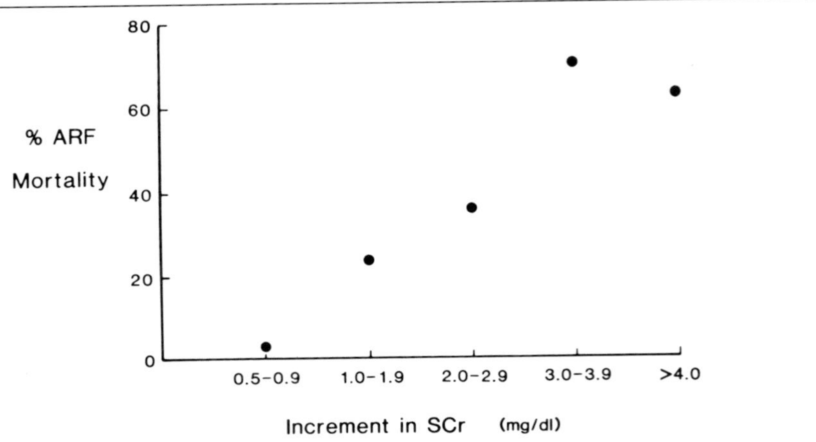

Fig. 48-5. Survival as a function of increment in serum creatine (SCr) in acute renal failure. (From [147].)

regression) to assess the impact of number and type of complications on the course of established ARF. In general, these analyses have shown somewhat similar results and the following general conclusions can be drawn: (1) Correctable pre- and postrenal forms of ARF have a better prognosis than ATN. (2) Patients in whom few or no clinical or biochemical complications develop during the course of ARF have a very favorable survival rate (> 90%). Unfortunately, these patients comprise fewer than 10 percent of all patients with ATN. (3) An inverse relationship exists between the number of organs that fail and the likelihood of survival with ARF. (4) The development of selected complications, such as respiratory failure, coma, cardiac failure, or sepsis, during the course of ARF portends a particularly bad outcome [239].

Bullock and collaborators [43] used a logistic regression analysis to examine prognostic factors in 462 patients with ATN who were seen during 7 years. Pulmonary complications (eightfold increased mortality), jaundice (four- to fivefold increased mortality), cardiovascular complications (three- to sixfold increased mortality), and hypercatabolism (twofold increased mortality) were the major identified risk factors.

Thus acute renal failure is a frequently encountered condition in many settings, with numerous associated complications and varied but high morbidity and mortality. The maximum effect of dialysis in this morbidity and mortality may already have been achieved. Consequently, future advances are awaited to provide a better understanding of the pathogenesis of the clinical entity acute tubular necrosis.

References

1. Abreo, K., Moorthy, A. V., and Osborne, M. Changing patterns and outcome of acute renal failure requiring hemodialysis. *Arch. Intern. Med.* 146: 1338, 1986.
2. Akmal, M., Goldstein, D. A., Telfer, N., et al. Resolution of muscle calcification in rhabdomyolysis and acute renal failure. *Ann. Intern. Med.* 89: 928, 1978.
3. Alexander, R. D., Berkes, S. L., and Abuleo, J. G. Contrast media-induced oliguric renal failure. *Arch. Intern. Med.* 138: 381, 1978.
4. Anderson, R. J. Radiocontrast nephrotoxicity. *West. J. Med.* 142: 685, 1985.
5. Anderson, R. J., and Gross, P. A. Acute Renal Failure and Toxic Nephropathy. In S. Klahr and S. G. Massry (eds.), *Contemporary Nephrology,* Vol. 1. New York: Plenum, 1981.
6. Anderson, R. J., Gross, P. A., and Gabow, P. Urinary chloride concentration in acute renal failure. *Miner. Electrolyte Metab.* 10: 92, 1984.
7. Anderson, R. J., Chung, H. M., Kluge, R., et al. Hyponatremia: A study of its incidence and pathogenetic role of vasopressin. *Ann. Intern. Med.* 102: 164, 1985.
8. Anderson, R. J., Linas, S. L., Berns, A. S., et al. Nonoliguric acute renal failure. *N. Engl. J. Med.* 296: 1134, 1977.
9. Ansari, E. R., Kazim, E., and Husain, I. Management of the choked ureter in obstructive renal failure due to uric acid lithiasis. *J. Urol.* 128: 257, 1981.
10. Anto, H. R., Chou, S. Y., Porush, J. G., et al. Infusion intravenous pyelography and renal function. Effect of hypertonic mannitol in patients with chronic renal insufficiency. *Arch. Intern. Med.* 141: 1652, 1981.
11. Arieff, A. I., and Carroll, H. J. Nonketotic hyperosmolar coma with hyperglycemia: Clinical features, pathophysiology, renal function, acid-base balance, plasma-cerebrospinal fluid equilibria and the effects of therapy in 37 cases. *Medicine* 51: 73, 1972.
12. Arieff, A. I., and Massry, S. G. Calcium metabolism of brain in acute renal failure. *J. Clin. Invest.* 53: 387, 1974.
13. Ault, B. H., Stapleton, F. B., Bager, L., et al. Acute renal failure during therapy with recombinant human gamma interferon. *N. Engl. J. Med.* 319: 1397, 1988.
14. Aurigemma, N. M., Feldman, N. T., Gottlieb, M., et al. Arterial oxygenation during hemodialysis. *N. Engl. J. Med.* 297: 871, 1977.
15. Babior, B. M. Villous adenoma of the colon. Study of a patient with severe fluid and electrolyte disturbances. *Am. J. Med.* 41: 615, 1966.
16. Badr, K. F., and Ichikawa, I. Prerenal failure: A deleterious shift from renal compensation to decompensation. *N. Engl. J. Med.* 319: 623, 1988.
17. Baek, S. M. Early prediction of acute renal failure and recovery: I. Sequential measurements of free water clearance. *Ann. Surg.* 177: 253, 1973.

18. Baek, S. M. Early prediction of acute renal failure and recovery: II. Renal function response to furosemide. *Ann. Surg.* 178: 604, 1973.
19. Baek, S. M., Makabali, G. G., and Shoemaker, W. C. Clinical determinants of survival from postoperative renal failure. *Surg. Gynecol. Obstet.* 140: 685, 1975.
20. Balslov, J. T., and Jorgensen, H. E. A survey of 499 patients with acute anuric renal insufficiency. Causes, treatment, complications, and mortality. *Am. J. Med.* 34: 75, 1963.
21. Banks, P. A., Sidi, S., and Gelman, M. L. Amylase-creatinine clearance ratios and serum amylase isoenzymes in moderate renal insufficiency. *J. Clin. Gastroenterol.* 1: 331, 1979.
22. Barton, C. H., Sterling, M. L., and Vaziri, N. D. Rhabdomyolysis and acute renal failure associated with phencyliden. *Arch. Intern. Med.* 140: 568, 1980.
23. Basten, A., and Opit, L. J. Severe sodium depletion with renal failure following common bile duct drainage. *Aust. N.Z. J. Surg.* 2: 105, 1966.
24. Baumelou, A., and Legrain, M. Medical nephrectomy with anti-inflammatory non-steroidal drugs. *Br. Med. J.* 1: 234, 1982.
25. Baxter, C. R., Zelditz, W. D., and Shires, G. T. High output acute renal failure complicating traumatic injury. *J. Trauma* 4: 567, 1964.
26. Beaman, M., Turney, J. H., Rodger, R. S., et al. Changing pattern of acute renal failure. *Q. J. Med.* 62: 15, 1987.
27. Beigelman, P. N. Severe diabetic ketoacidosis (diabetic "coma"). *Diabetes* 20: 490, 1971.
28. Beigelman, P. N., and Warner, N. E. Thirty-two fatal cases of severe diabetic ketoacidosis, including a case of mucormycosis. *Diabetes* 22: 847, 1973.
29. Bell, R. C., Coalson, J. J., Smith, J. D., et al. Multiple organ system failure and infection in adult respiratory distress syndrome. *Ann. Intern. Med.* 99: 293, 1983.
30. Berisa, F., Beaman, M., Adu, D., et al. Prognostic factors in acute renal failure following aortic aneurysm surgery. *Q. J. Med.* 76: 689, 1990.
31. Better, O. S., and Stein, J. H. Early management of shock and prophylaxis of acute renal failure in traumatic rhabdomyolysis. *N. Engl. J. Med.* 322: 825, 1990.
32. Bisivas, C. K., Milligan, D. A., Agte, S. D., et al. Acute renal failure and myopathy after epsilon aminocaproic acid. *Br. Med. J.* 281: 115, 1980.
33. Blachley, J. D., and Hill, J. B. Renal and electrolyte disturbances associated with cisplatin. *Ann. Intern. Med.* 95: 628, 1981.
34. Blackshear, J. L., Davidman, M., and Stillman, M. T. Identification of risk for renal insufficiency from nonsteroidal anti-inflammatory drugs. *Arch. Intern. Med.* 143: 1130, 1983.
35. Bleich, H. L., and Moore, M. J. Alcoholic myopathy in heart and skeletal muscle. *N. Engl. J. Med.* 301: 28, 1979.
36. Bluemle, L. W., Webster, G. D., and Elkinton, J. R. Acute tubular necrosis. *Arch. Intern. Med.* 104: 180, 1959.
37. Bohle, A., Christensen, J., Kokot, F., et al. Acute renal failure in man: New aspects concerning pathogenesis. *Am. J. Nephrol.* 10: 374, 1990.
38. Boswick, J. A., Jr., Thompson, J. D., and Kershner, C. J. Critical care of the burned patient. *Anesthesiology* 47: 164, 1977.
39. Boyd, R. E., Brennan, P. T., Deng, J. F., et al. Strychnine poisoning. *Am. J. Med.* 74: 507, 1983.
40. Boyer, T. D., Zia, P., and Reynolds, T. B. Effect of indomethacin and prostaglandin A_1 on renal function and plasma renin activity in alcoholic liver disease. *Gastroenterology* 77: 215, 1979.
41. Brown, R. Renal function in critically ill post-operative patients: Sequential assessment of creatinine osmolar and free water clearance. *Crit. Care Med.* 8: 68, 1980
42. Bull, G. M., Joekes, A. M., and Lowe, K. G. Renal function studies in acute tubular necrosis. *Clin. Sci.* 9: 379, 1950.
43. Bullock, M. L., Umen, A. J., Finkelstein, M., et al. The assessment of risk factors in 462 patients with acute renal failure. *Am. J. Kidney Dis.* 5(2): 97, 1985.
44. Bunning, R. D., and Barth, W. F. Sulindac. A potentially renal-sparing nonsteroidal anti-inflammatory drug. *J.A.M.A.* 248: 2864, 1982.
45. Burkett, E., and Anderson, R. J. Coexisting renal/respiratory failure: How to prevent and how to manage. *J. Crit. Illness* 6: 118, 1991.
46. Butler, W. T., Bennett, J. E., Alling, D. W., et al. Nephrotoxicity of amphotericin B. *Ann. Intern. Med.* 61: 175, 1964.
47. Byrd, L., and Sherman, R. L. Radiocontrast-induced acute renal failure: a clinical and pathophysiologic review. *Medicine* 58: 270, 1979.
48. Cadnapaphornchai, P., Dorfman, H., and McDonald, F. Differential Diagnosis of Acute Renal Failure. In H. Jacobson, G. Striker, and S. Klahr (eds.), *The Principles and Practice of Nephrology*. Philadelphia: Decker, 1991. P. 631.
49. Cadnapaphornchai, P., Taher, S., and McDonald, F. Acute drug-associated rhabdomyolysis. *Am. J. Med. Sci.* 280: 66, 1980.
50. Cameron, J. S. Disturbances of renal function in burnt patients. *Proc. R. Soc. Med.* 62: 49, 1969.
51. Cameron, J. S. Acute renal failure—the continuing challenge. *Q. J. Med.* 59: 337, 1986.
52. Cameron, J. S. Acute renal failure thirty years on. *Q. J. Med.* 74: 1, 1990.
53. Cameron, J. S., and Miller-Jones, C. M. H. Renal function and renal failure in badly burned children. *Br. J. Surg.* 54: 132, 1967.
54. Carpenter, C. C. J., Mitra, P. P., Sack, R. B., et al. Clinical studies in Asiatic cholera. III. Physiologic studies during treatment of the acute cholera patient: Comparison of lactate and bicarbonate in correction of acidosis; effects of potassium depletion. *Bull. Johns Hopkins Hosp.* 118: 197, 1966.
55. Carpenter, C. C. J., Mondal, A., Sack, R. B., et al. Clinical studies in Asiatic cholera. II. Development of 2:1 saline:lactate regimen. Comparison of this regimen with traditional methods of treatment, April and May, 1963. *Bull. Johns Hopkins Hosp.* 118: 174, 1966.
56. Cattell, W. R., McIntosh, C. S., Moseley, I. F., et al. Excretion urography in acute renal failure. *Br. Med. J.* 2: 275, 1973.
57. Charlson, M. E., MacKenzie, C. R., Gold, J. P., et al. Postoperative changes in serum creatinine. *Ann. Surg.* 209: 328, 1989.
58. Chrysant, S. G., Dunn, M., Marples, D., et al. Severe reversible azotemia from captopril therapy. *Arch. Intern. Med.* 143: 437, 1983.
59. Ciabattoni, G., Cinotti, G. A., Pierucci, A., et al. Effects of sulindac and ibuprofen in patients with chronic glomerular disease. *N. Engl. J. Med.* 310: 279, 1984.
60. Clark, A. S., and Mitch, W. E. Muscle protein turnover and glucose uptake in acutely uremic rats. *J. Clin. Invest.* 72: 836, 1983.
61. Cohen, A. H., Nost, C. C., Adler, S. G., et al. Clinical

utility of kidney biopsies in the diagnosis and management of renal disease. *Am. J. Nephrol.* 9: 309, 1989.
62. Colavita, R. D., Gaudio, K. M., and Siegel, N. J. Reversible reduction in renal function during treatment with captopril. *Pediatrics* 71: 839, 1983.
63. Collins, R., and Langman, M. Treatment with histamine H_2 antagonists in acute upper gastrointestinal hemorrhage. *N. Engl. J. Med.* 313: 660, 1985.
64. Conger, J. D., and Falk, S. A. Intrarenal dynamics in the pathogenesis and prevention of acute urate nephropathy. *J. Clin. Invest.* 59: 786, 1977.
65. Conger, J. D., Robinette, J. B., and Schrier, R. W. Smooth muscle calcium and endothelium-derived relaxing factor in the abnormal vascular response of acute renal failure. *J. Clin. Invest.* 82: 532, 1988.
66. Conger, J. D., Falk, S. A., Guggenheim, S. J., et al. A micropuncture study of the early phase of acute urate nephropathy. *J. Clin. Invest.* 58: 681, 1976.
67. Cooper, J. D., Lazarowitz, V. C., and Arieff, A. I. Neurodiagnostic abnormalities in patients with acute renal failure. *J. Clin. Invest.* 61: 1448, 1978.
68. Corwin, H. L., et al. Low FE_{Na} occurrence with hemoglobinuria and myoglobinuria. *Arch. Intern. Med.* 144: 981, 1984.
69. Corwin, H., Sprague, S. M., Deharia, G. A., et al. Acute renal failure associated with cardiac operations. *J. Thorac. Cardiovasc. Surg.* 98: 1107, 1989.
70. Corwin, H. L., Teplick, R. S., Schreiber, M. J., et al. Prediction of outcome in acute renal failure. *Am. J. Nephrol.* 7: 8, 1987.
71. Cosio, F. G., Zager, R. A., and Sharma, H. M. Atheroembolic renal disease causes hypocomplementemia. *Lancet* 2: 118, 1985.
72. Coulie, P., DePlaen, J. F., and van Ypersele de Strihou, C. Captopril-induced acute reversible renal failure. *Nephron* 35: 108, 1983.
73. Craddock, P. R., Fehr, J., Brigham, K. L., et al. Complement and leukocyte-mediated pulmonary dysfunction in hemodialysis. *N. Engl. J. Med.* 296: 769, 1977.
74. Crandell, W. B., Pappas, S. G., and MacDonald, A. Nephrotoxicity associated with methoxyflurance anesthesia. *Anesthesiology* 27: 591, 1966.
75. Crosbie, W. A., and Parsons, V. Cardiopulmonary responses to acute renal failure. *Kidney Int.* 9: 380, 1976.
76. Cunningham, E., Kohli, R., and Venuto, R. C. Influenza-associated myoglobinuric renal failure. *J.A.M.A.* 242: 2428, 1979.
77. Cunningham, R. J., Gilroil, M., Cowall, T., et al. Rapidly progressive glomerulonephritis in children: A report of thirteen cases and a review of the literature. *Pediatr. Res.* 14: 128, 1980.
78. Curry, N. S., Gobien, R. P., and Schabel, S. I. Minimal-dilatation obstructive nephropathy. *Radiology* 143: 531, 1982.
79. Curtis, J. J., Luke, R. G., Whelchel, J. D., et al. Inhibition of angiotensin-converting enzyme in renal-transplant recipients with hypertension. *N. Engl. J. Med.* 308: 377, 1983.
80. Danovitch, G., Carvounis, C., Weinstein E., et al. Nonoliguric acute renal failure. *Israel J. Med. Sci.* 15: 5, 1979.
81. Danziger, L. H., and Horn, J. R. Disopyramide-induced urinary retention. *Arch. Intern. Med.* 143: 1683, 1983.
82. Dash, H., Little, J. R., Zaino, R., et al. Metastatic periosteal osteosarcoma causing cardiac and renal failure. *Am. J. Med.* 75: 145, 1983.
83. Davenport, A., and Roberts, N. B. Accumulation of aluminum in patients with acute renal failure. *Nephron* 52: 253, 1989.
84. Delans, R. J., Ramirez, G., Farber, M. S., et al. Renal artery thrombosis: A cause of reversible acute renal failure. *J. Urol.* 128: 1287, 1982.
85. D'Elia, F. L., Brennan, R. E., and Brownstein, P. K. Acute renal failure secondary to ureteral obstruction by a gravid uterus. *J. Urol.* 128: 803, 1982.
86. D'Elia, J., Gleason, R. E., Alday, M., et al. Nephrotoxicity from angiographic contrast material. *Am. J. Med.* 72: 719, 1982.
87. Dentino, M., Luft, F. C., Yum, M. N., et al. Long-term effect of cis-diamminedichloride plantinum (CDDP) on renal function and structure in man. *Cancer* 41: 1274, 1978.
88. DeRay, G., Martinez, R., Kattama, C., et al. Foscarnet nephrotoxicity: Mechanism, incidence and prevention. *Am. J. Nephrol.* 9: 316, 1989.
89. de Torrente, A., Berl, T., Cohn, P. D., et al. Hypercalcemia of acute renal failure. *Am. J. Med.* 61: 119, 1976.
90. Diamond, J. R., and Yoburn, D. C. Nonoliguric acute renal failure associated with a low fractional excretion of sodium. *Ann. Intern. Med.* 96: 596, 1982.
91. Diamond, J. R., Cheung, J. Y., and Fang, L. S. Nifedipine-induced renal dysfunction. Alterations in renal hemodynamics. *Am. J. Med.* 77: 905, 1984.
92. Ditlove, J., Weidmann, P., Bernstein, M., et al. Methicillin nephritis. *Medicine* 56: 483, 1977.
93. Dixon, B. S., and Anderson, R. J. Nonoliguric acute renal failure. *Am. J. Kidney Dis.* 6: 71, 1985.
94. Dorfman, H. R., Sondheimer, J. H., and Cadnapaphornchai, P. Mannitol-induced acute renal failure. *Medicine* 69: 153, 1990.
95. Edwards, R. M. Segmental effects of norepinephrine and angiotensin II on isolated renal microvessels. *Am. J. Physiol.* 244: 526, 1983.
96. Eiser, A. R., Neff, M. S., and Slifkin, R. F. Acute myoglobinuric renal failure. A consequence of the neuroleptic malignant syndrome. *Arch. Intern. Med.* 142: 601, 1982.
97. Eliahou, H. E., Bata, A. The diagnosis of acute renal failure. *Nephron* 2: 287, 1965.
98. Ellis, E. N., and Arnold, W. C. Renal failure secondary to bilateral ureteric obstruction: review of 50 cases. *Can. Med. Assoc. J.* 127: 601, 1982.
99. Eneas, F., Schoenfeld, P. Y., and Humphreys, M. H. The effect of infusion of mannitol-sodium bicarbonate in the clinical course of myoglobinuria. *Arch. Intern. Med.* 139: 801, 1979.
100. Espinel, C. H. The FE_{Na} test use in the differential diagnosis of acute renal failure. *J.A.M.A.* 236: 579, 1976.
101. Espinel, C. H., and Gregory, A. W. Differential diagnosis of acute renal failure. *Clin. Nephrol* 13: 73, 1980.
102. Fang, L. S., Sirot, R. A., and Ebert, T. H. Low fractional excretion of sodium with contrast-media induced acute renal failure. *Arch. Intern. Med.* 140: 531, 1980.
103. Farese, R. V., Schambelan, M., Hollander, H., et al. Nephrogenic diabetes insipidus associated with foscarnet treatment of cytomegalovirus retinitis. *Ann. Intern. Med.* 112: 955, 1990.
104. Farley, K. F., Woo, K. T., Birch, D. F., et al. Triamterene-induced crystalluria and cylindruria: Clinical and experimental studies. *Clin. Nephrol.* 26: 169, 1986.
105. Feinstein, E. I., Akmal, M., Goldstein, D. A., et al. Hypercalcemia and acute widespread calcifications during the oliguric phase of acute renal failure due to rhabdomyolysis. *Miner. Electrolyte Metab.* 2: 193, 1979.

106. Figueroa, J. E. Acute renal failure: Its unusual causes and manifestations. *Med. Clin. North Am.* 51: 995, 1967.
107. Finn, W. F. Recovery from Acute Renal Failure. In B. M. Brenner and J. M. Lazarus (eds.), *Acute Renal Failure*. Philadelphia: Saunders, 1983. P. 753.
108. Fisher, R. P., Griffen, W. O., Resiser, M., et al. Early dialysis in the treatment of acute renal failure. *Surg. Gynecol. Obstet.* 123: 1019, 1966.
109. Flamenbaum, W., Gehr, M., Gross, M., et al. Renal Failure with Myoglobinuria and Hemoglobinuria. In B. M. Brenner, and J. M. Lazarus (eds.), *Acute Renal Failure*. Philadelphia: Saunders, 1983. P. 269.
110. Fong, H. J., and Cohen, A. H. Ibuprofen-induced acute renal failure with acute tubular necrosis. *Am. J. Nephrol.* 2: 28, 1982.
111. Fotino, S., and Spron, P. Nonoliguric acute renal failure after captopril therapy. *Arch. Intern. Med.* 143: 1252, 1983.
112. Frankel, M. C., Weinstein, A. M., and Stenzel, K. H. Prognostic patterns in acute renal failure: The New York Hospital, 1981–1982. *Clin. Exper. Dialysis Apheresis* 7 (1&2): 145, 1983.
113. Freston, J. W. Cimetidine. II. Adverse reactions and patterns of use. *Ann. Intern. Med.* 97: 728, 1982.
114. Furey, A. T. Hyponatremia after choledochostomy and T tube drainage. *Am. J. Surg.* 112: 850, 1966.
115. Fushimi, K., Schichiri, M., and Marumo, F. Decreased fractional excretion of urate as an indicator of prerenal azotemia. *Am. J. Nephrol.* 10: 489, 1990.
116. Fuss, M., Bagon, J., Dupont, E., et al. Parathyroid hormone and calcium blood levels in acute renal failure. *Nephron* 20: 196, 1978.
117. Gabow, P. A., Kaehny, W. D., and Kelleher, S. P. The spectrum of rhabdomyolysis. *Medicine* 61: 141, 1982.
118. Galpin, J. E., Shinaberger, J. H., Stanley, T. M., et al. Acute interstitial nephritis due to methicillin. *Am. J. Med.* 65: 756, 1978.
119. Gant, N. F. Non-oliguric renal failure—report of a case. *Obstet. Gynecol.* 34: 675, 1969.
120. Gellman, D. D. The renal complications of burns. *Can. Med. Assoc. J.* 97: 440, 1967.
121. Goldstein, D. A., and Massry, S. G. Effect of parathyroid hormone administration and its withdrawal on brain calcium and electroencephalogram. *Miner. Electrolyte Metab.* 2: 84, 1978a.
122. Goldstein, D. A., Chui, L. A., and Massry, S. G. Effect of parathyroid hormone and uremia on peripheral nerve calcium and motor nerve conduction velocity. *J. Clin. Invest.* 62: 88, 1978b.
123. Goodpastor, W. E., Levenson, S. M., and Tagnon, H. G. A clinical and pathologic study of the kidney in patients with thermal burns. *Surg. Gynecol. Obstet.* 82: 652, 1946.
124. Gornick, C. C., Jr., and Kjellstrand, C. M. Acute renal failure complicating aortic aneurysm surgery. *Nephron* 35: 145, 1983.
125. Graham, J. R., Suby, H. I., LeCompte, P. R., et al. Fibrotic disorders associated with methysergide therapy for headache. *N. Engl. J. Med.* 274: 359, 1966.
126. Graziani, G., Cantaluppi, A., and Casati, S. Dopamine and furosemide in oliguric acute renal failure. *Nephron* 37: 39, 1984.
127. Gross, P. A., and Anderson, R. J. Acute Renal Failure and Toxic Nephropathy. In S. Klahr and S. G. Massry (eds.), *Contemporary Nephrology*, Vol 2. New York: Plenum, 1983. P. 501.
128. Gross, P. A., and Anderson, R. J. Acute Renal Failure and Toxic Nephropathy. In S. Klahr and S. G. Massry (eds.), *Contemporary Nephrology*, Vol. 3. New York: Plenum, 1986.
129. Grossman, R. A., Hamilton, R. W., Morse, B. M., et al. Nontraumatic rhabdomyolysis and acute renal failure. *N. Engl. J. Med.* 291: 807, 1974.
130. Grundy, D. J., Rainford, D. J., and Silver, J. R. The occurrence of acute renal failure in patients with neuropathic bladders. *Paraplegia* 20: 35, 1982.
131. Halmos, P. B., Nelson, J. K., and Lowry, R. C. Hyperosmolar nonketoacidotic coma in diabetes. *Lancet* 1: 675, 1966.
132. Handa, S. P. Diagnostic indices in acute renal failure. *Can. Med. Assoc. J.* 96: 78, 1967.
133. Hansky, J. Effect of renal failure on gastrointestinal hormones. *World J. Surg.* 3: 463, 1979.
134. Hayes, D. M., Cvitkovic, E., Golbey, R. B. High dose cisplatinum diammine dichloride. Amelioration of renal toxicity by mannitol diuresis. *Cancer* 39: 1372, 1977.
135. Hays, R., Aquino, A., Lee, B. B., et al. Captopril-induced acute renal failure in a kidney transplant recipient. *Clin. Nephrol.* 19: 320, 1983.
136. Helzlsouer, K. J., Hayden, F. G., and Rogol, A. D. Severe metabolic complications in a cross-counter runner with sickle cell trait. *J.A.M.A.* 249: 777, 1983.
137. Henrich, W. L., Pettinger, W. A., and Cronin, R. E. The influence of circulating catecholamines and prostaglandins in canine renal hemodynamics during hemorrhage. *Circ. Res.* 48: 424, 1981.
138. Henrich, W. L., Anderson, R. J., Berns, A. S., et al. The role of renal nerves and prostaglandins in control of renal hemodynamics and plasma renin activity during hypotensive hemorrhage in the dog. *J. Clin. Invest.* 61: 744, 1978.
139. Henrich, W. L., Berl, T., McDonald, K. M., et al. Angiotensin II, renal nerves, and prostaglandins in renal hemodynamics during hemorrhage. *Am. J. Physiol.* 235(1): F46, 1978.
140. Hesdorffer, C. S., Milne, J. J., Meyers, A. M. et al. The value of Swan-Ganz catheterization and volume loading in preventing renal failure in patients undergoing abdominal aortic aneurysmectomy. *Clin. Nephrol.* 28: 272, 1987.
141. Hilton, P. J. Urinary osmolality in acute renal failure due to glomerulonephritis. *Lancet* 2: 655, 1969.
142. Hinglais, N., Garcia-Torres, and Kleinknecht, D. Long-term prognosis in acute glomerulonephritis. *Am. J. Med.* 56: 52, 1974.
143. Hoffman, L. M., and Suki, W. N. Obstructive uropathy mimicking volume depletion. *J.A.M.A.* 236: 2096, 1976.
144. Horgan, K. J., Ottaviano, Y. L., and Watson, A. J. Acute renal failure due to mannitol intoxication. *Am. J. Nephrol.* 9: 106, 1989.
145. Horl, W. H., and Heidland, A. Enhanced proteolytic activity. Cause of protein catabolism in acute renal failure. *Am. J. Clin. Nutr.* 33: 1423, 1980.
146. Horl, W. H., Gantert, C., Auer, I. O., et al. In vitro inhibition of protein catabolism by alpha$_2$-macroglobulin in plasma from a patient with post-traumatic acute renal failure. *Am. J. Nephrol.* 2: 32, 1982.
147. Hou, S. H., Bushinsky, D. A., Wish, J. B., et al. Hospital-acquired renal insufficiency: A prospective study. *Am. J. Med.* 74: 243, 1983.
148. Howell, S. B., and Carmody, J. Changes in glomerular filtration rate associated in high dose methohexate in adults. *Cancer Treat. Rep.* 61: 1389, 1977.
149. Hricik, D. E., and Dunn, M. J. Angiotensin-converting enzyme inhibitor–induced acute renal failure: Causes,

consequences and diagnostic uses. *J. Am. Soc. Nephrol.* 1: 845, 1990.
150. Hricik, D. E., Browning, P. J., Kopelman, R., et al. Captopril-induced functional renal insufficiency in patients with bilateral renal-artery stenosis or renal artery stenosis in a solitary kidney. *N. Engl. J. Med.* 308: 373, 1983.
151. Hussy, J. L., and Belzer, F. O. Cimetidine in renal transplant recipients. *Lancet* 1: 1089, 1979.
152. Imrie, C. W., and Whyte, A. S. A prospective study of acute pancreatitis. *Br. J. Surg.* 62: 490, 1975.
153. Ireland, G. W., and Cass, A. S. The recognition and management of acute high output renal failure. *J. Urol.* 108: 40, 1972.
154. Iseri, L. T., Batchelor, T. M., Boyle, A. J. Studies of fluid, electrolyte, and nitrogen balance in acute renal insufficiency. *Arch. Intern. Med.* 89: 188, 1952.
155. Jacobs, M. L., Daggett, W. M., and Ciretta, J. M. Acute pancreatitis: Analysis of factors influencing survival. *Ann. Surg.* 185: 43, 1977.
156. Jennings, A. E., Levey, A. S., and Harrington, J. T. Amoxapine-associated acute renal failure. *Arch. Intern. Med.* 143: 1525, 1983.
157. Jochimsen, F., Schafer, J. H., Maurer, A., and Distler, A. Impairment of renal function in medical intensive care: Predictability of acute renal failure. *Crit. Care Med.* 18: 480, 1990.
158. Johnson, M. W., Mitch, W. E., Heller, A. H., et al. The impact of an educational program on gentamicin use in a teaching hospital. *Am. J. Med.* 73: 9, 1982.
159. Johnston, P. A., Perrin, N. S., Bernard, D. B., et al. Control of rat renal vascular resistance at reduced renal perfusion pressure. *Circ. Res.* 48: 734, 1981.
160. Jones, D. B. Ultrastructure of human acute renal failure. *Lab. Invest.* 46: 254, 1982.
161. Jones, L. W., and Weil, M. H. Water, creatinine and sodium excretion following circulatory shock with renal failure. *Am. J. Med.* 51: 314, 1971.
162. Jones, R. H., Rudge, C. J., Bewick, M., et al. Cimetidine: Prophylaxis against upper gastrointestinal haemorrhage after renal transplantation. *Br. Med. J.* 1: 398, 1978.
163. Kalish, S. B., Tallman, M. S., Cook, F. V., et al. Polymicrobial septicemia associated with rhabdomyolysis, myoglobinuria, and acute renal failure. *Arch. Intern. Med.* 142: 133, 1982.
164. Kaptein, E. M., Levitan, D., Feinstein, E. I., et al. Alterations of thyroid hormone indices in acute renal failure and in acute critical illness with and without acute renal failure. *Am. J. Nephrol.* 1: 138, 1981.
165. Karatson, A., Johasz, J., and Hubler, J. Factors influencing the prognoses of acute renal failure (analysis of 228 cases). *Int. Urol. Nephrol.* 10: 321, 1978.
166. Kawamura, J., Okada, Y., Nishibuchi, S., et al. Transient anuria following administration of angiotensin I-converting enzyme inhibitor (SQ 14225) in a patient with renal artery stenosis of the solitary kidney successfully treated with renal autotransplantation. *J. Urol.* 127: 111, 1982.
167. Keidar, S., Kohan, R., Levy, J., et al. Non-oliguric acute renal failure after treatment with sulfinpyrazone. *Clin. Nephrol.* 17: 266, 1982.
168. Kelleher, S. P., and Berl, T. In B. M. Brenner, and J. M. Lazarus (eds.) *Acute Renal Failure.* Philadelphia: Saunders, 1983. P. 223
169. Kelleher, S. P., Robinette, J. B., and Conger, J. D. Sympathetic nervous system in the loss of autoregulation in acute renal failure. *Am. J. Physiol.* 246: F379, 1984.
170. Kelsen, D., Hilaris, B., Coonley, C., et al. Cisplatin, vindesine, and bleomycin chemotherapy of local-regional and advanced esophageal carcinoma. *Am. J. Med.* 75: 645, 1983.
171. Kelton, J., Kelley, W. N., and Holmes, E. W. A rapid method for the diagnosis of acute uric acid nephropathy. *Arch. Intern. Med.* 138: 612, 1978.
172. Kennedy, A. C., Burton, J. A., and Luke, R. G. Factors affecting the prognosis in acute renal failure. *J. Med.* 42: 73, 1973.
173. Kiley, J. E., Powers, S. R., and Beebe, R. T. Acute renal failure. Eighty cases of renal tubular necrosis. *N. Engl. J. Med.* 262, 481, 1960.
174. Kim, V., Kark, A. E., and Rudick, J. Factors influencing mortality in surgical treatment for massive gastroduodenal hemorrhage. *Am. J. Gastrointerol.* 62: 24, 1974.
175. Kimberly, R. P., Gill, J. R., and Bowden, R. E. Elevated urinary prostaglandin and the effect of aspirin on renal function in lupus erythematosus. *Ann. Intern. Med.* 89: 336, 1978.
176. Kjellstrand, C. M., Campbell, D. P., and Von Hartitzsch, B. Hyperuricemic acute renal failure. *Arch. Intern. Med.* 133: 347, 1974.
177. Kjellstrand, C. M., Ebben, J., and Davin, T. Time of death, recovery of renal function, development of chronic renal failure and need for chronic hemodialysis in patients with acute tubular necrosis. *Trans. Am. Soc. Artif. Intern. Organs* 27: 45, 1981.
178. Klahr, S. Renal failure after jejunoileal bypass for obesity. *Am. J. Med.* 69: 628, 1979.
179. Kleinknecht, D., and Ganeval, D. Preventive Hemodialysis in Acute Renal Failure: Its Effects on Mortality and Morbidity. In E. A. Friedman, and H. E. Eliahou (eds.), *Proceedings of the Conference on Acute Renal Failure,* DHEW Publ. No. (NIH) 74-608. Washington, D.C.: 1973. P. 165.
180. Klingbeil, T., Gise, H. V., and Bohle, A. Morphometric studies on acute renal failure in humans during the oligoanuric and polyuric phases. *Clin. Nephrol.* 20: 1, 1983.
181. Klintman, G. B. G., Iwatsuki, S., and Starzl, T. E. Nephrotoxicity of cyclosporin A in liver and kidney transplant patients. *Lancet* 1: 470, 1981.
182. Knaus, W. A., Draper, E. A., Wagner, D. R., et al. APACHE II: A severity of disease classification system. *Crit. Care Med.* 13: 818, 1985.
183. Knochel, J. P. Biochemical, Electrolyte, and Acid-Base Disturbances in Acute Renal Failure. In B. M. Brenner, and J. M. Lazarus (eds.), *Acute Renal Failure.* Philadelphia: Saunders, 1983. P. 568.
184. Koffler, A., Friedler, R. M., and Massry, S .G. Acute renal failure due to nontraumatic rhabdomyolysis. *Ann. Intern. Med.* 85: 23, 1976.
185. Kokot, F., and Kuska, J. The endocrine system in patients with acute renal insufficiency. *Kidney Int.* 10: S26, 1976.
186. Kovach, J. S., Moertel, C. G., Schutt, A. J., et al. Phase II of study of cis-diamminedichloroplatinum (NSC)-119875) in advanced carcinoma of the large bowel. *Canc. Chemother. Rep.* Part 1 57(3): 357, 1973.
187. Kovithavongs, T., Becker, F. O., and Ing. T. S. Parathyroid hyperfunction in acute renal failure. *Nephron* 9: 349, 1972.
188. Kraman, S., Khan, F., Patel, S., et al. Renal failure in the respiratory intensive care unit. *Crit. Care Med.* 7: 263, 1979.
189. Krug, H., Raszeja-Wanic, B., and Wochowiak, A. Intra-

vascular coagulation in acute renal failure after myocardial infarction. *Ann. Intern. Med.* 81: 494, 1974.
190. Kumar, R., Hill, C. M., and McGeown, M. G. Acute renal failure in the elderly. *Lancet* 1: 90, 1973.
191. Lam, M., and Kaufman, C. E. Fractional excretion of sodium as a guide to volume depletion during recovery from acute renal failure. *Am J. Kidney Dis.* 6: 18, 1985.
192. Lee, H. Y., Stretton, T. B., and Barnes, A. M. The lungs in renal failure. *Thorax* 30: 46, 1975.
193. Lemieux, G., Cuvelier, A. A., and Lefebvre, R. The clinical spectrum of renal insufficiency during acute glomerulonephritis in the adult. *Can. Med. Assoc. J.* 96: 1129, 1967.
194. Lennhoff, M., and Herrera, J. Acute renal failure in diabetic acidosis (letter). *Lancet* 1: 758, 1968.
195. Leonard, C. D., Nagle, R. B., and Striker, G. E. Acute glomerulonephritis with prolonged oliguria. *Ann. Intern. Med.* 73: 703, 1970.
196. Levine, J. A. Heat stroke in the aged. *Am. J. Med.* 47: 251, 1969.
197. Levitan, D., Massry, S. G., Romoff, M. S., and Campese, V. M. Autonomic nervous system dysfunction in patients with acute renal failure. *Am. J. Nephrol.* 2: 213, 1982.
198. Levitan, D., Moser, S. A., Goldstein, D. A., et al. Disturbances in the hypothalamic-pituitary-gonadal axis in male patients with acute renal failure. *Am. J. Nephrol.* 4: 99, 1984.
199. Lewis, E. J., Cavallo, T., Harrington, J. T., et al. An immunopathologic study of rapidly progressive glomerulonephritis in the adult. *Human Pathol.* 2: 185, 1971.
200. Lewy, J. E., Salina-Madrigal, L., Herdson, P. B., et al. Clinico-pathologic correlations in acute poststreptococcal glomerulonephritis. *Medicine* 50: 453, 1971.
201. Liano, F., Garcia-Martin, F., Gallego, A., et al. Easy and early prognosis in acute tubular necrosis: A forward analysis of 228 cases. *Nephron* 51: 307, 1989.
202. Lifschitz, M. D. Renal effects of nonsteroidal anti-inflammatory agents. *Lab. Clin. Med.* 102: 313, 1983.
203. Lijnen, P., Boelaert, J., van Eeghem, P., et al. Decrease in renal function due to sulphinpyrazine treatment early after myocardial infarction. *Clin. Nephrol.* 19: 143, 1983.
204. Lins, R. L., Verpoaten, G. A., DeClerck, D. S., et al. Urinary indices in acute interstitial nephritis. *Clin. Nephrol.* 26: 131, 1986.
205. Linton, A. L., Clark, W. F., Driedger, A. A., et al. Acute interstitial nephritis due to drugs. *Ann. Intern. Med.* 93: 735, 1980.
206. Lisker, W. H. Nonoliguric renal failure associated with zomepirac. *J.A.M.A.* 249: 1706, 1983.
207. Liu, E. T., Bristow, M. R., Stone, M. J., et al. Serum myoglobin, ionized calcium, and parathyroid function during rhabdomyolysis. *Arch. Intern. Med.* 143: 154, 1983.
208. Llach, F., Felsenfeld, A. J., and Haussler, M. R. Pathophysiology of altered calcium metabolism in rhabdomyolysis-induced acute failure. *N. Engl. J. Med.* 305: 117, 1981.
209. Lohr, J. W., McFarlane, M. J., and Grantham, J. J. A clinical index to predict survival in acute renal failure patients requiring dialysis. *Am. J. Kidney Dis.* 11: 254, 1988.
210. Lordon, R. E., and Burton, J. R. Post-traumatic renal failure in military personnel in Southeast Asia. *Am. J. Med.* 53: 137, 1972.
211. Luke, R. G., Briggs, J. D., and Allison, M. I. Factors determining response to mannitol in acute renal failure. *Am. J. Med. Sci.* 259: 166, 1970.
212. Lunding, M., Steiness, I. B., and Thaysen, J. H. Acute renal failure due to tubular necrosis. *Acta Med. Scand.* 176: 103, 1964.
213. Madias, N. E., and Harrington, J. T. Platinum nephrotoxicity. *Am. J. Med.* 65: 307, 1978.
214. Madias, N. E., and Harrington, J. T. Postischemic Acute Renal Failure. In B. M. Brenner, and J. M. Lazarus (eds.), *Acute Renal Failure*. Philadelphia: Saunders, 1983. P. 235.
215. Madias, N. E., Kwon, O. J., and Millan V. G. Percutaneous transluminal renal angioplasty. *Ann. Intern. Med.* 142: 693, 1982.
216. Maher, E. R., Robinson, K. N., Scoble, J. E., et al. Prognosis of critically ill patients with acute renal failure: APACHE II score and other predictive factors. *Q. J. Med.* 72: 857, 1989.
217. Maier, M., Stailinger, J., Wagner, M., et al. The effect of hemorrhagic hypotension on urinary kallikrein excretion, renin activity and renal cortical blood flow in the pig. *Cir. Res.* 48: 386, 1981.
218. Maillet, P. J., Pelle-Francoz, D., Laville, M., et al. Nondilated obstructive acute renal failure: Diagnostic procedures and therapeutic management. *Radiology* 160: 659, 1986.
219. Malhotra, M. S., Sharma, B. K., and Sivaraman, R. Requirements of sodium chloride during summer in the tropics. *J. Appl. Physiol.* 14: 823, 1959.
220. Mandal, A. K. Transmission electron microscopy of urinary sediment in renal disease. *Semin. Nephrol.* 6: 346, 1986.
221. Mandal, A. K., Sklar, A. H., and Hudson, J. B. Transmission electron microscopy of urinary sediment in human acute renal failure. *Kidney Int.* 28: 58, 1985.
222. Mandell, I., Krauss, E., and Millan, J. C. Oxalate-induced acute renal failure in Crohn's disease. *Am. J. Med.* 69: 628, 1980.
223. Mant, M. J., and King, E. G. Severe acute disseminated intravascular coagulation. *Am. J. Med.* 67: 557, 1979.
224. Martinez-Maldonado, M., Benobe, J., and Lopez-Nova, J. M. Acute Renal Failure Associated with Tubulointestitial Disease Including Papillary Necrosis. In B. M. Brenner, and J. M. Lazarus (eds.), *Acute Renal Failure*. Philadelphia: Saunders, 1983. P. 434.
225. Massry, S. G., Arieff, A. I., Coburn, J. W., et al. Divalent ion metabolism in patients with acute renal failure: Studies on the mechanism of hypocalcemia. *Kidney Int.* 5: 437, 1974.
226. Massry, S. G., Coburn, J. W., Lee, D. E. N., et al. Skeletal resistance to parathyroid hormone in renal failure: Studies of 105 human subjects. *Ann. Intern. Med.* 78: 357, 1973.
227. Massry, S. G., Dua, S., Garty, J., et al. Role of uremia in the skeletal resistance to the calcemic action of parathyroid hormone. *Miner. Eletrolyte Metab.* 1: 172, 1978.
228. Massry, S. G., Stein, R., Garty, J., et al. Skeletal resistance to the calcemic action of parathyroid hormone in uremia: Role of $1,25(OH)_2D_3$. *Kidney Int.* 9: 467, 1976.
229. Massry, S. G., Tuma, S., Dua, S., et al. Reversal of skeletal resistance to parathyroid hormone in uremia by vitamin D metabolites. *J. Lab. Clin. Med.* 94: 152, 1979.
230. Matzke, G. R., Lucarotti, R. L., and Shapiro, H. S. Controlled comparison of gentamicin and tobramycin nephrotoxicity. *Am. J. Nephrol.* 3: 11, 1983.
231. McCarthy, J. T., Shwartz, G. L., Blair, T. J., et al. Reversible nonoliguric acute renal failure associated with zomepirc therapy. *Mayo Clin. Proc.* 57: 351, 1982.

232. McCarthy, J. T., Torres, V. E., Romero, J. C., et al. Acute intrinsic renal failure induced by indomethacin. *Mayo Clin. Proc.* 57: 289, 1982.
233. McDonald, B. R., Kirmani, S., Vasquez, M., et al. Acute renal failure associated with the use of intraperitoneal carboplatin: A report of two cases and review of the literature. *Am. J. Med.* 90: 386, 1991.
234. McDougall, B. R., Baely, R. J., and Williams, R. H_2-receptor antagonists and antacids in the prevention of acute gastrointestinal hemorrhage in fulminant hepatic failure. *Lancet* 1: 616, 1977.
235. McInnes, E. G., Levy, D. W., Chaudhuri, M. D., et al. Renal failure in the elderly. *Q. J. Med.* 64: 583, 1987.
236. McLeish, K. R., Yum, M. N., and Luft, F. C. Rapidly progressive glomerulonephritis in adults: Clinical and histologic correlations. *Clin. Nephrol.* 10: 43, 1978.
237. McMurray, S. D., Luft, F. C., Maxwell, D. R., et al. Prevailing patterns and predictor variables in patients with acute tubular necrosis. *Arch. Intern. Med.* 138: 950, 1978.
238. McPhaul, J. J. Jr. Acute glomerular disease presenting as acute renal failure. *Semin. Nephrol.* 1: 21, 1981.
239. Mehler, P. S., Schrier, R. W., and Anderson, R. J. Clinical Presentation, Complications and Prognosis of Acute Renal Failure. In H. Jacobson, G. Striker, and S. Klahr (eds.), *The Principles and Practice of Nephrology.* Philadelphia: Decker, 1991. P. 660.
240. Meijer, S., Sleijfer, D. T., Mulder, N. H., et al. Some effects of combination chemotherapy with cis-platinum on renal function in patients with nonseminomotous testicular carcinoma. *Cancer* 51: 2035, 1983.
241. Melamed, I., Romem, Y., Keren, G., et al. March myoglobinemia. *Arch. Intern. Med.* 142: 1277, 1982.
242. Menashe, P. I., Ross, S. A., and Tottlieb, J. E. Acquired renal insufficiency in critically ill patients. *Crit. Care Med.* 16: 1106, 1988.
243. Meroney, W. H., Arney, G. K., and Segr, W. E. The acute calcification of damaged muscle, with particular reference to acute post-traumatic renal insufficiency. *J. Clin. Invest.* 36: 825, 1957.
244. Meroney, W. N., and Rubini, M. E. Kidney function during acute tubular necrosis: Clinical studies and therapy. *Metabolism* 8: 1, 1959.
245. Miller, P. D., Krebs, R. A., Neal, B. J., et al. Polyuric prerenal failure. *Arch. Intern. Med.* 140: 907, 1980.
246. Miller, F. C., Schorr, W. J., and Lacher, J. W. Zomepirac-induced renal failure. *Arch. Intern. Med.* 143: 1171, 1983.
247. Miller, T. R., Anderson, R. J., Berns, A. S., et al. Urinary diagnostic indices in acute renal failure. A prospective study. *Ann. Intern. Med.* 88: 47, 1978.
248. Minuth, A. N., Terrell, J. B., and Suki, W. N. Acute renal failure: A study of the course and prognosis of 104 patients and of the role of furosemide. *Am. J. Med. Sci.* 271: 317, 1976.
249. Misson, R. T., and Cutter, R. E. Radiocontrast-induced renal failure. *Western J. Med.* 142: 657, 1985.
250. Mitch, W. E., and Walker, W. G. Plasma renin and angiotensin II in acute renal failure. *Lancet* 1: 328, 1977.
251. Molitch, M. E., Rodman, E., Hirsch, C. A., et al. Spurious serum creatinine elevations in ketoacidosis. *Ann. Intern. Med.* 93: 280, 1980.
252. Mondon, C. E., Dolkas, C. B., and Reaven, G. M. The site of insulin resistance in acute uremia. *Diabetes* 27: 571, 1978.
253. Moran, M., and Kapsner, C. Acute renal failure associated with elevated plasma oncotic pressure. *N. Engl. J. Med.* 317: 150, 1987.
254. Moran, S. M., and Myers, B. D. Pathophysiology of protracted acute renal failure in man. *J. Clin. Invest.* 76: 1440, 1985.
255. Moran, S. M., and Myers, B. D. Course of acute renal failure studied by a model of creatinine kinetics. *Kidney Int.* 27: 928, 1985.
256. Morrin, P. A. F., Hinglais, N., Nabarra, B., et al. Rapidly progressive glomerulonephritis. *Am. J. Med.* 65: 446, 1978.
257. Mustonen, J., Pasternack, A., Helin, H., et al. Renal biopsy in acute renal failure. *Am. J. Nephrol.* 4: 27, 1984.
258. Muther, R. S., Potter, D. M., and Bennett, W. M. Aspirin-induced depression of glomerular filtration rate in normal humans: Role of sodium balance. *Ann. Intern. Med.* 94: 317, 1981.
259. Myers, B. D., and Moran, S. M. Hemodynamically mediated acute renal failure. *N. Engl. J. Med.* 314: 97, 1986.
260. Myers, B. D., Miller, D. C., and Mehigan, J. T. Nature of the renal injury following total ischemia in men. *J. Clin. Invest.* 73: 329, 1984.
261. Myers, B. D., Carrie, B. J., Yee, R. R., et al. Pathophysiology of hemodynamically mediated acute renal failure in man. *Kidney Int.* 18: 495, 1980.
262. Myers, B. D., Hilberman, M., Spencer, R. J., et al. Glomerular and tubular function in non-oliguric acute renal failure. *Am. J. Med.* 72: 642, 1982.
263. Myers, C., Roxe, B. M., and Hano, J. E. The clinical course of non-oliguric acute renal failure. *Cardiovasc. Med.* 4: 669, 1977.
264. Nadel, S. M., Jackson, J. W., and Ploth, D. W. Hypokalemic rhabdomyolysis and acute renal failure: Occurrence following total parenteral nutrition. *J.A.M.A.* 241: 2294, 1979.
265. Naidick, J. A., Rackson, M. E., Massey, R. T., et al. Nondilated obstructive uropathy: Percutaneous nephrostomy performed to reverse renal failure. *Radiology* 160: 653, 1986.
266. Nielson, O. J., and Thaysen, J. H. Erythropoietin deficiency in acute tubular necrosis. *J. Intern. Med.* 227: 373, 1990.
267. Nissenson, A. R., Baraff, L. J., Fine, L. N., and Knutson, D. W. Poststreptococcal acute glomerulonephritis: Fact and controversy. *Ann. Intern. Med.* 91: 76, 1979.
268. Nolan, C. R., Anger, M., and Kelleher, S. P. Eosinophiluria—A new method of detection and definition of the clinical spectrum. *N. Engl. J. Med.* 315: 1516, 1986.
269. Oliver, J. A., Sciacca, R. R., Pinto, J., et al. Role of the prostaglandins in norepinephrine release during augmented renal sympathetic nerve activity in the dog. *Circ. Res.* 48: 835, 1981.
270. O'Neill, W. M., Jr., Etheridge, W. B., and Bloomer H. A. High-dose corticosteroids. *Arch. Intern. Med.* 139: 514, 1979.
271. Oredugba, O., Mazumdar, D. C., Meyer, J. S., et al. Pulse methylprednisolone therapy in idiopathic, rapidly progressive glomerulonephritis. *Ann. Intern. Med.* 92: 504, 1980.
272. Owen, C. A., Mubarak, S. J., Hargens, A. R., et al. Intramuscular pressures with limb compression *N. Engl. J. Med.* 300: 1169, 1979.
273. Parker, M., Lee, W. H., Medina, N. et al. Functional renal insufficiency during long-term therapy with captopril and enalapril in severe chronic heart failure. *Ann. Intern. Med.* 106: 346, 1987.
274. Pascual, J., Orofino, L., Liano, F., et al. Incidence and prognosis of acute renal failure in older patients. *J. Am. Geriatr. Soc.* 38: 25, 1990.

275. Perlmutter, M. Unusual cases of acute tubular necrosis *Ann. Intern. Med.* 47: 81, 1957.
276. Perlmutter, M., Grossman, S. L., Rothenburg, S., et al. Urine-serum urea nitrogen ratio. *J.A.M.A.* 170: 1533, 1959.
277. Pietrek, J., Kokot, F., and Kuska, J. Serum 25-hydroxy vitamin D and parathyroid hormone in patients with acute renal failure. *Kidney Int.* 13: 178, 1978.
278. Pitman, S. W., and Frei, E. Weekly methotrexate-calcium leucovorum rescue: Effect of alkalinization on nephrotoxicity: pharmacokinetics in the CNS; and use in CNS non-Hodgkin's lymphoma. *Canc. Treat. Rep.* 61: 695, 1977.
279. Planas, M., Wachtel, T., Frank, H., et al. Characterization of acute renal failure in the burned patient. *Arch. Intern. Med.* 142: 2087, 1982.
280. Preibe, H. J., Skillman, J. J., Bushnell, L. S., et al. Antacid versus cimetidine in preventing acute gastrointestinal bleeding. *N. Engl. J. Med.* 302: 426, 1980.
281. Preston, R. A., Stemmer, C. L., Materson, B. J., et al. Renal biopsy in patients 65 years of age or older. *J. Am. Geriatr. Soc.* 38: 669, 1990.
282. Pru, C., and Kjellstrand, C. M. The FE_{Na} test is of no prognostic value in acute renal failure. *Nephron* 36: 20, 1984.
283. Puera, D. A., and Johnson, L. F. Cimetidine for prevention and treatment of gastroduodenal mucosal lesions in patients in an intensive care unit. *Ann. Intern. Med.* 103: 173, 1985.
284. Pumariega, A. J., Muller, B., and Rivers-Bulkeley, N. Acute renal failure secondary to amoxapine overdose. *J.A.M.A.* 248: 3141, 1982.
285. Pusey, C. D., Saltissi, D., and Bloodworth, L. Drug-associated acute interstitial nephritis: Clinical and pathological features and the response to high dose steroid therapy. *Q. J. Med.* 52: 194, 1983.
286. Rascoff, J. H., Golden, R. A., Spinowitz, B. S., et al. Nondilated obstructive nephropathy. *Arch. Intern. Med.* 143: 696, 1983.
287. Rasmussen, H. H., and Ibels, L. S. Acute renal failure. Multivariate analysis of causes and risk factors. *Am. J. Med.* 73: 211, 1982.
288. Ratner, S. J. Zomepirac and renal failure. *Ann. Intern. Med.* 96: 793, 1982.
289. Reubi, F. C. Hemodynamic changes in isotonic dehydration. *Contrib. Nephrol.* 21: 55, 1980.
290. Richet, G., Lopez, A., deNovales, E., et al. Drug intoxication and neurologic episodes in chronic renal failure. *Br. Med. J.* 2: 394, 1970.
291. Rigden, S. P. A., Barratt, T. M., Dillon, M. J., et al. Acute renal failure complicating cardiopulmonary bypass surgery. *Arch. Dis. Childh.* 57: 425, 1982.
292. Ritchie, J. P. Clinical Aspects of Urinary Tract Obstruction. In B. Brenner and J. M. Lazarus (eds.), *Acute Renal Failure.* Philadelphia: Saunders, 1983. P. 499.
293. Robinette, J. B., and Conger, J. C. Angiotensin and thromboxane in the enhanced renal adrenergic nerve sensitivity of acute renal failure. *J. Clin. Invest.* 86: 1532, 1990.
294. Ron, D., Taitelman, U., Michaelson, M., et al. Prevention of acute renal failure in traumatic rhabdomyolysis. *Arch. Intern. Med.* 144: 277, 1984.
295. Roscoe, M. H. Urine in acute and chronic renal failure. *Br. Med. J.* 1: 1084, 1964.
296. Roth, D., Alarcon, F. J., Fernandez, J. A., et al. Acute rhabdomyolysis associated with cocaine intoxication. *N. Engl. J. Med.* 319: 673, 1988.
297. Roy, S., Pitcock, J. A., and Etteldorf, J. N. Prognosis of acute poststreptococcal glomerulonephritis in childhood: Prospective study and review of the literature. *Adv. Pediatr.* 23: 453, 1976.
298. Rudnick, M. R., Bastl, C. P., Elfinbein, I. B., et al. The Differential Diagnosis of Acute Renal Failure. In B. M. Brenner, and M. J. Lazarus (eds.), *Acute Renal Failure.* Philadelphia: Saunders, 1983. P. 176.
299. Rupp, D. J., Seaton, R. D., and Wiegmann, T. B. Acute polyuric renal failure after aspirin intoxication. *Arch. Intern. Med.* 143: 1237, 1983.
300. Sawyer, M. H., Webb, D. E., Balow, J. E., et al. Acyclovir-induced renal failure. Clinical course of histology. *Am. J. Med.* 84: 1067, 1988.
301. Schorr, N., Ichikawa, I., and Brenner, B. M. Glomerular adaptations to chronic dietary salt restriction or excess. *Am. J. Physiol.* 238: F428, 1980.
302. Schrier, R. W., Henderson, H. S., Tisher, C. G., et al. Nephropathy associated with heat stress and exercise. *Ann. Intern. Med.* 67: 356, 1967.
303. Scully, R. E., Mark, E. J., and McNelley, B. U. Case records of the Massachusetts General Hospital. *N. Engl. J. Med.* 310: 244, 1984.
304. Serra, R. M., Engle, J. E., Jones, R. E., et al. Perianeurysmal retroperitoneal fibrosis. An unusual cause of renal failure. *Am. J. Med.* 68: 149, 1980.
305. Sevitt, S. Distal tubular necrosis with little or no oliguria. *J. Clin. Pathol.* 9: 12, 1956.
306. Shapira, N., Skillman, J. J., Steinman, T. I., et al. Gastric mucosal permeability and gastric acid secretion before and after hemodialysis in patients with chronic renal failure. *Surgery* 83: 528, 1978.
307. Shapiro, J. I., and Anderson, R. J. Urinary diagnostic indices in acute renal failure (letter). *AKF Nephrol.* 1: 13, 1984.
308. Shah, G. M., Alvarado, P., and Kirshenbaum, M. A. Symptomatic hypocalcemia and hypomagnesemia with renal magnesium wasting associated with pentamidine therapy in a patient with AIDS. *Am. J. Med.* 89: 380, 1990.
309. Shaw, A. B., and Gopalka, S. G. Renal artery thrombosis caused by antihypertensive treatment. *Br. Med. J.* 285: 1617, 1982.
310. Shen, S. C., and Ham, T. H. Studies on the destruction of red blood cells, III. Mechanism and complications of hemoglobinuria in patients with thermal burns: Spherocytosis and increased osmotic fragility of red blood cells. *N. Engl. J. Med.* 229: 701, 1943.
311. Sherman, R. A., and Byun, K. J. Nuclear medicine in acute and chronic renal failure. *Semin. Nucl. Med.* 12: 265, 1982.
312. Shin, B., Mackenzie, C., and Crowley, R. A. Changing patterns of posttraumatic acute renal failure. *Am. Surg.* 45: 182, 1979.
313. Shusterman, N., Strom, B. L., Murray, T. G., et al. Risk factors and outcome of hospital-acquired acute renal failure. *Am. J. Med.* 83: 65, 1987.
314. Silas, J. H., Klenka, Z., Solomon, S. A., et al. Captopril induced reversible renal failure: A marker of renal artery stenosis affecting a solitary kidney. *Br. Med. J.* 286: 1702, 1983.
315. Sirota, J. H. Carbon tetrachloride poisoning in man. I. The mechanisms of renal failure and recovery. *J. Clin. Invest.* 28: 1412, 1949.
316. Smith, V. T. Anaphylactic shock, acute renal failure and tubular dysfunction due to zomepirac therapy. *J.A.M.A.* 249: 396, 1982.

317. Smithies, M. N., and Cameron, J. S. Can we predict outcome in acute renal failure? *Nephron* 51: 297, 1989.
318. Solez, K., Morel-Maroger, L., and Sraer, J. D. The morphology of acute tubular necrosis in man: Analysis of 57 renal biopsies and a comparison with glycerol model. *Medicine* 58: 362, 1979.
319. Somerville, P. J., and Kaye, M. Resistance to parathyroid hormone in renal failure: Role of vitamin D metabolites. *Kidney Int.* 14: 245, 1978.
320. Somerville, P. J., and Kaye, M. Evidence that resistance to the calcemic action of parathyroid hormone in rats with acute uremia is caused by phosphate retention. *Kidney Int.* 16: 552, 1979.
321. Sos, T. A., Pickering, T. G., Phil, D., et al. Percutaneous transluminal renal angioplasty in renovascular hypertension due to atheroma or fibromuscular dysplasia. *N. Engl. J. Med.* 309: 274, 1983.
322. Sporn, I. N., Lancestremere, R. G., and Papper, S. Differential diagnosis of oliguria in aged patients. *N. Engl. J. Med.* 267: 130, 1961.
323. Sprung, C. L., and Portocarrero, C. J. Heat stroke (letter). *Ann. Intern. Med.* 91: 503, 1979.
324. Stecker, J. F., Jr., Rawls, H. P., Devine, C. J., et al. Retroperitoneal fibrosis and ergot derivatives. *J. Urol.* 112: 30, 1974.
325. Steiner, R. W. Low fractional excretion of sodium in myoglobinuric renal failure. *Arch. Intern. Med.* 142: 1216, 1982.
326. Steinman, T. I., and Lazarus, J. M. Organ-System Involvement in Acute Renal Failure. In B. M. Brenner and J. M. Lazarus (eds.), *Acute Renal Failure.* Philadelphia: Saunders, 1983. P. 586.
327. Stewart, R. B., Hale, W. E., and Marks, R. G. Effects of nonsteroidal anti-inflammatory drugs on renal function in the elderly. *South. Med. J.* 75: 824, 1982.
328. Stillman, M. T., and Schlesinger, P. A. Nonsteroidal anti-inflammatory drug nephrotoxicity. *Arch. Intern. Med.* 150: 268, 1990.
329. Stilmant, M. M., Boston, W. K., and Sturgill, B. C. Crescentic glomerulonephritis without immune deposits: Clinicopathologic features. *Kidney Int.* 15: 184, 1979.
330. Stott, R. B., Cameron, J. S., Ogg, C. S., et al. Why the persistently high mortality in acute renal failure? *Lancet* 2: 75, 1972.
331. Swann, R. C., and Merrill, J. P. The clinical course of acute renal failure. *Medicine* 32: 215, 1953.
332. Swartz, R. D., Rubin, J. E., Leeming, E. W., et al. Renal failure following major angiography. *Am. J. Med.* 65: 31, 1978.
333. Swenson, R. D., Golper, T. A., and Bennett, W. M. Acute renal failure and rhabdomyolysis after ingestion of phenylpropanolamine-containing diet pills. *Arch. Intern. Med.* 142: 601, 1982.
334. Swenson, R. S., Corell, W. F., and Redding, G. J. Differential diagnostic indices in early acute renal failure (abstract). *Clin. Res.* 23: 122, 1975.
335. Taylor, I. L., and Dockray, G. J. Hypergastrinemia in renal failure: The biological significance of molecular forms of gastrin. *Br. J. Surg.* 63: 657, 1976.
336. Taylor, W. H. Management of acute renal failure following surgical operation and head injury. *Lancet* 2: 703, 1957.
337. Taylor, W. H., and Reid, J. V. O. Acute uremic renal failure and head injury and surgical operation. *J. Clin. Pathol.* 9: 184, 1956.
338. Teschan, P., Post, R. S., Smith, L. H., et al. Posttraumatic renal insufficiency in military casualties: I. Clinical characteristics. *Am. J. Med.* 18: 172, 1955.
339. Textor, S. C., Margolin, K., Blayney, D., et al. Renal, volume and hormonal changes during therapeutic administration of recombinant interleukin-2 in man. *Am. J. Med.* 83: 1055, 1987.
340. Textor, S. C., Novick, A. C., Tarazi, R. C., et al. Critical perfusion pressure for renal function in patients with bilateral atherosclerotic renal vascular disease. *Ann. Intern. Med.* 102: 308, 1985.
341. Tungsanga, K., Boonwichit, D., Lekhakul, A., et al. Urine uric acid and urine creatinine ratio in acute renal failure. *Arch. Intern. Med.* 144: 934, 1984.
342. Turney, J. H., Marshall, D. H., Brownjohn, A. M., et al. The evolution of acute renal failure, 1956–1988. *Q. J. Med.* 74: 83, 1990.
343. Vaz, A. J. Low fractional excretion of urinary sodium in acute renal failure due to sepsis. *Arch. Intern. Med.* 143: 738, 1983.
344. Vertel, R. M., and Knochel, J. P. Acute renal failure due to heat injury. An analysis of ten cases associated with a high incidence of myoglobinuria. *Am. J. Med.* 43: 435, 1967.
345. Vertel, R. M., and Knochel, J. P. Non-oliguric acute renal failure. *J.A.M.A.* 200: 118, 1967.
346. Walshe, J. J., and Venuto, R. C. Acute oliguric renal failure induced by indomethacin: Possible mechanism. *Ann. Intern. Med.* 91: 47, 1979.
347. Ward, M. M. Factors predictive of acute renal failure in rhabdomyolysis. *Arch. Intern. Med.* 148: 1553, 1988.
348. Warshaw, A. L., and O'Hara, P. J. Susceptibility of the pancreas to ischemic injury in shock. *Ann. Surg.* 188: 197, 1978.
349. Waugh, W. H. Functional types of acute renal failure and their early diagnosis. *Arch. Intern. Med.* 103: 686, 1958.
350. Welt, L. G. *Clinical Disorders of Hydration and Acid-Base Equilibrium.* Boston: Little, Brown, 1955. P. 262.
351. Wesdorp, R. I. C., Falcao, H., and Banks, P. B. Gastrin and gastric acid secretion in renal failure. *Am. J. Surg.* 141: 334, 1981.
352. Wetherill, S. F., Guarino, M. J., and Cox, R. W. Acute renal failure associated with barium chloride poisoning. *Ann. Intern. Med.* 95: 187, 1981.
353. Wharton, J. M., Coleman, D. L., Wofsy, C. B., et al. Trimethoprim-sulfamethoxazole or pentamidine for *Pneumocystis carinii* pneumonia in the acquired immunodeficiency syndrome. *Ann. Intern. Med.* 1095: 37, 1986.
354. Wheeler, D. C., Feehally, J., and Walls, J. High risk acute renal failure. *Q. J. Med.* 61: 977, 1986.
355. Whelton, A., Stout, R. L., Spilman, P. E., et al. Renal effects of ibuprofen, piroxicam and sulindac in patients with asymptomatic renal failure. *Ann. Intern. Med.* 112: 568, 1990.
356. Wilkins, R. G., and Faragher, E. B. Acute renal failure in an intensive care unit: incidence, prediction and outcome. *Anesthesia* 38: 628, 1983.
357. Wilson, D. M., Turner, D. R., Cameron, J. S., et al. Value of renal biopsy in acute intrinsic renal failure. *Br. Med. J.* 2: 459, 1976.
358. Wise, W. J., Mamdani, B. H., Bakir, A. A., et al. Fibrinous pericarditis in hepatorenal failure. *Lancet* 2: 1336, 1980.

Acute Renal Vein Thrombosis

Francisco Llach
Bijan Nikakhtar

Thrombosis of the renal vein was originally thought to be a relatively uncommon vascular complication of the kidney. Although the first description of thrombosis of the renal vein was made by J. Hunter [35], it was Rayer who in 1840 was the first to make an association between renal vein thrombosis (RVT) and the nephrotic syndrome [64]. Much later, Abeshouse extensively reviewed the medical literature in regard to thrombolic disease of the renal vein [1]. Among the most important causes cited were infectious suppuration, malignancy, and trauma. It is important to note that in all of these patients reported to have RVT, the diagnosis was made postmortem. Later, with the development of more advanced radiographic techniques and selective catheterization, antemortem diagnosis of RVT was made possible, and the number of patients in the adult population diagnosed with RVT increased. Although RVT may be caused by trauma or tumor, it has become apparent that it occurs most commonly in the nephrotic patient.

Because of the early descriptions, emphasis was placed on the presence of lumbar pain with flank tenderness, edema, and the appearance of a lumbar mass. As a consequence, the early reports following this description focused attention on these symptoms, and it was generally assumed that RVT always presented suddenly with florid symptomatology. However, Harrison et al. in 1956 described two groups of patients with RVT [31]. The first, with complete acute thrombosis of the renal vein, was characterized by severe lumbar or abdominal pain, enlargement of the affected kidney, proteinuria, edema, and deterioration of renal function. A second group had only the nephrotic syndrome and absence of acute symptomatology. In the present chapter, we discuss the specific mechanisms and pathophysiology of RVT, concentrating primarily on the clinical aspects, diagnosis, and management of acute disease.

Etiology

The incidence of RVT in the adult population is difficult to establish. A review of 29,280 necropsy studies performed in the Mayo Clinic from 1920 to 1961 revealed 17 cases of bilateral RVT in adults, an incidence of approximately 0.6 percent per 1000 necropsies [56]. Among the 17 cases, only 2 had the nephrotic syndrome; however, during the last decade, prospective studies have evaluated the incidence of RVT in the nephrotic patient. This incidence has been found to be significant, although variable. In Table 49-1 are displayed various prospective studies evaluating the incidence of RVT in patients with the nephrotic syndrome and membranous nephropathy [10, 15, 50, 57, 60, 63, 82, 83, 84]. This table includes data only from prospective studies evaluating patients undergoing routine renal venograms regardless of the presence or absence of symptoms suggestive of RVT. It can be appreciated that the overall incidence of renal vein thrombosis in both the nephrotic syndrome and membranous nephropathy is significant; however, there are marked differences in this incidence, ranging from 5 to 62 percent. The reason for such differences is not clear. One possibility, in light of current immunologic advances, is that membranous nephropathy may include different immunologic entities and some may be more prone to develop RVT than others. Another possibility is that the duration of the nephrotic syndrome and the persistence and magnitude of the hypoalbuminemia may have varied in these studies. It is generally agreed that the most common underlying nephropathy associated with RVT is membranous nephropathy. A review of all .our patients with nephrotic syndrome is shown in Table 49-2. Of 151 patients with the syndrome, 33 had RVT, and of these, 20 had membranous nephropathy [51]. However, it can be appreciated that there are other causes such as membranoproliferative glomerulonephritis, lipoid nephrosis, and amyloidosis that may be associated with RVT. It should be emphasized that of our 33 patients with RVT, only 4 had an acute mode of presentation.

The concept of the relationship between renal vein thrombosis and the nephrotic syndrome has changed in the last two decades [46]. For many years, it was thought that RVT was the cause of the nephrotic syndrome, a belief that is no longer held. Several lines of evidence have seriously questioned this hypothesis. First, experimentally induced RVT causes only mild proteinuria, and the renal histology by immunofluorescent findings in these cases does not resemble that of membranous nephropathy [18–34]. Second, RVT has been reported in the surgical literature in the absence of the nephrotic syndrome [20–25,27,29–36]. Moreover, in autopsy studies of patients with RVT, nephrotic syndrome is present antemortem in only a few patients [56]. Third, most patients with RVT and nephrotic syndrome who have been subjected to renal morphologic study have exhibited an identifiable glomerulopathy most of the time—membranous nephropathy, which is responsible for the nephrotic syndrome [52]. Finally, it has recently been shown that RVT occurs after the onset of the nephrotic syndrome [49, 78]. Thus, the general view today is that the nephrotic syndrome provides a favorable milieu for the development of RVT.

Pathophysiology

An important factor in the causation of RVT in patients with the nephrotic syndrome is the presence of a hypercoagulable state. Profound clotting factor abnormalities have been observed in the nephrotic syndrome by various investigators. There are five major functional classes of coagulation components: (1) zymogens (factors II, V, IX, XI, and XII), which are activated by enzymes and cofactors (factors V and VIII) whose major role is to accelerate the role of enzymes; (2) fibrinogen and products

This work was supported in part by a grant from the Veterans Administration.

Table 49-1. Prospective studies evaluating the incidence of renal vein thrombosis (RVT) in patients with nephrotic syndrome (NS) and membranous glomerulopathy (MGN)

	Patients with RVT in NS	Incidence (%)	Patients with RVT in MGN	Incidence (%)
Bennett [10]			5/10	50
Noel et al. [60]			5/16	31
Wagoner et al. [84]			14/27	52
Cameron et al. [15]			2/15	13
Pohl et al. [63]	1/54	2	1/20	5
Llach et al. [50]	33/151	22	20/69	29
Monteon et al. [57]	15/53	28	15/24	62
Vosnides et al. [83]	7/44	16	5/30	17
Velasquez-Forero and Garcia-Prugue [82]	8/19	42	3/5	60

Modified from Llach [47].

Table 49-2. Etiology of the nephrotic syndrome in 151 patients

	Patients with renal vein thrombosis (no.)	Patients without renal vein thrombosis (no.)	Total
Renal Diagnosis			
Membranous nephropathy	20	49	69
Membranoproliferative glomerulonephritis	6	21	27
Lipoid nephrosis	2	8	10
Rapidly progressive glomerulonephritis	1	1	2
Amyloidosis	1	5	6
Focal sclerosis	1	3	4
Renal sarcoidosis	1	0	1
Lupus nephritis	1	10	11
Diabetic nephropathy	0	15	15
Focal glomerulonephritis	0	3	3
Acute poststreptococcal glomerulonephritis	0	2	2
End-stage renal disease	0	1	1
Total	33	118	151

From Llach et al. [50], with permission.

from the conversion of fibrinogen to fibrin; (3) the fibrinolytic system; (4) clotting inhibitors; and (5) components of the platelet reaction and thrombogenesis. Alterations in all of these coagulation components have been observed in the nephrotic patient.

Alterations in *zymogens and co-factors* include a decrease in the levels of factors IX, XI, and XII [28, 30, 33, 34, 44, 59, 71, 79, 80]. The low levels of these proteins most likely are due to urinary loss secondary to their small molecular size rather than to impaired protein synthesis. An increase in the levels of factor II and combined factors VII and X has also been described [40]. In general, most of these zymogen abnormalities tend to normalize with clinical remission of the nephrotic syndrome. Most consistently, increased levels of co-factors (factors V and VIII) have been noted in the nephrotic syndrome [37, 40, 77]. A number of studies have shown a correlation between increases in factors V and VIII with a fall in serum albumin [37, 44, 77]. It appears that these alterations in co-factors result from increased synthesis of these proteins by the liver; apparently, the mitochondria of the liver cells are the final sites of production of most of these proteins, and a decrease in plasma oncotic pressure and/or a decrease in serum albumin concentration may be sensed by these liver cells, which in turn respond with an increased production of different proteins [17].

During the earlier description of the hypercoagulable state of the nephrotic syndrome, the hypothesis was advanced that an increase in co-factors may lead to hypercoagulability and may explain the high incidence of thrombosis in these patients. However, two important points must be made regarding this hypothesis. First, all of these factors are normally present in great excess in the circulation with only a small amount of any given factor being activated during thrombus formation. Thus, it seems unlikely that high levels of any of these zymogens would lead to thrombosis or that reduced levels of some coagulation factors would be a sensitive marker of the presence of thrombosis. Second, there is no evidence suggesting that the increased level of co-factors may lead to thromboembolic phenomena. High levels of these factors are usually present during acute inflammatory responses because they are an acute-phase reactant protein. There is no current evidence that these conditions are associated with an increased risk of thrombosis.

An elevation of *plasma fibrinogen* level is a consistent and significant abnormality observed in nephrotic patients [5, 37, 77]. With the use of ^{131}I-labeled fibrinogen, the rate of fibrinogen catabolism is normal in these patients, and the observed increase in plasma fibrinogen is due to an increased liver synthesis that is proportional to the urinary protein loss [75]. In addition, there is a significant correlation between fibrinogen and cholesterol levels, and both are inversely related to the levels of serum albumin. The level of fibrinogen in nephrotic patients may be as high as 1 gm per deciliter and has been shown to alter plasma viscosity considerably [5]. Thus, increased plasma fibrinogen concentration reflects its increased hepatic synthesis; contracted intravascular distribution may be present, and there is a normal degradation rate of fibrinogen in the nephrotic patient. It is possible that the high fibrinogen levels, by increasing significantly blood viscosity, are important in the hypercoagulable state of nephrotic syndrome.

Various tests for determination of the products of fibrinogen to fibrin conversion have been developed for diagnosis of a prethrombotic state. An increase in the plasma concentration of fibrinogen degradation products (FDP) is not commonly observed in nephrotic patients but has been observed in the urine of patients with glomerulonephritis [17]. Some nephrotic patients have been found to have increased urinary levels of FDP [14]. However, these findings should not be taken as definite evidence for increased fibrinolysis in the systemic or renal vasculature, since in patients with nonselective proteinuria fibrinogen is filtered at the glomerulus and may undergo proteolytic degradation by protease. In this regard, gel chromatography clearly shows that material that has in the past been interpreted as FDP is actually filtered fibrinogen that has been degraded in the tubules [5, 29].

Alterations in the *fibrinolytic system* have also been observed in nephrotic patients [86]. The basic reaction of the fibrinolytic system is the conversion by plasminogen activators of a β-globulin, plasminogen, to an active serum protease, plasmin. This system is modulated by inhibitors of both plasminogen and plasmin. A number of clinical studies have reported an association between defective fibrinolysis and thrombosis; the association has included oral contraceptive ingestion [8], pregnancy [12], postoperative states [87], malignant disease [66], obesity [3], and the nephrotic syndrome [23]. The data in regard to the fibrinolytic abnormalities in nephrotic patients have shown in general a decrease in plasma plasminogen concentration [23, 32, 73] that is correlated with a low serum albumin and the magnitude of the proteinuria [23, 45, 49]. The clinical significance of this abnormality is not known, and a cause-effect relationship of these abnormalities and RVT has not been made. However, recently, Du and associates [21] have identified a plasmin inhibitor to be identical with α_2-antiplasmin. They evaluated 14 nephrotic patients with RVT together with 30 nephrotic patients without RVT. In both groups the level of total fibrinolytic activity was normal and that of the plasma inhibitor (α_2-antiplasmin) of plasminogen activation was elevated. However, the plasmin inhibitor was elevated in 13 of 14 patients with RVT and only in 12 of 30 patients without RVT. The authors suggested that the increased level of α_2-antiplasmin may be a factor in determining susceptibility to the development and persistence of RVT in the nephrotic patients. Further studies are needed to confirm the importance of these observations.

Alterations in *coagulation inhibitors* have been observed in nephrotic patients. The components of the coagulation system exist in the circulation as zymogens, and they are cleaved to form proteolytic enzymes. Activated clotting factors are inhibited by naturally occurring coagulation inhibitors [44, 59]. The most important physiologically of these inhibitors is antithrombin-III (AT-III). This is an α_2-globulin that is the main inhibitor of thrombin and also inhibits activated factors XII, IX, X, XI, and plasmin [24, 27, 55, 68, 69, 88]. The rate of inhibition of these enzymes by AT-III is markedly increased in the presence of heparin. In patients from families with an inherited deficiency of AT-III, an increased incidence of thromboembolic complications is generally observed when AT-III levels are below 75 percent of normal [24, 55].

Kauffman et al. have studied AT-III levels in 48 patients with proteinuria and their relationship with the occurrence of thromboembolic phenomena [39]. Nine patients had evidence of thrombosis, including 4 with RVT. In 8 of these 9 patients, the serum AT-III levels were below 70 percent of normal. There was a significant correlation between AT-III concentration and the urine protein excretion. Only 6 of the 32 patients who excreted less than 10 gm per 24 hours showed depressed AT-III levels below 85 percent, whereas 13 of 16 patients with a proteinuria higher than 10 gm per 24 hours showed depressed AT-III levels. Since the molecular weight of AT-III is relatively low, excretion in the urine would be expected in patients with proteinuria. Because of similar molecular weights, the renal clearance of AT-III and albumin were compared. A significant correlation was found between the plasma concentration of these two proteins. In addition, there was a significant correlation between the renal AT-III clearance and the degree of AT-III deficiency. It was concluded that thrombosis in nephrotic patients may be associated with deficiency of AT-III due to increased urinary loss and that low levels of AT-III may be insufficient to inactivate procoagulant factors, thus resulting in the development of thrombosis. These results are in apparent conflict with studies showing normal or increased antithrombin activity in nephrotic children [37, 77]. This finding may have been due to the nonspecific in vitro inhibition of thrombin by α_2-globulin and α_2-antitrypsin (two other clotting inhibitors), and therefore the apparent increment in AT-III activity may not have reflected a true increase in AT-

III levels. In addition, AT-III deficiency was generally reported by other investigators in association with serum albumin of less than 2 gm per deciliter [5, 38, 39], whereas in the earlier studies only a few patients had severe hypoalbuminemia. Recently, Panicucci et al. have reported normal levels of AT-III in spite of high urinary AT-III levels [62]. They suggested that increased AT-III synthesis compensated for its renal loss. Later, Vaziri et al. observed a significant decrease in AT-III plasma concentration and activity in 20 nephrotic patients compared with normal subjects [81]. Also, substantial urinary losses of AT-III were demonstrated in the nephrotic patients. Thus, although the rate of synthesis and degradation of AT-III and its distribution have not been determined, it is likely that renal losses of AT-III in nephrotic patients contribute to AT-III deficiency. It is possible that the danger of thromboembolic phenomena may arise with sudden changes in the activity of the renal disease, resulting in abrupt renal losses of AT-III while hepatic synthesis of AT-III has not yet increased. An interesting observation is the increase in AT-III levels in nephrotic children after steroid therapy [76].

Recently, important data about the role of coagulation inhibitors in the development of thrombosis have been reported. Protein C and protein S have been identified as potent anticoagulants. Protein C is a vitamin K–dependent serum protease zymogen, which is homologous with other known vitamin K–dependent serum proteases [74b]. This protein is an anticoagulant since it prolongs the clotting time of plasma in various clotting assays [40b]. The clinical role of protein C as an important antithrombotic regulatory molecule has been demonstrated recently by identifying a familial thrombotic disease that is associated with an inherited partial deficiency of protein C [28a]. Thus, families with a deficiency in plasma protein C have recurrent thrombosis. It appears that protein C levels below 50 percent result in thrombosis. While antithrombin-III appears to be a major regulatory protein in limiting the activity of procoagulant plasma enzymes, activated protein C may represent a major regulatory protein limiting the activity of activated procoagulant factor (factors V and VIII). In this respect, the anticoagulant properties of activated protein C and antithrombin-III are complementary.

Recently, the rate of inactivation of factor V by activated protein C has been found to be stimulated by another vitamin K–dependent protein, protein S [84b]. Protein S has no effect on factor V activity in the absence of activated protein C, indicating that it is not a protease. In a protein S–deficient plasma, the anticoagulant activity of activated protein C is reduced significantly, and, when protein S is added, the activity of protein C is restored. It appears that the complex between protein S and activated protein C is formed only in the presence of phospholipids [85]. Since protein S is required for the expression of the anticoagulant activity of activated protein C, it is not surprising that recently a deficiency of protein S has been found to predispose to recurrent thrombosis [17a]. Thus, Comp and Esmon [17a] have identified six unrelated persons with severe, recurrent venous thrombosis who were deficient in protein S, with levels between 15 and 37 percent. Early high protein C and S were observed in the nephrotic patients [19a].

Later, other investigators noted normal protein C in nephrotic patients [74]. However, still later, it was observed that the functional levels of protein S did not correlate with the immunologic levels. It was further described that protein S is found in two forms in plasma, as free and functionally active protein S and complexed to C4b-binding protein. When compared with control subjects, nephrotic patients had reduced functional levels of protein S despite having elevated levels of total protein S antigen [82a]. Decreased total protein S activity was caused by significant reductions in free (active) protein S levels due to selective urinary loss of free protein S and elevation of C4b-binding protein levels that favors complex formation. These authors also observed that the specific activity of protein C (activity-antigen ratio) was lower in nephrotic patients than in control subjects. The authors concluded that acquired protein S deficiency occurs in nephrotic syndrome and may be a risk factor for the development of the thromboembolic complications.

Platelet abnormalities have also been observed in nephrotic patients. Thus, thrombocytosis is often present [37, 40], and an increased platelet aggregation with adenosine diphosphate (ADP) and collagen but not with epinephrine has been observed [5, 9]. Remuzzi et al. have observed that the degree of platelet function abnormalities correlates with the degree of hypoalbuminemia and the severity of the proteinuria [65]. The levels of β-thromboglobulin, a specific protein released by platelets on aggregation, are significantly elevated in nephrotic patients and return to normal with clinical remission [2]. This suggests that nephrotic patients have an increase in platelet aggregation. However, normal β-thromboglobulin levels have also been reported in nephrotic patients [6]. A recent study of nephrotic patients has demonstrated that thrombotic complications occur only in patients with increased platelet aggregation and elevated β-thromboglobulin levels [43, 48]. In addition, these complications occurred primarily in patients with a serum albumin level of less than 2 gm/dl.

In summary, the hypercoagulable state of the nephrotic syndrome is characterized by low zymogen factors, a marked increase in co-factors, an increase in plasma fibrinogen levels, a decrease in the levels of AT-III and antiplasmin activity, thrombocytosis, increased platelet aggregation, and increased levels of β-thromboglobulin. The high levels of fibrinogen leading to increased plasma viscosity may be an important factor in the hypercoagulable state. A convincing relationship has been found between low AT-III and thrombosis, and it is likely that increased platelet aggregation may also be an important factor in hypercoagulability; the increased levels of β-thromboglobulin may be a reliable marker of platelet aggregation. The severity of the hypoalbuminemia, by increasing hepatic synthesis of fibrinogen and platelet aggregation, may play a pivotal role in the generation and maintenance of these abnormalities.

In regard to the role of a protein S deficiency in the

hypercoagulable state, additional studies in nephrotic patients with thrombosis are necessary to reach any conclusion. However, since protein S deficiency is an acquired problem, it should be determined in patients with thromboembolic complications.

In addition to hypercoagulability, other factors may be important in the pathogenesis of RVT. Thus, a persistent reduction in plasma volume, an important feature in some patients with the nephrotic syndrome, especially those with membranous nephropathy, may provide a milieu favorable to RVT. Theoretically, a sustained reduction in blood volume could lead to a decreased renal venous flow, thereby favoring the development of RVT. In this regard, we have been impressed by the marked decrease in washout time in renal venograms in patients with membranous nephropathy who do not have RVT [52]. Diuretics may enhance volume depletion and thus contribute to the thromboembolic phenomena of the nephrotic syndrome. Recent preliminary data presented by Cheng and associates [15a], in evaluating 97 nephrotic patients, strongly suggest that intensive diuretic therapy is associated with a high incidence of RVT. Third, the nature of the immunologic injury may also be important. A recent study investigating the relationship between membranous nephropathy and RVT has separated a subpopulation of patients with membranous nephropathy and RVT [61]. It is attractive to speculate that such complexes may be the triggering factor in the coagulation process. Recently, the presence of factor XII and prekallikrein in subepithelial deposits has been observed in 29 patients with membranous nephropathy [11]. It is tempting to relate the high incidence of RVT in membranous nephropathy to activation of factor XII, a factor that is at the crossroads of important proteolytic pathways. Clinically, it has been shown that patients with nephrotic syndrome and membranous nephropathy have a high incidence of other thromboembolic phenomena in addition to RVT [52]. Also, studies have shown that greater disturbances of hypercoagulability were noted in patients with membranous nephropathy than in those nephrotic patients with minimal change disease [53, 85]. Finally, the role of steroids in the pathogenesis of RVT has not yet been defined. Steroids have been shown to aggravate the hypercoagulable state [58], and historically the advent of steroid therapy coincided with observations of an increase in thromboembolic complications [19, 41, 54]. Again, the previously mentioned study by Cheng and co-workers [15a] indicated that steroid therapy was associated with a high incidence of RVT. Thus, these agents should be used cautiously in the treatment of nephrotic syndrome.

In summary, the pathogenesis of RVT in patients with nephrotic syndrome may be multifactorial. A general integrated scheme of the pathogenetic factors leading to RVT and other thromboembolic complications is displayed in Fig. 49-1.

Clinical Manifestations

The pattern and mode of clinical presentation of the nephrotic syndrome and RVT may differ from those mentioned in the early literature. Rayer's description of RVT included lumbar pain with tenderness, swelling, and the appearance of a lumbar mass [64]. Subsequent reports stressed the presence of flank pain and macroscopic hematuria in the clinical presentation of RVT. However, as more cases were described, it was noted that in many instances RVT did not have any local symptoms and signs. The clinical spectrum of RVT varies from patient to patient. The rapidity of venous occlusion and the development of venous collateral circulation determine the clinical presentation and subsequent renal function; however, in general, patients with RVT usually

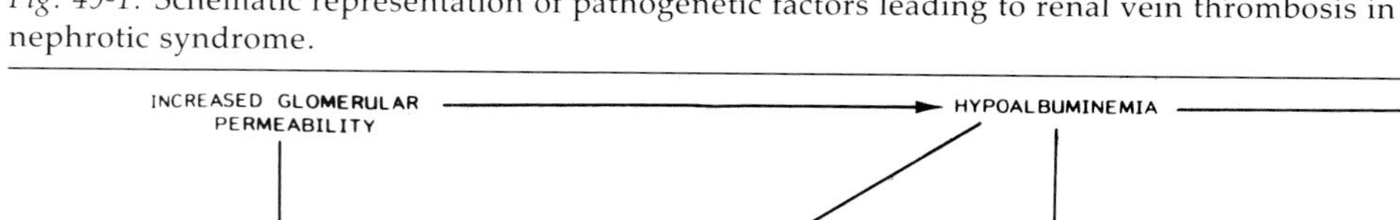

Fig. 49-1. Schematic representation of pathogenetic factors leading to renal vein thrombosis in nephrotic syndrome.

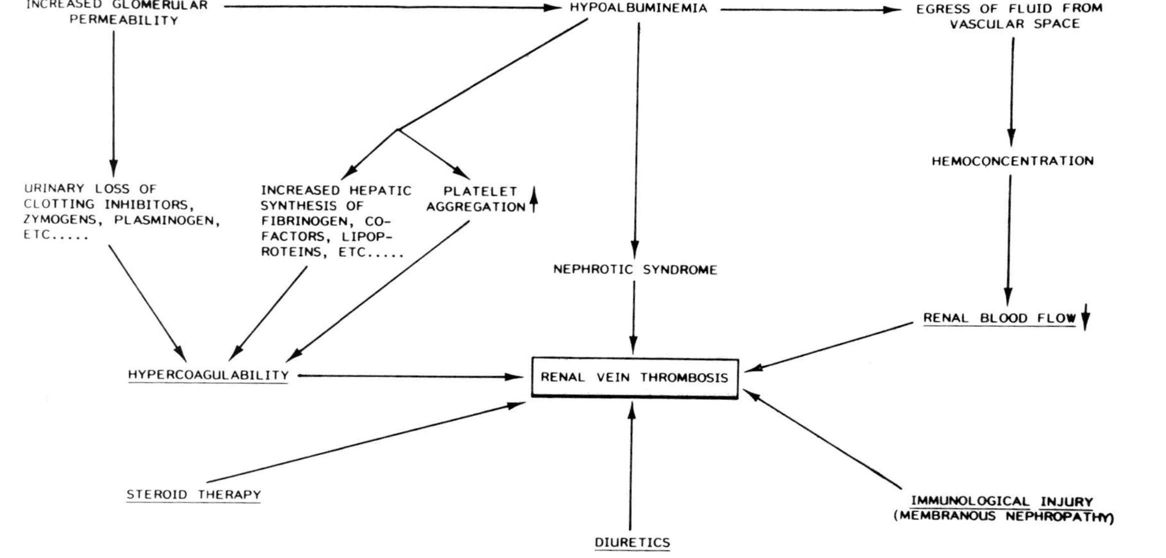

have two modes of clinical presentation: acute and chronic. The chronic presentation of RVT is observed most frequently and in general is asymptomatic. Acute RVT is characterized by sudden onset and usually occurs in younger patients complaining of persistent acute flank pain, which may be colicky at times; marked costovertebral angle tenderness and macroscopic hematuria are usually present. The following case is a representative example of acute RVT.

A 25-year-old white man came to the hospital with a year-long history of proteinuria and ankle swelling. Physical examination revealed no acute distress with normal blood pressure. The only physical finding was ankle edema. Urinary sediment demonstrated 3^{+} proteinuria. Biochemical data were consistent with the presence of nephrotic syndrome and normal renal function. Renal biopsy revealed early membranous nephropathy. Lung scan and intravenous pyelogram were within normal limits. An inferior vena cavogram as well as a left renal venogram were within normal limits. At the time the left renal venogram was performed, the patient experienced an acute left flank pain that lasted 4 to 5 hours and was accompanied by macroscopic hematuria and marked tenderness in the left costovertebral angle. The procedure was terminated and the patient was returned to the ward. A second intravenous pyelogram was obtained, and it showed marked enlargement of the left kidney with poor visualization of the pelvocalyceal system (Fig. 49-2). A selective left renal venogram obtained 1 week later revealed complete obstruction of the main renal vein. Creatinine clearance was reduced, and the patient was anticoagulated. In 2 days, the flank pain resolved completely, and creatinine clearances, after 6 months of anticoagulant therapy, increased from 40 to 90 ml per minute.

On occasion, acute RVT may be bilateral, resulting in marked oliguria and bilateral flank pain. The severity of the symptomatology and oliguria and the magnitude of renal function deterioration will depend on various factors. Thus, previously compromised renal function, absence of collateral circulation, and a large thrombus involving both renal veins may result in a florid clinical presentation as well as a rapid renal function deterioration [45a].

Other causes of acute RVT with or without the nephrotic syndrome are trauma, ingestion of oral contraceptive agents, dehydration (mostly in infants), and steroid administration.

Renal vein thrombosis secondary to trauma is usually accompanied by renal artery thrombosis. The history of the trauma, the severe acute flank pain, and a palpable mass are usually suggestive of this condition.

The use of oral contraceptives has been implicated occasionally as a cause of RVT. Thus, a young female on oral contraceptives without the nephrotic syndrome or any traumatic event developed acute RVT with florid clinical manifestations [74]. Whether there was a cause-effect relationship between the contraceptive agents and the RVT was not clear.

Dehydration has been clearly associated with RVT in infants [7]. In this condition thrombosis develops in the small renal veins, predominantly the arcuate or intralobular vein. The majority of these infants do not have nephrotic syndrome or even significant proteinuria. This syndrome develops initially in the clinical setting of diarrhea, vomiting, and often shock. Oliguria and hematuria rapidly ensue. Contributing factors are a history of maternal diabetes, congenital heart disease, and performance of angiocardiography. An enlarged palpable kidney may be found in 60 percent of cases. The common clinical presentation is a hyperosmolar hypovolemic syndrome. The mortality of RVT in infants is high. Fortunately, the frequency of this syndrome has diminished due to earlier therapy and control of volume-depleting events.

Steroid administration has been clearly associated with acute RVT as well as other thrombotic complications [19, 54]; however, the causative role of these agents

Fig. 49-2. Intravenous pyelogram of a patient with acute renal vein thrombosis. Note blurring and irregularities of the left pelvocalyceal system as well as marked enlargement of the left kidney. (From [47].)

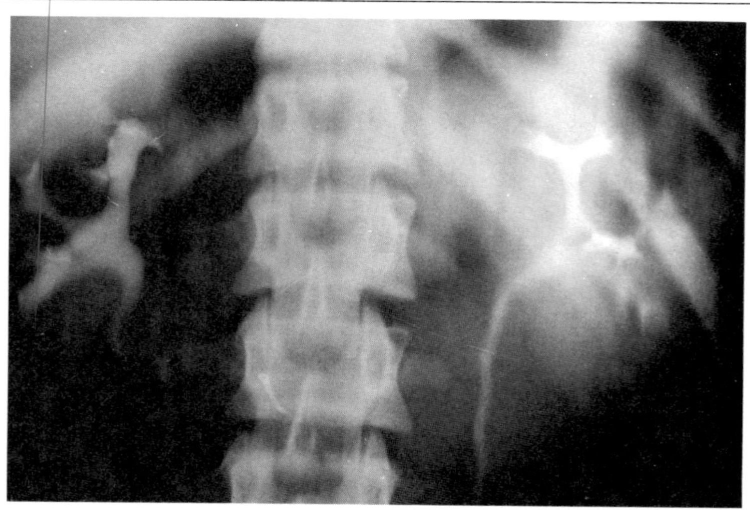

in RVT remains to be established. The role of steroids cannot be appraised until other factors influencing thrombus formation are understood. As mentioned earlier, Cheng and associates [15a] have presented preliminary data in 97 nephrotic patients prospectively evaluated. Of these, 44 patients were found to have RVT by routine renal venogram. Multivariate regression analysis revealed that steroid therapy was associated with a high tendency to RVT ($p < 0.01$).

Finally, abdominal tumors, especially hypernephroma, are a common cause of RVT; however, in the majority of these cases chronic rather than acute RVT is the common clinical presentation.

The radiologic manifestations of acute RVT are well defined and characteristic in contrast to those of chronic RVT, which often are minimal. Experimentally, with complete occlusion of the renal vein, the kidney increases rapidly in size within the first 24 hours, reaching a peak within 1 week of renal vein occlusion [41]. Thereafter, there is a progressive decrease in renal size over the next 2 months, resulting in a small, atrophic kidney. A progressive decrease in the caliber and length of the renal artery follows the occlusion.

Clinically, in a patient with acute RVT the plain film of the abdomen initially reveals an enlarged kidney (Fig. 49-2). In the intravenous pyelogram, if the obstruction is sudden and complete, there may not be any visualization of the collecting system. However, in most patients, due to the presence of some collateral circulation, there is renal enlargement and opacification of varying degree with some visualization of the kidney. Often the renal pelvis can be visualized and is usually stretched, distorted, and blurred (Fig. 49-2). This has been shown to be the result of severe interstitial edema and swelling of the pelvocalyceal system. At this stage the radiographic appearance has been compared to that observed in polycystic kidney disease, and on occasion it has led to this mistaken diagnosis. The acute symptomatology of RVT in association with this radiologic appearance establishes the diagnosis. Ureteral edema may progress to the point at which the collecting system is completely obliterated; there have been cases of complete ureteral obstruction in which during retrograde pyelography the catheter could not be advanced into the pelvis. A characteristic radiographic finding of RVT is notching of the ureter, which usually occurs when collateral veins in close relation to the ureters become tortuous as they dilate to form an alternative drainage route. Originally, the notching of the ureters was interpreted as representative of mucosal edema; however, more detailed radiographic studies have shown indentation of the ureters by the collateral venous circulation [80]. Notching of the ureter is a very infrequent finding in nephrotic patients with RVT and usually occurs only in a minority of patients with chronic rather than acute RVT [51].

Retrograde pyelography may be useful in the patient with complete RVT who does not excrete the contrast material. In such instances, retrograde pyelography may demonstrate a rectangular, linear mucosal pattern with irregular renal pelvic outlines similar to those described above with the intravenous pyelogram.

Inferior vena cavography with selective catheterization of the renal vein is the method of choice for the diagnosis of RVT. If the inferior vena cava is patent and free of filling defects and if a good streaming of unopacified renal blood is demonstrated to wash out contrast from the vena cava, a diagnosis of RVT is unlikely. The Valsalva maneuver is useful during vena cavography; by increasing the intraabdominal pressure the transit of contrast agent and blood from the inferior vena cava is slowed, the proximal part of the main renal vein may be opacified, and the patency of the lumen or even the outline of the thrombus may be demonstrated. On occasion, a lack of washout in the area of the renal vein may be suggestive of RVT; sometimes partial defects in the area of the renal vein, characteristic of renal venous thrombus extending into the inferior vena cava, may be demonstrated. In some instances partial or complete occlusion of the inferior vena cava is demonstrated. In the presence of complete inferior vena cava obstruction below the renal vein, it is desirable to demonstrate the proximal extent of the thrombus, and this can readily be accomplished by transbrachial catheterization with passage of the catheter into the inferior vena cava via the subclavian vein.

Often the inferior vena cavogram is not diagnostic, and selective catheterization of the renal vein must be performed. A normal renal venogram demonstrates the entire intralobular venous system to the level of the arcuate vein. In general, the use of epinephrine for better visualization of the smaller vessels is not necessary. However, in the presence of normal renal blood flow, all contrast material is washed out of the renal vein within 3 seconds or less, and occasionally only the main renal vein and major branches are visualized. Thus, in this situation there may be uncertainty about thrombi in major or smaller branches. Then the use of intrarenal arterial epinephrine by decreasing blood flow enhances retrograde venous filling and allows later visualization of the smaller intrarenal veins. An abnormal renal venogram usually demonstrates a thrombus within the lumen as a filling defect surrounded by contrast material (Fig. 49-3). In the presence of partial thrombosis, extensive collateral circulation can be demonstrated. Thus, the presence of such collaterals usually reflects the chronicity of the RVT and may explain the lack of renal functional deterioration.

Renal arteriography was considered originally by many investigators to be preferable to renal venography for the diagnosis of RVT. With renal arteriography, important information is obtained about the status of the renal parenchyma. In addition, the theoretical danger of dislodging the clot material from the renal vein during renal venography and precipitating a pulmonary embolism is avoided. However, this complication has not occurred following renal venography in several extensive radiographic series of patients with RVT [16, 51]. Renal arteriography may be useful in patients being evaluated for RVT associated with renal trauma or tumor because of the common involvement of the renal artery in these conditions. In addition, in the arterial phase, deviation and stretching of the interlobular arteries are usually ob-

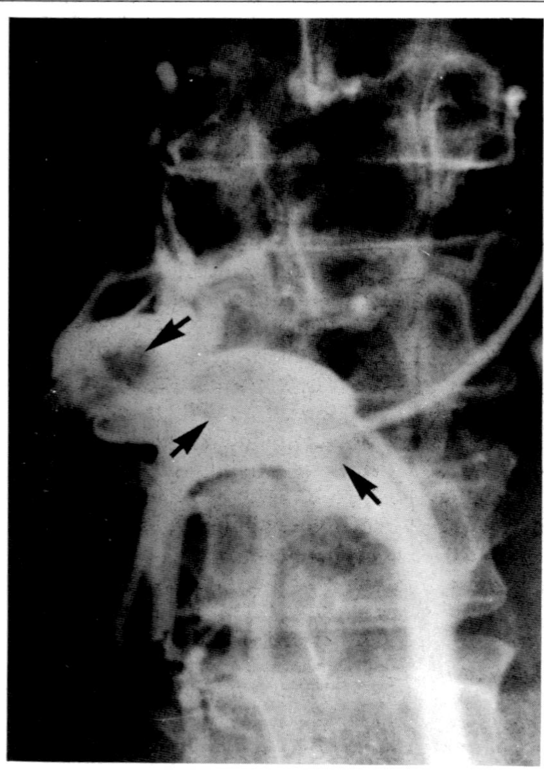

Fig. 49-3. Left renal venography from a patient with RVT. Note the arrows indicating filling defects, which reflect accumulation of thrombotic material surrounded by contrast material. There is complete obstruction of the main renal vein as well as of collateral circulation. (From [51].)

served in these conditions. In the nephrographic phase, the medullary pyramids are more densely opacified than the cortex, and instead of presenting the usual triangular appearance, they appear to bulge and sometimes are even ovoid in appearance.

Renal ultrasonography may be a useful potential diagnostic procedure for the diagnosis of RVT. The sonographic diagnosis of RVT is based on direct visualization of thrombi within the renal vein and inferior vena cava, demonstration of renal vein dilatation proximal to the point of occlusion, loss of normal renal structure, and increase in renal size during the acute phase. These ultrasonography findings, however, usually have to be confirmed with other diagnostic procedures.

Preliminary information has been advanced on the use of combined ultrasonic scanning and Doppler ultrasonography for the diagnosis of RVT. This is a noninvasive technique that essentially measures the renal venous flow velocity. The results of this approach are still very preliminary.

Computed tomography is the procedure of choice for the noninvasive evaluation of acute RVT. Lower attenuation density shows a thrombus and may be identified within the renal vein and inferior vena cava, or the venous diameter may be enlarged owing to obstruction. In general, intravenous infusion of contrast material, together with computed tomography, may help to visualize the thrombus. In the near future it is likely that noninvasive diagnosis of acute RVT may be possible using either ultrasonography and/or computed tomography together with clinical findings. The radiographic findings include enlargement and distention of the affected renal vein, with visualization of the clots within the vein and sometimes extension into the inferior vena cava [26]. Persistent parenchymal opacification with kidney enlargement is usually observed. Capsular venous collaterals, thickening of Gerota's fascia, and pericapsular "whiskering" are often observed.

Preliminary isolated observations suggest that magnetic resonance imaging (MRI) may be, in the future, the diagnostic procedure of choice in the noninvasive diagnosis of RVT. Since MRI produces high-contrast images between flowing blood, vascular walls, and surrounding tissues, vascular potency may be best determined by this technique. A major potential advantage in using this method is the avoidance of contrast material.

Clinical Course and Treatment

The experience to date on the course, prognosis, and treatment of RVT in nephrotic patients is limited. In 1963 Kowal et al. reviewed 65 patients with RVT [42]. Only 14 of these patients were alive after 2 years of follow-up. Unfortunately, clinical data and literature references were given only for the 14 surviving patients. Ten of these patients seemed to have acute RVT. Recurrent thromboembolic phenomena were cited as the most common cause of death. Later, Rosenmann et al. followed 11 of 15 nephrotic patients with RVT over a period of 24 to 115 months [70]. Only 4 of these patients had symptoms suggestive of acute RVT. The incidence of thromboembolic phenomena was high and was fatal in 7 patients. One or more episodes of pulmonary embolism occurred in 7 patients, and 4 had evidence of repeated episodes of thrombosis involving the renal venous system. Three patients received anticoagulant therapy and had no new episodes of pulmonary emboli. These data suggest that the prognosis for nephrotic patients with RVT is poor and is determined by the presence or absence of recurrent thrombotic complications.

In 1970 Richet and Meyrier reviewed 112 cases of RVT reported in the literature. Of the 112 patients, 72 had died, constituting a 64 percent mortality [67]. Earlier, McCarthy et al. estimated the average survival period after the onset of RVT to be 9 months [56]. These data, however, may not be representative of the present prognosis of this entity. First, most of the earlier data about the course and prognosis of RVT were obtained from autopsy studies. Thus, the mortality may have been overestimated. Second, renal insufficiency secondary to RVT was a common cause of death in these patients. Dialysis therapy has, of course, reduced uremic death considerably. Third, the new diagnostic techniques and better understanding of this entity together with better use of anticoagulant therapy have contributed to better management of these patients. Nevertheless, a serious complication in patients with RVT is still thromboembolic phenomena, most often pulmonary embolism.

Lavelle and associates [45a] have recently reevaluated 27 nephrotic patients with RVT, 10 of whom had acute lumbar pain and acute renal failure [53]. Eleven patients died within the first 6 months. Survivors were followed up from 6 months to 19 years. Nephrotic syndrome improved or even disappeared in 12 patients, and renal function did not worsen throughout the follow-up period. The main prognostic factors were initial renal function and type of nephropathy, that is, patients with membranous nephropathy had a significantly better renal function and a lower mortality than did patients with other nephropathies. Initial renal insufficiency was significantly associated with a poor prognosis. In fact, six of the eight patients with acute renal failure died; hemorrhagic complications were the major cause of death in these patients.

Renal function may dramatically improve in patients with acute RVT treated with anticoagulant therapy. Table 49-3 shows the follow-up data on patients with acute RVT compared with chronic RVT. Patients with acute RVT had significant improvement in renal function with anticoagulant therapy during the follow-up period, and it is recommended that these patients be maintained on long-term anticoagulant therapy. Convincing evidence has been gathered suggesting that anticoagulant therapy reduces the incidence of new thromboembolic episodes and often reverses the deterioration of renal function that occurs with acute RVT. Patients treated with anticoagulant therapy may have recanalization of the renal vein, and in some instances a total dissolution of the clot may occur [4]. Heparin is the initial therapy of choice. In patients with a large RVT and pulmonary embolism, the clearance of heparin is increased, and these patients may need higher doses of heparin in the early stages of therapy. Although the dosage of heparin varies from patient to patient, the aim is to maintain the clotting time of 2 to 2.5 times normal. In general, because of fewer complications, continued infusion of heparin is preferable to intermittent intravenous administration. Warfarin therapy is instituted once the patient has been treated with heparin for 5 to 7 days and the partial thromboplastin time is within the desired range. Warfarin is started orally with small loading doses. A common clinical problem with warfarin therapy is the drug interactions related to the kinetics of warfarin such as drug absorption, protein binding, metabolism, and excretion. These drug interactions are very common and may play an important role in the enhancement of or decrease in the anticoagulant effect of heparin. It should also be remembered that drugs such as aspirin and indomethacin may increase the risk of bleeding in these patients owing to the effect on the gastrointestinal mucosa and platelet aggregation. From all these observations, it is obvious that individualization of warfarin therapy is essential, and the clinical status, patient sensitivity, metabolism, and possible drug interactions must all be taken into consideration. Once oral anticoagulant therapy is established, the prothrombin time should be kept at about 1.5 to 2 times normal. The recommended duration of anticoagulant therapy in these patients is difficult to establish. The severity of the hypoalbuminuria is a good indicator of the magnitude of the hypercoagulability. Thus, the nephrotic patient should probably be treated with anticoagulants as long as serum albumin is below 2.5 gm per liter. Relapses with new episodes of acute RVT have been observed after cessation of anticoagulant therapy [13]. It is our belief that in general these patients should be on anticoagulation as long as they have the nephrotic syndrome. Intravenous urokinase or streptokinase has been used in isolated cases with success [45a], especially if these agents are directly infused within the affected renal vein [40a].

Surgical treatment for RVT is rarely used today because the role of thrombectomy in the treatment of RVT has not been established as beneficial. Although marked improvement in renal function has been occasionally observed after thrombectomy, the majority of these patients do not improve with surgery. This modality of therapy may be theoretically useful in patients with acute bilateral RVT who are not otherwise expected to survive the acute episode, especially when recurrent pulmonary emboli occur despite anticoagulation therapy.

Acknowledgment

The author thanks Ms. Lucille Sherrill for excellent secretarial assistance in the preparation of the manuscript.

References

1. Abeshouse, B. S. Thrombosis and thrombophlebitis of the renal veins. *Urol. Cutaneous Rev.* 49: 661, 1945.
2. Alder, A. J., Jundin, A. P., Feinroth, A. P., et al. β-thrombo-globulin levels in the nephrotic syndrome. *Am. J. Med.* 69: 551, 1980.
3. Almer, L. O., and Janzon, L. Low vascular fibrinolytic activity in obesity. *Thromb. Res.* 6: 171, 1975.

Table 49-3. Follow-up data on nephrotic patients with acute and chronic renal vein thrombosis (RVT)

Patients	Urine protein (gm/24 hr)	Creatinine clearance (ml/min)	Serum albumin (gm/dl)	Serum cholesterol (gm/dl)	No. of patients undergoing dialysis
29 with chronic RVT	5.9 ± 3.9* (4.8 ± 2.3)	71 ± 25* (65 ± 29)	2.4 ± 0.7* (2.9 ± 0.7)	370 ± 110* (360 ± 88)	4
4 with acute RVT	5.2 ± 1.2* (5.0 ± 1.2)	76 ± 19* (98 ± 8)**	2.1 ± 0.2* (2.3 ± 0.2)	347 ± 19* (332 ± 26)	0

*Initial laboratory data (mean + S.D.). Data obtained after anticoagulant therapy are shown in parentheses.
**$p<0.05$

4. Andrassy, K., and Ritz, R. Biochemie und klinische Bedeutung von Urokinase. *Dtsch. Med. Wochenschr.* 24: 1015, 1978.
5. Andrassy, K., Ritz, E., and Bommer, J. Hypercoagulability in the nephrotic syndrome. *Klin. Wochenschr.* 58: 1029, 1980.
6. Andrassy, K., Depperman, D., Walter, E., et al. Is beta thromboglobulin a useful indicator of thrombosis in nephrotic syndrome? *Thromb. Haemost.* 42: 486, 1979.
7. Arneil, G. C., MacDonald, A. M., Murphy, A. V., et al. Renal venous thrombosis. *Clin. Nephrol.* 1: 119, 1973.
8. Astedt, B., Issacson, S., Milsson, I. M. Thrombosis and oral contraceptives: Possible predisposition. *Br. Med. J.* 4: 631, 1973.
9. Bang, N., Tygstad, C., Schroeder, J., et al. Enhanced platelet function in glomerular renal disease. *J. Lab. Clin. Med.* 81: 651, 1973.
10. Bennett, W. M. Renal vein thrombosis and nephrotic syndrome. *Ann. Intern. Med.* 83: 577, 1975.
11. Berger, J., and Yneva, H. Hageman factor deposition in membranous nephropathy. *Transplant. Proc.* 3: 472, 1982
12. Bonnar, J., McNichol, G. P., and Douglas, A. S. Fibrinolytic enzyme system and pregnancy. *Br. Med. J.* 3: 387, 1969.
13. Briefel, G. R., Manis, T., Gordon, D. H., et al. Recurrent renal vein thrombosis consequent to membranous nephropathy. *Clin. Nephrol.* 10: 32, 1978.
14. Cade, R. Spooner, G., Juncos, L., et al. Chronic renal vein thrombosis. *Am. J. Med.* 63: 387, 1977.
15. Cameron, J. S., Ogg, C. S., and Wass, V. The complications of the nephrotic syndrome. In J. S. Cameron and R. J. Glassock (eds.), *The Nephrotic Syndrome*. New York: Marcel Dekker, 1988. Pp. 925–949.
15a. Cheng, H. F., Liu, Y. G., Pan, J. S., et al. A prospective study of renal vein thrombosis. XI International Congress of Nephrology, Tokyo, Japan, 1990. Abstracts, p. 6A.
16. Clark, R. A., Wyatt, G. M., and Colley, D. P. Renal vein thrombosis: An underdiagnosed complication of multiple renal abnormalities. *Diagn. Radiol.* 132: 43, 1979.
17. Clarkson, A., MacDonald, M., Petrie, J., et al. Şerum and urinary fibrinogen/fibrin degradation products in glomerulonephritis. *Br. Med. J.* 3: 447, 1971.
17a. Comp, P., and Esmon, C. T. Recurrent venous thromboembolism in patients with a partial deficiency of protein S. *N. Engl. J. Med.* 311: 1525, 1984.
18. Cornog, J. L., Rawson, A. J., Karp, L. A., et al. Immunofluorescent and ultrastructural study of the renal lesions observed in human renal vein thrombosis and the nephrotic syndrome. *Lab. Invest.* 18: 689, 1968.
19. Cosgriff, S. W., Diefenbach, A. F., and Vogt, W., Jr. Hypercoagulability of the blood associated with ACTH and cortisone therapy. *Am. J. Med.* 9: 752, 1950.
19a. Cosio, F. G., Harker, C., Batard, M. A., et al. Plasma concentrations of the natural anticoagulants protein C and protein S in patients with proteinuria. *J. Lab. Clin. Med.* 106: 218, 1985.
20. Deodhar, K. P., Bharlerao, R. A., Kelkar, M. D., et al. Inferior vena cava obstruction. *J. Postgrad. Med.* 25: 64, 1969.
21. Du, X. H., Glass-Greenwalt, P., Kank, K. S., et al. Nephrotic syndrome with renal vein thrombosis: Pathogenetic importance of a plasmin inhibitor. IX International Congress of Nephrology, Los Angeles, June, 1984. Abstracts, June, 1984. P. 84A.
22. Earley, L. E., Haule, R. J., Hopper, J., et al. Nephrotic syndrome. *Calif. Med.* 115: 12, 1971.
23. Edward, N., Young, D. P. G., and MacLeod, M. Fibrinolytic activity in plasma and urine in chronic renal disease. *J. Clin. Pathol.* 17: 365, 1961.
24. Egebert, O. Inherited antithrombin deficiency causing thrombophilia. *Thromb. Haemostas.* 13: 516, 1974.
25. Fisher, E. R., Sharkey, D., Pardo, V., et al. Experimental renal constriction. Its relation to renal lesions observed in human renal vein thrombosis and the nephrotic syndrome. *Lab. Invest.* 18: 689, 1968.
26. Gatewood, O. M., Siegelman, S. S., Fishman, E. K., et al. Renal vein thrombosis in patients with nephrotic syndrome. CT diagnosis. *Radiology* 159: 117, 1986.
27. Godal, H. C., Rygh, M., and Laake, K. Progressive inactivation of purified factor VIII by heparin and antithrombin III. *Thromb. Res.* 5: 773, 1974.
28. Green, D., Arruda, J., Honig, G., et al. Urinary loss of clotting factor due to hereditary membranous nephropathy. *Am. J. Clin. Pathol.* 65: 376, 1976.
28a. Griffin, J. H., Evatt, B., Zimmerman, T. S., et al. Deficiency of protein C in congenital thrombotic disease. *J. Clin. Invest.* 68: 1370, 1981.
29. Hall, C., Pejhan, N., Terry, J., et al. Urinary fibrin/fibrinogen degradation products in nephrotic syndrome. *Br. Med. J.* 1: 419, 1975.
30. Handley, D. A., and Lawrence, J. R. Factor IX deficiency in the nephrotic syndrome. *Lancet* 1: 1079, 1967.
31. Harrison, C. V., Milne, M. D., and Steiner, R. E. Clinical aspects of renal vein thrombosis. *Q. J. Med.* 25: 285, 1956.
32. Hedner, U., and Nilsson, I. M. Antithrombin III in a clinical material. *Thromb. Res.* 3: 631, 1973.
33. Honig, G. R., and Lindley, A. Deficiency of Hageman factor (factor XII) in patients with nephrotic syndrome. *J. Pediatr.* 78: 633, 1971.
34. Hruby, M. A., Honig, G. R., and Shapiro, E. Immunoquantitation of Hageman factor in the urine and plasma of children with nephrotic syndrome. *J. Lab. Clin. Med.* 96: 501, 1980.
35. Hunter, J. Guide to the Hunterian Collection, Part 1: Pathological Series in the Hunterian Museum. Specimen p. 389. A Case of Renal Vein Thrombosis (Lady Beauchamp). Edinburgh: Livingstone, 1966. P. 267.
36. Jackson, B. T., and Thomas, M. L. Post-thrombotic inferior vena cava obstruction. A review of 24 patients. *Br. Med. J.* 1: 18, 1970.
37. Kanfer, A., Fleinknetch, D., Broyer, M., et al. Coagulation studies in 45 cases of nephrotic syndrome without uremia. *Thromb. Diathes. Haemorrh.* 24: 562, 1970.
38. Kauffman, R. H., De Graeff, J., Brutel De La Rivierre, G., et al. Unilateral renal vein thrombosis and nephrotic syndrome. *Am. J. Med.* 60: 1048, 1976.
39. Kauffman, R. H., Veltkamp, J. J., Van Tilburg, N. H., et al. Acquired antithrombin III deficiency and thrombosis in the nephrotic syndrome. *Am. J. Med.* 65: 607, 1978.
40. Kendall, A. G., Lohmann, R. E., and Dossetor, J. B. Nephrotic syndrome: A hypercoagulable state. *Arch. Intern. Med.* 127: 1021, 1971.
40a. Kennedy, J. S., Gerety, B. M., Silverman, R., et al. Simultaneous renal arterial and venous thrombosis associated with idiopathic nephrotic syndrome: Treatment with intra-arterial urokinase. *Am. J. Med.* 90: 124, 1991.
40b. Kisiel, W., Canfield, W., Ericsson, L., and Davie, E. Anticoagulation properties of bovine plasma protein C following activation by thrombin. *Biochemistry* 16: 5824, 1977.
41. Koehler, P. R., Bowles, W. T., and McAlister, W. H. Renal arteriography in experimental renal vein occlusion. *Radiology* 86: 851, 1966.

42. Kowal, J., Figur, A., and Hitzig, W. M. Renal vein thrombosis and the nephrotic syndrome with complete remission. *J. Mt. Sinai Hosp.* 30: 47, 1963.
43. Kuhlmann, U., Stevrer, J., Rhyner, K., et al. Platelet aggregation and β-thromboglobulin levels in nephrotic patients with and without thrombosis. *Clin. Nephrol.* 15: 229, 1981.
44. Lange, L. G., III, Carvalho, A., Bagdasarian, A., et al. Activation of Hageman factor in the nephrotic syndrome. *Am. J. Med.* 56: 565, 1974.
45. Lau, S. O., Tkachuk, J. Y., Hasegawa, D. K., et al. Plasminogen and antithrombin III deficiencies in the childhood nephrotic syndrome associated with plasminogenuria and antithrombinuria. *J. Pediatr.* 96: 390, 1980.
45a. Lavelle, M., Aguilera, D., Maillet, P. J., et al. The prognosis of renal vein thrombosis: A reevaluation of 27 cases. *Nephrol. Dial. Transplantation* 3: 247, 1988.
46. Llach, F. Nephrotic Syndrome: Hypercoagulability, Renal Vein Thrombosis, and Other Thromboembolic Complications. In B. Brenner and J. Stein (eds.), *Contemporary Issues in Nephrology*, Vol. 9. New York: Churchill-Livingstone, 1982. Pp. 121–144.
47. Llach, F. Renal Vein Thrombosis and the Nephrotic Syndrome. In F. Llach, *Renal Vein Thrombosis*. Mount Kisco, N.Y.: Futura, 1983. P. 155.
48. Llach, F. The hypercoagulability and thrombotic complications of nephrotic syndrome (editorial review). *Kidney Int.* 28: 429, 1985.
49. Llach, F., Arieff, A. I., and Massry, S. G. Renal vein thrombosis and nephrotic syndrome: A prospective study of 36 adult patients. *Ann. Intern. Med.* 83: 8, 1975.
50. Llach, F., Koffler, A., and Massry, S. G. Renal vein thrombosis and the nephrotic syndrome. *Nephron* 19: 65, 1977.
51. Llach, F., Papper, S., Massry, S. G. The clinical spectrum of renal vein thrombosis: Acute and chronic. *Am. J. Med.* 69: 819, 1980.
52. Llach, F., Koffler, A., Finck, E., et al. On the incidence of renal vein thrombosis in the nephrotic syndrome. *Arch. Intern. Med.* 137: 33, 1977.
53. Lohman, R. C., Kendal, A. G., Dossetor, J. B., et al. The fibrinolytic system in the nephrotic syndrome. *Clin. Res.* 17: 333, 1969.
54. Luetscher, J. A., and Deming, Q. B. Treatment of nephrotics with cortisone. *J. Clin. Invest.* 29: 1576, 1950.
55. Marciniak, E., Farley, C. H., and Desimone, P. A. Familial thrombosis due to antithrombin III deficiency. *Blood* 43: 219, 1974.
56. McCarthy, L. J., Titus, J. L., and Daugherty, G. W. Bilateral renal vein thrombosis and the nephrotic syndrome in adults. *Ann. Intern. Med.* 58: 837, 1963.
57. Monteon, F., Trevino, A., Exaire, E., et al. Nephrotic syndrome with renal vein thrombosis treated with thrombectomy and anticoagulants. 8th International Congress of Nephrology, Athens, 1981. Abstracts, p. 82.
58. Mukherjee, A. P., Tog, B. H., and Chan, G. L. Vascular complications in nephrotic syndrome: Relationship to steroid therapy and accelerated thromboplastin generation. *Br. Med. J.* 4: 273, 1970.
59. Natelson, E. A., Lynch, E. C., Hettig, R. A., et al. Acquired factor IX deficiency in the nephrotic syndrome. *Ann. Intern. Med.* 73: 373, 1970.
60. Noel, L. H., Zannetti, M., Droz, D., et al. Long-term prognosis of idiopathic membranous glomerulonephritis: Study of 116 untreated patients. *Am. J. Med.* 66: 82, 1979.
61. Ooi, B. S., Ooi, Y. M., and Pollak, V. E. Circulating immune complexes in renal vein thrombosis. 11th Annual Meeting of the American Society of Nephrology, New Orleans, 1978. Abstracts, p. 24A.
62. Panicucci, F., Sagripanti, A., Pinori, E., et al. Comprehensive study of haemostasis in nephrotic syndrome. *Nephron* 33: 9, 1983.
63. Pohl, M. A., MacLaurin, J. P., and Alfidi, R. J. Renal vein thrombosis and the nephrotic syndrome. 10th Annual Meeting of the American Society of Nephrology, Washington, D.C. 1977. Abstracts, p. 20A.
64. Rayer, P. R. O. *Traite des Maladies des Reins et des Alterat Ions de la Secretions Urinaire*. Vol. 2. Paris: J, B. Baillière, 1840. Pp. 590–599.
65. Remuzzi, G., Mecca, G., Marchest, D., et al. Platelet hyperaggregability and the nephrotic syndrome. *Thromb. Res.* 16: 345, 1979.
66. Rennie, J., and Ogston, D. Fibrinolytic activity in malignant disease. *J. Clin. Pathol.* 28: 872, 1975.
67. Richet, G., and Meyrier, A. (eds.), *Liposclerose Retroperitoneal. Thrombose des Veines Renales. Deux Syndromes Retroperitoneaux*. Paris: Masson, 1970.
68. Rosenberg, J. S., McKeena, P., and Rosenberg, R. D. The inhibition of human factor IXa by human antithrombin-heparin cofactor. *J. Biol. Chem.* 250: 8883, 1975.
69. Rosenberg, R. D. Actions and interactions of antithrombin and heparin. *N. Engl. J. Med.* 292: 146, 1975.
70. Rosenmann, E., Pollak, V. E., and Pirani, C. L. Renal vein thrombosis in the adult: A clinical and pathological study based on renal biopsies. *Medicine* 47: 269, 1968.
71. Saito, K., Goodnough, L. T., Makker, S. P., et al. Urinary excretion of Hageman factor (factor XII) and presence of non-functional Hageman factor in the nephrotic syndrome. *Am. J. Med.* 70: 531, 1981.
72. Scanlon, G. T. Radiographic changes in renal vein thrombosis. *Radiology* 80: 208, 1963.
73. Scheinman, J. I., and Stiehm, E. R. Fibrinolytic studies on the nephrotic syndrome. *Pediatr. Res.* 5: 206, 1971.
74. Slick, G. L., Schnetzler, D. E., and Koloyanides, G. J. Hypertension, renal vein thrombosis and renal failure occurring in a patient on an oral contraceptive agent. *Clin. Nephrol.* 3: 70, 1975.
74a. Sorenson, P. J., Knudsen, F., Nielsen, A. H., and Dyerberg, T. Protein C activity in renal disease. *Thromb. Res.* 38: 243, 1985.
74b. Stenflo, J. A new vitamin K–dependent protein: Purification from bovine plasma and preliminary characterization. *J. Biol. Chem.* 251: 355, 1976.
75. Takeda, Y., and Chen, A. Fibrinogen metabolism and distribution in patients with the nephrotic syndrome. *J. Lab. Clin. Med.* 70: 678, 1967.
76. Thaler, E., Blazar, E., Kopsa, H., et al. Acquired antithrombin III deficiency in patients with glomerular proteinuria. *Hemostasis* 7: 257, 1978.
77. Thompson, C., Forbes, C. D., Prentice, C. R. M., et al. Changes in blood coagulation and fibrinolysis in the nephrotic syndrome. *Q. J. Med.* 43: 399, 1974.
78. Trew, P., Biava, C., Jacobs, R., et al. Renal vein thrombosis in membranous glomerulopathy: Incidence and association. *Medicine* 57: 69, 1978.
79. Van Royen, R. A., Deboer, J. E. G., Wilmink, J. M., et al. Acquired factor XII deficiency in a patient with nephrotic syndrome. *Acta Med. Scand.* 205: 535, 1979.
80. Vaziri, N. D., Ngo, J. C. T., Ibsen, K. H., et al. Deficiency and urinary losses of factor XII in adult nephrotic syndrome. *Nephron* 32: 342, 1982.
81. Vaziri, N. D., Paule, P., Toohey, J., et al. Acquired deficiency and urinary excretion of antithrombin III in nephrotic syndrome. *Arch. Intern. Med.* 144: 1802, 1984.

82. Velasquez-Forero, F., and Garcia-Prugue, N. Evaluation of asymptomatic renal vein thrombosis in patients with idiopathic nephrotic syndrome. 17th Annual Meeting of the American Society of Nephrology, Washington, D.C., December, 1984. Abstracts, p. 254A.

82a. Vigano-D'Angelo, S., D'Angelo, A., Kauffman, C. E., et al. Protein S deficiency occurs in the nephrotic syndrome. *Am. Inter. Med.* 107: 42, 1987.

83. Vosnides, G. R., Nicoloupoulon, N., Spanos, H., et al. Renal vein thrombosis in patients with nephrotic syndrome. IX International Congress of Nephrology, Los Angeles, June, 1984. Abstracts, p. 138A.

84. Wagoner, R. D., Stanson, A. W., Holley, K., et al. Renal vein thrombosis in idiopathic membranous glomerulopathy and the nephrotic syndrome. Incidence and significance. *Kidney Int.* 23: 368, 1983.

84a. Walker, F. J. Regulation of activated protein C by a new protein. *J. Biol. Chem.* 255: 5521, 1980.

84b. Walker, F. J. Regulation of activated protein C by protein S. *J. Biol. Chem.* 256: 11128, 1981.

85. Wardle, E. N., Memom, I. S., and Ratogi, S. P. Study of proteins and fibrinolysis in patients with glomerulonephritis. *Br. Med. J.* 2: 260, 1970.

86. Wu, K. K., and Hoak, J. C. Urinary plasminogen and chronic glomerulonephritis. *Am. J. Clin. Pathol.* 60: 915, 1973.

87. Ygge, J. Changes in blood coagulation and fibrinolysis during the post operative period. *Am. J. Surg.* 119: 225, 1970.

88. Yin, E. T., Wessler, S., and Stroll, P. J. Identity of plasma-activated factor X inhibitor with antithrombin III and heparin cofactor. *J. Biol. Chem.* 246: 3712, 1971.

Acute Interstitial Nephritis

Jean-Pierre Grünfeld
Dieter Kleinknecht
Dominique Droz

Acute interstitial nephritis (AIN) is characterized by the association of acute renal failure (i.e., abrupt clinical onset) and infiltration of the renal interstitium by inflammatory cells. This definition, however, needs further comments, since the clinical and pathologic picture may be more complex. Indeed, AIN may occasionally occur in patients with preexistent renal disease and may therefore result in acute exacerbation of preexisting renal failure. In addition, interstitial cell infiltration is commonly found in severe glomerulonephritis. It may also be difficult to clearly differentiate "acute tubulointerstitial nephropathy" comprising acute tubular necrosis, slight interstitial edema, and a few scattered cells in the renal interstitium, from AIN. In AIN, interstitial cell infiltration is usually associated with interstitial edema and mild and/or patchy tubular lesions. The presence of tubular changes in AIN, whatever their mechanism(s), explains why AIN is difficult to differentiate from acute tubular necrosis on clinical grounds.

The real incidence of AIN is unknown. Renal biopsy or autopsy findings are necessary to document the diagnosis. In three recent studies [124, 174, 215] the incidence of AIN in patients with acute renal failure (ARF) undergoing renal biopsy ranged from 8 to 14 percent. However, in two studies only 13 percent [215] and 22 percent [174] of the patients with ARF had renal biopsy. Acute interstitial nephritis represented 1.4 percent [215], 3 percent [173], and 8 percent [124] of all cases of ARF. The real incidence of AIN may have been underestimated in these series because its incidence is unknown in patients with reversible ARF who did not undergo renal biopsy. Wilson et al. emphasized that in none of the patients with AIN was the diagnosis suspected clinically before biopsy [215]. In the series of Buysen and associates [24], the diagnosis was clinically suspected in 11 of 18 patients, and was wrongly suspected in 14 additional cases. This underlines the absolute need for renal biopsy to establish the diagnosis of AIN, thus allowing adequate patient management.

The main causes of AIN are listed in Table 50-1. It is currently stated that drug-induced AIN predominates; however, numerous reports have been published that included fewer than 5 to 10 cases. Moreover, there is no clear information on the incidence of infectious AIN, especially in Asian or European countries where hemorrhagic fevers with acute renal involvement [208] are encountered with some frequency. Of interest, in the series of Richet et al. [174], acute pyelonephritis, mainly complicated with septicemia, represented almost 50 percent of the cases of AIN. In addition, it may be difficult to identify the mechanism involved in patients with systemic infection who receive antibiotics and are therefore exposed to the risk of drug-induced AIN.

Analysis of the renal cell infiltrate may provide an insight into the pathogenetic mechanism(s) involved in AIN and may afford a schematic classification. AIN due to bacterial infection is characterized by massive infiltration of polymorphonuclear neutrophils, whereas in drug-induced AIN, the infiltrate is composed of either mononuclear cells, lymphocytes, and/or plasma cells, or, more rarely, polymorphonuclear eosinophils. However, in AIN related to viral infection the interstitial infiltrate consists of mononuclear cells; eosinophils may predominate in some cases of idiopathic AIN. Thus, characterization of the interstitial cells affords useful but not definitive information on the cause of AIN. More precise typing of lymphocytes with monoclonal antibodies may provide additional clues to the pathogenesis. In addition, interstitial granulomas with epithelioid and giant multinucleated cells may be found in some cases (e.g., drug-induced, sarcoid, or idiopathic AIN). Finally, abundant interstitial cell infiltration is characteristic of acute rejection of a renal transplant (see Chap. 105).

Except for extrarenal symptoms characteristic of certain causes, the clinical renal features of AIN are nonspecific and may mimic those of acute tubular necrosis. The patients may be oliguric or nonoliguric. Kidneys are of normal size or enlarged if cell infiltration is diffuse and profuse. Marked renal uptake of gallium-67 (^{67}Ga) citrate has been noted in AIN [124, 219], but it has also been found in other renal diseases [124]. Few data are available on urinary indices in AIN. In some cases urinary sodium concentrations are in the intermediate range, from 20 to 60 mmol per liter [7, 31, 124], and fractional excretion of sodium is usually > 1, rarely < 1 [123]. Leukocyturia is frequently found [124]. Eosinophiluria is defined as more than 1 percent of urinary leukocytes being eosinophils. At least 200 white cells should be counted. Both Wright's stain and Hansel's stain have been employed. A report has suggested that Hansel's stain was superior in detecting eosinophiluria [152]. Eosinophils in AIN can be activated and lose some of their typical granules, including the major basic protein. Increased urinary levels of this protein were found in AIN [199]. Low percentages of eosinophils in the urine are not very specific and can be found in rapid progressive glomerulonephritis, chronic urinary tract infections, transplant rejection, and atheroembolic renal failure [201]. However, the predictive value of eosinophiluria, while poor at low levels ($< 5\%$), is 40 percent with > 5 percent and reaches 57 percent with > 10 percent urine eosinophils [46a].

Proteinuria is usually not detected. It is not uncommon, however, to find moderate proteinuria ranging from 0.5 to 2 gm per day but occasionally in the nephrotic range. The proteinuria is frequently associated with microscopic hematuria, more rarely with gross hematuria. It was thought that gross hematuria and the nephrotic syndrome were mainly restricted to methicillin-induced and nonsteroidal antiinflammatory drug (NSAID)-induced AIN, respectively, but these features

Table 50-1. Main causes of acute interstitial nephritis

Drug-induced (see Table 50-2)
Infections
- Septicemia
- Leptospirosis
- Hemorrhagic fevers
- Diphtheria, scarlet fever, streptococcal infections, pneumococcal infections, toxoplasmosis, typhoid fever, infectious mononucleosis, measles, brucellosis, syphilis, *Mycoplasma pneumoniae*, tuberculosis, Rocky Mountain spotted fever, Legionnaires' disease, *Campylobacter jejuni* enteritis, *Herpesvirus* infection, *Yersinia pseudotuberculosis* infection, human immunodeficiency virus (HIV) infection

Malignant cell infiltration
- Myeloma, lymphomas, acute leukemias

Systemic diseases
- Systemic lupus erythematosus, sarcoidosis, Sjögren's syndrome

Idiopathic
- With uveitis
- Isolated
- Megalocytic interstitial nephritis

were subsequently observed in other types of AIN as well [124, 173]. In various types of drug-induced or infectious AIN, for example, hemorrhagic fever with renal involvement [208], proteinuria was found to be transiently heavy in the early phase of the disease. The mechanism of proteinuria and hematuria has not been adequately explained, however. The association of proteinuria and hematuria in a patient with ARF may also suggest proliferative glomerulonephritis, particularly rapidly progressive glomerulonephritis with crescents, rather than AIN. This reemphasizes the value of renal biopsy for proper diagnosis.

Drug-Induced AIN

Drug-induced AIN is a rare but increasingly recognized cause of ARF. Nearly 100 drugs have been implicated in hypersensitivity reactions, but the most common are methicillin, ampicillin, sulfonamides, rifampicin, phenindione, and more recently, NSAID. Many other drugs may cause AIN, but the number of cases reported is low (Table 50-2). In many instances the responsibility of the drug is highly suspicious, while in other cases a combination of drugs has been used, or the clinical picture is confused by the symptoms and signs of the underlying disease. Detailed reviews can be found in the recent literature [27, 28, 45, 55, 74, 106].

INCIDENCE

The real incidence of drug-induced AIN is unknown. As stated above, renal biopsy is not performed in most patients with reversible ARF or in critically ill patients with multiple etiologic factors, including possible adverse renal effects due to drugs [124]. In a series of 976 patients presenting with ARF, renal biopsy was done in 218 cases for diagnostic purposes; drug-induced AIN was found in only 8 patients, that is, 3.6 percent of those in whom biopsies were done or 0.8 percent of all cases of ARF [174]. In another report, Linton et al. [124] stated that AIN associated with drugs may account for up to 8 percent of all cases of ARF seen. More recently, we conducted a multicenter 1-year report in 398 patients with drug-induced ARF; this figure represented 18.3 percent of all patients hospitalized with ARF during the same period [107]. Biopsies were done in 81 of these 398 patients, and AIN was proved in 20 patients; this is an incidence of 5 percent of patients with drug-induced ARF and 0.9 percent of all patients with ARF. In a very recent study from the Netherlands, 15 (2.5%) of 591 biopsied patients with ARF had drug-induced AIN [24] (Table 50-3).

A majority of cases of drug-induced AIN are due to antibiotics, mainly β-lactamines, but there is an increasing number of cases after use of NSAIDs [1, 6, 69].

CLINICAL AND PATHOLOGIC FEATURES AND CLINICAL COURSE

In spite of individual variations, drug-induced (hypersensitivity) AIN often has a characteristic clinical picture and course and distinctive renal pathologic changes. The most suggestive features are found in β-lactam–associated AIN, especially with methicillin [6, 74, 110]. The nephritis develops several days or weeks after the initiation of therapy and is not dose dependent. A rapidly progressive ARF is associated with fever, skin rash, arthralgias, sometimes liver involvement, gross hematuria, and blood eosinophilia. Such an onset is inconstantly found in AIN due to NSAIDs (Table 50-4). In an earlier study, the triad of fever, skin rash, and arthralgias was present in only 5 percent and gross hematuria in 10 percent of 19 patients with AIN due to a variety of drugs [110]. In a more recent collaborative study, the positive predictive value of fever, arthralgias, blood eosinophilia, and/or hepatocellular damage was only 0.60, since these symptoms were also present in 24 percent of patients with drug-induced acute tubular necrosis [107]. Eosinophiluria can be detected in some patients provided that the urine is alkalinized and examined with Hansel's stain [152]; however, as stated above, this finding is not specific of drug-induced AIN. Mild to moderate proteinuria and microscopic hematuria are common; a nephrotic syndrome is very rare in non-NSAID–induced AIN. ARF is often of the nonoliguric type, and dialysis was required in 31 percent of our patients.

On early renal biopsy specimens, the pathologic picture is well documented [45, 67, 82]. There is a diffuse or patchy infiltration of the renal interstitium by mononuclear cells, mainly lymphocytes and plasma cells, associated with edema but without marked fibrosis (Fig. 50-1). Eosinophils may be present, especially in the early phase, or absent. In the latter case, the discovery of noncaseating epithelioid granulomas with giant cells (Fig. 50-2) may be a clue to the diagnosis of drug hypersensitivity, especially when the clinical picture is not characteristic [74, 110, 128, 140]. Such granulomas are found in 28 to 45 percent of all patients with AIN [107, 109] (Table 50-5). Tubular lesions are common, ranging from minor changes to extensive necrosis or atrophy of tu-

Table 50-2. Drugs associated with acute interstitial nephritis

Antibiotics	NSAIDs	Other drugs
1. *Pencillin and derivatives*	1. *Propionic acid derivatives*	1. *Analgesics*
Penicillin*	Fenoprofen*	Aminopyrine*
Methicillin*	Ibuprofen*	Paracetamol*
Ampicillin*	Naproxen	Glafenin*
Amoxicillin	Ketoprofen	Floctafenin*
Carbenicillin	Pirprofen	Antrafenin
Oxacillin*	Benoxaprofen	Sulfinpyrazone
Nafcillin	2. *Indoleacetic derivatives*	2. *Diuretics*
Piperacillin	Indomethacin*	Thiazides*
2. *Cephalosporins*	Clometacin*	Triamterene*
Cephalothin	Tolmetin	Tienilic acid*
Cephalexin	Zomepirac	Chlorthalidone
Cephradine	Sulindac	Chlorazanil
Cefoxitin	3. *Anthranilic acid derivatives*	Bendrofluazide
Cefotaxime	Mefenamic acid	Furosemide
Cefaclor	Niflumic acid	3. *Anticonvulsive agents*
3. *Other antibiotics*	4. *Phenylacetic acid derivatives*	Diphenylhydantoin*
Rifampicin*	Diclofenac	Phenytoin
Sulfonamides*	Alclofenac	Phenobarbitone
Cotrimoxazole*	Fenclofenac	Carbamazepine
Polymyxin sulfate*	5. *Piroxicam*	Diazepam
Vancomycin*	6. *Pyrazolone derivatives*	Valproic acid
Erythromycin*	Phenylbutazone	4. *Others*
Spiramycin*	Phenazone	Phenindione*
Tetracyclines	7. *Salicylates*	Allopurinol*
Minocycline	Diflunisal*	Cimetidine*
Piromidic acid	Aspirin	Captopril*
Norfloxacin	Salicylazosulfapyridine	Bethanidine*
Ciprofloxacin	5-Aminosalicylic acid ?	Ajmaline
Ethambutol		Clofibrate
Isoniazid		Amphetamine
Gentamicin ?		Alpha methyldopa
Lincomycin ?		Alpha interferon
Acyclovir*		D-Penicillamine
		Warfarin sodium
		Paraaminosalicylic acid
		Gold and bismuth salts
		Azathioprine
		Radiocontrast agents
		Herbal medicines

*Sometimes with granulomas.

Table 50-3. Incidence of drug-induced acute interstitial nephritis in patients with acute renal failure

Study	Total number of patients with ARF	Patients with renal biopsy	Patients with biopsy-proven AIN	
			No.	Percent
Richet et al. [98]	976	218	8	0.8[a]
Linton et al. [124]	108	—	9	8.3[a]
French collaborative study [58]	2175	81[b]	20	0.9[a]
Buysen et al. [24]	—	591	15	2.5[c]

[a]Of total patients with ARF.
[b]Only 398 patients with drug-induced ARF were considered.
[c]Of biopsied patients with ARF.

Table 50-4. Comparison of some clinical features of β-lactam– and NSAID-associated acute interstitial nephritis

	β-lactam	NSAIDS
Number of cases	153	36
Age (yr)	Any age	64.6 ± 2.1
Male : female ratio	3 : 1	1 : 2
Duration of therapy	15 days	5.4 mo
Fever, rash, and/or eosinophilia	80%	19%
Eosinophiluria	83%	13%
Nephrotic syndrome	<1%	83%
Requirement for dialysis	17%	36%
Agent most commonly responsible	Methicillin (65%)	Fenoprofen (61%)

Source: Modified from [1], [3], and [40].

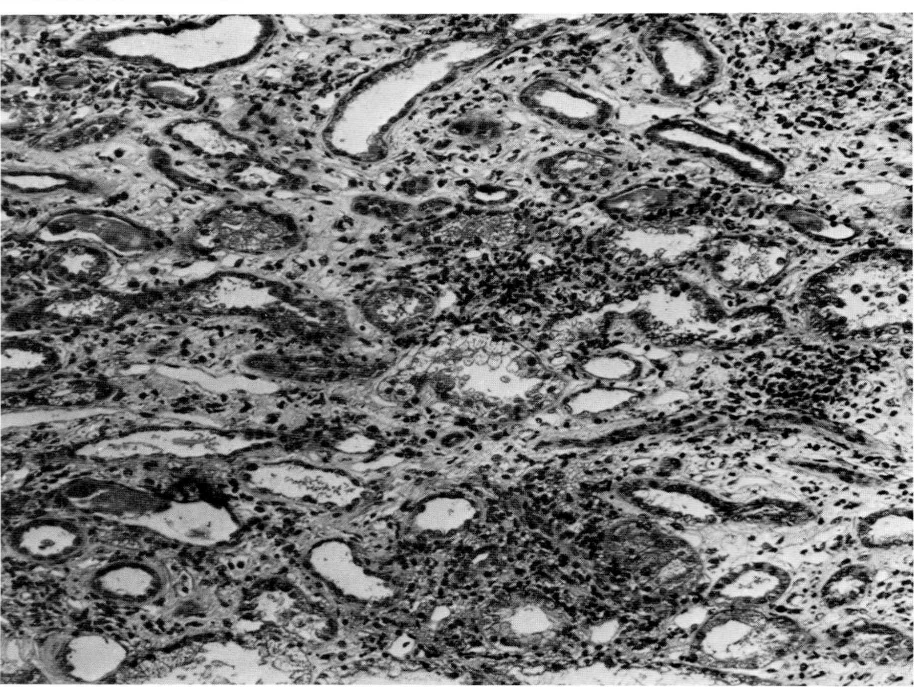

Fig. 50-1. AIN related to penicillin therapy. (Masson's trichrome, ×200.) The interstitial tissue is edematous and infiltrated by mononuclear cells and some neutrophils. Tubular cells are necrotic.

bular epithelial cells. Glomeruli and vessels are normal, except in rare cases with vasculitis or preexisting chronic renal disease. Immunofluorescence studies are generally negative. In a few cases, however, linear staining of IgG and/or C3 has been found along the tubular basement membrane (TBM), namely, in AIN after methicillin, ampicillin, phenylhydantoin, NSAIDs, and allopurinol [74]. On late renal biopsies (beyond the twentieth day), only signs of chronic interstitial nephritis may be present, including interstitial fibrosis, tubular atrophy, and occasional small lymphocyte infiltration [82, 113].

Laboratory tests for diagnosing hypersensitivity reaction do not have a high degree of sensitivity or specificity, excluding perhaps some tests done in AIN due to penicillins. A rise in serum IgE is found in only half of the reported cases. Circulating antibodies to the drug are sometimes found in patients with AIN due to penicillin, rifampicin, or glafenin and derivatives [110]. Circulating anti-TBM antibodies were detected in only a few cases due to methicillin, cephalothin, and diphenylhydantoin [74]. The lymphocyte transformation test and the lymphocyte migration test were inconstantly positive in some cases of AIN due to a variety of drugs [110].

Renal recovery is usual when the responsible drug is promptly withdrawn. Persistent renal failure or even death has been observed when the offending agent is continued or discontinued too late [67, 74, 104]. Recov-

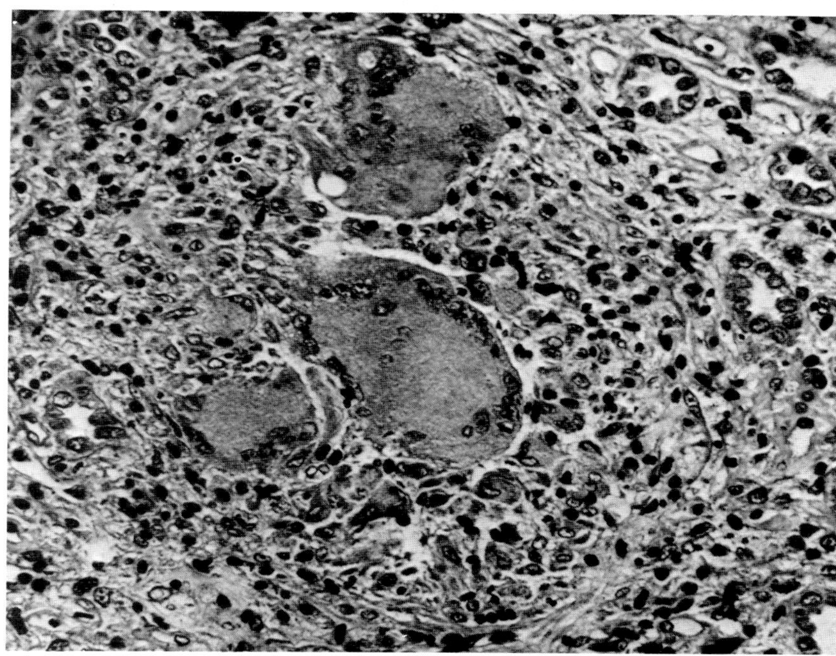

Fig. 50-2. Same patient as in Fig. 50-1. (Masson's trichrome, ×450.) Note presence of epithelioid and three giant cells in the interstitium. The granuloma is surrounded by lymphocytes and some neutrophils.

Table 50-5. Main clinical features and outcomes of acute interstitial nephritis with and without granulomas

	Granulomas	No granulomas
Number of cases	12	31
Drugs involved		
NSAID	8%	29%
Analgesics	50%	19%[a]
β-lactams	17%	26%
Others	25%	26%
Fever, rash, arthralgias, hematuria, and/or hepatic damage	33%	68%[a]
Eosinophilia	8%	32%
Oliguria	50%	29%
Permanent renal damage	50%	13%[b]

[a]$p<0.05$.
[b]$p<0.01$.
Source: Modified from [60].

ery is more frequent in nonoliguric than in oliguric patients and when severe tubular damage with basement membrane rupture is present [86]. A higher incidence of persistent renal impairment is also found in cases with renal granulomas than in those without granulomas [45, 109]. Recently, attention has been drawn to the possible mechanisms of interstitial fibrogenesis. Mediators and growth factors such as platelet-derived growth factors, which promote collagen fibrosis from fibroblasts, have been identified [52]. From experimental work performed in rats, it has also been proposed that increasing intrarenal ammonia may result in perpetuating tubulointerstitial damage through the activation of the alternate complement pathway [200].

Some reports suggest that steroids may improve the renal lesions and hasten recovery [20, 67, 74, 124, 165], whereas in other studies patients did not respond to steroid therapy [50, 74, 162]. Steroid therapy should be especially considered in cases of AIN with renal granulomas, since permanent renal damage is more frequently observed in these patients [109, 140, 205]. Galpin et al. [67], Laberke and Bohle [113], and Buysen and associates [24] observed a more complete return to baseline creatinine values in steroid-treated patients than in untreated patients. Linton et al. [124] treated 7 patients with AIN who did not recover promptly with 60 mg of prednisone daily for periods of 6 to 12 days; in all patients, renal function returned to baseline level within an average of 10 days. A prompt response within 72 hours was observed after short courses of high-dose methylprednisolone in 7 other patients who all regained normal renal function [165]. In another dialyzed patient, high-dose methylprednisolone (500 mg daily for 3 days) followed by a short course of prednisone therapy resulted in dramatic improvement; serum creatinine decreased to 2.0 mg per deciliter, and hemodialysis was no longer necessary [64]. Despite these favorable results, no controlled studies are available, and the indications for steroid therapy are still a matter of debate. It seems advisable to consider the risks and benefits of steroids in any individual patient with drug-induced AIN [6]. Neilson [145] believes that a limited course of high-dose prednisone is advisable for biopsy-proven AIN if renal failure has persisted for more than 1 week after removal of any inciting factor, and that steroids should be discontinued if no response is obtained after 3 to 4 weeks of therapy.

AIN ASSOCIATED WITH ANTIBIOTICS

β-*Lactamines*. These antibiotics, including penicillins and cephalosporins, often give the most characteristic picture of drug-induced AIN (Table 50-6).

METHICILLIN. About 150 cases of methicillin-induced AIN have been reported during the past 20 years in patients of all ages [67, 74], but unreported cases probably far exceed those reported. The true incidence of adverse renal reactions to methicillin would be 1 to 2 percent in all patients taking the drug but ranges from 12 to 20 percent in selected patients [6]. This incidence is much higher than that observed with any other antistaphylococcal antibiotic and does not seem to be related to the more widespread use of methicillin than of other β-lactamines. Methicillin is now much less prescribed, and very few cases of AIN due to this drug have been reported during the past few years [24, 74, 210].

Patients developing AIN received normal doses of methicillin for 10 to 20 days. The interval between the beginning of treatment and the appearance of renal symptoms ranges from 2 to 60 days. As defervescence following treatment of the infectious process is obtained, temperature rises again. High-grade fever, skin rash, and eosinophilia (10 to 60 percent of the leukocyte count) are found in only one third of total patients [74], indicating that the diagnosis of AIN should be considered in the absence of these symptoms. In most of the patients examined, the urinary sediment shows eosinophiluria, which ranged up to 33 percent of the urinary leukocytes in the study of Galpin et al. [67].

ARF is nonoliguric in two thirds of patients, with a high fractional excretion of sodium and a low urine-to-plasma creatinine concentration [7, 124]. Hemodialysis may be required. Tubular dysfunction has been described in nonoliguric patients, including impaired urinary concentration, impaired urinary acidification, and renal salt wasting with impaired ability to excrete potassium [74, 210].

Table 50-6. Acute interstitial nephritis associated with β-lactam antibiotics. Main clinical and pathologic features

1. Time of development ranges from 2 to 60 days
2. Fever, skin rash, hematuria, blood eosinophilia, and/or eosinophiluria are common
3. Nonoliguric renal failure with mild proteinuria is frequent
4. Renal biopsy shows interstitial infiltrates composed of lymphocytes, often eosinophils, sometimes epithelioid cell granulomas
5. Circulating anti-TBM antibodies are inconstantly found
6. Renal recovery is usual after withdrawal of the offending drug; steroid therapy seems effective in some cases

The renal histopathologic picture is characteristic of drug-induced AIN as described above. In some cases, extensive epithelioid cell granulomas may be responsible for persisting renal damage [74, 140]. In only a few patients, dimethoxyphenylpenicilloyl (DPO) hapten and linear IgG and C3 deposits were detected along the TBM, with IgG and DPO deposits along the glomerular basement membrane in one patient [74]. Circulating anti-TBM antibodies were also found in a few patients. Electron microscopy showed dense deposits within the TBM [6, 113] or extensive TBM damage [67]. Small- and medium-sized lymphocytes infiltrated between the tubular epithelial cells or between these cells and the TBM, which sometimes appeared ruptured. These lesions, called *tubulitis*, are not specific of AIN.

The outcome is favorable after withdrawal of therapy, and 90 percent of patients recover fully 1 year after the renal insult [74]. Persisting renal damage or death occurs in the remaining patients. A favorable effect of steroid therapy is suggested by several studies, the most convincing being that of Galpin et al. [67]. After withdrawal of methicillin, these authors compared the course of 8 patients receiving 60 mg of prednisone daily and that of 6 patients who received no steroids. In treated patients, serum creatinine returned to a baseline level in an average of 9.3 days, compared with 54 days in untreated patients. Moreover, in 6 of the 8 treated patients, serum creatinine returned to normal levels, whereas this was observed in only 2 of the 6 control patients.

PENICILLIN. Fewer than 20 cases of AIN due to penicillin have been reported, including only a few cases in the past 10 years [74, 79, 98, 107, 165]. We observed only 1 patient with penicillin-induced AIN out of 760 patients with ARF. Clinical and pathologic features (Figs. 50-1 and 50-2) are similar to those of methicillin-induced AIN. Large doses of penicillin have usually been prescribed, ranging from 12 to 60 million units per 24 hours for 7 to 21 days [74].

OTHER PENICILLIN DERIVATIVES. Some cases of AIN have appeared following the use of *ampicillin* [74, 110, 113, 124, 140, 165], *amoxicillin* [6, 24, 110, 161], *carbenicillin* [6, 74], *oxacillin* [6, 74, 161], *nafcillin* [74], and *piperacillin*. Symptoms suggesting a hypersensitivity reaction are less frequent than in methicillin- or penicillin-related AIN. Renal immunofluorescence sometimes shows linear deposits of immunoglobulins along the TBM. On electron microscopy, these deposits appear to be electron-dense and are located inside the TBM [6, 113]. Circulating antipenicillin antibodies were found in two instances [74, 110]. Since all antibiotics of the penicillin class seem capable of producing AIN, renal and extrarenal symptoms may recur when patients are given another penicillin derivative or even a cephalosporin [6, 74].

CEPHALOSPORIN. Cephalosporin antibiotics share a common β-lactam structural ring with penicillin and may also induce AIN. Some episodes have been attributed to *cephalothin* [6, 74, 110], *cephalexin* [6, 124, 161], *cephradine* [74], *cefoxitin*, *cefotaxime* [74], and *cefoteran* [150]. Cross-sensitization to penicillin or another penicillin derivative has sometimes been found [74, 110], whereas in other instances no reactivation of the disease occurred when patients were rechallenged with penicillins [6].

RIFAMPICIN AND ANTITUBERCULAR DRUGS. Since 1972, about 100 cases of ARF have been reported after rifampicin [110], but only a minority of these have had biopsy-proven AIN. The reason for rifampicin treatment was always tuberculosis, and in most instances patients were treated by an intermittent regimen (twice or thrice weekly) or discontinuously (resumption of therapy after a medication-free period). Such regimens are no longer used, and cases of AIN due to rifampicin have been rare during the past few years. Recent cases were more frequently seen with continuous daily therapy [37, 74, 149] than with accidental intermittent therapy [110].

Presenting symptoms appear a few hours to several days after taking the drug and include dizziness, chills, fever, lumbar pain, dark urine, myalgias, nausea, and vomiting. Skin rash, eosinophilia, thrombocytopenia, hemolysis, and hepatitis are uncommon but are possible features. Severe oliguric ARF of abrupt onset is frequent and requires dialysis, but renal failure may develop insidiously [74, 149]. Renal tubular dysfunction with glucosuria, potassium wasting, and an acidifying defect has been reported [37, 74, 166, 201]. Proliferative glomerulonephritis and nephrotic syndrome with fusion of epithelial cell foot processes were associated features in a few patients [83, 149].

Renal biopsies were available in half of the patients. Moderate interstitial infiltrates with mononuclear cells, rarely eosinophils, were frequent and were associated with focal tubular atrophy or necrosis. Renal interstitial granulomas are sometimes present [127a]. Severe and prominent tubular lesions with mild interstitial changes were seen in the remaining cases of ARF. Immunofluorescence studies were usually negative [6, 110].

By the indirect antiglobulin technique, high circulating levels of antirifampicin antibodies have been found in many patients; antibody titers decreased steadily after completion of therapy but could be detectable several months later [74]. The relationship between these antibodies and the onset of ARF remains obscure. Hemolysis and hypotension are documented in only a few cases.

Almost all patients recover normal renal function, but permanent renal damage has been observed [27, 74]. There is no proof that steroid therapy hastens recovery, and some patients developed AIN despite concomitant prednisone therapy [74].

AIN has been documented in a few patients simultaneously taking *isoniazid* and *ethambutol*, or isoniazid or ethambutol alone [74]. Rifampicin was associated in three instances [74] but was given twice as the renal function improved, and was reintroduced in another case without subsequent deterioration of renal function. It therefore seems unlikely that rifampicin could have initiated the renal damage in these patients.

SULFONAMIDES. AIN or granulomatous interstitial nephritis was described in the 1940s at autopsy of patients who had received sulfonamides shortly before death [6]. About 40 cases of AIN have appeared in the recent literature, following the use of normal or high doses of *cotrimoxazole* (trimethoprim and sulfamethoxazole) [23, 24, 47, 74, 107, 110, 113, 124, 140, 165]. Previous chronic renal insufficiency, without adequate reduction of cotrimoxazole dosage, may be a predisposing factor. Two renal transplant patients developed an adverse renal reaction despite ongoing therapy with methylprednisolone. Fever, rash, and blood eosinophilia are lacking in many patients, but on renal biopsy interstitial eosinophilic infiltrates or a granulomatous reaction is frequently seen. These patients often have immunologic evidence of an adverse reaction to the drug, with increased IgE levels, circulating immune complexes, positive lymphoblastic transformation tests, and positive skin tests [74, 110]. Renal recovery is not the rule.

OTHER ANTIBIOTICS. Biopsy-proven AIN from *vancomycin* has been reported in only one patient [43]. Fever, skin rash, eosinophilia, and/or eosinophiluria and renal failure developed in some patients after they received vancomycin. These signs reversed when vancomycin was stopped. AIN was suspected on a clinical basis, but renal biopsy was not done [74].

Tetracyclines [24, 113] and *minocycline* [74] have rarely been incriminated in AIN. Only one case of AIN following the use of *polymyxin B* is known [74]; on renal biopsy, the interstitial lesions were typical, showing eosinophils, but the responsibility of the concomitant use of methicillin cannot be excluded. Twenty years ago *polymyxin E* (colistin) was responsible for many cases of AIN; renal failure was dose dependent and occurred without any sign of hypersensitivity. Renal biopsies showed interstitial infiltrates composed of lymphocytes and plasma cells, without eosinophils.

AIN developed in four instances after *erythromycin* therapy [107, 124, 177, 187]; other drugs were also given concomitantly in two of these patients. *Spiramycin* induced an acute granulomatous interstitial reaction in one patient [140]. *Gentamicin* could have been responsible for two questionable cases of AIN; in the first, there was more evidence that cotrimoxazole was the offending agent, and in the second, lincomycin was an associated drug [74]. *Netilmicin*, another aminoglycoside, may possibly have induced granulomatous AIN in another case [107]. AIN has been associated with *quinolone derivatives*, such as *piromidic acid* [161, 179], *norfloxacin* [14], and *ciprofloxacin* [4, 81, 85, 175].

AIN ASSOCIATED WITH NONSTEROIDAL ANTIINFLAMMATORY DRUGS. NSAIDs can cause deterioration of renal function through a number of different mechanisms [1, 6, 28, 42, 46, 50, 69, 105] (see Chap. 44). The incidence of AIN due to NSAIDs is unknown. Renal abnormalities attributed to fenoprofen (the drug involved in one half to two thirds of patients with NSAID-induced AIN) were reported to be fewer than 1 case per 5300 patient years of treatment [20]. In one study, NSAID acute interstitial nephritis was diagnosed in 1 percent of 460 renal biopsies reviewed over an 18-month period [1]. In a collaborative study, the figures were 2 percent of 398 patients with drug-induced acute renal failure [107].

Acute interstitial nephritis may occur in patients taking any group of NSAIDs (see Table 50-2). *Propionic acid derivatives* have been the most frequently implicated, including *fenoprofen* [12, 28, 74, 79, 96, 108, 128, 192], naproxen [2, 12, 20, 24, 28, 74, 159, 171], ibuprofen [12, 24, 74, 108, 134, 159, 201], ketoprofen, pirprofen, and benoxaprofen [74]. The agents responsible in the remaining cases were *indomethacin* [24, 28, 73, 74, 79], tolmetin [12, 74], zomepirac [12, 48, 74, 135], phenylbutazone [74, 161], clometacin [108, 117, 118], diflunisal [74], mefenamic acid [2, 16, 21, 28, 74, 97, 98, 151], niflumic acid [110], noramidopyrine [110], diclofenac [28, 30, 178, 218], alclofenac [160], piroxicam [28, 62, 141, 182], aspirin [74], phenazone [74], and various pyrazolone derivatives [161]. Sometimes, two or more NSAIDs were given and it was not possible to identify the main offending agent [2, 108, 121, 184].

Careful analysis of well-documented cases shows that several features distinguish NSAID acute interstitial nephritis from β-lactam–induced AIN, the most common picture of allergic drug-induced AIN [1, 6, 42, 69] (Tables 50-4 and 50-7). Patients are older and predominantly female, and only few of them have evidence of an underlying renal disease. They are treated as ambulatory patients for a chronic disease, and renal insufficiency has a progressive onset, discovered several months or years after the initiation of NSAID treatment.

Presenting features include edema (68 percent of patients), oliguria or anuria, very rarely fever, rash, eosinophilia, and/or eosinophiluria. Heavy proteinuria within the nephrotic range occurred in 83 percent of patients with NSAID interstitial nephritis compared with a frequency of fewer than 1 percent in β-lactam–induced AIN when patients with an underlying glomerulonephritis are excluded [5]. The mean rate of protein excretion was 11.3 gm per 24 hours, with a range of 5 to 26 gm per 24 hours [69]. Renal failure is usually severe, requiring dialysis therapy in one third of patients, but nephrotic syndrome without renal failure has been reported [1, 32]. Extrarenal signs may occasionally be present. One patient taking diflunisal had erythroderma [74]. Hepatitis was commonly associated with clometacin nephrotoxicity [117, 118]. Vasculitis was reported in a few cases of AIN associated with the use of fenoprofen [63], indomethacin + niflumic acid [110], and diclofenac [121]. Most of the patients taking mefenamic acid had abdominal pain, diarrhea, and vomiting before renal failure was diagnosed [97, 151].

Renal histology findings showed that the interstitium was edematous, with either diffuse or focal mononuclear cell infiltrates and sometimes eosinophils (30 percent of biopsies), even in cases in which blood or urinary eosinophilia was absent [1, 6, 69]. Epithelioid cell granulomas were rarely found [74, 108, 110, 128, 184]. The tubules were focally atrophic or dilated. Extensive necrosis of the tubular epithelium was sometimes associated. Interestingly, in all cases with heavy proteinuria, the glomerular aspect was that of "minimal change" nephrotic syndrome with diffuse fusion of epithelial cell foot processes by electron microscopy. However, such diffuse fusion has been found in biopsies of some patients without significant proteinuria [74, 135]. Mild mesangial proliferation or mesangial electron-dense deposits have been observed in a few patients, sometimes associated with membranous and subendothelial deposits [1, 97, 134, 141]. Immunofluorescent staining is usually negative, and IgG and C3 granular staining along the TBM has been noted only in individual cases [12, 74].

Pathologic studies show that there is sometimes an overlap between AIN and structural renal lesions other than minimal change disease. Various degrees of superimposed interstitial inflammation have been reported in patients with acute tubular necrosis due to NSAID [96]. In other cases, AIN and membranous glomerulopathy were associated on renal biopsy specimens [30, 34, 40]. The pathophysiology of these findings is unclear.

These clinical and pathologic features are at variance with those found in the hemodynamic variety of ARF due to NSAID and attributed to prostaglandin synthesis inhibition (Table 50-8). NSAID interstitial nephritis may be easily suspected when the nephrotic syndrome and renal insufficiency appear together after a few days or weeks after drug exposure. In some cases, diagnosis

Table 50-7. Acute interstitial nephritis associated with NSAIDs: main clinical and pathologic features

1. Onset of renal failure is highly variable (often months after taking NSAIDs)
2. Heavy proteinuria with nephrotic syndrome is common
3. Rash, fever, hematuria, blood eosinophilia, and/or eosinophiluria are rare
4. Rapid decline in renal function with a nonoliguric course is common
5. Renal biopsy shows interstitial infiltrates with lymphocytes, sometimes eosinophils, rarely epithelioid cell granulomas; glomeruli often have only minimal changes
6. Circulating anti-TBM antibodies are absent
7. Renal recovery is usual; the efficacy of steroid therapy remains controversial

Table 50-8. Clinical features observed in the three major types of NSAID-associated acute renal failure

	Prerenal failure	Acute tubular necrosis	Acute interstitial nephritis
Groups	I	II	III
Mean age (yr)	73.2	61.9	60.2
Male : female ratio	2.7	2.1	2.1
Mean duration of the ARF period	8.4 days	4.5 days	13.8 days[a]
Heavy proteinuria	0%	21%	33%
Hypersensitivity signs	0%	31%	100%[b]
Reversibility of renal failure	89%	79%	25%[a]

[a] $p < 0.02$.
[b] $p < 0.001$.
Source: Modified from [59].

may be difficult when renal insufficiency is progressive and if more than one drug has been given. Other causes of nephrotic syndrome are then discussed. Features suggestive of an allergic reaction may be absent or may occur in patients with predominant acute tubular necrosis (Table 50-8). Therefore, when the clinical picture is nonspecific, a renal biopsy is mandatory.

In most cases AIN and the nephrotic syndrome resolve with the discontinuation of NSAIDs over a period ranging from several weeks to 1 year [45, 162]. However, in our experience, a high percentage of patients had permanent renal damage, compared to the outcome of those suffering from other types of NSAID-related renal lesions (Table 50-8). Persisting renal damage has also been documented by several workers [2, 16, 28, 108, 184]. Chronic dialysis was sometimes required [16, 74] and deaths were reported [2, 63, 74]. A beneficial effect of steroids on recovery is not clearly stated, since renal function frequently improves before steroid administration. At the present state of knowledge, steroid therapy seems no more beneficial than simply discontinuing the drug [6, 50, 162]. Since recurrence of AIN has been reported after use of the same [1, 118, 160, 167] or of a different NSAID [12], it seems preferable to avoid any future use of NSAIDs in these patients.

The nephrotic syndrome and AIN are frequently associated but may develop independently, suggesting that they represent two examples of glomerular and tubulointerstitial toxicity of NSAIDs. In this setting, the mechanism by which renal failure occurs remains speculative. It has been proposed that the decreased glomerular filtration rate seen in this type of NSAID nephropathy results from the additive effects of interstitial nephritis, reduced renal blood flow (by inhibition of prostaglandin synthesis), and reduced hydraulic permeability and/or surface area of the glomerular filtration barrier in cases of heavy proteinuria [1]. It is noteworthy that the association of nephrotic syndrome and AIN has been observed almost exclusively with NSAIDs, especially with propionic acid derivatives, and is likely to occur with any new NSAID. Only a few other drugs have been responsible in individual cases for this type of pathologic process, including ampicillin [172], a combination of amoxicillin and cefaclor [11], diphenylhydantoin [91], rifampicin [149], and alpha interferon [8].

A cell-mediated response to NSAID is suggested by the prolonged drug exposure, by the low incidence of clinical and laboratory signs of hypersensitivity, and by the finding that the predominant cells in the interstitial infiltrates are T lymphocytes with a high proportion of cytotoxic-suppressor (CD8) cells [12, 63, 192]. Cheng and associates [36] have found that the percentage of CD8 cells and the tubular expression of HLA-DR were greater in the early than in the late stages of NSAID interstitial nephritis. It has been postulated that inhibition of prostaglandin synthesis could facilitate lymphokine release by the infiltrating lymphocytes and the development of a delayed hypersensitivity reaction, by removing the inhibitory effect of prostaglandins on T-cell function or by shunting arachidonic catabolism toward the lipooxygenase pathway [42]. Proinflammatory substances, especially leukotrienes, are then produced and may explain the massive proteinuria. The additional necrotizing vasculitis found in a few patients could also occur through a T-cell–dependent mechanism [63].

AIN ASSOCIATED WITH OTHER DRUGS

Analgesics. With the widespread use of *paracetamol* (acetaminophen), many cases of reversible acute tubular necrosis with or without hepatic necrosis have been reported, but biopsy-proven AIN has been demonstrated in a few patients [110, 165, 187], including one with renal interstitial granulomas. Various drugs, however, were sometimes taken in association [187].

Glafenin, an aminochloroquinolein derivative, is a common cause of toxic ARF in Europe [110]. Like the NSAIDs, glafenin inhibits prostaglandin synthesis. The renal toxic damage is usually induced by supratherapeutic doses of glafenin and is possibly related to intratubular obstruction by a glafenin metabolite. However, several cases of documented AIN are also known, following either therapeutic [39, 110, 140] or supratherapeutic doses of glafenin [140]. Renal recovery is usual. Only one of our patients developed oliguric ARF unresponsive to steroid therapy and died from gastrointestinal hemorrhage. Circulating antiglafenin antibodies may be found in patients with AIN and a hemolytic reaction [140] but are usually absent in cases of direct nephrotoxicity [74]. Tests for humoral or cellular immunity are often positive [39, 110, 140]. Renal biopsy shows interstitial infiltrates with mononuclear cells, eosinophils, and often granulomas, with extensive tubular damage [108, 110, 140].

Proesmans et al. [164] reported the case of a young boy receiving repeated overdoses of glafenin who presented with recurrent episodes of ARF associated with eosinophilia, an increase in serum IgE level, and a positive Coombs test. Renal biopsy showed "acute tubulo-interstitial nephritis with a few foci of chronic interstitial inflammation."

Not surprisingly, we observed two cases of AIN with granulomas due to floctafenin, a glafenin derivative [110]. Circulating antibodies against floctafenin and glafenin were found, and a lymphocyte transformation test was positive for both drugs.

Sulfinpyrazone is a uricosuric analgesic used in treating gout and an antiplatelet agent sometimes prescribed after myocardial infarction. It also inhibits platelet prostaglandin synthesis and reduces the urinary excretion of PGE_2 and kallikrein [15], as do NSAIDs. Many reversible cases of ARF are due to this drug, but renal biopsy is usually not performed because of recent myocardial infarction. Nevertheless, some patients have had documented AIN due to sulfinpyrazone. Renal biopsy showed typical AIN with eosinophils [74] or only mild cellular infiltration of the interstitium and focal tubular necrosis [15]. There was no evidence of intratubular precipitation of uric acid crystals in the reported cases of AIN, but other mechanisms may have been operative as well, including inhibition of renal prostaglandin synthesis [15]. Renal function improved in all patients with discontinuation of sulfinpyrazone.

Diuretics. Few cases of AIN following the use of diuretics appeared until recently. During the 1970s, Lyons et al. [127] and Fuller et al. [66] reported 5 patients with proliferative or membranous glomerulonephritis who received *chlorothiazide/hydrochlorothiazide* or *furosemide,* or a combination of both, and who developed rash, fever, or blood eosinophilia. Renal biopsy showed intense interstitial infiltration with lymphocytes and numerous eosinophils superimposed on the preexisting glomerular lesions. Cessation of diuretics and institution of steroid therapy was followed by prompt improvement in renal function and return of serum creatinine to the previous baseline level. A hypersensitivity reaction was the favored diagnosis in one patient because of the immediate occurrence of fever, chills, and anuria after reinstitution of thiazide therapy [127]. The authors recalled that both thiazide diuretics and furosemide are chemical derivatives of sulfonamide, an agent that has been clearly recognized as a cause of allergic AIN. However, although hypersensitivity reactions are not uncommon after the use of thiazides and furosemide, the reported adverse reactions included allergic purpura with glomerulonephritis and renal vasculitis rather than AIN [127]. The agent to which the reaction was directed was also questionable. Since these first publications, biopsy-proven AIN was observed after chlorthalidone [74], hydrochlorothiazide alone [124, 129], and bendrofluazide [165] in patients without previous evidence of glomerular disease. These episodes suggest that thiazides rather than furosemide may be the responsible drug.

More recently, there have been several reports that renal failure may develop insidiously in patients treated with a combination of *hydrochlorothiazide* (or another thiazide) with *triamterene* [74, 110, 129, 199]. All patients had normal renal function prior to therapy and none had preexisting renal disease. ARF was often nonoliguric and developed several weeks after initiation of drug therapy. Fever and peripheral eosinophilia were frequently associated with ARF. Renal biopsy showed normal glomeruli and an intense mononuclear cell interstitial infiltrate with few eosinophils. In 12 of 16 patients who underwent biopsies, the prominent feature was the presence of noncaseating interstitial granulomas [107, 110, 129, 205]. In three biopsy specimens strong cytoplasmic immunoperoxidase staining for lysozyme (muramidase) was demonstrated in interstitial mononuclear cells but not in the epithelioid and multinucleated giant cells. Electron microscopy of the granulomas in two cases revealed that the epithelioid cells had "secretory" features characteristic of hypersensitivity granulomas, providing further evidence that cell-mediated immunity was involved in such instances [129]. Direct immunofluorescence studies were negative, and no electron-dense deposits were noted [129]. Withdrawal of the drug led to rapid renal recovery in each case. Although thiazides seem to be the main offending agent in these observations, it is possible that triamterene has a potentiating role, since some cases of AIN have appeared following the use of triamterene alone [74] or in combination with furosemide [129].

A number of cases with ARF due to *tienilic acid* (tricrynafen) have been reported; in most instances, renal failure was attributed to intratubular casts of uric acid. Only four cases of AIN due to this drug are known to us, including one patient who also received phenindione [6, 107, 110]. This diuretic was removed from the market in the United States because of liver and renal complications.

Other Agents. Several cases of AIN following the use of *cimetidine,* a potent H_2-receptor antagonist, are now documented [24, 74, 79, 124, 212]. Sulfinpyrazone was associated in one case [124]. Patients received therapeutic doses of cimetidine for duodenal ulcers or esophagitis. A few weeks later they complained of weakness, fever, and myalgia, leading to the discovery of nonoliguric renal insufficiency with peripheral eosinophilia or eosinophiluria. Renal biopsy showed typical AIN and eosinophils within the interstitium. Using monoclonal antibodies, Watson et al. [212] found a marked increase in the proportion of cytotoxic/suppressor T lymphocytes in the peripheral blood and in the inflammatory infiltrates found in both kidney and muscle; they hypothesized that the cell-mediated dysfunction might also have been responsible for the polymyositis associated with AIN in their patient. Renal improvement did not occur until cimetidine therapy was discontinued. Most patients regained normal renal function, but some residual renal damage was observed [74]. Rechallenge with cimetidine without prednisone resulted in prompt return of signs of AIN in one case. In another case, rechallenge with the drug occurred during prednisone therapy, and renal function continued to improve but worsened again when treatment with steroids was discontinued [74].

Severe hypersensitivity reactions to *allopurinol* with AIN have been described in several patients with previous renal dysfunction [6, 29, 75, 79, 130, 142]. Multisystem involvement with cutaneous vasculitis was frequent in these cases. Renal biopsy showed eosinophilic AIN and sometimes granulomas [142]; in one patient hepatitis with hepatic granulomas was an associated feature [142]. Circulating anti-TBM antibodies were found in one patient, but there were no anti-TBM deposits on renal biopsy examination [75]. A return to baseline renal function was observed after stopping allopurinol. The systemic reaction may have been favored by increased serum levels of allopurinol and of oxypurinol, a metabolite of allopurinol, since both renal insufficiency and diuretics decrease the urinary excretion of these compounds [142].

Only a few biopsy-proven cases of ATN due to *carbamazepine* have been reported [74]. Lymphocyte transformation tests and/or lymphocyte migration tests were positive to the drug but negative in control patients taking carbamazepine. Renal function improved after withdrawal of the drug, spontaneously or after prednisone therapy.

Allergic reactions associated with *diphenylhydantoin* (phenytoin), including renal vasculitis, have been discussed in numerous reports since the late 1930s. Cases of AIN have been more recently described [24, 91, 153]. Circulating anti-TBM antibodies were found in 2 patients, with linear deposits of immunoglobulins along the TBM on renal biopsies [91, 153]. In addition, Hyman et al. [91] were able to demonstrate in their patient the presence of diphenylhydantoin along the TBM, in the renal interstitium, and in the arteriolar walls, and a lymphocyte transformation test to the drug was positive. Undoubtedly, this case provides convincing evidence that the renal damage observed was associated with anti-TBM antibody formation as well as with cellular hypersensitivity.

Phenindione is now much less prescribed than in the 1960s, and this probably explains why no recent additional cases of AIN due to this drug have appeared. Patients usually presented with fever, rash, eosinophilia, oliguric ARF, and often jaundice. The outcome was severe, most patients dying from infection or from the consequences of the underlying illness. Chronic interstitial nephritis was reported in some surviving patients [74].

The possibility of *captopril*-induced AIN deserves more comment. Acute and reversible deterioration in renal function has been reported in many patients with renovascular hypertension treated with this angiotensin converting enzyme inhibitor; only hemodynamic factors seem involved in these cases. Membranous nephropathy without ARF has been documented in other patients, but ARF with a severe hypersensitivity reaction has been observed in very few instances. One hypertensive patient developed skin rash, Coombs-positive hemolytic anemia, peripheral eosinophilia, and ARF with eosinophiluria 7 weeks after the initiation of high doses of captopril therapy (300 mg/day) [74]; the patient also received furosemide and aspirin. Allergic AIN was diagnosed on a clinical basis, but renal biopsy was not performed. Another hypertensive patient presented with a generalized maculopapular rash after 3 weeks of captopril therapy. There was blood eosinophilia without eosinophiluria. Renal biopsy findings were compatible with acute tubular necrosis without evidence of allergic AIN [195]. Biopsy-proven AIN with prominent or occasional eosinophils developed in five other patients, often after usual doses of captopril (50–125 mg/day) given for a few days or weeks [26, 35, 84, 95, 190]. Allergic manifestations were usually present. Renal interstitial granulomas were found in one patient [95], and membranous nephropathy was an associated feature in another patient [26]. Except in the latter case, renal function improved promptly after discontinuation of captopril therapy, with or without steroids. After rechallenge with captopril, renal failure recurred on two occasions in a renal allograft recipient [84]. Subsequent antihypertensive treatment with enalapril did not deteriorate renal function, suggesting that the reaction was specific for captopril. This syndrome has not been reported with any of the other angiotensin converting enzyme inhibitors, but Barnes and associates [10] have described a reversible rash and eosinophilia in a patient treated with enalapril.

Acute interstitial nephritis may be related to the use of *antiviral agents*. Renal dysfunction associated with high bolus injections of *acyclovir* is usually due to crystalluria and obstructive nephropathy, although renal biopsy may reveal foci of interstitial inflammation without tubular necrosis [183]. In two patients with presumed herpes simplex encephalitis, severe but transient nonoliguric acute renal failure developed following slow acyclovir infusions; renal biopsy showed typical AIN with granulomas in one case [169]. AIN and a nephrotic syndrome have been observed in one woman receiving alpha *interferon* for mycosis fungoides [8], but not with the use of beta and gamma interferon. However, Ault and associates [7a] recently reported the case of a child in whom acute tubular necrosis without interstitial infiltrates developed after treatment with gamma interferon.

Other anecdotal reports of AIN were concerned with ajmaline [74, 205], clofibrate, fenofibrate, phenobarbital, azathioprine, amphetamines, alpha methyldopa, para-aminosalicylic acid, and possibly 5-aminosalicylic acid therapy [137, 221], gold and bismuth salts [74], D-penicillamine [61], and radiocontrast agents [74].

DIAGNOSIS

Excluding typical cases, it is sometimes difficult to differentiate drug-induced AIN from other types of AIN. Not uncommonly, the drug is given when the first manifestations of a bacterial or viral infection appear, and chronologic analysis of the manifestations may not be easy [206]. Moreover, more than one drug has sometimes been given [74, 104, 187].

The presence of extrarenal symptoms may be helpful, since most of the drugs capable of inducing AIN are frequently associated with allergic fever, cutaneous reactions (including vasculitis), eosinophilia, and/or hepatic damage. However, drug-induced multisystem involvement is rare in a given patient. AIN associated with vasculitis has been noted in only a few cases after penicillin [113], allopurinol [75], indomethacin [110], and fenoprofen [63]. Hepatic involvement has been particularly observed in AIN after clometacin [118], phenindione [74], rifampicin sometimes [110], and in individual cases after allopurinol [142] and salicylazosulfapyridine [74]. Some cases of hepatic damage without ARF due to clometacin have been reported from France, including acute and chronic active hepatitis, sometimes fatal; in most instances, there is evidence that an allergic mechanism may be operating, but it is not known why some patients develop hepatic rather than renal damage and vice versa. It must be stressed that reported drug-related multisystem damages without renal involvement are by no means a guarantee against a possible occurrence of AIN. Such a hazard has occasionally been observed many years after a drug is marketed.

When the clinical picture and laboratory tests are nonspecific, early renal biopsy may be a clue to the diagnosis of drug-induced AIN, and its indication should be liberal when this diagnosis is suspected. Undoubtedly, the discovery of interstitial infiltrates composed of eosinophils and/or epithelioid cell granulomas is a strong argument in favor of a hypersensitivity reaction to a drug, although granulomas may occasionally be found in AIN due to other causes. In AIN without eosinophilic or granulomatous interstitial infiltration, the pathologic picture may be similar to that observed in infectious AIN (see below). In some cases it is difficult to determine whether AIN is drug-induced, is of infectious origin, or is of unknown mechanism [113, 140].

Acute Interstitial Nephritis Associated with Systemic Infections

SEPTICEMIA

Acute interstitial nephritis complicating septicemia is characterized by diffuse or focal interstitial infiltration by polymorphonuclear neutrophils, which form microabscesses in some cases [74, 78, 173]. In most patients renal failure develops progressively. The high incidence of proteinuria above 2 gm per 24 hours without the nephrotic syndrome has been emphasized [173]. In other patients oligoanuria is the presenting manifestation [78, 173]. A CT scan with contrast enhancement shows typically wedge-shaped or round hypodense areas, probably due to focal ischemia, and diffuse nodular images, probably corresponding to regions with heavy cell infiltration or microabscesses [138]. Various microorganisms are involved, including *Escherichia coli, Staphylococcus, Proteus,* and *Candida albicans* [168]. The origin of infection lies within the urinary tract in many cases, and urinary tract obstruction is often found. However, AIN may follow extraurinary tract infections [173].

Renal function returns to normal only when infection is rapidly controlled by antibiotics and, if need be, by surgery. Uncontrolled infection resulted in extension of suppurative renal changes and in death in 30 percent of patients reported by Richet [173]. In other cases in which days or weeks were required to control infection, renal biopsies have shown clearing of neutrophils and microabscesses, infiltration by round lymphoplasmacytic cells, and interstitial fibrosis. The latter change may result in residual chronic renal failure [173]. In this regard, the conclusions drawn from the study of retrograde acute bacterial pyelonephritis in the rat may be relevant. It has been shown in this model that cell-mediated immunity is not involved in the subsequent development of chronic renal lesions (see ref. in [74]). Granulocytes rather than lymphocytes were responsible for the pathologic changes of chronic pyelonephritis resulting from acute kidney infection. Indeed, chronic kidney damage was a consequence of acute suppuration occurring in the first 3 days after onset of infection and not of persistent infection [72]. If the experimental results are applicable to humans, rapid control of acute infection would be of prime importance to prevent renal scarring.

Acute infectious interstitial nephritis may be superimposed on chronic renal disease (e.g., chronic pyelonephritis or chronic tubulointerstitial nephritis induced by analgesic abuse). In these cases, the duration of antibiotic therapy may be more critical than it is in patients without preexisting renal disease. The issue was recently discussed by Meyrier et al., who advocated long-term antibiotic therapy to eradicate infectious renal foci completely [139].

It should be emphasized that acute renal failure in septicemia may be related to various mechanisms [74, 78], including infectious AIN, glomerular proliferative changes, intraglomerular thrombi or immune deposits, drug nephrotoxicity, or drug-induced AIN. The exact diagnosis is based on careful analysis of the clinical features, and if necessary, on renal biopsy data.

LEPTOSPIROSIS

Leptospirosis is a rare cause of ARF in Western countries [78, 216]. Its incidence is approximately 60 per year in the British Isles [216]. In some tropical areas it accounts for almost 40 percent of ARF due to tropical diseases [188]. The *Leptospira interrogans* species comprises the pathogenic serotypes, all of which can induce ARF. In Europe, renal failure is more frequent in Icterohemorrhagiae infection. Rodents, mainly rats, are the most important reservoirs. Leptospires enter the host through abrasions of the skin or through the mucosa. The diagnosis is based either on identification of leptospires in blood or urine or on serologic tests.

Usually ARF is preceded by fever, myalgia, and jaundice (with mild abnormalities of liver tests) in subjects at risk from exposure to contaminated water. Oliguria or anuria accompanies renal failure, but nonoliguric forms are frequent. ARF is associated with severe hypercatabolism; the renal failure lasts 1 to 3 weeks and often requires dialysis. A polyuric phase heralds recovery. The disease may also include thrombocytopenia, petechiae, conjunctival suffusion, gastrointestinal hemorrhage, aseptic meningitis, and atrial fibrillation (due to myocarditis) [216]. Intensive supportive management and antibiotic administration (Herxheimer reaction has been reported after penicillin) [216] are required. Mortality can be as high as 50 percent in jaundiced elderly patients. Death is related to vascular collapse, hemorrhage, and cerebral complications. In contrast, AFR is milder in other cases not associated with jaundice and may be prerenal due to volume depletion [188]. In rare cases, renal involvement presents as a hemolytic-uremic syndrome [188].

Since 1929, it has been known that renal involvement in leptospirosis is characterized by tubulointerstitial lesions [78]. Interstitial edema and infiltration by mononuclear cells and a few eosinophils are observed; neutrophils may be present during the early stage [188]. Glomerular lesions are absent or discrete. Interstitial changes have long been considered secondary to acute tubular necrosis [78]. Recently Sitprija et al. [189] indicated that cell infiltration chronologically preceded tubular necrosis and was triggered by direct invasion of the kidney by leptospires. In experimental leptospirosis, leptospires gained first access to glomeruli through the bloodstream, causing transient and mild injury. Then leptospiral antigen was demonstrated in the interstitium and, in a later stage, in renal tubular epithelium [189]. Nonspecific effects of infection may be involved in ARF, such as hypovolemia, blood hyperviscosity, severe jaundice, or intravascular coagulation, or endotoxinemia for some serotypes [188]. In one patient with severe leptospirosis, anti-GBM antibodies were found in the blood, and linear fixation along the glomerular and tubular basement membranes was demonstrated by immunofluorescence [49]. In another patient with *Leptospira pomona* infection, complement deposits were seen in glomeruli by immunofluorescence [115].

HEMORRHAGIC FEVER WITH RENAL SYNDROME (HANTAVIRUS NEPHROPATHY)

Hemorrhagic fever with renal syndrome (HFRS) encompasses a large group of diseases observed in various parts of the world [208]. Korean HFRS attracted great attention during the Korean War. Its causative agent, an RNA virus, was first isolated in 1976 from the rodent *Apodemus agrarius* and from affected patients [119]. It was named Hantaan virus after the Hantaan river, which runs near the 38th parallel between North and South Korea [119]. HFRS is a major public health problem in Asia and in some European countries. Hemorrhagic nephrosonephritis in the Soviet Union and Songo fever or epidemic hemorrhagic fever in China have involved several thousand cases annually since 1913 [119]. Nephropathia epidemica has been observed in Scandinavia since 1934. Hemorrhagic fever has also been described in Eastern Europe, in the Balkan countries, and in Japan. "War nephritis," which affected thousands of soldiers in various wars, may be related to HFRS [119]. Recently, HFRS was recognized in Western European countries [207].

The Hantavirus group belongs to the Bunyaviridae family and comprises several viruses, of which Hantaan virus is the prototype; Seoul, Pummala (in Scandinavia and Western Europe), Leaky, Prospect Hill (in North America), and Fojnica (in the Balkans) are the other representative serotypes.

Various rodents (*Apodemus agrarius* in Korea, *Clethrionomys glareolus* in Scandinavia, and *Rattus*) are reservoirs of Hantaviruses. Humans are infected through inhalation of viruses eliminated by lungs, saliva, and urine of rodents. No interhuman contamination occurs. The disease develops predominantly in rural areas, but urban epidemics have been reported in Seoul and Osaka [119]. Epidemics have also been observed in research laboratories using infected rats in Asia and Europe [51]. The diagnosis is based on serologic tests. Specific antibodies to Hantavirus appear during the first week of symptoms, reach a peak at the end of the second week, and may persist indefinitely. This may allow retrospective diagnosis in patients labeled as affected by "acute epidemic glomerulonephritis" or leptospirosis on clinical grounds [208]. Seropositive subjects (and rodents) have been identified in the Americas, but human disease has not been reported so far [208].

In Scandinavia and Western Europe, HFRS predominates in males. The incubation period ranges from 9 to 35 days. Onset is marked by sudden fever and chills lasting 4 to 10 days. The presence of bradycardia (or the absence of tachycardia proportional to temperature) and of acute myopia has been stressed [116, 208]. Then loin pain, sometimes unilateral mimicking renal colic, occurs accompanied by digestive symptoms. Oliguria and renal failure appear on the fourth to the tenth day of the disease, when fever and loin pain have usually subsided. Heavy (1 to 30 gm/liter) and transient proteinuria is frequently found, associated with microhematuria. Kidneys are enlarged, but blood pressure is normal. Early and short-lived thrombocytopenia (in 20 to 50 percent of cases) is the most common extrarenal feature. Hemorrhage is minimal; conjunctival hemorrhage is found in fewer than 20 percent of patients. There is often a mild increase in serum transaminase and lactic dehydrogenase levels. Involvement of the central nervous system is rare, limited to headache, vomiting, sleepiness, and a slight increase in protein content of the cerebrospinal fluid.

Renal failure usually has a rapidly favorable course; hemodialysis is rarely needed. Proteinuria disappears between the ninth day and the second week and renal function returns to normal between the second and the sixth week of the disease. Mortality is below 1 or 0.5 percent. No significant late sequelae persist [114, 208].

The most prominent difference from East Asian HFRS resides in the mortality. In Asia, mortality ranges from 9 to 26 percent and is currently about 10 percent [22, 76, 119, 208]. Thrombocytopenia and hemorrhagic manifestations are more frequent, as are shock and neurologic and pulmonary symptoms [76, 208]. The more severe clinical course in Asia could be related to the higher virulence of the virus, which causes more widespread and intense capillary damage.

Renal biopsy shows mainly tubulointerstitial changes: tubular dilation, tubular cell atrophy, interstitial edema, medullary hyperemia or hemorrhages, and a cell infiltrate composed of lymphocytes and, less frequently, plasma and polymorphonuclear cells [206, 208]. Focal immune deposits have been found in glomeruli of patients in Scandinavia [100] but not in Western Europe [208].

VARIOUS INFECTIOUS DISEASES

The association of scarlet fever and diphtheria with acute interstitial nephritis was first described at the end of the nineteenth century [78]. In scarlet fever, early nephritis occurring in the first week or even in the first few days of the disease was characterized by diffuse or focal infiltration of the renal interstitial tissue by mononuclear cells [78]. Subsequently, since the antibiotic era, poststreptococcal AIN has been rarely reported [74]. Recently, Ellis et al. collected 13 cases of AIN in children, 10 of which were believed to be secondary to remote infection, including streptococcal infection in 7. Tubular dysfunction was demonstrated in 6 cases. All children recovered completely within approximately 2 months [56].

In addition to leptospirosis, streptococcal infections, and Hantavirus nephropathy, AIN has been described in association with other infectious diseases, such as typhoid fever [58], toxoplasmosis, infectious mononucleosis [111, 199], measles [6], brucellosis [143], syphilis [78, 143], *Mycoplasma* pneumonia, Rocky Mountain spotted fever [74], Legionnaires' disease [31, 158], *Yersinia pseudotuberculosis* infection [94], herpesvirus infection [186], tuberculosis [131], *Campylobacter* (or *Helicobacter*) *jejuni* enteritis [170], and human immunodeficiency virus (HIV) infection [151a].

Acute Interstitial Nephritis in Systemic Diseases

It should be stressed that renal interstitial cell infiltration is common in severe forms of glomerulonephritis, mainly with epithelial crescents. These cases, however, are beyond the scope of this review, since rapidly progressive renal failure is most probably ascribed to intense proliferative glomerular changes, although interstitial infiltration may also be contributive. In this regard, inflammatory cells and occasionally granulomas [140] may be found in the renal interstitium of patients with Wegener's granulomatosis and ARF, but these changes are consistently associated with severe glomerular lesions [28, 140].

In contrast, a few patients with *systemic lupus erythematosus* (SLE) presented with oligoanuric ARF related to prominent tubular and interstitial disease, with granular deposits of complement and IgG along the tubular basement membrane, whereas glomerular changes were slight and could not account for renal failure [103, 202]. One patient with *Sjögren's syndrome* developed focal TBM deposits of IgG and C3 and marked renal interstitial cell infiltration. Renal failure progressed in a few weeks and was then dramatically improved by prednisone and cyclophosphamide [217].

Sarcoid granulomatous nephritis may present as isolated rapidly progressive renal failure (see ref. in [80]). Serum calcium concentration is normal. Renal biopsy shows the interstitium to be infiltrated by noncaseating granulomas surrounded by lymphocytes and a few scattered plasma cells. Glomeruli are normal. Renal function is rapidly improved by corticosteroid therapy.

Acute granulomatous interstitial nephritis was recently reviewed by Mignon et al. [140]. Nine of their ten cases were related to drug hypersensitivity; in one patient, the mechanism was undetermined. Renal granulomas are characterized by the presence of epithelioid cells deriving from macrophages. In addition, granulomas may contain giant multinucleated cells formed by the fusion of macrophages. Cells other than those of the monocyte-macrophage system are also found. Granulomas are considered as markers of delayed-type hypersensitivity [140].

Acute Interstitial Nephritis in Malignancies

Infiltration of the kidneys by tumor cells is a frequent feature in lymphomas. It has been reported in 6 to 60 percent of cases in autopsy studies [44]. Rarely, in 0.5 percent of patients [44], it is responsible for rapidly progressive or acute renal failure in various lymphomas [44, 101], including Burkitt's lymphoma [185]. Both kidneys are enlarged by massive infiltration by tumor cells. Other causes of renal failure should be excluded (e.g., ureteric obstruction due to lymph node compression, ureteric wall infiltration, retroperitoneal fibrosis, renal artery or vein obstruction, hypercalcemia, amyloidosis, uric acid nephropathy or nephrolithiasis, or drug- or radiation-induced urinary tract damage). Kidney radiotherapy and/or chemotherapy may rapidly improve renal function when lymphomatous infiltration is involved [44, 101, 185]. Acute renal failure has also occasionally been ascribed to tumor cell infiltration in myeloma [68, 174] and in acute [126] or chronic lymphocytic leukemia [155, 203].

Idiopathic Acute Interstitial Nephritis

In some patients the cause of AIN could not be determined. Drug hypersensitivity and infections were not causative factors, and these cases have been reported as "idiopathic" [56, 157, 191, 213]. In other patients extrarenal features have been found. Hyun and Galen have described a case of AIN with elevated serum levels of IgG, IgM, and IgE (as in previously reported cases), persistent hypereosinophilia, and granular IgE and C3 deposits in renal tubules [93]. Dobrin et al. [53] first drew attention to the association of acute eosinophilic interstitial nephritis with anterior uveitis. They also noted the presence of bone marrow–lymph node granulomas in the 2 children studied. Nakamoto et al. later reported a similar association of acute eosinophilic interstitial nephritis with bone marrow granulomas in a 44-year-old male patient. Renal function improved with steroid therapy [144]. In idiopathic AIN, associated or not with uveitis, generalized proximal tubular dysfunction or isolated renal glycosuria may be found [90, 119a, 191]; it has even been observed in the absence of significant renal failure [95a].

The association of AIN with uveitis represents a relatively distinct clinical entity [53, 120, 196]. Uveitis, bilateral or unilateral, usually anterior but rarely posterior, may precede, occur concomitantly with, or follow nephritis. The disease has been observed in children [23, 120] and in adults [25, 196], mainly in female patients. The clinical course in an adult patient we observed in 1976 is depicted in Fig. 50-3. Interstitial infiltrate is composed of lymphocytes, plasma cells, and in approximately 50 percent of the cases, of eosinophils [103]. Mesangial immunoglobulin deposits have occasionally been

Fig. 50-3. Clinical course of AIN with uveitis in a 33-year-old woman. The first episode of anterior uveitis antedated and the second episode followed ARF. Renal failure improved dramatically concomitantly with prednisone administration.

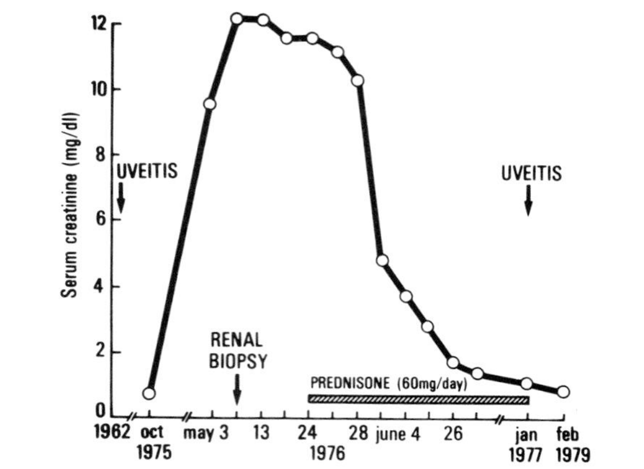

seen [120]. Corticosteroid therapy may lead to dramatic improvement in renal function [196], but spontaneous improvement has been described [25]. It should be recalled that AIN with uveitis may also occur in leptospirosis, in toxoplasmosis, and in sarcoidosis (see above).

Megalocytic interstitial nephritis, first described by Zollinger, is a quite exceptional cause of ARF [41]. On electron microscopy it is characterized by renal interstitial infiltration by large, round histiocytes containing crystalloid, electron-lucent, rod-shaped bodies in lysosomes. Its relationship with kidney malakoplakia and with xanthogranulomatous pyelonephritis has been discussed [57].

AIN and Acute Tubular Necrosis

When the interstitial infiltrates are moderate, it may be difficult to differentiate AIN from acute tubular necrosis (ATN). There is some overlap between the two entities [154]. Tubular changes are commonly observed in AIN, and it has been suggested that they contribute to the renal prognosis [112]. In some cases it is not clear whether ATN is primary with a prominent cellular interstitial reaction, or AIN is primary with secondary tubular lesions. Some drugs such as rifampicin, cephalosporins, and glafenin may induce pathologic pictures described as either AIN or ATN. Sex may also modulate the renal response, cell infiltration being more intense in female than in male rats after gentamicin administration [112]. Other nephrotoxins, such as those derived from the mushroom *Cortinarius orellanus,* induce "acute tubulointerstitial nephritis," since in early renal biopsy, both tubulorhexis and infiltration by lymphocytes and plasma cells are associated [60].

Pathophysiology

EXPERIMENTAL MODELS

Various experimental models (see reviews in [136, 145, 214]) have been devised to induce renal interstitial cell infiltration, with or without tubular change, but only a few mimic human AIN as defined above. The available models are schematically classified into two main groups: humorally mediated and cell mediated. There is, however, some overlap between these two groups.

Antitubular Basement Membrane (TBM) Disease. Steblay and Rudofsky first immunized guinea pigs with a crude preparation of rabbit tubular basement membranes in Freund's adjuvant. The animals developed tubular damage and interstitial infiltration by mononuclear and giant cells. Immunofluorescent study showed linear IgG fixation along the TBM, and circulating anti-TBM autoantibodies were found in the serum. Animals developed renal insufficiency. Linear fixation along the glomerular basement membrane (GBM) and circulating anti-GBM antibodies were also present in half of the animals, but the glomeruli were normal by light microscopy [194]. Strain differences in susceptibility were observed and shown to segregate with the major histocompatibility complex [92]. The disease was easily transferred with antibodies but not with immune cells, suggesting a prominent role for anti-TBM antibodies [209]. Both IgG_1 and IgG_2 isotypes transferred the disease and generated autoimmune amplification [77]. The injection of heterologous antiidiotypic antibodies inhibited anti-TBM antibody production and decreased tubulointerstitial damage. Guinea pig anti-TBM antibodies enhanced in vitro antibody-dependent cell-mediated cytotoxicity [148].

Anti-TBM disease has also been developed in Brown-Norway and in Lewis × Brown-Norway F_1 rats by immunization with Sprague-Dawley rat kidney homogenate or with bovine TBM [197]. Passive transfer of sensitized cells in normal rats resulted in mild tubulointerstitial nephritis (TIN). The characterization of renal inflammatory cells in Brown-Norway rats with anti-TBM disease showed sequential accumulation of T cells, with prevalence of T helper cells, then monocytes/macrophages after an initial polymorphonuclear leukocyte infiltration phase coincident with anti-TBM and complement deposition. Monocyte/macrophage interstitial infiltration increased after 2 weeks of the disease and constituted 40 percent of the total cells recovered from infiltrates when fibrosis and histologic evidence of chronicity of the lesions were apparent [132]. When given early and in high dose, daily cyclophosphamide administration impaired immune response and prevented TIN lesions or reduced progression when given in animals with established disease [3]. Administration of cyclosporin A or a stable analogue of prostaglandin E_1 (PGE_1) also impaired anti-TBM antibody production and reduced tubulointerstitial damage [71, 204].

Anti-TBM disease induced in mice differs from that in guinea pigs and rats by its delayed onset and by the predominant mechanism of cellular immunity. The severity of the lesions is related to the H-2 phenotype and not to the magnitude of the antibody response. The SJL mouse has been found to be the most susceptible [147, 181]. Much work has been done to determine the cell type involved in the antigen-recognition phase, immune-regulatory phase, and effector phase. Nephritogenic T helper cells producing interstitial nephritis are usually CD4+ and class II major histocompatibility complex (MHC) restricted. The effector cells can be either CD4+ or CD8+ but are usually CD8+ and class I MHC restricted. Effector T cells produce injury by two general mechanisms. They can induce a delayed-type hypersensitivity response, with the release of lymphokines and mediators, or they can produce cell-mediated cytotoxicity against a target by releasing proteases called perforins [133].

Using monoclonal antibody reactivity, the target antigen of anti-TBM disease has been characterized as a glycoprotein called 3M-1, of 48 kd molecular weight, secreted by proximal tubular cells and attached to the outer surface of the tubular basement membrane [38]. Although segments of this glycoprotein are preserved among different species, within a given species some polymorphism of expression occurs, and the first important determinant of susceptibility to anti-TBM disease is that the individual must express 3M-1 in order to focus the nephritogenic immune response. Very recently Butkowski and associates [23a] purified and characterized a new tubular basement membrane component—TIN antigen—of 58 kd, reactive with anti-TBM antibody–associated tubulointerstitial nephritis. Although 3M-1 and TIN antigen have distinct amino acid composition, these two molecules are presumably related since they react with the same human anti-TBM autoantibodies.

Immune Complex–Mediated Tubulointerstitial Nephritis. These models are characterized by granular deposits along the TBM or in the interstitium. None results in AIN, but all produce interstitial cell infiltrates. They can be triggered by either autologous or heterologous antigens [136, 145, 214].

Various autologous antigens have been used in rabbits to induce tubular atrophy, interstitial fibrosis, some cell infiltrates, and IgG, and C3 deposits along the TBM. Recently, tubulointerstitial lesions related to immune complex deposition have been induced in rats by immunization against Tamm-Horsfall protein (TH). There is a direct relationship between the serum level of anti-TH antibodies and the severity of the renal lesions. Immune deposits appeared to be a consequence of in situ formation of immune complexes [87]. Passive administration of antiserum to TH into normal rats produced tubulointerstitial disease. A similar experimental model raised in rabbits and using endotoxin-free TH resulted in chronic tubulointerstitial disease in the absence of anti-TH antibodies [13]. Although antibodies to TH have been found in humans with urinary tract infection, especially in those with vesicoureteral reflux, the relationship among these antibodies, tubular TH deposits, and renal interstitial inflammation is not clear [33]. Spontaneously, certain strains of autoimmune mice (NZB/W, MRL/1) developed, late in their diseases, deposits along the TBM, with mononuclear cell infiltration [5].

With regard to heterologous antigens, chronic immunization of rabbits with large doses of bovine serum albumin (BSA) led, in addition by membranous glomerulopathy, to the appearance of granular deposits containing BSA, immunoglobulin, and C3 along the TBM and in the interstitium [136].

Cell-Mediated Tubulointerstitial Diseases. Heterologous or autologous antigens have been used in animals. Injection into the renal cortex of heat-aggregated bovine gamma globulin in sensitized rats or guinea pigs resulted in local mononuclear cell infiltrates with tubular damage [136]. The reactivity to the antigen could be transferred with lymphocytes but not with serum. Only insoluble antigens could trigger a delayed-type hypersensitivity reaction in the renal interstitium. In other models in mice, heterologous antigens (such as lymphocytic choriomeningitis virus) were used and induced chronic tubulointerstitial damage via cell-mediated reactions [214].

With regard to autologous or homologous antigens, experiments were performed in Lewis rats [9, 198]. Within 2 weeks after immunization by Lewis or Brown-Norway rat renal basement membranes, renal insufficiency and severe tubulointerstitial lesions developed in these animals [198]. No immune deposits or anti-TBM antibodies were found. Cell infiltrates and tubular lesions were obtained by transfer of lymph node or spleen cells. The lesions could be obtained using renal basement membranes prepared from a number of rat strains, except Lewis and Wistar Furth rats, which are TBM antigen negative.

Interest has recently been renewed in the spontaneous chronic tubulointerstitial nephritis of kdkd mice. These mice developed, after 8 weeks of life, a fatal disease resembling human nephronophthisis. Despite the presence of severe tubulointerstitial changes, no antibodies directed against tubulointerstitial determinants were demonstrated. The development of the tubulointerstitial lesions in kdkd mice was markedly inhibited by T cell depletion induced by thymectomy or by treatment with adoptively transferred T cells from CBA/Ca mice [146]. The destructive renal lesions are mediated by tubular antigen-specific H2-K–restricted effector T cells of Ly T-2+ phenotype whose expression is facilitated by abnormal contrasuppression [102].

PATHOPHYSIOLOGY OF HUMAN AIN

Is human AIN an anti-TBM–mediated disease? Anti-TBM antibodies may be found, albeit rarely, in human AIN. Normal individuals who express the 3M-1 antigen (identified as the target of anti-TBM disease) are immunologically tolerant to this tubular molecule. This tolerance can be broken by impairing normal surveillance systems with immunosuppressive drugs, by introducing a foreign antigen that cross-reacts with a self-structure, or by creating a neoantigen. Such a mechanism of a hapten-carrier conjugate responsible for anti-TBM antibody production is possible in some cases of human AIN related to drugs. In fact, in a case of methicillin-associated AIN with anti-TBM antibodies, the DPO breakdown products of methicillin were bound to TBM together with IgG [17]. In a case of phenytoin-associated AIN with anti-TBM antibodies, phenytoin and IgG were present with a linear pattern along the TBM [91]. However, in the great majority of cases of AIN, evidence for anti-TBM–mediated disease is lacking. No correlation was found between titers or circulating anti-TBM antibodies (when present) and disease activity [153]. Moreover, the passive transfer of human anti-TBM antibodies failed to induce tubulointerstitial lesions in rats, whereas these antibodies were found to bind in vitro to rat or guinea pig TBM [19, 153]. Therefore, even though anti-TBM antibodies are observed in rare cases of AIN, there is little evidence that they are of pathogenic significance. This is emphasized by the observation of patients with a renal transplant who develop anti-TBM antibodies that bind to the graft tubules but do not significantly impair renal function [180].

Is human AIN an immune complex–mediated disease? Circulating immune complexes may be found in occasional patients [110]. Some rare cases of AIN with granular deposits of IgG along the TBM have been reported in SLE [202] as well as in Sjögren's syndrome [217]. In this latter condition, it has been observed that, whereas the interstitial infiltrate contains predominantly T cells, nodules of B cells are also present [176]. However, in the great majority of AIN cases, granular tubular deposits of IgG are not found. Scanty deposits of C3 can be seen along the TBM, but such deposits are also frequently observed in various renal diseases in the absence of tubulointerstitial damage (personal observations).

Very recently a new model of true AIN was induced in mice when animals with specific antibody were challenged with appropriate hapten-carrier antigen [99]. In this model humoral reactions with immune complex formation appear to play a major role in inducing the renal lesions and can be relevant to some human drug-induced AIN.

Is human AIN a cell-mediated disease? Several histopathologic findings favor cell-mediated mechanisms. Immunofluorescence studies are frequently negative. Interstitial infiltrates consist often of lymphocytes and mononuclear cells, although eosinophils and plasma cells may also be present. Epithelioid and giant-cell granulomas may be found, suggestive of a delayed-type hypersensitivity reaction. Positive skin tests with the offending drug or in vitro tests of cell-mediated reactivity have been reported in some cases [98, 110].

The use of monoclonal antibodies recognizing T- and B-cell subset surface antigens has allowed better characterization of the cells infiltrating the kidney in AIN. The majority of the interstitial lymphocytes are of the T lineage and are CD3 positive. With the exception of Sjögren's syndrome [176], few B cells are present, usually representing fewer than 10 percent of the cells. In the majority of the cases, CD4+ cells and CD8+ cells are present in the same sample in quite equal proportion or with a slight predominance of one phenotype over the other. Activation markers of the infiltrating T cells have been tested in some studies involving HLA class II molecules [18, 89] or CD25 (IL_2 receptor) expression [18]. Natural killer or large granular lymphocytes constitute a small proportion of the infiltrating lymphocytes [36]. The importance of the monocyte/macrophage population has been underlined, since up to 50 percent of the infiltrating cells are macrophages [18, 36].

On the basis of their morphologic expression (i.e., epithelioid and giant-cell granulomas and/or predominance of CD4-positive T cells and macrophages in the interstitium), cell-mediated reactions of delayed-type hypersensitivity may occur in cases of drug-related AIN, especially β-lactams [18, 128, 136], and in sarcoidosis [18]. On the other hand, cell-mediated cytotoxicity-type reactions mainly involve T cells of CD8 phenotype. The predominance of the CD8+ T-cell population in the infiltrates has been observed in AIN related to cimetidine [212], to NSAIDs [12, 18, 36, 117, 192], and in four of eight patients receiving antibiotics [70], suggesting cytotoxic T-cell injury in these cases. However, the phenotypic characteristics of the inflammatory cells do not always correlate with their functional status or effects. Furthermore, renal biopsy provides information only on a given moment during the course of an evolving process. Therefore, no definitive conclusion can be drawn from cell phenotypic analysis in AIN with regard to the primary mechanism(s) involved in tissue injury.

The use of monoclonal antibodies in studying renal biopsies has also pointed out the aberrant expression of HLA class II molecules by tubular cells in AIN [18, 36]. Such a phenomenon is not restricted to a particular cause of AIN and is also observed in other clinical conditions, such as lupus nephritis, vasculitis, and transplant rejection [18, 65]. Since antigen presentation takes place in a context of HLA class II molecules, DR-positive tubular cells would then be able to present antigen to T helper cells and thus to initiate or amplify local immune reaction and tissue damage.

References

1. Abraham, P. A., and Keane, W. F. Glomerular and interstitial disease induced by nonsteroidal anti-inflammatory drugs. *Am. J. Nephrol.* 4: 1, 1984.
2. Adams, D. H., Howie, A. J., Michael, J., et al. Non-steroidal anti-inflammatory drugs and renal failure. *Lancet* 1: 57, 1986.
3. Agus, D., Mann, R., Clayman, M., et al. The effects of daily cyclophosphamide administration on the development and extent of primary experimental interstitial nephritis in rats. *Kidney Int.* 29: 635, 1986.
4. Allon, M., Lopez, E. J., and Min, K. W. Acute renal failure due to ciprofloxacin. *Arch. Intern. Med.* 150: 2187, 1990.
5. Andrews, B. S., Eisenberg, R. A., Theofilopoulos, A. M., et al. Spontaneous murine lupus-like syndromes. Clinical and immunopathological manifestations in several strains. *J. Exp. Med.* 148: 1198, 1978.
6. Appel, G. B., and Kunis, C. L. Acute tubulo-interstitial nephritis. In R. S. Cotran, B. M. Brenner, and J. H. Stein (eds.), *Tubulo-interstitial nephropathies.* New York: Churchill, 1983. Pp. 151–185.
7. Appel, G. B., and Neu, H. C. Acute interstitial nephritis induced by β-lactam antibiotics. In J. P. Fillastre, A. Whelton, and P. Tulkens (eds.), *Antibiotic nephrotoxicity.* Paris: INSERM, 1982. Pp. 195–212.

7a. Ault, B. H., Stapleton, F. B., Gaber, L., et al. Acute renal failure during therapy with recombinant human gamma interferon. *N. Engl. J. Med.* 319: 1397, 1988.

8. Averbuch, S. D., Austin, H. A., III, Sherwin, S. A., et al. Acute interstitial nephritis with the nephrotic syndrome following recombinant leukocyte A interferon therapy for mycosis fungoides. *N. Engl. J. Med.* 310: 32, 1984.
9. Bannister, K. M., Ulich, T. R., and Wilson, C. B. Induction, characterization and cell transfer of autoimmune tubulointerstitial nephritis in the Lewis rats. *Kidney Int.* 32: 642, 1987.
10. Barnes, J. N., Davies, E. S., and Gent, C. B. Rash eosinophilia and hyperkalemia associated with enalapril. *Lancet* 2: 41, 1983.
11. Baum, M., Piel, C. F., and Goodman, J. R. Antibiotic-associated interstitial nephritis and nephrotic syndrome. *Am. J. Nephrol.* 6: 149, 1986.
12. Bender, W. L., Whelton, A., Beschorner, W. E., et al. Interstitial nephritis, proteinuria, and renal failure caused by nonsteroidal anti-inflammatory drugs. Immunologic characterization of the inflammatory infiltrate. *Am. J. Med.* 76: 1006, 1984.
13. Bierke, E. S., Mayrer, A. R., Miniter, P., et al. Tubulo-interstitial nephritis in rabbits challenged with homologous Tamm-Horsfall protein: The role of endotoxin. *Clin. Exp. Immunol.* 53: 562, 1983.
14. Boelaert, J., de Jaegere, P. P., Daneels, R., et al. Case report of renal failure during norfloxacin therapy. *Clin. Nephrol.* 25: 272, 1986.

15. Boelaert, J., Meyrier, A., Sraer, J. D., et al. Insuffisance rénale aiguë induite par la sulfinpyrazone. *Néphrologie* 2: 92, 1981.
16. Boletis, J., Williams, A. J., Shortland, J. R., et al. Irreversible renal failure following mefenamic acid. *Nephron* 51: 575, 1989.
17. Border, W. A., Lehman, D. H., Egan, J. D., et al. Antitubular basement-membrane antibodies in methicillin associated interstitital nephritis. *N. Engl. J. Med.* 291: 381, 1974.
18. Boucher, A., Droz, D., Adafer, E., et al. Characterization of mononuclear cell subsets in renal cellular interstitial infiltrates. *Kidney Int.* 29: 1043, 1986.
19. Brentjens, J. R., Matsuo, S., Fukatsu, A., et al. Immunologic studies in two patients with antitubular basement nephritis. *Am. J. Med.* 86: 603, 1989.
20. Brezin, J. H., Katz, S. M., Schwartz, A. B., et al. Reversible renal failure and nephrotic syndrome associated with nonsteroidal anti-inflammatory drugs. *N. Engl. J. Med.* 301: 1271, 1979.
21. Brunner, K., Burger, H. R., Greminger, P., et al. Mefenaminsäure (Ponstan)-induzierte, akute interstitielle Nephritis mit reversiblem, schwerem, nicht-oligurischem Nierenversagen. *Schweiz. Med. Wochenschr.* 115: 1730, 1985.
22. Bruno, P., Hassell, L. H., Brown, J., et al. The protean manifestations of hemorrhagic fever with renal syndrome. A retrospective review of 26 cases from Korea. *Ann. Intern. Med.* 113: 385, 1990.
23. Burghard, R., Brandis, M., Hoyer, P. F., et al. Acute interstitial nephritis in childhood. *Eur. J. Pediatr.* 142: 103, 1984.
23a. Butkowski, R. J., Langeveld, J. P. M., Wieslander, J., et al. Characterization of a tubular membrane component reactive with autoantibodies associated with tubulointerstitial nephritis. *J. Biol. Chem.* 265: 21091, 1990.
24. Buysen, J. G. M., Houthoff, H. J., Krediet, R. T., et al. Acute interstitial nephritis: A clinical and morphological study in 27 patients. *Nephrol. Dial. Transplant.* 5: 94, 1990.
25. Cacoub, P., Deray, G., Le Hoang, P., et al. Idiopathic acute interstitial nephritis associated with anterior uveitis in adults. *Clin. Nephrol.* 31: 307, 1989.
26. Cahan, D. H., and Ucci, A. A. Acute renal failure interstitial nephritis and nephrotic syndrome associated with captopril. *Kidney Int.* 25: 160, 1984.
27. Cameron, J. S. Allergic interstitial nephritis: Clinical features and pathogenesis. *Q. J. Med.* 66: 97, 1988.
28. Cameron, J. S. Immunologically-mediated interstitial nephritis: Primary and secondary. *Adv. Nephrol.* 18: 207, 1989.
29. Cameron, J. S., and Simmonds, H. A. Use and abuse of allopurinol. *Br. Med. J.* 294: 1504, 1987.
30. Campistol, J. M., Galofre, J., Botey, A., et al. Reversible membranous nephritis associated with diclofenac. *Nephrol. Dial. Transplant.* 4: 393, 1989.
31. Carlier, B., Lauwers, S., Cosyns, J. P., et al. Legionnaire's disease and acute renal failure. *Acta Clin. Belg.* 36: 12, 1981.
32. Carmichael, J., and Shenkel, S. W. Effects of nonsteroidal anti-inflammatory drugs on prostaglandins and renal function. *Am. J. Med.* 78: 992, 1985.
33. Chambers, R., Groufsky, A., Hunt, J. S., et al. Relationship of abnormal Tamm-Horsfall glycoprotein localization to renal morphology and function. *Clin. Nephrol.* 26: 21, 1986.
34. Champion de Crespigny, P. J., Becker, G. J., Ihle, B. Y., et al. Renal failure and nephrotic syndrome associated with sulindac. *Clin. Nephrol.* 30: 52, 1988.
35. Chauveau, P., Rouveix, B., and Kleinknecht, D. Insuffisance rénale aiguë d'origine immuno-allergique après captopril. *Néphrologie* 6: 193, 1985.
36. Cheng, H. F., Nolasco, F., Cameron, J. S., et al. HLA-DR display by renal tubular epithelium and phenotype of infiltrate in interstitial nephritis. *Nephrol. Dial. Transplant.* 4: 205, 1989.
37. Cheng, J. T., and Kahn, T. Potassium wasting and other renal tubular defects with rifampin nephrotoxicity. *Am. J. Nephrol.* 4: 379, 1984.
38. Clayman, M. D., Michaud, L., Brentjens, J., et al. Isolation of the target antigen of human anti-tubular basement membrane antibody-associated interstitial nephritis. *J. Clin. Invest.* 77: 1143, 1986.
39. Clèdes, J., Burtin, C., Hervé, J. P., et al. Rôle d'un mécanisme allergique dans l'insuffisance rénale aiguë induite par la glafénine. *Rev. Fr. Allergol.* 22: 71, 1982.
40. Clèdes, J., Gentric, A., Brière, J., et al. Glomérulonéphrite extramembraneuse au cours d'un traitement par le diclofénac. *Néphrologie* 9: 283, 1988.
41. Clèdes, J., Hervé, J. P., Le Roy, J. P., et al. Diminished bactericidal activity in megalocytic interstitial nephritis. *Clin. Nephrol.* 23: 101, 1985.
42. Clive, D. M., and Stoff, J. S. Renal syndromes associated with nonsteroidal antiinflammatory drugs. *N. Engl. J. Med.* 310: 563, 1984.
43. Codding, C. E., Ramseyer, L., Allon, M., et al. Tubulointerstitial nephritis due to vancomycin. *Am. J. Kidney Dis.* 14: 512, 1989.
44. Coggins, C. A. Renal failure in lymphoma. *Kidney Int.* 17: 847, 1980.
45. Colvin, R. B., and Fang, L. S. T. Interstitial Nephritis. In C. C. Tisher and B. M. Brenner (eds.), *Renal Pathology with Clinical and Functional Correlations* (vol. 1). Philadelphia: Lippincott, 1989. Pp. 728–776.
46. Corwin, H. L., and Bonventre, J. V. Renal insufficiency associated with nonsteroidal anti-inflammatory agents. *Am. J. Kidney Dis.* 4: 147, 1984.
46a. Corwin, H. L., and Haber, M. H. Award lectures and special reports. The clinical significance of eosinophiluria. *Am. J. Clin. Pathol.* 88: 520, 1987.
47. Cryst, C., and Hammer, S. P. Acute granulomatous interstitial nephritis due to cotrimoxazole. *Am. J. Nephrol.* 8: 483, 1988.
48. Cummings, D. M., McGehee, E. H., Dalmady, I. C., et al. Interstitial nephritis and proteinuria associated with zomepirac. *Clin. Pharmacol.* 3: 198, 1984.
49. Daoudal, P., Mahieu, P., Bloch, B., et al. Leptospirose avec immunisation anti-membrane basale glomérulaire. *Nouv. Presse Med.* 7: 3535, 1978.
50. Deray, G., Baumelou, A., Beaufils, H., et al. Néphropathies interstitielles d'origine médicamenteuse avec syndrome néphrotique. *Presse Méd.* 19: 1985, 1990.
51. Desmyter, J., Johnson, K. M., Deckers, C., et al. Laboratory rat associated outbreak of haemorrhage fever with renal syndrome due to Hantaan-like virus in Belgium. *Lancet* 2: 1445, 1983.
52. Deuel, T. F., and Senior, R. M. Growth factors in fibrotic diseases. *N. Engl. J. Med.* 317: 236, 1987.
53. Dobrin, R. S., Vernier, R. L., Fish, A. J., et al. Acute eosinophilic interstitial nephritis and renal failure with bone marrow-lymph node granulomas and anterior uveitis. *Am. J. Med.* 59: 325, 1975.
54. Dörner, O., Piper, C., Dienes, H. P., et al. Akute inter-

stitielle Nephritis nach Piperacillin. *Klin. Wochenschr.* 67: 682, 1989.

55. Eknoyan, G. Acute Renal Failure Associated with Tubulointerstitial Nephropathies. In B. M. Brenner and J. M. Lazarus (eds.), *Acute Renal Failure* (2nd ed.). New York: Churchill, 1988. Pp. 491–534.
56. Ellis, D., Fried, W. A., Yunis, E. J., et al. Acute interstitial nephritis in children: A report of 13 cases and review of the literature. *Pediatrics* 67: 862, 1981.
57. Esparza, A. R., McKay, D. B., Cronan, J. J., et al. Renal parenchymal malakoplakia. *Am. J. Surg. Pathol.* 13: 225, 1989.
58. Faierman, D., Ross, F. A., and Seckler, S. G. Typhoid fever complicated by hepatitis, nephritis, and thrombocytopenia. *J. Am. Med. Ass.* 221: 60, 1972.
59. Fasth, A., Bjure, J., Hjalmas, K., et al. Serum autoantibodies to Tamm-Horsfall protein and their relation to renal damage and glomerular filtration rate in children with urinary tract malformations. *Contr. Nephrol.* 39: 285, 1984.
60. Favre, H., Leski, M., Christeler, P., et al. Le Cortinarius orellanus: un champignon toxique provoquant une insuffisance rénale aiguë retardée. *Schweiz. Med. Wochenschr.* 106: 1097, 1976.
61. Feehally, J., Wheeler, D. C., MacKay, E. H., et al. Recurrent acute renal failure with interstitial nephritis due to D-penicillamine. *Renal Failure* 10: 55, 1987.
62. Fellner, S. K. Piroxicam-induced acute interstitital nephritis and minimal-change nephrotic syndrome. *Am. J. Nephrol.* 5: 142, 1985.
63. Finkelstein, A., Fraley, D. S., Stachura, I., et al. Fenoprofen nephropathy: lipoid nephrosis and interstitial nephritis. A possible T-lymphocyte disorder. *Am. J. Med.* 72: 81, 1982.
64. Frommer, P., Uldall, R., Fay, W. P., et al. A case of acute interstitial nephritis successfully treated after delayed diagnosis. *Canad. Med. Ass. J.* 121: 585, 1979.
65. Fuggle, S. V., McWinnie, D. L., Chapman, J. R., et al. Sequential analysis of HLA-class II antigens in human renal allografts: Induction of tubular class II antigens and correlations with clinical parameters. *Transplantation* 42: 144, 1986.
66. Fuller, T. J., Barcenas, C. G., and White, M. G. Diuretic-induced interstitial nephritis. *J. Am. Med. Ass.* 235: 1998, 1976.
67. Galpin, J. E., Shinaberger, J. H., Stanley, J. M., et al. Acute interstitial nephritis due to methicillin. *Am. J. Med.* 65: 756, 1978.
68. Ganeval, D., Jungers, P., Noël, L. H., et al. La néphropathie du myélome. In J. Hamburger, J. Crosnier, J. L. Funck-Brentano, J. F. Bach, and J. P. Grünfeld (eds.), *Actualités Néphrologiques de l'Hôpital Necker.* Paris: Flammarion, 1977. Pp. 309–347.
69. Garella, S., and Matarese, R. A. Renal effects of prostaglandins and clinical adverse effects of nonsteroidal anti-inflammatory agents. *Medicine* 63: 165, 1984.
70. Gimenez, A., and Mampaso, F. Characterization of inflammatory cells in drug-induced tubulointerstitial nephritis. *Nephron* 43: 239, 1986.
71. Gimenez, A., Leyva-Cobian, F., Fierro, C., et al. Effects of cyclosporin A on autoimmune tubulointerstitial nephritis in the Brown-Norway rat. *Clin. Exp. Immunol.* 69: 550, 1987.
72. Glauser, M. P., Lyons, J. M., and Braude, A. I. Prevention of chronic experimental pyelonephritis by suppression of acute suppuration. *J. Clin. Invest.* 61: 403, 1978.
73. Green, J., Yoffe, B., Barzilai, D., et al. Reversible acute interstitial nephritis associated with indomethacin. *Isr. J. Med. Sci.* 21: 142, 1985.
74. Grünfeld, J. P., Kleinknecht, D., and Droz, D. Acute interstitial nephritis. In R. W. Schrier and C. W. Gottschalk (eds.), *Diseases of the Kidney* (vol. 2, 4th ed.). Boston: Little, Brown, 1988. Pp. 1461–1487.
75. Grussendorf, M., Andrassy, K., Waldherr, R., et al. Systemic hypersensitivity to allopurinol with acute interstitial nephritis. *Am. J. Nephrol.* 1: 105, 1981.
76. Guang, M. Y., Liu, G. Z., and Cosgriff, J. M. Hemorrhage in hemorrhagic fever with renal syndrome in China. *Rev. Infect. Dis.* 2 (Suppl. 4): S884, 1989.
77. Hall, C. L., Colvin, R. B., Carey, K., et al., Passive transfer of autoimmune disease with isologous IgG1, and IgG2 antibodies to the tubular basement membrane in strain XIII guinea pigs. Loss of self-tolerance induced by autoantibodies. *J. Exp. Med.* 146: 1246, 1977.
78. Hamburger, J., Richet, G., Crosnier, J., et al. The kidney in septicemia and various infections. In *Nephrology,* vol. 2. Philadelphia: Saunders, 1968. Pp. 1014–1036.
79. Handa, S. P. Drug-induced acute interstitial nephritis: Report of 10 cases. *Can. Med. Assoc. J.* 135: 1278, 1986.
80. Hannedouche, T., Grateau, G., Noël, L. H., et al. Renal granulomatous sarcoidosis: Report of six cases. *Nephrol. Dial. Transplant.* 5: 18, 1990.
81. Helmink, R., and Benedkitsson, H. Ciprofloxacin-induced allergic interstitial nephritis. *Nephron* 55: 432, 1990.
82. Heptinstall, R. H. Renal complications of therapeutic and diagnostic agents, analgesic abuse, and addiction to narcotics. In *Pathology of the Kidney* (3rd ed.) Boston: Little, Brown, 1983. Pp. 1195–1255.
83. Hirsch, D. J., Bia, F. J., Kashgarian, M., et al. Rapidly progressive glomerulonephritis during antituberculous therapy. *Am. J. Nephrol.* 3: 7, 1983.
84. Hooke, D., Walker, R. G., Walter, N. M. A., et al. Repeated renal failure with use of captopril in a cystinotic renal allograft recipient. *Br. Med. J.* 285: 1538, 1982.
85. Hootkins, R., Fenves, A. Z., and Stephens, M. K. Acute renal failure secondary to oral ciprofloxacin therapy: A presentation of three cases and a review of the literature. *Clin. Nephrol.* 32: 75, 1989.
86. Hory, B., Chaillet, R., and Pérol, C. L'insuffisance rénale chronique terminale: Évolution inhabituelle d'une néphrite tubulointerstitielle aiguë. *Néphrologie* 8: 237, 1987.
87. Hoyer, J. R. Tubulointerstitial immune complex nephritis in rats immunized with Tamm-Horsfall protein. *Kidney Int.* 17: 284, 1980.
88. Hurault de Ligny, B., Prieur, J. P., Schmitt, J. L., et al. Ten new cases of HRFS in North-Eastern France. *Lancet* 2: 864, 1984.
89. Husby, G., Tung, K. S. R., and Williams, R. C. Characterization of renal tissue lymphocytes in patients with interstitial nephritis. *Am. J. Med.* 70: 31, 1981.
90. Huttunen, K., Grönhagen-Riska, C., and Fyhrquist, F. Acute renal failure presenting as Fanconi syndrome with lambda light chain proteinuria and interstitial nephritis. *Clin. Nephrol.* 31: 277, 1989.
91. Hyman, L. R., Ballow, M., and Knieser, M. R. Diphenylhydantoin interstitial nephritis. Roles of cellular and tumoral immunologic injury. *J. Pediatr.* 92: 915, 1978.
92. Hyman, L. R., Steinberg, A. D., Colvin, R. B., et al. Immunopathogenesis of autoimmune interstitial nephritis. II. Role of an immune response gene linked to the major histocompatibility complex. *J. Immunol.* 17: 1894, 1976.

93. Hyun, J., and Galen, M. A. Acute interstitial nephritis. A case characterized by increase in serum IgG, IgM, and IgE concentrations, eosinophilia and IgE deposition in renal tubules. *Arch. Intern. Med.* 141; 679, 1981.
94. Iijima, K., Yoshikawa, N., Sato, K., et al. Acute interstitial nephritis associated with *Yersinia pseudotuberculosis* infection. *Am. J. Nephrol.* 9: 236, 1989.
95. Islam, S., Dubigeon, M. P., and Guenel, J. Néphropathie interstitielle granulomateuse aiguë et réversible après traitement par le captopril. *Rev. Méd. Interne (Paris)* 11: 231, 1990.
95a. Itami, N., Akutsu, Y., Yasoshima, K., et al. Acute tubulointerstitial nephritis with uveitis. *Arch. Intern. Med.* 150: 688, 1990.
96. Jao, W. Iatrogenic renal disease as revealed by renal biopsy. *Semin. Diag. Pathol.* 5: 63, 1986.
97. Jenkins, D. A. S., Harrison, D. J., MacDonald, M. K., et al. Mefenamic acid nephropathy: An interstitial and mesangial lesion. *Nephrol. Dial. Transplant.* 2: 217, 1988.
98. Joh, K., Aizawa, S., Yamaguchi, Y., et al. Drug-induced hypersensitivity nephritis: Lymphocyte stimulation testing and renal biopsy in 10 cases. *Am. J. Nephrol.* 10: 222, 1990.
99. Joh, K., Shibasaki, T., Azuma, T., et al. Experimental drug-induced allergic nephritis mediated by antihapten antibody. *Int. Arch. Allergy Appl. Immunol.* 88: 337, 1989.
100. Jokinen, E. J., Lähdevirta, J., and Collan, Y. Nephropathia epidemica: immunohistochemical study of pathogenesis. *Clin. Nephrol.* 9: 1, 1978.
101. Kanfer, A., Vandewalle, A., Morel-Maroger, L., et al. Acute renal insufficiency due to lymphomatous infiltration of the kidneys. *Cancer* 38: 2588, 1976.
102. Kelly, C., and Neilson, E. G. Contrasuppression in autoimmunity. Abnormal contrasuppression facilitates expression of nephrotogenic effector T cells and interstitial nephritis in kdkd mice. *J. Exp. Med.* 165: 107, 1987.
103. Kenouch, S., and Méry, J. P. Les atteintes de l'interstitium rénal au cours des maladies systémiques. I & II. *Néphrologie* 9: 61, 1988.
104. Kida, H., Abe, T., Tomosugi, N., et al. Prediction of the long-term outcome in acute interstitial nephritis. *Clin. Nephrol.* 22: 55, 1984.
105. Kleinknecht, D. Kidney Diseases Caused by Non-steroidal Anti-inflammatory drugs. In J. H. Stewart (ed.), *Kidney Disease due to Analgesics and Anti-inflammatory Drugs.* Oxford: Oxford University Press. (in press).
106. Kleinknecht, D., and Droz, D. Acute Renal Failure from Interstitial Disease. In *Oxford Textbook of Clinical Nephrology.* Oxford: Oxford University Press. (in press).
107. Kleinknecht, D., Landais, P., and Goldfarb, B. Les insuffisances rénales aiguës associées à des médicaments ou à des produits de contraste iodés. Résultats d'une enquête coopérative multicentrique de la Société de Néphrologie. *Néphrologie* 7: 41, 1986.
108. Kleinknecht, D., Landais, P., and Goldfarb, B. Analgesic and nonsteroidal anti-inflammatory drug-associated acute renal failure: A prospective collaborative study. *Clin. Nephrol.* 25: 275, 1986.
109. Kleinknecht, D., Vanhille, Ph., and Druet, Ph. Néphrites interstitielles aiguës granulomateuses d'origine médicamenteuse. *Presse Méd.* 17: 201, 1988.
110. Kleinknecht, D., Vanhille, P., Morel-Maroger, L., et al. Acute interstitial nephritis due to drug hypersensitivity. An up-to-date review with a report of 19 cases. *Adv. Nephrol.* 12: 277, 1983.
111. Kopolovic, J., Pinkus, G., and Rosen, S. Interstitial nephritis in infectious mononucleosis. *Am. J. Kidney Dis.* 12: 76, 1988.
112. Kourilsky, O., Solez, K., Morel-Maroger, L., et al. The pathology of acute renal failure due to interstitial nephritis in man with comments on the role of interstitial inflammation and sex in gentamicin nephrotoxicity. *Medicine* 61: 258, 1982.
113. Laberke, H. G., and Bohle, A. Acute interstitial nephritis: Correlations between clinical and morphological findings. *Clin. Nephrol.* 14: 263, 1980.
114. Lädevirta, J. Clinical features of HFRS in Scandinavia as compared with East Asia. *Scand. J. Infect. Dis.* Suppl. 36: 93, 1982.
115. Lai, K. N., Aarons, I., Woodroffe, A. J., et al. Renal lesions in leptospirosis. *Aust. N.Z. J. Med.* 12: 276, 1982.
116. Lallement, P. Y., Morinière, B., Kaloustian, E., et al. Fièvre hémorragique avec syndrome rénal: Quatre cas autochtones. *Méd. Mal. Infect.* 14: 425, 1984.
117. Lang, Ph., Santelli, G., Benarbia, S., et al. Etude immunopathologique d'une néphropathie interstitielle aiguë induite par la clométacine. *Presse Méd.* 15: 915, 1986.
118. Lavaud, S., Mamez, B., Lavaud, F., et al. Insuffisance rénale aiguë par hypersensibilité à la clométacine. *Néphrologie* 5: 131, 1984.
119. Lee, H. W. Hemorrhagic fever with renal syndrome (HFRS). *Scand. J. Infect. Dis.* Suppl. 36: 82, 1982.
119a. Lessard, M., and Smith, J. D. Fanconi syndrome with uveitis in an adult woman. *Am. J. Kidney Dis.* 13: 158, 1989.
120. Lévy, M. Néphropathies Tubulo-interstitielles Immunologiques. In P. Royer, R. Habib, and H. Mathieu (eds.), *Néphrologie Pédiatrique.* Paris: Flammarion, 1983. Pp. 187–199.
121. Lévy, M., Prieur, A. M., Gubler, M. C., et al. Renal involvement in juvenile chronic arthritis: Clinical and pathologic features. *Am. J. Kidney Dis.* 9: 138, 1987.
122. Lin, C. Y., and Chiang, H. Sodium-valproate–induced interstitial nephritis. *Nephron* 48: 43, 1988.
123. Lins, R. L., Verpooten, G. A., DeClerck, D. S., et al. Urinary indices in acute interstitial nephritis. *Clin. Nephrol.* 26: 131, 1986.
124. Linton, A. L., Clark, W. F., Driedger, A. A., et al. Acute interstitial nephritis due to drugs. Review of the literature with a report of 9 cases. *Ann. Intern. Med.* 93: 735, 1980.
125. Linton, A. L., Richmond, J. M., Clark, W. F., et al. Gallium^{67} scintigraphy in the diagnosis of acute renal diseases. *Clin. Nephrol.* 24: 84, 1985.
126. Lunberg, W. B., Cadman, E. D., Finch, S. C., et al. Renal failure secondary to leukemic infiltration of the kidneys. *Am. J. Med.* 62: 636, 1977.
127. Lyons, H., Pinn, V. W., Cortell, S., et al. Allergic interstitial nephritis causing reversible renal failure in four patients with idiopathic nephrotic syndrome. *N. Engl. J. Med.* 288: 124, 1973.
127a. Mac-Moune Lai, F., Lai, K. N., and Chong, Y. M. Papillary necrosis associated with rifampicin therapy. *Austr. N.Z. J. Med.* 17: 68, 1987.
128. Magil, A. B. Drug-induced acute interstitial nephritis with granulomas. *Hum. Pathol.* 13: 36, 1983.
129. Magil, A. B., Ballon, H. S., Cameron, E. C., et al. Acute interstitial nephritis associated with thiazide diuretics. Clinical and pathologic observations in three cases. *Am. J. Med.* 69: 939, 1980.
130. Magner, P., Sweet, J., and Bear, R. A. Granulomatous

interstitial nephritis associated with allopurinol therapy. *Can. Med. Assoc. J.* 135: 496, 1986.

131. Mallinson, W. J. N., Fuller, R. W., Levison, D. A., et al. Diffuse interstitial renal tuberculosis. An unusual cause of renal failure. *Q. J. Med.* 50: 137, 1981.
132. Mampaso, F. M., and Wilson, C. B. Characterization of inflammatory cells in autoimmune tubulointerstitial nephritis in rats. *Kidney Int.* 23: 448, 1983.
133. Mann, R., Kelly, C. J., Clayman, M. D., et al. Effector T cell differentiation in experimental interstitial nephritis. I. Requirements for precursor cell development and effector lymphocyte maturation. *J. Immunol.* 138: 4200, 1987.
134. Marasco, W. A., Gikas, P. W., Azziz-Baumgartner, R., et al. Ibuprofen-associated renal dysfunction. Pathophysiologic mechanisms of acute renal failure, hyperkalemia, tubular necrosis, and proteinuria. *Arch. Intern. Med.* 147: 2107, 1987.
135. McCarthy, J. T., Schwartz, G. L., Blair, T. J., et al. Reversible nonoliguric acute renal failure associated with zomepirac therapy. *Mayo Clin. Proc.* 57: 351, 1982.
136. McCluskey, R. T. Immunologically-mediated tubulointerstitial nephritis. In Cotran R. S., Brenner, B. M., and Stein, J. H. (eds.), *Tubulointerstitial nephropathies.* New York: Churchill, 1983. Pp. 111–149.
137. Mehta, R. P. Acute interstitial nephritis due to S-aminosalicylic acid. *Can. Med. Assoc. J.* 143: 1031, 1990.
138. Meyrier, A., Condamin, M. C., Fernet, M., et al. Frequency of development of early cortical scarring in acute primary pyelonephritis. *Kidney Int.* 35: 696, 1989.
139. Meyrier, A., Jeanson, A., Mignon, F., et al. Néphrites interstitielles aiguës hématogènes à point de départ urinaire: facteur d'aggravation méconnu de l'insuffisance rénale chronique. *Néphrologie* 4: 48, 1983.
140. Mignon, F., Méry, J. P., Mougenot, B., et al. Granulomatous interstitial nephritis. *Adv. Nephrol.* 13: 219, 1984.
141. Mitnick, P. D., and Klein, W. J. Piroxicam-induced renal disease. *Arch. Intern. Med.* 144: 63, 1984.
142. Mousson, C., Justrabo, E., Tanter, Y., et al. Néphrite interstitielle et hépatite aiguë granulomateuses d'origine médicamenteuse. Rôle possible de l'association allopurinol-furosémide. *Néphrologie* 5: 199, 1986.
143. Muehrcke, R. C., Pirani, C. L., and Kark, R. M. Interstitial nephritis: A clinicopathological renal biopsy study. *Ann. Intern. Med.* 66: 1052, 1967.
144. Nakamoto, Y., Kida, H., and Mizumura, Y. Acute eosinophilic interstitial nephritis with bone marrow granulomas. *Clin. Immunol. Immunopathol.* 14: 379, 1979.
145. Neilson, E. G. Pathogenesis and therapy of interstitial nephritis. *Kidney Int.* 35: 1257, 1989.
146. Neilson, E. G., and Phillips, S. M. Cell-mediated immunity in interstitial nephritis. IV. Antitubular basement membrane antibodies can function in antibody-dependent cellular cytotoxicity reactions. Observation on a nephritogenic effector mechanism acting as an informational bridge between the humoral and cellular immune response. *J. Immunol.* 126: 1990, 1981.
147. Neilson, E. G., and Phillips, S. M. Murine interstitial nephritis. I. Analysis of disease susceptibility and its relationship to pleomorphic gene products defining both immune-response genes and a restriction requirement for cytotoxic T cells at H-2K. *J. Exp. Med.* 155: 1075, 1982.
148. Neilson, E. G., McCafferty, E., Feldman, A., et al. Spontaneous interstitial nephritis in kdkd mice. I. An experimental model of autoimmune renal disease. *J. Immunol.* 133: 2560, 1984.
149. Neugarten, J., Gallo, G. R., and Baldwin, D. S. Rifampin-induced nephrotic syndrome and acute interstitial nephritis. *Am. J. Nephrol.* 3: 38, 1983.
150. Nguyen, V. D., Nagelberg, H., and Agarwal, B. N. Acute interstitial nephritis associated with cefoteran therapy. *Am. J. Kidney Dis.* 16: 259, 1990.
151. Nicholls, A. J., Shortland, J. R., and Brown, C. B. Mefenamic acid nephropathy—a spectrum of renal lesions. *Proc. Eur. Dial. Transplant. Assoc.* 22: 991, 1985.
151a. Nochy, D., Glotz, D., Dosquet, P., et al. Renal disease associated with HIV infection: North American versus European experience. *Adv. Nephrol.* 22, 1993. (In press).
152. Nolan, C. R., III, Anger, M. S., and Kelleher, S. P. Eosinophiluria—a new method of detection and definition of the clinical spectrum. *N. Engl. J. Med.* 315: 1516, 1986.
153. Ooi, B. S., Ooi, Y. M., Mohini, R., et al. Humoral mechanisms in drug induced acute interstitial nephritis. *Clin. Immunol. Immunopathol.* 10: 330, 1978.
154. Olsen, T. S., Wassef, N. F., Olsen, H. J., et al. Ultrastructure of the kidney in acute interstitial nephritis. *Ultrastruct. Pathol.* 10: 1, 1986.
155. Pagniez, D. C., Fenaux, P., Delvallez, L., et al. Reversible renal failure due to specific infiltration in chronic lymphocytic leukemia. *Am. J. Med.* 85: 579, 1988.
156. Pagniez, D., Gosset, D., Hardouin, P., et al. Evolution vers la hyalinose segmentaire et focale d'un syndrome néphrotique à lésions glomérulaires minimes chez une patiente traitée par le sulindac. *Néphrologie* 9: 90, 1988.
157. Pamucku, R., Moorthy, A. V., Singer, J. R., et al. Idiopathic acute interstitial nephritis: characterization of the infiltrating cells in the renal interstitium as T helper lymphocytes. *Am. J. Kidney Dis.* 4: 24, 1984.
158. Paulter, N., Gabriel, R., Porter, K. A., et al. Acute interstitial nephritis complicating Legionnaire's disease. *Clin. Nephrol.* 15: 216, 1981.
159. Pirani, C. L., Valeri, A., D'Agati, V., et al. Renal toxicity of nonsteroidal anti-inflammatory drugs. *Contrib. Nephrol.* 55: 159, 1987.
160. Pirson, Y., and Van Ypersele de Strihou, Ch. Renal side effects of nonsteroidal anti-inflammatory drugs: Clinical relevance. *Am. J. Kidney Dis.* 8: 338, 1986.
161. Pommer, W., Offermann, G., Schultze, G., et al. Akute interstitielle Nephritis durch Medikamente. *Dtsch. Med. Wochenschr.* 108: 783, 1983.
162. Porile, J. L., Bakris, G. L., and Garella, S. Acute interstitial nephritis with glomerulopathy due to nonsteroidal anti-inflammatory agents. A review of its clinical spectrum and effects of steroid therapy. *J. Clin. Pharmacol.* 30: 468, 1990.
163. Power, D. A., Russell, G., Smith, F. W., et al. Acute renal failure due to continuous rifampicin. *Clin. Nephrol.* 20: 155, 1983.
164. Proesmans, W., Kyele Akumola Sina, J., Debucquoy, P., et al. Recurrent acute renal failure due to nonaccidental poisoning with glafenin in a child. *Clin. Nephrol.* 16: 207, 1981.
165. Pusey, C. D., Saltissi, D., Bloodworth, L., et al. Drug associated acute interstitial nephritis: clinical and pathological features and the response to high dose steroid therapy. *Q. J. Med.* 52: 194, 1983.
166. Quinn, B. P., and Wall, B. M. Nephrogenic diabetes insipidus and tubulointerstitial nephritis during continuous therapy with rifampin. *Am. J. Kidney Dis.* 14: 217, 1989.

167. Raftery, M. J., Forman, P., Farrington, K., et al. Fenclofenac induced interstitial nephritis confirmed by inadvertent rechallenge. *Br. Med. J.* 290: 1178, 1985.
168. Ramsay, A. G., Olesnicky, L., and Pirani, C. L. Acute tubulointerstitial nephritis from candida albicans with oliguric renal failure. *Clin. Nephrol.* 24: 310, 1985.
169. Rashed, A., Azadeh, B., and Abu Romeh, S. H. Acyclovir-induced acute tubulo-interstitial nephritis. *Nephron* 56: 436, 1990.
170. Rautelin, H. I., Outinen, A. V., and Kosunen, T. U. Tubulointerstitial nephritis as a complication of *Campylobacter jejuni* enteritis. *Scand. J. Urol. Nephrol.* 21: 151, 1987.
171. Ray, P. E., Rigolizzo, D., Wara, D. R., et al. Naproxen nephrotoxicity in a 2-year-old child. *Am. J. Dis. Child.* 142: 524, 1988.
172. Rennke, H. G., Roos, P. C., and Wall, S. G. Drug-induced interstitial nephritis with heavy glomerular proteinuria. *N. Engl. J. Med.* 302: 691, 1980.
173. Richet, G. Néphrites interstitielles aiguës avec insuffisance rénale. In *Proc. VIIth. Int. Congr. Nephrol.*, Montréal: Les Presses Universitaires de Montréal and Basel: Karger, 1978. Pp. 707–713.
174. Richet, G., Sraer, J. D., Kourilsky, O., et al. La ponction-biopsie rénale dans l'insuffisance rénale aiguë. *Ann. Méd. Interne (Paris)* 129: 335, 1978.
175. Rippelmeyer, D. J., and Synhavsky, A. Ciprofloxacin and allergic interstitial nephritis. *Ann. Intern. Med.* 109: 170, 1988.
176. Rosenberg, M. E., Schendel, P. B., McCurdy, F. A., et al. Characterization of immune cells in kidneys from patients with Sjögren's syndrome. *Am. J. Kidney Dis.* 11: 20, 1988.
177. Rosenfeld, J., Gura, V., Boner, G., et al. Interstitial nephritis with acute renal failure after erythromycin. *Br. Med. J.* 286: 938, 1983.
178. Rossi, E., Ferraccioli, G. F., Cavalieri, F., et al. Diclofenac-associated acute renal failure. Report of 2 cases. *Nephron* 40: 491, 1985.
179. Rossi, E., Silvestri, M. G., Manari, A., et al. Acute renal failure and piromidic acid. *Nephron* 32: 80, 1982.
180. Rotellar, C., Noël, L. H., Droz, D., et al. Role of antibodies directed against tubular basement membranes in human renal transplantation. *Am. J. Kidney Dis.* 7: 157, 1986.
181. Rudofsky, U. H., Dilwith, R. L., and Tung, K. S. K. Susceptibility differences of inbred mice to induction of autoimmune renal tubulointerstitial lesions. *Lab. Invest.* 43: 463, 1980.
182. Sarma, P. S. A. Fatal acute renal failure after piroxicam. *Clin. Nephrol.* 31: 54, 1989.
183. Sawyer, M. H., Webb, D. E., Balow, J. E., et al. Acyclovir-induced renal failure. Clinical course and histology. *Am. J. Med.* 84: 1067, 1988.
184. Schwarz, A., Krause, P. H., Keller, F., et al. Granulomatous interstitial nephritis after nonsteroidal anti-inflammatory drugs. *Am. J. Nephrol.* 8: 410, 1988.
185. Siegel, M. B., Alexander, L., Weintraub, L., et al. Renal failure in Burkitt's lymphoma. *Clin. Nephrol.* 7: 279, 1977.
186. Silbert, P. L., Matz, L. R., Christiansen, K., et al. Herpes simplex virus interstitial nephritis in a renal allograft. *Clin. Nephrol.* 33: 264, 1990.
187. Singer, D. R. J., Simpson, J. G., Catto, G. R. D., et al. Drug hypersensitivity causing granulomatous interstitial nephritis. *Am. J. Kidney Dis.* 11: 357, 1988.
188. Sitprija, V. Acute renal failure associated with leptospirosis. In V. E. Andreucci (ed.), *Acute Renal Failure*, The Hague: Martinns Nijhoff, 1984. Pp. 319–326.
189. Sitprija, V., Pipatanagul, V., Mertowidjojo, K., et al. Pathogenesis of renal disease in leptospirosis: Clinical and experimental studies. *Kidney Int.* 17: 827, 1980.
190. Smith, W. R., Neill, J., Cushman, W. C., et al. Captopril-associated acute interstitial nephritis. *Am. J. Nephrol.* 9: 230, 1989.
191. Spital, A., Panner, B. J., and Sterns, R. H. Acute idiopathic tubulointerstitial nephritis: Report of two cases and review of the literature. *Am. J. Kidney Dis.* 9: 71, 1987.
192. Stachura, I., Jayakumar, S., and Bourke, E. T and B lymphocyte subsets in fenoprofen nephropathy. *Am. J. Med.* 75: 9, 1983.
193. Stachura, I., Si, L., Madan, E., et al. Mononuclear cell subsets in human renal disease. Enumeration in tissue sections with monoclonal antibodies. *Clin. Immunol. Immunopathol.* 30: 262, 1984.
194. Steblay, R. W., and Rudofsky, U. Renal tubular disease and autoantibodies against tubular basement membrane induced in guinea-pigs. *J. Immunol.* 107: 589, 1971.
195. Steinman, T. I., and Silva, P. Acute renal failure, skin rash, and eosinophilia associated with captopril therapy. *Am. J. Med.* 75: 154, 1983.
196. Steinman, T. I., and Silva, P. Acute interstitial nephritis and iritis. Renal-ocular syndrome. *Am. J. Med.* 77: 189, 1984.
197. Sugisaki, T., Klassen, J., Milgrom, F., et al. Immunopathologic study of an autoimmune tubular and interstitial renal disease in Brown-Norway rats. *Lab. Invest.* 28: 658, 1973.
198. Sugisaki, T., Yoshida, T., McCluskey, R. T., et al. Autoimmune cell-mediated tubulointerstitial nephritis induced in Lewis rats by renal antigens. *Clin. Immunol. Immunopathol.* 15: 33, 1980.
199. Ten, R. M., Torres, V. E., Milliner, D. S., et al. Acute interstitial nephritis: Immunologic and clinical aspects. *Mayo Clin. Proc.* 63: 921, 1988.
200. Tolins, J. P., Hostetter, M. K., and Hostetter, T. H. Hypokalemic nephropathy in the rat. Role of ammonia in chronic tubular injury. *J. Clin. Invest.* 79: 1447, 1987.
201. Toto, R. D. Acute tubulointerstitial nephritis. *Am. J. Med. Sci.* 299: 392, 1990.
202. Tron, F., Ganeval, D., and Droz, D. Immunologically-mediated acute renal failure of nonglomerular origin in the course of systemic lupus erythematosus. *Am. J. Med.* 67: 529, 1979.
203. Tucker, B., Brown, A. L., d'Ardenne, A. J., et al. Reversible renal failure due to renal infiltration and associated tubulointerstitial disease in chronic lymphocytic leukaemia. *Nephrol. Dial. Transplant.* 5: 616, 1990.
204. Ulich, T. R., Nir, X., Gutman, G. A., et al. The effects of a stable analogue of PGE1 on the IgG subclass response to particulate bovine tubular basement membrane in the Brown-Norway rat. *Proc. Soc. Exp. Biol. Med.* 185: 441, 1987.
205. Vanhille, Ph., Kleinknecht, D., Dracon, M., et al. Néphrites interstitielles granulomateuses d'origine médicamenteuse. *Néphrologie* 8: 41, 1987.
206. Van Ypersele de Strihou, C. Acute oliguric interstitial nephritis. *Kidney Int.* 16: 751, 1979.
207. Van Ypersele de Strihou, C., and Méry, J. P. Hantavirus-related acute interstitial nephritis in Western Europe. Expansion of a world-wide zoonosis. *Q. J. Med.* 73: 941, 1989.

208. Van Ypersele de Strihou, C., Van der Groen, G., and Desmyter, J. Hantavirus nephropathy in Western Europe: Ubiquity of hemorrhagic fevers with renal syndrome. *Adv. Nephrol.* 15: 143, 1986.
209. Van Zwieten, M. J., Bahn, A. K., McCluskey, R. J., et al. Studies on the pathogenesis of experimental anti-tubular basement membrane nephritis in the guinea pig. *Am. J. Pathol.* 83: 531, 1976.
210. Vigeral, Ph., Kanfer, A., Kenouch, S., et al. Nephrogenic Diabetes Insipidus and Distal Tubular Acidosis in Methicillin-Induced Interstitial Nephritis. In A. Amerio and P. Coratelli (eds.), *Acute Renal Failure, Clinical and Experimental*. New York: Plenum Press, 1987. Pp. 129–134.
211. Volpi, A., Ferrario, G. M., Giordano, F., et al. Acute renal failure due to hypersensitivity interstitial nephritis induced by warfarin sodium. *Nephron* 52: 196, 1989.
212. Watson, A. J. S., Dalbow, M. H., Stachura, I., et al. Immunologic studies in cimetidine-induced nephropathy and polymyositis. *N. Engl. J. Med.* 308: 142, 1983.
213. Wilkinson, D. G., and Boyd, D. H. A. Recovery from acute interstitial nephritis. *Br. Med. J.* 1: 827, 1978.
214. Wilson, C. B. Study of the immunopathogenesis of tubulointerstitial nephritis using model systems. *Kidney Int.* 35: 938, 1989.
215. Wilson, D. M., Turner, D. R., Cameron, J. S., et al. Value of renal biopsy in acute intrinsic renal failure. *Br. Med. J.* 2: 459, 1976.
216. Winearls, C. G., Chan, L., Coghlan, J. D., et al. Acute renal failure due to leptospirosis: Clinical features and outcome in six cases. *Q. J. Med.* 53: 487, 1984.
217. Winer, R. L., Cohen, A. H., Sawhney, A. S., et al. Sjögren's syndrome with immune complex tubulointerstitial renal disease. *Clin. Immunol. Immunopathol.* 8: 494, 1977.
218. Wolters, J., and Van Breda Vriesman, P. J. Minimal change nephropathy and interstitial nephritis associated with diclofenac. *Neth. J. Med.* 28: 311, 1985.
219. Wood, B. C., Sharma, J. N., Germann, D. R., et al. Gallium citrate Ga^{67} imaging in noninfectious interstitial nephritis. *Arch. Intern. Med.* 138: 1665, 1978.
220. Zech, P., Geitner, S., Birraux, B., et al. Insuffisance rénale aiguë et syndrome néphrotique secondaires à la prise de fénoprofène. *Nouv. Presse Méd.* 11: 2227, 1982.
221. Zeier, M., Schmidt, R., Andrassy, K., et al. Idiopathic interstitial nephritis complicating ulcerative colitis. *Nephrol. Dial. Transplant.* 5: 901, 1990.

The Hepatorenal Syndrome

Ori S. Better
Robert W. Schrier

Synopsis

The hepatorenal syndrome (HRS) is a functional, potentially reversible renal failure that complicates advanced liver damage. It closely resembles prerenal failure with the exception that it does not respond to conventional volume replacement. It may remit, however, after spontaneous improvement of liver function or liver transplantation and, very rarely, following portacaval shunting or insertion of the LeVeen shunt.

The cause of death of most patients with HRS usually is "hepatic" (i.e., encephalopathy and variceal hemorrhage) rather than "uremic." The pathogenesis of HRS has not been clarified. There is no experimental model for HRS available. However, a combination of extreme renal vasoconstriction, peripheral vasodilatation, and pooling of blood in the splanchnic region diverts blood flow from the kidney and leads to renal cortical ischemia. Among the probable mediators of renal vasoconstriction in HRS are increased α-adrenergic tone, an increase in plasma arginine vasopressin, activation of the renin-angiotensin axis, endotoxinemia, and a possible increase in renal thromboxane A_2 synthesis coupled with reduced production of renal prostaglandin I_2 (PGI_2), prostaglandin E_2 (PGE_2), and kallikrein. There is no specific treatment for HRS short of improvement of the liver status. Exposure to nephrotoxic agents and acute perturbation of volume status in patients with advanced cirrhosis may precipitate HRS and should therefore be avoided.

Introduction

The HRS is defined as kidney failure in patients with severely compromised liver function in the absence of clinical, laboratory, or anatomic evidence of other known causes of renal failure [109]. The potentially reversible and functional nature of HRS is obvious from the following considerations: (1) The laboratory findings in the blood and urine resemble an extreme form of prerenal failure [109]; (2) transplantation of normal liver to patients suffering from HRS may reverse and resolve it [72]; (3) kidneys taken from patients who died with HRS may function normally following transplantation into recipients with normal liver [79]; (4) the striking angiographic renal vasoconstrictor pattern seen during life in patients with HRS disappears on postmortem angiography of these kidneys [53]; and (5) in most patients who died with HRS, kidney histology was preserved, and the minor anatomic changes occasionally seen cannot account for the renal failure [47, 109].

The purpose of this chapter is to review recent developments in the understanding of the pathophysiology and the management of HRS. This chapter does not deal with simultaneous injury of both the liver and the kidneys ("pseudo HRS") by toxins, coagulopathies, immunologic processes, and fulminant sepsis. These subjects were reviewed in depth and detail by Levenson, Skorecki, and Narins [87].

History

Over a century ago, Austin Flint noted that patients with advanced cirrhosis and ascites had severe oliguria as a preterminal phenomenon [58]. The term *hepatorenal syndrome* was first used some 55 years ago to designate what appears to have been acute renal failure complicating biliary surgery [67] and therefore is somewhat at variance with the present definition of HRS as presently used. The modern characterization of HRS occurred in the 1950s and is attributed to Sherlock [66] in Britain and Papper [108] in the United States. Hecker and Sherlock noted that patients in terminal stages of cirrhosis of the liver may suffer from renal failure associated with low urinary sodium excretion and absence of proteinuria [66]. Papper and his colleagues were the first to suggest that the cause of HRS is circulatory disturbance of an otherwise normal kidney [110]. On this background, they attempted to correct HRS with volume expansion. This, however, did not prove to be consistently fruitful [108, 110]. These findings were confirmed by Vesin [140] and by Baldus and associates [12], who stressed the functional nature of HRS.

Clinical Course

HRS may complicate any advanced chronic or acute liver failure whether due to cirrhosis, viral hepatitis [143], malignancy [97], or even massive partial resection of the liver [51]. In the United States and Europe, the great majority of cases of HRS occur in patients with advanced alcoholic (Laennec's) cirrhosis. On physical examination of patients with HRS, a striking contrast is seen between the conspicuous arterial hypotension (aggravated by orthostasis) and the warm, well-perfused extremities, suggesting a hyperdynamic circulation in HRS.

The most extensively documented experience with HRS is that of the late Solomon Papper [108–110]. In Papper's personal series of 200 patients with HRS [109], 90.5 percent had a tendency to arterial hypotension, 80.5 percent had hepatic encephalopathy, 75 percent had massive ascites, and 94 percent were oliguric. The renal failure developed within a period of observation of months or even days, and a triggering event could not be found in 24.5 percent. In 40 percent of the patients, HRS was associated with progressing jaundice. In some patients, HRS tended to follow acute volume disturbances such as gastrointestinal bleeding, abdominal paracentesis, and induced diuresis. In many patients, HRS apparently developed following hospitalization. Papper suspected that overzealous attempts at treatment in the hospital setting contributed to this phenomenon. Spon-

The research for this paper was supported in part by a grant from the National Council for Research and Development, Israel, and the G.S.F., Munich, West Germany. The authors express appreciation to Ms. R. Snyder Weiss for preparation of the manuscript.

taneous recovery occurred in only 1 percent of Papper's patients. Remission of HRS may occur following restoration of liver function such as that associated with recovery from viral hepatitis, alcohol withdrawal, or liver transplantation [72].

In the series of 203 patients with HRS of Bartoli et al. [15], the predominant cause of death was almost invariably a major episode of variceal bleeding on the background of an extreme degree of liver failure and an almost complete loss of coagulation factors from the blood. It appears, therefore, that the cause of death in most instances of HRS is not directly due to the renal failure. On some occasions, HRS may, however, lead to frank acute tubular necrosis [143]. Indeed, the relatively slow recovery of HRS kidneys following normalization of liver function by transplantation [72] suggests that the HRS in these kidneys had progressed to acute tubular necrosis. Acute tubular necrosis may, of course, occur in association with cadaver kidney transplantation in the absence of any liver disease in the donor. It has been speculated that the entire spectrum of kidney involvement in liver disease, from the preazotemic stage with avid renal sodium retention to frank HRS, is due to the same circulatory disorder, the nature of which will be discussed.

Under this scheme, early in cirrhosis of the liver, glomerular filtration rate (GFR) and renal plasma flow (RPF) are normal, and there is avid sodium retention, predominantly in the distal tubule. Ability to dilute the urine is normal, and the tendency toward sodium and fluid retention is readily responsive to treatment with spironolactone. With advancing cirrhosis there is a tendency for GFR and RPF to decrease. Exaggerated sodium reabsorption now also occurs in the proximal tubule, and the patient loses ability to "escape" from the sodium-retaining effects of hypermineralocorticism. Edema and ascites formation become increasingly resistant to loop diuretics and to spironolactone. With further deterioration of liver function, the hyperdynamic circulation becomes more pronounced and the HRS ensues. The cardinal lesson from clinical liver and kidney transplantation in this respect is that even in the extreme stages of this spectrum, renal failure is potentially reversible.

As noted by Papper, HRS may begin insidiously over a period of weeks to months [107] or appear suddenly and cause severe azotemia within days [109]. The rapid course is often the harbinger of death [5]. The common precipitating causes are deterioration of liver function, sepsis, the use of nephrotoxic antibiotics or nonsteroidal antiinflammatory drugs, overzealous use of diuretics, diarrhea, or gastrointestinal bleeding. Often, however, HRS occurs without any apparent precipitating cause [15]. In a given patient it is difficult to predict the onset of HRS [109]. There are no physical signs, blood chemistry determinations, or hemodynamic measurements that exclusively occur or are absent in the population of patients with HRS [15, 109] compared with nonazotemic patients with advanced cirrhosis. It is clear, however, that pretreatment hyponatremia and/or excretion of less than 20 percent of a 20 ml/kg water load in a stable cirrhotic patient carries a dire prognosis, with mortality reaching 75 to 90 percent over the next 6 to 12 months [41]. The cirrhotic patients with the highest plasma renin, aldosterone, and norepinephrine concentrations also have the highest incidence of HRS and mortality [9].

Blood urea nitrogen (BUN) and blood creatinine concentration usually grossly underestimate the decrease in glomerular filtration in chronic liver disease [107, 109]. Specifically, normal levels of BUN and blood creatinine may persist even when inulin clearance has decreased below 20 ml per minute [107]. The poor nutritional state and decreased muscular mass in cirrhotic patients are responsible for this decrease in BUN and blood creatinine concentration for a given glomerular filtration rate [107, 109] in the HRS.

Renal Function

The hallmark of HRS is oliguria with a urine osmolality that is two to three times the concentration of the plasma. Urinary sodium concentration is usually less than 10 mmol per liter and often less than 1 mmol per liter [109, 143]. The urine is generally acid, but impaired ability to lower urinary pH has been described in some patients with cirrhosis [24, 134].

Persistent and prolonged HRS may usher in acute tubular necrosis. This transition is reflected by an increase in urinary sodium concentration to above 40 mmol per liter and isosthenuria. Frequently, however, the patient with HRS dies of liver failure before the functional HRS progresses to acute tubular necrosis.

Glomerular filtration rate is grossly reduced in HRS. As mentioned previously, the degree of azotemia does not reflect the decline in GFR. In patients with HRS it is rare for blood creatinine to increase above 4 to 5 mg per deciliter before the patient's demise.

Renal blood flow is generally diminished in cirrhosis even in the early compensated stage [1, 17, 52, 73, 74, 109, 116, 117, 120]. This reduction in renal blood flow has been documented by paraaminohippurate (PAH) clearance [109], ^{133}xenon washout method [17, 52, 73, 74, 116, 117, 120], and renal angiography [17, 53]. Angiographic studies demonstrate that in HRS there is drastic renal cortical vasoconstriction involving the renal artery and its main branches [17, 53]. All these studies demonstrate preferential outer cortical renal ischemia. In general, the renal hypoperfusion parallels the decline in liver function and is particularly pronounced in the presence of hypoalbuminemia [117]. However, in a given patient, renal blood flow may be reduced without producing azotemia. Interestingly, tilting maneuvers resulted in appropriate reactivity of the renal circulation even in advanced stages of cirrhosis, despite the subnormal level of the renal blood flow [120].

Pathology

In the series of Papper [109] the kidneys of most of the patients dying with HRS were normal or showed minimal changes.

Eknoyan [47] has reviewed in depth 23 published re-

ports describing glomerular changes in patients with cirrhosis. Mild glomerular lesions were found in about 50 percent of 800 patients in postmortem studies and in 95 percent of patients with kidney biopsy studies. The changes noted on light microscopy were periglomerular fibrosis, glomerular sclerosis, glomerular basement membrane thickening, mesangial matrix thickening, and glomerular hypercellularity occasionally resembling proliferative glomerulonephritis. Electron microscopy almost invariably showed electron-dense deposits in the capillary wall and the mesangium, thickening of the basement membrane, and the presence of electron-dense osmiophilic deposits in the mesangial matrix and in the subendothelial aspect of the basement membrane. Immunofluorescence studies showed subendothelial and mesangial deposits of IgA, IgM, or C3. In general, however, there was no correlation between these anatomic changes and renal dysfunction.

In jaundiced patients with HRS, the tubuli may contain deposits of bile pigment ("cholemic nephrosis"). This lesion is also seen following chronic bile duct ligation in experimental animals [21]. In our experience, these deposits do not interfere with kidney function (with the exception of medullary damage in the Gunn rat with congenital nonconjugated hyperbilirubinemia [105]).

Pathogenesis

The etiology of HRS has not been elucidated despite extensive investigation. These studies have been hampered by the fact that models of chronic liver damage in animals such as those produced by CCl_4 or dimethylnitrosamine poisoning or chronic bile duct ligation [21], while leading usually to avid renal sodium and water retention, do not mimic frank HRS as seen in patients with advanced cirrhosis. The central enigma of the HRS remains: Why is there intense renal and cerebral [21, 55] vasoconstriction in the face of generalized vasodilatation? This striking pattern also differs from hypovolemic or hemorrhagic hypotension, in which total peripheral vascular resistance is increased. Renal vasoconstrictor stimuli originating in the portal and hepatic circulation as well as metabolic disturbances associated with liver failure [34, 66] and the direct exposure of the systemic circulation to metabolites absorbed from the gut but bypassing the liver [71, 76, 121] may act in concert to produce the extreme renal cortical ischemia of HRS. It is of interest that even under the highly artificial and isolated conditions of in vitro perfusion of the rat kidney, inclusion of a normal rat liver in the circulation improves renal function [101]. Such observations, as well as the distinct clinical impression that normal renal blood perfusion depends on adequate liver function [72, 79], raise the possibility that a humoral factor produced by the liver or present in the bloodstream but not inactivated by the diseased liver aggravates renal vasoconstriction.

In advanced liver failure the systemic circulation is grossly underfilled [23, 48, 96], and patients with HRS are frankly hypotensive [109]. This is due to (1) peripheral vasodilatation; (2) hypoalbuminemia leading to diminished plasma oncotic pressure and, consequently, loss of intravascular volume to the interstitial and peritoneal spaces; (3) pooling of blood in the massively engorged splanchnic circulation; (4) the presence of wide arteriovenous and portasystemic shunts; (5) diminished venous return [65]; and (6) most probably, impaired myocardial contractility also [63, 65, 95]. Such underfilling is sensed by the cardiopulmonary low-pressure mechanoreceptors as well as by the sinoaortic baroreceptors. These stimuli activate the sympathetic nervous system [62]. In addition to these systemic baroreceptors there are baroreceptors in the liver that may activate the sympathetic nervous system [104]. It is quite possible that intrahepatic hypertension [80] or even portal hypertension per se [2] may augment the sympathetic tone. The net result is that in cirrhosis the systemic underfilling and the intrahepatic hypertension lead to increased sympathetic tone as well as an increase in the level of blood catecholamines [25, 26, 68, 118, 120] (recently reviewed by Henriksen et al. [69] and DiBona [43]). Since RPF and GFR in cirrhosis are negatively correlated with plasma catecholamine levels, it has been assumed that activation of the sympathetic nervous system contributes to the renal vasoconstriction of HRS [9, 69]. It should be remembered, however, that HRS cannot be reversed by intrarenal infusion of adrenergic blocking agents or renal vasodilators [17, 53]. Even the avid sodium retention in moderate experimental liver disease cannot be overcome by renal denervation and pharmacologic renal α- and β-adrenergic blockade [35] or intrarenal infusion of the vasodilator acetylcholine [100]. Therefore, increased sympathetic tone by itself cannot totally explain the intense renal cortical ischemia of HRS, and additional other constrictor influences are evidently operative in HRS. The increased sympathetic tone in cirrhosis, as well as the activation of renal arteriolar baroreceptors by arterial hypotension, are powerful stimuli to renin production. The potential role of the renin-angiotensin system will therefore be discussed in a later section.

ROLE OF RENAL PROSTAGLANDIN PRODUCTION IN THE ETIOLOGY OF HRS

Interest in prostaglandins in HRS was kindled by the observation that administration of nonsteroidal antiinflammatory agents to patients with decompensated cirrhosis precipitated a reversible form of HRS [9, 33, 149]. These findings in humans were later confirmed in the dog with chronic bile duct ligation. Specifically, in this canine model administration of nonsteroidal antiinflammatory agents, in either the ascitic or preascitic model, resulted in a decrease in renal perfusion and GFR secondary to an increase in renal vascular resistance [92, 148]. It was further shown that indomethacin sensitivity in these animals was dependent on the presence of portal hypertension, a stimulated state of the renin-angiotensin axis, and increased renal kallikrein production [92]. Interestingly, the deterioration in renal function during the administration of nonsteroidal antiinflammatory agents occurred in parallel with an increase in

arterial blood pressure in the anesthetized dog with chronic bile duct ligation [148] and improvement in pressor response to angiotensin II in patients with cirrhosis [149]. These results suggest a role for prostaglandins in the peripheral vasodilatation and hypotension of chronic liver disease.

It has since been shown that in cirrhosis in humans in the pre-HRS [9] and in the dog with chronic bile duct ligation, there is an increase in urinary excretion of PGE_2. The rate of urinary excretion of PGE_2 in these patients correlated positively with glomerular filtration rate [9]. In patients with HRS, urinary excretion of the prostaglandin E series was low [45, 151]. Taken together, these data demonstrate that in chronic liver disease there is an increase in the production of renal vasodilatory prostaglandins, perhaps as a regulatory response to renal vasoconstriction or under the influence of the increased levels of circulating arginine vasopressin, angiotensin II, or catecholamines. Spontaneous or drug-induced reduction in renal prostaglandin synthesis resulted in an unopposed renal vasoconstriction and precipitation of HRS.

Zipser et al. [151] proposed an additional facet to the role of prostaglandins in HRS. They found that in patients with HRS, the drastic reduction in urinary PGE_2 excretion was associated with a sharp increase in urinary excretion of thromboxane B_2. This, in turn, may be viewed as reflecting enhanced renal synthesis of the potent vasoconstrictor thromboxane A_2. Assuming that renal thromboxane A_2 contributed to the renal vasoconstriction of HRS, they attempted to block its production selectively by the imidazole derivative dazoxiben. The results of this initial trial study on 8 patients with HRS were not fruitful [150]. Although urinary thromboxane levels were normalized, renal function was not improved despite the persistence of pre-dazoxiben levels of urinary PGE_2 and PGI_2. At present, therefore, the role of renal thromboxane A_2 production in the causation of the HRS has not been clarified. It is possible that renal ischemia per se stimulates synthesis and urinary excretion of thromboxane B_2 and its metabolites. Increase in urinary thromboxane B_2 excretion has been seen in other models of acute renal damage and may be a nonspecific sequel to acute renal ischemia rather than its cause. In a recent editorial, Dunn [45] expressed the opinion that a more potent inhibition of renal thromboxane A_2 production to subnormal levels may yet prove of value in the therapy of HRS. He also cites suggestions by others that dietary manipulations such as the use of eicosapentanoic acid, which is abundant in fish oils, may help to restore the normal balance between renal vasodilator and vasoconstrictor eicosanoids and thus may be useful in the management of the HRS.

In summary, in advanced cirrhosis of the liver, renal blood perfusion is critically dependent on increased renal synthesis of vasodilatory PGE_2 and PGI_2. This is apparently necessary to counteract the increased renal vasoconstrictor tone in cirrhosis secondary to activation of the α-adrenergic nervous system, renin-angiotensin axis, increased plasma arginine vasopressin level, and other undefined constrictor influences.

ROLE OF THE RENIN-ANGIOTENSIN-ALDOSTERONE AXIS (RAAA) IN THE ETIOLOGY OF HRS

The RAAA system is often highly stimulated in HRS, and intrarenal production of angiotensin II may contribute to the renal vasoconstriction as well as to the increased production of renal prostaglandins. The initial cause of increased renin production could be the stimulation of renal nerves and arteriolar baroreceptors by the arterial hypotension [133], hepatic venous congestion [88], portal hypertension [2], or alteration in distal delivery of sodium chloride to the macula densa. Some authors have postulated primary renal ischemia as a cause for the activation of the RAAA, since renal vasodilatation with dopamine may suppress the RAAA system in HRS [17]. Bosch et al. [32] and Arroyo et al. [6] have shown that in a large group of nonazotemic patients with cirrhosis, activation of the RAAA was a grave prognostic sign (50 percent survival at 6 months). Activation of the RAAA in advanced cirrhosis may help in the defense of maintaining arterial blood pressure [122, 131] in synergism with the action of increased circulating levels of catecholamines. However, activation of both the RAAA and the sympathetic nervous system intensifies renal vasoconstriction and contributes to the avid renal sodium reabsorption seen in this stage of cirrhosis.

In several large series of patients with cirrhosis and functional renal failure, plasma renin activity correlated negatively with creatinine clearance [14, 132, 145]. Conversely, various maneuvers that led to volume repletion (summarized in [5]) improved renal function and suppressed the RAAA in patients with cirrhosis. Berkowitz et al. [18, 19], noting that the renin substrate is low in the HRS, hypothesized that decreased renal angiotensin generation could directly cause HRS, perhaps by decreasing efferent glomerular arteriolar tone and thus reducing the filtration pressure. They observed improvement in renal function in HRS following administration of fresh frozen plasma to patients with HRS. This is supported by the finding of an increase in renin substrate prior to the restoration of kidney function following successful liver transplantation. In contrast, however, many other investigators could not reverse HRS with supplementation of the renin substrate by fresh frozen plasma.

In summary, the RAAA is almost invariably stimulated excessively in HRS. While participating in the defense of systemic arterial blood pressure, it most probably aggravates renal vasoconstriction and contributes to the initiation and maintenance of HRS. On the other hand, it may be one of the stimulators for renal vasodilatory renal PGE_2 and PGI_2 synthesis.

ROLE OF THE KALLIKREIN-KININ SYSTEM IN HRS

Infusion of kinins into humans and dogs augments renal blood flow and urinary sodium excretion [102, 136]. Since plasma prekallikrein and bradykinin levels are subnormal in cirrhosis [146], it has been suggested that suppression of this system may contribute to renal vasoconstriction in HRS. Indeed, recent data on the excretion of urinary kallikrein support this suggestion. Specifically, Perez-Ayuso et al. [113] found that patients with cirrhosis and normal renal function have supranor-

mal urinary excretion of both kallikrein and prostaglandin E_2. In patients with HRS there was a depression of both urinary kallikrein and prostaglandin E_2 on the background of activation of the RAAA and the sympathetic nervous system. The authors considered that this imbalance between intrarenal vasodilatory and vasoconstrictor influences was conducive to the emergence of HRS.

ROLE OF VASOACTIVE INTESTINAL PEPTIDES IN HRS

A vasoactive factor isolated from the small intestine (VIP) has biologic activity that mimics many of the associated circulatory and metabolic disorders of cirrhosis [76, 121]. Among these are peripheral vasodilatation, increased cardiac output, pulmonary shunting, and hyperventilation. Since this substance is inactivated by the liver [76], it has been suggested that in cirrhosis enough VIP may escape inactivation by the diseased liver to enter the systemic circulation, thereby contributing to the peripheral vasodilatation.

An additional powerful VIP, namely substance P, seems to be operative in patients with cirrhosis and hepatic coma who are prone to HRS [71]. When injected into volunteers, substance P causes a hyperdynamic circulation similar to that seen in advanced cirrhosis. Usually, substance P, an endecapeptide, is secreted by the gastrointestinal tract and is completely inactivated by passage through the liver. In advanced cirrhosis the degradative potential for this peptide is reduced, and it also bypasses the liver through portasystemic shunts. Hoertnagel et al. [71] found that in hepatic coma the levels of substance P increased more than 10-fold the normal level. Moreover, this increase was directly correlated with an increase in plasma noradrenaline levels and cardiac output and negatively correlated with systemic vascular resistance. Therefore, in patients with advanced cirrhosis and coma, extreme peripheral vasodilatation, partly caused by substance P, VIP, and possibly glucagon, may divert blood perfusion away from the kidney, thus aggravating HRS.

ROLE OF CHOLEMIA IN HRS

The hepatorenal syndrome is often associated with jaundice [109]. It is therefore surprising that there is only scant mention in the literature of the role of cholemia in the pathogenesis of the HRS. Classic studies suggested that bile compounds such as bilirubin [16, 42] or bile acids [3] were directly nephrotoxic. These studies did not, however, consider protein binding of these biliary components. Such binding would greatly reduce their nephrotoxicity. This is borne out by both experimental studies [1, 90] and clinical findings in humans that showed preservation of renal perfusion and GFR when hyperbilirubinemia is below 15 mg/dl in patients suffering from endemic cholangiocarcinoma in Thailand [135]. It appears that rather than being directly nephrotoxic, the "cholemic environment" disturbs volume regulation in at least two (prerenal) ways [22]: (1) depression of the entire cardiovascular system by an increase in circulating bile salts, an action reminiscent of myocardial beta-adrenergic blockade, as well as calcium channel blockade [30, 31, 56] and peripheral vascular alpha-adrenergic antagonism [27, 63, 64], and (2) the powerful natriuretic effect of bile salts causing obligatory salt wasting and volume depletion. Thus, the combination of cardiovascular depression and hypovolemia causes a circulatory embarrassment ("underfill") and interferes with normal constrictor and contractile defense mechanisms. The increased absolute cardiac output of HRS often is inadequate to meet metabolic and circulatory requirements, and may thus be a variant of high-output failure. Correction of the hypotension with exogenous constrictors may precipitate frank congestive heart failure and pulmonary edema [95].

Finally, in extreme hyperbilirubinemia (exceeding 30 mg/dl) direct "biliary" nephrotoxicity may eventually occur [135].

HRS AND LIVER TRANSPLANTATION

Acute renal failure is very common following liver transplantation, as reported in a recent review by McCauley and associates [98]. The presence of HRS before liver transplantation apparently does not influence the long-term outcome of this operation [98]. It is noteworthy that the hyperdynamism of the circulation may be corrected within 12 hours after successful liver engraftment [139]. This suggests that "abnormal hepatic environment" and attendant vasodilatory humoral influences, rather than preformed arteriovenous shunts, are the predominant mechanism for the increased cardiac output in the HRS.

ROLE OF ENDOTOXINEMIA IN HRS

Endotoxin is a lipopolysaccharide that is capable of causing peripheral vasodilatation, enhanced cardiac output, renal vasoconstriction, respiratory alkalosis, and, in large doses, myocardial depression. All these phenomena are seen in patients with HRS. Endotoxin is usually produced by bacteria in the gut and cleared by the liver. It is conceivable, therefore, that in patients with cirrhosis, endotoxinemia, even without bacteremia, may contribute to both the hyperkinetic circulation and HRS. Mounting evidence suggests that with the increasing severity of cirrhosis there is an increased incidence of endotoxinemia. Most authors [137, 142, 144] believe that endotoxinemia is one of the main causes of the renal vasoconstriction of HRS, although this matter is still debated [60]. In this respect, the elegant studies of Levy and Wexler [91] are illuminating.

They utilized osmotic minipumps that were able to infuse intravenously *Escherichia coli* endotoxin over a 7-day period. In normal dogs, doses of endotoxin of 50 μg per hour had no effect on systemic hemodynamics or kidney function. In cirrhotic dogs, in contrast, an endotoxin dose of 25 μg per hour caused a marked decline in GFR and renal plasma flow at a time when systemic hemodynamics were still normal. At a dosage of 50 μg per hour, cardiac output and arterial blood pressure declined. The selective renal vasoconstrictor effect of endotoxin in these cirrhotic dogs could not be abolished by α- or β-adrenergic blockade, thus mimicking HRS. Taken together, all these clinical and experimental find-

ings strongly suggest that endotoxinemia in advanced liver disease contributes to the causation of HRS. The known effects of endotoxin in enhancing aggregation of platelets and deposition of fibrin would aggravate its deleterious effect on kidney function [91, 142, 144].

ROLE OF FALSE NEUROTRANSMITTERS IN HRS

The presence of "false neurotransmitters," mainly octopamine, in the central and peripheral nervous systems has been invoked to explain the autonomic dysfunction, the hepatic coma including extrapyramidal changes, as well as the peripheral vasodilatation of cirrhosis [57]. According to this concept, the precursors of false neurotransmitters are produced in the bowel by bacterial degradation of protein. These compounds are usually cleared by the healthy liver, mainly due to catabolism by monoamine oxidase. However, in cirrhosis, these compounds may bypass the liver and enter the nervous system, where they are degraded locally by β-hydroxylation by relatively nonspecific enzymes. In the central nervous system they may replace normal neurotransmitters and thus interfere with normal synaptic transmission [83].

The role of false neurotransmitters in explaining HRS is questionable. In advanced liver disease blood catecholamines are elevated, suggesting overstimulation of the adrenergic nervous system. Moreover, false neurotransmitters would be expected to interfere with synaptic traffic and relieve renal vasoconstriction, thus ameliorating HRS.

PERIPHERAL ARTERIAL VASODILATION HYPOTHESIS

The classic "underfilling" hypothesis in cirrhosis proposes that ascites formation decreases plasma volume and thus leads to secondary renal sodium and water retention [46, 108]. However, plasma volume has been found to be expanded, not decreased, in cirrhosis [93, 94]; moreover, plasma volume has been shown to antecede ascites formation [89]. Thus, the "overflow" hypothesis was proposed, indicating that liver disease leads to primary renal sodium and water retention with plasma volume expansion [93]. This overflow hypothesis is in concert with the finding of plasma volume expansion in cirrhosis; in this context, ascites formation occurs secondary to the renal sodium and water retention and the portal hypertension. With the overflow hypothesis, however, total plasma volume expansion would be expected to suppress the neurohumoral profile, including plasma norepinephrine, renin, aldosterone, and vasopressin. Plasma renin and aldosterone have been found to be suppressed in some compensated patients with cirrhosis [5, 20]. This observation, however, has been associated with the supine position and an accompanying natriuresis, findings compatible with mobilization of splanchnic venous pooling with resultant central blood volume expansion. Moreover, with progression of cirrhosis from the compensated (no ascites) to decompensated (ascites) to hepatorenal syndrome, the neurohumoral profile is stimulated, not suppressed [26, 54, 103, 120]. Taken together, therefore, neither the underfill nor the overflow hypothesis provides an adequate explanation for the entire clinical spectrum of cirrhosis, which ultimately leads to the hepatorenal syndrome.

On this background, the peripheral arterial vasodilation hypothesis of sodium and water retention in cirrhosis has been proposed [127]. This hypothesis was formulated as an integral part of a unifying hypothesis of body fluid volume regulation in health and disease in which either a decrease in cardiac output (Fig. 51-1) or peripheral arterial vasodilation (Fig. 51-2) initiates arterial underfilling with secondary sodium and water retention [123, 124]. In cirrhosis, peripheral arterial vasodilation is proposed as the initiator of arterial underfilling and occurs in the splanchnic bed, but also in the skin, muscle, and lung [81, 141]. This peripheral arterial vasodilation hypothesis can explain the entire spectrum of cirrhosis (Fig. 51-3). The progressive plasma volume expansion occurs primarily in the venous circulation, while the relative underfilling of the arterial circulation occurs secondary to systemic arterial vasodilation. As shown in Fig. 51-2, there are several other sodium- and water-retaining states in which primary peripheral arterial vasodilation initiates renal sodium and water retention [123, 124]. The associated increase in cardiac output secondary to afterload reduction also contributes to the compensatory response. Thus, the ascites formation and the neurohumorally mediated renal vasoconstriction are adaptive responses, which in their advanced state may become maladaptive (Fig. 51-4). Specifically, the resultant ascites formation contributes to the predisposition of the cirrhotic patient to spontaneous bacterial peritonitis and sepsis, pulmonary complications, and generalized morbidity including anorexia. While the hepatic capillary fibrosis and resultant increased resistance to portal blood flow contribute to the portal hypertension, with the associated esophageal varices and variceal hemorrhage of cirrhosis, the increased splanchnic flow is also critical in causing the portal hypertension with its attendant complications. The renal vasoconstriction increases progressively as the systemic arterial vasodilation becomes more pronounced, and ultimately the hepatorenal syndrome may occur.

As discussed earlier, a number of potential humoral mediators of the systemic arterial vasodilation are associated with cirrhosis (Fig. 51-5). To date, however, the data are scarce in support of any specific mechanism [126]. Nevertheless, it is clear that in cirrhotic patients vasodilating prostaglandins attenuate the renal vasoconstriction [8] and the pressor response to angiotensin II [84]. Thus, cyclooxygenase inhibitors may cause renal functional deterioration, which mimics hepatorenal syndrome [8] and also raises blood pressure in cirrhotic animals and patients.

Endotoxin is absorbed from the gastrointestinal tract into the portal circulation and is then normally removed by the liver. However, in association with the portosystemic shunting, plasma endotoxin concentrations have been found to be elevated in cirrhosis [137]. Moreover, Radlomski, Palmer, and Moncada [115] have found that endotoxin induces a calcium-independent nitric oxide synthase in vascular smooth muscle. This enzyme is different from the constitutive nitric oxide synthase in en-

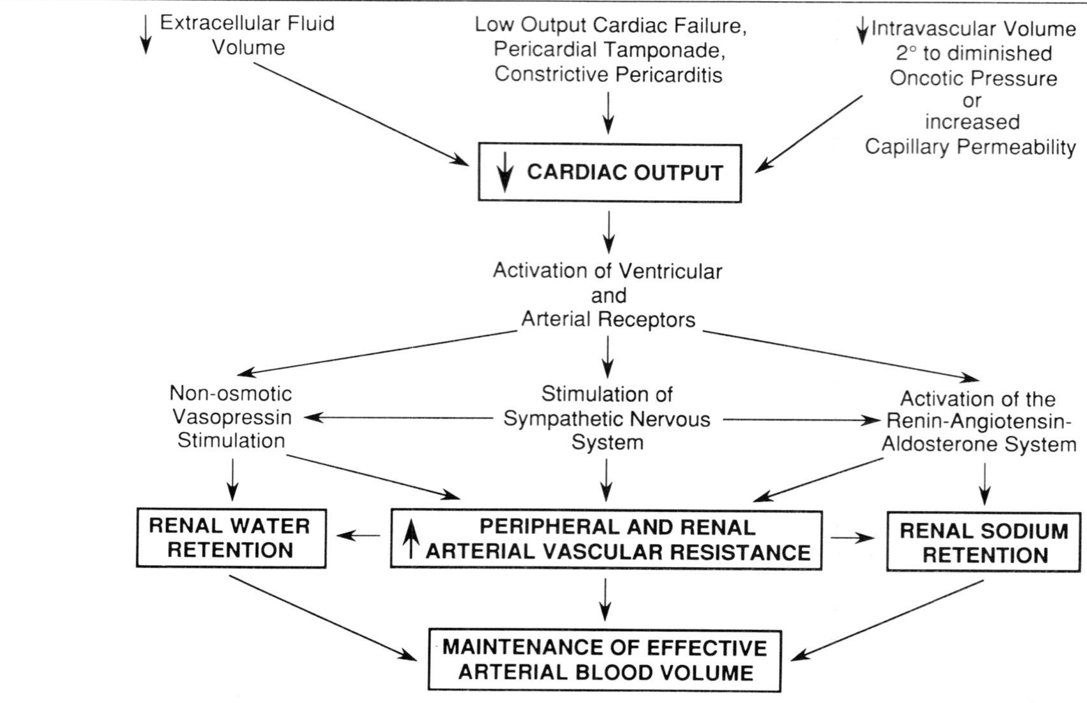

Fig. 51-1. Sequence of events in which reduced cardiac output initiates renal sodium and water retention. (From [124].)

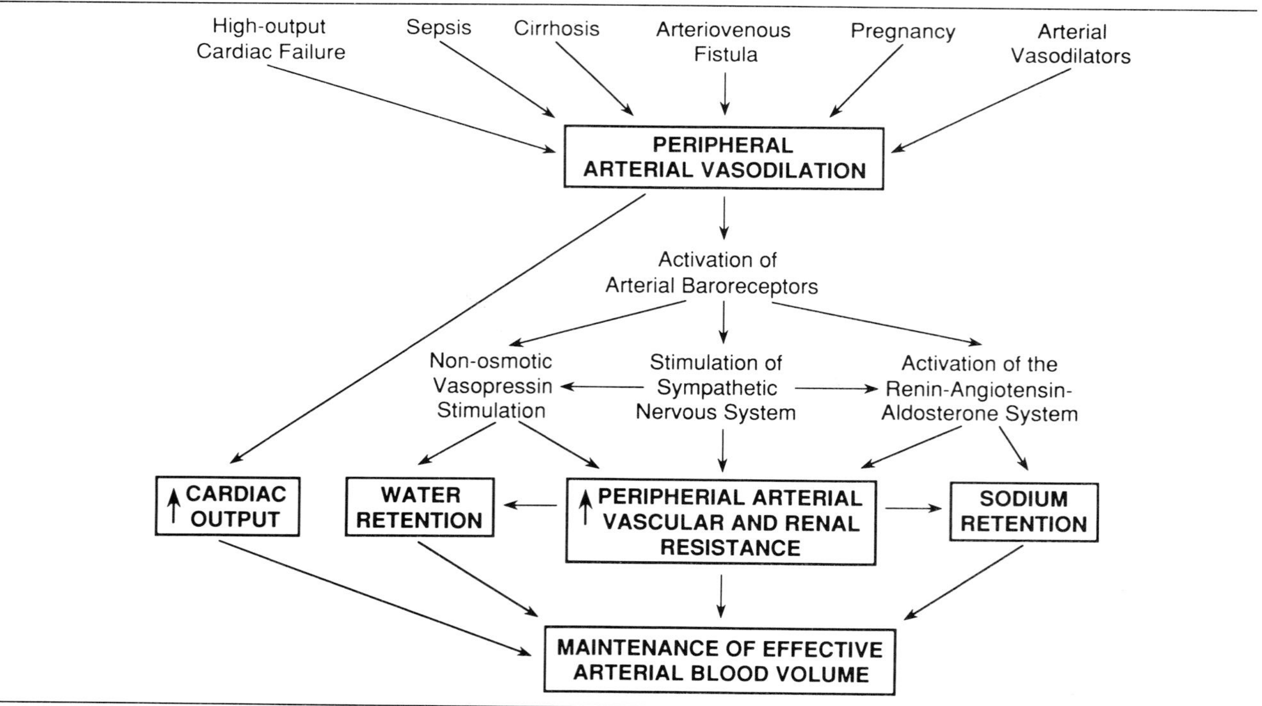

Fig. 51-2. Sequence of events in which peripheral arterial vasodilation initiates renal sodium and water retention. (From [124].)

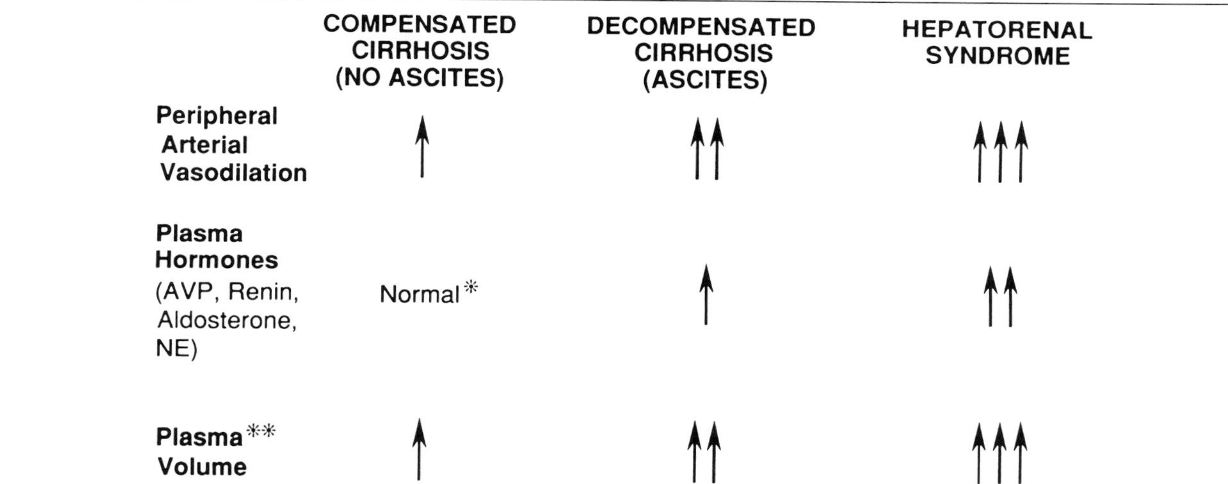

Fig. 51-3. Stages of progression of cirrhosis. AVP = arginine vasopressin; NE = norepinephrine. *Given the positive sodium and water balance that has occurred, these plasma hormones would be suppressed in normal subjects without liver disease. **The progressive renal sodium and water retention increases extracellular fluid, interstitial fluid, and plasma volume. However, the concomitant occurrence of hypoalbuminemia in decompensated cirrhosis and hepatorenal syndrome may attenuate the degree of plasma volume expansion. (From R. W. Schrier. The Edematous Patient. In R. W. Schrier (ed.), *Manual of Nephrology* (3rd ed.). Boston: Little, Brown, 1990. Pp. 1–19.)

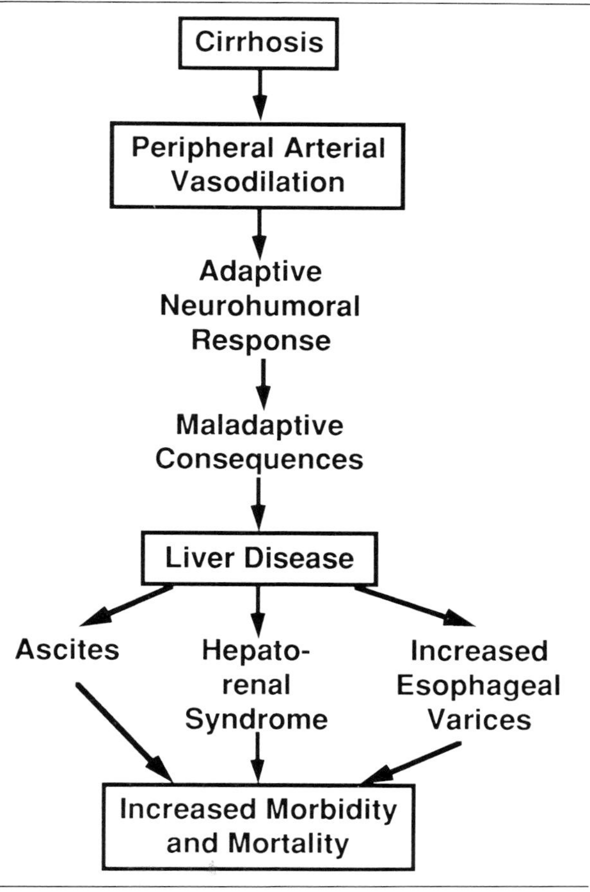

Fig. 51-4. Adaptive response to arterial underfilling may become maladaptive in cirrhosis.

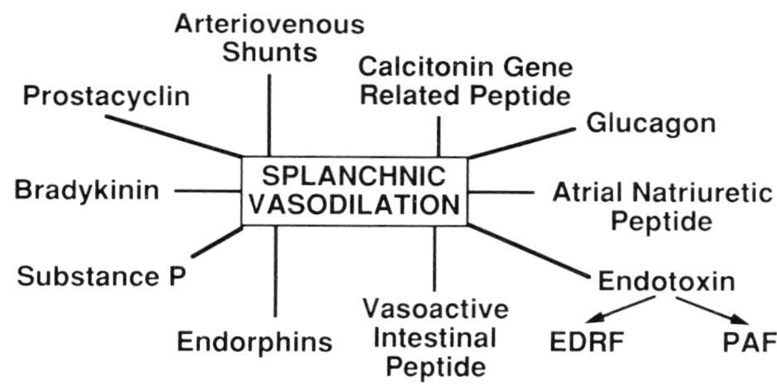

Fig. 51-5. Potential causes of splanchnic and nonsplanchnic vasodilation in cirrhosis. EDRF = endothelial relaxing factor; PAF = platelet activating factor.

dothelial cells, which is calcium dependent. These same workers found that nitric oxide antagonists, which are L-arginine analogues, will block the hypotension and improve survival in endotoxin shock. Vallance and Moncada [138] have further suggested that the peripheral arterial vasodilation in cirrhosis may be related to endotoxin-mediated nitric oxide. This possibility, however, remains to be examined.

Bradykinin antagonists are now also available for experimental use [44], but to date there are no results relating to a role of this hormone in the arterial vasodilation associated with cirrhosis. The availability of specific antagonists for atrial natriuretic peptide, substance P, and VIP will be necessary to examine a role of these hormones in the peripheral arterial vasodilation associated with cirrhosis.

There also seem to be physiologic shunts that are opened in cirrhosis by portal hypertension and perhaps

some neurohumoral events associated with cirrhosis. In experimental animals, shunting of 15 μ microspheres to the lung were shown to increase with temperature in both cirrhotic and control rats [85]. Moreover, the greater shunting to the lung in cirrhotic than control rats could be equalized with the combination of a 40°C temperature and alpha-adrenergic blockade [85].

Thus, taken together, the peripheral arterial vasodilation that has been proposed to initiate the renal sodium and water retention in cirrhosis may be multifactorial in nature. In any case, the use of a V_1 vasopressin agonist may attenuate the vasodilation in the splanchnic, muscle, and dermal beds [36]. The chances for the development of an orally active, nonpeptide V_1 agonist have been recently enhanced since such an orally active V_1 antagonist has already been developed [147]. In Fig. 51-4 is proposed a potential therapeutic strategy that would involve chronic therapy with an orally active V_1 agonist and a prophylactic LeVeen shunt. With prophylactic cephalosporin antibiotics, removal of ascites before the shunt insertion, and the use of a titanium connector to avoid thrombosis, the major complications of peritoneovenous shunting, including infection, thrombosis, and intravascular clotting, can be largely avoided.

Peripheral arterial vasodilation activates several vasoconstrictor pathways (see Fig. 51-2) that are known as mediators of renal vasoconstriction and sodium and water retention. As stated earlier, in advanced stages of decompensated cirrhosis these compensatory events may lead to the hepatorenal syndrome. Stimulation of the renal sympathetic nerves and circulating catecholamines are known to cause renal vasoconstriction. The evidence in cirrhosis for activation of the sympathetic nervous system in cirrhosis is now compelling and includes increased plasma norepinephrine concentrations [26, 120], increased norepinephrine secretion rates [103], and increased sympathetic discharges from peroneal nerve recordings [59]. Moreover, the highest concentrations of plasma renin, aldosterone, norepinephrine, and vasopressin are associated with the highest mortality [9]. The same poor prognosis is related to the degree of pretreatment hyponatremia, a state associated with the nonosmotic stimulation of vasopressin [41]. Henriksen and co-workers [70] also have shown an inverse correlation between plasma volume expansion and systemic vascular resistance in the various stages of cirrhosis (Fig. 51-5).

Henriksen and associates [68] have also shown in cirrhotic patients that renal venous norepinephrine concentration exceeds the renal arterial norepinephrine concentration. This finding is compatible with alpha-adrenergic renal vasoconstriction in cirrhosis. Plasma angiotensin II is also known to be elevated in cirrhosis and is a well-known, potent renal vasoconstrictor. Moreover, peripheral arterial vasodilation is known to stimulate the adrenergic nervous and renin-angiotensin-aldosterone systems [99].

In addition to causing a fall in GFR, and thus filtered sodium load, alpha-adrenergic stimulation [78] and angiotensin [37] are known to enhance sodium and water reabsorption in the proximal tubule. Taken together, these vascular and tubular epithelial events combine to

Fig. 51-6. Aldosterone escape in normal subjects (left side) and failure of aldosterone escape in patients with underfilling of the arterial circulation (right side). EABV = effective arterial blood volume; ECF = extracellular fluid. (From [124].)

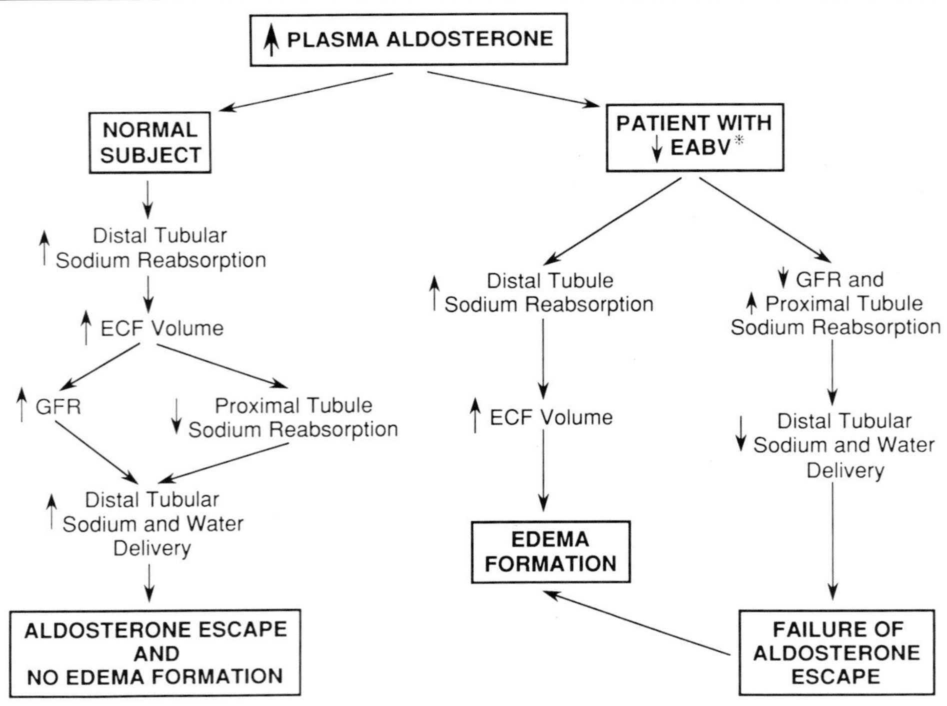

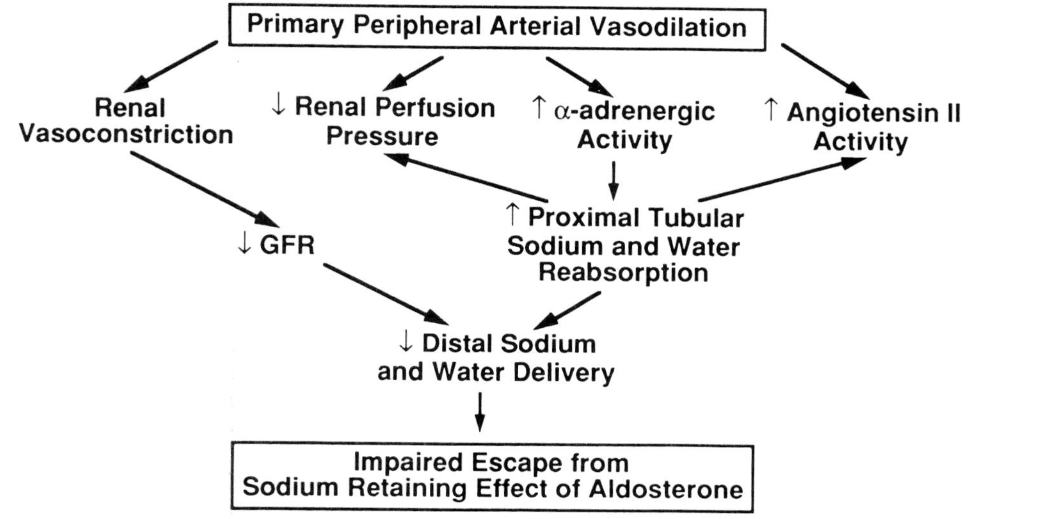

Fig. 51-7. Mechanisms whereby peripheral arterial vasodilation impairs escape from aldosterone in cirrhosis by decreasing distal sodium delivery. (From R. W. Schrier and O. S. Better. Pathogenesis of ascites formation: Mechanism of impaired aldosterone escape in cirrhosis. *Eur. J. Gastroenterol. Hepatol.*, 3:721, 1991.

decrease sodium and water excretion to the distal nephron, that is, the collecting duct, the site of action of vasopressin, aldosterone, and atrial natriuretic peptide (Fig. 51-6). We have recently published the rationale whereby the impaired aldosterone escape and the resistance to atrial natriuretic peptide are mediated by diminished distal sodium delivery. Lastly, it is well known that distal fluid delivery, as well as vasopressin, modulates solute-free water delivery. Thus, taken together, the peripheral arterial vasodilation hypothesis provides a framework to explain the spectrum of progressive severity of cirrhosis including the HRS.

Therapy of HRS

The HRS is usually a terminal complication in a patient with advanced liver disease. At this time, there is little that the internist can do to help the patient with HRS. The most important principles in the management of patients with HRS are avoidance of all measures that cause drastic perturbation in volume status and minimizing exposure to nephrotoxic drugs, nonsteroidal antiinflammatory agents, and contrast media. Oral neomycin, in the 6 gm per day dosage usually given to patients with hepatic pre-coma, may be absorbed from the gut in sufficient quantities to be nephrotoxic, and its dosage should therefore be reduced. One should particularly avoid excessive sudden volume losses due to diarrhea (e.g., treatment with lactulose), peritoneal taps, or induced diuresis. Volume replacement should be instituted gently to avoid rupture of varices. Since most patients with advanced liver disease have underfilling of the circulation and are hypotensive, an attempt should be made to correct volume deficits with salt-free albumin solution or normal saline until central venous pressure has risen to 8 to 10 cm water or pulmonary capillary wedge pressure has increased to 10 mm Hg. Tense ascites may increase intraabdominal and even intrathoracic pressure and interfere with venous return [65]. Therefore, tense ascites should be relieved with a slow tap to remove 500 ml two to three times a day [77]. Following this combined treatment, the responsiveness to diuretics may return.

Hemodialysis or peritoneal dialysis is of no value in the treatment of HRS [112], complicating irreversible liver damage. In certain cases, however, when the etiology of the renal failure in a patient with liver disease has not been clarified, one or two dialyses may be indicated. Such a procedure will "buy" time until a definite diagnosis of the variety of renal failure has been established. This procedure will also reduce the body pool of urea, which is a substrate for ammonia production by intestinal bacteria. In the future, the use of charcoal hemoperfusion [82] or hemodialysis with highly permeable polyacrylonitrile membrane may broaden the indication for this treatment in patients with HRS and hepatic coma [106].

On the other hand, conventional hemodialysis or, preferably, continuous arteriovenous hemoperfusion (CAVHP) has a definite place in the treatment of renal failure associated with reversible liver damage, such as that due to toxins, obstructive jaundice, cholangitis, or viral hepatitis [28, 111].

Pharmacologic intervention in an attempt to raise systemic blood pressure or reduce renal vascular resistance has been followed by only temporary success and does not change the inexorable course of HRS. Thus Cohn et al. [38, 39] achieved a temporary increase in renal cortical perfusion with the use of octapressin and renal vasodilators. Others have achieved a temporary increase in renal blood flow and GFR in HRS with dibenzyline [10, 11] or intravenous and intrarenal dopamine [13, 17]. Intrarenal phentolamine did not improve renal perfu-

sion in HRS but caused arterial hypotension [53]. Intravenous administration of prostaglandin A_1 and intrarenal infusion of prostaglandin E_2 did not resolve HRS [4, 152]. Thus, pharmacologic agents may temporarily increase renal perfusion in HRS, but usually this is not followed by diuresis.

In selected patients with HRS and stable liver function, the creation of a portacaval shunt may be followed by dramatic improvement including diuresis, increase in the GFR, normalization of the previously elevated plasma renin activity, and increase in plasma renin substrate [128, 130]. This result was thought to reflect correction of the systemic volume deficit following the portacaval shunt. In contrast, others could not find beneficial effects of the portacaval shunt on kidney function in patients with HRS [119]. Moreover, the operation of portacaval anastomosis may precipitate HRS [40, 61]. At present, therefore, portal decompressive surgery is not indicated for the management of most patients with HRS.

The LeVeen peritoneojugular shunt was introduced in 1974 as a treatment for refractory ascites [86]. This method is capable of redistributing the ascites into the systemic circulation, thus replenishing the depleted central volume and improving venous return to the heart. This is accomplished by decompression of the peritoneal cavity and the inferior vena cava. Insertion of the LeVeen shunt in patients with refractory ascites may cause dramatic improvement in central hemodynamics with an increase in GFR and RPF and brisk natriuresis leading to complete mobilization of the ascites [29]. Such salutary response is paralleled by normalization of the previously excessively stimulated renin-angiotensin-aldosterone axis (Fig. 51-7) [129]. Since this procedure may improve renal function in patients with advanced cirrhosis, it has been suggested that the LeVeen shunt can be used for the management of HRS [75, 114, 129]. Indeed, several well-documented cases are on record in which HRS was refractory to meticulous volume replacement but responded well to the introduction of the LeVeen shunt [129]. The initial enthusiasm for this method of treatment, however, has been tempered by the high rate of complications associated with it. In authoritative in-depth reviews of the subject, Epstein [49, 50] came to the following conclusions: Insertion of the LeVeen shunt is associated with operative mortality of 20 percent, and mechanical, metabolic, and hematologic complications occur in some two thirds of the patients thus treated. In most reported cases of the reversal of uremia by the LeVeen shunt, this occurred in patients in whom conservative measures such as volume replacement and combination of diuretics had not been tried. It is quite possible that these patients would have benefited from a less drastic treatment than the insertion of the LeVeen shunt. At present, therefore, the peritoneovenous shunt cannot be viewed as an established therapy for most patients with HRS. As discussed in the section entitled Peripheral Arterial Vasodilation Hypothesis, early insertion of a LeVeen shunt and an orally active V_1 agonist (when available) could prevent the progression to HRS.

Finally, a suggestion has been made that corticosteroid treatment may be useful in the management of the hepatorenal syndrome [142]. This steroid treatment may be most efficacious in younger patients with associated cirrhosis and alcoholic hepatitis.

References

1. Alon, U., Berant, M., Mordechovitz, D., et al. The effect of intrarenal infusion of bile on kidney function in the dog. *Clin. Sci.* 62: 431, 1982.
2. Anderson, R. J., Cronin, R. E., McDonald, K. M., et al. Mechanism of portal hypertension induced alteration in renal hemodynamics, renal water excretion and renin secretion. *J. Clin. Invest.* 58: 964, 1976.
3. Aoyagi, T., and Lowenstein, L. The effect of renal ischemia and bile acids on renal function. *J. Lab. Clin. Med.* 71: 686, 1968.
4. Arieff, A. I., and Chidsey, C. A. Renal function in cirrhosis and the effects of PGA_2. *Am. J. Med.* 56: 695, 1974.
5. Arroyo, V., Bosch, J., and Rodes, J. Should the Term "Hepatorenal Syndrome" Be Used? In E. Bartoli and L. Chiandussi (eds.), *Hepatorenal Syndrome.* Padova, Italy: Piccin Medical Books, 1979. Pp. 36–49.
6. Arroyo, V., Bosch, J., Gaya-Beltran, J., et al. Plasma renin activity and urinary sodium excretion as prognostic indicators in nonazotemic cirrhosis with ascites. *Ann. Intern. Med.* 94: 198, 1981.
7. Arroyo, V., Bosch, J., Mauri, M., et al. Renin, aldosterone and renal hemodynamics in cirrhosis with ascites. *Eur. J. Clin. Invest.* 9: 69, 1979.
8. Arroyo, V., Gines, P., Rimola, A., et al. Renal function abnormalities, prostaglandins, and effects of nonsteroidal anti-inflammatory drugs in cirrhosis with ascites. *Am. J. Med.* 81 (Suppl. 2B): 104, 1986.
9. Arroyo, V., Planas, R., Gaya, J., et al. Sympathetic nervous activity, renin-angiotensin system and renal excretion of prostaglandin E_2 in cirrhosis. Relationship to functional renal failure and sodium and water excretion. *Eur. J. Clin. Invest.* 13: 271, 1983.
10. Baldus, W. P. Etiology and management of renal failure in cirrhosis and portal hypertension. *Ann. N.Y. Acad. Sci.* 170: 267, 1969.
11. Baldus, W. P., Feichter, R. M., and Summerskill, W. H. J. The kidney in cirrhosis. I. Clinical and biochemical features of azotemia in hepatic failure. *Ann. Intern. Med.* 60: 353, 1964.
12. Baldus, W. P., Feichter, R. M., Summerskill, W. H. J., et al. The kidney in cirrhosis: II. Disorders of renal function. *Ann. Intern. Med.* 60: 366, 1964.
13. Barnardo, D. E., Baldus, W. P., and Maher, F. T. Effects of dopamine on renal function in patients with cirrhosis. *Gastroenterology* 58: 524, 1970.
14. Barnardo, D. E., Summerskill, W. H. J., Strong, C. G., et al. Renal function, renin activity and endogenous vasoactive substances in cirrhosis. *Am. J. Digest. Dis.* 15: 419, 1970.
15. Bartoli, E., Arras, S., Faedda, R., et al. Retrospective Analysis of the Incidence of the Hepatorenal Syndrome in Patients with Liver Disease. In E. Bartoli and L. Chiandussi (eds.), *Hepatorenal Syndrome.* Padova, Italy: Piccin Medical Books, 1979. Pp. 427–452.
16. Baum, M., Stirling, G. A., and Dawson, J. L. Further study into obstructive jaundice and ischemic renal damage. *Br. Med. J.* 2: 229, 1969.
17. Bennet, W. M., Keefe, E., Melnik, C., et al. Response to dopamine hydrochloride in the hepatorenal syndrome. *Arch. Intern. Med.* 135: 964, 1975.

18. Berkowitz, H. D. Renin Substrate in the Hepatorenal Syndrome. In M. Epstein (ed.), *The Kidney in Liver Disease*. New York: Elsevier, 1978. Pp. 254–270.
19. Berkowitz, H. D., Calvin, C., and Miller, L. D. Significance of altered renin substrate in the hepatorenal syndrome. *Surg. Forum* 23: 342, 1972.
20. Bernardi, M., Trevisani, F., Santini, C., et al. Aldosterone related blood volume expansions in cirrhosis before and during the early phase of ascites formation. *Gut* 24: 761, 1983.
21. Better, O. S. Bile Duct Ligation: An Experimental Model of Renal Dysfunction Secondary to Liver Disease. In M. Epstein (ed.), *The Kidney in Liver Disease* (2nd ed.). New York: Elsevier Biomedical, 1983. Pp. 295–311.
22. Better, O. S., and Bomzon, A. Effects of Jaundice on the Renal and Cardiovascular Systems. In M. Epstein (ed.), *The Kidney in Liver Disease* (3rd ed.). Baltimore: Williams & Wilkins, 1988. Pp. 508–534.
23. Better, O. S., and Schrier, R. W. Disturbed volume homeostasis in patients with cirrhosis of the liver. *Kidney Int.* 23: 303, 1983.
24. Better, O. S., Goldschmid, Z., Chaimovitz, C., et al. Defect in urinary acidification in cirrhosis. *Arch. Intern. Med.* 130: 77, 1972.
25. Bichet, D. G., Groves, B., and Schrier, R. W. Mechanism of improvement of water and sodium excretion by enhancement of central hemodynamics in decompensated cirrhotic patients. *Kidney Int.* 24: 788, 1983.
26. Bichet, D. G., Van Dutten, V. J., and Schrier, R. W. Potential role of increased sympathetic activity in impaired sodium and water excretion in cirrhosis. *N. Engl. J. Med.* 307: 1552, 1982.
27. Binah, O., Bomzon, A., Blendis, L. M., et al. Obstructive jaundice blunts myocardial contractile response to isoproterenol: A clue to the susceptibility of jaundiced patients to shock? *Clin. Sci.* 69: 647, 1985.
28. Bismuth, H., Kuntziger, H., and Coerlette, M. B. Cholangitis in acute renal failure. *Ann. Surg.* 181: 881, 1975.
29. Blendis, L. M., Greig, P. D., Langer, B., et al. The renal and hemodynamic effects of the peritoneovenous shunt for intractable hepatic ascites. *Gastroenterology* 77: 250, 1979.
30. Bomzon, A., Finberg, J. P. M., Tovbin, D., et al. Bile salts, hypotension and obstructive jaundice. *Clin. Sci.* 67: 177, 1984.
31. Bomzon, A., Gali, D., Better, O. S., et al. Reversible suppression of the vascular contractile response in rats with obstructive jaundice. *J. Lab. Clin. Med.* 105: 568, 1985.
32. Bosch, J., Arroyo, V., Betriv, A., et al. Hepatic hemodynamics and the renin-angiotensin-aldosterone system in cirrhosis. *Gastroenterology* 78: 92, 1980.
33. Boyer, T. D., Zia, P., and Reynolds, T. B. Effect of indomethacin and prostaglandin A_1 on renal function and plasma renin activity in alcoholic liver disease. *Gastroenterology* 77: 215, 1979.
34. Bradely, S. E. Hepatorenal and glomerulotubular imbalance. *N. Engl. J. Med.* 289: 1194, 1973.
35. Chaimovitz, C., Massry, S. G., Friedler, R. M., et al. Effect of renal denervation and alpha adrenergic blockade on sodium excretion in dogs with chronic ligation of the common bile duct. *Proc. Soc. Exp. Biol. Med.* 146: 764, 1974.
36. Claria, J., Jimenez, W., Arroyo, V., et al. The blockade of the vascular effect of antidiuretic hormone (ADH) decreases arterial pressure in experimental cirrhosis with ascites. *J. Hepatol.* 9: 519, 1989.
37. Cogan, M. D. Angiotensin II: A powerful controller of sodium transport in the early proximal tubule. *Hypertension* 15: 451, 1990.
38. Cohn, J. N., Tristani, F. E., and Khatri, I. M. Systemic vasoconstriction and renal vasodilator effects of PLV-2 (Octapressin) in man. *Circulation* 38: 151, 1964.
39. Cohn, J. N., Tristani, F. E., and Khatri, I. M. Renal vasodilator therapy in the hepatorenal syndrome. *Med. Ann. D.C.* 39: 1, 1970.
40. Conn, M. D. Rational approach to the hepatorenal syndrome. *Gastroenterology* 65: 321, 1973.
41. Cosby, R. L., Yee, B., and Schrier, R. W. New classification with prognostic value in cirrhotic patients. *Miner. Elect. Metab.* 15: 261, 1989.
42. Dawson, J. L. Acute postoperative renal failure in obstructive jaundice. *Ann. R. Coll. Surg.* 42: 163, 1968.
43. DiBona, G. F. Renal neural activity in the hepatorenal syndrome. *Kidney Int.* 25: 841, 1984.
44. Dixon, B. S., Breckon, R., Fortune, J., et al. Effects of kinins on cultured arterial smooth muscle. *Am. J. Physiol.* 258: C299, 1990.
45. Dunn, M. J. Role of eicosanoids in the control of renal function in severe hepatic disease. *Gastroenterology* 87: 1392, 1984.
46. Eisenmenger, W. J. Role of sodium in the formation and control of ascites in patients with cirrhosis. *Ann. Intern. Med.* 37: 261, 1952.
47. Eknoyan, G. Glomerular Abnormalities in Liver Disease. In M. Epstein (ed.), *The Kidney in Liver Disease* (2nd ed.). New York: Elsevier Biomedical, 1983. Pp. 119–146.
48. Epstein, F. M. Underfilling versus overflow in hepatic ascites. *N. Engl. J. Med.* 307: 1577, 1983.
49. Epstein, M. The LeVeen shunt for ascites and hepatorenal syndrome. *N. Engl. J. Med.* 302: 628, 1980.
50. Epstein, M. Peritoneovenous shunt in the management of ascites and the hepatorenal syndrome. *Gastroenterology* 82: 790, 1982.
51. Epstein, M., Oster, J. R., and deVelasco, R. E. Hepatorenal syndrome following hemihepatectomy. *Clin. Nephrol.* 5: 128, 1976.
52. Epstein, M., Schneider, N., and Befeler, B. Relationship of systemic and intrarenal hemodynamics in cirrhosis. *J. Lab. Clin. Med.* 89: 1175, 1977.
53. Epstein, M., Berk, D. P., Hollenberg, N. K., et al. Renal failure in the patient with cirrhosis. The role of active vasoconstriction. *Am. J. Med.* 49: 175, 1970.
54. Epstein, M., Levinson, R., Sancho, J., et al. Characterization of renin-aldosterone system in decompensated cirrhosis. *Circ. Res.* 41: 818, 1977.
55. Fazekas, J. F., Tictin, H. E., Ehrmantrant, W. R., et al. Cerebral metabolism in hepatic insufficiency. *Am. J. Med.* 21: 843, 1956.
56. Finberg, J. P. M., Syrop, H. A., and Better, O. S. Blunted pressor response to angiotensin and sympathomimetic amines in bile duct ligated dogs. *Clin. Sci.* 61: 535, 1981.
57. Fischer, J. E., and Baldessarini, R. J. False neurotransmitters and hepatic failure. *Lancet* 2: 75, 1971.
58. Flint, A. Clinical report on hydroperitoneum based on an analysis of 46 cases. *Am. J. Med. Sci.* 45: 306, 1863.
59. Floras, J. S., Legault, L., Morali, G. A., et al. Increased sympathetic outflow in cirrhosis and ascites: Direct evidence from intraneural recordings. *Ann. Intern. Med.* 114: 373, 1991.
60. Fulenwider, J. T., Sibley, C., Stein, F., et al. Endotoxemia in cirrhosis: An observation not substantiated. *Gastroenterology* 78: 1000, 1980.
61. Garett, J. G., Voorhees, A. B., and Sommers, S. C. Renal

failure following portasystemic shunt in patients with cirrhosis of the liver. *Ann. Surg.* 172: 218, 1970.

62. Gauer, O. H., and Henry, J. P. Neurohormonal Control of Plasma Volume. In A. C. Guyton and A. W. Cowley (eds.), *Neurohormonal Control of the Circulation*. International Review of Physiology II (Vol. 9). Baltimore: University Park Press, 1976. Pp. 145–190.
63. Green, J., Beyar, R., Bomzon, L., et al. Jaundice, the circulation and the kidney. *Nephron* 37: 145, 1984.
64. Green, J., Beyar, R., Sideman, S., et al. The "jaundiced heart." A possible explanation for postoperative shock in obstructive jaundice. *Surgery* 100: 14, 1986.
65. Guazzi, M., Polese, A., Margini, F., et al. Negative influence of ascites on the cardiac function of cirrhotic patients. *Am. J. Med.* 59: 165, 1975.
66. Hecker, R., and Sherlock, S. Electrolyte and circulatory changes in terminal renal failure. *Lancet* 2: 1121, 1956.
67. Helwig, F. C., and Schutz, C. B. A liver kidney syndrome. Clinical pathological and experimental studies. *Surg. Gynecol. Obstet.* 55: 570, 1932.
68. Henriksen, J. H., Christensen, N. J. H., and Ring-Larsen, H. Noradrenaline and adrenaline concentrations in various vascular beds in patients with cirrhosis. Relation to hemodynamics. *Clin. Physiol.* 1: 293, 1981.
69. Henriksen, J. H., Ring-Larsen, H., and Christensen, N. J. H. Sympathetic nervous activity in cirrhosis. A survey of plasma catecholamine studies. *J. Hepatology* 1: 55, 1984.
70. Henriksen, J. H., Bendtsen, F., Sorensen, T. I., et al. Reduced central blood volume in cirrhosis. *Gastroenterology* 97: 1506, 1989.
71. Hoertnagel, H., Lenz, K., Singer, E. A., et al. Substance P is markedly increased in plasma in patients with hepatic coma. *Lancet* 1: 480, 1984.
72. Iwatsuki, S., Popovtzer, M. M., Corman, J. L., et al. Recovery from "hepatorenal syndrome" after orthotopic liver transplantation. *N. Engl. J. Med.* 289: 1155, 1973.
73. Kew, M. C., Brunt, P. W., Varma, R. R., et al. Renal and intrarenal blood flow in cirrhosis of the liver. *Lancet* 2: 504, 1971.
74. Kew, M. C., Limbrick, C., Varma, R. R., et al. Renal and intrarenal blood flow in noncirrhotic portal hypertension. *Gut* 13: 763, 1972.
75. Kinney, M. J., Schneider, A., Wapnick, S., et al. The 'hepatorenal' syndrome and refractory ascites successful therapy with the LeVeen-type peritoneal-venous shunt and valve. *Nephron* 23: 228, 1979.
76. Kitamura, S., Yoshida, T., and Said, S. I. Vasoactive intestinal polypeptide. Inactivation in liver and potentiation in lung of anesthetized dogs. *Proc. Soc. Exp. Biol. Med.* 148: 25, 1975.
77. Knauer, C. M., and Lowe, H. M. Hemodynamics in the cirrhotic patient during paracentesis. *N. Engl. J. Med.* 276: 491, 1967.
78. Kopp, U. C., and DiBona, G. F. Catecholamines and Neurosympathetic Control of Renal Function. In J. W. Fisher (ed.), *Kidney Hormones* (vol. 3). London: Academic Press, 1986. P. 621.
79. Koppel, M. H., Coburn, J. W., Mims, M. M., et al. Transplantation of cadaveric kidneys from patients with hepatorenal syndrome. Evidence for functional nature of renal failure in advanced liver disease. *N. Engl. J. Med.* 280: 1367, 1969.
80. Kostreva, D. R., Castanar, A., and Kampire, J. P. Reflex effects of hepatic baroreceptors on renal and cardiac sympathetic nerve. *Am. J. Physiol.* 238: R390, 1980.
81. Kotelanski, B., Groszmann, R. J., and Cohn, J. N. Circulation times in the splanchnic and hepatic beds in alcoholic liver disease. *Gastroenterology* 53: 102, 1972.
82. Krumulovsky, F. A., del Greco, E., and Niederman, M. Prolonged hemoperfusion and hemodialysis in the management of hepatic failure and the hepatorenal syndrome. *Trans. Am. Soc. Artif. Intern. Organs* 24: 235, 1978.
83. Lam, K. C., Tall, A. R., Goldstein, G. B., et al. Role of false neurotransmitter, octopamine, in the pathogenesis of hepatic and renal encephalopathy. *Scand. J. Gastroenterol.* 8: 464, 1973.
84. Leehey, D. J. Prostaglandins modulate pressor sensitivity to angiotensin II in experimental liver cirrhosis. *Am. J. Physiol.*, in press.
85. Leehey, D. J., Betzelos, S., and Daugirdas, J. T. Arteriovenous shunting in experimental liver cirrhosis in rats. *J. Lab. Clin. Med.* 109: 687, 1987.
86. LeVeen, H. H., Christoudias, G., Ip, M., et al. Peritoneo-venous shunting for ascites. *Ann. Surg.* 180: 580, 1974.
87. Levenson, D. J., Skorecki, K. L., and Narins, R. G. Acute Renal Failure Associated with Hepatobiliary Disease. In B. M. Brenner and J. M. Lazarus (eds.), *Acute Renal Failure*. Philadelphia: Saunders, 1983. Pp. 467–498.
88. Levy, M. Renal function in dogs with acute selective hepatic venous outflow block. *Am. J. Physiol.* 227: 1073, 1974.
89. Levy, M. Sodium retention and ascites formation in dogs with experimental portal cirrhosis. *Am. J. Physiol.* 233: F572, 1977.
90. Levy, M., and Finestone, M. Renal response to four hours of biliary obstruction in the dog. *Am. J. Physiol.* 244: F516, 1983.
91. Levy, M., and Wexler, M. J. Subacute endotoxemia in dogs with experimental cirrhosis and ascites: Effect on kidney function. *Can. J. Physiol. Pharmacol.* 62: 673, 1984.
92. Levy, M., Wexler, M. J., and Fechner, C. Renal perfusion in dogs with experimental hepatic cirrhosis: Role of prostaglandins. *Am. J. Physiol.* 245: F521, 1983.
93. Lieberman, F. L., Denison, E. K., and Reynolds, T. B. The relationship of plasma volume, portal hypertension, ascites, and renal sodium and retention in cirrhosis: The "overflow" theory of ascites formation. *Ann. N.Y. Acad. Sci.* 170: 202, 1970.
94. Lieberman, F. L., Ito, S., and Reynolds, T. B. Effective plasma volume in cirrhosis with ascites: Evidence that a decreased volume does not account for renal sodium retention, a spontaneous reduction in glomerular filtration rate (GFR), and a fall in GFR during drug-induced diuresis. *J. Clin. Invest.* 48: 975, 1969.
95. Limas, C. J., Guiha, N. H., Lekagul, O., et al. Impaired left ventricular function in alcoholic cirrhosis with ascites. *Circulation* 69: 755, 1974.
96. Martinez-Maldonado, M. Edematous states (editorial). *Semin. Nephrol.* 3: 169, 1983.
97. Mass, A., Arroyo, V., Rodes, J., et al. Ascites and renal failure in primary liver carcinoma. *Br. Med. J.* 3: 629, 1975.
98. McCauley, J., Van Thiel, D. H., Starzl, T. E., et al. Acute and chronic renal failure in liver transplantation. *Nephron* 55: 121, 1990.
99. McDonald, K. M., Taher, M. S., and Schrier, R. W. Effect of Competitive Inhibitor of Angiotensin on Renin Release and Arterial Pressure. In P. Milliez and M. Safar (eds.), *Recent Advances in Hypertension* (vol. 1). Monte Carlo: Boehringer Ingelheim, 1975. P. 231.
100. Melman, A., and Massry, S. G. Role of renal vasodilatation in the blunted natriuresis of saline infusion in

dogs with chronic bile duct obstruction. *J. Lab. Clin. Med.* 89: 1053, 1977.
101. Mondon, C. E., Burton, S. D., and Ishidu, T. Functional status of isolated rat kidney perfused in combination with isolated liver (abstract). *Clin. Res.* 17: 168, 1969.
102. Nasjelleti, A., Celina-Chourio, J., and McGiff, J. C. Disappearance of bradykinin in the circulation of the dog: Effect of kininase inhibitors. *Circ. Res.* 37: 59, 1975.
103. Nicholls, K. M., Shapiro, M. D., Van Putten, V. J., et al. Elevated plasma norepinephrine concentrations in decompensated cirrhosis: Association with increased secretion rate, normal clearance rate and suppressibility by central blood volume expansion. *Circ. Res.* 56: 457, 1985.
104. Nijima, A. Afferent discharges from venous pressoreceptors in liver. *Am. J. Physiol.* 272: C76, 1977.
105. Odell, G. B., Natzschka, J. C., and Storey, G. N. B. Bilirubin nephropathy in the Gunn strain of rat. *Am. J. Physiol.* 212: 931, 1967.
106. Opolon, P., Lavallard, M. C., Huguet, C. L., et al. Hemodialysis versus cross hemodialysis in experimental hepatic coma. *Surg. Gynecol. Obstet.* 142: 845, 1976.
107. Papadakis, M. A., and Arieff, A. Hepatorenal syndrome: An expanded definition (abstract). *Proc. Am. Soc. Nephrol.* 16: 36A, 1983.
108. Papper, S. The role of the kidney in Laennec's cirrhosis of the liver. *Medicine* 37: 299, 1958.
109. Papper, S. The Hepatorenal Syndrome. In M. Epstein (ed.), *The Kidney in Liver Disease* (2nd ed.). New York: Elsevier Biomedical, 1983. Pp. 87–106.
110. Papper, S., Belsky, J. L., and Bleifer, K. H. Renal failure in Laennec's cirrhosis of the liver: (1) Description of clinical and laboratory features. *Ann. Intern. Med.* 51: 759, 1959.
111. Parsons, V., Wilkinson, S. P., and Weston, M. J. Use of dialysis in treatment of renal failure of liver disease. *Postgrad. Med. J.* 51: 515, 1975.
112. Perez, G. O., and Oster, J. R. A Critical Review of the Role of Dialysis in the Treatment of Liver Disease. In M. Epstein (ed.), *The Kidney in Liver Disease.* New York: Elsevier, 1978. Pp. 325–348.
113. Perez-Ayuso, R. M., Arroyo, V., Camps, J., et al. Renal kallikrein excretion in cirrhotics with ascites: Relationship to renal hemodynamics. *Hepatology* 4: 247, 1984.
114. Pladson, T. R., and Parrish, R. M. Hepatorenal syndrome: Recovery after peritoneovenous shunt. *Arch. Intern. Med.* 137: 1248, 1977.
115. Radlomski, M. W., Palmer, R. M. J., and Moncada, S. Glucocorticoids inhibit the expression of an inducible, but not the constitutive, nitric oxide synthase in vascular endothelial cells. *Proc. Natl. Acad. Sci. U.S.A.* 87: 10043, 1990.
116. Ring-Larsen, H. Renal blood flow in cirrhosis: Relation to systemic and portal hemodynamics and liver function. *Scand. J. Clin. Invest.* 37: 635, 1977.
117. Ring-Larsen, H. Renal Hemodynamics in the Hepatorenal Syndrome. Experimental Aspects. In E. Bartoli and L. Chiandussi (eds.), *Hepatorenal Syndrome.* Padova, Italy: Piccin Medical Books, 1979. Pp. 156–171.
118. Ring-Larsen, H., Henriksen, J. H., and Christensen, N. J. H. Increased sympathetic activity in cirrhosis. *N. Engl. J. Med.* 308: 1029, 1983.
119. Ring-Larsen, H., Hesse, B., and Stigsby, B. Effect of portacaval anastomosis on renal blood flow in cirrhosis. Preliminary results. *Postgrad. Med. J.* 51: 499, 1975.
120. Ring-Larsen, H., Hesse, B., Henriksen, J. H., et al. Sympathetic nervous activity and renal and systemic hemodynamics in cirrhosis: Plasma norepinephrine concentration, hepatic extraction and renal release. *Hepatology* 2: 304, 1982.
121. Said, S. I., and Mutt, V. Polypeptide with broad biological activity. Isolation from small intestine. *Science* 169: 1217, 1970.
122. Saito, I., Saruta, T., Eguchi, T., et al. Role of renin-angiotensin system in control of blood pressure and aldosterone in patients with cirrhosis and ascites. *Jpn. Heart J.* 19: 741, 1978.
123. Schrier, R. W. Pathogenesis of sodium and water retention in high-output and low-output cardiac failure, nephrotic syndrome, cirrhosis, and pregnancy. *N. Engl. J. Med.* 319: 1065 (Part 1) and 1127 (Part 2), 1988.
124. Schrier, R. W. Body fluid volume regulation in health and disease: A unifying hypothesis. *Ann. Intern. Med.* 113: 155, 1990.
125. Schrier, R. W., and Better, O. S. Pathogenesis of ascites formation: Mechanism of impaired aldosterone escape in cirrhosis. *Eur. J. Gastroenterol. Hepatol.* 3: 721, 1991.
126. Schrier, R. W., and Caramelo, C. Hemodynamic and Hormonal Alterations in Hepatic Cirrhosis. In M. Epstein (ed.), *The Kidney in Liver Disease* (3rd ed.). Baltimore: Williams & Wilkins, 1988. Pp. 265–285.
127. Schrier, R. W., Arroyo, V., Bernardi, M., et al. Peripheral arterial vasodilation hypothesis: A proposal for the initiation of renal sodium and water retention in cirrhosis. *Hepatology* 8: 1151, 1988.
128. Schroeder, E. T., and Anderson, G. H. Relation of the Renin-Angiotensin System to Hemodynamic Abnormalities in Cirrhosis: Studies Using Blockade of Angiotensin II. In M. Epstein (ed.), *The Kidney in Liver Disease.* New York: Elsevier, 1978. Pp. 239–250.
129. Schroeder, E. T., Anderson, G. H., Jr., and Smulyan, H. Effects of a portacaval or peritoneo-venous shunt on renin in the hepatorenal syndrome. *Kidney Int.* 15: 54, 1979.
130. Schroeder, E. T., Numann, P. J., and Chamberlain, B. E. Functional renal failure in cirrhosis. Recovery after portacaval shunt. *Ann. Intern. Med.* 72: 923, 1970.
131. Schroeder, E. T., Anderson, G. H., Goldman, S. H., et al. Effect of blockade of angiotensin II on blood pressure, renin and aldosterone in cirrhosis. *Kidney Int.* 9: 511, 1976.
132. Schroeder, E. T., Eich, R. H., Smulyan, H., et al. Plasma renin levels in hepatic cirrhosis: Relation to functional renal failure. *Am. J. Med.* 49: 186, 1970.
133. Shasha, S. M., Better, O. S., Chaimovitz, C., et al. Haemodynamic studies in dogs with chronic bile duct ligation. *Clin. Sci.* 50: 533, 1976.
134. Shear, L., Bonkowsky, H. L., and Gabuzda, G. J. Renal tubular acidosis in cirrhosis: A determinant of susceptibility to recurrent hepatic coma. *N. Engl. J. Med.* 280: 1, 1969.
135. Sitprija, V., Kashemsant, U., Sriratanaban, A., et al. Renal function in obstructive jaundice in man: Cholangiocarcinoma model. *Kidney Int.* 38: 948, 1990.
136. Stein, J. H., Congabalay, R. C., Karsh, D. L., et al. The effect of bradykinin on proximal tubular sodium reabsorption in the dog. Evidence for functional nephron heterogeneity. *J. Clin. Invest.* 51: 1709, 1972.
137. Tarao, K., So, K., Moroi, T., et al. Detection of endotoxin in plasma and ascitic fluid in patients with cirrhosis: Its clinical significance. *Gastroenterology* 73: 359, 1977.
138. Vallance, P., and Moncada, S. Hyperdynamic circulation in cirrhosis: A role for nitric oxide? *Lancet* 337: 776, 1991.

139. Vera, S. R., Williams, J. W., Peters, T. G., et al. Hemodynamic study following liver transplantation. *Transplant. Proc.* 21: 2302, 1989.
140. Vesin, P. Late Functional Renal Failure in Cirrhosis with Ascites: Pathophysiology, Diagnosis and Treatment. In G. A. Martini and S. Sherlock (eds.), *Aktuelle Probleme der hepatologie.* Stuttgart: Theime, 1962. Pp. 98–109.
141. Vorobioff, J., Bredfeldt, J. E., and Groszmann, R. J. Increased blood flow through the portal system in cirrhotic rats. *Gastroenterology* 87: 1120, 1984.
142. Wilkinson, S. P., and Williams, R. Endotoxin and renal failure in liver disease. In E. Bartoli and L. Chiandussi (eds.), *Hepatorenal Syndrome.* Padova, Italy: Piccin Medical Books, 1978. Pp. 230–255.
143. Wilkinson, S. P., and Williams, R. Defining the Hepatorenal Syndrome. In E. Bartoli and L. Chiandussi (eds.), *Hepatorenal Syndrome.* Padova, Italy: Piccin Medical Books, 1979. Pp. 21–33.
144. Wilkinson, S. P., Moodie, H., Stamatakis, V., et al. Endotoxinemia and renal failure in cirrhosis and obstructive jaundice. *Br. Med. J.* 2: 1415, 1976.
145. Wilkinson, S. P., Smith, I. K., and Williams, R. Changes in plasma renin activity in cirrhosis and reappraisal based on studies in 67 patients with "low renin" cirrhosis. *Hypertension* 1: 125, 1978.
146. Wong, P. Y., Colman, R. W., Talamo, R. C., et al. Kallikrein-bradykinin system in chronic alcoholic liver disease. *Ann. Intern. Med.* 77: 205, 1972.
147. Yamamura, Y., Ogawa, H., Chihara, T., et al. OPC-21268, an orally effective, nonpeptide vasopressin V1 receptor antagonist. *Science* 252: 572, 1991.
148. Zambraski, E. J., and Dunn, M. J. Importance of renal prostaglandins in control of renal function after chronic ligation of the common bile duct in dogs. *J. Lab. Clin. Med.* 103: 549, 1984.
149. Zipser, R. D., Hoefs, J. C., Speckart, P. F., et al. Prostaglandins: Modulators of renal function and pressor resistance in chronic liver disease. *J. Clin. Endocrinol. Metab.* 48: 895, 1979.
150. Zipser, R. D., Kronberg, I., Rector, W., et al. Therapeutic trial of thromboxane synthesis inhibition in the hepatorenal syndrome. *Gastroenterology* 87: 1228, 1984.
151. Zipser, R. D., Radvan, G., Kronberg, I., et al. Urinary thromboxane B_2 and prostaglandin E_2 in the hepatorenal syndrome: Evidence for increased vasoconstrictor and decreased vasodilator factors. *Gastroenterology* 84: 697, 1983.
152. Zusman, R. M., Axelrod, L., and Tolkoff, R. N. The treatment of the hepatorenal syndrome with intrarenal administration of PGE_1. *Prostaglandins* 13: 819, 1977.

Treatment of Acute Renal Failure

Carl M. Kjellstrand
Kim Solez

Acute renal failure most commonly occurs secondary to other diseases. In countries where sophisticated medicine is rarely practiced, it usually occurs secondary to trauma, snake bites, infections, abortions, or self-poisoning [7]. In countries with high-technology medicine, most instances of acute renal failure occur in the hospital, and develop most frequently as an iatrogenic complication. Acute renal insufficiency develops in 2 to 5 percent of all patients sent to tertiary-care hospitals. One half of these episodes are iatrogenic, and a quarter of the patients die [71, 86, 179].

Before the mid-1940s, when the artificial kidney was introduced into clinical practice, the mortality from severe acute renal failure was almost 100 percent. Dialysis reduced it to 50 percent, but since those early days, over four decades ago, no overall improvement has been achieved in survival, and lately the mortality is again increasing [2, 7, 25, 28, 66, 78, 195, 205, 210, 244, 247, 310, 332, 391, 409].

The methods for blood purification in acute renal failure include hemodialysis, peritoneal dialysis, hemofiltration, and hemodiafiltration. All these methods can be performed either intermittently or continuously.

In this chapter we first briefly review the incidence, pathophysiology, and clinical approach to the patient; the diagnostic evaluation; the mortality rates; and the causes of death. We discuss more extensively early etiologic treatment, conservative symptomatic treatment, and symptomatic treatment with dialysis.

Incidence of Acute Renal Failure and Need for Dialysis

The number of patients with severe acute renal failure, defined as renal failure needing dialysis, has been studied by several individual teams [109, 192, 233, 260, 394]. The incidence ranges from a low of approximately 20 per million per year in East Germany [192], to a high of 60 per million per year in Britain [394]. In a 1982 survey by the European Dialysis and Transplant Association drawn from 32 countries, a mean of 28.9 patients per million population per year requiring dialysis for acute renal failure was found. The range was 0.4 to 177.1 [414]. Since only centers performing chronic dialysis were questioned, the true incidence is probably higher. The clinical course of these patients is swift, typically requiring only four dialyses [205] before death or recovery occurs. Thus, in Western Europe, there is an estimated need of 200 dialyses per million population per year for acute renal failure.

For every patient with severe acute renal failure who requires dialysis, there are approximately 10 patients with milder forms of renal insufficiency who can be managed conservatively [86, 179].

Causes of Acute Renal Failure

The most common diseases leading to acute renal failure are listed in Fig. 52-1. Acute tubular necrosis is responsible for about 60 percent of such cases, and 18 percent are due to acute exacerbation of underlying chronic renal disease, a variant of acute tubular necrosis. Thus, acute tubular necrosis is the underlying pathology for almost four fifths of all cases of acute renal failure. Only 12 percent of patients with acute renal failure suffer from primary acute renal disease such as glomerulonephritis, lupus nephritis, vasculitis, acute interstitial nephritis, and so on. Since 1945, little change has been seen in the relative frequency of the diseases that cause acute renal failure [7, 25, 195, 205, 206]. In Western countries there has been a marked increase in acute tubular necrosis due to medical disease (Fig. 52-2). In the early years, surgery or trauma was the underlying cause in two thirds of such patients. Now, two thirds of the patients have iatrogenic renal failure, most often involving a combination of sepsis and nephrotoxic drugs [2, 7, 25, 195, 205, 206, 325]. In countries such as India, with developing medicine, acute renal failure following surgery is rapidly increasing [71].

Pathophysiology of Acute Tubular Necrosis

The exact pathophysiologic pathways through which the pathogenetic factors of ischemia and toxicity cause renal failure remain unknown (see also Chaps. 47 and 48). Most basic research into acute tubular necrosis has used animal models that are either purely ischemic or purely toxic [76, 169, 258, 289, 335, 367, 371]. However, the glycerol model contains elements of both types of injury [372] and some recent experimental work has combined toxic and ischemic insults [126, 263, 420].

Nevertheless, the clinical situation is considerably more complex. Most patients in whom acute tubular necrosis develops have coexistent ischemic and toxic insults. Rasmussen and associates [332], analyzing the renal insults in 145 patients who developed acute renal failure, found more than one insult in 74 percent, and others have had similar findings [86]. To confuse the clinical situation further, acute tubular necrosis and its most important differential diagnostic entity, prerenal failure, are often intermingled and may be impossible to distinguish in patients [325].

In order to prevent the occurrence of acute tubular necrosis, it is important to understand that one iatrogenic assault usually does not result in acute renal failure, but that repeated problems can often cause it. As was mentioned above, most patients in whom acute renal failure develops have had more than one assault [86, 332]. Similarly, Charlson and co-workers [66] found that if a mild degree of renal failure had occurred, another nephrologic insult, such as repeated surgery or intravenous contrast, almost always precipitated the patient into full-blown acute renal failure. Dehydration often precedes, and contributes to, acute tubular necrosis [86], and careful invasive volume monitoring may be preventive [170].

In almost every situation in which patients are involved, many factors cooperate to cause acute tubular necrosis. For example, in ruptured aortic aneurysm, de-

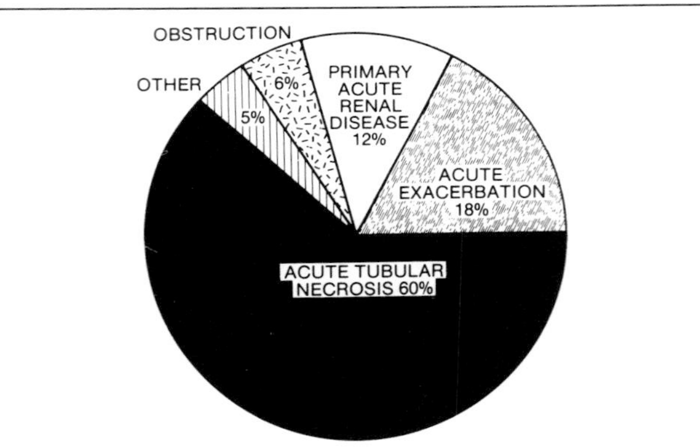

Fig. 52-1. Most patients (60%) with acute renal failure suffer from acute tubular necrosis; this is followed in frequency by acute exacerbations of chronic underlying renal failure (18%). This figure summarizes experience with 1381 patients dialyzed at the University of Lund and the University of Minnesota. There was no change in incidence in these categories from the mid-1950s through the late 1970s.

creased renal blood flow may preexist secondary to renal artery stenosis, which is aggravated by the sudden bleeding. The patient is then subject to the additional insult of radiographic contrast material through the angiogram, which is a necessary test for diagnosis. When blood flow to the legs is reestablished, myoglobin from ischemic muscles may damage the kidneys. Finally, nephrotoxic antibiotics such as aminoglycosides and cephalosporins are often used. Similarly, in medical sepsis, many factors will be operant. There will be a sudden increase in capacitance with relative hypovolemia. Increased capillary leakage of albumin aggravates the hypovolemia [133], and nephrotoxicity from necrosis of the tissues secondary to the infection as well as the antibiotics necessary for resuscitation then occurs [5, 401].

Mortality and Prognosis

MORTALITY

The mortality of patients suffering from severe acute renal failure who require dialysis is increasing and is now at 60 to 70 percent. Within the syndrome of acute renal failure, changes in mortality have occurred. Patients with primary uncomplicated renal disease such as glomerulonephritis currently have a mortality of approximately 24 percent; in the early days of dialysis, mortality was 50 percent. Similarly, acute exacerbation of chronic renal disease has shown a decrease in mortality from 86 to 27 percent. It is believed that this is a result of improved clinical dialysis techniques and the improved survival of patients receiving maintenance dialysis. By contrast, the mortality of patients with acute tubular necrosis increased from 55 percent in the 1950s and 1960s to 60 to 70 percent in the 1980s. The change in mortality

Fig. 52-2. A shift has occurred in the causes of acute tubular necrosis from surgery and trauma to medical problems, including decreased perfusion, sepsis, and toxin-induced and multifactorial renal failure. In the 1960s, patients with surgery and trauma made up two thirds of all patients with acute tubular necrosis. They now constitute one third and, instead, two thirds are due to medical disease.

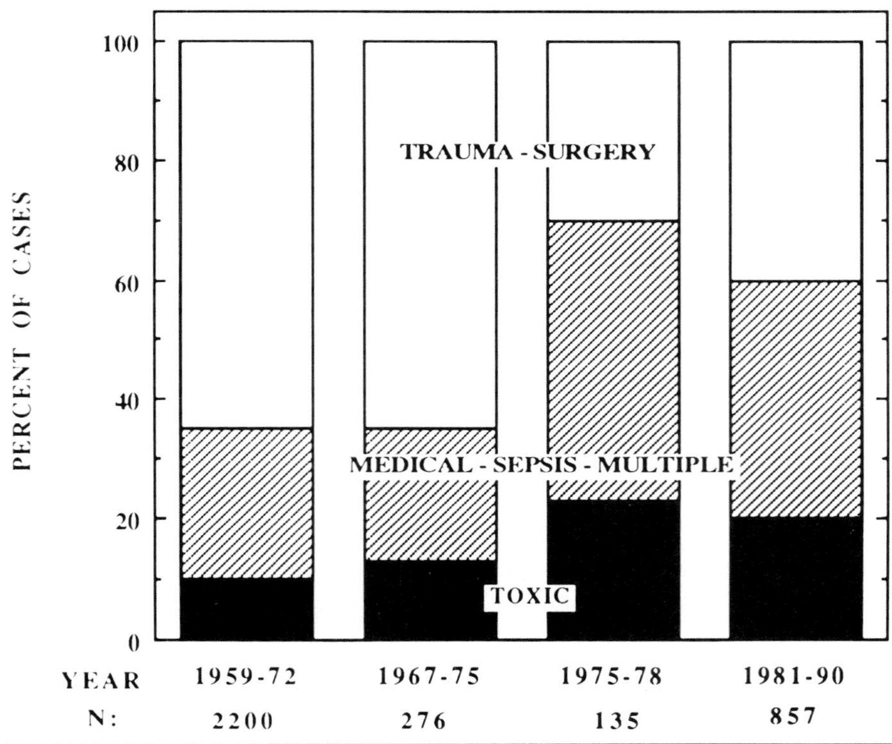

is not due to changes in mean age. Abreo and co-workers [2] have reported an increase in mortality with time, and this increase is entirely due to an increased death rate in patients younger than 60 years. One can speculate that the increased mortality is due to much more severe underlying disease. Simple dehydration-induced acute tubular necrosis seen after gastrointestinal infections in the late 1940s and 1950s has been replaced by more severe septic episodes that occur in immunosuppressed patients such as those with cancer [7, 195, 205, 206, 409].

CAUSES OF DEATH

The causes of death in patients who require dialysis for acute renal failure are outlined in Table 52-1, which summarizes the experience with approximately 3000 patients [6, 7, 25, 78, 148, 195, 198, 205, 206, 215, 231, 244, 247, 275, 310, 332, 366, 391, 409]. The most common cause of death in almost all series is infection. Infections are often complicated by progressive sequential system failure [103, 137, 318]. However, in 25 percent of the patients, sequential organ system failure occurs without evidence of infection [391]. The second most common cause of death is cardiac disease. Death occurs secondary to acute myocardial infarction, often caused by the stress of surgery, or irreversible cardiac failure in the elderly patient with a degenerative vascular disease. The third and fourth most common causes of death are gastrointestinal hemorrhage and pulmonary insufficiency. In particular, intestinal hemorrhage seems to have decreased with early and more frequent dialysis. Kleinknecht and associates [215] found that gastrointestinal hemorrhage decreased from 55 to 27 percent when hemodialysis was initiated earlier, and mean predialysis BUN decreased from 175 mg/dl to less than 100 mg/dl. A few patients die from irreversible central nervous system disease secondary to bleeding, brain edema, or unexplained coma. Even fewer patients die from hyperkalemia, digitalis intoxication, and technical dialysis mishaps. Although the latter tend to be underreported [317], they should occur in fewer than 1 of 50,000 dialyses [19, 136].

In summary, most patients die of infections, multiple organ failure, or irreversible underlying diseases. The exact role of each is difficult to establish, as infection often seems to bring on irreversible organ system failure.

Table 52-1. Causes of death in 3000 patients dialyzed for acute tubular necrosis

Cause of death	Percentage of patients
Infections	30–70%
Cardiac failure	5–30%
Intestinal hemorrhage and other disease	5–20%
Pulmonary emboli and insufficiency	1–10%
Central nervous system disease	1–5%
Hyperkalemia, technical dialysis problems	1–2%

PROGNOSTIC FACTORS FOR SURVIVAL

Demographic Factors. Gender is not a determining factor of the outcome in patients dialyzed for acute renal failure [52, 148].

The influence of age is controversial. Alwall [7] found a direct relationship between age and mortality, but his series was not corrected for underlying disease. A similar relationship was found in later analysis by Bullock and associates [52]. In the series by Alwall and Bullock, the mortality in patients below age 29 was 39 percent and rose to almost 80 percent in patients over the age of 80. Two groups have found a U-shaped relationship between survival and age; the lowest survival was encountered in the youngest and the very oldest patients [205, 276]. When corrected for underlying disease, age is usually of no importance [86, 148, 179, 310, 391].

The time period of dialysis is of no importance. Alwall [7], Gornick and Kjellstrand [148], and Abreo and associates [2] studied survival and found no improvement with time. Similarly, there has been no improvement in survival in war-induced acute renal failure. Thus, mortality was approximately 60 percent during the Korean War, the Vietnam War, and the Mideast crisis [26, 131, 255, 374].

Co-morbid Condition. Most have found a history of preexisting disease to be of no importance [2, 28, 247, 332].

Basic Underlying Disease. The basic disease seems to be the most important factor in determining survival. Gastrointestinal and cardiovascular surgery have always been associated with the highest mortality, usually approximately 80 percent. By contrast, the lowest mortality is encountered in patients with renal failure secondary to obstetric and gynecologic complications [7, 25, 198, 206, 276]. Acute renal failure secondary to obstruction and urologic surgery usually carries a low mortality. In military and civilian injuries followed by acute renal failure, those injuries affecting the lungs and chest carry the lowest mortality, and those involving the intestines and brain carry the highest [255, 271, 374].

Type and Degree of Renal Failure. There seems to be no difference in survival whether renal failure is toxic or ischemic [179]. Some have found better survival in nonoliguric renal failure than in oliguric renal failure. Thus, Anderson and co-workers [10] found a 26 percent mortality in nonoliguric patients compared with 50 percent mortality in those with oliguria. Similarly, Bullock and associates [52] found a 58 percent mortality in nonoliguric patients compared with 82 percent in anuric patients. None of these investigators stratified their patients according to basic disease. When this was done following aortic aneurysm and surgery, no difference was seen between oliguric renal failure and nonoliguric acute renal failure [148].

Hou and co-workers [179], in six factors studied, found the degree of renal failure to be the most impor-

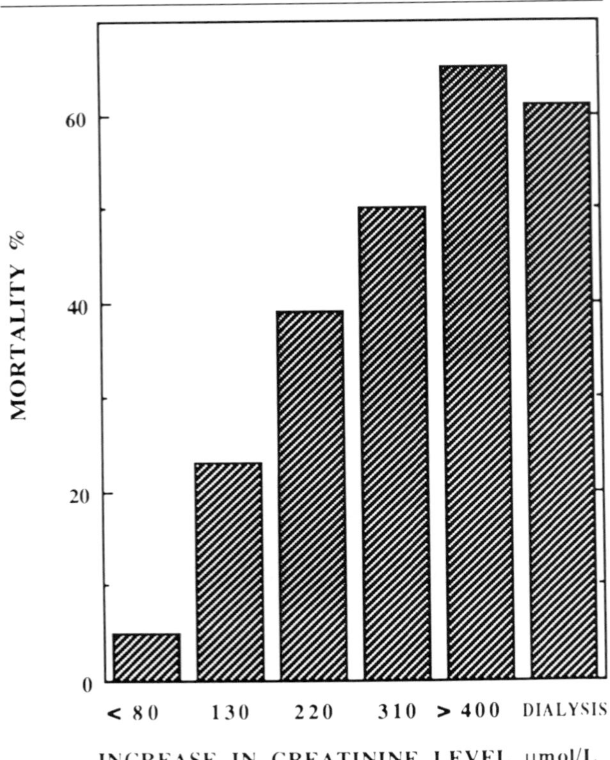

Fig. 52-3. The influence of the magnitude of the rise in serum creatinine on mortality in 188 patients in whom acute renal failure developed. In patients whose serum creatinine increased less than 80 μmol/liter, the mortality was 5 percent. It rose to 65 percent if the creatinine increased more than 400 μmol/liter and the patient did not undergo dialysis. Figure constructed from [86, 179].

tant factor associated with death. Others have made similar observations [86]. These observations of mortality and the rise of serum creatinine are summarized in Fig. 52-3.

Signs of Infections. As was already stated, infections are the most common cause of death in acute renal failure. McMurray and co-workers [275] showed a direct relationship between the number of infections and mortality. Survival was better than 80 percent in the noninfected patient and fell to less than 30 percent in patients with four or more infections. Gornick and Kjellstrand [148], in a study of 50 patients with acute renal failure after aortic aneurysm surgery, found a significant decreased survival time in patients who had a temperature over 100°F, or a white cell count over 10,000 leukocytes per cubic millimeter 2 weeks after the onset of renal failure. In Gornick's series patients showing positive blood cultures during antibiotic coverage did not survive.

Other Emerging Complications: Organ System Failure. The onset of organ system failure is an extremely grave prognostic sign in patients dialyzed for acute renal failure and is often secondary to severe infection [103, 137, 318]. If only the renal system showed signs of failure, 90 percent of the patients described by McMurray and associates survived, but fewer than 30 percent survived of those patients with more than seven organs failing. Bullock and co-workers [52] found that pulmonary complications, jaundice, and cardiovascular complications were all important predictors of death. Gornick found that a need for respiratory support, signs of central nervous system dysfunction, and pulmonary infiltrates were all significantly more common in patients who ultimately died than in those who survived [148]. He found no influence on survival of cardiac problems or gastrointestinal problems in his patients with acute renal failure after aortic aneurysm surgery. It is often difficult to know whether organ system failure is due to primary incurable disease or occurs secondary to infections, but 25 percent of the patients studied by Van Der Mere [391] died of multiple organ system failure, without any signs of infection. Perhaps this is a variant of nonbacteremic clinical sepsis, which usually starts with lung failure (adult respiratory distress syndrome, or ARDS) [87]. In a large review of 2719 patients, those patients who suffered failure of three or more organ systems for 5 days or more died [366].

Dialysis Procedure. With the advent of every-other-day hemodialysis and the early initiation of dialysis, there is no longer any difference in predialysis chemistries between patients who survive and patients who die [179, 271]. Mentzer and associates [278], using every-other-day dialysis, could not find any difference in survival at any time during the first 70 days between patients who had immediate renal function and those who needed dialysis for acute renal failure following transplantation. Similarly, Gillum and co-workers [143], in the only controlled study, comparing every-day to every-other-day hemodialysis, found no advantage in daily dialysis. Survival was only 41 percent in the daily dialysis group but 53 percent in the every-other-day group. Blood urea nitrogen was 60 mg/dl (21.4 mmol/liter), creatinine 5.3 mg/dl (469 μmol/liter), bicarbonate 23 mmol/liter, PO_4 4.3 mg/dl (1.4 mmol/liter), and pH 7.42 in the daily versus 101 mg/dl (36.1 mmol/liter), 9.1 mg/dl (80.5 μmol/liter), 18 mmol/liter, 6.7 mg/dl (2.2 mmol/liter), and 7.35, respectively. These findings strongly suggest that the dialysis procedure as such is almost never a cause of death, and that present every-other-day treatment schedules have probably achieved maximal survival benefit.

Multifactorial Analysis. As no single prognostic factor seems reliable, many teams have tried to use multifactorial analysis of several factors to arrive at some form of prognostic index. Table 52-2 summarizes several attempts at multifactorial analysis. Although the findings are divergent, perhaps two of them are important. First, preexisting disease, age, and gender, as well as the type of renal failure, seem to be of little importance in predicting outcome. It appears as if the complications occurring are the ones that set the stage for whether or not the patient will survive. Liano and Rasmussen and their

Table 52-2. Summary of multifactorial analyses for prognosis of acute renal failure

Reference no.:	[244]	[148]	[52]	[275]	[332]	[73]	[410]	[254]	[285]
Study									
Type	Prosp	Retro	Retro	Retro	Retro + prosp	Retro	Retro	Retro	Retro
No. of patients	228	47	462	276	148 + 113	65	100	125	57
RF	Cr > 2	Dialysis	Cr > 2.5	Dialysis	Cr > 2	Dialysis	Dialysis	Dialysis	Dialysis
Demography									
Age	No	No	Yes	No	No	Yes	Yes	No	Yes
Sex	No	No	No	No	No	Yes	No	No	No
Type renal failure									
Medical	No	—	No	—	No	—	No	—	No
Surgical	Yes	Only	No	—	No	Only	No	—	No
Toxic	Yes +	—	No	—	No	—	No	—	—
Oliguric	Yes	—	No	—	No	—	No	—	—
Complications									
Sepsis	No	Yes	No	Yes	No	No	—	Yes	Yes
BP/MI/ARR	Yes	No	Yes	Yes	Yes	Yes	No	Yes	No
Coma	Yes	Yes	?	—	Yes	—	—	Yes	No
Respirator	Yes	Yes	Yes	No	Yes	—	Yes	Yes	No
Pre-existing disease									
Hypertension	No	No			No			—	—
Diabetes	No	No			—			No	—
Heart	No	No			Yes			—	No
COPD	No	No			No			—	No
CRF	Yes	No			Yes			—	No
Cancer	No	No			Yes			—	—
PVD	Yes	No			Yes			—	—

Prosp = prospective; Retro = retrospective; RF = degree of renal failure in study; Cr = creatinine; dialysis = only dialyzed patients included; BP/MI/ARR = hypotension/infarct/arrhythmia; COPD = chronic obstructive pulmonary disease; CRF = chronic renal failure; PVD = peripheral vascular disease; yes = factor associated with higher mortality; no = factor not associated with mortality.

teams have devised the most sophisticated attempts to create multivariant projection formulas. Liano's discriminant score contains no preexisting or demographic variables. His discriminant score = 0.25 + 0.09 (oliguria) + 0.14 (respirator) + 0.2 (hypotension) + 0.27 (coma). No patient with a score of 0.9 or higher survived in Liano's series of 228 patients [244]. Rasmussen's formula was different. In his discrimination index 10 factors were associated with death. Three preexisting diseases—cancer, heart failure, and chronic renal failure—predicted death; the other seven factors predicting death were new complications: acute cardiac problems, oliguria, pancreatitis, trauma, surgery, CNS problems, and respiratory failure [332].

Nephrologists feel desperate because of the poor outcome and the poor prognostic indices available. Two leading articles [78, 366] review the problems and the confusion. Smithies and Cameron [366] summarize the dilemma well: "Such estimates show only that survival is unprecedented but not impossible. We all remember—perhaps too well—our exceptional patients who survived against the odds. . . . Only when we have a more rational basis can we judge when treatment is futile and our further efforts are likely to amount to nothing more than the bad management of a death."

Clinical Approach

The patient with acute renal failure presents the nephrologist with the most difficult clinical situation. The patient is usually extremely ill and iatrogenic elements are present. There is little margin for error, the differential diagnosis is difficult and sometimes impossible, and the time pressure is severe. Thus, it is necessary to take a strict logical approach to these desperately ill patients (Fig. 52-4). First resuscitate, next complete the differential diagnosis, then try etiologic treatment, and if that fails, prevent complications through the use of conservative therapy and dialysis treatment.

RESUSCITATION

The two most common causes of death in the early resuscitative phase of acute renal failure are overhydration with pulmonary edema and hyperkalemia [7]. Overhydration with pulmonary edema is almost always iatrogenically induced by futile attempts to restore urinary output and renal function by vigorous hydration. Hyperkalemia occurs secondary to an acidotic shift of potassium from the intracellular space to the extracellular space. Severe hyperkalemia tends to follow restoration of blood flow after temporary occlusion, as in the case of embolectomy or repair of an aortic aneurysm, crush

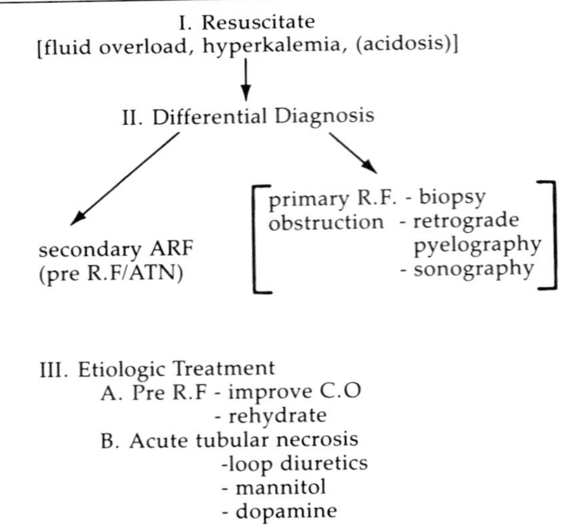

Fig. 52-4. Clinical approach to the patient in whom acute renal failure (ARF) develops. ATN = acute tubular necrosis. CO = cardiac output. Primary RF = renal parenchymal disease or vasculitis. Pre RF = prerenal (functional) failure.

injury with necrosis of large organs or body parts, or severe hyperthermia. Large amounts of potassium that have leaked from damaged tissue during ischemia are suddenly washed into the systemic circulation. In such cases, the potassium levels can be so elevated that vigorous conservative therapy is ineffective, and even continuous hemodialysis may have difficulty maintaining nonfatal potassium levels.

Fluid Overload. The assessment of hydration status is extremely important when kidney function, the most sensitive volume regulator, is absent. Daily weight measurement and careful monitoring of intake and output are essential. Unfortunately, patients frequently form or resorb third-spaced fluids and may have sudden changes in blood vessel capacitance as sepsis develops or is treated. Volume shifts secondary to such events are obviously not reflected in changes in body weight. Daily observations of mucous membranes, skin turgor, jugular vein filling, and auscultations are crude but clinically significant. More accurate, and absolutely necessary in the acute resuscitation phase, are frequent x-rays for pulmonary edema and, most important, invasive monitoring of pulmonary artery and wedged pressures [38, 105, 175]. The most dangerous complication of fluid overload is uremic pulmonary edema. Factors that place patients with acute renal failure at more risk for development of pulmonary edema include increased hydrostatic pressure and pulmonary capillary wedge pressure secondary to fluid overload; subtle capillary injury secondary to uremia, particularly in the perihilar region; and a decreased plasma oncotic pressure [7, 133, 259, 424]. the classic x-ray finding is the "butterfly" or "bat wing" edema (Fig. 52-5), thought to be caused by early leakage of fluid in the bronchial and large-vessel capillary beds in the hilus. At this early stage the only reliable diagnostic measure is chest x-ray because there may be few clinical signs. Rales and shortness of breath are often absent. The pulmonary edema then proceeds to diffuse fluid leakage through pulmonary capillaries, severe hypoxemia, and death. Several variants of the x-ray appearance of uremic pulmonary edema are important to know. Unilateral pulmonary edema, lobar pulmonary edema, and even patchy edema with "cannonball" lesions have been described, mimicking metastasis or fungal pulmonary infections [219]. Radiologic misdiagnoses probably occur in at least 30 percent of patients [7].

The immediate treatment of edema in the resuscitative phase of acute renal failure includes furosemide, which distributes fluid out of the lungs; morphine; and oxygen [8]. If the gastrointestinal tract is functional, large amounts of fluid can be removed by inducing diarrhea. Most effective in this respect is 70% sorbitol given in a dosage of approximately 2 ml/kg body weight orally, or as a 20% solution given 10 ml/kg body weight rectally through a retention edema. Sorbitol, a hexacarbon sugar, is not reabsorbed through the gastrointestinal tract. The effect of sorbitol is immediate and is later visible as watery diarrhea. Up to 5 kg per day of diarrhea can be created by sorbitol. The stool has a sodium content of 30 to 100 mEq per liter and a potassium concentration of 8 to 10 mEq per liter and is alkaline (average pH 7.5). Besides dehydration, one can thus expect serum sodium to rise, potassium to remain stable (although as potassium is lost in diarrhea an intracellular shift occurs secondary to a fall in pH), and blood bicarbonate concentration to become slightly lower [8]. An extremely rare complication has been colonic necrosis, which has occured when sodium polystyrene sulfonate (Kayexalate) has been added to the sorbitol enema [416]. If the patient's pulmonary edema is severe, emergency dialysis with ultrafiltration is indicated [7, 8, 105].

Hyperkalemia. Some degree of hyperkalemia develops in almost all patients with acute renal failure. In most, it is clinically insignificant, but in some patients it is intractably fatal. Disproportionate hyperkalemia, even in mild renal failure, has been reported to be particularly common in acute renal failure induced by nonsteroidal antiinflammatory agents [141].

The danger of hyperkalemia is caused by the cardiotoxic effects of a high extracellular to intracellular potassium concentration ratio. Changes on electrocardiograms induced by potassium are thought to be much more important than the actual serum concentration of potassium. Cardiotoxicity is illustrated in Fig. 52-6. The first change is tenting, followed by a high T wave. Serious toxicity is evident by a prolonged PR interval and a depressed ST segment. If auricular standstill and intraventricular block occur, cardiac arrest is imminent. Changes on the ECG caused by potassium that are indistinguishable from those of myocardial infarction and bundle branch block have also been described but are probably rare [181].

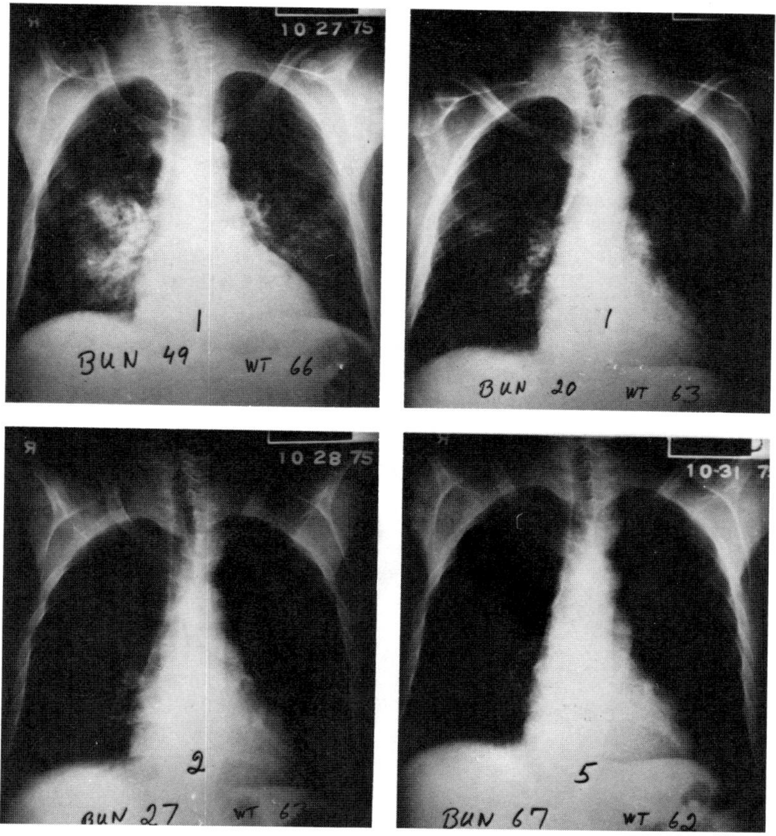

Fig. 52-5. Pulmonary edema in an anuric man. The perihilar appearance of the edema is apparent. The relationship to weight and the absence of relationship to the degree of uremia are also evident. (From [210].)

The treatment of hyperkalemia depends on the toxicity as evidenced by ECG changes. In the hyperacute clinical situation, with auricular standstill or ventricular fibrillation, calcium should be injected intravenously. Its effect is instantaneous but transient because calcium redistributes from blood to interstitial fluid. In less acute situations (PR prolongation and high T waves), potassium can be shifted from the extracellular to the intracellular space by a combination of insulin-glucose-bicarbonate or by the infusion or inhalation of β-adrenergic agonists such as albuterol [6, 285]. Finally, potassium can be removed by the use of exchange ion resins or dialysis. The ion exchange resins exchange sodium and hydrogen for potassium and calcium. A net gain of sodium occurs with a redistribution of water from the intracellular space to the extracellular space, and acidosis is aggravated. The details of treatment are outlined in Table 52-3 and a clinical example of treatment is given in Fig. 52-7.

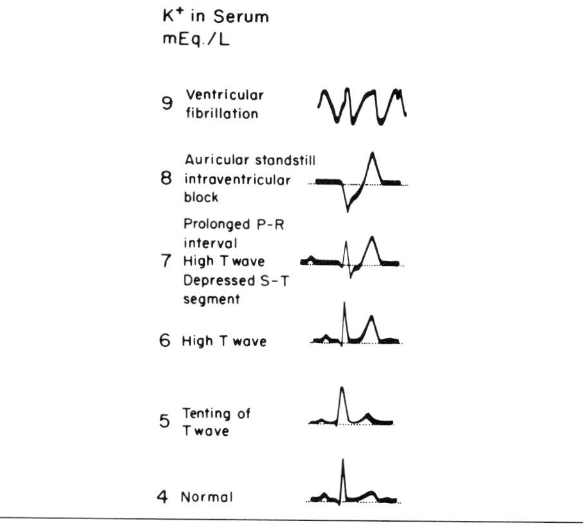

Fig. 52-6. Electrocardiographic changes of hyperkalemia. The tenting high T-wave and intraventricular conduction defects are evident. It is important to note that serum potassium levels and electrocardiographic changes may not correlate so closely as suggested in this figure. (From [210].)

DIFFERENTIAL DIAGNOSIS OF ACUTE RENAL FAILURE

In most instances the cause of acute renal failure can be identified by a combination of clinical history and examination. By far the most common cause of acute renal

Table 52-3. Treatment of hyperkalemia

Clinical level	Treatment	Dose	Mechanism	Time for effect
Hyperacute	Calcium IV	10 ml 10% calcium gluconate for 1–5 min until ECG improves	Antagonism	Immediate
Acute	A. Insulin-glucose bicarbonate	500 ml 30% dextrose, 30 units insulin, + 100 mEq Na-bicarbonate, 100 ml in first hr, then 20–30 ml/hr	Shifts K+ to intracellular space	30 min
	B. Bicarbonate	Fast infusion, dose based on blood bicarbonate level	—"—	30 min
	C. Albuterol	0.5 mg IV in 5 min or 10–20 mg nebulized and inhaled during 10 min	—"—	30 min
Less urgent	Exchange resin	30 gm Kayexalate orally in 100 ml sorbitol solution or 60 gm Kayexalate as an enema in 500 ml 10% sorbitol solution	Removes K+ from body	1–2 hr

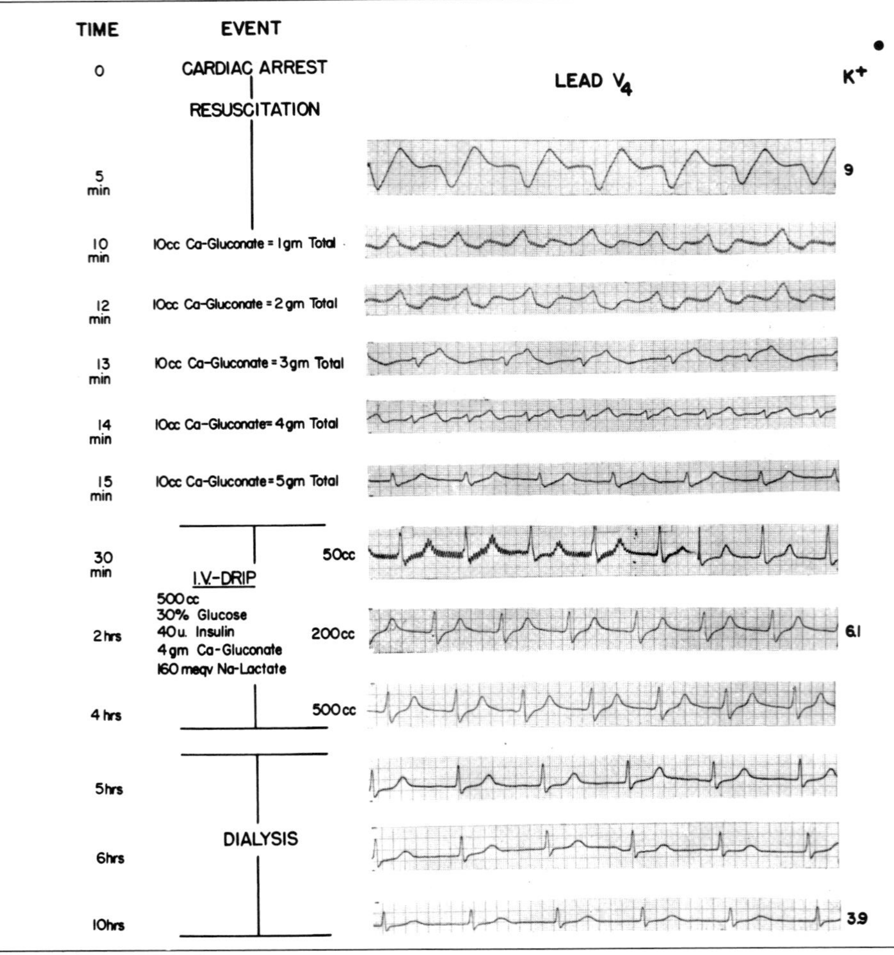

Fig. 52-7. Electrocardiographic changes occurring in a patient with hyperkalemia. The patient was initially treated with a rapid infusion of calcium gluconate, which antagonizes potassium toxicity, followed by a shift of potassium from extra- to intracellular fluid with the infusion of insulin, glucose, calcium, and lactate. The potassium level in serum fell from 9 mEq/liter to 6.1 mEq/liter, and was then further reduced to 3.9 mEq/liter by dialysis. (Reproduced with permission from Lea & Febiger.)

failure is acute tubular necrosis following administration of nephrotoxic agents, such as intravascular contrast media, aminoglycosides, or nonsteroidal antiinflammatory drugs, and infected, septic patients. In some cases it may be impossible to differentiate between acute renal failure secondary to prerenal failure and acute tubular necrosis. These diseases may often succeed each other and sometimes coexist in the same patient [324, 326]. In primary parenchymal renal disease, such as suspected glomerulonephritis, vasculitis, or interstitial nephritis, a renal biopsy should be performed. The renal biopsy may establish a diagnosis not suspected clinically and may significantly influence the choice of therapy and knowledge of prognosis [288, 332]. Other tests, such as serologic tests and nuclear scans, are often helpful in these patients (see Chaps. 47, 48, and 50, and Parts X and XI).

In cases of suspected obstruction, the patient should be investigated by ultrasonography or CT scans, or both. If in doubt, retrograde pyelography must be performed. Unilateral and silent obstruction may be particularly treacherous, as demonstrated in some patients reported to have had normal sonograms, intravenous pyelograms, and CT scans [110, 305, 314]. The diagnosis should be suspected when total anuria or intermittent anuria-polyuria exists. If the suspicion is strong, retrograde pyelography must be performed even if other tests are normal [69, 80, 98, 330]. Urinary chemistries and indices may be similar to those seen in prerenal failure in early obstruction and similar to acute tubular insufficiency after prolonged obstruction [305, 413].

The differential diagnosis of prerenal failure from acute tubular necrosis is sometimes very difficult or impossible. The treatment of one condition is often contraindicated in the other. Vigorous rehydration that may be curative of prerenal failure may kill the patient with acute tubular necrosis by inducing pulmonary edema [105]. If, on the other hand, fluid is withheld in the patient with prerenal failure, it may develop into acute tubular necrosis, with considerable morbidity and mortality. The diagnosis is of utmost importance, and yet it may be impossible to make because prerenal failure and acute tubular necrosis may occur successively or even coexist in the same patient [247, 326].

The differential diagnosis proceeds in a logical fashion. First, clinical data, such as weight and intake and output records, are reviewed. Although they are important, they cannot detect fluid shifts due to reabsorption or development of third spaces or changes in capacitance. Further clinical examination is then necessary, paying particular attention to the pressures in the pulmonary artery and pulmonary capillary bed [38, 170, 175].

A number of laboratory tests of urine chemistry or urine-blood ratios and indices have been devised to help in the differential diagnosis. These tests are outlined in Table 52-4 and have been recently reviewed [326]. Some of the tests may overlap between prerenal failure and acute tubular necrosis, particularly those that are only urine chemical. These tests include urinary specific gravity, urine osmolality, urine creatinine and urea, and urine sodium and potassium concentrations. Others, such as the urine-plasma osmolality ratio, the fractional excretion of sodium (FE_{Na}) test, and particularly sequential free water and creatinine clearances, may be more useful. This is true only if the tests are obtained before administration of diuretics and the patients do not suffer from underlying chronic renal failure or urinary tract obstruction [10, 11, 24, 49, 68, 108, 114, 161, 234, 272, 282, 284, 324–326, 355, 422]. However, even these tests may overlap, and the clearances are so time consuming that they are of little importance in the early decision making. They may, however, be valuable in the ongoing evaluation of the patient (Fig. 52-8).

The best clinical approach presently is to perform a clinical history and physical examination and x-ray of the lungs. These examinations have instantaneous results. At the same time, blood and urine are sent to the laboratory for the determinations necessary to do osmolar ratios and the FE_{Na} test. Treatment is then instituted, and the results and development are followed by sequential free water and creatinine clearances, which can be calculated based on the same tests that are used

Table 52-4. Differential diagnosis between prerenal failure and acute tubular necrosis

Test	Prerenal failure	Acute tubular necrosis
Urinary specific gravity	> 1.030	< 1.020
Urinary osmolality	> 400 mOsm/kg/H_2O	< 350 mOsm/kg/H_2O
Urine-plasma osmolal ratio	> 1.4	< 1.0
Urine-plasma creatinine ratio	> 30	< 20
Urine-plasma urea ratio	> 7	< 5
Serum urea N-creatinine ratio	> 10	Approximately 10
Urinary sodium concentration	< 30 mEq/liter	> 30 mEq/liter
FE_{Na}	< 1%	> 2%
Renal failure index	< 1	> 1
Free water clearance	Negative	Rising toward 0
2-hr creatinine clearance	Stable	Falling

FE_{Na} = fractional excretion of sodium.

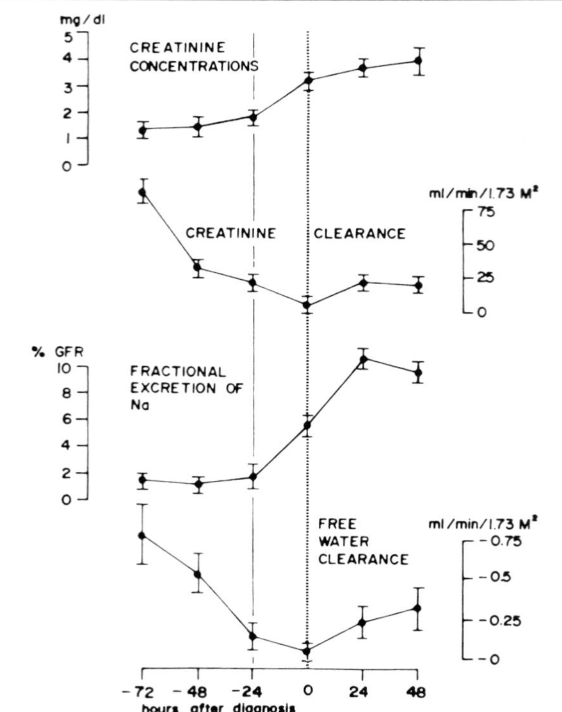

Fig. 52-8. Sequential change in renal function for 13 patients who were followed prospectively and in whom acute renal failure developed. The dotted vertical line indicates the time when 3 of the criteria for renal failure were met (free water clearance higher than 0 ml/min, creatinine clearance less than 30 ml/min; FE_{Na} greater than 3 percent; and persistently rising serum creatinine). The solid vertical line indicates the time, 24 hours earlier, when the diagnosis of acute renal failure was established by changes in creatinine clearance and free water clearance. These two latter parameters may therefore be earlier predictors of acute renal failure than FE_{Na} or serum creatinine concentration. GFR = glomerular filtration rate. (From [49].)

for the osmolar ratio and FE_{Na} test. The results of the clearance tests are then available as the patient is being reevaluated.

Etiologic Treatment

In this section we review extensively only the treatment of acute tubular necrosis. The etiologic treatment of dehydration is vigorous rehydration and, of obstruction, operative or percutaneous nephrostomy drainage (see Chap. 23). The multiple, dangerous, and poorly investigated treatments of acute renal failure due to parenchymal renal disease are discussed elsewhere in this book (see Parts VII, X, and XI). Because immunologic mechanisms seem to be a common etiology, they include treatment with corticosteroids, various cytotoxic drugs, anticoagulation, antiplatelet drugs, plasma infusion, plasmapheresis, and cytopheresis.

Two immediate treatments of etiologies should be applied in acute tubular necrosis. The first is a review of medications, followed by discontinuation of those that are nephrotoxic. The second is restoration of renal blood flow by improving cardiac dysfunction, reestablishment of euvolemia by control of bleeding and transfusion, and rehydration of the dehydrated patient. Once these treatments have been performed, the second line of defense is to stop any ongoing pathophysiologic development. Each sequential pathophysiologic step may create a hypothetical vicious feedback loop that perpetuates and aggravates the events that led to acute tubular necrosis [76, 169, 289, 335, 367]. Optimal therapy may therefore decrease both the progress of the renal failure and any feedback loops. Theoretically, the therapy should: (1) restore renal blood flow, (2) restore and increase tubular flow of urine, and (3) halt and repair ongoing intracellular injury. Any drug that increases renal blood flow is theoretically useful for treating developing acute tubular necrosis. The only drug presently used that has a large clinical experience is dopamine. Clinically, a dose of approximately 1 μg/kg/min has been thought, in uncontrolled clinical experiments, to decrease the severity or at least to convert oliguric to nonoliguric acute tubular necrosis [164, 246, 291].

Atrial natriuretic peptide is another potent renal vasodilator. Early animal studies were promising [292], but the first clinical studies are contradictory [116, 232, 333]. A worldwide multicenter study of the use of this agent in acute renal failure is presently taking place. The complication of hypotension can to some extent be circumvented by the simultaneous use of dopamine, or selective renal artery infusion [76, 246, 346]. Other potential agents to induce renal vasodilatation include calcitonin gene related peptide (CGRP), endothelial-derived relaxing factor (EDRF), and prostanoids. Clinical trials, however, are lacking.

Any drug that increases tubular flow and increases total sodium or chloride delivery to the macula densa may be effective in influencing the renin feedback loops. From a theoretical point of view, the loop diuretics and mannitol are particularly attractive. They both increase renal blood flow and tubular flow, and may thus inhibit feedback loops by both changing sodium delivery to the macula densa and by "flushing" out intratubular obstruction due to cellular debris. Loop diuretics may also minimize ischemic injury by inhibiting transport activity, thereby decreasing cellular oxygen demand [46].

Innumerable clinical studies with contradictory outcomes have been performed with these drugs [48, 58, 112, 200, 214]. They have been extensively reviewed by Levinsky and co-workers [242, 246]. The weighted clinical evidence indicates that these drugs often convert oliguria to nonoliguria and may decrease the need for dialysis. Whether they improve creatinine clearance remains very controversial. There is no evidence of improved mortality, but a prospective controlled study has yet to be performed.

Different timing of this intervention may be one reason why so much controversy exists [200]. Loop diuretics may be effective only in early acute tubular necrosis and patients respond with resolution of acute renal failure only if they are treated within 24 to 48 hours of renal insult and before the serum creatinine level exceeds 5 mg/dl [200]. Clinical and experimental studies indicate that dopamine and loop diuretics may exert a beneficial synergistic effect on acute tubular necrosis [246, 249, 250].

Theoretically, the final effect of ongoing intracellular damage can be attacked by the use of xanthine oxidase inhibitors [309], calcium channel blockers [347, 350], free oxygen radical scavengers [308], and infusions of intracellular substances, particularly magnesium chloride and nucleotides [306, 356, 376, 411], amino acids [1, 23, 303, 382] and epidermal growth factors [298]. The animal studies of these drugs remain controversial, and good clinical studies of most of these approaches are lacking. Many of them cannot be used in patients because of the risk of serious side effects such as magnesium intoxication. Exceptions are the use of intravenous amino acids and calcium channel blockers. Intravenous amino acids were found effective by Abel and co-workers and others [1, 22, 23] in both shortening the period of serum creatinine elevation and lowering mortality in patients with acute tubular necrosis. Several later investigators have failed to confirm this clinical finding [16, 237]. Experimental use of amino acids in acute renal failure has been reported to both improve and worsen renal function and to both lower and increase mortality [1, 22, 23, 303, 328, 382, 419, 421].

Several studies indicate that calcium channel blockers are effective in preventing or shortening acute tubular necrosis [125, 293, 400]. Others have found them useless [40]. Some of the differences may be dependent on the different timing of infusion and on the dissimilar action of various calcium channel blockers.

With such controversial experimental background, it is obvious that the clinical management of acute tubular necrosis is also subject to controversy. Many nephrologists believe that there is no true etiologic treatment and, after fluid volumes have been restored, will do nothing further. Others use dopamine, mannitol, and furosemide in a variety of combinations. We believe that a reasonable clinical approach is at least to try to treat the patient with a serum creatinine of below 5 mg/dl with a combination of dopamine infused at a rate of 1 μg/kg/min with rapidly escalating doses of furosemide, approximately 2 to 5 to 10 mg/kg infused at hourly intervals over a 15- to 20-minute period to decrease the ototoxicity of a high peak level. If diuresis is established, it can often be maintained by continued mannitol and furosemide infusion. The dose for a normal-sized, 60-kg adult would be a solution of 500 ml of 20% mannitol to which has been added the furosemide dose to which the patient responded, infused at a rate of 20 ml per hour. This will often maintain the diuresis and is sometimes associated with a fall in serum creatinine level. Even without the fall in serum creatinine, the diuresis considerably eases the conservative management of such a patient. If used, serum osmolality must frequently be checked by determinations of actual and calculated osmolality to avoid mannitol intoxication [42]. Other side effects of furosemide include pancreatitis and deafness [228, 327]. Some rare cases of acute oliguria resolve if increased abdominal pressure is reduced to normal [229, 365].

Symptomatic Conservative Treatment

If etiologic treatment fails, the patient enters a period of acute uremia, and the treatment now separates into conservative management to maintain homeostasis, and to prevent, detect, and treat complications that cause morbidity and mortality. In this section we address conservative treatment, and in the next, we discuss symptomatic treatment through various dialysis methods.

It is clear from the earlier section on mortality and prognosis in this chapter that infections are not only the most common cause of death in the patient with acute renal failure but also they are almost the only treatable factor. Infections often occur as a side effect of surgical complications, and both infections and surgical complications are thought to be increased if the patient becomes malnourished. In the rest of this section, we deal separately with infections, surgical complications, and nutrition, although they are interrelated. We also briefly discuss bleeding and other complications that may require conservative symptomatic treatment.

INFECTIONS

McMurray and co-workers have demonstrated that the more infections a patient with acute renal failure endures, the lower is the survival rate. In their series, 85 percent of patients without infections survived compared to only 25 percent of those with four infections [276].

Alwall [7] found signs of urinary tract infections in 80 percent of patients with acute renal failure, lung infections in 60 percent, clinical septicemia in 30 percent, and positive blood cultures in 15 percent. In several other series, none of the patients survived who developed positive blood cultures while they were receiving broad-spectrum antibiotics [62, 148, 271].

The diagnosis of infections is difficult in these patients. Urea is a strong antipyretic substance, and therefore the temperature response to infection is blunted [415] (Fig. 52-9). A patient with normal renal function will develop a temperature of over 103°F during culture-verified septicemia compared with only approximately 102°F in the patient with a creatinine clearance of less than 30 ml per minute.

In patients undergoing chronic dialysis, the white blood cell response to culture-verified septicemia is also blunted [147, 191, 313]. Thus, the segmented neutrophil count raised to over 5000 cells per cubic millimeter in only 5 of 17 patients studied by Peresecenschi and colleagues [313]. Peresecenschi demonstrated that nonsegmented neutrophils per cubic millimeter may be a more accurate sign of infection because in their series 13 of 17 patients achieved a count of more than 400 nonsegmented neutrophils per cubic millimeter. No studies have been performed on patients being dialyzed for acute renal failure, but it seems logical to assume a similar unreliability of the white count in such patients.

Patients with acute renal failure also show fewer clinical signs of infection. The abdominal examination is often normal in spite of abdominal catastrophes with severe peritonitis [224, 267].

Some of the tools, such as urinary tract catheters and

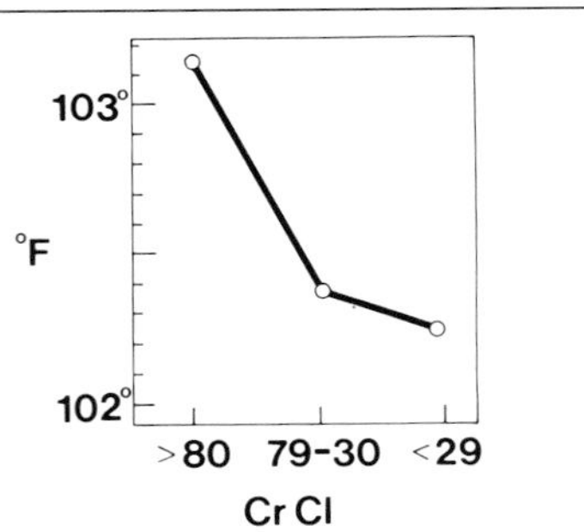

Fig. 52-9. Temperature in Fahrenheit versus creatinine clearance (CrCl) in patients with culture-verified septicemia. The more renal failure the patient has, the less the temperature will rise. (From [415].)

the indwelling pressure monitors used in the early resuscitation phase of the patient with acute renal failure, become increasingly dangerous if left in the patient's body. At the end of the week, there is an almost 100 percent incidence of positive urine cultures in the patient with an indwelling urinary catheter [53, 171, 386, 402]. If the patient is oliguric, a catheter is not needed. If the patient continues to produce urine, a Condome catheter should be attempted. If this is not possible, straight catheterization or at least a closed system should be utilized. Indwelling arterial and venous pressure monitoring devices also show high incidences of both infection and thromboembolic complications. Beyond the fourth day, 53 percent of patients with flow-directed pulmonary artery catheterization showed endocardial lesions [339]. The lessons learned from these studies are clear. Once the patient's condition is stabilized, indwelling catheters in the bloodstream and urinary tract should be removed. Beyond the fourth or fifth day, clinical examinations should suffice to judge fluid status. If changes occur, it is probably best to limit the studies through a reintroduced catheter to a few hours.

A special dilemma occurs if the patient needs hyperalimentation. It is difficult in the oliguric dialysis patient to perform this through peripheral sites. The safest approach is hyperalimentation through a Scribner shunt [54].

Because the lungs are often sites of infection, endotracheal tubes should be removed as soon as possible. Physical therapy, including breathing and coughing exercises, seems reasonable, although the value of these maneuvers is controversial [97, 150].

With the unreliability of clinical signs, temperature, and white blood counts, it is obvious that frequent, almost daily, blood, sputum, urine, and drain fluid cultures should be performed to allow early identification of an infectious agent. Because an association between early peak level of aminoglycoside antibiotics and survival of patients with gram-negative bacteremia has been established, monitoring of peak and trough levels of nephrotoxic antibiotics is required for the aggressive management of these infections [286].

Renal failure, major surgery, and malnutrition all induce immunologic deficiencies [56, 70, 83, 84, 197, 364]. Because most patients also have indwelling catheters and are treated with broad-spectrum antibiotics, unusual opportunistic infections and later fungal infection may also occur. Selective and time-limited antibiotic treatment should be used, and prophylaxis against fungal infections by nystatin or clotrimazole should be frequently administered either orally or through a nasogastric tube [60, 199]. Isolation of these patients is probably of little help because many infections are endogenous. Isolation tends to deprive patients of routine care such as mobilization. Close supervision is probably more important than the benefits derived from isolation [59, 60, 290]. A recent randomized double-blind study indicated that intravenous γ-globulin, 400 mg/kg/week, improves survival in acute renal failure. A larger study is presently under way [51].

In summary, infectious complications are the most common and perhaps the only truly treatable cause of death in patients who have acute renal failure. Clinical signs are often absent. Early prophylaxis should be instituted, including removal of catheters, repeated cultures, selective antibiotic treatment, and fungal prophylaxis. Intravenous γ-globulin may improve the survival.

SURGICAL COMPLICATIONS

Patients in whom acute renal failure develops after surgery have a very high incidence of complications that may be difficult to diagnose. The first thorough study was that by Marshall [267], who performed reoperations in 18 of 42 patients who had developed renal failure after surgery on the biliary tract, stomach, or large bowel. Of these patients, 17 (40%) had gross surgical complications. Fecal leak occurred in all 9 patients in whom acute tubular necrosis developed after large-bowel surgery. Marshall noted the absence of the usual clinical signs and the high incidence of postoperative septic shock in these patients as a presenting symptom.

Similarly, Kornhall [224], reviewing 298 surgical patients in whom postoperative acute tubular necrosis developed, found that 98 patients (33%) had neglected surgical complications. Eighty-eight of the 98 patients (90%) died. It is clear that aggressive surgery is indicated in these patients, and Marshall comments, "these patients are invariably too ill not to be operated on, rather than the reverse." In spite of reoperation, most patients in both series died. Such patients cannot survive without reoperation, but they also tolerate reoperation poorly. Perhaps the newer methods of percutaneous drainage of abscesses can improve this dismal state of affairs [34, 142, 392].

Intense diagnostic workup must be done continuously in the postoperative patient with acute renal failure. The new indium-labeled immunoglobulin scan, gallium and indium scans, ultrasound examinations, and CT scans of the operative areas of the body should be done early when acute renal failure develops [142, 217, 311, 343]. A baseline is thus obtained to use for comparison of later repeated studies. Changes in masses may then be detected early and can be further investigated by percutaneous aspirations.

CATABOLISM, NUTRITION, IMMUNOLOGIC PROBLEMS

Renal failure, malnutrition, and major surgery induce immunologic deficiencies in patients [56, 70, 84, 364]. Of these factors only malnutrition is treatable, and several investigators have found improvement of immunologic function with hyperalimentation [84, 91].

The gastrointestinal route of alimentation is much safer than the intravenous route and should be used whenever possible. Small-diameter soft nasogastric tubes and operative or percutaneous gastrostomy or ileostomy can be tried. A regular pureed diet is preferable to an elemental one because the osmolal load and diarrhea are less [100, 282, 345].

Patients with acute renal failure only develop extreme catabolism and may utilize 5000 calories and 200 gm protein per day [122]. The cause of catabolism is multifactorial and includes sepsis, trauma, and surgery. Contributing factors may include enhanced release of proteases or a reduction of protease inhibitors [74, 176–178]; increased levels of catecholamines, glucagon, and insulin [33, 185]; and the uremic state itself [64, 89, 134, 221, 284, 382, 383].

Many studies have been performed comparing hyperalimentation with a nonspecific nutritional regimen in patients with acute renal failure. Using glucose infusion as a control, Abel and associates [1] found both more rapid recovery of renal function and improved survival in the treatment group who received essential amino acid infusions. Similar results have been obtained by others [23, 287]. In contrast, Leonard and co-workers [237] found no difference in nitrogen balance in those patients using essential amino acid infusion and those patients receiving only dextrose. Several other investigators have not detected any effect on recovery or mortality by hyperalimentation [16, 122, 237].

The addition of nonessential amino acids to hyperalimentation in patients with acute renal failure was believed by one investigator to benefit patients and reduce mortality [22]. The results were confirmed, but only in the subgroup of patients with severe trauma [276]. Addition of nonessential amino acids was found by one investigator to decrease survival [135] and by another worker to be of no influence other than to increase negative nitrogen balance [121, 122]. It is noteworthy that some essential amino acids such as lysine are known to be nephrotoxic in some experimental settings [368]. The most thorough study, that by Feinstein and co-workers of nonessential amino acid (42 gm/day) or essential amino acid (21 gm/day) therapy with hypertonic dextrose compared with dextrose only, failed to find any improvement in recovery of renal function, survival, total serum concentration of albumin, total protein, or transferrin in the amino acid–treated patients [121, 122].

In view of these contradictory and discouraging results, some groups have suggested that benefit could be obtained by infusion of extremely high amounts of calories and amino acids, or "superalimentation" [274]. To date, there are no controlled studies of such an approach.

Hyperalimentation and superalimentation both induce metabolic and technical problems. Indwelling vascular catheters frequently become a source of infection. This problem can be partially circumvented through the use of a high-flow Scribner shunt with a T tube [54]. Unavoidable problems include a risk of fluid overload in anuric or oliguric patients and electrolyte disturbances. These negative factors must be weighed against the knowledge of malnutrition-induced immune deficiencies and clinical observations of spectacular decreases in urea appearance rate, potassium, phosphorus, and magnesium release after institution of hyperalimentation in severely ill patients with acute renal failure [84, 210]. A reasonable compromise is to avoid hyperalimentation in a patient with acute renal failure during the first several days. It is better at that time to achieve resuscitation and fluid and electrolyte control and homeostasis, and to start hyperalimentation after 1 week. The "best" solution to achieve hyperalimentation—whether protein hydrolysate, essential amino acids, or a mixture of essential and nonessential amino acids—is not known. Intestinal alimentation is always preferred, but if parenteral hyperalimentation is required, the shunt is probably the safest administration route. It is usually necessary to perform daily dialysis to remove the fluid load induced by hyperalimentation or to use continuous methods of dialysis, discussed later. The use of anabolic steroids can reduce catabolism in patients with acute renal failure, particularly women [37, 145].

BLEEDING

Bleeding complications of uremia are no longer common when dialysis treatment is used every other day or more. Kleinknecht and his co-workers observed that the incidence of gastrointestinal bleeding decreased from 59 to 15 percent when dialysis was initiated earlier and more frequently, and predialysis BUN was only 110 mg/dl compared with 190 mg/dl in their earlier series [215]. Although spontaneous bleeding in patients with acute renal failure is uncommon, it is important to recognize a bleeding tendency, particularly in patients who must undergo surgery between dialyses [193].

The more important known bleeding defects that occur in uremia are outlined in Table 52-5. It is not known how common the various abnormalities are and what clinical consequences each one has. Similarly, the exact pathogenesis behind the abnormalities remains obscure.

Table 52-5. Bleeding abnormalities in uremia

I. Platelets
    A. Reduced number
    B. Defective aggregation
    C. Decreased adhesiveness
    D. Decreased factor 3
II. Clotting cascade
    A. Vitamin K deficiency
    B. Liver disease
    C. Defective factor VIII
    D. Defective factor XIII
III. Blood vessels
    A. Increased prostacyclin

Important factors, particularly in the various platelet abnormalities, are small molecular toxins that interfere with platelets. Guanidinosuccinic acid and phenolic acid have been shown to decrease platelet production, adhesiveness, and factor III. Both are easily removed by dialysis. Exactly at what level of uremia these factors become important remains conjectural. Koppel and his coworkers [222] have shown that guanidinosuccinic acid levels are closely related to urea levels, and extrapolating from their research and that of others, one may reasonably assume that bleeding, correctable by dialysis, should not occur at BUN levels of less than 60 mg/dl, but may become more common if the BUN level exceeds 100 mg/dl [222]. Hemodialysis reduces platelet counts by a mean of 30 percent, and sometimes more, and may be associated with catastrophic bleeding [261, 398].

Some of the defects in the clotting cascade do not seem to be influenced by dialysis. If a normal bleeding time is not achieved by dialysis, the function of the clotting cascade can sometimes be normalized throughout the use of approximately 10 units of cryoprecipitate [186]. Deamino-arginine vasopressin, 0.3 μg/kg intravenously, has also been shown to correct bleeding time in uremic patients [265], as has the use of progesterone in high doses (10–30 mg daily) for several days [251]. An important observation is the influence of the hematocrit on hemostasis. Bleeding seems to be considerably more common if the hematocrit is less than 30 percent [83, 252]. Because other postoperative complications also escalate considerably if the hematocrit is below this level [83, 193], this hematocrit level should obviously be restored before patients are sent to surgery. Whether the increased prostacyclin that is found in blood vessel walls in patients on dialysis [334] is important for bleeding remains unknown because no clinical studies have examined this question. The usefulness of medications with antiprostaglandin activity thus remains speculative.

In summary, bleeding is no longer common in patients undergoing dialysis, but bleeding abnormalities may be catastrophic if not detected before surgery in such patients. The best clinical parameters to follow are platelet count, Ivy bleeding time, thrombin time, and prothrombin time. Before surgery vitamin K deficiencies should be corrected, hematocrit should be over 30 percent, and BUN should be brought to below 60 mg/dl by dialysis. If bleeding parameters remain abnormal, infusion of cryoprecipitate or deamino-arginine vasopressin, or use of progesterone, may restore them to normal.

OTHER COMPLICATIONS AND METABOLIC ABNORMALITIES

Gastrointestinal bleeding is not as common now as in the early days of dialysis. However, patients undergoing dialysis are often maximally stressed and have elevated gastrin levels [362, 380]. Sucralfate or aluminum hydroxide suspension, 15 to 60 ml several times a day, is therefore advocated prophylactically, and gastric acidity should be titrated to a pH above 3.5 [163, 410]. Sucralfate is as efficient as aluminum hydroxide and may decrease nosocomial pneumonia [385]. The antacids decrease gastric acidity and have the additional benefits of decreasing serum levels of phosphorus and hydrogen ion. If the patient has a nasogastric tube, he or she can be instilled through this and the tube clamped afterward. Side effects have included the formation of bezoar with both small- and large-bowel ischemia, perforation, and death [144, 344, 408]. If sorbitol is added to the solution, bringing it to a final concentration of 20%, this complication can be prevented. In some patients, phosphorus absorption by aluminum hydroxide leads to severe hypophosphatemia, particularly if the patient is also hyperalimented. In this case, aluminum phosphate antacid can be used instead. Magnesium-containing antacids should not be used unless serum magnesium levels are also monitored because serum magnesium may rise to toxic levels.

The exact role of histamine receptor inhibitors is unknown. These drugs are less effective than aluminum hydroxide antacids in stress ulceration [29, 36, 158, 240, 268, 323] and have more side effects [99, 119, 127, 294, 405]. The dose of histamine receptor antagonists must be reduced in uremia.

A number of metabolic problems occur with the onset of acute uremia. The serum calcium level immediately starts to fall and the serum phosphorus level to rise. Calcitonin and parathyroid hormone levels also increase [12, 162, 407]. Peripheral insulin sensitivity is decreased and many patients have hyperinsulinemia. There is, thus, a risk of decreased glucose metabolism with hyperglycemia. This occurs particularly if septicemia is also present. The metabolic problems with calcium and phosphorus are especially pronounced in rhabdomyolysis [4, 72, 90, 123, 153]. The cause of the decrease in serum calcium is intracellular migration; urinary calcium losses are not increased. Both calcium and magnesium intracellular concentrations increase, possibly contributing to the stupor and confusion that sometimes develop [13].

Most of the observed electrolyte abnormalities are ameliorated by dialysis, which will tend to restore blood levels of calcium, magnesium, and phosphorus to normal. Clinical symptoms of hypocalcemia such as muscle cramps or seizures are almost never observed. Since serum calcium levels tend to rebound during the recovery phase after acute tubular necrosis, it is probably best not to replace calcium unless clinically indicated by cramps or seizures. Erythropoietin production, which falls precipitously at the onset of acute tubular necrosis, may be suppressed long after recovery and contribute to the anemia [295].

DRUG USAGE

Most drug dosages need adjustment in patients with acute renal failure who are undergoing dialysis. Several drugs are normally excreted by the kidneys. They may also be removed by dialysis, and have different protein binding, distribution space, and even hepatic metabolism in patients with acute renal problems. Several of the excellent monographs [9, 31, 44] and frequently updated reviews [30, *Semin. Dial.*] should be consulted.

Symptomatic Dialysis Treatment

METHOD OF DIALYSIS

Three different methods of blood purification are available in acute uremia: hemodialysis, hemofiltration, and peritoneal dialysis, and there is a fourth combination of hemofiltration and hemodialysis, known as hemodiafiltration. Each method can be used either intermittently or continuously. The eight possible treatment modalities are summarized in Table 52-6.

There are no randomized clinical studies comparing one method with another. The only nonrandomized interinstitutional studies that have been performed have compared hemodialysis with intermittent peritoneal dialysis in patients with acute renal failure. They have all shown similar mortality [215, 266]. No comparison of mortality has been done for slow continuous hemofiltration, but the mortality reported for this procedure since 1985 has been higher than that reported for hemodialysis during the same time period. Of 870 patients treated with continuous hemofiltration/dialysis 650 (75%) died versus 559 of 834 (67%) patients treated with intermittent hemodialysis (unpublished observation). This may reflect a tendency to use slow continuous hemofiltration for the most seriously ill patients [225, 304, 375]. It is difficult to achieve satisfactory BUN clearance with hemofiltration, and in one series, morbidity was inversely related to BUN clearance of the hemofiltration [375]. In one randomized study of morbidity during slow continuous hemofiltration and hemodialysis, there were more side effects per treatment time during hemodialysis, but many more side effects per treatment efficiency (measured as total BUN clearance) with slow continuous hemofiltration [218]. There is only anecdotal experience with slow continuous hemodialysis, intermittent hemofiltration, or any method of hemodiafiltration in acute renal failure [358]. The relative indications for intermittent hemodialysis, peritoneal dialysis, or slow continuous hemofiltration/dialysis are therefore speculative.

The main advantage of hemodialysis is its efficiency—between 10 and 20 times that of peritoneal dialysis and slow continuous hemofiltration. Treatment times can, therefore, be kept short, and the patient is free to be mobilized and undergo other therapeutic or diagnostic procedures. The main disadvantages are the cardiovascular effects, and in particular hypotension, which occurs in 10 to 50 percent of treatments (see later in this chapter), and the intermittent cell edema, which to some degree seems to occur with each treatment. A relative disadvantage is the need for short-term anticoagulation during treatment. Some believe that the cardiovascular effects of intermittent hemodialysis may delay recovery of acute tubular necrosis [75].

The main advantages of peritoneal dialysis are that no anticoagulation is needed and there is minimal effect on the cardiovascular functions of the patients. The mechanical cleaning of the abdominal cavity may be an advantage in a patient with a soiled peritoneal cavity. The main disadvantages are its low efficiency, the requirement for an intact peritoneum, and the risk of peritonitis.

The main advantages of slow continuous hemofiltration or hemodiafiltration are the absence of cardiovascular effects, at least in the early phase of the treatment, and the ease with which clearance can be manipulated through the use of negative pressure. The main disadvantages include its relatively low efficiency [375], the need for continuous anticoagulation, the frequent manipulation of an infection-prone access, and possibly cardiovascular complications occurring later in treatment. Further problems are the large amount of time that the nurses need to spend on technical chores and fluid balance bookkeeping instead of patient care [404]. The procedure also ties the patient to the bed and is in the way of other important diagnostic and therapeutic procedures, which are then done too late or not at all.

The relative indications for the procedures can be discussed from two points of view, the timing of the procedure and the special complications of an individual patient. Most patients beginning dialysis show the greatest cardiovascular instability during the first several treatments [337]. Early in the treatment there would therefore be special advantages to using peritoneal dialysis or slow continuous hemofiltration/dialysis. Later, when the patients are more stable, it may be advantageous to mobilize them. Because mobilization is difficult with any continuous procedure, intermittent hemodialysis is better. Patients with a very unstable cardiovascular system may best be treated with peritoneal dialysis or slow continuous hemofiltration. For those whose conditions are stable, it is better to use intermittent hemodialysis. Considering only the risk of bleeding, peritoneal dialysis would be the best treatment, slow continuous hemofiltration by far the worst, and intermittent hemodialysis in between. The hypercatabolic patient may be treatable only with hemodialysis because of the low clearances of the other methods. The continuous methods make fluid and electrolyte balance much easier to maintain in the anuric patient who receives large amounts of intravenous fluids, such as during hyperal-

Table 52-6. List of possible dialysis methods

	Hemodialysis	Peritoneal dialysis	Hemofiltration	Hemodiafiltration
Intermittent	Most clinical experience "gold standard"	Results equal to intermittent hemodialysis	Anecdotal experience only; technically complicated	Anecdotal experience; very complicated
Continuous	Anecdotal experience; technically complicated	Anecdotal experience; many advantages	Large uncontrolled experience; technically simple; high mortality	Anecdotal experience; very complicated

imentation or superalimentation. Finally, the absence of brain edema and anticoagulation during continuous peritoneal dialysis probably makes this method preferable in the patient with brain damage [361].

In most instances the merits and advantages of various methods are trivial and the choice is best settled by the technical expertise of the treating center. The few individual exceptions have already been outlined. Some patients may best be treated with one method at one time of their disease and with another method later. For example, severely traumatized patients may need emergency hemodialysis to regulate homeostasis preoperatively, then continuous peritoneal dialysis to cleanse the peritoneal cavity and maintain them over a time of instability; later, they may return to hemodialysis when they can be mobilized.

WHEN TO START DIALYSIS

The experience from several large clinical studies, knowledge of protein catabolic rates, and quantitative considerations of dialysis clearance allow one to calculate when dialysis should be started and the frequency with which it should be applied. Based on 40 years of observations, it is clear that predialysis BUN should not exceed 100 to 120 mg/dl, usually achieved by every-other-day hemodialysis, "the gold standard." Gillum, Conger, and associates [143] are members of the only investigating team that has in recent times compared whether even more intense dialysis could further lower mortality. They randomized 34 patients to either "intense dialysis," done daily, in which the serum creatinine was kept below 5.1 mg/dl, or "ordinary dialysis," in which the mean predialysis serum creatinine was 9.1 mg/dl. They found no difference in mortality and no complications. Thus, assuming the usual 10:1 BUN-creatinine ratio, predialysis BUN levels should not exceed 100 mg/dl, and the creatinine should be kept below 9 to 10 mg/dl. Once these levels are reached, further lowering efforts seem futile. Others have made similar observations [62, 148, 271]. Indirectly, Mentzer and his co-workers [278] have come to the same conclusion. Comparing 236 patients who needed dialysis for acute renal failure immediately following renal transplantation with matched control subjects, they found no difference in mortality. This observation indicates that their dialysis, which was applied approximately every other day, had maximally lowered mortality.

One can easily calculate when continuous peritoneal and slow continuous hemofiltration should be started by comparing their clearance rates with those of intermittent hemodialysis. Both continuous methods have an approximate BUN clearance of 15 ml per minute. This is the same total clearance that one achieves with intermittent hemodialysis, used 4 hours every other day, with a blood flow that gives a BUN clearance of 180 ml per minute. Using the following formulas, one can calculate the frequency and duration needed for dialysis.

1. At a steady state: nitrogen production = nitrogen removal.
2. BUN removal = mean blood concentration of BUN × clearance of dialyzer × duration of dialysis = total body water × (predialysis − postdialysis BUN concentration).

With a protein catabolic rate (PCR) of 70 gm protein per day, the two continuous methods, with a BUN clearance of 15 ml per minute, would give a mean BUN concentration of 55 mg/dl. If the protein catabolic rate exceeds 120 gm per day, a constant BUN clearance of 15 ml per minute is insufficient to keep BUN concentration below 100 mg/dl. At such a PCR, one would need to dialyze approximately 3.5 hours every other day with intermittent hemodialysis, with a clearance of 180 ml per minute to keep the predialysis BUN concentration below 100 mg/dl, decreasing it to 45 mg/dl after dialysis. Two hours of daily dialysis would also keep predialysis BUN below 100 mg/dl. The need for dialysis at a BUN clearance of 3 ml/min/kg body weight versus PCR is illustrated in Fig. 52-10.

Practical conclusions from this reasoning suggest that hemodialysis should be initiated shortly before the patient's BUN level has reached 100 mg/dl and should be performed with a BUN clearance of 3 ml/min/kg body weight every day or every other day for 2 to 5 hours, depending on the catabolic rate. Continuous peritoneal dialysis or hemofiltration should be instituted when the BUN level is approximately 60 mg/dl. Because it is difficult to increase clearance further in continuous peritoneal dialysis, this method may not be sufficient if the urea nitrogen level continues to rise. It is possible to increase the BUN clearance with slow continuous hemofiltration by applying suction on the dialysate side [218], but then increasing problems will occur with very large fluid volume infusions and subsequent problems with fluid balance will follow. The efficiency can also be increased by combining it with dialysis [358].

HEMODIALYSIS

Vascular Access. Vascular access for acute hemodialysis is established either through percutaneous cannulation of the femoral or subclavian veins or through operative insertion of the Scribner shunt. Arteriovenous fistula or a vessel-bridging artificial blood vessel cannot be used because of the requirement for a maturing time. The Scribner shunt can be changed into an arteriovenous fistula at a later date should the patient fail to regain renal function [55]. Single-needle technique can be used with any access [395].

The fastest blood access is achieved by percutaneous cannulation. The safest route is the femoral vein. Potential lethal complications—perforation of the inferior vena cava and thrombosis of the femoral vein and pulmonary emboli—have a reported frequency of less than 1 percent [230]. Infectious complications and femoral thrombosis can probably be avoided completely by never leaving the catheter in for longer than 24 hours. Perforations of the vena cava, if they occur, have taken place during the cannulation procedure, but can be avoided by careful attention to resistance to the guide wire.

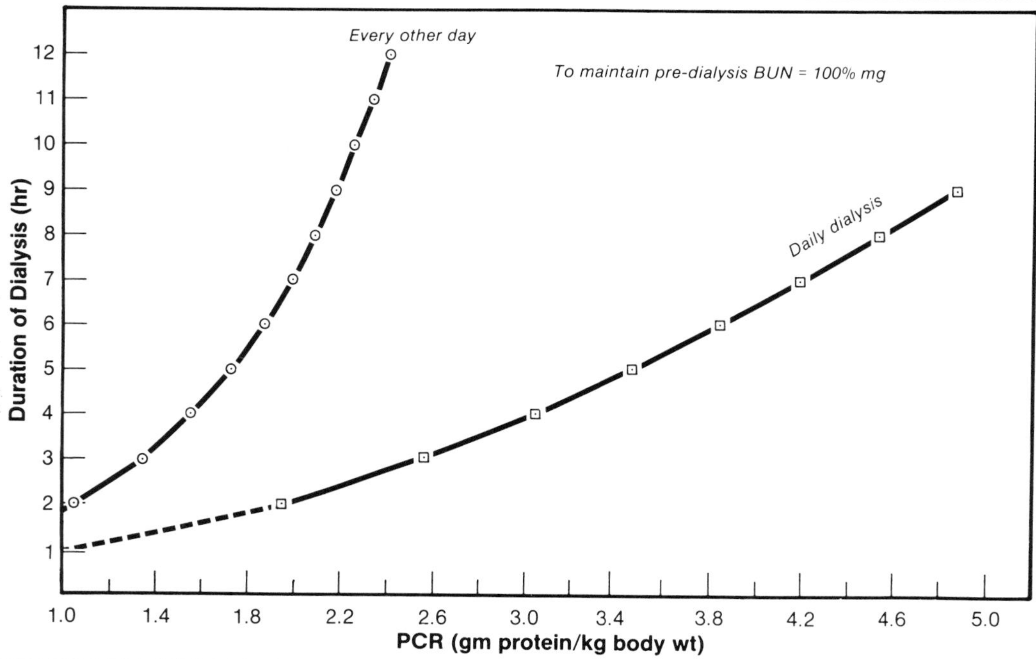

Fig. 52-10. The need for daily and every-other-day intermittent hemodialysis versus protein catabolic rate (PCR). In this example, a BUN clearance of 3 ml/min/kg body weight is used, and a fixed body water volume of 58 percent of body mass is assumed. The need for dialysis is calculated so predialysis BUN equals 100 mg/dl. Although the predialysis levels are equal, the postdialysis and mean BUN levels are lower in every-other-day dialysis. On the other hand, the oscillations in blood levels are much more pronounced with every-other-day dialysis, and this may cause more problems. (From [211]. Figure courtesy of Prakash Keshaviah, Ph.D.)

Subclavian vein catheterization has gained considerable popularity lately and is the most convenient but also the most dangerous method of achieving blood access. The incidence of complications is unknown, but several deaths have occurred from perforation of vena cava or the heart resulting in hemothorax both during and several days after insertion of the catheter [27, 160, 379]. Other complications include subclavian thrombosis [111] and septic complications [113, 354].

The safest method of blood vessel cannulation is operative insertion of a Scribner shunt. No lethal complications occur during insertion, infections are rare, and through the application of a T tube, it can be used for hyperalimentation and blood gas sampling, simplifying the care of the patient. Blood vessels are sacrificed, but they can be saved by later creation of an arteriovenous fistula after the vein has matured [55].

Dialyzer. The choice of dialyzer is not difficult. A dialyzer and its blood line should contain less than 10 percent of a patient's blood volume. Therefore, for pediatric patients or particularly small adult patients, special pediatric dialyzers should be used [173, 201, 210]. Flat-plate dialyzers as well as those made of the new synthetic membranes [184] are reputedly easier to anticoagulate, although this is a matter of controversy [63, 261, 397]. The newer membranes show less complement activation and neutropenia during dialysis, but there is no correlation between biocompatibility and clinical complications [3, 5, 363].

Dialysate. The dialysis solution should be adjusted based on considerations for individual patients, and the dialysate used for chronic dialysis (see Chap. 109) is not suitable for all acutely ill patients.

The *sodium* concentration should be approximately 140 mEq/per liter. Low sodium concentration, sometimes used for the treatment of hypertension in some chronically ill patients, is not suitable for the acutely ill patient [67, 120, 154, 241]. If the patient's sodium level is very high, it is advisable to add sodium to the dialysate to prevent cerebral edema secondary to idiogenic osmols known to be present in response to hyperosmolality [120]. Removal of idiogenic osmols is slow, and severe brain edema may result unless a high sodium dialysate is used [120]. Dialysate delivery systems are available that allow variation of the dialysate sodium concentration during therapy. The utility and benefits of such variations are controversial [67, 85, 269].

It is common to use a lower than normal *potassium* concentration if the patient is hyperkalemic. This may be dangerous in two clinical situations. If the patient is digitalized, a sudden decrease in potassium may precipitate digitalis intoxication. If the patient is markedly acidotic, rapid correction by dialysis may cause large shifts of potassium from the extracellular to the intracellular space that may result in severe, perhaps fatal, hypokalemia [412].

For most patients, the dialysate *calcium* concentration should be identical to normal plasma ionized calcium. Higher dialysate calcium concentrations have been advocated in some patients to better maintain blood pressure during dialysis [423]. Lower calcium concentrations may be useful for patients with hypoproteinemia or with hypercalcemia secondary to myeloma, hyperparathyroidism, or vitamin D intoxication [104]. Patients with very high serum phosphate levels should be dialyzed against a lower than normal calcium concentration in the dialysate to avoid soft tissue deposition of calcium phosphate, secondary to high calcium-phosphorus products. Hyperphosphatemia is particularly common in patients in whom acute tubular necrosis develops after rhabdomyolysis, lymphoma, or leukemia [72, 209].

Most patients with acute renal failure have *hyperphosphatemia*. However, acute renal failure secondary to heat stroke or burn injury may have associated hypophosphatemia [216, 300]. Hypophosphatemia may also occur secondary to successful hyperalimentation and the use of oral antacids. In these instances, phosphorus can be added directly to the dialysate if it is diluted before mixing with the calcium [94].

The dialysis fluid customarily contains a *magnesium* concentration close to normal plasma value. Some patients with alcoholism and those successfully hyperalimented may be hypomagnesemic, and more magnesium can then be conveniently added to the dialysate.

Bicarbonate should be used in dialysis of acute, often desperately ill patients. In selected patients with abnormally high bicarbonate levels, lower than normal bicarbonate dialysate should be used [21]. *Chloride* simply makes up the difference between cations and anions in dialysate.

Dextrose is added to the dialysate to prevent induction of a negative nitrogen balance secondary to gluconeogenesis [403] and other side effects of dialysis [238]. Very high dextrose levels, over 1000 mg/dl, should probably be avoided because postdialysis hypoglycemia and convulsions have been described with such solutions. A dialysate dextrose concentration close to 700 mg/dl may be optimal to inhibit gluconeogenesis, supply calories, cause only moderate elevation of blood sugar (50 mg/dl) at the end of dialysis, and minimize the disequilibrium syndrome [238, 336, 403].

Method of Dialysis. The first four dialyses, at least of chronic patients, are associated with three times as many side effects as later dialyses [337]. They probably result from intracellular fluid shifts secondary to rapid corrections of osmolality and changes in ionized calcium and other ionic shifts with correction of acidosis. Very rapid dialysis further increases these side effects [189, 212]. Very fast dialysis as presently used in some chronic dialysis patients should therefore be avoided [43]. Once a patient's condition is stabilized, a urea clearance based on the patient's body weight and equal to approximately 3 ml/min/kg is well tolerated [189, 212, 337] and if performed for at least 4 hours every other day, will offer an adequate amount of dialysis. If marked metabolic abnormalities are present (i.e., BUN > 120 mg/dl and marked acidosis), it is best to use a urea clearance of only 1 ml/min/kg body weight. Subsequent dialysis prescriptions can be increased by 0.5 ml/min/kg body weight per dialysis until a urea clearance of 3 ml/min/kg body weight is reached at the fifth dialysis [336].

Profound falls in osmolality can be counteracted by using a higher glucose concentration such as 700 mg/dl (see above) or by infusing mannitol in an approximate dose of 6 mOsm/kg (1.0 gm/kg) slowly during the entire dialysis. A similar dose can be infused during the second dialysis. Thereafter, a dose of 3 mOsm/kg body weight is used during dialysis three and four. Such an approach will reduce the osmolality fall during dialysis and will also decrease both the incidence of hypotension and other symptoms of disequilibrium [208, 336, 338]. It should not be used for more than four dialyses because of the risk of mannitol intoxication [42].

Anticoagulation. The mainstay of anticoagulation during dialysis remains heparin. The administration of a bolus of heparin as used in patients undergoing chronic dialysis should be avoided. If the patient is not at high risk for bleeding, a constant infusion of approximately 16 units/kg/hr of dialysis (4000 units of heparin totally during 4 hours to a 60-kg patient) is appropriate. If the patient is at high risk for bleeding, the heparin infusion is slower and is regulated by frequently performed clotting times [117, 204, 352]. Clotting times should not be allowed to rise more than 25 percent above baseline. Most patients can be anticoagulated with this schedule, which uses 1500 to 2000 units of heparin per therapy, and still have only a 2 to 5 percent incidence of dialyzer clotting. This approach will minimize bleeding even in very high-risk patients [204, 377].

Citrate has gained popularity as a form of regional anticoagulation during hemodialysis. With this procedure, heparin trisodium citrate is infused into the "arterial" blood line from the patient to the dialyzer. No calcium is added to the dialysate but calcium is infused into the venous return line from the dialyzer to the patient [316]. The method is somewhat cumbersome in that it involves a special dialysate and calibration of two constant infusion pumps. Metabolic problems include hyper- and hypocalcemia, hyperammonemia when used with cartridge urea removal systems, hypernatremia, and metabolic alkalosis. With this method it is clear that heparin-induced thrombocytopenia is avoided. The result in patients at high risk of bleeding appears equal to that of patients on low-heparin anticoagulation [277, 399]. In one prospective randomized study, less bleeding was found in patients anticoagulated with citrate than with heparin [132].

In patients with an extremely high risk for bleeding, one can occasionally use dialysis with no anticoagulation. Cellulose acetate dialyzers may be most suitable, although no controlled studies exist. No-heparin dialysis necessitates a high blood flow rate (over 300 ml/

min) and requires that the dialyzer be rinsed with 200 ml physiologic saline solution through the arterial segment every 20 minutes [61, 63, 184, 194, 245, 321].

Regional heparinization, involving simultaneous infusion of heparin into the arterial line and protamine into the venous line, is inferior to the methods previously described. The risk of rebound anticoagulation is high after dialysis has ceased because heparin is metabolized more slowly than protamine [159]. Comparisons of regional heparinization with low-dose heparin have shown that the incidence of bleeding is twice as high with regional heparinization and the incidence of dialyzer clotting is not improved [377].

Several other methods of anticoagulation have been described. They include prostacyclins [166, 167, 253, 426], ticlopidine [152], gabexate mesilate [378], and the new heparinoids [166, 167, 253]. There is little clinical experience with these anticoagulants and no controlled comparisons with heparin. Important indications may be for the occasional patient who cannot tolerate heparin. A major contribution would be the development of dialyzers requiring *no* anticoagulation [14].

Complications of Hemodialysis and Their Treatment. Hemodialysis is associated with considerable morbidity. During each dialysis, as a mean, one of the following complications will occur: hypertension, hypotension, headache, nausea, vomiting, or cramps. In chronically ill patients, the incidence of complications is three times as high during the first four dialyses, and it takes 1 month (15 dialyses) for a patient's condition to stabilize [202, 337]. The incidence of these side effects as reported in the literature is summarized in Table 52-7. The incidence in acutely ill patients is not known but is probably similar.

The pathogenesis of these effects is multifactorial, poorly understood, and a continuing source of controversy [211]. A great deal of confusion is semantic and results from failing to differentiate between pathogenesis, mediators, pathophysiology, and individual patient factors [196, 296]. Figure 52-11 is an attempt to summarize the present knowledge.

Isolated ultrafiltration usually does not cause hypotension, even when the ultrafiltrate volume equals the total circulating blood volume, unless diffusive dialysis is simultaneously performed [32, 146, 187, 197, 315].

Acute decreases in plasma osmolality contribute significantly to dialysis hypotension [93, 168, 203, 208, 211, 236, 338]. A decrease in plasma osmolality decreases extracellular fluid volume because water moves from the extracellular to the intracellular space [197] and because

Table 52-7. Mean frequency (percent) of side effects of hemodialysis

Hypotension	20–50%
Hypertension	15%
Nausea	15–30%
Vomiting	5–20%
Cramps	15–50%
Headache	2–25%

Fig. 52-11. Scheme of the mechanisms underlying dialysis-induced hypotension. At least five different pathogenetic factors may operate during dialysis. They affect one or several mediators, which, directly or through other mediators in turn, will decrease cardiac output or peripheral resistance. Several factors are also present in patients that may interfere with the defense against the dialysis-induced decrease in cardiac output or peripheral resistance.

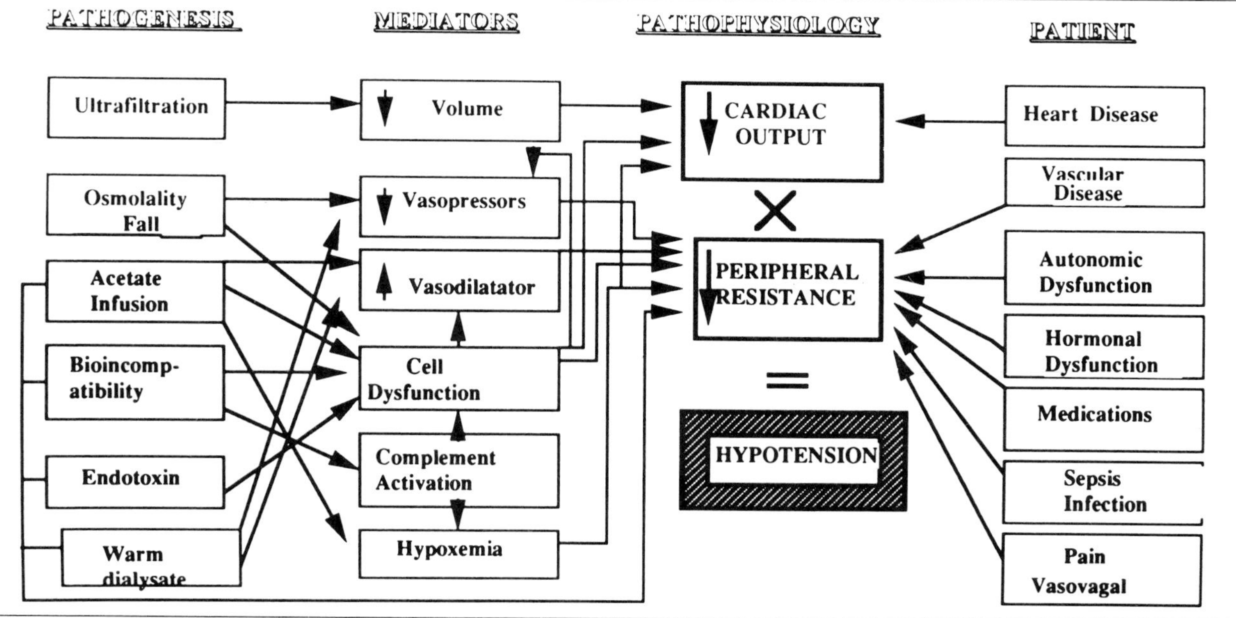

the increase in intracellular water results in cell dysfunction, which enhances the release of prostaglandin and vasodilatation and decreases vasopressin and vasoactive amine release in stress [118, 168, 236, 299, 348, 349, 417]. Although vasoactive amines are small molecules and easily dialyzable, most patients show no fall in epinephrine and norepinephrine blood levels during dialysis [45, 57, 223, 230, 425].

The infusion of acetate during dialysis has been shown to cause a fall in blood pressure, but only if dialysate sodium is low [35, 207, 406]. Dialysis may also aggravate dialysis-associated hypoxemia by removing carbon dioxide, which results in hypoventilation and hypoxemia from decreased minute ventilation. Some investigators believe hypoxemia may occur because of leukostasis in the pulmonary capillaries secondary to complement activation [86], but this pathogenetic mechanism remains controversial [18, 107, 301]. Oxygen consumption during acetate or bicarbonate dialysis is not different [273].

All currently available dialysis membranes are bioincompatible and induce complement activation, neutropenia, and thrombocytopenia [3, 5, 15, 79, 261]. The cellophane and cuprophane membranes are less biocompatible than cellulose acetate, polyacrylonitrile, and polycarbonate membranes [156]. There is no correlation between biocompatibility of the dialysis membrane and clinical symptoms during dialysis [363].

Certain medications may cause hypotension or interfere with blood pressure compensation during dialysis. These include blood pressure medications and phenothiazine [88]. Severe autonomic dysfunction obviously interferes with physiologic compensation mechanisms, counteracting hypotension [115, 196, 296].

The suggested treatment for dialysis hypotension is outlined in Table 52-8. A decrease in dialysis clearance will decrease the side effects of dialysis [201, 208, 338]. The dialyzer also should not have an excessive blood volume because this will increase side effects [212]. Some patients show allergic or sometimes fatal reactions to the dialyzer, particularly the hollow fiber, and one should therefore try flat-plate dialyzers if reactions occur [182]. Dialysis machines that use constant ultrafiltration also decrease hypotension during dialysis. Sequence dialysis/ultrafiltration has been found useless in decreasing dialysis hypotension if dialysis is performed immediately following ultrafiltration [187, 315]. It has been shown that at the end of the sequence, volume changes and hypotension are identical to simultaneous dialysis/ultrafiltration [315]. It may be more useful to do ultrafiltration every other day and dialysis every other day in the very susceptible patient, but this has not been tested [32, 187]. Decreasing the dialysate temperature to 35°C leads to better preservation of blood pressure during dialysis [248]. Some patients with profound cardiovascular abnormalities may best be treated by other methods, in particular, peritoneal dialysis.

Table 52-8. Treatment of dialysis hypotension

Technique	Decrease clearance Frequent dialysis Smaller dialyzer Different dialyzer Constant ultrafiltration Sequence dialysis/ultrafiltration Cooler dialysate (Peritoneal dialysis, hemofiltration)
Pharmacologic	Vasoactive amines Nasal oxygen Osmolal active agents Bicarbonate dialysate High calcium dialysate Albumin, hyperoncotic Prostaglandin inhibition
Patient factors	Medication interference (other)

A number of pharmacologic interventions can decrease dialysis hypotension. The use of hyperosmolar agents such as mannitol, sodium, or glucose, as mentioned previously, prevents or ameliorates dialysis hypotension [67, 93, 154, 208, 238, 241, 269, 338, 393]. Nasal oxygen was shown to decrease dialysis hypotension in one controlled study [262] but was ineffective in another [139]. Bicarbonate dialysate will also facilitate blood pressure stability, particularly if low-sodium dialysate has to be used [35, 329, 406]. Increasing dialysate calcium concentration may also improve blood pressure control but is contraindicated if hyperphosphatemia is present [423]. Infusions of vasoactive amines or hyperoncotic albumin are empirical treatment methods; the first treatment has predictable results, the second one unpredictable results [270]. Prostaglandin inhibition in one controlled crossover study in stable patients had no statistically significant effect on hypotension [41].

Most patient factors are untreatable, but medications such as antihypertensives and phenothiazines, which are known to aggravate hypotension, should be avoided [88].

SLOW CONTINUOUS HEMOFILTRATION/DIALYSIS

Slow continuous hemofiltration is the latest addition to the treatments of acute renal failure. The procedure is technically very easy to perform and requires no pumps or sophisticated monitoring equipment. Requirements include only an arteriovenous shunt, blood lines, filter, heparin infusion pump, and warmer for the intravenous replacement fluid. Equipment comparing rates of ultrafiltration to rates of intravenous fluid administration can consist of a simple balancing scale, which is desirable but not absolutely necessary [218, 227]. A small-volume, low-resistance hemofilter is connected without a blood pump to an arteriovenous shunt. The patient's arterial pressure and venous resistance produce a transmembrane pressure (TMP), which generates an ultrafiltrate at a rate of 10 to 15 ml per minute [124, 165, 190, 218, 226, 227, 235]. Low filtration rates secondary to hypotension or low venous resistance can be enhanced by connecting the filter to a simple wall suction negative-pressure outlet, which will provide filtration rates of up to 40 to 50 ml [218]. The low efficiency can also be overcome by adding dialysis [183, 358, 375], but this adds considerable technical complications. Different filters show marked individual variations in molecular rejection [124]. For small molecules such as urea, creatinine, or uric acid with membrane rejections of nearly zero, the clearance equals the ultrafiltration rate. Because of protein coating, this relationship is true only for molecules smaller than 1000 to 2000 daltons [124].

An advantage of the slow continuous methods is cardiovascular stability in the early hours of therapy. Blood pressure and pulse rate do not change [218, 307, 351]. Disadvantages of this therapy are related to the need for constant heparinization, constant supervision of changing fluid balance, and late changes in heart rate and blood pressure, which require a large commitment of nursing staff [92, 218, 404].

The survival results are lower than those obtained using intermittent hemodialysis. This may be because gravely ill patients have been selected for the procedure, or because slow continuous hemofiltration is inferior to hemodialysis in the therapy of acute renal failure. In one study, the mortality from slow continuous hemofiltration was inversely related to the ultrafiltration rate [375].

Access. For spontaneous filtration, an arteriovenous connection is necessary. The safest one is the Scribner arteriovenous shunt. Some investigators have used indwelling catheters in the femoral artery and femoral vein, but thrombosis of both vessels has been described and this route is probably best avoided [106, 174, 213, 225, 304]. If a vein-to-vein approach is used, a blood pump becomes necessary, requiring pressure meters and air detectors, and defeating the technical simplicity of the procedure.

Filter. Several filters with different membranes are clinically available [124, 218, 235]. All are highly biocompatible, each has different membrane characteristics, and there are marked variations in protein coating [124]. These variables are probably of no clinical relevance.

Anticoagulation. Continuous hemofiltration requires continuous anticoagulation. This poses a danger of bleeding, of which there are multiple reports [92, 190, 218, 225, 304]. In anecdotal cases, continuous filtration has been performed without anticoagulation [102]. In the future, hemofilters will probably be available that require no anticoagulation [14]. Currently, the need for continuous anticoagulation makes this method less safe than intermittent hemodialysis in patients who are at high risk for bleeding.

Complications. The main complication of slow continuous arteriovenous hemofiltration is bleeding [92, 190, 218, 225, 227]. Although the initial phase of hemofiltration is void of cardiovascular symptoms, this is not true if filtration proceeds for an extended time. In the only crossover study comparing slow continuous hemofiltration with intermittent hemodialysis in patients with acute renal failure, less hypotension and tachyarrhythmia occurred per time unit on slow continuous hemofiltration. However, when complications were more meaningfully normalized to BUN clearance, there were twice as many hypotensive and four times as many tachyarrhythmic episodes on slow continuous hemofiltration [92, 218]. It is presently unknown if the side effects caused by excessive ultrafiltration rates are inherent in the technique as such. The exact role of slow continuous hemofiltration in the treatment of severe acute renal failure has not been clearly determined.

CONTINUOUS PERITONEAL DIALYSIS (see also Chap. 106)

In studies of acute renal failure comparing intermittent peritoneal dialysis with hemodialysis, mortality has been identical [52, 215, 266]. There are as yet only small clinical studies of continuous peritoneal dialysis, which has replaced the inferior intermittent peritoneal dialysis, in acute renal failure [130, 320, 373]. The technique is simple and if the patient needs to be moved for other diagnostic or therapeutic procedures the continuous peritoneal dialysis is simply stopped and then resumed when the patient is returned to the ward.

The continuous peritoneal method has many advantages: There is no need for anticoagulation, there are no disequilibrium symptoms, and it is technically simple and can be performed anywhere in a hospital. Disadvantages include unpredictable electrolyte and glucose problems, a low BUN clearance insufficient to control uremia in hypercatabolic patients, and the risk of peritonitis. It is the best method for patients at high risk for bleeding, or for those who have severe head trauma, myocardial instability, or contaminated abdominal processes [271, 312, 361, 384, 388]. Peritoneal dialysis cannot be used in patients with large disruption of the peritoneal space, perforations of the diaphragm, or recent intestinal surgery because the peritoneal catheter may impair healing [384]. Patients with abdominal wall infections or hypercatabolism or those who need rapid correction of uremia and electrolyte abnormalities are best treated with intermittent hemodialysis.

Peritoneal Access. The best peritoneal access is achieved by placement of a soft Silastic catheter under direct visualization through a small minilaparotomy. With this technique, a perforation of the abdominal cavity can be avoided, the catheter drains better, and there is less associated pain. The stiff Teflon catheter can be placed percutaneously in the patient on the medicine ward, but this procedure carries a risk of bowel perforation, and outflow is sometimes compromised. Percutaneous placement techniques are therefore best avoided.

Peritoneal Dialysis Solution. The same peritoneal dialysate solutions used in the patient with chronic dialysis can be used in the patient with acute renal failure. The dextrose concentration of 1.5 gm/dl usually induces no net fluid removal from the patient. With a more concentrated solution, 4.25 gm/dl, 200 to 600 ml fluid is removed per hour depending on cycling techniques. Routine addition of heparin is no longer practiced. In the patient with an intact peritoneum, only small amounts of heparin are reportedly absorbed from the dialysate [146, 381]. However, if high concentrations are used, significant absorption can occur, resulting in severe anticoagulation and bleeding. It is customary to add heparin to the dialysis fluid to prevent obstruction of the catheter by fibrin if the patient has peritonitis.

Prophylactic antibiotics are of no value in preventing peritonitis [20]. For the patient with peritonitis antibiotics added to the dialysate may be curative and improve survival. The antibiotic concentration in the dialysis fluid should be similar to the concentration desired in plasma water [17, 20, 95, 264, 312, 353, 384, 389].

Several pharmacologic agents have been added to the dialysate to improve clearance or ultrafiltration rates. They include prostaglandins, prostaglandin precursors, dopamine, glucagon, isoproterenol, tolazoline, nitroprusside, and dipyridamole [155, 172, 297]. Most popular has been nitroprusside in a concentration of 4 to 5 μg per liter of dialysis fluid. It seems to have almost no systemic effect when used in this fashion. The increases in clearance, however, are usually trivial.

Complications. The complications of peritoneal dialysis are outlined in Table 52-9 and have been described in detail elsewhere [340, 390]. The most serious problems are perforations of abdominal organs. The presence of blood or fecal contamination in the return peritoneal dialysis fluid is diagnostic. Most perforations are simply treated by replacement of the catheter and the addition of antibiotics to the solution [342, 360]. A number of metabolic complications have been outlined elsewhere in this book (see Chap. 106). Monitoring of blood levels of electrolytes and glucose concentration is necessary. Hyperglycemia can be avoided by adding insulin to the dialysate [81, 151]. In occasional patients lactic acidosis may develop if the dialysate solution uses lactate as a buffer solution, and these patients must be treated with bicarbonate-containing solutions [396]. Protein and amino acids are sometimes lost in large amounts, particularly if the patient has peritonitis. Intravenous replacement is necessary in some patients [39, 341].

Adverse cardiovascular effects are rarely associated with peritoneal dialysis, but hypotension and arrhythmias have been described. These can be minimized by decreasing the volume of dialysate cycled or slowing the inflow rate, or both [149]. Pulmonary problems with atelectasis and hypostatic pneumonia are more common. Hydrothorax occurs in up to 10 percent of the patients [129, 256]. The most common and often disastrous complication is peritonitis. It is usually easy to recognize as turbidity of the dialysate, which is visually apparent to the personnel performing the dialysis. Earlier detection may be achieved by daily microscopic examination of the dialysate. More than 500 leukocytes per milliliter indicating impending peritonitis [180]. A test strip for leukocytes in the dialysate is also available [65].

Table 52-9. Complications of peritoneal dialysis

Mechanical	Hemorrhage Puncture of intraabdominal organ Leakage Inadequate drainage Dissection of fluid Wound/bowel suture problems Intraperitoneal catheter loss
Metabolic	Hypoglycemia or hyperglycemia Electrolyte abnormalities Fluid imbalance Acid-base problems Protein/amino acid loss
Cardiovascular/pulmonary	Pulmonary edema Hypotension Hypertension Arrhythmia/cardiac arrest Atelectasis Pneumonia Hydrothorax
Infectious complications	Abscess at puncture site Bacterial peritonitis Fungal peritonitis Sterile peritonitis

See also Chap. 106.

Recovery of Renal Function

Patients who require dialysis for acute tubular necrosis have a very rapid clinical course (Fig. 52-12). The median time from initiation of dialysis to recovery of renal function in the survivor is only 12 days, although occasional patients may recover after undergoing dialysis for several months [357]. For patients who die, the median time from the start of dialysis to death is only 5 days. Only four dialyses are usually necessary before the patient either has recovered enough renal function not to need dialysis or has died [205, 206]. At 1 month, 28 percent of the patients have regained renal function, 64 percent have died, and only 8 percent continue to need dialysis. Ultimately, only 1 percent of patients will need chronic dialysis. This outcome appears more common in patients who have acute renal failure secondary to aortic aneurysm [205, 206, 280]. Some have speculated that intermittent hemodialysis, by causing repeated hemodynamic instability, may delay renal recovery, but clinical data in support of this possibility are lacking [75].

Thus, two thirds of patients with severe acute tubular necrosis die and one third survive. Of the survivors, two thirds will have return of normal renal function, approximately 25 percent will have moderate renal insufficiency (creatinine 1.5–3 mg/dl), approximately 10 percent will be left with severe chronic renal failure (creatinine > 3 mg/dl), and 5 percent of the survivors (1% of all initiated on dialysis) will need continued chronic dialysis [205, 206, 280].

One month after the last dialysis, maximal renal function has occurred [205]. There are, however, anecdotes of recoveries that continue for many months after the last dialysis [47, 50, 101, 128, 138, 157, 239, 243, 322]. The recovery phase is usually gradual, but is occasionally accompanied by a period of tubular insufficiency characterized by large fluid and electrolyte losses in urine that

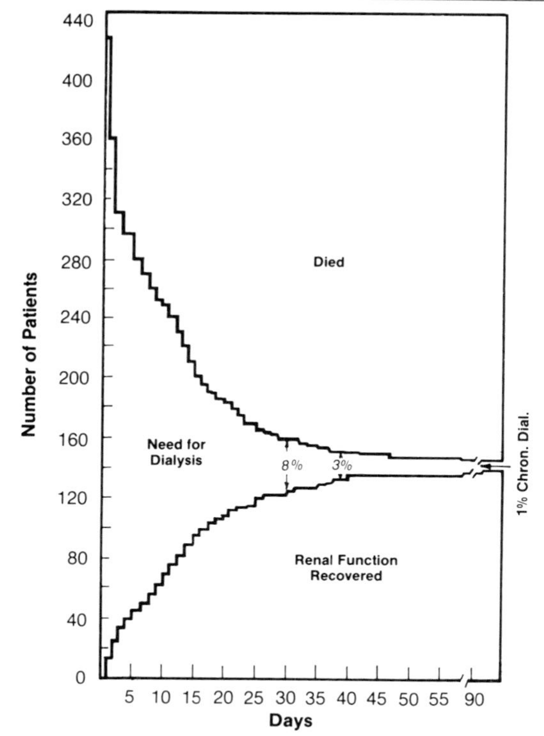

Fig. 52-12. Clinical course of 432 patients with acute tubular necrosis who needed dialysis. The median time for patients who recovered renal function is approximately 12 days, and for those who died, 5 days. By 30 days, 92 percent of the patients had either recovered renal function or died. At 40 days, only 3 percent of the patients remained on dialysis. Ultimately, only 1 percent of the patients started on dialysis (4% of those who survived) needed chronic dialysis. (From [205]. Reproduced with permission of the American Society for Artificial Internal Organs.)

require careful fluid and electrolyte replacement [7, 50, 101, 128, 205, 206].

The maximum renal function regained is independent of the duration of dialysis [128, 206]. The two most important variables are age of the patient and the presence or absence of urinary tract infections [138, 205]. In Figure 52-13 the return of renal function is outlined for 88 survivors of acute tubular necrosis who were known to have had normal renal function before dialysis. Only in patients over the age of 50 years did severe chronic renal failure occur. The effect of urinary tract infections was described by Fuchs and his co-workers, who found less recovery of paraaminohippuric acid and inulin clearances and less ability to concentrate the urine in patients who had severe urinary tract infections during acute renal failure [138].

Conclusions and Summary

Acute renal failure is an uncommon disease, occurring with a frequency of approximately 30 patients per million per year. The most common disease leading to acute renal failure is acute tubular necrosis. It is most often iatrogenic and carries a 50 to 75 percent mortality.

The pathophysiology of acute tubular necrosis remains obscure, but may include four vicious feedback loops: decreased prostaglandins, increased intrarenal release of renin, decreased tubular flow, and intracellular self-perpetuating damaging mechanisms.

The most common cause of death remains infections. Early problems include fluid overload and hyperkalemia.

The differential diagnosis is often easy but may be impossible. Even in the absence of diuretics, chronic renal failure, and obstruction, urinary indices are only moderately helpful in differentiating between prerenal azotemia and acute tubular necrosis. The etiologic treatment

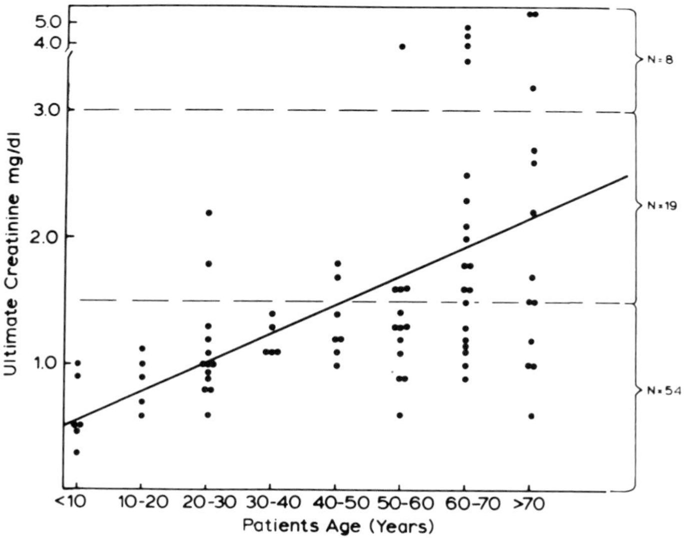

Fig. 52-13. Ultimate serum creatinine versus age of patients who needed dialysis for acute tubular necrosis. There is a direct relationship between ultimate serum creatinine level and age. Severe chronic renal failure occurs only in patients over the age of 50 years. (From [205]. Reproduced with permission of the American Society for Artificial Internal Organs.)

remains empirical and controversial, and includes loop diuretics, mannitol, dopamine, and calcium channel blockers, with trials of atrial natriuretic factor under way.

Symptomatic treatment includes early dialysis in which predialysis BUN should not be allowed to exceed 100 mg/dl during intermittent hemodialysis. If continuous hemofiltration or peritoneal dialysis methods are used, it is probably appropriate to keep the BUN level at 60 mg/dl. Lower blood values of BUN probably do not further increase survival. Symptomatic nondialysis treatment includes early reoperations in postoperative patients and a constant vigilance for infectious complications.

Intermittent hemodialysis, continuous peritoneal dialysis, and continuous hemofiltration/dialysis are the presently used clinical methods for blood purification. The choice of method is probably more technical or institutional than indicated by patient variables.

The clinical course is rapid, with a high percentage of patients dying. Most of the patients who recover renal function have no further clinical complications of renal failure.

References

1. Abel, R. M., Beck, C. H., Abbott, W. M., et al. Improved survival from acute renal failure after treatment with intravenous essential L-amino acids and glucose. *N. Engl. J. Med.* 288: 695, 1973.
2. Abreo, K., Moorthy, V., and Osborne, M. Changing patterns and outcome of acute renal failure requiring hemodialysis. *Arch. Intern. Med.* 146: 1338, 1986.
3. Agar, J. W., Hull, J. D., Kaplan, M., et al. Acute cardiopulmonary decompensation and complement activation during hemodialysis. *Ann. Intern. Med.* 94: 792, 1981.
4. Akmal, M., Goldstein, D. A., Telfer, N., et al. Resolution of muscle calcification in rhabdomyolysis and acute renal failure. *Ann. Intern. Med.* 89: 928, 1978.
5. Aljama, P., Bird, P. A. E., Ward, M. K., et al. Hemodialysis induced leucopenia and activation of complement: effects of different membranes. *Proc. Eur. Dial. Transplant Assoc.* 15: 144, 1978.
6. Allon, M., Dunlay, R., and Copkney, C. Nebulized albuterol for acute hyperkalemia in patients on hemodialysis. *Ann. Intern. Med.* 110: 6, 1989.
7. Alwall, N. *Therapeutic and Diagnostic Problems in Severe Renal Failure.* Copenhagen: Munksgaard, 1963.
8. Anderson, C. C., Shahvari, M. B. G., and Zimmerman, J. E. The treatment of pulmonary edema in the absence of renal function—a role for sorbitol and furosemide. *J.A.M.A.* 241: 1008, 1979.
9. Anderson, R. J., and Schrier, R. W. *Clinical Use of Drugs in Patients with Kidney and Liver Disease.* Philadelphia: Saunders, 1981.
10. Anderson, R. J., Gordon, J. A., Kim, J., et al. Renal concentration or defect following monoliguric acute renal failure in the rat. *Kidney Int.* 21: 583, 1982.
11. Anderson, R. J., Linas, S. L., Berns, A. S., et al. Nonoliguric Acute Renal Failure. *N. Engl. J. Med.* 296: 1134, 1977.
12. Ardaillou, R., Beaufilis, M., Nivers, M.-P., et al. Increased plasma calcitonin in early acute renal failure. *Clin. Sci. Mol. Med.* 49: 301, 1975.
13. Arieff, A. I., and Massry, S. G. Calcium metabolism of brain in acute renal failure. Effects of uremia, hemodialysis and parathyroid hormone. *J. Clin. Invest.* 53: 387, 1974.
14. Arnander, C., Hjelte, M. B., Lins, L. E., et al. Blood compatibility of a hollow-fiber dialyzer with a new coating of covalently bound heparin. *Proc. Eur. Soc. Artificial Organs* 9: 312, 1982.
15. Arnaout, M. D., Hakim, R. M., Todd, R. F., III, et al. Increased expression of an adhesion-promoting surface glycoprotein in the granulocytopenia of hemodialysis. *N. Engl. J. Med.* 312, 1985.
16. Asbach, H. W., Stoeckel, H., Schuler, H. W., et al. The treatment of hypercatabolic acute renal failure by adequate nutrition and haemodialysis. *Acta Anaesthesiol. Scand.* 18: 255, 1974.
17. Atkins, R. C., Scott, D. F., Holdsorth, S. R., et al. Prolonged antibiotic peritoneal lavage in the management of gross generalized peritonitis. *Med. J. Aust.* 1: 954, 1976.
18. Aurigemma, N. M., Feldman, N. T., Gottlieb, M., et al. Arterial oxygenation during hemodialysis. *N. Engl. J. Med.* 297: 871, 1977.
19. Avram, M. M., Pahilan, A., Altman, E., et al. A 15-year experience with intradialytic treatment mortality. *Abstr. Am. Soc. Artif. Organs* 11: 41, 1982.
20. Axelrod, J., Meyers, B. R., Hirschman, S. Z., et al. Prophylaxis with cephalothin in peritoneal dialysis. *Arch. Intern. Med.* 132: 368, 1973.
21. Ayus, J. C., Olivero, J. J., and Adrogue, H. J. Alkalemia associated with renal failure. *Arch. Intern. Med.* 140: 513, 1980.
22. Baek, S. M., Makabali, G. G., Bryan-Brown, C. W., et al. The influence of parenteral nutrition on the course of acute renal failure. *Surg. Gynecol. Obstet.* 141: 405, 1975.
23. Baek, S. M., Makabali, G. G., and Shoemaker, W. C. Clinical determinants of survival from postoperative renal failure. *Surg. Gynecol. Obstet.* 140: 685, 1975.
24. Baek, S. M., Makabali, G. G., and Shoemaker, W. C. Free-water clearance patterns as predictors and therapeutic guides in acute renal failure. *Surgery* 77: 632, 1975.
25. Balsolv, J. T., and Jorgensen, H. E. A survey of 499 patients with acute anuric renal insufficiency: Causes, treatment, complications and mortality. *Am. J. Med.* 34: 753, 1963.
26. Barsoum, R. S., Rihan, Z. E. B., Baligh, O. K., et al. Acute renal failure in the 1973 Middle East War; experience of a specialized base hospital: Effect of the site of injury. *J. Trauma* 20: 303, 1980.
27. Barton, B. R., Hermann, G., and Weil, R., III. Cardiothoracic emergencies associated with subclavian hemodialysis. *J.A.M.A.* 250: 2660, 1983.
28. Beauman, M., Turney, J. H., Rodger, R. S. C., et al. Changing pattern of acute renal failure. *Q. J. Med.* 62: 237, 1987.
29. Belliveau, P., Vas, S., and Himal, H. S. Septic induced acute gastric erosions: the role of cimetidine. *J. Surg. Res.* 24: 264, 1978.
30. Bennett, W. M., Aronoff, G. R., Morrison, G., et al. Drug prescribing in renal failure: Dosing guidelines for adults. *Am. J. Kidney Dis.* 3: 155, 1983.
31. Bennett, W. M., Porter, G. A., Bagby, S. P., et al. *Drugs and Renal Disease.* Edinburgh: Churchill-Livingstone, 1978.
32. Bergström, J., Asaba, H., Fürst, P., et al. Dialysis ultrafiltration and blood pressure. *Proc. Eur. Dial. Transplant Assoc.* 13: 293, 1976.
33. Bessey, P. Q., Watters, J. M., Aoki, T. T., et al. Com-

bined hormone infusion stimulates the metabolic response to injury. *Ann. Surg.* 200: 264, 1984.
34. Bia, M. J., Baggish, D., Katz, L., et al. Computed tomography in the diagnosis of pelvic abscesses in renal transplant patients. *J.A.M.A.* 246: 1435, 1981.
35. Bijaphala, S., Bell, A. J., Bennett, C. A., et al. Comparison of high and low sodium bicarbonate and acetate dialysis in stable chronic hemodialysis patients. *Clin. Nephrol.* 23: 179, 1985.
36. Bivens, B. A., Rogers, E. L., Rapp, R. P., et al. Clinical failure with cimetidine. *Surgery* 88: 417, 1980.
37. Blagg, C. R., and Parson, F. M. Earlier dialysis and anabolic steroids in acute renal failure. *Am. Heart J.* 61: 287, 1961.
38. Bland, R., Shoemaker, W. C., and Shabot, M. M. Physiologic monitoring goals for the critically ill patient. *Surg. Gynecol. Obstet.* 147: 833, 1978.
39. Blumenkrantz, M. J., Gahl, G. M., Kopple, J. D., et al. Protein losses during peritoneal dialysis. *Kidney Int.* 19: 593, 1981.
40. Bock, H. A., Brunne, F. P., et al. Failure of verapamil to protect from ischaemic renal damage. *Nephrology* 57: 299, 1991.
41. Borges, H. F., and Kjellstrand, C. M. The effect of prostaglandin inhibition on the clinical course of chronic hemodialysis. *Nephron* 42: 120, 1986.
42. Borges, H., Hocks, J., and Kjellstrand, C. Mannitol intoxication in patients with renal failure. *Arch. Intern. Med.* 142: 63, 1982.
43. Bosl, R., Shideman, J. R., Meyer, R. M., et al. Effects and complications of high efficiency dialysis. *Nephron* 15: 151, 1975.
44. Brater, D. C. *Drug Use in Renal Disease.* Sydney: Adis Health Science Press, 1983.
45. Brecht, H. M., Ernest, W., and Koch, K. M. Plasma noradrenaline levels in regular hemodialysis patients. *Proc. Eur. Dial. Transplant Assoc.* 12: 281, 1975.
46. Brezis, M., Rosen, S., Silva, P., et al. Renal ischemia: A new perspective. *Kidney Int.* 26: 375, 1984.
47. Briggs, J. D., Kennedy, A. C., Young, L. N., et al. Renal function after acute tubular necrosis. *Br. Med. J.* 3: 513, 1967.
48. Brown, C. B., Ogg, C. S., and Camerons, J. S. High dose furosemide in acute renal failure: A controlled trial. *Clin. Nephrol.* 15: 90, 1981.
49. Brown, R., Babcock, R., Talbert, J., et al. Renal function in critically ill postoperative patients: Sequential assessment of creatinine, osmolar and free water clearance. *Crit. Care Med.* 8: 68, 1980.
50. Bull, G. M., Joekes, A. M., and Lowe, K. G. Renal function studies in acute tubular necrosis. *Clin. Sci.* 8: 379, 1950.
51. Bullock, M. L., Hirata, C. A., Guay, D. R. P., et al. Efficacy of intravenous human immune globulin in patients with acute renal failure. *Abstr. Am. Soc. Nephrol.* 37: 478, 1990.
52. Bullock, M. L., Umen, A. J., Finkelstein, M., et al. The assessment of risk factors in 462 patients with acute renal failure. *Am. J. Kidney Dis.* 5: 97, 1985.
53. Burke, J. P., Garibaldi, R. A., Britt, M. R., et al. Prevention of catheter-associated urinary tract infections. *Am. J. Med.* 70: 655, 1981.
54. Buselmeier, T. J., Najarian, J. S., Simmons, R. L., et al. An A-V shunt for long term hyperalimentation in azotaemic patients. *Proc. Eur. Dial. Transplant Assoc.* 10: 516, 1973.
55. Buselmeier, T. J., Rynasiewicz, J. J., Howard, R. H., et al. Fistulization of shunt vasculature: A unique approach to fistula development. *Br. Med. J.* 2: 933, 1977.
56. Byron, P. R., Mallick, N. P., and Taylor, G. Immune potential in human uraemia. *J. Clin. Pathol.* 29: 770, 1976.
57. Cannella, G., Picotti, G. B., Mioni, G., et al. Blood pressure behaviour during dialysis and ultrafiltration. A pathogenic hypothesis on hemodialysis-induced hypotension. *Int. J. Artif. Organs* 1: 69, 1978.
58. Cantarovich, F., Galli, C., Benedetti, L., et al. High dose furosemide in established acute renal failure. *Br. Med. J.* 4: 449, 1973.
59. Caplan, E. S., and Hoyt, N. Infection surveillance and control in the severely traumatized patient. *Am. J. Med.* 70: 638, 1981.
60. Carpentieri, U., Haggard, M. E., and Lockhart, L. H. Clinical experience in prevention of candidiasis by nystatin in children with acute lymphocytic leukemia. *J. Pediatr.* 92: 593, 1978.
61. Caruana, R. J., and Raja, R. M. Heparin free dialysis: Comparative data and results in high risk patients. *Kidney Int.* 31: 1351, 1987.
62. Casali, R., Simmons, R. L., Najarian, J. S., et al. Acute renal insufficiency complicating major cardiovascular surgery. *Ann. Surg.* 181: 370, 1975.
63. Casati, S., Moia, M., Graziani, G., et al. Hemodialysis without anticoagulants: Efficiency and hemostatic aspects. *Clin. Nephrol.* 21: 102, 1984.
64. Cernacek, P., Spustova, V., and Dzurik, R. Inhibitor(s) of protein synthesis is uremic serum and urine: partial purification and relationship to amino acid transport. *Biochem. Med.* 27: 305, 1982.
65. Chan, L. K., and Oliver, D. O. Simple method for early detection of peritonitis in patients on continuous ambulatory peritoneal dialysis. *Lancet* 2: 1336, 1979.
66. Charlson, M. E., MacKenzie, C. R., et al. Postoperative changes in serum creatinine. *Ann. Surg.* 209: 3, 1989.
67. Chen, W. T., Ing, T. S., Daugirdas, J. T., et al. Hydrostatic ultrafiltration during hemodialysis using decreasing sodium dialysate. *Artif. Organs* 4: 187, 1980.
68. Chisholm, G. D., Charlton, C. A. C., and Orr, W. M. Urine-urea/blood-urea ratios in renal failure. *Lancet* 1: 20, 1966.
69. Chong, B. H., Trew, P., Meng, L., et al. Anuric renal failure due to encasement of the ureters by lymphoma-ureteric obstruction without dilatation. *Aust. N.Z. J. Surg.* 11: 542, 1981.
70. Christou, N. V., and Meakins, J. L. Delayed hypersensitivity in surgical patients: A mechanism for anergy. *Surgery* 86: 78, 1979.
71. Chugh, C., and Kjellstrand, C. M. The changing epidemiology of acute renal failure: Patterns in economically advanced and developing countries. *Int. Yearbook Nephrol.*, 1988. Pp. 207–226.
72. Chugh, K. S., Nath, I. V. S., Ubroi, H. S., et al. Acute renal failure due to non-traumatic rhabdomyolysis. *Postgrad. Med. J.* 55: 386, 1979.
73. Cioffi, W. G., Ashikaga, T., and Gamelli, R. L. Probability of surviving postoperative acute renal failure. *Ann. Surg.* 200: 205, 1984.
74. Clowes, G. H. A., Jr., George, B. C., Villee, C. A., Jr., et al. Muscle proteolysis induced by a circulating peptide in patients with sepsis or trauma. *N. Engl. J. Med.* 308: 545, 1983.
75. Conger, J. D. Does hemodialysis delay recovery from acute renal failure? *Semin. Dial.* 3: 3, 1990.

76. Conger, J. D., and Schrier, R. W. Renal hemodynamics in acute renal failure. *Annu. Rev. Physiol.* 42: 603, 1980.
77. Conger, J. D., Falk, S. A., Yuan, B. H., and Schrier, R. W. Atrial natriuretic peptide and dopamine in a rat model of ischemic acute renal failure. *Kidney Int.* 35: 1126, 1989.
78. Corwin, H. L., and Bonventre, J. V. Factors influencing survival in acute renal failure. Review Articles, *Semin. Dial.* 4: 220, 1989 (CMK 14).
79. Craddock, P. R., Fehr, J., Brigham, K. L., et al. Complement and leukocyte-mediated pulmonary dysfunction in hemodialysis. *N. Engl. J. Med.* 296: 769, 1977.
80. Creagh, F. M., Stone, T., Stephenson, T. P., et al. Retroperitoneal fibrosis with normal intravenous urogram. *Postgrad. Med. J.* 61: 183, 1985.
81. Crossley, K., and Kjellstrand, C. M. Intraperitoneal insulin for control of blood sugar in diabetic patients during peritoneal dialysis. *Br. Med. J.* 1: 269, 1971.
82. Cumming, A. D., Driedger, A. A., McDonald, J. W. D., et al. Vasoactive hormones in the renal response to systemic sepsis. *Am. J. Kidney Dis.* 11: 23, 1988.
83. Czer, L. S. C., and Shoemaker, W. C. Optimal hematocrit value in critically ill postoperative patients. *Surg. Gynecol. Obstet.* 147: 363, 1978.
84. Daly, J. M., Dudrick, S. J., and Copeland, E. M. Intravenous hyperalimentation: Effect on delayed cutaneous hypersensitivity in cancer patients. *Ann. Surg.* 192: 587, 1980.
85. Daugirdas, J. T., Al-Kudsi, R. R., Ing, T. S., et al. A double-blind evaluation of sodium gradient hemodialysis. *Am. J. Nephrol.* 5: 163, 1985.
86. Davidman, M., Olson, P., Kohen, J., et al. Iatrogenic renal disease. *Arch. Intern. Med.* 151: 1809, 1991.
87. DeCamp, M., and Demling, R. H. Posttraumatic multisystem organ failure: Concepts in emergency and critical care. *J.A.M.A.* 260: 530, 1988.
88. DeFremont, J. F., Coevoet, B., Andrejak, M., et al. Effects of antihypertensive drugs on dialysis-resistant hypertension, plasma renin and dopamine betahydroxylase activities, metabolic risk factors and calcium phosphate homeostasis: Comparison of metoprolol, alpha-methyldopa and clonidine in a cross-over trial. *Clin. Nephrol.* 12: 198, 1979.
89. Delaporte, C., and Gros, F. In vitro inhibition of protein synthesis by dialysates of plasma from uremic patients. *Eur. J. Clin. Invest.* 11: 139, 1981.
90. de Torrente, A., Berl, T., Cohn, P. D., et al. Hypercalcemia of acute renal failure: Clinical significance and pathogenesis. *Am. J. Med.* 61: 119, 1976.
91. Dionigi, R., Zonta, A., Dominioni, L., et al. The effects of total parenteral nutrition on immunodepression due to malnutrition. *Ann. Surg.* 185: 467, 1977.
92. Dodd, N. J., O'Donovan, R. M., Bennett-Jones, D. N., et al. Arteriovenous haemofiltration: A recent advance in the management of renal failure. *Br. Med. J.* 287: 1008, 1983.
93. Dumler, F., Grondin, G., and Levin, N. W. Sequential high/low sodium hemodialysis: An alternative to ultrafiltration. *Trans. Am. Soc. Artif. Intern. Organs* 25: 351, 1979.
94. Ebben, J., Streifel, A., Davin, T., et al. A system for adding poorly-soluble ions to dialysate. *Dialysis and Transplantation* 11: 899, 1982.
95. Editorial (anonymous). Antibiotic lavage for peritonitis. *Br. Med. J.* 2: 691, 1979.
96. Editorial (anonymous). Catheter-associated urinary tract infections. *Lancet* 2: 1033, 1978.
97. Editorial (anonymous). Chest physiotherapy under scrutiny. *Lancet* 2: 1241, 1978.
98. Editorial (anonymous). Diagnosing obstruction in renal failure. *Lancet* 2: 848, 1984.
99. Editorial (anonymous). Prevention or cure for stress-induced gastrointestinal bleeding? *Br. Med. J.* 281: 631, 1980.
100. Editorial. Current status of peripheral alimentation. *Ann. Intern. Med.* 95: 114, 1981.
101. Edwards, K. D. G. Recovery of renal function after acute renal failure. *Aust. Ann. Med.* 8: 195, 1959.
102. Eisele, G., and Paganini, E. P. Heparin-free continuous acute renal replacement therapy. *Artif. Organs* 14: 46, 1985.
103. Eiseman, B., Beart, R., and Norton, L. Multiple organ failure. *Surg. Gynecol. Obstet.* 144: 323, 1977.
104. Eisenberg, E., and Gotch, F. A. Normocalcemic hyperparathyroidism culminating in hypercalcemic crisis, treatment with hemodialysis. *Arch. Intern. Med.* 122: 258, 1968.
105. Eisenberg, P. R., Hansbrough, J. R., et al. A prospective study of lung water measurements during patient management in an intensive care unit. *Am. Rev. Respir. Dis.* 136: 662, 1987.
106. Eisenhauer, E. D., Derveloy, R. J., and Hastings, P. R. Prospective evaluation of central venous pressure (CVP) catheters in a large city-county hospital. *Ann. Surg.* 196(5): 560, 1982.
107. Eiser, A. R., Jayamanne, D., Koksong, C., et al. Contrasting alterations in oxygen consumption and respiratory quotient during acetate and bicarbonate hemodialysis. *Abstracts Am. Soc. Nephrol.* 13: 39, 1980.
108. Eliahou, H. E., and Bata, A. The diagnosis of acute renal failure. *Nephron* 2: 287, 1965.
109. Eliahou, H. A., Boichis, H., Bott-Kanner, G., et al. An epidemiologic study of renal failure. II. Acute renal failure. *Am. J. Epidemiol.* 101: 281, 1975.
110. Ellenbogen, P., Scheible, F., and Talner, L. Sensitivity of gray scale ultrasound in detecting urinary tract obstruction. *Am. J. Roentgenol.* 130: 731, 1978.
111. El-Nachef, R. F., Rashed, F., and Ricanati, E. S. Occlusion of the subclavian vein: A complication of indwelling subclavian venous catheters for hemodialysis. *Clin. Nephrol.* 24: 42, 1985.
112. Epstein, M., Schneider, N. S., and Befeler, B. Effect of intrarenal furosemide on renal function and intrarenal hemodynamics in acute renal failure. *Am. J. Med.* 58: 510, 1975.
113. Erben, J., Kvasnicka, J., Bastecky, J., et al. Long-term experience with the technique of subclavian and femoral vein cannulation in hemodialysis. *Artif. Organs* 3: 241, 1979.
114. Espinel, C. H., and Gregory, A. W. Differential diagnosis of acute renal failure. *Clin. Nephrol.* 13: 73, 1980.
115. Ewing, D. J., and Winney, R. Autonomic function in patients with chronic renal failure on intermittent haemodialysis. *Nephron* 15: 424, 1975.
116. Falk, S. A., and Conger, J. D. Effect of atrial natriuretic peptide (ANP) and dopamine in established ARF. *Kidney Int.* 37: 481, 1990.
117. Farrell, P. C., Ward, R. A., Schindhelm, K., et al. Precise anticoagulation for routine hemodialysis. *J. Lab. Clin. Med.* 92: 164, 1978.
118. Fasanella D'Amore, T., Wauters, J. P., Waeber, B., et al. Response of plasma vasopressin to changes in extracellular volume and/or plasma osmolality in patients on maintenance hemodialysis. *Clin. Nephrol.* 23: 299, 1985.
119. Feely, J., Wilkinson, G. R., and Wood, A. J. J. Reduction

of liver blood flow and propranolol metabolism by cimetidine. *N. Engl. J. Med.* 304: 692, 1981.
120. Feig, P. U., and McCurdy, D. K. The hypertonic state. *N. Engl. J. Med.* 294: 1444, 1977.
121. Feinstein, E. I. Parenteral nutrition in acute renal failure. *Am. J. Nephrol.* 5: 145, 1985.
122. Feinstein, E. I., Blumenkrantz, M. J., and Healy, M. Clinical and metabolic response to parenteral nutrition in acute renal failure. A controlled double blind study. *Medicine* 60: 124, 1981.
123. Feinstein, E. I., Akmal, M., Telfer, N., et al. Delayed hypercalcemia with acute renal failure associated with nontraumatic rhabdomyolysis. *Arch. Intern. Med.* 141: 753, 1981.
124. Feldhoff, P., Turnham, T., and Klein, E. Effect of plasma proteins on the sieving spectra of hemofilters. *Artif. Organs* 8: 186, 1984.
125. Ferguson, C. J., and Hillis, A. N. Calcium-channel blockers and other factors influencing delayed function in renal allografts. *Nephrol. Dial. Transplant.* 5: 816, 1990.
126. Fink, M. P., MacVittie, T. J., and Casey, L. C. Effects of nonsteroidal anti-inflammatory drugs on renal function in septic dogs. *J. Surg. Res.* 36: 516, 1984.
127. Finkelstein, W., and Isselbacher, K. J. Cimetidine. *N. Engl. J. Med.* 299: 992, 1978.
128. Finkenstaedt, J. T., and Merrill, J. P. Renal function after recovery from acute renal failure. *N. Engl. J. Med.* 254: 1023, 1956.
129. Finn, R., and Jowett, E. W. Acute hydrothorax complicating peritoneal dialysis. *Br. Med. J.* 2: 94, 1970.
130. Finn, W. F. Diagnosis and management of acute tubular necrosis. *Med. Clin. North Am.* 74: 4, 1990.
131. Fischer, R. P. High mortality of post-traumatic renal insufficiency in Vietnam: A review of 96 cases. *Am. Surg.* 40: 172, 1974.
132. Flanigan, M. J., Von Brech, J., et al. Reducing the hemorrhagic complications of hemodialysis: A controlled comparison of low-dose heparin and citrate anticoagulation. *Am. J. Kidney Dis.* 9: 2, 1987.
133. Fleck, A., Hawker, F., Wallace, P. I., et al. Increased vascular permeability: A major cause of hypoalbuminaemia in disease and injury. *Lancet* 1: 781, 1985.
134. Flugel-Link, R. M., Salusky, I. B., Jones, M. R., et al. Protein and amino acid metabolism in the posterior hemicorpus of acutely uremic rats. *Am. J. Physiol.* 244: 615, 1983.
135. Freund, H., Atamian, S., and Fischer, J. E. Comparative study of parenteral nutrition in renal failure using essential and nonessential amino acid containing solutions. *Surg. Gynecol. Obstet.* 151: 652, 1980.
136. Friedman, E. A., Manis, T., Delano, B. G., et al. Extraordinary safety of hemodialysis. *Abstracts Am. Soc. Artif. Intern. Organs* 11: 48, 1982.
137. Fry, D. E., Pearlstein, L., Fulton, R. L., et al. Multiple system organ failure. *Arch. Surg.* 115: 136, 1980.
138. Fuchs, H. J., Thelen, M., and Wilbrandt, R. Die Nierenfunktion nach akutem Nierenversagen-Eine Langzeitstudie an 70 Patienten (Renal function after acute renal failure—a long term study). *Dtsch. Med. Wochenschr.* 99: 1641, 1974 (in German).
139. Fujiware, Y., Hagihara, B., Yamauchi, A., et al. Hypoxemia and hemodialysis-induced symptomatic hypotension. *Clin. Nephrol.* 24: 9, 1985.
140. Furman, K. I., Gomperts, E. D., and Hockley, J. Activity of intraperitoneal heparin during peritoneal dialysis. *Clin. Nephrol.* 9: 15, 1978.
141. Galler, M., Folkert, V. M., and Schlondorff, D. Reversible acute renal insufficiency and hyperkalemia following indomethacin therapy. *J.A.M.A.* 246: 155, 1981.
142. Gerzof, S. G., Robbins, A. H., Johnson, W. C., et al. Percutaneous catheter drainage of abdominal abscesses. *N. Engl. J. Med.* 305: 653, 1981.
143. Gillum, D. M., Dixon, B. S., Yanover, M. J., et al. The role of intensive dialysis in acute renal failure. *Clin. Nephrol.* 25: 249, 1986.
144. Girotti, M. J., Ruddan, J., and Cohanim, M. Amphojeloma: Antacid impaction in a critically ill patient. *Can. J. Surg.* 271: 379, 1984.
145. Gjorup, S., and Thaysen, J. H. Anabolic steroids in the treatment of uraemia. *Lancet* 2: 886, 1958.
146. Glabman, S., Geronemus, R., von Albertini, B., et al. Clinical trial of maintenance sequential ultrafiltration and dialysis. *Trans. Am. Soc. Artif. Intern. Organs* 25: 394, 1979.
147. Goldblum, S. E., and Reed, W. P. Host defenses and immunologic alterations associated with chronic hemodialysis. *Ann. Intern. Med.* 93: 597, 1980.
148. Gornick, C. C., Jr., and Kjellstrand, C. M. Acute renal failure complicating aortic aneurysm surgery. *Nephron* 35: 145, 1983.
149. Gotloib, L., Mines, M., Garmizo, L., et al. Hemodynamic effects of increasing intraabdominal pressure in peritoneal dialysis. *Peritoneal Dial. Bull.* (Toronto, Can.). 1: 41, 1981.
150. Graham, W. G. B., and Bradley, D. A. Efficacy of chest physiotherapy and intermittent positive-pressure breathing in the resolution of pneumonia. *N. Engl. J. Med.* 299: 624, 1978.
151. Grodstein, G. P., Blumenkrantz, M. J., Kopple, J. D., et al. Glucose absorption during continuous ambulatory peritoneal dialysis. *Kidney Int.* 19: 564, 1981.
152. Gross, M. L., Bush, H., Weinger, R., et al. A comparison of ticlopidine and heparin on hemodialysis in dogs. *J. Lab. Clin. Med.* 100: 887, 1982.
153. Grossman, R. A., Hamilton, R. W., Morse, B. M., et al. Nontraumatic rhabdomyolysis and acute renal failure. *N. Engl. J. Med.* 291: 807, 1974.
154. Gurich, W., Mann, H., Stiller, S., et al. Sodium elimination and alterations of the EEG during dialysis. *Artif. Organs* 3: 15, 1979.
155. Gutman, R. A., Nixon, W. P., McRae, R. L., et al. Effect of intraperitoneal and intravenous vasoactive amines on peritoneal dialysis: Study in anephric dogs. *Trans. Am. Soc. Artif. Intern. Organs* 22: 570, 1976.
156. Hakim, R. M., Breillatt, J., Lazarus, J. M., et al. Complement activation and hypersensitivity reactions to dialysis membranes. *N. Engl. J. Med.* 311: 878, 1984.
157. Hall, J. W., Johnson, W. J., Maher, F. T., et al. Immediate and long-term prognosis in acute renal failure. *Ann. Intern. Med.* 73: 515, 1970.
158. Halter, F. Cimetidin versus Antazida. *Schweiz. Med. Wochenschr* 109: 497, 1979.
159. Hampers, C. L., Blaufox, M. D., and Merrill, J. P. Anticoagulation rebound after hemodialysis. *N. Engl. J. Med.* 275: 776, 1966.
160. Hansbrough, J. F., Narrod, J. A., and Stiegman, G. V. Cardiac perforation and tamponade from a malpositioned subclavian dialysis catheter. *Nephron* 32: 363, 1982.
161. Harrington, J. T., and Cohen, J. J. Measurement of urinary electrolytes; indications and limitations. *N. Engl. J. Med.* 293: 1241, 1975.
162. Hartenbower, D. L., Stella, F. J., Norman, A. W., et al.

Impaired vitamin D Metabolism in acute uremia. *J. Lab. Clin. Med.* 90: 760, 1977.
163. Hastings, P. R., Skillman, J. J., Bushnell, L. S., et al. Antacid titration in the prevention of acute gastrointestinal bleeding: a controlled, randomized trial in 100 critically ill patients. *N. Engl. J. Med.* 298: 1041, 1978.
164. Henderson, I. S., Beattie, T. J., and Kennedy, A. C. Dopamine hydrochloride in oliguric states. *Lancet* 2: 827, 1980.
165. Henderson, L. W., Colton, C. K., and Ford, C. A. Kinetics of hemodiafiltration: II. Clinical characterization of a new blood cleansing modality. *J. Lab. Clin. Med.* 85: 372, 1975.
166. Henny, Ch. P., TenCate, H., TenCate, J. W., et al. A randomized blind study comparing standard heparin and a new low molecular weight heparinoid in cardiopulmonary bypass surgery in dogs. *J. Lab. Clin. Med.* 106: 187, 1985.
167. Henny, Ch. P., TenCate, J. W., van Bronswijk, H., et al. Use of a new heparinoid as anticoagulant during acute haemodialysis of patients with bleeding complications. *Lancet* 1: 890, 1983.
168. Henrich, W. L., Woodard, T. D., Blachley, J. D., et al. Role of osmolality in blood pressure stability after dialysis and ultrafiltration. *Kidney Int.* 18: 480, 1980.
169. Hermreck, A. S., Ruiz-Ocana, F. M., Proberts, K. S., et al. Mechanisms for oliguria in acute renal failure. *Surgery* 82: 141, 1977.
170. Hesdorfe, C. S., Milne, J. F., et al. The value of Swan-Ganz catheterization and volume loading in preventing renal failure in patients undergoing abdominal aneurysmectomy. *Clin. Nephrology* 28: 6, 1987.
171. Hirsch, D. D., Fainstein, V., and Musher, D. M. Do condom catheter collecting systems cause urinary tract infection? *J.A.M.A.* 242: 340, 1979.
172. Hirszel, P., Lasrich, M., and Maher, J. F. Arachidonic acid increases peritoneal clearances. *Trans. Am. Soc. Artif. Intern. Organs* 27: 61, 1981.
173. Hodson, E. M., Kjellstrand, C. M., and Mauer, S. M. Acute renal failure in infants and children: Outcome of 53 patients requiring hemodialysis treatment. *J. Pediatr.* 93: 756, 1978.
174. Höfliger, N., Keusch, G., Baumann, P. C., et al. Die kontinuierliche arterio-venöse Hamofiltration zur Behandlung des akuten Nierenversagens. *Schweiz. Med. Wochenschr.* 115: 242, 1985.
175. Holliday, R. L., and Doris, P. J. Monitoring the critically ill surgical patient. *Can. Med. Assoc. J.* 121: 931, 1979.
176. Hörl, W. H., and Heidland, A. Enhanced proteolytic activity—cause of protein catabolism in acute renal failure. *Am. J. Clin. Nutr.* 33: 1423, 1980.
177. Hörl, W. H., Gantert, C., Auer, L. A., et al. In vitro inhibition of protein catabolism by alpha-2-macroglobulin in plasma from a patient with post-traumatic acute renal failure. *Am. J. Nephrol.* 2: 32, 1982.
178. Hörl, W. H., Stepinski, J., Schaefer, R. M., et al. Role of proteases in hypercatabolic patients with renal failure. *Kidney Int.* 16: 537, 1983.
179. Hou, S. H., Bushinsky, D. A., Wish, J. B., et al. Hospital-Acquired renal insufficiency: A prospective study. *Am. J. Med.* 74: 243, 1983.
180. Hurley, R. M., Muogbo, D., Wilson, G. W., et al. Peritoneal effluent cellularity: Predictor of bacterial peritonitis. *Kidney Int.* 8: 427, 1975.
181. Hylander, B. Survival of extreme hyperkalemia. *Acta Med. Scand.* 221: 121-3, 1987 (CMK 17).
182. Ing, T. S., Daugirdas, J. T., Popli, S., et al. First-use syndrome with cuprammonium cellulose dialyzers. *Int. J. Artif. Organs* 6: 235, 1983.
183. Ing, T. S., Purandri, V. V., Daugirdas, J. T., et al. Slow continuous hemodialysis. *Int. J. Artif. Organs* 7: 53, 1984.
184. Ivanovich, P., Xu, C. G., Kwaan, H. C., et al. Studies of coagulation and platelet functions in heparin-free hemodialysis. *Nephron* 33: 116, 1983.
185. Jaatela, J., Alho, A., Avikainen, V., et al. Plasma catecholamines in severely injured patients: A prospective study on 45 patients with multiple injuries. *Br. J. Surg.* 62: 177, 1975.
186. Janson, P. A., Jubelirer, S. J., Weinstein, M., et al. Treatment of the bleeding tendency in uremia with cryoprecipitate. *N. Engl. J. Med.* 303: 1318, 1980.
187. Jones, E. O., Ward, M. K., Hoenich, N. A., et al. Separation of dialysis and ultrafiltration—does it really help? *Proc. Eur. Dial. Transplant Assoc.* 14: 160, 1977.
188. Jubelirer, S. J. Hemostatic abnormalities in renal disease. *Am. J. Kidney Dis.* 5: 219, 1985.
189. Kaiser, B. A., Potter, D. E., Bryant, R. E., et al. Acid-base changes and acetate metabolism during routine and high-efficiency hemodialysis in children. *Kidney Int.* 19: 70, 1981.
190. Kaplan, A., Longnecker, R. E., and Folkert, V. W. Continuous arteriovenous hemofiltration. *Ann. Intern. Med.* 100: 358, 1984.
191. Kaplow, L. S., and Goffinet, J. A. Profound neutropenia during the early phase of hemodialysis. *J.A.M.A.* 203: 133, 1968.
192. Karatson, A., Juhasz, I., Koves, S., et al. Estimated frequency of acute and chronic renal insufficiencies in a transdanubian region of Hungary. *Int. Urol. Nephrol.* 7: 321, 1975.
193. Kasiske, B. L., and Kjellstrand, C. M. Perioperative management of patients with chronic renal failure and postoperative acute renal failure. *Urol. Clin. North Am.* 10: 35, 1983.
194. Keller, Seemann, J., et al. Risk factors of system clotting in heparin-free haemodialysis. *Nephrol. Dial. Transplant.* 5: 802, 1990.
195. Kennedy, A. C., Burton, J. A., Luke, R. G., et al. Factors affecting the prognosis in acute renal failure. A survey of 251 cases. *Q. J. Med.* 42: 73, 1973.
196. Kersh, E. S., Kronfield, S. J., Unger, A., et al. Autonomic insufficiency in uremia as a cause of hemodialysis-induced hypotension. *N. Engl. J. Med.* 290: 650, 1974.
197. Keshaviah, P., Ilstrup, K., Constantini, E., et al. The influence of ultrafiltration and diffusion on cardiovascular parameters. *Trans. Am. Soc. Artif. Intern. Organs* 26: 328, 1980.
198. Kirkland, K., Edwards, K. D. G., and Whyte, H. M. Oliguric renal failure: A report of 400 cases including classification, survival and response to dialysis. *Aust. Ann. Med.* 14: 275, 1965.
199. Kirkpatrick, C. H., and Alling, D. W. Treatment of chronic oral candidiasis with clotrimazole troches; a controlled clinical trial. *N. Engl. J. Med.* 299: 1201, 1978.
200. Kjellstrand, C. M. Ethacrynic acid in acute tubular necrosis. *Nephron* 9: 337, 1972.
201. Kjellstrand, C. M. Hemodialysis for Children. In E. A. Friedman (ed.), *Strategy in Renal Failure.* New York: Wiley, 1977. P. 149.
202. Kjellstrand, C. M. Can hypotension during dialysis be avoided? *Controv. Nephrol.* 2: 12, 1980.

203. Kjellstrand, C. M. Controversies and issues for future renal substitute therapy: sodium, acetate and bicarbonate. *Jpn. J. Artif. Organs* 12: 732, 1983.
204. Kjellstrand, C. M., and Buselmeier, T. J. A simple method for anticoagulation during pre- and postoperative hemodialysis, avoiding rebound phenomenon. *Surgery* 72: 630, 1972.
205. Kjellstrand, C. M., Ebben, J., and Davin, T. Time of death, recovery of renal function, development of chronic renal failure and need for chronic hemodialysis in patients with acute tubular necrosis. *Trans. Am. Soc. Artif. Intern. Organs* 27: 45, 1981.
206. Kjellstrand, C. M., Gornick, C., and Davin, T. Recovery from acute renal failure. *Clin. Exp. Dial. Apheresis* 5: 143, 1981.
207. Kjellstrand, C. M., Pru, C., and Borges, H. Acetate versus bicarbonate dialysis: A review of biochemical and clinical side effects. *Controv. Nephrol.* 3: 92, 1981.
208. Kjellstrand, C. M., Rosa, A. A., and Shideman, J. R. Hypotension during hemodialysis: osmolality fall is an important pathogenetic factor. *ASAIO J.* 3: 11, 1980.
209. Kjellstrand, C. M., Campbell, D. C., von Hartitzsch, B., et al. Hyperuricemic acute renal failure. *Arch. Intern. Med.* 133: 349, 1974.
210. Kjellstrand, C. M., Davin, T. J., Matas, A. J., et al. Postoperative Acute Renal Failure: Diagnosis, Etiologic and Symptomatic Treatment and Prognosis. In J. S. Najarian, and J. P. Delaney (eds.), *Critical Surgical Care.* New York: Stratton Intercontinental, 1977. P. 309.
211. Kjellstrand, C. M., Evans, R. L., Petersen, R. J., et al. The "unphysiology" of dialysis: A major cause of dialysis side effects? *Kidney Int.* 7: S30, 1975.
212. Kjellstrand, C. M., Mauer, S. M., Buselmeier, T. J., et al. Haemodialysis of premature and newborn babies. *Proc. Eur. Dial. Transplant Assoc.* 10: 349, 1973.
213. Kjellstrand, C. M., Merino, G. E., Mauer, S. M., et al. Complications of percutaneous femoral vein catheterizations for hemodialysis. *Clin. Nephrol.* 4: 37, 1975.
214. Kleinknecht, D., Ganeval, D., Gonzalez-Duque, L. A., et al. Furosemide in acute oliguric renal failure; a controlled trial. *Nephron* 17: 51, 1976.
215. Kleinknecht, D., Junger, P., Chanard, J., et al. Uremic and non-uremic complications in acute renal failure: Evaluation of early and frequent dialysis on prognosis. *Kidney Int.* 1: 190, 1972.
216. Knochel, J. P., and Caskey, J. H. The mechanism of hypophosphatemia in acute heat stroke. *J.A.M.A.* 238: 425, 1977.
217. Koehler, P. R., and Moss, A. A. Diagnosis of intraabdominal and pelvic abscesses by computerized tomography. *J.A.M.A.* 244: 49, 1980.
218. Kohen, J. A., Whitley, K. Y., and Kjellstrand, C. M. Continuous arteriovenous hemofiltration: A comparison with hemodialysis in acute renal failure. *Trans. Am. Soc. Artif. Organs* 31: 169, 1985.
219. Kohen, J. A., Opsahl, J. A., and Kjellstrand, C. M. Deceptive patterns of uremic pulmonary edema. *Am. J. Kidney Dis.* 7: 456, 1986.
220. Kone, B. C., Racusen, L. C., Solez, K., and Whelton, A. Renal morphology and function and urine electrolytes in experimental acute renal failure produced by cyclosporine and ischemia. *Uremia Invest.* 9: 119, 1986.
221. Kopple, J. D., Cianciaruso, B., and Massry, S. G. Does parathyroid hormone cause protein wasting? *Contrib. Nephrol.* 20: 138, 1980.
222. Kopple, J. D., Gordon, S. I., Wang, M., et al. Factors affecting serum and urinary guanidinosuccinic acid levels in normal and uremic subjects. *J. Lab. Clin. Med.* 90: 303, 1977.
223. Korchik, W. P., DeMaster, E. G., and Brown, D. C. Plasma norepinephrine and hemodialysis. *Kidney Int.* 12: 484, 1977.
224. Kornhall, S. Acute renal failure in surgical disease with special regard to neglected complications. *Acute Chir. Scand.* 419: 3, 1971.
225. Kramer, P., Bohler, J., Kehr, A., et al. Intensive care potential of continuous arteriovenous hemofiltration. *Trans. Am. Soc. Artif. Intern. Organs* 28: 28, 1982.
226. Kramer, P., Kaufhold, G., Grone, H. J., et al. Management of anuric intensive-care patients with arteriovenous hemofiltration. *Int. J. Artif. Intern. Organs* 3: 225, 1980.
227. Kramer, P., Wigger, W., Rieger, J., et al. Arteriovenous haemofiltration: A new and simple method for treatment of over-hydrated patients resistant to diuretics. *Klin. Wochenschr.* 55: 1121, 1977.
228. Kristensen, B. O., Skov, J., and Peterslund, N. A. Furosemide-induced increases in serum isoamylases. *Br. Med. J.* 2: 978, 1980.
229. Kron, I. L., Harman, P. K., and Nolan, S. P. The measurement of intra-abdominal pressure as a criterion for abdominal re-exploration. *Am. Surg.* 199: 28, 1984.
230. Ksiqzek, A. Dopamine-beta-hydroxylase activity and catecholamine levels in the plasma of patients with renal failure. *Nephron* 24: 170, 1979.
231. Kumar, R., Hill, C. M., and McGeown, M. G. Acute renal failure in the elderly. *Lancet* 1: 90, 1973.
232. Kurnik, B. R., Weisberg, L. S., et al. Effects of atrial natriuretic peptide versus mannitol on renal blood flow during radiocontrast infusion in chronic renal failure. *J. Lab. Clin. Med.* 116: 1, 1990.
233. Lachhein, L., Kielstein, R., Sauer, K., et al. Evaluation of 433 cases of acute renal failure. *Proc. Eur. Dial. Transplant Assoc.* 14: 628, 1977.
234. Landers, R. G., Lillehei, R. C., Lindsay, W. G., et al. Free-water clearance and the early recognition of acute renal insufficiency after cardiopulmonary bypass. *Ann. Thorac. Surg.* 22: 41, 1976.
235. Lauer, A., Saccaggi, A., Ronco, C., et al. Continuous arteriovenous hemofiltration in the critically ill patient. *Ann. Intern. Med.* 99: 455, 1983.
236. Leithner, C., Sinzinger, H., Stummvoll, H. K., et al. Enhanced 6-OXO-PGF_{1a} levels in plasma during hemodialysis. *Prostaglandins Med.* 5: 425, 1980.
237. Leonard, C. D., Luke, R. G., and Siegel, R. R. Parenteral essential amino acids in acute renal failure. *Urology* 6: 154, 1975.
238. Leski, M., Niethammer, T., and Wyss, T. Glucose-enriched dialysate and tolerance to maintenance hemodialysis. *Nephron* 24: 271, 1979.
239. Levin, M. L., Simon, N. M., Herdson, P. B., et al. Acute renal failure followed by protracted, slowly resolving chronic uremia. *J. Chronic Dis.* 25: 645, 1972.
240. Levine, B. A., Sirinek, K. R., McLeod, C. G., et al. The role of cimetidine in the prevention of stress induced gastric mucosal injury. *Surg. Gynecol. Obstet.* 148: 399, 1979.
241. Levine, J., Falk, B., Henriquez, M., et al. Effects of varying dialysate sodium using large surface area dialyzers. *Trans. Am. Soc. Artif. Intern. Organs* 24: 139, 1978.
242. Levinsky, N. G., Bernard, D. B., and Johnson, P. A. Enhancement of Recovery of Acute Renal Failure: Effect of

Mannitol and Diuretics. In B. Bienner and J. H. Stein (eds.), *Acute Renal Failure*. New York: Churchill Livingstone, 1980. P. 163.
243. Lewers, D. T., Mathew, T. H., Maher, J. F., et al. Long-term follow-up of renal function and histology after acute tubular necrosis. *Ann. Intern. Med.* 73: 523, 1970.
244. Liano, F., Garcia-Martin, F., Gallego, A., et al. Easy and early prognosis in acute tubular necrosis: A forward analysis of 228 cases. *Nephron* 51: 307, 1989.
245. Liboro, R., Schwartz, A. B., et al. Heparin free hemodialysis does not cause fibrin consumptive coagulopathy and maintains alternate pathway complement activation. *Trans. Am. Soc. Artif. Intern. Organs* XXXVI, 1990.
246. Lieberthal, W., and Levinsky, N. G. Treatment of acute tubular necrosis. *Semin. Nephrol.* 10: 6, 1990.
247. Lien, J., and Chan, V. Risk factors influencing survival in acute renal failure treated by hemodialysis. *Arch. Intern. Med.* 145: 2067, 1985.
248. Lindholm, T., Thysell, H., Yamamoto, Y., et al. Temperature and vascular stability in hemodialysis. *Nephron* 39: 130, 1985.
249. Lindner, A. Synergism of dopamine and furosemide in diuretic-resistant, oliguric acute renal failure. *Nephron* 33: 121, 1983.
250. Lindner, A., Cutler, R. E., and Goodman, W. G. Synergism of dopamine plus furosemide in preventing acute renal failure in the dog. *Kidney Int.* 16: 158, 1979.
251. Liu, Y. K., Kosfeld, R. E., and Marcum, S. G. Treatment of uraemic bleeding with conjugated oestrogen. *Lancet* 2: 887, 1984.
252. Livio, M., Marchesi, D., Remuzzi, G., et al. Uraemic bleeding: Role of anemia and beneficial effect of red cell transfusions. *Lancet* 2: 1013, 1982.
253. Ljungberg, B. A low molecular heparin fraction as an anticoagulant during hemodialysis. *Clin. Nephrol.* 24: 15, 1985.
254. Lohr, J. W., McFarlane, M. J., and Grantham, J. J. A clinical index to predict survival in acute renal failure patients requiring dialysis. *Am. J. Kidney Dis.* XI: 254, 1988.
255. Lordon, R. E., and Burton, J. R. Post-traumatic renal failure in military personnel in Southeast Asia: Experience at Clark USAF Hospital, Republic of the Philippines. *Am. J. Med.* 53: 137, 1972.
256. Lorentz, W. B. Acute hydrothorax during peritoneal dialysis. *J. Pediatr.* 94: 417, 1979.
257. Lowder, J. N., Lazarus, H. M., and Herzig, R. H. Bacteremias and fungemias in oncologic patients with central venous catheters. *Arch. Intern. Med.* 142: 1456, 1982.
258. Lucas, C. E. The renal response to acute injury and sepsis. *Surg. Clin. North Am.* 56: 953, 1976.
259. Lucas, C. E., Ledgerwood, A. M., Shier, M. R., et al. The renal factor in the post-traumatic "fluid overload" syndrome. *J. Trauma* 17: 667, 1977.
260. Lundberg, M. Dialysbehandling vid akut njurinsufficiens (Dialysis treatment in acute renal failure). *Lakartidningen* 67: 487, 1970 (in Swedish).
261. Lynch, R. E., Bosl, R. H., Streifel, A. J., et al. Dialysis thrombocytopenia: Parallel plate vs hollow fiber dialyzers. *Trans. Am. Soc. Artif. Intern. Organs* 24: 704, 1978.
262. Maierhofer, W., Maymon, H. L., Woods, M. P., et al. Hypoxemia during hemodialysis: Effects of hourly changes in bath composition. *Am. Soc. Nephrol.* 14: 46A, 1981.
263. Malis, C. D., Racusen, L. C., Solez, K., and Whelton, A. Nephrotoxicity of lysine and of a single dose of aminoglycoside in lysine-treated rats. *J. Lab. Clin. Med.* 103: 660, 1984.
264. Mandell, I. N., Ahern, M. J., Kliger, A. S., et al. Candida peritonitis complicating peritoneal dialysis: successful treatment with low dose amphotericin B therapy. *Clin. Nephrol.* 6: 492, 1976.
265. Mannucci, P. M., Remuzzi, G., Pusineri, F., et al. Deamino-8-o-arginine vasopressin shortens the bleeding time in uremia. *N. Engl. J. Med.* 308: 8, 1983.
266. Marshall, V. C. Acute renal failure in surgical patients. *Br. J. Surg.* 58: 17, 1971.
267. Marshall, V. Secondary surgical intervention in acute renal failure. *Aust. N.Z. J. Surg.* 44: 96, 1974.
268. Martin, L. F., Staloch, D. K., Simonowitz, D. A., et al. Failure of cimetidine prophylaxis in the critically ill. *Arch. Surg.* 114: 492, 1979.
269. Martin-Malo, A., Perez, R., Gomez, J., et al. Sequential hypertonic dialysis. *Nephron* 40: 458, 1985.
270. Marty, A. T. Hyperoncotic albumin therapy. *Surg. Gynecol. Obstet.* 139: 105, 1974.
271. Matas, A. J., Payne, W. D., Simmons, R. L., et al. Acute renal failure following blunt civilian trauma. *Ann. Surg.* 185: 301, 1977.
272. Mathew, O. P., Jones, A. S., James, E., et al. Neonatal renal failure: usefulness of diagnostic indices. *Pediatrics* 65: 57, 1980.
273. Mault, J. R., Dechert, R. E., Bartlett, R. H., et al. Oxygen consumption during hemodialysis for acute renal failure. *Trans. Am. Soc. Artif. Intern. Organs* 28: 510, 1982.
274. Mault, J. R., Kresowik, T. F., Dechert, R. E., et al. Continuous arteriovenous hemofiltration: The answer to starvation in acute renal failure. *Trans. Am. Soc. Artif. Intern. Organs* 30: 203, 1984.
275. McMurray, S. D., Luft, F. C., Maxwell, D. R., et al. Acute tubular necrosis; a multifactorial analysis of variables. *Proc. Clin. Dial. Transplant Forum* 6: 110, 1976.
276. McMurray, S. D., Luft, F. C., Maxwell, D. R., et al. Prevailing patterns and predictor variables in patients with acute tubular necrosis. *Arch. Intern. Med.* 138: 950, 1978.
277. Mehta, R. L., McDonald, B. R., et al. Regional citrate anticoagulation for continuous arteriovenous hemodialysis in critically ill patients. *Kidney Int.* 38: 976, 1990.
278. Mentzer, S. J., Fryd, D. S., and Kjellstrand, C. M. Why do patients with postsurgical acute tubular necrosis die? *Arch. Surg.* 120: 907, 1985.
279. Merino, G. E., Buselmeier, T. J., and Kjellstrand, C. M. Postoperative chronic renal failure: a new syndrome? *Ann. Surg.* 182: 37, 1975.
280. Michael, L., March, H. M., McMichan, J. C., et al. Infection of pulmonary artery catheters in critically ill patients. *J.A.M.A.* 245: 1032, 1981.
281. Michel, L., Serrano, A., and Malt, R. A. Nutritional support of hospitalized patients. *N. Engl. J. Med.* 304: 1147, 1981.
282. Miller, P. D., Krebs, R. A., Neal, B. J., et al. Polyuric prerenal failure. *Arch. Intern. Med.* 140: 907, 1980.
283. Miller, T. R., Anderson, R. J., Linas, S. L., et al. Urinary diagnostic indices in acute renal failure. *Ann. Intern. Med.* 88: 47, 1978.
284. Mitch, W. E. Amino acid release from the hindquarter and urea appearance in acute ureamia. *Am. J. Physiol.* 241: 415, 1981.
285. Montoliu, J., Lens, X. M., and Revert, L. Potassium-lowering of albuterol for hyperkalemia in renal failure. *Arch. Intern. Med.* 147: 713, 1987.
286. Moore, R. D., Smith, C. R., and Lietman, P. S. The association of aminoglycoside plasma levels with mortality in patients with gram-negative bacteremia. *J. Infect. Dis.* 149: 443, 1984.
287. Mullen, J. L., Buzby, G. P., Matthews, D. C., et al. Re-

duction of operative morbidity and mortality by combined preoperative and postoperative nutritional support. *Ann. Surg.* 192: 604, 1980.

288. Mustonen, J., Pasternack, A., Helin, H., et al. Renal biopsy in acute renal failure. *Am. J. Nephrol.* 4: 27, 1984.
289. Myers, B. D., Carrie, B. J., Yee, R. R., et al. Pathophysiology of hemodynamically mediated acute renal failure in man. *Kidney Int.* 18: 495, 1980.
290. Nauseef, W. M., and Maki, D. G. A study of the value of simple protective isolation in patients with granulocytopenia. *N. Engl. J. Med.* 304: 448, 1981.
291. Neiberger, R. E., and Passmore, J. C. Effects of dopamine on canine intrarenal blood flow distribution during hemorrhage. *Kidney Int.* 15: 219, 1979.
292. Neumayer, H. H., Blossei, N., et al. Amelioration of postischaemic acute renal failure in conscious dogs by human atrial natriuretic peptide. *Nephrol. Dial. Transplant.* 5: 32, 1990.
293. Neumayer, H. H., Junge, W., et al. Prevention of radiocontrast-media–induced nephrotoxicity by the calcium channel blocker nitrendipine: A prospective randomised clinical trial. *Nephrol. Dial. Tras.* 4: 1030, 1989.
294. Nichols, T. W. Phytobezoar formation. A new complication of cimetidine therapy. *Ann. Intern. Med.* 95: 70, 1981.
295. Nielsen, O. J., and Thaysen, J. H. Erythropoietin deficiency in acute tubular necrosis. *J. Int. Med. Res.* 227: 373, 1990.
296. Nies, A. S., Robertson, D., and Stone, W. J. Hemodialysis hypotension is not the result of uremic peripheral autonomic neuropathy. *J. Lab. Clin. Med.* 94: 395, 1979.
297. Nolph, K. D., Ghods, A. J., Van Stone, J., et al. The effects of intraperitoneal vasodilators on peritoneal clearances. *Trans. Am. Soc. Artif. Intern. Organs* 22: 586, 1976.
298. Nonclerq, D., Toubeau, G., et al. Redistribution of epidermal growth factor immunoreactivity in renal tissue after nephrotoxin-induced tubular injury. *Nephron* 57: 210, 1991.
299. Nord, E., and Danovitch, G. M. Vasopressin response in hemodialysis patients. *Kidney Int.* 16: 234, 1979.
300. Nordstrom, H., Lennquist, S., Lindell, B., et al. Hypophosphataemia in severe burns. *Acta Chir. Scand.* 143: 395, 1977.
301. O'Brien, T. F., Baxter, C. R., and Teschan, P. E. Prophylactic daily hemodialysis. *Trans. Am. Soc. Artif. Intern. Organs* 5: 77, 1959.
302. Oh, M. S., Uribarri, J. V., DelMonte, M. L., et al. Consumption of CO_2 in metabolism of acetate as an explanation for hypoventilation and hypoxemia during hemodialysis. *Abstracts Am. Soc. Nephrol.* 13: 125, 1980.
303. Oken, D. E., Sprinke, F. M., Kirschbaum, B. B., et al. Amino acid therapy in the treatment of experimental acute renal failure in the rat. *Kidney Int.* 17: 14, 1980.
304. Olbricht, C., Mueller, C., and Schurek, H. J. Treatment of acute renal failure in patients with multiple organ failure by continuous spontaneous hemofiltration. *Trans. Am. Soc. Artif. Intern. Organs* 28: 33, 1982.
305. Older, R. A., Van Moore, A., Foster, W. L., et al. Urinary tract obstruction, current methods of evaluation. *J.A.M.A.* 245: 1854, 1981.
306. Osias, M. B., Siegel, N. J., Chaudry, I. H., et al. Postischemic renal failure, accelerated recovery with adenosine triphosphate-magnesium chloride infusion. *Arch. Surg.* 112: 729, 1977.
307. Paganini, E. P., Fouad, F., Tarazi, R. C., et al. Hemodynamics of isolated ultrafiltration in chronic hemodialysis patients. *Trans. Am. Soc. Artif. Intern. Organs* 25: 422, 1979.
308. Paller, M. S. Free radical scavengers in mercuric chloride-induced acute renal failure in the rat. *J. Lab. Clin. Med.* 105: 459, 1985.
309. Paller, M. S., Hoidal, J. R., and Ferris, T. F. Oxygen free radicals in ischemic acute renal failure in the rat. *J. Clin. Invest.* 74: 1156, 1974.
310. Pascual, J., Orofino, L., Liano, F., et al. Incidence and prognosis of acute renal failure in older patients. *J.A.G.S.* 38: 25, 1990.
311. Patel, R., Tanaka, T., Mishkin, F., et al. Gallium-67 scan: Aid to diagnosis and treatment of renal and perirenal infections. *Urology* 16: 225, 1980.
312. Peloso, O. A., Floyd, V. T., and Wilkinson, L. H. Treatment of peritonitis with continuous postoperative peritoneal lavage using cephalothin. *Am. J. Surg.* 126: 742, 1973.
313. Peresecenschi, G., Blum, M., Aviram, A., et al. Impaired neutrophil response to acute bacterial infection in dialyzed patients. *Arch. Intern. Med.* 141: 1301, 1981.
314. Pfister, R., and Newhouse, J. Interventional percutaneous pyeloureteral techniques: Antegrade pyelography and ureteral perfusion. *Radiol. Clin. North Am.* 17: 314, 1979.
315. Pierides, A. M., Kurtz, S. B., and Johnson, W. J. Ultrafiltration followed by hemodialysis. A long-term trial and acute studies. *J. Dial.* 2: 325, 1978.
316. Pinnick, R. V., Wiegmann, T. B., and Diederich, D. A. Regional citrate anticoagulation for hemodialysis in the patient at high risk for bleeding. *N. Engl. J. Med.* 308: 258, 1983.
317. Plough, A. L., and Salem, S. Social and contextual factors in the analysis of mortality in end-stage renal disease patients: Implications for health policy. *Am. J. Public Health* 72: 1293, 1982.
318. Polk, H. C., Jr., and Shields, C. L. Remote organ failure: A valid sign of occult intra-abdominal infection. *Surgery* 81: 310, 1977.
319. Porter, G. A., and Bennett, W. M. Nephrotoxin-Induced Acute Renal Failure. In B. M. Brenner and J. H. Stein (eds.), *Acute Renal Failure.* New York: Churchill-Livingstone, 1980.
320. Posen, G. A., and Luiselto, J. Continuous equilibration peritoneal dialysis in the treatment of acute renal failure. *Peritoneal Dial. Bull.* 1: 6, 1980.
321. Preuschof, L., Keller, F., et al. Heparin-free hemodialysis with prophylactic change of dialyser and blood lines. *Int. J. Artif. Organs* 11: 4, 1988.
322. Price, J. D. E., and Palmer, R. A. A functional and morphological follow-up study of acute renal failure. *Arch. Intern. Med.* 105: 90, 1960.
323. Priebe, H. J., Skillman, J. J., Bushnell, L. S., et al. Antacid versus cimetidine in preventing acute gastrointestinal bleeding; a randomized trial in 75 critically ill patients. *N. Engl. J. Med.* 302: 426, 1980.
324. Pru, C., and Kjellstrand, C. M. On the clinical usefulness of the "FE_{Na}" test in acute renal failure: A critical analysis. *Proc. Clin. Dial. Transplant Forum* 10: 240, 1980.
325. Pru, C., and Kjellstrand, C. M. The FE_{Na} test is of no prognostic value in acute renal failure. *Nephron* 36: 20, 1984.
326. Pru, C., and Kjellstrand, C. M. Indices and urinary chemistries in the differential diagnosis of pre-renal failure and acute tubular necrosis. *Semin. Nephrol.* 5: 224, 1985.

327. Quick, C. A., and Hoppe, W. Permanent deafness associated with furosemide administration. *Ann. Otol. Rhinol. Laryngol.* 84: 94, 1975.
328. Racusen, L. C., Finn, W. F., Whelton, A., and Solez, K. Mechanism of lysine-induced nephrotoxicity in rats. *Kidney Int.* 27: 517, 1985.
329. Raja, R. M., Henriquez, M., Kramer, M. S., et al. Improved dialysis tolerance using Redy sorbent system with bicarbonate dialysate in critically ill patients. *Dial. Transplant* 8: 241, 1979.
330. Rascoff, J. H., Golden, R. A., Spinowitz, B. S., et al. Nondilated obstructive nephropathy. *Arch. Intern. Med.* 143: 696, 1983.
331. Rasmussen, H. H., and Lloyd, S. I. Acute renal failure. *Am. J. Med.* 73: 211, 1982.
332. Rasmussen, H. H., Pitt, E. A., Ibels, L. S., and McNeil, D. R. Prediction of outcome in acute renal failure by discriminant analysis of clinical variables. *Arch. Intern. Med.* 145: 2015, 1985.
333. Ratcliffe, P. J., and Richardson, A. J. Effect of intravenous infusion of atriopeptin 3 on immediate renal allograft function. *Kidney Int.* 39: 164, 1991.
334. Remuzzi, G., Marchesi, D., Cavenaghi, A. E., et al. Bleeding in renal failure: A possible role of vascular prostacyclin (PGI_2). *Clin. Nephrol.* 12: 127, 1979.
335. Reubi, F. C. The pathogenesis of anuria following shock. *Kidney Int.* 5: 106, 1974.
336. Rodrigo, F., Shideman, J., McHugh, R., et al. Osmolality changes during hemodialysis. Natural history, clinical correlations, and influence of dialysate glucose and intravenous mannitol. *Ann. Intern. Med.* 86: 554, 1977.
337. Rosa, A. A., Fryd, D. S., and Kjellstrand, C. M. Dialysis symptoms and stabilization in long-term dialysis, practical application of the CUSUM plot. *Arch. Intern. Med.* 140: 804, 1980.
338. Rosa, A. A., Shideman, J., McHugh, R., et al. The importance of osmolality fall and ultrafiltration rate on hemodialysis side effects. *Nephron* 27: 134, 1981.
339. Rowley, K. M., Clubb, K. S., Walker Smith, G. J., et al. Right-sided infective endocarditis as a consequence of flow-directed pulmonary-artery catheterization. *N. Engl. J. Med.* 311: 1152, 1984.
340. Roxe, D. M., Argy, W. P., Frost, B., et al. Complications of peritoneal dialysis. *South Med. J.* 69: 584, 1976.
341. Rubin, J., McFarland, S., Hellems, E. W., et al. Peritoneal dialysis during peritonitis. *Kidney Int.* 19: 460, 1981.
342. Rubin, J., Oreopoulos, D. G., Lio, T. T., et al. Management of peritonitis and bowel perforation during chronic peritoneal dialysis. *Nephron* 16: 220, 1976.
343. Rubin, R. H., Fischman, A. J., et al. In-labeled nonspecific immunoglobulin scanning in the detection of focal infection. *N. Engl. J. Med.* 321: 14, 1989.
344. Salmon, R., Aubert, P. H., David, R., et al. Aluminum gel causing large-bowel perforation. *Lancet* 1: 875, 1978.
345. Sargent, J. A., and Gotch, F. A. Nutrition and treatment of the acutely ill patient using urea kinetics. *Dial. Transplant* 10: 314, 1981.
346. Schrier, R. W., Klahr, S. The future of nephrology. *Am. J. Kidney Dis.* 16: 590, 1990.
347. Schrier, R. W., Arnold, P., and Burke, T. The calcium ion and calcium channel blockers in ischemic acute renal failure (ARF). *Trans. Am. Soc. Artif. Intern. Organs* 30: 707, 1984.
348. Schrier, R. W., Berl, T., and Anderson, R. J. Osmotic and nonosmotic control of vasopressin release. *Am. J. Physiol.* 236: F321, 1979.
349. Schultze, G., Maiga, M., Neumayer, H., et al. Prostaglandin E promotes hypotension on low-sodium hemodialysis. *Nephron* 37: 250, 1984.
350. Scriabine, A., Anderson, C. L., Janis, R. A., et al. Some recent pharmacological findings with nitrendipine. *J. Cardiovasc. Pharmacol.* 7: S937, 1984.
351. Shaldon, S., Beau, M. C., Deschodt, G., et al. Vascular stability during hemofiltration. *Trans. Am. Soc. Artif. Intern. Organs* 26: 391, 1980.
352. Shapiro, W. B., Faubert, P. F., Porush, J. G., et al. Low-dose heparin in routine hemodialysis monitored by activated partial thromboplastin time. *Artif. Organs* 3: 73, 1979.
353. Shear, L., Shinaberger, J. H., and Barry, K. G. Peritoneal transport of antibiotics in man. *N. Engl. J. Med.* 272: 666, 1964.
354. Sherertz, R. J., Falk, R. J., Huffman, K. A., et al. Infections associated with subclavian uldall catheters. *Arch. Intern. Med.* 143: 52, 1983.
355. Shin, B., Isenhower, N. N., McAslan, T. C., et al. Early recognition of renal insufficiency in postanesthetic trauma victims. *Anesthesiology* 50: 262, 1979.
356. Siegel, N. J., Glazier, W. B., Chaudry, I. H., et al. Enhanced recovery from acute renal failure by the postischemic infusion of adenine nucleotides and magnesium chloride in rats. *Kidney Int.* 17: 338, 1980.
357. Siegler, R. L., and Bloomer, H. A. Acute renal failure with prolonged oliguria; an account of five cases. *J.A.M.A.* 225: 133, 1973.
358. Sigler, M. H., Teehan, B. P., et al. Solute transport in continuous hemodialysis: A new treatment for acute renal failure. *Kidney Int.* 32: 562, 1987.
359. Silverstein, M. E., Ford, C. A., Lysaght, M. T., et al. Treatment of severe fluid overload by ultrafiltration. *N. Engl. J. Med.* 291: 747, 1974.
360. Simkin, E. P., and Wright, F. K. Perforating injuries of the bowel complicating peritoneal catheter insertion. *Lancet* 1: 64, 1968.
361. Sipkins, J. H., and Kjellstrand, C. M. Severe head trauma and acute renal failure. *Nephron* 28: 36, 1981.
362. Skillman, J. J., and Silen, W. Stress ulceration in the acutely ill. *Annu. Rev. Med.* 27: 9, 1976.
363. Skröder, R., Jacobson, S. H., Lins, L. E., and Kjellstrand, C. M. Biocompatibility of dialysis membranes is of no importance for objective or subjective symptoms during or after hemodialysis. *Trans. ASAIO* 36: 637, 1990.
364. Slade, M. S., Simmons, R. L., Yunis, E., et al. Immunodepression after major surgery in normal patients. *Surgery* 78: 363, 1975.
365. Smith, J. H., Merrell, R. C., and Raffin, T. A. Reversal of postoperative anuria by decompressive celiotomy. *Arch. Intern. Med.* 145: 553, 1985.
366. Smithies, M. N., and Cameron, J. S. Can we predict outcome in acute renal failure? *Nephron* 51: 297, 1989.
367. Smolens, P., and Stein, J. H. Pathophysiology of acute renal failure. *Am. J. Med.* 70: 479, 1981.
368. Solez, K. Amino acids in acute renal failure, the controversy between the experimental and clinical data. *Trans. Am. Soc. Artif. Intern. Organs* 30: 704, 1984.
369. Solez, K. Renal Interstitial, Glomerular, and Vascular Causes of Acute Renal Failure. In H. R. Jacobson, G. E. Striker, and S. Klahr (eds.), *The Principles and Practice of Nephrology.* Philadelphia: Decker, 1991.
370. Solez, K., and Racusen, L. C. Acute Renal Failure at a Crossroads. In D. Bihari and G. Neild (eds.), *Acute Renal Failure in the Intensive Therapy Unit.* New York: Springer-Verlag, 1990.
371. Solez, K., Morel-Maroger, L., and Sraer, J. D. The mor-

phology of "acute tubular necrosis" in man: Analysis of 57 renal biopsies and a comparison with the glycerol model. *Medicine* 58: 362, 1979.

372. Solez, K., Altman, J., Rienhoff, H. Y., et al. Early angiographic and renal blood flow changes after $HgCl_2$ or glycerol administration. *Kidney Int.* 10: 6, 153, 1976.
373. Steiner, R. W. Continuous equilibration peritoneal dialysis in acute renal failure (editorial). *Perit. Dial. Int.* 9: 1, 1989.
374. Stone, W. J., and Knepshield, J. H. Post-traumatic acute renal insufficiency in Vietnam. *Clin. Nephrol.* 2: 186, 1974.
375. Storck, M., Hartl, W. H., et al. Comparison of pump-driven and spontaneous continuous haemofiltration in postoperative acute renal failure. *Lancet* 337: 452, 1991.
376. Sumpio, B. E., Chaudry, I. H., and Baue, A. E. Reduction of the drug-induced nephrotoxicity by ATP-MgCl2. 1. Effects on the cis-diamminedichloroplatinum-treated isolated perfused kidneys. *J. Surg. Res.* 38: 429, 1985.
377. Swartz, R. D., and Port, F. K. Preventing hemorrhage in high-risk hemodialysis: Regional versus low-dose heparin. *Kidney Int.* 16: 513, 1979.
378. Taenaka, O., Shimada, Y., Hirata, T., et al. New approach to regional anticoagulation in hemodialysis using gabexate mesilate (FOY). *Crit. Care Med.* 10: 773, 1982.
379. Tapson, J. S., and Uldall, P. R. Delayed onset of hemothorax: An unusual complication of subclavian access for hemodialysis. *Nephron* 40: 495, 1985.
380. Tery, R. B., and Turner, M. D. Effect of acute hemorrhage on gastrin secretion rate and blood levels of gastrin and insulin in normal dogs and in dogs after vagotomy. *Surg. Gynecol. Obstet.* 142: 353, 1976.
381. Thayssen, P., and Pindborg, T. Peritoneal dialysis and heparin. *Scand. J. Urol. Nephrol.* 12: 73, 1978.
382. Toback, F. G. Amino acid enhancement of renal regeneration after acute tubular necrosis. *Kidney Int.* 12: 193, 1977.
383. Toback, F. G., Dodd, R. C., Mayer, E. R., et al. Amino acid administration enhances renal protein metabolism after acute tubular necrosis. *Nephron* 33: 238, 1983.
384. Tollhurst-Cleaver, C. L., Hopkins, A. D., and Kee Kwong, K. C. N. The effect of post-operative peritoneal lavage on survival, peritoneal wound healing and adhesion formation following fecal peritonitis: an experimental study in the rat. *Br. J. Surg.* 61: 601, 1974.
385. Tryba, M. Risk of acute stress bleeding and nosocomial pneumonia in ventilated intensive care unit patients: Sucralfate versus antacids. *Am. J. Med.* 83: 3B, 1987.
386. Turck, M., and Stamm, W. Nosocomial infection of the urinary tract. *Am. J. Med.* 70: 651, 1981.
387. Turney, J. H., Williams, L. C., Fewell, M. R., et al. Platelet protection and heparin sparing with prostacyclin during regular dialysis therapy. *Lancet* 2: 219, 1980.
388. Twardowski, Z. J. Peritoneal dialysis. Current technology and techniques. *Postgrad. Med.* 85: 5, 1985.
389. Tzamaloukas, A. H., Garella, S., and Chazan, J. A. Peritoneal dialysis for acute renal failure after major abdominal surgery. *Arch. Surg.* 106: 639, 1973.
390. Vaamonde, C. A., Michael, U. F., Metzger, R. A., et al. Complications of acute peritoneal dialysis. *J. Chronic Dis.* 28: 637, 1975.
391. Van Der Mere, W., and Collins, J. F. Acute renal failure in a critical care unit. N.Z. *Med. J.* 102: 96, 1989.
392. VanSonnenberg, E., Ferrucci, J. T., Jr., Mueller, P. R., et al. Percutaneous drainage of abscesses and fluid collections: Technique, results, and applications. *Radiology* 142: 1, 1982.
393. Van Stone, J. C., Carey, J., Meyer, R., et al. Hemodialysis with glycerol containing dialysate. *ASAIO J.* 2: 119, 1979.
394. Vaughan, G. Acute renal failure. *Br. Med. J.* 1: 1333, 1980.
395. Vaz, A. J. Subclavian vein single-needle dialysis in acute renal failure following vascular surgery. *Nephron* 25: 102, 1980.
396. Vaziri, N. D., Ness, R., Wellikson, L., et al. Bicarbonate-buffered peritoneal dialysis an effective adjunct in the treatment of lactic acidosis. *Am. J. Med.* 67: 392, 1979.
397. Vaziri, N. D., Toohey, J., Paule, P., et al. Effect of hemodialysis on contact group of coagulation factors, platelets, and leukocytes. *Am. J. Med.* 77: 437, 1984.
398. Vicks, S. L., Gross, M. L., and Schmitt, G. W. Massive hemorrhage due to hemodialysis-associated thrombocytopenia. *Am. J. Nephrol.* 3: 30, 1983.
399. Von Brecht, J. H., Flanigan, M. J., et al. Regional anticoagulation: Hemodialysis with hypertonic trisodium citrate. *Am. J. Kidney Dis.* 8: 3, 1986.
400. Wagner, K., Albrech, S., and Neumayer, H. H. Prevention of delayed graft function in cadaveric kidney transplantation by a calcium antagonist. Preliminary results of two prospective randomized trials. *Transplant. Proc.* XVIII: 3, 1986.
401. Walker, J. F., Lindsay, R. M., Sibbald, W. J., et al. Acute renal failure produced by non-hypotensive sepsis in a large animal model. *Am. J. Kidney Dis.* 8: 88, 1986.
402. Warren, J. W., Platt, R., Thomas, R. J., et al. Antibiotic irrigation and catheter-associated urinary-tract infections. *N. Engl. J. Med.* 299: 570, 1978.
403. Wathen, R., Keshaviah, P., Hommeyer, P., et al. Role of dialysate glucose in preventing gluconeogenesis during hemodialysis. *Trans. Am. Soc. Artif. Intern. Organs* 23: 393, 1977.
404. Watkinson, G. E. Chasing the bucket. A nurses view of continuous arteriovenous hemofiltration/dialysis. *J. Roy. Nav. Med. Serv.* 75: 13, 1990.
405. Weddington, W. W., Muelling, A. E., Moosa, H. H., et al. Cimetidine toxic reactions masquerading as delirium tremens. *J.A.M.A.* 245: 1058, 1981.
406. Wehle, B., Asaba, H., Castenfors, J., et al. The influence of dialysis fluid composition on the blood pressure response during dialysis. *Clin. Nephrol.* 12: 62, 1978.
407. Weinstein, R. S., and Hudson, J. B. Parathyroid hormone and 25-hydroxycholecalciferol levels in hypercalcemia of acute renal failure. *Arch. Intern. Med.* 140: 410, 1980.
408. Welch, J. P., Schweizer, R. T., and Bartus, S. A. Management of antacid impactions in hemodialysis and renal transplant patients. *Am. J. Surg.* 139: 561, 1980.
409. Wheeler, D. C., Feehally, J., and Walls, J. High risk acute renal failure. *Q. J. Med.* 61: 234, 977, 1986.
410. White, F. A., Clark, R. B., and Thompson, D. S. Preoperative oral antacid therapy for patients requiring emergency surgery. *South Med. J.* 71: 177, 1978.
411. Wickham, J. E. A., Fernando, A. R., Hendry, W. F., et al. Inosine in preserving renal function during ischaemic renal surgery. *Br. Med. J.* 2: 173, 1978.
412. Wiegand, C. F., Davin, T. D., Raij, L., et al. Severe hypokalemia induced by hemodialysis. *Arch. Intern. Med.* 141: 167, 1981.
413. Wilson, D. R. Renal function during and following obstruction. *Annu. Rev. Med.* 28: 329, 1977.
414. Wing, A. J., Broyer, M., Brunner, F. P., et al. Combined report on regular dialysis and transplantation in Europe, XIII, 1982. *Proc. Eur. Dial. Transplant Assoc.* 20: 5, 1983.

415. Wolk, P. J., and Apicella, M. A. The effect of renal function on the febrile response to bacteremia. *Arch. Intern. Med.* 138: 1084, 1978.
416. Wootton, F. T., Rhodes, D. F., et al. Colonic necrosis with Kayexalate-sorbitol enemas after renal transplantation. *Ann. Intern. Med.* 1111: 947, 1989.
417. Ylikorkala, O., Huttunen, K., Jarvi, J., et al. Prostacyclin and thromboxane in chronic uremia: effect of hemodialysis. *Clin. Nephrol.* 18: 83, 1982.
418. Zager R. A. A focus of tissue necrosis increases renal susceptibility to gentamicin administration. *Kidney Int.* 33: 84, 1988.
419. Zager, R. A., and Venkatachalam, M. A. Potentiation of ischemic renal injury by amino acid infusion. *Kidney Int.* 24: 620, 1983.
420. Zager, R. A., Sharma, H. M., and Johannes, G. A. Gentamicin increases renal susceptibility to an acute ischemic insult. *J. Lab. Clin. Med.* 101: 670, 1983.
421. Zager, R. A., Johannes, G., Tuttle, S. E., et al. Acute amino acid nephrotoxicity. *J. Lab. Clin. Med.* 101: 130, 1983.
422. Zager, R. A., Rubin, N. T., Ebert, T., et al. Rapid radioimmunoassay for diagnosing acute tubular necrosis. *Nephron* 26: 7, 1980.
423. Zawada, E. T., Bennett, E. P., Stinson, J. B., et al. Serum calcium in blood pressure regulation during hemodialysis. *Arch. Intern. Med.* 141: 657, 1981.
424. Zimmerman, J. E. Respiratory failure complicating posttraumatic acute renal failure: etiology, clinical features and management. *Ann. Surg.* 174: 12, 1971.
425. Zuccelli, P., Catizone, L., Esposti, E. D., et al. Influence of ultrafiltration on plasma renin activity and adrenergic system. *Nephron* 21: 317, 1978.
426. Zusman, R. M., Rubin, R. H., Cato, A. E., et al. Hemodialysis using prostacyclin instead of heparin as the sole antithrombotic agent. *N. Engl. J. Med.* 304: 934, 1981.

IX

Hypertension

Blood Pressure and the Kidney

Hugh E. de Wardener
Graham A. MacGregor

Brief Historical Survey

The notion that hypertension is in some way connected with the kidney was first proposed by Bright in 1836 [21]. He performed postmortem examinations on patients dying with "dropsy and coagulable urine," in whom he stated that there was always "some obvious derangement" in the kidneys. He also noted that the left ventricle was enlarged and the wall hypertrophied, and that in 22 patients out of 100 this hypertrophy was not accompanied by any abnormality of the large arteries. Bright concluded that "this leads us to look for some less local cause for the unusual efforts to which the heart has been impelled; and the two most readily solutions appear to be, either that the altered quality of the blood affords irregular and unwanted stimulus to the organ immediately; or that it so effects the minute and capillary circulation, as to render greater action necessary to force the blood through the distant sub-divisions of the vascular system." At first there was some confusion whether Bright was referring only to the "minute and capillary circulation of the kidney." This was clarified by Johnson in 1868 [90], who drew attention to the fact that all the minute arteries throughout the body were involved. He reported that in patients in whom the kidneys were diseased and the left ventricle was enlarged (i.e., Bright's disease) a Dr. Sanderson had measured the arterial pressure and found it to be raised and that he himself had observed that the walls of the very small arteries of the brain and pia mater, as well as the renal vasculature, were hypertrophied. Like Bright, he thought that this arterial change was due to an abnormality in the blood in that it was "contaminated by urinary excreta and otherwise deteriorated." The generalized nature of the arteriolar and capillary abnormalities in Bright's disease was confirmed by Gull and Sutton [77], who noted that in addition to the arterial hypertrophy there was "hyalinfibroid" formation of the walls of the minute arteries and a "hyalin granular change in the corresponding capillaries."

The next major step forward was that of Mahomed in 1879 [114]. He observed that "it is very common to meet people, apparently in good health, who have no albumin in the urine or any other sign of organic disease, who constantly present a condition of high arterial tension when examined by the aid of the sphygmograph." At postmortem examination he found that in such patients who had not had albuminuria the kidneys, though somewhat contracted, were "red" (i.e., they did not look very abnormal) rather than "yellow" like those who had died with albuminuria and dropsy. The patients without proteinuria had come under treatment for "symptoms of cerebral hemorrhage, heart disease, lung disease and sundry medical and surgical diseases." This is the first description of "primary" or essential hypertension (i.e., hypertension of unknown cause) in contrast to the hypertension associated with renal disease, which is now referred to as *secondary* hypertension (i.e., hypertension due to some obvious cause such as a visible abnormality of the kidney). Mahomed concluded that ". . . high pressure is a constant condition in the circulation of some individuals and that this condition is a symptom of a certain constitution or diathesis. . . . These persons appear to pass through life much as others do and generally do not suffer from their high blood pressures except in their petty ailments upon which it imprints itself . . . as age advances the enemy gains accession of strength . . . the individual has now passed 40 years of age, his lungs begin to deteriorate, he has a cough in the winter time, but by his pulse you will know him. . . . Alternatively headache, vertigo, epistaxis, a passing paralysis, a more severe apoplectic seizure, and then the final blow. . . . Of this I feel sure, that the clinical symptoms and the pathological changes resulting from high arterial pressure are frequently seen in cases in which slight, if any, disease is discoverable in the kidney."

Mahomed was also the first to observe that patients developing acute nephritis following scarlet fever might develop hypertension before the appearance of albumin in the urine [115]. He also observed that acute nephritis could lead to chronic Bright's disease.

These seminal observations were confirmed, elaborated, forgotten, and revived during the next 100 years. The next step forward was Volhard's demonstration in 1931 that primary hypertension could have either a benign or a malignant course [188]. The benign form of hypertension, though accompanied by enlargement of the heart, might remain unchanged for years (as Mahomed had noted), the patient eventually dying of heart failure or a cerebrovascular accident while renal function remained relatively unimpaired throughout. Malignant hypertension was heralded by acute retinal changes and then increasing renal functional deterioration, the patient rapidly dying of renal failure. Volhard considered that benign essential hypertension was due to a primary thickening of the arteriolar walls, which he called elastosis (i.e., full of elastic tissue) and thought was due to the effects of age on a genetic constitution. He thought that malignant hypertension in primary or secondary hypertension was due to the action of a pressor substance released because of renal ischemia, which was due either to severe "elastosis" of the renal arteries or, in nephritis, to the contracting kidney reducing the renal blood flow. He was also the first to suggest that vascular spasm of the renal vasculature produced by the pressor substance released by the kidney could lead to a vicious cycle effect that released more pressor substance. The concept of a circulating pressor substance was due to the work of Tigerstedt and Bergman, who had shown in 1898 [182] that saline extracts of fresh rabbit kidney or of an alcohol dried powder produced a prolonged rise of pressure when injected into lightly anesthetized rabbits with urethane; they had named this substance renin.

Volhard's hypothesis about the origin of malignant

hypertension was gradually supported, first by Goldblatt's observation in 1934 [68] that in dogs renal ischemia, induced by constricting either both renal arteries or only one if the other kidney had been removed, produced persistent hypertension that was due to some substance released from the kidney. It took another 20 years, however (a total of 56 years), before Tigerstedt and Bergman's experiments were confirmed, and horse angiotensin II was identified and structured by Skeggs et al. [175], and ox angiotensin II was similarly identified and structured by Peart et al. [152]. Volhard's vicious cycle hypothesis was supported by Wilson and Byrom's [195] experiments in rats, in which a partially occluding renal artery clip was placed on one renal artery while the other kidney was kept intact. In the first few weeks removal of the "clipped" kidney was associated with a return of the arterial pressure to normal, but later when the other kidney had suffered some irreversible vascular damage, removal of the clipped kidney no longer lowered the arterial pressure.

It is most important to note that except for malignant hypertension in which there is a persistent rise in renin and angiotensin, the cause of the rise of arterial pressure in the other forms of secondary hypertension remains obscure because plasma renin activity and angiotensin are rarely raised and are often low. Neither has the discovery of the renin-angiotensin system been of help in elucidating the initial cause of primary hypertension because in this form of hypertension plasma renin activity is inversely related to the arterial pressure.

It is obvious that in both primary and secondary hypertension other mechanisms are responsible for the rise in arterial pressure. A central mechanism common to both primary and secondary hypertension was revealed when the importance of dietary sodium on blood pressure was discovered. Ambard and Beaujard [3] were the first to draw attention to this connection when they found in 1904 that a reduction in salt intake in hypertensive men reduced arterial pressure. Salt intake as an initiator of hypertension was first unequivocally demonstrated by Meneely et al. [125], who fed groups of ordinary stock rats a range of dietary sodium intakes. At the end of a year the mean blood pressure of each batch was directly related to the intake of sodium. Dahl [35] confirmed these findings and made an additional observation of immense importance: In each batch of rats the blood pressure rose in some rats but not in others, and this "sensitivity" and "resistance" of the blood pressure to a high-salt diet was genetically determined. At about the same time Smirk and Hall [176] bred a strain of rats that became hypertensive with age on a normal sodium intake (the first strain of "spontaneously hypertensive" rat) and another strain that did not develop hypertension with age. The development of these hereditary forms of hypertension in rats provided the first animal models that closely resembled essential hypertension in humans. The remarkable demonstration that cross-transplantation of a kidney between hereditary hypertensive and normotensive strain rats causes the normotensive rat to develop hypertension and prevents the hypertensive rat from developing hypertension showed that in these hereditary forms of hypertension in the rat, the genetic lesion responsible for the rise in arterial pressure resides in the kidney [13, 36, 37, 91, 134, 157, 158]. If, as seems probable, hereditary hypertension in rats is due to the same mechanism as essential hypertension in humans, these cross-transplantation experiments support Borst and Borst de Geus's [19] and subsequently Guyton's [78] suggestion that in essential hypertension the kidney suffers from an inherited functional abnormality. Borst and Borst de Geus [19] defined this abnormality as an "unwillingness to excrete sodium." The evidence that in essential hypertension the kidney might have difficulty in excreting sodium came from many sources, including Dahl's [34] original observations that the prevalence of hypertension in various populations is related to dietary intake of sodium, and Grim et al.'s [72] demonstration that following a slow infusion of saline the normotensive relatives of hypertensive patients have a delayed urinary excretion of sodium.

In 1960 Losse et al. [106] were the first to show that the red cells from patients with essential hypertension had a high intracellular content of sodium. This observation initially led to the hypothesis that in essential hypertension there might be a genetically determined abnormality of cell membranes. In 1970 Clarkson et al. [30] and Buckalew et al. [25], who were studying the control of urinary sodium excretion in the normal dog, were the first to demonstrate that volume expansion was associated with a rise in the plasma concentration of a sodium transport inhibitor. Subsequently, Haddy and Overbeck [80] observed that a Na-K-ATPase inhibitor was present in excess in the plasma of certain forms of secondary hypertension in animals. Blaustein [18] then pointed out that theoretically a rise in the concentration of such a substance might increase the tone of vascular smooth muscle and be responsible for the hypertension. MacGregor et al. [113] in 1981 demonstrated that the plasma of patients with essential hypertension had a raised concentration of a Na-K-ATPase inhibitor and suggested that this was due to an inherited renal difficulty in excreting sodium. They suggested that the rise in the concentration of such a substance in secondary hypertension would presumably be due to the same reason—i.e., a difficulty in excreting sodium imposed by the experimental maneuver used to raise the blood pressure.

In contrast to the evidence favoring the proposition that hypertension is caused by an abnormality of the blood, which was an alternative first suggested by Bright, Folkow [58] has demonstrated that arterial wall thickening also contributes to the rise in arterial pressure in both primary and secondary hypertension, which is in line with Volhard's proposal that the rise in arterial pressure in benign hypertension might be due to a primary thickening of the arterial wall. At present, though it is not disputed that hypertension per se can cause arterial wall thickening, there is increasing interest in a phenomenon that supports Volhard's idea. It is that in various states of hypertension there appears to be a circulating substance that causes thickening of the peripheral vessels independently of an effect of the rise in pressure [148].

The Relation of Volume Expansion and Salt Intake to Hypertension

In order to understand certain important primary mechanisms that may cause a rise in arterial pressure, it is necessary to be aware of the relevance of certain phenomena that accompany an increase in body fluids (i.e., volume expansion). An acute transfusion of blood or saline or an increased intake of sodium will cause, among many other changes, an increase in the natriuretic capacity of the plasma, an increase in the plasma's ability to inhibit Na-K-ATPase, and an increase in the plasma's ability to increase vascular responses to vasoconstrictors such as noradrenaline and angiotensin [44]. These three changes may stem from two or more substances. The atrial natriuretic peptides are possibly one group of such substances [144], though there are probably other as yet unidentified natriuretic substances. The atrial natriuretic peptides, when injected intravenously, cause a brisk increase in sodium and water excretion of rapid onset and of short duration; and the concentration of plasma endogenous atrial natriuretic peptides rises with acute volume expansion. These peptides (1) stimulate particulate guanylate cyclase activity residing on the cell membrane [83], thus increasing the production of cyclic guanosine monophosphate (GMP), (2) inhibit the secretion of arginine vasopressin from the hypothalamus, and (3) suppress the secretion of aldosterone from the zona glomerulosa of the adrenal [40]. Atrial natriuretic peptides do not inhibit Na-K-ATPase [44] and have no generalized vascular effect except when given in high concentrations when they are vasodilators; they are inhibited by kallikreins. Atrial natriuretic peptides, when introduced into the brain, however, do increase the plasma's ability to inhibit Na-K-ATPase [177]. It is unlikely that the atrial natriuretic peptides are the only form of endogenous natriuretic substance. There are other observations in volume-expanded animals that demonstrate the presence in fresh plasma of a long-acting natriuretic substance with a very slow onset [44].

The extent of the rise in the plasma's ability to cause a natriuresis, to inhibit Na-K-ATPase, and to increase vascular reactivity when induced by an increase in salt intake, is magnified if the subject or animal has a persistent difficulty in excreting sodium. Such a difficulty in humans can be acquired, as in renal disease, primary aldosteronism, or renal artery stenosis, or it may be imposed experimentally in an animal by surgical reduction of renal mass, the placing of a renal artery clip (particularly if the other kidney is removed), and the administration of deoxycorticosterone acetate (DOCA) or aldosterone. These are all situations or procedures that cause secondary hypertension. In all of them the ability of the plasma to inhibit Na-K-ATPase and to increase vascular responses is enhanced, and in some an increased natriuretic capacity has also been observed. The possible relevance of the increased ability to inhibit Na-K-ATPase to the associated rise in blood pressure is discussed below.

In experiments in animals, as expected, the sudden imposition of a reduced ability to excrete sodium induces an initial rapid increase in blood volume, but it is of crucial importance that a few days or weeks later, although the imposed difficulty in excreting sodium continues, the blood volume returns to normal [14, 99]. This return is accompanied by a shift in the distribution of blood from the periphery to the center, so that the ratio of intrathoracic to total blood volume increases [63], and there is a tendency for intrathoracic venous pressure to rise. In these experimental or secondary forms of hypertension, therefore, a persistent tendency to retain sodium is usually accompanied by a normal or even low blood volume. In other words, a measurement of total blood volume in secondary hypertension usually gives no indication of the underlying tendency to retain sodium. By analogy, therefore, the usual finding that in primary hypertension the blood volume is normal or low does not exclude the possibility that in this form of hypertension the kidney also has difficulty excreting sodium. The evidence demonstrating that the kidneys in primary hypertension do have an "unwillingness" to excrete sodium is described below, as are the findings that the plasma has an increased capacity to inhibit Na-K-ATPase and to increase vascular reactivity. It is possible that the etiology of both primary and secondary hypertension stems from a difficulty in excreting sodium and that most forms of hypertension are "renal."

Relation of Salt Intake to Blood Pressure

AVAILABILITY OF SALT AND THE INSATIABLE HUMAN APPETITE FOR SALT

The human race is considered to have been on earth for about 3 million years and, except for the last 5,000 years, inland man has had to eat a low-salt diet. Evolution probably helped the human race to survive by, on the one hand, increasing the tongue's remarkable ability to detect and find intensely pleasurable minute quantities of salt and, on the other, conserving sodium by the ability to reduce sodium losses in the sweat and urine (it is possible to reduce 24-hour urine loss to less than 1 mmol). Man's salt intake rose as the idea of obtaining it from the sea and mines spread throughout the world, having originated in China. For a considerable time it was considered an expensive delicacy. It was one of the precious cargoes carried inland by camel caravans across the Arab and African deserts. The Roman army, which at first issued a monthly ration of salt to each man, eventually found it more convenient to pay the men an extra lump sum (a salary) with which it could be purchased. The insatiable human appetite for this scarce and delicious material made it an excellent object of commerce, especially for those countries that bordered on the sea or had salt mines. In the sixth century salt was mentioned as a chief article of Venetian commerce. Governments used man's avidity for salt as a source of revenue, much as they now use his liking for alcohol. The Chinese had a salt tax in the seventh century B.C. The demand for salt was so powerful and pervasive that smugglers took enormous risks to bypass the tax. In the seventeenth century about one-third of the galley slaves in France were persons sentenced for violation of the salt tax. It was the most hated of all taxes, and in the next century was one of the major causes of the French revolution [141].

Salt's almost magical property of preserving food caused it to be used increasingly. In 1850 it was estimated that salt consumption in England and France per capita was about 20 gm per day (330 mmol), half being added to the food at the table, the other half being present in the food. The introduction of refrigeration reversed this trend, and during the twentieth century salt consumption has tended to fall. Nevertheless, in Western communities it is still 100 to 400 mmol per day, with an average intake of 150 mmol in Europe and the United States. Less is now added at the table than in 1850, but processed foods are responsible for the greater proportion of the total intake. In addition to processed food containing sodium as sodium chloride, sodium is present as the glutamate, bicarbonate, or orthophosphate and many more additives.

THE EFFECT ON THE BLOOD PRESSURE OF INCREASING SODIUM INTAKE

Normal Animals. The prolonged ingestion of increased quantities of salt causes hypertension in the normal dog [2, 192], chicken [102], rabbit [64], baboon [28], and rat [38, 125, 168]. The rate of rise in blood pressure depends on the amount ingested. Hypertension usually comes on within a few weeks, is sustained thereafter, and is proportional to the intake. The effect is more marked in animals exposed just after birth [28, 38] and in males [28, 39]. In the baboon [28], the blood pressure returns to normal when the high salt intake is stopped after 1.5 years.

Normal Humans. A rise in sodium intake to less than a total of 420 mmol/day for 4 days to 4 weeks in young or middle-aged (< 47 years) normotensive subjects did not cause a rise in arterial pressure in four of five studies [26, 74, 95, 167, 179].

In another report [122], the administration of 640 mmol of sodium/day for 23 days to one young adult normal male subject, in addition to the salt contained in food taken at meals, caused a progressive rise in blood pressure from 110/75 to 135/88 mm Hg. In an extreme example of salt loading, Murray et al. [142] increased the oral intake of sodium to six normal young men from 10 to 300 and then to 800 mmol/day over only 9 days. For 3 further days, the 800 mmol of sodium by mouth was supplemented each day by an additional 700 mmol of sodium intravenously. There was a rise in mean blood pressure from 80 to 103 mm Hg, the relationship between systolic, diastolic, and mean blood pressures and sodium excretion being highly significant ($p < 0.001$). In another study [111] by the same group, intravenous saline was not used, the oral intake of sodium being raised to 1,200 mmol/day. In black subjects, an increase up to 600 to 800 mmol/day caused a rise in arterial pressure within 9 days. In white subjects, the sodium intake had to rise to 1,200 mmol/day before a rise in pressure was detectable within the 9-day period of study.

A most dramatic spontaneous demonstration of the effect of a high salt intake on a young normotensive individual, although admittedly not a normal subject, occurred in a boy suffering from diabetes with a craving for salt [123, 183]. On a sustained intake of 850 mmol/day he had severe hypertension. When switched to normal intake of 80 mmol/day, the pressure rapidly returned to normal. This phenomenon was confirmed in four other diabetic children and one normal child (aged between 13 and 15 years) by intentionally increasing sodium intake up to about 600 mmol/day for 2 weeks. In the normal boy the blood pressure rose from 120/70 to 145/100 mm Hg. There do not appear to be any studies, comparable with those made in animals, of the effect of a prolonged modest increase in salt intake on the blood pressure of young normal subjects. In older subjects (> 50 years) in whom it is normal for renal function to deteriorate [172], an impaired ability to excrete sodium becomes detectable and plasma renin falls; an increase in salt intake up to 340 mmol/day for 4 weeks has been shown to cause a rise in arterial pressure [75].

In view of the evidence that essential hypertension is a hereditary condition, study of the changes in urinary sodium excretion that occur with acute changes in sodium status in 37 pairs of monozygotic and 18 pairs of dizygotic normotensive twins is of interest. The twins were given 2 liters of saline intravenously during 4 hours, followed immediately by 120 mg of furosemide and a low-sodium diet. The results demonstrated that the induced changes in urinary sodium excretion were influenced by hereditary factors [73].

THE EFFECT ON THE BLOOD PRESSURE OF REDUCING SALT INTAKE

The effect of a reduction in salt intake on the arterial pressure of normal subjects has been studied in neonates, school-age children, and adults. The blood pressure in normal newborn babies was found to be particularly sensitive to a prolonged small reduction in sodium intake. Hofman et al. [86] allocated 476 babies into two groups, one of which had a normal sodium intake and the other a lower intake for 6 months. The normal intake was three times greater than the lower sodium intake. There was a progressive and increasing difference in systolic pressure between the two groups, so that the mean systolic pressure at 6 weeks was significantly higher in those on the higher sodium intake. In four studies in children the significance of the results was greatly influenced by the number of participants. In one study with a total of only 80 children, a reduction in sodium intake of 30 mmol/day to an intake of 56 mmol/day had no effect on the blood pressure at the end of 1 year [66]. In the second study with a total of 124 participants, a reduction in sodium intake of 65 mmol/day to an intake of 45 mmol/day for 24 days induced a nonsignificant fall in blood pressure [31]. In a third group of 149 subjects, a reduction in sodium intake of 55 mmol/day to an intake of 50 mmol/day induced a significant fall in blood pressure after 12 weeks but only after adjustment for age and weight [131]. With a total group of 750 children, however, a reduction in sodium intake of 39 mmol/day to an intake of 127 mmol/day induced a significant fall in blood pressure at 24 weeks [53].

In one study in 32 adults (aged around 40 years), a mean reduction in urinary sodium excretion from 153 to

70 mmol/day induced a significant fall in blood pressure at 12 weeks, the fall in pressure being correlated with the fall in urinary sodium excretion [130].

EPIDEMIOLOGIC STUDIES OF THE PREVALENCE OF HYPERTENSION VERSUS SALT INTAKE

Multiple population studies throughout the world have revealed that there is a close direct correlation between salt intake and blood pressure. In underdeveloped societies in which sodium intake is less than 60 mmol per day, the blood pressure does not rise with age. At the other end of the scale, in some areas of northern Japan, where the mean intake of sodium is 400 mmol per day, the prevalence of hypertension is about 50 percent [67, 112]. It has to be admitted that there are several other differences, apart from salt intake, when one is comparing underdeveloped societies to Western societies, particularly in their diet; for instance, the content of protein, calcium, and saturated fat is higher in Western diets, whereas the content of potassium and fiber is lower.

Studies of rural Oriental communities in which there is a wide range of salt intake and each individual's intake is relatively constant have repeatedly shown a direct relationship between 24-hour urinary sodium excretion and blood pressure [93, 94, 133, 171, 197]. In Western cultures, however, it has been difficult, until recently, to detect a significant relationship within populations. In addition, attempts to correlate data from international sources was criticized in that the various centers from which the data were obtained used different criteria, and there was a failure to take into account many confounding variables. Thus cross-center linear relationships between blood pressure and sodium intake, which were repeatedly demonstrated from data collected worldwide [33, 67], consistently failed to be universally convincing.

The results of a massive international epidemiologic study (the Intersalt Study), which avoided the weaknesses of previous investigations, have recently been published [89]. It was carried out in 10,079 men and women aged 20 to 59 years sampled from 52 centers around the world using a standardized protocol, central training, and a central laboratory [52]. After standardization for age, sex, body mass index, alcohol intake, and potassium excretion, within-center analyses showed that sodium excretion was significantly related to systolic pressure in individuals, and cross-center analyses showed that sodium excretion is significantly related to the rise in systolic and diastolic pressure with age (Fig. 53-1). A conservative estimate of the size of this effect is that, on average, a reduction in sodium intake of 100 mmol/day between the ages of 25 and 55 years corresponds to a 9 mm Hg lower rise in systolic pressure. This is likely to be an underestimate, as only one 24-hour sample of urine was analyzed for sodium excretion, but within-individual variations in daily sodium excretion may vary widely. In Western communities, it is necessary to sample 5 to 14 24-hour samples to obtain a correct regression coefficient [104, 110, 173, 189]. To try to adjust for this variability in the Intersalt Study, a coefficient of reliability was calculated from the results of two

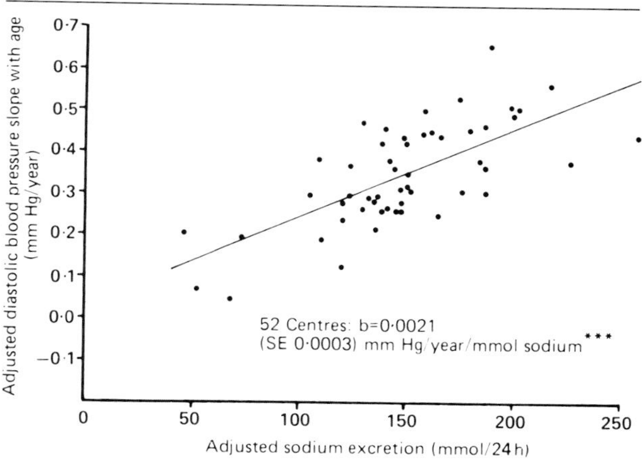

Fig. 53-1. Cross-center plots of diastolic blood pressure slope with age, and median sodium excretion and fitted regression lines standardized for age, sex, body mass index, and alcohol consumption for 52 centers. (From INTERSALT Cooperative Research Group. INTERSALT: An international study of electrolyte excretion and blood pressure. Results for 24-hour urinary sodium and potassium excretion. *Br. Med. J.* 297:319, 1988.)

24-hour urine samples collected from 807 participants at random.

Once again, the Intersalt Study demonstrated that in geographically isolated centers where urinary sodium excretion rates were below approximately 60 mmol/day, of which there were four in the Intersalt Study, the blood pressure does not rise with age and hypertension is rare. In the past, the applicability of such observations to other, and particularly to Western, societies have tended to be dismissed on the assumption that the general health and daily life patterns of such isolated unacculturated societies was probably more relevant to their low blood pressure than their intake of sodium [180]. It appears that this assumption is unwarranted. The local organizers at each of the four Intersalt centers with sodium intakes below 60 mmol/day have reported that the participants were physically active, appeared healthy, and showed no sign of malnutrition or protein deficiency [27]. The minor influence on the blood pressure of the daily life patterns of these isolated communities, in contrast to their intake of sodium, has been demonstrated in three further studies. One was in six Solomon Island communities with similar life patterns [149]. The physical fitness of the participants in all six islands was found to be "excellent." In three of the islands with sodium intakes below 30 mmol/day, the prevalence of hypertension was below 1 percent; in two islands where the inhabitants added salt to the cooking so that sodium intake varied between 50 and 130 mmol/day, the prevalence was 3.4 and 2.7 percent, and in the remaining island where they cooked in "copious amounts of sea water" it was 7.8 percent. The second study was in two tribes living on the shores of two adjoining southern tributaries of the Amazon [107]. One tribe, which was under the care of missionaries, regularly used table salt. In the men, there was a rising trend of arterial pressure with age; in the women, there was a similar, but statistically unimportant rise. In the other tribe, who ate native low-sodium food, there was no rise in blood pressure with age in either sex. The third study, which complements the others, was undertaken in an isolated nomadic tribe at a low level of acculturation in southern Iran [150]. Throughout the tribal area, which the tribe has inhabited for approximately 400 years, there are natural surface deposits of salt, which is used liberally in the baking of bread, in cooking, and at the table. The average urinary sodium excretion was 186 mmol/day in the men and 141 mmol/day in the women. The prevalence of hypertension in those over 30 years of age was 12 and 18 percent respectively, with no tendency for weight to increase with age.

Renal Mechanisms That Influence Arterial Pressure

The principal renal mechanisms that influence arterial pressure are:

1. The kidney's ability to excrete sodium
2. The renin-angiotensin system
3. Hypotensive hormones from the renal papilla
4. Renal control of interstitial space compliance

THE KIDNEY'S ABILITY TO EXCRETE SODIUM

Acquired or Imposed Restraints. FALL IN RENAL PERFUSION PRESSURE. Sodium excretion is directly related to the peritubular hydrostatic pressure [5, 17, 122]. A reduction in perfusion pressure therefore lowers sodium excretion. Such a reduction occurs initially in coarctation in the aorta and eventually in renal artery stenosis. In animals it can be imposed experimentally by forming a pseudocoarctation or by placing a clip on one or both renal arteries. It is also likely that the architectural chaos that accompanies most renal diseases, whether acquired in humans or imposed in animals, produces focal areas of diminished peritubular hydrostatic pressure.

A persistent reduction in arterial pressure therefore causes a persistent tendency toward sodium retention, but, as pointed out in the preceding section, this leads to a rise in the natriuretic capacity of the plasma, which opposes the tendency for sodium retention. This sequence of events can be demonstrated in experiments in which a persistent reduction in renal perfusion pressure is maintained [82]. Servo-controlled reductions of the perfusion pressure to both renal arteries in the dog have been continued for 1 week by partial occlusion of the aorta. There was a rise in arterial pressure above the occlusion. During the first 2 days the fall in renal perfusion pressure was accompanied by a fall in urinary sodium excretion and a rise in extracellular fluid volume. The blood volume was not measured. On the third day and thereafter, although the renal perfusion pressure remained low, urinary sodium excretion returned to control values, so that the extracellular fluid volume no longer continued to increase, but it remained raised. The return of urinary sodium excretion to normal, therefore, was independent of the renal perfusion pressure. It must have been due in part to the rise in the natriuretic capacity of the plasma, which would occur in these circumstances. Unfortunately, the renal nerves were still intact, and therefore it is not possible to exclude some neural influence. In the same way, it is probable that the rise in arterial pressure above the occlusion was due in part to the increased capacity of the plasma to increase vascular reactivity and to its increased capacity to inhibit Na-K-ATPase, both of which would also occur.

REDUCTION OF RENAL MASS. In humans, reduction of renal mass is the inescapable result of most renal diseases, which, in 80 percent of patients with advanced renal failure, are associated with hypertension. As the number of nephrons diminishes and renal failure develops, the ability to excrete a sodium load diminishes. Patients with renal failure, however, tend to continue to consume the same amount of salt, and, since they do not become edematous, urinary excretion of sodium must remain the same. This implies that a reduced number of nephrons are now excreting the same amount of sodium that was being excreted when the number of nephrons was normal. In other words, as nephrons disappear, each remaining nephron excretes, in absolute terms [44], an increasing amount of sodium. Theoretically, this might be achieved by either increasing single nephron filtration rate or diminishing tubular reabsorption of sodium. There is little evidence, however, that even when single nephron filtration rate does increase, that this is the mechanism whereby single nephron sodium excretion rate rises [84]. Persistent changes in glomerular filtration rate (GFR) do not influence sodium excretion. On the other hand, there is direct evidence that the increase in single nephron sodium excretion is due to diminished tubular reabsorption and that this is probably due to the associated observed increase in the plasma's natriuretic capacity. The extent of the diminution in sodium reabsorption can be calculated as the proportion of filtered sodium (GFR $\times$ plasma Na^+) that is excreted ($U_{Na} \times V$), which is otherwise known as the fractional excretion of sodium (Fe_{Na}). Normally, it is about 1 percent, whereas in chronic renal failure it can increase to over 10 percent.

HORMONAL RESTRAINT. The two principal sodium-retaining hormones are aldosterone and angiotensin. In normal animals sodium retention can be induced experimentally by subcutaneous administration of deoxycorticosterone acetate (DOCA). There is an initial period of sodium retention and weight gain followed within a few days by an increase in urinary excretion so that eventually there may be no detectable enlargement of the volume of extracellular fluid or blood volume or even a reduced blood volume. This phenomenon is usually known as the "escape" phenomenon. When it is prolonged in humans (primary aldosteronism) it is associated with hypertension and low plasma angiotensin and renin activity. In this condition and in its experimental counterpart in humans or animals, the plasma has increased natriuretic activity and sodium transport-inhibiting capacity [42]. While normal DOCA escape is associated with suppression of the renin-angiotensin system, continuous stimulation of the renin-angiotensin system occurs in edematous disorders. In the latter circumstance, angiotensin may increase sodium and water reabsorption in the proximal tubule and thus impair DOCA escape by limiting sodium delivery to the distal site of the aldosterone.

An interesting sequence of events occurs in humans who have an experimentally maintained rise in plasma angiotensin II (Fig. 53-2). In one experiment a continuous infusion of angiotensin II was given and adjusted so that it was sufficient to produce only a small rise in arterial pressure. At first 0.5 μg per minute was needed to produce this effect. During the first 4 days the antinatriuretic effect of the angiotensin II was such that urinary sodium excretion was less than sodium intake, and there was substantial sodium retention. There was then a rise in urinary sodium excretion, and for 2 days it was greater than intake; then, while the subject was still in positive sodium balance, urinary sodium excretion matched the intake of sodium. These changes in sodium balance were accompanied by a rapid diminution in the amount of angiotensin II needed to maintain the small rise in arterial pressure [98]. In other words, the volume expansion had, probably by means of the plasma Na-K-ATPase inhibitor and vascular reactivity factor, increased the vascular response to angiotensin II and by means of circulating natriuretic substances overcome the antinatriuretic properties of angiotensin II.

The same sequence can be seen in the experimental model in which a partially occluding "clip" is placed on one renal artery and the other kidney removed. There is then a sudden rise in plasma angiotensin II, acute sodium retention due to the fall in peritubular hydrostatic pressure and the raised plasma angiotensin II, followed by a rise in arterial pressure. The arterial pressure continues to rise very rapidly or stays raised, but the plasma angiotensin II falls, often to below normal level, and urinary sodium excretion of the clipped kidney returns to match the intake. With a clip on one renal artery and the contralateral kidney left in place the situation at first is different, but later it is often much the same as when the contralateral kidney is removed. At first the partial occlusion of the renal artery produces a brisk rise in plasma angiotensin II level with a rise in arterial pressure. At this time the natriuretic effect of the rise in arterial pressure on the intact kidney tends to overcome the sodium-retaining effects of the raised plasma angiotensin II level, and there is if anything a volume contraction. But with time the antinatriuretic effect of the angiotensin II often predominates, so that gradually

Fig. 53-2. Prolonged continuous angiotensin II infusion in a normal subject for 11 days. The dose of angiotensin II was adjusted to keep a mildly pressor response. Angiotensin II induced a marked and selective increase in the adrenal cortical secretion of aldosterone together with consequent sodium retention. As sodium was retained, angiotensin II became more pressor. Because of this increasing pressor sensitivity to angiotensin II, the dose was serially reduced to a point where aldosterone secretion returned to control levels. Thus the pressor sensitivity to angiotensin II increased as sodium retention progressed. The results indicate that angiotensin II can produce and then sustain hypertension with diminishingly small amounts as the tendency to volume increases the pressor effect of the angiotensin. (From J. H. Laragh. In J. Genest, O. Kuchel, P. Jamet, et al. [eds.], *Hypertension*. New York: McGraw Hill, 1983.)

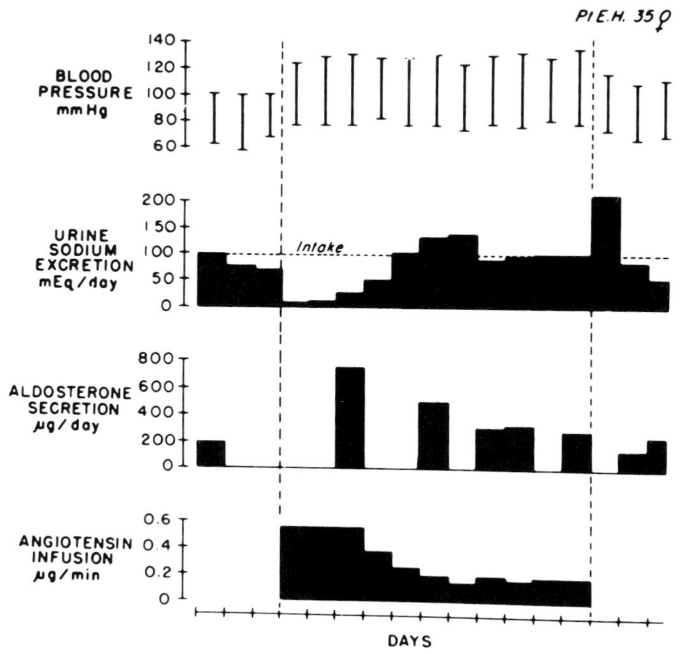

there is a tendency toward volume expansion, which, though it lowers the plasma angiotensin II sometimes to normal or near normal levels, causes an increase in vascular reactivity, so that the blood pressure remains raised. This situation is commonly seen in humans with unilateral renal artery stenosis and can cause much confusion in diagnosis.

Inherited Restraint on Sodium Excretion. There is evidence that in inherited forms of hypertension in humans and in the rat there is an inherited difficulty in excreting sodium. This evidence stems from experiments demonstrating that the genetic lesion responsible for the hypertension resides in the kidney [12], and other observations that the lesion consists of a diminished ability to excrete sodium.

IN THE RAT. Cross-transplantation experiments between a hypertensive-strain rat and a normotensive-strain rat have shown that the blood pressure of the recipient rat depends on the source of the donated kidney (see above). Some of these experiments have been performed before the rise in arterial pressure, which takes place from the sixth to the tenth week, depending on the strain. A bilateral nephrectomy is performed on both rats, and one kidney is then cross transplanted. As a result, when the recipient rat from the normotensive strain is given a kidney from a hypertensive rat it develops hypertension, whereas when a recipient rat from the hypertensive strain is given a kidney from a normotensive strain rat it does not develop hypertension. Two disconcerting but logical conclusions emerge from the cross-transplantation experiments in rats. The first is that in hereditary strains of hypertension the rise in arterial pressure stems from a genetic abnormality of the kidney. It does not follow that the genetic fault that leads to the functional hypertensinogenic renal disturbance is only present in the kidney. There is much evidence that in hereditary hypertension, in both rats and humans, there are generalized membrane abnormalities [96, 105, 145], including an increase in the density of β-adrenoceptors [126]. Nor does it follow that the same genetic abnormality is responsible for all forms of hereditary hypertension. The second conclusion that emerges from the cross-transplantation experiments is that genetic abnormalities in vascular smooth muscle, the brain, or sympathetic system in hereditary forms of hypertension, do not per se cause hypertension, for the blood pressure of a hypertensive strain rat does not rise in the presence of a normal kidney. Conversely, an imposed surgical procedure on a kidney can induce hypertension in an animal with no genetic abnormalities of its vascular smooth muscle or nervous system.

Direct evidence that the genetic renal abnormality is an impaired ability to excrete sodium comes from Tobian et al. [184] and Roman and Cowley [161], who perfused kidneys from prehypertensive and normotensive strains of Dahl and spontaneously hypertensive (SHR) rats. The kidneys from the hypertensive-strain rats excreted less sodium at each perfusion pressure than the kidneys of the sodium-resistant (normotensive-strain) controls. Less direct evidence comes from observations made in both the Milan and the stroke-prone spontaneously hypertensive Heidelberg strain that at about the sixth to the seventh week of life there is a transient period when the fractional excretion of sodium is lower and there is an increase in extracellular volume. At the end of this period the blood pressure of the salt-sensitive rat has risen considerably. Once the rat is adult there are no differences in sodium excretion or extracellular fluid volume, but plasma renin activity remains low as it does in the Dahl and Okamoto hypertensive strains.

Nature of Inherited Renal Abnormality Responsible for Impaired Sodium Excretion. IN THE RAT. It has been difficult to distinguish as inherited abnormality from one that has been acquired as a result of a rise in arterial pressure. The arterial pressure in inherited hypertensive rats tends to rise steeply around the sixth week of life. Therefore, the distinction between an inherited lesion and a lesion secondary to the rise in pressure has to be made in very young rats.

There is a scanning and electron microscopic study in 6-week-old spontaneously hypertensive rats (SHR) in which the arterial pressure was 131 mm Hg, as opposed to 121 mm Hg in control Wiston-Kyoto (WKY) rats [55]. The fenestrae of the glomerular capillary endothelium of the SHR were significantly smaller, and an increased number of cytoplasmic ridges and bulbous projections lay across the endothelial surface. These changes should reduce the filtration surface per unit area of endothelium. At 12 weeks, when the arterial pressure of the SHR was 175 mm Hg and that of the WKY rat was 138 mm Hg, these abnormalities were more pronounced, whereas the endothelium of the WKY rat was unchanged (in spite of the WKY rat having an arterial pressure slightly higher at 12 weeks than that of the SHR at 6 weeks). Not only is the filtration surface per unit area reduced, but some workers have also found that the SHR has a diminished number of nephrons [162].

In conformity with these structural abnormalities it has been found that the glomerulus of the young Milan hypertensive rat has a reduced glomerular ultrafiltration coefficient, a reduced glomerular filtration rate and single nephron filtration rate, and increased sodium reabsorption in the proximal tubule [6]. The net result is that the amount of sodium delivered to the distal tubule is reduced. The inability of the nephron to adjust sodium excretion to the reduced filtration rate therefore must be due to a functional abnormality of the distal and collecting tubule. This might be due to a relative resistance to the effect of circulating natriuretic substances. Alternatively, there is some evidence consistent with the idea that the distal tubule and collecting duct abnormality may be due to a fixed vascular resistance between the renal artery perfusion pressure and the peritubular capillaries of the distal tubule and collecting ducts that tends to keep the peritubular venous pressure at these sites below normal, thus causing an increase in sodium reabsorption at the site (see later).

As the arterial pressure rises, the difference in glomerular filtration rate between the SHR and the WKY rat at first disappears and is then reversed, so that in the young adult rat the glomerular filtration rate of the SHR is greater than that of the WKY rat [48]. Later still, the glomerular filtration rate of the spontaneously hypertensive rat gradually falls below that of the WKY rat.

IN HUMANS. The most suggestive evidence that the genetic lesion responsible for essential hypertension resides in the kidney has been provided by Curtis et al. [32]. Six patients with terminal renal failure from essential hypertension were studied in whom multiple renal biopsies, examined by an independent observer, had demonstrated that the renal histologic changes were only those that accompany a rise in arterial pressure. All 6 patients had their own kidneys removed and received a donor kidney. After an average follow-up period of 4.5 years all were normotensive. There is also the evidence of Guidi et al. [76] that the incidence of hypertension in recipients of human kidney grafts is related to the donor's family history of hypertension.

Observations in monozygotic and dizygotic twins have established that in normal subjects there are "strong heritable influences on the renal excretion of sodium which are most readily identified in the volume expanded state" [71]. Using a relatively slow infusion of saline (2 liters in 4 hours), it has also been demonstrated that normotensive, first-degree relatives of patients with essential hypertension excrete less sodium than control subjects [73]. Though highly suggestive, in view of the transplantation experiment, it must nevertheless be pointed out that this observation does not establish beyond question whether the difficulty is due to an intrinsic abnormality of the kidney or to an abnormality of those extrarenal factors that control sodium excretion. Probably the most suggestive evidence that the kidney in patients with essential hypertension has a "difficulty in excreting sodium" is the disputed finding that, as in inherited hypertension in the rat, patients with essential hypertension have been found to have a lowered lithium-creatinine clearance ratio, which indicates an increase in proximal tubule reabsorption [190].

Altered Relation of the Arterial Pressure to Urinary Sodium Excretion. The urinary sodium excretion of an isolated kidney is directly related to the perfusion pressure [5, 17, 121]. The change in pressure alters sodium excretion by changing the hydrostatic pressure of the venous capillaries surrounding the distal and collecting ducts, an effect that is independent of the glomerular filtration rate or of renal blood flow, which tends to remain unchanged throughout the autoregulatory range of perfusion pressure. The relation between urinary sodium excretion and renal perfusion pressure is sometimes referred to as a "pressure natriuresis" curve. Some isolated kidneys need a greater pressure to promote the same rate of sodium excretion, a change that can be referred to as a right shift of the pressure natriuresis curve.

There has been a tendency to assume that the fixity of the curves obtained in a perfused kidney also occurs with changes in arterial pressure when the kidney is in situ. This assumption, however, is complicated by the fact that changes in arterial pressure are produced by changes in overall vascular resistance that usually include the renal vasculature. For instance, a rise in arterial pressure due to an infusion of noradrenaline, which induces severe renal vasoconstriction, will have less effect on urinary sodium excretion than a similar rise in arterial pressure due to an infusion of dopamine, which tends to cause renal vasodilatation. Pressure natriuresis curves in vivo are therefore labile entities. The curve depends on the proportion of the change in pressure that is transmitted to the peritubular venous capillaries, while the angle of the slope of the pressure natriuresis curve also depends on the baseline urinary sodium excretion.

If the pressure natriuresis curve of an isolated kidney, perfused with blood from a normal animal, has shifted to the right, it is probable that there has been a rise in resistance in a vascular site between the arterial perfusion pressure and the peritubular venous capillaries. If this is true, it is evident that such a site of raised resistance is present in kidneys in situ in all forms of hypertension, otherwise hypertension would be accompanied by severe sodium depletion. Part of this rise in vascular resistance may be due to the well-known phenomenon of systemic autoregulation, in which a rise in arterial perfusion pressure induces an increase in vascular resistance as a direct result of the effect of the raised pressure on the vascular smooth muscle.

It has been proposed that in essential hypertension and inherited hypertension in the rat the shift of the natriuresis curve to the right is primary and is the cause of the kidney's difficulty in excreting sodium. The implication is that patients with essential hypertension are born with a fixed area of vascular resistance between the renal artery and the peritubular venous capillaries. There is no doubt that such a resistance is present in established essential hypertension because not only are patients with hypertension not sodium deficient, but the intrarenal venous pressure, which is an index of the peritubular venous capillary pressure, is normal [193]. But, because (see above) a normal kidney exposed to a raised arterial pressure will develop a shift of the "pressure site" curve to the right, the presence of such a curve in essential hypertension does not establish whether it was present in part before the rise in pressure. Tobian et al. [184] and Roman and Cowley [161], however, have shown that isolated kidneys of young prehypertensive salt-sensitive and spontaneously hypertensive Dahl rats have a shift to the right of the pressure natriuresis curve. It is possible, therefore, that the apparent difficulty of the distal and collecting duct of the SHR rat to reduce sodium reabsorption in order to compensate for the diminished delivery of sodium from the proximal tubule may be due to a low peritubular venous capillary pressure around this part of the nephron [42] due in turn to a documented abnormality of arachidonic acid metabolism that induces vasoconstricting substances [54]. This would result in a tendency toward sodium retention that would mobilize all those mechanisms mentioned earlier that are brought into play when there is a tendency to volume expansion. At first some of these compensatory natriuretic mechanisms will adjust urinary sodium excretion. Eventually the same or other mechanisms, brought into play by the persistent tendency toward volume expansion, may in part be responsible for the rise in arterial pressure (see below); however, it is clear from the chronic aortic occlusion experiments described earlier that the tendency toward sodium retention, perhaps caused by a reduced hydrostatic pressure, can be overcome without a rise in arterial pressure. This is presumably what occurs in the normotensive children of hypertensive parents. It is possible that the rise in arterial pressure, when it takes place, may also help to correct the tendency to retain sodium, but, because other mechanisms can perform this adjustment satisfactorily, it would appear that the possible natriuretic effect of the rise in pressure serves more as a back-up mechanism.

THE RENIN-ANGIOTENSIN SYSTEM

Factors Influencing Renin Secretion. Renin is secreted by the juxtaglomerular cells of the afferent arteriole into the lumen of the arteriole and into the surrounding interstitial tissue. Because of renin's capacity to convert angiotensinogen to angiotensin I, which is then converted into angiotensin II, it has a profound effect on many facets of hypertension. Several mechanisms influence renin secretion:

1. Intrarenal vascular receptors
2. Intracellular calcium concentration
3. Sympathetic nerves
4. Macula densa
5. Renal prostaglandins

INTRARENAL VASCULAR RECEPTOR AND INTRACELLULAR CALCIUM CONCENTRATION. The renin-secreting cells have myogenic properties and appear to respond to changes in perfusion pressure in the same manner as the whole renal vasculature; a fall in perfusion pressure causes dilatation, and an increase in pressure causes constriction. The cells secreting renin respond to changes in afferent arteriolar wall tension, so that decreased tension stimulates renin release [62]. Decreased tension of smooth muscle is associated with a lowered intracellular ionic concentration of calcium. It has also been shown that juxtaglomerular cells in vitro, when exposed to ouabain or to high calcium in the bathing solution, which raises intracellular ionic calcium, reduce renin excretion, whereas verapamil and low extracellular calcium concentrations increase renin secretion. Experiments on isolated kidneys perfused with perfusate of varying calcium concentrations have shown the same relationship. Similarly, the inhibitory effects of angiotensin II and ADH, which also increase intracellular calcium and therefore inhibit renin release in the isolated perfused kidney, require the presence of calcium in the perfusate. Therefore, it is possible that it is the lowered intracellular ionic calcium concentration in the vasodilating smooth muscle that stimulates renin release [60, 151, 153, 187]. This relationship is summarized in Table 53-1.

SYMPATHETIC NERVES. Renal sympathetic nerves terminate in the juxtaglomerular renin-secreting cells and in the smooth muscle of the arterioles and the renal tubules. The change in renin release induced by the direct action of the renal nerves, or catecholamines, on the juxtaglomerular cells is initiated by a β-adrenergic receptor mechanism. Stimulation of β-adrenergic receptors in smooth muscle leads to decreased concentration of intracellular ionic calcium and relaxation [49, 62]. The exact intracellular mechanism that leads to increased renin secretion in response to adrenergic stimulation is not clear, but it is very likely that stimulation of β-adrenergic receptors [92] of the juxtaglomerular cells has the same effect on these cells that it has on smooth muscle, lowering cytoplasmic calcium and causing increased renin release. Several indirect observations support this suggestion. For instance, ouabain, which inhibits Na-K-ATPase and raises intracellular calcium, blocks completely noradrenaline stimulation of renin release from cortical slices.

Table 53-1. Relation of intracellular ionic calcium concentration of juxtaglomerular apparatus and renin secretion

Intracellular ionic calcium concentration	Vessels	Renin secretion
Raised	Constricted	Low
Low	Dilated	High

Direct electrical stimulation of selected areas of the brain stem increases renin release, whereas stimulation of the hypothalamus reduces plasma renin activity. Both effects are abolished by renal denervation. Vagal cooling increases renin release and prevents the fall in renin release that occurs with left atrial distention, but the vagal effect is blocked by renal denervation [62].

MACULA DENSA. The vascular pole of each glomerulus has a small point of contact with the distal tubule belonging to that nephron [7]. It is well established that renin release from the juxtaglomerular cells, which abut onto the apposed distal tubule (the macula densa), is related *inversely* to the load of sodium chloride, and the resulting sodium chloride transport, which occurs in that area of distal tubule (e.g., an increased filtered load of sodium) is associated with an increased reabsorption of sodium and a decreased renin release [62]. There is also some evidence that the chloride ion contributes importantly to the signal perceived by the macula densa. Because the relation between sodium chloride delivery to the macula densa and renin release is inverse, the phenomenon of tubuloglomerular feedback, whereby a sudden increase in sodium load at the macula densa causes a sharp decrease in the filtration rate, is unlikely to be due to an increase in renin production and angiotensin II.

PROSTAGLANDINS. Prostaglandins locally manufactured in the kidney stimulate renin release both by a direct action on the juxtaglomerular cells and possibly by some other indirect action that influences the other renin release mechanisms discussed above. Numerous prostaglandins stimulate renin release including PGI and PGD, with which most of the investigations have been performed [170].

Multiple Effects of Angiotensin II. Angiotensin II (AII) has multiple actions, all of which tend to raise the blood pressure (Fig. 53-3).

MECHANISM OF ACTION. The cellular mechanism whereby angiotensin induces all these effects is not known. The vasoconstricting action, however, is probably effected by raising the intracellular ionic concentration of calcium in smooth muscle. The increased release and diminished uptake of noradrenaline that angiotensin induces in arteries, which results in an increased local concentration of noradrenaline, also increases the intracellular ionic concentration of calcium of the arterial smooth muscle.

The increase in sodium reabsorption induced by angiotensin is due to at least two mechanisms: (1) a direct effect on tubular sodium reabsorption, and (2) an increase in plasma aldosterone. The effect of a prolonged infusion of angiotensin over several days [4, 98] sufficient to maintain a small persistent increase in arterial pressure has been described above.

The effect of angiotensin II on increasing vascular reactivity to itself (and noradrenaline) is presumably due to sodium and water retention [4, 23] and is analogous to the increased vascular reactivity that occurs with a high sodium intake. There is, however, an alternative suggestion that the response to an acute dose of angiotensin is diminished or augmented by changes in sodium intake because more or fewer vascular receptors for angiotensin are occupied by endogenously produced angiotensin. It is pointed out that the response to an acute infusion of angiotensin in high and low sodium intake experiments is inversely related to the preceding endogenous concentration of angiotensin. Thus, a high sodium intake lowers plasma angiotensin, which denudes the receptors of angiotensin II and increases the number available for exogenous angiotensin. Therefore, the effect of an acute infusion of angiotensin at this time is greater. This hypothesis is supported by the finding that administration of a converting enzyme inhibitor (which blocks the formation of angiotensin II from angiotensin I) to a sodium-deprived dog with a high plasma renin suddenly increases the response to exogenous angiotensin. But when the converting enzyme inhibitor is given to a sodium-loaded animal with a low plasma angiotensin, the response to angiotensin is unchanged. In contrast to these experiments in which the response of the blood pressure is studied by infusing acute loads of angiotensin are the observations made during a continuous infusion of angiotensin reported above [98]. An increase in the response to angiotensin can be obtained in spite of the continuous infusion of exogenous angiotensin, which must not only saturate angiotensin receptors but also down-regulate the number of receptors. It is probable, therefore, that both hypotheses are correct and that the changes in vascular reactivity to angiotensin that occur with sodium intake may be due to changes in the concentration of a circulating vascular reactivity factor and the availability and number of receptors.

HYPOTENSIVE HORMONES FROM THE RENAL PAPILLA

If fragments of renal papilla (0.5 to 1 mm in size) from a healthy donor animal are transplanted subcutaneously or intraperitoneally into an animal suffering an experimentally induced form of hypertension, the blood pressure falls toward normal [137, 140, 196]. This observation has been made in renoprival hypertension in the dog and the rabbit and in one clip, one kidney hypertension in the rat [137, 165] (Fig. 53-4). The hypotensive effect is reversed by removal or rejection of the papillary transplant. In time the morphologic characteristics of the transplant change. The tubules disappear and the transplant consists mostly of renal interstitial cells embedded in a network of capillaries. Similar results have been obtained by injecting subcutaneously live monolayer cultures of renomedullary interstitial cells. In contrast, chemical ablation of the papillae in a rat on a normal diet

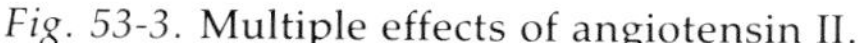
Fig. 53-3. Multiple effects of angiotensin II.

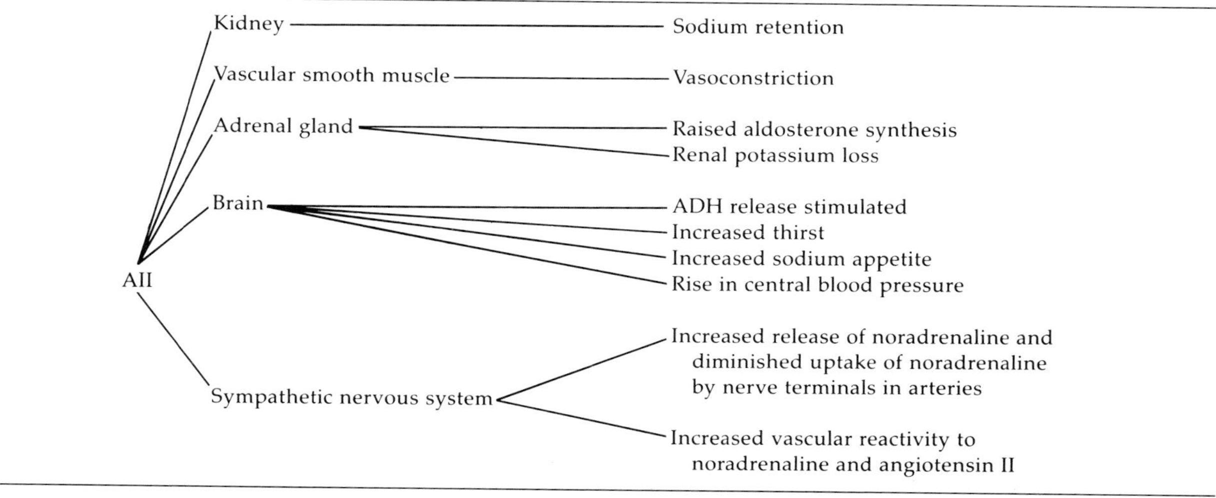

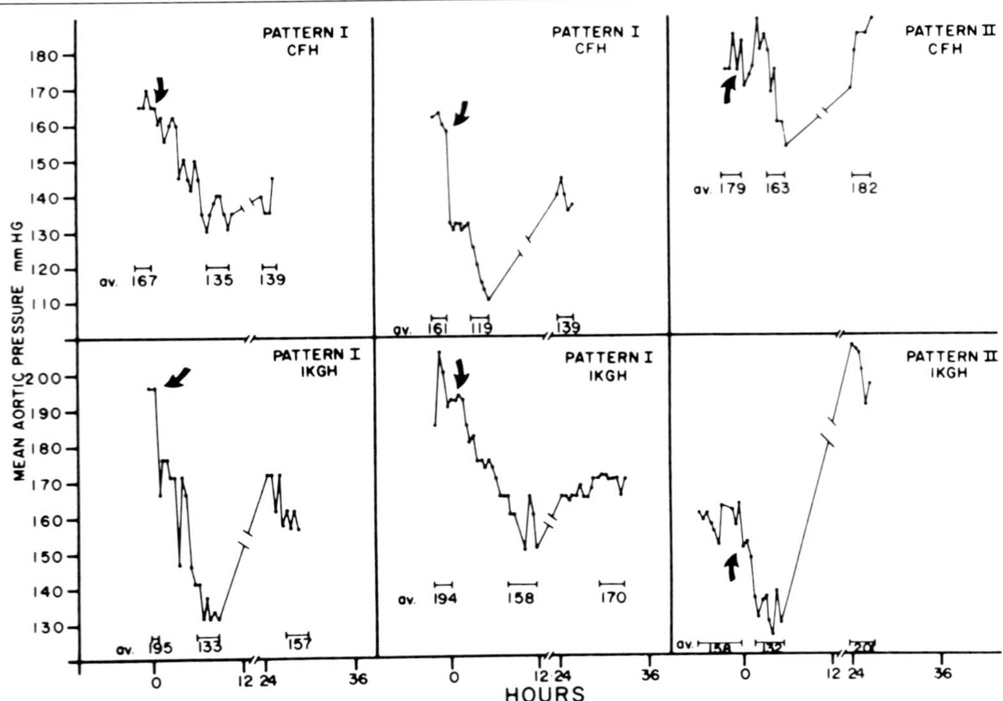

Fig. 53-4. Transplants of cultured renomedullary interstitial cells (RIC) in partial nephrectomy + salt (CFH) and one kidney Goldblatt (IKGH) hypertension. These are individual results. The transplant (30 M viable cells) was introduced at the arrow. The arterial pressure was lowered to a minimum by 6 to 12 hours. The figures under the bars are averages for the interval of the bar. (From E. E. Muirhead, W. A. Rightsel, B. E. Leech, et al. *Lab. Invest.* 36:162, 1977.)

leads to hypertension [16]. It has been concluded that the renal medullary cells induce this hypotensive effect by releasing into the circulation a substance or substances that cause vasodilation [138].

Renal medullalry cells lie alongside and between Henle's loop, the vasa recta, and the collecting ducts [137, 154]. They are surrounded by proteoglycans, which they secrete, and they extend cytoplasmic processes that touch adjoining structures. Renal interstitial cells contain lipid-containing granules that are a source of substrate for conversion into membrane lipid, prostaglandins, and possibly antihypertensive lipids. The granules per se, either intact or disrupted, however, do not have a hypotensive effect on their own when injected intravenously. Many forms of experimental hypertension are associated with a significant decrease in the lipid granules, which also show several degenerative changes. Such changes also occur in a papillary renal transplant or in cultured renal medullary cells when they are no longer able to lower the blood pressure.

Four groups of lipids that have hypotensive effects have been extracted from the renal medulla—prostaglandin, a renin inhibitor, and two other lipids, one of which is polar (APRL) and is an alkyl ether of phosphatidylcholine (AEPC) and the other of which appears chromatographically to be nonpolar (ANRL). Prostaglandins are local vasodilators but are unlikely to have generalized hypotensive effects. The renin inhibitor lowers the arterial pressure of animals in which hypertension is associated with a high plasma renin. The other two lipids, the antihypertensive polar renomedullary lipid (APRL) and the antihypertensive neutral renomedullary lipid (ANRL), have very similar biologic behaviors in that they both produce an acute and prolonged vasodepressor effect. It is possible that the neutral form may convert to the polar compound.

The prolonged hypotensive effect of these two lipids occurs without altering renal function or raising plasma renin [56], but the pressor activity of noradrenaline, angiotensin II, and vasopressin is markedly reduced [138]. ANRL has been obtained from renal venous blood immediately after unclipping a one kidney, one clip hypertensive rat or rabbit [69]. The amount of ANRL obtained at this time is much higher than that obtained from the renal veins of a sham-operated animal, which is the same concentration as vena caval blood. The sudden release of a hypotensive material from a clipped kidney on removal of the clip has also been demonstrated by extracorporeal perfusion of an isolated clipped kidney via an extracorporeal pump perfusion circuit in conscious normotensive rats. On removing the renal artery clip there is a significant fall in pressure of the normotensive rats from 125 mm Hg to 70 mm Hg within an hour without an associated rise in heart rate. The sudden appearance of ANRL in the renal venous blood as the blood pressure is falling is associated with an acute degranulation of the renomedullary interstitial cells of the kidney that has just been unclipped. It is concluded that the acutely released ANRL into the general circulation after unclipping the renal artery is an important factor in the fall of arterial pressure, which occurs for about 24 hours after the clip is removed. Maintenance of the low arterial pressure subsequently appears to be due to other mechanisms. Several additional observations reinforce this conclusion. For instance, it has been shown that release of a renal arterial clip in an animal in which the ureters have been implanted into the vena cava is associated with the usual fall in arterial pressure although sodium and water balance remains unchanged. In contrast, release of the clip in a hypertensive animal in which the renal papilla has been ablated chemically does not result in the usual fall of arterial pressure within the next 2 to 3 hours [136, 137].

The factors that control the release of the renal medullary hypotensive substances are not clear. What evidence there is suggests that during those forms of experimental hypertension that have been studied, the release of these hormones from the medulla is diminished. In the one clip, two kidney model of hypertension it appears that the unclipped kidney is failing to secrete its hypotensive hormones, because the arterial pressure can be lowered not only by removing the clip from the renal artery but also by removing the clipped kidney [137, 164]. The fall in arterial pressure occurs even if the animal is maintained in positive sodium balance. Therefore, the unclipped kidney has the power to reduce the blood pressure, and in some way this power is being prevented by the presence of the clipped kidney. To explain the inability of the unclipped or untouched kidney to prevent hypertension it has been proposed that the clipped kidney antagonizes the antihypertensive function of the opposite unclipped kidney.

Some observations suggest that this antagonism might be due to an inhibiting effect of the angiotensin II released by the clipped kidney. A bolus of the converting enzyme inhibitor captopril to the hypertensive one clip, two kidney rat often causes a transient depressor effect without a rise in heart rate [136, 137, 139], a response that is similar to that caused by the antihypertensive neutral renomedullary lipid (ANRL). This suggests that reducing the circulating concentration of angiotensin II stimulates release of the hypotensive lipids from the medulla. In addition, captopril increases the accumulation of large lipid granules of renomedullary interstitial cells [160]. Accordingly, angiotensin II and ANRL may be linked in a reciprocal manner as depicted in Fig. 53-5.

Renomedullary Interstitial Cells in Dahl Salt-Sensitive and Salt-Resistant Rats. The renomedullary interstitial cells of the salt-resistant rat are large, more numerous, and have prominent lipid granules, whereas the cells of the salt-sensitive rats are small, rounded, less numerous, and have fewer granules [184]. It is fascinating that these differences remain after multiple passages in cell cultures, suggesting that they are genetically determined. It is possible, therefore, that the salt-resistant rat's resistance to hypertension resides in having renal medullary interstitial cells that are more efficient at lowering the blood pressure, whereas the salt-sensitive rat has interstitial cells that are less efficient. This hypothesis suggests another possible genetic renal abnormality, in addition to those discussed earlier, in relation to the kidney's capacity to excrete sodium. It is, of course, compatible with the observation in cross-transplantation experiments in Dahl-strain rats that the blood pressure of the recipient rat is determined by the origin of the donor kidney. It is

Fig. 53-5. Relation of angiotensin II, sympathetic activity, vascular function, salt intake, urinary sodium excretion, and medullary vasodilatation. ANRL = antihypertensive neutral renomedullary lipid; APRL = antihypertensive polar renomedullary lipid. (From E. C. Muirhead and J. A. Pitcock. *J. Hypertension* 3:1, 1984; with permission.)

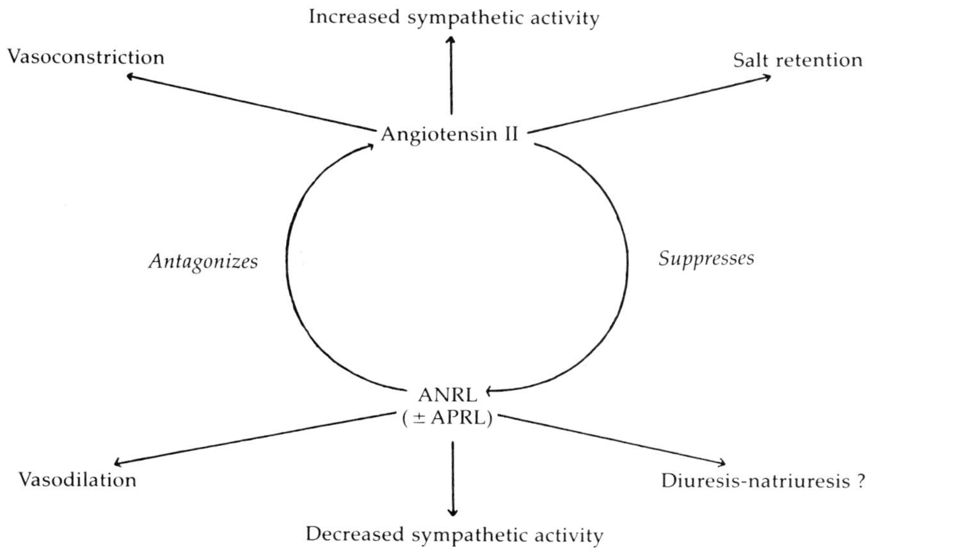

interesting to speculate whether these abnormalities of the medullary interstitial cells, which lie alongside the collecting ducts, might also impair the collecting ducts' control of sodium excretion. It will be remembered (see above) that inherited hypertension in the rat appears to be associated with diminished delivery of sodium into the distal nephron that is not compensated for normally, suggesting that there is an abnormality of the collecting duct.

RENAL CONTROL OF INTERSTITIAL SPACE COMPLIANCE

The compliance of the interstitial space determines the proportion of the extracellular fluid volume that is apportioned between the plasma and the interstitial space. Interstitial space compliance, therefore, is one determinant of blood volume, and blood volume, more particularly its distribution, is an important factor in the control of arterial pressure.

An index of the compliance of the interstitial space can be obtained by measuring the ratio of the plasma volume (PV) to the portion of the extracellular fluid volume (ECFV) that lies in the interstitial space (i.e., the interstitial fluid volume [IFV]); thus, IFV = ECFV − PV. Interstitial space compliance can also be assessed by measuring changes in interstitial fluid pressure, particularly during an acute infusion of saline. To maintain constant extracellular fluid osmolality, it is probable that changes in interstitial space compliance (i.e., its swelling to pressure characteristics) are accompanied by a change in the capacity of the space to bind sodium. Hyaluronic acid molecules can bind large amounts of sodium ions [146]. Changes in interstitial tissue compliance and its ability to bind sodium therefore probably represent a physiologic way to store water and sodium. These mechanisms can be demonstrated in some animals adapted to withstand heat and dehydration. There are studies of changes in body water and electrolytes after water deprivation and heat stress in Somali donkeys and Zebu cattle, animals that live under desert conditions for several days without drinking [108]. Donkeys lose up to 21 percent of body water and 29 percent of extracellular fluid but up to only 14 percent of plasma volume, while serum sodium concentration increases by only 7 percent. They can then drink large amounts of water and restore their total body water deficiency in a few minutes while serum sodium falls by only 5 percent [116].

The following observations suggest that the kidney controls the compliance of the interstitial space. Plasma volume–extracellular fluid volume ratio increases significantly more after bilateral nephrectomy than after unilateral nephrectomy and placement of the remaining ureter in the inferior vena cava. The interstitial pressure rises more after bilateral nephrectomy, though there is greater expansion of the interstitial fluid volume after unilateral nephrectomy and placement of the remaining ureter in the vena cava [57, 108, 109]. Interstitial space compliance was measured by measuring changes in IFV volume and tissue pressure 10 minutes after a saline infusion (compliance = IFV/TP, where TP = tissue pressure). After unilateral nephrectomy and placing the remaining ureter in the vena cava there was little change in compliance from values obtained after unilateral nephrectomy alone; following bilateral nephrectomy, however, compliance fell several-fold. Similar observations have been made 60 days after partial constriction of one renal artery with a clip and removal of the opposite kidney. Tissue pressure and venous pressure were significantly higher in rats that developed hypertension; in these animals plasma volume also increased, but interstitial fluid volume remained unchanged (i.e., the plasma volume to interstitial fluid volume [PV/IFV] ratio was higher). After removal of the clip, tissue pressure fell despite a rise in interstitial fluid volume, and there was a fall in PV/IFV.

A study of patients with chronic renal failure has yielded similar results [97]. Patients were divided into two groups, one with glomerular filtration rates greater than 32 ml per minute and the other with filtration rates less than 20 ml per minute. The PV/IFV ratio of the group with the lower glomerular filtration rates was significantly higher than that in the group with the higher filtration rate. On increasing salt intake, the PV/IFV ratio of the group with the lower glomerular filtration rose still higher, whereas in the patients with the higher filtration rate the ratio did not change. It was also noted that the associated rise in blood pressure induced by the increase in salt intake was directly related to the change in the PV/IFV ratio. In other words, the lower the renal mass, the less the compliance of the interstitial fluid space, so that with increasing sodium intake and the tendency to retain sodium (and water) associated with a reduced renal mass, a larger proportion of the extracellular fluid volume is apportioned to the plasma volume. The greater the plasma volume, the higher the arterial pressure, possibly through the mechanisms discussed earlier.

The nature of the substance responsible for the change in interstitial space compliance is not known. The experiments demonstrating its presence make it unlikely that the concentration of the substance is dependent on the excretory function of the kidney or on the kidney's ability to secrete renin. It is probable that it is a hormone, the rate of release of which is dependent on the amount of renal mass and its effective perfusion with blood.

Inherited Hypertension and the Kidney

Inherited hypertension in humans is usually called *essential hypertension.* There are several genetic strains of hypertensive rats; the name given to each usually stems from some historical or geographic association.

ESSENTIAL HYPERTENSION

Renal Function Abnormality. PRIMARY ABNORMALITY. The evidence suggesting that there is an inherited renal abnormality that impairs the urinary excretion of sodium has been discussed earlier.

SECONDARY ABNORMALITIES—BEFORE THE RISE IN ARTERIAL PRESSURE. The earliest changes in renal function are presumably induced by the difficulty in excreting sodium. They have been studied before the rise in arterial pressure in normotensive children of hypertensive parents. The most convincing studies have been done on normotensive children, both of whose parents had hypertension [11]. In such children renal blood flow and glomerular filtration rate are raised, while plasma renin activity is decreased. There is also a reduced urinary kallikrein excretion. The urinary response to intravenous sodium loads is also abnormal. If the saline is given rapidly (2 liters in 1 hour), the immediate rise in urinary sodium excretion that occurs is more extensive than that seen in children of normotensive parents (the phenomenon of accelerated natriuresis) [191].

IN THE EARLY HYPERTENSIVE STAGE. Changes in renal function due to hypertension have to be distinguished from those due to age and previous antihypertensive therapy. The following observations apply to patients below the age of 35 in whom these two variables have been excluded. Renal blood flow in such patients ranges from above normal to below normal [11, 100]. Interestingly, patients with the higher flows are not different in regard to age or duration of hypertension, but they do have significantly stronger family histories and are predominantly male, and their blood pressures are significantly lower. The whole group tends to have lower plasma renin activity, and in those with the higher renal blood flows the plasma renin activity is significantly lower than in the others. Glomerular filtration rate in early hypertension is usually in the normal range.

The phenomenon of accelerated natriuresis following a rapid intravenous sodium load is more pronounced than that seen in normotensive children of hypertensive parents, and the natriuresis is greatest in those with the lowest plasma renin activity [169]. The accelerated natriuresis is unrelated to changes in peritubular capillary hydrostatic or colloid osmotic pressure [193]. The phenomenon of accelerated natriuresis is highly suggestive of a state in which there is a continuing need to oppose a persistent tendency to retain sodium. It occurs in primary hyperaldosteronism [15] and in normal subjects given aldosterone, even when, as in essential hypertension, there is no measurable increase in extracellular fluid volume [163].

IN THE LATER STAGES OF HYPERTENSION. The decrease in renal blood flow with age is more rapid in patients with essential hypertension and becomes inversely related to the height of the blood pressure. There seems to be no further impairment of renal blood flow when the mean arterial pressure rises to more than 140 mm Hg unless malignant hypertension supervenes [100].

Glomerular filtration rate, in contrast to renal blood flow, tends to be well maintained until a late stage in the disease, though a rapid decline is often seen in malignant hypertension. The relative constancy of the filtration rate in the face of a falling plasma flow results in a rise in filtration fraction (i.e., that proportion of the renal plasma flow that is filtered through the glomeruli is increased) [100]. The exact mechanism responsible for this phenomenon is not known. Plasma renin activity in essential hypertension is inversely related to the arterial pressure but rises steeply in malignant hypertension [124]. Furthermore, in hypertensive patients with normal or low plasma renin, the rise in plasma renin with fluid deprivation is significantly less than that seen in normal subjects. Renal kallikrein excretion and prostaglandin production are reduced [117, 178]. In addition to the phenomenon of accelerated natriuresis, which also occurs at this later stage of hypertension, there are two further abnormalities of urinary sodium excretion—(1) an inverse diurnal rhythm in which the amounts of sodium excreted at night exceed the amount excreted during the day [103], and (2) the phenomenon of emotional natriuresis, in which a minor emotional stimulus causes a large sustained increase in sodium and water [128, 129]. It is interesting that all these abnormalities in urinary sodium excretion also occur in primary aldosteronism, which supports the proposal that their cause, in essential hypertension, derives from an impaired ability to excrete sodium that imposes a continuing need to oppose a tendency to volume expansion.

RAT STRAINS OF INHERITED HYPERTENSION

In general, the abnormalities of urinary sodium excretion described in patients with essential hypertension are also found in the inherited forms of hypertension in the rat. The Dahl salt-sensitive hypertensive rat has, by definition, an impaired ability to excrete sodium and a persistently low plasma renin value. On a normal sodium intake, however, the blood pressure tends to be normal. In the Milan [10] and Heidelberg [47] hypertensive strain rats there is a transient period ending about the sixth to the seventh week of life when the fractional excretion of sodium is lower, the cumulative retention of sodium is greater, and plasma renin activity is lower in the hypertensive strain than in the control normotensive rat. At the end of this period, the blood pressure of the hypertensive strain rat has risen considerably. The phenomenon of accelerated natriuresis is prominent in inherited hypertensive strains of rats and occurs, as in humans, both before and after the rise in arterial pressure [9, 194]. As in humans, it has been shown that the phenomenon of accelerated natriuresis in rats is unrelated to changes in peritubular capillary hydrostatic or colloid osmotic pressure [194].

Hypotheses on the Mechanism Responsible for the Rise in Pressure in Inherited Forms of Hypertension. The complexity of the subject, the number of variables involved in the control of normal blood pressure, and the numerous abnormalities that can be found in essential hypertension have given rise to the concept that essential hypertension is a multifactorial disease, implying that it may arise from several different primary causes. This convenient semantic refuge has diminished tension between the proponents of the various hypotheses advanced to explain the origins of essential hypertension, but its wholehearted acceptance tends to have a stultifying and inhibitory effect.

It is interesting that the two main proposals first suggested over 100 years ago to explain the primary mechanism responsible for a rise in arterial pressure still flourish—on the one hand, that the rise in pressure is due to some circulating substance, and on the other, that it is primarily due to a thickening of the arterial wall. It is possible that both these proposals are correct in that there is now evidence that in essential hypertension the plasma contains substances that in addition to influencing sodium transport and vascular reactivity may also increase vascular wall thickening [70]. This observation has been obtained in vessels of hypertensive animals that are not exposed to the raised arterial pressure (e.g., veins [70] and arteries below an experimentally induced lesion similar to that of a coarcted aorta [150]). Borst and Borst de Geus's [19] proposal that the primary abnormality in essential hypertension is an abnormal kidney that has an "unwillingness to excrete sodium" has also survived. If, as is likely, this turns out to be the truth, there would then be little difference between essential hypertension as described by Mahomed, in which the kidneys do not appear to be particularly affected, and the hypertension that follows gross renal disease as described by Bright. The only difference between "primary" hypertension (essential) and "secondary" hypertension would then be that in one the renal abnormality is inherited and difficult to detect and in the other it is acquired and conspicuous.

Two hypotheses have been suggested to explain how a congenital abnormality of the kidney's ability to excrete sodium might cause the arterial pressure to rise.

THE GUYTON HYPOTHESIS. It has been proposed that owing to the kidney's impaired ability to excrete sodium there are recurrent transient rises in fluid volume and central venous pressure that give rise to transient rises in cardiac output that raise the arterial pressure. After a few days the cardiac output returns to normal, but the arterial pressure now remains raised because of a rise in peripheral arterial resistance. It is suggested that the rise in peripheral arterial resistance is due to the arteriolar structural wall thickening that was induced by the initial phase of hypertension associated with the high cardiac output. Furthermore, it is proposed that the arterial pressure rises in order to induce some change in the kidney that will result in an increase in urinary sodium excretion. In this way, the initial retention of sodium is corrected and the patient returns to normal sodium balance but at a new point of equilibrium in the renal perfusion pressure to urinary sodium excretion relationship [78].

It is unfortunate that this alleged *structural* response of the arteriolar wall to a rise in arterial pressure has sometimes been referred to as an *autoregulatory* phenomenon. By usage, the term *circulatory autoregulation* is usually confined to the immediate *functional* response of a vascular bed to a change in perfusion pressure (i.e., when a sudden rise in arterial pressure causes within the next few seconds a rapid vasoconstriction that tends to prevent a change in blood flow).

There are so many examples of transitory spontaneous rises in cardiac output unaccompanied by a rise in arterial pressure that one questions whether a rise in cardiac output per se can cause a rise in arterial pressure [51]. Cardiac output can be increased experimentally in animals by a variety of procedures without producing chronic hypertension. In addition, the observation that in several long-term clinical and experimental forms of hypertension associated with severe structural changes the blood pressure returns to normal within minutes or hours of removal of the causal factor is difficult to reconcile with the proposition that structural changes in the arteries per se can cause a persistent rise in arterial pressure [65].

THE CONCEPT OF THE "NATRIURETIC HORMONE" AND INHERITED HYPERTENSION (ESSENTIAL HYPERTENSION AND THE VARIOUS HYPERTENSIVE STRAINS OF RATS). In this hypothesis it is proposed that in essential hypertension the congenitally abnormal kidney's difficulty in excreting sodium causes a persistent rise in the concentration of certain substances in the plasma that normally only rise when there is a tendency for the blood volume to increase [45, 80]. It is suggested that although these substances may succeed in keeping the blood volume normal, their persistently raised levels eventually cause the blood pressure to rise. The substances referred to are those responsible for the natriuretic capacity of the plasma, the plasma's ability to inhibit Na-K-ATPase activity, and the plasma's ability to control vascular reactivity. (These three phenomena are often referred to as being due to the "natriuretic hormone" as if they were all due to changes in the concentration of only one substance.)

There appear to be several Na-K-ATPase inhibitors. Using standard techniques, several different substances are being isolated. Ouabain itself has been identified in human plasma [118]. It is not yet known whether its concentration is raised in hypertension and volume expansion. Using a cytochemical bioassay, the plasma of patients with essential hypertension [113], of the SHR rat [132], and of the Milan hypertensive rat [87] contains a greatly increased capacity to inhibit Na-K-ATPase. There is also evidence suggesting that the cytochemically detectable substance originates in the hypothalamus [1, 79, 132, 135, 181] and that its concentration at this site rises with an increase in sodium intake [131, 181] and in acquired and inherited hypertension [88, 132]. It has been proposed that the raised plasma concentration may have a direct peripheral vasoconstrictive effect [18] and that the raised hypothalamic concentration may have a central hypertensinogenic effect [181]. The advantage of the cytochemical assays is that they have made it fairly certain that the substance they measure that causes the rise in the plasma's ability to inhibit Na-K-ATPase in the inherited forms of hypertension is the same substance as that which causes a similar rise in the plasma of normal subjects and animals after volume expansion. This provides additional support for the concept that in inherited hypertension there is a state of controlled volume expansion.

This concept is further supported by the observation that the plasma concentration of atrial natriuretic peptide is raised in essential hypertension and hypertensive strains of rats. There are also many observations that the plasma in inherited hypertension has an increased ability to increase vascular reactivity [127, 185]. It is theoretically possible that a Na-K-ATPase inhibitor increases vascular tone and might therefore be involved in raising the blood pressure [18], in which case a Na-K-ATPase inhibitor might be the same substance as that responsible for the increased capacity of the plasma to increase vascular reactivity; alternatively, the vascular reactivity factor may be another substance.

The main difficulty with this hypothesis is that all the substances responsible for the Na-K-ATPase inhibition and the increase in vascular reactivity have not yet been identified. Furthermore, it does not follow that because the concentration of any one of them is raised it is responsible for the rise in arterial pressure. There is a further difficulty. Blood volume in established essential hypertension and in the inherited forms of hypertension is usually normal or low, although it is raised in a minority of patients [59]. This appears inconsistent with the proposal that in essential hypertension the kidneys have a persistent difficulty in excreting sodium that leads to a persistent tendency toward volume expansion. It has been emphasized earlier, however, that in primary hyperaldosteronism, in which hypertension is certainly associated with a persistent tendency to retain sodium, the blood volume in the majority of patients is, as in essential hypertension, either normal or low [20] (Fig. 53-6). In only a minority of patients is it raised. Nevertheless, patients with essential hypertension and those with primary hyperaldosteronism both behave as if they were volume expanded. The phenomenon of accelerated natriuresis occurs in both, and the plasma of both has an increased capacity to inhibit Na-K-ATPase. The rise in

Fig. 53-6. Plasma volume values during normal dietary sodium intake in patients with primary hyperaldosteronism (1° Aldo) and essential hypertension (EH). Values are expressed as percent of normal. The cross-hatched area represents the variability of the method (that is, ± 8 percent). The open circles are primarily aldosteronism due to hyperplasia; the closed circles, aldosteronism due to adenomas. In primary aldosteronism, there were as many patients who were hypovolemic (25 percent) as there were those who were hypervolemic (30 percent). (From E. L. Bravo, R. C. Tarazi, H. A. Dustan, et al. *Am. J. Med.* 74[4]:641, 1983.)

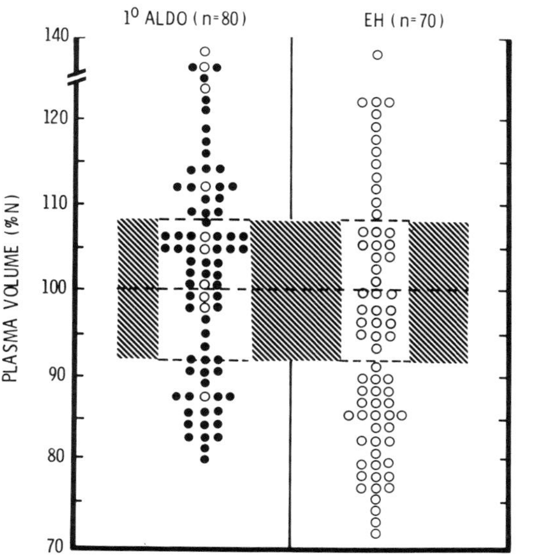

atrial natriuretic peptide in essential hypertension is certainly consistent with a central blood volume disturbance since the stimulus for the release of atrial natriuretic peptide release is distention of the auricles [46].

The discrepancy between having a normal or low total blood volume and yet responding to certain stimuli as if the blood volume were expanded is perhaps explained by the observation that in essential hypertension and in hypertensive strains of rats, there is an increase in tone of the venous vasculature with a diminished venous compliance and a shift of blood from the periphery to the thorax [166, 186]. Both in humans (M. Safar, personal communication) and the rat [159] these changes are accompanied by a rise in left auricular pressure. It is possible, therefore, that in essential hypertension a normal or even low blood volume may be associated with such a shift of blood to the chest that the intrathoracic venous pressure rises in spite of an overall fall in blood volume. This effect would be more marked if pulmonary vascular compliance were also reduced (Fig. 53-7).

OTHER POSSIBLE CONSEQUENCES OF A RAISED CONCENTRATION OF A CIRCULATING Na-K-ATPase INHIBITOR. Ouabain inhibits Na-K-ATPase in intact cells, and the documented effect it has on various organs suggests that perhaps some well-known but previously unexplained phenomena in essential hypertension may be due to a raised plasma concentration of an endogenous ouabain-like substance.

In vitro ouabain diminishes renin secretion in rat renal cortical slices [29], isolated glomeruli [8], and isolated perfused kidneys [61]. It is possible, therefore, that the low plasma renin activity in some patients with essential hypertension may be due not only to a central volume distention but also partly to the direct effect of the circulating Na-K-ATPase inhibitor. Ouabain in vitro also inhibits osteoclastic activity of parathyroid hormone. It is possible, therefore, that the slightly depressed concentration of plasma ionized calcium and raised plasma parathyroid hormone concentration claimed by some workers to occur in essential hypertension and in the SHR rat may be due to the effect of the endogenous Na-K-ATPase inhibitor on the skeleton. Ouabain in vitro increases noradrenaline output from the nerve terminal and reduces its reuptake, thus raising the amount of noradrenaline available to react with the receptor cells on the effector-cell membrane [41, 101, 143]. It is possible, therefore, that some of the changes in sympathetic activity repeatedly reported in essential hypertension and in the SHR rat are due to the raised concentration of the circulating Na-K-ATPase inhibitor. Similarly, platelets accumulate and store noradrenaline in subcellular granules in a way similar to that of neurons [156]. The high efflux rate of noradrenaline from platelets in hypertensive patients [120], or in normotensive close relatives of hypertensive patients [119], and the high intracellular ionic calcium concentration [24] may also be due to the circulating sodium transport inhibitor. Finally, potassium in concentrations within the *physiologic* range stimulates the activity of Na-K-ATPase [50], an effect opposite to that of ouabain. It is possible, therefore, that potassium lowers arterial pressure and *increases* nor-

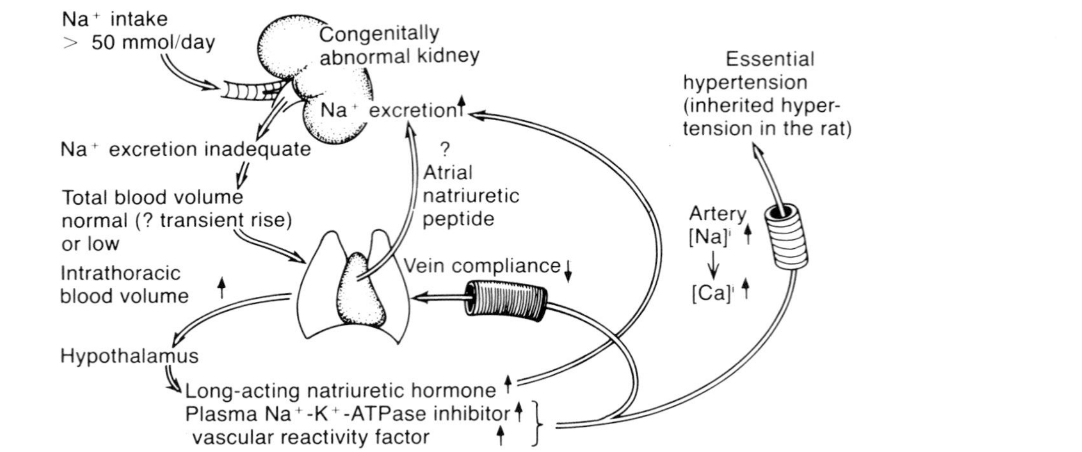

Fig. 53-7. Hypothesis explaining how a postulated inherited defect in the kidney's ability to excrete sodium (or an acquired difficulty in excreting sodium) and the dietary intake of sodium may be responsible for a rise in the plasma's natriuretic capacity and the observed increase in the plasma's ability to inhibit Na-K-ATPase activity and to increase vascular reactivity.

adrenaline uptake into the nerve terminal in inherited forms of hypertension by counteracting the effect of the raised concentration of a circulating Na-K-ATPase inhibitor.

Acquired Hypertension and the Kidney

Most of the acquired conditions that affect the kidney and produce hypertension involve a difficulty in excreting sodium; these include bilateral nephrectomy, coarctation of the aorta, diminution in renal mass, primary hyperaldosteronism, DOCA, uninephrectomy with renal artery stenosis, and uninephrectomy with perirenal fibrosis. All these conditions induce a permanent tendency for sodium retention that has to be controlled. In humans the difficulty in excreting sodium is due to disease and arises spontaneously. In animals the same conditions are imposed experimentally in order to study the mechanisms responsible for the hypertension. The commonest cause in humans is destruction of the renal parenchyma by pathologic conditions. Hyperaldosteronism in humans is usually reproduced in animals by administration of DOCA, and to speed and accentuate the process it is usual to also increase the salt intake. Coarctation of the aorta in humans can be surgically reproduced in dogs by an operation that narrows the aorta. The very rare human condition of renal artery stenosis usually occurs with a normal contralateral kidney. In animals the condition is reproduced by placing a partially constricting clip on one kidney and either leaving the other kidney intact or removing it. To accelerate the onset and increase the severity of the hypertension in such experimental maneuvers salt intake is often increased. The nearest experimental equivalent to a renin-producing tumor of the kidney is a slow chronic infusion of angiotensin II. Acromegaly is another form of hypertension with salt and water retention.

MECHANISM OF THE HYPERTENSION

Unlike the caution and reluctance with which many authorities view the relevance to essential hypertension of the information obtained from hypertensive strains of rats, there is a willingness to draw parallels between the mechanisms discovered in the many forms of experimental hypertension and their rare clinical counterparts in humans. Basically, however, it is probable that the mechanisms responsible for the rise in arterial pressure in the acquired forms of hypertension are much the same as those discussed for essential hypertension (Fig. 53-7). In general, these mechanisms tend to act for a shorter time and to be more pronounced, so that acquired hypertension develops more rapidly, and such mechanisms tend to be more obvious.

The relationship between the concentration of plasma angiotensin II and the state of fluid volume is particularly relevant in most forms of acquired hypertension. As stated earlier, in normal humans and animals there is a reciprocal relationship between, on the one hand, plasma angiotensin II and, on the other, the plasma concentration of the Na-K-ATPase inhibitor and the vascular reactivity factor. Normally, therefore, the effects of changes in blood volume or sodium intake on the arterial pressure are nicely balanced. Though blood volume expansion induces a marked fall in angiotensin II, it increases its effectiveness, so that the blood pressure shows only a mild change, while a contraction of the blood volume increases angiotensin II but reduces its effect.

With renal disease these relationships may become distorted and can then cause serious disturbances in blood pressure. Eighty percent of patients with diseased kidneys have a tendency to be volume expanded, while the distortion and architectural compression of the renal vascular tree causes a simultaneous *rise* in plasma renin activity and angiotensin II. This is the worst of all worlds. Because of the tendency toward volume expansion there is an *increased* vascular response to the *raised* levels of angiotensin II, presumably because of the associated rise in plasma Na-K-ATPase inhibitor and vascular reactivity factor. This is presumably why in most patients with chronic renal failure the blood pressure rises early, quickly, and often to heights that cause severe complications.

In primary hyperaldosteronism there is a persistent restraint on urinary sodium excretion. In experimental animals given DOCA or fludrocortisone or following a renal artery stenosis it can be shown that initially there is a brief period of positive sodium balance with a gain in weight, but it is usual for the weight gain to level out and then be restored to near its control value [14, 99, 174]. Edema does not occur. As in essential hypertension, systemic venous compliance diminishes, and there is also a tendency for the central blood volume to rise [147, 174, 196]. Edema does not form. Blood volume, like that in essential hypertension, tends to be normal or low or is raised in only a minority of patients [14, 174]. Total exchangeable sodium tends to be raised [14, 99]. Plasma renin is reduced, and it is possible that the hypertension is mainly due to the raised level of Na-K-ATPase inhibitor [81] and vascular reactivity factor [85, 127], but there is still insufficient information on this point.

In unilateral renal artery stenosis with the other kidney in situ plasma renin activity rises, and there is an initial sodium retention. Then, as mentioned earlier, the blood pressure rises, and sodium balance is adjusted by increasing the excretion of sodium through the unclipped kidney, perhaps because of the rise in arterial pressure but more probably because of a rise in central blood volume and an increase in plasma natriuretic activity. Then there is a continued rise in plasma renin that can be demonstrated to be an important cause of the rise in arterial pressure. With renal artery stenosis of a sole remaining kidney the eventual outcome is a tendency toward salt and water retention and a fall in plasma renin, so that the main hypertensive mechanisms are related to the volume retention.

HYPERTENSION AND DIALYSIS

Most patients on maintenance hemodialysis continue to fight a relentless battle against hypertension [43]. The mechanisms responsible for the rise in pressure are the same as those that caused the rise in pressure before dialysis, but now they are magnified and tend to be glaringly obvious. This is the reason why nephrologists have no difficulty in accepting the role of volume changes in the control of blood pressure. On the one hand, the gross reduction in daily urine volume inevitably causes a rapid increase in extracellular fluid volume between each dialysis (easily monitored as a gain in weight), and on the other hand, the severely diseased kidneys tend to secrete large amounts of renin. Furthermore, the need to lower the patient's weight at each dialysis by rapidly removing a considerable amount of fluid may cause a further brisk rise in plasma renin activity [22]. If this recurring see-saw reciprocal movement

Fig. 53-8. The effect of bilateral nephrectomy (B) on uncontrollable hypertension in a patient on maintenance hemodialysis with a very high plasma renin. There is an immediate fall in blood pressure, which is maintained though there is a rise in weight. At point (A) the patient had an attack of acute infectious hepatitis. (From J. J. Curtis, Lever, Robertson, et al. *Nephron* 6:329, 1969.)

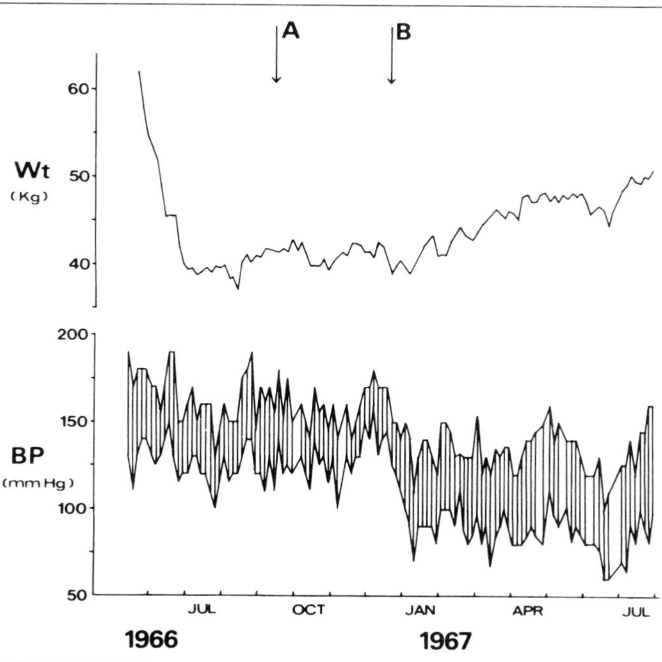

of extracellular fluid volume and renin release is sufficiently violent it eventually seems to resonate. Then the more one attempts to control the blood pressure by fluid removal, the greater the rise in renin and angiotensin II, so that at each dialysis the blood pressure, instead of falling, rises and becomes uncontrollable (Fig. 53-8). In one patient, in an attempt to control the hypertension, the weight was lowered from 60 kg to 40 kg in about 2 months [22]. This so reduced the extracellular fluid and blood volume that the patient fainted when he stood up, but his renin secretion was now so great that when he lay down he had severe hypertension with intolerable headaches and a tendency to develop acute pulmonary edema. The problem was resolved by bilateral nephrectomy, an operation that is now rarely performed to control hypertension.

Such cases are now rarely seen. Weight reductions are performed with more circumspection. By using measurements before and immediately after a dialysis, of blood volume, extracellular fluid volume, plasma renin activity, and substances that nullify the pressor effect of angiotensin II, it is now possible to show that hypertension in patients on maintenance hemodialysis is either volume dependent, angiotensin II dependent, or sometimes a combination of both.

In Fig. 53-9 is illustrated the findings in a patient whose blood pressure was volume dependent. Before dialysis, when the blood pressure was 200/100 mm Hg,

Fig. 53-9. Patient on maintenance hemodialysis with hypertension due to excess volume. Blood pressure (BP), weight, total blood volume (TBV), extracellular water (ECW), plasma renin activity (PRA), and the effect of an infusion of saralasin on the blood pressure, measured before and after the loss of 9.5 kg of weight in 17 days, are shown. Saralasin, a competitor of angiotensin II, was infused to gauge the dependency of the blood pressure on angiotensin II. On the first occasion, when the blood pressure was 200/100 mm Hg, the blood volume was obviously high, and there was a gross expansion of extracellular water, plasma renin activity was abnormally low, and the lack of effect of the infusion of saralasin on the blood pressure indicated that the blood pressure was not dependent on the plasma level of angiotensin II. On the second occasion, after the loss of weight, when the blood pressure was 128/78 mm Hg, blood volume, extracellular water, and plasma renin activity were now normal, and the saralasin infusion again demonstrated that the blood pressure was not dependent on angiotensin II.

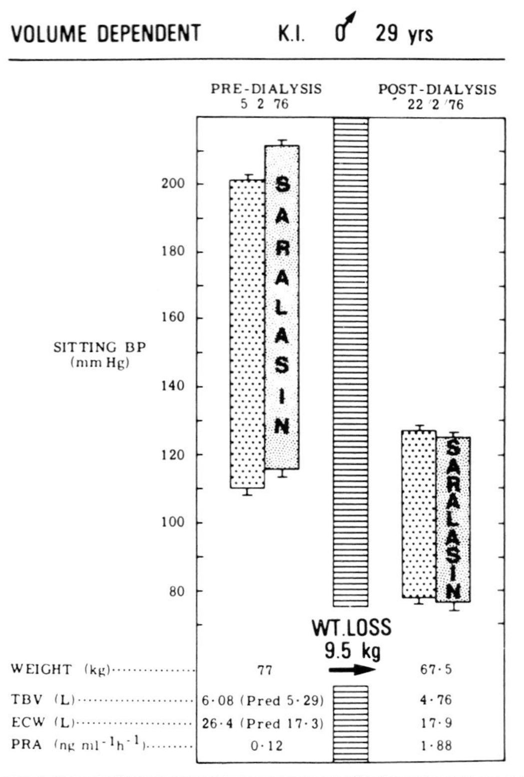

Fig. 53-10. Patient on maintenance hemodialysis with hypertension due to high plasma renin activity. Blood pressure (BP), weight, total blood volume (TBV), extracellular water (ECW), plasma renin activity (PRA), and the effect of an infusion of saralasin on the blood pressure measured before and after a loss of 2.5 kg of weight during a single dialysis of 7 hours are shown. Saralasin, a competitor of angiotensin II, was infused to gauge the dependency of the blood pressure on angiotensin II. Before dialysis, when the blood pressure was 180/100 mm Hg, the blood volume was normal, though the extracellular water was 2.5 kg greater than predicted (a not unusual gain in weight between dialyses), plasma renin activity was greatly raised, and the fall in blood pressure induced by the infusion of saralasin indicated that the blood pressure was under the influence of angiotensin II. After dialysis, having lost a "normal" amount of weight, the blood pressure was 170/95 mm Hg, the blood volume and extracellular water were normal, but the plasma renin activity was now extremely high, and the greater fall in blood pressure induced by saralasin infusion indicated that the blood pressure was even more dependent on angiotensin II.

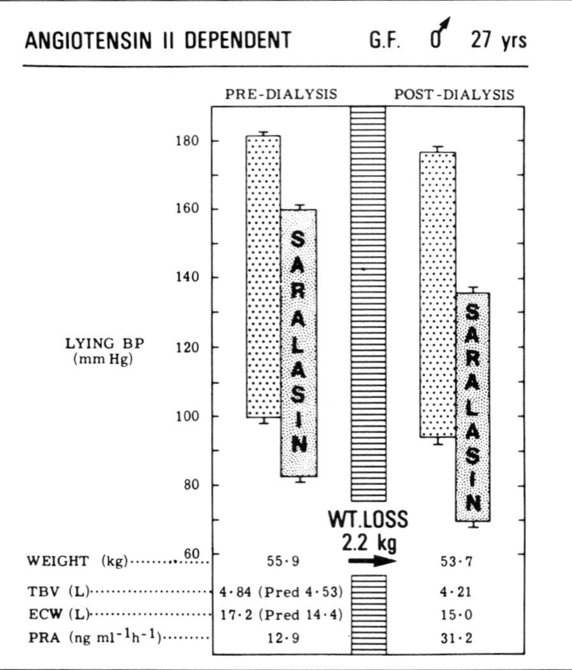

the blood volume was obviously high, and there was a gross expansion of extracellular water while plasma renin activity was abnormally low, and the lack of effect of an intravenous infusion of saralasin (a competitor of angiotensin II) on the blood pressure indicated that the blood pressure was not dependent on the plasma level of angiotensin II. After several dialyses, the patient lost 9.5 kg when the blood pressure was 128/78 mm Hg, and the blood volume, extracellular fluid volume, and plasma renin activity became normal, and the saralasin infusion again demonstrated that the blood pressure was not dependent on angiotensin II. It has recently been shown that after a dialysis that involves a loss of weight the plasma's capacity to inhibit Na-K-ATPase, which is raised initially, falls to normal.

In Fig. 53-10 are illustrated the findings in a patient in whom the blood pressure was dependent on a raised level of angiotensin II. Before dialysis, when the blood pressure was 180/100 mm Hg, the blood volume was normal, plasma renin activity was greatly raised, and the fall in pressure induced by saralasin indicated that the blood pressure was under the influence of angiotensin II. After a dialysis the patient lost 2.2 kg, the blood pressure fell to 170/95 mm Hg, the blood volume was still "normal" but the plasma renin activity was now extremely high, and the greater fall in blood pressure induced by the saralasin infusion indicated that the blood pressure was even more dependent on angiotensin II.

Renal Hypotension

Renal hypotension is a rare complication of some forms of renal disease and usually follows bilateral nephrectomy. The renal diseases that are most prone to this unusual complication are those that affect predominantly the renal medulla (e.g., reflux nephropathy, obstructive uropathy, and phenacetin nephropathy). Though the condition is sometimes referred to as *salt-losing nephritis*, it is rarely due to glomerular nephritis. The fall in arterial pressure is due to a urinary leak of sodium and occurs only with bilateral renal disease after the onset of renal failure. It is associated with a gross generalized hypertrophy of the juxtaglomerular apparati and the adrenals. Plasma renin activity and aldosterone are raised. Often there is hypokalemia due in part to the hyperaldosteronism and in part to the renal disease. The condition tends to fluctuate wildly. Exacerbations are often caused by an upper urinary tract infection when the combination of infection, hypotension, a fall in extracellular fluid volume, and hypokalemia may cause severe but usually entirely and easily reversible reductions in renal function. In spite of these alarming episodes these patients survive longer than other patients with renal failure whose progress is calmer but who develop hypertension. Survival of patients with renal hypotension depends on the skill and speed of reaction of those who look after them. The continuous administration of oral supplements of sodium chloride such as Slow Sodium (Ciba), repeated monitoring of the urine for infection, and prompt treatment of a relapse may prevent any progressive deterioration in renal function.

Renal hypotension is such a serious and frequent complication of the anephric state that, together with the accompanying extremely severe anemia, in which hemoglobin concentrations are often below 5 gm per deciliter, bilateral nephrectomy is no longer used for the treatment of intractable hypertension in patients on maintenance hemodialysis. After bilateral nephrectomy the relation between the arterial pressure and the blood volume is such that the volume has to be much greater than normal to maintain a normal blood pressure [43] (Fig. 53-11). Many anephric patients therefore live precarious lives of fluctuating hypotension in spite of an overexpanded extracellular fluid volume, sometimes to the point of demonstrable clinical edema and breathlessness. The low arterial pressure is presumably due primarily to the almost total absence of renin and angiotensin II, but there is suggestive evidence that it may also be due in part to the associated reduction in plasma aldosterone.

These two forms of hypotension beautifully illustrate the interdependence of angiotensin and extracellular fluid volume, and possibly therefore of the circulating sodium transport inhibitor, in the control of blood pressure. On the one hand, in "salt-losing nephritis" the urinary leak of sodium and the decrease in extracellular fluid volume are so great that the arterial pressure falls in spite of enormous rises in plasma renin activity. On the other hand, in the absence of angiotensin, gross overexpansion of the extracellular fluid volume barely prevents the arterial pressure from being intolerably low. Some workers have claimed that the relationship between fluid volume and arterial pressure after bilateral nephrectomy depends on whether the patient suffered from hypertension before the operation. Occasionally, amyloidosis of the sympathetic chains causes

Fig. 53-11. Blood volume versus mean lying blood pressure in patients on maintenance hemodialysis. At normal blood volumes the blood pressure of anephric patients (●) was lower than in patients whose kidneys were still in situ (○).

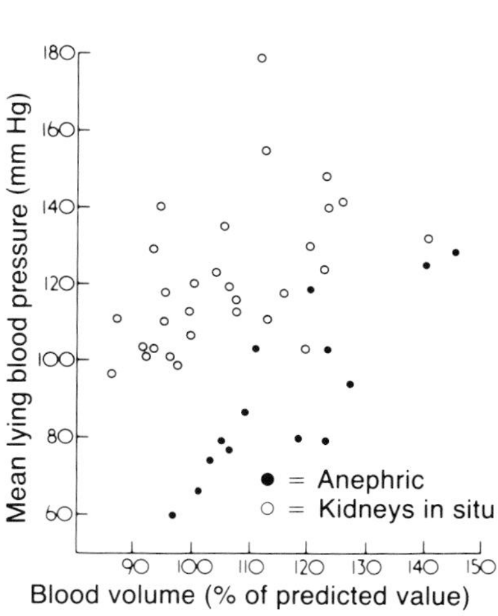

hypotension in a patient on dialysis. This is an intractable and irreversible condition that leads to endless difficulties and to death.

References

1. Alaghband-Zadeh, J., Fenton, S., Hancock, K., et al. Evidence that the hypothalamus may be a source of a circulating Na-K-ATPase inhibitor. *J. Endocrinol.* 98: 221, 1983.
2. Allen, F. M., and Cope, O. M. Influence of diet on blood pressure and kidney size in dogs. *J. Urol.* 47: 751, 1942.
3. Ambard, L., and Beaujard, E. Causes de l'hypertension arterielle. *Arch. Gen. Med.* 1: 520, 1904.
4. Ames, R. P., Borkowski, A. J., Sicinski, A. M., et al. Prolonged infusions of angiotensin II and norepinephrine and blood pressure, electrolyte balance, and aldosterone and cortisol secretion in normal man and in cirrhosis with ascites. *J. Clin. Invest.* 44: 1171, 1965.
5. Aperia, A. C., Broberger, C. G. O., and Soderlund, S. Relationship between renal artery perfusion pressure and tubular sodium reabsorption. *Am. J. Physiol.* 220: 1205, 1971.
6. Baer, P. G., and Bianchi, G. Renal micropuncture study of normotensive and Milan hypertensive rats before and after development of hypertension. *Kidney Int.* 13: 452, 1978.
7. Barajas, L. Anatomy of the juxtaglomerular apparatus. *Am. J. Physiol.* 237: F333, 1979.
8. Baumbach, L., and Skott, O. Renin release from isolated rat glomeruli. Seasonal variations and effects of D600 on the response to calcium deprivation. *J. Physiol.* 310: 285, 1981.
9. Ben-Ishay, D., Knudsen, K. D., and Dahl, L. K. Exaggerated response to isotonic saline loading in genetically hypertension prone rats. *J. Lab. Clin. Med.* 82: 597, 1973.
10. Bianchi, G., Baer, P. G., Fox, U., et al. The role of the kidney in the rat with genetic hypertension. *Postgrad. Med. J.* 53 (Suppl. 2): 123, 1977.
11. Bianchi, G., and Barlassina, C. Renal Function in Essential Hypertension. In J. Genest, O. Kuchel, P. Hamet, et al. (eds.), *Hypertension.* New York: McGraw Hill, 1983. P. 54.
12. Bianchi, G., Fox, U., Di Francesco, G. F., et al. The hypertensive role of the kidney in spontaneously hypertensive rats. *Clin. Sci. Mol. Med.* 45: 135s, 1973.
13. Bianchi, G., Fox, U., Di Francesco, G. F., et al. Blood pressure changes produced by kidney cross transplantation between spontaneously hypertensive rats and normotensive rats. *Clin. Sci. Mol. Med.* 47: 435, 1974.
14. Bianchi, G., Tilde-Tenconi, L., and Lucca, R. Effect in the conscious dog of constriction of the renal artery to a sole remaining kidney on haemodynamics, sodium balance, body fluid volumes, plasma renin concentration and pressor responsiveness to angiotensin. *Clin. Sci.* 38: 741, 1970.
15. Biglieri, E. G., and McIlroy, M. B. Abnormalities of renal function and circulatory reflexes in primary aldosteronism. *Circulation* 33: 78, 1966.
16. Bing, R. F., Russell, G. I., Swales, J. D., et al. Chemical renal medullectomy; effect upon reversal of two-kidney, one-clip hypertension in the rat. *Clin. Sci.* 61: 335s, 1981.
17. Blake, W. D., Wegria, R., Ward, H. P., et al. Effect of renal arterial constriction on excretion of sodium and water. *Am. J. Physiol.* 163: 422, 1950.
18. Blaustein, M. P. Sodium ions, calcium ions, blood pressure regulation and hypertension: a reassessment and a hypothesis. *Am. J. Physiol.* 232(3): C165, 1977.
19. Borst, J. G. G., and Borst de Geus, A. Hypertension explained by Starling's theory of circulatory homeostasis. *Lancet* 1: 677, 1963.
20. Bravo, E. L., Tarazi, R. C., Dustan, H. P., et al. The changing clinical spectrum of primary aldosteronism. *Am. J. Med.* 74(4): 641, 1983.
21. Bright, T. Tubular view of the morbid appearance in 100 cases connected with albuminous urine. With observations. *Guy's Hosp. Rep.* I: 380, 1836.
22. Brown, J. J., Curtis, J. R., Lever, A. F., et al. Plasma renin concentration and the control of blood pressure in patients on maintenance haemodialysis. *Nephron* 6: 329, 1969.
23. Brunner, H. R., Chang, P., Wallach, R., et al. Angiotensin II vascular receptors: Their avidity in relationship to sodium balance, the autonomic nervous system, and hypertension. *J. Clin. Invest.* 51: 58, 1972.
24. Bruschi, G., Bruschi, M. E., Caroppo, M., et al. Cytoplasmic free [Ca2 +] is increased in the platelets of spontaneously hypertensive rats and essential hypertensive patients. *Clin. Sci.* 68: 179, 1985.
25. Buckalew, V. M., Martinez, F. J., and Green, W. E. The effect of dialysates and ultrafiltrates of plasma of saline loaded dogs on toad bladder sodium transport. *J. Clin. Invest.* 49: 926, 1970.
26. Burstyn, P., Hornall, D., and Watchorn, C. Sodium and potassium intake and blood pressure. *Br. Med. J.* 2: 537, 1980.
27. Carvalho, J. J. M., Baruzzi, R. G., Howard, P. F., et al. Blood pressure in four remote populations in the Intersalt Study. *Hypertension* 14: 238, 1989.
28. Cherchovich, G. M., Capek, K., Jefremova, Z., et al. High salt intake and blood pressure in lower primates. *J. Appl. Physiol.* 40: 601, 1976.
29. Churchill, M. C., and Churchill, P. C. Separate and combined effects of ouabain and extracellular potassium on renin secretion from rat renal cortical slices. *J. Physiol.* 300: 105, 1980.
30. Clarkson, E. M., Talner, L. B., and de Wardener, H. E. The effect of plasma from blood volume expanded dogs on sodium, potassium and PAH transport of renal tubule fragments. *Clin. Sci.* 38: 617, 1970.
31. Cooper, R., van Horn, L., Liu, K., et al. Randomised trial on the effect of decreased dietary sodium intake on blood pressure in adolescence. *J. Hypertens.* 2: 361, 1984.
32. Curtis, J. J., Luke, R. G., Dustan, H. P., et al. Remission of essential hypertension after renal transplantation. *N. Engl. J. Med.* 309: 1009, 1983.
33. Dahl, L. K. Possible Role of Salt Intake in the Development of Essential Hypertension. In K. D. Brock and P. T. Cottier (eds.), *Essential Hypertension: Proceedings of an International Symposium.* London: Ciba, 1960. P. 53.
34. Dahl, L. K. Possible role of chronic excess salt consumption in the pathogenesis of essential hypertension. *Am. J. Cardiol.* 8: 571, 1961.
35. Dahl, L. K. Excessive salt intake and hypertension. A dietary and genetic interplay. *Brookhaven Lecture Ser.* 12: 22, 1962.
36. Dahl, L. K., and Heine, M. Primary role of renal homografts in setting chronic blood pressure levels in rats. *Circ. Res.* 36: 692, 1975.
37. Dahl, L. K., Heine, M., and Thompson, K. Genetic influence of renal homografts on the blood pressure of rats from different strains. *Proc. Soc. Exp. Biol. Med.* 140: 852, 1972.

38. Dahl, L. K., Knudsen, K. D., Heine, M. A., et al. Effects of chronic excess salt ingestion: Modification of experimental hypertension in the rat by variations in the diet. *Circ. Res.* 22: 11, 1968.
39. Dahl, L. K., and Shackow, E. Effects of chronic excess salt ingestion: Experimental hypertension in the rat. *Can. Med. Assoc. J.* 90: 155, 1964.
40. De Lean, A., Racz, K., Gutkowska, J., et al. Specific receptor-mediated inhibition by synthetic atrial natriuretic factor of hormone-stimulated steroidogenesis in cultured bovine adrenal cells. *Endocrinology* 115: 1636, 1984.
41. Dengler, H. J., Michaelson, I. A., Spiegel, H. E., et al. The uptake of labeled norepinephrine by isolated brain and other tissues of the cat. *Int. J. Neuropharmacol.* 1: 23, 1962.
42. de Wardener, H. E. Control of sodium excretion. *Am. J. Physiol.* 235(3): F163, 1978.
43. de Wardener, H. E. *The Kidney* (5th ed.). Edinburgh: Churchill-Livingstone, 1985. Chap. 16.
44. de Wardener, H. E., and Clarkson, E. M. Concept of natriuretic hormone. *Phys. Rev.* 65(3): 658, 1985.
45. de Wardener, H. E., and MacGregor, G. A. The relation of a circulating sodium transport inhibitor (the natriuretic hormone?) to hypertension. *Medicine* 62: 310, 1983.
46. Dietz, J. R. Release of natriuretic factor from rat heart-lung preparation by atrial distension. *Am. J. Physiol.* 247(16): R1093, 1984.
47. Dietz, R., Schömig, A., Haebara, H., et al. Studies on the pathogenesis of spontaneous hypertension of rats. *Circ. Res.* 43 (Suppl. 1): I-98, 1978.
48. Dilley, J. R., Stier, C. T., and Arendshorst, W. J. Abnormalities in glomerular function in rats developing spontaneous hypertension. *Am. J. Physiol.* 246(15): F12, 1984.
49. Donald, D. E. Studies on the release of renin by direct and reflex activation of renal sympathetic nerves. *Physiologist* 22: 39, 1979.
50. Dunham, E. T., and Glynn, I. M. Adenosine triphosphatase activity and the active movements of alkali metal ions. *J. Physiol.* 156: 274, 1961.
51. Dustan, H. P., and Tarazi, R. C. Cardiogenic hypertension. *Ann. Rev. Med.* 29: 485, 1978.
52. Elliott, P., and Stamler, R. Manual of operations for "Intersalt," an international cooperative study on the relation of sodium and potassium to blood pressure. *Controlled Clin. Trials* 9(Suppl.): 1, 1988.
53. Ellison, R. C., Capper, A. L., Stephenson, W. P., et al. Effects on blood pressure of a decrease in sodium use in institutional food preparation: The Exeter and Andover project. *J. Clin. Epidemiol.* 42: 201, 1989.
54. Escalante, B., Sessa, W. C., Falck, J. R., et al. Vasoactivity of 20-hydroxyeicostatetraenoic acid is dependent on metabolism by cyclooxygenase. *J. Pharmacol. Exp. Ther.* 248: 229, 1989.
55. Evan, A. P., Luft, F. C., Gattone, V., et al. The glomerular filtration barrier in the spontaneously hypertensive rat. *Hypertension* 3: I-154, 1981.
56. Faber, J. E., Barron, K. W., Bonham, A. C., et al. Regional hemodynamic effects of antihypertensive renomedullary lipids in conscious rats. *Hypertension* 6: 494, 1984.
57. Floyer, M. A. The Mechanism Underlying the Response of the Hypertensive Subject to a Saline Load. In P. Miliez (ed.), *L'Hypertension Arterielle.* Paris: L'Expansion Scientifique Francaise, 1966.
58. Folkow, B. Cardiovascular structural adaptation; its role in the initiation and maintenance of primary hypertension. The fourth Volhard Lecture. *Clin. Sci. Mol. Med.* 55: 3s, 1978.
59. Folkow, B. Physiological aspects of primary hypertension. *Physiol. Rev.* 62: 347, 1982.
60. Fray, J. C. S. Stimulation of renin release in perfused kidney by low calcium and high magnesium. *Am. J. Physiol.* 232(4): F377, 1977.
61. Fray, J. C. S. Mechanism by which renin secretion from perfused rat kidneys is stimulated by isoprenaline and inhibited by high perfusion pressure. *J. Physiol.* 308: 1, 1980.
62. Freeman, R. H., and Davis, J. O. Factors Controlling Renin Secretion and Metabolism. In J. Genest, O. Kuchel, P. Hamet, et al. (eds.), *Hypertension* (2nd ed.). New York: McGraw-Hill, 1983. P. 225.
63. Frolich, E. D., Kozul, V. J., Tarazi, R. C., et al. Physiological comparison of labile and essential hypertension. *Circ. Res.* 27(Suppl. 1): 1, 1970.
64. Fukuda, T. R. L'hypertension par le sel chez les lapins et ses relations avec la glande surrenale. *Union Med. Can.* 80: 1278, 1951.
65. Genest, J. Personal Views on the Mechanisms of Essential Hypertension. In J. Genest, O. Kuchel, P. Hamet, et al. (eds.), *Hypertension* (2nd ed.). New York: McGraw-Hill, 1983. P. 599.
66. Gillum, R. F., Elmer, P. J., and Prineas, R. J. Changing sodium intake in children. *Hypertension* 3: 698, 1981.
67. Gleiberman, L. Blood pressure and dietary salt in human populations. *Ecol. Food Nutr.* 2: 143, 1973.
68. Goldblatt, H., Lynch, J., Hanzal, R. F., et al. Studies on experimental hypertension; the production of persistent elevation of systolic blood pressure by means of renal ischemia. *J. Exp. Med.* 59: 347, 1934.
69. Gothberg, G., Lundin, S., and Folkow, B. An acute vasodepressor effect in normotensive rats following extracorporal perfusion of the declipped kidney of two-kidney, one clip hypertensive rats. *Hypertension* 4(Suppl. II): 101, 1982.
70. Greenberg, S., Gaines, K., and Sweatt, D. Evidence for circulating factors as a cause of venous hypertrophy in spontaneously hypertensive rats. *Am. J. Phys.* 241(10): H421, 1981.
71. Grim, C. E., Luft, F. C., Fineberg, N. S., et al. Responses to volume expansion and contraction in categorized hypertensive and normotensive man. *Hypertension* 1: 476, 1979.
72. Grim, C. E., Luft, F. C., Miller, J. Z., et al. Effects of sodium loading and depletion in normotensive first degree relatives of essential hypertensives. *J. Lab. Clin. Med.* 94: 764, 1979.
73. Grim, C. F., Miller, J. Z., Luft, F. C., et al. Genetic influences on renin, aldosterone, and the renal excretion of sodium and potassium following volume expansion and contraction in normal man. *Hypertension* 1: 583, 1979.
74. Gros, G., Weller, J. M., and Hoobler, S. W. Relationship of sodium and potassium intake to blood pressure. *Am. J. Clin. Nutr.* 24: 605, 1971.
75. Gudmundsson, O., and Berglund, G. Age and blood pressure response to increased salt intake (abstract). *Proc. IX Sci. Mtg. Int. Soc. Hypertens.* 1982. P. 158.
76. Guidi, E., Bianchi, G., Rivolta, E., et al. Hypertension in man with kidney transplant: Role of familial versus other factors. *Nephron* 41: 14, 1985.
77. Gull, W. W., and Sutton, H. G. On the pathology of the morbid state commonly called chronic Bright's disease with contracted kidney ("arteriocapillary fibrosis"). *R. Med. Chir. Trans.* 55: 273, 1872.

78. Guyton, A. C., Coleman, T. G., Cowley, A. W., et al. Arterial pressure regulation. Overriding dominance of the kidneys in long term regulation and in hypertension. *Am. J. Med.* 52: 584, 1972.
79. Haber, E., and Haupert, G. T. The search for a hypothalamic Na,K-ATPase inhibitor. *Hypertension* 9: 315, 1987.
80. Haddy, F. J., and Overbeck, H. W. The role of humoral agents in volume expanded hypertension. *Life Sci.* 19: 935, 1976.
81. Haddy, F. J., Pamnani, M. B., and Clough, D. L. Role of a Humoral Factor in Low Renin Hypertension. In B. Lichardus, R. W. Schrier, and J. Ponec (eds.), *Hormonal Regulation of Sodium Excretion*. Amsterdam: Elsevier, 1980. P. 379.
82. Hall, J. E., and Montani, J. P. Long-term autoregulation and adaptation to decreased renal perfusion pressure. *Proc. IXth International Congress of Nephrology*, 1984. P. 394A.
83. Hamet, P., Tremblay, J., Pang, S. C., et al. Effect of native and synthetic atrial natriuretic factor in cyclic GMP. *Biochem. Biophys. Res. Commun.* 123: 515, 1984.
84. Hayslett, J. P., Kashgarian, M., and Epstein, F. H. Mechanism of change in the excretion of sodium per nephron when renal mass is reduced. *J. Clin. Invest.* 48: 1002, 1969.
85. Hinke, J. A. M. In vitro demonstrations of vascular hyperresponsiveness in experimental hypertension. *Circ. Res.* 17: 359, 1965.
86. Hofman, A., Hazebroek, A., and Valkenburg, H. A. A randomized trial of sodium intake and blood pressure in newborn infants. *J.A.M.A.* 250: 370, 1983.
87. Holland, S., Millett, J., Alaghband-Zadeh, J., et al. Cytochemically assayable Na-K-ATPase inhibition by Milan hypertensive rat plasma. *Hypertension* 9(5): 498, 1987.
88. Holland, S., Millett, J., Alaghband-Zadeh, J., et al. Cytochemically detectable glucose-6-phosphate dehydrogenase-stimulating Na-K-ATPase inhibiting activity of plasma and hypothalamus in reduced renal mass hypertension. *Am. J. Hypertens.* 4: 315, 1991.
89. The Intersalt Study. *J. Hum. Hypertens.* 3: 279, 1989.
90. Johnson, G. On certain points in the anatomy and pathology of Bright's disease of the kidney. II. On the influence of the minute blood vessels upon the circulation. *R. Med. Chir. Trans.* 51: 57, 1868.
91. Kawabe, K., Watanabe, T. X., Shiono, K., et al. Influence on blood pressure of renal isografts between spontaneously hypertensive and normotensive rats utilizing the F1 hybrids. *Jpn. Heart J.* 19: 886, 1978.
92. Keeton, T. K., and Campbell, W. B. The pharmacologic alteration of renin release. *Pharmacol. Rev.* 31: 81, 1980.
93. Kesteloot, H., Huang, D. X., Yue-Lang, L., et al. The relationship between cations and blood pressure in the People's Republic of China. *Hypertension* 9: 654, 1987.
94. Kesteloot, H., Park, B. C., Lee, C. S., et al. A Comparative Study of Blood Pressure and Sodium Intake in Belgium and in Korea. In H. Kesteloot and J. V. Joosens (eds.), *Epidemiology and Arterial Blood Pressure*. The Hague: Martinus Nijhoff, 1980. P. 453.
95. Kirkendall, W. M., Conner, W. E., Abboud, F., et al. The effect of dietary sodium chloride on blood pressure, body fluids, electrolytes, renal function and serum lipids of normotensive man. *J. Lab. Clin. Med.* 87: 418, 1976.
96. Kobayashi, A., Nara, Y., Nisho, T., et al. Increased Na-H exchange activity in cultured vascular smooth muscle cells from stroke-prone spontaneously hypertensive rats. *J. Hypertens.* 8: 153, 1990.
97. Koomans, H. A., Roos, J. C., Boer, P., et al. Salt sensitivity of blood pressure in chronic renal failure. Evidence for renal control of body fluid distribution in man. *Hypertension* 4: 190, 1982.
98. Laragh, J. H. Personal Views on the Mechanisms of Hypertension. In J. Genest, O. Kuchel, P. Hamet, et al. (eds.), *Hypertension* (2nd ed.). New York: McGraw-Hill, 1983. P. 615.
99. Ledingham, J. M., and Cohen, R. D. Changes in extracellular fluid volume and cardiac output during development of experimental renal hypertension. *Can. Med. Assoc. J.* 90: 292, 1964.
100. Leeuw de, P. W., and Birkenhager, W. H. The renal circulation in essential hypertension. *J. Hypertension* 1: 321, 1983.
101. Leitz, F. H., and Stefano, F. J. E. Effect of ouabain and desipramine on the uptake and storage of norepinephrine and metaraminol. *Eur. J. Pharmacol.* 11: 278, 1970.
102. Lenel, R., Katz, L. N., and Rodbard, S. Arterial hypertension in the chicken. *Am. J. Physiol.* 152: 557, 1948.
103. Lennon, E. J., Ruetz, P. P., and Engstrom, W. W. Reversal of diurnal rhythm in excretion of water and salt in primary hyperaldosteronism. *Am. J. Med.* 30: 475, 1961.
104. Liu, K., Dyer, A. R., Cooper, R. S., et al. Can overnight urines replace 24-hour urine collections to assess salt intake? *Hypertension* i: 529, 1979.
105. Livne, A., Veitsch, R., Grinstein, S., et al. Increased platelet exchange rates in essential hypertension: Application of a novil test. *Lancet* i: 533, 1987.
106. Losse, H., Wehmeyer, H., and Wessels, F. The water and electrolyte content of erythrocytes in arterial hypertension. *Klin. Wochenschr.* 38: 393, 1960.
107. Lowenstein, F. W. Blood pressure in relation to age and sex in the tropics and sub-tropics: A review of the literature and an investigation in two tribes of Brazil Indians. *Lancet* i: 389, 1961.
108. Lucas, J., and Floyer, M. A. Renal control of changes in the compliance of the interstitial space; a factor in the aetiology of reno-prival hypertension. *Clin. Sci.* 44: 397, 1973.
109. Lucas, J., and Floyer, M. A. Changes in body fluid distribution and interstitial tissue compliance during the development and reversal of experimental renal hypertension in the rat. *Clin. Sci. Mol. Med.* 47: 1, 1974.
110. Luft, F. C., Fineberg, N. S., and Sloan, R. S. Estimating dietary sodium intake in individuals receiving a randomly fluctuating intake. *Hypertension* 4: 805, 1982.
111. Luft, F. C., Rankin, L. I., Bloch, R., et al. Cardiovascular and humoral responses to extremes of sodium intake in normal black and white men. *Circulation* 60: 697, 1979.
112. MacGregor, G. A. Sodium is more important than calcium in essential hypertension. *Hypertension* 7: 628, 1985.
113. MacGregor, G. A., Fenton, S., Alaghband-Zadeh, J., et al. An increase in a circulating inhibitor of Na,K,dependent ATPase: A possible link between salt intake and the development of essential hypertension. *Clin. Sci.* 61: 17s, 1981.
114. Mahomed, F. A. On chronic Bright's disease, and its essential symptoms. *Lancet* 1: 46, 1879.
115. Mahomed, F. A. Chronic Bright's disease without albuminuria. *Guy's Hosp. Rep.* 3rd Ser. 25: 295, 1881.
116. Maloiy, G. M. O., and Boarer, C. D. H. Response of the Somali donkey to dehydration: haematological changes. *Am. J. Phys.* 221: 37, 1971.
117. Margolius, H. S. Kallikrein and Kinins in Hypertension. In J. Genest, O. Kuchel, P. Hamet, et al. (eds.), *Hypertension* (2nd ed.). New York: McGraw Hill, 1983. P. 360.
118. Mathews, W. R., Ducharme, D. W., Hamlin, J. M., et al. Mass spectral characterization of an endogenous digi-

talis-like factor from human plasma. *Hypertension* 17: 930, 1991.
119. Mattiasson, I., and Hood, B. Efflux rate of noradrenaline from platelets in normotensive members of hypertensive families. *Clin. Sci.* 62: 151, 1982.
120. Mattiasson, I., Mattiasson, B., and Hood, B. The efflux rate of norepinephrine from platelets and its relation to blood pressure. *Life Sci.* 24: 2265, 1979.
121. McDonald, S. J., and de Wardener, H. E. The relationship between the renal arterial perfusion pressure and the increase in sodium excretion which occurs during an infusion of saline. *Nephron* 2: 1, 1965.
122. McDonough, J., and Wilhelmj, C. M. The effect of excess salt intake on human blood pressure in man. *Am. J. Dig. Dis.* 21: 180, 1954.
123. McQuarrie, I., Thompson, W. H., and Anderson, J. A. Effects of excessive ingestion of sodium and potassium salts on carbohydrate metabolism and blood pressure in diabetic children. *J. Nutr.* 11: 77, 1936.
124. Meade, T. W., Imeson, J. D., Gordon, D., et al. The epidemiology of plasma renin. *Clin. Sci.* 64: 273, 1983.
125. Meneely, G. R., Tucker, R. G., Darby, W. J., et al. Chronic sodium chloride toxicity: Hypertension, renal and vascular lesions. *Ann. Intern. Med.* 39: 991, 1953.
126. Michel, M. C., Insel, P. A., and Brodde, O.-E. Renal β-adrenergic receptor alterations: A cause of essential hypertension. *F.A.S.E.B. J.* 3: 139, 1989.
127. Michelakis, A. M., Mizukoshi, H., Huang, C., et al. Further studies on the existence of a sensitizing factor to pressor agents in hypertension. *J. Clin. Endocrinol. Metab.* 41: 90, 1975.
128. Miles, B. E., and de Wardener, H. E. Effect of emotion on renal function in normotensive and hypertensive women. *Lancet* 2: 539, 1953.
129. Miles, B. E., de Wardener, H. E., and McSwiney, R. R. Renal function during emotional diuresis. *Am. J. Med.* 12: 659, 1952.
130. Miller, J. Z., Daughtery, S. A., Weinberger, M. H., et al. Blood pressure responses to dietary sodium restriction in normotensive adults. *Hypertension* 5: 790, 1983.
131. Miller, J. Z., Weinberger, M. H., Daughtery, S. A., et al. Blood pressure response to dietary sodium restriction in healthy normotensive children. *Am. J. Clin. Nutr.* 47: 113, 1988.
132. Millett, J. A., Holland, S. M., Alaghband-Zadeh, J., et al. Na-K-ATPase inhibiting and glucose-6-phosphate dehydrogenase-stimulating activity of plasma and hypothalamus of the Okamoto spontaneously hypertensive rat. *J. Endocrinol.* 108: 69, 1986.
133. Mir, M. A., and Newcombe, R. The relationship of dietary salt and blood pressure in three farming communities in Kashmir. *J. Hum. Hypertens.* 2: 241, 1984.
134. Morgan, D. A., DiBona, G. F., and Mark, A. L. Effects of inter-strain renal transplantation on NaCl induced hypertension in Dahl rats. *Hypertension* 15: 436, 1990.
135. Morgan, K., Foord, S. M., Spurlock, G., et al. Release of an active sodium transport inhibitor from rat hypothalamic cells in culture. *Endocrinology* 115: 1642, 1984.
136. Muirhead, E. E. Antihypertensive functions of the kidney. *Hypertension* 2: 444, 1980.
137. Muirhead, E. E. The Renomedullary Antihypertensive System and Its Putative Hormone(s). In J. Genest, O. Kuchel, P. Hamet, et al. (eds.), *Hypertension* (2nd ed.). New York: McGraw-Hill, 1983. P. 394.
138. Muirhead, E. E., Folkow, B., Byers, L. W., et al. Cardiovascular effects of antihypertensive polar and neutral renomedullary lipids. *Hypertension* 5(Suppl. 1): 1, 1983.
139. Muirhead, E. E., Pitcock, J. A., Brooks, B., et al. Captopril in Angiotensin-Salt Hypertension: A Possible Linkage Between Angiotensin, Salt, Vascular Disease, and Renomedullary Interstitial Cells. In J. H. Laragh, F. R. Buhler, and D. W. Seldin (eds.), *Frontiers in Hypertension.* New York: Springer, 1981. P. 559.
140. Muirhead, E. E., Rightsel, W. A., Leach, B. E., et al. Antihypertensive lipid from tissue culture of renomedullary interstitial cells of the rat. *Clin. Sci. Mol. Med.* 51: 287S, 1976.
141. Multhauf, R. P. *Neptune's Gift. A History of Common Salt.* Baltimore: Johns Hopkins University Press, 1978.
142. Murray, R. H., Luft, F. C., Bloch, R., et al. Blood pressure responses to extremes of sodium intake in normal man (40364). *Proc. Soc. Exp. Biol. Med.* 159: 432, 1978.
143. Nakazato, Y., Ohga, A., and Onoda, Y. The effect of ouabain on noradrenaline output from peripheral adrenergic neurones of isolated guinea pig vas deferens. *J. Physiol.* 278: 45, 1978.
144. Needleman, P., Currie, M. G., Geller, D. M., et al. Atriopeptins: Potential mediators of an endocrine relationship between heart and kidney. *Trends Pharm. Sci.* 5: 506, 1984.
145. Ng, L. L., Dudley, C., Bomford, J., et al. Leucocyte intracellular pH and Na/H antiport activity in human hypertension. *J. Hypertens.* 7: 471, 1989.
146. Ogston, A. G., and Wells, J. D. The osmotic properties of sulphoethyl-Sephadex. A model for cartilage. *Biochem. J.* 128: 685, 1972.
147. Overbeck, H. W. Hemodynamics of early experimental renal hypertension in dogs. Normal limb blood flow, elevated limb vascular resistance and decreased venous compliance. *Circ. Res.* 31: 653, 1972.
148. Overbeck, H. W. Cardiovascular hypertrophy and "waterlogging" in coarctation hypertension. Role of sympathoadrenergic influences and pressure. *Hypertension* 1: 486, 1979.
149. Page, L. B., Damon, A., and Moellering, R. C. Antecedents of cardiovascular disease in six Solomon Island societies. *Circulation* 49: 1132, 1974.
150. Page, L. B., Vandevert, D. E., Nader, K., et al. Blood pressure of Quash'qai pastoral nomads in Iran in relation to culture, diet and body form. *Am. J. Clin. Nutr.* 34: 527, 1981.
151. Park, C. S., Han, D. S., and Fray, J. C. S. Calcium in the control of renin secretion: Ca2+ influx as an inhibitory signal. *Am. J. Physiol.* 240: F70, 1981.
152. Peart, W. S. The isolation of a hypertensin. *Biochem. J.* 62: 520, 1956.
153. Peart, W. S. Intrarenal factors in renin release. *Contrib. Nephrol.* 12: 5, 1978.
154. Pitcock, J. A., Rightsel, W. A., Brown, P., et al. Functional-morphological correlates of renomedullary interstitial cells. *Clin. Sci. Mol. Med.* 51: 291S, 1976.
155. Pitcock, J. A., Share, L., Rapp, J., et al. Major differences in the renomedullary interstitial cells of Dahl's S and R rats. A possible relation to the effects of salt. *Circulation* 64(Suppl. IV): 224, 1981.
156. Pletcher, A., and Laubescher, A. Use and Limitations of Platelets as Models of Neurones: Amine Release and Shape Change Reaction. In A. Rotman, F. A. Meyer, C. Giller, et al. (eds.), *Platelets: Cellular Response Mechanisms and Their Biological Significance.* London: John Wiley, 1980. P. 267.
157. Rettig, R., Folberth, C., Stauss, H., et al. Role of the kidney in primary hypertension: A renal transplantation study in rats. *Am. J. Physiol.* 258: F606, 1990.
158. Rettig, R., Stauss, H., Folberth, C., et al. Hypertension

transmitted by kidneys from stroke-prone spontaneously hypertensive rats. *Am. J. Physiol.* 257: F197, 1989.

159. Ricksten, S. E., Yao, T., and Thoren, P. Peripheral and central vascular compliances in conscious normotensive and spontaneously hypertensive rats. *Acta Physiol. Scand.* 112: 169, 1981.
160. Rightsel, W. A., Okamura, T., Inagami, T., et al. Juxtaglomerular cells grown as monolayer cell culture contain renin, angiotensin I converting enzyme, and angiotensins I and II/III. *Circ. Res.* 50: 822, 1982.
161. Roman, R. J., and Cowley, A. W., Jr. Abnormal pressure-diuresis-natriuresis response in spontaneously hypertensive rats. *Am. J. Physiol.* 248: F199, 1985.
162. Rosenberg, W., Palmieri, C., Schlager, G., et al. Quantitative structural aspects of the renal glomeruli of hypertensive mice. *Nephron* 30: 161, 1982.
163. Rovner, D. R., Conn, J. W., Knopf, R. F., et al. Nature of renal escape from the sodium-retaining effect of aldosterone in primary aldosteronism and in normal subjects. *J. Clin. Endocrinol. Metab.* 25: 53, 1965.
164. Russell, G. I., Bing, R. F., Swales, J. D., et al. Indomethacin or aprotinin infusion: Effect on reversal of chronic two-kidney, one-clip hypertension in the conscious rat. *Clin. Sci.* 62: 361, 1982.
165. Russell, G. I., Bing, R. F., Thurston, H., et al. Surgical reversal of two-kidney one clip hypertension during inhibition of the renin-angiotensin system. *Hypertension* 4: 69, 1982.
166. Safar, M. E., London, G. M., Levenson, J. A., et al. Rapid dextran infusion in essential hypertension. *Hypertension* 1: 615, 1979.
167. Sagnella, G. A., Markandu, N. D., Shore, A. C., et al. Plasma immunoreactive atrial natriuretic peptide and changes in dietary sodium intake in man. *Life Sci.* 40: 139, 1987.
168. Sapirstein, L. A., Brandt, W. L., and Drury, D. R. Production of hypertension in the rat by substituting hypertonic sodium chloride solutions for drinking water (17583). *Proc. Soc. Exp. Biol. Med.* 73: 82, 1950.
169. Schalekamp, M. A. D. H., Krauss, X. H., Schalekamp-Kuyken, M. P. A., et al. Studies on the mechanism of hypernatriuresis in essential hypertension in relation to measurements of plasma renin concentration, body fluid compartments and renal function. *Clin. Sci.* 41: 219, 1971.
170. Seymour, A. A., Davis, J. O., Freeman, R. H., et al. Renin release from filtering and nonfiltering kidneys stimulated by PGI2 and PGD2. *Am. J. Physiol.* 237(4): F285, 1979.
171. Shibata, H., and Hatano, S. A Salt Restriction Trial in Japan. In F. Gross and T. Strasser (eds.), *Mild Hypertension: Natural History and Management.* Bath: Pitman Medical, 1979. P. 147.
172. Shock, N. W., and Davies, D. F. Age changes in glomerular filtration rate, effective renal plasma flow and tubular excretory capacity in adult males. *J. Clin. Invest.* 29: 496, 1950.
173. Siani, A., Iacoviello, L., Giorgione, N., et al. Comparison of variability in urinary sodium, potassium and calcium in free living man. *Hypertension* 13: 38, 1989.
174. Simon, G. Altered venous function in hypertensive rats. *Circ. Res.* 38: 412, 1976.
175. Skeggs, L. T., Lentz, K. E., Kahn, J. R., et al. The amino acid sequence of hypertension. II. *J. Exp. Med.* 104: 193, 1956.
176. Smirk, F. H., and Hall, W. H. Inherited hypertension in rats. *Nature* 182: 727, 1958.
177. Songu-Mize, E., Bealer, S. L., and Hassid, A. I. Centrally administered ANF promotes appearance of a circulatory sodium pump inhibitor. *Am. J. Physiol.* 258: H1655, 1990.
178. Spokas, E. C., Quilley, J., and McGiff, J. C. Prostaglandins in Hypertension. In J. Genest, O. Kuchel, P. Hamet, et al. (eds.), *Hypertension* (2nd ed.). New York: McGraw-Hill, 1983. P. 373.
179. Sullivan, J. M., Ratts, T. E., Taylor, J. C., et al. Hemodynamic effects of dietary sodium in man. *Hypertension* 2: 506, 1980.
180. Swales, J. D. Salt saga continued. *Br. Med. J.* 297: 307, 1988.
181. Takahashi, H., Makoto, M., Suga, K., et al. Hypothalamic digitalis-like substance is released with sodium-loading in rats. *Am. J. Hypertens.* 1: 146, 1988.
182. Tigerstedt, R., and Bergman, P. G. Niere und Kreislauf. *Skand. Arch. Physiol.* 8: 223, 1898.
183. Tobian, L. Salt and Hypertension. In J. Genest, O. Kuchel, P. Hamet, et al. *Hypertension.* New York: McGraw Hill, 1983. P. 73.
184. Tobian, L., Lange, J., Azar, S., et al. Reduction of natriuretic capacity and renin release in isolated blood perfused kidneys of Dahl hypertension prone rats. *Circ. Res.* 43(Suppl. 1): 1, 1978.
185. Tobian, L., Pumper, M., Johnson S., et al. A circulating humoral pressor agent in Dahl S rats with salt hypertension. *Clin. Sci.* 57: 345S, 1979.
186. Tripoddo, N. C., Yamamoto, J., and Frolich, E. D. Whole body venous capacity and effective total tissue compliance in SHR. *Hypertension* 3: 104, 1981.
187. Vandongen, R., and Peart, W. S. Calcium dependence of the inhibitory effect of angiotensin on renin secretion in the isolated perfused kidney of the rat. *Br. J. Pharmacol.* 50: 125, 1974.
188. Volhard, P. Nieren und Ableitende Harnwege. In G. von Bergmann and R. Staehelin (eds.), *Hanbuch der inneren Medizin.* Berlin: Springer, 1931. Part 1.
189. Watson, R. L., and Langford, H. G. Usefulness of overnight urines in population groups. *Am. J. Clin. Nutr.* 23: 290, 1970.
190. Weder, A. B. Abnormal proximal tubular sodium reabsorption in essential hypertension. *Hypertension* 7: 847, 1985.
191. Wiggins, R. C., Basar, I., and Slater, J. D. H. Effect of arterial pressure and inheritance on the sodium excretory capacity of normal young men. *Clin. Sci. Mol. Med.* 54: 639, 1978.
192. Wilhelmj, C. M., Waldmann, E. B., and McGuire, T. F. Effect of prolonged high sodium chloride ingestion and withdrawal upon blood pressure of dogs (18784). *Proc. Soc. Exp. Biol. Med.* 77: 379, 1951.
193. Willassen, Y., and Ofstad, J. Renal sodium excretion and the peritubular capillary physical factors in essential hypertension. *Hypertension* 2: 771, 1980.
194. Willis, L. R., and Bauer, J. H. Aldosterone in the exaggerated natriuresis of spontaneously hypertensive rats. *Am. J. Physiol.* 234(1): F29, 1978.
195. Wilson, C., and Byrom, F. B. The vicious circle in chronic Bright's disease. Experimental evidence from the hypertensive rat. *Q. J. Med.* 10: 65, 1941.
196. Yamamoto, J., Trippodo, N. C., McPhee, A. A., et al. Decreased total venous capacity in Goldblatt hypertensive rats. *Am. J. Physiol.* 240: H487, 1981.
197. Yamori, Y., Kihara, M., Nara, Y., et al. Hypertension and diet: Multiple regression analysis in a Japanese farming community. *Lancet* i: 1204, 1981.

Nephrosclerosis

Robert G. Luke
John J. Curtis

DEFINITIONS

This chapter focuses on renal disease caused primarily by, or at least associated with, predominant changes in small intrarenal blood vessels, with the exclusion of arteritis and malignant hypertension. Either vascular narrowing in these small intrarenal vessels or its proximate cause leads eventually to glomerular and tubular damage with glomerular and tubulointerstitial atrophy and fibrosis. The most important pathogenic changes in nephrosclerosis occur at levels at and below the arcuate arteries—the interlobular artery and the afferent arteriole (*arteriolosclerosis*). Lesions of the main and segmental arteries—mainly atherosclerosis and fibrous dysplasia—which can lead to renovascular hypertension, renal or segmental infarction, and/or partial or complete ischemic atrophy of the kidney, are discussed elsewhere (Chap. 55).

Hypertensive nephrosclerosis is by far the most important cause of this type of progressive renal disease. The associated hypertension may be *essential* (idiopathic) or *secondary* to virtually all causes except possibly renal artery stenosis, in which protection of the vessels within the ipsilateral kidney distal to the lesion may occur. Thus nephrosclerosis complicates all renal parenchymal diseases that lead to hypertension. Since hypertension is present in 80 to 90 percent of such patients by the time end-stage renal disease is reached, nephrosclerosis is the rule in end-stage kidneys. Regardless of etiology, once high blood pressure develops, a vicious circle of hypertension, nephrosclerosis, increasing renal damage, and more hypertension can be established.

Indeed, as considered subsequently, it may be quite difficult, if the patient presents at end stage, to determine whether nephrosclerosis is the cause or the result of progressive renal parenchymal disease. Hypertensive nephrosclerosis, therefore, is both an important primary cause of chronic renal failure and a contributing factor to progression in other types of renal disease such as chronic glomerulonephritis.

Changes in small intrarenal vessels that mimic both malignant and "benign" hypertensive nephrosclerosis can be seen in the absence of hypertension in conditions such as the later phases of thrombotic microangiopathy including hemolytic uremic syndrome and postpartum renal failure [150], or in scleroderma [31]. This is termed *primary* nephrosclerosis. Again, hypertension frequently develops subsequently due to renal ischemia and loss of nephrons. Finally, nephrosclerosis is often regarded as a *phenomenon of aging,* which is very much accelerated by hypertension or diabetes mellitus.

Pathology

In the absence of renal infarction or ischemia due to occlusion or narrowing of the main renal artery or its segmental branches, kidneys with nephrosclerosis are symmetric and may be near normal or small in size [13] depending on the rate of loss of renal function—the more rapid the progression, the better preserved is renal size. In Bell's series, a severe reduction in size was seen in 10 percent of patients. The surfaces of the kidney are finely granular with occasional coarse scars but with a normal pelvicalyceal system. The arteriosclerotic and atherosclerotic narrowing of larger vessels that may accompany hypertensive arteriolosclerosis is probably responsible for the coarser scars and may contribute to nephron loss.

The two principal microscopic lesions [91, 115] are myointimal hypertrophy, most marked in the interlobular arteries, and hyaline arteriolosclerosis, most marked in the afferent arteriole and in vessels lacking an internal elastic lamina (Fig. 54-1). The interlobular arteries often also show reduplication of the internal elastic lamina and hypertrophy of the media (Fig. 54-1A). Hyaline change appears as an eosinophilic glassy thickening of the arteriolar wall and is prominent on PAS stains because it contains glycoproteins; there is associated atrophy of smooth muscle cells and narrowing of the lumen (Fig. 54-1B). Both lesions appear to contribute to glomerular fibrosis; the degree of glomerular damage tends to be more heterogeneous than in, for example, chronic glomerulonephritis. The glomerular capillaries characteristically show "wrinkling collapse" with thickening of the glomerular capillary wall; the former is best seen by silver stains (Fig. 54-1C). There is an associated increase in mesangial matrix, and collagenous thickening occurs inside Bowman's capsule. Eventually, the glomeruli tend to be small and atrophic with complete sclerosis. Secondary tubular atrophy, thickening of tubular basement membranes, and interstitial fibrosis become increasingly prominent. The blood supply of the tubules is postglomerular, and tubular atrophy may be prominent early even before glomerular ischemic changes are very marked. The effects of nephrosclerosis were previously often misdiagnosed as chronic pyelonephritis (reflux nephropathy) because of the severity of these tubulointerstitial changes, including the presence of thyroidlike areas. Nephrosclerosis, however, does not cause the coarse deep surface scars and associated pelvic inflammatory changes with caliectasis characteristic of that lesion. Nevertheless, on a histology section alone the differential diagnosis of primary vascular versus primary tubulointerstitial disease can be quite difficult: Attention to gross anatomic changes, which are usually obvious on radiologic study, is essential.

Heptinstall [91] has reviewed the available immunofluorescence studies of small vessels and glomeruli in nephrosclerosis. Apart from an increased prevalence of IgM in arterioles and in the mesangium, no specific pattern has been noted.

In both type I and type II diabetes mellitus the changes of nephrosclerosis are marked and include involvement of the efferent as well as the afferent arteriole. Involvement of the efferent arteriole can also be seen in hypertensive nephrosclerosis, but the changes are much less diffuse and prominent. Arteriolar renal

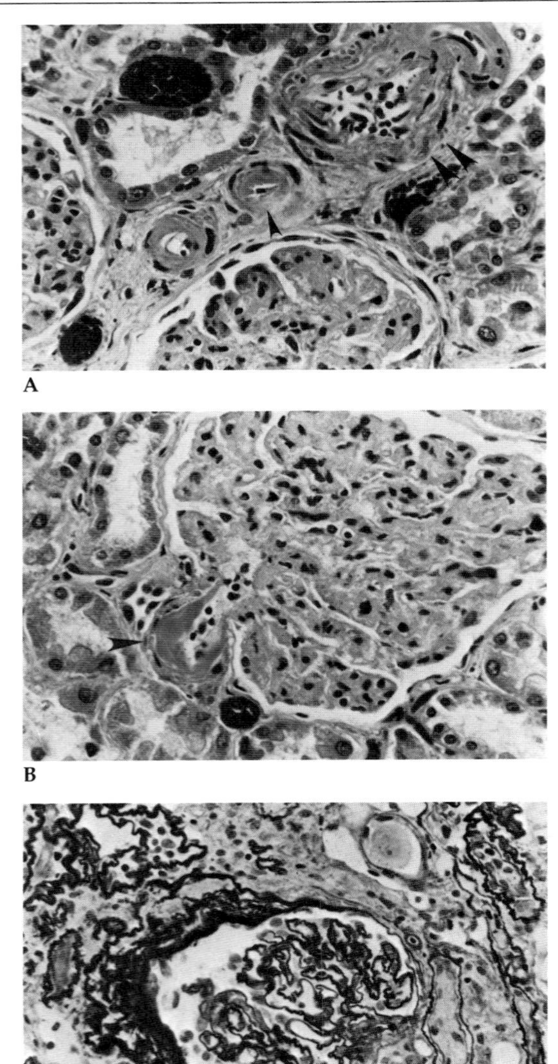

Fig. 54-1. A. Myointimal hypertrophy in an interlobular artery (*double arrows*) with marked hyaline changes in the adjacent arteriole (*single arrow*). (Hematoxylin and eosin, ×400.) B. Hyaline change in the afferent glomerular arteriole (*arrow*). (Hematoxylin and eosin, ×400.) C. This entire glomerulus has a collapsed, wrinkled appearance characteristic of advanced hypertension. (Jones silver methenamine, ×400.) (Courtesy of Ronald W. Alexander, M. D., Chief of Surgical Pathology at the University of Alabama at Birmingham.)

microaneurysms akin to those in the fundi have been observed with diabetes [156]. Although the glomerular changes characteristic of diabetes mellitus appear to be the dominant renal lesion [14], hypertension, at least experimentally, contributes importantly to that lesion, since in the two kidney-one clip renovascular hypertension model in hyperglycemic rats, both the glomerular and arteriolar lesions are much worse in the unclipped kidney, which is exposed to the full effects of systemic hypertension [145].

Fibrinoid necrosis and renal microinfarcts do not occur in so-called benign nephrosclerosis but are features of malignant or accelerated hypertension (Chap. 59). Nephrosclerosis leads to a slow atrophy and fibrosis, not to infarction of the glomeruli. While perhaps "benign" in relation to the effects of lesion of malignant hypertension, this adjective is clearly misused with nephrosclerosis.

The kidney is the most severely involved organ in arteriolosclerosis, but there is a correlation between renal arteriolar and retinal and pancreatic arteriolar involvement [201]. Even in the absence of hypertension, patchy microvascular changes characteristic of nephrosclerosis may be seen in the elderly normotensive patient. These changes are increasingly prevalent over the age of 60 years but virtually never cause end-stage renal disease in the absence of hypertension.

The lesions of nephrosclerosis occur as the sequelae of various diseases, even in the absence of hypertension. These include scleroderma (Chap. 73) [31], hemolytic uremic syndrome, and thrombotic microangiopathy in general, but also chronic radiation nephritis [140, 141], chronic allograft rejection [160, 177, 178], and some conditions associated with a normal blood pressure but with prolonged and marked elevation of angiotensin levels (see below). In the former conditions fibrinoid necrosis and lesions similar to malignant hypertension are often seen, especially if the clinical presentation is fulminant and leads to acute renal failure; however, changes more like those of benign nephrosclerosis can occur in partially recovered patients or in those who develop chronic renal failure [74].

Nephrosclerosis is also a feature of the pathology of all progressive parenchymal renal diseases associated with hypertension. Vascular changes are more severe in scarred areas in chronic pyelonephritis (reflux nephropathy) and have been attributed to arteritis at the time of acute pyelonephritic scarring [121]. Nephrosclerosis in the intervening normal areas, however, relates to the presence of hypertension [92, 121, 217]. The severe vascular narrowing in the scarred areas may contribute to severe renin-dependent hypertension in children and young adults even before any azotemia develops [93, 217]. Renal biopsies done as a follow-up of toxemia of pregnancy may also show scattered areas of arteriolonephrosclerosis [15, 176]. Marked hyaline arteriolosclerosis is sometimes seen in conjunction with focal segmental hyalinosis and glomerulosclerosis; a poor prognosis for progressive renal disease was associated with this finding in a group of young adults [24]. Myointimal hypertrophy may also be seen in the more chronic form of atheroembolic renal disease; sometimes organizing cholesterol microemboli can be seen in the layered intima [116, 199]. Baldwin and Neugarten [5] and Kincaid-Smith [122] have argued that the effect of hypertension on renal arterioles is enhanced by underlying chronic primary glomerular disease in general and that such lesions may occur even before the onset of secondary hypertension. Finally, severe intimal fibrosis of large and small renal vessels becomes increasingly prominent with duration of chronic dialysis in small end-stage kidneys [158].

PATHOGENESIS

The pathologic lesions of nephrosclerosis are most commonly associated with hypertension, and their extent and severity are in proportion to the severity and duration of hypertension [13, 33, 34, 98, 210]. Nevertheless, they can occur in histologically indistinguishable form in the absence of hypertension. Their occurrence in conditions associated with a chronically low ECF volume, *normotension*, renal or gut wasting of chloride (Bartter's syndrome or congenital chloridiarrhea), and very high renin-angiotensin levels for many years is of special interest [8, 32, 75, 165, 166]. It has been postulated that prolonged vasospasm of the renal arterioles secondary to elevated angiotensin II levels leads to endothelial and smooth muscle vascular injury and ultimately to nephrosclerosis. Similar nephrosclerotic-like lesions have been seen in chronic hypokalemic hypereninemia secondary to laxative abuse [47]. We have postulated [41] that even after successful transplantation high levels of renin production from old native kidneys may cause systemic hypertension and renal vasoconstriction in allografts and eventually may contribute to nephrosclerosis in the graft.

PRIMARY NEPHROSCLEROSIS

This appears to be a final common pathway for several mechanisms of injury to small intrarenal vessels (Table 54-1). The listed mechanisms are not proved. In some of these diseases features of both arteriolonecrosis and arteriolosclerosis are seen. The lesions are also seen, but to a much less severe degree, in aging, especially in patients over 60 years. Blood pressure does rise with age, and there is some evidence that the overall mean loss of glomerular filtration rate (GFR) with age (about 1 ml/min/year) is mainly due to those in the population who develop hypertension [133]. It is thus possible that hypertension also substantially accounts for nephrosclerosis and loss of nephrons with aging, or that those who develop primary nephrosclerosis due to aging per se—if such a mechanism exists—develop, as a consequence, both hypertension and loss of nephrons.

Table 54-1. Mechanisms of vascular damage in primary nephrosclerosis

Disease	Postulated mechanism
Thrombotic microangiopathy	Intravascular coagulation; endothelial damage or defective prostacyclin production
Scleroderma	Microcirculatory regulatory disturbance; overproduction of collagen
Barrter's syndrome	Prolonged vasospasm due to angiotensin II
Radiation nephritis	Direct toxic effect on endothelial cells
Chronic renal allograft rejection	Immune (?humoral) attack on endothelium

The presence of diabetes mellitus markedly increases nephrosclerosis in all age groups; indeed, it is associated with the most severe and diffuse lesions seen in any patients. Hypertension, if not initially present, soon develops in most patients. However, the glomerular lesion of diabetes mellitus, unlike that of hypertensive nephrosclerosis, does not seem to be dependent on the vascular lesion [14].

Conventional wisdom is that the vascular lesion in "hypertensive nephrosclerosis" is due to the high blood pressure. Extensive series of renal biopsies in patients with essential hypertension suggest that the incidence and severity of arteriolosclerosis increases with both the duration and the severity of hypertension; early in its course vascular lesions may be absent [33, 34, 90, 91, 201, 202]. In the two kidney-one clip model of hypertension, arteriolar lesions are much less severe, or absent, distal to the clamp, strongly supporting the view that these changes are due to the direct effects of hypertensive injury to arteriolar and small arterial vessel walls rather than to the effect of a systemic stimulus or of another proximate cause of hypertension [221]. The appearance of the lesions of arteriolosclerosis is not influenced by the etiology of the hypertension. Sommers et al. [200] hypothesized that arteriolar spasm in essential hypertension eventually led to deterioration of the elastic tissue, increased ground substance, and collagen formation and hyalinization. Recent studies in the early stages of essential hypertension in humans do support the presence of renal vasoconstriction [96, 97, 101, 135]. Cyclosporine produces renal vasoconstriction within hours, hypertension within weeks, and nephrosclerosis after years of ingestion. Thus, again, renal vasoconstriction may lead to systemic hypertension and eventually to nephrosclerosis [138].

A major problem in unraveling the pathogenesis of the lesion of hyaline arteriolosclerosis is lack of a good animal model unlike the lesion of fibrinoid necrosis [29]. In a review of the pathogenesis of hypertensive hyaline arteriolosclerosis, Kashgarian [115] suggests three possible sources for the hyaline material: increased passage of plasma macromolecules across the endothelium; increased formation of collagen and extracellular matrix substances; or fusion of basement membrane material in situ secondary to injured endothelial and smooth muscle cells. Increased formation of extracellular matrix material, including collagen and glycoproteins such as glycosaminoglycans, by cells in the arteriolar wall may be due to (1) mechanical injury to endothelial or arterial smooth muscle cells or (2) increased passage of circulating macromolecules into the matrix, which alters the milieu of the cells in the vessel wall and induces them to synthesize more matrix substances. The latter construct has been postulated to explain an increase in mesangial ground substance formation and focal glomerulosclerosis in the glomerular damage of hyperfusion nephropathy secondary to reduction in the number of remaining nephrons [159]. In experimental diabetes mellitus, which produces severe hyaline arteriolosclerosis, Rohrbach et al. [189] observed altered basement membrane formation with increased permeability to anionic protons, triggering the same sequence of events as in hypertension. Chronic volume expansion (see below) may induce smooth muscle hypertrophy independent of hypertension [83], perhaps through humoral mediators [181] and increased cell sodium [28].

In an interesting autopsy study, arteriolosclerosis correlated best with blood pressures prevailing in the weeks or months before death rather than with the previously higher levels [211]. The falls in blood pressure noted were not related to treatment but to such diseases as cancer. This suggests that the vascular lesions secondary to hypertension may be at least partly reversible; if true, this has important implications for the benefits of antihypertensive drug therapy.

Essential Hypertension

Idiopathic hypertension at present is responsible for about 85 to 90 percent of all hypertension in humans [114] and is by far the major cause of "benign" nephrosclerosis. An arbitrary definition of hypertension is a blood pressure exceeding 140 mm Hg systolic or 90 mm Hg diastolic pressure. Pickering [173] has argued against such a discrete separation and for a normal distribution of blood pressure in humans. There is no argument, however, about the association between increasing morbidity and mortality with increasing blood pressure even, in insurance population statistics, at levels from as low as 80 mm Hg diastolic pressure [173]. The major clinically significant sites targeted by hypertension are the heart, cerebral and retinal vasculature, and the kidneys. Hypertension is a major risk factor for atherosclerosis, myocardial infarction, congestive cardiac failure, and stroke; antihypertensive drug therapy has a major impact on reducing these risks, especially those of the latter two [70, 71, 110, 111, 214, 215]; the effectiveness of its role in preventing hypertensive nephrosclerosis will be discussed later.

By assessments employing *two* sequential screening blood pressure measurements [224], a minimum of approximately 16 million Americans in the age group 25 to 74 years have established diastolic hypertension (> 90 mm Hg). Such patients have a doubled risk for major cardiovascular and cerebrovascular disease events and are regarded as suitable for antihypertensive therapy. This recommendation was qualified by the statement that "because of the absence of adequate blood pressure risk-related data for blacks in the United States, the generalization of the recommendation in this report (on indications for treatment) to this important population group is limited. Documented higher prevalence and hypertension-related mortality in the black population emphasize the need for prospective studies of risk and progression of hypertension and its complications in blacks" [224]. Hypertension is twice as common in blacks as in whites [157], and it is also more severe [56, 73]. Thus for levels of diastolic blood pressure over 115 mm Hg, the ratio of black-white incidence is 5 : 1 for men and 7 : 1 for women [104]. The usual age of onset of essential hypertension is from 20 to 50 years; it is especially common during the fourth decade. However, in one large study, which included over 1,000 patients with essential hypertension with a diastolic blood pressure of over 90 mm Hg, onset, or at least recognition, occurred in 12 percent of patients under the age of 20 years and in 7 percent after 50 years of age [146]. A family history of hypertension is common. Most experimental animal and clinical data favor a polygenic mode of inheritance rather than a dominant single gene [69, 91, 173], although contrary views exist [153, 174].

Studies of renal function in the early stages of established essential hypertension have consistently shown varying degrees of reduced renal blood flow but with relatively well preserved GFR, presumably due to predominant efferent arteriolar vasoconstriction, so that the filtration fraction is elevated [37, 77, 96, 97]. An increased filtration fraction elevates oncotic pressure in peritubular blood, and this tends to increase net sodium reabsorption [25]. Reduced renal blood flow, especially in superficial cortical areas, has also been noted by xenon wash out and radiographic techniques [50, 96]. The concept that renal vasoconstriction causes an initially reversible (e.g., by vasodilators [77–79, 95, 96] increase in renal vascular resistance followed by an irreversible increase due to structural vascular narrowing has support [96, 200]. Most patients in whom renal biopsy is performed after 5 to 10 years of untreated essential hypertension do show slight-to-moderate arteriolosclerosis [33, 34], and there is a correlation between severity of sclerotic small vascular change and the degree of hypertension. Moreover, subsequent mortality also correlates with the severity of the benign arteriolar lesion on renal biopsy; specifically, mortality over 5 to 9 years of follow-up was 5 percent for patients with "no" vascular change versus 54 percent for "severe" nephrosclerosis in a series studied prior to the availability of drug treatment [34].

There is evidence [63, 131] of increased anatomic nephrosclerosis and reduction in renal blood flow in blacks compared with whites even at the same moderate (mean blood pressure 110 to 125 mm Hg) degree of severity of hypertension. Separate studies of cardiac output, plasma volume, and systemic peripheral resistance in matched hypertensive blacks and white patients, in contrast, showed no difference [148]. Normotensive black subjects excrete a sodium load more slowly than whites [137]. Hypertension and hypertensive nephrosclerosis are rare in rural blacks but common in urban blacks in South Africa [108]; in African blacks who migrate to cities urinary salt excretion and blood pressure increase [180]. These observations and the evidence that *all* causes of renal disease except congenital ones such as polycystic kidney disease progress more commonly to end-stage renal disease in blacks [191] certainly raise the possibility that, in this racial group, the renal vasculature responds abnormally, especially to environmental stimuli in a westernized culture [55, 56].

The natural history of untreated essential hypertension is available from studies prior to the availability of antihypertensive drugs and suggests that 1 to 7 percent [10, 11, 12, 123, 170] will enter the malignant phase and that 80 to 90 percent of untreated patients in that phase are dead within 1 year [173]. Malignant hypertension appears to be more frequent and to occur at an earlier age in blacks [91]. In patients who remain in the "benign" phase but die of hypertensive target organ disease, 40 percent die of heart disease, 15 percent of stroke, and 5 to 15 percent of uremia [12, 170, 173, 196] over a period of 10 to 20 years. Uremia is much more common in malignant hypertension. Mean survival in nonmalignant essential hypertension varies widely depending on severity [173]; in the series of Perera [170], it averaged 20 years but was only 9 years if the systolic blood pressure was over 200 or the diastolic over 120 mm Hg. In the study of Bechgaard [12], the mortality for essential hypertension was 60 percent over 16 to 22 years. In most untreated series women tolerated "benign" hypertension better than men. Other important prognostic factors are the level of blood pressure, the degree of hypertensive retinopathy, and the presence of proteinuria.

Unequivocal evidence of the efficacy of antihypertensive drug treatment in preventing strokes and heart disease is available for patients with diastolic pressures over 105 mm Hg [214, 215]; the evidence is suggestive in patients with diastolic pressure over 90 mm Hg [105]. In the Framingham study, an elevated systolic pressure was of equally serious prognostic import for heart disease and stroke [70, 71]. The efficacy of drug treatment in that condition, especially in the elderly (in whom isolated systolic hypertension is more common because of loss of elastic recoil in the aorta), is not yet proved; controlled prospective trials are currently ongoing in the United States. Although in most of the reported trials claims were made for the prevention of renal "events," these were, in fact, few in number in both treated and control groups (Table 54-2). Supporting data for efficacy in preventing progressive renal insufficiency and end-stage renal diseases by antihypertensive medications are, in fact, much less convincing than for prevention of cardiovascular disease, especially congestive heart failure [110] and stroke [111]. This is discussed in detail subsequently.

Laragh and co-workers [26] have claimed that an elevated plasma renin level, when interpreted in relation to the dietary sodium intake, is predictive of more target organ damage. This concept has not been sustained by other groups [112, 113, 162], and there is a significant fall in renin level with age in both normal and hypertensive patients [162]. It is likely, however, in both malignant hypertension and progressive hypertensive nephrosclerosis that small vessel disease within the kidney does activate renin release and contribute to vicious circle hypertension.

Despite a great deal of animal experimentation and human studies, the cause or causes of essential hypertension remain to be established. Guyton [81, 82, 83] has pointed out that, regardless of proximate cause, ultimately almost all varieties of chronic hypertension result

Table 54-2. Prospective controlled clinical trials: effect of treatment on progressive renal disease

	(Renal deterioration/ total patients)		
DBP (mm Hg)	Treated	Control	Ref. no.
115–129	0/70	3/73	214
90–114	0/194	2/186	215
90–104	7/3903	5/3922*	105

*Control group was referred to community physicians for routine care.

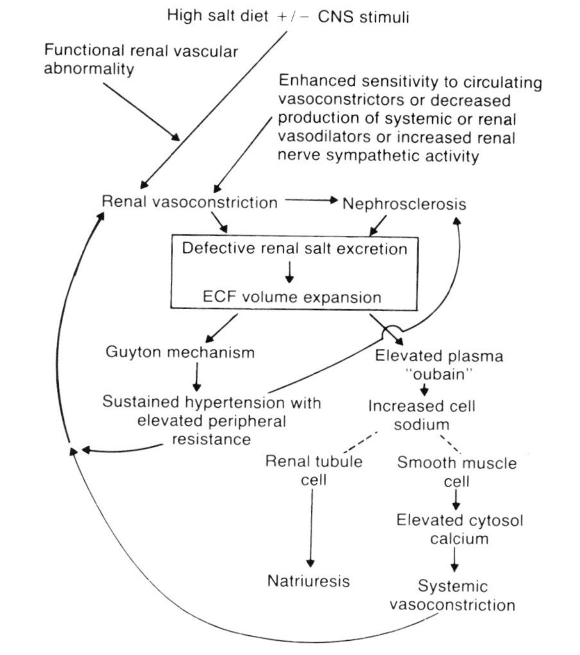

Fig. 54-2. Outline of possible renal mechanisms for development of "essential" hypertension.

from an inability of the kidney to excrete sodium chloride, reduce plasma and extracellular fluid (ECF) volume, and restore normotension (Figs. 54-2 and 54-3). He believes that long-term control of blood pressure is dependent on renal control of volume and that normally the signal has virtually infinite gain; that is, an increased intake of sodium chloride can be excreted by the normal kidney without any need for a sustained increase in blood pressure (Fig. 54-3). In contrast, in essential hypertension an extremely subtle, presumably genetically determined defect in excretion of sodium chloride, undetectable in short-term balance studies, leads, especially in the face of a high sodium chloride intake, to ECF volume expansion and a resulting increase in cardiac output. Perfusion through organs increases and, in a fundamental autoregulatory response, peripheral resistance increases, organ flow is reduced to normal, but blood pressure is increased, and cardiac output returns

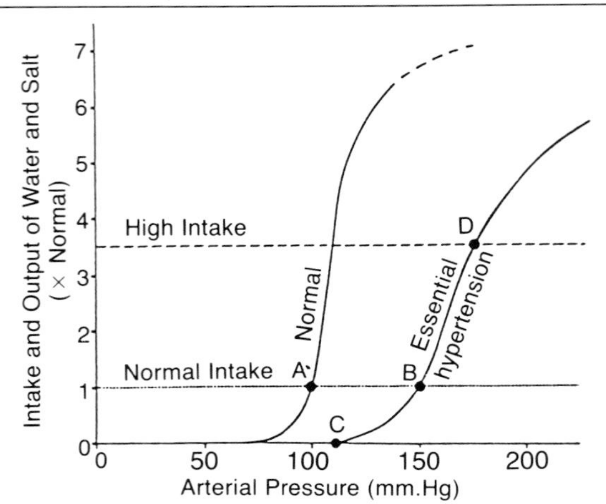

Fig. 54-3. Dr. Guyton's concept of elevated arterial pressure in essential hypertension. Point *A* represents normal steady state with balance between intake and output at a normal blood pressure, which increases almost undetectably at the new steady state on a high salt intake. In contrast, with essential hypertension at all intakes, an increasingly higher blood pressure is needed to maintain balance (points *C, B,* and *D*). (From A. C. Guyton, T. G. Coleman, A. W. Cowley, Jr., et al. Arterial pressure regulators: Overriding dominance of the kidneys in long-term regulation and in hypertension. *Am. J. Med.* 52:584:1972.)

to normal. Others have argued that the increase in cardiac output is an epiphenomenon and that the initiating change is the expansion of ECF volume, which leads, via humoral agents [86] or cardiogenic pressor reflexes [53], to hypertension. At the higher blood pressure and renal perfusion pressure, renal output of sodium chloride increases and now allows normal sodium balance but at the expense of persistently higher blood pressure (Fig. 54-3). The transition from labile hypertension with an elevated cardiac output and normal peripheral resistance to sustained hypertension with a normal cardiac output and elevated peripheral resistance has been observed in humans [58, 139, 219] as well as in dogs [35] and in experimental renovascular hypertension [129]. Expressed in another way, Guyton's hypothesis is that the renal natriuretic response to increasing perfusion pressure must be reset for hypertension to persist (Fig. 54-3).

Support for this hypothesis is also offered by the pathogenesis of surgically reversible hypertension in humans (e.g., renal artery stenosis, primary aldosteronism, Cushing's disease, and pheochromocytoma), in which some factor or factors have been demonstrated to interfere with normal renal sodium excretion—for example, lowered GFR, lowered hydrostatic pressure within the kidney, or inappropriately high ambient aldosterone, angiotensin II, or catecholamines levels. This is also true in experimental models, in nearly all of which hypertension is dependent on, or at least exacerbated by, a high intake of sodium chloride [84]. These models included Dahl salt-sensitive [43, 124] and spontaneously hypertensive rats (SHR) [19, 212], DOCA nephrectomy [54], and reduced renal mass [35] as well as one kidney-one clip and two kidney-one clip models [80]. In the latter case, the important antinatriuretic influences of circulating angiotensin II on the contralateral normal kidney have been recently highlighted [175]. In chronic renal failure, renin-angiotensin levels are abnormally high relative to the expanded ECF volume [16, 192, 216], presumably reflecting a diminished GFR, retention of sodium chloride, and abnormal renin release. However, in salt-wasting, progressive, primarily interstitial renal diseases, hypertension is either delayed or does not develop [21].

A recent modification of the Guyton hypothesis is the concept that ECF volume expansion stimulates production of a substance with a ouabain-like action that inhibits cellular Na-K-ATPase and hence decreases renal reabsorption of sodium chloride, thus restoring balance [20, 85, 86]. The ATPase-inhibiting effect also increases smooth muscle cytosol sodium, and this secondarily decreases passage of calcium out of cells via calcium-sodium exchange, since the latter is driven by the sodium gradient across the cell membrane. The resulting increase in smooth muscle calcium leads to increased muscle tone and elevated peripheral resistance [50, 73]. There is evidence of an increased sodium concentration in arteriolar walls in essential hypertension [209]. A red cell sodium transport defect leading to elevated red blood cell sodium has been described in hypertensive patients and their relatives and may have relevance for an associated similar transport defect in the kidney [1, 2].

The concept that essential hypertension may have a renal cause is certainly not new. Several investigators in the past have argued this case [65, 76, 152]. Indeed, Goldblatt's renal artery-clip animal models were intended by the investigator as a model for intrarenal small vessel narrowing as a cause of essential hypertension [76], an argument that Goldblatt himself continued to support. However, the consensus today is that the small vessel lesions are secondary rather than primary in essential hypertension [13, 34, 91, 173]. Thus it is argued that the lesions of arteriolosclerosis are identical to those acquired in primary glomerular renal disease as a result of secondary hypertension. A case could be made, however, for the proposition that, for example, in diabetes mellitus and focal glomerulosclerosis the associated hyperplastic arteriolosclerotic lesions may *primarily* contribute to the renal hypertension. The kidney arterioles in patients with essential hypertension also appear to be more extensively and earlier involved than those of other organs [210], although the vascular changes are sometimes slight or absent in established hypertension on biopsy [34] and even at autopsy when the whole kidneys are available for study.

Thus in some or all patients with essential hypertension, a primary hereditary abnormality of the renal vasculature, which may not have a structural correlate in the early stages of the disease, and may even be seen in normotensive relatives [18, 101], may cause selective renal vasoconstriction in response to certain environmental stimuli such as a high salt intake [94, 142] or environmental stress [78, 101] or exercise [167] (Fig. 54-2). This in turn leads to an impairment of renal salt excretion and, via Guyton's mechanisms, to systemic hypertension. The vasoconstriction and hypertension together could then lead ultimately to anatomic nephrosclerosis and a sustained increase in intrarenal vascular resistance [96]. It is intriguing that in SHR, which is probably the best animal model of essential hypertension, effective control of blood pressure by antihypertensive medications restored survival to control levels, prevented cardiac hypertrophy and *systemic* arteriolar changes, but failed to prevent progressive proteinuria or *renal* arteriolosclerosis [66]. The authors postulated a genetic defect in the vascular system of SHR, especially in the kidney. In the same model increased intrarenal vascular resistance [159], altered ion transport in smooth muscle [109] and red cell membranes [179], and diminished cortical Na-K-ATPase [203] have been observed, even prior to the onset of hypertension. This genetic ion transport abnormality might be related to the early increase in renal vascular resistance in SHR [68] by facilitating decreased calcium efflux from vascular smooth muscle cells through reduced sodium-calcium exchange [20].

A great deal of study is now aimed at elucidating the nature of the putative renal abnormality in idiopathic hypertension in these models and in humans. In general, the following described abnormalities or defects lead, either directly or in response to environmental stimuli [132], exercise [167], or an increased sodium chloride intake, to renal vasoconstriction and/or decreased sodium chloride excretion: (1) defective renal vasodilator and natriuretic prostaglandin production [184, 197, 198] or responsiveness [172]; (2) selectively increased renal efferent sympathetic nerve activity or sensitivity [52, 117]; (3) diminished production of the vasodilator bradykinin in response to sodium loading [84, 85, 130, 197, 198]; increased CNS or renal production of, or renal sensitivity to, circulating catecholamines [48, 52, 69]; diminished renal vasodilation and suppression of aldosterone in response to salt loading [99, 100, 220]; and increased susceptibility of the renal vasculature to injury or to angiotensin II [134]. Enhanced sensitivity to angiotensin II could lead to efferent arteriolar constriction [57, 72] and increased reabsorption of sodium in the proximal tubule and possibly in the loop of Henle. In patients with early essential hypertension [97] and in their normotensive relatives in response to stress [101], renal vasoconstriction with preservation of GFR and, presumably, efferent vasoconstriction have been shown. Enhanced vasodilatory responses to captopril in patients with essential hypertension compared with normal subjects with at least maintained GFR during both high and low salt intakes have been interpreted by Hollenberg et al. as further support for a pathogenetically important functional vascular abnormality in the kidney in the earlier stages of essential hypertension [99, 100]. The SHR model demonstrates, compared with normotensive controls, the antinatriuretic effects of the combination of a high sodium intake, environmental stress and enhanced renal sympathetic nerve activity [125]. It is important to note again that the initial abnormality may not be an anatomic or structural one within the kidney but rather may involve increased or decreased sensitivity to a humoral agent or lack of a hemodynamic response to salt loading. Thus the CNS-endocrine-renal axis, which maintains ECF volume in the face of environmental challenges such as increased stress or high intake of sodium chloride, may be functioning imperfectly.

One of the barriers to studying the pathogenesis of essential hypertension in humans is the long gestation period. Cyclosporine may offer a truncated-in-time iatrogenic model of "salt-dependent" essential hypertension in humans [41]; this drug not only leads to renal vasoconstriction with an elevated filtration fraction and to accelerated proximal tubule reabsorption of sodium chloride and water [128] but also directly and quickly leads to systemic vasoconstriction (compare with Fig. 54-2 for essential hypertension).

The pivotal pathogenetic role of the kidney in experimental rat hypertension is established by transplantation experiments between syngeneic rat strains. Thus hypertension or normotension can be transplanted with the kidney when accompanied by bilateral nephrectomy of the native kidneys, in three rat models of essential hypertension [19, 37, 43, 119, 120, 124].

We observed a similar response in humans to renal transplantation from normotensive donors in patients who reached end-stage renal disease (ESRD) because of hypertensive nephrosclerosis [39]. Six patients in whom classic clinical and pathologic data conclusively established that diagnosis had normal blood pressures a mean time of 4.5 years (range 1 to 8 years) after successful, immunologically well tolerated renal transplantation from a normotensive donor. An example of such a patient follows:

The patient was a 33-year-old black man who was told he had hypertension in 1966 during a physical examination for the armed forces. He did not receive therapy for his hypertension until 1976, when he was seen in a local emergency room for a laceration on his arm and was again found to be hypertensive. For 6 months his blood pressure was controlled with antihypertensive medications, but headaches developed, and he was seen at a local emergency room with a blood pressure of 188/120 mm Hg. He was admitted to that hospital and found to have left ventricular enlargement by chest radiography and electrocardiography; arteriolar narrowing and exudates were seen on funduscopic examination. His serum potassium level was 4 mmol per liter, his blood urea nitrogen level was 35 mg per deciliter (12 mmol per liter), and urinalysis was negative for protein. His blood pressure was better controlled with increases in his antihypertensive medications, and he was referred to another university hospital for evaluation of the cause of his hypertension. There he underwent intravenous pyelography and renal arteriography, the results of both of which were normal. Urinalysis revealed trace protein, and the 24-hour urinary protein excretion level was 500 mg. The 24-hour urinary excretion of catecholamines was also normal. The blood urea nitrogen level was 39 mg per deciliter (14 mmol per liter), and the patient was seen in consultation by members of the university nephrology service, who thought his longstanding hypertension, low level of proteinuria, and normal size kidneys were consistent with nephrosclerosis and recommended that he not undergo renal biopsy. The patient's mother and father were both hypertensive and required medication. One sister (age 30) was also taking antihypertensive medications, and a brother (age 23) had been told he was hypertensive and given prescriptions for medications.

The patient's antihypertensive medications were adjusted at the medical center, and he was discharged in 1976 with a diagnosis of essential hypertension, to be followed by his local physician. In 1978 he saw his physician again, admitted he had not taken his medications, and was noted to have a blood urea nitrogen level of 113 mg per deciliter and a creatinine level of 19 mg per deciliter. His blood pressure was 200/130 mm Hg, and he was started on hemodialysis therapy at this medical center. A bilateral nephrectomy was performed because the blood pressure could not be adequately controlled on dialysis. One month after nephrectomy, blood pressure control was improved. Detailed histologic and ultramicroscopic examinations of the kidneys showed nephrosclerosis without other primary renal disease. Mean arterial pressure was 113 ± 3 mm Hg on long-term dialysis. One year later (1979), the patient received a cadaveric renal transplant and did well. Three years later he was admitted to the clinical research center for studies. His blood pressure was 125/80 mm Hg (mean arterial pressure, 95 mm Hg) without antihypertensive medications [40].

The response of this and the other five patients in our clinical research center to a sequential normal, low and high salt intake over 9 days was virtually identical to that of an age- and sex-matched normotensive control group: blood pressure remained normal, and sodium balance, changes in the renin-angiotensin-aldosterone axis and in plasma catecholamines, plasma volume, cardiac output, and endogenous creatinine clearance were indistinguishable. After transplantation there was a striking decrease in left ventricular hypertrophy and improvement in the appearance of the retinal vessels in the previously hypertensive patients. When we then considered all patients in our transplant clinic who had nephrosclerosis as a cause of ESRD and previous native kidney nephrectomy, and had had successful renal transplantation at least 1 year previously with a serum creatinine of less than 2 mg per deciliter, 76 percent were normotensive, a percentage similar to that seen in patients with primary renal causes of ESRD [38]. It is, of course, possible that longer follow-up will reveal the development of hypertension in these patients, but it should also be remembered that they all receive chronic, although low-dose, steroid therapy as part of their immunosuppressive regimen.

We suggest that the findings support the hypothesis that the native kidneys must be involved in the etiology of "essential" hypertension, either directly or through interaction with another organ, humoral agent, or the sympathetic nervous system. The observations encourage pursuit of identification of the renal abnormality in high-risk, young, still normotensive siblings of patients with essential hypertension in an effort to identify such patients and prevent the development of this extremely common and important disease. It is, of course, quite possible that a specific renal etiology applies only to a subgroup of essential hypertensives.

In established essential hypertension *exaggerated natriuresis* in response to acute sodium loading compared with normotensive controls has been a consistent finding [4, 27, 36, 163]. This phenomenon is not altered by prior exposure to a low-salt diet [163], so it does not reflect prior sodium balance. Likewise, the hypertensive subjects do not have a defect of sodium conservation on a low sodium intake [204]. The excess natriuresis is also seen in response to acute volume expansion with non-sodium-containing fluids [30]. Support for the importance of hypertension and increased renal perfusion pressure per se in the pathogenesis of the exaggerated natriuresis is offered by the observation that normal subjects show it after pressor agents are used to elevate the blood pressure [143, 194, 213]; this has been confirmed in experimental animals. Enhanced natriuresis is associated in humans with enhanced wedged intrarenal vein pressure (and presumably peritubular capillary pressure) compared with normotensive controls [136]; it is quite possible that such altered physical factors diminish the net transport of sodium from the tubular lumen to the peritubular capillary. In experimental animals the phenomenon is seen in isolated perfused kidneys [37], thus excluding the necessity of involving circulating humoral agents or renal innervation. The nonspecificity of the finding for essential hypertension is also supported by its demonstration in *secondary* hypertension such as pheochromocytoma [87]. Since there is not an exaggerated increase in GFR [36, 163] or diminished renin-aldosterone responsiveness [127] compared with normotensives, tubular sodium absorption must be decreased. The site of the diminished sodium reabsorption is not established, but clearance studies in humans [27, 37, 44, 127] and micropuncture studies in rats [51, 205] suggest the loop of Henle as a likely site of the phenomenon. The possibility that this may relate to enhanced medullary solute washout has been suggested [127, 168, 194]; this would reduce the gradient for passive diffusion of sodium chloride from the thin ascending limb of the loop of Henle of juxtamedullary nephrons. An additional experimental finding has been a greater reduction of sympathetic nerve activity in response to the same volume load in hypertensive rats [188].

This acute, probably nonspecific, phenomenon of exaggerated natriuresis in response to an *acute* volume load in established hypertension is not to be confused with postulated defects in the ability to respond to *chronic* salt loads in the genesis of essential hypertension or of the established effect of chronic salt loading in worsening hypertension.

Hypertensive Nephrosclerosis

Hypertensive nephrosclerosis is present when essential hypertension produces evidence of renal dysfunction manifest by an elevation of serum creatinine or the development of significant proteinuria. Hypertensive nephrosclerosis is an important cause of ESRD in the United States and, to a lesser degree, in Europe [191, 222].

The patient may present with hypertension or its complications, such as left ventricular failure, or with symptoms of uremia, or because of positive findings on urinalysis or on measurement of BUN and serum creatinine at routine clinical screening (Table 54-3). In general, symptoms due to hypertension per se, as distinct from the effects of hypertension on target organs, are nonspecific. Presentation in the malignant phase is discussed in Chap. 59. A family history of hypertension is important, but a positive history may also be obtained in other familial renal diseases such as polycystic kidney disease and hereditary nephritis. Evidence of hypertensive changes in the retinal vessels and of left ventricular hypertrophy is usually present. Papilledema is a feature of malignant hypertension [123], and retinal exudates and hemorrhages are characteristic of severe, accelerated hypertension. An accentuated second aortic valve closure sound and presystolic atrial gallop may be found.

The age of onset of essential hypertension is, in general, between 25 and 45 years of age, and renal impairment as manifest by an elevation of serum creatinine is unusual until after at least 10 years of sustained "benign" hypertension. Previous histologic and radiographic studies have suggested that some degree of nephrosclerosis is usually present after 5 years of sustained hypertension [34, 96, 98].

Most patients who develop renal insufficiency secondary to essential hypertension in the third to fifth decade have a history of severe hypertension. Whether progressive renal failure ever develops in these age groups without the previous occurrence of the fully developed syndrome of malignant hypertension remains

Table 54-3. Features supporting a diagnosis of hypertensive nephrosclerosis

1. Black race
2. Positive family history; onset of hypertension between age 25 and 45
3. Long-standing or very severe hypertension
4. Evidence of hypertensive retinal damage
5. Evidence of hypertensive left ventricular hypertrophy
6. Onset of hypertension *prior* to development of proteinuria
7. Absence of any cause for primary renal disease
8. Biopsy evidence [7]; degree of glomerular ischemia and fibrosis compatible with degree of arteriolar and small arterial vascular disease

controversial [5, 91]. Although malignant hypertension is probably becoming less common [223] because of the increased availability, tolerability, and efficacy of treatment, there is still no evidence that hypertensive nephrosclerosis is diminishing in frequency as a cause of ESRD. Thus Rostand et al. [191] showed that nephrosclerosis accounted for a constant fraction of ESRD (about 20 percent) in Jefferson County, Alabama, between 1973 and 1978 without any downward trend, and data for this area for 1983 suggest that this percentage had not changed (Table 54-4). This is surprising in view of the increased utilization of antihypertensive drugs and raises the issue that such drug therapy may not prevent or reduce the incidence of hypertensive nephrosclerosis as a cause of ESRD, either because the medications are not taken effectively due to expense or side effects or, as discussed earlier, because the hypertension is the result and not the cause of a renal abnormality.

Nevertheless, most such patients give evidence of periods of accelerated or at least poorly controlled and quite severe diastolic hypertension, often due to episodes of noncompliance for economic or other reasons. In patients with mild-to-moderate essential hypertension development of ESRD occurs only after many years; usually such patients are elderly by the time ESRD is realized [91]. Lack of evidence of hypertensive disease in the fundi or of left ventricular hypertrophy, in the presence of a clear elevation of serum creatinine, should cause the clinician to carefully reconsider underlying primary renal rather than primary hypertensive disease. The incidence of hypertensive nephrosclerosis is much increased in blacks [186], especially in black males in the fourth decade [191]. Especially under the age of 30 years, the diagnosis of hypertensive nephrosclerosis in white patients should be treated with healthy skepticism; primary parenchymal renal disease is much more common. Clinical features supporting a diagnosis of hypertensive nephrosclerosis are listed in Table 54-3.

Urinalysis usually shows only modest proteinuria; in the absence of malignant hypertension, 24-hour urinary protein excretion is usually less than 1.5 to 2.0 gm except when severe right heart failure occurs. In untreated patients followed until death [170] proteinuria was noted in 42 percent. One report [155] describes higher amounts of proteinuria (up to 6.5 gm/24 hr) in patients with significant renal impairment due to severe "benign" hypertensive nephrosclerosis. Yamada et al. [225]

Table 54-4. Hypertensive nephrosclerosis as a cause of end-stage renal disease in Jefferson County, Alabama, 1974–1984

	1974[a]	1975[a]	1976[a]	1977[a]	1978[a]	1983[b]	1984[b]
Number of patients	11	20	10	10	20	41	45
Total ESRD patients	52	67	54	49	62	114	116
Percentage	21	30	19	20	32	36	39

[a]Data from Rostand et al. [191].
[b]Data from Health Care Financing Administration Medical Information System.
Note: Data from sources [a] and [b] are not strictly comparable since uniform criteria for diagnosis of hypertensive nephrosclerosis were strictly applied in [a]; furthermore, the ESRD population was older in 1983 and 1984 than before, with 50 percent of patients over the age of 50 years at the time of initiation of renal replacement therapy.

found mean proteinuria of 111 mg per deciliter at a mean diastolic of 117 mm Hg and 9 mg per deciliter at 108 mm Hg; proteinuria decreased significantly both with lesser severity of pretreatment blood pressure and subsequent to antihypertensive therapy. Formed elements on urinary microscopy are few, again except in the malignant phase. Specific tubular syndromes are rare except for renal tubular hyperkalemia due to hyporeninemic hypoaldosteronism, with which nephrosclerosis is one of the more commonly associated renal diseases after diabetic nephropathy [46]. This might relate in part to involvement of the juxtaglomerular cells by the hyaline arteriolosclerotic lesion of the afferent arteriole such that renin synthesis and release is impaired; ischemic tubular atrophy is also often marked in both conditions and may contribute by diminishing collecting duct tubular secretory capacity for potassium.

Renal size is usually symmetrically and modestly reduced. The renal calyces and pelves are normal, in contrast to papillary necrosis or reflux nephropathy. Asymmetry of size raises the possibility of complicating renovascular hypertension due to renal artery stenosis. Fortunately, a balanced, bilateral functionally significant renal artery stenosis with symmetric reduction in size of both kidneys is rare, or differential diagnosis between this condition and hypertensive nephrosclerosis would be more difficult. In addition, renal artery stenosis, especially the atherosclerotic type, is rare in blacks as a cause of hypertension [206]. Two additional diseases to be considered in differential diagnosis are gouty nephropathy and lead nephropathy. Many now argue that gouty nephropathy virtually never causes chronic renal failure in the absence of hypertension or recurrent uric acid stone disease with obstructive nephropathy [17, 185, 226] and that renal insufficiency in association with previous acute gout is, rather, usually [9] due to saturnine gout and chronic lead nephropathy. In the southeastern United States, this is commonly secondary to lead contamination of unbonded illicit alcohol, in which the alcohol is distilled in old car radiators, which are soldered with lead [6, 62]. Additional evidence of chronic lead exposure as a cause of subsequent chronic renal failure and hypertension is available from Australia in children chronically exposed to lead-containing paint [61, 88, 89]. Increased bone lead can be diagnosed [61] by demonstrating increased urinary excretion of lead after infusion of the chelating agent EDTA (ethylene diamine tetra-acetic acid). The renal diagnosis is difficult to establish, since no specific histologic change identifies chronic lead nephropathy. However, the possibility exists of "deleading" such patients, if renal fibrosis is not too far advanced, to arrest or retard the progress of the disease [9, 151]. More prospective studies are needed to establish this point, but creatinine clearance increased after deleading of patients with documented increased tissue lead stores after chronic industrial exposure to lead [9]. It is the author's clinical impression that hypertensive nephrosclerosis and lead nephropathy may occur together and that this combination of diseases may not be rare in the southeastern United States.

Differential diagnosis between hypertensive nephrosclerosis and bilateral parenchymal renal disease due to chronic glomerulonephritis with secondary renal hypertension, for example, can be quite difficult when chronic renal failure is advanced by the time the patient is first seen by the physician. Onset of proteinuria only after a period of sustained hypertension supports hypertensive nephrosclerosis and vice versa.

The diagnosis of hypertensive nephrosclerosis can be established only by careful exclusion of the various primary renal diseases. This requires a renal biopsy, but this invasive procedure is not usually performed when the clinical circumstances strongly support a diagnosis of nephrosclerosis (Table 54-3), just as biopsy is usually omitted in the appropriate clinical circumstances for the diagnosis of diabetic glomerulosclerosis. Nevertheless, hypertensive nephrosclerosis tends to be a much overused, poorly considered diagnosis, which is given especially to black patients with hypertension and renal insufficiency. The less strong the evidence for the long duration and severity of the hypertension, the less significant the family history, the more marked the proteinuria, the less appropriate the age of onset of diastolic hypertension for essential hypertension, and the less secure the evidence for hypertension prior to the onset of proteinuria, the more the physician should reconsider the diagnosis.

The mechanism of progressive nephron loss in hypertensive nephrosclerosis has been assumed to relate to glomerular and tubular ischemia secondary to narrowing of small vessels [91]. However, in various experimental animal models of essential hypertension intraglomerular pressure and plasma flow have been shown to be high [3, 54, 193], and glomerular damage with the lesions of focal sclerosis and widened mesangial areas has been attributed to these high pressures and flows [23]. A low-protein diet reduces systemic pressures, intraglomerular pressure and flow, proteinuria, and morphologic changes in the deoxycorticosterone (DOC) unilateral nephrectomy hypertensive model [54], as it does in experimental models of renal ablation [23] and chronic glomerulonephritis [5]. Brenner et al. [23] suggested on the basis of these experimental findings that hypertensive glomerular sclerosis is dependent on glomerular capillary hypertension with increased glomerular plasma flow. However, as Ferris has noted [67], it is possible that a component of afferent arteriolar constriction in essential hypertension protects the glomerular capillary bed from the potentially damaging effect of elevated glomerular pressures, in contrast to the compensatory afferent arteriolar dilatation seen in surviving glomeruli of kidneys with reduced renal mass. Thus Bank et al. [7] noted normal superficial nephron glomerular pressures despite systemic hypertension in SHR. In experimental hyperperfusion nephropathy in aging rats [23] and in human progressive primary interstitial renal disease such as reflux nephropathy, the characteristic glomerular lesion is focal glomerular sclerosis. However, focal glomerulosclerosis, although it does occur in hypertensive nephrosclerosis, is not as prominent a histologic feature as it is in reflux nephropathy. This suggests that glomerular atrophy in hypertensive nephrosclerosis in humans may result from both the primary injurious effects of glomerular ischemia and hyperperfusion nephropathy in surviving adapted hypertrophied nephrons; the latter may be modified if there is fixed vascular narrowing that does not allow increased plasma flow to that nephron. The relative preservation of GFR with an increased filtration fraction is characteristic of both clinical and experimental essential hypertension and supports the presence of efferent arteriolar vasoconstriction; others have argued that afferent or mesangial constriction may also contribute to the increased intrarenal vascular resistance [37, 83]. This seems especially likely at the afferent level as fixed vascular narrowing due to afferent arteriosclerosis develops.

Hypertension *secondary* to renal disease is believed to contribute to progression of both experimental and clinical glomerular renal disease, as reviewed by Baldwin and Neugarten [5]. It is hypothesized that, as nephrons are lost, a compensatory decrease in afferent arteriolar resistance to increased glomerular plasma flow in the remaining nephrons allows transmission of elevated systemic pressures to the glomerulus. Indeed, treatment of hypertension in experimental models of reduced nephron mass and in clinical diabetic glomerulosclerosis reduces histologic progression of the glomerular damage [102, 103, 164, 182]. If these experimental data are applicable to human hypertensive disease, then consideration of the effect of drug therapy on intraglomerular as well as systemic pressures will be necessary for optimum treatment [118]. In experimental hypertensive models, even a small rise in intraglomerular pressure in the presence of increased plasma flow is associated with glomerular damage [54].

Brenner and co-workers [23] have argued that the high-protein diet characteristic of western civilization contributes to hyperperfusion-induced glomerulosclerosis by increasing glomerular plasma flow and intraglomerular hydrostatic pressure in surviving nephrons that have hypertrophied after other nephrons have been destroyed. Nevertheless, recent preliminary studies of protein restriction in hypertensive nephrosclerosis with renal insufficiency showed no benefit, unlike the situation in patients with chronic pyelonephritis [60]; the authors attributed this to the predominant role of glomerular ischemia rather than hyperfiltration in hypertensive nephrosclerosis.

In hypertensive nephrosclerosis, antihypertensive drug therapy is mandatory. Indeed, for hypertension in general a serum creatinine of > 1.7 mg/dl and < 2.5 mg/dl is associated with increased mortality [195]. The prognostic significance of microalbuminuria in essential hypertension, however, remains to be determined in prospective studies. Hypertension is usually of significant degree when nephrosclerosis results, and vicious circle hypertension will ensue if hypertension is not treated. Furthermore, the evidence for the efficacy of drug treatment in protecting against cardiovascular disease and stroke is substantial. Likewise, in hypertension secondary to parenchymal renal disease, antihypertensive treatment will tend to prevent or retard the development of arteriolar nephrosclerosis, forestall entry into the malignant phase of hypertension (which is more likely than in essential hypertension), and probably assist in slowing the development of hyperperfusion nephropathy at the single nephron level as nephrons are lost. In support of the latter mechanism in essential hypertension is the reduction of subclinical albuminuria by antihypertensive drug therapy [169].

The evidence, however, that antihypertensive drug treatment of hypertensive nephrosclerosis prevents the development of progressive renal disease is not firm; certainly the evidence for prevention of kidney target organ damage is much less convincing than that for the heart and brain in nonmalignant essential hypertension (Table 54-2). Whether renal function may deteriorate in the long term in nonmalignant hypertension despite good blood pressure control remains controversial [149, 171, 190, 207]. Most of these studies were retrospective and lacked histologic confirmation of the absence of primary renal disease. The evidence for protection of renal function by therapy in malignant hypertension is strong [223].

In studies done prior to general acceptance of the view that not to treat established hypertension is unethical or at least unwise, the effect of 1 to 5 years of antihypertensive drug treatment on renal function in patients with moderate essential hypertension (diastolic blood pressure < 130 mm Hg) was compared with untreated patients [144, 152, 187]. No significant differences in changes in GFR and renal plasma flow (RPF) in treated and untreated groups were seen, but declines in these values were small in both groups. In a study of nineteen 49-year-old men before and 7 years after treatment of moderate essential hypertension compared with 15 age-matched normotensive controls, GFR fell 17 percent in the treated hypertensive group ($p < 0.05$) and 8 percent (p = NS) in normotensive controls [135].

Hypertensive nephrosclerosis accounts for one-third of ESRD in blacks in the United States and 5 to 10 percent of ESRD in whites in both Europe and the United States [191, 222]. Overall in the United States it accounts for 28 percent of ESRD patients [64]; there is as yet no evidence of a reduction in its incidence as a cause of ESRD in the United States (Table 54-4). This apparent failure to reduce the incidence of hypertensive nephrosclerosis has taken place against a background of increasing use of antihypertensive medications, according to recent data from the National Center for Health Statistics. Overall, the incidence of ESRD is four to five times greater in the black than in the white population [64, 126, 191]. This marked difference is explained only in part by the much higher incidence (an 18-fold increase) of nephrosclerosis in blacks, because the incidence over 5 years of every other cause of ESRD in Jefferson County, Alabama, a county of 700,000 people, was significantly increased in blacks (Table 54-5) except for congenital renal diseases such as polycystic kidney disease. Similar findings have been noted elsewhere in

Table 54-5. Race-specific risks for diseases causing end-stage renal disease in Jefferson County, Alabama, 1974–1978

	Yearly incidence per million population*				
	All	Black	White	Relative risk	p value <
All diseases	91	188	44	3.8	0.0001
Hypertension	23	64	4	18	0.0001
Glomerulonephritis	12	22	7	3	0.002
Diabetes mellitus	8	15	5	3	0.0013
Interstitial renal disease	20	38	12	3	0.001
Polycystic kidney disease	3	3	4	1	0.8
Unknown	21	41	11	4	0.001

*Numbers are rounded.
Source: Modified from S. G. Rostand, et al. Racial differences in the incidence of treatment for end-stage renal disease. *N. Engl. J. Med.* 306:1276, 1982.

the United States [218]. Since hypertension so commonly complicates these renal diseases, one explanation for this overall increased incidence may be an increased susceptibility in the kidneys of blacks to vascular damage as a result of hypertension or of the effects of a chronically expanded ECF volume. Additional evidence that black kidneys are an independent risk factor for progressive renal failure in primary hypertension has been provided by retrospective studies of treated patients [147, 190, 208].

We recently reexamined the prevalence of hypertensive nephrosclerosis as a cause of ESRD for the period 1983 to 1988 (i.e., 10 years after the first study) in Jefferson County, Alabama, using the same diagnostic criteria [183] (see Table 54-4). Again, there was no evidence of any reduction in hypertension as a cause for ESRD. There was, however, now evidence that antihypertensive therapy might be *delaying* progression to ESRD, because the peak incidence of ESRD due to hypertension had moved significantly from the age of 40 to 49 years in the 1970s to the age of 50 to 59 years in blacks in the 1980s.

If, indeed, antihypertensive treatment does not *prevent* progression of hypertensive nephrosclerosis to end stage, what are the possible explanations? First, at a certain stage of renal insufficiency (perhaps serum creatinine > 3 to 4 mg/dl) loss of nephrons may continue, even after the disappearance of the inciting cause for renal damage, by mechanisms related to increased solute excretion per nephron such as hyperperfusion nephropathy [102, 103] or tubulointerstitial deposition of calcium phosphate [107]. Second, the patient may not take the prescribed medications regularly, or the medications may not control the blood pressure sufficiently well; however, there is no evidence that blacks are being treated less than whites [106]. Third, although systemic hypertension may be treated, as discussed, glomerular hypertension may persist. Fourth, hypertension may be the result of a renal abnormality rather than the cause of it. It seems unlikely that this renal abnormality is nephrosclerosis per se because early in the course of hypertension the vascular lesions may be absent or minimal. However, *both* the vascular lesion and the hypertension could result from a common cause (e.g., a prolonged abnormal renal response to a high salt intake, central nervous stimuli, or ECF volume expansion [86]). Effective drug control of blood pressure in a rat model of spontaneous hypertension prevented cardiac hypertrophy but did not prevent renal vascular lesions [66]. Since to withhold antihypertensive drug therapy is unethical, only careful prospective studies of renal function in patients with histologically proven nephrosclerosis will answer this important question. These studies are now planned. Thus while the possibility of prevention of ESRD due to hypertensive nephrosclerosis by early detection and effective treatment of hypertension, especially in black patients, is a most attractive and desirable goal, its attainment may yet require more understanding of the pathogenesis of hypertensive nephrosclerosis.

The principles of treatment of hypertension in hypertensive nephrosclerosis do not differ markedly from those for hypertension treatment in general. In some patients renal function does deteriorate slightly at first as blood pressure is lowered; this is unpredictable but is usually mild and reversible with continued treatment [225]. Treatment of hypertension associated with severe chronic renal failure may even precipitate the need for dialysis; some recovery of renal function in such circumstances can occur in subsequent weeks or months and may allow cessation of dialysis at least for a prolonged period. In a study of 155 patients with essential hypertension, initiation of effective antihypertensive drug therapy significantly reduced proteinuria within a month [225]. Pretreatment urinary protein excretion and reduction in GFR was greatest in patients with higher diastolic blood pressure (DBP): in the most severe group DBP was 117 ± 3 mm Hg, urinary protein 1.1 ± 0.1 gm per liter, and creatinine clearance 78 ± 8 ml per minute; these data changed with treatment to 94 ± 3 ($p < 0.001$), 0.45 ± 0.1 gm per liter ($p < 0.001$), and 65 ± 7 ml per minute (p = NS), respectively. In general, antihypertensive treatment reduces albuminuria [169].

The renal effects of antihypertensive therapy have recently been succinctly reviewed [59]. We now believe that in hypertensive nephrosclerosis, as in primary renal disease, converting enzyme inhibitors and calcium channel blockers may offer the treatment of choice, although this is not proved by appropriate prospective studies. Both classes of drugs appear to increase renal blood flow, and this may be of special advantage in essential hypertension in which, as discussed, renal vasoconstriction may play a primary role. In a recent retrospective study of primary renal disease, treatment with calcium channel blockers slowed progression [22]. Converting enzyme inhibitors have at least the theoretic advantage of reducing intraglomerular hydrostatic pressure because of their predominant action on the *efferent* arteriole [54, 59, 100]. If the latter mechanism becomes critical for the maintenance of GFR, as when all nephrons are distal [42] to a functionally significant renal artery stenosis(es) or to very severe generalized afferent arteriolar nephrosclerosis [45], renal function may deteriorate abruptly if converting enzyme inhibitors are used. Recovery occurs quickly after converting enzyme inhibitors are discontinued. Hyperkalemia can also occur in severe renal insufficiency or in hyporeninemic hyperaldosteronism treated with converting enzyme inhibitors. In severe hypertension, calcium channel blockers and converting enzyme inhibitors can be combined effectively, if necessary; if renal function is substantially decreased, a loop diuretic may also be required. It should be emphasized that good control of blood pressure is more important than strict adherence to a particular class of drug. Issues of affordability and of individual side effects or preferences may necessitate use of other antihypertensives including minoxidil, peripheral α-antagonists, centrally acting α_2-agonists, or a cardioselective β-blocker.

References

1. Adragna, N. C., Canessa, M. L., Solomon, H., et al. Red cell lithium-sodium countertransport and sodium-potassium cotransport in patients with essential hypertension. *Hypertension* 4: 795, 1982.
2. Aronson, P. S. Red-cell sodium-lithium countertransport and essential hypertension. *N. Engl. J. Med.* 307: 317, 1982.
3. Azar, S., Johnson, M. A., Hertel, B., et al. Single nephron pressures, flows and resistances in hypertensive kidneys with nephrosclerosis. *Kidney Int.* 12: 28, 1977.
4. Baldwin, D. S., Biggs, A. W., Goldring, W., et al. Exaggerated natriuresis in essential hypertension. *Am. J. Med.* 24: 893, 1958.
5. Baldwin, D. S., and Neugarten, J. Treatment of hypertension in renal disease. *Am. J. Kidney Dis.* 5(4): A57, 1985.
6. Ball, G. V., and Sorensen, L. B. Pathogenesis of hyperuricemia in saturnine gout. *N. Engl. J. Med.* 280: 1199, 1969.
7. Bank, N., Alterman, L., and Aynedjian, H. S. Selective deep nephron hyperfiltration in uninephrectomized spontaneously hypertensive rats. *Kidney Int.* 24: 185, 1983.
8. Bartter, F. C., Pronove, P., Gill, J. R., et al. Hyperplasia of the juxtaglomerular complex with hyperaldosteronism and hypokalemic alkalosis. A new syndrome. *Am. J. Med.* 33: 811, 1962.
9. Batuman, V., Maesaka, J. K., Haddad, B., et al. The role of lead in gout nephropathy. *N. Engl. J. Med.* 304: 520, 1981.
10. Bechgaard, P. Arterial hypertension: A follow-up study of one thousand hypertonics. *Acta Med. Scand.* (Suppl.): 172, 1946.
11. Bechgaard, P. The Natural History of Benign Hypertension. In K. D. Bock and P. T. Cottier (eds.), *Essential Hypertension: An International Symposium.* Berlin: Springer, 1960. P. 198.
12. Bechgaard, P., Kopp, H., and Nielsen, J. One thousand hypertensive patients followed from 16–22 years. *Acta Med. Scand.* (Suppl.): 155, 1956.
13. Bell, E. T. *Renal Diseases* (2nd ed.). Philadelphia: Lea & Febiger, 1950.
14. Bell, E. T. Renal vascular disease in diabetes mellitus. *Diabetes* 2: 376, 1953.
15. Beller, F. K., Dame, W. R., and Whitting, C. L. Renal disease diagnosed by renal biopsy. In G. M. Eisenbach and J. Brod (eds.), *Contributions to Nephrology.* Vol. 25, *Kidney and Pregnancy.* Basel: Karger, 1981. Pp. 61–70.
16. Beretta-Piccoli, C., Weidmann, P., De Chatel, R., et al. Hypertension associated with early stage kidney disease: Complementary roles of circulating renin, the body sodium/volume state and duration of hypertension. *Am. J. Med.* 61: 739, 1976.
17. Berger, L., and Yu, T.-F. Renal function in gout. IV. An analysis of 524 gouty subjects including long-term follow-up studies. *Am. J. Med.* 59: 605, 1975.
18. Bianchi, G., Cusi, D., Gatti, M., et al. A renal abnormality as a possible cause of "essential" hypertension. *Lancet* 1: 173, 1979.
19. Bianchi, G., Fox, U., DiFrancesco, G. F., et al. Blood pressure changes by kidney cross-transplantation between spontaneously hypertensive rats and normotensive rats. *Clin. Sci. Mol. Med.* 47: 435, 1974.
20. Blaustein, M. P. Sodium ions, calcium ions, blood pressure regulation and hypertension: A reassessment and a hypothesis. *Am. J. Physiol.* 232: C165, 1977.
21. Blythe, W. B. Natural history of hypertension in renal parenchymal disease. *Am. J. Kidney Dis.* 5(4): A50, 1985.
22. Brazy, P. C., and Fitzwilliam, J. F. Progressive renal disease: Role of race and anti-hypertensive medications. *Kidney Int.* 37: 1113, 1990.
23. Brenner, M. B., Meyer, T. W., and Hostetter, T. H. Dietary protein intake and the progressive nature of kidney disease: the role of hemodynamically mediated glomerular injury in the pathogenesis of progressive glomerular sclerosis in aging, renal ablation and intrinsic renal disease. *N. Engl. J. Med.* 307: 652, 1982.
24. Brown, C. B., Cameron, J. S., Turner, D. R., et al. Focal segmented glomerulosclerosis with rapid decline in renal function ("malignant FSGS"). *Clin. Nephrol.* 10: 51, 1978.
25. Brown, J. J., Lever, A. F., and Robertson, J. I. S. Renal abnormality of essential hypertension. *Lancet* 2: 320, 1974.
26. Brunner, H. R., Laragh, J. H., Baer, L., et al. Essential hypertension. Renin and aldosterone, heart attack and stroke. *N. Engl. J. Med.* 286: 441, 1972.
27. Buckalew, V. M., Jr., Puschett, J. B., Kintzel, J. E., et al. Mechanism of exaggerated natriuresis in hypertensive man: Impaired sodium transport in the loop of Henle. *J. Clin. Invest.* 48: 1007, 1969.
28. Burns, P. C., and Rozengurt, E. Extracellular Na^+ and initiation of DNA synthesis: Role of intracellular pH and K^+. *J. Cell Biol.* 98: 1082, 1984.

29. Byrom, F. B. The pathogenesis of hypertensive encephalopathy and its relation to the malignant phase of hypertension. Experimental evidence from the hypertensive rat. *Lancet* 2: 201, 1954.
30. Cannon, P. J. Effects of five percent dextrose-water infusions in normal and hypertensive man. *Circulation* 37: 832, 1968.
31. Cannon, P. J., Hassar, M., Case, D. B., et al. The relationship of hypertension and renal failure in scleroderma (progressive systemic sclerosis) to structural and functional abnormalities of the renal cortical circulation. *Medicine* 53: 1, 1974.
32. Cannon, P. J., Leeming, J. M., Sommers, S. C., et al. Juxtaglomerular cell hyperplasia and secondary hyperaldosteronism (Bartter's syndrome). A reevaluation of the pathophysiology. *Medicine* 47: 107, 1968.
33. Castleman, B., and Smithwick, R. H. The relation of vascular disease to the hypertensive state based on a study of renal biopsies from one hundred hypertensive patients. *J.A.M.A.* 121: 1256, 1943.
34. Castleman, B., and Smithwick, R. H. The relation of vascular disease to the hypertensive state. II. The adequacy of the renal biopsy as determined from a study of 500 patients. *N. Engl. J. Med.* 239: 729, 1948.
35. Coleman, T. G., and Guyton, A. C. Hypertension caused by salt-loading in the dog. III. Onset transients of cardiac output and other circulatory variables. *Circ. Res.* 25: 153, 1969.
36. Cottier, P. T., Weller, J. M., and Hoobler, S. W. Effect of an intravenous sodium chloride load on renal hemodynamics and electrolyte excretion in essential hypertension. *Circulation* 17: 750, 1958.
37. Cowley, A. W., and Roman, R. J., Jr. Renal dysfunction in essential hypertension—implications of experimental studies. *Am. J. Nephrol.* 3: 59, 1983.
38. Curtis, J. J., Galla, J. H., Kotchen, T. A., et al. Prevalence of hypertension in a renal transplant population on alternate-day steroid therapy. *Clin. Nephrol.* 5: 123, 1976.
39. Curtis, J. J., Luke, R. G., Diethelm, A. G., et al. Benefits of removal of native kidneys in hypertension after renal transplantation. *Lancet* 2: 739, 1985.
40. Curtis, J. J., Luke, R. G., Dustan, H. P., et al. Remission of essential hypertension after renal transplantation. *N. Engl. J. Med.* 309: 1009, 1983.
41. Curtis, J. J., Luke, R. G., Jones, P., and Diethelm, A. G. Hypertension in cyclosporine-treated renal transplant recipients is sodium dependent. *Am. J. Med.* 85: 134, 1988.
42. Curtis, J. J., Luke, R. G., Whelchel, J. D., et al. Inhibition of angiotensin-converting enzyme in renal transplant recipients with hypertension. *N. Engl. J. Med.* 308: 377, 1983.
43. Dahl, L. K., and Heine, N. Primary role of renal homographs in setting chronic blood pressure levels in rats. *Circ. Res.* 36: 692, 1975.
44. Dal Canton, A., Conte, G., Fuiano, G., et al. Exaggerated natriuresis in the hypertensive man: Clinical evidence for intrarenal hemodynamic heterogeneity. *Nephron* 27: 122, 1981.
45. Davin, J. C., and Mahieu, P. R. Captopril-associated renal failure with endarteritis but not renal-artery stenosis in transplant recipient. *Lancet* I: 820, 1985.
46. De Fronzo, R. A. Hyperkalemia and hyporeninemic hypoaldosteronism. *Kidney Int.* 17: 118, 1980.
47. De Graeff, J., and Schuurs, M. A. M. Severe potassium depletion caused by the abuse of laxatives. *Acta Med. Scand.* 166: 407, 1960.
48. De Leeuw, P. W., Falke, H. E., Punt, R., et al. Noradrenaline secretion by the human kidney. *Clin. Sci. Mol. Med.* 55: 85s, 1978.
49. Dell, R. B., Sciacca, R., Lieberman, K., et al. A weighted least-squares technique for the analysis of kinetic data and its application to the study of renal ^{133}Xenon washout in dogs and man. *Circ. Res.* 32: 71, 1973.
50. De Wardener, H. E., and MacGregor, G. A. Dahl's hypothesis that a saluretic substance may be responsible for a sustained rise in arterial pressure: Its possible role in essential hypertension. *Kidney Int.* 18: 1, 1980.
51. DiBona, C. F., and Rios, L. L. Mechanism of exaggerated diuresis in spontaneously hypertensive rats. *Am. J. Physiol.* 235: F409, 1978.
52. DiBona, G. F. The kidney in the pathogenesis of hypertension: The role of renal nerves. *Am. J. Kidney Dis.* 5(4): A27, 1985.
53. Dustan, H. P., and Tarazi, R. C. Cardiogenic hypertension. *Ann. Rev. Med.* 29: 485, 1978.
54. Dworkin, L. D., Hostetter, T. H., Rennke, H. G., et al. Hemodynamic basis for glomerular injury in rats with desoxycorticosterone-salt hypertension. *J. Clin. Invest.* 73: 1448, 1984.
55. Editorial. Hypertension in blacks and whites. *Lancet* 2: 73, 1980.
56. Editorial. New evidence linking salt and hypertension. *Br. Med. J.* 282: 1993, 1981.
57. Edwards, R. M. Segmental effects of norepinephrine and angiotensin II on isolated renal microvessels. *Am. J. Physiol.* 13: F526, 1983.
58. Eich, R. H., Cuddy, R. P., Smulyan, H., et al. Hemodynamics in labile hypertension. A follow-up study. *Circulation* 34: 299, 1966.
59. Eknoyan, G., and Suki, W. N. Renal consequences of antihypertensive therapy. *Semin. Nephrol.* 11: 129, 1991.
60. El Nahas, A. M., Masters-Thomas, A., and Moorehead, J. F. Hyperfiltration or hypofiltration in chronic renal diseases. *Kidney Int.* 25(1): 243, 1984.
61. Emmerson, B. T. Chronic lead nephropathy: The diagnostic use of calcium EDTA and the association with gout. *Australas. Ann. Med.* 12: 310, 1963.
62. Emmerson, B. T. The clinical differentiation of lead gout from primary gout. *Arth. Rheum.* 11: 623, 1968.
63. Entwisle, G., Apostolides, A. Y., Hebel, J. R., et al. Target organ damage in black hypertensives. *Circulation* 55: 792, 1977.
64. Excerpts from United States Renal Data System 1991 Annual Report: III. Causes of end stage renal disease. *Am. J. Kidney Dis.* 2(Suppl.): 22, 1990.
65. Fahr, T. Über die beziehungen von arteriolensklerose, hypertonie und herzhypertrophie. *Virchows Arch. Pathol. Vanat. Physiol.* 239: 41, 1922.
66. Feld, L. G., Van Liew, J. B., Brentjens, J. R., et al. Renal lesions and proteinuria in the spontaneously hypertensive rat made normotensive by treatment. *Kidney Int.* 20: 606, 1981.
67. Ferris, T. F. Hypertension with renal disease. *Am. J. Kidney Dis.* 5(4): A48, 1985.
68. Fink, G. D., and Brody, M. J. Renal vascular resistance and reactivity in the spontaneously hypertensive rat. *Am. J. Physiol.* 237(2): F128, 1979.
69. Folkow, B. Physiological aspects of primary hypertension. *Physiol. Rev.* 62: 347, 1982.
70. Framingham Study: *An Epidemiological Investigation of*

Cardiovascular Disease. Section 30. *Some Characteristics Related to the Incidence of Cardiovascular Disease and Death: Framingham Study, 18-Year Followup.* Bethesda, MD: National Heart, Lung, and Blood Institute. DHEW Publication No. (NIH) 74-599, 1974.

71. Framingham Study: *An Epidemiological Investigation of Cardiovascular Disease. Section 31. The Results of the Framingham Study Applied to Four Other U.S.-Based Epidemiological Studies of Cardiovascular Disease.* Bethesda, MD: National Heart, Lung, and Blood Institute. DHEW Publication No. (NIH) 76-1083, 1976.
72. Frega, N. S., Davalos, M., and Leaf, A. Effect of endogenous angiotensin on the efferent glomerular arteriole of rat kidney. *Kidney Int.* 18: 323, 1980.
73. Freis, E. D. Age, race, sex, and other indices of risk in hypertension. *Am. J. Med.* 55: 275, 1973.
74. Gianantonio, C. A., Vitacco, M., Mendilaharzu, F., et al. The hemolytic-uremic syndrome. *Nephron* 11: 174, 1973.
75. Giese, J. Renin, Angiotensin and Hypertensive Vascular Damage: A Review. In J. H. Laragh (ed.), *Hypertension Manual.* New York: Dun-Donnelley, 1973. P. 371.
76. Goldblatt, H. The renal origin of hypertension. *Physiol. Rev.* 27: 120, 1947.
77. Goldring, W., Chasis, H., Ranges, H. A., et al. Effective renal blood flow in subjects with essential hypertension. *J. Clin. Invest.* 20: 637, 1941.
78. Gombos, E. A., Hulet, W. H., Bopp, D., et al. Reactivity of renal and systemic circulation to vasoconstrictor agents in normotensive and hypertensive subjects. *J. Clin. Invest.* 41: 203, 1962.
79. Gombos, E. A., Lee, T. H., Solinas, J., et al. Renal response to pyrogen in normotensive and hypertensive man. *Circulation* 36: 555, 1967.
80. Gross, F. The renin-angiotensin system and hypertension. *Ann. Intern. Med.* 75: 777, 1971.
81. Guyton, A. C., Coleman, T. G., Cowley, A. W., Jr., et al. Arterial pressure regulation: Overriding dominance of the kidneys in long-term regulation and in hypertension. *Am. J. Med.* 52: 584, 1972.
82. Guyton, A. C., Hall, J. E., Lohmeier, T. E., et al. Blood pressure regulation: Basic concepts. *Fed. Proc.* 40: 2252, 1981.
83. Guyton, A. C., Manning, R. D., Jr., Hall, J. E., et al. The pathogenic role of the kidney. *J. Cardiovasc. Pharmacol.* 6: S151, 1984.
84. Haddy, F. J. Mechanism, prevention and therapy of sodium dependent hypertension. *Am. J. Med.* 69: 746, 1980.
85. Haddy, F. J., and Pamnani, M. B. The kidney in the pathogenesis of hypertension: The role of sodium. *Am. J. Kidney Dis.* 5(4): A5, 1985.
86. Haddy, F. J., Pamnani, M. B., and Clough, D. L. The sodium-potassium pump in volume expanded hypertension. *Clin. Exp. Hypertension* 1: 295, 1978.
87. Hanenson, I. B., Taussky, H. H., Polasky, N., et al. Renal excretion of sodium in arterial hypertension. *Circulation* 20: 498, 1959.
88. Henderson, D. A. The aetiology of chronic nephritis in Queensland. *Med. J. Aust.* 1: 377, 1958.
89. Henderson, D. A., and Inglis, J. A. The lead content of bone in chronic Bright's disease. *Australas. Ann. Med.* 6: 145, 1957.
90. Heptinstall, R. H. Renal biopsies in hypertension. *Br. Heart J.* 16: 133, 1954.
91. Heptinstall, R. H. Hypertension: II. Essential Hypertension. In R. H. Heptinstall (ed.), *Pathology of the Kidney.* Vol. I (3rd ed.). Boston: Little, Brown, 1983. Chap. 5.
92. Heptinstall, R. H. Pyelonephritis: Pathologic Features. In R. H. Heptinstall (ed.), *Pathology of the Kidney.* Vol. III (3rd ed.). Boston: Little, Brown, 1983. Chap. 25.
93. Holland, N. H., Kotchen, T., and Bhathena, D. Hypertension in children with chronic pyelonephritis. *Kidney Int.* 8: S-243, 1975.
94. Hollenberg, N. K. The kidney in the pathogenesis of hypertension. A prologue. *Am. J. Kidney Dis.* 5(4): A2, 1985.
95. Hollenberg, N. K., and Adams, D. F. The renal circulation in hypertensive disease. *Am. J. Med.* 60:773, 1976.
96. Hollenberg, N. K., Adams, D. F., Solomon, H., et al. Renal vascular tone in essential and secondary hypertension. *Medicine* 54: 29, 1975.
97. Hollenberg, N. K., Boruchi, L. J., and Adams, D. F. The renal vasculature in early essential hypertension: Evidence for a pathogenetic role. *Medicine* 57: 167, 1978.
98. Hollenberg, N. K., Epstein, M., Basch, R. I., et al. "No man's land" of the renal vasculature. An arteriographic and hemodynamic assessment of the interlobar and arcuate arteries in essential and accelerated hypertension. *Am. J. Med.* 47: 845, 1969.
99. Hollenberg, N. K., Meggs, L. G., Williams, G. H., et al. Sodium intake and renal responses to captopril in normal man and in essential hypertension. *Kidney Int.* 20: 240, 1981.
100. Hollenberg, N. K., and Williams, G. H. Volume control and altered renal and adrenal responsiveness to angiotensin II in essential hypertension: Implication for treatment with converting enzyme inhibition. *J. Hypertension* (1 Suppl.): 119, 1983.
101. Hollenberg, N. K., Williams, G. H., and Adams, D. F. Essential hypertension: Abnormal renal vascular and endocrine responses to a mild psychological stimulus. *Hypertension* 3: 11, 1981.
102. Hostetter, T. H., Olson, J. L., Rennke, H. G., et al. Hyperfiltration in remnant nephrons: A potentially adverse response to renal ablation. *Am. J. Physiol.* 241: F85, 1981.
103. Hostetter, T. H., Rennke, H. G., and Brenner, B. M. The case for intrarenal hypertension in the initiation and progression of diabetic and other glomerulopathies. *Am. J. Med.* 72: 375, 1982.
104. Hypertension Detection and Follow-up Program. A program report. Hypertension Detection and Follow-up Program Cooperative Group. *Circ. Res.* 40(Suppl. 1): I-106, 1977.
105. Hypertension Detection and Follow-up Program Cooperative Group. Five-year findings of the Hypertension Detection and Follow-up Program. I. Reduction in mortality of persons with high blood pressure, including mild hypertension. *J.A.M.A.* 242: 2562, 1979.
106. *Hypertension Prevalence and the Status of Awareness, Treatment, and Control in the United States.* Final Report of the Subcommittee on Definition and Prevalence of the Joint National Committee on Detection, Evaluation and Treatment of High Blood Pressure, 1984.
107. Ibels, L. S., Alfrey, A. C., Haut, L., et al. Preservation of function in experimental renal disease by dietary restriction of phosphate. *N. Engl. J. Med.* 298: 122, 1978.
108. Isaacson, C. The pathology of hypertension in a tropical environment. *Clin. Cardiol.* 6: 195, 1983.
109. Jones, A. W. Altered ion transport in vascular smooth muscle from spontaneously hypertensive rats. *Circ. Res.* 33: 563, 1973.
110. Kannel, W. B., Castelli, W. P., McNamara, P. M., et al.

Role of blood pressure in the development of congestive heart failure. The Framingham Study. *N. Engl. J. Med.* 287: 781, 1972.
111. Kannel, W. B., Wolf, P. A., Verter, J., et al. Epidemiologic assessment of the role of blood pressure in stroke. The Framingham Study. *J.A.M.A.* 214: 301, 1970.
112. Kaplan, N. M. The prognostic implications of plasma renin in essential hypertension. *J.A.M.A.* 23: 167, 1975.
113. Kaplan, N. M. Renin profiles. The unfulfilled promises. *J.A.M.A.* 238: 611, 1977.
114. Kaplan, N. M. *Clinical Hypertension.* Baltimore: Williams & Wilkins, 1978.
115. Kashgarian, M. Pathology of small blood vessel disease in hypertension. *Am. J. Kidney Dis.* 5(4): A104, 1985.
116. Kassirer, J. P. Atheroembolic renal disease. *N. Engl. J. Med.* 280: 812, 1969.
117. Katholi, R. E. Renal nerves in the pathogenesis of hypertension in experimental animals and humans. *Am. J. Physiol.* 245: F1, 1983.
118. Kaufman, A. M., and Levitt, M. F. The effect of diuretics on systemic and renal hemodynamics in patients with renal insufficiency. *Am. J. Kidney Dis.* 5(4): A71, 1985.
119. Kawabe, K., Watanabe, T. X., Shiono, K., et al. Influence of blood pressure of renal isografts between spontaneously hypertensive and normotensive rats, utilizing the F_1 hybrids. *J. Heart J.* 19: 886, 1978.
120. Kawabe, K., Watanabe, T. X., Shiono, K., et al. Role of the kidney in the pathogenesis of SHR and other hypertensive rats determined by renal isografts. *J. Heart J.* 20 (Suppl. 1): 87, 1979.
121. Kincaid-Smith, P. Vascular obstruction in chronic pyelonephritic kidneys and its relation to hypertension. *Lancet* 2: 1263, 1955.
122. Kincaid-Smith, P. *The Kidney: A Clinico-Pathological Study.* Oxford: Blackwell Scientific, 1975. Pp. 212.
123. Kincaid-Smith, P., McMichael, J., and Murphy, E. A. The clinical course and pathology of hypertension with papilledema (malignant hypertension). *Q. J. Med.* 27: 117, 1958.
124. Knudsen, K. D., and Dahl, L. K. Essential hypertension: Inborn error of sodium metabolism. *Postgrad. Med. J.* 42: 148, 1966.
125. Koepke, J. P., and DiBona, G. F. High sodium intake enhances renal nerve and antinatriuretic responses to stress in spontaneously hypertensive rats. *Hypertension* 7: 357, 1985.
126. Krakauer, H., Grauman, J. S., McMullan, M. R., et al. The recent U.S. experience in the treatment of end-stage renal disease by dialysis and transplantation. *N. Engl. J. Med.* 308(26): 1558, 1983.
127. Kubo, S., Nishioka, A., Nishimura, H., et al. Studies on the mechanism of "exaggerated natriuresis" in essential hypertension. *J. Circ. J.* 45: 39, 1981.
128. Laskow, D. A., Curtis, J. J., Luke, R. G., et al. Cyclosporine-induced changes in glomerular filtration rate and urea excretion. *Am. J. Med.* 88: 497, 1990.
129. Ledingham, J. M., and Pelling, D. Cardiac output and peripheral resistance in experimental renal hypertension. *Circ. Res.* 20 and 21 (Suppl. 2): II-187, 1967.
130. Levy, S. B., Lilley, J. J., Frigon, R. P., et al. Urine kallikrein and plasma renin activity as determinants of renal blood flow. *J. Clin. Invest.* 60: 129, 1977.
131. Levy, S. B., Talner, L. B., Coel, M. N., et al. Renal vasculature in essential hypertension: Racial differences. *Ann. Intern. Med.* 88: 12, 1978.
132. Light, K. C., Koepke, J. P., Obrist, P. A., et al. Psychological stress induces sodium and fluid retention in men at high risk for hypertension. *Science* 220: 429, 1983.
133. Lindeman, R. D., Tobin, J. D., and Shock, N. W. Association between blood pressure and the rate of decline in renal function with age. *Kidney Int.* 26: 861, 1984.
134. Ljungman, S., Aurell, M., Hartford, M., et al. Effects of subpressor doses of angiotensin II on renal hemodynamics in relation to blood pressure. *Hypertension* 5: 368, 1983.
135. Ljungman, S., Aurell, M., Hartford, M., et al. Renal function and renal haemodynamics before and after 7 years' antihypertensive treatment in men with primary hypertension. *Acta Med. Scand.* Suppl. 693: 89, 1984.
136. Lowenstein, J., Beranbaum, E. R., Chasis, H., et al. Intrarenal pressure and exaggerated natriuresis in essential hypertension. *Clin. Sci.* 38: 359, 1970.
137. Luft, F. C., Grim, C. E., Higgins, J. T., Jr., et al. Differences in response to sodium administration in normotensive white and black subjects. *J. Lab. Clin. Med.* 90: 555, 1977.
138. Luke, R. G. Mechanism of cyclosporine induced hypertension. *Am. J. Hypertens.* 4: 468, 1991.
139. Lund-Johansen, P. Haemodynamics in essential hypertension. *Clin. Sci.* 59: 343s, 1980.
140. Luxton, R. W. Radiation nephritis. *Q. J. Med.* 22: 215, 1953.
141. Luxton, R. W. Radiation nephritis: A long-term study of 54 patients. *Lancet* 2: 1221, 1961.
142. MacGregor, G. A. Sodium is more important than calcium in essential hypertension. *Hypertension* 7: 4, 1985.
143. Mackenzie, H. S., Morrill, A. L., and Ploth, D. W. Pressure dependence of exaggerated natriuresis in two-kidney, one clip Goldblatt hypertensive rats. *Kidney Int.* 27: 731, 1985.
144. Magee, J. H., Unger, A. M., and Richardson, D. W. Changes in renal function associated with drug or placebo therapy of human hypertension. *Am. J. Med.* 36: 795, 1964.
145. Mauer, S. M., Steffes, M. W., Azar, S., et al. The effects of Goldblatt hypertension on the development of the glomerular lesions of diabetes mellitus in the rat. *Diabetes* 27: 738, 1978.
146. Maxwell, M. H. Cooperative study of renovascular hypertension: Current status. *Kidney Int.* 8: S-153, 1975.
147. McClellen, W., Tuttle, E., and Issa, A. Racial differences in the incidence of hypertension end-stage renal disease are not entirely explained by difference in the prevalence of hypertension. *Am. J. Kidney Dis.* 12: 285, 1988.
148. Messerli, F. H., DeCarvallho, J. G. R., Christie, B., et al. Essential hypertension in black and white subjects. Hemodynamic findings and fluid volume state. *Am. J. Med.* 67: 27, 1979.
149. Mitchell, H. C., Graham, R. M., and Pettinger, W. A. Renal function during long-term treatment of hypertension with Minoxidil. Comparison of benign and malignant hypertension. *Ann. Intern. Med.* 93: 676, 1980.
150. Morel-Maroger, L., Kanfer, A., Solez, K., et al. Prognostic importance of vascular lesions in acute renal failure with microangiopathic hemolytic anemia (hemolytic-uremic syndrome): Clinicopathologic study in 20 adults. *Kidney Int.* 15: 548, 1979.
151. Morgan, J. M., Hartley, M. W., and Miller, R. E. Nephropathy in chronic lead poisoning. *Arch. Intern. Med.* 118: 17, 1966.
152. Moritz, A. R., and Oldt, M. R. Arteriolar sclerosis in hypertensive and non-hypertensive individuals. *Am. J. Pathol.* 13: 679, 1937.

153. Morrison, S. L., and Morris, J. N. Epidemiological observations on high blood pressure without evident cause. *Lancet* 2: 864, 1959.
154. Moyer, J. H., Heider, C., Pevey, K., et al. The effect of treatment of the vascular deterioration associated with hypertension with particular emphasis on renal function. *Am. J. Med.* 24: 177, 1958.
155. Mujais, S. K., Emmanouel, D. S., Kasinath, B. S., et al. Marked proteinuria in hypertensive nephrosclerosis. *Am. J. Nephrol.* 5: 190, 1985.
156. Nakamoto, Y., Takazakura, E., Hayakawa, H., et al. Intrarenal microaneurysms in diabetic nephropathy. *Lab. Invest.* 42: 433, 1980.
157. National Health Survey: *Hypertension and Hypertensive Heart Disease in Adults. U.S. 1960–62.* Washington, D.C.: U.S. Dept. of Health, Education and Welfare, Vital and Health Statistics Series 11, No. 13. U.S. Government Printing Office, 1966.
158. Nishi, T., Bond, C., Jr., Brown, G., et al. A morphometric study of arterial intimal thickening in kidneys of dialyzed patients. *Am. J. Pathol.* 95: 597, 1979.
159. Nishiyama, K., Nishiyama, A., and Frohlich, E. D. Regional blood flow in normotensive and spontaneously hypertensive rats. *Am. J. Physiol.* 230: 691, 1976.
160. O'Connell, T. X., and Mowbray, J. F. Arterial intimal thickening produced by alloantibody and xenoantibody. *Transplantation* 15: 262, 1973.
161. Olson, J. L., Hostetter, T. H., Rennke, H. G., et al. Altered glomerular permselectivity in progressive sclerosis following extreme ablation of renal mass. *Kidney Int.* 22: 112, 1982.
162. Padfield, P. L., Brown, J. J., Lever, A. F., et al. Is low-renin hypertension a stage in the development of essential hypertension or a diagnostic entity? *Lancet* 1: 548, 1975.
163. Papper, S., Belsky, J. L., and Bleifer, K. H. The response to the administration of an isotonic sodium-chloride-lactate solution in patients with essential hypertension. *J. Clin. Invest.* 39: 876, 1960.
164. Parving, H. H., Smidt, U. M., Andersen, A. R., et al. Early aggressive antihypertensive treatment reduces rate of decline in kidney function in diabetic nephropathy. *Lancet* 1: 1175, 1983.
165. Pasternack, A., and Perheentupa, J. Hypertensive angiopathy in familial chloride diarrhoea. *Lancet* 2: 1047, 1966.
166. Pasternack, A., Perheentupa, J., Launiala, K., et al. Kidney biopsy findings in familial chloride diarrhoea. *Acta Endocrinol.* 55: 1, 1967.
167. Pedersen, E. B. Abnormal renal hemodynamics during exercise in young patients with mild essential hypertension without treatment and during long-term propranolol treatment. *Scand. J. Clin. Lab. Invest.* 38: 567, 1978.
168. Pederson, E. B., and Kornerup, H. J. Effect of sodium loading on the renin-aldosterone system in essential hypertension. *Acta Med. Scand.* Suppl. 625: 103, 1979.
169. Pedersen, E. B., and Mogensen, C. E. Effect of antihypertensive treatment on urinary albumin excretion, glomerular filtration rate, and renal plasma flow in patients with essential hypertension. *Scand. J. Clin. Lab. Invest.* 36: 231, 1976.
170. Perera, G. A. Hypertensive vascular disease. Description and natural history. *J. Chronic Dis.* 1: 33, 1955.
171. Pettinger, W. A., Lee, W. A., Reisch, J., et al. Long-term improvement in renal function after short-term strict blood pressure control in hypertensive nephrosclerosis. *Hypertension* 13: 766, 1989.
172. Pettinger, W. A., Umemura, S., and Smyth, D. D. The role of renal catecholamines in hypertension. *Am. J. Kidney Dis.* 5(4): A23, 1985.
173. Pickering, G. *High Blood Pressure* (2nd ed.). New York: Grune and Stratton, 1968.
174. Platt, R. Heredity in hypertension. *Lancet* 1: 899, 1963.
175. Ploth, D. W. Angiotensin-dependent renal mechanisms in 2-kidney 1-clip renal vascular hypertension. *Am. J. Physiol.* 245 (*Renal Fluid Electrolyte Physiology* 14): F131, 1983.
176. Pollak, V. E., and Nettles, J. B. The kidney in toxemia of pregnancy: A clinical and pathologic study based on renal biopsies. *Medicine* (Baltimore) 39: 469, 1960.
177. Porter, K. A. Renal Transplantation. In R. H. Heptinstall (ed.), *Pathology of the Kidney* (3rd ed.). Boston: Little, Brown, 1983. Chap. 27, p. 1455.
178. Porter, K. A., Dossetor, J. B., Marchioro, T. L., et al. Human renal transplants: I. Glomerular changes. *Lab. Invest.* 16: 153, 1967.
179. Postnov, Y. V., Orlov, S. N., Gulak, P., et al. Altered permeability of the erythrocyte membrane for sodium and potassium ions in spontaneously hypertensive rats. *Pfluegers Arch.* 365: 257, 1976.
180. Poulter, N., Khaw, K. T., Hopwood, B. E. C., et al. Salt and blood pressure in various populations. *J. Cardiovasc. Pharmacol.* 6: S197, 1984.
181. Preuss, H. G., and Goldin, H. Serum renotropic activity and renal growth in spontaneously hypertensive rats. *Kidney Int.* 23: 635, 1983.
182. Purkerson, M. L., Hoffsten, P. E., and Klahr, S. Pathogenesis of the glomerulopathy associated with renal infarction in rats. *Kidney Int.* 9: 407, 1976.
183. Qualheim, R. E., Rostand, S. T., Kirk, K. A., et al. Changing patterns of end-stage renal disease due to hypertension. *Am. J. Kidney Dis.* 18: 336, 1991.
184. Reid, G. M., and Dunn, M. J. Renal papillary collecting tubular (RPCT) cells differ in PGE_2 synthetic capacity in pre-hypertensive DAHL salt-sensitive (S) and salt-resistant (R) rats. *Kidney Int.* 27: 199, 1985.
185. Reif, M. C., Constantiner, A., and Levitt, M. F. Chronic gouty nephropathy: A vanishing syndrome? (Editorial) *N. Engl. J. Med.* 304(9): 535, 1981.
186. Relman, A. S. Race and end-stage renal disease. *N. Engl. J. Med.* 306: 1290, 1982.
187. Reubi, F. C. The Late Effects of Hypotensive Drug Therapy on Renal Functions of Patients with Essential Hypertension. In K. D. Bock and P. T. Cottier (eds.). *Essential Hypertension: An International Symposium*, Berne, June 7th–10th, 1960. Berlin: Springer-Verlag, 1960. P. 317.
188. Rickstein, S. E., Yao, K. T., DiBona, G. F., et al. Renal nerve activity and exaggerated natriuresis in conscious spontaneously hypertensive rats. *Acta Physiol. Scand.* 112: 161, 1981.
189. Rohrbach, D. H., Wagner, C. W., Star, V. L., et al. Reduced synthesis of basement membrane heparan sulphate proteoglycan in streptozotocin-induced diabetic mice. *J. Biol. Chem.* 258: 11672, 1983.
190. Rostand, S. G., Brown, G., Kirk, K. A., et al. Renal insufficiency in treated essential hypertension. *N. Engl. J. Med.* 320: 684, 1989.
191. Rostand, S. G., Kirk, K. A., Rutsky, E. A., et al. Racial differences in the incidence of treatment for end-stage renal disease. *N. Engl. J. Med.* 306: 1276, 1982.
192. Schalekamp, M. A., Beevers, D. G., Briggs, J. D., et al. Hypertension in chronic renal failure: An abnormal relation between sodium and the renin-angiotensin system. *Am. J. Med.* 55: 379, 1973.

193. Schweitzer, G., and Gertz, K. H. Changes in hemodynamics and glomerular ultrafiltration in renal hypertension of rats. *Kidney Int.* 15: 134, 1979.
194. Selkurt, E. E., Womack, I., and Dailey, W. N. Mechanism of natriuresis and diuresis during elevated renal arterial pressure. *Am. J. Physiol.* 209: 95, 1965.
195. Shulman, N. B., Ford, C. D., Hall, W. D., et al. Prognostic value of serum creatinine and effect of treatment of hypertension on renal function: Results from the Hypertension Detection and Follow-up Program. *Hypertension* 13 (Suppl. 1): I80, 1989.
196. Smith, D. E., Odel, H. M., and Kernohan, J. W. Causes of death in hypertension. *Am. J. Med.* 9: 516, 1950.
197. Smith, M. C., and Dunn, M. J. Renal Kallikrein, Kinins, and Prostaglandins in Hypertension. In B. M. Brenner and J. H. Stein (eds.), *Contemporary Issues in Nephrology.* Vol. 8, *Hypertension.* New York: Churchill-Livingstone, 1981. Chap. 7, p. 168.
198. Smith, M. C., and Dunn, M. J. The role of prostaglandins in human hypertension. *Am. J. Kidney Dis.* 5(4): A32, 1985.
199. Snyder, H. E., and Shapiro, J. L. Correlative study of atheromatous embolism in human beings and experimental animals. *Surgery* 49: 195, 1961.
200. Sommers, S. C., and Andersson, B. I. Vascular Morphologic Changes in Essential Hypertension. In G. Onesti, K. E. Kim, and J. H. Moyer (eds.), *Hypertension: Mechanisms and Management.* New York: Grune and Stratton, 1973.
201. Sommers, S. C., McLaughlin, R. J., and McAuley, R. L. Pathology of diastolic hypertension as a generalized vascular disease. *Am. J. Cardiol.* 9: 653, 1962.
202. Sommers, S. C., Relman, A. S., and Smithwick, R. H. Histologic studies of kidney biopsy specimens from patients with hypertension. *Am. J. Pathol.* 34: 685, 1958.
203. Sowers, J. R., Beck, F., Stern, N., et al. Reduced sodium-potassium dependent ATPase and its possible role in the development of hypertension in spontaneously hypertensive rats. *Clin. Exp. Hyper.* A5: 71, 1983.
204. Sporn, I. N., Lancestremere, R. G., Vaamonde, C. A., et al. Acute renal conservation of sodium in hypertension. *Arch. Intern. Med.* 111: 439, 1963.
205. Stumpe, K. O., Lowitz, H. D., and Ochwadt, B. Fluid reabsorption in Henle's loop and urinary excretion of sodium and water in normal rats and rats with chronic hypertension. *J. Clin. Invest.* 49: 1200, 1970.
206. Swinton, N. W., Jr. Clinical Presentation and Natural History of Renovascular Hypertension. In D. J. Breslin, N. W. Swinton, Jr., J. A. Libertino, et al. (eds.), *Renovascular Hypertension.* Baltimore: Williams & Wilkins, 1982. Chap. 5, p. 73.
207. Taverner, D., Bing, R. F., Heagerty, A., et al. Improvement of renal function during long-term treatment of severe hypertension with minoxidil. *Q. J. Med.* 206: 280, 1983.
208. Tierney, W. M., McDonald, C. J., and Luft, F. C. Renal disease in hypertensive adults: Effect of race and type II diabetes mellitus. *Am. J. Kidney Dis.* 13: 485, 1989.
209. Tobian, L., Jr., and Binion, J. T. Tissue cations and water in arterial hypertension. *Circulation* 5: 754, 1952.
210. Tracy, R. E. Hypertension and arteriolar sclerosis of the kidney, pancreas, adrenal gland and liver. *Virchows Arch.* 391: 91, 1981.
211. Tracy, R. E., and Toca, V. T. Nephrosclerosis and blood pressure II. Reversibility of proliferative arteriosclerosis. *Lab. Invest.* 30: 30, 1974.
212. Trippodo, N. C., and Frohlich. E. D. Similarities of genetic (spontaneous) hypertension. *Circ. Res.* 48: 309, 1981.
213. Vaamonde, C. A., Sporn, I. N., Lancestremere, R. G., et al. Augmented natriuretic response to acute sodium infusion after blood pressure elevation with metaraminol in normotensive subjects. *J. Clin. Invest.* 43: 496, 1964.
214. Veterans Administration Cooperative Study Group on Antihypertensive Agents. Effect of treatment on morbidity and mortality: Results in patients with diastolic blood pressures averaging 115 through 129 mm Hg. *J.A.M.A.* 202: 1028, 1967.
215. Veterans Administration Cooperative Study Group on Antihypertensive Agents. II. Results in patients with diastolic blood pressure averaging 90 through 114 mm Hg. *J.A.M.A.* 213: 1143, 1970.
216. Warren, D. J., and Ferris, T. F. Renin secretion in renal hypertension. *Lancet* 1: 159, 1970.
217. Weiss, S., and Parker, F., Jr. Pyelonephritis: Its relation to vascular lesions and to arterial hypertension. *Medicine* (Baltimore) 18: 221, 1939.
218. Weller, J. M., Wu, S-C. H., Ferguson, C. W., et al. End-stage renal disease in Michigan. Incidence, underlying causes, prevalence, and modalities of treatment. *Am. J. Nephrol.* 5: 84, 1985.
219. Wenting, G. J., Man in't Veld, A. J., Derkx, F. H. M., et al. Recurrence of hypertension in primary osteronism after discontinuation of spironolactone: Time course of changes in cardiac output and body fluid volumes. *Clin. Exp. Hyper.* A4: 1727, 1982.
220. Williams, G. H., and Hollenberg, N. K. Defect in Sodium-Mediated Adrenal Responsiveness to Angiotensin II in Essential Hypertension: Implications for Pathogenesis. In R. M. Carey, and C. Edwards (eds.), *Is Essential Hypertension an Endocrine Disease?* England: Butterworth, 1984.
221. Wilson, C., and Byrom, F. B. Renal changes in malignant hypertension. *Lancet* 1: 136, 1939.
222. Wing, A. J., Broyer, M., Brunner, F. P., et al. In A. M. Davison, and P. J. Guillou (eds.), *Proceedings of The European Dialysis and Transplant Association-European Renal Association,* Vol. 20. London: Pitman Publishing, 1983. P. 2.
223. Woods, J. E. Renal function in essential hypertension. *Semin. Nephrol.* 30: 30, 1983.
224. Working Group on Risk and High Blood Pressure (appointed by the National High Blood Pressure Education Program Coordinating Committee of NIH-NHLBI). An epidemiological approach to describing risk associated with blood pressure levels. *Hypertension* 7: 641, 1985.
225. Yamada, T., Ishihara, M., Ichikawa, K., et al. Proteinuria and renal function during antihypertensive treatment for essential hypertension. *J. Am. Geriat. Soc.* 28: 114, 1980.
226. Yu, T. F., Berger, L., Dorph, D. J., et al. Renal function in gout: V. Factors influencing the renal hemodynamics. *Am. J. Med.* 67: 766, 1979.

Renovascular Hypertension

Thomas G. Pickering
John H. Laragh
Thomas A. Sos

The exact prevalence of renovascular hypertension in the general population is not known, and it is probable that the diagnosis is missed in many patients. Clinically, it is an important diagnosis to make, first because it is the commonest curable form of hypertension at any age, and second because it is one of the few potentially reversible causes of chronic renal failure.

Pathophysiology of Renovascular Hypertension in Animals

The classic experiments on the production of renovascular hypertension were published in 1934 by Goldblatt et al. [65], who demonstrated that persistent hypertension could be produced in dogs by constricting either both renal arteries or one if the other kidney was removed. Goldblatt postulated that a humoral mechanism could be responsible for the hypertension, and this was later confirmed by the work of Houssay, Fasciolo, and Braun-Menendez [20], Pickering [147], and Page [144].

Despite the early work suggesting that hypersecretion of renin by the ischemic kidney was directly responsible for the raised blood pressure, later studies indicated that other factors were responsible for maintenance of the hypertension because the hyperreninemia often did not persist. Furthermore, the mechanism of the hypertension may differ according to whether the contralateral kidney is intact (one-clip, two-kidney Goldblatt hypertension, analogous to unilateral renal artery stenosis in humans) or removed (one-clip, one-kidney Goldblatt hypertension, analogous to bilateral renal artery stenosis in humans). The acute phase of the hypertension is probably the same in both cases. The overwhelming bulk of evidence favors a predominant role for the two limbs of the renin-angiotensin system—vasoconstriction and sodium retention—as shown in Fig. 55-1.

ACUTE PHASE

Constriction of a renal artery causes an immediate rise of blood pressure and also of renin and aldosterone. Administration of converting enzyme inhibitors or saralasin prevents this rise of blood pressure, indicating that it is a direct consequence of the hyperreninemia [185].

CHRONIC PHASE

After a few days, the blood pressure continues to rise, but renin and aldosterone concentration may return to normal. At this stage the course of the hypertension may differ somewhat depending on whether or not the contralateral kidney is present (see Table 55-1) and also on the species. Most of the experiments described below have been performed in rats.

One-Kidney One-Clip Hypertension. As the renin level falls, there is an expansion of the plasma volume, which occurs as a result of sodium retention [21]. If at this stage converting enzyme inhibitor is given, blood pressure falls little if at all [126]. If the animals are maintained on a low sodium diet throughout, the rise of pressure still takes place, but the mechanism is different: Renin levels remain elevated, but there is no sodium retention or increase of plasma volume [160]. These findings are consistent with experiments done by Gavras et al. [60] in rats, who found that acute saralasin infusion lowered the blood pressure of one-kidney one-clip hypertensive rats only if they were sodium depleted [60]. Thus it appears that this type of hypertension may be either renin-dependent or volume-dependent according to the sodium intake. Prolonged administration of captopril has a modest blood pressure-lowering effect, which is accompanied by a natriuresis and is more pronounced if the animals are in the malignant phase [11].

A role for the sympathetic nervous system in one-kidney one-clip hypertension has been suggested by several workers. Plasma norepinephrine levels are raised [36], and central sympatholytic interventions, such as administration of intracisternal 6-hydroxydopamine, may attenuate the hypertension [37]. Katholi et al. [93, 94] have suggested that renal afferent nerves are responsible for the sympathetic component of the hypertension, because renal denervation lowers blood pressure and plasma norepinephrine in the one-kidney model.

Two-Kidney One-Clip Hypertension. The main difference between one- and two-kidney Goldblatt hypertension is that in the latter there is less sodium retention [185, 196] (Fig. 55-2). Brunner et al. [22, 60] found that administration of either angiotensin antibody or saralasin produced a greater fall of pressure in two-kidney one-clip rats than in one-kidney rats, suggesting a greater degree of renin dependency in two-kidney hypertension. Prolonged administration of captopril also lowers blood pressure more in the two-kidney than in one-kidney Goldblatt rats, and without natriuresis [11]. In two-kidney Goldblatt hypertension the simplest explanation for the difference between one- and two-kidney hypertension is that in the latter case the contralateral kidney can excrete sodium normally, thereby preventing sodium retention. The contralateral kidney does not function entirely normally, however, because experiments using converting enzyme inhibitors indicate that there is an angiotensin-mediated vasoconstriction [81].

As the blood pressure rises following clipping, there is also a rise of peripheral plasma renin activity (PRA), but there is a closer correlation between renal vein renin activity from the ischemic kidney and blood pressure than between peripheral PRA and blood pressure [107]. The renin content of the contralateral kidney is correspondingly diminished [43]. These changes occurring in rats appear to parallel those observed in humans (see below).

VASOCONSTRICTION-VOLUME HYPOTHESIS AND THE RENIN AXIS

RENIN
ANGIOTENSIN I
ANGIOTENSIN II
ALDOSTERONE
SODIUM
VASOCONSTRICTION
VOLUME
BLOOD PRESSURE
---- Negative feedback

Fig. 55-1. The two major limbs of the renin-angiotensin system—angiotensin-mediated vasoconstriction and sodium retention—can account for most of the changes seen in renovascular hypertension.

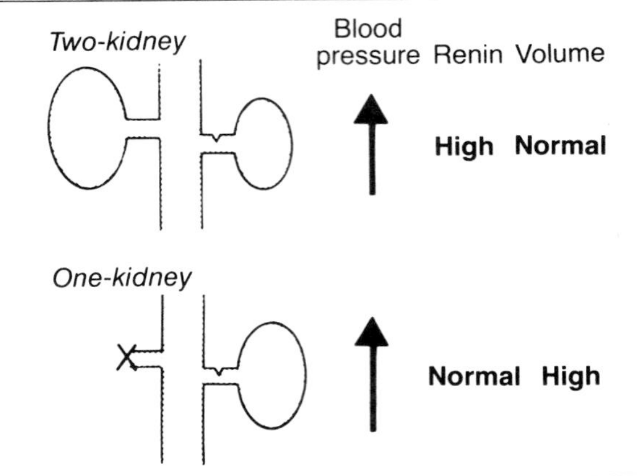

Fig. 55-2. Schema of the two types of renovascular hypertension. Two-kidney one-clip hypertension is mainly renin dependent, while one-kidney one-clip hypertension is mainly volume dependent.

After several months the hypertension in the one-kidney model may become less renin dependent, because prolonged infusion with saralasin has no effect, even though removing the constricting clip may still restore blood pressure to normal [194]. Despite the decline of plasma renin levels toward normal, plasma aldosterone may remain elevated, and this may contribute to the maintenance of the hypertension. In dogs with two-kidney Goldblatt hypertension, PRA returns to normal within a few days, and saralasin has no effect. This suggests that the renin-angiotensin system is not critical in the maintenance of two-kidney Goldblatt hypertension in the dog [202].

It has been suggested by Möhring et al. [130] that arginine vasopressin (AVP) may play a role in the pathogenesis of two-kidney one-clip hypertension in rats, particularly in the malignant phase, because AVP levels are usually raised and blood pressure is reduced by a specific vasopressin antibody. However, Rabito et al. [156] found that competitive vasopressin inhibitors had no effect on this form of hypertension.

As with one-kidney rats, denervating the kidneys of two-kidney one-clip hypertensive rats leads to a reduction of blood pressure and plasma norepinephrine levels, again suggesting a possible role for the sympathetic nervous system mediated by renal afferent nerves [94].

Prostaglandins mediate renin release in response to a decreased renal perfusion pressure or a decreased sodium chloride delivery to the macula densa [87], and in experimental hypertension produced by ligating the aorta between the renal arteries (analogous to two-kidney one-clip hypertension and also characterized by high renin levels) blockade of prostaglandin synthesis by indomethacin lowers the blood pressure [88].

EFFECTS OF UNCLIPPING THE ISCHEMIC KIDNEY

Although the majority of studies have investigated only the onset of renovascular hypertension, those that have studied its reversal are of greater relevance to the reversal of human renovascular hypertension by surgery or

Table 55-1. Changes in experimental Goldblatt hypertension during chronic phase

	One-clip, one-kidney	One-clip, two-kidney
Human equivalent	Bilateral stenoses	Unilateral stenosis
PRA	Normal	Raised (but less than in acute phase)
Plasma volume	Raised	Normal
Exchangeable Na	Raised	Normal
Plasma NE	Raised	Raised
AII antagonist effect on BP	Little change	Falls (less in chronic phase)
Unclipping		
Effect on BP	Falls	Falls
Effect on Na excretion	Rises	Falls
Effect on plasma NE	Falls	Falls

PRA = Plasma renin activity; NE = norepinephrine.

angioplasty. Once again, the response differs according to whether the contralateral kidney is present or absent, but in both cases there is a remarkably prompt fall of blood pressure following unclipping.

One-Kidney One-Clip Hypertension. In one-kidney one-clip Goldblatt hypertensive rats Liard and Peters [111] attributed the fall of pressure to natriuresis because they observed a correlation between these two factors after unclipping and also because if the ureter was ligated beforehand the pressure did not fall. Original attempts to prevent the fall of pressure by simply replacing urine loss were unsuccessful [136], perhaps because they did not allow for fluid loss from the lungs. More convincing support for the volume dependence of this type of hypertension was provided by Akahoshi and Carretero [1], who found that the fall of blood pressure following unclipping could be largely prevented by infusing saline to maintain plasma volume, whereas angiotensin II infusion had little effect. Lucas and Floyer [114] found that although venous pressure and plasma volume fell after unclipping, interstitial fluid volume rose, indicating that the major change was a redistribution of fluid within the circulation rather than a net loss. In the dog the fall of blood pressure may be more gradual, occurring over about 3 days [110]. As in the rat, however, removing the clip produces a negative sodium balance. Unclipping also produces a significant decrease of plasma norepinephrine levels [93].

Two-Kidney One-Clip Hypertension. Thurston et al. [195] examined the effects of removing the clip in rats with two-kidney one-clip hypertension, which is of course closely analogous to performing angioplasty in a patient with unilateral renal artery stenosis. The majority of their rats had high plasma renin levels before the clip was removed, whether or not they were in the early or chronic phase of the hypertension. Removal of the clip produced an acute fall of blood pressure to normal within 24 hours. More interestingly, there was also a fall of renin and a markedly positive sodium balance and a tendency for those animals showing the largest fall of blood pressure to show the greatest sodium retention, the exact opposite of what was observed by Liard and Peters in one-kidney rats [111]. Two important conclusions were possible from this study. First, the results do not support the view that the hypertension of the two-kidney Goldblatt rat is maintained by sodium retention, and second, the suddenness of the blood pressure fall cannot be attributed to structural changes in the vessels because these take weeks to reverse. The renin-angiotensin system thus seems to be the most important mechanism, although the authors raised the possibility that the unclipped kidney might release a vasodepressor substance into the plasma [195].

The possibility that active vasodilatation might contribute to the fall of pressure receives some support from hemodynamic studies, which have shown that the fall of pressure is due to an immediate fall of peripheral resistance to normal levels, with an increase in cardiac output [74, 162]. From these studies it is argued that, since there are structural changes that contribute to the raised peripheral resistance in such animals and that are not rapidly reversible, merely withdrawing vasoconstrictor influences by unclipping would not in itself be sufficient to normalize peripheral resistance. Muirhead et al. [133] have demonstrated increased quantities of an antihypertensive neutral renomedullary lipid, derived from renomedullary interstitial cells, following unclipping.

Russell et al. [161] sought to test the contribution of the renin-angiotensin system to the fall of pressure following unclipping by blocking the system with either saralasin or captopril before unclipping. Although both agents lowered the pressure to some extent, removing the clip produced a much bigger fall of pressure, the extent of which was similar whether or not the renin-angiotensin system had been blocked. These authors concluded that some other factors were responsible for the fall, again invoking the possibility of a vasodepressor substance released at the time of unclipping.

Pathophysiology of Renovascular Hypertension in Humans

ROLE OF THE RENIN-ANGIOTENSIN SYSTEM

It is far from clear whether renovascular hypertension in humans can be divided into the two types of renin-dependency and volume-dependency described in animals, but the following lines of evidence would be consistent with such a mechanism. First, plasma renin activity is usually normal or high in patients with renovascular hypertension but never low [21]. Second, the pattern of renin secretion from the ischemic and contralateral kidney is the same as that seen in experimental Goldblatt hypertension, that is, unilateral hypersecretion coupled with contralateral suppression. Third, in patients with unilateral renal artery stenosis, removal of the constriction or treatment with angiotensin-converting enzyme inhibitors often restores blood pressure to normal. Fourth, cardiac output is higher in patients with bilateral than with unilateral renal artery stenosis (see below). As shown in Fig. 55-3, the effects of angiotensin blockade and sodium depletion on the blood pressure of patients with bilateral renovascular hypertension are additive.

If a balloon-tipped catheter is placed in the renal artery of a normal subject and the balloon inflated there is a marked increase of renin secretion from the ischemic kidney with contralateral suppression, just as occurs in animal models [54]. Blood pressure does not rise within the first hour, however.

The normal PRA that occurs in some patients could occur because they are in a phase analogous to the chronic phase seen in animals, that is, the phase in which PRA is normalized as a result of sodium retention (in which case they should have a relatively high plasma volume), or it could exist because they have bilateral rather than unilateral disease. There is very little published information concerning the differences of PRA in patients with unilateral versus bilateral disease, although Bianchi et al. [16] found that both types of hypertension were characterized by high renin levels.

Another prediction that could be made from the ani-

Additive Effect of Sodium Depletion on Blood Pressure Reduction

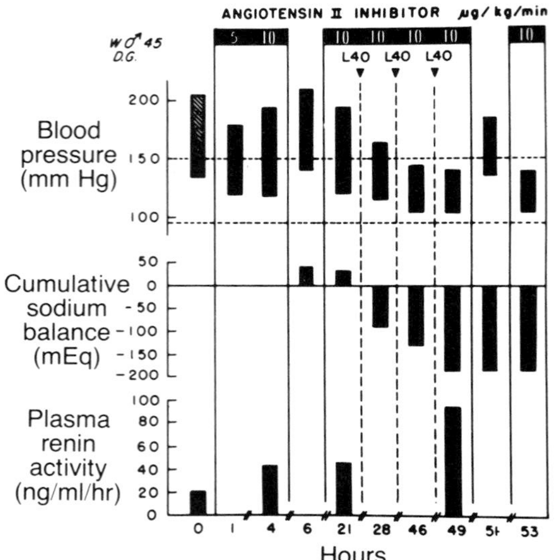

Fig. 55-3. Effects of angiotensin blockade by saralasin in a patient with bilateral renal artery stenosis. The effect on blood pressure is much greater following sodium depletion by 40 mg of furosemide (*L40*).

mal data is that when PRA is normal, blood volume should be high. This was indeed found to be true by Bianchi et al. [16], who also found that when PRA was high, there was no increase of plasma volume. This finding might reconcile some of the earlier confusing reports, for example, of Frohlich et al. [59], who found no difference of plasma volume in patients with essential or renovascular hypertension.

On the basis of the animal experiments reported above, plasma volume should be higher in patients with bilateral disease than in those with unilateral disease.

In a study reported by Davies et al. [38] it was found that total exchangeable sodium was normal in both essential and renovascular hypertension and that there was a weakly positive correlation between exchangeable sodium and blood pressure in the former but a strong negative correlation in the latter. They attributed the decrease of exchangeable sodium with increasing pressure in patients with unilateral renal artery stenosis to the effects of pressure natriuresis acting through the unaffected kidney, an interpretation consistent with the above animal data.

HEMODYNAMICS OF RENOVASCULAR HYPERTENSION

If sodium retention were the dominant mechanism underlying renovascular hypertension, it might be expected that hemodynamic measurements would reveal an increased cardiac output on the grounds that this has been reported in patients with primary aldosteronism [40], which is the classic example of volume-dependent hypertension. Frohlich et al. [59] found that cardiac output was higher in patients with renovascular than with essential hypertension, despite the fact that plasma volumes were no different. However, most of the renovascular patients were women, whereas the controls were mostly men.

We compared the hemodynamic patterns and degree of left ventricular hypertrophy in patients with essential and renovascular hypertension using echocardiography [200]. The patients with renovascular hypertension had significantly greater left ventricular dilatation and septal hypertrophy, and impaired fractional shortening. Cardiac output was higher in the patients with bilateral disease than in those with unilateral disease, a finding consistent with a state of relative volume overload in the former, as in one-clip one-kidney experimental hypertension.

THE ROLE OF POSTURE AND NEPHROPTOSIS IN RENOVASCULAR HYPERTENSION

The possibility that abnormal renal mobility or "nephroptosis" may be a causal factor in fibromuscular dysplasia has been entertained for many years [124], but conclusive data are lacking. Nephroptosis is commoner in women than in men and commoner on the right side than the left, differences that parallel the incidence of fibromuscular disease [19]. DeZeeuw et al. [45] measured renal mobility between the supine and upright positions in 234 patients undergoing intravenous pyelography, most of whom were hypertensive, and included 14 patients with fibromuscular dysplasia. Twelve of these fourteen patients had abnormally increased renal mobility, and this abnormality was always on the side that had the affected renal artery. These findings are consistent with those of Kaufman et al. [96], who reported nephroptosis in 70 percent of patients with fibromuscular dysplasia.

Despite this evidence for an apparent association between nephroptosis and hypertension, the physiologic mechanism remains obscure. It has been postulated that the renal mobility causes kinking of the renal artery leading to fibrosis and obstruction. This mechanism could be only contributory at best, since fibromuscular dysplasia also occurs in other, less mobile arteries (e.g., celiac artery), and other arteries subjected to much greater mobility (e.g., brachial artery) do not develop any similar lesions. Support for a functional significance of nephroptosis is derived from the results of a study by Bianchi et al. [15], which demonstrated that patients with nephroptosis show an exaggerated fall of glomerular filtration rate (GFR) on assuming the upright posture.

ROLE OF OTHER HORMONAL FACTORS

Many patients with renovascular hypertension have mild to moderate secondary hyperaldosteronism. However, in our experience, aldosterone excretion is generally less elevated for a given level of PRA than in other high-renin states (e.g., malignant hypertension). Two possible explanations for this observation are that there may be a dissociation between PRA and plasma levels of angiotensin II in some patients. The other, more likely hypothesis is that the state of sodium balance may alter the adrenal sensitivity to angiotensin II (AII), since it has been established that sodium depletion augments the aldosterone response to AII in isolated glomerulosa cells [27]. Thus the degree of hyperaldosteronism may be a marker of volume status.

Plasma catecholamines are probably normal in human renovascular hypertension [120] unless azotemia is present [103]. It has been suggested that the sympathetic nervous system contributes to short-term fluctuations of blood pressure because a positive correlation has been observed during a 24-hour period between plasma norepinephrine and blood pressure, and between plasma norepinephrine and renin [120].

Table 55-2. Anatomy of renal arteries (A) and veins (V)

Percent of subjects	Right kidney	Left kidney
38.5	1A, 1V	1A, 1V
31.5	1A, 1V	2A, 1V
10	2A, 1V	1A, 1V
9.5	1A, 2V	1A, 1V
28.5	Complex patterns	

Direct evidence of a role for prostaglandins in mediating renin release in human renovascular hypertension has been provided by Imanishi et al. [85], who demonstrated a close correlation between prostaglandin E_2 (PGE_2) and renin in the renal veins of the ischemic kidney. Furthermore, aspirin acutely lowered PGE_2, renin, and blood pressure in these patients.

ANATOMY AND PATHOLOGY OF RENAL ARTERIES

Normal Patterns. Although the most common pattern is a single renal artery and vein on each side, this in fact

Fig. 55-4. Aortogram of a patient with a unilateral atheromatous stenosis (A), which in the span of 2 months had progressed to complete occlusion (B).

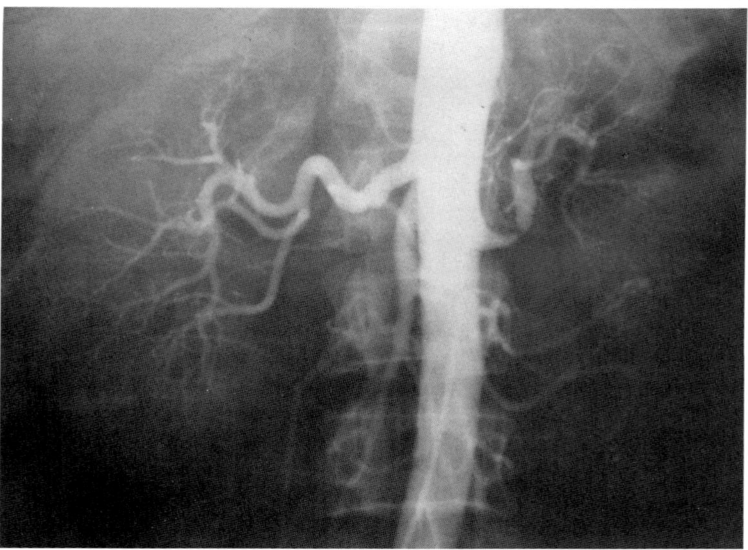

A

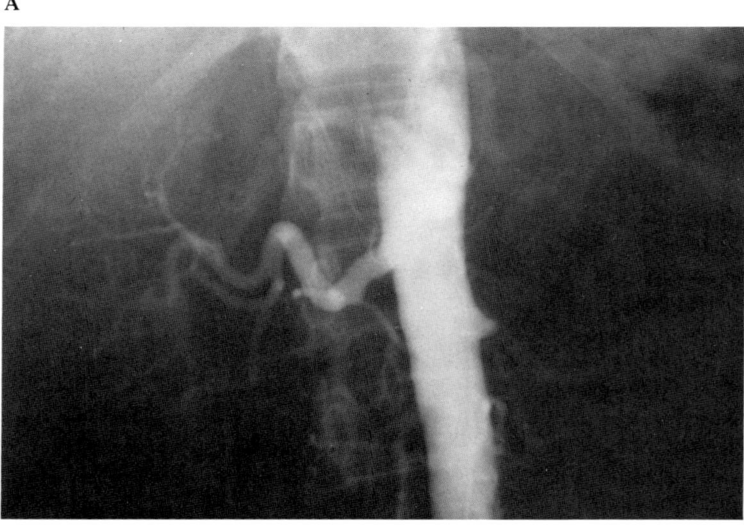

B

applies only to a minority (38.5 percent) of people [146], the majority of whom have either multiple renal arteries or veins on one side, as shown in Table 55-2.

Atheromatous Lesions. Atheromatous plaques occur most commonly in the proximal third of the renal artery, and in many cases plaques in the wall of the aorta may encroach on the ostium of the renal artery. If atheromatous lesions are left untreated, there is a high probability of progression to complete occlusion (Fig. 55-4). In one series the average rate of progression of the percentage of transluminal diameter stenosed was estimated to be about 1.5 percent per month [168]. Thus in patients with stenoses measuring 75 percent to 99 percent of luminal diameter at angiography, 40 percent had progressed to complete occlusion after 1 year.

Fibromuscular Dysplasia. Fibromuscular dysplasia of the renal arteries is the commonest cause of renovascular hypertension in younger patients and has been classified into four types according to pathologic differences in the lesions. Medial fibroplasia is the commonest variety in adults (accounting for 65 percent of cases) but is rare in children; it produces the classic beaded appearance on angiography due to areas of thickening of the media interspersed by areas of aneurysmal dilatation (Fig. 55-5). This type of lesion is not confined to the renal arteries because it may also occur in the carotid and cerebral arteries. Progression of these lesions to complete occlusion almost never occurs.

The next most common variety is perimedial fibroplasia (25 percent), in which there is proliferation of fibrous tissue in the outer half of the media. Radiographically, the appearance is also of beads, but because they are not aneurysmal they are of smaller diameter than the arterial lumen. The stenoses are often quite severe and may occasionally progress to complete occlusion [66].

Medial dissection (5 percent) is characterized by dissection of the intimal elastic membrane, which produces the appearance of a fusiform enlargement of the renal artery.

Medial hyperplasia and intimal fibroplasia (5 percent) are angiographically indistinguishable and may produce a single proximal stenosis that can resemble atheroma. The former is characterized histologically by increased smooth muscle in the media, the latter by proliferation of mesenchymal cells and connective tissue in the intima.

Arteritis. Takayasu's arteritis is a rare disease, affecting mainly young women, that can cause discrete stenosis of the aorta and major arteries, including the renal arteries.

Cholesterol Emboli. In patients who have diffuse atheroma, fragments of plaque may break off and cause embolization in the kidneys and other vascular beds. This may occur spontaneously or following aortic surgery and renal arteriography [75]. Pathologically, the lesions are characterized by microemboli of cholesterol crystals and amorphous debris, which are later replaced by foreign body giant cells and fibrosis.

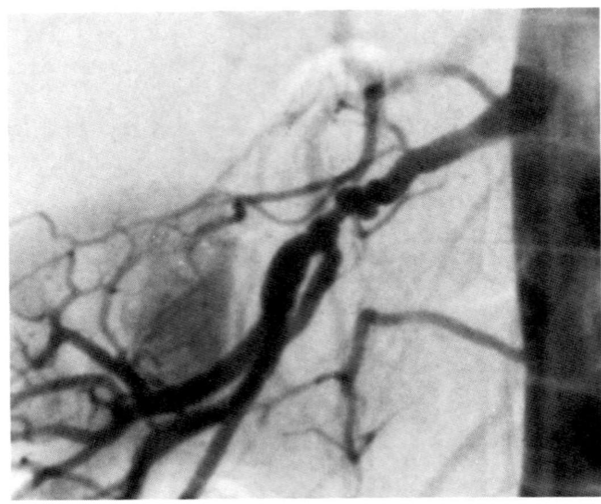

A

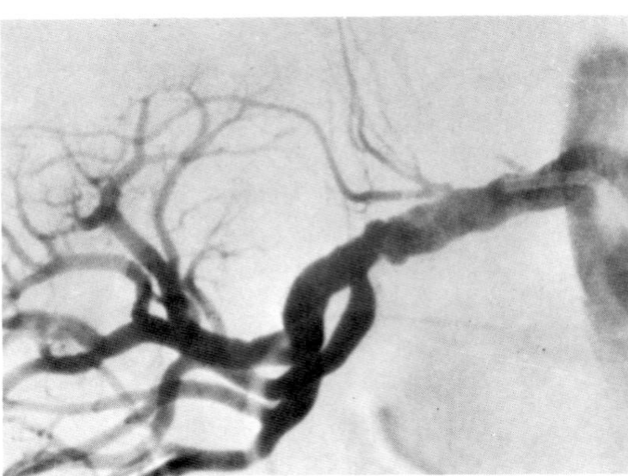

B

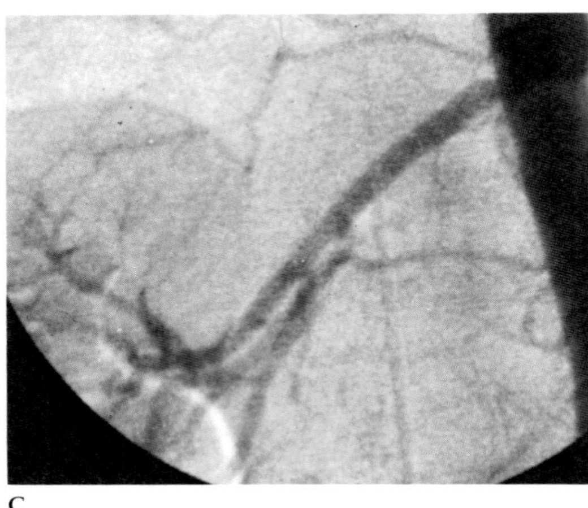

C

Fig. 55-5. A. Medical fibroplasia in a woman with renovascular hypertension. Note beaded appearance with aneurysmal dilatation. B. The same artery immediately after renal angioplasty. C. Five years later. Note remodeling with complete normalization of the arterial wall.

Clinically, the emboli are manifested by a deterioration of renal function and an exacerbation of the hypertension [92]. Other features include gastrointestinal bleeding, acute pancreatitis, and gangrene or livedo reticularis in the feet. The diagnosis may be suspected if these manifestations develop after an invasive procedure in a patient with known atheromatous disease over the age of 60 years, but it can be established with certainty only if the microemboli are visualized on a tissue biopsy.

The importance of cholesterol emboli as a cause of chronic renal failure has recently been emphasized by Meyrier et al. [125], who found a high prevalence on renal biopsy in azotemic patients who had angiographic evidence of diffuse atheromatous disease.

Clinical Features of Renovascular Hypertension

PREVALENCE

The prevalence of renovascular hypertension is unknown but is probably around 5 percent of the general hypertensive population [64], although for patients with more severe hypertension much higher figures have been reported. In a series of 123 patients with accelerated or malignant hypertension (grade III or IV retinopathy), Davis et al. [39] reported a prevalence of 43 percent in white patients and 7 percent in blacks. Anderson et al. [2] reported a prevalence ranging from less than 2 percent in patients less than 30 years of age to nearly 10 percent over the age of 60 years. It was also higher in patients with more severe hypertension. Most studies have reported a much lower prevalence in blacks than in whites [2, 39, 98], although one recent study found no difference when there were clinical clues suggestive of renovascular hypertension [184]. This study, however, did not report whether the clues themselves were equally prevalent in blacks and whites.

These results were all based on clinical studies, which, with one exception [39], did not utilize arteriography in all patients. The prevalence rates are therefore almost certainly an underestimate. However, the situation is complicated by the fact that the demonstration of an anatomic stenosis in the renal artery of a hypertensive patient does not imply that the lesion is causing the hypertension. In an autopsy series of 295 patients Holley et al. [78] found moderate or severe renal artery stenosis in 49 percent of normotensive subjects and 77 percent of hypertensives. In another series of 500 aortograms performed for investigations of peripheral vascular disease or hypertension, renal artery stenosis was detected in 32 percent of normotensives and in 62 percent of hypertensives [53].

CLINICAL SIGNS AND SYMPTOMS

Because of its relative frequency and curability, it is important not to miss the diagnosis of renovascular hypertension, and there may be many clues to its presence from the history and clinical examination. Some of the most important features that distinguish it from essential hypertension, and also the differences between the two commonest types, atheroma and fibromuscular dysplasia, are shown in Table 55-3.

In younger patients, and particularly in women, fibromuscular disease is the commonest cause of hypertension, but it is relatively rare in blacks. A family history of hypertension is less likely to be present than in cases of essential hypertension, although a familial occurrence of fibromuscular dysplasia has occasionally been described. Thus in a young white woman with a recent onset of hypertension and a negative family history, there should be a very high index of suspicion for fibromuscular disease. Women with fibromuscular dysplasia tend to be taller than those with essential hypertension or atheromatous renal artery stenosis [46]. Conversely, the finding of hypertension in a middle-aged man with other evidence of atheromatous disease such as coronary heart disease should raise the possibility of atheromatous renovascular hypertension. In hypertensive patients undergoing coronary angiography a surprisingly high prevalence of renovascular disease was detected [201].

In the physical examination there may also be clues to its presence. Abdominal bruits are present in about 40

Table 55-3. Clinical characteristics of renovascular hypertension

		Renovascular hypertension	
	Essential hypertension (%)	Atheroma (%)	Fibromuscular dysplasia (%)
Race (black)	29	7	10
Family history	67	58	41
Age at onset			
<20 years	12	2	16
>50 years	7	39	13
Duration <1 year	10	23	19
Obese	38	17	11
Abdominal bruit	7	41	57
High renin profile	15	80	80
Hypokalemia (<3.4 meq/L)	7	14	17
Smoking	42	88	71

Source: Data based on M. H. Maxwell, K. H. Bleefer, S. S. Franklin, et al. Cooperative Study of Renovascular Hypertension. Demographic analysis of the study. *J. A. M. A.* 220:1195, 1972.

percent of patients and usually signify the presence of renal artery stenosis, although they may originate from other vessels. Such bruits are of course most likely to be heard in thin patients.

Retinopathy may be particularly pronounced in patients with renovascular hypertension, perhaps because of its more brief and stormy course. In one series of patients with diastolic blood pressures above 125 mm Hg and hemorrhages or exudates in the fundi, renovascular hypertension was diagnosed in approximately one-third [39]. In our experience, pulmonary edema in a hypertensive patient is commonly associated with bilateral renal artery stenosis.

A history of smoking is another potential clue to the presence of renovascular hypertension. In our own series of patients with atheromatous renal artery stenosis, 88 percent were smokers compared with only 42 percent of patients with essential hypertension [137]. This finding is consistent with reports of an association between smoking and atheroma in other areas, for instance, coronary heart disease and peripheral vascular disease. Of more surprise was our finding of a higher than expected incidence of smokers in patients with fibromuscular disease.

Pulmonary Edema. We have recently been impressed by the relatively frequent occurrence of pulmonary edema in patients with advanced renovascular hypertension [150]. In a series of 55 consecutive patients who were also azotemic, pulmonary edema had occurred in 13 (25%). In the majority of these patients (92%), the renal artery stenosis was bilateral, or there was a solitary kidney with a stenosed artery. Successful revascularization of the ischemic kidney prevented further occurrence of the pulmonary edema. The occurrence of pulmonary edema was not related to the severity of the hypertension or renal failure. While it was commoner in patients who had associated coronary heart disease, this was not the most important predisposing factor, because it can also occur in patients with normal coronary arteries.

LABORATORY INVESTIGATIONS

Evidence of impaired renal function on routine biochemical tests, such as an elevated blood urea nitrogen (BUN) or creatinine level, suggests either that there is parenchymal disease or that, if there is renovascular disease, it is bilateral. In the U.S. Cooperative Study 15 percent of patients with atheromatous renal artery stenosis had an elevated serum creatinine compared with 11 percent of patients with essential hypertension and only 2 percent of patients with fibromuscular dysplasia [122].

A low serum potassium level is an occasional marker of renovascular disease; in the U.S. Cooperative Study about 15 percent of patients with either atheromatous or fibromuscular disease had a potassium value of below 3.4 mEq per liter. This occurs as a result of hyperreninemia stimulating angiotensin with a resultant rise in plasma aldosterone concentrations.

Urinalysis may show a slightly increased incidence of bacteriuria, and proteinuria may also be present, as described below.

PROTEINURIA IN RENOVASCULAR HYPERTENSION

Proteinuria is not an uncommon finding in patients with renovascular hypertension [173] and may occasionally be sufficiently pronounced to present as a nephrotic syndrome [14]. In our own experience proteinuria in excess of 500 mg per 24 hours usually signifies complete occlusion of a renal artery in patients with renovascular hypertension [207]. This proteinuria may be reversed by surgery or angioplasty.

RENAL SEGMENTAL INFARCTION

In occasional patients who present with an acute accelerated hypertension the underlying abnormality may be renal segmental infarction [51]. Clinically, it is characterized by abdominal or flank pain, sometimes associated with nausea, vomiting, and fever. Hematuria and proteinuria may also occur. The blood pressure may be very high, with retinopathy but with normal electrocardiogram (ECG) and renal function. Investigations show hyperreninemia with lateralizing renal vein renins. Intravenous pyelogram (IVP) and renal scans may show a decreased kidney size on one side, but the diagnosis is confirmed by arteriography, which shows characteristic defects in the nephrogram phase. The patients are typically young (e.g., 30 to 50 years old), and the underlying pathology is usually fibromuscular dysplasia with thrombosis occurring in an aneurysm. The hypertension is renin dependent and may respond dramatically to treatment with angiotensin-converting enzyme inhibitors. Surgery may not therefore be necessary.

RENOVASCULAR HYPERTENSION IN CHILDREN

Fibromuscular dysplasia is the commonest cause of renovascular hypertension in children and is usually of the intimal or perimedial type [139, 180]. In contrast to adults, medial fibroplasia is rare. The lesions are commonly ostial and bilateral and may be associated with neurofibromatosis or coarctation of the abdominal aorta.

Diagnosis of Renovascular Hypertension

SCREENING

The question of which patients should be screened for renovascular hypertension is an important one. Since many cases are not detected by routine evaluation, there is a definite need for a reliable and inexpensive screening test that could be performed in every patient. Unfortunately, it must be admitted that no such test exists at the present time. The main problem is that when a condition has a prevalence as low as 5 percent, the sensitivity and specificity of any screening test need to be greater than 95 percent, otherwise most of the cases that are detected by the test will be false positives. None of the currently available tests are this reliable.

There is no perfect screening test for the detection of renovascular hypertension. A large number of tests have been proposed, and the sensitivity and specificity of some of the more popular ones are given in Table 55-4. These tests can be classified into two categories: First are those that can be done in a physician's office, which are relatively simple to perform and inexpensive, but which do not indicate which kidney is involved. Measurement

Table 55-4. Screening tests for renovascular hypertension

Tests	Sensitivity	Specificity
Office tests		
Plasma renin activity	57%	66%
Captopril test	73–100%	72–100%
Tests of lateralization		
IVP	74–78%	86–88%
Renal scan	74%	77%
Captopril scan	92–94%	95–97%
Renal vein renin	62–80%	60–100%
Digital subtraction angiogram	88%	90%
Duplex Doppler imaging*	84–91%	95–97%
Exercise scan	?	?

*In patients in whom satisfactory recordings can be made.

Table 55-5. Criteria for a positive captopril test*

1. Stimulated PRA of 12 ng/ml/hr.
2. Absolute increase in PRA of ng/ml/hr or more.
3. Percent increase in PRA of 150% or more, or of 400% if baseline PRA is below 3 ng/ml/hr.

*All these criteria should be satisfied. Patients should be seated, not supine.

of peripheral plasma renin activity and the captopril test come into this category. Second are those tests that provide anatomic or functional information about each kidney and that cannot be routinely done in the office. Ideally, one or more of these tests should be done following the first-stage test.

Peripheral Plasma Renin Activity. Unilateral hypersecretion of renin should be the hallmark of potentially curable renovascular hypertension. We have found that peripheral PRA, measured in the morning in the seated position and when indexed against sodium excretion, is an excellent tool in identifying abnormally high renin secretion (Fig. 55-6). This high rate of secretion is present in about 75 percent of patients with proven renovascular hypertension [197]. In our experience, a low plasma renin level in an untreated patient virtually rules out the possibility of renovascular hypertension, but the sensitivity and specificity of a high peripheral PRA are inadequate to be of much value as a screening test.

Captopril Test. At the present time, the most sensitive office screening test for the diagnosis of renovascular hypertension is the captopril test. Case and Laragh [29] were the first to show that the reactive rise of renin following administration of captopril is greater in patients with renovascular than with essential hypertension. The criteria that we have found to be the most reliable for distinguishing patients with renovascular hypertension are shown in Table 55-5.

In a series of more than 200 patients we found that with these criteria the sensitivity and specificity of this test were better than 95 percent [134]. Other groups, however, have reported lower levels of sensitivity but have used somewhat different criteria [44, 84, 165, 183]. The range of disagreement concerning the usefulness of the captopril test is well illustrated by two recent studies. The first, by Postma et al. [155], reported a sensitivity of 39 percent and a specificity of 96 percent and concluded that the test is of little value. The second, by Fredrickson et al. [58], reported a sensitivity of 100 percent and a specificity of 80 percent and concluded that it is of value. This divergence may be partly due to differences in technique. The Postma study differed from both our original study and the confirmatory study of Frederickson in two important ways. First, the patients were studied supine, which means that the renin is likely to be less reactive to the captopril challenge than when the study is performed with the patient sitting; and second, the criterion for diagnosing renovascular hypertension was much looser. Postma et al. used an angiographic stenosis of more than 50 percent as the cutoff point, while we and Fredrickson used 75 percent.

In a study comparing the value of several screening tests (which included captopril renography and captopril-stimulated renal vein renins), Svetkey et al. [183] concluded that captopril-stimulated peripheral renin ac-

Fig. 55-6. Renin-sodium profiles in patients with unilateral renovascular hypertension before and after successful renal angioplasty. Cross-hatched area indicates normal range.

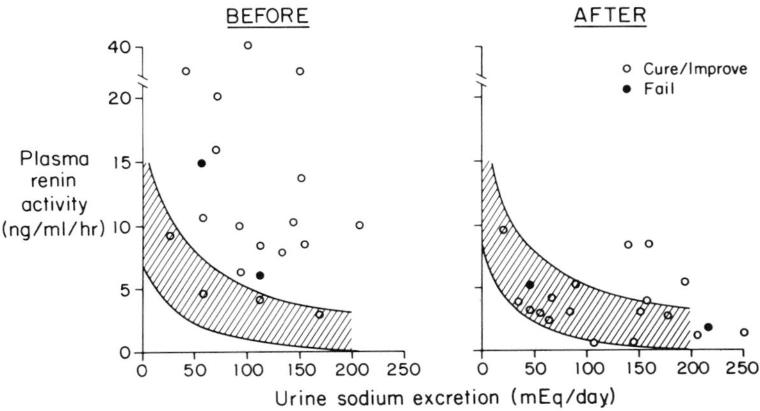

tivity had the highest sensitivity and specificity, although it was still not very good (73% and 72%, respectively). It is important to note that the renin response is a much more reliable marker than the blood pressure response. Although patients with renovascular disease tend to show a greater fall of blood pressure (average 18 mm Hg) than patients with essential hypertension (average 7 mm Hg) there is considerable overlap. The blood pressure response, however, may predict the blood pressure response to revascularization by surgery or angioplasty [164]. The test becomes less reliable in patients who are azotemic, although even here it is possible that patients who show a negative test may be less likely to benefit from renal revascularization. It does not discriminate between patients with unilateral versus bilateral disease, both of which groups usually show a positive response [44, 134].

Differential Renal Vein Renin Determinations. In patients with unilateral renal artery stenosis, hypersecretion of renin by the ischemic kidney is the hallmark of renovascular hypertension and can be evaluated by renal vein renin measurement. In the ideal situation, there is not only unilateral hypersecretion, but also contralateral suppression of renin secretion [153, 171, 197, 203]. This can be evaluated by comparing the renin level in each renal vein to the corresponding inferior vena cava (below the level of the renal veins), which has been shown to be the same as the level in the renal artery. Thus, when there is contralateral suppression of renin secretion, the renin level in the renal vein and inferior vena cava will be the same. Measuring the increment of renin (as V − A/A, where V and A are the levels in the renal vein and inferior vena cava) on each side has been shown to be superior to simply using the ratio between the two renal veins, because the latter cannot detect whether renin secretion is suppressed or not [197]. Renal vein renins tend to return to normal following successful revascularization (Fig. 55-7). The sensitivity of the test can be increased by repeating the measurements after acute administration of captopril, but false-negative results may still occur [116, 192].

In patients with stenoses of both renal arteries, the pattern of renal vein renins often shows the same degree of asymmetry as in patients with unilateral stenosis and usually lateralizes to the kidney that shows the greatest degree of stenosis on the arteriogram [151]. The most marked asymmetry is seen in patients who have complete occlusion of one renal artery, in whom a V − A/A of over 2 is commonly seen (Fig. 55-8). This may represent low flow through the kidney rather than hypersecretion of renin. Contralateral suppression of renin secretion may occur even in the presence of a severe stenosis of the contralateral renal artery. This asymmetry is less pronounced in the presence of azotemia. The test is thus of little value in patients with bilateral disease, except for identifying which kidney is most severely affected.

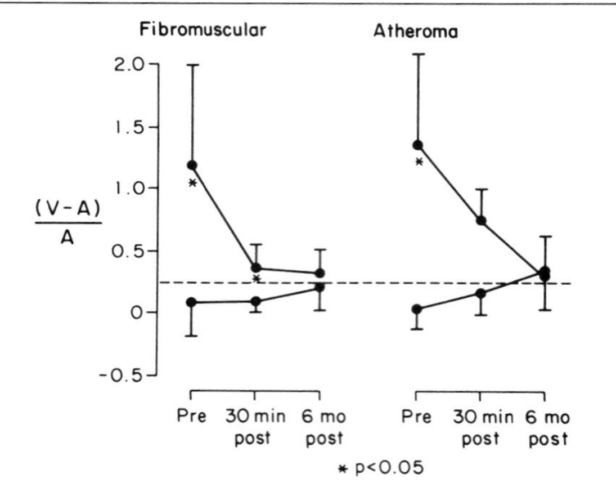

Fig. 55-7. Renal vein renin values (expressed as V-A/A) from ischemic (*upper points*) and contralateral kidneys (*lower points*) before, 30 minutes after, and 6 months after angioplasty. Dotted line indicates normal V-A/A of 0.24 on each side.

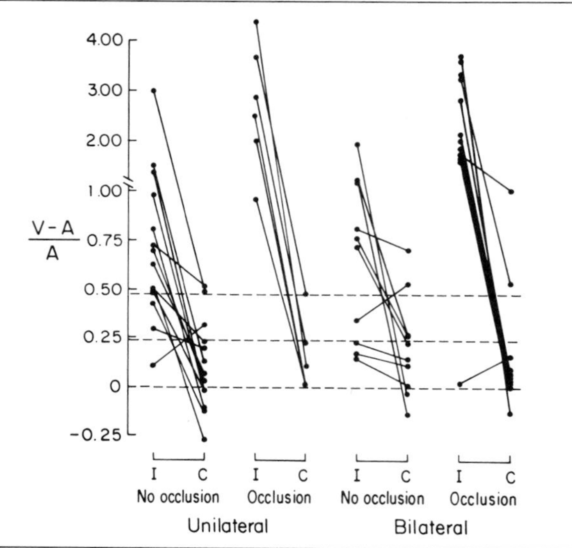

Fig. 55-8. Comparison of renal vein renin value in patients with unilateral and bilateral renal artery stenosis. *I* = more ischemic kidney; *C* = contralateral kidney. Occlusion = one renal artery totally occluded. Note similarity of patterns in unilateral and bilateral disease.

Intravenous Pyelogram. For many years the rapid-sequence IVP was used as the standard screening test. Surveys of its usefulness, however, have indicated that the number of hypertensive patients whose treatment is altered as a result of previously unsuspected abnormalities is very small, being 0.9 percent in one series [4], and 0.33 percent in another [7]. In the U.S. Cooperative series, the criteria for an abnormal IVP were delayed excretion, a difference in size of 1.5 cm or more between the two kidneys, and differences in dye concentration [18]. It was found that approximately 78 percent of patients with renovascular hypertension have an abnormal IVP, but there was a false-positive rate of 11 percent and a false-negative rate of 22 percent [193]. However, since the IVP was probably used to make the diagnosis of renovascular hypertension in many of these patients, the true sensitivity of the IVP is probably lower than the reported 78 percent; many of our patients with renovascular hypertension have had normal IVPs, and we no longer use it as a routine screening procedure.

Digital Subtraction Angiography. Digital subtraction angiography (DSA) represents a major advance in the evaluation of patients with suspected renovascular hypertension. Much of the information gained from conventional arteriography can now be gained from DSA, with much less expense and inconvenience to the patient. It can be performed as an outpatient investigation and, in our experience, can be conveniently combined with renal vein renin measurements.

Several studies have compared the reliability of DSA to arteriography [25, 31, 76, 205]. In about 80 percent of cases there is agreement between the two techniques, with DSA showing roughly 5 percent of false positives (i.e., lesions that are not detected on the arteriogram) and 10 percent of false negatives. In the latter case, lesions of branch renal arteries are particularly likely to be missed.

Because of the relatively large volume of dye needed, the technique is not suitable for use in azotemic patients, in whom there is a risk of dye-induced nephrotoxicity.

Renal Scans. Isotope renograms or renal scans have been available for many years but have not attained wide acceptance as screening tests because of their relatively low sensitivity and specificity [123]. The most widely used isotopes have been hippuran and DTPA (diethylene triamine penta-acetic acid); the former gives an approximate measure of renal blood flow, and the latter of GFR.

Two recent developments have given these techniques a new lease on life. The first is the development of more reliable quantitative evaluation of the renogram, and the second (described in the next section) the use of angiotensin converting enzyme (ACE) inhibitors to enhance the difference between normal and ischemic kidneys. An example of the improved quantification of DTPA scans is a recent study by Gruenewald et al. [72], who used deconvolution analysis to estimate parenchymal tracer transit (PTT) time through the kidney. In patients with atheromatous unilateral renal artery stenosis, a prolonged PTT was a highly specific predictor of the blood pressure response to angioplasty. These new methods of analysis require validation on a wider scale before their implications can be properly assessed.

Captopril Renography. A potentially interesting development of the conventional renal scan is to compare the renograms obtained before and after a single dose of captopril. The rationale for this is that the GFR of an ischemic kidney is dependent on the effects of angiotensin on the efferent glomerular arterioles, so that converting enzyme inhibition produces a marked fall in GFR (Fig. 55-9). Thus the characteristic effect of captopril in a kidney with a renal artery stenosis is to cause a decrease of DTPA uptake (a measure of GFR) with little change of hippuran uptake (a measure of renal blood flow), although the excretion phase of hippuran is delayed [55, 62].

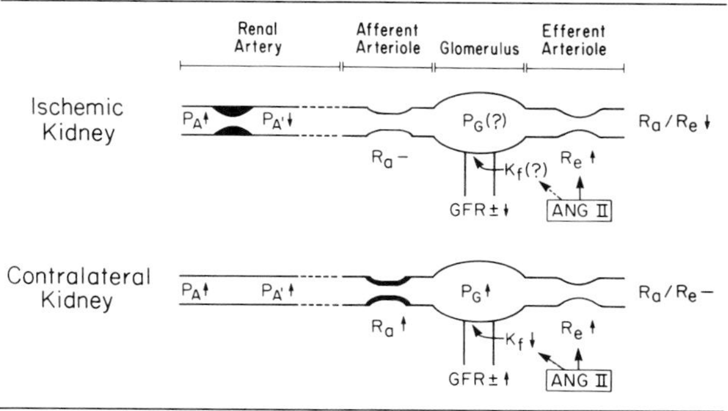

Fig. 55-9. Hypothetical changes in intrarenal hemodynamics in unilateral renal artery stenosis and the effects of angiotensin (ANG II). P_A and P_G represent pressures in renal artery and glomerular capillaries, respectively. R_a and R_e represent afferent and efferent arteriolar resistances. K_f = filtration coefficient. GFR = glomerular filtration rate.

Several recent studies have reported that the administration of captopril [35, 117] or enalapril [101] will increase both the sensitivity and specificity of renal scans. DTPA has been used most widely, although some have claimed that hippuran may be just as sensitive [52, 101]. Analytic techniques have included the estimation of PTT [101] and GFR [48] for examining the effects of captopril. We identified three criteria for diagnosing renal artery stenosis [117]: a percent uptake of DTPA by the affected kidney of less than 40 percent of the total, a time to peak uptake of DTPA of more than 5 minutes longer than in the contralateral kidney, and a prolonged retention of DTPA, expressed as the fraction of peak activity 15 minutes after DTPA administration, that is at least 20 percent greater than in the contralateral kidney. The sensitivity and specificity of these criteria were all greater for the post- than for the pre-captopril scan, but we did not find that the change induced by captopril had any additional diagnostic value. If this is confirmed in other studies, it suggests the possibility that the pre-captopril scan may be redundant in many instances. Captopril renography may prove particularly useful in discriminating between renovascular and parenchymal disease, although in our experience it does not work well in azotemic patients.

Exercise Renography. Another recent development of the conventional renal scan has been the recording of hippuran scans before and after exercise [32, 33]. In normal subjects, there is some delay in hippuran transport during exercise, probably occurring as a result of neurally mediated renal vasoconstriction. In patients with essential hypertension, there is a much more pronounced delay, which may be indicative of a transient cortical perfusion disturbance. The reasons for this are not clear but may possibly be due to structural changes occurring in the kidney. Patients with curable renovascular hypertension show a normal response to exercise. This test is potentially of interest, since it may be able to detect irreversible parenchymal changes, but it requires further evaluation.

Duplex Doppler Imaging. Another new technique currently being investigated is the use of Doppler ultrasound scanning to record velocity profiles from the renal arteries [89, 99]. A number of criteria have been developed for diagnosing renal artery stenosis [5, 67, 138]. The most reliable appears to be the ratio of peak systolic velocities in the renal artery and aorta. In patients in whom technically satisfactory readings can be obtained, a ratio of more than 3.5 predicts renal artery stenosis of 60 percent or greater with a sensitivity of 84 to 90 percent and a specificity of 95 to 97 percent [67, 138].

While these figures are encouraging, the technique has a number of limitations. First, up to 40 percent of examinations may be technically unsatisfactory because of inability to identify one or both renal arteries, because of factors such as obesity or excessive bowel gas [109]. It is usually only possible to obtain an adequate examination of the proximal end of the renal arteries, so lesions due to fibromuscular dysplasia may be missed. Another problem is the relatively common occurrence of multiple renal arteries, which may be overlooked. Further evaluation of this test is also needed.

Split Renal Function Studies. In 1953 Howard et al. [79] introduced split renal function studies to identify patients with surgically correctable renovascular hypertension. This remains one of the most accurate and reliable tests but has fallen into disfavor because of its relative invasiveness, as it necessitates cystoscopy and catheterization of both ureters.

ARTERIOGRAPHY

The demonstration of a stenosis in a renal artery in a hypertensive patient does not necessarily imply that the stenosis is causing the hypertension, particularly when it is atheromatous. Hypertension from any cause accelerates the development of atheroma, so that in some cases a stenosis in a renal artery may occur secondarily to essential hypertension. To cause renal ischemia and hypertension, a stenosis must occlude at least 75 percent of the arterial lumen, but the correlation between the arteriographic appearance and the degree of ischemia is poor [108, 172].

In one series in which the accuracy of arteriography in diagnosing the pathology of the renal arteries was estimated by comparison with the pathologic specimens removed at surgery, the sensitivity for distinguishing fibromuscular disease from atheroma was 82 percent [170]. The absence of abdominal aortic atherosclerosis was a reliable predictor of fibromuscular disease. Separation of the different types of fibromuscular disease could not be reliably assessed from the arteriogram, however.

SEQUENCE OF TESTING FOR EVALUATING RENOVASCULAR HYPERTENSION

Given the low overall prevalence of the disease, and the high cost and imperfect accuracy of the available screening tests, it is inappropriate to recommend routine screening in all hypertensive patients. By using simple clinical and demographic criteria, it is possible to identify a subgroup of patients in whom the probability of renovascular disease is quite high. In these patients an oral captopril test would be our next step, possibly combined with renography, if subsequent studies confirm its early promise. Duplex scanning of the renal arteries may also prove helpful, but while this test may provide anatomic information as to the presence of a stenosis, it can provide no information as to the effects of the stenosis on the kidney. An alternative approach, which we have used extensively in the past and which provides both fundamental and anatomic data, is a combined intravenous DSA and renal vein renin measurements.

It is ironic that most of the available tests work quite well in patients with "simple" renovascular hypertension, where there is a discrete unilateral stenosis and normal renal function, but none of them appears to work well in patients with "complex" renovascular hypertension, with bilateral stenoses and azotemia.

Treatment of Renovascular Hypertension

TREATMENT OPTIONS

There are three general modalities of treatment applicable to patients with renovascular hypertension: surgery, angioplasty, or medical treatment. Which is most appropriate depends on the etiology of the renal artery stenosis and the general condition of the patient. The two goals of treatment are to cure or improve the hypertension and to reverse or prevent impairment of renal function.

Both surgery and angioplasty yield a high cure rate and few complications in patients with fibromuscular dysplasia and are therefore almost always preferable to medical treatment. These patients also tend to be young, so that there is a good prospect of avoiding the costs and side effects of medical treatment over a period of many years.

With atheromatous lesions, the situation becomes much more murky. There is a relatively high probability that the lesions are coincidental to, or a consequence of the hypertension, rather than its original cause. Unlike the situation in the patient being considered for coronary or peripheral angioplasty, symptoms are of no help in deciding when treatment is indicated. In the patient with bilateral disease, the situation is further complicated by the fact that there is almost always some degree of nephrosclerosis in the less severely affected kidney. In such patients, therefore, it is unrealistic to expect that the hypertension can be cured, except on rare occasions. There is another consideration, however, which is that the progressive nature of the atherosclerotic process will eventually lead to an impairment of renal function. Once azotemia occurs, it develops at a more or less constant rate in individual patients, so that it is often possible to estimate when dialysis is going to be needed. Medical therapy is generally ineffective in preventing this relentless progression, and in some cases may make it worse, particularly if ACE inhibitors are used. There is now abundant evidence that revascularization by surgery or angioplasty can be achieved with safety in such patients and can result in an improvement or stabilization of their renal function.

Renovascular Hypertension in the Elderly. Improvements in diagnostic and interventional techniques, together with the aging of the general population, have resulted in increasing numbers of elderly patients with renovascular disease being detected and treated. They differ from younger patients in a number of ways: First, the renal artery stenosis is nearly always from atheroma; second, there is often significant atheromatous disease elsewhere, e.g., in the coronary and cerebral vascular beds; and third, it is often not clear whether the renal artery stenosis is the cause of the hypertension or has occurred coincidentally or consequently to it. Many patients are also azotemic. There is no doubt that revascularization can be achieved in such patients with acceptably low morbidity, both by surgery [9, 140] and by angioplasty [26, 175], and that this will improve the blood pressure. With a reticence rare among surgeons, and on the basis of what is probably the largest surgical series (919 patients) with the longest follow-up (up to 31 years), Lawrie et al. [105] have questioned the wisdom of surgical intervention in elderly patients. Their data showed that in younger patients a good blood pressure response appeared to improve survival, but this was not the case for the elderly. Furthermore, most of the deaths in the older patients were due to myocardial infarction, presumably from coexisting coronary heart disease.

If blood pressure is the only issue, therefore, a good case could be made for treating the elderly patient with renovascular hypertension medically rather than by surgery or angioplasty. However, many such patients are also azotemic, and as discussed below, there is evidence that revascularization can not only slow down the progression of renal failure, but also reverse it. If the disease process is too far advanced, however, the azotemia may be largely the result of cholesterol emboli to the kidney and hence irreversible [125].

SURGICAL MANAGEMENT

Techniques. The first operative cure of hypertension followed unilateral nephrectomy [79, 132]. Today, the indications for nephrectomy are limited, and a procedure to preserve renal function is preferable. Nephrectomy may still be appropriate (1) if there is poor or absent renal function, (2) if the patient is a poor surgical risk, (3) if there is uncorrectable vascular disease, or (4) following occlusion of an attempted revascularization. In many cases the blood pressure can be equally well controlled by the administration of converting enzyme inhibitors, provided that there is no stenosis in the renal artery of the other kidney. Partial nephrectomy can occasionally be performed if there is a stenosis of one or multiple renal arteries or of a branch. In patients with an occluded renal artery and a small (9 cm or less) kidney, nephrectomy may improve renal function, possibly because of elimination of the effect of angiotensin on the contralateral kidney [174].

Endarterectomy was the first revascularization procedure to be used as an alternative to nephrectomy. Its main application was for atheromatous lesions at the ostium of the renal artery.

Saphenous vein bypass grafting has become one of the most widely used techniques for revascularizing ischemic kidneys and is usually performed as an end-to-end anastomosis [182]. The results are usually very good, although stenoses may develop later on, either from fibrosis at the suture site or from thrombus forming in the lumen. Occasionally the graft may develop an aneurysmal dilatation, particularly in children, in whom it is not recommended.

Other revascularization techniques include the use of sections of autogenous artery, or synthetic Dacron or polytetrafluorethylene (PTFE) grafts. For patients with atheromatous renovascular disease, one of the most popular procedures is to perform a hepatorenal artery bypass on the right side and a splenorenal bypass on the left. These have the advantages of providing direct arterial end-to-end anastomoses and also of avoiding the necessity for manipulating the aorta, which may reduce the probability of cholesterol emboli.

Results with Surgery. In the U.S. Cooperative Study [45], which still serves as the benchmark in this field, the blood pressure response was categorized in three ways—as cured (blood pressure normal postoperative on no medication), improved (diastolic blood pressure less than 90 mm Hg postoperatively, or a decrease greater than 15%), or failed (no improvement). These criteria are still commonly used. In the U.S. Cooperative Study, 51 percent were cured, 15 percent were improved, and 34 percent were failures. Patients with fibromuscular disease had a favorable blood pressure response more commonly (80%) than patients with atheromatous disease (63%). Moreover, patients with bilateral atheromatous disease had a lower benefit rate (56%) and a high mortality (10%). The overall mortality was 6 percent, with a preponderance of deaths in patients with atheromatous disease (9.3%) in contrast to those with fibromuscular disease (3.4%). Other predictors of an unfavorable outcome included the presence of atherosclerotic coronary artery disease and serum creatinine above 1.4 mg/dl.

Since the time of the U.S. Cooperative Study, many other series have been reported, with generally better results, as shown in Table 55-6. There have been several important developments in the surgery of renovascular disease in recent years. First the population of patients has changed. The proportion of patients with fibromuscular dysplasia has decreased, because many are now treated with angioplasty, and there is a corresponding increase of elderly patients with atheromatous lesions [142]. This trend is likely to continue as the general population ages. The second major development is in surgical techniques, which has led to a much lower morbidity and mortality than reported in the U.S. Cooperative Study, particularly in patients with atheromatous renal artery disease. In earlier series the perioperative morbidity was to a large extent from associated cardiac or cerebrovascular disease, but improvements in diagnostic

Table 55-6. Results of surgical series for treatment of renovascular hypertension

References	Number of patients	Cured (%)	Improved (%)	Failed (%)
Fibromuscular dysplasia				
13, 56, 83, 104, 106, 140, 179, 181, 182, 190	663	59	30	11
Atheroma (focal)				
104, 106, 140, 167, 179	382	41	46	13
Atheroma (diffuse)				
106, 140, 167, 179	435	24	45	36

techniques, medical management, and where indicated, surgical correction before the renal artery surgery have made such complications much less common. In one recent series of patients with atheromatous renovascular hypertension over the age of 60 years, the perioperative mortality was 2.8 percent, and this was always associated with a septic process, not atherosclerotic complications [9]. Another development has been the avoidance of inserting grafts directly into the aorta, which in these patients tends to be severely diseased. By the use of procedures such as hepatorenal and splenorenal artery bypasses, the incidence of complications from cholesterol emboli can be greatly reduced.

REVASCULARIZATION TO PRESERVE RENAL FUNCTION

Revascularization of an ischemic kidney is one of the few situations in which chronic azotemia is reversible. In 1962, Morris et al. [132] described 8 patients with bilateral renal artery stenosis and azotemia in whom surgical revascularization was able to produce a sustained reduction in all but 2. Since then there have been several other reports describing similar benefits [42, 95, 141]. Ying et al. [204] studied 106 consecutive patients with refractory hypertension and diagnosed renovascular hypertension in 39 of these patients. Twenty-one of these were àlso azotemic, and in 10 the renal artery stenosis was bilateral. Surgical revascularization or angioplasty produced long-lasting improvement in the azotemia in all 10 patients.

Typically, such patients have severe hypertension in addition to renal failure. There is often complete occlusion of one renal artery and a tight stenosis of the other due to atheroma, which often involves the aorta and other vascular beds as well. In many of these patients treatment with angiotensin-converting enzyme inhibitors has resulted in a marked deterioration of renal function.

Renal angioplasty may also be of value in such patients (see below).

RENAL ANGIOPLASTY

The technique of transluminal balloon dilatation was pioneered by the work of Dotter and Judkins, who in 1964 first used coaxial catheters to produce progressive dilation of stenosed arteries [49], but at that time it did not find much popularity. Ten years later Grüntzig introduced the first successful balloon catheter [73], which has subsequently been further developed for use in several different arterial regions. In many centers, such as our own, renal angioplasty has become the treatment of first choice for patients with renovascular hypertension, particularly when the lesions are due to fibromuscular dysplasia.

Techniques. Before angioplasty is contemplated, it is our custom to consult a vascular surgeon. In a small proportion of cases emergency surgery is required either to repair a bleeding femoral artery at the site of the catheterization or to perform a renal bypass operation.

The fact that angioplasty can be performed at the same time as arteriography has led us to regard the arteriogram as a therapeutic rather than a diagnostic procedure. This means that the diagnosis should be reasonably certain before the arteriogram is performed.

The procedure is performed under local anesthesia in patients whose diastolic pressure is less than 110 mm Hg. The femoral approach is generally preferred [176], although some authors have favored using the axillary artery in patients whose renal artery originates from the aorta at a very acute angle. After the aortogram has been done to define the anatomy of the lesion, a thin guide wire is advanced across the stenosis. The deflated balloon catheter is then passed over the guide wire so that the midportion of the balloon straddles the stenosis. When this has been accomplished the balloon is inflated with contrast medium to a pressure of 5 or 6 atmospheres for about 30 seconds. Spot films are then taken to assess the adequacy of the dilation. This can also be assessed by measuring the pressure gradient across the stenosis before and after the procedure, bearing in mind the fact that the size of the catheter used to make this measurement (e.g., 5 French) may partially occlude the artery and hence overestimate the gradient.

One of the reasons for the low therapeutic success rate in some series may be because the diameter of the balloon is too small. It is our custom to use balloons whose diameter when inflated is at least as great as the diameter of the renal artery measured from the arteriogram, which in adults is typically 6 to 8 mm. Local arterial spasm may if necessary be relieved by administration of nifedipine.

Following the procedure, the patient is monitored for blood pressure, urine output, and bleeding from the arterial puncture site. With a successful angioplasty the blood pressure usually falls to a minimum level in about 4 to 6 hours.

Mechanisms of Angioplasty. It used to be thought that in atheromatous lesions the effect of angioplasty was to compress the plaque. Subsequent studies using animal models and cadaver arteries showed that it caused endothelial desquamation and intimal splitting of the plaque, with separation of the plaque from the tunica media [17, 206]. There is stretching and often rupture of the media of the arterial wall, with bulging of the adventitia, and an increase in the outer diameter. This may explain why better long-term results are produced by using the largest possible balloon diameter.

The angiogram taken immediately following angioplasty often shows an intimal flap or dissection. This usually is reabsorbed with time, and long-term follow-up often shows remodeling of the arterial lumen with a smoother appearance.

Hemodynamic and Hormonal Changes. Blood pressure begins to fall within 15 minutes of a successful angioplasty. This is accomplished in the presence of a transient increase of plasma renin activity, sympathetic nerve activity, and plasma norepinephrine [131]. The fact that these two pressor systems are activated in the face of a falling blood pressure would be accounted for by the release of vasodilator substance, of which Muirhead's renomedullary antihypertensive lipid [133] is one possible candidate. Plasma renin levels fall to normal within 24 hours.

Results with Angioplasty. There are now several published series of clinical results obtained with angioplasty, but as with surgery, it is appropriate to consider the results with atheroma and fibromuscular dysplasia separately. Success of the procedure can be gauged in two ways: first, the degree to which the lesion can be dilated, and second, the effects on the blood pressure. The criterion that we have used [175] for the former is that there should be a stenosis of at least 75 percent of the arterial lumen diameter on the arteriogram before angioplasty, and a successful dilation is one in which the residual stenosis is less than 50 percent. Partial success is defined as a residual stenosis of 50 to 70 percent, and failure occurs if no dilation of the lesion can be achieved. It should be emphasized that these criteria are somewhat crude because the lumen is commonly eccentric, and angiography is performed in only one plane.

The blood pressure response to angioplasty or surgery is usually classified as cured (that is, a diastolic pressure below 90 mm Hg without medication), improved (a decrease of at least 15 percent but still requiring medication), or failed (a decrease of less than 15 percent), according to the criteria originally developed for the U.S. Cooperative Study of surgery for renovascular hypertension [122].

The results of some of the larger published series are summarized in Table 55-7, which is based on a recent review by Ramsey and Waller [157]. This list is not comprehensive because we have excluded results in which the etiology of the stenosis was not specified and in which less than 10 patients were studied.

The results in patients with fibromuscular dysplasia are uniformly good and are comparable to those obtained with surgery. In the review of Ramsey and Waller [157], the average cure rate was 50 percent and the improvement rate 42 percent. In our experience, restenosis is very rare in these patients, and follow-up angiograms done up to 5 years after angioplasty often show no trace of any stenosis.

In the atheromatous group the results are not nearly so good, and there is a much wider scatter of success rates in the published series. In the largest series, of 100 atheromatous patients followed for 2 to 3 years after angioplasty, Canzanello et al. [26] reported a blood pressure benefit rate of 72 percent in unilateral and 45 percent in bilateral renal artery stenosis. The respective cure rates were 9 and 5 percent. The majority of therapeutic failures were due to restenosis of the dilated artery, which in many cases responded to repeat angioplasty. There are several reasons why the overall results are more diverse and generally not as good as in patients with fibromuscular dysplasia. One is the anatomy of the lesion. Ostial lesions, which originate in the aorta, can be less successfully dilated than lesions in the main renal artery, and Canzanello et al. [26] reported a benefit rate of 45 percent with the former and 87 percent with the latter. A second reason for the variability of the results relates to the technique of the radiologist. We believe that it is important to use as large a balloon as possible (Fig. 55-10). This is in accordance with the anatomic postmortem findings, which indicate that a functionally successful angioplasty usually results in tearing of the media and bulging of the adventitia of the stenosed artery [206]. Third, in many cases of atheromatous renal artery stenosis it is likely that the stenosis was not the original cause of the hypertension. Thus essential hypertension accelerates the formation of atheromatous plaques in the renal arteries just as in other regions. When the plaque reaches a critical size it may begin to add a renovascular component to the hypertension, and it is only this component that would be reversed by

Table 55-7. Results of angioplasty series for treatment of renovascular hypertension

	References	Number of patients*	Cured (%)	Improved (%)	Failed (%)
Fibromuscular dysplasia	10, 34, 62, 91, 119, 127, 175, 186	175	50	42	9
Atheroma (focal)	10, 34, 62, 91, 119, 127, 175, 186	391	19	52	30

*Refers to patients in whom angioplasty was technically successful

A

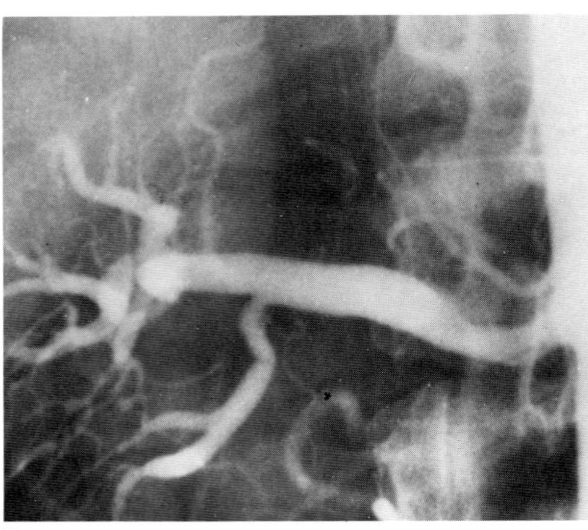

B

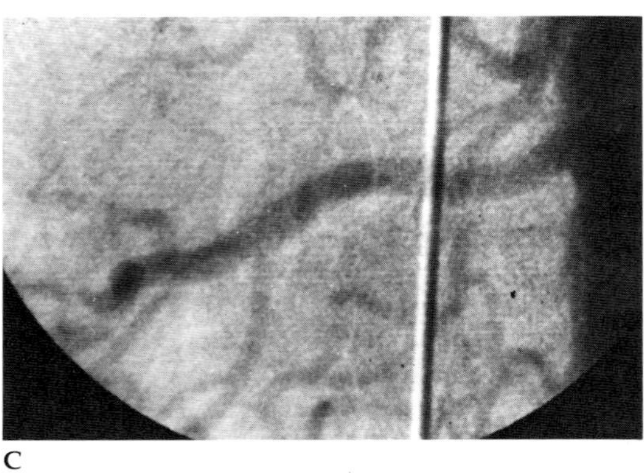

C

Fig. 55-10. A. Atheromatous stenosis in a patient with a solitary kidney. B. Following angioplasty using large-diameter balloon. C. Five years after angioplasty (digital subtraction angiogram).

angioplasty or surgical revascularization. In contrast, in fibromuscular dysplasia the patients are typically younger, the duration of the hypertension is often shorter, and there is a much greater degree of certainty that the stenosis is the original cause of the hypertension.

Another potential problem with atheromatous lesions is restenosis. No very precise figures are available, although it is considered by some to be a major problem [71]. One study reported a restenosis rate of 42 percent 19 months after angioplasty, but the same study reported a rate of 22 percent in fibromuscular lesions, which we would consider unacceptably high and may simply reflect inadequate dilation in the first place [100].

Angioplasty for the Preservation of Renal Function. In a smaller number of patients with renal failure we have also found that angioplasty can cause a significant improvement in renal function. We have seen this both in patients who have a critical stenosis of a solitary kidney and in patients who have severe bilateral stenoses. Such patients are notoriously difficult to treat with medications because a reduction of blood pressure is associated with a dramatic deterioration of renal function. This is most common when angiotensin-converting enzyme inhibitors are used [80]. If angioplasty can be achieved in this situation it is particularly rewarding because it can both improve renal function and make the blood pressure easier to control. However, we have seen other patients in whom renal function has not improved or has deteriorated despite a successful angioplasty. In other patients, who had grossly normal renal function, angioplasty can result in an increase in size of the kidney. In our series of 57 patients [152], all of whom had baseline serum creatinine values of above 2 mg per deciliter, 43 (75 percent) could be successfully dilated; 27 (63 percent) of these showed a decrease of creatinine, 5 (17 percent) showed no change, and 11 (26 percent) showed an increase.

Several other authors have reported improvement of renal function following angioplasty [10, 26, 100, 115]. This is, of course, mainly seen in patients who are azotemic to begin with [10, 155] and hence mainly applies to patients with atheromatous renal artery stenosis. In such patients the serum creatinine tends to increase progressively over time, and Canzanello et al. [26] reported that angioplasty may lower or stabilize it in 53 percent of patients with unilateral and 61 percent with bilateral disease.

A dramatic example of what can be achieved in this context was a patient with a single and totally occluded renal artery who had been anuric for 5 weeks and who had a successful angioplasty, with a subsequent creatinine clearance of 36 ml/minute [12].

Another advantage of angioplasty over surgery is that it can be undertaken in patients who would be turned down for surgery because of associated conditions such as coronary artery disease or cerebrovascular disease, both of which are of course common in patients with atheromatous renovascular hypertension.

Complications of Angioplasty. In all patients the potential benefits of angioplasty must be carefully weighed against the risks. It is our belief that the main risks are those of arteriography rather than of the angioplasty itself. Thus the commonest complications have been hematoma (in 4 percent of patients) and transient worsening of renal function from the dye load (in 2 percent). The latter has been much less common since the advent of digital subtraction angiography, with which much less dye is needed. Both of these complications have been seen only in patients with atheromatous renal artery stenosis who had extensive arterial disease. Dissection of the intima of the renal artery occurs in about 5 percent of cases and in most cases resolves spontaneously, although it may occasionally require emergency surgery [10, 26]. The most serious complication is cholesterol emboli, which may occasionally prove fatal [63]. This is seen mostly in patients with diffuse atheroma and is presumably the cause of the deterioration of renal function, which we saw in 9 percent of our series of azotemic patients [152]. The mortality related to the procedure is very low. In our own series of 57 high-risk patients it was zero [152], and in the larger series of Canzanello et al. [26] it was 2 percent.

Angioplasty Versus Surgery. There has not so far been any published study of a controlled randomized trial comparing surgery and angioplasty, although several authors have compared their results with the two procedures [68, 70, 127, 143]. They have generally concluded that surgery is preferable to angioplasty, but not too much weight should be put on such a conclusion. The patients treated with the different modalities were not necessarily comparable. In the study of Olin et al. [143], all patients treated with angioplasty had bilateral disease, whereas only two-thirds of those treated surgically did. Furthermore, although the benefit rate was higher for the surgical group, there were also more complications (two myocardial infarcts and one perioperative death). The data shown in Tables 55-4 and 55-5 suggest that the results with angioplasty are as good as with surgery for patients with fibromuscular dysplasia, and at a fraction of the cost and inconvenience to the patient. For patients with atheroma the overall success rate is somewhat better with surgery, but against this must be weighed the higher mortality and rate of nephrectomy.

It should be emphasized that both angioplasty and surgical revascularization are procedures that should be performed only in centers where there are teams experienced in their performance. With the possible exception of the very high risk patients with diffuse atheroma, we believe that when renovascular hypertension is diagnosed, one or the other form of revascularization should be attempted because in patients with fibromuscular dysplasia there is a high probability of a permanent cure, and in patients with atheromatous stenoses there may be progression of the lesion to complete occlusion of the renal artery if the patient is treated medically.

It is often stated that a clinical trial is needed to define the relative roles of angioplasty and surgery for the treatment of renovascular hypertension. We do not, however, regard the two forms of treatment as being mutually exclusive. Since in skilled hands angioplasty can be performed at the same time as the diagnostic arteriogram and with relatively little trauma, we usually prefer to attempt an angioplasty before proceeding to surgery.

For patients with fibromuscular dysplasia, the results with angioplasty are as good as those in any of the published surgical series. There also seems to be little doubt that the benefit is long lasting in these patients, and therefore angioplasty is the treatment of choice. For patients with localized atheroma (e.g., nonostial unilateral lesions), the benefit rate is somewhat lower than with surgery, but when angioplasty is successful, the savings of cost and trauma compared with surgery certainly make it worthwhile. If it is unsuccessful, there is still the option of a second attempt or of surgical revascularization. The greatest dilemma at the present time concerns the high-risk patients with diffuse atheroma and renal insufficiency (see above). Surgical morbidity in these patients is high, and these are also the patients most likely to develop complications after angioplasty. Nevertheless, we believe that angioplasty can benefit some of these patients, from the point of view of both their renal function and their blood pressure control. Further work is needed, however, to define which patients are the best candidates.

MEDICAL MANAGEMENT

While revascularization of the ischemic kidney by either surgery or angioplasty is the preferred method of treatment, there are some patients in whom these procedures are either unsuccessful or cannot be undertaken. In such patients medical management must be used.

The two main concerns with medical treatment of such patients are the progression of the renal artery stenosis and the hemodynamic effects of blood pressure reduction on renal function. In 1974 Hunt et al. [82] compared the retrospective, nonrandomized results of medically and surgically treated patients and reported a mortality over 7 to 14 years of 70 percent in the medically treated and 30 percent in the surgically treated patients. Most of the deaths were due to complications of atheroma, such as myocardial infarction or stroke, with only a minority dying from uremia. Blood pressures were, however, not comparably controlled in the two groups. In another series Dean et al. [41] followed 41 medically treated patients with atheromatous renovascular disease. Twelve percent progressed to complete occlusion, and 41 percent had deterioration of renal function.

There have been no randomized trials comparing medical and surgical treatment, but these above studies merely serve to underline the high probability of progression of atheromatous disease. Both of these studies were reported more than 10 years ago, however, and it seems likely that, just as with coronary artery disease, the mortality of medically treated patients with renal artery disease has improved. Recent advances that have improved medical management are the introductions of angiotensin-converting enzyme inhibitors and calcium antagonists.

β-Blockers. The majority of patients with renovascular hypertension have normal or high renin levels, and there is abundant evidence that all of the clinically available β-blockers lower plasma renin activity, and that this is a very important mechanism by which they lower blood pressure [23, 148]. Most β-blockers decrease renal blood flow little, if at all; nadolol has been reported to be particularly effective in this regard [188].

Although the mechanism by which β-blockers inhibit renin release is blockade of the sympathetic β-adrenergic receptors, it has been demonstrated that they lower renin in patients with renovascular hypertension as well as essential hypertension, although not to the same degree [24].

The Renin-Angiotensin System and the Control of Intrarenal Hemodynamics in Renovascular Hypertension. The clinical observation that converting enzyme inhibitors may cause a deterioration of renal function in some patients with renovascular hypertension can be accounted for by animal studies that have demonstrated the important effects of angiotensin on intrarenal hemodynamics. All of the components of the renin-angiotensin system—that is, renin, angiotensin I, converting enzyme, and angiotensin II—are present within the kidney, particularly in the region of the juxtaglomerular apparatus, and the concentrations of renin and angiotensin II are greater in renal lymph than in the renal veins [135]. One of the most important intrarenal effects of angiotensin II is to decrease renal blood flow, with a smaller decrease of glomerular filtration rate. Thus filtration fraction increases [113]. It has been proposed that these changes are brought about by a vasoconstriction of both afferent and efferent arterioles, the predominant effect being on the latter. Thus in the normal kidney, particularly when renin levels are high, angiotensin blockade increases renal blood flow, producing less consistent changes in glomerular filtration rate [77].

Angiotensin-Converting Enzyme Inhibitors (ACE). The introduction of ACE inhibitors represented a major advance for both the diagnosis and medical management of patients with renovascular hypertension. In our experience, a single-dose captopril test (see above) may be the best screening test for identifying the presence of renovascular disease.

There can be little question that ACE inhibitors are the most powerful antihypertensive agents in such patients. Although other mechanisms have occasionally been implicated, it is generally agreed that inhibition of angiotensin II formation is the most important mechanism by which they lower blood pressure, and a response to them identifies a renin-dependent component of an individual patient's hypertension. The acute blood pressure response to an ACE inhibitor is proportional to the baseline plasma renin activity [30], and patients with renovascular hypertension typically show a bigger response than those with essential hypertension. Patients with bilateral renal artery stenosis are just as likely to show a fall of blood pressure as those with a unilateral stenosis (see below). The long-term but not the acute response to an ACE inhibitor has been found to be a good predictor of the response to surgical revascularization [3, 177] and to renal angioplasty [178].

While the acute response to ACE inhibitors is of undoubted value in diagnosing renovascular hypertension (e.g., in the oral captopril test and captopril renography), their role in long-term treatment is more controversial. In patients with normal kidneys, ACE inhibitors may increase renal blood flow and GFR [77]. In patients with bilateral renal artery stenosis or with a stenosed artery and a solitary kidney, treatment with ACE inhibitors may cause a dramatic increase in the serum creatinine and BUN [80], sometimes resulting in acute renal failure [47]. It has been suggested that this occurs because of the loss of the effect of angiotensin on the efferent arterioles, which serves to maintain GFR in the presence of a reduced renal perfusion pressure.

Whether this phenomenon means that ACE inhibitors should not be used chronically in patients with renovascular hypertension is uncertain. There is some evidence that the impairment of renal function in the ischemic kidney is less pronounced with chronic (2 weeks) than with acute treatment [129] and that it may be reversible after as long as 2 years [163]. On the other hand, it has also been suggested that renal artery occlusion is more likely to occur in patients with renovascular disease treated with an ACE inhibitor, particularly in combination with a diuretic [154].

This phenomenon is not specific either to ACE inhibitors or to renovascular hypertension. Thus, azotemia induced by ACE inhibitors has been observed in patients with patent renal arteries [145], and nitroprusside infusion has been shown to cause a marked reduction of GFR in patients with bilateral renal artery stenosis [189].

It is also worth noting that there is evidence that ACE inhibitors may retard the progression of chronic renal failure and glomerulosclerosis in experimental animals [86] and of proteinuria in humans [97].

Calcium Antagonists. Calcium antagonists differ from some other vasodilators in that, in addition to lowering blood pressure, they may increase the GFR. This has been attributed to a selective vasodilator effect on the afferent arteriole [112]. In patients with renovascular hypertension, they do not cause the same deterioration of renal function that has been observed with ACE inhibitors [128, 159].

Clonidine. Administration of clonidine may produce an acute reduction of blood pressure in patients with renovascular hypertension; it occurs without any reduction of PRA but is associated with a decreased plasma norepinephrine level [121].

References

1. Akahoshi, M., and Carretero, O. Body fluid volume and angiotensin II in maintenance of one-kidney, one clip hypertension. *Hypertension* 14: 269, 1989.
2. Anderson, G. H., Blakeman, N., and Streeten, D. H. P. Prediction of renovascular hypertension: Comparison of clinical diagnostic indices. *Am. J. Hypertens.* 1: 301, 1988.
3. Atkinson, A. B., Brown, J. J., Cumming, A. M. M., et al. Captopril in renovascular hypertension: Long-term use in predicting surgical outcome. *Br. Med. J.* 284: 689, 1982.
4. Atkinson, A. B., and Kellet, R. J. Value of intravenous urography in investigating hypertension. *J. R. Coll. Physicians, London.* 8: 175, 1974.
5. Avasthi, P. S., Voyles, W. F., and Greene, E. R. Nonin-

vasive diagnosis of renal artery stenosis by echo-Doppler velocimetry. *Kidney Int.* 256: 824, 1984.
6. Ayers, C. R., Vaughan, E. D., Jr., Katholi, R. E., et al. Mechanism of renal arteriolar vasoconstriction and negative renin feedback in chronic one-kidney dog Goldblatt hypertension. *Clin. Res.* 24: 392A, 1976.
7. Bailey, S. M., Evans, D. W., and Fleming, H. A. Intravenous urography in investigation of hypertension. *Lancet* 2: 57, 1975.
8. Barger, A. C. The Goldblatt memorial lecture. I. Experimental renovascular hypertension. *Hypertension* 1: 447, 1979.
9. Bedoya, L., Ziegelbaum, M., Vidt, D. G., et al. Baseline renal function and surgical renovascularization in atherosclerotic renal arterial disease in the elderly. *Cleve. Clin. J. Med.* 56: 415, 1989.
10. Bell, G. M., Reid, J., and Buist, T. A. S. Percutaneous transluminal angioplasty improves blood pressure and renal function in renovascular hypertension. *Q. J. Med.* 63: 393, 1987.
11. Bengis, R. G., and Coleman, T. G. Antihypertensive effect of prolonged blockade of angiotensin formation in benign and malignant one- and two-kidney Goldblatt hypertensive rats. *Clin. Sci.* 57: 53, 1979.
12. Beraud, J. J., Calvet, B., Durand, A., and Mimran, A. Reversal of acute renal failure following percutaneous transluminal recanalization of an atherosclerotic renal artery occlusion. *J. Hypertens.* 7: 909, 1989.
13. Bergentz, S. E., Ericsson, B. F., and Husberg, B. Technique and complications in the surgical treatment of renovascular hypertension. *Acta Chir. Scand.* 145: 143, 1979.
14. Berlyne, G. W., Tarill, A. S., and Baker, S. B. C. Renal artery stenosis and the nephrotic syndrome. *Q. J. Med.* 33: 325, 1964.
15. Bianchi, C., Bonadio, M., and Andriole, V. T. Influence of postural changes on the glomerular filtration rate in nephroptosis. *Nephron* 16: 161, 1976.
16. Bianchi, G., Gampolo, L., Vegeto, A., et al. The value of plasma renin concentration per se, and in relation to plasma and extracellular fluid volume in diagnosis and prognosis of human renovascular hypertension. *Clin. Sci.* 39: 559, 1970.
17. Block, P. C., Myler, R., and Sterzer, S. Morphology after transluminal angioplasty in human beings. *N. Engl. J. Med.* 305: 382, 1981.
18. Bookstein, J. J., Abrams, H. L., Buenger, R. E., et al. Radiologic aspects of renovascular hypertension. Part 1. Aims and methods of Radiology Study Group. *J.A.M.A.* 220: 1218, 1972.
19. Braasch, W. F., Greene, L. F., and Goyanna, R. Renal ptosis and its treatment. *J.A.M.A.* 138: 399, 1948.
20. Braun-Menendez, E., Fasciolo, J. C., Leloir, L. F., et al. *Renal Hypertension.* Springfield, Ill.: Charles C Thomas, 1946.
21. Brown, J. J., Davies, D. L., Lever, A. F., et al. Plasma renin concentration in human hypertension. II. Renin in relation to aetiology. *Br. Med. J.* 2: 144, 1965.
22. Brunner, H. R., Kirshman, J. D., Sealey, J. E., et al. Hypertension of renal origin: Evidence for two different mechanisms. *Science* 1974: 1344, 1971.
23. Bühler, F. R., Laragh, J. H., Baer, L., et al. Propranolol inhibition of renin secretion: A specific approach to diagnosis and treatment of renin-dependent hypertensive diseases. *N. Engl. J. Med.* 287: 1209, 1972.
24. Bühler, F. R., Laragh, J. H., Vaughan, E. D., et al. Antihypertensive action of propranolol. Specific antirenin responses in high and normal renin forms of essential, renal, renovascular and malignant hypertension. *Am. J. Cardiol.* 32: 511, 1973.
25. Buonocore, E., Meaney, T. F., Borkowsky, G. P., et al. Digital subtraction angiography of the abdominal aorta and renal arteries. *Radiology* 139: 281, 1981.
26. Canzanello, V. J., Millan, V. G., Spiegel, J. E., et al. Percutaneous transluminal renal angioplasty in management of atherosclerotic renovascular hypertension: Results in 100 patients. *Hypertension* 13: 163, 1989.
27. Capponi, A. M., Aguilea, G., Fakunding, J. L., et al. Angiotensin II: Receptors and Mechanisms of Action. In R. L. Soffer (ed.), *Biochemical Regulation of Blood Pressure.* New York: Wiley, 1981. P. 205.
28. Carey, R. M., Vaughan, E. D., Jr., and Ackerly, J. A. The immediate pressor effect of saralasin in man. *J. Clin. Endocrinol. Metab.* 46: 36, 1978.
29. Case, D. B., and Laragh, J. H. Reactive hyperreninemia in renovascular hypertension after angiotensin blockade with saralasin or converting enzyme inhibitor. *Ann. Intern. Med.* 91: 153, 1979.
30. Case, D. B., Wallace, J. M., Keim, H. J., et al. Possible role of renin in hypertension as suggested by renin-sodium prófiling and inhibition of converting enzyme. *N. Engl. J. Med.* 296: 641, 1977.
31. Clark, R. A., and Alexander, E. S. Digital subtraction angiography of the renal arteries—prospective comparison with conventional arteriography. *Invest. Radiol.* 18: 6, 1983.
32. Clorius, J. H., Allenberg, J., Hupp, T., et al. Predictive value of exercise renography for presurgical evaluation of nephrogenic hypertension. *Hypertension* 10: 280, 1987.
33. Clorius, J. H., Mann, J., Schmidlin, P., et al. Clinical evaluation of patients with hypertension and exercise-induced renal dysfunction. *Hypertension* 10: 287, 1987.
34. Colapinto, R. F., Stronell, R. D., Harries-Jones, E. P., et al. Percutaneous transluminal diltation for the renal artery: Follow-up studies on renovascular hypertension. *A.J.R.* 139: 722, 1982.
35. Cuocolo, A., Esposito, S., Volpe, M., et al. Renal artery stenosis detection by combined Gates' technique and captopril test in hypertensive patients. *J. Nucl. Med.* 30: 51, 1989.
36. Dargie, J. H., Franklin, S. S., and Reid, J. L. Plasma noradrenaline concentrations in experimental renovascular hypertension in the rat. *Clin. Sci. Mol. Med.* 52: 477, 1977.
37. Dargie, J. H., Franklin, S. S., and Reid, J. L. The sympathetic nervous system in renovascular hypertension in the rat. *Br. J. Pharmacol.* 56: 365, 1975.
38. Davies, D. L., McElroy, K., Atkinson, A. B., et al. Relationship between exchangeable sodium and blood pressure in different forms of hypertension in man. *Clin. Sci.* 57: 69s, 1979.
39. Davis, B. A., Crook, J. E., Vestal, R. E., et al. Prevalence of renovascular hypertension in patients with Grade III or IV hypertensive retinopathy. *N. Engl. J. Med.* 301: 1273, 1979.
40. Davis, J. O., Freeman, R. H., Johnson, J. A., et al. Agents which block the action of the renin-angiotensin system. *Circ. Res.* 34: 279, 1974.
41. Dean, R. H., Kieffer, R. W., Smith, B. W., et al. Renovascular hypertension. Anatomic and renal functional changes during drug therapy. *Arch. Surg.* 116: 1408, 1981.
42. Dean, R. H., Lawson, J. D., Hollifield, J. W., et al. Re-

vascularization of the poorly functioning kidney. *Surgery* 85: 44, 1979.
43. DeJong, W. Release of renin by rat kidney slices; relationship by plasma renin after desoxycorticosteron and renal hypertension. *Proc. Soc. Exp. Biol. Med.* 130: 85, 1969.
44. Derkx, F. H. M., Tan-Tjiong, H. L., Wenting, G. J., et al. Captopril Test for Diagnosis of Renal Artery Stenosis. In N. Glorioso, J. H. Laragh, and A. Rappelli (eds.), *Renovascular Hypertension.* New York: Raven, 1987. Pp. 295–304.
45. DeZeeuw, D., Danker, A. J. M., Burema, J., et al. Nephroptosis and hypertension. *Lancet* 1: 213, 1977.
46. Dolgman, A. G., Varady, P. D., and Franklin, S. S. Body habitus and serum cholesterol in essential hypertension and renovascular hypertension. Cooperative study of renovascular hypertension. *J.A.M.A.* 221: 387, 1972.
47. Dominiczak, A., Isles, C., Gillen, G., and Brown, J. J. Angiotensin converting enzyme inhibition and renal insufficiency in patients with bilateral renovascular disease. *J. Hum. Hypertens.* 2: 53, 1988.
48. Dondi, M., Franchi, R., Levorato, M., et al. Evaluation of hypertensive patients by means of captopril enhanced renal scintigraphy with technetium-99m DTPA. *J. Nucl. Med.* 30: 615, 1989.
49. Dotter, C. T., and Judkins, M. P. Transluminal treatment of arteriosclerotic obstruction: Description of a new technique and a preliminary report of its applications. *Circulation* 30: 654, 1964.
50. Dustan, H. P., Tarazi, R. C., and Bravo, E. L. Physiologic Characteristics of Hypertension. In J. H. Laragh (ed.), *Hypertension Manual.* New York: Yorke, 1973.
51. Elkik, F., Corvol, P., Idatte, J.-M., et al. Renal segmental infarction: A cause of reversible malignant hypertension. *J. Hypertension* 2: 149, 1984.
52. Erbslöh-Möller, B., Dumas, A., Roth, D., et al. Furosemide-^{131}I-Hippuran renography after angiotensin-converting enzyme inhibition for the diagnosis of renovascular hypertension. *Am. J. Med.* 90: 23, 1991.
53. Eyler, W. R., Clark, M. D., Garman, J. E., et al. Angiography of the renal areas including a comparative study of renal arterial stenoses in patients with and without hypertension. *Radiology* 78: 379, 1962.
54. Fiorentini, C., Guazzi, M., Olivari, M. T., et al. Selective reduction of renal perfusion pressure and blood flow in man: Humoral and hemodynamic effects. *Circulation* 63: 973, 1981.
55. Fommei, E., Ghione, S., Palla, L., et al. Renal scintigraphic captopril test in the diagnosis of renovascular hypertension. *Hypertension* 10: 212, 1987.
56. Foster, J. H., Dean, R. H., Pinkerton, J. A., et al. Ten years experience with the surgical management of renovascular hypertension. *Ann. Surg.* 177: 755, 1973.
57. Foster, J. H., Maxwell, M. J., Franklin, S. S., et al. Renovascular occlusive disease: results of operative treatment. *J.A.M.A.* 231: 1043, 1975.
58. Fredrickson, E. D., Wilcox, C. S., Bucci, M., et al. Prospective evaluation of a simplified captopril test for the detection of renovascular hypertension. *Arch. Intern. Med.* 150: 569, 1990.
59. Frohlich, E. D., Urych, M., Tarazi, R. C., et al. A hemodynamic comparison of essential and renovascular hypertension. *Circulation* 34: 289, 1967.
60. Gavras, H., Brunner, H. R., Thurston, H., et al. Reciprocation of renin dependency in renal hypertension. *Science* 188: 1316, 1979.
61. Gavras, H., Brunner, H. R., Vaughan, E. D., Jr., et al. Angiotensin-sodium interaction in blood pressure maintenance of renal hypertensive and normotensive rats. *Science* 180: 1369, 1973.
62. Geyskes, G. G., Oei, H. Y., Puylaert, C. B. A. J., and Dorhout Mees, E. J. Unilateral Renal Failure after Captopril in Patients with Renovascular Hypertension. In N. Glorioso et al. (eds.), *Renovascular Hypertension.* New York: Raven, 1987. Pp. 281–294.
63. Geyskes, G. G., Puylaert, C. B. A., Dei, H. Y., et al. Follow-up study of 70 patients with renal artery stenosis treated by percutaneous transluminal dilatation. *Br. Med. J.* 287: 333, 1983.
64. Gifford, R. Evaluation of the hypertensive patient with emphasis on detecting curable causes. *Millbank Mem. Fund Q.* 47: 170, 1969.
65. Goldblatt, H., Lynch, J., Hanzal, R. F., et al. Studies on experimental hypertension. I. The production of persistent elevation of systolic blood pressure by means of renal ischemia. *J. Exp. Med.* 59: 347, 1934.
66. Goncharenko, V., Gerlock, A. J., Schaff, M. I., et al. Progression of renal artery fibromuscular dysplasia in 42 patients as seen on angiography. *Radiology* 139: 45, 1981.
67. Greene, E. R., Avasthi, P. S., and Hodges, J. W. Noninvasive Doppler assessment of renal artery stenosis and hemodynamics. *J. Clin. Ultrasound* 15: 653, 1987.
68. Greminger, P., Lüscher, T. F., Kuhlmann, U., et al. Surgery, transluminal dilatation and medical therapy in the management of renovascular hypertension. *Nephron* 44(Suppl. 1): 36, 1986.
69. Grim, C. E., Luft, F. C., and Yune, H. Y. Percutaneous transluminal dilatation in the treatment of renal vascular hypertension. *Ann. Intern. Med.* 95: 439, 1981.
70. Grim, C. E., Yune, H. Y., Donahue, J. P., et al. Treatment of Renal Vascular Hypertension: A Comparison of Patients Treated by Surgery or by Percutaneous Transluminal Angioplasty. In R. V. Schilfgaarde, et al. (eds.), *Clinical Aspects of Renovascular Hypertension.* Boston: Martinus Nijhoff, 1983. Pp. 238.
71. Grim, C. E., Yune, H. Y., Weinberger, M. H., et al. Balloon dilatation for renal artery stenosis causing hypertension: Criteria, concerns, and cautions. *Ann. Intern. Med.* 92: 117, 1980.
72. Gruenewald, S. M., Collins, L. T., Antico, V. F., et al. Can quantitative renography predict the outcome of treatment of atherosclerotic renal artery stenosis? *J. Nucl. Med.* 30: 1940, 1989.
73. Gruntzig, A., Kuhlmann, U., and Vetter, W. Treatment of renovascular hypertension with percutaneous transluminal dilatation of a renal artery stenosis. *Lancet* 1: 801, 1978.
74. Hallöack-Nordlander, M., Noresson, E., and Lundgren, Y. Haemodynamic alterations after reversal of renal hypertension in rats. *Clin. Sci.* 57: 15s, 1979.
75. Harrington, J. T., Sommers, S. C., and Kassirer, J. P. Atheromatous emboli with progressive renal failure. Renal arteriography as the probable inciting factor. *Ann. Intern. Med.* 68: 152, 1968.
76. Hillman, B. J., Ovitt, T. W., Nudelman, S., et al. Digital subtraction angiography of renal vascular abnormalities. *Radiology* 138: 271, 1981.
77. Hollenberg, N. K., Swartz, S. L., Passan, D. R., et al. Increased glomerular filtration rate after converting-enzyme inhibition in essential hypertension. *N. Engl. J. Med.* 301: 9, 1979.
78. Holley, K. E., Hunt, J. C., Brown, A. L., et al. Renal

artery stenosis. A clinical-pathologic study in normotensive and hypertensive patients. *Am. J. Med.* 37: 14, 1964.
79. Howard, J. E., Berthrong, M., Sloan, R. D., et al. Relief of malignant hypertension by nephrectomy in four patients with unilateral renal vascular disease. *Trans. Assoc. Am. Physicians* 66: 164, 1953.
80. Hricik, D. E., Browning, P. J., Kapelman, R., et al. Captopril-induced functional renal insufficiency in patients with bilateral renal-artery stenoses or renal-artery stenosis in a solitary kidney. *N. Engl. J. Med.* 308: 373, 1983.
81. Huang, W.-C., Ploth, D. W., Bell, P. D., et al. Bilateral renal function responses to converting enzyme inhibitor (SQ 20881) in two-kidney, one clip Goldblatt hypertensive rats. *Hypertension* 3: 285, 1981.
82. Hunt, J. C., Sheps, S. G., Harrison, E. G., et al. Renal and renovascular hypertension: A reasoned approach to diagnosis and management. *Arch. Intern. Med.* 133: 988, 1974.
83. Hunt, J. C., and Strong, C. G. Renovascular Hypertension. Mechanisms, Natural History and Treatment. In J. H. Laragh (ed.), *Hypertension Manual*. New York: Yorke, 1973. P. 509.
84. Idrissi, A., Fournier, A., Renard, N., et al. The captopril challenge test as a screening test for renovascular hypertension. *Kidney Int.* 34(Suppl. 25): S138, 1988.
85. Imanishi, M., Kawamura, M., Akabane, S., et al. Aspirin lowers blood pressure in patients with renovascular hypertension. *Hypertension* 14: 461, 1989.
86. Jackson, B., and Johnston, C. I. The contribution of systemic hypertension to progression of chronic renal failure in the rat remnant kidney: Effect of treatment with an angiotensin converting enzyme inhibitor or a calcium inhibitor. *J. Hypertens.* 6: 495, 1988.
87. Jackson, E. K. Relation between renin release and blood pressure response to nonsteroidal anti-inflammatory drugs in hypertension. *Hypertension* 14: 469, 1989.
88. Jackson, E. K., Oates, J. A., and Branch, R. A. Indomethacin decreases arterial blood pressure and plasma renin activity in rats with aortic ligation. *Circ. Res.* 49: 180, 1981.
89. Jenni, R., Vieli, A., Luscher, T. F., et al. Combined two-dimensional ultrasound Doppler technique: New possibilities for the screening of renovascular and parenchymatous hypertension? *Nephron* 44(Suppl. 1): 2, 1986.
90. Judson, W. E., and Helmer, O. M. Diagnostic and prognostic values of renin activity in renal venous plasma in renovascular hypertension. *Hypertension* 13: 79, 1965.
91. Kaplan-Pavlovcic, S., Koschi, M., Obrez, L., et al. Percutaneous transluminal renal angioplasty: Follow-up studies in renovascular hypertension. *Przegl. Lek.* 43: 342, 1985.
92. Kassirer, J. P. Atheroembolic renal disease. *N. Engl. J. Med.* 280: 812, 1969.
93. Katholi, R. E., Winternitz, S. R., and Oparil, S. Decrease in peripheral sympathetic nervous system activity following renal denervation or unclipping in the one-kidney one-clip Goldblatt hypertensive rat. *J. Clin. Invest.* 69: 55, 1982.
94. Katholi, R. E., Winthlow, P. L., Winternitz, S., et al. Importance of the renal nerves in established two-kidney, one-clip Goldblatt hypertension in the rat. *Hypertension* 4(Suppl. 2): 2, 1982.
95. Kaufman, J. J. Renal artery stenosis and azotemia. *Surg. Gynecol. Obstetr.* 137: 949, 1973.
96. Kaufman, J. J., Hanafee, W., and Maxwell, M. H. Upright renal arteriography in the study of renal hypertension. *J.A.M.A.* 187: 977, 1964.
97. Keane, W. F., Anderson, S., Aurell, M., et al. Angiotensin converting enzyme inhibitors and progressive renal insufficiency: Current experience and future directions. *Ann. Intern. Med.* 111: 503, 1989.
98. Keith, T. A. Renovascular hypertension in black patients. *Hypertension* 4: 438, 1982.
99. Kohler, T. R., Zierler, E., Martin, R. L., et al. Noninvasive diagnosis of renal artery stenosis by ultrasonic duplex scanning. *J. Vasc. Surg.* 4: 450, 1986.
100. Kremer Hovinga, T. K., de Jong, P. E., de Zeeuw, D., et al. Restenosis prevalence and long-term effects on renal function after percutaneous transluminal renal angioplasty. *Nephron* 44(Suppl. 1): 64, 1986.
101. Kremer Hovinga, T. K., de Jong, P. E., Piers, D. A., et al. Diagnostic use of angiotensin converting enzyme inhibitors in radioisotope evaluation of unilateral renal artery in stenosis. *J. Nucl. Med.* 30: 605, 1989.
102. Kulhmann, U., Greminger, P., Gruntzig, A., et al. Long-term experience in percutaneous transluminal dilatation of renal artery stenosis. *Am. J. Med.* 79: 692, 1985.
103. Lake, C. R., Chernow, B., Goldstein, D. S., et al. Plasma catecholamine levels in normal subjects and in patients with secondary hypertension. *Fed. Proc.* 43: 52, 1984.
104. Lankford, N. S., Donohue, J. P., Grim, C. E., et al. Results of surgical treatment of renovascular hypertension. *J. Urol.* 122: 439, 1979.
105. Lawrie, G. M., Morris, G. C., Glaeser, D. H., and De Bakey, M. E. Renovascular reconstruction: Factors affecting long-term prognosis in 919 patients followed up to 31 years. *Am. J. Cardiol.* 63: 1085, 1989.
106. Lawrie, G. M., Morris, G. C., Soussou, I. D., et al. Late results of reconstrictive surgery for renovascular disease. *Ann. Surg.* 191: 528, 1980.
107. Leenen, F. H. H., DeJong, W., and DeWied, D. Renal venous and periphreal plasma renin activity in renal hypertension in the rat. *Am. J. Physiol.* 225: 1514, 1973.
108. Levin, D. C., Beckmann, C. F., and Serur, J. R. Vascular resistance changes distal to progressive arterioal stenosis: A critical re-evaluation of the concept of vasodilator reverse. *Invest. Radiol.* 14: 120, 1980.
109. Lewis, B. D., and James, E. M. Current applications of duplex and color doppler ultrasound imaging: Abdomen. *Mayo Clin. Proc.* 64: 1158, 1989.
110. Liard, J. F., Cowley, A. W., McCaa, R. E., et al. Renin, aldosterone, body fluid volumes, and the baroreceptor reflex in the development and reversal of Goldblatt hypertension in conscious dogs. *Circ. Res.* 34: 549, 1974.
111. Liard, J. F., and Peters, G. Mechanism of the fall in blood pressure after "unclamping" in rats with Goldblatt-type hypertension. *Experientia* 26: 743, 1980.
112. Lin, H., and Young, D. B. The antihypertensive mechanism of verapamil: Alteration of glomerular filtration regulation. *Hypertension* 11: 639, 1988.
113. Lohmeier, T. E., and Cowley, A. W. Hypertensive and renal effects of chronic low level intrarenal angiotensin infusion in the dog. *Circ. Res.* 44: 154, 1979.
114. Lucas, J., and Floyer, M. A. Changes in body fluid distribution and interstitial tissue compliance during the development and reversal of experimental renal hypertension in the rat. *Clin. Sci. Mol. Med.* 47: 1, 1974.
115. Luft, F. R., Grim, C. E., and Weinberger, M. H. Intervention in patients with renovascular hypertension and renal insufficiency. *J. Urol.* 130: 645, 1983.
116. Lyons, D. F., Streck, W. F., Kem, D. C., et al. Captopril

stimulation of differential renins in renovascular hypertension. *Hypertension* 5: 615, 1983.
117. Mann, S. J., Pickering, T. G., Sos, T. A., et al. Captopril renography in the diagnosis of renal artery stenosis: Accuracy and limitations. *Am. J. Med.* 90: 30, 1991.
118. Martin, C. L., Price, R. B., Casarella, W. I., et al. Percutaneous angioplasty in clinical management of renovascular hypertension: Initial and long-term results. *Radiology* 155: 629, 1985.
119. Martin, E. D., Mattern, R. F., and Baer, L. Renal angioplasty for hypertension: Predictive factors for long-term success. *Am. J. Radiol.* 128: 951, 1981.
120. Maslowski, A. H., Nicholls, M. G., Espiner, E. A., et al. Mechanisms in human renovascular hypertension. *Hypertension* 5: 597, 1983.
121. Mathias, C. J., Wilkinson, A., Lewis, P. S., et al. Clonidine lowers blood pressure independently of renin suppression in patients with unilateral renal artery stenosis. *Chest* 83S: 357s, 1983.
122. Maxwell, M. H., Bleifer, K. H., Franklin, S. S., et al. Cooperative Study of Renovascular Hypertension. Demographic analysis of the study. *J.A.M.A.* 220: 1195, 1972.
123. Maxwell, M. H., Lupu, A. N., and Taplin, G. V. Radioisotope renogram in renal arterial hypertension. *J. Urol.* 100: 376, 1968.
124. McCann, W. S., and Romansky, M. J. Orthostatic hypertension: Effect of nephroptosis on renal blood flow. *J.A.M.A.* 115: 573, 1940.
125. Meyrier, A., Buchet, P., Simon, P., et al. Atheromatous renal disease. *Am. J. Med.* 85: 139, 1988.
126. Miller, E. D., Samuels, A. I., Haber, E., et al. Inhibition of angiotensin conversion and prevention of renal hypertension. *Am. J. Physiol.* 228: 448, 1975.
127. Miller, G. A., Ford, K. K., Braun, S. D., et al. Percutaneous transluminal angioplasty vs. surgery for renovascular hypertension. *A.J.R.* 144: 447, 1985.
128. Miyamori, I., Yasuhara, S., Matsubara, T., et al. Comparative effects of captopril and nifedipine on split renal function in renovascular hypertension. *Am. J. Hypertens.* 1: 359, 1989.
129. Miyamori, I., Yasuhara, S., and Takeda, R. Long-term effects of converting enzyme inhibitors on split renal function in renovascular hypertension. *Clin. Exp. Hypertens.* A9: 629, 1987.
130. Möhring, J., Möhring, B., Petri, M., et al. Plasma vasopressin concentrations and effects of vasopressin antiserum on blood pressure in rats with malignant two-kidney Goldblatt hypertension. *Circ. Res.* 42: 17, 1978.
131. Mörlin, C., Fagius, C., Hägg, A., et al. Continuous recording of muscle nerve sympathetic activity during percutaneous transluminal angioplasty in renovascular hypertension in man. *J. Hypertens.* 8: 239, 1990.
132. Morris, D. C., DeBakey, M. E., and Cooley, D. A. Surgical treatment of renal failure of renovascular origin. *J.A.M.A.* 182: 609, 1962.
133. Muirhead, E. E., Byers, L. W., Pitcock, J. A., et al. Denervation of neutral antihypertensive lipid from renal venous effluent in rats. *Clin. Sci.* 61: 331s, 1981.
134. Muller, F. B., Sealey, J. E., Case, C. B., et al. The captopril test for identifying renovascular disease in hypertensive patients. *Am. J. Med.* 80: 663, 1986.
135. Navar, L. G., and Rosivall, L. Contribution of the renin-angiotensin system to the control of intrarenal hemodynamics. *Kidney Int.* 25: 857, 1984.
136. Neubig, R. R., and Hoobler, S. W. Reversal of chronic renal hypertension: Role of salt and water excretion. *Proc. Soc. Exp. Biol. Med.* 150: 254, 1975.
137. Nicholson, J. P., Teichman, S. L., Alderman, M. H., et al. Cigarette smoking and renovascular hypertension. *Lancet* 2: 765, 1983.
138. Norris, C. S., Pfeiffer, J. S., Rittgers, S. E., and Barnes, R. W. Noninvasive evaluation of renal artery stenosis and renovascular resistance: Experimental and clinical studies. *J. Vasc. Surg.* 1: 192, 1984.
139. Novick, A. L., Straffon, R. A., Stewart, B. H., et al. Surgical treatment of renovascular hypertension in the pediatric patient. *J. Urol.* 119: 794, 1978.
140. Novick, A. C., Straffon, R. A., Stewart, B. H., et al. Diminished operative morbidity and mortality in renal revascularization. *J.A.M.A.* 246: 749, 1981.
141. Novick, A. C., Textor, S. C., Bodie, B., et al. Revascularization to preserve renal function in patients with atherosclerotic renovascular disease. *Urol. Clin. North Am.* 11: 477, 1984.
142. Novick, A. C., Ziegelbaum, M., Vidt, D. G., et al. Trends in surgical revascularization for renal artery disease: Ten years' experience. *J.A.M.A.* 257: 498, 1987.
143. Olin, J. W., Vidt, D. W., Gifford, R. W., and Novick, A. C. Renovascular disease in the elderly: An analysis of 50 patients. *J. Am. Coll. Cardiol.* 5: 1232, 1985.
144. Page, I. H., and Helmer, O. M. A crystalline pressor substance, angiotensin, resulting from reaction of renin and renin activator. *Proc. Soc. Clin. Invest.* 12: 17, 1939.
145. Pettinger, W., Mitchell, H. C., Lee, H. C., and Redman, H. C. Pseudo renal artery stenosis (PRAS) syndrome. *Am. J. Hypertens.* 2: 349, 1989.
146. Pick, J. W., and Anson, E. J. The renal vascular pedicle: Anatomical study of 430 body-halves. *J. Urol.* 44: 411, 1940.
147. Pickering, G. W. The role of the kidney in acute and chronic hypertension following renal artery constriction in the rabbit. *Clin. Sci.* 5: 229, 1945.
148. Pickering, T. G. Mechanisms of Beta Blockade Hypotension. In J. H. Laragh, et al. (eds.), *Frontiers in Hypertension Research*. New York: Springer Verlag, 1981. P. 458.
149. Pickering, T. G. Medical management of renovascular hypertension. *World J. Urol.* 7: 77, 1989.
150. Pickering, T. G., Devereux, R. B., James, G. D., et al. Recurrent pulmonary edema in hypertension due to bilateral renal artery stenosis: Treatment by angioplasty or surgical revascularization. *Lancet* 2: 551, 1988.
151. Pickering, T. G., Sos, T. A., James, G. D., et al. Comparison of renal vein renin activity in hypertensive patients with stenosis of one or both renal arteries. *J. Hypertens.* 3(Suppl. 3): S291, 1985.
152. Pickering, T. G., Sos, T. A., Saddekni, S., et al. Renal angioplasty in patients with azotemia and renovascular hypertension. *J. Hypertens.* 4(Suppl. 6): S667, 1986.
153. Pickering, T. G., Sos, T. A., Vaughan, E. D., Jr., et al. Predictive value and changes of renin secretion in hypertensive patients with unilateral renovascular disease undergoing successful renal angioplasty. *Am. J. Med.* 76: 398, 1985.
154. Postma, C. T., Hoefnagels, W. H. L., Barentz, J. O., et al. Occlusion of unilateral stenosed renal arteries: Relation to medical treatment. *J. Hum. Hypertens.* 3: 185, 1989.
155. Postma, C. T., Van der Streen, M. H., Hoefnagels, W. H. L., et al. The captopril test in the detection of renovascular disease in hypertensive patients. *Arch. Intern. Med.* 150: 625, 1990.
156. Rabito, S. F., Carretero, O. A., and Scicli, A. G. Evidence against a role of vasopressin in the maintenance

of high blood pressure mineralocorticoid and renovascular hypertension. *Hypertension* 3: 34, 1981.

157. Ramsay, L. E., and Waller, P. C. Blood pressure response to percutaneous transluminal angioplasty for renovascular hypertension: An overview of published series. *Br. Med. J.* 300: 569, 1990.
158. Re, R., Novelline, R., Escourrou, M.-T., et al. Inhibition of angiotensin-converting enzyme for diagnosis of renal artery stenosis. *N. Engl. J. Med.* 298: 582, 1978.
159. Ribstein, J., Mourad, G., and Mimran, A. Contrasting effects of captopril and nifedipine on renal function in renovascular hypertension. *Am. J. Hypertens.* 1: 239, 1988.
160. Rocchini, A. P., and Barger, A. C. Renovascular hypertension in sodium-depleted dogs: Role of renin and carotid sinus reflex. *Am. J. Physiol.* 236: H101, 1979.
161. Russell, G. I., Bing, R. F., Thurston, H., et al. Surgical reversal of two-kidney one clip hypertension during inhibition of the renin-angiotensin system. *Hypertension* 4: 69, 1982.
162. Russell, G. I., Brice, J. M., Bing, R. F., et al. Haemodynamic changes after surgical reversal of chronic two-kidney, one-clip hypertension in the rat. *Clin. Sci.* 61: 117s, 1981.
163. Salahudeen, A. K., and Pingle, A. Reversibility of captopril-induced renal insufficiency after prolonged use in an unusual case of renovascular hypertension. *J. Hum. Hypertens.* 2: 57, 1988.
164. Salvetti, A., Arzilli, F., Nuccorini, A., et al. Acute response to captopril as a predictive test for surgery in renovascular hypertension. *Nephron* 44(Suppl. 1): 87, 1986.
165. Salvetti, A., Arzilli, F., Nuccorini, A., et al. Does Humoral and Hemodynamic Response to Acute ACE Inhibition Identify True Renovascular Hypertension? In N. Glorioso, J. H. Laragh, and A. Rapelli (eds.), Renovascular Hypertension. New York: Raven, 1987. P. 305.
166. Schalekamp, M. A. D. H., and Derkx, F. H. M. Functional Diagnosis of Renovascular Hypertension, with Special Reference to Renin Measurements. In R. V. Schilfgaarde, et al. (eds.), *Clinical Aspects of Renovascular Hypertension.* Boston: Martinus Nijoff, 1983. P. 62.
167. Schilfgaarde, R. V., Bockel, J. H. V., Felthuis, W., et al. Clinical Results of Surgical Therapy for Renovascular Hypertension. In R. V. Schilfgaarde, et al. (eds.), *Clinical Aspects of Renovascular Hypertension.* Boston: Martinus Nijhoff, 1983. P. 150.
168. Schneider, M. J., Pohl, M. A., and Novick, A. C. The natural history of atherosclerotic and fibrous renal artery disease. *Urol. Clin.* 11: 383, 1984.
169. Schwarten, D. E., Yune, H. Y., Klatte, E. C., et al. Clinical experience with percutaneous transluminal angioplasty (PTA) of stenosed renal arteries. *Radiology* 135: 601, 1980.
170. Scott, J. A., Rabe, F. E., Becker, G. J., et al. Angiographic assessment of renal artery pathology: How reliable? *Am. J. Radiol.* 141: 1299, 1983.
171. Sealey, J. E., Buhler, F. R., Laragh, J. H., et al. The physiology of renin secretion in essential hypertension: Estimation of renin secretion rate and renal plasma flow from peripheral and renal vein renin levels. *Am. J. Med.* 55: 391, 1973.
172. Shipley, R. E., and Gregg, D. E. The effect of external constriction of a blood vessel on blood flow. *Am. J. Physiol.* 141: 287, 1944.
173. Simon, N., Franklin, S. S., Bleifer, K. H., et al. Clinical characteristics of renovascular hypertension. *J.A.M.A.* 220: 1209, 1972.
174. Sonkodi, S., Abraham, G., and Mohacsi, G. Effects of nephrectomy on hypertension, renin activity and total renal function in patients with chronic renal artery occlusion. *J. Hum. Hypertens.* 4: 277, 1990.
175. Sos, T. A., Pickering, T. G., Sniderman, K., et al. Percutaneous transluminal renal angioplasty in renovascular hypertension due to atheroma or fibromuscular dysplasia. *N. Engl. J. Med.* 309: 274, 1983.
176. Sos, T. A., and Sniderman, K. W. Percutaneous transluminal angioplasty. *Semin. Roentgenol.* 16: 26, 1981.
177. Staessen, J., Bulpitt, C., Fagard, R., et al. Long-term converting-enzyme inhibition as a guide to surgical curability of hypertension associated with renovascular disease. *Am. J. Cardiol.* 51: 1317, 1983.
178. Staessen, J., Wilms, G., Baert, A., et al. Blood pressure during long-term converting-enzyme inhibition predicts the inability of renovascular hypertension by angioplasty. *Am. J. Hypertens.* 1: 208, 1988.
179. Stanley, J. C. Renovascular Hypertension: The Surgical Point of View. In R. V. Schilfgaarde, et al. (eds.), *Clinical Aspects of Renovascular Hypertension.* Boston: Martinus Nijhoff, 1983. P. 259.
180. Stanley, J. C., and Fry, W. J. Pediatric renal artery occlusive disease and renovascular hypertension. Etiology, diagnosis, and operative treatment. *Arch. Surg.* 116: 669, 1981.
181. Stoney, R. J., DeLuccia, N., Ehrenfeld, W. K., et al. Aortorenal arterial autografts. *Arch. Surg.* 116: 1416, 1981.
182. Straffon, R., and Siegel, D. F. Saphenous bypass graft in the treatment of renovascular hypertension. *Urol. Clin. North Am.* 2: 337, 1975.
183. Svetkey, L. P., Himmelstein, S. I., Dunnick, N. R., et al. Prospective analysis of strategies for diagnosing renovascular hypertension. *Hypertension* 14: 247, 1989.
184. Svetkey, L. P., and Klotman, P. E. Racial differences in the prevalence of renovascular hypertension in clinically selected patients. *Am. J. Hypertens.* 3(Suppl.): 32A, 1990.
185. Swales, J. D., Thurston, H., Queiroz, F. P., et al. Dual mechanism for experimental hypertension. *Lancet* 2: 1181, 1971.
186. Tegtmyer, C. G., Dyer, R., and Teates, C. D. Percutaneous transluminal dilatation of renal arteries. *Radiology* 135: 589, 1980.
187. Tegtmeyer, C. J., Elson, J., and Glass, T. A. Percutaneous transluminal angioplasty: The treatment of choice for renovascular hypertension due to fibromuscular dysplasia. *Radiology* 143: 631, 1982.
188. Textor, S. L., Fouad, F. M., Bravo, E. L., et al. Redistribution of cardiac output to the kidneys during oral nadolol administration. *N. Engl. J. Med.* 307: 601, 1982.
189. Textor, S. C., Novick, A. C., Tarazi, R. C., et al. Critical perfusion pressure for renal function in patients with bilateral atherosclerotic renal vascular disease. *Ann. Intern. Med.* 102: 308, 1985.
190. Thevenet, A., Mary, H., and Boennec, M. Results following surgical correction of renovascular hypertension. *J. Cardiovasc. Surg.* 21: 517, 1980.
191. Thibonnier, M., Joseph, A., Sassano, P., et al. Improved diagnosis of unilateral renal artery lesions after captopril administration. *J.A.M.A.* 251: 56, 1984.
192. Thibonnier, M., Sassano, P., Joseph, A., et al. Diagnostic value of a single dose of captopril in renin- and aldosterone-dependent, surgically curable hypertension. *Cardiovasc. Rev. Rep.* 3: 1659, 1982.
193. Thornbury, J. R., Stanley, J. L., and Fryback, D. G. Limited use of hypertensive excretory urography. *Urol. Radiol.* 3: 209, 1982.

194. Thurston, H., Bing, R. F., Marks, E. S., et al. Response to chronic renovascular hypertension to surgical correction or prolonged blockade of the renin-angiotensin system by two inhibitors in the rat. *Clin. Sci.* 58: 15, 1980.
195. Thurston, H., Bing, R. F., and Swales, J. D. Reversal of two-kidney one-clip hypertension in the rat. *Hypertension* 2: 256, 1980.
196. Tobian, L., Coffee, K., and McCrea, P. Contrasting exchangeable sodium in rats with different types of Goldblatt hypertension. *Am. J. Physiol.* 217: 458, 1969.
197. Vaughan, E. D., Jr., Bühler, F. R., Laragh, J. H., et al. Renovascular hypertension: renin measurements to indicate hypersecretion and contralateral suppression, estimate renal plasma flow, and score for surgical curability. *Am. J. Med.* 55: 402, 1973.
198. Vaughan, E. D., Jr., Buhler, F. R., Laragh, J. H., et al. Hypertension and unilateral parenchymal renal disease: Evidence for abnormal vasoconstriction-volume interaction. *J.A.M.A.* 233: 1177, 1975.
199. Vecchio, T. J. Predictive value of a single diagnostic test in unselected populations. *N. Engl. J. Med.* 274: 1117, 1966.
200. Vensel, L., Devereux, R. B., Pickering, T. G., et al. Cardiac structure and function in human renovascular hypertension. Differences between unilateral and bilateral renal artery stenosis. (In press, 1986).
201. Vetrovec, G. W., Cowley, M. J., Landwehr, D. M., et al. High prevalence of renal artery stenosis in hypertensive patients with coronary artery disease. *JACC,* 3: 518, 1984.
202. Watkins, B. E., Davis, J. O., Hanson, R. C., et al. Incidence and pathophysiological changes in chronic two-kidney hypertension in the dog. *Am. J. Physiol.* 231: 954, 1976.
203. Woods, J. W., and Michelakis, A. M. Renal vein renin in renovascular hypertension. *Arch. Intern. Med.* 122: 382, 1968.
204. Ying, C. Y., Tifft, C. P. Gavras, H., et al. Renal revascularization in the azotemic hypertensive patient resistant to therapy. *N. Engl. J. Med.* 311: 1070, 1984.
205. Zabbo, A., and Novick, A. C. Digital subtraction angiography for noninvasive imaging of the renal artery. *Urol. Clin. North Am.* 11: 409, 1984.
206. Zarins, C. K., Chien-Tai, L., and Gewertz, B. Arterial disruption and remodeling following balloon dilatation. *Surgery* 92: 1089, 1982.
207. Zimbler, M. S., Pickering, T. G., Sos, T. A., and Laragh, J. H. Proteinuria in renovascular hypertension and the effects of renal angioplasty. *Am. J. Cardiol.* 59: 406, 1987.

The Syndrome of Primary Aldosteronism and Pheochromocytoma

Emmanuel L. Bravo

The Syndrome of Primary Aldosteronism

The hallmarks of primary aldosteronism are hypertension, aldosterone excess, and low plasma renin, usually associated with variable degrees of hypokalemic alkalosis. In the classic form (Conn's syndrome), aldosterone hypersecretion results from a unilateral adrenal cortical adenoma [37]. In a minority, perhaps about one-third of all patients, a tumor is not identified and the adrenal glands may show hyperplasia of the zona glomerulosa, with or without micronodular changes (idiopathic hyperaldosteronism) [27, 32, 45, 95, 97]. Rarely, the syndrome can result from either an adrenal [56, 150] or ovarian carcinoma. In a certain group of patients the hypertension and biochemical abnormalities can be corrected by dexamethasone suppression [74, 81, 107, 111, 144]. This glucocorticoid-remediable form of aldosteronism is, in all likelihood, not a primary adrenal cortical defect but may be due to a non-ACTH Proopiomelanocortin (POMC)–derived peptide that dexamethasone suppresses.

Primary aldosteronism is an uncommon cause of hypertension. Nevertheless, it is an important disorder to recognize in hypertensive patients for several reasons. First, the associated hypertension can be severe, and cardiovascular and renal complications are not uncommon. Second, removal of the tumor often results in cure of hypertension or at the very least renders it more responsive to medical therapy. Third, knowledge of the tumor's presence leads to rational and specific therapeutic regimen, resulting in better compliance and better blood pressure control. Reported prevalences of 20 percent of patients with apparent essential hypertension [40] and of 2 percent [141] and 12 percent [83] in selected patients are much too high. The prevalence among unselected patients with hypertension is probably closer to 1 percent.

Pathogenesis of Hypertension

The pathogenesis of mineralocorticoid hypertension is still unclear. Earlier studies have suggested that the salt and water retention with the expected increase in intravascular volume and subsequent cardiac output is primarily responsible for the initiation and maintenance of hypertension [50, 162]. Other studies in humans, however, have shown that hypervolemia is not a universal finding in primary aldosteronism [16, 28]. In addition, there is an inverse correlation between cardiac output and arterial blood pressure that indicates that peripheral resistance is probably more important than the elevated cardiac output in the maintenance of this hypertension [27, 115, 148]. Studies in intact conscious dogs treated with metyrapone also suggest that mineralocorticoid-induced hypertension is "resistance mediated" from its earliest stages and that the increase in sodium stores rather than volume expansion per se played the more important role in initiation of this hypertension. The mechanism of the increase in total peripheral resistance is uncertain, but several hypotheses have been proposed. Some studies have suggested that induction of hypertension with deoxycorticosterone acetate (DOCA) is related to changes of membrane properties of vascular smooth muscle leading to abnormal cation turnover, which in turn enhances vasoconstriction [12, 68, 90]. The structural changes (i.e., increased wall-to-lumen ratio) that follow further augment vascularity and reactivity responses to even normal stimuli [65], thus potentiating and maintaining the hypertensive process (Fig. 56-1). Another attractive possibility was advanced by the demonstration of a circulating "sodium pump inhibitor" in experimental volume-overload hypertension as well as in some patients with essential hypertension [20, 49, 83]. The consequent increase in intracellular sodium leads to increased intracellular calcium, which in turn could explain the increased vascular tone and even some of the cardiac hyperkinetic features of primary aldosteronism.

Clinical Features

AGE/SEX/RACE PREDILECTION

Primary aldosteronism can occur at all ages. In the series of Ferriss et al. [59, 159], ages ranged from 18 to 70 years, with a mean of 46.5 years. In our series [28] the age of diagnosis ranged from 20 to 67 years. In the reported series most patients were in their third, fourth, and fifth decades.

Aldosterone-producing adenomas occur more commonly in females than in males [7, 40, 59]. In contrast, idiopathic hyperaldosteronism is either equally frequent in men and women [7, 40] or more common in men [17, 158, 159]. Whites seem to be more subject to the disease than blacks.

SIGNS AND SYMPTOMS

The symptoms are usually related to hypokalemia or to the complications of hypertension. The most common complaints are proximal muscle weakness of the extremities, polyuria, nocturia, polydipsia, paresthesias, tetany, and muscle paralysis [40]. Often these symptoms may be precipitated by intake of potassium-wasting diuretics. Headaches, characterized as bifrontal and nagging, are common. However, many patients are completely asymptomatic and are detected at routine examination for serum electrolyte values and at assessment for diuretic-induced hypokalemia or refractory hypertension [28].

The hypertension of primary aldosteronism can range from mild to very high, although there are reports of patients with apparently normal blood pressure [132, 166]. In one series [59] of 136 patients the mean blood pressure was reported as 205/123 ± 28/13 mm Hg (SD). In our series [28] diastolic blood pressure was elevated mildly (less than 100 mm Hg) in 10 percent, moderately

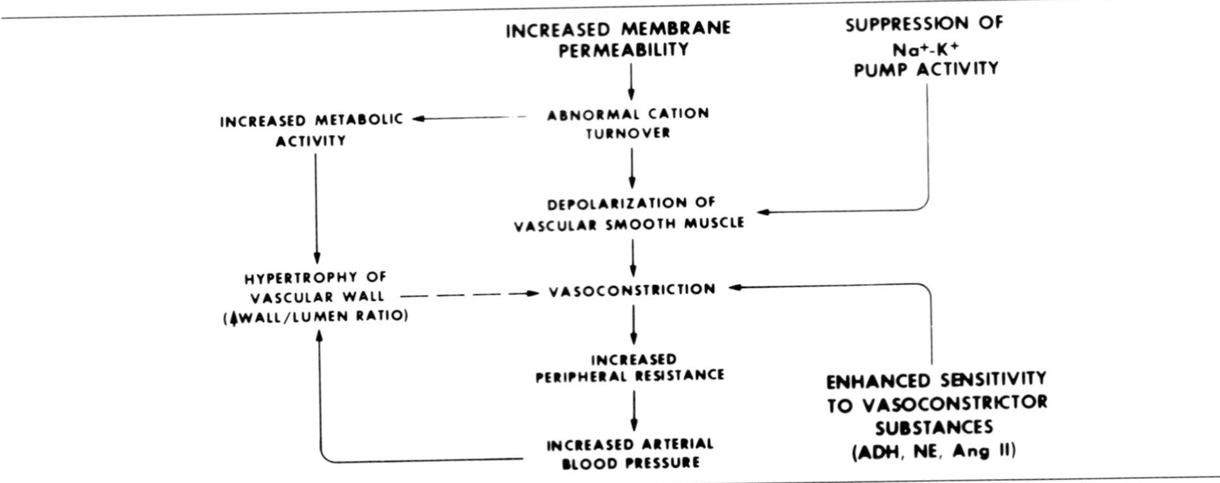

Fig. 56-1. A schematized diagram of the possible events leading to increased peripheral resistance in mineralocorticoid-induced hypertension. According to this hypothesis, hypertension is "resistance-mediated" from its onset and hypervolemia is not an essential element in the initiation and maintenance of the hypertension. ADH = antidiuretic hormone; NE = norepinephrine; Ang II = angiotensin II. (Modified from K. Onoyama, et al. Sodium extracellular fluid volume and cardiac output changes in the genesis of mineralcorticoid hypertension in the dog. *Hypertension* 1:331, 1979.)

increased (100 to 110 mm Hg) in 42 percent, moderately severe (greater than 120 mm Hg) in 18 percent. Arterial blood pressure does not differ between patients with adenoma and those with hyperplasia. There have been several reports of patients entering the malignant phase [59]. Vascular complications such as stroke and heart attacks occur in about one-fourth of all patients [11]. These observations suggest that the hypertension of primary aldosteronism is neither mild nor benign as previously indicated.

Screening for the Presence of Excessive Aldosterone Production

Classically, patients with this disorder have as diagnostic hallmarks the findings of hypokalemic alkalosis, suppressed plasma renin activity, and excessive aldosterone production. However, more recent studies suggest that a significant number of patients may not exhibit all these biochemical characteristics.

SERUM POTASSIUM CONCENTRATION

Hypokalemia, whether spontaneous or provoked, provides an important clue to the presence of excessive aldosterone production. However, a substantial number of patients do not present with spontaneous hypokalemia. Normal serum potassium concentration has been found in 7 to 38 percent of reported cases [38, 59, 73, 122]. In our own studies [28] 27.5 percent of the patients are normokalemic while receiving normal dietary sodium (Fig. 56-2). Of these, 12.5 percent did not develop hypokalemia despite salt loading for 3 days. Several factors can modify serum potassium concentration in the patient with primary aldosteronism. Previous therapy with potassium-sparing agents (e.g., spironolactone, amiloride, triamterene) and/or increased potassium intake (e.g., oral potassium chloride or salt substitutes rich in potassium) can cause repletion of total body potassium to such an extent that spontaneous hypokalemia does not develop as readily after discontinuance of these drugs. Because renal potassium wasting associated with excessive aldosterone production depends primarily on the amount of sodium reaching the sodium-for-potassium distal exchange sites, reducing sodium intake al-

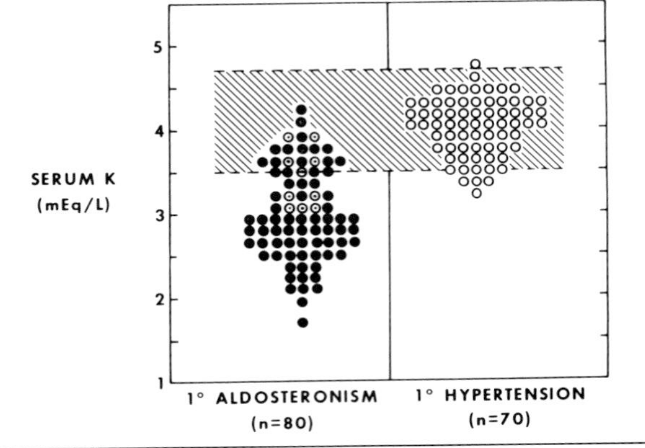

Fig. 56-2. Fasting, resting serum potassium values during normal dietary sodium intake. Each point represents the mean of at least three determinations. For patients with primary aldosteronism, the solid circles represent adenomas (n = 70), and the circles with dotted centers represent hyperplasia (n = 10). The cross-hatched area represents 95 percent confidence limits (3.5 to 4.6 mEq/L) of values obtained from 60 healthy subjects. (From E. L. Bravo, et al. The changing clinical spectrum of primary aldosteronism. *Am. J. Med.* 74:641, 1983.)

lows potassium retention and prevents the development of hypokalemia. Finally, renal disease can lead to renal tubular resistance to the effects of aldosterone. However, for reasons that are totally unclear, some patients have a normal aldosterone production. In such patients conventional diuretic therapy usually produces moderately severe hypokalemia (i.e., serum potassium ≤ 3.0 mEq/liter) that normalizes readily upon discontinuance of the drug.

PLASMA RENIN ACTIVITY

Measurement of plasma renin activity (PRA) under conditions of stimulation (sodium restriction, diuretic administration, and upright posture) has been used as a screening test to exclude primary aldosteronism. It is common practice not to pursue further investigation unless patients exhibit suppressed PRA values (less than 1.0 ng/ml/hr) that fail to increase above 2.0 ng/ml/hour after salt and water depletion. However, some patients may have clearly unsuppressed values during normal dietary sodium intake (Fig. 56-3), and a significant number may have stimulated PRA values (greater than 2 ng/ml/hr) (Fig. 56-4). In addition, about 40 percent of subjects with essential hypertension have suppressed PRA values during normal dietary sodium intake, 15 to 20 percent of whom have values below 2 ng/ml/hour under conditions of stimulation. Thus the large number of false-positive and false-negative results make PRA determination of limited use in screening patients for the presence of primary aldosteronism. In retrospect, since most hypertensive patients are treated with drugs that stimulate renin production and since pretreatment status is difficult to achieve after prolonged therapy, it is not surprising that some patients may present with unsuppressed and/or reactive PRA despite primary overproduction of aldosterone.

PLASMA ALDOSTERONE-RENIN RATIO

The ratio of aldosterone to renin is used to define the appropriateness of PRA for the circulating concentrations of aldosterone [101]. It is assumed that the volume expansion associated with the presence of an aldosterone-producing tumor inhibits the synthesis of renin without affecting the autonomous production of aldosterone. One serious drawback of this test is the inherent variability of plasma levels of aldosterone, even in the presence of a tumor, which translates into variability in the absolute value of the ratio. Another is the use of drugs that result in marked and prolonged stimulation of renin long after their discontinuation.

CAPTOPRIL TEST

The principle of the captopril test is similar to that of the plasma aldosterone-renin ratio test, but angiotensin II levels are lowered by pharmacologic blockade of angiotensin converting enzyme rather than by volume expansion [101, 109]. This test is subject to the same limitations as the plasma aldosterone-renin ratio.

Fig. 56-3. Plasma renin activity values after 3 to 5 days of normal dietary sodium intake. Patient identification as in Fig. 56-2. The cross-hatched area represents the 95 percent confidence limits (0.4 to 2.0 ng/ml/hr) of values obtained from 47 healthy subjects of similar age. Twelve patients (15 percent) with primary aldosteronism have values above 2.0 ng/ml/hr. Thirty patients (43 percent) with primary hypertension had values below 1.0 ng/ml/hr. (From E. L. Bravo, et al. The changing clinical spectrum of primary aldosteronism. *Am. J. Med.* 74:641, 1983.)

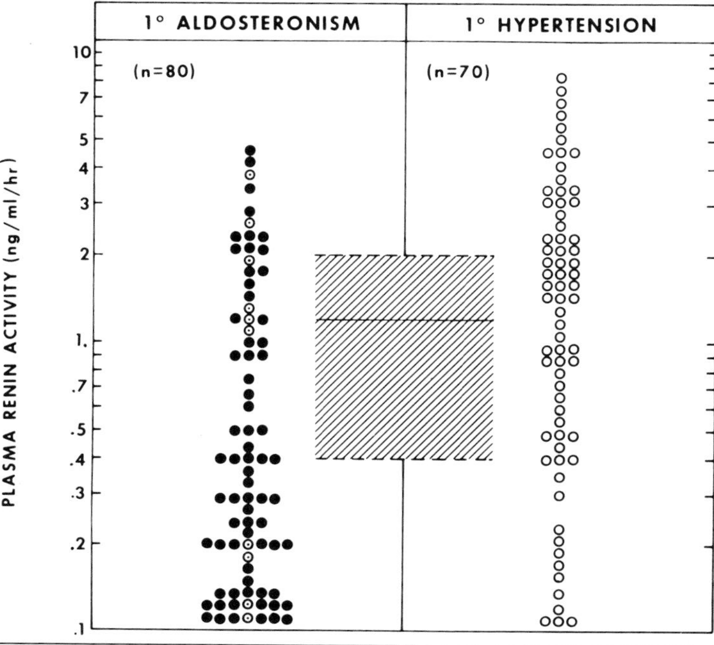

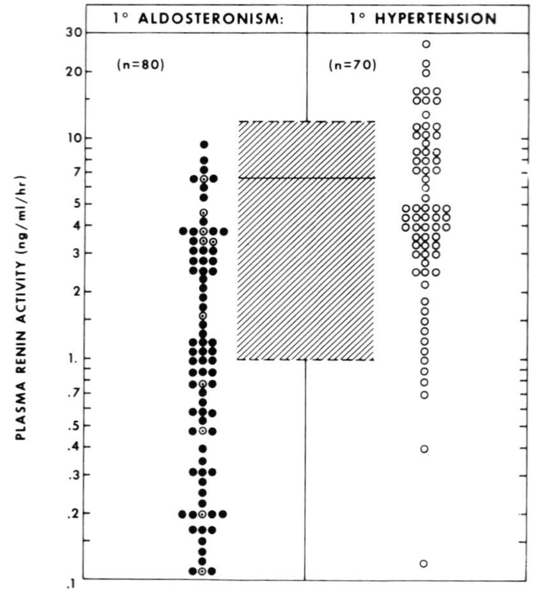

Fig. 56-4. Supine plasma renin activity values the morning after 4 days of sodium deprivation. Patient identification as in Fig. 56-2. The cross-hatched area represents the 95 percent confidence limits (1.06 to 12.18 ng/ml/hr) of values obtained from 47 healthy subjects. Twenty-nine patients (36 percent) with primary aldosteronism had values above 2.0 ng/ml/hr; 12 patients (17 percent) with primary hypertension had values below 2.0 ng/ml/hr. (From E. L. Bravo, et al. The changing clinical spectrum of primary aldosteronism. *Am. J. Med.* 74:641. 1983.)

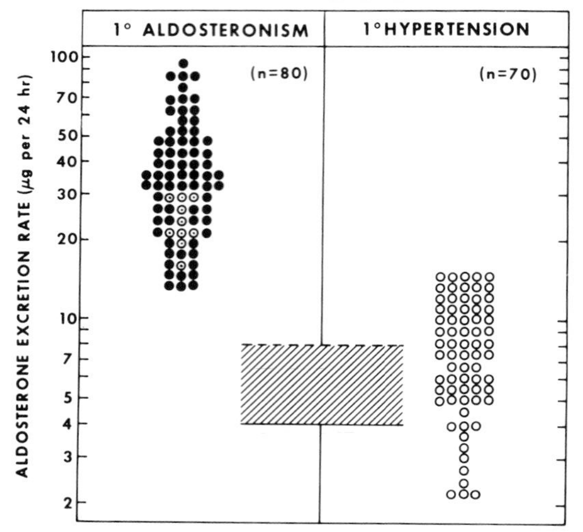

Fig. 56-5. Aldosterone excretion rate after 3 days of high sodium intake (urinary sodium ⩾ 250 mEq/24 hr). Patient identification as in Fig. 56-2. The cross-hatched area represents the mean (4.0 µg/24 hr) and + 2 S.D. above the mean (8.0 µg/24 hr) of values obtained from 47 healthy subjects. For patients with primary hypertension, the 95 percent upper confidence limit is 14 µg/24 hr. Six patients with adenoma had values that overlapped with the highest values obtained in patients with primary hypertension. (From E. L. Bravo, et al. The changing clinical spectrum of primary aldosteronism. *Am. J. Med.* 74:641, 1983.)

Confirmation of Inappropriate Aldosterone Production

Confirmation of the diagnosis of primary aldosteronism requires the demonstration of aldosterone values that are higher than in normal subjects or patients with essential hypertension and fail to suppress normally in response to administration of salt. In rare cases, aldosterone values are normal during normal dietary sodium intake but remain unaltered with high sodium intake.

Often the diagnosis can be established with relative ease. In the hypertensive patient on no treatment, the demonstration of significant hypokalemia (serum potassium < 3.0 mEq/liter) with inappropriate kaliuresis (24-hour urinary potassium > 30 mEq), PRA below 1.0 ng/ml, and elevated plasma or urinary aldosterone values makes the diagnosis incontrovertible. Often, however, the diagnosis is not obvious because of equivocal values; in such cases, multiple measurements during salt loading are needed.

The intravenous infusion of 2,000 ml of physiologic saline over 4 hours has been advocated as a quick and simple test to assess suppressibility of aldosterone production. Suppression of plasma aldosterone values to less than 10 ng/dl is considered a normal response. In one series of 51 patients with surgically proven primary aldosteronism, the sensitivity of the test was reported as 100 percent [159]. However, some studies report a false-positive rate as high as 20 percent [141]. One drawback of the test is the inherent variability of plasma levels of aldosterone. Another is the expected decrement of aldosterone production over the time taken to infuse the saline.

The single best test that identifies patients with primary aldosteronism is the measurement of aldosterone production after salt loading. In the studies shown (Fig. 56-5) an aldosterone excretion rate of greater than 14.0 µg per 24 hours clearly distinguishes most patients with primary aldosteronism from subjects with essential hypertension. Although 6 patients with primary aldosteronism have values that overlap with the highest values obtained in subjects with essential hypertension, the test provides far better sensitivity and specificity than either serum potassium concentration or plasma renin activity in identifying patients with primary aldosteronism.

The measurement of plasma aldosterone concentration is a much less sensitive test in the identification of patients with primary aldosteronism. As shown in Fig. 56-6, 2 patients have values that fall within the 95 percent normal range, and 17 (39 percent) of the patients have values that fall within the range of values obtained in patients with essential hypertension. In the series of Ferriss and co-workers [59] plasma aldosterone levels were persistently elevated in 22 of 54, but only intermittently raised in 32 of 54 cases.

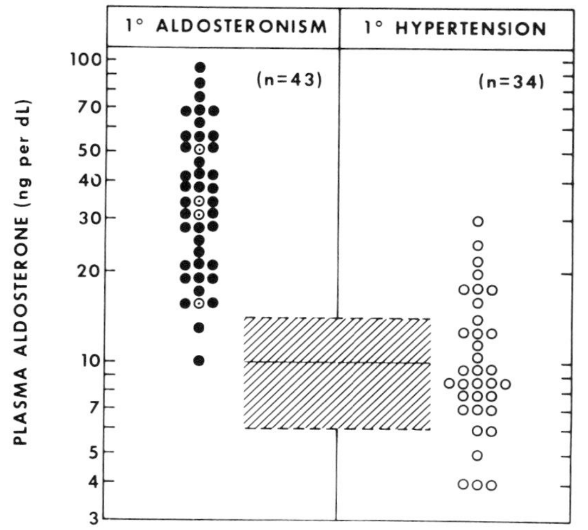

Fig. 56-6. Fasting, supine plasma aldosterone concentration the morning after 3 days of high sodium intake (urinary sodium ≥ 250 mEq/24 hr). Patient identification as in Fig. 56-2. The cross-hatched area represents the 95 percent confidence limits of values (5.3 to 13.7 ng/dl) obtained from 47 healthy subjects. For primary hypertension the 95 percent upper confidence limit is 21.8 ng/dl. Seventeen patients (39 percent) with primary aldosteronism had values that fell within the range of values obtained in patients with primary hypertension. (From E. L. Bravo, et al. The changing clinical spectrum of primary aldosteronism. *Am. J. Med.* 74:641, 1983.)

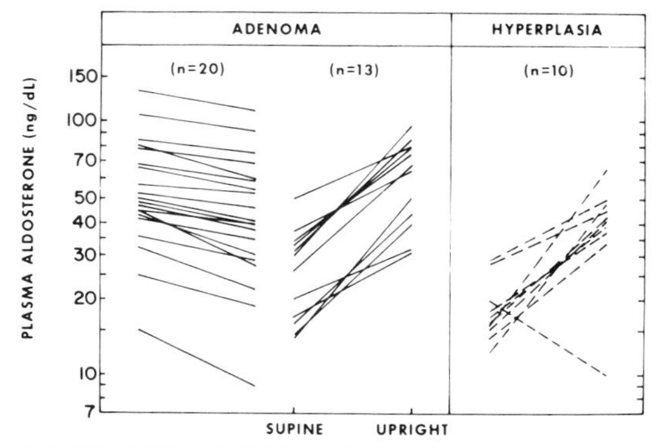

Fig. 56-7. Postural response of plasma aldosterone concentration in pateints with adenoma and hyperplasia during normal dietary sodium intake. Supine, fasting values were obtained at 8:00 A.M., and upright values at 11:00 A.M. after 2 hours of ambulation. Thirteen of thirty-three patients with adenoma had false-negative test results; one of 10 patients with hyperplasia had a false-positive test result. (From E. L. Bravo, et al. The changing clinical spectrum of primary aldosteronism. *Am. J. Med.* 74:641, 1983.)

Biochemical Distinction Between Adenoma and Hyperplasia

Since only patients with adenoma respond favorably to surgery, differentiation between the two forms of the disease is of prime clinical importance. Persistently low serum potassium concentrations during a normal sodium intake appear to favor the presence of an adenoma. In 15 separate reports involving 504 patients [28], a serum potassium concentration of less than 3.5 mEq per liter was found in 80 percent of patients with adenomas and in only 42 percent of those with hyperplasia. In our own series [28], spontaneous hypokalemia below 3.0 mEq per liter was always associated with a tumor; no patient with hyperplasia had basal serum potassium values below 3.0 mEq per liter. It is notable, however, that 24 percent of our patients with adenoma exhibited normokalemia during normal dietary sodium intake and that 8.5 percent remained normokalemic despite high sodium intake for 3 consecutive days.

Ganguly and co-workers [70] first described the anomalous postural decrease in plasma aldosterone concentrations as a reliable test to differentiate adrenal adenoma from adrenal hyperplasia. This was subsequently confirmed by Biglieri and co-workers [16]. However, as experience with the test grew, it became clear that it did not provide the reliability and precision that investigators had hoped. Six separate studies [16, 28, 61, 141, 157, 159] involving 160 proven cases reported false-negative results ranging from 21 to 56 percent and false-positive results from 0 to 30 percent. In our own series, 13 of 33 patients (39 percent) with adenomas exhibited an increase rather than a decrease in plasma aldosterone concentration with ambulation (Fig. 56-7). Of 10 patients with hyperplasia, 1 had a decrease rather than an increase in plasma aldosterone concentration. From this and other studies, it can be concluded that the postural decrease in plasma aldosterone concentration, when present, is a valuable clue to the presence of the tumor. However, an increase in plasma aldosterone concentration does not exclude its presence.

Recently, Biglieri and Schambelan [15] described the measurement of plasma 18-hydroxycorticosterone as a useful aid in differentiating adenoma from hyperplasia. These investigators reported that overnight recumbent values greater than 100 ng per deciliter are considered pathognomonic of an adenoma. This conclusion has been confirmed by others [105]. We [28] also showed that lower values between 50 and 100 ng per deciliter may be just as precise in differentiating between the two pathologic conditions (Fig. 56-8).

Ulick and co-workers [153] have recently identified yet another steroid, 18-hydroxycortisol, in the urine of patients with primary aldosteronism. Their initial studies suggest that it may serve to distinguish tumor from bilateral hyperplasia with even better precision than the measurements of plasma 18-hydroxycorticosterone concentration.

A final means of differentiating a tumor from hyperplasia might be the response to adrenocorticotropic hormone (ACTH) and to angiotensin II infusion [67]. Adenoma patients show a greater than normal aldosterone response to ACTH infusion, whereas the response to infused angiotensin II is poor or absent. Unlike patients

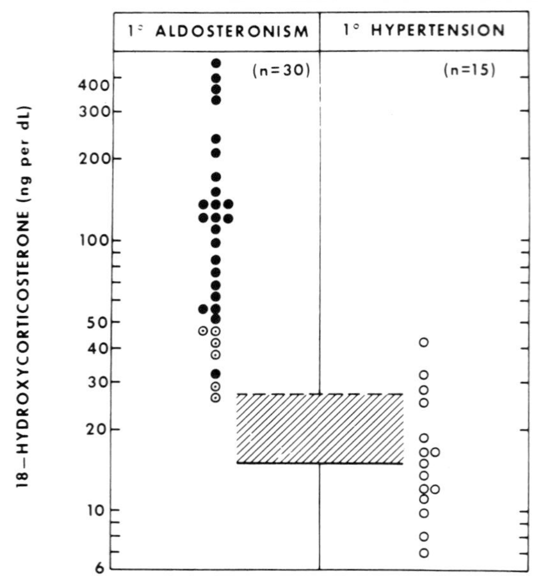

Fig. 56-8. Overnight recumbent values of plasma 18-hydroxycorticosterone during normal dietary sodium intake. Patient identification as in Fig. 56-2. Cross-hatched area represent the means (14.5 ng/dl) and + 2 S.D. (26 ng/dl) of values obtained in 20 normal subjects. One patient with an adenoma had a value that fell within the range obtained in patients with hyperplasia. Plasma values greater than 50 ng/dl identified 97 percent (29 of 30) of patients with adenoma. (From E. L. Bravo, et al. The changing clinical spectrum of primary aldosteronism. *Am. J. Med.* 74:641, 1983.)

with adenoma, patients with idiopathic hyperaldosteronism show increased adrenal sensitivity to infused angiotensin II.

In summary, a patient with the clinical features of primary aldosteronism is more likely to have an adenoma in the presence of moderately severe spontaneous hypokalemia (serum potassium ≤ 3.0 mEq/L), an anomalous postural fall in plasma aldosterone concentration during ambulation, an overnight recumbent plasma 18-hydroxycorticosterone concentration greater than 100 ng per deciliter, and a greater than normal response to ACTH infusion contrasted with a poor or absent response to infused angiotensin II.

Localization of Aldosterone-Producing Tumors

Preoperative localization of an adenoma simplifies the surgical procedure and significantly reduces mortality. Confirmation of the presence and ultimate location of an adenoma has been accomplished by computed tomographic (CT) scan of the adrenal glands, scintigraphy with radiolabeled iodocholesterol [39], adrenal venography, and measurement of aldosterone concentration in adrenal venous effluent.

ADRENAL CT SCAN

Because of its noninvasive nature, the adrenal CT scan should be considered the initial step in localization (Figs. 56-9 and 56-10). All adenomas 1.5 cm in diameter or larger can be accurately located on CT scans. However, only 60 percent of nodules measuring 1.0 to 1.4 cm in diameter are detected by CT, and nodules smaller than 1.0 cm in diameter are very difficult if not impossible to demonstrate. The overall sensitivity of localizing adenomas by high resolution CT scan exceeds 90 percent [72, 100, 163].

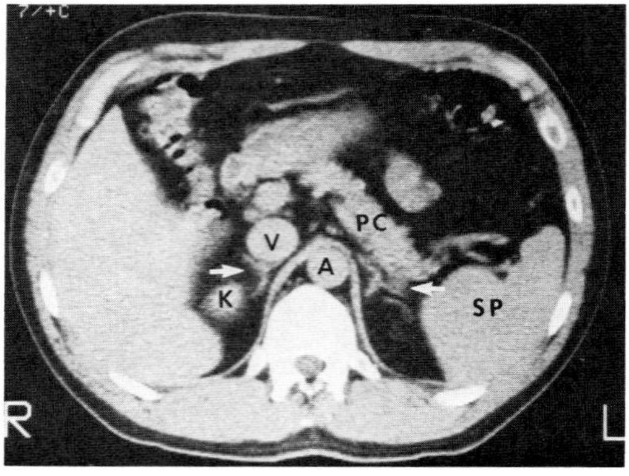

A

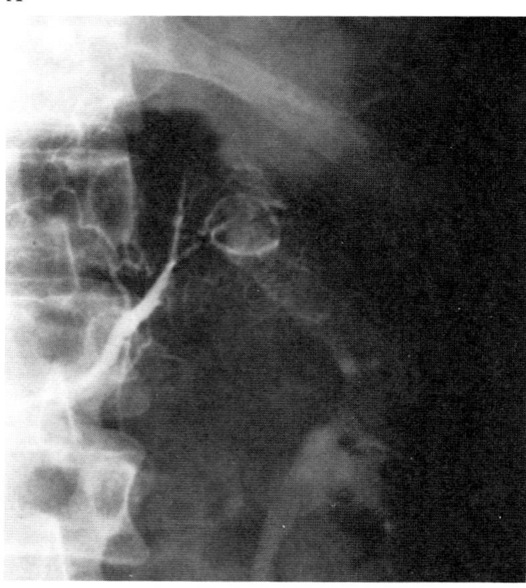

B

Fig. 56-9. A. An adrenal CT scan showing a 1.0-cm mass with a very low attenuation originating from the lateral limb of the left adrenal gland (*arrow*). SP = spleen; PC = pancreas; K = kidney; V = vena cava; A = aorta. B. An adrenal venography of (A) showing a solitary space-consuming mass in the same area of the left adrenal gland on CT scan. Surgery revealed a mass with characteristics of an aldosterone-producing tumor.

SCINTIGRAPHY WITH RADIOLABELED IODOCHOLESTEROL

Adrenal imaging with iodocholesterol (^{131}I-6β-iodomethyl-19-norcholesterol, NP-59) provides a noninvasive means of differentiating patients with an aldosterone-producing adenoma from those with idiopathic hyperaldosteronism and also for identifying the site of an adenoma when present [123]. It accurately localizes an al-

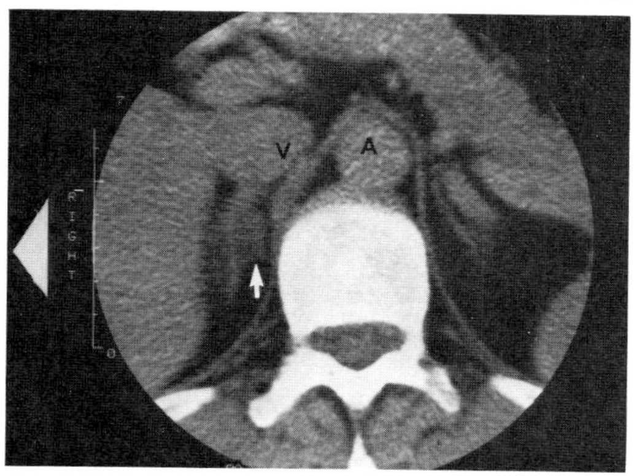

A

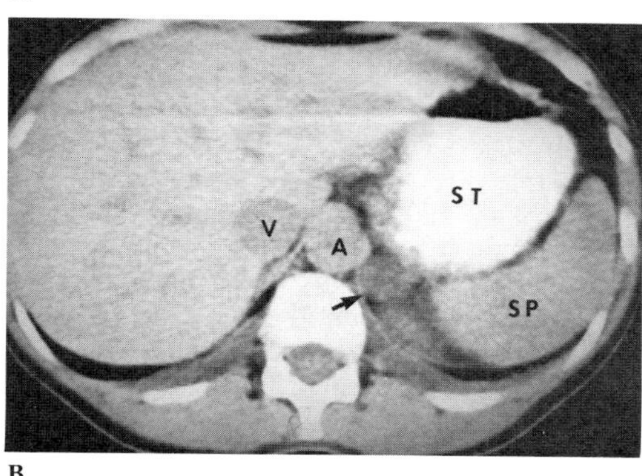

B

Fig. 56-10. A. An adrenal CT scan showing a mass originating from the medial limb of the right adrenal gland (*arrow*). This mass was an aldosterone-producing tumor that measured 0.8 cm in its greatest diameter at pathologic examination. V = vena cava; A = aorta. B. An adrenal CT scan showing a low attenuation left suprareal mass. This was an aldosterone-producing tumor that measured 2.5 cm in diameter at pathologic examination. V = vena cava; A = aorta; ST = stomach with contrast dye; SP = spleen.

dosterone-producing adenoma in more than 90 percent of patients. Because NP-59 accumulates rapidly in the adrenals, it permits scintigraphy within 5 days of administration. Patients with adenoma concentrate radioactivity at the site of the tumor, whereas patients with idiopathic hyperaldosteronism usually show diffuse uptake or bilaterally reduced activity. Some patients in the latter group may show asymmetric uptake, but dexamethasone will suppress uptake bilaterally in these cases and will also enhance the early difference in uptake between the two sides in patients with adenoma [39]. A small adenoma that is less than 1.0 cm in diameter may be missed, and aldosterone-producing carcinomas show little or no radioactivity. Imaging with NP-59 may supplant adrenal vein catheterization for diagnosis and localization in primary aldosteronism. However, some false-negative results have been observed [105].

ADRENAL VEIN SAMPLING FOR PLASMA ALDOSTERONE CONCENTRATION

Adrenal venous aldosterone levels should be measured when the results of the adrenal CT scan and scintigraphy are ambiguous. Bilateral adrenal venous sampling for the measurement of aldosterone concentration is still the most accurate test in localizing aldosterone-producing tumors. However, the procedure is invasive, technically demanding, and requires considerable skill and experience. There is an appreciable incidence of complications including adrenal and iliac vein thrombosis and extravasation of dye into the gland, leading to adrenal insufficiency. However, when technically successful and when both adrenal veins are entered, the accuracy of comparative adrenal venous aldosterone levels in confirming either a tumor or hyperplasia exceeds 95 percent [28, 72, 86, 87, 105, 106, 159]. Normal adrenal venous aldosterone concentration is 200 to 600 ng per deciliter. The ratio of ipsilateral to contralateral aldosterone is usually greater than 10 to 1. Correct placement of the catheter in the adrenal vein is essential. The accuracy of placement can best be evaluated by obtaining simultaneous ACTH-stimulated selective adrenal venous cortisol levels [159]. An aldosterone ratio greater than 10 to 1 in the presence of symmetric ACTH-induced cortisol response is diagnostic of an aldosterone producing-adenoma.

Mineralocorticoid Excess Syndromes Mimicking Primary Aldosteronism

There are several circumstances in which hypertension with hypokalemia and suppressed PRA may occur in the absence of excessive aldosterone production. These include deoxycorticosterone (DOC) excess syndromes, and "apparent mineralocorticoid excess" (AME) syndromes.

The best defined circumstances in which DOC excess plays a significant role in hypertension are with the syndromes in which there is deficiency of 11β- [165] or 17α-hydroxylation of steroids [14]. These disorders are usually congenital in nature but may be induced by excessive production of estrogen/androgen from either a benign or malignant tumor [126, 133]. Deficiency of either 11β- or 17α-hydroxylation decreases cortisol production, which results in disinhibition of ACTH release. The excessive circulating ACTH leads to stimulation of DOC. Excess DOC may also contribute to the hypertension in certain cases of Cushing's syndrome (particularly with ectopic ACTH production) and in DOC-producing adrenocortical adenomas [88].

In the syndrome of AME, no known mineralocorticoids are present in elevated amounts. Liddle et al. [99] first described such a condition in 1963, a hypertensive syndrome that responds to sodium deprivation or triamterene but not to spironolactone. The abnormality has been defined as a non-aldosterone-dependent enhanced sodium reabsorption at distal renal tubular sites leading to hypertension and suppression of PRA, and thus of aldosterone biosynthesis. In the 1970s, several children were described with a similar clinical picture, but who responded to spironolactone [164]. In-depth studies of steroid production in these patients revealed deficient 11β-hydroxysteroid dehydrogenase (11β-OHSD), the enzyme that converts cortisol to cortisone, in conjunction with decreased steroid 5β-reductase and normal activity of 5α-reductase [154, 155]. This attenuated metabolism results in increased cortisol half-life, but plasma cortisol remains normal because of reduced cortisol secretion rate (brought about by the negative ACTH feedback mechanism). Since reduced 11β-OHSD is associated with loss of normal specificity for the type I receptor (in the kidney), cortisol acts in preference to aldosterone on this receptor. Therefore, cortisol under these circumstances may act as a potent mineralocorticoid [55]. Acquired inhibition of 11β-OHSD (by glycyrrhetenic acid) has been proposed to explain the mineralocorticoid excess syndrome that results from chronic intake of licorice [139].

Other rare forms of hypertension associated with excess aldosterone production include glucocorticoid-remediable aldosteronism, aldosterone-producing adrenal carcinoma, and aldosterone-producing ovarian carcinoma.

In glucocorticoid-remediable aldosteronism, patients usually present with all of the typical features of primary aldosteronism. Unlike primary aldosteronism, however, glucocorticoids produce a sustained reversal of all the abnormalities within 2 weeks of dexamethasone treatment. In mild cases, hypokalemia may be minimal or absent. As in patients with aldosterone-producing adenomas, the plasma aldosterone concentration may fall on assuming an upright posture [69]. Plasma ACTH and cortisol levels are usually within the normal range. Some patients have been shown to have an exaggerated plasma aldosterone response to infused ACTH [81]; however, this has not been confirmed in all patients. Surgical exploration has revealed hyperplasia of the zona glomerulosa without tumor [144]. These cases may be familial with an autosomal dominant transmission, but they are not HLA-linked [110]. The cause of the abnormalities remains unknown.

Patients with hyperaldosteronism resulting from secretion by an adrenocortical carcinoma exhibit certain clinical features that readily distinguish them from those with benign tumors. Fever, muscle weakness, and abdominal pain are common. These tumors are usually larger than 5.0 cm in diameter, have ill-defined margins, may invade contiguous organs, and show increased vascularity. Benign, aldosterone-producing tumors are usually nonvascular. Excessive production of adrenal corticosteroids other than aldosterone is common. Less commonly, corticosterone and/or 11-deoxycorticosterone may be produced in large amounts and are primarily responsible for the manifestations of the syndrome of hypermineralocorticoidism [18, 19]. There have also been reports of patients in whom the only steroid abnormality is excessive aldosterone production [149].

Aldosterone-producing ovarian carcinoma is an even rarer cause of hyperaldosteronism and hypokalemia. There are only two cases reported in the literature. One patient was a 9-year-old girl with precocious puberty in whom a Serotoli cell tumor was found [56]. The other presented with a widely metastasizing arrhenoblastoma [150]. In each, aldosterone was extracted from tumor tissue, and the adrenal glands appeared normal.

ASSOCIATED ENDOCRINE DISORDERS

Primary aldosteronism and acromegaly have occurred together in individual patients [51, 140]. Primary aldosteronism and primary hyperparathyroidism have also been associated [62, 108, 113, 140]. Recently, Barkan et al. [10] described a patient with primary hyperparathyroidism who exhibited biochemical evidence of primary aldosterone excess that remitted after removal of a parathyroid adenoma. They speculated that prolonged hypercalcemia might produce changes in the renin-angiotensin-aldosterone system that mimic those of primary aldosteronism. However, the plasma concentrations of total renin, angiotensin II, and aldosterone are usually normal in patients with primary hyperparathyroidism [60]. Ferriss and co-workers [60] were also unable to find evidence of hyperparathyroidism in any of their 25 patients with primary aldosteronism.

Diagnosis

SENSITIVITY AND SPECIFICITY OF SCREENING TESTS IN THE DIAGNOSIS OF PRIMARY HYPERALDOSTERONISM

Serum potassium concentration, either spontaneous or provoked, gives a low sensitivity (73 percent and 86 percent, respectively) but a very high specificity (94 percent and 96 percent, respectively). Suppressed plasma renin activity (less than 2.0 ng/ml/hr after low sodium intake for 4 days) provides a sensitivity of only 64 percent and a specificity of 86 percent. Nonsuppressible plasma aldosterone concentration (greater than 22 ng/dl after 3 days of salt loading) gives a sensitivity of only 72 percent but a much higher specificity at 91 percent. An aldosterone excretion rate greater than 14 μg per 24 hours after 3 days of salt loading provides the highest sensitivity (96 percent) and specificity (93 percent) in identifying patients with primary aldosteronism (Table 56-1). The combination of excessive aldosterone production, spontaneous or provoked hypokalemia, and/or suppressed plasma renin activity makes the diagnosis of primary aldosteronism virtually assured.

Table 56-2 shows the responses of aldosterone excretion, plasma renin activity, and plasma aldosterone concentration to dietary sodium manipulation.

RECOMMENDED APPROACH TO THE PATIENT SUSPECTED OF HAVING PRIMARY HYPERALDOSTERONISM

Priority of evaluation should be given to patients with a history of spontaneous hypokalemia, marked sensitivity to potassium wasting diuretics, and those with "refractory hypertension." Based on the sensitivity and specificity of screening tests, it is recommended that patients suspected of having primary hyperaldosteronism have as the initial screening test the determination of aldosterone excretion rate during prolonged salt loading (Fig. 56-11). This evaluation can be accomplished in the outpatient unit by adding 10 to 12 gm of sodium chloride to the patient's daily intake and determining the values of serum potassium concentration and the 24-hour urinary excretion of sodium, potassium, and aldosterone after 5 to 7 days of high salt intake. Serum and urinary potassium values indicate whether inappropriate kaliuresis

Table 56-1. Sensitivity and specificity of various screening tests for primary aldosteronism

Test	Standard	Sensitivity (number of patients)	Specificity (number of patients)
Serum potassium[a]	Spontaneous (< 3.5 mEq/L)	0.73 (58/80)	0.94 (66/70)
Serum potassium[b]	Provoked (< 3.5 mEq/L)	0.86 (70/80)	0.96 (67/70)
Plasma renin activity	Suppressed (< 2.0 ng/ml/hr)	0.64 (51/80)	0.83 (58/70)
Aldosterone excretion rate[b]	Nonsuppressible (> 14 μg/24 hr)	0.96 (77/80)	0.93 (65/70)
Plasma aldosterone concentration[b]	Nonsuppressible (> 22 ng/dl)	0.72 (31/43)	0.91 (31/34)

[a]Normal sodium intake for 3 to 5 days.
[b]High sodium intake for 3 days.
Low sodium intake for 4 days.
Sensitivity = percent of subjects with the disease that have positive results. Specificity = percent of subjects without disease that have negative results. Standards for aldosterone excretion rate and plasma aldosterone concentration represent the upper 95 percent range of values obtained in subjects with essential hypertension. *Source:* From E. L. Bravo, R. C. Tarazi, H. P. Dustan, et al. The changing clinical spectrum of primary aldosteronism. *Am. J. Med.* 74:641, 1983.

Table 56-2. Responses to dietary sodium manipulation

Measurements	Adrenal adenoma (n = 70)	Adrenal hyperplasia (n = 10)	Essential hypertension (n = 70)	Normal control subjects (n = 47)
Aldosterone excretion (μg/24hr)				
Normal	33 ± 16[a]	27 ± 11[a]	11 ± 5	7 ± 2
Low	42 ± 18	63 ± 36[b]	42 ± 32	58 ± 24
High	37 ± 20	24 ± 4	8 ± 3	4 ± 2
Plasma renin activity (ng/ml)				
Normal	0.62 ± 0.87[a]	1.31 ± 1.06	1.84 ± 1.76	1.18 ± 0.37
Low	1.61 ± 1.83	3.27 ± 3.02	6.68 ± 5.83	6.62 ± 2.78
High	0.64 ± 0.89	0.70 ± 0.78	1.08 ± 0.96	0.87 ± 0.57
Plasma aldosterone (ng/dl)	(n = 39)	(n = 4)	(n = 34)	
Normal	44.8 ± 36.6[a]	41.0 ± 14.4[a]	15.1 ± 6.6	12.7 ± 4.9
Low	56.2 ± 56.6	56.3 ± 20.3	33.9 ± 18.6	44.7 ± 24.4
High	45.5 ± 42.3	32.5 ± 13.2	10.8 ± 5.5	9.5 ± 2.1

[a]Significantly different from essential hypertension values.
[b]Significantly different from essential hypertension and adenoma values.
Significantly different from essential hypertension values and from each other.
All values are expressed as mean ± 1 SD. Normal, low, and high = daily sodium intake.
Source: From E. L. Bravo, R. C. Tarazi, H. P. Dustan, et al. The changing clinical spectrum of primary aldosteronism. *Am. J. Med.* 74:641, 1983.

(serum potassium less than 3.0 mEq/L with a urinary potassium greater than 30 mEq/24 hr) occurs during salt loading. A 24-hour urinary sodium value of at least 250 mEq per day gives some assurance that the patient has ingested the prescribed salt intake. Under these conditions, patients who fail to suppress their aldosterone excretion rate below 14 μg per 24 hours are prime candidates for additional studies. The presence of hypokalemia and/or suppressed plasma renin activity provides corroborative data, but their absence does not preclude the diagnosis. The demonstration of an anomalous postural decrease in plasma aldosterone concentration and increased plasma 18-hydroxycorticosterone values indicate the presence of an adenoma.

For localization, an adrenal CT scan should be performed first and considered diagnostic if an adrenal mass is clearly identified. When the results of the computed tomographic scan are inconclusive, adrenal scintigraphy should be done with NP-59. Adrenal venous aldosterone levels should be measured when the results of both the adrenal CT scan and scintigraphy are ambiguous.

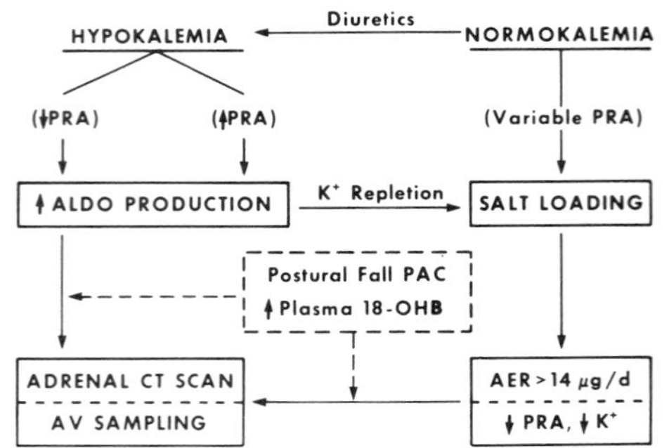

Fig. 56-11. A recommended approach to the patient with suspected primary aldosteronism. PRA = plasma renin activity; ALDO = aldosterone; AER = aldosterone excretion rate; PAC = plasma aldosterone concentration.

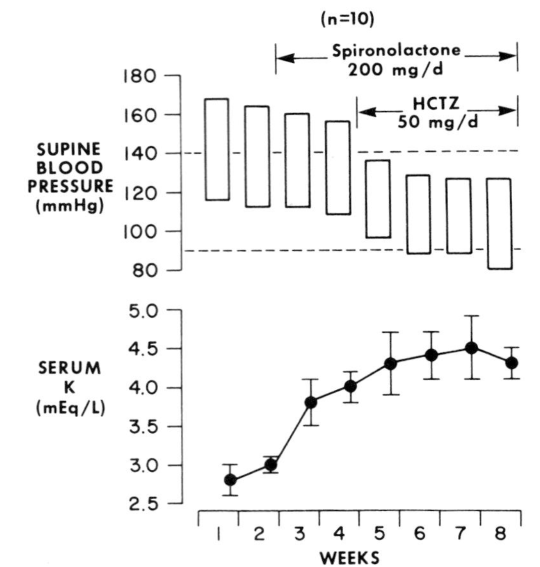

Fig. 56-12. The effect of spironolactone plus hydrochlorothiazide (HCTZ) on the serum potassium and blood pressure of patients with aldosterone-producing adenoma. (From E. L. Bravo, et al. Spironolactone as a nonspecific treatment for primary aldosteronism. *Circulation* 48:491, 1973.)

Management of Primary Aldosteronism

In most cases the hypertension can be managed adequately with salt and water depletion. The combination of 200 mg per day of spironolactone (to correct the hypokalemia) and conventional doses of either hydrochlorothiazide or furosemide have been successful in correcting both the metabolic abnormality and the hypertension (Fig. 56-12) [23]. Either amiloride or triamterene [105] may be substituted for spironolactone if the necessity arises.

However, unless there are absolute contraindications, tumors confined to one gland are best treated surgically since the prospects of cure in this group are significant. At the very least, surgery renders arterial pressure easier to control with medications. In addition, neither the duration and the severity of hypertension nor the degree of end-organ target involvement has any relation to the arterial pressure response after surgery [24]. On the other hand, bilateral hyperplasia is best managed medically because not only is the cure rate low, but also there is the risk of producing adrenal insufficiency if too much adrenal tissue is resected in an effort to reduce aldosterone production.

Before surgery, patients with adenoma should receive drug treatment, both to decrease arterial pressure and to correct the metabolic abnormalities, for at least 8 to 10 weeks. Unilateral adrenalectomy is highly successful in treating aldosterone-producing adenoma. One year postoperatively, about 70 percent of patients are normotensive, but 5 years postoperatively, only 53 percent remain normotensive [17, 105]. The restoration of normal potassium homeostasis is permanent. However, in idiopathic hyperaldosteronism, bilateral adrenalectomy relieves hypertension in only one-third of patients. Not only are the results far from ideal, but substituting the problems of adrenal insufficiency for those of primary aldosteronism is an unwelcome trade-off.

Pheochromocytoma

The term *pheochromocytoma* refers to a tumor of cells of neuroectodermal origin that have an affinity for chromium salts. Immersion in a chromium salt fixative (Zenker's or potassium dichromate solution) changes the tumor from its usual pale gray appearance to a dark black color as cytoplasmic catecholamines are oxidized. These catecholamine-producing cells occur predominantly in the adrenal medulla. They may also be found in rests of chromaffin tissue along the abdominal aorta or its main branches, at the sites of the paravertebral sympathetic ganglia within the posterior mediastinum or retroperitoneal space, the organ of Zuckerkandl, the bladder wall, and spermatic cord. Similar tumors may originate in the neck at the site of the carotid body or beneath the jugular foramen (glomus jugulare tumors).

The true prevalence of pheochromocytoma is not known. It is estimated that at least 0.1 percent of patients with diastolic hypertension have this tumor. Assuming that 35 million people in this country have hypertension, that the prevalence of pheochromocytoma is 0.1 percent of patients with sustained diastolic hypertension, and that 50 percent of patients with pheochromocytoma have paroxysmal hypertension, it can be calculated that approximately 70,000 persons in this country have pheochromocytoma. It occurs in one of every 20,000 to 50,000 patients admitted to hospital. About 1,000 new cases are found annually in the United States.

Early recognition, accurate localization, and appropriate management of these tumors usually result in complete cure in almost all patients with benign tumors. Unrecognized, these tumors are potentially lethal; hypertensive crises and/or shock and arrhythmias or cardiac arrest leading to death have been precipitated by drugs, anesthetic agents, parturition, or surgery for an unrelated condition.

Pheochromocytoma can occur at any age but is most frequent in the fourth and fifth decades. In children, about two-thirds of cases occur in boys; in adults, 53 to 60 percent are women. About 10 percent of patients with pheochromocytoma have relatives with the disease. It may become manifest for the first time during pregnancy.

Pathophysiology

REGULATION OF BLOOD PRESSURE

Of all the secondary forms of hypertension, the mechanism of elevated blood pressure in patients with pheochromocytoma seems to be the most straightforward. However, about 15 percent of patients may be normotensive [154]. In addition, no relationship exists between the prevailing levels of plasma catecholamines and the height of arterial blood pressure [39] (Fig. 56-13). Indeed, normotension in the face of increased circulating catecholamines is not uncommon.

Several factors could conceivably alter the response of the vascular smooth muscle to circulating catecholamines. One factor is blood volume. Hypovolemia has been shown to diminish blood pressure response to circulating pressor agents. However, hypovolemia is not a universal finding in this disorder [147]. In addition, blood volume is inversely related to the height of diastolic blood pressure, a relationship that would be direct if the height of arterial blood pressure depended on the level of intravascular volume. Alternatively, increased production of vasodilator agents may protect against the hypertensive action of norepinephrine. Louis and coworkers [102] have raised the possibility that concomitant secretion of dopa may counteract the vasoconstrictive effect of norepinephrine. The demonstration that epinephrine itself enhances prostaglandin synthesis provides yet another possible reason [54].

Prolonged stimulation of tissues by adrenergic agonists can lead to diminished responsiveness of the tissue to subsequent activation by catecholamine; this phenomenon has been termed desensitization or tachyphylaxis. Tsujimoto and co-workers [151] examined the in vivo consequences of prolonged stimulation of vascular α-adrenergic receptors in rats harboring norepinephrine-producing tumors. They found that in the early stages of the disease, loss of sensitivity was observed for both α_1- and α_2-adrenergic agonists, whereas responsiveness to Arg-vasopressin and angiotensin II was intact (homologous desensitization). Additionally, radioligand binding studies showed that the α_1-adrenergic receptor number decreased 36 percent in mesenteric artery plasma membrane for these rats, whereas α_2-adrenergic receptor number was unaltered. It has also been reported that fat cells from patients with pheochromocytoma are relatively resistant to β-adrenergic stimulation of lypolysis [130]. In addition, the ability of agonists to stimulate cyclic adenosine monophosphate (AMP) production in lymphocytes from patients with pheochromocytoma is blunted [81]. In rats with pheochromocytoma, selective down-regulation of β_1-receptors has been shown in the heart, lungs, kidneys, and fat cells [131, 152]. The decline in β_1-receptors in fat cells is accompanied by a decreased cyclic AMP response to stimulation by isoproterenol [131].

NEURAL REGULATION OF BLOOD PRESSURE

It has always been assumed that in pheochromocytoma an increase in sympathetic nerve activity would be depressed reflexly due to the high circulating catecholamines. However, there is both clinical and experimental evidence suggesting that the sympathetic nervous

Fig. 56-13. Relationship of the height of arterial blood pressure to circulating plasma catecholamines in pheochromocytoma. (From E. L. Bravo, et al. Circulating and urinary catecholamines in pheochromocytoma: Diagnostic and pathophysiologic implications. *N. Engl. J. Med.* 301:682, 1979.)

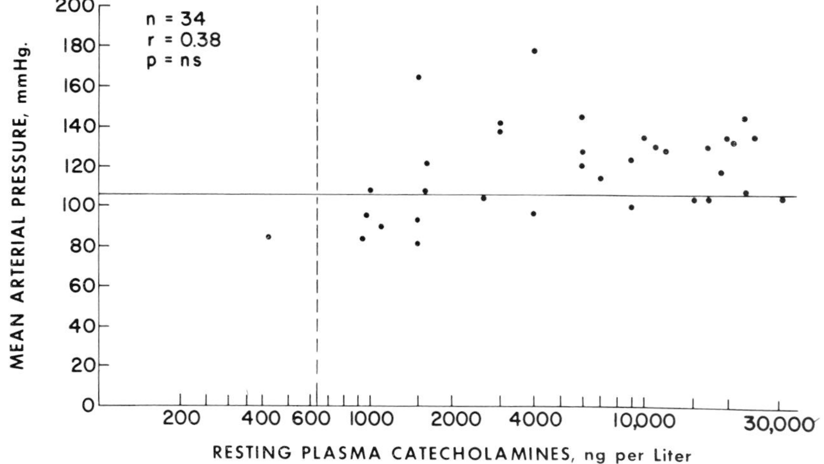

system may play a significant role in the maintenance of hypertension in patients with pheochromocytoma. Informative clinical data in this regard come from studies of the effects of orally administered clonidine in patients with either essential hypertension or pheochromocytoma [30]. Clonidine is a centrally-acting α_2-agonist that inhibits neurally mediated catecholamine release. Clonidine decreases blood pressure in both essential hypertension and pheochromocytoma patients to the same degree. These results suggest that the sympathetic nervous system is intact in pheochromocytoma. In essential hypertension, the fall in blood pressure is associated with decreases in circulating catecholamines, but in pheochromocytoma there is no change in plasma catecholamine levels (Fig. 56-14). The demonstration that blood pressure in pheochromocytoma was lowered despite high levels of circulating catecholamines suggests that the norepinephrine released from axon terminals of sympathetic postganglionic neurons is biologically more significant than circulating catecholamines. This difference could be related to the easier access of norepinephrine released from preganglionic neurons to its effector site at effector cells.

Neural control of blood pressure has also been demonstrated in rats harboring pheochromocytoma. Eliminating sympathetic nerve activity by pithing caused a greater reduction of blood pressure in pheochromocytoma-bearing rats than in age-matched, unimplanted rats [151]. Additionally, Prokocimer and co-workers [119] found that both clonidine and chlorisondamine, a ganglion blocker, markedly decreased blood pressure in intact rats with pheochromocytoma. However, the observation that the blood pressure in pithed pheochromocytoma rats is further reduced by phentolamine, an α-adrenergic antagonist, suggests that high concentration of circulating catecholamines are also involved in the maintenance of the elevated blood pressure.

Thus, the hypertension in pheochromocytoma is a complex process influenced by both the sympathetic nervous system and circulating catecholamines, as well as alterations in cardiovascular responses to catecholamines.

Clinical Recognition

SIGNS AND SYMPTOMS

The detection of pheochromocytoma requires a high degree of clinical alertness. Patients come to the clinician in a variety of settings. They may arrive at the emergency room with a transient ischemic attack or even completed stroke or with a surgical abdomen. They may present with accelerated or malignant hypertension or with the signs and symptoms of diabetes mellitus, hyperthyroidism, hypercalcemia, congestive heart failure, myocardial infarction, or shock. They may have classic attacks characterized by diaphoresis, tachycardia, and headaches, or they may have the identical clinical and physical findings of patients with the syndrome of β-adrenergic hyperresponsiveness.

Elevation of blood pressure is the most consistent manifestation of this disorder. Sustained hypertension occurs in about half of all patients, and paroxysmal episodes of hypertension in about a third. Approximately a fifth have no hypertension at all. Most patients are symptomatic and some dramatically so. The most common symptoms include headache, which is characteristically, but not always, pounding and severe; palpitations with or without tachycardia; and excessive and inappropriate perspiration. In a series of 76 patients with pheochromocytoma, all but 3 had one or more of these three symptoms and 55 had at least two [75]. In a

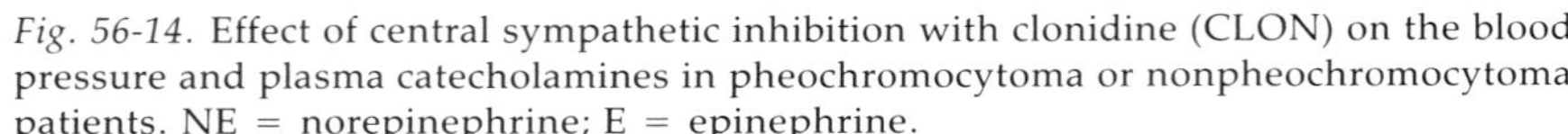
Fig. 56-14. Effect of central sympathetic inhibition with clonidine (CLON) on the blood pressure and plasma catecholamines in pheochromocytoma or nonpheochromocytoma patients. NE = norepinephrine; E = epinephrine.

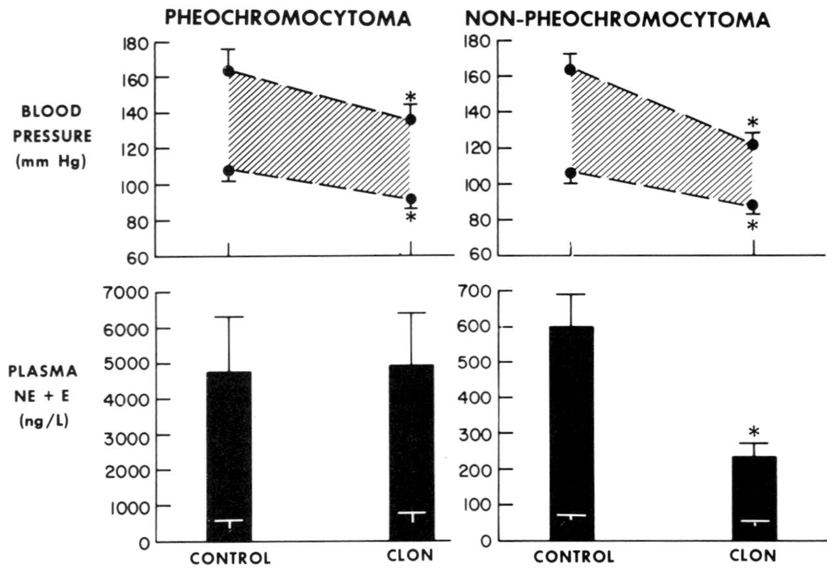

recent report the symptomatic triad of sweating attacks, tachycardia, and headaches in a hypertensive patient was found to have a specificity of 93.8 percent, a sensitivity of 90.9 percent, and an exclusion value of 99.9 percent in the diagnosis of pheochromocytoma [118].

Postural hypotension occurs in 50 to 75 percent of patients. Its occurrence has been ascribed to several mechanisms: decreased plasma volume [129], norepinephrine metabolites acting as false neurotransmitters, decreased adrenergic receptor sensitivity, or release of vasodilator substances [47]. Glucose intolerance may be present and is probably related to catecholamine-induced suppression of insulin release [85]. The glucose intolerance is reversed by pharmacologic blockade of α-adrenergic receptor and remits with removal of the tumor. Patients with epinephrine-secreting pheochromocytomas may present with supine hypotension [116]. Severe cardiomyopathies have been reported. Recent studies suggest that norepinephrine-secreting tumors tend to be associated with hypertrophic cardiomyopathy, whereas epinephrine-secreting tumors produce congestive cardiomyopathy [44].

Less commonly encountered symptoms include anxiety, tremors, pallor, nausea, weakness, exhaustion, fatigue, chest or abdominal pain, and weight loss. Obesity and flushing are rarely associated with pheochromocytoma.

Finally, certain prescribed drugs may precipitate a hypertensive crisis in the presence of pheochromocytoma. These include tricyclic antidepressants, imipramine and desipramine [2], antidopaminergic agents, sulpiride and metoclopramide [3], and naloxone [21].

ASSOCIATED CLINICAL SYNDROMES

Pheochromocytoma usually occurs as a sporadic event in patients without related disease. However, there are well-documented associations occurring in several family members: (1) von Recklinghausen's neurofibromatosis, (2) von Hippel-Lindau's disease (angiomata of the retina with cystic hemangioblastoma of the cerebellum), (3) Werner's syndrome or multiple endocrine adenomatosis (MEN) type I (hyperparathyroidism, pancreatic tumors secreting gastrin, insulin, glucagon, or vasoactive intestinal peptide [VIP] and pituitary tumors), (4) Sipple's syndrome or MEN type IIA (bilateral adrenal tumors, medullary carcinoma of the thyroid, and hyperparathyroidism), (5) mucocutaneous neuromas with bilateral adrenal tumors, medullary carcinoma of the thyroid, and glanglioneuromas of the visceral autonomic plexuses (MEN type IIB). There have also been reports of pheochromocytoma associated with acromegaly [93] or with Cushing's syndrome (pheochromocytoma secreting excessive amounts of ACTH) [66].

CLINICAL SETTINGS LIKELY TO BE CONFUSED WITH PHEOCHROMOCYTOMA

Unrelated disorders that are likely to be confused with pheochromocytoma are listed in Table 56-3. Clonidine withdrawal is associated with marked hypertension and plasma catecholamine concentrations and urinary catecholamine metabolite values that approximate those found in pheochromocytoma. Another condition that may mimic the signs and symptoms associated with pheochromocytoma occurs when patients receiving a monoamine oxidase inhibitor ingest tyramine, ephedrine, or amphetamine. Any of these substances can release the rich stores of norepinephrine in postganglionic sympathetic neurons that accumulate with chronic inhibition of monoamine oxidase. Some foods (pickled herring, chicken livers, aged cheese, especially cheddar) and certain beverages (Chianti wine and foreign beers) contain enough tyramine to trigger such a reaction. Factitious self-administration of sympathomimetic agents can also mimic pheochromocytoma symptomatically and biochemically. A history of drug ingestion and the circumstances under which the crisis occurs should provide clues for the proper diagnosis. Moreover, catecholamines and their urinary metabolites should return to normal within 24 to 48 hours after a crisis and should remain normal thereafter. Other than acute hypoglycemia [43] and vasodilator therapy with minoxidil, none of the other conditions listed are associated with catecholamine values in plasma or urine that approximate those observed in pheochromocytoma.

Prevalence of Undiagnosed Pheochromocytoma

The many ways in which a pheochromocytoma can manifest explain why many tumors are often missed. In a series from the Mayo Clinic [145], 76 percent of the 54

Table 56-3. Clinical settings likely to be confused with pheochromocytoma

β-Adrenergic hyperresponsiveness	Acute drug withdrawal
Acute state of anxiety	Clonidine
Angina pectoris	β-Adrenergic blockade
Acute infections	α-Methyldopa
Autonomic epilepsy	Alcohol
Hyperthyroidism	Vasodilator therapy
Idiopathic orthostatic hypotension	Hydralazine
Cerebellopontine angle tumors	Minoxidil
Acute hypoglycemia	Factitious administration of sympathomimetic agents
	Tyramine ingestion in patients on monoamine oxidase (MAO) inhibitors
	Menopausal syndrome with migraine headaches

autopsy-proven cases were clinically unsuspected during life. Only 17 percent were correctly diagnosed before death; 7 percent were incidentally discovered at laparotomy for unrelated conditions. Of those diagnosed after death, only 54 percent had hypertension and headaches (27%); diaphoresis (17%) and palpitations (17%) were less common compared to those whose disease was diagnosed before death. Twelve patients were over 68 years old; in 9 of these elderly patients the clinical diagnosis was unsuspected. A retrospective study from Australia [86] showed that of 46 proven cases, 29 (63%) were diagnosed and treated during life, while 17 (37%) were diagnosed at autopsy. Of the latter, 7 were found incidentally at post mortem, and most were found in patients 60 years or older. Stenstrom and co-workers [136] reviewed their experience in 439 patients with pheochromocytoma registered in Sweden from 1958 to 1981. The incidence of pheochromocytoma increased continuously with advancing age for both men and women. In 40 percent of all patients, the diagnosis was made at autopsy. Pheochromocytoma was an incidental finding in 14 percent of the series. The overall average age at diagnosis was 56 years, but it was significantly lower (48.5 years old) in those with clinically diagnosed disease compared to those diagnosed at autopsy, whose mean age was 65.8 years. Of the older age group, pheochromocytoma was an incidental finding in 33 percent. Similarly, Krane [96], reporting on experience at the Henry Ford Hospital, found that of 32 patients with pathologically confirmed tumors, 11 (34%) of them had tumors that were clinically unsuspected. Of these, 9 patients were considered asymptomatic during their lifetimes.

These observations indicate that a large number of patients with pheochromocytoma may present with relatively minor signs and symptoms. In addition, the elderly patient appears to present a special diagnostic dilemma. A contributory factor to the rarity of the antemortem diagnosis of pheochromocytoma in the elderly may be a decrease in sensitivity to catecholamines with age. Additionally, most elderly patients have concomitant diseases whose signs and symptoms may detract from the diagnosis of pheochromocytoma. For example, cardiac and neurologic symptoms may be attributed to coronary artery and cerebrovascular disease from atherosclerosis. Of note is that acute ischemic heart disease and stroke (from any etiology) are associated with high circulating catecholamines, which may confuse the diagnosis of pheochromocytoma.

Diagnostic Considerations

The diagnosis of pheochromocytoma is usually suspected on the basis of clinical manifestations, but the definitive diagnosis rests primarily on laboratory test results. In the ensuing discussion, a brief survey of the biochemistry and metabolism of catecholamines and the biochemical and pathophysiologic characteristics of pheochromocytoma will be described, thereby laying the foundation on which the rationale and limitations of the diagnostic procedures are based.

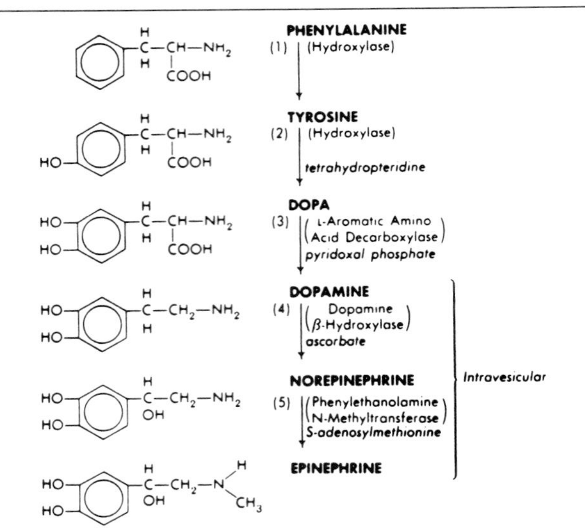

Fig. 56-15. Steps involved in the biosynthesis of norepinephrine and epinephrine. (From S. E. Mayer, *The Pharmacological Basis of Therapeutics* [6th ed.]. New York: McGraw-Hill, 1980.)

BIOCHEMISTRY OF CATECHOLAMINES

The catecholamines are the products of the amino acid tyrosine (Fig. 56-15). The initial step in the sequence is the hydroxylation of tyrosine to L-dopa by the action of the rate-limiting enzyme tyrosine hydroxylase. The next step in synthesis is conversion of L-dopa to dopamine. When hydroxylated, dopamine yields the sympathetic neurotransmitter norepinephrine. This reaction is catalyzed by dopamine-β-hydroxylase (DBH). As norepinephrine is released by sympathetic neural transmission, a small amount of DBH is also released and reaches the systemic circulation [108].

All of the preceding steps from tyrosine to norepinephrine take place within adrenergic neurons. However, in the adrenal medullary chromaffin cell, an additional step occurs: the conversion of norepinephrine to epinephrine. The enzyme phenylethanolamine-*N*-methyltransferase (PNMT) catalyzes this step. In a normal adrenal medulla the concentration of epinephrine is about four times that of norepinephrine, and the same ratio is found in the adrenal venous effluent. Thus the principal secretion of a normal adrenal medulla is epinephrine [43]. *The epinephrine fraction of normal adrenal vein blood ranges from 54.3 to 83.3 percent. The epinephrine fraction from adrenal veins draining pheochromocytomas is 9.3 to 47.7 percent* [64].

The catecholamines are metabolized principally by two enzymes (Fig. 56-16): monoamine oxidase (MAO) and catechol-O-methyltransferase (COMT). MAO is found within adrenergic neurons and in several nonneural tissues. COMT is localized for the most part in nonneural tissues. The action of COMT leads to the formation of metanephrines, the methylated metabolites of norepinephrine and epinephrine. The combined O-methylation by COMT and oxidation of the amines by

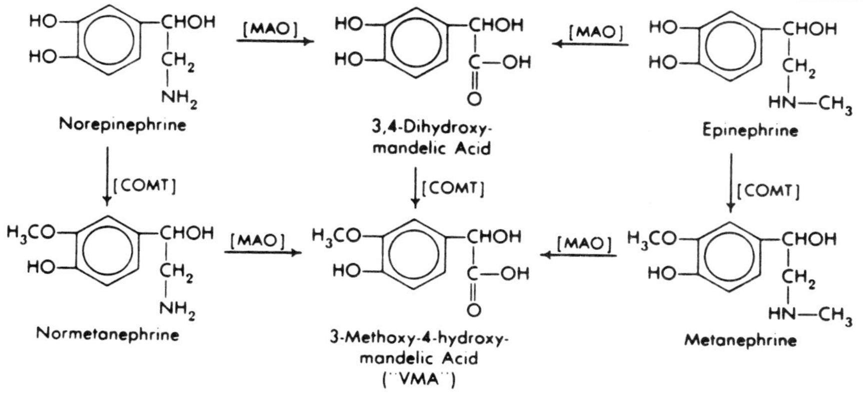

Fig. 56-16. Metabolism of norepinephrine and epinephrine. COMT = catechol-O-methyltransferase; MAO = monoamine oxidase. (Modified from S. E. Mayer, *The Pharmacological Basis of Therapeutics* [6th ed.]. New York: McGraw-Hill, 1980.)

MAO results in the formation of vanillylmandelic acid (VMA). The major metabolites of the catecholamines, the metanephrines and VMA, are the major excretory products in urine and are commonly assayed to assess sympthoadrenomedullary activity [76].

In the plasma of normal subjects, norepinephrine concentration is about 8 to 10 times that of epinephrine. The overflow of norepinephrine released from adrenergic nerve endings accounts for most of the circulating norepinephrine. Adrenomedullary secretion of catecholamines accounts for all of the circulating epinephrine but only 2 percent of circulating norepinephrine [34].

Norepinephrine released from peripheral sympathetic nerves diffuses across the synaptic cleft between the nerve ending and the effector cell, where it interacts with specific adrenergic receptors and initiates a series of biochemical events ultimately resulting in a characteristic biologic response. The major portion of released norepinephrine never reaches the effector cell but is retaken up into the axon terminals. Much of the norepinephrine transported to the effector cell is catabolized to normetanephrine by COMT, the dominant degradative mechanism outside the neuron. Only a very small fraction of locally released norepinephrine escapes the recapture mechanism and diffuses into the circulation as free unconjugated norepinephrine, where it would be reflected in a plasma norepinephrine level or indirectly by urinary catecholamine metabolites. From these physiologic mechanisms, it follows that (1) transport of norepinephrine via the circulation is not required to explain its actions, and (2) physiologically effective release of norepinephrine from axon terminals may be reflected in relatively small increments in plasma norepinephrine concentrations. Thus in the immediate postdischarge period, a steep norepinephrine concentration gradient exists from the synaptic cleft to the plasma. From this it also follows that the cleft concentration required to produce biologic effects is much greater than the plasma norepinephrine concentration and that if sufficient norepinephrine were either released (as in pheochromocytoma) or exogenously introduced into the circulation to produce biologically active cleft norepinephrine concentration, plasma norepinephrine concentrations would be expected to be substantially higher than normal plasma norepinephrine levels.

BIOCHEMISTRY OF PHEOCHROMOCYTOMA

In pheochromocytoma the activities of the enzymes involved in catecholamine synthesis (tyrosine hydroxylase, aromatic amino acid decarboxylase, and DBH) are markedly enhanced, whereas the activities of the enzymes involved in catecholamine catabolism (MAO and COMT) are reduced [90]. Thus excess amounts of newly synthesized norepinephrine that cannot be stored in the filled catecholamine storage vesicles may not be degraded and could diffuse from the pheochromocytoma into the circulation. This could result in large amounts of circulating norepinephrine with relatively small increases in urinary catecholamine metabolites.

Crout and Sjoerdsma [41] have also demonstrated that the size of the tumor might be an important determinant of the relative amounts of catecholamine excretory products. They reported that small tumors weighing less than 50 gm have rapid turnover rates with small catecholamine content. These tumors release mainly unmetabolized catecholamines into the circulation as reflected by a relatively low ratio of concentrations of metabolites to free catecholamines in the urine. On the other hand, large tumors weighing more than 50 gm have slow turnover rates with large catecholamine content. These tumors release mainly metabolized catecholamines into the circulation as deduced by a relatively high ratio of metabolites to free catecholamines in the urine. Tumors classified in the small tumor group had a mean rate of catecholamine turnover that was eight times greater than that of the tumors in the large tumor group. The classification of pheochromocytomas into small tumors with rapid catecholamine turnover rates and large tumors with slow catecholamine turnover rates is graphically illustrated in Fig. 56-17. These observations may

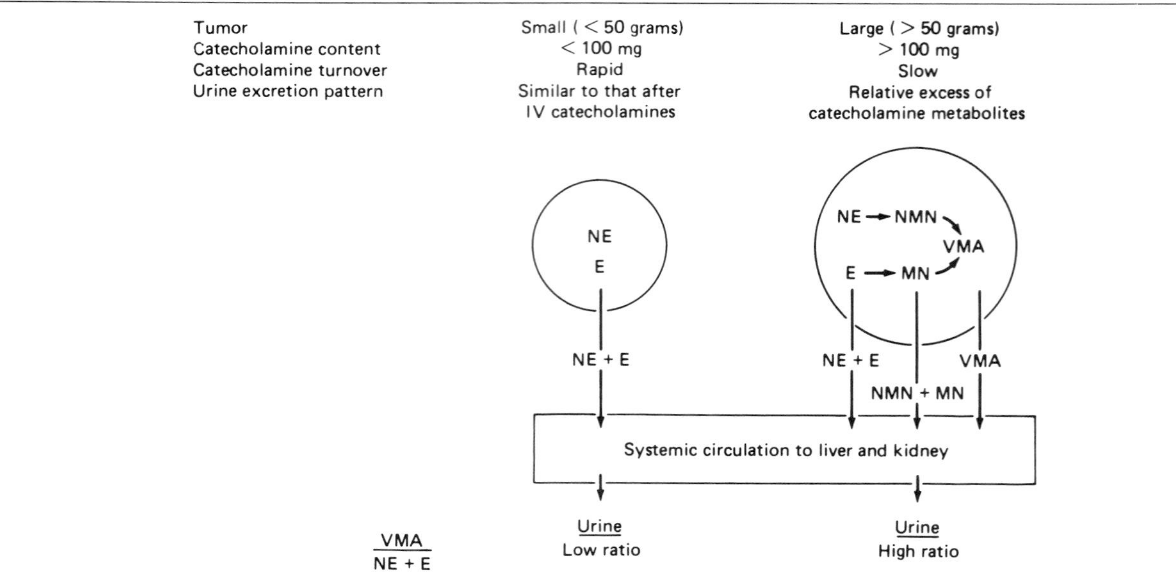

Fig. 56-17. Relationship of tumor size to catecholamine excretory products in urine (see text for explanation). NE = norepinephrine; E = epinephrine; NMN = normetanephrines; MN = metanephrines; VMA = vanillylmandelic acid. (From J. R. Crout, et al. Turnover and metabolism of catecholamine in patients with pheochromocytoma. *J. Clin. Invest.* 43:94, 1964.)

have important diagnostic implications. Small tumors, since they release free unmetabolized catecholamines into the circulation, may tend to produce more symptoms and are best diagnosed by the measurement of plasma catecholamines. On the other hand, patients who have large tumors that metabolize most of the secreted catecholamines tend to have less symptoms, have relatively lower circulating free catecholamines, but high urinary catecholamine metabolites.

PATHOPHYSIOLOGIC CORRELATIONS

It is reasonable to assume that the sympathetic nerve terminals in patients with pheochromocytoma have accumulated excessive stores of catecholamines such as occurs in patients receiving norepinephrine infusion [98]. In addition, the easier access of norepinephrine released from the postganglionic neurons to its receptor site at effector cells can result in marked symptoms with relatively small increments in circulating norepinephrine. Therefore, any direct or reflexly mediated stimulus to the sympathetic nervous system could release excessive quantities of catecholamines into the synaptic cleft and produce a hypertensive crisis. These observations have important clinical implications. They can account not only for the observation that spontaneous or evoked rises in blood pressure (pain, hyperventilation, anesthesia) can occur without detectable increases in plasma catecholamines but also for the demonstration that blood pressure may be normal despite high circulating levels of catecholamines. Those patients with a pheochromocytoma who are tested at a time when their blood pressure is increased invariably have striking elevations of plasma norepinephrine concentrations. Normal or even moderately elevated levels in the face of hypertension exclude this diagnosis. However, normal plasma catecholamine levels in a normotensive patient do not exclude the diagnosis, since in some cases there is true intermittent secretion by the tumor.

Biochemical Diagnostic Tests

PLASMA CATECHOLAMINES

Clinically, the term *catecholamines* is usually used to refer to norepinephrine and epinephrine. Three assay methods for determination of plasma catecholamine levels are commercially available today. The isotope derivative (or radioenzymatic) method utilizes enzymatic conversion of catecholamines to tritium-labeled O-methyl derivatives, metanephrine and normetanephrine, by COMT, followed by extensive purification of the derivatives by thin layer chromatography [117]. This assay is sensitive to 5.0 pg per 50 μl of plasma for either catecholamine and is highly reproducible. Although technically demanding, it has been used extensively in research and clinical studies. A second method employs high pressure liquid chromatography to separate the catecholamines in a plasma extract, with measurement by electrochemical detection [80]. Results from this assay correlate well with those of the radioenzymatic assay. Although less sensitive, it is acceptable for clinical applications. A third method is a radioimmunoassay procedure that uses antiserum to metanephrine [120]. Only limited data comparing this method with the others are available.

Because of the lability of plasma catecholamines, rigidly controlled environmental conditions must be ensured during patient sampling and subsequent storage of samples. Basal levels are preferably drawn by means of an indwelling 21-gauge butterfly needle and kept patent with heparinized saline following an overnight fast and 20 minutes of supine rest. No coffee, tea, or smoking should be allowed for at least 3 hours prior to testing.

Heparin and 10 percent acid-citric-dextrose (ACD) are equally useful as anticoagulants. No loss of norepinephrine occurs when freshly drawn blood is immediately diluted with 10 percent ACD, or is heparinized, put on ice, and centrifuged at 4°C within 1 hour. Plasma stored at 20°C will lose 30 percent of the norepinephrine content after 6 months and 75 percent after 12 months compared with identical samples assayed on the day blood is drawn or stored at −70°C. If the plasma proteins are immediately precipitated with perchloric acid, the resultant acidic supernatant can be stored at −20°C without loss of norepinephrine.

Some drugs alter plasma norepinephrine concentrations. Drugs that inhibit central sympathetic outflow (e.g., clonidine, methyldopa, bromocriptine, haloperidol) decrease plasma catecholamines in normal and hypertensive subjects but have little effect on the excessive catecholamine secretion by pheochromocytoma. Drugs that tend to increase plasma catecholamines (e.g., phenoxybenzamine, phentolamine, prazosin, labetalol, theophylline, β-blockers, diuretics) do so only slightly and rarely approach values usually encountered in pheochromocytoma. There are, however, two drug-related clinical situations that could easily be confused with pheochromocytoma: (1) during sudden clonidine withdrawal, and (2) during vasodilator therapy, especially with minoxidil. In both situations, plasma catecholamines can rise to very high levels (> 2,000 pg per ml) and are usually associated with a hyperdynamic circulation.

In Fig. 56-18 are depicted plasma catecholamine levels in a group of patients with documented pheochromocytoma [25]. It is clear that the majority of patients with pheochromocytoma have markedly elevated plasma catecholamine levels that are far above those seen in other conditions. Four patients had values that fell within the upper 95 percent confidence limits for values obtained in patients with essential hypertension. None had values that fell within the range for age- and sex-matched normotensive subjects. Engelman et al. [57], Geffen and co-workers [71], Cryer [42], and Ball [9] reported consistently good results similar to ours. Plasma epinephrine is not as useful in differentiating extra-adrenal from adrenal pheochromocytoma as originally thought.

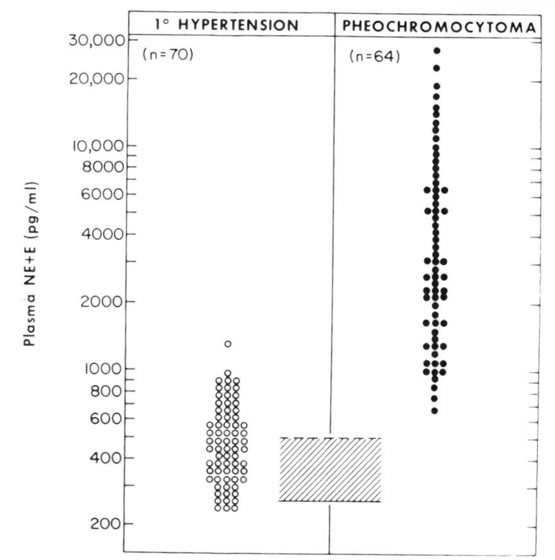

Fig. 56-18. Supine resting plasma catecholamine values in patients with essential hypertension or pheochromocytoma. The cross-hatched area represents the mean (260 pg/ml) + 2 S.D. (500 pg/ml) of values in 47 normotensive healthy adults with an age and sex distribution similar to that of the two patient groups. For subjects with essential hypertension the mean and + 2 S.D. is 516 and 950 pg per milliliter, respectively; 4 patients with pheochromocytoma had levels that fell within the range of values in patients with essential hypertension. NE + E denotes norepinephrine plus epinephrine. (From E. L. Bravo, and R. W. Gifford. Pheochromocytoma: Diagnosis, localization and management. *N. Engl. J. Med.* 311:1298, 1973.)

URINARY CATECHOLAMINE AND METABOLITES

The most useful urine tests are those that measure concentrations of metanephrines, VMA, and free (unconjugated) catecholamines. These tests have been compared in patients with confirmed pheochromocytoma and hypertensive patients without the tumor. Bravo and Gifford [25] showed that in 43 patients, the false-negative rates were 30 percent for urinary VMA and 10 percent for urinary metanephrines. Duncan and co-workers [53] reported in 25 patients a false-negative rate of 0 percent for urinary free norepinephrine. Thus, assays of 24-hour urinary catecholamines and metanephrines are adequate to diagnose pheochromocytoma in most patients. However, 24-hour urine collections are difficult and cumbersome to obtain and hospitalization may even be required to ensure completeness, rigid dietary control, and proper collection. Such specimens are extraordinarily difficult to obtain in children. Some investigators have used "bracketed" 2- to 4-hour collections and overnight collections to obviate the need for 24-hour specimens [94, 143]. The results are expressed as concentrations of the metabolite per milligram of creatinine. It is claimed that these measurements are as accurate as those in 24-hour specimens for the diagnosis of pheochromocytoma.

Table 56-4 shows the effects of various drugs on simultaneously measured urinary catecholamine metabolites and plasma catecholamines. Of the three determinations, urinary VMA appears to be subject to the greatest error, urinary metanephrines next, and plasma catecholamines least.

Problems with urine collections and spurious results from drug or dietary interference aside, reliance on urinary determinations alone as indexes of catecholamine production can be misleading. In pheochromocytoma the amounts of excreted free catecholamines and their metabolites vary depending on the levels of synthesizing and metabolizing enzymes within the tumor [90]. Their amounts in urine also depend on the excretory

Table 56-4. Effect of various drugs in simultaneously measured plasma catecholamines and urinary catecholamine metabolites

Drugs	Plasma catecholamines	Urinary VMA	Urinary NMN + MN
X-ray contrast	No change	Decrease	Decrease
Nalidixic acid	No change	Increase	Decrease
Clofibrate	No change	No change	Decrease
Robaxin	No change	Increase	No change
Glyceryl guaiacolate	No change	Increase	No change
α-Methyldopa	Increase	No change	?
Labetalol	Increase	Increase	Increase

VMA = Vanillylmandelic acid; NMN = normetanephrines; MN = metanephrines.

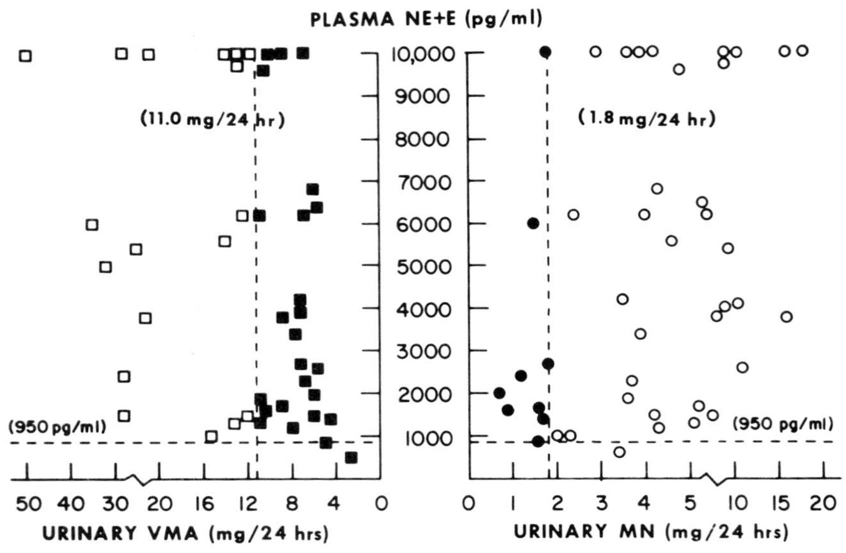

Fig. 56-19. Comparison of simultaneously measured indexes of catecholamine production in 43 patients with surgically confirmed pheochromocytoma. The horizontal broken lines represent the 95 percent upper confidence limits of values for urinary vanillylmandelic acid (VMA) (i.e., 11 mg/24 hr) and urinary metanephrines (MN), (i.e., 1.8 mg/24 hr) in 30 subjects with essential hypertension. NE + E denotes norepinephrine plus epinephrine. Solid symbols denote false negative tests. (From E. L. Bravo, and R. W. Gifford. Pheochromocytoma: Diagnosis, localization and management. *N. Engl. J. Med.* 311:1298, 1984.)

function of the kidneys [8]. These factors may account for reported false-positive and false-negative test results in a number of studies [31, 46, 121, 125]. Fig. 56-19 shows the results of comparing simultaneously measured plasma catecholamines and urinary catecholamine metabolites in patients who had surgically confirmed pheochromocytoma [25]. Using measurements in patients with essential hypertension as reference values, it can be shown that 25 of the 43 patients had false-negative results for urinary vanillylmandelic acid. On the other hand, only 9 had false-negative results for urinary metanephrines. In 1 patient all three biochemical determinants were within the range of values in patients with essential hypertension. In 1 patient an elevated level of urinary metanephrines was the only biochemical abnormality, and in 3 the only abnormal result was an elevated level of plasma catecholamines. These findings are in accord with current indications that of the urinary indexes of catecholamine production, urinary metanephrines provide a more reliable clue to the presence of pheochromocytoma than either urinary vanillylmandelic acid or free catecholamines [76]. Furthermore, the results suggest that plasma catecholamine measurements are at least as reliable as the measurement of urinary metanephrines in predicting the presence of pheochromocytoma.

OTHER BIOCHEMICAL TESTS

Plasma chromogranin A concentration has been proposed as a diagnostic test for pheochromocytoma, the plasma levels of which are about tenfold higher than those found in other hypertensive patients [114]. Chromogranin A is a soluble protein contained in catecholamine storage vesicles. Since it is co-released with norepinephrine, its level in plasma reflects sympathoadrenal activity [161]. However, chromogranin A is also found in blood of patients with other neuroendocrine tumors [133].

Table 56-5. Sensitivity and specificity of various biochemical tests

Biochemical test	Standard	Sensitivity (% range)*	Specificity (% range)*
Plasma NE + E	> 950 pg/ml	88–100	93–101
Urinary NMN + MN	> 1.8 mg/24 hr	67–91	83–103
Urinary VMA	> 11.0 mg/24 hr	28–56	98–102

*Values are expressed as ± 2 SE. Upper 95 percent confidence limits obtained from essential hypertension subjects under basal conditions. NE + E = norepinephrine plus epinephrine; NMN + MN = normetanephrine plus metanephrine; VMA = vanillylmandelic acid.

Table 56-6. Catecholamine values in normotensive and hypertensive subjects

Biochemical measurements	Normotensive subjects	Hypertensive subjects
Plasma norepinephrine	218 ± 92 pg/ml*	425 ± 193 pg/ml*
Plasma epinephrine	42 ± 18 pg/ml*	59 ± 38 pg/ml*
Urinary VMA	< 6.8 mg/24 hr	< 11.0 mg/24 hr
Urinary NMN + MN	< 1.3 mg/24 hr	< 1.8 mg/24 hr
Urinary catecholamines	< 100 μg/24 hr	< 156 μg/24 hr

*Values are mean ± 1 SD. VMA = Vanillylmandelic acid; NMN = normetanephrines; MN = metanephrines.

Platelets concentrate catecholamines [1], and patients with pheochromocytoma have increased platelet norepinephrine and epinephrine content. Zweifler and Julius [167] have suggested that platelet catecholamine content might discriminate patients with pheochromocytoma from other hypertensives. However, a recent study [13] showed that the usefulness of platelet catecholamine in the diagnosis of pheochromocytoma is limited because of the high false-positive rates—35.5 percent for platelet norepinephrine and 19.4 percent for platelet epinephrine.

The simultaneous measurement of urinary norepinephrine and 3,4-dihydroxyphenylglycol (DHPG) has been proposed as a means of increasing the specificity of urine testing. Norepinephrine that is released by neurons is retaken up and converted to DHPG [79]. Therefore, DHPG levels reflect the extent of neuronal traffic. In patients with pheochromocytoma, however, norepinephrine is released directly into the circulation and results in higher ratios of norepinephrine/DHPG than observed in other hypertensives [33]. However, measuring free norepinephrine in urine has been shown to be as accurate as the norepinephrine/DHPG ratio [53].

SENSITIVITY AND SPECIFICITY OF VARIOUS BIOCHEMICAL TESTS

On the basis of the author's experience the sensitivity and specificity of various biochemical tests to detect pheochromocytoma are as follows (Table 56-5): Measurement of plasma catecholamines appears to have the highest sensitivity, and measurement of urinary vanillylmandelic acid the lowest. However, when values are elevated, all three tests provide excellent specificity. It must be kept in mind that some methods for the measurement of urinary vanillylmandelic acid are notoriously nonspecific.

Debate about the relative merits of these various tests will continue. It seems likely that if reliably carried out, one test will serve as well as another provided that the investigator is aware of the limitations and pitfalls of some of the methods of analysis. However, because the metabolism of catecholamines in patients with pheochromocytoma may be modified by either a lack or excess of metabolizing enzymes, both plasma catecholamines and catecholamine metabolites in urine should be measured in equivocal cases. Finally, it must be emphasized that the reliable diagnosis of pheochromocytoma is ultimately based on careful biochemical studies in an appropriate clinical setting. Table 56-6 refers to catecholamine values in normotensive and hypertensive subjects.

Pharmacologic Diagnostic Tests

The diagnostic dilemma in the workup of pheochromocytoma is to separate pheochromocytoma patients with relatively low levels of synthetic activity from nonpheochromocytoma patients with secondarily activated sympathetic nervous systems. Pharmacologic tests are designed to either provoke secretion by a pheochromocytoma or to suppress excessive activity of the sympathetic nervous system. A provocative test is usually employed when the clinical findings are highly suggestive of pheochromocytoma but the blood pressure is normal or only slightly increased (BP ≥ 160/100 mm Hg) and catecholamine production is nearly normal. In patients with moderate increases in catecholamines (between 1,000 and 2,000 pg/ml) with or without hypertension, a suppression test is employed.

The *glucagon stimulation* test [98] is widely used as a provocative agent because it has fewer side effects. Glucagon is given as an intravenous bolus dose of 1.0 to 2.0 mg after determination of the patient's pressor response to a cold pressor test. A positive glucagon test requires a clear increase (at least threefold or over 2,000 pg/ml) in plasma catecholamines, 1 to 3 minutes after drug administration (Fig. 56-20). A simultaneous increase in blood pressure of at least 20/15 mm Hg above the pressor response to a cold pressor test is desirable but not essential.

The *clonidine suppression test* [29] uses the ability of clonidine, a centrally acting α-adrenergic agonist, to suppress the release of neurogenically mediated catecholamine release. The test is based on the principle that normal increases in plasma catecholamines are mediated through activation of the sympathetic nervous system, whereas in patients with pheochromocytoma, the increases result from diffusion of excess catecholamines from the tumor into the circulation, bypassing normal storage and release mechanisms. Therefore, clonidine should not be expected to suppress the release of catecholamines in patients with pheochromocytoma. This expectation was borne out by earlier studies; plasma catecholamines in patients with essential hypertension were suppressed with clonidine, whereas they were unaltered in subjects with pheochromocytoma.

Fig. 56-21 shows the results of the clonidine suppression test in 32 patients with proven pheochromocytoma. The results were compared with those in 70 sex- and age-matched subjects with essential hypertension. Of the 32 patients, 21 had adrenal pheochromocytoma and 11 had extraadrenal pheochromocytoma. After clonidine had been administered, plasma catecholamine values fell below 500 pg per milliliter in all but one hypertensive patient. All but one patient with pheochromocytoma had plasma catecholamine values above 500 pg per milliliter. Based on this experience, a normal clonidine suppression test should consist of a fall in the basal values of plasma norepinephrine plus epinephrine to a level below 500 pg per milliliter or 3 hours after the oral administration of 0.3 mg of clonidine.

Since clonidine exerts its antihypertensive action by inhibiting central sympathetic outflow, it reduces blood pressure in both patients with essential hypertension and those with pheochromocytoma (refer to Fig. 56-14). Thus a potential hazard during the performance of the test is hypotension. Experience with the test over the years indicates that in the untreated patient, symptomatic hypotension is not a problem. All cases of severe hypotension requiring treatment have occurred in patients who were receiving antihypertensive medications or had other conditions that would tend to augment the effects of any antihypertensive agent [35, 77]. In particular, marked volume depletion should be avoided, and any β-adrenergic blocking agent should be discontinued about 48 hours before test performance. Since clonidine has a potent vagotonic effect, concomitant β-adrenergic blockade could lead to marked bradycardia, with further decreases in stroke volume and cardiac output resulting in severe hypotension.

Certain pitfalls must be avoided when performing the clonidine suppression test. Beta-adrenergic blockers can prevent the plasma catecholamine-lowering effect of clonidine in a patient without pheochromocytoma because of the ability of such agents to interfere with hepatic clearance of catecholamines [58]. Radioimmunoassays that measure both free and conjugated catecholamines give false-positive results [5]. Circulating conjugated catecholamines have a long half-life that is influenced by even moderate degrees of renal dysfunction. Therefore, during the clonidine suppression test, the measured levels of plasma catecholamines remain high, giving a false-positive result. For this reason, only assays that measure free catecholamines should be used; the radioenzymatic

Fig. 56-20. The glucagon stimulation test in pheochromocytoma. Three patients had no increases in blood pressure despite marked increases in simultaneously measured plasma catecholamine levels. NE + E denotes norepinephrine plus epinephrine. (From E. L. Bravo and R. W. Gifford. Pheochromocytoma: Diagnosis, localization and management. *N. Engl. J. Med.* 311:1298, 1984.)

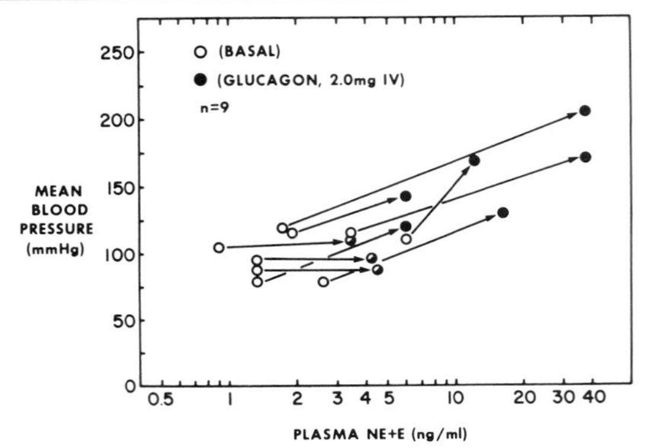

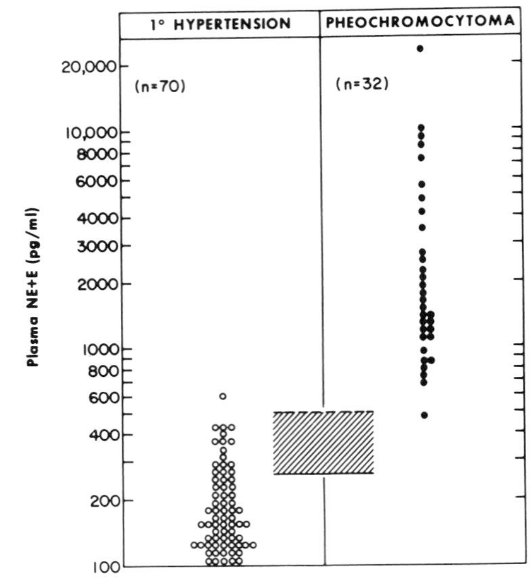

Fig. 56-21. The clonidine suppression test in essential hypertension or pheochromocytoma. Values shown represent the lowest values reached (at either 2 or 3 hours) after administration of 0.3 mg oral clonidine. The cross-hatched area represents the mean + 2 S.D. of basal values in normotensive control subjects. NE + E denotes norepinephrine plus epinephrine. (From E. L. Bravo and R. W. Gifford. Pheochromocytoma: Diagnosis, localization and management. *N. Engl. J. Med.* 311:1298, 1973.)

assay with catechol-O-methyltransferase is recommended because it measures both free norepinephrine and epinephrine with precision.

Pentolinium, 2.5 mg given intravenously, has been used by Brown and co-workers [34] to detect small pheochromocytomas in patients. They found that the plasma epinephrine concentration, which was invariably increased in these patients, was not suppressed by pentolinium administration. However, this drug, which can produce acute urinary retention in susceptible persons, is not available in the United States.

Preoperative Localization of Pheochromocytoma

Once the diagnosis has been confirmed, anatomic localization is mandatory. Fig. 56-22 depicts the frequency with which this tumor appears in various sites. Ninety-seven percent are found in the abdominal region. Less likely sites are the thorax (2 to 3 percent) and the neck (1 percent). The majority are found in the adrenal glands. Multiple tumors may arise in 10 percent of adults. Familial pheochromocytomas are frequently bilateral or arise from multiple sites. Pheochromocytomas occurring in children are more commonly bilateral and more frequently lie outside the adrenal than in adults.

Tumor localization not only serves to confirm the diagnosis of pheochromocytoma but also assists the surgeon in planning the surgical strategy. Advances in noninvasive imaging techniques now provide safe and reliable means of localizing pheochromocytomas anywhere in the body. *Computed tomographic (CT) scanning* is the most widely applied and accepted modality for the anatomic localization of pheochromocytoma [78]; it appears to detect tumors larger than 1.0 cm accurately (Fig. 56-23) and has a localizing precision of about 96 percent [138]. The tumor size lends itself to visualization in virtually every instance in which the tumor is in the adre-

Fig. 56-22. Possible sites of pheochromocytoma.

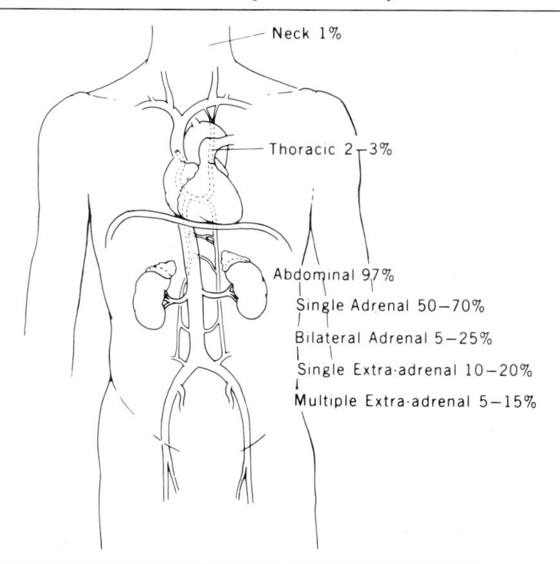

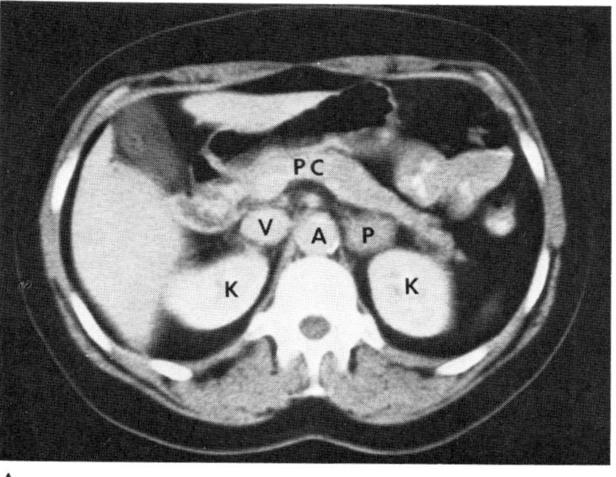

A

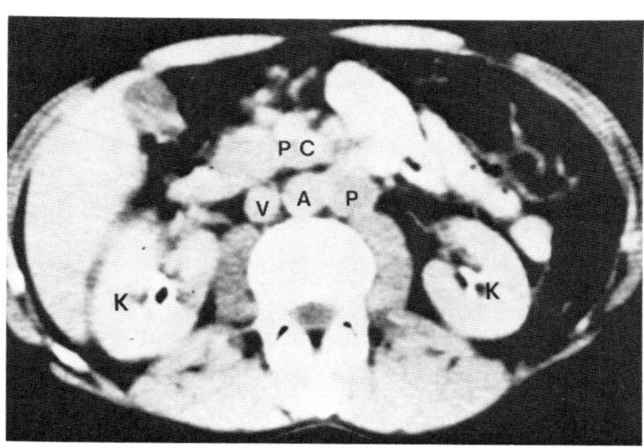

B

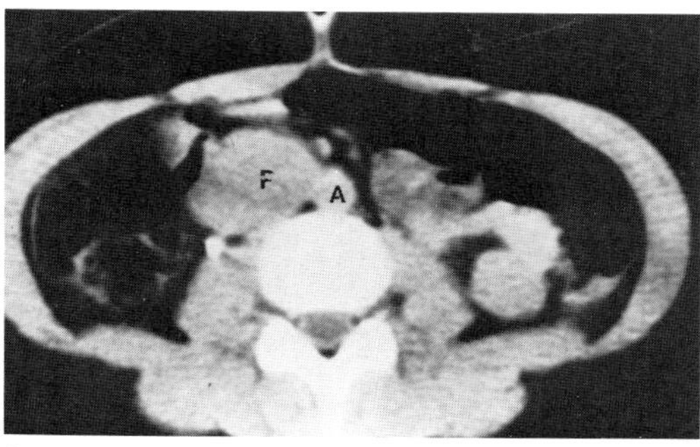

C

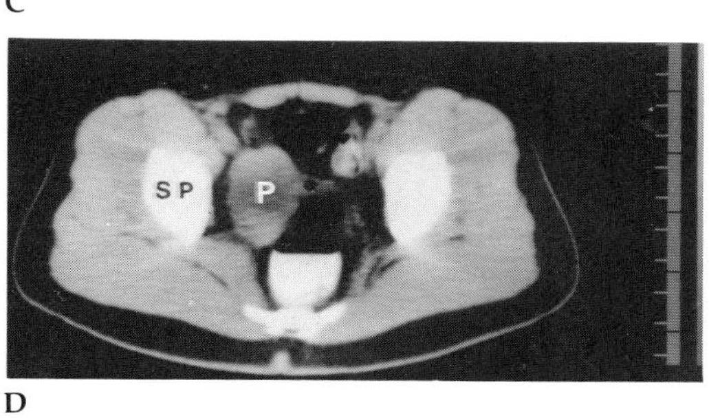

D

Fig. 56-23. Localization of pheochromocytoma by computed tomographic scan. A. Left adrenal pheochromocytoma. B. Paraaortic extraadrenal pheochromocytoma. C. Pelvic pheochromocytoma. D. Urinary bladder pheochromocytoma.

nal gland. *Magnetic resonance imaging (MRI)* is an alternative to CT scanning in the detection and localization of pheochromocytoma [63]. MRI has several advantages over CT scanning. First, it is a nonionizing imaging technique, and therefore, there is no radiation exposure. It is the procedure of choice in pregnant women (because it poses no danger to the fetus) and in patients with surgical clips that interfere with CT. Second, it allows the presentation of cross-sectional anatomy in transaxial, coronal, and sagittal planes with equal resolution (Fig. 56-24). Third, it has the capacity to differentiate tumor masses from surrounding vascular tissues, eliminating the need to administer contrast material intravenously. Fourth, it lends itself to in vivo tissue characterization; pheochromocytomas demonstrate high signal intensity on T-2 weighted image, unlike a benign tumor, which has a low signal intensity [52, 63]. *Scintigraphic localization with radioiodinated* ^{131}*I-metaiodobenzylguanidine (MIBG)* provides both anatomic and functional characterization of a tumor [127] (Fig. 56-25). MIBG is actively concentrated in sympathomedullary tissue through the catecholamine pump, and the administration of drugs that block the reuptake mechanism may therefore result in false-negative tests. Tricyclic antidepressants, guanethidine, and labetolol may interfere with the test. Phenoxybenzamine, prazosin, propranolol, and calcium antagonists do not interfere with MIBG uptake.

A comparison of the three imaging techniques is shown in Table 56-7. This was a prospective study involving 109 patients suspected of having a pheochro-

Fig. 56-24. Localization of pheochromocytoma by MRI. Images are from the same patients. A. Coronal MRI scan of the abdomen. L = liver; St = stomach; Sp = spleen; T = tumor; k = kidneys. B. Transverse abdominal T-1 weighted MRI scan of the abdomen. L = liver; V = inferior vena cava; A = aorta; St = stomach; Sp = spleen; T = tumor. Adjacent vascular structures are depicted. The tumor is isointensive relative to the liver. C. Transverse abdominal T-2 weighted MRI scan of the abdomen. L = liver; V = inferior vena cava; A = aorta; T = tumor; Sp = spleen. The tumor is hyperintense to the liver.

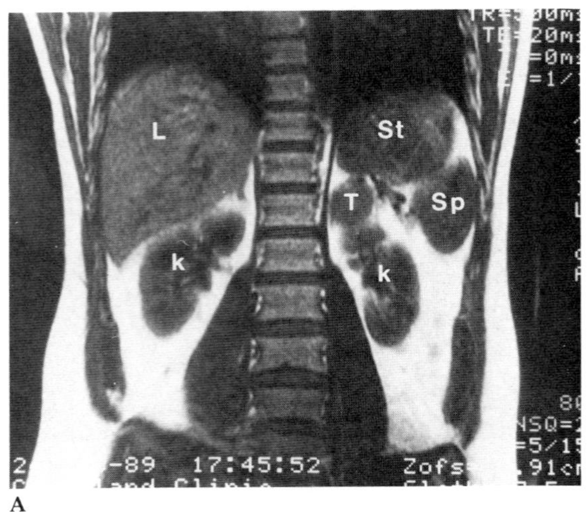

A

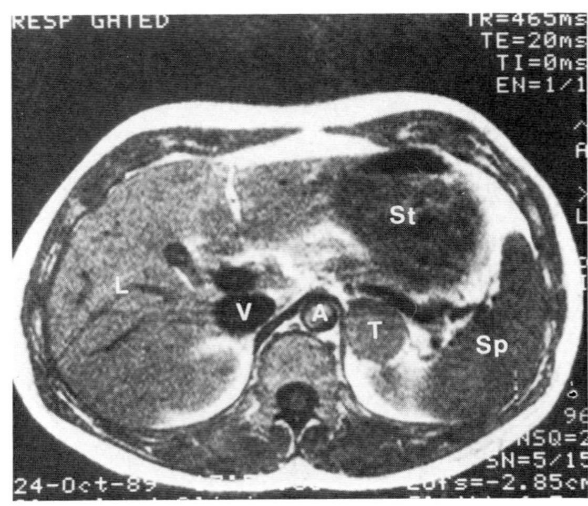

B

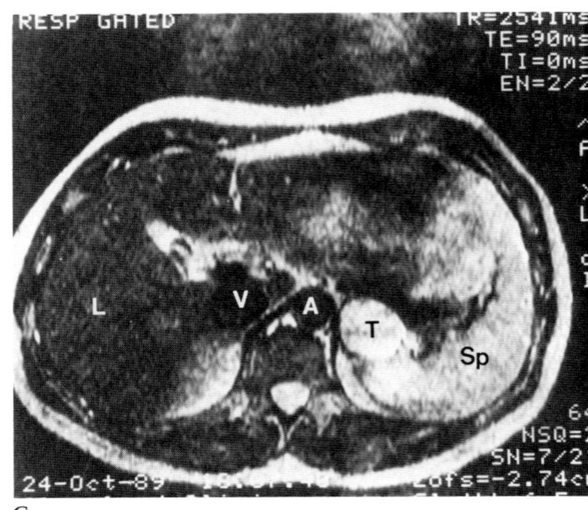

C

mocytoma [26]. All the patients had CT scanning and MIBG scintigraphy; 40 patients with tumor masses had, in addition, an MRI as a third localizing procedure. Forty-five patients had surgically proven pheochromocytoma, 20 had nonpheochromocytoma adrenal masses, and the remaining 44 were considered free of the disease after repeated biochemical testing and long-term follow-up. Based on the sensitivity, specificity, and predictive

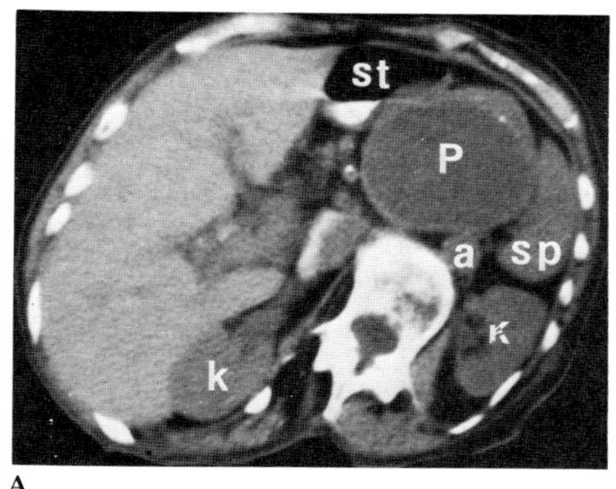

A

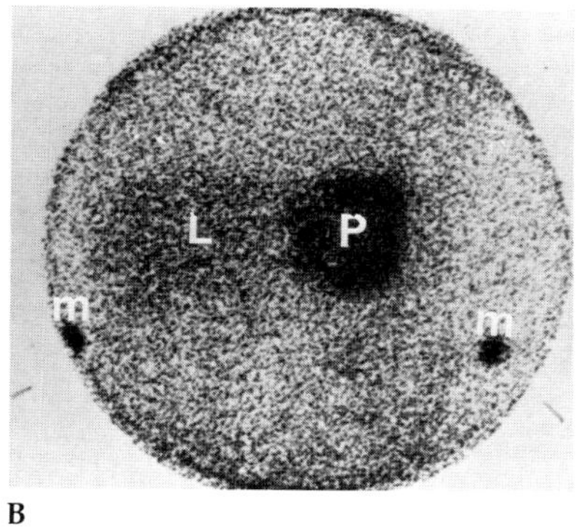

B

Fig. 56-25. Localization of pheochromocytoma employing ^{131}I-metaiodobenzylguanidine (MIBG). A. A large extraadrenal pheochromocytoma (P) shown by CT scan bordered by the stomach (st), spleen (sp), and aorta (a). k = kidney. B. Uptake of ^{131}I-MIBG (m) by the same tumor (P) 72 hours after injection of the radioactive isotope.

Table 56-7. Accuracy of three imaging techniques in the localization and diagnosis of pheochromocytoma

Parameter	CT (%)	MRI (%)	MIBG (%)
Sensitivity	98	100	78
Specificity	70	67	100
PV (+)	69	83	100
PV (−)	98	100	87

PV = predictive value.
Source: E. L. Bravo, G. Saha, and R. Go. Preoperative localization of pheochromocytome: A prospective comparison of ^{131}I-metaiodobenzylguanidine and abdominal computed tomography. Program of the Fourth European Meeting on Hypertension, Milan, Italy, June 1989.

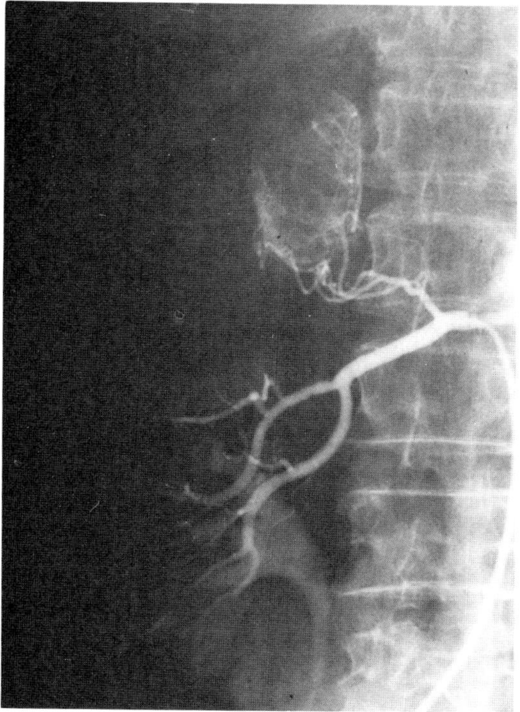

A

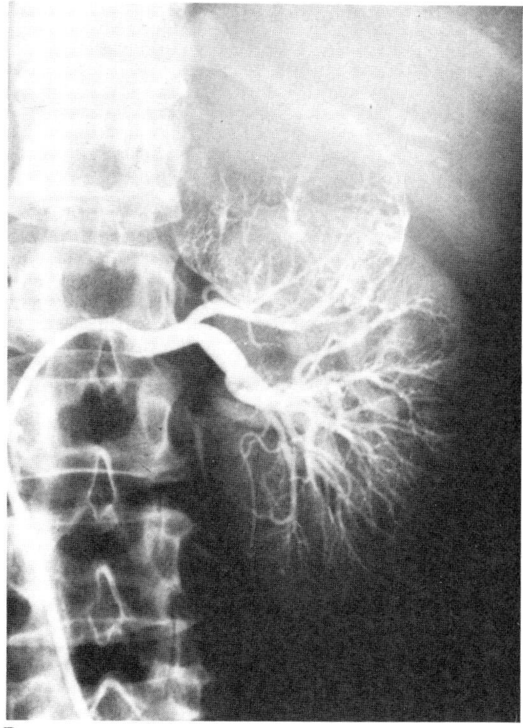

B

Fig. 56-26. Localization of pheochromocytoma by selective arteriogram. A. Right adrenal pheochromocytoma. B. Left adrenal pheochromocytoma.

value of each of the three imaging techniques, the following sequence of localization is recommended. An efficient sequence might begin with an abdominal CT/MRI (including the pelvic region) with special attention to the adrenal gland. This is appropriate, since 97 percent of pheochromocytomas are located in the abdominal area and 90 percent are intraadrenal. MIBG scintigraphy is performed in patients without demonstrable tumors. However, even if a primary adrenal pheochromocytoma is identified, MIBG may be useful in locating occult secondary or metastatic sites, which may be present in about 10 percent of cases. Venous catheterization with selective sampling of blood for measurement of plasma catecholamine concentration at various sites along the superior and inferior vena cava is reserved for patients whose clinical and biochemical findings are strongly suggestive of pheochromocytoma but whose radiologic studies fail to locate the tumor [4]. Arteriography is reserved for patients in whom the arterial supply of the tumor requires better definition (Fig. 56-26).

Evaluation of the Patient with Suspected Pheochromocytoma

Priority of evaluation (Fig. 56-27) is given to patients with the signs or symptoms described previously. Concentrations of total plasma catecholamines are measured after the patient has rested in a supine position for at least 30 minutes. Values over 2,000 pg per milliliter are considered pathognomonic of pheochromocytoma. When patients have values between 1,000 and 2,000 pg per milliliter, a *clonidine suppression test* is performed. An abdominal CT scan is then performed in patients with clinical and biochemical features suggestive of pheochromocytoma.

A small percentage (about 9 percent) of patients may have moderate elevations in plasma catecholamine levels—that is, less than 1,000 pg per milliliter. Therefore, whenever the clinical presentation is suggestive of pheochromocytoma and plasma catecholamine levels are only slightly or moderately increased, further evaluation should be performed. *Repeat testing including the measurement of urinary catecholamine metabolites should be done for confirmation.* Such cases will require either a provocative test or a suppression test for a more definitive diagnosis. However, a provocative test should not be performed when the arterial blood pressure is 160/100 mm Hg or higher or when the patient has concomitant problems that might make sudden increases in blood pressure risky. In these cases, the clonidine suppression test may be employed.

Fig. 56-27. An algorithm recommended as an approach to patients with suspected pheochromocytoma.

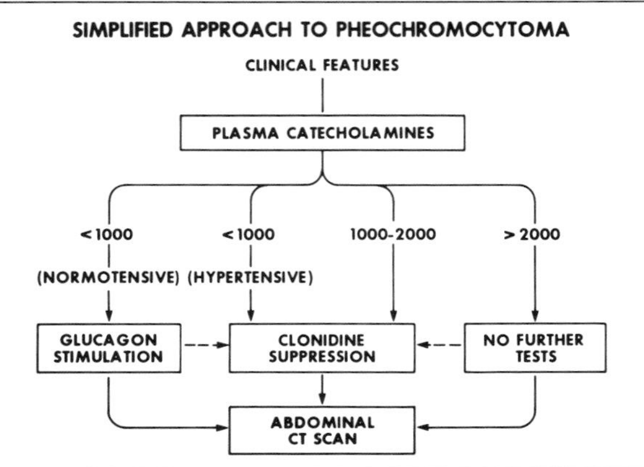

Management of Pheochromocytoma

Pheochromocytomas have a low level of malignancy. As with other endocrine tumors, the adverse effects of the tumor are due to secreted catecholamines rather than to the tumor burden itself. Therefore, the treatment of choice is surgical, and removal of the tumor is curative in most cases.

MEDICAL MANAGEMENT

The goals of therapy are to treat or prevent cardiovascular complications and to prepare the patient for surgical intervention. The most frequently used therapeutic agent is phenoxybenzamine, a long-acting, noncompetitive α-adrenergic blocker. Typically, dosing is initiated at 20 mg/day and increased stepwise to 80 to 100 mg/day as tolerated according to the severity of postural signs and symptoms. Prazosin hydrochloride, a shorter-acting α-blocking agent has also been used with some success [112]. Calcium antagonists are attractive agents because they are not only effective in controlling blood pressure but also useful in managing cardiovascular complications [124]. They attenuate the pressor response to norepinephrine and may also prevent catecholamine-induced coronary spasm and myocarditis. In addition, they have none of the complications associated with chronic use of α-adrenergic blockers. β-Adrenergic blockers are added as needed to control tachycardia and arrhythmias. If β-blockade is absolutely contraindicated, either lidocaine or amiodarone [134] may be used in its place. Hypertensive crises may be managed with the parenteral administration of either phentolamine hydrochloride or sodium nitroprusside. Nifedipine, 10 mg sublingually or orally, has also been used with success.

SURGICAL MANAGEMENT

The preoperative management of pheochromocytoma has been dominated by attempts to minimize the dramatic increases in blood pressure often encountered during surgery because of the sudden release of large quantities of catecholamines into the circulation. Phenoxybenzamine has been the drug of choice. Its theoretic advantages relate to its ability to permit vascular volume repletion and to block α-receptors noncompetitively, making it difficult for released catecholamines during surgery to overcome its blocking effect [136, 160]. It is recommended to control blood pressure for at least 2 to 4 weeks before the surgical procedure. The criteria proposed [48] to ensure adequate preoperative preparation with α-blockade are (1) arterial pressure not greater than 160/90 mm Hg for 48 hours, (2) orthostatic hypotension present but not exceeding 80/45 mm Hg, (3) electrocardiogram free of ST-segment or T-wave changes for at least 2 weeks, and (4) no more than one premature ventricular contraction (PVC) every 5 minutes.

However, in a recent review of 60 patients with pheochromocytoma who underwent a total of 63 surgical procedures, Boutros and co-workers [22] found that these patients can undergo consistently successful surgical outcomes without preoperative profound and long-lasting α-adrenergic blockade. Of 29 patients who did not receive α-adrenergic blockade, there were no recorded deaths or clinically documented cerebral or cardiac complications. In addition, 80 percent of the patients required neither vasopressors nor vasodilators in the immediate postoperative period. Further, there were no differences in the length of stay in the PACU or in the duration of postoperative hospitalization between patients who received α-blockers and those who did not. These favorable outcomes reflect the modern advances in anesthetic and monitoring techniques and the availability of fast-acting drugs capable of correcting sudden changes in cardiovascular variables.

Expansion of intravascular volume with 1 or 2 units of whole blood within 12 to 18 hours before the operation and generous replacement of blood lost during the procedure will greatly reduce the frequency and severity of postoperative hypotension.

Anesthetic management includes monitoring of intraarterial pressure by a catheter in a large artery to avoid false readings that may result from spasm of smaller vessels. Either phentolamine, nitroglycerin, or sodium nitroprusside is given intravenously to manage the hypertensive crises that arise during induction of anesthesia, intubation, or surgical manipulation of the tumor. To lower heart rate, either propranolol or esmolol, a rapidly-acting β-adrenergic blocking agent, is given intravenously.

There are some postoperative complications that require emphasis. The first is hypotension. This is attributed to withdrawal of catecholamines in the face of diminished receptor sensitivity to endogenous catecholamines, which results in marked arterial and venous dilatation. This can be compounded by previous preoperative α-blockade and inadequate volume repletion. Volume replacement, rather than use of vasopressors, is the primary treatment. Second, persistence of hypertension beyond 10 to 14 days after tumor excision should raise concern about residual or metastatic pheochromocytoma. If plasma catecholamines are still elevated at this time, a clonidine suppression test will determine whether the hypertension is neurogenically mediated. Third, hypoglycemia may develop postoperatively [36]. This is due to excessive insulin release that has previously been inhibited by high circulating catecholamines. Hypoglycemia can manifest as persistent hypotension despite adequate volume repletion and use of vasopressor agents.

FOLLOW-UP

Postoperatively, periodic biochemical assessment at 6-month intervals during the first 5 years and at 12-month intervals thereafter is desirable. This facilitates early detection of any recurrence.

MALIGNANT PHEOCHROMOCYTOMA

Malignant pheochromocytomas are, in general, slow-growing tumors. Evidence of malignancy may occur years (median 5.6 years) after successful surgical excision of an apparently benign pheochromocytoma. The 5-year survival of patients with malignant pheochromocytoma is about 44 percent, but some patients have survived for 20 years or longer [121]. Since these tumors respond poorly to either chemotherapy or radiotherapy, the long-term goals of treatment are to counteract the effects of increased circulating catecholamines with α- or β-adrenergic blocking drugs and/or calcium antagonists and to decrease synthesis of catecholamines by the tumor with metyrosine, a "false" catecholamine precursor that inhibits tyrosine hydroxylase, the first and rate-limiting enzyme in catecholamine synthesis [92]. Whenever possible, surgical excision or debulking of accessible tumors should be performed to reduce the mass of tumor tissue. This often helps to decrease the levels of circulating catecholamines and to provide easier control of blood pressure and other manifestations. Combination chemotherapy with cyclophosphamide, vincristine, and dacarbazine has been used in patients with advanced malignancy [30] and found to be effective in suppressing the activity of some tumors. However, the effect is only temporary. The administration of ^{131}I-MIBG to ablate primary and metastatic sites is presently being explored [128]. Initial results, however, are disappointing.

References

1. Abrams, W. B., and Solomon, H. M. The human platelet as a pharmacologic model for the adrenergic neurone: The uptake and release of norepinephrine. *Clin. Pharmacol. Ther.* 10: 702, 1969.
2. Achong, M. R., and Keane, P. M. Pheochromocytoma unmasked by desipramine therapy. *Ann. Intern. Med.* 94: 358, 1981.
3. Agabiti-Rosei, E., Alicandri, C. I., and Corea, I. Hypertensive crises in patients with pheochromocytoma given metoclopramide. *Lancet* 1: 600, 1977.
4. Allison, D. J., Brown, M. J., Jones, D. H., et al. Role of venous sampling in locating a pheochromocytoma. *Br. Med. J.* 286: 1122, 1983.
5. Aron, D. C., Bravo, E. L., and Kapcala, L. P. Erroneous plasma norepinephrine levels in radioimmunoassay. *Ann. Intern. Med.* 98: 1023, 1983.
6. Averbuch, S. D., Steakley, C. S., Young, R. C., et al. Malignant pheochromocytoma: Effective treatment with a combination of cyclophosphamide, vincristine, and dacarbazine. *Ann. Intern. Med.* 109: 267, 1988.
7. Baer, L., Sommers, S. C., Krakoff, L. R., et al. Pseudo-primary aldosteronism: An entity distinct from true primary aldosteronism. *Circ. Res.* 26–27(Suppl. I): 203, 1970.
8. Baines, A. D., Craan, A. A., Chan, W., et al. Tubular secretion and metabolism of dopamine, norepinephrine, methoxytyramine and normetanephrine by the rat kidney. *J. Pharmacol. Exp. Ther.* 208: 144, 1979.
9. Ball, S. G. In J. I. S. Robertson (ed.), *Handbook of Hypertension*, Vol. 2. *Clinical Aspects of Secondary Hypertension*. New York: Elsevier, 1983. Pp. 238–275.
10. Barkan, A., Marilus, R., Winkelsberg, G., et al. Primary hyperparathyroidism: Possible cause of primary aldoste-

ronism in a 60 year old woman. *J. Clin. Endocrinol. Metab.* 51: 144, 1980.
11. Beevers, D. G., Brown, J. J., Ferriss, J. B., et al. Renal abnormalities and vascular complications in primary hyperaldosteronism. Evidence on tertiary hyperaldosteronism. *Q. J. Med.* 45: 764, 1978.
12. Berecek, K. H., and Bohr, D. F. Whole body vascular reactivity during the development of deoxycorticosterone acetate hypertension in the pig. *Circ. Res.* 42: 764, 1978.
13. Berent, H., Uchman, B., and Wocial, B. Platelet norepinephrine and epinephrine concentration in patients with pheochromocytoma. *Am. J. Hypertens.* 3: 618, 1990.
14. Biglieri, E. G., Herron, M. A., and Brust, N. 17-Hydroxylation deficiency in man. *J. Clin. Invest.* 45: 1946, 1966.
15. Biglieri, E. G., and Schambelan, M. The significance of elevated levels of plasma 18-hydroxycorticosterone in patients with primary aldosteronism. *J. Clin. Endocrinol. Metab.* 49: 87, 1979.
16. Biglieri, E. G., Schambelan, M., Brust, N., et al. Plasma aldosterone concentration: Further characterization of aldosterone-producing adenomas. *Circ. Res.* 34(Suppl. I): 1183, 1974.
17. Biglieri, E. G., Schambelan, M., Slaton, P. E., et al. The intercurrent hypertension of primary aldosteronism. *Circ. Res.* 26–27(Suppl. I): 195, 1970.
18. Biglieri, E. G., Slaton, P. E., Schambelan, M., et al. Hypermineralocorticoidism. *Am. J. Med.* 45: 170, 1968.
19. Biglieri, E. G., Stockigt, J. R., and Schambelan, M. Adrenal mineralocorticoids causing hypertension. *Am. J. Med.* 52: 623, 1972.
20. Blaustein, M. P. Sodium ions, calcium ions, blood pressure regulation, and hypertension: A reassessment and a hypothesis. *Am. J. Physiol.* 232: C165, 1977.
21. Bouloux, P. M. G., Grossman, A., and Besser, G. M. Naloxone provokes catecholamine release in pheochromocytomas and paragangliomas. *Clin. Endocrinol.* 24: 319, 1986.
22. Boutros, A. R., Bravo, E. L., Zanettin, G., et al. Perioperative management of 63 patients with pheochromocytoma. *Cleve. Clin. J. Med.* 57: 613, 1990.
23. Bravo, E. L., Dustan, H. P., and Tarazi, R. C. Spironolactone as a nonspecific treatment for primary aldosteronism. *Circulation* 48: 491, 1973.
24. Bravo, E. L., Fouad-Tarazi, F. M., Tarazi, R. C., et al. Clinical implications of primary aldosteronism with resistant hypertension. *Hypertension* 11(Suppl. I): I-207, 1988.
25. Bravo, E. L., and Gifford, R. W., Jr. Pheochromocytoma: Diagnosis, Localization and Management. *N. Engl. J. Med.* 311: 1298, 1984.
26. Bravo, E. L., Saha, G., and Go, R. Preoperative localization of pheochromocytoma: A prospective comparison of ^{131}I-metaiodobenzylguanidine and abdominal computed tomography. Program of the Fourth European Meeting on Hypertension, Milan, Italy, June 1989.
27. Bravo, E. L., Tarazi, R. C., and Dustan, H. P. Multifactorial analysis of chronic hypertension induced by electrolyte-active steroids in trained unanesthetized dogs. *Circ. Res.* 40(Suppl. I): 140, 1977.
28. Bravo, E. L., Tarazi, R. C., Dustan, H. P., et al. The changing clinical spectrum of primary aldosteronism. *Am. J. Med.* 74: 641, 1983.
29. Bravo, E. L., Tarazi, R. C., Fouad, F. M., et al. Clonidine-Suppression: A Useful Aid in the Diagnosis of Pheochromocytoma. *N. Engl. J. Med.* 305: 623, 1981.
30. Bravo, E. L., Tarazi, R. C., Fouad, F. M., et al. Blood pressure regulation in pheochromocytoma. *Hypertension* 4(Suppl. II): II–193, 1982.
31. Bravo, E. L., Tarazi, R. C., Gifford, R. W., et al. Circulating and urinary catecholamines in pheochromocytoma: Diagnostic and pathophysiologic implications. *N. Engl. J. Med.* 301: 682, 1979.
32. Brown, J. J., Chinn, R. H., Davies, D. L., et al. Plasma electrolytes, renin and aldosterone in the diagnosis of primary hyperaldosteronism, with a note on plasma corticosterone concentration. *Lancet* 2: 55, 1968.
33. Brown, M. J. Simultaneous assay of noradrenaline and its deaminated metabolite, dihydroxyphenylglycol, in plasma: Simplified approach to the exclusion of phaeochromocytoma in patients with borderline elevation of plasma noradrenaline concentration. *Eur. J. Clin. Invest.* 14: 67, 1984.
34. Brown, M. J., Allison, D. J., Jenner, D. A., et al. Increased sensitivity and accuracy of phaeochromocytoma diagnosis achieved by use of plasma-adrenaline estimations and a pentolinum-suppression test. *Lancet* 1: 174, 1981.
35. Burris, J. F., and D'Angelo, L. J. Complications of clonidine suppression test for pheochromocytoma. *N. Engl. J. Med.* 307: 756, 1982.
36. Chambers, S., Espiner, E. A., Donald, R. A., et al. Hypoglycaemia following removal of phaeochromocytoma: Case report and review of the literature. *Postgrad. Med. J.* 58: 503, 1982.
37. Conn, J. W. Primary aldosteronism: A new clinical syndrome. *J. Lab. Clin. Med.* 45: 6, 1955.
38. Conn, J. W. The evaluation of primary aldosteronism: 1954–1967. *Harvey Lect.* 62: 257, 1967.
39. Conn, J. W., Cohen, E. L., and Herwig, K. R. Primary aldosteronism: A non-invasive procedure for tumor localization as well as distinction from bilateral hyperplasia. *Adv. Nephrol.* 7: 137, 1964.
40. Conn, J. W., Knopf, R. F., and Nesbit, R. M. Clinical characteristics of primary aldosteronism from an analysis of 145 cases. *Am. J. Surg.* 107: 159, 1964.
41. Crout, J. R., and Sjoerdsma, A. Turnover and metabolism of catecholamine in patients with pheochromocytoma. *J. Clin. Invest.* 43: 94, 1964.
42. Cryer, P. Pheochromocytoma and autonomic dysfunction. *Arch. Intern. Med.* 137: 783, 1977.
43. Cryer, P. E. Physiology and pathophysiology of the human sympathoadrenal neuroendocrine system. *N. Engl. J. Med.* 303: 436, 1980.
44. Darsee, J. R., and Nutter, D. O. Two distinct catecholamine cardiomyopathies from norepinephrine and epinephrine secreting pheochromocytomas (abstr.). *Circulation* 62: 317, 1980.
45. Davis, W. W., Newsome, H. H., Wright, L. D., et al. Bilateral adrenal hyperplasia as a cause of primary aldosteronism with hypertension, hypokalemia and suppressed renin activity. *Am. J. Med.* 42: 642, 1967.
46. DeOreo, G. A., Jr., Stewart, B. A., Tarazi, R. C., et al. Preoperative blood transfusion in the safe surgical management of pheochromocytoma: A review of 46 cases. *J. Urol.* 111: 715, 1974.
47. DeQuattro, V., and, Campese, V. M. Pheochromocytoma: Diagnosis and Therapy. In L. DeGroot (ed.), *Endocrinology.* New York: Grune and Stratton, 1979. Pp. 1279–1288.
48. Desmonts, J. M., and Marty, J. An anesthetic management of patients with pheochromocytoma. *Br. J. Anesth.* 56: 781, 1984.
49. De Wardener, H. E., and MacGregor, G. A. Dahl's hy-

pothesis that a saluretic substance may be responsible for a systemic rise in arterial pressure: Its possible role in essential hypertension. *Kidney Int.* 18: 1, 1980.
50. Distler, A., Just, H. J., and Phillip, T. H. Studies on the mechanism of aldosterone-induced hypertension in man. *Clin. Sci. Mole. Med.* 45: 743, 1973.
51. Dluhy, R. G., and Williams, G. H. Primary aldosteronism in a hypertensive acromegalic patient. *J. Clin. Endocrinol. Metab.* 29: 1319, 1969.
52. Doppman, J. L., Reinig, J. W., Dwyer, A. J., et al. Differentiation of adrenal masses by magnetic resonance imaging. *Surgery* 102: 1018, 1987.
53. Duncan, M. W., Compton, P., Lazarus, L., et al. Measurement of norepinephrine and 3,4-dihydroxyphenylglycol in urine and plasma for the diagnosis of pheochromocytoma. *N. Engl. J. Med.* 319: 136, 1988.
54. Dunn, M. J., and Hood, V. L. Prostaglandin and the kidney. *Am. J. Physiol.* 233: F169, 1977.
55. Edwards, C. R. W., Stewart, P. M., Burt, D., et al. Localization of 11β-hydroxysteroid dehydrogenase tissue specific protector of the mineralocorticoid receptor. *Lancet* 11: 986, 1988.
56. Ehrlich, E. N., Dominguez, O. V., Samuels, L. T., et al. Aldosteronism and precocious puberty due to an ovarian andoblastoma (Sertoli cell tumor). *J. Clin. Endocrinol. Metab.* 23: 358, 1963.
57. Engelman, K., Portnoy, B., Sjoerdsma, A. Plasma catecholamine concentrations in patients with hypertension. *Circ. Res.* 26 and 27: 1, 1970.
58. Esler, M., Jackman, G., Leonard, P., et al. Effect of propranolol on noradrenaline kinetics in patients with essential hypertension. *Br. J. Clin. Pharm.* 12: 375, 1981.
59. Ferriss, J. B., Beevers, D. G., Brown, J. J., et al. Clinical, biochemical and pathological features of low renin ("primary") hyperaldosteronism. *Am. Heart J.* 95: 375, 1978a.
60. Ferriss, J. B., Brown. J. J., Cumming, A. M. M., et al. Primary hyperparathyroidism associated with primary hyperaldosteronism. *Acta Endocrinol.* 103: 365, 1983.
61. Ferriss, J. B., Brown, J. J., Fraser, R., et al. Hypertension with aldosterone excess and low plasma renin: Preoperative distinction between patients with and without adrenocortical tumor. *Lancet* 2: 995, 1970.
62. Fertig, A., Webley, M., and Lynn, J. A. Primary hyperparathyroidism in a patient with Conn's syndrome. *Postgrad. Med. J.* 56: 45, 1980.
63. Fink, I. J., Reinig, J. W., Dwyer, A. J., et al. MR imaging of pheochromocytoma. *J. Comput. Assist. Tomogr.* 9: 454, 1985.
64. Fiorica, V., Galloway, D. C., Males. J. L., et al. Epinephrine fraction of adrenal vein blood in pheochromocytoma. *Am. J. Med. Sci.* 284: 9, 1982.
65. Folkow, B., and Oberg, B. The effect of functionally induced changes of wall/lumen ratio on the vasoconstrictor response to standard amounts of vasoactive agents. *Acta Physiol. Scand.* 47: 131, 1959.
66. Forman, B. H., Marban, E., Kayne, R., et al. Ectopic ACTH syndrome due to pheochromocytoma. *Yale J. Biol. Med.* 52: 181, 1979.
67. Fraser, R., Beretta-Piccoli, C., Brown, J. J., et al. Response of aldosterone and 18-hydroxycorticosterone to angiotensin II in normal subjects and patients with essential hypertension. Conn's syndrome and non-tumorous hyperaldosteronism. *Hypertension* 3(Suppl. I): 87, 1981.
68. Friedman, S. M., and Fredman, C. L. Cell permeability, sodium transport and the hypertensive process in the rat. *Circ. Res.* 39: 433, 1976.
69. Ganguly, A., Grim, C. E., and Weinberg, M. H. Anomalous postural aldosterone response in glucocorticoid-suppressible hyperaldosteronism. *N. Engl. J. Med.* 305: 991, 1981.
70. Ganguly, A., Melada, G. A., Luetscher, J. A., et al. Control of plasma aldosterone in primary aldosteronism: Distinction between adenoma and hyperplasia. *J. Clin. Endocrinol. Metab.* 37: 765, 1973.
71. Geffen, L. B., Rush, R. A., Louis, W. J., et al. Plasma dopamine β-hydroxylase and noradrenaline amounts in essential hypertension. *Clin. Sci.* 44: 617, 1973.
72. Geisinger, M. A., Zelch, M. A., Bravo, E. L., et al. Primary hyperaldosteronism: comparison of CT, adrenal venography, and venous sampling. *Am. J. Roentgenol.* 141: 299, 1983.
73. George, J. M., Wright, L., Bell, N. H., et al. The syndrome of primary aldosteronism. *Am. J. Med.* 48: 343, 1970.
74. Giebink, G. S., Golin, R. W., Biglieri, E. G., et al. A kindred with familial glucocorticoid-suppressible aldosteronism. *J. Clin. Endocrinol. Metab.* 36: 715, 1973.
75. Gifford, R. W., Jr., Kvale, W. F., et al. Clinical features, diagnosis, and treatment of pheochromocytoma: A review of 76 cases. *Mayo Clin. Proc.* 39: 281, 1964.
76. Gitlow, S. E., Mendlowitz, M., and Bertani, L. M. The biochemical techniques for detecting and establishing the presence of a pheochromocytoma. *Am. J. Cardiol.* 26: 270, 1970.
77. Given, B. D., Taylor, T., Lilly, L. S., et al. Symptomatic hypotension following clonidine suppression test for pheochromocytoma. *Arch. Intern. Med.* 143: 2195, 1983.
78. Glazer, G. M., Francis, I. R., and Quint, L. E. Imaging of the adrenal glands. *Invest. Radiol.* 23: 3, 1988.
79. Goldstein, D. S., Eisenhofer, G., Stull, R., et al. Plasma dihydroxyphenylglycol and the intraneuronal disposition of norepinephrine in humans. *J. Clin. Invest.* 82: 213, 1988.
80. Goldstein, D. S., Fenerstein, G. I., Izzo, J. L., Jr., et al. Validity and reliability of fluid chromatography with electrochemical detection for measuring plasma levels of norepinephrine and epinephrine in man. *Life Sci.* 28: 467, 1981.
81. Greenacre, J. K., and Conolly, M. E. Desensitization of the beta-adrenoceptor of lymphocytes from normal subjects and patients with pheochromocytoma: Studies in vivo. *Br. J. Clin. Pharmacol.* 5: 191, 1978.
82. Grim, C. E., Weinberger, M. H., and Anad, S. K. Familial, dexamethasone-suppressible normokalemic hyperaldosteronism. In M. I. New and L. S. Levine (eds.), *Juvenile Hypertension.* New York: Raven Press, 1977. Pp. 109–122.
83. Grim, C. E., Weinberger, M. H., Higgins, J. T., et al. Diagnosis of secondary forms of hypertension. *J.A.M.A.* 237: 1331, 1977.
84. Haddy, F. J., and Overbeck, H. W. The role of humoral agents in volume expanded hypertension. *Life Sci.* 19: 935, 1976.
85. Hamaji, M. Pancreatic α and β cell function in pheochromocytoma. *J. Clin. Endocrinol. Metab.* 49: 322, 1979.
86. Hartley, L., and Perry-Keene, D. Phaeochromocytoma in Queensland: 1970–83. *Aust. N.Z. J. Surg.* 55: 471, 1985.
87. Herwig, K. R. Primary aldosteronism: Experience with thirty-eight patients. *Surgery* 86: 470, 1979.
88. Horton, R., and Finck, E. Diagnosis and localization in primary aldosteronism. *Ann. Intern. Med.* 76: 885, 1972.
89. Irony, I., Biglieri, E. G., Perloff, D., et al. Pathophysiol-

ogy of deoxycorticosterone-secreting adrenal tumors. *Clin. Endocrinol. Metab.* 65(5): 836, 1987.

90. Jarrott, B., and Louis, W. J. Abnormalities in enzymes involved in catecholamine synthesis and catabolism in pheochromocytoma. *Clin. Sci. Mol. Med.* 53: 529, 1977.
91. Jones, A. W., and Hart, R. G. Altered ion transport in aortic smooth muscle during deoxycorticosterone acetate hypertension in the rat. *Circ. Res.* 37: 333, 1975.
92. Jones, N. F., Walker, G., Ruthven, C. R. J., et al. α-Methyl-*p*-tyrosine in the management of pheochromocytoma. *Lancet* 2: 1105, 1968.
93. Kalin, M. T., and Mullon, D. A. Pheochromocytoma with hypertension—report of a patient with acromegaly. *J.A.M.A.* 188: 74, 1964.
94. Kaplan, N., Kramer, N., Holland, B., et al. Single-voided urine metanephrine assays in screening for pheochromocytoma. *Arch. Intern. Med.* 137: 190, 1977.
95. Katz, F. H. Primary aldosteronism with suppressed plasma renin activity due to bilateral nodular adrenocortical hyperplasia. *Ann. Intern. Med.* 67: 1035, 1967.
96. Krane, N. K. Clinically unsuspected pheochromocytoma: Experience at Henry Ford Hospital and a review of the literature. *Arch. Intern. Med.* 146: 54, 1986.
97. Laragh, J. H., Ledingham, J. G. G., and Sommers, S. C. Secondary aldosteronism and reduced plasma renin in hypertensive disease. *Trans. Assoc. Am. Physicians* 80: 168, 1967.
98. Lawrence, A. M. Glucagon provocative test for pheochromocytoma. *Ann. Intern. Med.* 66: 1091, 1967.
99. Liddle, G. W., Bledsoe, T., and Coppage, W. S. A Familial Renal Disorder Simulating Primary Aldosteronism but with Negligible Aldosterone Secretion. In E. E. Baulieu and P. Robel (eds.), *Aldosterone*. Oxford: Blackwell, 1964. P. 353.
100. Linde, R., Coulam, C., Battin, R., et al. Localization of aldosterone-producing adenoma by computed tomography. *J. Clin. Endocrinol. Metab.* 49: 642, 1979.
101. Lins, P. W., and Adamson, U. Plasma aldosterone-plasma renin activity ratio: A simple test to identify patients with primary aldosteronism. *Acta Endocrinol.* (Copenh.) 113: 564, 1986.
102. Louis, W. J., Doyle, A. E., and Heath, W. C. Secretion of dopa in pheochromocytoma. *Br. Med. J.* 4: 325, 1972.
103. Lyons, D. F., Kem, D. C., Brown, R. D., et al. Single dose captopril as a diagnostic test for primary aldosteronism. *J. Clin. Endocrinol. Metab.* 57: 892, 1983.
104. Madhavan, T., Frame, B., and Block, M. A. Influence of surgical correction of primary hyperparathyroidism on associated hypertension. *Arch. Surg.* 100: 212, 1970.
105. Melby, J. C. Primary aldosteronism. *Kidney Int.* 26: 769, 1984.
106. Melby, J. C., Spark, R. F., Dale, S., et al. Diagnosis and localization of aldosterone-producing adenomas by adrenal vein catheterization. *N. Engl. J. Med.* 277: 1050, 1967.
107. Miura, K., Yoshinaga, K., Goto, K., et al. A case of glucocorticoid-responsive hyperaldosteronism. *J. Clin. Endocrinol. Metab.* 28: 1807, 1968.
108. Molinoff, P. B., and Axelrod, J. Biochemistry of catecholamines. *Ann. Rev. Biochem.* 40: 465, 1971.
109. Murtani, H., Abe, I., Tomita, Y., et al. Is single oral administration of captopril beneficial in screening for primary aldosteronism? *Am. Heart J.* 112: 361, 1986.
110. New, M. I., Oberfield, S. E., Levine, L. S., et al. Autosomal dominant transmission and absence of HLA linkage in dexamethasone suppressible hyperaldosteronism. *Lancet* 1: 550, 1980.
111. New, M. I., Siegal, E. J., and Peterson, R. E. Dexamethasone-suppressible hyperaldosteronism. *J. Clin. Endocrinol. Metab.* 37: 93, 1973.
112. Nicholson, J. P., Vaughn, E. D., Jr., Pickering, T. G., et al. Pheochromocytoma and prazosin. *Ann. Intern. Med.* 99: 477, 1983.
113. Novak, L. P., Strong, C. G., and Hunt, J. C. Body composition in primary and secondary hypertension. In J. Genest and E. Koiw (eds.), *Hypertension*. New York: Springer-Verlag, 1972. Pp. 444–459.
114. O'Connor, D. T., and Deftos, L. J. Secretion of chromogranin A by peptide producing endocrine neoplasms. *N. Engl. J. Med.* 314: 1145, 1986.
115. Onoyama, K., Bravo, E. L., and Tarazi, R. C. Sodium extracellular fluid volume and cardiac output changes in the genesis of mineralocorticoid hypertension in the dog. *Hypertension* 1: 331, 1979.
116. Page, L. B., Raker, J. W., and Berberich, F. R. Pheochromocytoma with predominant epinephrine secretion. *Am. J. Med.* 47: 648, 1969.
117. Peuler, J. D., and Johnson, G. A. Simultaneous single isotope radioenzymatic assay of plasma norepinephrine, epinephrine, and dopamine. *Life Sci.* 21: 625, 1977.
118. Plouin, P. F., Degoulet, P., Tugay'e, A., et al. Screening for pheochromocytoma. A semilogical study of 2585 patients, including 11 patients with pheochromocytoma. *Nouv. Presse Med.* 10: 869, 1981.
119. Prokocimer, P. G., Maze, M., and Hoffman, B. B. Role of the sympathetic nervous system in the maintenance of hypertension in rats harboring pheochromocytoma. *J. Pharmacol. Exp. Ther.* 241: 870, 1987.
120. Raum, W. J., and Swerdloff, R. S. A radioimmunoassay for epinephrine and norepinephrine in tissues and plasma. *Life Sci.* 28: 2819, 1981.
121. Remine, W. H., Chong, G. C., van Heerdeen, J. A., et al. Current management of pheochromocytoma. *Ann. Surg.* 179: 740, 1974.
122. Rhamy, R. F., McCoy, R. M., Scott, H. W., et al. Primary aldosteronism: Experience with current diagnosis criteria and surgical treatment in fourteen patients. *Ann. Surg.* 167: 718, 1968.
123. Sarkar, S. D., Cohen, L. E., Beierwaltes, W. H., et al. A new and superior adrenal imaging agent. ^{131}I-b-beta-iodometyl-19-nor-cholesterol (NP-59); evaluation in humans. *J. Clin. Endocrinol. Metab.* 45: 353, 1977.
124. Serfas, D., Shoback, D. M., and Lorell, B. H. Pheochromocytoma and hypertrophic cardiomyopathy: Apparent suppression of symptoms and noradrenaline secretion by calcium-channel blockade. *Lancet* 2: 711, 1983.
125. Sheps, S. G., Tyce, G. M., Flock, E. V., et al. Current experience in the diagnosis of pheochromocytoma. *Circulation* 34: 473, 1966.
126. Siegler, R. L., and Rallison, M. L. Hypertension with virilizing adrenal tumor. *Pediatrics* 61: 925, 1978.
127. Sisson, J. C., Frager, M. S., Valk, T. W., et al. Scintigraphic localization of pheochromocytoma. *N. Engl. J. Med.* 305: 12, 1981.
128. Sisson, J. C., Shapiro, B., Beierwaltes, W. H., et al. Radiopharmaceutical treatment of malignant pheochromocytoma. *J. Nucl. Med.* 25: 197, 1984.
129. Sjoerdsma, A., Engelman, K., Waldmann, T. A., et al. Current concepts of diagnosis and treatment. *Ann. Intern. Med.* 65: 1302, 1966.
130. Smith, U., Sjostrom, L., Stenstrom, G., et al. Studies on the catecholamine resistance in fat cells from patients with pheochromocytoma. *Eur. J. Clin. Invest.* 7: 355, 1977.

131. Snavely, M. D., Mahan, L. C., O'Connor, D. T., et al. Selective down-regulation of adrenergic receptor subtypes in tissue from rats with pheochromocytoma. *Endocrinology* 113: 354, 1983.
132. Snow, M. H., Nicol, P., Wilkinson, R., et al. Normotensive primary aldosteronism. *Br. Med. J.* 1: 1125, 1976.
133. Sobol, R. E., Memoli, V., and Deftos, L. J. Hormone-negative, chromogranin A-positive endocrine tumors. *N. Engl. J. Med.* 320: 444, 1989.
134. Solares, G., Ramos, F., Martin-Duran, R., et al. Amiodarone, phaeochromocytoma and cardiomyopathy. *Anaesthesia* 41: 186, 1986.
135. Solomon, S. S., Swersie, S. P., Paulsen, C. A., et al. Feminizing adrenocortical carcinoma with hypertension. *J. Clin. Endocrinol. Metab.* 28: 608, 1968.
136. Stenstrom, G., Haljamae, H., and Tissell, L. E. Influence of pre-operative treatment with phenoxybenzamine on the incidence of adverse cardiovascular reactions during anesthesia and surgery of phaeochromocytoma. *Acta Anaesthiol. Scand.* 29: 797, 1985.
137. Stenstrom, G., and Svardsudd, K. Pheochromocytoma in Sweden 1958–1981: An analysis of the National Cancer Registry Data. *Acta Med. Scand.* 220: 225, 1986.
138. Stewart, B. H., Bravo, E. L., Haaga, J., et al. Localization of pheochromocytoma by computed tomography. *N. Engl. J. Med.* 299: 460, 1978.
139. Stewart, P. M., Wallace, A. M., Valentino, R., et al. Mineralocorticoid activity of liquorice: 11β-hydroxysteroid dehydrogenase deficiency comes of age. *Lancet* ii:821, 1987.
140. Strauch, G., Vallotton, M. B., Touitou, Y., et al. The renin-angiotensin-aldosterone system in normotensive and hypertensive patients with acromegaly. *N. Engl. J. Med.* 287: 795, 1972.
141. Streeten, D. H. P., Tomyca, N., and Anderson, G. H. Reliability of screening methods for the diagnosis of primary aldosteronism. *Am. J. Med.* 67: 403, 1979.
142. Stromblad, B. C. R., and Nickerson, M. Accumulation of epinephrine and norepinephrine by some rat tissues. *J. Pharmacol. Exp. Ther.* 113: 154, 1961.
143. Sullivan, J., and Solomon, H. The diagnosis of pheochromocytoma—overnight secretion of catecholamine metabolites. *J.A.M.A.* 231: 618, 1975.
144. Sutherland, D. J. A., Ruse, J. L., and Laidlaw, J. C. Hypertension, increased aldosterone secretion and low plasma renin activity relieved by dexamethasone. *Can. Med. Assoc. J.* 95: 1109, 1966.
145. Sutton, M. G., Sheps, S. G., and Lie, J. T. Prevalence of clinically unsuspected pheochromocytoma. Review of a 50-year autopsy series. *Mayo Clin. Proc.* 56: 354, 1981.
146. Swensen, S. J., Brown, M. L., Sheps, S. G., et al. Use of ^{131}I-MIBG scintigraphy in the evaluation of suspected pheochromocytoma. *Mayo Clin. Proc.* 60: 299, 1985.
147. Tarazi, R. C., Dustan, H. P., Frohlich, E. D., et al. Plasma volume and chronic hypertension. *Arch. Intern. Med.* 125: 835, 1970.
148. Tarazi, R. C., Ibrahim, M. M., Bravo, E. L., et al. Hemodynamic characteristics of primary aldosteronism. *N. Engl. J. Med.* 289: 1330, 1973.
149. Taylor, H. C., Douglas, J. G., Berg, G. J., et al. Primary aldosteronism caused by adrenal cortical carcinoma. *Endocrinol. Jpn.* 29: 701, 1982.
150. Todesco, S., Terribile, V., Borsatti, A., et al. Primary aldosteronism due to a malignant ovarian tumour. *J. Clin. Endocrinol. Metab.* 41: 809, 1975.
151. Tsujimoto, G., Honda, K., Hoffman, B. B., et al. Desensitization of postjunctional α_1- and α_2-adrenergic receptor-mediated vasopressor responses in rat harboring pheochromocytoma. *Circ. Res.* 61: 86, 1987.
152. Tsujimoto, G., Manger, W. M., and Hoffman, B. B. Desensitization of adrenergic receptors by pheochromocytoma. *Endocrinology* 114: 1272, 1984.
153. Ulick, S., and Chu, M. D. Hypersecretion of a new corticosteroid. 18-hydroxycortisol, in two types of adrenocortical hypertension. *Clin. Exp. Hypertens. (A) Theory and Practice A4* 9 and 10: 1771, 1982.
154. Ulick, S., Levine, L. S., Guncler, P., et al. A syndrome of apparent mineralocorticoid excess associated with defects in the peripheral metabolism of cortisol. *J. Clin. Endocrinol. Metab.* 49: 757, 1979.
155. Ulick, S., Ramirez, L. C., and New, M. I. An abnormality in steroid reductive metabolism in a hypertensive syndrome. *J. Clin. Endocrinol. Metab.* 44: 799, 1979.
156. Van Heerden, J. A., Sheps, S. G., Hamberger, B., et al. Pheochromocytoma: Current status and changing trends. *Surgery* 91: 367, 1982.
157. Vaughan, N. J. A., Jowett, T. P., Slater, J. D. H., et al. The diagnosis of primary hyperaldosteronism. *Lancet* 1: 120, 1981.
158. Vetter, H., Siebenschein, R., Studer, A., et al. Primary aldosteronism: Inability to differentiate unilateral from bilateral adrenal lesions by various routine clinical and laboratory data and by peripheral plasma aldosterone. *Acta Endocrinol.* 89: 710, 1978.
159. Weinberger, M. H., Grim, C. E., Hollifield, J. W., et al. Primary aldosteronism: Diagnosis localization and treatment. *Ann. Intern. Med.* 90: 386, 1979.
160. Weiner, N. Drugs that Inhibit Adrenergic Nerves and Block Adrenergic Receptors. In A. G. Gilman et al. (eds.), *The Pharmacologic Basis of Therapeutics.* New York: Macmillan, 1985. Pp. 181–124.
161. Weinshilbaum, R. M. Serum dopamine β-hydroxylase. *Pharmacol. Rev.* 30: 133, 1979.
162. Wenting, G. J., Veld, A. J. M., Verhoeven, R. P., et al. Volume-pressure relationships during development of mineralocorticoid hypertension in man. *Circ. Res.* 40 (Suppl. 1): 163, 1977.
163. White, E. A., Schambelan, M., Rost, C. R., et al. Use of computed tomography in diagnosing the cause of primary aldosteronism. *N. Engl. J. Med.* 303: 1503, 1980.
164. Winter, J. S. D., and McKenzie, J. K. A Syndrome of Low-Renin Hypertension in Children. In M. I. New and L. S. Levine (eds.), *Juvenile Hypertension.* New York: Raven Press, 1977. Pp. 123–131.
165. Zachmann, M., Tassinari, D., and Prader, A. Clinical and biochemical variability of congenital adrenal hyperplasia due to 11β-hydroxylase deficiency: A study of 25 patients. *J. Clin. Endocrinol. Metab.* 56: 222, 1983.
166. Zipser, R. D., and Speckart, P. F. "Normotensive" primary aldosteronism. *Ann. Intern. Med.* 88: 655, 1978.
167. Zweifler, A. J., and Julius, S. Increased platelet catecholamine content in pheochromocytoma. *N. Engl. J. Med.* 306: 890, 1982.

Hypertension and Pregnancy

John M. Davison
Marshall D. Lindheimer

Hypertension complicates 1 in 10 pregnancies, and although advances in perinatal care have markedly improved both maternal and fetal prognoses, the hypertensive disorders of pregnancy remain a significant cause of morbidity in mother and baby [114, 229]. This chapter describes our understanding of blood pressure control and vascular reactivity in normal pregnancy as well as aberrations and their cause(s) in gestations complicated by hypertension, with special focus on the pathophysiology of preeclampsia, the disorder most apt to be associated with serious and life-threatening complications. The final section reviews the status of antihypertensive drugs currently administered to pregnant women and discusses a number of disputes related to the management of high blood pressure in pregnant women.

Control of Blood Pressure in Normal Pregnancy

An appropriate definition of hypertension requires cognizance of blood pressure changes in normal pregnancy so that the criteria decided on will truly establish a dividing line between normal and abnormal levels. In fact, mean blood pressure decreases early in pregnancy, reaching a nadir by midtrimester when diastolic levels are often 10 mm Hg below values measured postpartum [84, 154, 196]. Blood pressure then increases gradually, approaching nonpregnant values near term and small rises may also be observed in the immediate puerperium [287]. These changes have been observed in patients in large epidemiologic surveys [84, 196] as well as in those studied under rigidly standardized conditions in a quiet environment [154]. Since cardiac output rises quickly during the first trimester (to 140 to 160 percent of nonpregnant values) and remains relatively constant thereafter until term, the decrease in blood pressure is due to a marked decrement in peripheral vascular resistance. This is greatest in the uterine vasculature, which becomes a large "low resistance shunt," but vasodilatation occurs in other organ systems including the kidney and skin. The return of mean blood pressure from a midtrimester nadir toward nonpregnant values near term is of interest because it demonstrates that increasing vasoconstrictor tone is a feature of late normal pregnancy.

Given the above normal alterations in pregnancy, what constitutes high blood pressure? The American College of Obstetricians and Gynecologists, for instance, has specified four criteria for diagnosing hypertension in pregnancy: (1) an increment of 30 or more mm Hg in systolic and (2) 15 or more mm Hg in diastolic blood pressure as well as (3) systolic and (4) diastolic pressures of 140/90 mm Hg or greater. These abnormalities must be present on two or more occasions separated by intervals of at least 6 hours. Such criteria, however abnormal, may require revision, and this is further underscored by the results of two epidemiologic surveys. In the Collaborative Perinatal Project, 38,806 women were studied prospectively, and it was discovered that significant fetal morbidity was already present when diastolic blood pressure was 85 mm Hg [84]. In another survey involving 12,954 pregnancies, perinatal mortality increased significantly when mean blood pressure ([diastolic × 2 plus systolic] divided by 3) exceeded 90 mm Hg in the second and 95 mm Hg in the third trimester, respectively [196]. Thus while 90 mm Hg is designated as the upper limit of normal diastolic pressure, levels of 75 mm Hg in midtrimester and 85 mm Hg in the third trimester should be viewed suspiciously.

When reviewing the literature, one notes differences in the reporting of diastolic blood pressure. Many utilize Korotkoff sound IV (muffling or decrease in intensity, which is the designation of the World Health Organization [WHO] and the British Hypertension Society [298]). Others use phase V (disappearance). The latter has been designated as diastolic pressure in the National Institutes of Health's recent Consensus Report [184a]. The recording of phase IV can be quite variable [277] and may overestimate intraarterial pressures by as much as 10 mm Hg. Thus Korotkoff V is our personal choice; phase IV should be recorded only in the < 10 percent of normal gravidas in whom the discrepancy between muffling and disappearance becomes quite large.

VASCULAR REACTIVITY IN NORMAL PREGNANCY

Renin-Angiotensin System. The plasma concentrations of renin (in both its active and its inactive form), its substrate, and angiotensin I and II all increase substantially during pregnancy [9, 25, 112, 289, 295]. Furthermore, normal gravidas are highly resistant to the pressor effects of infused angiotensin II, and this remarkable diminution in vascular responsiveness is already present by the tenth week of pregnancy [91]. There is also renal resistance to this peptide, since at equipressor doses, renal hemodynamics and sodium excretion decrease less in gravidas than in nonpregnant subjects [39]. Although early reports [39] suggest the pressor response to norepinephrine may be unaltered, Nissel et al. [186] have shown that this may be due to greater increases in cardiac output during pregnancy, counterbalancing vessel refractoriness to catecholamines.

This marked change in sensitivity may relate to down-regulation of angiotensin receptors, perhaps due to the gestational rise in circulating angiotensin II levels [10]. Another explanation is that the resistance is due to increases in the production of vasodilator prostaglandins (see below).

In nonpregnant subjects, angiotensin II exerts a feedback control on renin production. For instance, a woman ingesting an oral contraceptive containing estrogen and progestogen experiences increments in the production of both renin substrate and angiotensin II [35]. How-

This work was supported by the Medical Research Council, England, and the National Institutes of Health.

ever, the latter hormone inhibits renin secretion, and the concentration of the enzyme decreases. This does not occur in pregnancy, and plasma renin concentration, which is already quite elevated in the first trimester, remains increased throughout gestation despite increments in estrogen, progesterone, and angiotensin II production [35].

It might be asked whether the changes observed in the renin-angiotensin system in pregnancy play a physiologic role or whether renin-angiotensin levels are increased secondarily and excessively, due in part to increments in the secretions of other hormones such as estrogen and progesterone. Thus it is of interest that despite "high" concentrations, maneuvers such as sodium restriction and alterations in posture result in further increases in renin activity [141], while administration of converting enzyme inhibitors to first-trimester subjects may produce exaggerated hypotension [9].

Elevated angiotensin II levels and vascular resistance to its effects are reminiscent of conditions that prevail in sodium-depleted persons and in patients with Bartter's syndrome, in whom the increments in the renin-angiotensin system are believed to be compensatory in nature. However, the situation that prevails during pregnancy is complex, and some of the observations are currently difficult to explain. For example, the increases in circulating angiotensin II and the vascular refractoriness to its action occur in the face of a "physiologic hypervolemia" and renal hyperemia. In this respect, earlier studies in which angiotensin blockers were administered to pregnant rodents suggested an important role for angiotensin II in the maintenance of blood pressure in pregnancy [82]. However, studies in awake and chronically catheterized rats using both saralasin and captopril have failed to confirm this observation [15, 142]. Of further note, infusion of whole blood or isotonic saline, a maneuver that decreases maternal renin activity, does not alter the pressor refractoriness to infused angiotensin II [94].

Overall the studies of pressor responsiveness in animal models have proved equivocal. Although most investigators have reported pressor refractoriness to angiotensin II in sheep, rabbits, rats, and guinea pigs [48, 105, 135, 141], the responses to catecholamines and vasopressin have been less consistent, with both refractoriness to these agents and increments in blood pressure similar to those of the nonpregnant animal being reported [135, 141, 156, 198, 199, 276]. Of interest in this respect are two reports. Quillen et al. [213] suggest that investigators have failed to take into account the volume of distribution (increased in pregnancy) into which the administered pressors must diffuse. These authors studied guinea pigs and claimed that when the pressor response to angiotensin II was related to its levels rather than to the quantity of peptide infused, the blood pressure response in pregnant and nonpregnant animals was similar. More recently, Hines, Lindheimer, and Barron [109] observed that total autonomic blockade eliminated the attenuated pressor response to angiotensin II in rats. They suggest that differences in blood pressure responses may reflect alterations in central nervous system influences on the control of blood pressure during gestation (see below).

Uterine Renin. Renin is present in the uterus of pregnant women and animals, and the highest renin concentrations have been recorded in amniotic fluid [5, 34, 262]. The source of the enzyme found in the uterus and products of conception, although disputed, appears to be the decidua [5, 9, 242, 262]; whether uterine renin is identical to renal renin or whether it represents an isoenzyme is not clear. Furthermore, it has been suggested that much of the renin measured in the peripheral blood or amniotic fluid of gravidas is of the higher-molecular-weight "inactive" form [5, 9, 25, 112, 262]. The role of uterine renin has remained obscure, and it has been claimed by some that it enters the maternal circulation only after nonphysiologic procedures such as bilateral nephrectomy. There is some evidence that it may play a role in regulating blood flow to the uterus, especially during pregnancy. For example, angiotensin II infused into the uterine artery of pregnant dogs, rabbits, or primates increases blood flow, an effect mediated by both β-adrenergic receptors and the synthesis of a prostaglandin E-like substance. Moreover, converting enzyme inhibition may decrease uterine blood flow in pregnant rabbits [9, 74, 268].

Prostaglandins. Prostaglandins (PGs) are potent vasodilators. The metabolism of these hormones is extremely rapid, and their activity may be limited to the immediate vicinity of the tissue synthesizing them [80, 117]. Thus reports that circulating levels of PGs are increased are difficult to interpret.

Urinary excretion and plasma levels of prostaglandin E_2 (PGE_2) increase during human pregnancy [80, 141]. Elevated levels of 6-keto-$PGF_{1\alpha}$, the major metabolite of prostacyclin (PGI), have also been observed in the urine and blood of gravidas. PGI is a potent vasodilator and an inhibitor of platelet aggregation. Ingestion of indomethacin (a cyclooxygenase inhibitor) by normal pregnant women increases their sensitivity to infused angiotensin II to values similar to those measured in nonpregnant subjects, whereas infusions of PGE_2 blunt vasopressor response to coinfusion of angiotensin II [25, 80, 94].

During pregnancy the uterus becomes a rich source of both PGE_2 and PGI; large quantities of these hormones may egress through the uterine veins, into the systemic circulation [74, 80, 96, 99]. But the placenta contains high concentrations of degrading enzymes [117], which in theory should inactivate most of the locally produced PGs. Still it has been suggested that it is PGI, not PGE_2 that escapes inactivation by the uterus and lung and is responsible for the decreased blood pressure. It has further been suggested that prostaglandins may play an important role in modulating uterine blood flow [74].

Other Hormones. The concentration of several hormones that may alter vascular reactivity directly by affecting smooth muscle or indirectly by influencing salt metabolism is increased in normal pregnancy gestation [42, 111, 141]. These hormones include estrogen, progesterone, prolactin, aldosterone, and vasoactive intestinal polypeptide (VIP). Estrogens, for instance, cause marked hyperemia in the nonpregnant uterus, and progesterone may increase renal plasma flow. Vasopressin levels are unaltered in pregnancy, but their influence on blood pressure maintenance in gestation remains to be elucidated [138].

Neurogenic Factors. In gravidas the sympathetic nervous system appears to have an important role in maintaining arteriolar and venous tone, particularly that of the capacitance vessels [7, 30, 149]. For instance, autonomic blockade with tetraethylammonium chloride or spinal anesthesia of a degree that only minimally affects recumbent nonpregnant subjects may produce severe hypotension in supine gravidas. Similar data emphasizing the importance of sympathetic tone in pregnancy have been observed in gravid sheep. In the gravid rat, although blockade of the actions of angiotensin II, vasopressin (AVP), and catecholamines produces decrements in blood pressure similar to nonpregnant animals, it is the autonomic nervous system that is the major defense against hypotensive stress [199].

Little is known about neurally mediated catecholamine release during pregnancy. Studies describing plasma catecholamine levels in pregnant women often relate to a single measurement only, but generally plasma catecholamine levels are similar in normotensive gravidas and nonpregnant subjects. However, only a few critical evaluations of the catecholamine response to physiologic maneuvers (e.g., upright posture) or pharmacologic intervention (e.g., clonidine administration) have been undertaken in pregnant populations, and reports suggest that the norepinephrine response to stress, such as upright posture and exercise, may be decreased in human gestation [13, 186, 187].

Despite these studies, baroreceptor function has really been poorly evaluated during pregnancy, and much more needs to be learned about high- and low-pressure receptors, including such basic information as normal traffic to and from these structures. Any future work in this area should take cognizance of a recent review of maternal volume homeostasis in pregnancy by Dürr [62], who notes that high- and low-pressure receptors are more responsive to pulsatile stimuli than changes in mean pressure per se. As pregnancy mimics a state of systemic shunting, there will be increased pulsatile venous return, a steep rise and increased atrial v-wave amplitude, and greater receptor activity, even if pressure is minimally affected. Similarly, since aortic compliance may be enhanced during gestation [107], aortic pulsation is tolerated at a lower mean arterial pressure. The author [62] uses this hypothesis to explain the resetting of volume-AVP secretory relationship [138] (nonosmotic hormone release is under baroreceptor control) and to argue against those who consider the circulation of gravidas underfilled or their effective arterial volume decreased, in which case baroreceptor function should be depressed.

Blood Vessel Wall Factors. As well as vasodilation being due to circulating factors or their imbalances, there could be alterations between the endothelin (constrictor)–endothelium-derived relaxing factor (EDRF) (dilator) interaction innate to the blood vessel wall [275]. In normal pregnancy, enhanced EDRF production could be responsible for both the decrease in blood pressure and pressor refractoriness. For instance, the aorta of gravid rats produces more EDRF than that of controls, but admittedly studies that have examined whether EDRF is responsible for the decreased basal blood pressure or for the pressor resistance in pregnant animals have yielded conflicting data [116, 169, 272, 293].

Both in vitro and in situ studies have been performed on conduit resistance vessels. Some appear to confirm the decreased responsiveness to pressors in pregnancy [51, 141, 164, 170], while in others results were similar in gravid and nonpregnant animals [106, 294]. Conrad and colleagues [47] have noted attenuation of myoinositol uptake, phosphoinositide turnover, and inositol phosphate production (changes that could affect cell signalling) in the aortas of pregnant rats, suggesting a biochemical basis for vasodilatation and reduced vascular reactivity in gestation. Also of interest are recent preliminary data from in vitro experiments on mesenteric resistance-sized arterioles indicating that gestation may evoke alterations in structural components (decreased collagen content [155]), and mechanical (increased distensibility [174]), and electrical properties (hyperpolarization [168]) of such vessels.

Venous Factors. More data are needed on venous physiology during pregnancy because the capacitance vessels determine cardiac preload and thus play a key role in regulating cardiac output. Forearm distensibility appears to be increased in normal gravidas, a change that reverses prior to and during the appearance of hypertension [14, 202, 259]. Whether this alteration also affects other vascular beds (e.g., the critical splanchnic circulation) is, however, unknown.

Finally, and as suggested above, alterations in vascular responsiveness may reflect differences in reflex responses via the central nervous system, an interesting and understudied area that remains to be explored in gravid models [109].

VOLUME HOMEOSTASIS

Average weight gain in first pregnancy is 12.5 kg and 1 kg less during subsequent gestations. Much of the increment in weight is fluid, because total body water increases 6 to 8 liters, 4 to 6 of which are extracellular. Included in these alterations are increments in maternal plasma volume and interstitial space. In essence, there is measurable maternal hypervolemia in normal pregnancy [141].

Sodium is the major solute and determinant of the extracellular space, and approximately 950 mEq is cumu-

Table 57-1. Factors affecting sodium excretion during pregnancy[a]

Causing increased excretion	Causing decreased excretion
Increased GFR	Increased plasma aldosterone levels
Increased progesterone production[b]	Increased levels of other salt-retaining hormones [estrogen, cortisol, human placental lactogen (hPL), and prolactin]
Antidiuretic hormone	Physical factors
Physical factors	Filtration fraction increased (postglomerular oncotic pressure)
Decreased plasma albumin (postglomerular oncotic pressure)	Placenta simulating an AV shunt
Decreased vascular resistance	Exaggerated influence of upright posture
Natriuretic hormone(s)	Increased ureteral pressure
?Increased neurophysins, prostaglandins and melanocyte-stimulating hormone	Increased renin activity
?Increased renin activity	
?Increased "ouabain-like" inhibitors of Na-K-ATPase	
?Increased atrial natriuretic factor(s)	

[a]See Chap. 83 for more complete details.
[b]Since progesterone is converted to deoxycorticosterone by extraadrenal mechanisms, increased production of this hormone may also lead to sodium retention.

latively retained during pregnancy, distributed between the products of conception and the maternal extracellular volume. However, the gravida's volume receptors sense these substantial gains in sodium in her intravascular and interstitial spaces as normal, and when salt restriction or diuretic therapy limits this hypervolemia, the maternal response is similar to that of salt-depleted nonpregnant subjects. In Table 57-1 are listed the effects of the various hormonal and hemodynamic changes that may modulate urinary sodium excretion in pregnancy. The role of the kidney in volume homeostasis is described further in Chap. 83.

Classification of the Hypertensive Disorders in Pregnancy

There are many classifications of the hypertensive disorders of pregnancy, some quite complex and confusing. In this chapter we will utilize the terminology suggested by the American College of Obstetricians and Gynecologists and recently endorsed by a National Institutes of Health working group [184a] because it is both sound and concise; it considers hypertension associated with pregnancy in only four categories:

1. Preeclampsia-eclampsia
2. Chronic hypertension (of whatever cause)
3. Chronic hypertension with superimposed preeclampsia
4. Late or transient hypertension

One reason the literature is controversial and confusing lies in the difficulty of distinguishing clinically between preeclampsia, essential or secondary hypertension, renal disease, and combinations of these entities [39, 78, 209]. The problem arises in part because certain women with undiagnosed essential hypertension experience the physiologic decrement in blood pressure early in pregnancy, and normal levels may be recorded when they are initially examined. They are then erroneously labeled as having preeclampsia when frankly elevated blood pressures are recorded near term. In other instances, an accelerated phase of essential hypertension (albeit unusual in pregnancy) and certain forms of renal disease such as glomerulonephritis and lupus erythematosus (SLE) may mimic preeclampsia.

These diagnostic dilemmas are best illustrated in reports in which the cause of high pressure complicating pregnancy was determined with the aid of renal biopsies. In one study [209] in which an academic obstetrician and a nephrologist recorded their impressions prior to biopsy, an accurate diagnosis was made by clinical criteria in only 58 percent of the patients. Our own experience is [78] summarized in Table 57-2, which demonstrates the pathologic diagnosis on postpartum renal biopsy of 176 patients hospitalized at The University of Chicago Medical Center between 1958 and 1976. In most instances the clinicians thought the patient had preeclampsia (or "toxemia"), because proteinuria and edema usually accompanied the hypertension, but such a diagnosis proved incorrect in 24 percent of the nulliparas and was wrong more often than not in multiparas. Of further interest was the presence of a substantial number of patients with unsuspected parenchymal renal disease. Such data underscore the problems inherent in interpreting reports in which diagnosis is based on clinical criteria alone; most suspect are series in which many of the patients labeled *preeclamptic* or *toxemic* were multiparas.

Since there are few antepartum indications for renal biopsy, investigators [reviewed in 140] have attempted to differentiate pure or superimposed preeclampsia from other hypertensive disorders using biochemical markers such as plasma levels of urate [220], antithrombin III [291, 292], and urinary excretion of calcium [264]. Others have analyzed changes in platelet count [71], circulating Fe^{2+} and carboxyhemoglobin levels [68], and even antibodies to laminin [81]. All these tests lack morphologic correlations, which makes it difficult to assess their true sensitivity and specificity.

PREECLAMPSIA-ECLAMPSIA

Other terms for preeclampsia include *pregnancy-induced hypertension* (PIH), *hypertension peculiar to pregnancy*, and *pregnancy-associated hypertension*, and this category accounts for over 50 percent of the hypertensive disorders complicating gestation. Preeclampsia is characterized by

Table 57-2. Renal pathology in 176 hypertensive gravidas diagnosed clinically as having preeclampsia

Biopsy diagnosis	Number of patients	Primigravidas	Multiparas
Preeclampsia*	96	79	17
With nephrosclerosis	13	6	7
With renal disease	3	1	2
With both	2	1	1
Nephrosclerosis	19	3	16
With renal disease	4	2	2
Renal disease	31	12	19
Normal histology	8	0	8

*Only glomerular capillary endotheliosis on biopsy. Modified from Fisher et al. [78].

hypertension, proteinuria, edema, and, at times, coagulation and/or liver abnormalities. It occurs primarily in nulliparas, usually after the twentieth gestational week and most often near term. The disease has, however, been recorded prior to midgestation, often in association with hydatidiform mole and nonimmune fetal hydrops [39]. When the disease progresses to a convulsive phase it is termed *eclampsia*. Although third-trimester hypertension is defined by diastolic pressures exceeding 90 mm Hg, increments in blood pressure of 30 and 15 mm Hg over previous systolic or diastolic levels, respectively, are also considered abnormal, especially when such increases occur rapidly. These latter criteria are important because a young gravida may have had earlier diastolic levels of 50 mm Hg, in which case a rise to 85 mm Hg could represent potentially serious disease.

Women with preeclampsia may show an interesting reversal of the diurnal blood pressure rhythm that normally occurs in pregnant and nonpregnant populations (i.e., morning peaks and nighttime nadirs). In preeclampsia, the magnitude of the variation may decrease, and in severe disease the rhythm may be abolished or even reversed, with the highest pressures occurring at night [141, 219]. This has implications for antihypertensive therapy (see below).

Proteinuria is defined as the excretion of 0.3 gm or greater in a 24-hour specimen. While this may correlate with 30 mg/dl ("1+" dipstick) or greater in a random urine sample, most require the qualitative values from random samples to be "2+" or greater. Proteinuria can be a late sign in the course of preeclampsia; although it is nonspecific, its appearance greatly endorses the diagnosis of preeclampsia, and its absence makes the diagnosis suspect.

In the past excessive weight gain or edema was considered an ominous sign. There are, however, large variations in the weight increase during normal pregnancy, and leg edema occurs in up to 80 percent of normotensive pregnant women. Neither edema nor maternal weight gain alone can be correlated with poor fetal outcome.

Eclamptic convulsions are dramatic and life-threatening. Although these fits are usually preceded by various premonitory signs including headache, severe epigastric pain, and hyperreflexia, eclampsia can appear suddenly and without warning in a seemingly stable patient manifesting only minimal blood pressure elevations. This is why attempts to categorize preeclampsia as "mild" or "severe" (i.e., diastolic and systolic levels of 110 and 170 mm Hg or greater, heavy proteinuria, and neurologic symptoms) may be misleading. Many authorities stress that de novo third trimester hypertension in a nullipara, whether or not other signs are present, is sufficient reason to consider hospitalization and treatment as if the patient were preeclamptic [139–141, 184a].

Last, some discussion about the term *toxemia* is relevant. A "toxin" has never been isolated from the blood. Furthermore, *toxemia* has been misused in the literature and has included such entities as hyperemesis gravidarum and essential hypertension; the latter condition is not, of course, specific to pregnancy.

CHRONIC HYPERTENSION (OF WHATEVER CAUSE)

This category includes approximately one-third of all cases of high blood pressure complicating gestation. In most cases the underlying pathology is essential hypertension, but in some patients the elevated blood pressure is secondary to such conditions as coarctation of the aorta, renal artery stenosis, primary aldosteronism, cocaine addiction, or chronic renal disease (reviewed in [40, 140, 141]). Pregnant women with chronic hypertension may be more prone to develop superimposed preeclampsia, but otherwise gestation seems to have little influence on the course of their underlying disease. Fetal outcome in these patients appears to be related to the extent of end-organ damage prior to conception and to the occurrence of superimposed preeclampsia, its timing and severity.

Exceptions to the predictions above are pheochromocytoma, scleroderma (usually with renal involvement), and periarteritis nodosa, in which pregnancy may have a devastating effect. Fortunately, these conditions are uncommon. Pheochromocytoma can have a catastrophic outcome in pregnancy, and maternal mortality rates of 40 percent or more have been recorded [132, 140, 141, 237]. Most of the deaths were due to diagnostic failures in which a fulminating clinical picture was labeled preeclampsia and its true nature was unsuspected. There are now many cases in which both maternal outcome and pregnancy have been successful because a prenatal diagnosis of pheochromocytoma was made quickly and

A

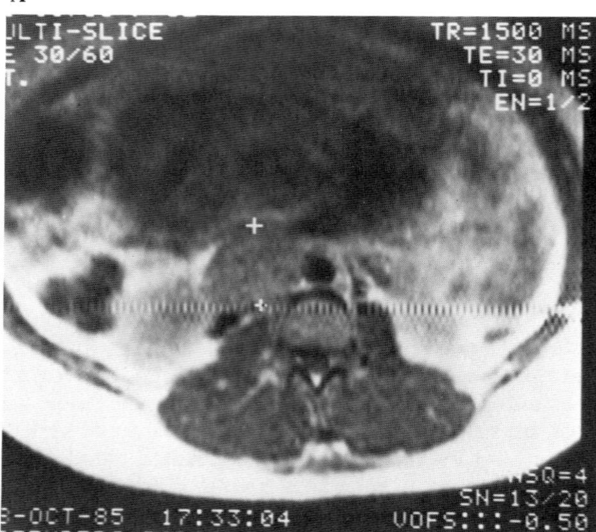

B

Fig. 57-1. Magnetic resonance images of an extraadrenal pheochromocytoma in a 27-week pregnant patient who presented during gestational week 19 with severe hypertension (240/140 mm Hg) alternating with hypotension (80/50 mm Hg) even when lying in bed. Plasma norepinephrine levels exceeded 8,000 pg per milliliter in this patient, who was managed with phenoxybenzamine and propranolol through gestational week 36, at which time a 2,900-gm healthy boy was delivered by cesarean section followed by extirpation of the tumor.

Coronal section (A) demonstrating a tumor (4–5 cm in diameter between the two + marks) located above the bifurcation of the aorta. (B) Transverse view. This tumor was posterior to the uterus and just anterior of the vena cava and aorta. This well-encapsulated pheochromocytoma presented few problems at surgery despite its proximity to the great vessels. (From [100].)

the tumor was resected or managed medically (with α-adrenergic antagonists) through term (Fig. 57-1) [32, 100, 132, 237]. Thus if they were not evaluated previously, measurement of plasma catecholamine levels and/or urinary catecholamine or vanillylmandelic acid secretion should be considered whenever hypertension predated pregnancy or was discovered early in pregnancy. Fetal outcome also appears poor in the rare pregnant patient with Cushing's disease [6].

In contrast to the complications noted above, normalization of blood pressure and amelioration of potassium wasting have been described during pregnancy in patients with primary aldosteronism [140]; potassium sparing is ascribed to increases in circulating progesterone levels that accompany pregnancy. Also, the vascular refractoriness to angiotensin II, characteristic of the pregnant state, may reduce blood pressure in some gravid hypertensives with renal artery stenosis [65].

CHRONIC HYPERTENSION WITH SUPERIMPOSED PREECLAMPSIA

Some 20 to 40 percent of women with chronic hypertension may experience rapid rises in blood pressure late in pregnancy, often associated with proteinuria, and there is evidence from renal biopsy material that many of these cases are due to superimposed preeclampsia. However, such a presentation may be misleading, especially in women with preexisting renal disease [78]. For example, in a survey of pregnancy in 89 women with underlying parenchymal renal disease, "superimposed preeclampsia" was diagnosed by their physicians on clinical grounds in 12 patients and eclampsia in 1, all of whom underwent postpartum renal biopsies [123]. The characteristic glomerular changes of preeclampsia were present in only 7 of these gravidas, including the 1 with eclampsia.

A substantial number of hypertensive patients with superimposed preeclampsia are multiparas, who may present early in the last trimester. If their pregnancies are allowed to continue they often manifest extremes of hypertension (frequently resistant to therapy), heavy proteinuria, coagulation abnormalities, and liver dysfunction and can develop sudden oliguria. Also intrauterine fetal death may suddenly occur. In elderly multiparas who already manifest end-organ damage, superimposed preeclampsia can be life-threatening; furthermore, if these patients conceive again, there is a tendency for this acute condition to recur [39].

LATE OR TRANSIENT HYPERTENSION

The category of late or transient hypertension includes a number of patients otherwise difficult to classify. These women develop hypertension late in pregnancy or in the immediate puerperium, but their blood pressure returns to normal within 10 days after delivery. However, nulliparas who manifest this condition may be preeclamptic patients who have not had other signs of the disease, and it is always prudent to manage them as such.

Patients in the transient hypertension category often develop high blood pressure in two or more pregnancies, becoming normotensive within 10 days after delivery (an entity once called *recurrent toxemia*). Some of these women may be representative of patients whose blood pressure increases on ingestion of oral contraceptives. In such patients, the transient hypertension could be related to increments in estrogen production during pregnancy. However, severe contraceptive-induced hypertension has been noted in patients who subsequently remained normotensive throughout gestation. Thus knowledge that oral contraceptives have caused increments in blood pressure in a given patient cannot be considered evidence that hypertension will complicate a future pregnancy.

Patients with transient hypertension probably represent women destined to develop essential hypertension later in life, analogous to women with gestational hyperglycemia who often become frankly diabetic. In essence, transient pregnancy hypertension defines a population in whom close scrutiny will lead to the early detection of high blood pressure one to three decades later.

Awareness of two uncommon entities in normotensive gravidas is important: "late postpartum eclampsia" (hypertension and convulsions occurring days to weeks after delivery), the existence of which is debated [27, 245], and "postpartum hypertension" [76]. The latter condition, characterized by abnormal increments in blood pressure 2 weeks to 6 months after delivery, is rather benign because the blood pressure increment rarely requires treatment and usually returns to normal within 1 year. Of note is a syndrome resembling both of these entities that has been reported to occur in women ingesting the dopamine agonist bromocriptine, a drug commonly used to suppress lactation [210].

SUMMARY

The incidence of hypertension complicating gestation is about 10 percent of all pregnancies [38–41, 141, 181, 184a], and approximately 50 to 60 percent of the patients have preeclampsia (Table 57-3). There is an increased frequency of preeclampsia in first pregnancies. Other conditions that predispose to preeclampsia are chronic hypertension, renal disease, extremes of age, hydatidiform mole, fetal hydrops, and α-thalassemia. The last three conditions are often associated with early preeclampsia, occurring before or at midpregnancy.

The Pathophysiology of Preeclampsia

While often decreased, cardiac output may be unchanged in preeclampsia (see below). Therefore, hypertension in preeclamptic women is essentially the result of an increment in peripheral resistance. The hypertension is characterized by its lability, a reflection of the intense vascular sensitivity these women have to their own endogenous pressor peptides and amines.

VASCULAR REACTIVITY

Renin-Angiotensin System. Whereas normal gravidas are quite resistant to the pressor effects of infused angiotensin II, those destined to develop preeclampsia manifest increased pressor responsiveness to this peptide many weeks prior to the appearance of abnormal blood pressure or other signs of the disease [91]. In women with chronic essential hypertension, sensitivity to infused angiotensin II also increases prior to the development of superimposed preeclampsia [92]. Inevitably, this has led to the suggestion that the renin-angiotensin system may be involved in the altered vascular reactivity. Most investigators [1, 9, 25, 26, 289, 295] note that renin concentration, renin activity, and angiotensin II are decreased in preeclampsia when compared with their measurements during normal pregnancy. However, some authors [26] have noted increments in both plasma renin activity and angiotensin II levels, the latter correlating with the degree of maternal hypertension [261]. Even if concentrations do decrease, these pressor substances may still have a pathogenic role, especially when the exquisite sensitivity of the vasculature is considered [91], related, perhaps, to up-regulation of angiotensin receptors [10]. Also, when overt disease does occur (in the last

Table 57-3. Combined incidence and prevalence of hypertension in pregnancy in Brooklyn, New York, hospitals participating in the obstetric statistical cooperative during 1979

	All hypertension		Preeclampsia-eclampsia		Perinatal mortality		
Hospital	Cases	Percentage	Cases	% of hypertensives	Cases	No. with hypertension	% with hypertension
Kings County	434	10.1	255	58.7	89	13	14.6
University	163	8.8	79	48.5	52	9	17.3
Maimonides	123	2.7	69	56.1	48	7	14.6
Brooklyn-Cumberland	267	6.6	114	42.7	65	1	1.5
Brooklyn Jewish	221	10.9	162	73.3	26	3	11.5
Greenpoint	161	14.1	145	90.1	14	1	7.1
Totals and Weighted Means	1369	7.8	824	60.0	294	34	11.6

Source: From Chesley, L. C. [40]. With permission.

few weeks of pregnancy), the vasculature is exposed to more hormone than when the patient is not pregnant, since these patients usually have concentrations of angiotensin II that are still greater than those of nonpregnant women.

Prostaglandins. Preeclamptics display several aberrations in eicosinoid metabolism, which has led to the suggestion that preeclampsia is due to a relative or absolute PG deficiency [4, 79, 80, 139, 141, 189, 225]. The belief is that an imbalance occurs between the vasodilatory PGs and vasoconstrictor influences of angiotensin and/or thromboxane. According to one hypothesis, increased PG production is required during normal pregnancy to counteract the vasoconstrictor actions of the elevated angiotensin II levels. In keeping with this view are several observations: (1) Ingestion of aspirin or indomethacin at doses that completely inhibit the cyclooxygenase enzyme decreases the vascular resistance of normal gravidas to infused angiotensin II to the levels observed and in both nongravid subjects and women with preeclampsia; (2) infusion of PG into gravidas blunts their vasopressor response to coinfusion of angiotensin II; (3) PG inhibition increases blood pressure in pregnant animals; and (4) dietary restriction of essential fatty acid precursors of PGs in pregnant animals leads to increased sensitivity toward angiotensin II.

There is evidence that circulating levels of prostacyclin (or excretion of its metabolites) decrease, while thromboxane synthesis increases in preeclampsia [79, 80, 225]. In addition, levels or production of vasodilatory PGs is decreased in the placenta, decidua, chorion, and amnion in women with preeclampsia, and there is reduced prostacyclin generation in the maternal and fetal vessels of such patients [79, 80, 158, 225, 284, 285]. The decrement in umbilical PGI generation is greater than that in the maternal vasculature, and this has been suggested as evidence that fetomaternal blood flow is more impaired than maternal uteroplacental flow. Of interest, also, is the presence of increased levels of PGI-stimulating activity in plasma from preeclamptics in comparison with those having a normal pregnancy. This, too, has been interpreted as a compensatory mechanism in response to subnormal PGI synthesis in preeclampsia.

Several studies in animal models and humans further suggest a critical role for PG. Inhibition of thromboxane synthesis or action seems to have reversed the hypertension provoked by aortic constriction in dogs [300] or by fasting in ewes [125]. However, the most remarkable observations in relation to this topic have been that low-dose aspirin (60–150 mg) appears to protect against the development of both intrauterine growth retardation and preeclampsia, a subject that will be discussed further in the section devoted to prevention. Furthermore, such therapy may enhance vascular resistance to infused angiotensin II in women at risk of developing preeclampsia, effects attributed to the fact that low-dose aspirin primarily inhibits production of platelet thromboxane [20, 238, 257].

There are some aberrations in fatty acid metabolisms that could relate to the alterations in PG described in preeclampsia. For instance, decrements in placental and fetal arachidonic acid levels as well as increases in the maternal concentrations of this fatty acid have been reported in preeclampsia [113, 191]. These findings are further reinforced by observations that the ratio of 5-8-11 eicosatrienoic to arachidonic acid is increased in the umbilical cord blood from infants born from hypertensive mothers [192]. This has been interpreted as evidence of essential fatty acid deficiency and suggests that dietary problems could underlie the generalized prostacyclin deficiency claimed to occur in preeclampsia. Furthermore, 5-8-11 eicosatrienoic acid is a substrate for lipoxygenase enzymes, the products of which include monhydroxy fatty acids and leukotrienes. The latter have physiologic effects on vascular smooth muscle and capillary permeability and also cause edema.

Free radical oxidation products, which may be related to the synthesis of some PGs and their vasoactive derivatives, are increased during pregnancy [113]. A diene-conjugated isomer of linoleic acid 18:2(9,11) is formed by free radical isomerization of 18:2(9,12) linoleic acid, and measurement of the former is an index of free radical activity. Finally the ratio of 18:2(9,11) to 18:2(9,12) linoleic acid is significantly higher in hypertensive pregnancies compared with normals as early as the twenty-eighth gestational week, often prior to overt signs of preeclampsia [70].

Other Hormones. Other hormones implicated in preeclampsia include progesterone, prolactin, vasopressin (antidiuretic hormone), the catecholamines, VIP, circulating inhibitors of cellular membrane pumps, and levels of newly identified vasoconstrictors (e.g., endothelin).

PROGESTERONE. It was suggested that production of progesterone, a vasodilator hormone with natriuretic action, may be decreased in preeclampsia. This suggestion was based on measurement of the urinary metabolites of this hormone, but more recently circulating levels of progesterone have been reported to be unaltered in preeclampsia [reviewed in 141]. Still, infusions of the progesterone metabolite, 5-hydroxyprogesterone, into women with preeclampsia did abolish their increased sensitivity to angiotensin II, their response to the pressor peptide becoming similar to that of normal gravidas [94].

PROLACTIN. This hormone is purported to antagonize the effect of circulating pressor substances, but levels of this hormone in preeclampsia vary and have been reported as decreased, normal, and elevated [141, 223].

VASOPRESSIN. Arginine vasopressin, suspected almost 50 years ago of playing a role in so-called toxemia, has been implicated in the blood pressure rise seen in several experimental animals as well as in nonpregnant humans. In one report, levels of antidiuretic hormone measured by radioimmunoassay were lower in preeclamptics than in normal gravidas, thus the role of this hormone in preeclampsia is not clear [295].

VIP. VIP is a regulator peptide with potent vasodilatory and muscle-relaxing effects widely distributed in the human body. A relative abundance of VIP immunoreactivity, mainly representing VIP in nerve fibers, have been demonstrated in the female genital tract [193]. Plasma VIP concentrations are substantially increased in preeclampsia [111], but there are no differences between mild and severe disease nor between women having small and normal weight babies. Nevertheless, it has been postulated that the increased levels of VIP in preeclampsia may represent a compensatory mechanism attempting to restore vascular perfusion of various organs, including the uterus and the placenta.

SEROTONIN. Serotonin, which may be released from platelets, has also been postulated to play a pathogenic role in the augmented pressor reactivity, as well as the vasoconstriction characteristic of preeclampsia. This subject has been reviewed by Weiner [290]. There is at present, however, little evidence to support the hypothesis.

CATECHOLAMINES. Urinary and uterine tissue norepinephrine and the pressor effects of this catecholamine increase in preeclampsia, but data concerning plasma norepinephrine and epinephrine levels are fragmentary and conflict [39, 140, 141, 186, 187, 201, 208]. Urinary dopamine excretion appears unaltered in this disease.

While plasma catecholamines normally increase during labor, greater increments may occur in preeclampsia [201]. On the other hand, norepinephrine levels that were initially the same increase similarly in normotensive and hypertensive proteinuric gravidas subjected to isometric exercise or to cold pressor tests [186, 187].

Mendlowitz, who in 1961 noted that digital reactivity to norepinephrine is increased at midpregnancy in women who later developed "toxemia" [172], proposed in 1980 an intriguing hypothesis for the role of catecholamines in increased blood pressure during preeclampsia [173]. There is a considerable literature describing (in nonpregnant hypertensives) membrane transport abnormalities characterized by increased intracellular calcium in smooth muscle, which sensitizes it to constrictor stimuli. Thus Mendlowitz suggested that preeclampsia occurs in gravidas who manifest a temporary defect in their calcium transport system. In this formulation, gestation is an anabolic state in which some women fail to produce sufficient calcium-transporting protein. Early reports noting that there are decrements in sodium-potassium adenosinetriphosphatase (ATPase) of cord blood erythrocytes from preeclamptic women and that their plasma decreases the short-circuit current in toad bladder (a measure of sodium transport) and contains ouabain-like substances that inhibit Na-K-ATPase were of interest, because a defect in the sodium pump has been postulated in the pathogenesis of the cellular calcium transport effect described above. We cite the Mendlowitz hypothesis in view of current interest focusing on the role of calcium in the hypertensive disorders of pregnancy.

Calcium and Magnesium. Disturbances in mineral homeostasis, such as a low intake or increased excretion of calcium, have been implicated in both human and experimental hypertension during the nonpregnant state. This cation is also under investigation in relation to its possible role in preeclampsia (and gestation hypertension in general) [18, 139, 141]. Belizan et al. [18, 19] have reviewed several epidemiologic surveys and animal data that suggested that decreased calcium intake is associated with hypertension during gestation, while calcium supplements reduce mean blood pressure in normotensive gravidas. Also of interest is a report by Taufield et al. [264], who studied 40 third-trimester subjects, of which 30 had various forms of hypertension. The women with pure or superimposed preeclampsia had markedly lower 24-hour urinary calcium excretion rates than those with transient or chronic hypertension or normotensive gravidas. Similarly, Sanchez-Ramos et al. [236] have observed that patients with preeclampsia have significantly less excretion of total calcium (130 ± 19 mg [SEM]/24 hours) than normotensives (284 ± 12 mg/24 hours) or those with gestational hypertension (233 ± 22 mg/24 hours), calculating a urine calcium threshold of 12 mg/dl as a predictor for the development of preeclampsia (sensitivity of 85% and specificity of 91%). Also of note are two reports. In one [124], a 600-mg calcium supplement enhanced pressor resistance to angiotensin II. Second, Zemel et al. [302] suggest that an intrinsic biochemical marker for subsequent development of preeclampsia is a marked increase in sensitivity of platelets to increase their intracellular calcium levels when stimulated in vitro by AVP, an effect that occurs quite early in gestation. The current status of trials designed to prevent preeclampsia by calcium supplementation are discussed in the section devoted to prevention. Lastly, magnesium has been linked to the hypertensive disorders of pregnancy, but in one carefully conducted study magnesium supplementation failed to decrease the incidence of preeclampsia [251].

Unknown Humoral Substances, Infection, Membrane Pump Inhibitors, and Endothelin. The literature abounds with reference to "unknown humoral substances" because plasma obtained from preeclamptics has been shown to have vasoconstrictor properties in nonpregnant subjects [205]. Many of these reports await confirmation and further clarification.

There is an infection theory of preeclampsia, and in the early 1980s one group of workers claimed to have identified various forms of a parasitic helminth in the blood of preeclamptic patients and women with trophoblastic disease. The parasite was also identified in the placentas and cord blood of the offspring of patients with preeclampsia-eclampsia, and in trophoblastic tumor tissue [3, 150]. It was also claimed that inoculates of this organism, *Hydatoxi lualba,* induced a toxemia-like syndrome in pregnant beagles and that intrauterine transmission of the parasite occurred, explaining the fact that there is a higher incidence of preeclampsia in the daughters of mothers who have had the disease. Subsequent studies, however, revealed that the suggested organisms were artefacts created by cotton or other cellulose fibers and glove talc, introduced during the preparation of the microscope slides [95, 146].

Finally, natriuretic factors, various membrane pump inhibitors (e.g., of Na^+-K^+-ATPase, Na-Li co-transport, Na-H exchange) or the activity of these pumps or exchangers, and potent vasoconstrictors such as endothelin have all been implicated in the preeclamptic syndrome. Data as yet are inconsistent, and the reader should consult references [139], [141], and [226] for further details.

VOLUME HOMEOSTASIS AND SODIUM RETENTION

Preeclamptic patients usually have an impaired ability to excrete sodium, but preeclampsia can occur in the absence of fluid retention. Even when edema is present, plasma volume (when compared with that of a normal gravida) is usually decreased [39, 87, 141, 255].

In fact, severe disease can occur in the absence of edema (the "dry preeclamptic") [39]. The cause of sodium retention in preeclampsia is obscure. The glomerular filtration rate (GFR) does decrease, but the decrement seems insufficient to explain the positive salt balance. Aldosterone levels in early or midpregnancy in gravidas destined to develop hypertension in the third trimester are similar to those in women who remain normotensive, and concentrations actually decrease in frank preeclampsia [1, 9, 39, 141, 254, 289, 295]. The metabolism of other mineralocorticoids that may cause sodium retention has scarcely been evaluated in preeclampsia. Deoxycorticosterone (DOC) levels increase in normal pregnancy and are not suppressible by physiologic maneuvers such as sodium loading, suggesting that this mineralocorticoid could play a role in maintaining edema in preeclampsia [141]. Also of interest is that progesterone, whose levels increase in normal pregnancy, and remain unchanged in preeclampsia, is converted to DOC at extraadrenal sites in the mother, possibly in the vicinity of its renal receptor. This conversion may be enhanced in preeclamptics [reviewed in 141].

The decrement in plasma volume in preeclampsia is the basis of a major controversy in the management of the disease [8, 141]. Some investigators believe that decreased intravascular volume is the primary event in preeclampsia, perhaps responsible for the rise in blood pressure (i.e., placental hypoperfusion may induce release of a pressor substance from the uterus, or relative hypovolemia may result in excessive instead of compensatory secretion of catecholamines and other pressor hormones). This has led to the recommendation of volume expansion therapy for preeclampsia, an approach rejected by traditional hypertension experts. The latter believe that decrements in volume are secondary to vasoconstriction as well as to the effect of the hypertension on renal sodium excretion (the so-called pressure natriuresis). They note that if myocardial performance is compromised and capillary wedge pressure normal or elevated, treatment with volume expanders could be dangerous, leading to aggravation of the hypertension as well as to pulmonary edema [8]. Consequently, opponents of volume expansion therapy advocate primarily the use of vasodilating drugs (and some diuretics). Data in the literature, however, suggest that in preeclampsia the decrease in plasma volume precedes the occurrence of hypertension [39, 87] and that cardiac output is usually decreased, while pulmonary capillary wedge and central venous pressures are low normal or also decreased [103, 141, 279, 281] (the latter varying inversely with the severity of the blood pressure elevation [121]). The controversy will be further discussed in the section on management (see below).

PLATELETS AND COAGULATION ABNORMALITIES

During normal pregnancy, profound changes occur in both the coagulation and the fibrinolytic systems [39, 139, 291]. Several clotting factors, including factors VII, VIII, X, and fibrinogen, increase and reach peak values in the third trimester [291]. At the same time, fibrinolytic activity, as measured by the levels of circulating plasminogen, is depressed. This combination of changes suggests that the gravida is particularly susceptible to the development of intravascular coagulation; indeed, some suggest that normal pregnancy is a chronic state of intravascular fibrin formation and that this stage is exaggerated in preeclampsia.

There is controversy concerning the incidence and significance of coagulation abnormalities in preeclampsia, including their role in the etiology of the disorder [71]. Some have claimed that a decrement in platelet count and often a defect in platelet function (collagen-induced synthesis of thromboxane B_2) is the earliest sign of preeclampsia and can occur weeks before clinical signs are evident [126]. Indeed, there are reports of the unwary clinician mistakenly diagnosing idiopathic thrombocytopenic purpura [97, 239]. Decrements in antithrombin III have also been suggested as an early indicator of preeclampsia [291, 292].

The possibility that coagulation problems and deficient PG production may be linked in this disease has also been suggested, because the appropriate balance between vascular PGI and platelet thromboxane synthesis is considered important for normal clotting. It has been suggested that even when the diagnosis of preeclampsia is a remote consideration an immediate platelet count is mandatory because severe thrombocytopenia may remain undiagnosed.

Contrasting with these views are studies that do not ascribe a primary role to coagulation abnormalities in the pathogenesis of preeclampsia. Pritchard and colleagues performed a battery of five tests (platelet count, plasma fibrinogen and its degradation products, fibrin monomer, and thrombin time) and found evidence of disordered coagulation in only a minority of their eclamptic patients [211], which is the experience at the University of Chicago as well. Pritchard also notes that in abruptio placentae (an obstetric syndrome that may be associated with marked intravascular coagulation), hypertension, convulsions, and other manifestations seen in preeclampsia are usually absent. Decrements in the level of clotting factors in preeclampsia could also be due to liver involvement in this disease (see below), which on occasion may be quite severe and may produce marked jaundice.

Etiology of Preeclampsia

Preeclampsia can still justifiably be called the disease of theories [38, 39]. The previous section has discussed several factors that are suspected of playing a fundamental role in the pathophysiology (e.g., sensitivity to angiotensin II, impaired PG synthesis, coagulation defects, hypovolemia). The following discussion focuses on the possible initiating causes of preeclampsia.

DECREASED UTEROPLACENTAL PERFUSION

Proponents of this theory hypothesize that decrements in uteroplacental perfusion trigger hypertensive mechanisms, possibly by increasing uterine venous efflux of a vasopressor substance or decreasing the outflow of a vasodilator hormone. The cause of reduced arterial flow is not known, but nonpregnant human uterine arteries and veins studied in vitro respond to endothelin with a slowly developing and long-lasting vasoconstriction, and neuropeptide Y has a similar but slightly weaker effect [83].

Animal experiments indicate that acute reductions in uteroplacental flow are accompanied by decreased amounts of PG-like material in the uterine veins. There are also several animal models of hypertension in pregnancy produced by decreasing blood flow to the uterus, and there is an interesting observation in humans that high altitude increases the incidence of preeclampsia [39, 141, 179, 300]. There are no human data comparable to the animal studies cited above to which to refer, but the healthy human placenta must function normally over a range of perfusing pressures, including the 15 percent decrease in mean arterial pressure that occurs at night during sleep [219]. Certainly, a convincing animal model of preeclampsia would be a useful step toward understanding this disease.

ENDOTHELIAL CELL DAMAGE

Normal endothelium has many functions, including inhibition and modification of the contractile activity of the adjacent vascular smooth muscle [275]. As already mentioned, endothelial cells produce several hormones and autocoids including prostacyclin, the local vasodilatory EDRF (synonymous with nitric oxide), and the potent vasoconstrictor endothelin. There is a growing body of morphologic and biochemical data suggesting that endothelial dysfunction or damage is an early and important feature of preeclampsia, responsible for several signs of this disease including vasoconstriction and coagulation abnormalities [182, 226, 227, 230]. The primary renal lesion involves the glomerular endothelium (see below), and there is evidence of endothelial damage in placentas of preeclamptic women [241]. Biochemical alterations in preeclampsia include increments in circulating levels of fibronectin produced exclusively by endothelial cells ($ED1^+$), factor VIII antigens, and endothelial cell antibodies [145, 226, 227]. EDRF release may be impaired from umbilical vessels of fetuses born to hypertensive women, which could reflect a decrease in EDRF release through the maternal circulation [204], perhaps due to the presence of elevated serum endothelial cytotoxins, mitogens, or lipid peroxides [113]. Of even greater interest are preliminary data that sera from preeclamptic patients are cytotoxic and mytogenic and increase the transcription and production of a growth factor(s) by endothelial cells in culture [182, 226, 227, 230, 266, 267]. This latter factor(s), in the process of being characterized [266], appears to be heat and acid labile and has been dubbed by the group researching it as ELMER (Endogenous Ligand conferring MitogEnic Response).

Finally, given that decreased uteroplacental perfusion may trigger hypertensive mechanisms (see earlier), it is of interest that in the perfused human fetoplacental circulation there is a capacity to generate nitric oxide intracellularly. Nitric oxide can act as a vasodilator, and its basal release probably contributes to vascular resistance in this circulation [102, 183].

IMMUNOLOGIC MECHANISMS

There is evidence to suggest that severe preeclampsia may have an immunologic basis [17, 21, 67, 81a, 128, 222]. Circulating immune complexes, which have been found in preeclampsia in higher concentrations than in normal pregnancy, could trigger the disseminated intravascular coagulation (DIC) that has been reported to occur in preeclampsia by some investigators. High levels of IgG and IgM antibodies to laminin, a glycoprotein present in both trophoblast and glomerular basement membrane, have been detected in sera from preeclamptic women [81a]. Immune complexes have been found in preeclamptic vascular lesions of the placental bed and the kidney, the density of renal immunoglobulin deposits correlating with the severity of the disease. Perhaps these lesions could account for other abnormalities, for example, decreased placental blood flow resulting from vascular lesions; this might explain the decreased placental PGE concentrations observed in preeclampsia, which in turn may account for the increased vascular responsiveness to angiotensin II. Although these theories are interesting, they do not explain the basic immunologic abnormality.

At first consideration it would seem unlikely for severe preeclampsia to have an immunologic basis because it is most common in first pregnancies, in contrast to the best-documented immunologic condition in pregnancy, rhesus isoimmunization. However, preeclampsia may be the result not of an excessive immune response but of an inadequate response [21], the protective immune response possibly being less efficient in first than in later pregnancies. Evidence for an impaired immune response in preeclampsia compared with normal pregnancy comes from studies of lymphocyte DNA synthesis, lymphocyte response to phytohemagglutinin, lymphocytotoxic antibody titers, and reduced T-helper and T-suppressor cytotoxic cell percentages during labor [11, 17, 258]. The decrease in T-helper cell count can occur several weeks before the development of clinical preeclampsia [11].

Pregnancy always suppresses a mother's immune response to some extent, since rejection of an antigenically foreign fetus needs to be prevented, but this physiologic immunosuppression may be greater than usual in preeclampsia. This could account for the increased evidence of the disease in conditions such as twin pregnancy and molar pregnancy, in which there are high plasma concentrations of human chorionic gonadotropin (hCG), a likely immunosuppressive agent.

Why should women with preeclampsia have a defective immune response? It is interesting that no particular maternal HLA antigen is associated with preeclampsia, nor is there excessive maternal-fetal HLA incompatibility. However, what is apparent in some investigations is that preeclamptic gravidas have increased homozygosity for human leukocyte antigens (HLA) antigens: Those who are homozygous for HLA-A and HLA-B antigens are more likely to have severe preeclampsia [222]. This would account for the apparently increased HLA compatibility between mothers and fetuses, and also the decreased immune response. HLA genes are thought to be closely linked to immune-response genes at adjacent loci, and Redman and colleagues [222] have suggested that homozygosity of HLA genes in a given patient therefore would imply that the adjacent immune-response genes are almost certainly homozygous as well, suggesting the operation of a recessive gene in preeclampsia.

GENETIC FACTORS

One hypothesis is that there is homozygosity for recessive maternal immune-response genes linked to HLA (most recently DR4 [128]) and that genetic control of severe preeclampsia may depend on mendelian inheritance of a single recessive gene [41, 49, 128, 222]. Because preeclampsia is manifest only in pregnancy, the two obvious possibilities for the determining factor are the genotype of either the mother or the fetus. If there is recessive inheritance, these two possibilities will not be distinguished by study of mother-daughter pairs. Instead, it is necessary to know the incidence of preeclampsia in sisters of affected women (higher than expected incidence if maternal genotype hypothesis is correct) or in the husband's female relatives (higher than expected incidence if the fetal hypothesis is correct). Cooper and Liston [49] re-analyzed the family data collected by Chesley [41] and found that the incidence to "toxemia" in the sisters, the daughters, and the sisters-in-law of eclamptic women proved to fit closely with the notion of maternal homozygosity for a recessive gene. However, when they extended their analysis to two further sets of their own data, evidence for the fetal-genotype hypothesis was apparent; thus, as to be expected, there was a significant deficit of preeclamptic illness in sisters of affected women. Thus a final decision on this matter was deferred.

Any hypothesis on the etiology of preeclampsia has to account for the first-pregnancy preponderance. If preeclampsia depended on the fetal gene, the influence of parity would be extremely difficult to explain. It is easier to accept the Chesley data and the re-analysis with the suggestion that the evidence in favor of the fetal-genotype hypothesis may be biased by problems of underascertainment. Parous women who conceive for the first time by a new partner seem to have an increased risk of preeclampsia, thus behaving as primigravidas [240]. This leads to the concept that preeclampsia results from an absent or deficient maternal immune response to the fetus, which is necessary for normal pregnancy and is more likely to be imperfectly developed in first exposure to fetal antigens [21, 240].

Thus the first-pregnancy preponderance of preeclampsia, its familial occurrence, and the HLA data can be gathered together by one genetic hypothesis; the putative gene and its function have not been identified, but circumstantial evidence suggests that it may be an immune-response gene.

Clinical Sequelae of Hypertension

THE KIDNEYS

With hypertension in pregnancy, renal hemodynamics decrease by approximately 25 percent compared with normal pregnancy. Since renal hemodynamics increase 30 to 50 percent in normal gestation, the GFR and effective renal plasma flow (ERPF) of preeclamptic women often remain above prepregnancy values. Occasionally, functional impairment is quite severe, and preeclampsia can cause both tubular and cortical necrosis.

Uric acid clearance, which also increases during normal pregnancy, decreases markedly in preeclampsia [39, 58, 141, 220]. The decrement is earlier and greater than that of GFR (although there is disagreement about this conclusion), and elevated serum uric acid levels may be the first sign of the disease (although this is also debatable [71]); serum values of 4.5 mg per deciliter or more during pregnancy are abnormal and are associated with a poor fetal outcome [reviewed in 141].

Abnormal proteinuria that is moderately unselective is a hallmark of preeclampsia. The increments in urinary protein excretion may be minimal to large. Preeclampsia is the most common cause of nephrotic syndrome in pregnancy [77, 78] (see also Chap. 83).

Preeclampsia is accompanied by a characteristic renal lesion termed *glomerular capillary endotheliosis* [78, 85]. The renal pathology of preeclampsia is illustrated and discussed in Chap. 83 and will be briefly summarized here. The glomerular swelling is due to a characteristic hypertrophy of the intracapillary cells involving mainly the endothelial and less commonly the mesangial cells. These swollen cells, which contain a variety of vacuoles and lipid clusters, encroach on the capillary lumen, thus creating the appearance of a bloodless glomerulus. On occasion, the glomerular swelling results in herniation of the tuft into the initial segment of the proximal tubule, a pattern termed *pouting* by Sheehan and Lynch [243]. The basement membrane is usually normal. Some authors stress the occurrence of mesangial proliferation leading to its interposition in the basement membrane and a "tramline" image in the glomerulus [reviewed in 85, 243]. This is unusual in our experience [78, 85]. Similarly, while some state that focal glomerular sclerosis occurs de novo in pure preeclampsia, we believe that such changes, when present, have predated the disease [85].

Occasionally small endothelial deposits (thought to represent accumulation of protein) and tactoids of fibrin or a fibrinlike material may be seen. Such images may be due in part to the accumulation of several basement membrane proteins including laminin, type IV collagen, fibronectin, and a proteoglycan in the glomeruli of preeclamptics [81a].

The tubules are usually intact. The significance of immunoglobulins and fibrin deposition that are present in the glomeruli of preeclamptic patients is disputed and is discussed in detail elsewhere [78, 85]. Of interest, though, is the report by Packham et al. [195] in which biopsies performed prior to delivery contained substantially more fibrin deposition than those obtained postpartum, suggesting that mobilization of deposits postpartum occurs more rapidly than was originally appreciated.

THE LIVER

Preeclampsia is probably the most common cause of liver function abnormalities in pregnancy, but elevations of transaminases are usually mild. One should be aware, however, of a variant that can appear deceptively benign because the patient presents with minimal changes in blood pressure, small decrements in platelet counts, mild elevations in liver enzymes, and little or no renal dysfunction, thus tempting the physician to temporize. This form of the disease may progress rapidly and become a life-threatening syndrome characterized by hemolysis with liver (transaminase and lactic acid dehydrogenases rising to 1,000 IU) and coagulation (platelets considerably below 100,000 per mm^3) abnormalities. This uncommon form of preeclampsia has been termed the HELLP syndrome (acronym for hemolysis, elevated liver enzymes, and low platelet counts; often just *ellp*) and constitutes an emergency requiring termination of the pregnancy [159, 161, 162, 246, 249]. Furthermore, while postpartum recovery is usually rapid, the disease may persist for almost a week. Some authors have had to do a plasma exchange in a few of these patients [163], but this is not our experience, and perhaps some of the women treated by exchange had thrombotic thrombocytopenic purpura—extremely rare, but associated with pregnancy.

Whether there is a characteristic liver lesion for preeclampsia is debated, its most enthusiastic proponent being the pathologist Sheehan [243]. Fibrin deposition has also been noted in liver biopsies, and subcapsular hematomas and rupture into the abdomen are a dangerous complication of preeclampsia.

THE PLACENTA

When establishing hemochorial placentation, the nonvillous trophoblast breaches the spiral arteries in the basal decidua and later migrates down the arteries, reaching the radial arteries in the myometrium. The interaction between endovascular trophoblasts and the tissues of the maternal vessel wall adapts these arteries to the uteroplacental arteries, so that large-caliber vessels empty into the intervillous space. Loss of reactive musculoelastic tissue results in a dilated vessel, which permits increased blood flow into the intervillous space. In women destined to develop preeclampsia, there is a variable inhibition of the secondary endovascular trophoblastic migration in the second trimester, so that myometrial segments of the uteroplacental arteries remain narrowed and responsive [203, 228]. In addition, a necrotizing arteriopathy or "acute atherosis" may affect the small muscular arteries in the placental bed.

In preeclampsia, placental blood flow, as determined by the placental clearance or accumulation of various injected radiolabels, is reduced, with a concomitant decrement in intervillous blood oxygen saturation [144]. Obviously, there are several structural features that could cause or may be associated with reduced placental blood flow, and as will be discussed later, these will not themselves be reversed by medical treatment (see below).

THE CENTRAL NERVOUS SYSTEM

Eclampsia is the convulsive phase of preeclampsia and may occur at any time prior to, during, or after delivery. As many as one-third of the reported cases present on the first postpartum day. Hypertension and convulsions have also been reported days to weeks into the puerperium and have been termed *late postpartum eclampsia*, but whether or not these patients in fact had preeclampsia is controversial [27, 245].

Cerebral hemorrhage is the major cause of maternal death from preeclampsia or eclampsia (Table 57-4) [114, 243]. As well as large hemorrhages, diffusely scattered infarcts, cortical petechiae, smaller subcortical hemorrhages, and necrotic arterioles (some containing fibrin thrombi) are found [243]. The large hemorrhages can be similar to those found in hypertension in nonpregnant individuals, and the other changes are like the autopsy findings seen in hypertensive encephalopathy. To equate eclampsia with hypertensive encephalopathy, however, is not strictly correct because although eclampsia usually correlates with the severity of the hypertension, it may also occur when blood pressure elevations are mild [139–141]. For example, in 22 percent of eclamptic patients originally described by Dieckman, systolic levels never exceeded 140 mm Hg [reviewed in 39], and similar observations were reported by Sheehan and Lynch in their large series [243]. It could be argued that such women had experienced large and sudden increments from previously low values and that it is the magnitude of the change in pressure that is responsible for the convulsion. However, it is not unusual to observe a gravida suddenly develop proteinuria and hyperreflexia and even convulse over a short period of time even though the blood pressure differs little from that recorded 24 hours previously. Furthermore, retinal exudates, hemorrhages, and/or papillary edema, which are hallmarks of hypertensive encephalopathy, are infrequent in preeclampsia-eclampsia, in which funduscopic changes are minimal. Another possible cause of the convulsion (and transient blindness) is brain edema [256], but whereas some authors have offered selective evidence of such pathology—usually by computerized tomography (CT) scanning—many women who convulse have normal findings by CT scans [245].

In summary, the pathogenesis of the eclamptic con-

Table 57-4. Maternal deaths in England and Wales

Period	All maternal deaths	Deaths attributable to eclampsia (% of all deaths)	Eclamptic deaths with significant cerebral hemorrhage (% of all eclamptic deaths)
1961–1963	692	40 (5.8%)	13 (32.5%)
1964–1966	579	40 (6.9%)	14 (36.0%)
1967–1969	455	41 (9.0%)	10 (24.4%)
1970–1972	355	29 (8.2%)	16 (55.2%)
1973–1975	235	21 (8.9%)	11 (52.4%)
1976–1978	217	13 (5.9%)	8 (61.5%)
1979–1981	176	20 (11.4%)	7 (35.0%)
1982–1984	138	14 (10.1%)	7 (50.0%)
1985–1987	139	12 (8.6%)	4 (33.3%)

Source: From *Reports on Confidential Enquiries into Maternal Deaths in England and Wales*. London: Her Majesty's Stationery Office, 1966, 1969, 1972, 1975, 1979, 1982, 1986, 1989, and 1991 [114].

vulsion is poorly understood. Advocates of hypertensive encephalopathy invoke acute pressure-induced injury of the cerebral arterioles, which, on losing their ability to remain in protective spasm and participate in autoregulatory control, then expose the more peripheral vessels to high-pressure hyperfiltration and permeability changes affecting the blood-brain barrier. Others attribute convulsions to DIC characterized by platelet fibrin clots that obstruct the cerebral microcirculation [167]. Sheehan and Lynch [243], who performed most of their autopsies between 15 minutes and 2 hours after death, ascribe the cerebral changes to the vasoconstriction itself. There is also a high percentage of frank cerebral bleeding in autopsy material from women dying of eclampsia, but according to Sheehan and Lynch, most of these episodes occur after the initial convulsion.

CARDIOVASCULAR HEMODYNAMICS

The statement that cardiac output and pulmonary capillary wedge pressure (PCWP) are lower in preeclamptics compared to normotensive gravidas was a simplified synthesis of current information that avoided considerable controversy on this subject. Actually, cardiac output has been variably described as decreased, unchanged, and increased in this disease, and there are similar contrasting data regarding alterations in PCWP. Resolution of these discrepancies, important for therapeutic strategy (i.e., volume loading versus diuretics, vasodilators, etc.) would seem easy to resolve with the advent of percutaneous catheterization technology, but results continue to conflict [153, 279, 281]. Two reasons for these discrepancies are that investigators often report data from mixed populations, including women with severe forms of essential hypertension, and that measurements are frequently reported only after therapeutic interventions, including substantial volume loading.

The studies of Wallenburg [279, 281], Hankins [103], and their respective colleagues are exceptions to the above and form the basis for the view we favor. The first group, who studied large numbers of nulliparous proteinuric hypertensives (most would be true preeclamptics) prior to any form of treatment included normotensive third-trimester subjects in their study. Cardiac output was decreased while PCWP was low-normal in the preeclamptic women compared to the controls. Hypertension was thus maintained by a marked increase in systemic vascular resistance. Hankins et al. [103] evaluated primigravid *eclamptics* whose fluid was restricted to 75 ml/hour (in the absence of renal biopsy, convulsion in a nullipara is good evidence of pure preeclampsia). In these patients, PCWPs were definitely low, ranging from 1 to 5 cm H_2O initially. Lang et al. [133], using noninvasive echocardiography, studied primigravid proteinuric hypertensives and normotensive pregnant controls at term, and again after the puerperium. These authors confirmed that the cardiac output was decreased and systemic vascular resistance markedly increased in the preeclamptics; these values returned to normal 6 weeks postpartum. Another finding of this latter study was that load-independent left ventricular contractility was unaltered in preeclampsia.

In contrast, Mabie et al. [153] described a large group of hypertensive gravidas who underwent pulmonary artery catheterization at term. They analyzed retrospectively a subgroup of nulliparous women, studied before any substantial therapeutic maneuvers had been undertaken, and noted a variety of central hemodynamic values in which cardiac output was typically normal to high, while PCWP was often normal. Resolution of all the discrepancies listed above may be provided by studies of Easterling and colleagues [64], who prospectively measured cardiac output throughout gestation using noninvasive echocardiographic techniques. These authors claim that cardiac output is initially "excessively" increased and peripheral resistance low in women destined to develop preeclampsia. Resistance increases while cardiac output falls as frank disease develops. Measurements made at various stages of this crossover period may explain the broad spectrum of results. The serial observations of Easterling et al. require confirmation, and some believe that future preeclamptics develop increased peripheral resistance very early in gestation.

Also it appears to us that those with the most obvious or severe disease have low cardiac output and markedly increased resistances.

The Hypertensive Gravida Without Preeclampsia

There is substantial literature documenting the increased risk associated with pregnancy in women with chronic hypertension [reviewed in 39]. Complications include superimposed preeclampsia, accelerated rise of pressure to a malignant phase, abruptio placentae [2], acute renal tubular and cortical necrosis, intrauterine growth retardation, and midtrimester fetal death. Such events seem to correlate with the age of the gravida and the duration of her high blood pressure. Thus the majority of these complications occur in women 30 years of age or over, or in those whose preexistent hypertension has caused end-organ damage (primarily nephrosclerosis). On the other hand, over 85 percent of patients with essential hypertension have uncomplicated gestations.

Women with chronic essential hypertension often manifest reductions in blood pressure by midpregnancy that may exceed those observed in normotensive gravidas [39]. In fact, failure of this decrement to occur or increments in blood pressure in early pregnancy or midtrimester portend a reserved prognosis.

Fetal outcome is poorer in hypertensive women with superimposed preeclampsia than in previously normotensive women with this complication, and it is the combination of chronic hypertension and preeclampsia that seems responsible for most cases of cerebral hemorrhage in pregnancy. The marked increase in morbid events, however, is due primarily to the specific pathophysiology of preeclampsia.

Assessment and Management of Hypertension in Pregnancy

GENERAL AIMS OF ANTENATAL CARE

The aims of management are the maintenance of maternal well-being and the delivery of an infant who will survive and develop normally. There have been phenomenal improvements in fetal prognosis in the past decade due to more aggressive and careful antenatal care, so that morbidity and mortality have substantially decreased in patients with chronic hypertension (who may develop superimposed preeclampsia) and those prone to develop preeclampsia. This has been possible by greater reliance on judicious and deliberate preterm delivery and the skills of the neonatologists [224]. We note here, however, that the approach to the hypertensive gravida has historically been (and may still be) quite controversial, with major disputes on managing the hypertension and preventing or treating convulsions in preeclamptics. In these respects an important breakthrough is the report of the Working Group on High Blood Pressure in Pregnancy, convened by the National High Blood Pressure Program at the National Institutes of Health (U.S.A.), where perhaps for the first time obstetricians and internists have reached agreements on a number of controversial issues [184a].

A first and crucial step in approaching the gravida with hypertension is to differentiate preeclampsia (pure or superimposed) from essential hypertension (chronic or transient) (Table 57-5). Since the latter usually do well, temporization is less risky. Preeclampsia, however, is always potentially dangerous and explosive, and the signs and symptoms listed in Table 57-6 are especially ominous.

Table 57-7 lists the guidelines for the initial evaluation

Table 57-5. Differential Diagnosis of Preeclampsia and Chronic Hypertension

	Preeclampsia	Chronic Hypertension
Age	Extremes of age	More often older
Parity	Nulliparous	Multiparous
Onset	Rare before 20 wk	May have BP elevation noted before 20 wk gestation
History	Negative	Positive, often with hypertension in previous pregnancy
Fundi	Retinal edema, arteriolar spasm	May have chronic changes of arteriosclerosis
Cardiac status	Usually normal	Ventricular hypertrophy if disease is long-standing
Deep tendon reflexes	Hyperactive	Normoactive
Proteinuria	Increased	May be absent or minimal
Uric acid	Elevated	Normal
Liver function	May have right upper quadrant pain/tenderness and increased transaminases	Normal
Hematologic tests	May have variable degrees of thrombocytopenia, intravascular coagulation, and hemolytic anemia	Normal

Source: W. M. Barron. Hypertension. In W.M. Barron and M. D. Lindheimer (eds.), *Medical Disorders During Pregnancy*. St. Louis: Mosby-Year Book, 1991.

Table 57-6. Warning signs and symptoms in women with preeclampsia

Preeclampsia is always potentially dangerous but particularly ominous may be:

- Blood pressure ≥ 160 mm Hg systolic or ≥ 110 mm Hg diastolic.
- New onset proteinuria of ≥ 2 gm/24 hours (or ≥ 2+ qualitatively).
- Increasing serum creatinine levels (especially > 177 μmol/liter [2 mg/dl], unless known to be elevated previously).
- Platelet count < 10 × 10^9/liter or evidence of microangiopathic hemolytic anemia (e.g., schistocytes, and/or increased lactic acid dehydrogenase and direct bilirubin).
- Upper abdominal pain (especially epigastric and right upper quadrant).
- Headache, visual disturbances, or other cerebral signs.
- Cardiac decompensation (e.g., pulmonary edema). Usually associated with underlying heart pathology or chronic hypertension.
- Retinal hemorrhages, exudates, or papilledema. (These are extremely rare in the absence of other of the above indications of severity and, when present, almost always denote underlying chronic hypertension.)
- Presence of intrauterine growth retardation and decreasing urine volumes also require added vigilance.

Source: Modified from [184a].

Table 57-7. Guidelines for initial evaluation of pregnant patients with chronic hypertension

1. Detection of end-organ damage	Presence of end-organ involvement suggests a poorer maternal and fetal prognosis. Careful funduscopy and cardiac examination are necessary, and if cardiac hypertrophy is suspected echocardiography may be undertaken (x-rays and electrocardiograms are usually not informative in these situations).
2. Detection of secondary causes of hypertension	a. Screening test for pheochromocytoma (plasma catecholamines, urinary catecholamines or vanillylmandelic acid) b. Renal disease (urinalysis, serum creatinine, or its clearance) Presence of qualitative proteinuria should be followed by measurement of 24-hr excretion patterns. c. Mineralocorticoid excess hypertension (serum potassium)
3. Data base that may help detect superimposed preeclampsia at a later date	a. Hematologic parameters: (Hct, Hb, platelet count) Optional: antithrombin III b. Renal system: Serum creatinine and uric acid levels, urinalysis Optional:24 hr protein c. Liver function, bilirubin, transaminases d. Miscellaneous: Serum albumin

in early pregnancy for women with chronic hypertension. As for managing a woman in whom high blood pressure accelerates to a severe state or in whom an acute hypertensive crisis appears de novo the following guidelines are suggested: In general, induction is the therapy of choice near term, whereas attempts can be made to postpone action if pregnancy is at an earlier stage (mainly before 34 weeks). If a decision is made to temporize, several antihypertensive agents considered safe and effective in pregnancy are available (discussed later; see Tables 57-8 and 57-9). However, if severe hypertension (diastolic levels above 105 mm Hg in most women; some allow 110 mm Hg in chronic hypertensives) persists after 24 to 48 hours of treatment, delivery is usually indicated regardless of the stage of gestation, since the mother is at risk and further delay rarely saves the fetus. Advances in neonatology have been such that most infants weighing 1500 gm or more survive better in a premature nursery than in the womb of a woman with preeclampsia. The appearance of clotting abnormalities, decreasing renal function, and signs of impending convulsions (headache, epigastric pain, and hyperreflexia) are indications for termination of pregnancy.

FETAL SURVEILLANCE AND DECISIONS CONCERNING DELIVERY

Delivery is delayed until, but usually not past, term unless hypertensive control is not readily achieved, hypertension recurs after initial improvement, or there is evidence of fetal jeopardy as determined by contemporaneous techniques of fetal surveillance. If complications do arise, the judicious moment for intervention and the method of delivery must be decided with the aim of minimizing neonatal morbidity and mortality and the hazards of prematurity. The administration of corticosteroids (even in severe hypertension) to induce fetal pulmonary maturity is debated. During labor, the fetus should be monitored carefully, with close cooperation between the obstetrician, the anesthetist and the pediatrician.

Table 57-8. Blood pressure (BP) levels used in recent trials of antihypertensive agents in pregnancy (1976–1985)

Study	BP (mm Hg) entry criteria
Methyldopa versus placebo Redman et al. [221]	BP between 140/90 and 170/110 before twenty-eighth week of pregnancy on two separate occasions
Labetalol versus methyldopa Lamming et al. [131]	Normotensive before twentieth week of pregnancy but thereafter 140/90 or greater, remaining elevated for 3 consecutive days after hospitalization
Oxprenolol versus methyldopa Gallery et al. [88, 89]	Diastolic BP at least 95 on two separate occasions at least 24 hours apart or greater than 105 on one occasion
Atenolol versus placebo Rubin et al. [235]	BP between 140 and 170 systolic or between 90 and 110 diastolic (after 10-minute rest supine or after 5 minutes standing) on two occasions separated by 24 hours
Oxprenolol versus methyldopa Fidler et al. [75]	As defined by Gallery and co-workers
Labetalol versus methyldopa Redman [217]	BP equal to or exceeding 170 systolic or 110 diastolic on two separate occasions

Table 57-9. Food and drug administration pregnancy risk classification

A: *Controlled studies show no risk.* Well-designed studies in humans have failed to demonstrate risk to the fetus.

B: *No evidence of risk in humans.* Either (a) animal studies demonstrate risk but human findings do not or (b) if no adequate human studies have been done, animal findings are negative.

C: *Risk cannot be ruled out.* Human studies are lacking, and animal studies are either positive for fetal risk or have not been performed. However, potential benefits may justify the potential risk.

D: *Positive evidence of risk.* Investigational or post-marketing data show risk to the fetus. Nevertheless, potential benefits may outweigh the risks (e.g., for treatment of serious disease for which safer alternatives are not available).

X: *Contraindicated in pregnancy.* Studies in animals or humans (or post-marketing reports) have shown fetal risk that clearly outweighs any potential benefit to the patient.

SPECIAL CONSIDERATIONS

Invasive hemodynamic monitoring may be required intrapartum or during the immediate puerperium in severe or complicated cases, especially during operative procedures [115]. There have been published indications for invasive monitoring [43], which we consider too broad, and a view shared by the NIH Consensus Group and the American College of Obstetricians and Gynecologists [115]. It is our experience that the need for Swan-Ganz catheterization (a procedure with a certain morbidity) is uncommon, and virtually all cases can be managed using clinical acumen. Patients with marked coagulation changes and severe right upper quadrant pain should be considered for ultrasonic or (postpartum) CT scanning of the liver, which may reveal subcapsular hemorrhages that can rupture, resulting in an acute emergency [159].

Role of Antihypertensive Therapy

The controversial nature of "treating" the hypertension was demonstrated in the early 1980s by mail surveys in which attempts were made to determine how clinicians were managing their hypertensive gravidas [36, 136]. The approach in the United States was different compared with practice in the United Kingdom, and there were disagreements about the level of blood pressure to be treated (Table 57-8), the use of diuretics, the place of antithrombotic therapy, and the level to which blood pressure should be reduced.

There can, however, be no denying that several special features of hypertension in pregnancy, especially that in preeclampsia, do affect decisions about the use of antihypertensive drugs. For example, hypertension is often short-lived and potentially curable (by delivery), and the need for and/or the deleterious effects of treatment on fetal well-being must also be considered.

There seem to be three situations in which antihypertensive agents have been widely used in pregnancy: (1) to control blood pressure in women with essential hypertension, often as a continuation of treatment started before conception, (2) to temporize in situations where pure or superimposed preeclampsia occurs when the fetus is still quite immature, and (3) during acute hypertensive emergencies, usually those due to preeclampsia at term. While all agree that moderate and severe hypertension must be treated, there is a debate about whether mild hypertension [defined here as diastolic levels between 90 and 100 mm Hg (Korotkoff V)] should be treated [73, 139–141, 184]. Any decision on the use of antihypertensive drugs can be taken only after answering three basic questions: (1) What are the adverse consequences of the level of hypertension under consideration? (2) What are the potential benefits of treatment and what is the evidence? (3) What are the possible adverse effects of treatment and what is the evidence?

Any benefits must be weighed against possibly adverse effects on the offspring, short- and long-term. There is a paucity of data and there are no standards for drug testing, including criteria for prehuman testing in animal models, that encompasses (1) effects of the agent on the ability of the fetus to withstand hypoxic stress, (2) thorough analyses of structural and functional variables in the neonate, and (3) long-term assessment of intellectual and physical well-being of the offspring.

The U.S. Food and Drug Administration has suggested a "risk assessment classification" that theoretically assigns an individual drug according to risk posed to the fetus or neonate (Table 57-9). Most drugs have not been "risk assessed" by the manufacturers, so variable categorization may occur between different authors. Furthermore, clinicians may be lulled into a false sense of security about drug prescribing during pregnancy because of a notation that "no fetal or reproductive side effects have been described."

There have been very few studies of even crude markers of drug safety let alone any subtle effects. The teratogenicity of all antihypertensives remains virtually unknown, since drug trials of even the best-studied agents (such as methyldopa) have generally included women only when they are beyond the first trimester. Since virtually all drugs prescribed to pregnant women reach the fetus, the above considerations serve as a reminder that therapeutic agents of any kind should be prescribed to pregnant women with the utmost caution.

MILD OR MODERATE HYPERTENSION

If hypertension in pregnancy is not severe, or if its severity has been reduced but drug treatment is required for continued control, the need for ongoing treatment must be decided. Merely treating a physical sign and restoring blood pressure to normal levels is not sufficient reason for treatment.

Maternal Benefits. The risks to the mother of mild or moderate hypertension are unclear. It may be considered that the woman should be treated with long-term antihypertensive therapy on the same grounds that she would be treated if she were not pregnant (i.e., to protect her from the long-term vascular problems of hypertension). Whereas there is reasonable evidence that treatment of moderate hypertension will reduce these complications, it is questionable whether treatment is indicated for mild hypertension [184, 184a]. Furthermore, the treatment and potential gains are long-term considerations, and postponing treatment until after pregnancy may be reasonable.

Preventing Preeclampsia. Patients who develop hypertension in early pregnancy are probably at increased risk of preeclampsia later on. If chronic hypertension has a causal role in the development of preeclampsia, then treatment of the hypertension early in pregnancy might prevent later superimposed preeclampsia, and this has been claimed [22, 234, 235]. However, critical review of the evidence [184, 248] indicates to us that apart from lowering blood pressure antihypertensive agents do not affect the development of proteinuria nor any of the other features of preeclampsia.

Uteroplacental Blood Flow. The possible effect on the uteroplacental circulation and hence on the fetal lifeline is an important consideration when deciding whether or not the blood pressure of a hypertensive gravida should be reduced [139]. We do not yet know the answers. There are two premises: (1) The uterine artery behaves as a rigid conduit (or is maximally dilated), and any reductions in maternal blood pressure concomitantly decrease uteroplacental perfusion; consequently, large reductions in maternal blood pressure are guarded against, especially when acute hypertension develops near term. (This is important in relation to the arguments that placental ischemia is the cause, rather than the consequence, of the hypertension.) (2) The uteroplacental blood flow autoregulates rapidly and completely; therefore, aggressive lowering of blood pressure should be the aim. If it is assumed that autoregulation does take place in humans, a critical but unanswered question is how quickly it occurs, because the fetus may be compromised by trivially brief periods of ischemia.

Uteroplacental perfusion appears to be normal or even increased with mild to moderate maternal hypertension, becoming abnormal only when severe preeclampsia and/or intrauterine growth retardation is present [93, 144], consistent with the fact that pregnancies complicated by mild to moderate hypertension often exhibit no evidence of fetal compromise [248].

There have been detailed discussions of the control and effects of antihypertensive agents on uterine blood flow in experimental animals. It appears that most studied measurements included perfusion of uterine tissues (nonplacental flow) as well as the placental bed, so it is difficult to determine whether the changes observed were in the former, the latter, or both.

Fetal Benefits. If therapy cannot be rationalized on the basis of improvement of the so-called uteroplacental unit, another index might be the effects on fetal salvage. There are claims [221, 252] disputed [248] that early maternal hypertension is associated with a predisposition to midtrimester fetal death. Fetal outcome in later pregnancy is closely linked to the presence of preeclampsia, and in pregnancies complicated by hypertension without preeclampsia, fetal outcome appears no worse than in normal pregnancies [37].

One must be circumspect in interpreting results in hypertensives who demonstrate improvement over previous gestations because superimposed preeclampsia (in which there is a higher incidence of fetal mortality) occurs most often in the first pregnancy only, and a gravida is more likely to be compliant if a previous gestation was complicated.

Conclusions. We suggest an intermediate approach toward therapy in mild or moderate hypertension. Antihypertensive agents are not given during pregnancy as long as maternal blood pressure is only mildly elevated. The Consensus Group [184a] concluded that therapy can be withheld until diastolic pressures reach 100 mm Hg, a view with which we concur. Exceptions, though, include individuals with end-organ damage, including those with renal disease, as well as selected gravidas whose initial levels were very low and increased rapidly. In these groups, treatment should be more aggressive. All these approaches take into account both the mother's safety and the fetal outcome. Finally, rest or a sedate environment can be important, and it is common to encounter patients whose blood pressure is controlled by hospitalization alone but who experience a striking exacerbation on discharge [28, 108].

Antihypertensive Agents. Several antihypertensive agents are in current usage (Table 57-10), including the following (see [184a], [225], and [260] for details):

METHYLDOPA (ALDOMET). This is a centrally acting drug and an α_2-receptor agonist that reduces sympathetic tone and is effective in maintaining blood pressure at safe levels in most cases of essential hypertension and, for a time, in the many women with preeclampsia. However, preeclampsia is a progressive disorder, and methyldopa may eventually become inadequate for proper control. Intermittent acute treatment can be added if necessary, but the woman should usually be delivered without delay at this stage.

Methyldopa is the hypotensive drug whose long-term safety for the newborn has been most satisfactorily assessed [44, 184, 194]. In carefully controlled studies there were no significant adverse effects on fetal or neonatal outcome except for a small transient reduction in neonatal blood pressure. Follow-up of the infants at 7 years has revealed no abnormality in development. This is the NIH Consensus Group's [184a] drug of choice.

Methyldopa treatment should be started by administration of 0.5 to 0.75 gm per day and can be increased to 3.0 to 4.0 gm per day; the latter amounts, which are greater than those given to nonpregnant women, are tolerated and may be required in pregnancy because there is increased hepatic clearance of the drug. Lethargy and some drowsiness are very common when therapy is started, but these usually disappear within a few days, and significant depression is unusual in pregnancy.

BETA-ADRENERGIC BLOCKING AGENTS. The use of β-adrenergic blocking agents (β-blockers) in pregnancy was initially condemned [reviewed in 184a, 225, 233, 260]. However, as a larger experience has accrued, more and more authorities are recommending their use in pregnant women. Beta-adrenoceptor antagonists have been used most widely in women with mild to moderate essential hypertension in pregnancy, where they are effective as antihypertensives, but the benefits of treatment are uncertain [75, 89, 90, 234, 235]. Whether or not β-blocking drugs reduce the frequency of preeclampsia is controversial: For instance, significant reductions in proteinuria have been reported by one group [235], but in these studies the incidence of proteinuria in the placebo group was extremely high, given the selection criteria for mild hypertension. Furthermore, neither birth weight nor perinatal survival was affected in the placebo group, which is suspect given the high incidence of their complications in true proteinuric preeclampsia. Thus in this often quoted study, the benefit seems to be nonspecific suppression of proteinuria, not a known action of β-blockers, rather than a blunting of the progression of preeclampsia. Beta-adrenoceptor antagonists alone may not be adequate to maintain control of severe hypertension, and the addition of an α-blocking drug has been effective, albeit in uncontrolled studies [147, 148].

Earlier, anecdotal reports suggested that β-blockers were associated with adverse neonatal outcomes, but these have not been confirmed in larger controlled trials

Table 57-10. Antihypertensive drugs in pregnancy

α_2-Receptor agonists	Methyldopa is the most extensively used drug in this group, its safety and efficacy supported in randomized trials, and there is a 7-yr follow-up study of children born to treated mothers. *Methyldopa is the drug of choice recommended by the N.I.H. Working Group* [184a].
β-Receptor antagonists	These drugs, especially atenolol and metoprolol, appear safe and efficacious in late pregnancy, but fetal growth retardation has been noted when treatment was started in early or mid-gestation. Fetal bradycardia can occur, and animal studies suggest the fetus' ability to tolerate hypoxic stress may be compromised.
α- and β-Receptor antagonists	Labetalol appears as effective as methyldopa, but follow-up studies of children are unreported, and there is concern for maternal hepatotoxicity.
Arteriolar vasodilators	Hydralazine is used frequently as adjunctive therapy with methyldopa and β-receptor antagonists. Rarely, neonatal thrombocytopenia has been reported. Trials with calcium channel blockers look promising. Experience with minoxidil is limited; this drug is not recommended.
Converting enzyme inhibitors	Captopril causes fetal death in diverse animal species, and several converting enzyme inhibitors have been associated with renal failure in the newborn when administered to humans [231]. *Do not use in pregnancy.*
Diuretics	Many authorities discourage their use, but others continue these medications if they were prescribed before gestation, or if a chronic hypertensive appears quite salt sensitive. *The latter views have been endorsed by the N.I.H. Working Group* [184a].

Source: Modified from Cunningham and Lindheimer, *N. Engl. J. Med.* 326:927, 1992. (See Remuzzi et al. [225] and Sturgiss et al. [260] for further discussion.)

[233–235]. Although no adverse effects on fetal outcome have been seen, the reported benefits have been inconsistent. Gallery and her colleagues [89, 90] reported a significantly greater birth weight and placental weight in oxprenolol-treated patients compared with those treated with methyldopa. However, in a similar but larger study, Fidler and co-workers [75] reported no difference in birth weight or any other parameter of fetal or maternal outcome; these authors also noted that the birth weights in the methyldopa group described by Gallery and her colleagues were unusually small compared with those in several other studies. Finally, in a recently reported controlled (but limited) trial, Butters and colleagues [33] have suggested that β-blockers, when commenced in early gestation actually provoke intrauterine growth retardation.

Although β-blockers appear to be safe in the context of mild to moderate hypertension in pregnancy, there remains a concern that these drugs may impair the capacity of the fetus to cope with intrauterine stress, as observed in animal studies [118]; and in human pregnancy, β-blockade may attenuate the usual signs of fetal distress [147]. Fetal jeopardy is likely to occur most commonly in the context of severe preeclampsia; experience with β-blocking drugs in this situation is more limited, and no controlled studies of such a group of patients are available. Also, the fetus may develop bradycardia when these drugs are used, which may be misinterpreted as fetal distress.

Several β-blockers have been used in pregnancy, and doses differ [225, 260]. Side effects of β-blocker therapy are unusual as long as the contraindications to their use are observed.

LABETALOL. This is a combined α- and β-adrenoceptor blocking agent. Randomized controlled trials of labetalol and methyldopa have revealed that labetalol can be a useful drug in the control of maternal hypertension. One group treated moderate hypertension and concluded that side effects were fewer than with methyldopa and that labetalol improved renal function significantly with a markedly lower incidence of proteinuria [131]. The experience of two larger studies [217, 248], however, is that methyldopa and labetalol are equally effective in treating hypertension in pregnancy.

It should be noted that labetalol has theoretical advantages, particularly for the uteroplacental circulation [151, 152] possibly because of its α-blocking action and possibly its ability to counteract platelet aggregation [280], but these effects should not lead one, as has been suggested, to raise the drug's status to that "of choice." When used it is usually started at 100 mg three or four times daily and can be increased to a total of 1,200 mg daily. Side effects are usually minor and include headache and tremulousness. Some disturbing features, however, are observation of an increase in retroplacental clots, noted in the study at Oxford, and recent reports that chronic use in nonpregnant populations is associated with hepatotoxicity.

The infants born to mothers who have received labetalol apparently show little evidence of clinically significant neonatal β-blockade. Systolic blood pressure can be lower by 10 mm Hg at 2 hours after delivery, but gradually normalizes by 24 hours.

HYDRALAZINE. This vasodilator has greater activity on arteries than veins; it is said to increase renal, cerebral, and uteroplacental perfusion; and it does not have known deleterious effects on the fetus. A potential problem with this drug, however, is the appearance of tachycardia, which may exaggerate the physiologic hyperdynamic state of pregnancy. Also, while hydralazine appears reasonably safe for the fetus, thrombocytopenia of uncertain etiology has been reported in a few babies [299] and there are no long-term follow-up studies on children exposed to this drug in utero. When given orally, if the dose is started at 10 mg three times daily and increased gradually, hemodynamic stresses are rare. Hydralazine has also been used quite successfully combined with methyldopa. Finally, the reversible SLE-like syndrome reported to complicate hydralazine therapy should not occur if the daily dose is kept below 200 mg.

SEVERE HYPERTENSION

This section deals with drug treatment when high blood pressure accelerates a situation most often encountered near term and often in the intrapartum period (Table 57-11).

Antihypertensive treatment will reduce the risk only of those complications that are a direct consequence of high blood pressure; the other complications of severe preeclampsia need to be specifically managed in their own right. Thus the major aim of treating severe hypertension in pregnancy is the prevention of acute cerebrovascular injury. Blood pressures of 170/110 and 180/120 mm Hg represent mean arterial pressures of 130 and 140 mm Hg, respectively, levels at which vascular decompensation and end-organ damage occur, and in pregnant women damage may conceivably occur at even lower levels of pressure. It is essential to avoid elevations of blood pressure to or above these levels, even for short periods, and in our hospitals we try to maintain diastolic levels below 100 mm Hg in teenage gravidas and below 105 mm Hg in all others. Even when delivery is expedited, high blood pressure often does not disappear immediately and it may be necessary to use drug treatment in the immediate puerperium.

Bearing in mind our earlier discussion, the main theoretical disadvantage of lowering arterial pressure is the decrement in perfusion pressure (especially when such decrements are precipitous) [57] in the uteroplacental circulation. Thus ideal agents should act quickly, but reduce blood pressure in a controlled manner. They should not decrease cardiac output (to avoid catecholamine release), should reverse uteroplacental vascular constriction, and should have minimal adverse effects on mother and fetus [184, 184a].

Antihypertensive Agents. HYDRALAZINE. Because most preeclamptics are vasoconstricted and have low cardiac output and intravascular volume, parenteral hydralazine

Table 57-11. Guidelines for treating severe hypertension near term or during labor

1. The degree to which blood pressure should be decreased is disputed. The NIH Consensus Group recommends levels between 90 and 105 mm Hg (see text).
2. Drug therapy
   a. Hydralazine administered intravenously is the drug of choice. Start with low doses (5 mg IV bolus), then administer 5–10 mg q20–30 min, to avoid precipitous decreases. Side effects include tachycardia and headache. Neonatal thrombocytopenia has been reported.
   b. Diazoxide is recommended for the occasional patient whose hypertension is refractory to hydralazine. Use 30-mg miniboluses, as precipitous hypotension can occur with higher doses. Side effects include arrest of labor and neonatal hypoglycemia.
   c. Experience with labetalol is growing, and some use this agent, instead of diazoxide, as a second-line drug (see also Table 57-10).
   d. Favorable results have also been reported with calcium channel blockers. However, if magnesium sulfate is being infused, the magnesium may potentiate the effect of the calcium channel blockers, resulting in precipitous and severe hypotension.
   e. Refrain from using nitroprusside (fetal cyanide poisoning has been reported in animal models). However, in final analysis, maternal well-being will dictate choice of therapy.
3. The National Institutes of Health Working Group [184a] recommends parenteral magnesium sulfate as the drug of choice for preventing impending eclamptic convulsions. Therapy should continue for 12–24 hours into the puerperium, since one-third of patients with eclampsia have their convulsion after childbirth.

Source: Modified from Cunningham and Lindheimer, *N. Engl. J. Med.* 326:927, 1992.

should be administered cautiously. A loading dose should be limited to 10 mg, usually given intravenously. Thereafter, 5- or 10-mg doses can be repeated approximately every 30 minutes until the diastolic pressure is reduced to its desired end point. Others utilize a constant intravenous infusion (40 to 60 mg of hydralazine dissolved in a liter of intravenous fluid, *not* dextrose, according to the manufacturer's instructions), again adjusting the rate to keep diastolic blood pressure at about 100 mm Hg. It should be remembered that the onset of action of hydralazine is delayed by 20 to 30 minutes after intravenous and 30 to 40 minutes after intramuscular or subcutaneous administration. Thus the full effect of the drug will not be apparent for 30 to 45 minutes, and it is probably for this reason that "overreduction" of blood pressure can be a problem when the dose is repeated at too short intervals or constant infusions are used. Some have advocated determining the patient's baseline hemodynamic setting, as assessed by echocardiography, before deciding on the dose of parenteral hydralazine to be used [130], a course that is neither practical nor appears cost-effective to us and may delay the onset of treatment. Generally, gravidas with a low cardiac output and high vascular resistance are more susceptible to precipitous hypotension with use of vasodilating agents, and, as noted, one should proceed cautiously starting with low doses of hydralazine.

The duration of effect is relatively short, often no more than 2 to 3 hours, so that small doses at 1- to 2-hourly intervals are better than larger doses delayed until blood pressure is rising out of control. Blood pressure can be reduced to an acceptable level with this regimen, but occasionally there is some symptomatic distress—headache, tremor, tachycardia, flushing, nausea and vomiting—symptoms that mimic impending eclampsia, possibly prompting the unwary clinician to terminate the pregnancy earlier than might otherwise be necessary [184]. On the very rare occasions when adequate control cannot be achieved, additional small, intermittent doses of diazoxide appear to be more satisfactory than very large doses of hydralazine.

Hydralazine has been reported to produce vasodilation in the uteroplacental circulation [119], but there is also evidence that uterine blood flow may decrease after hydralazine in some preeclamptic women, and there are case reports of fetal distress after low doses [115, 278]. In chronically hypertensive women, a decrease in the metabolic clearance of dehydroisoandrosterone sulfate was seen after hydralazine, also suggesting that uteroplacental perfusion may have been reduced. Intravenous hydralazine may increase plasma norepinephrine concentrations for periods that exceed its relatively short hypotensive action; hence, it may be catecholamine-induced uteroplacental vasoconstriction that is responsible for the reduced placental perfusion rather than a reduction in perfusion pressure alone [184]. If hydralazine is administered concurrently with methyldopa (which reduces sympathetic responses to hydralazine), the reduction in plasma catecholamines, and the avoidance of an unnecessary reduction in arterial pressure, will help reduce the incidence of fetal distress after this treatment.

LABETALOL. Although β-blockade is the predominant action at low to moderate doses, labetalol appears to induce vasodilation. Indeed, by reducing uterine vascular resistance it could produce an increase in uteroplacental perfusion, the opposite of the effects of hydralazine. With intravenous administration it has a relatively rapid and smooth onset of action, a 50-mg bolus reaching maximal effect within 20 minutes (sustained for about 3 hours) [152] compared with a delay of 30 minutes after 100 mg given orally [280]. Some claim that repeating these doses every 20 to 30 minutes as necessary is so safe and effective that constant infusions are not necessary.

Intravenous labetalol has been compared with intravenous hydralazine (using dextrose as the vehicle for labetalol, contrary to the manufacturer's instructions), and it has been suggested that hydralazine has an unacceptably high incidence of side effects as well as causing unpredictable decrements in blood pressure [57]. The dose of hydralazine used in this study, however, was much higher than the approach we recommend.

DIAZOXIDE. This vasodilator acts more rapidly than hydralazine or labetalol, producing its maximal effect within 2 to 5 minutes after an intravenous dose and lasting several hours. In the past it was recommended that diazoxide be administered as a rapid 300-mg intravenous bolus, and in most reports of its use in pregnancy, it was prescribed in this way [175, 176]. This irretrievable injection of an arbitrary dose, however, can cause an uncontrolled fall in blood pressure, with fetal distress as well as uterine atony, acute cerebral ischemia, and even maternal death. These problems can be avoided if the blood pressure is reduced in a controlled manner, by titrating dose against response. This involves either miniboluses (30 to 60 mg intravenously) repeated every 5 minutes [214] or a slow intravenous infusion (10 mg/min) until the desired effect is seen [269].

Diazoxide appears to be a very suitable drug for the immediate control of severe hypertension. The effect on placental perfusion is not known, but fetal well-being appears to be unimpaired if excessive falls in blood pressure are avoided [12]. The initial adverse reports have tended to restrict its usage, and we feel it should be limited to the occasional patient whose hypertension does not respond adequately to reasonable doses of hydralazine. Further studies are needed before it can be promoted for primary management.

NIFEDIPINE. This calcium-channel blocker inhibits the slow channel influx of calcium ions in vascular smooth muscle. Walters and Redman [286] have shown that after a single oral dose of 5 to 10 mg, significant reduction of mean systolic and diastolic blood pressures ensued within 30 minutes and persisted for 4 to 8 hours. There were no serious side effects or sequelae, but the authors concluded that further studies were needed on this category of drug (particularly it use concurrently with other drugs) before firm recommendations could be made. There have been several limited studies since then, most of which are quite encouraging. In one [72], a "quasi" randomized and controlled trial in 44 women, nifedipine appeared superior to hydralazine; there was better control of blood pressure and less fetal distress. However, the hydralazine bolus was quite large, and 4 versus 1 of the women receiving nifedipine experienced decrements in GFR and increments in proteinuria.

In animal studies, nifedipine administered to *normotensive* sheep and monkeys reduced blood pressure but caused significant decrements in uteroplacental flow and some cases of fetal acidosis [63, 104, 200]. This does not seem to be the experience in pregnant women, in whom studies with radionucleotides or analyses of Doppler ultrasound results suggest little effect on uteroplacental blood flow and proportional reductions in vascular resistances and perfusion pressures [103a, 160, 207].

ANGIOTENSIN CONVERTING ENZYME (ACE) INHIBITORS. These have not been assessed in controlled trials in human pregnancy. There are, however, a considerable number of reports of anuric renal failure in babies exposed to this category of drug in utero [231] and high rates of fetal wastage in animal studies. These data strongly suggest that converting enzyme inhibitors must be avoided during pregnancy, a view emphasized in the NIH Consensus Report [184a].

ALPHA-ADRENERGIC BLOCKERS. Prazosin (specifically an α_1-receptor antagonist) has been used in uncontrolled studies of chronic hypertension and pheochromocytoma complicating pregnancy [225, 260]. No specific untoward effects have been identified; however, given the lack of data and lack of benefit over other, better studied agents, there is little reason to use this drug for hypertension during pregnancy except for patients with a pheochromocytoma.

SEROTONIN (TYPE II) BLOCKERS. Drugs such as kentanserin have been used in severe preeclampsia with variable success and cannot be recommended until considerably more data accrue [177, 290].

SODIUM NITROPRUSSIDE. This potent vasodilator has been used in very few pregnant women, usually in an emergency situation such as pulmonary edema or life-threatening hypertension unresponsive to more conventional therapy [225, 250, 260]. This drug, which is metabolized to cyanide and thiocyanate, crosses the placenta, thus the concern regarding potential fetal toxicity. Although brief infusions of relatively low doses (4 mg/kg/min) have not been associated with maternal or fetal cyanide levels in the toxic range or with clinically evident toxicity, nitroprusside remains a drug of last resort during pregnancy and should be avoided. Nonetheless, maternal safety takes precedence, and nitroprusside should not be withheld in the rare gravida with life-threatening hypertension unresponsive to more conventional therapy.

Prevention and Treatment of the Eclamptic Convulsion

MAGNESIUM SULFATE

Because the pathogenesis of the eclamptic convulsion is poorly understood, it is not surprising that controversy concerning its prevention and management exists [59, 122, 139, 141, 245]. While magnesium sulfate is the obstetrician's choice in North America, neurologists questioning magnesium's efficacy recommend phenytoin [122], while in Europe a variety of narcotics, barbiturates, and benzodiazepine derivatives are prescribed. We believe there is a mistaken tendency in the literature to equate the eclamptic convulsion with hypertensive lenephalopathy, since it can arise in a seemingly stable patient manifesting only minimal blood pressure elevation. In fact, this is why most North American obstetricians initiate therapy when women with suspected preeclampsia are in labor, even if premonitory signs are absent. Critics of the use of magnesium sulfate stress that it fails to cross the blood-brain barrier (recently disputed) and has little effect on electroencephalographic abnormalities [245]. Supporters cite evidence that magnesium gates central *N*-methyl-D-aspartate receptors in mice [188], evidence that levels of this divalent cation similar to those in treated preeclamptics (as well as plasma from treated patients) increases prostacyclin release by cultured endothelial cells from human umbilical veins [288], and most important, a large body of empirical data attesting to its successful use [39, 40, 212, 245]. The NIH Consensus Group recommended that parenteral magnesium sulfate remain the drug of choice for prevention and treatment of the eclamptic convulsion, but noted that, while the success of such therapy seemed documented in several large series [39, 212, 245], it had never undergone a definitive controlled trial.

At the University of Chicago's Lying-In Hospital an intravenous regimen is used. Four to 6 gm of $MgSO_4$ in a 10% solution is infused during a 10- to 20-minute period (never as a bolus), after which a sustaining infusion of 24 gm of $MgSO_4$ in 1 liter of 5% dextrose solution is given at a rate of 1 gm per hour. The patient is constantly observed, magnesium levels are periodically measured, and calcium gluconate is kept by the bedside as an antidote for magnesium toxicity. On occasion, a patient remains hyperreflexic with this regimen, and supplemental loading doses or judicious increments in the infusion rate may be required. In other centers, the intravenous loading dose is followed by periodic intramuscular injections, an approach that also seems to maintain therapeutic levels.

As the controversy regarding preventing and treating eclampsia seems incompletely resolved, review of some more recent data on magnesium, diazepam, and phenytoin is in order.

DIAZEPAM

Diazepam (10-mg IV bolus followed by an intravenous infusion) was recently compared to magnesium sulfate (4-gm IV bolus followed by 10 gm intramuscularly) in the management of 51 women with eclampsia [54]. Overall maternal morbidity (defined as recurrent convulsions, cardiopulmonary problems, coagulation failure, and renal failure) was nonsignificantly lower in the magnesium group (29%) than in women treated with diazepam (52%). Recurrent convulsions after stabilization (1 hour of treatment) were commoner in the diazepam group (4 cases versus 1), and furthermore the patient in the magnesium group who convulsed did not receive the correct maintenance dosage as stated in the protocol. Three women in the diazepam group developed pneumonia, and one patient experienced respiratory depression, whereas none treated with magnesium had respiratory complications. Diminished urine output was less common in magnesium-treated women (3 cases versus 12). Babies born to mothers receiving magnesium sulfate had significantly higher Apgar scores at 1 and 5 minutes and required less frequent intubation, intermittent positive-pressure ventilation, and admission to the neonatal intensive care unit. The study, however, was undertaken in a busy obstetric unit in the developing world, and the authors mentioned that patient supervision (and especially titration of intravenous diazepam) may have been less than ideal.

There are concerns for the fetus when diazepam is administered that also must not be neglected. This drug, which crosses the placenta, is slowly metabolized by the newborn, and significant circulating levels persist for up to 8 days after delivery [53]. Doses of 20 to 30 mg or more to the mother have resulted in delayed breathing at birth, as well as shallow and inadequate respirations in the neonate. Other side effects have included floppiness, impaired thermogenesis, and poor sucking ability [166, 224]. While some have underscored low calcium levels in infants of mothers receiving magnesium, few side effects have been recorded.

A large-scale controlled, randomized trial of magnesium sulfate versus diazepam after eclampsia is now being promoted by the World Health Organization. It is scheduled to start in 1992, and its results should be of considerable interest.

PHENYTOIN

Intravenous infusion of phenytoin was used for seizure prophylaxis in 24 women with moderate to severe preeclampsia and 2 women with eclampsia in one study [253]; the authors noted that none convulsed and the drug was well tolerated. However, one woman had a hypotensive episode (130/80 to 95/50 mm Hg), which resolved without any therapy or adjustment of the infusion rate, and one neonate developed a cephalhematoma. Phenytoin has been used alone or in combination with diazepam, furosemide, and hydralazine, and the main benefit of adding phenytoin was greater reduction of blood pressure and less maternal sedation [180]. Of concern, though, are several reports of women having further seizures after phenytoin, and in some the serum phenytoin levels were apparently in the therapeutic range [247, 271]. In one, a comparative study of phenytoin and magnesium sulfate administered to 22 eclamptic women, further convulsions occurred in 4 of the 11 receiving phenytoin (compared to none of those receiving magnesium sulfate) [60]. Two of the women with recurrent convulsions had low-borderline phenytoin levels (45 and 46 μmol/liter), but the other two had levels of 65 and 70 μmol/liter. There are other problems with phenytoin—discomfort at the infusion site, the requirement for continuous maternal heart rate monitoring, and the effect of serum albumin on levels of free unbound "active" drug. For such reasons we cannot recommend phenytoin and thus endorse the NIH Consensus Group's conclusions on this issue.

Roles of Anticoagulation, Volume Expansion Therapy, and Infused Prostaglandins

ANTICOAGULANT THERAPY

There have been isolated and conflicting reports on the use of heparin in the management of preeclampsia [140, 291]. The use of anticoagulants in patients whose hypertensive disease may be associated with cerebral bleeding and subcapsular hematoma of the liver appears too hazardous to us, especially when other approaches can be successful. The antithrombotic potential of aspirin is discussed later.

VOLUME EXPANSION

Normal pregnancy is accompanied by increases in plasma volume, and it has been claimed that such increments are important for a successful pregnancy [39, 141]. In preeclampsia, there is intravascular volume depletion compared with normal pregnancy, and plasma volume in patients with essential hypertension may be intermediate, falling between that of normal gravidas and preeclamptic patients. Reduced plasma volume, the reported low central venous or pulmonary capillary wedge pressures, and the possibility that vasoconstriction may be due to overcompensation of the sympathetic or other pressor systems to intravascular volume depletion, all provide the basis for a controversy [8, 23, 39, 86–88, 139]. One view is that decreased intravascular volume is the primary event that may be responsible for the rise in blood pressure. The other, that of traditional hypertension experts, is that decrements in intravascular volume are secondary to vasoconstriction, with the volume merely fitting a contracted vascular bed.

Reviewing the literature, the findings are equivocal and unconvincing [61, 140]. The ongoing experience of Gallery and associates is an exception [86–88]. These authors have carefully studied hospitalized hypertensive pregnant women whose blood pressure remained elevated despite 48 hours of bed rest. Plasma volume and extracellular spaces were measured with Evans blue dye and mannitol, respectively, and the patients were infused with 500 ml of a commercial stable-protein substitute over 15 to 20 minutes. Rapid decreases in both systolic and diastolic pressure occurred and persisted for about 48 hours. Remeasurements of intravascular and extracellular compartments demonstrated that the decrement in pressure was accompanied by restoration of an initially low plasma volume to values normal for pregnancy, the increment in intravascular volume being due to mobilization of fluid from the interstitial space. The authors acknowledged the possibility that the decrement in pressure may be due to contamination of the plasma protein infusate with vasodilatory peptides (i.e., bradykinin) but believe that if such were the case, the decrease in blood pressure would be transient, whereas that observed by them persisted for 48 hours. Furthermore, they reproduced this work, though less elegantly, with infusions of albumin [88].

While the results of the elegant studies described above are impressive, most of the patients had only moderate hypertension, and effects were quite transient. We caution against plasma expansion therapy for the following reasons: Myocardial performance may be compromised in some women with severe preeclampsia and especially in those in whom the disease is superimposed on chronic hypertension. Volume expansion, especially with saline, may enhance vascular reactivity. Furthermore, infusion of crystalloids alone decreases the oncotic pressure, which is already quite low in most preeclamptics (Fig. 57-2). Since central volumes and pressures tend to rise postpartum, the liberal use of saline may result in decrements in oncotic levels to a point where pulmonary and cerebral edema may then ensue [50, 303]. It is of interest that many of the complications occur during the first postpartum day when oncotic pressure is reaching its nadir (Fig. 57-2) and pulmonary capillary wedge pressure, initially low in preeclampsia, is rising; therefore, crystalloid therapy during labor should be kept to below 75 ml per hour if possible [103, 303].

PROSTAGLANDIN THERAPY

The suggestion that preeclampsia is a state of generalized PGI deficiency and increased thromboxane A_2 (TXA_2) activity has resulted in therapeutic approaches that include stimulation of PGI production and/or inhibition of TXA_2 production [270, 274]. Dietary supple-

Fig. 57-2. Intrapartum and postpartum plasma colloid oncotic pressure in 9 normotensive gravidas (upper curve). (From M. Zinaman, J. Rubin, and M. D. Lindheimer. Serial plasma oncotic pressure levels and echoencephalography during and after delivery in severe preeclampsia. *Lancet* 1:1245, 1985 [303].)

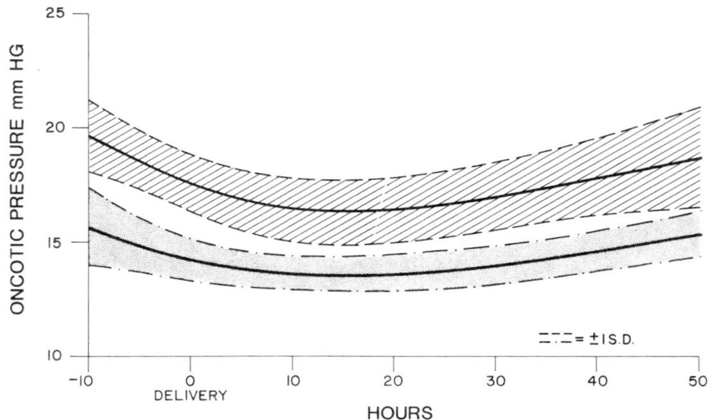

mentation with essential fatty acid precursors has been reported not to decrease the incidence of preeclampsia, but larger studies are needed. The results of direct infusion of PGI in women with severe preeclampsia have also not been encouraging. The short plasma half-life of PGI necessitates continuous infusion and, although PGI_2 infusions are effective in lowering blood pressure, side effects including weakness, nausea, headache, hypotension, and bradycardia are seen, and fetal demise may occur, perhaps as a result of reduced uteroplacental perfusion secondary to maternal peripheral vasodilation.

It has been claimed that the incidence of preeclampsia is lower in women who take any aspirin in pregnancy compared with those who do not [52]. Low-dose aspirin (< 100 mg/day), which inhibits the cyclooxygenase enzyme of TXA_2-generating platelets more effectively than the cyclooxygenase of PGI_2-generating endothelial cells, may therefore be beneficial in preeclampsia. The role of low-dose aspirin in preventing preeclampsia is discussed in a subsequent section; however, there are little data on whether such therapy is effective once hypertension occurs.

Anesthesia, Analgesia, and Blood Transfusion

ANESTHESIA AND ANALGESIA

There is debate on the safest and most effective analgesia and anesthesia for patients with severe preeclampsia. The recent NIH Consensus Group unfortunately avoided detailed discussion of these controversies, but perhaps a future working group will give this topic greater priority. The major dispute involves general anesthesia versus epidural analgesia, especially for operative interventions. Concerns regarding general anesthesia (the choice of several leading experts in obstetrics) have centered around the marked hypertensive response to laryngoscopy, intubation, airway suctioning, and extubation [56, 110, 190]. On the other hand, epidural analgesia (preferred by most anesthesiologists) may be associated with precipitous hypotension and volume overload [24, 56, 121].

Intubation may provoke transient, but severe hypertension, which in theory may increase intracranial pressure, enhancing the danger of cerebral edema or hemorrhage, and precipitating cardiac arrhythmias or failure. Drugs used to limit this pressor response [discussed in 56] include hydralazine, labetalol, nitroglycerin, nitroprusside, trimethaphan, and fentanyl-droperidol. Some of these agents produce vasodilation, which may decrease uteroplacental blood flow, and compromise the fetus, and as noted, certain preeclamptics already have substantial preexisting placental insufficiency.

Proponents of the epidural approach cite its record of safety and claim that this form of analgesia increases intervillous blood flow in the placenta [120] (although optimal methodology to demonstrate this has not been achieved). Epidural analgesia produces hypotension in 12 to 32 percent of normotensive gravidas, but authorities stress this can be prevented with rapid infusion of crystalloid. Nevertheless, in one study [24], 32 percent of 538 gravidas still manifested hypotension despite rapid intravenous prehydration, "prophylactic" ephedrine decreasing this to only 25 percent. Given the hemoconcentration characteristic of severe preeclampsia, decisions to use epidural analgesia require caution and the presence of experienced obstetric anesthesiologists (a view in a technical bulletin issued by the American College of Obstetricians and Gynecologists [190]).

BLOOD TRANSFUSION

A gravida with a shrunken intravascular compartment is less tolerant of blood loss than is the normal pregnant woman [263]. Blood replacement must therefore be initiated sooner, but at the same time very carefully, to guard against the dangers of underfilling and overfilling. Close monitoring of the central venous pressure (CVP) or pulmonary capillary wedge pressure may be required in extremely severe and complicated cases, especially during operative procedures.

Prevention of Preeclampsia

Several approaches for the prevention of preeclampsia have been proposed, including administration of diuretics, aggressive treatment of women with mild hypertension (to prevent superimposed preeclampsia), low-dose aspirin, and calcium or magnesium supplementation.

DIURETICS

Prophylactic use of diuretics was investigated in the 1960s, when it was postulated that sodium retention was etiologically related to the disorder. In 1985 Collins and colleagues [46] published a meta-analysis of nine prospective, randomized trials of diuretics, administered primarily for edema or rapid weight gain, and concluded that such treatment had marginal benefits in that it significantly decreased the incidence of hypertension and edema. However, despite inclusion of over 7,000 women in the analysis, there was no difference in the incidence of hypertension plus proteinuria (presumably preeclampsia) in diuretic ingestors and controls. Furthermore, many of the women in these investigations were multiparas, which makes the data and conclusions difficult to interpret. When one combines such information with case reports of diuretic-induced neonatal thrombocytopenia and jaundice, as well as maternal electrolyte imbalance, several instances of pancreatitis, and even death, we conclude that the balance of risk-benefit considerations does not favor the use of prophylactic diuretics during pregnancy.

TREATMENT OF HYPERTENSION

Another approach is based on the premise that early treatment of hypertension may forestall the appearance of the manifestations of preeclampsia. This was discussed earlier, where it was noted that much of the literature fails to support this approach. Still it may be of interest to settle this issue and also to determine if treatment of mild hypertension decreases the frequency of hospitalizations, studies that will require large multicenter trials to resolve.

CALCIUM

There have been reports [18, 19] that calcium supplementation prevents preeclampsia, but in one large randomized trial only a small reduction in gestational hypertension occurred, while decrements in the incidence of preeclampsia failed to reach significance [18]. Another large, randomized multicenter study was commenced by the National Institutes of Health in 1992.

LOW-DOSE ASPIRIN

One of the more promising approaches, ingestion of low-dose aspirin (~ 60 mg/day) starting shortly after gestational week 12, is based on the rationale that this dosage produces greater inhibition of thromboxane, thus protecting against vasoconstriction and pathologic clotting. A meta-analysis [45] of 13 limited trials has already demonstrated reduction in "proteinuric preeclampsia," and as of 1992 several large multicenter trials were nearing completion. The excitement they have generated warrants review of some of the findings. In one [238], aspirin treatment of high-risk pregnancies reduced thromboxane concentration by almost one-half and the ratio of thromboxane to prostacyclin by one-third, while in women receiving placebos the ratio increased by 51 percent. Also, women in the aspirin group who did develop hypertension had smaller reductions in this ratio than women remaining normotensive. In another report [20], which involved women with poor obstetric histories or chronic hypertension, platelet generation of thromboxane (at 24 weeks and term) was reduced by over 80 percent, but urinary excretion of a prostacyclin metabolite was unaltered. In this same study, there was a greater reduction in the urinary excretion of thromboxane metabolites (thought to originate purely from platelets) than those compounds that reflect more generalized production, suggesting that low-dose aspirin is inhibiting platelet thromboxane to a far greater degree than it does other sources of thromboxane synthesis.

Fetal, Neonatal, and Maternal Risks. What are the possible risks of aspirin treatment? There are theoretic concerns that such treatment might lead to an increased incidence of fetal hemorrhagic complications. There are anecdotal reports linking aspirin to certain cardiac malformations and delayed closure of the ductus arteriosus, which could lead to postnatal pulmonary hypertension and severe neonatal hypoxemia. There is also concern that aspirin might be administered to mothers with subclinical bleeding disorders and that some patients with preeclampsia already have acquired platelet defects. First, one should note that most data in the literature reflect events where women were receiving 150 to 300 mg/day, not "low-dose" aspirin. Secondly, when treatment is started after the twelfth gestational week, the mother has passed the teratogenic period. In addition, a recent case-controlled study [296] has failed to confirm older observations linking aspirin to cardiac anomalies. More important, published studies [16, 20, 45, 171, 238, 273] to date, some of which include ultrasound examination of the neonate to detect intracranial bleeding, have failed to demonstrate adverse effects. Also, two large ongoing trials have now recruited over 8,000 women, and their safety monitoring committees have found no reason to halt these studies.

One important question to be resolved is the following: If the meta-analyses are so encouraging, should we not administer aspirin to all gravidas? In fact, one group of experts have already suggested using aspirin in high-risk pregnancy (e.g., repeated midtrimester severe disease) [55]. In this respect, we close this discussion with the recommendations of the *Oxford Data Base for Perinatal Trials,* where the meta-analysis of aspirin studies are updated periodically and reported via an electronic publication [45]. Their conclusions as of February 1991 were as follows: "The routine use of antiplatelet therapy cannot yet be recommended for any identifiable group of women. The significance of the promising but inconclusive evidence . . . will not be clear until sufficiently large numbers of women have participated in randomized trials to allow an assessment . . . on substantive outcomes of pregnancy." Much of their conclusions reflect the fact that we still have little evidence that perinatal loss is effected or that there are major impacts on maternal morbidity. Furthermore, although no disturbing side effects have been observed (or reported), there is still the opinion that safety has yet to be "proved." For example, the studies reviewed by them, so far, have been too small to have the power to demonstrate rare but serious side effects. Consequently, we agree with them that one should await the results of the large ongoing trials (one organized by the Medical Research Council of England, the other by the National Institutes of Child Health and Development of NIH) before a decision to use aspirin in pregnancy is made.

Remote Prognosis

There is debate about the remote prognosis of preeclampsia-eclampsia [39, 40, 69, 78, 140]. One view [69] is that these women have an increased incidence of cardiorenal disorders later in life, which might relate to the duration of the disease during pregnancy. Another view [39, 40, 78] is that the remote prognosis for preeclamptic gravidas is no different from that for normotensives, and that women who manifest hypertensive cardiovascular disorders later in life are those who were destined to develop essential hypertension anyway.

The validity of the second view seems to have been confirmed by Chesley and co-workers over the years [39, 40]. In the most thorough epidemiologic survey published through 1976, they have periodically reexamined 267 of 270 women surviving eclampsia during the years 1931 to 1951. Some of these women were followed as long as 40 years after their eclamptic episode. The remote mortality in white patients who convulsed during their first pregnancy was not greater than that of age-matched unselected women, whereas white multiparous patients who convulsed had a remote mortality two to five times that expected. The prevalence of later hypertension was increased in women who were eclamptic as multigravidas, and this increment seems to account for their death rate. In contrast, the prevalence of hypertension or the distribution of systolic and diastolic blood pressure levels in women who were eclamptic as primigravidas was also similar to those reported in several large epidemiologic surveys. Furthermore, the prevalence of hypertension was greater in women eclamptic as primigravidas who manifested high blood pressure in subsequent gestations than in those who were normotensive in all later pregnancies.

Chesley concluded that eclampsia is neither a predictive sign nor a cause of essential hypertension and suggested that women eclamptic as multigravidas were more apt to have both preeclampsia and latent essential hypertension, the latter being responsible for their poorer prognosis. Similar conclusions were reached by Bryans and Torpin [31], who studied a large group of black women with eclampsia.

Others who have observed an increased incidence of remote hypertension in "toxemic" women have criticized the conclusions of Chesley and Bryans and their respective colleagues, stating that such studies use reference populations and fail to survey "control groups" of normotensive gravidas. Chesley, however, has countered that because pregnancy frequently induces transient increments in the blood pressure of women destined to have essential hypertension later in life, the choice of only normotensive gravidas as "controls" creates a population with an abnormally low remote incidence of high blood pressure. If such were the case, then eclamptics, who are presumably a less selected population, would always demonstrate more hypertension when reexamined years later in life.

Our studies support Chesley's thesis: We reexamined 53 biopsy-proved preeclamptic black gravidas an average of 68 months after their index pregnancies and found their incidence of high blood pressure (9 percent) to be similar to an age- and race-matched group of women selected from the survey of the National Institutes of Health [78]. However, each preeclamptic patient was also compared with an age-, race-, and parity-matched woman whose normotensive gestation occurred within 6 months of the index preeclamptic's pregnancy. The latter group had an incidence of remote hypertension that was abnormally lower than the biopsied preeclamptics or the population at large. Use of data from women normotensive during pregnancy would have led to the erroneous conclusion that preeclamptics have a higher incidence of remote hypertension. Thus normotension throughout one or more pregnancies suggests that a woman will remain normotensive for life.

Summary and Conclusions

Hypertension remains a major problem in pregnancy that jeopardizes both mother and fetus. The most serious of the hypertensive complications is preeclampsia, a potentially explosive condition that can enter a convulsive phase (eclampsia) even when blood pressure is only mildly elevated.

The initial approach to any gravida requires cognizance of the normal physiologic changes that occur during pregnancy. Blood pressure falls early in pregnancy, returning toward normal near term; thus although a level ≥ 90 mm Hg is viewed as the start of abnormal diastolic pressure, levels above 75 mm Hg in the second trimester and 85 mm Hg in the third trimester are already suspect. Plasma volume normally increases during pregnancy, and gravidas may handle salt-restricted diets poorly; inadequate volume expansion has been linked to poor fetal outcome. This must be taken into account when managing hypertensive gravidas who may have both decreased intravascular volumes and compromised fetoplacental perfusion.

There are many gaps in our knowledge concerning the pathophysiology of preeclampsia, but recent observations, e.g., that the disease is caused by an imbalance between vasodilating and vasoconstricting prostaglandins and/or is due to endothelial dysfunction, may help explain, prevent, and treat this disorder. The disease is characterized by extreme vasoconstriction, enhanced vascular reactivity to pressor peptides and amines, and decreased intravascular volume (despite an increased interstitial space). Other manifestations include decreased renal hemodynamics and nonselective proteinuria, which may be in the nephrotic range. Preeclampsia is not only a hypertensive disorder, but a systemic disease as well. Some patients manifest variable signs of coagulopathy, which range from mild abnormalities in coagulation factors to severe disseminated intravascular coagulation, and in others the clotting problems are accompanied by severe liver dysfunction. There is a decrease in uteroplacental blood flow, a factor that certainly contributes to the increased fetal loss and morbidity associated with preeclampsia. The pathogenesis of the diverse manifestations of preeclampsia is controversial, so it is no surprise that views on management differ so much.

The course of most women with chronic essential hypertension, especially younger women without end-organ damage, is rather benign. Presence of end-organ involvement and superimposed preeclampsia, however, increase both maternal and fetal risk substantially. Any hypertensive complication occurring after the thirty-fourth gestational week is usually best treated by delivery. In cases of early preeclampsia (pure or superimposed), temporization may be tried (that is, blood pressure reduction) but is often unsuccessful. The presence of clotting or liver abnormalities, however, is a sign of an impending emergency, and one should end such gestations regardless of blood pressure control. Only a few antihypertensive agents have been subjected to control testing in gravid women, and these are the ones that should be utilized in pregnancies. Finally, the many controversies led the National Institutes of Health, through its National High Blood Pressure Education Program, to convene a working party; the report [184a] should be read by all who manage pregnant women with hypertension.

References

1. Aalkjaer, R., Danielsen, H., Johannesen, P., et al. Abnormal vascular function and morphology in preeclampsia: A study of isolated resistance vessels. *Clin. Sci.* 69: 477, 1985.

2. Abdella, T. N., Sibai, B. M., Hays, J. M., et al. Relationship of hypertensive disease to abruptio placentae. *Obstet. Gynecol.* 63: 365, 1984.
3. Aladjem, S., Lueck, J., and Brewer, J. I. Experimental induction of a toxemia-like syndrome in the pregnant beagle. *Am. J. Obstet. Gynecol.* 145: 27, 1983.
4. Alam, N. A., Clary, P., and Russell, P. T. Depressed placental prostaglandin E1 metabolism in toxemia of pregnancy. *Prostaglandins* 4: 363, 1973.
5. Alhenc-Gelas, F., Tache, A., Saint-Andre, J. P., et al. The renin angiotensin system in pregnancy and parturition. *Adv. Nephrol.* 15: 25, 1986.
6. Aron, D. C., Schnall, A. M., and Scheeler, L. R. Cushing's syndrome and pregnancy. *Am. J. Obstet. Gynecol.* 162: 244, 1990.
7. Assali, N. S., and Brinkman, C. R., III. Disorders of Maternal Circulating and Respiratory Adjustments. In N. S. Assali (ed.), *Pathophysiology of Gestational Disorders,* Vol. 1. New York: Academic Press, 1972.
8. Assali, N. S., and Vaughan, D. L. Blood volume in preeclampsia: Fantasy and reality. *Am. J. Obstet. Gynecol.* 129: 355, 1977.
9. August, P., and Sealey, J. E. The Renin-Angiotensin System in Normal and Hypertensive Pregnancy and in Ovarian Function. In J. H. Laragh and B. M. Brenner (eds.), *Hypertension: Pathophysiology, Diagnosis, and Management.* New York: Raven, 1990.
10. Baker, P. N., Broughton-Pipkin, F., and Symonds, E. M. Platelet angiotensin II binding sites in normotensive and hypertensive women. *Br. J. Obstet. Gynaecol.* 98: 436, 1991.
11. Bardeguez, A. D., McNerney, R., Frieri, M., et al. Cellular immunity in preeclampsia: Alterations in T-lymphocyte subpopulations during early pregnancy. *Obstet. Gynecol.* 77: 859, 1991.
12. Barr, P. A., and Gallery, E. D. M. Effect of diazoxide on the antepartum cardiotocograph in severe pregnancy-associated hypertension. *Aust. N.Z. J. Obstet. Gynaecol.* 21: 11, 1981.
13. Barron, W. M., Mujias, S. K., Zinaman, M., et al. Plasma catecholamine responses to physiologic stimuli in normal human pregnancy. *Am. J. Obstet. Gynecol.* 154: 80, 1986.
14. Barwin, B. N., and Roddie, I. C. Venous distention during pregnancy determined by graded venous congestion. *Am. J. Obstet. Gynecol.* 125: 921, 1976.
15. Baylis, C., and Collins, R. C. Angiotensin II inhibition on blood pressure and renal hemodynamics in pregnant rats. *Am. J. Physiol.* 250: F308, 1986.
16. Beaufils, M., Uzan, S., Donsimoni, R., et al. Prevention of preeclampsia by early antiplatelet therapy. *Lancet* 1: 840, 1985.
17. Beer, A. E. Possible immunologic basis of preeclampsia/eclampsia. *Semin. Perinatol.* 2: 39, 1978.
18. Belizan, J. M., Villar, J., Gonzales, L., et al. Calcium supplementation to prevent hypertensive disorders of pregnancy. *N. Engl. J. Med.* 325: 1399, 1991.
19. Belizan, J. M., Villar, J., and Repke, J. The relationship between calcium intake and pregnancy-induced-hypertension: Up-to-date evidence. *Am. J. Obstet. Gynecol.* 158: 898, 1988.
20. Benigni, A., Gregorini, G., Frusca, T., et al. Effect of low-dose aspirin on fetal and maternal generation of thromboxane by platelets in women at risk for pregnancy-induced hypertension. *N. Engl. J. Med.* 321: 357, 1989.
21. Birkeland, S. A., and Kristofferson, K. Pre-eclampsia: A state of mother-fetus immune imbalance. *Lancet* 2: 720, 1979.
22. Blake, S., and MacDonald, D. The prevention of maternal manifestation of preeclampsia by intensive antihypertensive treatment. *Br. J. Obstet. Gynaecol.* 98: 244, 1991.
23. Boekkooi, P. F., Verkeste, C. M., and Peeters, L. L. H. The effect of volume expansion on placental blood flow in awake hypovolemic rats in late pregnancy. *Am. J. Obstet. Gynecol.* 164: 921, 1991.
24. Brizgys, R. V., Dailey, P. A., Schinder, S. M., et al. The incidence and neonatal effects of maternal hypotension during epidural anesthesia for cesarean section. *Anesthesiology* 67: 782, 1987.
25. Broughton-Pipkin, F. The Renin-Angiotensin System in Normal and Hypertensive Pregnancies. In P. C. Rubin (ed.), *Handbook of Hypertension.* Vol. 10, Hypertension in Pregnancy. Amsterdam: Elsevier, 1988.
26. Broughton-Pipkin, F., and Symonds, E. M. The renin-angiotensin system in the maternal and fetal circulation in pregnancy hypertension. *Clin. Obstet. Gynecol.* 4: 651, 1977.
27. Brown, C. E., Cunningham, F. G., and Pritchard, J. A. Convulsions in proteinuric primiparas more than 24 hours after delivery. Eclampsia or some other cause? *J. Reprod. Med.* 32: 499, 1987.
28. Brown, M. A. Non-pharmacological management of pregnancy-induced hypertension. *J. Hypertens.* 8: 295, 1990.
29. Brown, M. A., Broughton-Pipkin, F., and Symonds, E. M. The effects of intravenous angiotensin II upon blood pressure and sodium and urate excretion in human pregnancy. *J. Hypertens.* 6: 457, 1988.
30. Brust, A. A., Assali, N. S., and Ferris, E. B. Evaluation of neurogenic and humoral factors in blood pressure maintenance in normal and toxemic pregnancy using tetraethylammonium chloride. *J. Clin. Invest.* 27: 717, 1948.
31. Bryans, C. I., Jr., and Torpin, R. A follow-up study of two hundred forty-three cases of eclampsia for an average of twelve years. *Am. J. Obstet. Gynecol.* 58: 1054, 1949.
32. Burgess, G. E. Alpha blockade and surgical intervention of pheochromocytoma in pregnancy. *Obstet. Gynecol.* 53: 266, 1979.
33. Butters, L., Kennedy, S., and Rubin, P. C. Atenolol in essential hypertension during pregnancy. *Br. Med. J.* 301: 587, 1990.
34. Carretero, O. A. The Properties and Possible Role of Renin-like Enzymes in the Uterus and Amniotic Fluid. In M. D. Lindheimer, A. I. Katz, and F. P. Zuspan (eds.), *Hypertension in Pregnancy.* New York: Wiley, 1976.
35. Catt, K. J., Bankal, A., and Ashburn, M. The Renin-Angiotensin System During Oral Contraceptive Therapy and Pregnancy. In M. J. Fregly and M. S. Fregly (eds.), *Oral Contraceptives and High Blood Pressure.* Gainesville, FL: Dolphin Press, 1973.
36. Chamberlain, G. V., Lewis, P. J., De Swiet, M., et al. How obstetricians manage hypertension in pregnancy. *Br. Med. J.* 1: 626, 1978.
37. Chamberlain, G. V., Phillip, E., and Howlett, B. *British Births 1970,* Vol. 2. London: Heinemann, 1978.
38. Chesley, L. C. False Steps in the Study of Preeclampsia. In M. D. Lindheimer, A. I. Katz, and F. P. Zuspan (eds.), *Hypertension in Pregnancy.* New York: Wiley, 1976.
39. Chesley, L. C. *Hypertensive Disorders in Pregnancy.* New York: Appleton-Century-Crofts, 1978.

40. Chesley, L. C. Hypertension in Pregnancy. In D. P. Goldstein, and D. M. Levanthal (eds.), *Current Problems in Obstetrics and Gynecology*. Chicago: Year Book, 1981.
41. Chesley, L. C., and Cooper, D. W. Genetics of hypertension in pregnancy: Possible single gene control of preeclampsia and eclampsia in the descendants of eclamptic women. *Br. J. Obstet. Gynaecol.* 93: 898, 1986.
42. Chesley, L. C., and Tepper, I. H. Effects of progesterone and estrogen on the sensitivity to angiotensin II. *J. Clin. Endocrinol. Metab.* 27: 576, 1967.
43. Clark, S. L., and Cotton, D. B. Clinical indications for pulmonary artery catheterization in the patient with severe preeclampsia. *Am. J. Obstet. Gynecol.* 158: 453, 1988.
44. Cockburn, J., Moar, V. A., Ounsted, M., et al. Final report of study on hypertension during pregnancy: The effects of specific treatment on the growth and development of the children. *Lancet* 1: 647, 1982.
45. Collins, R. Antiplatelet Agents in IUGR and Pre-eclampsia. In I. Chalmers (ed.), *Oxford Data Base for Perinatal Trials*. Version 1.2, Disk issue 5, 1991, Record 4000, 1991. (If electronic publications unavailable see Collins, R., and Wallenberg, H. C. S., Pharmacological Prevention and Treatment of Hypertensive Disorders in Pregnancy. In I. Chalmers, M. Enkin, and M. J. N. C. Keirse (eds.), *Effective Care in Pregnancy and Childbirth*. Oxford: Oxford University Press, 1989.
46. Collins, R., Yusuf, S., and Peto, R. Overview of randomised trials of diuretics in pregnancy. *Br. Med. J.* 290: 17, 1985.
47. Conrad, K. P., Barrera, S. A., Freidman, P. A., et al. Evidence of attenuation of myo-inositol uptake, phosphoinositide turnover and inositol phosphate production in aortic vasculature of rats during pregnancy. *J. Clin. Invest.* 87: 1700, 1991.
48. Conrad, K. P., and Colpoys, M. C. Evidence against the hypothesis that prostaglandins are the vasodepressor agents of pregnancy. Serial studies in chronically instrumented, conscious rats. *J. Clin. Invest.* 77: 236, 1986.
49. Cooper, D. W., and Liston, W. A. Genetic control of severe preeclampsia. *J. Med. Genet.* 16: 409, 1979.
50. Cotton, D. B., Gonik, B., Spillman, T., et al. Intrapartum to postpartum changes in colloid osmotic pressure. *Am. J. Obstet. Gynecol.* 149: 174, 1984.
51. Crandall, M. E., Keve, T. M., and McLaughlin, M. K. Characterization of norepinephrine sensitivity in the maternal splanchnic circulation during pregnancy. *Am. J. Obstet. Gynecol.* 162: 1296, 1990.
52. Crandon, A. J., and Isherwood, D. M. Effect of aspirin on incidence of preeclampsia. *Lancet* 1: 356, 1979.
53. Cree, J. E., Meyer, J., and Hailey, D. M. Diazepam in labour: Its metabolism and effect on the clinical condition and thermogenesis of the newborn. *Br. Med. J.* 4: 251, 1977.
54. Crowther, C. Magnesium sulphate versus diazepam in the management of eclampsia: A randomized controlled trial. *Br. J. Obstet. Gynaecol.* 97: 110, 1990.
55. Cunningham, F. G., and Gant, N. F. Prevention of preeclampsia: A reality? *N. Engl. J. Med.* 321: 606, 1989.
56. Cunningham, F. G., MacDonald, P. C., and Gant, N. F. Analgesia and Anaesthesia. In *Williams Obstetrics* (18th ed.). Norwalk, CT: Appleton & Lange, 1988.
57. Davey, D. A., Dommisse, J., and Garden, A. Intravenous Labetalol and Intravenous Dihydralazine in Severe Hypertension in Pregnancy. In A. Riley, E. M. Symonds (eds.), *The Investigation of Labetalol in the Management of Hypertension in Pregnancy*. Amsterdam: Excerpta Medica, 1982.
58. Davison, J. M., and Dunlop, W. Changes in renal hemodynamics and tubular function induced by normal pregnancy. *Semin. Nephrol.* 4: 198, 1984.
59. Dinsdale, H. B. Does magnesium sulfate treat eclamptic seizures? Yes. *Arch. Neurol.* 45: 1360, 1988.
60. Dommisse, J. Phenytoin sodium and magnesium sulphate in the management of eclampsia. *Br. J. Obstet. Gynaecol.* 97: 104, 1990.
61. Duncan, S. L. Does volume expansion in pre-eclampsia help or hinder? *Br. J. Obstet. Gynaecol.* 96: 634, 1989.
62. Dürr, J. A. Maternal Fluid Adaptation to Pregnancy. In R. A. Brace, M. G. Ross, and J. E. Robillard (eds.), *Reproductive and Perinatal Medicine*. Vol. XI, Fetal and Neonatal Body Fluids. Ithaca, NY: Perinatology Press, 1989.
63. Dusay, C. A., Cook, M. J., and Veille, J. C. Cardiorespiratory Effects of Calcium Channel Blocker Tocolysis in Pregnant Rhesus Monkeys. In C. T. Jones and P. W. Nathanielsz (eds.), *The Physiological Development of the Fetus and Newborn*. London: Academic, 1985. Pp. 423–428.
64. Easterling, T. R., Benedetti, T. J., Schmucker, B. C., et al. Maternal hemodynamics in normal and pre-eclamptic pregnancies: A longitudinal study. *Obstet. Gynecol.* 77: 647, 1991.
65. Easterling, T. R., Goldman, M. L., Strandness, D. E., et al. Renal vascular hypertension during pregnancy. *Obstet. Gynecol.* 78: 921, 1991.
66. Editorial. Inheriting pre-eclampsia. *Br. Med. J.* 1: 1557, 1980.
67. Editorial. Genetic control of pre-eclampsia. *Lancet* 1: 634, 1980.
68. Entman, S. S., Kambam, J. R., Bradley, C. A., et al. Increased levels of carboxyhemoglobin and serum iron as an indication of increased red cell turnover in preeclampsia. *Am. J. Obstet. Gynecol.* 156: 1169, 1987.
69. Epstein, F. H. Late vascular effects of toxemia of pregnancy. *N. Engl. J. Med.* 271: 391, 1964.
70. Erskine, K. J., Iversen, S. A., and Davies, R. An altered ratio of 18 : 2(9,11) to 18 : 2(9,12) linoleic acid in plasma phospholipids as a possible predictor of preeclampsia. *Lancet* 1: 554, 1985.
71. Fay, R. A., Bromhan, D. R., Brooks, J. A., et al. Platelets and uric acid in the prediction of preeclampsia. *Am. J. Obstet. Gynecol.* 152: 1038, 1985.
72. Fenakel, K., Fenakel, G., Appelman, Z., et al. Nifedipine in the treatment of severe preeclampsia. *Obstet. Gynecol.* 77: 331, 1991.
73. Ferris, T. F. Hypertension During Pregnancy. In J. C. Hunt, T. Cooper, E. D. Frohlich, et al. (eds.), *Hypertension Update: Mechanisms, Epidemiology, Evaluation, Management*. Bloomfield, N. J.: Health Learning Systems, 1980.
74. Ferris, T. F., and Weiss, E. K. Effect of captopril on uterine blood flow and prostaglandin E synthesis in the pregnant rabbit. *J. Clin. Invest.* 71: 809, 1983.
75. Fidler, J., Smith, V., Fayers, P., et al. Randomised controlled comparative study of methyldopa and oxprenolol in treatment of hypertension in pregnancy. *Br. Med. J.* 286: 1927, 1983.
76. Finnerty, F. A., Bucholtz, J. H., and Guillandeu, R. L. A pressor phenomenon with the postpartum period. *J.A.M.A.* 165: 778, 1957.
77. Fisher, K. A., Ahuja, S., Luger, A., et al. Nephrotic proteinuria with preeclampsia. *Am. J. Obstet. Gynecol.* 129: 643, 1977.
78. Fisher, K. A., Luger, A., Spargo, B. H., et al. Hypertension in pregnancy: Clinical pathological correlations and remote prognosis. *Medicine* 60: 267, 1981.
79. Fitzgerald, D. J., and Fitzgerald. G. A. Eicosanoids in

the Pathogenesis of Preeclampsia. In J. H. Laragh and B. M. Brenner (eds.), *Hypertension: Pathophysiology, Diagnosis and Management*. New York: Raven, 1990.

80. Fitzgerald, D. J., Rocki, W., Murray, R., et al. Thromboxane A_2 synthesis in pregnancy-induced hypertension. *Lancet* i: 751, 1990.

81. Foidart, J. M., Hunt, J., Lapiere, C. M., et al. Antibodies to laminin in preeclampsia. *Kidney Int.* 29: 1050, 1986.

81a. Foidart, J. M., Nochy, D., Nusgens, B. et al. Accumulation of several basement membrane proteins in glomeruli of patients with preeclampsia and other hypertensive syndromes of pregnancy. *Lab. Invest.* 49: 250, 1983.

82. Fowler, W. L., Jr., Johnson, J. A., Kurz, K. D., et al. Role of the renin-angiotensin system in maintaining arterial pressure in conscious pregnant rats. *Endocrinology* 109: 290, 1981.

83. Fried, G., and Samuelson, U. Endothelin and neuropeptide Y are vasoconstrictors in human uterine blood vessels. *Am. J. Obstet. Gynecol.* 164: 1330, 1991.

84. Friedman, E. A., and Neff, R. K. Pregnancy Hypertension. In E. A. Friedman and R. K. Neff (eds.), *A Systematic Evaluation of Clinical Diagnostic Criteria*. Littleton, MA: PSG Publishing, 1977.

85. Gaber, L. W., Spargo, B. H., and Lindheimer, M. D. The Nephropathy of Preeclampsia-Eclampsia. In C. C. Tisher and B. M. Brenner (eds.), *Renal Pathology*. Philadelphia: Lippincott, 1989.

86. Gallery, E. D. M. Volume homeostasis in normal and hypertensive human pregnancy. *Semin. Nephrol.* 4: 221, 1984. (See also *Clin. Obstet. Gynaecol.* 1: 835, 1987.)

87. Gallery, E. D. M., Delprado, W., Györy, A. Z., et al. Plasma volume contraction: A significant factor in both pregnancy-associated hypertension (preeclampsia) and chronic hypertension in pregnancy. *Q. J. Med.* 48: 593, 1979.

88. Gallery, E. D. M., Delprado, W., and Györy, A. Z. Antihypertensive effect of plasma volume expansion in pregnancy-associated hypertension. *Aust. N.Z. J. Med.* 11: 20, 1981.

89. Gallery, E. D. M., Ross, M. R., and Györy, A. Z. Antihypertensive treatment in pregnancy: Analysis of different responses to oxprenolol and methyldopa. *Br. Med. J.* 291: 563, 1985.

90. Gallery, E. D. M., Saunders, D. M., Hunyor, S. N., et al. Randomised comparison of methyldopa and oxprenolol for treatment of hypertension in pregnancy. *Br. Med. J.* 1: 1591, 1979.

91. Gant, N. F., Daley, G. L., Chand, S., et al. A study of angiotensin II pressor response throughout primigravid pregnancy. *J. Clin. Invest.* 52: 2682, 1973.

92. Gant, N. F., Jimenez, J. M., Whalley, P. J., et al. A prospective study of angiotensin II pressor responsiveness in pregnancies complicated by essential hypertension. *Am. J. Obstet. Gynecol.* 127: 369, 1977.

93. Gant, N. F., Madden, J. D., and Siiteri, P. K. The metabolic clearance rates of dehydroisoandrosterone sulfate. IV. Acute effects of induced hypertension, hypotension and natriuresis in normal and hypertensive pregnancies. *Am. J. Obstet. Gynecol.* 124: 143, 1976.

94. Gant, N. F., Worley, R. J., Everett, R. B., et al. Control of vascular responsiveness during human pregnancy. *Kidney Int.* 18: 253, 1980.

95. Gau, G. S., Bhundia, J. P., Napier, K. A., et al. Observations on an organism reported to be associated with gestational pathology. *J. Obstet. Gynaecol.* 4: 209, 1984.

96. Gerber, J. G., Payne, N. A., Murphy, R., et al. Prostacyclin produced by the pregnant uterus in the dog may act as a circulating vasodepressor substance. *J. Clin. Invest.* 67: 632, 1981.

97. Goldenberg, R. L., Huddleston, J. F., Davis, R. O., et al. Toxemia of pregnancy masquerading as idiopathic thrombocytopenic purpura. *Obstet. Gynecol.* 62: 32S, 1983.

98. Goodlin, R. C. Preeclampsia as the great imposter. *Am. J. Obstet. Gynecol.* 164: 1577, 1991.

99. Goodman, R. P., Killam, R. P., Brush, A. R., et al. Prostacyclin production during pregnancy: Comparison of production during normal pregnancy and pregnancy complicated by hypertension. *Am. J. Obstet. Gynecol.* 142: 817, 1982.

100. Greenberg, M., Moawad, A. H., Wietes, B. M., et al. Extraadrenal pheochromocytoma: Detection during pregnancy using MR imaging. *Radiology* 161: 475, 1985.

101. Greiss, F. C. J. Pressure-flow relationship in the gravid uterine vascular bed. *Am. J. Obstet. Gynecol.* 96: 41, 1966.

102. Griggs, K. C., Mackey, K. R., and McLaughlin, M. K. Human chorionic plate arteries lack an endothelium-dependent relaxation response. *Clin. Exp. Hypertens.* [B]10: 21, 1991.

103. Hankins, G. D. P., Wendel, G. D., Jr., Cunningham, F. G., et al. Longitudinal evaluation of hemodynamic changes in eclampsia. *Am. J. Obstet. Gynecol.* 150: 506, 1984.

103a. Hanretty, K. P., Whittle, M. J., Howie, C. A., et al. Effect of nifedipine on Doppler flow velocity waveforms in severe pre-eclampsia. *Br. Med. J.* 299: 1205, 1989.

104. Harake, B., Gilbert, R. D., Ashwal, S., et al. Nifedipine: Effects on fetal and maternal hemodynamics in pregnant sheep. *Am. J. Obstet. Gynecol.* 157: 1003, 1987.

105. Harrison, G. L., and Moore, L. G. Blunted vasoreactivity in pregnant guinea pigs is not restored by meclofenamate. *Am. J. Obstet. Gynecol.* 160: 258, 1989.

106. Hart, J. L., Freas, W., and Muldoon, S. M. Neurovascular function in the rat during pregnancy. *Am. J. Physiol.* 251: H1000, 1986.

107. Hart, M. V., Morton, M. J., Hosenpud, J. D., et al. Aortic function during normal human pregnancy. *Am. J. Obstet. Gynecol.* 154: 887, 1986.

108. Hauth, J. C., Cunningham, F. G., and Whalley, P. J. Management of pregnancy-induced hypertension in the nullipara. *Obstet. Gynecol.* 48: 253, 1976.

109. Hines, T., Lindheimer, M. D., and Barron, W. M. Total autonomic blockade eliminates the attenuated vascular response to angiotensin II (AII) in the pregnant rat (abstract). *Clin. Res.* 39: 694A, 1991.

110. Hodgkinson, R., Husain, F. J., and Hyashi, R. H. Systemic and pulmonary blood pressure during cesarean section in parturients with gestational hypertension. *Can. Anesth. Soc. J.* 27: 389, 1980.

111. Holst, N., Øian, P., Anne, B., et al. Increased plasma levels of vasoactive intestinal polypeptide in pre-eclampsia. *Br. J. Obstet. Gynaecol.* 98: 803, 1991.

112. Hsueh, W. A., Leutscher, J. A., Carlson, E. J., et al. Changes in active and inactive renin in pregnancy. *J. Clin. Endocrinol. Metab.* 54: 1010, 1982.

113. Hubel, C. A., Roberts, J. M., Taylor, R. N., et al. Lipid peroxidation in pregnancy: New perspectives on pre-eclampsia. *Am. J. Obstet. Gynecol.* 161: 1025, 1989.

114. Hypertensive Disease in Pregnancy. In *Report on Confidential Inquiry in Maternal Deaths in England and Wales 1982–1984*. London: Her Majesty's Stationery Office, 1989.

115. Invasive hemodynamic monitoring in obstetrics and gynecology. *Technical Bull.* 128, American College of Obstetrics and Gynecology, 1988.
116. Jansakul, C., Boura, A. L. A., and King, R. G. Effects of endothelial cell removal on constrictor and dilator responses of aortae or pregnant rats. *J. Auton. Pharmacol.* 9: 93, 1989.
117. Jarabak, J., Watkins, J. D., and Lindheimer, M. D. In vitro activity of nicotinamide adenine dinucleotide–and nicotinamide adenine dinucleotide phosphate–linked 15-hydroxyprostaglandin dehydrogenases in placentas from normotensive and preeclamptic/eclamptic pregnancies. *J. Clin. Invest.* 80: 936, 1987.
118. Joelsson, I., and Barton, M. D. The effect of blockade of the beta receptors of the sympathetic nervous system of the fetus. A preliminary report. *Acta Obstet. Gynecol. Scand.* 48(Suppl. 3): 75, 1969.
119. Johnson, T., and Clayton, C. G. Diffusion of radioactive sodium in normotensive and preeclamptic pregnancies. *Br. Med. J.* 1: 312, 1957.
120. Joupilla, P., Jouppila, R., Holmen, A., et al. Lumbar epidural anesthesia to improve intervillous blood flow during labor and severe preeclampsia. *Obstet. Gynecol.* 59: 158, 1982.
121. Joyce, T. H., Debnath, K. S., and Baker, E. A. Preeclampsia: Relationship of CVP and epidural analgesia. *Anesthesiology* 51: S297, 1979.
122. Kaplan, P. W., Lesser, R. P., Fisher, R. S., et al. No, magnesium sulfate should not be used in treating eclamptic seizures. *Arch. Neurol.* 45: 1361, 1988.
123. Katz, A. I., Davison, J. M., Hayslett, J. P., et al. Pregnancy in women with kidney disease. *Kidney Int.* 18: 192, 1980.
124. Kawasaki, N., Matsui, K., Ito, M., et al. Effect of calcium supplementation on the vascular sensitivity to angiotensin II in pregnant women. *Am. J. Obstet. Gynecol.* 153: 576, 1985.
125. Keith, J. C., Miller, K., Eggleston, M. K., et al. Effects of thromboxane synthetase inhibition on maternal fetal homeostasis in gravid ewes with ovine pregnancy-induced hypertension. *Am. J. Obstet. Gynecol.* 161: 1305, 1989.
126. Kelton, J. G., Hunter, D. J. S., and Neame, P. B. A platelet function defect in preeclampsia. *Obstet. Gynecol.* 65: 107, 1985.
127. Killam, A. P., Dillard, S. H., Patton, R. C., et al. Pregnancy induced hypertension complicated by acute liver disease and disseminated intravascular coagulation. Five case reports. *Am. J. Obstet. Gynecol.* 123: 823, 1975.
128. Kilpatrick, D. C., Liston, W. A., Gibson, F., et al. Association between susceptibility to pre-eclampsia within families and HLA DR4. *Lancet* ii: 1063, 1989.
129. Koch-Weser, J. Drug therapy-hydralazine. *N. Engl. J. Med.* 295: 320, 1976.
130. Kuzniar, J., Skret, A., Piela, A., et al. Hemodynamic effects of intravenous hydralazine in pregnant women with severe hypertension. *Obstet. Gynecol.* 66: 453, 1985.
131. Lamming, G. D., Broughton-Pipkin, F., and Symonds, E. M. Comparison of the alpha and beta blocking drug, labetalol, and methyldopa in the treatment of moderate and severe pregnancy-induced hypertension. *Clin. Exp. Hypertens.* 2: 865, 1980.
132. Lamming, G. D., Symonds, E. M., and Rubin, P. C. Phaeochromocytoma in pregnancy: Still a cause of maternal death. *Clin. Exp. Hypertens.* [B] 9: 57, 1990.
133. Lang, R. M., Pridjian, G., Fedlman, T., et al. Alterations in left ventricular mechanics in pregnancy-induced hypertension. *Am. Heart J.* 121: 1768, 1991.
134. Lederman, R. P., McCann, D. S., Work, B., et al. Endogenous plasma epinephrine and norepinephrine in last trimester of pregnancy and labor. *Am. J. Obstet. Gynecol.* 129: 5, 1977.
135. Lee, M. I., Oakes, G. K., Lam, R., et al. The rabbit: A suitable model for investigation of vascular responsiveness during pregnancy. *Clin. Exp. Hypertens.* [B] 1: 429, 1982.
136. Lewis, P. J., Bulpitt, C. J., and Zuspan, F. P. A comparison of current British and American practice in the management of hypertension in pregnancy. *Am. J. Obstet. Gynecol.* 1: 78, 1982.
137. Lin, M. S., McNay, J. L., and Shepherd, A. M. M. Increased plasma norepinephrine accompanies persistent tachycardia after hydralazine. *Hypertension* 5: 257, 1983.
138. Lindheimer, M. D., Barron, W. M., and Davison, J. M. Osmoregulation of thirst and vasopressin release in pregnancy. *Am. J. Physiol.* 257: F159, 1989.
139. Lindheimer, M. D., and Katz, A. I. Preeclampsia: Pathophysiology, diagnosis, and management. *Annu. Rev. Med.* 40: 233, 1989.
140. Lindheimer, M. D., and Katz, A. I. The Kidney and Hypertension in Pregnancy. In B. M. Brenner and R. O. Rector, Jr. (eds.), *The Kidney* (4th ed.). Philadelphia: Saunders, 1991.
141. Lindheimer, M. D., and Katz, A. I. Renal Physiology and Disease in Pregnancy. In D. W. Seldin and G. Giebish (eds.), *The Kidney: Physiology and Pathophysiology* (2nd ed.). New York: Raven, 1992.
142. Lindheimer, M. D., Katz, A. I., Koppen, B. M., et al. Kidney function and sodium handling in the pregnant spontaneously hypertensive rat. *Hypertension* 5: 498, 1983.
143. Lindow, S. W., Davies, N., Davey, D. A., et al. The effect of sublingual nifedipine on uteroplacental blood flow in hypertensive pregnancy. *Br. J. Obstet. Gynaecol.* 95: 1276, 1988.
144. Lippert, T. H., Cloeren, S. E., and Fridrich, R. Assessment of uteroplacental hemodynamics in complicated pregnancy. *Int. J. Gynaecol. Obstet.* 16: 274, 1978.
145. Lockwood, C. J., and Peters, J. H. Increased levels of $ED1^+$ cellular fibronectin precede the clinical signs of preeclampsia. *Am. J. Obstet. Gynecol.* 162: 358, 1990.
146. Long, E. G., Tsin, T., Reinarz, J. A., et al. "Hydatoxoi lualba" identified. *Am. J. Obstet. Gynecol.* 149: 462, 1984.
147. Lubbe, W. F. More on beta-blockers in pregnancy. *N. Engl. J. Med.* 307: 753, 1982.
148. Lubbe, W. F., and Hodge, J. V. Combined alpha- and beta-adrenoceptor antagonism with prazosin and oxprenolol in control of severe hypertension in pregnancy. *N.Z. Med. J.* 94: 169, 1981.
149. Lucas, W. E., Kirschbaum, T. H., and Assali, N. S. Effects of autonomic blockade with spinal anesthesia on uterine and fetal hemodynamics and oxygen consumption in the sheep. *Biol. Neonate* 10: 166, 1966.
150. Lueck, J., Brewer, J. I., Alajam, S., et al. Observation of an organism found in patients with gestational trophoblastic disease and in patients with toxemia of pregnancy. *Am. J. Obstet. Gynecol.* 145: 15, 1983.
151. Lunell, N. O., Hjemdahl, P., Fredholm, B. B., et al. Acute Effects of Labetalol on Maternal Metabolism and Uteroplacental Circulation in Hypertension of Pregnancy. In A. Riley and E. M. Symonds (eds.), *The Inves-*

tigation of Labetalol in the Management of Hypertension in Pregnancy. Amsterdam: Excerpta Medica, 1982.

152. Lunell, N. O., Lewander, R., and Mamoun, I. Uteroplacental blood flow in pregnancy induced hypertension. *Scand. J. Clin. Lab. Invest.* 169(Suppl.): 28, 1984.
153. Mabie, W. C., Ratts, T. E., and Sibai, B. M. The central hemodynamics of severe preeclampsia. *Am. J. Obstet. Gynecol.* 161: 1443, 1989.
154. MacGillivray, I., Rose, G. A., and Rowe, B. Blood pressure survey in pregnancy. *Clin. Sci.* 37: 395, 1969.
155. Mackey, K., Stirewalt, W. S., Hibbert, S. R., et al. Pregnancy-induced changes in structural components of resistance-sized mesenteric arteries from rats (abstract). In *Proceedings of the Society of Gynecologic Investigation*, 37th Annual Meeting, 1990. P. 182.
156. Magness, R. R., and Rosenfeld, C. R. Systemic and uterine responses to adrenergic stimulation in pregnant and nonpregnant ewes. *Am. J. Obstet. Gynecol.* 155: 897, 1986.
157. Makila, U. M., Jouppila, P., Kirkinen, P., et al. Relation between umbilical prostacyclin production and blood flow on the fetus. *Lancet* 1: 728, 1983.
158. Makila, U. M., Viinikka, L., and Ylikorkala, O. Evidence that prostacyclin deficiency is a specific feature in preeclampsia. *Am. J. Obstet. Gynecol.* 148: 772, 1984.
159. Manas, K. J., Welsh, J. D., and Rankin, R. A. Hepatic rupture without hemorrhage in preeclampsia. *N. Engl. J. Med.* 312: 424, 1985.
160. Mari, G., Kirshon, B., Moise, K. J., et al. Doppler assessment of the fetal and utero placental circulation during nifedipine therapy for preterm labor. *Am. J. Obstet. Gynecol.* 161: 1514, 1989.
161. Martin, J. N., Jr., Blake, P. G., Lowry, S. L., et al. Pregnancy complicated by preeclampsia-eclampsia with the syndrome of hemolysis, elevated liver enzymes, and low platelet count: How rapid is postpartum recovery? *Obstet. Gynecol.* 76: 737, 1990.
162. Martin, J. N., Jr., Blake, P. G., Perry, K. G., Jr., et al. The natural history of HELLP syndrome: Patterns of disease progression and regression. *Am. J. Obstet. Gynecol.* 164: 1500, 1991.
163. Martin, J. N., Jr., Files, J. C., Blake, P. G., et al. Plasma exchange for preeclampsia: I. Postpartum use for persistently severe preeclampsia-eclampsia with HELLP syndrome. *Am. J. Obstet. Gynecol.* 162: 126, 1990.
164. Massicotte, G., St. Louis, J., Parent, A., et al. Decreased in vitro responses to vasoconstrictors during gestation in normotensive and spontaneously hypertensive rats. *Can. J. Physiol. Pharmacol.* 65: 2466, 1987.
165. Matthews, D. D., Agarwal, V., and Shuttleworth, T. P. A randomised controlled trial of complete bed rest versus ambulation in the management of proteinuric hypertension during pregnancy. *Br. J. Obstet. Gynaecol.* 89: 128, 1982.
166. McCarthy, G. T., O'Connell, B., and Robinson, A. E. Blood levels of diazepam in infants of two mothers given large doses of diazepam during labour. *J. Obstet. Gynaecol. Br. Commonw.* 80: 349, 1973.
167. McKay, D. G. Chronic intravascular coagulation in normal pregnancy and pre-eclampsia. *Contrib. Nephrol.* 25: 108, 1981.
168. McLaughlin, M. K., and Brayden, J. E. Pregnancy results in the hyperpolarization of the vascular smooth muscle of maternal mesenteric resistance arteries (abstract). In *Proceedings of the Society of Gynecologic Investigation*, 37th Annual Meeting, 1990. P. 183.
169. McLaughlin, M. K., Griggs, K., and Crandall, M. E. Pregnancy enhances endothelium-dependent relaxation (abstract). In *Proceedings of the Society of Gynecologic Investigation*, 36th Annual Meeting, 1989. P. 171.
170. McLaughlin, M. K., and Keve, T. M. Pregnancy-induced changes in resistance blood vessels. *Am. J. Obstet. Gynecol.* 155: 1296, 1986.
171. McParland, P., Pearce, J. M., and Chamberlain, G. V. P. Doppler ultrasound and aspirin in recognition and prevention of pregnancy-induced hypertension. *Lancet* i: 1552, 1990.
172. Mendlowitz, M. Digital vascular reactivity to L-norepinephrine in the second trimester of pregnancy as a test for latent essential hypertension and toxemia. *Am. J. Obstet. Gynecol.* 81: 643, 1961.
173. Mendlowitz, M. Toxemia of pregnancy and eclampsia. *Obstet. Gynecol. Surv.* 35: 327, 1980.
174. Meyer, M. C., and McLaughlin, M. K. Pregnancy-associated changes in mechanics, myogenicity and reactivity in resistance-sized mesenteric arteries (abstract). In *Proceedings of the Society of Gynecologic Investigation*, 37th Annual Meeting, 1990. P. 184.
175. Michael, C. A. Intravenous diazoxide in the treatment of severe pre-eclamptic toxaemia and eclampsia. *Aust. N.Z. J. Obstet. Gynaecol.* 13: 143, 1973.
176. Michael, C. A., and Potter, J. M. A Comparison of Labetalol with Other Antihypertensive Drugs in the Treatment of Hypertensive Disease of Pregnancy. In A. Riley, and E. M. Symonds (eds.), *The Investigation of Labetalol in the Management of Hypertension in Pregnancy*. Amsterdam: Excerpta Medica, 1982.
177. Montenegro, R., Knuppel, R. A., Shah, D., et al. The effect of serotonergic blockade in postpartum preeclamptic patients. *Am. J. Obstet. Gynecol.* 153: 130, 1985.
178. Moodley, J., Norman, R. J., and Reddi, K. Central venous concentrations of immunoreactive prostaglandins E, F, and 6-keto-prostaglandin F1α in eclampsia. *Br. Med. J.* 288: 1487, 1984.
179. Moore, L. G., Hershey, D. W., Jahnigen, D., et al. The incidence of pregnancy-induced hypertension is increased among Colorado residents at high altitude. *Am. J. Obstet. Gynecol.* 144: 423, 1982.
180. Moosa, S. M., and El Zayat, S. G. Phenytoin infusion in severe pre-eclampsia. *Lancet* ii: 1147, 1987.
181. Moutquin, J. M., Rainville, C., Giroux, L., et al. A prospective study of blood pressure in pregnancy: Prediction of preeclampsia. *Am. J. Obstet. Gynecol.* 151: 191, 1985.
182. Musci, T. J., Roberts, J. M., Rogers, G. M., et al. Mitogenic activity is increased in the sera of preeclamptic women before delivery. *Am. J. Obstet. Gynecol.* 159: 1446, 1988.
183. Myatt, L., Brewer, A., and Brockman, D. E. The action of nitric oxide in the perfused human fetal-placental circulation. *Am. J. Obstet. Gynecol.* 164: 687, 1991.
184. Naden, R. P., and Redman, C. W. G. Antihypertensive drugs in pregnancy. *Clin. Perinatol.* 12: 521, 1985.
184a. National High Blood Pressure Education Program Working Group Report on High Blood Pressure in Pregnancy ("Consensus Report"). *Am. J. Obstet. Gynecol.* 163: 1689, 1990. (Also NIH Pub. No. 90-3029, August 1990, U.S. Dept. Health and Human Services, Washington.)
185. Nelson, D. M., and Walsh, S. W. Aspirin differentially affects thromboxane and prostacyclin production by trophoblast and villous core compartments of human placental villi. *Am. J. Obstet. Gynecol.* 161: 1593, 1989.
186. Nisell, H., Hjemdahl, P., and Linde, B. Cardiovascular

responses to circulating catecholamines in normal pregnancy and in pregnancy-induced hypertension. *Clin. Physiol.* 5: 479, 1985.

187. Nisell, H., Hjemdahl, P., Linde, B. L., et al. Sympathoadrenal and cardiovascular reactivity in pregnancy-induced hypertension. I: Responses to isometric exercise and cold pressor test. *Br. J. Obstet. Gynaecol.* 92: 722, 1985.
188. Nowak, L., Bregestovsky, P., Ascher, P., et al. Magnesium gates glutamate activated channels in mouse central neurones. *Nature* 307: 462, 1984.
189. O'Brien, P. M. S., and Broughton-Pipkin, F. The effects of deprivation of prostaglandin precursors on vascular sensitivity to angiotensin II and on the kidney in the pregnant rabbit. *Br. J. Pharmacol.* 65: 29, 1979.
190. Obstetric analgesia and anesthesia. *Technical Bull.* 112, American College of Obstetrics and Gynecology, 1988.
191. Ogburn, P. L., Williams, P. P., Johnson, S. B., et al. Serum arachidonic acid levels in normal and preeclamptic pregnancies. *Am. J. Obstet. Gynecol.* 148: 5, 1984.
192. Ongari, M. A., Ritter, J. M., Orchard, M. A., et al. Correlation of prostacyclin synthesis by human umbilical artery with status of essential fatty acids. *Am. J. Obstet. Gynecol.* 149: 455, 1984.
193. Otteson, B. Vasoactive intestinal polypeptide as a neurotransmitter in the female genital tract. *Am. J. Obstet. Gynecol.* 147: 208, 1983.
194. Ounsted, M. K., Moar, V. A., Good, F. J., et al. Hypertension during pregnancy with and without specific treatment; the children at the age of 4 years. *Br. J. Obstet. Gynaecol.* 87: 19, 1980.
195. Packham, D. K., Mathews, D. C., Fairley, K. F., et al. Morphometric analysis of preeclampsia in women biopsied in pregnancy and in the post-partum. *Kidney Int.* 34: 704, 1988.
196. Page, E. W., and Christianson, R. The impact of mean arterial pressure in the middle trimester upon the outcome of pregnancy. *Am. J. Obstet. Gynecol.* 125: 740, 1976.
197. Paller, M. S. Mechanism of decreased pressor responsiveness of Ang II, NE and vasopressin in the conscious pregnant rat. *Am. J. Physiol.* 247: H100, 1984.
198. Paller, M. S., Gregorini, G., and Ferris, T. F. Pressor responsiveness in pseudopregnant and pregnant rats: Role of maternal factors. *Am. J. Physiol.* 257: R866, 1989.
199. Pan, Z. R., Lindheimer, M. D., Bailin, J., et al. Regulation of blood pressure in pregnancy: Pressure system blockade and stimulation. *Am. J. Physiol.* 258: H1559, 1990.
200. Parisi, V. M., Salinas, J., and Stockmar, E. J. Placental vascular responses to nicardipine in the hypertensive ewe. *Am. J. Obstet. Gynecol.* 161: 1039, 1989.
201. Pederson, E. B. Autonomic Nervous System and Vascular Reactivity in Normal and Hypertensive Pregnancy. In P. C. Rubin (ed.), *Handbook of Hypertension.* Vol. 10, Hypertension in Pregnancy. Amsterdam: Elsevier, 1988.
202. Pickles, C. J., Brinkman, C. R., Stainer, K., et al. Changes in peripheral venous tone before onset of hypertension in women with gestational hypertension. *Am. J. Obstet. Gynecol.* 160: 678, 1989.
203. Pijneborg, R., Anthony, J., Davey, D. A., et al. Placental bed spiral arteries in the hypertensive disorders of pregnancy. *Br. J. Obstet. Gynaecol.* 98: 648, 1991.
204. Pinto, A., Sorrentino, R., Sorrentino, P., et al. Endothelial-derived relaxing factor released by endothelial cells of human umbilical vessels and its impairment in pregnancy-induced hypertension. *Am. J. Obstet. Gynecol.* 164: 507, 1991.
205. Pirani, B. B., and MacGillivray, I. The effect of plasma retransfusion on the blood pressure in the puerperium. *Am. J. Obstet. Gynecol.* 121: 221, 1975.
206. Pircon, R. A., Lagrew, D. C., Towers, C. V., et al. Antepartum testing in the hypertensive patient: When to begin. *Am. J. Obstet. Gynecol.* 164: 1563, 1991.
207. Pirhonen, J. P., Erkkola, R. U., and Ekbald, U. Uterine and fetal flow velocity waveforms in hypertensive pregnancy: The effect of a single dose of nifedipine. *Obstet. Gynecol.* 76: 37, 1990.
208. Poland, M. L., and Lucas, C. P. Plasma Epinephrine and Norepinephrine in Normotensive and Pregnancy: Induced Hypertensive Pregnancies. In J. Bonnar, I. MacGillivray, and E. M. Symonds (eds.), *Pregnancy Hypertension.* Lancaster, England: MTP Press, 1980.
209. Pollak, V. E., and Nettles, J. B. The kidney in toxemia of pregnancy: A clinical and pathologic study based on renal biopsies. *Medicine* 39: 469, 1960.
210. Postpartum hypertension seizures, strokes reported with bromocriptine. *FDA Drug Bull.* 14: 1, 1984.
211. Pritchard, J. A., Cunningham, F. G., and Mason, R. A. Does Coagulation Have a Causative Role in Eclampsia? In M. D. Lindheimer, A. I. Katz, and F. P. Zuspan (eds.), *Hypertension in Pregnancy.* New York: Wiley, 1976.
212. Pritchard, J. A., Cunningham, F. G., and Pritchard, S. A. The Parkland Memorial Hospital protocol for treatment of eclampsia: Evaluation of 245 cases. *Am. J. Obstet. Gynecol.* 148: 951, 1984.
213. Quillen, E. W., Jr., Delfier, J. C., Archambault, D., et al. Blood volume and angiotensin II effect on the angiotensin pressor response of pregnant guinea pigs (abstract). In *Proceedings of the Society of Gynecologic Investigation,* 35th Annual Meeting, 1988.
214. Ram, C. V. S., and Kaplan, N. M. Individual titration of diazoxide dosage in the treatment of severe hypertension. *Am. J. Cardiol.* 43: 627, 1979.
215. Ramos-Santos, E., Devoe, L. D., Wakefield, M. L., et al. The effects of epidural anesthesia on the Doppler velocimetry of umbilical and uterine arteries in normal and hypertensive patients during active term labor. *Obstet. Gynecol.* 77: 20, 1991.
216. Rappaport, V. J., Jirata, G., Yap, H. K., et al. Antivascular endothelial cell antibodies in severe preeclampsia. *Am. J. Obstet. Gynecol.* 162: 138, 1990.
217. Redman, C. W. G. A Controlled Trial of the Treatment of Hypertension in Pregnancy: Labetalol Compared with Methyldopa. In A. Riley, and E. M. Symonds (eds.), *The Investigation of Labetalol in the Management of Hypertension in Pregnancy.* Amsterdam: Excerpta Medica, 1982.
218. Redman, C. W. G. Platelets and the beginnings of preeclampsia. *N. Engl. J. Med.* 327: 238, 1990.
219. Redman, C. W. G., Beilin, L. J., and Bonnar, J. Variability of Blood Pressure in Normal and Abnormal Pregnancy. In M. D. Lindheimer, A. I. Katz, and F. P. Zuspan (eds.), *Hypertension in Pregnancy.* New York: Wiley, 1976.
220. Redman, C. W. G., Beilin, L. J., and Bonnar, J. Renal function in preeclampsia. *J. Clin. Pathol.* 29(Suppl. 10): 91, 1976.
221. Redman, C. W. G., Beilin, L. J., Bonnar, J., et al. Fetal outcome in trial of antihypertensive treatment in pregnancy. *Lancet* 2: 753, 756: 1976.
222. Redman, C. W. G., Bodner, J. G., Bodner, W. F., et al.

HLA antigens in severe pre-eclampsia. *Lancet* 2: 397, 1978.

223. Redman, C. W. G., Bonnar, J., Beilin, L. J., et al. Prolactin in hypertensive pregnancy. *Br. Med. J.* 1: 304, 1975.
224. Rementeria, J. L., and Bhatt, K. Withdrawal symptoms in neonates from intrauterine exposure to diazepam. *J. Pediatr.* 90: 123, 1977.
225. Remuzzi, G., and Ruggenenti, P. Prevention and treatment of pregnancy associated hypertension: What have we learned in the last 10 years? *Am. J. Kidney Dis.* 18: 285, 1991.
226. Roberts, J. M., Taylor, R. N., and Goldfein, A. Clinical and biochemical evidence of endothelial cell dysfunction in the pregnancy syndrome preeclampsia. *Am. J. Hypertens.* 4: 700, 1991.
227. Roberts, J. M., Taylor, R. N., Musci, T. J., et al. Preeclampsia: An endothelial disorder. *Am. J. Obstet. Gynecol.* 161: 1200, 1988.
228. Robertson, W. B., Brosens, I., and Dixon, G. Maternal Uterine Vascular Lesions in the Hypertensive Complications of Pregnancy. In M. D. Lindheimer, A. I. Katz, and F. P. Zuspan (eds.), *Hypertension in Pregnancy*. New York: Wiley, 1976.
229. Rochat, R. W., Koonen, L. M., Atrash, H. K., et al. Maternal mortality in the United States: Report from the Maternal Mortality Collaborative. *Obstet. Gynecol.* 151: 110, 1988.
230. Rodgers, G. M., Taylor, R. N., and Roberts, J. M. Preeclampsia is associated with a serum factor cytotoxic to human endothelial cells. *Am. J. Obstet. Gynecol.* 159: 908, 1988.
231. Rosa, F. W., Bosco, L. A., Graham, C. F., et al. Neonatal anuria with maternal angiotensin converting enzyme inhibition. *Obstet. Gynecol.* 74: 371, 1989.
232. Rosenfeld, J., Bott-Kanner, G., Boner, G., et al. Treatment of hypertension during pregnancy with hydralazine monotherapy or with combined therapy with hydralazine and pindolol. *Eur. J. Obstet. Gynecol. Reprod. Biol.* 22: 197, 1986.
233. Rubin, P. C. Beta-blockers in pregnancy. *N. Engl. J. Med.* 305: 1323, 1981.
234. Rubin, P. C., Butters, L., Clark, D., et al. Obstetric aspects of the use in pregnancy-associated hypertension of the beta-adrenoceptor antagonist atenolol. *Am. J. Obstet. Gynecol.* 150: 389, 1984.
235. Rubin, P. C., Butters, L., Clark, D. M., et al. Placebo-controlled trial of atenolol in treatment of pregnancy-associated hypertension. *Lancet* 1: 431, 1983.
236. Sanchez-Ramos, L., Sandroni, S., Andres, F. J., et al. Calcium excretion in preeclampsia. *Obstet. Gynecol.* 77: 510, 1991.
237. Schenker, J. G., and Granat, M. Pheochromocytoma and pregnancy—an updated appraisal. *Aust. N.Z. J. Obstet. Gynecol.* 22: 1, 1982.
238. Schiff, E., Peleg, E., Goldenberg, M., et al. The use of aspirin to prevent pregnancy-induced hypertension and lower the ratio of thromboxane A_2 to prostacyclin in relatively high risk pregnancies. *N. Engl. J. Med.* 321: 351, 1989.
239. Schwartz, M. L., and Brenner, W. Toxemia in a patient with none of the standard signs and symptoms of preeclampsia. *Obstet. Gynecol.* 66: 19S, 1985.
240. Scott, J. S., Jenkins, D. M., and Need, J. A. Immunology of preeclampsia. *Lancet* 1: 704, 1978.
241. Shanklin, D. R., and Sibai, B. M. Ultrastructural aspects of preeclampsia: I. Placental bed and uterine boundary vessels. *Am. J. Obstet. Gynecol.* 161: 735, 1989.
242. Shaw, K. J., Do, Y. S., Kjos, S., et al. Human decidua is a major source of renin. *J. Clin. Invest.* 83: 2085, 1989.
243. Sheehan, H. L., and Lynch, J. B. Pathology of Toxaemia of Pregnancy. In H. L. Sheehan, and J. B. Lynch (eds.), *Pathology of Toxaemia of Pregnancy*. Baltimore: Williams and Wilkins, 1973.
244. Shoemaker, C. T., and Meyers, M. Sodium nitroprusside for control of severe hypertensive disease of pregnancy: A case report and discussion of potential toxicity. *Am. J. Obstet. Gynecol.* 149: 171, 1984.
245. Sibai, B. H. Eclampsia. In P. C. Rubin (ed.), *Handbook of Hypertension*. Vol. 10, Hypertension in Pregnancy. Amsterdam: Elsevier, 1988.
246. Sibai, B. M. The HELLP syndrome (hemolysis, elevated liver enzymes, and low platelets): Much ado about nothing? *Am. J. Obstet. Gynecol.* 162: 311, 1990.
247. Sibai, B. M. Magnesium sulfate is the ideal anticonvulsant in preeclampsia-eclampsia. *Am. J. Obstet. Gynecol.* 162: 1141, 1990.
248. Sibai, B. M., Mabie, W. C., Shamsa, F., et al. A comparison of no medication versus methyldopa or labetalol in chronic hypertension during pregnancy. *Am. J. Obstet. Gynecol.* 162: 960, 1990.
249. Sibai, B. M., Nazar, E., Taslimini, M. M., et al. Maternal-perinatal outcome associated with the syndrome of hemolysis, elevated liver enzymes and low platelets in severe preeclampsia-eclampsia. *Am. J. Obstet. Gynecol.* 155: 501, 1986.
250. Sibai, B. M., Taslimi, M., Abdella, T. N., et al. Maternal and perinatal outcome of conservative management of severe preeclampsia in midtrimester. *Am. J. Obstet. Gynecol.* 152: 32, 1985.
251. Sibai, B. M., Villar, M. A., and Bray, E. Magnesium supplementation during pregnancy: A double blind randomized controlled clinical trial. *Am. J. Obstet. Gynecol.* 161: 115, 1989.
252. Silverstone, A., Trudinger, B. J., Lewis, P. J., et al. Maternal hypertension and intrauterine fetal death in mid-pregnancy. *Br. J. Obstet. Gynaecol.* 87: 457, 1980.
253. Slater, R. M., Wilcox, F. L., Smith, W. D., et al. Phenytoin infusion in severe pre-eclampsia. *Lancet* i: 1417, 1987.
254. Smeaton, T. A., Andersen, G. J., and Fulton, I. S. Study of aldosterone levels in plasma during pregnancy. *J. Clin. Endocrinol. Metab.* 44: 1, 1977.
255. Soffronoff, E. C., Kaufmann, B. M., and Connaughton, J. F. Intravascular volume determinations and fetal outcome in hypertensive diseases of pregnancy. *Am. J. Obstet. Gynecol.* 127: 4, 1977.
256. Sonnenberg, C. M., Bermans, M. G. M., Arts, N. F. T., et al. Transient blindness in preeclampsia: Two cases and a review of literature. *Clin. Exp. Hypertens.* [B]8: 593, 1989.
257. Spitz, B., Magness, R. R., Cox, S. M., et al. Low-dose aspirin I: Effect on angiotensin II pressor responses and blood prostaglandin concentrations in pregnant women sensitive to angiotensin II. *Am. J. Obstet. Gynecol.* 159: 1035, 1988.
258. Sridma, V., Yang, S., Moawad, A., et al. T cell subsets in patients with preeclampsia. *Am. J. Obstet. Gynecol.* 147: 566, 1983.
259. Stainer, K., Morrison, R., Pickles, C., et al. Abnormalities of peripheral venous tone in women with pregnancy induced hypertension. *Clin. Sci.* 70: 155, 1986.
260. Sturgiss, S. N., Lindheimer, M. D., and Davison, J. M. Treatment of Hypertension During Pregnancy: Drugs to Be Avoided and Drugs to Use. In V. E. Andreucci, and

L. G. Fine (eds.), *International Year Book of Nephrology 1992*. London: Springer Verlag, 1991.
261. Symonds, E. M. The Renin-Angiotensin System and Sodium Excretion During Gestation. In M. D. Lindheimer, A. I. Katz, and F. P. Zuspan (eds.), *Hypertension in Pregnancy*. New York: Wiley, 1976.
262. Symonds, E. M., Stanley, M. A., and Skinner, S. L. Production of renin by in vitro cultures of human chorion and uterine muscle. *Nature* 217: 1152, 1968.
263. Tatum, H. J., and Mule, J. G. Puerperial vasomotor collapse in patients with toxemia of pregnancy: A new concept of the etiology and rational plan of treatment. *Am. J. Obstet. Gynecol.* 71: 492, 1956.
264. Taufield, P. A., Ales, K., Resnick, L., et al. Hypocalciuria in preeclampsia. *N. Engl. J. Med.* 316: 715, 1987.
265. Taylor, R. N., Heilbron, D. C., and Roberts, J. M. Growth factor activity in the blood of women in whom preeclampsia develops is elevated from early pregnancy. *Am. J. Obstet. Gynecol.* 163: 1839, 1990.
266. Taylor, R. N., Musci, T. J., Kuhn, R. W., et al. Partial characterization of a novel growth factor from the blood of women with preeclampsia. *J. Clin. Endocrinol. Metab.* 70: 1285, 1990.
267. Taylor, R. N., Musci, T. J., Rodgers, G. M. et al. Preeclamptic sera stimulate increased platelet derived growth factor mRNA and protein expression by cultured human endothelial cells. *Am. J. Reprod. Immunol.* 25: 105, 1991.
268. Terragno, N. A., Terragno, D. A., and McGiff, J. C. The Role of Prostaglandins in the Control of Uterine Blood Flow. In M. D. Lindheimer, A. I. Katz, and F. P. Zuspan (eds.), *Hypertension in Pregnancy*. New York: Wiley, 1976.
269. Thien, T. H., Koene, R. A. P., and Schijf, C. L. Infusion of diazoxide in severe hypertension during pregnancy. *Eur. J. Obstet. Gynecol. Reprod. Biol.* 10: 367, 1980.
270. Toppozada, M. K., Darwish, E., and Barakat, A. A. T. Management of severe preeclampsia detected in early labor by prostaglandin A_1 or dihydralazine infusions. *Am. J. Obstet. Gynecol.* 164: 1229, 1991.
271. Tuffnell, D., O'Donovan, P., Lilford, R. J., et al. Phenytoin in preeclampsia. *Lancet* i: 273, 1989.
272. Umans, J. G., Lindheimer, M. D., and Barron, W. M. Pressor effect of endothelium derived relaxing factor inhibition in conscious virgin and gravid rats. *Am. J. Physiol.* 259: F293, 1990.
273. Uzan, S., Beaufils, M., Breart, G., et al. Prevention of fetal growth retardation with low-dose aspirin: Findings of the EPREDA trial. *Lancet* i: 1427, 1991.
274. Van Assche, F. A., Spitz, B., Vermylen, J., et al. Preliminary observations on treatment of pregnancy induced hypertension with a thromboxane synthetase inhibitor. *Am. J. Obstet. Gynecol.* 148: 216, 1984.
275. Vane, J. R., Anggard, E. E., and Botting, R. M. Regulatory functions of the vascular endothelium. *N. Engl. J. Med.* 323: 27, 1990.
276. Venuto, R., Min, I., Barone, P., et al. Blood pressure control in pregnant rabbits: Norepinephrine and prostaglandin interactions. *Am. J. Physiol.* 247: R786, 1984.
277. Villar, J., Repke, J., Markush, L., et al. The measuring of blood pressure during pregnancy. *Am. J. Obstet. Gynecol.* 161: 1019, 1989.
278. Vink, G. J., and Moodley, J. The effect of low-dose dihydrallazine on the fetus in the emergency treatment of hypertension in pregnancy. *S. Afr. Med. J.* 62: 475, 1982.
279. Visser, W., and Wallenburg, H. C. S. Central hemodynamic observations in untreated preeclamptic patients. *Hypertension* 17: 1072, 1991.
280. Walker, J. J., Crooks, A., Erwin, L., et al. Labetalol in Pregnancy-Induced Hypertension: Fetal and Maternal Effects. In A. Riley, and E. M. Symonds (eds.), *The Investigation of Labetalol in the Management of Hypertension in Pregnancy*. Amsterdam: Excerpta Medica, 1982.
281. Wallenburg, H. C. S. Hemodynamics in Hypertensive Pregnancy. In P. C. Rubin (ed.), *Handbook of Hypertension*. Vol. 10, Hypertension in Pregnancy. New York: Elsevier, 1988.
282. Wallenburg, H. C. S., Dekker, G. A., Makovitz, J. W., et al. Low-dose aspirin prevents pregnancy-induced hypertension and preeclampsia in angiotensin-sensitive gravidae. *Lancet* i: 1, 1986.
283. Wallenburg, H. C. S., Dekker, G. A., Makovitz, J. W., et al. Effect of low dose aspirin on vascular refractoriness to angiotensin-sensitive primigravid women. *Am. J. Obstet. Gynecol.* 164: 1169, 1991.
284. Walsh, S. W. Preeclampsia: An imbalance in placental prostacyclin and thromboxane production. *Am. J. Obstet. Gynecol.* 152: 335, 1985.
285. Walsh, S. W., Behr, M. J., and Allen, N. H. Placental prostacyclin production in normal and toxemic pregnancies. *Am. J. Obstet. Gynecol.* 151: 110, 1985.
286. Walters, B. N. J., and Redman, C. W. G. Treatment of severe pregnancy-associated hypertension with the calcium antagonist nifedipine. *Br. J. Obstet. Gynaecol.* 91: 330, 1984.
287. Walters, B. W. J., Thompson, M. E., Lee, A., et al. Blood pressure in the puerperium. *Clin. Sci.* 71: 589, 1986.
288. Watson, K. V., Moldow, C. F., Ogburn, P. L., et al. Magnesium sulfate: Rationale for its use in preeclampsia. *Proc. Natl. Acad. Sci.* 83: 1075, 1986.
289. Weinberger, M. H., Kramer, N. J., Peterson, L. P., et al. Sequential Changes in the Renin-Angiotensin-Aldosterone Systems and Plasma Progesterone Concentration in Normal and Abnormal Human Pregnancy. In M. D. Lindheimer, A. I. Katz, and F. P. Zuspan (eds.), *Hypertension in Pregnancy*. New York: Wiley, 1976.
290. Weiner, C. P. The role of serotonin in the genesis of hypertension in preeclampsia. *Am. J. Obstet. Gynecol.* 156: 885, 1987.
291. Weiner, C. P. Clotting Alterations with the Pre-eclampsia/Eclampsia Syndrome. In P. C. Rubin (ed.), *Handbook of Hypertension*. Vol. 10, Hypertension in Pregnancy. Amsterdam: Elsevier, 1988.
292. Weiner, C. P., Kwaan, H. C., Xu, C., et al. Antithrombin III activity in women with hypertension during pregnancy. *Obstet. Gynecol.* 65: 302, 1985.
293. Weiner, C. P., Martinez, E., Chestnut, D. H., et al. Effect of pregnancy on uterine and carotid artery response to norepinephrine, epinephrine, and phenylephrine in vessels with documented functional endothelium. *Am. J. Obstet. Gynecol.* 161: 1605, 1989.
294. Weiner, C., Martinez, E., Zhu, L. K., et al. In vitro release of endothelium-derived relaxing factor by acetylcholine is increased during guinea pig pregnancy. *Am. J. Obstet. Gynecol.* 161: 1599, 1989.
295. Weir, R. J., Doig, A., Fraser, R., et al. Studies of the Renin-Angiotensin-Aldosterone System, Cortisol, DOC and ADH in Normal and Hypertensive Pregnancy. In M. D. Lindheimer, A. I. Katz, and F. P. Zuspan (eds.), *Hypertension in Pregnancy*. New York: Wiley, 1976.
296. Werler, M. M., Mitchell, A. A., and Shapiro, S. The relation of aspirin use during the first trimester of pregnancy to congenital cardiac defects. *N. Engl. J. Med.* 321: 1639, 1989.
297. Whittaker, P. G., Gerrard, J., and Lind, T. Catechol-

amine response to changes in posture during human pregnancy. *Br. J. Obstet. Gynaecol.* 92: 586, 1985.

298. WHO Study Group. *The Hypertensive Disorders of Pregnancy.* Technical Report Series 758. Geneva: World Health Organization, 1987.
299. Widerlov, E., Karlman, I., and Storsater, J. Hydralazine-induced neonatal thrombocytopenia. *N. Engl. J. Med.* 303: 1235, 1980.
300. Woods, L. L. Importance of prostaglandins in hypertension during reduced uteroplacental perfusion pressure. *Am. J. Physiol.* 257: R1558, 1989.
301. Woods, L. L., Mizelle, H. L., and Hall, J. E. Autoregulation of renal blood flow and glomerular filtration rate in the pregnant rabbit. *Am. J. Physiol.* 252: R69, 1987.
302. Zemel, M. B., Zemel, P. C., Berry, S., et al. Altered platelet calcium metabolism as an early predictor of increased peripheral vascular resistance and preeclampsia in urban black women. *N. Engl. J. Med.* 323: 434, 1990.
303. Zinaman, M., Rubin, J., and Lindheimer, M. D. Serial plasma oncotic pressure levels and echoencephalography during and after delivery in severe preeclampsia. *Lancet* 1: 1245, 1985.

Hypertension in Cushing's Syndrome

Bruce A. Scoggins
Judith A. Whitworth

Cushing, in his classic text on the pituitary body and its disorders [23], associated for the first time adrenal pathology with symptoms associated with pituitary dysfunction. In a group of patients of his and of others published prior to 1910, all of whom had amenorrhea, adiposity, hirsutism, and a pituitary abnormality, adenomatous or hyperplastic adrenal glands were found. Cushing concluded, "It will thus be seen that we may perchance be on the way toward recognition of the consequences of hyperadrenalism. Heretofore the only recognizable clinical state associated with primary adrenal disease has been the syndrome of Addison, and the grouping of these cases may possibly add one more to the series of clinical conditions related to primary maladies of the ductless glands." Cushing also noted that hyperadrenalism was present in two of his patients with high blood pressure.

Cushing's syndrome is now recognized as one of a number of clinical syndromes characterized by adrenocortical steroid excess and hypertension. In a number of these syndromes such as Cushing's disease both steroid and adrenocorticotropic hormone (ACTH) secretion are increased. Clearly, under these circumstances the hypersecretion of ACTH plays a pivotal role in the development of the clinical features of the disease.

Classification

Cushing's syndrome has been defined as the clinical features associated with prolonged exposure to elevated glucocorticoid hormone. A classification of Cushing's syndrome is shown in Table 58-1. Cushing's disease accounts for some two-thirds of cases, ectopic ACTH 15 percent, adrenal adenoma 9 percent, and adrenal carcinoma 8 percent [36].

ACTH-DEPENDENT CUSHING'S SYNDROME

Pituitary ACTH Excess (Cushing's Disease). The majority of cases of Cushing's syndrome are due to an abnormality in the hypothalamic-pituitary-adrenal axis, resulting in excess ACTH (and β-lipotropin) secretion [57] and bilateral adrenal hyperplasia. Plasma ACTH levels are frequently elevated.

Some 10 percent of cases are associated with discrete pituitary enlargement due to adenomas, either of the chromophobe variety or basophil, as originally described by Cushing. Microadenomas are found in the pituitary in the majority of cases.

The studies on which this chapter was based were supported by the National Health and Medical Research Council of Australia, the Life Insurance Medical Research Fund of Australia and New Zealand, the National Heart Foundation of Australia, the William Buckland Trust, and the Potter Foundation.

Ectopic ACTH Production. Production of excess ACTH (or its precursor proopiomelancortin, or corticotropin-releasing factor, CRF) by nonendocrine (e.g., oat cell tumor of the lung) or endocrine tumors (e.g., islet cell tumor of the pancreas, medullary carcinoma of the thyroid) is associated with suppression of pituitary ACTH secretion and bilateral adrenal hyperplasia. Rarely, ectopic ACTH secretion may be due to a pheochromocytoma [46]. It commonly affects males and produces severe hypokalemic alkalosis, weakness, and pigmentation in the absence of classic signs of Cushing's syndrome. Hypertension is a feature in some but is less frequent than in pituitary-dependent ACTH excess [99], and the electrolyte abnormalities appear to be more closely correlated to secretion of deoxycorticosterone (DOC) and corticosterone than to cortisol or related glucocorticoids. The reason for the reduced incidence of hypertension is not clear but may relate in part to the poor general condition of patients with this disease who have uncontrolled malignancy.

Exogenous ACTH. Following the introduction of ACTH for the treatment of rheumatic diseases, hypertension was soon recognized as a complication of treatment. Hench and colleagues [45] reported a moderate (20 to 40 mm Hg) elevation of blood pressure in 2 women receiving ACTH for rheumatoid arthritis. Perera [89] found a rise in blood pressure with ACTH administration in the majority of a heterogeneous group of 13 patients, including hypertensives and patients with rheumatoid arthritis and related disorders. Savage et al. [98] reported a rise in blood pressure in 28 of 105 (27 percent) of rheumatoid patients treated with long-term ACTH compared with 17 percent of patients receiving cortisone. In 4 ACTH-treated patients hypertension necessitated drug withdrawal, and this was followed by return of blood pressure to normal levels. Treadwell et al. [115] reported "mild" hypertension (diastolic blood pressure 100 to 110 mm Hg) developing in 5 of 68 patients (7 percent) on long-term cortisone compared with 10 of 68 (15 percent) treated with ACTH, and hypertension with diastolic pressures of over 110 mm Hg in 6 percent of both ACTH and cortisone-treated patients. ACTH has also been used in the management of infantile spasms and in some infants therapy has been limited by the development of hypertension [48].

ACTH-INDEPENDENT CUSHING'S SYNDROME (ADRENAL CUSHING'S SYNDROME)

Adrenal Adenoma. Adrenal adenoma accounts for about 10 percent of cases of Cushing's syndrome. These tumors are usually single and (through pituitary ACTH suppression) are associated with atrophy of both the contralateral adrenal and ipsilateral normal adrenal tissue.

Adrenal Carcinoma. Adrenal carcinoma is less common than adenoma, usually occurring in infants and children. Hypokalemic alkalosis and hypertension may be prominent features.

Table 58-1. Classification of Cushing's syndrome

ACTH-dependent Cushing's syndrome
Pituitary ACTH excess (Cushing's disease)
Ectopic ACTH
Exogenous ACTH
Adrenal Cushing's syndrome
Adrenal adenoma
Adrenal carcinoma
Exogenous glucocorticoid

Exogenous Glucocorticoid Administration. Hypertension is said to occur in only 20 percent of patients with iatrogenic Cushing's syndrome [98, 115], but synthetic glucocorticoids probably invariably increase pressure to some degree. Severe hypertension may occur and has been reported also with topical steroids [3].

ALCOHOL-INDUCED PSEUDO-CUSHING'S SYNDROME

A "pseudo-Cushing's syndrome" has been reported in patients who abuse alcohol [109]. The abnormality is reversed if alcohol is withdrawn [66]. These subjects are usually hypertensive, and it has been suggested that the well-recognized association between hypertension and alcohol consumption [52] might be related to abnormalities of the hypothalamic-pituitary-adrenal axis.

GLUCOCORTICOID-SUPPRESSIBLE HYPERTENSION

Familial glucocorticoid suppressible hypertension was originally described by Sutherland et al. [113] and New and Peterson [80]. The condition is characterized by benign hypertension, hypokalemia, and increased aldosterone secretion rate, with a fall in aldosterone on standing, suppressed plasma renin activity, expanded plasma volume, and reversal of these abnormalities on administration of synthetic glucocorticoids in low dosage, classically dexamethasone 2 mg per day. Aldosterone is suppressed to very low levels by dexamethasone. Spironolactone has no effect on the blood pressure. New et al. [81] failed to reproduce hypertension in a dexamethasone-suppressed patient by infusion of aldosterone 1 mg per day, 18-OH-DOC 1 mg per day, or DOC 30 mg per day for 5 days. ACTH or oral metyrapone, however, produced hypertension within 5 days. The metyrapone effect was eliminated by aminoglutethimide, suggesting that an 11-deoxysteroid is responsible for the hypertension. It thus seems unlikely that the elevated aldosterone secretion seen in patients with dexamethasone-suppressible hypertension is responsible for the elevated blood pressure. The mode of inheritance of this form of hypertension is not known but may be autosomal dominant [34]. Grim, Weinberger, and Anad [38] reported a family with dexamethasone-suppressible hypertension in whom hypokalemia was not a consistent finding. Without measurement of renin levels these patients would have been said to have essential hypertension.

Steroids in Cushing's Syndrome

Apart from the well-documented cortisol excess, a variety of other plasma steroids are elevated in Cushing's syndrome.

11-Deoxycortisol (S) is raised [85]. Aldosterone is low or normal in the great majority of cases [29] but rarely is increased in patients with adrenal adenoma [39]. Corticosterone (B) is increased in a proportion of patients [12, 85, 99]. Deoxycorticosterone is increased in a proportion of patients with all varieties of Cushing's syndrome [10, 21, 85], and 18-OH-DOC also has been reported to be increased [72]. Dihydroepiandrostenedione sulfate has been reported to be elevated or normal in Cushing's disease and decreased in adenoma [135].

Clinical Features of Cushing's Syndrome

Hypertension occurs in 80 percent of patients with idiopathic Cushing's syndrome. Other classic clinical features include glucose intolerance, menstrual disorders, sterility, loss of libido, hirsutism, acne, red and depressed striae, osteoporosis, weakness and muscle wasting, purpura and easy bruising, mental disturbance, edema, polyuria, ocular changes, peptic ulceration, nephrocalcinosis, renal stones, reduced resistance to infection, and poor wound healing [95]. In a survey of 70 patients Ross and Linch [94] identified ecchymoses, myopathy, and hypertension as the clinical features of greater discriminatory value.

The spontaneous disease is relatively rare, predominantly affecting adult women (the ratio of women to men is 4:1) in the third and fourth decades. The iatrogenic variety is becoming increasingly common with the use of glucocorticoids in transplant patients and patients with a variety of immunologic and inflammatory disorders.

Insidious onset of Cushing's syndrome suggests Cushing's disease, whereas a rapid onset suggests carcinoma, either of the adrenal, or association with ectopic ACTH production.

Patients very commonly have abnormally high fasting blood glucose concentrations, impaired glucose tolerance, and hyperlipidemia. They usually show neutrophilia, lymphopenia, and eosinopenia and may be hypokalemic.

Cushing's Syndrome in Pregnancy

Because most women with Cushing's syndrome are amenorrheic or anovulatory, the association with pregnancy is rare. Pregnancy itself has some of the features of Cushing's syndrome, for example, striae, obesity, and glucose intolerance in some patients. However, although cortisol production and plasma cortisol concentrations are increased during pregnancy, the normal pregnant woman demonstrates a diurnal rhythm for cortisol, and cortisol is suppressed by dexamethasone. Plasma ACTH may be slightly decreased in pregnancy. Plasma cortisol levels are elevated in patients taking oral contraceptives.

Diagnosis

Cushing's syndrome is characterized by cortisol excess, with increased cortisol secretion and urinary excretion of free cortisol. Urinary 17-hydroxycorticoids are usually raised, and 17-ketogenic steroids are raised less frequently. These steroids, however, are also raised with obesity, thyrotoxicosis, acromegaly, and stress. Plasma cortisol may be high, and circadian rhythm tends to be abolished.

Pituitary-dependent adrenal hyperplasia is characterized by increased plasma ACTH levels, increased cortisol response to ACTH, suppression of plasma cortisol with dexamethasone, and a marked increase in 17-ketogenic steroids following metyrapone administration. Ectopic ACTH is distinguished by very high ACTH levels, normal cortisol response to ACTH, and partial suppression of plasma cortisol with dexamethasone. Adrenal adenomas show normal ACTH levels, less marked suppression of plasma cortisol with dexamethasone, and a decrease in 17-ketogenic steroids following metyrapone. In patients with adrenal carcinoma, there is usually marked elevation of urinary 17-ketosteroids and no increase of plasma cortisol with ACTH.

Diagnosis of Cushing's syndrome (Fig. 58-1) has historically been based on the findings of elevated urinary 17-hydroxycorticosteroids, elevated urinary free cortisol, loss of diurnal rhythm of plasma cortisol concentrations, and failure of plasma cortisol to suppress after a single dose (1 mg) of dexamethasone overnight [83]. Measurement of urinary 17-hydroxycorticosteroids may give both false-positive results in obese subjects and false-negative results in patients with Cushing's syndrome [22], and obese and acromegalic subjects may not suppress with the overnight suppression test [47]. The low-dose dexamethasone suppression test [60] (0.5 mg every 6 hours for 2 days) separates patients with Cushing's syndrome from normal subjects. Classically, measurements of urinary steroids have been used in the low-dose dexamethasone suppression test, but results of serum cortisol measurements are simpler and appear as reliable [51].

The most direct method of demonstrating an increase in cortisol secretion involves injection of ^{3}H-cortisol with determination of the specific activity of a completely converted metabolite as described by Melby [71], but this is rarely used except as a research procedure.

Once a diagnosis of Cushing's syndrome is made, the etiology must be determined. The high-dose dexamethasone suppression test (2 mg every 6 hours for 2 days) distinguishes Cushing's disease (pituitary-dependent), which suppresses, from adrenal tumor, which does not. Metapyrone, an 11β-hydroxylase inhibitor, in a dose of 750 mg every 4 hours for 24 hours, blocks conversion of 11-deoxycortisol to cortisol and thus increases ACTH secretion in normal subjects and Cushing's disease with a consequent increase in urinary 17-hydroxysteroids and 17-ketogenic steroids. In patients with adrenal tumor, no such increase is seen. Measurement of plasma ACTH [7] distinguishes patients with ectopic ACTH secretion (high levels) and Cushing's disease (high or normal levels) from patients with adrenal tumor (undetectable or low levels). ACTH stimulation (25 IU intravenously over 8 hours) increases plasma cortisol and 17-hydroxysteroids in adenoma but not in carcinoma. In practice, the results of these investigations are not always clear-cut. Recently, Van Cauter and Refetoff [116] reported dimin-

Fig. 58-1. Flow chart of the tests used for the diagnosis of Cushing's syndrome.

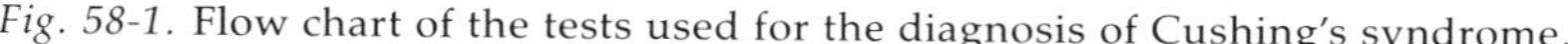

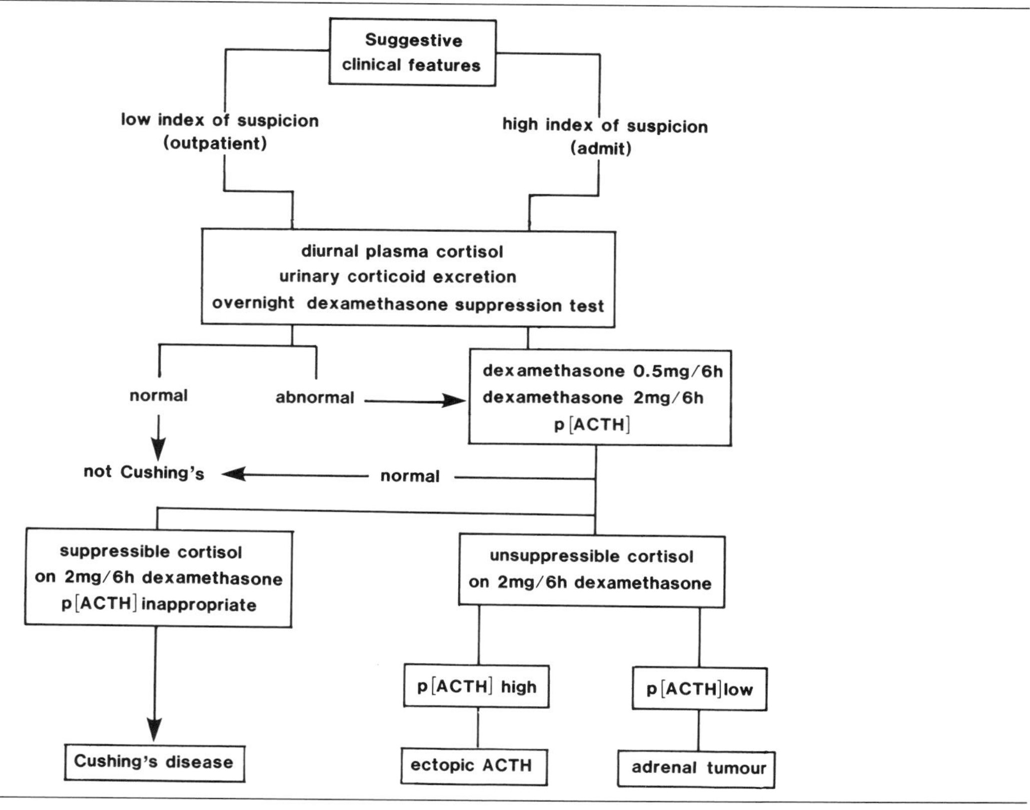

ished episodic variations in plasma cortisol in patients with adenoma compared with Cushing's disease and suggested that repeated sampling may be of value diagnostically. They further subdivided patients with Cushing's disease into two groups, those who were hypopulsatile and those who were hyperpulsatile, and suggested that the former might represent excess pituitary secretion of ACTH and the latter increased hypothalamic release of (or increased pituitary responsiveness to) CRF. Further, Hale et al. [43] reported a case of pituitary-dependent Cushing's disease with clinical and biochemical features of the ectopic ACTH syndrome.

The role of CRF in diagnosis remains to be established. Plasma ACTH and cortisol are increased in patients with Cushing's disease following CRF administration [86], and successful transsphenoidal surgery led to lack of CRF responsiveness. No such response is seen in patients with adrenal adenoma [15].

Although ectopic ACTH production from a pheochromocytoma is rare, accurate diagnosis is vital because appropriate preoperative management may be critical for a successful outcome. It is thus appropriate to screen patients with Cushing's syndrome due to an adrenal tumor for catecholamine excess [45].

LOCALIZATION

The right adrenal lies above the upper pole of the right kidney, behind the inferior vena cava and between the crus of the right hemidiaphragm and the liver. The left adrenal is slightly medial to the upper pole of the left kidney near the tail of the pancreas and behind the splenic vein.

Localization of the lesion usually involves tomography of the pituitary fossa, cerebral and abdominal computed tomography (CT), and, on occasion, selective sampling for plasma ACTH and/or cortisol by venography.

Fig. 58-2. CT scan: coronal view of a pituitary macroadenoma (>1 cm in diameter). (Courtesy of Dr. Brian Tress.)

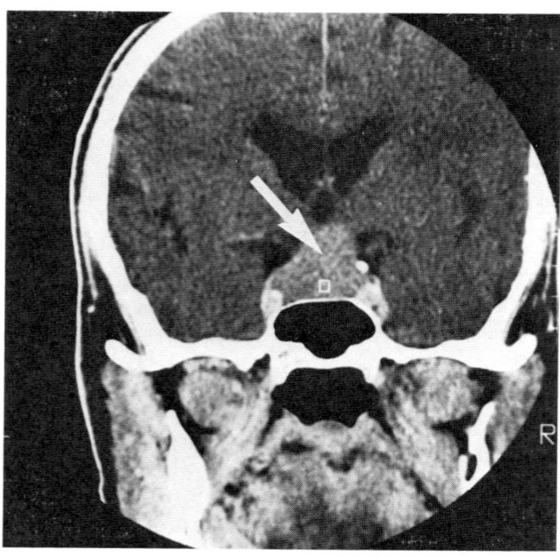

About 10 percent of patients with Cushing's disease have an abnormal pituitary fossa on skull x-ray, and with tomography this proportion increases to around 20 percent [63]. Cerebral CT scanning is more likely to reveal a pituitary tumor (Fig. 58-2) and with high resolution can also detect microadenomas (Fig. 58-3).

CT of the adrenals may show a tumor or bilaterally enlarged glands (Fig. 58-4), particularly in patients with ectopic ACTH, but in some 50 percent of patients with Cushing's disease no abnormality of the adrenals can be detected.

Iodocholesterol uptake by the adrenal has been reported to separate reliably bilateral adrenal hyperplasia from cortical adenoma in over 95 percent of cases [97] but has been less rewarding in other hands.

Selective venous sampling is useful in distinguishing

Fig. 58-3. CT scan: sagittal reformatted (reconstructed) image of pituitary microadenoma. The adenoma is hypodense relative to the normal pituitary tissue and is situated within the posteroinferior aspect of the gland. (Courtesy of Dr. Brian Tress.)

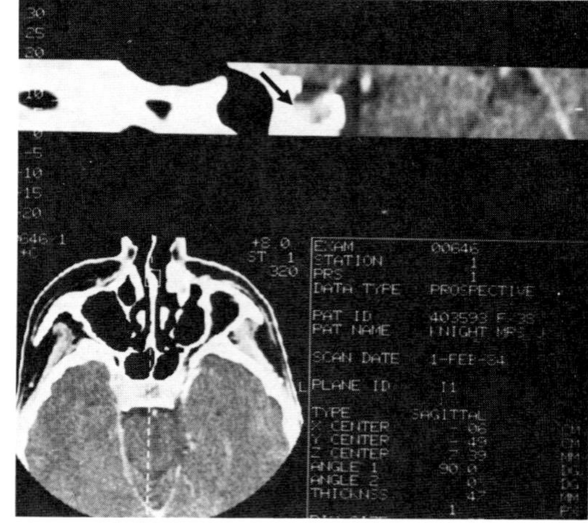

Fig. 58-4. CT scan showing diffuse bilateral adrenal gland enlargement. (Courtesy of Dr. Terry Doyle.)

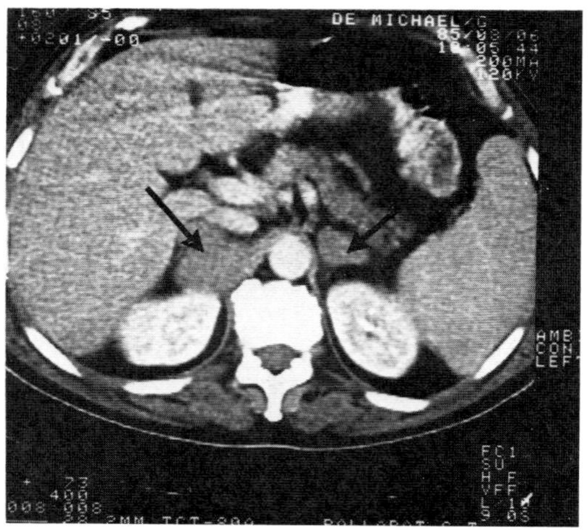

ectopic ACTH from Cushing's disease. Both inferior petrosal sinuses should be sampled. The ratio of sinus to peripheral plasma ACTH concentration is more than 2 in Cushing's disease and less than 1.5 in ectopic ACTH [31]. Sampling at various levels in the vena cava may help identify the site of ectopic ACTH secretion [28].

Management

Untreated Cushing's syndrome has a very poor prognosis, with only a 50 percent 5-year survival [90]. Even when treatment has achieved a permanent biochemical remission, mortality is still four times that of the general population [94], largely due to cardiovascular disease. Cardiovascular risk factors in these patients include hypertension, hyperlipidemia, glucose intolerance, and obesity.

CUSHING'S DISEASE

For many years bilateral adrenalectomy was the favored method of treatment [87]. With total bilateral adrenalectomy, virtually 100 percent of patients are cured [87] compared with subtotal adrenalectomy in which hypertension was relieved in only 59 percent [91]. Bilateral adrenalectomy, however, necessitates permanent steroid replacement therapy, and a proportion of patients will subsequently develop Nelson's syndrome. More recently, selective excision of pituitary adenomas by a transsphenoidal approach has been used, even when the adenoma has not been demonstrated radiologically [96, 133], and this is now widely regarded as the treatment of choice [14].

A variety of drugs have been used in medical treatment of Cushing's disease, with varying degrees of success. These include the 11β-hydroxylase inhibitor metyrapone [114], the serotonergic antagonist cyproheptadine [56], reserpine [77], the dopaminergic agonists bromocriptine [59] and lisuride [11], aminoglutethimide [32], *o,p'*-DDD [87], trilostane, an inhibitor of 3β-hydroxysteroid dehydrogenase [54], hydrogenase [54], ketoconazole [84], and sodium valproate [27], which acts by inhibiting GABA-transaminase. The use of relatively specific glucocorticoid antagonists is currently under clinical investigation.

Pituitary irradiation has been used in adults [50] and is regarded by many as the preferred treatment for children and adolescents [70]. Approximately one-third of patients with Cushing's disease treated by bilateral adrenalectomy develop pituitary macroadenoma with increased skin and mucosal pigmentation (Nelson's syndrome). Pituitary irradiation is commonly undertaken following pituitary surgery to prevent recurrence or following adrenal surgery to prevent Nelson's syndrome.

ADRENAL TUMOR

Adrenal malignancy is best treated surgically, but the results are poor. In patients with extensive adrenal carcinoma, medical therapy may be of some benefit; the drugs used include aminoglutethimide and mitolane (*o,p'*-DDD) [6]. Results of removal of adrenal adenoma by unilateral adrenalectomy are excellent [87, 91]. Postoperatively, patients may require temporary adrenal replacement therapy.

The majority of ectopic ACTH-secreting tumors are malignant and nonresectable, and medical therapy is used.

HYPERTENSION IN CUSHING'S SYNDROME

Cushing's syndrome is a rare cause of hypertension. It affects about 0.1 percent of the population in autopsy studies or 1 in 300 to 400 hypertensives. On the other hand, hypertension is very common in idiopathic Cushing's syndrome, affecting some 80 percent of patients [37, 90, 95, 110].

Patients with Cushing's syndrome rarely present to the clinician with hypertension for investigation because the diagnosis of Cushing's syndrome is often apparent on clinical grounds. A more common problem in the hypertension clinic is the differential diagnosis between Cushing's syndrome and the obese hypertensive patient.

The prevalence and severity of the hypertension may differ depending on the etiology of Cushing's syndrome, although this has been disputed [110]. In the series of Greminger et al. [37] 64 percent of patients with Cushing's disease were hypertensive (mean blood pressure 158/100 mm Hg), compared with 83 percent of patients with adenoma (mean blood pressure 164/100 mm Hg) and 100 percent with carcinoma (184/114 mm Hg). Ross et al. [95] found that 87 percent of patients with hyperplasia were hypertensive, and all of his 15 patients with adenoma or carcinoma were hypertensive. In a series from Britain, 93 percent of patients with Cushing's syndrome were hypertensive, and the incidence and severity were not affected by sex, nature of the underlying lesion, or duration or severity of symptoms [119]. Compared with age- and sex-matched normals, blood pressure was raised 43/29 mm Hg. Forty percent of the patients had cardiovascular complications.

The proportion of patients with ectopic ACTH production who are hypertensive is usually lower [99], but whether this reflects the relatively short duration of the disease, a consequence of a malignant disease, or a different pattern of steroid production, is not clear.

The prevalence of hypertension is only 20 percent in iatrogenic Cushing's syndrome [98, 115], presumably because of differences between naturally occurring and synthetic steroids.

Hypertension is an important cause of morbidity and mortality in Cushing's syndrome, and its complications are similar to those of hypertension of other etiologies including stroke, hypertensive heart failure, myocardial infarction, and cases of accelerated hypertension and renal failure [65].

MANAGEMENT OF HYPERTENSION

Appropriate treatment of Cushing's syndrome as outlined above may be sufficient to normalize the blood pressure. In some 40 percent of cases, however, hypertension persists, and in these cases antihypertensive treatment is indicated.

Experimental Studies in Humans

ACTH ADMINISTRATION

Short-term ACTH administration increases blood pressure in both normal and hypertensive children [93] and adults [19, 130] (Fig. 58-5) but not in addisonian subjects [130] (Fig. 58-6). Doses as low as 1 μg/kg/day (by IV infusion) are sufficient to raise blood pressure [125].

In studies in adult subjects receiving 100 mmol of sodium and potassium daily, ACTH administration, 1 mg/day for 5 days, raises systolic pressure 22 ± 4 mm Hg (n = 12). Subsequent studies in subjects receiving 200 to 300 mmol of sodium and free potassium daily have shown that ACTH can produce substantial rises in pressure over 5 days, 35 ± 11 mm Hg systolic pressure [129], whereas on a low sodium intake of 15 mmol/day the rise in pressure was only 9 ± 4 mm Hg [20] (Fig. 58-7).

ACTH administration is characterized by a rise in plasma sodium concentration, a fall in plasma potassium concentration, initial urinary sodium retention, a rise in fasting blood glucose, and a rise in body weight [130].

Plasma cortisol, 11-deoxycortisol, deoxycorticosterone, and corticosterone are increased, and aldosterone

Fig. 58-5. Blood pressure and metabolic effects of ACTH (1 mg/day) in normal subjects.

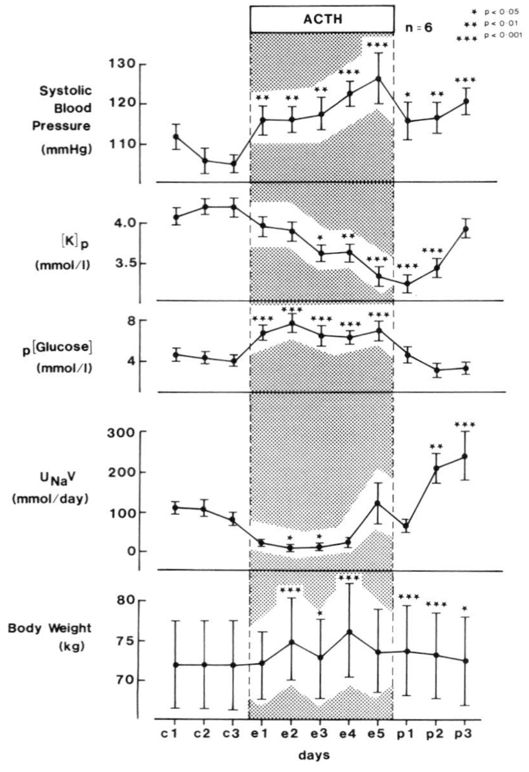

Fig. 58-6. Change in systolic blood pressure with ACTH (1 mg/day) in normotensive, hypertensive, and addisonian subjects; ***$p < 0.001$.

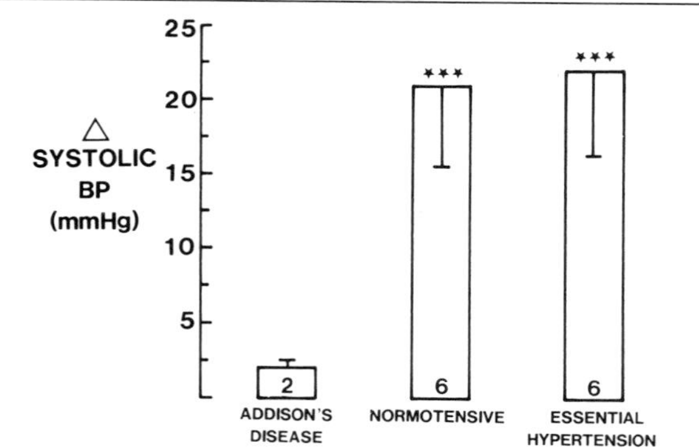

Fig. 58-7. Effect of sodium intake on blood pressure response to ACTH (1 mg/day); **$p < 0.01$.

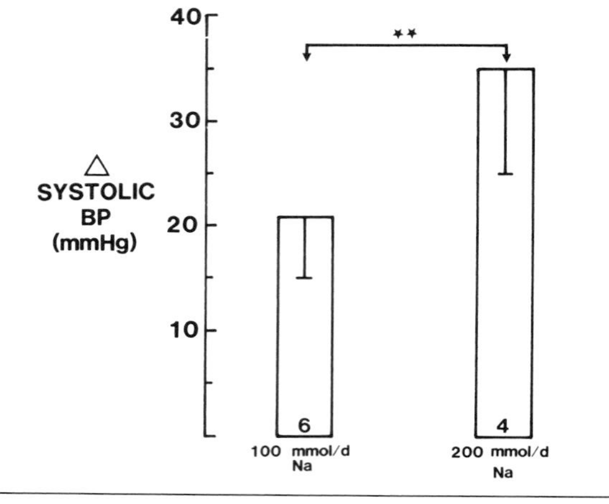

Fig. 58-8. Hormonal effects of ACTH (1 mg/day) in normal subjects. PRC = plasma renin concentration.

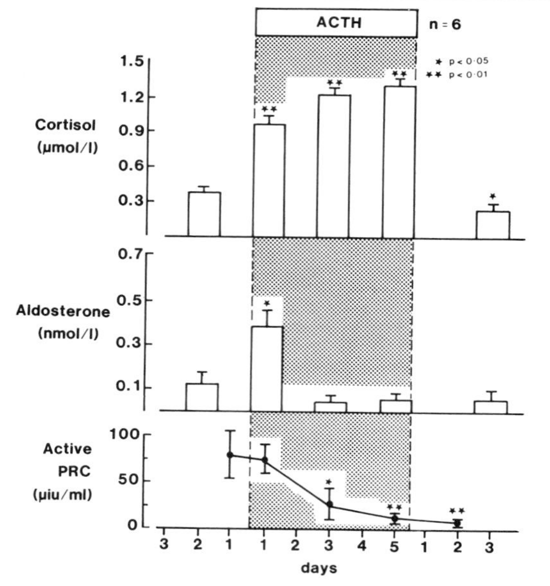

is increased transiently [9, 130] (Fig. 58-8). Plasma 17α-hydroxyprogesterone and 17α,20α-dihydroxyprogesterone, which have been shown to be hypertensinogenic in sheep [101], are also increased by ACTH in humans [130]. Plasma renin substrate rises with ACTH treatment, plasma renin concentration falls [130] (Fig. 58-8), and urinary kallikrein activity is increased [132]. Plasma noradrenaline concentrations fall, and atrial natriuretic peptide levels are increased [19].

ACTH administration produced increases in cardiac index, but peripheral resistance was unchanged [127] (Fig. 58-9). Plasma volume increased [130], as did extracellular fluid volume, exchangeable sodium, and inulin clearance [19]. Pressor responsiveness to phenylephrine was also increased [123].

STEROID INFUSIONS

To determine which steroid(s) was responsible for the blood pressure-raising effects of ACTH in humans, cortisol (6 to 8 mg/day, n = 7) and deoxycorticosterone (1 mg/day, n = 6) were infused at rates that produced blood concentrations of steroid appropriate for conditions of ACTH stimulation [128]. Cortisol infusion for 5 days reproduced the blood pressure and metabolic effects of ACTH administration (Fig. 58-10), whereas deoxycorticosterone infusion produced a small fall in diastolic blood pressure, initial urinary sodium retention, and an increase in body weight (Fig. 58-11). Cortisol administration also reproduces the haemodynamic, volume, and hormonal [19] effects of ACTH as well as the alterations in pressor responsiveness [121, 122] with no increase in sympathetic activity [112]. It thus appears that the rise in blood pressure seen with short-term ACTH administration in humans is due to the increased secretion of cortisol (Fig. 58-12).

It is speculative to what degree these observations are relevant to Cushing's syndrome. Patients with Cushing's disease often have ACTH concentrations that are normal or only mildly elevated, with decreased sensitivity to cortisol feedback suppression of ACTH [134]. In our experimental studies, ACTH and cortisol increased plasma sodium and decreased plasma potassium concentrations and suppressed renin, features that are not prominent in Cushing's disease.

The extent to which other steroids that are increased by ACTH, such as deoxycorticosterone, corticosterone, or 17α,20α-dihydroxyprogesterone, might contribute to the blood pressure-raising effects of ACTH is not clear. The experimental evidence, however, suggests that cortisol alone is sufficient to cause substantial increases in blood pressure.

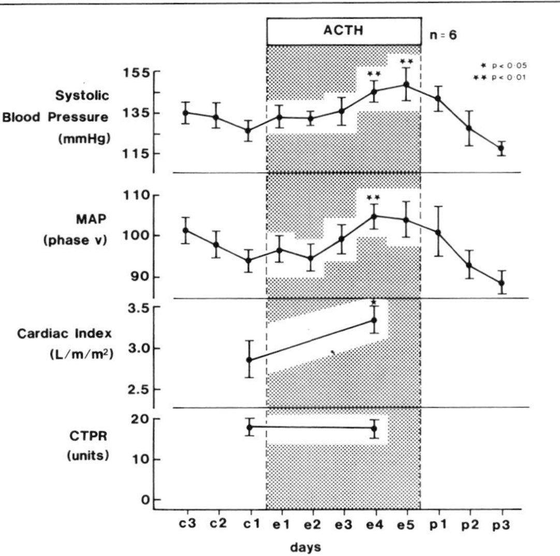

Fig. 58-9. Hemodynamic effects of ACTH (1 mg/day) in patients with essential hypertension. MAP = mean arterial pressure; CTPR = calculated total peripheral vascular resistance.

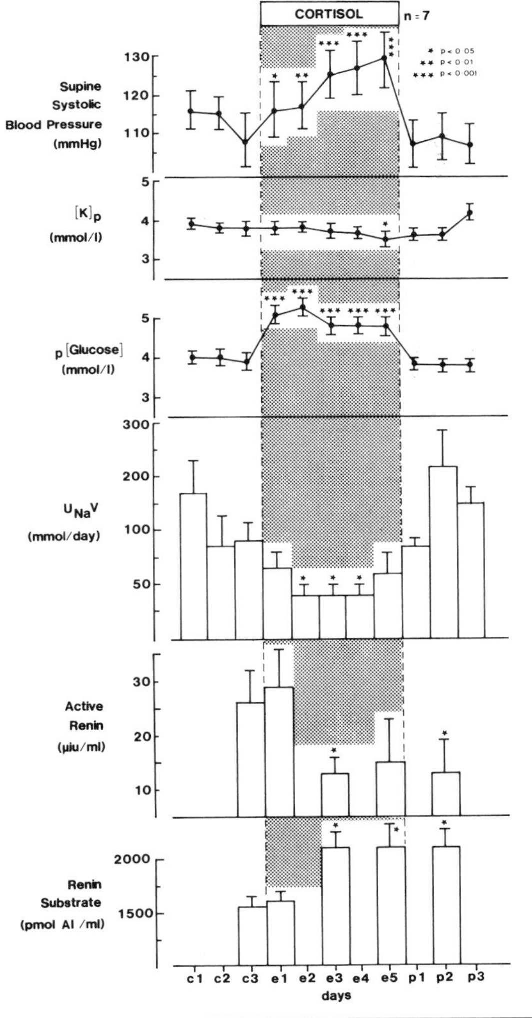

Fig. 58-10. Blood pressure and metabolic effects of cortisol infusion (6–8 mg/hr).

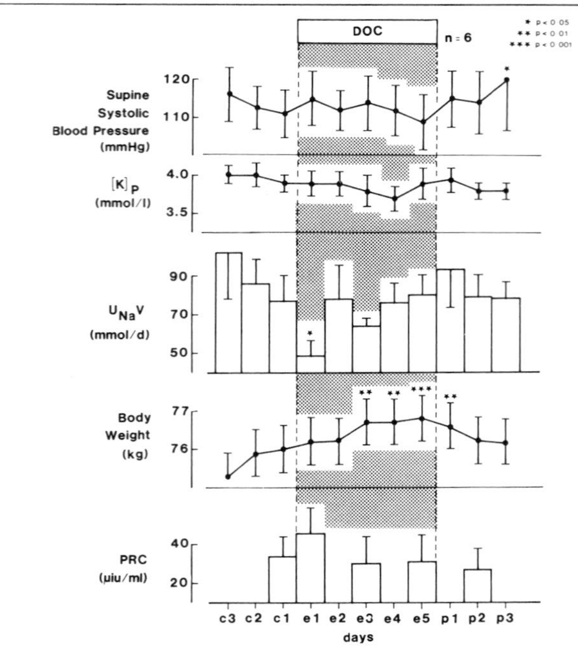

Fig. 58-11. Blood pressure and metabolic effects of deoxycorticosterone (DOC) infusion (1 mg/day). PRC = plasma renin concentration.

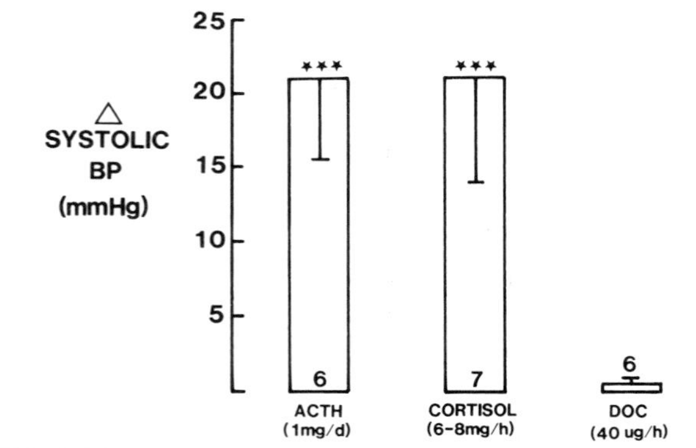

Fig. 58-12. Comparison of changes in systolic blood pressure with ACTH, cortisol, and deoxycorticosterone (DOC); ***p < 0.001.

Physiologic Mechanisms Involved in the Hypertension of Adrenocortical Steroid Excess

Since the first demonstration in animals of the blood pressure-raising effects of steroids such as cortisone [35] and deoxycorticosterone [58], many different mechanisms have been proposed as being involved in the production of the hypertension. These have been reviewed in detail for ACTH-dependent hypertension by Scoggins et al. [104] and Lohmeier and Kastner [62]. Detailed studies in sheep [104], rat [33, 40, 126], and dog [62] have described the physiologic changes associated with ACTH administration. However, the majority of experiments have examined the effect of individual naturally occurring or synthetic steroids. These studies have usually been in the rat. On many occasions the animals have had a unilateral nephrectomy, and their drinking water has been substituted by saline. These two procedures amplify the hypertensive effects of adrenocortical steroids but do little to resolve the mechanism because the procedures exacerbate both sodium and non-sodium-dependent types of hypertension [104].

The physiologic mechanisms by which steroids with primarily "glucocorticoid" activity raise blood pressure are thought to be different from those associated with "mineralocorticoid" administration. However, studies in sheep have led us to propose that the pressor effects of all steroids may be mediated via a common mechanism involving "hypertensinogenic" activity of the steroids [106]. The evidence for this novel class of steroid hormone activity has been described in detail and is based on studies examining ACTH-induced hypertension in sheep and the finding that the pressor effects of naturally occurring and synthetic steroids can be dissociated from their glucocorticoid and mineralocorticoid activity [106]. Not all glucocorticoids raise blood pressure, and responses vary from species to species. For example, although 6α-methylprednisolone produces hypertension in the rat [55], it has no effect in either the sheep [79] or the dog [44]. Further, although cortisol at a high rate of infusion (20 mg/hr) is pressor in sheep [120], it lowers blood pressure in the dog [62]. Structure activity studies have shown that there is no simple relationship between the features of the molecule that endow in vivo glucocorticoid activity and effects on blood pressure [102].

A number of physiologic effects of glucocorticoids on the circulation have been described. These include:

1. *Changes in body fluid distribution.* It has been reported that in the rat corticosterone increases plasma volume as a result of a shift of fluid from the intracellular to the extracellular compartment [41]. In sheep glucocorticoids may raise the plasma volume without change in the extracellular fluid volume (ECFV) or body weight [105].

   It is clear that the change in plasma volume is not necessary for the development of ACTH-induced hypertension in the sheep because blood pressure is increased in animals subjected to acute sodium depletion (−450 mmol sodium) in which plasma volume is falling as blood pressure is increased [104].
2. *Changes in vascular response to norepinephrine.* Although increased pressor responsiveness to norepinephrine is a widely reported feature of mineralocorticoid administration, similar changes following ACTH or glucocorticoid administration have not been observed in sheep [69] or in 6α-methylprednisolone-treated rats [55]. In the dog ACTH greatly enhances the pressor effects of chronic norepinephrine infusion, an effect not reproduced by either cortisol or aldosterone [61]. However, it has been proposed that glucocorticoids may inhibit phospholipase A_2 and prostanoid production leading to increased vasoconstrictor responses to

norepinephrine without changing the plasma norepinephrine concentration [92]. Increased pressor responses to norepinephrine have also been seen in corticosterone-treated rats [100] and in Cushing's syndrome [73]. In ACTH-treated sheep, pressor responsiveness to other agonists such as angiotensin II, tyramine, serotonin, and arginine vasopressin (AVP) is also unchanged [104].

A possible role for reduced prostacyclin production arising from glucocorticoid action and increased effects of the steroid on vascular tone has been proposed as the mechanism of the hypertension of Cushing's syndrome by Axelrod [4]. In the ACTH-treated sheep, experiments involving acute and chronic indomethacin infusion and prostacyclin infusion [67] suggest that prostanoids may modulate the severity of adrenocortical hypertension but are unlikely to play a primary role in the development of the hypertension.

3. *Changes in the renin-angiotensin system.* Although glucocorticoids increase renin substrate [130] and although plasma renin activity may remain in the normal range during the early stages of steroid administration, at later stages in the hypertensive animal, as in humans, renin concentration or activity or plasma angiotensin II levels are suppressed [41]. In sheep treated with ACTH, the suppressed renin levels are unresponsive to stimulation by sodium depletion, isoprenaline, or prostacyclin infusion [104]. It has been reported that the renin-angiotensin system may play a role in the development of 6α-methylprednisolone hypertension in the rat [55]. However, it is possible that the reduced sodium status of these animals may be responsible for their observed increased angiotensin II dependency. More recently, this group found that the angiotensin converting enzyme inhibitor captopril produced smaller falls in blood pressure in 6α-methylprednisolone-treated rats than in control animals on a similar low sodium diet [30]. In sheep, captopril had no effect on the development of ACTH-induced hypertension [111]. In Cushing's syndrome, although the angiotensin II antagonist saralasin has been reported to lower blood pressure [24], others have not confirmed this with either saralasin [117] or captopril [37].
4. *Changes in adrenergic activity.* There have been few studies on the role of either the central or peripheral sympathetic nervous system in glucocorticoid-treated animals. There is, however, considerable evidence for involvement of the sympathetic nervous system in mineralocorticoid hypertension [16]. In ACTH-treated sheep there is no change in plasma catecholamines [106]. Further "total" autonomic blockade or ganglion blockade does not prevent the development of ACTH hypertension [106]. Renal denervation is also without effect in this type of hypertension [120]. Recently, Majewski and Rand have proposed that epinephrine may be a mediator of steroid or "stress"-induced hypertension [64]. It is proposed that epinephrine of adrenal medullary or sympathetic nerve origin acts on the prejunctional β-adrenoreceptor, leading to increased norepinephrine release and raised blood pressure. It is of interest that increased pressor responses to subpressor doses of epinephrine were observed in cortisol-treated dogs [1]. In the ACTH-treated sheep there is no change in plasma epinephrine levels, and adrenal denervation has no effect on the development of the hypertension [108].

   Hemodynamic studies examining the onset of the effect of ACTH on blood pressure in sheep have established that cardiac output is increased within 60 minutes. However, total peripheral resistance falls at this time, and it is only when resistance returns to normal at 4 to 6 hours that blood pressure starts to rise (unpublished observations). Further evidence supporting an important role for changes in peripheral resistance has been obtained from studies in which nisoldipine or minoxidil have been infused. Both these drugs prevent the development of ACTH hypertension (unpublished observations).
5. *Role of the preoptic hypothalamic area and AVP.* Although lesions of the anteroventral region of the third ventricle prevent the development of DOC hypertension in the rat [13], they have no influence on the development of ACTH hypertension in sheep [103]. Although subsequent studies in the rat have suggested that inhibition of AVP release by the lesion may play an important role in the development of the steroid hypertension [5], ACTH has only a very small effect on plasma AVP, and there is no change in pressor responsiveness to infused AVP [18].
6. *Changes in membrane ion transport.* Mitchell and Bohr [76] have speculated that mineralocorticoids such as DOC produce changes in membrane ion transport in the central nervous system that lead to increased intracellular [Na], increased Na-K-ATPase, a reset of the cardiovascular regulatory center, and hypertension. Differences in the effects of mineralocorticoids and glucocorticoids on Na-K-ATPase have been reported [88]. In volume-expanded hypertension an inhibitor of the sodium pump has been proposed [42]. In contrast, in the dexamethasone-treated rat there is an increase in Na-K-ATPase [42]. It is of interest that the observed effects of mineralocorticoids on sodium pump activity in arterial tissue are opposite to the effect of the steroids on the same enzyme in the kidney [17]. Glucocorticoids also increase renal Na-K-ATPase activity [17]. In Cushing's syndrome there is an increase in erythrocyte Na-K-ATPase. Studies in ACTH-treated rats suggest that changes in membrane ion transport are more closely related to the sodium-volume status of the animal than to the rise in blood pressure [107]. It is of interest that in steroid-treated animals changes are observed in the activity of the sodium pump. In patients with essential hypertension the abnormalities of membrane transport are usually found in the cotransport or countertransport mechanisms [118].
7. *Effects of sodium and potassium status.* The sodium dependency of mineralocorticoid-induced hypertension is well known [105], and this type of hypertension has recently been shown in the sheep to be sensitive to

potassium intake. An increase in dietary potassium intake from 200 to 800 mmol per day prevents DOC-induced rises in blood pressure [74]. Glucocorticoid-induced hypertension is less sodium dependent [53], and increases in blood pressure in the rat can be obtained without reduction in renal mass and increased sodium intake. In the sheep, acute sodium depletion of 15 to 20 percent of exchangeable sodium over the 48 hours prior to infusion of cortisol resulted in a reduction in the pressor response (unpublished observation). Similar reductions in sodium status have little effect on the development of ACTH hypertension in sheep [106]. Dietary sodium restriction also fails to prevent ACTH-induced increases in blood pressure in sheep. However, if sodium intake is reduced to less than 2 mmol per day, the rise in blood pressure is significantly less [49].

Increased dietary intake of potassium did not prevent the development of either ACTH or cortisol-induced hypertension in sheep [74]. However, the rise in blood pressure after 5 days is slightly less than that seen on a normal potassium diet.

Overall, it is clear that both sodium and potassium status may play an important role in modulating the severity of glucocorticoid-induced hypertension.

Conclusion

In summary, the mechanism(s) whereby ACTH and cortisol raise blood pressure in humans are not clear. Although there are features of a glucocorticoid type of hypertension, it is possible the steroids may be exerting their effects through a "hypertensinogenic" activity. In sheep, the hypertensinogenic effects of steroids can be separated from their mineralocorticoid or glucocorticoid effects [101, 105, 106]. It may be that, in contrast to the sheep, this hypertensinogenic action is seen in humans only at rates of steroid (or ACTH) administration that also have demonstrable glucocorticoid and/or mineralocorticoid effects.

References

1. Anderson, W. P., and Harris, D. T. Blood pressure responses to prolonged infusions of adrenaline and noradrenaline in conscious dogs. *Clin. Exp. Hypertens.* 6: 1469, 1984.
2. Anderson, W. P., and Ramsey, B. E. Blood pressure responses to ACTH and adrenaline infusion in dogs. *Clin. Exp. Hypertens.* 7: 525, 1985.
3. Armbruster, H., Vetter, W., Reck, G., et al. Severe arterial hypertension caused by chronic abuse of a topical mineralocorticoid. *Int. J. Clin. Pharmacol.* 12: 170, 1975.
4. Axelrod, L. Inhibition of prostaglandin production mediates permissive effect of glucocorticoids on vascular tone. *Lancet* 1: 904, 1983.
5. Berecek, K. H., Barron, K. W., Webb, R. L., et al. Vasopressin-central nervous system interactions in the development of DOCA hypertension. *Hypertension* 4: 131, 1982.
6. Bergenstal, D. M., Hertz, R., Lipsett, M. B., et al. Chemotherapy of adrenocortical cancer with O,P′-DDD. *Ann. Intern. Med.* 53: 672, 1960.
7. Berson, S. A., and Yalow, R. S. Radioimmunoassay of ACTH in plasma. *J. Clin. Invest.* 47: 2725, 1968.
8. Biglieri, E. G., Hane, S., Slaton, P. E., et al. In-vivo and in-vitro studies of adrenal secretions in Cushing's syndrome and primary aldosteronism. *J. Clin. Invest.* 42: 516, 1963.
9. Biglieri, E. G., Schambelan, M., and Slaton, P. E. Effect of adrenocorticotropin on DOC, corticosterone and aldosterone excretion. *Clin. Endocrinol.* 19: 1090, 1969.
10. Biglieri, E. G., Stockigt, J. R., and Schambelan, M. Adrenal mineralocorticoids causing hypertension. *Am. J. Med.* 52: 623, 1972.
11. Boscaro, M., Merola, G., Seratini, E., et al. Effect of short and long-term administration of lisuride on Cushing's disease. *J. Endocrinol. Invest.* 8: 13, 1985.
12. Boscaro, M., Scaroni, C., Masarotto, P., et al. Circadian secretion of ACTH, cortisol and mineralocorticoids in Cushing's syndrome. *Clin. Exp. Hypertens.* 4: 1779, 1982.
13. Brody, M. J., Fink, G. D., Buggy, J., et al. The role of anteroventral third ventricle region in experimental hypertension. *Circ. Res.* 43: I-2, 1978.
14. Burch, W. Cushing's disease. *Arch. Intern. Med.* 145: 1106, 1985.
15. Catania, A., Cantalamessa, A., Orsatti, A., et al. Plasma ACTH-response to the corticotropin releasing factor in patients with Cushing's disease. *Metabolism* 33: 478, 1984.
16. Chalmers, J. P. Nervous system and hypertension. *Clin. Sci. Mol. Med.* 55: 45s, 1978.
17. Charney, A. N., Silva, P., Besarab, A., et al. Separate effects of aldosterone, DOCA and methylprednisolone on renal Na-K-ATPase. *Am. J. Physiol.* 227: 345, 1974.
18. Coghlan, J. P., Denton, D. A., Graham, W. F., et al. Effect of ACTH administration on the haemodynamic response to arginine-vasopressin in sheep. *Clin. Exp. Pharmacol. Physiol.* 7: 559, 1980.
19. Connell, J. M. C., Whitworth, J. A., Davies, D. L., et al. Effects of ACTH and cortisol administration on blood pressure, electrolyte metabolism, atrial natriuretic peptide and renal function in normal man. *J. Hypertens.* 5: 425, 1987.
20. Connell, J. M. C., Whitworth, J. A., Davies, D. L., et al. Haemodynamic, hormonal and renal effects of ACTH in sodium restricted man. *J. Hypertens.* 6: 17, 1988.
21. Crane, M. G., and Harris, J. J. Desoxycorticosterone secretion rates in hyperadrenocortism. *J. Clin. Endocrinol. Metab.* 26: 1135, 1966.
22. Crapo, L. Cushing's syndrome: A review of diagnostic tests. *Metabolism* 28: 955, 1979.
23. Cushing, H. *The Pituitary Body and Its Disorders.* London: Lippincott, 1912.
24. Dalakos, T. G., Elias, A. N., Anderson, G. H., et al. Evidence for an angiotensinogenic mechanism of the hypertension of Cushing's syndrome. *J. Clin. Endocrinol. Metab.* 46: 114, 1978.
25. Distler, A., Just, H. J., and Philipp, T. H. Studies on the mechanism of aldosterone-induced hypertension in man. *Clin. Sci.* 45: 743, 1973.
26. Distler, A., and Philipp, T. H. On the Mechanism of Mineralocorticoid-Induced Hypertension. Effect of 9α-Fluorocortisone on Haemodynamics in Man. In W. Kaufman and O. K. Krause (eds.), *Central Nervous Control of Sodium Balance: Relations to the Renin-Angiotensin System.* Stuttgart: Georg Thieme, 1976.
27. Dornhurst, A., Jenkins, J. S., Lamberts, S. W. J., et al. The evaluation of sodium valproate in the treatment of

Nelson's syndrome. *J. Clin. Endocrinol. Metab.* 56: 985, 1983.
28. Drury, P. L., Tarrer, S., Tomlin, S., et al. Experience with selective venous sampling in the diagnosis of ACTH-dependent Cushing's syndrome. *Br. Med. J.* 284: 9, 1982.
29. Dyrenfurth, I., Sybulski, S., Notchev, V., et al. Urinary corticosteroid excretion patterns in patients with adrenocortical dysfunction. *J. Clin. Endocrinol. Metab.* 18: 391, 1958.
30. Elijovich, F., and Krakoff, L. R. Mechanism of the response to captopril in glucocorticoid hypertension. *Clin. Exp. Hypertens.* 4: 1795, 1982.
31. Findling, J. W., Aron, D. C., Tyrell, J. B., et al. Selective venous sampling for ACTH in Cushing's syndrome. *Ann. Intern. Med.* 94: 647, 1981.
32. Fishman, L. M., Liddle, G. W., Island, D. P., et al. Effects of aminoglutethimide on adrenal function in man. *J. Clin. Endocrinol. Metab.* 27: 481, 1967.
33. Freeman, R. H., Davis, J. O., and Fullerton, D. Chronic ACTH administration and the development of hypertension in rats. *Proc. Soc. Exp. Biol. Med.* 163: 473, 1980.
34. Ganguly, A. New insights and questions about glucocorticoid-suppressible hyperaldosteronism. *Am. J. Med.* 72: 851, 1982.
35. Gaudino, N. M. Las suprarenales en la hipertension arterial nefrogna. *Rev. Soc. Argent de Biol.* 20: 470, 1944.
36. Gold, E. M. The Cushing's syndromes: Changing views of diagnosis and treatment. *Ann. Intern. Med.* 90: 829, 1979.
37. Greminger, P., Tenschert, W., Vetter, W., et al. Hypertension in Cushing's Syndrome. In F. Mantero, E. G. Biglieri, and C. R. W. Edwards (eds.), *Endocrinology of Hypertension.* London and New York: Academic Press, 1982.
38. Grim, C. E., Weinberger, M. H., and Anand, S. K. Familial, Dexamethasone Suppressible Normokalaemic Hyperaldosteronism. In M. I. New and L. S. Levine (eds.), *Juvenile Hypertension.* New York: Raven Press, 1977.
39. Guthrie, G. P., and Kotchen, T. A. Hypertension and aldosterone overproduction without renin suppression in Cushing's syndrome from an adrenal adenoma. *Am. J. Med.* 67: 524, 1979.
40. Haack, D., Engel, R., and Vecsei, P. The effect of chronic ACTH treatment on blood pressure and urinary excretion of steroids in the rat. *Klin. Wochenschr.* 56: Suppl. I-183, 1978.
41. Haack, D., Mohring, J., Mohring, B., et al. Comparative study on development of corticosterone and DOCA hypertension in rats. *Am. J. Physiol.* 233: F403, 1977.
42. Haddy, F. J. Mechanism, prevention and therapy of sodium-dependent hypertension. *Am. J. Med.* 69: 746, 1980.
43. Hale, A. C., Millar, J. B. G., Ratter, S. J., et al. A case of pituitary dependent Cushing's disease with clinical and biochemical features of ectopic ACTH syndrome. *Clin. Endocrinol.* 22: 479, 1985.
44. Hall, J. E., Morse, C. L., Smith, M. J., et al. Control of arterial pressure and renal function during glucocorticoid excess in dogs. *Hypertension* 2: 139, 1980.
45. Hench, P. S., Kendall, E. C., Slocumb, C. H., et al. The effect of a hormone of the adrenal cortex (17-OH,11-dehydrocorticosterone: compound E) and of pituitary adrenocorticotrophic hormone on rheumatoid arthritis. *Proc. Staff Meet. Mayo Clin.* 24: 181, 1949.
46. Hoffman, L., Martin, F. R., Buchanan, M. R. C., et al. Cushing's syndrome due to an ACTH-secreting adrenal medullary tumour. *Aust. N.Z. J. Med.* 10: 654, 1980.
47. Holdaway, I. M., Evans, M. C., and Ibbertson, H. K. Experience with a short test of pituitary-adrenal function. *Aust. N.Z. J. Med.* 3: 507, 1973.
48. Hrachovy, R. A., Frost, J. D., Kellaway, P., et al. A controlled study of ACTH therapy in infantile spasms. *Epilepsia* 21: 631, 1980.
49. Humphrey, T. J., Fan, J. S. K., Coghlan, J. P., et al. Interrelationships between sodium and potassium intake and the blood pressure effects of ACTH in sheep. *J. Hypertension* 1: 19, 1983.
50. Jennings, A. S., Liddle, G. W., and Orth, D. N. Results of treating childhood Cushing's disease with pituitary irradiation. *N. Engl. J. Med.* 297: 957, 1977.
51. Kennedy, L., Atkinson, A. B., Johnston, H., et al. Serum cortisol concentrations during low dose dexamethasone suppression test to screen for Cushing's Syndrome. *Br. Med. J.* 289: 1188, 1984.
52. Klatsky, A. L. L., Friedman, G. C., Seiglaub, M. S., et al. Alcohol consumption and blood pressure. *N. Engl. J. Med.* 296: 1194, 1977.
53. Knowlton, A. I., Loeb, E. N., and Stoerk, N. C. Effect of synthetic analogues of hydrocortisone on the blood pressure of adrenalectomized rats on sodium restriction. *Endocrinology* 60: 768, 1957.
54. Komanicky, P., Spark, R. F., and Melby, J. C. Treatment of Cushing's syndrome with trilostane (WIN 24,540), an inhibitor of adrenal steroid biosynthesis. *J. Clin. Endocrinol. Metab.* 47: 1042, 1978.
55. Krakoff, L. R., Selvadurai, R., and Sutter, E. Effect of methylprednisolone upon arterial pressure and the renin angiotensin system in the rat. *Am. J. Physiol.* 228: 613, 1975.
56. Kreiger, D. T., Amorosa, L., and Linick, F. Cyproheptadine-induced remission of Cushing's disease. *N. Engl. J. Med.* 293: 893, 1975.
57. Kreiger, D. T., Liotta, A. S., Suda, T., et al. Human plasma immunoreactive lipotropin and adrenocorticotropin in normal subjects and in patients with pituitary-adrenal disease. *J. Clin. Endocrinol. Metab.* 48: 566, 1979.
58. Kuhlmann, D., Ragan, C., Ferrebee, J. W., et al. Toxic effects of desoxycorticosterone esters in dogs. *Science* 90: 496, 1939.
59. Lamberts, S. W. J., Timmermans, H. A. T., Dejong, F. H., et al. The role of dopaminergic depletion in the pathogenesis of Cushing's disease and the possible consequences for medical therapy. *J. Clin. Endocrinol.* 7: 185, 1977.
60. Liddle, G. W. Tests of pituitary-adrenal suppressibility in the diagnosis of Cushing's syndrome. *J. Clin. Endocrinol.* 20: 1539, 1960.
61. Lohmeier, T. E., and Carroll, R. G. Chronic potentiation of vasoconstrictor hypertension by adrenocorticotropic hormone. *Hypertension* 4: 138, 1982.
62. Lohmeier, T. E., and Kastner, P. R. Chronic effects of ACTH and cortisol excess in arterial pressure in normotensive and hypertensive dogs. *Hypertension* 4: 652, 1982.
63. MacErlean, C. P., and Doyle, F. H. The pituitary fossa in Cushing's syndrome. *Br. J. Radiol.* 49: 820, 1976.
64. Majewski, H., and Rand, M. J. Adrenaline-mediated hypertension: A clue to the antihypertensive effect of β-adrenoceptor blocking drugs? *Trends Pharm. Sci.* 2: 24, 1981.
65. Mannix, H., and Glenn, F. Hypertension in Cushing's syndrome. *J.A.M.A.* 180: 225, 1962.
66. Marks, V., and Wright, J. W. Endocrinological and metabolic effects of alcohol. *Proc. R. Soc. Med.* 70: 337, 1977.

67. Mason, R. T., Allen, K. J., Coghlan, J. P., et al. The haemodynamic effects of prostacyclin infusions in normotensive and ACTH-induced hypertensive conscious sheep. *Prostaglandins Leukotrienes Med.* 16: 57, 1984.
68. Mason, R. T., Coghlan, J. P., Denton, D. A., et al. Prostaglandin synthesis inhibition with indomethacin in ACTH-induced hypertension. *J. Cardiovasc. Pharmacol.* 6: 288, 1984.
69. McDougall, J. G., Barnes, A. M., Coghlan, J. P., et al. The effect of corticotrophin (ACTH) administration on the pressor action of angiotensin II, noradrenaline and tyramine in sheep. *Clin. Exp. Pharm. Physiol.* 5: 449, 1978.
70. McHardy, K. Suspected Cushing's syndrome. *Br. Med. J.* 289: 1519, 1984.
71. Melby, J. C. Assessment of adrenocortical function. *N. Engl. J. Med.* 285: 735, 1971.
72. Melby, J. D., Dale, S. L., Grekin, R. J., et al. 18-hydroxy-11-deoxycorticosterone(18-OH-DOC) secretion in experimental and human hypertension. *Recent Prog. Horm. Res.* 28: 287, 1972.
73. Mendlowitz, M., Gitlow, S., and Naftchi, N. Work of digital vasoconstriction produced by infused norepinephrine in Cushing's syndrome. *J. Appl. Physiol.* 13: 252, 1958.
74. Mills, E. H., Coghlan, J. P., Denton, D. A., et al. The effect of potassium on the hypertensive and electrolyte responses to ACTH administration in sheep. *Clin. Exp. Hypertension* 6: 1613, 1984.
75. Mills, E. H., Coghlan, J. P., Denton, D. A., et al. The cardiovascular and renal effects of potassium loading in conscious sheep. In F. Mantero, E. Biglieri, J. Funder, and B. Scoggins (eds.), *The Adrenal Gland and Hypertension, Serono Symposium.* New York: Raven Press, 1985.
76. Mitchell, J., and Bohr, D. F. Mechanisms of Mineralocorticoid-Induced Hypertension. In W. Kaufmann, G. Wambach, A. Helber, et al. (eds.), *Mineralocorticoids and Hypertension.* Berlin: Springer Verlag, 1983.
77. Miura, K., Aida, M., Mihara, A., et al. Treatment of Cushing's disease with reserpine and pituitary irradiation. *J. Clin. Endocrinol. Metab.* 41: 511, 1975.
78. Nelson, M. A., Coghlan, J. P., Denton, D. A., et al. Total autonomic blockade does not modify the hypertensive response to ACTH in the sheep. *Proc. XXIXth Int. Union. Physiol. Sci., Sydney,* 339: 11, 1983.
79. Nelson, M. A., Coghlan, J. P., Denton, D. A., et al. Metabolic and blood pressure effects of 6α-methylprednisolone in the conscious sheep. *Clin. Exper. Hypertension* 6: 1067, 1984.
80. New, M. I., and Peterson, R. E. A new form of congenital adrenal hyperplasia. *J. Clin. Endocrinol. Metab.* 27: 300, 1967.
81. New, M. I., Saenger, P. H., Levine, L. S., et al. New evidence for a steroid hormone capable of producing hypertension in man. *Bull. N.Y. Acad. Med.* 51: 1180, 1975.
82. Nomura, K., Demura, H., Imaki, T., et al. Concomitant falls of plasma cortisol and ACTH levels in a case of Cushing's disease during treatment with trilostane. *Acta Endocrinol.* 105: 93, 1984.
83. Nugent, C. A., Nichol, T., and Tyler, F. J. Diagnosis of Cushing's syndrome. Single dose dexamethasone suppression test. *Arch. Intern. Med.* 116: 172, 1965.
84. Oates, J. A., and Wood, A. J. J. The use of ketoconazole as an inhibitor of steroid production. *N. Engl. J. Med.* 317: 812, 1987.
85. Oddie, C. J., Coghlan, J. P., and Scoggins, B. A. Plasma deoxycorticosterone levels in man with simultaneous measurement of aldosterone, corticosterone, cortisol and 11-deoxycortisol. *J. Clin. Endocrinol. Metab.* 34: 939, 1972.
86. Orth, D. N., De Bold, C. R., De Cherney, G., et al. Pituitary microadenomas causing Cushing's disease respond to corticotrophin releasing factor. *J. Clin. Endocrinol. Metab.* 55: 1017, 1982.
87. Orth, D., and Liddle, G. Results of treatment in 108 patients with Cushing's syndrome. *N. Engl. J. Med.* 285: 243, 1971.
88. Pamnani, M. B., Clough, D. L., and Haddy, F. J. Altered activity of the sodium-potassium pump in arteries of rats with steroid hypertension. *Clin. Sci. Mol. Med.* 55: 41s, 1978.
89. Perera, G. A. Modification of Blood Pressure by Corticosterone and ACTH in Normotensives and Hypertensives. In J. R. Mote (ed.), *Proc. 1st ACTH Conference,* Lakiston, Chicago, 1950.
90. Plotz, C., Knowlten, A., and Ragan, C. The natural history of Cushing's syndrome. *Am. J. Med.* 13: 597, 1952.
91. Racker, J., Cope, O., and Ackerman, I. Surgical experience with the treatment of hypertension of Cushing's syndrome. *Am. J. Surg.* 107: 153, 1964.
92. Rascher, W., Dietz, R., Schomig, A., et al. Modulation of sympathetic vascular tone by prostaglandins in corticosterone-induced hypertension in rats. *Clin. Sci.* 57: 235s, 1979.
93. Rauh, W., Levine, L. S., Gottesdiener, K., et al. Mineralocorticoids, salt balance and blood pressure after prolonged ACTH administration in juvenile hypertension. *Klin. Wochenschr.* 56: 161, 1978.
94. Ross, E. J., and Linch, D. C. Cushing's syndrome—Killing disease: Discriminatory value of signs and symptoms aiding early diagnosis. *Lancet* 2: 646, 1982.
95. Ross, E. J., Marshall-Jones, P., and Friedman, M. Cushing's syndrome. Diagnostic criteria. *Q. J. Med.* 35: 149, 1966.
96. Salassa, R. M., Laws, E., Carpenter, P. C., et al. Transsphenoidal removal of pituitary microadenomata in Cushing's disease. *Mayo Clin. Proc.* 53: 24, 1978.
97. Sarkar, S. D., Cohen, E. L., Bierwaltes, W. H., et al. A new and superior adrenal imaging agent ^{131}I-6β-iodimethyl-19-norcholesterol (NP-59): Evaluation in humans. *J. Clin. Endocrinol. Metab.* 45: 353, 1977.
98. Savage, O., Copeman, W. S. C., Chapman, L., et al. Pituitary and adrenal hormones in rheumatoid arthritis. *Lancet* 1: 232, 1962.
99. Schambelan, M., Slaton, P. E., and Biglieri, E. G. Mineralocorticoid production in hyperadrenocorticism. *Am. J. Med.* 51: 299, 1971.
100. Schomig, A., Luth, B., Dietz, R., et al. Changes in vascular smooth muscle sensitivity to vasoconstrictor agents induced by corticosteroids, adrenalectomy and differing salt intake in rats. *Clin. Sci. Mol. Med.* 51: 61s, 1976.
101. Scoggins, B. A., Butkus, A., Coghlan, J. P., et al. Adrenocorticotropic hormone-induced hypertension in sheep: A model for the study of the effect of steroid hormones on blood pressure. *Circ. Res.* 43: 176, 1978.
102. Scoggins, B. A., Butkus, A., Coghlan, J. P., et al. The Role of "Mineralocorticoids," "Glucocorticoids" and "Hypertensinogenic" Steroids in ACTH-Induced Hypertension. In W. Kaufman, G. Wambach, A. Helber, et al. (eds.), *Mineralocorticoids and Hypertension.* Berlin: Springer-Verlag, 1983.
103. Scoggins, B. A., Coghlan, J. P., Congiu, M., et al. Alterations in osmotic but not pressor responses to ACTH by optic recess lesions in sheep. *Hypertension* 4: II-154, 1982.

104. Scoggins, B. A., Coghlan, J. P., and Denton, D. A. ACTH-Induced Hypertension in Sheep. In W. de Jong (ed.), *Handbook of Hypertension 4*. Amsterdam: Elsevier Science, 1984.
105. Scoggins, B. A., Coghlan, J. P., Denton, D. A., et al. A Review of Mechanisms Involved in the Production of Steroid-Induced Hypertension with Particular Reference to ACTH-Dependent Hypertension. In F. Mantero, E. G. Biglieri, and C. R. W. Edwards (eds.), *Endocrinology of Hypertension*. London: Academic Press, 1982.
106. Scoggins, B. A., Coghlan, J. P., Denton, D. A., et al. How do adrenocortical steroid hormones produce hypertension? *Clin. Exp. Hypertens.* A6: 315, 1984.
107. Shinholster, D. L., Jones, A. W., and Freeman, R. H. Action of ACTH infusion in rats on blood pressure, plasma aldosterone and aortic ^{42}K fluxes. *Fed. Proc.* 40: 501, 1981.
108. Shulkes, A. A., Coghlan, J. P., Denton, D. A., et al. The effect of adrenal denervation on ACTH-induced hypertension in sheep. *Clin. Exp. Pharmacol. Physiol.* 1: 479, 1974.
109. Smals, A. G., Kloppenborg, P. W., Njo, K. T., et al. Alcohol-induced Cushingoid syndrome. *Br. Med. J.* 2: 1298, 1976.
110. Soffer, L., Iannacore, A., and Gabrilove, J. Cushing's syndrome. *Am. J. Med.* 30: 129, 1961.
111. Spence, C. S., Coghlan, J. P., Denton, D. A., et al. Angiotensin converting enzyme inhibition does not prevent development of ACTH-induced hypertension in sheep. *Clin. Exp. Pharmacol. Physiol.* 12: 181, 1985.
112. Sudhir, K., Jennings, G. L., Esler, M. D., et al. Hydrocortisone induced hypertension in humans: Pressor responsiveness and sympathetic function. *Hypertension* 13: 416, 1989.
113. Sutherland, D. J. A., Ruse, J. L., and Laidlaw, J. C. Hypertension, increased aldosterone secretion and low plasma renin activity relieved by dexamethasone. *Can. Med. Assoc. J.* 95: 1109, 1966.
114. Temple, T. E., and Liddle, G. W. Inhibitors of adrenal steroid biosynthesis. *Ann. Rev. Pharmacol.* 10: 199, 1970.
115. Treadwell, B. L. J., Sever, E. D., Savage, O., et al. Side effects of long term treatment with corticosteroids and corticotrophin. *Lancet* 1: 1121, 1964.
116. Van Cauter, E., and Refetoff, S. Evidence for two subtypes of Cushing's disease based on the analysis of episodic cortisol secretion. *N. Engl. J. Med.* 312: 1343, 1985.
117. Vetter, W., Vetter, H., Beckerhoff, R., et al. The effect of saralasin (1-sar-8-ala-angiotensin II) on blood pressure in patients with Cushing's syndrome. *Klin. Wochenschr.* 54: 661, 1976.
118. Wambach, G., Helber, A., Allolio, B., et al. Increased activity of the Na-K-ATPase in red cell-ghosts of patients with Cushing's syndrome: possible significance for the pathogenesis of glucocorticoid-induced hypertension. *Klin. Wochenschr.* 58: 485, 1980.
119. Welbourn, R. B., Montgomery, D. A. D., and Kennedy, T. L. The natural history of treated Cushing's syndrome. *Br. J. Surg.* 58: 1, 1971.
120. Whitworth, J. A., Coghlan, J. P., Denton, D. A., et al. Comparison of the effects of "glucocorticoid" and "mineralocorticoid" infusions on blood pressure in sheep. *Clin. Exp. Hypertension* 1: 649, 1979.
121. Whitworth, J. A., Connell, J. M. C., Gordon, D., and Scoggins, B. A. Effects of indomethacin on steroid induced changes on pressor responsiveness in man. *Clin. Exp. Pharmacol. Physiol.* 15: 305, 1988.
122. Whitworth, J. A., Connell, J. M. C., Lever, A. F., and Fraser, R. Pressor responsiveness in steroid induced hypertension in man. *Clin. Exp. Pharmacol. Physiol.* 13: 353, 1986.
123. Whitworth, J. A., Denton, D. A., Graham, W. F., et al. The effect of renal denervation on ACTH-induced hypertension in sheep. *Clin. Exp. Pharmacol. Physiol.* 8: 203, 1981.
124. Whitworth, J. A., Gordon, D., Andrews, J., and Scoggins, B. A. The hypertensive effect of synthetic glucocorticoids in man: Role of sodium and volume. *J. Hypertens.* 7: 537, 1989.
125. Whitworth, J. A., Gordon, D., and Scoggins, B. A. Dose response relationships for adrenocorticotrophin induced hypertension in man. *Clin. Exp. Pharmacol. Physiol.* 14: 65, 1987.
126. Whitworth, J. A., Hewitson, T. D., Wilson, R. S., et al. ACTH hypertension in the rat: Haemodynamic, metabolic and morphologic characteristics. *J. Hypertens.* 8: 27, 1990.
127. Whitworth, J. A., Saines, D., Andrews, J., et al. Haemodynamic response to ACTH administration in essential hypertension. *Clin. Exp. Pharmacol. Physiol.* 8: 553, 1981.
128. Whitworth, J. A., Saines, D., and Scoggins, B. A. Blood pressure and metabolic effects of cortisol and deoxycorticosterone in man. *Clin. Exp. Hypertension* 6: 795, 1984.
129. Whitworth, J. A., Saines, D., and Scoggins, B. A. Potentiation of ACTH hypertension in man with salt loading. *Clin. Exp. Pharmacol. Physiol.* 12: 239, 1985.
130. Whitworth, J. A., Saines, D., Thatcher, R., et al. Blood pressure and metabolic effects of ACTH in normotensive and hypertensive man. *Clin. Exp. Hypertension* 5: 501, 1983.
131. Whitworth, J. A., and Scoggins, B. A. Hypertensinogenic class of steroid hormone activity in man? *Clin. Exp. Pharmacol. Physiol.* 17: 163, 1990.
132. Whitworth, J. A., Van Leeuwen, B. H., Hannah, M. C., et al. Effect of ACTH administration on urinary kallikrein excretion in man. *Clin. Exp. Pharmacol. Physiol.* 11: 87, 1984.
133. Wilson, C. G., and Dempsey, L. C. Transsphenoidal surgical removal of 250 pituitary adenomas. *J. Neurosurg.* 48: 13, 1978.
134. Wolfson, A. R., and Odell, W. D. The dose-response relationship of ACTH and cortisol in Cushing's disease. *Clin. Endocrinol.* 12: 557, 1980.
135. Yamaji, T., Ishibashi, M., Teramoto, A., et al. Hyperprolactinemia in Cushing's disease and Nelson's syndrome. *J. Clin. Endocrinol. Metab.* 58: 790, 1984.

Malignant Hypertension and Other Hypertensive Crises

Charles R. Nolan III
Stuart L. Linas

The Clinical Spectrum of Severe Hypertension

In most patients, hypertension begins insidiously and is asymptomatic for many years until complications due to atherosclerosis, cerebrovascular disease, or congestive heart failure supervene. In a minority of patients this "benign" course is interrupted by a hypertensive crisis.

A *hypertensive crisis* is defined as the turning point in the course of an illness at which acute management of the elevated blood pressure plays a decisive role in the eventual outcome. The urgency with which the elevated blood pressure must be controlled varies with each crisis. However, the crucial role of hypertension in the disease process must be identified and a plan for management of the blood pressure successfully implemented if the outcome is to be optimal.

The absolute level of diastolic blood pressure is *not* the most important factor in determining the existence of a hypertensive crisis. In children, pregnant women, and other previously normotensive individuals in whom moderate hypertension develops suddenly, crisis may occur at a diastolic blood pressure normally well tolerated by adults with chronic hypertension (i.e., 100 to 110 mm Hg). Furthermore, in patients with only modest hypertension, a crisis may occur in the setting of concomitant acute organ system dysfunction involving the brain or heart. In contrast, the finding of severe hypertension does not always imply that a hypertensive crisis is present. In patients with severe hypertension that is not accompanied by acute end-organ dysfunction or evidence of malignant hypertension (vide infra), eventual complications due to stroke, myocardial infarction, or congestive heart failure occur over a time-frame of months to years rather than hours to days. Although long-term control of blood pressure may prevent these complications, a hypertensive crisis cannot be diagnosed, since there is no evidence that acute reduction of blood pressure results in an improvement in long-term prognosis. The spectrum of hypertensive crises and other categories of severe hypertension is outlined in Table 59-1.

Malignant hypertension is a clinical syndrome characterized by marked elevation of blood pressure with widespread acute arteriolar injury. Funduscopy reveals hypertensive neuroretinopathy with striate (flame-shaped) hemorrhages, cotton-wool (soft) exudates, and often papilledema. Regardless of the degree of blood pressure elevation, malignant hypertension cannot be diagnosed in the absence of hypertensive neuroretinopathy [383, 575]. Some authors have defined *malignant hypertension* by the presence of papilledema and have used the term *accelerated hypertension* when hemorrhages and cotton-wool spots are present in the absence of papilledema [280]. However, recent studies have shown that the prognosis is the same in patients with striate hemorrhages and cotton-wool spots whether or not papilledema is present [4, 350]. In this regard, the World Health Organization has recommended that *accelerated hypertension* and *malignant hypertension* be regarded as synonymous terms for the same disease [575].

Hypertensive neuroretinopathy is an important clinical finding that points to the presence of a widespread hypertension-induced arteriolitis that may involve the central nervous system, heart, and kidneys. Untreated, there is a rapid and relentless progression to death in less than 1 year. The majority of untreated patients can be expected to die from uremia unless death occurs earlier from hypertensive encephalopathy, intracerebral hemorrhage, or congestive heart failure.

Hypertensive encephalopathy is a medical emergency in which cerebral malfunction is attributed to the severe elevation of blood pressure. It is one of the most serious complications of malignant hypertension. However, malignant hypertension (neuroretinopathy) need not be present for hypertensive encephalopathy to develop. It may also occur with severe hypertension of any cause, especially when acute blood pressure elevation occurs in a previously normotensive individual with eclampsia, acute glomerulonephritis, pheochromocytoma, or drug-withdrawal hypertension. Clinical features include severe headache, blurred vision or blindness, nausea, vomiting, and mental confusion. If treatment is withheld, symptoms may progress to stupor, convulsions, and death within hours. The *sine qua non* of hypertensive encephalopathy is the prompt and dramatic clinical response to antihypertensive therapy.

On occasion, hypertension that is not in the malignant phase may still qualify as a hypertensive crisis when acute end-organ dysfunction occurs in the presence of even moderate hypertension. The term *benign hypertension with acute complications* includes hypertension complicating acute pulmonary edema, acute myocardial infarction or unstable angina, active bleeding, acute aortic dissection, or central nervous system catastrophe (hypertensive encephalopathy, intracerebral or subarachnoid hemorrhage, or severe head trauma). In each case, control of the blood pressure is the cornerstone of successful therapy.

Catecholamine excess states, as in pheochromocytoma crisis, monoamine oxidase inhibitor–tyramine interaction, phenylpropanolamine overdose, and abrupt withdrawal of clonidine, methyldopa, or guanabenz may produce a life-threatening hypertensive crisis. The clinical presentation usually includes marked elevation of blood pressure with headache, profound diaphoresis, and tachycardia. With the severe acute elevation of blood pressure a number of complications may occur including hypertensive encephalopathy, intracerebral hemorrhage, or acute left ventricular failure. Thus, catecholamine-related hypertensive crises require prompt recognition and control of blood pressure to avert disaster.

Table 59-1. The clinical syndromes of severe hypertension

- I. Hypertensive crises
  - A. Malignant hypertension (hypertensive neuroretinopathy present)
  - B. Hypertensive encephalopathy
  - C. Benign hypertension with acute complications (acute organ system dysfunction but no hypertensive neuroretinopathy)
    - 1. Acute pulmonary edema
    - 2. Atherosclerotic coronary vascular disease
      - a. Acute myocardial infarction
      - b. Unstable angina
    - 3. Acute aortic dissection
    - 4. Active bleeding including postoperative bleeding
    - 5. Central nervous system catastrophe
      - a. Hypertensive encephalopathy
      - b. Intracerebral hemorrhage
      - c. Subarachnoid hemorrhage
      - d. Severe head trauma
  - D. Catecholamine excess states
    - 1. Pheochromocytoma crisis
    - 2. Monoamine oxidase inhibitor/tyramine interactions
    - 3. Antihypertensive drug withdrawal syndromes
    - 4. Phenylpropanolamine overdose
  - E. Preeclampsia and eclampsia
  - F. Poorly controlled hypertension in a patient requiring emergency surgery
  - G. Severe postoperative hypertension
  - H. Scleroderma renal crisis
  - I. Miscellaneous hypertensive crises
    - 1. Severe hypertension complicating extensive burn injury
    - 2. High-dose cyclosporine in children after bone marrow transplantation
    - 3. Autonomic hyperreflexia in quadriplegic patients
    - 4. Severe hypertension with acute rejection or transplant renal artery stenosis in renal allograft recipients
    - 5. Hypoglycemia in patients receiving β-adrenergic receptor blockers
- II. Benign hypertension with chronic stable complications (chronic end-organ dysfunction but no hypertensive neuroretinopathy)
  - A. Chronic renal insufficiency due to primary renal parenchymal disease
  - B. Chronic congestive heart failure
  - C. Atherosclerotic coronary vascular disease
    - 1. Stable angina
    - 2. Previous myocardial infarction
  - D. Cerebrovascular disease
    - 1. Transient ischemic attacks
    - 2. Prior cerebrovascular accident
- III. Severe uncomplicated hypertension (severe hypertension without hypertensive neuroretinopathy or end-organ dysfunction)

Preeclampsia is a hypertensive disorder unique to pregnancy that usually presents after the twentieth week of gestation with proteinuria, edema, and hypertension. Eclamptic seizures may ensue and without treatment may result in death. Hypertensive disorders of pregnancy and their management are discussed in Chap. 57.

Poorly controlled hypertension in patients requiring emergency surgery is a hypertensive crisis because of the increased cardiovascular risk that accompanies inadequate preoperative blood pressure control. Surgical manipulation of the carotid arteries or open heart surgery (especially coronary artery bypass) is occasionally followed by severe hypertension in the immediate postoperative period. *Severe postoperative hypertension* represents a crisis requiring immediate blood pressure control, since it may cause hypertensive encephalopathy or intracerebral hemorrhage or jeopardize the integrity of vascular suture lines, leading to postoperative hemorrhage.

In patients with progressive systemic sclerosis, *scleroderma renal crisis* may occur with sudden onset of hypertension that may enter the malignant phase. There is a rapid progression to end-stage renal disease in 1 to 2 months unless the vicious cycle of hypertension and renal damage is interrupted.

Severe acute hypertension may also occur in patients with extensive burns or in children receiving high-dose cyclosporine for allogenic bone marrow transplantation. In quadriplegic patients, hypertensive crises may develop due to autonomic hyperreflexia resulting from stimulation of nerves below the level of the spinal cord injury. Hypertensive crises may also develop due to acute rejection or transplant renal artery stenosis in patients with renal allografts. In each of these instances, a sudden increase in blood pressure may cause acute pulmonary edema, hypertensive encephalopathy, cerebrovascular accident, or death.

Severe or complicated hypertension does not always represent a true hypertensive crisis requiring immediate control of the blood pressure. Patients with benign hypertension (no hypertensive neuroretinopathy) and chronic stable end-organ dysfunction do not require emergent reduction of blood pressure, although a long-term lack of adequate blood pressure control often results in further end-organ deterioration. The term *benign hypertension with chronic stable complications* includes hypertension occurring in the setting of chronic renal insufficiency due to primary renal parenchymal disease, chronic congestive heart failure, atherosclerotic coronary vascular disease (stable angina pectoris or prior myocardial infarction), or cerebrovascular disease (prior transient ischemic attacks or cerebrovascular accident).

Severe uncomplicated hypertension is defined by the presence of diastolic blood pressure over 115 mm Hg without evidence of malignant phase (no hypertensive neuroretinopathy) or signs of end-organ dysfunction. Although this is not a hypertensive crisis as defined above, it is a common form of severe hypertension. Severe uncomplicated hypertension is usually found in patients with chronic essential hypertension who are undiagnosed, undertreated, or noncompliant. While the severe elevation of blood pressure is often discovered incidentally in an asymptomatic patient, many patients complain of headache. However, there is no evidence of hypertensive encephalopathy or other acute end-organ dysfunction. The fundus does not show striate hemorrhages, cotton-wool spots, or papilledema. Complications of severe uncomplicated hypertension occur over a period of weeks to months rather than hours to days. The common practice of acute reduction of blood pressure with oral antihypertensive agents prior to discharge from the acute care setting has recently been questioned [155, 159, 582]. Instead, the goal of treatment should be the gradual reduction of blood pressure to normotensive levels over a few days in conjunction with frequent outpatient follow-up visits to modify the antihypertensive regimen and reinforce the importance of lifelong compliance with therapy. In the past, this entity has been termed *urgent* hypertension. We favor the more descriptive term, *severe uncomplicated hypertension,* since the urgency of treatment is not nearly as great as in patients with true hypertensive crisis.

Malignant Hypertension

HISTORICAL PERSPECTIVE

In 1836, 75 years before a blood pressure-measuring device was available, Bright [53] recognized the association between hypertrophy of the heart and contraction of the kidney. The myocardial change was thought to be the result of the increased work required to force blood through a vascular tree constricted by irritating humoral substances accumulated in renal failure.

Johnson [267] and Gull and Sutton [210] described patients with cardiac hypertrophy who died of uremia, heart failure, or apoplexy. Morphologically, a granular contracted kidney was commonly found, and the disease came to be called "red granular kidney" or "contracted granular kidney." Johnson (1868) [267] described muscular hypertrophy of the arteriolar walls in the kidney and various organs and thought it was due to sustained overaction in opposing the heart. The diseased kidney was thought to cause retention of noxious substances, and the vasculature of various organs was postulated to be constricted to restrict the passage of impure blood. The left ventricle was thought to hypertrophy because of the increased effort required to propel the blood.

Gull and Sutton (1872) [210] did not find muscular hypertrophy of arteriolar walls but described a hyaline-fibroid change in the small arteries (now called *hyaline arteriosclerosis*) not only in the kidney but also in numerous organs throughout the body. The hyaline-fibroid changes in the arterioles were postulated to result in a loss of elasticity. The loss of elasticity necessitated an increase in cardiac work and eventually led to ventricular hypertrophy. In addition, the renal arteriolar changes were postulated to lead to atrophy of the kidney (contracted granular kidney). In addition, Gull and Sutton made the important observation that, in many cases, the arteriolar changes and cardiac hypertrophy were present in the absence of an impairment in renal excretory function. On the basis of these observations, they concluded that the hyaline-fibroid change in the arterioles was the primary event, with contraction of the kidney being a secondary and much later phenomenon.

In the late nineteenth century it was widely held that increased blood pressure in chronic Bright's disease was caused by toxic products that accumulated following primary renal injury. Mahomed (1879) [337] objected to this view and proposed that the converse was true; namely, that high blood pressure was the primary event leading to cardiovascular changes and, in some instances, to secondary renal involvement. He emphasized that the largest proportion of deaths in patients with chronic Bright's disease with contracted kidneys occurred not from renal failure but from cardiovascular diseases.

Allbutt (1915) [5] was the first to describe essential hypertension without renal involvement as a unique entity distinct from chronic nephritis with hypertension. He recognized the primary importance of hypertension as a cause of cardiac and cerebral failure and felt that essential hypertension, even in fatal cases, did not result in uremic symptoms.

The separation of essential hypertension in which significant clinical renal involvement was uncommon from secondary hypertension in which high blood pressure was caused by chronic nephritis marked a great advance. During subsequent years, however, controversy arose. One group of patients with hypertension did not fit either of these categories. This group appeared initially to have essential hypertension without renal involvement but eventually developed fulminant renal failure. This is now recognized as the syndrome of malignant hypertension.

Volhard and Fahr (1914) [552] introduced the descriptive terms *benign* and *malignant,* aimed at separating renal arteriosclerosis into two distinct types. The type without renal failure was called *benign nephrosclerosis* and was characterized pathologically by arteriosclerosis of the kidney. The type with renal failure was called *malignant nephrosclerosis* and was characterized by necrotizing arteriolitis with inflammatory changes in the glomeruli in addition to the arteriosclerosis seen in the benign form [156]. Volhard [551] later abandoned the concept of inflammatory changes and substituted prolonged ischemia secondary to vascular spasm as the cause of the renal lesion in the malignant type.

The prognostic importance of eye ground changes in hypertensive patients has long been recognized. *Albuminuric retinitis* was the term used by Liebreich (1859) [319] to describe the retinal changes in some advanced cases of Bright's disease, which were characterized by papilledema, ill-defined white exudates, a macular star, and linear hemorrhages. Volhard [551, 552] noted that the appearance of albuminuric retinitis was often the first sign heralding a transition from the benign to the malignant phase of nephrosclerosis.

Keith and Wagener (1928) [281] coined the term *malignant hypertension* to describe a clinical syndrome characterized by severe hypertension with arteriolopathy manifest by papilledema, hemorrhages, and exudates (grade IV retinopathy). The vast majority of these patients died within 1 year of various combinations of brain, heart, and kidney failure. Interestingly, at the time of presentation with severe hypertension and grade IV retinopathy, the majority of these patients had normal or only mildly impaired renal function.

By 1935 the concept had emerged that the clinical syndrome of malignant hypertension was not due to a single etiology but to a variety of different etiologies. Derow and Altschule (1935) [120, 121] pointed out that malignant hypertension occurred in association with essential hypertension as well as secondary forms of hypertension such as chronic glomerulonephritis, chronic pyelonephritis, Cushing's syndrome, pheochromocytoma, renal artery stenosis, and polyarteritis nodosa.

During the last 30 years, it has been recognized that regardless of the underlying etiology of malignant hypertension, the relentless progression of the disease can be slowed or even reversed by reduction of blood pressure with any one of a number of methods, including sympathectomy [237, 573], pyrogens [418], rice diet [282], excision of a unilaterally diseased kidney, adrenal resection in Cushing's syndrome [436], excision of a pheochromocytoma [214], or a variety of drugs that lower arterial pressure [436, 505].

UNTREATED PROGNOSIS AND NATURAL HISTORY

A review of the survival statistics in the era before effective antihypertensive drugs became available reveals the reason why this disorder was called "malignant" hypertension. Keith, Wagener, et al. [280, 281] described 81 patients with grade III or grade IV retinopathy in whom initial renal involvement was mild. Even in the absence of significant nephropathy, the short-term prognosis was grave. Their classic mortality curve is shown in Fig. 59-1. They reported 1-year death rates in hypertensive patients grouped on the basis of initial funduscopic findings. In group I (mild arteriolar narrowing or sclerosis of retinal vessels), the 1-year death rate was 10 percent; in group II (moderate sclerosis with increased light reflex and arteriovenous compression or localized arteriolar narrowing), 12 percent; in group III (retinal hemorrhages and exudates), 35 percent; and in group IV (hemorrhages and exudates plus papilledema), 80 percent.

Many other series of untreated hypertensive patients with severe retinopathy have also shown this dismal prognosis. Ellis [147] reported 46 patients with an average survival of 1 year from the first symptom until death. In the series of Kincaid-Smith et al. [288], 55 per-

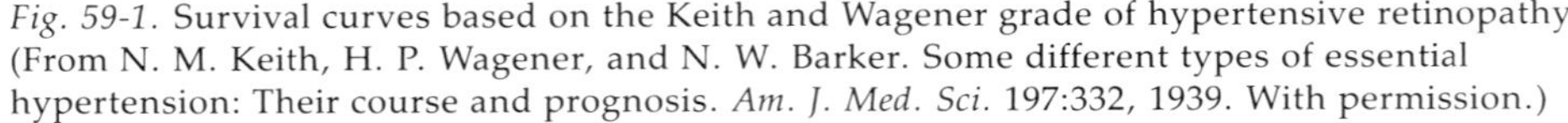
Fig. 59-1. Survival curves based on the Keith and Wagener grade of hypertensive retinopathy. (From N. M. Keith, H. P. Wagener, and N. W. Barker. Some different types of essential hypertension: Their course and prognosis. *Am. J. Med. Sci.* 197:332, 1939. With permission.)

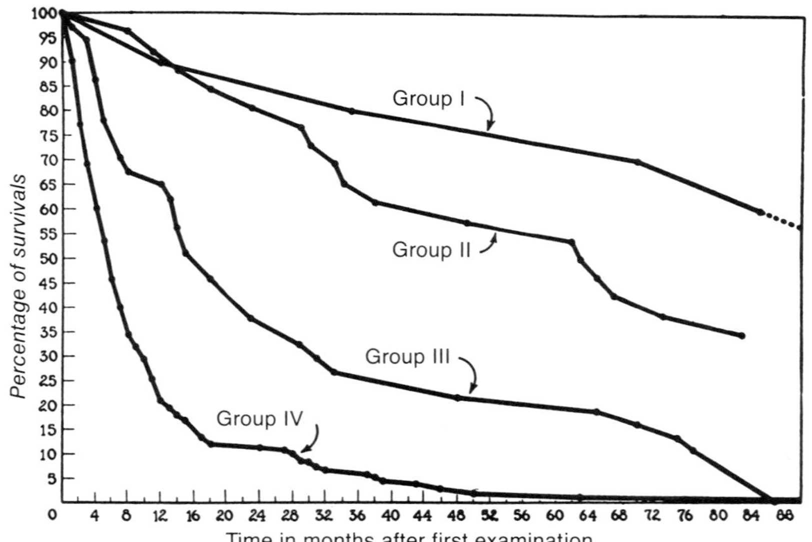

cent of untreated patients died within 2 months and 90 percent within 1 year. Schottstaedt and Sokolow [482] reported a mean survival of 8.7 months from the time of diagnosis of grade IV retinopathy to death. Milliez et al. [366] found mean survival of 11 months after diagnosis of grade IV funduscopic changes.

The reported causes of death in untreated patients with malignant hypertension were similar in most series. Keith and Wagener [280] concluded that the terminal picture was often obscure due to simultaneous rapid failure of the brain, heart, and kidney. In Heptinstall's series [226], 70 percent of patients died secondary to uremia. The causes of death among the patients of Kincaid-Smith et al. [288] included uremia plus heart failure, 48 percent; uremia alone, 17 percent; heart failure alone, 13 percent; cerebrovascular accident, 20 percent; aortic dissection, 1 percent; and acute myocardial infarction, 1 percent. Milliez et al. [366] found that 72 percent of patients died from uremia while 28 percent had a fatal cerebromeningeal hemorrhage. Among the 60 patients reported by MacMahon and Pratt [336] 58 percent died from uremia, 20 percent from cerebral hemorrhage, 17 percent from congestive heart failure, and 3 percent from aortic rupture.

Ellis [148] outlined four different clinical courses in patients with severe hypertension and hypertensive neuroretinopathy. In the *cerebral* type, patients died due to an intracerebral hemorrhage or hypertensive encephalopathy. In the *cardiac* type, severe congestive heart failure with attacks of acute pulmonary edema dominated the clinical picture. With the *renal* type, death was the result of terminal uremia. In the *combined* type, patients succumbed with manifestations of both congestive heart failure and uremia. Each type showed evidence of widespread vasculopathy and a rapidly fatal course.

Thus, the majority of untreated patients with malignant hypertension can be expected to die from uremia within 1 year. Congestive heart failure is often present. Some patients, however, succumb earlier due to hypertensive encephalopathy or intracerebral hemorrhage at a time when renal involvement may not be pronounced.

The most important *prognostic factor* in untreated patients with malignant hypertension was the level of renal function at the time of diagnosis. Kincaid-Smith et al. [288] found no prognostic significance in relation to age, sex, cardiac, or neurologic involvement. However, the level of blood urea at presentation had a significant negative effect on survival time. In Schottstaedt and Sokolow's series [482], patients with malignant hypertension and initially satisfactory renal function (less than 4 plus albuminuria, and phenolsulfonphthalein excretion greater than 50 percent in 2 hours) had a mean survival of 16 months, whereas survival for the whole group was only 8 months.

ETIOLOGIES OF MALIGNANT HYPERTENSION

Hypertension of virtually any etiology may enter a malignant phase (Table 59-2). Derow and Altschule [120, 121] were the first to note that malignant hypertension was not a single disease entity but rather a syndrome in which hypertension could be either primary (essential) or secondary to one of any number of different etiologies. Moreover, in the individual patient with malignant hypertension, on clinical grounds it was often difficult to distinguish whether the underlying hypertension was primary or secondary.

Table 59-2. Etiologies of malignant hypertension

Primary (essential) malignant hypertension*
Secondary malignant hypertension
Primary renal disease
Chronic glomerulonephritis*
Chronic pyelonephritis*
Acute glomerulonephritis
Analgesic nephropathy
Radiation nephritis
Ask-Upmark kidney
Renovascular hypertension*
Oral contraceptives
Chronic lead poisoning
Endocrine hypertension
Pheochromocytoma
Aldosterone-producing adenoma
Cushing's syndrome
Congenital adrenal hyperplasia
Renal cholesterol embolization
Scleroderma renal crisis

*Most common underlying etiologies.

Malignant hypertension usually develops in patients with preexisting poorly controlled or undiagnosed hypertension. However, occasional patients have been described who apparently had an abrupt onset of so-called *de novo malignant hypertension* without a preceding phase of benign hypertension [366, 427]. The presence of de novo malignant hypertension almost always indicates an underlying secondary cause of hypertension [366].

Primary (Essential) Malignant Hypertension. In the era prior to the introduction of antihypertensive drugs, the most common cause of malignant hypertension was essential hypertension that had evolved into a malignant phase. Primary malignant hypertension was found in 57 percent of patients in the series of Milliez et al. [366] and in 49 percent of Heptinstall's patients [226]. However, more recent series have found a much lower incidence of primary malignant hypertension, most likely reflecting prevention of malignant phase through effective antihypertensive therapy in patients with essential hypertension [208, 579]. In a series of patients studied between 1979 and 1985, primary malignant hypertension was found in only 20 percent of cases [579]. This observation may not apply to blacks with malignant phase, among whom essential hypertension continues to represent the most common etiology [367, 385, 439]. Essential hypertension appears to be a rare cause of malignant hypertension in children. Secondary causes of hypertension such as chronic pyelonephritis, chronic glomerulonephritis, and renal artery stenosis are much more common in this age group.

Secondary Malignant Hypertension. Malignant hypertension may develop due to a variety of underlying conditions. The most common secondary cause is primary renal parenchymal disease. *Chronic glomerulonephritis* has been reported to underlie the development of malignant hypertension in up to 20 percent of cases [226, 579]. Unless a history of an acute nephritic episode or long-standing hematuria or proteinuria is available, the underlying glomerulonephritis may be apparent only if a renal biopsy is performed [579]. Recently, IgA nephropathy has been reported as a frequent cause of malignant hypertension in series from Spain and Australia [428, 526, 579]. For example, in one series of 66 patients with IgA nephropathy, 10 percent developed malignant hypertension [526].

Chronic pyelonephritis has been reported as a cause of malignant hypertension in 9 to 16 percent of patients in recent series [208, 579]. In children, chronic atrophic pyelonephritis may be the most frequent cause of malignant hypertension [236, 516]. Children with chronic atrophic pyelonephritis due to reflux nephropathy may present with either hypertensive encephalopathy or malignant hypertension [236].

In Australia, malignant hypertension may complicate up to 7 percent of cases of *analgesic nephropathy*. Transient malignant hypertension responsive to volume expansion, an entity that is rare with other causes of malignant hypertension, may occur in the setting of analgesic nephropathy [286]. It has been suggested that the salt-wasting state caused by tubulomedullary dysfunction may contribute to the pathogenesis of malignant hypertension by causing severe volume depletion and activation of the renin-angiotensin system [395].

Malignant hypertension has been reported as both an early and late complication of *radiation nephritis* [288, 330]. In a series of patients treated for seminoma with radiotherapy to the posterior lymph nodes, acute radiation nephritis occurred in 13 patients with a latent period of 6 to 12 months. It was characterized by hypertension, anemia, albuminuria, and renal insufficiency. Hypertensive neuroretinopathy (striate hemorrhages, cotton-wool spots, and papilledema), indicating the development of malignant hypertension, occurred in 5 of these patients, of whom 3 died as a consequence of congestive heart failure, hypertensive encephalopathy, and uremia [330]. In some patients, malignant hypertension developed with a latent period of 1.5 to 11.0 years after radiotherapy, in the absence of a history of prior acute radiation nephritis. However, at autopsy, there was evidence of chronic radiation nephritis with ill-defined hyaline obliteration of capillary loops, as well as diffuse interstitial fibrosis and tubular atrophy [330].

Congenital unilateral renal hypoplasia (Ask-Upmark kidney) is a rare cause of malignant hypertension in children and adolescents. This entity is characterized by unilateral renal hypoplasia with an enlarged and deformed renal pelvis that has one or more recesses that end blindly near the surface of the kidney. There is debate as to whether this represents a distinct clinicopathologic entity [471, 584] or is simply the result of chronic pyelonephritis in a congenitally hypoplastic kidney [435].

Renovascular hypertension due to either fibromuscular dysplasia or atherosclerotic disease is a well-recognized cause of malignant hypertension. Its frequency, however, varies in the different series. Kincaid-Smith et al. [288] reported a 3 percent incidence, while Milliez et al. [366] found a 4 percent incidence of underlying renovascular hypertension among patients with malignant hypertension. A 10 percent incidence of renal artery stenosis has been reported among children with severe hypertension [516]. In contrast to these series, others have reported a very high incidence of renovascular hypertension among patients with malignant hypertension [115, 567]. In a series of 123 patients with malignant hypertension, renovascular hypertension was found in 43 percent of white patients and 7 percent of black patients. The prevalence of renovascular hypertension was the same when the group with hemorrhages and exudates without papilledema was analyzed separately from the group with papilledema [115].

Although hypertension is usually mild to moderate in patients with *polyarteritis nodosa* [116], malignant hypertension has been reported [203]. In polyarteritis, even in normotensive individuals, lesions indistinguishable from primary malignant nephrosclerosis may be seen in the interlobular arteries (proliferative endarteritis) and afferent arterioles (fibrinoid necrosis). However, the finding of healed and active lesions in larger medium-sized muscular arteries of the kidney (arcuate and larger), mesentery, lungs, pancreas, and adrenals is unusual in primary malignant hypertension and suggests the diagnosis of polyarteritis nodosa [226].

In women of childbearing age, *oral contraceptives* have been reported as a common cause of malignant hypertension [220, 235, 320, 430]. In most of the reported cases, the patients were normotensive prior to the initiation of oral contraceptives, although several patients had gestational hypertension during a prior pregnancy. In the absence of underlying renal disease, with discontinuation of oral contraceptives, the long-term prognosis is excellent [320].

Severe hypertension, which may enter the malignant phase, has been described as a complication of *renal cholesterol embolization syndrome* [108, 270, 464, 468]. In patients with severe aortic atherosclerotic disease undergoing aortic angiography, cardiac catheterization, or vascular surgery, evidence of cholesterol embolization may develop immediately after the procedure with lower extremity livedo reticularis and purple toes, abdominal pain, eosinophilia, eosinophiluria, and acute renal failure. Severe hypertension is often present and may enter the malignant phase. Alternatively, the patient may present with malignant hypertension weeks to months after the inciting procedure, at a time when peripheral evidence of cholesterol embolization has entirely resolved.

Scleroderma renal crisis is the most acute and life-threatening manifestation of progressive systemic sclerosis. It is characterized by malignant hypertension and rapidly progressive renal failure and is uniformly fatal without treatment [513]. In one large series, scleroderma renal crisis occurred in 7 percent of white patients and 21 percent of black patients with progressive systemic sclerosis [540]. The renal histology in scleroderma renal crisis is often virtually indistinguishable from primary malignant nephrosclerosis [111]. However, in progressive systemic sclerosis, renal vasculature disease, with proliferative endarteritis involving the interlobular arteries and fibrinoid necrosis of the afferent arterioles, may be a primary event that precedes either hypertension or renal insufficiency [71]. The renal ischemia that results from these lesions causes hypertension through activation of the renin-angiotensin system, leading to a vicious cycle of severe hypertension and renal ischemic injury. Treatment with converting enzyme inhibitors has dramatically improved survival in this disorder [513].

Malignant hypertension may rarely complicate the course of IgG myeloma. Although the pathogenesis is not known, hyperviscosity has been implicated [476]. Moreover, we have seen a patient with IgG myeloma, malignant hypertension, and progressive renal insufficiency in whom the renal histology was consistent with immunotactoid glomerulopathy.

Patients with *chronic lead poisoning* may develop severe hypertension and the neuroretinopathy typical of malignant hypertension [120].

A number of endocrine disorders may cause secondary malignant hypertension. Malignant hypertension is a rare complication of *pheochromocytoma* [77, 221, 557]. Although malignant hypertension secondary to *aldosterone-producing adenoma* is rare, several cases have been described [6, 119, 274]. However, a diagnosis of primary hyperaldosteronism must be made with caution in patients with a history of malignant hypertension. Following successful treatment of malignant hypertension, plasma renin activity usually returns rapidly to normal, whereas aldosterone secretion may remain elevated for up to a year. This observation has been attributed to the development of adrenal hyperplasia due to long-standing hyperreninemia with disordered feedback control (tertiary hyperaldosteronism) [347]. During this period, hypokalemia, metabolic alkalosis, and hyperaldosteronism may persist, despite suppressed plasma renin activity, thereby mimicking primary hyperaldosteronism. In patients with this condition, bilateral nodular adrenal hyperplasia has been found at surgery [94, 307]. Although adrenalectomy alleviates hypokalemia in this setting, there is no improvement in blood pressure [94, 307].

Cushing's syndrome with bilateral adrenal hyperplasia is most often associated with benign hypertension, although occasional cases of malignant hypertension have been reported [288, 335]. *Congenital adrenal hyperplasia* in patients with 11β-hydroxylase deficiency [212] or 17α-hydroxylase deficiency [379] has been reported to cause malignant hypertension.

EPIDEMIOLOGY OF MALIGNANT HYPERTENSION

Incidence. Although malignant hypertension is often a complication of preexisting hypertension, the risk of its development in hypertensive patients is difficult to estimate. Bechgaard (1956) [29, 30] found a 1 percent incidence among 1,000 patients followed for 16 to 22 years. Kincaid-Smith et al. (1958) [288] used a complicated formula to estimate the incidence of malignant hypertension in the British population at 1 percent. Perera (1955) [426] reported an incidence of 7 percent, but this estimate was based on a referral population and probably overestimated the true incidence. In the era of effective antihypertensive therapy for benign hypertension, there are few data on the incidence of malignant hypertension. A review of death certificates in New York City between 1958 and 1974 revealed that the overall mortality due to malignant hypertension had declined by 78 percent from 2.25 to 0.48 deaths per 100,000 population [315]. Although some of the decreased mortality was probably due to successful treatment of patients with malignant hypertension with antihypertensive drugs and dialysis, the authors speculated that the overall incidence of malignant hypertension had declined to less than 1 percent due to successful treatment of benign hypertension.

Age. The malignant phase tends to occur more frequently in younger subjects. The mean age of patients with malignant hypertension has been reported to be 40 to 50 years with 57 percent of the patients between 30 and 50 years old [366]. No difference has been found in the age of onset in men compared to women or in blacks compared to whites [264, 288, 366, 427, 482]. Pickering [435] suggested that the age dependency of malignant hypertension could be related to the increased frequency of secondary, more severe forms of hypertension in the young. Bechgaard [29] proposed that hypertension in patients with essential hypertension destined to enter the malignant phase was more rapidly progressive from the onset, so that the disease would be expected to occur predominantly in younger patients. Malignant hypertension has been reported to be a rare development in patients beyond the age of 65 [288]. The declining incidence of malignant hypertension in patients with essential hypertension relative to age is in marked contrast to the overall incidence of benign hypertension, which reaches a peak in the eighth decade [288]. In patients over 60 years old who develop malignant hypertension, the majority have underlying renovascular hypertension or primary renal parenchymal disease [205].

Gender. In most series of patients with malignant hypertension, males predominate over females by as much as 2 to 1 [226, 264, 288, 426, 427, 482].

Race. Blacks have an increased incidence of essential hypertension compared to whites. Moreover, several studies have demonstrated that blacks also have an increased risk of entering the malignant phase. In a population in which 31 percent of all hypertensive patients were black, 46 percent of 200 patients with malignant hypertension were found to be black [427]. In a recent study of 135 pairs of black and white hypertensive patients matched for age and gender, 4.4 percent of the blacks had hypertensive retinopathy consistent with malignant hypertension, whereas only 0.74 percent of the white patients had these funduscopic findings [389]. The increased frequency of malignant hypertension in blacks has been postulated to reflect the fact that (1) blacks presented later in the course of essential hypertension; (2) antihypertensive therapy in blacks was inadequate to prevent the transition from the benign to the malignant phase; or (3) essential hypertension may be a more aggressive disease in blacks than in whites [176].

Preceding Duration of Benign Hypertension. Although there are occasional case reports in which the malignant phase began de novo, the majority of patients show evidence of a variable period of benign hypertension before onset of the malignant phase. Milliez et al. [366] reported a preceding duration of benign hypertension of 7.7 years [366]. Kincaid-Smith et al. [288] detailed the duration of hypertension preceding the malignant phase in 77 patients: 0 to 6 months, 4 percent; 6 months to 1 year, 10 percent; 1 to 2 years, 12 percent; 2 to 4 years, 23 percent; 4 to 6 years, 16 percent; 6 to 8 years, 17 percent; and 8 to 10 years, 4 percent. Only 14 percent had more than 10 years of benign hypertension prior to onset of the malignant phase.

Smoking As a Risk Factor. The risk of malignant hypertension has been shown to be higher among hypertensive patients who smoke [46, 146, 254]. In one series, 82 percent of the patients with malignant hypertension were smokers versus 50 percent of inpatients and 43 percent of outpatients with benign hypertension and 52 percent of normotensive control subjects [254]. The relative risk for developing malignant hypertension was five times higher in hypertensive patients who smoked. In patients with malignant hypertension, at initial presentation, renal insufficiency was more common among smokers. The mean serum creatinine in nonsmokers was 1.2 mg/dl compared to 2.5 mg/dl in smokers. Moreover, of the 18 patients with a serum creatinine over 2.8 mg/dl, 17 were smokers and 1 was an ex-smoker [254].

In contrast to the findings with regard to smoking risk, no significant difference has been found for the prevalence or quantity of alcohol consumption in groups of patients with benign or malignant hypertension [146].

CLINICAL FEATURES OF MALIGNANT HYPERTENSION

The clinical features of malignant hypertension as outlined by Volhard and Fahr in 1914 [552] are still valid today: (1) elevation of diastolic blood pressure, usually fixed and severe; (2) funduscopic changes of hypertensive neuroretinopathy with striate hemorrhages, cotton-wool spots, and papilledema; (3) renal insufficiency; (4) rapid progression to a fatal outcome, usually due to uremia; and (5) renal histology demonstrating malignant nephrosclerosis with fibroid necrosis of afferent arterioles and proliferative endarteritis of interlobular arteries [552]. Unless hypertensive neuroretinopathy is present, malignant hypertension cannot be diagnosed regardless of the height of the arterial blood pressure [383, 575]. However, the other features need not be present initially to substantiate a diagnosis of malignant hypertension. For example, there is no critical level of diastolic blood pressure that defines the presence of malignant hypertension. An acute increase in blood pressure in previously normotensive individuals can precipitate the malignant phase at a diastolic blood pressure as low as 100 to 110 mm Hg. Conversely, very high diastolic blood pressures may persist for many years in patients with essential hypertension without the development of malignant hypertension [285].

Although with untreated malignant hypertension, severe renal impairment inevitably occurs, there may be minimal renal involvement at the time of presentation. Moreover, histologic malignant nephrosclerosis may be absent in patients dying early in the course of malignant hypertension due to cerebrovascular accident or congestive heart failure.

Some authors have distinguished *accelerated hypertension* (hemorrhages and cotton-wool spots) from *malignant hypertension* (papilledema). However, since the finding of striate hemorrhages and cotton-wool spots has the same prognostic significance whether or not papilledema is present [4, 350], it has been recommended that accelerated hypertension and malignant hypertension be regarded as synonymous terms for a clinical syndrome in which there is widespread hypertension-induced acute arteriolar injury [575]. We favor exclusive use of the term *malignant hypertension* to describe this disease process. The term *accelerated hypertension* should probably be abandoned, since this term is now commonly used to describe patients who develop increasingly severe or resistant hypertension independent of the funduscopic findings that characterize true accelerated or malignant hypertension.

Presenting Symptoms. The most common presenting complaints in patients with malignant hypertension are headache, blurred vision, and weight loss [288, 366, 453, 482]. Less common presenting symptoms include dyspnea, fatigue, malaise, gastrointestinal complaints (nausea, vomiting, epigastric pain), polyuria, nocturia, and gross hematuria [366, 416, 482]. In many series, the onset of symptoms was noted to be remarkably sudden, such that it could often be dated precisely [366, 427, 482]. In contrast, Kaplan [275] has noted that an *"asymptomatic" presentation* of malignant hypertension is not uncommon, especially in young black males who deny any prior symptoms when they present in the end-stage of the hypertensive process with florid failure of the brain, heart, and kidneys.

Headache is the most frequent presenting complaint in patients with malignant hypertension. Unfortunately, headache is a nonspecific finding that occurs frequently in patients with benign hypertension. However, when patients with severe hypertension experience recent onset of headaches or the intensification of an existing headache pattern, the possibility of a transition from the benign to the malignant phase of hypertension should be carefully considered [288].

In one large series, *visual symptoms* were present at initial diagnosis in 76 percent of patients, and 90 percent of patients eventually developed visual problems [482]. The most common complaints were blurred vision and decreased visual acuity. Sudden blindness occurred in 14 percent of cases. Scotoma, diplopia, and hemianopsia were also reported.

Weight loss is a very common symptom early in the course of malignant hypertension and often occurs before the onset of anorexia or uremia [281, 288, 416, 427, 453]. In many patients, at least a portion of the weight loss can be attributed to volume depletion resulting from a spontaneous natriuresis with the onset of the malignant phase [25, 189, 395].

Level of Blood Pressure. There is apparently no absolute level of blood pressure above which malignant hypertension invariably occurs. In most series of patients with malignant hypertension, the average diastolic blood pressure was greater than 120 to 130 mm Hg [281, 366, 482]. However, two series have found considerable overlap of blood pressure levels in patients with benign and malignant hypertension (Fig. 59-2) [40, 288].

Funduscopic Manifestations. Examination of the ocular fundus is of great importance in the assessment of patients with severe hypertension, especially with regard to prognosis [132, 164, 290, 435, 481]. Although there had been earlier reports on the funduscopic changes in hypertension, Keith and Wagener's description of the prognosis of hypertensive patients based on a grading system for hypertensive retinopathy was the landmark study in this field [281]. They graded retinal findings in untreated hypertensive patients as follows: grade I—mild narrowing or sclerosis of arterioles; grade II—moderate sclerosis with an increased light reflex and arteriovenous compression; grade III—retinal hemorrhages and exudates; grade IV—the findings in grade III plus papilledema. The presence of papilledema was associated with the worst prognosis and became synonymous with the term *malignant hypertension*. In subsequent years, the term *accelerated hypertension* was adopted to describe patients with grade III retinopathy [60].

Although widely accepted, the usefulness of the Keith and Wagener classification has recently been questioned [4, 290, 350]. It is extremely difficult to quantitate arteriolar narrowing [290]. Moreover, there is observer bias such that patients with mild hypertension and questionable narrowing are inevitably placed in this group [290]. Thus, the finding of grade I changes is of limited usefulness. There is also great interobserver variability with regard to the definition of arteriovenous crossing changes [128]. Another objection to the Keith and Wagener classification is that it does not clearly distinguish between the retinal changes of benign and malignant hypertension [435]. For example, the clinical significance of a large, ill-defined white exudate (cotton-wool spot)

Fig. 59-2. Systolic and diastolic blood pressure in patients with malignant hypertension compared with age- and sex-matched patients with severe benign hypertension. (From P. Kincaid-Smith. Malignant hypertension: Mechanisms and management. *Pharmacol. Ther.* 9:245, 1980. With permission.)

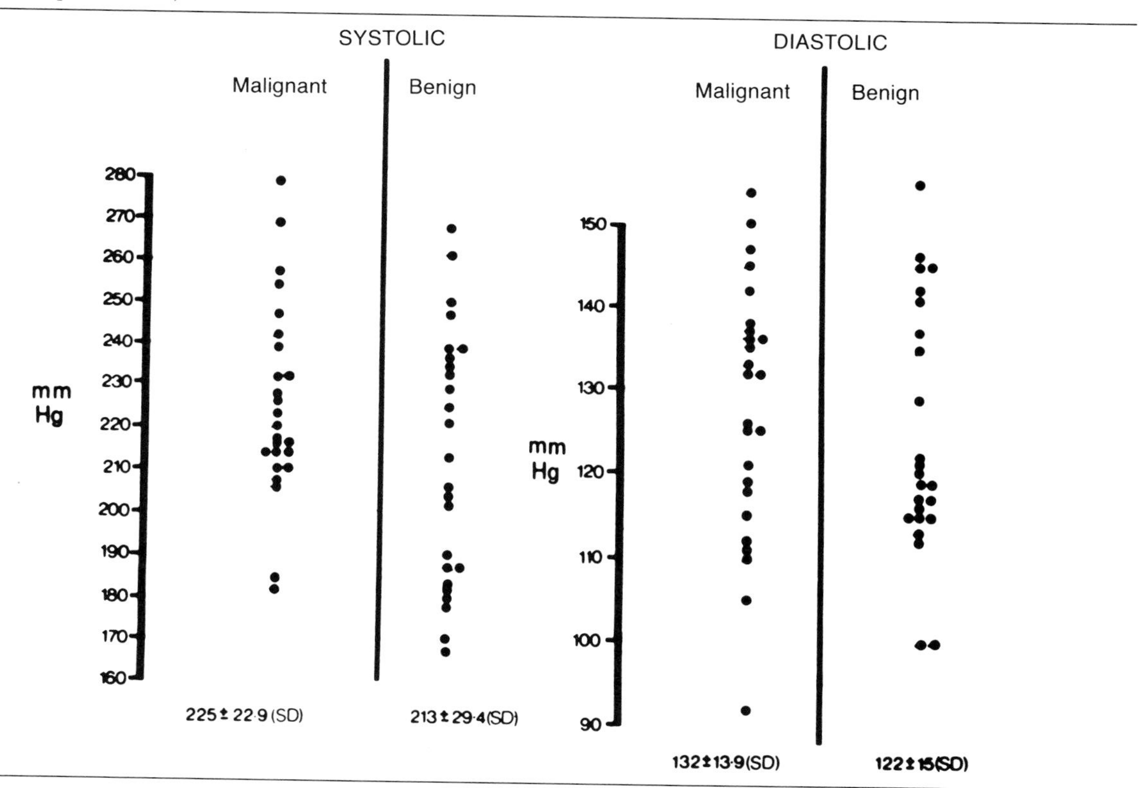

Table 59-3. Retinal changes in hypertension

Retinal arteriosclerosis and arteriosclerotic retinopathy
Arteriolar narrowing (diffuse)
Focal arteriolar narrowing
Arteriovenous crossing changes
Broadening of the light reflex
Copper or silver wiring
Perivasculitis
Solitary round hemorrhages
Hard exudates
Central or branch venous occlusion
Hypertensive neuroretinopathy
Generalized arteriolar narrowing
Striate (flame-shaped) hemorrhages*
Cotton-wool spots (soft exudates)*
Bilateral papilledema*
Macular star

*Features that distinguish retinal arteriosclerosis (characteristic of benign hypertension) from hypertensive neuroretinopathy (characteristic of malignant hypertension).

appearing in the fundus of a young man with severe hypertension is quite different from the clinical significance of a sharply defined glistening hard exudate in a 60-year-old patient with moderate hypertension. In the first example, the cotton-wool spot and the clinical circumstances suggest the onset of malignant hypertension. In the older patient, the retinal picture is consistent with retinal arteriosclerosis characteristic of benign hypertension [435]. The therapeutic and prognostic implications of these two types of exudates are clearly different, although both would be assigned to grade III in the Keith and Wagener classification.

A number of authorities have recommended abandonment of the Keith and Wagener classification in favor of the hypertensive retinopathy classification initially proposed by Fishberg and Oppenheimer [164]. This classification draws a distinction between *retinal arteriosclerosis with arteriosclerotic retinopathy,* which is characteristic of benign hypertension, and *hypertensive neuroretinopathy,* which defines the presence of malignant hypertension (Table 59-3).

Retinal arteriosclerosis with or without arteriosclerotic retinopathy is seen in patients with long-standing benign hypertension from either primary or secondary causes. Retinal arteriosclerosis (arteriolosclerosis) is characterized histologically by the accumulation of hyaline material. In the early stages, the material is deposited beneath the endothelium, while in older lesions deposits extend into the media and ultimately the entire vessel wall is affected. Funduscopic changes reflecting retinal arteriosclerosis include irregularity of the lumen and focal narrowing, arteriovenous crossing changes, broadening of the light reflex, copper or silver wiring, perivasculitis (parallel white lines around blood columns), and generalized arteriolar narrowing (Fig. 59-3). *Arteriosclerotic retinopathy,* which results from this arteriosclerotic process, is manifest by the presence of hemorrhages and hard exudates. These hemorrhages are usually solitary, round or oval, and are confined to the periphery of the fundus (Fig. 59-4). They are caused by

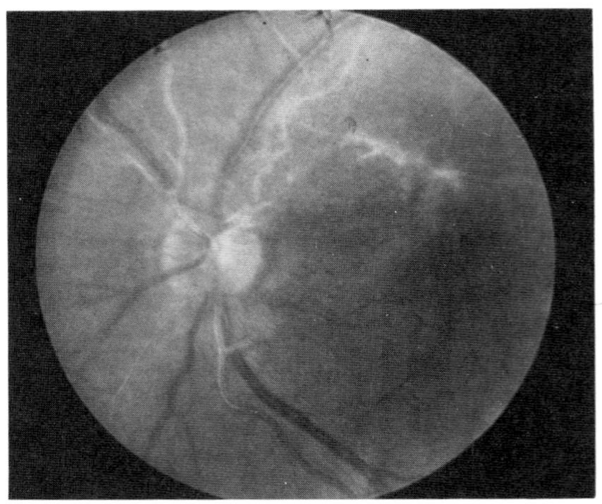

Fig. 59-3. Retinal arteriosclerosis in benign hypertension with arteriolar narrowing, mild arteriovenous crossing changes, copper wiring, and perivasculitis (parallel white lines around blood columns). The striate hemorrhages, cotton-wool spots, and papilledema characteristic of malignant hypertension are absent. (Courtesy of Daniel J. Mayer, M.D.)

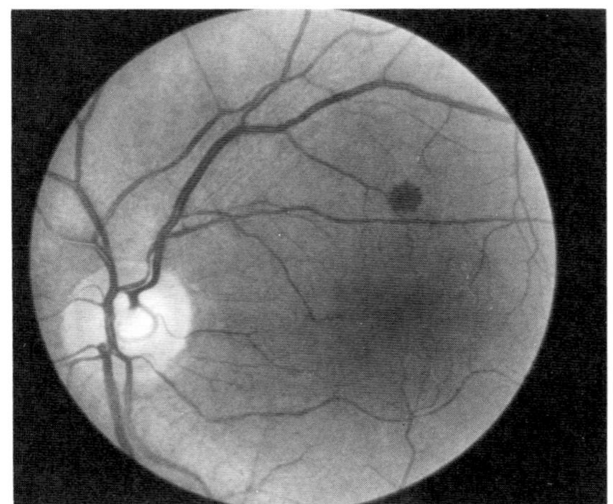

Fig. 59-4. Arteriosclerotic retinopathy in a 52-year-old woman with benign hypertension, demonstrating a solitary round hemorrhage. (Courtesy of Daniel J. Mayer, M.D.)

venous or arterial occlusion [290]. Hard exudates may appear as multiple small white dots that give a powdery appearance to the retina, or they may appear as large glistening spots that are sharply defined from the adjacent retina. Arteriosclerotic retinopathy may also cause localized areas of retinal edema and hemorrhage due to occlusion of small branch veins. However, the principal findings of hypertensive neuroretinopathy—namely, striate hemorrhages, cotton-wool spots, and papilledema—are absent (Table 59-3).

The finding of retinal arteriosclerosis in hypertensive patients often does not imply a poor prognosis. Even patients with severe arteriosclerotic retinopathy may live for many years before the development of morbid events due to coronary artery disease, congestive heart failure, or cerebrovascular accident. Furthermore, the presence of retinal arteriosclerosis in patients with essential hypertension is usually not associated with significant renal impairment. This observation is in sharp contrast to patients with hypertensive neuroretinopathy in whom renal impairment, if not already present, is imminent without treatment.

The prognostic significance of retinal arteriosclerosis in hypertensive patients with regard to the risks of coronary atherosclerosis and cerebrovascular disease has been questioned [132, 290, 481]. Most of the arteries visualized with the ophthalmoscope are technically arterioles, since they are 0.1 mm or less in diameter [290]. Moreover, hyaline arteriolosclerosis of the retina is an entity that is entirely separate and distinct from the atherosclerotic process that may affect larger muscular arteries. Thus, the retinal arteriolar changes are often not predictive of the presence or absence of atherosclerotic disease of the coronary or cerebral vessels or other major arterial branches of the aorta [132]. The prognostic significance of retinal changes in benign hypertension has also been questioned on the basis of the observation that normotensive control subjects between the ages of 40 and 60 have a high incidence of retinal arteriosclerosis, presumably reflecting age-related vascular changes [545].

In a recent study designed to assess the usefulness of ophthalmoscopy in mild to moderate hypertension, 25 patients with untreated essential hypertension were evaluated with direct ophthalmoscopy, assessment of fundus photographs, ambulatory blood pressure monitoring, estimation of left ventricular mass by electrocardiography and two-dimensional echocardiography, and measurement of urinary microalbumin excretion. No statistical relation was found between either clinic or ambulatory blood pressure readings and the severity of retinal arteriosclerosis as defined by the presence of arteriolar narrowing or arteriovenous crossing changes. Moreover, there was no independent relationship between retinal changes and age, measures of left ventricular mass, creatinine clearance, or urinary microalbumin excretion. The authors concluded that the finding of retinal arteriosclerosis was not clinically useful in the evaluation of mild to moderate hypertension [128].

The lack of significance of retinal arteriosclerosis in hypertensive patients contrasts markedly with the importance and prognostic significance of the finding of *hypertensive neuroretinopathy*. The appearance of striate hemorrhages and cotton-wool spots with or without papilledema closely parallels the development of severe arteriolar damage (fibrinoid necrosis or proliferative endarteritis) in the circulation of other organs including the brain and kidneys. Hypertensive neuroretinopathy is the clinical *sine qua non* of malignant hypertension and therefore signifies a far more ominous prognosis than the finding of retinal arteriosclerosis.

The appearance of small *striate hemorrhages* is often the first sign that hypertension has entered the malignant phase. These hemorrhages are linear or flame-shaped and are most commonly observed in a radial arrangement around the optic disc [132, 290] (Figs. 59-5 and 59-6). They arise from superficial capillaries in the nerve fiber bundles, which have a high intravascular pressure because they are perfused directly by arterioles [132]. The hemorrhages extend along nerve fibers parallel to the retinal surface. They often have a frayed distal border due to extravasation between nerve fiber bundles. Even when widespread, hemorrhages are rarely seen lateral to the macula in hypertensive neuroretinopathy. Striate hemorrhages often occur adjacent to cotton-wool spots (Fig. 59-5) and most likely arise from capillary microaneurysms at the margins of the spots. Since hemoglobin absorbs fluorescein, hemorrhages appear black with fluorescein angiography [132]. Striate hemorrhages

Fig. 59-5. Hypertensive neuroretinopathy in a 44-year-old woman with malignant hypertension demonstrating linear (striate) hemorrhages, cotton-wool spots, and early papilledema. (Courtesy of Daniel J. Mayer, M.D.)

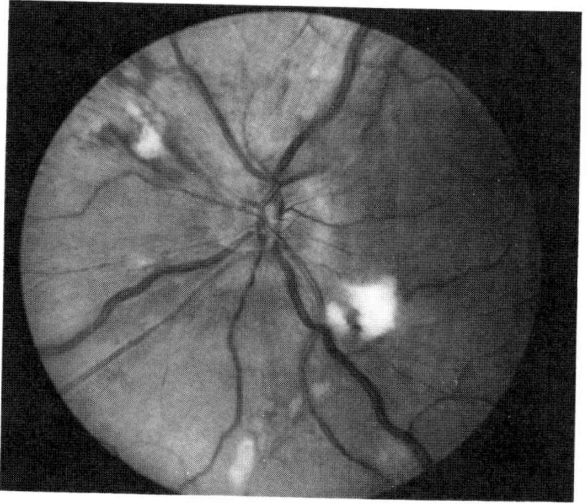

Fig. 59-6. Hypertensive neuroretinopathy in a 30-year-old man with malignant hypertension demonstrating linear (striate) hemorrhages, cotton-wool spots, papilledema, and a star figure at the macula. (Courtesy of Daniel J. Mayer, M.D.)

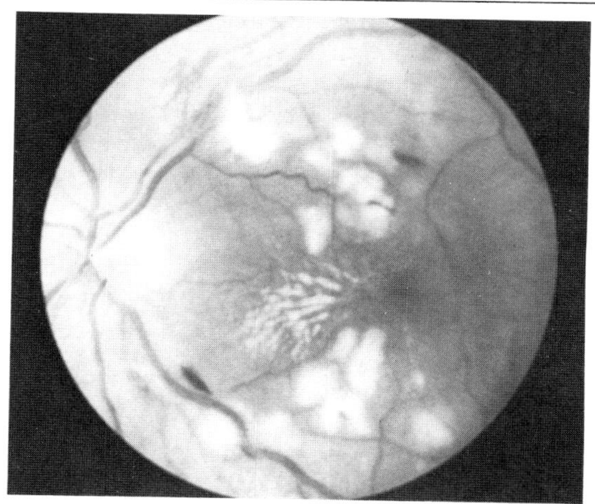

can usually be distinguished from the hemorrhages due to retinal arteriosclerosis, which are solitary, round, and confined to the periphery of the fundus [290].

Cotton-wool spots are the most characteristic features of malignant hypertension and are the result of ischemic infarction of nerve fiber bundles caused by arteriolar occlusion. They usually surround the optic disc and most commonly occur within 3 disc diameters of the optic disc (Figs. 59-5 and 59-6). Cotton-wool spots begin as grayish-white discolorations of the retina, but within 24 hours they become shiny white with fluffy margins. Red dots may be seen in the bed of the exudate (microaneurysms). The occluded vessel can sometimes be seen as an outpouching from a large vessel [132]. Cotton-wool spots are not specific for hypertensive neuroretinopathy and can also be seen with diabetic retinopathy, retinal emboli, and central and branch retinal vein occlusion. However, differentiation of these disorders from malignant hypertension is usually not difficult.

A *star figure at the macula* represents hard exudates that are arranged in a radial fashion from the central fovea (Fig. 59-6). Although a star figure can occasionally be seen in arteriosclerotic retinopathy, it more often develops in conjunction with florid retinal changes in malignant hypertension. In hypertensive neuroretinopathy, the exudates form lines or sheets around the macula rather than the discrete dots around the macula that occur in arteriosclerotic retinopathy [435].

Papilledema may occur in hypertensive neuroretinopathy, but it is not invariably present. The detection of mild papilledema is subject to large interobserver variability [350]. When papilledema occurs, it is usually accompanied by striate hemorrhages and cotton-wool spots (Fig. 59-6). When papilledema occurs alone, the possibility of a primary intracranial process such as a tumor or cerebrovascular accident should be considered [435].

Hypertensive neuroretinopathy almost always precedes clinically apparent damage in other end-organs, but there are occasional reports of malignant nephrosclerosis appearing before the onset of hypertensive neuroretinopathy [56, 198]. It should also be noted that the findings of striate hemorrhages, cotton-wool spots, and papilledema are not specific for malignant hypertension. Funduscopic findings that are indistinguishable from those of hypertensive neuroretinopathy may occur in severe anemia, subacute bacterial endocarditis, systemic lupus erythematosus, polyarteritis, temporal arteritis, and scleroderma [435]. In these disorders, the retinopathy may develop even in the absence of hypertension. Central retinal vein occlusion may also mimic florid hypertensive neuroretinopathy but is normally unilateral, whereas hypertensive neuroretinopathy is bilateral.

Severe hypertension may also affect the choroidal as well as the retinal circulation. *Hypertensive choroidopathy* may occur in malignant hypertension and is manifest by lesions known as acute *Elschnig's spots,* which are white areas of retinal pigment epithelial necrosis with overlying localized serous detachments of the retina (Fig. 59-7) [123].

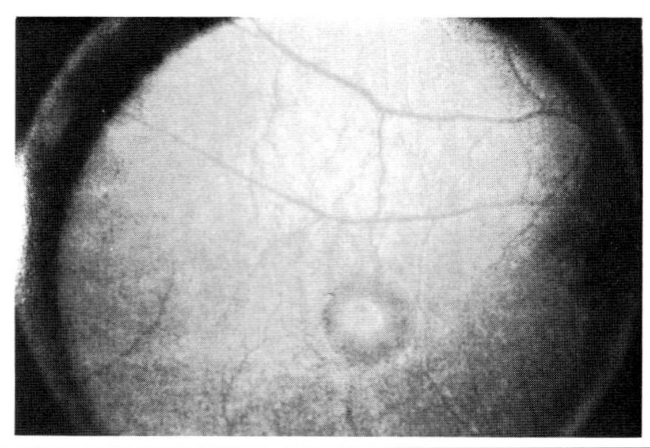

Fig. 59-7. Hypertensive choroidopathy in malignant hypertension demonstrating focal serous detachment of the sensory retina with a whitish lesion at the level of the retinal pigment epithelium (acute Elschnig's spot). (From G. de Venecia and L. M. Jampol. The eye in accelerated hypertension: II. Localized serous detachments of the retina in patients. *Arch. Ophthalmol.* 102:68, 1984. Copyright 1984, American Medical Association. With permission.)

The serous retinal detachments may vary from ⅓ to 6 disc diameters. Fluorescein angiography reveals staining of the damaged pigment epithelium and leakage into the subretinal space [123]. Although most patients with this hypertensive choroidopathy also have typical changes of hypertensive neuroretinopathy with striate hemorrhages and cotton-wool spots, if the elevation of blood pressure is relatively sudden, the changes of hypertensive choroidopathy may predominate [123].

In the past, accelerated hypertension and malignant hypertension were regarded as distinct clinical entities [280]. Accelerated hypertension was defined by the presence of hemorrhages and exudates (grade III), and the diagnosis of malignant hypertension was reserved for patients who also had papilledema (grade IV). However, recent studies have shown that the prognosis is equally grave in patients with severe hypertension accompanied by striate hemorrhages and cotton-wool spots whether or not papilledema is present [4, 350]. Therefore, papilledema should not be regarded as an essential requirement for the diagnosis of malignant hypertension. By life-table analysis, 10-year survival was 46 percent in patients with hemorrhage and exudates and 48 percent when papilledema was also present [350]. The lack of association between papilledema and the length of survival was confirmed using the Cox's proportional hazards model, which revealed associations between survival and age ($p = 0.06$), smoking habit ($p = 0.03$), initial serum creatinine concentration ($p = 0.01$), and the level of blood pressure control achieved with therapy ($p < 0.01$), but no association was found with papilledema ($p = 0.48$). When other covariates were controlled simultaneously, no association was found between the presence of papilledema and survival (Fig. 59-8). The failure of recent studies to find a difference in survival between grade III and grade IV retinopathy as previously described by Keith et al. [280],

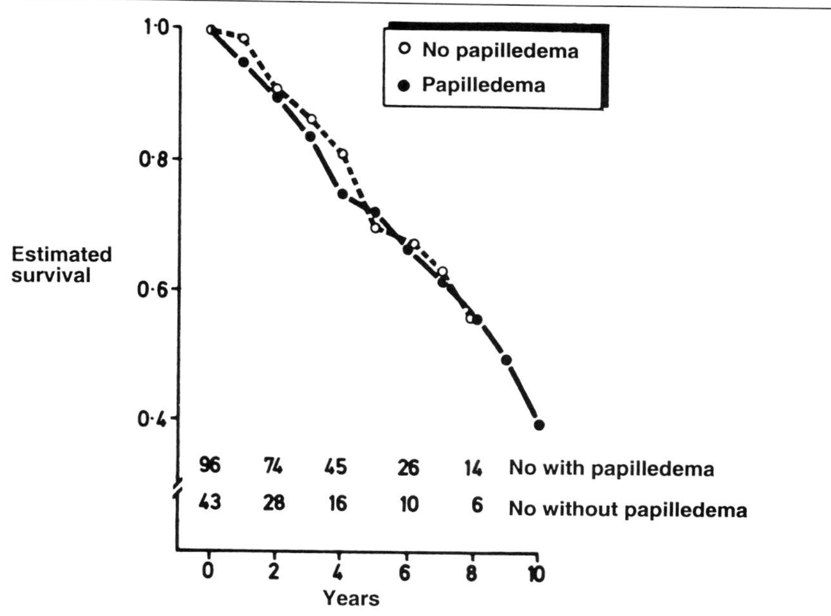

Fig. 59-8. Relation between papilledema and survival in 139 hypertensive patients with bilateral retinal hemorrhages and exudates after controlling for age, gender, smoking habit, initial serum creatinine concentration, and initial and achieved blood pressure by multivariate analysis. Failure of papilledema to influence prognosis was confirmed by likelihood ratio test ($x^2 = 0.89$, 1 df, $p = 0.34$). (From E. McGregor, C. G. Isles, J. L. Jay, et al. Retinal changes in malignant hypertension. *Br. Med. J.* 292:233, 1986. With permission.)

may be due to the fact that the earlier study involved untreated patients. Papilledema may be associated with a worse prognosis only when the hypertension is untreated or ineffectively treated [350].

There is no evidence to indicate that the apparent severity of hypertensive neuroretinopathy is predictive of a more severe hypertensive vasculopathy or more aggressive end-organ destruction. Papilledema is not always present even when there is severe malignant nephrosclerosis presenting as oliguric acute renal failure. In four series with a total of 25 patients with malignant hypertension and acute renal failure, 14 patients had papilledema. However, 11 patients had hemorrhages and cotton-wool spots but no papilledema [96, 339, 345, 492].

The lack of a difference in prognosis in patients with hypertensive neuroretinopathy with or without papilledema suggests that accelerated hypertension and malignant hypertension are really synonymous and should be regarded as the same disease [4, 350, 575]. In this regard, one study found arteriolar fibrinoid necrosis in eight patients with severe hypertension who had retinal hemorrhage and cotton-wool spots but who lacked papilledema [57]. Moreover, recent evidence indicates that cotton-wool spots and papilledema share a similar pathogenesis [352, 353].

The diagnosis of malignant hypertension may be made in the setting of severe hypertension when only a single cotton-wool spot is observed. The approach to the treatment of hypertension in this setting should be just as aggressive as in patients with full-blown hypertensive neuroretinopathy with extensive striate hemorrhages and cotton-wool spots with bilateral papilledema. Moreover, since the funduscopic findings in patients with malignant hypertension may sometimes be subtle, the evaluation of patients with severe hypertension should include a careful ophthalmologic examination after pupillary dilation with 1% tropicamide [514]. Since the presence of even mild hypertensive neuroretinopathy has important therapeutic and prognostic implications, if adequate visualization of the retina cannot be accomplished, formal ophthalmologic evaluation with indirect ophthalmoscopy should be considered.

Renal Manifestations. Malignant hypertension is a progressive systemic vasculopathy in which renal involvement is a secondary and relatively late development [147, 336, 390]. Thus, patients with malignant hypertension may present with a spectrum of renal involvement ranging from minimal albuminuria with normal renal function to severe renal failure indistinguishable from that seen in patients with end-stage renal disease due to primary renal parenchymal disease [147, 264, 281, 366].

The first sign of renal involvement in malignant hypertension is often the abrupt appearance of proteinuria. About 20 percent of patients also have painless gross hematuria, while 50 percent have microhematuria [198]. Pickering [435] regarded the appearance of blood or more than a trace of protein in the urine of patients with essential hypertension to be an indication of the onset of malignant nephrosclerosis, since significant proteinuria and hematuria have been found to be rare in benign nephrosclerosis [198]. However, recent reports suggest that nephrotic range proteinuria may sometimes occur with severe benign nephrosclerosis [378, 387, 396].

Quantitation of *24-hour protein excretion* in patients with malignant hypertension has revealed less than 2 gm in one-third, between 2 and 4 gm in one-third, and over 4 gm in one-third of patients [482]. The level of protein excretion has been found to be of little value in the differentiation of primary (essential) malignant hypertension from malignant hypertension due to secondary causes [264, 288, 437].

Hematuria is a very important clinical finding in patients with essential hypertension. In the absence of renal parenchymal disease or a urologic source, the onset of hematuria is virtually diagnostic of malignant nephrosclerosis [435]. In one series, hematuria was found in 100 percent of patients with malignant hypertension [264]. However, the absence of hematuria does not exclude the diagnosis [416]. Of interest is the fact that *red blood cell casts* have been described in patients with malignant hypertension who had no evidence of glomerulonephritis at renal biopsy [345].

Pyuria has been reported in 75 percent of patients with malignant hypertension. However, the presence of pyuria did not differentiate between primary and secondary malignant hypertension [482].

Renal size is variable and depends on the duration of prior benign hypertension. In patients with primary (essential) hypertension, the kidneys may be normal or only slightly reduced in size. There may be little reduction in renal size even when patients develop terminal renal failure [288].

The *spectrum of clinical renal involvement* in malignant hypertension is variable. Four clinical renal syndromes have been described:

1. *Progressive subacute deterioration to end-stage renal disease (ESRD).* In patients presenting with malignant hypertension and initially normal to mildly impaired renal function, in the absence of adequate treatment, it is common to observe deterioration of renal function with progression to ESRD over a period of weeks to months. The salient clinical features in this group include abrupt onset of albuminuria with microhematuria; isosthenuria, polyuria, and nocturia followed by oliguria in the terminal stages; progressive development of uremic signs and symptoms; and progression to death within 1 year [336].
2. *Transient deterioration of renal function with initial control of blood pressure.* This is a well-described entity that occurs in patients presenting with mild to moderate renal impairment. It is reviewed in detail in the later section on Treatment of Malignant Hypertension.
3. Occasionally, patients with malignant hypertension present with *established renal failure.* The close similarity between the terminal stage of primary malignant nephrosclerosis and chronic nephritis with superimposed malignant hypertension has long been recognized. In this regard, it may not be possible to ascertain whether a patient presenting with hypertensive neuroretinopathy, severe hypertension, and renal failure has primary or secondary malignant hypertension [435]. While a history of an acute nephritic episode or long-standing proteinuria or hematuria may suggest underlying primary renal parenchymal disease, the distinction between primary malignant nephrosclerosis and chronic nephritis often requires a renal biopsy [120, 163, 292, 435].
4. *Oliguric acute renal failure.* Mattern et al. [345] have described 4 cases of malignant hypertension characterized by diastolic blood pressure greater than 130 mm Hg; advanced hypertensive neuroretinopathy; marked weight loss; normal to slightly decreased kidney size; active urine sediment with proteinuria, hematuria, and red blood cell casts; and evidence of microangiopathic hemolytic anemia. Although the initial blood urea nitrogen (BUN) was less than 60 mg/dl, in each case oliguric renal failure occurred that necessitated the initiation of dialysis within a few days of admission. Despite dialytic therapy, the blood pressure was extremely difficult to control and each patient died. Renal histology revealed malignant nephrosclerosis with fibrinoid necrosis and proliferation endarteritis. The glomeruli were normal except for evidence of ischemic changes. Multifocal tubular necrosis was present and presumed to be secondary to ischemia. Pitcock et al. [439] and Sevitt et al. [492] have described similar cases. In most of these cases, the diagnosis of malignant hypertension was delayed because the patients were initially considered to have rapidly progressive glomerulonephritis or systemic vasculitis, which were treated with high-dose steroids. The diagnosis of malignant hypertension was not suspected until renal histology revealed malignant nephrosclerosis.

Neurologic Manifestations. Clarke and Murphy [86] have detailed the neurologic findings among 190 patients with malignant hypertension. Central nervous system involvement was present at some time during the course in 42 percent of patients. In the 65 patients for whom a cause of death could be ascertained, 33 suffered a fatal neurologic event. Of the total deaths 20 percent were due to a neurologic cause. *Intracerebral hemorrhage* occurred in 23 patients. Episodes of focal brain ischemia, presumed to be due to *cerebral thrombosis,* occurred in 35 patients. Generalized *seizures* occurred in 11 patients and focal seizures in 8. Bell's palsy occurred in 7 patients. Primary *subarachnoid hemorrhage* occurred in 4 patients. The incidence of *headache* was comparable in patients with and without neurologic abnormality. Thus, the presence of headache did not necessarily imply central nervous system involvement. In this series, *hypertensive encephalopathy* was found in only 1 percent of patients; however, other series have reported a higher incidence [411]. The clinical presentation, pathophysiology, and treatment of hypertensive encephalopathy are discussed in detail in a separate section to follow.

The *cerebrospinal fluid* (CSF) findings in patients with malignant hypertension are variable. Even among patients with papilledema, CSF pressure was greater than 200 mm water in only 65 percent [86, 482]. In contrast, Pickering [434] found that patients with malignant hypertension had higher CSF pressures than patients with benign hypertension and that there was a direct correlation between the height of the blood pressure and the CSF pressure. Blood-stained or xanthochromic fluid has been reported only in patients with intracerebral or subarachnoid hemorrhage [86]. Protein concentration was greater than 60 mg per deciliter in 69 percent of patients (range, 11 to 307 mg/dl). No pleocytosis was reported. Although Clarke et al. [86] reported no complications from lumbar puncture, others have reported a 12 percent incidence of complications including severe headache, sudden blindness, coma, and death due to cerebellar herniation [482].

Gastrointestinal Manifestations. The most common gastrointestinal manifestations of malignant hypertension are nonspecific symptoms including *nausea, vomiting,* and *epigastric pain* [198, 453]. However, *acute pancreatitis* has been reported as a rare complication [23]. In this series of 42 patients with malignant hypertension, 7 developed severe acute pancreatitis that could not be attributed to gallstones or alcohol abuse. All of the patients were black and were on maintenance hemodialysis for renal failure caused by malignant nephrosclerosis. The blood pressure was poorly controlled in each patient. In another series reporting on the frequency of pancreatitis in a dialysis population, the majority of patients were found to have hypertensive nephrosclerosis as the cause of ESRD [16]. It has been proposed that acute pancreatitis occurs with increased frequency in patients with malignant hypertension because of the use of hemodialysis. Although dialysis prevents death from uremia, if the blood pressure remains poorly controlled, hypertensive vasculopathy could continue in other organs such as the pancreas. Moreover, the use of heparin might precipitate this complication by causing hemorrhage into inflamed pancreatic tissue [23].

Cases have been described in which patients with malignant hypertension presented with an *acute abdomen.* Abdominal exploration revealed necrotic bowel with involvement of the distal ileum and ascending colon. Pathologic examination revealed fibrinoid necrosis and thrombotic occlusion of the small arteries of the bowel wall [414]. *Gastrointestinal hemorrhage* has also been reported in patients with malignant hypertension due to hypertension-induced necrotizing mesenteric arteriolitis [198, 497].

Hematologic Manifestations. A variety of hematologic findings have been reported in patients with malignant hypertension. *Elevation of the erythrocyte sedimentation rate* has been reported [288]. The *hemoglobin concentration* at the time of presentation may correlate with the etiology of the malignant phase. A hemoglobin concentration greater than 12.5 gm/dl was more often associated with primary malignant hypertension, while a lower value was more often associated with chronic glomerulonephritis or pyelonephritis [288, 482].

There are numerous reports of *microangiopathic hemolytic anemia* in association with malignant hypertension. In one series of 24 patients with malignant hypertension, 16 were found to have evidence of microangiopathic hemolysis [323]. Other significant abnormalities reported in malignant hypertension include thrombocytopenia, increased fibrin degradation products, increased factor VIII levels, increased fibrinogen, and increased urokinase sensitivity consistent with decreased fibrinolysis [183].

Blood viscosity has also been reported to be significantly increased in patients with malignant hypertension [255]. The significance of this abnormality is unknown.

Cardiac Manifestations. Congestive heart failure may be a presenting feature of malignant hypertension. Moreover, heart failure alone or in combination with uremia was a common cause of death prior to the advent of effective antihypertensive drugs [366, 453, 482]. Heart failure in malignant hypertension has been reported to be predominantly left-sided with pulmonary congestion resulting in orthopnea, paroxysmal nocturnal dyspnea, cardiac asthma, and recurrent episodes of acute pulmonary edema. Peripheral venous congestion with dependent edema or hepatic congestion was found to be minimal or absent even when death resulted from congestive heart failure [147]. The management of acute pulmonary edema in patients with malignant hypertension is discussed in the section on Hypertension Complicated by Acute Pulmonary Edema.

Angina and myocardial infarction, though common in long-standing benign hypertension, are uncommon in malignant hypertension [288]. Aortic dissection is also rare in patients with malignant hypertension [288].

Abnormalities of the Renin-Angiotensin-Aldosterone Axis. Evidence of activation of the renin-angiotensin-aldosterone axis is present in many, but not all, patients with malignant hypertension [32]. Among 53 patients with malignant hypertension not secondary to renal artery stenosis, 55 percent had increased plasma renin activity (PRA), while 45 percent had PRA in the normal range [57]. Among 25 patients with malignant hypertension secondary to renal artery stenosis, PRA was consistently elevated to levels above those seen with renovascular hypertension in the benign phase [57].

Aldosterone secretion rate (ASR) has been studied in patients with malignant hypertension [307]. There was a marked increase in ASR in 7 of 8 patients with malignant hypertension (papilledema present) and in 5 of 8 patients with accelerated hypertension (retinal hemorrhages without papilledema). The ASR in these patients was often higher than that seen in patients with aldosterone-producing adenoma. Postmortem examination of the adrenal glands in 7 cases of malignant hypertension revealed bilateral areas of focal hyperplasia, especially in the region of the zona glomerulosa [307]. In a subsequent study, ASR in malignant hypertension was found to correlate with PRA, suggesting that the hyperaldosteronism was secondary to hyperreninemia [306]. Mc-

Allister et al. [347] studied PRA and ASR in 22 patients with malignant hypertension at presentation and then at varying intervals during treatment. Since only 36 percent of patients had elevated PRA at presentation, they concluded that malignant hypertension could occur in the absence of increased PRA. Of interest, among patients with elevated PRA and ASR, there was often a transient period during therapy in which PRA returned to normal yet ASR remained elevated. This dissociation often persisted for months. The authors postulated that with prolonged hyperreninemia, hyperplasia of the zona glomerulosa occurred. When renin levels reverted back to normal with therapy, persistent hyperplasia of the zona glomerulosa and a delay in resetting feedback control mechanisms could have led to oversecretion of aldosterone despite normal PRA (tertiary hyperaldosteronism) [347].

Electrolyte Abnormalities. Hypokalemic metabolic alkalosis has been reported in up to 50 percent of patients with malignant hypertension, presumably reflecting a state of hyperreninemia and secondary hyperaldosteronism [307]. After effective therapy, aldosterone hypersecretion may persist long after volume depletion is corrected and renin levels have returned to normal. Thus, the findings of hypokalemia, increase urinary potassium losses, and aldosterone hypersecretion with suppressed PRA may mimic the findings of primary hyperaldosteronism [347].

Hyponatremia is not uncommon in patients with malignant hypertension, particularly when sodium restriction is instituted. In an analysis of 127 patients with malignant hypertension treated with a rice diet, in 33 patients the diet had to be abandoned because of severe, progressive hyponatremia [401].

Patients with malignant hypertension due to renal artery stenosis may occasionally present with the striking *hyponatremic hypertensive syndrome* [15, 56, 233]. The characteristic features of this syndrome include severe hypertension, hypertensive neuroretinopathy, polyuria, polydipsia, weight loss, and salt craving. Biochemical changes include hyponatremia, hypokalemia, and low total exchangeable sodium and potassium, with markedly elevated PRA, angiotensin II, aldosterone, and arginine vasopressin levels. Atkinson et al. [15] have proposed that this syndrome may result from the action of angiotensin II, which produces hypertension and marked pressure natriuresis from the contralateral kidney.

PATHOLOGIC FINDINGS IN MALIGNANT HYPERTENSION

Renal Pathology. With malignant nephrosclerosis, small pinpoint petechial hemorrhages may be present on the cortical surface, giving the kidney a peculiar *flea-bitten* appearance. The renal size varies depending on the duration of preexisting benign hypertension or the presence of underlying primary renal parenchymal disease. When terminal renal failure occurs in patients with primary malignant hypertension, the kidneys may be normal in size [285]. However, when secondary malignant hypertension is superimposed on primary renal disease, the kidneys may be small.

Fibrinoid necrosis of the afferent arteriole has traditionally been regarded as the hallmark of malignant nephrosclerosis (Fig. 59-9) [288, 482]. The characteristic finding is the deposition in the arteriolar wall of a granular material that appears bright pink with hematoxylin and eosin stain. On trichrome staining, this granular material has a deep red color. This fibrinoid material is usually found

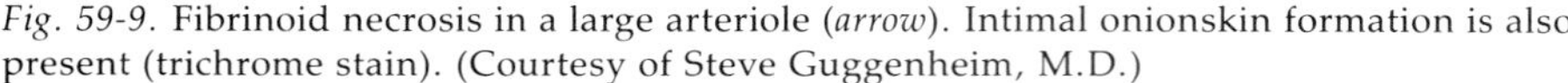

Fig. 59-9. Fibrinoid necrosis in a large arteriole (*arrow*). Intimal onionskin formation is also present (trichrome stain). (Courtesy of Steve Guggenheim, M.D.)

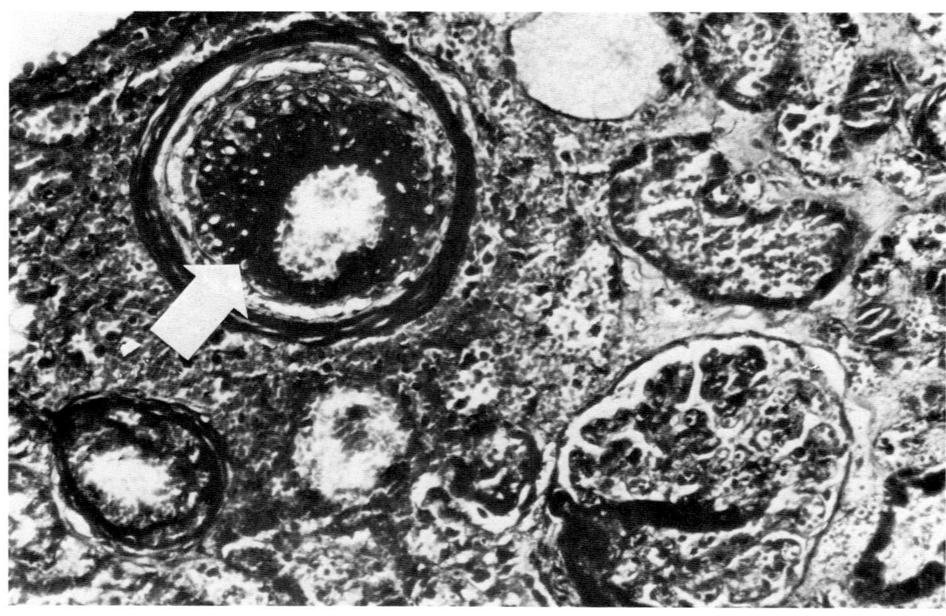

in the media, but it may also be present in the intima. Histochemical and immunofluorescent techniques have identified this material as fibrin. Within the media, muscle fibers cannot be identified. Cell nuclei are lost or fragmented. Whole or fragmented erythrocytes may be extravasated into the arteriolar wall. The hemorrhages that occur may account for the petechiae observed on the cortical surface. The arteriolar lumen may be reduced in size as a result of wall thickening and intraluminal fibrin thrombi. Infrequently, polymorphonuclear leukocytes and monocytes may infiltrate arterioles, giving the appearance of a necrotizing arteriolitis.

The *interlobular arteries* reveal characteristic lesions variously referred to as *proliferative endarteritis, productive endarteritis, endarteritis fibrosa,* or the *onionskin lesion.* The typical finding is intimal thickening that causes moderate to severe luminal narrowing. In severely affected vessels, the luminal diameter may be reduced to the size of a single red blood cell. Occasionally there is complete obliteration of the lumen by a fibrin thrombus.

Traditionally, three patterns of intimal thickening have been described [501]. The *onionskin* pattern consists of pale layers of elongated, concentrically arranged myointimal cells and delicate connective tissue fibrils that give rise to a lamellated appearance (Fig. 59-10). The media often appears as an attenuated layer stretched around the expanded intima. *Mucinous* intimal thickening consists of a sparsely cellular lesion containing a lucent, faintly basophilic staining, amorphous material (Fig. 59-11). In *fibrous* intimal thickening, there are hyaline deposits, reduplicated bands of elastica, and coarse layers of pale connective tissue with the staining properties of collagen (Fig. 59-12). In rare cases, fibrinoid necrosis may also be apparent in the interlobular arteries [501].

In blacks with malignant hypertension Pitcock et al. [385, 439] do not find fibrinoid necrosis of the afferent arterioles. Instead, they report a marked degree of arteriolar hyalinization. In addition, they describe a prominent and characteristic finding in the interlobular arteries and larger arterioles known as *musculomucoid intimal hyperplasia* (Fig. 59-13). The arterial walls are thickened by hyperplastic smooth muscle cells. A small amount of myxoid material, which stains light blue with hematoxylin and eosin, is observed between the cells. With periodic acid–Schiff staining, this material resembles basement membrane. Staining for acid mucopolysaccharide suggests the presence of chondroitin sulfate and possibly hyaluronic acid.

By electron microscopy, in each pattern of intimal thickening, the characteristic cellular element is a modified smooth muscle cell designated as the *myointimal cell.* In these cells there are smooth muscle–like ultrastructural features including cytoplasmic myofilaments and abundant rough endoplasmic reticulum [245, 501]. In the pure onionskin variant, the intercellular space is occupied by multiple strands of nonperiodic fibrils with the ultrastructural features of basement membrane [501]. In the mucinous variant, broad electron-lucent

Fig. 59-10. Onionskin lesion consisting of pale layers of elongated, concentrically arranged myointimal cells and delicate connective tissue fibrils that produce a lamellated appearance. The media is attenuated and stretched around the thickened intima (hematoxylin and eosin stain, × 350). (From R. A. Sinclair, T. T. Antonovych, and F. K. Mostofi. Renal proliferative arteriopathies and associated glomerular changes. A light and electron microscopic study. *Hum. Pathol.* 7:565, 1976. With permission.)

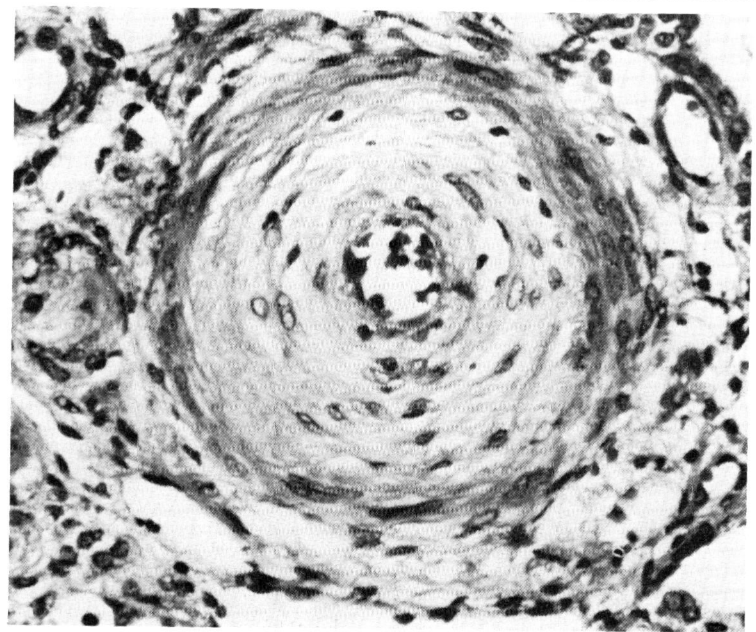

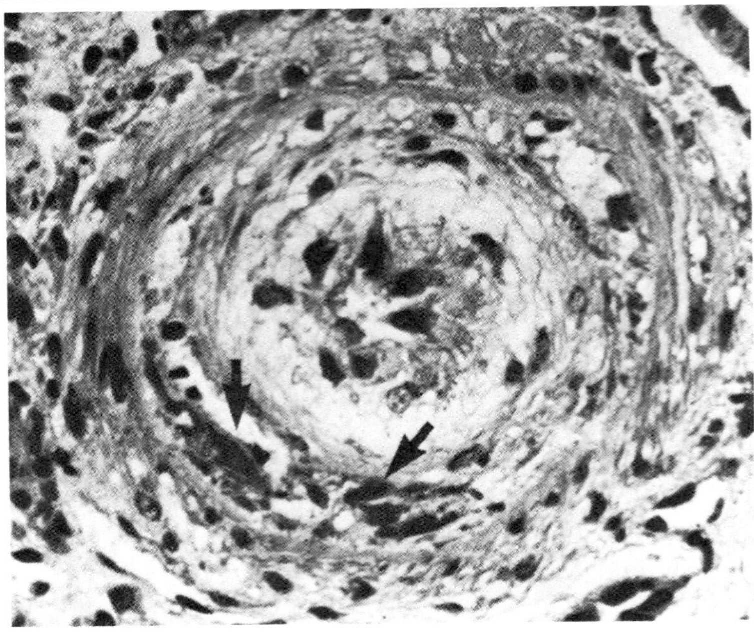

Fig. 59-11. Mucinous intimal thickening. The lesion is sparsely cellular and consists mainly of a lucent, faintly basophilic-staining amorphous material. There are small foci of fibrinoid necrosis (*arrows*) deep within the intima (hematoxylin and eosin stain, × 350). (From R. A. Sinclair, T. T. Antonovych, and F. K. Mostofi. Renal proliferative arteriopathies and associated glomerular changes. A light and electron microscopic study. *Hum. Pathol.* 7:565, 1976. With permission.)

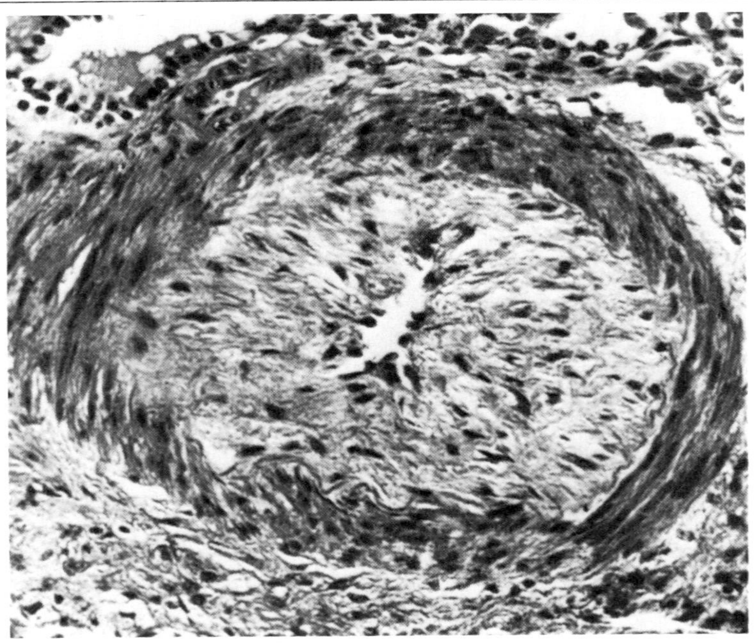

Fig. 59-12. Fibrous intimal thickening. The lesion consists of a thick layer of connective tissue, which stains for collagen and elastin (hematoxylin and eosin stain, × 300). (From R. A. Sinclair, T. T. Antonovych, and F. K. Mostofi. Renal proliferative arteriopathies and associated glomerular changes. A light and electron microscopic study. *Hum. Pathol.* 7:565, 1976. With permission.)

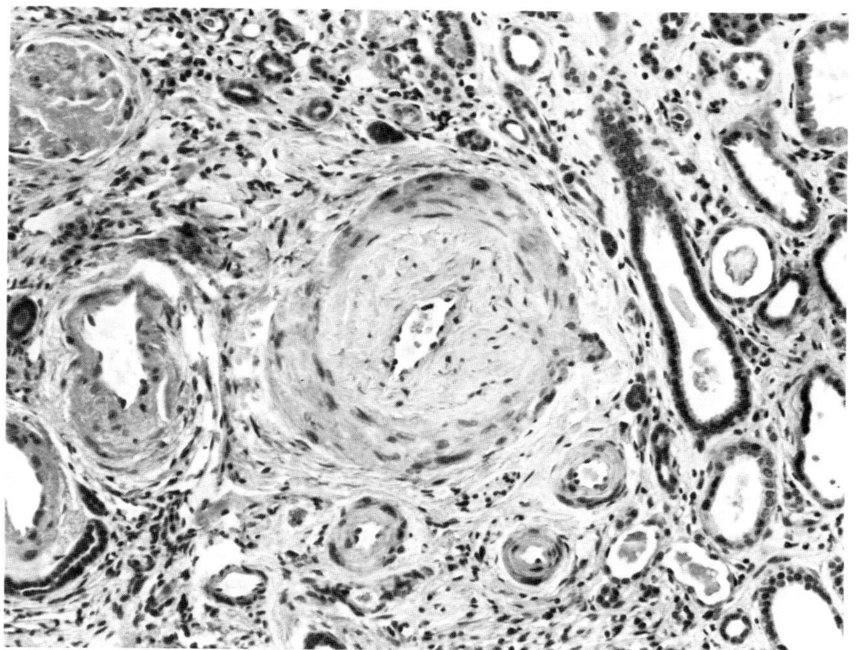

Fig. 59-13. Musculo-mucoid intimal hyperplasia of an interlobular artery. The arterial walls are thickened by hyperplastic smooth muscle cells. A small amount of myxoid material is seen between the smooth muscle cells (hematoxylin and eosin stain, × 170). (From J. A. Pitcock, J. G. Johnson, F. E. Hatch, et al. Malignant hypertension in blacks. Malignant intrarenal arterial disease as observed by light and electron microscopy. *Hum. Pathol.* 7:333, 1976. With permission.)

zones with scattered finely granular material are found in the intercellular space [245]. With the fibrous variant, numerous bundles of collagen, recognizable by the characteristic banding, are dispersed between the myointimal cells [501].

There are no characteristic changes in the arcuate and larger renal arteries in malignant hypertension. However, fibrous thickening and elastic reduplication may be found if long-standing benign hypertension is also present.

In large autopsy series from the pretreatment era, *focal and segmental fibrinoid necrosis* was the typical *glomerular* finding [228]. Glomerular lesions often occurred in continuity with a necrotic afferent arteriole. Glomerular crescent formation and segmental proliferation in areas of necrosis were also found. Rupture of these necrotic capillaries gave rise to hemorrhage into the glomerular or tubular space accounting for some of the petechiae seen grossly. The occurrence of this necrotizing glomerulonephritis led Volhard and Fahr [552] to propose that malignant nephrosclerosis was due to arteriosclerosis with superimposed exogenous nephritis. However, even in cases of terminal uremia, the percentage of involved glomeruli was found to be only 5 to 30 percent [228]. The focal and segmental nature of the glomerular lesion in primary malignant hypertension could be used to distinguish this entity from chronic glomerulonephritis with superimposed malignant phase in which glomerular involvement is diffuse and global [228].

The focal and segmental necrotizing lesions that were originally described in autopsy cases of untreated malignant hypertension are now rarely seen in tissue obtained at renal biopsy in treated patients [269, 439]. This observation might be due to the sampling error inherent in closed renal biopsy. Alternatively, these lesions may rapidly resolve with initiation of antihypertensive therapy and thus may not be apparent if renal biopsy is delayed.

In patients who have received antihypertensive therapy, as well as blacks with treated or untreated malignant hypertension, the most characteristic glomerular lesion found in malignant nephrosclerosis is *accelerated glomerular obsolescence* secondary to the intense ischemia produced by the obliterative arterial lesions [269, 439]. The earliest glomerular changes consist of thickening and wrinkling of the basement membrane (Fig. 59-14) [269, 439]. Later, there is shrinkage of the tuft such that it does not fill Bowman's space. There is laminar reduplication of Bowman's capsule around the shrunken glomerulus [501]. The end-stage is the *obsolescent glomerulus,* which is an avascular wrinkled glomerular tuft surrounded by a collagenous scar that fills Bowman's space (Fig. 59-15).

By electron microscopy, the lamina densa of the glomerular capillary basement membrane is thickened and wrinkled (Fig. 59-16) [269]. Eventually, the entire basement membrane becomes thickened. These glomerular changes are not specific for malignant nephrosclerosis,

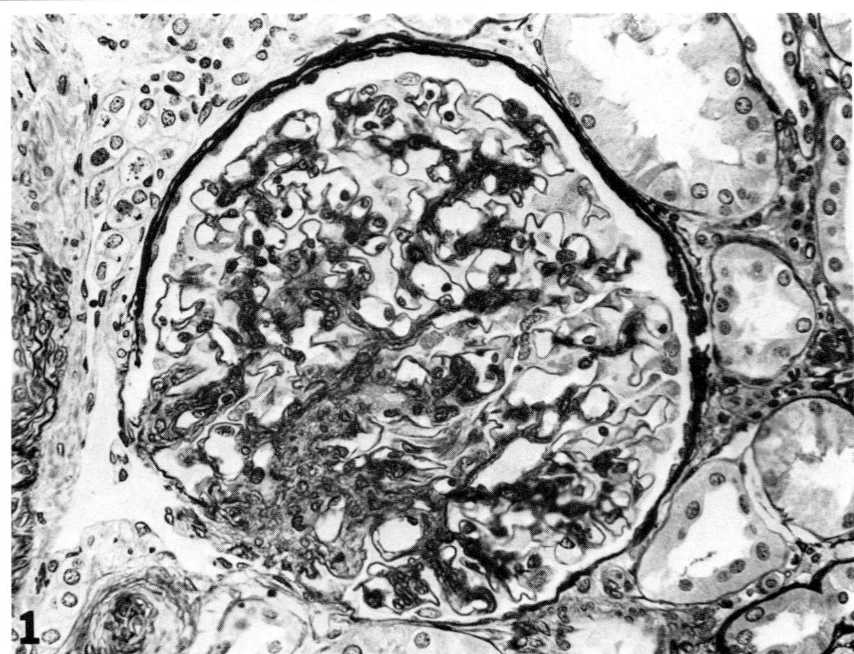

Fig. 59-14. The earliest ischemic glomerular change in malignant hypertension consists of some basement membrane wrinkling, particularly in areas adjacent to the mesangium, with a slight increase in mesangial matrix (periodic acid-silver methenamine stain, × 250). (From J. A. Pitcock, J. G. Johnson, F. E. Hatch, et al. Malignant hypertension in blacks. Malignant intrarenal arterial disease as observed by light and electron microscopy. *Hum. Pathol.* 7:333, 1976. With permission.)

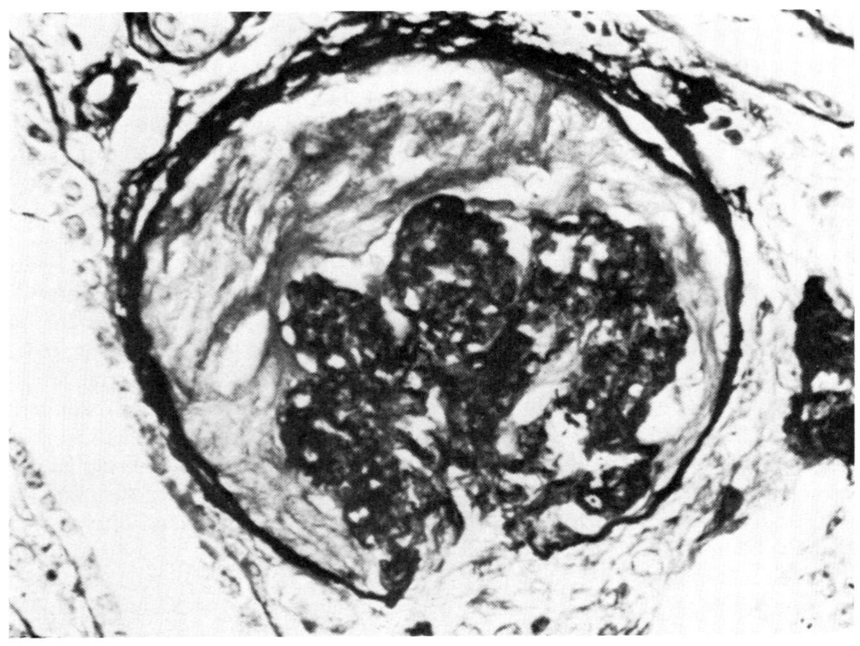

Fig. 59-15. Glomerular obsolescence in malignant hypertension. The collapsed, avascular glomerular tuft consists predominantly of markedly convoluted basement membranes. The sclerosed tuft is partially enclosed within a collar of hyaline filling Bowman's space (periodic acid-silver methenamine stain, × 485). (From R. A. Sinclair, T. T. Antonovych, and F. K. Mostofi. Renal proliferative arteriopathies and associated glomerular changes. A light and electron microscopic study. *Hum. Pathol.* 7:565, 1976. With permission.)

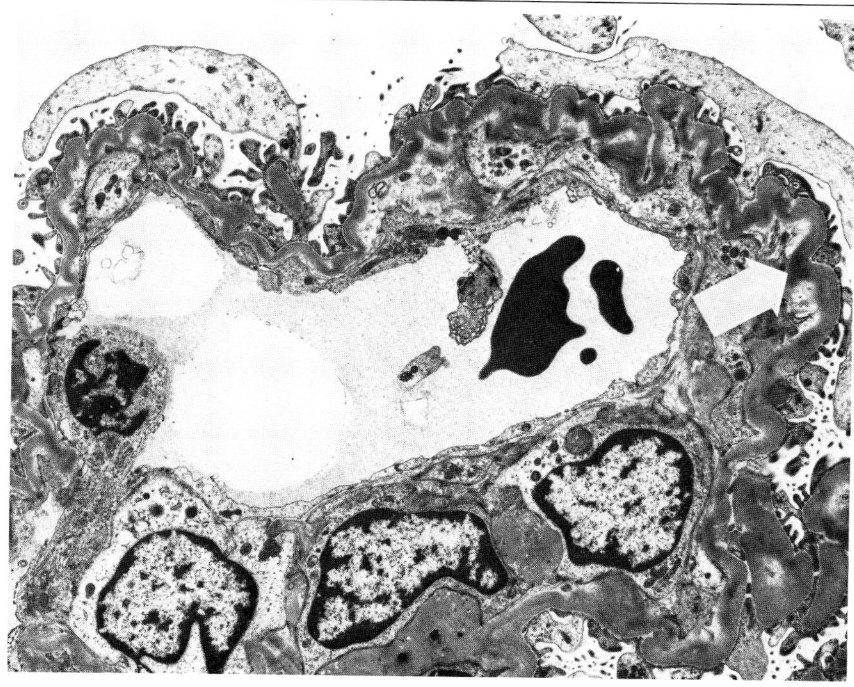

Fig. 59-16. Accelerated glomerular obsolescence in malignant hypertension. The glomerular capillaries show striking basement membrane wrinkling (*arrow*) and some reduplication of the inner basement membrane (uranyl acetate and lead citrate, ×4250). (From D. B. Jones. Arterial and glomerular lesions associated with severe hypertension. Light and electron microscopic studies. *Lab. Invest.* 31:303, 1974. With permission.)

since they may also occur in scleroderma renal crisis, hemolytic uremic syndrome, and even severe benign nephrosclerosis. However, the glomerular changes in malignant nephrosclerosis differ from the simple ischemic obsolescence observed in benign hypertension. In addition to the wrinkled basement membrane observed in benign nephrosclerosis, there is constriction of the glomerular vascular bed in malignant nephrosclerosis due to the deposition of a new subendothelial layer of basement membrane material inside the original basement membrane [269] (Fig. 59-17). The new capillary lumen formed by this process is smaller, resulting in a decreased blood volume in the ischemic glomerulus.

In malignant nephrosclerosis, the *tubules* may be atrophied and focally destroyed in areas supplied by severely narrowed arteries. Occasional tubules may be dilated and filled with eosinophilic cast material [228]. In the *interstitium* in these areas, there may be a fine reticular fibrosis and chronic inflammatory cells. In malignant hypertension, as in other renal parenchymal processes, renal insufficiency apparently appears to correlate best with the degree of tubular atrophy [439].

Immunofluorescence microscopy in patients with malignant nephrosclerosis demonstrates deposition of gamma globulin, fibrinogen, albumin, and sometimes complement in the walls of arterioles that have fibrinoid necrosis by light microscopy [421]. Some of the glomeruli, especially those with focal necrosis, contain gamma globulin, albumin, and complement. Fibrinogen is found diffusely along capillary basement membranes. Fibrinogen may be found in the intima of the interlobular arteries that by light microscopy show cellular or mucinous thickening [228].

Striking *juxtaglomerular hyperplasia* has been reported in patients with malignant hypertension [67, 269, 351]. This ultrastructural finding is consistent with the high-renin state often noted clinically [67].

Effective antihypertensive therapy may alter the pathology of malignant hypertension [218, 287, 348]. Within days, there may be resolution of fibrinoid necrosis, which leaves behind residual hyaline deposits in the arteriolar wall. In contrast to benign hypertension in which arteriolar hyaline change is often subendothelial, in treated malignant hypertension the hyaline material may be present throughout the entire vessel wall. Fibrosis of the arterioles with collagen replacement of the arteriolar muscle and elastica may also occur. Within several weeks after initiation of therapy, the segmental fibrinoid glomerular necrosis may also resolve, leaving behind an area of hyaline deposition. Furthermore, with treatment, in the intima of the interlobular arteries there may be an evolution from cellular hyperplasia to a more fibrous form of intimal thickening. A newly formed internal elastic lamina often separates this new collagen from the narrowed lumen. Heptinstall [228] has postulated that the cellular lesion is an early finding implying active disease, whereas the acellular fibrotic lesion is a later process often reflecting a response to treatment. These modifications in the interlobular arteries that occur following treatment may not be accompanied by any

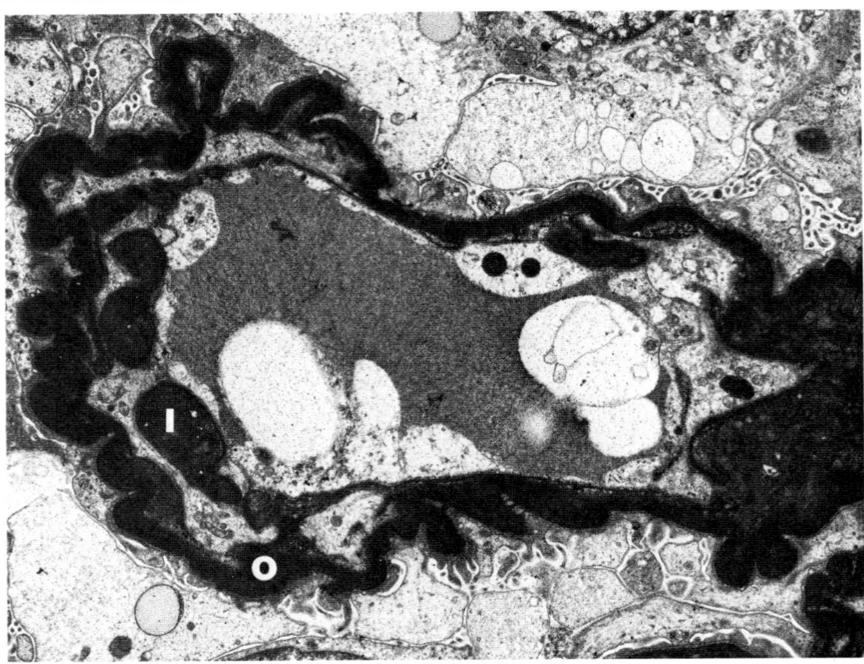

Fig. 59-17. Accelerated glomerular obsolescence in malignant hypertension. The outer basement membrane (O) is thickened and wrinkled. There is a reduplicated inner basement membrane (I) with the capillary lumen still patent (uranyl acetate and lead citrate stain, × 4250). (From D. B. Jones. Arterial and glomerular lesions associated with severe hypertension. Light and electron microscopic studies. *Lab. Invest.* 31:303, 1974. With permission.)

increase in the caliber of the lumen. Severely narrowed interlobular arteries often do not improve, and the renal parenchyma distal to these arteries undergoes severe ischemic atrophy and scarring [287]. However, the nephrons supplied by interlobular arteries of normal caliber may undergo substantial hypertrophy following treatment of malignant hypertension. This pathologic finding may explain the improvement in renal function that occurs in some patients following institution of antihypertensive therapy with resolution of the malignant phase.

In summary, although fibrinoid necrosis was the hallmark of malignant nephrosclerosis in untreated patients at autopsy, it is now rarely observed. In treated patients with malignant hypertension or blacks with malignant hypertension, closed renal biopsy most often reveals marked intimal hyperplasia of the interlobular arteries in association with accelerated glomerular obsolescence [269, 385, 439].

Renal Pathology in Secondary Malignant Hypertension. A variety of primary renal parenchymal diseases may cause secondary malignant hypertension. Although it is often impossible to differentiate primary (essential) malignant hypertension from secondary malignant hypertension by clinical criteria, the distinction can usually be made by renal biopsy.

Malignant hypertension may develop during the course of *chronic glomerulonephritis.* When glomerulonephritis causes malignant hypertension, there is usually evidence of diffuse glomerulonephritis in addition to the vascular lesions seen in malignant nephrosclerosis. In contrast to the focal and segmental glomerular lesions seen in primary malignant hypertension, in secondary malignant hypertension due to chronic glomerulonephritis, diffuse and global changes usually involve more than 90 percent of glomeruli [228, 240, 336].

Chronic pyelonephritis may also cause secondary malignant hypertension. The pyelonephritic process may be unilateral or bilateral. There is coarse irregular scarring of the kidney(s), as well as difference in the size and shape of the two kidneys [288]. The cortex is affected in a patchy fashion with alternating areas of scarred and normal-appearing tissue. Histologically, alternating areas of sharply demarcated normal and scarred parenchyma are observed [226]. In scarred areas, there are dilated, colloid-filled tubules, crowded hyalinized glomeruli, and periglomerular fibrosis. In the interstitium, there is severe fibrosis with a chronic inflammatory infiltrate. Vascular lesions indistinguishable from malignant nephrosclerosis may be seen in scarred areas, even in normotensive subjects with chronic pyelonephritis. However, with superimposed malignant hypertension, vascular lesions of malignant hypertension are found in nonscarred areas of the kidney [226, 560]. Moreover, in unilateral pyelonephritis with superimposed malignant hypertension, histologic findings of malignant hypertension occur in the contralateral kidney [226].

In the microscopic form of *polyarteritis nodosa* (PAN), fibrinoid necrosis of the afferent arterioles and proliferative endarteritis of the interlobular arteries may occur in the absence of malignant hypertension. However, secondary malignant hypertension has been reported in patients with PAN [226, 288]. Primary malignant hypertension and secondary malignant hypertension due to PAN can be differentiated histologically. In PAN, there is usually diffuse glomerular involvement as well as an active cellular infiltrate in the necrotic vascular and glomerular lesions [228]. In addition, there are often healed and active necrotizing lesions typical of PAN in larger, medium-sized muscular arteries of the kidney, mesentery, pancreas, and adrenals. Involvement of vessels of this size in primary malignant hypertension is rarely observed [226].

In *scleroderma renal crisis*, changes in the renal vessels may be virtually identical to primary malignant hypertension [71]. The characteristic extrarenal manifestations of progressive systemic sclerosis must be used to differentiate these two entities.

Distribution of Vascular Lesions in Malignant Hypertension. Malignant hypertension is a diffuse hypertension-induced vasculopathy, and in its terminal stages, widespread arterial and arteriolar lesions are found in a variety of organs [288, 554]. These vascular changes are similar to those seen in the kidney, namely, proliferative endarteritis of small arteries and fibrinoid necrosis of arterioles. The vascular beds of the pancreas, gastrointestinal tract, and liver are most frequently involved [279]. However, similar vascular lesions have been described in the retina [83], brain [83, 147], myocardium [279], prostate [288], and skeletal muscle [554]. The pathologic changes in the various organs and tissues are secondary to ischemia caused by these obliterative vascular changes.

Ophthalmic Pathology. Chester et al. [83] found that among 17 patients with malignant hypertension, thickening and hyalinization of the walls of the arterioles and capillaries of the retina and choroid were present in every case. Fibrinoid necrosis was seen in 8 patients. Fibrin thrombi in the arterioles were seen in 13 patients. Microaneurysms at or near the occluded segments of capillaries were found in 8 patients. Small ischemic infarcts of the retina (cytoid bodies), corresponding to the cotton-wool spots seen clinically, were present in 16 patients. They were located in the nerve fiber and ganglion cell layers of the retina in the vicinity of vascular lesions. The arterioles supplying the optic nerve were thickened and hyalinized to varying degrees, and fibrinoid necrosis was found in 7 patients.

Cardiac Pathology. Left ventricular hypertrophy with normal chamber size is the predominant finding in most patients with malignant hypertension [288, 482]. Severe coronary atherosclerosis is a rare finding in these patients [288, 482].

Pulmonary Pathology. In the era before effective antihypertensive therapy, uremic edema of the lung was frequently found in fatal cases of malignant hypertension [135]. Gross examination of the lungs revealed widespread gelatinous consolidation, which was most intense in the perihilar region.

Adrenal Pathology. Fibrinoid necrosis of the small arterioles of the adrenal glands is observed in up to 50 percent of fatal cases of malignant hypertension [288]. The adrenal glands are often enlarged with multiple macroscopic nodules. This adrenal hyperplasia reflects activation of the renin-angiotensin-aldosterone axis [307].

Gastrointestinal Pathology. Significant arteriolopathy of the mesenteric vessels is a frequent finding in patients with malignant hypertension [279]. In addition, among 100 cases of malignant hypertension, 60 percent had proliferative endarteritis of the pancreatic arterioles [244]. Pancreatic lesions were frequently found, including infarcts associated with arterial thrombosis, focal parenchymal necrosis, and foci of atrophy and fibrosis.

PATHOPHYSIOLOGY OF MALIGNANT HYPERTENSION

On the basis of the clinical presentation, natural history, and vascular and renal pathology, it can be concluded that benign and malignant hypertension are distinct clinicopathologic entities rather than a spectrum of the same disease. However, the mechanism that initiates the transition from the benign to the malignant phase is not entirely clear and remains the subject of considerable controversy. The primary function of the microcirculation is to ensure that the cardiac output is distributed to a variety of tissues, which vary widely in metabolic requirements. The arterioles control the blood flow to the capillary network through the process of autoregulation. It is not surprising, therefore, that the arterioles are the major target of the acute vascular damage in malignant hypertension. However, the central question is whether severe hypertension alone is sufficient to cause the vascular injury characteristic of the malignant phase or whether additional co-factors are required to produce the vascular injury.

Role of Increased Blood Pressure Per Se (The Pressure Hypothesis). According to the pressure hypothesis, the development of fibrinoid necrosis and proliferative endarteritis is a direct consequence of the mechanical stress placed on the vessel walls by severe hypertension [34, 65, 163, 228, 435]. Several lines of evidence support the hypothesis that severe hypertension is the fundamental pathophysiologic process underlying the malignant phase. In this regard, the malignant phase may occur in hypertension of diverse etiologies, the common denominator being severe hypertension. Regardless of etiology, the malignant phase is reversible given adequate blood pressure control [436]. The transition from the benign to the malignant phase is usually accompanied by a dramatic rise in blood pressure [435]. In addition, the occurrence of fibrinoid necrosis tends to correlate with the height of the arterial pressure. Heptinstall [227] studied the arterial lesions in renal biopsies obtained at the time of sympathectomy for blood pressure control. Although there was overlap, the frequency distribution of diastolic blood pressures differed between patients with and without arteriolar necrosis. Arterial necrosis appeared at a diastolic blood pressure of around 150 mm Hg and became progressively more severe as the arterial pressure increased.

Another finding supporting the crucial role of severe hypertension in the development of the vascular lesions of malignant hypertension is the absence of these lesions in vascular beds protected from the elevated blood pressure. In the two-kidney, two-clip model of malignant hypertension in the dog, vascular necroses were found in mesenteric arterioles and other vessels exposed to the high pressure, but not in renal arterioles that were protected from the high perfusion pressure [191]. Likewise, in rats with two-kidney, one-clip malignant hypertension, there were vascular necrotic lesions in the nonclipped kidney and the systemic circulation but not in the clipped kidney [564]. Patients with unilateral renal artery stenosis and malignant hypertension have been reported in whom arteriolar necrosis occurred in the contralateral kidney but not in the stenotic kidney [479].

A number of experimental models of malignant hypertension lend support to the pressure hypothesis. Brief overdistention of the arteriolar system by forceful injection of saline into the aorta was shown to result in a sudden increase in mean arterial pressure of 80 to 90 mm Hg accompanied by the development of fibrinoid necrosis in the interlobular arteries and afferent arterioles of the kidney [66]. Fibrinoid necrosis failed to develop if the kidney was protected from the sudden rise in pressure.

Byrom [63] utilized windows in the skull and abdominal wall to view the microcirculation in rats with one-kidney, one-clip malignant hypertension. Cerebral and mesenteric arterioles developed focal constrictions and dilatations, giving rise to a string of beads or *sausage string pattern.* Intravenous injection of trypan blue resulted in patchy leakage of dye in the dilated regions but not in constricted regions. These dilated areas were found to be the site of fibrinoid necrosis [64].

Giese found that the sausage string pattern developed rapidly in mesenteric arterioles in the rat when the blood pressure was raised acutely with angiotensin or norepinephrine [186, 187]. When colloidal carbon particles were injected, carbon was deposited in the walls of dilated segments but not constricted segments. He concluded that the abnormal vascular pattern was the direct result of elevated blood pressure and that the dilated segments represented the earliest site of vascular damage as manifest by increased permeability to plasma proteins.

Goldby and Beilin [193] found that the extent of carbon deposition was related to the height of arterial pressure rather than to the type of pressor substance infused (i.e., angiotensin, norepinephrine, or renal extract). If the increase in blood pressure was prevented by the administration of hydralazine, the sausage string pattern failed to develop and carbon was not deposited in the vascular walls. The authors concluded that the abnormal permeability in dilated segments was the result of hypertension-induced structural damage to the vessel wall. They found no evidence to support the concept of a direct vasculotoxic effect of angiotensin or norepinephrine independent of their pressor effect.

These sausage string lesions were evaluated using electron microscopy [194]. In dilated segments, breaks in the endothelium were observed as a result of disruption of intracellular junctions or destruction of the cell body. These lesions gave rise to gaps in the endothelium that were permeable to intravenously injected colloidal carbon particles. Amorphous deposits consisting of plasma, carbon particles, and fibrin-like material were seen in the media. These deposits displaced and destroyed smooth muscle cells. The vascular lesions did not appear to be caused by a direct vasculotoxic effect of angiotensin because identical results were reported with deoxycorticosterone acetate (DOCA)-salt hypertension, a model in which angiotensin levels are suppressed [192].

Based on these experiments, it was concluded that the mechanical stress of severe hypertension was the central cause of fibrinoid necrosis in the malignant phase. All of the vascular changes could be attributed to the indirect pressor effect of the infused substances rather than to any direct effect of these substances on vascular permeability. The following mechanism for the development of fibrinoid necrosis was proposed [64, 186, 187, 194]. When the arterial pressure is sufficiently increased by whatever means, local areas of the arterial wall are unable to withstand the mechanical stress and become dilated. Since smooth muscle may not be uniformly distributed along arterioles, some areas are unable to withstand mechanical stress and are forcibly vasodilated. By the law of LaPlace, as the radius increases in dilated segments, wall tension increases proportionately. As a consequence, the endothelium may become stretched, damaged, and abnormally permeable. Plasma proteins and fibrinogen then pass into the vessel wall, compressing and destroying smooth muscle. Local fibrinogen deposition occurs, producing fibrinoid necrosis.

The Vasculotoxic Theory. The major criticism of the pressure hypothesis is that there is substantial overlap between the levels of blood pressure observed in patients with benign hypertension and those with malignant hypertension [40, 288]. Moreover, occasional patients sustain severe diastolic hypertension for long periods without ever progressing to the malignant phase [285]. The abrupt change from an asymptomatic patient with severe hypertension to a critically ill patient with a multisystem disease suggests that factors in addition to blood pressure may contribute to the transition from the benign to the malignant phase [286]. According to the vasculotoxic theory, severe hypertension is necessary but not sufficient to cause the malignant phase.

The vasculotoxic theory proposes that humoral factors cause the vascular damage observed in malignant hypertension. Based on his classic dog model of renovascular hypertension, Goldblatt [191] felt that renal failure was a necessary cofactor for the development of the malignant phase. He proposed that a vasculotoxic factor accumulated in severe renal disease. However, it has subsequently been demonstrated, in both humans and experimental animals, that malignant hypertension can develop in the absence of uremia and even before the vascular lesions of malignant nephrosclerosis develop in the kidney [148, 281].

Others have suggested that vascular permeability factors of renal origin (renin or angiotensin), catecholamines, or vasopressin may cause vascular damage independent of their pressor effects. For example, administration of rat kidney extracts to nephrectomized rats produced a lethal syndrome characterized by large pleural and peritoneal effusions, edema of the pancreas, and the arteriolar fibrinoid necrosis characteristic of malignant hypertension [14]. To explain these findings, the presence of a vascular permeability factor of renal origin was postulated. Identical findings have been produced by constriction of both renal arteries and by the administration of semipurified hog renin to nephrectomized rats [186, 187]. In addition, there are reports of acute vascular lesions produced in rats and dogs by the injection of renal extracts [316, 394, 568].

Each of these experiments purported to demonstrate that a vascular permeability factor of renal origin, presumably the renin-angiotensin system, caused the arteriolar necrosis. Unfortunately, blood pressure was not measured in these studies. Thus it is also possible that arteriolar necrosis occurred as a consequence of the pressor response to these maneuvers [344].

Robertson and Khairallah [465] have provided convincing evidence that angiotensin II does have a direct effect on the vascular endothelium to increase permeability. In these studies Evans blue dye was administered intravenously in rabbits, and a segment of abdominal aorta was isolated between temporary ligatures. The injection of 100 pgm of angiotensin II into the isolated segment caused a diffuse increase in permeability of the aortic endothelium as evidenced by staining with blue dye. Areas of the aorta not exposed to angiotensin II showed no increase in permeability. Injections of Ringer's solution (vehicle) produced no blue staining of the aortic endothelium. Evaluation of the areas exposed to angiotensin II by electron microscopy revealed rounding and shortening of the endothelial cells with widening of spaces between endothelial cells.

Studies of dermal capillary permeability in response to vasoactive agents have confirmed the fact that there appears to be a direct effect of angiotensin II on vascular endothelium [465]. When norepinephrine or angiotensin I was injected into the dermis, there was no extravasation of Evans blue dye. However, when angiotensin II was injected in low concentrations, there was severe capillary leak. The increased permeability could be prevented by simultaneous administration of angiotensin II receptor antagonists but not by antihistamines. The authors concluded that angiotensin II increased vascular permeability independent of a pressor response by causing contraction of endothelial cells [465].

Role of the Renin-Angiotensin Axis in Malignant Hypertension. In patients with malignant hypertension there is often evidence of activation of the renin-angiotensin system [32, 307]. At the time of presentation, some but not all patients have elevated PRA [347]. There is often hyperplasia of the juxtaglomerular apparatus [351]. The adrenal glands frequently reveal hyperplasia and nodularity of the zona glomerulosa [307].

In patients with malignant hypertension, activation of the renin-angiotensin system may be primary or secondary. For example, activation of the renin-angiotensin system could be a critical step in the conversion from the benign to the malignant phase through either direct (vasculotoxic) or indirect (hypertensive) effects on the vasculature. Conversely, hyperreninemia may be a secondary phenomenon occurring in response to renal ischemia produced by the malignant arteriolar lesions. These two processes are not mutually exclusive. In fact, both may occur simultaneously, resulting in a vicious cycle of hypertension-induced vascular damage causing renal ischemia, which leads to enhanced renin release, which may exacerbate the hypertensive process.

Möhring et al. [375] have extensively studied the course of malignant hypertension in rats using the two-kidney, one-clip model of renal hypertension [375]. Onset of the malignant phase occurs after 3 to 5 weeks. The course of hypertension was predictable and followed a typical pattern. Following application of a sufficiently small clip to the renal artery, the renin-angiotensin system was activated. When the systolic blood pressure surpassed a critical level of 180 to 190 mm Hg, spontaneous natriuresis and diuresis occurred. Water intake increased, but weight loss and hyponatremia ensued. Eventually, renal function deteriorated, and the microscopic findings of malignant nephrosclerosis were apparent in the contralateral kidney. The rats eventually died of renal failure, heart failure, or cerebral hemorrhage. In this model of malignant hypertension, it was apparent that a vicious cycle developed following activation of the renin-angiotensin system. Renal ischemia resulted in activation of the renin-angiotensin system with the development of hypertension. The severe hypertension caused natriuresis, diuresis, and volume depletion. Volume depletion further stimulated the renin-angiotensin system. As the gain on this cycle increased, hypertension induced vascular damage or the direct vasculotoxic effect of angiotensin induced vascular damage and deterioration of renal function [372]. Volume depletion was pivotal in the pathogenesis of this model of malignant hypertension. Rats with malignant hypertension, given a choice of deionized water or normal saline, exhibited compulsive saline drinking [376]. During the first 24 hours of saline drinking, there was a marked decrease in blood pressure and an increase in body weight. Moreover, there was correction of the abnormal levels of hematocrit, serum sodium, renin, and angiotensin II. With continued saline drinking for 2 to 7 days, the blood pressure increased to the previous high levels, but signs of malignant hypertension did not recur. If saline was withdrawn at that time, within 2 days the cycle of natriuresis, activation of the renin-angiotensin system, and malignant hypertension recurred. Thus the pathogenesis of malignant hypertension in this model appears to be critically dependent on spontaneous natriuresis, volume depletion, and activation of the renin-angiotensin system.

Gross et al. [206] investigated the role of the contralateral kidney in the spontaneous natriuresis and diuresis. In rats with one-kidney, one-clip hypertension, there was no phase of renal salt loss. Likewise, in rats with two-kidney, two-clip hypertension, the phase of salt loss did not occur. However, if one clip was removed, there was an immediate onset of a salt-losing state associated with the syndrome of malignant hypertension and fibrinoid necrosis in the unclipped kidney. The authors concluded that the spontaneous natriuresis of malignant hypertension was mediated by the contralateral kidney in the two-kidney, one-clip model.

Evidence of involvement of the renin-angiotensin system in the development of the malignant phase was also found in the experimental model of hypertension produced by complete aortic ligation between the renal arteries [80, 85]. The relation between blood pressure, PRA, and interlobular arterial lesions in the nonischemic kidney was studied in rats undergoing aortic ligation. After surgery, rats drank either ad lib tap water or normal saline. In the group on tap water, mean arterial pressure correlated with the increase in PRA, and blood pressure and PRA correlated with the extent of histologic damage. In the group on normal saline, however, mean arterial pressure did not correlate with PRA, and there was no correlation between the level of pressure and the extent of histologic damage. In contrast, there was a correlation between PRA and the degree of vascular injury. The authors concluded that the level of PRA, independent of its effect on pressure, correlated with the vascular change in malignant hypertension. This effect was presumed to be mediated by a direct vasculotoxic effect of renin or angiotensin II.

Whereas activation of the renin-angiotensin system may be crucial in the development of the malignant phase in some experimental models and some patients with malignant hypertension, the clinical and pathologic features of malignant hypertension may occur in the absence of activation of the renin-angiotensin system [347]. For example, widespread necrotizing arteriolar disease occurs in hypertension caused by bilateral nephrectomy in experimental animals [386].

Dietz et al. [126] studied a number of models of malignant hypertension and concluded that the mechanical load on the vascular system caused by the height of the blood pressure or by the rapidity of the increase in blood pressure was more important in the genesis of the vasculopathy than were hormonal factors such as the renin-angiotensin system. For example, in the two-kidney, one-clip and one-kidney, one-clip models of renal hypertension, they were able to demonstrate that malignant hypertension developed at a time when the renin-angiotensin system was suppressed. Furthermore, they found that the administration of DOCA to animals with two-kidney, one-clip benign hypertension resulted in suppression of PRA but caused the transition to the malignant phase.

In summary, neither hypersecretion of renin nor the presence of kidneys are necessary for the development of malignant hypertension. On the other hand, a high concentration of angiotensin II may be an aggravating factor or, in some circumstances, may actually trigger the transition from the benign to the malignant phase. Activation of the renin-angiotensin system by renal ischemia may contribute to the vicious cycle of malignant hypertension.

Role of Vasopressin in Malignant Hypertension. Gavras et al. [182] studied the model of malignant hypertension resulting from administration of DOCA and salt to unilaterally nephrectomized rats. The animals were in positive sodium balance for 3 to 4 weeks with a progressive increase in weight and blood pressure. At the time when blood pressure had reached a maximum, there were no arteriolar lesions in the kidney compatible with malignant nephrosclerosis. Over the ensuing weeks, there occurred periods of spontaneous natriuresis and diuresis as evidenced by hemoconcentration. These findings marked the onset of the malignant phase with fibrinoid necrosis in the kidney. Plasma renin activity was markedly suppressed throughout the experiment, and infusion of angiotensin II inhibitors failed to cause a depressor response. Möhring et al. [373] extended these observations and demonstrated a role for vasopressin in the DOCA-salt model of malignant hypertension. At the time of the development of the malignant phase, they found that plasma arginine vasopressin (AVP) levels were 10 times higher than those in control animals and three times higher than those in animals with benign hypertension. In addition, the administration of biologically active AVP antisera resulted in a transient reduction in blood pressure to normal or subnormal levels. Since AVP and norepinephrine levels have been shown to be elevated in DOCA hypertension, it has been postulated that AVP and perhaps catecholamines may be important in DOCA-salt hypertension [458].

Möhring et al. [374] have also reported data that suggest a possible role for AVP in the two-kidney, one-clip model of malignant hypertension. They have found AVP to be three times higher than in rats with benign hypertension and four to five times higher than in normotensive control rats. The administration of AVP antisera resulted in a reduction of blood pressure to normal values in 4 of 8 animals. The authors hypothesized that the spontaneous natriuresis, diuresis, and volume depletion that activate the renin axis in malignant hypertension may also stimulate vasopressin release. They concluded that both the renin-angiotensin system and AVP may contribute to the development of the malignant phase.

In contrast to studies demonstrating a role for AVP in malignant hypertension, there are a number of studies suggesting that malignant hypertension can occur independent of AVP. In both the DOCA-salt and the two-kidney, one-clip malignant hypertension model, Rabito et al. [449] found that the administration of vasopressin antagonists did not cause a significant fall in blood pressure. Woods et al. observed that malignant hypertension developed in AVP-deficient Brattleboro rats after aortic ligation [572]. Padfield et al. [415] measured vasopressin levels in 29 patients with untreated malignant hypertension prior to antihypertensive therapy. Although plasma vasopressin levels were higher than in normal subjects (13 ± 2 versus 5.8 ± 0.2 pg/ml), there was no correlation between vasopressin levels and the height of the blood pressure. Moreover, the infusion of AVP into normal volunteers to obtain AVP levels greater than those found in patients with malignant hypertension did not increase blood pressure. In addition, they were not able to identify an increase in blood pressure in any of 28 patients with the syndrome of inappropriate antidiuretic hormone secretion due to bronchogenic carcinoma who had an average vasopressin level of 40 pg per milliliter. The authors concluded that vasopressin excess does not contribute to blood pressure elevation or to the syndrome of malignant hypertension in humans. These data, however, do not entirely exclude a pathogenetic role for AVP in malignant hypertension. It is possible that there is an increased sensitivity to the pressor effect of AVP or that AVP exerts a permissive effect by enhancing the pressor response to angiotensin II or catecholamines. Also, their data do not exclude a direct vasculotoxic effect of AVP in patients with malignant hypertension.

Role of Volume Depletion in Malignant Hypertension. In several experimental models, spontaneous natriuresis appears to be the initiating event in the transition from the benign to the malignant phase of hypertension [140, 182, 325, 372, 375]. In patients with malignant hypertension, an abrupt onset of weight loss early in the course of the disease has been reported [133, 147, 281, 288, 366, 453]. In the series of Kincaid-Smith et al. [288], the transition from the benign to the malignant phase often appeared suddenly. With little change in blood pressure, the patients became suddenly ill with weakness, wasting, and profound weight loss. The rapidity of the weight loss could only be explained by the loss of total body salt and water and may be the human counterpart of Möhring's two-kidney, one-clip renovascular hypertension model of malignant hypertension in which spontaneous natriuresis preceded the onset of the malignant phase [372, 375]. Barraclough [25] has reported a well-documented case of malignant hypertension caused by unilateral renal artery stenosis in which sudden and profound weight loss and natriuresis developed at the time of onset of the malignant phase. When the ischemic kidney was revascularized, the malignant phase resolved.

Travis et al. [541] and Gill et al. [189] described patients with malignant hypertension who were unable to conserve sodium on a low sodium intake. Excessive quantities of sodium were lost in the urine, and hypovolemic hyponatremia developed. When the hypertension was effectively controlled, the defect in sodium conservation resolved. In analgesic nephropathy, volume depletion has been found to precipitate the malignant phase, whereas restoration of volume reduced blood pressure and reversed the malignant phase [395].

In summary, it appears that volume depletion due to spontaneous natriuresis is often associated with the transition from the benign to the malignant phase of hypertension in both experimental and human malignant hypertension. The mechanism of the spontaneous salt wasting is not known. In the isolated, perfused kidney, an acute increase in arterial perfusion pressure results in increased urine flow rate and sodium excretion [490]. Since glomerular filtration rate and renal blood flow remain unchanged, the natriuresis has been attributed to inhibition of tubular sodium resorption by elevated blood pressure. Angiotensin II also influences sodium excretion independent of its effect on blood pressure. The net effect of angiotensin II on renal sodium handling may be dose dependent. Small doses of angiotensin reduce sodium excretion. The increase in efferent arteriolar resistance caused by angiotensin II causes a fall in hydrostatic pressure and an increase in oncotic pressure in the peritubular capillaries, which results in enhanced sodium reabsorption. Angiotensin II also directly stimulates proximal tubular sodium reabsorption [86a]. In contrast, large doses of angiotensin II may increase sodium excretion [58, 423]. These observations suggest that there may be a threshold level of activity of the renin-angiotensin system for sodium metabolism above which sodium wasting occurs. Perhaps in the setting of severe hypertension, renin production from the ischemic kidney is in excess of this threshold. However, the mechanism of spontaneous natriuresis in malignant hypertension remains obscure.

Role of Localized Intravascular Coagulation in Malignant Hypertension. Evidence of microangiopathic hemolytic anemia and disorders of coagulation and fibrinolysis has been reported in experimental models of malignant hypertension [548]. This anemia is characterized by red cell fragmentation and evidence of intravascular hemolysis (hemoglobinuria and iron in the renal tubules).

Since intravascular coagulation is found in malignant hypertension, it has been postulated to be important in the pathogenesis of the malignant phase. Severe hypertension, perhaps augmented by vasculotoxic factors, injures arteriolar walls. This injury leads to an increase in endothelial permeability to fibrinogen and other plasma proteins. The clotting cascade is initiated by tissue thromboplastin and fibrin deposited in the wall and the lumen of the vessel. Platelets are deposited, and microangiopathic hemolytic anemia is produced by fragmentation of red blood cells as they traverse intravascular fibrin strands. The lysis of platelets and red blood cells produces adenosine diphosphate (ADP) and thromboplastin, which aggravate intravascular coagulation and produce a vicious cycle of hemolysis and fibrin deposition. Tissue ischemia is produced by a combination of intravascular fibrin deposition and arteriolar wall thickening, which constrict the vessel lumen.

In this scheme, intravascular coagulation is the consequence of hypertension-induced vascular injury. It has also been postulated that the coagulation abnormalities may be the primary event that causes the transition from the benign to the malignant phase [183]. This theory is based on the observation that renal vascular lesions identical to those in primary malignant nephrosclerosis can occur in idiopathic postpartum renal failure and the hemolytic uremic syndrome. In these disorders, abnormalities of coagulation and fibrinoid necrosis often preceded the development of hypertension [48].

Role of Prostacyclin in Malignant Hypertension. Abnormal prostacyclin (PGI_2) metabolism has recently been postulated to play a role in the pathogenesis of malignant hypertension in cigarette smokers and women taking oral contraceptives [430]. Enhanced PGI_2 synthesis by vessel walls may be a protective mechanism that limits the vascular injury caused by hypertension [475]. For example, PGI_2 may limit the extent of thrombus formation at sites of endothelial injury. Both oral contraceptives [578] and cigarette smoking [355] are associated with lower concentrations of 6-keto-$PGF_{1\alpha}$, a stable metabolite of PGI_2. Impaired vessel wall synthesis of PGI_2 in hypertensive cigarette smokers or women taking oral contraceptives may predispose to the development of malignant hypertension [430]. Moreover, absence of the protective effect of PGI_2 could amplify the vascular endothelial injury caused by severe hypertension.

Role of Intracellular Calcium in Malignant Hypertension. Increased availability of free calcium in vascular smooth muscle may be important in the pathogenesis of hypertension. Moreover, it has recently been suggested that an excess of cytosolic calcium may be a crucial step in the development of malignant hypertension and that this deleterious calcium overload may be activated or inhibited independent of the arterial blood pressure [277].

Dahl salt-sensitive rats on a high-salt diet develop fulminant hypertension with a necrotizing vasculopathy in the kidney. However, treatment with nifedipine, which inhibits calcium influx via activated membrane calcium channels, prevents the rise in blood pressure and the occurrence of necrotizing vascular lesions. A similar protective effect has been described with nisoldipine and nitrendipine but not with captopril [277].

The stroke-prone spontaneously hypertensive rat (SHR-SP) is another experimental model of malignant hypertension that mimics the renal and vascular changes of human essential malignant hypertension [406]. In salt-loaded SHR-SP rats, treatment with either nimodipine or parathyroidectomy dramatically reduces vascular injury and mortality despite an insignificant effect on the level of blood pressure [277]. Since hypertension-induced vascular injury can be prevented by manipulation of calcium influx into cells, it has been postulated that vascular injury in malignant hypertension may be mediated by calcium overload in vascular smooth muscle cells.

Patients with malignant hypertension, when compared to normotensive controls or patients with nonmalignant hypertension, have been found to have abnormalities of erythrocyte sodium transport leading to elevated intra-erythrocyte sodium concentration [230]. Although the cause of this abnormal sodium transport is unknown, the resulting increase in cellular sodium content may cause an increase in cytosolic calcium, which in vascular smooth muscle would lead to vasoconstriction and increased peripheral resistance [45]. The increase in cytosolic calcium may also mediate vascular injury as discussed above.

Role of Dietary Potassium in Malignant Hypertension. It has been shown that in Dahl salt-sensitive rats on a high-salt diet, supplementation of dietary potassium intake can prevent the hypertension-induced intimal thickening of the interlobular arteries without a concomitant reduction in blood pressure [537]. A high-potassium diet has also been shown to prevent the intimal thickening of mesenteric and cerebral arteries, independent of an effect on blood pressure, in the stroke-prone spontaneously hypertensive rat model of malignant hypertension [536].

Tobian [535] has proposed that the low-potassium diet characteristically consumed by blacks in the southern United States may exacerbate the hypertension-induced endothelial injury in the interlobular arteries leading to the development of pronounced musculomucoid intimal hyperplasia (malignant nephrosclerosis). He has suggested that low dietary potassium intake may, at least in part, explain the high frequency of end-stage renal disease due to hypertension among blacks.

Role of Glucocorticoids in Malignant Hypertension. Chatelain et al. [79] proposed that elevated glucocorticoid secretion is important in the pathogenesis of experimental malignant hypertension. They utilized the aortic ligation model to study the patterns of glucocorticoid secretion and arterial connective tissue metabolism in rats with either benign or malignant hypertension. In this model, immediately following aortic ligation there was a period of weight loss associated with elevated levels of plasma corticosterone. After 9 days there were marked differences between animals that had persistent benign hypertension and those that entered the malignant phase. In animals with benign hypertension, corticosterone levels normalized, body growth resumed, and there was marked connective tissue proliferation in the aorta, akin to the findings described in other experimental models of hypertension. However, in animals that developed malignant hypertension, there was continued weight loss, and plasma corticosterone levels remained elevated. In contrast to animals with benign hypertension, there was no proliferation of connective tissue in the aorta. The authors postulated that glucocorticoids were important in the pathogenesis of the abnormalities in arterial connective tissue metabolism in malignant hypertension. It is unclear whether these findings are applicable to the pathophysiology of malignant hypertension in humans.

Role of Immunologic Mechanisms in Malignant Hypertension. Gudbrandsson et al. [209] have suggested a possible role of immunologic mechanisms in the pathogenesis of arterial lesions in malignant hypertension. In studies of immunologic parameters in 20 patients who had survived the malignant phase of essential hypertension, they demonstrated increased T-lymphocyte reactivity against human arterial antigens compared with age- and sex-matched normotensive control subjects. Since the response to mitogens such as phytohemagglutinin and concanavalin-A was not different between the two groups, the data suggested a specific increase in reactivity against arterial antigens in malignant hypertension.

The presence of specific T-lymphocyte reactivity against arterial antigens suggests that immunologic abnormalities may contribute to the vascular damage of malignant hypertension. However, it is not known whether these immunologic changes are primary or merely a consequence of arterial damage that has led to arterial antigen exposure and a secondary immunologic response. Whether primary or secondary, the increased T-lymphocyte reactivity against the arterial wall components might be expected to aggravate arterial wall injury.

Study of HLA phenotypes suggests a possible genetic predisposition to malignant hypertension [170]. HLA-Bw35 and Cw4 antigens were found to be significantly more frequent in a group of 32 patients with malignant hypertension and terminal uremia than in a control group of healthy blood donors. In contrast, the frequency of these antigens in a group of 60 nonuremic patients with biopsy proven glomerulonephritis without malignant hypertension was similar to the control group. The authors speculated that these HLA antigens might in some way be related to the vascular response to severe hypertension.

Role of the Kallikrein-Kinin System in Malignant Hypertension. In addition to enhanced activity of vasopressor hormones, decreased activity of vasodilator hormone systems may be involved in the pathogenesis of malignant hypertension. Kinins are potent vasodilators that exert a marked influence on renal salt and water excretion. Ribeiro et al. [462] have reported that plasma levels of kininogen were markedly decreased in patients with malignant hypertension compared with either patients with benign hypertension or normotensive controls. The decrease in kininogen levels in malignant hypertension could not be explained by renal insufficiency, changes in hematocrit or fibrinogen levels, or alteration in prekallikrein or kallikrein levels.

Role of Endothelium-Derived Relaxing Factors and Endothelin in Malignant Hypertension. Recent studies have shown that hypertension is associated with various functional changes of the vascular endothelium including decreased formation of endothelium-derived relaxing factor (EDRF) and increased release of contracting factors such as endothelin. This dysfunction of the hypertensive endothelial organ may contribute to the elevation of peripheral resistance and the development of hypertensive complications in the cerebral, coronary, or renal circulations [329, 496, 546]. However, the precise role of these local vascular hormones in the pathogenesis of malignant hypertension has not yet been defined.

Mechanism of Production of Fibrinoid Necrosis and Proliferative Endarteritis. In experimental models of malignant hypertension, vascular damage from either the mechanical stress of hypertension or vasculotoxic hormones leads to endothelial injury that is manifest by the sausage string pattern and accompanied by seepage of plasma proteins including fibrinogen into the vessel wall. Contact of plasma constituents with smooth muscle cells activates the coagulation cascade, and fibrin is deposited in the wall. Fibrin deposits cause necrosis of smooth muscle cells and the development of *fibrinoid necrosis*.

Two theories have been advanced to explain the occurrence of *proliferative endarteritis*. Kincaid-Smith [286] has postulated that smooth muscle proliferation in the intima is the result of organization of a thrombus in the vessel wall. Schwartz et al. [485] have proposed that sudden, severe elevation of blood pressure produces forced vasodilation of the interlobular arteries with denudation of the vascular endothelium. Attachment of platelets at the sites of endothelial injury is accompanied by the synthesis and release of platelet-derived growth factor (PDGF), which stimulates proliferation of medial smooth muscle cells with chemotaxis toward the intima. The intimal proliferation of smooth muscle cells is accompanied by deposition of mucopolysaccharide and later collagen, leading to the lesions characteristic of proliferative endarteritis or musculomucoid intimal hyperplasia.

Summary of the Pathophysiology of Malignant Hypertension. Based on the foregoing discussion, it is clear that the exact pathophysiologic mechanism underlying the transition from the benign to the malignant phase of hypertension is not fully understood. Undoubtedly a marked increase in blood pressure is pivotal. Severe hypertension is the common element in malignant hypertension in humans and in each of the animal models of malignant hypertension. Moreover, reduction of the blood pressure reverses the malignant phase regardless of the underlying etiology. Thus increased blood pressure is *necessary* for the development and progression of the malignant phase. The major issue is whether the mechanical stress of severe hypertension alone is *sufficient* to cause the transition to the malignant phase. Since there is considerable overlap in the levels of blood pressure seen in patients with benign and malignant hypertension, it is likely that severe hypertension is *not sufficient* to cause the malignant phase in all patients. In some patients, additional factor(s) probably participate in the development of malignant hypertension. These cofactors are not necessarily the same in every case. For example, activation of the renin-angiotensin system may be important in some patients but not in others. In these patients, perhaps vasopressin, catecholamines, or activation of the clotting cascade interacts with hypertension to produce the malignant phase.

The vicious cycle of malignant hypertension is best demonstrated in the kidneys but applies equally well to the vascular beds of the pancreas, gastrointestinal tract, retina, and brain (Fig. 59-18). In this scheme, severe hy-

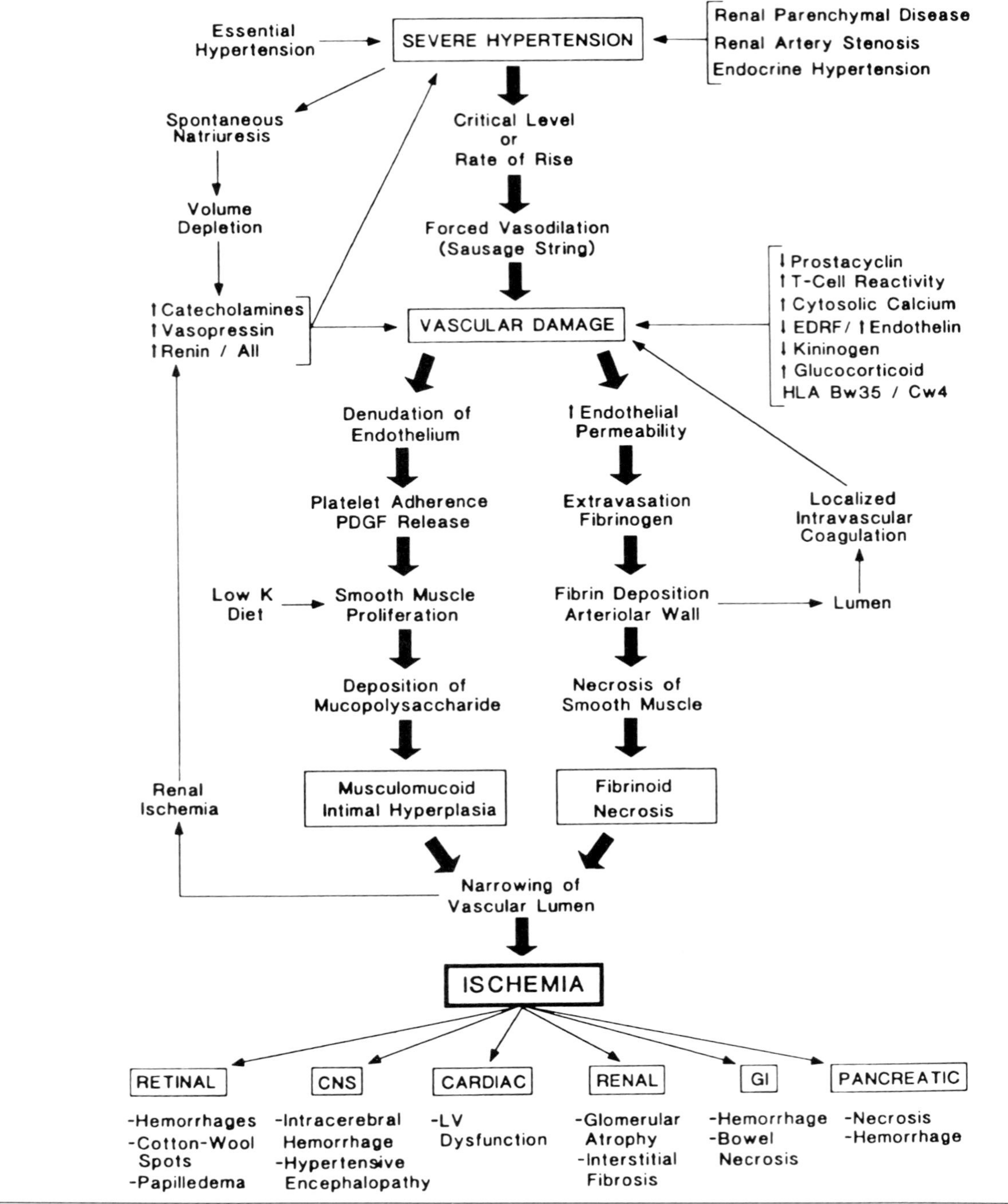

Fig. 59-18. Pathophysiology of malignant hypertension. AII = angiotensin II; EDRF = endothelium-derived relaxing factor; PDGF = platelet-derived growth factor; LV = left ventricular.

pertension is central. Hypertension may be essential or secondary to any one of a variety of disorders. The interaction between the level of blood pressure and the adaptive capacity of the vasculature may be important. Chronic hypertension results in thickening and remodeling of arterial walls, which may be an adaptive mechanism to prevent vascular damage from mechanical stress [28]. However, when the blood pressure rises to a level or at a rate that is excessive, the adaptive mechanism may be overwhelmed, resulting in vascular damage. Focal segments of the vascular system become dilated, producing the sausage string pattern as the result of the mechanical stress of increased transmural pressure. Other hormonal factors may act synergistically with hypertension to damage the arterial vasculature. For example, spontaneous natriuresis at some critical level of blood pressure may result in volume depletion with elevation of renin-angiotensin, vasopressin, or catecholamine levels, which further elevate blood pressure. In addition, these hormones may be directly vasculotoxic. Fibrinogen and other plasma proteins may permeate the damaged vascular wall and activate the intrinsic clotting system, causing deposition of fibrin in the vessel wall and lumen, leading to fibrinoid necrosis. The onset of localized intravascular coagulation may cause a cycle in which red blood cells and platelets are deposited on intravascular strands with release of adenosine diphosphate and thromboplastin with further activation of the clotting cascade. Platelet adherence to damaged endothelium with release of PDGF leads to myointimal proliferation in the interlobular arteries, which results in proliferative endarteritis. The wall thickening and luminal narrowing in the interlobular arteries and afferent arterioles may cause glomerular ischemia, accelerated glomerular obsolescence, and renal insufficiency. Resulting renal ischemia may cause activation of the renin-angiotensin system, which may cause further increases in blood pressure, vascular damage, and pressure-induced natriuresis, such that a vicious cycle of hypertension, vascular damage, and renal insufficiency develops.

Other factors, although less certain, may also be important in the transition from the benign to the malignant phase. Low dietary potassium may predispose to hypertensive arterial injury in black patients with severe hypertension. Abnormalities in membrane sodium transport and cytosolic calcium may mediate hypertension-induced vascular injury. Activation of T-cell immunity to vascular antigens may further aggravate vascular injury. Cigarette smoking or oral contraceptives may decrease prostacyclin production and inhibit repair of hypertensive vascular damage. Altered glucocorticoid metabolism or abnormalities in the kallikrein-kinin system may also be important in some cases.

Pathophysiology of Hypertensive Neuroretinopathy. Retinal arteriolar vasculopathy in malignant hypertension leads to obliterative occlusion of vessels or to rupture of vessels resulting in striate hemorrhages, cotton-wool spots, and papilledema. Hypertensive neuroretinopathy is not caused by renal failure. In this regard, hypertensive neuroretinopathy may occur in malignant hypertension prior to the onset of clinically significant renal disease [164]. It also appears that hypertensive neuroretinopathy frequently occurs in the absence of increased intracranial pressure [164].

The retinal circulation is under autoregulatory control and does not have a sympathetic nerve supply. As the systemic blood pressure increases, if autoregulation is intact, the retinal arterioles constrict to maintain retinal blood flow constant. The appearance of hypertensive neuroretinopathy implies that autoregulation has failed [132].

Striate hemorrhages result from bleeding from superficial capillaries in the nerve fiber bundles near the optic disc. These capillaries originate from arterioles, so that when autoregulation fails, the high systemic pressure is transmitted directly to the capillaries. This leads to breaks in the continuity of the capillary endothelium with subsequent hemorrhage [132].

Cotton-wool spots result from ischemic infarction of nerve fibers due to arteriolar occlusion [132]. Fluorescein angiography demonstrates that cotton-wool spots are areas of retinal nonperfusion [234]. Embolization of the pig retina with glass beads produced immediate intracellular edema and later accumulation of mitochondria and other subcellular organelles in the ischemic nerve fibers [493]. McLeod et al. [353] observed that cotton-wool spots occurred in areas where a large number of nerve fibers were ischemic. They postulated that the normal axoplasmic flow of subcellular organelles was disrupted by ischemia, so that the accumulation of organelles in ischemic areas resulted in a visible white patch. Cotton-wool spots tend to distribute around the optic disc because the nerve fiber bundles are most dense in this region.

The pathogenesis of *papilledema* in malignant hypertension has been controversial. Pickering [434] suggested that papilledema resulted from increased intracranial pressure. However, intracranial pressure is not always increased in malignant hypertension [164]. Papilledema was produced in rhesus monkeys by occlusion of the long posterior ciliary artery that supplies the optic disc [223]. Subsequent observations have confirmed that papilledema, like cotton-wool spots, results from ischemia of the nerve fibers in the disc [224, 352].

TREATMENT OF MALIGNANT HYPERTENSION

It is well established that malignant hypertension must be treated expeditiously to prevent complications such as hypertensive encephalopathy, intracerebral hemorrhage, acute pulmonary edema, and renal failure. The hypertensive patient with hypertensive neuroretinopathy (hemorrhages, cotton-wool spots with or without papilledema) should be hospitalized for intensive medical therapy. Initiation of appropriate therapy should not be delayed pending extensive laboratory and roentgenographic examinations aimed at defining a potential underlying etiology. The work-up for secondary causes should be deferred until the blood pressure has been controlled and the patient stabilized.

The traditional therapeutic approach to patients with malignant hypertension has been the initiation of therapy with rapidly acting parenteral hypotensive agents such as sodium nitroprusside, trimethaphan, or diazoxide [10, 294]. Table 59-4 lists the settings in which the use of parenteral antihypertensive agents is recommended for the initial management of malignant hypertension. In general, parenteral therapy should be utilized in patients who have evidence of acute end-organ damage or who are unable to tolerate oral medications. The management of patients with acute pulmonary edema, hypertensive encephalopathy, or intracerebral

Table 59-4. Indications for parenteral therapy in malignant hypertension

Patient unable to tolerate oral therapy due to intractable vomiting
Hypertensive encephalopathy
Rapidly failing vision
Intracerebral hemorrhage
Acute pulmonary edema
Acute myocardial infarction
Rapid deterioration of renal function
Acute pancreatitis
Gastrointestinal hemorrhage
Acute abdomen secondary to mesenteric vasculitis

hemorrhage is discussed in separate sections on each of these topics.

The drug of choice for the management of patients with malignant hypertension requiring parenteral therapy is sodium nitroprusside. Trimethaphan is an alternative, but a number of significant adverse effects limit its usefulness. Diazoxide, employed in a minibolus fashion, may be advantageous in selected patients for whom monitoring in an intensive care unit is not available. Minibolus injections of labetalol have also been utilized for the treatment of malignant hypertension [565].

There are no absolute guidelines for the goal level of blood pressure during parenteral therapy. The theoretical risks of rapid reduction of blood pressure are discussed in the section on The Controversy Over Gradual Versus Rapid Reduction of Blood Pressure. As a general rule, it is safe to reduce the mean arterial pressure initially by 20 percent or to a level of 160 to 170/100 to 110 mm Hg [175]. During the reduction of blood pressure with parenteral antihypertensives, the patient should be closely monitored for evidence of cerebral or myocardial hypoperfusion. The use of a short-acting agent such as sodium nitroprusside has obvious advantages because the blood pressure can be quickly stabilized at a higher level if complications develop during rapid blood pressure reduction. If there is no evidence of vital organ hypoperfusion following this initial reduction of blood pressure, the diastolic blood pressure can gradually be lowered to 90 mm Hg over a period of 12 to 36 hours.

Oral antihypertensive agents should be initiated as soon as possible so that the duration of parenteral therapy can be minimized. However, a common error in the management of patients with malignant hypertension is the abrupt discontinuation of parenteral therapy immediately after oral therapy has been initiated. With this approach, severe rebound hypertension often develops before the oral antihypertensive regimen becomes effective. Ideally, oral antihypertensives should be initiated as soon as the patient has been stabilized and is able to tolerate medications by mouth. The nitroprusside infusion should be continued until the oral agents have taken effect and have been titrated to an effective dose. The nitroprusside infusion can then be weaned as the oral regimen is gradually increased.

Although other agents may be effective in the long-term management of patients with malignant hypertension, the cornerstone of initial oral therapy should be an arteriolar vasodilator such as hydralazine, sustained-release nifedipine, or minoxidil. Vasodilators may reflexly activate the adrenergic system and cause tachycardia with an increase in cardiac output that can blunt the hypotensive response [295]. Therefore, treatment with β-adrenergic blockers is usually also required. Direct-acting vasodilators also cause renal salt and water retention, fluid overload, and the development of pseudotolerance to the hypotensive effect of the drug. Thus, although diuretics may not be required for the initial management of patients with malignant hypertension, they are usually required as a part of the long-term maintenance antihypertensive regimen.

The regimen that follows has proved to be generally effective in the conversion from parenteral to oral therapy. After the blood pressure has been controlled with nitroprusside and while the infusion is continued, hydralazine (50 mg) and propranolol (40 mg) are administered orally. As the oral agents become effective and the blood pressure declines, the nitroprusside infusion is tapered. Brief interruption of the nitroprusside infusion can be used to assess the hypotensive response to the oral agents. If after 6 to 8 hours the diastolic blood pressure remains over 100 mm Hg, a second dose of hydralazine (100 mg) should be given. The propranolol dose is increased as needed to maintain adequate β-blockade (heart rate 60 to 80 beats/min). The usual dose of propranolol is 80 to 120 mg administered twice a day, but occasionally larger doses may be required. If the blood pressure is not controlled with hydralazine at a dose of 100 mg twice daily, minoxidil should be substituted for hydralazine. The starting dose of minoxidil (2.5 mg) is increased by 2.5 to 5.0 mg every 6 to 8 hours until the blood pressure is adequately controlled. The usual effective dose is 5 to 10 mg twice a day. Treatment with a β-blocker is recommended as for hydralazine. As the blood pressure is brought under control with oral agents, the sodium nitroprusside infusion is gradually weaned. When the convalescing patient is mobilized, the upright blood pressure should be carefully monitored to avoid orthostatic hypotension. A diuretic, usually furosemide at a starting dose of 40 mg twice a day, is added to either the hydralazine or minoxidil regimen when it becomes evident that salt and water retention has occurred.

Volume Status and the Role of Diuretics. It has traditionally been taught that patients with malignant hypertension require potent parenteral diuretic therapy during the initial phase of treatment along with a potent parenteral vasodilator [275, 294]. However, there is now evidence suggesting that routine parenteral diuretic therapy during the acute phase of treatment for malignant hypertension may actually be deleterious [286]. Overdiuresis may result in deterioration of renal function due to superimposed prerenal azotemia. Moreover, volume depletion may activate the renin-angiotensin axis and other pressor hormone systems.

Even patients with malignant hypertension and pulmonary edema may not be total body salt and water overloaded. Pulmonary congestion in this setting may result from an increase in left ventricular filling pressure due to a decrease in the compliance of the left ventricle rather than an increase in left ventricular volume. With severe hypertension, the ventricle may become noncompliant due to the excessive workload imposed by the elevated systemic vascular resistance (SVR). As a result, left ventricular end-diastolic pressure (LVEDP) increases dramatically even though left ventricular end-diastolic volume (LVEDV) may be near normal. With vasodilator therapy, SVR decreases, left ventricular compliance improves, LVEDP decreases, and LVEDV may actually increase [91]. Despite the increase in LVEDV, pulmonary congestion improves because of the reduction in pulmonary capillary pressure. Thus even in patients with malignant hypertension complicated by pulmonary edema, afterload reduction rather than vigorous diuretic therapy should be the mainstay of therapy.

Some patients with malignant hypertension may benefit from a cautious trial of volume expansion. Intravascular volume depletion in patients with malignant hypertension is manifested by the finding of exquisite sensitivity to vasodilator therapy with a precipitous drop in the blood pressure at relatively low infusion rates. Patients with an underlying salt-losing nephropathy due to chronic interstitial nephritis caused by analgesic nephropathy are particularly prone to be severely volume depleted at presentation [286, 395].

In summary, the need for diuretic therapy during the initial phase of treatment for malignant hypertension depends on an assessment of volume status. Unless obvious fluid overload is present, diuretics should not be given initially. Although vasodilator therapy will eventually result in salt and water retention by the kidney, an increase in total body sodium content cannot occur unless the patient is given sodium. Thus in the initial phase of treatment, patients should be placed on a no-added salt diet with close monitoring of intravenous fluid administration. However, as mentioned above, during subsequent long-term treatment with oral vasodilators, the use of diuretics is usually essential to prevent fluid retention and adequately control blood pressure.

Management of Malignant Hypertension Complicated by Renal Insufficiency. All patients with malignant hypertension should receive aggressive antihypertensive therapy to prevent further renal damage, regardless of the degree of renal impairment. Control of blood pressure in patients with malignant hypertension and renal insufficiency occasionally precipitates oliguric acute renal failure, especially when the initial glomerular filtration rate is less than 20 ml per minute. However, this is not a contraindication to aggressive antihypertensive therapy aimed at normalization of the blood pressure. Control of hypertension protects other vital organs such as the brain and heart whose function cannot be replaced. Moreover, with tight blood pressure control, even patients who appear to have end-stage renal disease due to malignant nephrosclerosis have recovered renal function [2, 18, 22, 43, 96, 125, 145, 257, 327, 339, 356, 370, 500, 558]

In patients in whom aggressive control of hypertension precipitates the need for dialysis, dialysis is utilized to correct serum chemistries, treat uremia, and correct fluid overload. However, since dialysis alone rarely results in adequate control of blood pressure in patients with malignant hypertension, antihypertensive drug therapy is almost always required. A regimen with minoxidil and propranolol has proved to be particularly efficacious in this setting [96, 257, 321, 327, 339, 356, 370, 431].

Role of Nephrectomy in Malignant Hypertension. In the past, the use of bilateral nephrectomy to control severe hypertension in patients with malignant hypertension and azotemia was advocated [136, 311, 338]. In many patients with malignant hypertension and uremia accompanied by encephalopathy, bilateral nephrectomy was lifesaving [311]. In 1972, Lazarus et al. [311] proposed a role for urgent bilateral nephrectomy for patients with malignant hypertension who had life-threatening complications such as cerebrovascular accident, rapidly progressive congestive heart failure, or encephalopathy. The authors suggested that nephrectomy might be of value if performed early, even before the development of ESRD. Patients were sometimes nephrectomized with serum creatinine levels as low as 7.0 mg/dl.

Following the introduction of minoxidil, however, the role of nephrectomy in the management of malignant hypertension with azotemia was questioned [382]. Eleven patients with malignant hypertension were reported who had been refractory to maximal doses of conventional antihypertensive agents. Seven of these patients had advanced renal failure and were candidates for nephrectomy to control blood pressure. Institution of a regimen of minoxidil combined with diuretics or dialysis to control fluid retention and propranolol to control reflex tachycardia resulted in blood pressure reduction to normotensive levels in all patients with remarkably few side effects [431]. Thus, even in patients with renal failure requiring dialysis, hypertension can usually be controlled with minoxidil [321, 356, 382, 431]. Given the proven efficacy of minoxidil, bilateral nephrectomy is rarely, if ever, indicated to control refractory hypertension. Nephrectomy should clearly be a last resort, since delayed recovery of renal function is possible in some cases.

In summary, the long-term management of patients with ESRD secondary to malignant hypertension should include vigorous antihypertensive therapy with the goal of sustained normotension. Dramatic recovery of renal function may occasionally occur. Even if renal function fails to recover, adequate control of the blood pressure is essential to prevent the potentially fatal complications of malignant hypertension such as hypertensive encephalopathy, intracerebral hemorrhage, congestive heart failure, and hemorrhagic pancreatitis [16, 23].

Initial Oral Therapy for Malignant Hypertension. While many patients with malignant hypertension require prompt treatment with parenteral antihypertensive agents, some patients may not yet have evidence of cerebral or cardiac complications or rapidly deteriorating renal function and therefore do not require instantaneous control of the blood pressure [9, 10, 256, 275, 286]. These patients may be safely managed with an intensive oral regimen designed to bring the blood pressure under control over a period of 12 to 24 hours.

In patients with malignant hypertension, a multidrug oral regimen is often required to achieve adequate blood pressure control. The most useful combinations include a diuretic, a β-adrenergic blocker, and an arteriolar vasodilator. Minoxidil appears to be particularly well suited for the initial management of malignant hypertension that requires prompt but not immediate blood pressure reduction [7, 9, 409]. Alpert and Bauer [7] have described the use of a triple regimen of minoxidil, propranolol, and furosemide in 9 patients with blood pressure greater than 120 mm Hg. Seven of these patients had malignant hypertension. Furosemide (40 mg) and propranolol (40 mg) were given initially by mouth. Two hours later, if the diastolic pressure was greater than 120 mm Hg, a loading dose of minoxidil (20 mg) was administered. If the diastolic pressure was still over 100 mm Hg 4 hours after the loading dose, a booster dose of minoxidil was given. The amount of the booster dose was estimated based on the magnitude of the response to the loading dose. Maintenance therapy with minoxidil was begun with one-half the sum of the loading and booster doses given twice daily, with adjustment of β-blocker and diuretic dose as necessary for control of heart rate and fluid balance. Following the booster dose of minoxidil, a sustained decrease in blood pressure was seen in all patients. No overshoot hypotension or other adverse effects were encountered. During long-term therapy, they were able to substitute hydralazine for minoxidil in 5 patients. However, the remaining 4 patients required chronic minoxidil therapy for adequate blood pressure control [9].

Initial oral therapy with sustained-release nifedipine has recently been shown to be effective in the management of malignant hypertension in black patients who did not require parenteral therapy for hypertensive encephalopathy or acute pulmonary edema [256]. No precipitous decreases in blood pressure or neurologic complications were encountered. However, despite adequate control of blood pressure during the first 24 hours with sustained-release nifedipine, all patients eventually required one or more additional drugs for long-term blood pressure control. Although treatment with sublingual or oral nifedipine capsules has also been recommended for the initial management of malignant hypertension [39, 150, 178], the sustained-release nifedipine preparation may be preferable because there appears to be less risk of overshoot hypotension [256].

The converting enzyme inhibitors have also been reported to be effective in the treatment of malignant hypertension. However, converting enzyme inhibitors can produce profound hypotension in volume-depleted patients, so they should be used with caution during the initial phase of treatment. Moreover, they may not always be effective in the acute management of malignant hypertension [160].

Oral loading regimens with clonidine have been reported to be useful in severe uncomplicated (urgent) hypertension [11, 87, 510]. However, there is limited information about the use of oral clonidine loading in initial management of malignant hypertension. Clonidine loading can cause significant sedation, which may interfere with the assessment of potential neurologic complications during acute blood pressure reduction. Moreover, common side effects such as sedation and dry mouth may have a negative impact on compliance in patients treated long-term with clonidine. Thus, we do not recommend oral clonidine loading regimens for the initial management of malignant hypertension.

Long-Term Management of Malignant Hypertension. After the immediate crisis has resolved and the blood pressure has been brought under control with parenteral and/or oral therapy, lifelong surveillance of the blood pressure is essential. Close follow-up and aggressive treatment are mandatory because noncompliance or inadequate therapy may have devastating consequences. If blood pressure control becomes inadequate, the malignant phase may recur even after years of successful antihypertensive therapy. In a study of the quality of care provided to patients with a history of malignant hypertension who subsequently died, only 27 percent of patients had an average treated diastolic blood pressure of less than 110 mm Hg [144]. Thus meticulous long-term treatment of hypertension is imperative in patients with a history of malignant hypertension. Triple therapy with a diuretic, a β-blocker, and a vasodilator is often required to achieve satisfactory blood pressure control.

RESPONSE TO THERAPY IN MALIGNANT HYPERTENSION

In the absence of adequate blood pressure control, malignant hypertension has a uniformly poor prognosis. Without treatment, the 1-year mortality rate approaches 80 to 90 percent, and uremia is the most common cause of death [288, 482]. Since the introduction of potent antihypertensive agents, numerous studies have shown that with control of the blood pressure survival can be substantially prolonged.

In 1959 Harington et al. [218] reported 82 patients with malignant hypertension who were treated with ganglionic blocking agents (hexamethonium, pentolinium, and mecamylamine). Because of side effects, patients seldom tolerated doses of medications that resulted in sustained normotension. The objective of therapy was to reduce the standing systolic blood pressure to less than 160 mm Hg. The survival curve for these 82 treated patients in contrast to the survival curve for a series of patients from the pretreatment era is shown in Fig. 59-19. In the treated group, overall survival was 50 percent at 1 year, 33 percent at 2 years, and 25 percent at 4 years.

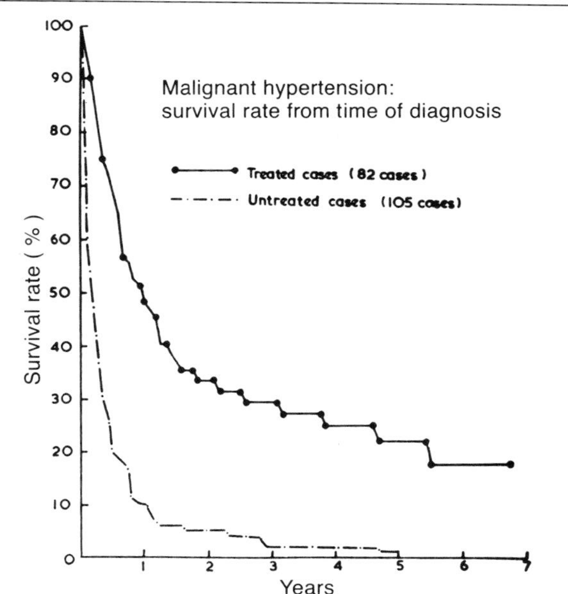

Fig. 59-19. Survival in patients with malignant hypertension. Treated patients received ganglionic blocking agents. Untreated patients are historical controls from the pre-treatment era. (From M. Harington, P. Kincaid-Smith, and J. McMichael. Results of treatment in malignant hypertension. A seven year experience in 94 cases. *Br. Med. J.* 2:969, 1959. With permission.)

In the untreated group, survival was only 10 percent at the end of the first year. Adequacy of blood pressure control was found to be an important prognostic factor. Patients with adequate blood pressure control had a 38 percent 5-year survival compared to 18 percent in the inadequately treated patients.

Mohler and Fries reported 64 patients with malignant hypertension treated with ganglionic blockers, hydralazine, and rauwolfia derivatives [371]. They found an 80 percent 1-year survival and a 22 percent 5-year survival. Again patient survival was directly related to the adequacy of blood pressure control. Although pretreatment blood pressures were identical among patients who survived 5 years or longer, the average blood pressure after 5 years of treatment was 147/99 mm Hg. In patients who died before 5 years, the last available blood pressure was 192/119 mm Hg.

Hood et al. [239] reported survival statistics for patients with malignant hypertension treated during the period from 1950 to 1962. Among 128 patients with grade IV funduscopic changes, the 5-year survival was 50 percent, while among 177 with grade III changes, the 5-year survival was 61 percent. Other series of treated patients from the 1960s also demonstrated a 5-year survival of around 50 percent [24, 50].

In a more recent series of 83 treated patients collected between 1979 and 1985, 1-year and 5-year patient survival rates were 94 percent and 75 percent, respectively. Renal survival, defined as patients surviving with native renal function, was 66 percent at 1 year and 51 percent at 5 years [579]. The improved patient survival in recent years has been attributed to a decrease in uremic deaths due not only to the availability of dialysis but also to prevention of end-stage renal disease through adequate blood pressure control [208, 579].

In contrast to studies in the pretreatment era [280], the most recent studies have failed to demonstrate a difference in patient or renal survival between patients with grade III and grade IV hypertensive retinopathy [4, 350, 579].

Prognostic Importance of Renal Function at the Time of Diagnosis. Numerous series have documented the prognostic significance of the level of renal function at the time of the initial presentation of malignant hypertension. Harington et al. [218] demonstrated that the greatest mortality occurred during the first year of treatment, mainly in patients who had grossly impaired renal function at the time of diagnosis. Those patients with an initial blood urea level greater than 60 mg per deciliter (BUN > 30 mg/dl or 11 mmol/liter) had a 13 percent 1-year survival compared with a 73 percent 1-year survival among those with an initial blood urea level of less than 60 mg per deciliter (Fig. 59-20). With antihypertensive therapy, renal function tended to remain normal in patients with good renal function at presentation. In contrast, despite blood pressure control, renal function often deteriorated in patients with renal insufficiency at presentation. The authors concluded that hypotensive therapy did not halt the progression of established renal insufficiency and that a good long-term prognosis could be anticipated only in patients with nonuremic malignant hypertension.

Fig. 59-20. Survival in treated patients with malignant hypertension according to the level of renal function at the time of initial presentation. (From M. Harington, P. Kincaid-Smith, and J. McMichael. Results of treatment in malignant hypertension. A seven year experience in 94 cases. *Br. Med. J.* 2:969, 1959. With permission.)

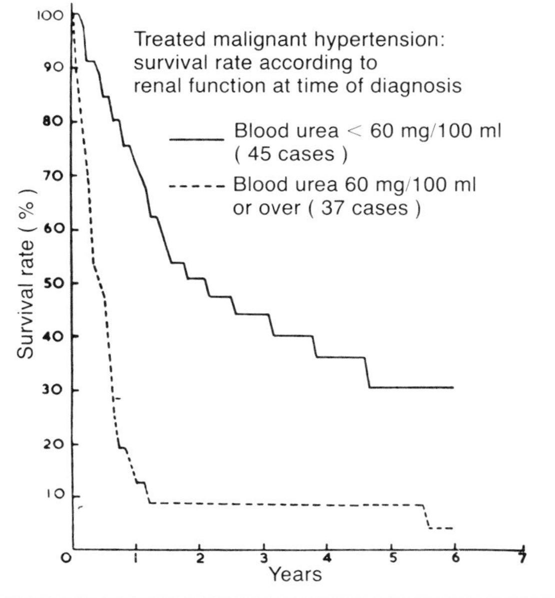

Perry et al. [429] reported on the response to therapy in 316 patients with an initial diastolic blood pressure over 110 mm Hg who were treated with ganglionic blocking agents and hydralazine beginning in 1951. The patients were divided into four groups based on the presence of hypertensive neuroretinopathy and end-organ damage at the time of presentation. Patients with hemorrhages, exudates, and papilledema were divided into those with a nonprotein nitrogen level of > 30 mg per deciliter (11 mmol/liter) (malignant azotemic) and those with a nonprotein nitrogen level of < 30 mg per deciliter (malignant nonazotemic). Patients without neuroretinopathy were divided into those with congestive heart failure or prior cerebrovascular complications (benign complicated) and those without complications (benign uncomplicated). The survival curves for the four groups differed markedly (Fig. 59-21). The 7- to 13-year survival rate was 69 percent in benign uncomplicated, 20 percent in benign complicated, 41 percent in malignant nonazotemic, and 8 percent in malignant azotemic. Of note was the observation that malignant nonazotemic patients had a better survival than those in the benign complicated group. This finding was explained on the basis of the shorter duration of hypertension and its atherosclerotic complications in the malignant nonazotemic group. Despite adequate blood pressure control in the benign complicated group, mortality due to myocardial infarction, stroke, or aortic dissection remained high, presumably reflecting the presence of irreversible atherosclerotic disease.

Fig. 59-21. Survival in patients with initial diastolic blood pressure greater than 110 mm Hg who were intensively treated with ganglionic blocking agents and hydralazine. Patients with hypertensive neuroretinopathy were divided into those with nonprotein nitrogen > 30 mg/dl (malignant azotemic) and those with nonprotein nitrogen < 30 mg/dl (malignant nonazotemic). Patients without neuroretinopathy were divided into those with cerebrovascular complications or congestive heart failure (benign complicated) and those without complications (benign uncomplicated). (From H. M. Perry, H. A. Schroeder, F. J. Catanzaro, et al. Studies on the control of hypertension. VIII. Morbidity, mortality and remissions during twelve years of intensive therapy. *Circulation* 33:958, 1966. With permission.)

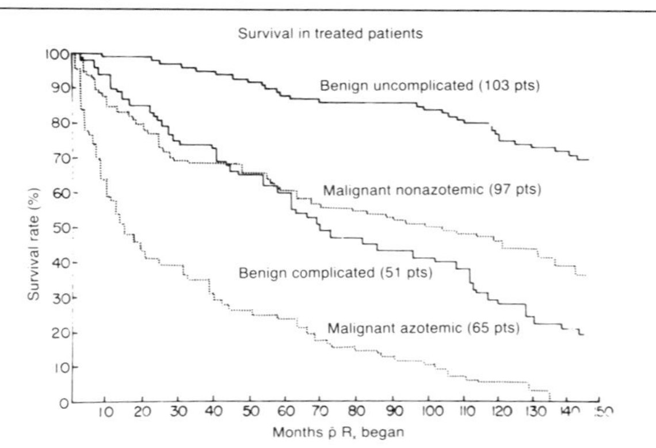

Based on the experience between 1950 and 1965, most published series concluded that aggressive treatment of malignant hypertension in patients with renal insufficiency often resulted in worsening of renal function and sometimes even precipitated ESRD. As recently as the mid-1960s, it was routinely stated that azotemic patients with malignant hypertension should be managed conservatively and that if the BUN were greater than 60 mg per deciliter (21.5 mmol/liter), no antihypertensive therapy should be undertaken [304, 359]. "Treatment may be epitomized as being mandatory but disastrous in the uremic malignant hypertensive patient—mandatory, for the necrotizing arteriolitis will not heal unless the blood pressure is lowered and disastrous because the BUN almost always increases markedly on hypotensive therapy" [359].

However, in 1967 Woods and Blythe reported their encouraging experience with the treatment of malignant hypertension complicated by severe renal insufficiency [570, 571]. They examined the effect of aggressive antihypertensive therapy, undertaken regardless of the initial effect on renal function, in a group of patients with malignant hypertension and an initial BUN of > 50 mg per deciliter (18 mmol/liter). Twenty patients were treated with methyldopa to attain a recumbent diastolic blood pressure of < 100 mm Hg. Two patients died during the initial hospital course, and 9 patients died within 6 months. However, 11 patients (55 percent) survived 1 year, 4 (20 percent) survived 5 years, and 2 (10 percent) survived 7 years. Woods and Blythe postulated that further improvement in survival might be possible in patients with malignant hypertension and severe renal impairment if dialytic support was provided in conjunction with aggressive treatment of hypertension. They predicted that with time, control of hypertension might lead to healing of the vascular lesions with recovery of renal function. They recommended that the blood pressure be reduced to normal in these patients and that a transient worsening of renal function should not necessitate discontinuation of therapy.

Mroczek et al. subsequently demonstrated the value of aggressive therapy in patients with malignant hypertension and azotemia [384]. They treated 25 patients with diazoxide and furosemide followed by conventional oral therapy in an attempt to maintain diastolic blood pressure at < 100 mm Hg. At the time of diagnosis, the average BUN was 62 mg per deciliter (22 mmol/liter) and the average creatinine was 6.9 mg per deciliter (610 μmol/liter). Three patients died with uremia during the first 2 weeks despite adequate blood pressure control. In the remaining 22 patients, there was a transient decline in renal function. Within 3 months, however, in association with adequate blood pressure control, there was an improvement in renal function with a reduction in the mean creatinine by 2.8 mg per deciliter (250 μmol/liter). After 6 months, the average creatinine was 3.3 ± 0.2 mg per deciliter (290 ± 18 μmol/liter). At 12 months, the mean creatinine had decreased to 2.8 ± 0.6 mg per deciliter (250 ± 50 μ/liter). Among long-term survivors, only one uremic death occurred in a patient who discontinued therapy and developed relapse of malignant hypertension.

Herlitz et al. [229] reported 24 patients who survived the malignant phase of hypertension. The patients were divided into two groups, 7 patients who developed terminal renal failure and 17 patients who maintained renal function. In the patients who developed renal failure, renal insufficiency was present at the time of diagnosis with a mean serum creatinine of 448 ± 105 μmol per liter (5.1 ± 1.2 mg/dl). It was not possible to attain adequate blood pressure control in any of these patients. In the patients in whom renal function was preserved with therapy, serum creatinine was 169 ± 19 μmol per liter (1.9 ± 0.2 mg/dl). In these patients, the blood pressure was controlled with three or more drugs and at the time of follow-up, the mean serum creatinine was 132 ± 8 μmol per liter (1.5 ± 0.1 mg/dl). Glomerular filtration rate had increased in 55 percent and had remained stable in 45 percent. Although the results highlight the prognostic value of the level of renal function at presentation, there was considerable overlap in the initial level of renal function between patients who progressed and those who did not. The crucial factor in determining the risk of progression appeared to be the adequacy of long-term blood pressure control.

A more recent study has confirmed the prognostic value of the initial serum creatinine concentration in patients with malignant hypertension [579]. Among 33 patients with initial serum creatinine < 300 μmol/liter (< 3.4 mg/dl), 85 percent had stable or improved renal function during long-term follow-up. Only 3 patients progressed to end-stage renal disease. In a second group of 32 patients with initial serum creatinine > 300 μmol/liter, all but 3 patients had deterioration of renal function during follow-up. Dialysis was eventually required in 76 percent of these patients.

Mroczek has concluded that there are two distinct groups of patients with malignant hypertension and renal insufficiency [383, 384]. In one group, malignant hypertension is secondary to underlying renal parenchymal disease. Renal biopsy reveals fibrinoid necrosis and proliferative endarteritis superimposed on underlying chronic glomerulonephritis or pyelonephritis. In this group, initial control of blood pressure may result in a transient worsening of renal function, but within 2 to 16 weeks renal function gradually returns to baseline. Despite adequate blood pressure control, however, eventually the underlying renal disease slowly progresses to end stage. In the other group, primary malignant hypertension is present and renal biopsy reveals only malignant nephrosclerosis. In these patients, intensive antihypertensive therapy may result in an improvement in renal function, especially if initial renal impairment is mild to moderate. Even in patients with severe renal impairment, recovery of renal function may sometimes occur during sustained normotension. However, many months of therapy may be required before recovery of renal function is apparent, presumably reflecting the time required for resolution of the vascular lesions.

Recently, the observation was made that the combined length of the two kidneys at presentation (combined renal length) was predictive of the chance for recovery of renal function in patients with malignant hypertension and severe renal failure [403]. The mean combined renal length was 20.2 cm in the group that recovered renal function and 14.2 in the group with persistent renal failure despite strict blood pressure control.

Lawton studied the time course for the recovery of renal function in patients with malignant hypertension and azotemia and found that most patients who were destined to recover renal function began to demonstrate improvement within the first 2 weeks of antihypertensive therapy [310].

However, there have been a number of recent reports describing dramatic recovery of renal function in patients with presumed ESRD due to malignant nephrosclerosis, even after many months to years of maintenance hemodialysis. Recovery of renal function in these cases has been attributed to strict control of blood pressure. These reports have challenged the notion that established renal failure in malignant hypertension is irreversible [2, 18, 22, 43, 96, 125, 145, 257, 327, 339, 356, 370, 500, 558]. In the majority of these reports, recovery of renal function has been associated with the use of the potent peripheral vasodilator minoxidil in combination with a β-adrenergic blocking drug and dialysis. Often patients who had refractory hypertension or disabling side effects while taking maximal doses of conventional antihypertensive agents eventually became normotensive with minimal side effects after the initiation of this regimen [321, 431]. Recovery of renal function with strict control of blood pressure has been reported up to 26 months after the initiation of maintenance hemodialysis [339]. In most of the reports describing the recovery of renal function after prolonged maintenance dialysis, the initial clinical presentation has been that of oliguric acute renal failure [257]. This observation is encouraging because the oliguric acute renal failure presentation had previously been reported to carry a grim prognosis despite treatment [345]. As predicted by Woods and Blythe, recovery of renal function in malignant hypertension may occur if the blood pressure is strictly controlled, even if temporary replacement of renal function is required for patients in whom renal failure occurs with initial normalization of the blood pressure [570, 571].

The long-term course in patients with primary malignant hypertension who recover from renal failure requiring dialysis has recently been reported [20]. Ten black patients (8 male) with renal failure due to primary malignant nephrosclerosis were treated with dialysis and strict blood pressure control. Renal function improved and dialysis was discontinued at 6 ± 2 months. During long-term follow-up, 5 patients maintained good renal function at 2 years (group I), whereas 5 patients developed progressive renal insufficiency culminating in a return to dialysis at 16 ± 6 months (group II). At initial presentation, the serum creatinine was lower in group I than in group II, 800 ± 110 μmol/liter (9 ± 1.2 mg/dl) and 1150 ± 150 μmol/liter (13 ± 1.7 mg/dl), respectively.

Renal function deteriorated in all patients and dialysis was initiated 8 ± 4 days after admission in group I and 38 ± 28 days after admission in group II. Renal function recovered, and dialysis was terminated after 4 ± 1.5 months in group I and 8 ± 4 months in group II. With recovery, the nadir of serum creatinine was lower in group I at 170 ± 30 μmol/liter (1.9 ± 0.3 mg/dl) versus 500 ± 120 μmol/liter (5.7 ± 1.4 mg/dl) in group II. There was no difference between the groups with regard to age, duration of hypertension, initial blood pressures, severity of retinopathy, renal size, or the prevalence of minoxidil use. However, the blood pressure was poorly controlled in group II, largely as a result of poor compliance with medical therapy.

Mechanism of Recovery of Renal Function. The mechanism of recovery of renal function after prolonged renal failure in malignant hypertension is uncertain. Extensive tubular damage resembling acute tubular necrosis has been reported in patients with oliguric acute renal failure [257, 345]. This tubular damage was thought to result from ischemia caused by the obliterative vascular lesions of malignant nephrosclerosis. In this regard, it has been postulated that the mechanism of recovery is the resolution of tubular necrosis [257]. However, unexplained is the observation that the need for dialysis persisted well beyond the usual time-frame for resolution of ischemia-induced acute tubular necrosis.

Kincaid-Smith has postulated that the initial loss of renal function results from glomerular ischemia due to narrowing of the interlobular arteries by proliferative endarteritis [286]. Although the endarteritis may be arrested by adequate blood pressure control, narrowing of the arterioles may persist. Improvement in renal function, therefore, may not result from the resolution of arteriolar lesions but from hypertrophy of the remaining nephrons supplied by patent interlobular arteries.

Regardless of the mechanism underlying recovery of renal function, it is clear that aggressive antihypertensive therapy with maintenance of normotension is pivotal with regard to eventual recovery of renal function.

Reversal of Hypertensive Neuroretinopathy. The funduscopic changes associated with hypertensive neuroretinopathy are reversible with control of blood pressure [47, 132]. Striate hemorrhages cease to form as soon as the blood pressure is controlled. Clearance of existing hemorrhages takes 2 to 8 weeks. Cotton-wool spots may continue to form for several days after the blood pressure is controlled. The cellular (axonal) debris that comprises cotton-wool spots is cleared away within 2 to 12 weeks. Hard exudates clear more slowly. A macular star may require over a year to resolve completely. Papilledema often continues to increase for the first few days of treatment. In the majority of patients, however, it resolves slowly over several weeks. In contrast, the changes reflecting retinal arteriosclerosis, such as arteriolar narrowing, arteriovenous crossing defects, and changes in the light reflexes, usually persist despite adequate control of blood pressure [47].

EVALUATION FOR SECONDARY CAUSES OF MALIGNANT HYPERTENSION

The various secondary causes of malignant hypertension have been discussed earlier in the section Etiology of Malignant Hypertension. Whereas, less than 5 percent of patients with benign hypertension have an underlying secondary cause of hypertension, malignant hypertension may be associated with a secondary cause in up to 50 percent of patients. For example, among patients with benign hypertension, the incidence of renovascular hypertension is less than 0.5 percent [574]. In contrast, there is a substantial incidence of renovascular hypertension (43 percent in whites, 7 percent in blacks) among patients with malignant hypertension [115]. Thus, after malignant hypertension has been successfully treated, the possibility of underlying renovascular hypertension should be investigated. Noninvasive screening tests such as rapid-sequence intravenous pyelography and radionuclide renal scans are of little value because of the high frequency of false-positive and false-negative results [574]. Renal arteriography is the procedure of choice to exclude the possibility of anatomic renal artery stenosis. The diagnosis and treatment of renovascular hypertension are discussed in detail in Chap. 55.

Pheochromocytoma is a rare cause of malignant hypertension. However, given the likelihood of surgical cure or amelioration of hypertension, pheochromocytoma should be excluded. The approach to the diagnosis of pheochromocytoma is discussed in Chap. 56.

Primary hyperaldosteronism due to an adrenal aldosterone-producing adenoma is an extremely rare cause of malignant hypertension. However, the biochemical abnormalities in patients with malignant hypertension may mimic those of primary hyperaldosteronism [347]. Long after the malignant phase has resolved, hypokalemia with inappropriate urinary potassium wasting, increased aldosterone secretion, and suppressed plasma renin activity may persist. This phenomenon has been postulated to represent a form of tertiary hyperaldosteronism [347]. With sustained treatment of hypertension, this hyperaldosteronism eventually resolves. Since primary hyperaldosteronism is an unusual cause of malignant hypertension, an evaluation for primary hyperaldosteronism should not be undertaken unless these abnormalities persist for over a year after the malignant phase has resolved.

The role of renal biopsy in the diagnosis of possible underlying primary renal parenchymal disease in patients with malignant hypertension is controversial. In patients presenting with malignant hypertension and renal failure, it may not be possible on clinical grounds to distinguish primary malignant hypertension from chronic glomerulonephritis or chronic interstitial nephritis with superimposed malignant nephrosclerosis. A renal biopsy may be required to make this distinction. When the kidneys appear small with ultrasonography, a biopsy is not indicated, since it is unlikely that the results of the biopsy will alter therapy. In contrast, when the kidneys are normal in size, a renal biopsy may provide useful information. If primary malignant nephrosclerosis with ischemic but viable glomeruli is found, then aggressive antihypertensive therapy may be associated with the eventual recovery of renal function, even after months of maintenance dialysis. Conversely, the finding of chronic glomerulonephritis or chronic interstitial nephritis with superimposed malignant nephrosclerosis suggests a less favorable long-term outcome.

Malignant hypertension may mimic acute glomerulonephritis or vasculitis. Patients may present with severe hypertension and oliguric acute renal failure with a nephritic sediment [345]. In this setting, a renal biopsy is essential, since acute glomerulonephritis or vasculitis may require specific therapy in addition to antihypertensive treatment.

Since uremia and severe hypertension predispose to serious hemorrhagic complications after renal biopsy, it is prudent to manage the patient with aggressive dialysis and blood pressure control for 1 to 3 weeks prior to performance of a percutaneous renal biopsy. Unfortunately, this delay in obtaining tissue may make the diagnosis of malignant nephrosclerosis more difficult, since the lesions of fibrinoid necrosis may heal rapidly with the institution of antihypertensive treatment, leaving a residual hyaline or fibrous scar [218, 348]. Moreover, given the sampling error inherent in closed renal biopsy, the patchy necrotic lesions of malignant nephrosclerosis may be missed. Thus, diagnosis of malignant nephrosclerosis is often made on the basis of the findings of accelerated glomerular obsolescence and marked intimal hyperplasia of the arterioles [269].

Unilateral renal disease from atrophic pyelonephritis may occasionally cause malignant hypertension in both children and adults [236, 288, 516]. However, the experience with unilateral nephrectomy for hypertension control has been disappointing [506]. In hypertensive patients with a unilaterally small scarred kidney on intravenous pyelography, Kaplan [275] has proposed that nephrectomy should be reserved for those patients who fulfill the following criteria: severe hypertension, marked loss of renal function on the affected side, normal function of the contralateral kidney, and lateralizing renal vein renin ratios. In children, cure of malignant hypertension has been reported after partial nephrectomy of a scarred segment if high renin values are documented on segmental renal vein catheterization [262, 441].

BENIGN VERSUS MALIGNANT HYPERTENSION

Since the original description by Volhard and Fahr [552], two forms of essential hypertension have been recognized, benign and malignant. It is worth emphasizing that these two forms of hypertension should be conceptualized as distinct clinical and pathologic entities. In benign hypertension, there is usually a long asymptomatic phase, with death resulting from complications of cerebrovascular disease, atherosclerotic disease, or congestive heart failure, rather than renal disease [30, 426, 427]. In benign essential hypertension (i.e., hypertension without a malignant phase or underlying primary renal disease), only rarely does end-stage renal failure occur [198, 228, 284, 285, 336]. In contrast, malignant hypertension, if untreated, uniformly progresses to end-stage renal disease (ESRD).

There is much controversy in the field of hypertension regarding the frequency with which benign hypertension (benign arteriolar nephrosclerosis), in the absence of a superimposed malignant phase, causes ESRD. Goldring and Chasis [198] extensively evaluated renal function in a large group of patients with essential hypertension. Most patients with long-standing essential hypertension had anatomic lesions in kidneys consistent with hyaline arteriolar nephrosclerosis. Moreover, the majority had demonstrable renal abnormalities including abnormal urinalysis with hyaline and granular casts, low-grade proteinuria (less than 1 gm/day), decreased tubular maximum for para-aminohippurate, decreased renal blood flow, normal to slightly decreased glomerular filtration rate, and increased filtration fraction. However, they found that ESRD rarely occurred in patients with benign hypertension. Among 150 hypertensive patients with ESRD, only one was found to have benign nephrosclerosis as the sole underlying etiology [198]. They concluded that, in benign hypertension, functional failure occurred earlier in the heart and brain than in the kidney and that death from renal failure without a superimposed malignant phase was a rare event.

In contrast to these early reports, which were based principally on renal histologic findings at autopsy, in more recent series *hypertensive nephrosclerosis* is listed as a common cause of ESRD, especially among black patients. For example, Easterling [142] and Rostand et al. [473] found that the overall rate of ESRD was four times higher in blacks than whites. Both studies suggest that much of the excess risk of ESRD among blacks can be explained by an extraordinarily high rate of renal failure from hypertensive nephrosclerosis. The relative risk of hypertensive nephrosclerosis was 17 to 18 times higher in blacks than whites [142, 473]. Moreover, it has been estimated that on a national scale, 29 percent of blacks with ESRD have hypertension as the primary cause [142, 473]. However, in these recent studies, classification of the causes of ESRD was based on clinical rather than histologic evidence. Furthermore, in these studies it is not clear whether the term *hypertensive nephrosclerosis* refers to benign or malignant nephrosclerosis. In the few available studies detailing the pathologic findings in blacks with ESRD due to hypertension, the characteristic findings have been those of malignant nephrosclerosis, namely, musculomucoid intimal hyperplasia of the interlobular arteries and accelerated glomerular obsolescence [439, 535].

The widely held notion that benign hypertension with benign nephrosclerosis is a common cause of ESRD is difficult to support [21, 285, 562]. In contrast to the large body of literature relating mild to moderate benign hypertension to excessive cardiovascular morbidity, there is surprisingly little information available regarding the corresponding risk of significant renal disease [562]. Autopsy studies in patients with documented benign hypertension suggest that significant renal damage due to benign nephrosclerosis is rare except in the presence of renal artery stenosis (ischemic nephropathy) or superimposed malignant hypertension [198, 285]. Kincaid-Smith [285, 289] has stated that in the patient with hypertension and renal impairment, if renal artery stenosis and malignant hypertension have been excluded, the most likely diagnosis is underlying primary renal parenchymal disease rather than benign nephrosclerosis.

An analysis of the data from three recent large clinical trials in patients with essential hypertension revealed that less than 1 percent of 10,000 patients developed advanced renal failure during the 4 to 6 years of follow-up [60, 61, 258, 301]. A very low incidence of clinically significant deterioration of renal function was also noted in the Hypertension Detection and Follow-up Program [498]. Moreover, a study of untreated patients with mild to moderate essential hypertension found only minor declines in glomerular filtration rate (1.6 percent per year) and renal blood flow (2.1 percent per year), which did not differ from the renal function decline associated with aging in normotensive individuals [461]. Even severe untreated hypertension (diastolic blood pressure 120 to 150 mm Hg), in the absence of a malignant phase, caused only a minor decrement in glomerular filtration rate (1.7 percent per year) [461].

In contrast to these studies, a provocative recent study found that mild to moderate benign hypertension did cause renal insufficiency that progressed despite adequate blood pressure control [472]. However, since renal biopsies were not performed, the data do not exclude the possibility of occult primary renal parenchymal disease in patients demonstrating progressive renal insufficiency [291].

In summary, while it is clear that malignant hypertension is a frequent cause of ESRD, especially among blacks, there remains controversy regarding the commonly held belief that benign hypertension per se causes ESRD. The critical issue that has yet to be resolved is why blacks constitute a disproportionately high percentage of patients with ESRD in the United States [459, 473]. Epidemiologic studies suggest that essential hypertension occurs more frequently in blacks and is associated with more severe cardiovascular end-organ damage for any given level of blood pressure [151, 176]. In angiographic studies of patients with mild to moderate essential hypertension and normal renal function, blacks tended to have more severe angiographic evidence of nephrosclerosis than whites [318]. Tobian [535] has postulated that the low-potassium diet characteristically consumed by blacks in the United States (30 mmol/day versus 65 mmol/day in the general population) accelerates the intimal thickening of the renal vasculature that occurs due to hypertensive damage. He has proposed that this may account for the increased risk of progressive renal insufficiency due to hypertension in blacks.

There are several other plausible explanations for the high frequency with which hypertensive nephrosclerosis is reported as a cause of ESRD in the black population. Since most of the available data are based on clinical diagnoses, there may be a tendency on the part of physicians to identify hypertension as the cause of ESRD given the known high prevalence of hypertension in blacks, even when a primary renal parenchymal disease cannot be excluded on clinical grounds [562]. Another possibility is that blacks with essential hypertension tend to develop more severe benign nephrosclerosis that, unlike benign nephrosclerosis in whites, results in progressive renal insufficiency and ESRD. Finally, it is possible that recurrent bouts of unrecognized or inadequately treated malignant hypertension are the actual cause of the increased incidence of ESRD. In this regard, a recent study of 100 patients admitted to an inner-city New York hospital with a diagnosis of hypertensive emergency showed that two-thirds had malignant hypertension based on funduscopic findings [35]. These patients were predominantly young, male, black or Hispanic individuals of lower socioeconomic status. At least 93 percent of these patients had been previously diagnosed as hypertensive, and at least 83 percent were aware of their diagnosis of hypertension. At least 87 percent were known to have received prior pharmacologic treatment for hypertension. However, no source of regular health care could be documented in 60 percent of cases. More than 50 percent were noted to have stopped their antihypertensive medications more than 30 days prior to admission, and only 24 percent had taken any medication on the day of admission. If the overrepresentation of young blacks with ESRD is due to undiagnosed or inadequately treated malignant hypertension, this would have tremendous public health implications, since malignant hypertension is clearly preventable and even significant renal dysfunction is potentially reversible with early and aggressive antihypertensive therapy.

Hypertensive Encephalopathy

Most of the deleterious effects of hypertension on the brain are the result of long-standing mild to moderate elevations of blood pressure, including atherothrombotic infarction, lacunar infarction, and intracerebral hemorrhage. Occasionally, severe acute hypertension can produce dramatic and life-threatening cerebral complications. *Hypertensive encephalopathy* is an acute cerebral syndrome that develops in association with a sudden and sustained elevation of blood pressure [411]. It may occur with malignant hypertension or severe hypertension that is not in the malignant phase. Hypertensive encephalopathy is a medical emergency that demands prompt diagnosis and rapid control of blood pressure to prevent irreversible brain damage or death. The clinical *sine qua non* of hypertensive encephalopathy is the prompt resolution of symptoms when the blood pressure is brought under control. Although hypertensive encephalopathy is a distinct clinicopathologic entity, in the past the term has sometimes been used inappropriately to describe any cerebrovascular event that occurs in association with hypertension, including transient ischemic attacks, cerebral infarction or hemorrhage, senile dementia, or cortical atrophy.

CLINICAL PRESENTATION

The diagnosis of hypertensive encephalopathy is usually made on clinical grounds. The appearance of cerebral symptoms usually follows the *sudden onset* of hypertension in previously normotensive individuals or the *abrupt increase* in blood pressure in patients with chronic hypertension. The abrupt blood pressure elevation usually occurs 12 to 48 hours before the onset of symptoms, although this is often difficult to document. Symptoms may appear at lower levels of blood pressure in previously normotensive individuals than in those with chronic hypertension. For example, in children with acute glomerulonephritis or pregnant women with eclampsia, hypertensive encephalopathy may occur when the blood pressure is no greater than 160/100 [188]. However, the syndrome rarely occurs in chronically hypertensive individuals at pressures less than 200/120 mm Hg and may not occur until the blood pressure is greater than 250/150 mm Hg.

The initial symptom of hypertensive encephalopathy is usually a severe, generalized *headache* that increases steadily in severity [129]. Unfortunately, headache is a nonspecific symptom, and even among patients with malignant hypertension it does not necessarily imply central nervous system damage [86]. *Weakness, nausea,* and *vomiting* (sometimes projectile) are often present. *Neck stiffness* is an occasional finding. *Loss of vision* is another common feature. Visual loss may be caused by the retinal edema and hemorrhages that accompany hypertensive neuroretinopathy, or as the result of *cortical (occipital) blindness* [263]. Denial of visual loss or loss of vision in the presence of a normal light reflex suggests cortical blindness.

Altered mental status is a prominent clinical feature of hypertensive encephalopathy. Apathy, somnolence, and confusion are the initial manifestations and usually appear several hours to days after the onset of headache. If treatment is not instituted, coma and death may occur. Recurrent *seizures* are common and may be either generalized or focal.

There is controversy regarding whether *focal neurologic deficits* occur in hypertensive encephalopathy. There are numerous reports of transient focal neurologic disturbances in patients with hypertensive encephalopathy including fleeting paresthesias and numbness in extremities, transient paralysis, and aphasia [263, 411]. Others have suggested that focal deficits in patients with severe hypertension always imply underlying ischemic infarct or hemorrhage [86, 225, 585]. Chester et al. [83] reported a clinicopathologic study of 20 patients with malignant hypertension and hypertensive encephalopathy. Eight patients developed focal neurologic signs in addition to the typical features of hypertensive encephalopathy [83]. After the blood pressure was controlled, the nonfocal cerebral symptoms of hypertensive encephalopathy resolved dramatically; however, the focal neurologic deficits persisted. At postmortem examination, intracerebral hemorrhage, lacunar infarcts, and larger ischemic infarcts were found in addition to pathologic changes attributed to hypertensive encephalopathy. Thus, focal neurologic deficits do not necessarily exclude the diagnosis of hypertensive encephalopathy.

Hypertensive neuroretinopathy (striate hemorrhages, cotton-wool spots, and papilledema) is present when hypertensive encephalopathy occurs in patients with malignant hypertension. However, neuroretinopathy may be absent when hypertensive encephalopathy develops in the setting of acute glomerulonephritis, eclampsia, pheochromocytoma, monoamine oxidase inhibitor–tyramine interactions, or antihypertensive drug withdrawal syndromes [188, 263].

Many authors have cautioned that *lumbar puncture* should be avoided in patients with suspected hypertensive encephalopathy because of the risk of cerebellar herniation [129, 482]. When performed, lumbar puncture has revealed elevated cerebrospinal fluid (CSF) pressure in most patients ranging from 230 to 560 mm water [83, 263]. CSF protein is usually moderately elevated (48 to 90 mg/dl) but may be normal. The cell count is usually normal [83, 263].

Electroencephalography performed during the acute stage of hypertensive encephalopathy may reveal suppression of alpha activity and the appearance of rhythmic slow delta activity in the occipital leads. These abnormalities resolve with control of the blood pressure [263].

Computed tomography may show compression of the lateral ventricles, which is an indication of cerebral edema. Symmetric, well-demarcated, low-density areas may occur in the white matter and probably represent edema because they resolve following control of the blood pressure [129].

ETIOLOGIES OF HYPERTENSIVE ENCEPHALOPATHY

Although hypertensive encephalopathy may complicate malignant hypertension [83, 411], not all patients with hypertensive encephalopathy have malignant hypertension. In fact, it most commonly occurs in previously normotensive individuals who experience sudden, severe hypertension (Table 59-5). The reported causes of hy-

Table 59-5. Etiologies of hypertensive encephalopathy

Malignant hypertension of any cause
Acute glomerulonephritis
Eclampsia
Renovascular hypertension
Post–coronary artery bypass hypertension
Abrupt withdrawal of antihypertensive therapy
Monoamine oxidase inhibitor–tyramine interactions
Pheochromocytoma
Phencyclidine (PCP) poisoning
Phenylpropanolamine overdose
Acute renal artery occlusion
Acute lead poisoning in children
High-dose cyclosporine in children
Transplant renal artery stenosis or acute rejection
Femoral lengthening procedures
Acute or chronic spinal cord injuries

pertensive encephalopathy include *acute glomerulonephritis, eclampsia* [129, 263], *renovascular hypertension* [188], *post–coronary artery bypass hypertension* [95], *clonidine withdrawal* [457], *monoamine oxidase inhibitor–tyramine interactions* [190], *pheochromocytoma* [201], *phencyclidine (PCP) poisoning* [143], *phenylpropanolamine overdose* [302, 425], *acute renal artery occlusion* [263], *acute lead poisoning* [263], *high-dose cyclosporine* therapy after bone marrow transplantation in children [271, 326], *transplant renal artery stenosis or acute rejection* [349, 531], or *femoral lengthening procedures* in children [364]. Hypertensive encephalopathy may also occur in patients with *acute or chronic spinal cord injuries* if there is excessive autonomic stimulation due to bowel or bladder distention [153, 392]. It may also complicate rebound hypertension that follows diagnostic *saralasin infusion* in patients with renovascular hypertension [278].

PATHOLOGIC FINDINGS IN HYPERTENSIVE ENCEPHALOPATHY

In the initial case reports that described pathology in fatal cases of hypertensive encephalopathy, the brain was frequently normal except for the finding of *diffuse cerebral edema* [411]. However, in two large series, definite pathologic findings characteristic of this syndrome have been identified [83, 470].

The brain weight was increased in only 2 of 20 patients, and cerebellar herniation was found in only 1 case of hypertensive encephalopathy. There was no evidence that cerebral edema was a prominent manifestation of hypertensive encephalopathy.

There were characteristic changes in the cerebral microvasculature. *Fibrinoid necrosis* of the cerebral arterioles was found in 13 of 20 patients with malignant hypertension complicated by hypertensive encephalopathy (Fig. 59-22). The arteriolar walls were swollen and stained bright red with hematoxylin and eosin and deep blue or purple with phosphotungstic acid-hematoxylin (PTAH). *Fibrin thrombi* occluded the lumens of necrotic or intact arterioles in 12 cases. In addition, there were *focal or segmental irregularities* in the walls of arterioles in each patient with hypertensive encephalopathy. These consisted of marked *fibrous thickening* and *hyalinization, occlusion of the lumen* by fibrous or hyaline masses, and *endothelial hyperplasia*. In addition to these vascular abnormalities, characteristic parenchymal changes were frequently found. There were *miliary zones of infarction* from 100 microns to 2 mm in diameter, which were associated with vessels containing fibrinoid necrosis and fibrin occlusion (Fig. 59-23). In advanced stages, the lesions took the form of microglial nodules. In the chronic stages, the reaction consisted mainly of fibrous and gemistocytic astrocytes [83]. The vascular and parenchymal lesions were distributed diffusely in the brain stem, basal ganglia, diencephalon, cerebral white matter, cerebral cortex, and spinal cord, in descending order of frequency. The extent and severity of the lesions varied but tended to correlate with the severity of the neurologic manifestations and the level of blood pressure [83].

The authors conclude that the pathology characteristic of hypertensive encephalopathy is fibrinoid necrosis of cerebral arterioles in combination with miliary infarcts and microglial nodules [83]. However, this study has been criticized because the pathologic findings might have been due to recurrent, partially treated bouts of malignant hypertension rather than a manifestation of the changes corresponding to acute hypertensive en-

Fig. 59-22. Pons. Arteriole with fibrinoid necrosis phosphotungstic acid–hematoxylin stain, × 430. (From E. M. Chester, D. P. Agamanolis, B. Q. Banker, and M. Victor. Hypertensive encephalopathy: A clinicopathologic study of 20 cases. *Neurology* 28:928, 1978. With permission.)

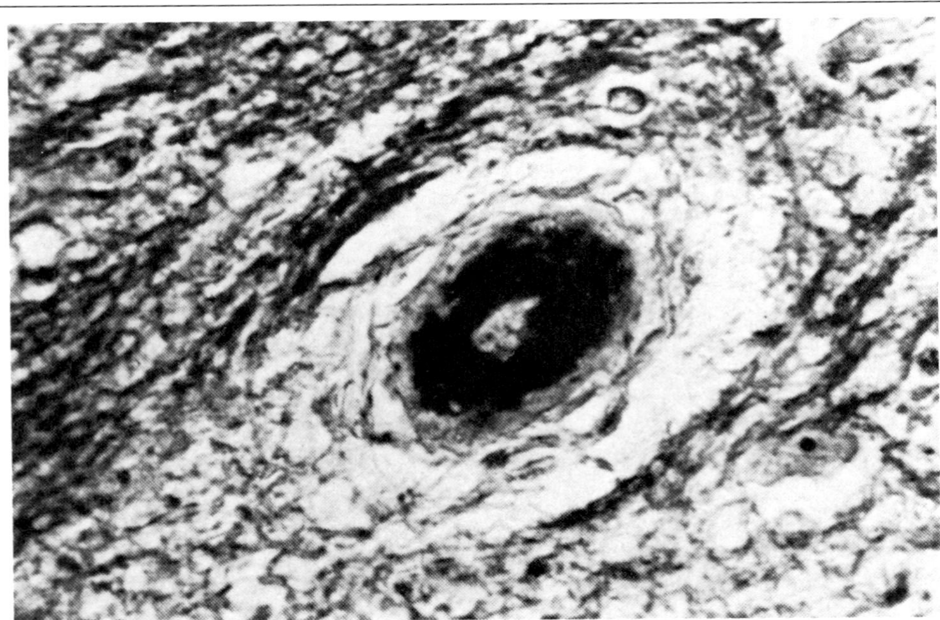

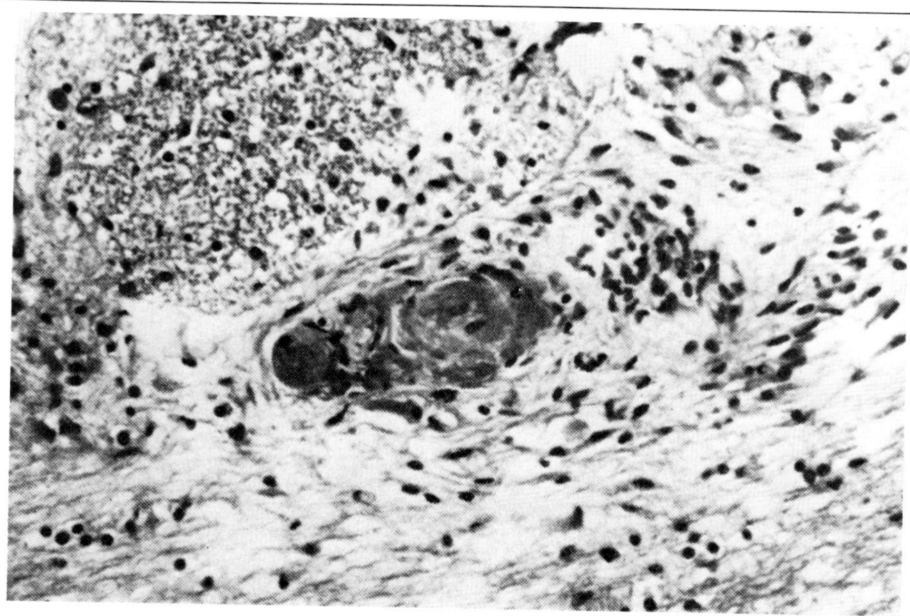

Fig. 59-23. Medulla. Arteriole with fibrinoid necrosis and thrombosis surrounded by a microinfarct (hematoxylin and eosin, × 170). (From E. M. Chester, D. P. Agamanolis, B. Q. Banker, and M. Victor. Hypertensive encephalopathy: A clinicopathologic study of 20 cases. *Neurology* 28:928, 1978. With permission.)

cephalopathy [130]. These pathologic findings may not be present in cases of hypertensive encephalopathy due to acute, severe hypertension that is not in the malignant phase [411].

THE PATHOGENESIS OF HYPERTENSIVE ENCEPHALOPATHY

The Overregulation Theory of Hypertensive Encephalopathy. The traditional theory on the pathogenesis of hypertensive encephalopathy was originally proposed by Oppenheimer and Fishberg [411] (Fig. 59-24). They proposed that in response to a rapid severe increase in blood pressure, there was intense reflex *cerebral vasoconstriction.*This intense spasm was thought to lead to *decreased cerebral blood flow* (*overregulation*) and *ischemia.* The vasoconstriction and ischemia were thought to account for the development of increased capillary permeability, fibrinoid necrosis, and capillary hemorrhage. Moreover, damage to the blood-brain barrier was felt to cause cerebral edema in some cases.

Continued support for the overregulation theory of hypertensive encephalopathy derives from the fact that increased cerebral blood flow and cerebral edemas, which are central features of the breakthrough theory, are rare findings in patients with hypertensive encephalopathy [162, 188].

The Breakthrough Theory of Hypertensive Encephalopathy. The breakthrough theory originally proposed by Lassen and Angoli [308] is summarized in Fig. 59-25. Under normal circumstances, there is autoregulation of the cerebral microcirculation such that, over a wide range of perfusion pressures, cerebral blood flow remains constant. It has been proposed that in the setting of a sudden, severe increase in blood pressure, autoregulatory vasoconstriction fails, and there is *forced vasodilation.* The dilatation is initially segmental (sausage string pattern) but eventually becomes diffuse. The endothelium in the dilated segments becomes abnormally permeable, and there is extravasation of plasma components with the development of *cerebral edema.* This theory may explain the clinical observation that hypertensive encephalopathy develops at a much lower level of blood pressure in previously normotensive individuals than it does in those with chronic hypertension. With long-standing hypertension, structural changes and remodeling of the cerebral arterioles may lead to a shift in the autoregulatory curve such that much higher levels of perfusion pressure can be tolerated before forced vasodilation and breakthrough of autoregulation occur [522, 524].

Strandgaard et al. [520, 521] have reported studies on the regulation of cerebral blood flow in baboons with acute hypertension. Cerebral blood flow was measured using the xenon washout technique as the blood pressure was gradually increased during angiotensin II infusion. Cerebral blood flow remained constant up to a mean arterial blood pressure (MAP) of 130 to 139 mm Hg by virtue of an increase in cerebrovascular resistance (intact autoregulation). However, at this level of MAP, cerebrovascular resistance reached a maximum value. At higher levels of MAP, cerebral blood flow increased significantly as cerebrovascular resistance decreased, consistent with a breakthrough of autoregulation. There was no evidence of spasm or decreased cerebral blood flow (overregulation theory) in response to severe hypertension.

Despite the evidence of an overall increase in cerebral

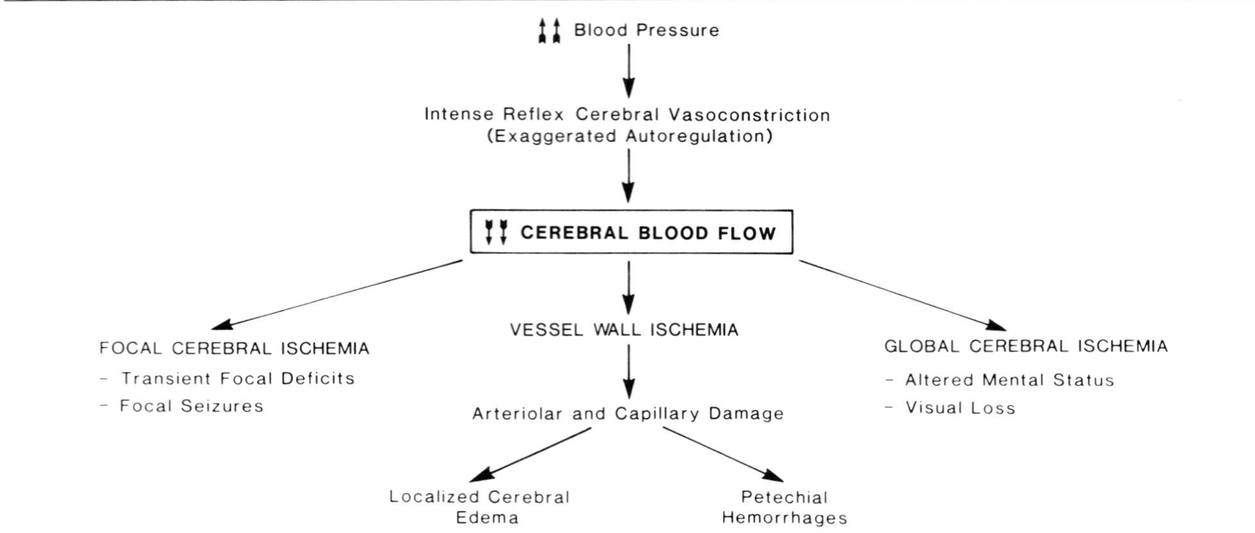

Fig. 59-24. The overregulation theory of hypertensive encephalopathy.

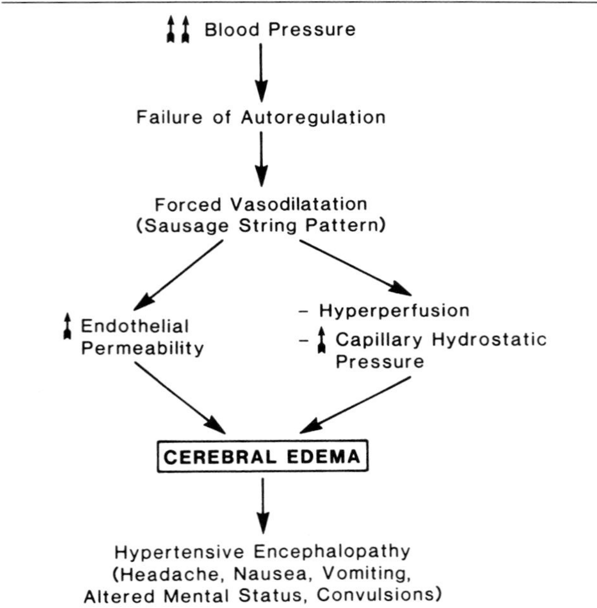

Fig. 59-25. The breakthrough theory of hypertensive encephalopathy.

blood flow at high mean arterial pressures, it has been argued that blood flow could nonetheless be decreased in highly localized areas of the brain and that these areas of reduced flow might not be identified by techniques used to measure global cerebral blood flow [131]. To address this concern, MacKenzie et al. [334] studied the effects of acute hypertension on pial arteriolar caliber, local cerebral blood flow, and the blood-brain barrier in cats. Changes in pial arteriolar caliber were observed directly through a craniotomy window with a stereomicroscope. Changes in local cerebral blood flow were measured by a hydrogen clearance technique with electrodes inserted into specific segments of the brain. As the blood pressure was increased with angiotensin II, the pial arterioles constricted up to a MAP of 160 mm Hg. At approximately 180 mm Hg, there were focal areas of vasodilation and constriction in the arterioles. However, the caliber of constricted areas was no smaller than it was at 160 mm Hg, which suggested that the sausage string pattern resulted from focal areas of forced vasodilation rather than from areas of further constriction. After approximately 20 minutes, the entire arteriole became dilated. Local cerebral blood flow remained constant until the MAP exceeded 160 mm Hg. Above this level, the cerebral blood flow increased in proportion to the MAP. There was no evidence of a local or global reduction in blood flow.

Johansson et al. [265] have demonstrated that hypertension-induced damage to the blood-brain barrier develops within minutes of a sudden, severe increase in blood pressure [265]. The injury was postulated to result from overstretching of vessels rather than from spasm and ischemia, since hypoxic injury to the blood-brain barrier requires several hours to develop.

In a rat model of hypertensive encephalopathy due to one-kidney, one-clip renovascular hypertension, the sausage string pattern developed in pial vessels in response to severe hypertension. Injection of colloidal carbon particles demonstrated that there was increased vascular permeability in the dilated segments [186, 187].

Structural damage to the blood-brain barrier may not be required for the formation of cerebral edema in response to sudden severe hypertension. Nag et al. [393] have shown that cerebral arterioles and capillaries become abnormally permeable to protein-bound dyes within seconds after induction of severe hypertension [393]. Pinocytotic vessels were observed to transport these large molecular markers through the structural components of the blood-brain barrier during periods of acute hypertension. It was proposed that passage of protein molecules by pinocytosis results in the extravascular accumulation of protein-rich fluid and water (cerebral edema).

The Structural Theory of Hypertensive Encephalopathy. In both the overregulation and breakthrough theories, hypertensive encephalopathy is conceptualized as a functional derangement of the cerebral circulation, which is reversible when the blood pressure is lowered. Although structural alteration of the arterioles and brain parenchyma have been reported in both humans [83, 188] and experimental animals [65, 405, 529], their role in the pathogenesis of hypertensive encephalopathy remains unclear.

Chester et al. [83] have proposed a modification of the breakthrough theory that is consistent with the pathophysiology of malignant hypertension in other vascular beds (Fig. 59-26). They proposed that a sudden increase in blood pressure results in forced overdistention of cerebral arterioles, increased endothelial permeability, extravasation of fibrinogen and other plasma proteins, and development of fibrinoid necrosis. These necrotic lesions may result in petechial hemorrhages, intracerebral hemorrhage, and ischemic miliary infarcts. They proposed that the clinical findings in hypertensive encephalopathy might be caused by these focal structural lesions. Multiple small lesions that are diffusely distributed could cause damage to the reticular activating system with depression of consciousness. Small cortical lesions could trigger seizures. Microinfarcts of the brain stem or spinal cord could cause focal neurologic signs.

TREATMENT OF HYPERTENSIVE ENCEPHALOPATHY

The optimal management of hypertensive encephalopathy does not depend on resolution of the controversy regarding pathogenesis. Prompt reduction of the blood pressure is indicated regardless of whether spasm, breakthrough, or structural damage underlies the cerebral dysfunction.

When the diagnosis of hypertensive encephalopathy seems likely, antihypertensive therapy should be initiated prior to obtaining the results of time-consuming laboratory and radiologic examinations. The goal of therapy, especially in the previously normotensive patient with acute hypertension, should be the reduction of blood pressure to normal or near normal levels as promptly as possible [188]. Although theoretically cerebral blood flow may be jeopardized by the rapid reduction of blood pressure in patients with chronic hypertension in whom the lower limit of autoregulation is shifted to a higher level of blood pressure [522, 524], clinical experience has shown that the prompt reduction of blood pressure with the avoidance of frank hypotension is beneficial in patients with hypertensive encephalopathy [188]. Of the conditions in the differential diagnosis of hypertension with acute cerebral dysfunction, only cerebral infarction might be adversely affected by the abrupt reduction of blood pressure [99]. Pharmacologic agents that have a rapid onset and short duration of action, such as sodium nitroprusside, should be utilized so that the blood pressure can be carefully titrated with close observation of the patient's neurologic status. The clinical *sine qua non* of hypertensive encephalopathy is a prompt clinical response to antihypertensive therapy. Conversely, when blood pressure reduction is associated with the development of new or progressive neurologic deficits, other diagnoses should be considered, and the blood pressure should be stabilized at a higher level.

Fig. 59-26. The structural theory of hypertensive encephalopathy.

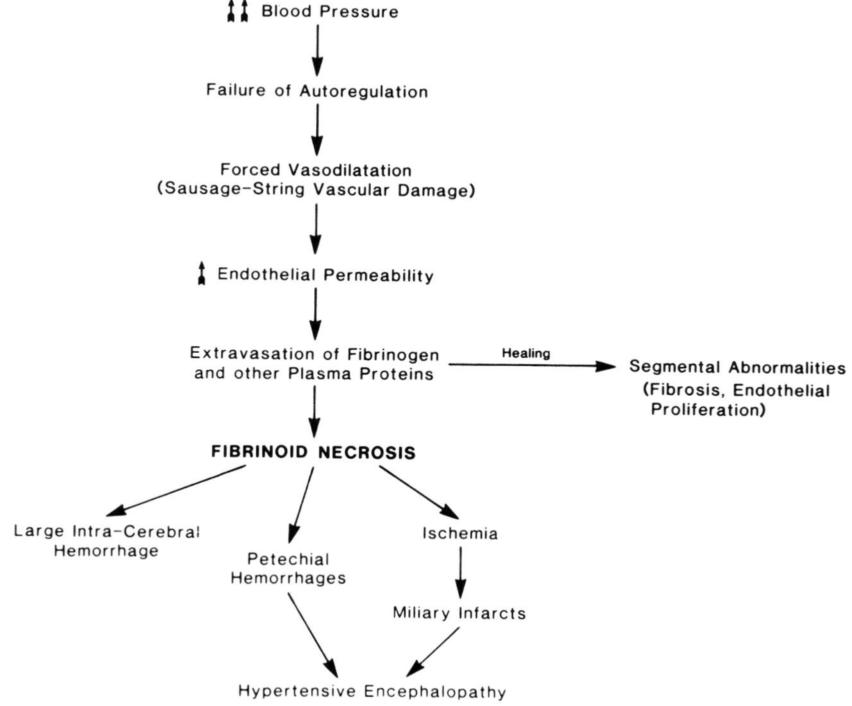

In women with eclampsia, convulsions and other neurologic manifestations occur that are indistinguishable from those observed in nonpregnant individuals with hypertensive encephalopathy, except that they occur at lower blood pressures. Eclampsia is associated with extreme risk to both the mother and the fetus. Although delivery of the fetus is the definitive cure in most cases, rapid control of the blood pressure and encephalopathic manifestations is essential before the induction of labor or performance of a cesarean section [8].

Hypertension Complicated by Acute Pulmonary Edema

Both malignant hypertension and severe benign hypertension may be complicated by acute pulmonary edema. Acute fulminant pulmonary edema was a frequent cause of death among patients with malignant hypertension in the pre-antihypertensive treatment era [226, 288, 336]. Historically, in untreated patients with benign hypertension, the development of left ventricular failure was associated with a mean survival of only 1.8 years [163]. However, with the advent of effective antihypertensive therapy, the prognosis for hypertensive patients with left ventricular failure has improved dramatically. With adequate control of blood pressure, long-term survival is possible. However, the treatment of hypertension varies depending on whether patients present with evidence of chronic congestive heart failure or a hypertensive crisis with acute pulmonary edema.

Traditionally, congestive heart failure has been equated with systolic dysfunction in which there is an inability of the myofibrils to shorten against a load such that the left ventricle loses its ability to eject blood into the high-pressure aorta [512]. The end result is a dilated, poorly contractile left ventricle with a low ejection fraction and a reduced cardiac output. In recent years, however, there has been increasing recognition that abnormalities in the diastolic function of the left ventricle may result in symptoms of congestive heart failure despite the presence of normal ejection fraction and cardiac output [137, 324, 508, 512]. *Diastolic dysfunction* implies that the ventricle cannot fill normally at low filling pressures. Ventricular filling is slow, delayed, or incomplete unless the atrial pressure increases [324, 512]. A compensatory increase in filling pressure occurs that is sufficient to maintain normal systolic function but at the expense of pulmonary and systemic venous congestion. Thus, signs and symptoms of pulmonary or systemic venous congestion are not always the result of systolic dysfunction; instead, they may result from isolated abnormalities of the diastolic properties of the left ventricle [137, 324, 508, 512].

Hypertensive patients with chronic congestive heart failure manifest by dyspnea and symptoms of pulmonary and systemic venous congestion are not infrequently found to have intact systolic function but abnormal diastolic function as defined by echocardiographic or radionuclide evaluation of diastolic filling [137, 508, 538]. The left ventricular hypertrophy that develops in response to chronic systemic hypertension may cause abnormal myocardial relaxation and increased left ventricular chamber stiffness, which lead to the impairment in diastolic filling that characterizes diastolic dysfunction. In clinical practice, the presence of dyspnea, pulmonary rales, and radiographic evidence of pulmonary venous congestion despite a normal ejection fraction should suggest the possibility of diastolic dysfunction [512]. Recent evidence suggests that the traditional treatment for congestive heart failure with digitalis and arterial vasodilators may be deleterious in patients with isolated diastolic dysfunction due to hypertensive heart disease [538]. This type of *chronic diastolic dysfunction* in hypertensive patients is best managed with β-blockers, calcium channel blockers, or both. These drugs decrease heart rate and improve the balance between myocardial oxygen supply and demand and thus may improve myocardial relaxation and overall diastolic function. Classes of drugs that are associated with regression of left ventricular hypertrophy, such as angiotensin converting enzyme inhibitors, nondihydropyridine calcium channel blockers, β-blockers, and centrally acting α-adrenergic agonists, may result in an improvement in diastolic function as the hypertrophy regresses [559]. Diuretics and salt restriction may be used to treat congestive symptoms, but care should be taken to avoid excessive preload reduction, which may compromise systolic function [512]. Venodilatation and preload reduction with nitrates may also improve symptoms of pulmonary congestion [512].

Isolated diastolic dysfunction is also the pathophysiologic process that underlies the development of acute pulmonary edema in patients with either malignant hypertension or severe benign hypertension. However, in the setting of this *acute hypertensive heart failure,* the compromise of left ventricular diastolic function is due to the markedly increased work load imposed on the heart as a result of a pronounced elevation in systemic vascular resistance [89]. Hypertension complicated by acute pulmonary edema represents a crisis requiring immediate control of blood pressure with potent peripheral vasodilators, such as sodium nitroprusside, to quickly reduce the high systemic vascular resistance that is the proximate cause of this disorder.

The hemodynamic derangements in acute hypertensive heart failure were defined in a study that compared 5 patients with severe long-standing essential hypertension complicated by acute pulmonary edema with a control group of 5 patients of similar age who had long-standing hypertension of equal severity but who never had evidence of congestive heart failure [91, 467]. The subjects in both groups had electrocardiographic evidence of left ventricular hypertrophy and chest radiographic evidence of cardiomegaly with left ventricular prominence. However, pulmonary venous engorgement was evident only in the group with heart failure. The hemodynamic findings in the two groups of severely hypertensive patients are displayed in Fig. 59-27. The levels of mean arterial pressure, heart rate, cardiac index, and stroke work index were the same in both groups. The left ventricular end-diastolic volume (LVEDV) was similarly elevated in both groups. In fact, the only hemodynamic difference between the two groups was a

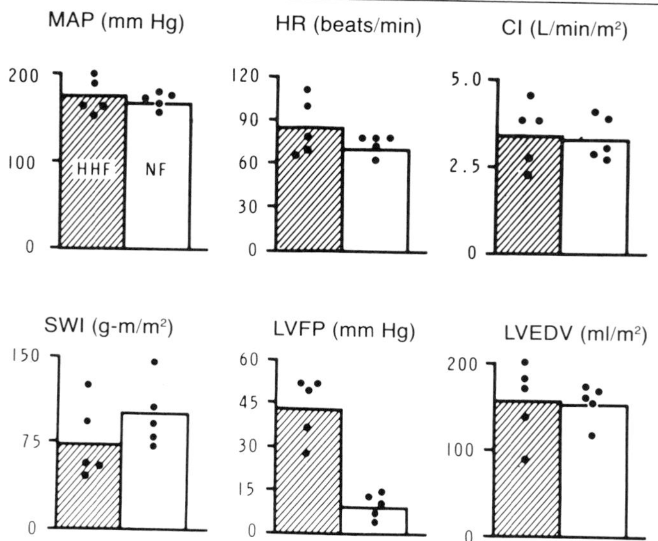

Fig. 59-27. Pretreatment hemodynamics in patients with acute hypertensive heart failure (HHF) and those with severe hypertension but without heart failure (NF). MAP = mean arterial pressure; HR = heart rate; CI = cardiac index; SWI = stroke work index; LVFP = left ventricular filling pressure; LVEDV = left ventricular end-diastolic volume. The MAP, HR, SWI, and LVEDV were the same in both groups. The only difference between the groups was a significant elevation of LVFP in the patients with HHF. These findings suggest a decrease in left ventricular compliance in the patients with HHF, since the LVFP was significantly increased even though the LVEDV was the same as in patients without heart failure. (From J. N. Cohn, E. Rodriguera, and N. H. Guiha. Hypertensive Heart Disease. In O. Onesti, K. E. Kim, and J. H. Moyer (eds.), *Hypertension: Mechanisms and Management*. New York: Grune & Stratton, 1973. With permission.)

significant elevation of left ventricular filling pressure (pulmonary capillary wedge pressure) in the patients with acute heart failure. In this small series of patients with acute hypertensive heart failure, systolic function was normal as evidenced by the normal resting cardiac index. The finding of elevated left ventricular end-diastolic pressures (LVEDP) despite normal ejection fractions and cardiac indices suggested the presence of isolated diastolic dysfunction. The increase in LVEDP was not the result of volume overload since the LVEDV was the same in both groups (Fig. 59-27). The increase in left ventricular filling pressure despite a similar end-diastolic volume could only be explained on the basis of a *decrease in left ventricular compliance* in the patients with acute hypertensive heart failure [91]. The pathophysiologic role of decreased left ventricular compliance was confirmed through observation of the hemodynamic responses to vasodilator therapy [91, 467]. Sodium nitroprusside infusion was utilized to reduce mean arterial pressure and systemic vascular resistance. This resulted in prompt relief of congestive symptoms in the acute hypertensive heart failure patients, with dramatic decreases in LVEDP from a mean of 43 mm Hg to 18 mm Hg. The decrease in left ventricular filling pressure was not due to venodilation and decreased venous return, since the LVEDV actually increased during sodium nitroprusside infusion. It was concluded that the beneficial effect of sodium nitroprusside was mediated through decreases in systemic vascular resistance, which led to improvement in left ventricular compliance. The signs and symptoms of pulmonary congestion were improved because there were reductions in LVEDP. The reductions in pressure occurred despite increases in left ventricular volume because of improvements in ventricular compliance.

A schematic representation of the changes in the left ventricular end-diastolic pressure-volume relationship in patients with acute hypertensive heart failure treated with sodium nitroprusside is displayed in Fig. 59-28. The diastolic pressure-volume relationship is considered to be an index of left ventricular compliance. In acute hypertensive heart failure, the pressure-volume curve is shifted up and to the left, reflecting a decrease in compliance such that a higher LVEDP is required to achieve any level of LVEDV. Normal systolic function is maintained but at the expense of a very high wedge pressure, which results in acute pulmonary edema. Treatment with sodium nitroprusside causes a reduction in the high systemic vascular resistance. The concomitant decrease in impedance to left ventricular ejection results in an improvement in compliance such that a lower filling pressure is required to maintain systolic function. Symptoms of pulmonary edema resolve as a result of the reduction in LVEDP despite the fact that the LVEDV actually increases during sodium nitroprusside infusion.

Compliance is only one index of diastolic performance. Aortic cross-clamp experiments in the canine model have been used to study the effects of acute increases in systemic vascular resistance (afterload) on other indices of left ventricular diastolic function [586].

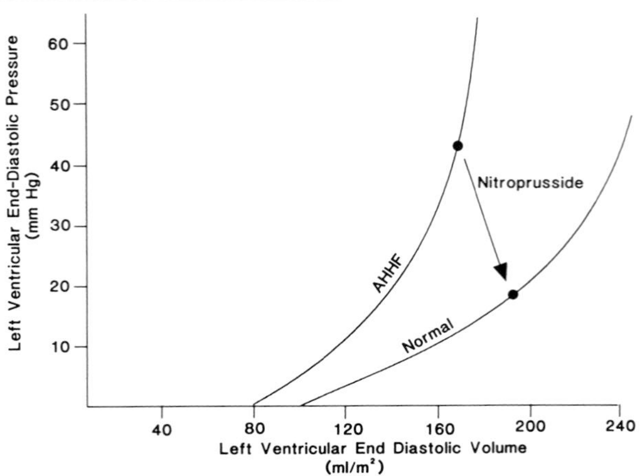

Fig. 59-28. Schematic representation of the left ventricular end-diastolic pressure-volume relationship in a patient with acute hypertensive heart failure (AHHF) treated with sodium nitroprusside. In AHHF, the pressure volume curve is shifted up and to the left, reflecting a decrease in left ventricular (LV) compliance. A higher than normal left ventricular end-diastolic pressure (LVEDP) is required to achieve any level of left ventricular end-diastolic volume (LVEDV,. Normal LV systolic function is maintained but at the expense of a very high wedge pressure, which results in acute pulmonary edema. Treatment with sodium nitroprusside causes a reduction in the high systemic vascular resistance with a concomitant decrease in impedance to LV ejection. As a result, LV compliance improves. Pulmonary edema resolves due to a reduction in LVEDP despite the fact that LVEDV actually increases during sodium nitroprusside infusion.

During acute aortic cross-clamping, the isovolemic relaxation rate and early diastolic filling rate were found to be inversely proportional to the left ventricular systolic pressure. Thus, an acute increase in systolic load resulted in instantaneous changes in left ventricular diastolic function. The authors postulate that in patients with severe hypertension complicated by acute pulmonary edema, an acute increase in left ventricular systolic load due to increased systemic vascular resistance may lead to abnormal myocardial relaxation and diastolic filling, resulting in an elevation of filling pressure and pulmonary congestion [586].

It is not clear why some patients with long-standing, severe hypertension do not develop heart failure, while in other patients, it develops as a relatively early complication of hypertension. The rate of rise of blood pressure may be important. Sudden worsening of preexisting hypertension, as occurs in patients with malignant hypertension superimposed on chronic essential hypertension, may precipitate heart failure. Moreover, acute hypertension in previously normotensive patients, as occurs in the setting of toxemia of pregnancy or acute glomerulonephritis, may cause left ventricular failure even though the blood pressure is only modestly elevated. In contrast, more severe hypertension, which develops gradually, may be tolerated for years without cardiac decompensation.

It is possible that with long-standing hypertension, the development of left ventricular hypertrophy may be a compensatory mechanism that serves to decrease left ventricular wall stress in the face of the increased impedance to left ventricular ejection [91]. However, when the onset of hypertension is abrupt or there is a sudden worsening of chronic hypertension, compensatory mechanisms may not be fully developed. Under these circumstances, precipitous left ventricular dysfunction with pulmonary and systemic venous congestion occur [91].

Thus, available evidence suggests that acute hypertensive heart failure results from primary increases in systemic vascular resistance, which cause increases in aortic impedance or resistance to left ventricular ejection. Systolic dysfunction (low cardiac output) does not occur because there is an increase in left ventricular wall tension that is sufficient to overcome the impedance to ejection. However, acute pulmonary edema develops because abnormalities of diastolic function such as delayed myocardial relaxation, decreased early diastolic filling, and reduced left ventricular compliance result in an increase in LVEDP that is transmitted to the pulmonary capillaries, resulting in transudation of fluid into alveoli [91, 586].

These pathophysiologic considerations have important therapeutic implications in the treatment of hypertensive patients with *acute pulmonary edema.* Since the proximate cause of the impaired diastolic performance in acute hypertensive heart failure is the contraction load imposed on the ventricle by increases in systemic vascular resistance, potent peripheral vasodilators are clearly the treatment of choice [89]. The initial clinical challenge is to distinguish patients in whom acute pulmonary edema is secondary to severe hypertension from those in whom hypertension is a reflex response to acute respiratory distress. A history of chronic hypertension, diastolic blood pressure over 120 to 130 mm Hg, funduscopic changes of hypertensive neuroretinopathy, or most importantly, failure of the hypertension to respond rapidly to the administration of oxygen, potent diuretics, and morphine are findings that suggest severe hypertension has resulted in acute pulmonary edema. Furthermore, in patients with suspected reflex hypertension, if hypertension persists after institution of therapy with preload reducing agents, parenteral antihypertensive agents are indicated.

Sodium nitroprusside is the preferred drug for the management of acute hypertensive heart failure because it reduces both preload and afterload. There is no absolute goal level of blood pressure. The dose of sodium nitroprusside should be increased until signs and symptoms of pulmonary congestion subside or the arterial pressure falls to hypotensive levels. However, it is rarely necessary to lower the blood pressure to this extent, since reduction to levels still within the hypertensive range is usually associated with dramatic improvement in symptoms. Although hemodynamic monitoring is not always required, it is essential in patients in whom concomitant myocardial ischemia or compromised cardiac output is suspected.

After the acute episode of hypertension with acute pulmonary edema has resolved, oral therapy can be substituted as the sodium nitroprusside infusion is weaned. Unfortunately, guidelines for long-term antihypertensive treatment in patients with a history of acute hypertensive heart failure are not well-defined. Despite the fact that direct-acting vasodilators may sustain or even promote left ventricular hypertrophy, in some patients with severe or resistant hypertension, adequate blood pressure control may require use of hydralazine or minoxidil in conjunction with β-blockers to control reflex tachycardia and diuretics to prevent reflex salt and water retention. However, as in the treatment of hypertensive patients with chronic symptoms of congestive heart failure due to diastolic dysfunction, agents such as β-blockers or calcium channel blockers, which not only decrease blood pressure but also improve diastolic function, may represent the most logical first-line therapy. Moreover, control of blood pressure with β-blockers, calcium channel blockers, converting enzyme inhibitors, or central α-adrenergic agonists may lead to a regression of left ventricular hypertrophy [559]. However, it is not clear whether regression of left ventricular hypertrophy leads to a long-term improvement in diastolic function, congestive symptoms, or prognosis. Furthermore, it is conceivable that regression of left ventricular hypertrophy might predispose to subsequent episodes of acute hypertensive heart failure if severe hypertension suddenly recurs due to noncompliance with antihypertensive therapy.

Hypertension Complicating Cerebrovascular Accident

The importance of hypertension as a risk factor for cerebrovascular accident is well established. The Framingham study showed that hypertension is associated with an increased incidence of atherothrombotic and hemorrhagic stroke in patients of either sex at all ages [273]. Several prospective, randomized clinical trials have demonstrated that long-term antihypertensive drug therapy results in a significant reduction in morbidity and mortality from cerebrovascular accident [106]. Despite the proven benefits of blood pressure control in the prevention of stroke, the role of treatment of hypertension in the acute phase of stroke remains controversial. Whether antihypertensive therapy is indicated depends not only on the magnitude of the blood pressure elevation, but also on the type of cerebrovascular accident. The management of hypertension accompanying cerebral infarction is different than for hypertension complicating either intracerebral hemorrhage or subarachnoid hemorrhage.

CEREBRAL INFARCTION

In the cerebral circulation, the sites of predilection for atherosclerosis are the bifurcations of the common carotid arteries, the carotid siphons, the origins of the vertebral and basilar arteries, the circle of Willis, and the proximal parts of the cerebral arteries [432]. Cerebral infarction may result from partial or complete occlusion of an artery by a plaque or embolization of atherothrombotic debris from a plaque. Infarction produced by one of these mechanisms (atherothromboembolism) typically involves the cerebral or cerebellar cortex or the pons [432]. In contrast, hypertension-induced lipohyalinosis of the small penetrating cerebral end arteries is the principal cause of the small, deep infarcts known as lacunes that occur in the basal ganglia, pons, thalamus, cerebellum, and deep hemispheric white matter [432].

Hypertension is common in the setting of acute cerebral infarction. In a series of 334 consecutive admissions for acute stroke, the blood pressure was elevated in 84 percent of the patients on the day of admission. Even without specific antihypertensive treatment, the blood pressure decreased spontaneously an average of 20 mm Hg systolic and 10 mm Hg diastolic in the 10 days following the acute event [556]. This early elevation in blood pressure most likely represents a physiologic response to brain ischemia. Decreases in blood pressure accompany recovery of brain function.

Because of the known benefits of antihypertensive therapy with regard to stroke prevention, it has been assumed that reduction in blood pressure would benefit patients with acute cerebral infarction. Unfortunately, since treatment of hypertension in this setting has never been evaluated in a prospective, randomized trial, there are no good data to guide management. Moreover, there is no evidence to suggest that rapid reduction of blood pressure is beneficial. In fact, several cases have been reported in which worsening of the patient's neurologic status was apparently precipitated by emergency treatment of hypertension [54, 309]. The rationale for not treating hypertension in acute ischemic strokes is based on concerns regarding an impairment in autoregulation of cerebral blood flow in this setting [309, 361, 577]. In normal individuals, cerebral blood flow is maintained constant at mean arterial pressures ranging between 60 and 120 mm Hg. In patients with chronic hypertension, as well as elderly patients, however, the curve is shifted such that the lower limit of autoregulation occurs at a higher mean arterial pressure. Furthermore, there is evidence that local autoregulation of cerebral blood flow is disturbed in the so-called ischemic penumbra that surrounds the area of infarction [361]. Without intact autoregulation, the regional blood flow becomes critically dependent on the perfusion pressure. Thus, to some extent, the presence of hypertension may be protective, and reduction of blood pressure may cause a regional reduction in blood flow with extension of the infarct.

Since there is no evidence that mild to moderate hypertension has a deleterious effect on the outcome of cerebral infarction during the acute stage, it is probably wise to allow the blood pressure to seek its own level during the first few days to weeks after the event. In most cases, the hypertension tends to resolve spontaneously over the first week without specific therapy [556]. If hypertension persists in the patient with a completed stroke (over 3 weeks after the acute event), reduction of blood pressure into the normal range can safely be accomplished [219]. Although the goal of long-term antihypertensive treatment in hypertensive stroke survivors is the prevention of stroke recurrence, its efficacy remains uncertain. Whereas some studies demonstrated a reduction in risk of stroke recurrence [33, 75], others did not find a benefit from blood pressure reduction in this regard [251, 357].

Although benign neglect of mild to moderate hypertension is prudent in the setting of acute cerebral infarction, there may be certain indications for active treatment of hypertension [509]. If the diastolic blood pressure is sustained at over 130 mm Hg, many authorities recommend cautious reduction of the blood pressure to the 160 to 170 over 100 to 110 mm Hg range with a short-acting parenteral agent [309, 313, 509, 524]. Stroke accompanied by other hypertensive crises such as acute myocardial ischemia or left ventricular dysfunction with acute pulmonary edema is also an indication for cautious blood pressure reduction [309, 509]. Stroke due to carotid occlusion caused by aortic dissection mandates aggressive blood pressure reduction to prevent propagation of the dissection [309, 509]. In some patients with severe hypertension, it may be impossible to distinguish between hypertensive encephalopathy and cerebral infarction on clinical grounds. Since rapid lowering of the blood pressure may be lifesaving in the patient with hypertensive encephalopathy, a cautious diagnostic trial of blood pressure reduction with a short-acting parenteral antihypertensive agent, such as sodium nitroprusside, may be indicated [509, 577]. In stroke patients requiring anticoagulation therapy, moderate control of severe hypertension into the 160 to 170 over 100 to 110 mm Hg range may be prudent. In the severely hypertensive patient with progressing stroke in whom continued deterioration is felt to be secondary to cerebral edema, cautious blood pressure reduction may be warranted. Appropriate management of such patients may require continuous intracranial as well as intraarterial pressure monitoring so that cerebral perfusion pressure can be optimized [509].

In the setting of acute cerebral infarction, hypertension tends to be very labile and exquisitely sensitive to hypotensive therapy. Even modest doses of oral antihypertensive agents may cause profound and devastating overshoot hypotension [54]. Antihypertensive treatment, when indicated, should be initiated with extreme caution using small doses of short-acting agents such as sodium nitroprusside.

INTRACEREBRAL HEMORRHAGE

Hypertension is a major risk factor for intracerebral hemorrhage. The small-diameter penetrating cerebral end arteries are especially vulnerable to the deleterious effects of hypertension because they arise directly from the main arterial trunks [432]. The most common sites of hypertension-associated hemorrhage include the basal ganglia, pons, thalamus, cerebellum, and deep hemispheric white matter [104]. Lacunar infarcts arise from the same vessels and are similarly distributed.

Hypertensive hemorrhage most often occurs in patients over 50 years of age. Intracerebral hemorrhage characteristically begins abruptly with headache and vomiting followed by steadily increasing focal neurologic deficits and alteration of consciousness [104]. More than 90 percent of hemorrhages rupture through brain parenchyma into the ventricles, producing a bloody cerebrospinal fluid [104]. Hypertension is uniformly present upon presentation. In fact, the finding of a normal or low blood pressure makes the diagnosis of intracerebral hemorrhage unlikely [104]. In contrast to cerebral infarction, the blood pressure does not tend to decrease spontaneously during the first week after the event [556]. Once the hemorrhage has occurred, the patient's condition worsens steadily over a period of minutes to days until the neurologic deficit either stabilizes or the patient dies [104]. When death occurs, it is most often due to herniation caused by the expanding hematoma and surrounding edema.

Small hemorrhages, which may be clinically indistinguishable from cerebral infarction, probably require no specific therapy [432]. The issue of treatment of hypertension in the setting of a large intracerebral hemorrhage (greater than 3 cm) is controversial. There is almost always a rise in intracranial pressure that is accompanied by a reflex increase in systemic blood pressure [556]. Because cerebral perfusion pressure is a function of the difference between systemic arterial pressure and intracranial pressure, reduction of blood pressure may compromise cerebral perfusion. Furthermore, the hematoma impairs the local autoregulatory response in the surrounding area of marginal ischemia [309]. Since there is no good evidence that persistent hypertension promotes further bleeding, some authorities strongly advise against treating hypertension in patients with intracerebral hemorrhage [68, 577]. On the other hand, cerebral vasogenic edema may develop as a consequence of an abrupt, severe increase in blood pressure [432]. Treatment of hypertension may thus be beneficial by virtue of a reduction in cerebral edema and intracranial pressure. Thus, in deciding to treat hypertension, a precarious balance must be struck between beneficial reduction of cerebral edema on the one hand and deleterious reduction of cerebral blood flow on the other. In a study of 8 patients with intracerebral hemorrhage treated with trimethaphan, cerebral blood flow measurements revealed that the cerebral autoregulation curve was intact but shifted such that the lower limit of autoregulation was at 80 percent of the initial level of blood pressure [272]. Thus, a 20 percent decrease in mean arterial pressure should be considered the maximal reduction of blood pressure during the acute stage. Active treatment of the blood pressure should only be undertaken in the intensive care environment where intracranial pressure and intraarterial pressure can be closely monitored [432].

The drug of choice for the management of hypertension in the setting of intracerebral hemorrhage is a matter of debate. Sodium nitroprusside has traditionally been regarded as the best agent, since its brief duration of action allows for rapid titration with avoidance of the catastrophic consequence of sustained overshoot hypotension [68, 313, 432]. Recently, concern has been expressed that since sodium nitroprusside induces an increase in venous capacitance as well as cerebral arterial vasodilation, the resulting increase in cerebral blood volume may cause a further elevation of intracranial pressure [70, 523, 544]. Other cerebral vasodilators such as intravenous nitroglycerin, hydralazine, or calcium channel blockers may also cause potentially deleterious elevations of intracranial pressure in patients with compromised intracranial compliance due to intracranial disease [544]. Since labetalol or urapidil, a postsynaptic α-receptor blocker, may not alter intracranial pressure, they have been recommended for treatment of hypertension in neurosurgical patients [544]. Unfortunately, these agents have the potential to cause overshoot hypotension, which may be difficult to reverse quickly. In the authors' opinion, despite the theoretic risk of intracranial pressure elevation, sodium nitroprusside remains the treatment of choice when severe hypertension must be treated in patients with intracerebral hemorrhage because its short duration of action allows for cautious, graded blood pressure reduction that can be quickly reversed if the patient's neurologic status deteriorates or a further increase in intracranial pressure occurs. Of interest, some patients with cerebral infarction or hemorrhage have extreme elevations of catecholamine levels, which may render hypertension refractory to sodium nitroprusside in the absence of concomitant β-blocker therapy [157].

Cerebellar hemorrhage represents a neurosurgical emergency requiring prompt diagnosis and treatment [231]. Typically, patients present complaining of the sudden onset of dizziness, nausea, vomiting, headache, and difficulty walking. Truncal ataxia, nystagmus, and ipsilateral sixth nerve paresis may be present [231]. If the process continues unchecked, brain stem compression or herniation produces progressive stupor and coma. The untreated mortality is extremely high. The diagnosis can usually be confirmed by computed tomography (CT) scan. Treatment consists of emergent suboccipital craniotomy with evacuation of the hematoma [231].

SUBARACHNOID HEMORRHAGE

Subarachnoid hemorrhage accounts for less than 10 percent of all cerebrovascular accidents. Rupture of a congenital aneurysm is the most common cause of subarachnoid hemorrhage. Rupture is heralded by the sudden onset of a profound headache and is often followed by brief syncope. If the mass of the hemorrhage is large, patients rapidly become comatose. As the hemorrhage diffuses throughout the subarachnoid space, the patient may awaken and experience headache, nausea, vomiting, and seizures. Within 24 hours, nuchal rigidity and other meningeal signs develop. Initially, neurologic findings are nonfocal. CT scan can be used to confirm the diagnosis.

Delayed cerebral ischemia due to *cerebral arterial vasospasm* is the most important cause of morbidity after subarachnoid hemorrhage [232]. Vasospasm, which is probably caused by the irritating effects of blood in the subarachnoid space closely opposed to the large arteries, usually develops between 4 and 12 days after the acute event. Symptoms include a gradual deterioration of the level of consciousness, accompanied by focal neurologic deficits [232].

Recurrent hemorrhage is another potential complication that is associated with a high mortality. The presence of hypertension is associated with an increase risk of rebleeding during the 30 days after the initial rupture [402]. However, whether treatment of hypertension after subarachnoid hemorrhage reduces the risk of rebleed or improves prognosis is uncertain. In the setting of elevated intracranial pressure and cerebral arterial vasospasm, hypertension may be protective, since it helps to maintain cerebral perfusion pressure. Thus, reduction of the blood pressure could conceivably result in aggravation of cerebral vasospasm and ischemia.

In the face of these conflicting clinical imperatives, no treatment scheme has been proved to have a clear advantage. Recently, an aggressive approach has been advocated that calls for the initial use of antihypertensive therapy to reduce the risk of rebleeding. Treatment of hypertension is accomplished in conjunction with vigorous attempts to reduce the elevated intracranial pressure by means of external cerebrospinal fluid drainage. The objective is to keep the cerebral perfusion pressure (mean arterial pressure minus mean intracranial pressure) in the normal range (80–90 mm Hg) [440]. Surgical clipping of the aneurysm is undertaken as soon as possible to prevent rebleeding [440]. Postoperatively, there is evidence that intravascular volume expansion with crystalloid and colloid, in conjunction with induction of arterial hypertension using dopamine or dobutamine, may be an effective means of reversing the ischemic neurologic deficits caused by cerebral vasospasm, provided that cerebral infarction has not already occurred [276].

Nimodipine, a 1,4-dihydropyridine calcium channel blocker, has recently been approved for the treatment of cerebral ischemia caused by subarachnoid hemorrhage. Nimodipine is highly lipid soluble and readily crosses the blood-brain barrier [305]. It dilates cerebral blood vessels at lower concentrations than required for dilatation of the peripheral vasculature [305]. Thus, it may improve cerebral blood flow at doses that do not result in a significant reduction in mean arterial pressure. Furthermore, inhibition of calcium uptake by neurons may also protect against ischemic injury at the cellular level, independent of an effect on cerebral blood flow [305]. Several studies have shown that both intravenous and oral nimodipine treatment result in a significant reduction in the incidence of cerebral infarction caused by delayed vasospasm in the setting of subarachnoid hemorrhage [407, 433]. The optimal timing of surgery in nimodipine-treated patients has not yet been defined.

HYPERTENSION COMPLICATING SEVERE HEAD TRAUMA

Systemic hypertension may contribute to the increase in intracranial pressure that often accompanies traumatic head injury [161]. In patients with severe head injury, the degree of intracranial hypertension correlates with mortality. If the intracranial pressure is less than 20 mm

Hg, mortality is about 20 percent. However, if the intracranial pressure exceeds 40 mm Hg, mortality is over 80 percent [365]. The primary danger of intracranial hypertension is a compromise of cerebral blood with secondary ischemic injury. Severe, uncontrolled intracranial hypertension can result in rapid brain death due to global cerebral ischemia. The minimum cerebral perfusion pressure (mean arterial pressure minus intracranial pressure) necessary to prevent secondary cerebral ischemia is 50 mm Hg [161].

A major goal of treatment in the head-injured patient is to maintain intracranial pressure at levels less than 30 mm Hg. However, effective treatment requires measurement of intracranial pressure with a device such as a ventricular catheter, subarachnoid bolt, or epidural transducer. The major treatments for reducing elevated intracranial pressure are hyperventilation, osmotic diuretics, removal of cerebrospinal fluid, corticosteroids, high-dose barbiturates, and *control of arterial blood pressure* [161].

Autoregulation of cerebral blood flow is impaired in patients with severe head injury such that changes in mean arterial pressure will cause parallel changes in intracranial pressure through alterations in cerebral blood volume. Moreover, severe hypertension may cause a breakthrough of cerebral autoregulation with cerebral edema in a manner analogous to hypertensive encephalopathy. On the other hand, some increase in blood pressure may be beneficial with regard to maintenance of cerebral perfusion pressure in the face of increased intracranial pressure.

Rational treatment of hypertension in the setting of severe head trauma requires continuous monitoring of mean arterial pressure, intracranial pressure, pulmonary capillary wedge pressure, and cardiac output. Frequent neurologic examinations must be performed to assess response to therapy. The choice of antihypertensive agent is also important. Vasodilators, when used alone, tend to be relatively ineffective, so the patient should be pretreated with β-adrenergic receptor blockers. A vasodilator such as sodium nitroprusside or intravenous nitroglycerin is the treatment of choice [161]. If an increase in intracranial pressure accompanied by compromise of cerebral perfusion pressure occurs with vasodilator therapy, intravenous labetalol represents an alternative option. Diuretics should be avoided because a decrease in intravascular volume reduces cardiac output and increases sympathetic tone.

Hypertension Complicating Acute Myocardial Infarction

Transient systemic hypertension is a frequent occurrence during the early stages of acute myocardial infarction, even among previously normotensive patients. This postinfarction hypertension has been attributed to a hyperadrenergic state resulting from release of catecholamines from infarcted myocardium or to an increase in sympathetic tone in response to stress, pain, or anxiety. Serial measurements of plasma epinephrine and norepinephrine in patients with acute myocardial infarction have revealed a significant direct correlation between plasma catecholamines and systolic blood pressure [499]. A cardiogenic hypertensive chemoreflex has been described. Injection of serotonin into the left atrium or branches of the proximal left coronary artery in dogs produced an intense pressor response that was dependent on vagal afferent impulses to the central nervous system and was blocked by the α-adrenergic blocking agent phentolamine. By histologic examination, a small structure resembling a chemoreceptor was identified. This chemoreceptor received its blood supply from the left coronary artery [261]. It has been postulated that in the setting of acute myocardial infarction, platelet deposition in stenosed vessels results in the release of serotonin and activation of the chemoreceptor. The chemoreceptor reflex results in increased sympathetic tone and systemic hypertension [499].

In most patients, postinfarction hypertension is a transient finding early in the course of acute myocardial infarction that resolves without specific therapy other than pain control and sedation. The short-term changes in blood pressure in untreated patients with acute myocardial infarction have been well-characterized [184]. During the first hour of hospitalization the mean systolic blood pressure (SBP) was 150 ± 30.7 mm Hg, and SBP of ≥ 160 mm Hg was present in 30 percent of patients. The mean diastolic blood pressure (DBP) was 92 ± 18.7, and DBP ≥ 100 mm Hg was present in 42 percent of patients. Overall, 45 percent of patients had a blood pressure of ≥ 140/90 mm Hg and 32 percent had a blood pressure of ≥ 160/100 mm Hg during the first hour of hospitalization. However, during the subsequent 6 hours, the blood pressure spontaneously normalized in the majority of patients. By the sixth hour of hospitalization, SBP had fallen to 130 ± 24 mm Hg, and DBP decreased to 81 ± 15.5 mm Hg. Among the patients with initial BP of ≥ 140/90 mm Hg, only 25 percent were still hypertensive by 6 hours. Patients with an initial BP of ≥ 160/100 mm Hg demonstrated a similar fall in blood pressure, so that only 20 percent remained above this level at 6 hours. The authors found no difference in the clinical course of the patients with and without hypertension. They concluded that in early uncomplicated acute myocardial infarction, no specific therapy of hypertension is indicated other than attention to relief of pain and adequate sedation [184].

In contrast, there are a number of studies indicating that hypertension in the setting of acute myocardial infarction signifies a less favorable prognosis. In a study of 143 patients with acute myocardial infarction, high systolic blood pressure on admission was found to indicate a worse prognosis for 2-year survival [328]. In another study of 106 patients with acute myocardial infarction who had systolic blood pressure of ≥ 170 mm Hg that persisted for at least 30 minutes, the blood pressure fell spontaneously to less than 150 mm Hg within 72 hours in all patients [172]. No antihypertensive therapy was employed. The control group consisted of 106 patients with acute myocardial infarction who had SBP of 120 to 150 mm Hg and DBP of ≤ 100 mm Hg. Mean peak aspartate aminotransferase (AST) levels were significantly higher in the systolic hypertension group than in the normotension group. The duration of SBP of ≥ 170 mm Hg before return to normotension correlated with the mean peak AST and presumably infarct size. The overall mortality, incidence of major arrhythmias, and incidence of cardiac failure were higher in the hypertensive group.

Postinfarction hypertension has been reported to be the most important risk factor for cardiac rupture [391]. Although the incidence of chronic hypertension prior to acute myocardial infarction was similar in patients with and without rupture, 40 percent of the patients with cardiac rupture had postinfarction hypertension (DBP ≥ 90 mm Hg) compared with 15 percent of patients without cardiac rupture.

A major objective of therapy in acute myocardial infarction is to minimize myocardial infarct size [477]. The extent of ischemic damage is dependent on the balance between myocardial oxygen supply and demand. In experimental models, factors that increase myocardial oxygen demand have been shown to increase infarct size, and conversely, infarct size can be minimized by reducing myocardial oxygen consumption [110, 174]. The heart rate, wall tension, and myocardial contractility are the major determinants of myocardial oxygen consumption.

Treatment with β-adrenergic receptor blockers leads to a reduction in myocardial oxygen demand through a reduction in heart rate, systemic vascular resistance, and myocardial contractility [31]. In addition, β-blockers counter the excess production of catecholamines commonly seen in patients with acute myocardial infarction. They also have antiarrhythmic properties. When given intravenously within the first few hours after the acute event, β-blockers have been shown to reduce both infarct size and early in-hospital mortality [253]. It has been recommended that intravenous β-blocker therapy be considered in all patients with acute myocardial infarction unless contraindications such as severe bradycardia, heart block, systemic hypotension, severe congestive heart failure, or reactive airway disease are present [31]. Secondary prevention trials have shown that chronic β-blocker treatment after myocardial infarction reduces both nonfatal reinfarction rate and long-term mortality [197, 580].

During the first few days after an acute myocardial infarction, the systemic arterial pressure is the most important determinant of LVEDP [173]. Accordingly, it has been proposed that in the setting of postinfarction hypertension, reduction of the blood pressure with arteriolar vasodilators might prevent extension of ischemia by reducing LVEDP, wall tension, and myocardial oxygen demand. Studies of vasodilator therapy with sodium nitroprusside, intravenous nitroglycerin, or trimethaphan in patients with hypertension complicating acute myocardial infarction have demonstrated improved cardiac performance with decreased LVEDP and stable or increased cardiac output, findings that should be associated with a reduction in myocardial oxygen demand [13, 17, 81, 298, 388, 495].

In the setting of acute myocardial infarction, patients with a blood pressure greater than 160/100 mm Hg that lasts longer than 1 hour and that is unresponsive to intravenous β-blocker therapy, should be considered candidates for treatment with parenteral vasodilators to decrease systemic vascular resistance, afterload, and myocardial oxygen demand. Since systemic hemodynamics may change rapidly in the setting of acute myocardial infarction, the use of agents with a short duration of action is recommended. Sodium nitroprusside, intravenous nitroglycerin, and trimethaphan are preferred in this setting. Nitroglycerin may have theoretical advantages as a vasodilator in the setting of acute myocardial infarction because it dilates intercoronary collaterals and improves blood flow to the ischemic myocardium [74, 84, 165, 332, 341]. Methyldopa and reserpine are not recommended because they have a delayed onset of action and an unpredictable hypotensive effect. Diazoxide and hydralazine are contraindicated because their use can result in reflex activation of the adrenergic system, resulting in increases in heart rate, cardiac output, and myocardial oxygen demand. Recent reports have described the successful use of intravenous labetalol in selected patients with hypertension complicating acute myocardial infarction [72, 343, 460].

Acute reduction of blood pressure in patients with acute myocardial infarction necessitates careful monitoring of filling pressure and cardiac output. Definition of an arbitrary goal level of blood pressure is impossible. The blood pressure should be gradually reduced over a period of 10 to 15 minutes with frequent checks of systemic hemodynamics. The goal of therapy should be the reduction of systemic vascular resistance so that LVEDP is reduced to the range of 15 to 18 mm Hg without reflex tachycardia or compromise of cardiac output [81, 90]. The blood pressure may be reduced to normotensive levels as long as cardiac output remains stable or increases, the heart rate does not increase, and there is no evidence of increased myocardial ischemia (pain or increased ischemic changes on electrocardiogram). Vasodilator therapy can usually be weaned within 24 hours as the hypertension resolves.

Despite the fact that afterload reduction may improve myocardial performance and decrease myocardial oxygen demands, it should be undertaken with great caution. Myocardial blood flow is critically dependent on coronary perfusion pressure, and overshoot hypotension may worsen ischemia and extend the infarct [181]. Afterload reduction should be restricted to patients with increased LVEDP (wedge pressure ≥ 15 mm Hg) [81, 90]. The use of vasodilator therapy in patients with normal or reduced filling pressure may cause a decrease in cardiac output and reflex tachycardia, which may worsen myocardial ischemia [81, 90].

Aortic Dissection

Acute aortic dissection is a hypertensive crisis requiring immediate antihypertensive therapy aimed at halting the progression of the dissecting hematoma. Patients with acute aortic dissection should be stabilized with intensive antihypertensive therapy to prevent life-threatening complications prior to diagnostic evaluation with angiography.

Aortic dissection is initiated by a small intimal tear. In

60 to 65 percent of cases the intimal tear arises in the ascending aorta within a few centimeters of the aortic valve. In 30 to 35 percent it begins in the descending thoracic aorta just distal to the origin of the left subclavian artery, while in 5 to 10 percent of cases the dissection originates in the transverse aortic arch [561]. DeBakey et al. [117] have defined three types of aortic dissection. Type I begins in the ascending aorta and extends for a variable distance into the descending aorta. It may involve the entire aorta. Type II begins in the ascending aorta and is confined to this segment. Type III originates in the descending aorta and propagates distally for a variable distance, with type IIIA stopping above the diaphragm and type IIIB extending below the diaphragm. A type III dissection may also extend in a retrograde fashion into the ascending aorta. A more clinically useful classification is based on the presence or absence of involvement of the ascending aorta regardless of the site of the original intimal tear [107] (Fig. 59-29). *Proximal (type IIIA) dissections* include all dissections that involve the ascending aorta, including those that begin in the descending aorta and propagate retrograde into the ascending aorta. *Distal (type IIIB) dissections* involve only the descending aorta. In general, the type of dissection, proximal or distal, defines whether management should be accomplished with drug therapy plus surgery or intensive drug therapy alone. Another important aspect of classification is the duration of the dissection at the time of first presentation. Dissections are defined as *acute* if presentation occurs within 2 weeks of onset of symptoms and *chronic* if more than 2 weeks have elapsed [122]. The importance of this temporal classification lies in the fact that 60 to 70 percent of patients with untreated dissection die within the first 2 weeks after onset.

Fig. 59-29. Classification of aortic dissection based on the presence or absence of involvement of the ascending aorta. The dissection is defined as proximal (type IIIA) if there is involvement of the ascending aorta. The primary intimal tear in proximal dissection may arise in the ascending aorta (1), transverse aortic (2), or descending aorta (3). In distal (type IIIB) dissections, the process is confined to the descending aorta; the ascending aorta is not involved. The primary intimal tear occurs most commonly just distal to the origin of the left subclavian artery. Proximal dissections account for approximately 67 percent and distal dissections 43 percent of all acute aortic dissections. (Adapted from M. W. Wheat, Jr. Acute dissecting aneurysms of the aorta: Diagnosis and treatment, 1979. *Am. Heart. J.* 99:373, 1980.)

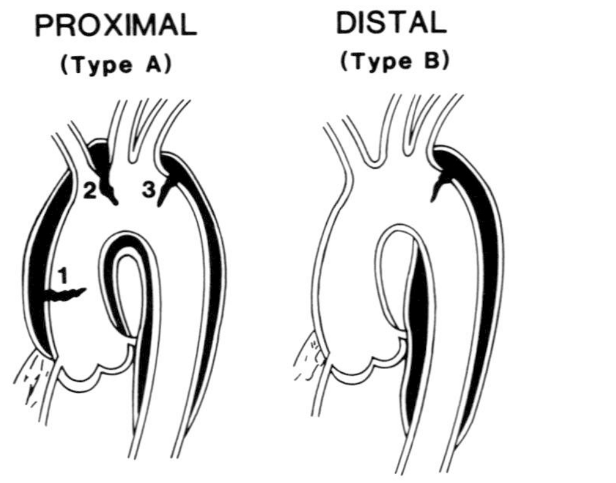

Degenerative changes in the aortic media underlie most cases of aortic dissection. This medial degeneration is believed to be the result of chronic stress on the aortic wall. Chronic hypertension is the most important risk factor for the development of aortic dissection. In a series of 124 patients with acute dissection, there was a history of long-standing hypertension in 49 percent of those with proximal dissection and 78 percent of patients with distal dissection. Moreover, even in the absence of a known history of hypertension, 65 percent of patients with proximal dissection and 96 percent of those with distal dissection had left ventricular hypertrophy suggesting the presence of underlying hypertension [504]. Less common factors predisposing to aortic dissection include Marfan and Ehler-Danlos syndromes, bicuspid aortic valve, coarctation of the aorta, and pregnancy [503].

Following an initial tear in the intima, a column of blood driven by the force of arterial pressure enters the aortic wall and destroys the media while stripping the intima for a variable distance along the length of the aorta. The extent of propagation of the dissecting hematoma is determined by several mechanical factors including systolic blood pressure, velocity or shearing forces, turbulence of blood flow, and steepness of the pulse wave (dp/dt) [561]. Experimental evidence suggests that the two most important factors are the blood pressure and the steepness of the pulse wave [377, 442]. Without therapy, acute aortic dissection is almost always fatal. In a review of survival in untreated patients, one-quarter died within 24 hours, one-half died within 1 month, and more than 90 percent died within 1 year. There are three major complications of aortic dissection, including rupture of the aorta, occlusion of major arterial branches arising from the aorta, and acute aortic insufficiency [561]. The most frequent mechanism of death is a through and through rupture of the weakened aortic adventitia [561]. The most common site of rupture is the ascending aorta. Since the parietal pericardium is attached to the aorta just proximal to the origin of the innominate artery, rupture of any portion of the ascending aorta leads to hemopericardium and pericardial tamponade. Rupture of the aortic arch causes hemorrhage into the mediastinum; the descending thoracic aorta, into the left pleural space; and the abdominal aorta, into the retroperitoneum [561].

Extension of the dissecting hematoma into the ostia of any artery arising from the aorta may lead to occlusion with ischemia of distal organs and tissues. Occlusion of renal artery ostia may be signaled by the development of virtually uncontrollable hypertension due to renin release from the ischemic kidney [122]. Occlusion of coronary ostia can lead to acute myocardial infarction. Cerebral ischemia and infarction occur with involvement of the cephalic vessels. Mesenteric artery occlusion may cause intestinal ischemia or infarction. Extension into a common iliac artery leads to ischemia of the lower extremity. Ischemic neurologic complications include cerebral infarction, paraparesis due to occlusion of spinal arteries, and ischemic peripheral neuropathy [561].

Acute aortic insufficiency may develop with proximal dissection due to dilatation of the aortic root or widening of the annulus by the dissecting hematoma so that the valve leaflets fail to oppose during diastole [122].

Slater and DeSanctis [503] have reviewed the clinical features of acute aortic dissection. Men predominate over women by a ratio of 3 : 1. The peak incidence is in the sixth and seventh decades. The pain is usually cataclysmic in onset and maximal at its inception in contrast to the crescendo nature of pain seen with acute myocardial infarction. The pain is often described as tearing, ripping, or stabbing. Another characteristic of the pain is its tendency to migrate from the point of origin along the path followed by the dissecting hematoma. The location of the pain is suggestive of the site of origin. Pain felt maximally in the anterior thorax is more frequently due to proximal dissection, whereas pain felt maximally in the interscapular area is more common in distal dissections. Vasovagal symptoms such as diaphoresis, apprehension, nausea, and vomiting are common. Less common presenting symptoms included syncope (usually due to cardiac tamponade) or acute pulmonary edema (secondary to acute aortic insufficiency) [503].

Although the majority of patients with aortic dissection have evidence of long-standing hypertension, the blood pressure may fall such that hypertension is absent at the time of presentation. Fifty-six percent of patients with distal dissections were hypertensive at the time of presentation compared with 9 percent of patients with proximal dissections [503]. True hypotension, which is more common with proximal dissections, is attributable to rupture of the dissection with cardiac tamponade or hemorrhage into the pleural space or retroperitoneum [503]. *Pseudohypotension* may be caused by compromise of flow through either or both subclavian arteries [503].

Although the chest roentgenogram may show widening of the mediastinum, this sign is present in only 40 to 50 percent of cases [561]. The mediastinum bulges to the right with involvement of the ascending aorta and to the left with involvement of the descending thoracic aorta. At the aortic knob, a greater than 1-cm separation of the intimal calcification from the adventitial border, the so-called calcium sign, is highly suggestive but not diagnostic of aortic dissection [122]. A left pleural effusion may also occur.

Aortic angiography, which is the most definitive method for confirming the diagnosis of aortic dissection, has a diagnostic accuracy of 95 to 99 percent [122, 141]. The presence or absence of involvement of the ascending aorta is used to define the dissection as proximal or distal. Aortography also provides other important information including the site of the intimal tear, the extent of the dissection, and the effects of the dissection on the arterial trunks. The aortic root can be evaluated to quantitate aortic insufficiency, if present. These data are crucial for planning surgical intervention.

Recently, *transesophageal Doppler echocardiography* has been reported to be a sensitive and accurate method for the diagnosis of aortic dissection [152, 222, 528]. Further evaluation is required to determine whether this less invasive technique can replace angiography as the procedure of choice for the diagnosis and evaluation of aortic dissection [141].

Noninvasive techniques such as M-mode and two-dimensional ultrasonography [474], CT scanning [534], and magnetic resonance imaging [283] are inferior to angiography in the definitive evaluation of patients with acute aortic dissection [122]. However, these modalities may be useful in the evaluation of patients with suspected chronic dissection and in the long-term follow-up of medically and surgically treated survivors of aortic dissection [122]. They may also be used to screen patients in whom the likelihood of acute dissection is not high but the diagnosis must be excluded [122].

TREATMENT OF ACUTE AORTIC DISSECTION

Intensive medical therapy should be instituted in patients with suspected acute dissection, preferably even before definitive diagnostic procedures are begun. The initial therapeutic goal is the elimination of pain (which correlates with a halting of the dissection process) and reduction of systolic blood pressure to the 100 to 120 mm Hg range or the lowest level compatible with maintenance of adequate renal, cardiac, and cerebral perfusion. Even in the absence of hypertension, therapy should be instituted. Antihypertensive therapy should be designed not only to lower blood pressure but also to decrease the steepness of the pulse wave. The most commonly used treatment regimen consists of an intravenous β-adrenergic blocking drug such as propranolol in combination with sodium nitroprusside [122, 503]. Propranolol should be initiated prior to nitroprusside to prevent an adrenergic-mediated reflex increase in cardiac contractility, which could further propagate the dissection. After an initial test dose of 0.5 mg, propranolol is administered in 1-mg increments over 5 minutes until there is adequate β-blockade as evidenced by a pulse rate of approximately 60 beats/minute [504]. However, the total dose should not exceed 0.15 mg/kg. Subsequent propranolol doses of 0.05 to 0.15 mg/kg should be given every 4 to 6 hours to maintain β-blockade [122]. Pretreatment with intravenous esmolol or metoprolol is also acceptable [141]. After pretreatment with β-blocker, sodium nitroprusside is administered to lower the systolic blood pressure into the 100 to 120 mm Hg range.

Trimethaphan is considered by some to be the preferred drug for the treatment of acute aortic dissection [419, 561]. In animal models, doses of propranolol much larger than those necessary to produce bradycardia were required to prevent the reflex increase in dp/dt associated with the use of nitroprusside [419]. In contrast, trimethaphan is not associated with reflex increases in heart rate and contractility because it blocks the adrenergic system. Unfortunately, the prolonged use of trimethaphan is limited by its sympathoplegic side effects as well as the rapid development of tachyphylaxis [122].

Labetalol, by virtue of its combined α_1- and β-blocking properties, may be useful in the management of patients with acute dissection. However, its long duration of hypotensive action may not be desirable in critically ill patients with acute aortic dissection who may require urgent surgical intervention. Selective arteriolar vasodilators such as diazoxide and hydralazine, which activate the adrenergic system, are contraindicated in acute aortic dissection.

After the blood pressure is controlled and the patient is pain free, angiography is performed. In deciding between medical and surgical therapy, the most important angiographic finding is involvement of the ascending aorta. Collective results from six long-term follow-up (> 1 year) studies indicate that surgical therapy is superior to medical therapy alone in proximal dissections. In patients with proximal dissection treated surgically, the overall survival rate was 70 percent compared with only 26 percent in medically treated patients [561]. Conversely, in distal dissections, intensive drug therapy led to a survival of 80 percent compared with 50 percent survival in surgically treated patients [561].

Surgical therapy is advantageous in patients with proximal dissection because progression of the dissecting hematoma may result in devastating consequences including aortic rupture with cardiac tamponade, acute aortic insufficiency, or neurologic compromise [503]. However, patients with acute proximal dissection arising from the aortic arch represent an exception. In these patients, medical therapy is preferred because of the exceedingly high morbidity and mortality associated with surgery in this region [122]. Likewise, there are a number of explanations for the advantages of medical therapy in acute distal dissection. These patients are generally at greater surgical risk because they are older and have a higher incidence of advanced atherosclerosis and coexistent cardiopulmonary disease [503]. Moreover, the risk of life-threatening complications such as cardiac tamponade, aortic insufficiency, or cerebrovascular accident is less than with proximal dissections. Although medical therapy is generally the treatment of choice in distal dissection, there are situations in which surgery is required. These include inability to control blood pressure, inability to control pain (which implies continued propagation), compromise or occlusion of a major branch of the aorta, or development of a saccular aortic aneurysm during long-term medical therapy. There is also general agreement that acute distal dissection in patients with Marfan's syndrome should be managed surgically [122].

Patients who present with chronic dissections have already survived the most life-threatening period of aortic dissection, and they are best managed medically unless complications such as aortic insufficiency or saccular aortic aneurysm are present [122].

LONG-TERM MEDICAL MANAGEMENT OF AORTIC DISSECTION

After aortography, patients with uncomplicated distal dissection should be continued on propranolol and nitroprusside or trimethaphan infusions. A transition to oral antihypertensive therapy should be initiated after the blood pressure has stabilized and clinical evidence of progression or complications of dissection has subsided. Survivors of surgical intervention should also receive long-term medical therapy. The preferred antihypertensive agents for the long-term management of patients with aortic dissection are those that have a negative inotropic effect such as β-blockers without intrinsic sympathomimetic activity, verapamil, diltiazem, labetalol, methyldopa, reserpine, or guanethidine. Vasodilators such as prazosin, hydralazine, or minoxidil, which cause a reflex increase in sympathetic tone, should be avoided. Nifedipine and isradipine can cause a reflex increase in heart rate and cardiac output and should probably be avoided or used only in combination with a β-blocker [141]. Converting enzyme inhibitors have been recommended for long-term medical management of aortic dissection; however, experience with their use in this setting is limited [141]. The objective of therapy should be to maintain the systolic blood pressure below 130 mm Hg. Even patients without hypertension should be given β-adrenergic blocking drugs postoperatively if at all possible [122].

Reoperation may be required for late complications including progressive aortic insufficiency, localized saccular aneurysm formation, and redissection [122]. In a long-term study of surgically treated survivors of aortic dissection, 29 percent of all late deaths were due to the development and eventual rupture of a localized saccular aneurysm [118]. Thus, close lifelong monitoring of treated survivors of aortic dissection is required. Routine chest roentgenograms should be obtained every 3 months for the first year of follow-up and at least twice annually thereafter [122]. A semi-annual CT scan should be considered in patients with Marfan's syndrome, since they are at high risk for late aneurysm formation [122].

Hypertensive Crises in the Surgical Patient

POORLY CONTROLLED HYPERTENSION IN THE PATIENT REQUIRING SURGERY

Hypertension in the preoperative patient is a common problem. In a series of 1,000 patients over the age of 40 presenting for surgery, 28 percent were hypertensive [196]. The benefits of preoperative control of blood pressure were demonstrated in a study that evaluated intraoperative systemic hemodynamics in patients with either preoperative normotension, adequately treated hypertension, or inadequately treated hypertension [447]. During anesthesia, cardiac output decreased by 30 percent in all three groups. In normotensive and adequately treated hypertensives, there were only minor changes in systemic vascular resistance, resulting in modest decreases in mean arterial pressure of 23 percent and 33 percent, respectively. In contrast, the inadequately treated hypertensives experienced, on average, a 27 percent decrease in systemic vascular resistance, which, coupled with the declines in cardiac output, resulted in reduction of mean arterial pressure by 45 percent during anesthesia. Electrocardiographic changes consistent with myocardial ischemia were commonly observed in the latter group [447].

Poor control of preoperative hypertension, with a diastolic blood pressure over 110 mm Hg, is a relative contraindication to elective surgery [195]. In patients with diastolic blood pressure over 110 mm Hg, perioperative morbidity and mortality were found to be increased due to a high incidence of intraoperative hypotension accompanied by myocardial ischemia and postoperative acute renal failure [195].

It should be noted, however, that these data were collected in patients hospitalized for preoperative evaluation in whom multiple blood pressure readings were available to document persistently poor preoperative blood pressure control. It is not clear whether these criteria should be applied to patients presenting for outpatient surgery who are found to have a diastolic blood pressure over 110 mm Hg. The finding of elevated blood pressure in this circumstance may not necessarily be reflective of long-term inadequate blood pressure control. In this setting, if there is no history of long-standing inadequate blood pressure control and if the blood pressure responds satisfactorily to sedation, sublingual nifedipine, or minibolus labetalol, it may be possible to proceed with elective outpatient surgery.

Malignant hypertension presents an excessive surgical risk, and all but lifesaving emergency surgery should be deferred until the blood pressure can be controlled and organ function stabilized [342].

Some authorities believe that mild to moderate, uncomplicated, preoperative hypertension (diastolic blood pressure $\leq$ 110 mm Hg) does not significantly increase the risk of surgery and is therefore not a reason to postpone elective surgery [51, 195]. However, patients with mild to moderate hypertension and preexisting complications, such as ischemic heart disease, cerebrovascular disease, congestive heart failure, or chronic renal insufficiency, represent a subgroup with a significantly increased perioperative risk [195]. In these patients, adequate preoperative control of blood pressure is imperative [444, 456]. Even though the blood pressure in patients with severe or complicated hypertension can usually be controlled within hours using aggressive parenteral therapy, such precipitous control of hypertension carries the risk of significant complications such as hypovolemia, electrolyte abnormalities, and marked intraoperative and postoperative blood pressure lability. These risks predispose to myocardial ischemia, cerebrovascular accidents, and acute renal failure [342]. In these high-risk groups, if possible, elective surgery should be postponed and blood pressure brought under control for a few weeks before surgery [342, 456]. Ideally, good preoperative blood pressure control should be the aim in all hypertensive patients [342, 444, 456].

In patients with adequately treated hypertension, antihypertensive and antianginal medications should be continued up to and including the morning of surgery. Such treatment decreases intraoperative blood pressure lability and protects against the hypertensive response associated with endotracheal intubation and other noxious stimuli during surgery [444, 446]. Oral administration of blood pressure medications with a small amount of water (15–20 ml) a few hours before surgery has not been shown to increase the risk of gastric aspiration during anesthesia induction [342]. Since hypovolemia increases the risk of intraoperative hypotension and postoperative acute renal failure, diuretics should be withheld for 1 to 2 days preoperatively except in patients with overt heart failure or fluid overload. Adequate potassium supplementation should be provided to correct hypokalemia well in advance of surgery. Drugs such as clonidine, which carry the potential for withdrawal reactions or hypertensive rebound during the postoperative period, may be electively tapered and replaced with other medications over 1 to 2 weeks preoperatively. Alternatively, the clonidine transdermal therapeutic system has been recommended for the perioperative management of patients receiving long-term centrally-acting α_2-agonist therapy [268]. Clonidine may also be given by the sublingual or rectal routes of administration.

Although, theoretically, β-adrenergic blockers could cause hemodynamic instability in the face of surgical stress, blood loss, and the myocardial depression caused by anesthetics, studies have shown that elective withdrawal of β-blockers preoperatively is not only unnecessary but may also be deleterious in patients with underlying coronary artery disease. Continuation of oral propranolol until a few hours before general anesthesia did not appear to impair hemodynamic function [297]. Furthermore, patients pretreated with β-blockers had less hypertension, tachycardia, myocardial ischemia, and dysrhythmia during endotracheal intubation than did patients who did not receive β-blockers [445].

The use of converting enzyme inhibitors in the preoperative management of the hypertensive patient is controversial [369]. The current consensus is that patients receiving chronic therapy with a converting enzyme inhibitor should continue the drug up until surgery and then restart therapy as soon as possible postoperatively. However, studies in animals suggest that pretreatment with captopril inhibits recovery of blood pressure and renal perfusion pressure after acute hypovolemic hypotension induced by moderate hemorrhage [576, 583]. Given the physiologic role of the renin-angiotensin system in patients subjected to a hypovolemic insult intraoperatively, concern has been raised regarding the risk of intraoperative hemodynamic instability in patients undergoing extensive surgical procedures involving large amounts of blood loss or fluid shifts. There is a recent report of prolonged hypotension in patients undergoing surgery who were treated with converting enzyme inhibitor preoperatively [489].

In contrast, there are data that suggest that converting enzyme inhibitors may be beneficial in patients undergoing coronary artery bypass. Comparison of systemic hemodynamics and renal function in patients pretreated with either captopril or placebo showed that renal plasma flow, glomerular filtration rate, and urinary sodium excretion were higher in patients treated with captopril [93].

The choice of anesthetic technique in the hypertensive patient should be individualized [342, 446]. For peripheral procedures, regional nerve block involves minimal physiologic stress and may be the procedure of choice. Although spinal anesthesia for lower extremity and certain abdominal procedures minimizes myocardial depression and is not associated with sympathetic discharge during endotracheal intubation, the concomitant sympathetic blockade is not quickly reversible and may lead to cardiovascular collapse in high-risk hypertensive patients [342]. For general anesthesia, most of the commonly used anesthetics are acceptable for use in the hypertensive patient. However, drugs such as ketamine that provoke hypertensive responses should be avoided. During anesthesia, there are often wide and rapid fluctuations in blood pressure, which require close monitoring, often by the direct intraarterial method [342]. Continuous electrocardiographic monitoring is essential to monitor for evidence of myocardial ischemia. Accurate measurement of urine output is a helpful indirect measure of the adequacy of renal perfusion. Patients with severe hypertension undergoing upper abdominal or thoracic surgery may require central venous pressure monitoring as a guide to fluid replacement. Monitoring of cardiac output and wedge pressure should be considered in patients with a history of left ventricular failure or ischemic heart disease and in those undergoing major thoracic or cardiovascular procedures [342].

The hypertensive surge during endotracheal intubation can be managed with infusion of sodium nitroprusside, esmolol, or minibolus labetalol [102, 317, 342, 456]. In complicated patients with a history of cardiovascular disease or congestive heart failure, intraoperative and postoperative hypertension should be managed with short-acting agents such as sodium nitroprusside until the preoperative oral antihypertensive regimen can be resumed. Given the benefits of intravenous nitroglycerin with regard to coronary vasospasm and the collateral circulation, it may be a useful agent for the management of perioperative hypertension in patients with coronary artery disease undergoing either noncardiac surgery or coronary artery bypass [167].

In uncomplicated patients, intermittent intravenous labetalol injections may be useful in the management of mild to moderate intraoperative and postoperative hypertension [127, 412]. Parenteral furosemide, β-blockers, hydralazine, and sublingual nifedipine have also been recommended for management of uncomplicated postoperative hypertension until oral therapy can be resumed [3, 456]. Many patients with long-standing severe hypertension require much smaller doses of antihypertensive medications in the early postoperative course. Thus, the preoperative regimen should not be automatically restarted. Routine measurements of supine and standing blood pressure should be utilized as a guide to dosage adjustments during the postoperative recovery period. In most instances, the requirement for antihypertensive medications will gradually increase over a few days to weeks to eventually equal the preoperative requirement.

POSTCORONARY BYPASS HYPERTENSION

Paroxysmal hypertension in the immediate postoperative period is a frequent and serious complication of cardiac surgery. It is the most common complication of coronary artery bypass surgery, occurring in 30 to 50 percent of patients [154]. Postbypass hypertension is mediated by increases in systemic vascular resistance. The heightened systemic vascular resistance increases cardiac work and myocardial oxygen demand. The accompanying increase in LVEDP impairs subendocardial perfusion and may cause myocardial ischemia in patients with limited coronary reserve. The acute increase in afterload may also impair cardiac performance and precipitate acute pulmonary edema. In addition, hypertension increases the incidence and severity of postoperative bleeding in recently heparinized patients. Therefore, postbypass surgery hypertension should be diagnosed and rapidly treated.

There are numerous precipitating factors for hypertension in the postoperative setting including emergence from anesthesia, tracheal or nasopharyngeal irritation from the endotracheal tube, pain, hypothermia with shivering, ventilator asynchrony, hypoxemia, hypercarbia, myocardial ischemia, or withdrawal phenomena resulting from preoperative discontinuation of antihypertensive medications [154]. Hypervolemia, though often cited as the mechanism of postoperative hypertension, is a rare cause of hypertension in this setting except in patients with renal failure [154]. Marked sympathetic overreaction to hypovolemia is a common, often unrecognized cause of severe postoperative hypertension and impaired tissue perfusion [88, 216].

Hypertension after myocardial revascularization occurs as frequently in previously normotensive patients as in those with chronic hypertension [171]. The increase in blood pressure usually occurs during the first 4 hours after surgery and tends to resolve 6 to 12 hours postoperatively. The hypertension, which results from a rise in the systemic vascular resistance (SVR) without any change in cardiac output, may be related to an increase in sympathetic tone due to the activation of pressor reflexes from the heart, great vessels, or coronary arteries [154, 171].

The initial management of postbypass hypertension should include attempts to ameliorate reversible causes of hypertension previously mentioned. Hypertension from pain and anxiety can be managed with analgesics or sedatives. Hypothermia should be treated with warming blankets; intravenous fluids should be heated to 37°C. Patients with paradoxical hypertension in response to volume depletion are exquisitely sensitive to vasodilator therapy and may develop precipitous hypotension even with low-dose infusions of sodium nitroprusside or nitroglycerin. Hypertension in this setting should be treated using careful volume expansion with crystalloid or transfusion as required [88]. If these general measures fail to control the hypertension, further therapy should be guided by measurement of systemic hemodynamics. Parenterally administered vasodilators are the treatment of choice for postbypass hypertension. Sodium nitroprusside or intravenous nitroglycerin may be utilized to provide controlled reduction of the SVR and blood pressure. Intravenous nitroglycerin is as effective as nitroprusside for hypertension in this setting [167]. Nitroglycerin may be the preferred drug, since it dilates intercoronary collaterals and causes less intrapulmonary shunting than does nitroprusside. Postbypass hypertension is usually transient and resolves over 6 to 12 hours, after which the vasodilator can be weaned. The hypertension does not usually recur after the initial episode in the immediate postoperative period [171].

An intravenous β-blocker such as propranolol is occasionally recommended for control of hypertension in surgical patients with tachycardia. However, β-blocking agents are generally not indicated in the setting of postbypass hypertension because the hypertension is usually secondary to increased SVR rather than to increased cardiac output [154, 171]. Moreover, β-blocker therapy may be detrimental, since these agents compromise cardiac output and increase SVR. Esmolol, a short-acting β-blocker, has occasionally been used in hypertensive postoperative patients with a high cardiac output and normal left ventricular function. Its brief duration of action is a major advantage in this situation, where hemodynamic parameters may change rapidly [527]. However, labetalol may cause a significant reduction in cardiac index in patients with hypertension following bypass surgery [358].

POST-CAROTID ENDARTERECTOMY HYPERTENSION

Hypertension in the immediate postoperative period is extremely common after carotid endarterectomy. In one large series, 58 percent of patients developed post-carotid endarterectomy hypertension as defined by an increase in systolic blood pressure greater than 35 mm Hg or systolic blood pressure requiring treatment with sodium nitroprusside [502]. A history of hypertension and, in particular, poor control of hypertension preoperatively dramatically increased the risk of postoperative hypertension [539]. Severe postoperative hypertension following carotid endarterectomy was associated with an increased incidence of focal neurologic deficits as well as an increased postoperative mortality rate [539]. Moreover, the risk of intracerebral hemorrhage following carotid endarterectomy was dramatically increased by the presence of postoperative hypertension [73].

The mechanism of post-carotid endarterectomy hypertension is poorly understood. The incidence of hypertension is the same whether or not the carotid sinus nerves are preserved [539]. A mechanism for the development of postoperative intracerebral hemorrhage due to hypertension has been proposed [73]. In patients with high-grade carotid artery stenosis, the distal cerebral bed has been protected from systemic hypertension by the stenosis. Following removal of the obstructing lesion, a relative increase in perfusion pressure occurs in the previously protected arteriocapillary bed. Especially in the setting of postoperative hypertension, cerebral autoregulation may fail such that there is overperfusion and rupture resulting in hemorrhagic infarction.

Since poor preoperative blood pressure control increases the risk of postoperative hypertension, strict blood pressure control is mandatory prior to elective carotid endarterectomy. Furthermore, intraarterial blood pressure should be monitored intraoperatively and in the immediate postoperative period. Ideally, the patient should be awake and extubated prior to reaching the recovery room so that serial neurologic examinations can be used to assess the development of focal deficits. When the systolic blood pressure exceeds 200 mm Hg, an intravenous infusion of sodium nitroprusside should be initiated to maintain systolic blood pressure between 160 and 200 mm Hg [539]. The use of a short-acting parenteral agent is imperative to avoid overshoot hypotension and cerebral hypoperfusion.

HYPERTENSIVE CRISES AFTER REPAIR OF AORTIC COARCTATION

During the first week after repair of coarctation of the aorta, severe systemic hypertension often develops [185]. This so-called *paradoxical hypertension* usually resolves spontaneously if the repair has been satisfactory. There are two distinct phases to the paradoxical hypertensive response: an acute rise in systolic blood pressure during the first postoperative day and a later rise in the diastolic pressure from the second through fourth postoperative days [185, 487]. The immediate postoperative increase in systolic blood pressure lasts 8 to 12 hours and is similar in mechanism to the postmyocardial revascularization hypertension described above. The second phase of hypertension, which is accompanied by abdominal pain and signs of an acute abdomen, causes considerable morbidity and mortality due to the development of mesenteric endarteritis [549].

After repair of the coarctation, the decline in blood pressure in the upper body results in baroreceptor inactivation. The release of the sympathetic axis from tonic baroreceptor inhibition results in a "vasomotor storm" with a markedly increased heart rate and blood pressure. The renin-angiotensin axis may also be activated by the increase in sympathetic tone [185], and angiotensin-mediated vasoconstriction may account for part of the pressor response. The mesenteric vessels that had been exposed to the low pressure distal to the coarctation are suddenly exposed to severe hypertension. This may cause endarteritis and vascular necrosis with intestinal ischemia and infarction.

Prophylactic oral propranolol, 1.5 mg/kg/day in divided doses for 2 weeks before surgery, may prevent paradoxical postcoarctectomy hypertension [185]. Sodium nitroprusside and parenteral β-blockers have also been successfully used to treat postcoarctectomy hypertension. The goal of therapy should be to maintain systolic blood pressure in the range of 120 to 150 mm Hg. As soon as possible, oral propranolol should be instituted as the sodium nitroprusside infusion is weaned [563]. Intravenous labetalol has also been recommended for control of hypertension following coarctation repair [49].

HYPERTENSION COMPLICATING POSTOPERATIVE BLEEDING

Hypertension in the postoperative period may result in severe and intractable bleeding from vascular suture lines. Hypertension may also aggravate bleeding in the setting of severe epistaxis and tracheal, gastrointestinal, or urinary tract hemorrhage. Retroperitoneal hemorrhage after closed renal biopsy may be exacerbated by hypertension. In each situation, control of the blood pressure is required for normal hemostasis. Sodium nitroprusside is utilized for immediate and precise control of the blood pressure. In postoperative patients, trimethaphan is contraindicated because of its tendency to produce bowel and bladder atony.

Catecholamine-Related Hypertensive Crises

HYPERTENSIVE CRISES WITH PHEOCHROMOCYTOMA

The diagnosis and treatment of pheochromocytoma are discussed in detail in Chap. 56. Our comments here are restricted to treatment of hypertensive crises in patients with pheochromocytoma with emphasis on the perioperative management of hypertension. In the majority of cases, pheochromocytoma causes sustained hypertension, which occasionally enters the malignant phase. In roughly 30 percent of cases, paroxysmal hypertension is present. Paroxysms usually occur spontaneously and consist of severe hypertension, headache, profuse diaphoresis, pallor of the face, coldness of the hands and feet, palpitations, and abdominal discomfort. Metoclopramide infusion can precipitate hypertensive crises in patients with pheochromocytoma, possibly due to its presynaptic dopaminergic blocking effect, which may result in increased catecholamine release [1]. Marked elevation of blood pressure may lead to intracerebral hemorrhage, hypertensive encephalopathy, or acute pulmonary edema [450]. Prompt reduction of blood pressure is mandatory to prevent these life-threatening complications [450]. Although the nonselective α-adrenergic receptor blocker phentolamine is often cited as the treatment of choice for pheochromocytoma-related hypertensive crises, sodium nitroprusside is equally effective [247, 494]. Phentolamine is given in 5- to 10-mg intravenous boluses every 5 minutes as necessary to control blood pressure. Given its short duration of action, a continuous infusion of phentolamine may be utilized. After the blood pressure has been controlled with sodium nitroprusside or phentolamine, intravenous β-adrenergic receptor blockers such as esmolol or propranolol may be used to control tachycardia or arrhythmias. After resolution of the hypertensive crisis, oral antihypertensive agents should be instituted as the parenteral agents are weaned.

Skillful preoperative management of blood pressure and volume status is clearly a prerequisite to successful surgical intervention [247, 438, 494]. Usually, the nonselective α-blocker phenoxybenzamine is administered for 1 to 2 weeks prior to elective surgery. The initial dose of 10 mg twice daily is increased every other day until normotension, accompanied by moderate (15 mm Hg) asymptomatic orthostatic hypertension, has been attained and paroxysms are well-controlled [247, 494]. The last dose of phenoxybenzamine is usually administered at 10:00 P.M. on the evening before surgery. After adequate α-blockade has been achieved, oral β-blocker therapy may be initiated if needed to control tachycardia. Oral or intravenous β-blockers should never be administered before adequate α-adrenergic blockade has been achieved. Administration of β-blocker to patients with catecholamine-secreting tumors can lead to severe hypertension with acute pulmonary edema as the result of intense α-adrenergic-mediated vasoconstriction that is no longer opposed by β-adrenergic vasodilatory stimuli. Prazosin, a selective α_1-antagonist, has been reported to be as effective as phenoxybenzamine for preoperative management of hypertension [101]. However, hypertensive crises responsive to low-dose phenoxybenzamine have been reported in patients receiving apparently adequate α-blockade with prazosin [293]. Labetalol has also been advocated for the preoperative management of hypertension in patients with pheochromocytoma [469]. However, hypertensive crises precipitated by the use of labetalol have been reported [398]. The paradoxical increase in blood pressure was attributed to the fact that labetalol is a more potent β-blocker than it is an α-blocker.

Careful attention to *volume status* is imperative in the preoperative period [438, 494]. Alleviation of the chronic state of catecholamine-induced vasoconstriction by α-blockade results in increases in both arterial and venous capacitance. Preoperative volume expansion guided by measurements of central venous pressure or wedge pressure has been advocated to reduce the severity of intraoperative hypotension [438]. However, other authors maintain that a high-salt diet or infusions of crystalloid are usually not necessary in the majority of patients during the preoperative period, since treatment with α-adrenergic blockade for 1 to 2 weeks alleviates the chronic state of vasoconstriction and allows for spontaneous restoration of normal plasma volume [247]. Moreover, caution has been advised if intravenous fluids are administered during the preoperative period, since pulmonary edema may occur if an underlying catecholamine-induced cardiomyopathy is present [247].

Cardiac status should be carefully evaluated in the preoperative period. Approximately 25 percent of patients with catecholamine-secreting tumors have some degree of cardiomyopathy with biventricular dysfunction caused either by a direct toxic effect of catecholamines on the myocardium or indirectly by chronic hypertension [247, 486]. This catecholamine-induced cardiomyopathy is associated with an increased risk of sudden death from arrhythmias, as well as increased operative risk. Thus, preoperative evaluation should include echocardiography to assess ventricular function. The cardiomyopathy is usually reversible with adequate preoperative adrenergic blockade. Operative intervention should generally be deferred until serial echocardiograms confirm that ventricular function has improved in response to treatment with adrenergic blocking drugs.

During surgery, rapid and wide fluctuation in blood pressure should be anticipated [494]. Adequate premedication should be used to minimize the risk of sympathetic activation during endotracheal intubation and induction of anesthesia. Diazepam and short-acting barbiturates are the agents of choice for premedication [494]. Droperidol, phenothiazines, and morphine are contraindicated because they may cause catecholamine release. Atropine should be avoided because its vagolytic effect results in tachycardia in the setting of high circulating catecholamine levels.

Careful intraoperative monitoring of intraarterial blood pressure, cardiac output, wedge pressure, and SVR is required to manage rapid swings in blood pressure [494]. Despite adequate preoperative α-blockade with phenoxybenzamine, severe hypertension may occur during intubation or intraoperatively due to catecholamine release during tumor manipulation. Although intermittent bolus phentolamine has been advocated in this setting, prolonged α-blockade may predispose to significant hypotension following tumor devascularization [494]. Therefore, sodium nitroprusside, with its immediate onset and short duration of action, is the agent of choice for controlling acute hypertension during pheochromocytoma surgery [494]. Infusions of esmolol, propranolol, or lidocaine can be used for short-term control of arrhythmias [247, 494].

At the opposite end of the spectrum, *severe intraoperative hypotension* may occur. Hypotension or even frank shock may supervene following isolation of tumor venous drainage from the circulation with a resultant abrupt decrease in circulating catecholamine levels. This hypotension is caused by a precipitous reduction in vascular tone, which may be further aggravated by operative blood loss, down-regulation of adrenergic receptors in response to a chronic increase in catecholamines, α-adrenergic blockade, or impaired heart rate response resulting from β-adrenergic blocking drugs [494]. Volume expansion with crystalloid, colloid, or blood as needed is the recommended treatment for intraoperative hypotension [494]. Volume repletion should be guided by measurements of wedge pressure and cardiac output. Pressors should only be employed if hypotension is unresponsive to adequate volume repletion [494]. The risk of hypotension due to hypovolemia extends into the postoperative period, during which close monitoring of volume status is essential. In the postoperative period, required volume replacement not uncommonly exceeds measured fluid losses [494].

HYPERTENSIVE CRISES SECONDARY TO WITHDRAWAL OF ANTIHYPERTENSIVE THERAPY

Abrupt discontinuation of high doses of centrally acting antihypertensive agents such as clonidine [238, 241, 457], methyldopa [62, 177], and guanabenz [241, 451] can produce a withdrawal syndrome characterized by sympathetic overactivity [180]. Symptoms consisting of headache, nausea, restlessness, agitation, insomnia, and tremor usually begin 12 to 72 hours after the discontinuation of the drug. Occasionally, this withdrawal syndrome is accompanied by a rapid increase in the blood pressure to above pretreatment levels (overshoot hypertension) [400]. The abrupt rise in blood pressure may precipitate a hypertensive crisis with hypertensive encephalopathy or acute pulmonary edema. The development of malignant hypertension as evidenced by hypertensive neuroretinopathy on funduscopic examination has been reported [177, 525].

The symptoms that develop following cessation of centrally acting α-receptor agonists are suggestive of sympathetic overactivity. It has been postulated that the syndrome may be related to excessive circulating catecholamine levels [180]. Since the antihypertensive action of central α-agonists is due to reduction in catecholamine release from nerve terminals, abrupt discontinuation may provoke a sudden catecholamine surge. Increased plasma and urine catecholamine levels have been found after abrupt discontinuation of high-dose clonidine [217, 457]. The renin-angiotensin system may also be involved in the withdrawal phenomenon. Since clonidine and methyldopa suppress PRA, it is possible that a rebound increase in PRA and angiotensin II could mediate the hypertensive overshoot following drug withdrawal [525].

In general, withdrawal symptoms or rebound hypertension occurs only after cessation of large doses of drugs. Withdrawal symptoms rarely appear after discontinuation of clonidine in doses less than 1.2 mg per day [238]. The dose of guanabenz in the reported cases of withdrawal syndrome was 48 mg per day [451]. However, the withdrawal syndrome can occasionally be precipitated by cessation of lower doses of drugs. This is especially apt to occur in patients with underlying renal insufficiency or renovascular hypertension [525]. Patients treated with β-blockers may be predisposed to develop severe hypertension during withdrawal of centrally acting α-agonists [19]. Beta-adrenergic receptor blockade inhibits the vasodilatory effect of β_2-receptors on the peripheral vasculature, leaving vasoconstrictor α_1-receptors unopposed.

Treatment of antihypertensive drug withdrawal syndromes should be individualized. In patients with generalized symptoms of sympathetic overactivity but without excessive blood pressure elevation, reinstitution of the previously administered drug is usually all that is required [180]. However, if the withdrawal syndrome is associated with severe hypertension, hypertensive encephalopathy, or acute pulmonary edema, rapid control of the blood pressure with parenteral antihypertensive agents is imperative. Sodium nitroprusside or phentolamine is the agent of choice for the management of these hypertensive crises. After the blood pressure is controlled with phentolamine or sodium nitroprusside, oral clonidine, guanabenz, or methyldopa is reinstated. The offending drug should then be gradually withdrawn with close monitoring for withdrawal symptoms and rebound hypertension. Another oral antihypertensive regimen, preferably without a β-blocker, should be initiated simultaneously.

HYPERTENSIVE CRISES SECONDARY TO MONOAMINE OXIDASE INHIBITOR INTERACTIONS

Severe paroxysmal hypertension complicated by intracerebral or subarachnoid hemorrhage, hypertensive encephalopathy, acute pulmonary edema, or even death may occur in patients receiving monoamine oxidase (MAO) inhibitors after the ingestion of certain foods or drugs [44, 190].

Although catechol-O-methyltransferase is important in the metabolism of circulating catecholamines, MAO is required for the degradation of intracellular amines including epinephrine, norepinephrine, and dopamine [199]. Since MAO normally limits intracellular amine accumulation, MAO inhibitors cause an increase in the quantity of amines within storage granules. The amino acid tyramine releases these stores of catecholamines from nerve endings, causing a profound pressor response. Certain foods contain substantial amounts of tyramine including natural or aged cheeses, Chianti wines, certain beers, pickled herring, chicken liver, yeast, soy sauce, fermented sausage, coffee, avocados, bananas, chocolate, and canned figs [44]. As a result of hepatic MAO inhibition, tyramine escapes oxidative degradation in the liver and causes release of norepinephrine from nerve endings. Sympathomimetic amines in nonprescription cold remedies can also provoke neurotransmitter release. A hyperadrenergic state resembling pheochromocytoma then ensues.

In a large series of patients treated with MAO inhibitors, symptoms typically began within 10 minutes to 2 hours of the ingestion of the offending food or drug. Symptoms included sudden onset of a severe pounding headache, palpitations, throbbing vessels in the neck, flushing or pallor, profuse diaphoresis, nausea, vomiting, and extreme prostration. The onset of marked hypertension was a characteristic finding. The mean increase in blood pressure was 55 mm Hg systolic and 30 mm Hg diastolic. Complications included intracerebral hemorrhage, subarachnoid hemorrhage, hypertensive encephalopathy, and acute pulmonary edema. The duration of the attacks varied from 10 minutes to 6 hours [44].

Sodium nitroprusside and phentolamine are drugs for management of the crisis. Since most patients are normotensive prior to the onset of the hypertensive crisis, the goal of treatment should be normalization of the blood pressure. Intravenous β-blockers may be required for control of heart rate and tachyarrhythmias. Since the hypertensive crises with MAO inhibitor/tyramine interactions are usually self-limited, the sodium nitroprusside or phentolamine infusion can be weaned without institution of an oral antihypertensive agent.

HYPERTENSIVE CRISES DUE TO NONPRESCRIPTION SYMPATHOMIMETIC AMINES

Phenylpropanolamine, ephedrine, and pseudoephedrine are sympathomimetic amines that are available in a wide variety of over-the-counter drug preparations, which are marketed as nasal decongestants, appetite suppressants, or stimulants. Although there is mounting evidence of the safety of these drugs when used at recommended doses [299, 448], toxic effects may result from overdose [302, 425]. Moreover, there may be substantial abuse potential for use as amphetamine substitutes [425]. A recent study in healthy, normotensive subjects found that 150 mg of phenylpropanolamine (the amount contained in a double dose of an over-the-counter appetite suppressant) substantially elevated blood pressure [303]. Review of adverse drug effect case reports suggests that overdose of phenylpropanolamine can cause a significant increase in blood pressure, which may be complicated by severe headache, hypertensive encephalopathy, intracerebral hemorrhage, seizures, and even death [302]. In patients who present with hypertensive encephalopathy of unknown origin, the possibility of recent ingestion of phenylpropanolamine-containing drugs should be investigated. Hypertensive crises secondary to phenylpropanolamine should be treated with a rapid-acting agent such as sodium nitroprusside or phentolamine. This is generally the only treatment that is required because the drug is rapidly excreted in the urine and the duration of the toxic reaction is usually less than 6 hours [425].

Miscellaneous Hypertensive Crises

Hypertensive crises have been reported in a wide variety of clinical settings. Patients with extensive *second- or third-degree burns* may develop hypertensive crises 3 to 4 days after hospitalization [55]. Hypertensive crises have been reported as idiosyncratic reactions to a number of drugs including *amphotericin B* [138], *lithium* [363], *amitriptyline* [139], and *metrizamide* [466]. Severe hypertension with hypertensive encephalopathy has been reported to occur in a dose-related fashion in children treated with *high-dose cyclosporine* for allogenic bone marrow transplantation [271, 326]. Hypertensive crises may also complicate the use of *recreational drugs* including cocaine hydrochloride or "crack" [202, 454], and phencyclidine hydrochloride (PCP) [143].

In each of these conditions, sudden elevation of blood pressure in previously normotensive individuals may cause hypertensive encephalopathy, intracerebral hemorrhage, or acute pulmonary edema. Sodium nitroprusside is the treatment of choice for the management of hypertension in these diverse settings.

Hypertensive crises may occur in quadriplegic patients, especially those with a spinal cord lesion above the origin of the thoracolumbar preganglionic sympathetic neurons (T_5 or above) [392]. *Autonomic hyperreflexia* is a clinical syndrome that develops episodically in up to 85 percent of patients with chronic spinal cord injury [27, 153, 392, 533]. The syndrome consists of paroxysmal episodes of severe headache with diaphoresis, facial flushing, piloerection, and pallor below the level of the cord lesion. There is a sudden, marked increase in blood pressure accompanied by profound bradycardia [392]. Since quadriplegic patients are usually hypotensive, the sudden elevation of blood pressure can cause hypertensive encephalopathy, intracerebral hemorrhage, and even death.

Autonomic hyperreflexia is usually triggered by noxious stimuli in the dermatomes, muscles, or viscera supplied by nerves below the level of the spinal cord injury. Stimuli related to distention of a hollow viscus are particularly effective in eliciting this response [27, 533]. Therefore, bladder distention and fecal impaction are frequent inciting stimuli [153]. Urinary catheter insertion, cystoscopy, bladder irrigation, and transurethral resection of the prostate may also precipitate hypertensive crises. Paraplegic patients undergoing abdominal or bladder surgery are also at high risk. Hypertensive crises, presumably due to autonomic hyperreflexia, have also been reported in patients with Guillain-Barré syndrome [113].

Autonomic hyperreflexia is the result of massive sympathetic discharge in response to noxious stimuli. Afferent impulses from nerves below the level of the cord lesion cause excess stimulation of preganglionic sympathetic neurons. The result is reflex sympathetic outflow via the splanchnic nerves. In normal individuals, this reflex outflow is inhibited by input from higher centers. However, in patients with spinal cord lesions above the major splanchnic outflow (T_5 and above), this inhibitory input is blocked and reflex sympathetic output continues unabated, resulting in intense vasoconstriction with severe hypertension [27, 533]. The sudden increase in blood pressure results in bradycardia due to aortic arch and carotid baroreceptor-mediated parasympathetic nervous system activation.

Management of hypertensive crises due to autonomic hyperreflexia requires prompt recognition with correction of precipitating causes. Relief of bladder or bowel distention may be all that is required to alleviate the crises [153]. Sodium nitroprusside or phentolamine is useful for the management of intraoperative hypertensive crises in patients with spinal cord lesions [27, 533].

Hypertensive crises have been reported in patients with insulin-induced hypoglycemia concomitantly treated with β-blockers [340]. It has been postulated that epinephrine release induced by hypoglycemia, in the presence of vascular β_2-receptor blockade by propranolol, causes severe hypertensive reactions due to unopposed α_1-receptor-mediated vasoconstriction.

Hypertensive crises may develop in *renal allograft recipients* due to acute rejection, high-dose glucocorticoid treatment, or transplant renal artery stenosis [349, 483, 531]. Refractory hypertension complicated by hypertensive encephalopathy may also occur in patients with chronic allograft rejection who have returned to dialysis. This complication tends to develop during tapering of immunosuppressive therapy and may be caused by superimposed acute allograft rejection. Allograft nephrectomy may be indicated for the long-term control of blood pressure in this setting.

The Controversy Over Gradual Versus Rapid Reduction of Blood Pressure

Over the last several years, some authors have cautioned against rapid lowering of blood pressure in patients with hypertensive crises and have recommended a more gradual reduction of blood pressure [26, 249, 313, 314]. The case for gradual reduction of blood pressure is based largely on the finding of altered autoregulation of cerebral blood flow in hypertensive patients and scattered case reports of serious neurologic sequelae resulting from overly aggressive reduction of blood pressure in patients with severe hypertension or hypertensive crises [98, 200, 211, 215, 248, 300, 443, 519].

In both hypertensive and normotensive individuals, cerebral blood flow is maintained constant, at approximately 50 ml/min/100 gm of brain tissue, over a wide range of perfusion pressures, by virtue of various intrinsic and neurohumoral autoregulatory mechanisms. The *lower limit of cerebral blood flow autoregulation* is the blood pressure below which autoregulatory vasodilation becomes maximal and cerebral blood flow decreases. In normotensive subjects, the lower limit of autoregulation is a mean arterial pressure of 60 to 70 mm Hg. In chronically hypertensive patients, the lower limit of autoregulation is shifted so that autoregulation fails and cerebral blood flow decreases at a higher level of blood pressure [522, 524]. This effect may be the result of hypertension-induced changes in the cerebral arterioles. Animal models have shown that chronic hypertension causes hypertrophy of the walls of cerebral vessels with a reduction in internal diameter. Moreover, during chronic hypertension, cerebral arterioles undergo structural remodeling that results in a smaller external diameter and encroachment on the vascular lumen [28].

On the one hand, these structural changes are protective in that the thickened cerebral arterioles are able to maintain constant cerebral blood flow at a higher perfusion pressure than would be tolerated by normotensive individuals. In this regard, in chronically hypertensive individuals, the mean arterial pressure at which autoregulatory vasoconstriction gives way to pressure-induced forced vasodilation and hyperperfusion (the *upper limit of cerebral blood flow autoregulation*) is shifted to a higher level compared to normotensive individuals (see discussion of breakthrough theory of hypertensive encephalopathy) [522, 524]. As a consequence of these structural changes, however, the arterioles are not able to dilate fully at low levels of mean arterial pressure, which could predispose hypertensive patients to cerebral ischemia if the blood pressure is lowered excessively.

Fortunately, with long-term control of blood pressure, these changes in cerebral arterioles appear to be at least partially reversible given the observation that patients with previously severe but adequately treated hypertension have a lower limit of autoregulation that is shifted toward the range for normotensive subjects (Table 59-6) [517].

The upward shift in the autoregulatory curve in patients with chronic hypertension is one of the major arguments put forward by those who favor gradual reduction of blood pressure in patients with hypertensive crises [249, 313]. However, the clinical importance and therapeutic implications of this shift in the autoregulatory curve may have been overemphasized. The demonstration of hypertensive adaptation of cerebral autoregulation should not be interpreted to mean that acute reduction of blood pressure in hypertensive crises is unwise [524]. In the various hypertensive crises in which rapid reduction of blood pressure is indicated, the proven benefits of acute reduction of blood pressure (i.e., decreased risk of intracerebral hemorrhage, hypertensive encephalopathy, or acute pulmonary edema) clearly outweigh the theoretical risk of blood pressure reduction (i.e., possible cerebral ischemia).

In practice, moderate, controlled reduction of blood pressure in hypertensive crises rarely causes cerebral ischemia [524]. This clinical observation may be explained by the fact that even though the autoregulatory curve is shifted toward a higher level of blood pressure in chronically hypertensive patients, there is still a considerable difference between the presenting level of blood pressure and the lower limit of autoregulation (Table 59-6) [517]. Strandgaard [517] studied the autoregulation of cerebral blood flow during controlled hy-

Table 59-6. Autoregulation of cerebral blood flow during trimethaphan-induced hypotension

Group	MAP mm Hg			% Resting MAP	
	Resting level	Autoregulation	Tolerated MAP	Autoregulation	Tolerated
Uncontrolled severe hypertensives (n = 13)	145 ± 17	113 ± 17*†	65 ± 10*	79 ± 10	45 ± 6
Controlled hypertensives (n = 9)	116 ± 18	96 ± 17	53 ± 18	72 ± 29	46 ± 16
Normotensives (n = 10)	98 ± 10	73 ± 9	43 ± 8	74 ± 12	45 ± 12

Values given as mean ± SD.
MAP = mean arterial pressure; *$p < 0.01$ for difference between normotensives and uncontrolled hypertensives; † = $p < 0.01$ for difference between controlled and uncontrolled hypertensives.
Source: Adapted from R. W. Gifford, Jr. Effect of reducing elevated blood pressure on cerebral circulation. *Hypertension* 5 (Suppl. III):III-17, 1983.

potension produced with trimethaphan and a 25-degree head-up tilt in 13 patients with untreated or ineffectively treated hypertension. At least 8 of these patients had grade III or grade IV changes on funduscopy consistent with the diagnosis of malignant hypertension. The control groups included 10 normotensive subjects and 9 patients who had been severely hypertensive in the past but whose blood pressure was effectively controlled at the time of the study. Baseline mean arterial pressure in the three groups was 145 ± 17, 116 ± 18, and 98 ± 10 mm Hg, respectively (Table 59-6). The lower limit of mean arterial pressure at which autoregulation of cerebral blood flow failed was 113 ± 17 mm Hg in uncontrolled hypertensives, 96 ± 17 mm Hg in controlled hypertensives, and 73 ± 9 mm Hg in normotensive individuals. Although the absolute level at which autoregulation failed differed substantially in the three groups, the percentage reduction of mean arterial pressure at which autoregulation failed was similar. The mean arterial pressure at the lower limit of autoregulation was 79 ± 10 percent of the resting mean arterial pressure in the uncontrolled hypertensives, 72 ± 29 percent in the controlled hypertensive group, and 74 ± 12 percent in the normotensive group. Thus, a reduction in mean arterial pressure of approximately 20 to 25 percent from the baseline level was required in each group to reach the lower limit of autoregulation. Therefore, even in uncontrolled hypertensive patients, there was a considerable safety margin before the limit of autoregulation was reached.

Another important observation from this study was that symptoms of cerebral hypoperfusion did not occur until the blood pressure was reduced substantially below the lower limit of autoregulation [517]. Studies have shown that with normal cerebral blood flow, oxygen extraction is not maximal, since oxygen saturation in the jugular venous blood at rest is normally 60 to 70 percent. Thus, even when the mean arterial pressure is reduced below the lower limit of autoregulation, cerebral metabolism can be maintained and ischemia prevented by increasing oxygen extraction from the blood [524]. The *lowest tolerated blood pressure,* which was defined as the level at which mild symptoms of brain hypoperfusion were encountered (yawning, nausea, and hyperventilation with hypocapnia), was 65 ± 10 mm Hg in patients with uncontrolled hypertension, 53 ± 18 mm Hg in patients with controlled hypertension, and 43 ± 8 mm Hg in normotensive subjects. These values were 45 ± 6 percent, 46 ± 16 percent, and 45 ± 12 percent of the resting baseline mean arterial pressures, respectively. Thus, symptoms of cerebral hypoperfusion did not occur until the mean arterial pressure was reduced by an average of 55 percent from the resting level (Table 59-6).

In summary, with regard to the shift in cerebral autoregulation in chronically hypertensive patients, there is a therapeutic threshold above which the blood pressure can be safely reduced in patients with hypertensive crises who require immediate control of hypertension. Strandgaard [517, 518] concluded that the upward shift in cerebral autoregulation should not be taken as a warning against aggressive antihypertensive therapy in hypertensive crises. It merely implies that the initial treatment should be aimed at partial reduction but not complete normalization of blood pressure.

The second argument used to support the recommendation for gradual reduction of blood pressure is based on case reports of the occurrence of acute neurologic sequelae during rapid blood pressure reduction in the treatment of severe hypertension or hypertensive crises [98, 200, 211, 215, 248, 300, 314, 443, 519].

Franklin [175] has reviewed 19 reported cases of neurologic complications following aggressive antihypertensive therapy. The average age was 36 years. All the patients had evidence of severe antecedent hypertension with an average mean arterial pressure of 188 ± 19 mm Hg. Malignant hypertension, based on the finding of hypertensive neuroretinopathy, was present in 79 percent, and hypertensive encephalopathy was present in 53 percent of these patients. Aggressive antihypertensive treatment resulted in a reduction of mean arterial pressure to 84 ± 18 mm Hg. This represented a 56 percent decrease from the baseline blood pressure level, a level clearly below the predicted autoregulatory range for hypertensive patients. The time course of blood pressure reduction was within minutes in 26 percent and over many hours in 74 percent of patients. However, the most critical factor in the development of neurologic sequelae appeared to be the long duration of induced overshoot hypotension, which varied from a period of hours to days. Neurologic complications consisted of permanent blindness in 47 percent, coma in 32 percent, pyramidal tract signs in 32 percent, residual neurologic deficits after therapy in 58 percent, and death in 3 patients. The majority of these patients (80 percent) had received a large intravenous bolus of diazoxide. Three patients received no parenteral agents but had sustained hypotension induced with multiple oral agents. Franklin [175] concluded that rather than the rapidity with which blood pressure was reduced, the duration of excessive hypotension was the factor that correlated best with the development of neurologic complications.

In summary, the data suggest that in the treatment of patients with hypertensive crises who require prompt control of blood pressure, potent parenteral agents can be used safely if excessive lowering of blood pressure is avoided. The studies of Strandgaard [517, 518] suggest that autoregulation of cerebral blood flow can be maintained in hypertensive patients as long as the mean arterial pressure is not reduced below 120 mm Hg. This value is two standard deviations above the average mean arterial pressure at which patients in the reported series developed neurologic sequelae.

In general, an initial blood pressure reduction to 160 to 170 over 100 to 110 mm Hg or to a mean arterial pressure of 120 to 130 mm Hg can be safely accomplished in patients who require immediate control of blood pressure in hypertensive crises [175]. Alternatively, the initial antihypertensive therapy can be individualized based on the pretreatment level of blood pressure. In the individual patient, reduction of the mean arterial pressure by 20 percent should be the initial therapeutic goal. At this level, the blood pressure should still be above the predicted autoregulatory lower limit. Once this goal is obtained, the patient should be carefully evaluated for evidence of cerebral hypoperfusion. Further reduction of blood pressure can then be undertaken if necessary in a controlled fashion based on the overall status of the patient. In previously normotensive individuals who develop acute hypertensive crises, such as patients with acute glomerulonephritis complicated by hypertensive encephalopathy, the autoregulatory curve may not yet be shifted, and the initial goal of therapy may be normalization of the blood pressure.

The use of potent parenteral agents with a rapid onset and short duration of action, such as sodium nitroprusside, has obvious advantages. If overshoot hypotension or neurologic sequelae develop, they can be quickly reversed by allowing the blood pressure to stabilize at a higher level. Agents with a long duration of action have an inherent disadvantage in that excessive reduction of blood pressure cannot be easily reversed. Thus, diazoxide, labetalol, minoxidil, hydralazine, converting enzyme inhibitors, calcium channel blockers, and central α-agonists should be used with extreme caution in patients requiring rapid blood pressure reduction in order to avoid prolonged overshoot hypotension.

Although in the great majority of hypertensive patients cautious blood pressure reduction can be undertaken without a significant risk of causing cerebral hypoperfusion, it should be noted that there is one clinical setting in which there is a significant risk of causing cerebral ischemia even with moderate blood pressure reduction. In patients with *acute cerebral infarction,* because of failure of autoregulation in the surrounding marginally ischemic zone, even moderate blood pressure reduction may be detrimental. Therefore, in acute cerebral infarction, the above considerations regarding the general safety of acute blood pressure reduction may not apply. The management of hypertension complicating acute cerebral infarction has been discussed in the section on Hypertension Complicating Cerebrovascular Accident.

Pharmacology of Drugs Useful in the Treatment of Hypertensive Crises

SODIUM NITROPRUSSIDE

In 1929, Johnson demonstrated that intravenous administration of the color indicator sodium nitroprusside lowered blood pressure [266]. However, concern that the hypotensive action was related to the release of cyanide led to a delay in the introduction of the drug. In 1955 Page et al. showed that intravenous infusion of the drug provided a safe and effective method for achieving short-term blood pressure control [417]. In 1974 sodium nitroprusside (Nipride) was approved for clinical use. Over the last 20 years it has remained the drug of choice for the management of virtually all hypertensive crises. Sodium nitroprusside is useful for the management of hypertensive crises due to malignant hypertension, pheochromocytoma, and other catecholamine-related hypertensive crises, hypertensive encephalopathy, acute pulmonary edema, intracerebral hemorrhage, aortic dissection (in combination with propranolol), and perioperative hypertension [90].

Mechanism of Action. Sodium nitroprusside is a potent intravenous hypotensive agent with an immediate onset and brief duration of action. The site of action is the vascular smooth muscle. It has no direct effect on the myocardium, although it may indirectly affect cardiac performance through alterations in systemic hemodynamics. In therapeutic doses it has no effect on uterine or duodenal smooth muscle [417]. It lacks a central nervous system effect. Sodium nitroprusside causes vasodilation of both arteriolar resistance vessels and venous capacitance vessels. Its hypotensive action is the result of a decrease in systemic vascular resistance. Venodilation results in a decrease in venous return, hence preload is reduced. The combined decrease in preload and afterload reduces left ventricular wall tension and myocardial oxygen demand.

The net effect of sodium nitroprusside on cardiac output and heart rate depends on the intrinsic state of the myocardium [199, 419]. In the absence of congestive heart failure, venodilation and preload reduction may result in a small decrease in cardiac output with a reflex increase in sympathetic tone and heart rate [41, 82, 530]. In contrast, in patients with left ventricular dysfunction and elevated left ventricular end-diastolic volume and/or pressure, sodium nitroprusside causes an increase in stroke volume and cardiac output as the result of a reduction in afterload and impedance to left ventricular ejection. There is usually a reduction in heart rate as the result of improved cardiac performance [41, 82, 530].

The cellular mechanism of action of nitroprusside has been well defined [207, 252]. The rapid onset and brief duration of action support the hypothesis that the drug rather than its metabolites (cyanide, thiocyanate) is the mediation of vasodilation. Nitroprusside is an iron coordinator complex with five cyanide moieties and a nitroso group. The action of sodium nitroprusside, as well as that of other nitrogen oxide-containing vasodilators, is mediated by a reaction with cysteine to form nitrosocysteine (and other short-acting S-nitrosothiols). Nitrosocysteine, a potent activator of guanylate cyclase, causes cyclic guanosine monophosphate accumulation and relaxation of vascular smooth muscle [207, 252].

Pharmacokinetics. The hypotensive effect of sodium nitroprusside appears within seconds and is immediately reversible when the infusion is stopped. It is rapidly metabolized, with a reported half-life of 3 to 4 minutes. Cyanide is formed, as a short-lived intermediate product, by direct combination of sodium nitroprusside with sulfhydryl groups in red cells and tissue [417]. The cyanide groups are rapidly converted to thiocyanate by the liver mitochondrial enzyme rhodanase in a reaction in which thiosulfate acts as a sulfur donor. Thiocyanate is excreted unchanged by the kidney with a half-life of 1 week in patients with normal renal function [419].

Dosage and Administration. The contents of a 50-mg sodium nitroprusside vial should be dissolved in 2 ml of dextrose in water. No other diluent should be used. The stock solution is diluted in 250 ml of dextrose in water to yield a concentration of 200 μg/ml. The container is immediately wrapped in aluminum foil to prevent decomposition on exposure to light. A small portion of the tubing may be left uncovered to observe the solution for color changes during administration. The freshly prepared solution has a faint brownish tint. The nitroprusside molecule reacts with a wide variety of organic and inorganic substances to yield highly colored reaction products. Therefore, the infusion fluid should not be used as a vehicle for the delivery of other drugs. If a color change occurs, the solution should be replaced. Regardless, the solution should be changed every 24 hours.

In patients who are not on other antihypertensives, the average effective dose is 3.0 μg/kg/min (range, 0.5 to 10 μg/kg/min). The initial infusion rate should be 0.5 μg/kg/min. The flow-rate should be increased in increments of 1 μg/kg/min every 2 to 3 minutes until the desired hypotensive response is obtained. The solution should be administered by infusion pump or microdrip regulator to allow for precise measurement of flow rate. The blood pressure should be monitored every 30 to 60 seconds during the initial titration and every 15 minutes thereafter. To avoid excessive accumulation of thiocyanate and the risk of cyanide toxicity, the infusion rate should not be increased above 10 μg/kg/min. Sodium nitroprusside failures are extremely rare, and tachyphylaxis does not occur. Concomitant oral antihypertensive agents should be initiated as soon as possible and the sodium nitroprusside infusion weaned as they become effective.

Adequate facilities, equipment, and personnel must be available for close monitoring of blood pressure during sodium nitroprusside administration. Auscultatory pressures are usually adequate, so that intraarterial pressure monitoring is not routinely required [90]. However, in hypertensive patients with acute myocardial infarction or acute pulmonary edema, hemodynamic monitoring may be required for assessment of left ventricular filling pressure and cardiac output [90].

Adverse Effects. Nitroprusside is the most effective parenteral agent for the management of hypertensive crises. When properly administered in an intensive care unit setting it is also very safe, and clinically significant adverse reactions are uncommon. Overshoot hypotension may result from accidental bolus infusion, faulty infusion equipment, or failure to monitor the blood pressure frequently. However, the hypotensive action is evanescent and hypotension can be easily reversed by slowing or discontinuing the infusion.

The most frequent side effects of sodium nitroprusside administration include anorexia, nausea, vomiting, abdominal cramps, diaphoresis, headache, apprehension, restlessness, and palpitations. Most of these adverse reactions result from rapid blood pressure reduction, and they usually disappear if the infusion is slowed.

Thiocyanate accumulation and toxicity may occur when a high dose or prolonged infusion is required, especially in the setting of renal insufficiency. When these risk factors are present, thiocyanate levels should be monitored and the infusion reduced or discontinued if the level exceeds 10 mg per deciliter. Thiocyanate toxicity is rare in patients with normal renal function requiring less than 3 μg/kg/min for less than 72 hours. Symptoms of thiocyanate toxicity include fatigue, anorexia, weakness, tinnitus, blurred vision, and disorientation, which may progress to frank organic psychosis with hallucinations. Seizures have also been reported. Treatment consists of discontinuing the infusion. Thiocyanate is also readily removed by both peritoneal and hemodialysis [419].

Cyanide poisoning is a very rare complication of sodium nitroprusside use. Since the liver enzyme rhodanase may be deficient in patients with severe liver disease [90] and in rare conditions such as Leber's optic atrophy or tobacco amblyopia [566], the use of sodium nitroprusside is contraindicated in these settings. Most of the reported deaths from cyanide have occurred when very high doses (20 μg/kg/min) have been required for the control of refractory hypertension or in normotensive patients in whom very large doses were used to induce deliberate surgical hypotension [92, 114]. The cyanide ion combines with cytochrome-C and inhibits aerobic metabolism so that lactic acidosis results. Cyanide toxicity most often occurs within the first 6 to 8 hours of therapy. Cyanide toxicity should be considered if there appears to be increased tolerance to the drug. Tachyphylaxis and an increased anion gap metabolic acidosis are the most reliable early signs of cyanide toxicity. Other signs include the smell of bitter almonds on the breath, anxiety, headache, stiffness of the lower jaw, dyspnea, and widely dilated pupils. Coma, seizures, and death may follow. Treatment of cyanide toxicity consists of amyl nitrite inhalation, and sodium nitrite, thiosulfate, and hydroxycobalamin infusions [90, 97].

The safe use of sodium nitroprusside in pregnancy has not been established. In animals nitroprusside readily crosses the placenta. Naulty et al. [397] found that in 5 of 8 normotensive pregnant ewes, high doses of nitroprusside (mean 25 μg/kg/min) were required to reduce blood pressure by 20 percent for 1 hour. In this group, a marked accumulation of maternal cyanide occurred. Fetal blood levels of cyanide were even higher, and all of these fetuses died. However, in 3 of 8 ewes, hypotension was achieved with low doses of sodium nitroprusside (< 1 μg/kg/min). All the fetuses in this group survived, and umbilical cord blood cyanide levels were low.

Ellis et al. [149] used sodium nitroprusside to achieve normotension for 50 minutes in pregnant ewes with norepinephrine-induced hypertension. The mean infusion rate required to control blood pressure was only 2.3 μg/kg/min, and no fetal or maternal deaths occurred. Neither maternal nor fetal blood samples contained greater than 50 μg per liter of cyanide (toxic levels in humans, 5,000 μg/liter).

There are few reports that describe the safe use of sodium nitroprusside for hypertensive crises in pregnant women [134, 463, 515]. Berkowitz [37] has recommended that the use of sodium nitroprusside for hypertensive crises in pregnancy be restricted to patients who are unresponsive to intravenous hydralazine or diazoxide. When nitroprusside is required, it should only be used briefly to manage the acute crisis, and delivery should be performed as quickly as possible.

In summary, sodium nitroprusside has several characteristics that make it nearly the ideal drug for the short-term management of hypertensive crises including rapid onset of action, immediate reversibility, specific effects on resistance and capacitance vessels with no direct effect on the myocardium or central nervous system, lack of tachyphylaxis, and high potency. It is also a very safe drug when used as outlined above. It is the most useful and consistently effective drug available for parenteral use in the treatment of hypertensive crises.

DIAZOXIDE

Diazoxide (Hyperstat) is structurally related to the thiazide diuretics but its pharmacologic effect is direct relaxation of smooth muscle (arteriolar, uterine, and gastrointestinal). The major role of diazoxide is in the treatment of malignant hypertension or hypertensive encephalopathy in situations in which administration of sodium nitroprusside is not feasible and also in the management of acute obstetrical hypertensive emergencies refractory to hydralazine [250, 362, 424, 478].

Diazoxide lowers blood pressure by relaxing arteriolar smooth muscle and reducing systemic vascular resistance. It has no effect on venous capacitance vessels. Although diazoxide has no direct cardiac effect, it does produce reflex sympathetic activation. Heart rate increases, and the cardiac output may double [41]. In patients with preexisting atherosclerotic disease, diazoxide may cause myocardial ischemia as a result of the increase in myocardial oxygen demand [381]. Moreover, given the reflex increase in heart rate and contractility, use of diazoxide is contraindicated in patients with aortic dissection.

Diazoxide, like other arterial vasodilators, causes avid renal salt and water retention [296]. With prolonged use, fluid retention can cause pseudotolerance. This has led to the recommendation that loop diuretics be given concomitantly with diazoxide [295]. However, the routine use of diuretics at the initiation of diazoxide therapy is not recommended. Since patients with malignant hypertension may be volume depleted, the combined use of furosemide and diazoxide can lead to overshoot hypotension. Unless there is obvious fluid overload, diuretic use should be avoided.

Following a bolus injection of 50 to 300 mg of diazoxide, a hypotensive response begins within 1 minute and reaches a peak within 5 minutes. Thereafter, the duration of the hypotensive effect ranges from 4 to 20 hours. This rapid onset and long duration of action may be an advantage. Continuous infusion is not required and once the desired blood pressure has been achieved, continuous monitoring is not required. The long half-life results from extensive protein binding of the drug. Approximately 50 percent of the drug is eliminated unchanged by the kidney, while the other 50 percent undergoes hepatic metabolism. The hypotensive response to diazoxide is increased in uremia because the drug is displaced from plasma protein binding sites. Thus, in uremic patients the dose of diazoxide must be reduced [410, 422].

Diazoxide activates adenosine triphosphate–sensitive K^+ channels, which hyperpolarizes smooth muscle cells leading to vasodilation [511]. It has a generalized effect on smooth muscle because myometrium and gastrointestinal smooth muscle are also affected.

Recent studies suggest that diazoxide is effective in over 90 percent of patients when it is administered as a series of small injections rather than a single large injection [452, 547]. In the past, diazoxide was administered as a 300-mg bolus over 15 seconds, given the belief that a large bolus was necessary to saturate plasma protein binding sites so that a sufficient quantity of free drug would be available to interact with vascular smooth muscle [296, 491]. The sustained hypotensive effect was felt to be caused by irreversible binding to vascular receptors. Unfortunately, the large bolus injection technique was associated with a significant risk of severe, sustained overshoot hypotension [98, 300, 314]. More recently, it has been shown that the plasma diazoxide concentration directly correlates with its hypotensive action independent of the method of administration [452, 547]. Therefore, the use of the large (300-mg) single bolus injection technique is no longer recommended.

Through the use of multiple small injections of diazoxide, the blood pressure can be more carefully titrated. In the minibolus technique, 50 to 100 mg is rapidly injected over 15 to 30 seconds every 10 to 15 minutes until the desired hypotensive response is obtained. The hypotensive action lasts 4 to 20 hours. Repeated small bolus injections of 50 to 100 mg every 4 to 6 hours can then be utilized to maintain the hypotensive response. Most patients respond after total doses of 150 to 450 mg, although some require as much as 600 mg or more [452, 547]. Slow continuous infusion of diazoxide at 15 mg/minute for 20 to 30 minutes (5 mg/kg total dose) has also been shown to be safe and effective treatment for severe hypertension [250]. The diazoxide solution is very alkaline (pH 11.6), and extravasation may cause severe local pain and cellulitis.

Although myocardial infarction, angina, arrhythmias, electrocardiographic abnormalities, strokes, coma, and seizures have all been reported with diazoxide, most of these adverse events have occurred in patients with precipitous hypotension induced by the rapid administration of a 300-mg bolus, especially in patients with underlying cardiovascular and cerebrovascular disease. Precipitous hypotension is more likely to occur in patients who are volume depleted due to prior diuretic administration or are receiving other antihypertensive agents. Diazoxide is contraindicated in patients with acute myocardial infarction or aortic dissection [404]. Since diazoxide may precipitate cerebral ischemia, it is contraindicated in patients with cerebrovascular disease or intracerebral hemorrhage [294, 296].

Diazoxide causes hyperglycemia by inhibiting insulin release from pancreatic islet cells [204]. The hyperglycemia is usually mild and rarely requires therapy, but the blood glucose should be closely monitored in patients with renal insufficiency or type II diabetes mellitus. Failure to recognize and treat hyperglycemia has been reported to lead to diabetic ketoacidosis and nonketotic hyperosmolar coma [78, 543].

The use of diazoxide to treat pregnancy-related hypertensive crises is controversial but has been recommended as an alternative to hydralazine [250, 380, 399]. Since diazoxide relaxes uterine smooth muscle, uterine hypotonia and cessation of labor may occur. However, this effect can be overcome with oxytocin. The drug crosses the placenta and may cause neonatal hyperglycemia and hyperbilirubinemia [368]. Overshoot hypotension, which may compromise ureteroplacental blood flow and result in fetal bradycardia, is usually reversible with fluid administration [250].

TRIMETHAPHAN

Trimethaphan camsylate (Arfonad) is a potent parenteral ganglionic blocking agent that is utilized infrequently now that other parenteral agents with fewer side effects have become available. However, some authors consider trimethaphan to be the drug of choice for the management of acute aortic dissection [420]. It has also been used for the management of hypertensive encephalopathy, subarachnoid hemorrhage, and hypertension complicated by acute pulmonary edema. It is useful in the management of autonomic hyperreflexia in patients with spinal cord injuries [27, 533].

The antihypertensive effect of trimethaphan is produced by ganglionic blockade. It blocks both sympathetic and parasympathetic autonomic ganglionic transmission by occupying postsynaptic receptor sites, thereby preventing binding of acetylcholine liberated from presynaptic terminals [199]. The sympathetic blockade causes dilation of arteriolar resistance vessels. In addition, there is venodilation, so that venous return and preload are reduced. Unlike nitroprusside and other peripheral vasodilators that may cause reflex sympathetic stimulation, trimethaphan blocks sympathetic reflexes so that peripheral vasodilation is not accompanied by a reflex increase in inotropy or chronotropy. Therefore, trimethaphan does not cause an increase in cardiac output in patients with normal left ventricular function, since preload is reduced and sympathetic reflexes are blocked. In contrast, in patients with left ventricular dysfunction, the cardiac output may increase and the heart rate decrease in response to the decrease in afterload and impedance to left ventricular ejection.

The onset of action of trimethaphan occurs within minutes. After the infusion is stopped, the duration of the hypotensive effect is 5 to 15 minutes. The metabolic fate of trimethaphan is unclear. The relatively brief duration of action is believed to be due to destruction of trimethaphan by cholinesterase [532].

Tachyphylaxis often develops with prolonged use of the drug, usually after 24 to 48 hours, so that the dose may have to be increased to maintain the hypotensive response. In addition, pseudotolerance may be caused by renal salt and water retention. In this circumstance, responsiveness can be reestablished by parenteral diuretic administration.

Trimethaphan is available in 10-ml vials containing 500 mg of the drug, which should be diluted in 500 ml of 5% dextrose in water to achieve a final concentration of 1 mg per milliliter. The drug should be administered by an infusion pump or microdrip regulator. The initial infusion rate is 0.5 mg per minute. The infusion rate should be increased every 3 to 5 minutes until the desired blood pressure is obtained. The typical dosage requirement is 0.5 to 5 mg per minute. Doses larger than 5 mg per minute should not be utilized because respiratory arrest has been reported [109]. Continuous monitoring of the blood pressure is required every 30 seconds during the initial titration and every 10 to 15 minutes thereafter. The decrease in pressure is posture dependent. Thus the amount of drug required to lower blood pressure can be minimized by the use of a tilt bed. To reduce the duration of therapy, concomitant oral antihypertensives should be initiated as soon as possible, and the trimethaphan infusion weaned as they become effective.

Most of the side effects of trimethaphan are those expected of parasympathetic blockade. Blurred vision results from paralysis of accommodation and mydriasis. The use of trimethaphan is contraindicated in patients with glaucoma. Paralytic ileus results from decreased tone and motility of the gastrointestinal tract. Thus it should not be used for the postoperative management of hypertension. Urinary retention occurs with use of trimethaphan for over 48 hours. Despite bladder distention, patients experience no urge to void. Thus a bladder catheter is required in most patients. Ganglioplegia results in inactivation of pupillary reflexes. This may cause confusion in the evaluation of comatose neurologic patients with hypertensive encephalopathy, head injury, or intracerebral hemorrhage. Since hypoventilation and respiratory arrests have been described in association with the curare-like action at the neuromuscular junction, trimethaphan is contraindicated in patients with respiratory insufficiency. The use of trimethaphan in pregnancy can lead to meconium ileus in the newborn [213].

INTRAVENOUS NITROGLYCERIN

Intravenous nitroglycerin is particularly useful for the management of hypertension complicating acute myocardial infarction and hypertension occurring after coronary artery bypass. Nitroglycerin causes relaxation of vascular smooth muscle. The predominant effect at lower doses is venodilation. At higher doses, both venous and arterial dilation occur in a dose-dependent fashion [168]. As with nitroprusside and trimethaphan, the effects of intravenous nitroglycerin on stroke volume and cardiac output vary depending on the presence or absence of left ventricular dysfunction [166]. In patients without heart failure, the reduction in preload usually predominates and stroke volume falls. In contrast, in patients with left ventricular failure, a decrease in afterload predominates, and stroke volume is maintained despite a reduction in preload.

For the treatment of hypertension complicating acute myocardial infarction or postbypass hypertension, nitroglycerin may have an advantage over sodium nitroprusside [165]. Chiariello et al. [84] studied 10 patients with acute myocardial infarction treated with nitroprusside at a rate that lowered the mean arterial pressure by 25 mm Hg. All of the patients developed an increase in ST segment elevation by precordial mapping, suggesting a worsening of regional myocardial ischemia. In 5 of the patients, subsequent use of sublingual nitroglycerin reduced mean arterial pressure by 14 mm Hg. However, there was a concomitant decrease in ST segment elevation, suggesting an improvement in regional ischemia.

Recent studies have suggested that nitroglycerin and nitroprusside may have different effects on regional myocardial blood flow [74, 332, 341]. Although both drugs dilate coronary vessels, nitroglycerin has a predominant effect on large coronary conductance arteries, including intercoronary collaterals, and relatively little effect on small resistance arterioles. In contrast, sodium nitroprusside predominantly dilates the resistance vessels and has less effect on intercoronary collaterals. In the setting of regional myocardial ischemia, resistance vessels in the ischemic region are already maximally dilated. Thus sodium nitroprusside may dilate resistance vessels in nonischemic areas and shunt blood away from ischemic areas (coronary steal). In contrast, nitroglycerin, by predominantly dilating conductance vessels, improves blood flow to the ischemic region. Given the potentially deleterious effects of nitroprusside on regional myocardial blood flow, Flaherty [166] has recommended that intravenous nitroglycerin be used in preference to nitroprusside for the treatment of hypertension or left ventricular dysfunction in association with acute myocardial infarction.

The cellular mechanism of action of nitrates has been reviewed by Zelis [581]. Nitrates produce vasodilation through the formation of the free radical nitric oxide, which activates guanylate cyclase. There appears to be a tight coupling between cyclic guanosine monophosphate (cGMP) production and smooth muscle relaxation. A cGMP-dependent protein kinase is stimulated that results in alterations in the phosphorylation of various proteins in smooth muscle. Dephosphorylation of the light chain of myosin leads to smooth muscle relaxation [555].

Intravenous nitroglycerin has a rapid onset and brief duration of action with a half-life of 1 to 4 minutes. It is metabolized in the liver by a glutathione-dependent organic nitrate reductase. Intravenous nitroglycerin is supplied in 10-ml bottles containing 50 mg, which should be diluted in 5% dextrose in water or 0.9% sodium chloride. Usually one bottle is diluted in a 250-ml volume to yield a final concentration of 200 μg per milliliter. Nitroglycerin interacts with many types of plastic. Thus the drug should be diluted only in glass parenteral solution bottles. Special infusion sets have been developed that absorb less nitroglycerin than standard polyvinyl chloride tubing. The initial infusion rate should not exceed 5 μg per minute. The dose is titrated in 5-μg per minute increments every 3 to 5 minutes until the desired hypotensive response is achieved. There is no standard optimal dose of nitroglycerin. There tends to be great variability in response from patient to patient. Blood pressure should be monitored every 30 seconds during the titration phase and every 15 minutes thereafter. As with nitroprusside, close monitoring in an intensive care unit setting is required. In the setting of acute myocardial infarction, monitoring of cardiac output and wedge pressure is essential.

LABETALOL

Intravenous labetalol has been reported to be of value in a variety of hypertensive crises including malignant hypertension [565], hypertension complicating acute myocardial infarction [72, 460], hypertensive encephalopathy [100, 565], aortic dissection [103], and hypertensive crises in pregnancy [103].

Labetalol has selective α_1- and nonselective β-blocking properties [331, 354]. The ratio of β- to α-blocking potency is 7 : 1 for intravenous labetalol. The acute antihypertensive effect after intravenous administration appears to be caused by a decrease in systemic vascular resistance without an appreciable change in cardiac output [354]. The β-blocking effect offsets the baroreceptor-mediated sympathetic response to hypotension. Thus heart rate remains unchanged or decreases slightly.

After intravenous injection, the full antihypertensive effect occurs within 5 to 10 minutes, and the blood pressure gradually rises to pretreatment levels over 16 to 18 hours. The duration of action, defined as the time from the last injection until the diastolic blood pressure rises 10 mm Hg above the nadir pressure, ranges from 2 to 6.5 hours [565]. The major route of elimination is via glycuronide conjugation in the liver. Thus the labetalol dose must be decreased in patients with liver dysfunction but need not be modified in patients with renal failure.

Labetalol is supplied in 20-ml ampules containing 100 mg of the drug. It is usually administered by repeated minibolus injections through an intravenous line. The initial dose is 20 mg (4 ml) injected slowly over a 2-minute period. The maximum hypotensive response usually occurs within 5 minutes of the injection. If the desired hypotensive response is not obtained after 10 minutes, a 40-mg bolus is administered over 2 minutes. Additional injections of 40 to 80 mg can be given at 10-minute intervals until the desired hypotensive response is obtained or the maximum total dose of 300 mg has been given.

Labetalol may also be given by slow continuous infusion. The contents of 2 ampules (200 mg, 40 ml) are added to 160 ml of diluent to yield a volume of 200 ml with a final concentration of 1 mg per milliliter. The infusion is begun at 2 mg per minute. The infusion is continued until the desired response is obtained and then discontinued. Again, the maximum total dose of 300 mg should not be exceeded.

After the pressure has been controlled with either the minibolus or continuous infusion technique, it has been recommended that oral therapy be initiated with labetalol as soon as the supine diastolic blood pressure increases by 10 mm Hg above the minimum obtained with parenteral therapy. The initial oral dose is 200 mg. Thereafter the oral dose is titrated beginning at 200 mg twice daily and increased to 600 mg twice daily as required. The addition of a diuretic often enhances the long-term blood pressure response.

As with other parenteral antihypertensive agents, intravenous labetalol can cause precipitous hypotension, which may result in cerebral ischemia. Exaggerated hypotensive responses have usually been reported when the initial injection is large (1.5 to 2.0 mg/kg); however, overshoot hypotension may also develop with either the minibolus or continuous infusion technique.

Other side effects of labetalol are related to its nonselective β-blocking properties. Labetalol should be avoided in patients with severe sinus bradycardia, heart block greater than first degree, bronchial asthma, or congestive heart failure.

Labetalol may cause a significant reduction in cardiac index when used in the setting of hypertension after open heart surgery [358]. The hypotensive action of the drug appeared to result from a decrease in cardiac output rather than from a decrease in systemic vascular resistance. Thus use of nitroglycerin or sodium nitroprusside is preferred in this setting.

Although there are reports of preoperative management of pheochromocytoma with labetalol [455, 469], β-blockade could result in exacerbation of hypertension if α-blockade is incomplete. In this regard, there have been reports of paradoxical hypertension when labetalol was used to treat pheochromocytoma [52]. Therefore, the routine use of labetalol for the preoperative management of pheochromocytoma is not recommended.

In summary, although intravenous labetalol has been used to treat a variety of hypertensive crises, its long duration of action is a major disadvantage. For this reason, sodium nitroprusside usually represents a more logical choice for the acute management of patients with hypertensive crises requiring parenteral therapy.

PHENTOLAMINE

Phentolamine is useful in the management of catecholamine-related hypertensive crises including pheochromocytoma, monoamine oxidase inhibitor/tyramine interactions, and clonidine, methyldopa, or guanabenz withdrawal reactions. It is not consistently effective in other hypertensive crises. In fact, phentolamine has largely been replaced by sodium nitroprusside in the management of catecholamine-related hypertensive crises.

Phentolamine is a nonselective α-adrenergic blocking agent that competitively inhibits the effect of norepinephrine on vascular smooth muscle α_1-receptors. It does not have β-blocking activity and therefore does not block the cardiac effects associated with β_1-receptor activation by catecholamines. Phentolamine produces dilation of both arteriolar resistance vessels and venous capacitance vessels [112, 199].

The intravenous injection of 1 to 5 mg produces a hypotensive effect within 2 to 3 minutes; however, the duration of action may last only 15 to 30 minutes, so that frequent dosing is required to control blood pressure. Phentolamine is supplied in ampules containing 5 mg. The initial dose should be 1 mg. Subsequent boluses of 1 to 5 mg are administered up to a total dose of 20 to 30 mg or until the blood pressure is controlled. After the desired blood pressure is achieved, intermittent injections are given as necessary to maintain the response [488].

Side effects due to phentolamine are common. Tachycardia and arrhythmias may occur due to β-adrenergic cardiac stimuli that are not blocked by phentolamine. Gastrointestinal side effects include abdominal pain, nausea, vomiting, and diarrhea. Exacerbation of peptic ulcer disease can occur, so phentolamine should be used with caution in patients with a history of gastritis or peptic ulcer disease [199].

HYDRALAZINE

In the past, parenteral hydralazine was frequently used for the treatment of hypertensive crises. Many obstetricians still consider hydralazine to be the drug of choice for the management of hypertensive crises in pregnancy [37]. However, aside from its use in pregnancy, hydralazine has been largely replaced by other agents in the treatment of hypertensive crises.

The hypotensive response to either intramuscular or intravenous hydralazine is unpredictable. The onset of action occurs 10 to 30 minutes after a parenteral dose. The duration of action is 3 to 9 hours. The dose and frequency of administration needed to control the blood pressure are highly variable [295, 530]. Profound and sustained hypotension may occur with an intravenous dose as low as 10 mg. Hydralazine is a direct-acting arteriolar vasodilator. It causes reflex activation of the adrenergic nervous system [530]. Because venous capacitance vessels are not affected, venous return is maintained. In association with activation of the adrenergic system, there are increases in heart rate and stroke volume [530]. Hydralazine is contraindicated in the treatment of aortic dissection because the increase in myocardial contractility may result in propagation of the dissection. It is also contraindicated in patients with ischemic heart disease because the increased myocardial oxygen demand can precipitate angina or myocardial infarction.

Parenteral hydralazine is still used in acute hypertensive crises of pregnancy. In the majority of patients, hydralazine reduces the blood pressure to acceptable levels and is well tolerated by both mother and fetus, despite reflex activation of the adrenergic system [37]. Dosing guidelines for the use of parenteral hydralazine in pregnancy are well established [105]. Since maternal hypertension helps to maintain placental perfusion, there is concern that aggressive treatment aimed at normalization of blood pressure might further compromise placental perfusion to the detriment of the fetus. Therefore, hydralazine treatment is usually instituted if the diastolic blood pressure is over 110 mm Hg and the goal of therapy is a diastolic pressure in the 90 to 100 mm Hg range. After an initial intravenous dose of 5 mg, additional 5- to 10-mg doses are administered every 15 to 20 minutes until the desired response is obtained. Since preeclampsia is associated with intravascular volume depletion, it is important to initiate therapy with a low dose to avoid overshoot hypotension. Intramuscular injection of hydralazine is unsatisfactory because uptake from this location in patients with a labile peripheral vascular bed is erratic [488].

NIFEDIPINE

The numerous studies that have assessed the clinical use of nifedipine in severe uncomplicated hypertension and hypertensive crises have recently been reviewed [178, 242, 507]. Nifedipine appears to produce a consistent, prompt, and usually predictable fall in systemic arterial pressure after a single dose administered by either the oral, sublingual, buccal, or rectal route.

Nifedipine and other calcium channel blockers inhibit the movement of extracellular calcium through the cell membrane and the release of calcium from sarcoplasmic reticulum into the cell cytoplasm. The decrease in available calcium reduces the activity of calcium-dependent adenosine triphosphatase, which results in uncoupling of excitation-contraction [169]. The antihypertensive effect results from arteriolar vasodilation with a decrease in systemic vascular resistance. Nifedipine produces a prompt reduction in systolic, diastolic, and mean arterial pressures of about 25 percent below baseline values in most patients [507]. The magnitude of the hypotensive response tends to be proportional to the height of the initial pressure. A mild increase in heart rate occurs in most patients. With the decrease in afterload, stroke volume and cardiac output increase. In patients with left ventricular dysfunction, pulmonary capillary wedge pressure may decrease.

Nifedipine is usually administered as a 10-mg sublingual, buccal, or oral dose. The onset of action occurs 5 to 10 minutes after sublingual or buccal administration of the liquid drug, which has been squeezed or aspirated with a needle and syringe from the capsule. With oral or rectal administration of the intact capsule, the onset of action occurs at 15 to 20 minutes. However, a recent study showed that absorption of nifedipine from the oral mucosa is negligible and that most absorption occurs in the stomach [346]. The rapid onset of action when the liquid is administered by the sublingual route is explained by the absorption of swallowed liquid from the stomach. The lag in onset of action when the intact capsule is swallowed is due to the time required for dissolution of the capsule. The most reliable method of administration of the drug may be to bite and swallow the capsule [346]. The peak effect occurs in 20 to 30 minutes. The duration of action is 4 to 6 hours regardless of the route of administration [178, 507].

The major acute side effects of nifedipine include a burning sensation in the face and legs, facial flushing, headache, and palpitations. Overshoot hypotension has been reported, especially in hypovolemic patients or patients pretreated with diuretics [39, 178, 408, 553]. Exaggerated hypotension has been reported to cause myocardial ischemia in patients with underlying coronary atherosclerosis [408].

Sublingual or oral nifedipine may be useful in the management of patients with malignant hypertension who do not have an absolute indication for parenteral antihypertensive therapy. Sustained release nifedipine (Procardia XL) may also be useful in this setting [256]. However, in patients with hypertensive crises requiring careful moment-to-moment titration of the hypotensive response, the prolonged duration of action and the potential risk of overshoot hypotension with nifedipine are major disadvantages. The use of sodium nitroprusside is clearly preferable in these patients.

The role of nifedipine in the acute treatment of severe uncomplicated hypertension in the emergency room setting prior to discharge is discussed under Severe Uncomplicated Hypertension.

MINOXIDIL

Minoxidil is a potent antihypertensive agent which is available only for oral use. In combination with a potent diuretic and a β-blocker, it has proved very useful in the control of hypertension refractory to conventional antihypertensive regimens. The efficacy of a triple-drug regimen with minoxidil in the management of the patient with malignant hypertension and azotemia has already been discussed. Minoxidil is frequently employed for the long-term control of blood pressure in patients with hypertensive crises after initial control of the blood pressure with parenteral medications. Furthermore, in some crises not requiring immediate blood pressure reduction, an oral triple-drug regimen consisting of minoxidil, a β-blocker and a loop diuretic can effectively control the blood pressure over a period of hours to days and thereby eliminate the need for parenteral antihypertensive therapy (see Treatment of Malignant Hypertension).

Minoxidil is a direct-acting arteriolar vasodilator. Its antihypertensive effect results from a decrease in systemic vascular resistance [322]. It has no effect on venous capacitance vessels. The hypotensive response to minoxidil is accompanied by a baroreceptor-mediated reflex increase in sympathetic tone which results in an increase in heart rate, contractility, and cardiac output. Unopposed, the cardiac output may increase three- to four-fold and attenuate the fall in blood pressure [69, 322]. The resulting increase in myocardial oxygen demand may precipitate ischemia in patients with limited coronary reserve. For this reason, minoxidil is usually given concomitantly with a β-adrenergic blocking drug.

As with other peripheral vasodilators, minoxidil induces profound renal salt and water retention [322]. This fluid retention is probably related to the hypotensive effect of the drug. A similar antinatriuresis occurs with both hydralazine and diazoxide. Minoxidil causes more fluid retention because it is a more potent vasodilator. Several factors enhance the renal salt and water retention [69]. Decreased peritubular capillary pressure is a potent stimulus for salt and water resorption in the proximal tubule. Increased adrenergic tone also enhances proximal tubular salt and water resorption. Like other vasodilators, minoxidil increases renin release, which leads to increased aldosterone production and enhanced distal sodium resorption [322]. Pseudotachyphylaxis to the original hypotensive effect of minoxidil may occur if either β-blockade or diuretic therapy is inadequate.

The serum half-life of minoxidil is 4½ hours; however, the duration of action is longer than the half-life would predict [69]. After oral administration, the antihypertensive effect of minoxidil begins within 30 to 60 minutes, reaches a maximum in 2 to 4 hours, and slowly abates over the next 12 to 18 hours. The prolonged hypotensive effect is probably due to the persistent binding of minoxidil at the site of action in the vascular smooth muscle. About 15 percent of the parent compound is excreted in the urine, while the remainder is metabolized in the liver by glucuronide conjugation [69].

Although the serum half-life is 4 hours, the persistent hypotensive effect allows for a twice daily dosing schedule. Prior to the initiation of minoxidil, all other antihypertensives except diuretics and β-blockers should be discontinued. Minoxidil is started at a dose of 2.5 mg twice a day and is increased in 5 mg per day increments every 2 to 3 days until the desired response is obtained. The usual effective dose is 10 to 40 mg per day. The doses of loop diuretic and β-blocker are titrated to maintain dry weight and prevent tachycardia, respectively.

When more rapid control of arterial pressure is required, incremental changes in minoxidil dosage can be made every 6 hours. The initial 2.5-mg dose is doubled every 6 hours up to a maximum dose of 20 mg or until the desired response is obtained. The effective dose should then be administered every 12 hours and the dose of diuretic and β-blocker titrated as necessary [69].

The dose of β-blocker required in conjunction with minoxidil therapy to prevent reflex tachycardia is often in excess of the usual β-blocking dose. This is because the sympathetic nervous system is activated by minoxidil, and β-blockers compete with catecholamines for receptor binding [69]. The starting dose of β-blocker should be propranolol 160 mg per day or equivalent. The dose is then titrated to maintain resting heart rate at 70 to 80 beats/minute.

In general, thiazide diuretics are not potent enough to counteract minoxidil-induced antinatriuresis, especially if renal insufficiency is present. The starting dose of furosemide is 40 mg twice a day. However, a daily dose of 300 to 400 mg/day may be required to prevent fluid retention and maintain dry weight.

The most common side effects of minoxidil are related to its pharmacologic properties. Fluid retention can lead to weight gain, edema, anasarca, congestive heart failure, and pericardial effusion. With inadequate β-blockade, reflex sympathetic stimulation may lead to angina or myocardial infarction in patients with underlying coronary artery disease. Electrocardiographic changes have been reported following the initiation of minoxidil. Over 90 percent of patients develop flattening or inversion of T waves [69]. Although often marked, these changes do not necessarily indicate myocardial ischemia, and they usually resolve with continued therapy [69, 322].

Pericardial effusions have been reported with minoxidil; however progression to cardiac tamponade is rare. The cause of the effusion is unknown, but it occurs most commonly in patients with renal failure, collagen vascular diseases, or inadequate diuretic therapy. A hemodynamically insignificant effusion is not necessarily a reason to discontinue minoxidil, but the patient should be treated aggressively with diuretics and followed closely for signs of tamponade [69, 322]. Patients on dialysis should have a trial of intensive daily dialysis with a vigorous attempt to achieve and maintain dry weight.

Reversible hypertrichosis of the face, back, and arms occurs in almost all patients on minoxidil and is the most frequent reason for discontinuation of the drug, especially among female patients. Calcium thioglycolate depilatory agents and shaving are used to control this cosmetic side effect.

Triple therapy with minoxidil, a β-blocker, and a loop diuretic is often dramatically effective in the long-term management of severe or malignant hypertension, even when conventional antihypertensive regimens are unsuccessful or produce intolerable side effects [36, 124, 321, 333, 356, 431].

OTHER DRUGS FOR THE TREATMENT OF SEVERE HYPERTENSION

Converting Enzyme Inhibitors. Captopril has been used successfully in the treatment of hypertensive crises. Both oral and sublingual routes of administration have been described [42, 76, 480, 542]. Converting enzyme inhibitors are clearly the treatment of choice for scleroderma renal crisis [513].

Unfortunately, first-dose hypotension has been reported as a significant risk in the treatment of hypertensive crises with converting enzyme inhibitors [179]. Hypotension is most likely to occur in patients with high levels of angiotensin II, underlying renovascular hypertension, or intravascular volume depletion resulting from spontaneous natriuresis in malignant hypertension or from prior diuretic treatment. In addition, the use of converting enzyme inhibitors in the initial management of patients with renal insufficiency may lead to confusion if the renal dysfunction persists or worsens, since bilateral renal artery stenosis may underlie the development of the malignant phase. Use of converting enzyme inhibitors in pregnancy is contraindicated, since they may cause acute renal failure in the neonate [484].

Although malignant hypertension is often characterized by high plasma renin activity, this is not invariably the case. Therefore, converting enzyme inhibitors may not be effective in all patients with malignant hypertension. Moreover, although converting enzyme inhibitors may be useful in the long-term management of patients with malignant hypertension, captopril has not been shown to be superior to other antihypertensive agents in preventing the recurrence of malignant hypertension [160].

Thus, although converting enzyme inhibitors may be useful in the long-term management of hypertension in patients with a history of malignant hypertension or other hypertensive crises, for the reasons outlined above we do not recommend converting enzyme inhibitors for the initial management of hypertensive crises except in patients with scleroderma renal crisis.

Methyldopa. In the past, parenteral methyldopa was often recommended for the treatment of hypertensive crises. However, it has several disadvantages including a delayed onset of action, unpredictable hypotensive effect, and central nervous system sedation. It has virtually been replaced by more rapidly acting and predictable parenteral agents such as sodium nitroprusside and diazoxide.

Reserpine. Intramuscular reserpine in a dose of 1 to 5 mg was widely utilized in the past for the treatment of hypertension complicating acute pulmonary edema, pheochromocytoma, toxemia of pregnancy, and aortic dissection [246]. However, with the advent of more reliable agents with fewer side effects, the use of reserpine for the management of hypertensive crises can no longer be recommended [10].

Clonidine. Oral clonidine loading has been recommended for the management of severe hypertension that is *not* accompanied by evidence of end-organ dysfunction [11, 12, 87, 510]. However, oral clonidine loading is *not recommended* for the management of the true hypertensive crises outlined in Table 59-1. Thus, if hypertension is accompanied by hypertensive neuroretinopathy (malignant hypertension), hypertensive encephalopathy, congestive heart failure, acute myocardial infarction, aortic dissection, or central nervous system catastrophe, the use of oral clonidine loading is not recommended [11]. For example, in patients with hypertensive encephalopathy or another central nervous system catastrophe, clonidine may cause sedation, which would interfere with the assessment of mental status. Moreover, the relatively long duration of action represents a disadvantage in the treatment of hypertensive crises requiring moment-to-moment titration of blood pressure. The oral clonidine loading regimen was described specifically for the management of severe hypertension that is not associated with end-organ dysfunction, an entity known as *urgent hypertension* or *severe uncomplicated hypertension* [11]. There has been an unfortunate tendency to utilize this type of regimen for the treatment of true hypertensive crises in which the use of the potent parenteral medications described above is clearly indicated. The use of oral clonidine loading in the outpatient setting for the management of severe uncomplicated hypertension is discussed in the next section.

Severe Uncomplicated Hypertension

The benefits of acute reduction of blood pressure in the setting of true hypertensive crises are obvious. Fortunately, hypertensive crises are relatively rare events that never affect the vast majority of hypertensives. Another type of presentation that is more common among hypertensive patients than true hypertensive crisis is severe hypertension (diastolic blood pressure over 115 mm Hg) in the absence of the hypertensive neuroretinopathy or other acute end-organ damage that would signify a true crisis. This entity, which is known as *severe uncomplicated hypertension*, is very common in the emergency department setting. In a recent study of severe uncomplicated hypertension treated in an emergency room, 60 percent of the patients were entirely asymptomatic and had presented for prescription refills or routine blood pressure checks or were found to have elevated blood pressure during routine examinations. The other 40 percent presented with nonspecific symptoms such as headache, dizziness, or weakness (in the absence of evidence of acute end-organ dysfunction), which were possibly related to the elevated blood pressure [260].

In the past, this entity has been referred to as *urgent hypertension*, reflecting the widely accepted notion that acute reduction of blood pressure, over a few hours prior to discharge from the emergency room, was essential to minimize the risk of short-term complications from the severe hypertension [11, 12, 68, 259]. Commonly used treatment regimens included oral clonidine loading or sublingual nifedipine given to acutely reduce the blood pressure prior to initiation of a maintenance antihypertensive regimen [12, 243, 260].

In recent years, however, the urgency of treatment in patients with severe uncomplicated hypertension has been questioned [155, 159, 582]. While it is clear that, in comparison to patients with mild or moderate hypertension, patients with severe uncomplicated hypertension are at increased long-term risk of cardiovascular complications [550], they are infrequently in any immediate danger of an untoward event [159]. The argument supporting the acute reduction of blood pressure is based on the following assumptions: (1) it is important to reduce blood pressure immediately to avoid complications; (2) oral antihypertensive loading prior to initiation of maintenance therapy improves immediate and long-term blood pressure control; and (3) there are no adverse consequences of this form of treatment [155]. Two studies provide some useful information regarding the need to reduce blood pressure immediately with the aim of preventing hypertensive complications. In the Veteran's Administration Cooperative Study of patients with severe hypertension [550], there were 70 untreated patients who had no evidence of malignant hypertension or significant end-organ dysfunction despite the presence of diastolic blood pressure averaging 121 mm Hg. Among these patients, 27 experienced morbid events at an average of 11 $\pm$ 8 months into follow-up. The earliest morbid event was after 2 months [550]. Likewise, a similar study in Baltimore showed that among 42 untreated patients with severe but uncomplicated hypertension, 19 patients experienced morbid events (congestive heart failure, onset of malignant hypertension, cerebrovascular accident, or evidence of declining renal function) at a mean of 12 $\pm$ 7 months into follow-up. The earliest morbid event occurred at 2 months [569]. These data suggest that patients who have severe but uncomplicated hypertension need not be exposed to the risk of "urgent" blood pressure reduction in the emergency room setting, since hypertensive complications tend to occur over a matter of months to years rather than hours to days.

A recent study has addressed the question of whether antihypertensive loading prior to initiation of maintenance therapy improves or hastens blood pressure control. Sixty-four asymptomatic patients with severe hypertension were randomized to treatment with (1) hourly doses of clonidine followed by maintenance therapy, (2) an initial dose of clonidine followed by hourly placebo and then subsequent maintenance therapy, or (3) initiation of maintenance therapy without prior antihypertensive loading. There was no difference between the first two groups with regard to the time required to achieve acceptable blood pressure control during loading therapy. Furthermore, there was no difference between the three groups with regard to adequacy of blood pressure control at 24 hours or 1 week. The authors concluded that sustained blood pressure control resulted solely from maintenance therapy and that the time to adequate control and eventual level of blood pressure were independent of the administration of an initial loading dose of antihypertensive drug. They suggested that the common practice of acute oral antihypertensive loading to treat severe, asymptomatic hypertension should be reconsidered [582]. In this regard, a recent study of 32 patients with severe uncomplicated hypertension found that a significant decrease in blood pressure frequently occurred in the emergency department even before pharmacologic intervention was initiated. Without treatment, over a 50-minute period, the mean arterial pressure decreased by 6 percent [312]. The authors suggest that, given a short period of observation, many patients with severe uncomplicated hypertension will experience a fall in blood pressure to mildly or moderately hypertensive levels, which would clearly make acute blood pressure reduction with an antihypertensive loading regimen unnecessary.

Although generally safe, the oral antihypertensive loading regimens occasionally cause significant adverse effects. Sublingual nifedipine can produce severe headache and profound overshoot hypotension [553]. The marked blood pressure reduction can exacerbate underlying ischemic heart disease, resulting in angina or myocardial infarction [408]. Loading doses of clonidine cause sedation in 60 percent of patients, and some of these patients are difficult to awaken and require assistance in returning home [260]. Furthermore, the recommended conversion from the oral loading dose to a twice daily dose of clonidine [11] may present special problems in the treatment of patients with severe uncomplicated hypertension. Clonidine produces a number of common side effects, including dry mouth, drowsiness, and constipation, that may interfere with long-term compliance with medical therapy. The risk of hypertensive rebound upon abrupt discontinuation of clonidine [241] should be considered, since many patients with this form of hypertension are noncompliant [582].

While the acute reduction of blood pressure in patients with severe uncomplicated hypertension using sublingual nifedipine or oral clonidine loading regimens is the standard of care in many emergency rooms around the country, this practice is often an emotional response on the part of the treating physician to the dramatic elevation of blood pressure [159]. This aggressive approach may also be motivated by fear of medicolegal repercussions in the unlikely event that an untoward hypertensive complication occurs shortly after the emergency room visit [159]. Although observing and documenting the dramatic fall in blood pressure prior to discharge is a satisfying therapeutic maneuver, there is no scientific basis for this approach, and it is not clear that even the small but definite risks of acute blood pressure reduction are justified. There is, at present, no literature to support the notion of an absolute level of blood pressure above which the acute reduction of blood pressure is mandatory before the patient can be discharged from the acute care setting. In the authors' experience, for asymptomatic patients with severe uncomplicated hypertension, acute reduction of blood pressure in the emergency room is often counterproductive, since it may produce untoward symptoms that render the patient less likely to comply with long-term drug therapy. Since the available data suggest that the risks to the patient are not immediate, therapeutic intervention should focus on tailoring an effective, well-tolerated maintenance antihypertensive regimen with emphasis on patient education to enhance compliance [582]. Therefore, oral antihypertensive loading in this setting is of little value. If the patient has simply run out of medications, reinstitution of the previous regimen should suffice. If the patient is thought to be compliant with an existing drug regimen, a sensible change in therapy such as an increase in a suboptimal dosage of an existing drug or the addition of a drug of another class is appropriate. Addition of a low dose of a thiazide diuretic as a second-step agent to existing monotherapy with converting enzyme inhibitor, calcium channel blocker, β-blocker, or central α_2-agonist is often efficacious. Another essential goal of the intervention should be to arrange for suitable outpatient follow-up within a few days. Gradual reduction of blood pressure to normotensive levels over the next few days to a week should be accomplished in conjunction with frequent outpatient follow-up visits to modify drug regimens and reinforce the importance of lifelong compliance with therapy. Though less dramatic than the acute reduction of blood pressure in the emergency room, this type of approach to the treatment of this chronic disease is more likely to prevent long-term hypertensive complications as well as recurrent bouts of severe uncomplicated hypertension.

Finally, an important entity that may masquerade as severe uncomplicated hypertension deserves special mention. *Pseudohypertension* is a condition in which indirect measurement of arterial pressure using a cuff sphygmomanometer is artificially high in comparison to direct intraarterial pressure measurements [413]. Failure to recognize pseudohypertension may result in unwarranted and sometimes frankly dangerous treatment. Pseudohypertension may result from Mönckeberg's medial calcification (a clinically benign form of arterial calcification), advanced atherosclerosis with widespread calcification of intimal plaques, or azotemic arteriopathy (metastatic vascular calcification in patients with end-stage renal disease) [413]. In these entities, stiffening of the arterial wall may prevent its collapse by externally applied pressure, resulting in artificially high indirect blood pressure readings affecting both systolic and diastolic measurements. Pseudohypertension should be suspected in the patient with severe hypertension in the absence of significant target organ damage. The presence of a positive Osler's maneuver, in which the radial or brachial artery remains clearly palpable despite being made pulseless by proximal inflation of a cuff above systolic blood pressure, is an important physical examination finding that should suggest the diagnosis [360]. Roentgenograms of the extremities will frequently reveal calcified vessels [413]. However, the diagnosis can only be made definitively by direct measurement of intraarterial pressure. If unrecognized, pseudohypertension may result in unwarranted treatment with sublingual nifedipine or oral clonidine loading. Patients with pseudohypertension are often elderly and therefore may have critical limitations of blood flow to the brain or heart such that inappropriate blood pressure reduction may precipitate life-threatening ischemic events [413].

References

1. Abe, M., Orita, Y., Nakashima, Y., and Nakamura, M. Hypertensive crisis induced by metoclopramide in patient with pheochromocytoma. *Angiology* 35: 122, 1984.
2. Adelman, R. D., and Russo, J. Malignant hypertension: Recovery of renal function after treatment with antihypertensive medication and hemodialysis. *J. Pediatr.* 98: 766, 1981.
3. Adler, A. G., Leahy, J. J., and Cressman, M. D. Management of perioperative hypertension using sublingual nifedipine: Experience in elderly patients undergoing eye surgery. *Arch. Intern. Med.* 146: 1927, 1986.
4. Ahmed, M. E. K., Walker, J. M., Beevers, D. G., and Beevers, M. Lack of difference between malignant and accelerated hypertension. *Br. Med. J.* 292: 235, 1986.
5. Allbutt, I. C. *Diseases of the Arteries Including Angina Pectoris.* London: Macmillan, 1915.
6. Aloia, J. F., and Beutow, G. Malignant hypertension with aldosterone-producing adenoma. *Am. J. Med. Sci.* 268: 241, 1974.
7. Alpert, M. A., and Bauer, J. H. Rapid control of severe hypertension with minoxidil. *Arch. Intern. Med.* 142: 2099, 1982.
8. Alpert, M. A., and Bauer, J. H. Hypertensive emergencies: Recognition and pathogenesis. *Cardiovasc. Rev. Rep.* 6(4): 407, 1985.
9. Alpert, M. A., and Bauer, J. H. Hypertensive emergencies: Management. *Cardiovasc. Rev. Rep.* 6(5): 602, 1985.
10. AMA Committee on Hypertension. The treatment of malignant hypertension and hypertensive emergencies (editorial). *J.A.M.A.* 228: 1673, 1974.
11. Anderson, R. J., Hart, G. R., Crumpler, C. P., et al. Oral clonidine loading in hypertensive urgencies. *J.A.M.A.* 246: 848, 1981.
12. Anderson, R. J., and Reed, W. G. Current concepts in treatment of hypertensive urgencies. *Am. Heart J.* 111: 211, 1986.
13. Armstrong, P. W., Walker, D. C., Burton, J. R., et al. A vasodilator therapy in acute myocardial infarction. A comparison of sodium nitroprusside and nitroglycerin. *Circulation* 52: 1118, 1975.
14. Asscher, A. W., and Anson, S. G. A vascular permeability factor of renal origin. *Nature* 198: 1097, 1963.
15. Atkinson, A. B., Brown, J. J., Davies, D. L., et al. Hyponatremic hypertensive syndrome with renal artery occlusion corrected by captopril. *Lancet* 2: 606, 1979.
16. Avram, M. M. High prevalence of pancreatic disease in chronic renal failure. *Nephron* 18: 68, 1977.
17. Awan, N. A., Miller, R. R., Vera, Z., et al. Reduction of ST segment elevation with infusion of nitroprusside in patients with acute myocardial infarction. *Am. J. Cardiol.* 38: 435, 1976.
18. Bacon, B. R., and Ricanati, E. S. Severe and prolonged renal insufficiency. *J.A.M.A.* 239: 1159, 1978.
19. Bailey, R. R., and Neale, T. J. Rapid clonidine withdrawal with blood pressure overshoot exaggerated by beta blockade. *Br. Med. J.* 1: 942, 1976.
20. Bakir, A. A., Bazilinski, N., and Dunea, G. Transient and sustained recovery from renal shutdown in accelerated hypertension. *Am. J. Med.* 80: 172, 1986.
21. Baldwin, D. S., and Neugarten, J. Treatment of hypertension in renal disease. *Am. J. Kidney Dis.* 5: A57, 1985.
22. Barcenas, C. G., Eigenbrodt, E., Long, D. L., et al. Recovery from malignant hypertension with anuria after prolonged hemodialysis. *South. Med. J.* 69: 1230, 1976.
23. Barcenas, C. G., Gonzales-Molina, M., and Hall, A. R. Association between acute pancreatitis and malignant hypertension with renal failure. *Arch. Intern. Med.* 138: 1254, 1978.
24. Barnett, A. J., and Silverberg, F. G. Long-term results of the treatment of severe hypertension. *Med. J. Aust.* 2: 960, 1973.
25. Barraclough, M. A. Sodium and water depletion with acute malignant hypertension. *Am. J. Med.* 40: 265, 1966.
26. Barry, D. I. Cerebrovascular aspects of antihypertensive treatment. *Am. J. Cardiol.* 63: 14C, 1989.
27. Basta, J. W., Niejadlik, K., and Pallares, V. Autonomic hyperreflexia: Intraoperative control with pentolinium tartrate. *Br. J. Anaesth.* 49: 1087, 1977.
28. Baumbach, G. L., and Heistad, D. D. Remodeling of cerebral arterioles in chronic hypertension. *Hypertension* 13: 968, 1989.

29. Bechgaard, P. Arterial hypertension: Follow-up study of 1000 hypertensives. *Acta Med. Scand.* (Suppl.) 127: 3, 1946.
30. Bechgaard, P., Kopp, H., and Nielsen, J. One thousand hypertensive patients followed 16–22 years. *Acta Med. Scand.* (Suppl.) 312: 175, 1956.
31. Becker, R. C., and Alpert, J. S. Current management of acute myocardial infarction. *Curr. Probl. Cardiol.* 14(9): 501, 1989.
32. Beevers, D. G., Brown, J. J., Fraser, R., et al. The clinical value of renin and angiotensin estimations. *Kidney Int.* 8(Suppl.): S181, 1975.
33. Beevers, D. G., Hamilton, M., Fairman, M. J., et al. Antihypertensive treatment and the course of established cerebral vascular disease. *Lancet* 1: 1407, 1973.
34. Beilin, L. J., and Goldby, F. S. High arterial pressure versus humoral factors in the pathogenesis of the vascular lesions of malignant hypertension: The case for pressure alone. *Clin. Sci. Molec. Med.* 52: 111, 1977.
35. Bennett, N. M., and Shea, S. Hypertensive emergency: Case criteria, sociodemographic profile, and previous care of 100 cases. *Am. J. Public Health* 78: 636, 1988.
36. Bennett, W. M., Golper, T. A., Muther, R. S., et al. Efficacy of minoxidil in the treatment of severe hypertension in systemic disorders. *J. Cardiovasc. Pharmacol.* 2(Suppl. 2): S142, 1980.
37. Berkowitz, R. L. The Management of Hypertensive Crises During Pregnancy. In R. L. Berkowitz (ed.), *Critical Care of the Obstetric Patient*. New York: Churchill Livingstone, 1983.
38. Bertel, O., and Conen, L. D. Treatment of hypertensive emergencies with the calcium channel blocker nifedipine. *Am. J. Med.* 79(Suppl. 4A): 31, 1985.
39. Bertel, O., Conen, D., Radii, E. W., et al. Nifedipine in hypertensive emergencies. *Br. Med. J.* 286: 19, 1983.
40. Bevan, A. T., Honour, A. J., and Stott, F. H. Direct arterial pressure recording in unrestricted man. *Clin. Sci.* 36: 329, 1969.
41. Bhatia, S. K., and Frolich, E. D. Hemodynamic comparison of agents useful in hypertensive emergencies. *Am. Heart J.* 85: 367, 1973.
42. Biollaz, J., Waeber, B., and Brunner, H. R. Hypertensive crisis treated with orally administered captopril. *Eur. J. Clin. Pharmacol.* 25: 145, 1983.
43. Bischel, M. D., Gans, D. S., and Barbour, B. H. Bilateral nephrectomy for hypertension. *Ann. Intern. Med.* 77: 656, 1972.
44. Blackwell, B., Marley, E., Price, J., et al. Hypertensive interactions between monoamine oxidase inhibitors and food stuffs. *Br. J. Psychiatry* 113: 349, 1967.
45. Blaustein, M. P. Sodium ions, calcium ions, blood pressure regulation: A reassessment and a hypothesis. *Am. J. Physiol.* 232: C165, 1977.
46. Bloxham, C. A., Beevers, D. G., and Walker, J. M. Malignant hypertension and cigarette smoking. *Br. Med. J.* 1: 581, 1979.
47. Bock, K. D. Regression of retinal vascular changes by antihypertensive therapy. *Hypertension* 6(Suppl. III): III-158, 1984.
48. Bohle, A., Grund, K. E., Helmchen, U., et al. Primary malignant nephrosclerosis. *Clin. Sci. Molec. Med.* 51(Suppl.): 23S, 1976.
49. Bojar, R. M., Weiner, B., and Cleveland, R. J. Intravenous labetalol for the control of hypertension following repair of coarctation of the aorta. *Clin. Cardiol.* 11: 639, 1988.
50. Breckenridge, A., Dollery, C. T., and Parry, E. H. O. Prognosis of treated hypertension changes in life expectancy and causes of death between 1952 and 1967. *Q. J. Med.* 39: 411, 1970.
51. Breslin, D. J., and Swinton, N. W. Elective surgery in hypertensive patients—preoperative considerations. *Surg. Clin. North Am.* 50(3): 585, 1970.
52. Briggs, R. S. J., Britwell, A. J., and Pohl, J. E. F. Hypertensive response to labetalol in pheochromocytoma. *Lancet* 1: 1045, 1978.
53. Bright, R. Cases and observations of renal disease with secretion of albuminous urine. *Guy's Hosp. Reports* 1: 338, 1836.
54. Britton, M., de Faire, U., and Helmers, C. Hazards of therapy for excessive hypertension in acute stroke. *Acta Med. Scand.* 207: 253, 1980.
55. Brizio-Molteni, L., Molteni, A., Cloutier, L. C., and Rainey, S. Incidence of post burn hypertensive crisis in patients admitted to two burn centers and a community hospital in the United States. *Scand. J. Plast. Reconstr. Surg.* 13: 21, 1979.
56. Brown, J. J., Davies, D. L., Lever, A. F., et al. Plasma renin concentrations in human hypertension I: Relationship between renin, sodium and potassium. *Br. Med. J.* 2: 144, 1965.
57. Brown, J. J., Davies, D. L., Lever, A. F., et al. Plasma renin concentrations in human hypertension III: Renin in relation to complications of hypertension. *Br. Med. J.* 1: 505, 1966.
58. Brown, J. J., and Peart, W. S. The effect of angiotensin on urine flow and electrolyte excretion in hypertensive patients. *Clin. Sci.* 22: 1, 1962.
59. Bulpitt, C. J. Prognosis of treated hypertension 1951–1981. *Br. J. Clin. Pharmacol.* 13: 73, 1982.
60. Bulpitt, C. J. Mortality and morbidity results from the European Working Party on High Blood Pressure in the Elderly trial. *Drugs* 31(Suppl. 1): 29, 1986.
61. Bulpitt, C. J., Beevers, D. G., Butler, A., et al. The survival of treated hypertensive patients and their causes of death: A report from the DHSS Hypertensive Care Computing Project (DHCCP). *J. Hypertens.* 4: 93, 1986.
62. Burden, A. C., and Alexander, C. P. T. Rebound hypertension after methyldopa withdrawal. *Br. Med. J.* 1: 1056, 1976.
63. Byrom, F. B. The pathogenesis of hypertensive encephalopathy and its relation to malignant phase of hypertension. Experimental evidence from the hypertensive rat. *Lancet* 2: 201, 1954.
64. Byrom, F. B. The evolution of acute hypertensive arterial disease. *Prog. Cardiovasc. Dis.* 17: 31, 1974.
65. Byrom, F. B. Tension and the artery: The experimental elucidation of pseudo-uremia and malignant nephrosclerosis. *Clin. Sci. Molec. Med.* 51(Suppl.): 3s, 1976.
66. Byrom, F. B., and Dodson, L. F. The causation of acute arterial necrosis in hypertensive disease. *J. Pathol. Bacteriol.* 60: 357, 1948.
67. Cain, H., and Kraus, B. The juxtaglomerular apparatus in malignant hypertension of man. *Virchows Arch.* [*A*] 372: 11, 1976.
68. Calhoun, D. A., and Oparil, S. Treatment of hypertensive crisis. *N. Engl. J. Med.* 323: 1177, 1990.
69. Campese, V. M. Minoxidil: A review of its pharmacologic properties and therapeutic use. *Drugs* 22: 257, 1981.
70. Candia, G. J., Heros, R. C., Lavyne, M. H., et al. Effect of intravenous sodium nitroprusside on cerebral blood flow and metabolism. *Neurosurgery* 3: 50, 1978.
71. Cannon, P. J., Hassar, M., Case, D. B., et al. The relationship of hypertension and renal failure in sclero-

derma (progressive systemic sclerosis) to structural and functional abnormalities of the renal cortical circulation. *Medicine* 53: 1, 1974.

72. Cantelli, I., and Bracchetti, D. Hemodynamic effects of intravenous labetalol in patients with acute myocardial infarction and systemic arterial hypertension. *Curr. Ther. Res.* 30: 1043, 1981.
73. Caplan, L. R., Skillman, J., Ojemann, R., and Fields, W. S. Intracerebral hemorrhage following corotid endarterectomy: A hypertensive complication? *Stroke* 9: 457, 1978.
74. Cappuro, N. L., Kent, N. M., and Epstein, S. E. Comparison of nitroglycerin, nitroprusside and phentolamine induced changes in coronary collateral function in dogs. *J. Clin. Invest.* 60: 295, 1972.
75. Carter, A. B. Strokes and hypertension. *Am. Heart J.* 82: 131, 1971.
76. Case, D. B., Atlas, S. A., Sullivan, P. A., et al. Acute and chronic treatment of severe and malignant hypertension with oral angiotensin-converting enzyme inhibitor, captopril. *Circulation* 64: 765, 1981.
77. Chamovitz, J., and Fanger, H. Malignant pheochromocytoma and hypertension (a case report). *Am. J. Clin. Pathol.* 19: 243, 1949.
78. Charles, M. A., and Danforth, E. Nonketoacidotic hyperglycemia and coma during intravenous diazoxide therapy in uremia. *Diabetes* 20: 501, 1971.
79. Chatelain, R. E., Bumpus, F. M., Chernicky, C. L., et al. Differing patterns of altered glucocorticoid secretion in experimental malignant and benign hypertension. Influences upon the lymphoid system and on arterial connective tissue metabolism. *J. Pathol.* 139: 69, 1983.
80. Chatelain, R. E., DiBellow, P. M., and Ferrario, C. M. Experimental benign and malignant hypertension with malignant nephrosclerosis. *Br. J. Exp. Pathol.* 61: 401, 1980.
81. Chatterjee, K., Parmley, W. W., Ganz, W., et al. Hemodynamic and metabolic responses to vasodilator therapy in acute myocardial infarction. *Circulation* 48: 1183, 1973.
82. Chen, R. Y. Z., Fan, F., Schuessler, G. B., et al. Baroreflex control of heart rate in humans during nipride induced hypotension. *Am. J. Physiol.* 243: R18, 1982.
83. Chester, E. M., Agamanolis, D. P., Banker, B. Q., et al. Hypertensive encephalopathy: A clinicopathologic study of 20 cases. *Neurology* 28: 928, 1978.
84. Chiarielo, M., Gold, H. K., Leinbach, R. C., et al. Comparison between the effects of nitroprusside and nitroglycerin on ischemic injury during acute myocardial infarction. *Circulation* 54: 766, 1976.
85. Chusilp, S., and Kincaid-Smith, P. Accelerated hypertension in the rat: Relation between renin, renal vascular lesions, salt intake and blood pressure. *Clin. Sci. Molec. Med.* 51: 69S, 1976.
86. Clarke, E., and Murphy, E. A. Neurologic manifestation of malignant hypertension. *Br. Med. J.* 2: 1319, 1956.
86a. Cogan, M. G. Angiotensin II: A powerful controller of sodium transport in the early proximal tubule. *Hypertension* 15: 451, 1990.
87. Cohen, I. M., and Katz, M. A. Oral clonidine loading for rapid control of hypertension. *Clin. Pharmacol. Ther.* 24: 11, 1978.
88. Cohn, J. N. Paroxysmal hypertension and hypovolemia. *N. Engl. J. Med.* 275: 643, 1966.
89. Cohn, J. N. Blood pressure and cardiac performance. *Am. J. Med.* 55: 351, 1973.
90. Cohn, J. N., and Burke, L. P. Nitroprusside. *Ann. Intern. Med.* 91: 752, 1979.
91. Cohn, J. N., Rodriguera, E., and Guiha, N. H. Hypertensive Heart Disease. In O. Onesti, K. E. Kim, J. H. Moyer (eds.), *Hypertension: Mechanisms and Management.* New York: Grune & Stratton, 1973.
92. Cole, P. The safe use of sodium nitroprusside. *Anesthesia* 33: 473, 1978.
93. Colson, P., Ribstein, J., Mimran, A., et al. Effect of angiotensin converting enzyme inhibition on blood pressure and renal function during open heart surgery. *Anesthesiology* 72: 23, 1990.
94. Conn, J. W. Aldosteronism in man. Some clinical and climatological aspects. Part II. *J.A.M.A.* 183: 871, 1963.
95. Conomy, J. P. Impact of arterial hypertension in the brain. *Postgrad. Med. J.* 68(2): 86, 1980.
96. Cordingley, F. T., Jones, N. F., Wing, A. J., et al. Reversible renal failure in malignant hypertension. *Clin. Nephrol.* 14: 98, 1980.
97. Cottrell, J. E., Casthely, P., Brodie, J. D., et al. Prevention of nitroprusside induced cyanide toxicity with hydroxycobalamin. *N. Engl. J. Med.* 298: 809, 1978.
98. Cove, D. H., Seddon, M., Fletcher, R. F., et al. Blindness after treatment for malignant hypertension. *Br. Med. J.* 2: 245, 1979.
99. Cressman, M. D., and Gifford, R. W., Jr. Hypertension and stroke. *J. Am. Coll. Cardiol.* 1: 521, 1983.
100. Cressman, M. D., Vidt, D. G., Gifford, R. W., et al. Intravenous labetalol in the management of severe hypertension and hypertensive emergencies. *Am. Heart J.* 107: 980, 1984.
101. Cubeddu, L. X., Zarate, N. A., Rosales, C. B., and Zschaeck, D. W. Prazosin and propranolol in preoperative management of pheochromocytoma. *Clin. Pharmacol. Ther.* 32: 156, 1982.
102. Cucchiara, R. F., Benefiel, D. J., Matteo, R. S., et al. Evaluation of esmolol in controlling increases in heart rate and blood pressure during endotracheal intubation in patients undergoing carotid surgery. *Anesthesiology* 65: 528, 1986.
103. Cummings, A. M., and Davies, D. L. Intravenous labetalol in hypertensive emergency. *Lancet* 1: 929, 1979.
104. Cuneo, R. A., and Caronna, J. J. The neurologic complications of hypertension. *Med. Clin. North Am.* 61(3): 565, 1977.
105. Cunningham, F. G., MacDonald, P. C., and Gant, N. F. *Williams Obstetrics* (15th ed.). Norwalk, CT: Appleton & Lange, 1989. Pp. 683–684.
106. Cutler, J. A., MacMahon, S. W., and Furberg, C. D. Controlled clinical trials of drug treatment for hypertension: A review. *Hypertension* 13(Suppl. I): I-36, 1989.
107. Daily, P. O., Trueblood, H. W., Stinson, E. B., et al. Management of acute aortic dissection. *Ann. Thorac. Surg.* 10: 237, 1970.
108. Dalakos, T. G., Streeten, D. H. P., Jones, D., et al. Malignant hypertension resulting from athermatous emboli predominantly involving one kidney. *Am. J. Med.* 57: 135, 1974.
109. Dale, R. C., and Schroeder, E. T. Respiratory paralysis during treatment of hypertension with trimethaphan camsylate. *Arch. Intern. Med.* 136: 816, 1976.
110. DaLuz, P. L., Forrester, J. S., and Wyatt, H. L., et al. Hemodynamic and metabolic effects of sodium nitroprusside on the performance and metabolism of regional ischemic myocardium. *Circulation* 52: 400, 1975.
111. D'Angelo, W. A., Fries, J. F., Masi, A. T., et al. Pathologic observations in progressive systemic sclerosis (scleroderma). A study of 58 autopsy cases and 58 matched controls. *Am. J. Med.* 46: 428, 1969.

112. Das, P. K., and Parratt, J. R. Myocardial and hemodynamic effects of phentolamine. *Br. J. Pharmacol.* 41: 437, 1971.
113. Davidson, D. L. W., and Jellinek, E. H. Hypertension and papilloedema in the Guillain-Barré syndrome. *J. Neurol. Neurosurg. Psychiatry* 40: 144, 1977.
114. Davies, D. W., Kadar, D., Steward, D. J., et al. A sudden death associated with the use of sodium nitroprusside for induction of hypotension during surgery. *Can. Anesth. Soc. J.* 22: 547, 1975.
115. Davis, B. A., Crook, J. E., Vestal, R. E., et al. Prevalence of renovascular hypertension in patients with grade III or grade IV hypertensive retinopathy. *N. Engl. J. Med.* 31: 1273, 1979.
116. Davson, J., Ball, J., and Platt, R. The kidney in periarteritis nodosa. *Q. J. Med.* 17: 175, 1948.
117. DeBakey, M. E., Henly, W. S., Cooley, D. A., et al. Surgical management of dissecting aneurysms of the aorta. *J. Thorac. Cardiovasc. Surg.* 49: 130, 1965.
118. DeBakey, M. E., McCollum, C. H., Crawford, E. S., et al. Dissection and dissecting aneurysms of the aorta: Twenty-year follow-up of five hundred twenty-seven patients treated surgically. *Surgery* 92: 1118, 1982.
119. DelGreco, F., Dolkart, R., Skom, J., et al. Association of accelerated (malignant) hypertension in a patient with primary aldosteronism. *Clin. Endocrinol.* 26: 808, 1966.
120. Derow, H. A., and Altschule, M. J. Malignant hypertension. *N. Engl. J. Med.* 213: 951, 1935.
121. Derow, H. A., and Altshule, M. D. The nature of malignant hypertension. *Ann. Intern. Med.* 14: 1768, 1941.
122. DeSanctis, R. W., Doroghazi, R. M., Austen, W. G., and Buckley, M. J. Aortic dissection. *N. Engl. J. Med.* 317: 1060, 1987.
123. De Venecia, G., and Jampol, L. M. The eye in accelerated hypertension: II. Localized serous detachments of the retina in patients. *Arch. Ophthalmol.* 102: 68, 1984.
124. Devine, B. L., Fife, R., and Trust, P. M. Minoxidil for severe hypertension after failure of other hypotensive agents. *Br. Med. J.* 2: 667, 1977.
125. Dichoso, C. C., Minuth, A. N. W., and Eknoyan, G. Malignant hypertension. Recovery of kidney function after renal allograft failure. *Arch. Intern. Med.* 135: 300, 1975.
126. Dietz, R., Haebara, H., Lüth, B., et al. Does the renin-angiotensin system contribute to vascular lesions in renal hypertensive rats? *Clin. Sci. Molec. Med.* 51(Suppl. 3): 33S, 1976.
127. Dimich, I., Lingham, R., Gabrielson, G., et al. Comparative hemodynamic effects of labetalol and hydralazine in the treatment of postoperative hypertension. *J. Clin. Anesth.* 1: 201, 1989.
128. Dimmitt, S. B., West, J. N. W., Eames, S. M., et al. Usefulness of ophthalmoscopy in mild to moderate hypertension. *Lancet* 1: 1103, 1989.
129. Dinsdale, H. B. Hypertensive encephalopathy. *Stroke* 13: 717, 1982.
130. Dinsdale, H. B. Hypertensive encephalopathy. *Neurol. Clin.* 1(1): 3, 1983.
131. Dinsdale, H. B., Robertson, D. M., and Hass, R. A. Cerebral blood flow in acute hypertension. *Arch. Neurol.* 31: 80, 1974.
132. Dollery, C. T. Hypertensive Retinopathy. In J. Genest, O. Kuchel, P. Hamet, et al. (eds.), *Hypertension: Pathophysiology and Treatment*. New York: McGraw-Hill, 1983. Pp. 723–732.
133. Dollery, C. T., and Shackman, R. Malignant hypertension cured by nephrectomy. *Br. Med. J.* 2: 1367, 1959.
134. Donchin, Y., Amiraw, B., Sahar, A., et al. Nipride for aneurysm surgery in pregnancy. Report of a case. *Br. J. Anesthesiol.* 50: 849, 1978.
135. Doniach, I. Uremic edema of the lungs. *Am. J. Roentgenol.* 58: 620, 1947.
136. Donohue, J. P., Bohnert, W. W., and Shires, D. L. Bilateral nephrectomy: Its role in the management of malignant hypertension of end-stage renal disease. *J. Urol.* 106: 488, 1971.
137. Dougherty, A. H., Naccarelli, G. V., Gray, E. L., et al. Congestive heart failure with normal systolic function. *Am. J. Cardiol.* 54: 778, 1984.
138. Dukes, C. S., and Perfect, J. R. Amphotericin B–induced malignant hypertensive episodes. *J. Infect. Dis.* 161: 588, 1990.
139. Dunn, F. G. Malignant hypertension associated with use of amitriptyline hydrochloride. *South. Med. J.* 75: 1124, 1982.
140. Dzau, V. J., Siwek, L. G., Rosen, S., et al. Sequential renal hemodynamics in experimental benign and malignant hypertension. *Hypertension* 3(Suppl. I): I-63, 1981.
141. Eagle, K. A., and DeSanctis, R. W. Aortic dissection. *Curr. Probl. Cardiol.* 14(5): 229, 1989.
142. Easterling, R. E. Racial factors in the incidence and causation of end-stage renal disease. *Trans. Am. Soc. Artif. Intern. Organs* 23: 28, 1977.
143. Eastman, J. W., and Cohen, S. N. Hypertensive crisis and death associated with phencyclidine poisoning. *J.A.M.A.* 231: 1270, 1975.
144. Editorial. Hypertensive encephalopathy. *Br. Med. J.* 2: 1387, 1979.
145. Eknoyan, G., and Siegel, M. B. Recovery from anuria due to malignant hypertension. *J.A.M.A.* 215: 1122, 1971.
146. Elliot, J. M., and Simpson, F. O. Cigarettes and accelerated hypertension *N. Z. Med. J.* 91: 447, 1980.
147. Ellis, A. Malignant hypertension. *Lancet* 1: 977, 1938.
148. Ellis, L. B. The clinical course of malignant hypertension. *Med. Clin. North Am.* 15: 1025, 1932.
149. Ellis, S. C., Wheeler, A. S., James, F. M., et al. Fetal and maternal effects of sodium nitroprusside used to counteract hypertension in gravid ewes. *Am. J. Obstet. Gynecol.* 143: 766, 1982.
150. Ellrodt, A. G., Ault, M. J., Riedinger, M. S., and Murata, G. H. Efficacy and safety of sublingual nifedipine in hypertensive emergencies. *Am. J. Med.* 79(Suppl. 4A): 19, 1985.
151. Entwisle, G., Apostolides, A. Y., Hebel, J. R., and Henderson, M. M. Target organ damage in black hypertensives. *Circulation* 55: 792, 1977.
152. Erbel, R., Engberding, R., Daniel, W., et al. Echocardiography in the diagnosis of aortic dissection. *Lancet* 1: 457, 1989.
153. Erickson, R. P. Autonomic hyperreflexia: Pathophysiology and medical management. *Arch. Phys. Med. Rehabil.* 61: 431, 1980.
154. Estafanous, F. G., and Tarazi, R. C. Systemic arterial hypertension associated with cardiac surgery. *Am. J. Cardiol.* 46: 685, 1980.
155. Fagan, T. C. Acute reduction of blood pressure in asymptomatic patients with severe hypertension: An idea whose time has come—and gone. *Arch. Intern. Med.* 149: 2169, 1989.
156. Fahr, T. H. Ueber die Beziehungen von Arteriolensklerose, Hypertonie und Herzhypertrophie. *Virchows. Arch. Pathol. Anat.* 239: 41, 1922.

157. Feibel, J. H., Baldwin, C. A., and Joynt, R. J. Catecholamine-associated refractory hypertension following acute intracranial hemorrhage: Control with propranolol. *Ann. Neurol.* 9: 340, 1981.
158. Ferguson, R. K., and Vlasses, P. H. Hypertensive emergencies and urgencies. *J.A.M.A.* 255: 1607, 1986.
159. Ferguson, R. K., and Vlasses, P. H. How urgent is "urgent" hypertension? *Arch. Intern. Med.* 149: 257, 1989.
160. Ferguson, R. K., Vlasses, P. H., and Rotmensch, H. H. Clinical applications of angiotensin-converting enzyme inhibitors. *Am. J. Med.* 77: 690, 1984.
161. Fink, M. E. Emergency management of the head-injured patient. *Emerg. Med. Clin. North Am.* 5(4): 783, 1987.
162. Finnerty, F. A. Hypertensive encephalopathy. *Am. J. Med.* 52: 672, 1972.
163. Fishberg, A. M. *Hypertension and Nephritis* (5th ed.). Philadelphia: Lea & Febiger, 1954.
164. Fishberg, A. M., and Oppenheimer, B. S. The differentiation and significance of certain ophthalmoscopic pictures in hypertensive diseases. *Arch. Intern. Med.* 46: 901, 1930.
165. Flaherty, J. T. Comparison of intravenous nitroglycerin and sodium nitroprusside in acute myocardial infarction. *Am. J. Med.* 74(Suppl. 6B): 53, 1983.
166. Flaherty, J. T., Come, P. C., et al. Effects of intravenous nitroglycerin on left ventricular function and ST segment changes in acute myocardial infarction. *Br. Heart J.* 38: 612, 1976.
167. Flaherty, J. T., Magee, P. A., Gardner, T. J., et al. Comparison of intravenous nitroglycerin and sodium nitroprusside for the treatment of acute hypertension developing after coronary artery bypass surgery. *Circulation* 65: 1072, 1982.
168. Flaherty, J. T., Reid, P. R., Kelly, D. T., et al. Intravenous nitroglycerin in acute myocardial infarction. *Circulation* 51: 132, 1975.
169. Fleckenstein, A. Specific pharmacology of calcium in myocardium, cardiac pacemakers, and vascular smooth muscle. *Ann. Rev. Pharmacol. Toxicol.* 17: 149, 1977.
170. Forsberg, B., and Löw, B. Malignant hypertension and HLA antigens. *Tissue Antigens* 22: 155, 1983.
171. Fouad, F. M., Estatanous, F. G., and Tarazi, R. C. Hemodynamics of postmyocardial revascularization hypertension. *Am. J. Cardiol.* 41: 564, 1978.
172. Fox, K. M., Tomlinson, I. W., Portal, R. W., et al. Prognostic significance of acute systolic hypertension after myocardial infarction. *Br. Med. J.* 3: 128, 1975.
173. Franciosa, J. A., Guiha, N. H., and Limas, C. J. Arterial pressure as a determinant of left ventricular filling pressure after acute myocardial infarction. *Am. J. Cardiol.* 34: 506, 1974.
174. Franciosa, J. A., Notargiacomo, A. V., and Cohn, J. N. Comparative hemodynamics and metabolic effects of vasodilator and inotropic agents in experimental myocardial infarction. *Cardiovasc. Res.* 12: 294, 1978.
175. Franklin, S. S. Hypertensive Emergencies: The Case for Rapid Reduction of Blood Pressure. In R. G. Narins (ed.), *Controversies in Nephrology and Hypertension*. New York: Churchill-Livingstone, 1984.
176. Freis, E. D. Age, race, sex, and other indices of risk in hypertension. *Am. J. Med.* 55: 275, 1973.
177. Frewin, D. B., and Penhall, R. K. Rebound hypertension after sudden discontinuation of methyldopa therapy. *Med. J. Aust.* 1: 659, 1977.
178. Frishman, W. H., Weinberg, P., Peled, H. B., et al. Calcium entry blockers for the treatment of severe hypertension and hypertensive crises. *Am. J. Med.* 77(2B): 35, 1984.
179. Frolich, E. D., Cooper, R. A., and Lewis, E. J. Review of the overall experience of captopril in hypertension. *Arch. Intern. Med.* 144: 1441, 1984.
180. Garbus, S. B., Weber, M. A., Priest, R. T., et al. The abrupt discontinuation of antihypertensive treatment. *J. Clin. Pharmacol.* 19: 476, 1979.
181. Gascho, J. A., Mahanes, M. S., Flanagan, T. L., and Beller, G. A. Effects of nitroglycerin-induced hypotension on myocardial blood flow in a two vessel occlusion-stenosis anesthetized canine model. *J. Am. Coll. Cardiol.* 6: 856, 1985.
182. Gavras, H., Brunner, H. R., Laragh, J. H., et al. Malignant hypertension resulting from deoxycorticosterone acetate and salt excess. *Circ. Res.* 36: 300, 1975.
183. Gavras, H., Oliver, N., Aitchison, J., et al. Abnormalities of coagulation and the development of malignant phase hypertension. *Kidney Int.* 8(Suppl.): S252, 1975.
184. Gibson, T. C. Blood pressure levels in acute myocardial infarction. *Am. Heart J.* 96: 475, 1978.
185. Gidding, S. S., Rocchini, A. P., Beekman, R., et al. Therapeutic effect of propranolol on paradoxical hypertension after repair of coarctation of the aorta. *N. Engl. J. Med.* 312: 1224, 1985.
186. Giese, J. Acute hypertensive vascular disease. I. Relation between blood pressure changes and vascular lesion in different forms of acute hypertension. *Acta Pathol. Microbiol. Scand.* 62: 481, 1964.
187. Giese, J. Acute hypertensive vascular disease. 2. Studies on vascular reaction patterns and permeability changes by means of vital microscopy and colloidal tracer techniques. *Acta Pathol. Microbiol. Scand.* 62: 497, 1964.
188. Gifford, R. W., Jr., and Westbrook, E. Hypertensive encephalopathy: mechanisms, clinical features, and treatment. *Prog. Cardiovasc. Dis.* 17: 115, 1974.
189. Gill, J. R., George, J. M., Solomon, A., et al. Hyperaldosteronism and renal sodium loss reversed by drug treatment for malignant hypertension. *N. Engl. J. Med.* 270: 1088, 1964.
190. Glazener, F. S., Morgan, W. A., Simpson, J. M., et al. Pargyline, cheese, and acute hypertension. *J.A.M.A.* 188: 754, 1964.
191. Goldblatt, H. Studies on experimental hypertension VII. The production of the malignant phase of hypertension. *J. Exp. Med.* 67: 809, 1938.
192. Goldby, F. S. The arteriolar lesions of steroid hypertension in rats. *Clin. Sci. Molec. Med.* 51(Suppl.): 31s, 1976.
193. Goldby, F. S., and Beilin, L. J. Relationship between arterial pressure and the permeability of arterioles to carbon particles in acute hypertension in the rat. *Cardiovasc. Res.* 6: 384, 1972.
194. Goldby, F. S., and Beilin, L. J. How an acute rise in arterial pressure damages arterioles. Electron microscopic changes during angiotensin infusion. *Cardiovasc. Res.* 6: 569, 1972.
195. Goldman, L., and Caldera, D. L. Risk of general anesthesia and elective surgery in hypertensive patients. *Anesthesiology* 50: 285, 1979.
196. Goldman, L., Caldera, D. L., Nussbaum, S. R., et al. Multifactorial index of cardiac risk in noncardiac surgical procedures. *N. Engl. J. Med.* 297: 845, 1977.
197. Goldman, L., Sia, S. T. B., Cook, E. F., et al. Costs and effectiveness of routine therapy with long-term beta-adrenergic antagonists after acute myocardial infarction. *N. Engl. J. Med.* 319: 152, 1988.

198. Goldring, W., and Chasis, H. *Hypertension and Hypertensive Disease.* New York: Commonwealth Fund, 1944.
199. Goodman, L. S., Gilman, A., Wall, T. R., et al. (eds.). *Goodman and Gilman's The Pharmacological Basis of Therapeutics* (8th ed.). New York: Pergamon Press, 1990.
200. Graham, D. I. Ischemic brain damage of cerebral perfusion failure type after treatment of severe hypertension. *Br. Med. J.* 4: 739, 1975.
201. Graham, J. B. Pheochromocytoma and hypertension. An analysis of 207 cases. *Int. Abstracts Surg./Surg. Gynecol. Obstet.* (Suppl.) 92: 105, 1951.
202. Grannis, F. W., Bryant, C., Caffaratti, J. D., and Turner, A. F. Acute aortic dissection associated with cocaine abuse. *Clin. Cardiol.* 11: 572, 1988.
203. Grant, R. T. Observations on periarteritis nodosa. *Clin. Sci.* 4: 245, 1939–1942.
204. Greenwood, R. H., Mahler, R. F., and Hales, C. N. Improvement in insulin secretion after diazoxide. *Lancet* 1: 444, 1976.
205. Grimm, C. E. Emergency treatment of severe and malignant hypertension. *Geriatrics* 35(12): 57, 1980.
206. Gross, R., Dietz, R., Mast, G. J., and Szokol, M. Salt loss as a possible mechanism eliciting an acute malignant phase in renal hypertensive rats. *Clin. Exp. Pharmacol. Physiol.* 2: 323, 1975.
207. Gruetter, C. A., Gruetter, D. Y., Lyon, J. E., et al. Relationship between cyclic guanosine 3′-5′ monophosphate formation and relaxation of coronary artery smooth muscle by glyceryl trinitrate, nitroprusside, nitrite, and nitric oxide: Effects of methylene blue and methemoglobin. *J. Pharmacol. Exp. Ther.* 219: 181, 1981.
208. Gudbrandsson, T., Hansson, L., Herlitz, H., and Andrén, L. Malignant hypertension—improving prognosis in a rare disease. *Acta Med. Scand.* 206: 495, 1979.
209. Gudbrandsson, T., Hansson, L., Herlitz, H., et al. Immunological changes in patients with previous malignant essential hypertension. *Lancet* 1: 406, 1981.
210. Gull, W., and Sutton, H. On the pathology of the morbid state commonly called Bright's disease with contracted kidney (arterio-capillary fibrosis). *Trans. Medico. Chir. Soc.* (London) 55: 273, 1872.
211. Haas, D. C., Streeten, D. H. P., Kim, D. C., et al. Death from cerebral hypoperfusion during nitroprusside treatment of acute angiotensin-dependent hypertension. *Am. J. Med.* 75: 1071, 1983.
212. Hague, W. M., and Honour, J. W. Malignant hypertension in congenital adrenal hyperplasia due to 11β-hydroxylase deficiency. *Clin. Endocrinol.* 18: 505, 1983.
213. Hallum, J. L., and Hatchuel, W. L. F. Congenital paralytic ileus in a premature baby as a complication of hexamethonium therapy for toxemia of pregnancy. *Arch. Dis. Child.* 29: 354, 1954.
214. Hamilton, M., Litchfield, J. W., Peart, W. S., et al. Pheochromocytoma. *Br. Heart J.* 15: 241, 1953.
215. Hankey, G. J., and Gubbay, S. S. Focal cerebral ischemia and infarction due to antihypertensive therapy. *Med. J. Aust.* 146: 412, 1987.
216. Hanson, E. L., Kane, P. B., Askanazi, J., et al. Comparison of patients with coronary artery or valve disease. Intra-operative differences in blood volume and observations of the vasomotor response. *Ann. Thorac. Surg.* 22: 343, 1976.
217. Hansson, L., Hunyor, S. N., Julius, S., et al. Blood pressure crisis following withdrawal of clonidine with special reference to arterial and urinary catecholamine levels and suggestions for acute management. *Am. Heart J.* 85: 605, 1973.
218. Harington, M., Kincaid-Smith, P., and McMichael, J. Results of treatment in malignant hypertension. A seven year experience in 94 cases. *Br. Med. J.* 2: 969, 1959.
219. Harmsen, P., Kjaerulff, J., and Skinhøj, E. Acute controlled hypotension and EEG in patients with hypertension and cerebrovascular disease. *J. Neurol. Neurosurg. Psychiatry* 34: 300, 1971.
220. Harris, P. W. R. Malignant hypertension associated with oral contraceptives. *Lancet* 2: 466, 1969.
221. Harrison, T. S., Birbari, A., and Seaton, J. F. Malignant hypertension in pheochromocytoma: correlation with plasma renin activity. *Johns Hopkins Med. J.* 130: 329, 1972.
222. Hashimoto, H., Kumada, T., Osakada, G., et al. Assessment of transesophageal Doppler echography in dissecting aortic aneurysm. *J. Am. Coll. Cardiol.* 14: 1253, 1989.
223. Hayreh, S. S., and Baines, J. A. Occlusion of the posterior ciliary artery III. Effects on the optic nerve head. *Br. J. Ophthalmol.* 56: 754, 1972.
224. Hayreh, S. S., Servais, G. E., and Virdi, P. S. Fundus lesions in malignant hypertension: V. Hypertensive optic neuropathy. *Ophthalmology* 93: 74, 1986.
225. Healton, E. B., Brust, J. C., Feinfeld, D. A., et al. Hypertensive encephalopathy and the neurologic manifestations of malignant hypertension. *Neurology* 32: 127, 1982.
226. Heptinstall, R. H. Malignant hypertension: A study of fifty-one cases. *J. Pathol. Bacteriol.* 65: 423, 1953.
227. Heptinstall, R. H. Renal biopsies in hypertension. *Br. Heart J.* 16: 133, 1954.
228. Heptinstall, R. H. *Pathology of the Kidney* (3rd ed.). Boston: Little, Brown, 1983.
229. Herlitz, H., Gudbrandsson, T., and Hansson, L. Renal function as an indicator of prognosis in malignant essential hypertension. *Scand. J. Urol. Nephrol.* 16: 51, 1982.
230. Herlitz, H., Hilme, E., Jonsson, O., et al. Erythrocyte sodium transport in malignant hypertension. *J. Intern. Med.* 228: 133, 1990.
231. Heros, R. C. Cerebellar hemorrhage and infarction. *Stroke* 13: 106, 1982.
232. Heros, R. C., Zervas, N. T., and Varsos, V. Cerebral vasospasm after subarachnoid hemorrhage: An update. *Ann. Neurol.* 14: 599, 1983.
233. Heslop, H., Richards, A. M., Nicholls, M. G., et al. Hyponatraemic-hypertensive syndrome due to unilateral renal ischaemia in women who smoke heavily. *N.Z. Med. J.* 98: 739, 1985.
234. Hodge, J. V., and Dollery, C. T. Retinal soft exudates. A clinical study by color and fluorescence photography. *Q. J. Med.* 33: 117, 1964.
235. Hodsman, G. P., Robertson, J. I. S., Semple, P. F., et al. Malignant hypertension and oral contraceptives: Four cases, with two due to the 30 microgram estrogen pill. *Eur. Heart J.* 3: 255, 1982.
236. Holland, N. H., Kotchen, T., and Bhathena, D. Hypertension in children with chronic pyelonephritis. *Kidney Int.* 8(Suppl.): S243, 1975.
237. Hollenhorst, R. W., and Wagener, H. P. The ocular fundus in relation to operations for hypertensive cardiovascular disease. *Am. J. Med. Sci.* 218: 225, 1949.
238. Hoobler, S. W., and Kashima, T. Central nervous system action of clonidine in hypertension. *Mayo Clin. Proc.* 52: 395, 1977.
239. Hood, B., Orndahl, G., and Björk, S. Survival and mortality in malignant (grade IV) and grade III hyperten-

sion. Trends in consecutive, actively treated groups. *Acta Med. Scand.* 187: 291, 1970.
240. Horn, H., Klemperer, P., and Steinberg, M. F. Vascular phase of chronic diffuse glomerulonephritis. A clinicopathologic study. *Arch. Intern. Med.* 70: 260, 1942.
241. Houston, M. C. Abrupt cessation of treatment in hypertension: Consideration of clinical features, mechanisms, prevention and management of the discontinuation syndrome. *Am. Heart J.* 102: 415, 1981.
242. Houston, M. C. Treatment of hypertensive urgencies and emergencies with nifedipine. *Am. Heart J.* 111: 963, 1986.
243. Houston, M. C. Treatment of severe hypertension and hypertensive crises with nifedipine. *West. J. Med.* 146: 701, 1987.
244. Hranilovich, G. T., and Baggenstoss, A. H. Lesions of the pancreas in malignant hypertension. *Arch. Pathol.* 55: 443, 1953.
245. Hsu, H.-C., and Churg, J. The ultrastructure of mucoid "onionskin" intimal lesions in malignant nephrosclerosis. *Am. J. Pathol.* 99: 67, 1980.
246. Hughes, W. M., Moyer, J. H., and Daeschner, W. C. Parenteral reserpine in the treatment of hypertensive emergencies. *Arch. Intern. Med.* 95: 563, 1955.
247. Hull, C. J. Phaeochromocytoma: Diagnosis, preoperative preparation, and anaesthetic management. *Br. J. Anaesth.* 58: 1453, 1956.
248. Hulse, J. A., Taylor, D. S. I., and Dillon, M. J. Blindness and paraplegia in severe childhood hypertension. *Lancet* 2: 553, 1979.
249. Hurtig, H. I. Hypertensive Emergencies: The Case for Gradual Reduction of Blood Pressure. In R. G. Narins (ed.), *Controversies in Nephrology and Hypertension.* New York: Churchill-Livingstone, 1984. Pp. 213–219.
250. Huysmans, F. T. M., Thein, T., and Koene, R. A. Acute treatment of hypertension with slow infusion of diazoxide. *Arch. Intern. Med.* 143: 882, 1983.
251. Hypertension-Stroke Cooperative Study Group. Effect of antihypertensive treatment on stroke recurrence. *J.A.M.A.* 229: 409, 1974.
252. Ignarro, L. J., Lippton, H., Edwards, J. C., et al. Mechanism of vascular smooth muscle relaxation by organic nitrates, nitrites, nitroprusside and nitric acid: Evidence for the involvement of S-nitrosothiols as active intermediates. *J. Pharmacol. Exp. Ther.* 218: 739, 1981.
253. ISIS-1 (First International Study of Infarct Survival) Collaborative Group. Randomized trial of intravenous atenolol among 16,027 cases of suspected acute myocardial infarction: ISIS-1. *Lancet* 2: 57, 1986.
254. Isles, C., Brown, J. J., Cumming, A. M. M., et al. Excess smoking in malignant phase hypertension. *Br. Med. J.* 1: 579, 1979.
255. Isles, C., Lowe, G. D. O., Drummond, M. M., et al. Blood rheology in malignant phase hypertension. *Scand. J. Clin. Lab. Invest.* 41(Suppl. 156): 175, 1981.
256. Isles, C. G., Johnson, A. O. C., and Milne, F. J. Slow release nifedipine and atenolol as initial treatment in blacks with malignant hypertension. *Br. J. Clin. Pharmacol.* 21: 377, 1986.
257. Isles, C. G., McLay, A., and Boulton-Jones, J. M. Recovery in malignant hypertension presenting as acute renal failure. *Q. J. Med.* 53: 439, 1984.
258. Isles, C. G., Walker, L. M., Beevers, G. D., et al. Mortality in patients of the Glasgow Blood Pressure Clinic. *J. Hypertens.* 4: 141, 1986.
259. Jackson, R. E. Hypertension in the emergency department. *Emerg. Med. Clin. North Am.* 6(2): 173, 1988.
260. Jaker, M., Atkin, S., Soto, M., et al. Oral nifedipine vs. oral clonidine in the treatment of urgent hypertension. *Arch. Intern. Med.* 149: 260, 1989.
261. James, T. N., Isobe, J. H., and Urthaler, F. Analysis of components in a cardiogenic hypertensive chemoreflex. *Circulation* 52: 179, 1975.
262. Javadpour, N., Doppman, J. L., Scardino, P. T., et al. Segmental renal vein assay and segmental nephrectomy for correction of renal hypertension. *J. Urol.* 115: 580, 1976.
263. Jellinek, E. H., Painter, M., Prineas, J., et al. Hypertensive encephalopathy with cortical disorders of vision. *Q. J. Med.* 33: 239, 1964.
264. Jhetams, D., Dansey, R., Morar, C., et al. The malignant phase of essential hypertension in Johannesberg blacks. *S. Afr. Med. J.* 61: 899, 1982.
265. Johansson, B., Li, C. L., Olsson, Y., et al. The effect of acute arterial hypertension on the blood brain barrier and protein tracers. *Acta Neuropathol. (Berlin).* 16: 117, 1970.
266. Johnson, C. C. The toxicity and actions of sodium nitroprusside. *Arch. Int. Pharmacol. Ther.* 35: 480, 1929.
267. Johnson, G. On certain points in the anatomy and pathology of Bright's disease of the kidney. On the influence of the minute blood vessels upon the circulation. *Medico-Chirurg. Trans.* 51: 57, 1868.
268. 1988 Joint National Committee. The 1988 report of the Joint National Committee on Detection, Evaluation, and Treatment of High Blood Pressure. *Arch. Intern. Med.* 148: 1023, 1988.
269. Jones, D. B. Arterial and glomerular lesions associated with severe hypertension. Light and electron microscopy studies. *Lab. Invest.* 31: 303, 1974.
270. Jones, D. B., and Iannoccone, P. M. Atheromatous emboli in renal biopsies. *Am. J. Pathol.* 78: 261, 1975.
271. Joss, D. V., Barrett, A. J., Kendra, J. R., et al. Hypertension and convulsions in children receiving cyclosporin A. *Lancet* 1: 906, 1982.
272. Kaneko, T., Sawada, T., Niimi, et al. Lower limit of blood pressure in treatment of acute hypertensive intracranial hemorrhage. *J. Cereb. Blood Flow Metab.* 3(Suppl. 1): S51, 1983.
273. Kannel, W. B., Wolf, P. A., Verter, J., et al. Epidemiologic assessment of the role of blood pressure in stroke. The Framingham study. *J.A.M.A.* 214: 301, 1970.
274. Kaplan, N. M. Primary aldosteronism with malignant hypertension. *N. Engl. J. Med.* 269: 1282, 1963.
275. Kaplan, N. M. *Clinical Hypertension.* Baltimore: Williams and Wilkins, 1982. Pp. 193–209.
276. Kassell, N. F., Peerless, S. J., Durward, Q. J., et al. Treatment of ischemic deficits from vasospasm with intravascular volume expansion and induced arterial hypertension. *Neurosurgery* 11: 337, 1982.
277. Kazda, S., Garthoff, B., and Luckhaus, G. Calcium and malignant hypertension in animal experiment: Effects of experimental manipulation of calcium influx. *Am. J. Nephrol.* 6(Suppl. 1): 145, 1986.
278. Keim, H. J., Drayer, J. I., Case, D. B., et al. A role for renin in rebound hypertension and encephalopathy after infusion of saralasin acetate (Sar^1 - Ala^8 - angiotensin II). *N. Engl. J. Med.* 295: 1175, 1976.
279. Keith, N. M., Odel, H. M., Morlock, C. G., et al. Pathologic studies of the arterial system in severe hypertension. *Proc. Staff Meet. Mayo Clin.* 14: 209, 1939.
280. Keith, N. M., Wagener, H. P., and Barker, N. W. Some different types of essential hypertension: their course and prognosis. *Am. J. Med. Sci.* 197: 332, 1939.
281. Keith, N. W., Wagener, H. P., and Kernohan, J. W. The

syndrome of malignant hypertension. *Arch. Intern. Med.* 41: 141, 1928.
282. Kempner, W. Treatment of hypertensive vascular disease with rice diet. *Am. J. Med.* 4: 545, 1948.
283. Kersting-Sommerhoff, B. A., Higgins, C. B., White, R. D., et al. Aortic dissection: Sensitivity and specificity of MR imaging. *Radiology* 166: 651, 1988.
284. Kimmelstiel, P., and Wilson, C. Benign and malignant hypertension and nephrosclerosis. A clinical and pathologic study. *Am. J. Pathol.* 12: 45, 1936.
285. Kincaid-Smith, P. *The Kidney: A Clinicopathologic Study.* Oxford: Blackwell Scientific, 1975. Pp. 205–221.
286. Kincaid-Smith, P. Malignant hypertension: Mechanisms and management. *Pharmacol. Ther.* 9: 245, 1980.
287. Kincaid-Smith, P. Renal pathology in hypertension and the effects of treatment. *Br. J. Clin. Pharmacol.* 13: 107, 1982.
288. Kincaid-Smith, P., McMichael, J., and Murphy, E. A. The clinical course and pathology of hypertension with papilledema (malignant hypertension). *Q. J. Med.* 27: 117, 1958.
289. Kincaid-Smith, P., and Whitworth, J. A. Pathogenesis of hypertension in chronic renal disease. *Semin. Nephrol.* 8: 155, 1988.
290. Kirkendall, W. M. Retinal Changes of Hypertension. In F. A. Mausolf (ed.), *The Eye in Systemic Disease.* St. Louis: C. V. Mosby Co., 1975. Pp. 212–222.
291. Klahr, S. The kidney in hypertension—villain and victim. *N. Engl. J. Med.* 320: 731, 1989.
292. Klemperer, P., and Otani, S. "Malignant nephrosclerosis" (Fahr). *Arch. Pathol.* 11: 60, 1931.
293. Knapp, H. R., and Fitzgerald, G. A. Hypertensive crisis in prazosin-treated pheochromocytoma. *South. Med. J.* 77: 535, 1984.
294. Koch-Weser, J. Hypertensive emergencies. *N. Engl. J. Med.* 290: 211, 1974.
295. Koch-Weser, J. Vasodilator drugs in the treatment of hypertension. *Arch. Intern. Med.* 133: 1017, 1974.
296. Koch-Weser, J. Diazoxide. *N. Engl. J. Med.* 294: 1271, 1976.
297. Kopriva, C. J., Brown, A. C. D., and Pappas, G. Hemodynamics during general anesthesia in patients receiving propranolol. *Anesthesiology* 48: 28, 1978.
298. Kotter, V., VonLeitner, E. R., Wunderlich, J., et al. Comparison of hemodynamic effects of phentolamine, sodium nitroprusside and glyceryl trinitrate in acute myocardial infarction. *Br. Heart J.* 39: 1196, 1977.
299. Kroenke, K., Omori, D. M., Simmons, J. O., et al. The safety of phenylpropanolamine in patients with stable hypertension. *Ann. Intern. Med.* 111: 1043, 1989.
300. Kumar, G. K., Dastoor, F. C., Rabayo, J. R., et al. Side effects of diazoxide. *J.A.M.A.* 235: 275, 1976.
301. Labeeuw, M., Zech, P., Pozet, N., et al. Renal failure in essential hypertension. *Contrib. Nephrol.* 71: 90, 1989.
302. Lake, C. R., Gallant, S., Masson, E., and Miller, P. Adverse drug effects attributed to phenylpropanolamine: A review of 142 case reports. *Am. J. Med.* 89: 195, 1990.
303. Lake, C. R., Zaloga, G., Bray, J., et al. Transient hypertension after two phenylpropanolamine diet aids and the effects of caffeine: A placebo-controlled follow-up study. *Am. J. Med.* 86: 427, 1989.
304. Langford, H. G., and Bonar, J. R. Treatment of the uremic hypertensive patient. *Modern Treat.* 3: 62, 1966.
305. Langley, M. S., and Sorkin, E. M. Nimodipine: A review of its pharmacodynamic and pharmacokinetic properties, and therapeutic potential in cerebrovascular disease. *Drugs* 37: 669, 1989.
306. Laragh, J. H., Sealy, J. E., and Sommers, S. C. Patterns of adrenal secretion and urinary excretion of aldosterone and plasma renin activity in normal and hypertensive subjects. *Circulation* 18(Suppl. I): I–158, 1966.
307. Laragh, J. H., Ulick, S., Januszewicz, V., et al. Aldosterone secretion and primary malignant hypertension. *J. Clin. Invest.* 39: 1091, 1960.
308. Lassen, N. A., and Angoli, A. The upper limit of autoregulation of cerebral blood flow on the pathogenesis of hypertensive encephalopathy. *Scand. J. Clin. Lab. Invest.* 30: 113, 1972.
309. Lavin, P. Management of hypertension in patients with acute stroke. *Arch. Intern. Med.* 146: 66, 1986.
310. Lawton, W. J. The short-term course of renal function in malignant hypertensives with renal insufficiency. *Clin. Nephrol.* 17: 277, 1982.
311. Lazarus, J. M., Hampers, C. L., and Bennett, A. H. Urgent bilateral nephrectomy for severe hypertension. *Ann. Intern. Med.* 76: 733, 1972.
312. Lebby, T., Paloucek, F., DeLa Cruz, F., and Leikin, J. B. Blood pressure decrease prior to initiating pharmacological therapy in nonemergent hypertension. *Am. J. Emerg. Med.* 8: 27, 1990.
313. Ledingham, J. G. G. Management of hypertensive crises. *Hypertension* 5(Suppl. III): III–114, 1983.
314. Ledingham, J. G. G., and Rajogoplan, B. Cerebral complications in the treatment of accelerated hypertension. *Q. J. Med.* 48: 25, 1979.
315. Lee, T. H., and Alderman, M. H. Malignant hypertension. Declining mortality rate in New York City, 1958 to 1974. *NY State J. Med.* 78: 1389, 1978.
316. Leiter, L., and Eichelberger, L. Pressor kidney extracts ("renin") and the production of cardiac and gastrointestinal hemorrhages and necroses in dogs with abnormal renal circulation. *J. Mount Sinai Hosp. (NY)* 8: 744, 1942.
317. Leslie, J. B., Kalayjian, R. W., McLoughlin, T. M., and Plachetka, J. R. Attenuation of the hemodynamic responses to endotracheal intubation with preinduction intravenous labetalol. *J. Clin. Anesth.* 1: 194, 1989.
318. Levy, S. B., Talner, L. B., Coel, M. N., et al. Renal vasculature in essential hypertension: Racial differences. *Ann. Intern. Med.* 88: 12, 1978.
319. Liebreich, R. Ophthalmoskopischer Befund bei morbus Brightii. *Albrecht. Graefes. Arch. Ophthalmol.* 5: 265, 1859.
320. Lim, K. G., Isles, C. G., Hodsman, G. P., et al. Malignant hypertension in women of childbearing age and its relation to the contraceptive pill. *Br. Med. J.* 294: 1057, 1987.
321. Limas, C. J., and Freis, E. D. Minoxidil in severe hypertension with renal failure. Effect of its addition to conventional antihypertensive drugs. *Am. J. Cardiol.* 31: 355, 1973.
322. Linas, S. L., and Nies, A. S. Minoxidil. *Ann. Intern. Med.* 94: 61, 1981.
323. Linton, A. L., Gavras, H., Gleadle, R. I., et al. Microangiopathic hemolytic anemia and the pathogenesis of malignant hypertension. *Lancet* 1: 1277, 1969.
324. Little, W. C., and Downes, T. R. Clinical evaluation of left ventricular diastolic performance. *Prog. Cardiovasc. Dis.* 32: 273, 1990.
325. Lohmeier, T. E., Tillman, L. J., Carroll, R. G., et al. Malignant hypertensive crisis induced by chronic intrarenal norepinephrine infusion. *Hypertension* 6(Suppl. I): I-177, 1984.
326. Loughran, R. P., Deeg, H. J., Jr., Dahlberg, S., et al. Incidence of hypertension after marrow transplantation among 112 patients randomized to either cyclosporine or

methotrexate as graft-versus-host disease prophylaxis. *Br. J. Haematol.* 59: 547, 1985.

327. Luft, F. C., Block, R., Szwed, J. J., et al. Minoxidil treatment of malignant hypertension. Recovery of renal function. *J.A.M.A.* 240: 1985, 1978.
328. Luria, M. H., Knoke, J. D., Margolis, R. M., et al. Acute myocardial infarction: Prognosis after recovery. *Ann. Intern. Med.* 85: 561, 1976.
329. Lüscher, T. F., Bock, H. A., Yang, Z., and Diederich, D. Endothelium-derived relaxing and contracting factors: Perspectives in nephrology. *Kidney Int.* 39: 575, 1991.
330. Luxton, R. W. Radiation nephritis. *Q. J. Med.* 22: 215, 1953.
331. MacCarthy, E. P., and Bloomfield, S. S. Labetalol: A review of its pharmacology, pharmacokinetics, clinical uses and adverse effects. *Pharmacotherapy* 3: 193, 1983.
332. Macho, P., and Vatner, S. F. Effects of nitroglycerin and nitroprusside on large and small coronary vessels in conscious dogs. *Circulation* 64: 1101, 1981.
333. MacKay, A., Isles, C., Henderson, I., et al. Minoxidil in the management of intractable hypertension. *Q. J. Med.* 50: 175, 1981.
334. MacKenzie, E. T., Strandgaard, S., Graham, D. I., et al. Effects of acutely induced hypertension in cats, on pial arteriolar caliber, local cerebral blood flow and the blood brain barrier. *Circ. Res.* 39: 33, 1976.
335. MacMahon, H. E., Close, G. H., and Hass, G. Cardiovascular renal changes with basophil adenoma of the anterior lobe of the pituitary (Cushing's syndrome). *Am. J. Pathol.* 10: 177, 1934.
336. MacMahon, H. E., and Pratt, J. H. Malignant nephrosclerosis (malignant hypertension). *Am. J. Med. Sci.* 189: 221, 1935.
337. Mahomed, F. A. Some of the clinical aspects of chronic Bright's disease. *Guy's Hosp. Rep.* 24:(series III): 363, 1879.
338. Mahony, J. F., Storey, B. G., and Gibson, G. R. Bilateral nephrectomy for malignant hypertension. *Lancet* 1: 1036, 1972.
339. Madani, B. H., Lim, V. S., Mahurkar, S. D., et al. Recovery from prolonged renal failure in patients with accelerated hypertension. *N. Engl. J. Med.* 291: 1343, 1974.
340. Mann, S. J., and Krakoff, L. R. Hypertensive crisis caused by hypoglycemia and propranolol. *Arch. Intern. Med.* 144: 2427, 1984.
341. Mann, T., Cohn, P. F., Holman, B. L., et al. Effects of nitroprusside on regional myocardial blood flow in coronary disease: Results in 25 patients and comparison with nitroglycerin. *Circulation* 57: 732, 1978.
342. Martin, D. E., and Kammerer, W. S. The hypertensive surgical patient: Controversies in management. *Surg. Clin. North Am.* 63(5): 1017, 1983.
343. Marx, P. G., and Reid, D. S. Labetalol infusion in acute myocardial infarction with systemic hypertension. *Br. J. Clin. Pharmacol.* 8: 233S, 1979.
344. Masson, G. M. C., McCormack, L. J., Dustan, H. P., et al. Hypertensive vascular disease as a consequence of increased arterial pressure. Quantitative study in rats with hydralazine treated renal hypertension. *Am. J. Pathol.* 34: 817, 1958.
345. Mattern, W. D., Sommers, H. C., and Kassirer, J. P. Oliguric renal failure in malignant hypertension. *Am. J. Med.* 52: 187, 1972.
346. McAllister, R. G. Kinetics and dynamics of nifedipine after oral and sublingual doses. *Am. J. Med.* 81(Suppl. 6A): 2, 1986.
347. McAllister, R. G., Van Way, C. W., Dayani, K., et al. Malignant hypertension: Effects of therapy on renin and aldosterone. *Circ. Res.* 28 and 29(Suppl. II): 160, 1971.
348. McCormack, L. J., Beland, J. E., Schneckloth, R. E., et al. Effect of antihypertensive treatment on the evolution of renal lesions in malignant nephrosclerosis. *Am. J. Pathol.* 34: 1011, 1958.
349. McGonigle, R. J. S., Trafford, J. A. P., Bewick, M., and Parsons, V. Hypertensive encephalopathy complicating transplant renal artery stenosis. *Postgrad. Med. J.* 60: 356, 1984.
350. McGregor, E., Isles, C. G., Jay, J. L., et al. Retinal changes in malignant hypertension. *Br. Med. J.* 292: 233, 1986.
351. McLaron, K. M., and MacDonald, M. K. Histologic and ultrastructural studies of the human juxtaglomerular apparatus in benign and malignant hypertension. *J. Pathol.* 139: 41, 1983.
352. McLeod, D., Marshall, J., and Kohner, E. M. Role of axoplasmic transport in the pathophysiology of ischaemic disc swelling. *Br. J. Ophthalmol.* 64: 247, 1980.
353. McLeod, D., Marshall, J., Kohner, E. M., et al. The role of axoplasmic transport in the pathogenesis of retinal cotton wool spots. *Br. J. Ophthal.* 61: 177, 1977.
354. Mehta, J., Feldman, R. L., Marx, J. D., et al. Systemic, pulmonary and coronary hemodynamic effects of labetalol in hypertensive subjects. *Am. J. Med.* 75(4A): 32, 1983.
355. Mehta, P., and Mehta, J. Effect of smoking on platelet and plasma thromboxane-protacyclin balance in man. *Prostaglandins Leukotrienes Med.* 9: 141, 1982.
356. Mehta, P. K., Mandani, B., Shansky, R., et al. Severe hypertension. Treatment with minoxidil. *J.A.M.A.* 233: 249, 1975.
357. Meissner, I., Whisnant, J. P., and Garraway, W. M. Hypertension management and stroke recurrence in a community (Rochester, Minnesota, 1950–1979). *Stroke* 19: 459, 1988.
358. Meretoja, O. A., Allonen, H., Arola, M., et al. Combined alpha and beta-blockade with labetatol in post open heart surgery hypertension. Reversal of hemodynamic deterioration with glucagon. *Chest* 78: 810, 1980.
359. Merril, J. P. Hypertensive Vascular Disease. In T. R. Harrison, R. D. Adams, and J. L. Bennett, Jr. *Principles of Internal Medicine*. New York: McGraw-Hill, 1962.
360. Messerli, F. H., Ventura, H. O., and Amodeo, C. Osler's maneuver and pseudohypertension. *N. Engl. J. Med.* 312: 1548, 1985.
361. Meyer, J. S., Shimazu, K., Fukuuchi, Y., et al. Impaired neurogenic cerebrovascular control and dysautoregulation after stroke. *Stroke* 4: 169, 1973.
362. Michael, C. A. The control of hypertension in labour. *Aust. N.Z. J. Obstet. Gynaecol.* 12: 48, 1972.
363. Michaeli, J., Ben-Ishay, D., Kidron, R., and Dasberg, H. Severe hypertension and lithium intoxication. *J.A.M.A.* 251: 1680, 1984.
364. Miller, A., and Rosman, M. A. Hypertensive encephalopathy as a complication of femoral lengthening. *Can. Med. Assoc. J.* 124: 296, 1980.
365. Miller, J. D., Becker, D. P., Ward, J. D., et al. Significance of intracranial hypertension in severe head injury. *J. Neurosurg.* 47: 503, 1977.
366. Milliez, P., Tcherdakoff, P., Samarq, P., et al. The Natural Course of Malignant Hypertension. In K. D. Boch (ed.), *Essential Hypertension: An International Symposium* Berlin: Springer, 1960. Pp. 214–239.
367. Milne, F. J., James, S. H., and Veriava, Y. Malignant hy-

pertension and its renal complications in black South Africans. *S. Afr. Med. J.* 76: 164, 1989.
368. Milsap, R. L., and Auld, P. A. M. Neonatal hyperglycemia following maternal diazoxide administration. *J.A.M.A.* 243: 144, 1980.
369. Mirenda, J. V., and Grissom, T. E. Anesthetic implications of the renin-angiotensin system and angiotensin-converting enzyme inhibitors. *Anesth. Analg.* 72: 667, 1991.
370. Mitchell, H. C., Graham, R. M., and Pettinger, W. A. Renal function during long-term treatment of hypertension with minoxidil. Comparison of benign and malignant hypertension. *Ann. Intern. Med.* 93: 676, 1980.
371. Mohler, E. R., and Freis, E. D. Five-year survival with malignant hypertension treated with antihypertensive agents. *Am. Heart J.* 60: 329, 1960.
372. Möhring, J., Möhring, B., Näumann, H., et al. Salt and water balance and renin activity in renal hypertension of rats. *Am. J. Physiol.* 228: 1847, 1975.
373. Möhring, J., Möhring, B., Petri, M., et al. Vasopressor role of ADH in the pathogenesis of malignant DOC hypertension. *Am. J. Physiol.* 232: F260, 1977.
374. Möhring, J., Möhring, B., Petri, M., et al. Plasma vasopressor concentrations and effects of vasopressin antiserum on blood pressure in rats with malignant two-kidney Goldblatt hypertension. *Circ. Res.* 42: 17, 1978.
375. Möhring, J., Möhring, B., Petri, M., et al. Studies on the pathogenesis of the malignant course of renal hypertension in rats. *Kidney Int.* 8(Suppl.): S-175, 1971.
376. Möhring, J., Petri, M., Szokol, M., et al. Effects of saline drinking on malignant course of renal hypertension in rats. *Am. J. Physiol.* 230: 849, 1976.
377. Moran, J. F., Derkac, W. M., and Conkle, D. M. Pharmacologic control of acute dissection in hypertensive dogs. *Surg. Forum* 29: 231, 1978.
378. Morduchowicz, G., Boner, G., Ben-Bassat, M., and Rosenfeld, J. B. Proteinuria in benign nephrosclerosis. *Arch. Intern. Med.* 146: 1513, 1986.
379. Morimoto, I., Maeda, R., Izumi, M., et al. An autopsy cause of 17-alpha hydroxylase deficiency with malignant hypertension. *J. Clin. Endocrinol. Metab.* 56: 915, 1983.
380. Morris, J. A., Arce, J. T., Hamilton, C. J., et al. The management of severe preeclampsia and eclampsia with intravenous diazoxide. *Obstet. Gynecol.* 49: 675, 1977.
381. Moser, M. Diazoxide—an effective vasodilator in accelerated hypertension. *Am. Heart J.* 87: 791, 1974.
382. Mroczek, W. J. Malignant hypertension: Kidneys too good to be extirpated. *Ann. Intern. Med.* 80: 754, 1974.
383. Mroczek, W. J. Malignant hypertension. *Angiology* 28: 444, 1977.
384. Mroczek, W. J., Davidov, M., Gavrilovich, L., et al. The value of aggressive therapy in the hypertensive patient with azotemia. *Circulation* 40: 893, 1969.
385. Muirhead, E. E., and Pitcock, J. A. Histopathology of severe renal vascular damage in blacks. *Clin. Cardiol.* 12: IV-58, 1989.
386. Muirhead, E. E., Vanatta, J., and Grollman, A. Hypertensive cardiovascular disease: An experimental study of tissue changes in bilaterally nephrectomized dogs. *Arch. Pathol.* 48: 234, 1949.
387. Mujais, S. K., Emmanouel, D. S., Kasinath, B. S., and Spargo, B. H. Marked proteinuria in hypertensive nephrosclerosis. *Am. J. Nephrol.* 5: 190, 1985.
388. Mukherjee, D., Feldman, M. S., and Helfant, R. H. Nitroprusside therapy: Treatment of hypertensive patients with recurrent chest pain: ST segment elevation and ventricular arrhythmias. *J.A.M.A.* 235: 2406, 1976.
389. Munro-Faure, A. D., Beilin, L. J., Bulpitt, C. J., et al. Comparison of black and white patients attending hypertension clinics in England. *Br. Med. J.* 1: 1044, 1979.
390. Murphy, F. D., and Grill, J. So-called malignant hypertension: A clinical and morphologic study. *Arch. Intern. Med.* 46: 75, 1930.
391. Naeim, F., de la Maza, L. M., and Robbins, S. L. Cardiac rupture during myocardial infarction. *Circulation* 45: 1231, 1972.
392. Naftchi, N. E., Demeny, M., Lowman, E. W., and Tuckman, J. Hypertensive crises in quadriplegic patients. *Circulation* 57: 336, 1978.
393. Nag, S., Robertson, D. M., and Dinsdale, H. B. Cerebral-cortical changes in acute experimental hypertension. An ultrastructural study. *Lab. Invest.* 36: 150, 1977.
394. Naim, R. C., Masson, G. M. C., and Corcoran, A. C. The production of serous effusions in nephrectomized animals by the administration of renal extracts and renin. *J. Pathol. Bacteriol.* 71: 155, 1956.
395. Nanra, R. S., Stuart-Taylor, J., DeLeon, A. H., et al. Analgesic nephropathy: etiology, clinical syndrome and clinicopathologic correlations in Australia. *Kidney Int.* 13: 79, 1978.
396. Narvarte, J., Privé, M., Saba, S. R., and Ramirez, G. Proteinuria in hypertension. *Am. J. Kidney Dis.* 10: 408, 1987.
397. Naulty, J., Cefalo, R. R., and Lewis, P. E. Fetal toxicity of nitroprusside in the pregnant ewe. *Am. J. Obstet. Gynecol.* 139: 708, 1981.
398. Navaratnarajah, M., and White, D. C. Labetalol and pheochromocytoma. *Br. J. Anaesth.* 56: 1179, 1984.
399. Neuman, J., Weiss, B., Rabello, Y., et al. Diazoxide for the acute control of severe hypertension complicating pregnancy: A pilot study. *Obstet. Gynecol.* 53(Suppl.): 50S, 1979.
400. Neusy, A. J., and Lowenstein, J. Blood pressure and blood pressure variability following withdrawal of propranolol and clonidine. *J. Clin. Pharmacol.* 29: 18, 1989.
401. Newborg, J. C., and Kempner, W. Analysis of 177 cases of hypertensive vascular disease with papilledema. One hundred twenty-six patients treated with rice diet. *Am. J. Med.* 19: 33, 1955.
402. Nibbelink, D. W. Cooperative aneurysm study: Antihypertensive and Antifibrinolytic Therapy Following Subarachnoid Hemorrhage From Ruptured Intracranial Aneurysm. In J. P. Whisnant, and B. A. Sandok (eds.), *Cerebral Vascular Diseases (Ninth Conference).* New York: Grune & Stratton, 1975.
403. Nicholson, G. D. Long-term survival after recovery from malignant nephrosclerosis. *Am. J. Hypertens.* 1: 73, 1988.
404. O'Brien, K. P., Grigor, R. R., and Taylor, P. M. Intravenous diazoxide in the treatment of hypertension associated with recent myocardial infarction. *Br. Med. J.* 4: 74, 1975.
405. Ogata, J., Fujishima, M., Tamaki, K., et al. Stroke prone spontaneously hypertensive rats as an experimental model of malignant hypertension. A light and electron microscopic study of the brain. *Acta Neuropathologica* (Berlin). 51: 179, 1980.
406. Ogata, J., Fujishima, M., Tamaki, K., et al. Stroke prone spontaneously hypertensive rats as an experimental model of malignant hypertension. A pathologic study. *Virchows Arch. Pathol. Anat.* 394: 185, 1982.
407. Öhman, J., Servo, A., and Heiskanen, O. Long-term effects of nimodipine on cerebral infarcts and outcome after aneurysmal subarachnoid hemorrhage and surgery. *J. Neurosurg.* 74: 8, 1991.
408. O'Mailia, J. J., Sander, G. E., and Giles, T. D. Nifedi-

pine-associated myocardial ischemia or infarction in the treatment of hypertensive urgencies. *Ann. Intern. Med.* 107: 185, 1987.

409. O'Malley, K., and McNay, J. L. A method for achieving blood pressure control expeditiously with oral minoxidil. *Clin. Pharmacol. Ther.* 18: 39, 1975.
410. O'Malley, K., Velasco, M., Prutt, A., et al. Decreased plasma protein binding of diazoxide in uremia. *Clin. Pharmacol. Ther.* 18: 53, 1975.
411. Oppenheimer, B. S., and Fishberg, A. M. Hypertensive encephalopathy. *Arch. Intern. Med.* 41: 264, 1928.
412. Orlowski, J. P., Vidt, D. G., Walker, S., and Haluska, J. F. The hemodynamic effects of intravenous labetalol for postoperative hypertension. *Cleve. Clin. J. Med.* 56: 29, 1989.
413. Oster, J. R., and Materson, B. J. Pseudohypertension: A diagnostic dilemma. *J. Clin. Hypertens.* 4: 307, 1986.
414. Padfield, P. L. Malignant hypertension presenting with acute abdomen. *Br. Med. J.* 3: 353, 1975.
415. Padfield, P. L., Brown, J. J., Lever, A. F., et al. Blood pressure in acute and chronic vasopressin excess. Studies of malignant hypertension and the syndrome of inappropriate antidiuretic hormone secretion. *N. Engl. J. Med.* 304: 1067, 1981.
416. Page, I. H. A clinical study of malignant hypertension. *Ann. Intern. Med.* 12: 978, 1939.
417. Page, I. H., Corcoran, A. C., Dustan, H. P., et al. Cardiovascular actions of nitroprusside in animals and hypertensive patients. *Circulation* 11: 188, 1955.
418. Page, I. H., and Taylor, R. D. Pyrogens in the treatment of malignant hypertension. *Mod. Concepts Cardiovasc. Dis.* 18: 51, 1949.
419. Palmer, R. F., and Lasseter, K. C. Sodium nitroprusside. *N. Engl. J. Med.* 292: 294, 1975.
420. Palmer, R. F., and Lasseter, K. C. Nitroprusside and aortic dissection. *N. Engl. J. Med.* 294: 1403, 1976.
421. Paronetto, F. Immunocytochemical observations on the vascular necrosis and renal glomerular lesions of malignant nephrosclerosis. *Am. J. Pathol.* 46: 901, 1965.
422. Pearson, R. M., and Breckenridge, A. M. Renal function, protein binding and pharmacological response to diazoxide. *Br. J. Clin. Pharmacol.* 3: 169, 1976.
423. Peart, W. S., and Brown, J. J. Effect of angiotensin (hypertensin or angiotensin) on urine flow and electrolyte excretion in hypertensive patients. *Lancet* 1: 28, 1961.
424. Pennington, J. C., and Picker, R. H. Diazoxide in the treatment of the acute hypertensive emergency in obstetrics. *Med. J. Aust.* 2: 1051, 1972.
425. Pentel, P. Toxicity of over-the-counter stimulants. *J.A.M.A.* 252: 1898, 1984.
426. Perera, G. A. Hypertensive vascular disease: Description and natural history. *J. Chron. Dis.* 1: 33, 1955.
427. Perera, G. A. The accelerated form of hypertension—a unique entity. *Trans. Assoc. Am. Physicians* 71: 62, 1958.
428. Perez-Fontan, M., Miguel, J. L., Picazo, M. L., et al. Idiopathic IgA nephropathy presenting as malignant hypertension. *Am. J. Nephrol.* 6: 482, 1986.
429. Perry, H. M., Schroeder, H. A., Catanzaro, F. J., et al. Studies on the control of hypertension VIII. Mortality, morbidity, and remissions during twelve years of intensive therapy. *Circulation* 33: 958, 1966.
430. Petitti, D. B., and Klatsky, A. L. Malignant hypertension in women age 15–44 years and its relation to cigarette smoking and oral contraceptives. *Am. J. Cardiol.* 52: 297, 1983.
431. Pettinger, W. A., and Mitchell, H. C. Minoxidil–an alternative to nephrectomy for refractory hypertension. *N. Engl. J. Med.* 289: 167, 1973.
432. Phillips, S. J. Pathogenesis, diagnosis, and treatment of hypertension-associated stroke. *Am. J. Hypertens.* 2: 493, 1989.
433. Pickard, J. D., Murray, G. D., Illingworth, R., et al. Effect of oral nimodipine on cerebral infarction and outcome after subarachnoid haemorrhage: British aneurysm nimodipine trial. *Br. Med. J.* 298: 636, 1989.
434. Pickering, G. W. The cerebrospinal fluid pressure in arterial hypertension. *Clin. Sci.* 1: 397, 1934.
435. Pickering, G. W. *High Blood Pressure* (2nd Ed.). New York: Grune & Stratton, 1968.
436. Pickering, G. W. Reversibility of malignant hypertension. Follow-up of three cases. *Lancet* 1: 413, 1971.
437. Pillay, V. K. G., Schwartz, F. D., and Kark, R. M. Proteinuria in malignant hypertension. *Lancet* 2: 1263, 1968.
438. Pinaud, M., Desjars, P., Tasseau, F., and Cozian, A. Preoperative acute volume loading in patients with pheochromocytoma. *Crit. Care Med.* 13: 460, 1985.
439. Pitcock, J. A., Johnson, J. G., Hatch, F. E., et al. Malignant hypertension in blacks. Malignant intrarenal arterial disease as observed by light and electron microscopy. *Human Pathol.* 7: 333, 1976.
440. Plets, C. Arterial hypertension in neurosurgical emergencies. *Am. J. Cardiol.* 63: 41C, 1989.
441. Poutasse, E. F., Stecker, J. F., Ladaga, L. E., et al. Malignant hypertension in children secondary to chronic pyelonephritis: Laboratory and radiologic indications for partial or total nephrectomy. *J. Urol.* 119: 264, 1978.
442. Prokop, E. K., Wheat, M. W., Jr., and Palmer, R. F. Hydrodynamic focus in dissecting aneurysm: In vitro studies in a tygon model and in dog aortas. *Circ. Res.* 27: 121, 1970.
443. Pryor, J. S., Davies, P. D., and Hamilton, D. Blindness and malignant hypertension. *Lancet* 2: 803, 1979.
444. Prys-Roberts, C. Hypertension and anesthesia—fifty years on. *Anesthesiology* 50: 281, 1979.
445. Prys-Roberts, C., Foëx, P., Biro, G. P., and Roberts, J. G. Studies on anaesthesia in relation to hypertension: V. Adrenergic beta-receptor blockade. *Br. J. Anaesth.* 45: 671, 1973.
446. Prys-Roberts, C., and Meloche, R. Management of anesthesia in patients with hypertension or ischemic heart disease. *Int. Anesthesiol. Clin.* 18(4): 181, 1980.
447. Prys-Roberts, C., Meloche, R., and Foëx, P. Studies on anaesthesia in relation to hypertension: I. Cardiovascular responses of treated and untreated patients. *Br. J. Anaesth.* 43: 122, 1971.
448. Puder, K. S., and Morgan, J. P. Persuading by citation: An analysis of the references of fifty-three published reports of phenylpropanolamine's clinical toxicity. *Clin. Pharmacol. Ther.* 42: 1, 1987.
449. Rabito, S. F., Carretero, O. A., and Scicli, A. G. Evidence against a role of vasopressin in the maintenance of high blood pressure in mineralocorticoid and renovascular hypertension. *Hypertension* 3: 34, 1981.
450. Ram, C. V. Pheochromocytoma. *Cardiol. Clin.* 6(4): 517, 1988.
451. Ram, C. V. S., Holland, O. B., Fairchild, C., et al. Withdrawal syndrome following cessation of guanabenz therapy. *J. Clin. Pharmacol.* 19: 148, 1979.
452. Ram, C. V. S., and Kaplan, N. M. Individual titration of diazoxide dosage in the treatment of severe hypertension. *Am. J. Cardiol.* 43: 627, 1979.

453. Ramos, O. Malignant hypertension: The Brazilian experience. *Kidney Int.* 25: 209, 1984.
454. Ramoska, E., and Sacchetti, A. D. Propranolol-induced hypertension in treatment of cocaine intoxication. *Ann. Emerg. Med.* 14: 1112, 1985.
455. Reach, G., Thibonnier, M., Chevillard, C., et al. Effect of labetalol on blood pressure and plasma catecholamine concentrations in patients with pheochromocytoma. *Br. Med. J.* 280: 1300, 1980.
456. Reichgott, M. J. Hypertension in the Perioperative Patient. In D. R. Goldmann, F. N. Brown, W. K. Levy, et al. (eds.), *Medical Care of the Surgical Patient: A Problem-Oriented Approach to Management.* Philadelphia: J. B. Lippincott, 1982. Pp. 78–86.
457. Reid, J. L., Wing, L. M. H., Dargie, H. L., et al. Clonidine withdrawal hypertension. *Lancet* 1: 1171, 1977.
458. Reid, J. L., Zivin, J. A., and Kopin, I. J. Central and peripheral adrenergic mechanism in the development of deoxycorticosterone-saline hypertension in the rat. *Circ. Res.* 37: 569, 1975.
459. Relman, A. S. Race and end-stage renal disease. *N. Engl. J. Med.* 306: 1290, 1982.
460. Renard, M., Riviere, A., Jacobs, P., et al. Treatment of hypertension in acute stage of myocardial infarction. Hemodynamic effects of labetalol. *Br. Heart J.* 49: 522, 1983.
461. Reubi, F. C. The Late Effects of Hypotensive Drug Therapy on Renal Functions of Patients with Essential Hypertension. In K. D. Bock and P. Cottier (eds.), *Essential Hypertension: An International Symposium.* Berlin: Springer-Verlag, 1960. Pp. 317–331.
462. Ribeiro, A. B., Schwarzwalder, S. R., Saragoca, M. A. S., et al. Malignant hypertension: A syndrome accompanied by plasmatic diminution of low and high molecular weight kininogens. *Hypertension* 5(Suppl. V): V158, 1983.
463. Rigg, D., and McDonogh, A. Use of sodium nitroprusside for deliberate hypotension during pregnancy. *Br. J. Anesthesiol.* 53: 985, 1981.
464. Ritz, E., Bommer, J., Andrassy, K., and Waldherr, R. Acute renal failure, hypertension and skin necrosis in a patient with streptokinase therapy. *Am. J. Nephrol.* 4: 193, 1984.
465. Robertson, A. L., and Khairallah, P. A. Effects of angiotensin II and some analogues on vascular permeability in the rabbit. *Circ. Res.* 31: 923, 1971.
466. Rodman, M. D., and White, W. B. Accelerated hypertension associated with the central nervous system toxicity of metrizamide. *Drug Intell. Clin. Pharmacol.* 20: 62, 1986.
467. Rodriguera, E., Guiha, N., and Cohn, J. N. Left ventricular function in hypertensive heart failure. *Circulation* 44(Suppl. II): II–129 (Abstr. 476), 1971.
468. Rosansky, S. J. Multiple cholesterol emboli syndrome. *South. Med. J.* 75: 677, 1982.
469. Rosei, E. A., Brown, J. J., et al. Treatment of pheochromocytoma and of clonidine withdrawal hypertension with labetalol. *Br. J. Clin. Pharmacol.* 3(Suppl.): 809, 1976.
470. Rosenberg, E. F. The brain in malignant hypertension: A clinicopathological study. *Arch. Intern. Med.* 65: 545, 1940.
471. Rosenfeld, J. B., Cohen, L., Garty, I., et al. Unilateral renal hypoplasia with hypertension (Ask-Upmark kidney). *Br. Med. J.* 2: 217, 1973.
472. Rostand, S. G., Brown, G., Kirk, K. A., et al. Renal insufficiency in treated essential hypertension. *N. Engl. J. Med.* 320: 684, 1989.
473. Rostand, S. G., Kirk, K. A., Rutsky, E. A., et al. Racial differences in the incidence of treatment for end-stage renal disease. *N. Engl. J. Med.* 306: 1276, 1982.
474. Roudant, R. P., Billes, M. A., Gosse, P., et al. Accuracy of m-mode and two-dimensional echocardiography in the diagnosis of aortic dissection: An experience with 128 cases. *Clin. Cardiol.* 11: 553, 1988.
475. Roy, L., Mehta, J., and Mehta, P. Increased plasma concentration of prostacyclin metabolite 6-keto PGF_1-alpha in essential hypertension. *Am. J. Cardiol.* 51: 464, 1983.
476. Rubio-Garcia, R., Garcia-Diaz, J., Ortiz, M. C., and Praga, M. IgG myeloma with hyperviscosity presenting as malignant hypertension. *Am. J. Med.* 87: 119, 1989.
477. Rude, R. E., Muller, J. E., and Braunwald, E. Efforts to limit the size of myocardial infarcts. *Ann. Intern. Med.* 95: 736, 1981.
478. Sankar, D., and Moodley, J. Low-dose diazoxide in the emergency management of severe hypertension in pregnancy. *S. Afr. Med. J.* 65: 279, 1984.
479. Saphir, O., and Ballinger, J. Hypertension (Goldblatt) and unilateral malignant nephrosclerosis. *Arch. Intern. Med.* 66: 541, 1940.
480. Saragoca, M. A., Homsi, E., Ribeiro, A. B., et al. Hemodynamic mechanism of blood pressure response to captopril in human malignant hypertension. *Hypertension* 5(Suppl. I): I–53, 1983.
481. Scheie, H. G. Evaluation of ophthalmoscopic changes of hypertension and arteriolar sclerosis. *Arch. Ophthalmol.* 49: 117, 1953.
482. Schottstaedt, M. F., and Sokolow, M. The natural history and course of hypertension with papilledema (malignant hypertension). *Am. Heart J.* 45: 331, 1953.
483. Schramek, A., Better, O. S., Adler, O., et al. Hypertensive crisis, erythrocytosis, and uraemia due to renal-artery stenosis of kidney transplants. *Lancet* 1: 70, 1975.
484. Schubiger, G., Flury, G., and Nussberger, J. Enalapril for pregnancy-induced hypertension: Acute renal failure in a neonate. *Ann. Intern. Med.* 108: 215, 1988.
485. Schwartz, S. M., Campbell, G. R., and Campbell, J. H. Replication of smooth muscle cells in vascular disease. *Circ. Res.* 58: 427, 1986.
486. Scully, R. E., Mark, E. F., McNeely, W. F., and McNeely, B. U. Case records of the Massachusetts General Hospital: Case 15-1988. *N. Engl. J. Med.* 318: 970, 1988.
487. Sealy, W. C. Coarctation of the aorta and hypertension. *Ann. Thorac. Surg.* 3: 15, 1967.
488. Segal, J. L. Hypertensive emergencies: Practical approach to treatment. *Postgrad. Med. J.* 68(2): 107, 1980.
489. Selby, D. G., Richards, J. D., and Marshman, J. M. Ace inhibitors (letter). *Anaesth. Int. Care* 17: 110, 1989.
490. Selkurt, E. E. Effect of pulse pressure and mean arterial pressure modification on renal hemodynamics and electrolyte and water excretion. *Circulation* 4: 541, 1951.
491. Sellers, E. M., and Koch-Weser, J. Protein binding and vascular activity of diazoxide. *N. Engl. J. Med.* 281: 1141, 1969.
492. Sevitt, L. H., Evans, D. J., and Wrong, O. M. Acute oliguric renal failure due to accelerated (malignant) hypertension. *Q. J. Med.* 40: 127, 1971.
493. Shakig, M., and Ashton, N. Ultrastructural changes in focal retinal ischaemia. *Br. J. Ophthal.* 50: 325, 1966.
494. Shapiro, B., and Fig, L. M. Management of pheochromocytoma. *Endocrinol. Metab. Clin. North Am.* 18(2): 443, 1989.
495. Shell, W. E., and Sobel, B. E. Protection of jeopardized ischemic myocardium by reduction of ventricular afterload. *N. Engl. J. Med.* 291: 481, 1974.

496. Shichiri, M., Hirata, Y., Ando, K., et al. Plasma endothelin levels in hypertension and chronic renal failure. *Hypertension* 15: 493, 1990.
497. Shin, M. S., and Ho, K. J. Malignant hypertension as a cause of massive intestinal bleeding. *Am. J. Surg.* 133: 742, 1977.
498. Shulman, N. B., Ford, C. E., Hall, W. D., et al. Prognostic value of serum creatinine and effect of treatment of hypertension on renal function: Results from the Hypertension Detection and Follow-up Program. *Hypertension* 13(Suppl. I): I-80, 1989.
499. Siggers, D. C., Slater, C., and Fluck, D. C. Serial plasma adrenalin and nonadrenalin levels in myocardial infarction using a new double isotope technique. *Br. Heart J.* 33: 878, 1971.
500. Simon, N. M., Graham, M. B., Kyser, F. A., et al. Resolution of renal failure with malignant hypertension in scleroderma. Case report and a review of the literature. *Am. J. Med.* 67: 533, 1979.
501. Sinclair, R. A., Antonovych, T. T., and Mostofi, F. K. Renal proliferative arteriopathies and associated glomerular changes. A light and electron microscopic study. *Human Pathol.* 7: 565, 1976.
502. Skydell, J. L., Machleder, H. I., Baker, J. D., et al. Incidence and mechanism of post-carotid endarterectomy hypertension. *Arch. Surg.* 122: 1153, 1987.
503. Slater, E. E., and DeSanctis, R. W. The clinical recognition of dissecting aortic aneurysm. *Am. J. Med.* 60: 625, 1976.
504. Slater, E. E., and DeSanctis, R. W. Dissection of the aorta. *Med. Clin. North Am.* 63(1): 141, 1979.
505. Smirk, F. H., and Alstad, K. S. Treatment of arterial hypertension by penta and hexamethonium salts. *Br. Med. J.* 1: 1217, 1951.
506. Smith, H. W. Unilateral nephrectomy in hypertensive disease. *J. Urol.* 76: 685, 1956.
507. Sorkin, E. M., Clissold, S. P., and Brogden, R. N. Nifedipine: A review of its pharmacodynamic and pharmacokinetic properties, and therapeutic efficacy, in ischaemic heart disease, hypertension and related cardiovascular disorders. *Drugs* 30: 182, 1985.
508. Soufer, R., Wohlgelernter, D., Vita, N. A., et al. Intact systolic left ventricular function in clinical congestive heart failure. *Am. J. Cardiol.* 55: 1032, 1985.
509. Spence, J. D., and Del Maestro, R. F. Hypertension in acute ischemic strokes—treat. *Arch. Neurol.* 42: 1000, 1985.
510. Spitalewitz, S., Parush, J. G., and Oguagha, C. Use of oral clonidine for rapid titration of blood pressure in severe hypertension. *Chest* 83: 404, 1983.
511. Standen, N. B., Qualye, J. M., Davies, N. W., et al. Hyperpolarizing vasodilators activate ATP-sensitive K^+ channels in arterial smooth muscle. *Science* 245: 177, 1989.
512. Stauffer, J. C., and Gaasch, W. H. Recognition and treatment of left ventricular diastolic dysfunction. *Prog. Cardiovasc. Dis.* 32: 319, 1990.
513. Steen, V. D., Costantino, J. P., Shapiro, A. P., and Medsger, T. A. Outcome of renal crisis in systemic sclerosis: Relation to availability of angiotensin converting enzyme (ACE) inhibitors. *Ann. Intern. Med.* 113: 352, 1990.
514. Steinmann, W. C., Millstein, M. E., and Sinclair, S. H. Pupillary dilation with tropicamide 1% for funduscopic screening. *Ann. Intern. Med.* 107: 181, 1987.
515. Stempel, J. E., O'Grady, J. P., Morton, M. J., and Johnson, K. A. Use of sodium nitroprusside in complications of gestational hypertension. *Obstet. Gynecol.* 60: 533, 1982.
516. Still, J. L., and Cottom, D. Severe hypertension in childhood. *Arch. Dis. Child.* 42: 34, 1967.
517. Strangaard, S. Autoregulation of cerebral blood flow in hypertensive patients. The modifying influence of prolonged antihypertensive treatment on the tolerance to acute, drug induced hypotension. *Circulation* 53: 720, 1976.
518. Strandgaard, S. Cerebral blood flow in hypertension. *Acta Med. Scand.* (Suppl.) 678: 11, 1983.
519. Strandgaard, S., Andersen, G. S., Ahlgreen, P., and Nielsen, P. E. Visual disturbances and occipital brain infarct following acute, transient hypotension in hypertensive patients. *Acta Med. Scand.* 216: 417, 1984.
520. Strandgaard, S., MacKenzie, E. T., Jones, J. V., et al. Studies on the cerebral circulation of the baboon in acutely induced hypertension. *Stroke* 7: 287, 1976.
521. Strandgaard, S., MacKenzie, E. T., Sengupta, D., et al. Upper limit of autoregulation of cerebral blood flow in the baboon. *Circ. Res.* 34: 435, 1974.
522. Strandgaard, S., Olesen, J., Skinhoj, E., and Lassen, N. A. Autoregulation of brain circulation in severe arterial hypertension. *Br. Med. J.* 1: 507, 1973.
523. Strandgaard, S., and Paulson, O. B. Cerebral autoregulation. *Stroke* 15: 413, 1984.
524. Strandgaard, S., and Paulson, O. B. Cerebral blood flow and its pathophysiology in hypertension. *Am. J. Hypertens.* 2: 486, 1989.
525. Strauss, T. G., Franklin, S. S., Lewin, A. J., et al. Withdrawal of antihypertensive therapy. Hypertensive crises in renovascular hypertension. *J.A.M.A.* 238: 16: 1737, 1977.
526. Subias, R., Botey, A., Darnell, A., et al. Malignant or accelerated hypertension in IgA nephropathy. *Clin. Nephrol.* 27: 1, 1987.
527. Sum, C. Y., Yacobi, A., Kartzinel, R., et al. Kinetics of esmolol, an ultra-short-acting beta blocker, and of its major metabolite. *Clin. Pharmacol. Ther.* 34: 427, 1983.
528. Taams, M. A., Gussenhoven, W. J., Schippers, L. A., et al. The value of transoesophageal echocardiography for diagnosis of thoracic aorta pathology. *Eur. Heart J.* 9: 1308, 1988.
529. Tamaki, K., Sadoshima, S., Baumbach, G. L., et al. Evidence that disruption of the blood brain barrier precedes reduction in cerebral blood flow in hypertensive encephalopathy. *Hypertension* 6(Suppl. I): I–75, 1984.
530. Tarazi, R. C., Dustan, H. P., Bravo, E. L., et al. Vasodilating drugs: Contrasting hemodynamic effects. *Clin. Sci. Molec. Med.* 51: 575S, 1976.
531. Tejani, A. Post-transplant hypertension and hypertensive encephalopathy in renal allograft recipients. *Nephron* 34: 73, 1983.
532. Tewfik, G. I. Trimethaphan: Its effect on the pseudocholinesterase level of man. *Anaesthesia* 12: 326, 1957.
533. Texter, J. H., Reece, R. W., and Hranowsky, N. Pentolinium in the management of autonomic hyperreflexia. *J. Urol.* 116: 350, 1976.
534. Thorsen, M. K., San Dretto, M. A., Lawson, T. L., et al. Dissecting aortic aneurysms: Accuracy of computer tomographic diagnosis. *Radiology* 148: 773, 1983.
535. Tobian, L. Hypothesis: Low dietary k may lead to renal failure in blacks with hypertension and severe intimal thickening. *Am. J. Med. Sci.* 295: 384, 1988.
536. Tobian, L., Lange, J., Ulm, K., et al. Potassium reduces cerebral hemorrhage and death rate in hypertensive rats, even when blood pressure is not lowered. *Hypertension* 7(Suppl. I): I-110, 1985.
537. Tobian, L., MacNeill, D., Johnson, M. A., et al. Potas-

sium protection against lesions of the renal tubules, arteries, and glomeruli and nephron loss in salt-loaded hypertensive Dahl S rats. *Hypertension* 6(Suppl. I): I-170, 1984.

538. Topol, E. J., Traill, T. A., and Fortuin, N. J. Hypertensive hypertrophic cardiomyopathy of the elderly. *N. Engl. J. Med.* 312: 277, 1985.
539. Towne, J. B., and Bernhard, V. M. The relationship of postoperative hypertension to complications following carotid endarterectomy. *Surgery* 88: 575, 1980.
540. Traub, Y. M., Shapiro, A. P., Rodnan, G. P., et al. Hypertension and renal failure (scleroderma renal crisis) in progressive systemic sclerosis. *Medicine* 62: 335, 1983.
541. Travis, R. H., Garst, J. B., and Jelliffe, R. Urinary aldosterone and hypertension. *Circulation* 24: 592, 1961.
542. Tschollar, W., and Belz, G. G. Sublingual captopril in hypertensive crisis. *Lancet* 2: 34, 1985.
543. Updike, S. J., and Harrington, A. R. Acute diabetic ketoacidosis—a complication of intravenous diazoxide for refractory hypertension. *N. Engl. J. Med.* 280: 768, 1969.
544. Van Aken, H., Cottrell, J. E., Anger, C., and Puchstein, C. Treatment of intraoperative hypertensive emergencies in patients with intracranial disease. *Am. J. Cardiol.* 63: 43C, 1989.
545. VanBuchem, F. S. P., Heuvel-Aghira, J. W. M., and Heuvel, J. E. A. Hypertension and changes of the fundus oculi. *Acta Med. Scand.* 176: 539, 1964.
546. Vanhoutte, P. M. Endothelium and control of vascular function. *Hypertension* 13: 658, 1989.
547. Velasco, M., Gallardo, E., Plaja, J., et al. A new technique for safe and effective control of hypertension with intravenous diazoxide. *Curr. Therapeutic Res.* 19: 185, 1976.
548. Venkatachalam, M. A., Jones, D. B., and Nelson, D. A. Microangiopathic hemolytic anemia in rats with malignant hypertension. *Blood* 32: 278, 1968.
549. Verska, J. J., DeQuattro, V., and Wooley, M. M. Coarctation of the aorta: The abdominal pain syndrome and paradoxical hypertension. *J. Thorac. Cardiovasc. Surgery* 58: 746, 1969.
550. Veterans Administration Cooperative Study Group on Antihypertensive Agents. Effects of treatment on morbidity in hypertension. I. Results in patients with diastolic blood pressure averaging 115–129 mm Hg. *J.A.M.A.* 202: 1028, 1967.
551. Volhard, F. Der arterielle Hochdruck. *Verh. Dt. Ges. Inn. Med.* 35: 134, 1923.
552. Volhard, F., and Farh, T. *Die Brightische Neirenkrankheit, Klinik Pathologie und Atlas.* Berlin: Julius Springer, 1914.
553. Wachter, R. M. Symptomatic hypotension induced by nifedipine in the acute treatment of severe hypertension. *Arch. Intern. Med.* 147: 556, 1987.
554. Wagener, H. P., and Keith, N. M. Diffuse arteriolar disease with hypertension and the associated retinal lesions. *Medicine* (Baltimore) 18: 317, 1939.
555. Waldman, S. A., and Murad, F. Cyclic GMP synthesis and function. *Pharmacol. Rev.* 39: 163, 1987.
556. Wallace, J. D., and Levy, L. L. Blood pressure after stroke. *J.A.M.A.* 246: 2177, 1981.
557. Washington, E. L., Callahan, W. P., and Edwards, E. W. Pheochromocytoma of the adrenal medulla. Its role in the pathogenesis of malignant hypertension. *J. Clin. Endocrinol.* 6: 688, 1946.
558. Wauters, J. P., and Brunner, H. R. Discontinuation of chronic hemodialysis after control of arterial hypertension, long term follow-up. *Proc. Eur. Dial. Transplant. Assoc.* 19: 182, 1982.
559. Weber, J. R. Left ventricular hypertrophy: Its prime importance as a controllable risk factor. *Am. Heart J.* 116: 272, 1988.
560. Weiss, S., and Parker, F. Pyelonephritis: Its relation to vascular lesions and to arterial hypertension. *Medicine* (Baltimore) 18: 221, 1939.
561. Wheat, M. W., Jr. Acute dissecting aneurysms of the aorta: Diagnosis and treatment, 1980. *Am. Heart J.* 99: 373, 1980.
562. Whelton, P. K., and Klag, M. J. Hypertension as risk factor for renal disease: Review of clinical and epidemiological evidence. *Hypertension* 13(Suppl. I): I-19, 1989.
563. Will, R. J., Walker, O. M., Traugott, R. C., et al. Nitroprusside and propranolol therapy for management of post-coarctectomy hypertension. *J. Thorac. Cardiovasc. Surg.* 75: 722, 1978.
564. Wilson, C., and Byrom, F. B. The vicious circle in chronic Bright's disease. Experimental evidence from the hypertensive rat. *Q. J. Med.* 10: 65, 1941.
565. Wilson, D. J., Wallin, J. D., Vlachakis, N. D., et al. Intravenous labetalol in the treatment of severe hypertension and hypertensive emergencies. *Am. J. Med.* 75 (Suppl. 4A): 95, 1983.
566. Wilson, J. Leber's hereditary optic atrophy: A possible defect of cyanide metabolism. *Clin. Sci.* 29: 505, 1965.
567. Wilson, L., Dustan, H. P., Page, I. H., et al. Diagnosis of renal artery lesions. *Arch. Intern. Med.* 112: 168, 1963.
568. Winternitz, M. C., Mylar, E., Waters, L. L., et al. Studies on the relation of the kidney to cardiovascular disease. *Yale J. Biol. Med.* 12: 623, 1939.
569. Wolff, F. W., and Lindeman, R. D. Effects of treatment in hypertension: Results of a controlled study. *J. Chronic Dis.* 19: 227, 1966.
570. Woods, J. W., and Blythe, W. B. Management of malignant hypertension complicated by renal insufficiency. *N. Engl. J. Med.* 277: 57, 1967.
571. Woods, J. W., Blythe, W. B., and Huffines, W. D. Management of malignant hypertension complicated by renal insufficiency. A follow-up study. *N. Engl. J. Med.* 291: 10, 1974.
572. Woods, R. L., Abrahams, J. M., Kincaid-Smith, P., et al. Vascular lesions and angiotensin in malignant hypertension in the absence of vasopressin. *Clin. Exp. Pharmacol. Physiol.* 9: 297, 1982.
573. Woods, W. W., and Peet, M. M. The surgical treatment of hypertension. II. Comparison of mortality following operation with that of Wagener-Keith medically treated control series. *J.A.M.A.* 117: 1508, 1941.
574. Working Group on Renovascular Hypertension. Detection, evaluation, and treatment of renovascular hypertension. *Arch. Intern. Med.* 147: 820, 1987.
575. World Health Organization. Arterial hypertension—report of the WHO expert committee. *WHO Tech. Rep. Ser.* (Geneva) 628, 1978.
576. Yamashita, M., Oyama, T., and Kudo, T. Effect of the inhibitor of angiotensin I converting enzyme on endocrine function and renal perfusion in haemorrhagic shock. *Can. Anaesth. Soc. J.* 24: 695, 1977.
577. Yatsu, F. M., and Zivin, J. Hypertension in acute ischemic stroke: Not to treat. *Arch. Neurol.* 42: 999, 1985.
578. Ylikorkala, U., Puolakka, J., and Viinikka, L. Oestrogen-containing oral contraceptives decrease prostacyclin production (letter). *Lancet* 1: 42, 1981.
579. Yu, S. H., Whitworth, J. A., and Kincaid-Smith, P. S. Malignant hypertension: Aetiology and outcome in 83 patients. *Clin. Exp. Hypertens.* [A] 8: 1211, 1986.

580. Yusuf, S., Peto, R., Lewis, J., et al. Beta blockade during and after myocardial infarction: An overview of the randomized trials. *Prog. Cardiovasc. Dis.* 27: 335, 1985.
581. Zelis, R. Mechanism of vasodilatation. *Am. J. Med.* 74 (Suppl. 68): 3, 1983.
582. Zeller, K. R., Kuhnert, L. V., and Matthews, C. Rapid reduction of severe asymptomatic hypertension. *Arch. Intern. Med.* 149: 2186, 1989.
583. Zerbe, R. L., Feurestein, G., and Kopin, I. J. Effect of captopril on cardiovascular, sympathetic and vasopressin responses to hemorrhage. *Eur. J. Pharmacol.* 72: 391, 1981.
584. Zezulka, A. V., Arkell, D. G., and Beevers, D. G. The association of hypertension, the Ask-Upmark kidney and other congenital abnormalities. *J. Urol.* 135: 1000, 1986.
585. Ziegler, D. K., and Zilele, T. Hypertensive encephalopathy. *Arch. Neurol.* 12: 472, 1965.
586. Zile, M. R., and Gaasch, W. H. Mechanical loads and the isovolumic and filling indices of left ventricular relaxation. *Prog. Cardiovasc. Dis.* 32: 333, 1990.

X

Chronic Glomerulonephritis and Chronic Interstitial Nephritis

Immunopathology of Glomerular and Interstitial Disease

Charles D. Pusey
D. Keith Peters

Since the last edition of this book, there have been rapid advances in the understanding of immunologic processes, based on the development of cellular and molecular biology. The aim of this chapter is to review the mechanisms underlying the development of nephritis, in the context of current concepts in immunology. This approach cannot be comprehensive and is not intended to duplicate the contents of the previous edition [351], although much of relevance has been retained. Emphasis is given to what has been learned from experimental models of nephritis and how this relates to human disease.

There is increasing evidence for the role of autoimmunity in several forms of nephritis, including some in which the deposition of circulating immune complexes was believed to be important. For example, in Heymann nephritis, a model of membranous nephropathy in the rat, it has been shown that autoantibodies to glomerular epithelial cell antigens are responsible for the appearance of granular immune deposits—said to be characteristic of "immune complex" nephritis [55]. Similarly, exogenous antigens may be planted in glomerular capillaries and serve as the focus for local or "in-situ" immune complex formation.

There is considerable evidence that autoimmune responses generally depend on the interaction of peptides derived from self-antigens with class II major histocompatibility complex (MHC) gene products on antigen-presenting cells, followed by recognition of this complex by the T cell receptor on autoreactive Th lymphocytes (Fig. 60-1), and subsequent recruitment of effector T or B cells [454]. Proof that this mechanism operates in human renal disease, and understanding of the interactions involved, will depend on molecular characterization of the individual components. There are examples, such as antiglomerular basement membrane (anti-GBM) disease, where progress has been made in identifying the autoantigen and MHC genes concerned [467]. In many other forms of nephritis, an association with MHC genes or identification of autoantigens suggests a similar pathogenesis.

There have also been major advances in the understanding of immunologically mediated inflammation; this topic is considered in detail in Chap. 71. There is increasing evidence for the role of T lymphocytes and macrophages in glomerular injury and for the importance of the cytokines that they release. Glomerular mesangial and endothelial cells can respond to, and produce, various cytokines and are likely to be involved directly in modulation of renal inflammation, rather than being passive targets of injury [269].

Nephritis in Experimental Models

We shall consider three separate categories of experimental nephritis, with emphasis on recent findings: (1) disease resulting from administration of foreign antibody and/or antigen; (2) induction of autoimmunity by antigen administration or polyclonal activation; and (3) spontaneous nephritis occurring in certain species.

NEPHRITIS INDUCED BY EXOGENOUS ANTIBODY OR ANTIGEN

Much of our knowledge of the immunopathologic mechanisms in nephritis is based on the use of classic models such as nephrotoxic nephritis [469] and serum sickness [169]. These have led to the development of two broad categories of experimental nephritis: (1) those induced by passive administration of antibodies directed against various renal antigens and (2) those involving the planting of antigen or antibody in the glomerulus with subsequent local immune complex formation. These models do not directly contribute to understanding autoimmune processes in renal disease but are of value in confirming the role of certain antibody-antigen systems and in examining mechanisms of renal injury.

Nephrotoxic Nephritis. The administration to animals of heterologous antibody raised to GBM preparations results in a biphasic disease [469]. In the first or heterologous phase, there is binding of foreign antibody to the GBM followed within a few days by neutrophil accumulation and proteinuria. In the second or autologous phase, which follows within 2 weeks, there is production of host antibodies to the foreign immunoglobulin (Ig) on the GBM. This phase leads to mesangial and endothelial cell proliferation and macrophage infiltration. The speed and severity of the autologous stage of the disease can be increased by preimmunization with appropriate Ig, resulting in the accelerated or "telescoped" model of nephrotoxic nephritis.

This experimental system has been used to investigate mechanisms of antibody-mediated glomerular injury. It is clear from studies of the heterologous phase that the amount of antibody bound, the rate of deposition, and the characteristics of the antibody (e.g., avidity, complement-fixing ability) are determinants of tissue injury [469]. There is also considerable variation in species susceptibility. Under certain circumstances, antibody deposition alone may be sufficient to cause proteinuria [414]. However, a multiplicity of mediator systems have been identified using variations of the basic model (Fig. 60-2), and it seems likely that several of these will be simultaneously engaged in spontaneous disease. They include (1) neutrophil-dependent injury, which is usually mediated via C3, but which may occur independently of complement [83, 305, 342, 451]; (2) complement-dependent injury as a direct effect of the membrane attack complex [183, 452]; (3) macrophage-dependent injury, which generally requires deposition of fibrin in Bowman's space and which may result from signals generated by antibody deposition or by T cells [53, 203, 404, 450, 453].

The mechanisms of tissue injury are considered elsewhere in this book, but those found in nephrotoxic ne-

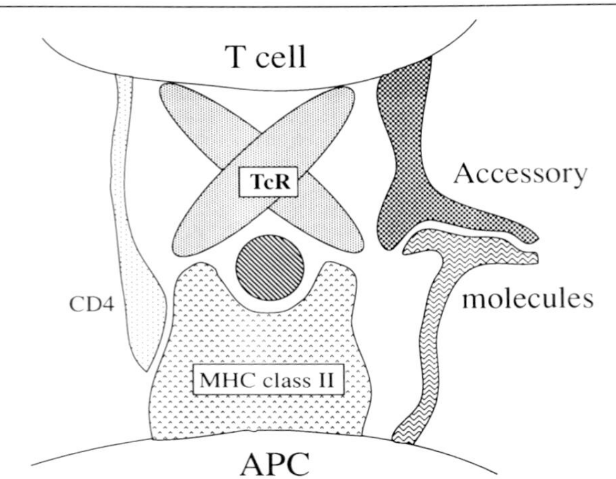

Fig. 60-1. Diagrammatic representation of antigen presentation by a major histocompatibility complex (MHC) class II bearing antigen-presenting cell (APC) to a T helper lymphocyte. (Drawn by Dr. R. I. Lechler.)

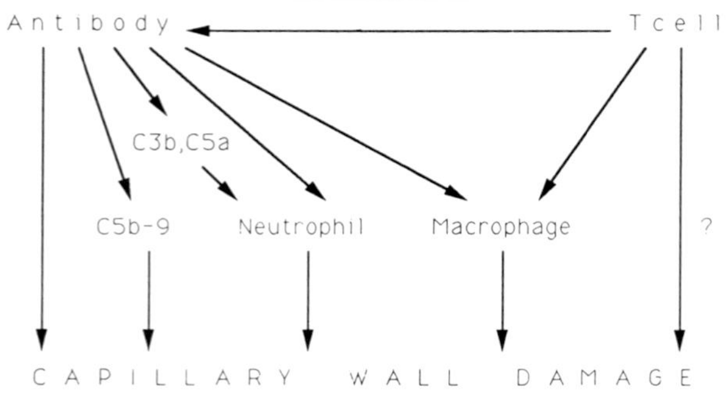

Fig. 60-2. Effector mechanisms recognized in experimental models of glomerulonephritis (see text for details).

phritis will be discussed briefly. There is increasing evidence that neutrophil-mediated injury depends, at least in part, on the production of reactive oxygen species [52]. In addition, both leukotrienes (LTB4) and hydroxyeicosatetraenoic acids (5-HETE) are produced by glomeruli from nephritic rats [263]. Their production is complement dependent and may represent an important proinflammatory stimulus [262]. Prostaglandin E_1 has been shown to protect rats with autologous phase nephrotoxic nephritis [73, 245]. The role of cytokines is not yet clear, although the severity of the heterologous phase can be increased by subnephrotoxic doses of lipopolysaccharide or by tumor necrosis factor (TNF) or interleukin-1 (IL-1) [460]. The effects of these cytokines are synergistic and can be prevented by appropriate anticytokine antibodies. These studies may well explain the nonspecific enhancement of glomerular injury provoked by intercurrent infection.

Immune Complex Nephritis. The notion that glomerulonephritis could result from the deposition of circulating immune complexes was based largely on experiments involving models of serum sickness. In acute serum sickness, the single intravenous injection of an antigen such as bovine serum albumin in rabbits is followed by the development of proliferative glomerulonephritis and extrarenal vasculitis at the time of immune elimination, when complexes are detectable in the circulation and in tissue deposits [169]. The strength of the immune response, which determines the characteristics of the immune complexes, is a major factor in severity of disease [499]. Localization to the kidney may depend on reactions between antigen or complexes and sites in the glomerulus. In chronic serum sickness, repeated injections of antigen result in a range of histologic changes, from membranous to diffuse proliferative nephritis [124, 171]. Variations in the strength of the immune response determine the development of disease. Animals failing to generate an immune response do not develop nephritis, those with a high response clear immune complexes sufficiently rapidly to avoid nephritis, and those with an intermediate response develop immune complexes accompanied by nephritis [170, 500]. The characteristics of these complexes depend on properties of the antigen (size, number of reactive sites) and antibody (avidity, concentration, Fc function) and on the ratio of antigen to antibody [7, 82, 123, 212]. In general, larger complexes containing high-affinity antibody were found to localize in the mesangium or subendothelium, whereas smaller complexes containing low-affinity antibody deposited on the subepithelial side of the basement membrane [260]. Immunologic mediator systems similar to those involved in nephrotoxic nephritis have been identified in models of serum sickness.

These observations on the nature of immune complex nephritis may need reinterpretation in light of the "planted antigen" mechanism, discussed below, and increasing knowledge of the factors that influence disposal of immune complexes (Fig. 60-3) (reviewed in [401]). These include: (1) inhibition of precipitation and solubilization of complexes, mediated respectively by the classic and alternative pathways of complement; (2) uptake of complement-reacted complexes by the complement receptor CR1 on erythrocytes (in primates), which also

Fig. 60-3. Mechanisms involved in the disposal of immune complexes in primates (see text for details). Ag = antigen; Ab = antibody; C = complement; CR1 = complement receptor 1; MPS = mononuclear phagocytic system; EV = extravascular compartment; IV = intravascular compartment.

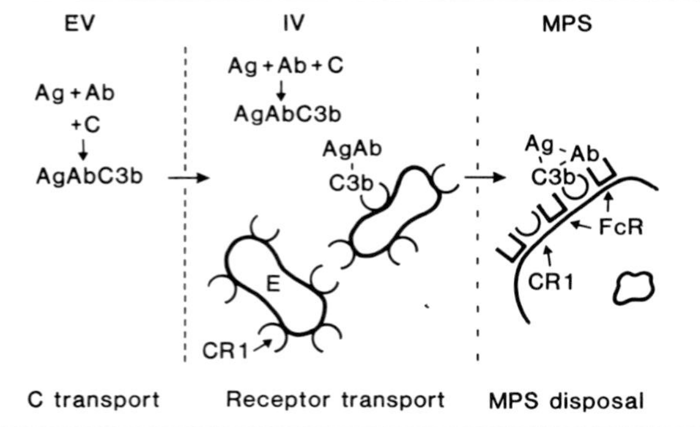

acts as a cofactor for cleavage of C3b by factor I; and (3) clearance of complexes from CR1 by mononuclear cells in the liver and spleen, which probably depends on their higher density of C3b and/or Fc receptors. It follows that abnormalities of the complement proteins, CR1 receptors or mononuclear phagocytic system, may lead to faulty clearance of immune complexes and thereby predispose to disease.

Planted Antigens. Localization of antigens, antibodies, or immune complexes to sites in the glomerulus can serve as the initial event in the development of immune deposits [101, 283]. Several experimental models have been described in which administration of an antigen, followed by antibody to it, leads to "immune complex" nephritis. Experiments using the isolated perfused rat kidney are of particular interest, since this approach excludes effects of the intact immune system; in one such study, accumulation of immune deposits was achieved by alternating perfusion with antigen and antibody [156]. Antigens such as lectins, DNA, and Ig may be "planted" in the glomerulus as a result of their physicochemical affinity for glomerular components [4, 176, 213]. The role of charge has received considerable attention since it was appreciated that many cationic molecules are localized to the glomerular capillary wall and mesangium by the array of anionic sites on glycosaminoglycans [47, 162, 167, 328, 484]. Neutralization of these sites by positively charged molecules, such as protamine, prevents localization of cationic antigen or antibodies and subsequent development of nephritis [5].

The site of localization of immune deposits within the glomerulus (Fig. 60-4) is relevant both to the mechanisms initiating aggregation and to the inflammatory mediators engaged [382]. Reaction of antibody and antigen in the subepithelial space necessarily occurs locally, since preformed complexes cannot readily traverse the intact glomerular capillary wall. A membranous pattern of nephritis results, in which there is complement-dependent, leukocyte-independent injury due mainly to the membrane attack complex. Limitation of the effects of leukocytes could be due to their restricted access to this site or to the inability of chemotaxins to diffuse against the flux of ultrafiltration. Subendothelial deposits may contain preformed immune complexes and generally lead to proliferative nephritis with complement-dependent, leukocyte-mediated injury. Immune deposits can be cleared rapidly from this site, with accompanying resolution of injury, whereas subepithelial deposits are more persistent [160].

IgA-Dependent Experimental Nephritis. The role of IgA containing immune complexes in mesangial nephritis has been examined in several experimental models. Mice bearing an IgA myeloma specific for dinitrophenol (DNP) conjugated bovine serum albumin (BSA) were

Fig. 60-4. Diagrammatic representation of the localization of immune deposits in the glomerulus (see text for details). GBM = glomerular basement membrane; MM = mesangial matrix; 1 = large subepithelial deposits seen in acute post-streptococcal glomerulonephritis; 2 = subendothelial deposits seen in MCGN type I; 3 = fine subepithelial deposits seen in membranous nephropathy; 4 = mesangial deposits seen in IgA nephropathy. (Drawn by C. J. Derry.)

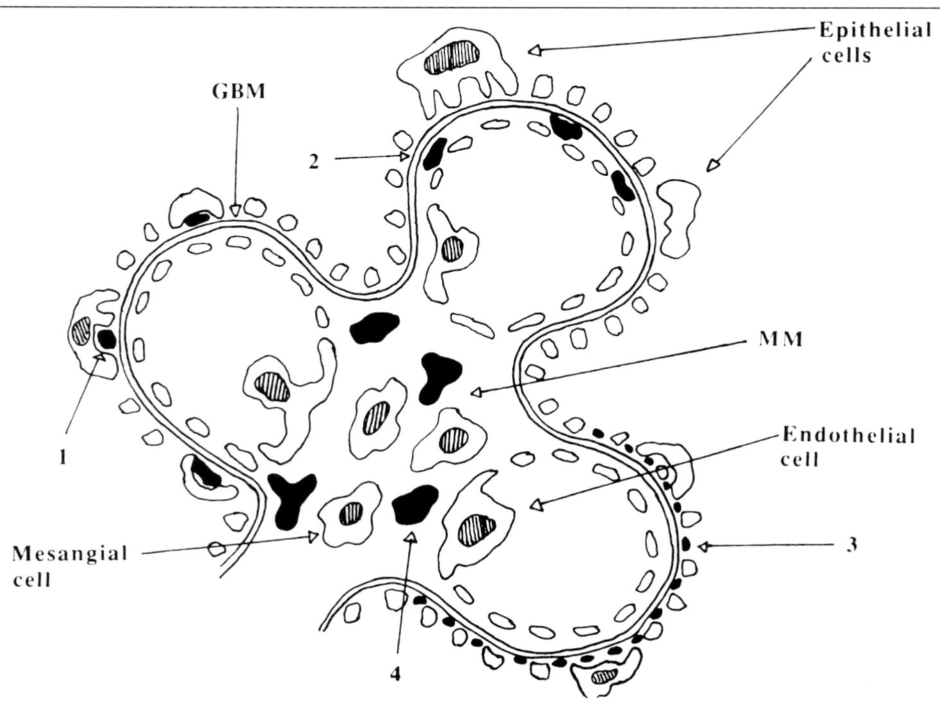

used to develop a model in which passive administration of preformed IgA-DNP-BSA complexes resulted in mesangial deposits of IgA but minimal injury [363]. This system was used to demonstrate that polymeric IgA was necessary for development of disease and that the nature of the antigen was important in complement activation [361, 362]. In another model, chronic immunization of mice with dextrans leads to mesangial proliferation with IgA deposits, and both the size and charge of the dextrans were found to influence complement activation and injury [211]. Certain orally administered antigens (including ovalbumin, gammaglobulin, ferritin) can also induce mesangial IgA nephritis in mice [136]. Blockade of the reticuloendothelial system in this model results in increased IgA deposition and glomerular injury [390]. More recent experiments, involving intravenous challenge with the previously administered oral antigen, show that codeposition of IgG or IgM (or of "complement-activating" antigens) is necessary for both complement deposition and nephritis [138]. This suggests that deposition of IgA alone is insufficient to induce mesangial nephritis. The relationship between liver disease and IgA nephropathy has been examined by inducing liver damage with carbon tetrachloride or by bile-duct ligation [180, 289]. In both of these models there was mesangial deposition of IgA but without major histologic changes.

Antibodies to Glomerular Cells. There is increasing evidence that renal injury may be caused by antibodies to specific cell types in the glomerulus [55]. The best characterized is the model of "passive Heymann nephritis," which involves antibodies to epithelial cells [148]. In Heymann nephritis (see below), rats immunized with homologous renal tubular cell preparations (Fx1A) develop membranous nephropathy with granular immune deposits [132]. It was believed that these deposits arose from deposition of circulating immune complexes; however, it has now been shown that they result from the binding of antibodies to cell surface antigens (including gp330) common to tubular and glomerular epithelial cells [102, 228, 472].

The administration of heterologous antibodies to Fx1A or gp330 reproduces the immunofluorescence pattern and to a varying extent the glomerular injury [21, 148]. These antibodies react with gp330 in the clathrin-coated pits of the podocytes of epithelial cells, and this is followed by capping and shedding of the resulting "in situ" immune complexes [70, 230]. Proteinuria in the early passive phase of this model depends on the membrane attack complex of complement, although in the later autologous phase, decomplementation does not fully abrogate proteinuria, suggesting the involvement of other mechanisms [383].

The possible role of antiendothelial cell antibodies has been investigated following their detection in systemic lupus erythematosus [80] and primary systemic vasculitis [152]. Antibodies to angiotensin converting enzyme (ACE), expressed on glomerular endothelial cells, can cause transient endothelial injury in rabbits. However, this model is complicated by the later development of subepithelial immune deposits. The possibility that mesangial cells are the target for autoantibodies in human mesangial proliferative nephritis [24] has been investigated using antibodies to Thy1.1, a mesangial cell antigen in the rat. Heterologous anti-Thy1.1 antibodies bind to mesangial cells in vivo and lead to early mesangiolysis, followed in a few days by mesangial hypercellularity and proteinuria in susceptible strains [20]. The binding of these antibodies was accompanied by complement deposition, and the initial lytic lesion was shown to be complement dependent [512]. Further in vitro studies demonstrated that the membrane attack complex was responsible for lysis of anti-Thy1.1–treated cultured mesangial cells. Recently, it has been reported that nephritis in this model is accompanied by increased production of TGF-β1, an inducer of extracellular matrix formation, and that the histologic changes can be inhibited by anti-TGF-β1 antisera [46].

INDUCTION OF AUTOIMMUNITY

Animal models of autoimmune nephritis allow the analysis of mechanisms involved in the induction and regulation of autoimmunity, as well as study of the modulation of renal injury. Of particular interest is that they are suitable for the investigation of various approaches to specific immune intervention [510]. The principal features of selected models are shown in Table 60-1.

Steblay Nephritis. An antigen-induced model of anti-GBM disease was first described by Steblay in 1962, who demonstrated that sheep immunized with heterologous or homologous GBM in adjuvant developed linear deposits of IgG and C3 along the basement membrane accompanied by crescentic proliferative nephritis [426]. The pathogenic role of circulating anti-GBM antibodies was demonstrated by both cross-circulation and passive transfer experiments [429].

A similar type of experimental autoimmune glomerulonephritis (EAG) has subsequently been induced in numerous species, including mice [19], rats [347, 381, 438], rabbits [470], guinea pigs [103], and monkeys [427]. In general, immunization with heterologous GBM in adjuvant has been required, and in this situation the response of T cells to antigens to which the animal is not tolerant may lead to stimulation of autoreactive B cells. There are considerable species differences in the severity of nephritis produced, and it has proved difficult to induce disease (as opposed to autoantibodies) in small animals appropriate for thorough immunologic investigation. However, both BN and WKY/NCrj rats are susceptible to a single injection of homologous or heterologous GBM. These strains develop sustained anti-GBM antibody synthesis, with linear deposits of IgG on the GBM, focal necrotizing glomerulonephritis, and proteinuria [347, 381]. Nephritis can be transferred by antibodies from immunized animals [380]. However, the role of T cells is suggested by the therapeutic effect of cyclosporin A on antibody production and proteinuria [358] and by cell transfer experiments that demonstrate

Table 60-1. Principal immunopathologic features of experimental autoimmune nephritis

Disease	Stimulus	Species	Strain	Serology	Immunohistology	Pathogenesis	Regulation
Anti-GBM nephritis (Steblay)	GBM + CFA	Sheep	—	Anti-GBM Ab	Linear IgG ± C3 on GBM	Transfer by Ab	—
		Rat	BN, WKY	Anti-GBM Ab	Linear IgG on GBM	Transfer by Ab Priming by MC	CsA
		Chicken	SC (bursec-tomized)	—	—	Transfer by MC	—
Membranous nephritis (Heymann)	Fx1A + CFA	Rat	LEW, PVG	Anti-brush-border Ab Anti-gp330 Ab	Granular IgG ± C3 along capillary wall	Transfer by Ab	Ts cells Anti-id Ab CsA
Interstitial nephritis	TBM + CFA	Guinea pig	XIII	Anti-TBM Ab	Linear IgG ± C3 on TBM	Transfer by Ab	Anti-id Ab
		Rat	BN	Anti-TBM Ab	Linear IgG ± C3 on TBM	Transfer by Ab MC required	Anti-id Ab CsA, Cyclo
		Mouse	SJL	Anti-TBM Ab	Linear IgG ± C3 on TBM	Transfer by Tdth cells Mild form by Ab	Ts cells (id and anti-id)
Toxic nephropathy	Hg, Au, penicillamine	Rat	BN	Anti-GBM Ab Common idiotype Polyclonal activation with other auto-Ab	Linear IgG on GBM (later granular IgG)	Transfer by Th cells	Ts cells Anti-id Ab (in vitro) Cyclo, CsA
"Lupus" nephritis	Spontaneous	Mouse	NZB/W, BXSB MRL/Ipr	Anti-DNA Ab Polyclonal activation	Granular Ig + C3 on GBM	—	Anti-id Ab Anti-MHC Ab Anti-T cell Ab Anti-IL-2R Ab

GBM = glomerular basement membrane; Ab = antibody; MC = mononuclear cell; id = idiotype; CsA = cyclosporin A; TBM = tubular basement membrane; Cyclo = cyclophosphamide.

the priming effect of Th lymphocytes from animals with EAG (Reynolds et al., unpublished observation). More direct evidence for the role of T cells in mediation as well as initiation of the disease comes from an interesting model of EAG in the chick [43, 465]. Bursectomized chicks immunized with heterologous GBM developed nephritis in the absence of detectable anti-GBM antibodies, and furthermore the disease could be transferred to syngeneic SN chicks by T lymphocytes [42a].

The relationship between renal and pulmonary disease, the cardinal features of Goodpasture's syndrome, has been investigated in various models. Immunization with GBM can induce alveolar hemorrhage [347, 381], while alveolar basement membrane can induce nephritis [428]. These observations support studies in humans, which demonstrate that the same antigen is present in both target organs (see below). The development of lung hemorrhage may depend on the permeability of alveolar capillaries, which normally limit access of antibody to basement membrane antigens. This idea is supported by experiments in nephrotoxic nephritis, in which exposure to toxic concentrations of oxygen [217] or to gasoline [513] allow binding of anti-GBM antibodies to the alveolar basement membrane.

Chemically Induced Glomerulonephritis. The administration of polyclonal activators, such as $HgCl_2$ or penicillamine, can induce anti-GBM antibodies in rats [127, 388] and rabbits [371]. The best characterized model is that induced by repeated subcutaneous injections of $HgCl_2$ in BN rats. This leads to a biphasic disease, in which linear deposits of IgG on the GBM are replaced by granular deposits. Proteinuria accompanies this response, but histologic changes in the glomerulus are slight [129]. Recent observations in this model suggest that extrarenal injury may be more common than previously appreciated [280a]. $HgCl_2$-treated BN rats develop necrotizing vasculitis in the gut, pancreas, and possibly lung and also have antibodies to myeloperoxidase, suggesting that this disease may also form a useful experimental model of primary systemic vasculitis.

A number of observations on the mechanisms of induction and regulation of nephritis have been made in this model: (1) Anti-GBM antibodies are formed as part of a polyclonal response, which includes the presence of other autoantibodies, e.g., to collagen, thyroglobulin, and DNA [202, 345]. (2) The response is T cell dependent and involves the induction of anti-Ia Th lymphocytes [336]. The mechanism remains unclear but could involve chemical alteration of MHC class II molecules. The disease can be transferred by T cells from affected animals [337] and can be inhibited by cyclosporin A [27]. (3) Susceptibility to the disease is strain dependent and is linked to the MHC, as well as one or two other genes [128]. (4) The autoimmune response is self-limiting, despite continued injection of $HgCl_2$, with anti-GBM antibodies peaking at around 2 weeks and becoming undetectable by 4 weeks [51, 345]. Animals in which $HgCl_2$ is discontinued remain resistant to further challenge for several months, and there is evidence for the role of both T suppressor cells [51] and anti-idiotypic interactions [78]. (5) Anti-GBM antibodies and proteinuria can be suppressed by a single injection of cyclophosphamide, although very low doses may paradoxically increase antibody levels, perhaps by a selective effect on Ts lymphocytes [346]. Animals treated with higher doses of cyclophosphamide remain resistant to rechallenge with $HgCl_2$ for up to a year, an observation that may be of relevance to the development of treatment based on the idea of "stimulation-deletion" of B cell clones.

It is of interest that a similar form of anti-GBM nephritis occurs as part of the polyclonal B cell response in murine graft-versus-host disease (GVHD) [370] and host-versus-graft disease [177]. In both instances, the autoimmune response may occur as a result of semi-allogeneic T-B cell interactions. It has recently been shown that rats with GVHD produce anti-GBM antibodies that share a common cross-reactive idiotype with antibodies in $HgCl_2$, gold, or penicillamine-treated animals [185]. Thus several different stimuli involving the induction of anti-class II T cells may lead to the activation of similar B cell clones.

Heymann Nephritis. In this model of membranous glomerulonephritis, first described by Heymann in 1959, rats immunized with kidney homogenates in adjuvant developed granular immune deposits along with glomerular capillary wall accompanied by proteinuria [196]. The antigen involved was originally characterized as a fraction (Fx1A) of the brush border of proximal tubular cells and later as a more purified 28s lipoprotein (RTEα5) [132]. At least one antigenic component has now been identified as a glycoprotein (gp330) found on proximal tubular and glomerular epithelial cells, where it is localized to clathrin-coated pits [228]. A cDNA clone encoding a major pathogenic domain of gp330 has now been isolated, and the resulting fusion protein can be used to induce Heymann nephritis [341].

Heymann nephritis was originally regarded as an example of "immune complex" nephritis, but it is now clear that it represents an autoimmune disorder in which antibodies bind to gp330, followed by capping and shedding of the antibody-antigen complex into the subepithelial space (Fig. 60-5) [230]. Disease can be passively transferred by antibodies to Fx1A or gp330, and perfusion of isolated kidneys with these antibodies results in the typical immune deposits [102, 228, 472]. Interestingly, administration of antibodies to gp330, or active immunization with gp330, leads to less severe nephritis than when a cruder preparation is used. This finding supports the suggestion that more than one antigen-antibody system is involved in the original Heymann model [21, 220, 290, 372, 479]. For example, antibodies to dipeptidyl-peptidase IV (present in Fx1A) may contribute to glomerular injury, although they are unlikely to initiate it [309].

The induction of Heymann nephritis is strain dependent and linked to the MHC. Susceptible strains include LEW, AS, and WG rats, whereas BN rats (susceptible to anti-GBM disease) are resistant [79, 433]. As in EAG, cyclosporin A is protective, suggesting a role for T cells in initiation of the disease [184]. Resistance to disease can

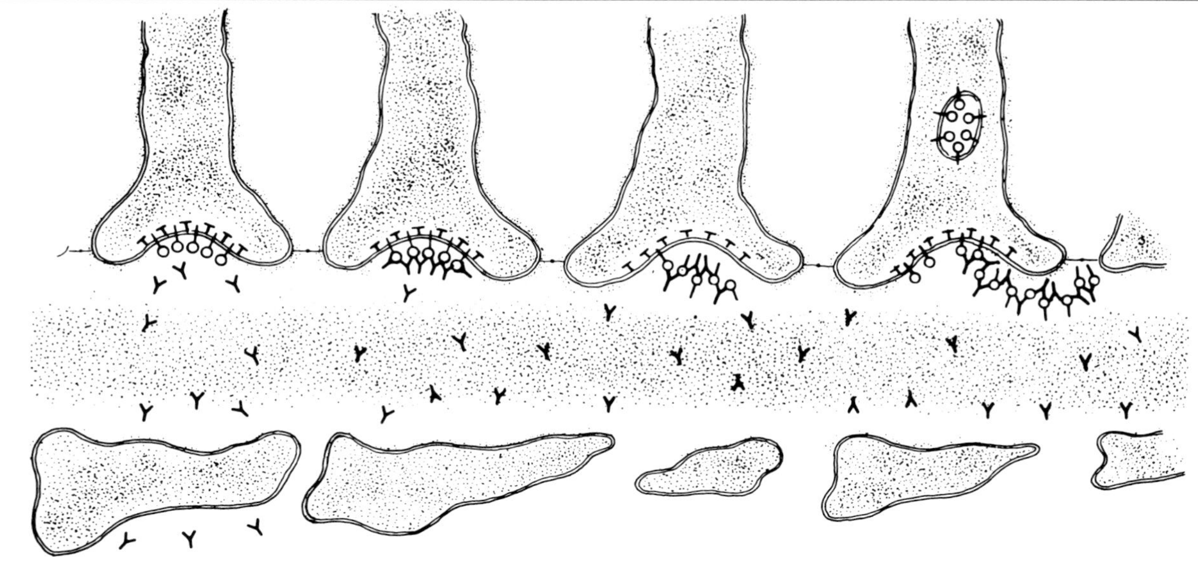

Fig. 60-5. Diagrammatic representation of in situ immune complex formation in Heymann nephritis (see text for details). T = clathrin coat, ⚲ = gp330, Y = anti-gp330 IgG. (Courtesy of Prof. D. Kerjaschki.)

be transferred by Ts cells [79, 119, 266] and also by the induction of anti-idiotypic antibodies [131]. Renal injury is reduced by complement depletion in the early stages of the disease, but not by neutrophil depletion [383, 384]. There is mounting evidence that the membrane attack complex of complement is responsible for glomerular damage [106, 118, 231, 334].

Interstitial Nephritis. Tubulointerstitial nephritis (TIN) can be induced in several species, including mice, rats, guinea pigs, and rabbits, by the administration of tubular basement membrane (TBM) preparations in adjuvant. The role of various immunopathologic mechanisms, including autoantibodies, immune complexes, and T cells, has been demonstrated in different models, although none corresponds directly to the common drug-induced acute interstitial nephritis in humans [285].

Steblay and Rudofsky [430] first established a reproducible model of TIN in guinea pigs immunized with rabbit TBM in adjuvant. Linear deposition of IgG along the TBM was accompanied by severe interstitial inflammation with lymphocytes, monocytes, and giant cells. The disease could be transferred by anti-TBM antibodies, but not by lymphoid cells [431]. The severity of renal injury was reduced by both complement depletion with cobra venom factor (CVF) [378] and leukocyte depletion using irradiation [377]. As in other autoimmune models, genetic susceptibility linked to the MHC was demonstrated, in that strain XIII guinea pigs developed TIN more readily than strain II animals [208]. Of possible therapeutic interest is the observation that the disease could be inhibited by heterologous anti-idiotypic sera [58].

The use of rat and mouse models of TIN has allowed more detailed analysis of the immune mechanisms involved. In susceptible BN rats, the administration of homologous or heterologous TBM in adjuvant leads to linear deposition of IgG and C3 along the proximal TBM in 2 to 3 weeks [255, 439]. This is initially accompanied by neutrophil infiltration and later by accumulation of lymphocytes and monocytes. Several weeks after injection of rat (but not bovine) TBM, granular deposits of Ig are seen in the glomerular capillaries, in a distribution similar to that found in Heymann nephritis. A mild form of the disease can be transferred by anti-TBM antibodies [323, 439], but not by lymphocytes, although cell-mediated mechanisms have been implicated in the disease [277].

Two distinct elements determining genetic susceptibility have been identified: the development of an adequate autoimmune response and the presence of immunoreactive TBM antigen. Certain strains (F344, AUG) do not produce sufficient anti-TBM antibodies, whereas others (LEW, MAXX) develop circulating antibody but lack the target antigen. The susceptible BN strain both produces a strong antibody response and possesses the autoantigen [255, 311]. Interestingly, transplantation of kidneys from a strain with the nephritogenic antigen into animals lacking it is followed by development of anti-TBM disease in the recipient [254].

The development of TIN in the rat can be prevented by administration of heterologous anti-idiotypic antibodies [516] and also by maneuvers leading to an auto-anti-idiotypic response—e.g., immunization with TBM-reactive T lymphoblasts [317]. It has been suggested that the failure of auto-anti-idiotypic immunity may underlie susceptibility [315]. The disease can be prevented by high doses of cyclophosphamide, whereas lower doses appear to exacerbate disease (as in the $HgCl_2$-induced model) [8]. Cyclosporin A can also prevent and ameliorate disease, supporting a role for T cells [173, 411]. In other experiments, a stable analogue of prostaglandin E_1 (PGE_1)–inhibited anti-TBM production and prevented interstitial nephritis [468], perhaps via effects on the induction of effector T cells [227].

A similar model of TIN in mice can be induced by injection of rabbit TBM in adjuvant [316, 376]. Susceptibility depends on the MHC haplotype (H-2K) and on immunoglobulin genes (Igh-1) [313]. The disease can be transferred by T cells with delayed type hypersensitivity function, and a milder form can be induced by passive transfer of anti-TBM antibodies [515]. Immunoregulation has been achieved by immunization with tubular antigen "derivatized" lymphocytes. This induces a T suppressor cell system involving both idiotypic and anti-idiotypic Ts cells, restricted by MHC (I-J) and immunoglobulin (IgH-V) genes [314]. The target of the anti-TBM response has been identified as a glycoprotein of 42 kd in the rat and 30 kd in the mouse. The antigen was isolated by the use of a monoclonal antibody reactive with proximal TBM of BN but not LEW rats [81], since the latter do not express the nephritogenic antigen (see above) [255]. The autoantigen, known as 3M-I, is localized to the lateral aspect of the TBM and is capable of inducing the disease. A cDNA clone encoding 3M-I has now been isolated from a murine tubular epithelial cell library [318] and should allow more precise definition of T cell responses in different strains of mouse.

SPONTANEOUS NEPHRITIS

Glomerulonephritis develops spontaneously in a number of domestic and laboratory animals. We shall consider only what has been learned from the nephritis of murine systemic lupus erythematosus (SLE) and progressive tubulointerstitial nephritis.

Murine SLE. Three separate lupus-prone strains of mice have been well characterized: NZB/NZW F1, BXSB, and MRL/lpr (reviewed in [448, 449]). They share the common feature of polyclonal B cell activation, which includes production of autoantibodies to native DNA. Anti-DNA antibodies of restricted idiotype can be eluted from the kidneys of nephritic mice and are believed to play a pathogenetic role through in situ formation or deposition of immune complexes [12]. The polyclonal activation is T cell dependent, and various immunoregulatory defects have been proposed in different strains, including impaired Ts cell function (NZB/W), over production of Th factors (MRL/lpr), and over-responsiveness of certain B cell populations (BXSB, NZB/W) [448]. Both genetic and environmental factors influence the severity of disease, including male chromosomal sex (BXSB), the lymphoproliferative gene (MRL/lpr), female sex hormones (NZB/W) and viral infections. Studies of immunoglobulin and TCR genes have not revealed specific abnormalities associated with autoimmunity, although the NZB TCR β gene is unusual. It has been established that self-reactive T cells are normally deleted in the thymus of NZB/W and MRL/lpr mice. However, a role for double-negative (CD4−, CD8−), α/β TCR–bearing T cells has been proposed in both NZB/W and MRL/lpr strains [449].

This model has been widely used in studies of immunotherapy. Immunization of NZB/W mice with a monoclonal anti-DNA antibody induces a protective anti-idiotypic response [190]. However, monoclonal antibodies to a cross-reactive idiotype only resulted in transient suppression of disease, due to the production of anti-DNA antibodies bearing different idiotypes [191]. This approach was not successful in MRL/lpr mice [444]. Monoclonal antibodies to Th cells can prevent or ameliorate disease in all strains [505, 506], and experiments using $F(ab)_2$ fragments showed that this does not depend on T cell depletion [71]. Furthermore, monoclonals to the IL-2 receptor (present on activated T cells) are also effective [437]. Finally, monoclonal antibodies to MHC class II gene products (I-A) can suppress disease in the NZB/W strain [3].

Murine Progressive TIN. A spontaneous form of progressive TIN occurs in kdkd mice, a substrain of the CDA strain [271, 312]. The disease is inherited in an autosomal recessive pattern and has been considered as a model of human nephronophthisis. Affected mice develop severe peritubular mononuclear cell infiltrates by about 8 weeks, followed by progressive tubular damage and fibrosis. No autoantibodies have been identified, but the disease can be transferred by MHC class I restricted ($H\text{-}2K^k$) CD8+ T cells [225]. Susceptibility is thought to depend on the presence of antigen-specific contrasuppressor cells, and T cells from non-disease-prone CDA mice can prevent TIN in the kdkd strain [226].

Human Nephritis

In this section, we consider the immunopathology of the better defined histologic types of glomerulonephritis and of acute interstitial nephritis in humans. Understanding of these diseases is incomplete and still relies heavily on analogies with experimental models; caution is needed to avoid inappropriate extrapolation. For convenience, we group the different types of human glomerulonephritis into (1) those where there is reasonable evidence for the involvement of circulating or deposited immune reactants (antibodies and complement) and (2) those in which such evidence is inconsistent or lacking. In the latter group it remains possible that immune mechanisms are involved, but that immune deposits are not seen because they are rapidly cleared, or that local or distant T cell–mediated responses are involved. A brief and necessarily incomplete summary of the immunology of human nephritis, with and without immune deposits, is given in Table 60-2. The clinicopathologic features and natural history of these disorders have been reviewed elsewhere [65, 175] and are considered in the relevant chapters in this book.

NEPHRITIS WITH IMMUNE DEPOSITS

Anti-GBM Disease. The combination of rapidly progressive glomerulonephritis (RPGN) and alveolar hemorrhage is termed Goodpasture's syndrome [425, 501]. Various systemic diseases may produce this clinical picture, so the term anti-GBM disease (or Goodpasture's *disease*)

Table 60-2. Principal immunopathologic features of human glomerulonephritis

Disease	MHC association	Serology	Immunohistology	Pathogenesis	Treatment
Anti-GBM disease	DR2, DR4	Anti-GBM Ab	Linear IgG ± C3 on GBM	Auto-Ab to GBM	PE + Pred + Cyclo
Membranous nephropathy	DR3 (DR2 in Japan)	Variable IC	Subepithelial fine granular IgG ± C3	?Auto-Ab to epithelial cells ?Planted Ag	Pred + chlorambucil
MCGN I	—	Variable IC, low C3	Subendothelial granular IgG + C3 (± IgM)	?IC disease	—
MCGN II	?DR7	NeF, low C3	Linear C3 on GBM	?Auto-Ab to C3bBb	—
IgA nephropathy	DR4, DQw7	Variable raised IgA ± IgA – IC ?Anti-mesangial cell Ab	Mesangial IgA + C3 (± IgG)	?IC disease ?Auto-Ab to mesangial cells	?Cyclo + anticoagulants ?Pred in nephrotic syndrome
Poststreptococcal GN	DR4 (DR1 in Japan)	Anti-strep Ab Variable raised Ig + IC Low C3 ± C4	Subepithelial coarse granular IgG + C3 (± other Ig)	?Planted Ag	—
SLE	DR3	Anti-DNA Ab Anti-Sm Ab Polyclonal increase Ig ± IC Low C4 ± C3	Subepithelial, subendothelial, and mesangial IgG + IgM + IgA + C3	?Autoimmune ?Planted Ag ?IC disease	Pred ± Cyclo or Aza ?PE or pulse MP (severe)
EMC II	—	Cryoglobulins Paraprotein (IgM) IC + RF Low C4	Subendothelial granular IgM + IgG + C3	IC disease	PE ± Pred ± Cyclo
Minimal change nephropathy	DR7 (DR8 in Japan)	Sometimes raised IgM	Negative or sparse mesangial IgM	Not known ?Role of T cell factors	Pred Cyclo or CsA (relapse)
Focal necrotizing GN	?DR2, DQw7	ANCA Variable raised Ig + IC	Negative or variable scattered IgG ± IgM ± C3	?Autoimmune	Pred + Cyclo (induction) Pred + Aza (maintenance) PE or pulse MP (severe)

GBM = glomerular basement membrane; MCGN = mesangiocapillary glomerulonephritis; GN = glomerulonephritis; Ab = antibody; Ag = antigen; IC = immune complex; Cyclo = cyclophosphamide; Aza = Azathioprine; CsA = cyclosporin A; Pred = prednisolone; PE = plasma exchange; MP = methylprednisolone; EMC = essential mixed cryoglobulinemia.

is preferred for those cases with anti-GBM antibodies. The detection of linear deposits of IgG on the GBM on immunofluorescence, similar to the pattern observed in nephrotoxic nephritis, first prompted the notion that this disease was antibody mediated [130, 396]. The pathogenicity of these antibodies was subsequently demonstrated by Lerner et al. [257], who showed that anti-GBM antibodies eluted from patients' kidneys could be used to induce proliferative nephritis in squirrel monkeys. The diagnosis of Goodpasture's disease can readily be made by sensitive solid-phase immunoassays for circulating anti-GBM antibodies [50, 275, 494], as well as by direct immunohistology of renal biopsy specimens (Fig. 60-6).

Immunohistologic studies, using eluted anti-GBM antibodies and a murine monoclonal antibody (PI) to the Goodpasture antigen, have demonstrated that the same target antigen is present in GBM, distal TBM, and alveolar basement membrane. Thus, the same antibody-antigen interaction is likely to account for both major aspects of the disease [346a], and the variability of pulmonary hemorrhage reflects the involvement of other factors (see below). The Goodpasture antigen is also detectable in basement membranes of the choroid plexus, lens capsule, retina/choroid, cochlea, and certain endocrine glands [72, 237]. Its distribution coincides with that of type IV collagen but is considerably more restricted. One- and two-dimensional Western blotting studies have shown that the same antigenic components of GBM, cationic glycoproteins of 26 to 58 kd, are recognized by sera from all patients, as well as by monoclonal antibodies to the Goodpasture antigen, demonstrating the restricted specificity of this autoimmune response [122, 346a].

The autoantigen forms part of the noncollagenous globular domain (NC1) of type IV collagen [206a]. The monomeric and dimeric components recognized on Western blotting represent single or linked C-terminal regions of α(IV) procollagen molecules [60, 495]. Amino acid sequences obtained from immunoreactive monomers suggest that the antigenic site is located on one or more novel α(IV) chains, rather than on the well-characterized α1 and α2 chains [61, 62, 392]. Recently, the identity of the antigen has been confirmed as the α3 chain of type IV collagen by the isolation of cDNA clones from bovine [300] and human [466] kidney libraries.

Fig. 60-6. Direct immunoperoxidase of renal biopsy from a patient with anti-GBM disease demonstrating linear deposition of IgG along the GBM. (Courtesy of Dr. E. M. Thompson.)

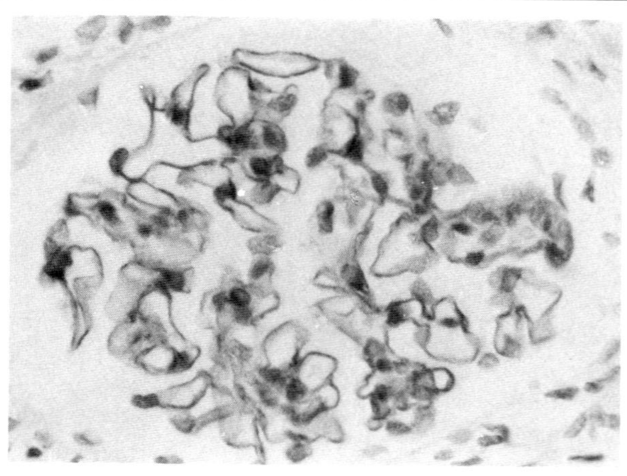

Susceptibility to the disease depends on genetic and environmental factors. Identical twins with anti-GBM disease have been reported [113], and there is a strong association with MHC genes. Serologic typing techniques revealed that the development of anti-GBM disease was strongly associated with HLA-DR2 and that patients also possessing B7 developed more severe nephritis [357]. Recent studies using restriction fragment length polymorphism (RFLP) analysis and allele specific oligonucleotide subtyping have confirmed a strong association with the DRw15(DR2) allele and revealed a weaker association with DR4 [59]. No unique disease-associated sequences have been identified, and it is possible that a normal sequence common to DRw15 and DR4 is involved. An association with immunoglobulin Gm allotypes has also been reported [355].

Environmental factors in anti-GBM disease have proved difficult to identify, although there are reports of associations with influenza A2 infection [34] and hydrocarbon exposure [31]. However, these stimuli could have provoked presentation of the disease rather than causing it. There are also several observations of clusters of cases, supporting the involvement of an environmental agent, but no clear precipitant was identified in these studies [338, 497]. There is good evidence for the relationship between cigarette smoking and the development of lung hemorrhage [126], as well as reports of hemorrhage being provoked by infection or fluid overload [356, 415]. Increased pulmonary capillary permeability may allow antibody binding to the alveolar basement membrane in these situations.

Anti-GBM antibodies are known to be pathogenic from transfer experiments [257], and this finding is supported by the observation that their concentration generally correlates with severity of disease [339, 394]. However, the events leading to tissue injury are not fully understood and may also involve cellular mechanisms. The work of Bonsib [44] suggests that the development of breaks in the glomerular capillary wall may be fundamental to the crescent formation that characterizes severe anti-GBM nephritis (Fig. 60-7). Immunofluorescence of renal biopsies almost invariably demonstrates the presence of IgG on the GBM, with IgM and/or IgA in about 10 percent of cases [394, 498]. Deposition of complement C3 is found in only one-third to one-half of cases, suggesting that non-complement-dependent injury may also be important. As in other types of crescentic nephritis, T cell [424] and macrophage [17] infiltration of the glomeruli and adjacent interstitium has been reported. Many studies reveal a predominance of CD4+ T cells, although smaller numbers of CD8+ cells can be detected [42b, 310, 325]. It has been suggested that T cell infiltration occurs at an early stage of the dis-

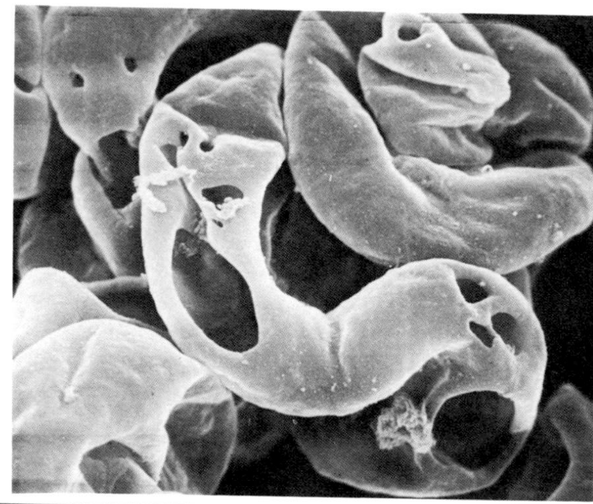

Fig. 60-7. Scanning electron micrograph of an acellular glomerulus from a patient with crescentic nephritis demonstrating "perforations" in the glomerular capillaries. (Courtesy of Dr. S. M. Bonsib.)

ease, preceding macrophage influx. These observations, however, provide only indirect evidence for participation of the mediation systems concerned.

Treatment with a combination of plasma exchange, prednisolone, and cyclophosphamide has been shown to be effective in reducing anti-GBM antibody levels [339, 348]. Antibody usually becomes undetectable by 8 weeks in treated patients, whereas it persists for around a year in untreated patients on dialysis. Solid-phase immunoassays for circulating anti-GBM antibodies have proved of value in monitoring treatment and also allow the selection of dialysis-dependent patients for transplantation, since rapid recurrence occurs in cases transplanted in the presence of circulating antibody [10, 415, 501]. The redevelopment of anti-GBM antibody after adequate treatment is exceptional, and maintenance therapy is not required, suggesting that immune tolerance has been reestablished. The outcome for renal function depends largely on the severity of renal injury at the time of treatment. The majority of patients treated before reaching dialysis show an improvement in renal function, whereas dialysis-dependent patients only rarely improve [218, 394, 486]. This outcome nonetheless represents a great improvement in the natural history of the disease [501].

Membranous Nephropathy. This condition commonly presents with isolated proteinuria or the nephrotic syndrome and progresses to renal failure in approximately 30 percent of cases by 10 years. It was long regarded as an example of "immune complex" nephritis because of the characteristic immunofluorescence findings of fine granular deposits of IgG and C3, occasionally with IgM and IgA, along the glomerular capillary wall (Fig. 60-8) [63]. Electron microscopy shows that these immune deposits are predominantly subepithelial. The striking similarity to Heymann nephritis (see above) has prompted suggestions that these deposits represent "in situ" complexes formed between circulating autoantibodies and epithelial cell antigens, although a similar antibody-antigen system has proved difficult to identify in humans. The presence of antibodies to "brush border" antigens has been reported in isolated patients [308, 517], but their specificity is different from that in Heymann nephritis [89]. Indeed, a gp330-like molecule has been identified in human proximal tubules but not in the glomerulus [229]. Recently, it has been reported that antibodies raised to human glomerular epithelial cells lead to the development of subepithelial deposits in vivo in monkeys and in the isolated perfused human kidney [161]. An alternative explanation for the immune deposits in this disorder is that a "planted antigen" is involved. There have been several reports of the detection of specific antigens in the deposits of membranous glomerulonephritis, although these findings have not been widely confirmed and would not in any case provide good evidence for the pathogenicity of such antigens [32].

The same immunohistologic findings are present in primary membranous nephropathy and in cases occurring in association with other diseases. Membranous nephritis has been related to (1) malignancy, especially of lung, gut, breast, and kidney [29, 331, 374]; (2) infection, including hepatitis B and several chronic bacterial and protozoal infections [90, 201, 259]; (3) drugs, particularly gold, penicillamine, and captopril [215, 461]; (4) autoimmune disease, most commonly SLE [23, 182] and rarely thyroid disorders [204, 218a] and anti-GBM nephritis [234, 246]; and (5) sickle cell anemia [333]. Although the "planted antigen" hypothesis provides an attractive explanation for these associations, many of the above conditions could also lead to disordered regulation of immunity, and hence to autoantibody-mediated disease.

Fig. 60-8. Direct immunoperoxidase of renal biopsy from a patient with membranous nephropathy demonstrating fine granular deposits of IgG along the glomerular capillary wall. (Courtesy of Dr. E. M. Thompson.)

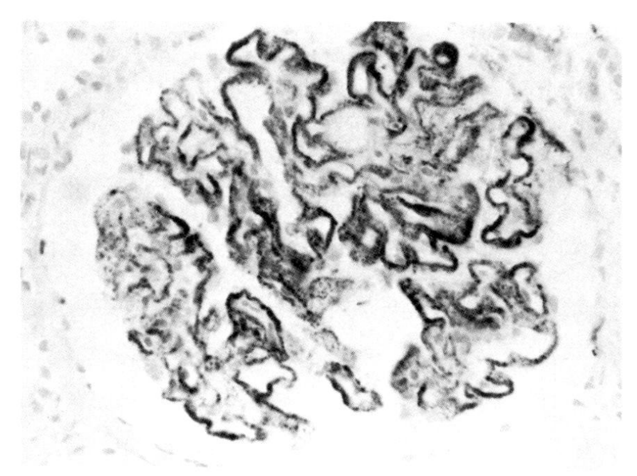

Strong associations with HLA-DR3 are reported in whites with primary membranous nephropathy [165, 238, 303, 366] and with the secondary form complicating gold and penicillamine therapy [509]. However, the main association in Japanese is with HLA-DR2 [197], suggesting either that the MHC gene responsible is in linkage disequilibrium with different alleles in the two populations or that the diseases involve intrinsically different glomerular antigens. The former suggestion is supported by the finding that a DQA1 allele identified by RFLP, and inherited with DR3 and DR5, was more strongly associated with the disease than DR3 itself [478]. Severity of the nephritis may also depend on genetic influences, although this has not been convincingly demonstrated. One study suggested that patients with the haplotype DR3 B18 BfF1 had a worse prognosis than those with other DR3-bearing haplotypes [412]. However, another report does not confirm this finding and suggests that the haplotype DR3 B8 BfS is associated with a worse outcome [332].

The therapeutic effect of immunosuppressive drugs provides further evidence that membranous nephropathy may be immunologically mediated. The use of high-dose steroids alone was of marginal benefit in one study [84], but not in another [65a]. However, the combination of prednisolone with chlorambucil [344] or cyclophosphamide [492] appears to have a considerable effect on the natural history of the disease. Ponticelli et al. [344] reported that both proteinuria and progressive renal impairment could be modified by treatment with alternating months of prednisolone and chlorambucil for 6 months. Most patients in this trial were treated early and had grossly normal renal function. A modification of this regimen was later used in an uncontrolled study of patients with impaired renal function and resulted in a marked short-term improvement [281].

Mesangiocapillary (Membranoproliferative) Glomerulonephritis. This condition usually presents with a combination of hematuria and proteinuria, or with nephrotic syndrome, and progresses to renal failure in about 50 percent of cases by 10 years. There are two principal subtypes, with similar clinical features and light-microscopic appearances, but different immunohistology (Fig. 60-9) and electron microscopy [187]. In type I mesangiocapillary glomerulonephritis (MCGN) there are subendothelial immune deposits, whereas in type II there are linear "dense deposits" along the GBM (Fig. 60-10). Type I MCGN has therefore been regarded as an "immune complex" disease, which is consistent with the location of the deposits, whereas the immunopathology of type II remains uncertain. The majority of cases are idiopathic [67, 188], although the histologic appearances of type I MCGN have been noted in association with various infections [114], including subacute infective endocarditis, "shunt nephritis," and leprosy, and with malignancy. It is the commonest pattern of nephritis in essential mixed cryoglobulinemia and forms part of the spectrum of nephritis due to SLE. It also occurs in the presence of genetic complement deficiencies [37, 88, 232, 340, 352].

Of particular immunologic interest is the finding of a

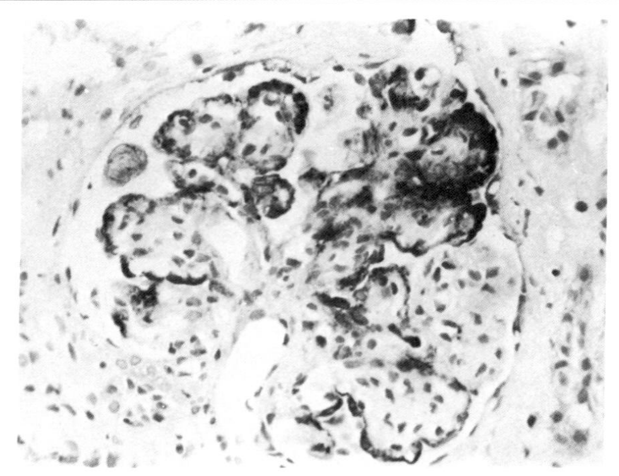

Fig. 60-9. Direct immunoperoxidase of renal biopsy from a patient with type I mesangiocapillary nephritis demonstrating course granular deposits of IgG in peripheral capillary loops. (Courtesy of Dr. E. M. Thompson.)

specific autoantibody, nephritic factor (NeF), in association with type II and rarely type I MCGN [67, 399, 422]. Nephritic factor is an IgG antibody with specificity for determinants on the alternative pathway C3 convertase C3bBb and renders this normally labile enzyme resistant to its inhibitors, factors H and I [108, 407]. As a result, there is persistent complement activation with marked lowering of C3, but sparing of the early components of the classical pathway. Nephritic factor has a slightly higher molecular weight than most IgG molecules due to glycosylation; this appears to be important for its activity, which can be inhibited in vitro by neuraminidase [107, 117, 406]. The use of sensitive assay systems has allowed the demonstration of NeF in some normocomplementemic patients with type II MCGN. It is also found in patients with partial lipodystrophy, who are particularly prone to develop type II and less commonly type I MCGN [420].

Atypical C3 nephritic factors have been described that cause only weak fluid phase C3 conversion, yet stabilize cell-bound C3bBb [320]. They are associated with decreased levels of C5 and increased activation of the terminal complement pathway in vivo [296]. The molecular basis for this difference in activity remains unknown. Considerably less common than C3NeF are antibodies that stabilize the classical pathway C3 convertase C4b2b; these have been described in post-streptococcal glomerulonephritis [192] and SLE [109].

The evidence for a genetic predisposition to the development of NeF is not strong, although there was a predominance of HLA-DR7 in one small series of patients with MCGN and NeF [354a]. Another report suggests that patients with MCGN bearing the HLA B8 DR3 haplotype are more likely to develop renal failure than others [490]. MCGN with partial lipodystrophy has also been related to partial complement deficiency due to inherited hypomorphism of C3f [287]. The relationship between NeF and the development of nephritis is not understood, although there are two broad categories of

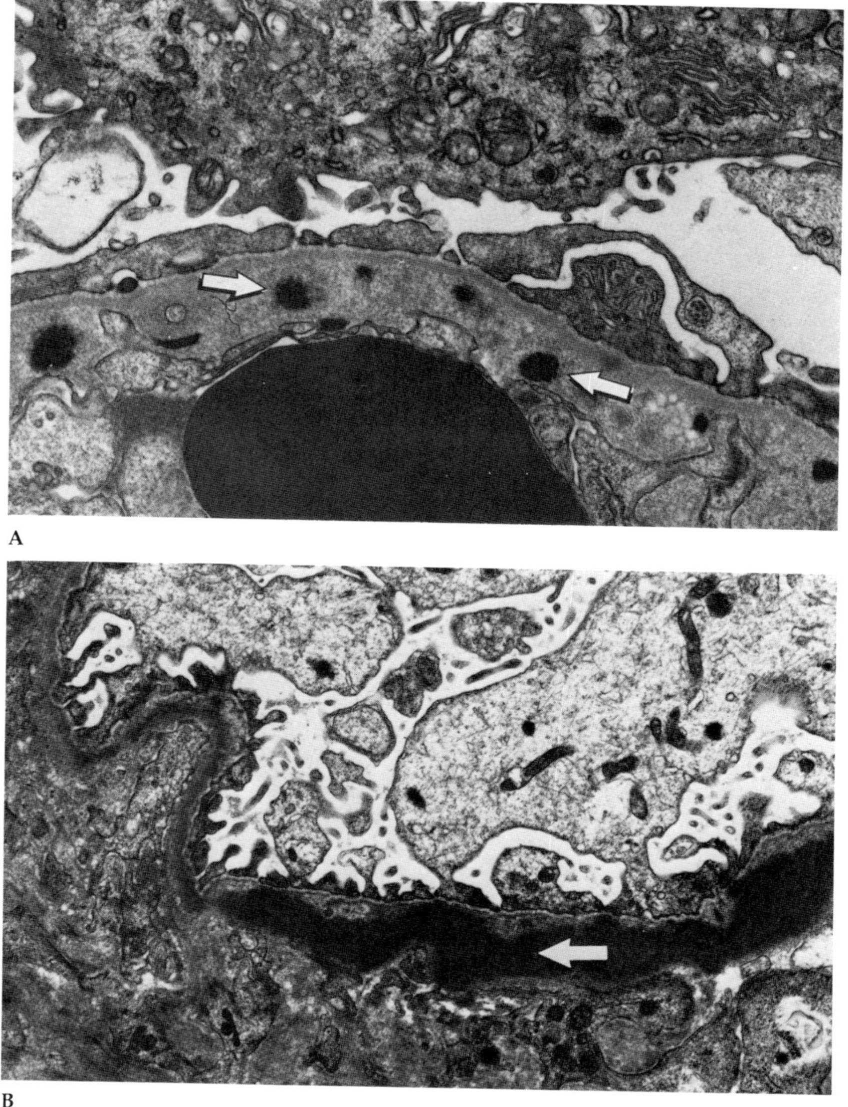

Fig. 60-10. Electron microscopy of renal biopsies from patients with (A) type I mesangiocapillary nephritis demonstrating discrete subendothelial deposits and (B) type II mesangiocapillary nephritis demonstrating linear "dense deposits" within the GBM. Immune deposits indicated by arrows. (Courtesy of Prof. D. J. Evans.)

explanation: (1) The complement deficiency induced by NeF leads to nephritis by mechanisms similar to those found in genetic complement deficiency, and (2) persistent activation of complement, under certain undefined circumstances, is nephrotoxic. There is little direct evidence in support of either of these suggestions; nephritis in complement deficiency generally has features of immune complex as opposed to dense deposit disease, and prolonged complement activation in experimental animals has consistently failed to produce nephritis [416, 480]. The nature of the dense deposits is not known; they are closely associated with C3 but not usually with immunoglobulin deposition.

Treatment of mesangiocapillary nephritis has generally been unsuccessful. In one uncontrolled series, early steroid therapy was associated with an improved outcome as compared with historical controls [491], but controlled trials of steroids and of cyclophosphamide with anticoagulants and antiplatelet drugs [74] have failed to demonstrate significant benefit.

IgA-Associated Glomerulonephritis. Mesangial proliferative glomerulonephritis with IgA deposition, also known as Berger's disease [36], is now one of the commonest forms of nephritis in developed countries [110]. One reason for this could be the increased tendency to obtain biopsies from patients with mild disease [146]. Presentation is frequently recurrent episodes of macroscopic hematuria, sometimes accompanied by proteinuria, and renal failure develops in 10 to 20 percent of cases by 10 to 20 years. Similar histologic and immunologic findings occur in Henoch-Schönlein purpura (HSP), which has prompted suggestions that IgA nephritis represents a limited form of HSP [137].

The distinctive immunologic feature of these conditions is mesangial deposition of IgA (Fig. 60-11), usually accompanied by IgG and the alternative pathway complement components C3 and properdin [137, 307]. Similar deposits have been reported in skin in both IgA nephritis and HSP [464]. The nature of the IgA in deposits has been extensively studied; the consensus view is that it is mainly IgA-1, with a predominance of λ light chains, and is usually polymeric with J-chain but without secretory component [92, 143, 249, 268, 457, 471]. There is often a high circulating concentration of IgA and an altered κ/λ ratio of light chains in both IgA and IgG. IgA-containing immune complexes are reported in one-third to two-thirds of cases [134, 508].

Since IgA forms the majority of antibody in epithelial secretions, considerable efforts have been made to implicate IgA antibodies to dietary and other environmental antigens in the formation of immune complexes in IgA nephropathy. Despite several studies in favor of this notion [157, 163, 304, 385], there are also many negative reports. The possible role of immunity to gliadin has received much attention, and IgA binding to gliadin occurs in a variable proportion of cases. In addition, there is in vitro evidence that gluten can form complexes with mesangial cells, allowing the possibility of "in situ" immune complex formation. An alternative explanation is that there is polyclonal activation of IgA- and IgG-secreting B cells and that the antibodies produced react directly with intrinsic or planted mesangial antigen [193, 397, 473]. There are a number of reports of abnormal regulation of immunoglobulin synthesis in IgA nephropathy, but no single coherent mechanism has been identified [97, 144, 511]. The proposed autoimmune mechanism is supported by observations that IgA eluted from renal biopsies recombines with autologous kidney [456] and that IgA from patients' sera binds to glomerular constituents including collagen, fibronectin, and laminin; however, this binding was not shown to be $F(ab)_2$ dependent [75, 76]. Of interest is the report that IgG autoantibodies reactive with mesangial cells are found in IgA nephropathy and HSP [24]. It has been suggested that the IgA rheumatoid factors present in this disorder [391, 418] could react with IgG deposited in the mesangium, thus accounting for the IgA-containing deposits; this possibility requires further investigation.

Fig. 60-11. Direct immunoperoxidase of renal biopsy from a patient with mesangial IgA nephritis demonstrating mesangial deposits of IgA. (Courtesy of Dr. E. M. Thompson.)

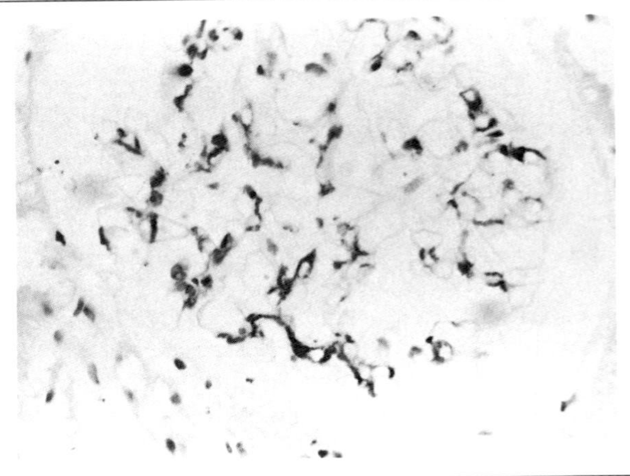

The role of genetic factors in susceptibility to IgA nephropathy has proved difficult to define. Familial cases have been reported, although family studies did not reveal MHC linkage [219, 223, 379]. An association with HLA-DR4 has been reported in some European [35, 133, 142] and most Japanese [198, 221, 306] studies, although other European and American series failed to confirm this finding [145, 194]. A recent study using RFLP analysis and oligonucleotide subtyping revealed a strong association with the DQw7 allele at the DQB locus; there was a weaker association with DR4 and DR5, both of which are linked to DQw7 allele [261]. It is therefore possible that the principal association is with the DQB1 locus and that the varying reports of DR4 frequency reflect varying linkage disequilibrium in different populations. Recently, an association with immunoglobulin heavy-chain allotypes has also been reported [120].

Environmental factors are also likely to be involved in IgA nephropathy, and the role of dietary antigens has already been considered. It is clear that infections, usually of the upper respiratory tract, may provoke episodes of macroscopic hematuria [112]; however, this could represent nonspecific enhancement of inflammation rather than stimulation of an immune response. Deposition of IgA in the mesangium also accompanies cirrhosis of the liver and certain enteropathies [222, 324, 386, 419]. In these circumstances, however, the characteristics of the immune deposits are different than those in primary IgA nephritis, and the development of clinically significant renal injury is rare.

The role of treatment for IgA nephropathies remains uncertain, and since many cases pursue a benign course specific therapy is often unnecessary. The use of steroids alone has been reported to induce remission of nephrotic syndrome, but not to alter progression of renal failure [250]. Another uncontrolled study involved a course of steroids for up to 2 years, followed by antiplatelet agents; treatment was reported to reduce both proteinuria and the rate of decline of renal function [240]. In one controlled trial, involving the use of cyclophosphamide together with antiplatelet agents and warfarin, treated patients showed less proteinuria and less decline in renal function [507]. In the occasional patients who develop crescentic nephritis on a background of IgA disease or HSP, there are uncontrolled reports of benefit from immunosuppressive drugs and plasma exchange [93, 321].

Postinfective Nephritis. Poststreptococcal nephritis was the first form of renal disease in which immunologic mechanisms were implicated, because of the serum sickness-like latent period followed by hypocomplementemia and development of immune deposits in the glomeruli. The characteristic presentation is acute nephritis 2 to 3 weeks after a group A streptococcal infection of the respiratory tract or skin. Certain M serotypes are particularly associated with development of the disease [368]. The natural history is of resolution, and second attacks and progression to renal failure are rare. Poststreptococcal nephritis remains an important cause of glomerular disease in less-developed countries but is now uncommon in North America and Western Europe.

Immunofluorescence of renal biopsies reveals discrete granular deposits of immunoglobulin and complement along the capillary walls, and electron microscopy demonstrates the presence of large subepithelial immune aggregates sometimes termed "humps" [150, 200]. Assays for circulating immune complexes are often positive, there is generally a polyclonal rise in IgG and IgM, and complement levels are reduced. Most patients show a reduction in C3 concentration, whereas reduction in early classical pathway components is less frequent; these usually return to normal in about 2 months [367, 474]. A raised antibody titer to streptococcal antigens (e.g., streptolysin O) is found in a large proportion of patients.

This disease was originally considered to be due to deposition of circulating immune complexes. However, early studies of epidemic streptococcal infection weakened this argument, since microscopic hematuria was demonstrated at the onset of infection in those who would later develop the characteristic syndrome, suggesting some affinity of streptococcal antigens for the kidney [434]. It now appears likely that nephritogenic streptococcal antigens act as "planted antigens" for subsequent local immune complex formation. The precise nature of the antigens concerned is not yet clear, although there are several candidates [251, 482, 483]. Evidence for the role of these antigens includes their isolation from nephritogenic streptococci, their detection in renal biopsies, and the presence of antibodies to them in patients. Recent work supports the involvement of "endostreptosin"—a 45-kd molecule extracted from the cytoplasm of group A streptococci—as a major immunogen [105]. The development of poststreptococcal glomerulonephritis appears to depend on genetic susceptibility, as well as the characteristics of the infecting organism. This was initially suggested by family studies [369], and various MHC associations have been reported, notably with HLA-DR4 in South America [252] and with DR1 [306] and D"En" [389] in Japan.

Many other persistent infections—bacterial, viral, fungal, and protozoal—have been associated with proliferative glomerulonephritis. These have been reviewed elsewhere [186] and will not be considered in detail. The best characterized examples include organisms responsible for infective endocarditis (*Staphylococcus albus, Streptococcus faecalis* and *viridans, Coxiella burnetii*) [115, 286, 319], ventriculoatrial shunt infection (*S. albus*) [125, 398], and visceral abscesses (*Staphylococcus aureus, Pseudomonas aeruginosa*) [30].

Systemic Lupus Erythematosus. Systemic lupus erythematosus (SLE) has been widely regarded as the prototype human immune complex disease [242], with renal involvement as one of the most serious clinical features. The spectrum of lupus nephritis includes most of the clinically and histologically defined patterns of glomerulonephritis [13, 182]. Attempts have been made to classify renal involvement in SLE on a morphologic basis, and although some patients do show a consistent pattern of histology, in others the pattern differs between individual glomeruli in a single biopsy and can change considerably between sequential biopsies.

Immunofluorescence generally reveals plentiful deposits of IgG, IgM, IgA, and complement components C3, C4, and C1q in a subendothelial and/or mesangial distribution in proliferative nephritis and in a subepithelial location in membranous nephritis. Sometimes deposits are found in all sites across the capillary wall [182, 365]. Deposition of the C3 breakdown product C3d, and of the membrane attack complex of complement, has also been reported [40, 141]. Although eluted immune deposits have been shown to contain DNA and anti-DNA antibodies, this antigen-antibody system can only account for a small proportion of the immune complexes present [241].

Serologic abnormalities are widespread and include hyperglobulinemia, a variety of autoantibodies (including the diagnostic anti-dsDNA and anti-Sm antibodies), hypocomplementemia involving C1q, C4, and C3, and circulating immune complexes [6, 66, 94, 299]. However, the pathogenetic role of these autoantibodies and immune complexes and their value in monitoring activity of disease remain uncertain. In general, there is a poor correlation between anti-dsDNA antibodies, complement components, or immune complexes with severity of nephritis. In certain patients, however, the sequential changes in these factors are useful in predicting the course of the disease.

There has been considerable interest in the relationship between the characteristics of anti-dsDNA antibodies and development of nephritis. High concentrations of high-avidity precipitating antibodies have been linked to subendothelial deposits with proliferative nephritis and lower levels of nonprecipitating antibody to subepithelial deposits with membranous nephritis [16, 159, 463]. However, there is still a lack of direct evidence for the pathogenicity of anti-DNA antibodies or the immune complexes they form. Another area of interest is that normal immune complex clearance mechanisms are compromised in SLE, which could predispose to tissue deposition of potentially phlogistic complexes [401]. Abnormalities are present at all three major stages of clearance: (1) hypocomplementemia leads to impaired inhibition of precipitation, solubilization, and opsonization of complexes [294, 400, 440]; (2) there is depletion of erythrocyte receptors (CRI) for complement-reacted complexes, which form the usual route of transport in the circulation [224, 295, 489, 502]; (3) there is impairment of the capacity of the mononuclear phagocytic system to clear antibody-coated red cells or soluble immune complexes [158, 267, 488]. Although there are inherited differences in erythrocyte CRI expression, it seems likely that most of these phenomena are acquired rather than of primary pathogenic importance; they could nonetheless contribute toward disease.

Alternative explanations for the development of nephritis in SLE include the "planting" of various antigens in the glomerulus and direct reactivity of autoantibodies with antigens on glomerular components. It has been observed that DNA has an affinity for GBM and for collagen V and might therefore act as a focus for local immune deposits [168, 213]. Other work shows that monoclonal antibodies to DNA can bind directly to normal glomeruli [273]. It is also possible that histones, which have a high affinity for GBM, serve as the focus for DNA–anti-DNA aggregates [402]. Many of these studies are difficult to interpret, since anti-DNA antibodies may carry small fragments of DNA, which could be involved in binding. Antibodies to endothelial cells have also been identified in patients with SLE [80], although their reactivity with glomerular capillaries has not yet been demonstrated. Another potential target for autoimmunity is the lupus-associated membrane protein (LAMP), which is found in coated pits of the glomerular epithelial cells [214].

Genetic, hormonal, and environmental factors are important in the development of lupus but will not be considered in detail here. There is an increased incidence of disease in relatives of patients [487], and over 50 percent of monozygotic (but not dizygotic) twins are concordant for SLE [15, 42]. There are associations with HLA-DR3 [41, 77] and with null alleles of C2 and C4 [154]. A lupus-like immune complex disease is associated with genetic deficiencies of complement components, especially of C2. Functional deficiency of C4, due to inhibition of its binding to C1 by hydralazine, has been suggested as a factor in the development of SLE associated with this drug [413]. However, the factors that determine whether nephritis develops, and that influence its severity, remain to be clarified.

There is no doubt that the treatment of lupus nephritis with immunosuppressive drugs has considerably improved the outlook in this condition. Treatment with steroids was a major advance, and the introduction of azathioprine or cyclophosphamide has further improved prognosis [151]. Controlled studies of the treatment of diffuse proliferative nephritis from the National Institutes of Health reveal a better long-term outcome in patients treated with cyclophosphamide (particularly as intravenous boluses) and prednisolone, than with prednisolone alone [18]. The addition of azathioprine to prednisolone also appeared to confer benefit, although this was not statistically significant. Overall, it seems reasonable to use steroids alone for mild histologic lesions but to add a second drug for more severe disease. In life-threatening cases, high doses of intravenous methylprednisolone [233] or plasma exchange [195, 253] has been used successfully, but in these rare patients there are insufficient data to draw firm conclusions about indications or benefit.

Cryoimmunoglobulinemia. Cryoglobulinemia is frequently accompanied by nephritis, most often with a mesangiocapillary pattern [96, 179, 442]. There are three immunologically distinct forms of cryoglobulinemia [57]. Type I is the result of a paraprotein that has the property of precipitation in the cold; this type is not usually associated with clinically important nephritis and will not be considered further. Mixed cryoglobulins consist of rheumatoid factors (usually IgM) complexed with other immunoglobulins and complement; they are termed essential when there is no apparent underlying disorder. In type II cryoglobulinemia, the rheumatoid factor is monoclonal (often IgMκ), whereas in type III, rheumatoid factors are polyclonal. The physicochemical basis for cryoprecipitation is poorly understood, but this phenomenon is presumably a gross reflection of the molecular interactions that lead to in vivo immune aggregation [503].

Essential mixed cryoglobulinemia (EMC) is perhaps the best example of a human "immune complex" disease, in which nephritis occurs as part of a systemic vasculitis. There is generally profound lowering of early components of the classical pathway of complement, C1, C4, and C2, but with no (or less) change in C3 levels [111, 265, 441]. Immunofluorescence of renal tissue reveals coarse granular deposits of the constituents of the cryoglobulin (IgM, IgG, and complement) along the capillary wall. Electron microscopy in patients with a monoclonal component reveals subendothelial deposition of material with distinctive ultrastructural characteristics, similar to those that can be generated in vitro [95, 149].

The monoclonal rheumatoid factors in type II cryoglobulinemia have been found to bear common cross-reactive idiotypes, which are highly conserved and likely to represent Ig gene products in germ-line configuration [2, 244, 329]. It has been suggested that these rheumatoid factors result from paraneoplastic changes in B cells that form part of a "primitive" immune defense system, in which their role is to bind IgG Fc pieces and thus enhance opsonization of foreign antigens. The relatively high incidence of B cell lymphoma in our series of patients with type II EMC supports the notion that this is essentially a lymphoproliferative disorder [158a]. Type III cryoglobulins, on the other hand, are often associated with chronic infection, autoimmune disease, and nonlymphoid malignancy [57, 179, 442], and the polyclonal rheumatoid factors produced could therefore result from chronic antigenic stimulation or abnormalities of immune regulation.

Management of these disorders has proved unsatisfactory, but plasma exchange effectively reduces cryoglobulin levels in association with short-term clinical improvement [153]. In patients with a rapid rate of resynthesis of the cryoglobulin, the addition of cytotoxic drugs to plasmapheresis may be of value [417]. In view of the generally indolent nature of the disease, management by intermittent plasma exchange alone seems the best initial choice for many patients.

NEPHRITIS WITHOUT IMMUNE DEPOSITS

Minimal Change Nephropathy and Focal Glomerulosclerosis. These conditions generally present with nephrotic syndrome and are much commoner in childhood and early adult life. Light microscopy reveals no change or minor mesangial proliferation only in minimal change nephropathy (MCN), but shows focal and segmental areas of sclerosis in focal glomerulosclerosis (FGS) [189]. However, there are widespread ultrastructural abnormalities of glomerular epithelial cells, notably podocyte fusion, in both disorders. Some authors have adopted an operational approach to these conditions depending on their responsiveness to steroids, and it is apparent that there is considerable overlap between steroid-sensitive MCN and steroid-resistant FGS [14, 68, 446]. There are reported cases of evolution from MCN to FGS, but the presence of mild focal lesions at the time of the earlier biopsy cannot be excluded. Because of the uncertainty about the nature of these conditions, it seems appropriate to consider them together.

Although their pathogenesis remains unknown, there is strong circumstantial evidence for an immune etiology. Several disease associations have been reported, more frequently in MCN than in FGS. These include atopy [288, 462], various allergies (pollen, cow's milk, pork, drugs, and insect stings) [205, 247, 360, 387, 504], and lymphoma, notably Hodgkin's disease [100, 298, 514]. There are reports in which successful treatment of lymphoma or control of allergy has led to a favorable response of the nephrotic syndrome. However, the best evidence for an immune etiology comes from the response to immunosuppressive drugs (see below). Familial cases are well-recognized and account for approximately 3 percent of cases in Europe [493]. There are several reports of an association with HLA-DR7 in white children [9, 301, 327, 375], together with increased frequency of HLA-DQw2 and, in one report, a negative association with DR2 [327]. An association with HLA-DR8 has been found in Japan [243].

The lack of immune reactants on renal biopsy prompted the hypothesis, elaborated by Shalhoub [409], that T cells were important in pathogenesis. Despite considerable efforts, this hypothesis has not yet been confirmed. The identification of lymphocyte-derived permeability factors in various experimental systems has been widely reported; however, the evidence for their role in disease remains incomplete, and no "factor" has yet been fully characterized [248, 330, 458]. It is also possible that lymphocytes or monocytes from patients with MCN are responsible for the production of factors that affect the charge of the glomerular capillary wall. Neutralization of glomerular polyanions would reduce the charge barrier for molecules such as albumin and account for the highly selective proteinuria seen in MCN. One group has suggested a more generalized abnormality of membrane charge, following the observation of a reduction in negatively charged sites on erythrocytes and platelets [258]. These findings have not been confirmed, and there is controversy over the methodology [147].

There are also many reports of abnormal lymphocyte function in MCN, including impaired mitogen responses in vitro, decreased T suppressor cell activity, and raised IgM and/or lowered IgG concentrations [172, 297, 405, 459]. A variety of effects of sera from nephrotic patients have been recorded in different systems, including inhibition of mitogenic responses and of T suppressor cell function [209, 278, 297, 443]. In many instances, however, similar findings are obtained with sera from patients with other causes of nephrotic syndrome, and no clear overall picture has emerged. Of interest with regard to infection in MCN is that the ability of B lymphocytes to respond to antigen in a plaque-forming assay is impaired by soluble immune response suppressors (SIRS) produced by T suppressor lymphocytes, the concentration of which correlates well with disease activity [403].

The rapid response of MCN to corticosteroids is well-known, but relapse after reduction or withdrawal of therapy is common [210, 423]. Cyclophosphamide and chlorambucil are both effective in frequently relapsing patients, although toxicity is a particular concern in the young [28, 69, 447]. Of both therapeutic and immunologic interest are reports of the effectiveness of cyclosporin A in MCN, although relapse often follows withdrawal [206, 291, 445]. Since the main action of cyclosporin is to inhibit the production of IL-2 by activated T cells, its therapeutic effect provides further indirect support for the role of T lymphocytes in the pathogenesis of MCN. Recently, FK506 has also been used successfully in steroid-resistant FGS [284].

It has become apparent that FGS is by far the commonest histologic pattern found in AIDS (HIV)–associated nephropathy [353]. This disorder commonly presents with nephrotic syndrome, followed by rapid progression to end-stage renal failure. In North America, it is most frequent in black males, especially intravenous drug users. Light microscopic findings are similar to those of idiopathic FGS, although there are distinctive features, including hyperplastic and vacuolated visceral epithelial cells and severe tubulointerstitial lesions [85]. Immunofluorescence generally shows focal glomerular deposits of IgM and C3. There is still controversy over the relationship between HIV-associated nephropathy and heroin-associated nephropathy (also characterized by an FGS-like lesion) [354], since both may occur in similar groups of patients. However, HIV-associated nephropathy has been reported in children of HIV-infected mothers [436] and in recipients of contaminated blood products [49], in whom drug abuse was not a factor. The pathogenesis of HIV-associated nephropathy is not understood, but the demonstration of proviral HIV DNA in renal cells suggests a direct viral etiology [86]. This does not, however, exclude the possible role of immunologic mechanisms.

Systemic Vasculitis and Focal Necrotizing Glomerulonephritis. Focal necrotizing glomerulonephritis (FNGN) with crescent formation generally presents as rapidly progressive nephritis associated with a small-vessel vasculitis such as Wegener's granulomatosis or microscopic polyarteritis [142a, 343, 373, 395, 408]. A histologically indistinguishable form of glomerulonephritis may occur in isolation, and this is often referred to as idiopathic RPGN [25, 99, 435]. There is increasing evidence that isolated FNGN represents a localized form of small-vessel vasculitis [98, 104, 347a, 496], and we shall consider the immunology of this group of disorders together.

Despite the severity of tissue injury, there is little evidence for the involvement of humoral immune factors. Sparse granular deposits of immunoglobulins and complement are found on biopsy in a variable proportion of patients, although these are generally localized to necrotic or sclerosed glomeruli [373, 408]. Some authors have used the terms "pauci-immune" and "no immune deposit" glomerulonephritis in this context, although there is no evidence that the lesion behaves differently whether or not a few deposits are detected. Because of the presence of vasculitis in classic studies of serum sickness in animals [359], it was long presumed that immune complex mechanisms were important in human systemic vasculitis; however, despite considerable efforts, evidence for their involvement is still lacking. The lack of detectable immune deposits could be explained by their rapid clearance from the site of inflammation or by the insensitivity of methods of detection. A variety of serologic abnormalities such as circulating complexes, raised immunoglobulin concentrations, and rheumatoid factor are found in one-third to two-thirds of patients [373, 408].

More recently, interest has focused on the presence of antibodies to neutrophil cytoplasmic antigens (ANCA), first described by Davies et al. in patients with vasculitis thought to be due to viral infection [116]. It is now recognized that these autoantibodies are found in the great majority of patients with active Wegener's granulomatosis and microscopic polyarteritis [395a, 476] as well as in cases of idiopathic RPGN [140]. Two different patterns of ANCA can be recognized by indirect immunofluorescence of patients' sera on ethanol-fixed normal neutrophils (Fig. 60-12): (1) diffuse granular cytoplasmic staining, known as C-ANCA, and (2) perinuclear staining, known as P-ANCA. Although there is some overlap in most studies, C-ANCA are generally associated with Wegener's granulomatosis (and some cases of microscopic polyarteritis), and P-ANCA with microscopic polyarteritis and idiopathic RPGN [216, 326, 475]. The antigenic targets of these autoantibodies have not been conclusively identified. However, there is increasing evidence that most C-ANCA recognize a neutrophil serine proteinase (proteinase 3) [178, 270, 322] and that P-ANCA generally recognize myeloperoxidase [140]. Whether ANCA have a pathogenic role in systemic vasculitis remains uncertain, although they have proved of value in monitoring disease activity [326, 421] and predicting patients at risk of relapse [87, 166]. It is also re-

Fig. 60-12. Indirect immunofluorescence of ethanol-fixed normal human neutrophils demonstrating (A) granular cytoplasmic staining (C-ANCA) with serum from a patient with Wegener's granulomatosis and (B) perinuclear staining (P-ANCA) with serum from a patient with microscopic polyarteritis.

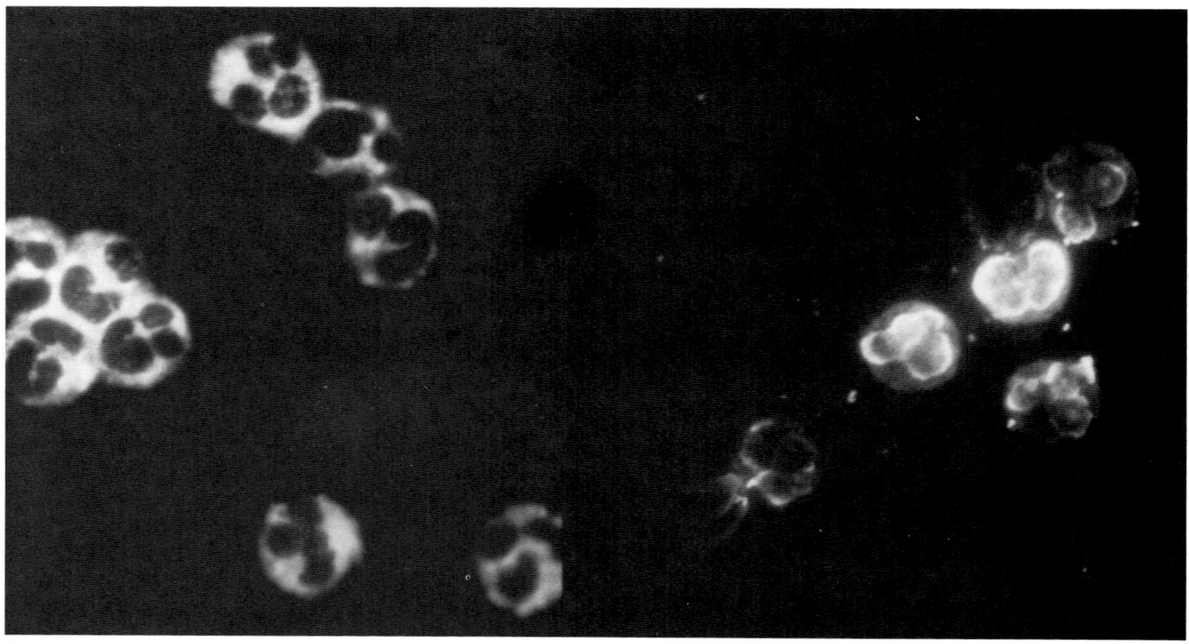

ported that they can induce neutrophil degranulation and oxygen radical production in vitro [141a], which could lead to enhanced neutrophil cytotoxicity to endothelial cells. There are recent reports of antibodies binding to endothelial cells in ELISA systems [152, 393], which are apparently not cross-reactive with ANCA, of antibodies that cause lysis of endothelial cells in vitro [54], and of antibodies binding to glomerular endothelial and epithelial cells in culture [1].

The relative lack of immune deposits in this disorder has prompted suggestions that T cells are directly involved in glomerular injury in FNGN. Immunohistology using monoclonal antibodies to T cell subsets has confirmed the presence of both CD4- and CD8-bearing T lymphocytes in the glomeruli and adjacent interstitium [42b, 325, 424]. The CD4+ cells could be involved in signaling to macrophages, which are the predominant inflammatory cells in crescentic nephritis [48, 274]. However, the mechanisms of glomerular inflammation in FNGN remain uncertain, and there is as yet no good animal model (see above).

Genetic factors are likely to be important in susceptibility to disease. There are several pairs of siblings with Wegener's granulomatosis, and in one report they had lived apart for years, making a common environmental cause unlikely [239]. An association with HLA-DR2 (defined serologically) has been reported in both Wegener's granulomatosis [135], and idiopathic RPGN [302], although these studies involved small numbers. More recently, a study using RFLP analysis and oligonucleotide typing has demonstrated a strong positive association with DQw7, a weaker association with DR4, and a negative association with DR3 [421a]. Environmental factors may also be involved in the etiology of systemic vasculitis. Polyarteritis has been associated with hepatitis B [292], there is a history of long-standing respiratory or pulmonary disease in many patients with Wegener's granulomatosis [343], there are several reports of drug-associated systemic vasculitis [26, 279], and crescentic nephritis may also be associated with neoplasia [39] and deep-seated visceral abscesses [30].

This group of disorders generally shows an excellent response to immunosuppressive drugs. The use of steroids alone led to only a slight improvement in the prognosis of systemic vasculitis. However, the addition of cyclophosphamide resulted in benefit in the majority of cases [25, 142a]. It now seems clear that renal disease improves in almost all patients (with Wegener's granulomatosis or microscopic polyarteritis) treated with oral prednisolone and cyclophosphamide, unless they are already on dialysis. In patients with advanced disease, the addition of plasma exchange has been shown to lead to an improved renal outcome [199, 349]. Uncontrolled studies suggest that high-dose intravenous methylprednisolone may also confer short-term benefit in this situation [42c]. Reports of the benefit of co-trimoxazole in indolent or limited Wegener's granulomatosis require confirmation, since it is possible that such treatment acts by control of infection (known to exacerbate disease) rather than on the underlying vasculitis [121]. There are also a few reports of the successful use of cyclosporin A [181], although these require confirmation.

Acute Interstitial Nephritis. This clinicopathologic syndrome presents with a generally self-limiting form of acute renal failure, which is accompanied histologically by interstitial infiltration with lymphocytes, plasma cells, macrophages, and sometimes eosinophils. The great majority of cases in developed countries are associated with allergic reactions to drugs, most commonly antibiotics (penicillins, sulphonamides, and rifampicin), nonsteroidal anti-inflammatory agents, diuretics, and anticonvulsants [33, 64, 236, 350]. Interestingly, patients with interstitial nephritis related to nonsteroidal drugs may also develop nephrotic syndrome with minimal change glomerular histology [155]. Evidence that these reactions involve hypersensitivity mechanisms includes (1) frequent presence of rash and eosinophilia, particularly in antibiotic-associated cases; (2) occurrence in only a small number of patients exposed to normal (nontoxic) doses of the drug; (3) recurrence on reexposure to the drug in a few reported cases; and (4) response to corticosteroid therapy. However, the mechanisms involved remain unknown, and there is no comparable experimental model of TIN (see above).

There are a few early reports suggesting the involvement of humoral mechanisms, for example, circulating and fixed anti-TBM antibodies [45, 207, 410], and immune deposits containing penicillin-derived antigens and immunoglobulin [22, 45], but these have not been detected in many more similar cases. The histologic findings are suggestive of the predominant role of cell-mediated mechanisms, and several studies have identified both CD4+ and CD8+ lymphocytes in the interstitial infiltrate [33, 155, 174]. In a few cases, specific drug sensitivity has been suggested by in vitro studies of lymphocyte function [91, 207, 410]. Although there are no controlled data, the usual rapid response to steroids is impressive and provides indirect evidence for the involvement of immune mechanisms [164, 350].

Interstitial nephritis also occurs in association with infections, historically most often streptococcal and diphtherial, but a range of different organisms has been implicated [64]. In some cases, the microorganism may have a direct pathogenic effect, but others are probably due to the resulting immune reaction. Several systemic diseases and primary glomerulonephritides are associated with immune deposits on the TBM and interstitial nephritis. These include SLE, EMC, Sjögren's syndrome, anti-GBM disease, and MCGN [11, 56, 256, 276, 285, 502a]. Whether the tubular lesions are due to deposition of immune reactants similar to those responsible for the glomerular lesions is not known. There are also rare but well-documented instances of isolated "anti-TBM" disease, in which circulating and fixed anti-TBM antibodies have been demonstrated [38, 73a, 235, 335]; some of these have followed renal transplantation. The antigenic target of anti-TBM antibodies has been isolated as a 48-kd glycoprotein from collagenase-solubilized human TBM [81a]. A granulomatous interstitial nephritis may occur in sarcoidosis and is occasionally the presenting feature [272, 293]. A recently described and rare oculorenal syndrome of unknown etiology is acute TIN with uveitis [432, 477].

Conclusions

Despite the explosive growth of immunology, and more recently molecular biology, there have been relatively few important advances in the immunotherapy of nephritis. This reflects in part our incomplete knowledge of the molecular basis of autoimmune reactions affecting the kidney, as well as a lack of new and clinically applicable immunotherapeutic agents. However, what has been learned clearly points the way to the development of techniques of specific immune intervention. The majority of diseases discussed in this chapter are now perceived as autoimmune, and a central role for T lymphocytes in their induction, if not in mediation of tissue injury, seems highly probable. There is increasing evidence from experimental autoimmune diseases, including some models of nephritis described above, that methods of blocking the interaction between MHC class II gene products, autoantigenic peptides, and the T-cell receptor can be therapeutically effective [510]. The development of monoclonal antibodies to these components—"humanized" by recombinant DNA technology—offers considerable promise for the control of autoimmunity in humans. A successful example of this approach, using monoclonal antibodies to T cells, has recently been reported in a patient with vasculitis [280]. Knowledge of the effector mechanisms involved in glomerular inflammation, particularly the role of various cytokines, is also increasing rapidly. Whether antibodies to or antagonists of proinflammatory cytokines would be effective in limiting renal injury, as in experimental nephritis, is not yet known. Although we have seen major advances in understanding the immunopathology of nephritis since the last edition of this book, it remains disappointing that these have not yet led to more therapeutic innovations.

References

1. Abbott, F., Jones, S., Lockwood, C. M., and Rees, A. J. Autoantibodies to glomerular antigens in patients with Wegener's granulomatosis. *Nephrol. Dial. Transplant.* 4: 1, 1989.
2. Abraham, G. N., Podell, D. N., Welch, E. H., et al. Idiotypic relatedness of human monoclonal IgG cryoglobulins. *Immunology* 48: 315, 1983.
3. Adelman, N., Watting, D., and McDevitt, H. O. Treatment of NZB/W F1 disease with monoclonal anti-I-A antibodies. *J. Exp. Med.* 158: 1350, 1983.
4. Adler, S., Salant, D. J., Dittmer, J. E., et al. Mediation of proteinuria in membranous nephropathy due to a planted glomerular antigen. *Kidney Int.* 23: 807, 1983.
5. Adler, S. G., Wang, H., Ward, H. J., et al. Electrical charge. Its role in the pathogenesis and prevention of experimental membranous nephropathy in the rabbit. *J. Clin. Invest.* 71: 487, 1983.
6. Adu, D., Dobson, J., and Williams, D. G. DNA-anti-DNA circulating complexes in the nephritis of systemic lupus erythematosus. *Clin. Exp. Immunol.* 43: 605, 1981.
7. Agodoa, L. Y., Gauthier, V. J., and Mannik, M. Precipitating antigen–antibody systems are required for the formation of subepithelial electron-dense immune deposits in rat glomeruli. *J. Exp. Med.* 158: 1259, 1983.
8. Agus, D., Mann, R., Clayman, M., et al. The effects of daily cyclophosphamide administration on the development and extent of primary experimental interstitial nephritis in rats. *Kidney Int.* 29: 635, 1986.
9. Alfifer, C. A., Roy, L. P., Doran, T., et al. HLA-DR7 and steroid responsive nephrotic syndrome. *Clin. Nephrol.* 14: 71, 1980.
10. Almquist, R. D., Buckalew, V. M., Hirszel, P., et al. Recurrence of antiglomerular basement membrane antibody mediated glomerulonephritis in an isograft. *Clin. Immunol. Immunopathol.* 18: 54, 1981.
11. Andres, G., Brentjens, J., Kohli, R., et al. Histology of human tubulo-interstitial nephritis associated with antibodies to renal basement membranes. *Kidney Int.* 13: 480, 1978.
12. Andrzejewski, C., Rauch, J., Lafer, E. M., et al. Antigen binding diversity and idiotypic cross-reactions among hybridoma autoantibodies to DNA. *J. Immunol.* 126: 226, 1980.
13. Appel, G. B., Silva, F. G., and Pirani, C. L. Renal involvement in systemic lupus erythematosus (SLE): A study of 56 patients emphasising histologic classification. *Medicine* 57: 371, 1978.
14. Arbus, G. S., Poncell, S., Bachagie, G. S., et al. Focal segmental glomerulosclerosis with idiopathic nephrotic syndrome. *J. Pediatr.* 101: 40, 1982.
15. Arnett, F. C., and Schulman, L. E. Studies in familial systemic lupus erythematosus. *Medicine* 55: 313, 1976.
16. Asano, Y., and Nakamoto, Y. Avidity of anti-native DNA antibody and glomerular immune complex localisation in lupus nephritis. *Clin. Nephrol.* 10: 134, 1978.
17. Atkins, R. C., Holdsworth, S. R., Glasgow, E. F., et al. The macrophage in human rapidly progressive glomerulonephritis. *Lancet* 1: 830, 1976.
18. Austin, H. A., Klippel, J. H., Balow, J. E., et al. Therapy of lupus nephritis: Controlled trial of prednisolone and cytotoxic drugs. *N. Engl. J. Med.* 514: 614, 1986.
19. Avasthi, P. S., Avasthi, P., Tokuda, S., et al. Experimental glomerulonephritis in the mouse. I. The model. *Clin. Exp. Immunol.* 9: 667, 1971.
20. Bagchus, W. M., Hoedemaeker, P. J., Rozing, J., and Bakker, W. W. Glomerulonephritis induced by monoclonal anti-Thy 1.1 antibodies: A sequential histological and ultrastructural study in the rat. *Lab. Invest.* 55: 680, 1986.
21. Bagchus, W. M., Vos, J. T. W. M., Hoedemaeker, P. J., and Bakker, W. W. The specificity of nephritogenic antibodies: III. Binding of anti-FxIA antibodies in glomeruli is dependent on dual specificity. *Clin. Exp. Immunol.* 63: 639, 1986.
22. Baldwin, D. S., Levine, B. B., McCluskey, R. T., et al. Renal failure and interstitial nephritis due to penicillin and methicillin. *N. Engl. J. Med.* 279: 1245, 1968.
23. Baldwin, D. S., Lowenstein, J., Rothfield, N. F., et al. The clinical course of the proliferative and membranous forms of lupus nephritis. *Ann. Intern. Med.* 73: 929, 1970.
24. Ballardie, F. W., Brenchley, P. E. C., and Williams, S. Autoimmunity in IgA nephropathy. *Lancet* 2: 598, 1988.
25. Balow, J. E. Renal vasculitis. *Kidney Int.* 27: 954, 1985.
26. Banfi, G., Imbasciati, E., and Guerra, L. Extracapillary glomerulonephritis with necrotizing vasculitis in D-penicillamine treated rheumatoid arthritis. *Nephron* 33: 56, 1983.
27. Baran, D., Vendeville, B., Vial, M. C., et al. Effect of cy-

closporin A on mercury-induced autoimmune glomerulonephritis in the Brown Norway rat. *Clin. Nephrol.* 25: 175, 1986.
28. Barratt, T. M., Burcowsky, A., Osafsky, S. G., et al. Cyclophosphamide treatment in steroid-sensitive nephrotic syndrome of childhood. *Lancet* 1: 55, 1975.
29. Barton, C. K., Vazin, N. D., and Spear, G. S. Nephrotic syndrome associated with adenocarcinoma of the breast. *Am. J. Med.* 68: 308, 1980.
30. Beaufils, M., Morel-Maroger, L., Sraer, J. D., et al. Acute renal failure of glomerular origin during visceral abscesses. *N. Engl. J. Med.* 295: 185, 1976.
31. Beirne, G. J., and Brennan, J. T. Glomerulonephritis associated with hydrocarbon solvents. *Arch. Environ. Health* 25: 365, 1972.
32. Bellon, B., Belair, M. F., Kuhn, J., et al. Trapping of circulating proteins in immune deposits of Heymann nephritis. *Lab. Invest.* 46: 306, 1982.
33. Bender, W. L., Whetton, A., Beschormer, W. E., et al. Interstitial nephritis, proteinuria and renal failure caused by non-steroidal anti-inflammatory drugs. *Am. J. Med.* 76: 1006, 1984.
34. Benoit, F. L., Rulon, C. B., Theil, G. B., et al. Goodpasture's syndrome. A clinicopathologic entity. *Am. J. Med.* 37: 424, 1964.
35. Berger, J. IgA mesangial nephropathy 1968–1983. *Contrib. Nephrol.* 40: 4, 1984.
36. Berger, J., and Hinglais, N. Les depots intercapillaires d'IgA-IgG. *J. Urol. Nephrol.* 74: 694, 1968.
37. Berger, M., Balow, J. E., Wilson, C. B., et al. Circulating immune complexes and glomerulonephritis in a patient with congenital absence of the third component of complement. *N. Engl. J. Med.* 308: 1009, 1983.
38. Bergstein, J., and Litman, N. Interstitial nephritis with anti-tubular basement membrane antibody. *N. Engl. J. Med.* 292: 875, 1975.
39. Biara, C. G., Gonwa, T. A., Naughton, J. L., and Hopper, J. R. Crescentic glomerulonephritis associated with non-renal malignancies. *Am. J. Nephrol.* 4: 208, 1984.
40. Biesecker, G., Katz, S. M., and Koffler, D. Renal localization of the membrane attack complex in systemic lupus erythematosus nephritis. *J. Exp. Med.* 154: 1779, 1981.
41. Black, C. M., Welsh, K. I., Fielder, A., et al. HLA antigens and Bf allotypes in SLE: Evidence for the association being with specific haplotypes. *Tissue Antigens* 19: 115, 1982.
42. Block, S. R., Winfield, J. B., Lockshin, M. D., et al. Studies of twins with systemic lupus erythematosus: A review of the literature and presentation of 12 additional sets. *Am. J. Med.* 59: 533, 1975.
42a. Bolton, W. K., Chandra, M., Tyson, T. M., et al. Transfer of experimental glomerulonephritis in chickens by mononuclear cells. *Kidney Int.* 34: 598, 1988.
42b. Bolton, W. K., Innes, D., Sturgill, B. C., and Kaiser, D. L. T cells and macrophages in rapidly progressive glomerulonephritis: Clinicopathological correlations. *Kidney Int.* 32: 869, 1987.
42c. Bolton, W. K., and Sturgill, B. C. Methylprednisolone therapy for acute crescentic rapidly progressive nephritis. *Am. J. Nephrol.* 9: 368, 1989.
43. Bolton, W. K., Tucker, F. L., and Sturgill, B. C. New avian model of experimental glomerulonephritis consistent with mediation by cellular immunity. *J. Clin. Invest.* 73: 1263, 1984.
44. Bonsib, S. M. Glomerular basement membrane necrosis and crescent organisation. *Kidney Int.* 33: 966, 1988.
45. Border, W. A., Lehman, D. H., Egon, J. D., et al. Antitubular basement membrane antibodies in methicillin-associated interstitial nephritis. *N. Engl. J. Med.* 291: 381, 1974.
46. Border, W. A., Okuda, S., Languino, L. R., et al. Suppression of experimental glomerulonephritis by antiserum against transforming growth factor B1. *Nature* 346: 371, 1990.
47. Border, W. A., Ward, H. J., Kamil, E. S., et al. Induction of membranous nephropathy in rabbits by administration of an exogenous cationic antigen. *J. Clin. Invest.* 69: 451, 1982.
48. Boucher, A., Droz, D., Adafer, E., and Noel, L. H. Relationship between the integrity of Bowman's capsule and the composition of crescents in human crescentic glomerulonephritis. *Lab. Invest.* 56: 526, 1987.
49. Bourgoignie, J. J., Meneses, R., Ortiz, C., et al. The clinical spectrum of renal disease associated with human immunodeficiency virus. *Am. J. Kidney Dis.* 12: 131, 1988.
50. Bowman, C., and Lockwood, C. M. Clinical application of a radio-immunoassay for auto-antibodies to glomerular basement membrane. *J. Clin. Lab. Immunol.* 17: 197, 1985.
51. Bowman, C., Mason, D. W., Pusey, C. D., et al. Autoregulation of autoantibody synthesis in mercuric chloride nephritis in the Brown Norway rat. I. A role for T suppressor cells. *Eur. J. Immunol.* 14: 464, 1984.
52. Boyce, N. W., and Holdsworth, S. R. Hydroxyl radical mediation of immune renal injury by desferrioxamine. *Kidney Int.* 30: 813, 1986.
53. Boyce, N. W., and Holdsworth, S. R. Macrophage Fc-receptor affinity: Role in cellular mediation of antibody initiated glomerulonephritis. *Kidney Int.* 36: 537, 1989.
54. Brasile, L., Kremer, J. M., Clarke, J. L., and Cerilli, J. Identification of an autoantibody to vascular endothelial cell-specific antigens in patients with systemic vasculitis. *Am. J. Med.* 87: 74, 1989.
55. Brentjens, J. R., and Andres, G. Interaction of antibodies with renal cell surface antigens. *Kidney Int.* 35: 954, 1989.
56. Brentjens, J. R., Sepulveda, M., Baliah, T. J., et al. Interstitial immune complex nephritis in patients with systemic lupus erythematosus. *Kidney Int.* 7: 342, 1975.
57. Brouet, J.-C., Clanvel, J.-P., Danon, F., et al. Biologic and clinical significance of cryoglobulins: A report of 86 cases. *Am. J. Med.* 57: 775, 1974.
58. Brown, A. C., Carey, K., and Colvin, R. B. Inhibition of autoimmune tubulointerstitial nephritis in guinea pigs by heterologous antisera containing anti-idiotype antibodies. *J. Immunol.* 123: 2102, 1979.
59. Burns, A., So, A., Pusey, C. D., and Rees, A. J. The susceptibility to Goodpasture's syndrome (abstract). *Q. J. Med.* 77: 1094, 1990.
60. Butkowski, R. J., Langeveld, J. P. M., Wieslander, J., et al. Localization of the Goodpasture epitope to a novel chain of basement membrane collagen. *J. Biol. Chem.* 262: 7874, 1987.
61. Butkowski, R. J., Shen, G.-Q., Wieslander, J., et al. Characterisation of type IV collagen NC1 monomers and Goodpasture antigen in human renal basement membranes. *J. Lab. Clin. Med.* 115: 365, 1990.
62. Butkowski, R. J., Weislander, J., Wisdom, B. J., et al. Properties of the globular domain of Type IV collagen and its relationship to the Goodpasture antigen. *J. Biol. Chem.* 260: 3739, 1985.
63. Cameron, J. S. Pathogenesis and treatment of membranous nephropathy. *Kidney Int.* 15: 88, 1979.

64. Cameron, J. S. Allergic interstitial nephritis: Clinical features and pathogenesis. *Q. J. Med.* 66: 97, 1988.
65. Cameron, J. S. The Long Term Outcome of Glomerular Diseases. In R. W. Schrier and C. W. Gottschalk (eds.), *Diseases of the Kidney* (4th ed.). Boston: Little, Brown, 1988. P. 2127.
65a. Cameron, J. S., Healey, M. J. R., and Adu, D. The MRC trial of short term high dose alternate day prednisolone in idiopathic membranous nephropathy with nephrotic syndrome in adults. *Q. J. Med.* 74: 133, 1990.
66. Cameron, J. S., Lessoff, M. H., Ogg, C. S., et al. Disease activity in the nephritis of systemic lupus erythematosus in relation to serum complement concentrations. *Clin. Exp. Immunol.* 25: 418, 1976.
67. Cameron, J. S., Turner, D. R., Heaton, J., et al. Idiopathic mesangiocapillary glomerulonephritis. *Am. J. Med.* 74: 175, 1983.
68. Cameron, J. S., Turner, D. R., Ogg, C. S., et al. The long term prognosis of patients with focal segmental glomerulonephritis. *Clin. Nephrol.* 10: 213, 1978.
69. Cameron, J. S., Turner, D. R., Ogg, C. S., et al. The nephrotic syndrome in adults with 'minimal change' glomerular lesions. *Q. J. Med.* 43: 461, 1984.
70. Camussi, G., Brentjens, J. R., Noble, B., et al. Antibody-induced redistribution of Heymann antigen on the surface of cultured glomerular visceral epithelial cells: Possible role in the pathogenesis of Heymann glomerulonephritis. *J. Immunol.* 135: 2409, 1985.
71. Carteron, N. L., Schimenti, C. L., and Wofsy, D. Treatment of murine lupus with $F(ab)_2$ fragments of monoclonal antibody to L3T4. *J. Immunol.* 142: 1470, 1989.
72. Cashman, S. J., Pusey, C. D., and Evans, D. J. Extraglomerular distribution of immunoreactive Goodpasture antigen. *J. Pathol.* 155: 61, 1988.
73. Cattel, V., Smith, J., and Cook, H. T. Prostaglandin E_1 suppresses macrophage infiltration and ameliorates injury in an experimental model of macrophage-dependent glomerulonephritis. *Clin. Exp. Immunol.* 79: 260, 1990.
73a. Cattran, D. C. Circulating anti-tubular basement membrane antibody in a variety of human renal diseases. *Nephron* 26: 13, 1980.
74. Cattran, D. C., Cardella, C. J., Roscoe, J. M., et al. Results of a controlled drug trial in membranoproliferative glomerulonephritis. *Kidney Int.* 27: 436, 1985.
75. Cederholm, B., Wieslander, J., and Bygren, P. Patients with IgA nephropathy have circulating anti-basement membrane antibodies reacting with structures common to collagen I, II and IV. *Proc. Natl. Acad. Sci. U.S.A.* 83: 6151, 1986.
76. Cederholm, B., Wieslander, J., and Bygren, P. Circulating complexes containing IgA and fibronectin in patients with primary IgA nephropathy. *Proc. Natl. Acad. Sci. U.S.A.* 85: 4865, 1988.
77. Celada, A., Barras, C., Benzonana, G., et al. Increased frequency of HLA-DRw3 in systemic lupus erythematosus. *Tissue Antigens* 15: 283, 1980.
78. Chalopin, J. M., and Lockwood, C. M. Auto-regulation of auto-antibody synthesis in mercuric chloride nephritis in the Brown Norway rat II: Presence of antigen augmentable plaque forming cells in the spleen is associated with humoral factors behaving as auto-anti-idiotypic antibodies. *Eur. J. Immunol.* 14: 470, 1984.
79. Cheng, I. K. P., Dorsch, S. E., and Hall, B. M. The regulation of autoantibody production in Heymann's nephritis by T lymphocyte subsets. *Lab. Invest.* 59: 780, 1988.
80. Cines, D. B., Lyss, A. P., Reeber, M. B., and De Horatius, R. J. Presence of complement-fixing anti-endothelial cell antibodies in systemic lupus erythematosus. *J. Clin. Invest.* 73: 611, 1984.
81. Clayman, M., Martinez-Hernandez, A., Michaud, L., et al. Isolation and characterisation of the nephritogenic antigen producing anti-tubular basement membrane disease. *J. Exp. Med.* 161: 290, 1985.
81a. Clayman, M. D., Michaud, L., Bretjens, J., et al. Isolation of the target antigen in human anti-tubular basement membrane nephritis. *J. Clin. Invest.* 77: 1143, 1986.
82. Cochrane, C. G., and Koffler, D. Immune complex disease in experimental animals and man. *Adv. Immunol.* 16: 185, 1973.
83. Cochrane, C. G., Unanue, E. R., and Dixon, F. J. A role of polymorphonuclear leucocytes and complement in nephrotoxic nephritis. *J. Exp. Med.* 122: 99, 1965.
84. Coggins, C. H. A controlled study of short-term prednisolone treatment in adults with membranous nephropathy. *N. Engl. J. Med.* 301: 1301, 1979.
85. Cohen, A. H., and Nast, C. C. HIV-associated nephropathy: A unique combined glomerular, tubular and interstitial lesion. *Mod. Pathol.* 1: 87, 1988.
86. Cohen, A. H., Sun, N. C. J., Shapshak, P., et al. Demonstration of human immunodeficiency virus in renal epithelium in HIV-associated nephropathy. *Mod. Pathol.* 2: 125, 1989.
87. Cohen-Tervaert, J. W., van der Woude, F. J., Fauci, A. S., et al. Prevention of relapse in Wegener's granulomatosis by treatment based on anti-neutrophil cytoplasmic antibody titre. *Lancet* 336: 709, 1990.
88. Coleman, T. H., Forristal, J., Kosaka, T., et al. Inherited complement component deficiencies in membranoproliferative glomerulonephritis. *Kidney Int.* 24: 681, 1983.
89. Collins, A. B., Andres, G., and McCluskey, R. T. Lack of evidence for a role of renal tubular antigen in human membranous glomerulonephritis. *Nephron* 27: 197, 1981.
90. Collins, A. B., Bhan, A. K., Dienstag, J. L., et al. Hepatitis B immune complex glomerulonephritis: Simultaneous glomerular deposition of hepatitis B surface and e antigens. *Clin. Immunol. Immunopathol.* 26: 137, 1983.
91. Colvin, R. B., Burton, J. R., Hyslop, M. E., et al. Penicillin-associated interstitial nephritis. *Ann. Intern. Med.* 81: 404, 1974.
92. Conley, M. E., Cooper, M. D., and Michael, A. F. Selective deposition of IgA_1 in immunoglobulin A nephropathy, anaphylactoid purpura nephritis and systemic lupus erythematosus. *J. Clin. Invest.* 66: 1432, 1980.
93. Coppo, R., Basolo, B., and Grachino, O. Plasmapheresis in a patient with rapidly progressive idiopathic IgA nephropathy: Removal of IgA containing circulating immune complexes and clinical recovery. *Nephron* 40: 488, 1985.
94. Coppo, R., Bosticardo, G. M., Basoli, B., et al. Clinical significance of the detection of circulating immune complexes in lupus nephritis. *Nephron* 32: 320, 1982.
95. Cordonnier, D., Martin, H., Groslambert, P., et al. Mixed IgG-IgM cryoglobulinaemia with glomerulonephritis. *Am. J. Med.* 59: 867, 1975.
96. Cordonnier, D., Vialtel, P., Renversez, J. C., et al. Renal diseases in 18 patients with mixed type II IgM-IgG cryoglobulinaemia: Monoclonal lymphoid infiltration (2 cases) and membranoproliferative glomerulonephritis (14 cases). *Adv. Nephrol.* 12: 177, 1983.
97. Cosio, F. G., Lam, S., Folami, A. O., et al. Immune regulation of immunoglobulin production in IgA nephropathy. *Clin. Immunol. Immunopathol.* 23: 430, 1982.

98. Couser, G. W. Rapidly progressive glomerulonephritis: Classification, pathogenetic mechanisms and therapy. *Am. J. Kidney Dis.* 6: 449, 1988.
99. Couser, W. G. Idiopathic rapidly progressive glomerulonephritis. *Am. J. Nephrol.* 2: 57, 1982.
100. Couser, W., Badger, A., Cooperband, S., et al. Hodgkin's disease and lipoid nephritis. *Lancet* 1: 912, 1977.
101. Couser, W. G., and Salant, D. J. In situ immune complex formation and glomerular injury. *Kidney Int.* 17: 1, 1980.
102. Couser, W. G., Steinmuller, D. R., Stilmant, M. M., et al. Experimental glomerulonephritis in the isolated perfused rat kidney. *J. Clin. Invest.* 62: 1275, 1978.
103. Couser, W. G., Stilmant, M., and Lewis, E. J. Experimental glomerulonephritis in the guinea pig. I. Glomerular lesions associated with antiglomerular basement antibody deposits. *Lab. Invest.* 29: 236, 1973.
104. Croker, B. P., Lee, T., Cauille Gunnell, S. J., et al. Clinical and pathologic features of polyarteritis nodosa and its renal-limited variant: Primary crescentic and necrotizing glomerulonephritis. *Hum. Pathol.* 18: 38, 1987.
105. Cronin, W., Deal, H., Azadegan, A., and Lange, K. Endostreptosin: Isolation of the probable immunogen of acute post-streptococcal glomerulonephritis. *Clin. Exp. Immunol.* 76: 198, 1989.
106. Cybulsky, A. V., Quigg, R. J., and Salant, D. J. The membrane attack complex in complement-mediated glomerular epithelial cell injury: Formation and stability of C5b-9 and C5b-7 in rat membranous nephropathy. *J. Immunol.* 137: 1511, 1986.
107. Daha, M., Austen, K. F., and Fearon, D. T. Heterogeneity, polypeptide chain composition and antigenic reactivity of C3 nephritic factor. *J. Immunol.* 120: 1389, 1978.
108. Daha, M., Fearon, D. T., and Austen, K. F. C3 nephritic factor (C3 NeF): Stabilisation of fluid phase and cell bound alternative pathway convertase. *J. Immunol.* 116: 1, 1976.
109. Daha, M. R., Hazevoet, H. M., Van Es, L. A., et al. Stabilization of the classical pathway C3 convertase C42 by a factor F42 isolated from serum of patients with systemic lupus erythematosus. *Immunology* 40: 417, 1980.
110. D'Amico, G. The commonest glomerulonephritis in the world: IgA nephropathy. *Q. J. Med.* 64: 709, 1987.
111. D'Amico, G., Ferrario, F., Colosanti, G., and Bucci, A. Glomerulonephritis in essential mixed cryoglobulinaemia. *Proc. Eur. Dial. Transplant. Assoc.* 21: 527, 1984.
112. D'Amico, G., Imbasciati, E., Barbians di Belgioioso, G., et al. Idiopathic IgA mesangial nephropathy: Clinical and histological study of 374 patients. *Medicine* 64: 49, 1985.
113. D'Apice, A. J. F., Kincaid-Smith, P., Becker, G. J., et al. Goodpasture's syndrome in identical twins. *Ann. Intern. Med.* 88: 61, 1978.
114. Date, A., Neela, P., and Shastry, J. C. M. Membranoproliferative glomerulonephritis in a tropical environment. *Ann. Trop. Med. Parasitol.* 77: 279, 1983.
115. Dathan, J. R. E., and Heyworth, M. F. Glomerulonephritis associated with *Coxiella burnetii* endocarditis. *Br. Med. J.* 1: 326, 1975.
116. Davies, D. J., Moran, J. E., Niall, J. F., and Ryan, G. B. Segmental necrotising glomerulonephritis with antineutrophil antibody: Possible arbovirus aetiology. *Br. Med. J.* 285: 606, 1982.
117. Davis, A. E., Ziegler, J. B., Gelfand, E. W., et al. Heterogeneity of nephritic factor and its identification as an immunoglobulin. *Proc. Natl. Acad. Sci. U.S.A.* 74: 3980, 1977.
118. De Heer, E., Daha, M. R., Bhakdi, S., et al. Possible involvement of terminal complement complex in active Heymann nephritis. *Kidney Int.* 27: 388, 1985.
119. De Heer, E., Daha, M. R., and Van Es, L. A. The autoimmune response in active Heymann's nephritis in Lewis rats is regulated by T lymphocyte subsets. *Cell. Immunol.* 92: 254, 1985.
120. Demaine, A. G., Rambausek, M., and Knight, J. F. Relation of mesangial IgA glomerulonephritis to polymorphism of immunoglobulin heavy chain switch region. *J. Clin. Invest.* 81: 611, 1988.
121. De Remee, R. A., McDonald, T. J., and Welland, L. H. Wegener's granulomatosis: Observations on treatment with antimicrobial agents. *Mayo Clin. Proc.* 60: 27, 1985.
122. Derry, C. J., Dunn, M. J., Rees, A. J., and Pusey, C. D. Restricted specificity of the autoantibody response in Goodpasture's syndrome demonstrated by two-dimensional Western blotting. *Clin. Exp. Immunol.* 86: 457, 1991.
123. Devey, M. E., Bleasdale, K., Stanley, C., et al. Failure of affinity maturation leads to increased susceptibility to immune complex glomerulonephritis. *Immunology* 52: 377, 1984.
124. Dixon, F. J., Feldman, J. D., and Vazquez, J. J. Experimental glomerulonephritis. The pathogenesis of a laboratory model resembling the spectrum of human glomerulonephritis. *J. Exp. Med.* 113: 899, 1961.
125. Dobrin, R. S., Day, N. K., Quie, P. G., et al. The role of complement, immunoglobulin and bacterial antigen in coagulase-negative staphylococcal shunt nephritis. *Am. J. Med.* 59: 660, 1975.
126. Donaghy, M., and Rees, A. J. Cigarette smoking and lung haemorrhage in glomerulonephritis caused by autoantibodies to glomerular basement membrane. *Lancet* 2: 1390, 1983.
127. Donker, A. J., Venuto, R. C., Vladutin, A. O., et al. Effects of prolonged administration of D-penicillamine or captopril in various strains of rats. *Clin. Immunol. Immunopathol.* 30: 142, 1984.
128. Druet, E., Sapin, C., Fournie, G., et al. Genetic control of susceptibility to mercury-induced immune nephritis in various strains of rat. *Clin. Immunol. Immunopathol.* 25: 203, 1982.
129. Druet, P., Druet, E., Potdevin, F., et al. Immune type glomerulonephritis induced by $HgCl_2$ in the Brown Norway rat. *Ann. Immunol. (Paris)* 129C: 777, 1978.
130. Duncan, D. A., Drummond, K. N., Michael, A. F., et al. Pulmonary hemorrhage and glomerulonephritis. Report of six cases and study of the renal lesion by fluorescent antibody technique and electron microscopy. *Ann. Intern. Med.* 62: 920, 1965.
131. Ebert, T. H., McCluskey, R. T., Collins, A. B., et al. Modulation of autologous immune complex nephritis (AIC) by preimmunisation with autoantibodies or sensitised cells. *Kidney Int.* 19: 181, 1981.
132. Edgington, T. S., Glassock, R. J., and Dixon, F. J. Autologous immune complex nephritis induced with renal tubular antigens. I. Identification and isolation of the pathogenetic antigen. *J. Exp. Med.* 127: 555, 1968.
133. Egido, J., Jillian, B. A., and Wyatt, R. J. Genetic factors in primary IgA nephropathy. *Nephrol. Dial. Transplant.* 2: 134, 1987.
134. Egido, K., Sancho, J., Rivera, F., et al. The role of IgA and IgG immune complexes in IgA nephropathy. *Nephron* 36: 52, 1984.
135. Elkon, K. B., Sutherland, D. C., Rees, A. J., et al. HLA antigen frequencies in systemic vasculitis: Increase in

HLA-DR2 in Wegener's granulomatosis. *Arthritis Rheum.* 26: 98, 1983.
136. Emancipator, S. N., Gallo, F., and Lamm, M. E. Experimental IgA nephropathy induced by oral immunisation. *J. Exp. Med.* 157: 572, 1983.
137. Emancipator, S. N., Gallo, G. R., and Lamm, M. E. IgA nephropathy: Perspective on pathogenesis and classification. *Clin. Nephrol.* 24: 161, 1985.
138. Emancipator, S. N., Ovary, Z., and Lamm, M. E. The role of mesangial complement in the haematuria of experimental IgA nephropathy. *Lab. Invest.* 57: 269, 1987.
139. Evans, D. J., Williams, D. G., Peters, D. K., et al. Glomerular deposition of properdin in Henoch Schönlein syndrome and idiopathic focal nephritis. *Br. Med. J.* 3: 326, 1973.
140. Falk, R., and Jennette, J. C. Antineutrophil cytoplasmic antibodies with specificity for myeloperoxidase in patients with systemic vasculitis and idiopathic necrotising and crescentic glomerulonephritis. *N. Engl. J. Med.* 318: 1651, 1988.
141. Falk, R. J., Dalmasso, A. P., Kim, Y., et al. Neoantigen of the polymerised ninth component of complement. Characterisation of a monoclonal antibody and immunohistochemical localisation in renal disease. *J. Clin. Invest.* 72: 560, 1983.
141a. Falk, R. J., Terrell, R. S., Charles, L. A., and Jennette, J. C. Anti-neutrophil cytoplasmic autoantibodies induce neutrophils to degranulate and produce oxygen radicals in vitro. *Proc. Natl. Acad. Sci. U.S.A.* 87: 4115, 1990.
142. Faucet, R., Le Pogamp, P., Genetet, B., et al. HLA-DR4 antigen and IgA nephropathy. *Tissue Antigens* 16: 405, 1980.
142a. Fauci, A. S., Haynes, B. F., Katz, P., et al. Wegener's granulomatosis: Prospective clinical and therapeutic experience with 85 patients for 21 years. *Ann. Intern. Med.* 98: 76, 1983.
143. Feehally, J. Immune mechanisms in glomerular IgA deposition. *Nephrol. Dial. Transplant.* 3: 361, 1988.
144. Feehally, J., Beattie, J. T., and Brenchley, P. E. C. Sequential studies of the IgA system in relapsing IgA nephropathy. *Kidney Int.* 30: 924, 1986.
145. Feehally, J., Dyer, P. A., Davidson, J. A., et al. Immunogenetics of IgA nephropathy: Experience in a U.K. centre. *Dis. Markers* 2: 493, 1984.
146. Feehally, J., O'Donoghue, D. J., and Ballardie, F. W. Current nephrological practice in the investigation of haematuria: Relationship to incidence of IgA nephropathy. *J. R. Coll. Physicians* 23: 228, 1989.
147. Feehally, J., Samanta, A., Kinghorn, H., et al. Red cell charge in glomerular disease. *Lancet* 2: 635, 1986.
148. Feenstra, K., Lee, R. V. D., Greben, H. A., et al. Experimental glomerulonephritis in the rat induced by antibodies directed against tubular antigens. I. The natural history: A histologic and immunohistologic study at the light microscopic and ultrastructural level. *Lab. Invest.* 32: 235, 1975.
149. Feiner, H., and Gallo, G. Ultrastructure in glomerulonephritis associated with cryoglobulinaemia. *Am. J. Pathol.* 88: 145, 1977.
150. Feldmann, J. D., Mardiney, M. R., and Schuler, S. E. Immunology and morphology of acute post-streptococcal glomerulonephritis. *Lab. Invest.* 15: 283, 1966.
151. Felson, D. J., and Anderson, J. Evidence for the superiority of immunosuppressive drugs and prednisolone over prednisolone alone in lupus nephritis: Results of a pooled analysis. *N. Engl. J. Med.* 311: 1528, 1984.
152. Ferraro, G., Meroni, P. L., Tincani, A., et al. Anti-endothelial cell antibodies in patients with Wegener's granulomatosis and micropolyarteritis. *Clin. Exp. Immunol.* 79: 47, 1990.
153. Ferri, C., Moriconi, L., Gregnai, G., et al. Treatment of renal involvement in mixed essential cryoglobulinaemia with prolonged plasma exchange. *Nephron* 43: 246, 1986.
154. Fielder, A. H. H., Walport, M. J., Batchelor, J. R., et al. Family study of the major histocompatibility complex in patients with systemic lupus erythematosus: Importance of null alleles of C4A and C4B in determining disease susceptibility. *Br. Med. J.* 286: 425, 1983.
155. Finkelstein, A., Fraley, D. S., Stachura, I., et al. Fenoprofen nephropathy: Lipoid nephrosis and interstitial nephritis. A possible T lymphocyte disorder. *Am. J. Med.* 72: 81, 1982.
156. Fleuren, G., Grond, J., and Hoedemaeker, P. J. In situ formation of subepithelial glomerular immune complexes in passive serum sickness. *Kidney Int.* 17: 631, 1980.
157. Fornasieri, A., Sinico, R. A., and Madifassi, P. IgA-antigliadin antibodies in IgA mesangial nephropathy (Berger's disease). *Br. Med. J.* 295: 78, 1988.
158. Frank, M. M., Hamburger, M. I., Lawley, T. J., et al. Defective reticuloendothelial system Fc-receptor function in systemic lupus erythematosus. *N. Engl. J. Med.* 300: 518, 1979.
158a. Frankel, A. H., et al. Type II essential mixed cryoglobulinaemia: Presentation, treatment and outcome in 13 patients. *Q. J. Med.* 82: 101, 1992.
159. Friend, P. S., Kim, Y., Michael, A. F., et al. Pathogenesis of membranous nephropathy in systemic lupus erythematosus: Possible role of non-precipitating DNA antibody. *Br. Med. J.* 1: 25, 1977.
160. Fries, J. W. U., Mendrick, D. L., and Rennke, H. G. Determinants of immune complex-mediated glomerulonephritis. *Kidney Int.* 32: 333, 1988.
161. Fukatsu, A., Yuzawa, Y., Olson, L., et al. Interaction of antibodies with human glomerular epithelial cells. *Lab. Invest.* 61: 389, 1989.
162. Gallo, G. R., Caulin-Glaser, T., Emancipator, S. N., et al. Nephritogenicity and differential distribution of glomerular immune complexes related to immunogen charge. *Lab. Invest.* 48: 353, 1983.
163. Gallo, J. H., Russell, M. W., Hammond, D., et al. Environmental antigens in IgA nephropathy. *Kidney Int.* 27: 210, 1985.
164. Galpin, J. E., Shinaberger, J. H., Stanley, T. M., et al. Acute interstitial nephritis due to methicillin. *Am. J. Med.* 65: 756, 1978.
165. Garovoy, M. R. Idiopathic Membranous Glomerulonephritis (IMGN): An HLA Associated Disease. In P. I. Terasaki (ed.), *Histocompatibility Workshop 1980*. Los Angeles: University of California Press, 1980. P. 129.
166. Gaskin, G., Savage, C. O. S., Ryan, J. J., et al. Anti-neutrophil cytoplasmic antibodies and disease activity during long-term follow-up of 70 patients with systemic vasculitis. *Nephrol. Dial. Transplant.* 6: 689, 1991.
167. Gauthier, V. J., Mannik, M., and Striker, G. W. Effect of cationised antibodies in preformed immune complexes on deposition and persistence in renal glomeruli. *J. Exp. Med.* 156: 766, 1982.
168. Gay, S., Losman, M. J., Koopman, W. J., and Miller, E. J. Interaction of DNA with connective tissue matrix proteins reveals preferential binding to type V collagen. *J. Immunol.* 135: 1097, 1985.

169. Germuth, F. G. A comparative histologic and immunologic study in rabbits of induced hypersensitivity of the serum sickness type. *J. Exp. Med.* 97: 257, 1953.
170. Germuth, F. G., Senterfit, L. B., and Dressman, G. R. Immune complex disease. V. The nature of the circulating complexes associated with glomerular alterations in the chronic BSA-rabbit system. *Johns Hopkins Med. J.* 130: 344, 1972.
171. Germuth, F. G., Senterfit, L. B., and Pollack, A. D. Immune complex disease. 1. Experimental acute and chronic glomerulonephritis. *Johns Hopkins Med. J.* 120: 225, 1967.
172. Giangiacomo, J., Cleary, T. G., Cole, B. R., et al. Serum immunoglobulins in the nephrotic syndrome. *N. Engl. J. Med.* 8: 12, 1975.
173. Gimenez, A., Leyva-Cobian, F., Fierro, C., et al. Effect of cyclosporin A on autoimmune tubulointerstitial nephritis in the Brown Norway rat. *Clin. Exp. Immunol.* 69: 550, 1987.
174. Gimenez, A., and Mampaso, F. Characterisation of inflammatory cells in drug induced tubulo-interstitial nephritis. *Nephrol.* 43: 239, 1986.
175. Glassock, R. J. Natural history and treatment of primary proliferative glomerulonephritis: A review. *Kidney Int.* 28: 5136, 1985.
176. Golbus, S. M., and Wilson, C. B. Experimental glomerulonephritis induced by in situ formation of immune complexes in glomerular capillary wall. *Kidney Int.* 16: 148, 1979.
177. Goldman, M., Feng, H. M., Engers, H., et al. Autoimmunity and immune complex disease after neonatal induction of tolerance in mice. *J. Immunol.* 131: 251, 1983.
178. Goldschmeding, R., Van der Schoot, C. E., Ten Bokkel Huinink, D., et al. Wegener's granulomatosis autoantibodies identify a novel diisopropylfluorophosphate-binding protein in the lysozomes of normal human neutrophils. *J. Clin. Invest.* 84: 1577, 1989.
179. Gorevic, P. D., Kassab, H. J., Levo, Y., et al. Mixed cryoglobulinaemia: Clinical aspects and long-term follow up of 40 patients. *Am. J. Med.* 69: 287, 1980.
180. Gormly, A. A., Seymour, A. E., Clarkson, A. R., and Woodroffe, A. J. IgA glomerular deposits in experimental cirrhosis. *Am. J. Pathol.* 104: 50, 1981.
181. Gremmel, F., Druml, W., Schmidt, P., and Graninger, W. Cyclosporin in Wegener's granulomatosis. *Ann. Intern. Med.* 108: 491, 1988.
182. Grishman, E., Gerber, M. A., and Churg, J. Patterns of renal injury in systemic lupus erythematosus: Light and fluorescence microscopic observations. *Am. J. Kidney Dis.* 4: 135, 1982.
183. Groggel, G. C., Salant, D. J., Darby, C., et al. Role of terminal complement pathway in the heterologous phase of anti-glomerular basement membrane nephritis. *Kidney Int.* 27: 643, 1985.
184. Gronhagen-Riska, C., Von Willebrand, E., Tikkanen, E., et al. The effect of cyclosporin A on interstitial mononuclear cell infiltration and the induction of Heymann's nephritis. *Clin. Exp. Immunol.* 79: 266, 1990.
185. Guery, J.-C., Tournade, H., Pelletier, L., et al. Rat anti-glomerular basement membrane antibodies in toxin-induced autoimmunity and in chronic graft versus host reaction share recurrent idiotypes. *Eur. J. Immunol.* 20: 101, 1990.
186. Guttman, R. A., Morel-Maroger Striker, L., Striker, G. E. Glomerulonephritis with Bacterial Endocarditis, Shunts and Abdominal Abscesses. In R. W. Schrier and C. W. Gottschalk (eds.), *Diseases of the Kidney* (4th ed.). Boston: Little, Brown, 1988. P. 1885.
187. Habib, R., Gubler, M.-C., Loirat, C., et al. Dense deposit disease: A variant of membranoproliferative glomerulonephritis. *Kidney Int.* 7: 204, 1975.
188. Habib, R., Kleinknecht, C., Gubler, M. C., et al. Idiopathic membranoproliferative glomerulonephritis in children. Report of 105 cases. *Clin. Nephrol.* 1: 194, 1973.
189. Habib, R., Levy, M., and Gubler, M. C. Clinicopathologic correlations in the nephrotic syndrome. *Pediatrician* 8: 325, 1979.
190. Hahn, B. H., and Ebling, F. M. Suppression of NZB/NZW murine nephritis by administration of a syngeneic monoclonal antibody to DNA. Possible role of anti-idiotypic antibodies. *J. Clin. Invest.* 71: 1728, 1983.
191. Hahn, B. H., and Ebling, F. M. Suppression of murine lupus nephritis by administration of an anti-idiotypic antibody to anti-DNA. *J. Immunol.* 132: 187, 1984.
192. Halbwachs, L., Leveille, M., Lesavre, P., et al. Nephritic factor of the classical pathway of complement. Immunoglobulin G autoantibody directed against the classical pathway C3 convertase enzyme. *J. Clin. Invest.* 65: 249, 1980.
193. Hale, G., McIntosh, S. L., and Hiki, Y. Evidence for IgA specific B cell hyperreactivity in patients with IgA nephropathy. *Kidney Int.* 29: 718, 1986.
194. Hanly, P., Garrett, P., Spencer, S., and O'Dwyer, W. F. HLA -A, -B and -DR antigens in IgA nephropathy. *Tissue Antigens* 23: 270, 1984.
195. Haworth, S. J., Pusey, C. D., and Lockwood, C. M. Plasma exchange in lupus nephritis. *Proc. Eur. Dial. Transplant. Assoc.* 22: 699, 1985.
196. Heymann, W., Hackel, D. B., Harwood, S., et al. Production of nephrotic syndrome in rats by Freund's adjuvant and rat kidney suspension. *Proc. Soc. Exp. Biol. Med.* 100: 660, 1959.
197. Hiki, Y., Kobayashi, Y., Itoh, I., and Kashiwagi, N. Strong association of HLA-DR2 and MTI with idiopathic membranous nephropathy in Japan. *Kidney Int.* 25: 953, 1984.
198. Hiki, Y., Kobayashi, T., Tateno, S., et al. Strong association of HLA-DR4 with benign IgA nephropathy. *Nephron* 32: 222, 1982.
199. Hind, C. R. K., Paraskevakou, H., Lockwood, C. M., et al. Prognosis after immunosuppression of patients with crescentic nephritis requiring dialysis. *Lancet* 1: 263, 1983.
200. Hinglais, N., Garcia-Torres, R., and Kleinknecht, D. Long term prognosis in acute glomerulonephritis. The predictive value of early clinical and pathological features observed in 65 patients. *Am. J. Med.* 56: 52, 1974.
201. Hirose, H., Udo, K., Kojima, M., et al. Deposition of hepatitis B e antigen in membranous glomerulonephritis—Identification by $F(ab')_2$ fragments of monoclonal antibody. *Kidney Int.* 26: 338, 1984.
202. Hirsch, F., Couderc, J., Sapin, C., et al. Polyclonal effect of $HgCl_2$ in the rat, its possible role in an experimental autoimmune disease. *Eur. J. Immunol.* 12: 620, 1982.
203. Holdsworth, S. R., Neale, T. J., and Wilson, C. B. Abrogation of macrophage dependent injury in experimental glomerulonephritis in the rabbit. *J. Clin. Invest.* 68: 698, 1981.
204. Horvath, F., Trague, P., Gaffrey, E. F., et al. Thyroid antigen associated immune complex glomerulonephritis in Graves' disease. *Am. J. Med.* 67: 901, 1979.
205. Howanietz, H., and Lubec, G. Idiopathic nephrotic syn-

drome treated with steroids for five years, found to be allergic reaction to pork. *Lancet* 2: 450, 1985.

206. Hoyer, P. F., Knell, F., and Brodehl, J. Cyclosporin in frequently relapsing minimal change nephrotic syndrome. *Lancet* 1: 335, 1986.

206a. Hudson, B. G., Weislander, J., Wisdom, B. J., and Noclken, M. E. Goodpasture's syndrome: Molecular architecture and function of basement membrane antigen. *Lab. Invest.* 61: 256, 1989.

207. Hyman, L. R., Ballow, M., and Knieser, M. R. Diphenylhydantoin interstitial nephritis. Roles of cellular and humoral immunological injury. *J. Pediatr.* 92: 915, 1978.

208. Hyman, L. R., Colvin, R. B., and Steinberg, A. D. Immunopathogenesis of autoimmune tubulo-interstitial nephritis. I. Demonstration of different susceptibility in strain II and strain XIII guinea pigs. *J. Immunol.* 116: 327, 1976.

209. Iitaka, K., and West, C. D. A serum inhibitor of blastogenesis in idiopathic nephrotic syndrome transferred by lymphocytes. *Clin. Immunol. Immunopathol.* 12: 62, 1979.

210. Imbasciati, E., Gusmano, R., Edeonti, A., et al. Controlled trial of methyl prednisolone and low dose oral prednisolone for the minimal change nephrotic syndrome. *Br. Med. J.* 291: 1305, 1985.

211. Isaacs, K. L., and Miller, F. Role of antigen size and charge in immune complex glomerulonephritis. *Lab. Invest.* 47: 198, 1982.

212. Iskander, S. S., and Jennette, J. C. Influence of antibody avidity on glomerular immune complex localization. *Am. J. Pathol.* 112: 155, 1983.

213. Izui, S., Lambert, P. H., and Miescher, P. A. In vitro demonstration of a particular affinity of glomerular basement membrane and collagen for DNA: A possible basis for a local formation of DNA-anti-DNA complexes in systemic lupus erythematosus. *J. Exp. Med.* 144: 428, 1976.

214. Jacob, L., Lety, M. A., Choquette, D., et al. Presence of antibodies against a cell-surface protein, cross-reactive with DNA, in systemic lupus erythematosus: A marker of the disease. *Proc. Natl. Acad. Sci. U.S.A.* 84: 2956, 1987.

215. Jaffe, I. A., Treser, G., Suzuki, Y., et al. Nephropathy induced by penicillamine. *Ann. Intern. Med.* 69: 549, 1968.

216. Jennette, J. C., Wilkman, A. S., and Falk, R. J. Anti-neutrophil cytoplasmic autoantibody associated glomerulonephritis and vasculitis. *Am. J. Pathol.* 135: 921, 1989.

217. Jennings, L., Roholt, O. A., Pressman, D., et al. Experimental anti-alveolar basement membrane antibody-mediated pneumonitis: I. The role of increased permeability of the alveolar capillary wall induced by oxygen. *J. Immunol.* 127: 129, 1981.

218. Johnson, J. P., Moore, J., Austin, H. A., et al. Therapy of anti-glomerular basement membrane antibody disease: Analysis of prognostic significance of clinical, pathologic and treatment factors. *Medicine* 64: 219, 1985.

218a. Jordan, S. C., Buckingham, B., Sakai, R., et al. Studies of immune-complex glomerulonephritis mediated by human thyroglobulin. *N. Engl. J. Med.* 304: 1212, 1981.

219. Julian, B. A., Quiggins, P. A., Thompson, J. S., et al. Familial IgA nephropathy. Evidence of an inherited mechanism of disease. *N. Engl. J. Med.* 312: 202, 1985.

220. Kamata, K., Baird, L. G., Erikson, M. E., et al. Characterization of antigens and antibody specificities induced in Heymann nephritis. *J. Immunol.* 135: 2400, 1985.

221. Kasahara, M., Hamada, K., Okuyama, T., et al. Role of the HLA in IgA nephropathy. *Clin. Immunol. Immunopathol.* 25: 189, 1982.

222. Katz, A., Dyck, R. F., and Bear, R. A. Coeliac disease associated with immune complex glomerulonephritis. *Clin. Nephrol.* 11: 39, 1979.

223. Katz, A., Karanicolas, S., and Falk, J. A. Family study in IgA glomerulonephritis: The possible role of HLA antigens. *Transplantation* 29: 505, 1980.

224. Kazatchkine, M. D., Fearon, D. T., Appay, M. D., et al. Immunohistochemical study of the human glomerular C3b receptor in normal kidney and in seventy-five cases of renal diseases. Loss of C3b receptor antigen in focal hyalinosis and in proliferative nephritis of systemic lupus erythematosus. *J. Clin. Invest.* 69: 900, 1982.

225. Kelly, C. J., Korngold, R., Mann, R., et al. Characterization of a tubular antigen specific H-2K restricted Lyt-2+ effector T cell that mediates destructive tubulointerstitial injury. *J. Immunol.* 136: 526, 1986.

226. Kelly, C. J., and Neilson, E. G. Contrasuppression in autoimmunity: Abnormal contrasuppression promotes the expression of nephritogenic effector T cells and histologic interstitial nephritis in kdkd mice. *J. Exp. Med.* 165: 107, 1987.

227. Kelly, C. J., Zunier, R. B., Krakauer, K. A., et al. Prostaglandin E_1 inhibits effector T cell induction and tissue damage in experimental murine interstitial nephritis. *J. Clin. Invest.* 79: 782, 1987.

228. Kerjaschki, D., and Farquhar, M. G. The pathogenic antigen of Heymann nephritis is a membrane glycoprotein of the renal proximal tubule brush border. *Proc. Natl. Acad. Sci. U.S.A.* 79: 5557, 1982.

229. Kerjaschki, D., Horvat, R., Binder, S., et al. Identification of a 400kD protein in the brush borders of human kidneys that is similar to gp330, the nephritogenic antigen of rat Heymann nephritis. *Am. J. Pathol.* 129: 183, 1987.

230. Kerjaschki, D., Miettirien, A., and Farquhar, M. G. Initial events in the formation of immune deposits in passive Heymann nephritis. *J. Exp. Med.* 166: 109, 1987.

231. Kerjaschki, D., Schultze, M., Binder, S., et al. Transcellular transport and membrane insertion of the C5b-9 membrane attack complex of complement by glomerular epithelial cells in experimental membranous nephropathy. *J. Immunol.* 143: 546, 1989.

232. Kim, Y., Friend, P. S., Dresner, I. G., et al. Inherited deficiency of the 2nd component of complement (C2) with membranoproliferative glomerulonephritis. *Am. J. Med.* 62: 765, 1977.

233. Kimberly, R. D., Locshin, M. D., Sherman, R. L., et al. High dose intravenous methylprednisolone pulse therapy in systemic lupus erythematosus. *Am. J. Med.* 70: 817, 1981.

234. Klassen, J., Elwood, C., Grossberg, A., et al. Evolution of membranous nephropathy into anti-glomerular basement membrane glomerulonephritis. *N. Engl. J. Med.* 290: 1340, 1974.

235. Klassen, J., Kano, K., Milgrom, F., et al. Tubular lesions produced by autoantibodies to tubular basement membrane in human renal allografts. *Int. Arch. Allergy Appl. Immunol.* 45: 675, 1973.

236. Kleinknecht, D., Kenfer, A., Morel-Maroger, L., et al. Immunologically mediated drug-induced acute renal failure. *Contrib. Nephrol.* 10: 42, 1978.

237. Kleppel, M. M., Santi, P. A., Cameron, J. D., et al. Human tissue distribution of novel basement membrane collagen. *Am. J. Pathol.* 134: 813, 1989.

238. Klouda, P. T., Manos, J., Acheson, E. J., et al. Strong association between idiopathic membranous nephropathy and HLA-DRw3. *Lancet* 2: 770, 1979.
239. Knudsen, B. B., Joergensen, T., and Munch-Jensen, B. Wegener's granulomatosis in a family. *Scand. J. Rheumatol.* 17: 225, 1988.
240. Kobayashi, Y., Fujii, K., Hiki, Y., and Tateno, S. Steroid therapy in IgA nephropathy: A prospective pilot study in moderate proteinuric cases. *Q. J. Med.* 61: 985, 1986.
241. Koffler, D. Immunopathogenesis of systemic lupus erythematosus. *Annu. Rev. Med.* 25: 149, 1974.
242. Koffler, D., Agnello, V., Thoburn, R., et al. Systemic lupus erythematosus: Prototype of immune complex disease in man. *J. Exp. Med.* 134: 169, 1971.
243. Komori, K., Nose, Y., Inouye, H., et al. Immunogenetical study in patients with chronic glomerulonephritis. *Tokai J. Exp. Clin. Med.* 8: 135, 1983.
244. Kunkel, H. G., Agnello, V., Joslin, F. G., et al. Cross-idiotypic specificity among monoclonal IgM proteins with anti-γ-globulin activity. *J. Exp. Med.* 137: 331, 1973.
245. Kuntel, S. L., Zanetti, M., and Sapin, C. Suppression of nephrotoxic serum nephritis in rats by prostaglandin E_1. *Am. J. Pathol.* 108: 240, 1982.
246. Kurki, P., Helve, T., von-Bonsdorff, M., et al. Transformation of membranous glomerulonephritis into crescentic glomerulonephritis with glomerular basement membrane antibodies. Serial determinations of anti-GBM before the transformation. *Nephron* 38: 134, 1984.
247. Lagrue, G., Laurent, J., Belghiti, D., and Sainte-Laudy, J. Food sensitivity and idiopathic nephrotic syndrome. *Lancet* 2: 777, 1985.
248. Lagrue, G., Xheneumont, S., Branellec, A., et al. Lymphokines and nephrotic syndrome. *Lancet* 1: 271, 1975.
249. Lai, K.-N., Chui, S.-H., and Lai, F. M. Predominant synthesis of IgA with lambda light chains in IgA nephropathy. *Kidney Int.* 33: 584, 1988.
250. Lai, K.-N., Lai, E. M., and Ho, C. P. Corticosteroid therapy in IgA nephropathy with nephrotic syndrome: A long-term controlled trial. *Clin. Nephrol.* 26: 174, 1986.
251. Lange, K., Seligson, G., and Cromin, W. Evidence for the in situ origin of post-streptococcal glomerulonephritis: Glomerular localisation of endostreptosin and the clinical significance of the subsequent antibody response. *Clin. Nephrol.* 19: 3, 1983.
252. Layrisse, Z., Rodriguez-Iturbe, B., Garcia, R., et al. Family studies of the HLA system in acute post-streptococcal glomerulonephritis. *Hum. Immunol.* 7: 177, 1983.
253. Leaker, B. R., Becker, G. J., Dowling, J. P., and Kincaid-Smith, P. Rapid improvement in severe lupus glomerular lesions following intensive plasma exchange associated with immunosuppression. *Clin. Nephrol.* 25: 236, 1986.
254. Lehman, D. H., Lee, S., Wilson, C. B., et al. Induction of antitubular basement membrane antibodies in rats by renal transplantation. *Transplantation* 17: 429, 1974.
255. Lehman, D. H., Wilson, C. B., and Dixon, F. J. Interstitial nephritis in rats immunised with heterologous tubular basement membrane. *Kidney Int.* 5: 187, 1974.
256. Lehman, D. H., Wilson, C. B., and Dixon, F. J. Extraglomerular immunoglobulin deposits in human nephritis. *Am. J. Med.* 58: 765, 1975.
257. Lerner, R., Glassock, R. J., and Dixon, F. J. The role of anti-glomerular basement membrane antibody in the pathogenesis of human glomerulonephritis. *J. Exp. Med.* 126: 989, 1967.
258. Levin, M., Smith, C., Walters, M. D. S., et al. Steroid-responsive nephrotic syndrome: A generalised disorder of membrane charge. *Lancet* 2: 239, 1985.
259. Levy, M., and Kleinknecht, C. Membranous glomerulonephritis and hepatitis B virus infection. *Nephron* 26: 259, 1980.
260. Lew, A. M., Staines, N. A., and Steward, M. W. Glomerulonephritis induced by pre-formed immune complexes containing monoclonal antibodies of defined affinity and isotype. *Clin. Exp. Immunol.* 57: 413, 1984.
261. Li, P. K., Burns, A. P., So, A. K. L., et al. The DQw7 allele at the HLA-DQB locus is associated with susceptibility to IgA nephropathy in Caucasians. *Kidney Int.* 39: 961, 1991.
262. Lianos, E. A. Synthesis of hydroxyeicosatetranoic acids and leukotrienes in rat nephrotoxic serum glomerulonephritis. *J. Clin. Invest.* 82: 427, 1988.
263. Lianos, E. A., Andres, G. A., and Dunn, M. J. Glomerular prostaglandin and thromboxane synthesis in rat nephrotoxic serum nephritis: Effects on renal hemodynamics. *J. Clin. Invest.* 72: 1439, 1983.
264. Liebowitch, J., Leveille, M., Halbwachs, L., et al. Glomerulonephritides and hypocomplementemia: Pathophysiology and pathogenetic implications. *Adv. Nephrol.* 9: 295, 1980.
265. Linscott, W. D., and Kane, J. P. The complement system in cryoglobulinaemia. *Clin. Exp. Immunol.* 21: 510, 1975.
266. Litwin, A., Bash, J. A., Adams, L. E., et al. Immunoregulation of Heymann nephritis. I. Induction of suppressor cells. *J. Immunol.* 122: 1029, 1979.
267. Lockwood, C. M., Worlledge, S., Nicholas, A., et al. Reversal of impaired splenic function in patients with nephritis or vasculitis (or both) by plasma exchange. *N. Engl. J. Med.* 300: 524, 1979.
268. Lomax Smith, J. D., Zabrowarny, L. A., Howarth, G. S., et al. The immunochemical characterisation of mesangial IgA deposits. *Am. J. Pathol.* 113: 359, 1983.
269. Lovett, D. H., and Sterzl, R. B. Cell culture approaches to the analysis of glomerular inflammation. *Kidney Int.* 30: 246, 1986.
270. Ludemann, J., Utecht, B., and Gross, W. L. Anti-neutrophil antibodies in Wegener's granulomatosis recognize an elastinolytic enzyme. *J. Exp. Med.* 357: 362, 1990.
271. Lyon, M. F., and Hulse, E. V. An inherited kidney disease of mice resembling human nephronophthisis. *J. Med. Genet.* 8: 41, 1971.
272. MacScarraigh, E. T., Doyle, C. T., Twomey, M., et al. Sarcoidosis with renal involvement. *Postgrad. Med. J.* 54: 528, 1978.
273. Madaio, M. P., Carlson, J. A., and Hodder, S. Monoclonal anti-DNA antibodies (MaDNA) bind directly to intrinsic glomerular antigens and form immune deposits. (Abstract) *Kidney Int.* 27: 216, 1985.
274. Magil, A. B., and Wadsworth, L. D. Monocyte involvement in glomerular crescents: A histochemical and ultrastructural study. *Lab. Invest.* 47: 160, 1982.
275. Mahieu, P., Lambert, P. H., and Miescher, P. A. Detection of anti-glomerular basement membrane antibodies by a radioimmunological technique. Clinical application in human nephropathies. *J. Clin. Invest.* 54: 128, 1974.
276. Makker, S. P. Tubular basement membrane antibody induced nephritis in systemic lupus erythematosus. *Am. J. Med.* 69: 949, 1980.
277. Mampaso, F. M., and Wilson, C. B. Characterisation of

inflammatory cells in autoimmune tubulointerstitial nephritis in rats. *Kidney Int.* 23: 448, 1983.

278. Martini, A., Vitiello, M. A., Siena, S., et al. Multiple serum inhibitors of lectin-induced lymphocyte proliferation in nephrotic syndrome. *Clin. Exp. Immunol.* 45: 178, 1981.

279. Mason, P. D., and Lockwood, C. M. Rapidly progressive nephritis in patients taking hydralazine. *J. Clin. Lab. Immunol.* 20: 151, 1986.

280. Mathieson, P. W., Cobbold, S. P., Hale, G., et al. Monoclonal antibody therapy in systemic vasculitis. *N. Engl. J. Med.* 323: 250, 1990.

280a. Mathieson, P. W., Thiru, S., and Oliveira, D. B. G. Mercuric chloride-treated Brown Norway rats develop widespread tissue injury including necrotizing vasculitis. *Lab. Invest.* (in press).

281. Mathieson, P. W., Turner, A. N., Maidment, C. G. H., et al. Prednisolone and chlorambucil treatment in idiopathic membranous nephropathy with deteriorating renal function. *Lancet* 2: 869, 1988.

282. Matsuo, S., Fukatsu, A., Taub, M. L., et al. Glomerulonephritis induced in the rabbit by anti-endothelial antibodies. *J. Clin. Invest.* 79: 1798, 1987.

283. Mauer, S. M., Sutherland, D. E. R., Howard, R. J., et al. The glomerular mesangium. III. Acute immune mesangial injury: A new model of glomerulonephritis. *J. Exp. Med.* 137: 553, 1973.

284. McCauley, J., Tzakis, A. G., Fung, J. J., et al. FK506 in steroid-resistant focal sclerosing glomerulonephritis of childhood. *Lancet* 335: 674, 1990.

285. McCluskey, R. T., and Colvin, R. B. Immunological aspects of renal tubular and interstitial disease. *Annu. Rev. Med.* 29: 191, 1978.

286. McKenzie, P. E., Hawke, D., Woodroffe, A. J., et al. Serum and tissue immune complexes in infective endocarditis. *J. Clin. Lab. Immunol.* 4: 125, 1980.

287. McLean, R. H., and Hoefnagel, D. Partial lipodystrophy and familial C3 deficiency. *Hum. Hered.* 30: 149, 1980.

288. Meadows, S. R., Sarsfield, J. K., Scott, D. G., and Rajah, S. M. Steroid-responsive nephrotic syndrome and allergy: Immunological studies. *Arch. Dis. Child.* 56: 517, 1981.

289. Melvin, T., Burke, B., Michael, A. F., et al. Experimental IgA nephropathy in bile duct ligated rats. *Clin. Immunol. Immunopathol.* 27: 369, 1983.

290. Mendrick, D. L., and Rennke, H. G. Epitope specific induction of proteinuria by monoclonal antibodies. *Kidney Int.* 33: 831, 1988.

291. Meyrier, A., Simon, P., Perret, G., and Condamin-Meyrier, M.-C. Remission of idiopathic nephrotic syndrome after treatment with cyclosporin A. *Br. Med. J.* 292: 789, 1986.

292. Michalak, T. Immune complexes of hepatitis B surface antigen in the pathogenesis of periarteritis nodosa. A study of seven necropsy cases. *Am. J. Pathol.* 90: 619, 1978.

293. Mignon, F., Mery, J.-P., Mougenot, B., et al. Granulomatous interstitial nephritis. *Adv. Nephrol.* 13: 219, 1984.

294. Miller, G. W., and Nussenzweig, V. A new complement function: Solubilisation of antigen—antibody aggregates. *Proc. Natl. Acad. Sci. U.S.A.* 72: 418, 1975.

295. Miyakawa, Y., Yamada, A., Kosaka, K., et al. Defective immune adherence (C3b) receptor on erythrocytes from patients with systemic lupus erythematosus. *Lancet* 2: 493, 1981.

296. Mollnes, T. E., Ng, Y. C., Peters, D. K., et al. Effect of nephritic factor on C3 and on the terminal pathway of complement in vivo and in vitro. *Clin. Exp. Immunol.* 65: 73, 1986.

297. Moorthy, A. V., Zimmerman, S. W., and Burtholder, P. M. Inhibition of lymphocyte blastogenesis by plasma of patients with minimal change nephrotic syndrome. *Lancet* 1: 1160, 1976.

298. Moorthy, A. V., Zimmerman, S. W., and Burkholder, P. M. Nephrotic syndrome in Hodgkin's disease: Evidence for pathogenesis alternative to immune complex deposition. *Am. J. Med.* 61: 471, 1976.

299. Morimoto, C., Sano, H., Ave, T., et al. Correlation between clinical activity of systemic lupus erythematosus and the amounts of DNA in DNA/anti-DNA antibody immune complexes. *J. Immunol.* 129: 1960, 1982.

300. Morrison, K. K., Germino, G. G., and Reeders, S. T. Use of the polymerase chain reaction to clone and sequence a cDNA encoding the bovine alpha 3 chain of type IV collagen. *J. Biol. Chem.* 266: 34, 1991.

301. Mouzon-Cambon, A., Bouisson, F., Dutau, G., et al. HLA-DR7 in children with idiopathic nephrotic syndrome. Correlation with atopy. *Tissue Antigens* 17: 518, 1981.

302. Muller, G. A., Gebhardt, M., Kompf, J., et al. Association between rapidly progressive glomerulonephritis and the properdin factor BfF and different HLA-D region products. *Kidney Int.* 25: 115, 1984.

303. Muller, G. A., Muller, C., Liebau, G., et al. Strong association of idiopathic membranous nephropathy with HLA-DR3 and MT-2 without involvement of HLA-B18 and no association to BfF1. *Tissue Antigens* 17: 332, 1981.

304. Nagy, J., Scott, H., and Brandtzaeg, P. Autoantibodies to dietary antigens in IgA nephropathy. *Clin. Exp. Immunol.* 29: 274, 1988.

305. Naish, P. F., Thomson, N. M., Simpson, I. J., et al. Role of polymorphonuclear leucocytes in the autologous phase of nephrotoxic nephritis. *Clin. Exp. Immunol.* 22: 102, 1975.

306. Naito, S., Kohara, M., and Arakawa, K. Association of class II antigens of HLA with primary glomerulonephritis. *Nephron* 45: 111, 1987.

307. Nakamoto, Y., Asano, Y., and Dohi, D., et al. Primary IgA glomerulonephritis and Schönlein-Henoch purpura nephritis; clinicopathological and immuno-histological characteristics. *Q. J. Med.* 47: 495, 1978.

308. Naruse, T., Kitanura, K., Miyakawa, Y., et al. Deposition of renal tubular epithelial antigen along the glomerular capillary walls of patients with membranous glomerulonephritis. *J. Immunol.* 110: 1163, 1973.

309. Natori, Y., Hayakawa, I., and Stibata, S. Role of dipeptidyl peptidase IV (p108) in passive Heymann nephritis. *Am. J. Pathol.* 134: 405, 1989.

310. Neale, T. J., Tipping, P. G., Carson, S. D., and Holdsworth, S. R. Participation of cell mediated immunity in deposition of fibrin in glomerulonephritis. *Lancet* 2: 421, 1988.

311. Neilson, E. G., Gasser, D. I., McCafferty, E., et al. Polymorphism of genes involved in anti-tubular basement membrane disease in rats. *Immunogenetics* 17: 55, 1983.

312. Neilson, E. G., McCafferty, E., Feldmann, A., et al. Spontaneous interstitial nephritis in kdkd mice: An experimental model of autoimmune renal disease. *J. Immunol.* 133: 2560, 1984.

313. Neilson, E. G., McCafferty, E., Mann, R., et al. Murine interstitial nephritis. III. The selection of phenotypic

(Lyt and L3T4) and idiotypic (RE-Id) T cell preferences by genes in Igh-I and H2-K characterises the cell mediated potential for disease expression: Susceptible mice provide a unique effector T cell repertoire in response to tubular antigen. *J. Immunol.* 134: 2375, 1985.
314. Neilson, E. G., McCafferty, E., Mann, R., et al. Tubular antigen-derivatised cells induce a disease-protective, antigen-specific, and idiotype-specific suppressor T cell network restricted by I-J and IgH-V in mice with experimental interstitial nephritis. *J. Exp. Med.* 162: 215, 1985.
315. Neilson, E. G., McCafferty, E., Phillips, S. M., et al. Anti-idiotypic immunity in interstitial nephritis. II. Rats developing anti-tubular basement membrane disease fail to make an anti-idiotypic regulatory response: The modulatory role of an RT7.1$^+$, OX8$^-$ suppressor T cell mechanism. *J. Exp. Med.* 159: 1009, 1984.
316. Neilson, E. G., and Phillips, S. M. Murine interstitial nephritis: I. Analysis of disease susceptibility and relationship to pleomorphic gene products defining both immune-response genes and a restrictive requirement for cytotoxic T cells at H-2K. *J. Exp. Med.* 155: 1075, 1982.
317. Neilson, E. G., and Phillips, S. M. Suppression of interstitial nephritis by auto-anti-idiotypic immunity. *J. Exp. Med.* 155: 179, 1982.
318. Neilson, E. G., Sun, M. J., Emery, J., et al. Molecular cloning of the 3M-1 nephritogenic antigen. *Kidney Int.* 35: 358, 1989.
319. Neugarten, J., and Baldwin, D. S. Glomerulonephritis in bacterial endocarditis. *Am. J. Med.* 77: 297, 1984.
320. Ng, Y. C., and Peters, D. K. C3 nephritic factor (C3NeF): Dissociation of cell-bound and fluid phase stabilisation of alternative pathway C3 convertase. *Clin. Exp. Immunol.* 65: 450, 1986.
321. Nicholls, K., Becker, G., Walker, R., et al. Plasma exchange in progressive IgA nephropathy. *J. Clin. Apheresis* 5: 122, 1990.
322. Niles, J. L., McCluskey, R. T., Ahmed, M. F., and Arnaout, M. A. Wegener's granulomatosis autoantigen is a novel neutrophil serine proteinase. *Blood* 74: 1888, 1989.
323. Noble, B., Mendrick, D. L., Brentjens, J. R., et al. Antibody mediated injury in proximal tubules in the rat kidney induced by passive transfer of homologous anti-brush border serum. *Clin. Immunol. Immunopathol.* 19: 289, 1981.
324. Nochy, D., Callard, P., and Bellon, B. Association of overt glomerulonephritis and liver disease: A study of 34 patients. *Clin. Nephrol.* 6: 422, 1976.
325. Nolasco, F. E., Cameron, J. S., Hartley, B., et al. Intraglomerular T cells and monocytes in nephritis: Study with monoclonal antibodies. *Kidney Int.* 31: 1160, 1987.
326. Nolle, B., Specks, U., Ludemann, J., et al. Anticytoplasmic autoantibodies: Their immunodiagnostic value in Wegener's granulomatosis. *Ann. Intern. Med.* 111: 28, 1989.
327. Nunex-Roldon, A., Villechenous, E., Fernadez-Andrade, C., and Martin-Govantes, J. Increased HLA-DR7 and decreased DR2 in steroid-responsive nephrotic syndrome. *N. Engl. J. Med.* 306: 366, 1982.
328. Oite, T., Batsford, S. R., Mihatsch, M. J., et al. Quantitative studies of in situ immune complex glomerulonephritis in the rat induced by planted, cationized antigen. *J. Exp. Med.* 155: 460, 1982.
329. Ono, M., Winearls, C. G., Amos, N., et al. Monoclonal antibodies to restricted and cross-reactive idiotopes on monoclonal rheumatoid factors and their recognition of idiotopic positive cells. *Eur. J. Immunol.* 17: 343, 1987.
330. Ooi, B. S., Orlina, A. R., and Masaitas, L. Lymphocytotoxins in primary renal disease. *Lancet* 2: 1348, 1974.
331. Ozawa, T., Pluss, R., Lacher, J., et al. Endogenous immune complex nephropathy associated with malignancy: I. Studies on the nature and immunopathogenic significance of glomerular bound antigen and antibody. Isolation and characterisation of tumour specific antigen and antibody and circulating immune complexes. *Q. J. Med.* 64: 523, 1975.
332. Papiha, S. S., Pareck, S. K., Rodger, R. S. C., et al. HLA-A, B, DR and Bf allotypes in patients with idiopathic membranous nephropathy. *Kidney Int.* 31: 130, 1987.
333. Pardo, V., Strauss, J., Kramer, H., et al. Nephropathy associated with sickle cell anaemia: An autologous immune complex nephritis. II. Clinicopathological study of seven patients. *Am. J. Med.* 59: 650, 1975.
334. Parkinson, D. T., Baker, P. J., Couser, W. G., et al. Membrane attack complex deposition in experimental glomerular injury. *Am. J. Pathol.* 120: 121, 1985.
335. Paul, L. C., Stuffers-Heiman, M., van Es, L. A., et al. Antibodies directed against brush border antigens of proximal tubules in renal allograft recipients. *Clin. Immunol. Immunopathol.* 14: 238, 1979.
336. Pelletier, L., Pasquier, R., Hirsch, F., et al. Autoreactive T cells in mercury-induced autoimmune disease: In vitro demonstration. *J. Immunol.* 137: 2548, 1986.
337. Pelletier, L., Pasquier, R., Rossert, J., et al. Autoreactive T cells in mercury-induced autoimmunity: Ability to induce the autoimmune disease. *J. Immunol.* 140: 750, 1988.
338. Perez, G. O., Bjornsson, S., Ross, A. H., et al. A mini-epidemic of Goodpasture's syndrome: Clinical and immunological studies. *Nephron* 13: 161, 1974.
339. Peters, D. K., Rees, A. J., Lockwood, C. M., et al. Treatment and prognosis in anti-GBM antibody-mediated nephritis. *Transplant. Proc.* 14: 513, 1982.
340. Pickering, R. J., Michael, A. F., Herdman, R. C., et al. The complement system in chronic glomerulonephritis. Three newly associated aberrations. *J. Pediatr.* 78: 30, 1971.
341. Pietromonaco, S., Kerjaschki, D., Binder, S., et al. Molecular cloning of a cDNA encoding a major pathogenic domain of the Heymann nephritis antigen gp330. *Proc. Natl. Acad. Sci. U.S.A.* 87: 1811, 1990.
342. Pilia, P. A., Boackle, R. J., Swain, R. P., et al. Complement independent nephrotoxic serum nephritis in Munich Wister rats. *Lab. Invest.* 48: 585, 1983.
343. Pinching, A. J., Lockwood, C. M., Pussell, B. A., et al. Wegener's granulomatosis: Observations on 18 patients with severe renal disease. *Q. J. Med.* 52: 435, 1983.
344. Ponticelli, C., Zucchelli, P., Imbasciati, E., et al. Controlled trial of methyl prednisolone and chlorambucil in idiopathic membranous nephropathy. *N. Engl. J. Med.* 310: 946, 1984.
345. Pusey, C. D., Bowman, C., Morgan, A., et al. Kinetics and pathogenicity of autoantibodies induced by mercuric chloride in the Brown Norway rat. *Clin. Exp. Immunol.* 81: 76, 1990.
346. Pusey, C. D., Bowman, C., Peters, D. K., et al. Effect of cyclophosphamide on auto-antibody synthesis in the Brown Norway rat. *Clin. Exp. Immunol.* 54: 697, 1983.
346a. Pusey, C. D., Dash, A., Kershaw, M. J., et al. A single autoantigen in Goodpasture's syndrome identified by a

monoclonal antibody to human glomerular basement membrane. *Lab. Invest.* 56: 28, 1987.
347. Pusey, C. D., Holland, M. J., Cashman, S. J., et al. Experimental autoimmune glomerulonephritis induced by homologous and isologous glomerular basement membrane in Brown Norway rats. *Nephrol. Dial. Transplant.* 6: 457, 1991.
347a. Pusey, C. D., and Lockwood, C. M. Autoimmunity in rapidly progressive glomerulonephritis. *Kidney Int.* 35: 929, 1989.
348. Pusey, C. D., Lockwood, C. M., and Peters, D. K. Plasma exchange and immunosuppressive drugs in the treatment of glomerulonephritis due to antibodies to the glomerular basement membrane. *Int. J. Artif. Organs.* 6: 15, 1983.
349. Pusey, C. D., Rees, A. J., Evans, D. J., et al. Plasma exchange in focal necrotizing glomerulonephritis without anti-GBM antibodies. *Kidney Int.* 40: 757, 1991.
350. Pusey, C. D., Saltissi, D., Bloodworth, L., et al. Drug associated acute interstitial nephritis: Clinical and pathological features and the response to high dose steroid therapy. *Q. J. Med.* 52: 194, 1983.
351. Pusey, C. D., Venning, M. C., and Peters, D. K. Immunopathology of Glomerular and Interstitial Disease. In R. W. Schrier and C. W. Gottschalk (eds.), *Diseases of the Kidney* (4th ed.). Boston: Little, Brown, 1988. P. 1827.
352. Pussell, B. A., Bourke, E., Nayef, M., et al. Complement deficiency and nephritis. *Lancet* 1: 675, 1980.
353. Rao, T. K. S., and Friedman, E. A. AIDS (HIV)-associated nephropathy: Does it exist? An in-depth review. *Am. J. Nephrol.* 9: 441, 1989.
354. Rao, T. K. S., Nicastri, A. D., and Friedman, E. A. Natural history of heroin-associated nephropathy. *N. Engl. J. Med.* 290: 19, 1974.
354a. Rees, A. J. The HLA complex and susceptibility to glomerulonephritis. *Plasma Ther. Transfus. Technol.* 5: 455, 1984.
355. Rees, A. J., Demaine, A. G., and Welsh, K. I. The association between immunoglobulin allotypes with autoantibodies to glomerular basement membrane and their titre. *Hum. Immunol.* 10: 213, 1984.
356. Rees, A. J., Lockwood, C. M., and Peters, D. K. Enhanced allergic tissue injury in Goodpasture's syndrome by intercurrent bacterial infection. *Br. Med. J.* 2: 723, 1977.
357. Rees, A. J., Peters, D. K., Amos, N., et al. The influence of HLA-linked genes on the severity of anti-GBM antibody-mediated nephritis. *Kidney Int.* 26: 444, 1984.
358. Reynolds, J., Cashman, S. J., Evans, D. J., and Pusey, C. D. Cyclosporin A in the prevention and treatment of experimental autoimmune glomerulonephritis in the Brown Norway rat. *Clin. Exp. Immunol.* 85: 28, 1991.
359. Rich, A. R., and Gregory, J. E. The experimental demonstration that periarteritis nodosa is a manifestation of hypersensitivity. *Bull. Johns Hopkins Hosp.* 72: 65, 1943.
360. Richards, W., Olson, D., and Church, J. A. Improvement of idiopathic nephrotic syndrome following allergy treatment. *Ann. Allergy* 39: 332, 1977.
361. Rifai, A., Chen, A., and Imai, H. Complement activation in experimental IgA nephropathy: An antigen-mediated process. *Kidney Int.* 32: 838, 1987.
362. Rifai, A., and Millard, K. Glomerular deposition of immune complexes prepared with monomeric or polymeric IgA. *Clin. Exp. Immunol.* 60: 363, 1985.
363. Rifai, A., Small, P. A., Teague, P. O., et al. Experimental IgA nephropathy. *J. Exp. Med.* 150: 1161, 1979.
364. Roberts, J. L., Schwartz, M. M., and Lewis, E. J. Hereditary C2 deficiency and systemic lupus erythematosus associated with severe glomerulonephritis. *Clin. Exp. Immunol.* 31: 328, 1978.
365. Roberts, J. L., Wyatt, R. J., Schwartz, M. M., et al. Differential characteristics of immune-bound antibodies in diffuse proliferative and membranous forms of lupus glomerulonephritis. *Clin. Immunol. Immunopathol.* 29: 223, 1983.
366. Roccatello, D., Coppo, R., Amoroso, A., et al. Failure to relate mononuclear phagocyte system function to HLA-A, A, C.DR, DQ antigens in membranous nephropathy. *Am. J. Kidney Dis.* 31: 130, 1987.
367. Rodriguez-Iturbe, B. Epidemic post-streptococcal glomerulonephritis. *Kidney Int.* 25: 129, 1984.
368. Rodriguez-Iturbe, B., Castillo, L., Valbuena, B., et al. Acute post-streptococcal glomerulonephritis: A review of recent developments. *Paediatrician* 8: 307, 1979.
369. Rodriguez-Iturbe, B., Rubio, L., and Garcia, R. Attack rate of post-streptococcal nephritis in families. *Lancet* 1: 401, 1981.
370. Rolink, A. G., Gleichmann, H., and Gleichmann, E. Diseases caused by reactions of T lymphocytes to incompatible structures of the major histocompatibility complex. VII. Immune-complex glomerulonephritis. *J. Immunol.* 130: 209, 1983.
371. Roman-Franco, A. A., Turiello, M., Albini, B., et al. Anti-basement membrane antibodies and antigen–antibody complexes in rabbits injected with mercuric chloride. *Clin. Immunol. Immunopathol.* 9: 464, 1978.
372. Ronco, P., Neale, T. J., Wilson, C. B., et al. An immune pathological study of a 330kd protein defined by monoclonal antibodies and reactive with anti-RTEα5 antibodies and kidney eluates from active Heymann nephritis. *J. Immunol.* 136: 125, 1986.
373. Ronco, P., Verroust, P., Mignon, F., et al. Immunopathological studies of polyarteritis nodosa and Wegener's granulomatosis: A report of 43 patients with 51 renal biopsies. *Q. J. Med.* 52: 212, 1983.
374. Row, P. G., Cameron, J. S., Turner, D. R., et al. Membranous nephropathy. Long term follow-up and association with neoplasia. *Q. J. Med.* 44: 207, 1975.
375. Ruder, H., Scharer, K., Lenhard, V., et al. HLA phenotypes and idiopathic nephrotic syndrome in children. *Proc. Eur. Dial. Transplant. Assoc.* 19: 602, 1982.
376. Rudofsky, U. H., Dilwith, R. L., and Tung, K. S. K. Susceptibility differences of inbred mice to induction of autoimmune renal tubulointerstitial lesions. *Lab. Invest.* 43: 463, 1980.
377. Rudofsky, U. H., and Pollara, B. Studies on the pathogenesis of experimental autoimmune renal tubulointerstitial disease in guinea-pigs. II. Passive transfer of renal lesions by anti-tubular basement membrane autoantibody and non-immune bone marrow cells to leukocyte-depleted recipients. *Clin. Immunol. Immunopathol.* 6: 107, 1976.
378. Rudofsky, U. H., Steblay, R. W., and Pollara, B. Inhibition of experimental autoimmune renal tubulointerstitial disease in guinea-pigs by depletion of complement with cobra venom factor. *Clin. Immunol. Immunopathol.* 3: 396, 1975.
379. Sabatier, J. C., Genin, C., Assenat, H., et al. Mesangial IgA glomerulonephritis in HLA identical brothers. *Clin. Nephrol.* 11: 35, 1979.
380. Sado, T., Naito, I., and Okigaki, T. Transfer of anti-glomerular basement membrane antibody-induced glomerulonephritis in inbred rats with isologous antibodies from the urine of nephritic rats. *J. Pathol.* 158: 325, 1989.

381. Sado, T., Okigaki, T., Takamiya, H., et al. Experimental autoimmune glomerulonephritis with pulmonary haemorrhage in rats. The dose-effect relationship of the nephritogenic antigen from bovine glomerular basement membrane. *J. Clin. Lab. Immunol.* 15: 199, 1984.
382. Salant, D. J., Adler, S., Darby, C., et al. Influence of antigen distribution on the mediation of immunological glomerular injury. *Kidney Int.* 27: 938, 1985.
383. Salant, D. J., Belok, S., Madaio, M. P., et al. A new role for complement in experimental membranous nephropathy in rats. *J. Clin. Invest.* 66: 1339, 1980.
384. Salant, D. J., Quigg, R. J., and Cybulsky, A. V. Heymann nephritis: Mechanisms of renal injury. *Kidney Int.* 35: 976, 1989.
385. Sancho, J., Egido, J., Rivera, F., et al. Immune complexes in IgA nephropathy: Presence of antibodies against diet antigens and delayed clearance of specific polymeric IgA immune complexes. *Clin. Exp. Immunol.* 54: 194, 1983.
386. Sancho, J., Egido, J., Sanchez-Crespo, M., et al. Detection of monomeric and polymeric IgA containing immune complexes in serum and kidney from patients with alcoholic liver disease. *Clin. Exp. Immunol.* 47: 327, 1982.
387. Sandberg, D. H., McIntosh, R. M., Bernstein, C. W., et al. Severe steroid-responsive nephrosis associated with hypersensitivity. *Lancet* 1: 388, 1977.
388. Sapin, C., Druet, E., and Druet, P. Induction of antiglomerular basement membrane antibodies in the Brown Norway rat by mercuric chloride. *Clin. Exp. Immunol.* 28: 173, 1977.
389. Sasazuki, T., Hayase, R., Iwanoto, I., and Tsuchida, H. HLA and acute poststreptococcal glomerulonephritis. *N. Engl. J. Med.* 301: 1184, 1979.
390. Sato, M., Ideura, T., and Koshikawa, S. Experimental IgA nephropathy in mice. *Lab. Invest.* 54: 377, 1986.
391. Saulsbury, F. T. The role of IgA rheumatoid factor in the formation of IgA-containing immune complexes in Henoch-Schönlein purpura. *J. Clin. Lab. Immunol.* 23: 123, 1987.
392. Saus, J., Wieslander, J., Langeveld, J. P. M., et al. Identification of the Goodpasture antigen as the α3(IV) chain of collagen IV. *J. Biol. Chem.* 263: 13374, 1988.
393. Savage, C. O. S., Pottinger, B. E., Gaskin, G., et al. Vascular damage in Wegener's granulomatosis and microscopic polyarteritis: Presence of anti-endothelial cell antibodies and their relation to anti-neutrophil cytoplasmic antibodies. *Clin. Exp. Immunol.* 85: 14, 1991.
394. Savage, C. O. S., Pusey, C. D., Bowman, C., et al. Antiglomerular basement membrane antibody mediated disease in the British Isles 1980–1984. *Br. Med. J.* 292: 301, 1986.
395. Savage, C. O. S., Winearls, C. G., Evans, D. J., et al. Microscopic polyarteritis: Presentation, pathology and prognosis. *Q. J. Med.* 56: 467, 1985.
395a. Savage, C. O. S., Winearls, C. G., Jones, S., et al. Prospective study of radioimmunoassay for antibodies against neutrophil cytoplasm in diagnosis of systemic vasculitis. *Lancet* 1: 1389, 1987.
396. Scheer, R. L., and Grossman, M. A. Immune aspects of the glomerulonephritis associated with pulmonary hemorrhage. *Ann. Intern. Med.* 60: 1009, 1964.
397. Schena, F. P., Mastrolitti, G., and Frasasso, A. R. Increased immunoglobulin secreting cells in the blood of patients with active idiopathic IgA nephropathy. *Clin. Nephrol.* 26: 163, 1986.
398. Schena, F. P., Pertosa, G., Pastore, A., et al. Circulating immune complexes in infected ventriculoatrial and ventriculoperitoneal shunts. *J. Clin. Immunol.* 3: 173, 1983.
399. Schena, F. P., Pertosa, G., Stanziale, P., et al. Biological significance of the C3 nephritic factor in membranoproliferative glomerulonephritis. *Clin. Nephrol.* 18: 240, 1982.
400. Schifferli, J. A., Bartolotti, S. R., and Peters, D. K. Inhibition of immune precipitation by complement. *Clin. Exp. Immunol.* 42: 387, 1980.
401. Schifferli, J. A., and Taylor, R. P. Physiological and pathological aspects of circulating immune complexes. *Kidney Int.* 35: 993, 1989.
402. Schmiedeke, T. M. J., Stockl, F. W., Weber, R., et al. Histones have high affinity for the glomerular basement membrane: Relevance for immune complex formation in lupus nephritis. *J. Exp. Med.* 169: 1879, 1989.
403. Schnaper, H. W., and Aune, T. M. Identification of the lymphokine soluble immune response suppressor in urine of nephrotic children. *J. Clin. Invest.* 76: 341, 1985.
404. Schreiner, G. F., Cottran, R. S., Pando, V., et al. A mononuclear cell component in experimental immunological glomerulonephritis. *J. Exp. Med.* 147: 369, 1978.
405. Schulte-Wisserman, H., Lemmel, E. M., Reitz, M., et al. Nephrotic syndrome of childhood and disorder of T cell function. *Eur. J. Pediatr.* 124: 121, 1977.
406. Scott, D. M., Amos, N., and Bartolotti, S. R. The role of carbohydrate in the structure and function of nephritic factor. *Clin. Exp. Immunol.* 46: 120, 1981.
407. Scott, D. M., Amos, N., Sissons, J. G. P., et al. The immunoglobulin nature of nephritic factor (Nef). *Clin. Exp. Immunol.* 32: 12, 1978.
408. Serra, A., Cameron, J. S., Turner, D. R., et al. Vasculitis affecting the kidney: Presentation, histopathology and long-term outcome. *Q. J. Med.* 53: 181, 1984.
409. Shalhoub, R. J. Pathogenesis of lipoid nephrosis. A disorder of T cell function. *Lancet* 2: 556, 1974.
410. Sheth, K. J., Casper, J. T., and Good, T. A. Interstitial nephritis due to phenytoin hypersensitivity. *J. Pediatr.* 91: 438, 1977.
411. Shih, W., Hines, W. H., and Neilson, E. G. Effects of cyclosporin A on the development of immune-mediated interstitial nephritis. *Kidney Int.* 33: 1113, 1988.
412. Short, C. D., Dyer, P. A., Cairns, S. A., et al. A major histocompatibility system haplotype associated with poor prognosis in idiopathic membranous nephropathy. *Disease Markers* 1: 189, 1983.
413. Sim, E., Gill, E. W., and Sim, R. B. Drugs that induce systemic lupus erythematosus inhibit complement component C4. *Lancet* 2: 422, 1984.
414. Simpson, I. J., Amos, N., Evans, D. J., et al. Guinea-pig nephrotoxic nephritis. I. The role of complement and polymorphonuclear leucocytes and effect of antibody subclass and fragments in the heterologous phase. *Clin. Exp. Immunol.* 19: 499, 1975.
415. Simpson, I. J., Doak, P. B., Williams, L. C., et al. Plasma exchange in Goodpasture's syndrome. *Am. J. Nephrol.* 2: 301, 1982.
416. Simpson, I. J., Moran, J., Evans, D. J., et al. Prolonged complement activation in mice. *Kidney Int.* 13: 467, 1978.
417. Singer, D. R. J., Venning, M. C., Lockwood, C. M., and Pusey, C. D. Cryoglobulinaemia: Clinical features and response to treatment. *Ann. Med. Interne* (Paris) 137: 251, 1986.
418. Sinico, R. A., Fornasieri, A., and Ureni, M. Polymeric IgA rheumatoid factor in idiopathic IgA mesangial nephropathy (Berger's disease). *J. Immunol.* 137: 536, 1986.

419. Sinniah, R. Heterogeneous IgA glomerulonephropathy in liver cirrhosis. *Histopathology* 8: 947, 1984.
420. Sissons, J. G. P., West, R. J., Fallows, J., et al. The complement abnormalities of lipodystrophy. *N. Engl. J. Med.* 294: 461, 1976.
421. Specks, U., Wheatley, C. L., McDonald, T. J., et al. Anticytoplasmic antibodies in the diagnosis and follow-up of Wegener's granulomatosis. *Mayo Clin. Proc.* 64: 28, 1989.
421a. Spencer, S. J. W., et al. HLA class II specificities in vasculitis with antibodies to neutrophil cytoplasmic antigens. *Kidney Int.* 41: 1059, 1992.
422. Spitzer, R. E., Vallota, E. H., Forristal, J., et al. Serum C3 lytic system in patients with glomerulonephritis. *Science* 164: 436, 1969.
423. Srivastava, R. N., Agarwal, R. K., Mondgil, A., and Bhuyan, U. N. Late resistance to corticosteroids in nephrotic syndrome. *J. Pediatr.* 108: 66, 1986.
424. Stachura, I., Si, L., and Whiteside, T. L. Mononuclear-cell subsets in human idiopathic crescentic glomerulonephritis (ICGN): Analysis in tissue sections with monoclonal antibodies. *J. Clin. Immunol.* 4: 202, 1984.
425. Stanton, M. C., and Tange, J. D. Goodpasture's syndrome: Pulmonary haemorrhage associated with glomerulonephritis. *Austr. Ann. Med.* 7: 132, 1958.
426. Steblay, R. W. Glomerulonephritis induced in sheep by injections of heterologous glomerular basement membrane and Freund's complete adjuvant. *J. Exp. Med.* 116: 253, 1962.
427. Steblay, R. W. Glomerulonephritis induced in monkeys by injections of heterologous glomerular basement membrane and Freund's adjuvant. *Nature* 197: 1173, 1963.
428. Steblay, R. W., and Rudofsky, U. Autoimmune glomerulonephritis induced in sheep by injections of human lung and Freund's adjuvant. *Science* 160: 204, 1968.
429. Steblay, R. W., and Rudofsky, U. In vitro and in vivo properties of autoantibodies eluted from kidneys of sheep with autoimmune glomerulonephritis. *Nature* 218: 1269, 1968.
430. Steblay, R. W., and Rudofsky, U. Renal tubular disease and autoantibodies against tubular basement membrane induced in guinea pigs. *J. Immunol.* 107: 589, 1971.
431. Steblay, R. W., and Rudofsky, U. Transfer of experimental autoimmune renal cortical tubular and interstitial disease in guinea pigs by serum. *Science* 180: 966, 1973.
432. Steinman, T. I., and Silva, P. Acute interstitial nephritis and iritis: Reno-ocular syndrome. *Am. J. Med.* 77: 189, 1984.
433. Stenglein, B., Thoenes, G. H., and Gunther, E. Genetic control of susceptibility to autologous immune complex glomerulonephritis in inbred rat strains. *Clin. Exp. Immunol.* 33: 88, 1978.
434. Stetson, C. A., Rammelkamp, C. H., Krause, R. M., et al. Epidemic acute nephritis: Studies on etiology, natural history and prevention. *Medicine* 34: 431, 1955.
435. Stilmant, M. M., Bolton, W. K., Sturgill, B. C., et al. Crescentic glomerulonephritis without immune deposits: Clinicopathological features. *Kidney Int.* 15: 184, 1979.
436. Strauss, J., Pardo, V., Scott, G., et al. A spectrum of histological changes in children with ARC/AIDS and nephrotic syndrome. *Kidney Int.* 33: 210, 1988.
437. Strom, T. B., and Kelly, V. E. Towards more selective therapies to block undesired immune responses. *Kidney Int.* 35: 1026, 1989.
438. Stuffers-Heiman, M., Gunther, E., and Van Es, L. A. Induction of autoimmunity to antigens of the glomerular basement membrane in inbred Brown Norway rats. *Immunology* 36: 759, 1979.
439. Sugisaki, T., Klassen, J., Milgrom, F., et al. Immunologic study of an autoimmune tubular and interstitial renal disease in Brown Norway rats. *Lab. Invest.* 28: 658, 1973.
440. Takata, Y., Tamura, N., and Fujita, T. Interaction of C3 with antigen–antibody complexes in the process of solubilization of immune precipitates. *J. Immunol.* 132: 2531, 1984.
441. Tarantino, A., Anelli, A., Costantino, A., et al. Serum complement pattern in essential mixed cryoglobulinaemia. *Clin. Exp. Immunol.* 32: 77, 1978.
442. Tarantino, A., De Vecchi, A., Montagnino, G., et al. Renal disease in essential mixed cryoglobulinaemia. *Q. J. Med.* 50: 1, 1981.
443. Taube, D., Chapman, S., Brown, Z., and Williams, D. G. Depression of normal lymphocyte transformation by sera of patients with minimal change nephropathy and other forms of nephrotic syndrome. *Clin. Nephrol.* 15: 286, 1981.
444. Teitlebaum, D., Rauch, J., Stollar, B. D., et al. In vivo effects of antibodies against a high frequency idiotype of anti-DNA antibodies in MRL mice. *J. Immunol.* 132: 1282, 1984.
445. Tejani, A., Butt, K., Trachtman, H., et al. Cyclosporin induced remission of relapsing nephrotic syndrome in children. *J. Pediatr.* 111: 1056, 1987.
446. Tejani, A., Nicastri, A. D., Sen, D., et al. Long term evaluation of children with nephrotic syndrome and focal segmental glomerulonephritis. *Nephron* 35: 225, 1983.
447. Tejani, A., Phadke, K., Nicastri, A., et al. Efficacy of cyclophosphamide in steroid sensitive nephrotic syndrome with different morphological lesions. *Nephron* 41: 170, 1985.
448. Theofilopoulos, A. N., and Dixon, F. J. Murine models of systemic lupus erythematosus. *Adv. Immunol.* 37: 269, 1985.
449. Theofilopoulos, A. N., Kofler, R., Singer, P. A., and Dixon, F. J. Molecular genetics of murine lupus models. *Adv. Immunol.* 46: 61, 1989.
450. Thomson, N. M., Holdsworth, S. R., Glasgow, E. F., et al. The macrophage in the development of experimental crescentic glomerulonephritis. *Am. J. Pathol.* 94: 223, 1979.
451. Thomson, N. M., Naish, P. F., Simpson, I. J., et al. The role of C3 in the autologous phase of nephrotoxic nephritis. *Clin. Exp. Immunol.* 24: 464, 1976.
452. Tipping, P. G., Boyce, N. W., and Holdsworth, S. R. Relative contributions of chemoattractant and terminal components of complement to anti-glomerular basement membrane (GBM) glomerulonephritis. *Clin. Exp. Immunol.* 78: 444, 1989.
453. Tipping, P. C., Neale, T. J., and Holdsworth, S. R. T lymphocyte participation in antibody induced experimental glomerulonephritis. *Kidney Int.* 27: 530, 1985.
454. Todd, J. A., Acha-Orbea, H., Bell, J. I., et al. A molecular basis for MHC class II associated autoimmunity. *Science* 240: 1003, 1988.
455. Tolkoff-Rubin, N. E., Cosimi, A. B., Fuller, T., et al. IgA nephropathy in HLA identical siblings. *Transplantation* 26: 430, 1978.
456. Tomino, Y., Endoh, M., Nomoto, Y., et al. Specificity of eluted antibody from renal tissues of patients with IgA nephropathy. *Am. J. Kidney Dis.* 1: 276, 1982.
457. Tomino, Y., Sakai, H., Miura, M., et al. Detection of polymeric IgA in glomeruli from patients with IgA nephropathy. *Clin. Exp. Immunol.* 49: 419, 1982.

458. Tomizawa, S., Mariiyama, K., Nagasawa, N., et al. Studies of vascular permeability factor derived from T lymphocytes and inhibitory effect of plasma on its production in minimal change nephrotic syndrome. *Nephron* 41: 157, 1985.
459. Tomizawa, S., Suzuki, S., Oguri, M., and Kuroume, T. Studies of T lymphocyte function and inhibitory factors in minimal change nephrotic syndrome. *Nephron* 24: 179, 1979.
460. Tomosugi, N. I., Cashman, S. J., Hay, H., et al. Modulation of antibody-mediated glomerular injury in vivo by bacterial lipopolysaccharide, tumour necrosis factor and IL-1. *J. Immunol.* 142: 3083, 1989.
461. Tornroth, T., and Skrifvars, B. Gold nephropathy prototype of membranous glomerulonephritis. *Am. J. Pathol.* 75: 573, 1974.
462. Trompeter, R. S., Barratt, T. M., Kay, R., et al. HLA, atopy and cyclophosphamide in steroid responsive childhood nephrotic syndrome. *Kidney Int.* 17: 113, 1980.
463. Tron, F., and Bach, J. F. Relationships between antibodies to native DNA and glomerulonephritis in systemic lupus erythematosus. *Clin. Exp. Immunol.* 28: 426, 1977.
464. Tsai, C. D., Giangiacomo, J., and Zuckner, J. Dermal IgA deposits in Henoch Schönlein purpura and Berger's nephritis. *Lancet* 1: 342, 1975.
465. Tucker, F. L., Sturgill, B. C., and Bolton, W. K. Ultrastructural studies of experimental autoimmune glomerulonephritis in normal and bursectomised chicks. *Lab. Invest.* 53: 563, 1985.
466. Turner, N., et al. Molecular cloning of the human Goodpasture antigen demonstrates it to be the α_3 chain of type IV collagen. *J. Clin. Invest.* 89: 592, 1992.
467. Turner, A. N., and Pusey, C. D. Anti-glomerular Basement Membrane Disease. In C. D. Pusey (ed.), *Immunology of Renal Diseases*. Lancaster: Kluwer, 1991. P. 229.
468. Ulrich, T. R., and Ni, R.-X. Inhibition of experimental autoimmune tubulointerstitial nephritis in Brown Norway rats by (155)-15-methyl prostaglandin E_1. *Am. J. Pathol.* 124: 286, 1986.
469. Unanue, E. R., and Dixon, F. J. Experimental glomerulonephritis: Immunological events and pathogenetic mechanisms. *Adv. Immunol.* 6: 1, 1967.
470. Unanue, E. R., Dixon, F. J., and Feldmann, J. D. Experimental allergic glomerulonephritis induced in the rabbit with homologous renal antigens. *J. Exp. Med.* 125: 163, 1967.
471. Valentijin, R. M., Radi, J., Haaijman, J. J., et al. Circulating and mesangial secretory component binding IgA-1 in primary IgA nephropathy. *Kidney Int.* 26: 760, 1984.
472. Van Damme, B. J. C., Fleuren, G. J., Bakker, W. W., et al. Experimental glomerulonephritis in the rat induced by antibodies directed against tubular antigens. V. Fixed glomerular antigens in the pathogenesis of heterologous immune complex glomerulonephritis. *Lab. Invest.* 38: 502, 1978.
473. Van den Wall Bake, A. W., Daha, M. R., Haaijman, J. J., et al. Elevated production of polymeric and monomeric IgA_1 by the bone marrow in IgA nephropathy. *Kidney Int.* 35: 1400, 1989.
474. Van de Rijn, I., Fillit, H., Brandeis, W. E., et al. Serial studies on circulating immune complexes in post-streptococcal sequelae. *Clin. Exp. Immunol.* 34: 318, 1978.
475. Van der Woude, F. J., Daha, M. R., and Van Es, L. A. The current status of anti-neutrophil cytoplasmic antibodies. *Clin. Exp. Immunol.* 78: 143, 1989.
476. Van der Woude, F. J., Rasmussen, N., Lobatto, S., et al. Autoantibodies against neutrophils and monocytes: Tool for diagnosis and marker of disease activity in Wegener's granulomatosis. *Lancet* 1: 425, 1985.
477. Van Haesebrouck, P., Carton, D., DeBel, C., et al. Acute tubular interstitial nephritis and uveitis syndrome (TINU syndrome). *Nephron* 40: 418, 1985.
478. Vaughan, R. W., Demaine, A. G., and Welsh, K. I. A DQA1 allele is strongly associated with idiopathic membranous nephropathy. *Tissue Antigens* 34: 261, 1989.
479. Verroust, P. J., Ronco, P. M., and Chatelet, F. Monoclonal antibodies and identification of glomerular antigen. *Kidney Int.* 30: 649, 1986.
480. Verroust, P. J., Wilson, C. B., and Dixon, F. J. Lack of nephritogenicity of systemic activation of the alternative complement pathway. *Kidney Int.* 6: 157, 1974.
481. Vignon, J. D., Houssin, A., Soulillou, J. P., et al. HLA antigens and Berger's disease. *Tissue Antigens* 16: 108, 1980.
482. Villareal, H., Fischetti, V. A., Van de Rijn, I., et al. The occurrence of a protein in the extracellular products of streptococci isolated from patients with acute glomerulonephritis. *J. Exp. Med.* 149: 459, 1979.
483. Vogt, A., Batsford, S., Rodriguez-Iturbe, B., et al. Cationic antigens in poststreptococcal glomerulonephritis. *Clin. Nephrol.* 20: 271, 1983.
484. Vogt, A., Rohrbach, R., Shimizu, F., et al. Interaction of cationised antigen with rat glomerular basement membrane. In situ immune complex formation. *Kidney Int.* 22: 27, 1982.
485. Waldo, B. F., Beischel, L., and West, C. D. IgA synthesis by lymphocytes from patients with IgA nephropathy and their relatives. *Kidney Int.* 29: 1229, 1986.
486. Walker, R. G., Scheinkesterl, C., Becker, G. J., et al. Clinical and morphological aspects of the management of crescentic anti-glomerular basement membrane (GBM) nephritis/Goodpasture's syndrome. *Q. J. Med.* 54: 75, 1985.
487. Walport, M. J., Black, C. M., and Batchelor, J. R. The immunogenetics of SLE. *Clin. Rheum. Dis.* 8: 3, 1982.
488. Walport, M. J., Peters, A. M., Elkon, K. B., et al. The splenic extraction ratio of antibody coated erythrocytes and its response to plasma exchange and pulse methylprednisolone. *Clin. Exp. Immunol.* 60: 465, 1985.
489. Walport, M. J., Ross, G. D., Mackworth-Young, C., et al. Family studies of erythrocyte complement receptor type I levels: Reduced levels in patients with SLE are acquired, not inherited. *Clin. Exp. Immunol.* 59: 547, 1985.
490. Welch, T. R., Beischel, L., Balakrishnan, K., et al. Major-histocompatibility-complex extended haplotypes in membranoproliferative glomerulonephritis. *N. Engl. J. Med.* 314: 1476, 1986.
491. West, C. D. Childhood membranoproliferative glomerulonephritis: An approach to management. *Kidney Int.* 29: 1077, 1986.
492. West, M. L., Jindal, K. K., Bear, R. A., and Goldstein, M. B. A controlled trial of cyclophosphamide in patients with membranous glomerulonephritis. *Kidney Int.* 32: 579, 1987.
493. White, R. H. R. The familial nephrotic syndrome: I. A European survey. *Clin. Nephrol.* 1: 215, 1973.
494. Wieslander, J., Bygren, P. G., and Heinegard, D. Antibasement membrane antibody: Immunoenzymic assay and specificity of antibodies. *Scand. J. Clin. Invest.* 41: 763, 1981.
495. Wieslander, J., Bygren, P., and Heinegard, D. Isolation of the specific glomerular basement membrane antigen

involved in Goodpasture's syndrome. *Proc. Natl. Acad. Sci. U.S.A.* 81: 1544, 1984.

496. Wilkowski, M. J., Velosa, J. A., Holley, K. E., et al. Risk factors in idiopathic renal vasculitis and glomerulonephritis. *Kidney Int.* 36: 1133, 1989.
497. Williams, P. S., Davenport, A., McDickens, I., et al. Increased incidence of anti-glomerular basement membrane antibody (anti-GBM) nephritis in the Mersey region September 1984–October 1985. *Q. J. Med.* 68: 727, 1988.
498. Wilson, C. B. Nephritogenic antibody mechanisms involving antigens within the glomerulus. *Immunol. Rev.* 55: 257, 1981.
499. Wilson, C. B., and Dixon, F. J. Antigen quantitation in experimental immune complex glomerulonephritis. *J. Immunol.* 105: 279, 1970.
500. Wilson, C. B., and Dixon, F. J. Quantitation of acute and chronic serum sickness in the rabbit. *J. Exp. Med.* 134: 75, 1971.
501. Wilson, C. B., and Dixon, F. J. Anti-glomerular basement membrane antibody-induced glomerulonephritis. *Kidney Int.* 3: 74, 1973.
502. Wilson, J. G., Wong, W. W., Schur, P. H., and Fearon, D. T. Mode of inheritance of decreased C3b receptors on erythrocytes of patients with systemic lupus erythematosus. *N. Engl. J. Med.* 307: 981, 1982.

502a. Winer, R. L., Cohen, A. H., Sawhrey, A. S., and Gorman, J. T. Sjogren's syndrome with immune complex tubulointerstitial renal disease. *Clin. Immunol. Immunopathol.* 8: 494, 1977.

503. Winfield, J. B. Cryoglobulinaemia. *Hum. Pathol.* 14: 350, 1983.
504. Wittig, H. J., and Goldman, A. S. Nephrotic syndrome associated with inhaled allergens. *Lancet* 1: 542, 1970.
505. Wofsy, D., Ledbetter, J. A., Hendlar, P. L., et al. Treatment of murine lupus with monoclonal anti-T cell antibody. *J. Immunol.* 134: 852, 1985.
506. Wofsy, D., and Seaman, W. E. Successful treatment of autoimmunity in NZB/NZW F1 mice with monoclonal antibody to L3T4. *J. Exp. Med.* 161: 378, 1986.
507. Woo, K. T., Edmondson, R. P. S., and Yap, H. K. Effects of triple therapy on the progression of mesangial proliferative glomerulonephritis. *Clin. Nephrol.* 27: 56, 1987.
508. Woodroffe, A. J., Gormly, A. A., McKenzie, P. E., et al. Immunologic studies in IgA nephropathy. *Kidney Int.* 18: 366, 1980.
509. Wooley, P. H., Griffin, J., Panayi, G. S., et al. HLA-DR antigens and toxic reaction to sodium aurothiomalate and D-penicillamine in patients with rheumatoid arthritis. *N. Engl. J. Med.* 303: 300, 1980.
510. Wraith, D. C., McDevitt, H. O., Steinman, L., and Acha-Orbea, H. T cell recognition as the target for immune intervention in autoimmune disease. *Cell* 57: 709, 1989.
511. Wyatt, R. J., Valenski, W., and Stapleton, F. B. Immunoregulatory studies in patients with IgA nephropathy. *J. Clin. Lab. Immunol.* 25: 109, 1988.
512. Yamamoto, T., and Wilson, C. B. Complement dependence of antibody-induced mesangial cell injury in the rat. *J. Immunol.* 138: 3758, 1987.
513. Yamamoto, T., and Wilson, C. B. Binding of anti-basement membrane antibody to alveolar basement membrane after intratracheal gasoline instillation in rabbits. *Am. J. Pathol.* 126: 497, 1987.
514. Yum, M. N., Edwards, J. L., and Kleit, S. Glomerular lesions in Hodgkin's disease. *Arch. Pathol.* 99: 645, 1975.
515. Zakheim, B., McCafferty, E., Phillips, S. M., et al. Murine interstitial nephritis. II. The adoptive transfer of disease with immune T lymphocytes produces a phenotypically complex interstitial lesion. *J. Immunol.* 133: 234, 1984.
516. Zanetti, M., Mampaso, F., and Wilson, C. B. Anti-idiotype as a probe in the analysis of autoimmune tubulointerstitial nephritis in the Brown Norway rat. *J. Immunol.* 131: 1268, 1983.
517. Zanetti, M., Mandet, C., Duboust, A., et al. Demonstration of a passive Heymann nephritis-like mechanism in a human kidney transplant. *Clin. Nephrol.* 15: 272, 1981.

Glomerulonephritis with Bacterial Endocarditis, Ventriculovascular Shunts, and Visceral Infections

Sharon G. Adler
Arthur H. Cohen

Bacterial Endocarditis

CLINICAL PERSPECTIVES

The renal lesions and nephrologic clinical presentations of bacterial endocarditis are numerous and varied (Table 61-1). Patients with endocarditis may present with gross hematuria as a manifestation of renal infarction due to emboli. The "flea-bitten" kidneys, appreciated in the late nineteenth and early twentieth centuries [36, 85], are the pathologic counterparts of this clinical event. Septic emboli may lead to renal abscesses. Associated septicemia may cause disseminated intravascular coagulation or hypotension, leading to acute tubular necrosis and acute renal failure. Antibiotic therapy may induce hypersensitivity acute tubulointerstitial nephritis or acute renal failure due to drug nephrotoxicity. Finally, glomerulonephritis as a complication of bacterial endocarditis was highlighted at the turn of the century by Harbitz [34] and Löhlein [48] and later by Baehr [3, 4]. These early investigators believed that endocarditis-associated glomerulonephritis was caused by emboli. However, this assumption has been effectively challenged by the clear documentation of glomerulonephritis in patients with right-sided endocarditis who did not have right-to-left shunts [5]. The immune-mediated basis of this glomerulonephritis is now well accepted [6] and is supported by the findings of circulating immune complexes [7], glomerular immunoglobulin and complement deposition [31], and detection of bacterial antigen in glomerular immune complexes [15, 67, 95].

The frequency with which glomerulonephritis complicates bacterial endocarditis is difficult to determine with precision, as no prospective study has been performed in which all patients with endocarditis undergo renal biopsy regardless of the clinical manifestations. Autopsy studies may overestimate the occurrence of glomerulonephritis, since azotemia predisposes to higher morbidity and mortality in endocarditis [40, 43]. Alternatively, it has been suggested that autopsy studies may sometimes decrease the appreciation of glomerulonephritis, since antibiotic therapy may contribute to its resolution prior to the patient's death. Reports derived from studies on renal biopsies tend to exaggerate the severity and underestimate the prevalence of glomerulonephritis because biopsies are usually performed in patients with the most extreme clinical features. Thus patients with mild or fleeting clinical manifestations of glomerulonephritis are likely to remain undiagnosed. Studies that depend on urinalysis to diagnose glomerulonephritis may overestimate its presence, mistaking the hematuria of embolic infarction or the leukocyturia and hematuria of tubulointerstitial nephritis for glomerular disease. Despite the shortcomings in assessing prevalence, it appears that the frequency with which glomerulonephritis complicates bacterial endocarditis is decreasing. In the preantibiotic era, focal glomerulonephritis was reported in as many as 50 percent of patients dying of endocarditis [3, 12, 79], and diffuse glomerulonephritis was present in 30 to 60 percent [12, 39, 79]. With the advent of penicillin, Spain and King [79] reported a precipitous decrement in endocarditis-associated glomerulonephritis at autopsy, from 81 percent to 25 percent in their population.

In a series reported by Neugarten et al. [58], the incidence of glomerulonephritis was 22 percent, of which 8 percent was focal and 14 percent was diffuse. The decline in the frequency of glomerulonephritis likely relates both to the changing nature of bacterial endocarditis as it is currently seen and to changes in treatment strategies. Early cases of endocarditis were more likely to be "subacute," with less virulent organisms such as *Streptococcus viridans* infecting congenitally abnormal valves or valves damaged by rheumatic fever. In this clinical setting, it was argued that the duration of bacteremia was prolonged, thus predisposing patients to the development of immunologically mediated complications [32]. Because of the declining occurrence of rheumatic fever and the advent of prophylactic antibiotics for patients with known valvular disease, subacute bacterial endocarditis is less common at the present time. Instead, acute endocarditis associated with intravenous drug abuse is increasing and is most frequent with *Staphylococcus aureus* bacteremia involving previously normal heart valves, often the tricuspid or pulmonic. Despite the "acuteness" of the clinical illness, the involvement of right-sided valves, and the availability of antibiotic therapy, glomerulonephritis is a frequent occurrence in such patients [59]. This has led some investigators to suggest that in this setting, the duration of clinical illness may be less a predisposing factor to the development of glomerulonephritis than the nature of the infecting organism. *S. aureus* is estimated to cause approximately one-third of the current cases of infectious endocarditis but is present in more than half of the patients with associated glomerulonephritis [44, 59, 62]. Occasionally unusual organisms, such as *Actinobacillus,* may be responsible for endocarditis and be associated with glomerulonephritis [77]. Nonimmune activation of the alternate complement pathway by staphylococcal antigen has been suggested as one explanation for the high incidence of glomerulonephritis in some patients [59], especially those lacking glomerular immunoglobulin deposits [69]. However, other workers have postulated that the occasional observation of glomerular complement without immunoglobulin in this setting may instead be due to rapid antibiotic-associated immune complex clearance from glomeruli, with a more prolonged clearance time for complement [54].

There are two common patterns of glomerular injury: focal and diffuse glomerulonephritis. Both forms present clinically in a spectrum from completely asymptomatic to severe. The focal lesion is usually manifested by

Table 61-1. Renal complications of bacterial endocarditis

Emboli
Infarction
Abscesses
Associated with septicemia
Shock-induced acute tubular necrosis
Disseminated intravascular coagulation
Associated with antibiotic therapy
Nephrotoxic acute tubular necrosis
Hypersensitivity-induced acute tubulointerstitial nephritis
Immune complex–mediated lesions
Focal glomerulonephritis
Diffuse glomerulonephritis
Membranoproliferative glomerulonephritis

microscopic hematuria and nonnephrotic proteinuria [59]. Autopsy studies indicate that focal proliferative glomerulonephritis can be present without premortem urinary abnormalities [54]. Although clinically mild, focal proliferative glomerulonephritis may occasionally present with gross hematuria [22], nephrotic syndrome [74], and renal insufficiency or renal failure [17, 18, 46, 92], especially when bacteriologic cure is not achieved [68]. Hypertension is uncommon [59]. In one study, the serum creatinine exceeded 2 mg/dl only when other factors (e.g., hypotension, radiocontrast media administration) were present; renal dysfunction did not result in the need for dialysis nor did it contribute to patient mortality [59]. Diffuse proliferative glomerulonephritis was more likely to be diagnosed premortem [59] because of its tendency to manifest severe clinical features that lead to the performance of a renal biopsy. Excluding patients in whom contrast or hypotension produced acute renal failure, the majority of individuals with diffuse proliferative glomerulonephritis had peak serum creatinines prior to the initiation of antibiotic therapy and recovery of renal function with resolution of infection. Failure to resolve infection was associated with worsening renal function and, in some cases, dialysis dependence. It is unclear whether uremia contributed to the inability to control the infectious process or whether the severity of the infection caused the more serious renal disease. In any case, renal failure is a poor prognostic feature, often presaging a fatal outcome [59].

Microscopic hematuria is a near universal finding [59], although gross hematuria [59, 84] and red blood cell casts [65] may also be noted. Pyuria is evident in approximately two-thirds of patients, and proteinuria occurs in all, with nephrotic syndrome in approximately 25 percent [59]. Fifteen to 30 percent have positive urine cultures [42, 55].

Numerous serologic abnormalities are present. Rheumatoid factor has been reported in 10 to 70 percent of cases. Although its titer tends to fall with successful antibiotic therapy, its relationship to pathogenesis or course of glomerulonephritis is controversial [65, 78]. Circulating immune complexes are present in approximately 90 percent of patients with endocarditis [6, 19, 38, 53, 92]. High levels of circulating immune complexes have been associated with less virulent organisms, protracted courses, and right-sided valvular lesions [6, 19, 38]. Some investigators have suggested that the finding of circulating immune complexes identifiable by the C1q binding and Raji cell assays correlate with glomerulonephritis [35, 38]. Mixed cryoglobulinemia is frequent, declines with therapy, and is unrelated to the presence or absence of glomerulonephritis [19, 37]. Hypocomplementemia is frequent but not invariable. Complement activation occurs most often via the direct pathway, although the possibility of alternate pathway activation has been suggested [9, 38, 62]. Normalization of complement levels is observed with bacteriologic cure and resolution of glomerulonephritis [22, 70, 92].

With antibiotic therapy, urinary sediment abnormalities and azotemia (when present) normalize within days to weeks. Rarely, microscopic hematuria and proteinuria persist for months to years [59]. Occasionally, the continued clinical signs of glomerulonephritis suggest failure to eradicate the underlying infection; this is frequently the case in Q fever endocarditis [68]. While effective antibiotic therapy generally results in rapid recovery of renal function, in some instances renal failure progresses despite bacteriologic cure [59]. The patients with progressive renal disease often have a high proportion of glomerular crescents on renal biopsy [6, 7, 52, 70]. Some workers have suggested that immunosuppressive therapy, including plasma exchange, corticosteroids, and/or cytotoxic therapy, may be useful in the occasional patient whose renal disease progresses despite appropriate antibiotic or surgical therapy [6, 51, 52, 72]. Recommendations for immunosuppressive therapy in this setting are thus based on anecdotal case reports. Use of such therapy should be tempered by the possible risk of exacerbation of the underlying infectious process, as well as by the other side effects common to employment of immunosuppressive strategies.

PATHOLOGIC CHANGES

The major glomerular abnormalities are the result of immune complex deposits; the antigen is presumed of bacterial origin. The form of injury varies depending on severity of the immunologic process but is characterized by some degree of increased glomerular hypercellularity.

The less severe abnormalities, usually occurring in *S. viridans* subacute endocarditis, are termed focal glomerulonephritis. This implies "focal" glomerular involvement; lesions in the abnormal glomeruli are segmental, with increased cells in portions of the tufts (mesangial, endothelial, leukocytes) (Fig. 61-1) and occasionally segmental crescents. Capillary walls are thin and single contoured and are disrupted in the face of crescent formation. Depending on the duration of the crescent, healing by organization occurs; fibrocellular or fibrotic crescents with collapse or sclerosis of the capillary tufts ensue. Diffuse increase in glomerular cellularity (diffuse glomerulonephritis) (Fig. 61-2) is more common in staphylococcal endocarditis as compared to streptococcal infection. The hypercellularity results from increased mesangial and endothelial cells as well as accumulation

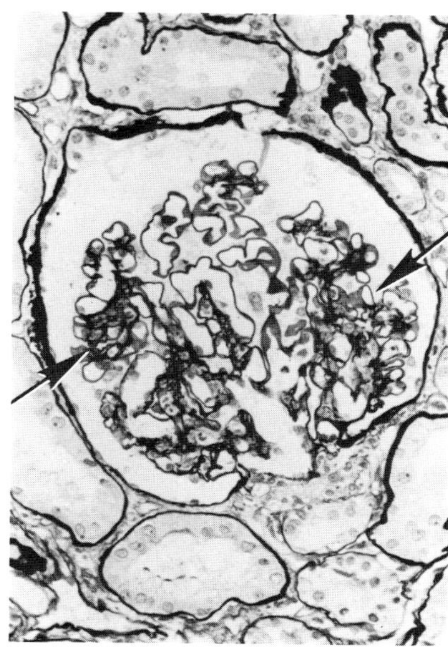

Fig. 61-1. Glomerulonephritis in bacterial endocarditis. There is segmental increase in mesangial cellularity involving two lobules (*arrows*). This less severe involvement is also known as focal glomerulonephritis. (Periodic acid–methenamine silver, ×190.)

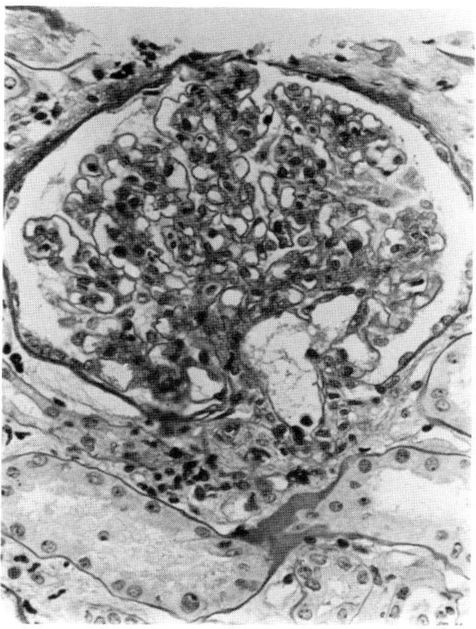

Fig. 61-2. Diffuse glomerulonephritis in intravenous heroin user with staphylococcal endocarditis. Numerous leukocytes in many capillaries account for the increased cellularity. (Periodic acid–Schiff, ×185.)

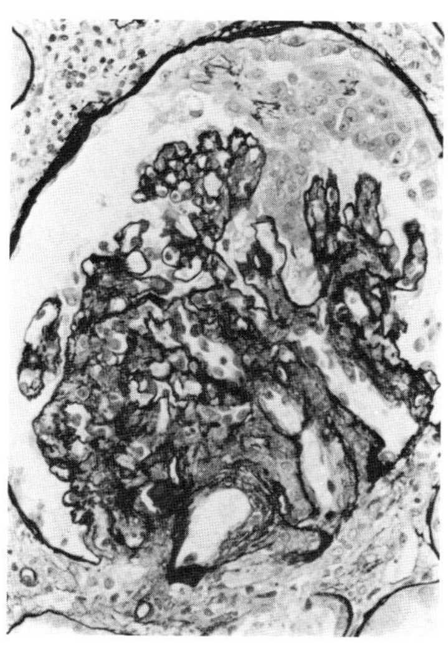

Fig. 61-3. Glomerulus from patient with similar history as in Fig. 61-2. There is a segmental cellular crescent. (Periodic acid–methenamine silver, ×170.)

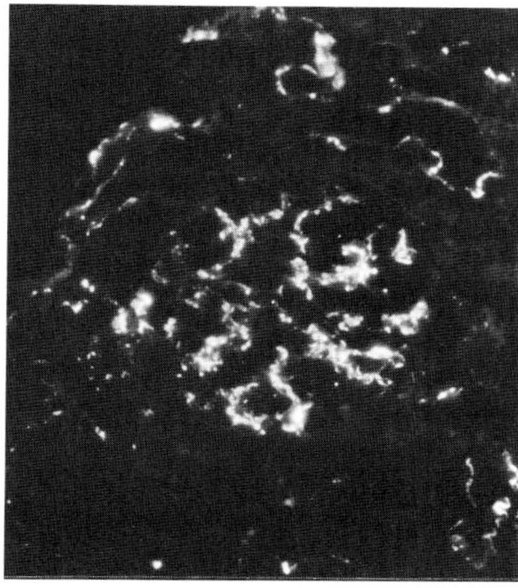

Fig. 61-4. Immunofluorescence demonstrating granular capillary wall and mesangial deposits. (Anti-C3, ×250.)

of neutrophils and monocytes. Double contours of capillary walls are present to varying degrees, and crescents are not uncommon (Fig. 61-3), although they rarely affect more than 50 percent of the glomeruli [9, 17, 29, 31, 32, 59]. The interstitium is often edematous and infiltrated by mononuclear leukocytes. Whether this last lesion is an integral part of the endocarditis-associated renal injury or is the consequence of antibiotic-induced hypersensitivity is controversial [23].

Regardless of the light microscopic pattern of glomerular injury (focal versus diffuse hypercellularity), the immunofluorescence findings are the same. Granular mesangial and capillary wall immunoglobulins (most commonly IgG and/or IgM) and complement (C3 predominantly, C1q less frequently) are regularly observed in all glomeruli (Fig. 61-4). Fibrin is in the urinary spaces and in capillaries when crescents are present [9, 29, 31, 32, 54] (Fig. 61-5). Extraglomerular deposits are infrequent; we have observed granular deposits in tubular basement membranes and the interstitium in a small number of renal biopsies. In keeping with the systemic nature of this immune complex disease, we documented granular deposits in splenic sinuses in a patient with concomitant glomerulonephritis [57].

As pointed out by Gutman and colleagues [31], the ultrastructural findings are identical to those of postinfectious (streptococcal) glomerulonephritis. There are electron-dense deposits in mesangial regions and in capillary walls. While the deposits are characteristically in subepithelial locations as large, hump-shaped structures (Fig. 61-6), they are also small and discrete in subendothelial sites and in the mesangium (Fig. 61-7). The foot processes of visceral epithelial cells are usually effaced. Peripheral migration and interposition of mesangium are variably present although these are an uncommon finding [29, 31, 32].

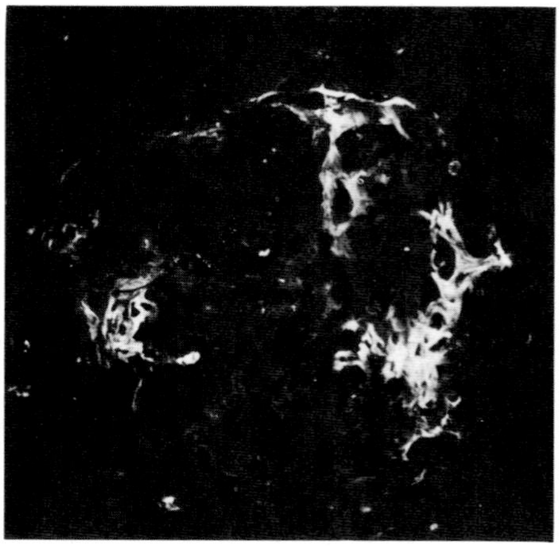

Fig. 61-5. Immunofluorescence for fibrin, which is in the urinary space of this glomerulus with a crescent. (×320.)

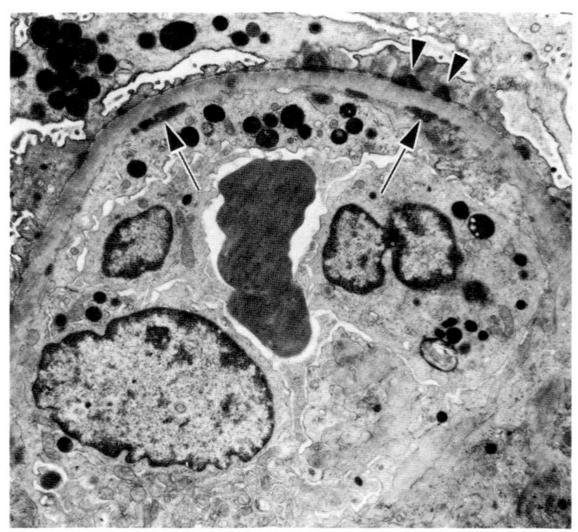

Fig. 61-7. Electron micrograph demonstrating multiple small subendothelial deposits (*arrows*) along with small subepithelial deposits (*arrowheads*). (×4,000.)

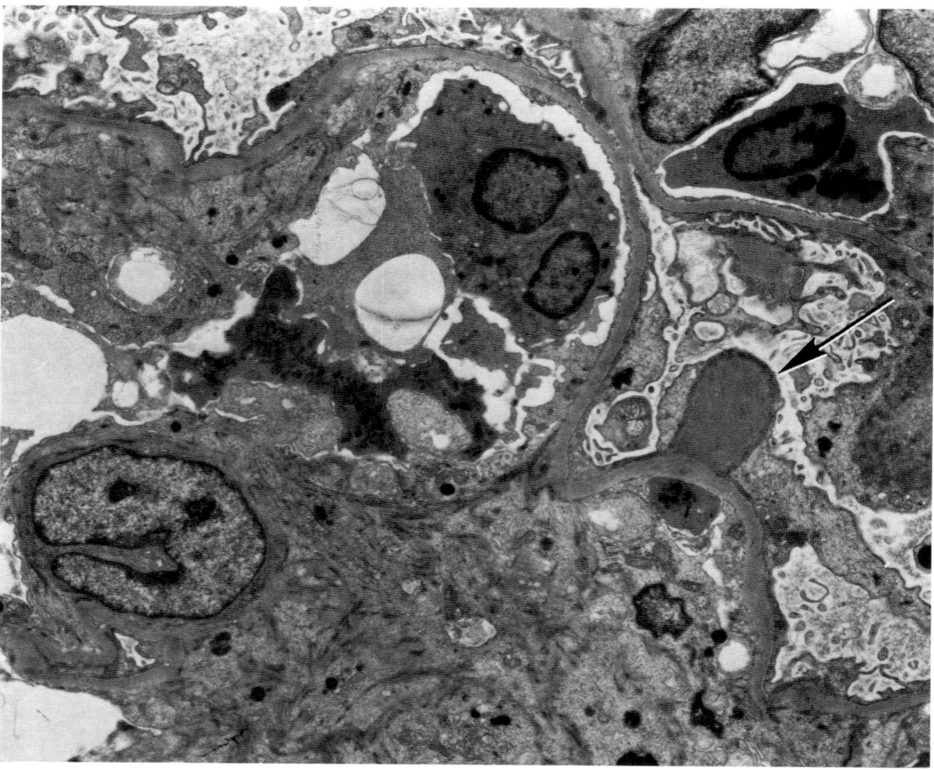

Fig. 61-6. Electron micrograph depicting many leukocytes in capillary lumina and mesangium and a large subepithelial, hump-shaped dense deposit (*arrow*). (×3,750.)

Studies in which information is available on kidney tissue examined following successful treatment of infective endocarditis [9] have indicated almost complete resolution of the glomerular abnormalities. As with other forms of postinfectious glomerulonephritis, residual mesangial expansion and completely sclerotic glomeruli may be the only evidence of prior injury.

Ventriculovascular Shunts

CLINICAL PERSPECTIVES

Although not frequently employed today, ventriculoatrial, vena caval, and jugular shunts were once commonly placed for the surgical treatment of hydrocephalus. As many as 6 to 27 percent of these ventriculovascular shunts became colonized with microorganisms [11, 13, 20, 27, 33, 76]—75 percent with *Staphylococcus albus,* 8 percent with diphtheroids, 3 percent with *S. aureus,* and the remainder with *Listeria monocytogenes, Bacillus subtilis, Peptococcus, Serratia, Corynebacterium bovis,* and a variety of fungi [14, 20, 28, 56, 64, 66, 76, 80, 81]. Glomerulonephritis occurred in 1 to 4 percent of patients with infected shunts [76]. In contrast, ventriculoperitoneal shunts are more resistant to colonization and infection, and associated glomerulonephritis is rare [26, 60].

The majority of patients with glomerulonephritis are children, although a number of reported cases involve adolescents or adults [2, 14, 66, 83]. Fever is the most common presenting manifestation and occurs in 84 percent of patients. Blood and sometimes cerebrospinal fluid cultures may be negative, and bacterial identification may be possible only after culture of the removed shunt. Symptoms of glomerulonephritis may occur as early as a few weeks or as late as 14 years after initial shunt placement [2, 66]. Hematuria is almost universal, with gross hematuria in up to 50 percent of patients.

Nephrotic range proteinuria occurs in approximately 50 to 60 percent of patients. Hepatosplenomegaly and anemia are common, as are purpura, arthralgias, and adenopathy. Hypertension, leukopenia, and thrombocytopenia are uncommon [26, 64, 80, 87]. Nonspecific hyperglobulinemia is characteristic [2], and the presence of serum cryoglobulins, rheumatoid factor, and circulating immune complexes are in keeping with an immunologic pathogenesis [14, 81].

Hypocomplementemia has been noted with ventriculovascular-associated glomerulonephritis but not with uncomplicated shunt colonization or infection [45]. Serial measurements of serum complement levels have been suggested as a means of monitoring the activity of the glomerulonephritis, for normalization corresponds with resolution of the glomerular process [93].

On initial presentation with glomerulonephritis, 25 percent of patients have normal renal function but have an abnormal urinary sediment or proteinuria. Fifty percent demonstrate mild to moderate renal impairment, and 25 percent have severe renal insufficiency. Treatment usually requires early surgical removal of the shunt along with antibiotic therapy, although improvement of the renal disease has been occasionally reported with antibiotic treatment alone [14, 20, 30, 45, 94]. Some workers have suggested that delay in shunt removal may result in irreparable renal damage [52]. With eradication of infection, one-half to two-thirds of patients experience a full renal recovery [2, 89]. However, approximately one-third demonstrate persistent renal insufficiency marked by azotemia, proteinuria, microhematuria, and rarely, hypertension. Progression to end-stage renal disease has been reported [2]. Steroids and cytotoxic agents have not been beneficial in anecdotal reports [80].

PATHOLOGIC ASPECTS

The glomerular lesion is most commonly a membranoproliferative glomerulonephritis pattern, with increased mesangial cellularity, double contoured capillary walls, and lobular architecture. This may be complicated by crescents [83]. Other patterns of tuft injury include diffuse proliferative glomerulonephritis similar to acute postinfectious glomerulonephritis, and infrequently mesangial hypercellularity. Immunofluorescence discloses granular glomerular capillary wall and mesangial deposits with a preponderance of IgM and C3, with lesser frequency, in descending order, of IgG, C1q, IgA, and C4. Electron microscopy demonstrates subendothelial deposits, often in association with peripheral migration and interposition of mesangium. Centrilobular mesangial deposits are also present [2, 29, 32, 45, 87, 89].

Visceral Infections

CLINICAL PERSPECTIVES

In 1976, Whitworth et al. [90] and Beaufils et al. [10] described a number of patients with glomerulonephritis and visceral abscesses. Although some had endocarditis, a significant number had infections elsewhere, including appendicitis with abscess of Douglas' pouch and peritonitis, septic pleuritis with pulmonary abscess, maxillary sinus abscess, and infection of aortofemoral bypass grafts [8, 10]. Since then, glomerulonephritis has been reported coincident with a number of subacute or chronic infections, including septic abortion [16], tuberculosis [16, 61, 71, 82], pneumonia [16, 27, 75, 86, 91], *Campylobacter (Helicobacter) jejuni* enteritis [1, 50], *Salmonella–Schistosoma mansoni* infection [41], bronchiectasis [16] and lung abscess [25], osteomyelitis [15, 16], malaria [16], hepatitis B antigenemia [16, 24, 47], sinusitis [16, 63], and typhoid fever [21, 73]. It is also likely that "trench nephritis," occurring among World War I soldiers who fought in trenches, was a postinfectious glomerulonephritis; while the organism(s) was not identified, it is likely a virus. A similar epidemic was described among troops in the American Civil War [49]. Although the causal link between these above infections and glomerulonephritis is less well established than the association between glomerulonephritis and endocarditis or shunt infections, certain features, nevertheless, suggest an immunopathogenetic relationship. These include the presence of immunoglobulin and/or complement (and sometimes bacteria-associated antigen) [28, 41] in glomeruli and the parallel course of the infectious process and the glomerulonephritis.

Clinically, renal involvement is heralded by the onset of hematuria, which was macroscopic in 3 of 7 patients with this syndrome described by Beaufils et al. [10] and was often accompanied by red blood cell casts. Abnormal proteinuria was present in all nonoliguric patients. Acute renal failure with rapid renal functional loss is a typical feature of this syndrome, often causing diagnostic confusion with acute tubular necrosis or acute interstitial nephritis [8, 10]. Usually, hematuria may distinguish glomerulonephritis from acute tubular necrosis, but further distinction from interstitial nephritis may occasionally be difficult without a renal biopsy. Oliguria and hypertension are present in approximately 50 percent of patients.

On presentation, many patients are severely ill, have high fever, and are catabolic with considerable weight loss. In the initial report of Beaufils et al. [10], infection was present from 2 weeks to 3 years at the time of the diagnosis of glomerulonephritis. Extrarenal manifestations included lower extremity purpura with hypersensitivity angiitis, necrotic cutaneous lesions, and arthralgias. Blood cultures were frequently negative, a fact that may be explained by antecedent antibiotic therapy.

Mixed cryoglobulinemia, present at onset, resolves with eradication of infection [8, 10]. Total serum complement is normal in the majority of affected patients, although a C3 nephritic factor has been identified occasionally. Circulating immune complexes may be present in a minority of patients. Rheumatoid factor is not present, a feature distinguishing this syndrome from glomerulonephritis and endocarditis or shunt infection [10].

Renal prognosis is most clearly associated with eradication of the infection, and complete remission of glomerulonephritis is thereby achievable [8, 10, 16]. However, delay in treatment or unsuccessful treatment can result in either patient death or survival with significant renal impairment [10].

PATHOLOGIC ASPECTS

The glomerular abnormalities are varied but are characterized by hypercellularity as the basic feature. The lesions include mesangial proliferative glomerulonephritis, membranoproliferative glomerulonephritis often with numerous polymorphonuclear leukocytes in capillary lumina (Fig. 61-8), and diffuse proliferative (exudative) glomerulonephritis with or without crescents. Immunofluorescence typically discloses granular mesangial and capillary wall C3 deposits. Immunoglobulins are infrequently identified; IgG is most commonly noted. Ultrastructural studies are not commonly reported; electron-dense deposits are in the mesangium and occasionally in subepithelial locations as humps [8, 10, 16, 29, 32].

Fig. 61-8. Membranoproliferative glomerulonephritis in patient with abdominal abscess. The tuft is lobular, and there are leukocytes in capillaries. (Periodic acid–methenamine silver, ×160.)

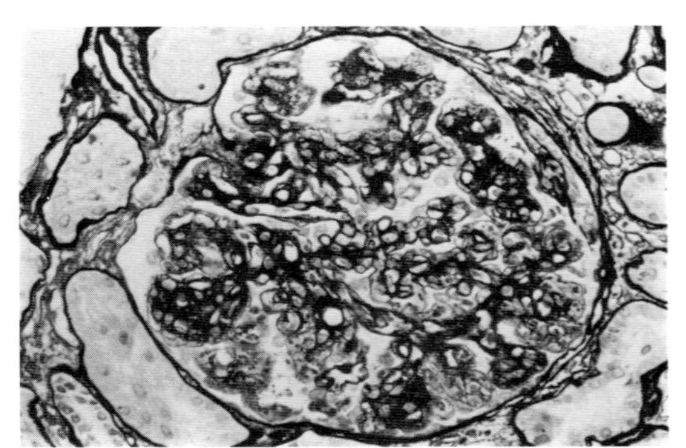

References

1. Andrews, P. I., Kainer, G., Yong, L. C. J., et al. Glomerulonephritis, pulmonary hemorrhage and anemia associated with *Campylobacter jejuni* infection. *Aust. N.Z. J. Med.* 19: 721, 1989.
2. Arze, R. S., Rashid, H., Morley, R., et al. Shunt nephritis: Report of two cases and review of the literature. *Clin. Nephrol.* 19(1): 48, 1983.
3. Baehr, G. Glomerular lesion of subacute bacterial endocarditis. *J. Exp. Med.* 15: 330, 1912.
4. Baehr, G., and Lande, H. Glomerulonephritis as a complication of subacute *Streptococcus* endocarditis. *J.A.M.A.* 75: 789, 1920.
5. Bain, R. C., Edwards, J. E., Shiefley, C. H., et al. Right-sided bacterial endocarditis and endarteritis: A clinical and pathological study. *Am. J. Med.* 24: 98, 1958.
6. Bayer, A. S., and Theofilopoulos, A. N. Immunopathogenetic aspects of infective endocarditis. *Chest* 97: 204, 1990.
7. Bayer, A. S., Theofilopoulos, A. N., Eisenberg, R., et al. Circulating immune complexes in infective endocarditis. *N. Engl. J. Med.* 295(27): 1500, 1976.
8. Beaufils, M. Glomerular disease complicating abdominal sepsis. *Kidney Int.* 19: 609, 1981.
9. Beaufils, M., Gilbert, C., Morel-Maroger, L., et al. Glomerulonephritis in severe bacterial infections with and without endocarditis. *Adv. Nephrol.* 7: 217, 1978.
10. Beaufils, M., Morel-Maroger, L., Sraer, J.-D., et al. Acute renal failure of glomerular origin during visceral abscesses. *N. Engl. J. Med.* 295: 185, 1977.
11. Beeler, B. A., Crowder, J. A., Smith, J. W., et al. *Propionibacterium acnes:* Pathogen in central nervous system shunt infection. Report of three cases including immune complex glomerulonephritis. *Am. J. Med.* 61: 935, 1976.
12. Bell, E. J. The glomerular lesion associated with endocarditis. *Am. J. Pathol.* 8: 639, 1932.
13. Black, J. A., Challacombe, D. N., and Ockenden, B. G. Nephrotic syndrome associated with bacteraemia after shunt operations for hydrocephalus. *Lancet* II: 921, 1965.
14. Bolton, W. K., Sande, M. A., Normansell, D. E., et al. Ventriculojugular shunt nephritis with *Corynebacterium bovis*. *Am. J. Med.* 59: 417, 1975.
15. Boonshaft, B., Maher, J. F., and Schreiner, G. E. Nephrotic syndrome associated with osteomyelitis without secondary amyloidosis. *Arch. Intern. Med.* 125: 320, 1970.
16. Boulton-Jones, J. M., and Davison, A. M. Persistent infection as a cause of renal disease in patients submitted to renal biopsy: A report from the glomerulonephritis registry of the United Kingdom MRC. *Q. J. Med.* 58: 123, 1986.
17. Boulton-Jones, J. M., Sissons, J. G. P., Evans, D. J., et al. Renal lesions of subacute infective endocarditis. *Br. Med. J.* 2: 11, 1974.
18. Boyarsky, S., Burnett, J. M., and Barker, W. H. Renal fail-

ure in embolic glomerulonephritis as a complication of subacute bacterial endocarditis. *Bull. Johns Hopkins Hosp.* 84: 207, 1949.

19. Cabane, J., Godeau, P., Herreman, G., et al. Fate of circulating immune complexes in infective endocarditis. *Am. J. Med.* 66: 277, 1979.
20. Caron, C., Luneau, C., Gervais, M. H., et al. La glomerulonephrite de shunt: Manifestations cliniques et histopathologiques. *Can. Med. Assoc. J.* 120: 557, 1979.
21. Chowdhury, K. L., Saproo, R. K., Bhat, M. Y., et al. Typhoid nephritis. *J. Assoc. Phys. Ind.* 36: 447, 1988.
22. Christian, H. A. The kidney in subacute *Streptococcus viridans* endocarditis. *J. Mt. Sinai Hosp.* 8: 427, 1942.
23. Colvin, R. B., and Fang, L. S. T. Interstitial Nephritis. In C. C. Tisher and B. M. Brenner (eds.), *Renal Pathology with Clinical and Functional Correlations.* Philadelphia: Lippincott, 1989. Pp. 728–776.
24. Combes, B., Stastny, P., Shorey, J., et al. Glomerulonephritis with deposition of Australia antigen-antibody complexes in glomerular basement membrane. *Lancet* 2: 234, 1971.
25. Danovitch, G. M., Nord, E. P., Barki, Y., et al. Staphylococceal abscess and acute glomerulonephritis. *Isr. J. Med. Sci.* 15: 840, 1979.
26. Dobrin, R. S., Day, N. K., Quie, P. G., et al. The role of complement, immunoglobulin and bacterial antigen in coagulase-negative staphylococcal shunt nephritis. *Am. J. Med.* 59: 660, 1975.
27. Forrest, D. M., and Cooper, D. G. W. Complications of ventriculoatrial shunts: A review of 455 cases. *J. Neurosurg.* 29: 506, 1968.
28. Forrest, J. W., John, F., Mills, L. R., et al. Immune complex glomerulonephritis associated with *Klebsiella pneumoniae. Clin. Nephrol.* 7: 76, 1977.
29. Gallo, G. R., Neugarten, J., and Baldwin, D. S. Glomerulonephritis Associated with Systemic Bacterial and Viral Infections. In C. C. Tisher and B. M. Brenner (eds.), *Renal Pathology with Clinical and Functional Correlations.* Philadelphia: Lippincott, 1989. Pp. 548–574.
30. Groeneveld, A. B. J., Nommensen, F. E., Mullink, H., et al. Shunt nephritis associated with *Propionibacterium acnes* with demonstration of the antigen in the glomeruli. *Nephron* 32: 365, 1982.
31. Gutman, R. A., Striker, G. E., Gilliland, B. C., et al. The immune complex glomerulonephritis of bacterial endocarditis. *Medicine* 51: 1, 1972.
32. Gutman, R. A., Striker, L. M.-M., and Striker, G. E. Glomerulonephritis with Bacterial Endocarditis, Shunts, and Abdominal Abscesses. In R. W. Schrier and C. W. Gottschalk (eds.), *Diseases of the Kidney.* (4th ed.) Boston: Little, Brown, 1988. Pp. 1885–1901.
33. Halmagyi, G. M., and Horvath, J. S. Acute glomerulonephritis in an adult with infected ventriculoatrial shunt. *Med. J. Aust.* 1: 136, 1979.
34. Harbitz, F. Studien Uber Endocarditis. *Dtsch. Med. Wochenschr.* 25: 121, 1899.
35. Hooper, D. C., Bayer, A. S., Karchmer, A. W., et al. Circulating immune complexes in prosthetic valve endocarditis. *Arch. Intern. Med.* 143: 2081, 1983.
36. Horder, T. J. Infective endocarditis with an analysis of 150 cases with special reference to the chronic form of the disease. *Q. J. Med.* 2: 289, 1909.
37. Hurwitz, D., Quismorio, F. P., and Friou, G. J. Cryoglobulinaemia in patients with infective endocarditis. *Clin. Exp. Immunol.* 19: 131, 1975.
38. Kauffman, R. H., Thompson, J., Valentijn, R. M., et al. The clinical implications and the pathogenetic significance of circulating immune complexes in infective endocarditis. *Am. J. Med.* 71: 17, 1981.
39. Keefer, C. S. Subacute bacterial endocarditis: Active cases without bacteremia. *Ann. Intern. Med.* 11: 714, 1937–1938.
40. Kerr, A. *Subacute Bacterial Glomerulonephritis.* Springfield, Ill.: C. C. Thomas, 1955.
41. Lambertucci, J. R., Godoy, P., Neves, J., et al. Glomerulonephritis in *Salmonella–Schistosoma mansoni* association. *Am. J. Trop. Med. Hyg.* 38: 97, 1988.
42. Lee, B. K., Crossley, K., and Gerding, D. N. L. The association between *Staphylococcus aureus* bacteremia and bacteriuria. *Am. J. Med.* 65: 303, 1978.
43. Lerner, P. I., and Weinstein, L. Infective endocarditis in the antibiotic era. *N. Engl. J. Med.* 274: 199, 1966.
44. Levine, D. P., Cushing, R. D., Jui, J., et al. Community-acquired methicillin-resistant *Staphylococcus aureus* endocarditis in the Detroit Medical Center. *Ann. Intern. Med.* 97: 330, 1982.
45. Levy, M., Gubler, M.-C., and Habib, R. Pathology and Immunopathology of Shunt Nephritis in Children: Report of 10 Cases. In W. Zurukzoglu, M. Papadimitriou, M. Pyrpasopoulos, et al. (eds.), *Proceedings of the 8th International Congress of Nephrology.* Basel: Karger, 1981. P. 290.
46. Levy, R. L., and Hong, R. The immune nature of subacute bacterial endocarditis (SBE) nephritis. *Am. J. Med.* 54: 645, 1973.
47. Lin, C. Y. Hepatitis B virus associated membranous nephropathy: Clinical features, immunologic profiles and outcomes. *Nephron* 55: 37, 1990.
48. Lohlein, M. Ueber hamorrhagische nierenaffectionen bei schronischer uizerozer endokarditis. *Med. Klin.* 6: 375, 1910.
49. Maher, J. F. Trench nephritis: A retrospective perception. *Am. J. Kidney Dis.* 7: 355, 1986.
50. Maidment, C. G., Evans, D. B., Couldon, R. A., et al. *Campylobacter* enteritis complicated by glomerulonephritis. *J. Infect.* 10: 177, 1985.
51. McKenzie, P. E., Taylor, A. E., Woodroffe, A. J., et al. Plasmapheresis in glomerulonephritis. *Clin. Nephrol.* 12: 97, 1979.
52. McKinsey, D. S., McMurray, T. I., and Flynn, J. M. Immune complex glomerulonephritis associated with *Staphylococcus aureus* bacteremia: Response to corticosteroid therapy. *Rev. Infect. Dis.* 12: 125, 1990.
53. Mohammed, I., Ansell, B. M., Holborow, E. J., et al. Circulating immune complexes in subacute infective endocarditis and post-streptococcal glomerulonephritis. *J. Clin. Pathol.* 30: 308, 1977.
54. Morel-Maroger, L., Sraer, J.-D., Herreman, G., et al. Kidney in subacute endocarditis. *Arch. Pathol.* 94: 205, 1972.
55. Musher, D. M., and McKenzie, S. O. Infections due to *Staphylococcus aureus. Medicine* 56: 383, 1978.
56. Narchi, H., Taylor, R., Azmy, A. F., et al. Shunt nephritis. *J. Pediatr. Surg.* 23: 839, 1988.
57. Nast, C. C., Colodro, I., and Cohen, A. H. Splenic immune deposits in bacterial endocarditis. *Clin. Immunol. Immunopathol.* 40: 209, 1986.
58. Neugarten, J., and Baldwin, D. S. Glomerulonephritis in bacterial endocarditis. *Am. J. Med.* 77: 297, 1984.
59. Neugarten, J., Gallo, G. R., and Baldwin, D. S. Glomerulonephritis in bacterial endocarditis. *Am. J. Kidney Dis.* 5: 371, 1984.
60. Noe, H. N., and Roy, S. Shunt nephritis. *J. Urol.* 125: 731, 1981.
61. O'Brien, A. A. J., Kelly, P., Gaffney, E. F., et al. Immune

complex glomerulonephritis secondary to tuberculosis. *Ir. J. Med. Sci.* 159: 187, 1990.

62. O'Connor, D. T., Weisman, M. H., and Fierer, J. Activation of the alternate complement pathway in *Staph. aureus* infective endocarditis and its relationship to thrombocytopenia, coagulation abnormalities, and acute glomerulonephritis. *Clin. Exp. Immunol.* 34: 179, 1978.
63. Patel, Y., Drews, M. H., and Latos, D. L. Glomerulonephritis and sinusitis: Hypocomplementemic glomerulonephritis associated with coagulase-negative staphylococcal pansinusitis and subdural empyema. *W. Va. Med. J.* 85: 186, 1989.
64. Peeters, W., Mussche, M., Becaus, I., et al. Shunt nephritis. *Clin. Nephrol.* 9: 122, 1978.
65. Pelletier, L. L., Jr., and Petersdorf, R. G. Infective endocarditis: A review of 125 cases from the University of Washington Hospitals, 1963–72. *Medicine* 56(4): 287, 1977.
66. Pereira, B. J. G., Kumari, S., Gupta, K. L., et al. Shunt nephritis associated with *Staphylococcus aureus* septicaemia. *J. Assoc. Phys. Ind.* 35: 796, 1987.
67. Perez, G. O., Rothfield, N., and Williams, R. C. Immune-complex nephritis in bacterial endocarditis. *Arch. Intern. Med.* 136: 333, 1976.
68. Perez-Fontan, M., Huarte, E., Tellez, A., et al. Glomerular nephropathy associated with chronic Q fever. *Am. J. Kidney Dis.* 11: 298, 1988.
69. Pertschuk, L. P., Woda, B. A., Vuletin, J. C., et al. Glomerulonephritis due to *Staphylococcus aureus* antigen. *Am. J. Clin. Pathol.* 65: 301, 1976.
70. Phair, J. P., and Clarke, J. Immunology of infective endocarditis. *Prog. Cardiovasc. Dis.* 22: 137, 1979.
71. Rodriguez-Garcia, J. L., Fraile, G., Mampaso, F., et al. Pulmonary tuberculosis associated with membranous nephropathy. *Nephron* 55: 218, 1990.
72. Rovzar, M. A., Logan, J. L., Ogden, D. A., et al. Immunosuppressive therapy and plasmapheresis in rapidly progressive glomerulonephritis associated with bacterial endocarditis. *Am. J. Kidney Dis.* 7: 428, 1986.
73. Sarma, P. S. Typhoid glomerulonephritis. *J. Assoc. Physicians India* 36: 733, 1988.
74. Savin, V., Siegel, L., and Schreiner, G. E. Nephropathy in Heroin Addicts with Staphylococcal Septicemia. In P. Kincaid-Smith, T. M. Matthew, and E. L. Becker (eds.), *Glomerulonephritis, Morphology, Natural History and Treatment.* New York: Wiley, 1973. Pp. 397–404.
75. Schachter, J., Pomeranz, A., Berger, I., et al. Acute glomerulonephritis secondary to lobar pneumonia. *Int. J. Pediatr. Nephrol.* 8: 211, 1987.
76. Schoenbaum, S. C., Gardner, P., and Shillito, J. Infections of cerebrospinal fluid shunts: Epidemiology, clinical manifestations, and therapy. *J. Infect. Dis.* 131: 543, 1975.
77. Shah, G. M., and Winer, R. L. Glomerulonephritis associated with endocarditis caused by *Actinobacillus actinomycetemcomitans. Am. J. Kidney Dis.* 1: 113, 1981.
78. Sheagren, J. N., Tuazon, C. V., Griffin, C., et al. Rheumatoid factor in acute bacterial endocarditis. *Arthritis Rheum.* 19: 887, 1976.
79. Spain, D. M., and King, D. W. The effect of penicillin on the renal lesion of subacute bacterial endocarditis. *Ann. Intern. Med.* 36: 1086, 1952.
80. Stickler, G. B., Shin, M. H., Burke, E. C., et al. Diffuse glomerulonephritis associated with infected ventriculoatrial shunt. *N. Engl. J. Med.* 279: 1077, 1968.
81. Strife, C. F., McDonald, B. M., Ruley, E. J., et al. Shunt nephritis: The nature of the serum cryoglobulins and their relation to the complement profile. *J. Pediatr.* 88: 403, 1976.
82. Teruel, J. L., Matesanz, R., Mampaso, F., et al. Pulmonary tuberculosis, cryoglobulinemia, and immune complex glomerulonephritis. *Clin. Nephrol.* 27: 480, 1987.
83. Toth, T., Redl, J., and Beregi, E. Shunt nephritis with crescent formation. *Int. J. Pediatr. Nephrol.* 8: 231, 1987.
84. Vatanabunaborn, C., and Jan, J. S. Diagnostic difficulties of staphylococcal endocarditis in geriatric patients. *Geriatrics* 28: 168, 1973.
85. Virchow, R. *Cellular Pathology.* London: Churchill, 1860.
86. Vitallo, B. B., O'Regan, S., de Chadorevian, J. P., et al. *Mycoplasma* pneumonia associated with acute glomerulonephritis. *Nephron* 21: 284, 1978.
87. Wakabayashi, Y., Kobayashi, Y., and Shigemat, H. Shunt nephritis: Histological dynamics following removal of the shunt. Case report and review of literature. *Nephron* 40: 111, 1985.
88. Wald, S. L., and McLaurin, R. L. Shunt-associated glomerulonephritis. *Neurosurgery* 3: 146, 1978.
89. Wegmann, W., and Leumann, E. P. Glomerulonephritis associated with infected ventriculoatrial shunt: Clinical and morphological findings. *Virchows Arch.* [*A*] 359: 185, 1973.
90. Whitworth, J. A., Morel-Maroger, L., Mignon, F., et al. The significance of extracapillary proliferation. *Nephron* 16: 1, 1976.
91. William, D. K., Takeshio, O., Marvin, I. S., et al. Acute nephritis and pulmonary alveolitis following pneumococcal pneumonia. *Arch. Intern. Med.* 138: 806, 1978.
92. Williams, R. C., Jr., and Kunkel, H. G. Rheumatoid factor, complement, and conglutinin aberrations in patients with subacute bacterial endocarditis. *J. Clin. Invest.* 41(3): 666, 1962.
93. Wyatt, R. J., Walsh, J. W., and Holland, N. H. Shunt nephritis: Role of complement system in its pathogenesis and management. *J. Neurosurg.* 55: 99, 1981.
94. Yeh, B. P. Y., Young, H. F., Schatzki, P. F., et al. Immune complex disease associated with an infected ventriculojugular shunt: A curable form of glomerulonephritis. *South. Med. J.* 70: 1141, 1977.
95. Yum, M. N., Wheat, L. J., Maxwell, D., et al. Immunofluorescent localization of *Staphylococcus aureus* antigen in acute bacterial endocarditis nephritis. *Am. J. Clin. Pathol.* 70(5): 832, 1978.

Rapidly Progressive Glomerulonephritis

Robert C. Atkins
Napier M. Thomson

Rapidly progressive glomerulonephritis (RPGN) is one of the most calamitous of nephrologic conditions, and patients can progress from normal renal function to end-stage renal failure within weeks. RPGN is a syndrome and consists clinically of sudden and relentless deterioration in renal function associated with the pathologic finding on renal biopsy of extensive crescent formation surrounding most glomeruli.

Many types of glomerulonephritis can exhibit crescent formation and sometimes renal failure. These types are listed in Table 62-1 and include both primary glomerular disease and systemic disease with a glomerular component. Consequently, the definition of RPGN has been difficult and the terminology has varied over the years, incorporating either the clinical or pathologic components, or both.

Crescents were first described by Langhans, now over 100 years ago (Fig. 62-1) [141]. Volhard and Fahr [237] used the term *extracapillary glomerulonephritis* in 1914 because of the glomerular crescents surrounding the capillary tuft, and Löhlein called this type of glomerulonephritis a *stormy course* because of the renal failure that led to death [153]. Ellis [75] coined the phrase *rapidly progressive type 1,* but the disease has also since been referred to as *malignant* [96], *acute necrotizing* [30], *acute anuric* [28], *proliferative, with crescents* [194], and *nonstreptococcal rapidly progressive glomerulonephritis* [19]. The most commonly used synonym for RPGN today is *idiopathic crescentic glomerulonephritis* [110].

Therefore, in this chapter, *RPGN* is used to describe this relatively rare syndrome, consisting clinically of an acute glomerulonephritis, with a rapid and progressive deterioration in renal function, and, pathologically, of extensive crescent formation surrounding the majority of glomeruli in the absence of another type of primary glomerulonephritis or systemic disease. In spite of these restrictions, RPGN is still a heterogeneous entity and can be divided further on immunopathogenetic criteria into subgroups with different prognoses and responses to treatment.

Pathology

The pathognomonic feature of RPGN is the presence of crescents within Bowman's capsule (Figs. 62-2 and 62-3). A glomerular crescent may be defined as an aggregation of cells, at least two layers deep, which can occupy a small or large segment of Bowman's space and can extend virtually to obliterate the glomerular-capillary tuft. Cases of widespread crescent formation usually are associated with oliguric renal failure. In general, those patients with the most rapid progression and most severe renal failure have a greater number of glomerular crescents [170, 242]. There is no agreement concerning the percentage of glomeruli that need to be involved before the term RPGN can be used. The studies vary from 20 percent of glomeruli involved [222] to more than 80 percent [242]. Nield et al. [182], in a recent and extensive review of the Guy's Hospital experience, introduced the concept of the importance of the degree of the glomerular circumferential involvement. They defined the pathologic criteria for RPGN as greater than 60 percent of circumferential involvement of more than 60 percent of glomeruli.

The cells that constitute the crescent are large, pale staining, and elongated, with an occasional mitotic figure being evident (Figs. 62-2 and 62-3). It was traditional belief that these cells were derived from proliferated epithelial cells, and the term *epithelial crescent* was used [19, 110, 169]. However, as will be described later, it has now been shown, using monoclonal antibodies as specific markers, that epithelial cells are only a minor component of the crescent and the major identifiable cell type is of macrophage origin [98]. A cellular crescent also frequently contains erythrocytes, polymorphonuclear leukocytes, and deposits of fibrin (Fig. 62-3). Often, the crescent is composed entirely of cells—the cellular crescent (Figs. 62-2 and 62-3)—whereas others contain, in addition, connective tissue. The fibrocellular crescent (Fig. 62-4) and others are made up almost entirely of fibrous tissue—the sclerosed crescent. In general, this progression from a cellular to a sclerosed crescent is related to the duration and activity of the disease process, with the fibrocellular and then, finally, the sclerosed crescent being seen as the disease process evolves. Various degrees and stages of crescent formation can be seen in different glomeruli within the same biopsy.

Most patients also have glomerular tuft involvement, with sometimes focal and segmental necrosis of glomerular capillaries and often marked fibrin deposition (Fig. 62-3). Particularly with extensive crescent formation, the glomerular tuft can be almost completely compressed, and changes within glomerular capillaries may be masked (Fig. 62-3). However, there may be proliferation of endothelial and mesangial cells and an infiltration of polymorphonuclear leukocytes and monocytes (Figs. 62-2 and 62-3). Multinucleated giant cells also have been found [129]. Proliferation of intrinsic glomerular cells and infiltration by leukocytes has been assessed by light microscopy [26], electron microscopy [33, 167], tissue culture of isolated glomeruli [12–14], enzymatic labels [100], and monoclonal antibody marker identification [14, 15, 119, 217], and these have been reviewed recently [17].

Glomerular culture studies [11, 84] rekindled interest in the role of the macrophage in RPGN. It was demonstrated that the culture outgrowth from glomeruli that were isolated from renal biopsies from patients with crescentic glomerulonephritis contained macrophages in greater numbers than cultures from normal glomeruli or, indeed, glomeruli from biopsies that showed other forms of glomerulonephritis [11–13]. In Fig. 62-5 is demonstrated macrophages in a culture outgrowth from an isolated glomerulus of a patient with RPGN. Culture outgrowths from crescentic glomeruli demonstrated an increased number of mesangial cells, though fewer epithelial cells, than outgrowths from normal glomeruli [12, 13].

With the advent of monoclonal antibodies [137] that can be used as specific markers for both leukocytes [29] and intrinsic glomerular cells [17, 101, 102, 171, 223], it is now possible to assess the number of individual glomerular cells and infiltrating leukocytes in situ. Glomeruli from patients with RPGN have increased numbers of macrophages and polymorphs within glomeruli [15, 37, 118, 119, 149, 172, 184, 217].

Table 62-1. Types of glomerulonephritis that can be associated with rapid deterioration in renal function and glomerular crescent formation

PRIMARY RENAL DISEASES
RPGN—anti-GBM without lung involvement
RPGN—immune complex deposition
RPGN—without immune deposit
Membranoproliferative glomerulonephritis [91, 163]
Membranous nephropathy [133, 168, 183]
IgA disease [145]
Hereditary nephritis [105]
SYSTEMIC DISEASES
Goodpasture's syndrome (Chap. 68)
Postinfectious
Poststreptococcal (Chap. 63)
Endocarditis (Chap. 61)
Shunt nephritis (Chap. 61)
Abscess (Chap. 61)
Henoch-Schönlein disease (Chap. 67)
Lupus nephritis (Chap. 72)
Polyarteritis (Chap. 76)
Wegener's granulomatosis (Chap. 76)
Cryoglobulinemia (Chap. 78)
Scleroderma (Chap. 73)
Relapsing polychondritis [181]
Malignancy [31, 191]
Malignant hypertension [216] (Chap. 59)

Recently, intraglomerular T cells have been demonstrated in glomeruli of patients with crescentic glomerulonephritis [37, 149, 172, 184, 217]. Such T cells are functionally active, as demonstrated by their association with activated monocytes and fibrin, the other components of cell-mediated immunity [180], and their expression of receptors for interleukin 2 (IL-2R) denoting immune activation [148, 149].

Animal studies have provided evidence that sensitized T cells are capable of inducing glomerular injury and crescent formation. Bolton et al. [35, 39] depleted chickens of B cells and induced antiglomerular basement membrane (anti-GBM) disease with crescent formation by injection of heterologous glomeruli. This was associated with intraglomerular T cells and furthermore was also induced in naive chickens by transfer of T cells from affected, but not control, hosts. Studies in sequential anti-GBM disease in rats have shown that T cells precede monocytic infiltrations into glomeruli [234], produce lymphokines [45], and express IL-2R, indicating functional activation [139].

Two recent studies have demonstrated that crescentic glomerulonephritis can be induced by cellular immune response to exogenous antigens lodged in the glomerulus, in the absence of antibody. Otie et al. [188] produced sensitized T cells in rats by injection of hapten TNP. Renal arterial injection of this hapten coupled to cationized

Fig. 62-1. Reproduction of drawings from Langhans' paper, over 100 years ago, which first described crescents within Bowman's space and inferred an epithelial cell origin [141].

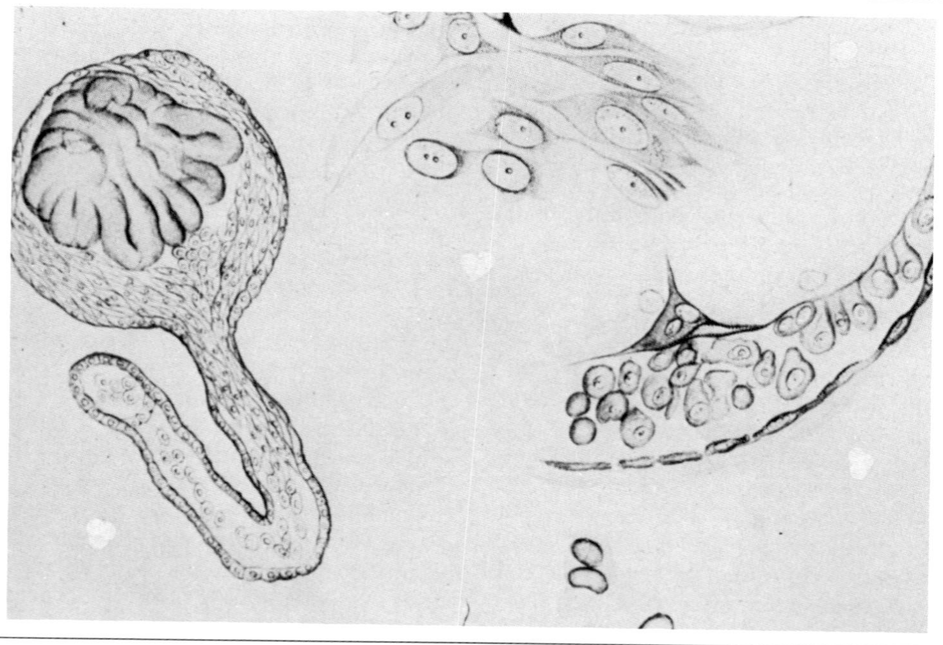

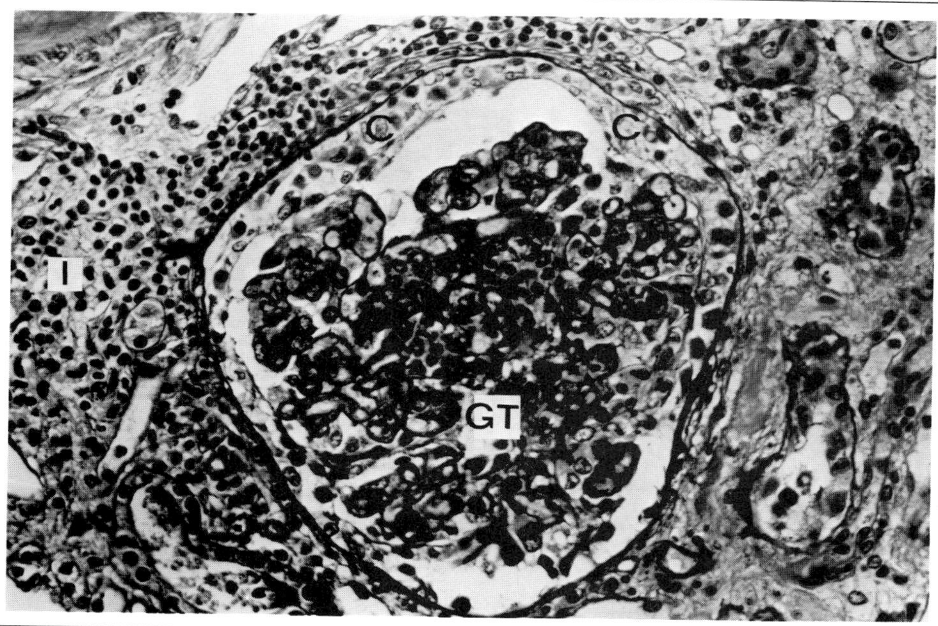

Fig. 62-2. A small cellular crescent (C) surrounding a glomerular tuft (GT) from a 67-year-old patient with RPGN. The glomerulus shows some mesangial and endothelial cell proliferation. There is a pronounced interstitial cellular infiltrate (I). (Silver-Masson trichrome, ×400.)

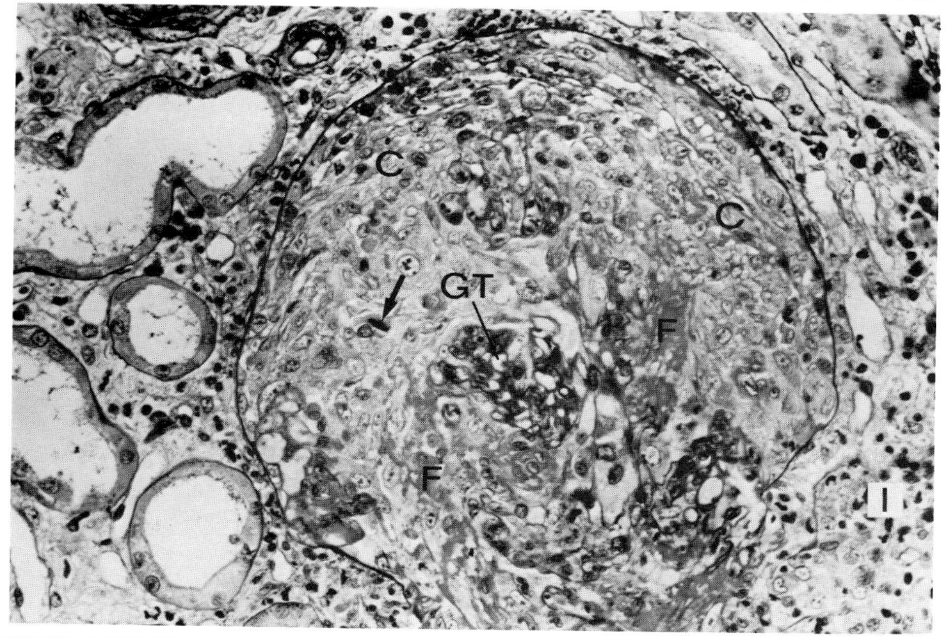

Fig. 62-3. An extensive cellular crescent (C) from the same biopsy as Figs. 62-2 and 62-7b. There is virtual obliteration of the glomerular tuft (GT). There are large areas of fibrin deposition (F) within the crescent. A mitotic figure can be seen within the crescent (*arrow*). An interstitial mononuclear cell infiltrate (I) surrounds the glomerulus. (Silver-Masson trichrome, ×400.)

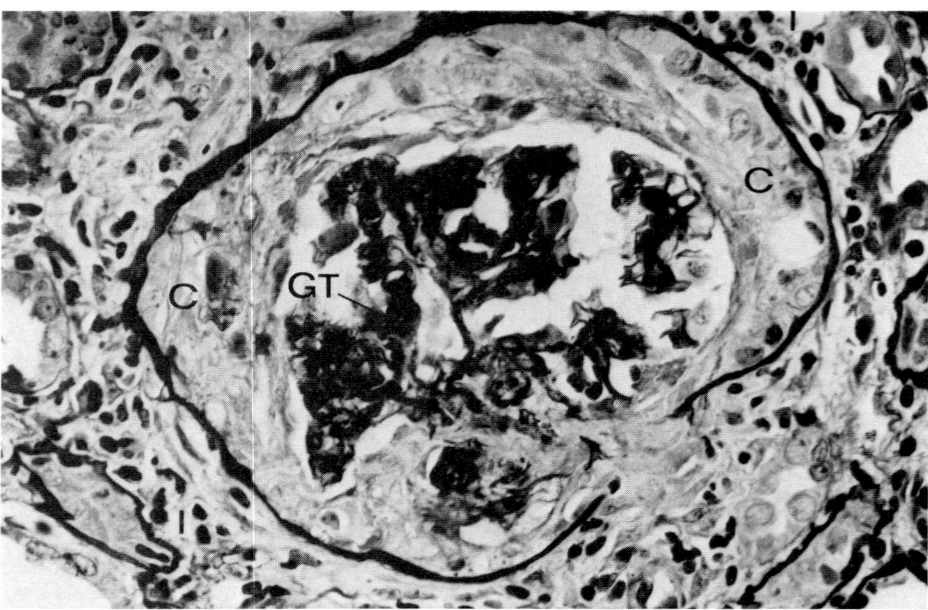

Fig. 62-4. A glomerulus showing a fibrocellular crescent (C) surrounding the glomerular tuft (GT) from a patient with RPGN, 90-percent crescent formation, and no immunoglobulin deposition. Interstitial infiltration with mononuclear cells is present (I). The patient is the same as in Fig. 62-6. (Silver-Masson trichrome, ×400.)

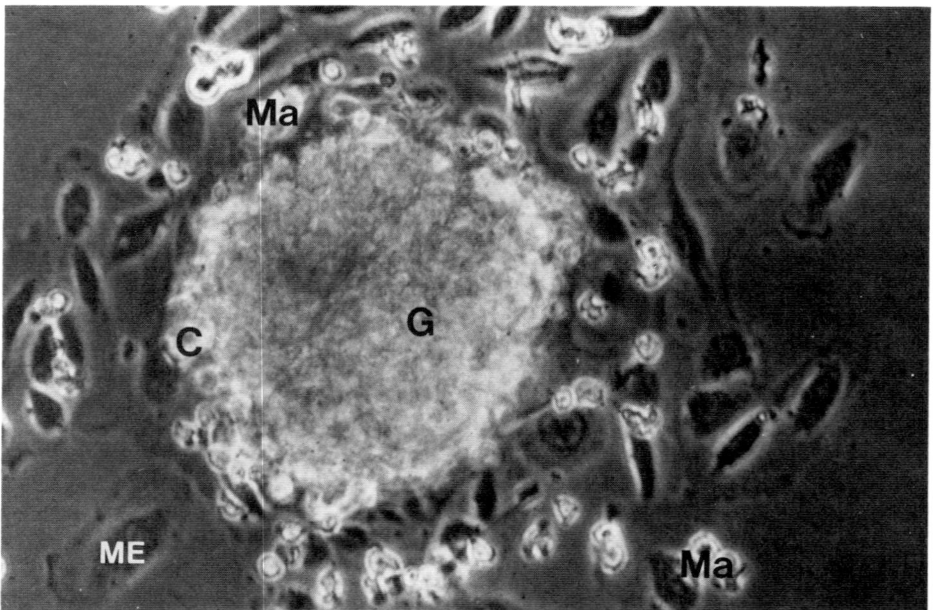

Fig. 62-5. Phase-contrast photomicrograph of an isolated glomerulus (G) in tissue culture from a patient with RPGN and 100-percent crescent formation. A large population of macrophages (Ma) is seen within the crescent (C) and egressing into the culture. Mesangial cells (ME) also are present in the culture outgrowth, but no epithelial cells are evident. (×150.)

albumin into sensitized rats produced a proliferative glomerulonephritis with crescent formation. Rennke et al. [199] induced a severe crescentic glomerulonephritis with marked interstitial involvement in a similar model, but in addition transferred sensitized T cells to naive recipients and following antigen injection into the renal artery, producing a focal crescentic glomerulonephritis. These studies provide conclusive evidence that T cells alone can induce proliferative crescentic glomerulonephritis in a variety of experimental models of glomerulonephritis. Even so, it is still unclear how T cells induce glomerular damage. They could recruit and activate monocytes as in the classic delayed-type hypersensitivity reaction; release cytokines that cause cell injury or stimulate intrinsic glomerular cells to proliferate and secrete inflammatory mediators. Perhaps cytotoxic T cells themselves could also cause renal injury [16, 162].

In most cases of RPGN, there is hypercellularity in the glomerular tuft, which is composed of proliferated intrinsic glomerular cells and infiltrating leukocytes. It is now realized that the three intrinsic glomerular cells—mesangial, endothelial, and epithelial cells—are all capable of an active role in the glomerulonephritis process. The cytokine interrelationships of the resident glomerular cells and infiltrating cells are just beginning to be unravelled [10]. The technical ability to obtain and grow pure isolates of these intrinsic glomerular cells in culture has enabled controlled manipulation of their properties [3, 20, 107, 155, 166, 197] and has provided insight into their behavior in the glomerulonephritis process in vivo. Even so, glomerular hypercellularity needs further study to elucidate the contribution of cell proliferation, matrix production, and the effects of recombinant proteins, especially the inflammatory cytokines, to RPGN. In a minority of cases of RPGN, however, there is no apparent glomerular tuft hypercellularity at all [30, 170, 222].

In most renal biopsies of patients with RPGN, there is a prominent interstitial inflammatory cell infiltrate [110]. It is usually widespread throughout the interstitium but is often most marked surrounding Bowman's capsule (Figs. 62-2, 62-3, and 62-4). The severity of the infiltrate may be related to the underlying pathogenesis of the RPGN, and Andres [6] has demonstrated an increased interstitial infiltration of leukocytes in the presence of antitubular basement-membrane (anti-TBM) antibodies. The interstitial changes in RPGN may well relate more to the outcome of the disease than to the glomerular changes [224]. It has been shown that there is a highly significant correlation between the degree of interstitial mononuclear cell infiltration and impairment of renal function, whereas there is minimal correlation between glomerular cell numbers and renal function [118]. All these findings suggest that the interstitial mononuclear cell infiltrate may be a more important component of the renal response to glomerular injury than has been recognized previously [10, 18].

Two very recent studies using monoclonal antibodies as leukocyte subset markers have, for the first time, evaluated the composition of the interstitial leukocytic infiltration in RPGN [118, 217]. Hooke et al. [118] compared the interstitial cell infiltrate in 14 patients with RPGN with 84 other types of glomerulonephritis using a sensitive four-layer peroxidase-antiperoxidase (PAP) technique for leukocyte localization [100]. This study found that the interstitial leukocyte numbers were greater in the RPGN group of patients, that the T lymphocyte was the major cell involved (64%), and that the T4 : T8 ratio (i.e., T helper cell to T cytotoxic/suppressor cell) was 1.0, which was the same as in other glomerulonephritides and in normal biopsies. Remaining cells were monocytes (22%), B cells (10%), and granulocytes (2%). A typical interstitial leukocytic infiltrate, stained by the monoclonal antibody PHM1, which recognizes a cell-membrane antigen that is present on all human leukocytes [22], is shown in Fig. 62-6.

Stachura et al. [217] have published similar interstitial findings in 16 patients with RPGN using an Avidin-Biotin-immunoperoxidase cell localization technique. They found that the mononuclear interstitial infiltrate con-

Fig. 62-6. A cryostat section of a biopsy from the patient with RPGN in Fig. 62-4. Leukocytes are identified by the monoclonal antibody PHM1 [16] and a four-layer PAP technique [82], giving black staining. The total infiltrating leukocyte population is identified by PHM1 as it recognizes a leukocyte common antigen. Large numbers of interstitial leukocytes (I) can be seen, particularly surrounding the glomerulus (GT). There are also mononuclear leukocytes identified within the glomerulus tuft (GT). Many cells in the crescent (C) are also stained (×125). (Courtesy D. Hooke.)

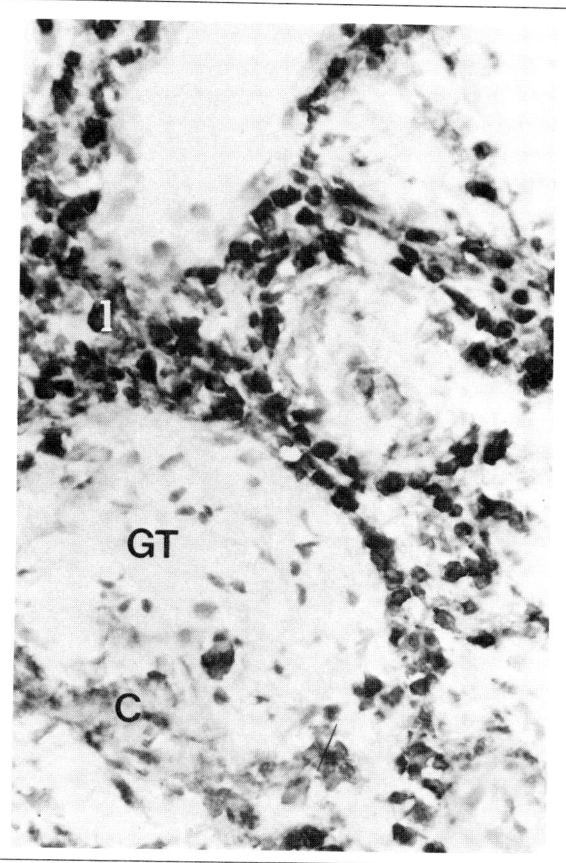

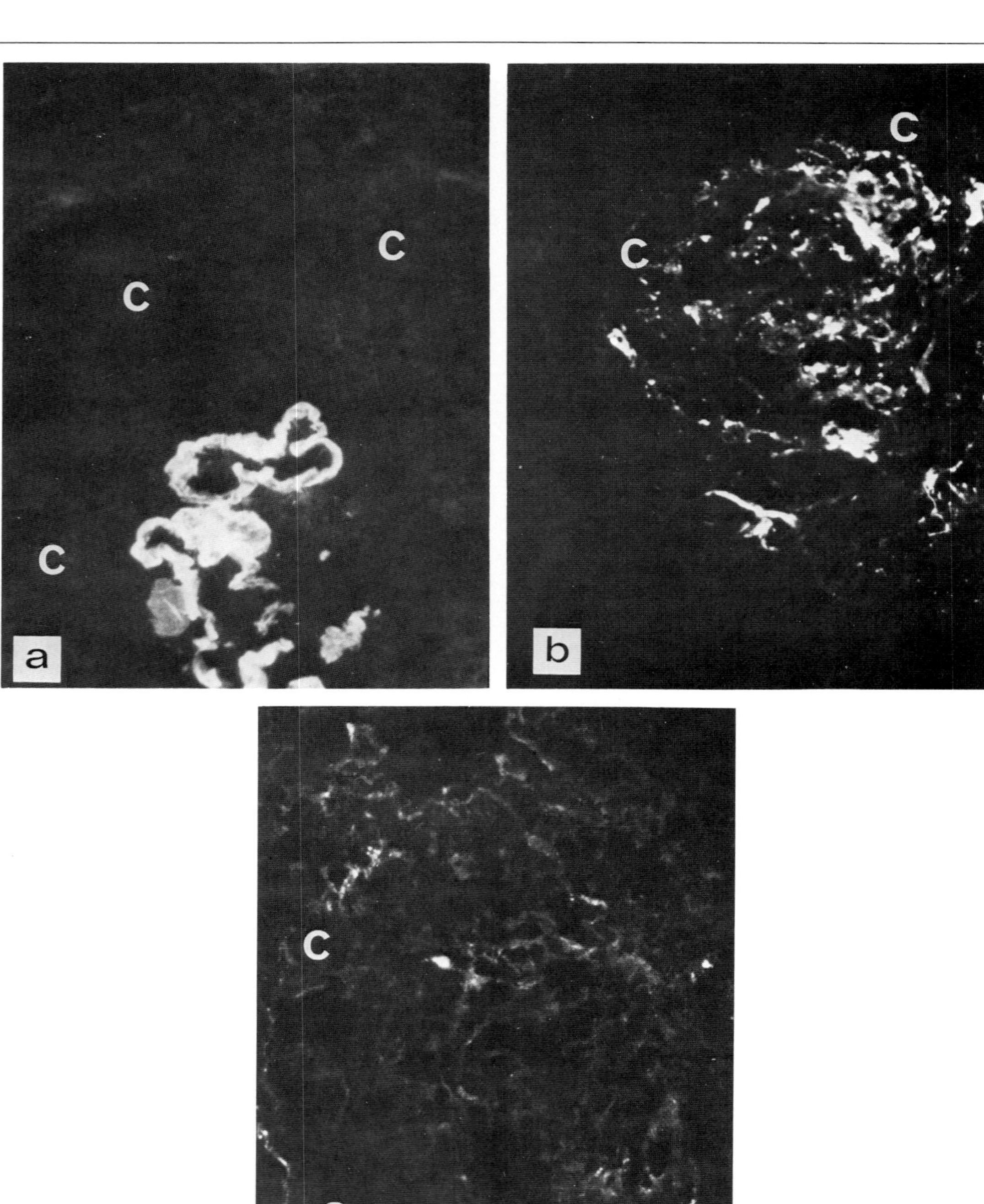

Fig. 62-7. Immunofluorescence micrographs of renal biopsies from three different patients with RPGN demonstrate the three underlying immunopathogenic mechanisms. The crescents (C) are identified. (a) Linear pattern of IgG deposition along the glomerular basement membrane of a patient with anti-GBM RPGN. (b) Granular fluorescence of IgG along the capillary loops of the same patient with RPGN as in Figs. 62-2 and 62-3, due to immune-complex deposition. (c) No definite immunofluorescence deposition is seen within the capillary tuft, but some deposits of C_3 are evident on the visceral layer of Bowman's capsule in a patient with idiopathic or no immune-deposit RPGN.

sisted mainly of T lymphocytes (80%) and monocytes (19%) and very small numbers of B cells and natural killer cells. The majority of the T lymphocytes, both in the interstitium as well as in glomeruli, were of the helper (T4) phenotype in normal patients as well as in patients with RPGN. These studies again raise the possibility that the cellular arm of the immune response is involved in the pathogenesis of RPGN, as discussed later. In recent studies we demonstrated that a high proportion of interstitial mononuclear cells, approximately 20 percent, expressed IL-2R [148], thus demonstrating that they had undergone immune activation. In addition, there was a relationship between glomerular crescentic activity and interstitial leukocyte infiltration. In IgA disease, a denser interstitial infiltration of leukocytes occurred in biopsies from patients with glomerular crescents than from those without crescent formation [149].

We have also determined the relationship between glomerular and interstitial leukocytic involvement in a rat crescentic model of accelerated anti-GBM disease [139]. Within 15 minutes of disease induction, leukocytes appeared within the glomerular and surrounded the efferent and afferent arterioles of the periglomerular stalk. Over the ensuing days the leukocytes increased in number, surrounded the glomerulus by the third day, and appeared throughout the interstitium by day 7. However, the leukocytic profile differed between glomerulus and interstitium, the glomerular leukocytes being mainly monocytes and a few T cells and the periglomerular and interstitial infiltrate made up of 50 percent monocytes and 50 percent T cells. Again many of these mononuclear leukocytes exhibited IL-2R positivity but only 7 days after disease induction and solely in the interstitium. It could well be that this hilar accumulation of leukocytes results from cytokine dispersal from an inflamed glomerular tuft.

The nature of the immune deposits (immunoglobulin and complement) in crescentic glomerulonephritis, as detected by immunofluorescence or an immunoperoxidase technique, depends on the underlying type of glomerulonephritis. In RPGN, three basic patterns are described [66, 85], which reflect the different immunopathogenesis of this disease, as discussed more fully later in the chapter. These are (1) linear GBM deposition of immunoglobulins (anti-GBM antibody), with or without complement (C3) (Fig. 62-7a), (2) granular deposition of immunoglobulin and complement along capillary loops and mesangium, suggesting an immune complex disease (Fig. 62-7b), and (3) no or very scanty immunoglobulin or complement deposition (Fig. 62-7c). The proportion of cases in each individual group varies markedly from one series to another [7, 24, 27, 66, 69, 82, 126, 146, 147, 165, 170, 174, 182, 190, 242]. In very general terms, however, about 30 percent of cases of RPGN account for each category of immunopathogenesis. In addition, there seems to be a great geographic variation. In the United States and Australia, anti-GBM disease is relatively common, while in Europe, it is uncommon. In a series of 75 biopsies from patients from various disease areas and containing more than 50 percent crescents, 12 percent of the patients had anti-GBM

Fig. 62-8. Transmission electron micrograph of part of a glomerulus from a renal biopsy of a 12-year-old male with RPGN, illustrating an early crescent (C) adjacent to the urinary space in which a macrophage (M) can be seen. Bowman's capsule (BC) surrounds the glomerulus. Some capillary loops (L) remain patent, but there are areas of marked endocapillary cell proliferation (P), one of which is adjacent to the early crescent (×3,000). (Courtesy Prof. E. F. Glasgow.)

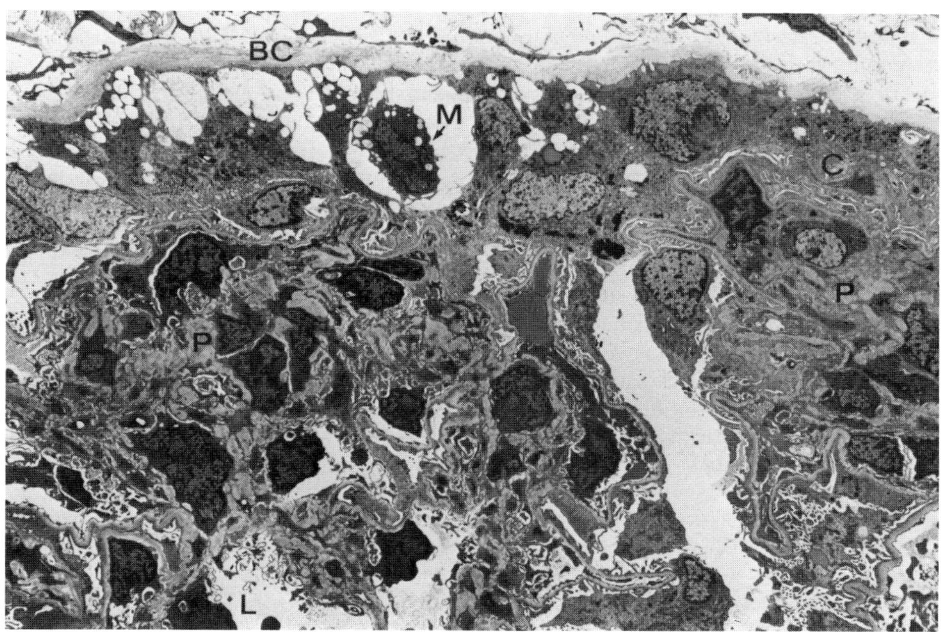

disease, 38 percent had immune complex glomerulonephritis, and 50 percent had pauci-immune (no immune deposits) glomerulonephritis [127]. In our experience of 11 cases of RPGN, 5 were caused by anti-GBM disease, 2 were caused by immune complex deposits, and 4 had no immune deposits [98]. Fibrin/fibrinogen deposition is usually detected within both the crescent and the capillary tuft, and its presence seems to be unrelated to the underlying immunopathogenesis.

Electron microscopy will confirm the presence or absence of mesangial or capillary loop immune deposits in immune complex crescentic glomerulonephritis. Collapse of the capillary wall and necrosis of glomerular cells within the tuft are frequently seen [19, 26, 33, 78, 165, 169, 170, 214, 225], and ruptures in the capillary loops are common and may be important in crescent formation [167]. Electron microscopy also commonly demonstrates macrophages, epithelioid cells, and epithelial cells in the crescent [33, 156], although this technique is not really suited to the determination of the relative proportion of each of these cell types within the crescent. Fibrin is normally seen between the cells of the crescent and, as the crescent evolves, basement-membrane material and collagen fibers may also be seen. In Fig. 62-8 is shown an electron micrograph that illustrates many of these features in a crescent from a patient with RPGN.

Pathogenesis

Our current understanding of the immunopathogenesis of this disease has come largely from the study of the glomerular immune deposits in patients and the study of experimentally induced RPGN in animals. The histologic pattern and clinical course of the entity of RPGN results from three underlying immunopathogenic mechanisms. However, it is even possible that these mechanisms can coexist and perhaps may be variations within a spectrum of disease [47, 66, 127, 196].

GLOMERULAR DEPOSITION OF ANTI-GBM ANTIBODY

In about one-third of patients with RPGN, linear deposition of immunoglobulin (predominantly IgG) along the GBM is detected. In these patients, anti-GBM antibody is also detected in the circulation, particularly if a sensitive and specific radioimmunoassay is used to detect the antibody [117]. In some patients, this antibody also reacts with the pulmonary basement membrane and results in pulmonary hemorrhage [115] (Goodpasture's syndrome; see Chap. 68). The anti-GBM antibody also can cross-react with renal tubular basement membrane, and this has been linked to a more severe interstitial component [6]. The "Goodpasture antigen" has been now identified as the noncollagenous globular domain NCI of collagen IV, various monometric substances have been characterized [48], and the distribution within various known basement membranes has been established [241].

RPGN caused by anti-GBM antibody can be induced in animals, notably in sheep, by the repeated injection of particulate heterologous (e.g., rabbit) or homologous (i.e., sheep) GBM in complete Freund's adjuvant, causing Steblay's nephritis [219]. If serum from sheep with anti-GBM glomerulonephritis (induced by rabbit GBM) is injected IV into rabbits, then the anti-GBM antibody will fix to the rabbit GBM, inducing proteinuria (heterologous phase of nephrotoxic nephritis). With the development 5 to 6 days later of a rabbit antibody response to the sheep antibody on the rabbit GBM, a rapidly progressive crescentic glomerulonephritis develops in the rabbit (autologous phase of nephrotoxic nephritis) [159]. Studies of both these models of crescentic glomerulonephritis have provided considerable insight into the pathogenesis of this disease as well as the mechanisms by which the glomerulus is damaged and the crescent formed.

GLOMERULAR IMMUNE-COMPLEX DEPOSITION

A granular deposition of immunoglobulin and complement along the capillary loops and in the mesangium is seen in about one-third of patients with RPGN. This pattern strongly suggests an immune-complex pathogenesis, although circulating immune complexes are not commonly detected in these patients. The actual antigen(s) involved are not known. The possibility of a viral etiology has been suggested by the demonstration of type IV nuclear bodies in the kidney of some patients with crescentic glomerulonephritis [87]. RPGN due to deposition of immune complexes can be induced in animals, especially the rabbit, by the daily injection IV of bovine serum albumin (BSA) in a dose according to the animal's antibody response to the BSA (chronic serum sickness). Immune complexes of BSA—anti-BSA are produced in the circulation in large amounts and deposit in the glomerular capillary loops and mesangium [23].

ABSENT GLOMERULAR IMMUNE DEPOSITS

In some patients with RPGN, significant immune deposits are not detected in the glomeruli [222]. Thus it has been difficult to incriminate humoral immune mechanisms in these patients. However, 80 percent of these patients have circulating antineutrophil cytoplasmic antibodies [125, 126, 127], and it has been suggested that the patients have systemic vasculitis but without systemic clinical manifestations [207]. The possibility exists that cell-mediated immunity plays a role in this situation, with injury occurring either through recruitment of inflammatory cells by lymphokine release or by the direct effect of cytotoxic T cells [80, 157, 162, 234]. This concept was supported by studies performed 20 years ago [202], in which lymphocytes from patients with RPGN showed in vitro delayed-type hypersensitivity responses (e.g., liberation of migration inhibition factor) in the presence of GBM. However, similar findings were seen in patients with other forms of proliferative glomerulonephritis as well as in patients with RPGN due to anti-GBM antibody or deposition of immune complexes. It may be that the finding of a cell-mediated response to GBM in these patients is a consequence of the glomerular injury rather than the cause. The detection of large numbers of macrophages in the glomeruli and the interstitium in RPGN would be consistent with a cell-mediated delayed hypersensitivity reaction, although macrophages also can accumulate in an inflammatory reaction due to humoral immunity. The presence of T cells within glomeruli found by Stachura [37, 148, 149, 172, 180, 184, 217] and the marked T cell infiltration in the interstitium (particularly of the T4 helper phenotype), as described earlier, adds credence to the cellular immune hypothesis [118, 217].

Theoretically, crescentic glomerulonephritis without immune deposits might be due to nonimmune mechanisms, and crescent formation has been reported in association with extensive glomerular capillary necrosis due to malignant hypertension [216].

Over the past 5 years, however, a specific serologic marker for the RPGN lacking glomerular immunoglobulin deposits (sometimes categorized as "pauci-immune") has been described (see Chap. 76). Antineutrophil cytoplasmic antibodies (ANCAs), first described by Davies et al. in 1982 [70], are a marker for "idiopathic" glomerulonephritis when it occurs with no evidence of extrarenal disease and in glomerulonephritis associated with systemic necrotizing arteritides including polyarteritis nodosa and Wegener's granulomatosis [5, 77, 88, 94, 126, 127, 150, 235, 239].

ANCAs have been detected in about 80 percent of patients with pauci-immune crescentic glomerulonephritis in one center [77, 126, 127], and Jayne et al. [123] found that the sera of 28 percent of 889 consecutive patients with suspected RPGN were positive for ANCA. Cohen et al. [62] reviewed 35 consecutive patients with crescentic glomerulonephritis without glomerular immunoglobulin deposition and concluded that both vasculitis-associated and idiopathic crescentic glomerulonephritis were specifically associated with ANCA to myeloid lysosomal enzymes. Thus, it may be that idiopathic crescentic RPGN without glomerular immune deposits is just part of a spectrum of the vasculitides. Although there are obviously ANCAs to various antigens [62, 123, 127], it may be that C-ANCA (cytoplasmic staining to serine protease) occurs in Wegener's granulomatosis and microscopic polyarteritis and P-ANCA (against myeloperoxidase) is found in patients with crescentic glomerulonephritis who have no glomerular immune deposits and manifest no extrarenal disease. It has been postulated that ANCAs not only are diagnostic markers of disease but may be involved in pathogenetic mechanisms causing crescentic glomerulonephritis [127].

The Mechanism of Crescent Formation

The initial histologic studies describing crescent formation were done over 100 years ago by Langhans [141], and his sketches are reproduced in Fig. 62-1. Since then, the crescent has traditionally been considered to be composed of proliferated epithelial cells. This belief has been based primarily on light and ultrastructural studies of cells of the crescents [19, 169, 185]. However, several investigators, while supporting the epithelial concept of crescent formation, noted cells in crescents that had phagocytic capacity and morphologic features that might be suggestive of macrophages [33, 167]. Magil and Wadsworth [156] in 1982, in a histochemical, immunopathologic, and ultrastructural study, concluded that monocytes participate in crescent formation but that epithelial cell proliferation is more important, particularly in immune complex disease.

The initial evidence suggesting a role of macrophages in crescent formation in patients with RPGN came from tissue-culture studies of glomeruli isolated from renal biopsies [11], which demonstrated an increase in the number of macrophages. Later studies also showed a reduction in the number of epithelial cells in culture outgrowth from crescentic glomeruli [12, 13]. These observations suggested that epithelial cell proliferation was not a major factor in crescent formation, but that macrophages probably played an important role.

The initial supporting experimental evidence for the hypothesis that crescents are formed from accumulated infiltrating macrophages rather than proliferation of either visceral or parietal epithelial cells came from earlier studies of Kondo et al. [138] where, in a morphologic evaluation of experimental crescentic nephritis in rabbits (nephrotoxic nephritis), large numbers of clear cells in the crescent and glomerular tuft, with the features of monocytes, were described. Further morphologic support came from studies on serial renal biopsies of animals developing crescentic nephritis [227]. The initial event of crescent formation was shown to be the deposition of fibrin within Bowman's space. This was followed by an influx of mononuclear cells into Bowman's space, where they phagocytosed fibrin. Epithelioid and giant-cell transformation then occurred. These morphologic observations suggest that crescent formation is a result of the transformation of infiltrating macrophages (Fig. 62-9). In Fig. 62-10 is a scanning electron micrograph of an isolated glomerulus in tissue culture from a rabbit with nephrotoxic nephritis and illustrates macrophages within the crescent.

In experimental RPGN induced either by anti-GBM antibodies [113] or immune complexes [23], enzyme histochemistry has demonstrated that most crescentic cells have an enzymatic profile consistent with a macrophage origin. Elegant studies of Cattell and Aldrige [56], using irradiation to induce leukocyte depletion, also suggested that the crescents originate from circulating leukocytes. In recent ultrastructural analysis of crescent formation in both rats and rabbits with nephrotoxic nephritis, Clarke et al. [59, 60] concluded that the crescent cells evolve predominantly from circulating macrophages.

In order to definitely identify the origin of the crescent cells in patients with RPGN, we developed specific monoclonal antibodies to human epithelial cells [97] and to macrophages and monocytes [22, 103], and we used a sensitive immunoperoxidase technique for the localization of these monoclonal antibodies in renal biopsy specimens from patients with RPGN [100]. In order to identify and quantitate the cell types during different stages of the evolution of the crescent, 12 patients with RPGN, 9 with cellular, and 3 with sclerosed crescents were examined [98]. Cellular crescents consisted of 35 percent macrophages, 12 percent polymorphonuclear leukocytes, and 10 percent epithelial cells. Sclerosed crescents contained few macrophages (5%) but similar proportions of polymorphonuclear leukocytes (11%) and epithelial cells (12%). Many of the crescent cells

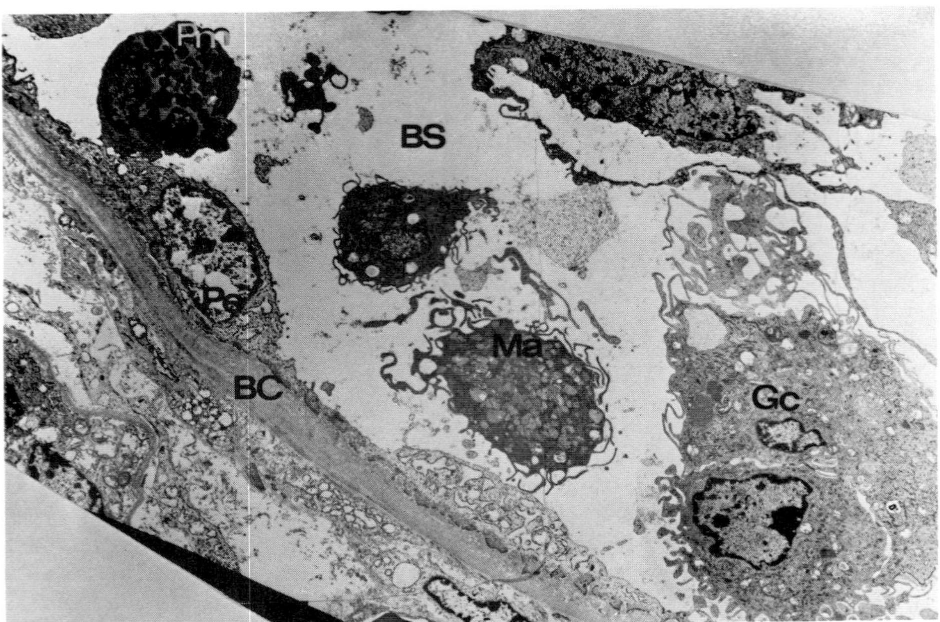

Fig. 62-9. Transmission electron micrograph depicting a glomerulus from a rabbit with nephrotoxic nephritis at day 10 of the disease (i.e., the stage of early crescent formation). Bowman's space (BS), bounded on one side by Bowman's capsule (BC) and a parietal epithelial cell (Pe), contains a number of exudative macrophages (Ma) and a polymorphonuclear leukocyte (Pm). A macrophage that has undergone giant-cell (Gc) transformation can be seen (×4,800). (Courtesy Prof. E. F. Glasgow.)

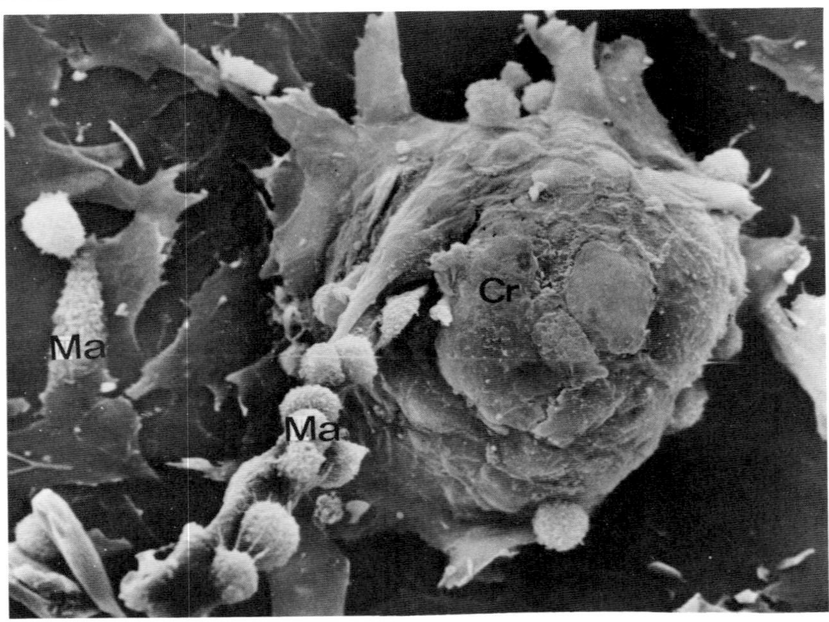

Fig. 62-10. Scanning electron micrograph of a nephrotoxic glomerulus in tissue culture. The glomerulus itself is covered by a cellular crescent (Cr) and from which macrophages (Ma) are emerging. (Courtesy Prof. E. F. Glasgow.)

were unlabeled, but we felt that they probably were fibroblasts because of their morphologic appearance and the expression of surface fibronectin. In Fig. 62-11a and b is demonstrated the complementary staining of epithelial cells and macrophages within the glomerular tuft as well as the crescent in the renal biopsy of a patient with RPGN.

This conclusion was confirmed by the unique study of Schiffer and Michael [209]. Two human female kidney grafts, which were transplanted into male recipients, developed crescentic glomerulonephritis. As demonstrated by the presence of Y-body positivity, 35 percent of cells in the crescents were infiltrating leukocytes from the recipient. Thus the human studies are consistent with the animal observations that macrophages are the predominant cells in the early stages of crescent formation and that, as the crescent evolves and becomes fibrosed, fewer macrophages are seen. Following activation, macrophages themselves may even promote further fibrin deposition by the secretion of procoagulant and other factors [72, 99, 143].

Several studies have approached the problem of identification of crescent cells using a battery of various monoclonal antibodies and concluded that the predominant cell type was the epithelial cell rather than macrophage [89, 124, 248]. The explanation for the discrepant results could in part be explained by the study of Boucher et al. in 1987 [43]. They related the cellular composition of human crescents to the integrity of Bowman's capsule. When Bowman's capsule was intact, the majority of the crescent cells were identified as parietal epithelial cells. When Bowman's capsule was disrupted, few epithelial cells were found and the crescents were composed of macrophage and some T cells. We have confirmed these observations on the relationship between Bowman's capsule integrity and crescent composition in experimental anti-GBM glomerulonephritis in the rat [139]. Such observations could explain some of the discrepancies in crescent composition in the literature. In addition we previously have shown that cellular composition of crescents is dependent on the stage of evolution of the crescent, macrophages being dominant in early and active formation [98].

There is a very prominent interstitial periglomerular infiltration of leukocytes associated with crescentic glomerulonephritis in both human [68, 118, 158] and experimental crescentic glomerulonephritis [139, 199]. We have recently determined the relationship between the glomerular inflammatory process and the interstitial leukocytic infiltration, which begins at the hilus in experimental anti-GBM disease [139]. It may well be that many leukocytes forming crescents in Bowman's space enter from the interstitium as well as via the ruptured capillary tuft. Our sequential studies demonstrated that Bowman's capsule is ruptured after the accumulation of periglomerular leukocytes and that aggregation of leukocytes within Bowman's space then follows [139].

Because crescents can be found in many types of glomerulonephritis with various pathogenic mechanisms (see Table 62-1), there is probably an underlying common pathway of crescent formation. The experiments of Vassali and McCluskey [236] provided evidence that the basic stimulus to crescent formation might be the presence of fibrin in Bowman's space. Min et al. [167] suggested that breaks in the capillary basement membrane allowed fibrin to leak into the urinary space, causing proliferation of epithelial cells. Our morphologic studies [23, 227] of crescent formation in rabbits are consistent with fibrin leakage. In these models, the immune reaction (the deposition of anti-GBM antibody or immune complexes), results in cellular infiltration by polymorphonuclear leukocytes and macrophages within the glomerular tufts. The resultant damage to the GBM leads to proteinaceous exudation, including fibrinogen and fibrin, into Bowman's space. Macrophages, probably under the chemotactic influence of fibrin, migrate into Bowman's space, phagocytose fibrin, and are transformed into epithelioid cells, the accumulation of which results in crescent formation. This sequence is outlined in simplified diagrammatic form in Fig. 62-12. If the fibrin deposition is prevented by defibrination of animals with ancrod, then crescent formation does not occur, although the inflammatory reaction and macrophage accumulation within the glomerular tuft is unaltered [116]. This observation highlights the pivotal role that fibrin has in the attraction of macrophages into Bowman's space. Such a role for fibrin would be in accord with the observation in humans that fibrin is most commonly found in freshly formed crescents and tends to disappear as the crescents become sclerotic [174]. Furthermore, since fibrin-related antigens are usually present in crescents and factor VIII is absent, an independent mechanism (i.e., not the contact-initiated intrinsic pathway of coagulation) has been suggested [121]. Recently, these authors, using a model of rat anti-GBM glomerulonephritis, found that factor VIII was present early in crescent formation and postulated that fibrin persisted because of a less effective clearance mechanism [213]. However, in experimental nephritis in rabbits, macrophages have been shown to be responsible for the glomerular fibrin deposition and express augmented procoagulant activity [233].

The importance of fibrin in progression of crescentic disease was recently demonstrated by Zoja et al. [250]. Recombinant plasminogen activator, which causes lysis of fibrin clots by activating plasminogen to plasmin, reduced glomerular fibrin deposition and crescent formation together with prevention of renal failure in experimental anti-GBM nephritis.

As mentioned previously, monocytes, when activated, express on their surface a procoagulant molecule—tissue factor—which activates the extrinsic pathway of coagulation [99]. We demonstrated in 10 patients with crescentic glomerulonephritis that all macrophages within the crescent have tissue factor expressed on their surface, as recognized by a specific monoclonal antibody, and that all are associated with fibrin deposition [99]. Thus not only may the presence of fibrin attract monocytes into Bowman's space but, when activated, monocytes may contribute further to the fibrin deposition.

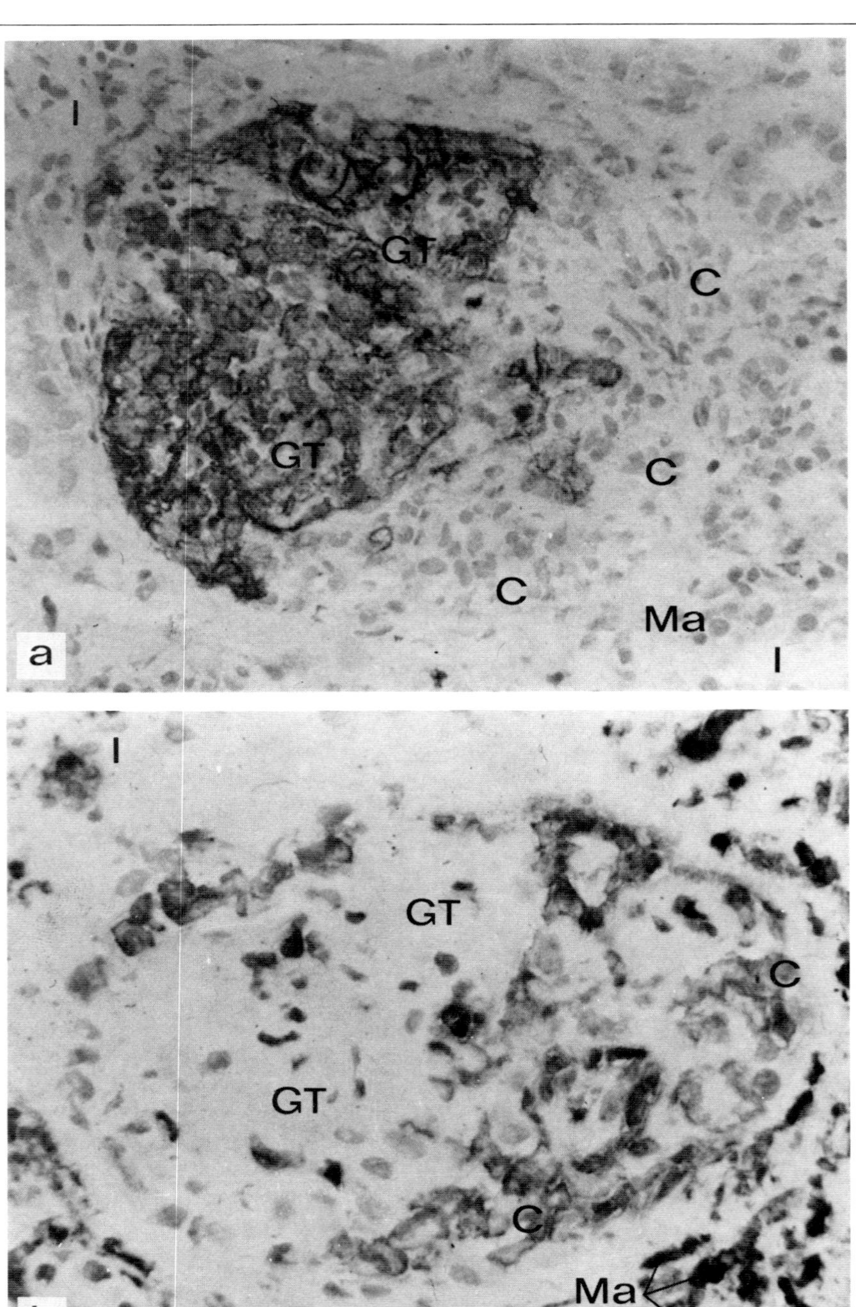

Fig. 62-11. Serial cryostat sections from the renal biopsy of a patient with RPGN, with immunohistochemical labeling of monoclonal antibodies by the four-layer PAP technique [97]. In both a and b, the glomerular tuft (GT) has been compressed into the left half of Bowman's space by the crescent (C) that occupies the right half. (a) The epithelial cells of the glomerulus (GT) are stained using the antiglomerular epithelial cell marker PHM5 [100]. This labels all the epithelial cells in the compressed glomerular tuft (GT) but virtually none of the cells of the crescent (C). (b) Macrophages (Ma) are stained using monoclonal antibodies to monocyte/macrophages FMC32 [84]. Over 90 percent of the cells in the crescent are stained together with many macrophages (Ma) in the interstitium (I) surrounding the glomerulus. (H&E ×250.)

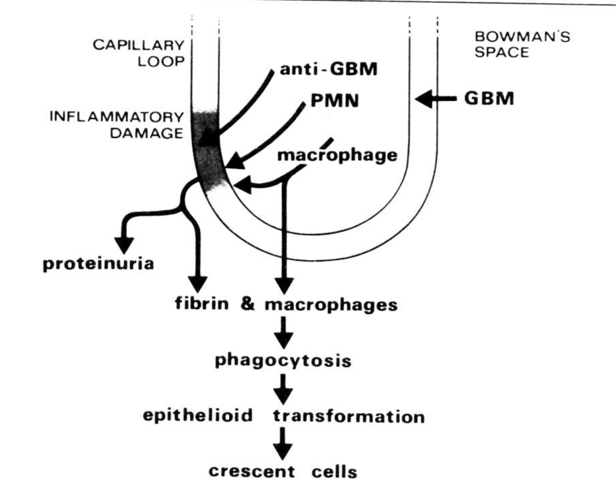

Fig. 62-12. Simple representation of the pathway of mediation of injury in RPGN, leading to crescent formation. This schema summarizes the studies of many workers, including ourselves. Fibrin released into Bowman's space attracts macrophages, which undergo epithelial transformation to form the cells of the crescent. This sequence is probably similar no matter what the underlying cause of the inflammatory insult—in this case, anti-GBM disease.

Table 62-2. Clinical features of rapidly progressive glomerulonephritis

Age: median: fifth and sixth decades
Sex: M : F = 2 : 1
Prodromal illness: common (upper respiratory infection, "flu-like" illness, fever)

Presenting features:	Percent of patients
Nonspecific symptoms of malaise, lethargy	>90
Symptoms of renal failure	60
Oliguria	>60
Edema	60–70
Macroscopic hematuria	20–30
Nephrotic syndrome	10–30
Acute nephritic syndrome	10–20
Hypertension	10–20

Clinical Features

RPGN is an uncommon disease, comprising about 2 percent of all cases of glomerulonephritis, although the reported incidence varies from 2 to 5 percent [6, 24, 58, 69, 85, 214, 242, 243]. This variation is, in part, explained by referral patterns and possibly by true variation from one country to another. The disease is predominantly seen in the third to sixth decade, with a reported median age ranging from 39 to 58 years [19, 24, 110, 144, 160, 165, 170, 210, 214, 222, 224, 242]. Occurrence in childhood is very rare [4, 67, 90, 215]. Patients with RPGN associated with anti-GBM antibody or endocapillary cell proliferation tend to be younger than those without immune deposits or endocapillary proliferation [24, 170]. In contrast, severe crescentic glomerulonephritis of poststreptococcal etiology is most frequent in children [4, 110, 144], while crescentic disease in the elderly is not infrequently associated with systemic vasculitis, particularly with the microscopic form of polyarteritis [71, 106, 110]. Males are more commonly affected than females (2 : 1) [24, 110, 165, 170, 214, 222, 224, 242], and this ratio is higher in patients with anti-GBM disease [24]. There is a genetic predisposition to RPGN in that there is a susceptibility to anti-GBM antibody synthesis in patients who are HLA-DR2. The resultant glomerulonephritis is more severe when it is associated with HLA-B7 [198].

Despite the varying underlying immunopathogenesis of RPGN, the clinical features are remarkably similar in all three subgroups (Table 62-2). However, the signs and symptoms depend on the stage of the disease at presentation. Usually, the onset is insidious and patients present with nonspecific symptoms for several weeks [19, 28, 54, 58, 81, 106, 142, 144, 160, 195, 204, 210, 214, 224, 242]. These symptoms include malaise, lethargy, weakness, anorexia, and nausea. At presentation, many have symptoms of renal failure. Most patients are oliguric and some are anuric—these being poor prognostic features, as discussed in the following section. Occasionally, the onset is very acute, with features of an acute nephritic syndrome, and advanced renal failure develops over a few days. Macroscopic hematuria is not uncommon and microscopic hematuria is invariable. Edema is seen in most patients, and the nephrotic syndrome is seen in 10 to 30 percent [19, 144, 224, 242]. Hypertension, if present, is mild when not due to sodium and water retention [24, 144, 170]. In about 50 percent of patients, an upper respiratory or influenza-like illness precedes the other symptoms; however, only rarely has a specific viral etiology been established. Aronson and Phillips found evidence of infection with Coxsackie virus B5 in six patients with acute oliguric renal failure [8], and an outbreak of influenza A2 has been associated with RPGN with anti-GBM antibody [25, 245]. A greater than expected association with exposure to hydrocarbon solvents also has been reported [24, 249], and other authors have noticed an increased association of preceding myocardial infarction [146, 222], malignancy [120, 222], and membranous glomerulonephritis [24].

By way of contrast, patients with crescentic glomerulonephritis associated with vasculitis usually have prominent systemic symptoms, such as a recurring fever, skin rash, arthritis–arthralgia, mucosal ulceration, and respiratory symptoms, including dyspnea and hemoptysis. Similarly, patients with crescentic glomerulonephritis associated with systemic lupus erythematosus (SLE), endocarditis, or Henoch-Schönlein disease will have the systemic features of these diseases.

Frank hemoptysis suggests Goodpasture's disease (glomerulonephritis and pulmonary hemorrhage associated with anti-GBM antibody), but this can also be a prominent feature of systemic vasculitis [236]. Thus presenting symptoms may be relatively nonspecific and variable and, apart from a rapid deterioration in renal function, have little to alert the clinician to the seriousness of this relatively rare disease.

While it has been known for some time that RPGN can recur posttransplantation [243], it has only been reported recently that RPGN can occur de novo in a transplanted kidney [44, 122]. This occurrence may have some implications concerning the effectiveness of immunosuppressive treatment in this condition (discussed later).

Laboratory Findings

Microscopic hematuria is invariable, the red cells being dysmorphic, indicating a glomerular pathology [32]. Red cell, granular, and leukocyte casts are frequent, although the urine sediment correlates poorly with the severity of disease. Proteinuria is always present, though, in the nephrotic range, in only 10 to 30 percent [19, 144, 224, 242]. More severe disease is less likely to be associated with heavy proteinuria, which simply reflects the low glomerular filtration rate. Fibrin degradation products may be elevated in both the serum and the urine [57, 72, 74, 130, 221].

Most patients have elevated serum creatinine and BUN levels at presentation and are often in severe renal failure, with a serum creatinine elevated to more than 50 mg/dl and a creatinine clearance that is less than 10 percent of normal. The degree of renal failure at presentation depends on the chronicity and severity of the renal lesion. However, as discussed in the following section, most patients progress to end-stage renal failure within several weeks or months.

A normochromic, normocytic anemia is frequently observed and is often more profound than expected from the degree of renal failure. The erythrocyte sedimentation rate is usually elevated; however, if it is very high (> 100 mm in the first hour), an underlying systemic disease should be suspected. Serum complement levels are not depressed [7, 19, 147], in contrast to the hypocomplementemia seen in crescentic glomerulonephritis of both poststreptococcal glomerulonephritis and SLE. As already mentioned, in the third of the patients with RPGN who have linear deposition of antibody along the GBM, circulating anti-GBM antibody is usually detected [154, 157], particularly if a specific and sensitive radioimmunoassay is used [117, 244]. Circulating immune complexes are present in 20 to 30 percent of patients with immune deposits within glomeruli, suggesting an immune complex etiology for their disease [41, 49, 152, 247]. However, circulating immune complexes also have been described in sera of patients with no glomerular immune deposits [152, 218]. The presence of circulating cryoglobulin has been reported in some patients [2, 164]. Hyperglobulinemia and the presence of rheumatoid factor are unusual, while anti-DNA antibodies are not found. The presence of antineutrophil cytoplasmic antibodies suggests an underlying vasculitis [125, 126, 127]. Laboratory investigation thus helps to exclude other primary or secondary crescentic glomerulonephritides. The laboratory findings are summarized in Table 62-3.

Table 62-3. Laboratory features of rapidly progressive glomerulonephritis

Urine:	Microscopic hematuria (dysmorphic): 100% of patients Casts (red cell, granular, leukocyte): common Proteinuria: 100% (>3 gm/24 hr: 10–30%)
Renal function:	Impaired: 100% Creatinine clearance < 20 ml/min: (30%)
Normal renal size	
Normocytic normochronic anemia	
Erythrocyte sedimentation rate: moderate rise (< 100 mm first hour)	
Circulating anti-GBM antibody (30%)	
Circulating immune complexes (10–15%)	
Serum complement components: normal	
Anti-DNA antibody: negative	
Antistreptolysin 0 titer: no rise	
Antineutrophil cytoplasmic antibody (80% if absent glomerular immune deposits)	

Natural History

As mentioned previously, most patients have severe renal failure at the time of presentation, reflecting extensive glomerular damage. Thus prognosis is already predetermined, at least in part, by the degree of irreversible renal damage. Studies of experimentally induced crescentic glomerulonephritis have shown that even if the inflammatory/immune insult is ceased in established disease, many animals will die from progressive renal failure, reflecting the severity of irreversible glomerular damage that is frequently present [228, 229].

In several reported series [7, 19, 109, 147] of patients with RPGN, the authors have attempted to determine prognostic factors and the effect of treatment. These series are not strictly comparable, because there are variations in the criteria for diagnosis—the underlying immunopathogenetic processes, the extent of crescent formation (> 30% crescents, > 50% crescents, or > 80% crescents), and the inclusion or exclusion of clinically suspected microscopic vasculitis or Goodpasture's syndrome. Moreover, a valid life table analysis of persistence of renal function and survival of patients has rarely been undertaken. However, a synthesis of these reports indicates that about 20 percent of patients present with permanent end-stage renal failure. About 50 percent progress to end-stage renal failure by one year; and 75 percent, by two years (see Table 62-4). A variety of patterns of deterioration or improvement in renal function are seen. Some patients show spontaneous rapid improvement in renal function soon after presentation. In a few patients, this improvement is sustained and in others it is temporary, with the patients drifting into renal failure within months. Other patients show progressive decline in renal function after presentation, while others maintain stable renal function. These various patterns of outcome probably reflect a number of

Table 62-4. Prognosis of rapidly progressive glomerulonephritis according to urine output at presentation

Percentage of patients with renal function at 12 months				
Author	No. of patients	All patients (%)	Nonoliguric (%)	Oliguric (%)
Sonsino (1972) [214]	56	48	79	26
Whitworth (1976) [242]	60	72	87	53
Beirne (1977) [24]	23	31	61	22
Morrin (1978) [170]	29	31	59	20
Neild (1983) [182]	19	52	100	10
Heilman (1987) [109]	24	40	78	22
	Mean =	46	78	25

events, including the persistence or loss of the causative factors, the degree of initial renal damage, the severity of the scarring process that subsequently evolves (e.g., fibrosis of crescents and interstitial fibrosis), and the development or absence of vascular damage and hypertension. In addition, these patterns also may be altered by the several therapeutic measures used in this disease.

URINE OUTPUT AT PRESENTATION

It has become evident that the presence of oliguria at presentation of RPGN is associated with a significantly poorer outcome than is seen in patients who have maintained good urine output. In Table 62-4 are summarized the results from six large recently reported series of patients with RPGN [24, 109, 170, 182, 214, 242], and the persistence of renal function at 12 months, in patients who presented with or without oliguria, is listed. Although there is a wide variation, each series shows a significant difference in survival between oliguric and nonoliguric patients. Temporary or sustained recovery of renal function was seen in only 26 percent of patients who were oliguric at presentation. On the other hand, 78 percent of nonoliguric patients were alive at 12 months with adequate renal function.

Patients who are anuric at presentation rarely recover renal function. The poor outcome associated with oligoanuria reflects the degree of crescent formation, because in 80 percent of oligoanuric patients, more than 80 percent of the glomeruli are involved.

EXTENT OF CRESCENT FORMATION

Several studies have shown a positive correlation between the percentage of glomeruli affected by crescent formation and the severity of initial and subsequent renal failure [106, 144, 160, 165, 170, 182, 186, 218, 222, 242]. In three studies, all patients with crescents in 100 percent of the glomeruli progressed rapidly to end-stage renal failure [106, 170, 214], while other authors have reported the recovery of renal function in less than 10 percent of patients [24, 144, 177, 178]. Habib [90, 92] found a similar incidence of end-stage renal failure in patients with more than 80 percent crescents. Morrin et al. [170] found that 39 percent of patients with more than 80 percent crescents showed some recovery of renal function compared to 90 percent of patients with less than 60 percent crescents. Neild et al. [182] have reviewed 11 published series of RPGN, totaling 200 patients, and have confirmed the findings that the more extensive the crescent formation, the less there is a chance of recovery of renal function (Table 62-5).

The development of crescents in other forms of primary glomerulonephritis (especially IgA glomerulonephritis and membranoproliferative glomerulonephritis) and in glomerulonephritis of a systemic disease is also associated with a poor outcome.

CHANGES IN THE GLOMERULAR TUFT

Endocapillary cell proliferation (glomerular hypercellularity) has been reported as a good prognostic feature compared to normocellularity of the glomerular tuft [170, 182, 214, 224]. Morrin et al. [170] reported recovery of renal function in only 30 percent of patients with RPGN who had normal glomerular tuft cellularity compared to 50 percent of patients with hypercellular glomerular tufts. However, in Morrin's series, glomerular hypercellularity also was associated with less compact glomerular crescents, and necrosis of the tuft was less evident, both findings also being possible factors in better renal function. Moreover, endocapillary cell proliferation is seen in postinfectious glomerulonephritis, a

Table 62-5. Improvement in renal function following rapidly progressive glomerulonephritis according to the extent of crescent formation

	100%	90–99%	80–89%	70–79%	60–69%
Number of patients (total 200)	66	43	36	35	20
Number of patients with improvement in renal function	10	14	18	20	11
Percentage	15%	32%	50%	56%	55%

From Neild et al., 1983 [182].

disease with a better prognosis than RPGN. It is thus possible that some of the studies included some patients with postinfectious glomerulonephritis, although this assumption does not seem to be true in Morrin's series.

Glomerular tuft necrosis is thought to be a poor prognostic feature [46, 144, 170, 214, 224]. This notion is supported by the observation that in the microscopic form of polyarteritis, where segmental or diffuse tuft necrosis is very prominent, severe renal failure may be present with minimal crescent formation. Global glomerular sclerosis and gaps in Bowman's capsule are also bad prognostic features [173].

INTERSTITIAL FIBROSIS AND TUBULAR ATROPHY

It has been reported that the extent of interstitial fibrosis correlates with the severity of initial and ultimate renal dysfunction [173, 215, 224]. Striker et al. [224] found that if interstitial fibrosis involved more than 30 percent of the biopsy tissue, then recovery of renal function was unusual, and the patients were often anuric at presentation.

IMMUNOPATHOGENESIS

The group of patients with little or no immune deposits in the glomeruli seem to have the best prognosis [24, 165, 222], although this has not been the experience of all authors [242]. The lack of immune deposits may represent resolution of the initial immune insult, and thus recovery of function may be more likely.

Granular immune deposits also have been reported as indicative of a better prognosis [24, 170], with renal function being recovered in more patients than expected, given the histologic and clinical severity of the disease. On the other hand, other authors reported a poor prognosis for patients with granular immune deposits [165, 242]. Again, this conflict of findings may reflect the inclusion, in some series, of patients with poststreptococcal crescentic glomerulonephritis. Thus it is still not clear if immune complex RPGN has a better prognosis than RPGN as a whole.

The group with RPGN associated with anti-GBM antibody has the worst prognosis [24, 26, 129, 165, 170, 182, 243]. The reason for this occurrence is not clear except that these patients may show glomerular deposition of anti-GBM antibody and circulating anti-GBM antibody for many months after detection of the disease. Thus chronicity of the immune insult may explain the worse prognosis. Urine protein excretion, degree of interstitial cellular infiltration, and age show a weak correlation with outcome [109]. A summary of the factors determining the outcome of RPGN is outlined in Table 62-6.

Treatment

Many therapeutic regimens have been used in the treatment of RPGN, and the relative benefits of these regimens are very much in dispute. Because of the rarity of RPGN, there have been no controlled trials comparing either one treatment regimen with another or with no treatment. Many studies have simply compared outcome associated with a treatment to outcome in historic controls. This is not a valid comparison, particularly given the advances made in the minimization of progression of renal disease with nonspecific therapy, such as control of hypertension, hyperphosphatemia, diet, and the more successful management of renal failure, including temporary dialysis. It is also important to note that many of the therapies used to treat RPGN have the potential to induce serious complications, including sepsis, hemorrhage, sterility, and malignancy.

On the other hand, because controlled trials have not been undertaken, neither have the various therapeutic regimens been proved to be ineffective. Further evaluation of the various therapies should, therefore, continue. It also must be said that several authors have noted spectacular recovery from RPGN in an appreciable number of patients given immunosuppressive and anticoagulative agents, in whom the expected recovery rate would be nil (e.g., advanced renal failure with 100 percent crescents). These observations have been sufficient evidence for many renal physicians to routinely use this therapy for such patients. The various regimens used, either alone or in combination ("cocktail"), in the treatment of RPGN are listed in Table 62-7. The basis for these therapies, which are directed at the immune and the inflammatory processes, lies in studies of the nature of the immune and inflammatory events in both human and experimental crescentic glomerulonephritis.

CORTICOSTEROIDS

Because of their anti-inflammatory properties, corticosteroids are frequently used in the treatment of RPGN. There are very little published data on the use of corticosteroids in experimental crescentic glomerulonephritis. However, two reports have demonstrated marked improvement in renal function with intravenous meth-

Table 62-6. Factors determining the outcome of rapidly progressive glomerulonephritis

Factors	Poorer prognosis	Better prognosis
Urine output at presentation	Oliguric	Nonoliguric
Extent of crescent formation	> 80%	50–80%
The glomerulus	Fibrinoid necrosis	Endocapillary cell proliferation
Glomerular immune deposits	Linear deposition (anti-GBM)	Granular deposition (immune complex) or no immune reactants
Interstitium	Interstitial fibrosis and tubular atrophy	

Table 62-7. Therapeutic regimens used in crescentic glomerulonephritis, either alone or in combination

Corticosteroids	Oral prednisolone/prednisone
Methylprednisolone	Intravenous
Cytotoxic agents	Cyclophosphamide Azathioprine Chlorambucil Nitrogen Mustard
Anticoagulants	Heparin Warfarin Ancrod Streptokinase/t-PA
Antiplatelet agents	Dipyridamole, sulfinpyrazone Aspirin
Antilymphocyte globulin	
Plasma exchange	

ylprednisolone [135, 201]. Holdsworth and Tipping have shown [114, 232] that glomerular injury induced by macrophages in rabbits can be reduced substantially by corticosteroids, while injury induced by polymorphonuclear leukocytes is unaffected. As discussed earlier, both polymorphonuclear leukocytes and macrophages are thought to be injurious in crescentic glomerulonephritis.

There is no evidence that oral steroids alone are of benefit in RPGN [28, 50, 106, 144, 177]. Their use is usually in conjunction with immunosuppressive and anticoagulant agents. The lack of benefit from steroids alone is strikingly different from their often dramatic effect in necrotizing crescentic glomerulonephritis associated with vasculitis [61, 192, 211]. However, several reports indicate that high-dose intravenous "pulse" therapy of methylprednisolone, given daily or alternate daily for three to six doses, can lead to dramatic and sustained improvement in renal function in RPGN [34, 36, 63, 79, 186, 187, 220, 222, 246]. Bolton et al. [36, 38] found this benefit only in patients with RPGN that was not caused by anti-GBM antibody. All these investigators have commented on the low incidence of side effects of intravenous "pulse" steroid therapy.

CYTOTOXIC AGENTS

Immunosuppression with either azathioprine or cyclophosphamide (or, occasionally, chlorambucil) is commonly used in the treatment of crescentic glomerulonephritis, again usually in combination with anticoagulation and steroids and, more recently, plasma exchange.

Experimental evidence provides some foundation for the use of immunosuppressives. Naisch et al. [176] showed that nitrogen mustard substantially prevented the development of crescents in experimental crescentic nephritis, but this occurrence required the induction of neutropenia.

There appears to be little or no evidence to support the use of either cyclophosphamide or azathioprine on their own. Several authors have reported substantial benefit from the combination of cyclophosphamide with anticoagulation, steroids, and antiplatelet drugs, while others have been unable to demonstrate benefit [24, 46, 53, 178, 181]. The use of intravenous cyclophosphamide in the treatment of RPGN has only rarely been reported [231] unlike its use in lupus nephritis.

ANTICOAGULANTS

For a number of years, it has been appreciated that glomerular fibrin deposition is prominent in crescentic glomerulonephritis, within the glomerular tuft, and especially within Bowman's space and the crescent [57, 71, 110]. The role of the coagulation process in development of the crescent in experimental glomerulonephritis has already been discussed. Several studies in experimental glomerulonephritis have shown that anticoagulation with heparin, prior to the onset of the glomerular injury, can reduce the formation of crescents and severity of renal failure [95, 134, 230], although other authors have failed to demonstrate a significant change [40, 41]. Anticoagulation with warfarin also has been shown to reduce, to a smaller degree, crescent formation [42, 236]. However, although intravenous heparin has been shown to reduce glomerular fibrin deposition, crescent formation, and renal failure in nephrotoxic nephritis in rabbits, enormous doses were required, rendering blood unclottable [230]. Moreover, despite the use of such massive doses of heparin, some glomerular fibrin deposition still occurred. This finding suggests that the pathogenetic mechanisms occurring locally within the glomerulus are capable of producing local coagulation, overriding the effects of circulating anticoagulants. This occurrence could possibly result from a failure of heparin, a small but highly charged molecule, to penetrate the mesangium and Bowman's space. Another explanation for the relative ineffectiveness of heparin is that the fibrin deposition results from thrombin-independent mechanisms, as discussed previously.

By contrast, defibrination with ancrod, a purified coagulant enzyme [76], in experimental crescentic glomerulonephritis due to either anti-GBM antibody or immune complex deposition, virtually prevents any glomerular fibrin deposition and crescent formation and results in preservation of renal function [175, 229, 230]. The reported benefit of plasma exchange in the treatment of idiopathic crescentic glomerulonephritis may, in part, be related to the induction of fibrinogen depletion by the technique. The benefit of anticoagulation in established crescentic glomerulonephritis is less obvious. However, defibrination with ancrod or fibrinolysis with streptokinase in experimental glomerulonephritis have been shown to result in more rapid and effective resolution of crescents and recovery from renal failure, provided that irreversible renal damage has not already occurred [228]. There has been only limited experience with the use of ancrod in human RPGN [193, 212].

Similarly, human recombinant tissue plasminogen activator (t-PA) when given to rabbits developing crescentic glomerulonephritis markedly reduces glomerular fibrin deposition, crescent formation, and renal failure [250]. t-PA has the advantage of activating plasminogen to plasmin mainly within clots, unlike streptokinase. Human studies with t-PA have yet to be reported.

Anticoagulation with heparin for human RPGN was

first reported by Kincaid-Smith et al. in 1968 [132]. The subsequent use of heparin in this disease usually has been in combination with one or more other drugs, including steroids, immunosuppressives, and antiplatelet agents [46, 51, 52, 53, 54, 85, 111, 225]. It has thus been difficult to determine the relative benefit of the anticoagulation, and even now there is still no clear-cut evidence that their use is beneficial.

ANTIPLATELET AGENTS

Platelets are potential mediators for glomerular injury, particularly through the release of vasoactive amines. However, little direct evidence exists that they are involved in crescentic glomerulonephritis, although a role in the coagulation process in the glomerulus has not been excluded [51, 83, 189]. Antiplatelet agents, such as dipyrimadole and sulfinpyrazone, have been used in the disease as part of the "cocktail," with no proven benefit.

PLASMA EXCHANGE

Since the demonstration of the benefit of plasma exchange for patients with Goodpasture's syndrome [131, 140, 150, 208, 238], the technique has been used widely in a variety of types of glomerulonephritis, including RPGN [9, 21, 64, 104, 108, 112, 152, 200, 206, 226, 240], usually in conjunction with immunosuppression. Glockner et al. [86] reported in 1988 a randomized study of plasma exchange in 26 patients with RPGN, also given steroids and immunosuppression, and was unable to demonstrate drug difference in outcome of renal function after 8 weeks. However, no large randomized study has been made of the "benefit" of plasma exchange, with or without immunosuppression, to immunosuppression alone. Nevertheless, many physicians feel that plasma exchange is beneficial, particularly in nonoliguric anti-GRM RPGN. The role of plasma exchange and its mechanisms of action are fully detailed in Chap. 67.

RENAL TRANSPLANTATION

Successful transplantation is possible in patients with RPGN [73, 243]. The disease can recur in the allograft [73, 93, 160], but this is unusual if transplantation is delayed until the circulating anti-GBM antibody, if present, has disappeared.

FACTORS TO BE CONSIDERED IN THE TREATMENT OF RPGN

The simple diagnosis of RPGN alone is not sufficient to determine the type of treatment. Several other factors are likely to be relevant to the potential benefit, or not, of treatment: (1) The acute or chronic nature of the glomerular lesion; the presence of acute cellular crescents with extensive fibrin deposition is more indicative of a likely positive response to immunosuppression and anticoagulation than disease in which crescents are undergoing fibrosis and in which glomerulosclerosis and interstitial fibrosis are prominent. (2) The presence of segmental glomerular capillary loop necrosis should raise the possibility of an underlying vasculitis and thus a greater chance of a response to immunosuppression. Similarly, the presence of systemic symptoms other than those of renal failure should suggest the possibility of vasculitis. (3) Immunosuppression, anticoagulation, and the use of plasma exchange all have the potential for inducing severe and, occasionally, fatal side effects [128, 203, 205]. It could be argued that the patient particularly at risk from these side effects (e.g., the elderly, infected, or patients with peptic ulceration) is better treated by aggressive control of hypertension and renal failure rather than by immunosuppression. If immunosuppression is to be successful, early diagnosis of RPGN is essential before irreparable damage has occurred. Early diagnosis depends on urinalysis and assessment of renal function in any patient presenting to a general practitioner with persistent nonspecific symptoms [55].

The author's personal approach to the treatment of RPGN is to treat all patients, unless renal biopsy shows irreversible damage, with a trial of immunosuppression, consisting of corticosteroids and cyclophosphamide, usually without heparin. Pulse methylprednisolone is given IV (1 gm) on each of three successive days, followed by oral prednisolone at a dose of 60 mg per day for 2 to 3 weeks and then reduced rapidly to a maintenance of 10 to 15 mg per day, which is sustained for 6 months to 1 year, depending on the clinical progress. Cyclophosphamide is used at 2 to 3 mg/kg of body weight, usually for 1 to 3 months. Anticoagulation with heparin is not used routinely nor is dipyridamole or other antiplatelet agents. If renal function continues to deteriorate despite the immunosuppression, plasma exchange of 3 to 4 liters on alternate days is begun and continued for 2 to 3 weeks.

Failure of response to these measures leads to an early rather than late cessation of therapy, in order to minimize complications. Maintenance dialysis remains the alternative for those patients who are not treated or are not responding to treatment.

References

1. Abbott, F., Jones, S., Lockwood, C. M., et al. Autoantibodies to glomerular antigens in patients with Wegener's granulomatosis. *Nephrol. Dial. Transplant.* 4(1): 1, 1989.
2. Adam, C., Morel-Maroger, L., and Richet, G. Cryoglobulins in glomerulonephritis not related to systemic disease. *Kidney Int.* 3: 334, 1973.
3. Adler, S., Chen, X., and Eng, B. Control of rat glomerular epithelial cell growth in vitro. *Kidney Int.* 37: 1048, 1990.
4. Anand, S. K., Trygstad, C. W., Sharma, H. M., et al. Extracapillary proliferative glomerulonephritis in children. *Pediatrics* 56: 434, 1975.
5. Andrassy, K., Koderisch, J., Waldherr, R., et al. Diagnostic significance of anticytoplasmic antibodies (ACPA/ANCA) in detection of Wegener's granulomatosis and other forms of vasculitis. *Nephron* 49: 257, 1988.
6. Andres, G., Brentjens, J., Kohli, R., et al. Histology of human tubulo-interstitial nephritis associated with antibodies to renal basement membrane. *Kidney Int.* 13: 480, 1978.
7. Arieff, A. I., and Pinggera, W. F. Rapidly progressive glomerulonephritis treated with anticoagulants. *Arch. Intern. Med.* 129: 77, 1972.
8. Aronson, M. D., and Philips, C. A. Coxsackie virus B5

infections in acute oliguric renal failure. *J. Infect. Dis.* 131: 303, 1975.

9. Asaba, H., Rekola, S., Bergestrand, A., et al. Clinical trial of plasma exchange with a membrane filter in treatment of crescentic glomerulonephritis. *Clin. Nephrol.* 14: 60, 1980.
10. Atkins, R. C. Pathogenesis of Glomerulonephritis. In M. Hatano, *Proceedings of XIth International Congress of Nephrology,* New York: Springer-Verlag, Vol. 1, pp. 14–17, 1991.
11. Atkins, R. C., Glasgow, E. F., Holdsworth, S. R., et al. The macrophage in human rapidly progressive glomerulonephritis. *Lancet* I: 830, 1976.
12. Atkins, R. C., Glasgow, E. F., Holdsworth, R. S., et al. Glomerular Cells in Glomerulonephritis. In P. Kincaid-Smith, A. d'Apice, and R. C. Atkins (eds.), *Progress in Glomerulonephritis.* New York: Wiley, 1979. Pp. 91–105.
13. Atkins, R. C., Glasgow, E. F., Holdsworth, S. R., et al. Tissue culture of isolated glomeruli from patients with glomerulonephritis. *Kidney Int.* 17: 515, 1980.
14. Atkins, R. C., Hancock, W. W., Hooke, D. H., et al. The Cellular Participants in Human Glomerulonephritis. In G. I. Becker, R. C. Atkins, and P. Kincaid-Smith (eds.), *Proceedings of the Second Asian Pacific Congress of Nephrology.* Melbourne: Dominion Press, 1984. Pp. 141–145.
15. Atkins, R. C., Hancock, W. W., Stow, J. L., et al. Macrophage Identification in Human and Experimental Glomerulonephritis. *Proceedings of the VIIIth International Congress of Nephrology.* Basil: Karger, 1981. Pp. 865–871.
16. Atkins, R. C., and Holdsworth, S. R. Cellular Mechanisms of Immune Glomerular Injury. In B. Brenner and Stein (eds.), *Cellular Mechanisms of Injury in GN.* New York: Churchill Livingstone, 1988. Pp. 111–135.
17. Atkins, R. C., Holdsworth, S. R., Hancock, W. W., et al. Cellular immune mechanisms in human glomerulonephritis: The role of mononuclear leukocytes. *Springer Semin. Immunopathol.* 5: 269, 1982.
18. Atkins, R. C., Lan, H. Y., and Paterson, D. J. Pathogenic mechanisms of interstitial leucocyte infiltration in glomerulonephritis. In G. D'Amico and G. Colasanti, *Issues in Nephrosciences* Milan: Wichtig, 1991. P. 123.
19. Bacani, R. A., Velasquez, F., Kanter, A., et al. Rapidly progressive (nonstreptococcal) glomerulonephritis. *Ann. Intern. Med.* 69: 463, 1968.
20. Ballerman, B. J. Regulation of bovine glomerular endothelial cell growth in vitro. *Am. J. Physiol.* 256(1): C182, 1988.
21. Becker, G. J., d'Apice, A. J. F., Walker, R. G., et al. Plasmapheresis in the treatment of glomerulonephritis. *Med. J. Aust.* 2: 693, 1977.
22. Becker, G. J., Hancock, W. W., Kraft, N., et al. Monoclonal antibodies to human macrophage and leucocyte common antigen. *Pathology* 13: 669, 1981.
23. Becker, G. J., Hancock, W. W., Stow, J. L., et al. The involvement of the macrophage in experimental chronic immune complex glomerulonephritis. *Nephron* 32: 227, 1982.
24. Beirne, G. J., Wagnild, J. P., Zimmerman, S. W., et al. Idiopathic crescentic glomerulonephritis. *Medicine* (Baltimore) 56: 349, 1977.
25. Benoit, F. L., Rulon, D. B., Theil, G. B., et al. Goodpasture's syndrome: A clinico-pathologic entity. *Am. J. Med.* 37: 424, 1964.
26. Berg, R., Bergstrand, A., Bergstrom, J., et al. Rapidly progressive glomerulonephritis with antibodies against glomerular basement membranes in serum and kidneys. *Clin. Nephrol.* 5: 37, 1976.
27. Berger, J., Yaneva, H., and Hinglais, N. *Immunohistochemistry of Glomerulonephritis: Advances in Nephrology,* Vol. 1. Chicago: Year Book, 1971. Pp. 11.
28. Berlyne, G. M., and Baker, S. B. de C. Acute anuric glomerulonephritis. *Q. J. Med.* 33: 105, 1964.
29. Bernard, A., Boumsell, L., Dausset, J., et al. *Leucocyte Typing—Human Leucocyte Differentiation Antigens Detected by Monoclonal Antibodies.* New York: Springer-Verlag, 1984.
30. Bialestock, D., and Tange, J. D. Acute necrotizing glomerulitis: The clinical features and pathology in nine cases. *Aust. Ann. Med.* 8: 281, 1959.
31. Biava, C. G., Gonwa, T. A., Naughton, J. L., et al. Crescentic glomerulonephritis associated with non-renal malignancies. *Am. J. Nephrol.* 4: 208, 1984.
32. Birch, D. F., Fairley, K. F., Whitworth, J. A., et al. Urinary erythrocyte morphology in the diagnosis of glomerular hematuria. *Clin. Nephrol.* 20: 78, 1983.
33. Bohman, S. O., Olsen, S., and Petersen, V. P. Glomerular ultrastructure in extracapillary glomerulonephritis. *Acta Pathol. Microbiol. Scand.* [A] 82 (Suppl. 249): 29, 1974.
34. Bolton, W. K. Pulse Methyl Prednisolone Therapy of Rapidly Progressive Glomerulonephritis. In G. Schreiner (ed.), *Controversies in Nephrology,* Vol. 3. Washington: Georgetown University, 1981. P. 213.
35. Bolton, W. K., Chandra, M., Tyson, T. M., et al. Transfer of experimental glomerulonephritis in chickens by mononuclear cells. *Kidney Int.* 34(5): 598, 1988.
36. Bolton, W. K., and Couser, W. G. Intravenous pulse methylprednisolone therapy of acute crescentic rapidly progressive glomerulonephritis. *Am. J. Med.* 66: 495, 1979.
37. Bolton, W. K., Innes, D. G., Sturgill, B. C., et al. T cells and macrophages in rapidly progressive glomerulonephritis: Clinicopathological correlations. *Kidney Int.* 32: 869, 1987. P. 876.
38. Bolton, W. K., and Sturgill, B. Pulse methylprednisolone therapy of rapidly progressive glomerulonephritis—10 years experience. *Kidney Int.* 29: 180, 1985.
39. Bolton, W. K., Tucker, F. L., and Sturgill, B. C. New avian model of experimental GN consistent with mediation by cellular immunity. *J. Clin. Invest.* 73: 1263, 1984.
40. Bone, J., Saldess, A., Germuth, F., et al. Heparin therapy in anti-basement membrane nephritis. *Kidney Int.* 8: 72, 1975.
41. Border, W., Wilson, C., and Dixon, F. Failure of heparin to affect two types of experimental glomerulonephritis in rabbits. *Kidney Int.* 8: 140, 1975.
42. Borrero, J., Todd, M. E., Becker, C. G., et al. Masugi nephritis: The renal lesion and the coagulation process. *Clin. Nephrol.* 1: 86, 1972.
43. Boucher, A., Droz, D., Adafer, E., et al. Relationship between the integrity of Bowman's capsule and the composition of cellular crescents in human crescentic glomerulonephritis. *Lab. Invest.* 56(5): 526, 1987.
44. Boyce, N., Holdsworth, S., Dowling, J., et al. Denovo anti-GBM antibody inducing glomerulonephritis in a renal transplant. *Clin. Nephrol.* 23: 148, 1985.
45. Boyce, N. W., Tipping, P. G., and Holdsworth, S. R. Lymphokine (MIF) production by glomerular T lymphocytes in experimental glomerulonephritis. *Kidney Int.* 30: 673, 1986.
46. Brown, C. B., Wilson, D., Turner, D., et al. Continued immunosuppression and anticoagulation in rapidly progressive glomerulonephritis. *Lancet* 2: 1166, 1974.
47. Bruijn, J. A., Hoedemaeker, P. J., and Fleuren, G. J.

Pathogenesis of antibasement membrane glomerulopathy and immune complex glomerulonephritis: Dichotomy dissolved. *Lab. Invest.* 61: 480, 1989.
48. Butkowski, R. J. M., Shen, G. Q., Wieslander, J., et al. Characterization of type IV collagen NC1 monomers and Goodpasture antigen in human renal basement membranes. *J. Lab. Clin. Med.* 115: 365, 1990.
49. Cairns, S., London, R., Mallick, N., et al. The significance of circulating immune complexes in idiopathic glomerulonephritis. *Kidney Int.* 16: 911, 1979.
50. Cameron, J. Immunosuppressant agents in the treatment of glomerulonephritis: II. Cytotoxic drugs. *J. R. Coll. Physicians Lond.* 5: 301, 1971.
51. Cameron, J. S. Platelets and glomerulonephritis. *Nephron* 18: 253, 1977.
52. Cameron, J. The Natural History of Glomerulonephritis. In P. Kincaid-Smith, A. J. d'Apice, and R. C. Atkins (eds.), *Progress in Glomerulonephritis.* New York: Wiley, 1979. P. 1.
53. Cameron, J., Gill, D., Turner, D., et al. Combined immunosuppression and anticoagulation in rapidly progressive glomerulonephritis. *Lancet* II: 923, 1975.
54. Cameron, J. S., and Ogg, C. S. Rapidly Progressive Glomerulonephritis with Extensive Crescents. In P. Kincaid-Smith, T. H. Mathew, and E. L. Becker (eds.), *Glomerulonephritis: Morphology, Natural History and Treatment.* New York: Wiley, 1973. P. 473.
55. Cassidy, M. J. D., Gaskin, G., Savill, J., et al. Towards a more rapid diagnosis of rapidly progressive glomerulonephritis. *Br. Med. J.* 301: 329, 1990.
56. Cattell, V., and Arlidge, S. The origin of proliferating cells in glomeruli and Bowman's capsule in nephrotoxic serum nephritis: Effect of unilateral renal irradiation. *Br. J. Exp. Pathol.* 62: 669, 1981.
57. Chirawong, P., Nanra, R. S., and Kincaid-Smith, P. Fibrin degradation products and the role of coagulation in "persistent" glomerulonephritis. *Ann. Intern. Med.* 74: 853, 1971.
58. Churg, J., Morita, T., and Suzuki, Y. Glomerulonephritis with Fibrin and Crescent Formation. In P. Kincaid-Smith, T. H. Matthew, and E. L. Becker (eds.), *Glomerulonephritis: Morphology, Natural History and Treatment.* New York: Wiley, 1973. P. 677.
59. Clarke, B. E., Ham, K. N., Tange, J. D., et al. Macrophages and glomerular crescent formation. Studies with rat nephrotoxic nephritis. *Pathology* 15: 75, 1983.
60. Clarke, B. E., Ham, K. N., Tange, J. D., et al. Origin of glomerular crescents in rabbit nephrotoxic nephritis. *J. Pathol.* 139: 247, 1983.
61. Cohen, R. D., Conn, D. L., and Ilstrup, D. M. Clinical features, prognosis, and response to treatment in polyarteritis. *Mayo Clin. Proc.* 55: 146, 1980.
62. Cohen Tervaert, J. W., Goldschmeding, R., Elema, J. D., et al. Autoantibodies against myeloid lysosomal enzymes in crescentic glomerulonephritis. *Kidney Int.* 37(2): 799, 1990.
63. Cole, B. R., Blocklebank, J. T., Kinestra, R. A., et al. "Pulse" methylprednisolone therapy in the treatment of severe glomerulonephritis. *J. Pediatr.* 88: 307, 1976.
64. Cole, E. Plasma exchange in rapidly progressive glomerulonephritis. *Apheresis* 1:257, 1990.
65. Couser, W. Goodpasture's syndrome: A response to nitrogen mustard. *Am. J. Med. Sci.* 268: 175, 1975.
66. Couser, W. G. Rapidly progressive glomerulonephritis: Classification, pathogenetic mechanisms and therapy. *Am. J. Kidney Dis.* 11: 449, 1988.
67. Cunningham, R. J., III, Gilfoil, M., Cavallo, T., et al. Rapidly progressive glomerulonephritis in children: A report of thirteen cases and a review of the literature. *Pediatr. Res.* 14: 128, 1980.
68. D'Amico, G. Role of interstitial infiltration of leukocytes in glomerular diseases. *Nephrol. Dial. Transplant.* 3(5): 596, 1988.
69. Dash, S. C., Malhotra, K. K., Sharma, R. K., et al. Spectrum of rapidly progressive (crescentic) glomerulonephritis in Northern India. *Nephron* 30: 45, 1982.
70. Davies, D. J., Moran, J. E., Niall, J. F., et al. Segmental necrotizing glomerulonephritis with antineutrophil antibody: Possible arbovirus aetiology? *Br. Med. J.* 285: 606, 1982.
71. Davson, J., and Platt, R. A clinical and pathological study of renal disease: I. Nephritis. *Q. J. Med.* 18: 149, 1949.
72. Dayer, J. M., and Demcsuk, S. Cytokines and other mediators in rheumatoid arthritis. *Springer Semin. Immunopathol.* 7: 387, 1984.
73. Dixon, F. J., McPhaul, J. J., Jr., and Lerner, R. S. The contribution of kidney transplantation to the study of glomerulonephritis: The recurrence of glomerulonephritis in renal transplants. *Transplant. Proc.* 1: 194, 1969.
74. Dotremont, G., Vermylen, J., Donati, M. B., et al. Urinary Excretion of Fibrinogen-Fibrin Related Antigen in Glomerulonephritis. In P. Kincaid-Smith, T. H. Matthew, and E. L. Becker (eds.), *Glomerulonephritis: Morphology, Natural History, and Treatment.* New York: Wiley, 1973. P. 829.
75. Ellis, A. Natural history of Bright's disease: Clinical, histological and experimental observations. *Lancet* 1:1, 1942.
76. Esnouf, M. P., and Tunnah, G. W. The isolation and properties of the thrombin-like activity from *Ancistrodon rhodostoma* venom. *Br. J. Haematol.* 13: 581, 1967.
77. Falk, R. J., and Jennette, J. C. Anti-neutrophil cytoplasmic autoantibodies with specificity for myeloperoxidase in patients with systemic vasculitis and idiopathic necrotizing and crescentic glomerulonephritis. *Clin. Nephrol.* 29: 1, 1988.
78. Farquhar, M. G., Vernier, R. L., and Good, R. A. An electron microscope study of the glomerulus in nephrosis, glomerulonephritis and lupus erythematosus. *J. Exp. Med.* 106: 649, 1957.
79. Ferraris, J. R., Gallo, G. E., Ramirez, J., et al. "Pulse" methylprednisolone therapy in the treatment of acute crescentic glomerulonephritis. *Nephron* 34: 207, 1983.
80. Fillit, H. M., and Zabriskie, J. B. Cellular immunity in glomerulonephritis. *Am. J. Pathol.* 109: 227, 1982.
81. Forland, M., Jones, R. E., Easterling, R. E., et al. Clinical and renal biopsy observations in oliguric glomerulonephritis. *J. Chronic Dis.* 19: 163, 1966.
82. Gartner, H. V., Wehner, H., and Bohle, A. The immunohistological findings in various forms of glomerulonephritis: A comparative investigation based on 335 renal biopsies. Part II: Minimal proliferating intercapillary glomerulonephritis (with nephrotic syndrome), focal sclerosing, epi-extraperimembranous, membranoproliferative and extracapillary (rapidly progressive) glomerulonephritis. *Pathol. Res. Pract.* 162: 198, 1978.
83. George, C. R. P., Clark, W. F., and Cameron, J. S. The Role of Platelets in Glomerulonephritis. In J. Hamburger, J. Crosnier, and M. H. Maxwell (eds.), *Advances in Nephrology.* Chicago: Year Book, 1975. P. 19.

84. Glasgow, E. F., Hancock, W. W., and Atkins, R. C. The Technique of Glomerular Culture. In D. Allen and J. P. Dowling (eds.), *Techniques of Nephropathology*. Fla.: C. R. C. Press, 1981. P. 87.
85. Glassock, R. J. A clinical and immunopathological dissection of rapidly progressive glomerulonephritis. *Nephron* 22: 253, 1978.
86. Glockner, W., Sieberth, H., Wichmann, H., et al. Plasma exchange and immunosuppression in rapidly progressive glomerulonephritis: A controlled, multicentre study. *Clin. Nephrol.* 29: 1, 1988.
87. Graham, A. R., Payne, C. M., and Nagle, R. B. A quantitative light and electron-microscopic study of Type IV nuclear bodies in crescentic glomerulonephritis. *Am. J. Pathol.* 102: 359, 1981.
88. Gross, W. L., Landemann, G., Kiefer, G., et al. Anticytoplasmic antibodies in Wegener's granulomatosis. *Lancet* 1: 806, 1986.
89. Guettier, C., Nochy, D., Jacquot, C., et al. Immunohistochemical demonstration of parietal epithelial cells and macrophages in human proliferative extracapillary lesions. *Virchows Arch.* 409(5): 739, 1986.
90. Habib, R. Classification anatomique des nephropathies glomerularies. *Paediatr. Fort.* 28: 81, 1970.
91. Habib, R., Kleinknecht, C., Gubler, M. C., et al. Idiopathic membranoproliferative glomerulonephritis in children: Report of 105 cases. *Clin. Nephrol.* 1: 194, 1973.
92. Habib, R., and Levy, M. Contribution of immunofluorescent microscopy to classification of glomerular diseases. In P. Kincaid-Smith, A. J. F. d'Apice, and R. C. Atkins (eds.), *Progress in Glomerulonephritis*. New York: Wiley, 1979. P. 119.
93. Halgrimson, C. G., Wilson, C. B., Dixon, F. J., et al. Goodpasture's syndrome: Treatment with nephrectomy and transplantation. *Arch. Surg.* 103: 283, 1970.
94. Hall, J. B., Wadham, B. M., Wood, C. J., et al. Vasculitis and glomerulonephritis: A subgroup with an antineutrophil cytoplasmic antibody. *Aust. N.Z. J. Med.* 14: 277, 1984.
95. Halpern, B., Millez, P., Lagrue, G., et al. Protective action of heparin in experimental immune nephritis. *Nature* 105: 257, 1965.
96. Hamburger, J. Les Glomerulo-nephrites Malignes. In *Entretiens de Bichat*, Vol. 1. Paris: Expansion, 1956.
97. Hancock, W. W., and Atkins, R. C. Monoclonal antibodies to human glomerular cells: A marker for glomerular epithelial cells. *Nephron* 33: 83, 1983.
98. Hancock, W. W., and Atkins, R. C. Cellular composition of crescents in human rapidly progressive glomerulonephritis identified using monoclonal antibodies. *Am. J. Nephrol.* 3: 177, 1984.
99. Hancock, W. W., and Atkins, R. C. Application of Coagulation Pathways and Fibrin Deposition in Human Glomerulonephritis. In R. Cotran (ed.), *Seminars in Nephrology* 5: 69, 1985.
100. Hancock, W. W., Becker, G. J., and Atkins, R. C. A comparison of fixatives and immunohistochemical techniques for use with monoclonal antibodies to cell surface antigens. *Am. J. Clin. Pathol.* 78: 825, 1982.
101. Hancock, W. W., Jackson, A. E., Hooke, D. H., et al. Monoclonal Antibodies to Human Renal Antigens. In G. J. Becker, R. C. Atkins, and P. Kincaid-Smith (eds.), *Proceedings of the Second Asian Pacific Congress of Nephrology*. Melbourne: Dominion Press, 1984. P. 115.
102. Hancock, W. W., Kraft, N., Clarke, F., et al. Production of monoclonal antibodies to fibronectin, type IV collagen and other antigens of the human glomerulus. *Pathology* 16: 197, 1984.
103. Hancock, W. W., Zola, H., and Atkins, R. C. Antigenic heterogeneity of human mononuclear phagocytes—Immunohistological analysis using monoclonal antibodies. *Blood* 62: 1271, 1983.
104. Harmer, D., Finn, R., Goldsmith, H. J., et al. Plasmapheresis in fulminating crescentic nephritis. *Lancet* 1: 679, 1979.
105. Harris, J. P., Rakowski, T. A., Argy, W. P., Jr., et al. Alport's syndrome presenting as crescentic glomerulonephritis: A report of two siblings. *Clin. Nephrol.* 10: 245, 1978.
106. Harrison, C. V., Loughridge, L. W., and Milne, M. D. Acute oliguric renal failure in acute glomerulo-nephritis and polyarteritis nodosa. *Q. J. Med.* 33: 39, 1964.
107. Hawkins, N. J., Wakefield, D., and Charlesworth, J. A. The role of mesangial cells in glomerular pathology. *Pathology* 22: 24, 1990.
108. Heaf, J., Jorgenson, F., and Nielsen, L. Treatment and prognosis of extracapillary glomerulonephritis. *Nephron* 35: 217, 1983.
109. Heilman, R. L., Offord, K. P., Holley, K. E., and Velosa, J. A. Analysis of risk factors for patients and renal survival in crescentic glomerulonephritis. *Am. J. Kidney Dis.* 9(2): 98, 1987.
110. Heptinstall, R. H. *Pathology of the Kidney*, 3rd ed. Boston: Little, Brown, 1983. P. 443.
111. Herdman, R., Edson, J., Pickering, R., et al. Anticoagulants in renal disease in children. *Am. J. Dis. Child.* 119: 27, 1970.
112. Hind, C. R. K., Lockwood, C. M., Peters, D. K., et al. Prognosis after immunosuppression of patients with crescentic nephritis requiring dialysis. *Lancet* 1: 263, 1983.
113. Holdsworth, S. R., Allen, D., Thomson, N. M., et al. Histochemistry of glomerular cells in animal models of crescentic glomerulonephritis. *Pathology* 12: 339, 1980.
114. Holdsworth, S. R., and Bellomo, R. Differential effects of steroids on leukocyte-mediated glomerulonephritis. *Kidney Int.* 26: 162, 1984.
115. Holdsworth, S. R., Boyce, N., Thomson, N. M., et al. The clinical spectrum of acute glomerulonephritis and lung haemorrhage (Goodpasture's syndrome). *Q. J. Med.* 216: 75, 1985.
116. Holdsworth, S. R., Thomson, N. M., Glasgow, E. F., et al. The effect of defibrination on macrophage participation in rabbit nephrotoxic nephritis: Studies using glomerular culture and electron microscopy. *Clin. Exp. Immunol.* 37: 38, 1979.
117. Holdsworth, S. R., Wischusen, N. J., and Dowling, J. P. A radioimmunoassay for the detection of circulating anti-GBM antibodies. *Aust. N.Z. J. Med.* 13: 15, 1983.
118. Hooke, D. H., Gee, D. C., and Atkins, R. C. Leukocyte analysis using monoclonal antibodies in human glomerulonephritis. *Kidney Int.* 31: 964, 1987.
119. Hooke, D. H., Hancock, W. W., Gee, D. C., et al. Monoclonal antibody analysis of glomerular hypercellularity in human glomerulonephritis. *Clin. Nephrol.* 22: 163, 1984.
120. Hopper, J., Biava, C., and Naughton, C. Glomerular extracapillary proliferation (crescentic glomerulonephritis) associated with non-renal malignancies. *Kidney Int.* 10: 554, 1976.
121. Hoyer, J. R., Michael, A. F., and Hoyer, L. W. Immunofluorescent localization of antihemophilic factor anti-

gen and fibrinogen in human renal diseases. *J. Clin. Invest.* 53: 1375, 1974.

122. Ihle, B. U., d'Apice, A. J. F., Dowling, J., et al. De Novo crescentic glomerulonephritis in a renal transplant. *Transplant. Proc.* XV: 2147, 1983.
123. Jayne, D. R. W., Marshall, P. D., Jones, S. J., et al. Autoantibodies to GBM and neutrophil cytoplasm in rapidly progressive glomerulonephritis. *Kidney Int.* 37: 965, 1990.
124. Jennette, J. C., and Hipp, C. G. The epithelial antigen phenotype of glomerular crescent cells. *Am. J. Clin. Pathol.* 86: 274, 1986.
125. Jennette, J. C., and Falk, R. J. Diagnosis and management of glomerulonephritis and vasculitis presenting as acute renal failure. *Med. Clin. North Am.* 74(4): 893, 1990.
126. Jennette, J. C., and Falk, R. J. Anti-neutrophil cytoplasmic autoantibodies and associated diseases: A review. *Am. J. Kidney Dis.* 15(6): 517, 1990.
127. Jennette, J. C., Wilkman, A. S., and Falk, R. J. Anti-neutrophil cytoplasmic autoantibody-associated glomerulonephritis and vasculitis. *Am. J. Pathol.* 135: 921, 1989.
128. Johnson, J. P., Moore, L., Austin, H. A., et al. Therapy of antiglomerular basement membrane antibody disease: Analysis of prognostic significance of clinical pathologic and treatment factors. *Medicine* 64: 219, 1985.
129. Kalowski, S., McKay, D. G., Howes, E. L., Jr., et al. Multinucleated giant cells in antiglomerular basement membrane antibody-induced glomerulonephritis. *Nephron* 16: 415, 1976.
130. Katmitsuji, H., Tani, K., and Taniguchi, A. Urinary fibrin-fibrinogen degradation products and intraglomerular fibrin-fibrinogen deposition in various renal diseases. *Thromb. Res.* 21: 285, 1981.
131. Kincaid-Smith, P., and d'Apice, A. J. F. Plasmapheresis in rapidly progressive glomerulonephritis. *Am. J. Med.* 65: 564, 1978.
132. Kincaid-Smith, P., Saker, B., and Fairley, K. Anticoagulants in "irreversible" acute renal failure. *Lancet* II: 1360, 1968.
133. Klassen, J., Elwood, C., Grossberg, A. L., et al. Evolution of membranous nephropathy into anti-glomerular-basement-membrane glomerulonephritis. *N. Engl. J. Med.* 290: 1340, 1974.
134. Kleinerman, J. Effects of heparin on experimental nephritis in rabbits. *Lab. Invest.* 3: 495, 1980.
135. Kobayashi, Y., Shigematsu, H., Masaki, Y., et al. *Virchows Arch.* [*Cell. Pathol.*] 35: 45, 1980.
136. Koelz, A., Morley, A., Uldall, P., et al. A controlled trial of Cyclophosphamide in the treatment of proliferative glomerulonephritis. *Proc. Eur. Dial. Transplant Assoc.* 11: 491, 1975.
137. Kohler, G., and Milstein, C. Continuous cultures of fused cells secreting antibody of predefined specificity. *Nature* 256: 495, 1975.
138. Kondo, Y., Shigematsu, H., and Kobayashi, Y. Cellular aspects of rabbit Masugi nephritis. II. Progressive glomerular injuries with crescent formation. *Lab. Invest.* 27: 620, 1972.
139. Lan, H. Y., Paterson, D. J., and Atkins, R. C. Evolving pattern of the interstitial leukocyte infiltrate in experimental anti-GBM glomerulonephritis (abstract). *Kidney Int.* 36: 1176, 1989.
140. Lang, C. H., Brown, D. C., Staley, N., et al. Goodpasture syndrome treated with immunosuppression and plasma exchange. *Arch. Intern. Med.* 137: 1076, 1977.
141. Langhans, T. Uber die veranderungen der glomeruli bei der nephritis nebst einigen Bemerkungen uber die Entshehung der Fibrinzylinder. *Arch. Pathol. Physiol. Klin. Med.* 76: 85, 1879.
142. Lawrence, J. R. Glomerulonephritis with Fibrin and Crescent Formation. In P. Kincaid-Smith, T. H. Matthew, and E. L. Becker (eds.), *Glomerulonephritis: Morphology, Natural History and Treatment*. New York: Wiley, 1973. P. 739.
143. Leibovich, S. J., and Ross, R. A macrophage dependent factor that stimulates the proliferation of fibroblasts in vitro. *Am. J. Pathol.* 84: 501, 1976.
144. Leonard, C. D., Nagle, R. B., Striker, G. E., et al. Acute glomerulonephritis with prolonged oliguria. An analysis of 29 cases. *Ann. Intern. Med.* 73: 703, 1970.
145. Levy, M., Beaufils, H., Gubler, M. C., et al. Idiopathic recurrent macroscopic hematuria and mesangial IgA-IgG deposits in children (Berger's disease). *Clin. Nephrol.* 1: 63, 1973.
146. Lewis, E. J., Busch, G. J., and Schur, P. H. Gamma G globulin subgroup composition of the glomerular deposits in human renal diseases. *J. Clin. Invest.* 49: 1103, 1970.
147. Lewis, E. J., Cavallo, T., Harrington, J. T., et al. An immunopathologic study of rapidly progressive glomerulonephritis in the adult. *Hum. Pathol.* 2: 185, 1971.
148. Li, H. L., Hancock, W. W., Dowling, J. P., and Atkins, R. C. Activated (IL-2R$^+$) Intraglomerular mononuclear cells are associated with decreased renal function in patients with crescentic glomerulonephritis. *Kidney Int.* 39: 793, 1991.
149. Li, H. L., Hancock, W. W., Hooke, D. H., et al. Mononuclear cell activation and decreased renal function in IgA nephropathy with crescents. *Kidney Int.* 37: 1552, 1990.
150. Lockwood, C. M., Bakes, D., Jones, S., et al. Association of alkaline phosphatase with an autoantigen recognized by circulating anti-neutrophil antibodies in systemic vasculitis. *Lancet* 1: 716, 1987.
151. Lockwood, C. M., Boulton-Jones, J. M., Lowenthal, R. M., et al. Recovery from Goodpasture's syndrome after immunosuppressive treatment and plasmapheresis. *Br. Med. J.* 2: 252, 1975.
152. Lockwood, C., Rees, A., Pinching, A., et al. Plasma exchange and immunosuppression in the treatment of fulminating immune complexes crescentic glomerulonephritis. *Lancet* 1: 63, 1977.
153. Lohlein, M. Uber Nephritis nach dem heutigen Stande der pathologischanatomischen forschung. *Ergeb. Inn. Med. Kinderheilkd.* 5: 411, 1910.
154. Macanovic, M., Evans, D. J., and Peters, D. K. Allergic response to glomerular basement membrane in patients with glomerulonephritis. *Lancet* 2: 207, 1972.
155. MacKay, K., Striker, B. J., Elliot, S., et al. Glomerular epithelial, mesangial and endothelial cell lines from transgenic mice. *Kidney Int.* 33: 677, 1988.
156. Magil, A. B., and Wadsworth, L. D. Monocyte involvement in glomerular crescents: A histochemical and ultrastructural study. *Lab. Invest.* 47: 160, 1982.
157. Mahieu, P., Lambert, P. H., and Miescher, P. A. Detection of anti-glomerular basement membrane antibodies by a radioimmunological technique: Clinical application in human nephropathies. *J. Clin. Invest.* 54: 128, 1974.
158. Markovic-Lipkovski, J., Muller, C. A., Risler, T., et al. Association of glomerular and interstitial mononuclear leukocytes with different forms of glomerulonephritis. *Nephrol. Dial. Transplant.* 5: 10, 1990.
159. Masugi, M. Uber die experimentalle glomerulonephritis durch das spezifische antinieren serum. Ein beitrag

zur pathogenese der diffusen glomerulonephritis. *Beitr. Path. Anat.* 92: 429, 1934.

160. Matthew, T. H., and Kincaid-Smith, P. Severe Fibrin and Crescent Glomerulonephritis. In P. Kincaid-Smith, T. H. Matthew, and E. L. Becker (eds.), *Glomerulonephritis: Morphology, Natural History and Treatment.* New York: Wiley, 1973. P. 727.
161. McCluskey, R. T., and Bhan, A. K. Cell-mediated mechanisms in renal diseases. *Kidney Int.* 21 (Suppl. 11): S6, 1982.
162. McCluskey, R. T., and Bhan, A. K. Cell mediated immunity in renal disease. *Hum. Pathol.* 17: 146, 1986.
163. McCoy, R. C., Clapp, J., and Seigler, H. F. Membranoproliferative glomerulonephritis: Progression from the pure form to the crescentic form with recurrence after transplantation. *Am. J. Med.* 59: 288, 1975.
164. McIntosh, R. M., Griswold, W. R., Chernack, W. B., et al. Cryoglobulins. III. Further studies on the nature, incidence, clinical, diagnostic, prognostic and immunopathologic significance of cryoproteins in renal disease. *Q. J. Med.* 44: 285, 1975.
165. McLeish, K. R., Yum, M. N., and Luft, F. C. Rapidly progressive glomerulonephritis in adults: Clinical and histologic correlations. *Clin. Nephrol.* 10: 43, 1978.
166. Mene, P., Simonson, M. S., and Dunn, M. J. Physiology of the mesangial cell. *Physiol. Rev.* 69: 1347, 1989.
167. Min, K. W., Gyorkey, F., Gyorkey, P., et al. The morphogenesis of glomerular crescents in rapidly progressive glomerulonephritis. *Kidney Int.* 5: 47, 1974.
168. Moorthy, A. V., Zimmerman, S. W., Burkholder, P. M., et al. Association of crescentic glomerulonephritis with membranous glomerulonephropathy: A report of 3 cases. *Clin. Nephrol.* 6: 319, 1976.
169. Morita, T., Suzuki, Y., and Churg, J. Structure and development of the glomerular crescent. *Am. J. Pathol.* 72: 349, 1973.
170. Morrin, P. A. F., Hinglais, N., Nabarra, B., et al. Rapidly progressive glomerulonephritis: A clinical and pathologic study. *Am. J. Med.* 65: 446, 1978.
171. Muller, G. A., and Muller, C. Characterisation of renal antigens on distinct part of the human nephron by monoclonal antibodies. *Klin. Wochenschr.* 61: 893, 1983.
172. Muller, G. A., Muller, C. A., Markovic-Lipkovski, J., et al. Renal major histocompatability complex antigens and cellular components in rapidly progressive glomerulonephritis identified by monoclonal antibodies (with 1 colour plate). *Nephron* 49: 132, 1988.
173. Muller, G. A., Seipel, L., and Risler, T. Treatment of non-anti-GBM antibody mediated rapidly progressive glomerulonephritis by plasmapheresis and immunosuppression. *Klin. Wochenschr.* 64: 231, 1986.
174. Nagai, T., Tamura, T., and Kawai, C. Immunohistologic findings in the glomerular crescents in various renal diseases. *Jpn. Circ. J.* 43: 83, 1979.
175. Naish, P., Penn, G. B., Evans, D. J., et al. The effect of defibrination of nephrotoxic serum nephritis in rabbits. *Clin. Sci.* 42: 643, 1972.
176. Naish, P. F., Thomson, N. M., Simpson, I. J., et al. The role of polymorphonuclear leucocytes in the autologous phase of nephrotoxic nephritis. *Clin. Exp. Immunol.* 22: 102, 1975.
177. Nakamoto, S., Dunea, G., Kolff, W. J., et al. Treatment of oliguric glomerulonephritis with dialysis and steroids. *Ann. Intern. Med.* 63: 359, 1965.
178. Nakamoto, Y., Dohi, K., Fujioka, M., et al. Combined anticoagulant and immunosuppressive treatment in rapidly progressive glomerulonephritis: A long term follow-up study. *Jpn. J. Med.* 18: 210, 1979.
179. Nassberger, L., Sjoholm, A. G., Bygren, P., et al. Circulating anti-neutrophil cytoplasm antibodies in patients with rapidly progressive glomerulonephritis and extracapillary proliferation. *J. Intern. Med.* 225: 191, 1989.
180. Neale, T. J., Tipping, P. G., Carson, S. D., et al. Participation of cell-mediated immunity in deposition of fibrin in glomerulonephritis. *Lancet* II: 421, 1988.
181. Neild, G. H., Cameron, J. S., Lessof, M. H., et al. Relapsing polychondritis with crescentic glomerulonephritis. *Br. Med. J.* 1: 743, 1978.
182. Neild, G. H., Cameron, J. S., Ogg, C. S., et al. Rapidly progressive glomerulonephritis with extensive glomerular crescent formation. *Q. J. Med.* 207: 395, 1983.
183. Nicholson, G. D., Amin, U. F., and Alleyne, G. A. O. Membranous glomerulonephropathy with crescents. *Clin. Nephrol.* 5: 198, 1975.
184. Nolasco, F. E. B., Cameron, J. S., Hattley, B., et al. Intraglomerular T cells and monocytes in nephritis: Study with monoclonal antibodies. *Kidney Int.* 31: 1160, 1987.
185. Olsen, S. Extracapillary glomerulonephritis: A semiquantitative light microscopical study of 59 patients. *Acta Pathol. Microbiol. Scand.* [*A*] (Suppl. 249)82: 7, 1974.
186. O'Neill, W. M., Jr., Etheridge, W. B., and Bloomer, H. A. High-dose corticosteroids: Their use in treating idiopathic rapidly progressive glomerulonephritis. *Arch. Intern. Med.* 139: 514, 1979.
187. Oredugba, O., Mazumdar, D. C., Meyer, J., et al. Pulse methylprednisolone therapy in idiopathic, rapidly progressive glomerulonephritis. *Ann. Intern. Med.* 92: 504, 1980.
188. Otie, T., Shimuzu, F., Kagami, S., et al. Hapten-specific cellular immune response producing glomerular injury. *Clin. Exp. Immunol.* 76(3): 463, 1989.
189. Parbtani, A., and Cameron, J. S. Platelet and plasma serotonin concentrations in glomerulonephritis. II. *Thromb. Res.* 15: 109, 1979.
190. Pettersson, E. E., and Colvin, R. B. Cold-insoluble globulin (fibronectin, LETS protein) in normal and diseased human glomeruli: Papain-sensitive attachment to normal glomeruli and deposition in crescents. *Clin. Immunol. Immunopathol.* 11: 425, 1978.
191. Petzel, R. A., Brown, D. C., Staley, N. A., et al. Crescentic glomerulonephritis and renal failure associated with malignant lymphoma. *Am. J. Clin. Pathol.* 71: 728, 1979.
192. Pirofsky, B., and Bardana, E. J., Jr. Immunosuppressive therapy in rheumatic disease. *Med. Clin. North Am.* 61: 419, 1977.
193. Pollack, V. E., Glueck, H. I., Weiss, M. A., et al. Defibrination with ancrod in glomerulonephritis: Effect on clinical and histologic findings and on blood coagulation. *Am. J. Nephrol.* 2: 195, 1982.
194. Pollack, V. E., and Mendosa, N. Rapidly progressive glomerulonephritis. *Med. Clin. North Am.* 55: 1397, 1971.
195. Proesmans, W. Proliferative glomerulonephritis with crescents. *Proceedings of the 2nd International Symposium of Paediatric Nephrology, Paris.* 1971. P. 91.
196. Pusey, C. D., and Lockwood, C. M. Autoimmunity in rapidly progressive glomerulonephritis. *Kidney Int.* 35: 929, 1989.
197. Raychowdhury, R., Hiles, J. L., McCluskey, R. T., et al. Autoimmune target in Heymann nephritis is a glycoprotein with homology to the LDL receptor. *Science* 244: 1163, 1989.

198. Rees, A. J., Peters, D. K., Amos, N., et al. The influence of HLA-linked genes on the severity of anti-GBM antibody mediated nephritis. *Kidney Int.* 26: 444, 1984.
199. Rennke, H. G., Klein, P. S., and Mendrick, D. L. Cell-mediated immunity (CMI) in hapten-induced interstitial nephritis and glomerular crescent formation in the rat (abstract). *Kidney Int.* 37: 428, 1990.
200. Rifle, G., Chalopin, J. M., Zech, P., et al. Treatment of idiopathic acute crescentic glomerulonephritis by immunodepression and plasma-exchange. *Proc. Eur. Dial. Transplant. Assoc.* 18: 493, 1980.
201. Robson, A., Giangiacomo, J., and Germuth, F. Efficacy of methyl-prednisolone pulses in the treatment of experimental glomerulonephritis. *Kidney Int.* 14: 660, 1978.
202. Rocklin, R., Lewis, E., and David, J. In vitro evidence for cellular hypersensitivity to glomerular-basement-membrane antigens in human glomerulonephritis. *N. Engl. J. Med.* 283: 497, 1970.
203. Rondeau, E., Levy, M., Dosquet, P., et al. Plasma exchange and immunosuppression for rapidly progressive glomerulonephritis: Prognosis and complications. *Nephrol. Dial. Transplant.* 4: 196, 1989.
204. Rosen, S. Crescentic Glomerulonephritis: Occurrence, Mechanisms and Prognosis. In S. C. Sommers (ed.), *Pathology Annual,* Vol. 10. New York: Appleton, Century, Crofts, 1975. P. 37.
205. Rubenstein, W. D., Wall, R. F., Wood, G. S., and Edwards, M. A. Complications of therapeutic apheresis including a fatal case with pulmonary vascular disease. *Am. J. Med.* 75: 171, 1983.
206. Russ, G. R., and d'Apice, A. J. F. Plasma exchange and immunosuppression in crescentic glomerulonephritis. *Proceedings of the 8th International Congress of Nephrology,* 1981. P. 661.
207. Salant, D. J. Immunopathogenesis of crescentic glomerulonephritis and lung purpura. *Kidney Int.* 32: 408, 1987.
208. Savage, C., Pusey, C., Bowman, C., et al. Antiglomerular basement membrane antibody mediated diseases in the British Isles 1980–1984. *Br. Med. J.* 292: 301, 1986.
209. Schiffer, M. S., and Michael, A. F. Renal cell turnover studied by Y chromosomes (Y body) staining of the transplanted human kidney. *J. Lab. Clin. Med.* 92: 841, 1978.
210. Schreiner, G. E., Rakowski, T. A., Argy, W. P., Jr., et al. Natural History of Oliguric Glomerulonephritis. In P. Kincaid-Smith, T. H. Matthew, and E. L. Becker (eds.), *Glomerulonephritis: Morphology, Natural History, and Treatment.* New York: Wiley, 1973. P. 711.
211. Scott, D. G. I., Bacon, P. A., Elliott, P. J., et al. Systemic vasculitis in a district general hospital, 1972–1980. Clinical and laboratory features, classification and prognosis of 80 cases. *Q. J. Med.* 51: 292, 1982.
212. Segastothy, M., Kong, C. T., Morad, Z., and Suleiman, A. B. Rapidly progressive glomerulonephritis: Treatment with combined immunosuppression and anticoagulation with Arvin. *Singapore Med. J.* 27: 422, 1986.
213. Silva, F. G., Hoyer, J. R., and Pirani, C. L. Sequential studies of glomerular crescent formation in rats with anti-GBM induced glomerulonephritis and the role of coagulation factors. *Lab. Invest.* 51: 404, 1984.
214. Sonsino, E., Nabarra, B., Kazatchkine, M., et al. Extracapillary Proliferative Glomerulonephritis, So-Called Malignant Glomerulonephritis. In J. Hamburger, J. Crosnier, and M. H. Maxwell (eds.), *Advances in Nephrology.* Chicago: Year Book, 1972. P. 121.
215. Southwest Pediatric Nephrology Study Group. A clinpathologic study of crescentic glomerulonephritis in 50 children. *Kidney Int.* 27: 450, 1985.
216. Spargo, B. H., Seymoor, A. E., and Ordonez, N. G. (eds.). *Renal Biopsy Pathology with Diagnostic and Therapeutic Implications.* New York: Wiley, 1980. P. 177.
217. Stachura, I., Si, L., and Whiteside, T. L. Mononuclear-cell subsets in human idiopathic crescentic glomerulonephritis (ICGN): Analysis in tissue sections with monoclonal antibodies. *J. Clin. Immunol.* 4: 202, 1984.
218. Stachura, I., Whiteside, T., and Kelley, R. Circulating and deposited immune complexes in patient with glomerular disease. Immunopathologic correlations. *Am. J. Pathol.* 103: 21, 1981.
219. Steblay, R. W. Glomerulonephritis induced in sheep by injections of heterologous glomerular basement membrane and Freund's complete adjuvant. *J. Exp. Med.* 116: 253, 1962.
220. Stevens, M. E., McConnell, M., and Bone, J. M. Aggressive treatment with pulse methylprednisolone or plasma exchange is justified in rapidly progressive glomerulonephritis. *Proc. Eur. Dial. Transplant. Assoc.* 19: 724, 1982.
221. Stichm, E. R., Kuplic, L. S., and Uehling, D. T. Urinary fibrin split products in human renal disease. *J. Lab. Clin. Med.* 77: 843, 1971.
222. Stilmant, M. M., Bolton, W. K., Sturgill, B. C., et al. Crescentic glomerulonephritis without immune deposits. Clinicopathologic features. *Kidney Int.* 15: 184, 1979.
223. Striker, G. E., and Atkins, R. C. Monoclonal Antibodies as Probes of Normal and Abnormal Renal Structure. In R. R. Robinson (ed.), *Proceedings of the IXth International Society of Nephrology.* New York: Springer-Verlag, 1984. P. 575.
224. Striker, G. E., Cutler, R. E., Huang, T. W., et al. Renal Failure, Glomerulonephritis and Glomerular Epithelial Cell Hyperplasia. In P. Kincaid-Smith, T. H. Matthew, and E. L. Becker (eds.), *Glomerulonephritis: Morphology, Natural History, and Treatment.* New York: Wiley, 1973. P. 657.
225. Suc, J. M., Durand, D., Conte, J., et al. The use of heparin in the treatment of idiopathic rapidly progressive glomerulonephritis. *Clin. Nephrol.* 5: 9, 1976.
226. Swainson, C. P., Winney, R. J., Urbaniak, S. J., et al. Plasma exchange in severe glomerulonephritis—Who benefits? *Proc. Eur. Dial. Transplant. Assoc.* 19: 732, 1982.
227. Thomson, N. M., Holdsworth, S. R., Glasgow, E. F., et al. The macrophage in the development of experimental crescentic glomerulonephritis: Studies using tissue culture electron microscopy. *Am. J. Pathol.* 94: 223, 1979.
228. Thomson, N. M., Moran, J., Simpson, I. J., et al. Defibrination with Ancrod in nephrotoxic nephritis in rabbits. *Kidney Int.* 10: 343, 1976.
229. Thomson, N. M., Simpson, I. J., Evans, D. J., et al. Defibrination with Ancrod in experimental chronic immune complex nephritis. *Clin. Exp. Immunol.* 20: 527, 1975.
230. Thomson, N. M., Simpson, I. J., and Peters, D. K. A quantitative evaluation of anticoagulants in experimental nephrotoxic nephritis. *Clin. Exp. Immunol.* 19: 301, 1975.
231. Tietjen, D. P., and Moore, W. J. Treatment of rapidly progressive glomerulonephritis due to Behcet's syndrome with intravenous cyclophosphamide. *Nephron* 55: 69, 1990.
232. Tipping, P., and Holdsworth, S. R. The mechanism of action of corticosteroids on glomerular injury in acute serum sickness. *Clin. Exp. Immunol.* 59: 555, 1985.

233. Tipping, P. G., Lowe, M. G., and Holdsworth, S. R. Glomerular macrophages express augmented procoagulant activity in experimental fibrin-related glomerulonephritis in rabbits. *J. Clin. Invest.* 82(4): 1253, 1988.
234. Tipping, P. G., Neale, T. J., and Holdsworth, S. R. T lymphocyte participation in antibody-induced experimental glomerulo-nephritis. *Kidney Int.* 27: 530, 1985.
235. van der Woude, F. J., Basmussen, N., Lobatto, S., et al. Autoantibodies against neutrophils and monocytes: Tool for diagnosis and marker of disease activity in Wegener's granulomatosis. *Lancet* 1: 425, 1985.
236. Vassalli, P., and McCluskey, R. T. The pathogenic role of the coagulation process in rabbit Masugi nephritis. *Am. J. Pathol.* 45: 653, 1964.
237. Volhard, F., and Fahr, T. *Die Brightsche nierenkrankheit.* Berlin: Springer, 1914. P. 115.
238. Walker, R. G., d'Apice, A. J. F., Kincaid-Smith, P., et al. Plasmapheresis in Goodpasture's syndrome with renal failure. *Med. J. Aust.* 1: 875, 1977.
239. Walters, M. D. S., Savage, C. O. S., Dillon, M. J., et al. Antineutrophil cytoplasm antibody in crescentic glomerulonephritis. *Arch. Dis. Child.* 63: 814, 1988.
240. Warren, S. E., Mitas, J. A., Golbus, S. M., et al. Recovery from rapidly progressive glomerulonephritis: Improvement of the plasmapheresis and immunosuppression. *Arch. Intern. Med.* 141: 175, 1981.
241. Weber, M., Pullig, O., and Kohler, H. Distribution of Goodpasture antigens within various human basement membranes. *Nephrol. Dial. Transplant.* 5: 87, 1990.
242. Whitworth, J. A., Morel-Maroger, L., Mignon, F., et al. The significance of extracapillary proliferation: Clinicopathological review of 60 patients. *Nephron* 16: 1, 1976.
243. Wilson, C. B., and Dixon, F. J. Antiglomerular basement membrane antibody-induced glomerulonephritis. *Kidney Int.* 3: 74, 1973.
244. Wilson, C. B., Marquardt, H., and Dixon, F. J. Radioimmunoassay for circulating antiglomerular basement membrane antibody (Abstract). *Kidney Int.* 6: 114A, 1974.
245. Wilson, C. B., and Smith, R. C. Goodpasture's syndrome associated with influenza A infection. *Ann. Intern. Med.* 76: 91, 1972.
246. Wing, E., Bruns, F., Fraley, D., et al. Infectious complications with plasmapheresis in rapidly progressive glomerulonephritis. *J.A.M.A.* 244: 2423, 1980.
247. Woodroofe, A. J., Border, W. A., Theofilopoulos, A. N., et al. Detection of circulating immune complexes in glomerulonephritis. *Kidney Int.* 12: 268, 1977.
248. Yoshioka, K., Takemura, T., Matsubara, K., et al. Immunohistochemical studies of reflux nephropathy: The role of extracellular matrix membrane attack complex and immune cells in glomerular sclerosis. *Am. J. Pathol.* 129(2): 223, 1987.
249. Zimmerman, S. W., Groehler, K., and Beirne, G. J. Hydrocarbon exposure and chronic glomerulonephritis. *Lancet* 2: 199, 1975.
250. Zoja, C., Corna, D., Macconi, D., et al. Tissue plasminogen activator therapy of rabbit nephrotoxic nephritis. *Lab. Invest.* 62: 34, 1990.

Acute Poststreptococcal Glomerulonephritis

Bernardo Rodríguez-Iturbe

Infections with group A β-hemolytic streptococcus are a well-known cause of acute glomerulonephritis. The clinical presentation of poststreptococcal nephritis is not uniform, but since the acute nephritic syndrome consisting of edema, hypertension, hematuria, and oliguria is the most common and best recognized, the terms *acute glomerulonephritis, poststreptococcal nephritis,* and *acute nephritic syndrome* are sometimes used interchangeably. Nevertheless, in its strictest sense, the term *glomerulonephritis* corresponds to pathologic characteristics that may not always be manifested by the acute nephritic syndrome, and only when the nature of the preceding infections is known, should the nephritis be labeled poststreptococcal.

Historically, the initial observations associating the convalescence of scarlet fever with "dropsy and suppression of the urine" and swelling were made during the epidemics in Florence in 1717. The first detailed reports of this complication were published in the late eighteenth century, when separate monographs by Borsieri and von Plenciz emphasized the latent period that followed infection, the noninflammatory nature of the edema, and the dark and scanty urine [18]. In 1812, Wells [172] published the classic paper he had delivered 6 years earlier to the Society for the Improvement of Medical and Chirurgical Knowledge, in which he defined time limits of the latent period, gave detailed accounts of the characteristics of the edema, presented evidence that the urine contained both "the red matter" as well as "the serum" of the blood, and emphasized that this complication occurred more frequently in siblings of index cases than in the general population. In 1836, the landmark paper of Richard Bright [17] on glomerulonephritis was published, and in 1905 Reichel [117] emphasized the glomerular changes in fatal cases of postscarlatinal nephritis.

Epidemiology

Poststreptococcal glomerulonephritis (PSGN) is decreasing in the United States, Central Europe, and Great Britain [88] but continues to be a significant cause of morbidity worldwide as indicated by reports from Alaska, Africa, Australia, the Middle East, the Caribbean islands, South America, and New Zealand (reviewed in [121]). In Papua New Guinea, Malaysia, Pakistan, and India, acute endocapillary glomerulonephritis is the most common histologic presentation of primary renal disease, and poststreptococcal etiology is strongly suspected in some of these countries [116].

Children between the ages of 2 and 12 are most commonly affected, but PSGN may occur at any age. In areas where the disease is endemic, 5 percent of the patients are younger than 2 years, and about 10 percent are older than 40 years of age [130]. There is a 2:1 male predominance in the clinical cases of PSGN; however, both sexes are affected with equal frequency when subclinical nephritis is included in the analysis [133].

The preceding infection is usually located in the skin or upper respiratory tract. When impetigo and pharyngitis are present at the same time, the latter usually represents secondary contamination from the skin [4]. Pharyngitis and tonsillitis are common sites of infection in the winter and spring in temperate climates, while in the tropics peak incidence of postpyoderma PSGN is frequently in the summer months [13, 31].

Sporadic cases tend to occur in clusters in rural or urban communities of low socioeconomic status with poor hygienic conditions and crowded homes [110, 130]. Not surprisingly, patients with PSGN have a high incidence of malnutrition, anemia, and intestinal parasitosis [130]. Epidemics occur in "close" communities [119, 179] and reappear at periodic intervals in certain areas such as Trinidad [110], the Red Lake Indian Reservation in Minnesota [3], and Maracaibo in Venezuela [130]. The epidemic and endemic incidence of the disease in different areas of the same city are closely correlated [129]. In Great Britain, isolated outbreaks have resulted from infected skin abrasions in rugby team members [80].

The risk of developing glomerulonephritis after infection with a nephritogenic streptococcus is extremely variable, depending on a variety of factors, including the site of infection. The throat infection with streptococcus M type 49 carries a 5 percent risk of nephritis, while the same infection in the skin carries a risk 5 times larger. Overall, the risk of nephritis after a nephritogenic streptococcal infection has been estimated to be about 15 percent [30].

Etiopathogenesis

The biologic and epidemiologic differences observed between rheumatic fever and acute glomerulonephritis, as well as the time-honored observation that both poststreptococcal diseases rarely coexist in the same patient, led Seegal and Earle [146] and Rammelkamp, Weaver, and Dingle [114] to postulate the existence of nephritogenic streptococcal strains. This notion [155] appears still to be valid because bacteriologic studies in populations where both rheumatic fever and glomerulonephritis are endemic, such as in Kuwait [83, 84] and Chile [9], have shown differences in the M and T types of the isolates in these poststreptococcal complications. Nevertheless, what makes a streptococcus nephritogenic remains undefined.

Group A streptococci of M types 1, 2, 4, 6, 12, 18, 25, 31, 49, 51, 52, 55, 57, 59, 60, and 61 have been isolated from patients with glomerulonephritis, some of them such as M types 4, 12, 49, and 57 during the course of epidemics. Specific M types such as 47, 49, 55, 57, and 60 are associated with impetigo resulting in nephritis [28]. In sporadic cases of poststreptococcal glomerulonephritis, nontypeable strains are common. The relevant nephritogenic fraction in many strains associated with glomerulonephritis remains a matter of controversy.

We shall discuss separately the streptococcal antigens, the existence of autoimmune reactivity, and the participation of humoral as well as cellular immune mechanisms in the pathogenesis of the renal lesion.

STREPTOCOCCAL ANTIGENS

Repeated injections of M protein alone or in association with fibrinogen result in nephritis and localization of injected M protein-fibrinogen complexes in the glomeruli [59, 63]. Furthermore, there is cross-reactivity between M protein and glomerular basement membrane [85]. Nevertheless, it appears unlikely that M protein per se is the relevant antigen in nephritis; the large number of nephritogenic M types contrasts with the notion of a single nephritogen, as suggested by the observation that the disease seems to induce a long-lasting immunity and second attacks of nephritis, if they occur at all, are extremely rare. Further evidence in this regard was obtained by Treser et al. [159], who showed that convalescent sera, presumably containing specific antibody to the putative nephritogenic antigen, binds to free antigenic sites in biopsies obtained early in the course of the disease, and this reactivity was independent of the M type of the initial infection.

Considerable efforts have been devoted to isolate antigenic fractions from nephritogenic streptococci and to show their localization in renal biopsies from patients with nephritis. These efforts were summarized in 1973 by Zabriskie et al. [177]. In many instances, results were inconclusive or difficult to repeat, a fact attributed by Treser et al. [160] to the variable timing of biopsies; early in the course of the disease, free antigenic sites are more likely to be present, while at a later date, such sites are covered with antibody and therefore unavailable for detection probes.

The New York Medical College group [71, 176] isolated an antigen (endostreptosin, water-soluble preabsorbing antigen) that showed affinity for the glomerular basement membrane from pressure-disrupted streptococci of groups A, C, and G [147]. This antigen was identified because it could block the capacity of fluorescein-labeled IgG, obtained from convalescent patients, to stain early biopsies [71]; however, the specificity of the glomerular binding of IgG obtained from patients is open to question, since reactivity to normal human IgG has been shown to occur in poststreptococcal glomerulonephritis [90]. Lange et al. [73] have suggested that endostreptosin acts as a planted antigen for in situ reaction in the glomeruli.

Villarreal et al. [163] isolated a protein from cultured supernatants of nephritogenic strains (nephritis strain-associated protein). This protein is antigenically similar to streptokinase, in particular to a variant produced at 32°C [56, 57]. The New York Medical College antigen and the nephritis strain-associated protein have similar molecular weights of about 43,000 to 50,000 daltons and have been found in renal biopsies of patients with poststreptococcal nephritis; in addition, antibody titers to both these antigenic fractions are present in the serum of a vast majority of patients with PSGN, as well as in a significant number of normal individuals [103, 147]. Recently, Cronin and Lange [25] have suggested that endostreptosin is similar to the antigen studied by Villarreal et al. [163].

Another antigen currently under study is a cationic proteinase that was isolated by Vogt and co-workers [166] from cultured supernatants of nephritis-associated streptococcus and its presence is demonstrated in renal biopsies of patients with poststreptococcal nephritis. This cationic proteinase has been cloned [45], and subsequent studies [14] have shown that it is related to the streptococcal erythrogenic toxin. This nephritogen shares epitopes with the glomerular basement membrane [14]. Cationic molecules can easily penetrate the negatively charged polyanionic filtration barrier in the basement membrane and are readily localized in the subepithelial surface [167], a typical site of localization of electron-dense immune deposits in poststreptococcal nephritis. Antibody response to cationic proteinase and its precursor, zymogen, has been found in 82 percent of patients with poststreptococcal nephritis and appears to be a better marker for the disease than anti-DNase B, antihyaluronidase, or antistreptokinase [178].

Recently, Yoshimoto et al. [174] reported that patients with PSGN have high levels of serum antibodies directed against antigens in the cell membrane of streptococcus T type 12; since such antibody response was not found in streptococcal pharyngitis without nephritis, they suggested that this immune response had nephritogenic relevance. Bergey and Stinson [8] studied two solubilized surface proteins of M type 6 streptococcus of molecular weights of 6,000 and 15,000, which in vitro bind selectively to the proteoglycan-rich regions of the glomerular basement membrane. This binding was competitively inhibited by heparin, and a potential nephritogenicity of these polypeptides was suspected.

AUTOIMMUNE REACTIVITY

Autoantibodies may play a pathogenic role in poststreptococcal nephritis. Anti-IgG reactivity was first postulated by McIntosh et al. [91], who showed that antiglobulin formation and nephritis could be induced experimentally by the injection of autologous IgG depleted of sialic acid by exposure to streptococcal neuraminidase (salidase). Following this lead, anti-immunoglobulin reactivity was investigated in serum and renal biopsies of patients with PSGN. High rheumatoid factor titers have been found in 33 to 43 percent of the patients with PSGN [120, 148]. Sesso et al. [148] have found that IgG–rheumatoid factor is two times more common than IgM–rheumatoid factor in poststreptococcal nephritis. Interestingly, IgG–rheumatoid factor is not found in patients with IgA nephropathy and membranoproliferative nephritis type I, diseases in which IgM–rheumatoid factors may be present [37]. Anti–human IgG deposits have been detected in 19 of 22 renal biopsies of patients with acute nephritis [90], and IgG with anti-IgG reactivity was eluted from the kidneys of a fatal case of the disease [135].

Two mechanisms may be responsible for the production of anti-immunoglobulins. The first mechanism involves the antigenic potential of autologous IgG with modifications of its carbohydrate composition induced by neuraminidase [91]. Mosquera et al. [95, 96] demonstrated neuraminidase production by 16 of 20 streptococcal strains isolated from patients with nephritis and showed that immunoglobulins, in particular IgM, were substrates relatively sensitive to the action of this bacterial enzyme [96]. Neuraminidase activity and free neuraminic acid have been found in the serum of patients with acute PSGN by us [132] and others [5]. Mosquera et al. [97] provided further evidence in favor of a role for neuraminidase by the demonstration of glomerular binding sites for peanut agglutinin, presumably indicating free galactosamine radicals exposed by the loss of sialic acid from deposited immunoglobulin. Streptococcal neuraminidase may have an additional pathogenetic influence, since it could remove sialic acid from the epithelial and endothelial cell surfaces in the glomerular basement membrane, thereby facilitating the penetration of anionic streptococcal antigens that otherwise could be repelled by the negative electrostatic filtration barrier. In fact, perfusion of the kidney with neuraminidase has been shown to induce a size and charge permeability defect in the basement membrane [60, 61].

Another mechanism for the production of anti-immunoglobulins in poststreptococcal nephritis is suggested by the existence of type II receptors in the wall of group A streptococci demonstrated by Kronvall [70] and isolated by Grubb et al. [49]. These receptors bind the Fc immunoglobulin fragment, and the immunogenic potential of this binding is shown by the fact that anti-IgG antibodies are systematically induced in rabbits by injection with group A streptococci cultured in media containing autologous serum [141]. However, affinity for light kappa chains and human serum albumin, rather than for IgG, is more characteristic of nephritogenic strains [142]. Schroder et al. [144] have identified another type of streptococcal receptors that have affinity for IgM–rheumatoid factor, suggesting a potential mechanism for autoimmune reactivity in PSGN.

Autoimmune reactivity in poststreptococcal nephritis is not confined to anti-Ig production, since DNA–anti-DNA complexes have also been found in these patients [162].

In addition, the sera of patients with PSGN have antibodies against glomerular basement membrane components such as heparan sulfate proteoglycans [41], collagen type IV, and laminin [64].

NEPHRITOGENICITY OF THE IMMUNE REACTION

In 1907, Bela Schick [143] attributed the latent interval between scarlet fever and nephritis to the development of lowered resistance or hypersensitivity reactions, and 4 years later, von Pirquet [169] postulated that altered reactivity ("allergy") was due to antibodies developed in convalescence, in a manner similar to the events responsible for serum sickness.

Traditional explanations of the pathogenesis of PSGN gave a central role to immune complexes formed in circulation and eventually deposited in the glomeruli, where they recruited the complement cascade and inflammatory cells, thereby triggering a phlogogenic reaction. This hypothesis derived from the similarities between PSGN and the acute serum sickness model of glomerulonephritis, developed in classic studies of Germuth [46] and Dixon and his co-workers [32]. In this model, a single large dose of bovine serum albumin was given to rabbits, and subsequent determinations showed that antigen levels decreased slowly as the antibody response developed, until a level of equivalence was reached. At this time, usually occurring 7 to 14 days after the administration of antigen, there was a rapid period of antigen elimination that coincided with the fall in serum complement and the development of proteinuria; complement and Ig were deposited afterward in the glomerular basement membrane. Similarities between this experimental model and PSGN included the immunohistologic and ultramicroscopic appearance, the decrease in serum complement, and the rapid resolution of the disease.

Damage mediated by humoral immune mechanisms is assumed to require the participation of inflammatory cells, particularly neutrophils, recruited to a large extent by the chemotactic properties of the terminal components of the complement cascade. However, it was well recognized that proteinuria occurred before the immune deposits became prominent, and subsequent investigations showed that acute serum sickness nephritis was not prevented by decomplementation with cobra venom factor [50] or with depletion of neutrophils [68]; furthermore, the disease, albeit with somewhat diminished intensity, occurs in C6-deficient rabbits [108].

Accumulated evidence now suggests that mechanisms of cellular immunity have a determinant role in the nephritis of acute serum sickness. Hunsicker et al. [54] have shown that proteinuria correlates with glomerular monocyte infiltration, and Holdsworth et al. [53] demonstrated that proteinuria was suppressed almost completely with antimacrophage serum. The role of lymphocytes, presumably promoting the monocyte infiltration in the glomeruli, has been underlined by the work of Neild et al. [100], who showed that treatment with cyclosporin A prevented proteinuria in the acute serum sickness model. More recently, Parra et al. [105] showed that supernatants of glomerular cultures had migration inhibition factor (MIF) activity that correlated with the intensity of proteinuria and with monocyte and lymphocyte intraglomerular accumulation; moreover, MIF activity of glomerular supernatants was suppressed if glomeruli were preincubated with specific antilymphocytic monoclonal antibody.

In human renal biopsies taken during the acute period of PSGN, Parra et al. [106] have shown intraglomerular accumulation of CD4+ lymphocytes and monocytes, and other studies [102] have reported correlation between monocyte and T lymphocyte infiltration with proteinuria in postinfectious nephritis, as well as extravasation of monocytes with disruption of the capillary wall [86]. Therefore, it seems reasonable to suspect that cellular immunity is also critically involved in the pathogenesis of PSGN.

The site of antigen-antibody reactivity leading to nephritis is also open to question. As early as 1976, it was suggested [120] on the basis of the detailed data obtained by Wilson and Dixon [173] that most of the antibody present in the kidney likely met its antigen in situ, rather than in circulation; indeed, these authors found the same amount of radioactive antigen in the kidney before and after antibody deposition, and therefore, it seemed unlikely that significant amounts of antigen arrived complexed with antibody to the kidney. Additional reasons to question the circulating immune-complex pathogenesis have been discussed by Vogt and colleagues [165, 168], who reviewed why large immune complexes should be excluded by the size filtration barrier and the lack of significant nephritogenicity found with the intravenous injection of preformed immune complexes. These considerations, taken together with the fact that cationic antigens regularly induce subepithelial immune deposits [167], are reasons that make the cationic streptococcal proteinase [166] a particularly attractive putative nephritogen in PSGN.

GENETIC ASPECTS

Almost two centuries ago, Wells [172] noted that cases of postscarlatinal nephritis appeared in clusters in affected families. These observations have stood the test of time: Dodge et al. [35] noted that 20 percent of the siblings of affected families had clinical evidence of PSGN, and we found in prospective studies [136] involving 22 families that 38 percent of the siblings of index cases developed clinical or subclinical glomerulonephritis. This familial incidence is higher than the attack rate in the population at risk during epidemics, which has been estimated to be 28.3 percent for throat infections and 4.5 percent for nephritogenic impetigo [4]. An intriguing finding that awaits confirmation is that after correction for incomplete selection, the calculation of familial incidence gives a proportion of 0.260 ± 0.016, suggestive of autosomal recessive inheritance [133].

Understandably, genetic associations have been investigated, in particular with HLA antigens, but results have been inconclusive. Layrisse et al. [74] did not find significant differences between the families with nephritis and the general population, and only the DRW4 antigen showed increased frequency in unrelated patients with the disease. More recently, in Japan, Naito et al. [98] has found associations between DR1 antigen and PSGN.

Clinical Manifestations

STREPTOCOCCAL INFECTION

The usual locations of streptococcal infection are the skin and throat, but other sites are also possible [101, 130].

Streptococcal impetigo characteristically appears in exposed areas as small vesicles that break easily and leave a thick crust. Regional lymphadenopathy is present in 90 percent of the cases [29] and is frequently superimposed on lesions caused by scratching associated with scabies. The association with scabiosis is particularly frequent in epidemics reported in the tropics [110, 130], and a history of itching in other family members should raise this suspicion. The latent period of postimpetigo nephritis is 3 to 6 weeks.

Streptococcal pharyngitis can cause few symptoms or be associated with cervical lymphadenopathy, fever, and tonsillar purulent exudate, alone or in combination. Only 3 percent of the pharyngitis without any of these three findings is streptococcal. Scarlatinal rash on the face and neck is present if the bacteria produces erythrogenic toxin. The latent period after upper respiratory tract infections is 1 to 3 weeks.

During the latent period, the patient is asymptomatic, but the urinary sediment shows microscopic hematuria and mild albuminuria in one-third of the patients; those presenting with hematuria are more likely to develop symptomatic nephritis [154].

NEPHRITIS

Glomerulonephritis is subclinical in the majority of the cases and is manifested by microscopic hematuria and a fall in serum complement with or without hypertension, in a patient who had an antecedent streptococcal infection. Estimates of the incidence of subclinical disease vary considerably. Sharrett et al. [149] studied household members in the homes of index cases and found that clinical disease was more common, but since serial testing was not done, subclinical nephritis was likely underestimated. In fact, every other study [4, 34, 136, 138] has indicated that asymptomatic disease is 1.5 [4] to 19 times [138] more frequent than clinical nephritis. Our own studies [136] prospectively following family members of index cases gives a subclinical-clinical ratio of 4.0, reasonably close to the value of 5.3 found by Dodge et al. [34]. In Fig. 63-1, subclinical disease is shown to have an incidence of 90 percent, as an average of several prospective studies in the literature [4, 34, 136, 138]. Clinical nephritis is manifested in children by the same features of the acute nephritic syndrome in about 96 percent of the cases; about 4 percent of the patients have a full-blown nephrotic syndrome, and less than 1 percent of the patients develop rapidly progressive azotemia with exocapillary proliferation.

Table 63-1 shows the relative frequency of the clinical manifestations in 1,610 patients, almost all children, with acute PSGN [123]. The complete clinical picture of the acute nephritic syndrome (edema, hematuria, hy-

Fig. 63-1. Clinical presentations of acute poststreptococcal glomerulonephritis. The incidence of subclinical disease is an estimate obtained from several prospective studies [4, 34, 136, 138]. The incidences of acute nephritic syndrome (ANS), nephrotic syndrome (NS), and rapidly progressive glomerulonephritis (RPGN) are taken from data in children. In adults, the incidence of NS is significantly higher (see text).

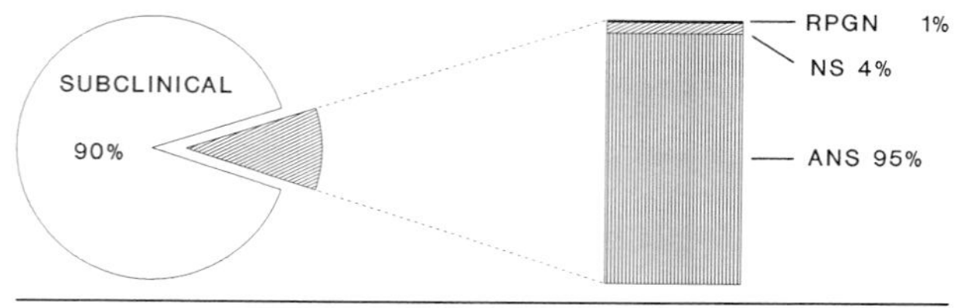

Table 63-1. Clinical findings in acute poststreptococcal glomerulonephritis[a]

Clinical manifestation	Frequency (%)
Hematuria	100 (31% macroscopic)
Edema	89 (62% chief complaint)
Hypertension	82 (52% severe)[b]
Proteinuria	80 (10% more than 2 gm/day)
Oliguria	50 (15% less than 200 ml/day)
General malaise, weakness, anorexia	55
Nausea, vomiting	15
Dull lumbar pain	5

[a]Clinical findings at admission of 1,610 patients with poststreptococcal glomerulonephritis and laboratory findings.
[b]Severe hypertension = diastolic blood pressure more than 20 mm Hg above the age-corrected normal value.
Source: Modified from Rodríguez-Iturbe [123].

pertension, and oliguria) was present in 40 percent of these patients [121, 123].

Hematuria is present in practically all patients. Only exceptionally [22, 48] the diagnosis of glomerulonephritis may be made if the urinary sediment is normal. Glomerular hematuria is manifested by red cell casts and by dysmorphism in 80 percent or more of the red blood cells found in the urine [39]. The usefulness of evaluating the shape and appearance of erythrocytes as a marker of renal parenchymal disease has been questioned recently, and in addition, two observers were found to differ in their interpretation in 38 percent of the occasions [113]. Emphasis should be placed on the use of freshly voided samples for urine sediment analysis because red cells are rapidly destroyed, especially in alkaline urine.

Edema is the chief complaint in almost two-thirds of the patients. Generalized edema is found in 36 percent of the children between the ages of 2 and 6 years [130]. Ascites is uncommonly associated with the nephritic syndrome, a fact noted by Wells [172] in the early nineteenth century.

Blood pressure is elevated in 82 percent of the patients, and diminished urinary output is noticed by patients or relatives in about half of the cases. Congestive heart failure is a complication related to excessive fluid retention. Somnolence, convulsions, and coma in association with severe arterial hypertension are characteristic of hypertensive encephalopathy; papilledema and increased cerebrospinal fluid pressure are not always present, and local vasoconstriction has been implicated in the pathogenesis of this complication [19].

Malaise, weakness, and anorexia were present in 55 percent of the patients, and nausea, vomiting, and a dull lumbar aching are less common [123].

Proteinuria is found in 80 percent of the patients with PSGN, but only in 10 percent of them is it in excess of 2 gm/day. As noted earlier, the full picture of the nephrotic syndrome is found in 4 percent of the children with the disease. In some series [65, 78], however, heavy proteinuria is reported to occur in 20 to 30 percent of the cases. In older patients, heavy proteinuria occurs 5 times more frequently than in children [93].

Increased serum concentrations of cholesterol and triglycerides have been found in as many as 40 percent of the patients, independently of the levels of serum albumin [51].

The manifestations of the acute nephritic syndrome begin to improve after 4 to 7 days, and the child is usually free of edema and normotensive 1 to 2 weeks afterwards. Microscopic hematuria may persist for a year, and during this time it may be intensified during febrile episodes; this finding does not carry a worse long-term prognosis.

SEROLOGIC FINDINGS

The serologic findings in acute PSGN include the detection of antistreptococcal antibodies, increase in the levels of serum immunoglobulins, anti-immunoglobulins, and immune complexes, and depression of serum complement.

Interest in serologic evidence of streptococcal infection dates from the 1920s when Dick [27] and Dochez and Sherman [33] established that β-hemolytic streptococcus was the etiologic agent of scarlet fever. Increase in the titers of antistreptolysin O (ASO), antihyaluronidase, and anti-DNase B are well-known markers of recent streptococcal infection. It is well known that the severity of nephritis and the level of antistreptococcal antibody titers are not related. ASO titers begin to increase 1 to 3 weeks after infection, reach a maximum at 3 to 5 weeks, and return slowly to normal levels in the following months [81, 87]. Following upper respiratory infection, ASO titers are elevated in 60 to 80 percent of the patients, but early antibiotic therapy decreases this incidence to 30 percent [66]. ASO response after skin infections is poor, possibly due to the effects of skin lipids minimizing the antigenicity of streptolysin O [62]; an antibody response to hyaluronidase or DNase B are far more common in streptococcal impetigo [12, 31, 171].

Recently, Zaum et al. [178] have studied the relative frequency of the antibody response to extracellular streptococcal antigens in the serum of 77 patients with poststreptococcal nephritis. As shown in Table 63-2, anticationic proteinase titers, most frequently directed against its precursor, zymogen, occur in 82 percent of our patients, and this antibody response appears to be a better marker for infection with nephritogenic streptococci than antihyaluronidase or anti-DNase B.

Antibodies directed to streptococcal M protein are type specific and play a role in short-term specific immunity [156]. Anti–M protein antibodies appear 4 to 6 weeks after infection but last for years, and therefore, they are important in the retrospective investigations of epidemics.

Serum levels of IgG and IgM are increased in more than 80 percent of the patients (Table 63-2) and return to normal 1 to 2 months afterward [127]. IgA levels are normal in most patients with PSGN [127], a finding that

Table 63-2. Serologic findings in the first week of acute PSGN

	%	Positive/total
Antistreptococcal antibodies		
Anticationic proteinase	82	63/77
Anti-DNase B	73	56/77
Antihyaluronidase	38	29/77
Antistreptolysin O	33	25/77
Antistreptokinase	7	5/77
Serum C3 < 100 mg/dl	93	112/120
Serum IgM > 150 mg/dl	86	94/110
Serum IgG > 1,600 mg/dl	85	102/120
C1q BA > 15%	60	29/48
Serum rheumatoid factor > 1:32	43	47/110

C1q BA = C1q binding activity.
Source: Data from Zaum et al. [178]. Immunologic data updated from [125].

clearly differs from the elevated IgA levels found in 80 percent of the cases of rheumatic fever [112].

Circulating immune complexes as detected by the C1q binding activity are found in almost two-thirds of the patients in the first week of acute PSGN, and the incidence of this finding and the levels detected decrease in subsequent weeks; after the third week, circulating immune complexes are rarely found [127, 150, 175]. This finding per se is not specific, since comparable incidence and similar molecular weight were found in circulating immune complexes of rheumatic fever and PSGN [161] and in nonnephritogenic upper respiratory [161, 175] and skin [94] infections. Despite the lack of specificity of the finding, Lin [79] has reported that immune complexes continue to be present for 6 to 9 months in patients with persistent hematuria and proteinuria.

Serum complement is depressed in 93 percent of the patients with the disease (Table 63-2). Serum levels of properdin, C2, and C4 are depressed, suggesting that both the alternative pathway and the classical pathway are activated in some cases [20, 76, 92]. C1 activation has been found to be a feature of both lupus erythematosus and PSGN [170]. Endre et al. [38] have shown that C3 synthesis is depressed in association with changes in the metabolic rate similar to those found in hypocomplementemic nephritis; yet, in contrast with that disease, C5 levels were decreased in correlation with C3 levels [38]. These authors [38] suggested that in PSGN complement was activated by a surface-bound convertase, probably located in the glomerular basement membrane, capable of cleaving C5 and C3.

The levels of complement return to normal after 2 months in 94 percent of the patients with uncomplicated PSGN [20], and persistence of a low level should raise the possibility of a diagnosis other than PSGN, such as systemic lupus erythematosus or mesangioproliferative hypocomplementemic glomerulonephritis.

Increased rheumatoid factor titers have been detected in 32 to 43 percent of the patients with PSGN [121, 148]. High rheumatoid factor titers are more common in the first week of nephritis, and they are part of the autoimmune reactivity in PSGN.

Pathophysiology of the Acute Nephritic Syndrome

The initial event in acute glomerulonephritis is a decrease of the glomerular filtration rate, which is due to the inflammatory damage at the glomerular capillary. The ultrafiltration coefficient, which is the product of intrinsic hydraulic permeability and filtration surface area, is reduced; in addition, there is shunting of the circulation between glomerular capillaries. The fall in glomerular filtration rate is associated with normal or increased renal plasma flow [16, 36]; therefore, the filtration fraction is diminished. Several experimental studies have indicated that in glomerulonephritis, for each level of glomerular filtration rate, the absolute proximal reabsorption is correspondingly decreased [55], a finding interpreted as a compensatory mechanism for the diminished volume of filtrate reaching this area. Therefore, the fall in glomerular filtration is a determining factor resulting in decreased distal delivery of filtrate. Diminished distal delivery associated with maintained distal reabsorption results in the sodium and water retention associated with the acute nephritic syndrome. Renal vasoconstriction with intact tubular function is the event responsible for the typical urinary findings in acute glomerulonephritis: fractional reabsorption of sodium < 1 percent and urinary-plasma creatinine ratio > 40.

The elevated blood pressure is the result of extracellular expansion due to sodium and water retention. Plasma volume, cardiac output, and peripheral vascular resistance are increased in the majority of these patients [134]. The severity of hypertension is directly related to the degree of fluid retention [11, 126].

Volume-sensitive hormonal systems responding appropriately in a compensatory response to an expanded extracellular compartment have been studied extensively. The renin-angiotensin-aldosterone is suppressed in these patients (Fig. 63-2) [126], and atrial natriuretic factor is increased in direct correlation with the weight gain in the acute nephritic syndrome [128]. This is in contrast with the lack of correlation between fluid retention and levels of atrial natriuretic factor in patients with the nephrotic syndrome (Fig. 63-3).

Renal vasodilatory hormones are depressed. Urinary levels of kallikrein and prostaglandins are decreased by 70 percent and 50 percent, respectively, during the acute episode [23]. The reasons for the changes in the renal hormones are not clear, but it is unlikely that they play a determinant role in the clinical picture because the urinary excretion of kallikrein and prostaglandin E (PGE) persist at low levels when the renal hemodynamic features of acute glomerulonephritis are no longer present [23]. Congruent with these interpretations, Godon and Damas [47] found that kallikrein did not participate in the sodium retention induced by saline overload in experimental nephritis.

Adrenergic neural activity may play a role in fluid retention in the nephrotic syndrome, since plasma levels of norepinephrine are increased during edema forma-

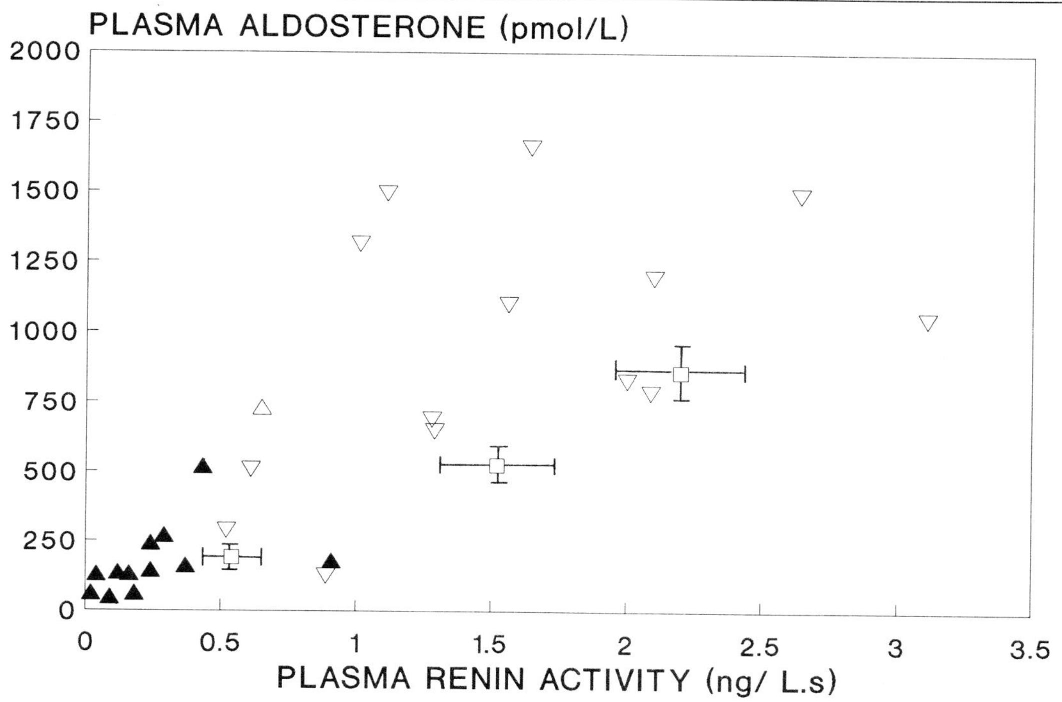

Fig. 63-2. Plasma renin activity and plasma aldosterone in acute nephritic syndrome. Patients studied during the acute nephritic syndrome (▲) and after recovery with low Na diet (▽) are compared with control subjects (mean ± SEM) on diets of 10, 150, and 300 mEq of Na per day. (Data modified and updated from [126].)

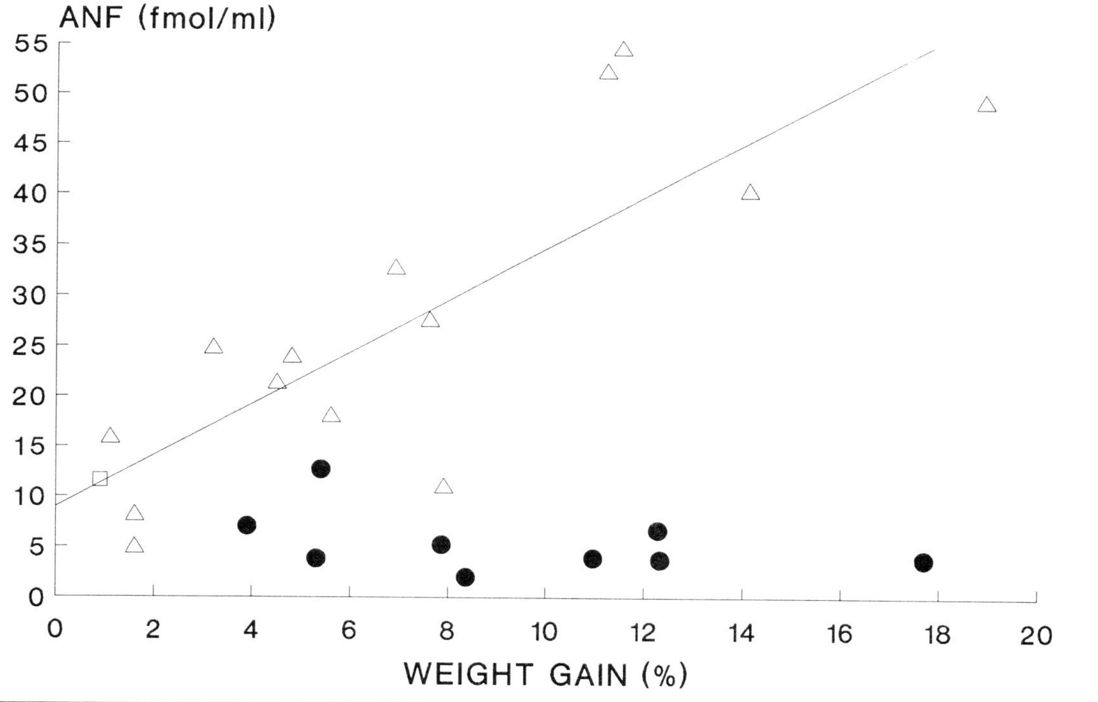

Fig. 63-3. Relationship between plasma atrial natriuretic factor (ANF) and weight gain (calculated as the difference between admission weight and dry weight) expressed as percent change of dry weight. The correlation in patients with acute glomerulonephritis (△) is highly significant ($r = 0.825$, $p < 0.001$, $Y = 9.37 + 2.55X$) but is not present in patients with nephrotic syndrome (●). Mean data in control subjects on a diet of 300 mEq of Na per day are shown as open square. (From [128].)

tion [115]; it is so far unknown if adrenergic tone is also increased in patients with the acute nephritic syndrome.

Differential Diagnosis of the Acute Nephritic Syndrome

Determination of serum complement has been suggested as a first-line test in evaluating patients with acute glomerulonephritis [82] because a normal serum complement would make unlikely the diagnosis of postinfectious glomerulonephritis, lupus nephritis, membranoproliferative glomerulonephritis types I and II, or subacute bacterial endocarditis. Urinary protein excretion, if considered in association with complement levels, could give additional help in the diagnosis of the acute nephritic syndrome [125]. As shown in Table 63-3, proteinuria in the nephrotic range is rare in PSGN, subacute bacterial endocarditis, IgA nephropathy, Henoch-Schönlein purpura, polyarteritis, and uremic hemolytic syndrome.

Pathology

The kidneys in acute PSGN are slightly enlarged and pale with a smooth surface. The typical microscopic changes are those of diffuse endocapillary glomerulonephritis: Increased numbers of mesangial and endothelial cells are found in the glomerular tuft, which seems to fill Bowman's space (Fig. 63-4A). In early biopsies, sometimes the neutrophil infiltration is particularly intense, a finding sometimes referred to as "exudative" glomerulonephritis. The mononuclear cell population infiltrating the glomeruli has been studied by Parra et al. [106] using monoclonal probes, which showed that monocytes and CD4+ lymphocytes (Fig. 63-4B) are increased in number in biopsies taken less than a month after the beginning of nephritis (Table 63-4).

Immunoglobulin G and M and components of the complement cascade, including the C5b-C9 membrane attack complex, are localized in the glomeruli of almost all patients with PSGN. IgA and IgE deposits are almost never present. The results of our biopsy material are shown in Table 63-5. The demonstration of membrane attack complex along capillary walls in renal biopsies of patients with PSGN [106], as well as in other glomerulopathies [40], is relevant because of recent evidence (reviewed in [24]) suggesting that the terminal components of the complement system may induce damage to the basement membrane by cell-independent mechanisms. These mechanisms are probably related to chemical mediators of inflammation produced by platelets, macrophages, and mesangial cells, which are stimulated by the C5b-C9 membrane attack complex.

Anti-immunoglobulin deposits may be found in almost one-third of the renal biopsies. The pattern of immune deposition in postinfectious glomerulonephritis has been analyzed by Sorger and co-workers in a series of papers [151, 152, 153]. In the first week, a finely granular pattern with the appearance of a "starry sky" is characteristically present and corresponds to deposits of immunoglobulins and complement components located predominantly in the capillary walls and to a lesser degree in the mesangial areas. In biopsies taken 4 to 6 weeks later, a so-called mesangial pattern is frequently found, consisting of irregular complement deposits without immunoglobulins. A third type of confluent IgG and C3 deposits predominantly located in the capillary loops constitute the "garland pattern"; this pattern has no relationship with the time of biopsy. The garland pattern is associated with large numbers of subepithelial electron-dense deposits and with massive proteinuria.

Ultrastructural studies have shown electron-dense deposits in subepithelial, endothelial, and intramembranous locations. Deposits in the subepithelial position have a dome-like appearance and are called "humps" (Fig. 63-4C) from the classic description of Kimmelstiel [67]; they are characteristic, but not exclusive, of PSGN. Electron-dense subepithelial deposits are more common in early biopsies and tend to disappear after 6 weeks [77]. Immunoglobulin G has been identified in the humps [145, 176]. Recently, Lee et al. [75] have studied the basement membrane and concluded that segmental abnormalities were present in 45 percent of their biopsy material, and they were more frequent in late biopsies and in areas adjacent to the humps.

Exocapillary proliferation with extensive crescent for-

Table 63-3. Serum complement and proteinuria in the diagnosis of the acute nephritic syndrome

	Proteinuria > 3 g per day		
Serum complement	Probable (70–90%)	Unlikely (< 10%)	No help (40–60%)
Normal (> 90%)	Visceral abscesses	IgA nephropathy Henoch-Schönlein purpura Microscopic PAN Uremic hemolytic syndrome	Anti-GBM disease
Low (> 90%)	MPGN I and II Lupus nephritis Shunt nephritis	Acute poststreptococcal GN SBE Essential cryoglobulinemia	

MPGN = membranoproliferative glomerulonephritis; PAN = polyarteritis nodosa; SBE = subacute bacterial endocarditis; GBM = glomerular basement membrane.
Source: Rodríguez-Iturbe [125].

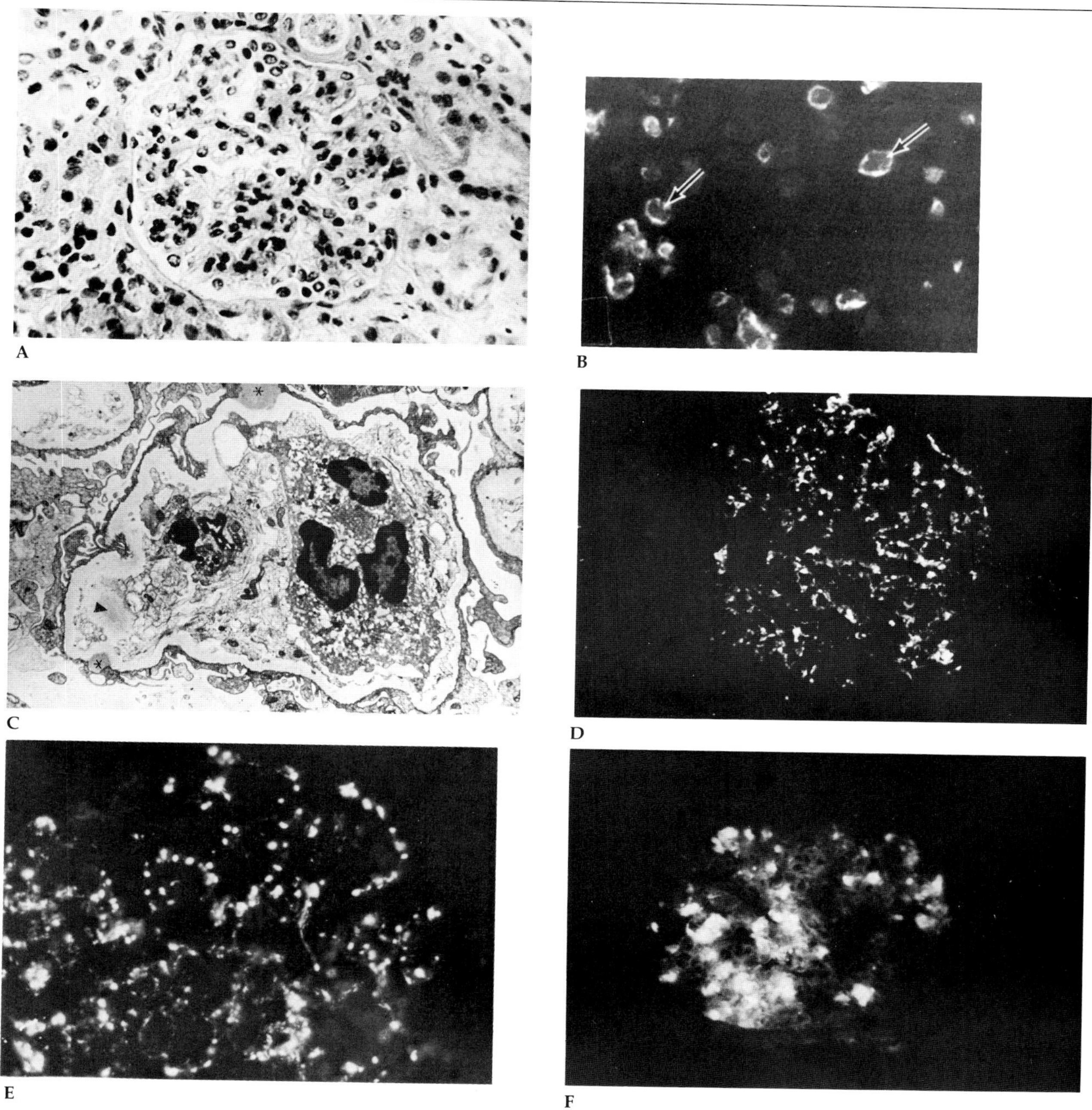

Fig. 63-4. Pathology of poststreptococcal glomerulonephritis. A. Endocapillary proliferation with increased number of mesangial cells and glomerular infiltration with neutrophils (PMN). Biopsy taken 10 days after the beginning of symptoms. (H&E, ×500.) B. Intraglomerular cells reactive with OKM1 monoclonal antibody (*arrows*) in a biopsy obtained 14 days after the initial symptoms. Monocytes and neutrophils are recognized by the antibody, and reactivity with antihuman lactoferrin (which identifies PMN) in serial sections was used to define glomerular monocyte infiltration. (From [106].) C. Glomerular capillary loop with polymorphonuclear leukocytes in the lumen. Electron-dense deposits are present in subepithelial ("humps") (*) and subendothelial (▶) locations. (×12,000.) D. C3 deposits (+1) in the glomerular basement membrane and mesangium. (FITC-labeled antihuman C3, ×500.) E. Glomerular deposition of the membrane attack complex of complement in a biopsy obtained 16 days after onset identified with monoclonal Poly-C9 antibody, which recognizes a neoantigen on C9. Pattern and localization of deposits is similar to the one found for C3 and C5. (From [106].) F. Antiimmunoglobulin G deposits (+2) in the mesangium. (FITC-labeled human IgG, ×500.)

Table 63-4. Glomerular infiltrating cells in poststreptococcal glomerulonephritis

		Cells per 100 glomerular cells	
Cells	(Normal)	< 1 month	> 1 month
Neutrophils	(0.1)	4.94	2.62
Monocytes	(0)	3.35	1.06
CD4+ lymphocytes	(0)	0.25	0.19
CD8+ lymphocytes	(0.06)	0.07	0.39
CD4/CD8 ratio	(−)	3.57	0.48

Source: Data from Parra et al. [106].

Table 63-5. Immune deposits and infiltrating cells in acute poststreptococcal glomerulonephritis

Immune deposits	Positive/total biopsies*
Complement C3	53/53
C5b-C9	6/7
IgG	32/52
IgM	38/50
IgA	1/40
IgE	0/34
Antihuman IgG	16/55

*Data obtained from biopsies taken less than 1 month after the beginning of symptoms.
Source: Data from Parra et al. [106].

mation has been found in some cases, which usually are characterized clinically by a progressive nitrogen retention. In Natal, South Africa, PSGN is the commonest cause of crescentic glomerulonephritis [104]. It has been stated that crescentic glomerulonephritis of poststreptococcal origin has a better prognosis than others [2, 7, 99], but this contention was not substantiated by the work of Bhuyan et al. [10]. This worker documented that outcome in PSGN was correlated with the extent of the crescents and the proportion of glomeruli affected, rather than with the etiology of nephritis.

Prognosis

The mortality of acute PSGN is low; only 5 to 8 cases in 1,000 die as a result of complications such as pulmonary edema, hypertensive encephalopathy, or rapidly progressive exocapillary proliferation with irreversible renal failure [121]. Melby et al. [93] have emphasized recently that PSGN is considerably more dangerous in elderly patients than in children. Congestive heart failure is 8 times more common in these patients than in children, and early mortality may be as high as 25 percent. Poorer prognosis may be due to coexistence of diabetes or cardiovascular or liver disease in elderly individuals. Follow-up studies reported from several groups of investigators [35, 78, 109, 111, 154, 158] suggested that prognosis was excellent in those patients who recover from the initial acute episode, although progression to chronicity was known to occur in some cases [140].

The debate of the long-term prognosis started after Baldwin and his co-workers [6, 42, 139] challenged this optimistic outlook, providing detailed data, both histologic and clinical, that indicated that about 50 percent of the patients presented histologic evidence of renal damage, mostly mesangial sclerosis, in the absence of urinary abnormalities or alteration in renal function. Due to their careful studies [6, 42, 139] to a large extent, it is now well established that the incidence of glomerular sclerosis is considerably higher than urinary or renal function abnormalities. Because of this fact, and depending on whether histologic criteria are used to define chronicity, the incidence of persisting disease ranges in the literature from 60 percent [6] to 3.5 percent [111]. Our own initial studies [129] confirmed that glomerular sclerosis, sometimes impressively intense, frequently in association with IgG and C3 deposits, is present in most renal biopsies obtained 5 to 6 years after the acute episode. Nevertheless, only one of these patients developed azotemia in a 12-year follow-up study [44], and the clinical significance of the pathologic changes remains questionable. Furthermore, we analyzed serum rheumatoid factor titers, cryoglobulins, and immunoglobulin levels during the postacute course of our patients, and no correlation between abnormal urinary findings and any of the serologic parameters tested could be found [44]. We have now extended our follow-up observations in epidemic as well as sporadic PSGN, including a cohort of children who had subclinical nephritis [43]. When compared with the corresponding adult or schoolchildren control populations, no significant differences were detected with respect to the incidence of hypertension, proteinuria, or decreased creatinine clearance; only microscopic hematuria was found more frequently in the follow-up of a subgroup of patients with sporadic glomerulonephritis [43].

Because the renal function appeared well preserved in these patients, we [131] tested their response to an acute protein load and found that patients with postacute nephritis had a 60 percent reduction in their capacity to increase their creatinine clearance after a protein meal. In contrast, four patients with subclinical disease responded normally, suggesting that renal functional reserve may be better preserved after a milder initial attack. Similar reductions in renal reserve capacity have been found after single nephrectomy without progressive functional deterioration, and therefore, the relevance of this finding as a prognostic marker is presently in doubt [124].

To address the question of abnormal findings other than those demonstrable by histologic analysis, I have pooled the data collected by Perlman et al. [109], Travis et al. [158], Potter et al. [111], Baldwin et al. [6], Garcia et al. [44], Lien et al. [78], Vogl et al. [164], and Clark et al. [21], corresponding to a total of 1,032 patients, in follow-ups ranging from 5 to 19 years (Table 63-6). It must be recognized that data from some individual series differ substantially from the rest, and the reasons for that variability remain unclear. It is possible that discrepancies could be due to the differences in the clinical char-

Table 63-6. Long-term prognosis of poststreptococcal glomerulonephritis

	Present %	Positive/Total
Symptomatic PSGN (endemic and epidemic)		
Any abnormality	17.4	174/998
Proteinuria	13.8	137/991
Hypertension	13.7	137/998
Hematuria	2.3	23/991
Azotemia	1.3	14/1032
Subclinical PSGN	?	

Source: Data collected from Perlman et al. (n = 61) [109]; Travis et al. (n = 54) [158]; Potter et al. (n = 534) [111]; Baldwin et al. (n = 176) [6]; García et al. (n = 71) [44]; Lien et al. (n = 34) [78]; Vogl et al. (n = 72) [164]; and Clark et al. (n = 30) [21], concerning patients with 5 to 19 years of follow-up.

acteristics of the initial nephritis, since the cases reported in some series [6, 44], but not in others [111], represented disease severe enough to require admission to the hospital.

The prognosis appears to be different in children and adults. Studies by Hinglais et al. [52], Garcia et al. [44], and Vogl et al. [164], which have clearly established age differences, indicate that 30 to 55 percent of adults have abnormal urine sediment or proteinuria or low creatinine clearance up to 15 years postacute PSGN. In children, these abnormal findings are 10 times less frequent. Reid et al. [118] have reported that lymphocyte reactivity to group A streptococcal antigens is significantly depressed in patients older than 10 years and have suggested that suppressor activity in the adherent cell population of older patients may be a factor in progression to chronicity.

A subset of adult patients who have massive proteinuria, with or without the full clinical picture of the nephrotic syndrome, have a particularly bad prognosis, since 77 percent of them develop chronic renal failure [164].

Treatment

STREPTOCOCCAL INFECTIONS

All patients with acute PSGN should be treated as if they had active infection. Oral penicillin G, 125 mg every 6 hours for 7 to 10 days, or oral benzyl penicillin, 200,000 units every 6 hours for 7 to 10 days, should eradicate the infection. Better compliance and equal results can be achieved with a single injection of 1.2 million units of benzathine penicillin, or half this dose if the patient weighs less than 30 kg. In persons allergic to penicillin, erythromycin (250 mg every 6 hours in adults and 40 mg/kg in children, for 7–10 days) is an appropriate alternative.

Throat culture remains the best way to establish the streptococcal etiology of pharyngitis, but this test has a 10 percent false-negative and 30 to 50 percent false-positive rate, representing streptococcal carriers. Stollerman [157] has emphasized the importance of a negative culture; assuming a 50 percent prevalence, 90 percent sensitivity, and 85 percent specificity, the negative predictive value of the throat culture is 97 percent. Komaroff et al. [69] have noted that certain clinical clues are helpful in deciding when to rely on culture results for the treatment of a sore throat. Fever, tonsillar exudate, and cervical adenitis are more frequent in streptococcal pharyngitis; when these three signs are present the likelihood of streptococcal etiology is 40 to 50 percent, and when all three are absent the probability of such etiology is 3 percent. Because of the false-positive and false-negative rates in throat cultures, patients who have fever, tonsillar exudate, and adenitis should be treated, while patients without any of these signs should not be treated, irrespective of culture results. The majority of the patients are not in any of these two categories, and in these patients throat culture is useful because they should receive treatment only if results are positive.

Prophylactic antibiotic therapy is advisable in patients at risk during epidemics, and based on the high attack rate of PSGN in families [72, 136], the siblings of index cases should also be treated preventively.

ACUTE NEPHRITIC SYNDROME

All patients benefit from restriction of sodium and fluid intake. Our practice is to withhold oral intake in the first 24 hours, since, as noted by de Wardener [26], it is necessary to know the urine output before deciding on fluid allowance. Loop diuretics may be administered parenterally on admission to patients who require hospitalization. With the use of this medication, the return to dry weight and normal blood pressure may be reduced from 7 to 13 days to 4 to 6 days [134]. About 50 percent of the patients will need antihypertensive medication. The oral angiotensin converting enzyme inhibitor captopril, 75 to 100 mg in a single dose, should decrease the blood pressure within 1 hour, but serum potassium should be closely monitored [107]; alternatively, 10 mg of nifedipine may be given sublingually after breaking the capsule and repeated within 1 hour if necessary. Parenteral diazoxide, hydralazine, or sodium nitroprusside is an appropriate choice if hypertensive encephalopathy is present; if repeated convulsions occur, deep sedation and intubation may be needed.

Pulmonary edema, if present, should be treated with ancillary methods of morphine, oxygen, tourniquets, and diuretics. Digitalis is contraindicated because it is ineffective and frequently associated with intoxication. Uremia and hyperkalemia may necessitate dialysis treatment.

On rare occasions, rising concentrations of blood urea and creatinine and persisting oliguria may indicate the development of rapidly progressive crescentic glomerulonephritis. This circumstance is an indication for renal biopsy, and treatment with intravenous pulse steroid therapy, as has been suggested for other causes of acute crescentic glomerulonephritis [15], may be attempted. Infectious processes, if present, are a contraindication to steroid therapy. Other therapy, such as quintuplet drug treatment (prednisone, azathioprine, cyclophosphamide, dypiridamole, and heparin followed by warfarin), offers no advantage over supportive treatment alone [137]. There is no evidence that enforced bed rest improves the prognosis of the disease [1, 58, 89].

References

1. Akerren, Y., and Lindgren, M. Investigations concerning early rising in acute hemorrhagic nephritis. *Acta Med. Scand.* 151: 419, 1955.
2. Anand, S. K., Trygstad, C. M., Sharma, H. M., et al. Extracapillary proliferative glomerulonephritis in children. *Pediatrics* 56: 434, 1975.
3. Anthony, B. F., Kaplan, E. L., Chapman, S. S., et al. Epidemic acute nephritis with reappearance of type 49 streptococcus. *Lancet* 2: 787, 1967.
4. Anthony, B. F., Kaplan, E. L., Wannamaker, L. W., et al. Attack rates of acute nephritis after type 49 streptococcal infection of the skin and of the respiratory tract. *J. Clin. Invest.* 48: 1697, 1969.
5. Asami, T., Tanaka, T., Gunji, T., and Sakai, K. Elevated serum and urine sialic acid levels in renal diseases of childhood. *Clin. Nephrol.* 23: 112, 1985.
6. Baldwin, D. S., Melvin, C., Gluck, M. C., et al. The long-term course of poststreptococcal glomerulonephritis. *Ann. Intern. Med.* 80: 342, 1974.
7. Beirne, G. J., Wagnild, J. P., Zimmerman, S. W., et al. Idiopathic crescentic glomerulonephritis. *Medicine* 56: 349, 1977.
8. Bergey, E. J., and Stinson, M. W. Heparin-inhibitable basement membrane-binding protein of *Streptococcus pyogenes*. *Infect. Immun.* 56(7): 1715, 1988.
9. Berrios, X., Quesney, F., Morales, A., et al. Acute rheumatic fever and poststreptococcal glomerulonephritis in an open population: Comparative studies of epidemiology and bacteriology. *J. Lab. Clin. Med.* 108(6): 535, 1986.
10. Bhuyan, U. N., Dash, S. C., Srivastava, R. N., et al. Immunopathology, extent and course of glomerulonephritis with crescent formation. *Clin. Nephrol.* 18: 280, 1982.
11. Birkenhager, W. H., Schalekamp, M. A., Schalekamp-Kuyen, M. A., et al. Interrelations between arterial pressure, fluid volumes and plasma renin concentration in the course of acute glomerulonephritis. *Lancet* 1: 1086, 1970.
12. Bisno, A. L., Nelson, K. E., Waytz, P., et al. Factors influencing serum antibody response in streptococcal pyoderma. *J. Lab. Clin. Med.* 81: 410, 1973.
13. Bisno, A. L., Pierce, I. A., Wall, H. P., et al. Contrasting epidemiology of acute rheumatic fever and acute glomerulonephritis. Nature of the antecedent streptococcal infection. *N. Engl. J. Med.* 283: 561, 1970.
14. Bohus, M., Batsford, S., and Vogt, A. Cationic streptococcal proteinase and human renal basement membrane have common epitopes. *Xth Lancefield International Symposium on Streptococci and Streptococcal Diseases*. Cologne, Germany, 1987. P. 79.
15. Bolton, W. K. Use of Pulse Methylprednisolone in Primary and Multisystem Glomerular Disease. In R. R. Robinson (ed.), *Nephrology*. New York: Springer-Verlag, 1984. Vol. II, pp. 1464–1473.
16. Bradley, S. E., Bradley, G. P., Tyson, C. J., et al. Renal function in renal disease. *Am. J. Med.* 9: 766, 1950.
17. Bright, R. Cases and observations, illustrations of renal disease accompanied with secretion of albuminous urine. *Guy's Hosp. Rep.* 1: 338, 1836.
18. Burserius de Kanifeld, J. B. *The Institutions and Practice of Medicine*. Edinburgh: Cadell and Davies, 1801; Von Plenciz, M. A. *Tractus III de Scarlatina*. Vienna: J. A. Trattner, 1792; Cited by Becker, C. G., and Murphy, G. E. The experimental induction of glomerulonephritis like that in man by infection with group A streptococcus. *J. Exp. Med.* 127: 1, 1968.
19. Byrom, F. B. The pathogenesis of hypertensive encephalopathy and its relation to the malignant phase of hypertension. Experimental evidence from the hypertensive rat. *Lancet* 2: 201, 1954.
20. Cameron, J. S., Vick, R. M., Ogg, C. S., et al. Plasma C3 and C4 concentrations in the management of glomerulonephritis. *Br. Med. J.* 3: 668, 1973.
21. Clark, G., White, R. H. R., Glasgow, E. F., et al. Poststreptococcal glomerulonephritis in children: Clinicopathological correlations and long-term prognosis. *Pediatr. Nephrol.* 2: 381, 1988.
22. Cohen, J. A., and Levitt, M. F. Acute glomerulonephritis with few urinary abnormalities. Report of two cases proven with renal biopsy. *N. Engl. J. Med.* 268: 749, 1963.
23. Colina-Chourio, J. A., Rodríguez-Iturbe, B., Baggio, B., et al. Urinary excretion of prostaglandins (PGE2 and PGF2a) and kallikrein in acute glomerulonephritis. *Clin. Nephrol.* 20: 217, 1983.
24. Couser, W. G., Baker, P. J., and Adler, S. Complement and the direct mediation of immune glomerular injury: A new perspective. *Kidney Int.* 28: 879, 1985.
25. Cronin, W. J., and Lange, K. Immunologic evidence for the in situ deposition of a cytoplasmic streptococcal antigen (endostreptosin) on the glomerular basement membrane in rats. *Clin. Nephrol.* 34(4): 143, 1990.
26. De Wardener, H. E. Treatment of acute glomerular nephritis. *Am. Heart J.* 98: 523, 1979.
27. Dick, G. F., and Dick, G. H. Experimental scarlet fever. *J.A.M.A.* 81: 1166, 1923.
28. Dillon, H. C. Pyoderma and nephritis. *Annu. Rev. Med.* 18: 207, 1967.
29. Dillon, H. C. Impetigo contagiosa: Suppurative and non-suppurative complications. I. Clinical, bacteriologic and epidemiologic characteristics of impetigo. *Am. J. Dis. Child.* 115: 530, 1968.
30. Dillon, H. C. Streptococcal Infection of the Skin and Its Complications: Impetigo and Nephritis. In C. W. Wannamaker and J. M. Matsen (eds.), *Streptococci and Streptococcal Diseases*. New York: Academic Press, 1972. P. 571.
31. Dillon, H. C., and Reeves, M. S. A. Streptococcal immune responses in nephritis after skin infections. *Am. J. Med.* 56: 333, 1974.
32. Dixon, F. J., Feldman, J. D., and Vasquez, J. J. Experimental glomerulonephritis: The pathogenesis of a laboratory model resembling the spectrum of human glomerulonephritis. *J. Exp. Med.* 113: 889, 1961.
33. Dochez, A. R., and Sherman, L. The significance of *Streptococcus hemolyticus* in scarlet fever and the preparation of a specific antiscarlatinal serum by immunization of the horse to *Streptococcus hemolyticus* scarlatinae. *J.A.M.A.* 82: 542, 1924.
34. Dodge, W. F., Spargo, B. F., and Travis, L. B. Occurrence of acute glomerulonephritis in sibling contacts of children with sporadic acute glomerulonephritis. *Pediatrics* 40: 1028, 1967.
35. Dodge, W. F., Spargo, B. H., Travis, L. B., et al. Poststreptococcal glomerulonephritis. A prospective study in children. *N. Engl. J. Med.* 286: 273, 1972.
36. Earle, D. P., Farber, J. J., Alexander, J. D. A., et al. Renal function and electrolyte metabolism in acute glomerulonephritis. *J. Clin. Invest.* 30: 421, 1951.

37. Endoh, M., Suga, T., and Sakai, H. IgG, IgA and IgM rheumatoid factors in patients with glomerulonephritis. *Nephron* 39(4): 330, 1985.
38. Endre, Z. H., Pusell, B. A., Charlesworth, J. A., et al. C3 metabolism in acute glomerulonephritis: Implications for sites of complement activation. *Kidney Int.* 25: 937, 1984.
39. Fairley, K., and Birch, D. F. Hematuria: A simple method for identifying glomerular bleeding. *Kidney Int.* 21: 105, 1982.
40. Falk, R. J., Dalmasso, A. P., Kim, Y., et al. Neoantigen of the polymerized ninth component of complement characterization of a monoclonal antibody and immunohistochemical localization in renal disease. *J. Clin. Invest.* 72: 560, 1983.
41. Fillit, H., Damle, S. P., Gregory, J. D., et al. Sera from patients with poststreptococcal glomerulonephritis contain antibodies to glomerular heparan sulfate proteoglycan. *J. Exp. Med.* 161(2): 277, 1985.
42. Gallo, G. R., Feiner, H. D., Steel, J. M., Jr., et al. Role of intrarenal vascular sclerosis in progression of poststreptococcal glomerulonephritis. *Clin. Nephrol.* 13: 449, 1980.
43. García, R., Rubio, L., Molina, E., et al. Long-term course of clinical and subclinical poststreptococcal glomerulonephritis (PSGN). *Xth Lancefield International Symposium on Streptococci and Streptococcal Diseases.* Cologne, Germany, 1987. P. 54.
44. García, R., Rubio, L., and Rodríguez-Iturbe, B. Long-term prognosis of epidemic poststreptococcal glomerulonephritis in Maracaibo: Follow-up studies 11–12 years after the acute episode. *Clin. Nephrol.* 15: 291, 1981.
45. Gassman, G. S., Vogt, A., and Ulf, B. G. Expression of the streptococcal protease gene in *Escherichia coli. Xth Lancefield International Symposium on Streptococci and Streptococcal diseases.* Cologne, Germany, 1987. P. 97.
46. Germuth, F. J. Comparative histologic and immunologic study in rabbits of induced hypersensitivity of serum sickness type. *J. Exp. Med.* 97: 257, 1953.
47. Godon, J. P., and Damas, J. The kallikrein-kinin system in normal and glomerulonephritis rats. *Arch. Int. Physiol. Biochim.* 82: 273, 1974.
48. Goorno, W., Ashworth, C. T., and Carter, N. W. Acute glomerulonephritis with absence of abnormal urinary findings. *Ann. Intern. Med.* 66: 345, 1967.
49. Grubb, A., Grubb, R., Christensen, P., et al. Isolation of an IgG-Fc Binding Protein from Group A Streptococci Type 15. In S. E. Holm and P. Christensen (eds.), *Basic Concepts of Streptococci and Streptococcal Diseases.* Surrey, England: Reedbooks, 1982. P. 203.
50. Henson, P. M., and Cochrane, C. G. Acute immune complex disease in rabbits: The role of complement and of a leucocyte-dependent release of vasoactive amines from platelets. *J. Exp. Med.* 133: 554, 1970.
51. Heyman, W., and Wilson, S. G. G. Hyperlipemia in early stages of acute glomerulonephritis. *J. Clin. Invest.* 38: 117, 1966.
52. Hinglais, N., García-Torres, R., and Kleinknecht, D. Long-term prognosis in acute glomerulonephritis. The predictive value of early clinical and pathologic features observed in 65 patients. *Am. J. Med.* 56: 52, 1974.
53. Holdsworth, S. R., Neale, T. J., and Curtis, C. B. Abrogation of macrophage dependent injury in experimental glomerulonephritis in the rabbit. Use of antimacrophage serum. *J. Clin. Invest.* 68: 686, 1981.
54. Hunsicker, L. G., Shearer, T. P., Plattner, S. B., et al. The role of monocytes in serum sickness nephritis. *J. Exp. Med.* 150: 413, 1979.
55. Ichikawa, I., Hoyer, J. R., Seiler, M. W., and Brenner, B. M. Mechanisms of glomerulotubular balance in the setting of heterogeneous glomerular injury. *J. Clin. Invest.* 69: 185, 1982.
56. Johnson, K. H., Kulisek, E. S., Zabriskie, J. B., et al. Antigenic variation of streptokinases from groups A, C and G streptococci and relation to the nephritis strain associated protein. *Xth Lancefield International Symposium on Streptococci and Streptococcal Diseases.* Cologne, Germany, 1987. P. 27.
57. Johnson, K. H., and Zabriskie, J. B. Purification and partial characterization of the nephritis strain-associated protein from streptococcus pyogenes. *J. Exp. Med.* 163: 697, 1986.
58. Joseph, M. C., and Polani, P. A. The effect of bed rest on acute hemorrhagic nephritis in children. *Guys Hosp. Rep.* 107: 413, 1958.
59. Kantor, F. S. Fibrinogen precipitation by streptococcal M protein. II. Renal lesions induced by intravenous injections of M protein into mice and rats. *J. Exp. Med.* 121: 861, 1965.
60. Kanwar, Y. S. and Farquhar, M. G. Detachment of endothelium and epithelium from the glomerular basement membrane produced by kidney perfusion with neuraminidase. *Lab. Invest.* 43: 375, 1980.
61. Kanwar, Y. S., and Rosenzweig, L. J. Altered glomerular permeability as a result of focal detachment of the visceral epithelium. *Kidney Int.* 21: 565, 1982.
62. Kaplan, E. L., and Wannamaker, L. W. Suppression of host response to streptolysin O by the skin lipids and its clinical implications. *Pediatr. Res.* 7: 375, 1973.
63. Kaplan, M. H. Localization of streptococcal antigens in tissues. Histologic distribution and persistence of M protein types 1, 5, 12, and 19 in tissues of the mouse. *J. Exp. Med.* 121: 849, 1965.
64. Kefalides, N. A., Pegg, M. T., Ohno, N., et al. Antibodies to basement membrane collagen and to laminin are present in sera from patients with poststreptococcal glomerulonephritis. *J. Exp. Med.* 163(3): 588, 1986.
65. Khuffash, F. A., Sharda, D. C., and Majeed, H. A. Sporadic pharyngitis-associated acute poststreptococcal nephritis: A four-year prospective clinical study of the acute episode. *Clin. Pediatr.* (Phila.) 25(4): 181, 1986.
66. Kilbourne, E. D., and Loge, J. P. The comparative effects of continuous and intermittent penicillin therapy on the formation of antistreptolysin in hemolytic streptococcal pharyngitis. *J. Clin. Invest.* 27: 418, 1948.
67. Kimmelstiel, P. The hump—a lesion of acute glomerulonephritis. *Bull. Pathol.* 6: 187, 1965.
68. Kniker, W. T., and Cochrane, C. G. Pathogenic factors in the vascular lesions of experimental serum sickness. *J. Exp. Med.* 122: 83, 1965.
69. Komaroff, A. L., Pass, T. M., Aronson, M. D., et al. The prediction of streptococcal pharyngitis in adults. *J. Gen. Intern. Med.* 1: 1, 1986.
70. Kronvall, G. A surface component of A, C, and G streptococci with non-immune reactivity for immunoglobulin G. *J. Immunol.* 111: 1401, 1973.
71. Lange, K., Ahmed, U., Kleinberger, H., et al. A hitherto unknown streptococcal antigen and its probable relation to acute poststreptococcal glomerulonephritis. *Clin. Nephrol.* 5: 207, 1976.
72. Lange, K., Azadegan, A. A., Seligson, G., et al. Asymptomatic poststreptococcal glomerulonephritis in relatives of patients with symptomatic glomerulonephritis: Diagnostic value of endostreptosin. *Chil. Nephrol. Urol.* 9: 11, 1988–1989.

73. Lange, K., Seligson, G., and Cronin, W. Evidence for the in-situ origin of poststreptococcal glomerulonephritis: Glomerular localization of endostreptosin and clinical significance of the subsequent antibody response. *Clin. Nephrol.* 19: 3, 1983.
74. Layrisse, Z., Rodríguez-Iturbe, B., García, R., et al. Family studies of the HLA system in acute poststreptococcal glomerulonephritis. *Hum. Immunol.* 7: 177, 1983.
75. Lee, H. S., Choi, Y., Oh, H. Y., and Koh, H. I. Abnormalities of glomerular basement membrane in acute postinfectious glomerulonephritis. *Clin. Nephrol.* 31(5): 239, 1989.
76. Lewis, J. E. Patterns of circulating complement in renal diseases. *Annu. Rev. Med.* 30: 445, 1979.
77. Lewy, J. E., Salinas-Madrigal, L., Herdson, P. B., et al. Clinico-pathological correlations in acute poststreptococcal glomerulonephritis. *Medicine* 50: 453, 1971.
78. Lien, J. K. W., Mathew, T. H., and Meadows, R. Acute poststreptococcal glomerulonephritis in adults: A long-term study. *Q. J. Med.* 189: 99, 1979.
79. Lin, C. Y. Serial studies of circulating immune complexes in poststreptococcal glomerulonephritis. *Pediatrics* 70(5): 725, 1982.
80. Ludlam, H., and Cookson, B. Scrum kidney: Epidemic pyoderma caused by a nephritogenic *Streptococcus pyogenes* in a rugby team. *Lancet* 2: 331, 1986.
81. Lyttle, J. D., Seegal, D., Loeb, E. N., et al. The serum anti-streptolysin titer in acute glomerulonephritis. *J. Clin. Invest.* 17: 632, 1938.
82. Madaio, M. P., and Harrigton, J. T. The diagnosis of acute glomerulonephritis. *N. Engl. J. Med.* 309: 1299, 1983.
83. Majeed, H. A., Khuffash, F. A., Sharda, D. C., et al. Children with acute rheumatic fever and acute poststreptococcal glomerulonephritis and their families in a subtropical zone: A three-year prospective comparative epidemiological study. *Int. J. Epidemiol.* 16(4): 561, 1987.
84. Majeed, H. A., Khuffash, F. A., Yousof, A. M., et al. The concurrent associations of group A streptococcal serotypes in children with acute rheumatic fever or pharyngitis-associated glomerulonephritis and their families in Kuwait. *Zentralbl. Bakteriol. Mikrobiol. Hyg. [A]* 262(3): 346, 1986.
85. Makowitz, A. S., and Lange, C. F. Streptococcal related glomerulonephritis. I. Isolation, immunochemistry and comparative chemistry of soluble fractions from type 12 nephritogenic streptococci and human glomeruli. *J. Immunol.* 94: 565, 1964.
86. Mazzucco, G., and Monga, G. Monocyte escape through a glomerular capillary basement membrane gap: An ultrastructural observation in a case of acute glomerulonephritis. *Nephron* 39(3): 272, 1985.
87. McCarty, M. The Antibody Response to Streptococcal Infections. In M. McCarty (ed.), *Streptococcal Infections*. New York: Columbia University Press, 1954. P. 130.
88. McCarty, M. The streptococcus and human disease. *Am. J. Med.* 65: 717, 1978.
89. McCrory, W. W., Fleisher, D. S., and Sohn, W. B. Effects of early ambulation on the course of nephritis in children. *Pediatrics* 24: 395, 1959.
90. McIntosh, R. M., García, R., Rubio, L., et al. Evidence for an autologous immune complex pathogenic mechanism in acute poststreptococcal glomerulonephritis. *Kidney Int.* 14: 501, 1978.
91. McIntosh, R. M., Kaufman, D. B., McIntosh, J. R., et al. Glomerular lesions produced in rabbits by autologous serum and autologous IgG modified by treatment with a culture of hemolytic streptococcus. *J. Med. Microbiol.* 4: 535, 1972.
92. McLean, R. H., and Michael, A. F. Properdin and C3 proactivator: Alternate pathway components in human glomerulonephritis. *J. Clin. Invest.* 52: 634, 1973.
93. Melby, P. C., Musick, W. D., Luger, A. M., and Khanna, R. Poststreptococcal glomerulonephritis in the elderly. *Am. J. Nephrol.* 7: 235, 1987.
94. Mezzano, S., Olavarria, F., Ardiles, L., and Lopez, M. I. Incidence of circulating immune complexes in patients with acute glomerulonephritis and in patients with streptococcal impetigo. *Clin. Nephrol.* 26: 61, 1986.
95. Mosquera, J. A., Katiyar, V. N., Coello, J., et al. Neuraminidase production by streptococci isolated from patients with glomerulonephritis. *J. Infect. Dis.* 151: 259, 1985.
96. Mosquera, J., and Rodríguez-Iturbe, B. Extracellular neuraminidase production of streptococci associated with acute nephritis. *Clin. Nephrol.* 21: 21, 1984.
97. Mosquera, J. A., and Rodríguez-Iturbe, B. Glomerular binding sites for peanut agglutinin in acute poststreptococcal glomerulonephritis. *Clin. Nephrol.* 26: 227, 1986.
98. Naito, S., Hohara, M., and Arakawa, K. Associations of class II antigens of HLA with primary glomerulopathies. *Nephron* 45: 111, 1987.
99. Neild, G. H., Cameron, J. S., Ogg, C. S., et al. Rapidly progressive glomerulonephritis with extensive glomerular crescent formation. *Q. J. Med.* 207: 395, 1983.
100. Neild, G. H., Ivory, K., Hiramatsu, M., et al. *Clin. Exp. Immunol.* 52: 586, 1983.
101. Nissenson, A. R., Baraff, L. J., Fine, R. N., et al. Poststreptococcal acute glomerulonephritis. Fact and controversy. *Ann. Intern. Med.* 91: 76, 1979.
102. Nolasco, F. E. B., Cameron, J. S., Hartley, B., et al. Intraglomerular T cells and monocytes in nephritis: Study with monoclonal antibodies. *Kidney Int.* 31: 1160, 1987.
103. Ohkuni, H., Friedman, J., van de Rijn, I., et al. Serological Studies on Streptococcal Nephritis Patients with an Extracellular Protein Associated with Nephritogenic Streptococci. In S. H. Holm and P. Christensen (eds.), *Basic Concepts of Streptococci and Streptococcal Diseases*. Surrey, England: Reedbooks, 1982. P. 263.
104. Parag, K. B., Naran, A. D., Seedat, Y. K., et al. Profile of crescentic glomerulonephritis in Natal: A clinicopathological assessment. *Q. J. Med.* 68(256): 629, 1988.
105. Parra, G., Mosquera, J., and Rodríguez-Iturbe, B. Migration inhibition factor in acute serum sickness nephritis. *Kidney Int.* 38: 1118, 1990.
106. Parra, G., Platt, J. L., Rodríguez-Iturbe, B., et al. Cell populations and membrane attack complex in glomeruli of patients with poststreptococcal glomerulonephritis: Identification using monoclonal antibodies by indirect immunofluorescence. *Clin. Immunol. Immunopathol.* 33: 324, 1984.
107. Parra, G., Rodríguez-Iturbe, B., Colina-Chourio, J., and García, R. Short-term treatment with captopril in hypertension due to acute glomerulonephritis. *Clin. Nephrol.* 29: 58, 1988.
108. Parra, G., Takekoshi, Y., Vernier, R. L., and Michael, A. F. Acute serum sickness (AcSS) in NZW and complement (C6) deficient (C6D) rabbits: Role of terminal components. *Xth International Congress of Nephrology*, 1987. P. 351.
109. Perlman, L. V., Herdman, R. C., Kleinman, H., et al. Poststreptococcal glomerulonephritis. A ten year follow-up of an epidemic. *J.A.M.A.* 194: 175, 1965.
110. Poon-King, T., Mohammed, I., Cox, R., et al. Recurrent

epidemic nephritis in South Trinidad. *N. Engl. J. Med.* 277: 728, 1967.
111. Potter, E. V., Lipschultz, S. A., Abidh, S., et al. Twelve to seventeen-year follow-up of patients with poststreptococcal acute glomerulonephritis in Trinidad. *N. Engl. J. Med.* 307: 725, 1982.
112. Potter, E. V., Shaughnessy, M. A., Poon-King, T., et al. Serum immunoglobulin A and antibody to M-associated protein in patients with acute glomerulonephritis or rheumatic fever. *Infect. Immun.* 37: 227, 1982.
113. Raman, G. V., Pead, L., Lee, H. A., and Maskell, R. A blind controlled trial of phase contrast microscopy by two observers for evaluating the source of haematuria. *Nephron* 44: 304, 1986.
114. Rammelkamp, C. H., Weaver, R. S., and Dingle, J. H. Significance of the epidemiologic differences between acute nephritis and acute rheumatic fever. *Trans. Assoc. Am. Physicians* 65: 168, 1952.
115. Rascher, W., and Tulassay, T. Hormonal regulation of water metabolism in children with nephrotic syndrome. *Kidney Int.* 32(Suppl. 21): 583, 1987.
116. Rastegar, A., Sitprija, V., and Rocha, H. Tropical Nephrology. In R. W. Schrier and C. W. Gottschalk (eds.), *Diseases of the Kidney* (4th ed.). Boston: Little, Brown, 1988. Pp. 2583–2613.
117. Reichel, H. Uber Nephritis bei Scharlach. *Z. Heilk.* 6: 72, 1905.
118. Reid, H. F. M., Read, S. E., Zabriskie, J. B., et al. Suppression of cellular reactivity in group A streptococcal antigens in patients with acute poststreptococcal glomerulonephritis. *J. Infect. Dis.* 149: 841, 1984.
119. Reinstein, C. R. Epidemic nephritis at Red Lake, Minnesota. *J. Pediatr.* 47: 25, 1965.
120. Rodríguez-Iturbe, B. Glomerulonephritis as a Consequence of Bacterial Disease: Considerations on Etiology and Pathogenesis. In R. Kluthe, A. Vogt, and S. Batsford (eds.), *Glomerulonephritis.* Stuttgart: Georg Thieme, 1976. P. 19.
121. Rodríguez-Iturbe, B. Nephrology Forum: Epidemic poststreptococcal glomerulonephritis. *Kidney Int.* 25: 129, 1984.
122. Rodríguez-Iturbe, B. Poststreptococcal Glomerulonephritis. In R. Robinson (ed.), *Nephrology Today.* New York: Springer-Verlag, 1985. P. 623.
123. Rodríguez-Iturbe, B. Acute Poststreptococcal Glomerulonephritis. In R. W. Schrier and C. W. Gottschalk (eds.), *Diseases of the Kidney* (4th ed.). Boston: Little, Brown, 1988. Pp. 1929–1947.
124. Rodríguez-Iturbe, B. The renal response to an acute protein load in man: Clinical perspective. *Nephrol. Dial. Transplant.* 5: 1, 1990.
125. Rodríguez-Iturbe, B. Acute Endocapillary Glomerulonephritis. In J. S. Cameron, A. M. Davison, J. Grunfeld, et al. (eds.), *Oxford Textbook of Clinical Nephrology.* Oxford: Oxford University Press, 1992.
126. Rodríguez-Iturbe, B., Baggio, B., Colina-Chourio, J., et al. Studies on the renin–aldosterone system in the acute nephritic syndrome. *Kidney Int.* 19: 47, 1981.
127. Rodríguez-Iturbe, B., Carr, R. I., García, R., et al. Circulating immune complexes and serum immunoglobulins in acute poststreptococcal glomerulonephritis. Evidence for circulating immune complex pathogenesis. *Clin. Nephrol.* 13: 1, 1980.
128. Rodríguez-Iturbe, B., Colic, C., Parra, G., et al. Atrial natriuretic factor in the acute nephritic and nephrotic syndromes. *Kidney Int.* 38: 512, 1990.
129. Rodríguez-Iturbe, B., García, R., Rubio, L., et al. Epidemic glomerulonephritis in Maracaibo. Evidence for progression to chronicity. *Clin. Nephrol.* 5: 197, 1976.
130. Rodríguez-Iturbe, B., García, R., Rubio, L., and Cuenca, L. Características clínicas y epidemiológicas de la glomerulonefritis postestreptocóccica en la región Zuliana. *Invest. Clín.* 26: 191, 1985.
131. Rodríguez-Iturbe, B., Herrera, J., and García, R. Response to acute protein load in kidney donors and in apparently normal postacute glomerulonephritis patients: Evidence for glomerular hyperfiltration. *Lancet* II: 461, 1985.
132. Rodríguez-Iturbe, B., Katiyar, V. N., and Coello, J. Neuraminidase activity and free sialic acid levels in the serum of patients with acute poststreptococcal glomerulonephritis. *N. Engl. J. Med.* 304: 1506, 1981.
133. Rodríguez-Iturbe, B., Moreno-Fuenmayor, H., Rubio, L., et al. Mendelian recessive ratios in acute poststreptococcal glomerulonephritis. *Experientia* 38: 981, 1982.
134. Rodríguez-Iturbe, B., and Parra, G. Loop Diuretics and Angiotensin Enzyme Inhibitors in Acute Nephritic Syndrome. In J. B. Puschett and A. Greenberg (eds.), *Diuretics: II. Chemistry, Pharmacology and Clinical Applications.* New York: Elsevier, 1987. Pp. 536–541.
135. Rodríguez-Iturbe, B., Rabideau, D., García, R., et al. Characterization of the glomerular antibody in acute poststreptococcal glomerulonephritis. *Ann. Intern. Med.* 92: 478, 1980.
136. Rodríguez-Iturbe, B., Rubio, L., and García, R. Attack rate of poststreptococcal glomerulonephritis in families. A prospective study. *Lancet* 1: 401, 1981.
137. Roy, S., Murphy, W. M., and Arant, B. S., Jr. Poststreptococcal crescentic glomerulonephritis in children: Comparison of quintuple therapy versus supportive care. *J. Pediatr.* 98: 403, 1981.
138. Sagel, I., Treser, G., Ty, A., et al. Occurrence and nature of glomerular lesions after group A streptococcal infection in children. *Ann. Intern. Med.* 79: 492, 1973.
139. Schacht, R. G., Gallo, G. R., Gluck, M. C., et al. Irreversible disease following acute poststreptococcal glomerulonephritis in children. *J. Chronic Dis.* 32: 515, 1979.
140. Schacht, R. G., Gluck, M. C., Gallo, G. R., et al. Progression to uremia after remission of acute poststreptococcal glomerulonephritis. *N. Engl. J. Med.* 295: 977, 1976.
141. Schalen, C., Burova, L. A., Christensen, P., et al. Aspects of induction of anti-IgG in rabbits by immunization with group A streptococci. *IX Lancefield International Symposium on Streptococci and Streptococcal Diseases.* Lake Yamanaka, Japan, 1984. P. 128.
142. Schalen, C., Christensen, P., Kurl, D., et al. Strong binding of aggregated immunoglobulin light chains and serum albumin in type M12 and some other group A streptococci: Possible relation to nephritogenicity. *IX Lancefield International Symposium on Streptococci and Streptococcal Diseases.* Lake Yamanaka, Japan, 1984. P. 121.
143. Schick, B. Die Nachkrankheiten des Scharlach. *Jahrb. Kinderheilk.* 65(Suppl.): 132, 1907.
144. Schroder, A. K., Christensen, P., Ghravi, A. E., et al. Molecular interactions between human IgG, IgM–rheumatoid factor (RF) and streptococcal IgG Fc receptors. *Xth Lancefield International Symposium on Streptococci and Streptococcal Diseases.* Cologne, Germany, 1987. P. 82.
145. Seegal, B. C., Andres, J. A., Hsu, K. C., et al. Studies on the pathogenesis of acute and progressive glomerulonephritis in man by immunofluorescein and immunoferritin techniques. *Fed. Proc.* 24(Part 1): 100, 1965.
146. Seegal, D., and Earle, D. P. A consideration of certain

biological differences between glomerulonephritis and rheumatic fever. *Am. J. Med. Sci.* 201: 528, 1941.

147. Seligson, G., Lange, K., Majeed, H. A., et al. Significance of endostreptosin antibody titers in poststreptococcal glomerulonephritis. *Clin. Nephrol.* 24: 69, 1985.
148. Sesso, R. C. C., Ramos, O. L., and Pereira, A. B. Detection of IgG–rheumatoid factor in sera of patients with acute poststreptococcal glomerulonephritis and its relation with circulating immunocomplexes. *Clin. Nephrol.* 26: 55, 1986.
149. Sharrett, A. R., Poon-King, T., Potter, E. V., et al. Subclinical nephritis in South Trinidad. *Am. J. Epidemiol.* 94: 231, 1971.
150. Solling, J. Circulating immune complexes in glomerulonephritis: A longitudinal study. *Clin. Nephrol.* 20: 177, 1983.
151. Sorger, K. Postinfectious glomerulonephritis: Subtypes, clinico-pathological correlations, and follow-up studies. *Veroff. Pathol.* 125(9): 1, 1986.
152. Sorger, K., Balun, J., Hubner, F. K., et al. The garland type of acute postinfectious glomerulonephritis: Morphological characteristics and follow-up studies. *Clin. Nephrol.* 20: 17, 1983.
153. Sorger, K., Gessler, U., Hubner, F. K., et al. Subtypes of acute postinfectious glomerulonephritis: Synopsis of clinical and pathological features. *Clin. Nephrol.* 20: 177, 1983.
154. Stetson, C. A., Rammelkamp, C. H., Krause, R. M., et al. Epidemic acute nephritis: Studies on etiology, natural history and prevention. *Medicine* 34: 431, 1955.
155. Stollerman, G. H. Nephritogenic and rheumatogenic group A streptococci. *J. Infect. Dis.* 120: 258, 1969.
156. Stollerman, G. H. Streptococcal immunology: Protection versus injury. *Ann. Intern. Med.* 88: 422, 1978.
157. Stollerman, G. H. Global changes in group A streptococcal diseases and strategies for their prevention. *Adv. Intern. Med.* 27: 373, 1982.
158. Travis, L. B., Dodge, W. F., Beathard, G. A., et al. Acute glomerulonephritis in children: A review of the natural history with emphasis on prognosis. *Clin. Nephrol.* 1: 169, 1973.
159. Treser, G., Semar, M., Sagel, I., et al. Independence of the nephritogenicity of group A streptococci from their M types. *Clin. Exp. Immunol.* 9: 57, 1971.
160. Treser, G., Semar, M., Ty, A., Sagel, I., et al. Partial characterization of antigenic streptococcal plasma membrane components in acute glomerulonephritis. *J. Clin. Invest.* 49: 762, 1970.
161. Van de Rijn, I., Fillit, H., Brandeis, W. E., et al. Serial studies on circulating immune complexes in poststreptococcal sequelae. *Clin. Exp. Immunol.* 34: 318, 1978.
162. Vilches, A. R., and Williams, D. G. Persistent anti-DNA antibodies and DNA-anti DNA complexes in poststreptococcal glomerulonephritis. *Clin. Nephrol.* 22: 97, 1984.
163. Villarreal, H., Jr., Fischetti, V. A., van de Rijn, I., et al. The occurrence of a protein in the extracellular products of streptococci isolated from patients with acute glomerulonephritis. *J. Exp. Med.* 149: 459, 1979.
164. Vogl, W., Renke, M., Mayer-Eichberger, D., et al. Long-term prognosis for endocapillary glomerulonephritis of post streptococcal type in children and adults. *Nephron* 44: 58, 1986.
165. Vogt, A. New aspects of the pathogenesis of immune complex glomerulonephritis: Formation of subepithelial deposits. *Clin. Nephrol.* 21: 15, 1984.
166. Vogt, A., Batsford, S., Rodríguez-Iturbe, B., et al. Cationic antigens in poststreptococcal glomerulonephritis. *Clin. Nephrol.* 20: 271, 1983.
167. Vogt, A., Rohrbach, R., Shimizu, F., et al. Interaction of cationized antigen with rat glomerular basement membrane: In situ immune complex formation. *Kidney Int.* 2: 27, 1982.
168. Vogt, A., Schmiedeke, F., Stockl, F., et al. The role of cationic proteins in the pathogenesis of immune complex glomerulonephritis. *Nephrol. Dial. Transplant.* [Suppl.] 1: 6, 1990.
169. Von Pirquet, C. E. Allergy. *Arch. Intern. Med.* 7: 424, 1911.
170. Waldo, F. B., and West, C. D. Quantitation of (C1INH)2 C1r-C1s complexes in glomerulonephritis as an indicator of C1 activation. *Clin. Immunol. Immunopathol.* 42(2): 239, 249, 1987.
171. Wannamaker, L. W. Medical progress: Difference between streptococcal infections of the throat and of the skin. *N. Engl. J. Med.* 282: 78, 1970.
172. Wells, W. C. Observation on the dropsy which succeeds scarlet fever. *Trans. Soc. Imp. Med. Chir. Knowledge* 3: 167, 1812.
173. Wilson, C. B., and Dixon, F. J. Quantitation of acute and chronic serum sickness in the rabbit. *J. Exp. Med.* 134: 75, 1971.
174. Yoshimoto, M., Hosoi, S., Fujisawa, S., et al. High levels of antibodies to streptococcal cell membrane antigens specifically bound to monoclonal antibodies in acute poststreptococcal glomerulonephritis. *J. Clin. Microbiol.* 25(4): 680, 1987.
175. Yoshizawa, N., Treser, G., McClung, J. A., et al. Circulating immune complexes in patients with acute poststreptococcal glomerulonephritis. *Am. J. Nephrol.* 3: 23, 1983.
176. Yoshizawa, N., Treser, G., Sagel, I., et al. Demonstration of antigenic sites in glomeruli of patients with acute poststreptococcal glomerulonephritis by immunofluorescein and immunoferritin technics. *Am. J. Pathol.* 70: 131, 1973.
177. Zabriskie, J. B., Utermohlen, V., Read, S. E., et al. Streptococcus-related glomerulonephritis. *Kidney Int.* 3: 100, 1973.
178. Zaum, R., Vogt, A., and Rodríguez-Iturbe, B. Analysis of the immune response to streptococcal proteinase in poststreptococcal disease. *Xth Lancefield International Symposium on Streptococci and Streptococcal Diseases.* Cologne, Germany, 1987. P. 88.
179. Zimmerman, R., Cross, M., Miller, D. R., et al. A streptococcal epidemic in an isolated civilian population with institution of mass prophylaxis. *J. Pediatr.* 69: 40, 1966.

Nephrotic Syndrome: Minimal Change Disease, Focal Glomerulosclerosis, and Related Disorders

H. William Schnaper
Alan M. Robson

The term *nephrotic syndrome* refers to the presence in a patient of proteinuria, hypoproteinemia, edema, and hyperlipidemia. Although an interrelationship between some of these findings was recognized as early as the fifteenth century [31], the term *nephrosis* first achieved widespread acceptance in the early part of this century, when Volhard and Fahr employed it as one of the major divisions of bilateral kidney disease [579]. Later developments, notably the advent of percutaneous renal biopsy, have facilitated further delineation of the many forms of kidney disease that result in the nephrotic syndrome. We have divided these diseases into three general categories, as shown in Table 64-1: (1) primary nephrotic syndrome, without a morphologic explanation for the disease; (2) inflammatory lesions or systemic diseases affecting the glomerulus; and (3) other diseases affecting the kidney. This categorization is not meant to imply that all patients in any one group have the same disease process. In most of these conditions, the pathogenesis remains poorly understood. Pathologic findings may represent a common end result of many different pathogenetic mechanisms. However, all of these diseases share a common denominator in that each causes proteinuria of sufficient severity to produce hypoproteinemia. Typically, when the serum albumin concentration falls below a critical level of approximately 2 gm/dl, the other clinical features of the nephrotic syndrome appear.

The prevalence of the different renal diseases that cause nephrotic syndrome is age-related. About 80 percent of nephrotic children, but only 25 percent of adult patients, have primary nephrotic syndrome. Glomerulonephritis is responsible for more than half of the cases of nephrotic syndrome in adults but only 10 to 15 percent of childhood cases. These glomerulonephritides may result from a systemic disease, such as systemic lupus erythematosus, or they may be idiopathic, i.e., the underlying disease process may not be known, such as in membranous glomerulonephritis. The remaining cases of nephrotic syndrome are associated with such diseases as diabetes mellitus or amyloidosis. They account for up to 20 percent of adult cases but a very small percentage of childhood cases. This general pattern of causes for nephrotic syndrome is observed in most industrial countries; different patterns of disease are seen in developing nations [8, 476, 528, 587]. For example, the glomerulopathy associated with malaria is a major cause of nephrotic syndrome in many African countries [273].

In recent years, a proliferation of terms has resulted in considerable confusion in terminology. In this discussion, we employ *primary nephrotic syndrome* to describe the clinical picture of nephrotic syndrome that occurs in the absence of evidence for glomerulonephritis or systemic disease, such as diabetes mellitus. Primary nephrotic syndrome is seen in adults but most often occurs in childhood; it usually responds to treatment with steroids and often recurs. It includes patients who have been described as having lipoid nephrosis, "nil" disease, idiopathic nephrotic syndrome of childhood, minimal change nephrotic syndrome, and steroid-sensitive or steroid-responsive nephrotic syndrome. A spectrum of renal histologic findings has been described in these patients. In each instance the histology is characterized by little or no inflammatory response in the glomeruli. In the majority of patients, the only apparent abnormality is fusion of the epithelial podocytes; this lesion is classified here as minimal change nephrotic syndrome (MCNS). In some cases of primary nephrotic syndrome, there may be slight deposition of IgM in the glomeruli, which usually is interpreted by the pathologist as being insignificant; some biopsies reveal mesangial hypercellularity; in others, focal segmental glomerulosclerosis (FSGS) may be identified. Increasing evidence suggests that these represent variations of the same disease process rather than being separate entities. Thus several of these changes may be present in the same biopsy. Alternatively, a patient diagnosed as having MCNS on an initial biopsy may be found to have FSGS subsequently [655]. To further complicate the issue, some of the patients, irrespective of the underlying pathology, respond to treatment with steroids; others, with an apparently identical histologic lesion, are resistant to steroid therapy, whereas a third group may respond to steroids initially but become steroid-resistant in later relapses.

This chapter focuses on primary nephrotic syndrome, including the clinical features and management of patients with this entity. The mechanisms by which the renal lesion translates into the clinical features of the nephrotic syndrome are reviewed, as well as current observations on the pathogenesis of primary nephrotic syndrome.

Clinical Aspects of Nephrotic Syndrome

CLINICAL FEATURES

History and Physical Findings. Minimal change nephrotic syndrome (MCNS) is typically thought of as a pediatric disease. Indeed, it is the second most common primary renal parenchymal disease in children aged 15 years or less. Two to 7 new cases occur annually per 100,000 children [287], and the prevalence is about 15 cases per 100,000 of the pediatric population [46]. Although most children with MCNS achieve permanent remission of symptoms by the time they reach puberty, some cases persist into adulthood. In addition, MCNS may present in adults. New cases have been reported in as late as the eighth decade of life [346]. However, the relative incidence of MCNS as the etiology of nephrotic syndrome

Table 64-1. Some causes of the nephrotic syndrome and their relative frequencies in pediatric and adult patients

	Relative incidence (%)*	
	Children	Adults
Primary Nephrotic Syndrome	79	24
Minimal change nephrotic syndrome (MCNS)		
MCNS with IgM deposits		
Mesangial hypercellularity		
Focal segmental glomerulosclerosis (FSGS)		
Nephrotic Syndrome Associated with Glomerulopathy		
Idiopathic glomerulopathy	13	52
Membranous glomerulonephritis		
Membranoproliferative glomerulonephritis		
Proliferative glomerulonephritis		
Others		
Secondary glomerulopathy	7	24
Systemic lupus erythematosus		
Diabetes mellitus		
Amyloidosis		
Others		
Other Diseases	< 1	< 1
Congenital nephrotic syndrome (Finnish and other varieties)		
Diffuse mesangial sclerosis		
Others		

*Data derived from ISKDC [306] and from Glassock [239].

Table 64-2. Drugs and other factors reported to have precipitated primary nephrotic syndrome

Drugs
Gold [208]
Penicillamine [193]
Ampicillin [542]
Mercury-containing compounds [48]
Nonsteroidal anti-inflammatory agents
Sulindac [413]
Tolmetin sodium [196]
Fenprofen [148]
Trimethadione, paramethadione [277]
Atopy
Pollen [535]
Food allergy
Milk [568]
Pork [286]
House dust [388]
Contact dermatitis (poison ivy and oak) [564]
Bee stings [565]
Tumors
Lymphoma [104, 214]
Others [176]
Infections
Various viral infections [257]
Schistosomiasis [425]
Guillain-Barré (as an epiphenomenon) [209]
Immunizations [265]
Obesity [313]
Dermatitis herpetiformis [213]

decreases with age in both children and adults [384, 689]. Although it is not clear that adult-onset disease represents the same entity as that found in childhood or that all patients with the clinical picture of MCNS have an identical disease, the clinical course and outcome of pediatric and adult cases appear to be sufficiently similar to consider all cases together.

Minimal change disease can appear in the first year of life, but it is more common after this age, with a peak incidence at age 2 years. It occurs twice as often in male as in female children but has an equal incidence in male and female adults [111]. Although no precipitating cause may be apparent in many children, it is not unusual for the development of edema and proteinuria to be preceded by an upper respiratory tract infection, an allergic reaction to a bee sting, or the use of certain drugs (Table 64-2). In adult patients, malignancies, especially Hodgkin's disease, have been associated with the development of MCNS.

Within a few days of the inciting event, the patient develops edema. Typically, facial edema is noted first, with few other indications of an ongoing disease process. This, especially if associated with an upper respiratory tract infection, may be confused with allergic symptoms. Edema usually increases gradually. It becomes detectable in the adult only when several liters of fluid has accumulated, so that by the time medical advice is sought, the patient has pitting edema involving the sacrum and the lower extremities. When anasarca is present, periorbital edema can be so severe that the eyelids are swollen shut, scrotal or vulval edema may be marked, and there may be significant abdominal distention. Respiratory embarrassment may occur from accumulation of either pleural or ascitic fluid, although the infrequency of dyspnea or orthopnea in the face of massive fluid retention is striking. This reflects the absence of increased pulmonary capillary wedge pressure generating pulmonary edema. Headaches and irritability are common accompanying complaints of edema. The patient may note vague symptoms, such as malaise, easy fatigability, irascibility, and depression. Typically, these symptoms do not dominate the clinical picture. The development of cellulitis, peritonitis, or pneumonia may be the first indication of an underlying nephrotic syndrome. The pallor resulting from edema may be misinterpreted as indicating anemia. Gross hematuria may be the presenting sign in patients with FSGS or mesangial hypercellularity [265, 607].

On physical examination, dependent edema is the most prominent finding. The retina has a characteristic "wet" appearance. Subungual edema may reverse the usual color pattern on the fingernails—the normally white lunulae may be pink and the rest of the nailbed white. Horizontal white lines may be seen on both the finger- and toenails and are referred to as Muehrcke's lines. Inguinal and umbilical hernias may be present, especially if the patient has had severe ascites for a prolonged period of time. The elasticity of the cartilage in the ear appears to be decreased.

Blood pressure in patients with MCNS typically is normal, but elevated systolic pressure has been recorded in 21 percent and elevated diastolic pressure in 14 percent of the children reported by the International Study of Kidney Diseases in Children (ISKDC) [304]. Hypertension is seen more commonly in adult patients with MCNS [151] and in all patients with FSGS or glomerulonephritis as a cause for the nephrotic syndrome, regardless of age.

Growth failure may be found in children, most often in those who have had multiple relapses of MCNS requiring frequent courses of steroids [5a]. Evidence for infection, especially peritonitis, cellulitis, or pneumonia, should be sought as part of the physical examination. These infections may be associated with septicemia and shock.

Nephrotic Syndrome and Malignancy. Several glomerulopathies, notably membranous glomerulonephritis, have been associated with neoplasia. A significant number of patients with cancer-related nephrotic syndrome, however, have MCNS (Table 64-3). The relationship between MCNS and lymphomatous disorders, particularly Hodgkin's disease, is especially striking [214]. In a survey of the literature, 33 of 134 patients with cancer-related nephrotic syndrome had MCNS on biopsy [176]. Of the patients with MCNS, 26 had Hodgkin's disease and an additional two had non-Hodgkin's lymphoma. In another review [104], 36 of 44 patients who had Hodgkin's disease and the nephrotic syndrome had MCNS and only two had membranous glomerulonephritis. There was a much higher incidence of nephritic diseases in patients with other types of neoplasia. Nonlymphomatous tumors associated with MCNS include renal oncocytoma [207], embryonal cell tumors [176], pancreatic carcinoma [670], nephroblastoma [409], Waldenström's macroglobulinemia [284], and bronchogenic carcinoma [390, 472].

Evidence suggests that in these cases the tumor may be involved directly in the pathogenesis of the MCNS. In several reports, MCNS was the initial presenting sign of a lymphomatous disorder [231, 520, 656] and may have preceded clinical evidence of lymphoma by several years [289]. With appropriate and successful antineoplastic therapy, either medical or surgical, the proteinuria in tumor-related MCNS resolves, renal function remains normal, and the nephrotic syndrome remits [176, 207, 472]. The relationship between relapse of the tumor and of the nephrotic syndrome [297, 522] also strongly suggests an etiologic role for the tumor in the pathogenesis of MCNS in these patients. These observations indicate the importance of considering a malignancy as an underlying cause in any adult patient who presents with nephrotic syndrome [347, 474]. In such cases, it is essential to treat the primary neoplasm rather than the renal disease.

Atopy and MCNS. A relationship between allergy and MCNS has long been suspected. Anecdotal experience suggests that exposure to allergens may precipitate the nephrotic syndrome [213, 286, 535, 547]; rhinorrhea and allergic skin reactivity frequently precede relapses [453], and a high prevalence of allergic symptoms has been observed in nephrotic patients. In a controlled study, patients who had a pathologic diagnosis of MCNS on renal biopsy experienced a decrease in proteinuria when placed on an elemental diet and did not require treatment with corticosteroids. Challenge with milk led to a decrease in serum C3 and increased protein excretion, strongly suggesting that hypersensitivity was causally linked to proteinuria [568]. The administration of an antihistamine/decongestant preparation has been reported to result in an improved sense of well-being [205]. Furthermore, a human basophil degranulation test was reported to be positive in 16 of 28 adults with MCNS and 14 of 18 with FSGS; in contrast, only 5 of 29 patients with glomerulonephritis and 1 of 11 normal donors showed a positive response [521]. In addition, atopy and MCNS have been associated with the increased frequency of expression of HLA-B12 and DRw7 antigens [160, 630].

Despite a wide range of values, mean serum IgE levels have been found to be significantly elevated in patients with MCNS compared to those with other renal prob-

Table 64-3. Nephrotic syndrome in patients with malignancy

	Renal histology*		
Type of malignancy	Minimal change disease	Membranous nephropathy	Membranoproliferative glomerulonephritis
Hodgkin's lymphoma	26	4	0
Non-Hodgkin's lymphoma	2	2	1
Leukemia	1	4	1
Multiple myeloma	0	0	1
Carcinoma	3	33	4
Benign or embryonal tumors	1	1	0

*Only cases with defined renal pathology and without amyloidosis are shown. Data taken from Eagen and Lewis [176].

lems [254]; elevated levels also have been associated with frequent relapse in children [454]. More than 50 percent of adult MCNS patients were found to have serum IgE levels greater than two standard deviations above the normal mean; of these, more than 70 percent had associated allergic symptoms [371, 375]. Other investigators have made similar observations but have sought to draw a distinction between primary allergic disease and the elevated IgE levels found in nephrotic syndrome. They have suggested that since IgE deposition in the glomerulus is rare [228], elevated serum IgE could represent not the causal factor in MCNS but, rather, evidence of more generalized derangement in the immune system [586]. This concept is supported by a finding that increases in serum IgE may persist even with remission. If this view is correct, it could explain why attempts to treat MCNS in atopic patients with inhaled disodium cromoglycate [640] or an orally administered analogue [452] have been unsuccessful.

These apparently conflicting observations may be resolved by study of specific antigens. Thus a majority of adult nephrotic patients were reported to have detectable elevations of specific IgE titers, with the most common sensitizing agent being house dust or dust mites. After remission induced by institution of specific desensitization and sodium cromolyn, several of these patients relapsed on reexposure to the allergen [372, 388, 389].

Patterns of Inheritance. There may be a familial incidence of MCNS. In a survey from Europe, which excluded cases of the congenital nephrotic syndrome [671], it was found that 63 of 1,877 nephrotic children had affected family members. This prevalence of 3.35 percent was higher than that predicted from the frequency with which MCNS occurs in the general population. Most often siblings were affected. The similarity of pathologic findings and clinical course for affected members within a family was striking [468], although, in at least one other report, siblings showed differences in these features [355]. Familial nephrotic syndrome in children has been divided into two broad categories: (1) patients with an infantile onset and a poor prognosis regardless of renal morphology and (2) patients with a juvenile onset and a generally good response to conventional therapy, provided MCNS is found on renal biopsy. Other forms of primary nephrotic syndrome that may have a familial occurrence include congenital diffuse mesangial sclerosis, which has been reported in identical twins as well as a third sibling [348], and in two siblings who were born from consanguineous parents and had concomitant ocular, neurologic, and other abnormalities [239]. Among other forms of primary nephrotic syndrome, FSGS has been reported in siblings with associated deficient T-cell function [618] or with sickle cell and thalassemia hemoglobinopathies [123].

An indication of a possible genetic predisposition for development of MCNS is the reported association of MCNS, and in some cases atopy [630, 638], with certain histocompatibility-complex antigens. The two most commonly cited are HLA-B12 (now refined to its B44 component) and DRw7. Not all studies have confirmed these associations. Indeed, a variety of other HLA antigens have been associated with MCNS (Table 64-4) and negative associations have been reported, too. HLA-B8 was found frequently in families with more than one case of childhood nephrosis [449]. In one study, the combined occurrence of B8 with DR3 and DR7 produced a relative risk of 21.5 [562]. In another study, DR7 was linked to steroid-sensitive disease and DR3 to steroid-resistant disease. The differences among results from these studies may be due in part to racial or geographical differences, or both.

The recent observation that two extended HLA haplotypes (HLA-A1, B8, DR3, DRw52, SCO1; and HLA-B44, DR7, DRw53, FC31) occurred with greater than expected frequency in children with steroid-sensitive, frequently relapsing MCNS provides the strongest evidence to date for a genetic predisposition to the disease, perhaps through an immunogenetic mechanism [375]. In support of this concept is the finding that variability in C4 gene number or expression occurs more frequently in nephrotic children than in controls [450].

The association between HLA type and MCNS has been made primarily in children, with many studies being unable to make similar correlations in adult patients. This finding suggests that MCNS in adult and pediatric patients could represent different diseases that share common pathologic and clinical features. For example, HLA-DR7, which has been linked to MCNS (Table 64-4), was observed in only 18 percent of adult MCNS patients, a frequency not different from that of controls. However, if the data were analyzed according to age of onset of the nephrotic syndrome, 45 percent of patients in whom onset was before the age 15 years were HLA-DR7, whereas the equivalent incidence in adult-onset patients was only 7 percent [387]. More recently, a study from Japan has linked MCNS in adult patients to HLA-DRw8 and DQw3 [357].

Focal segmental sclerosis has been linked to HLA type DRw8 in nephrotic children of Hispanic origin [446, 626] and B8 combined with DR3 and DR7 in German children [562]. One study of adult patients with FSGS found an increased incidence of HLA-DR4 in both black and white subjects [242]. HLA-Bw53 was increased in black male adult patients with FSGS secondary to heroin nephropathy [270].

LABORATORY FINDINGS

Urinalysis. Most urines from nephrotic patients foam when voided into a receptacle. This is due to marked proteinuria, which on a dipstick characteristically reads 3+ to 4+. Other edema-forming, hypoalbuminemic states, such as malnutrition and protein-losing enteropathy, may mimic nephrotic syndrome but do not manifest significant proteinuria. The amount of protein in the urine of nephrotic patients may range from less than 1 to more than 25 gm per day. The value for adult patients is usually between 3 and 16 gm per day; that for children typically is lower than this amount, even when allowances are made for body size [161], and averages about 50 mg/kg of body weight per day [265]. Since

Table 64-4. Relationship between MCNS and HLA type

Author [ref.]	Year	Country of origin	No. of patients	HLA association	Relative risk	Children	Comments
Thomson et al. [630]	1976	England	71	B12	6.3	Yes	Relative risk with B12 and atopy—13
Trompeter et al. [638]	1980	England	116	B12	3.1	Yes	Could not confirm atopy data
O'Regan et al. [504]	1980	Ireland	54	B8 B18	3.5 3.16	Yes	
Alfiler et al. [11]	1980	Australia	42	DRw7	5.9	Yes	MCNS—confirmed by biopsy; decreased DR2
Noss et al. [495]	1981	Germany	45	B8	2.81	Yes	
DeMouzan-Cambon et al. [160]	1981	France	54	DRw7	4.4	Yes	Related to atopy; decreased DR2
Nunez-Roldan et al. [496]	1982	Spain	50	DRw7	4.5	Yes	Decreased DR2
Kobayashi et al. [357]	1985	Japan	40	DRw8 DQw3	3.74 1.11	No	Studied adult subjects
Cambon-Thomsen et al. [105]	1986	France	72 27	DR7 DR3	6.9 3.0	Yes	Steroid-sensitive Steroid-resistant
Lagueruela et al. [375]	1990	United States	32	A1, B8, DR3, DRw52, SCO1 and/or B44, DR7, DRw53, FC31	— —	Yes	Steroid-sensitive Frequently relapsing
Ruder et al. [562]	1990	Germany	91	B8, DR3, DR7	21.5	Yes	Steroid-sensitive

urine protein is proportional to plasma protein concentration [129], children with MCNS, who frequently have serum albumin levels of 1 gm/dl or less, may have amounts of proteinuria as low as 100 to 200 mg per day. This finding also reflects removal of much of the filtered protein from the glomerular filtrate as it traverses the proximal convoluted tubule [140]. In most children with FSGS, the quantity of proteinuria is much higher, typically 4 to 6 gm per day [607]. As a consequence of proteinuria, the urine specific gravity is characteristically high, exceeding 1.025 and often 1.035 or higher. The exception is the patient with nephrotic syndrome and renal failure, where lower (but not isosthenuric) values for urine specific gravity are found.

The pattern of protein excretion depends on the renal disease responsible for the nephrotic syndrome. In primary nephrotic syndrome, most of the urine protein is albumin; in other diseases, such as glomerulonephritis, both albumin and globulins are lost in increased amounts. This occurrence has led to determinations of "protein selectivity" being proposed as a noninvasive method to separate MCNS from other causes of nephrotic syndrome, such as glomerulonephritis [69, 108, 316]. By comparing clearance of albumin to that of larger molecules, such as IgG or transferrin, a curve can be generated, indicating whether the proteinuria is *selective* and restricted to small molecules or *nonselective*, consisting of both large and small molecules. Characteristically, patients with MCNS show selective proteinuria, while those with other causes for the nephrotic syndrome have nonselective proteinuria. Unfortunately, this generalization is limited by considerable overlap in results from patients in different diagnostic categories, so that the test has limited value for individual patients. This may be due to factors other than molecular size that also affect entry of proteins into the glomerular filtrate and differences in tubular function, which modify reabsorption of filtered protein [518].

The urine sediment from nephrotic subjects often contains oval fat bodies. Lipiduria is better diagnosed, however, using a microscope equipped with polarized light to demonstrate doubly refractile fat bodies ("Maltese crosses") in degenerative fatty vacuoles in the cytoplasm of desquamated renal epithelial cells or free in the urine as neutral fat droplets. Characteristically, urines with heavy proteinuria also contain hyaline casts.

Other urinary findings vary with the cause of the disease. One-third of patients with MCNS may have mild microscopic hematuria, e.g., 10 red blood cells per high-power field in a centrifuged urine sample. Gross hematuria is rarely observed in uncomplicated MCNS. By contrast, it is seen more commonly in patients with prominent mesangial proliferation [73]. In addition, hematuria, particularly gross hematuria, is more likely to be seen in FSGS [607]. In patients with nephrotic syndrome secondary to glomerulonephritis, the urine shows more abnormalities, with cellular elements and granular, cellular, and mixed hyaline casts being present. However, patients with MCNS cannot always be differentiated from those with glomerulonephritis on the basis of urine sediment abnormalities alone.

Blood Studies. Hypoproteinemia is common to all nephrotic patients and is caused, primarily, by hypoalbuminemia. Total serum protein is characteristically reduced to between 4.5 and 5.5 gm/dl; serum albumin concentrations usually fall to below 2 gm/dl and, in children with MCNS, may be less than 1 gm/dl [47]. Although albumin concentrations are usually decreased, those of total globulins are remarkably well preserved despite massive proteinuria. Typically, serum α_1-globulin concentrations are normal or slightly decreased, whereas levels of serum α_2- and β-globulins are increased. Although the concentration of gamma globulin determined by electrophoresis is normal or reduced, the levels of individual components vary. In MCNS [233], serum IgG levels average approximately 20 percent of normal, whereas IgA levels are less severely reduced; IgM and IgE levels are increased. The changes in serum IgG and IgA concentrations are less pronounced in patients with other causes for the nephrotic syndrome, and IgM and IgE typically are normal in these subjects [233].

Hyperlipidemia comprises part of the definition of the nephrotic syndrome. Serum total cholesterol is usually elevated, especially when the serum albumin has fallen to 2 gm/dl or less [54]. Values average 400 mg/dl, but levels in excess of 1,000 mg/dl have been recorded. Other changes in plasma lipids are summarized later in this chapter.

Most often, serum electrolyte concentrations are within the normal range even when anasarca is present, indicating proportionate retention of sodium and water. Mild reductions in the serum sodium concentration to about 130 mEq/L have been reported in the presence of marked hyperlipidemia. This pseudohyponatremia results from the nonaqueous, nonsodium-containing component of the serum or plasma being increased due to hyperlipidemia. It does not require treatment, since the sodium concentration in the aqueous phase of blood is normal, as is plasma osmolality. This artifact is not observed when sodium levels are determined by the newer techniques that measure sodium activity with ion-specific electrodes. Rarely, patients may manifest profound hyponatremia, mediated by elevated plasma vasopressin [635] and by high water ingestion relative to dietary sodium intake [513]. This problem may be exacerbated by diuretic therapy. A decreased anion gap is associated with decreased total serum protein or albumin. This finding is common to all hypoalbuminemic states and is not a direct reflection of either renal dysfunction or altered serum lipid levels [483, 596]. Serum calcium may be low, mainly as a result of the hypoproteinemia. Normally, 40 percent of total serum calcium is bound to protein, primarily albumin. A decrease in serum albumin concentration of 1 gm/dl results in a decrease in total serum calcium of 0.8 mg/dl. In contrast, 1 gm globulin binds only 0.16 mg calcium. In some cases, the hypocalcemia may be out of proportion to the hypoalbuminemia and is caused by a reduction of ionized calcium levels [16] by as much as 5 to 20 percent, possibly because of urinary loss of 25-OH vitamin D (see below). Symptoms of hypocalcemia rarely occur. Total and ionized serum calcium levels return to normal with remission. Serum phosphorus is normal unless the nephrotic syndrome is associated with renal insufficiency.

Blood urea nitrogen and serum creatinine values are characteristically normal in MCNS. Mild elevations of blood urea nitrogen (BUN) occur because of either increased intrarenal urea circulation or increased protein catabolism if the patient has received steroids. Glomerular filtration rate (GFR) measured by inulin clearance is reduced to an average of 80 percent of normal [68]; occasionally, values are reduced to 20 to 30 percent of normal. This may represent the development of acute renal failure secondary to hypovolemia. Reduced GFR at the onset of MCNS is reversible and does not imply an unfavorable outcome [76]. Unfortunately, the presence or absence of azotemia cannot be used as a reliable indicator in the differential diagnosis of the nephrotic syndrome.

Hemoglobin levels and hematocrits may be normal or even increased if there is hemoconcentration secondary to hypoproteinemia. This factor may help to differentiate patients with MCNS from those with severe renal insufficiency from parenchymal disease, in whom anemia is more typical.

Measured levels of serum complement and its components are generally considered to be normal in MCNS as well as in FSGS. Although urinary losses cause decreases in low-molecular-weight complement components, serum concentrations of the components measured to detect activation of the complement cascade are unchanged [614]. Thus, reduced levels of the third component of complement (β-1-C globulin) or C4 indicate that a glomerulonephritis underlies the nephrotic syndrome; conversely, such changes do not occur invariably with glomerulonephritis. Circulating immune complexes may be elevated in MCNS or in FSGS [103, 399]. Plasma renin activity will be discussed later.

Other Studies. In MCNS, the chest radiograph usually shows a normal or small heart size; pleural effusions may be present, as may pneumonitis or pneumonic changes in the lung fields. The presence of an increased heart size and congestive changes in the hilar regions suggests that the nephrotic syndrome is secondary to glomerulonephritis.

Indications for Renal Biopsy. The indications for and benefits of a renal biopsy in patients with nephrotic syndrome remain controversial [223]. The diagnosis of MCNS often can be made by exclusion of other diseases using the clinical and laboratory features just discussed. Thus a renal biopsy is not indicated in every patient with nephrotic syndrome. Children 1 to 6 years of age with all the features of MCNS and no atypical features (Table 64-5) may be given a therapeutic trial of steroids without prior histologic confirmation of the diagnosis. Induction

Table 64-5. Features suggesting that nephrotic syndrome is caused by a disease other than minimal change nephrotic syndrome

History
- Onset: before 1 year or after 6 years of age*
- Past history: skin rashes, joint pains, "nephritis," or hematuria*
- Family history: family member with Alport's syndrome or development of end-stage renal disease*

Physical examination
- General: clinical features of collagen vascular disease
- Blood pressure: marked elevation or evidence of vascular changes in fundi*
- Skin: purpura*
- Subcutaneous tissue: lipodystrophy

Laboratory findings
- Urine: dilute urine
  - urine sediment containing more than 10 red blood cells per high-power field; cylinduria*; nonselective proteinuria*
- Renal function: markedly decreased*
- Chest x-ray: enlarged heart, vascular engorgement, pulmonary edema
- Serology: decreased C3 or C4
  - ANA or anti-DNA positive
- Serum cholesterol: only mild increase*
- Plasma protein: only mild decrease in albumin*
  - markedly decreased or increased globulin

*While these features are unusual for MCNS, their presence does not exclude the lesion.

Table 64-6. Indications for renal biopsy in patients with nephrotic syndrome

At onset
- Features suggesting a diagnosis other than MCNS
- Nephrotic syndrome presenting in the first year of life (especially after third month of life)
- Nephrotic syndrome presenting after age 6 years

Intermediate
- Failure to respond to 28-day course of prednisone given in adequate dosage

Later
- Frequently relapsing nephrotic syndrome
- Steroid-dependent nephrotic syndrome
- Development of steroid resistance
- Change in clinical course, e.g., development of features of glomerulonephritis
- Prior to beginning treatment with a course of cytotoxic drugs

of a complete remission by steroids in such patients is considered to be adequate confirmation of the diagnosis of MCNS [307], although other benign conditions may occasionally appear to respond to steroid therapy [274]. A histologic diagnosis by renal biopsy is recommended in all patients who present with nephrotic syndrome in the first year of life or after the age of 6 years. However, risk–benefit analysis has suggested that biopsy may not be diagnostically superior to a therapeutic trial of steroids even in adults [384]. Other patients who require a biopsy (Table 64-6) are those who are steroid-resistant, who have frequent relapses, or who are candidates for therapy with immunosuppressive drugs.

Frequently, a renal biopsy is technically difficult to perform if the patient has anasarca; surrounding fluid allows the kidney to be ballotted by the biopsy needle. In such subjects, it is preferable to delay the attempted biopsy until after a spontaneous or drug-induced diuresis has occurred and most of the ascites has resolved.

HISTOPATHOLOGY OF PRIMARY NEPHROTIC SYNDROME

Minimal Change Nephrotic Syndrome. The morphologic classification of nephrotic syndrome in childhood derives from classic papers by Churg et al. [133] and White et al. [672]. The term *minimal change nephrotic syndrome* describes a pathologic appearance on light microscopy in which there are no definitive changes from normal in glomeruli (Fig. 64-1), although the degree of change that may be considered significant remains the subject of some controversy. Other terms that have been used to describe this entity include "nil" disease, lipoid nephrosis, and steroid-responsive nephrotic syndrome. Changes in the proximal tubule cells reflect increased reabsorption of protein. These cells may contain apparent vacuoles that are doubly refractile and are similar to the fine lipid droplets seen in oval fat bodies in the urine. The presence of this pathologic abnormality generated the term *lipoid nephrosis.* There is no tubular atrophy, and the renal interstitium is normal. Older patients may show some globally fibrosed glomeruli with associated nephron loss. This is rare in children and should not involve more than 5 to 10 percent of glomeruli even in elderly patients [239]. Typically, there is reduced staining in the glomerular tufts for glomerular polyanion if sections are stained with Alcian blue, colloidal iron, or ruthenium red. Staining with immunofluorescence techniques reveals the absence of immunoglobulin or complement deposition. Electron microscopy (Fig. 64-1) reveals only glomerular epithelial cell foot-process fusion [194]. Recent advances may permit this finding to be visualized on high-resolution light microscopy [279]. The diffuse effacement of the podocytes that frequently contain protein-reabsorptive droplets typically results in the appearance of an almost continuous layer of cytoplasm on the urinary side of the glomerular basement membrane (GBM). There may be apparent segmental detachment of the epithelial cells, producing denuded areas of the GBM. The GBM itself, however, appears normal. There are no electron-dense deposits present adjacent to the GBM [132]. Up to 85 percent of children with primary nephrotic syndrome have this lesion [304], compared to a prevalence of about 20 percent in adults.

Variations in Histopathology. IGM DEPOSITION. Some patients with all the clinical features of MCNS may have minor morphologic differences from those described already. A common variation is the presence of IgM in the glomerular mesangium. An early report [136] suggested that this variant represented a separate entity, which was termed *mesangial IgM nephropathy.* All of the patients, whose ages range from 1.5 to 59 years, showed a

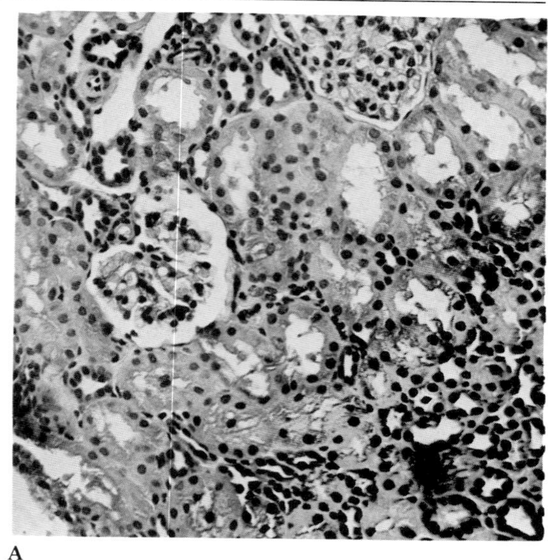

A

Fig. 64-1. Findings on renal biopsies from three children with the clinical features of primary nephrotic syndrome. A. Light microscopy of a patient with minimal change nephrotic syndrome (MCNS). Portions of two glomeruli are shown. Cellularity is normal and the capillary loops are patent. Tubular and interstitial structures are normal in appearance (magnification for all light microscopy, ×350). B. Electron microscopy from the same patient. The endothelial cells (En) lining the capillary loop show a normal fenestrated structure; the glomerular basement membrane (GBM) is uniform in thickness and structure. The epithelial cell (Ep) layer shows characteristic fusion of the epithelial foot processes, with the podocytes being in continuous contact with the GBM. Proteinaceous material and a nucleated cell are present in the capillary lumen (CAP).

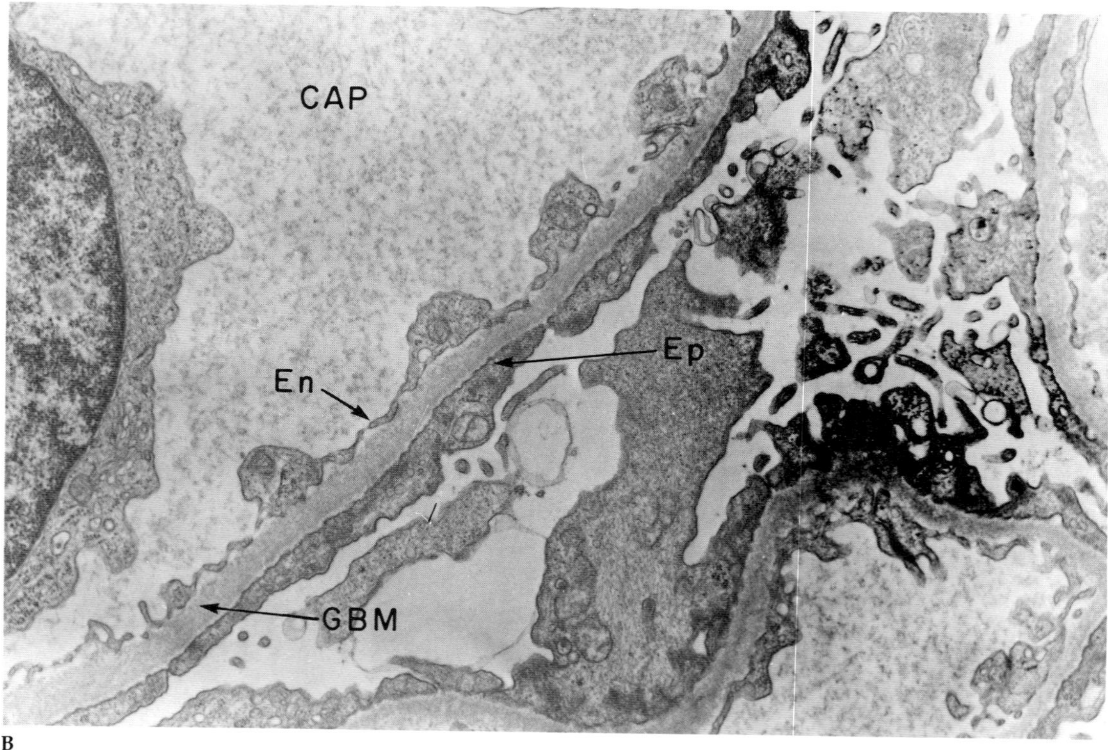

B

slight increase in mesangial matrix and, in addition to the IgM deposits, some had C3 and rare IgA deposition. Dense mesangial deposits were noted on electron microscopy in 9 of the 12 subjects. More recent observations do not support this as being a separate entity. In one study, 40 percent of 149 consecutive patients with the clinical picture of primary nephrotic syndrome were found on biopsy to have mesangial IgM deposits. Of these, 20 had mostly or entirely IgM without complement. They could not be differentiated clinically from other MCNS patients [480]. Because the presence of mesangial deposits of IgM in patients with clinical MCNS does not appear to affect either the patient's response to treatment or disease outcome [510], it is now believed that this finding has little significance.

Recently, a group of adult patients has been described as having steroid-responsive nephrotic syndrome with intercapillary foam cells adherent to Bowman's capsule in a tuft near the tubular origin (the glomerular tip lesion). Although this adhesion is irreversible, the patients appear to have a good prognosis [58].

OTHER IMMUNOGLOBULIN DEPOSITS. Mesangial IgM de-

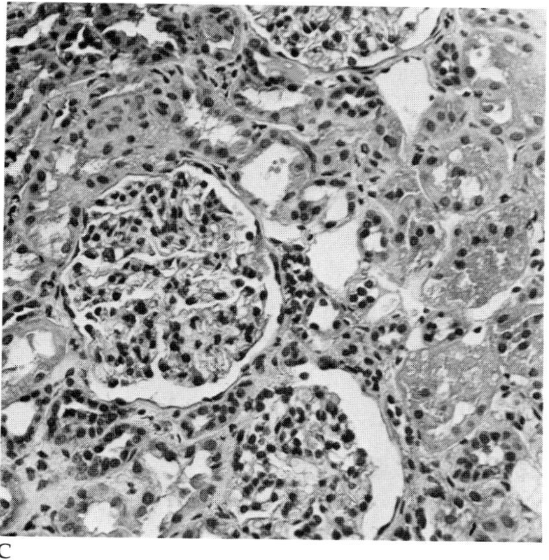

C

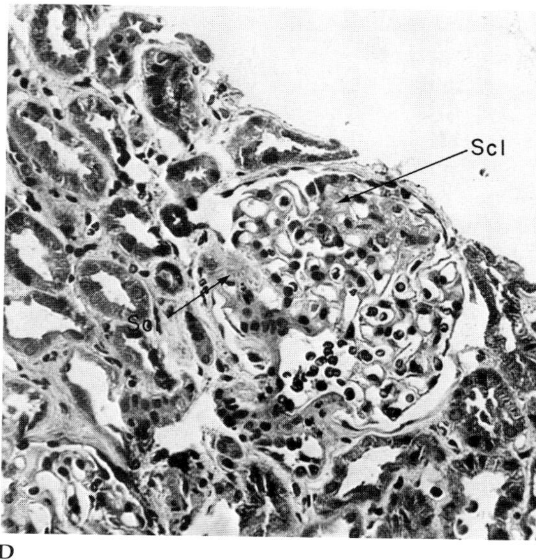

D

Fig. 64-1 (continued) C. Light microscopy in a patient with mesangial hypercellularity. The tubular and glomerular capillary structures are normal, but an increased number of nuclei are present in the mesangial areas of the glomeruli. Immunofluorescent microscopy was negative for immunoglobulins and C3. The patient behaved clinically as one with MCNS. D. Focal segmental glomerulosclerosis. Two focal areas of sclerosis (Scl) are present in the glomerulus; other areas of the glomerulus are normal. No hyalinosis in the glomerulus or tubular atrophy is apparent. (Histology courtesy of Dr. John M. Kissane.)

posits in apparent MCNS may, in some cases, be associated with immune complexes [119]. Since deposits are often found in patients who are biopsied after receiving a trial of corticosteroid therapy, it is of interest that experimental models of immune complex metabolism have suggested that steroid administration may prolong the systemic half-life of larger complexes and enhance and prolong their appearance in a mesangial pattern in the glomerulus [261]. The presence in the glomeruli of immunoglobulins in addition to IgM usually indicates a diagnosis of a disease other than MCNS [381]. A group of patients with a clinical diagnosis of MCNS has been described in which there is some glomerular proliferation associated with immunoglobulin deposits, primarily IgG, in the glomeruli. This lesion is more often observed in black patients [647]. Although they may respond to treatment with steroids initially, their subsequent course is one of frequent relapses or the development of resistance to treatment.

MESANGIAL PROLIFERATION. Some patients with otherwise typical MCNS have increased numbers of mesangial cells in the glomeruli. One study that correlated glomerular morphometry with the patient's clinical course found increased numbers of mesangial nuclei and smaller nuclear size in patients who relapsed frequently. The authors proposed that this indicated mesangial cell activation. They cautioned, however, that disease duration could play a role in the development of this finding, since the frequently relapsing patients had a 4-year course compared to 1.4 years in the population with infrequent relapses [212]. Based on the finding of identical immunohistochemistry in patients with or without mesangial proliferation, it has been argued that mesangial IgM deposition does not appear to play a role in the induction of the mesangial cell response [315]. It has been suggested that mesangial hypercellularity is associated with a decreased response to steroid therapy [15, 218, 240, 509], frequent relapse [15, 288], steroid dependency [643], or a poorer prognosis [278, 655]. The International Study of Kidney Disease in Children (ISKDC) found that approximately 2.5 percent of children with nephrotic syndrome had mesangial hypercellularity [308]. The significance of this finding for patients with focal sclerosis is discussed in the section on Relationship Among Histopathologic Variants.

FOCAL SEGMENTAL GLOMERULOSCLEROSIS (FSGS). In contrast to the preceding variations of MCNS, most of which do not appear to have major clinical significance, the lesion of FSGS strongly influences clinical management and patient outcome. Synonyms for this lesion include focal and segmental glomerulosclerosis with hyalinosis, focal sclerosing glomerulonephritis, and focal sclerosing glomerulopathy. The entity should be distinguished from the finding of occasional globally sclerosed (obsolescent) glomeruli, a benign pattern that is seen in 2 percent or less of glomeruli in childhood but increases somewhat in frequency with age [184].

Rich [545] is generally credited with the initial observation that some patients develop FSGS. Juxtamedullary glomeruli appear particularly susceptible, especially early in the course of the disease, although not all studies have confirmed this observation [259]. The lesion subsequently progresses centrifugally to affect the outer cortical glomeruli. As a consequence, an early, superficial renal biopsy might miss the lesion. Typically, the pathologic abnormalities affect only some glomeruli (focal) with only part of the glomerular tuft involved (segmental). On light microscopy, the segmental sclerosis spreads from the glomerular hilus and is associated with an increase in mesangial matrix. The capillary lumina are collapsed in the affected segments, and there is accumulation of acellular hyaline subendothelial deposits. Special stains have shown these areas to be composed largely of collapsed basement membranes and associated mesangial matrix adherent to Bowman's capsule [262]. Tubular atrophy and interstitial, but not glomerular, inflammatory infiltrates also may be observed [133]. Immunofluorescent microscopy demonstrates IgM and C3 deposits in a granular pattern. Unaffected glomerular areas may reveal IgM and C3 in a mesangial distribution. IgG is usually not present, although both this immunoglobulin and IgA have been reported to be present in some cases [475]. Electron microscopy shows epithelial cell foot-process fusion that, in patients with heavy proteinuria, is diffuse and involves areas of the glomeruli that do not demonstrate sclerosis. Paramesangial and subendothelial, finely granular electron-dense deposits may be seen. Mesangial hypercellularity is present variably.

Development of renal failure is more common in FSGS than in MCNS [296, 607]. In patients in whom advanced renal failure has developed, renal pathology often shows a nonspecific, chronic sclerosing glomerulonephritis, the etiology of which is unclear.

There are numerous differences in descriptions of the clinical and pathologic features of FSGS as well as its prognosis. The incidence of FSGS in patients originally diagnosed as having MCNS has varied from under 10 percent to more than 40 percent in individual studies [456], which may reflect whether the report presents a primary or referral population. Further, there are many causes for the pathologic changes described as FSGS (Table 64-7). Thus it is found in the nephropathy associated with human immunodeficiency virus infection, in heroin abuse, in association with reflux nephropathy, and in a variety of other disorders [246].

Table 64-7. Diseases other than primary nephrotic syndrome that have been associated with the development of focal glomerular sclerosis

Acquired immunodeficiency syndrome [17, 87, 533]
Obstructive uropathy [660]
Decreased nephron mass
Unilateral renal agenesis [350]
Experimental [91]
Drugs
Analgesics [484]
Heroin [146]
Glomerulopathy associated with malignancies [176, 665]
Glomerulonephritis
Poststreptococcal glomerulonephritis [39]
Experimental [627]
Congenital diseases
Familial dysautonomia [512]
Oligomeganephronia [64]
Segmental hypoplasia [246]
Transplantation
Recurrence [401]
De novo [127]
Diabetes mellitus
In humans [386]
Experimental [285]
Aging
Human [83]
Experimental [181]
Miscellaneous
Radiation nephritis [653]
Sickle cell disease [492]
Obesity [135]
Experimental hypertension [175]

Relationship Among Histopathologic Variants. It remains unresolved whether MCNS and FSGS are different diseases or whether they represent a spectrum of presentations of the same disease process. According to the latter view, patients with only a single episode of MCNS constitute the most benign form of the disease; those who have FSGS and progress to end-stage renal failure represent the most malignant variant; and patients with relapsing MCNS and those with steroid-resistant FSGS but stable renal function would represent intermediate forms. In support of this concept are the observations that the clinical presentation of primary nephrotic syndrome in patients with either MCNS or FSGS may be the same; immunofluorescence is identical and ultrastructural findings are similar [557]. Some authors believe that patients may have different histopathologic findings at different times in the disease course, so that findings may change in sequential biopsies. There are documented cases in which apparent MCNS developed into FSGS [271], although it has been suggested that FSGS may have been missed in the early biopsies either because of a sampling error or because no juxtamedullary glomeruli were obtained. In contrast, the marked differences in response to steroid therapy between MCNS and FSGS, as well as the higher frequency of chronic renal failure in the latter, suggest that these represent two distinct disease entities [98].

Consideration of the presence or absence of mesangial proliferative changes in the relationship between MCNS and FSGS must also be taken into account. This pathologic finding may represent a specific entity, a reactive response, or a transitional form between uncomplicated MCNS and FSGS [278]. Both MCNS and FSGS may occur with or without mesangial proliferation. Rather than reflecting a different disease entity, mesangial proliferation could simply indicate a less common and perhaps less benign systemic response to the disease process. This would explain the observation that mesangial proliferation has been found to be an indicator of relatively poor outcome [583]. Alternatively, poorer outcome may imply that mesangial proliferative changes indicate a different pathogenetic process. By this hypothesis, mesangial proliferative glomerulonephritis has histopathologic and physiologic elements similar to MCNS but, in its relative resistance to steroid therapy and the increased risk of azotemia, may represent a different disease [85].

Although there is strong evidence for a relationship among these entities, clinical differences may exist even among patients with the same pathologic findings. For example, two clinical patterns of FSGS have been described: a progressive form presenting on initial development of nephrotic syndrome and a more indolent form in which nephrotic syndrome develops after proteinuria of considerable duration [329]. The authors of this paper proposed a continuum of disease, with varying outcome; this has subsequently been supported by clinicopathologic correlation indicating that predominance of hilar sclerosis and tubulointerstitial disease indicate a poor prognosis in otherwise identical patients [607, 688]. However, the data are equally consistent with the existence of a heterogeneous group of diseases that have the common pathologic finding of FSGS. Certainly, a wide range of diseases have been reported to cause FSGS (Table 64-7). Habib and colleagues [557, 655] have suggested that MCNS, FSGS, and diffuse mesangial proliferation represent variations of primary nephrotic syndrome, which may be found alone or in combination. As indicated in Fig. 64-2, the renal biopsy findings may vary at different stages of the disease. Thus MCNS, FSGS, and mesangial proliferation could be seen alone or in any combination in sequential biopsies in the same patient. To illustrate this point, a patient with FSGS entered remission at age 2 years following steroid therapy. Twenty years later, nephrotic syndrome recurred following treatment with ibuprofen for an unrelated illness. Biopsy showed MCNS that proved to be steroid-responsive [147].

Newer techniques in the evaluation of biopsy material could further elucidate the relationship among the pathologic variants seen in primary nephrotic syndrome. Morphometric analysis may show subtle changes in light microscopy that were previously undetectable [35]. In addition, ultrastructural study has identified increased numbers of dense deposits and microfilamentous structures in focal sclerosis [687], and scanning electron microscopy of isolated glomeruli has identified globular structures adjacent to cells that may be unique to FSGS [489]. Further study using these and other [537] techniques may provide insight into the pathogenesis of the morphologic variants of MCNS and the relationship between them.

MECHANISM OF MESANGIAL CHANGES. Intrinsic kidney cells and cells migrating into the kidney as part of the inflammatory response release factors that regulate mesangial cell proliferation. Mesangial cells produce platelet-derived growth factor (PDGF), a stimulant of endothelial growth and wound healing [1]; prostacyclin and thromboxane, produced by a variety of cells, are stimulatory cofactors for mesangial cell growth [458]. In addition, two autocrine growth mechanisms have been defined. The first involves interleukin-1 (IL-1). Mesangial cells in culture secrete a mesangial cell growth factor with characteristics identical to those of IL-1 [419]. Indeed, these cells express mRNA for IL-1 in vivo [668]. The second autocrine system involves IL-6. Mesangial cell–derived IL-6 stimulates mesangial cell growth in vitro [563]. Moreover, mice transgenic for the human IL-6 gene show marked mesangial proliferation [615]. In human disease, urinary excretion of IL-6 and mesangial staining of biopsy material for IL-6 have been associated with mesangial proliferation by some [283], but not all, authors [546]. Since mesangial proliferative changes are associated with steroid resistance, it is noteworthy that IL-6-induced cell activation is not inhibited by steroids [680]. Finally, negative regulation of mesangial cell growth may be provided by GBM itself, since proliferation of mesangial cells is decreased by heparan sulfate [253].

Mesangial cell activation may have functional implications for both extracellular matrix composition and development of sclerosis. IL-1 stimulates mesangial cell synthesis of prostaglandins, prostacyclin, thromboxane, and type IV collagenase activity [417, 418], perhaps through activation of a protein kinase [417]. Transforming growth factor (TGF)–β increases proteoglycan secretion by cultured mesangial cells [86], and expression of

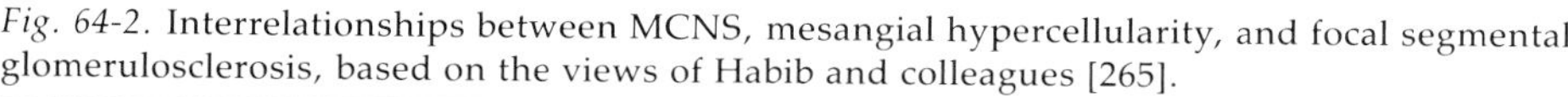
Fig. 64-2. Interrelationships between MCNS, mesangial hypercellularity, and focal segmental glomerulosclerosis, based on the views of Habib and colleagues [265].

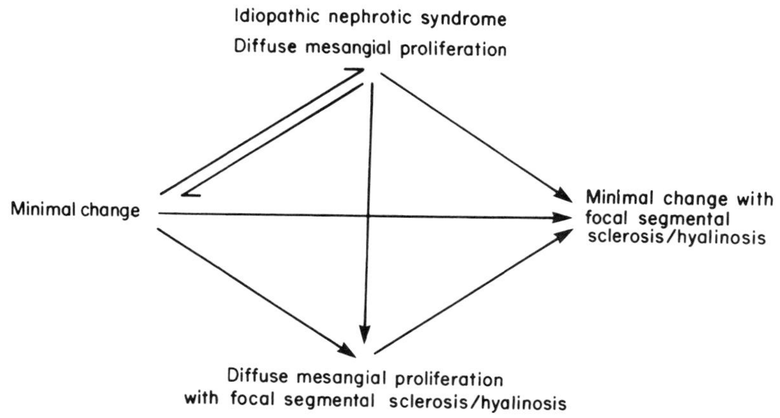

TGF-β by cultured glomeruli correlates with disease severity in an animal model of increased glomerular matrix synthesis [499]. Although this last model represents a disease triggered by inflammation, it can be presumed that regulation of matrix synthesis by endogenously produced TGF-β represents a more generalizable control mechanism. Thromboxane, which is produced by a variety of activated glomerular cells, has recently been reported to stimulate synthesis of laminin, fibronectin, and type IV collagen. This effect was independent of any stimulatory effect on cell division [100a].

MECHANISM OF PROGRESSION TO FSGS. Many explanations have been proposed to explain the development of glomerular sclerosis in some patients with apparent MCNS and for the progression of this lesion to end-stage renal failure. The most widely held theory is that glomerulosclerosis results from the continuing passage of large amounts of plasma proteins across the GBM or directly into the mesangium [539] and is exacerbated by the consistently high-protein dietary intake of modern civilization [91]. Indeed, reports have shown that a low-protein diet may retard the progression of chronic renal insufficiency [300, 353, 500]. In an experimental nephrotic syndrome in rats, a significant correlation was found between the percentage of focally sclerotic glomeruli and the degree of proteinuria that occurred. Unilateral nephrectomy markedly exacerbated the sclerotic process in the remaining kidney, suggesting an accelerating effect of increased protein load per nephron [238]. A high-protein diet accelerates nephron loss in animals with 5/6 nephrectomy [344], and a low-protein diet prevents sclerosis in doxorubicin-treated rats [541]. In humans, four patients who had undergone uninephrectomy for nonnephrotic disease were found to have FSGS on renal biopsy when investigated for the development of proteinuria several years later [692]. However, long-term follow-up studies of sizeable populations of kidney donors have not confirmed that hyperfiltration damages the remaining kidney [266]. Moreover, many patients with chronically relapsing or steroid-resistant MCNS have massive proteinuria, but only a limited number develop FSGS. Thus additional factors may be important in the genesis of glomerular sclerosis.

There is considerable experimental evidence in animals that hemodynamic changes play a role in the development of FSGS. A strain of male Wistar rats develops spontaneous glomerulosclerosis as they age. The lesions begin in the juxtaglomerular region. A low-sodium diet significantly retards the development of the pathology and progression of the proteinuria [181]. The association of hypertension and vascular disease with FSGS in another animal model also implicates hemodynamic factors [3]. Control of glomerular hypertension appears to limit progression of scarring in rat models [20, 538]. In humans, meclofenamate administration slowed progression of disease in recurrent FSGS in a renal transplant recipient, presumably by altering renal hemodynamics [634]. The possibility that hemodynamics may mediate the lesion as well as causing progression [175] is supported by the observation that glomerular hypertrophy in patients with apparent MCNS is frequently predictive of subsequent development of FSGS [204].

A hypercoagulable state may also contribute to the development of FSGS and its progression to end-stage renal failure. Coagulation abnormalities, present in patients with nephrotic syndrome (see below), resolve when the patient enters remission [14]. Persistence of these abnormalities in patients who are unresponsive to therapy could result in the development of FSGS. Indeed, fibrin has been found in both sclerosed and nonsclerosed segments of glomeruli in FSGS [649]. Furthermore, treatment with anticoagulants has been shown to reverse coagulation abnormalities and improve the prognosis for both patients and experimental animals with a variety of progressive glomerulopathies that are often associated with glomerular sclerosis [169, 210, 528, 552]. Recent observations have suggested, however, that the role of heparin may be as an inhibitor of growth of arteriolar smooth muscle after injury rather than as an anticoagulant [117]. It is possible that the inciting event for the coagulation changes could be visceral cell injury, which results from protein overload [246]. Fibrin deposition would then lead to sclerotic changes, a process that could become self-perpetuating [107].

Analysis of renal biopsy material from 472 patients, most of whom were nephrotic, suggested that retarded mesangial transport of immune complexes resulted in their accumulation, especially in the paraarterial regions and the afferent arteriole. Supplemental experimental studies suggested that these changes predisposed to the development of focal sclerosis [437]. This finding is consistent with the suggestion that the rapidly progressive form of FSGS may represent a vascular disease [98] and supports the hypothesis that different clinical patterns in FSGS represent different etiologies.

Other factors intrinsic to the glomerulus may be involved in disease progression. In young rats subjected to subtotal nephrectomy and evaluated for development of sclerosis, the greatest increase in single-nephron GFR occurred in superficial nephrons, but sclerosis was greatest in the deeper (juxtamedullary) nephrons [302]. This sclerosis may be mediated by alterations in matrix synthesis, with increased expression of laminin and collagen but decreased heparan sulfate proteoglycans observed in one model [177]. A number of transgenic models of FSGS have been developed to investigate intrinsic regulatory processes in the glomerulus. These include a portion of human immunodeficiency virus (HIV) DNA [7, 358a] and mice overexpressing growth hormone [423]. In a model in which mice are transgenic for the viral SV-40 large T antigen, which is associated with increased cellular proliferation, glomerular size increase was accompanied by sclerosis; this suggested that regulation of growth within the glomerulus is important in the development of FSGS [167]. In another model, only mice homozygous for a transgenic retrovirus developed focal sclerosis. Because all the affected animals in this model had a common insertion point for the proviral DNA, the insertion may have interrupted expression of a gene responsible for normal glomerular morphogenesis or function [666]. Other genetic factors may be equally significant [3].

Lipid nephrotoxicity [471] may also affect both the development and progression of FSGS (see the section on Hyperlipidemia). This hypothesis is supported by both the similarity of the FSGS lesion to that of atherosclerosis [34] and hemodynamic alterations induced by hyperlipidemia [19]. Intrarenal release of arachidonic acid metabolites [529], perhaps by mononuclear leukocytes [566] could also mediate hemodynamic and proliferative changes. It is apparent that progression of glomerular scarring is multifactorial [163]; the specific mechanisms involved in idiopathic FSGS remain to be elucidated.

NEPHROTIC SYNDROME IN THE FIRST YEAR OF LIFE

Nephrotic syndrome may occur in the first year of life and can result from MCNS. Much more frequently, however, it is due to congenital nephrotic syndrome, especially that associated with infantile microcystic disease [267, 294]. This lesion is most commonly found in Finland and in people of Finnish ancestry, but it has been described as well in many other ethnic groups throughout Europe and North America. The disease is inherited as an autosomal recessive trait. Affected infants typically have a large placenta, with the placental-to-fetal weight ratio ranging from 0.25 to 0.43 compared to a normal 0.14. They often are born prematurely, may show signs of perinatal asphyxia, and have a high perinatal mortality rate. Indeed, the incidence of early death from congenital nephrotic syndrome may be higher than that reported, since edema and failure to thrive may not become apparent for several weeks or months, even though proteinuria is present from birth. The course in infancy is usually one of progressive deterioration with hypoalbuminemia, edema, and wasting dominating the clinical picture. Renal function is usually decreased but renal failure does not occur. Half of the patients die before 6 months of age and few survive past 2 years. In the past, dialysis and renal transplantation were not thought to be beneficial in these patients. A recent report showed that aggressive medical management, combined with nephrectomy to prevent protein loss (and improve intractible edema and nutritional status), and renal transplantation dramatically improved the outlook. More than two-thirds of the patients survived, and there was a marked increase in growth rate [427].

Histologic changes of the congenital nephrotic syndrome can be subtle in the newborn. They include dilated cortical tubules from which the entity derives its name (i.e., infantile microcystic disease), mesangial hypercellularity, and glomerulosclerosis, none of which is pathognomonic for the congenital nephrotic syndrome of the Finnish type. An inherited metabolic defect in basement-membrane synthesis has been postulated as the cause of the disease, and a significant reduction in the number of negative charge sites in the GBM has been reported [651] in support of this thesis. Prenatal diagnosis can be confirmed by finding increased α-fetoprotein levels in the amniotic fluid.

Other idiopathic types of congenital nephrotic syndrome have been described. These are less well defined and probably represent a heterogeneous group of diseases, most of which do not appear to be inherited [366]. They are distinguished from the Finnish type by the combination of clinical characteristics and histologic picture. Most have a poor prognosis, but the clinical course is often more protracted. Attempts have been made to classify these lesions according to the dominant pathologic findings. According to this approach, the presence of microcystic disease has been used to diagnose the Finnish type of congenital nephrotic syndrome. In the absence of microcystic tubules, the disease has been classified on the basis of the most prominent glomerular lesion, for example, mesangial proliferation, focal segmental glomerulosclerosis, or global glomerular sclerosis. In the absence of such changes, the patient is diagnosed as having MCNS. A recent study has summarized the problems of this classification system. It emphasizes that microcystic tubules are neither specific nor diagnostic for the Finnish lesion and may be acquired as a consequence of severe proteinuria in the immature kidney [598]. In an effort to distinguish among these types of infantile nephrosis and identify abnormal basement membrane synthesis, the ratio of urinary heparan sulfate to chondroitin sulfate was measured in 37 patients and 17 healthy controls. However, patients with Finnish-type disease, diffuse mesangial sclerosis and focal sclerosis had elevated ratios, whereas children with MCNS had studies similar to normal subjects [311a].

Diffuse mesangial sclerosis may be the dominant pathologic picture in some infants with nephrotic syndrome. Prognosis is poor, irrespective of whether the onset of disease is congenital or infantile. Congenital glomerulosclerosis characterized by hyalinized glomeruli in otherwise normal kidneys also has been found in infants developing nephrotic syndrome and renal failure early in life. Evidence has been presented suggesting that such lesions are the consequence of intrauterine infections [57]. Other entities that have been associated with the nephrotic syndrome in the first year of life are summarized in Table 64-8.

The importance of diagnosing congenital nephrotic syndrome of the Finnish type is that is permits genetic counselling. Establishing an exact histologic diagnosis in other patients appears to be less important in developing a treatment regimen and predicting outcome. Rather, age at presentation is a more important factor. An extensive analysis [598] found that 97 percent of 177 patients died or subsequently required care for end-stage renal disease if they presented with nephrotic syndrome in the first 3 months of life. In contrast, death or end-stage disease occurred in only 31 percent of patients with onset of nephrotic syndrome between the ages of 3 and 12 months. A pathologic diagnosis in these infants is helpful, since some of the lesions, especially MCNS, benefit from treatment with corticosteroid drugs.

TREATMENT

Treatment of MCNS and Related Disorders. The optimal treatment for this group of diseases is still evolving. It is

Table 64-8. Causes of the nephrotic syndrome in the first year of life

Relatively common
- Congenital nephrotic syndrome of the Finnish (inherited) variety [267, 294]
- Other congenital nephrotic syndromes [326, 598]

Less common
- Diffuse mesangial sclerosis [263, 366, 598]
- Focal segmental glomerulosclerosis, congenital glomerulosclerosis, and hyalinosis [57]
- MCNS
- Acquired immunodeficiency syndrome

Rare
- Wilms' tumor [409]
- Nail-patella syndrome [601]
- Pseudohermaphroditism [250, 608]
- XY gonadal dysgenesis [226]
- Mercury intoxication [675]
- Hemolytic uremic syndrome [232]
- Syphilis [327, 619]
- Toxoplasmosis [591]
- Cytomegalic inclusion disease [158]
- Renal vein thrombosis [402]

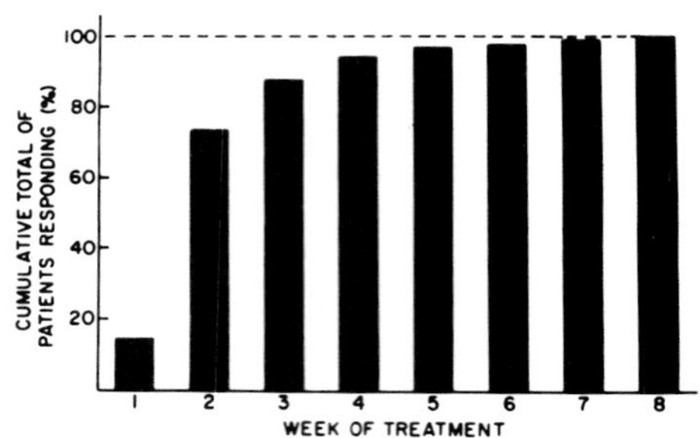

Fig. 64-3. The cumulative rate of response to treatment with prednisone of children with primary nephrotic syndrome. Only steroid-sensitive patients are included in this analysis. The majority of patients respond in the second or third week of treatment. A small percentage, however, may take 7 or 8 weeks to respond. (Data derived from ISKDC [307].)

noteworthy that in the era before current drugs were available, 25 percent of children with idiopathic nephrotic syndrome underwent a spontaneous remission [139]. Even today, a careful history will often suggest that prior to the presenting episode, the nephrotic patient has had one or more periods of edema that resolved without treatment. The association between MCNS and both allergy and malignancy has been reviewed already. An occasional patient with frequently relapsing MCNS may enter long-term remission only when a dietary allergen is withdrawn [286] or an underlying malignancy is identified and treated [656, 665]. Thus the possibility that either of these conditions is responsible for the patient's symptoms should be considered before any drug therapy is instituted.

Before 1940, the mortality rate in nephrotic syndrome was 40 percent; the major cause of death was infection [45]. The introduction of antibiotics reduced mortality by more than 50 percent. The development of corticosteroids has further reduced mortality to between 3 and 7 percent [133, 265, 673]. The major benefits of steroids, however, may well be the faster induction of a remission and reduction of morbidity, although this has never been subjected to a controlled trial. In the older adult nephrotic patient, the risk of undesirable side effects of steroids could outweigh the benefits of these drugs [134]. Despite these caveats, adrenocorticosteroids remain the main therapeutic agent for primary nephrotic syndrome.

PREDNISONE. Cessation of proteinuria in response to the oral administration of prednisone is virtually diagnostic of MCNS in children aged 1 to 6 years who present with all the clinical features of this disease. The standard dosage regimen for inducing a remission is 2 mg/kg of body weight per day or 60 mg/m^2 surface area per day given in a single daily dose [448]. We prefer this to the alternate approach of giving the same total dose in three divided doses per day. In our experience, the single daily dose is more effective, perhaps because it achieves higher peak blood levels, and short-term side effects are fewer. In addition, it is more convenient to administer, with a lesser chance of missed doses. The daily dose is rounded up to the nearest multiple of 20 mg, never exceeding 100 mg/day. It should be ascertained that the patient does not have subclinical pulmonary tuberculosis before therapy with prednisone is begun.

Typically, patients respond with a diuresis and resolution of proteinuria. In most instances, response can be considered to have occurred if the patient has had protein-free urine for at least 3 days (Table 64-9). This occurs within 2 weeks of starting treatment in 75 percent of cases (Fig. 64-3) and in over 90 percent by 4 weeks. According to the definitions derived by the ISKDC and others (Table 64-9), patients who do not respond by this time are considered to be steroid-resistant. However, response may be delayed for up to 8 or more weeks in a small percentage of cases, so that approximately 95 percent of patients eventually will be found to be steroid-responsive. Serum albumin levels may not return to normal for up to 3 months [501], and serum lipid abnormalities may persist for protracted periods, too [691].

The persistence of proteinuria does not always indicate steroid resistance. Postural proteinuria may persist in a minority of patients [40] and, in others, contraction of blood volume consequent upon a brisk diuresis may result in renin-mediated proteinuria [82]. In either case, the degree of proteinuria is moderate, typically registering 1+ to 2+ on dipstick or being less than 1 gm per day. This should not be misinterpreted as partial responsiveness and should not be used to justify continuing steroid therapy in high dosage. Alternatively, failure to respond to steroids may indicate the presence of an occult infection [448] or frequent relapse may relate to poor adrenal function in the patient [392]. This latter conclusion was based on adrenocorticotropic hormone (ACTH) stimulation tests performed on children with MCNS before or after completion of therapy. The average duration of remission was longer in patients who showed an intact endogenous response at all times, as

Table 64-9. Some definitions used to describe patients with minimal change nephrotic syndrome*

Relapse
Proteinuria (> 1+ on dipstick or > 4 mg/hr/m² surface area) for at least 1 week
Response
Protein-free urine (< 1+ on dipstick or < 4 mg/hr/m² surface area) for at least 3 days
Steroid responsive
Response to prednisone (≥ 60 mg/m² surface area per day) within 8 weeks of starting treatment†
Frequent relapsing nephrotic syndrome
Initially responsive to prednisone: at least two relapses in a subsequent 6-month period or five in 18 months
Steroid dependent nephrotic syndrome
Initially responsive to prednisone:
Either two consecutive relapses during period of steroid taper
Or two consecutive relapses, each occurring within 2 weeks of ending a course of corticosteroid therapy

*Derived from [26, 303–310, 456].
†Some studies define steroid-responsive patients as those responding within 4 weeks of starting treatment. Those responding between 5 and 8 weeks are referred to as late responders.

indicated by cortisol production. While virtually all children with decreased responses relapsed within 1 year, only half of children with normal responses did so [393]. Early relapse in the children with poor adrenal function was prevented by low-dose maintenance cortisol administration [391, 392]. This finding is supported by observations from others, even though adrenal function was not evaluated in their patients [582]. The data from patients tested before treatment suggest that the endocrine abnormality may, in some patients, reflect the underlying disease process as well as the effect of exogenous steroid administration.

After response to treatment, the dose of steroids is reduced in stepwise fashion during the next 4 to 12 weeks, depending on the preference of individual centers. Irrespective of the length of time used to taper steroid dosage, the goal should be to start an alternate-day schedule within 4 weeks of response. The purpose of this approach is to reduce the incidence of steroid-induced side effects. Alternate-day therapy has been found to be more effective than the use of intermittent therapy in which steroids are given on three successive days in each 7-day period [96, 282] and is less disruptive to the pituitary-adrenal axis.

One widely used regimen administers prednisone, 60 mg/m²/day for 4 weeks, followed by 40 mg/m² every other day for 4 weeks and then discontinuation [25, 96]. It has been our practice to taper therapy over 10 or 12 weeks to decrease the likelihood of relapse, which is higher when shorter tapering periods are employed [28, 305]. For a patient who is treated initially with prednisone 60 mg per day, the dose is reduced to 40 mg per day after response and 2 weeks later to 40 mg on alternate days. The dose subsequently is reduced by 50 percent every 2 weeks. Finally, prednisone, 5 mg on alternate days, is given for 2 weeks, after which the drug is discontinued.

Although earlier reports suggested that as many as 50 percent of steroid-responsive children do not relapse after the initial episode of nephrotic syndrome, recent observations indicate that this figure approximates only 25 percent [257, 287]. The difference could be due to an altering pattern of disease but more likely reflects the types of patients being referred to reporting centers. Comparable figures for adults with MCNS are not readily available. Another 25 to 30 percent of children have infrequent relapses and usually respond well to further courses of steroids, as already described. The remaining patients have either frequently relapsing or steroid-dependent nephrotic syndrome (Table 64-9). These latter two groups of patients are most prone to develop serious and unacceptable steroid side effects, because attempts to control relapses of their disease with steroids result in protracted use of these drugs. In an effort to minimize these side effects, alternative regimens using smaller doses of steroids have been proposed. The lower response and higher relapse rate associated with these approaches may result eventually in the use of higher cumulative doses of steroids and may not be justified [28]. Indeed, a recent study has suggested that, for some frequently relapsing patients, maintenance on daily rather than alternate-day steroids while tapering the dosage results in less frequent relapse and equal or lesser cumulative steroid dose [677]. Generally, development of severe side effects from steroids in the frequently relapsing or steroid-dependent nephrotic patient should be an indication to treat the disease by some other therapeutic regimen (see the following discussion).

A small but significant percentage of MCNS patients who are steroid-responsive initially will become steroid-resistant after one or more subsequent relapses. This development is an indication for renal biopsy and frequently denotes the presence of FSGS.

Several attempts have been made to correlate pathology with response to steroids or with the pattern of relapses. Frequency of relapse showed no correlation with histopathology in a study by the ISKDC [309] but early relapse after the initial episode was predictive of more frequent relapses subsequently. In another study, this same group found that delaying the change from daily to alternate-day dosage schedule for frequently relapsing patients prolonged the duration of remission [305].

The presence of IgM deposits does not appear to have an effect on response to steroids [349]. Although initial observations suggested that patients with mesangial hypercellularity respond to treatment in a manner similar to that seen in MCNS [100], recent studies indicate that a considerable proportion of these patients may be steroid unresponsive [14, 218]. However, evaluation of large groups of children indicates that persistence of proteinuria is only weakly predictive of mesangial hypercellularity on biopsy [65, 308].

In general, the response rate to steroids in adult MCNS patients is comparable to that reported in children [111, 689]. Adult patients, however, may be particularly prone to complications consequent upon prednisone therapy [68].

OTHER STEROID THERAPY. Alternative steroid regimens have been attempted in an effort to improve response to therapy. High-dose pulses of intravenous methylprednisolone have been utilized in a small series of patients and appeared to decrease frequency of relapses [524]. Remission was reported to occur in 5 of 8 corticosteroid-resistant children treated with methylprednisolone pulses, although this therapy did not benefit corticosteroid-dependent subjects [479]. In yet another experience, methylprednisolone pulses reduced proteinuria but did not result in remission in patients resistant to oral steroids given in conventional doses [556]. Methylprednisolone pulses were less effective than standard therapy in adult patients [685].

An occasional patient who does not respond to oral steroid therapy will respond to an equivalent dose of the drug given as methylprednisolone by intramuscular injection. The patient's weekly dose of prednisone is calculated and given as a long-acting preparation of methylprednisolone in either weekly or twice weekly injections. It is not clear whether this improved response to injection of steroids relates to the patient's compliance, to poor absorption of oral drugs, or to the metabolism of steroids by the liver. The routine measurement of prednisolone kinetics, however, does not appear to help in the management of children with MCNS [560].

CYCLOPHOSPHAMIDE. It was reported in 1958 that nitrogen mustard, given at the end of a course of ACTH, enhanced the duration of remission in patients with MCNS [669]. Subsequent studies have confirmed the efficacy of nitrogen mustard analogues. However, the potentially severe side effects of these drugs have limited their use. Cyclophosphamide and related drugs are usually recommended only in frequently relapsing and steroid-dependent nephrotic patients, especially in those with marked steroid side effects [400]. It is our recommendation that histologic confirmation of MCNS should be obtained before the drug is used. An alternative view argues that initial [443a] or continued [585] steroid responsiveness eliminates the need to obtain a biopsy. The original regimen of cyclophosphamide utilized dosages of 5 mg/kg per day but was associated with a high incidence of leukopenia, loss of hair, and cystitis [445] and is no longer recommended. Most centers obtain satisfactory results with a dosage of 2 mg/kg per day given for no more than 90 consecutive days; others have reported equally good results with 2.5 mg/kg per day for 8 weeks [50, 110, 309, 445]. At a dose of 2 mg/kg/day, an 8-week course of cyclophosphamide is followed by a higher relapse rate [26]. In children with steroid-dependent nephrotic syndrome, prolonging the course to 12 weeks increases the likelihood of a prolonged remission [27]. It has been suggested that frequently relapsing adults are more responsive than children to cyclophosphamide [494].

The use of cyclophosphamide alone has been reported to be effective in the treatment of adult patients with MCNS [13]. The majority of centers, however, prefer to utilize cyclophosphamide in conjunction with steroids [109]. Certainly, the induction of a remission with steroids before instituting therapy with cyclophosphamide permits a liberal fluid intake to induce a high urine flow rate during treatment with the immunosuppressive agent, reducing the risk of cystitis [170].

Cyclophosphamide therapy is often effective for frequent relapse. Approximately 65 percent of such patients remain in remission for at least 5 years after treatment [109, 447], and permanent remissions have been reported in 50 percent of patients [174]. Response to cyclophosphamide may be predictable from the pattern of relapse after steroids. Of those patients who relapse immediately after tapering of steroids, two-thirds also relapse quickly after cyclophosphamide. Conversely, frequently relapsing patients who can maintain remission more than 14 days after stopping steroids have longer remissions and suffer fewer relapses after cyclophosphamide [26].

It is rare to see acute side effects with the current drug regimens using cyclophosphamide, although white blood cell counts should be monitored at least weekly, especially early in the course of therapy. The frequency of cystitis, alopecia, or leukopenia due to cyclophosphamide has been reduced markedly by institution of smaller daily and cumulative doses of the drug than were utilized initially. The gonadal toxicity of cyclophosphamide also appears to be dose-related; testicular and ovarian toxicity are uncommon if the total dose is below 200 mg/kg [190, 395]. However, such doses do decrease sperm counts [639]. Higher doses lead to more significant testicular dysfunction [75]. Female patients treated with a mean total dose of 439 mg/kg at an average age of 8.7 years were followed for a mean of 12.3 years. All had normal pubertal development and regular menstrual patterns. Hormonal studies did not show obvious ovarian or pituitary-gonadal dysfunction, and two patients had borne normal children [74]. In children, the drug is usually given well before puberty in an effort to minimize the risk of gonadal toxicity, although it has been suggested that prepubertal males are more sensitive than pubertal males [511]. Concern has been expressed about the potential for cyclophosphamide to induce malignancies. It remains uncertain whether this is a major risk of current therapeutic regimens used in nephrotic syndrome, although leukemia has been reported in at least one child treated for nephrotic syndrome with prednisone and cyclophosphamide [368]. Furthermore, the use of cyclophosphamide may be associated with findings of increased sister chromatid exchange [185] and long-lasting immunosuppressive effects [126]. The development of infections, especially varicella, during the period of treatment with cyclophosphamide is of concern, although effective treatment with acyclovir has been reported [523].

CHLORAMBUCIL. Many of the side effects of cyclophosphamide are shared by chlorambucil; the major advantage of this latter drug is that it does not induce cystitis. Unlike cyclophosphamide, it has been reported to produce seizures in some patients [673] and may induce electroencephalographic changes in the absence of seizures in others [438]. At least three nephrotic children treated with this drug have developed malignancies [356, 478]. However, the overall incidence of serious complications with chlorambucil is low, especially when it is used in a dose of 0.1 to 0.2 mg/kg per day for an 8-week course [514]. It has been reported to produce a more stable remission than cyclophosphamide [258, 674] and to be effective in some steroid-dependent and cyclophosphamide-resistant children with nephrotic syndrome [186].

CYCLOSPORINE. In preliminary studies, cyclosporin A has been reported to be effective in certain adult and pediatric cases of steroid-unresponsive, steroid-dependent, or frequently relapsing nephrotic patients [352, 460, 491, 624]. Currently it is suggested that this drug, in a dosage ranging around 150 mg/m^2/day, is effective in inducing and sustaining remission in steroid-responsive MCNS and allows steroid medication to be discontinued. After termination of the cyclosporine, however, the patients again experience a high rate of relapse. Using this dosage, no nephrotoxicity and minimal other side effects were observed. The major advantage of this drug appears, at present, to be the reduction of side effects in steroid-toxic patients [95]. Preliminary data suggest that a combination of cyclosporin A and prednisone, both given in low doses for protracted periods of time, may produce prolonged remission [491].

OTHER DRUGS. Levamisole, an antihelmintic drug and immunopotentiating agent, has been used to successfully treat children with MCNS [621]. In one study [490], 30 children with frequently relapsing nephrotic syndrome were treated with oral levamisole, 2.5 mg/kg body weight twice a week for a mean period of 9.9 months. In 16 children, corticosteroid dose could be reduced significantly without relapse, while the drug was ineffective in the remaining 14 children. The only side effects noted were a decrease in neutrophil count in 7 of the patients who responded to the drug and transient granulocytopenia in 3. A recent study indicates that levamisole may be a useful steroid-sparing maintenance drug in steroid dependent patients [93b].

Therapy with nonsteroidal anti-inflammatory drugs has been attempted in patients with MCNS with variable results [171, 221]. Some of the patients selected for this therapy were unresponsive to all standard forms of treatment and may represent a recalcitrant population, accounting for the disappointing results [221]. Although indomethacin and other nonsteroidal anti-inflammatory agents have a theoretical use in protecting against progressive nephron loss, administration of indomethacin to nephrotic patients has led to a high incidence of irreversible renal failure [354]. Reversible acute renal failure [92, 413] and the development of nephrotic syndrome [147, 148, 200] also have been described following the use of these drugs to treat other diseases.

SYMPTOMATIC TREATMENT. Many, but not all, patients with nephrotic syndrome respond to the acute use of diuretics, with marked increases of urinary losses of sodium and water. Although diuretics may be effective, there are limited indications for their use in the acute treatment of nephrotic subjects, especially children. The degree of diuresis and natriuresis they induce is small compared to that observed when the patient responds to treatment with steroids. Thus these drugs may not reduce significantly the patient's morbidity or length of stay in the hospital. Furthermore, it is possible that diuretic use, by depleting intravascular as well as interstitial fluid volume, may contribute to the development of shock seen in some patients with MCNS [683]. In addition, a diuretic-induced increase in urine output may complicate the interpretation of whether steroids are inducing a remission, the first sign of which typically is an increased urine output [501]. Diuretic therapy may be less effective in patients with idiopathic nephrotic syndrome than in most other patients, in part because of a combination of factors resulting in physiologically decreased ability to excrete sodium (see section on Consequences of Proteinuria). This is especially true of the loop diuretics such as furosemide. The efficacy of furosemide may also be inhibited by its binding to albumin present in the tubular lumen [350a]. Although spironolactone enhances distal nephron sodium delivery, its delayed onset of action and relatively weak potency limit its utility to a potentiating agent with loop diuretics. Metolazone, which impedes both proximal and late distal nephron sodium absorption [59], may be the most effective oral diuretic in patients with sodium retention secondary to nephrotic syndrome.

However, if the patient has anasarca, if respiratory embarrassment results from ascites, if scrotal edema is sufficiently severe to threaten perforation [667], or if peritonitis is present, then more aggressive therapy to decrease the amount of edema is warranted. A useful regimen consists of oral spironolactone, 1 mg/kg per day given in three divided doses, and daily intravenous infusions of albumin: 0.5 gm/kg initially, increasing, if well tolerated, to 1 gm/kg per day. The albumin infusion should be preceded by the intravenous infusion of furosemide 0.5 mg/kg. A repeat dose of diuretic is given toward the end of the albumin infusion. Blood pressure should be monitored throughout the albumin infusion to help avoid complications from rapid mobilization of edema fluid into the circulation, although the regimen is usually free from significant side effects when used in children and young adults.

Patients with steroid-unresponsive or steroid-dependent nephrotic syndrome may be controlled symptomatically on a chronic basis with dietary sodium restriction and diuretics. Oral furosemide or metolazone, used alone or in combination, or in conjunction with spironolactone, is usually effective. Most patients learn to individualize their dosage. Unless there is evidence for progressive loss of renal function, this regimen probably is preferable to attempting control of the nephrotic syndrome with longer-term steroid therapy because of the significant complication rate of this latter approach. However, progressive interstitial nephritis has been reported in nephrotic patients chronically treated with diuretics, especially furosemide [456].

IMMUNIZATION. Because patients often develop bacterial peritonitis (see Complications of Nephrotic Syndrome), some clinicians support immunization with pneumococcal polysaccharide vaccines. However, concern regarding possible poor response to immunogens in nephrotic patients, and the potential for an immunogenic stimulus to trigger a relapse, has made the issue of childhood immunization a controversial one. A recent survey of North American pediatric nephrologists [574] indicated that most modified their approach to immunization but that there was little evidence to strongly support recommendations regarding any specific practices.

Treatment of Patients with Steroid-Resistant MCNS. A small percentage of patients with MCNS appear resistant to standard approaches to inducing remission. We have found that, in several patients, a tapered course of parenteral sustained-release, intramuscular methylprednisolone and prolonged chlorambucil (4 months at a dose sufficient to decrease the peripheral white blood count to less than 5,000/mm^3) may either induce remission or decrease proteinuria sufficiently that the patient may be edema-free with little or no additional diuretic therapy. This treatment must be employed cautiously after full consideration of its potential long-term side effects such as risk of neoplasm. Alternatively, patients may be maintained on a regimen of sodium and fluid restriction combined with judicious use of diuretics. Balancing the desire to minimize tissue edema against the importance of avoiding intravascular volume depletion is a rigorous challenge for the clinician.

Nonsteroidal anti-inflammatory drugs such as indomethacin and meclofenamate will reduce proteinuria in some patients and have been suggested in the management of nephrotic proteinuria. They are ineffective in about one-third of patients, are not always well tolerated, and may cause a decrease in renal function [354, 464]. Most studies have evaluated treatment in membranous and membranoproliferative disease [61]. However, one study evaluated use of these drugs in children with frequently relapsing or steroid-resistant MCNS; some patients showed a reduction in proteinuria, but all remained nephrotic [221].

Angiotensin converting enzyme inhibitors decrease proteinuria in diabetic patients and in those with various renal diseases, including children with steroid-resistant nephropathies [464, 636]. The mechanism appears to relate to decreased glomerular filtration pressure [272]. In some patients, the response is sufficient to reduce or eliminate the need for diuretics, and the reduction of proteinuria is sustained. The drug is usually well tolerated and may thus have a role in treatment of steroid-resistant children.

Treatment of Focal Segmental Glomerulosclerosis (FSGS). Analyzing the response to treatment of patients with FSGS is complicated by the fact that this pathologic lesion may be seen with a variety of disorders in addition to primary nephrotic syndrome. In general, few adult patients respond to treatment with either steroids or cytotoxic drugs alone. Although it is stated that only a minority of FSGS patients unresponsive to steroids will respond to alkylating agents [426], a compilation of reported cases has demonstrated a significant increase in remission rate for patients receiving prednisone plus alkylating agents compared to patients receiving no treatment at all [523]. Thus with appropriate consideration of the potential risks, a limited course of treatment with cytotoxic therapy may have a role in management of adults with FSGS.

The response of children with FSGS to treatment with cytoxic drugs has been better documented and is somewhat more favorable. A review of nine series involving children [456] revealed that 23 percent of 247 children with FSGS were steroid-responsive; 70 of the patients were treated with cytotoxic drugs, of whom 30 percent responded; at the time of their last examination, 19.5 percent of the 247 children were in remission. It was not possible to determine how many of these children had FSGS documented when they presented with nephrotic syndrome and how many were found to have this lesion only when they became steroid-resistant after having previous episodes of steroid-responsive nephrotic syndrome. These latter children usually prove resistant to all forms of treatment, including the use of cyclophosphamide [306]. Although it has been reported that chlorambucil may be effective [41], this has not been evaluated in a larger, prospective controlled trial.

Alternative therapeutic approaches have been sought. In an uncontrolled pilot study, the nonsteroidal anti-inflammatory agent, meclofenamate, was found to reduce urine protein by 40 percent without decreasing GFR in more than half of the 30 steroid-resistant nephrotic adults studied, 16 of whom had FSGS [650]. In another study, patients with FSGS who were unresponsive to prednisone and cyclophosphamide were given prednisone plus dipyridamole or aspirin as a platelet inhibitor, with or without systemic anticoagulants. Platelet half-life was increased and proteinuria was decreased [210]. Creatinine clearance was better preserved over time with use of platelet antagonists compared to controls [211].

A recently described protocol [251] has been employed in an effort to induce more frequent remission in children with prednisone-resistant FSGS. Methylprednisolone was initiated at 30 mg/kg (maximum 1,000 mg) intravenously every other day for 6 doses, followed by the same dose weekly for 10 weeks, with similar boluses thereafter on a tapering schedule. This was supplemented by oral prednisone, 2 mg/kg every other day. Some patients also received alkylating agents. Of 23 children treated, 12 entered remission, 6 had decreased proteinuria, and 4 remained nephrotic. One child developed renal failure [457]. This treatment leads to significant steroid side effects but represents a markedly improved response rate compared to other protocols.

Adjunct Therapy. Management of the patient with nephrotic syndrome due to either MCNS or FSGS should include dietary restriction. During relapse, dietary sodium intake should be reduced to about 0.5 gm/day, which is approximately equivalent to a 1-gm salt diet or about 20 mEq sodium per day. Such severe dietary restriction is difficult to accomplish even in a hospital setting, in which diets are designed by dietitians. It is important to emphasize that severe restriction of sodium intake will not result in weight loss when nephrotic patients are in the sodium-retaining phase of their disease. In such patients, the normal extrarenal losses of sodium amount to less than 10 mEq per day; both the urine output and urine sodium concentrations are so low that urinary sodium loss frequently is less than 5 mEq per day. Consequently, daily sodium losses in these patients amount to 15 mEq or less. Thus severe dietary sodium restriction is intended to prevent further accumulation of edema. Use of a salt substitute may facilitate compliance with the sodium-restricted diet, but in patients with renal insufficiency, it must be limited because these preparations consist of potassium and ammonium salts.

At home, most patients can rarely manage dietary restriction below that of a no-added-salt diet. This provides a sodium intake of 40 to 60 mEq per day depending on the patient's size. It should be employed not only to lessen the risk of edema formation if the patient has not responded to steroid therapy or if a relapse occurs but, also, to reduce side effects from steroid administration.

Although there is some debate regarding this approach, we feel that fluid intake also should be restricted. If intake equals insensible fluid losses plus urinary output, the patient's weight will remain stable without further accumulation of edema. To accomplish loss of weight, fluid intake must be reduced below this level. Some nephrotic patients experience intense thirst. If sodium, but not fluid, intake is limited in these subjects, they can become hyponatremic and remain edematous.

Anecdotal experience suggests that bed rest may potentiate a diuresis, perhaps by redistribution of fluid from the peripheral to the central circulation, increasing renal blood flow. Bed rest also may accelerate response to steroids and, when practical, should be advised for patients with anasarca. Other therapies that may facilitate a diuresis in some patients include local pressure using surgical elastic stockings or immersion up to the neck in warm water [365]. After remission is induced, a high-protein diet may increase the rate at which plasma protein concentration returns to normal [70].

COMPLICATIONS OF NEPHROTIC SYNDROME

Most of the complications observed in patients with nephrotic syndrome are secondary to therapy. Steroid-induced side effects are well known and include the typical changes in facies, obesity, hirsutism, striae, and pseudotumor cerebri. Hypertension may occur but is seen less frequently if patients adhere to a sodium-restricted diet. Growth retardation may be seen in children, especially if they have received high doses of steroids for protracted periods of time [295]. Catch-up growth often occurs when steroid therapy is discontinued [202]. Patients with steroid-responsive nephrotic syndrome who had received repeated courses of high-dose steroids during childhood and who had completed growth were found to have a mean height equivalent to the fortieth percentile [206]; total corticosteroid dose, however, correlated only weakly with the height scores. Corticosteroid-induced cataracts have been found in a high percentage of children [94], even when visual acuity is not impaired. The complications of cytotoxic drugs have been discussed previously.

Peritonitis is a particularly important complication of nephrotic syndrome in children [363]. Patients who have one such episode appear to be at increased risk for subsequent episodes. Peritonitis typically occurs during relapses of the disease associated with gross edema and ascites. Clinical evidence of peritoneal irritation usually is present even in patients receiving steroids. The most common infecting agent remains *Streptococcus pneumoniae*, which is found in approximately half of the cases [363]; *Escherichia coli* is cultured in a further 25 percent; a variety of other organisms, including *Hemophilus influenzae* may be found in a small percentage of patients, and the peritoneal fluid is culture negative in the remaining cases.

Infections were responsible for the majority of deaths in nephrotic patients in the preantibiotic era. Although infections occur with much less frequency now, they are still seen. For example, in a report on long-term outcome of treatment from the ISKDC in which 389 children with MCNS were followed for 5 to 15 years, 6 of the 10 deaths were due to infections. Other causes of death included one episode of dural sinus thrombosis and one incident of cardiorespiratory failure following infusion of salt-poor albumin. One child died in chronic renal failure after development of FSGS not seen on initial biopsy, and one death was from uncertain causes. Five of the deaths occurred in initially nonresponsive patients, and four occurred in patients manifesting early relapse. The number of fatalities among nonresponders was particularly striking; it constituted 20 percent of all initial nonresponders in the study [310]. Nonrenal causes of death not mentioned in this study but which may be encountered include other thromboembolic phenomena, hemorrhagic pancreatitis [265], and hypovolemic shock.

Patients with FSGS show a high incidence of severe complications of pregnancy, including spontaneous abortion, stillbirth, and neonatal death [110]. In general, no significant increase in complications of pregnancy has been reported in patients with MCNS [110, 617], although late recurrence of MCNS in association with pregnancy has been described [527].

OUTCOME

Although late relapses of patients with MCNS have been reported [147, 527], the majority of children with MCNS enter permanent remission either before or at puberty. Their long-term prognosis is good, with at least 70 percent entering adult life without renal or urinary abnormalities. This finding contrasts with the much less favorable outcome if the nephrotic syndrome is associated with glomerulonephritis [569]. A minority of pediatric patients who are initially steroid-responsive may eventually progress to renal failure [637, 655]. Most are found to have developed FSGS [637, 655], although this lesion is not always present [444]. In addition, after a period of relative stability, an occasional child will follow a fulminant, rather than an indolent, course, characterized by rapid loss of renal function, a microangiopathic hemolytic anemia, and crescentic glomerulonephritis [364].

There have been many attempts to predict the long-term course either from renal histology or from patterns of response to treatment with steroids. For example, in children, the presence of mesangial hypercellularity and immune complexes in the glomeruli has been associated with an increased relapse rate [15]. In contrast, the ISKDC [309] was unable to correlate frequency of relapse with (1) the histopathologic subgroups of MCNS, (2) clinical or laboratory characteristics present at the time of diagnosis, (3) the time of initial response, or (4) the interval between the initial response and the first relapse. Frequent relapses in the first 6 months, however, were highly predictive of frequent relapses subsequently.

Adult patients with MCNS also have a good prognosis; in one series (Fig. 64-4), more than 90 percent survived for 10 or more years without development of end-stage renal disease [111]. It has been reported that adult patients who showed even partial response to steroids had good renal function over the long term, whereas 16 of 44 patients with no response had progressed to renal failure within 3 years. Although the presence of minimal changes indicated a good prognosis, steroid response was an equally valid predictor of outcome [299].

Fig. 64-4. Long-term survival rates for adults and children with various causes for the nephrotic syndrome. Prognosis for minimal change nephrotic syndrome (MCNS) is better than for either focal segmental glomerulosclerosis (FSGS) or membranoproliferative glomerulonephritis (MPGN). (Data derived from Cameron et al. [111, 112], Koskimies et al. [361], and Glassock et al. [239].)

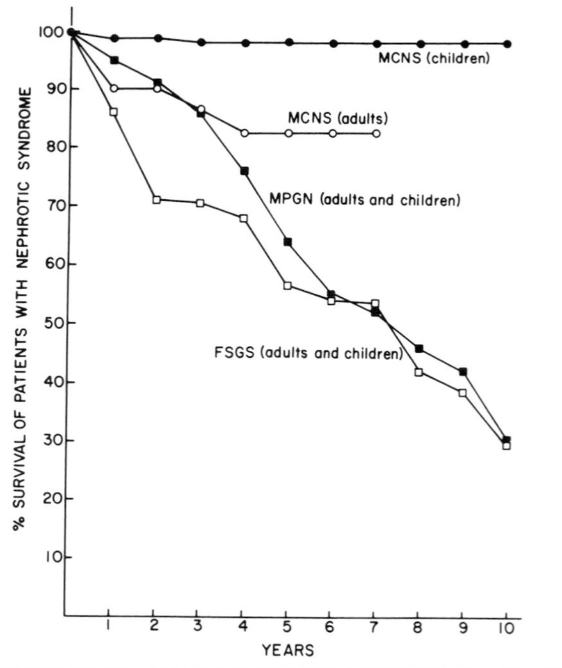

The prognosis in FSGS often has been reported to be uniformly grave. However, not all FSGS patients will develop renal insufficiency. In one series, more than 40 percent of FSGS patients survived for more than 10 years without end-stage renal disease (Fig. 64-4). The prognosis may be somewhat worse in adult than in pediatric patients [487]. In a follow-up study ranging from 7 to 217 months, the Southwest Pediatric Nephrology Study Group reported that 21 percent of their children with FSGS developed end-stage renal disease, another 23 percent had reduced GFR, and 37 percent had persistent proteinuria only; 11 percent were in remission and 8 percent were lost to follow-up [607]. In another study, only a minority of patients with FSGS were found to have decreased renal function 8 to 10 years after biopsy and diagnosis [599].

Certain characteristics on renal biopsy may help to identify FSGS patients who will have progressive disease and a poor prognosis. These include the presence of crescents [532], interstitial infiltrates [607], and mesangial hypercellularity [278, 469, 655]. For example, in a group of FSGS patients followed for 1 to 10 years, 10 of 13 who had mesangial accentuation and proliferation in nonsclerotic portions of the glomeruli had values for GFR reduced to less than 90 ml/min per 1.73 m^2; four of these patients had advanced renal failure. In contrast, none of the 11 patients without mesangial involvement had similar reductions in renal function [583]. Not all studies agree with such a conclusion. It has been suggested that most patients with FSGS will develop mesangial hypercellularity at some stage in their disease course and that this pathologic abnormality does not correlate with prognosis [607].

The prognosis for long-term renal function in FSGS also may be forecast from the patients' response to treatment. In one study utilizing such a criterion [29], three distinct groups of patients were identified. The first group entered remission with steroid or cytotoxic therapy and never experienced progression to renal failure. The second group failed to respond to treatment and had a high incidence of progression to end-stage disease. In the third group, a portion of the initial responders became resistant to treatment within 18 months of diagnosis and many subsequently lost renal function. Thus the authors cautioned that a good prognosis could not be predicted until patients had been followed for at least 18 months. It also has been suggested that prognosis may be worse for patients in whom FSGS is diagnosed on initial presentation than for those who develop focal sclerotic changes after years of proteinuria. While the more indolent form of the disease may progress to renal failure [485], patients with early appearance of FSGS more frequently follow a rapid downhill course [329].

Transplantation. Recurrence of both uncomplicated MCNS [444] and FSGS [401, 429] in renal transplants is an accepted hazard in these patients. MCNS may be a complication of transplantation, unrelated to initial renal diagnosis, as suggested by two reports of occurrence in children with end-stage renal disease secondary to congenital nephrotic syndrome [379, 600]. Habib and colleagues have considered whether the transplant lesion in FSGS is identical to the initial disease or represents a different process. Their findings of recurrence in 26 of 229 transplant patients might indicate that these patients have a systemic process inducing focal sclerosis, regardless of histocompatibility considerations [264]. In another report, a large percentage of patients who developed chronic renal failure within 3 years of onset of FSGS also experienced recurrence in their transplanted kidneys. Half of these patients lost the graft secondary to disease recurrence [520]. The lesion appears to begin with focal segmental epithelial proliferation, followed by later scarring [359]. The association of recurrence with the aggressive form of FSGS [396] would again suggest that the rapidly progressive form may represent a disease caused by a systemic factor, whereas the more chronic form may be a distinct entity resulting from damage induced by prolonged proteinuria.

Pathophysiology of the Nephrotic Syndrome

Virtually every abnormality observed in primary nephrotic syndrome can be traced directly or indirectly to the occurrence of proteinuria. The following section reviews (1) the renal mechanisms thought to be responsible for this proteinuria, (2) the systemic consequences of the loss of proteins in the urine, and (3) the immunologic abnormalities that have been associated with primary nephrotic syndrome, some of which have been proposed to relate to the pathogenesis of the renal lesion.

MECHANISMS FOR PROTEINURIA

Renal Handling of Macromolecules. The glomerular barrier to filtration consists of three layers: fenestrated endothelial cells, the trilaminar glomerular basement membrane (GBM), and the epithelial cell layer (Fig. 64-5). The epithelium does not constitute a continuous layer; rather, the interdigitating extensions from adjacent epithelial cells or podocytes are separated by spaces readily apparent on electron microscopy. Attention has focused on the GBM as being the major barrier to filtration [118]. Experimental evidence supports both the possibility that the GBM is a thixotropic gel (one containing spicules that retard the passage of macromolecules through it) [603] and that it is a porous structure through which molecules pass subject to steric hindrance [89]. In addition to the presence of the basement membrane, epithelial slit diaphragms have been identified, joining the bases of adjacent podocytes. These diaphragms have rectangular pores [581] that could constitute a further filter and have been suggested to be the limiting barrier structure [580]. Permselectivity curves that plot the renal clearance of macromolecules, relative to GFR, against molecular radius, describe a sigmoid shape (Fig. 64-6) between approximately 20 and 50 Å in humans [156]. Thus some restriction in filtration of dextran molecules occurs with molecules of about 20-Å radius; restriction increases with increasing molecular size and approaches 100 percent for molecules of radius of 50 Å [658]. In addition to size, the ability of macromolecules to cross the glomerular barrier is affected by molecular configuration, shape, deformability, and flexibility [544]. Permselectivity also is modified by glomerular hemodynamic factors, since glomerular filtration occurs by both convection and diffusion [88].

Electrostatic charge also modifies the movement of macromolecules across the glomeruli. The glomerular filter contains negatively charged sialoglycoproteins [467] present at regularly spaced intervals in the lamina rarae of the basement membrane [325], at the endothelial fenestrae [382], and lining the epithelial podocytes [383]. Collectively, these comprise the glomerular polyanion (Fig. 64-5). The presence of such negative charge sites is believed to be responsible for both the facilitated transport of polycations [80] and the restricted transport of polyanions [124] relative to that of neutral molecules of comparable size (Fig. 64-7). Thus the determinants of glomerular permeability for a given particle are steric hindrance, glomerular hemodynamics, and electrostatic charge [88].

Proteins are handled by the kidney in a manner similar to that for inert macromolecules [543]. However, clearances of proteins tend to be less than those of similarly charged dextrans of comparable size [544]. This is particularly true for albumin, which has an effective molecular radius of 36 Å. Its clearance by the normal kidney is considerably less than that of equivalent-sized neutral dextran molecules but only slightly less than that of similarly sized dextran carrying a negative charge [90].

Fig. 64-5. The glomerular barrier. The distribution of glomerular polyanion in the glomerular basement membrane and on the endothelial and epithelial cell layers is shown.

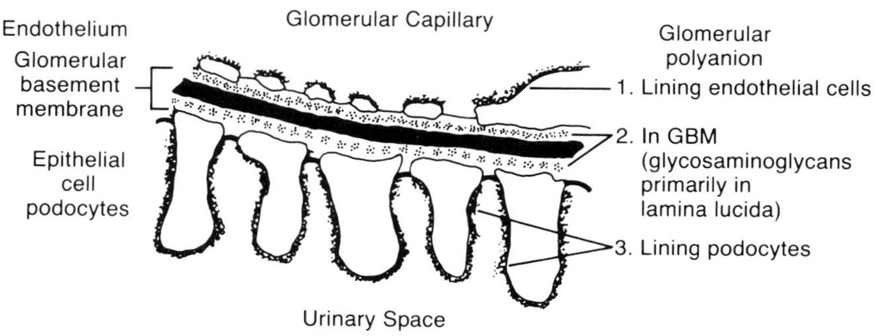

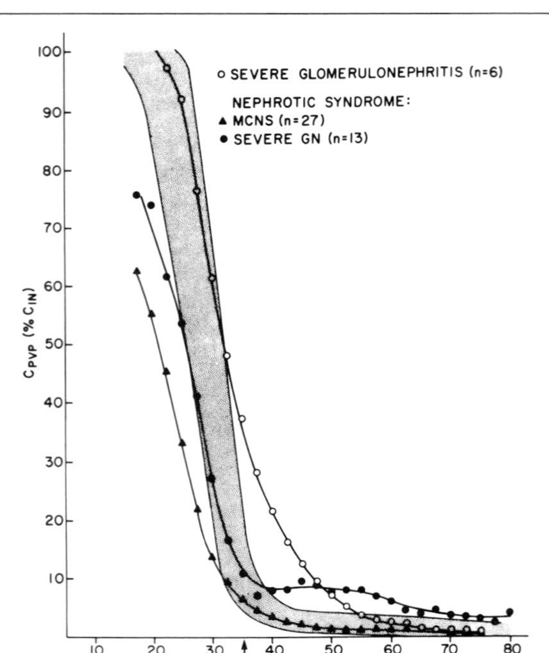

Fig. 64-6. Permselectivity curves for patients with severe proliferative glomerulonephritis and for those with nephrotic syndrome secondary either to the minimal change lesion (MCNS) or to glomerulonephritis. Normal values are depicted by the shaded area. The arrow indicates the molecular size of albumin. The fractional clearance of larger macromolecules is increased in severe glomerulonephritis. In MCNS, the fractional clearances of smaller molecules is decreased. Patients with nephrotic syndrome secondary to glomerulonephritis show a hybrid curve. (Data modified from Robson and Cole [551].)

Permselectivity patterns obtained in patients with MCNS [551, 553] (Fig. 64-6) or animal models of albuminuria [81, 125] show a relative decrease in macromolecular clearance even in the presence of marked proteinuria. In contrast, patients with glomerulonephritis show increased macromolecular clearances (Fig. 64-6), presumably due to the structural damage in the GBM, which may be visible on renal biopsy in these disease states; this concept is supported by work in animals [342]. Thus the mechanisms for proteinuria in primary nephrotic syndrome and in glomerulonephritis appear to be distinct. In the former, proteinuria is primarily selective for albumin and occurs even though clearance of macromolecules comparable in size to albumin is decreased. In the latter, permselectivity of macromolecules that are 25 Å or larger is increased, resulting in poorly selective proteinuria. Patients with nephrotic syndrome secondary to glomerulonephritis show a pattern of permselectivity (Fig. 64-6) that is a hybrid between those found in primary nephrotic syndrome and in glomerulonephritis [551]. In these patients, as in MCNS, clearances of smaller molecules are relatively decreased. However, in contrast to the situation in MCNS, the relative clearance of larger molecules is increased. Similar hybrid curves have been described in diabetic glomerulosclerosis [156].

Initially, it was held that macromolecule handling could be accounted for by an isoporous model for glomerular filtration, one in which steric hindrance of glomerular passage of macromolecules results from the presence of uniform pores in the barrier, each with a radius of approximately 50 Å. The size of these pores may be increased in models of increased permeability of the GBM [93a]. However, it has become apparent that a heteroporous model may be more appropriate. In this model, there are two pathways: one subject to classic

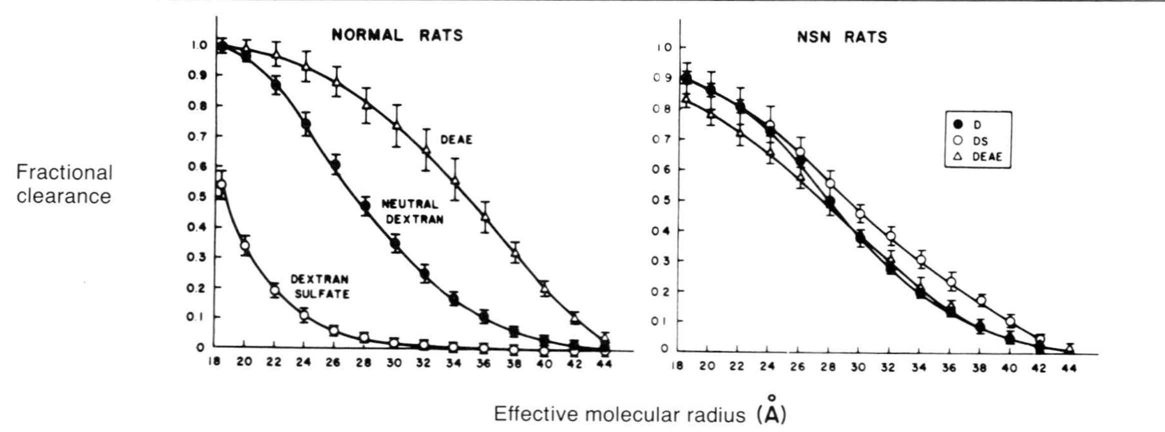

Fig. 64-7. Clearance of neutral dextran (D), negatively charged dextran sulfate (DS), and positively charged DEAE dextran of varying molecular size in normal rats and in those made albuminuric by treatment with nephrotoxic serum (NSN). In normal animals, clearance of negatively charged dextrans is retarded, that of cationic dextrans is enhanced, demonstrating charge selectivity by the glomerular filter. In NSN, charge discrimination is lost. (Reprinted from Bohrer et al. [82], by copyright permission of the American Society for Clinical Investigation.)

steric hindrance, and a "shunt" pathway unaffected by size selectivity [594]. As demonstrated by clearance of very large dextrans, glomerular filtration of macromolecules through this second pathway is enhanced in nephrosis and is ameliorated by antihypertensive therapy [12], pressor doses of angiotensin II [414], or indomethacin [243]. These manipulations decrease transglomerular passage of all macromolecules. Thus, although a significant portion of the proteinuria of nephrosis is caused by enhanced utilization of this shunt pathway, it is not clear whether these findings represent a cause or a result of glomerular hyperfiltration. The effect of this shunt is most noticeable for large molecules (over 60 Å); its effect on albumin clearance remains to be determined.

Role of Glomerular Electrostatic Charge in Nephrosis. There is a significant body of evidence suggesting that proteinuria in MCNS and its variants result from alterations in glomerular charge sites. This proteinuria is highly selective and consists primarily of albumin, which carries a negative charge under normal physiologic conditions. Renal clearances of proteins carrying other charges are not increased comparably despite massive proteinuria. Renal biopsy material from patients with nephrotic syndrome provides an explanation for this observation, since there is decreased staining for glomerular polyanion [71, 114, 428]. Indeed, studies in MCNS patients have suggested that albuminuria results from a reduction of fixed negative charge by approximately 50 percent [93]. Depletion of polyanion also has been documented in congenital nephrotic syndrome [651], where a semiquantitative technique has revealed a significant decrease in glycosaminoglycan content of the GBM. These reports indicate that disparate mechanisms can cause depletion or alteration of charge sites in nephrosis.

Although differences among models [66, 67] dictate caution in generalizing to human disease, studies in animals with experimental forms of nephrotic syndrome support a role for decreased glomerular negative charge. Rats with nephrotic syndrome induced by puromycin aminonucleoside (PAN) have predominantly albuminuria.

Glomeruli in these animals show decreased staining by cationic dyes [461] and decreased sialic acid content [72]. Animals with PAN nephrotic syndrome [81] as well as those with acute heterologous nephrotoxic serum nephritis [90] show increased clearance of negatively charged dextrans, with permselectivity curves approximating those of neutral dextrans. Intravenous infusion of various polycations into animals results in loss of staining for glomerular polyanion, increased porosity of the glomerular filter, and heavy proteinuria [44, 291, 648]. Unilateral renal artery infusion of the polycation protamine sulfate causes ipsilateral albuminuria and depletion of glomerular polyanion. In this model, the only significant morphologic change is foot-process fusion. Neither this nor hemodynamic changes were sufficient to account for the degree of proteinuria observed [648]. These findings indicate that loss of charge selectivity may lead to a selective increase in albumin excretion. It remains unresolved whether the loss of glomerular charge sites is directly responsible for increased albuminuria or whether it results in anatomic derangement of the GBM, which permits the increased transglomerular passage of protein [291].

The cause of depletion or neutralization of negative charges in human disease is unknown. Intraglomerular release of platelet factor 4, which has been shown to bind to glomerular polyanion by an ionic reaction [43], could cause proteinuria by a mechanism analogous to that seen with polycation infusions. Studies in patients suggest that neutralization of anionic charges may be systemic in nature [397, 398] rather than confined to the kidney. This could result from effects of a protease present in circulation [38]. A variety of immunologic factors represent additional potential mechanisms for inducing albuminuria in MCNS and are discussed later in the chapter. Once initiated, proteinuria could be perpetuated by additional mechanisms, such as alterations in arachidonic acid metabolism, with increased thromboxane production in the kidney [540].

In addition to increasing albuminuria, depletion of glomerular negative charge also may cause the morphologic finding of epithelial foot-process fusion. Electron micrographs of renal tissue obtained after protamine sulfate infusion sufficient to deplete glomerular polyanion show podocyte alterations identical to those seen in nephrotic syndrome [589]. This finding suggests that electrostatic effects of the negatively charged coating may be responsible for the normal separation of adjacent podocytes. Since albuminuria itself may cause foot-process fusion [561], it may be argued that the effect of charge neutralization is not a direct one. However, chemical removal of the sialic acid coating also causes foot-process fusion [23], and perfusion of the kidney with heparin after infusion of polycation results in reestablishment of the normal podocyte structure [588].

Regardless of its origin, alteration of podocyte architecture also may account for the generally decreased clearance of macromolecules in nephrotic syndrome cited previously. It has been suggested that simplification of foot processes makes the glomerular pore less complex, allowing for increased clearance of some long, narrow, rigid molecules. However, most proteins are prolate ellipsoids (cigar-shaped) and show decreased clearance [422]. The effective pore radius has been found to be decreased in both MCNS and FSGS [676]. In this study, the ratio of total pore area to pore length was found to be reduced by over 50 percent. This finding would account for decreased macromolecular clearance but not enhanced albumin clearance. The latter would result directly from decreased electrostatic hindrance to filtration of albumin.

CONSEQUENCES OF PROTEINURIA

It is generally accepted that the central feature of the nephrotic syndrome, irrespective of its underlying renal cause, is hypoalbuminemia resulting from urinary loss of albumin. Studies have shown that there is increased fractional catabolism of albumin in nephrotic syndrome [237], mostly within the renal tubule after increased filtration of plasma proteins [215]. Rates of hepatic synthesis of albumin are increased [314], but this increase is inadequate to compensate for urinary losses [657]. Although gastrointestinal losses are possible through transudation of albumin across the bowel wall, these are unlikely to contribute significantly to decreased plasma albumin concentrations.

However, urinary losses cannot be considered as an isolated phenomenon; it is apparent that a special relationship exists among protein synthetic capability, urinary loss of protein, and plasma protein concentrations in nephrotic syndrome. For example, patients on chronic peritoneal dialysis lose "nephrotic range" amounts of protein, yet they have close to normal serum albumin concentrations [173]. In nephrosis, the rate of hepatic albumin synthesis is related to dietary protein intake. However, increasing protein intake leads to glomerular hyperfiltration [312, 466] and enhanced loss of protein in the urine, resulting in lower serum albumin concentrations in patients on high-protein diets [335]. The increase in dietary intake appears to stimulate selective hepatic expression of mRNA for albumin, indicating that the stimulus is specific for albumin production and not generalized to other proteins as well [337]. The dietary stimulus can be dissociated from potential stimulatory effects of alterations in plasma oncotic pressure [338]. Although the mechanism of such an effect is not clear, several liver-specific transcription regulatory factors have been identified for albumin [403, 679]. Although specific plasma amino acid content is unchanged, nitrogen balance is rendered more positive by angiotensin converting enzyme inhibition [168], which decreases hyperfiltration and thus the amount of protein lost in the urine. Indeed, enalapril decreases $U_{albumin}V$ and fractional catabolism of albumin in normal or nephrotic rats on high-protein diets [292, 293]. Thus, low plasma albumin concentrations may reflect hemodynamic effects of increased protein turnover rather than simply the effects of failure of the glomerular barrier to limit protein passage.

Edema Formation. One of the major consequences of hypoalbuminemia is edema formation. The major forces that maintain vascular volume are believed to be those described by Starling [612], namely, the algebraic sum of hydrostatic and oncotic pressures acting at the level of the capillary beds (Fig. 64-8). Hydrostatic pressure is the dominant force at the arteriolar end of the capillary, where it is generated by arterial blood pressure. Pressure is lower in the capillaries (40 to 45 mm Hg) than in the arterial system, but it is markedly higher than tissue pressure, which ranges from 2 to 5 mm Hg. Hydrostatic pressure is opposed by plasma oncotic pressure (the osmotic pressure generated by colloidal solutes), which is 25 to 30 mm Hg in health. The resulting net force (10 to 15 mm Hg) drives an ultrafiltrate of blood from the capillaries into the interstitial fluid space. By the venous end of the capillary, hydrostatic pressure has been further dissipated (Fig. 64-8) and is exceeded by oncotic pressure, so there is a net force for return of fluid into the capillaries. In health, the loss of fluid at the arteriolar end of the capillaries exceeds the amount resorbed at the venous end. The difference is returned to the circulation through the lymphatic system [550].

Albumin, because of its relatively small molecular size, is the plasma protein primarily responsible for the generation of oncotic pressure. Because of the mathematical relationship between plasma albumin concentration and oncotic pressure [378], a decrease in the former,

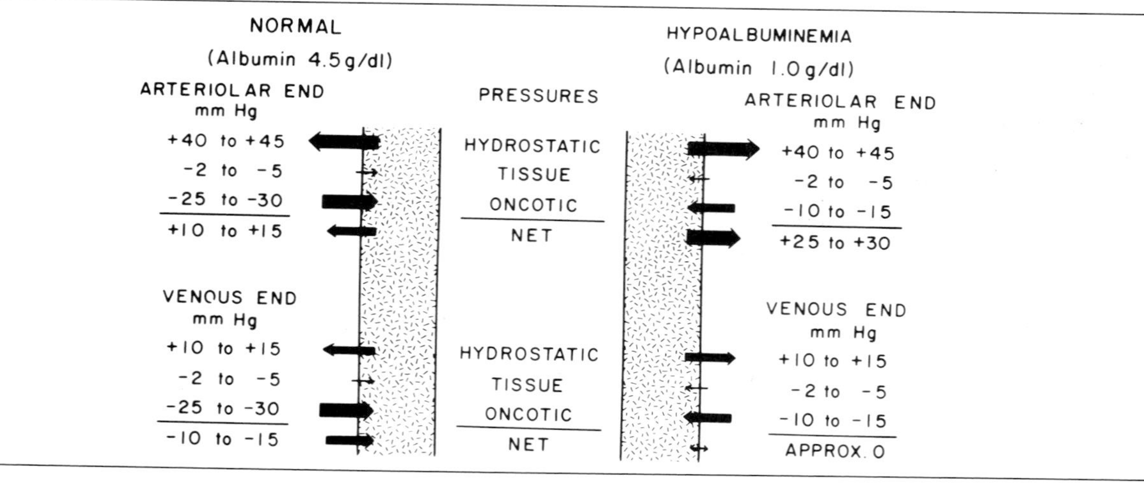

Fig. 64-8. The forces that govern the movement of fluid across the capillary walls in healthy persons and in patients with MCNS. The shaded area represents the lumina of the capillaries. The size and direction of the arrows are in proportion to the magnitude and direction of the force described by that arrow. In MCNS, hypoalbuminemia causes a marked reduction in oncotic pressure. This increases the driving force for fluid out of the arteriolar end of the capillary and decreases the forces available for return of fluid at the venous end. The result is the development of increased amounts of fluid in the interstitial space and the beginning of edema formation. See text for more details. [From A. M. Robson, Edema and Edema Forming States. In S. Klahr (ed.), *The Kidney and Body Fluids in Health and Disease*. New York: Plenum, 1984. Pp. 119–146.]

as in nephrotic syndrome, results in an even greater decrease in oncotic pressure, so that the net driving force for loss of fluid at the arteriolar end of the capillary bed is increased and that for return of fluid at the venous end is reduced. In consequence, fluid accumulates in the interstitial space, initiating edema formation. This accumulation occurs first where tissue pressure is lowest, for example, in the eyelids or in the scrotum; it also appears in the most dependent parts of the body, because venous pressure is highest at these sites and is transmitted to the venous end of the capillaries.

The translocation of fluid from the vascular to the interstitial fluid spaces as edema forms should decrease blood volume. It has been proposed that the physiologic responses precipitated by such a reduction are important factors in producing the massive amounts of edema often seen in nephrotic syndrome. These changes include the release of antidiuretic hormone (ADH), the release of renin with increased production of angiotensin II, and decreases in renal blood flow and GFR [77, 553]. All these changes favor renal retention and positive balances of both sodium and water unless intakes are decreased. Indeed, patients may exhibit increased thirst, which is probably stimulated both by angiotensin II [318] and by the decrease in blood volume monitored through baro- and volume-receptors. Retained sodium and water does not remain in the vascular space. Because of the hypoalbuminemia, it adds to the edema.

The pathophysiology of edema formation in nephrotic syndrome is probably more complex than this traditional concept. Animal studies have documented that hypoproteinemia alone does not result in edema [339]. Such studies must be interpreted with care, since traditional means of calculating colloid osmotic pressure in animals, as opposed to direct measurement, may be inaccurate [463]. In humans, some patients with congenital analbuminemia do not develop edema and have a normal plasma volume even in the virtual absence of serum albumin [341]. Furthermore, if the traditional theory is correct, patients in relapse of nephrotic syndrome should have decreased blood volumes and values should return to normal in remission from the disease. Although reduced values for blood volume have been reported [642], normal or even increased levels have been documented, too [180, 225]. A survey of the literature [172] found that only 38 percent of nephrotic subjects had measurements indicating blood volumes reduced by 10 percent or more from normal; 48 percent had normal values, and 14 percent had increased values. Furthermore, patients with carefully documented MCNS studied in relapse and again in remission have not shown a consistent increase in blood volumes; indeed, in most, the values did not change [172, 501].

There are several possible explanations for these variable results. One is that not all of the reported patients had MCNS. Nephrotic syndrome secondary to glomerulonephritis is usually associated with a normal or expanded blood volume [455]. A second explanation is that some patients were receiving treatment when studied. Natriuretic therapy reduced both blood and interstitial fluid volume in nephrotic subjects [222]. A third possibility is that measurements of blood volume are difficult to interpret because of methodologic problems. Labeled red cells may not circulate ideally in volume-depleted states, so that peripheral hematocrit may not reflect total-body hematocrit; labeled albumin may have an increased volume of distribution in nephrotic syndrome, especially if vascular integrity to albumin is decreased [201]. Thus both methods could be subject to errors [455]. Indeed, if the suggestion that nephrotic syndrome results from a generalized loss of negative charge sites [397, 554] proves to be correct, loss of such charge sites in capillary beds could cause increased losses of albumin into edema fluid, as suggested by recent studies [646]. This occurrence would not only alter the apparent volume distribution of albumin, but it would also decrease oncotic pressure at the level of the capillaries. Support for this hypothesis is found in the observation that large changes in extracellular fluid volume caused little change in plasma volume [358].

An attractive explanation for the variations in reported blood volume is that nephrotic patients have been studied in different phases of their disease process. Blood volume could be reduced early in relapse of MCNS but return to normal as anasarca develops. Thus the decrease in plasma volume after experimental depletion of serum proteins can be prevented by massive expansion of the extracellular fluid with saline [659]. Nephrotic subjects progress through a sodium-retaining phase but eventually enter into a new steady state, in which they no longer accumulate edema and once again demonstrate the ability to excrete a sodium load [77]. With this new steady state, sodium and water retention may have been so marked and edema accumulation so massive that tissue pressure is increased and blood volume is returned to normal. This may explain reports in which nephrotic subjects could be separated into those with high and those with low urine sodium concentrations [501].

Studies of the renin-angiotensin system also have not produced consistent support for the traditional hypothesis about edema formation. Earlier work suggested that fluid redistribution resulted in aldosterone-mediated sodium retention designed to replenish vascular volume [421, 459]. Accordingly, aldosterone activity was thought to be more important in the genesis of fluid retention than either serum albumin or colloid osmotic pressure [501]. The current view is that increased tubular sensitivity to the hormone [593] enhances edema formation and explains why therapy with aldosterone antagonists in nephrotic patients may induce a significant diuresis.

The inconsistencies in plasma renin activity (PRA) results that have been reported could be due to clinical factors similar to those that confound interpretation of blood-volume measurement. They include different stages of both disease process and sodium balance as well as variations in therapeutic regimen. For example, immunofluorescent staining of renin-producing cells in renal biopsy material from nephrotic patients has shown that increased numbers of these cells are found in hypoalbuminemic states. However, the increase correlated with a number of variables, most notably the presence of vascular disease [493]. In an attempt to standardize some of these variables, renin-sodium profiles were performed on patients with nephrotic syndrome [455]. Two groups of patients were identified. In keeping with the traditional concepts, the "classic" form was typically seen in patients with MCNS, where high levels of PRA and aldosterone activity were associated with vasoconstriction and hypoalbuminemia; values were further stimulated rather than suppressed by salt loading and decreased spontaneously before the occurrence of steroid-induced diuresis. In the hypervolemic, or "overfilling," form, seen typically with chronic glomerulonephritis and renal insufficiency, low renin activity was associated with sodium retention and increased normally with sodium depletion. Other recent studies have correlated PRA with plasma volume, serum albumin concentration [99], or the state of sodium balance [172]. Natriuresis in MCNS was associated with an increase in PRA and presumably a decrease in plasma volume [172], whereas that induced by water immersion, presumably mediated by an increase in blood volume, was associated with a measured decrease in PRA [365]. Thus PRA appears to correlate better with plasma volume than with rate of urinary sodium excretion.

Difficulties in confirming a definitive role for the renin-angiotensin system in the genesis of nephrotic edema are similar to those in explaining edema formation in cirrhosis [188]. A multiplicity of interacting factors may be responsible in both of these disease states. Thus plasma renin levels could be controlled tightly by a variety of feedback mechanisms so that subtle changes, too small to be detected by current laboratory methods, are all that occur to maintain the altered homeostasis. In addition to renin, other factors affecting volume status may include abnormal vascular tone [683], altered levels of catecholamines [502], volume-mediated increases in ADH secretion [642], and altered prostaglandin metabolism. Elevated levels of PGE_2 were found in the sera of patients with nephrotic syndrome, the majority of whom had MCNS [220]. The highest values were observed when the patients had clinically apparent edema. Urinary PGE_2 levels were increased in patients with idiopathic nephrotic syndrome who had a low urine sodium concentration as well as elevated plasma renin-aldosterone activity [30]. The observation that the administration of indomethacin to nephrotic patients results in an increase in body weight and decrease in GFR suggests that prostaglandins may play a role in either maintenance of GFR or amelioration of edema in nephrotic syndrome. Indomethacin also decreased proteinuria and plasma renin activity [30]. Response to indomethacin is dependent on concurrent sodium intake. When given to nephrotic patients on sodium-restricted diets, it resulted in a decrease in GFR; a similar drug regimen for patients with more liberal sodium intake did not affect renal hemodynamics [260].

Because atrial natriuretic factor (ANF) causes renal vasodilatation, increase in GFR, and increased sodium excretion [486], it has been suggested that abnormal metabolism of this hormone could be involved in events mediating sodium retention in nephrosis. The acute increase of plasma volume following albumin infusion in nephrotic children is accompanied by a fivefold increase in ANF levels [641]. However, this may simply reflect low plasma volume status before beginning the infusion. Plasma concentrations of ANF were determined to be low in nephrotic patients compared to those in patients who had acute glomerulonephritis, and ANF levels correlated well with the degree of edema in nephritis but not in nephrosis [555]. Thus, regulation of ANF appeared to be appropriate for presumed volume status. In rats with doxorubicin-induced nephrotic syndrome, changes in GFR after infusion of ANF were similar to those in control animals, indicating that nephrosis does not alter glomerular filtration by a mechanism related to ANF [516]. In a similar model, no change was detected in ANF receptor density in nephrotic kidneys [517]. Nephrotic patients respond physiologically to ANF infusion [690], although the mechanism by which this occurs may be different from that in normal subjects [519]. It has been proposed that ANF mediates the diuretic response of head-out immersion in nephrosis [189], but the effect of ANF infusion is, unlike that of immersion, blocked by enalapril [530]. Taken together, these findings suggest that, while secretion of ANF may in part mediate diuresis, physical factors are of greatest importance in the fluid retention of nephrosis, with abnormalities of ANF representing appropriate responses for the patient's physiology.

These physical factors may include a significant intrarenal component. Children with MCNS have mild decreases in both GFR and filtration fraction [60, 77, 553]. This decrease in GFR could be due to a decrease in the ultrafiltration coefficient, causing a reduction in single-nephron GFR [298], and has been suggested to result from foot-process fusion of the glomerular epithelial cells [79]. Alternatively, the decreased GFR could be the consequence of a raised intratubular hydrostatic pressure in the proximal tubule secondary to the presence of filtered albumin, an increase in resistance to tubular flow [369], or decreased proximal reabsorption of tubular fluid as a result of a reduction in peritubular capillary oncotic pressure [298]. There also may be a local role for the renin-angiotensin system, since saralasin infusion in experimental unilateral PAN-induced nephrotic syndrome resulted in an increase in single-nephron GFR in the experimental, but not the control, kidney [298]. In another animal model of nephrotic syndrome, that of nephrotoxic serum nephritis, the ultrafiltration coefficient was reduced, but compensatory mechanisms maintained renal blood flow, whole kidney, and single-nephron GFR. These responses appeared to be intrarenal in origin and caused an increase in glomerular capillary pressure [567].

Unexplained alterations in renal physiology in the nephrotic syndrome include an increase in distal renal tubular sodium delivery [77, 507] and decreased solute-free water reabsorption in children with MCNS, although the capacity to generate solute-free water remains intact [78].

Other Physiologic Changes in Fluid and Electrolyte Metabolism. A curious phenomenon in primary nephrotic syndrome, perhaps related to decreased filtration fraction, is the occurrence of reversible or permanent renal failure unexplained by the underlying disease process. This has been reported in association with both MCNS [152, 604, 613] and FSGS [531]. Some cases were associated with the use of nonsteroidal anti-inflammatory drug therapy [92, 631]. These episodes occur in the absence of renal vein thrombosis (vide infra) or other systemic symptoms. Since fractional excretion of sodium also has been reported to be low in these cases [290], it is likely that the marked decrease in GFR occurs for hemodynamic reasons [178] rather than because of acute tubular necrosis and vasomotor nephropathy. In a study of 15 patients with MCNS and renal failure, GFR measured by inulin clearance was decreased out of proportion to clearance of PAH, with filtration fraction reduced to between 3 and 9 percent [420]. Improvement of renal function occurred in association with diuretic therapy either with or without albumin infusions. In patients who improved with pharmacologic diuresis, the creatinine again rose on return to an edematous state. The authors postulated that glomerular hemodynamics were altered by the presence of intrarenal edema, which occurred when the patients developed peripheral edema.

Other circulatory abnormalities have been observed in patients with nephrotic syndrome. The occurrence of hypovolemic shock and hypotension has been related to a variety of medical procedures [682]. However, some cases occur spontaneously. These episodes usually are seen in patients in relapse, who have an intercurrent illness, such as emesis or diarrhea, causing fluid loss. The patients usually show marked responsiveness to small amounts of intravenous saline, which are insufficient to replenish all fluid losses, suggesting a failure in maintenance of vascular tone. Recovery usually occurs if this complication is identified early and treated promptly. Sequelae may include acute tubular necrosis, renal vein thrombosis, or death.

Hyperlipidemia. Lipemic serum has long been recognized as a cardinal feature of the nephrotic syndrome [187]. Abnormalities in postprandial lipid metabolism were described more than 30 years ago [52]. Biochemical evaluation has shown that all lipid components of the plasma are increased, with cholesterol increasing more rapidly than phospholipid. Thus, as acute severity of the disease worsens, the ratio of cholesterol to phospholipid increases [63]. Triglycerides are relatively normal at the initiation of relapse but increase rapidly as the disease course lengthens [53]; lactescence occurs when the plasma triglyceride content exceeds 400 mg/dl. Hyperlipidemia may persist well into remission [691].

Depending on the classification employed, the most common patterns of hyperlipoproteinemia seen in nephrosis are types II and IV [131] or types IIa, IIb, and V [488]. Low-density lipoproteins (LDL) and very low–density lipoproteins (VLDL) show the greatest increase in concentration. Values for high-density lipoprotein (HDL) cholesterol have been reported to be elevated [462, 497], normal [113, 498], or decreased [53, 121, 229]. This variation may relate to the age of the patients studied, the underlying cause of the nephrotic syndrome, patient treatment, and whether renal insufficiency was present. Studies of lipoprotein cholesterol have produced conflicting results [53, 113, 121, 229, 462, 497, 498]. The ratio of cholesterol to phospholipid or triglyceride in various lipoproteins is altered, indicating abnormalities in quality as well as quantity of lipoproteins.

The cause of these abnormalities is under intensive investigation. Lipid metabolism is normally accomplished through a series of complex steps (Fig. 64-9). Through the action of 3-hydroxy-3-methylglutaryl-coenzyme A (HMG CoA) reductase, mevalonate is produced from acetate in the liver. This in turn is used to make cholesterol, which is incorporated into lipoproteins. The greater the triglyceride content of the lipoprotein, the less dense it is. Dietary fat absorbed from the intestine is formed into chylomicrons by being surrounded with a coat of apolipoprotein that is critical for transport of the hydrophobic lipid. The triglyceride content of the chylomicron is reduced in the periphery (mainly by the action of lipoprotein lipase [LPL]), and the chylomicron remnant binds to the hepatocyte via a receptor for apolipoprotein B-48 [548a]. VLDL is synthesized in the liver and metabolized in the periphery through the action of LPL to intermediate-density lipoprotein (IDL) and then to LDL. LDL is bound to apolipoprotein B-100, which is then taken up by the hepatocyte LDL receptor [334, 548a]. This brings additional cholesterol back to the liver, suppressing HMG CoA reductase activity and decreasing new cholesterol synthesis. The liver also produces HDL, which participates as a transport protein in catabolism of lower-density moieties, being regenerated by lecithin-cholesterol acyltransferase (LCAT). HDL also carries apolipoprotein C-II, which activates lipoprotein lipase. Abnormalities at any step of this pathway from lipid uptake to the enterohepatic secretion of bile could result in the hyperlipidemia of nephrosis. Likely contributing factors include increased hepatic synthesis of lipoprotein, abnormal transport of lipid through the metabolic pathway, and abnormal catabolism secondary to decreased enzyme activity.

LIPOPROTEIN SYNTHESIS. It is clear that hepatic synthesis of lipoproteins is increased in nephrotic patients [63, 340, 434, 435]. The signal for this event appears to be related to hypoalbuminemia, since daily infusion of albumin into nephrotic patients, sufficient to raise serum levels, also decreases serum lipids, triglycerides, and cholesterol [236]. Increasing the plasma oncotic pressure in nephrotic patients or animals, by infusion of dextrans, also decreases hepatic lipoprotein synthesis [54, 159]. Additional laboratory studies have suggested that the regulatory signal could be viscosity rather than oncotic pressure [24, 155, 684]. Cholesterol biosynthesis has also been investigated [247, 249]. These studies showed increased incorporation of ^{14}C from labeled mevalonate into cholesterol by the liver in experimental nephrosis. Although this result is consistent with the interpretation that rates of hepatic cholesterol synthesis are increased in nephrosis, artifactual changes due to addition of exogenous substrate (mevalonate) could not be ruled out in these experiments.

LIPID TRANSPORT. Several aspects of lipid transport may be impaired in nephrosis. The major cholesterol-transporting protein associated with the LDL in the

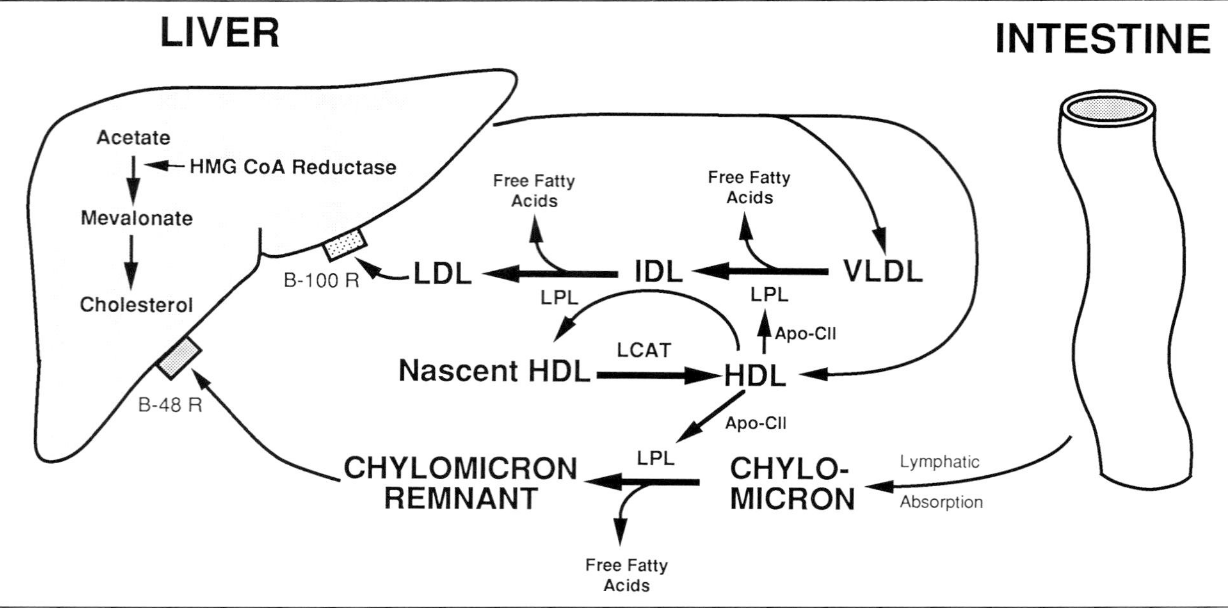

Fig. 64-9. Normal pathways of lipid metabolism. HDL = high-density lipoprotein; IDL = intermediate-density lipoprotein; LDL = low-density lipoprotein; VLDL = very low–density lipoprotein; apo-CII = apolipoprotein C-II; HMG CoA reductase = 3-hydroxy-3-methylglutaryl coenzyme A reductase; LPL = lipoprotein lipase; LCAT = lecithin-cholesterol acyltransferase; B-48 R = apolipoprotein B-48 receptor; B-100 R = apolipoprotein B-100 (LDL) receptor.

plasma is apolipoprotein B-100 [256]. This has also been implicated as the significant apolipoprotein in atherogenesis. Elevated serum concentrations of cholesterol, triglycerides, and phospholipids were found mostly in apolipoprotein B-100–containing lipoproteins in a recent study of nephrotic patients. The size of the apolipoprotein B-100 pool in patients was two to three times that found in normal subjects or in patients in remission. Fractional catabolism was only slightly decreased, suggesting that the major problem was overproduction rather than decreased breakdown [322]. Hepatic uptake of LDL may be decreased [661] if the structural composition of LDL in the circulating pool is abnormal, or if systemic neutralization of membrane negative charge leads to less efficient uptake of the largely cationic liposomes [471a]; this would exacerbate hypercholesterolemia by decreasing negative feedback affecting hepatic synthesis. Alternatively, decreased hepatic uptake of LDL could result from, rather than cause, hepatic overproduction of cholesterol [256].

METABOLISM OF LIPIDS. Interest regarding catabolism of lipids in nephrosis has focused on two enzymes: LPL, which facilitates the breakdown of ester bonds in glycerides, and LCAT, which catalyzes the reaction of lecithin and cholesterol to form lysolecithin and cholesterol ester [137]. In nephrotic children, elevated serum lipid levels correlate with decreased post-heparin LPL activity [681]. In another study of nephrotic patients, most of whom had MCNS, hepatic LPL activity was normal, but serum and adipose tissue LPL activity were decreased in association with elevated plasma triglycerides [497]. Decreased hepatic [217] and adipose tissue [681] LPL activity in experimental rat models of nephrosis may contribute to altered lipoprotein levels in these animals. LCAT activity is also decreased in experimental nephrosis [590], with levels appearing to correlate with serum albumin concentration [199].

Activity of these enzymes may be affected both directly and indirectly by urinary protein loss. Albumin binds to free fatty acids (FFA); decreases in serum albumin concentration lead to FFA accumulation, inhibiting LPL activity [236]. LCAT activity is inhibited by accumulation of triglyceride and cholesterol esters [199], suggesting that abnormal LCAT activity could be a result, rather than a cause, of nephrotic hyperlipidemia. However, lysolecithin, a reaction product that binds to albumin, inhibits LCAT activity in vitro; this feedback mechanism is blocked by addition of physiologic levels of albumin [165, 199]. LPL activity may be inhibited by cholesterol [198]. Thus, urinary loss of albumin may lead to inhibition of lipolytic enzyme function.

Albumin loss does not account entirely for the elevated lipid levels, however. While infusion of albumin decreased serum lipids in an acute animal model of nephrotic syndrome, normalization occurs only after simultaneous infusion of heparin. This suggests the need for an additional factor, which aids in clearing lipid from the plasma [559]. In further experiments with this model, nephrectomy results in greater improvement of the hyperlipidemia than does albumin infusions alone [558], indicating that the factor may be lost in the urine. Further support for loss of a specific regulatory molecule(s) in the urine is provided by the observation that alteration of dietary protein intake markedly modulates hepatic albumin synthetic rate but does not alter hepatic synthesis of lipoproteins [336]. In this study, lipoprotein synthesis correlated directly with urinary clearance of albumin, suggesting that albumin, or another substance lost in parallel with albumin, was needed to suppress lipoprotein synthesis. Experiments with analbuminemic rats indicated that albumin itself was not likely to be the critical molecule [153]. It has been suggested that the lost factor is LCAT [63]. HDL, which plays an essential role in catabolism of VLDL, also has been reported to be lost in the nephrotic urine [197, 230]. Conversely, other studies have indicated that HDL excretion is decreased [159], especially in MCNS [415]. Apolipoprotein C-II also may be lost in the urine [255, 329a].

CLINICAL SIGNIFICANCE. Regardless of the cause, the clinical significance of the lipid abnormalities in nephrosis is uncertain. Hyperlipidemia has been associated with cardiovascular disease in otherwise healthy young adults, but studies evaluating such a correlation in nephrotic patients have produced conflicting results. Premature coronary atherosclerosis [323] and a high incidence of myocardial infarction and other cardiovascular diseases [10, 62] have been described in nephrotic subjects, as has a higher incidence of hypertension in male nephrotics than in controls [663]. In this respect, the observation that macrophage morphology and function is altered by the hyperlipidemia of nephrosis [51] could relate to the development of atheromatous plaques. In contrast, other studies have not confirmed a predisposition to atherosclerosis in nephrosis [234, 652]. The discrepant results may reflect limitations of population base or preselecting factors. In the studies that did not demonstrate an increased risk, it is unclear whether stratification of the patients into cohorts according to the degree of lipid abnormality would have shown an increased risk in patients with the highest consistent elevations in lipoprotein levels. Age, underlying diagnosis, disease course, and incidence of other complicating factors such as hypertension also may be important. Another significant consideration is the possible ameliorating effect of HDL on hyperlipidemia [431, 662]. In several studies [415, 497], HDL levels were normal or increased in MCNS. This could have a protective effect and decrease the likelihood of cardiovascular complications. Further study of larger groups of nephrotic patients would allow differentiation among patients with various cardiac risk factors in addition to the potential hazard of elevated serum lipids.

A second risk involves the role of lipids in causing or enhancing the progression of the renal disease itself. Rats with PAN nephrosis fed high-cholesterol diets develop mesangial foam cells and mesangial proliferative changes [164]. The relationship of systemic hypertension and hyperlipidemia to atherosclerosis parallels the relationship of intraglomerular hypertension and high lipid levels to focal sclerosis [164]. Effective therapy of hyperlipidemia ameliorates single-nephron hyperfiltration [330a] and retards progression of renal failure in obese Zucker rats [330] and in nephrotic rats with reduced renal mass [269]. A recent study in obese Zucker rats suggests that a relative decrease in polyunsaturated fatty acids (PUFA), rather than high cholesterol levels, may be the most important lipid-related factor in progression of renal disease, since dietary supplementation with n-6 PUFA (sunflower oil) or n-3 PUFA (fish oil) both slowed progression of renal disease, but only fish oil decreased serum cholesterol [331].

In view of these considerations and the fact that treatments for nephrosis such as steroids and diuretics may exacerbate hyperlipidemia, clinicians have invested increasing effort in controlling the lipid abnormalities of nephrosis. Traditional dietary therapy is of marginal value and may actually worsen the hyperlipidemia [256]. Cholestyramine may, by increasing secretion of cholesterol into the bile, predispose toward development of cholesterol gallstones [255]. Nicotinic acid has significant side effects and has not been studied extensively. Probucol may cause concomitant loss of HDL [256]. However, it has been shown experimentally to reverse lipid-mediated vasoconstriction [328]. Two classes of drugs recently found to be effective in treating nephrotic hyperlipidemia are fibric acids and HMG CoA reductase inhibitors. Gemfibrozil, a fibric acid, caused a 51 percent reduction in serum triglyceride levels but only a 15 percent decrease in cholesterol when given at a dose of 600 mg twice a day to adult nephrotic patients; a 26 percent reduction in apolipoprotein B was achieved [252]. Lovastatin, an inhibitor of HMG CoA reductase, causes a 27 to 29 percent reduction in total cholesterol, LDL cholesterol, and apolipoprotein B at a dose of 20 mg twice daily in adult patients with nephrosis due to diseases other than MCNS [332]. In patients with nephrotic-range proteinuria, doses up to 40 mg twice daily caused similar decreases regardless of whether the patients were on corticosteroid therapy. A slight increase was noted in serum HDL concentrations [248]. Kinetic studies showed that lovastatin enhances catabolism of VLDL triglycerides and lowers LDL cholesterol by decreasing input rates for LDL [645].

Disorders of Hemostasis. The association between nephrotic syndrome and intravascular coagulation has been known for more than a century, but it was not until 1948 that a thrombotic diathesis in nephrotic patients was proposed [5]. In a review of 3,377 children with the nephrotic syndrome, the incidence of thromboembolic complications was 1.8 percent [179]. The prevalence of such complications in adult nephrotic subjects is much higher and averaged 26 percent in 8 series of patients [410]. Thrombosis may occur at any stage during the course of the nephrotic syndrome, but it is most frequent in the early months.

Deep vein thrombosis of the leg is the most common complication in the nephrotic adult and was responsible for one-third of the thromboembolic complications in the largest published series of nephrotic children [179]. Other reported sites of venous thromboses include the subclavian, axillary, external jugular, portal, splenic, hepatic, and mesenteric veins as well as the superficial cerebral cortical sinus, where thrombosis has been described in both children and adults and often is fatal [106]. Arterial thrombosis occurs less frequently and is seen primarily in children. Thrombosis of the aorta and of the mesenteric, axillary, femoral, ophthalmic, carotid, cerebral, renal, pulmonary, and coronary arteries has been reported as has intracardiac thrombosis [106]. The pulmonary [319] and femoral arteries are particularly susceptible, the latter usually as a complication of attempted blood sampling from the femoral vein. Although recanalization of the artery does occur, a high proportion of patients with arterial thrombi die [106].

The lesion that has attracted the most attention, however, is renal vein thrombosis (RVT). It is seen most frequently with membranous glomerulonephritis [654] and is now thought to be a complication (rather than the cause) of the glomerulonephritis. The reported frequency of RVT in patients with membranous glomerulonephritis has ranged from 4 to 51 percent, depending on the methods used to establish the diagnosis of RVT and to select the patient population for study [101]. The mean prevalence is 12 percent. There is a high incidence of RVT in mesangiocapillary glomerulonephritis and the nephritis of systemic lupus erythematosus (SLE), and it can complicate numerous other renal diseases [106]. It is uncommon in nephrotic children except in those with the congenital nephrotic syndrome of the Finnish variety [106, 402]. The interesting suggestion has been made that loss of inhibitors of coagulation in the urine may predispose blood in the renal venous system to thrombosis [182].

The thrombosis may involve only the renal venous system or it may extend into the inferior vena cava. Thus it is not surprising that about 40 percent of adult patients with RVT develop pulmonary emboli, although this complication occurs rarely in children. Death from pulmonary emboli is uncommon [106, 179].

Diagnosis of acute RVT is suggested by flank pain, costovertebral angle tenderness, gross hematuria, and acute reduction in renal function; intravenous pyelography may show ureteral notching or pelvocalyceal irregularities [101]. Ultrasonography may demonstrate only a large kidney or can visualize the thrombus if it extends into the renal vein or inferior vena cava. A more chronic form of RVT may be asymptomatic and may be identifiable only by venography [101, 411]. The mode of presentation of other thromboses depends on their site. Diagnosis can be difficult and the existence of arterial thrombosis may not be realized until autopsy. Ultrasonography and angiography are the preferred studies at this time.

Many causes for the high incidence of thromboembolic complications in nephrotic syndrome have been proposed. These include alterations in blood levels of the various factors involved in the coagulation and fibrinolytic systems (Fig. 64-10), venous stasis, hemoconcentration, increased blood viscosity, and possibly the administration of steroids. Numerous observations in patients with nephrotic syndrome document alterations of blood concentrations of the factors involved in the production and inhibition of fibrin formation, in cross-linking of fibrin (factor XIII), and in fibrinolysis. These are discussed in detail elsewhere [106, 410]; only a summary is presented here.

Most studies have shown decreased blood levels of factors IX, XI, and XII [644]. Such changes are believed to result from increased urinary losses of these proteins, which are of relatively low molecular weight. In contrast, blood levels of factors II, V, VII, VIII, X, and XIII are typically increased [138, 343, 629]. The magnitude of these increases, especially those of the co-factors (factors V and VIII), correlates with the degree of reduction in serum albumin and are thought to result from increased hepatic synthesis of the factors, stimulated by hypoalbuminemia [324]. There is no direct evidence that any of these changes are responsible for the hypercoagulable state. Indeed, the alterations in blood levels of these factors frequently are inconsistent and of minor degree. Most of the changes in concentration of these zymogen factors reverse with clinical remission of the nephrotic syndrome.

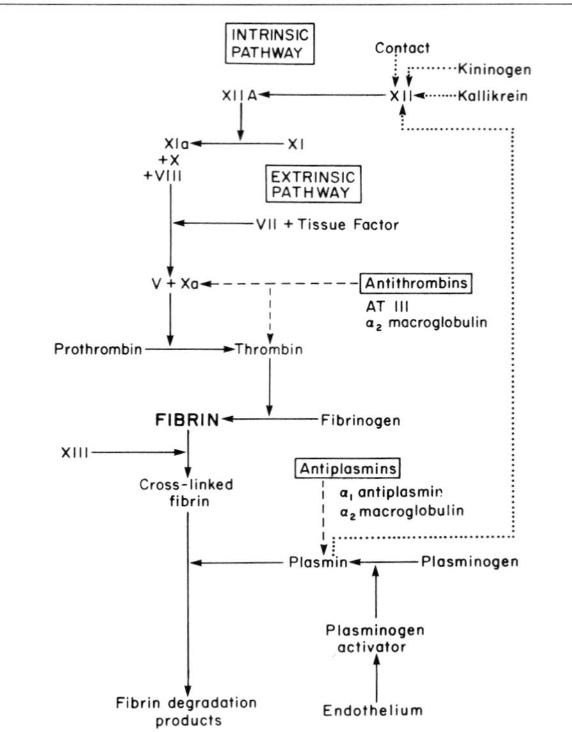

Fig. 64-10. A schema outlining the normal system for fibrin formation and for fibrinolysis. The solid lines indicate known pathways; the dotted lines, proposed pathways; and the hatched lines, inhibitory pathways. The major abnormalities described in these systems in the nephrotic syndrome are discussed in the text.

The most direct evidence for a hypercoagulable state is provided by studies of fibrinogen metabolism. Plasma fibrinogen is consistently elevated in nephrotic syndrome due to increased hepatic synthesis. Plasma fibrinogen chromatography demonstrates increased polymerization of the plasma fibrinogen; proteolytic derivatives of fibrinogen or fibrin are also present in increased concentration. These changes reverse as patients with nephrotic syndrome enter remission [14]. This evidence for increased intravascular fibrin formation is supported by the finding of increased plasma levels of fibrinopeptide A, at least in FSGS [14].

Alterations in the concentrations of several of the

components of both the fibrinolytic and antithrombin systems have been documented, too [570]. Such changes provide indirect evidence for a hypercoagulable state; most have not been correlated with the development of thrombotic complications. Decreased fibrinolytic activity has been associated with hypertriglyceridemia [602]. Of the individual components of the fibrinolytic system, decreased concentrations of plasminogen have been found [597]; levels of plasminogen activator are elevated [106]. Varying levels of α_2-antiplasmin have been reported [14, 106], possibly depending on whether thrombosis has occurred. Of the serine protease inhibitors that modulate both the fibrinolytic and thrombin systems, levels of α_2-macroglobulin are increased [629], and those of α_1-antitrypsin are decreased [629]. With regard to the antithrombins, several studies have documented low plasma concentrations of antithrombin III (AT III) in nephrotic syndrome [84, 320, 333, 385, 628]. This was presumed to be due to urinary loss of AT III, which has a relatively low molecular weight. Indeed, nephrotic syndrome plasma AT III levels correlate well with those of serum albumin and with the renal clearance of AT III. Since hereditary AT III deficiency is associated with frequent thrombosis, it was hypothesized that the low plasma AT III levels were insufficient to inactivate procoagulant factors and were the major cause for the hypercoagulable state and the development of thrombosis in nephrotic syndrome [333]. However, only patients with plasma albumin levels below 2 gm/dl show significant reductions in plasma AT III levels [22], while hypercoagulability may be present in patients with albumin levels exceeding this value. Further, normal plasma levels of AT III have been found in nephrotic subjects who had loss of AT III in the urine and who had thromboembolic complications [508]. Indeed, decreases in AT III levels may be compensated for by increased plasma levels of α_2-macroglobulin [629] and protein C [142], leading to increased total antithrombin activity [14].

Platelets may play a key role in the genesis of the coagulopathy of nephrotic syndrome. Several abnormalities have been documented. Thrombocytosis is commonly found and there is evidence for increased platelet activity. Thus platelet aggregability is increased and platelet degranulation has been described [548]. In addition, plasma levels of the platelet release substance β-thromboglobulin are increased [6], although levels of another of these factors, platelet factor 4, are reportedly normal [21].

The mechanisms responsible for the changes in platelet function have been examined. Platelet hyperaggregability correlated with the degree of proteinuria as well as with plasma cholesterol levels. It could be reversed by the addition of urine protein [22]. These findings suggest that the urinary loss of albumin [367] or some factor that normally inhibits platelet aggregation was responsible for the changes seen in nephrotic syndrome. Alternatively, hyperlipidemia could result in the changes, since platelet aggregation is increased in patients with type II hyperlipoproteinemia to a degree that is comparable to that seen in nephrotic syndrome [116]. Altered platelet function could be a response to hypoalbuminemia, since the conversion of arachidonic acid released from platelet phospholipids or elsewhere into metabolites that aggregate platelets is known to be regulated by albumin [321, 686]. Thus platelets from normal or nephrotic patients show greater production of thromboxane B_2 and malondialdehyde in nephrotic plasma than in normal plasma when challenged with arachidonic acid. Addition of albumin to the nephrotic plasma corrects this abnormality [571]. Finally, it is possible that alterations in platelet membranes could be responsible for increased platelet activity. Platelet membranes contain a sialoglycoprotein with a pK of 1.8 to 2.2 [515]. This may be important in preventing spontaneous platelet aggregation or platelet interaction with the vessel wall [227]. These negative charge sites have been shown to be reduced in relapses of nephrotic syndrome [398], perhaps by the same mechanism responsible for reduction of negative charge sites in the GBM.

Increased blood viscosity may also contribute to generation of thromboembolic complications [412]. Both children and adults with MCNS and well-preserved renal function may have marked hemoconcentration with elevated values for both hematocrit and hemoglobin concentration. Such changes are associated with disproportionate increases in viscosity and could be aggravated by the therapeutic use of diuretics, especially if they cause further hemoconcentration [592]. In addition, when plasma fibrinogen levels increase, especially to values as high as 1 gm/dl, as may be seen in nephrotic syndrome, they cause increased erythrocyte aggregation and marked increases in plasma viscosity [506].

Steroid administration is known to increase the concentrations of several clotting factors and to modify coagulation mechanisms [106]. Moreover, a high incidence of thromboses was recorded after these drugs were first used to treat nephrotic syndrome [141]. However, both arterial and venous thrombosis have been found in nephrotic subjects not receiving steroids. Furthermore, a hypercoagulable state is present in untreated MCNS patients, and levels of the coagulation factors do not change after steroid treatment is implemented [14].

Infections. It has long been known that patients with MCNS have increased susceptibility to infection. This increased risk may well be related to the prolonged presence of gross edema or ascites, which are composed of fluids that represent ideal culture media for bacterial growth. It may be potentiated by therapy with steroids or immunosuppressive drugs, although the high incidence of infections was noted in the era before these drugs were available. Humoral responses to bacteria also may be defective. Plasma concentrations of IgG are markedly reduced [233] and the ability of MCNS patients to generate specific antibodies is impaired [610], especially during relapses of the disease. Although the role of these abnormalities in predisposing nephrotic subjects to infections remains to be elucidated, it may be significant that boys with MCNS respond poorly to hepatitis B vaccine [377]. This same population has a higher incidence of chronic HB_s antigenemia than found in a control population [376]. Another factor that could contribute to a high rate of infections in the nephrotic subject is a decreased serum level of alternate complement pathway factor B. Absence of this factor has been linked to defective opsonization of *E. coli* in nephrotic patients [451] and to defective neutrophil function [18]. Serum levels of hemolytic factor D also are decreased in patients in relapse and return to normal with remission [40]. Levels of both of these factors correlate strongly with serum albumin concentration, suggesting that decreased serum levels result from urinary loss.

Consequences of Loss of Other Proteins. Numerous proteins in addition to albumin are lost in the urine. In most instances, these proteins are similar to or smaller in size than albumin. Such losses could alter function in the endocrine system or in metabolic pathways. Thus loss of insulin-like growth factors could contribute to poor growth in some nephrotic children [219]. The urinary loss of thyroxine-binding globulin (TBG) has been shown to correlate well with total urinary protein [224]. In addition to TBG, losses of thyroxine (T_4) and triiodothyronine (T_3) have been documented in nephrotic urine and are associated with decreased serum levels of T_3 and TBG. However, most of the patients studied were clinically euthyroid and their serum levels of free thyroxine and thyroid stimulating hormone (TSH) did not differ from those in normal control subjects [9]. In addition, their values for T_3 uptake were normal. Another study documented urinary losses, but normal serum concentrations, of TBG [481]. The patients had low or low-normal thyroxine levels. Such differences in findings could well relate to the underlying cause for nephrotic syndrome, whether it is associated with selective or nonselective proteinuria and whether it is accompanied by uremia. For example, impaired peripheral conversion of T_4 to T_3 has been observed in chronic renal failure [609], so that low serum T_3 values would be expected in nephrotic patients who are uremic. Children with MCNS have serum T_4 or free T_4 levels that are marginally low. They have been interpreted as having mild thyroid failure based on increased baseline TSH levels and their response to thyrotropin-releasing hormone [157].

Total serum calcium is markedly reduced, primarily because of hypoalbuminemia and the consequent decrease in protein-bound calcium referred to previously. Ionized serum calcium levels may be reduced as well [404, 433], even in nephrotic subjects with normal renal function; this may result in symptomatic hypocalcemia. Ionized serum calcium decreases about 0.2 mg/dl for each 1 gm/dl fall in serum albumin. It is now believed that at least some of the reduction in ionized calcium is the consequence of loss of 25-OH vitamin D_3 in nephrotic urine [49, 245]; other metabolites of vitamin D may be lost, too [122]. Low plasma levels of 25-OH D_3, 1,25-$(OH)_2$ D_3, and 24,25-$(OH)_2$ D_3 have been reported in patients with nephrotic syndrome [245] and intestinal absorption of calcium is reduced, too [405]; serum PTH levels are increased [433]. From these observations, it has been postulated [244] that urinary loss of vitamin D complex results in decreased absorption of intestinal calcium, skeletal resistance to parathyroid hormone, and reduced serum calcium levels. In turn, these changes cause increased parathyroid hormone production and could result in defective bone mineralization, although it has not been proved that the changes described cause significant bone disease [360]. It is likely that the maintenance of nephrotic patients on high-dose steroid medication may exacerbate a tendency to develop osteopenia, possibly because of altered vitamin D metabolism [128].

Carbohydrate metabolism also may be deranged. Of 38 adult nephrotic patients who had not received any drugs, including glucocorticoids, for at least 2 months, 14 had oral glucose tolerance tests that were similar to those found in diabetic patients [416]. Affected patients had increased insulin secretion that was felt to be secondary to increased growth hormone levels. The initiating event for these changes was not determined. There was no correlation of these findings with either serum albumin levels or renal histopathology.

Alterations in trace metal metabolism may be due to urinary losses of either the metals or their carrier proteins. Decreased serum levels of both iron and copper, associated with a low serum iron-binding capacity and low erythrocyte copper content, have been described in nephrotic syndrome [115]. Serum levels of copper, but not iron, were improved by oral administration of the metal. Urinary iron and copper concentrations correlated with protein excretion. The intravenous infusion of albumin led to increased albuminuria and increased metal excretion. In each case, the abnormalities appear to be related to urinary protein loss. A nephrotic child has been reported who developed anemia secondary to transferrin loss in the urine [183], and children with other causes for nephrotic syndrome also have been documented to have profound urinary loss of transferrin and iron [549]. Serum zinc levels are low in nephrotic syndrome, but urinary excretion of zinc is not elevated. Zinc binds to albumin so that serum zinc levels change with alterations in albumin levels, regardless of the etiology of the nephrotic syndrome. However, decreased zinc content in the hair of these patients suggests that other aspects of zinc metabolism also may be deranged [536].

Many drugs are protein-bound in the plasma. Hypoalbuminemia will decrease the number of drug-binding sites and could well result in increased toxicity of drugs that normally are bound to protein. For example, digoxin is 25 percent bound to proteins in the plasma, digitoxin is 90 percent bound, hydrochlorothiazide is 60 percent bound, and furosemide is 96 percent bound; hydralazine, prazosin, and diazoxide are all approximately 90 percent bound, whereas the binding of barbiturates varies from 5 to 80 percent, depending on molecular structure [235].

IMMUNOLOGIC ABNORMALITIES IN PRIMARY NEPHROTIC SYNDROME

It has long been recognized that immunogenic stimuli may precipitate presentation or relapse of MCNS. In addition to the frequent association with atopy discussed previously, relapse episodes may follow upper respiratory infections, bee stings, or diseases linked with abnormal immune responses. The relationship of immunogenic events to onset of disease and the finding of abnormalities of immune responses in these patients led Shalhoub [592] to propose a unifying hypothesis relating MCNS to the immune system. He cited four points: (1) evidence for abnormal humoral immune responsiveness; (2) marked sensitivity of the disease process to treatment with corticosteroids or immunosuppressive agents; (3) remission of MCNS on infection with measles, an inhibitor of cell-mediated immunity; and (4) the high incidence of MCNS in Hodgkin's disease. In view of the lack of significant morphologic evidence of renal damage, he suggested that MCNS represented the renal manifestation of a systemic immunologic abnormality rather than a primary renal disorder. Although subsequent investigation has not yet demonstrated a causal immunologic event, numerous abnormalities in both humoral and cellular immune responses [572] have been described in nephrotic patients (Table 64-10). These may, in time, provide a pathogenetic mechanism.

Immunoglobulin Synthesis. Clinical and in vitro assays have shown impaired immunoglobulin synthesis in MCNS. Serum IgG levels are decreased significantly in children with MCNS, while IgM levels are markedly increased [216, 233, 276, 534]. These values return toward normal with remission, although the IgM levels remain elevated. Not all studies have found an equal tendency toward normalization with remission, nor is this abnormality confined to MCNS in all cases [120, 269]. Although nephrotic syndrome due to diseases that cause nonselective proteinuria may be associated with urinary loss of IgG, such losses are insufficient to explain low serum IgG levels in MCNS [97]. This pattern of increased IgM and decreased IgG levels in the serum is also associated with some other immune-deficient states, most notably X-linked immunodeficiency disease [97].

Table 64-10. Immunologic abnormalities that have been described in nephrotic syndrome

Defective opsonization
- Decreased factor B [451]
- Decreased factor D [40]
- Decreased neutrophil chemiluminescence [18]
- Abnormal reticuloendothelial function [154]

Circulating immune complexes [103, 399, 424, 606]

Abnormal immunoglobulin production
- Altered serum immunoglobulin levels [97, 216, 233, 276, 543]
- Decreased specific antibody reactivity [377, 380, 470, 610]
- Decreased synthesis stimulated in vitro [150, 275, 276]
- Increased spontaneous in vitro synthesis [56, 97]

Alterations in cell surface markers [32, 150, 275, 345, 442, 620]

Altered cellular immunity
- Toxicity to renal tubular epithelium [191]
- Proliferation to glomerular basement membrane [192]
- Decreased delayed-type hypersensitivity [203, 408, 442]
- Decreased experimental local graft-versus-host disease [443]
- Increased β_2 microglobulin production [549a]
- Decreased IL-1 and IL-Z synthesis [277a, 439a]
- Decreased induced blast transformation [126, 440, 465]
- Increased inducible suppressor-cell activity [505]

Humoral immune abnormalities
- Serum toxicity to lymphocytes [503]
- Inhibition of rosette formation by serum [154, 605, 633]
- Altered antibody-dependent cellular cytotoxicity [406]
- Suppressor lymphokines [42, 301, 436]
  - Monocyte migration inhibitory factor [192, 432]
  - Vascular permeability factor [370, 374, 632]
  - Soluble immune response suppressor [575]
  - Tumor necrosis factor [616]

Depression of specific antibody titers, such as those to the common streptococcal antigens, endostreptosin, streptolysin O, and streptozyme, has been found in children and adults with idiopathic nephrotic syndrome [380]. Levels were low during active disease, remained low for up to 20 years afterwards, and were not changed by steroid therapy. Patients who were nephrotic from chronic glomerulonephritis, SLE, membranous glomerulonephritis, diabetes mellitus, or amyloidosis did not have depressed titers. These data suggest a chronic, specific impairment of response in patients with MCNS. Inability to generate [610] or to maintain [280, 470] specific titers against pneumococcal polysaccharide has been described in MCNS, but not all studies have confirmed this observation [625]. Thus depression of specific antibody titers may be restricted to certain patients or certain antigens.

In vitro secretion of immunoglobulins by lymphocytes activated with lectins has been evaluated by several groups. Correlating with the decrease in serum IgG levels, pokeweed mitogen-stimulated synthesis of IgG by patient lymphocytes has been found to be decreased in MCNS during the active stage of disease, returning toward normal with remission [150, 275, 276]. Unstimulated secretion of immunoglobulin may be increased [56, 97], suggesting spontaneous activation of lymphocytes in MCNS. Studies of IgA and IgM synthesis and of lymphocytes obtained from patients with other causes for the nephrotic syndrome have produced more variable results [407]. Decreased immunoglobulin production in vitro or in vivo could result from either abnormalities of lymphocytes or the presence of inhibitory agents systemically or on the cell surface. Evidence suggests that both mechanisms may be present in MCNS.

Studies of Lymphocyte Surface Marker Expression. These studies have been employed to determine whether the immunoglobulin abnormalities in MCNS reflect some form of immune cell dysfunction. Cells infiltrating the renal interstitium in MCNS have been found to be predominantly T lymphocytes [611]. The ratio of helper cells to suppressor cells may be similar to that found in lymphocytes in the peripheral circulation [611] or vary from one patient to another [482]. Circulating lymphocyte subsets in MCNS generally have been reported to show no significant alterations in helper-to-suppressor cell ratios [102]. Studies of B- and T-cell subpopulations have produced conflicting data, regardless of whether patients with MCNS or FSGS were studied [150, 275,

442, 620]. A potential increase in cells co-expressing B-cell and T-cell surface markers has been reported, comparable to findings in X-linked immunodeficiency [345]. However, in most studies of lymphocyte subpopulations in primary nephrotic syndrome, there are few significant changes. The meaning of the differences that have been found remains to be determined. In general, studies showing alterations in lymphocyte subpopulations may be useful in suggesting the possible presence of immune derangement, but inferences of a potential role for these changes in disease pathogenesis should be made with caution unless corroborated by accompanying functional analysis. Some progress in this direction is provided by a preliminary report indicating that circulating activated total T cells and suppressor T cells are increased, while activated helper T cells are decreased, in relapse [32].

Cellular Immunity. In studies of delayed-type hypersensitivity to common antigens, MCNS patients in relapse have been reported to have decreased skin reactivity to PPD, *Candida,* live varicella vaccine, streptokinase-streptodornase, and topical dinitrochlorobenzene [203, 408, 442]. Reactivity returns when the patients enter remission [203]. In addition, MCNS patient lymphocytes manifest decreased local graft-versus-host activity when injected into rats [443], a finding that can be normalized by preincubation of the cells with thymic humoral factor [440]. These observations may not be restricted to MCNS [439, 441].

In vitro studies also have shown abnormal cellular responses in nephrotic patients. Lymphocytes from MCNS patients, but not from normal controls or patients who were nephrotic secondary to proliferative glomerulonephritis, were found to be toxic to cultured renal tubular epithelial cells [191]. Lymphocytes from some patients also proliferated on exposure to glomerular basement membrane [192]. It is not clear from these papers whether the findings represent a primary process or the result of immunologic sensitization after renal damage. Blast transformation of patient lymphocytes has been found to be decreased in the presence of control or nephrotic sera [465], returning to normal after entry of the patient into remission [442]. Other results have shown that MCNS is associated with increased concanavalin A-activated suppressor cell activity. This finding demonstrates at least the potential for exaggerated suppressor lymphocyte responses and is not consistently found in other renal diseases [407, 505, 678].

Evidence for Abnormal Lymphokine Activity in Nephrotic Syndrome. This evidence includes the observations that sera from adult nephrotic patients inhibit leukocyte migration in the presence of renal antigens [432], that serum monocyte migration inhibitory factor activity present during relapse of MCNS disappears with remission of the disease [192], and that sera from most patients with MCNS as well as some with diffuse proliferative glomerulonephritis are lymphocytotoxic, whereas those from patients with acute tubular necrosis or urologic disease are not [503]. Sera from nephrotic patients also may inhibit the ability of cells to form rosettes [605, 633], although this is not specific for MCNS, and patient sera do not support in vitro antibody-dependent cell-mediated cytotoxicity (ADCC) assays [406]. Decreased splenic uptake of radiolabeled complexes has been correlated with deficient Fc receptor function in nephrotic patients and could be due to the presence of an inhibitory protein that attaches to cell surfaces [154]. Finally, several studies have demonstrated a suppressive effect of patient sera on blastogenesis by normal lymphocytes [55, 436, 473, 623]. The specificity of this phenomenon for MCNS has varied from one study to another. Efforts to attribute suppressive activity in nephrotic sera to a lymphokine should attempt to exclude the possibility that the observed effects are caused by nonspecific toxicity to immune responses, resulting from the biochemical abnormalities that occur in nephrotic syndrome. For example, the suppressive activity in plasma from nephrotic children segregates in the lipid-rich fraction [394]. It could thus be derived from constituents of LDL and VLDL lipoproteins that are present in increased concentrations in nephrotic plasma and suppress in vitro cellular immune responses [130, 149]. However, this finding is also consistent with migration of a suppressor lymphokine in the lipid-rich fraction.

Several studies that have partially characterized the suppressive activity suggest that production of a suppressor lymphokine may mediate suppression. A heat-stable substance, present in the sera of nephrotic patients, inhibits lymphocyte proliferation. It binds to lymphocytes in the assay system and is not removed by washing [301]. A heat-stable inhibitory substance has been described in another study in the plasma of 76 percent of 67 children with MCNS and 6 of 9 children with FSGS [42]. Only one sample from 7 patients with membranous glomerulonephritis or 31 normal adults or children showed similar activity. The factor was toxic to normal lymphocytes and was between 100,000 and 300,000 daltons in size. The preliminary finding of tumor necrosis factor (TNF) in sera of some patients may potentially be related to suppressive activity [616].

Urines and sera from children with steroid-responsive nephrotic syndrome, but not other causes for proteinuria, were reported [575] to contain the lymphokine, soluble immune response suppressor (SIRS). This factor, which inhibits antibody production [578] and delayed-type hypersensitivity responses [576], is secreted by patient lymphocytes without a requirement for exogenous stimulating agents. SIRS production could thus account for suppression of immune responses seen in nephrotic patients. Suppressive activity disappears from the urine after initiation of corticosteroid therapy but before proteinuria decreases significantly. Patient serum activates normal lymphocytes to produce SIRS by a steroid-sensitive process [577], and a regulatory mechanism has been proposed by which CD4+ T lymphocytes from patients in relapse secrete a protein that activates CD8+ T cells to produce SIRS [574]. Although the parallel between the sensitivity of SIRS production to steroids and steroid-responsiveness of nephrotic proteinuria in patients who produce SIRS is striking, there is no evidence to indicate that SIRS itself causes nephrotic proteinuria [573]. It is instead likely to serve as a marker for steroid-sensitive mechanisms of proteinuria. The means by which SIRS acts on immune responses is not known.

Circulating Immune Complexes. A variety of glomerulonephritides have been associated with soluble circulating immune complexes (CIC). It has been reported that the circulating complexes are similar to those found in the kidney; patients with MCNS had little or no IgG or IgA complexes but did have marked variation with regard to circulating IgM complexes [166]. Although CICs have been documented in some patients with MCNS or FSGS [606], not all studies have confirmed this observation [424]. A possible reason for this variation is use of different assay systems [103]. In screening studies that employed liquid- and solid-phase C1q binding and Raji-cell assays, at least one assay was positive in serum from 11 of 14 adults with MCNS, 13 of 27 patients with FSGS, and 26 of 55 patients with membranous nephropathy. Prednisone treatment did not affect the prevalence of CICs in this study [4]. In another report, 17 of 18 MCNS patients had IgG immune complexes that did not bind to C1q; in 7 of 9 patients followed serially, immune complexes disappeared within 6 weeks of entry into remission [399]. This temporal relationship and the absence of IgG in the glomerulus in patients with MCNS suggest that CICs could be a result rather than a cause of the disease, a concept supported by the observation that most known human renal diseases may involve in situ immune complex formation rather than deposition of CICs [144]. Although they may not cause the disease, some CICs could account for the apparently nonspecific presence of IgM in the mesangium of some patients. In support of this is the finding that large, neutral, or anionic complexes show focal to diffuse mesangial localization [311, 351]. Complexes containing IgM tend to be large. In contrast, low-avidity, polycationic, and small immune complexes tend to deposit in capillary or mesangiocapillary distribution.

Other Findings. Further evidence of a potential role for the immune system in MCNS is the possible relationship between this disease and allergic phenomena, already discussed, as well as the unique association between MCNS and tumors of immune-cell origin. Impaired lymphocyte blast transformation has been reported in the presence of plasma from patients with MCNS and Hodgkin's disease [474, 595]; in vitro responses improve significantly after antitumor therapy [145]. The strong association of lymphoid tumor, abnormal cellular immune responses, and MCNS would support the hypothesis that deranged immunity may play a role in the pathogenesis of at least some cases of nephrotic syndrome.

Relationship of the Immunologic Abnormality to Disease Pathogenesis. Despite all of these studies, Shalhoub's hypothesis has not yet been proved. There is strong support, however, for the concept that cellular immunity may be a mediator of proteinuria. There is increasing evidence that monocytes or macrophages are important in the pathogenesis of some forms of glomerulonephritis [584] and in the genesis of proteinuria [281, 362]. These studies imply a role for mononuclear cells but do not explain how they may act. One possibility is through release of the lymphokine, vascular permeability factor (VPF), which is produced by activated lymphocytes from some nephrotic subjects and which when injected intradermally causes increased permeability of vessels to macromolecules [370, 374]. More recently, VPF has been detected in supernatants of unstimulated cultures of patients' cells but not those of normal controls [632]. A VPF-like serine protease in patient serum has been found to decrease staining for polyanion when used to treat normal glomerular tissue [36]. However, the effect of VPF does not appear to be specific for permeability of albumin, making it an unlikely cause of selective proteinuria. Furthermore, a similar substance has been described in IgA nephropathy, even in the absence of nephrotic syndrome [37], indicating that VPF activity could be secondary to renal disease rather than a cause of proteinuria. A recently described substance produced by T-cell hybridomas derived from nephrotic patients' lymphocytes may be a more selective permeability factor [361a].

Despite the absence of proof for Shalhoub's hypothesis, the indirect evidence of an immunogenic basis for many cases of MCNS remains compelling [430]. Onset is frequently preceded by an immunogenic stimulus. Measles, which induces remission, inhibits lymphokine production but not proliferation by lymphocytes [317]. Studies of drug-related cases of MCNS induced by nonsteroidal anti-inflammatory drugs [200] or cimetidine [664] indicate that the disease may be associated with abnormal T-cell function. The relationship of disease to altered immunity is particularly striking with regard to suppressor-cell activity. A good therapeutic response to cyclophosphamide has been reported to be associated with decreased suppressor-cell activity after treatment [622], although others were unable to confirm this finding [195]. Further, as described previously, cellular and humoral immune responses are suppressed in MCNS. Thus it is intriguing that recombinant leukocyte interferon A, an agent that induces production of SIRS, has been reported to cause nephrotic syndrome with minimal glomerular changes in a patient with T-lymphocyte malignancy [33] and that the antihelminthic agent levamisole, which inhibits SIRS activity [578], has been used successfully to treat MCNS [490, 621]. Despite the evidence suggesting that cytokines may be involved in promoting vascular permeability [2], the data regarding lymphokines do not address their role as a pathogenic agent in nephrosis and are equally consistent with the interpretation that production of these substances is an epiphenomenon of the derangement that causes albuminuria. Further, the existence of differences between studies or even within a patient group in a given study suggests that multiple etiologies may exist for MCNS, only one (or several) of which may be immunologic. Considerable work remains to be done in this area.

Conclusion

From the previous discussion, several conclusions can be drawn regarding the group of diseases under consideration. First, nephrotic syndrome represents a complex of symptoms resulting from urinary protein loss rather than a disease entity characterized by specific pathology. The abnormalities found include not only the hypoalbuminemia, edema, and hyperlipidemia classically associated with nephrotic syndrome but also derangements of hemostasis, metabolism, and endocrine function. Second, the majority of children and a significant subgroup of adults with the nephrotic syndrome show insufficient histopathologic abnormalities to account for the loss of protein in the urine on the basis of disruption of the glomerular filter. Proteinuria, instead, may result from depletion or neutralization of fixed negative charges within the glomerulus. Because of the absence of significant glomerulopathy, we refer to these cases as having *primary nephrotic syndrome*. Third, primary nephrotic syndrome is characterized by heterogeneity of therapeutic response and prognosis. Although certain histopathologic variants may be associated more frequently with specific patterns of response to treatment and outcome, such categorizations are not absolute. This suggests heterogeneity of pathogenetic mechanisms, even within a given histopathologic subgroup. One potential mechanism that has received considerable attention involves abnormalities of the immune system. However, despite evidence linking immunologic abnormalities to primary nephrotic syndrome, no direct evidence has demonstrated a pathogenetic role for the associated immunologic derangements.

Finally, the heterogeneity described by these observations suggests that the relationship among histopathologic variants may best be described by a modified Venn diagram (Fig. 64-11). The majority of patients will have MCNS on biopsy. Patients with FSGS comprise an intersecting set; some cases are excluded from the MCNS group because they occur in association with other forms of renal disease (Table 64-7). Most of the patients with MCNS and some of those with FSGS are steroid-responsive. The remaining patients with MCNS and a larger proportion of those with FSGS are steroid-resistant. A smaller group of patients who have only mild mesangial proliferation (MesPGN) is found entirely within the MCNS circle. Since this pathologic finding is weakly associated with poor response to steroids, a portion of the group is included in the steroid-resistant category. Further, since patients with both FSGS and MesPGN may have a relatively poor prognosis, a majority of those patients with both findings are in the steroid-resistant category. It should be noted that mesangial proliferation is likely to be a reactive process, and diseases other than idiopathic nephrotic syndrome may manifest a mesangial proliferative component. Another subgroup within MCNS, showing mesangial deposition of IgM, may or may not have a segment belonging to the steroid-resistant population.

Fig. 64-11. Relationships among the histopathologic variants of primary nephrotic syndrome. See text for details. MCNS = minimal change nephrotic syndrome; FSGS = focal segmental glomerulosclerosis; MesPGN = mesangial hypercellularity; IgM = MCNS in which glomerular deposits of IgM are noted.

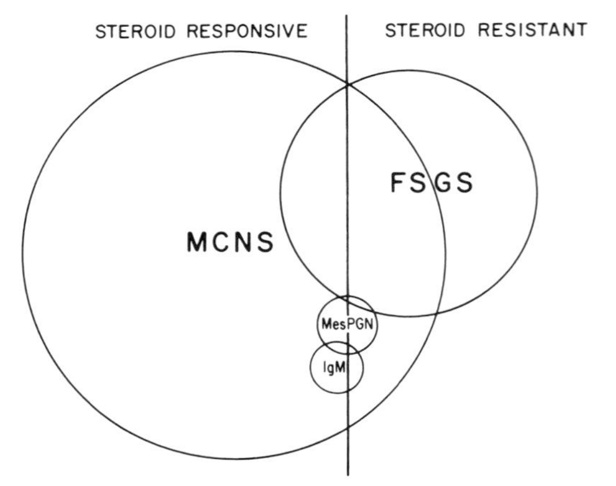

It should be clear that all the patients having a poor prognosis with regard to long-term renal function are in the steroid-resistant group. Further, changes from one form of pathology to another are possible, since all are contained within a single diagnostic entity. Finally, multiple pathogenic mechanisms are possible within this categorization. It is presumed that steroid-responsive and steroid-resistant disease involve separate pathogeneses. Some cases may be precipitated by a steroid-sensitive mechanism but eventually become resistant to steroids with the advent of a second, supervening mechanism. However, it is quite probable that several mechanisms are involved for steroid-responsive disease and several for steroid-resistant disease, accounting for the morphologic heterogeneity observed.

References

1. Abboud, H. E., Poptic, E., and DiCorleto, P. Production of platelet-derived growth factorlike protein by rat mesangial cells in culture. *J. Clin. Invest.* 80: 675, 1987.
2. Abe, Y., Sekiya, S., Yamasita, T., et al. Vascular hyperpermeability induced by tumor necrosis factor and its augmentation by IL-1 and IFN-γ is inhibited by selective depletion of neutrophils with a monoclonal antibody. *J. Immunol.* 145: 2902, 1990.
3. Abramowsky, C. R., Aikawa, M., Swinehart, G. L., et al. Spontaneous nephrotic syndrome in a genetic rat model. *Am. J. Pathol.* 117: 400, 1984.
4. Abrass, C. K. Circulating immune complexes in adults with idiopathic nephrotic syndrome. *Kidney Int.* 17: 545, 1980.
5. Addis, T. *Glomerular Nephritis, Diagnosis and Treatment.* New York: MacMillan, Vol. 1, 1948. P. 216.

5a. Adhikari, M., Manikkam, N. E. G., and Coovadia, H. M. Effect of repeated courses of daily steroids and of persistent proteinuria. On linear growth in children with nephrotic syndrome. *Pediatr. Nephrol.* 6: 4, 1992.

6. Adler, A. J., Lundin, A. P., Feinroth, M. V., et al. β-Thromboglobulin levels in the nephrotic syndrome. *Am. J. Med.* 69: 551, 1980.
7. Adler, S. H., Kopp, J. B., Dickie, P., et al. Enhanced renal extracellular matrix protein accumulation in mice

transgenic for HIV genes (abstract). *J. Am. Soc. Nephrol.* 1: 513, 1990.
8. Adu, D., Anin-Addo, Y., Foll, A. K., et al. The nephrotic syndrome in Ghana: Clinical and pathological aspects. *Q. J. Med.* 50: 297, 1981.
9. Afrasiabi, M. A., Vaziri, N. D., Gwinup, G., et al. Thyroid function studies in the nephrotic syndrome. *Ann. Intern. Med.* 90: 335, 1979.
10. Alexander, J. H., Schapel, G. J., and Edwards, D. G. Increased incidence of coronary heart disease associated with combined elevation of serum triglyceride and cholesterol concentrations in the nephrotic syndrome in man. *Med. J. Aust.* 2: 119, 1974.
11. Alfiler, C. A., Roy, L. P., Doran, T., et al. HLA-DRw7 and steroid-responsive nephrotic syndrome of childhood. *Clin. Nephrol.* 14: 71, 1980.
12. Alfino, P. A., Neugarten, J., Schacht, R. G., et al. Glomerular size-selective barrier dysfunction in nephrotoxic serum nephritis. *Kidney Int.* 34: 151, 1988.
13. Alkhader, A. A., Lien, J. W., and Aber, G. M. Cyclophosphamide alone in the treatment of adult patients with minimal change glomerulonephritis. *Clin. Nephrol.* 11: 26, 1979.
14. Alkjaersig, N., Fletcher, A. P., Narayanan, M., et al. Course and resolution of the coagulopathy in nephrotic children. *Kidney Int.* 31: 772, 1987.
15. Allen, W. R., Travis, L. B., Cavallo, T., et al. Immune deposits and mesangial hypercellularity in minimal change nephrotic syndrome: Clinical relevance. *J. Pediatr.* 100: 188, 1982.
16. Alon, U., and Chan, J. C. M. Calcium and vitamin D metabolism in nephrotic syndrome. *Int. J. Pediatr. Nephrol.* 4: 115, 1983.
17. Alpers, C. E., Harawi, S., and Rennke, H. G. Focal glomerulosclerosis with tubuloreticular inclusions: Possible predictive value for acquired immunodeficiency syndrome (AIDS). *Am. J. Kidney Dis.* 12: 240, 1988.
18. Anderson, D. C., York, T. L., Rose, G., et al. Assessment of serum factor B, serum opsonins, granulocyte chemotaxis and infection in nephrotic syndrome of children. *J. Infect. Dis.* 140: 1, 1979.
19. Anderson, S., King, A. J., and Brenner, B. M. Hyperlipidemia and glomerular sclerosis: An alternative viewpoint. *Am. J. Med.* 87: 5-34N, 1989.
20. Anderson, S., Meyer, T. W., Rennke, H. G., et al. Control of glomerular hypertension limits glomerular injury in rats with reduced renal mass. *J. Clin. Invest.* 76: 612, 1985.
21. Andrassy, K., Depperman, D., Ritz, E., et al. Different effects of renal failure on beta-thromboglobulin and high affinity platelet factor 4 (HA-PF4) concentrations. *Thromb. Res.* 18: 469, 1980.
22. Andrassy, K., Ritz, E., and Bommer, J. Hypercoagulability in the nephrotic syndrome. *Klin. Wochenschr.* 58: 1029, 1980.
23. Andrews, P. M. Glomerular epithelial alterations resulting from sialic acid surface coat removal. *Kidney Int.* 15: 376, 1979.
24. Appel, G. B., Blum, C. B., Chien, S., et al. The hyperlipidemia of the nephrotic syndrome. Relation to plasma albumin concentration, oncotic pressure and viscosity. *N. Engl. J. Med.* 312: 1544, 1985.
25. Arbeitsgemeinschaft fur Padiatrische Nephrologie. Alternate-day vs. intermittent prednisone in frequently relapsing nephrotic syndrome. *Lancet* 1: 401, 1979.
26. Arbeitsgemeinschaft fur Padiatrische Nephrologie. Effect of cytoxic drugs in frequently relapsing nephrotic syndrome with and without steroid dependence. *N. Engl. J. Med.* 306: 451, 1982.
27. Arbeitsgemeinschaft fur Padiatrische Nephrologie. Cyclophosphamide treatment of steroid dependent nephrotic syndrome: Comparison of eight week with 12 week course. *Arch. Dis. Child.* 62: 1102, 1987.
28. Arbeitsgemeinschaft fur Padiatrische Nephrologie. Short versus standard prednisone therapy for initial treatment of idiopathic nephrotic syndrome in children. *Lancet* i: 380, 1988.
29. Arbus, G. S., Poucell, S., Bacheyie, G. S., et al. Focal segmental glomerulosclerosis with idiopathic nephrotic syndrome: Three types of clinical response. *J. Pediatr.* 101: 40, 1982.
30. Arisz, I., Donker, A. J. M., Brentjens, J. R. H., et al. The effect of indomethacin on proteinuria and kidney function in the nephrotic syndrome. *Acta Med. Scand.* 199: 121, 1976.
31. Arneil, G. C. The nephrotic syndrome. *Pediatr. Clin. North Am.* 18: 547, 1971.
32. Arnold, W. C., Fisher, R. T., Carlton, R. K., et al. Two-color flow cytometric analysis of T-lymphocyte subsets in pediatric minimal change nephrotic syndrome. *J. Am. Soc. Nephrol.* 1: 557, 1990.
33. Averbuch, S. D., Austin, H. A., III, Sherwin, S. A., et al. Acute interstitial nephritis with the nephrotic syndrome following recombinant leukocyte A interferon therapy for mycosis fungoides. *N. Engl. J. Med.* 310: 32, 1984.
34. Avram, M. M. Similarities between glomerular sclerosis and atherosclerosis in human renal biopsy specimens: A role for lipoprotein glomerulopathy. *Am. J. Med.* 87: 5-39N, 1989.
35. Baak, J. P., and Wehner, H. A multivariate morphometric analysis of the glomeruli in the normal and pathologically changed human kidney. *Virchows Arch [A] [Pathol. Anat.]* 399: 105, 1983.
36. Bakker, W. W., Baller, J. F. W., van Luijk, W. H. J., et al. A kallikrein-like molecule and vasoactivity in minimal change disease: Increased turnover in relapse vs. remission. *Contrib. Nephrol.* 67: 31, 1988.
37. Bakker, W. W., Beukhof, J. R., VanLuijh, W. H., et al. Vascular permeability increasing factor (VPF) in IgA nephropathy. *Clin. Nephrol.* 18: 165, 1982.
38. Bakker, W. W., and van Luijk, W. H. J. Do circulating factors play a role in the pathogenesis of minimal change nephrotic syndrome? *Pediatr. Nephrol.* 3: 341, 1989.
39. Baldwin, D. S. Chronic glomerulonephritis: Nonimmunologic mechanisms of progressive glomerular damage. *Kidney Int.* 21: 109, 1982.
40. Ballow, M., Kennedy, T. L., Gaudio, K. M., et al. Serum hemolytic factor D values in children with steroid-responsive idiopathic nephrotic syndrome. *J. Pediatr.* 100: 192, 1982.
41. Baluarte, H. J., Gruskin, A. B., Polinsky, M. S., et al. Chlorambucil Therapy in the Nephrotic Syndrome. In A. B. Gruskin and M. Norman (eds.), *Pediatric Nephrology.* Boston: Martinus Nyhoff, 1981. P. 429.
42. Barna, B. P., Makker, S., Kallen, R., et al. A lymphocytotoxic factor(s) in plasma of patients with minimal change nephrotic syndrome: Partial characterization. *Clin. Immunol. Immunopathol.* 27: 272, 1983.
43. Barnes, J. L., Levine, S. P., and Venkatachalam, M. A. Binding of platelet factor four (PF4) to glomerular polyanion. *Kidney Int.* 25: 759, 1984.
44. Barnes, J. L., Radnik, R. A., Gilchrist, E. P., et al. Size and charge selective permeability defects induced in glo-

merular basement membrane by a polycation. *Kidney Int.* 25: 11, 1984.

45. Barness, L. A., Moll, G. H., and Janeway, C. A. Nephrotic syndrome. I. Natural history of the disease. *Pediatrics* 5: 486, 1949.
46. Barnett, H. L., Schoeneman, M., Bernstein, J., et al. Minimal Change Nephrotic Syndrome. In C. M. Edelmann (ed.), *Pediatric Kidney Disease*. Boston: Little, Brown, 1978. P. 695.
47. Barnett, H. L., Schoeneman, M., Bernstein, J., et al. The Nephrotic Syndrome. In C. M. Edelmann (ed.), *Pediatric Kidney Disease*. Boston: Little, Brown, 1978. P. 679.
48. Barr, R. D., Rees, P. H., Cordy, P. E., et al. Nephrotic syndrome in adult Africans in Nairobi. *Br. Med. J.* 2: 131, 1972.
49. Barragry, J. M., France, M. W., Carter, N. D., et al. Vitamin D metabolism in nephrotic syndrome. *Lancet* 2: 629, 1977.
50. Barratt, T. M., and Soothill, J. F. Controlled trial of cyclophosphamide in steroid-sensitive relapsing nephrotic syndrome of childhood. *Lancet* 2: 479, 1970.
51. Bass, J. E., Fisher, E. A., Prack, M. M., et al. Macrophages from nephrotic rats regulate apolipoprotein E biosynthesis and cholesterol content independently. *J. Clin. Invest.* 87: 470, 1991.
52. Baxter, J. H. Hyperlipoproteinemia in nephrosis. *Arch. Intern. Med.* 109: 742, 1962.
53. Baxter, J. H., Goodman, H. C., and Allen, J. C. Effects of infusions of serum albumin on serum lipids and lipoproteins in nephrosis. *J. Clin. Invest.* 40: 490, 1961.
54. Baxter, J. H., Goodman, H. C., and Havel, R. J. Serum lipid and lipoprotein alterations in nephrosis. *J. Clin. Invest.* 39: 455, 1960.
55. Beale, M. G., Hoffsten, P. E., Robson, A. M., et al. Inhibitory factors of lymphocyte transformation in sera from patients with minimal change nephrotic syndrome. *Clin. Nephrol.* 13: 271, 1980.
56. Beale, M. G., Nash, G. S., Bertovich, M. J., et al. Immunoglobulin synthesis by peripheral blood mononuclear cells in minimal change nephrotic syndrome. *Kidney Int.* 23: 380, 1983.
57. Beale, M. G., Strayer, D. S., Kissane, J. M., et al. Congenital glomerulosclerosis and nephrotic syndrome in two infants. *Am. J. Dis. Child.* 133: 842, 1979.
58. Beaman, M., Howie, A. J., Hardwicke, J., et al. The glomerular tip lesion: A steroid responsive nephrotic syndrome. *Clin. Nephrol.* 27: 217, 1987.
59. Bennett, W. M., and Porter, G. A. Efficacy and safety of metolazone in renal failure and the nephrotic syndrome. *J. Clin. Pharmacol.* 13: 357, 1973.
60. Berg, U., and Bohlin, A. B. Renal hemodynamics in minimal change nephrotic syndrome in childhood. *Int. J. Pediatr. Nephrol.* 3: 187, 1982.
61. Bergstein, J. M. Prostaglandin inhibitors in the treatment of nephrotic syndrome. *Pediatr. Nephrol.* 5: 335, 1991.
62. Berlyne, G. M., and Mallick, N. P. Ischaemic heart disease as a complication of nephrotic syndrome. *Lancet* ii: 399, 1969.
63. Bernard, D. B. Metabolic Abnormalities in Nephrotic Syndrome: Pathophysiology and Complications. In B. M. Brenner and J. H. Stein (eds.), *Contemporary Issues in Nephrology. IX. Nephrotic Syndrome*. New York: Churchill Livingstone, 1982. P. 85.
64. Bernstein, J. Renal Hypoplasia and Dysplasia. In C. M. Edelmann (ed.), *Pediatric Kidney Disease*. Boston: Little, Brown, 1978. Pp. 541–556.
65. Bernstein, J., Jr., and Edelmann, C. M., Jr. Minimal change nephrotic syndrome. Histopathology and steroid responsiveness (Editorial). *Arch. Dis. Child.* 57: 816, 1982.
66. Bertolatus, J. A., Abuyousefy, M., and Hunsicker, L. G. Glomerular sieving of high molecular weight proteins in proteinuric rats. *Kidney Int.* 31: 1257, 1987.
67. Bertolatus, J. A., and Hunsicker, L. G. Glomerular sieving of anionic and neutral bovine albumins in proteinuric rats. *Kidney Int.* 28: 467, 1985.
68. Black, D. A. K. Controlled trial of prednisone in adult patients with the nephrotic syndrome. *Br. Med. J.* 3: 421, 1970.
69. Blainey, J. D. High protein diets in the treatment of the nephrotic syndrome. *Clin. Sci.* 13: 567, 1954.
70. Blainey, J. D., Brewer, D. B., Hardwicke, J., et al. The nephrotic syndrome: Diagnosis by renal biopsy and biochemical and immunologic analyses related to the response to steroid therapy. *Am. J. Med.* 29: 235, 1960.
71. Blau, E. B., and Haas, J. E. Glomerular sialic acid and proteinuria in human renal disease. *Lab. Invest.* 38: 477, 1973.
72. Blau, E. B., and Michael, A. F. Rat glomerular glycoprotein composition and metabolism in aminonucleoside nephrosis. *Proc. Soc. Exp. Biol. Med.* 141: 164, 1972.
73. Bluett, N. H., Chantler, C., and Huges, D. T. Failure of doxantrole in steroid-sensitive nephrotic syndrome. *Lancet* 1: 809, 1977.
74. Bogdanovic, R., Banicevic, M., and Cvoric, A. Pituitary-gonadal function in women following cyclophosphamide treatment for childhood nephrotic syndrome: Long-term follow-up study. *Pediatr. Nephrol.* 4: 455, 1990.
75. Bogdanovic, R., Banicevic, M., and Cvoric, A. Testicular function following cyclophosphamide treatment for childhood nephrotic syndrome: Long-term follow-up study. *Pediatr. Nephrol.* 4: 451, 1990.
76. Bohlin, A.-B. Clinical course and renal function in minimal change nephrotic syndrome. *Acta Paediatr. Scand.* 73: 631, 1984.
77. Bohlin, A.-B., and Berg, U. Renal sodium handling in minimal change nephrotic syndrome. *Arch. Dis. Child.* 59: 825, 1984.
78. Bohlin, A.-B., and Berg, U. Renal water handling in minimal change nephrotic syndrome. *Int. J. Pediatr. Nephrol.* 2: 93, 1984.
79. Bohman, S.-O., Jeremko, G., Bohlin, A.-B., et al. Foot process fusion and glomerular filtration rate in minimal change nephrotic syndrome. *Kidney Int.* 25: 696, 1984.
80. Bohrer, M. P., Baylis, C., Humes, H. D., et al. Permselectivity of the glomerular capillary wall. Facilitated filtration of circulating polycations. *J. Clin. Invest.* 61: 72, 1978.
81. Bohrer, M. P., Baylis, C., Robertson, C. R., et al. Mechanism of the puromycin-induced defects in the transglomerular passage of water and macromolecules. *J. Clin. Invest.* 60: 152, 1977.
82. Bohrer, M. P., Deen, W. M., Robertson, C., et al. Mechanism of angiotensin II-induced proteinuria in the rat. *Am. J. Physiol.* 233: F13, 1977.
83. Bolton, W. K., Westervelt, F. B., and Sturgill, B. C. Nephrotic syndrome and focal glomerular sclerosis in aging man. *Nephron* 20: 307, 1978.
84. Boneu, B., Boissou, F., Abbal, M., et al. Comparison of progressive antithrombin activity and the concentration of three thrombin inhibitors in nephrotic syndrome. *Thromb. Haemost.* 46: 623, 1981.

85. Border, W. A. Distinguishing minimal change disease from mesangial disorders. *Kidney Int.* 34: 419, 1988.
86. Border, W. A., Okuda, S., Languino, L. R., et al. Transforming growth factor-β regulates production of proteoglycans by mesangial cells. *Kidney Int.* 37: 689, 1990.
87. Bourgoignie, J. J., Meneses, R., Ortiz, C., et al. The clinical spectrum of renal disease associated with human immunodeficiency virus. *Am. J. Kidney Dis.* 12: 131, 1988.
88. Brenner, B. M., Bohrer, M. P., Baylis, C., et al. Determinants of glomerular permselectivity: Insights derived from observations *in vivo*. *Kidney Int.* 12: 229, 1977.
89. Brenner, B. M., Hostetter, T. H., and Humes, H. D. Glomerular permselectivity: Barrier function based on discrimination of molecular size and charge. *Am. J. Physiol.* 234: F455, 1978.
90. Brenner, B. M., Hostetter, T. H., and Humes, H. D. Molecular basis of proteinuria of glomerular origin. *N. Engl. J. Med.* 298: 826, 1978.
91. Brenner, B. M., Meyer, T. W., and Hostetter, T. H. Dietary protein intake and the progressive nature of kidney disease: The role of hemodynamically mediated glomerular injury in the pathogenesis of progressive glomerulosclerosis in aging, renal ablation, and intrinsic renal disease. *N. Engl. J. Med.* 307: 652, 1982.
92. Brezin, J. H., Katz, S. M., Schwarts, A. B., et al. Reversible renal failure and nephrotic syndrome associated with non-steroidal anti-inflammatory drugs. *N. Engl. J. Med.* 301: 1271, 1979.
93. Bridges, C. R., Myers, B. D., Brenner, B. M., et al. Glomerular charge alterations in human minimal change nephropathy. *Kidney Int.* 22: 677, 1982.
93a. Bridges, C. R., Rennke, H. G., Deen, W. M., et al. Reversible hexadimethrine-induced alterations in glomerular structure and permeability. *J. Am. Soc. Nephrol.* 1: 1095, 1991.
93b. British Association for Pediatric Nephrology. Levamisole for corticosteroid-dependent nephrotic syndrome in childhood. *Lancet* 337: 1555, 1991.
94. Brockelbank, J. T., Harcourt, R. B., and Meadow, S. R. Corticosteroid-induced cataracts in idiopathic nephrotic syndrome. *Arch. Dis. Child.* 53: 30, 1982.
95. Brodehl, J., and Hoyer, P. F. Ciclosporin in idiopathic nephrotic syndrome of children. *Am. J. Nephrol.* 9(Suppl. 1): 61, 1989.
96. Brodehl, J., Krohn, H. P., and Ehrich, J. H. The treatment of minimal change nephrotic syndrome (lipoid nephrosis): Cooperative studies of the Arbeitsgemeinschaft fur Padiatrische Nephrol (APN). *Klin. Paediatr.* 194: 162, 1982.
97. Brouhard, B. H., Goldblum, R. M., Bunce, H., III, et al. Immunoglobulin synthesis and urinary IgG excretion in the idiopathic nephrotic syndrome of children. *Int. J. Pediatr. Nephrol.* 2: 163, 1981.
98. Brown, C. B., Cameron, J. S., Turner, D. R., et al. Focal segmental glomerulosclerosis with rapid decline in renal function ("malignant FSGS"). *Clin. Nephrol.* 10: 51, 1978.
99. Brown, E. A., Markandu, N. D., Roulston, J. E., et al. Is the renin-angiotensin system involved in the sodium retention in the nephrotic syndrome? *Nephron* 32: 102, 1982.
100. Brown, E. A., Upadhyaya, K., Hayslett, J. P., et al. The clinical course of mesangial proliferative glomerulonephritis. *Medicine* (Baltimore) 58: 295, 1979.
100a. Bruggeman, L. A., Horigan, E. A., Horikoshi, S., et al. Thromboxane stimulates synthesis of extracellular matrix proteins in vitro. *Am. J. Physiol.* 261: F488, 1991.
101. Cade, R., Spooner, G., Juncos, L., et al. Chronic renal vein thrombosis. *Am. J. Med.* 63: 387, 1977.
102. Cagnoli, L., Tabacchi, P., Pasquali, S., et al. T cell subset alterations in idiopathic glomerulonephritis. *Clin. Exp. Immunol.* 50: 70, 1982.
103. Cairns, S. A., London, R. A., and Mallick, N. P. Circulating immune complexes in idiopathic glomerular disease. *Kidney Int.* 21: 507, 1982.
104. Cale, W. F., Ullrich, I. H., and Jenkins, J. J. Nodular sclerosing Hodgkin's disease presenting as nephrotic syndrome. *South Med. J.* 75: 604, 1982.
105. Cambon-Thomsen, A., Boissou, F., Abbal, M., et al. HLA et Bf dans le syndrome nephrotique idiopathique de l'enfant: Differences entre les formes corticosensibles et corticoresistantes. *Pathol. Biol.* (Paris) 34: 725, 1986.
106. Cameron, J. S. Coagulation and thromboembolic complications in the nephrotic syndrome. *Adv. Nephrol.* 13: 75, 1984.
107. Cameron, J. S. Mechanisms of progression in glomerulonephritis. *Proc. Eur. Dial. Transplant. Assoc.* 19: 617, 1983.
108. Cameron, J. S., and Blandford, G. The simple assessment of selectivity in heavy proteinuria. *Lancet* ii: 242, 1966.
109. Cameron, J. S., Chantler, C., Ogg, C. S., et al. Long-term remission in nephrotic syndrome after treatment with cyclophosphamide. *Br. Med. J.* 4: 7, 1974.
110. Cameron, J. S., and Hicks, J. Pregnancy in patients with pre-existing glomerular disease. *Contrib. Nephrol.* 37: 149, 1984.
111. Cameron, J. S., Turner, D. R., Ogg, C. S., et al. The nephrotic syndrome in adults with "minimal change glomerular lesion." *Q. J. Med.* 43: 461, 1974.
112. Cameron, J. S., Turner, D. R., Ogg, C. S., et al. The long-term prognosis of patients with focal segmental glomerulosclerosis. *Clin. Nephrol.* 10: 213, 1978.
113. Cameron, J. S., Wass, V., Jarrett, R. J., et al. Nephrotic syndrome and cardiovascular disease. *Lancet* ii: 1017, 1979.
114. Carrie, B. J., Salyer, W. R., and Myers, B. D. Minimal change nephropathy: An electrochemical disorder of the glomerular membranes. *Am. J. Med.* 70: 262, 1981.
115. Cartwright, G. E., Gubler, C. J., and Wintrobe, M. M. Studies on copper metabolism. XI. Copper and iron metabolism in the nephrotic syndrome. *J. Clin. Invest.* 33: 685, 1954.
116. Carvalho, A., Colman, R., and Lees, R. Platelet function in hyperlipoproteinemia. *N. Engl. J. Med.* 290: 434, 1974.
117. Castellot, J. J., Beeler, D. L., Rosenberg, R. D., et al. Structural determinants of the capacity of heparin to inhibit the proliferation of vascular smooth muscle cells. *J. Cell. Physiol.* 120: 315, 1984.
118. Caulfield, J. P., and Farquhar, M. G. The permeability of glomerular capillaries to graded dextrans. Identification of the basement membranes as the primary filtration barrier. *J. Cell Biol.* 63: 883, 1974.
119. Cavallo, T., and Johnson, M. P. Immunopathologic study of minimal change of glomerular disease with mesangial IgM deposits. *Nephron* 27: 281, 1981.
120. Chan, M. K., Chan, K. W., and Jones, B. Immunoglobulins (IgG, IgA, IgM, IgE) and complement components (C_3, C_4) in nephrotic syndrome due to minimal change and other forms of glomerulonephritis: A clue for steroid therapy? *Nephron* 47: 125, 1987.
121. Chan, M. K., Persaud, J. W., Ramdial, L., et al. Hyperlipidemia in untreated nephrotic syndrome, increased

production or decreased removal? *Clin. Chim. Acta* 117: 317, 1981.

122. Chan, Y. L., Mason, R. S., Parmentier, M., et al. Vitamin D metabolism in nephrotic rats. *Kidney Int.* 24: 336, 1983.
123. Chandra, M., Mouradian, J., and Hoyer, F. R. Familial nephrotic syndrome and focal segmental glomerulosclerosis. *J. Pediatr.* 98: 556, 1981.
124. Chang, R. L. S., Deen, W. M., Robertson, C. R., et al. Permselectivity of the glomerular capillary wall: III. Restricted transport of polyanion. *Kidney Int.* 8: 212, 1975.
125. Chang, R. L. S., Deen, W. M., Robertson, C. R., et al. Permselectivity of the glomerular capillary wall. Studies of experimental glomerulonephritis in the rat using neutral dextran. *J. Clin. Invest.* 57: 1272, 1976.
126. Chapman, S., Taube, D., Brown, Z., et al. Impaired lymphocyte transformation in minimal change nephropathy in remission. *Clin. Nephrol.* 18: 34, 1982.
127. Cheigh, J. S., Mouradian, J., Soliman, M., et al. Focal segmental glomerulosclerosis in renal transplants. *Am. J. Kidney Dis.* 2: 449, 1983.
128. Chesney, R. F., Hamstra, A., Rose, P., et al. Vitamin D and parathyroid hormone status in children with the nephrotic syndrome and chronic mild glomerulonephritis. *Int. J. Pediatr. Nephrol.* 5: 1, 1984.
129. Chinard, F. P., Lauson, H. D., Eder, H. A., et al. A study of the mechanism of proteinuria in patients with the nephrotic syndrome. *J. Clin. Invest.* 33: 621, 1954.
130. Chisari, F. V. Immunoregulatory properties of human plasma in very low density lipoproteins. *J. Immunol.* 119: 2129, 1977.
131. Chopra, J. S., Mallick, N. P., and Stone, M. C. Hyperlipoproteinemias in the nephrotic syndrome. *Lancet* i: 317, 1971.
132. Churg, J., Grishman, E., Goldstein, M. H., et al. Idiopathic nephrotic syndrome in adults. *N. Engl. J. Med.* 272: 165, 1965.
133. Churg, J., Habib, R., and White, R. H. R. Pathology of the nephrotic syndrome in children. A report for the International Study of Kidney Disease in Children. *Lancet* i: 1299, 1970.
134. Coggins, C. H. Minimal Change Nephrosis in Adults. In *Proceedings of the 8th International Congress of Nephrology.* Basel: Karger, 1981. P. 336.
135. Cohen, A. H. Massive obesity and the kidney. *Am. J. Pathol.* 81: 117, 1975.
136. Cohen, A. H., Border, W. A., and Glassock, R. J. Nephrotic syndrome with glomerular mesangial IgM deposits. *Lab. Invest.* 38: 610, 1978.
137. Cohen, L., Cramp, D. G., Lewis, A. D., et al. The mechanism of hyperlipidemia in nephrotic syndrome—Role of low albumin and the LCAT reaction. *Clin. Chim. Acta* 104: 393, 1980.
138. Coppola, R., Guerra, L., Ruggeri, Z. M., et al. Factor VIII/von Willebrand factor in glomerular nephropathies. *Clin. Nephrol.* 16: 217, 1981.
139. Cornfeld, D., and Schwartz, M. W. Nephrosis: A long-term study of children treated with corticosteroids. *J. Pediatr.* 68: 507, 1966.
140. Cortney, M. A., Sawin, L. L., and Weiss, D. D. Renal tubular protein absorption in the rat. *J. Clin. Invest.* 49: 1, 1970.
141. Cosgriff, S. W. Thromboembolic complications associated with ACTH and cortisone therapy. *J.A.M.A.* 147: 924, 1951.
142. Cosio, F. G., Harker, C., Batard, M. A., et al. Plasma concentrations of the natural anticoagulants protein C and protein S in patients with proteinuria. *J. Lab. Clin. Med.* 106: 218, 1985.
143. Cotran, R. S. Glomerulosclerosis in reflux nephropathy. *Kidney Int.* 21: 528, 1982.
144. Couser, W. G. What are circulating immune complexes doing in glomerulonephritis? *N. Engl. J. Med.* 304: 1230, 1981.
145. Crowley, J. P., Ree, H. J., and Esparza, A. Monocyte-dependent serum suppression of lymphocyte blastogenesis in Hodgkin's disease: An association with nephrotic syndrome. *J. Clin. Immunol.* 2: 270, 1982.
146. Cunningham, E. E., Brentjens, J. R., Zielezny, M. A., et al. Heroin nephropathy: A clinicopathologic and epidemiology study. *Am. J. Med.* 68: 47, 1980.
147. Cuoghi, D., Evangelista, A., Baraldi, A., et al. Relapse of nephrotic syndrome following remission for 20 years. *Int. J. Pediatr. Nephrol.* 4: 211, 1983.
148. Curt, G. A., Kaldany, A., and Whitley, L. G. Reversible rapidly progressive renal failure with nephrotic syndrome due to fenoprofen calcium. *Ann. Intern. Med.* 92: 72, 1980.
149. Curtiss, L. K., and Edgington, T. S. Regulatory serum lipoproteins: Regulation of lymphocyte stimulation by a species of low density lipoprotein. *J. Immunol.* 118: 1452, 1976.
150. Dall'Aglio, P. Minimal change glomerulonephritis and focal glomerulosclerosis markers and *'in vitro'* activity of peripheral blood mononuclear cells. *Proc. Eur. Dial. Transplant. Assoc.* 19: 673, 1982.
151. Danielsen, H., Kornerup, H. J., Olsen, S., et al. Arterial hypertension in chronic glomerulonephritis. An analysis of 310 cases. *Clin. Nephrol.* 19: 284, 1983.
152. Dash, S. C., Molhotra, K. K., Sharma, R. K., et al. Reversible acute renal failure in idiopathic nephrotic syndrome with minimal change nephropathy. *J. Assoc. Physicians India* 30: 399, 1982.
153. Davies, R. W., Staprans, I., Hutchison, F. N., et al. Proteinuria, not altered albumin metabolism, affects hyperlipidemia in the nephrotic rat. *J. Clin. Invest.* 86: 600, 1990.
154. Davin, J. C., Foidart, J. B., and Mahieu, P. R. Fc receptor function in minimal change nephrotic syndrome of childhood. *Clin. Nephrol.* 20: 280, 1983.
155. Davis, R. A., Engelhorn, S. C., Weinstein, D. B., et al. Very low density lipoprotein secretion by cultured rat hepatocytes. Inhibition by albumin and other macromolecules. *J. Biol. Chem.* 255: 2039, 1980.
156. Deen, W. M., Myers, B. D., and Brenner, B. M. The Glomerular Barrier to Macromolecules: Theoretical and Experimental Considerations. In B. M. Brenner and J. H. Stein (eds.), *Contemporary Issues in Nephrology. IX. Nephrotic Syndrome.* New York: Churchill Livingstone, 1982. P. 1.
157. DeLuca, F., Gemelli, M., Pandullo, E., et al. Changes in thyroid function tests in infantile nephrotic syndrome. *Horm. Metab. Res.* 15: 258, 1983.
158. DeLuca, G., Delinid, N., and D'Andrea, S. Un raro caso di nefrosi congenita e malattia de inclusioni citomegalicho. *Minerva Pediatr.* 16: 1164, 1964.
159. deMendoza, S. G., Kashyap, M. L., Chen, C. Y., et al. High density lipoproteinuria in nephrotic syndrome. *Metabolism* 25: 1143, 1976.
160. deMouzon-Cambon, A., Bouissou, F., Dutau, G., et al. HLA-DR7 in children with idiopathic nephrotic syndrome. Correlation with atopy. *Tissue Antigens* 17: 518, 1981.

161. Dennis, V. W., and Robinson, R. R. Proteinuria. In C. M. Edelmann (ed.), *Pediatric Kidney Disease*. Boston: Little, Brown, 1978. P. 306.
162. Diamond, J. R. Effects of dietary interventions on glomerular pathophysiology. *Am. J. Physiol.* 258: F1, 1990.
163. Diamond, J. R., and Karnovsky, M. J. Exacerbation of chronic aminonucleoside nephrosis by dietary cholesterol supplementation. *Kidney Int.* 32: 671, 1987.
164. Diamond, J. R., and Karnovsky, M. J. Focal and segmental glomerulosclerosis: Analogies to atherosclerosis. *Kidney Int.* 33: 917, 1988.
165. Dixit, V. M., and Hettiaratchi, E. S. The mechanism of hyperlipidemia in the nephrotic syndrome. *Med. Hypotheses* 5: 1327, 1979.
166. Doi, T., Kanatsu, K., Sekita, K., et al. Circulating immune complexes of IgG, IgA and IgM classes in various glomerular diseases. *Nephron* 32: 335, 1982.
167. Doi, T., Striker, L. J., Quaife, C., et al. Progressive glomerulosclerosis develops in transgenic mice expressing growth hormone and growth hormone releasing factor but not in those expressing insulinlike growth factor-1. *Am. J. Pathol.* 131: 398, 1988.
168. Don, B. R., Wada, L., Kaysen, G. A., et al. Effect of dietary protein restriction and angiotensin converting enzyme inhibition on protein metabolism in the nephrotic syndrome. *Kidney Int.* 36(Suppl. 27): S-163, 1989.
169. Donadio, J. V., Jr. Primary glomerular disease: To treat or not to treat. *Contrib. Nephrol.* 33: 86, 1982.
170. Donadio, J. V., Anderson, C. F., Mitchell, J. C., et al. Membranoproliferative glomerulonephritis. A prospective clinical trial of platelet inhibitor therapy. *N. Engl. J. Med.* 310: 1421, 1984.
171. Donker, A. J. M., Brentjens, J. R. H., van der Hem, et al. Treatment of the nephrotic syndrome with indomethacin. *Nephron* 22: 374, 1978.
172. Dorhout Mees, E. J., Roos, J. C., Boer, P., et al. Observations on edema formation in the nephrotic syndromes in adults with minimal lesion. *Am. J. Med.* 67: 378, 1979.
173. Dulaney, J. T., and Hatch, F. E., Jr. Peritoneal dialysis and loss of protein: A review. *Kidney Int.* 26: 253, 1984.
174. Dundon, S., O'Callaghan, U., and Raftery, J. Stability of remission in minimal lesion nephrotic syndrome after treatment with prednisone and cyclophosphamide. *Int. J. Pediatr. Nephrol.* 1: 22, 1980.
175. Dworkin, L. D., Hostetter, T. H., Rennke, H. G., et al. Evidence for a hemodynamic basis for glomerular injury in hypertension. *Kidney Int.* 21: 229, 1982.
176. Eagen, J. W., and Lewis, E. J. Glomerulopathies of neoplasia. *Kidney Int.* 11: 297, 1977.
177. Ebihara, I., Nakamura, T., Suzuki, S., et al. Altered expression of matrix genes in glomeruli with focal glomerular sclerosis (FGS) (abstract). *J. Am. Soc. Nephrol.* 1: 349, 1990.
178. Editorial. More about minimal change. *Lancet* 1: 1298, 1981.
179. Egli, F., Eiminger, P., and Stalder, G. Thromboembolism in the nephrotic syndrome. *Pediatr. Res.* 8: 903, 1974.
180. Eisenberg, S. Blood volume in persons with the nephrotic syndrome. *Am. J. Med. Sci.* 255: 320, 1968.
181. Elema, J. D., and Arends, A. Focal and segmental glomerular hyalinosis and sclerosis in the rat. *Lab. Invest.* 33: 554, 1975.
182. Elliott, G. B., Grant-Tyrell, J., and Ringer, G. Congenital lipoid nephrosis with left renal vein thrombosis and Chiari's syndrome. *J. Can. Assoc. Radiol.* 30: 175, 1979.
183. Ellis, D. Anemia in the course of nephrotic syndrome secondary to transferrin depletion. *J. Pediatr.* 90: 953, 1977.
184. Ellis, D., Kapur, S., Antonovych, T., et al. Focal glomerulosclerosis in children: Correlation of histology with prognosis. *J. Pediatr.* 93: 762, 1978.
185. Elzouki, A. Y., Al-Nassar, K., Al-Ali, M., et al. Sister chromatid exchange analysis in monitoring chlorambucil therapy in primary nephrotic syndrome of childhood. *Pediatr. Nephrol.* 5: 59, 1991.
186. Elzouki, A. T., and Jaiswal, O. P. Evaluation of chlorambucil therapy in steroid-dependent and cyclophosphamide-resistant children with nephrosis. *Pediatr. Nephrol.* 4: 459, 1990.
187. Epstein, A. A. The nature and treatment of chronic parenchymatous nephritis (nephrosis). *J.A.M.A.* 69: 444, 1917.
188. Epstein, E. H. Underfilling vs. overflow in hepatic ascites. (Editorial) *N. Engl. J. Med.* 307: 1577, 1982.
189. Epstein, M., Loutzenhiser, R., Friedland, E., et al. Relationship of increased plasma atrial natriuretic factor and renal sodium handling during immersion-induced central hypervolemia in normal humans. *J. Clin. Invest.* 79: 738, 1987.
190. Etteldorf, J. N., West, C. D., Pitcock, J. A., et al. Gonadal function, testicular histology and meiosis following cyclophosphamide. *J. Pediatr.* 88: 206, 1976.
191. Eyres, K., Mallick, N. P., and Taylor, G. Evidence for cell-mediated immunity to renal antigens in minimal-change nephrotic syndrome. *Lancet* i: 1158, 1976.
192. Eyres, K., Mallick, N. P., and Taylor, G. Studies of cellular immune responses in patients with minimal change nephropathy. *Dial. Transplant. Nephrol.* 11: 533, 1976.
193. Falck, H. M., Tornroth, T., Kock, B., et al. Fatal renal vasculitis and minimal change glomerulonephritis complicating treatment with penicillamine. Report on two cases. *Acta Med. Scand.* 205: 133, 1979.
194. Farquhar, M. G., Vernier, R. L., and Good, R. A. An electron microscope study of the glomerulus in nephrosis, glomerulonephritis, and lupus erythematosus. *J. Exp. Med.* 106: 649, 1957.
195. Feehally, J., Beattie, T. J., Brenchley, P. E. C., et al. Modulation of cellular immune function by cyclophosphamide in children with minimal change nephropathy. *N. Engl. J. Med.* 310: 415, 1984.
196. Feinfeld, D. A., Olesnicky, L., Pirani, C. L., et al. Nephrotic syndrome associated with use of the nonsteroidal anti-inflammatory drugs. Case report and reviews of the literature. *Nephron* 37: 174, 1984.
197. Felts, J. M., and Mayerle, J. A. Urinary loss of plasma high density lipoprotein—A possible cause of hyperlipidemia in the nephrotic syndrome. *Circulation* 49/50 (Suppl. III): 263, 1974.
198. Fielding, C. J. Human lipoprotein lipase inhibition of activity by cholesterol. *Biochim. Biophys. Acta* 218: 221, 1970.
199. Fielding, C. J., Shore, V. G., and Fielding, P. E. Lecithin: cholesterol acyltransferase: Effects of substrate upon enzyme activity. *Biochim. Biophys. Acta* 270: 513, 1972.
200. Finkelstein, A., Fraley, D. S., Stachura, I., et al. Fenprofen nephropathy: Lipoid nephrosis and interstitial nephritis. A possible T-lymphocyte disorder. *Am. J. Med.* 72: 81, 1982.
201. Fleck, A., Raines, G., Hawker, F., et al. Increased vascular permeability: A major cause of hypoalbuminemia in disease and injury. *Lancet* ii: 781, 1985.

202. Fleisher, D. S., McCrory, W. W., and Rapoport, M. The effects of intermittent doses of adrenocortical steroids on the statural growth of nephrotic children. *J. Pediatr.* 57: 192, 1960.
203. Fodor, P., Saitua, M. T., Rodriguez, E., et al. T-cell dysfunction in minimal-change nephrotic syndrome of childhood. *Am. J. Dis. Child.* 136: 713, 1982.
204. Fogo, A., Hawkins, E. P., Berry, P. L., et al. Glomerular hypertrophy in minimal change disease predicts subsequent progression to focal glomerular sclerosis. *Kidney Int.* 38: 115, 1990.
205. Fontana, V. J., Spain, W. C., and Desanctis, A. G. The role of allergy in nephrosis. *N.Y. State J. Med.* 56: 3907, 1956.
206. Foote, K. D., Brocklebank, J. T., and Meadow, S. R. Height attainment in children with steroid-responsive nephrotic syndrome. *Lancet* ii: 917, 1985.
207. Forland, M., and Bannayan, G. A. Minimal-change lesion nephrotic syndrome with renal oncocytoma. *Am. J. Med.* 75: 715, 1983.
208. Francis, K. L., Jenis, E. H., Jensen, G. E., et al. Gold-associated nephropathy. *Arch. Pathol. Lab. Med.* 108: 234, 1984.
209. Froelich, C. J., Searles, R. P., Davis, L. E., et al. A case of Guillain-Barré syndrome with immunologic abnormality. *Ann. Intern. Med.* 93: 563, 1980.
210. Futrakul, P. A new therapeutic approach to nephrotic syndrome associated with focal segmental glomerulosclerosis. *Int. J. Pediatr. Nephrol.* 1: 18, 1980.
211. Futrakul, P., Porhyachinda, M., and Mitrakul, C. Focal sclerosing glomerulonephritis. A kinetic evaluation of hemostasis and the effect of anticoagulant therapy: A controlled study. *Clin. Nephrol.* 10: 180, 1978.
212. Fydryk, J., Waldherr, R., Mall, G., et al. Mesangial alterations in steroid-responsive minimal change nephrotic syndrome. *Virchow's Arch.* [*Pathol. Anat.*] 397: 193, 1982.
213. Gaboardi, F., Perletti, L., Cambie, M., et al. Dermatitis herpetiformis and nephrotic syndrome. *Clin. Nephrol.* 20: 49, 1983.
214. Gagliano, R. G., Costanzi, J. J., Beathard, G. A., et al. The nephrotic syndrome associated with neoplasia: An unusual paraneoplastic syndrome. *Am. J. Med.* 60: 1026, 1976.
215. Galaske, R. G., Baldamus, C. A., and Stolte, H. Plasma protein handling in the rat kidney: Micropuncture experiments in the acute heterologous phase of anti-GBM nephritis. *Pfluegers Arch.* 375: 269, 1978.
216. Ganguly, N. K., Singhal, P. C., Tewari, S. C., et al. Serum immunoglobulins in glomerulonephritis with a special reference to minimal lesion glomerulonephritis. *J. Assoc. Physicians India* 27: 1003, 1979.
217. Garber, D. W., Gottleib, B. A., Marsh, J. B., et al. Catabolism of very low density lipoproteins in experimental nephrosis. *J. Clin. Invest.* 74: 1375, 1984.
218. Garin, E. H., Donnelly, W. H., Geary, D., et al. Nephrotic syndrome and diffuse mesangial proliferative glomerulonephritis in children. *Am. J. Dis. Child.* 137: 109, 1983.
219. Garin, E. H., Grant, M. B., and Silverstein, J. H. Insulin-like growth factors in patients with active nephrotic syndrome. *Am. J. Dis. Child.* 143: 865, 1989.
220. Garin, E. H., Sausville, P. J., and Richard, G. A. Plasma prostaglandin E2 concentration in nephrotic syndrome. *J. Pediatr.* 103: 253, 1983.
221. Garin, E. H., Williams, R. L., Rennell, R. S., III, et al. Indomethacin in the treatment of idiopathic minimal lesion nephrotic syndrome. *J. Pediatr.* 93: 138, 1978.
222. Garnett, E. S., and Webber, C. E. Changes in blood-volume produced by treatment of the nephrotic syndrome. *Lancet* ii: 798, 1967.
223. Gault, M. H., and Muehrcke, R. C. Renal biopsy: Current views and controversies (Editorial). *Nephron* 34: 1, 1983.
224. Gavin, L. A., McMahon, F. A., Castle, J. N., et al. Alterations in serum hormones and serum thyroxine-binding globulin in patients with nephrosis. *J. Clin. Endocrinol. Metab.* 46: 125, 1978.
225. Geers, A. B., Koomans, H. A., Roos, J. C., et al. Functional relationships in the nephrotic syndrome. *Kidney Int.* 26: 324, 1984.
226. Gentner, J. M., Kauschowsky, A., Gresher, D. W., et al. XY gonadal dysgenesis associated with the congenital nephrotic syndrome. *Obstet. Gynecol.* 35: 655, 1980.
227. George, J. N., Nurden, A. T., and Phillips, D. R. Molecular defects in interactions of platelets with the vessel wall. *N. Engl. J. Med.* 311: 1084, 1984.
228. Gerber, M. A., and Paronetto, F. IgE in glomeruli of patients with nephrotic syndrome. *Lancet* i: 1097, 1971.
229. Gherardi, E., Rota, E., Calandra, S., et al. Relationship among the concentrations of serum lipoproteins and changes in their chemical composition in patients with untreated nephrotic syndrome. *Eur. J. Clin. Invest.* 7: 563, 1977.
230. Gherardi, E., Vecchia, L., and Calandra, S. Experimental nephrotic syndrome in the rat induced by puromycin aminonucleoside. Plasma and urinary lipoproteins. *Exp. Mol. Pathol.* 32: 128, 1980.
231. Ghosh, L., and Muehrcke, R. C. The nephrotic syndrome: A prodrome to lymphoma. *Ann. Intern. Med.* 72: 379, 1970.
232. Gianantonio, C., Vitacco, M., Mendilaharzu, F., et al. The hemolytic uremic syndrome. *J. Pediatr.* 64: 478, 1964.
233. Giangiacomo, J., Cleary, T. G., Cole, B. R., et al. Serum immunoglobulins in the nephrotic syndrome. A possible cause of minimal change nephrotic syndrome. *N. Engl. J. Med.* 293: 8, 1975.
234. Gilboa, N. Incidence of coronary heart disease associated with the nephrotic syndrome. *Med. J. Aust.* 1: 207, 1976.
235. Gilman, A. G., Goodman, L. S., Rall, T. W., et al. (eds.). Goodman and Gilman's, *The Pharmacological Basis of Therapeutics*, 7th Ed. New York: Macmillan, 1985. Pp. 1668–1713, Table A-II-1.
236. Gitlin, D., Cornwell, D. G., Nakasato, D., et al. Studies on the metabolism of plasma proteins in the nephrotic syndrome. II. The lipoproteins. *J. Clin. Invest.* 37: 172, 1958.
237. Gitlin, D., Janeway, C. A., and Farr, L. E. Studies on the metabolism of plasma proteins in the nephrotic syndrome. I. Albumin, γ-globulin and iron-binding globulin. *J. Clin. Invest.* 35: 44, 1956.
238. Glasser, R. J., Velosa, J. A., and Michael, A. F. Experimental model of focal sclerosis. I. Relationship to protein excretion in aminonucleoside nephrosis. *Lab. Invest.* 36: 519, 1977.
239. Glassock, R. J. The nephrotic syndrome. *Hosp. Pract.* 14(11): 105, 1979.
240. Glassock, R. J. Immunosuppressive treatment in the prevention of renal failure in primary glomerular diseases. *Clin. Exp. Dial. Apheresis.* 5: 21, 1982.

241. Glastre, C., Cochat, P., Bouvier, R., et al. Familial infantile nephrotic syndrome with ocular abnormalities. *Pediatr. Nephrol.* 4: 340, 1990.
242. Glicklich, D., Haskell, L., Senitzer, D., et al. Possible genetic predisposition to idiopathic focal segmental glomerulosclerosis. *Am. J. Kidney Dis.* 12: 26, 1988.
243. Golbetz, H., Black, V., Shemesh, O., et al. Mechanism of the antiproteinuric effect of indomethacin in nephrotic humans. *Am. J. Physiol.* 256: F44, 1989.
244. Goldstein, D. A., Haldimann, B., Sherman, D., et al. Vitamin D metabolites and calcium metabolism in patients with nephrotic syndrome and normal renal function. *J. Clin. Endocrinol. Metab.* 52: 116, 1981.
245. Goldstein, D. A., Oda, Y., Kurokawa, K., et al. Blood levels of 25-hydroxyvitamin D in nephrotic syndrome. *Ann. Intern. Med.* 87: 664, 1977.
246. Goldszer, R. C., Sweet, J., and Cotran, R. S. Focal segmental glomerulosclerosis. *Annu. Rev. Med.* 35: 429, 1984.
247. Golper, T. A., Feingold, K. R., Fulford, M. H., et al. The role of circulating mevalonate in nephrotic hypercholesterolemia. *J. Lipid Res.* 27: 1044, 1976.
248. Golper, T. A., Illingworth, R., Morris, C. D., et al. Lovastatin in the treatment of multifactorial hyperlipidemia. *Am. J. Kidney Dis.* 13: 312, 1989.
249. Golper, T. A., and Swartz, S. H. Impaired renal mevalonate metabolism in nephrotic syndrome: A stimulus for increased hepatic cholesterogenesis independent of GFR and hypoalbuminemia. *Metabolism* 31: 471, 1982.
250. Gottloib, L., London, R., and Rosenmann, E. Infantile nephrotic syndrome due to glomerulonephritis in a male pseudohermaphrodite. *Isr. J. Med. Sci.* 12: 52, 1976.
251. Griswold, W. R., Tune, B. M., Reznik, V. M., et al. Treatment of childhood prednisone-resistant nephrotic syndrome and focal segmental glomerulosclerosis with intravenous methylprednisolone and oral alkylating agents. *Nephron* 46: 73, 1987.
252. Groggel, G. C., Cheung, A. K., Ellis-Benigni, K., et al. Treatment of nephrotic hyperlipoproteinemia with gemfibrozil. *Kidney Int.* 36: 266, 1989.
253. Groggel, G. C., Marinides, G. N., Hovingh, P., et al. Inhibition of rat mesangial cell growth by heparan sulfate. *Am. J. Physiol.* 258: F259, 1990.
254. Groshong, T., Mendelson, L., Mendoza, S., et al. Serum IgE in patients with minimal-change nephrotic syndrome. *J. Pediatr.* 83: 767, 1973.
255. Grundy, S. M. Management of hyperlipidemia of kidney disease. *Kidney Int.* 37: 847, 1990.
256. Grundy, S. M., and Vega, G. L. Rationale and management of hyperlipidemia of the nephrotic syndrome. *Am. J. Med.* 87: 5-3N, 1989.
257. Grupe, W. E. Childhood nephrotic syndrome: Clinical associations and response to therapy. *Postgrad. Med.* 65: 229, 1979.
258. Grupe, W. E., Makker, S. P., and Ingelfinger, I. R. Chlorambucil treatment of frequently relapsing nephrotic syndrome. *N. Engl. J. Med.* 295: 746, 1976.
259. Gubler, M.-C., Broyer, M., and Habib, R. Signification des lésions de sclerose/hyalinose segmentaire et focale (S/HSF) dans la nephrose. In *Proceedings of the VIIIth International Congress of Nephrology*. Basel: Karger, 1978. P. 437.
260. Gutierrez Millet, V., Ruilope, L. M., Alcazar, J. M., et al. Effect of indomethacin administration upon renal function, proteinuria, renin-angiotensin-aldosterone axis, and urinary prostaglandin E2 in nephrotic syndrome. *Kidney Int.* 22: 213, 1982.
261. Haakenstad, A. O., Case, J. B., and Mannik, M. Effect of cortisone on the disappearance kinetics and tissue localization of soluble immune complexes. *J. Immunol.* 113: 1153, 1975.
262. Habib, R. Focal glomerulosclerosis. *Kidney Int.* 4: 355, 1973.
263. Habib, R., and Bois, E. Heterogeneite des syndromes nephrotiques a debut precoce du nourisson (syndrome nephrotique "infantile"). *Helv. Paediatr. Acta* 28: 91, 1973.
264. Habib, R., Hebert, D., Gagnadoux, M. F., et al. Transplantation in idiopathic nephrosis. *Transplant. Proc.* 14: 489, 1982.
265. Habib, R., and Kleinknecht, C. The Primary Nephrotic Syndrome in Childhood. Classification and Clinicopathologic Study of 406 Cases. In S. C. Somers (ed.), *Pathology Annual*. New York: Appleton-Century-Crofts, 1971. P. 417.
266. Hakim, R. M., Goldszer, R. C., and Brenner, B. M. Hypertension and proteinuria: Long-term sequelae of uninephrectomy in humans. *Kidney Int.* 25: 930, 1984.
267. Hallman, N., Norio, R., and Rapola, J. Congenital nephrotic syndrome. *Nephron* 11: 101, 1973.
268. Harris, H. W., Umetsu, D., Geha, R., et al. Altered immunoglobulin status in congenital nephrotic syndrome. *Clin. Nephrol.* 25: 308, 1986.
269. Harris, K. P. G., Purkerson, M. L., Yates, J., et al. Lovastatin ameliorates the development of glomerulosclerosis and uremia in experimental nephrotic syndrome. *Am. J. Kidney Dis.* 15: 16, 1990.
270. Haskell, L. P., Glicklich, D., and Senitzer, D. HLA associations in heroin-associated nephropathy. *Am. J. Kidney Dis.* 12: 45, 1988.
271. Hayslett, J. P., Krasser, L. S., Bensch, K. G., et al. Progression of "lipid nephrosis" to renal insufficiency. *N. Engl. J. Med.* 281: 181, 1969.
272. Heeg, J. E., de Jong, P. E., van der Hem, G. K., et al. Efficacy and variability of the antiproteinuric effect of ACE inhibition by lisinopril. *Kidney Int.* 36: 272, 1989.
273. Hendrickse, R. G., Glasgow, E. F., Adenyi, A., et al. Quartan malarial nephrotic syndrome. A collaborative clinicopathologic study in Nigerian children. *Lancet* i: 1143, 1972.
274. Herdman, R. C., Michael, A. F., and Good, R. A. Postural proteinuria. Response to corticosteroid therapy. *Ann. Intern. Med.* 65: 286, 1966.
275. Herrod, H. G., Stapleton, F. B., Trouy, R. L., et al. Evaluation of T lymphocyte subpopulations in children with nephrotic syndrome. *Clin. Exp. Immunol.* 52: 581, 1983.
276. Heslan, J. M., Lautie, J. P., Intrator, L., et al. Impaired IgG synthesis in patients with the nephrotic syndrome. *Clin. Nephrol.* 18: 144, 1982.
277. Heymann, W. Nephrotic syndrome after use of trimethadione and paramethadione in petit mal. *J.A.M.A.* 202: 127, 1967.
277a. Hinoshita, F., et al. Decreased production and responsiveness of interleukin-2 in lymphocytes of patients with nephrotic syndrome. *Nephron* 54: 122, 1990.
278. Hirszel, P., Yamase, H. T., Carney, W. R., et al. Mesangial proliferative glomerulonephritis with IgM deposits. *Nephron* 38: 100, 1984.
279. Hoffmann, E. O. The detection of effaced podocytes by high resolution light microscopy. *Am. J. Clin. Pathol.* 78: 508, 1982.

280. Hogg, R. J. Unpublished observation.
281. Holdsworth, S. R., Neale, T. J., and Wilson, C. B. Abrogation of macrophage-dependent injury in experimental glomerulonephritis in the rabbit. *J. Clin. Invest.* 68: 686, 1981.
282. Hopper, J., Jr., Ryan, P., and Lee, J. C. Lipoid nephrosis in 31 adult patients: Renal biopsy study by light, electron and fluorescence microscopy with experience in treatment. *Medicine* 49: 321, 1970.
283. Horii, Y., Muraguchi, A., Iwano, M., et al. Involvement of IL-6 in mesangial proliferative glomerulonephritis. *J. Immunol.* 143: 3949, 1989.
284. Hory, B., Saunier, F., Wolff, R., et al. Waldenstrom macroglobulinemia and nephrotic syndrome with minimal change lesion. *Nephron* 45: 68, 1987.
285. Hostetter, T. H., Troy, J. L., and Brenner, B. M. Glomerular hemodynamics in experimental diabetes mellitus. *Kidney Int.* 19: 410, 1981.
286. Howanietz, H., and Lubec, G. Idiopathic nephrotic syndrome, treated with steroids for five years, found to be allergic reaction to pork. *Lancet* ii: 450, 1984.
287. Hoyer, J. R. Idiopathic Nephrotic Syndrome with Minimal Glomerular Changes. In B. M. Brenner and J. H. Stein (eds.), *Contemporary Tissues in Nephrology. IX. Nephrotic Syndrome.* New York: Churchill Livingstone, 1982. P. 145.
288. Hui, A., Poucell, S., Thorner, P., et al. Clinical features and glomerular immunofluorescent of biopsies from children with nephrotic syndrome due to minimal change glomerulonephritis. *Int. J. Pediatr. Nephrol.* 5: 5, 1984.
289. Huisman, R. M., deJong, P. E., de Zeeuw, D., et al. Nephrotic syndrome preceding Hodgkin's disease by 42 months. *Clin. Nephrol.* 26: 311, 1986.
290. Hulter, H. N., and Bonner, E. L., Jr. Lipoid nephrosis appearing as acute oligenic renal failure. *Arch. Intern. Med.* 140: 403, 1980.
291. Hunsicker, L. G., Shearer, T. P., and Shaffer, S. J. Acute reversible proteinuria induced by infusion of the polycation hexadimethrine. *Kidney Int.* 20: 7, 1981.
292. Hutchison, F. N., Martin, V. I., Jones, H. Jr., et al. Differing actions of dietary protein and enalapril on renal function and proteinuria. *Am. J. Physiol.* 258: F126, 1990.
293. Hutchison, F. N., Schambelan, M., and Kaysen, G. A. Modulation of albuminuria by dietary protein and converting enzyme inhibition. *Am. J. Physiol.* 253: F719, 1987.
294. Huttunen, N. P. Congenital nephrotic syndrome of the Finnish type: Study of 75 patients. *Arch. Dis. Child.* 51: 344, 1976.
295. Hyams, J. S., and Carey, D. E. Corticosteroids and growth. *J. Pediatr.* 113: 249, 1988.
296. Hyman, L. R., and Burkholder, P. M. Focal sclerosing glomerulonephropathy with segmental hyalinosis: A clinicopathologic analysis. *Lab. Invest.* 28: 533, 1973.
297. Hyman, L. R., Burkholder, P. M., and Joo, P. A. Malignant lymphoma and nephrotic syndrome. A clinicopathologic analysis with light, immunofluorescence and electron microscopy of the renal lesion. *J. Pediatr.* 82: 207, 1973.
298. Ichikawa, I., Rennke, H. G., Hoyer, J. R., et al. Role for intrarenal mechanisms in the impaired salt excretion of experimental nephrotic syndrome. *J. Clin. Invest.* 71: 91, 1983.
299. Idelson, B. A., Smithline, N., and Smith, G. W. Prognosis in steroid-treated idiopathic nephrotic syndrome in adults. *Arch. Intern. Med.* 137: 891, 1977.
300. Ihle, B. U., Becker, G. J., Whitworth, J. A., et al. The effect of protein restriction on the progression of renal insufficiency. *N. Engl. J. Med.* 321: 1773, 1989.
301. Iitaka, K., and West, C. D. A serum inhibitor of blastogenesis in idiopathic nephrotic syndrome transferred by lymphocytes. *Clin. Immunol. Immunopathol.* 12: 62, 1979.
302. Ikoma, M., Yoshioka, T., Ichikawa, I., et al. Mechanism of the unique susceptibility of deep cortical glomeruli of maturing kidneys to severe focal glomerular sclerosis. *Pediatr. Res.* 28: 270, 1990.
303. International Study of Kidney Disease in Children. Prospective, controlled trial of cyclophosphamide therapy in children with the nephrotic syndrome. *Lancet* ii: 423, 1974.
304. International Study of Kidney Disease in Children. Nephrotic syndrome: Prediction of histopathology from clinical and laboratory characteristics at time of diagnosis. *Kidney Int.* 13: 159, 1978.
305. International Study of Kidney Disease in Children. Nephrotic syndrome in children: A randomized trial comparing two prednisone regimens in steroid-responsive patients who relapse early. *J. Pediatr.* 95: 239, 1979.
306. International Study of Kidney Disease in Children. A controlled therapeutic trial of cyclophosphamide plus prednisone vs. prednisone alone in children with focal segmental glomerulonephritis. *Pediatr. Res.* 14: 1006, 1980.
307. International Study of Kidney Disease in Children. The primary nephrotic syndrome in children. Identification of patients with minimal change nephrotic syndrome from initial response to prednisone. *J. Pediatr.* 98: 561, 1981.
308. International Study of Kidney Disease in Children. Primary nephrotic syndrome in children: Clinical significance of histopathologic variants of minimal change and of diffuse mesangial hypercellularity. *Kidney Int.* 20: 765, 1981.
309. International Study of Kidney Disease in Children. Early identification of frequent relapsers among children with minimal change nephrotic syndrome. *J. Pediatr.* 101: 514, 1982.
310. International Study of Kidney Disease in Children. Minimal change nephrotic syndrome in children: Deaths during the first 5 to 15 years' observation. *Pediatrics* 73: 497, 1984.
311. Isaacs, K. L., and Miller, F. Antigen size and charge in immune complex glomerulonephritis. *Am. J. Pathol.* 111: 298, 1983.
311a. Jadresic, L. P., Filler, G., and Barratt, T. M. Urine glycosaminoglycans in congenital and acquired nephrotic syndrome. *Kidney Int.* 40: 280, 1991.
312. Jaffa, A. A., Harvey, J. N., Sutherland, S. E., et al. Renal kallikrein responses to dietary protein: A possible mediator of hyperfiltration. *Kidney Int.* 36: 1003, 1989.
313. Jennette, J. C., Charles, L., and Grubb, W. Glomerulomegaly and focal segmental glomerulosclerosis associated with sleep-apnea syndrome. *Am. J. Kidney Dis.* 10: 470, 1987.
314. Jensen, H., Rossing, N., Andersen, S. B., et al. Albumin metabolism in the nephrotic syndrome in adults. *Clin. Sci.* 33: 445, 1967.
315. Ji-Yun, Y., Melvin, T., Sibley, R., et al. No evidence for a specific role of IgM in mesangial proliferation of idiopathic nephrotic syndrome. *Kidney Int.* 25: 100, 1984.
316. Joachim, G. R., Cameron, J. S., Schwartz, M., et al. Selectivity of protein excretion in patients with the nephrotic syndrome. *J. Clin. Invest.* 43: 2332, 1964.
317. Joffe, M. I., and Rabson, A. R. Dissociation of lympho-

kine production and blastogenesis in children with measles infection. *Clin. Immunol. Immunopathol.* 10: 335, 1978.

318. Johnson, A. K., Mann, J. F. E., Rascher, W., et al. Plasma angiotensin II concentrations and experimentally induced thirst. *Am. J. Physiol.* 240: R229, 1981.
319. Jones, C. L., and Hebert, D. Pulmonary thrombo-embolism in the nephrotic syndrome. *Pediatr. Nephrol.* 5: 56, 1991.
320. Jørgensen, K. A., and Stofferson, E. Antithrombin III and the nephrotic syndrome. *Scand. J. Haematol.* 22: 442, 1979.
321. Jørgensen, K. A., and Stofferson, E. On the inhibitory effect of albumin on platelet aggregation. *Thromb. Res.* 17: 13, 1980.
322. Joven, J., Villabona, C., Vilella, E., et al. Abnormalities of lipoprotein metabolism in patients with the nephrotic syndrome. *N. Engl. J. Med.* 323: 579, 1990.
323. Kallen, R. J., Byrnes, R. K., Aronson, A. J., et al. Premature coronary atherosclerosis in a 5-year-old with corticosteroid-refractory nephrotic syndrome. *Am. J. Dis. Child.* 131: 976, 1977.
324. Kanfer, A., Kleinknecht, D., Broyer, M., et al. Coagulation studies in 45 cases of nephrotic syndrome without uremia. *Thromb. Diathes. Haemorrh.* 24: 562, 1970.
325. Kanwar, Y. S., and Farquhar, M. G. Anionic sites in the glomerular basement membrane. *In vivo* and *in vitro* localization to the laminase rarae by cationic probes. *J. Cell Biol.* 81: 137, 1979.
326. Kaplan, B. S., Bureau, M. A., and Drummond, K. N. The nephrotic syndrome in the first year of life: Is a pathological classification possible? *J. Pediatr.* 85: 615, 1974.
327. Kaplan, B. S., Wiglesworth, F. W., Marks, M. I., et al. The glomerulopathy of congenital syphilis: An immune deposit disease. *J. Pediatr.* 81: 1154, 1972.
328. Kaplan, R., Aynedjian, H. S., Schlondorff, D., et al. Renal vasoconstriction caused by short-term cholesterol feeding is corrected by thromboxane antagonist or probucol. *J. Clin. Invest.* 86: 1707, 1990.
329. Kashgarian, M., Hayslett, J. P., and Seigel, N. J. Lipoid nephrosis and focal sclerosis: Distinct entities or spectrum of disease. *Nephron* 13: 105, 1974.
329a. Kashyap, M. L., Srivastava, L. S., and Hynd, B. A. Apolipoprotein C-II and lipoprotein lipase in human nephrotic syndrome. *Atherosclerosis* 35: 29, 1980.
330. Kasiske, B. L., O'Donnell, M. P., Cleary, M. P., et al. Effects of reduced renal mass on tissue lipids and renal injury in hyperlipidemic rats. *Kidney Int.* 35: 40, 1989.
330a. Kasiske, B. L., O'Donnell, M. P., Garvis, W. J., et al. Pharmacologic treatment of hyperlipidemia reduces glomerular injury in rat 5/6 nephrectomy model of chronic renal failure. *Circ. Res.* 62: 367, 1988.
331. Kasiske, B. L., O'Donnell, M. P., Lee, H., et al. Impact of dietary fatty acid supplementation in obese Zucker rats. *Kidney Int.* 39: 1125, 1991.
332. Kasiske, B. L., Velosa, J. A., Halstenson, C. E., et al. The effects of lovastatin in hyperlipidemic patients with the nephrotic syndrome. *Am. J. Kidney Dis.* 15: 8, 1990.
333. Kauffmann, R. H., Veltkamp, J. J., and vanTilburg, N. Acquired antithrombin III deficiency and thrombosis in the nephrotic syndrome. *Am. J. Med.* 65: 607, 1978.
334. Kaysen, G. A. Hyperlipidemia in the nephrotic syndrome. *Am. J. Kidney Dis.* 12: 548, 1988.
335. Kaysen, G. A., Gambertoglio, J., Jimenez, I., et al. Effect of dietary protein intake on albumin homeostasis in nephrotic patients. *Kidney Int.* 29: 572, 1986.
336. Kaysen, G. A., Gambertoglio, J., Felts, J., et al. Albumin synthesis, albuminuria and hyperlipemia in nephrotic patients. *Kidney Int.* 31: 1368, 1987.
337. Kaysen, G. A., Jones, H., Jr., and Hutchison, F. N. High protein diets stimulate albumin synthesis at the site of albumin mRNA transcription. *Kidney Int.* 36(Suppl. 27): S-168, 1989.
338. Kaysen, G. A., Jones, H., Jr., Martin, V., et al. A low-protein diet restricts albumin synthesis in nephrotic rats. *J. Clin. Invest.* 83: 1623, 1990.
339. Kaysen, G. A., Paukert, T. T., Menke, D. J., et al. Plasma volume expansion is necessary for edema formation in the rat with Heymann nephritis. *Am. J. Physiol.* 248: F247, 1985.
340. Kekki, M., and Nikkila, E. A. Plasma triglyceride metabolism in the adult nephrotic syndrome. *Eur. J. Clin. Invest.* 1: 345, 1971.
341. Keller, H., Morell, A., Noseda, G., et al. Analbuminämie Pathophysiológische Untersuchungen an einem Fall. *Schweiz. Med. Wochenschr.* 102: 71, 1972.
342. Kelley, V. E., and Cavallo, T. Glomerular permeability. Ultrastructural studies in New Zealand black/white mice using polyanionic. *Lab. Invest.* 37: 265, 1977.
343. Kendall, A. G. Nephrotic syndrome: A hypercoagulable state. *Arch. Intern. Med.* 127: 1021, 1971.
344. Kenner, C. H., Evan, A. P., Blomgren, P., et al. Effect of protein intake on renal function and structure in partially nephrectomized rats. *Kidney Int.* 27: 739, 1985.
345. Kerpen, H. O., Bhat, J. G., Kantor, R., et al. Lymphocyte subpopulations in minimal change nephrotic syndrome. *Clin. Immunol. Immunopathol.* 14: 130, 1979.
346. Khokhar, N., Akavaram, N. R., and Quinones, E. M. Lipoid nephrosis in the elderly. *South. Med. J.* 73: 790, 1980.
347. Kiely, J. M., Wagoner, R. D., and Holley, K. E. Renal complications of lymphoma. *Ann. Intern. Med.* 71: 1159, 1969.
348. Kikuta, Y., Yoshimura, M., Saito, T., et al. Nephrotic syndrome with diffuse mesangial sclerosis in identical twins. *J. Pediatr.* 102: 586, 1983.
349. Kim, P. K., Kim, N. A., Kim, K. S., et al. Steroid effects on minimal lesion nephrotic syndrome with and without immune deposits. *Int. J. Pediatr. Nephrol.* 3: 257, 1983.
350. Kiprov, D. D., Colvin, R. B., and McCluskey, R. T. Focal and segmental glomerulosclerosis and proteinuria associated with unilateral renal agenesis. *Lab. Invest.* 46: 275, 1982.
350a. Kirchner, K. A., Voelker, J. R., and Brater, D. C. Binding inhibitors restore furosemide potency in tubule fluid containing albumin. *Kidney Int.* 40: 418, 1991.
351. Kiskander, S. S., and Jennette, J. C. Influence of antibody avidity on glomerular immune complex formation. *Am. J. Pathol.* 112: 155, 1983.
352. Kitano, Y., Yoshikawa, N., Tanaka, R., et al. Ciclosporin treatment in children with steroid-dependent nephrotic syndrome. *Pediatr. Nephrol.* 4: 474, 1990.
353. Klahr, S., Buerkert, J., and Purkerson, M. L. Role of dietary factors in the progression of renal disease. *Kidney Int.* 24: 579, 1983.
354. Kleinknecht, C., Broyer, M., Gubler, M.-C., et al. Irreversible renal failure after indomethacin in steroid-resistant nephrosis (Letter). *N. Engl. J. Med.* 302: 691, 1980.
355. Kleinknecht, C., Gonzales, G., and Gubler, M. C. Familial nephrosis. (Abstract) *Pediatr. Res.* 14: 1003, 1980.
356. Kleinknecht, C., Guesry, P., Lenoir, G., et al. High-cost

benefit of chlorambucil in frequently relapsing nephrotic syndrome. *N. Engl. J. Med.* 296: 48, 1977.

357. Kobayashi, Y., Chen, X.-M., Hiki, Y., et al. Association of HLA-DRw8 and DQw3 with minimal change nephrotic syndrome in Japanese adults. *Kidney Int.* 28: 193, 1985.
358. Koomans, H. A., Braam, B., Geers, A. B., et al. The importance of plasma protein for blood volume and blood pressure homeostasis. *Kidney Int.* 30: 730, 1986.
358a. Kopp, J. B., et al. Progressive glomerulosclerosis and enhanced renal accumulation of basement membrane components in mice transgenic for human immunodeficiency virus type I genes. *Proc. Natl. Acad. Sci.* 89: 1577, 1992.
359. Korbet, S. M., Schwartz, M. M., and Lewis, E. J. Recurrent nephrotic syndrome in renal allografts. *Am. J. Kidney Dis.* 11: 270, 1988.
360. Korkor, A., Schwartz, J., Bergfeld, M., et al. Absence of metabolic bone disease in adult patients with the nephrotic syndrome and normal renal function. *J. Clin. Endocrinol. Metab.* 56: 496, 1983.
361. Koskimies, O., Vilska, J., Rapola, J., et al. Long-term outcome of primary nephrotic syndrome. *Arch. Dis. Child.* 57: 544, 1982.
361a. Koyama, A., Fuijisak, M., Kobayashi, M., et al. A glomerular permeability factor produced by human T cell hybridomas. *Kidney Int.* 40: 453, 1991.
362. Kreisberg, J. E., Wayne, D. B., and Karnovsky, M. J. Rapid and focal loss of negative charge associated with mononuclear cell infiltration early in nephrotoxic serum nephritis. *Kidney Int.* 16: 290, 1979.
363. Krensky, A. M., Inglefinger, J. R., and Gruge, W. E. Peritonitis in childhood nephrotic syndrome. *Am. J. Dis. Child.* 136: 732, 1982.
364. Krensky, A. M., Ingelfinger, J. R., Grupe, W. E., et al. Hemolytic uremic syndrome and crescentic glomerulonephritis complicating childhood nephrosis. *Clin. Nephrol.* 19: 99, 1983.
365. Krishna, G. G., and Danovitch, G. M. Effects of water immersion and renal function in the nephrotic syndrome. *Kidney Int.* 21: 395, 1982.
366. Kristal, H., and Lichtig, C. Infantile nephrotic syndrome. Clinicopathological study of 11 cases. *Isr. J. Med. Sci.* 19: 626, 1983.
367. Kuhlmann, U., Steurer, J., and Rhyner, K. Platelet aggregation and beta thromboglobulin levels in nephrotic patients with and without thrombosis. *Clin. Nephrol.* 15: 229, 1981.
368. Kuis, W., DeKraker, J., Kuijten, R. H., et al. Acute lymphoblastic leukemia after treatment of nephrotic syndrome with immunosuppressive drugs. *Helv. Paediatr. Acta* 31: 91, 1976.
369. Kuroda, S., Aynedjian, H. S., and Bank, N. A micropuncture study of renal sodium retention nephrotic syndrome in rats: Evidence for increased resistance to tubular fluid flow. *Kidney Int.* 16: 561, 1979.
370. Lagrue, G., Branellec, A., Blanc, C., et al. A vascular permeability factor in lymphocyte culture supernatants from patients with nephrotic syndrome. II. Pharmacological and physiochemical properties. *Biomedicine* 23: 73, 1975.
371. Lagrue, G., and Laurent, J. Is lipoid nephrosis an "allergic" disease? *Transplant. Proc.* 14: 485, 1982.
372. Lagrue, G., and Laurent, J. Allergy and lipoid nephrosis. *Adv. Nephrol.* 12: 151, 1983.
373. Lagrue, G., Laurent, G., Hirbec, G., et al. Serum IgE in primary glomerular disease. *Nephron* 36: 5, 1984.
374. Lagrue, G., Xheneumont, S., Branellec, A., et al. A vascular permeability factor elaborated from lymphocytes. I. Demonstration in patients with nephrotic syndrome. *Biomedicine* 23: 37, 1975.
375. Lagueruela, C. C., Buettner, T. L., Cole, B. R., et al. HLA extended haplotypes in steroid-sensitive nephrotic syndrome of childhood. *Kidney Int.* 38: 145, 1990.
376. La Manna, A., Polito, C., Del Gado, R., et al. Hepatitis B surface antigenaemia and glomerulopathies in children. *Acta Paediatr. Scand.* 74: 122, 1985.
377. La Manna, A., Polito, C., and Foglia, A. C. Reduced response to HBV vaccination in boys with steroid sensitive nephrotic syndrome. *Pediatr. Nephrol.*, in press, 1992.
378. Landis, E. M., and Pappenheimer, J. R. Exchange of Substances Through the Capillary Walls. In W. F. Hamilton and P. Dow (eds.), *Handbook of Physiology*, Section Z, Circulation, Vol. II, Chap. 29. Washington, D.C.: American Physiological Society, 1963. P. 961.
379. Lane, P. H., Schnaper, H. W., Vernier, R. L., et al. Steroid-dependent nephrotic syndrome following renal transplant for congenital nephrotic syndrome. *Pediatr. Nephrol.* 5: 300, 1991.
380. Lange, K., Ahmed, U., Seligson, G., et al. Depression of endostreptosin, streptolysin O and streptozyme antibodies in patients with idiopathic nephrosis with and without nephrotic syndrome. *Clin. Nephrol.* 15: 279, 1981.
381. Larsen, S. Immunofluorescent microscopy findings in minimal or no change disease and slight generalized mesangioproliferative glomerulonephritis. Fluorescent microscopy results correlated to symptoms and clinical cause. *Acta Pathol. Microbiol. Scand.* 86A: 531, 1978.
382. Latta, H., and Johnston, W. H. The glycoprotein inner layer of glomerular capillary basement membrane as a filtration barrier. *J. Ultrastruct. Res.* 57: 65, 1976.
383. Latta, H., Johnston, W. H., and Stanley, T. M. Sialoglycoproteins and filtration barriers in the glomerular capillary wall. *J. Ultrastruct. Res.* 51: 354, 1975.
384. Lau, J., Levey, A. S., Kassirer, J. P., et al. Idiopathic nephrotic syndrome in a 53 year old woman. Is a kidney biopsy necessary? *Med. Decision Making* 2: 497, 1982.
385. Lau, S. O., Tkachuck, M. T., Hasegawa, D. K., et al. Plasminogen and antithrombin III deficiencies in the childhood nephrotic syndrome associated with plasminogenuria and antithrombinuria. *J. Pediatr.* 96: 390, 1980.
386. Laufer, A., and Stein, O. The exudative lesion in diabetic glomerulosclerosis. *Am. J. Clin. Pathol.* 32: 56, 1959.
387. Laurent, J., Ansquer, J. C., deMouzon-Cambon, A., et al. Adult onset lipoid nephrosis is not DR7 associated. *Tissue Antigens* 22: 229, 1983.
388. Laurent, J., Lagrue, G., Belghiti, D., et al. Is house dust allergen a possible causal factor for relapses in lipoid nephrosis? *Allergy* 39: 231, 1984.
389. Laurent, J., Rostoker, G., Robeva, R., et al. Is adult idiopathic nephrotic syndrome food allergy? Value of oligoantigenic diets. *Nephron* 47: 7, 1987.
390. Lee, J. C., Yamauchi, H., and Hopper, J., Jr. The association of cancer and the nephrotic syndrome. *Ann. Intern. Med.* 64: 41, 1966.
391. Leisti, S., Koskimies, O., Perheentupa, J., et al. Idiopathic nephrotic syndrome: Prevention of early relapse. *Br. Med. J.* 1: 892, 1978.
392. Leisti, S., Koskimies, O., Rapola, J., et al. Association of post-medication hypocortisolism with early first relapse of idiopathic nephrotic syndrome. *Lancet* 2: 795, 1977.
393. Leisti, S., Vilska, J., and Hallman, N. Adrenocortical in-

sufficiency and relapsing in the idiopathic nephrotic syndrome of childhood. *Pediatrics* 60: 334, 1977.

394. Lenarsky, C., Jordan, S. C., and Ladisch, S. Plasma inhibition of lymphocyte proliferation in nephrotic syndrome: Correlation with hyperlipidemia. *J. Clin. Immunol.* 2: 276, 1982.
395. Lentz, R. D., Bergstein, J., Steffes, M. W., et al. Postpubertal evaluation of gonadal function following cyclophosphamide therapy before and during puberty. *J. Pediatr.* 91: 385, 1977.
396. Leumann, E. P., et al. Recurrence of focal segmental glomerular sclerosis in the transplanted kidney. *Nephron* 25: 65, 1980.
397. Levin, M., Gascoine, P., Turner, M. W., et al. A highly cationic protein in plasma and urine of children with steroid-responsive nephrotic syndrome. *Kidney Int.* 36: 867, 1989.
398. Levin, M., Smith, C., Walters, M. D. S., et al. Steroid-responsive nephrotic syndrome: A generalised disorder of membrane negative charge. *Lancet* 2: 239, 1985.
399. Levinsky, R. J., Malleson, P. N., Barratt, T. M., et al. Circulating immune complexes in steroid-responsive nephrotic syndrome. *N. Engl. J. Med.* 298: 126, 1978.
400. Lewis, E. J. Chlorambucil for childhood nephrotic syndrome. A word of caution. *N. Engl. J. Med.* 302: 963, 1980.
401. Lewis, E. J. Recurrent focal sclerosis after renal transplantation. *Kidney Int.* 22: 315, 1982.
402. Lewy, P. R., and Jao, W. Nephrotic syndrome in association with renal vein thrombosis in infancy. *J. Pediatr.* 85: 359, 1974.
403. Lichsteiner, S., and Schibler, U. A glycosylated liver-specific transcription factor stimulates transcription of the albumin gene. *Cell* 57: 1179, 1989.
404. Lim, P., Jacob, E., Chio, L. F., et al. Serum ionized calcium in nephrotic syndrome. *Q. J. Med.* 179: 421, 1976.
405. Lim, P., Jacob, E., Tock, E. P. C., et al. Calcium and phosphorus metabolism in nephrotic syndrome. *Q. J. Med.* 46: 327, 1977.
406. Lin, C.-Y. Decreased antibody-dependent cellular cytotoxicity in minimal change nephrotic syndrome. *Pediatr. Nephrol.* 2: 224, 1988.
407. Lin, C.-Y., Chen, C.-H., and Lee, P.-P. In vitro B-lymphocyte switch disturbance from IgM into IgG in IgM mesangial nephropathy. *Pediatr. Nephrol.* 3: 254, 1989.
408. Lin, T.-Y., Wang, Y. M., and Lin, S.-T. Application of a live varicella vaccine in children with acute leukemia or nephrotic syndrome. *J. Formosan Med. Assoc.* 70: 683, 1981.
409. Lines, D. R. Nephrotic syndrome and nephroloblastoma. Report of a case. *J. Pediatr.* 72: 264, 1968.
410. Llach, F. Hypercoagulability, renal vein thrombosis, and other thrombotic complications of nephrotic syndrome. *Kidney Int.* 28: 429, 1985.
411. Llach, F., Arieff, A. I., and Massry, S. G. Renal vein thrombosis and nephrotic syndrome: A prospective study of 36 adult patients. *Ann. Intern. Med.* 83: 8, 1975.
412. Llach, F., Papper, S., and Massry, S. G. The clinical spectrum of renal vein thrombosis. Acute and chronic. *Am. J. Med.* 69: 819, 1980.
413. Lomwardia, S., Pinn, V. W., Wadhwa, M. L., et al. Nephrotic syndrome associated with sulindac. *N. Engl. J. Med.* 304: 424, 1981.
414. Loon, N., Shemesh, O., Morelli, E., et al. Effect of angiotensin II infusion on the human glomerular filtration barrier. *Am. J. Physiol.* 257: F608, 1989.
415. Lopes-Virella, M., Virella, G., Debeukelaer, M., et al. Urinary high density lipoprotein in minimal change glomerular disease and chronic glomerulopathies. *Clin. Chim. Acta* 94: 73, 1979.
416. Loschiavo, C., Lupo, A., Valvo, E., et al. Carbohydrate metabolism in patients with nephrotic syndrome and normal renal function. *Nephron* 33: 257, 1983.
417. Lovett, D. H., Martin, M., Bursten, S., et al. Interleukin 1 and the glomerular mesangium: III. IL-1-dependent stimulation of mesangial cell protein kinase activity. *Kidney Int.* 34: 26, 1988.
418. Lovett, D. H., Resch, K., and Gemsa, D. Interleukin 1 and the glomerular mesangium: II. Monokine stimulation of mesangial cell prostanoid secretion. *Am. J. Pathol.* 129: 543, 1987.
419. Lovett, D. H., Szamel, M., Ryan, J. L., et al. Interleukin 1 and the glomerular mesangium: I. Purification and characterization of a mesangial cell-derived autogrowth factor. *J. Immunol.* 136: 3700, 1986.
420. Lowenstein, J., Schacht, R. G., and Baldwin, D. S. Renal failure in minimal change nephrotic syndrome. *Am. J. Med.* 70: 227, 1981.
421. Luetscher, J. A., Jr., and Johnson, B. B. Chromatographic separation of the sodium-retaining corticoid from the urine of children with nephrotic syndrome, compared with observations in normal children. *J. Clin. Invest.* 33: 276, 1954.
422. Luke, R. L. Permselectivity: Relation between foot process simplification and macromolecular configuration. *Renal Physiol.* 7: 129, 1984.
423. MacKay, K., Striker, L. J., Stauffer, J. W., et al. Relationship of glomerular hypertrophy and sclerosis: Studies in SV40 transgenic mice. *Kidney Int.* 37: 741, 1990.
424. Madalinski, K., Wyszynska, T., Mikulska, B., et al. Immune complexes in children with different forms of glomerulonephritis. *Arch. Immunol. Ther. Exp.* (Warsz.) 7: 129, 1984.
425. Magalhaes-Filho, A. G., Barbosa, A. V., and Ferreira, T. C. Glomerulonephritis in schistosomiasis with mesangial IgM deposits. *Mem. Inst. Oswaldo Cruz* 76: 181, 1981.
426. Maggiore, Q., and Martorano, C. Immunosuppressive therapy in primary glomerulonephritides. *Contrib. Nephrol.* 34: 55, 1982.
427. Mahan, J. D., Mauer, S. M., Sibley, R. K., et al. Congenital nephrotic syndrome: Evaluation of medical management and results of renal transplantation. *J. Pediatr.* 105: 549, 1984.
428. Mahan, J. D., Sisson, S. P., and Vernier, R. L. Altered glomerular basement membrane (GBM) anionic sites in the minimal change nephrotic syndrome (MCNS) in man (Abstract). *Kidney Int.* 27: 217, 1985.
429. Malekzadeh, M. H., Heuser, E. T., Ettinger, R. B., et al. Focal glomerulosclerosis and renal transplantation. *J. Pediatr.* 95: 249, 1979.
430. Mallick, N. P. The pathogenesis of minimal change nephropathy. *Clin. Nephrol.* 7: 87, 1977.
431. Mallick, N. P., and Short, C. D. The nephrotic syndrome and ischaemic heart disease. *Nephron* 27: 54, 1981.
432. Mallick, N. P., Williams, R. J., McFarlane, H., et al. Cell-mediated immunity in nephrotic syndrome. *Lancet* i: 507, 1972.
433. Malluche, H. H., Goldstein, D. A., and Massry, S. G. Osteomalacia and hyperparathyroid bone disease in patients with nephrotic syndrome. *J. Clin. Invest.* 63: 494, 1979.
434. Marsh, J. B., and Sparks, C. E. Hepatic secretion of li-

poproteins in the rat and the effect of experimental nephrosis. *J. Clin. Invest.* 64: 1229, 1979.
435. Marsh, J. B., and Sparks, C. E. Lipoproteins in experimental nephrosis: Plasma levels and composition. *Metabolism* 28: 1040, 1979.
436. Martini, A., Vitiello, M. A., Siena, S., et al. Multiple serum inhibitors of lectin-induced lymphocyte proliferation in nephrotic syndrome. *Clin. Exp. Immunol.* 45: 178, 1981.
437. Masugi, Y., Masuda, Y., Sato, S., et al. Retarded mesangial transport and its pathomorphologic sequelae in human and experimental renal diseases. *Acta Pathol. Jpn.* 33: 219, 1983.
438. Matsui, A., Takezawa, N., Suzuki, K., et al. Neurotoxicity of chlorambucil and cyclophosphamide therapy in steroid-dependent and/or frequently relapsing nephrotic syndrome. *Pediatr. Nephrol.* 3: C167, 1989.
439. Matsumoto, K. Impaired local graft-versus host reaction in lipoid nephrosis (Letter). *Nephron* 31: 281, 1982.
439a. Matsamoto, K. Decreased production of interleukin by monocytes from patients with lipoid nephrosis. *Clin. Nephrol.* 31: 292, 1989.
440. Matsumoto, K., Katayama, H., and Hatano, M. Effect of thymic humoral factor on a local graft-versus-host reaction of lymphocytes in patients with lipoid nephrosis (Letter). *Nephron* 32: 279, 1982.
441. Matsumoto, K., Osakabe, K., Harada, M., et al. Impaired cell-mediated immunity in lipoid nephrosis. *Nephron* 29: 190, 1981.
442. Matsumoto, K., Osakabe, K., and Hatano, M. Impaired cell-mediated immunity in idiopathic membranous nephropathy mediated by suppressor cells. *Clin. Nephrol.* 19: 213, 1983.
443. Matsumoto, K., Osakabe, K., Katayama, H., et al. Defective cell-mediated immunity in lipoid nephrosis. *Int. Arch. Allergy Appl. Immunol.* 73: 370, 1984.
443a. Mattoo, T. K. Kidney biopsy prior to cyclohexamide therapy in primary nephrotic syndrome. *Pediatr. Nephrol.* 5: 617, 1991.
444. Mauer, S. M., Hellerstein, S., Cohen, R. A., et al. Recurrence of steroid-responsive nephrotic syndrome after renal transplantation. *J. Pediatr.* 95: 261, 1979.
445. McCrory, W. W., Shibuya, M., Lu, W.-H., et al. Therapeutic and toxic effects observed with different dosage programs of cyclophosphamide in treatment of steroid-responsive but frequently relapsing nephrotic syndrome. *J. Pediatr.* 82: 614, 1973.
446. McCurdy, F. A., Butera, P. J., and Wilson, M. The familial occurrence of focal segmental glomerular sclerosis. *Am. J. Kidney Dis.* 10: 467, 1987.
447. McDonald, J., Murphy, A. V., and Arneil, G. C. Long-term assessment of cyclophosphamide therapy for nephrosis in children. *Lancet* ii: 980, 1974.
448. McEnery, P. T., and Strife, C. F. Nephrotic syndrome in childhood. Management and treatment in patients with minimal change disease, mesangial proliferation, or focal glomerulosclerosis. *Pediatr. Clin. North Am.* 29: 875, 1982.
449. McEnery, P. T., and Welch, T. E. Major histocompatibility complex antigens in steroid-responsive nephrotic syndrome. *Pediatr. Nephrol.* 3: 33, 1989.
450. McLean, R. H., Bias, W. B., Tina, L., et al. Variability of C4 gene number in the nephrotic syndrome (Abstract). *Kidney Int.* 33: 165, 1988.
451. McLean, R. H., Forsgren, A., Bjorksten, B., et al. Decreased serum factor B concentration associated with decreased opsonization of *Escherichia coli* in the idiopathic nephrotic syndrome. *Pediatr. Res.* 11: 910, 1977.
452. Meadow, S. R., Brocklebank, J. T., and Wainscott, G. Anti-allergic drugs in idiopathic nephrotic syndrome of childhood. *Lancet* i: 1200, 1978.
453. Meadow, S. R., and Sarsfield, J. K. Steroid-responsive nephrotic syndrome and allergy: Clinical studies. *Arch. Dis. Child.* 56: 509, 1981.
454. Meadow, S. R., Sarsfield, J. K., Scott, D. G., et al. Steroid-responsive nephrotic syndrome and allergy: Immunological studies. *Arch. Dis. Child.* 56: 517, 1981.
455. Meltzer, J. I., Keim, H. J., Laragh, J. H., et al. Nephrotic syndrome: Vasoconstriction and hypervolemia types indicated by renin-sodium profiling. *Ann. Intern. Med.* 91: 688, 1979.
456. Melvin, T., Sibley, R., and Michael, A. F. Nephrotic Syndrome. In B. M. Tune and S. A. Mendoza (eds.), *Contemporary Issues in Nephrology. XII. Pediatric Nephrology.* New York: Churchill Livingstone, 1984. P. 191.
457. Mendoza, S. A., Reznik, V. M., Griswold, W. R., et al. Treatment of steroid-resistant focal segmental glomerulosclerosis with pulse methylprednisolone and alkylating agents. *Pediatr. Nephrol.* 4: 303, 1990.
458. Mene, P., Abboud, H. E., and Dunn, M. J. Regulation of mesangial cell growth in culture by thromboxane A_2 and prostacyclin. *Kidney Int.* 38: 232, 1990.
459. Metcoff, J., and Janeway, C. A. Studies on the pathogenesis of nephrotic edema. *J. Pediatr.* 58: 640, 1961.
460. Meyrier, A., Simon, P., Perett, G., et al. Remission of idiopathic nephrotic syndrome after treatment with cyclosporin A. *Br. Med. J.* 292: 789, 1986.
461. Michael, A. F., Blau, E., and Vernier, R. L. Glomerular polyanion: Alteration in aminonucleoside nephrosis. *Lab. Invest.* 23: 649, 1970.
462. Michaeli, J., Bar-On, H., and Shafrir, E. Lipoprotein profiles in a heterogeneous group of patients with nephrotic syndrome. *Isr. J. Med. Sci.* 17: 1001, 1981.
463. Miller, P. L., and Meyer, T. W. Plasma protein concentration and colloid osmotic pressure in nephrotic rats. *Kidney Int.* 34: 1988.
464. Milliner, D. S., and Morganstern, B. S. Angiotensin converting enzyme inhibitors for reduction of proteinuria in children with steroid-resistant nephrotic syndrome. *Pediatr. Nephrol.* 5: 587, 1991.
465. Minchin, M. A., Turner, K. J., and Bower, G. D. Lymphocyte blastogenesis in nephrotic syndrome. *Clin. Exp. Immunol.* 42: 241, 1980.
466. Mizuiri, S., Hayashi, I., Ozawa, T., et al. Effects of an oral protein load on glomerular filtration rate in healthy controls and nephrotic patients. *Nephron* 48: 101, 1986.
467. Mohos, S. C., and Skoza, L. Glomerular sialoprotein. *Science* 164: 1519, 1967.
468. Moncrieff, M. W., White, R. H. R., Glasgow, E. F., et al. The familial nephrotic syndrome: II. A clinicopathologic study. *Clin. Nephrol.* 1: 220, 1973.
469. Mongeau, J. G., Corneille, L., Robitaille, P., et al. Primary nephrosis in childhood associated with focal glomerulosclerosis: Is long-term prognosis that severe? *Kidney Int.* 20: 743, 1981.
470. Moore, D. H., Shackelford, P. G., Robson, A. M., et al. Recurrent pneumococcal sepsis and defective opsonization after pneumococcal capsular polysaccharide vaccine in a child with nephrotic syndrome. *J. Pediatr.* 96: 882, 1980.
471. Moorehead, J. F., Chan, M. K., El-Nahas, M., et al. Lipid nephrotoxicity in chronic progressive glomerular and tubulointerstitial disease. *Lancet* ii: 1309, 1982.

471a. Moorehead, J. F., Wheeler, D. C., and Varghese, Z. Glomerular structures and lipids in progressive renal disease. *Am. J. Med.* 87: 5N, 1989.

472. Moorthy, A. V. Minimal change glomerular disease: A paraneoplastic syndrome in two patients with bronchogenic carcinoma. *Am. J. Kidney Dis.* 3: 58, 1983.

473. Moorthy, A. V., Zimmerman, S. W., and Burkholder, P. M. Inhibition of lymphocyte blastogenesis by plasma of patients with minimal-change nephrotic syndrome. *Lancet* i: 1160, 1976.

474. Moorthy, A. V., Zimmerman, S. W., and Burkholder, P. M. Nephrotic syndrome in Hodgkin's disease: Evidence for pathogenesis alternative to immune complex deposition. *Am. J. Med.* 61: 471, 1976.

475. Morel-Maroger, L., Leathem, A., and Richet, G. Glomerular abnormalities in non-systemic diseases. Relationship between findings by light microscopy and immunofluorescence in 433 renal biopsy specimens. *Am. J. Med.* 53: 170, 1972.

476. Morgan, A. G., Shah, D. J., Williams, W., et al. Proteinuria and glomerular disease in Jamaica. *Clin. Nephrol.* 21: 205, 1984.

477. Morganstern, S. J., Bruns, F. J., Fraley, D. S., et al. Ibuprofen-associated lipoid nephrosis without interstitial nephritis. *Am. J. Kidney Dis.* 14: 50, 1989.

478. Müller, W., and Brandis, M. Acute leukemia after cytotoxic treatment for nonmalignant disease in childhood. A case report and review of the literature. *Eur. J. Pediatr.* 136: 105, 1981.

479. Murnaghan, K., Vasmant, D., and Bensman, A. Pulse methylprednisolone therapy in severe idiopathic childhood nephrotic syndrome. *Acta Paediatr. Scand.* 73: 733, 1984.

480. Murphy, M. J., Bailey, R. R., and McGiven, A. R. Is there an IgM nephropathy? *Aust. N.Z. J. Med.* 13: 35, 1983.

481. Musa, B. U., Seal, U. S., and Doe, R. P. Excretion of corticosteroid-binding globulin, thyroxine-binding globulin and total protein in adult males with nephrosis: Effect of sex hormones. *J. Clin. Endocrinol.* 27: 768, 1967.

482. Nagata, K., Platt, J. L., and Michael, A. F. Interstitial and glomerular immune cell populations in idiopathic nephrotic syndrome. *Kidney Int.* 25: 88, 1984.

483. Nanji, A. A., Campbell, D. J., and Pudek, M. R. Decreased anion gap associated with hypoalbuminemia and monoclonal gammopathy. *J.A.M.A.* 246: 859, 1981.

484. Nanra, R. S., Stuart-Taylor, J., DeLeon, A. H., et al. Analgesic nephropathy: Etiology, clinical syndrome, and clinicopathologic correlations in Australia. *Kidney Int.* 13: 79, 1978.

485. Nash, M. A., Bakare, M. A., D'Agati, V., et al. Late development of chronic renal failure in steroid-responsive nephrotic syndrome. *J. Pediatr.* 101: 411, 1982.

486. Needleman, P., Adams, S. P., Cole, B. R., et al. Atriopeptins as cardiac hormones. *Hypertension* 7: 469, 1985.

487. Newman, W. J., Tisher, C. C., McCoy, R. C., et al. Focal glomerular sclerosis: Contrasting clinical patterns in children and adults. *Medicine* 55: 67, 1978.

488. Newmark, S. R., Anderson, C. F., Donadio, J. V., et al. Lipoprotein profiles in adult nephrotics. *Mayo Clin. Proc.* 50: 359, 1975.

489. Ng, W. L., Chan, K. W., and Ma, L. A scanning electron microscope study of isolated glomeruli in glomerulonephritis. *Pathology* 15: 139, 1983.

490. Niaudet, P., Drachman, R., Gagnadoox, M. F., et al. Treatment of idiopathic nephrotic syndrome with levamisole. *Acta Paediatr. Scand.* 73: 637, 1984.

491. Niaudet, P., Habib, R., Tete, M. J., et al. Cyclosporin in the treatment of idiopathic nephrotic syndrome in children. *Pediatr. Nephrol.* 1: 566, 1987.

492. Nicastri, A. D., Tejani, A., Manis, T., et al. Renal lesions in sickle cell nephropathy (Abstract). *Kidney Int.* 23: 131, 1983.

493. Nochy, D., Barres, D., Camilleri, J. P., et al. Abnormalities of renin-containing cells in human glomerular and vascular renal diseases. *Kidney Int.* 23: 375, 1983.

494. Nolasco, F., Cameron, J. S., Heywood, E. F., et al. Adult-onset minimal change nephrotic syndrome: A long-term follow-up. *Kidney Int.* 29: 1215, 1986.

495. Noss, G., Bachmann, H. J., and Olbing, H. Association of minimal change nephrotic syndrome (MCNS) with HLA-B8 and B-13. *Clin. Nephrol.* 15: 172, 1981.

496. Nunez-Roldan, A., Villechenous, E., Fernandez-Andrade, C., et al. Increased HLA-DR7 and decreased DR2 in steroid-responsive nephrotic syndrome. *N. Engl. J. Med.* 306: 366, 1982.

497. Oetliker, O. H., Mordasini, R., Lutschg, J., et al. Lipoprotein metabolism in nephrotic syndrome in childhood. *Pediatr. Res.* 14: 64, 1980.

498. Ohta, T., and Matsuda, I. Lipid and apolipoprotein levels in patients with nephrotic syndrome. *Clin. Chim. Acta* 117: 133, 1981.

499. Okuda, S., Languino, L. R., Ruoslahti, E., et al. Elevated expression of transforming growth factor-β and proteoglycan production in experimental glomerulonephritis: Possible role in expansion of extracellular matrix. *J. Clin. Invest.* 86: 453, 1990.

500. Oldrizzi, L., Rugiu, C., Valvo, E., et al. Progression of renal failure in patients with renal disease of diverse etiology on protein-restricted diet. *Kidney Int.* 27: 553, 1985.

501. Oliver, W. J. Physiologic responses associated with steroid-induced diuresis in the nephrotic syndrome. *J. Lab. Clin. Med.* 62: 449, 1963.

502. Oliver, W. J., Kelsch, R. C., and Chandler, J. P. Demonstration of increased catecholamine excretion in the nephrotic syndrome. *Proc. Soc. Exp. Biol. Med.* 125: 1176, 1967.

503. Ooi, B. S., Orlina, A. R., and Masaitis, L. Lymphocytotoxins in primary renal disease. *Lancet* ii: 1348, 1974.

504. O'Regan, D., O'Callaghan, U., Dundon, S., et al. HLA antigens and steroid responsive nephrotic syndrome of childhood. *Tissue Antigens* 16: 147, 1980.

505. Osakabe, K., and Matsumoto, K. Concanavalin A-induced suppressor cell activity in lipoid nephrosis. *Scand. J. Immunol.* 14: 161, 1981.

506. Ozanne, P., Francis, R. B., and Meiselman, H. J. Red blood cell aggregation in nephrotic syndrome. *Kidney Int.* 23: 519, 1983.

507. Paller, M. S., and Schrier, R. W. Pathogenesis of sodium and water retention in edematous disorders. *Am. J. Kidney Dis.* 2: 241, 1982.

508. Panicucci, F., Sagripanti, A., Vispi, M., et al. Comprehensive study of haemostasis in nephrotic syndrome. *Nephron* 33: 9, 1983.

509. Papadopoulou, Z. L., Jenis, E. H., Tina, L. V., et al. Chronic relapsing minimal change nephrotic syndrome with or without mesangial deposits: Long term follow-up. *Int. J. Pediatr. Nephrol.* 3: 179, 1982.

510. Pardo, V., Reisgo, I., Zilleruello, G., et al. The clinical significance of mesangial IgM deposits and mesangial hypercellularity in minimal change nephrotic syndrome. *Am. J. Kidney Dis.* 3: 264, 1984.

511. Parra, A., Santos, D., Cervantes, C., et al. Plasma go-

nadotropins and gonadal steroids in children treated with cyclophosphamide. *J. Pediatr.* 92: 117, 1978.

512. Pearson, J., Gallo, G., Gluck, M., et al. Renal disease in familial dysautonomia. *Kidney Int.* 17: 102, 1980.
513. Pedersen, E. B., Danielsen, H., Sorenson, S. S., et al. Renal water excretion before and after remission of nephrotic syndrome: Relationship between free water clearance and kidney function, arginine vasopressin, angiotensin II and aldosterone in plasma before and after water loading. *Clin. Sci.* 71: 97, 1986.
514. Pennisi, A. J., Grushkin, C. M., and Lieberman, E. Gonadal function in children with nephrosis treated with cyclophosphamide. *Am. J. Dis. Child.* 129: 315, 1975.
515. Pepper, D. S., and Jamieson, G. A. Studies on glycoproteins. III. Isolation of sialoglycopeptides from human platelet membranes. *Biochemistry* 8: 3362, 1969.
516. Perico, N., Delaini, F., Lupini, C., et al. Renal response to atrial peptides is reduced in experimental nephrosis. *Am. J. Physiol.* 252: F654, 1987.
517. Perico, N., Delaini, F., Lupini, C., et al. Blunted excretory response to atrial natriuretic peptide in experimental nephrosis. *Kidney Int.* 36: 57, 1989.
518. Pesce, A. J., Gaizutis, M., and Pollak, V. E. Selectivity of proteinuria: An evaluation of the immunochemical gel filtration techniques. *J. Lab. Clin. Med.* 75: 586, 1970.
519. Peterson, C., Madsen, B., Perlman, A., et al. Atrial natriuretic peptide and the renal response to hypervolemia in nephrotic humans. *Kidney Int.* 34: 825, 1988.
520. Pinto, J., Lacerda, G., Cameron, J. S., et al. Recurrence of focal segmental glomerulosclerosis in renal allografts. *Transplantation* 32: 83, 1981.
521. Pirotzky, E., Hieblot, C., Benveniste, J., et al. Basophil sensitization in idiopathic nephrotic syndrome. *Lancet* 1: 358, 1982.
522. Plager, J., and Stutzman, L. Acute nephrotic syndrome as a manifestation of active Hodgkin's disease. Report of four cases and review of the literature. *Am. J. Med.* 50: 56, 1971.
523. Ponticelli, C., Banfi, G., Imbasciati, E., et al. Immunosuppressive therapy in primary glomerulonephritis. *Contrib. Nephrol.* 34: 33, 1982.
524. Ponticelli, C., Imbasciati, E., Case, N., et al. Intravenous methylprednisolone in minimal change nephrotic syndrome. *Br. Med. J.* 1: 685, 1980.
525. Prathap, K., and Looi, L. M. Morphological patterns of glomerular disease in renal biopsies from 1,000 Malaysian patients. *Ann. Acad. Med. Singapore* 11: 52, 1982.
526. Prober, C. G., Kirk, L. E., and Keeney, R. E. Acyclovir therapy of chickenpox in immunosuppressed children—A collaborative study. *J. Pediatr.* 101: 622, 1982.
527. Pru, C., Kjellstrand, C. M., Cohn, R. A., et al. Late recurrence of minimal lesion nephrotic syndrome. *Ann. Intern. Med.* 100: 69, 1984.
528. Purkerson, M. L., Joist, J. H., Greenberg, J. M., et al. Inhibition by anticoagulant drugs of the progressive hypertension and uremia associated with renal infarction in rats. *Thromb. Res.* 26: 227, 1982.
529. Purkerson, M. L., Joist, J. H., Yates, J., et al. Inhibition of thromboxane synthesis ameliorates the progressive kidney disease of rats with subtotal renal ablation. *Proc. Natl. Acad. Sci. U.S.A.* 82: 193, 1985.
530. Rabelink, T. J., Koomans, H. A., Boer, P., et al. Role of ANP in natriuresis of head-out immersion in humans. *Am. J. Physiol.* 257: 375, 1989.
531. Raij, L., Keane, W. F., Leonard, A., et al. Irreversible acute renal failure in idiopathic nephrotic syndrome. *Am. J. Med.* 61: 207, 1976.
532. Ramirez, F., Travis, L. B., Cunningham, R. J., et al. Focal segmental glomerulosclerosis, crescent, and rapidly progressive renal failure. *Int. J. Pediatr. Nephrol.* 3: 175, 1982.
533. Rao, T. K. S., Filippone, E. J., Nicastri, A. D., et al. Associated focal and segmental glomerulosclerosis in the acquired immunodeficiency syndrome. *N. Eng. J. Med.* 310: 669, 1984.
534. Rashid, H., Skillen, A. W., Morley, A. R., et al. Serum immunoglobulins in minimal change nephrotic syndrome—A possible defect in T-cell function. *Bangladesh Med. Res. Council Bull.* 8: 15, 1982.
535. Reeves, W. G., Cameron, J. S., Johansson, S. G. O., et al. Seasonal nephrotic syndrome. Description and immunological findings. *Clin. Allergy* 5: 121, 1975.
536. Reimold, E. W. Changes in zinc metabolism during the course of nephrotic syndrome. *Am. J. Dis. Child.* 134: 46, 1980.
537. Remuzzi, A., Pergolizzi, R., Mauer, M. S., et al. Three-dimensional morphometric analysis of segmental glomerulosclerosis in the rat. *Kidney Int.* 38: 851, 1990.
538. Remuzzi, A., Puntorieri, S., Battaglia, C., et al. Angiotensin converting enzyme inhibition ameliorates glomerular filtration of macromolecules and water and lessens glomerular injury in the rat. *J. Clin. Invest.* 85: 541, 1990.
539. Remuzzi, G., and Bertani, T. Is glomerulosclerosis a consequence of altered glomerular permeability to macromolecules? *Kidney Int.* 38: 384, 1990.
540. Remuzzi, G., Imberti, L., Rossini, M., et al. Increased glomerular thromboxane synthesis as a possible cause of proteinuria in experimental nephrosis. *J. Clin. Invest.* 75: 94, 1985.
541. Remuzzi, G., Zoja, C., Remuzzi, A., et al. Low-protein diet prevents glomerular damage in Adriamycin-treated rats. *Kidney Int.* 28: 21, 1985.
542. Rennke, H. G., Roos, P. C., and Wall, S. G. Drug-induced interstitial nephritis with heavy glomerular proteinuria. *N. Engl. J. Med.* 302: 691, 1980.
543. Rennke, H. G., and Venkatachalam, M. A. Glomerular permeability: *In vivo* tracer studies with polyanionic and polycationic ferritins. *Kidney Int.* 11: 44, 1977.
544. Rennke, H. G., and Venkatachalam, M. A. Glomerular permeability of macromolecules. Effect of molecular configuration on the fractional clearance of uncharged dextran and neutral horseradish peroxidase in the rat. *J. Clin. Invest.* 63: 713, 1979.
545. Rich, A. R. A hitherto undescribed vulnerability of the juxtamedullary glomeruli in lipoid nephrosis. *Bull. Johns Hopkins Hosp.* 100: 173, 1957.
546. Richards, N. T., Gordon, C., Richardson, K., et al. Urinary IL-6: A marker for mesangial proliferation? *J. Am. Soc. Nephrol.* 1: 566, 1990.
547. Richards, W., Olson, D., and Church, J. A. Improvement of idiopathic nephrotic syndrome following allergy therapy. *Ann. Allergy* 39: 332, 1977.
548. Richman, A. V., and Kasnic, G., Jr. Endothelial and platelet reactions in the idiopathic nephrotic syndrome: An ultrastructural study. *Hum. Pathol.* 13: 548, 1982.

548a. Rifai, N. Lipoproteins and apolipoproteins: Composition, metabolism, and association with coronary heart disease. *Arch. Pathol. Lab. Med.* 110: 694, 1986.

549. Rifkind, D., Kravetz, H. M., Knight, V., et al. Urinary excretion of iron-binding protein in nephrotic syndrome. *N. Engl. J. Med.* 265: 115, 1961.

549a. Robeva, R., et al. Enhanced B_2-microglobulin levels in lymphocyte culture supernatants from patients with idiopathic nephrotic syndrome: Inhibition of lymphocyte activation by cyclosporine. *Clin. Nephrol.* 30: 211, 1988.

550. Robson, A. M. Edema and Edema-Forming States. In S. Klahr (ed.), *The Kidney and Body Fluids in Health and Disease.* New York: Plenum, 1983. P. 119.
551. Robson, A. M., and Cole, B. R. Pathologic and Functional Correlations in the Glomerulopathies. In N. B. Cummings, A. F. Michael, and C. B. Wilson (eds.), *Immune Mechanisms in Renal Disease.* New York: Plenum, 1982. P. 109.
552. Robson, A. M., Cole, B. R., Kienstra, R. A., et al. Severe glomerulonephritis complicated by coagulopathy: Treatment with anticoagulant and immunosuppressive drugs. *J. Pediatr.* 90: 881, 1977.
553. Robson, A. M., Giangiacomo, J., Kienstra, R. A., et al. Normal glomerular permeability and its modification by minimal change nephrotic syndrome. *J. Clin. Invest.* 54: 1190, 1974.
554. Robson, A. M., and Vehaskari, V. M. The Role of Charge Sites in Vascular Permeability. In J. Brodehl and J. H. H. Ehrich (eds.), *Pediatric Nephrology.* New York: Springer-Verlag, 1983.
555. Rodriguez-Iturbe, B., Colic, D., Parra, G., et al. Atrial natriuretic factor in the acute nephritic and nephrotic syndromes. *Kidney Int.* 38: 512, 1990.
556. Rose, G. M., Cole, B. R., and Robson, A. J. The treatment of renal glomerulopathies in children using high dose intravenous methylprednisolone pulses. *Am. J. Kidney Dis.* 1: 148, 1981.
557. Rosen, S., Galvanek, E., Levy, M., et al. Glomerular disease. *Hum. Pathol.* 12: 964, 1981.
558. Rosenman, R. H., Byers, S. O., and Friedman, M. Plasma lipid interrelationships in experimental nephrosis. *J. Clin. Invest.* 36: 1558, 1957.
559. Rosenman, R. H., and Friedman, M. *In vivo* studies of the role of albumin in endogenous heparin-activated lipaemia clearing in nephrotic rats. *J. Clin. Invest.* 36: 700, 1957.
560. Rostin, M., Barthe, P., Houin, G., et al. Pharmacokinetics of prednisolone in children with the nephrotic syndrome. *Pediatr. Nephrol.* 4: 470, 1990.
561. Roy, L. P., Vernier, R. L., and Michael, A. F. Effect of protein-load proteinuria on glomerular polyanion. *Proc. Soc. Exp. Biol. Med.* 141: 870, 1972.
562. Ruder, H., Scharer, K., Opelz, G., et al. Human leukocyte antigens in idiopathic nephrotic syndrome in children. *Pediatr. Nephrol.* 4: 478, 1990.
563. Ruef, C., Budde, K., Lacy, J., et al. Interleukin 6 is an autocrine growth factor for mesangial cells. *Kidney Int.* 38: 249, 1990.
564. Rytand, D. A. Fatal anuria, the nephrotic syndrome and glomerular nephritis as sequels of the dermatitis of poison oak. *Am. J. Med.* 5: 548, 1948.
565. Rytand, D. A. Onset of the nephrotic syndrome during a reaction to bee sting. *Stanford Med. Bull.* 13: 224, 1955.
566. Saito, T., and Atkins, R. C. Contribution of mononuclear leukocytes to the progression of experimental focal glomerular sclerosis. *Kidney Int.* 37: 1076, 1990.
567. Sakai, T., Harris, F. H., Jr., Marsh, D. J., et al. Extracellular fluid expansion and autoregulation in nephrotoxic serum nephritis in rats. *Kidney Int.* 25: 619, 1984.
568. Sandberg, D. H., McIntosh, R. M., Bernstein, C. W., et al. Severe steroid-responsive nephrosis associated with hypersensitivity. *Lancet* i: 388, 1977.
569. Schärer, K., and Minges, U. Long-term prognosis of the nephrotic syndrome in childhood. *Clin. Nephrol.* 1: 182, 1973.
570. Scheinman, K. I., and Stiehm, E. R. Fibrinolytic studies in the nephrotic syndrome. *Pediatr. Res.* 5: 206, 1971.
571. Schieppati, A., Dodesini, P., Benigni, A., et al. The metabolism of arachidonic acid by platelets in nephrotic syndrome. *Kidney Int.* 25: 671, 1984.
572. Schnaper, H. W. The immune system in minimal change nephrotic syndrome. *Pediatr. Nephrol.* 3: 101, 1989.
573. Schnaper, H. W. The soluble immune response suppressor pathway in nephrotic syndrome. *Semin. Nephrol.* 9: 107, 1989.
574. Schnaper, H. W. A regulatory system for soluble immune response suppressor production in steroid-responsive nephrotic syndrome. *Kidney Int.* 38: 151, 1990.

574a. Schnaper, H. W. Immunization practices in childhood nephrotic syndrome: A survey of North American pediatric nephrologists. *Pediatr. Res.* 29: 350A, 1991.

575. Schnaper, H. W., and Aune, T. M. Identification of the lymphokine soluble immune response suppressor in urine of nephrotic children. *J. Clin. Invest.* 76: 341, 1985.
576. Schnaper, H. W., and Aune, T. M. Suppression of immune responses to sheep erythrocytes by the lymphokine soluble immune response suppressor (SIRS) in vivo. *J. Immunol.* 137: 863, 1986.
577. Schnaper, H. W., and Aune, T. M. Steroid-sensitive mechanism of soluble immune response suppressor production in patients with steroid-responsive nephrotic syndrome. *J. Clin. Invest.* 79: 254, 1987.
578. Schnaper, H. W., Pierce, C. W., and Aune, T. M. Identification and initial characterization of concanavalin A- and interferon-induced human suppressor factors: Evidence for a human equivalent of murine soluble immune response suppressor (SIRS). *J. Immunol.* 132: 2429, 1984.
579. Schnaper, H. W., and Robson, A. M. Minimal Change Nephrotic Syndrome: New Look at An Old Problem. In A. J. Moss (ed.), *Pediatrics Update. Reviews for Physicians,* 1985 Edition. New York: Elsevier, 1985. P. 81.
580. Schneeberger, E. E. Glomerular permeability to protein molecules—Its possible structural basis. *Nephron* 13: 7, 1974.
581. Schneeberger, E. E., Levey, R. H., McCluskey, R. T., et al. The isoporous substructures of the human glomerular slit diaphragm. *Kidney Int.* 8: 48, 1975.
582. Schoeneman, M. J. Minimal change nephrotic syndrome: Treatment with low doses of hydrocortisone. *J. Pediatr.* 102: 791, 1983.
583. Schoeneman, M. J., Bennett, B., and Greifer, I. The natural history of focal segmental glomerulosclerosis with and without hypercellularity in children. *Clin. Nephrol.* 9: 45, 1978.
584. Schreiner, F. G., Cotran, R. S., Pardo, V., et al. A mononuclear cell component in experimental immunologic glomerulonephritis. *J. Exp. Med.* 47: 369, 1978.
585. Schulman, S. L., Kaiser, B. A., Polinsky, M. S., et al. Predicting the response to cytotoxic therapy for childhood nephrotic syndrome: Superiority of response to corticosteroid therapy over histopathologic patterns. *J. Pediatr.* 113: 996, 1988.
586. Schulte-Wisserman, H., Gortz, W., and Straub, E. IgE in patients with glomerulonephritis and minimal-change nephrotic syndrome. *Eur. J. Pediatr.* 131: 105, 1979.
587. Seggie, J., Davies, P. G., Ninin, D., et al. Patterns of glomerulonephritis in Zimbabwe: Survey of disease characterized by nephrotic proteinuria. *Q. J. Med.* 53: 109, 1984.
588. Seiler, M. W., Rennke, H. G., Venkatachalam, M. A., et

al. Pathogenesis of polycation-induced alterations ("fusion") of glomerular epithelium. *Lab. Invest.* 36: 48, 1977.
589. Seiler, M. W., Venkatachalam, M. A., and Cotran, R. S. Glomerular epithelium: Structural alterations induced by polycations. *Science* 189: 390, 1975.
590. Sestak, T. L., Alavi, N., and Subbaiah, P. V. Plasma lipids and acyltransferase activities in experimental nephrotic syndrome. *Kidney Int.* 36: 240, 1989.
591. Shahin, B., Papadopoulou, Z. L., and Jenis, E. H. Congenital nephrotic syndrome associated with congenital toxoplasmosis. *J. Pediatr.* 85: 366, 1974.
592. Shalhoub, R. J. Pathogenesis of lipoid nephrosis: A disorder of T-cell function. *Lancet* ii: 556, 1974.
593. Shapiro, M., Hasbargen, J., Cosby, R., et al. Role of aldosterone in the Na retention of patients with nephrotic syndrome. *Kidney Int.* 29: 203, 1986.
594. Shemesh, O., Deen, W. M., Brenner, B. M., et al. Effect of colloid volume expansion on glomerular barrier size selectivity in humans. *Kidney Int.* 29: 916, 1986.
595. Sherman, R. L., Susin, M., and Wexler, M. E. Lipoid nephrosis in Hodgkin's disease. *Am. J. Med.* 52: 699, 1972.
596. Sheth, K. J., and Kher, K. K. Anion gap in nephrotic syndrome. *Int. J. Pediatr. Nephrol.* 2: 89, 1984.
597. Shimamatsu, K., Onoyama, K., Maeda, T., et al. Massive pulmonary embolism occurring with corticosteroid and diuretics therapy in a minimal-change nephrotic patient. *Nephron* 32: 78, 1982.
598. Sibley, R. K., Mahan, J., Mauer, S. M., et al. A clinicopathologic study of forty-eight infants with nephrotic syndrome. *Kidney Int.* 27: 544, 1985.
599. Siegel, N. J., Kashgarian, M., Spargo, B. H., et al. Minimal change and focal sclerotic lesions in lipoid nephrosis. *Nephron* 13: 125, 1974.
600. Sigstrom, L., Hansson, S., and Jodal, U. Long term survival of girl with congenital nephrotic syndrome and recurrence of proteinuria after renal transplantation. *Pediatr. Nephrol.* 3: C169, 1989.
601. Similä, S., Vesa, L., and Wasz-Höckert, O. Hereditary onycho-osteodysplasia (nail-patella syndrome) with nephrosis-like renal disease in a newborn boy. *Pediatrics* 46: 61, 1970.
602. Simpson, H. C. R., Mann, J. I., Meade, I. W., et al. Hypertriglyceridaemia and hypercoagulability. *Lancet* i: 786, 1983.
603. Simpson, L. O. Glomerular permeability: An alternate to the pore theory. *Lancet* ii: 251, 1981.
604. Sjoberg, R. J., McMillan, V. M., Bartram, L. S., et al. Renal failure with minimal change nephrotic syndrome: Reversal with hemodialysis. *Clin. Nephrol.* 20: 98, 1983.
605. Smith, M. D., Barratt, T. M., Hayward, A. R., et al. The inhibition of complement-dependent lymphocyte rosette formation by the sera of children with steroid-sensitive nephrotic syndrome and other renal diseases. *Clin. Exp. Immunol.* 21: 236, 1975.
606. Sølling, J. Molecular weight of immune complexes in patients with glomerulonephritis. *Nephron* 30: 137, 1982.
607. Southwest Pediatric Nephrology Study Group. Focal segmental glomerulosclerosis in children with idiopathic nephrotic syndrome. *Kidney Int.* 27: 442, 1985.
608. Spear, G. S., Hyde, T. P., Gruppo, R. A., et al. Pseudohermaphroditism, glomerulonephritis with the nephrotic syndrome, and Wilms' tumor in infancy. *J. Pediatr.* 79: 677, 1971.
609. Spector, D. A., Davis, P. J., Helderman, H., et al. Thyroid function and metabolic state in chronic renal failure. *Ann. Intern. Med.* 85: 724, 1976.
610. Spika, J. S., Halsey, N. A., Fish, A. J., et al. Serum antibody response to pneumococcal vaccine in children with nephrotic syndrome. *Pediatrics* 69: 219, 1982.
611. Stachura, I., Si, L., Madan, E., and Whiteside, T. Mononuclear cell subsets in human renal disease. Enumeration in tissue sections with monoclonal antibody. *Clin. Immunol. Immunopathol.* 30: 362, 1984.
612. Starling, E. H. On the absorption of fluids from the connective tissue space. *J. Physiol.* (Lond.) 19: 312, 1986.
613. Steele, B. T., Bacheyie, G. S., Baumal, R., et al. Acute renal failure of short duration in minimal lesion nephrotic syndrome of childhood. *Int. J. Pediatr. Nephrol.* 3: 59, 1982.
614. Strife, C. F., Jackson, E. C., Forristal, J., et al. Effect of the nephrotic syndrome on the concentration of serum complement components. *Am. J. Kidney Dis.* 8: 37, 1986.
615. Suematsu, S., Matsuda, T., Aozasa, K., et al. IgG1 plasmacytosis in interleukin 6 transgenic mice. *Proc. Natl. Acad. Sci. U.S.A.* 86: 7547, 1989.
616. Suranyi, M. G., Quiza, C., Gausch, A., et al. Cytokine levels in patients with the nephrotic syndrome (Abstract). *Kidney Int.* 37: 445, 1990.
617. Surian, M., Imbasciati, E., Cosci, P., et al. Glomerular disease and pregnancy. A study of 123 pregnancies in patients with primary and secondary glomerular diseases. *Nephron* 36: 101, 1984.
618. Tabin, R., Guignard, J.-P., Gautier, E., et al. Corticoresistant nephrotic syndrome associated with T-cell deficiency in two sisters. *Pediatrics* 71: 93, 1983.
619. Taitz, L. S., Isaacson, C., and Stein, H. Acute nephritis associated with congenital syphilis. *Br. Med. J.* 2: 152, 1961.
620. Tani, Y., Kida, H., Abe, T., et al. β-lymphocyte subset patterns and their significance in idiopathic glomerulonephritis. *Clin. Exp. Immunol.* 48: 201, 1982.
621. Tanphaichitr, P., Tanphaichitr, D., Sureeratanan, J., et al. Treatment of nephrotic syndrome with levamisole. *J. Pediatr.* 96: 490, 1980.
622. Taube, D., Brown, Z., and Williams, D. G. Long-term impairment of suppressor-cell function by cyclophosphamide in minimal-change nephropathy and its association with therapeutic response. *Lancet* 1: 235, 1981.
623. Taube, D., Chapman, S., Brown, Z., et al. Depression of normal lymphocyte transformation by sera of patients with minimal change nephropathy and other forms of nephrotic syndrome. *Clin. Nephrol.* 15: 286, 1981.
624. Tejani, A., Butt, K., Khawar, R., et al. Cyclosporin induced remission of relapsing nephrotic syndrome in children (Abstr.). *Kidney Int.* 29: 206, 1986.
625. Tejani, A., Fikrig, S., Schiffman, G., et al. Persistence of protective pneumococcal antibody following vaccination in patients with the nephrotic syndrome. *Am. J. Nephrol.* 4: 32, 1984.
626. Tejani, A., Nicastri, A., Phadke, K., et al. Familial focal segmental glomerulosclerosis. *Int. J. Pediatr. Nephrol.* 4: 231, 1983.
627. Teodoru, C. V., Saifer, A., and Frankel, H. Conditioning factors influencing evolution of experimental glomerulonephritis in rabbits. *Am. J. Physiol.* 196: 457, 1959.
628. Thaler, E., Balzar, E., Kopsa, H., et al. Acquired antithrombin III deficiency in patients with glomerular proteinuria. *Haemostasis* 7: 257, 1978.
629. Thomson, C., Forbes, C. D., Prentice, C. R., et al. Changes in blood coagulation and fibrinolysis in the nephrotic syndrome. *Q. J. Med.* 43: 399, 1974.
630. Thomson, P. D., Barratt, T. M., Stokes, C. R., et al. HLA antigens and atopic features in steroid-responsive nephrotic syndrome of childhood. *Lancet* ii: 765, 1976.

631. Thysell, H., Brun, C., Larsen, S., et al. Plasma exchange in two cases of minimal change nephrotic syndrome with acute renal failure. *Int. J. Artif. Organs* 6(Suppl.): 75, 1983.

632. Tomizawa, S., Maruyama, K., Nagasawa, N., et al. Studies of vascular permeability factor derived from T lymphocytes and inhibitory effect of plasma on its production in minimal change nephrotic syndrome. *Nephron* 41: 157, 1985.

633. Tomizawa, S., Suzuki, S., Oguri, M., et al. Studies of T lymphocyte function and inhibitory factors in minimal change nephrotic syndrome. *Nephron* 24: 179, 1979.

634. Torres, V. E., Velosa, J. A., Holley, K. E., et al. Meclofenamate treatment of recurrent idiopathic nephrotic syndrome with focal segmental glomerulosclerosis after renal transplant. *Mayo Clin. Proc.* 59: 146, 1984.

635. Trachtman, H., and Gauthier, B. Platelet vasopressin levels in childhood idiopathic nephrotic syndrome. *Am. J. Dis. Child.* 142: 1313, 1988.

636. Trachtman, H., and Gauthier, B. Effect of angiotensin converting enzyme inhibitor therapy on proteinuria in children with renal disease. *J. Pediatr.* 112: 295, 1988.

637. Trainin, E. B., and Gomez-Leon, G. Development of renal insufficiency after long-standing steroid-responsive nephrotic syndrome. *Int. J. Pediatr. Nephrol.* 3: 55, 1982.

638. Trompeter, R. S., Barratt, T. M., Kay, R., et al. HLA, atopy and cyclophosphamide in steroid-responsive childhood nephrotic syndrome. *Kidney Int.* 17: 113, 1980.

639. Trompeter, R. S., Evans, P. R., and Barratt, T. M. Gonadal function in boys with steroid-responsive nephrotic syndrome treated with cyclophosphamide for short periods. *Lancet* i: 1177, 1981.

640. Trompeter, R. S., Thomson, P. D., Barratt, T. M., et al. Controlled trial of disodium cromoglycate in prevention of relapse of steroid-responsive nephrotic syndrome of childhood. *Arch. Dis. Child.* 53: 430, 1978.

641. Tulassay, T., Rascher, W., Lang, R. E., et al. Atrial natriuretic peptide and other vasoactive hormones in nephrotic syndrome. *Kidney Int.* 31: 1391, 1987.

642. Usberti, M., Federico, S., Meccariello, S., et al. Role of plasma vasopressin in the impairment of water excretion in nephrotic syndrome. *Kidney Int.* 25: 422, 1984.

643. Vangelista, A., Frasca, G., Biagini, G., et al. Long-term study of mesangial proliferative glomerulonephritis with IgM deposits. *Proc. Eur. Dial. Transplant. Assoc.* 18: 503, 1981.

644. Vaziri, N. D., Ngo, J.-C. T., Ibsen, K. H., et al. Deficiency and urinary loss of factor XII in nephrotic syndrome. *Nephron* 32: 342, 1982.

645. Vega, G. L., and Grundy, S. M. Lovastatin therapy in nephrotic hyperlipidemia: Effects on lipoprotein metabolism. *Kidney Int.* 33: 1160, 1988.

646. Vehaskari, V. M., Chang, C. T. C., Stevens, J. K., et al. The effect of polycation on vascular permeability in the rat: A proposed role for charge sites. *J. Clin. Invest.* 73: 1053, 1984.

647. Vehaskari, V. M., and Robson, A. M. The nephrotic syndrome in children. *Ann. Pediatr.* 10: 42, 1981.

648. Vehaskari, V. M., Root, E. R., Germuth, F. G., et al. Glomerular charge and urinary protein excretion: Effects of systemic and intrarenal polycation infusion in the rat. *Kidney Int.* 22: 127, 1982.

649. Velosa, J. A., Glasser, R. J., Nevins, T. E., et al. Experimental model of focal sclerosis. II. Correlation with immunopathologic changes, macromolecular kinetics and polyanion loss. *Lab. Invest.* 36: 527, 1977.

650. Velosa, J. A., Torres, V. E., Donadio, J. V., et al. Treatment of severe nephrotic syndrome with meclofenamate: An uncontrolled pilot study. *Mayo Clin. Proc.* 60: 586, 1985.

651. Vernier, R. L., Klein, D. J., Sisson, S. P., et al. Heparan sulfate-rich anionic sites in the human glomerular basement membrane. Decreased concentrations in congenital nephrotic syndrome. *N. Engl. J. Med.* 309: 1001, 1983.

652. Vosnides, G., and Cameron, J. S. Hyperlipidemia in renal disease (Letter). *Med. J. Aust.* 2: 855, 1974.

653. Wachtel, L. N., Cole, J., and Rosen, V. J. X-ray induced glomerulosclerosis in rats: Modification of lesions by food restriction, uninephrectomy and age. *J. Gerontol.* 21: 442, 1966.

654. Wagoner, R. D., Stanson, A. W., and Holley, K. E. Renal vein thrombosis in idiopathic membranous glomerulopathy and nephrotic syndrome: Incidence and significance. *Kidney Int.* 23: 368, 1983.

655. Waldherr, R., Gubler, M. C., Levy, M., et al. The significance of pure diffuse mesangial proliferation in idiopathic nephrotic syndrome. *Clin. Nephrol.* 10: 171, 1978.

656. Walker, F., O'Neill, S., Carmody, M., et al. Nephrotic syndrome in Hodgkin's disease. *Int. J. Pediatr. Nephrol.* 4: 39, 1983.

657. Walker, W. A., Lowman, J. T., and Hong, R. A. Measuring albumin turnover rates in patients with hypoproteinemia. *Am. J. Dis. Child.* 125: 51, 1973.

658. Wallenius, G. Renal clearance of dextran as a measure of glomerular permeability. *Acta Soc. Med. Ups.* [Suppl.] 4: 1, 1954.

659. Warren, J. V., Merrill, A. J., Stead, E. A., Jr. Role of extracellular fluid in maintenance of normal plasma volume. *J. Clin. Invest.* 22: 635, 1943.

660. Warshaw, B. L., Edelbrock, H. H., Ettinger, R. B., et al. Progression to end-stage renal disease in children with obstructive uropathy. *J. Pediatr.* 100: 183, 1982.

661. Warwick, G. L., Caslake, M. J., Boulton-Jones, J. M., et al. Low-density lipoprotein metabolism in the nephrotic syndrome. *Metabolism* 34: 10, 1990.

662. Wass, V. J., and Cameron, J. S. Cardiovascular disease and the nephrotic syndrome: The other side of the coin. *Nephron* 27: 58, 1981.

663. Wass, V. J., Jarrett, R. J., Chilvers, C., et al. Does the nephrotic syndrome increase the risk of cardiovascular disease? *Lancet* ii: 664, 1979.

664. Watson, A. J. S., Dalbow, M. H., Stachura, I., et al. Immunologic studies in cimetidine-induced nephropathy and polymyositis. *N. Engl. J. Med.* 308: 142, 1983.

665. Watson, A., Stachura, I., Fragola, J., et al. Focal segmental glomerulosclerosis in Hodgkin's disease. *Am. J. Nephrol.* 3: 228, 1983.

666. Weiher, H., Noda, T., Gray, D. A., et al. Transgenic mouse model of kidney disease: Insertional inactivation of ubiquitously expressed gene leads to nephrotic syndrome. *Cell* 62: 425, 1990.

667. Welch, T. R., Gianis, J., and Sheldon, C. A. Perforation of the scrotum complicating nephrotic syndrome. *J. Pediatr.* 113: 336, 1988.

668. Werber, H. I., Emancipator, S. N., Tykocinski, M. L., et al. The interleukin 1 gene is expressed by rat glomerular mesangial cells and is augmented in immune complex glomerulonephritis. *J. Immunol.* 138: 3207, 1987.

669. West, C. D. Use of combined hormone and mechlorethamine (nitrogen mustard) therapy in lipoid nephrosis. *Am. J. Dis. Child.* 95: 498, 1958.

670. Whelan, T. V., and Hirszel, P. Minimal-change nephropathy associated with pancreatic carcinoma. *Arch. Intern. Med.* 148: 975, 1988.

671. White, R. H. R. The familial nephrotic syndrome. I. A European survey. *Clin. Nephrol.* 1: 215, 1973.
672. White, R. H. R., Glasgow, E. F., and Mills, R. J. Clinicopathologic study of nephrotic syndrome in childhood. *Lancet* i: 1353, 1970.
673. Williams, S. A., Makker, S. P., and Grupe, W. E. Seizures: A significant side effect of chlorambucil therapy in children. *J. Pediatr.* 93: 516, 1978.
674. Williams, S. A., Makker, S. P., Inglefinger, J. R., et al. Long-term evaluation of chlorambucil plus prednisone in the idiopathic nephrotic syndrome of childhood. *N. Engl. J. Med.* 302: 929, 1980.
675. Wilson, V. K., Thomson, M. L., and Hohlzel, A. Mercury nephrosis in young children. *Br. Med. J.* 1: 359, 1952.
676. Winetz, J. A., Robertson, C. R., Golbetz, H. V., et al. The nature of the glomerular injury in minimal change and focal sclerosing glomerulopathies. *Am. J. Kidney Dis.* 1: 91, 1981.
677. Wingen, A.-M., Muller-Wiefel, D. E., and Scharer, K. Comparison of different regimens of prednisone therapy in frequently relapsing nephrotic syndrome. *Acta Paediatr. Scand.* 79: 305, 1990.
678. Wu, M. J., and Moorthy, A. V. Suppressor cell function in patients with primary glomerular disease. *Clin. Immunol. Immunopathol.* 22: 442, 1982.
679. Wuarin, J., and Schibler, U. Expression of the liver-specific transcriptional activator protein DBP follows a stringent circadian rhythm. *Cell* 63: 1257, 1990.
680. Xu, H.-W., Jevnikar, A. M., Brennan, D. C., et al. Dexamethasone prevents proximal tubular Ia antigen but not ICAM-1 expression in mice protected from autoimmune nephritis (Abstract). *J. Am. Soc. Nephrol.* 1: 546, 1990.
681. Yamada, M., and Matsuda, I. Lipoprotein lipase in clinical and experimental nephrosis. *Clin. Chim. Acta* 30: 787, 1970.
682. Yamauchi, H., and Hopper, J., Jr. Hypovolemic shock and hypotension as a complication in the nephrotic syndrome: Report of ten cases. *Ann. Intern. Med.* 60: 242, 1964.
683. Yamauchi, H., Hopper, J., Jr., and McCormack, K. Blood volume and fainting in nephrosis (Abstract). *Clin. Res.* 8: 195, 1960.
684. Yedgar, S., Weinstein, D. B., Patsch, W., et al. Vicosity of culture medium as a regulation of synthesis and secretion of very low density lipoproteins by cultured hepatocytes. *J. Biol Chem.* 257: 2188, 1982.
685. Yeung, C. K., Wong, K. L., and Ng, W. L. Intravenous methylprednisolone pulse therapy in minimal change nephrotic syndrome. *Aust. N.Z. J. Med.* 13: 349, 1983.
686. Yoshida, A., and Aoki, N. Release of arachidonic acid from human platelets. A key role for the potentiation of platelet aggregating ability in normal subjects as well as in those with nephrotic syndrome. *Blood* 52: 969, 1978.
687. Yoshikawa, N., Cameron, A. H., and White, R. H. Ultrastructure of the nonsclerotic glomeruli in childhood nephrotic syndrome. *J. Pathol.* 136: 133, 1982.
688. Yoshikawa, N., Ito, H., Akamatsu, R., et al. Focal segmental glomerulosclerosis with and without nephrotic syndrome in children. *J. Pediatr.* 109: 65, 1986.
689. Zech, P., Colon, S., Pointet, P., et al. The nephrotic syndrome in adults aged over 60: Etiology, evolution, and treatment of 76 cases. *Clin. Nephrol.* 17: 232, 1982.
690. Zietse, R., and Schalekamp, M. A. Effect of synthetic human atrial natriuretic peptide (102-126) in nephrotic humans. *Kidney Int.* 34: 717, 1988.
691. Zilleruelo, G., Hsia, S. L., Freundlich, M., et al. Persistence of serum lipid abnormalities in children with idiopathic nephrotic syndrome. *J. Pediatr.* 104: 61, 1984.
692. Zucchelli, P., Cagnoli, L., Casanova, S., et al. Focal glomerulosclerosis in patients with unilateral nephrectomy. *Kidney Int.* 24: 649, 1983.

Membranous Nephropathy

Cecil H. Coggins

Historical Introduction

Membranous nephropathy (also called *idiopathic membranous nephropathy, membranous glomerulonephritis, extramembranous glomerulonephritis,* and *epimembranous nephropathy*) is a glomerular disease that is characterized clinically by proteinuria. In many series, it is the most common glomerular disease underlying nephrotic syndrome in adults. Historically, the accurate definition of membranous nephropathy (MN) awaited the development of sensitive histologic techniques, since the pathology is far more specific than the clinical picture. In the 1930s, Bell [27] and Dunn [99] noted thickening of the glomerular capillary walls in many nephrotic patients. Their techniques did not allow them to discern the cause of the thickening nor to distinguish mild membranous change from lipoid nephrosis or mild proliferative glomerulonephritis. Membranous nephropathy was included in type II in Ellis' classification [105] along with lipoid nephrosis and other noninflammatory diseases of the glomerulus, and in 1950, they were still grouped as a cause of nephrotic syndrome [11, 28]. With the introduction of silver tissue stains [193], thin sections and, especially with the introduction of electron and immunofluorescence microscopy in the 1950s, the current definition of MN was elucidated along with its clear separation from lipoid nephrosis.

Pathology

The most specific identifying characteristic in the pathology of membranous nephropathy is the presence of subepithelial deposits, which are electron dense when viewed by electron microscopy. Other histologic changes may be characteristic but not specific. On gross examination, the kidneys of a patient with membranous nephropathy have a pale appearance and tend to be rather large. Only in advanced chronic renal failure do they gradually become small.

LIGHT MICROSCOPY

Under light microscopy using hematoxylin and eosin (H & E) or periodic acid–Schiff (PAS) stains, glomeruli show a regular thickening of the capillary wall (Fig. 65-1). This change is diffuse, involving all glomeruli, and usually global, involving the whole glomerulus. The endothelial cells appear normal. The mesangial cells are usually normal in number, although some mesangial hypercellularity can be seen even in the absence of lupus [127, 354] (see the following discussion). Hyaline droplets may be present in some of the epithelial cells, which tend to be normal in number. The parietal epithelial cells may be enlarged and, rarely, crescents are present [127]. With the H & E stain, the capillary wall appears as a uniform eosinophilic band, but silver stains show densely staining projections extending from the endothelial side into the basement membrane as a series of "spikes." Presumably, these spikes represent normal basement membrane extending between the subepithelial deposits [102]. In some cases, no thickening of the capillary wall may be seen by H & E and PAS stains, and membranous nephropathy may be confused with minimal change disease [393]. The use of immunofluorescence microscopy or electron microscopy, therefore, may be essential to identify the correct process. When the membrane is extremely thick, the spikes may spread and meet in the subepithelial region, giving the membrane a bilaminar or split appearance. This occurrence also may lead to difficulties in diagnosis by light microscopy alone. In advanced cases, the capillary wall thickening may become so severe as to occlude the lumen, with resulting total glomerular sclerosis and accompanying tubular atrophy. Tubulointerstitial lesions are, in general, encountered in more advanced stages of the disease. An increase in T lymphocytes of both helper/inducer and suppressor/cytotoxic types [10, 167] and monocytes are seen in the interstitium, but a marked interstitial infiltrate may suggest an associated disease process, such as renal vein thrombosis (see the following discussion) or drug-related interstitial nephritis. Vascular changes also occur, mostly at later stages, especially when accompanied by hypertension. Intimal proliferation and hyaline changes occur in the arteries and arterioles. Proteinaceous casts may be present in the tubules. The tubular cells may show the characteristic changes of nephrotic syndrome with hyaline droplets and lipid vacuoles. A few interstitial foam cells may be present.

ELECTRON MICROSCOPY

Electron microscopy shows a general enlargement of the glomerulus [15], confirms the mild changes in the epithelial and mesangial cells, and discloses subepithelial electron-dense deposits of varying sizes and shapes (Figs. 65-2 through 65-6). Four pathologic stages have been described by Ehrenreich and Churg [102], which were originally thought to reflect the course of the disease. A stage 1 lesion includes small scattered subepithelial deposits associated with spike-like irregularities of the epithelial surface of the basement membrane and swollen and distorted epithelial foot processes. The deposits may be quite few in number. In stage 2 lesions, the subepithelial deposits are more numerous, larger, and have a more uniform distribution throughout the glomerular tuft—even in "submesangial" regions. Epithelial spikes are prominent and foot processes are markedly obliterated. In stage 3, the electron-dense deposits become completely encircled by lateral extensions

The author is most grateful for the patient and intelligent help of Ms. Robin L. Parsons in the preparation of this manuscript.

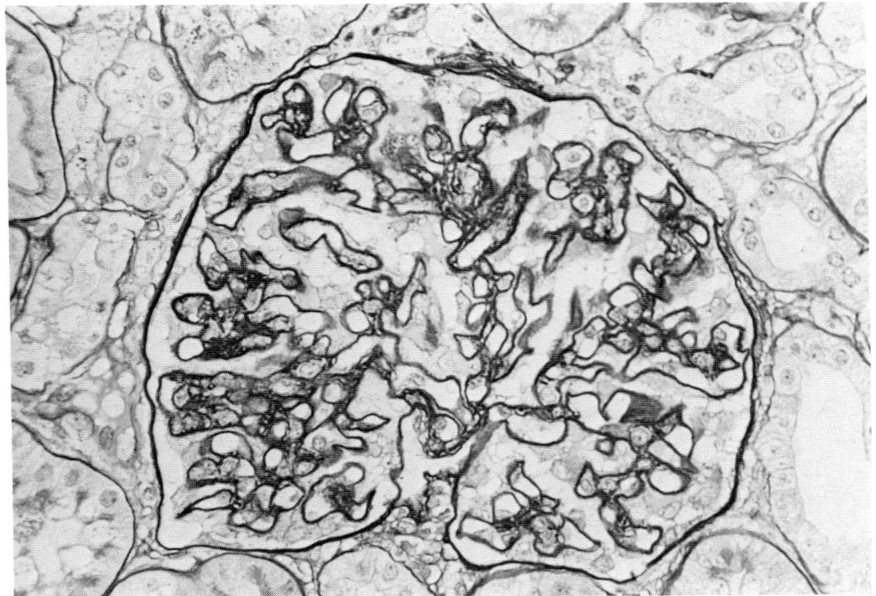

Fig. 65-1. Light microscopy of a glomerulus from a patient with fully developed membranous nephropathy. There is a moderate thickening of the glomerulus basement membrane that stains intensely positive with PAS. Cellular elements are not increased in number. The interstitium shows a minimal increase in connective tissue and edema. (PAS stain.) All figures are reproduced with permission from M. Arnaout, H. Rennke, and R. Cotran, Membranous Glomerulonephritis. In *Nephrotic Syndrome—Contemporary Issues in Nephrology,* Vol. 9. (New York: Churchill Livingstone, 1982.)

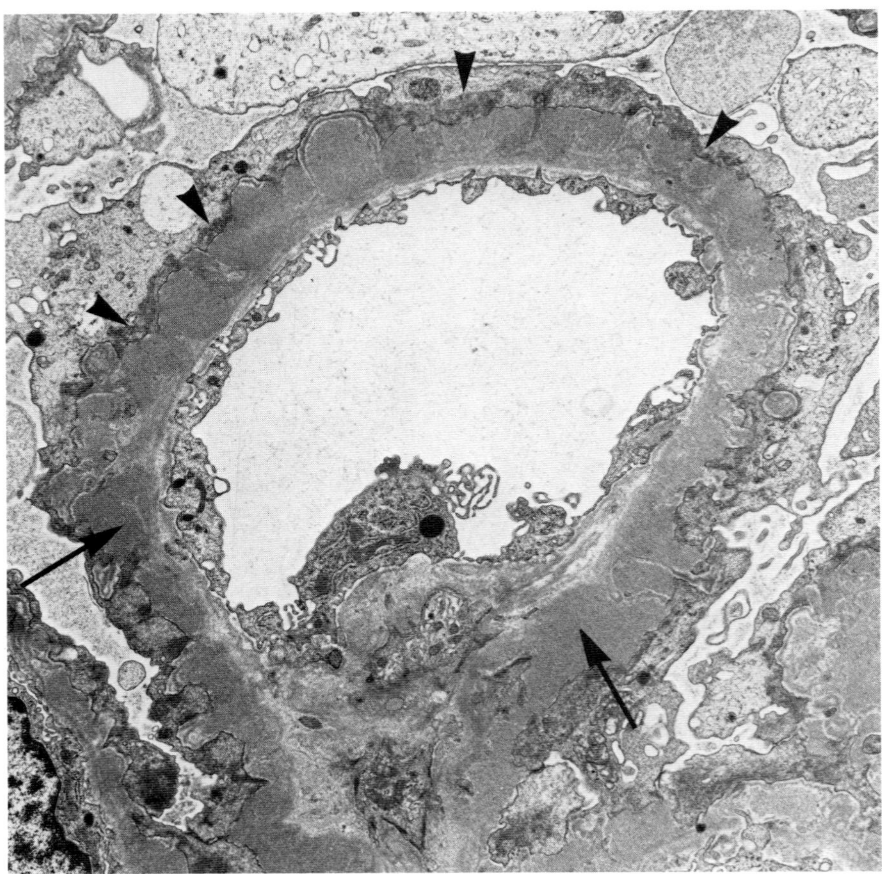

Fig. 65-2. Electron micrograph of a glomerular capillary loop from a patient with stage I–II membranous nephropathy. Subepithelial electron-dense deposits that are often confluent are seen (*arrows*); basement membrane-like material is slightly increased. The epithelial cells show marked condensation of the cytoplasm adjacent to the immune deposits (*arrowheads*).

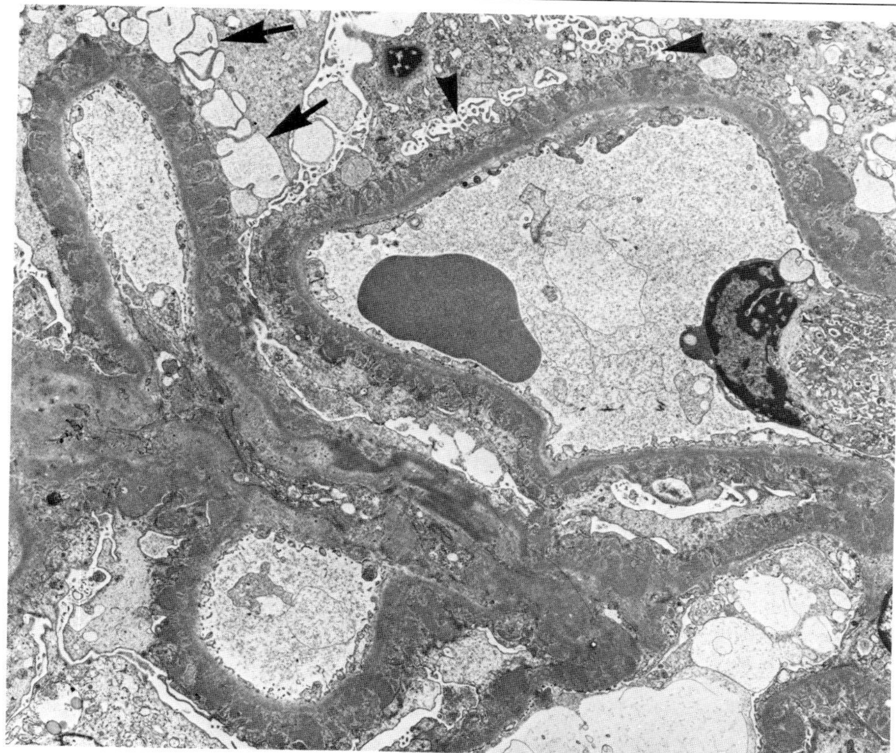

Fig. 65-3. Electron micrograph illustrating ultrastructural changes in fully developed membranous nephropathy. Electron-dense deposits are distributed diffusely throughout the subepithelial aspect of the glomerular basement membrane. Mesangial deposits are absent in most idiopathic cases. Conspicuous vacuolar changes (*arrows*) and microvillous transformation (*arrowheads*) are seen in epithelial cells that, in addition, show diffuse obliteration of foot processes.

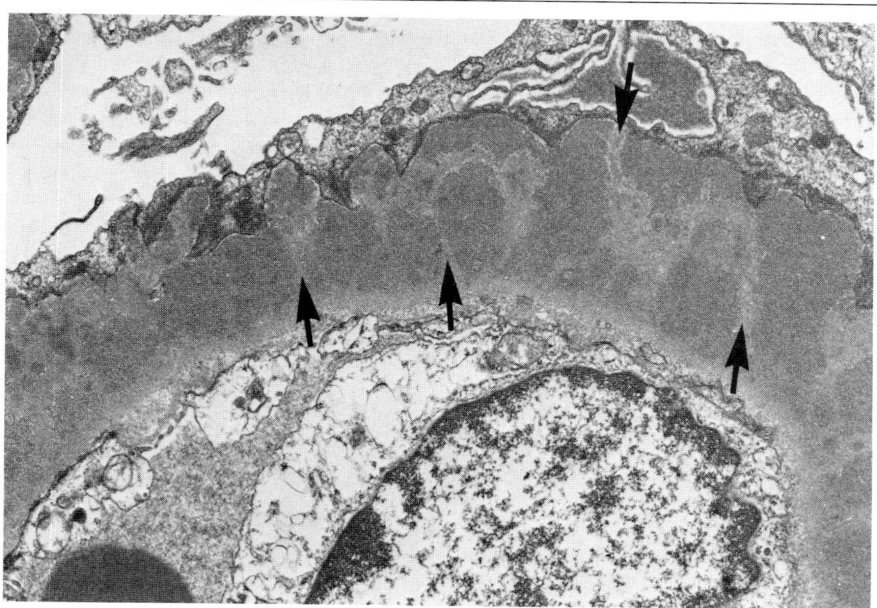

Fig. 65-4. Fully developed (stage II) membranous nephropathy, demonstrating immune deposits separated by basement-membrane projections (*arrows*). Deposits rearranged in a double layer.

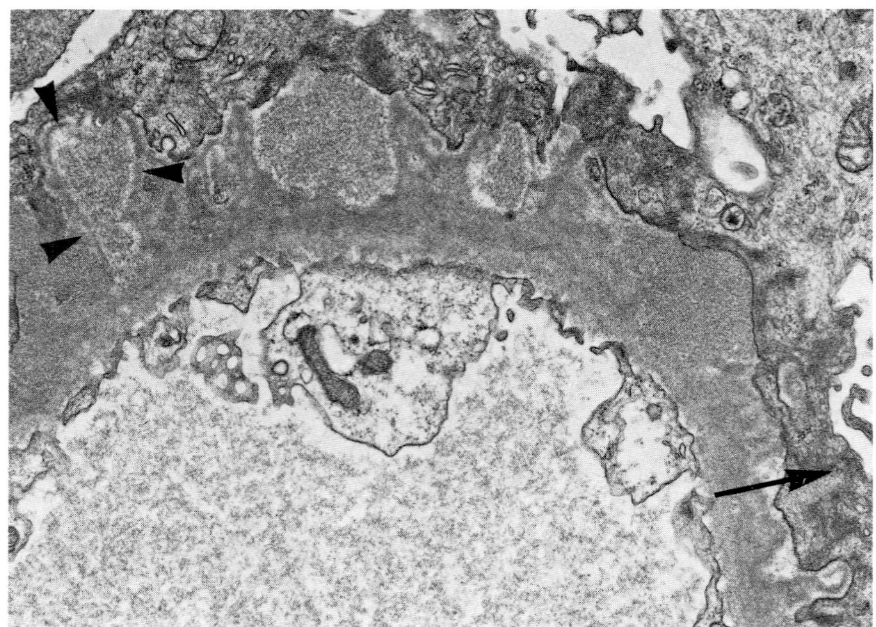

Fig. 65-5. High-power electron micrograph, showing finely granular immune deposits with a prominent increase of basement-membrane material separating adjacent densities. On the left is shown a deposit almost completely incorporated into the basement membrane (*arrowheads*). Note complete obliteration of foot processes (*arrow*).

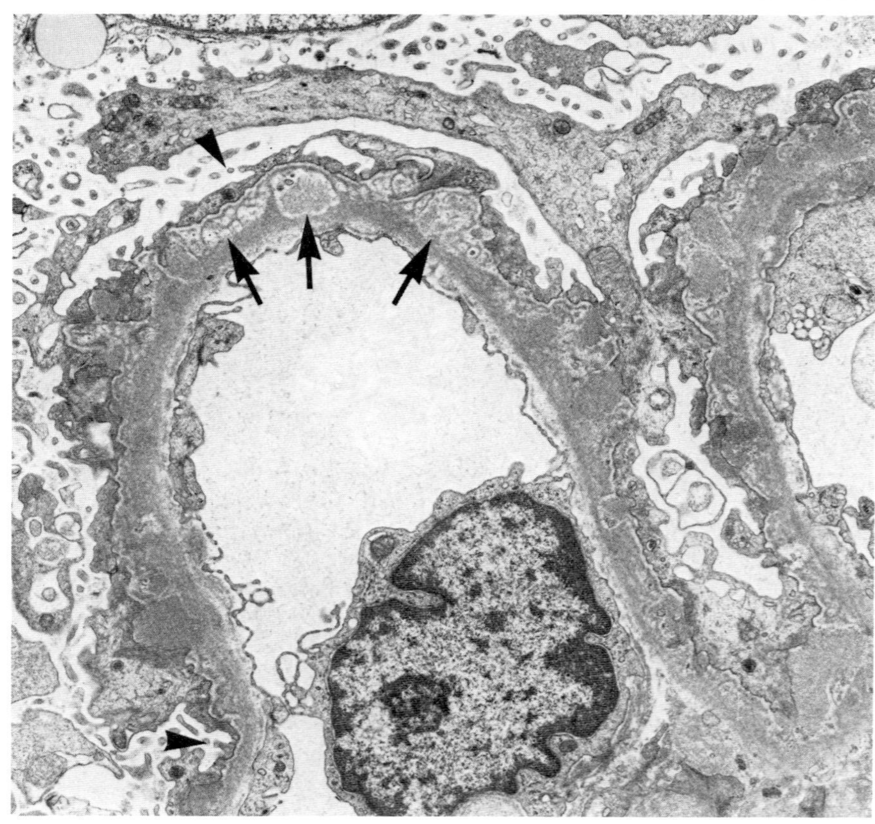

Fig. 65-6. Ultrastructural changes in a moderately advanced (stage II–III) case of membranous nephropathy. Numerous electron-lucent deposits (*arrows*) impart a "moth-eaten" appearance to the basement membrane. Microvillous projections of epithelial cell membrane are prominent in the upper and left portions of the micrograph (*arrowheads*).

of the subepithelial basement membrane spike and are incorporated into the membrane. This is the so-called membranous transformation. Stage 4 shows a definite rarefaction of the former electron-dense deposits, together with extremely variable thickening of the basement membrane. In idiopathic membranous nephropathy, electron-dense deposits are only occasionally encountered in the mesangial region [165, 354].

IMMUNOFLUORESCENCE MICROSCOPY

Immunofluorescence microscopy shows diffuse, finely granular deposits containing IgG in all capillary walls, probably corresponding to the electron-dense deposits on electron microscopy (Fig. 65-7). Studies by Doi et al. [91] and by Noel and co-workers [287] of the IgG subclasses showed that IgG 4 was present in the capillary loops of almost all patients with membranous nephropathy, accompanied sometimes by a small amount of IgG 1. IgG 2 and 3 were not seen in contrast to the findings in patients with lupus or membranoproliferative glomerulonephritis. C3 is not as uniformly present as is IgG, particularly in early cases. Mesangial deposits are very infrequent. In 42 patients studied by Cameron et al. [51], 100 percent had IgG deposits; 75 percent, C3; 30 percent, IgA or IgM; 30 percent, fibrin; and 20 percent, C1q or C4. Albumin, IgG, and C3 also have been found within the cytoplasm of tubular epithelial cells. Immunofluorescence studies demonstrate an abnormal distribution of type IV collagen and laminin in the outer portion of the basement membrane [122].

Studies utilizing polyethyleneimine as a cationic probe [291] and phosphotungstic acid staining [316] demonstrate a loss of anionic sites along the lamina rara externa of the basement membrane and on the surface of the epithelial cells, presumably correlating with loss of the glomerular protein barrier.

ATYPICAL PATHOLOGY

Membranous Lupus Nephritis. Whereas mesangial dense deposits, subendothelial dense deposits, tubuloreticular inclusions in glomerular structures, prominent IgA or IgM deposits by immunofluorescence, and even the presence of tubular basement-membrane deposits can be seen in idiopathic membranous glomerulonephropathy [145, 188, 237, 294, 354, 355], they are more suggestive of the membranous form of lupus nephritis. When Jennette et al. [188] studied a group of 170 patients with membranous nephropathy, including 22 patients with lupus at the time of biopsy and 6 patients later developing clinical lupus, these histologic findings had the following predictive values for lupus: tubular basement-membrane deposits, 100 percent; subendothelial dense deposits, 77 percent; mesangial dense deposits, 63 percent; and tubuloreticular inclusions, 61 percent.

Renal Vein Thrombosis. Renal vein thrombosis, which occurs frequently in association with membranous nephropathy (see the following section), may be suspected when marked interstitial edema, interstitial inflammatory infiltrate, and margination of the polymorphonuclear leukocytes in the glomerular capillaries are present.

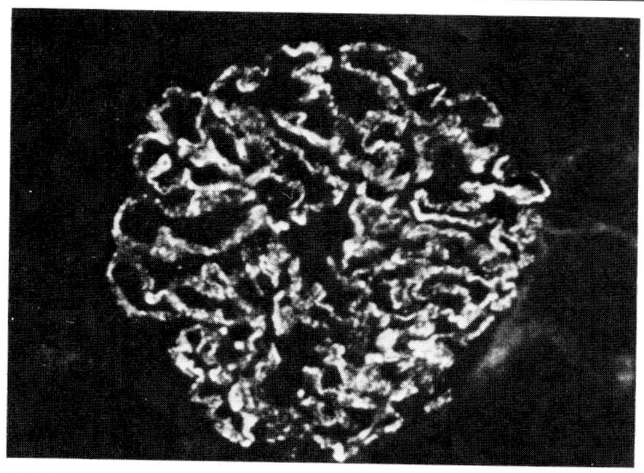

Fig. 65-7. Fluorescence micrograph of a glomerulus with membranous nephropathy. The frozen section was reacted with monospecific fluorescein-conjugated anti-human IgG. There is diffuse granular staining along the glomerular capillary wall.

Secondary Membranous Nephropathy. The patients who have membranous nephropathy secondary to some systemic disease, infection, or toxin tend to have fewer subepithelial deposits [144] and more numerous mesangial deposits [165]. In the study by Graham and Nagel [144], patients with idiopathic membranous nephropathy had subepithelial deposits occupying 48 percent of the surface of their glomerular basement membrane, whereas those whose disease was secondary had deposits that occupied an average of only 12 percent of the surface.

Focal segmental membranous glomerulonephritis has been described accompanying other renal diseases as an epiphenomenon [32] as well as a stage of partially resolved MN [126]. It may be seen in patients with more severe disease [397, 398] as well as those with milder courses [12].

The coexistence of MN and IgA nephropathy has been noted [212], sometimes with hematuria [189] or accompanying hepatitis B [220].

Gaps in the basement membrane, visible on electron microscopy, have been thought to allow the passage of red blood cells, which are frequently found in the urine in this condition.

Pathogenesis of Membranous Nephropathy

CIRCULATING IMMUNE COMPLEX HYPOTHESIS

Several decades of investigation into the immunologic cause of glomerulonephritis were culminated by the work of Dixon [88] and of Germuth [134]. (See Chap. 60 for a general discussion of the immunopathology of renal disease.) They felt that there were two major types of immune-mediated glomerular disease: In the first type, circulating immune complexes formed by the combination of exogenous or endogenous antigen, with its resulting antibody, become lodged in glomeruli with resulting glomerular damage. In the second type, a presumed antigen that shares determinants with structures on the glomerular basement membrane leads to the formation of an antibody, which, in turn, damages the glomerular basement membrane. The glomerular disease associated with Goodpasture's syndrome was presumed to be an example of the second, while membranous nephropathy, with deposition of immunoglobulin and complement in the capillary walls, and its known frequent relationship to foreign antigen seemed to be an excellent candidate for a circulating immune complex disease. It was reasoned that relatively small complexes formed under conditions of antigen excess would lead to subepithelial deposits in distinction to the mesangial or subendothelial locations of larger complexes. Conditions of antigen excess might exist when antigen production has continued for prolonged periods in the body or as a result of continued antigen administration in experimental models [135].

THE HEYMANN MODEL

The Heymann model of experimental nephritis in rats seemed to support this hypothesis [155]. In this model, autologous kidney mixed with complete Freund's adjuvant was injected into rats. The resulting pattern of nephritis resembled human membranous nephropathy, with subepithelial deposits in the glomerular capillary walls. Glassock, Edgington, and their co-workers [140] and Grupe and Kaplan [148] demonstrated that the immunizing antigen (Fx-1A) was derived from the brush border of proximal tubular cells. The glomeruli contained IgG directed against the brush-border antigen as well as the complement; and proteinuria was observed. It was considered that circulating immune complexes became trapped in the glomerular capillary wall, leading to damage, with an increased permeability for protein. The detection of circulating immune complex in human disease tended to support this hypothesis [198, 369, 373, 431]. Indeed small, cationic circulating immune complexes containing antibodies to brush-border or tubular antigens have been found in the sera of untreated patients with MN as well as in post-transplant de novo MN [416]. In active Heymann nephritis in the rat, circulating complexes have been identified that contain the same tubular antigen that is found in the glomerular deposits [177].

Other studies of circulating immune complexes in this disease, however, are not substantiating [2, 49, 142, 216, 298, 299, 325, 365, 366]. Complexes often were found only transiently, although disease activity persisted. Complexes detected by one technique were absent by another. Patients with membranous nephropathy did not exhibit a higher percentage of circulating immune complexes than other forms of glomerular disease. In fact, further study of the elements of this model cast more doubt that circulating immune complexes are the cause of membranous nephropathy. For example, the injection of rabbit antibodies to rat brush-border antigen (passive Heymann nephritis) will produce subepithelial deposits and proteinuria, while the injection of preformed immune complexes will not [113].

IN SITU FORMATION OF IMMUNE COMPLEXES

Although Evans had proposed in 1974 that antigens and antibodies might meet in the glomerular capillary wall to cause disease [108], it was in the laboratories of Couser [72, 73] and Hoedemaeker [113] and Golbus and Wilson [143] that the process of in situ formation of immune complexes became clear. Rat kidneys perfused directly with sheep anti-Fx-1A [73] or Fab fragments [339] showed a direct localization of the antibody in a subepithelial position, suggesting that the glomerular basement membrane possesses an antigen similar to brush-border antigen. When rat kidneys were perfused alternately with antigen and antibody and never exposed to circulating complexes, similar subepithelial deposits were demonstrated [113]. Other antigens, including cationized ferritin [25], cationized bovine serum albumin [37], and antibrush-border antibody eluted from a Heymann nephritis kidney [253] were all shown to localize at the subepithelial space with subsequent production of glomerulonephritis resembling membranous nephropathy.

The glomerular localization of antibodies (which may subsequently become antigens in an autoimmune phase) also appears to be influenced by charge, cationic antibodies being preferentially bound [250]. Even isolated glomeruli in vitro can bind anti-Fx-1A antibody [338]. Antibodies directed against a single glycoprotein in proximal tubule cell membrane (GP-330) bind to clathrin-coated pits on epithelial cell surfaces and can reproduce most of the results obtained with the cruder Fx-1A in the rat [201, 202] but not mouse [16]. The GP-330 antigen has not been found in the human. This has been recently reviewed by Verroust [408].

Although most of these studies were performed in the rat, a similar localization of antibrush-border antibody can be seen in the mouse [17].

It appears then that in the Heymann model for membranous nephropathy, immune complexes form in situ in a subepithelial position in the glomerular capillary wall and lead to proteinuria and reduction in glomerular filtration [123, 124]. Although the antibodies have been formed in response to a proximal tubular brush-border antigen, they react with an apparently related antigen in the glomeruli.

The in situ formation of complexes also appears likely in human membranous glomerulopathy, although the antigen involved is completely unknown. In a very unusual case, maternal circulating IgG antibodies against tubular brush-border antigen led to MN and transient renal failure in a newborn [282]. The in situ formation of immune complexes can involve not only antigens endogenous to the glomerular capillary wall but also "planted" antigens, including Fx-1A [1]. It is interesting that in the rat with Heymann nephritis, five-sixths nephrectomy markedly worsens proteinuria and progression and adds the histologic changes of focal sclerosis [292].

PHYSICAL PROPERTIES OF DEPOSITED ANTIGENS

The localization of a "planted" antigen to a subepithelial position in the basement membrane would seem to require that the antigen has appropriate size and electrical charge characteristics. As noted above, cationized proteins with isoelectric pHs higher than 7 will often localize in a subepithelial position—probably because their charge enables them to permeate more proximal layers of basement membrane and to bind with the strongly anionic subepithelial layers. The use of cationized bovine serum albumin [6, 37], human IgG [290], ferritin [25], and other cationized proteins [411] have supported this theory. Protamine sulfate, a polycation that also binds to glomerular basement membrane, can prevent the glomerular lesions produced in rabbits by cationic bovine serum albumin, perhaps by occupying and neutralizing the anionic sites in the capillary wall. Proteinuria also was significantly reduced in animals [6] with this disease model.

ROLE OF COMPLEMENT

Recent studies from Couser's laboratory have clarified the role of complement in experimental membranous nephropathy. In passive Heymann nephritis in rats, removing complement (with cobra venom factor) did not interfere with the formation of IgG deposits in the glomerular basement membrane but did prevent the appearance of proteinuria [337]. Complement (but not cells) must also be present for the production of proteinuria when heterologous antigens are planted in rat [7] or rabbit [161] glomeruli. The formation of the C5b-9 membrane attack complex appears to mediate the damage to the glomerular capillary wall with ensuing proteinuria in rat models [19, 77, 124]. It is present in the membrane deposits, into which it may be inserted by the glomerular epithelial cells [203] and is accompanied by the generation of the prostanoids PGE_2 and thromboxane B_2. An inhibitor of thromboxane did not, however, prevent proteinuria [370].

In patients with idiopathic MN, glomerular localization of the C5b-9 complex is regularly found, but it is less frequent in hepatitis-associated MN [8, 221].

If this animal model reflects human disease, it is puzzling to note that some patients with membranous nephropathy have no C3 complement demonstrable in their glomeruli by fluorescence microscopy. A study of 16 patients by Doi et al. [90] showed that while all 16 had IgG deposits, only 8 showed C3. All patients, however, showed deposits of the complement degradation product C3d. It may be that C3 is invariably deposited in glomeruli with MN but is then degraded and seen only as C3d in some. It was notable that the patients demonstrating C3 deposits had larger quantities of proteinuria than did the others in this study. There appears to be no generalized abnormality in the modulation of complement activation in MN [274].

To summarize, on the basis of these laboratory studies, it seems likely that human MN occurs as a result of the formation of immune complexes and subsequent activation of the complement in situ in the glomerular capillary wall. The antigens involved could be either endogenous glomerular antigens or exogenous antigens, either native or foreign, which became deposited in a subepithelial position by virtue of their size and electrical charge. Explaining the presence of disease in patients would involve either unusual host susceptibility or exposure to unusual antigens.

HOST SUSCEPTIBILITY

Ooi et al. [297] found that lymphocytes from patients with MN, when stimulated with pokeweed mitogen, produced less IgG and IgM than did control patients. They suggested that a suppressor of lymphocyte function may be present in these patients. The IgG response to tetanus toxoid immunization also seems to be impaired [110]. A lymphocyte defect also was detected in a patient whose MN was related to mercuric chloride poisoning [57]. MN patients may have less skin reactivity to PPD tests than do controls. They may have a low ratio of T/B lymphocytes [260]. Studies with concanavalin A suggested an increase in suppressor-cell activity in some studies [259, 261] but not in others [383]. Other investigators have not shown consistent changes in OKT4/OKT8 ratios [33, 225, 260, 306, 332]. A reduced splenic uptake of sensitized red cells has been demonstrated by several investigators [20, 33, 225, 326, 401]. Thus it is possible that abnormalities in cellular immunity or phagocytic function might predispose to MN [10], but details remain unclear. It is also uncertain which abnormalities of lymphocyte function may be the result rather than the cause of the nephrotic state [306, 383].

IMMUNOGENETICS

If certain patients are immunologically more likely to develop MN, then genetic markers might identify them. This possibility was raised when a distribution of histocompatibility antigens in MN patients appeared to be different from that in the general population. The Manchester, United Kingdom, group found first an association of MN with HLA DRw3 and then noted that DRw3, B18, and B8 also had higher-than-expected frequencies in the MN population. The circulating complement component, properdin factor BfF1, was also associated with MN, as was, in particular, the haplotype B18-BfF1-DR3 [48, 59, 211, 254]. Patients possessing all three components seemed to be at greatest risk for progressive disease and least likely to have remissions of proteinuria.

Investigators in other countries have confirmed some of these observations but have failed to confirm others [303]. French studies found an increased incidence of DR3 and B8, but not B18, and found no notable clinical correlates [33, 225, 231]. In Germany, HLA DR3 was found, but not B18 or BfF1 in a study of 21 patients [275]. A review from the United States, including some of the European patients among the 176 reported, concluded that HLA DR3 contributed a relative risk for contracting MN of about 4:1 and seemed to be a stronger risk factor in the United Kingdom and Spain than in the United States [130, 131]. Rashid et al. [321] showed a relationship between MN and DR3 and B8 in 34 patients. An association with MT 2 also has been described [130, 131, 275]. These associations have also been noted in genomic DNA [403].

It is notable that in Japan, different frequencies appear to exist. Tomura et al. [391] and Hiki et al. [158] found the predominant association to be with HLA DR2 and MT 1. In China, however, DR3 seems predominant [180].

Immunoglobulin typing by Demaine et al. [82, 83] suggested unusual patterns in MN patients, but the Manchester group considered that variations in the IgG molecule did not describe major risk factors for MN [41].

In summary, it appears that there may be genetic markers for the susceptibility for MN, but the resulting immunologic abnormalities, if any, have not been delineated clearly. It is interesting that other diseases, including gluten enteropathy, dermatitis herpetiformis, Sjögren's syndrome, Graves' disease, and diabetes mellitus may share an association with HLA DR3 [274].

POSSIBLE CAUSATIVE ANTIGENS

Brush-Border Antigens. The cause of human MN might involve an immunologic predisposition, as noted in the previous section. It might, however, be more related to exposure to specific antigens that have the ability to initiate the pathologic process. By analogy to Heymann nephritis, the animal model most resembling human MN, a search for renal tubular epithelial brush-border antigens (RTE antigen) in the diseased glomeruli has been made by several investigators. In 1973, Naruse et al. [280, 281] found an antigen that resembles renal tubular epithelial antigen in the glomeruli of MN patients. Attempts to confirm this finding have so far been unsuccessful. Zager et al., in 1979 [438], found no free or immune complexed antibodies to renal tubular epithelial antigens. Thorpe and Cavallo [439] found no RTE antigens in glomerular deposits or eluates therefrom. Gilboa [137] found neither RTE antigens nor antibodies in blood or glomeruli (though the antigen *was* apparent in the glomeruli of patients with proliferative lupus nephritis!). Crosson et al. [75], using an antiserum prepared specifically against the Fx-1A antigen, found none in the glomeruli of MN patients. Niles et al. [286], however, in preliminary studies found that antibody eluted from glomeruli with MN reacted with a glycoprotein antigen on renal tubular cell membranes.

It has been speculated that the MN, which occurs occasionally following gold therapy for rheumatoid arthritis, may result from renal tubular damage by the heavy metal, with release of immunologically active tubular antigens, leading to a Heymann-like nephropathy [368]. Gold itself has not been found in glomerular capillary walls, but it does appear in cellular deposits [7, 333]. RTE antigens or antibodies have not been reported in glomerular subepithelial deposits.

It is interesting that a patient reported by Zanetti et al. [439], when in end-stage renal failure (not from MN), showed plasma antibodies that reacted in vitro with rat kidney brush border. After transplantation, the antibodies disappeared, and proteinuria appeared, followed by failure of the graft. The transplanted kidney showed de novo MN, and eluates from it produced antibodies reactive against rat brush border. Thus Heymann-like mechanisms may have been involved.

Thyroid Antigens. Membranous nephropathy occurs occasionally in thyroid disease, and thyroid-related antigens have been sought in the glomerular deposits as early as 1976 [300]. Thyroglobulin-containing antigens have been demonstrated in the kidneys of patients with MN and autoimmune (Hashimoto's) thyroiditis [185, 196, 420]. Associated antithyroglobulin, antimicrosomal antibodies [185], and circulating immune complexes containing thyroglobulin [194] also have been shown.

Hepatitis Antigens. The frequent association of the hepatitis virus carrier state with MN, particularly among children and in Far East populations, led to a search for glomerular deposition of hepatitis antigens. HBsAg has been found by some investigators [163, 361], including a patient in whom the MN appeared to be associated with rheumatoid arthritis [409]. Others [210, 234], however, failed to demonstrate the antigen. It may be that co-deposited immunoglobulins block direct immunofluorescence of the HBsAg [251]. Slusarczyk et al. [363] demonstrated hepatitis B core antigen (HBcAg) in two-thirds of 98 children with MN; only half of these children simultaneously showed HBsAg. More recently, the presence of hepatitis Be antigen (HBeAg) was demonstrated in the glomeruli of the great majority of patients with hepatitis-associated MN [162, 179, 221, 226, 270, 279, 378, 437]. It may be that this antigen (and perhaps HBeAg-HBeAb complexes [150]) are more directly related to the pathogenesis of MN in these patients.

DNA Antigens. In patients with the membranous form of lupus nephropathy, DNA/anti-DNA complexes have been demonstrated in both the circulation and in the glomeruli. It is notable that in comparison to patients with proliferative lupus nephritis, the membranous histology is associated with much lower titers of circulating antibody; and the antibody is almost completely nonprecipitating in nature [117, 118]. During 30 months of high-dose steroid treatment, one patient's histologic transformation from proliferative to membranous was accompanied by a change in circulating anti-DNA antibody from high-titer precipitating to low-titer nonprecipitating [120, 230]. It may be that nonprecipitating antibody is less readily removed from the circulation by the reticuloendothelial system or by renal mesangial cells and is available to traverse the basement membrane to form subepithelial immune complexes. An alternative explanation might be that it possesses favorable size and charge characteristics for subepithelial deposition. Although anti-DNA antibodies are not present in idiopathic MN, this general principle may apply to MN.

Tumor Antigens. Although nephrotic syndrome with membranous nephropathy has been seen in association with many tumors (see the following discussion), only rarely have specific tumor antigens been identified in the glomeruli. Lewis et al. [236], in 1972, described a patient with bronchial carcinoma and membranous nephropathy in whom immunoglobulins eluted from glomeruli reacted specifically with surface plasma membranes of the tumor cells. Costanza et al. [70] described a patient with colon cancer and MN in whom carcinoembryonic antigen (CEA) was found in the blood and in a granular pattern in the glomerular capillary walls. Couser et al. [74] also described a patient with colon cancer and MN in whom CEA was found in the blood but not in the glomeruli. A week after resection of the tumor, however, an antibody was discovered in the blood, which reacted with an antigen in the glomerular basement membrane. This antibody could be absorbed by the tumor.

Other Antigens. In addition to hepatitis, some patients with MN associated with systemic infections may have evidence of infectious antigens in their glomeruli. Antigens associated with hydatid disease have been found in glomerular deposits [341, 410] and, in one case, the removal of an echinococcus cyst resulted in a resolution of the nephrosis [410]. Treponemal antigen and antitreponemal antibody were found in glomerular subepithelial deposits in a baby with congenital syphilis [247]. Treponemal antigens and antibodies [129] also have been demonstrated in acquired syphilis. Antigens related to quartan malaria have been found in glomeruli of some nephrotic patients with renal histology that is somewhat atypical for MN [154].

Immune deposits resembling IgG–anti-IgG rheumatoid factor complexes were found in a patient who developed posttransplant de novo MN. Hageman factor (XII) and prekallikrein were found in subepithelial deposits in 24 of 49 MN patients by Berger and Yaneva [31]. There appeared to be no correlation between the deposits and cause or course of the disease.

Clinical Membranous Nephropathy

INCIDENCE

In most series of biopsied adults with nephrotic syndrome, membranous nephropathy is the most common diagnosis. In collected series totaling 920 biopsied adult nephrotic patients [34, 36, 66, 115, 151, 268, 289, 334], 227, or 25 percent, of patients showed membranous histology, with individual fractions ranging from 8 to 42 percent. In a Canadian study of 948 patients [56] biopsied because of glomerular disease, 11 percent had membranous histology, with approximately similar fractions having a diagnosis of focal sclerosis, focal proliferative glomerulonephritis, and membranoproliferative glomerulonephritis. A series from Tampa, Florida of 970 renal biopsies included 128 patients with MN, 28 percent of the total glomerular disease group [45].

The incidence in a particular study may vary not only with geographic location but also with the local indications for biopsy. A population survey in southeast England, which presumably avoided this selection factor, showed the appearance of about nine new adult nephrotic patients per million of population each year. A nearly equal number with substantial proteinuria did not meet the strict definition of nephrotic syndrome. Twelve percent of the adult nephrotic patients showed membranous histology compared to 30 percent with minimal change disease [352]. In a study of nephrectomies done in patients presenting for transplantation, Schwartz and Cotran [343] found only 2 patients with recognizable membranous histology among 47 with glomerular disease of various types.

In any group of patients with MN, some will have idiopathic disease, while in others, the renal pathology is secondary to some systemic disease or toxicity. In a French study of 92 patients, 27 were secondary to such conditions as drugs, toxins, neoplasms, parasitic infestations, and systemic lupus [58]. In a British series, 10 of 66 were secondary to neoplasms, gold, mercury, and hepatitis [334], while in another [52] about 20 percent of 267 patients were secondary to lupus, drugs, malignancy, and other diseases. In a California study, 18 of 100 were secondary to rheumatoid arthritis (or its drug treatment) or to neoplasms [176].

AGE AND SEX

MN occurs most commonly in adults between 30 and 50 years of age but extends into extremes of childhood and old age. Row et al. [334] found two peaks of incidence at ages 35 and 55, but most other series have a relatively even distribution. Children with MN are much less numerous than those with minimal change disease and are relatively older, forming a continuous age distribution with young adults.

Male patients are more numerous than females in most series, composing 83 percent of 267 [52] and 66 percent of 140 [93] in two recent studies.

GEOGRAPHY

The incidence of membranous histology is unusually high in Japanese children with nephrotic syndrome, a finding that seems to be completely attributable to the presence of hepatitis B infection in this population [379] (see the following discussion).

In some populations in Africa, the incidence in adults is also remarkably high—an occurrence that has been attributed to the use of skin-lightening creams that contain organic mercury compounds [345, 418]. An association of MN with malaria of *Plasmodium malariae* and *Plasmodium falciparum* types has been made [429], but the histology is often found to have a degree of proliferation as well as membranous change; and the simultaneous presence of hepatitis infection frequently complicates interpretation [95, 429].

In South Africa, membranous histology appears to be relatively common in blacks [95] and is present in 26 percent of biopsied Bantu nephrotic children compared with 11 percent of Indian children—without known cause for the difference. In an area free of malaria, Seedat et al. [347] found membranous nephropathy to be common, but proliferative histology was more common still. In New Guinea, both membranous and minimal change diseases appear to be uncommon, while proliferative histology is common [314].

MEMBRANOUS NEPHROPATHY IN CHILDHOOD

Although minimal change disease is by far the dominant cause of nephrotic syndrome in childhood, membranous nephropathy is not uncommon, especially among older children. The incidence seems to reflect, in part, the prevalence of hepatitis in the population. (See Chap. 87 for a general discussion of childhood glomerular disease.) In a French series, 37 nephrotic children with membranous histology were seen in a group that also contained 35 with focal segmental glomerular sclerosis and 209 with minimal change disease [149]. The youngest of these patients was 9 months old. There were 29 boys compared with 8 girls in the series.

In an expansion of this study [209, 210], 30 of 85 children with membranous nephropathy appeared to have underlying systemic disease, including lupus and sickle cell disease, and 11 patients had hepatitis virus infection. Clinical remissions of proteinuria in the hepatitis patients occurred in about 50 percent—the same as in other subgroups.

In a Canadian study [224], 14 of 1,025 children biopsied for renal disease had membranous nephropathy, and 11 of these children had nephrotic range proteinuria. Their prognosis was similar to adults with the disease. In a series from New York [293], the younger children did well, with frequent remissions, while the older children had more progressive disease.

In England, in the study of Row et al. [334], membranous nephropathy was found in 2.7 percent of biopsied nephrotic children; 11 children accompanied 66 adults in the same population.

In an international study [241], 2 of 127 nephrotic children had membranous nephropathy.

Hepatitis is a frequent cause of membranous nephropathy in children. In Warsaw [363], 21 of 98 children biopsied for glomerular disease had membranous histology and all 21 were associated with hepatitis! Much of the African membranous nephropathy is associated with hepatitis or malaria [3, 4, 348, 429] as is also the case in Japan [379, 435] and in Taiwan [178], where 14 of 63 children with glomerulonephritis had membranous histology and all of these children had hepatitis.

Childhood MN is thought to have more frequent hematuria and less frequent renal vein thrombosis as compared to adults [52].

HEREDITARY MEMBRANOUS NEPHROPATHY

The occurrence of membranous nephropathy has been recorded in families [98, 266, 342, 379, 400, 404], but it seems often to be an atypical variety. In one family both mother and child had the disease and were infected with hepatitis B virus [379], and in another, tubulointerstitial disease and antitubular basement-membrane antibodies were present.

SELECTIVITY OF PROTEINURIA

The proteinuria in MN is not, in general, highly selective. The ratio of clearances of IgG to transferrin tends to fall in the moderately or poorly selective range, from 0.5 to 0.3, rather than in the highly selective range, below 0.05. The vast bulk of patients with MN have selectivity above 0.1. Thus a highly selective urinary protein tends to exclude MN, while a less-selective finding is of little help [50, 269].

MEMBRANOUS NEPHROPATHY WITH ASYMPTOMATIC PROTEINURIA

Some patients with membranous nephropathy on biopsy have proteinuria below the usual nephrotic range and no appreciable edema or other manifestations of nephrotic syndrome. The frequency of this finding naturally depends on specific indications for biopsy. An investigation in which Hungarian schoolchildren, athletes, and pregnant women had routine screening urinalyses resulted in biopsy of 260 patients with membranous histology [29]. The majority of these patients were asymptomatic. In an English population survey, 5 of 11 adults with membranous histology were nonnephrotic [352]. In a report by Noel et al. [288], 28 of 116 were nonnephrotic as were 9 of 34 studied by Pierides et al. [308], 12 of 66 studied by Row et al. [334], 17 of 100 studied by Hopper et al. [193], 41 of 267 in the British Medical Research Council study [53], and 24 of 140 seen at the Mayo Clinic [93].

In general, the patients with asymptomatic proteinuria seem to have frequent remissions and are much less likely to progress to renal failure [176, 206, 288, 289, 308].

Associations with Systemic Disease, Drugs, and Toxins

ASSOCIATION WITH MALIGNANCY

The relationship of tumor antigens in the pathogenesis of membranous nephropathy has been discussed in the section entitled Pathogenesis.

Various tumors, including carcinoma of the lung, esophagus, stomach, breast, colon, and carotid body as well as lymphomas, have been found in about 5 percent of patients with MN reported in several series [45, 47, 53, 58, 96, 103, 174, 197, 334, 353]. In addition, associations have been found with oat cell cancer of the lung associated with dermatomyositis [329], malignant melanoma [425], neuroblastoma [440], and renal cell cancer [76, 204]. Two patients with colon cancer had MN associated with elevated circulating titers of CEA [70, 236].

In some cases, nephrotic syndrome will resolve spontaneously after the removal or treatment of the tumor. This occurrence has been noted with breast [24] and stomach [54] lesions as well as in squamous cell lung carcinoma and colon cancer [434]. Although nephrotic syndrome occurring in lymphoma patients is more frequently of the minimal change variety, membranous histology is also seen in some patients with Hodgkin's disease and particularly in non-Hodgkin's lymphoma [128, 265, 331]. Chronic lymphocytic leukemia, perhaps particularly when accompanied by the T-lymphocyte surface antigen T-65 [427], has been accompanied by membranous nephropathy as has multicentric angiofollicular lymph node hyperplasia. Surgical removal of abdominal giant lymph node hyperplasia led to clinical and pathologic remission in a young woman with MN [336] as did removal of a benign ovarian tumor in a 7-year-old girl [26].

It would be particularly useful to know how often an accompanying tumor was not immediately apparent at the time of diagnosis of the nephrotic syndrome. This would enable the physician to know how vigorous a search should be made for an accompanying malignancy in MN patients. In six of eight patients reported by Lee et al. [228], the symptoms of nephrotic syndrome preceded the tumor diagnosis (by periods of 1, 2, 8, 10, 13, and 19 months). It is not stated how often the diagnosis of membranous nephropathy was made substantially before the diagnosis of tumor.

In a careful study involving epidemiologic surveillance with searches of hospital and tumor registry records [45], 4 of 128 patients with MN were found to have accompanying malignancy. All 4 were discovered within 13 months postbiopsy, and all occurred among 52 patients older than 50 years, for an incidence of 8 percent in this group. The authors expected an annual incidence of diagnosis of malignancy of about 1 percent in equivalent populations.

It seems likely that approximately 5 percent of adult patients with membranous nephropathy might have an underlying malignancy that is not obvious at the time of the diagnosis of the nephrotic syndrome. This percentage might be expected to be somewhat higher in older populations and also should be interpreted in relation to the frequency of malignancies in patients of similar age but without nephrotic syndrome.

ASSOCIATION WITH INFECTION

A note has already been made of the discovery of some infectious antigens in glomeruli of patients with MN. The associated systemic infections have included quartan malaria [174], in which the MN often appears histologically atypical, schistosomiasis [13], leprosy [360], syphilis (both congenital and acquired) [129, 247], hydatid disease [341, 410], filarial worms causing loiasis [22, 58], scabies and threadworms with accompanying eosinophilia [85], miliary tuberculosis [327], and rectal abscess [272].

The most frequently reported dissociated infection, however, is hepatitis B. Although MN has been reported in association with liver disease when the hepatitis antigen has not been discovered, such as in patients with primary biliary cirrhosis [317, 323], juvenile cirrhosis [328], and nodular regenerative hyperplasia [263], more frequently some evidence of the hepatitis B virus can be demonstrated in patients with MN and liver disease [41]. Particularly in childhood, a very large fraction of patients with MN appear to have associated hepatitis B. The association has been made in a number of countries, including Italy [81], France [210, 233, 234], and particularly in Taiwan [178], Malaysia [415], and Japan [162, 184, 279, 378, 379]. It has been stressed that very sensitive techniques for the identification of virus antigen may show evidence of infection in patients who are otherwise totally asymptomatic. Some patients have evidence of circulating core antigen [222, 265] or e antigen [162, 184, 270, 279, 378, 437] sometimes in the absence of HBsAg. HBeAg is regularly found in glomerular deposits [179, 221, 437] sometimes in association with HBe antibody [150].

Horizontal transmission of hepatitis among these children from siblings and age mates appears to be more common than vertical spread from parents [178].

ASSOCIATION WITH RHEUMATOID ARTHRITIS

Although membranous nephropathy is frequently reported in association with arthritis, it is uncommonly reported in patients with rheumatoid arthritis who have not also received drug therapy [157, 167, 340]. Thus it is usually unclear whether the renal disease results from the arthritis or from its treatment. Two cases in ankylosing spondylitis [38, 218] have been reported in patients who apparently were not receiving drugs likely to cause nephrotic syndrome. It is of note that both patients were HLA type-B27 and one was, in addition, a DR4.

Most of the patients with rheumatoid arthritis who have had accompanying nephrotic syndrome with membranous nephropathy have been simultaneously receiving gold, penicillamine, or nonsteroidal anti-inflammatory prostaglandin inhibitors.

ASSOCIATION WITH DRUGS

Gold. Proteinuria is not uncommon in patients with rheumatoid arthritis undergoing gold therapy; it occurs in perhaps 1 to 3 percent [106, 227]. (See Chap. 46 for a general discussion of heavy metals and renal diseases.) The full-blown nephrotic syndrome is less common, occurring in less than 1 percent of patients in most series [150], but it may occasionally be more frequent [362, 368]. Of patients with membranous nephropathy, 1 of 66 in the series of Rowe et al. [334] and 4 of 90 in the series of Samuels et al. [340] had received gold. In most cases, the histologic picture resembles that of idiopathic membranous nephropathy [7, 144, 333, 340, 349, 368, 419] but, occasionally, it varies [116]. As discussed in the section on pathogenesis, gold inclusions may be found in glomerular and tubular cells but not in the subepithelial location associated with the immune complex deposits, and the pathogenesis of gold nephropathy is not clear. Renal failure may occur and can be reversible [35].

Penicillamine. Another explanation for the association of membranous nephropathy with rheumatoid arthritis is the fact that such patients are frequently treated with penicillamine. Between 5 and 20 percent of such patients develop proteinuria [80, 161, 424], and the possible occurrence of MN has been noted with the related drug bucillamine [200] and 2-mercaptopropionylglycine [241]. The proteinuria seems more likely to appear near the onset of therapy [182] and when the dose is abruptly raised or given at a very high level [160, 161, 248]. Proteinuria with membranous nephropathy is similarly seen when penicillamine is used for other diseases, such as Wilson's disease [414] or hepatitis [191]. Occasionally, glomerular disease of other types is associated with penicillamine, including minimal change disease [18, 87, 109], renal vasculitis [109], and crescentic glomerulonephritis [136, 372]. Of patients with rheumatoid arthritis treated with penicillamine who developed proteinuria, about one-third became frankly nephrotic [147].

As with idiopathic MN, a large fraction of patients in whom penicillamine induces proteinuria have the HLA haplotype DR3 [302].

Captopril. Soon after the introduction of this converting enzyme inhibitor for the treatment of hypertension, an association with proteinuria was noted [170, 171, 315]. Some of these patients were nephrotic and when biopsied showed the histologic changes of membranous nephropathy [144, 170, 374, 377]. Discontinuing the drug frequently led to resolution of the nephrosis, although histologic lesions sometimes continued to persist [170]. The likelihood of severe proteinuria and impairment of renal function appeared more likely to occur in patients with preexisting renal disease [195, 386] and when higher doses of the drug were used.

In view of the presence of sulfur in both penicillamine and the gold salts, it is of note that captopril also contains a sulfhydryl group. Lewis comments, however [235], that the incidence of nephrosis following captopril (about 1½%) is approximately the same as that following the use of the similar converting enzyme inhibitor enalapril, which does not contain a sulfhydryl group. He regards the incidence of nephrosis following the use of these drugs as not being much greater than that occurring with other treatments of rheumatoid arthritis and hence feels their association with membranous nephropathy is not well substantiated.

Nonsteroidal Prostaglandin Antagonists. A fourth class of drugs used frequently in the treatment of patients with rheumatoid arthritis is the family of nonsteroidal prostaglandin antagonists. Nephrotic syndrome and the histologic appearance of membranous nephropathy may appear in rheumatoid patients taking ibuprofen and indomethacin [344], diclofenac [97, 181] indomethacin alone [152], ketoprofen [350], and tolmetin and naproxen [112].

SICKLE CELL DISEASE

Patients with sickle cell disease may develop nephrotic syndrome and be found to have a histologic picture resembling MN. This topic is covered in Chap. 84.

THYROID DISEASE

The presence of thyroid antigens in glomeruli has already been noted. The clinical association with membranous nephropathy is usually an autoimmune thyroiditis of Hashimoto's type [9, 185, 194, 300, 420, 421]. A high incidence of patients with the HLA haplotype DR3 was noted in one group of such patients [421].

MERCURY

Exposure to mercury is also quite well established as a cause of membranous nephropathy. In Africa, the use of mercury-containing cosmetics for the purpose of skin lightening was associated with a near epidemic of membranous nephropathy and nephrotic syndrome [23, 44, 205, 345, 418] and still occasionally occurs outside of Africa [295]. Drug and industrial exposure [399] also has been noted. In an industrial case, mercury could be identified in renal tubular cells but not in glomeruli [399]. It is interesting that mercury toxicity in the cat also has been associated with membranous nephropathy [359].

DIABETES MELLITUS

Churg and Ehrenreich [64] called attention to the frequent association of MN with diabetes mellitus—an observation made by a number of others as well [187, 213, 405, 417, 436]. The onset of the two conditions could be nearly simultaneous [187, 405] or separated by as much as 20 years [417]. The histologic lesion of membranous nephropathy was sometimes accompanied by more typical diabetic nephropathy and was sometimes present by itself. It would appear reasonable to suspect a nondiabetic cause of nephrotic syndrome if the onset of the nephrosis occurred soon after the onset of diabetes, was unaccompanied by retinopathy or other evidence of diabetic microvascular disease, and occurred in the presence of normal glomerular filtration rate. Membranous nephropathy also has been associated with diabetes in the dog [186].

MISCELLANEOUS ASSOCIATIONS

Nephrotic syndrome with histologic membranous nephropathy has been reported in association with hemolytic uremic syndrome [85], dermatitis herpetiformis [68, 381], and eosinophilic lymphofolliculosis of skin [367, 433] (13 of 175 such patients were reported to have nephrosis). Myasthenia gravis [60], chronic progressive demyelinating neuropathy [430], Guillain-Barré syndrome [277, 285, 380], Weber Christian panniculitis [100], Fanconi's syndrome [232], primary sclerosing cholangitis [407], small intestine enteropathy [279], and systemic mastocytosis [223] have also been associated with MN.

Although drug addicts more frequently have focal sclerosing and other glomerular abnormalities, they occasionally have an atypical sort of membranous nephropathy [264]. Four patients exposed to volatile hydrocarbons in the plastics industry developed membranous nephropathy [104].

At least 10 patients have been reported to have the association of MN with sarcoidosis [192, 256, 296, 384, 385].

LUPUS ERYTHEMATOSUS

The renal manifestations of systemic lupus are covered in Chap. 72. Some patients without clinical or serologic evidence of lupus but with membranous histology may ultimately prove to have lupus—sometimes after years of observation. Libit et al. [237] stress that, in children, one might particularly suspect lupus if the child is female, has a low serum complement concentration, and has evidence of IgA deposition in the glomeruli. Evidence of mesangial deposits or of subendothelial deposits would similarly raise suspicion (see Pathology).

RENAL VEIN THROMBOSIS

The frequent occurrence of thromboses in nephrotic patients has long been appreciated (see Chap. 49). A particular example is the occurrence of renal vein thrombosis in certain histologic groups, particularly membranous nephropathy.

The exact incidence is difficult to determine, because most renal vein studies have been done in patients who already had evidence of thrombosis or embolization. In the first of a series of studies by Llach et al. [244, 245], 50 percent of patients with membranous histology had renal vein thrombosis. In a later study, Llach reported a 29-percent incidence [246]. This relatively high incidence contrasts with 4 percent noted by Row and Cameron [334] and 7 percent noted by Trew et al. [394]. A prospective study by Wagoner et al. [412], using renal venography accompanied by intrarenal artery epinephrine in 27 of 33 consecutive patients, demonstrated renal vein thrombi in 13. These thromboses had been clinically suspected in only 2 of the group.

The incidence of complications of renal vein thrombosis in membranous nephropathy is similarly clouded by the process of selecting patients for study. Pulmonary emboli occurring in 10 of 11 patients with renal vein thromboses in one study [39] undoubtedly reflected the criteria for performing the renal venogram. In no study in which prospective investigations disclosed renal vein thromboses were patients allowed to remain without anticoagulation. A thrombosis of the entire pulmonary artery has been reported as a complication of MN [271].

The cause of these thromboses is discussed elsewhere in this volume, but the existence of a hypercoagulable state [243, 412], perhaps associated with accelerated thromboplastin generation, has been postulated [274].

The classic symptoms of acute renal vein thrombosis are flank pain and gross hematuria. The majority of patients with renal vein thrombosis complicating membranous nephropathy do not seem to have these symptoms [63, 246, 412]. The thromboses are more commonly discovered either by prospective study or following evidence of a complication, such as pulmonary embolus [42, 91].

It is interesting that in a group of 18 patients with MN, only the 5 with renal vein thrombosis had demonstrable circulating immune complexes (shown by both C1q and Raji methods) [298]. Renal vein thrombosis may occur in patients with secondary membranous histology (e.g., gold nephropathy) as well as in those with primary disease [283].

The treatment of renal vein thrombosis in membranous nephropathy has evolved from surgical embolectomy followed by anticoagulation [111] to anticoagulation alone. Patients who had pulmonary emboli appear to remain free of emboli during anticoagulation [42, 252, 412], but if anticoagulation is discontinued while the nephrotic syndrome persists, then the likelihood of recurrent pulmonary emboli is fairly good [42]. In many cases, renal function is unaffected by the renal vein thrombosis [91, 412].

TRANSFORMATIONS

Membranous nephropathy has been reported in association with IgA mesangial proliferative nephritis [89]. Poststreptococcal glomerulonephritis was found to be superimposed on MN in one patient [432], and Richet et al. [324] reported a transformation of proliferative glomerulonephritis into membranous nephropathy in four patients.

By far the most frequently reported transformation or association is of membranous with crescentic glomerulonephritis [61, 208, 215, 217, 273, 284, 305, 382]. The presence of crescents often implies a rapidly deteriorating course [284, 382]. Although the crescents are usually superimposed on an immune complex type of glomerulonephritis, in at least four patients [208, 217, 273], the picture was one of antiglomerular basement membrane disease. It has been suggested that damage to the glomerular capillary wall occurring in MN may release antigens into the circulation with the resultant formation of anti-GBM antibodies.

Transplantation

Nephrotic syndrome occurring after transplantation is not common. When it does occur, however, a sizeable proportion of cases are explained as a manifestation of allograft rejection [59, 168]. The remainder are caused largely by recurrent or de novo glomerulonephritis. Although focal glomerulosclerosis and membranoproliferative glomerulonephritis have a relatively high incidence of recurrence, membranous nephropathy, both de novo and recurrent, is probably the most frequent diagnosis in posttransplant glomerulopathy, occurring in perhaps 1 percent of transplants, and is certainly the most frequent type to occur de novo. A number of such patients have been reported [14, 21, 43, 59, 71, 75, 86, 125, 153, 157, 164, 168, 199, 238, 278, 335, 364, 371, 406, 413, 416], of which perhaps one-third appeared to have recurrent disease and two-thirds represent membranous nephropathy occurring de novo in the allograft. In de novo occurrences, the pretransplant renal diseases included focal glomerular sclerosis [59, 71, 86, 371, 375], membranoproliferative and other chronic glomerulonephritis [43, 59], crescentic rapidly progressive glomerulonephritis (including antiglomerular basement membrane disease) [371], medullary sponge kidney [43], cystinuria [86], and amyloid [86, 153, 159]. A patient who had MN with crescents prior to transplant developed MN with crescents posttransplantation [159]. Although recurrent proteinuria may appear as soon as 7 days posttransplantation [238, 335], in most cases, several months pass before the return of proteinuria, and the graft renal function remains quite stable or deteriorates slowly [59, 75]. On occasion the histologic findings of MN are present before proteinuria occurs [14]. In one study [164], an unusually high rate of de novo MN occurred in patients with ureteral obstruction, possibly representing rejection of the transplanted ureter. In another [21], MN appeared during pregnancy in a kidney donated by a conjoint twin. As mentioned earlier, small cationic circulating immune complexes containing antibodies related to brush border antigens have been identified in some patients with de novo post-transplant MN [416]. MN has also been described in the native kidneys of a bone-marrow transplant recipient [155].

The frequency of MN posttransplantation suggests that the immunosuppressive programs used in such patients are not completely effective in preventing the development of MN, although an occasional patient in renal failure from MN regains some native function in the posttransplant setting [62, 114]. It has been suggested, in fact, that the altered immunologic state of the treated transplant recipients may favor the specific subepithelial localization of immune complexes in these patients

[406]. In one case, the glomerular deposits appeared to consist of IgG/IgG-rheumatoid factor complexes [375].

The Course of Membranous Nephropathy

(See also Chap. 69.)

REMISSIONS

Although complete remission of proteinuria is much more characteristic of minimal change disease, it is not uncommon in membranous nephropathy. Even repeated remissions with subsequent relapses, apparently associated with corticosteroid therapy, are seen occasionally [66, 147], and the prevalence of remissions seems to be higher in steroid-treated groups [66]. In a group reported by Suki et al. [376], 18 of 23 patients remitted. All but 2 of these patients' remissions were associated with vigorous steroid and cytotoxic therapy. Hopper et al. [176] also found remissions to be more frequent with prednisone treatment; they also noted a higher incidence of remissions in women than in men. In the French series of Noel et al. [288], 23 percent of patients went into remission without prednisone treatment. This group included 24 percent patients with asymptomatic proteinuria in whom the remissions were more frequent. Patients with membranous nephropathy secondary to systemic disease, such as lupus, neoplasms, drugs, toxins, and infections, appear to be more likely to have remissions as the underlying condition is controlled. More recent studies have confirmed the occurrence of as many as 38 percent spontaneous remissions in MN patients with nephrotic range proteinuria [55].

Remissions may be even more frequent in children. In a series reported by Habib et al. [149], 16 of 37 patients were in complete remission at last follow-up, while 10 had asymptomatic proteinuria and only 8 remained nephrotic; 3 were in renal failure.

RENAL FAILURE

The favorable course of patients with remissions is mirrored by the progression toward renal failure in other patients with membranous nephropathy. Cameron [51] has proposed that if a group of patients with membranous nephropathy is followed over 10 to 15 years, eventually about half will have developed renal failure, half will be in remission or have mild proteinuria, and almost none will remain nephrotic (see also Chap. 69). This notion is roughly borne out in a number of studies. It is of further interest that the group with remission remains almost completely separate from the group that develops renal failure. In other words, the occurrence of a complete remission appears to identify a patient as one with a good prognosis, even if a relapse occurs later. Pierides et al. [308] found 7 of 25 adult nephrotic patients in renal failure at 8 years of follow-up, while 9 were in remission. Of 54 nephrotic patients reported by Row et al. [334], 9 were in terminal renal failure at 5.4 years. Seven of 41 adult nephrotic patients followed by Noel et al. [288] for 4 years had creatinine levels above 3 mg %. Kida et al. [206] noted steady functional deterioration in half of 75 patients followed for 10 years. In the United States' collaborative study, 29 percent of untreated patients doubled their serum creatinine levels during a period of observation that averaged 2 years, in contrast to only 6 percent of treated patients [66].

Davison et al. [79] found that about half of a group of untreated patients with MN had a steady decline in renal function, with serum creatinine levels doubling at an average of 30 months.

Hopper et al. [176] noted 30 patients in renal failure compared to 22 in remission at 8.3 years follow-up. In distinction to the predominance of female patients in remission, most of the patients in renal failure were men.

More recent studies have generally shown more favorable outcomes. Kida et al. [207] estimated almost normal renal function in 45 percent of patients with MN and nephrotic range proteinuria after 15 years. Cattran et al. [55] found 70 percent of MN patients retained at least 75 percent of their entry creatinine clearance at 3 years of follow-up. The Medical Research Council [53] trial showed 31 percent of 103 patients to have normal serum creatinine at average 4.5 years of follow-up, while 27 percent had moderate creatinine elevations and 25 percent had severe elevations or were on dialysis. In the Mayo Clinic series [93], 20 percent were in end-stage renal failure at 5 years.

PATHOLOGY CORRELATIONS

Attempts to correlate the histologic staging obtained from electron microscopy with clinical severity or prognosis have usually been unsuccessful, with most investigators finding no relationship between stages and outcome [58, 66, 224, 288, 334, 393]. This has also been true in children [224], although in one study of children, stages III and IV appeared to progress more rapidly [318]. In adults, Beregi and Varga [29] found stage I more frequently in patients who were young and female, with few clinical symptoms and with good outcomes. Fuiano et al. [121] found a better outcome in stage I patients compared to stage II following 6 months of steroid therapy. Minimal abnormalities on electron microscopy also were associated with a benign course in patients of Tu et al. [395]. Zucchelli et al. [441] found patients with stage I and II pathology were more likely to achieve sustained remissions than III and IV and that stage V represented a healing phase found in prolonged remission. Noel et al. [288] felt that "early" stages might correlate with disease of short duration, but without relationship to severity or outcome. Tornroth et al. [393] described 7 patients who were completely normal on light microscopy, while representing all electron microscopic stages without spikes or membrane thickening. All had spontaneous remissions. These investigators feel that formation of deposits correlates with active disease and that their transformation into intramembranous lucencies corresponds to periods of remission [392]. It is interesting that in 29 transplanted patients followed by Antignac et al. [14] the histologic findings of MN preceded the appearance of proteinuria by months to years.

Some investigators have pointed out a better correlation between severe disease and the total volume of interstitial space in the renal biopsy. Glomerular hypercellularity with prominence of the parietal epithelial cells was thought to indicate a poor prognosis in another study [127]. A rapid decline in renal function may indicate a transformation to (or addition of) crescentic nephritis [215, 284], but the presence of crescents does not invariably imply a decline in function [133].

When patients in remission are rebiopsied, the histologic abnormalities of membranous nephropathy usually persist [255, 262, 288] but, occasionally, complete histologic remission occurs [288, 301, 434].

PROGNOSTIC FACTORS

To summarize factors mentioned previously, a relatively benign prognosis, with the occurrence of remissions or with less likelihood of progression to end-stage renal failure, is suggested by female gender, initial nonnephrotic ("asymptomatic") proteinuria, mild glomerular changes on electron microscopy, and underlying systemic disease or drug-associated MN.

In addition, the occurrence of a remission (or even a partial remission with proteinuria decreasing to 2 gm per day or less) suggests a good outcome [66, 93, 183, 304] for glomerular filtration rate.

A greater likelihood of persistent proteinuria and progressive loss of renal function is seen with the male sex, heavy initial proteinuria, and increased serum creatinine at biopsy. It is not clear which of these variables are independent and which might not withstand multivariate analysis of large groups of MN patients. Other histologic changes including increased interstitial volume [422] and the occurrence of capsular drops (inspissated protein "crescents") may accompany more severe disease.

HLA haplotypes and other pathologic findings, as mentioned earlier, also may have predictive value, but their reliability is less well substantiated [53, 303]. It has been suggested [442] that patients with milder disease have higher ratios of peripheral helper/inducer to suppressor/cytotoxic T cells.

Treatment of Membranous Nephropathy

GENERAL TREATMENT

Patients with nephrotic syndrome due to membranous nephropathy will, of course, benefit from general therapy, including salt restriction, adequate dietary protein, and appropriate use of diuretics. In addition, the use of nonsteroidal anti-inflammatory agents, such as indomethacin, has been shown to reduce proteinuria in some patients with membranous nephropathy in a number of studies [94, 267, 356, 389, 394, 402]. This reduction in proteinuria is usually accompanied by a fall in glomerular filtration rate, which is probably hemodynamically mediated and returns to baseline when the medication is discontinued [389]. It is accompanied by a fall in urinary prostaglandins [356] and appears to be most effective when used in patients with high renin and angiotensin levels, such as following the use of diuretics and a low-salt diet [94]. Indomethacin and meclofenamate [394] have been the agents most studied. Whether it is possible to alter the long-term outcome of the disease through drug therapy has been the subject of much discussion [51, 65, 78, 138].

CORTICOSTEROID THERAPY

Corticosteroid therapy without the addition of immunosuppressive agents has been a frequently recommended approach. The use of prednisone in uncontrolled studies has been reported from 1959 onward [139, 351]. Complete and partial responses of proteinuria and enhanced survival have been claimed by proponents of corticosteroid therapy [36, 103, 190, 322, 376]. In particular, Hopper et al., in a series of papers [173–176] describing the course of 83 nephrotic patients with membranous histology who were followed an average of 100 months, noted that 27 of 61 steroid-treated patients improved, with complete remissions for a year or longer in 14. He emphasizes [172] that high doses (as much as 200 mg every second day) for prolonged periods may be necessary.

As demonstrated in one study, even patients with declining renal function may respond to intensive corticosteroid therapy. Fifteen patients with rising serum creatinine concentrations were treated with 1-gm pulses of intravenous methylprednisolone daily for 5 days followed by 100 mg on alternate days tapered to 0 over 6 months [358]. In 13 patients the creatinine trend was reversed, but in some of these the effect was temporary.

It has been suggested [121] that histologic stage I responds to corticosteroid treatment, while stage II does not.

Comparing the outcome in treated with untreated patients in uncontrolled series is hazardous, however, because of the influence of such variables as age, gender, quantity of proteinuria at onset, remissions, glomerular filtration rate at onset, and the presence of associated systemic diseases. In addition, there appear to be other, so far unrecognized, variables that influence outcome and may be responsible for the great geographical and institutional variability seen. Without knowing the probable outcome of an identical group of untreated patients, it is impossible to assess the affect of treatment. In particular, the generally excellent outcome of some groups of untreated patients, such as those reported by Noel et al. [288] and Donadio et al. [93], should lead to caution in attributing a good outcome to steroid therapy.

Some general statements can be made despite this uncertainty:

1. Many patients have satisfactory courses, leading gradually to remission without any steroid or immunosuppressive therapy.
2. The occurrence of a complete remission during the course of corticosteroids (such as is usually seen in minimal change disease of childhood) is uncommon in membranous nephropathy unless prolonged intensive therapy is undertaken [66, 107], but repeated remissions and relapses are seen in an occasional (usually treated) patient.
3. A minority of patients with this disease progress

steadily and rather quickly to irreversible failure. If a benefit is to be derived from therapy, it may be in this group.

Five prospective controlled studies of the use of corticosteroids in the treatment of this disease are available for review. These are the two studies of the British Medical Research Council [34, 53], the United States' collaborative study [66], a Canadian collaborative study [55], and a Japanese study [214].

In the British Medical Research Council Study, directed by Professor Black [34], 19 adult patients with MN were randomly allocated to prednisone therapy (an average of 32 mg per day, gradually diminishing to 14 mg per day at 12 months) or to no therapy. Fourteen patients were followed for nearly 3 years. The treated patients had more remissions and a lower average serum creatinine value during the follow-up period, but these trends did not reach the 0.05 percent level of statistical significance.

In the United States' Collaborative Study of the Adult Idiopathic Nephrotic Syndrome [66], 72 adult patients with membranous nephropathy and nephrotic proteinuria were randomly allocated either to alternate-day prednisone 125 mg q.o.d. for 2 months, with an additional month taper, or to placebo. The placebo and treatment groups were comparable with respect to age, sex, duration of disease, severity of nephrotic syndrome, and histologic findings. The prevalence of complete and partial remissions was significantly increased in the treatment group. More relapses occurred in the prednisone group, however, so that there were no differences in remissions present at the end of the study. Remissions of proteinuria occurred earlier and more frequently in the treated group as compared to the placebo group; however, no patient sustained a complete remission of proteinuria during the initial prednisone treatment. More importantly, progressive impairment of glomerular filtration rate (GFR) was much less frequent in the treated group. A progressive fall in GFR occurred in a sizable proportion of the placebo group during the first 2 years of follow-up. The deterioration could not be explained readily by clinically detectable renal vein thrombosis or interstitial nephritis. Thus treatment of these patients seldom led to a stable permanent remission of proteinuria but did reduce the propensity for the development of progressive renal failure over 2 to 3 years follow-up in a subset of patients (approximately one-fourth) with membranous nephropathy.

In a prospective and sequentially controlled, but not randomized, study of patients with membranous histology and nonnephrotic proteinuria from Japan [214], Kobayashi et al. studied the effect of prednisone treatment, tapering from an initial dose of 30 mg per day down to 0 over a 2-year period. Eight of 9 treated patients had complete remissions of proteinuria at 1 year compared to 0 of 9 untreated patients.

In the Toronto area, Cattran et al. [55] studied 158 patients with idiopathic MN, of whom 120 had nephrotic range proteinuria. They were randomly assigned to 45 mg/m^2 prednisone on alternate days for 6 months or to placebo. Although there was a trend toward reduced proteinuria and better preserved creatinine clearance in the treated group in early months of follow-up, no significant difference between the groups was noted at the end of follow-up (mean duration 48 months).

A second MRC sponsored study was conducted in Great Britain under the direction of Dr. J. S. Cameron [53]. From 267 total candidates (which included secondary disease, low-grade proteinuria, etc.), 107 adult nephrotic patients with MN histology were selected. They were randomly allocated to 125 mg of prednisone every second day for 8 weeks, or to placebo. Again, during the early months of follow-up there was a trend toward reduced proteinuria in the treated group, but at 36 months of follow-up there was no difference in proteinuria or in creatinine clearance between the groups.

Thus from the data available, it would seem that perhaps some patients with membranous nephropathy may benefit from corticosteroid therapy (especially in the short term); but when large groups are studied with careful controls, alternate-day steroids administered either for 2 months in high dose or for 6 months in moderate dose fail to produce long-term benefit.

Very prolonged or very intense (e.g., "pulse" infusions) administration of corticosteroids could offer benefit but have not yet been adequately studied.

CYTOTOXIC THERAPY

Several uncontrolled studies combining cytotoxic agents with corticosteroids have had a remarkable number of complete remissions [103, 151, 206, 307, 320, 334, 376, 402].

Even patients with deteriorating creatinine clearance and elevated serum creatinine can sometimes respond. Eleven consecutive such patients were treated with cyclophosphamide for 1 year (accompanied by alternate-day prednisone during the first months) and showed improvement [46]. Another group of 8 such patients was treated with 6 months of alternating prednisone and chlorambucil therapies (see Ponticelli regimen, below), and 6 had improved creatinine clearance [258]. Pulse methylprednisolone followed by oral steroids and azathioprine or cyclophosphamide in 10 patients [428] improved creatinine clearance in 6, slowed progression in 3, and had no effect in one. Shearman et al. [353], however, in a retrospective review of 67 Australian patients could find no difference in outcome between alternate-day prednisone, a cyclophosphamide-dipyridamole-warfarin combination, and no therapy at all. Without careful observation of strictly comparable control groups, it is difficult to evaluate the risk-benefit of such therapy.

In a study with concurrent, but nonrandomized controls [426], nine patients with MN, nephrotic proteinuria, and elevated serum creatinine concentration were treated with cyclophosphamide (mean dose 1.5 mg/kg/day) for a mean of 23 months. At a total follow-up of mean 49 months, the treated patients were improved as compared to the controls in serum creatinine levels, serum albumin, and proteinuria.

Controlled randomized studies of cytotoxic therapy

have had varying results [307]. In a small study from Canada [69], four patients treated with azathioprine did not differ significantly from five controls. Eleven patients treated with cyclophosphamide by Donadio et al. did not do better than eleven controls at 1 year [92] or at 3.5 years. In this study, most, but not all, patients had well-preserved renal function at onset. GFR was generally stable in both groups. There were no significant differences in remission rates between the two groups. The fact that some of the patients (not specified as to number or group) had previously received corticosteroid therapy complicates the interpretation.

Lagrue et al. [218] prospectively treated 11 patients with azathioprine (3 mg/kg per day for 6 months followed by 2 mg/kg per day for 6 months) and 16 patients with chlorambucil (0.2 mg/kg per day for 6 months followed by 0.1 mg/kg per day for 6 months), with 14 untreated patients serving as controls. The azathioprine group did not differ significantly from the control group. The chlorambucil group did significantly better, however, with 13 of 16 having a partial or complete remission compared to only 3 of 14 control patients.

In an Australian study, combined cyclophosphamide, dipyridamole, and warfarin reduced proteinuria in a group of patients with MN, but only at the cost of serious side effects [390].

Ponticelli et al. [311–313] studied the effects of a 6-month program in which steroids and chlorambucil were alternated. The 6-month treatment consisted of three cycles of a 2-month therapy. The 2-month therapy began with three 1-gm pulses of intravenous methylprednisolone followed by daily oral methylprednisolone (0.4 mg/kg per day) or prednisone (0.5 mg/kg per day) for a month. At the end of the first month, the steroid was stopped and chlorambucil (0.2 mg/kg per day) was given for 1 month. The dose was adjusted if the leukocyte count fell below 5,000/mm^3. This 2-month cycle was then repeated for a total of three courses.

Eighty-one patients were randomly assigned either to this program or to supportive therapy alone. After follow-up of median 5 years, there were significant differences in proteinuria and plasma creatinine in favor of the treated group, with few treatment side effects.

Most, but not all, of these data suggest that chlorambucil or cyclophosphamide, when added to prednisone, may have a beneficial effect on the course of membranous nephropathy in some patients. Whether the net benefits outweigh the risks of cytotoxic therapy (including increased susceptibility to infection and to malignancies) remains for longer-term observations to disclose. No therapy so far reported has had a convincing benefit in patients who had severe impairment of renal function at the onset of treatment.

In an interesting, but so far unconfirmed observation, Palla et al. [301], after 6 months' observation, gave 9 patients with MN a course of repeated intravenous pulses of mixed human IgG. Three sets of three daily pulses of 0.4 gm/kg were given at 21-day intervals, followed by 1 pulse each 21 days for a total treatment of 1 year. Eight patients showed clinical and histologic benefit when evaluated at the end of the treatment period.

With persisting uncertainty about the effectiveness of these therapies and their potential risks, the choice for many patients requires art and individualization as well as science. For patients who are relatively asymptomatic or who have only modest proteinuria and have had stable renal function over an extended period of time, the natural history of the untreated disease will probably be benign, and the risks of therapy will outweigh the benefits. This might be true particularly in young female patients who appear to have a particularly good prognosis [176].

Therapy may be beneficial for patients whose risk profile suggests a graver outcome (e.g., male patients with large amounts of proteinuria and hypertension, particularly if a trend toward increased serum creatinine is evident). Combinations of prednisone with cyclophosphamide or chlorambucil as described above appear to be effective for many patients, even if mild renal insufficiency has begun. Intravenous immunoglobulins may offer promise but have not yet been adequately tested.

References

1. Abrass, C. K., and Cohen, A. H. The role of circulating antigen in the formation of immune deposits in experimental membranous nephropathy. *Proc. Soc. Exp. Biol. Med.* 183(3): 348, 1986.
2. Abrass, C. K., Hall, C. L., Border, W. A., et al. Circulating immune complexes in adults with idiopathic nephrotic syndrome. Collaborative study of the adult idiopathic nephrotic syndrome. *Kidney Int.* 17: 545, 1980.
3. Adhikari, M., Coovadia, H. M., and Chrystal, V. Extramembranous nephropathy in black South African children. *Ann. Trop. Paediatr.* 3: 17, 1983.
4. Adhikari, M., Coovadia, H. M., and Loening, W. E. The nephrotic syndrome in children. *S. Afr. Med. J.* 50: 39, 1976.
5. Adler, S., Salant, D. J., Dittmer, J. E., et al. Mediation of proteinuria in membranous nephropathy due to a planted glomerular antigen. *Kidney Int.* 23: 807, 1983.
6. Adler, S. G., Wang, H., Ward, H. J., et al. Electrical charge. Its role in the pathogenesis and prevention of experimental membranous nephropathy in the rabbit. *J. Clin. Invest.* 71: 487, 1983.
7. Ainsworth, S. K., Swain, R. P., Watabe, N., et al. Gold nephropathy. Ultrastructural, fluorescent, and energy-dispersive x-ray microanalysis study. *Arch. Pathol. Lab. Med.* 105: 373, 1981.
8. Akano, N., Yoshioka, K., Aya, N., et al. Immunoelectron microscopic localization of membrane attack complex and hepatitis B e antigen in membranous nephropathy. *Virchows Arch.* 414(4): 325, 1989.
9. Akikusa, B., Kondo, Y., Lemoto, Y., et al. Hashimoto's thyroiditis and membranous nephropathy developed in progressive systemic sclerosis (PSS). *Am. J. Clin. Pathol.* 81: 260, 1984.
10. Alexopoulos, E., Seron, D., Hartley, R. B., et al. Immune mechanisms in idiopathic membranous nephropathy: The role of the interstitial infiltrates. *Am. J. Kidney Dis.* 13(5): 404, 1989.
11. Allen, A. C. *The Kidney*. New York: Grune & Stratton, 1951.
12. Amenta, P. S., Swartz, C., and Katz, S. M. Concurrent

focal segmental glomerulosclerosis and membranous nephropathy. *Clin. Nephrol.* 32(4): 173, 1989.

13. Andrade, Z. A., and Rocha, H. Schistosomal glomerulopathy. *Kidney Int.* 16: 23, 1979.
14. Antignac, C., Hinglais, N., Gubler, M. C., et al. De novo membranous glomerulonephritis in renal allografts in children. *Clin. Nephrol.* 30(1): 1, 1988.
15. Aparicio, S. R., Woolgar, A. E., Aparicio, S. A., et al. An ultrastructural morphometric study of membranous glomerulonephritis. *Nephrol. Dial. Transplant.* 1(1): 22, 1986.
16. Assmann, K. J., Ronco, P., Tangelder, M. M., et al. Involvement of an antigen distinct from the Heymann antigen in membranous glomerulonephritis in the mouse. *Lab. Invest.* 60(1): 138, 1989.
17. Assman, K. J., Tangelder, M. M., Lane, W. P., et al. Membranous glomerulonephritis in the mouse. *Kidney Int.* 24: 303, 1983.
18. Bacon, P., Tribe, C. R., Machenzie, J. C., et al. Penicillamine in rheumatoid arthritis. A clinical pathological and immunological study. *Q. J. Med.* 45: 661, 1976.
19. Baker, P. J., Ochi, R. F., Schulze, M., et al. Depletion of C6 prevents development of proteinuria in experimental membranous nephropathy in rats. *Am. J. Pathol.* 135(1): 185, 1989.
20. Bannister, K. M., Hay, J., and Clarkson, A. R. Fc-specific reticulo-endothelial clearance in systemic lupus erythematosus and glomerulonephritis. *Am. J. Kidney Dis.* 3: 287, 1984.
21. Bansal, V. K., Kozeny, G. A., Fresco, R., et al. De novo membranous nephropathy following renal transplantation between conjoint twins. *Transplantation* 41(3): 404, 1986.
22. Bariety, J., Barbier, M., Laigre, M. C., et al. Proteinurie et loase. Etude histologique, optique et electronique d'un cas. *Bull. Soc. Med. Paris* 118: 1015, 1967.
23. Barr, R. D., Rees, P. H., Cordy, P. E., et al. Nephrotic syndrome in Adult Africans in Nairobi. *Br. Med. J.* 2: 131, 1972.
24. Barton, C. H., Vaziri, N. D., and Spear, G. S. Nephrotic syndrome associated with adenocarcinoma of the breast. *Am. J. Med.* 68: 308, 1980.
25. Batsford, S. R., Takamyra, H., and Vogt, A. A model of in-situ immune complex glomerulonephritis in the rat employing cationized ferritin. *Clin. Nephrol.* 14: 211, 1980.
26. Beauvais, P., Vaudour, G., Boccon-Gibod, L., et al. Membranous nephropathy associated with ovarian tumor in a young girl: Recovery after removal. *Eur. J. Pediatr.* 148(7): 624, 1989.
27. Bell, E. T. Lipoid nephrosis. *Am. J. Pathol.* 5: 587, 1929.
28. Bell, E. T. *Renal Diseases,* 2nd ed. Philadelphia: Lea & Febiger, 1950.
29. Beregi, E., and Varga, I. Analysis of 260 cases of membranous glomerulonephritis in renal biopsy material. *Clin. Nephrol.* 2: 215, 1974.
30. Berger, B. E., Vincenti, F., Biava, C., et al. De novo and recurrent membranous glomerulopathy following kidney transplantation. *Transplantation* 35: 315, 1983.
31. Berger, J., and Yaneva, H. Hageman factor deposition in membranous glomerulopathy. *Transplant. Proc.* 14: 472, 1982.
32. Bertani, T., Appel, G. B., Cagati, V., et al. Focal segmental membranous glomerulonephropathy associated with other glomerular diseases. *Am. J. Kidney Dis.* 2: 439, 1983.
33. Berthoux, F. C., Laurent, B., le Petit, J. C., et al. Immunogenetics and immunopathology of human primary membranous splenic macrophage Fc-receptors and peripheral blood T-lymphocyte subpopulations. *Clin. Nephrol.* 22: 15, 1984.
34. Black, D. S., Rose, G., and Brewer, D. B. Controlled trial of prednisone in adult patients with the nephrotic syndrome. *Br. Med. J.* 3: 421, 1970.
35. Blum, M., and Aviram, A. Nephrotic syndrome with reversible severe renal failure after gold therapy. *Int. J. Clin. Pharmacol. Ther. Toxicol.* 10: 562, 1984.
36. Bolton, W. K., Atuk, N. O., Sturgill, B. C., et al. Therapy of the idiopathic nephrotic syndrome with alternate day steroids. *Am. J. Med.* 62: 60, 1977.
37. Border, W. A., Ward, H. J., and Kamiz, E. S. Induction of membranous nephropathy in rabbits by administration of an exogenous cationic antigen. *J. Clin. Invest.* 69: 451, 1982.
38. Botey, A., Torras, A., and Revert, L. Membranous nephropathy in ankylosing spondylitis (Letter). *Nephron* 29: 203, 1981.
39. Bradley, W. G., Jr., Jacobs, R. P., Trew, P. A., et al. Renal vein thrombosis: Occurrence in membranous glomerulonephropathy and lupus nephritis. *Radiology* 139: 571, 1981.
40. Breathnach, S. M., Dutt, M. K., and Black, M. M. A severe bullous eruption occurring in a patient with chronic active hepatitis and glomerulonephritis. *Arch. Dermatol.* 116: 1060, 1980.
41. Brenchley, P., Feehally, J., Dore, P., et al. Gm allotypes in membranous nephropathy (Letter). *N. Engl. J. Med.* 309: 556, 1985.
42. Briefel, G. R., Manis, T., Gordon, D. H., et al. Recurrent renal vein thrombosis consequent to membranous glomerulonephritis. *Clin. Nephrol.* 10: 32, 1978.
43. Briner, J., Binswanger, U., and Largiader, F. Recurrent and de novo membranous glomerulonephritis in renal cadaver allotransplants. *Clin. Nephrol.* 13: 189, 1980.
44. Brown, K. G. E., Abrahams, C., and Meyers, A. M. The nephrotic syndrome in Malawian blacks. *S. Afr. Med. J.* 52: 275, 1977.
45. Brueggemeyer, C. D., and Ramirez, G. Membranous nephropathy: A concern for malignancy. *Am. J. Kidney Dis.* 9(1): 23, 1987.
46. Bruns, F. J., Adler, S., Fraley, D. S., et al. Sustained remission of membranous glomerulonephritis after cyclophosphamide and prednisone. *Ann. Intern. Med.* 114: 725, 1991.
47. Cahen, R., Francois, B., Trolliet, P., et al. Aetiology of membranous glomerulonephritis: A prospective study of 82 adult patients. *Nephrol. Dial. Transplant.* 4(3): 172, 1989.
48. Cairns, S., Klouda, P., Dyer, P., et al. Role of the major histocompatibility complex system in idiopathic membranous nephropathy: Prediction of outcome and response to treatment. Abstract of the Renal Association. *Kidney Int.* 18: 802, 1980.
49. Cairns, S. A., London, R. A., and Mallick, N. D. Circulating immune complexes in idiopathic glomerular diseases. *Kidney Int.* 21: 507, 1982.
50. Cameron, J. S. Histology, protein clearances and response to treatment in the nephrotic syndrome. *Br. Med. J.* 627: 352, 1968.
51. Cameron, J. S. Pathogenesis and treatment of membranous nephropathy. *Kidney Int.* 15: 88, 1979.
52. Cameron, J. S. Membranous nephropathy in childhood and its treatment. *Pediatr. Nephrol.* 4(2): 193, 1990.

53. Cameron, J. S., Healy, M. J., and Adu, D. The Medical Research Council trial of short-term high-dose alternate day prednisolone in idiopathic membranous nephropathy with nephrotic syndrome in adults. *Q. J. Med.* 74(274): 133, 1990.
54. Catane, R., Kaugman, J. H., Douglass, H. O., et al. Nephrotic syndrome associated with gastric cancer. *J. Surg. Oncol.* 9: 207, 1977
55. Cattran, C. C., Delmore, T., Roscoe, J., et al. A randomized controlled trial of prednisone in patients with idiopathic membranous nephropathy. *N. Engl. J. Med.* 320(4): 210, 1989.
56. Central Committee of the Toronto Glomerulonephritis Registry. Regional program for the study of glomerulonephritis. *Can. Med. Assoc. J.* 124: 158, 1981.
57. Charpentier, B., Moullot, P., Faux, N., et al. T lymphocyte functions in mercuric chloride-induced membranous glomerulonephritis in man. Evidence for a defect of presentation of the histocompatibility class II molecules at the cell surface. *Nephrologie* 2: 153, 1981.
58. Chavaz, A., Mignon, F., and Morel-Maroger, L. Glomerulites extramembraneuses. A propose de 92 observations. *Schweiz. Med. Wochenschr.* 107: 899, 1977.
59. Cheigh, J. S., Mouradian, J., Susin, M., et al. Kidney transplant nephrotic syndrome: Relationship between allograft histopathology and natural course. *Kidney Int.* 18: 358, 1980.
60. Chen, W. Y., Wang, R. H., Yen, T. S., et al. Membranous glomerulonephritis and myasthenia gravis. *Taiwan I Hsueh Hui Tsa Chih* 79: 667, 1980.
61. Cheong, I. K., Chong, S. M., Singh, N., et al. Extensive crescent formation in idiopathic membranous glomerulonephritis. A case report. *Med. J. Malaysia* 36: 8, 1981.
62. Chopra, S., Kaufman, J. S., Hamburger, R. J., et al. Membranous nephropathy with chronic renal failure: Partial native renal function recovery after unsuccessful renal transplant. *Arch. Intern. Med.* 140: 437, 1980.
63. Chugh, K. S., Malik, N., Uberoi, H. S., et al. Renal vein thrombosis in nephrotic syndrome—A prospective study and review. *Postgrad. Med. J.* 57: 566, 1981.
64. Churg, J., and Ehrenreich, T. Membranous Nephropathy. In P. Kincaid-Smith, T. H. Mathew, and E. L. Becker (eds.), *Glomerulonephritis I.* New York: Wiley, 1973. Pp. 443–448.
65. Coggins, C. H. Is membranous nephropathy treatable? *Am. J. Nephrol.* 1: 219, 1981.
66. Collaborative Study of the Adult Idiopathic Nephrotic Syndrome. A controlled study of short-term prednisone treatment in adults with membranous nephropathy. *N. Engl. J. Med.* 301: 1301, 1979.
67. Collins, A. B., Andres, G. A., and McCluskey, R. T. Lack of evidence for a role of renal tubular antigen in human membranous glomerulonephritis. *Nephron* 27: 297, 1981.
68. Combs, R. C., and Hazelrigg, D. W. Dermatitis herpetiformis and membranous glomerulonephritis. *Cutis* 25: 660, 1980.
69. Controlled trial of azathioprine in the nephrotic syndrome secondary to idiopathic membranous glomerulonephritis. *Can. Med. Assoc. J.* 115: 1209, 1976.
70. Costanza, M. E., Pinn, V. W., Schwartz, R. S., et al. Carcinoembryonic antigen-antibody complexes in a patient with colonic carcinoma and nephrotic syndrome. *N. Engl. J. Med.* 289: 520, 1973.
71. Cosyns, J. P., Pirson, Y., Van Ypersele de Srihou, C., et al. Recurrence of de novo graft membranous glomerulonephritis. *Nephron* 29: 142, 1981.
72. Couser, W. G., and Salant, D. J. In situ immune complex formation and glomerular injury. *Kidney Int.* 17: 1, 1980.
73. Couser, W. G., Steinmuller, D. R., and Stilmant, M. M. Experimental glomerulonephritis in the isolated perfused rat kidney. *J. Clin. Invest.* 62: 1275, 1978.
74. Couser, W. G., Wagonfeld, J. V., and Spargo, B. H. Glomerular deposition of tumor antigen in membranous nephropathy associated with colonic carcinoma. *Am. J. Med.* 57: 962, 1974.
75. Crosson, J. T., Wathen, L., and Raif, L. Recurrence of idiopathic membranous nephropathy in a renal allograft. *Arch. Intern. Med.* 135: 1101, 1975.
76. Cudkowicz, M. E., Sayegh, M. H., and Rennke, H. G. Membranous nephropathy in a patient with renal cell carcinoma. *Am. J. Kidney Dis.* 17(3): 349, 1991.
77. Cybulsky, A. V., Rennke, H. G., Feintzeig, I. D., et al. Complement-induced glomerular epithelial cell injury: Role of the membrane attack complex in rat membranous nephropathy. *J. Clin. Invest.* 77(4): 1096, 1986.
78. D'Achiardi-Rey, R., and Pollak, V. E. Membranous glomerulonephropathy: There is no significant effect of treatment with corticosteroids. *Am. J. Kidney Dis.* 1: 386, 1982.
79. Davison, A. M., Cameron, J. S., Kerr, D. N. S., et al. The natural history of untreated idiopathic membranous glomerulonephritis in adults. Abstr. CN-196. *Clin. Nephrol.* 22: 61, 1984.
80. Day, A. T., Golding, J. R., Lee, P. N., et al. Penicillamine in rheumatoid disease. A long-term study. *Br. Med. J.* 1: 180, 1974.
81. DelVecchio-Blanco, C., Polito, C., Caporaso, N., et al. Membranous glomerulopathy and hepatitis B virus (HBV) infection in children. *Int. J. Pediatr. Nephrol.* 4: 235, 1983.
82. Demaine, A. G., Cameron, J. S., Taube, D. T., et al. Immunoglobulin (Gm) allotype frequencies in idiopathic membranous nephropathy and minimal change nephropathy. *Transplantation* 37: 507, 1984.
83. Demaine, A. G., Vaughan, R. W., Taube, D. H., et al. Association of membranous nephropathy with T-cell receptor constant beta chain and immunoglobulin heavy chain switch region polymorphisms. *Immunogenetics* 27(1): 19, 1988.
84. Desanto, N. G., Capodicasa, G., and Giordano, C. Treatment of idiopathic membranous nephropathy unresponsive to methylprednisolone and chlorambucil with cyclosporin. *Am. J. Nephrol.* 7(1): 74, 1987.
85. Dische, F. E., Culliford, E. J., and Parsons, V. Haemolytic uraemic syndrome and idiopathic membranous glomerulonephritis. *Br. Med. J.* 1: 1112, 1978.
86. Dische, F. E., Herbertson, B. M., Melcher, D. H., et al. Membranous glomerulonephritis in transplant kidneys: Recurrent or de novo disease in four patients. *Clin. Nephrol.* 15: 154, 1981.
87. Dische, F. E., Svensson, D. R., Hamilton, E. B. D., et al. Immunopathology of penicillamine-induced glomerular disease. *J. Rheumatol.* 3:145, 1976.
88. Dixon, F. J. The pathogenesis of glomerulonephritis (Editorial). *Am. J. Med.* 44: 493, 1968.
89. Doi, T., Kanatsu, K., Nagai, H., et al. An overlapping syndrome of IgA nephropathy and membranous nephropathy? *Nephron* 35: 24, 1983.
90. Doi, T., Kanatsu, K., Nagai, H., et al. Demonstration of C3d deposits in membranous nephropathy. *Nephron* 37: 232, 1984.
91. Doi, T., Mayumi, M., Kanatsu, K., et al. Distribution of

IgG subclasses in membranous nephropathy. *Clin. Exp. Immunol.* 58: 57, 1984.
92. Donadio, J. V., Jr., Holley, K. E., Anderson, C. R., et al. Controlled trial of cyclophosphamide in idiopathic membranous nephropathy. *Kidney Int.* 6: 431, 1974.
93. Donadio, J. V., Jr., Torres, V. E., Velosa, J. A., et al. Idiopathic membranous nephropathy: The natural history of untreated patients. *Kidney Int.* 33(3): 708, 1988.
94. Donker, A. J., Brentjens, J. R., Van Der Hem, G. K., et al. Treatment of the nephrotic syndrome with indomethacin. *Nephron* 22: 374, 1978.
95. Dreyer, L. The frequency of hepatitis B surface antigen in membranous nephropathy in black and white South Africans. *S. Afr. Med. J.* 65: 166, 1984.
96. Ducret, F., Pointet, P., Bonnet, P., et al. Membranous glomerulonephritis associated with esophageal carcinoma. *Praxis* 70: 519, 1981.
97. Ducret, F., Pointet, P., and Pichot, C. Membranous glomerulonephritis during rheumatoid arthritis. Probable toxicity of diclofenac. *Nephrologie* 1: 143, 1980.
98. Dumas, R., Dumas, M. L., Baldet, P., et al. Membranous glomerulonephritis in two brothers associated in one with tubulo-interstitial disease. Fanconi syndrome and anti-TBM antibodies (author's translation). *Arch. Fr. Pediatr.* 39: 75, 1982.
99. Dunn, J. S. Nephroxis or nephrites. *J. Pathol. Bacteriol.* 39: 1, 1934.
100. Dupont, A. G., Verbeelen, D. L., and Six, R. D. Weber-Christian panniculitis with membranous glomerulonephritis. *Am. J. Med.* 75: 527, 1983.
101. Dyer, P. A., Klouda, P. T., Harris, R., et al. Properdin factor B alleles in patients with idiopathic membranous nephropathy. *Tissue Antigens* 15: 505, 1980.
102. Ehrenreich, T., and Churg, J. Pathology of membranous nephropathy. *Pathol. Annu.* 3: 145, 1968.
103. Ehrenreich, T., Porush, J. G., Churg, J., et al. Treatment of idiopathic membranous nephropathy. *N. Engl. J. Med.* 295: 741, 1976.
104. Ehrenreich, T., Yunis, S. L., and Churg, J. Membranous nephropathy following exposure to volatile hydrocarbons. *Environ. Res.* 14: 35, 1977.
105. Ellis, A. Natural history of Bright's disease: Clinical, histological and experimental observations. *Lancet* 1: 1, 34, 72, 1942.
106. Empire Rheumatism Council Research Subcommittee. Gold therapy in rheumatoid arthritis. Report of a multicenter controlled trial. *Ann. Rheum. Dis.* 19: 95, 1960.
107. Erwin, D. T., Donadio, J. V., and Holley, K. E. The clinical course of membranous nephropathy. *Mayo Clin. Proc.* 48: 697, 1973.
108. Evans, D. J. Pathogenesis of membranous nephropathy. *Lancet* 1: 1143, 1974.
109. Falck, H. M., Tornroth, T., Kock, B., et al. Fatal renal vasculitis and minimal change glomerulonephritis complicating treatment with penicillamine. Report on two cases. *Acta Med. Scand.* 205: 133, 1979.
110. Feehally, J., Brenchley, P. E., Coupes, B. M., et al. Impaired IgG response to tetanus toxoid in human membranous nephropathy: Association with HLA-DR3. *Clin. Exp. Immunol.* 63(2): 376, 1986.
111. Fein, R. L., Chait, A., and Leviton, A. Renal vein thrombectomy for the treatment of renal vein thrombosis associated with the nephrotic syndrome. *J. Urol.* 99: 1 1968.
112. Figueroa, J. E., and Waxman, J. Membranous nephropathy in rheumatoid arthritis. *South. Med. J.* 75: 480, 1982.
113. Fleuren, G. J., Grond, J., and Hoedemaeker, Ph. J. Insitu formation of subepithelial glomerular immune complexes in passive serum sickness. *Kidney Int.* 17: 631, 1980.
114. Ford, A. R. Improvement of renal failure due to membranous glomerulonephritis after unsuccessful renal transplantation. *Nephron* 20: 304, 1978.
115. Forland, M., and Spargo, B. H. Clinicopathological correlations in idiopathic nephrotic syndrome with membranous nephropathy. *Nephron* 6: 498, 1969.
116. Francis, K. S., Jenis, E. H., Jensen, G. E., et al. Gold associated nephropathy. *Arch. Pathol. Lab. Med.* 108: 234, 1984.
117. Franklin, W. A., Jennings, R. B., and Earle, D. P. Membranous glomerulonephritis: Long-term serial observations on clinical course and morphology. *Kidney Int.* 4: 36, 1973.
118. Friend, P. S. A unique antibody response associated with the development of membranous nephropathy in systemic lupus erythematosus. *Am. Heart J.* 95: 672, 1978.
119. Friend, P. S., Kim, Y., and Michael, A. F. Pathogenesis of membranous nephropathy in systemic erythematosus: Possible role of nonprecipitating DNA antibody. *Br. Med. J.* 1: 25, 1977.
120. Friend, P. S., and Michael, A. F. Hypothesis: Immunologic rationale for the therapy of membranous lupus nephropathy. *Clin. Immunol. Immunopathol.* 10: 35, 1978.
121. Fuiano, G., Stanziale, P., Balletta, M., et al. Effectiveness of steroid therapy in different stages of membranous nephropathy. *Nephrol. Dial. Transplant.* 4(12): 1022, 1989.
122. Fukatsu, A., Matsuo, S., Killen, P. D., et al. The glomerular distribution of type IV collagen and laminin in human membranous glomerulonephritis. *Hum. Pathol.* 19(1): 64, 1988.
123. Gabbai, F. B., Gushwa, L. C., Wilson, C. B., et al. An evaluation of the development of experimental membranous nephropathy. *Kidney Int.* 31(6): 1267, 1987.
124. Gabbai, F. B., Mundy, C. A., Wilson, C. B., et al. An evaluation of the role of complement depletion in experimental membranous nephropathy in the rat. *Lab. Invest.* 58(5): 539, 1988.
125. Gaffney, E. Allograft membranous glomerulonephritis (Letter). *Arch. Pathol. Lab. Med.* 105: 559, 1981.
126. Gaffney, E. F., Alexander, R. W., and Donnelly, W. H. Segmental membranous glomerulonephritis. *Arch. Pathol. Lab. Med.* 106: 409, 1982.
127. Gaffney, E. F., and Panner, B. J. Membranous glomerulonephritis: Clinical significance of glomerular hypercellularity and parietal epithelial abnormalities. *Nephron* 29: 209, 1981.
128. Gagliano, R. G., Costanzi, J. J., Beathard, G. A., et al. The nephrotic syndrome associated with neoplasia. *Am. J. Med.* 60: 1026, 1976.
129. Gamble, C. N., and Reardon, J. B. Immunopathogenesis of syphilitic glomerulonephritis. Elution of antitreponemal antibody from glomerular immune complex deposits. *N. Engl. J. Med.* 292: 449, 1975.
130. Garovoy, M. R. Idiopathic membranous glomerulonephritis: An HLA-associated disease. Histocompatibility testing 1980—Report of the Eighth International Histocompatibility Workshop. University of California at Los Angeles, 1980. Pp. 673–680.
131. Garovoy, M. R., Braun, W. B., and Duquesnoy, R. Idiopathic membranous glomerulonephritis: Associated

with a new B-cell antigen system in the major histocompatibility complex. *Clin. Res.* 28: 445A, 1980.
132. Gartner, H. V., Fischbach, H., Wehner, H., et al. Comparison of clinical and morphological features of peri- (epi extra-) membranous glomerulonephritis. *Nephron* 13: 288, 1974.
133. Gerhardt, R. E., Peskoe, S. T., Rao, R. N., et al. Spontaneous remission in idiopathic membranous glomerulonephritis with crescents. *South. Med. J.* 75(3): 356, 1982.
134. Germuth, F. G., and Rodriguez, E. *The Immunopathology of the Renal Glomerulus.* Boston: Little, Brown, 1973.
135. Germuth, F. G., Taylor, T. J., Siddiqui, S. Y., et al. Immune complex disease VI: Some determinants of the varieties of glomerular lesions in the chronic bovine serum albumin-rabbit system. *Lab. Invest.* 37: 162, 1977.
136. Gibson, T., Burry, H. C., and Ogg, C. Goodpasture's syndrome and D-penicillamine. *Ann. Intern. Med.* 84: 100, 1976.
137. Gilboa, N. Membranous nephropathy: Further evidence against the involvement of renal tubular epithelial antigen (Letter). *Nephron* 27: 323, 1981.
138. Glassock, R. J. Corticosteroid therapy is beneficial in adults with idiopathic membranous glomerulopathy. *Am. J. Kidney Dis.* 1: 376, 1982.
139. Glassock, R. J. The therapy of idiopathic membranous glomerulonephritis. *Semin. Nephrol.* 11: 138, 1991.
140. Glassock, R. J., Edgington, T. S., Watson, J. I., et al. Autologous immune complex nephritis induced with renal tubular antigen. II. The pathogenic mechanism. *J. Exp. Med.* 127: 573, 1968.
141. Gluck, M. C., Gallo, G., Lowenstein, J., et al. Membranous glomerulonephritis. *Ann. Intern. Med.* 78: 1, 1973.
142. Gluckman, J. C., Jacob, N., Beaufils, H., et al. Clinical significance of circulating immune complexes detection in chronic glomerulonephritis. *Nephron* 22: 1, 138, 1978.
143. Golbus, S., and Wilson, C. B. Glomerulonephritis (GN) produced by the in situ formation of immune complexes on the glomerular basement membrane (Abstract). *Kidney Int.* 13: 61A, 1978.
144. Graham, A. R., and Nagle, R. B. Quantitative electron microscopic study of membranous glomerulopathy. *Am. J. Clin. Pathol.* 80: 816, 1983.
145. Griffel, B., and Bernheim, J. Glomerular deposits in idiopathic membranous glomerulopathy. *Arch. Pathol. Lab. Med.* 104: 56, 1980.
146. Grizzle, W. E., and Johnson, K. H. Membranous nephropathy in a renal allograft. Its occurrence in a patient with previous anti-glomerular basement membrane disease. *Arch. Pathol. Lab. Med.* 105: 71, 1981.
147. Groggel, G. C., Adler, S., Rennke, H. G., et al. Role of the terminal complement pathway in experimental membranous nephropathy in the rabbit. *J. Clin. Invest.* 72: 1948, 1983.
148. Grupe, W. E., and Kaplan, M. H. Demonstration of an antibody to proximal tubule antigen in the pathogenesis of experimental autoimmune nephrosis in rats. *J. Lab. Clin. Med.* 74: 400, 1969.
149. Habib, R., and Kleinknecht, C. The primary nephrotic syndrome of childhood. Classification and clinicopathologic study of 406 cases. *Pathol. Annu.* 6: 417, 1971.
150. Hattori, S., Furuse, A., and Matsuda, I. Presence of HBe antibody in glomerular deposits in membranous glomerulonephritis is associated with hepatitis B virus infection. *Am. J. Nephrol.* 8(5): 384, 1988.
151. Hayslett, J. P., Kashgarian, M., and Bensch, K. G. Clinicopathological correlations in the nephrotic syndrome due to primary renal disease. *Medicine* 52: 93, 1973.
152. Heaney, D. J., Kupor, L. R., Gyorkey, F., et al. Membranous nephropathy associated with rheumatoid arthritis. *South Med. J.* 71: 467, 1978.
153. Helin, H., Pasternack, A., Falck, H., et al. Recurrence of renal amyloid and de novo membranous glomerulonephritis after transplantation. *Transplantation* 32: 6, 1981.
154. Hendrickse, R. G. The quartan malarial nephrotic syndrome. *Adv. Nephrol.* 6: 229, 1976.
155. Heymann, W., Hackel, D. B., Harwood, J., et al. Production of nephrotic syndrome in rats by Freund's adjuvants and rat kidney suspension. *Proc. Soc. Exp. Biol. Med.* 100: 660, 1959.
156. Hiesse, C., Goldschmidt, E., Santelli, G., et al. Membranous nephropathy in a bone marrow transplant recipient. *Am. J. Kidney Dis.* 11(2): 188, 1988.
157. Higuchi, A., Suzuki, Y., and Okada, T. Membranous glomerulonephritis in rheumatoid arthritis unassociated with gold or penicillamine treatment. *Ann. Rheum. Dis.* 46(6): 488, 1987.
158. Hiki, Y., Kobayashi, Y., Itoh, I., et al. Strong association of HLA-DR2 and MT1 with idiopathic membranous nephropathy in Japan. *Kidney Int.* 25: 953, 1984.
159. Hill, G. S., Robertson, J., Grossman, R., et al. An unusual variant of membranous nephropathy with abundant crescent formation and recurrence in the transplanted kidney. *Clin. Nephrol.* 10(3): 114, 1978.
160. Hill, H., Hill, A., and Davison, A. M. Resumption of treatment with penicillamine after proteinuria. *Ann. Rheumatol. Dis.* 38: 229, 1979.
161. Hill, H. H., Hill, A. G. S., Day, A. T., et al. Maintenance dose of penicillamine in rheumatoid arthritis: A comparison between a standard and a response-related flexible regimen. *Ann. Rheumatol. Dis.* 38: 429, 1979.
162. Hirose, H., Udo, K., Kojima, M., et al. Deposition of hepatitis B e antigen in membranous glomerulonephritis: Identification by $F(ab')_2$ fragments of monoclonal antibody. *Kidney Int.* 26: 338, 1984.
163. Hirsch, H. Z., Ainsworth, S. K., Debeukelaer, M., et al. Membranous glomerulonephritis in a child asymptomatic for hepatitis B virus. Concomitant seropositivity for HBSAG and anti-HBS. *Am. J. Clin. Pathol.* 75: 597, 1981.
164. Hoitsma, A. J., Kroon, A. A., Wetzels, J. F., et al. Association between ureteral obstruction and de novo membranous nephropathy in renal allografts. *Transplant. Proc.* 22(4): 1388, 1990.
165. Honig, C., Mouradian, J. A., Montoliu, J., et al. Mesangial electron-dense deposits in membranous nephropathy. *Lab. Invest.* 42: 427, 1980.
166. Honkanen, E. Survival in idiopathic membranous glomerulonephritis. *Clin. Nephrol.* 25(3): 122, 1986.
167. Honkanen, E., Gronhagen-Riska, C., von-Willebrand, E., et al. Renal mononuclear inflammatory cell populations in membranous glomerulonephritis: A fine-needle aspiration biopsy study. *Clin. Nephrol.* 28(5): 232, 1987.
168. Honkanen, E., Tornroth, T., Pettersson, E., et al. Glomerulonephritis in renal allografts: Results of 18 years of transplantations. *Clin. Nephrol.* 21: 210, 1984.
169. Honkanen, E., Tornroth, T., Pettersson, E., et al. Membranous glomerulonephritis in rheumatoid arthritis not related to gold or D-penicillamine therapy: A report of four cases and review of the literature. *Clin. Nephrol.* 27(2): 87, 1987.

170. Hoorntje, S. J., Donker, A. J., Prins, E. J., et al. Membranous glomerulopathy in a patient on captopril. *Acta Med. Scand.* 208: 325, 1980.
171. Hoorntje, S. J., Weening, J. J., Kallenberg, C. G., et al. Serum-sickness-like syndrome with membranous glomerulopathy in patient on captopril (Letter). *Lancet* 2: 1297, 1979.
172. Hopper, J. Prednisone in the treatment of idiopathic membranous nephropathy. *N. Engl. J. Med.* 321(4): 260, 1989.
173. Hopper, J., Jr. Letter. *Ann. Intern. Med.* 79: 285, 1973.
174. Hopper, J., Jr., Biava, L. G., and Tu, W. H. Membranous nephropathy: High-dose alternate-day therapy with prednisone. *West. J. Med.* 135: 1, 1981.
175. Hopper, J., Lee, J. C., Lewis, M. L., et al. Membranous nephropathy treatment with glucocorticoids. *Proceedings of the Vth International Congress of Nephrology,* 1972. P. 101.
176. Hopper, J., Jr., Trew, P. A., and Biava, C. G. Membranous nephropathy: Its relative benignity in women. *Nephron* 29: 18, 1981.
177. Hori, M. T., and Abrass, C. K. Isolation and characterization of circulating immune complexes from rats with experimental membranous nephropathy. *J. Immunol.* 144(10): 3849, 1990.
178. Hsu, H. C., Lin, G. H., Chang, M. H., et al. Association of hepatitis B surface (HBs) antigenemia and membranous nephropathy in children in Taiwan. *Clin. Nephrol.* 20: 121, 1983.
179. Hsu, H. C., Wu, C. Y., Lin, C. Y., et al. Membranous nephropathy in 52 hepatitis B surface antigen (HBsAg) carrier children in Taiwan. *Kidney Int.* 36(6): 1103, 1989.
180. Huang, C. C. Strong association of HLA-DR3 in Chinese patients with idiopathic membranous nephropathy. *Tissue Antigens* 33(3): 425, 1989.
181. Hurault de Ligny, B., Faure, G., Bene, M. C., et al. Extra-membranous glomerulonephritis during the treatment of rheumatoid polyarthritis with diclofenac (Letter). *Nephrologie* 5: 135, 1984.
182. Huskisson, E. C. Penicillamine and the rheumatologist: A review. *Pharmatherapeutica* 1: 24, 1976.
183. Idelson, B. A., Smithline, N., and Smith, G. W. Prognosis in steroid treated idiopathic nephrotic syndrome in adults. *Arch. Intern. Med.* 137: 891, 1977.
184. Ito, H., Hattori, S., Matusda, T., et al. Hepatitis B e antigen-mediated membranous glomerulonephritis. Correlation of ultrastructural changes with HBEAG in the serum and glomeruli. *Lab. Invest.* 44: 214, 1981.
185. Iwaoka, T., Umeda, T., Nakayama, M., et al. A case of membranous nephropathy associated with thyroid antigens. *Jpn. J. Med. Biol.* 21: 29, 1982.
186. Janle-Swain, E., Thornhill, J. A., Carter, J. M., et al. Case study of a diabetic dog with chronic membranous glomerulopathy treated with continuous intraperitoneal insulin infusion. *Am. J. Vet. Res.* 43: 2044, 1982.
187. Jennette, J. C., and Huffman, K. A. Concurrent membranous glomerulopathy and diabetes mellitus (Letter). *Arch. Intern. Med.* 141: 1386, 1981.
188. Jennette, J. C., Iskandar, S. S., and Dalldorf, F. G. Pathologic differentiation between lupus and nonlupus membranous glomerulopathy. *Kidney Int.* 24: 377, 1983.
189. Jennette, J. C., Newman, W. J., and Diaz-Buxo, J. A. Overlapping IgA and membranous nephropathy. *Am. J. Clin. Pathol.* 88(1): 74, 1987.
190. Jensen, H., and Jensen, E. Steroid treatment of the nephrotic syndrome in adults. *Acta Med. Scand.* 182: 741, 1967.
191. Jezersek, P., and Ferluga, D. Nephrotic syndrome induced by D-penicillamine therapy. *Int. Urol. Nephrol.* 11: 349, 1979.
192. Jones, B., and Fowler, J. Membranous nephropathy associated with sarcoidosis. *Nephron* 52(1): 101, 1989.
193. Jones, D. B. Nephrotic glomerulonephritis. *Am. J. Pathol.* 33: 313, 1957.
194. Jordan, S. C., Buckingham, B., Sakai, R., et al. Studies of immune-complex glomerulonephritis mediated by human thyroglobulin. *N. Engl. J. Med.* 304: 1212, 1981.
195. Joyce, D. A., Beilin, L. J., and Vandongen, R. Captopril induced nephrotic syndrome (Letter). *Med. J. Aust.* 1: 190, 1981.
196. Kallen, R. J., Lee, S.-K., and Aronson, A. J. Idiopathic membranous glomerulopathy preceding the emergence of systemic lupus erythematosus in two children. *J. Pediatr.* 90: 72, 1977.
197. Kaplan, B. S., Klassen, J., and Gault, M. H. Glomerular injury in patients with neoplasia. *Annu. Rev. Med.* 27: 117, 1976.
198. Kasai, N., Parbtani, A., Cameron, J. S., et al. Platelet-aggregating immune complexes in idiopathic glomerulonephritis and SLE. *Proc. Eur. Dial. Transplant. Assoc.* 17: 621, 1980.
199. Katz, S. M., Swartz, C., Pitone, J., et al. Membranous glomerulonephritis in renal allografts (Letter). *N. Engl. J. Med.* 302: 1206, 1980.
200. Kawano, M., Nomura, H., Iwainaka, Y., et al. Bucillamine-associated membranous nephropathy in a patient with rheumatoid arthritis. *Nippon Jinzo Gakkai Shi* 32(7): 817, 1990.
201. Kerjaschki, D., and Farqhuar, M. G. The pathogenic antigen of Heymann nephritis is a membrane glycoprotein of the renal proximal tubular brush border. *Proc. Natl. Acad. Sci. U.S.A.* 79: 5557, 1982.
202. Kerjaschki, D., and Farqhuar, M. G. Immunocytochemical localization of the Heymann nephritis antigen (GP 330) in glomerular epithelial cells of normal Lewis rats. *J. Exp. Med.* 157: 667, 1983.
203. Kerjaschki, D., Schulze, M., Binder, S., et al. Transcellular transport and membrane insertion of the C5b-9 membrane attack complex of complement by glomerular epithelial cells in experimental membranous nephropathy. *J. Immunol.* 143(2): 546, 1989.
204. Kerpen, H. O., Bhat, J. G., Feiner, H. D., et al. Membranous nephropathy associated with renal cell carcinoma. Evidence against a role of renal tubular or tumor antibodies in pathogenesis. *Am. J. Med.* 64: 863, 1978.
205. Kibukamusoke, J. W., Davies, D. R., and Hutt, M. S. R. Membranous nephropathy due to skin-lightening cream. *Br. Med. J.* 2: 646, 1974.
206. Kida, H., Asamoto, T., and Hattori, N. Long-term prognosis of membranous nephropathy. Abstr. CN-073, *8th International Congress of Nephrology,* Athens, June 7–12, 1981.
207. Kida, H., Asamoto, T., Yokoyama, H., et al. Long-term prognosis of membranous nephropathy. *Clin. Nephrol.* 25(2): 64, 1986.
208. Klassen, J., Elwood, C., and Grossberg, A. L. Evolution of membranous nephropathy into anti-glomerular-basement-membrane glomerulonephritis. *N. Engl. J. Med.* 290: 1340, 1974.
209. Kleiknecht, C., Levy, M., Gagnadoux, M. F., et al. Membranous glomerulonephritis with extrarenal disorders in children. *Medicine* 58: 219, 1979.
210. Kleinknecht, C., Levy, M., Peix, A., et al. Membranous glomerulonephritis and hepatitis B surface antigen in

children. *J. Pediatr.* 95: 946, 1979.
211. Klouda, P. T., Manos, J., Acheson, E. J., et al. Strong association between idiopathic membranous nephropathy and HLA-DRW3. *Lancet* 2:770, 1979.
212. Kobayashi, Y., Fujii, K., Hiki, Y., et al. Coexistence of IgA nephropathy and membranous nephropathy. *Acta Pathol. Jpn.* 35(5): 1293, 1985.
213. Kobayashi, K., Harada, A., Onoyama, K., et al. Idiopathic membranous glomerulonephritis associated with diabetes mellitus: Light, immunofluorescence and electron microscopic study. *Nephron* 28: 163, 1981.
214. Kobayashi, Y., Tateno, S., Shigematsu, H., et al. Prednisone treatment in non-nephrotic patients with idiopathic membranous nephropathy. *Nephron* 30: 210, 1982.
215. Koethe, J. D., Gerig, J. S., Glickman, J. L., et al. Progression of membranous nephropathy to acute crescentic rapidly progressive glomerulonephritis and response to pulse methylprednisolone. *Am. J. Nephrol.* 6(3): 224, 1986.
216. Koyama, A., Niwa, Y., Shigematsu, H., et al. Studies on passive serum sickness. II. Factors determining the localization of antigen–antibody complexes in the murine renal glomerulus. *Lab. Invest.* 38: 253, 1978.
217. Kurki, P., Helve, T., von Bonsdorff, M., et al. Transformation of membranous glomerulonephritis into crescentic glomerulonephritis with glomerular basement membrane antibodies. Serial determinations of anti-GBM before the transformation. *Nephron* 38: 134, 1984.
218. Lagrue, G., Bernard, D., Bariety, J., et al. Traitment par le chlorambucil et l'azathioprine dans les glomerulonephritis primitives. *J. Urol. Nephrol.* (Paris) 9: 655, 1975.
219. Lai, F. M., Tam, J. S., Li, P. K., et al. Replication of hepatitis B virus with corticosteroid therapy in hepatitis B virus related membranous nephropathy. *Virchows Arch.* 414(3): 279, 1989.
220. Lai, K. N., Lai, F. M., Lo, S. T., et al. IgA nephropathy and membranous nephropathy associated with hepatitis B surface antigenemia. *Hum. Pathol.* 18(4): 411, 1987.
221. Lai, K. N., Lo, S. T., and Lai, F. M. Immunohistochemical study of the membrane attack complex of complement and S-protein in idiopathic and secondary membranous nephropathy. *Am. J. Pathol.* 135(3): 469, 1989.
222. Lai, K. N., Tam, J. S., Lin, H. J., et al. The therapeutic dilemma of the usage of corticosteroid in patients with membranous nephropathy and persistent hepatitis B virus surface antigenaemia. *Nephron* 54(1): 12, 1990.
223. Lal, S. M., Brooks, C. S., Luger, A. M., et al. Systemic mastocytosis associated with membranous nephropathy and peripheral neuropathy. *Am. J. Kidney Dis.* 12(6): 538, 1988.
224. Latham, P., Poucell, S., Koresaar, A., et al. Idiopathic membranous glomerulopathy in Canadian children: A clinicopathologic study. *J. Pediatr.* 101: 682, 1982.
225. Laurent, B., Berthoux, F. C., LePetit, J. C., et al. Immunogenetics and immunopathology of human membranous glomerulonephritis. *Proc. Eur. Dial. Transplant. Assoc.* 19: 629, 1983.
226. Lee, H. S., and Koh, H. I. Hepatitis B e antigen-associated membranous nephropathy. *Nephron* 52(4): 356, 1989.
227. Lee, J. C., Dushkin, M., Eyring, E. J., et al. Renal lesions associated with gold therapy. Light and electron microscopic studies. *Arthritis Rheum.* 8: 1, 1965.
228. Lee, J. C., Yamauchi, H., and Hopper, J. The association of cancer and the nephrotic syndrome. *Ann. Intern. Med.* 64: 41, 1966.
229. Lemmer, J. P., and Irby, W. R. Coexistence of HLA-B27 ankylosing spondylitis and DR4 seropositive nodular rheumatoid arthritis in patient with membranous nephropathy. *J. Rheumatol.* 8: 661, 1981.
230. Lentz, R. D., Michael, A. F., and Friend, P. S. Membranous transformation of lupus nephritis. *Clin. Immunol. Immunopathol.* 19: 131, 1981.
231. Le Petit, J. C., Laurent, B., and Berthoux, F. C. HLA-DR3 and idiopathic membranous nephritis (IMN) association. *Tissue Antigens* 20: 227, 1982.
232. Levy, M., Gagnadoux, M. F., Beziau, A., et al. Membranous glomerulonephritis associated with anti-tubular and anti-alveolar basement membrane antibodies. *Clin. Nephrol.* 10: 158, 1978.
233. Levy, M., and Kleinknecht, C. Membranous glomerulonephritis and hepatitis B virus infection. *Nephron* 26: 259, 1980.
234. Levy, M., Kleinknecht, C., and Peix, A. Membranous nephropathy and HBs Ag (Letter). *Lancet* 1: 113, 1979.
235. Lewis, E. J. Captopril and membranous glomerulopathy (Letter). *J.A.M.A.* 252: 900, 1984.
236. Lewis, M. G., Loughridge, L. W., and Phillips, T. M. Immunological studies in nephrotic syndrome associated with extrarenal malignant disease. *Lancet* ii: 134, 1972.
237. Libit, S. A., Burke, B., and Michael, A. F. Extramembranous glomerulonephritis in childhood: Relationship to systemic lupus erythematosus. *J. Pediatr.* 88: 394, 1976.
238. Lieberthal, W., Bernard, D. B., Donohoe, J. F., et al. Rapid recurrence of membranous nephropathy in a related renal allograft. *Clin. Nephrol.* 12: 222, 1979.
239. Lin, C. Y., and Lo, S. C. Treatment of hepatitis B virus–associated membranous nephropathy with adenine arabinoside and thymic extract. *Kidney Int.* 39(2): 301, 1991.
240. Lin, J. T., Wada, H., Maeda, H., et al. Mechanism of hematuria in glomerular disease. An electron microscopic study in a case of diffuse membranous glomerulonephritis. *Nephron* 35: 68, 1983.
241. Lindell, A., Dennebert, T., Enestrom, S., et al. Membranous glomerulonephritis induced by 2-mercaptopropionylglycine (2-MPG). *Clin. Nephrol.* 34(3): 108, 1990.
242. Linshaw, M. A., Gruskin, A. B. Management of the nephrotic syndrome. *Clin. Pediatr.* 13: 45, 1974.
243. Llach, F. Thromboembolic complications in nephrotic syndrome. Coagulation abnormalities, renal vein thrombosis, and other conditions. *Postgrad. Med.* 1: 111, 116, 121, 1984.
244. Llach, F., Arieff, A. I., and Massry, S. Renal vein thrombosis and nephrotic syndrome. *Ann. Intern. Med.* 83: 8, 1975.
245. Llach, F., Koffler, A., Finck, E., et al. On the incidence of renal vein thrombosis in the nephrotic syndrome. *Arch. Intern. Med.* 137: 333, 1977.
246. Llach, F., Papper, S., and Massry, S. G. The clinical spectrum of renal vein thrombosis: Acute and Chronic. *Am. J. Med.* 69: 819, 1980.
247. Losito, A., Bucciarello, E., Massi-Benedetti, F., et al. Membranous glomerulonephritis in congenital syphilis. *Clin. Nephrol.* 12: 32, 1979.
248. Lyle, W. H. Penicillamine. *Clin. Rheum. Dis.* 5: 569, 1979.
249. MacTier, R., Boulton-Jones, J. M., Payton, C. D., et al. The natural history of membranous nephropathy in the West of Scotland. *Q. J. Med.* 60(232): 793, 1986.
250. Madaio, M. P., Adler, S., Groggel, G. C., et al. Charge selective properties of the glomerular capillary wall in-

fluence antibody binding in rat membranous nephropathy. *Clin. Immunol. Immunopathol.* 39(1): 131, 1986.

251. Maggiore, Q., Bartolomeo, F., and L'Abbate, A. Hepatitis B antigen glomerular deposits in glomerulonephritis: Fact or artifact? *Kidney Int.* 19: 579, 1981.
252. Mailloux, L. U., Susin, M., Stein, H. L., et al. Nephrotic syndrome, membranous nephropathy, and renal vein thrombosis. Long-term follow-up. *N.Y. State J. Med.* 78: 1873, 1978.
253. Makker, S. P., and Moorthy, B. In situ immune complex formation in isolated perfused kidney using homologous antibody. *Lab. Invest.* 44: 1, 1981.
254. Mallick, N. P., Short, C. D., and Manos, J. Clinical membranous nephropathy. *Nephron* 34: 209, 1983.
255. Manos, J., Short, C. D., Acheson, E. J., et al. Relapsing idiopathic membranous nephropathy. *Clin. Nephrol.* 18: 286, 1982.
256. Mariani, A. F., Clifton, S., Davies, D. J., et al. Membranous glomerulonephritis associated with sarcoidosis. *Aust. N.Z. J. Med.* 8: 420, 1978.
257. Martini, A., Scotta, M. S., Notarangelo, L. D., et al. Membranous glomerulopathy and chronic small-intestinal enteropathy associated with autoantibodies directed against renal tubular basement membrane and the cytoplasm of intestinal epithelial cells. *Acta Paediatr. Scand.* 72: 931, 1983.
258. Mathieson, P. W., Turner, A. N., and Maidment, C. G. Prednisolone and chlorambucil treatment in idiopathic membranous nephropathy with deteriorating renal function. *Lancet* 2(8616): 869, 1988.
259. Matsumoto, K., Osakabe, K., and Hatano, M. Impaired cell-mediated immunity in idiopathic membranous nephropathy mediated by suppressor cells. *Clin. Nephrol.* 19: 213, 1983.
260. Matsumoto, K., Osakabe, K., Katayama, H., et al. Cell-mediated immunity in idiopathic membranous nephropathy. *Int. Arch. Allergy Appl. Immunol.* 66: 310, 1981.
261. Matsumoto, K., Osakabe, K., Katayama, H., et al. Concanavalin-A-induced suppressor cell activity in idiopathic membranous nephropathy. *Int. Arch. Allergy Appl. Immunol.* 69: 26, 1982.
262. McCluskey, R. T., Ingelfinger, J. Membranous remission in persistent pathogenesis. *N. Engl. J. Med.* 294: 127B, 1976.
263. McCulloch, A. J., Morley, A. R., Wilkinson, R., et al. Nodular regenerative hyperplasia of the liver with membranous glomerulonephritis. *Postgrad. Med. J.* 57: 402, 1981.
264. McGinn, J. T., McGinn, T. G., Cherubin, C. E., et al. Nephrotic syndrome in drug addicts. *N.Y. State J. Med.* 74: 92, 1974.
265. McLeish, K. R., Smith, M. R., and Gohara, A. F. Non-Hodgkin's lymphoma and membranous nephropathy in mixed connective tissue disease. *Am. J. Med. Sci.* 290(40): 152, 1985.
266. Meroni, M., Volpi, A., Usberti, M., et al. Two brothers with idiopathic membranous nephropathy and familial sensorineural deafness. *Am. J. Kidney Dis.* 15(3): 269, 1990.
267. Michielsen, P., Vanrenterghem, Y., and Roels, L. Treatment of Chronic Glomerulonephritis with Indomethacin. In R. Kluthe, A. Vogt, and S. R. Batsford (eds.), *Glomerulonephritis.* New York: Wiley, 1977. P. 49.
268. Miller, R. B., Harrington, J. T., and Ramos, C. P. Long term results of steroid therapy in adults with idiopathic nephrotic syndrome. *Am. J. Med.* 46: 919, 1969.
269. Miller, W. E., Vidt, D. G., Deodhar, S. D., et al. Selectivity index as a guide to treatment in heavy proteinuria. *Am. J. Med. Sci.* 258: 386, 1969.
270. Milner, L. S., Dusheiko, G. M., Jacobs, D., et al. Biochemical and serological characteristics of children with membranous nephropathy due to hepatitis B virus infection: Correlation with hepatitis B e antigen, hepatitis B DNA and hepatitis D. *Nephron.* 49: 184, 1988.
271. Min, K. W., Song, J., Flynn, C. T., et al. Membranous glomerulonephropathy (MGN) with pulmonary arterial thrombosis: A case report. *Iowa Med.* 74: 63, 1984.
272. Mitas, J. A., II, Frank, L. R., Swerdlin, A. R., et al. Crescentic glomerulonephritis complicating idiopathic membranous glomerulonephropathy. *South. Med. J.* 76: 664, 1983.
273. Moorthy, A. V., Zimmerman, S., and Burkholder, P. M. Association of crescentic glomerulonephritis with membranous glomerulonephropathy: A report of three cases. *Clin. Nephrol.* 6: 320, 1976.
274. Moseley, H. L., and Whaley, K. Control of complement activation in membranous and membranoproliferative glomerulonephritis. *Kidney Int.* 17: 535, 1980.
275. Muller, G. A., Muller, C., Liebau, G., et al. Strong association of idiopathic membranous nephropathy (IMN) with HLA-DR 3 and MT-2 without involvement of HLA-B 1B and no association to DR3 and MT-2 without involvement of HLA-B 1B and no association to BfF1. *Tissue Antigens* 17: 332, 1981.
276. Murphy, B. F., Fairley, K. F., and Kincaid-Smith, P. S. Idiopathic membranous glomerulonephritis: Long-term follow-up in 139 cases. *Clin. Nephrol.* 30(4): 175, 1988.
277. Murphy, B. F., Gonzales, M. F., Ebeling, P., et al. Membranous glomerulonephritis and Landry-Guillain-Barré syndrome. *Am. J. Kidney Dis.* 8(4): 267, 1986.
278. Muthuswami, S. G., Tannen, R. L., and Gikas, P. W. Membranous glomerulonephritis in renal allografts (Letter). *N. Engl. J. Med.* 302: 1207, 1980.
279. Nagata, K., Fujita, M., Aoyama, R., et al. A case of membranous glomerulonephritis in which positive to negative change of hepatitis B e antigen in glomeruli was observed. *Int. J. Pediatr. Nephrol.* 2: 103, 1981.
280. Naruse, T., Kitamure, K., Miyakawa, Y., et al. Deposition of renal tubular epithelial antigen along with the glomerular capillary walls of patients with membranous glomerulonephritis. *J. Immunol.* 110: 1163, 1973.
281. Naruse, T., Miyakawa, Y., Kitamura, K., et al. Membranous glomerulonephritis mediated by renal tubular epithelial antigen–antibody complex. *J. Allergy Clin. Immunol.* 45: 311, 1974.
282. Nauta, J., de-Heer, E., Baldwin, W. M., 3rd., et al. Transplacental induction of membranous nephropathy in a neonate. *Pediatr. Nephrol.* 4(2): 111, 1990.
283. Nelson, D. C., and Birchmore, D. A. Renal vein thrombosis associated with nephrotic syndrome and gold therapy in rheumatoid arthritis. *South. Med. J.* 72: 1616, 1979.
284. Nicholson, G. D., Amin, U. F., and Alleyne, G. A. O. Membranous glomerulonephropathy with crescents. *Clin. Nephrol.* 5: 198, 1975.
285. Nicholson, G. D., Prussia, P. R., Sirarajan, S., et al. Membranous glomerulonephritis and the nephrotic syndrome in a patient with Landry-Guillain-Barré-Strohl syndrome. *West Indian Med. J.* 38(1): 51, 1989.
286. Niles, J., Collins, B., Baird, L., et al. Antibodies with a renal glycoprotein and deposits in membranous nephritis (Abstract). *Kidney Int.* 31: 338, 1987.

287. Noel, L. H., Aucouturier, P., Monteiro, R. C., et al. Glomerular and serum immunoglobulin G subclasses in membranous nephropathy and anti-glomerular basement membrane nephritis. *Clin. Immunol. Immunopathol.* 46(2): 186, 1988.
288. Noel, L. H., Zanetti, M., Droz, D., and Barbanel, C. Long-term prognosis of idiopathic membranous glomerulonephritis. Study of 116 untreated patients. *Am. J. Med.* 66: 82, 1979.
289. Nyberg, M., Petterson, E., Tallqvist, G., et al. Survival in idiopathic glomerulonephritis. *Acta Pathol. Microbiol. Scand.* [*A*] 88: 319, 1980.
290. Oite, T., Shimizu, F., Kihara, I., et al. An active model of immune complex glomerulonephritis in the rat employing cationized antigen. *Am. J. Pathol.* 112: 185, 1983.
291. Okada, K., Kawakami, K., Miyao, M., et al. Ultrastructural alterations of glomerular anionic sites in idiopathic membranous glomerulonephritis. *Clin. Nephrol.* 26(1): 7, 1986.
292. Okuda, S., Oh, Y., Tsuruda, H., et al. Rapidly progressive renal deterioration in partially nephrectomized rats with experimental membranous nephropathy. *Nephron* 41(4): 359, 1985.
293. Olbing, H. J., Greifer, I., and Bennett, B. P. Idiopathic membranous nephropathy in children. *Kidney Int.* 3: 381, 1973.
294. Olesnicky, L., Doty, S. B., Bertani, T., et al. Tubular microfibrils in the glomeruli of membranous nephropathy. *Arch. Pathol. Lab. Med.* 108: 902, 1984.
295. Oliveira, D. B., Foster, G., and Savill, J. Membranous nephropathy caused by mercury-containing skin lightening cream. *Postgrad. Med. J.* 63(738): 303, 1987.
296. Oliver-Rotellar, J. A., Garcia-Ruiz, C., and Martinez-Vea, A. Response to prednisone in membranous nephropathy associated with sarcoidosis. *Nephron* 54(2): 195, 1990.
297. Ooi, B. S., Ooi, Y. M., and Hsu, A. Diminished synthesis of immunoglobulin by peripheral lymphocytes of patients with idiopathic membranous glomerulonephropathy. *J. Clin. Invest.* 65: 789, 1980.
298. Ooi, B. S., Ooi, Y. M., and Pollak, V. E. Identification of circulating immune complexes in a subpopulation of patients with membranous glomerulonephropathy. *Clin. Immunol. Immunopathol.* 16: 447, 1980.
299. Ooi, Y. M., Ooi, B. S., and Pollak, V. E. Relationship of levels of circulating immune complexes to histologic patterns of nephritis: A comparative study of membranous glomerulopathy and diffuse proliferative glomerulonephritis. *J. Lab. Clin. Med.* 90: 891, 1977.
300. O'Regan, S., Fong, J. S. C., DeChadarevian, J. P., et al. Treponemal antigens in congenital and acquired syphilitic nephritis. *Ann. Intern. Med.* 85: 235, 1976.
301. Palla, R., Cirami, C., Panichi, V., et al. Intravenous immunoglobulin therapy of membranous nephropathy: Efficacy & safety. *Clin. Nephrol.* 35: 98, 1991.
302. Panayi, G. S., Wooley, P., and Batchelor, J. R. Genetic basis of rheumatoid diseases. HLA antigens, disease manifestations and toxic reactions to drugs. *Br. Med. J.* 2: 1326, 1978.
303. Papiha, S. S., Pareek, S. K., Rodger, R. S., et al. HLA-A, B, DR and Bf allotypes in patients with idiopathic membranous nephropathy. *Kidney Int.* 31(1): 130, 1987.
304. Passerini, P., Pasquali, S., Cesana, B., et al. Long-term outcome of patients with membranous nephropathy after complete remission of proteinuria. *Nephrol. Dial. Transplant.* 4(6): 525, 1989.
305. Pettersson, E., Tornroth, T., and Miettinen, A. Simultaneous anti-glomerular basement membrane and membranous glomerulonephritis case report and literature reviews. *Clin. Immunol. Immunopathol.* 31: 171, 1984.
306. Pettersson, E., von-Willebrand, E., and Honkanen, E. Immunological mechanisms in glomerulonephritis. *Scand. J. Urol. Nephrol.* [*Suppl.*] 90: 29, 1985.
307. Pierides, A. M., and Kerr, D. N. Idiopathic membranous nephropathy. *Nephron* 20: 301, 1978.
308. Pierides, A. J., Malasit, P., and Morley, A. R. Idiopathic membranous nephropathy. *Q. J. Med.* 46: 163, 1977.
309. Pohl, M. A., MacLaurin, J. P., and Alfidi, R. J. Renal vein thrombosis and the nephrotic syndrome. *Kidney Int.* 12: 472, 1977.
310. Pollak, V. E., Rosen, S., Pirani, C. L., et al. Natural history of lipoid nephrosis and of membranous glomerulonephritis. *Ann. Intern. Med.* 69: 1171, 1968.
311. Ponticelli, C., Zucchelli, P., Imbasciati, E., et al. Controlled trial of monthly alternated courses of steroid and chlorambucil for idiopathic membrane nephropathy. *Proc. Eur. Dial. Transplant. Assoc.* 19: 717, 1983.
312. Ponticelli, C., Zucchelli, P., Imbasciati, E., et al. Controlled trial of methylprednisolone and chlorambucil in idiopathic membranous nephropathy. *N. Engl. J. Med.* 310: 946, 1984.
313. Ponticelli, C., Zucchelli, P., Passerini, P., et al. A randomized trial of methylprednisolone and chlorambucil in idiopathic membranous nephropathy. *N. Engl. J. Med.* 320(1): 8, 1989.
314. Powell, K. C., and Meadows, R. The nephrotic syndrome in New Guinea—A clinical and histological spectrum. *Aust. N.Z. J. Med.* 1: 363, 1971.
315. Prins, E. J. L., Hoorntje, S. J., Weening, J. J., et al. Nephrotic syndrome in patients on captopril. *Lancet* 2: 306, 1979.
316. Quatacker, J., Praet, M., and Matthys, E. Ultrastructural alterations in the sialic acid distribution in minimal change disease and membranous glomerulonephritis. *Pathol. Res. Pract.* 182(2): 188, 1987.
317. Rai, G. S., Hamlyn, A. N., Dahl, M. G., et al. Primary biliary cirrhosis, cutaneous capillaritis, and IgM-associated membranous glomerulonephritis. *Br. Med. J.* 1: 817, 1977.
318. Ramirez, F., Brouhard, B. H., Travis, L. B., et al. Idiopathic membranous nephropathy in children. *J. Pediatr.* 101: 677, 1982.
319. Ramzy, M. H., Cameron, J. S., and Turner, D. R. The long-term outcome of idiopathic membranous nephropathy. *Clin. Nephrol.* 16: 13, 1981.
320. Randall, R. E., Tung, M. Y., Abukurah, A. R., et al. Responsiveness of adult idiopathic membranous nephropathy to cyclophosphamide. *Abstracts* (Fourth Annual Meeting), *Am. Soc. Nephrol.*, 1970. P. 65.
321. Rashid, H. U., Papiha, S. S., Agroyannis, B., et al. The associations of HLA and other genetic markers with glomerulonephritis. *Hum. Genet.* 63: 38, 1983.
322. Rastogi, S. P., Hart-Mercer, J., and Kerr, D. N. S. Idiopathic membranous glomerulonephritis in adults. Remission following steroid therapy. *Q. J. Med.* 38: 335, 1969.
323. Reitsma, D., Gratama, S., and Vroom, T. M. Clinical remission of membranous glomerulonephritis in primary biliary cirrhosis with cutaneous vasculitis. *Br. Med. J.* [*Clin. Res.*] 288: 27, 1984.
324. Richet, G., Fillastre, J. P., Morel-Maroger, L., et al. Change from diffuse proliferative to membranous glo-

merulonephritis. Serial biopsy in four cases. *Kidney Int.* 5: 5771, 1976.

325. Robinson, M. F., Roberts, J. L., Jones, J. V., et al. Circulating immune complex assays in patients with lupus and membranous glomerulonephritis. *Clin. Immunol. Immunopathol.* 14: 348, 1979.
326. Roccatello, D., Coppo, R., Amoroso, A., et al. Failure to relate mononuclear phagocyte system function to HLA-A, B, C, DR, DQ antigens in membranous nephropathy. *Am. J. Kidney Dis.* 9(6): 470, 1987.
327. Rodriguez-Soriano, I., Fidalgo, I., Camarero, C., et al. Juvenile cirrhosis and membranous glomerulonephritis in child with alpha-I antitrypsin deficiency PiSz. *Acta Pediatr. Scand.* 67: 793, 1978.
328. Rodriguez-Soriano, J., Fidalgo, I., Camarero, C., et al. Juvenile cirrhosis and membranous glomerulonephritis in child with alpha-1 antitrypsin deficiency PiSz. *Acta Pediatr. Scand.* 67: 793, 1978.
329. Rose, J. D. Membranous glomerulonephritis, dermatomyositis, and bronchial carcinoma. *Br. Med. J.* 2: 641, 1979.
330. Rosemann, E., Pollak, V. E., and Pirani, C. L. Renal vein thrombosis in the adult: A clinical and pathologic study based on renal biopsies. *Medicine* 47: 269, 1968.
331. Rosenmann, E., Brisson, M. L., Bercovitch, D. D., et al. Atypical membranous glomerulonephritis with fibrillar subepithelial deposits in a patient with malignant lymphoma. *Nephron* 48(3): 226, 1988.
332. Rothschild, E., and Chatenoud, L. T-cell subset modulation of immunoglobulin production in IgA nephropathy and membranous glomerulonephritis. *Kidney Int.* 25: 557, 1984.
333. Rovenska, E., Kapeller, K., and Rossmann, P. Gold nephropathy in rheumatoid arthritis and in juvenile chronic arthritis. *Czech. Med.* 125, 1979.
334. Row, P. G., Cameron, J. S., Turner, O. R., et al. Membranous nephropathy: Long-term follow-up and association with neoplasia. *Q. J. Med.* (New Series) 44: 207, 1975.
335. Rubin, R. J., Pinn, V. W., and Barnes, B. A. Recurrent idiopathic membranous glomerulonephritis. *Transplantation* 24: 4, 1977.
336. Ruggieri, G., Barsotti, P., Coppola, G., et al. Membranous nephropathy associated with giant lymph node hyperplasia: A case report with histological and ultrastructural studies. *Am. J. Nephrol.* 10(4): 323, 1990.
337. Salant, D. J., Belok, S., Madaio, M. P., et al. A new role for complement in experimental membranous nephropathy in rats. *J. Clin. Invest.* 66: 1339, 1980.
338. Salant, D. J., Darby, C., and Couser, W. G. Experimental membranous glomerulonephritis in rats. Quantitative studies of glomerular immune deposit formation in isolated glomeruli and whole animals. *J. Clin. Invest.* 66: 71, 1980.
339. Salant, D. J., Madaio, M. D., Adler, S., et al. Altered glomerular permeability induced by $F(ab^{+})_2$ and Fab′ antibodies to rat renal tubular epithelial antigen. *Kidney Int.* 21: 36, 1981.
340. Samuels, B., Lee, J. C., Engleman, E. P., et al. Membranous nephropathy in patients with rheumatoid arthritis: Relationship to gold therapy. *Medicine* 57: 319, 1978.
341. Sanchez Ibarrola, A., Sobrini, B., Guisantes, J., et al. Membranous glomerulonephritis secondary to hydatid disease. *Am. J. Med.* 70: 311, 1981.
342. Sato, K., Oguchi, H., Hora, K., et al. Idiopathic membranous nephropathy in two brothers. *Nephron* 46(2): 174, 1987.
343. Schwartz, M. M., and Cotran, P. S. Primary renal disease in transplant recipients. *Hum. Pathol.* 7: 455, 1976.
344. Schwartzberg, M., Burnstein, S. L., Calabro, J. J., et al. The development of membranous glomerulonephritis in a patient with rheumatoid arthritis and Sjogren's syndrome. *J. Rheumatol.* 6: 65, 1979.
345. Seedat, Y. I. C., Simjez, A. E., and Naido, D. R. Nephrotic syndrome due to cosmetics containing mercury. *S. Afr. Med. J.* 47: 506, 1973.
346. Seedat, Y. K. The nephrotic syndrome in Bantu and Indian patients. A clinicopathological study. *S. Afr. Med. J.* 47: 2237, 1973.
347. Seedat, Y. K. Nephrotic syndrome in the Africans and Indians of South Africa. A ten year study. *Trans. R. Soc. Trop. Med. Hyg.* 12: 506, 1978.
348. Seggie, J., Nathoo, K., and Davies, P. G. Association of hepatitis B (HBs) antigenaemia and membranous glomerulonephritis in Zimbabwean children. *Nephron* 38: 115, 1984.
349. Sellars, L., Siamopoulos, K., Wilkinson, R., et al. Renal biopsy appearances in rheumatoid disease. *Clin. Nephrol.* 20: 114, 1983.
350. Sennesael, J., Van-den-Houte, K., and Verbeelen, D. Reversible membranous glomerulonephritis associated with ketoprofen. *Clin. Nephrol.* 26(4): 213, 1986.
351. Sharpe, A. R., and Unger, A. M. The nephrotic syndrome. *Arch. Intern. Med.* 104: 684, 1959.
352. Sharpstone, P., Ogg, C. S., and Cameron, J. S. Nephrotic syndrome due to primary renal disease in adults. *Br. Med. J.* 2: 533, 1969.
353. Shearman, J. D., Yin, Z. G., Aarons, I., et al. The effect of treatment with prednisolone or cyclophosphamide-warfarin-dipyridamole combination on the outcome of patients with membranous nephropathy. *Clin. Nephrol.* 30(6): 320, 1988.
354. Shearn, M. A., Biava, C., and Hopper, J., Jr. Mesangial deposits (by electron microscopy) in idiopathic membranous glomerulonephritis. (Letter) *N. Engl. J. Med.* 301: 212, 1979.
355. Shearn, M. A., Hopper, J., and Biava, C. G. Membranous lupus nephropathy initially seen as idiopathic membranous nephropathy. *Arch. Intern. Med.* 140: 1521, 1980.
356. Shehadeh, I. H., Demers, L. M., Abt, A. B., et al. Indomethacin and the nephrotic syndrome. *J.A.M.A.* 241: 1264, 1979.
357. Short, C. D., Feehally, J., Gokal, R., et al. Familial membranous nephropathy. *Br. Med. J.* 289: 1500, 1984.
358. Short, C. D., Solomon, L. R., Gokal, R., et al. Methylprednisolone in patients with membranous nephropathy and declining renal function. *Q. J. Med.* 65(247): 929, 1987.
359. Shull, R. M., Stowe, C. M., Osborne, C. A., et al. Membranous glomerulonephropathy and nephrotic syndrome associated with iatrogenic metallic mercury poisoning in a cat. *Vet. Hum. Toxicol.* 23: 1, 1981.
360. Shwe, T. Immune complexes in glomeruli of patients with leprosy. *Lepr. Rev.* 42: 282, 1972.
361. Silver, M. M., Rance, C. F., Middleton, P. J., et al. Hepatitis B-associated membranous glomerulonephritis in a child. *Am. J. Clin. Pathol.* 72: 1034, 1979.
362. Silverberg, D. S., Kidd, E. G., Schnitka, T. K., et al. Gold nephropathy, a clinical and pathologic study. *Arthritis Rheum.* 13: 812, 1970.
363. Slusarczyk, J., Michalak, T., Nazarewica-de Mezer, T., et al. Membranous glomerulopathy associated with hepatitis B core antigen immune complexes in children. *Am.*

J. Pathol. 98: 29, 1980.
364. Smith, W. E., and McMorrow, R. B. Membranous glomerulonephritis in renal allografts (Letter). *N. Engl. J. Med.* 302: 1207, 1980.
365. Solling, J. Circulating immune complexes in glomerulonephritis: A longitudinal study. *Clin. Nephrol.* 20: 177, 1983.
366. Solling, J., and Olsen, S. Circulating immune complexes in glomerulonephritis. *Clin. Nephrol.* 16: 63, 1981.
367. Sonkodi, S., Jarmay, K., Korom, I., et al. Membranous nephropathy accompanied by angiolymphoid hyperplasia of the skin. *Nephron* 47(1): 32, 1987.
368. Srifvars, B. Hypothesis for the pathogenesis of sodium aurothiomalate (myocrisin) induced immune complex nephritis. *Scand. J. Rheumatol.* 8: 113, 1979.
369. Stachura, I., Whiteside, T. L., and Kelly, R. Circulating and deposited immune complexes in patients with glomerular diseases: Immunopathologic correlations. *Am. J. Pathol.* 103: 21, 1981.
370. Stahl, R. A., Adler, S., Baker, P. J., et al. Enhanced glomerular prostaglandin formation in experimental membranous nephropathy. *Kidney Int.* 31(5): 1126, 1987.
371. Steinmuller, D. R., Stilmant, M. M., Idelson, B. A., et al. DeNovo development of membranous nephropathy in cadaver renal allografts. *Clin. Nephrol.* 9: 210, 1978.
372. Sternlieb, I., Bennett, B., and Scheinberg, I. H. D-Penicillamine induced Goodpasture's syndrome in Wilson's disease. *Ann. Intern. Med.* 82: 673, 1975.
373. Stuhlinger, W. D., Verroust, P. J., and Morel-Maroger, L. Detection of circulating immune complexes in patients with various renal diseases. *Immunology* 30: 43, 1976.
374. Sturgill, B. C., and Shearlock, K. T. Membranous glomerulopathy and nephrotic syndrome after captopril therapy. *J.A.M.A.* 250: 2343, 1983.
375. Sugisaki, T., Kano, K., Brentjens, J. R., et al. Immune complexes in a renal allograft with de novo membranous nephropathy. *Transplantation* 34: 90, 1982.
376. Suki, W. N., and Chavez, A. Membranous nephropathy: Response to steroids and immunosuppression. *Am. J. Nephrol.* 1: 11, 1981.
377. Sunderrajan, S., Luger, A., and Bauer, J. H. Captopril-induced membranous glomerulopathy. *South. Med. J.* 76: 1294, 1983.
378. Takekoshi, Y., Tanaka, M., Miyakawa, Y., et al. Free "small" and IgG-associated "large" hepatitis B e antigen in the serum and glomerular capillary walls of two patients with membranous glomerulonephritis. *N. Engl. J. Med.* 300: 814, 1979.
379. Takekoshi, Y., Tanaka, M., Shida, N., et al. Strong association between membranous nephropathy and hepatitis-B surface antigenaemia in Japanese children. *Lancet* 2: 1065, 1978.
380. Tálamo, T. S., and Borochovitz, D. Membranous glomerulonephritis associated with the Guillain-Barré syndrome. *Am. J. Clin. Pathol.* 78: 563, 1982.
381. Tan, C. Y., Davies, M. G., and Marks, R. Co-existing dermatitis herpetiformis and membranous glomerulonephritis. *Clin. Exp. Dermatol.* 5: 177, 1980.
382. Tateno, S., Sakai, T., Kobayashi, Y., et al. Idiopathic membranous glomerulonephritis with crescents. *Acta Pathol. Jpn.* 31: 211, 1981.
383. Taube, D., Brown, Z., and Williams, D. G. Impaired lymphocyte and suppressor cell function in minimal change nephropathy, membranous, membranous nephropathy and focal glomerulosclerosis. *Clin. Nephrol.* 22: 176, 1984.
384. Taylor, T. G., Fisher, C., and Hoffbrand, B. I. Sarcoidosis and membranous glomerulonephritis: A significant association. *Br. Med. J.* 284: 1297, 1982.
385. Taylor, T. K., Senekjian, H. O., Knight, T. F., et al. Membranous nephropathy with epithelial crescents in a patient with pulmonary sarcoidosis. *Arch. Intern. Med.* 139: 1183, 1979.
386. Textor, S. C., Gephard, T. G. N., Bravo, E. L., et al. Membranous glomerulopathy associated with captopril therapy. *Am. J. Med.* 74: 705, 1983.
387. Thaiss, F., Schoeppe, W., Willaredt-Stoll, J. G., et al. Cyclosporin A prevents proteinuria in an active model of membranous nephropathy in rats. *Lab. Invest.* 61(6): 661, 1989.
388. Thorpe, L. W., and Cavallo, T. Renal tubule brush border antigens: Failure to confirm a pathogenetic role in human membranous glomerulonephritis. *J. Clin. Lab. Immunol.* 3: 125, 1980.
389. Tiggeler, R. G. W. L., Hulme, B., and Wijdereld, P. G. A. B. Effect of indomethacin on glomerular permeability in the nephrotic syndrome. *Kidney Int.* 16: 312, 1979.
390. Tiller, D. J., Clarkson, A. R., Mathew, T., et al. A prospective randomized trial in the use of cyclophosphamide, dipyridamole and warfarin in membranous and mesangiocapillary glomerulonephritis. *Proceedings of the 8th International Congress of Nephrology,* Athens, June 7–12, 1981. Pp. 345–351.
391. Tomura, S., Kashiwabara, H., Tuchida, H., et al. Strong association of idiopathic membranous nephropathy with HLA-DR2 and MT1 in Japanese. *Nephron* 36: 242, 1984.
392. Tornroth, T., Honkanen, E., and Pettersson, E. The evolution of membranous glomerulonephritis reconsidered: New insights from a study on relapsing disease. *Clin. Nephrol.* 28(3): 107, 1987.
393. Tornroth, T., Tallqvist, G., Pasternack, A., et al. Nonprogressive, histologically mild membranous glomerulonephritis appearing in all evolutionary phases as histologically "early" membranous glomerulonephritis. *Kidney Int.* 14: 511, 1978.
394. Trew, P. A., Biava, C. G., and Jacobs, R. D. Renal vein thrombosis in membranous glomerulonephropathy: Incidence and association. *Medicine* 57: 69, 1978.
395. Tu, W. H., Petitti, D. B., Biava, C. G., et al. Membranous nephropathy predictors of terminal renal failure. *Nephron* 36: 118, 1983.
396. Tubbs, R. R., Gephardt, G. N., McMahon, J. T., et al. Membranous glomerulonephritis associated with industrial mercury exposure. Study of pathogenetic mechanisms. *Am. J. Clin. Pathol.* 77: 409, 1982.
397. Van-Damme, B., Tardanico, R., Vanrenterghem, Y., et al. Adhesions, focal sclerosis, protein crescents, and capsular lesions in membranous nephropathy. *J. Pathol.* 161(1): 47, 1990.
398. Van-Damme, B., Tardanico, R., Vanrenterghem, V., et al. Comment on "Concurrent Focal Segmental Glomerulosclerosis and Membranous Nephropathy" by Amenta et al. *Clin. Nephrol.* 33(3): 152, 1990.
399. Van Der Woude, F. J., Piers, D. A., Van Der Giessen, M., et al. Abnormal reticuloendothelial function in patients with active vasculitis and idiopathic membranous glomerulopathy. A study with 99 mTc-labeled heat-damaged autologous red blood cells. *Eur. J. Nucl. Med.* 8: 60, 1983.
400. Vangelista, A., Tazzari, R., and Bonomini, V. Idiopathic membranous nephropathy in 2 twin brothers. *Nephron* 50(1): 79, 1988.
401. Vanrenterghem, Y., Roels, L., Verberckmoes, R., et al.

Treatment of chronic glomerulonephritis with a combination of indomethacin and cyclophosphamide. *Clin. Nephrol.* 4: 218, 1975.

402. Vasmant, D., Bensman, A., Baudon, J. J., et al. Global pancreatic and gastric deficiency after a familial membranous glomerulonephritis in a child treated by corticoids and chlorambucil for a long time (author's translation). *Ann. Med. Interne* 133: 276, 1982.
403. Vaughan, R. W., Demaine, A. G., and Welsh, K. I. A DQA1 allele is strongly associated with idiopathic membranous nephropathy. *Tissue Antigens* 34(5): 261, 1989.
404. Velosa, J. A., Torres, V. E., Wochos, D. N., et al. Treatment of nephrotic syndrome (NS) and focal segmental glomerulosclerosis (FSGS) or idiopathic membranous glomerulopathy (MGP) with meclofenamate (MCF). Preliminary experience. *Abstracts of the International Congress of Nephrology, 1984.* P. 138A.
405. Venkateswara, K., and Crosson, J. T. Idiopathic membranous glomerulonephritis in diabetic patients: Report of three cases and review of the literature. *Arch. Intern. Med.* 140: 624, 1980.
406. Verani, R., and Dan, M. Membranous glomerulonephritis in renal transplant. A case report and review of the literature. *Am. J. Nephrol.* 2: 316, 1982.
407. Verresen, L., Waer, M., Verberckmoes, R., et al. Primary sclerosing cholangitis associated with membranous nephropathy. *Ann. Intern. Med.* 108(6): 909, 1988.
408. Verroust, P. J. Kinetics of immune deposits in membranous nephropathy. *Kidney Int.* 35(6): 14118, 1989.
409. Via, C. S., Hasbargen, J. S., Moore, J., Jr., et al. Rheumatoid arthritis and membranous glomerulonephritis: A role for immune complex dissociative technique. *J. Rheumatol.* 11: 342, 1984.
410. Vialtel, P., Chenais, F., Desgeorges, P., et al. Membranous nephropathy associated with hydatid disease (Letter). *N. Engl. J. Med.* 304: 610, 1981.
411. Vogt, A., Schmidt, H. U., Takamiya, H., et al. 'In situ' immune complex nephritis and basic proteins. *Proc. Eur. Dial. Transplant. Assoc.* 17: 613, 1980.
412. Wagoner, R. D., Stanson, A. W., Holley, K. E., et al. Renal vein thrombosis in idiopathic membranous glomerulopathy and nephrotic syndrome: Incidence and significance. *Kidney Int.* 23: 368, 1983.
413. Wakabayashi, T., Akiyama, N., Ohtsubo, O., et al. Renal allografts with glomerulonephritic change and proteinuria. *Acta Pathol. Jpn.* 34: 1017, 1984.
414. Walshe, J. M. Toxic reactions to penicillamine in patients with Wilson's disease. *Postgraduate Med. J.* 44(Suppl.): 6, 1968.
415. Wang, F., Menon, A., Murugasu, R., et al. Membranous glomerulonephritis and chronic hepatitis. *Med. J. Malaysia* 32: 78, 1977.
416. Ward, H. J., and Koyle, M. A. Immunopathologic features of de novo membranous nephropathy in renal allografts. *Transplantation* 45(3): 524, 1988.
417. Warms, P. C., Rosenbaum, B. J., Michelis, M. F., et al. Idiopathic membranous glomerulonephritis occurring with diabetes mellitus. *Arch. Intern. Med.* 132: 735, 1973.
418. Warnhin, D. M., Rees, P. H., and Barr, R. D. Nairobi nephrosis; the nephrotic syndrome and skin lightening cream. *East Afr. Med. J.* 51: 953, 1974.
419. Watanabe, I., Whittier, F. C., Moore, J., et al. Gold nephropathy. Ultrastructural fluorescence and microanalytic studies of two patients. *Arch. Pathol. Lab. Med.* 100: 632, 1976.
420. Weber, J. P., Jr., and Cawley, L. P. Membranous glomerulonephropathy: Thyroid antigen-antibody immune complex MGN. *J. Kans. Med. Soc.* 82: 397, 1981.
421. Weetman, A. P., Pinching, A. J., Pussel, B. A., et al. Membranous glomerulonephritis and autoimmune thyroid disease. *Clin. Nephrol.* 15: 50, 1981.
422. Wehrmann, M., Bohle, A., Bogenschutz, O., et al. Long-term prognosis of chronic idiopathic membranous glomerulonephritis: An analysis of 334 cases with particular regard to tubulo-interstitial changes. *Clin. Nephrol.* 31(2): 67, 1989.
423. Weisenburger, D. D. Membranous nephropathy. Its association with multicentric angiofollicular lymph node hyperplasia. *Arch. Pathol. Lab. Med.* 103: 591, 1979.
424. Weiss, A. S., Markenson, J. A., Weiss, M. S., et al. Toxicity of DL-penicillamine in rheumatoid arthritis. A report of 63 patients including two with aplastic anemia and one with the nephrotic syndrome. *Am. J. Med.* 64: 114, 1978.
425. Weksler, M. E., Carey, T., Day, N., et al. Nephrotic syndrome in malignant melanoma. Demonstration of melanoma antigen–antibody complexes. *Kidney Int.* 6: 112a, 1974.
426. West, M. L., Jindal, K. K., and Bear, R. A. A controlled trial of cyclophosphamide in patients with membranous glomerulonephritis. *Kidney Int.* 32(4): 579, 1987.
427. White, C. A., Dillman, R. O., and Royston, I. Membranous nephropathy associated with an unusual phenotype of chronic lymphocytic leukemia. *Cancer* 52: 2253, 1983.
428. Williams, P. S., and Bone, J. M. Immunosuppression can arrest progressive renal failure due to idiopathic membranous glomerulonephritis. *Nephrol. Dial. Transplant.* 4(3): 181, 1989.
429. Wing, A. J., Hutt, M. S., and Kibukamusoke, J. W. Progression and remission in the nephrotic syndrome associated with quartan malaria in Uganda. *Q. J. Med.* 163: 273, 1972.
430. Witte, A. S., and Burke, J. F. Membranous glomerulonephritis associated with chronic progressive demyelinating neuropathy. *Neurology* 37(2): 342, 1987.
431. Woodroffe, A. J., Border, W. A., Theofilopoulos, A. N., et al. Detection of circulating immune complexes in patients with glomerulonephritis. *Kidney Int.* 12: 268, 1977.
432. Wu, M. J., Osanloo, E. D., Molnar, Z. V., et al. Poststreptococcal crescentic glomerulonephritis in a patient with preexisting membranous glomerulonephropathy. *Nephron* 35: 62, 1983.
433. Yamada, A., Mitsuhashi, K., Miyakawa, Y., et al. Membranous glomerulonephritis associated with eosinophilic lymphofolliculosis of the skin (Kimura's disease): Report of a case and review of the literature. *Clin. Nephrol.* 18: 211, 1982.
434. Yamauchi, H., Linsey, M. S., Biava, C. G., et al. Cure of membranous nephropathy after resection of carcinoma. *Arch. Intern. Med.* 145(11): 2061, 1985.
435. Yoshikawa, N., Ito, H., Yamada, Y., et al. Membranous glomerulonephritis associated with hepatitis B antigen in children: A comparison with idiopathic membranous glomerulonephritis. *Clin. Nephrol.* 23: 28, 1985.
436. Yoshikawa, Y., Truong, L. D., Mattioli, C. A., et al. Membranous glomerulonephritis in diabetic patients: A study of 15 cases and review of the literature. *Mod. Pathol.* 3(1): 36, 1990.
437. Zacchello, G., Zancan, L., Alberti, A., et al. Membranous nephropathy associated with chronic hepatitis caused by B virus. *Pediatr. Med. Chir.* 8(3): 311, 1986.

438. Zager, R. A., Couser, W. G., Andrews, B. S., et al. Radioimmunologic search for anti-tubular epithelial antibodies and circulating immune complexes in patients with membranous nephropathy. *Nephron* 24: 10, 1979.
439. Zanetti, M., Mandet, C., Duboust, A., et al. Demonstration of a passive Heymann nephrotic-like mechanism in a human kidney transplant. *Clin. Nephrol.* 15: 272, 1981.
440. Zheng, H. L., Maruyama, T., Matsuda, S., et al. Neuroblastoma presenting with the nephrotic syndrome. *J. Pediatr. Surg.* 14: 414, 1979.
441. Zucchelli, P., Cagnoli, L., Pasquali, S., et al. Clinical and morphologic evolution of idiopathic membranous nephropathy. *Clin. Nephrol.* 25(6): 282, 1986.
442. Zucchelli, P., Ponticelli, C., Cagnoli, L., et al. Prognostic value of T lymphocyte subset ratio in idiopathic membranous nephropathy. *Am. J. Nephrol.* 8(1): 15, 1988.

Membranoproliferative Glomerulonephritis

James V. Donadio, Jr.

Membranoproliferative glomerulonephritis (MPGN), also called *mesangiocapillary glomerulonephritis,* has been described in several distinct morphologic forms as primary glomerular disease and in association with a variety of clinical disorders. Systemic immune-complex diseases (including hereditary complement deficiencies), neoplastic diseases, infections, chronic liver disease, and a variety of other disorders can be associated with an important glomerulopathy represented as MPGN. The primary glomerular disease can recur in a kidney transplant and as a new disease in the allograft. Idiopathic MPGN is divided into type I, type II, and several type IIIs, and these types are characterized by histopathologic patterns on conventional light, electron, and immunofluorescent microscopic examination. During the last two decades, the various types of MPGN and their clinical features have been identified and reported both in primary and associated diseases, so that a classification of MPGN can be constructed (Table 66-1).

In this chapter, the idiopathic forms and those disorders associated with MPGN are reviewed.

Pathology

Idiopathic MPGN has several distinctive histopathologic and immunopathologic features [30, 83, 85, 157, 161]. As more series of patients with MPGN are reported, variations and subtypes are added to the pathologic descriptions.

DIFFUSE MEMBRANOPROLIFERATIVE OR MESANGIOCAPILLARY GLOMERULONEPHRITIS; TYPE I MPGN

The essential morphologic features of this lesion are (1) endocapillary cellular proliferation, (2) mesangial expansion, (3) capillary wall thickening, and (4) demonstration of immune complexes in the mesangium and along capillary walls. The extent of each of these alterations may vary from one glomerulus to another and from one glomerular lobule to another. This variability relates, in part, to the stage or duration of the renal disease and to the severity of the immunologic injury [3]. Also, finding atypical morphologic lesions suggests the possibility of associated diseases, such as systemic lupus erythematosus, mixed essential cryoglobulinemia, or neoplastic disease, although, at times, these associated diseases also may have typical or classic lesions [30, 83, 85, 93, 157].

LIGHT MICROSCOPY

Cellular Proliferation. Endocapillary cellular proliferation is predominantly mesangial, with lesser degrees of endothelial cell increase and swelling (Fig. 66-1A). Also contributing to the cellular increase is the presence of varying numbers of polymorphonuclear leukocytes, sometimes similar to that seen in early postinfectious glomerulonephritis (the so-called exudative feature). In addition, extracapillary proliferation of glomerular parietal epithelium or crescent formation is common. Generally, such proliferation is segmental in distribution and may be found in biopsy samples taken from both children and adults and in all the morphologic subtypes of MPGN. It also should be mentioned that prominent glomerular parietal epithelium is also found in patients with diabetes, acute glomerulonephritis, focal glomerulosclerosis, and diffuse proliferative lupus nephritis, and such changes are associated commonly with interstitial fibrosis, tubular atrophy, and vascular thickening and is associated with a bad prognosis [66]. On occasion, circumferential crescents involving nearly all of the glomeruli may be the primary morphologic feature.

Mesangial Expansion. Mesangial expansion is the result of cellular proliferation, matrix increase, and, to a lesser extent, immune deposits (Fig. 66-1A). These features may be segmental, as is the case with cellular proliferation. However, in general, they involve most of the lobules within the glomeruli. Review of serial sections is important in this assessment. The increase in mesangial cells and matrix leads to an extenuation of the normal lobular architecture of the glomerulus—a feature that helps to characterize this lesion. In addition to the mesangial cells, occasional polymorphonuclear leukocytes and monocytes may be present within the mesangium. In some instances, cellular mesangial nodules will be prominent, leading to a designation of *lobular glomerulonephritis* [112]. It is now appreciated that this lobular lesion may be a feature of either type I or type II MPGN and is not a discrete morphologic entity.

Membranous Thickening. Capillary wall thickening is primarily due to mesangial interposition (Fig. 66-1B). This morphologic alteration may be a feature of any mesangial expansive lesion, but it is particularly expressed in type I MPGN. Both mesangial cells and matrix extend or protrude along the subendothelial aspect of the lamina densa and beneath the plasma membrane of the endothelial cells. Further contributions to this widening of the capillary wall are made by immune deposits and inflammatory cells, generally polymorphonuclear leukocytes. A feature of the interposition is the formation of a new basement membrane between the interposed cellular and matrix material and the endothelial cell plasma membrane. This basement-membrane-like material is similar to that present in the mesangium, it stains positively with periodic acid–Schiff reagent, and is argyrophilic with periodic acid–methenamine silver stains. Two positive staining tracks producing a double contour, or "tram-track," are formed, delimiting the interposed mesangial matrix. The original basement membrane is easily recognized and generally is not altered

Table 66-1. Classification of membranoproliferative glomerulonephritis

- I. Idiopathic
  - A. Diffuse membranoproliferative or mesangiocapillary glomerulonephritis; type I MPGN
  - B. Intramembranous dense deposit glomerulonephritis or dense deposit disease; type II MPGN
  - C. Morphologic variants; type III MPGN
- II. Associated disorders
  - A. Systemic immune-complex diseases
    1. Systemic lupus erythematosus
    2. Mixed cryoimmunoglobulinemia
    3. Hereditary deficiency of complement components
  - B. Neoplastic diseases
    Light-chain nephropathy (monoclonal bone marrow plasmacytosis, multiple myeloma, lymphocytic and large-cell lymphoma, lymphoplasmacytic lymphoma [Waldenström]); monoclonal cryoimmunoglobulinemia (with and without chronic lymphocytic leukemia); Hodgkin's disease; non-Hodgkin's lymphoma; individual patients with metastatic prostate carcinoma, metastatic melanoma, esophageal carcinoma, and Wilms' tumor.
  - C. Infectious diseases
    Bacteremia with visceral abscesses; subacute bacterial endocarditis; infected ventriculoatrial shunts; tropical diseases: *Schistosoma mansoni* and *hematobium*, bancroftian filariasis, lepromatous leprosy, *P. malariae*, tropical pulmonary eosinophilia; hyperglobulinemia E with recurrent infections; acute mycoplasma infections, *Candida* endocrinopathy syndrome (type II MPGN).
  - D. Chronic liver disease
    Chronic acute hepatitis, seropositive for HB_sAG, HB_cAG, HB_eAg, and/or anti-HB_c; non-A, non-B hepatitis; cirrhosis; α-1-antitrypsin deficiency, phenotype ZZ, and cirrhosis.
  - E. Other disorders
    Partial lipodystrophy, C3NeF, recurrent infections, and type II MPGN; immunoglobulin deficiency (IgG, IgM, and IgA) and type I MPGN; retroperitoneal lymphoid angiofollicular hyperplasia (Castleman's pseudotumor) and type I MPGN; sarcoidosis; scleroderma; sickle cell disease; renal and intestinal artery stenosis and nephrotic syndrome; chronic Talwin abuse; Turner's syndrome, 46X, del(x), low C3, and type I MPGN; congenital cyanotic heart disease, nonimmune deposit glomerular changes—"pseudo MPGN."

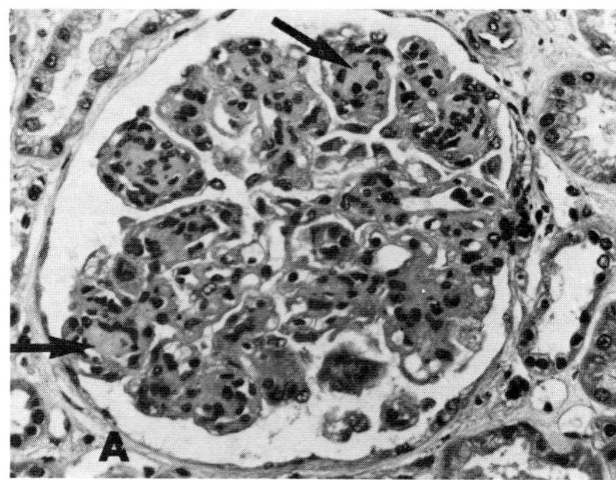

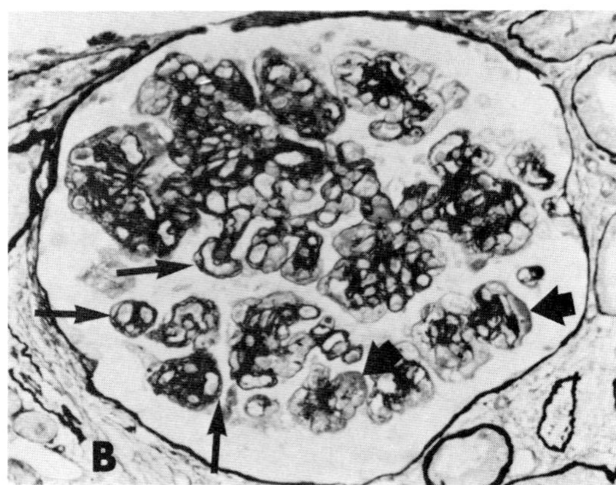

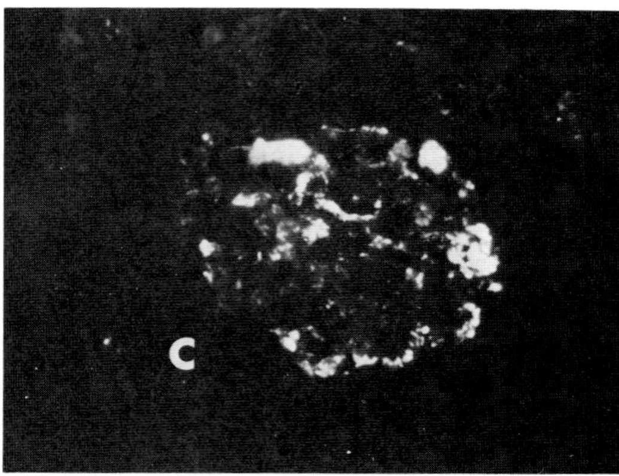

Fig. 66-1. Type I MPGN. (A) Endocapillary cellular proliferation, with prominent lobular accentuation and early mesangial nodules (*arrows*). Thickened peripheral capillary walls (hematoxylin and eosin; ×250). (B) Circumferential mesangial interposition (*long arrows*), subendothelial deposits (*short arrows*), and lobular accentuation (periodic acid–methenamine silver; ×250). (C) Immunofluorescence, showing granular capillary-wall staining and irregular, mesangial granular staining. Note nodular feature (antihuman C3; ×300).

significantly. The inner or new basement membrane is usually discontinuous and has a variable thickness. True splitting of the lamina densa does not occur. This new basement-membrane material is a product of the mesangial cells.

IMMUNOFLUORESCENCE

Because type I MPGN is likely a chronic immune complex-mediated glomerulopathy, an essential element in diagnosis is the demonstration of deposits within the subendothelial area (more accurately, the subendomem-

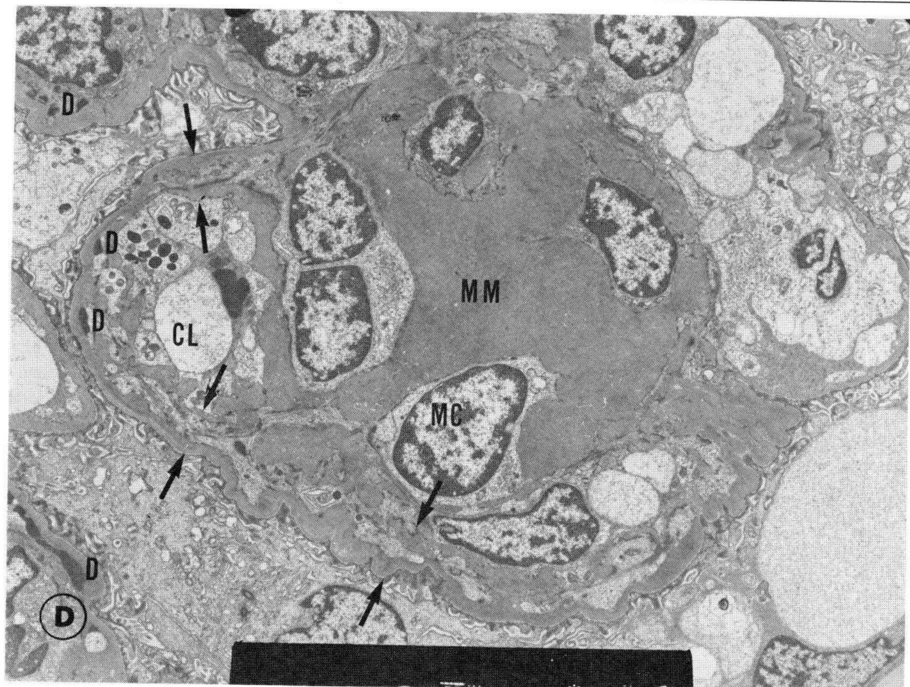

Fig. 66-1 (continued). (D) Well-developed mesangial nodule (MM), small subendothelial deposits (D), and circumferential mesangial interposition (*between arrows*);
CL = capillary lumen, MC = mesangial cell (×2,500). (From J. V. Donadio and K. E. Holley, Membranoproliferative glomerulonephritis. *Semin. Nephrol.* 2:214, 1982. By permission from Grune & Stratton, Inc.)

branous region) and mesangium. The most common pattern seen on immunofluorescence is the demonstration of immunoglobulins, IgG (IgG3 subclass in a recent study [8]), IgM, and IgA, and components of complement, C3, C1q, and C4, each in descending order, in a coarse, granular pattern along the glomerular capillary walls and within the mesangium (Fig. 66-1C). In some cases, C3 may be demonstrated alone or with only traces of immunoglobulins. A characteristic peripheral capillary wall staining pattern is noted. Properdin is commonly demonstrated in association with the deposition of C3. Fibronectin by immunofluorescence also has been demonstrated in glomerular capillary loops [177].

Failure to demonstrate complement or immunoglobulins along the capillary wall and mesangium should lead one to question the diagnosis of idiopathic type I MPGN, even in the presence of well-developed mesangial interposition. Secondary or associated diseases may be responsible for an immunofluorescent-negative lesion.

ELECTRON MICROSCOPY

Electron microscopy confirms the information gained by careful light microscopy and immunofluorescent examinations. In some instances of early type I MPGN, higher resolution allows more accurate assessment of the capillary walls and mesangium and is essential to a complete evaluation of the glomerular structure (Fig. 66-1D). In some cases, subepithelial deposits are demonstrated. When these deposits are prominent, the lesion has been referred to as *type III MPGN* [19]. Also, electron-dense deposits associated with cryoglobulinemia and systemic lupus erythematosus have characteristic staining and location that are helpful to the final morphologic assessment [31, 85, 157]. In lesions involving hepatitis B virus infections, viral particles may be associated with immune deposits.

In summary, the morphologic diagnosis of type I MPGN can be made only when the elements of endocapillary proliferation, mesangial expansion, circumferential interposition, and immune complexes are identified in sufficient numbers of lobules and glomeruli to permit these changes to characterize a glomerular response.

INTRAMEMBRANOUS DENSE-DEPOSIT GLOMERULONEPHRITIS OR DENSE-DEPOSIT DISEASE; TYPE II MPGN

Much discussion has taken place in the literature concerning the continued consideration of this lesion with idiopathic membranoproliferative glomerulonephritis [30, 83, 85, 93, 157]. Most authors acknowledge that the similarity which type II MPGN has with type I relates primarily to the clinical presentation and the morphologic appearance of the glomeruli viewed in hematoxylin and eosin preparations, that is, the combination of endocapillary proliferation, mesangial expansion, and mesangial interposition. There is dissimilarity when the glomerular lesions are studied by special stains, immunofluorescence, and electron microscopic techniques [30, 83, 85, 157].

Type II MPGN is diagnosed by demonstrating intramembranous dense deposits, either segmentally or diffusely, usually in a discontinuous pattern, not only within the glomerular basement membrane but also in the basement membranes of Bowman's capsule and convoluted tubules and occasionally within the walls of capillaries and small arterioles [30, 51, 68, 81, 83, 85, 106, 115, 157, 172]. This lesion may be considered a nephropathy rather than a glomerulopathy.

LIGHT MICROSCOPY

Endocapillary cellular proliferation may be less extensive; however, mesangial cells predominate and polymorphonuclear leukocytes are usually more numerous in the capillary lumens of type II than of type I lesions (Fig. 66-2A through C). Crescents are more frequently seen in type II lesions, and the basement-membrane disruption may be seen associated with fibrin deposits (necrosis). In a recent study, intrarenal cross-linked fibrin deposits were observed in the mesangium and in sclerotic areas in glomeruli both in MPGN and in other severe proliferative types of nephritis [94].

Further emphasis should be placed on the great variability in the morphologic expression of this lesion. Some biopsy specimens show little proliferation, while others will mimic the most florid endocapillary proliferative lesions. Mesangial expansion is also variable, and mesangial nodular formation may occur, as in type I MPGN. Additionally, glomerular lesions of pure mesangial cell proliferation or focal segmental glomerulosclerosis and normal morphology by light microscopy have been described in which intramembranous dense deposits also were present [153].

Thickening of capillary walls is due not only to mesangial interposition, as in type I, but also to a characteristic expansion of the lamina densa secondary to accumulation of homogeneous intramembranous material. Periodic acid–Schiff, periodic acid–methenamine silver, or toluidine blue stains allow the demonstration of characteristic wavy, ribbon-like capillary basement membranes, often interrupted with small segments of normal basement membranes. Distribution of these lesions may be segmental or diffuse. Similar changes in the basement membrane are noted in Bowman's capsule, convoluted tubular basement membranes [25], and the walls of small arteries and capillaries. These deposits do not occur in the basement membranes of collecting ducts. Some deposits are argyrophilic only with prolonged silver impregnation, appearing more brown with the usual staining times. Careful examination of thin sections by light microscopy utilizing appropriate special stains usually leads to the correct diagnosis. However, one should utilize electron microscopy for final assessment.

Recently, the dense deposit material was shown to stain with thioflavin T, a histochemical stain that is commonly used for amyloid [40]. There was no reaction to the dense deposit material against anti-SAA amyloid protein, but there has been described a distinctive abnormal immunofluorescent staining pattern with anti-SAP amyloid protein [53], which is also a constituent of normal human glomerular basement membrane. Abnormal staining patterns with anti-SAP also have been observed in the glomerular basement membranes of biopsy samples from patients with diabetes, membranous nephropathy, systemic vasculitis, and Goodpasture's syndrome [53]. Its specificity for pathogenesis remains unknown.

IMMUNOFLUORESCENCE

The immunohistologic pattern is unique in that no specific immunoglobulin deposition is present, and C3 gives a characteristic linear, smooth, capillary basement-membrane staining (Fig. 66-2D). By high-resolution epifluorescence technique, deposition of C3 can be demonstrated along the outer and inner rims of normal lamina densa and around the negative staining intramembranous dense deposit material [99]. Similarly, by epifluorescence, there is a splitting of Goodpasture's antigen by GBM dense deposits into a double linear array along the endothelial and epithelial margins of the GBM [148]. Further, a particular granular mesangial immunofluorescence, termed *mesangial rings,* is present [99]. The centers of mesangial deposits are dark and represent dense deposit material, while the outer rims of this material stain with C3. A similar linear, smooth immunofluorescence pattern with C3 is found in Bowman's capsule, tubular basement membranes, and vessel walls, where dense deposit material also is located. Staining for immunoglobulins, C1q, C4, and properdin is infrequent and variable.

ELECTRON MICROSCOPY

Electron microscopic appearance shows a typical homogenous material in basement membranes, which lacks the granular features of immune deposits (Fig. 66-2E). Distribution can be segmental, discontinuous, or diffuse. Silver impregnation techniques also have proved useful in electron microscopic studies to characterize further this material and distinguish it from other intramembranous material. Rarely should confusion exist in differ-

Fig. 66-2. Type II MPGN (dense deposit disease). (A and B) Endocapillary cellular proliferation and lobular accentuation are variable (hematoxylin and eosin; ×250). (C) Note irregular thickened peripheral basement membranes (*closed arrows*). Similar intramembranous material is within basement membrane of Bowman's capsule and convoluted tubules (*open arrows*). Segmental crescent (C) (periodic acid–methenamine silver; ×250). (D) Immunofluorescence, showing smooth peripheral capillary-wall staining and mesangial "rings" (anti-C3 complement; ×1,000). (E) Note variability of intramembranous dense deposits with gaps (*arrows*). Dense deposits are present in mesangium (D). Prominent nodular mesangial interposition (MI); P = polymorphonuclear leukocytes (×3,750). (From J. V. Donadio and K. E. Holley, Membranoproliferative glomerulonephritis. *Semin. Nephrol.* 2:214, 1982. By permission from Grune & Stratton, Inc.)

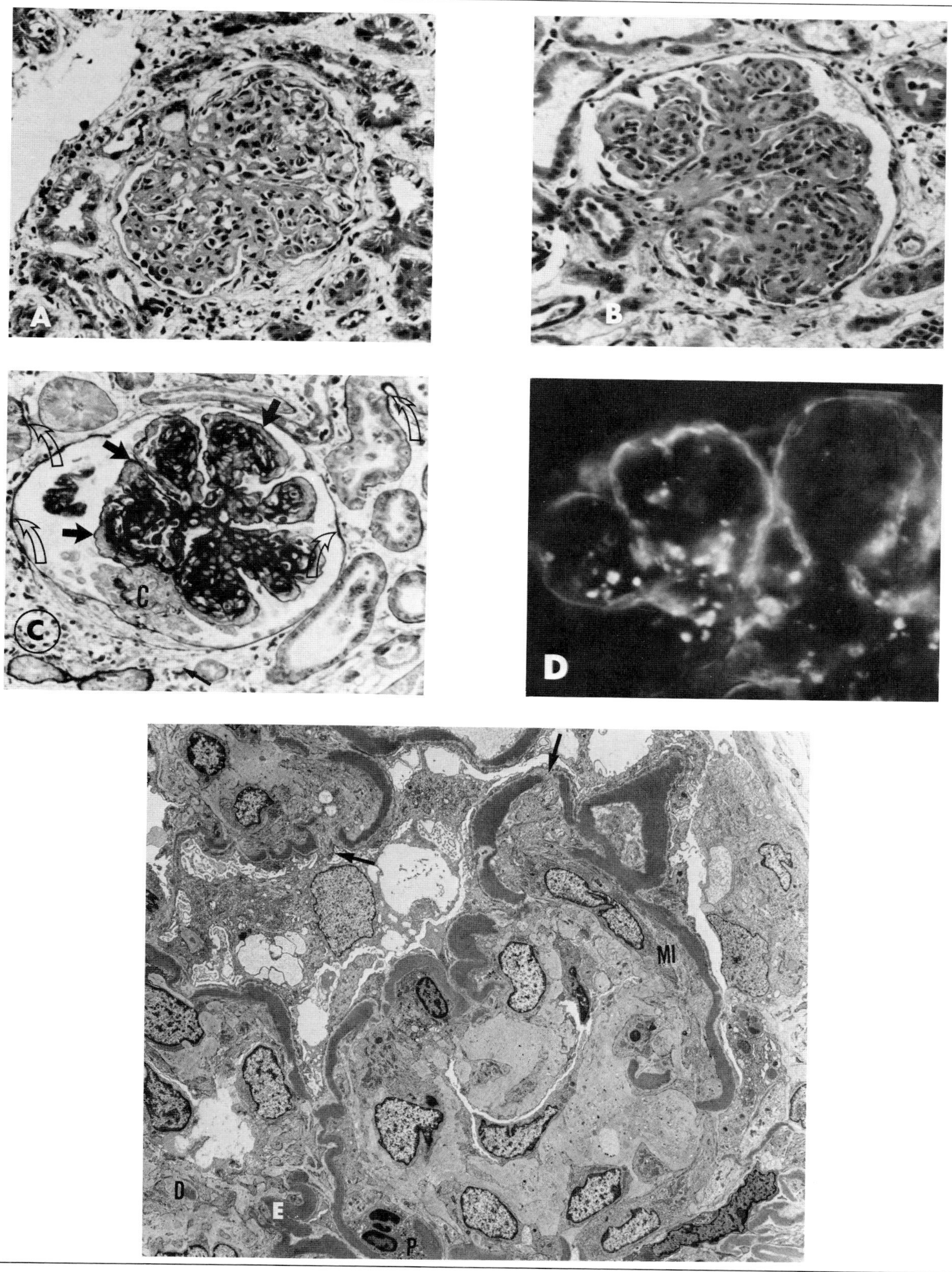
A
B
C
C
D
MI
D
E
P

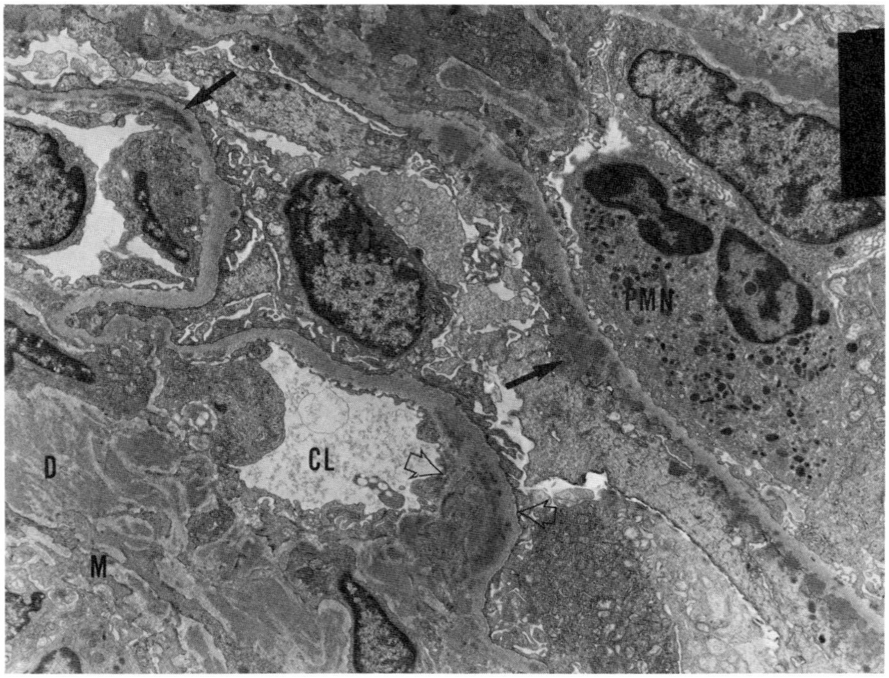

Fig. 66-3. MPGN with subepithelial deposits (type III, Burkholder). Expanded mesangium (M) with numerous deposits (D), paramesangial interposition (*open arrows*), and subendothelial, intramembranous, and epimembranous deposits (*closed arrows*) (×8,250). (From J. V. Donadio and K. E. Holley, Membranoproliferative glomerulonephritis. *Semin. Nephrol.* 2:214, 1982. By permission from Grune & Stratton, Inc.)

entiating the intramembranous dense deposits of MPGN from other intramembranous deposits when all features of the morphologic lesion are considered [19]. Scattered subepithelial deposits are more frequently seen in type II than in type I lesions.

MORPHOLOGIC VARIANTS; TYPE III MPGN

Burkholder et al. [19] described a lesion that was termed type III MPGN and differed from type I MPGN by the presence of numerous subepithelial deposits, with a reaction by the lamina densa, similar to the lesions seen in membranous glomerulopathy (Fig. 66-3). Anders and Thoenes [4] and Strife et al. [162] characterized another variant that they also called type III MPGN by utilizing silver impregnation staining techniques of ultrathin sections of tissue and electron microscopy. The lamina densa was disrupted, and there was an accumulation of new basement-membrane material arranged in layers. Electron-dense deposits were noted within short segments of basement membranes of glomerular capillaries, Bowman's capsule, and convoluted tubules in association with other electron-dense deposits that were more reminiscent of immune complexes. The presence of variants should not be unexpected in a chronic immune complex glomerulopathy. Their presence in no way diminishes the need to utilize strict morphologic and immunologic criteria in the diagnosis of types I and II MPGN [30, 83, 85, 93, 157].

Pathogenesis

The pathogenesis of MPGN is poorly understood. Immune-complex mediation is suggested on the basis of several clinicopathologic associations. Chronic antigenemia probably occurs in many of the infections in which MPGN is particularly associated (Table 66-1). Moreover, in idiopathic MPGN, activation of the complement system is a hallmark [57, 79, 130, 178, 179], complement components are invariably found in the glomeruli by direct immunofluorescence (with immunoglobulins to a lesser extent) [24, 41, 49, 81, 82, 98, 106, 172], and circulating immune complexes are found in a high percentage of patients [42, 138, 156], adding support to the concept of an immune complex pathogenesis. Also, MPGN has been described in young Finnish Landrace lambs who are C3-deficient [5] and in human beings with various hereditary deficiencies of complement components [33, 97, 109, 137], leading to the hypothesis that such complement component deficiencies predispose to immune-complex glomerulonephritis. Yet in both type I and type II MPGN, specific antigens have not been identified, pathogenetic events seem to be more complicated, and mechanisms of complement activation are not yet fully understood [98].

COMPLEMENT SYSTEM AND MPGN

When discussing the pathogenesis of MPGN, it is necessary to consider involvement of the complement system. Activation of both classic and alternative (properdin) pathways and of the amplification loop mechanism (by means of the amplification C3 convertase or C3bBb) has been described in primary MPGN with certain distinctions between types I and II [57, 130, 180].

In type I MPGN, at the time of diagnosis, one-third to one-half of patients have low concentrations of C3 and CH_{50} [24, 41, 49, 82, 98, 99, 130, 176]. During follow-up observations, serum complement levels have varied considerably, remaining low in most but also normalizing, including the presence of normal values throughout a course of observation. Concentrations of C1q and C4 and of factor B and properdin may be borderline or low, indicating activation of both classic and alternative pathways, respectively [99, 130, 178]. Increased levels of early complement components of the classical (C1q, C4) and the alternative (factor B, properdin) pathway also have been observed, suggesting overproduction after a period of increased complement consumption [147]. Immunopathologic studies usually show glomerular deposition of C3 and properdin in the capillary loops and in the mesangium, while C1q, C4, and immunoglobulins (IgG, IgA, and IgM) are found with varying frequency in these locations. In one study of serum concentrations of complement components in patients with type I MPGN, low levels of serum properdin were found that correlated significantly with serum concentrations of C1q, C4, and C3 [130]. The authors also found positive glomerular immunofluorescence with properdin, C1q, and C3.

These findings suggest the following mechanisms of complement activation in type I MPGN. First, classic pathway activation occurs by way of immune complex formation and deposition. It must be remembered, however, that specific antigens have not been identified, and there are discrepancies in the results of studies that examine patients with MPGN for circulating immune complexes [42, 156]. Second, alternative pathway activation occurs by way of the C1 bypass that involves C1, properdin, and factor B. There is experimental proof of the C1 bypass with properdin and immune complexes in which sensitized sheep red blood cells with Forssman antibody became lysed when they were later incubated with serum deficient in C4 and C2 [130]. Third, the alternative pathway also might be activated through the amplification loop by means of interaction between properdin and the other alternative pathway proteins, leading to the formation of a C3-cleaving enzyme that, in turn, recruits the other properdin factors [57]. The exact molecular mechanism by which this occurs is still under investigation.

The reason that serum complement is persistently low, or only low at times, might be explained further by the results of turnover studies of radiolabeled C3, which demonstrate increased breakdown and reduced synthesis of C3 in some patients with types I and II MPGN [23, 35]. Increased turnover of factor B has been found in patients with MPGN who also had decreased levels of C3 [28]. There appears to be no generalized deficiency in modulation of complement activation when three controlling proteins of the complement system—C1 inhibitor (C1-INH), C3b inactivator (C3b-INA), and beta-1H—were examined in serum and renal tissue of patients with MPGN and were found to be in concordance with their corresponding complement proteins [126, 183].

NEPHRITIC FACTOR

In type II MPGN, serum levels of C3 are nearly always low and more persistently so than in type I [24, 41, 49, 81, 82, 106, 172]. C1q and C4 concentrations are usually normal. Direct immunofluorescence demonstrates C3 in linear, smooth patterns along the capillary walls and in the mesangium, whereas properdin, C1q, and C4 immunoreactants are negative. A unique IgG autoantibody, called *nephritic factor* or *C3NeF* [39, 149, 166, 181], has been found in 43 to 70 percent of the sera of patients with type II MPGN, in 20 to 30 percent of patients with type I MPGN, and in up to 50 percent of sera from patients with MPGN accompanying mixed cryoglobulinemia, systemic lupus erythematosus (SLE), and so-called shunt nephritis [42, 57, 130, 147, 178]. C3NeF binds to the amplification C3 convertase (C3bBb) and prevents the decay of its C3b-cleaving activity by the C3b inactivator [39, 57, 149]. This occurrence results in further breakdown of C3 and the completion of the effector sequence of C5 through C9. This action is similar to the stimulation of complement activity through the alternative pathway by properdin; however, C3NeF is a protein distinct from properdin. C3NeF appears not to be a kidney-dependent factor in that it can be measured in the circulation of patients after nephrectomy, along with persistently low levels of C3 and CH_{50} [51, 57]. There is also dissociation between C3NeF, C3, and factor B levels, indicating that many factors are probably influencing the levels of these proteins over and above the modulating effect of C3NeF [147, 170, 178]. Further evidence that C3NeF itself may not be nephritogenic is found in the reports of patients who had partial lipodystrophy and hypocomplementemia, which was accompanied by C3NeF and alternative pathway activation by means of the amplification loop, but who had no glomerulonephritis [154]. On the other hand, the association of partial lipodystrophy, C3NeF and low serum C3, and type II MPGN also has been well documented [133].

HEREDITARY COMPLEMENT DEFICIENCIES

Additional support for an immune-complex pathogenesis comes from a description of families with hereditary deficiencies of complement components, some of whom had type I MPGN but no other systemic disease [33, 97, 109, 137]. A hypothesis for an immune-complex disease is that these persons are predisposed to viral and bacterial infections to which they can mount an antibody response. But because of the complement deficiency states, there is interference with clearance of antigen-antibody complexes, which leads to the development of glomerulonephritis. In newborn C3-deficient Finnish Landrace lambs [5], a form of progressive glomerulonephritis similar to type I MPGN develops. The early lesions show predominantly C3 glomerular deposits, while, later, more developed lesions show a progressive increase in amounts of deposited immunoglobulins (IgM, IgA, and later IgG), leading to a more generalized immune-complex disease.

Another hypothesis is that the complement deficiency might be a "marker" and not a cause of disease by relating to impaired function of closely linked B-cell alloantigens (also referred to as *Ia antigens*), whose functions are concerned with genetic control of specific immunologic responses—the recognition of antigen and the ability to respond or not to respond to that antigen. Recently, Friend et al. [62] described a B-lymphocyte surface antigen that was strongly associated with MPGN, and Sakai et al. [146] found an increase in IgM-bearing peripheral blood lymphocytes in patients with both types I and II, whose family members had no renal disease. Berry et al. [13] described MPGN in two sibships. In one, a brother had type III and a sister, type I. In the second family, two brothers had type I with similar clinical manifestations. These observations suggest both an immunogenetic and familial predisposition to the development of this glomerulopathy. Clearly, more systematic study is necessary to define these observations further.

NATURE OF DENSE DEPOSITS IN TYPE II

In type II MPGN, the nature of the electron-dense deposits located in the renal basement membranes is unknown. The dense deposit material does not react with antisera directed against immunoglobulins, complement components, glomerular basement membranes, or collagen. Galle and Mahieu [68] have questioned the generally accepted idea that the changes in the renal basement membranes represent deposits. They suggest that such changes are an accumulation of a glycoprotein-membrane material that contains a greater amount of sialic acid than normal glomerular basement membrane.

CELLULAR IMMUNE FUNCTION

In three studies of cellular immune function in patients with idiopathic MPGN (type unspecified), T-lymphocyte subsets were examined using monoclonal antibodies OKT3 (peripheral T-cells), OKT4 (helper/inducer cells), and OKT8 (suppressor/cytotoxic T-cells). In two of these studies, Chatenoud and Bach [29] and Fornasieri et al. [60] found no significant alterations of either total peripheral T-cells or the percentage or ratio of OKT4/OKT8. On the other hand, Brando et al. [14] described reduction in the OKT4/OKT8 ratios and in OKT8 suppressor-cell function in hypocomplementemic patients who were not nephrotic and who had normal renal function. Because of the few studies reported, and conflicting results, it is unclear whether there is significant alteration in T-lymphocyte immunoregulation in MPGN.

PLATELETS AND MPGN

Renewed interest in the participation by platelets in the pathogenesis of glomerulonephritis stems from earlier work that has been enhanced by recent experimental and clinical studies [22]. Part of this information has a bearing on the glomerular injury in MPGN.

In models of experimental glomerulonephritis, platelets may participate in glomerular injury, together with other mediators, by complex mechanisms [21]. Platelets show an effect on proteinuria in autologous/accelerated anti-GBM nephritis and in models of acute and chronic immune-complex nephritis. The important recent information concerning platelets as mediators of glomerular injury are (1) that the potent mitogenic protein—platelet-derived growth factor—can recruit and mitogenically stimulate mesenchymal cells [128, 145], and (2) along with the platelet-specific protein—platelet factor$_4$ (PF_4)—possesses chemotactic activity for monocytes and neutrophils [44, 45].

Intact platelets or their fragments are not often found in the biopsy samples of diseased kidneys. Perhaps platelets disrupt after contact with injured glomerular capillaries and other vessel walls. Localization of platelet antigens using rabbit antibody to human platelets has been found in significant amounts in glomerular capillaries and vascular walls in kidney tissue from patients with both types I and II MPGN (also hemolytic-uremic syndrome [HUS] and diabetic glomerulopathy) [52, 122]. The problem with using platelet immunofluorescence is that the structural basis of many platelet antigens is unknown, and it is difficult to know which (if any) of the deposited antigens is pathogenic to the glomerulus.

Platelet-specific proteins, beta transforming growth factor (β-TG) and PF_4, and concentrations in intraplatelet versus plasma serotonin have been measured, testing their alterations as indicators of increased platelet activation in a variety of glomerular diseases [131, 132]. Both increased and normal values for both β-TG and PF_4 have been found in various studies, and the effects of retention in uremic serum, the nephrotic state, or occult thrombosis limit their use as monitors of platelet activation in glomerular disease. Reduced intraplatelet concentration of serotonin and increased free plasma 5-OH indol (serotonin) were found in patients with MPGN (also in membranous nephropathy, focal glomerulosclerosis, systemic vasculitis, and lupus nephritis) [131, 132]. There was some correlation with disease activity. However, there was considerable overlap between normal and abnormal values in those with stable and progressive disease both in terms of platelet-to-plasma serotonin ratios and platelet serotonin levels.

Shortened platelet survival by in vivo platelet labeling techniques has been demonstrated in patients with a variety of glomerular diseases. The platelet survival test measures the interaction of platelets with surfaces, with the resultant removal of platelets from the circulation by incorporation into aggregates or through removal of altered platelets in the spleen or other organs [65]. On this basis, it may be concluded that a thrombotic state (or a glomerulopathy) might be associated with increased utilization of platelets and that platelet survival time may be reduced in such states. George et al. [76] showed selective platelet consumption in MPGN, HUS, glomerulosclerosis, early transplant rejection, diabetic nephropathy, and crescentic glomerulonephritis. We demonstrated shortened platelet survival in 70 percent of patients studied with MPGN [46] and diabetic nephropathy [47], and we improved or stabilized the glomerular filtration rate after treatment with platelet inhibitors (dipyridamole and aspirin).

In summary, platelets are implicated in the pathogenesis of glomerular disease, as evidenced in structural and functional cellular studies, in the dissection of experimental models of glomerulonephritis, and in clinical studies in which shortened platelet survival can be demonstrated and favorable effects shown with platelet inhibitor regimens, with MPGN being among the glomerular diseases studied. However, the true importance of platelet interaction in the initiation and continuation of glomerular injury remains unknown.

Clinical Manifestations of Idiopathic MPGN

After Gotoff et al. [79] and West [178] first emphasized the association between persistent hypocomplementemia and membranoproliferative glomerulonephritis, there arose an increasing interest and recognition of the disorder among nephrology groups throughout the world. Over the past 20 years, the clinical features of types I and II disease have been described in a number of clinical studies and reviews of the subject, in which currently accepted histopathologic and immunopathologic criteria for diagnosis have been fulfilled [6, 9, 24, 41, 49–51, 79, 81, 82, 86, 98, 106, 111, 112, 164, 172, 179]. As a primary glomerular disease, MPGN generally occurs in older children and young adults. In a few persons, the disease develops during the first 5 years of life [82, 86, 98, 106] and in the sixth decade and beyond [24, 49, 111, 164]. There is a variably reported predominance of sex in individual series of patients that equalizes in the cumulative experience, and there is a predilection for the white race. Generally, both types of MPGN are progressive, sustained remissions are uncommon, and there are no essential differences in outcome between children and adults, with exceptions to be discussed.

In *type I MPGN,* the nephrotic syndrome is the presenting illness in two-thirds or more of the patients. Less commonly, an abnormal urine sediment containing erythrocytes (RBC), dysmorphic RBCs, and RBC casts, accompanied by qualitative proteinuria, acute nephritis, or recurrent episodes of macroscopic hematuria may be the presenting clinical findings. Often, these clinical presentations overlap with one another. Clinical renal abnormalities are preceded by infections, usually upper respiratory in type, and more commonly in children with type II MPGN [6, 41, 81]. Some infections are streptococcal in origin, with positive throat cultures for beta-hemolytic streptococci associated with elevated antistreptolysin 0 titers. The urinary excretion of N-acetyl-beta-glucosaminidase (NAG) and beta-2-microglobulin (beta 2M) has been found to be elevated in patients with MPGN, as in many forms of nephropathy, suggesting either renal tubular injury or dysfunction [90, 152]. Caution is advised in interpreting results of increased urinary NAG levels in that, when NAG excretion is related to creatinine excretion, levels of NAG vary inversely with glomerular filtration rate irrespective of the type of renal parenchymal disease [90].

Usually, the disease is slowly progressive, with estimated survival rates of 50 to 60 percent after about 10 years. In some of these estimates, mortality is used to denote patient deaths and the development of advanced renal failure, and different authors use different starting points to calculate the time course, for example, from the clinical onset of disease or from the time of morphologic diagnosis. In children, Habib et al. [82] estimated a survival rate of 50 percent approximately 11 years after diagnosis. In a mixed population of children and adults with type I MPGN, Cameron et al. [24] calculated a survival rate of 50 percent 10 years from the onset of disease. In mostly adults, Droz et al. [50] found a 60-percent survival rate in patients with what they termed *the pure form* of type I MPGN and in 36 percent of those with the lobular form 10 years after diagnosis. The disease also may remain stable for years beyond these estimates and in spite of persistent proteinuria. Prolonged clinical remissions have been described, ranging from 5.7 to 20 percent in six clinical reports, in which data were provided [27, 41, 50, 82, 98, 164]. It is to be noted that patients entered remission spontaneously as well as after various forms of treatment. Clinical remission was accompanied by morphologic regression in several studies in which follow-up renal biopsies also were obtained [50, 82, 116].

Type II MPGN is considerably less common than type I. In studies in which consecutive patients with both types have been described, type II lesions usually have constituted the lower percentage (15–35%) of the total number of patients described with MPGN [24, 49, 81]. As a more graphic example of the infrequent occurrence of this form of MPGN, 128 patients with type II lesions were reported from six separate nephrology referral groups that reviewed a cumulative total of 90 years of biopsy experience [24, 41, 49, 81, 106, 153].

The presenting illness in type II MPGN is similar to that in type I, with some investigators reporting a more frequent appearance of acute nephritis or recurrent macroscopic hematuria at onset [24, 81]. Antoine and Faye [6] reported complete reversal of acute nephritic episodes (transient renal failure, edema, microscopic hematuria, and hypertension) nine times in eight patients, with the nephritis most often occurring during the clinical onset of disease [6]. On the other hand, we found that all patients with acute nephritis at onset either experienced end-stage renal disease or had progressive renal insufficiency (4 patients with type II and 12 patients with type I lesions) [49].

Type II MPGN may be a more aggressive disease than type I MPGN though some patients can maintain stable renal function and mild proteinuria for many years. Clinical remissions are apparently very uncommon, as evidenced in the reports by Habib et al. [81], who described 1 of 44 children, and by Cameron et al. [24], who showed 1 of 35 patients entering remission. The 50-percent statistical mortality has been variably estimated: in

Table 66-2. Clinical parameters at diagnosis, indicating poor prognosis in idiopathic MPGN

Hypertension [9, 49]
Reduced renal function [9, 49, 82, 164]
Nephrotic syndrome [6, 9, 24, 82, 164]
Cellular crescents in renal biopsy [24, 123, 164]

one study, between the ninth and tenth year after diagnosis in children [81], in another study, at about the eighth year [24], and, in another study, between the eleventh and twelfth years [6] after onset in a mixture of children and adults.

In both types of idiopathic MPGN, hypertension, impaired renal function, nephrotic syndrome, and the presence of epithelial cell crescents in renal biopsy, samples are usually associated with a poor outcome (Table 66-2). In several studies, a clearly more progressive course was found in patients with nephrotic syndrome and the mortality rate was two times or more that of patients with nonnephrotic proteinuria, both from actuarial survival curves and specific, long-term follow-up information [6, 9, 24, 82, 164]. On the other hand, in a paper highlighting clinical remissions, Droz et al. [50] reported seven patients with nephrotic syndrome among 13 who had spontaneous remissions of their disease from 2 to 16 years after onset. Azotemia presaged a poor prognosis in four reports, because the majority of patients who presented with impaired renal function showed progression to advanced renal failure [9, 49, 82, 164]. Also, hypertension was associated with progressive renal failure in two studies [9, 49]. Although finding extracapillary proliferation is common in both types I and II MPGN, the presence of crescents affecting 20 to 40 percent or more of the glomeruli tends to be associated with a higher proportion of such patients developing advanced renal failure [24, 123, 164].

Macroscopic hematuria has not been shown to have prognostic value, with one exception, and that is in the report by Habib et al. [82], in which more children developed renal failure who had gross hematuria than those who did not. Activation of the complement system already has been discussed, and no correlation was noted between the serum levels of complement or C3NeF and the progression of glomerular disease either in type I or type II MPGN [51, 57, 82, 130, 178]. Davis et al. [42] reported serial measurements of circulating immune complexes, measured by solid-phase C1q assay, in patients with various types of MPGN. At the time of diagnosis, complexes were present in increased amounts in about one-half of the patients. The levels correlated in an opposite manner from what might be expected with clinical status. Complexes were absent in patients whose disease had progressed to renal failure, while they were increased when there was no renal function impairment. Perhaps the complexes detected by this method are not nephritogenic or complexes of different size, composition, and low concentration might have escaped detection by the C1q assay. In another study in which serial measurements of circulating immune complexes were made, complexes were found intermittently, transiently, or consistently in patients with type I MPGN, without correlation with disease progression [156].

Argument continues whether type I and type II MPGN represent different diseases. Type II does differ from type I in several respects. (1) In type II MPGN, there is a younger age at onset: the overwhelming majority of patients are less than 20 years old at the onset of their disease; occasionally, however, older patients are reported [6, 115]. (2) Serum C3 concentrations are more persistently lowered [24, 41, 49, 81, 82, 106, 172]. (3) C3NeF is present in most patients in whom it is measured [39, 149, 166, 181]. (4) The morphologic and immunopathologic alterations are distinctive [51, 81, 99, 106, 172]. (5) The association of partial lipodystrophy, low serum C3 levels, and intramembranous dense deposit disease is well established [133]. (6) Type II MPGN appears with more regularity in renal allografts than does type I disease [20, 23, 38, 81].

However, when one examines the studies in which long-term data are provided and outcomes were compared between morphologic groups and between children and adults, few differences were found (Table 66-3). When the two outcomes of death from any cause and advanced renal failure were considered together, Cameron et al. [24] found no differences between types I and II MPGN. However, the subgroup of adults with type I had more renal failure than did children with type I MPGN. In the study by Magil et al. [111], all adult males, but no women, were either dead or in renal failure after an average time of only 17.7 months in comparison with 43 percent of children (both males and females) who were in renal failure after an average time of 51.6 months. No important differences in either patient survival or kidney failure between morphologic groups, ages, or both were described in any of the other studies listed in the table.

Regarding *type III MPGN,* in the original series by Burkholder et al. [19] and in a more recent report of nine patients [1], there was a mixture of children and adults, the nephrotic syndrome was the usual presenting illness, and the clinical course was variable. Nephrotic syndrome, hypertension, and impaired renal function at diagnosis related to a poor outcome. Serum C3 levels were reduced in about one-half of the patients and did not correlate with progressive disease. In the type III disease described by Anders and Thoenes [4] and Strife et al. [162], the latter group of authors recently provided long-term follow-up of 17 children [160]. Seven of 17 patients presented with the nephrotic syndrome. C3, properdin, and C5 levels were reduced; C3NeF was notably absent. Progression was variable, occurring mainly in patients who were initially nephrotic in contrast to those persons with nonnephrotic proteinuria at presentation, most of whom remained stable or improved. In follow-up renal biopsies, there was less mesangial proliferation found in those patients who were stable.

There is debate whether or not the morphologic variants, or type IIIs, should be considered separately from type I MPGN or perhaps with another chronic glomer-

Table 66-3. Differences in outcomes between types I and II MPGN

Groups compared	Study [reference]	Differences in outcomes[a]	Follow-up (years)
Types I and II; children and adults	[6]	None[b]	N/A[c]
	[164]	None	5–22
	[24]	Worse in adults (Type I only)	2–21
Types I and II; children	[82]	None	5
	[41]	None	N/A
Type I; children and adults	[111]	Worse in adult males[d]	0.5–10

[a]Outcomes are defined in studies as combinations of death from any cause and terminal renal failure.
[b]Shorter survival in patients with lobular pattern.
[c]Not available.
[d]Renal failure defined as serum creatinine $\geqslant$ 2 mg/dl.

ulopathy. For example, Habib and Lévy [83] suggested that lesions showing widespread subepithelial deposits might be an unusual variant of membranous nephropathy. Yet morphologic lesions of mesangial proliferation and subendothelial and mesangial deposits, activation of the complement system by means of alternative (properdin) pathway, and similar clinical characteristics mitigate against separating these variants from the type I MPGN group. Perhaps such variants should be recognized by their morphologic characteristics only.

Treatment

Treatment of patients with MPGN remains an unsettled issue. Five randomized clinical trials have studied the effects of treatment in both children and adults with MPGN (Table 66-4). The follow-up periods were relatively short, ranging from 1 to 4 years, and the results have not provided convincing evidence for the effectiveness of any treatment.

Two clinical trials used triple-drug therapy with cyclophosphamide, dipyridamole, and warfarin, which had been shown previously in an uncontrolled study by Kincaid-Smith [100] to benefit patients with MPGN. In one of these trials, Cattran et al. [27] studied 59 patients with types I and II MPGN. After 18 months, treatment had no significant effects on proteinuria or renal function. Small numbers of patients with type II disease were entered into the trial; thus, the statistical power was insufficient to allow conclusions regarding this type of treatment in type II disease. In the second clinical trial, the Australian Working Party in Glomerulonephritis [167] reported their results with these agents in 37 patients with type I MPGN. No beneficial effect was noted in treated patients compared with control subjects who completed 36 months of treatment. The Australian group also reported a high dropout rate related to drug toxicity. Hemorrhagic cystitis, other bleeding complications, and bone marrow depression were the main reasons for withdrawal from the study. Thus, the earlier uncontrolled observations by Kincaid-Smith were not confirmed by these two prospective, randomized trials examining the use of this combination of agents.

Because there is evidence for platelet activation and increased platelet consumption in the pathogenesis of MPGN, two additional prospective trials examined the usefulness of platelet inhibitors. Zimmerman et al. [185] combined antiplatelet drug treatment using dipyridamole (400 mg per day) with an anticoagulant, sodium warfarin, in 18 adult patients (17 with type I, 1 with type II). All patients completed either a control or treatment

Table 66-4. Effects of treatment of MPGN in randomized, controlled clinical trials

Drugs tested	Study [reference]	Duration of renal disease before treatment, years	Number of patients, disease type, ages	Effect of treatment on	
				Renal function	Proteinuria
Cyclophosphamide, dipyridamole and warfarin	[27]	1+	59; 47 I, 12 II; children and adults	N/S[a]	N/S
	[167]	NA[b]	37 I; ages not given	N/S	N/S
Dipyridamole and warfarin	[185]	3.2	18; 17 I, 1 II; adults	Stabilized[c]	N/S
Dipyridamole and aspirin	[47]	3	40 I; children and adults	Stabilized[d]	N/S
Prednisone	[143]	NA	37 I; children	N/S	N/S

[a]Not significant.
[b]Not available.
[c]In unpaired analysis, comparing slopes of reciprocal serum creatinine values during control year first with treatment year first (< 0.03).
[d]Comparing iothalamate clearance slopes for 12 months ($p < 0.02$).

year, and 13 completed both a control and treatment year in a crossover study design. Renal function was found to be preserved better in the treated group by determining the slopes of reciprocal serum creatinine values during control and treatment years, but only in the unpaired analysis of 18 patients, comparing a control year first with a treatment year first. In the paired analysis of renal function changes in the 13 patients who completed both a control and a treatment year, differences in slopes of reciprocal creatinine, favoring treatment, were noted only for 6 patients who demonstrated a change in renal function during one of the years of observation. Also, the complication rate was high; significant hemorrhagic problems occurred in 37 percent of the treated patients, and one death was due to intracerebral hemorrhage during treatment. In another prospective, randomized, double-blind, placebo-controlled study, we studied 40 patients with type I MPGN who were treated for 1 year with dipyridamole (225 mg/day) and aspirin (975 mg/day) [46]. Glomerular filtration rate (GFR), as estimated by iothalamate clearance, was stabilized, and shortened platelet survival was improved in the treatment group, suggesting a relationship between platelet consumption and the glomerular disease. The blinded conditions of our clinical trial ended after 1 year of treatment, and subsequently all patients were followed up regularly, including determinations of serum creatinine or iothalamate clearance. Data on survival analysis will be shown in a subsequent discussion that addresses the long-term treatment studies.

Another form of treatment that has received considerable attention is the long-term use of steroids in children. In a series of studies, McAdams, McEnery and West [116, 117] and Strife et al. [160] treated children with types I, II, and III disease with alternate-day prednisone in an uncontrolled fashion. The alternate-day regimen consisted of prednisone, 2.0 to 2.5 mg/kg (maximum 80 mg) as a single dose on alternate days. Treatment regarding the average daily dose and tapering schedules varied considerably. Many of the children had improved renal function and glomerular morphology. In an attempt to substantiate these long-term uncontrolled studies, the International Study of Kidney Disease in Children conducted a randomized, controlled clinical trial of alternate-day prednisone therapy in 37 children with type I MPGN [143]. Using a 50 percent decline in GFR as an end point, the authors found that the GFR was maintained but was not significantly different in the steroid-treated versus the placebo-treated patients. When treatment success was judged by the lack of either a reduction of GFR or a severe toxic reaction, for example, severe hypertension or seizures related to steroid use, there were no differences between the two treatment groups. The authors concluded that although alternate-day steroid therapy may slow the rate of progression of type I MPGN, long-term treatment is associated with substantial side effects. In a further follow-up of this study, Edelmann [55] suggested that the long-term use of low-dose prednisone improved survival. However, treatment failures with respect to renal failure were similar between the prednisone and control groups, and details of this longer follow-up are not available (both reports from the International Study have been published in abstract form only [55, 143]).

In addition to the randomized clinical trials, three long-term, uncontrolled treatment studies [105, 117, 129] and the long-term observations in our clinical trial of platelet inhibitor therapy [48] are available (Table 66-5). Treatments included alternate-day prednisone in children [117]; combinations of prednisone and cyclophosphamide, prednisone, cyclophosphamide, dipyridamole, and warfarin, and dipyridamole and nonsteroidal anti-inflammatory drugs in adults [129]; various nonsteroidal anti-inflammatory drugs in adults [105]; and dipyridamole and aspirin in a cohort of children and adults [46]. When survival curves from the onset of clinical illness were constructed, the 10-year cumulative survivals free of renal failure ranged from 60 to 85 percent in the various treatment groups (Table 66-5). In earlier published studies of children and adults with MPGN, many of whom were not treated or were treated in uncontrolled fashion with corticosteroids alone or in com-

Table 66-5. Survival free of renal failure 10 years after clinical onset of disease in patients receiving various nonplacebo treatments for MPGN

Patient group [ref]	No. of patients	Treatment (no. of patients)	10-year survival*
Children [117]	45	Alternate-day prednisone (31) + dipyridamole-aspirin or mechlorethamine (14)	74%
Adults [129]	107	Prednisone + cyclophosphamide (57) Prednisone + cyclophosphamide + dipyridamole + warfarin (29) Dipyridamole + nonsteroidal anti-inflammatory drug (19)	60%–80%
Adults [105]	53	Nonsteroidal anti-inflammatory drug (53)	85%
Children and adults [48]	21	Dipyridamole + aspirin (21)	70%

*Life-table analysis using treated patients in each treatment group.
Source: Modified from J. V. Donadio, Jr. and K. P. Offord. Reassessment of treatment results in membranoproliferative glomerulonephritis, with emphasis on life-table analysis. *Am. J. Kidney Dis.* 14:445, 1989. By permission from W. B. Saunders Co.

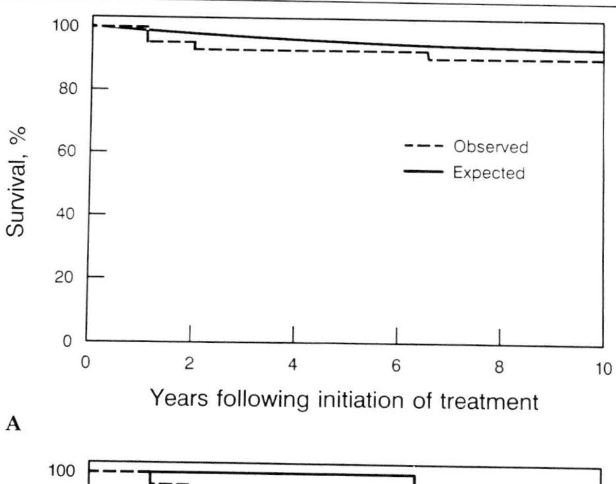

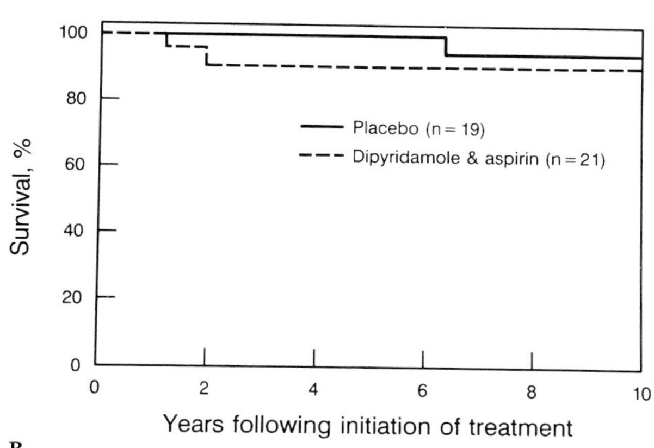

Fig. 66-4. Observed survival of patients with MPGN after initiation of treatment. A. Comparison of overall survival with expected survival of age- and sex-matched Upper Midwest (life-table) population. B. Comparison of observed survival in group treated with dipyridamole and aspirin versus placebo-treated group (difference was not significant by log-rank test comparing entire survival experience). (Adapted from J. V. Donadio, Jr. and K. P. Offord, Reassessment of treatment results in membranoproliferative glomerulonephritis, with emphasis on life-table analysis. *Am. J. Kidney Dis.* 14:445, 1989, by permission from W. B. Saunders Co.)

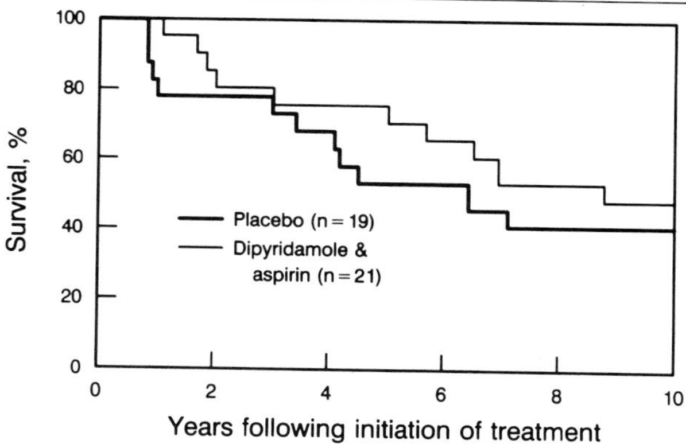

Fig. 66-5. Cumulative survival free of renal failure in patients with MPGN after initiation of treatment with dipyridamole and aspirin versus placebo (not significantly different by log-rank test comparing entire survival experience). (Adapted from J. V. Donadio, Jr. and K. P. Offord, Reassessment of treatment results in membranoproliferative glomerulonephritis, with emphasis on life-table analysis. *Am. J. Kidney Dis.* 14:445, 1989, by permission from W. B. Saunders Co.)

bination with cytotoxic drugs, antimalarial drugs, or nonsteroidal anti-inflammatory drugs, the 10-year cumulative survival was approximately 50 percent or less. The authors of the more recent studies [105, 117, 129] concluded that the observed improved survival was due to the treatments that were given.

Unfortunately, life-table analyses used to support this contention are not comparable because treatment was not started concurrently with the clinical onset in any of the patients. In fact, because in many patients treatment was begun many years after clinical onset, survival curves included the time before treatment was even begun. The only way improved survival can be predicated on a given therapy is to compare survival with that of a contemporaneous, randomly assigned, suitably matched control group and plot survival curves from the beginning of treatment. Studies that advocated alternate-day prednisone, the various combinations of prednisone and cyclophosphamide, dipyridamole, warfarin, and nonsteroidal anti-inflammatory drugs, and nonsteroidal anti-inflammatory drugs alone were uncontrolled and, therefore, did not have a control group with which to compare outcome. In our randomized clinical trial of dipyridamole and aspirin, survival curves were plotted from the beginning of treatment (Figs. 66-4 and 66-5). Overall, the observed 10-year patient survival was 92% ± 4.5% (mean ± SEM), compared with an expected survival of 94% ± 4% in the general population (Fig. 66-4A); survival was 90% ± 6.5% in patients treated with dipyridamole and aspirin and 94% ± 6% in the placebo-treated group (Fig. 66-4B). These differences are not significant. The 10-year cumulative survival free of renal failure was 49% ± 11.5% in the platelet inhibitor–treated group and 41% ± 11% in the placebo group, a difference that is not statistically significant (Fig. 66-5).

In conclusion, no treatment for children and adults with idiopathic MPGN has been proven effective. According to life-table analysis with time zero as the date from clinical onset, survival in the more recently studied patients is better than that reported in earlier studies. However, the improvement cannot be attributed to the different treatments that have been used because of the major flaw in constructing survival curves starting from the time of the detected onset of disease, which may be months to years before any therapy was started in many patients. Controlled clinical trials are still needed to test promising new therapies for this and other forms of chronic glomerulopathy.

Associated Disorders

In many of the associated disorders described (Table 66-1), the glomerular lesions resemble idiopathic MPGN in various ways on the basis of their histopathologic and immunopathologic features. There are usually mesangiocapillary features with mesangial proliferation, thickened capillary walls related to mesangial interposition and new basement-membrane formation, or lobular patterns on light microscopy. Immunofluorescence also can be similar to that observed in idiopathic MPGN. There can be granular, coarse, or segmental linear glomerular capillary wall staining and variable mesangial immunofluorescence with IgG, IgM, C3, and the early components of complement, C1q, and C2. In some of the disorders, type II MPGN has been the associated glomerulopathy.

SYSTEMIC IMMUNE-COMPLEX DISEASES

Systemic Lupus Erythematosus (SLE). An uncommon renal morphologic lesion similar to idiopathic MPGN occurs in SLE. It is categorized as a variant of type IV diffuse glomerulonephritis under the WHO morphologic classification of renal lesions in SLE [31]. It is a lesion that is particularly noted in patients who have been treated with corticosteroid, immunosuppressive drugs, or both. Occasionally, a patient with SLE shows a renal lesion of intramembranous dense deposit disease [61].

The clinical situation allows the clinician and renal pathologist to narrow a differential diagnosis when examining a renal biopsy sample. Although at times the morphologic changes are quite similar to the idiopathic disease, clinical features of SLE with laboratory confirmation (elevated anti-DNA antibodies, reduced complement, and its components in the serum), and findings of RBCs and RBC casts, proteinuria, and variably impaired renal function characterize the illness as SLE.

Mixed Cryoimmunoglobulinemia. The classification of cryoimmunoglobulinemia into types I, II, and III, the physical-chemical characteristics of the cryoprecipitates, and the diseases frequently associated with these different types are shown in Table 66-6 [15–17].

Prior to 1966, most recognized immunoglobulins were type I. It is now appreciated that "mixed" cryoimmunoglobulins (especially type III) occur more frequently. Mixed cryoimmunoglobulins have been found not only associated with B-cell proliferative disorders (usually type II) but also in various infections, autoimmune disorders, and hepatic and renal diseases (usually type III). These cryoimmunoglobulins are thought to be circulating immune complexes, with an IgM (less frequently IgG or IgA) antibody directed against another immunoglobulin (usually IgG), that are modified by or bound to an antigen in some way related to the underlying disease. The presence of these circulating cryoimmunoglobulins in different diseases has been considered an exacerbation of a normal physiologic process because, when sufficiently large amounts of blood are adequately analyzed for the presence of cryoimmunoglobulins, low levels (< 80 μg/ml) can be found in many healthy persons [37]. Tissue deposition of circulating cryoimmunoglobulins undoubtedly contributes to the underlying disease process in some cases [59] but, in others, the finding of small amounts of mixed cryoimmunoglobulins might have no pathogenetic consequence [74].

More than 50 percent of the patients with essential mixed cryoglobulinemia have evidence of renal involvement sometime during the course of their illness. The onset of the renal manifestations usually coincides with the development of extrarenal symptoms, and medical attention is frequently sought because of symptoms related to the kidney. In most patients, however, the renal manifestations occur after the onset of purpura, with an average delay of approximately 4 years. Nearly all patients with renal involvement have microhematuria, frequently with RBC casts and proteinuria—in the nephrotic range in approximately one-fourth of the patients. Episodes of acute glomerulonephritis with renal insufficiency are less common, but complete and sustained remissions are possible. Morphologically, the renal involvement in essential mixed cryoglobulinemia is characterized by a membranoproliferative glomerulonephritis, similar to idiopathic type I, with mesangial cell proliferation and expansion, subendothelial and mesangial deposits of immunoglobulins and complement, and occasional formation of pseudothrombi [174]. The afferent arterioles and interlobular arteries can show evidence of vasculitis. Hypertension is present in 50 percent or more of the patients with renal involvement. Less frequent renal manifestations of essential mixed cryoglobulinemia are ARF due to massive precipitation of cryoglobulins after cold exposure [26] and papillary necrosis, presumably from necrotizing angiitis of the vasa recta [102].

Hereditary Deficiency of Complement Components. Hereditary complement deficiencies can occur in healthy persons, but frequently these deficiencies carry a predisposition for the development of specific disorders, especially bacterial infections and immune-complex diseases. It is difficult to establish whether the coexistence of two different disorders is due to true association or just coincidence. Deficiencies of complement components, except for C1 inhibitor (C1-INH) and C2, are very rare. C1-INH deficiency is a common cause of angioneurotic edema, and two patients have been reported with MPGN—one lobular form and one type II—which may be a coincidental association [89]. The association of homozygous C2 deficiency with SLE is established beyond doubt [2]. The frequencies of homozygous and heterozygous C2 deficiencies are 0.0025 and 1 percent, respectively. Homozygous C2 deficiency also has been reported in some cases of MPGN [97, 109, 155] and anaphylactoid purpura [75]. Heterozygous C2 deficiency is also unusually frequent in SLE [2]. Patients with C2 deficiency and SLE have a low incidence of renal involvement. Deficiencies of C1, C4, C5, C7, and C8 also have been associated with SLE. It has been suggested that weaker inflammatory reactions can result from complement component deficiencies, and, in most instances, the renal disease in the associated immune-complex glomerulonephritis is mild. The occasional patient with C2 deficiency has been reported with severe MPGN, including recurrence in a renal allograft [109]. There are also scattered reports of MPGN, IgA nephropathy, and rapidly progressive glomerulonephritis associated with

Table 66-6. Classification of cryoimmunoglobulins [15–17]

	Ig type	Concentration	Temperature of initial cryoprecipitation	Associated diseases
Type I (monoclonal)	IgG or IgM Rarely IgA or light chains	High (90% > 1 mg/ml, 60% > 5 mg/ml)	Variable, often high (15–37°C)	Multiple myeloma, Waldenström's macroglobulinemia, monoclonal gammopathy of undetermined significance (essential monoclonal cryoimmunoglobulinemia)
Type II (mixed, monoclonal–polyclonal)	IgM–IgG IgM–IgG IgG_3–IgG_2 IgA–IgG	Intermediate (80% > 1 mg/ml, 40% > 5 mg/ml)	Intermediate	Multiple myeloma, Waldenström's macroglobulinemia, lymphoproliferative disease, essential mixed cryoimmunoglobulinemia, others, as in type III
Type III (mixed, polyclonal–polyclonal)	IgM–IgG IgM–IgG–IgA IgA–IgG	Low (80% < 1 mg/ml, 0% 5 mg/ml)	Variable, often low (18–33°C)	Connective tissue diseases, infections,* essential mixed cryoimmunoglobulinemia

*Epstein-Barr virus, cytomegalovirus, trypanosomiasis, lymphogranuloma venereum, primary and secondary syphilis, leprosy, subacute bacterial endocarditis, poststreptococcal glomerulonephritis, and so forth.

deficiencies of C1, C3, and factor H [137, 182]. In a recent study, partial complement deficiencies were observed in 22.7 percent of 44 patients with type I or type III MPGN [33]. This frequency was significantly higher than in the normal population. The deficiencies were present over long periods, were found in family members, and involved C2, C3, factor B, C6, C7, and C8. The authors suggested that the complement deficiencies are a predisposing factor in the pathogenesis of the disease. Most reports of the association of glomerulonephritis and complement deficiency have been in patients less than 20 years old. Hereditary complement deficiencies, therefore, should be suspected in young patients who have a low total complement and complement components that either are normal or have a single reduction. Some of these patients have siblings with similar problems or a history of recurrent infections.

NEOPLASTIC DISEASES

Light-chain nephropathy occurs in association with monoclonal B-cell proliferative disorders that are characterized by benign or malignant proliferation of a single clone of B lymphocytes or plasma cells. A nephropathy occurs when such neoplasms produce free monoclonal immunoglobulin light chains, with or without a complete serum monoclonal immunoglobulin. Moreover, a hematologic abnormality may be entirely inapparent. The conditions associated with light-chain nephropathy that have been reported include nodular, poorly differentiated lymphocytic lymphoma, diffuse large cell lymphoma, lymphoplasmacytic lymphoma (Waldenström), multiple myeloma, and monoclonal marrow plasmocytosis, which may initially appear insignificant or may evolve into frank myeloma [56, 69, 70, 72].

With the use of monospecific antisera for light-chain determinants, light-chain nephropathy has been described as a cause of renal failure associated with nodular mesangial and tubular basement-membrane deposition of monoclonal immunoglobulin light chains [142, 150, 168]. While usually restricted to renal tissue, this deposition may occur systemically in a manner similar to primary amyloidosis [72]. Kappa light chain is identified in the majority of cases (lambda light chains infrequently), producing a nodular glomerulosclerosis morphologically similar to that described in diabetes by Kimmelstiel and Wilson [3, 142, 150, 168].

The pathology and clinical manifestations of light-chain nephropathy are distinct from the much more common renal manifestations of multiple myeloma [43] and amyloidosis [135] and from the precipitation of cryoglobulin in Waldenström's macroglobulinemia [10]. Morphologically, the principal differential considerations are diabetes [72, 150], amyloidosis [135], and types I and II MPGN [3, 142].

Type I MPGN accounts for the most common diagnostic error and can be excluded by normal serum complement, the absence of evidence of immune complex deposition by immunofluorescence, a lack of true mesangial cell proliferation, and variable mesangiocapillary interposition.

Type II MPGN may occasionally resemble light-chain nephropathy when linear deposition predominates, although the electron-dense deposits of light-chain nephropathy tend to be more coarsely granular and subendothelial in location rather than the electron-dense homogeneous basement-membrane deposits of type II MPGN, which stain for C3 by immunofluorescence [3, 142].

Amyloid is excluded by negative Congo red, thioflavin T, metachromatic stains, and by the ultrastructural distinctions between the 80 to 100 Å diameter fibrils of amyloid and the granular electron-dense appearance of light-chain protein deposits.

Finally, diabetes can be excluded readily on clinical and biochemical grounds.

The onset of renal failure may supervene during the course of one of the associated monoclonal B-cell proliferative disorders, or it may occur primarily, with the subsequent diagnosis of an underlying hematologic disease. The common feature that links the hematologic and renal pathology is the secretion of monoclonal immunoglobulin light chains, which are deposited and can be demonstrated immunohistologically within renal tissue [3, 56, 70, 72, 168].

The cause of light-chain deposition is speculative, although there is good evidence that the nephrotoxicity of light chains is qualitative rather than quantitative. As an example, among patients with myeloma, Bence Jones proteinuria, which may be massive even in the absence of renal disease, is common; yet direct tissue deposition of immunologically recognizable light chains is rare [70]. Detailed studies of circulating and secreted light chains in patients with primary amyloidosis have shown abnormal light chains (usually lambda) as well as fragments and polymers of light chains [78, 103]. In vitro enzymatic degradation of certain light chains has been shown to produce amyloid fibrils, while other studies have shown a correlation between light-chain isoelectric points and renal tubular cast formation [32, 104].

There is also considerable evidence to suggest that light-chain nephropathy may relate to some intrinsic physical or chemical light-chain characteristics. Unlike amyloidosis in light-chain nephropathy, kappa light chains predominate [3, 142, 150, 168], although lambda chains have been reported [168], as have single cases of IgA kappa deposition [3] and another showing that production and deposition of proteins that have both lambda-chain and IgG Fc fragment determinants [56]. Clearly, only small amounts of light chain are required to produce the renal lesion, as evidenced by the frequent nonsecretory plasma-cell dyscrasias reported in association with light-chain nephropathy as compared to an incidence of less than 1 percent of all cases of myeloma [69, 70, 72, 150]. In most reports, the marrow plasmocytosis is monoclonal kappa, corresponding to the glomerular kappa-chain deposition [72, 150].

In *monoclonal cryoimmunoglobulinemia,* proliferative glomerulonephritis or MPGN and the nephrotic syndrome are uncommon [7, 11, 77, 96, 108, 136] in comparison to that seen in mixed cryoimmunoglobulinemia. It is questionable, however, whether some of the patients reported have monoclonal cryoimmunoglobulinemia or whether they have mixed cryoimmunoglobulinemia, with a large monoclonal and a small undetected polyclonal component. The presence of more than one immunoglobulin class in the glomerular deposits, examined by immunofluorescence in two patients, and the presence of rheumatoid factor activity in the serum or cryoprecipitate of four patients, cast some doubts on the monoclonal character of the cryoglobulinemia. Furthermore, the detection of mixed IgG–IgG cryoimmunoglobulins might be very difficult, since the monoclonal immunoglobulin may account for almost all the protein in the cryoprecipitate, and the latex test for rheumatoid factor is frequently negative [80]. Nevertheless, there are potential pathogenetic mechanisms by which cryoprecipitation of a monoclonal immunoglobulin can result in complement activation and an inflammatory reaction. These mechanisms may explain not only the exceptional cases of monoclonal cryoglobulinemia with glomerulonephritis but also other symptoms more commonly observed, such as cold-induced urticaria.

An occasional patient with *Hodgkin's disease* will have an associated nephrotic syndrome and MPGN. The association of the nephrotic syndrome (unrelated to amyloidosis) with Hodgkin's disease occurs in less than 1 percent of the cases, with fewer than 100 cases having been reported. In approximately 80 percent of the patients, the renal histology is consistent with minimal change disease [124].

The association of the nephrotic syndrome with *chronic lymphocytic leukemia* (with or without a monoclonal IgG cryoimmunoglobulin) or *non-Hodgkin's lymphomas* has been observed in several patients who had histologic glomerular changes that were consistent with MPGN (as well as other glomerulopathies, including segmental proliferative or sclerosing glomerulonephritis and, rarely, membranous glomerulopathy) [58, 77, 163].

Since the initial report by Lee et al. [107] in 1966, the association of *carcinomas* and nephrotic syndrome, unrelated to renal amyloidosis or renal vein thrombosis, has been reported frequently [55, 95]. In 70 percent of the patients, histologic examination of the kidney revealed membranous glomerulopathy. In the remaining 30 percent, other lesions are observed, including MPGN, minimal change disease, and crescentic glomerulonephritis. Because of this association, some authors have recommended evaluation of nephrotic adult patients, especially in the older age groups for occult malignancies.

INFECTIOUS DISEASES

A number of infectious diseases associated with MPGN have been described, usually as individual case reports or clinical studies containing a few patients. Among the chronic bacterial infections, type I MPGN is frequently associated with infected ventriculoatrial shunts, especially with *Staphylococcus epidermidis* [141, 158, 184]. Both improvement in renal function and reduction in proteinuria occur after replacement or revision of the infected shunt [184]. Another common association between infection and MPGN has been described in patients with *Schistosoma mansoni* infection in Brazil, in which it also has been observed that MPGN is a frequent glomerulopathy in adult patients with nephrotic syndrome in that country [140]. The lesion of MPGN varies from the description of the usual idiopathic types in that electron-dense deposits are located predominantly in the mesangium. Gardenswartz et al. [73] described MPGN, among several glomerulopathies, in patients with acquired immune deficiency syndrome (AIDS) who also demonstrated proteinuria, renal insufficiency, or both. The group with glomerulopathy also had a high incidence of other infections, including candidiasis, other fungal infections, and a high mortality. The described etiologic agent of AIDS, the so-called human T-cell lymphotropic virus type III (HTLV-III) [71], has not been associated with any other renal disorder.

What may be common between each of the infections listed in Table 66-1 and their association with MPGN is that the pathogenesis of the glomerular lesion relates to an apparent chronic antigenemia, resulting in an immune-complex glomerulopathy.

CHRONIC LIVER DISEASE

The association of glomerular disease with cirrhosis of the liver and hepatitis is well described. Evidence of clinical or serologic hepatitis B viral infection, or both, has been found in 0 to 50 percent of glomerulonephritic patients who have immune-complex deposits, especially those who have membranous glomerulopathy and, less frequently, those with MPGN and mesangiopathic glomerulonephritis [36, 127]. The association of hepatitis B viral antigens and membranous glomerulopathy has been especially frequent in pediatric populations [18, 64, 101, 110], in which membranous glomerulopathy is a rare cause of nephrotic syndrome, and in reports from Poland, Hungary, and Japan [18, 127, 165]. However, the association in the United States appears to be rare. Three viral antigens have been reported to be present in the deposits: HBsAg, HBcAg, and HBeAg [34, 165]. HBsAg might also be important in the pathogenesis of mixed cryoimmunoglobulinemia and vasculitis.

Glomerular lesions are common in cirrhosis of the liver. Generally, these lesions are clinically silent, but some patients may have microhematuria, proteinuria, or the nephrotic syndrome. The glomerular lesions observed are those of mesangiopathy or MPGN, often with deposits of IgA [12, 63, 113]. Deposits of aggregated IgA and immune complexes containing viral, bacterial, or dietary antigens and autoantigens have been suspected in the pathogenesis of these lesions. Eight patients with α_1-antitrypsin deficiency, phenotype ZZ, cirrhosis, and associated nephrotic syndrome have been described [125, 143, 159, 175]. The glomerular changes have most frequently been those of MPGN, and, in two cases, α_1-antitrypsin was demonstrated in the deposits by immunofluorescence [125, 175]. Nevertheless, deposits of IgA consistently seen in these patients and glomerulonephritis in α_1-antitrypsin deficiency is more likely related to chronic liver disease rather than to the presence of an abnormal protease inhibitor [159].

OTHER DISORDERS

A variety of unrelated diseases and clinical syndromes with which MPGN has been associated have been reported in individual or several case studies (Table 66-1). A clinical syndrome that has received much attention is one in which C3NeF was found in patients with partial lipodystrophy alone [154], with recurrent infections [154] and with intramembranous dense deposit disease [133, 154, 170, 181]. Such studies led to the isolation of C3NeF from the sera of these patients and further identified the nephritic factor as an immunoglobulin (IgG) that had the ability to break down C3 in normal human serum in vitro [39, 148, 166, 181]. Many of the other disorders listed suggest an association with a chronic glomerulopathy, such as MPGN, through chronic antigenemia, although a true immunologic pathogenesis has not been shown clearly in any of these disorders.

MPGN in Renal Allografts

Although it was recognized that glomerular changes frequently developed in a human allograft in the early experience of renal transplantation [84, 91], the differential diagnosis between chronic allograft rejection and recurrent and de novo glomerulonephritis is often difficult to make based on clinicopathologic studies. The reported incidence of recurrent MPGN in renal allografts varies considerably [20, 23, 38, 114, 118, 169]. This difference can be explained, in part, by the different methods of approach to the study of patients who have undergone renal transplantation. In some transplant centers, systematic renal biopsy specimens are taken, while in most centers, biopsy specimens are selective and based on finding increased urinary protein excretion (usually in the nephrotic range) or progressive loss of renal function (or both) in a patient that is not explained by rejection episodes. An important corollary to documenting recurrent glomerulonephritis of any kind in a renal allograft is the availability of an accurate morphologic diagnosis of the primary renal disease before transplantation [151].

Recurrence has been most frequently found in type II MPGN, especially by recognizing the presence of the characteristic intramembranous dense deposits of electron microscopy both with and without a membranoproliferative glomerulonephritis [20, 67, 81, 169]. Intramembranous dense deposits have been noted in 50 to 100 percent of allograft biopsy specimens taken several weeks to many years after the kidney was transplanted. In a review by Cameron [20], 42 (88%) of 48 renal allografts that were biopsied from patients with type II showed dense deposits in glomerular basement membrane. However, renal failure in the allograft due to recurrent type II MPGN is far less common than the reported incidence of recurrence of dense deposits [20, 23, 38]. Occasionally, fulminant MPGN with necrotizing and crescentic lesions and intramembranous dense deposits can produce early and rapid loss of graft function, usually accompanied by the nephrotic syndrome. Recurrence of type I MPGN is less frequent and is estimated to be about 25 to 30 percent [23, 38, 114, 169]. Documented allograft loss owing to a recurrent type I lesion is as uncommon as is the case with type II lesions (estimates in both instances of about 10%) [20]. Even when recurrent MPGN has been documented, most allograft renal failure is due to rejection [23, 114, 118, 169].

Several years after successful transplantation and stabilized renal function, the appearance of an abnormal urine sediment, progressive decline in renal function, and, especially, nephrotic-range proteinuria presents two further diagnostic considerations in addition to recurrence of a primary glomerular disease and chronic allograft rejection. These conditions are what have been called *glomerular transplant disease*, or *allograft glomerulonephritis*, and a true de novo *glomerulonephritis* [23, 88, 134]. Glomerular structural changes in allograft glomerulonephritis are nonuniform. They include thickening of the glomerular basement membrane, such as is seen in membranous nephropathy; mesangiocapillary interposition involving both endothelial and mesangial cells, and mesangial proliferation that is usually more focal and segmental than in idiopathic MPGN; focal, segmental sclerosing lesions, such as is seen in focal segmental glomerulosclerosis; and deposition of immunoglobulins, C3, and fibrinogen in mixed granular and linear capillary wall and mesangial patterns. Thus it is not surprising that it is difficult to distinguish between allograft glomerulonephritis and a true de novo glomerulonephritis. De novo type I MPGN has been documented only rarely [88, 139] and type II de novo glomerulonephritis has never been reported. Conditions for making a diagnosis of de novo MPGN require that rigid diagnostic features be fulfilled, including elimination of MPGN as the primary disease in the native kidneys, classic histologic and immunopathologic findings of MPGN in the allograft, and, preferably, low serum C3 levels. Clinically, the patient would most likely have a nephrotic syndrome.

Several pathogenetic mechanisms have been proposed for the development of allograft glomerulonephritis, including (1) various exogenous antigens, such as cytomegalic inclusion virus (CMV), antilymphocyte globulin, or HBsAg [23], (2) renal antigens that were produced under certain host conditions established either by rejection episodes and renal injury (analogous to the experimentally produced Heymann nephritis) [87], or (3) by soluble HLA antigen-antibody complexes [92]. None of these mechanisms has been demonstrated convincingly in patients with allograft glomerulonephritis. Finally, vesicoureteral reflux into transplanted kidneys is a frequent complication that has been infrequently associated with a glomerulopathy that resembles MPGN, with changes of mesangiocapillary interposition and expansion—changes that are also consistent with allograft glomerulonephritis [119].

References

1. Abreo, K., and Moorthy, A. V. Type 3 membranoproliferative glomerulonephritis: Clinicopathologic correlations and long-term follow-up in nine patients. *Arch. Pathol. Lab. Med.* 106: 413, 1982.
2. Angello, V. Association of systemic lupus erythematosus and SLE-like syndromes with hereditary and acquired complement deficiency states. *Arthritis Rheum.* Suppl. 21: 146, 1978.
3. Alpers, C. E., Tu, W.-H., Hopper, J., Jr., et al. Single light chain subclass (kappa chain) immunoglobulin deposition in glomerulonephritis. *Hum. Pathol.* 16: 294, 1985.
4. Anders, D., and Thoenes, W. Basement membrane-changes in membranoproliferative glomerulonephritis: A light and electron microscopic study. *Virchows Arch.* [*A*] [*Pathol. Anat.*] 369: 87, 1975.
5. Angus, K. W., Gardiner, A. C., Mitchell, B., et al. Mesangiocapillary glomerulonephritis in lambs: The ultrastructure and immunopathology of diffuse glomerulonephritis in newly born Finnish landrace lambs. *J. Pathol.* 131: 65, 1980.
6. Antoine, B., and Faye, C. The clinical course associated with dense deposits in the kidney basement membranes. *Kidney Int.* 1: 420, 1972.
7. Avasthi, P. S., Erickson, D. G., Williams, R. C., Jr., et al. Benign monoclonal gammaglobulinemia and glomerulonephritis. *Am. J. Med.* 62: 324, 1977.
8. Bannister, K. M., Howarth, G. S., Clarkson, A. R., et al. Glomerular IgG subclass distribution in human glomerulonephritis. *Clin. Nephrol.* 19: 161, 1983.
9. Barbiano di Belgiojoso, G., Tarantino, A., Colasanti, G., et al. The prognostic value of some clinical and histological parameters in membranoproliferative glomerulonephritis (MPGN): Report of 112 cases. *Nephron* 19: 250, 1977.
10. Beaufils, M., and Morel-Maroger, L. Pathogenesis of renal disease in monoclonal gammopathies: Current concepts. *Nephron* 20: 125, 1978.
11. Bengtsson, U., Larsson, O., Lindstedt, G., et al. Monoclonal IgG cryoglobulinemia with secondary development of glomerulonephritis and nephrotic syndrome. *Q. J. Med.* 44: 491, 1975.
12. Berger, J., Yaneva, H., and Nabarra, B. Lésions Glomérulaires des Cirrhotiques. In *Actualités Néphrologiques de l'Hôpital Necker.* Paris: Flammarion Medicine Sciences, 1977. Pp. 165–167.
13. Berry, P. L., McEnery, P. T., McAdams, A. J., et al. Membranoproliferative glomerulonephritis in two sibships. *Clin. Nephrol.* 16: 101, 1981.
14. Brando, B., Busnach, G., Bertoli, S., et al. T-suppressor cell abnormalities in type I membranoproliferative glomerulonephritis. *Proc. Eur. Dial. Transplant. Assoc.* 19: 669, 1983.
15. Brouet, J. C., Clauvel, J. P., and Danon, F. Cryoglobulins: Clinicobiological Correlations. In F. Chenais (ed.), *Cryoproteines.* Villars-de-Lans: Françoise Chenais, 1978. Pp. 159–170.
16. Brouet, J.-C., Clauvel, J.-P., Danon, F., et al. Biologic and clinical significance of cryoglobulins: A report of 86 cases. *Am. J. Med.* 57: 775, 1974.
17. Brouet, J. C., Danon, F., and Seligmann, M. Immunochemical Classification of Human Cryoglobulins. In F. Chenais (ed.), *Cryoproteines.* Villars-de-Lans: Françoise Chenais, 1978. Pp. 13–20.
18. Brzosko, W. J., Krawczyński, K., Nazarewicz, T., et al. Glomerulonephritis associated with hepatitis-B surface antigen immune complexes in children. *Lancet* 2: 477, 1974.
19. Burkholder, P. M., Marchand, A., and Krueger, R. P. Mixed membranous and proliferative glomerulonephritis: A correlative light, immunofluorescence, and electron microscopic study. *Lab. Invest.* 23: 459, 1970.
20. Cameron, J. S. Glomerulonephritis in renal transplants. *Transplantation* 34: 237, 1982.
21. Cameron, J. S. The Pathogenesis of Glomerulonephritis. In T. Bertani, and G. Remuzzi (eds.), *Glomerular Injury 300 Years After Morgagni.* Milano: Wichtig Editore, 1983. P. 18.
22. Cameron, J. S. Platelets in glomerular disease. *Annu. Rev. Med.* 35: 175, 1984.
23. Cameron, J. S., and Turner, D. R. Recurrent glomerulonephritis in allografted kidneys. *Clin. Nephrol.* 7: 47, 1977.

24. Cameron, J. S., Turner, D. R., Heaton, J., et al. Idiopathic mesangiocapillary glomerulonephritis: Comparison of types I and II in children and adults and long-term prognosis. *Am. J. Med.* 74: 175, 1983.
25. Campbell-Boswell, M. V., Linder, D., Naylor, B. R., et al. Kidney tubule basement membrane alterations in type II membranoproliferative glomerulonephritis. *Virchows Arch.* [A] [*Pathol. Anat.*] 382: 49, 1979.
26. Carloss, H. W., and Tavassoli, M. Acute renal failure from precipitation of cryoglobulins in a cool operating room. *J.A.M.A.* 244: 1472, 1980.
27. Cattran, D. C., Cardella, C. J., Roscoe, J. M., et al. Results of a controlled drug trial in membranoproliferative glomerulonephritis. *Kidney Int.* 27: 436, 1985.
28. Charlesworth, J. A., Williams, D. G., Sherington, E., et al. Metabolic studies of the third component of complement and the glycine-rich beta glycoprotein in patients with hypocomplementemia. *J. Clin. Invest.* 53: 1578, 1974.
29. Chatenoud, L., and Bach, M.-A. Abnormalities of T-cell subsets in glomerulonephritis and systemic lupus erythematosus. *Kidney Int.* 20: 267, 1981.
30. Churg, J., and Sobin, L. H. *Renal Disease: Classification and Atlas of Glomerular Diseases.* Tokyo: Igaku-Shoin, 1982. Pp. 83–110.
31. Churg, J., and Sobin, L. H. *Renal Disease: Classification and Atlas of Glomerular Diseases.* Tokyo: Igaku-Shoin, 1982. Pp. 127–149.
32. Clyne, D. H., Pesce, A. J., and Thompson, R. E. Nephrotoxicity of Bence Jones proteins in the rat: Importance of protein isoelectric point. *Kidney Int.* 16: 345, 1979.
33. Coleman, T. H., Forristal, J., Kosaka, T., et al. Inherited complement component deficiencies and membranoproliferative glomerulonephritis. *Kidney Int.* 24: 681, 1983.
34. Collins, A. B., Bhan, A. K., Dienstag, J. L., et al. Hepatitis B immune complex glomerulonephritis: Simultaneous glomerular deposition of hepatitis B surface and e antigens. *Clin. Immunol. Immunopathol.* 26: 137, 1983.
35. Colten, H. R., Levey, R. H., Rosen, F. S., et al. Decreased synthesis of C3 in membranoproliferative glomerulonephritis. (Abstract) *J. Clin. Invest.* 52: 20A, 1973.
36. Combes, B., Stastny, P., Shorey, J., et al. Glomerulonephritis with deposition of Australia antigen–antibody complexes in glomerular basement membrane. *Lancet* 2: 234, 1971.
37. Cream, J. J. Cryoglobulins in vasculitis. *Clin. Exp. Immunol.* 10: 117, 1972.
38. Curtis, J. J., Wyatt, R. J., Bhathena, D., et al. Renal transplantation for patients with type I and type II membranoproliferative glomerulonephritis: Serial complement and nephritic factor measurements and the problem of recurrence of disease. *Am. J. Med.* 66: 216, 1979.
39. Daha, M. R., and van Es, L. A. Further evidence for the antibody nature at C3 nephritic factor (C3NeF). *J. Immunol.* 123: 755, 1979.
40. Date, A., Neela, P., and Shastry, J. C. Thioflavin T fluorescence in membranoproliferative glomerulonephritis. *Nephron* 32: 90, 1982.
41. Davis, A. E., Schneeberger, E. E., Grupe, W. E., et al. Membranoproliferative glomerulonephritis (MPGN Type I) and dense deposit disease (DDD) in children. *Clin. Nephrol.* 9: 184, 1978.
42. Davis, C. A., Marder, H., and West, C. D. Circulating immune complexes in membranoproliferative glomerulonephritis. *Kidney Int.* 20: 728, 1981.
43. DeFronzo, R. A., Cooke, C. R., Wright, J. R., et al. Renal function in patients with multiple myeloma. *Medicine* (Baltimore) 57: 151, 1978.
44. Deuel, T. F., Senior, R. M., Chang, D., et al. Platelet factor 4 is chemotactic for neutrophils and monocytes. *Proc. Natl. Acad. Sci. U.S.A.* 78: 4584, 1981.
45. Deuel, T. F., Senior, R. M., Huang, J. S., et al. Chemotaxis of monocytes and neutrophils to platelet-derived growth factor. *J. Clin. Invest.* 69: 1046, 1982.
46. Donadio, J. V., Jr., Anderson, C. F., Mitchell, J. C., III, et al. Membranoproliferative glomerulonephritis: A prospective clinical trial of platelet-inhibitor therapy. *N. Engl. J. Med.* 310: 1421, 1984.
47. Donadio, J. V., Ilstrup, D. M., Holley, K. E., et al. Platelet-inhibitor treatment of diabetic nephropathy: Ten years of prospective study. *Mayo Clin. Proc.* 63: 3, 1988.
48. Donadio, J. V., and Offord, K. P. Reassessment of treatment results in membranoproliferative glomerulonephritis, with emphasis on life-table analysis. *Am. J. Kidney Dis.* 14: 445, 1989.
49. Donadio, J. V., Jr., Slack, T. K., Holley, K. E., et al. Idiopathic membranoproliferative (mesangiocapillary) glomerulonephritis: A clinicopathologic study. *Mayo Clin. Proc.* 54: 141, 1979.
50. Droz, D., Noel, L. H., Barbanel, C., et al. Evolution à long terme des glomérulonéphrites membranoprolifératives de l'adulte: Rémission spontanée durable chez 13 malades avec étude de biopsies rénales itératives dans 5 cas. *Nephrologie* 3: 6, 1982.
51. Droz, D., Zanetti, M., Noël, L.-H., et al. Dense deposits disease. *Nephron* 19: 1, 1977.
52. Duffus, P., Parbtani, A., Frampton, G., et al. Intraglomerular localization of platelet related antigens, platelet factor 4 and β-thromboglobulin in glomerulonephritis. *Clin. Nephrol.* 17: 288, 1982.
53. Dyck, R. F., Evans, D. J., Lockwood, C. M., et al. Amyloid P-component in human glomerular basement membrane: Abnormal patterns of immunofluorescent staining in glomerular disease. *Lancet* 2: 606, 1980.
54. Eagen, J. W., and Lewis, E. J. Glomerulopathies of neoplasia. *Kidney Int.* 11: 297, 1977.
55. Edelmann, C. M. Long-term low-dose prednisone ameliorates the course of membranoproliferative glomerulonephritis (MPGN): A report of the International Study of Kidney Disease in Children (Abstract). *Pediatr. Res.* 21: 474A, 1987.
56. Fang, L. S. T. Light-chain nephropathy. *Kidney Int.* 27: 582, 1985.
57. Fearon, D. T., Daha, M. R., Strom, T. B., et al. Pathways of complement activation in membranoproliferative glomerulonephritis and allograft rejection. *Transplant. Proc.* 9: 729, 1977.
58. Feehally, J., Hutchinson, R. M., Mackay, E. H., et al. Recurrent proteinuria in chronic lymphocytic leukemia. *Clin. Nephrol.* 16: 51, 1981.
59. Feiner, H. D. Relationship of tissue deposits of cryoglobulin to clinical features of mixed cryoglobulinemia. *Hum. Pathol.* 14: 710, 1983.
60. Fornasieri, A., Sinico, R., Fiorini, G., et al. T-lymphocyte subsets in primary and secondary glomerulonephritis. *Proc. Eur. Dial. Transplant. Assoc.* 19: 635, 1983.
61. Friedman, A. L., Chesney, R. W., Oberley, T. D., et al. Clinical systemic lupus erythematosus with dense deposit disease. *Int. J. Pediatr. Nephrol.* 4: 171, 1983.
62. Friend, P. S., Yunis, E. J., Noreen, H. J., et al. B-cell alloantigen associated with Chronic mesangiocapillary glomerulonephritis. *Lancet* 1: 562, 1977.

63. Fukuda, Y. Renal glomerular changes associated with liver cirrhosis. *Acta Pathol. Jpn.* 32: 561, 1982.
64. Furuse, A., Hattori, S., Terashima, T., et al. Circulating immune complex in glomerulonephropathy associated with hepatitis B virus infection. *Nephron* 31: 212, 1982.
65. Fuster, V., and Chesebro, J. H. Antithrombotic therapy: Role of platelet-inhibitor drugs. I. Current concepts of thrombogenesis: Role of platelets (first of three parts). *Mayo Clin. Proc.* 56: 102, 1981.
66. Gaffney, E. F. Prominent parietal epithelium: A common sign of renal glomerular injury. *Hum. Pathol.* 13: 651, 1982.
67. Galle, P., Hinglais, N., and Crosnier, J. Recurrence of an original glomerular lesion in three renal allografts. *Transplant. Proc.* 3: 368, 1971.
68. Galle, P., and Mahieu, P. Electron dense alteration of kidney basement membranes: A renal lesion specific of a systemic disease. *Am. J. Med.* 58: 749, 1975.
69. Gallo, G. R., Feiner, H. D., and Buxbaum, J. N. The kidney in lymphoplasmacytic disorders (part 1). *Pathol. Annu.* 17: 291, 1982.
70. Gallo, G. R., Feiner, H. D., Katz, L. A., et al. Nodular glomerulopathy associated with nonamyloidotic kappa light chain deposits and excess immunoglobulin light chain synthesis. *Am. J. Pathol.* 99: 621, 1980.
71. Gallo, R. C., Salahuddin, S. Z., Popovic, M., et al. Frequent detection and isolation of cytopathic retroviruses (HTLV-III) from patients with AIDS and at risk for AIDS. *Science* 224: 500, 1984.
72. Ganeval, D., Mignon, F., Preud'Homme, J. L., et al. Visceral deposition of monoclonal light chains and immunoglobulins: A study of renal and immunopathologic abnormalities. *Adv. Nephrol.* 11: 25, 1982.
73. Gardenswartz, M. H., Lerner, C. W., Seligson, G. R., et al. Renal disease in patients with AIDS: A clinicopathologic study. *Clin. Nephrol.* 21: 197, 1984.
74. Garin, E. H., Fennell, R. S., Shulman, S. T., et al. Clinical significance of the presence of cryoglobulins in patients with glomerulopathies not associated with systemic disease. *Clin. Nephrol.* 13: 5, 1980.
75. Gelfand, E. W., Clarkson, J. E., and Minta, J. O. Selective deficiency of the second component of complement in a patient with anaphylactoid purpura. *Clin. Immunol. Immunopathol.* 4: 269, 1975.
76. George, C. R. P., Slichter, S. J., Quadracci, L. J., et al. A kinetic evaluation of hemostasis in renal disease. *N. Engl. J. Med.* 291: 1111, 1974.
77. Gilboa, N., Durante, D., Guggenheim, S., et al. Immune deposit nephritis and single-component cryoglobulinemia associated with chronic lymphocytic leukemia: Evidence for a role of circulating IgG-anti-IgG immune complexes in the pathogenesis of the renal lesion. *Nephron* 24: 223, 1979.
78. Glenner, G. G., Ein, D., Eanes, E. D., et al. Creation of "amyloid" fibrils from Bence Jones proteins in vitro. *Science* 174: 712, 1971.
79. Gotoff, S. P., Fellers, F. X., Vawter, G. F., et al. The $beta_{1C}$ globulin in childhood nephrotic syndrome: Laboratory diagnosis of progressive glomerulonephritis. *N. Engl. J. Med.* 273: 524, 1965.
80. Grey, H. M., Kohler, P. F., Terry, W. D., et al. Human monoclonal γG-cryoglobulins with anti-γ-globulin activity. *J. Clin. Invest.* 47: 1875, 1968.
81. Habib, R., Gubler, M.-C., Loirat, C., et al. Dense deposit disease: A variant of membranoproliferative glomerulonephritis. *Kidney Int.* 7: 204, 1975.
82. Habib, R., Kleinknecht, C., Gubler, M. C., et al. Idiopathic membranoproliferative glomerulonephritis in children. Report of 105 cases. *Clin. Nephrol.* 1: 194, 1973.
83. Habib, R., and Lévy, M. Membranoproliferative Glomerulonephritis. In J. Hamburger, J. Crosnier, J.-P. Grünfeld (eds.), *Nephrology*. New York: Wiley, 1979. Pp. 507–534.
84. Hamburger, J., Crosnier, J., and Dormont, J. Observations in patients with a well-tolerated homotransplanted kidney: Possibility of a new secondary disease. *Ann. N.Y. Acad. Sci.* 120: 558, 1964.
85. Heptinstall, R. H. *Pathology of the Kidney*, 3rd ed., Vol. 1. Boston: Little, Brown, 1983. Pp. 479–518.
86. Herdman, R. C., Pickering, R. J., Michael, A. F., et al. Chronic glomerulonephritis associated with low serum complement activity (chronic hypocomplementemic glomerulonephritis). *Medicine* (Baltimore) 49: 207, 1970.
87. Heymann, W., Hackel, D. B., Harwood, S., et al. Production of nephrotic syndrome in rats by Freund's adjuvants and rat kidney suspensions. *Proc. Soc. Exp. Biol. Med.* 100: 660, 1959.
88. Honkanen, E., Törnroth, T., Pettersson, E., et al. Glomerulonephritis in renal allografts: Results of 18 years of transplantations. *Clin. Nephrol.* 21: 210, 1984.
89. Hory, B., Panouse-Perrin, J., Saint-Hillier, Y., et al. Déficit héréditaire en inhibiteur de la C1 estérase: Lupus et glomérulonéphrite. *Rev. Med. Interna* 4: 57, 1983.
90. Hultberg, B., and Ravnskov, U. The excretion of N-acetyl-β-glucosaminidase in glomerulonephritis. *Clin. Nephrol.* 15: 33, 1981.
91. Hume, D. M., Sterling, W. A., Weymouth, R. J., et al. Glomerulo-nephritis in human renal homotransplants. *Transplant. Proc.* 2: 361, 1970.
92. Jeannet, M., Pinn, V. W., Flax, M. H., et al. Humoral antibodies in renal allotransplantation in man. *N. Engl. J. Med.* 282: 111, 1970.
93. Jones, D. B. Membranoproliferative glomerulonephritis: One or many diseases? *Arch. Pathol. Lab. Med.* 101: 457, 1977.
94. Kamitsuji, H., Kusumoto, K., Taira, K., et al. Localization of intrarenal cross-linked fibrin in children with various renal diseases. *Nephron* 35: 94, 1983.
95. Kaplan, B. S., Klassen, J., and Gault, M. H. Glomerular injury in patients with neoplasia. *Annu. Rev. Med.* 27: 117, 1976.
96. Kaplan, N. G., and Kaplan, K. C. Monoclonal gammopathy, glomerulonephritis, and the nephrotic syndrome. *Arch. Intern. Med.* 125: 696, 1970.
97. Kim, Y., Friend, P. S., Dresner, I. G., et al. Inherited deficiency of the second component of complement (C2) with membranoproliferative glomerulonephritis. *Am. J. Med.* 62: 765, 1977.
98. Kim, Y., Michael, A. F., and Fish, A. J. Idiopathic membranoproliferative glomerulonephritis. *Contemp. Issues Nephrol.* 9: 237, 1982.
99. Kim, Y., Vernier, R. L., Fish, A. J., et al. Immunofluorescence studies of dense deposit disease: The presence of railroad tracks and mesangial rings. *Lab. Invest.* 40: 474, 1979.
100. Kincaid-Smith, P. The treatment of chronic mesangiocapillary (membranoproliferative) glomerulonephritis with impaired renal function. *Med. J. Aust.* 2: 587, 1972.
101. Kleinknecht, C., Levy, M., Gagnadoux, M.-F., et al. Membranous glomerulonephritis with extra-renal disorders in children. *Medicine* (Baltimore) 58: 219, 1979.
102. Koelz, A. M., and Bourke, E. Cryoglobulinaemic nephropathy with papillary necrosis. *Nephron* 19: 242, 1977.

103. Kyle, R. A., and Bayrd, E. D. Amyloidosis: Review of 236 cases. *Medicine* (Baltimore) 54: 271, 1975.
104. Kyle, R. A., and Greipp, P. R. The laboratory investigation of monoclonal gammopathies. *Mayo Clin. Proc.* 53: 719, 1978.
105. Lagrue, G., Laurent, J., and Belghiti, D. Renal survival in membranoproliferative glomerulonephritis (MPGN): Role of long-term treatment with non-steroid anti-inflammatory drugs (NSAID). *Int. Urol. Nephrol.* 20: 669, 1988.
106. Lamb, V., Tisher, C. C., McCoy, R. C., et al. Membranoproliferative glomerulonephritis with dense intramembranous alterations: A clinicopathologic study. *Lab. Invest.* 36: 607, 1977.
107. Lee, J. C., Yamauchi, H., and Hopper, J., Jr. The association of cancer in the nephrotic syndrome. *Ann. Intern. Med.* 64: 41, 1966.
108. Lockwood, C. M. Lymphoma, cryoglobulinemia, and renal disease. *Kidney Int.* 16: 522, 1979.
109. Loirat, C., Levy, M., Peltier, A. P., et al. Deficiency of the second component of complement: Its occurrence with membranoproliferative glomerulonephritis. *Arch. Pathol. Lab. Med.* 104: 467, 1980.
110. López Gómez, J. M., Canals, M. J., Rengel, M., et al. Asociación del antígeno de superficie del virus de la hepatitis B (AgHBs) con la nefropatía membranosa en la infancia. *Rev. Clin. Esp.* 164: 153, 1982.
111. Magil, A. B., Price, J. D. E., Bower, G., et al. Membranoproliferative glomerulonephritis type 1: Comparison of natural history in children and adults. *Clin. Nephrol.* 11: 239, 1979.
112. Mandalenakis, N., Mendoza, N., Pirani, C. L., et al. Lobular glomerulonephritis and membranoproliferative glomerulonephritis. *Medicine* (Baltimore) 50: 319, 1971.
113. Manigand, G., Taillandier, J., Morel-Maroger, L., et al. La néphropathie glomérulaire des cirrhoses du foie. *Ann. Med. Interne (Paris)* 132: 178, 1981.
114. Mathew, T. H., Mathews, D. C., Hobbs, J. B., et al. Glomerular lesions after renal transplantation. *Am. J. Med.* 59: 177, 1975.
115. Mazzucco, G., Barbiano di Belgiojoso, G., et al. Glomerulonephritis with dense deposits: A variant of membranoproliferative glomerulonephritis or a separate morphological entity? Light, electron microscopic and immunohistochemical study of eleven cases. *Virchows Arch.* [*A*] [*Pathol. Anat.*] 387: 17, 1980.
116. McAdams, A. J., McEnery, P. T., and West, C. D. Mesangiocapillary glomerulonephritis: Changes in glomerular morphology with long-term alternate-day prednisone therapy. *J. Pediatr.* 86: 23, 1975.
117. McEnery, P. T., McAdams, A. J., and West, C. D. The effect of prednisone in a high-dose, alternate-day regimen on the natural history of idiopathic membranoproliferative glomerulonephritis. *Medicine* 64: 401, 1985.
118. McLean, R. H., Geiger, H., Burke, B., et al. Recurrence of membranoproliferative glomerulonephritis following kidney transplantation: Serum complement component studies. *Am. J. Med.* 60: 60, 1976.
119. McMorrow, R. G., Curtis, J. J., Lucas, B. A., et al. Does vesicoureteric reflux result in renal allograft failure? *Clin. Nephrol.* 14: 89, 1980.
120. Michielsen, P., Van Damme, B., Dotremont, G., et al. Indomethacin Treatment of Membranoproliferative and Lobular Glomerulonephritis. In P. Kincaid-Smith, T. H. Mathew, and E. L. Becker (eds.), *Glomerulonephritis: Morphology, Natural History, and Treatment.* New York: Wiley, 1973. Pp. 611–631.
121. Michielsen, P., and Varenterghem, Y. Proteinuria and nonsteroid anti-inflammatory drugs. *Adv. Nephrol.* 12: 139, 1983.
122. Miller, K., Dresner, I. G., and Michael, A. F. Localization of platelet antigens in human kidney disease. *Kidney Int.* 18: 472, 1980.
123. Miller, M. N., Baumel, R., Poucell, S., et al. Incidence and prognostic importance of glomerular crescents in renal diseases of childhood. *Am. J. Nephrol.* 4: 244, 1984.
124. Moorthy, A. V., Zimmerman, S. W., and Burkholder, P. M. Nephrotic syndrome in Hodgkin's disease: Evidence for pathogenesis alternative to immune complex deposition. *Am. J. Med.* 61: 471, 1976.
125. Moroz, S. P., Cutz, E., Balfe, J. W., et al. Membranoproliferative glomerulonephritis in childhood cirrhosis associated with alpha$_1$-antitrypsin deficiency. *Pediatrics* 57: 232, 1976.
126. Moseley, H. L., and Whaley, K. Control of complement activation in membranous and membranoproliferative glomerulonephritis. *Kidney Int.* 17: 535, 1980.
127. Nagy, J., Bajtai, G., Brasch, H., et al. The role of hepatitis B surface antigen in the pathogenesis of glomerulopathies. *Clin. Nephrol.* 12: 109, 1979.
128. Nakashima, Y., Hirose, S., and Hamashima, Y. Proliferation of cultured rabbit renal glomerular cells stimulated by platelet factor. *Acta Pathol. Jpn.* 30: 1, 1980.
129. Narita, M., and Koyama, A. Therapeutic and Prognostic Studies in Renal Disease, part 2. In S. Tojo (Director), *1987's Annual Report of Progressive Renal Lesions.* Japan: Ministry of Health and Welfare, 1988. Pp. 244–253.
130. Ooi, Y. M., Vallota, E. H., and West, C. D. Classical complement pathway activation in membranoproliferative glomerulonephritis. *Kidney Int.* 9: 46, 1976.
131. Parbtani, A., Frampton, G., and Cameron, J. S. Platelet and plasma serotonin concentrations in glomerulonephritis, II. *Clin. Nephrol.* 14: 112, 1980.
132. Parbtani, A., Frampton, G., Yewdall, V., et al. Platelet and plasma serotonin in glomerulonephritis. III: The nephritis of systemic lupus erythematosus. *Clin. Nephrol.* 14: 164, 1980.
133. Peters, D. K., Williams, D. G., Charlesworth, J. A., et al. Mesangiocapillary nephritis, partial lipodystrophy, and hypocomplementaemia. *Lancet* 2: 535, 1973.
134. Petersen, V. P., Olsen, T. S., Kissmeyer-Nielsen, F., et al. Late failure of human renal transplants: An analysis of transplant disease and graft failure among 125 recipients surviving for one to eight years. *Medicine* (Baltimore) 54: 45, 1975.
135. Pirani, C. L. Tissue Distribution of Amyloid. In O. Wegelius and A. Pasternack (eds.), *Amyloidosis.* New York: Academic Press, 1976. Pp. 33–46.
136. Ponticelli, C., Imbasciati, E., Tarantino, A., et al. Acute anuric glomerulonephritis in monoclonal cryoglobulinaemia. *Br. Med. J.* 1: 948, 1977.
137. Pussell, B. A., Bourke, E., Nayef, M., et al. Complement deficiency and nephritis: A report of a family. *Lancet* 1: 675, 1980.
138. Pussell, B. A., Lockwood, C. M., Scott, D. M., et al. Value of immune-complex assays in diagnosis and management. *Lancet* 2: 359, 1978.
139. Pommer, W., Schultze, G., Bohl, D., et al. De novo membrano-proliferative glomerulonephritis in a renal allograft. *Int. Urol. Nephrol.* 15: 359, 1983.
140. Queiroz, F. P., Brito, E., and Martinelli, R. Influence of regional factors in the distribution of the histologic patterns of glomerulopathies in the nephrotic syndrome. *Nephron* 14: 466, 1975.

141. Rames, L., Wise, B., Goodman, J. R., et al. Renal disease with *Staphylococcus albus* bacteremia: A complication in ventriculoatrial shunts. *J.A.M.A.* 212: 1671, 1970.
142. Randall, R. E., Williamson, W. C., Jr., Mullinax, F., et al. Manifestations of systemic light chain deposition. *Am. J. Med.* 60: 293, 1976.
143. Report of the International Study of Kidney Disease in Children. Alternate day steroid therapy in membranoproliferative glomerulonephritis: A randomized controlled clinical trial. (Abstract) *Kidney Int.* 21: 150, 1982.
144. Rodriguez-Soriano, J., Fidalgo, I., Camarero, C., et al. Juvenile cirrhosis and membranous glomerulonephritis in a child with alpha$_1$-antitrypsin deficiency PiSZ. *Acta Paediatr. Scand.* 67: 793, 1978.
145. Ross, R., Glomset, J., Kariya, B., et al. A platelet-dependent serum factor that stimulates the proliferation of arterial smooth muscle cells *in vitro*. *Proc. Natl. Acad. Sci. U.S.A.* 71: 1207, 1974.
146. Sakai, H., Nomoto, Y., Arimori, S., et al. Increase of IgM-bearing peripheral blood lymphocytes in patients with idiopathic membranoproliferative glomerulonephritis (MPGN) and their family members. *Clin. Nephrol.* 12: 210, 1979.
147. Schena, F. P., Pertosa, G., Stanziale, P., et al. Biological significance of the C3 nephritic factor in membranoproliferative glomerulonephritis. *Clin. Nephrol.* 18: 240, 1982.
148. Schiffer, M. S., Michael, A. F., Kim, Y., et al. Distribution of glomerular basement membrane antigens in diseased human kidneys. *Lab. Invest.* 44: 234, 1981.
149. Schreiber, R. D., Götze, O., and Müller-Eberhard, H. J. Nephritic factor: Its structure and function and its relationship to initiating factor of the alternative pathway. *Scand. J. Immunol.* 5: 705, 1976.
150. Schubert, G. E., and Adam, A. Glomerular nodules and long-spacing collagen in kidneys of patients with multiple myeloma. *J. Clin. Pathol.* 27: 800, 1974.
151. Schwartz, M. M., and Cotran, R. S. Primary renal disease in transplant recipients. *Hum. Pathol.* 7: 455, 1976.
152. Sherman, R. L., Drayer, D. E., Leyland-Jones, B. R., et al. *N*-acetyl-β-glucosaminidase and β_2-microglobulin: Their urinary excretion in patients with renal parenchymal disease. *Arch. Intern. Med.* 143: 1183, 1983.
153. Sibley, R. K., and Kim, Y. Dense intramembranous deposit disease: New pathologic features. *Kidney Int.* 25: 660, 1984.
154. Sissons, J. G. P., West, R. J., Fallows, J., et al. The complement abnormalities of lipodystrophy. *N. Engl. J. Med.* 294: 461, 1976.
155. Sobel, A. T., Moisy, M., Hirbec, G., et al. Hereditary C2 deficiency associated with nonsystemic glomerulonephritis. *Clin. Nephrol.* 12: 132, 1979.
156. Sølling, J. Circulating immune complexes in glomerulonephritis: A longitudinal study. *Clin. Nephrol.* 20: 177, 1983.
157. Spargo, B. H., Seymour, A. E., and Ordóñez, N. G. *Renal Biopsy Pathology with Diagnostic and Therapeutic Implications*. New York: Wiley, 1980. Pp. 120–151.
158. Stickler, G. B., Shin, M. H., and Burke, E. C. Diffuse glomerulonephritis associated with infected ventriculoatrial shunt. *N. Engl. J. Med.* 279: 1077, 1968.
159. Strife, C. F., Hug, G., Chuck, G., et al. Membranoproliferative glomerulonephritis and α_1-antitrypsin deficiency in children. *Pediatrics* 71: 88, 1983.
160. Strife, C. F., Jackson, E. C., and McAdams, A. J. Type III membranoproliferative glomerulonephritis: Long-term clinical and morphologic evaluation. *Clin. Nephrol.* 21: 323, 1984.
161. Strife, C. F., McAdams, A. J., and West, C. D. Membranoproliferative glomerulonephritis characterized by focal, segmental proliferative lesions. *Clin. Nephrol.* 18: 9, 1982.
162. Strife, C. F., McEnery, P. T., McAdams, A. J., et al. Membranoproliferative glomerulonephritis with disruption of the glomerular basement membrane. *Clin. Nephrol.* 7: 65, 1977.
163. Strippoli, P., De Marco, S., Marinosci, A., et al. Chronic lymphocytic leukemia and membranoproliferative glomerulonephritis. *Haematologica (Pavia)* 67: 805, 1982.
164. Swainson, C. P., Robson, J. S., Thomson, D., et al. Mesangiocapillary glomerulonephritis: A long-term study of 40 cases. *J. Pathol.* 141: 449, 1983.
165. Takekoshi, Y., Tanaka, M., Miyakawa, Y., et al. Free "small" and IgG-associated "large" hepatitis B e antigen in the serum and glomerular capillary walls of two patients with membranous glomerulonephritis. *N. Engl. J. Med.* 300: 814, 1979.
166. Thompson, R. A. C3 inactivating factor in the serum of a patient with chronic hypocomplementaemic proliferative glomerulo-nephritis. *Immunology* 22: 147, 1972.
167. Tiller, D. J., Clarkson, A. R., Mathew, T., et al. A Prospective Randomized Trial in the Use of Cyclophosphamide, Dipyridamole and Warfarin in Membranous and Mesangiocapillary Glomerulonephritis. In W. Zurukzoglu, M. Papadimitriou, M. Pyrpasopoulos, et al. (eds.), *Proceedings of the 8th International Congress of Nephrology. Advances in Basic and Clinical Nephrology*. Basel: Karger, 1981. Pp. 345–351.
168. Tubbs, R. R., Gephardt, G. N., McMahon, J. T., et al. Light chain nephropathy. *Am. J. Med.* 71: 263, 1981.
169. Turner, D. R., Cameron, J. S., Bewick, M., et al. Transplantation in mesangiocapillary glomerulonephritis with intramembranous dense "deposits": Recurrence of disease. *Kidney Int.* 9: 439, 1976.
170. Vallota, E. H., Forristal, J., Davis, N. C., et al. The C3 nephritic factor and membranoproliferative nephritis: Correlation of serum levels of the nephritic factor with C3 levels, with therapy, and with progression of the disease. *J. Pediatr.* 80: 947, 1972.
171. Varenterghem, Y., Roels, L., Verberckmoes, R., et al. Treatment of chronic glomerulonephritis with a combination of indomethacin and cyclophosphamide. *Clin. Nephrol.* 4: 218, 1975.
172. Vargas, A. R., Thomson, K. J., Wilson, D., et al. Mesangiocapillary glomerulonephritis with dense "deposits" in the basement membranes of the kidney. *Clin. Nephrol.* 5: 73, 1976.
173. Velosa, J. A., Torres, V. E., Donadio, J. V., Jr., et al. Treatment of severe nephrotic syndrome with meclofenamate: An uncontrolled pilot study. *Mayo Clin. Proc.* 60: 586, 1985.
174. Verroust, P., Mery, J.-P., Morel-Maroger, L., et al. Glomerular lesions in monoclonal gammopathies and mixed essential cryoglobulinemias IgG-IgM. *Adv. Nephrol.* 1: 161, 1971.
175. Ward, A. M., Pickering, J. D., and Shortland, J. R. The Renal Manifestations of PiZ. In J.-P. Martin (ed.), *L'Alpha-1-Antitrypsine et le Systéme Pi*. Paris: INSERM, 1975. Pp. 131–134.
176. Watson, A. R., Poucell, S., Thorner, P., et al. Membranoproliferative glomerulonephritis type I in children: Correlation of clinical features with pathologic subtypes.

Am. J. Kidney Dis. 4: 141, 1984.

177. Weiss, M. A., Ooi, B. S., Ooi, Y. M., et al. Immunofluorescent localization of fibronectin in the human kidney. *Lab. Invest.* 41: 340, 1979.
178. West, C. D. Pathogenesis and approaches to therapy of membranoproliferative glomerulonephritis. *Kidney Int.* 9: 1, 1976.
179. West, C. D., McAdams, A. J., McConville, J. M., et al. Hypocomplementemic and normocomplementemic persistent (chronic) glomerulonephritis: Clinical and pathologic characteristics. *J. Pediatr.* 67: 1089, 1965.
180. Whaley, K., Ward, D., and Ruddy, S. Modulation of the properdin amplification loop in membranoproliferative and other forms of glomerulonephritis. *Clin. Exp. Immunol.* 35: 101, 1979.
181. Williams, D. G., Bartlett, A., and Duffus, P. Identification of nephritic factor as an immunoglobulin. *Clin. Exp. Immunol.* 33: 425, 1978.
182. Wyatt, R. J., Julian, B. A., Weinstein, A., et al. Partial H (β1H) deficiency and glomerulonephritis in two families. *J. Clin. Immunol.* 2: 110, 1982.
183. Wyatt, R. J., McAdams, A. J., Forristal, J., et al. Glomerular deposition of complement-control proteins in acute and chronic glomerulonephritis. *Kidney Int.* 16: 505, 1979.
184. Yeh, B. P.-Y., Young, H. F., Schatzki, P. F., et al. Immune complex disease associated with an infected ventriculojugular shunt: A curable form of glomerulonephritis. *South Med. J.* 70: 1141, 1977.
185. Zimmerman, S. W., Moorthy, A. V., Dreher, W. H., et al. Prospective trial of warfarin and dipyridamole in patients with membranoproliferative glomerulonephritis. *Am. J. Med.* 75: 920, 1983.

IgA Nephropathy and Henoch-Schönlein Purpura

Anthony R. Clarkson
Andrew J. Woodroffe
Ian Aarons

IgA nephropathy is now regarded as the most common form of glomerulonephritis in the world [47]. Its "discovery" in 1968 by Berger and Hinglais [17, 18] depended on the systematic application of fluorescein conjugated antibodies to IgA to human renal biopsies for the first time and was promoted so assiduously by Jean Berger that the entity became eponymously linked to him—Berger's disease. In the original series, 25 percent of 300 biopsies fluoresced strongly for IgA. While a small number of these biopsies were from patients with systemic lupus erythematosus (SLE), Henoch-Schönlein purpura (HSP), and other systemic diseases, the majority came from patients suffering recurring bouts of macroscopic hematuria or hematuria detected only by urine microscopy and with no overt systemic symptoms. In these patients, the IgA fluorescence was mesangial and accompanied by IgG and C3.

Since the original reports, there has been progressively wider interest in the natural history, pathology, and immunology of IgA nephropathy despite a skeptical reception to it initially. Doubts concerning the specificity of the IgA antisera used and the alarmingly high incidence of the disease in France have been dispelled over the ensuing 23 years in all countries where renal biopsy is practiced extensively.

Progress in understanding the pathogenesis has been slow, although recently acquired knowledge of the biology of immunoglobulin A has spurred research. In addition to its function in mucosal immunity at the level of the upper and lower respiratory, gastrointestinal, and genitourinary tracts, the roles of secretory component and the enterohepatic circulation and the various cytokines in the regulation of IgA synthesis have attracted wide attention. Recognition of secondary forms of IgA nephropathy in which derangements of IgA biology clearly contribute to the development of renal disease likewise has pointed to possible pathogenetic mechanisms in the primary disease.

The disease is not nearly so benign as initially thought. As more knowledge is acquired of the natural history, estimates of 15 to 20 percent of cases progressing to end-stage renal failure have been revised upward to 25 to 40 percent. Furthermore, IgA nephropathy recurs in kidneys transplanted to recipients with the disease and disappears from kidneys inadvertently transplanted from donors suffering from IgA nephropathy into recipients not likewise afflicted. Positive immunofluorescence for IgA is not limited to the glomerular mesangium in IgA nephropathy. It has also been described in capillaries of the dermis [7], lung, liver, and gut. These observations suggest strongly that the disease is systemic in nature and the probability of immune-complex mediation has been supported by many authors [40, 48, 57, 65, 83, 116, 145, 183, 212, 213, 234]. Many workers also have emphasized the almost identical immunopathologic features of HSP and question the separate identity of these conditions. Historically HSP is a much older disease than IgA nephropathy. It is a clinical syndrome readily recognized because of the overt purpura, arthritis, gut manifestations, and glomerulonephritis. While Schönlein [192] in 1837 associated the purpura and arthritis, and Henoch in 1874 [87] later recognized the gastrointestinal and renal manifestations, the first clinical description of the disease was probably by Heberden in 1806 [85].

Until the 1970s, most accounts of HSP were descriptive, but once again, the advent of immunofluorescence technology allowed exploration of possible immunopathogenetic mechanisms. As with IgA nephropathy, positive IgA immunofluorescence occurs in the glomerular mesangium, skin (especially in purpuric lesions) [6], and other organs; IgA-containing immune complexes are present in the circulation [76, 103, 234]; there are primary and secondary forms; and similar aberrations exist in the control of IgA production. While the clinical features, incidence, and age of onset tend to vary, the many similarities of these two conditions suggest that they may represent a spectrum of the same systemic disease. Their combined frequencies in many communities is high, higher even than SLE. When, in addition, its poor prognosis is taken into account, the relative importance of this worldwide problem can be placed in its true perspective. There still is lacking, however, a unifying diagnostic marker such as the LE cell or antinuclear antibody.

Nomenclature

It should be recognized that the "diseases" under discussion are more correctly syndromes and that any name or label attached to them (it) will be imprecise. The term *IgA nephropathy* is hallowed by common usage, but belies the systemic nature of the "disease," does not encompass secondary forms, and is not descriptive. Inclusion of HSP under the same umbrella awaits the proof of unity, which, if obtained, would demand a totally new approach to nomenclature. Synonyms other than IgA nephropathy should be remembered and include *mesangial IgA disease, IgA mesangial glomerulonephritis, IgA mesangial nephropathy,* and similar variations. *Berger's disease* may still be the most appropriate name, but as with many other medical eponyms, the original description does not embrace current knowledge. In like manner, *Henoch-Schönlein purpura* (a term frequently used by nephrologists) and *Schönlein-Henoch purpura* (favored by chronologists and dermatologists) are used interchangeably with *anaphylactoid purpura,* which is a misnomer.

Diagnosis

"Les dépôts intercapillaires d'IgA-IgG" was the title of Berger and Hinglais's [18] original article describing IgA nephropathy. Save for the variable presence of IgG immunofluorescence, this remains an accurate description of the principal diagnostic criterion of IgA nephropathy. None of the clinical, biochemical, or serologic associations is specific, and thus the diagnosis may not be easy when the renal disease is advanced, when IgA mesangial glomerulonephritis occurs secondary to other diseases, or when associated renal pathology supervenes. Thus the diagnosis can be made conclusively only by observing predominant mesangial IgA immunofluorescence on renal biopsy. HSP, on the other hand, is clearly a clinical syndrome, consisting of palpable purpura, arthritis, abdominal pain, and glomerulonephritis. All features are not necessarily present in every case, and it is not uncommon to find occasional patients with primary IgA nephropathy who intermittently experience one or more features of HSP associated with an exacerbation of glomerulonephritis.

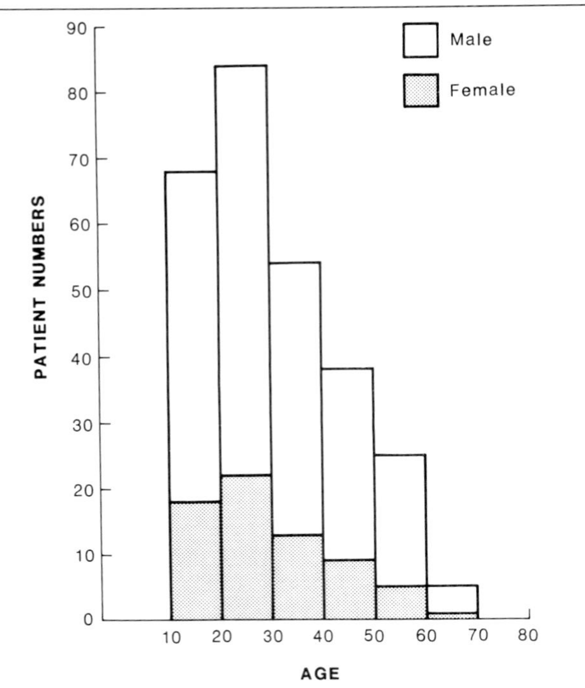

Fig. 67-1. Age and sex of patients with primary IgA nephropathy admitted to an adult hospital over 10 years.

Geographic Distribution

IgA nephropathy is probably the commonest form of glomerulonephritis in the world. This is certainly the case in first-world countries where postinfectious glomerulonephritis now is distinctly uncommon. In the United States [70, 129, 235] and the United Kingdom [204], the reported incidence has been lower than in France [53, 60, 61], Italy [46, 125], Spain [44, 80], Finland [164], Germany [78], and Singapore [202], although some reports from the U.S. and U.K. [165, 206] indicate isolated areas in these countries where the incidence is much higher. Whether these observations are true or merely reflect different biopsy policies is still not resolved. In Australia [35] where the population is heterogeneous and includes many immigrants from third-world countries, all racial groups seem to be affected equally apart from Aborigines. A similar low incidence is seen in American blacks [75]. Provided, therefore, that environmental and racial factors are not found to play a major role in pathogenesis, it would seem on this evidence that the disease also may be common in underdeveloped countries.

Incidence

Figures on the incidence of IgA nephropathy depend entirely on renal biopsies studied by immunofluorescence. They vary from one country to another, being approximately 10 percent in biopsy series from the United States and Canada, 20 to 25 percent in Europe and Australia, and more than 30 percent in Japan. The possibility exists that the true incidence is indeed higher. General population studies in Germany and France have suggested an incidence of 2 cases per 10,000 population (0.02%) [167, 197, 198]. This figure may, however, represent only the tip of the iceberg, as necropsy studies in Singapore [201] and Germany [228] indicate that as many as 2.0 to 4.8 percent of the population may be afflicted.

While the disease occurs at all ages, it is most common in the second and third decades and is 3 to 6 times more frequent in males than in females. In Fig. 67-1 are shown the age and sex incidence at presentation of patients in our unit, which is representative of many other studies. Corresponding data from patients with HSP are not available, although Fig. 67-2 indicates a schema of the relatively high incidence of HSP in children. The prevalence of glomerular disease in patients with HSP, especially in children, varies from 20 to 100 percent [132] depending on how carefully evidence for it is sought.

Clinical Features at Presentation

IgA NEPHROPATHY

The clinical manifestations of IgA nephropathy are protean, but the symptom most likely to attract immediate medical attention is macroscopic hematuria (Table 67-1). Characteristically there is a close temporal relationship between its onset and an upper respiratory tract infection, especially pharyngitis or tonsillitis, the hematuria often coinciding with or occurring within 1 to 2 days of the sore throat. Less frequently, such hematuria also will accompany infections of other IgA mucosal surfaces, e.g., gastroenteritis and urinary tract infections. The hematuria is painless but often is associated with systemic symptoms such as fever, malaise, fatigue, dif-

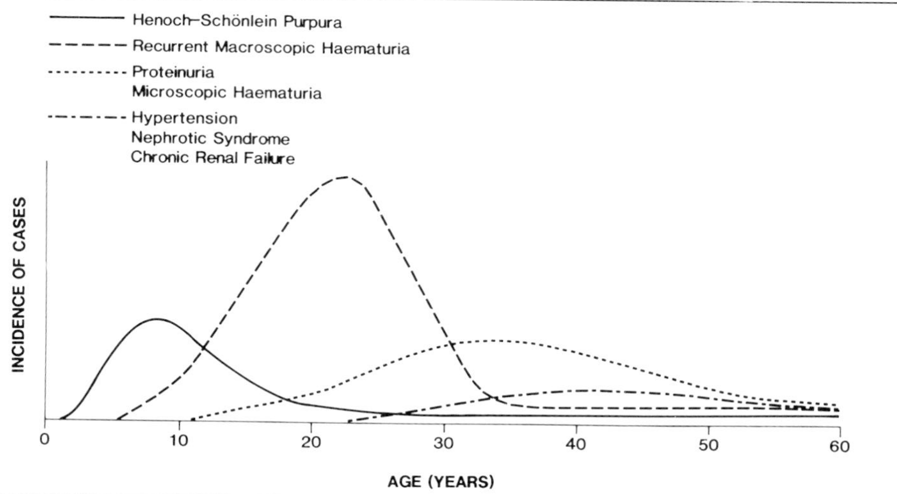

Fig. 67-2. The age distribution of patients with mesangial IgA nephritis and the various presenting clinical features. (Reproduced from *IgA Mesangial Nephropathy*, p. 188, with permission of the publishers, S. Karger, Basel.)

Table 67-1. Presenting features in patients with mesangial IgA glomerulonephritis

Features	Percent
Macroscopic hematuria ± loin pain	30
Microscopic hematuria ± proteinuria (intermittent)	8
Proteinuria + microscopic hematuria	24
Hypertension	8
Malignant hypertension	3
Chronic renal failure	10
Acute renal failure	2
Nephrotic syndrome	3
Acute nephritis	2
HSP	10

fuse muscle aches, and abdominal [230] and dull loin pain [123]. It is usually short-lived, lasting 1 to 5 days, and its disappearance coincides with resolution of the systemic symptoms. Differentiation from other causes of macroscopic hematuria is important, because frequent and unnecessary radiographic and urologic investigations may ensue if the true cause is not recognized. Macroscopic hematuria due to IgA nephropathy occurs far more frequently in children and young adults than in middle-aged or elderly patients, in whom such a symptom should raise the suspicion of urinary tract malignancy or stones. Of paramount importance, however, is examination of the centrifuged urinary sediment, which will display dysmorphic red blood cells (of glomerular origin) and granular and red cell casts. Under these circumstances, renal biopsy is the appropriate first diagnostic procedure. Urine in postinfectious (streptococcal) glomerulonephritis rarely is so deeply blood-stained, but rather is generally smoky or dark. Furthermore, the hematuria occurs consistently between 8 and 14 days after the streptococcal infection and thus can be distinguished from the "synpharyngitic" hematuria of IgA nephropathy. Moreover, the latter is often recurrent, and careful history may reveal similar episodes in the past. Hypertension and edema, so commonly associated with postinfectious glomerulonephritis, usually are not features of the early hematuric phase of IgA nephropathy; however, acute deterioration of renal function may occur in both.

As IgA nephropathy has become more widely recognized, the true incidence of macroscopic hematuria has become clearer. Initially it was thought to be the presenting symptom in the majority of patients; this is, however, only the case in 30 to 35 percent, although it may occur subsequently in another 10 to 15 percent.

In our experience, an equal number of patients (30–35%) present for investigation of asymptomatic proteinuria that is usually accompanied by microscopic hematuria. The presence of glomerulonephritis in these patients may be further suspected because of coexisting hypertension. Proteinuria and microscopic hematuria certainly persist between episodes of macroscopic hematuria, but the reasons why so many patients with IgA nephropathy never suffer macroscopic urinary blood loss are not clear.

A further one-third of patients experience a variety of symptom complexes, including acute nephritis, nephrotic syndrome, acute or chronic renal failure, or malignant hypertension. Although nephrotic syndrome, which may be reversible with corticosteroid therapy, appears to be a distinct subset of IgA nephropathy [146], presentation with the nephrotic syndrome in other patients may simply indicate advanced glomerular disease [102]. This is also the case in those patients who present with end-stage renal disease, malignant hypertension, or both. As indicated previously, acute deterioration of

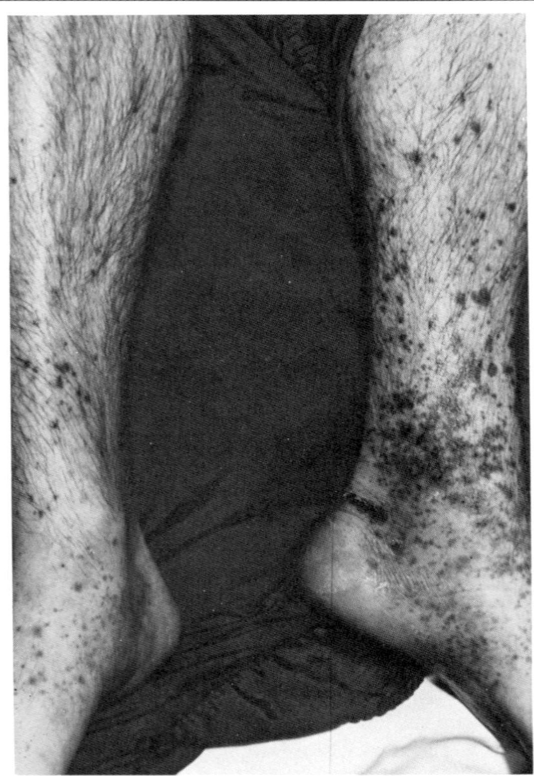

Fig. 67-3. The characteristic "vasculitic" rash of Henoch-Schönlein purpura. The thighs and buttocks are frequently involved, but appearance of the rash on trunk and upper limbs is unusual.

renal function may occur in association with episodes of macroscopic hematuria. We have encountered 10 such patients who have required temporary dialysis [35]. As reported by Kincaid-Smith et al. [105], we have found these episodes to be reversible without the need for "specific" therapy.

HENOCH-SCHÖNLEIN PURPURA

The characteristic rash (Fig. 67-3), joint, and gastrointestinal involvement usually make the syndrome of HSP clearly identifiable in children and adults; however, some adults initially thought to be suffering from HSP later may develop features characteristic of polyarteritis nodosa [74]. Although these symptoms may cause much acute morbidity, recovery is usual. Glomerulonephritis, on the other hand, is responsible for the mortality rate of 1 to 3 percent, and its presence must be sought in all cases. Renal involvement is usually apparent within 4 weeks of diagnosis, although many cases are described in which the overt features of glomerulonephritis develop much later [133]. As with IgA nephropathy, intermittent macroscopic hematuria or persisting microscopic hematuria is the most common finding. Likewise, more severe cases develop significant proteinuria, nephrotic syndrome, hypertension, and renal impairment. The clinical similarity between the nephritis of HSP and IgA nephropathy can be extended when factors provoking acute disease or exacerbations of HSP are considered. In the past, hypersensitivity to various allergens, infecting organisms [27], food [2], and drugs [128] has been implicated, but the majority of cases occur following a nonspecific upper respiratory, gastrointestinal, or urinary tract infection. For many years before the advent of immunofluorescence microscopy, many investigators believed that both conditions were variants of poststreptococcal glomerulonephritis. The serologic evidence obtained by Ayoub and Hoyer [5] demonstrated no relation between streptococcal infections and HSP; this and subsequent studies demonstrating conclusive immunopathologic differences served to dispel any confusion.

Clinical Course

Analysis of available evidence suggests a remarkable similarity between the clinical course and outcome of groups of patients with the nephritis of HSP and IgA nephropathy [16, 35, 46, 60, 132, 149]. The prognosis in individual patients, however, is difficult to predict. The subject is dealt with in another chapter, but it is pertinent here to examine those factors, both clinical and pathologic, that contribute to a poor prognosis. Most authors agree that the presence, either initially or during the course of the disease, of sustained hypertension, persistent proteinuria, or nephrotic syndrome and continued renal function impairment is unfavorable. These patients have correspondingly more severe changes on renal biopsy, especially glomerulosclerosis, interstitial scarring, and hypertensive vascular changes. Controversy remains concerning the significance of recurring heavy bouts of hematuria (associated with recurring purpura in HSP) and the presence of crescents on the initial biopsy. Bennett and Kincaid-Smith [16] suggest that these are associated with a poor prognosis. As is emphasized [16], however, macroscopic hematuria may be an early (and easily recognizable) diagnostic feature and a prelude to a long, slow and otherwise featureless course toward renal failure, whereas in other patients the disease onset is not clearly identifiable. Only late in the disease process will significant proteinuria, hypertension, and renal impairment develop. Statistics indicate that the majority of patients (approximately 70%) with HSP nephritis and IgA nephropathy have an excellent prognosis. Current data reveal that this majority will reach their expected life span, but at the expense of hypertension, its consequences and treatment, and moderately impaired renal function. There is a general agreement among most workers that the remaining 30 percent will progress to chronic renal failure, requiring dialysis or causing death within 1 to 40 years.

Classification and Associated Diseases

IgA nephropathy has a clear association with other disease states, particularly those affecting mucosal surfaces and where there is a demonstrable immunoglobulin response of the IgA class (Table 67-2) [143]. The impor-

Table 67-2. Classification of the IgA nephropathies

PRIMARY
Isolated mesangial IgA nephritis (IgA nephropathy)
Henoch-Schönlein purpura
SECONDARY
Alcoholic liver disease [20, 29, 154, 234]
Portal systemic shunts [234]
Celiac disease [86, 101, 139]
Dermatitis herpetiformis [49, 86, 139, 161]
IgA monoclonal gammopathy [58, 91]
Mycosis fungoides [168]
Mucin-secreting and other carcinomas [28, 144, 200]
Leprosy [226]
Pulmonary hemosiderosis [237]
Ankylosing spondylitis [8, 96, 134]
Cyclical neutropenia [150]

tance of these observations resides in (1) the ability to classify IgA nephropathy into primary and secondary forms, (2) the provision of clues provided by these associated conditions for potential pathogenetic mechanisms in the primary disease, and (3) clinical recognition of the potentially serious significance of some associated conditions. Careful analysis of our own series of adult patients with HSP suggests similar relationships.

Laboratory Features

There is no specific serologic test for HSP or IgA nephropathy. Most accounts of both conditions describe an elevation of serum IgA concentrations in up to 50 percent of cases [35, 39, 109, 118]. Serum complement components C1q and C2-9 are uniformly normal or elevated [35, 67, 79, 98, 118, 136], as are factor B, properdin, B1H, C3b INA, and C1 esterase inhibitor. Detailed studies [98] indicate the occasional presence of partial familial deficiencies in single complement components. In addition to IgA and C3, properdin [67, 175, 176] and B1H [98, 136] have been demonstrated in the mesangial deposits, suggesting strongly that local activation of the alternative complement pathway occurs. The findings of Miyazaki et al. [136] of mesangial C4 binding protein (C4bp) in 60 percent, C4 in 30 percent, and elevated serum C4bp concentrations suggest that at least in some patients the classical pathway also may be involved.

The finding of circulating IgA-containing immune complexes in IgA nephropathy [40, 48, 55, 57, 65, 79, 83, 116, 145, 147, 159, 183, 212, 213, 224, 234] and HSP [40, 103, 117, 234] has been confirmed widely with various techniques. Most authors agree that circulating immune complexes (CIC) are present only intermittently and correlate with episodes of clinical activity, e.g., macroscopic hematuria. In addition, sequential studies [116] indicate that recurrence of IgA nephropathy in patients with renal transplants correlates with the detection by conglutinin assay of CIC containing IgA. The presence of CIC does not correlate with serum IgA concentrations.

However, IgA with antiglobulin activity (IgA rheumatoid factor) has been detected in serum [45, 203], and antibodies have also been detected that have affinity for glomerular mesangium [214, 217] or glomerular basement membrane components [31]. Recently autoantibodies against glomerular [10] and endothelial cell [72] antigens have been found and the autoantigens partially characterized [158]. While it has been suggested that the findings of these autoantibodies may be associated with disease activity and progression, their presence is intermittent and of little diagnostic importance. Antibodies have also been found against a wide range of environmental, dietary, and infective antigens, but, again, their presence is thought to be nonspecific.

As with mesangial deposits, CIC may contain IgG and IgM in addition to IgA and are intermediate in size [116, 234]. IgA immune complexes are phagocytosed primarily in the liver [172, 173], but other components of the reticuloendothelial system and peripheral blood polymorphonuclear leukocytes may also contribute [212].

IgA nephropathy has been described in identical twins [178], HLA identical siblings [210], and families [32, 97, 137]. It is not surprising, therefore, that HLA associations have been described. The data, however, are not consistent. Associations have been described with BW35 [22, 155], B12, and DR4 [68, 89, 99, 100]. Other large series have not confirmed these observations [26, 32, 145, 235]. Notwithstanding this confusion, and unequal racial distribution of IgA nephropathy and HSP, familial predisposition may have an important role in the clinical expression of IgA-associated glomerular disease [75, 97]. Furthermore, studies of the switch regions of the immunoglobulin heavy-chain genes of patients with IgA nephropathy using restriction fragment length polymorphism has disclosed that genes within the immunoglobulin heavy-chain loci may be important in the pathogenesis [52]. Unfortunately these observations, as yet, have no diagnostic value.

Transplantation

There are two intriguing facts relating to renal transplantation in patients with IgA nephropathy and HSP. First, the disease recurs in grafts whether derived from living or cadaver [9, 19, 21, 30, 120, 126, 141, 195] donors. Recurrence is not related to HLA matching or mismatching and affects approximately half of the patients from 6 months to 4 years following transplantation. Clinically, the recurrent disease is mild. Macroscopic hematuria and cutaneous lesions are unusual. None of the 17 patients described by Berger [19] had developed renal insufficiency after 10 years, although we have noted this occurrence in isolated cases. Disease recurrence in grafts correlates well with reappearance in the circulation of IgA containing CIC [116]. As the recurrent disease seems so mild, transplantation in patients with IgA nephropathy and HSP is not contraindicated. Second, IgA deposits have disappeared from kidneys that are already diseased with IgA nephropathy that inadvertently have been transplanted into patients without IgA nephropathy or HSP [184, 196]. This observation has focused attention on host factors that are responsible for initiation and perpetuation of the diseases.

Pathology

LIGHT MICROSCOPY

The spectrum of glomerular disease is highly variable, although the morphologic features are virtually identical in patients with HSP and IgA nephropathy, the hallmark of each being segmental mesangial proliferation (Fig. 67-4). Overall, the changes in patients with HSP are described as more severe, with a greater tendency for necrotizing lesions [207, 233].

In their mildest forms, the mesangial changes may be quite focal as well as segmental. Appreciable numbers of glomerular tufts may appear to be quite normal, and even in those affected, the mesangial cells and matrix changes may be quite marginal (Fig. 67-5). Classically, however, the disease is diffuse, although the tuft changes may be segmental or global in distribution. As a result of mesangial proliferation, the tuft stalk expands and becomes accentuated (Fig. 67-6), often markedly so (Fig. 67-7), an appearance described as "arborization."

Tiny hyaline and fibrinoid globules may be apparent in the mesangial matrix in appropriately stained sections, and these represent the deposits seen ultrastructurally. Capillary loops are usually patent, with a normal configuration of capillary walls. However, in more florid disease, mesangial proliferative activity results in the matrix extending peripherally and circumferentially within the capillary walls, resulting in double-contouring or "tram-line" effect, usually with lumen narrowing. A diffuse mesangiocapillary (membranoproliferative) glomerulonephritis type I pattern has been described in the more severe forms of HSP [207], but it is rarely seen in patients with IgA nephropathy.

In active disease, there may be tuft necrosis associated with an exudate of fibrin and infiltration of neutrophils, some of which may show karyorrhexis. This occurrence is associated with crescent formation (Fig. 67-8) in up to one-third of initial biopsies (90 percent of those with macroscopic hematuria in one series) [67] and usually affects up to 25 percent of sampled glomeruli. Circumferential crescents are not unusual in both conditions when overt renal disease is present, but involvement of greater than 85 percent of glomeruli (rapidly progressive glomerulonephritis) is distinctly uncommon [16, 88, 118, 119].

In long-standing disease, areas of segmental tuft collapse and sclerosis (Fig. 67-9), sometimes with overlying hyalinosis, are seen, related to which usually are broad synechiae (Fig. 67-10). In progressive disease, the end result is total glomerular obsolescence and sclerosis (Fig. 67-11). The presence in one biopsy of all the lesions described is not infrequent and probably indicates persisting and long-standing disease activity. The glomerular lesions in HSP have been classified according to the following grades [43]:

Fig. 67-4. Three glomeruli, showing varying degrees of mesangial proliferation. The worst affected shows early segmental sclerosis. The tubules are normal, as is the interstitium (silver H&E, ×200).

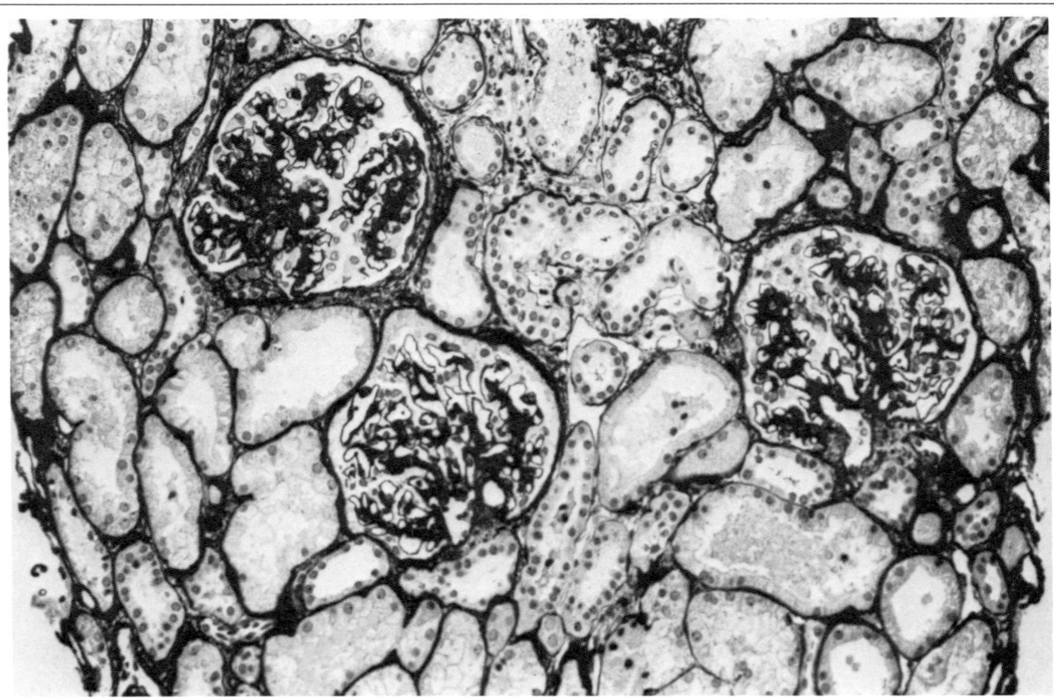

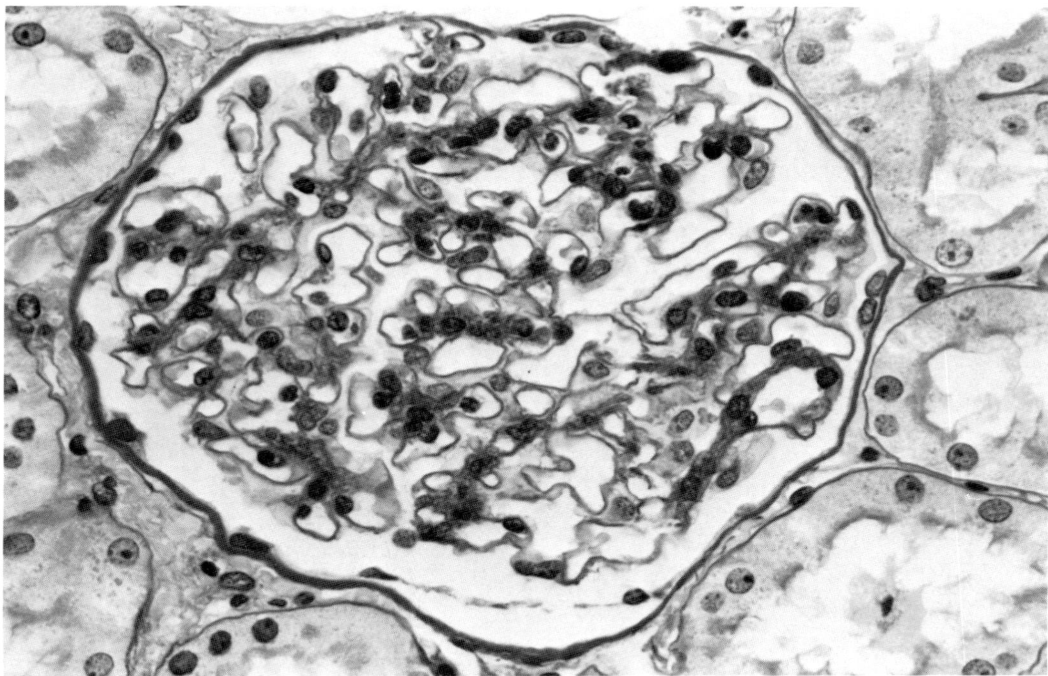

Fig. 67-5. Mild segmental mesangial proliferation with slight hypercellularity. Capillaries are patent with normal walls (PAS, ×630).

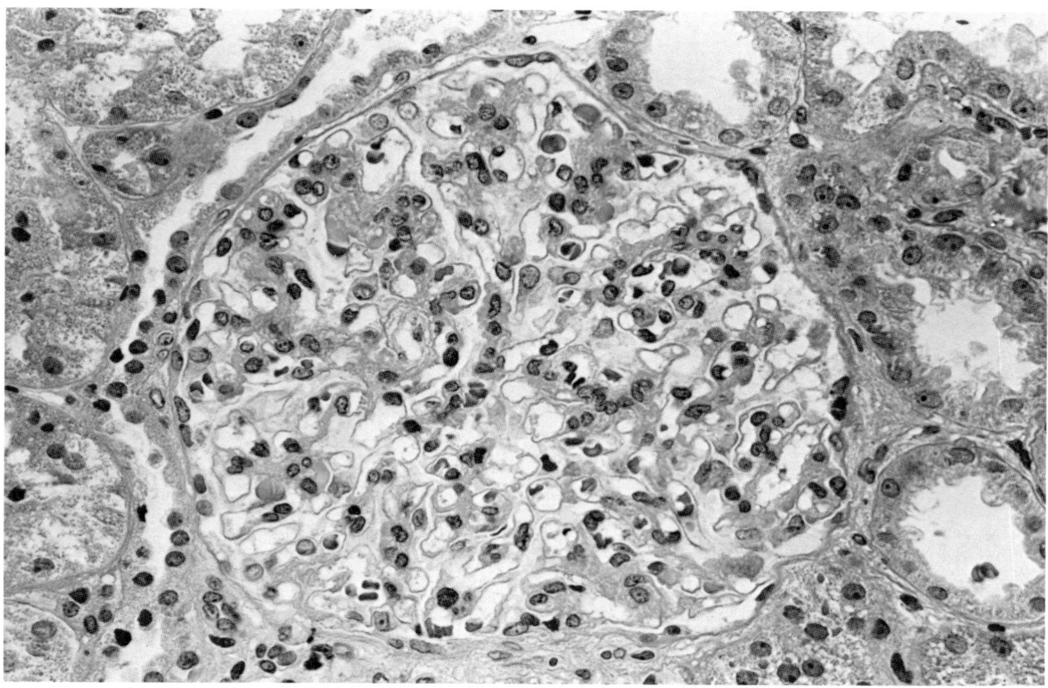

Fig. 67-6. Glomerulus, showing moderate mesangial cell and matrix proliferation, with broadening of the tuft stalk. Neutrophils in the tuft add to the hypercellularity. Most capillary loops are patent, though early double contouring is present peripherally (at 10 o'clock) (H&E, ×400).

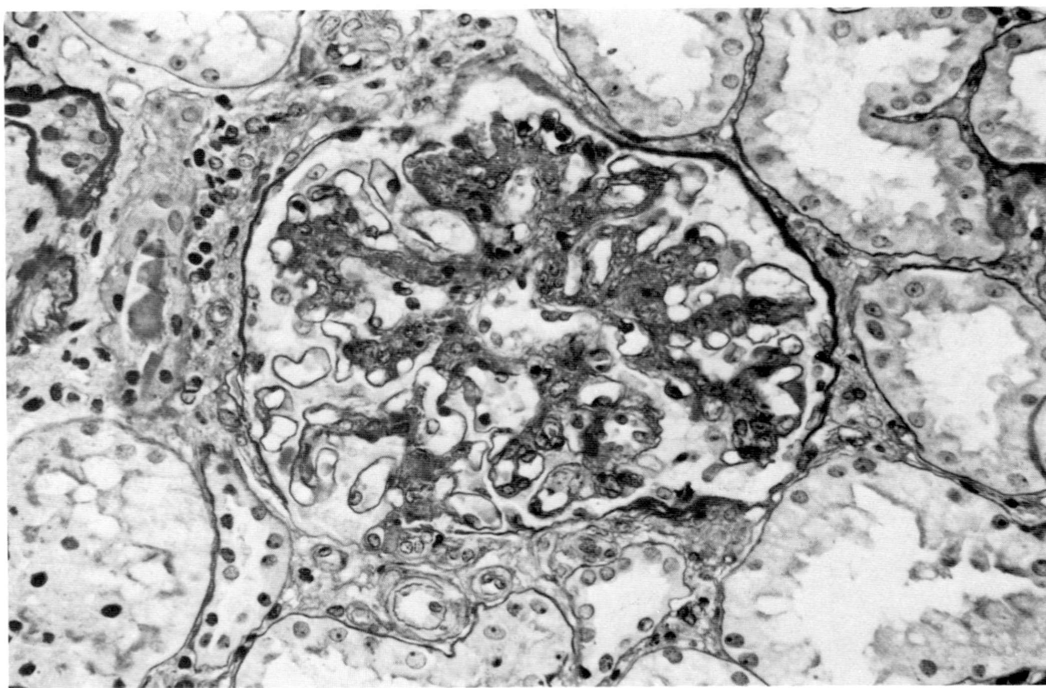

Fig. 67-7. Glomerulus, presenting prominent mesangial proliferation, resulting in "arborization" of the tuft. There is some double contouring and narrowing of capillary loops, patchy interstitial tissue fibrosis, and tubular atrophy (PAS, ×400).

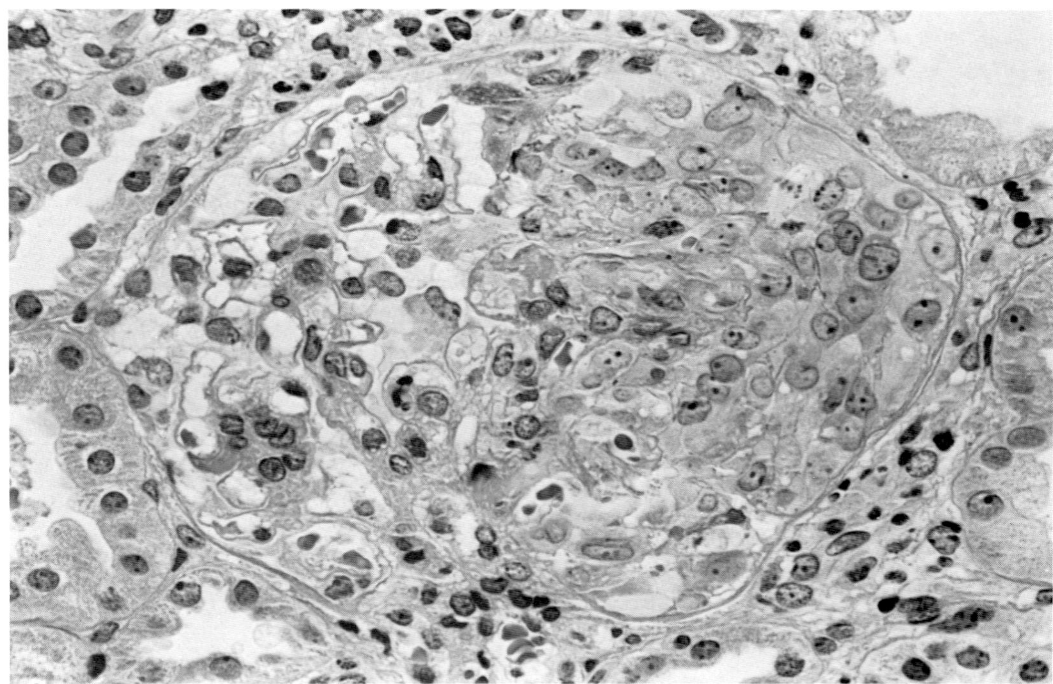

Fig. 67-8. Glomerulus, containing a large recent active crescent, displacing and distorting the tuft, which also shows segmental mesangial proliferation. Periglomerular inflammation with karyorrhexis is present (H&E, ×630).

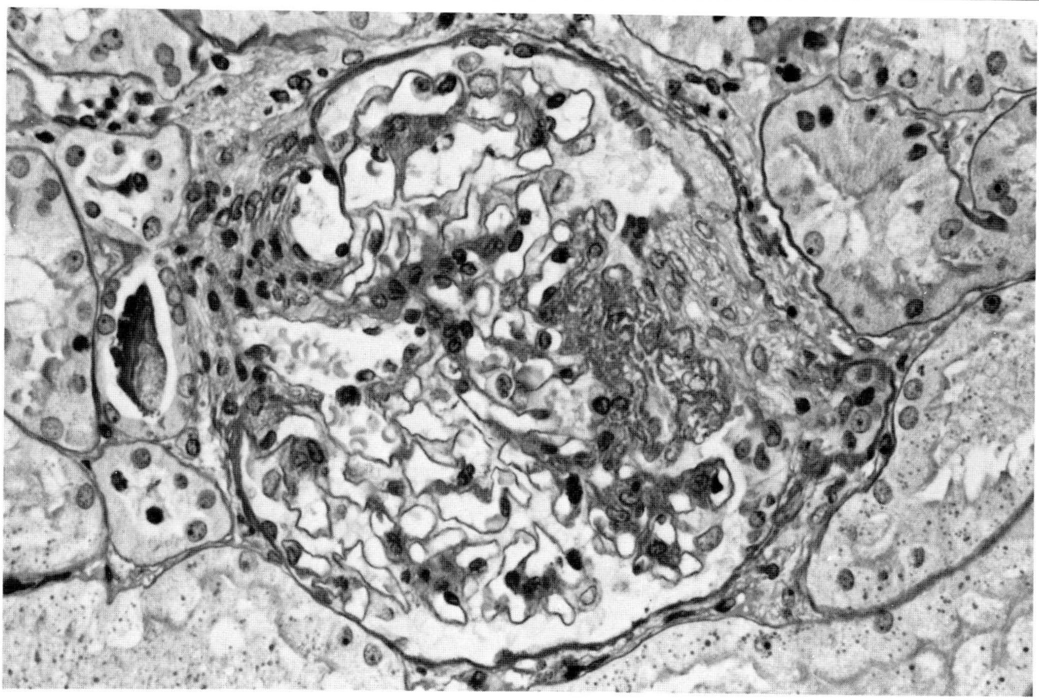

Fig. 67-9. Glomerulus, showing segmental tuft collapse and sclerosis associated with broad synechia formation. The remainder of the tuft shows mild mesangial proliferation only (H&E, ×630).

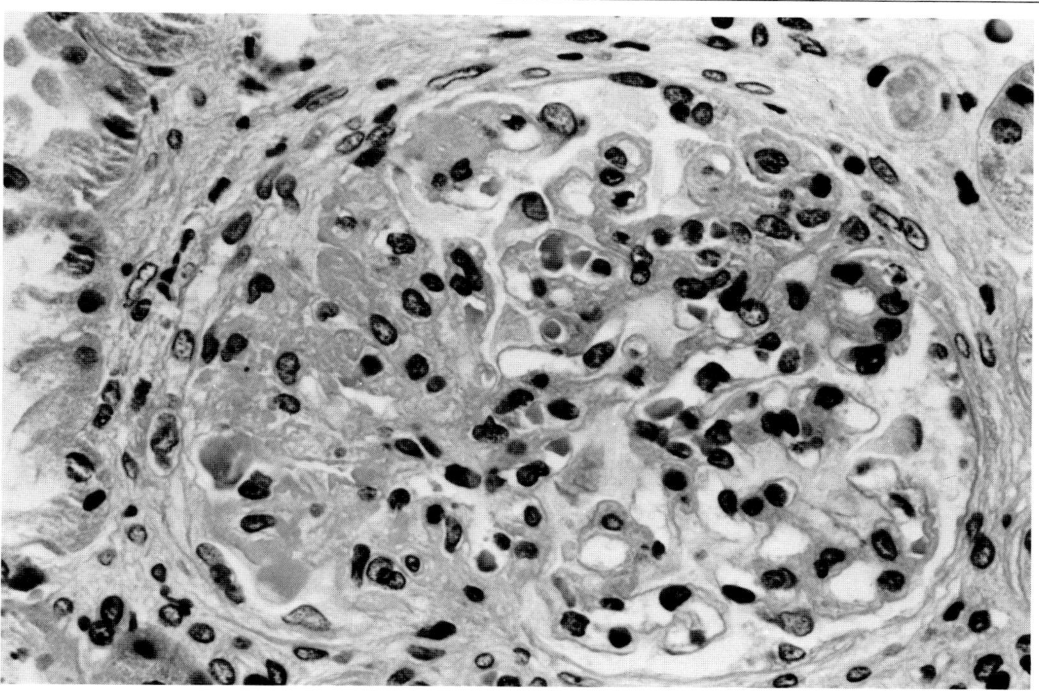

Fig. 67-10. Glomerulus, presenting early, though extensive, segmental tuft sclerosis associated with hyalinosis and several synechiae. The areas of hyalinosis appear as small, glassy homogeneous spheres. Double contouring is readily evident in the still-viable portion of the tuft (H&E, ×630).

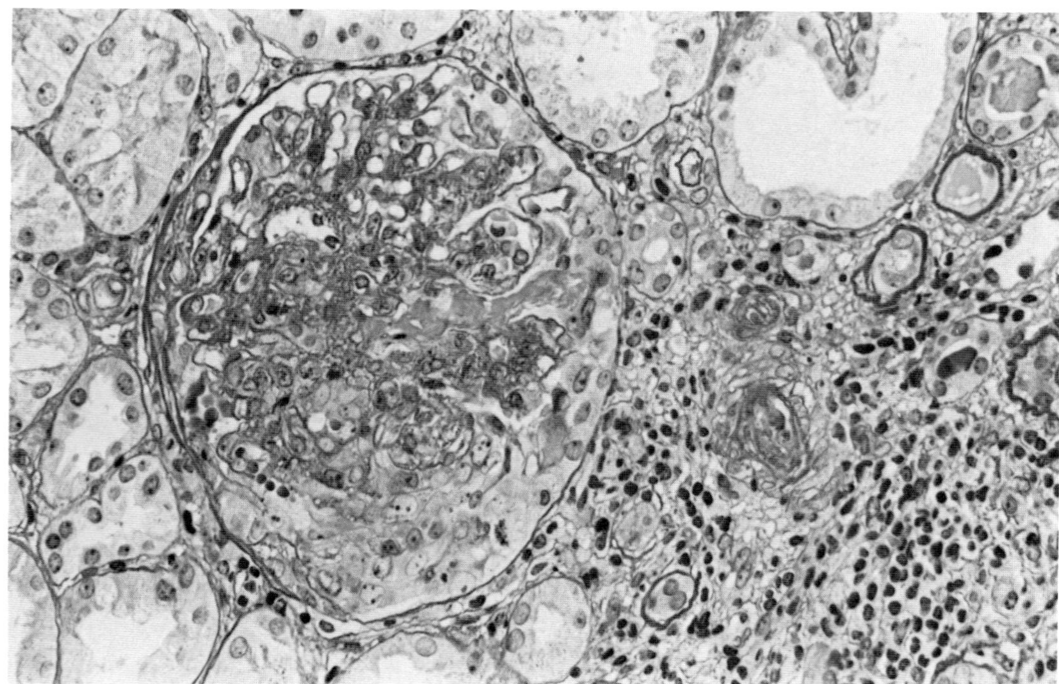

Fig. 67-11. A glomerulus, showing near-total sclerosis associated with crescent formation. There is marked interstitial fibrosis, with inflammatory cell infiltrate, tubular atrophy, and marked hypertensive arteriolosclerosis with lumen narrowing (PAS, ×400).

Grade

I. Minimal alteration
II. Pure mesangial proliferation
III. a. Focal mesangial proliferation; b. Diffuse mesangial proliferation — With less than 50 percent crescents
IV. a. Focal mesangial proliferation; b. Diffuse mesangial proliferation — 50–70 percent crescents
V. a. Focal mesangial proliferation; b. Diffuse mesangial proliferation — Greater than 75 percent crescents
VI. Pseudo-membranoproliferative glomerulonephritis

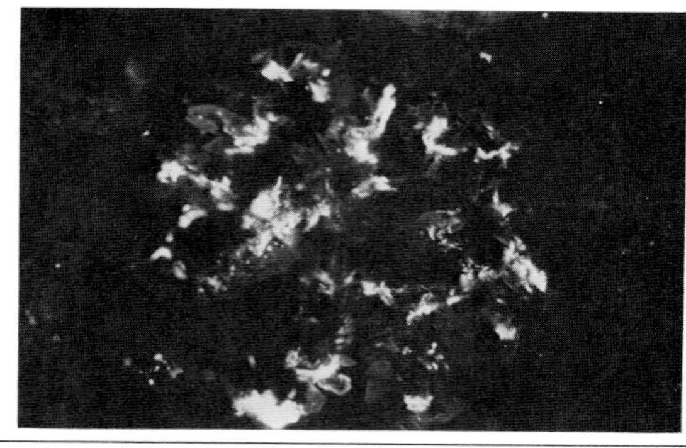

Fig. 67-12. Glomerulus, with brightly fluorescing, granular mesangial deposits of IgA (anti-human IgA, ×400).

This classification has been modified [84] by adding (a) focal and (b) diffuse categories to grade II, thus ensuring that the quite frequent group of focal segmental glomerulonephritis without crescents is not entered into grade III. A similar grading is appropriate for IgA nephropathy, but it should be reiterated that, in both conditions, such groupings are arbitrary and do not take into account the likelihood of many, if not all, grades being present in the one biopsy.

Proportional to the degree of glomerular damage, there may be tubulointerstitial disease. When active glomerular disease is present, there is often interstitial edema associated with a mild to moderate infiltrate of mononuclear cells and scattered neutrophils. Secondary tubular damage also may be evident. Interstitial scarring and tubular atrophy are features of advanced disease (Fig. 67-11).

Hypertensive changes complicate advanced cases, and related vascular lesions become evident (Fig. 67-11). On the other hand, arteriolar hyalinization unrelated to hypertension or age is frequent [35, 46, 70]. Vasculitis within the kidney is rarely seen in either disorder, which is surprising in view of the skin, gut, and joint pathology in HSP.

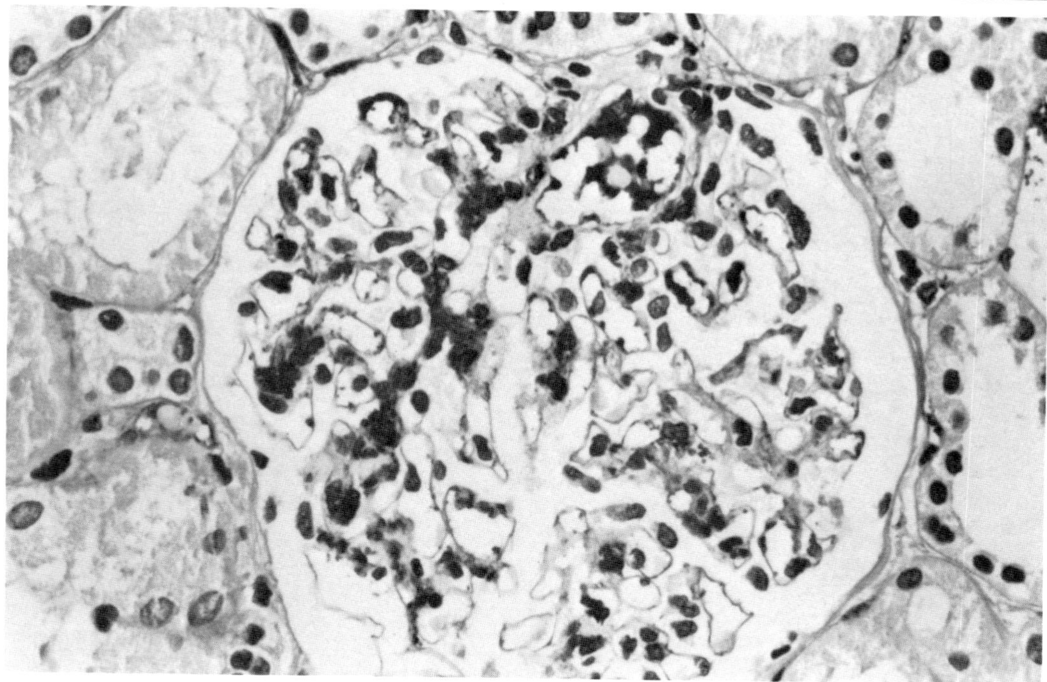

Fig. 67-13. Immunoperoxidase reaction, showing segmentally distributed granular deposits of IgA in the mesangium. Capillary loops are free of deposits (immunoperoxidase stain, ×630).

IMMUNOLOGIC STUDIES

A definitive diagnosis of both disorders can only be made with the aid of immunofluorescent or immunoperoxidase techniques [199] applied to renal tissue. Both techniques give identical results. Both IgA nephropathy and HSP present essentially similar glomerular features; granular deposition of IgA and C3 are present predominantly in the mesangium, even in apparently normal or minimally affected glomeruli (Figs. 67-12 and 67-13). While an early report indicated the presence of predominantly IgA2 subclass in mesangial deposits [3], this has not subsequently been verified; most workers find polymeric IgA1 [14, 37, 108, 121, 142, 211, 215, 225]. Recent work by Lai et al. [111] but not others demonstrates that the mesangial IgA is predominantly with lambda light chains despite the fact that the kappa light chain is present in higher concentrations in the serum. In addition, there may be variable deposits of IgG, IgM, or both, frequently fluorescing with lesser intensity [18, 35, 46]. C1q and C4-binding protein are found rarely; B1H and properdin are common in the mesangial areas [67, 136, 175, 176].

Capillary loop fluorescence for IgA (Fig. 67-14) is observed most commonly when active disease is present. Such cases also may show mesangial and capillary wall fibrinogen; the latter is also present in crescents. IgM frequently is seen in mesangia. It also is present in areas of sclerosis in addition to insudated proteins. Walls of small- and medium-sized blood vessels may contain abundant granular C3, particularly if the patient is hypertensive. Fibrinogen and other insudative proteins

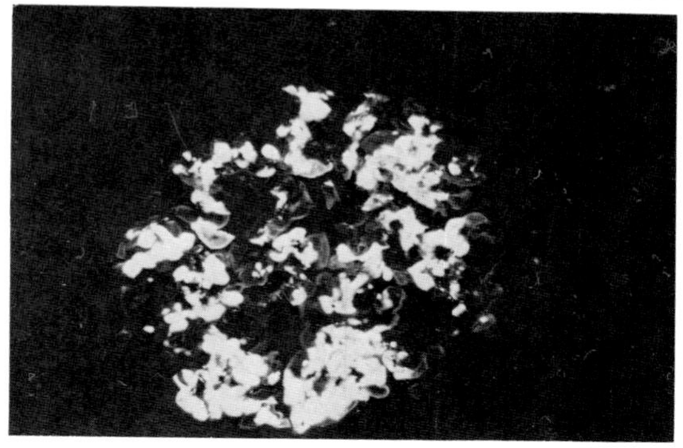

Fig. 67-14. Glomerulus, showing extensive mesangial and capillary loop deposits of IgA. The deposits are particularly prominent in several areas of segmental sclerosis (anti-human IgA, ×400).

may be present in vessel walls if vasculitis is present, but this is an uncommon event. Recently attention has been drawn to the presence of tubulointerstitial deposits that contain C3 and occasionally IgG and IgA [73]. In 19 of 51 patients, significant correlation was observed between the presence of these deposits, tubulointerstitial damage, and a decrease in renal function on follow-up visits.

ELECTRON MICROSCOPY

Both IgA nephropathy and HSP present similar ultrastructural features [135]. There is a varying degree of ex-

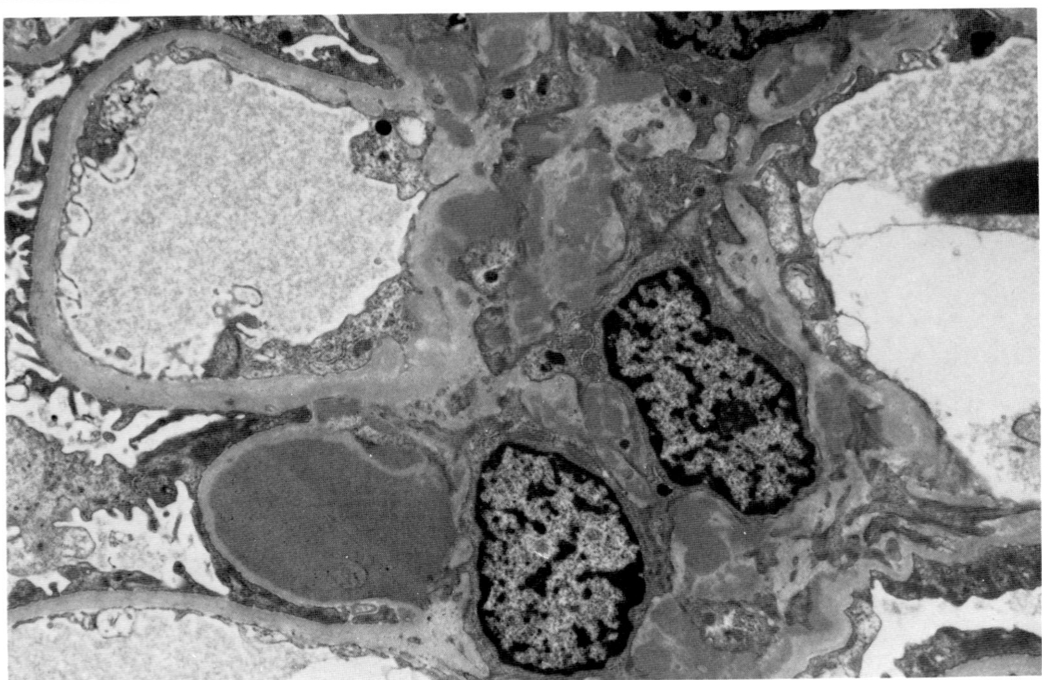

Fig. 67-15. Glomerulus, showing prominent, frequently large, electron-dense deposits in the mesangial matrix and paramesangial regions. Capillary loops are patent, with normal basement membranes and podocytes (×3,800).

pansion and proliferation of both mesangial cells and matrix; electron-dense deposits of differing sizes and amounts are present in the matrix (Fig. 67-15). Not infrequently, the deposits are particularly evident in paramesangial regions or even localized to this site. Immunoelectron microscopic studies using both peroxidase and gold techniques have shown a good correlation with immunofluorescence with respect to the distribution and nature of the deposits [54, 62, 157]. Corresponding to the segmental nature of the disease process, the distribution and amount of deposits may be quite patchy. Some mesangial sites may be distinctly free of deposits, yet others within the same glomerulus may be packed with them. The deposits are usually solid and homogeneous, but granular forms have been described [151]. Massive globular forms, usually distorting the paramesangial areas and corresponding to prominent glassy, strongly PAS-positive globules, as seen by conventional microscopy, may be found. Their presence may suggest alcohol-induced IgA nephropathy.

Subepithelial and intramembranous deposits occasionally may be evident, particularly in those patients with more florid renal symptoms (Fig. 67-16). Very rarely, a pattern suggestive of membranous nephropathy may be found. An overlapping syndrome of IgA nephropathy and membranous nephropathy has been described [56], while nephrotic syndrome with the clinical and pathologic features of minimal change disease also has been noted in patients with IgA nephropathy [146].

Capillary loops are usually patent with basement membranes of normal width. Not infrequently, isolated subepithelial notchings or nippings are seen (Fig. 67-17), but only occasionally are there full-thickness breakages of the basement membranes (Fig. 67-18). Sometimes these appear to be related to areas of resorbed subepithelial deposits, and the visceral epithelial cytoplasm is condensed at this site (Fig. 67-19). Scanning electron microscopic studies have demonstrated localized perforations of capillary loops [152]. Basement membrane irregularity, thinning, splitting, and lamellation have also been noted frequently [104, 140, 194, 208] (see Figs. 67-16 and 67-17). Occasionally glomerular basement membranes are uniformly thin, and this observation probably signifies the presence together of two common conditions, IgA nephropathy and thin-membrane nephropathy. Fragmentation of the basement membrane associated with exudation of fibrin occurs in relation to crescent formation. Peripheral circumferential interposition of the mesangial matrix also may be seen in progressive lesions; electron-dense deposits are carried forward by this process (Fig. 67-20). Unlike type I membranoproliferative glomerulonephritis, however, this process is quite focal and segmental. Fibrin and fibrin-like deposits may be observed [193, 207]. Segmental capillary loop collapse, hyalinosis (Fig. 67-21), and tuft collagenization (Fig. 67-22) probably represent the end stage of the inflammatory process. Podocytes may show patchy and localized effacement, particularly related to underlying basement-membrane changes.

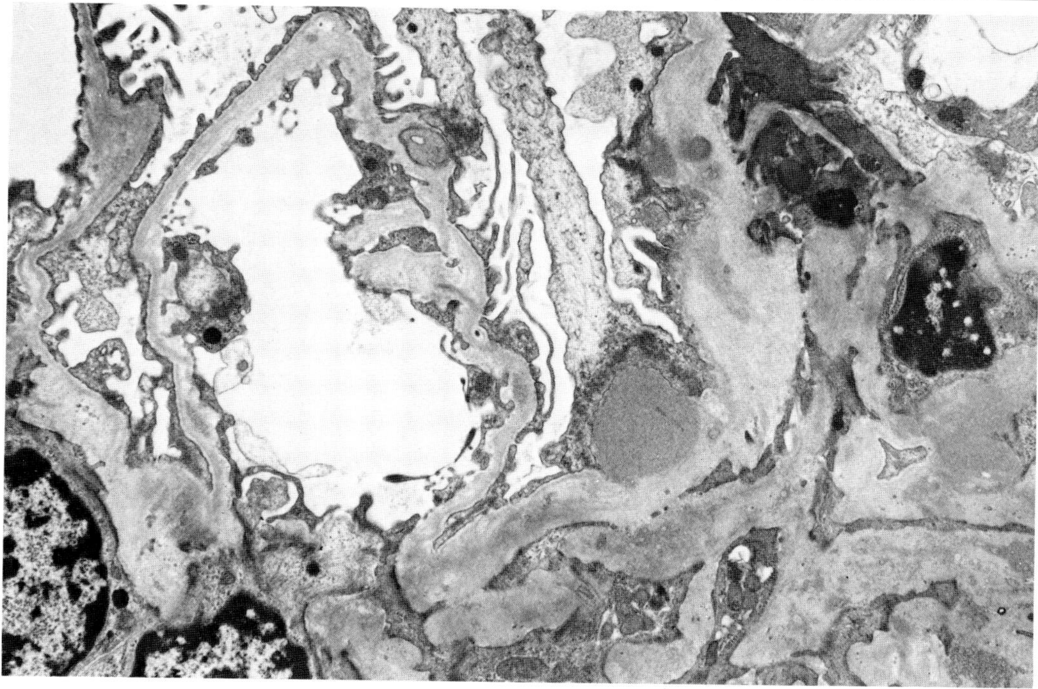

Fig. 67-16. Glomerulus, with subepithelial and intramembranous electron-dense deposits, also seen paramesangially and in proliferated mesangial matrix. The glomerular basement membrane is irregular, frayed, and lamellated (×3,800).

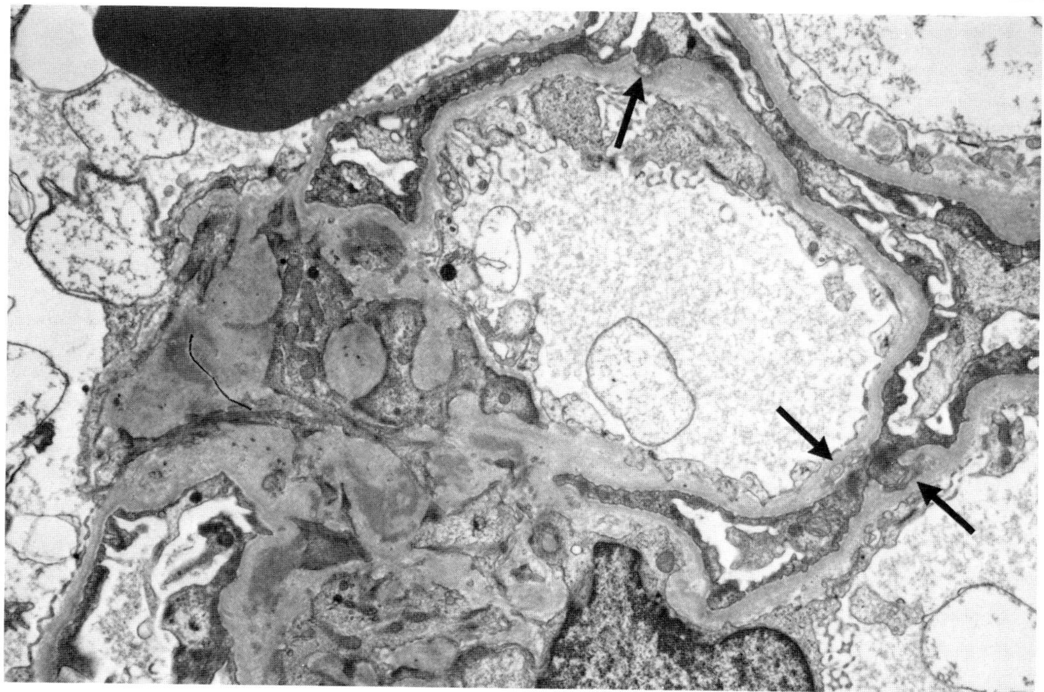

Fig. 67-17. Irregular, frayed glomerular basement membrane, showing several subepithelial notchings or nippings (*arrows*). At least one appears to be related to an area of resorbed deposit (×4,200).

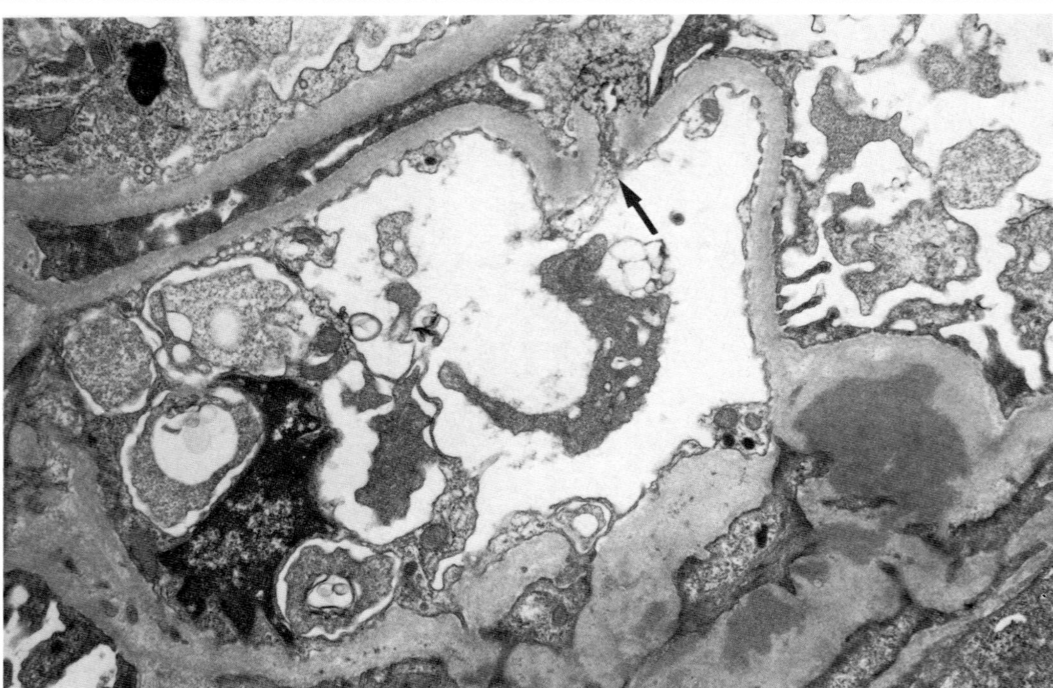

Fig. 67-18. Glomerular capillary, presenting a complete break of the basement membrane (*arrow*). Large electron-dense deposits are present paramesangially (×4,200).

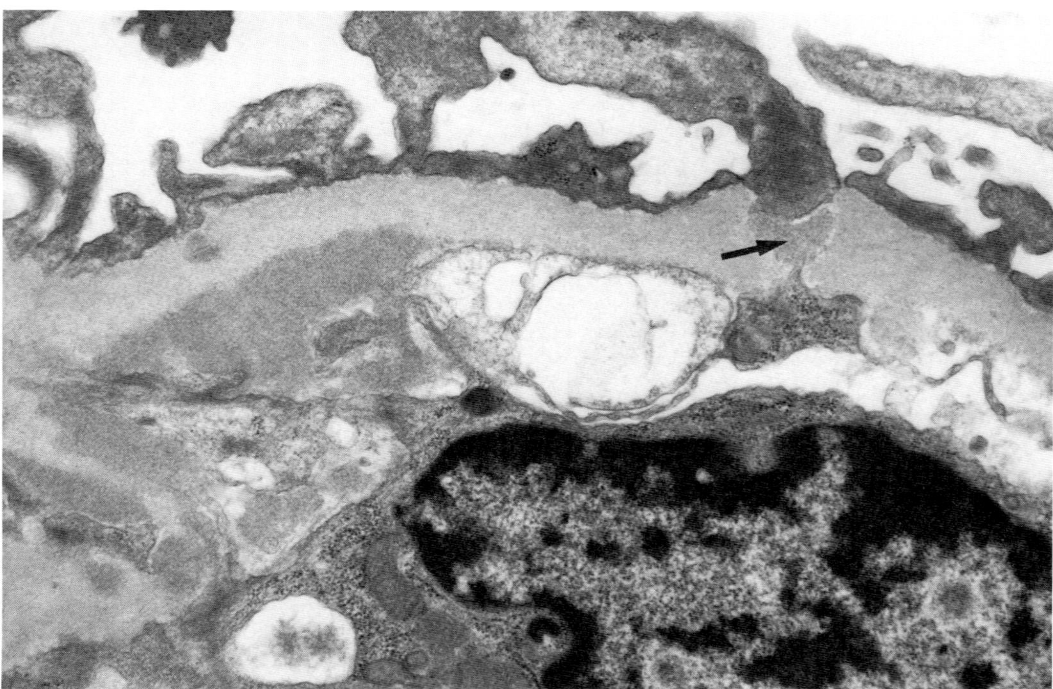

Fig. 67-19. Complete break of a glomerular basement membrane (*arrow*) related to a resorbing deposit (×14,800).

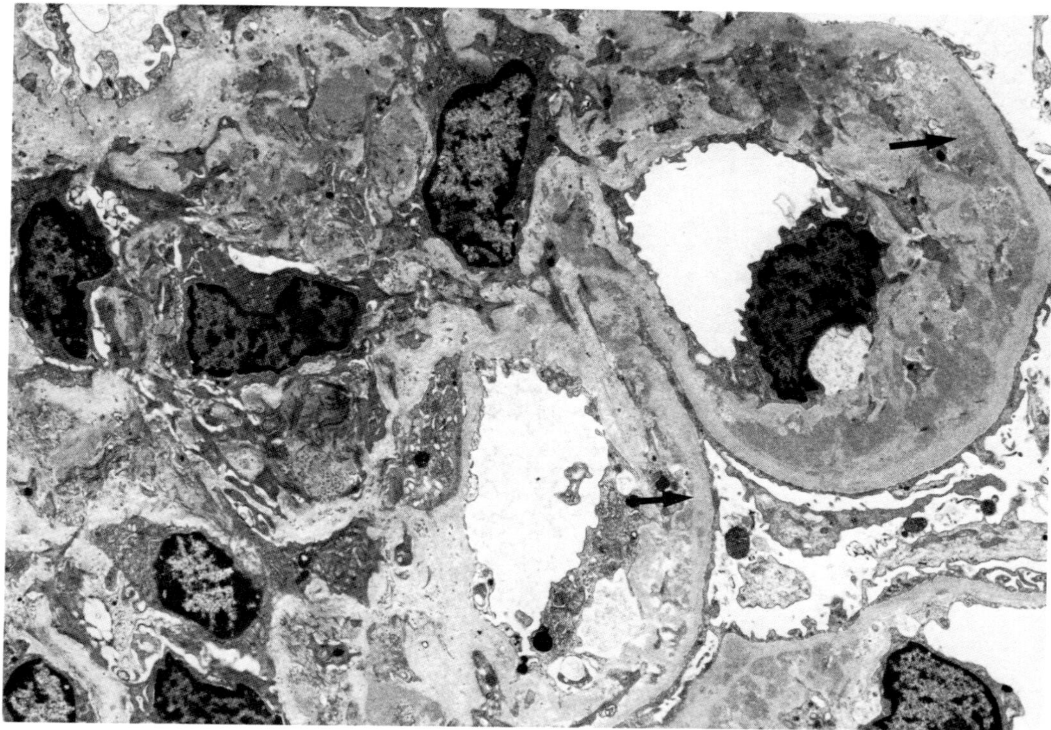

Fig. 67-20. Marked mesangial matrix proliferation, resulting in extensive peripheral circumferential interposition affecting two capillary loops with lumen narrowing (*arrow*). Abundant electron-dense deposits present in the matrix have been carried forward by the process (*arrow*) (× 2,600).

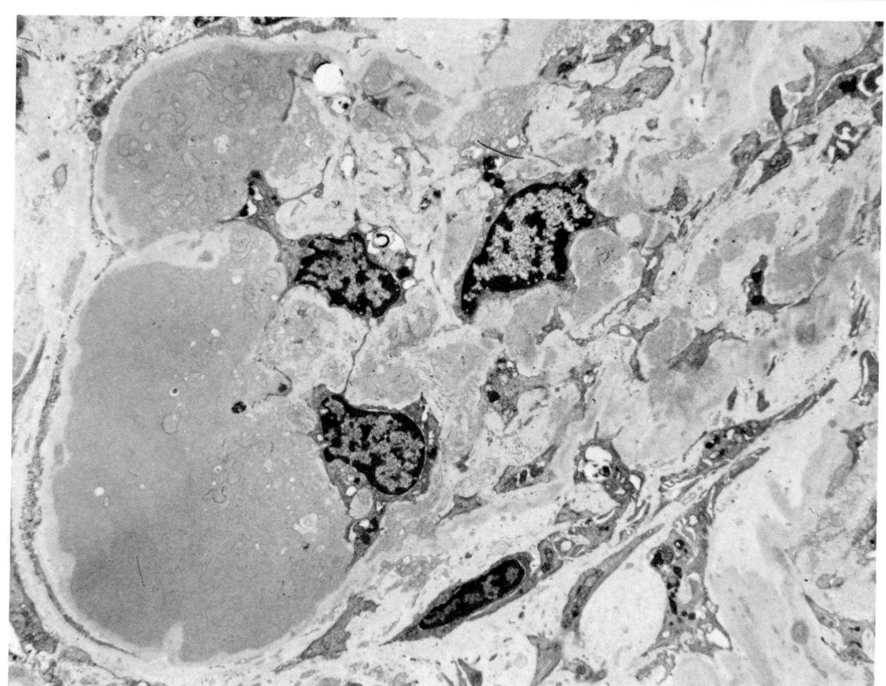

Fig. 67-21. Massive electron-dense deposits in an area of severe mesangial matrix proliferation and capillary loop obliteration, which corresponds to an area of segmental sclerosis and hyalinosis (× 1,850).

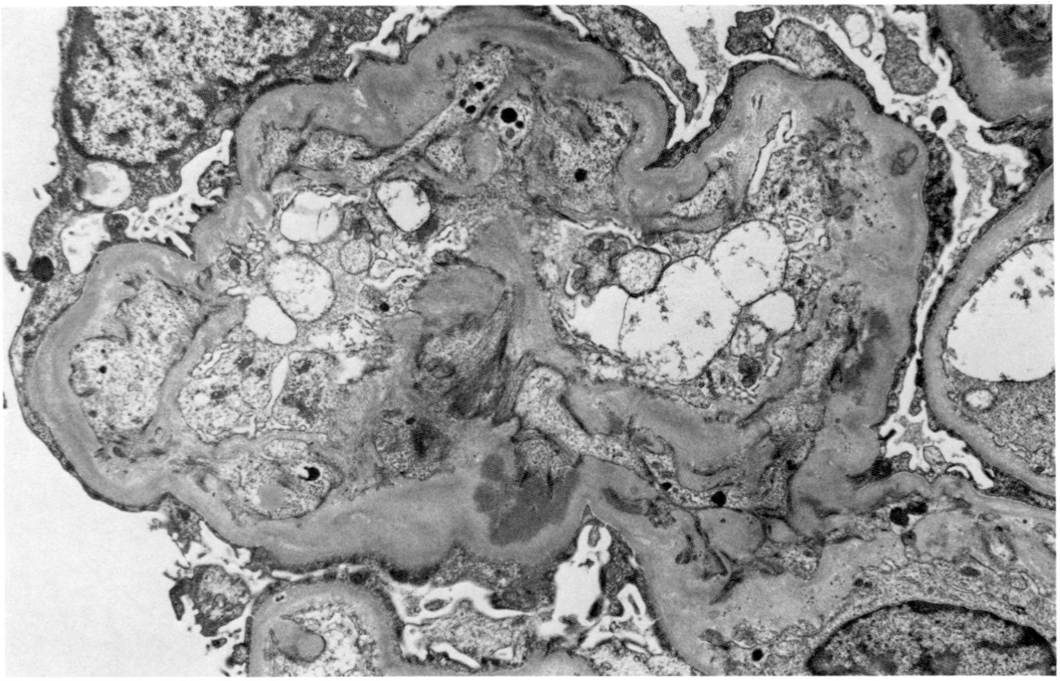

Fig. 67-22. Electron microscopy of a segment of a glomerular tuft, showing capillary loop obliteration and early collagenization (×3,800).

Vasculitis

In patients with HSP, most clinical features are a reflection of a systemic leukocytoclastic vasculitis, characteristically affecting the skin, gastrointestinal tract, and joints. It is a disease of the small blood vessels, particularly the postcapillary venules [1] and probably the result of immune complex deposition, with activation of complement and consequent leukotaxis. Neutrophils attracted to the site frequently undergo karyorrhexis, resulting in the nuclear dusting that gives the disorder its name. There is variable endothelial cell proliferation, mural fibrin, and, in severe cases, fibrinoid necrosis [181]. In addition to neutrophils, there are eosinophils and mononuclear cells both in the vessel walls and perivascular regions (Fig. 67-23). Variable hemorrhages also may occur. In severe cases, there may be cutaneous infarction with ulcer formation. Deposits of C3, frequently associated with IgA and IgM, may be found in blood vessel walls (Fig. 67-24). Electron-dense deposits and fibrin have been demonstrated in early lesions [24]. Immune complexes also have been detected in the cytoplasm of associated neutrophils, indicating phagocytic activity of these cells. These changes may be found not

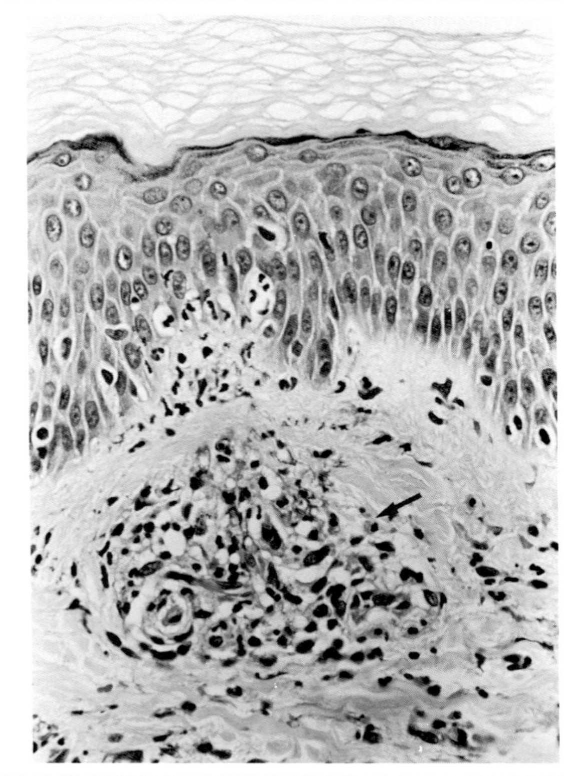

Fig. 67-23. Skin in leukocytoclastic vasculitis. Small dermal blood vessels show endothelial cell proliferation, and there is a prominent perivascular mixed inflammatory cell infiltrate with karyorrhexis. The inflammation affects the overlying epidermis, which also shows spongiosis (H&E, ×400).

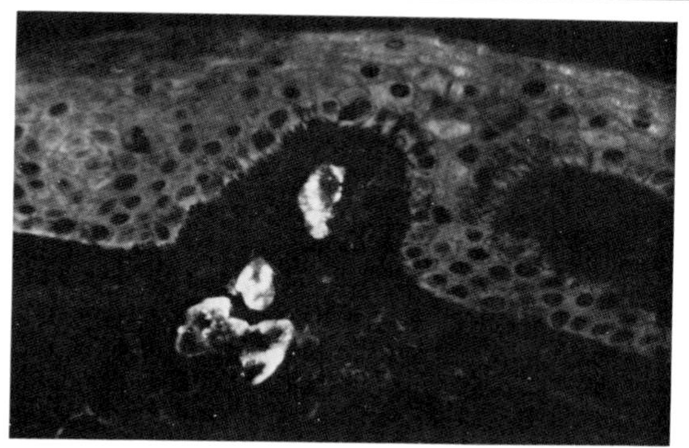

Fig. 67-24. Skin immunofluorescence. There are brightly fluorescing granular deposits of IgA in the small dermal blood vessels. A similar pattern is also seen with C3 (anti-human IgA, ×400).

only in the vessels of purpuric areas but also in healthy skin. By contrast, the skin changes in IgA nephropathy are by no means so dramatic, since vasculitis is not a feature. However, deposits of IgA are found in the dermal blood vessels in most cases of IgA nephropathy, and a small number of cases also have deposits of IgM, C3, and fibrin [7, 209].

Clinicopathologic Correlation

The major clinicopathologic correlations are shown in Table 67-3. Most are not controversial, but the relative contribution of glomerular crescents to hematuria, acute renal failure, and chronic renal failure is not clear.

Table 67-3. Correlation of clinical with pathologic features in the IgA nephropathies

Macroscopic hematuria	Basement membrane breaks, crescents
Microscopic hematuria	Basement membrane nips, irregularities
Proteinuria	Basement membrane and podocyte changes; glomerular tuft collapse and sclerosis; ? mesangial dysfunction
Nephrotic syndrome	Diffuse basement membrane changes, glomerular sclerosis, diffuse podocyte expansion (minimal change) and epimembranous deposits (rare)
Acute renal failure	Acute tubular necrosis; tubular plugging by red cells; glomerular crescents
Hypertension	Sclerotic and hypertensive vascular changes, glomerular sclerosis
Chronic renal failure	Glomerular sclerosis and obsolescence; hypertensive vascular changes; tubulointerstitial scarring; tubular atrophy; glomerular crescents
HSP (skin, gut, joint)	Immune complex vasculitis

Pathogenesis*

IMMUNOBIOLOGY OF IgA

A detailed description of the immunobiology of IgA is beyond the scope of this chapter, and a recent review by McGhee et al. [130] is recommended for detailed study. A working knowledge is, however, important to understand the nuances of pathogenesis, animal models, and secondary forms of the disease. IgA is the major immunoglobulin in external body secretions but is present in relatively low concentrations in serum. Serum IgA is 90 percent monomeric, while that found in secretions is mostly polymeric. Dimers or polymers of IgA contain a bridging or joining polypeptide—the J chain. Secretory component (SC) synthesized in glandular epithelial cells joins to dimeric IgA at mucosal surfaces to provide local immunity. Secretory IgA (sIgA) is more stable at these sites than serum IgA, which is readily degraded. IgM also exists as polymers linked by J chain. J chain is responsible for binding to SC of both polymeric IgA and IgM. Two subclasses of IgA (IgA1 and IgA2) exist in serum and secretions, IgA1 accounting for 90 percent of serum IgA, whereas IgA2 composes 60 percent of IgA in secretions. The subclasses differ antigenically, in their metabolic properties, chemical content, and the lengths of their hinge regions.

Serum IgA is derived from B cells in bone marrow, spleen, and peripheral lymph nodes as well as those at mucosal sites, e.g., bronchial, gastrointestinal, and urinary tracts. Cells at all those sites are capable of producing monomeric and polymeric forms of IgA and are under the influence of T helper and T suppressor cells. The relative contributions of these production sites to the serum IgA pool probably vary from time to time and in individuals, although the vast numbers of IgA-producing cells within the lamina propria of the intestine suggest that the contribution from this site may be significant. The small size (7S) of monomeric IgA allows its diffusion into lymphatics from intestinal sites, from where it passes into the circulation. Polymeric IgA (10–21S), on the other hand, may enter the portal circulation to be transported to the liver, where it is preferentially catabolized [223].

The molecular and cellular interactions that regulate the differentiation of lymphoid cells into IgA production are only partially understood. T cells and T cell cytokines profoundly influence the isotype-specific differentiation of B cells but only following the homing of B and T cells to mucosal effector sites. Commitment of B cells to produce the IgA isotype is influenced by the heavy-chain gene family. Switching of production from one isotype to another (e.g., IgM to IgA) involves a DNA recombination event between DNA sequences that occurs in tandem in specific switch regions on the heavy-chain gene. Whether T helper cell products interleukin-4 (IL-4), IL-5, and IL-6 induce B cells to switch to IgA production is not known, but they are of great impor-

*Parts of this section were reproduced with permission from A. J. Woodroffe, IgA Nephropathy: Toward an Understanding of Its Pathogenesis. In C. B. Wilson, B. M. Brenner, S. H. Stein (eds.), *Immunopathology of Renal Disease*. New York: Churchill Livingstone, 1988.

tance in B cell growth and proliferation. In addition, IL-7 as well as IL-4, IL-5, and IL-6 probably regulate positively or negatively the terminal differentiation of mature B cells into antibody secreting plasma cells.

GENETIC FACTORS

A genetic predisposition is likely given the apparent racial differences in prevalence of IgA nephropathy, instances of the occurrence of disease in first-degree relatives (with many others having similar immune abnormalities in vitro) [32, 137, 178, 210], in some studies an association with DR4 [68, 89, 99, 100], and also on chromosome 6, with complement genes (C4A and C4B null phenotypes) [97, 131] and in others with the immunoglobulin "switch region" on chromosome 14 [52]. Further studies including those with DQ genes [138] are in progress in this area, and more definitive associations are likely to be found. These will almost certainly confirm the genetic susceptibility for the condition through overproduction of IgA and just possibly could provide a discrete diagnostic marker.

ENVIRONMENTAL AGENTS

In a genetically determined "IgA over-responder," any mucosally presented antigen could in theory be responsible for IgA immune complex formation and tissue deposition. This is borne out by studies that implicate viral antigens (Epstein-Barr virus [222], herpes simplex and adenoviruses [219], hepatitis B virus [94, 114]), bacterial antigens (pneumococcus [59], *Escherichia coli* [234]), and dietary antigens (bovine serum albumin [234], ovalbumin and soybean protein [185], gluten [41]) in the facilitation of IgA nephropathy. Having said this, it must be acknowledged that identification of such antigens within the mesangial deposits has been the exception rather than the rule. It should also be stressed that the lectin binding activities of IgA may be just as important as true antigen-antibody complex formation [38].

Finally it is likely that alcohol can facilitate the process firstly by increasing gut permeability to macromolecules and secondly, in established alcoholic liver disease, by reducing immune clearance (see below).

INCREASED IgA PRODUCTION

The results of cell culture studies of immunoglobulin production in IgA nephropathy patients have been quite variable. Some describe increased IgA production in both unstimulated and stimulated cultures, others in only one or the other, and others not at all [11, 64, 82, 163, 174]. The discrepancies may be technical but are more likely a function of disease heterogeneity and patient selection. Several mechanisms for increased IgA production are possible: (1) a defect in IgA-specific suppressor T cell activity [180], (2) an increase in IgA-specific helper T cell activity and in T α4 cells [179, 236] (interleukin 6 appears to be important in mediating the latter [13]), (3) IgA-specific B cell hyperactivity [82], and (4) increased stimulus to IgA production through a function of macrophages [163]. Each of these has been described, but at present there is neither consensus regarding the precise immunoregulatory abnormality or abnormalities, nor any relationship to activity of disease. In longitudinal studies, we have found no consistent relationship between in vitro IgA synthesis and clinical evidence of disease activity [82]. However, others describe increases in IgA-bearing B lymphocytes, T helper-suppressor ratios, and pokeweed mitogen-induced IgA production during relapse [69].

There have been more limited studies of IgA production by mucosally derived cells, but these have also shown an increase and the IgA is polymeric [15, 63]. Other studies support the bone marrow as the site of increased IgA production [227].

High IgA responders have also been found in a group of patients with IgA nephropathy by studying serum IgA antibodies after subcutaneous immunization with influenza vaccines [66], mumps vaccination [162], and oral polio immunization [229].

HUMORAL IMMUNE ABNORMALITIES

Remote from the glomerulus, a number of abnormalities have been described in IgA nephropathy that might be centrally significant. Thus the serum IgA concentration is elevated in 40 to 50 percent of patients [35, 40, 109, 118], albeit not correlating with disease activity or prognosis. Investigators have reported increased amounts of polymeric serum IgA [122], and some have shown a correlation between this parameter and active disease [224]. IgA class immune complexes are also frequently detected by conglutinin binding, IgA inhibition, and Raji cell assays [40, 65, 83, 116, 224], and in some reports, the complexed IgA is polymeric [65, 224]. This latter observation is totally consistent with a murine model of IgA nephropathy in which the IgA must be both polymeric and complexed to produce mesangial deposits [170]. Some investigators have shown a correlation between the concentration of IgA class immune complexes and disease activity [40] and, of special interest, a significant delay in the postprandial clearance of such complexes in IgA nephropathy patients [40]. In some instances, these complexes have been shown to contain food antigens [183]. Studies have indicated that the circulating "macromolecular" (10–21S) IgA is of the IgA1 subclass [224], but as pointed out earlier, this does not help to define where the IgA is being produced.

Autoantibodies have also been reported in patients with IgA nephropathy. These include antibodies to immunoglobulins [45, 203], nucleoproteins [156], vascular endothelial cells [72], glomerular cells [158], and glomerular basement membrane antigens [31]. However, not all are of IgA class, and if of IgG class, there is seemingly a lack of correlation with the concomitant presence of glomerular IgG deposits. Preliminary reports of serum IgA anti-IgA antibodies may be of more interest in this respect.

DEFECTIVE IMMUNE CLEARANCE

Hepatobiliary clearance of IgA polymers is about 50 times less important in humans than in rats [51]. The expression of SC on hepatocytes has been correlated with hepatobiliary IgA clearance and is low in guinea pigs, dogs, and humans, but high in rats, rabbits, and mice. However, SC is present on human bile duct cells and lumens and may contribute to the clearance of polymeric IgA. The clearance of polymeric IgA is known to be delayed in patients with alcoholic cirrhosis [50], a condition frequently associated with mesangial deposits of IgA [232].

Binding of C3b-containing immune complexes to red cells via their complement receptors (CR1) is an important mechanism in delivery to the fixed macrophage system. One study has reported normal or high concentrations of CR1 in patients with IgA nephropathy, in contrast to SLE in which CR1 is reduced [95]. Another reports that the quantity of IgA immune complexes bound to red cells is too small to be important [127]. The expression of glomerular C3b receptors [205] is variably reduced in renal biopsies from patients with IgA nephropathy. Fc-mediated (splenic) and C3-mediated (hepatic) clearance studies have also been performed [12, 153, 171]. Delayed clearance was observed in a proportion of these patients, sometimes correlating with the results of immune complex determinations [171]. Similar findings have been seen in in vitro studies [173]. Rather than being a primary event, however, these features may well be due to saturation of receptors by IgA and C3.

Finally, one group has reported a decreased capacity of IgA nephropathy patients' sera to solubilize glomerular immune deposits in an in vitro test system [218]. It was considered that this solubilization capacity was complement mediated, perhaps implying the existence of a subtle abnormality in the complement pathway in those patients. These authors have subsequently tested the capacity of Danazol to correct the abnormality [216].

MEDIATION OF GLOMERULAR INJURY

It is still not clear how the IgA deposits lead to glomerular injury. The traditional mediators (e.g., complement, neutrophils, platelets, superoxide radicals) may be operative in acute exacerbations but seem unlikely to be responsible for the indolent, noninflammatory chronic lesions. There is no numerical increase in intraglomerular macrophages or T cells, although the interstitium often contains increased numbers of these cells with an increased CD4/CD8 ratio [4]. In IgA nephropathy, there is increased B cell function with production of excessive quantities of polymeric IgA [188]. This B cell hyperactivity most likely is T helper cell induced. As T and B cell function is in large part determined by the activity of various interleukins, and immunoglobulin secretion is regulated by lymphokines produced by activated T cells, the pathogenesis of glomerular changes in IgA nephropathy may in part be related to consequences of these abnormalities. Conceptually there may be an overproduction of one or more of these lymphokines, or increased response by the T and B cells to the lymphokines. Much recent work has concentrated on these aspects. High concentrations of IL-2 and soluble IL-2 receptor have been found in the supernatant of cultured peripheral blood mononuclear cells and in sera from patients with IgA nephropathy [115, 189]. Studies have also demonstrated that IL-6 may be an autocrine growth factor responsible for proliferation of mesangial cells [93, 177]. In IL-6 transgenic mice, the mesangial proliferation is associated with heavy proteinuria and polyclonal rise in immunoglobulins. In these studies, antibody to human IL-6 diminished mesangial cell proliferation and improved renal function [92]. Thus abnormally regulated production of IL-6 either by mesangial cells or by infiltrating T cells may be responsible for the mesangial cell proliferation in IgA nephropathy. In support of this concept is the finding of increased IL-6 concentrations in the urine of patients with IgA nephropathy [93].

Other potential mediators include interleukin-1 (which has an autocrine role in mesangial proliferation) [33], platelet-derived growth factor [71], and possibly low-density lipoproteins [231].

It is possible that glomerular sclerosis develops simply as a reaction to mesangial occlusion by the immune deposits and fibrin. It is also possible that these glomerular lesions are a consequence of vasoconstriction mediated by the disordered local production of angiotensin and prostaglandins (PGE). The mesangial cell has receptors for angiotensin II [160]. The cell contracts in the presence of angiotensin, thus reducing glomerular filtration area. Angiotensin has also been shown to increase the glomerular uptake of macromolecules [166]. PGE is produced by mesangial cells and causes relaxation/dilatation [187]. The combined effect of an increase in angiotensin and decrease in PGE could account for the observed functional and structural abnormalities (Fig. 67-25). Studies are required to evaluate this hypothesis but a down-regulation of glomerular angiotensin II receptors in IgA nephropathy [81] and reduced plasma prostacyclin metabolite concentrations in patients with HSP have already been reported [220]. Lastly, hyperfiltration no doubt plays a role in the progression of disease once nephron damage is established. In one study with dopamine infusion used to assess the renal functional reserve, it was found that the kidneys of patients with IgA nephropathy were already maximally hyperfiltering when the glomerular filtration rate was less than 73 ml/minute [23].

SUMMARY (Fig. 67-26)

Our current understanding of the pathogenesis of IgA nephropathy is imperfect, but some general conclusions can be made. It is reasonably well established that the mesangial deposits are derived from circulating IgA immune complexes in which the IgA is polymeric and predominantly of the IgA1 subclass. Antigen exposure at mucosal surfaces, increased production of IgA1, to-

Fig. 67-25. Hypothetical scheme for the role of angiotensin II (AII) in glomerular injury from IgA nephropathy. (Modified from [166].)

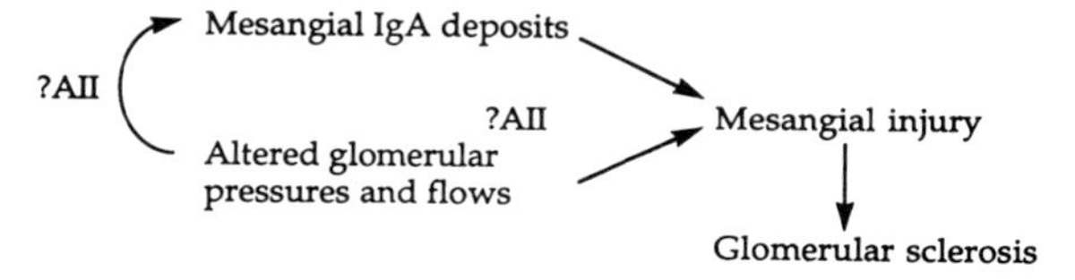

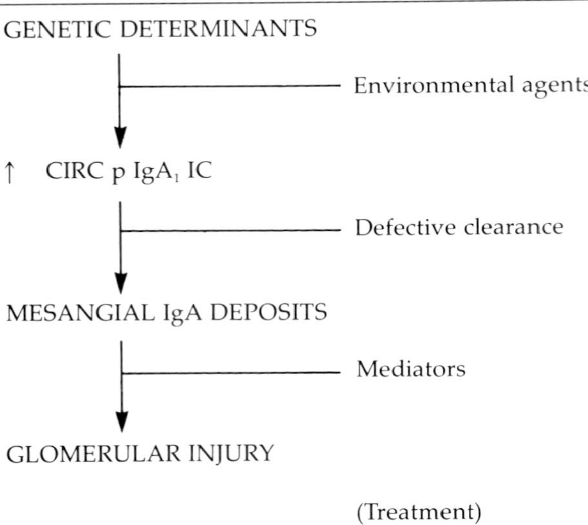

Fig. 67-26. Broad outline of possible pathogenetic mechanisms in IgA nephropathy. CIRC p IgA_1 IC = Circulatory polymere IgA_1 Immune Complexes.

gether with the formation of immune complexes and decreased immune clearance may jointly or separately be responsible. It is likely that these mechanisms are operative to different extents in different individuals with IgA nephropathy, hence the subsets that are being defined by laboratory tests. Less is known about the mediation of injury, although the role of cytokines produced in excess locally or by activated T cells has attracted increasing attention with respect to mesangial proliferation. These cytokines may also be responsible in part for the indolent but progressive vascular and sclerotic lesions that develop in patients destined to have a bad prognosis. It is suggested, however, that alteration of glomerular hemodynamics may also be important in this respect.

Treatment

Until the pathogenesis of IgA nephropathy and HSP is clarified, there will be no specific curative treatment for these conditions. Management, often over long periods, is therefore determined by careful definition of risk factors and complications. Often this can be performed during initial assessment of the patient. Variables such as age, persistent proteinuria, hypertension, renal dysfunction, glomerular crescents and sclerosis, interstitial fibrosis, and vascular lesions are important considerations when constructing a management policy. A poor prognosis, which can be predicted in approximately 30 percent of patients based on the presence of the above abnormalities, evokes a different therapeutic response than in the remaining 70 percent in whom regular but infrequent visits for confirmation of the good prognosis may be all that is required.

HYPERTENSION

Adequate treatment of hypertension is thought to delay the progression of renal impairment, and angiotensin converting enzyme inhibitors and calcium channel blocking drugs may be more effective than other hypotensive agents in view of their favorable action on glomerular hemodynamics.

DIET

The role of hemodynamically mediated progressive glomerular sclerosis may be particularly important in augmenting renal function loss. Specific dietary protein restriction has been impressive in halting the decline of renal function in some patients, perhaps because of the associated improvement of glomerular hypertension [25]. The effect of adequate control of systemic hypertension, hyperlipidemia, and associated salt restriction also may be important.

SYSTEMIC SYMPTOMS

The presence of skin rash, arthritis, gastrointestinal symptoms, and nephritis may evoke a more alarmist response from the physician. For example, corticosteroids have been used widely in patients with HSP but do not seem to influence the course of nephritis, rash, or arthritis. Response of the gastrointestinal lesions, particularly intramural hematomas may, however, be dramatic. Similar observations have been made following plasma exchange therapy.

MACROSCOPIC HEMATURIA

It is considered wise to measure renal function during an episode of macroscopic hematuria. Such episodes are frequently associated with glomerular crescent formation [16] and occasionally with acute renal failure [35]. The decreased renal function found during these episodes is frequently reversible spontaneously and apart from temporary dialysis requires no specific therapy. The use of corticosteroids and immunosuppressive and anticoagulant drugs has not proved beneficial [34].

PRIMARY OR SECONDARY DISEASE

In Table 67-2 is shown our classification of the diseases into primary and secondary forms. Differentiation is of general therapeutic importance because removal of inciting factors such as alcohol in cirrhotic patients, gluten from the diet in celiac disease and dermatitis herpetiformis, and so on, may interfere with factors significant in the development of renal disease.

MEASURES DIRECTED AGAINST PATHOGENETIC FACTORS

Based on the preceding information regarding pathogenesis (Fig. 67-26), approaches to therapy have included decreased antigen exposure (antibiotics [106], tonsillectomy [110], dietary manipulation [41, 42]) and antigen entry (alcohol, sodium cromoglycate [186]), decreased IgA production (phenytoin [36, 39], immunosuppression with corticosteroids [107] and cyclosporin A [113]), increased clearance of IgA polymers and complexes with plasma exchange, and blocking the mediators of glomerular injury with anticoagulants and antiplatelet drugs. In general, no definite evidence of short-

or long-term clinical, pathologic, or biochemical improvement has been obtained for any of these treatments.

References

1. Ackerman, A. B. *Histologic Diagnosis of Inflammatory Skin Diseases. A Method by Pattern Analysis.* London: Lea & Febiger, 1978.
2. Ackroyd, J. F. Allergic purpura, including purpura due to food, drugs and infections. *Am. J. Med.* 14: 605, 1953.
3. Andre, C., Berthoux, F. C., Andre, F., et al. Prevalence of IgA_2 deposits in IgA nephropathies. *N. Engl. J. Med.* 303: 1343, 1980.
4. Atkins, R. C., Boyce, N. W., Tipping, P. G., et al. Cellular Mediators in Glomerular Injury. In K. T. Woo, A. Y. P. Wu, and C. H. Lim (eds.), *Proceedings of the 3rd Asian Pacific Congress of Nephrology,* Singapore, October 1986. P. 395.
5. Ayoub, E. M., and Hoyer, J. Anaphylactoid purpura: Streptococcal antibody titers and B_1C globulin levels. *J. Pediatr.* 75: 193, 1969.
6. Baart de la Faille-Kuyper, E. H., Kater, L., Kooiker, C. J., et al. IgA deposits in cutaneous blood vessel walls and mesangium in Henoch-Schönlein syndrome. *Lancet* 1: 892, 1973.
7. Baart de la Faille-Kuyper, E. H., Kuitjen, R. H., et al. Occurrence of vascular IgA deposits in clinically normal skin of patients with renal disease. *Kidney Int.* 9: 424, 1976.
8. Bailey, R. R., Burry, A. F., McGiven, A. R., et al. A renal lesion in ankylosing spondylitis. *Nephron* 26: 171, 1980.
9. Baliah, T., Kim, K. H., Anthone, S., et al. Recurrence of Henoch-Schönlein purpura glomerulonephritis in transplanted kidneys. *Transplantation* 18: 343, 1974.
10. Ballardie, F. W., Brenchley, P. E., Williams, S., et al. Autoimmunity in IgA nephropathy. *Lancet* 2: 588, 1988.
11. Bannister, K. M., Drew, P. A., Clarkson, A. R., et al. Immunoregulation in glomerulonephritis, Henoch-Schönlein purpura and lupus nephritis. *Clin. Exp. Immunol.* 53: 384, 1983.
12. Bannister, K. M., Hay, J., Clarkson, A. R., et al. Fc-specific reticulo-endothelial clearance in systemic lupus erythematosus and glomerulonephritis. *Am. J. Kidney Dis.* 3: 287, 1984.
13. Beagley, K. W., Eldridge, J. H., Lee, F., et al. Interleukins and IgA synthesis: Human and murine interleukin 6 induce high rate IgA secretion in IgA committed B cells. *J. Exp. Med.* 169: 2133, 1989.
14. Bene, M., Faure, G., and Duheille, J. IgA nephropathy: Characterization of the polymeric nature of mesangial deposits by "in vivo" binding of free secretory component. *Clin. Exp. Immunol.* 47: 527, 1982.
15. Bene, M. C., Faure, G., Hurault de Ligny, B., et al. Immunoglobulin A nephropathy. Quantitative immunohistomorphometry of the tonsillar plasma cell evidences an inversion of the Immunoglobulin A versus Immunoglobulin G secreting cell balance. *J. Clin. Invest.* 71: 1342, 1983.
16. Bennett, W. M., and Kincaid-Smith, P. S. Macroscopic haematuria in mesangial IgA nephropathy. Correlation with glomerular crescents and renal dysfunction. *Kidney Int.* 23: 393, 1983.
17. Berger, J. IgA glomerular deposits in renal disease. *Transplant. Proc.* 1: 939, 1969.
18. Berger, J., and Hinglais, N. Les dépôts intercapillaires d'IgA-IgG. *J. Urol.* 74: 694, 1968.
19. Berger, J., Noel, L. H., and Nabarra, B. Recurrence of mesangial IgA nephropathy after renal transplantation. *Contrib. Nephrol.* 40: 195, 1984.
20. Berger, J., Yaneva, H., and Nabarra, B. Glomerular changes in patients with cirrhosis of the liver. *Adv. Nephrol.* 7: 3, 1978.
21. Berger, J., Yaneva, H., Nabarra, B., et al. Recurrence of mesangial deposition of IgA after renal transplantation. *Kidney Int.* 7: 232, 1975.
22. Berthoux, F. C., Gagne, A., Sabatier, J. C., et al. HLA-BW35 and mesangial IgA glomerulonephritis. *N. Engl. J. Med.* 298: 1034, 1978.
23. Beukhof, H. R., Ter Wee, P. M., Sluiter, W. J., and Donker, A. J. M. Effect of low-dose dopamine on effective renal plasma flow and glomerular filtration rate in 32 patients with IgA nephropathy. *Am. J. Nephrol.* 5: 267, 1985.
24. Brauerman, I. M., and Yen, A. Demonstration of immune complexes in spontaneous and histamine induced lesions and in normal skin of patients with leukocytoclastic angiitis. *J. Invest. Dermatol.* 64: 105, 1975.
25. Brenner, B. M., Meyer, T. W., and Hostetter, T. H. Dietary protein intake and the progressive nature of kidney disease: The role of hemodynamically mediated glomerular injury in the pathogenesis of progressive glomerular sclerosis in aging, renal ablation and intrinsic renal disease. *N. Engl. J. Med.* 307: 652, 1982.
26. Brettle, R., Peters, D. K., and Batchelor, J. R. Mesangial IgA glomerulonephritis and HLA antigens. *N. Engl. J. Med.* 298: 1034, 1978.
27. Bywaters, E. G. L., Isdale, I., and Kempton, J. J. Schönlein-Henoch purpura; evidence for a group of A betahaemolytic streptococcal infection. *Q. J. Med.* 26: 161, 1957.
28. Cairns, S. A., Mallick, N. P., Lawler, W., et al. Squamous cell carcinoma of the bronchus presenting with Henoch-Schönlein purpura. *Br. Med. J.* 2: 474, 1978.
29. Callard, P., Feldmann, G., Prandi, D., et al. Immune complex type glomerulonephritis in cirrhosis of the liver. *Am. J. Pathol.* 80: 329, 1975.
30. Cameron, J. S. Glomerulonephritis in renal transplants. *Transplantation* 34: 237, 1982.
31. Cederholm, B., Weislander, J., Bygren, P., et al. Patients with IgA nephropathy have circulating anti-basement membrane antibodies reacting with structures common to collagen I, II and IV. *Proc. Natl. Acad. Sci. U.S.A.* 83: 6151, 1986.
32. Chan, S. H., Ku, G., and Sinniah, R. HLA and Chinese IgA mesangial glomerulonephritis. *Tissue Antigens* 17: 351, 1981.
33. Chen, X. M., Tian, J., and Li, L. S. IL-1B gene expression and IL-1 production of mouse mesangial cells and the effects of interleukins on proliferation of mesangial cells. *Proceedings of the XIth International Congress of Nephrology,* Tokyo 1990. P. 371A.
34. Clarkson, A. R., Seymour, A. E., Chan, Y.-L., et al. Clinical, Pathological and Therapeutic Aspects of IgA Nephropathy. In P. Kincaid-Smith, A. J. F. d'Apice, and R. C. Atkins (eds.), *Progress in Glomerulonephritis.* New York: Wiley, 1979. P. 247.
35. Clarkson, A. R., Seymour, A. E., Thompson, A. J., et al. IgA nephropathy, a syndrome of uniform morphology, diverse clinical features and uncertain prognosis. *Clin. Nephrol.* 8: 459, 1977.
36. Clarkson, A. R., Seymour, A. E., Woodroffe, A. J., et al. Controlled trial of phenytoin therapy in IgA nephropathy. *Clin. Nephrol.* 13: 215, 1980.

37. Conley, M. F., Cooper, M. D., and Michael, A. F. Selective deposition of Immunoglobulin A_1 in Immunoglobulin A nephropathy, anaphylactoid purpura nephritis and systemic lupus erythematosus. *J. Clin. Invest.* 66: 1432, 1980.
38. Coppo, R., Amore, A., Roccatello, D., et al. IgA antibodies to dietary proteins and IgA lectin binding in sera from Italian, Australian and Japanese IgA nephropathy patients. *Proceedings of the 26th Congress EDTA*, 1989.
39. Coppo, R., Basolo, B., Bulzomi, M. R., et al. Ineffectiveness of phenytoin treatment on IgA-containing circulating immune complexes in IgA nephropathy. *Nephron* 36: 275, 1984.
40. Coppo, R., Basolo, B., Martina, G., et al. Circulating immune complexes containing IgA, IgG and IgM in patients with primary IgA nephropathy and with Henoch-Schönlein nephritis. Correlation with clinical and histologic signs of activity. *Clin. Nephrol.* 18: 230, 1982.
41. Coppo, R., Basolo, B., Rollino, C., et al. Mediterranean diet and primary IgA nephropathy. *Clin. Nephrol.* 26: 72, 1986.
42. Coppo, R., Roccatello, D., Amore, A., et al. Effects of a gluten free diet in primary IgA nephropathy. *Clin. Nephrol.* 33: 72, 1990.
43. Counahan, R., Winterborn, M. H., White, R. H. R., et al. Prognosis of Henoch-Schönlein nephritis in children. *Br. Med. J.* 2: 11, 1977.
44. Covarsi, A., Flors, R., Barcelo, P., et al. Glomerulonephritis per depositōs mesangialis de 'IgA (enfermedad de Berger) parametros evolutivos. *Nefrologia* 1: 1, 1981.
45. Czerkinsky, C., Koopman, W. J., Jackson, S., et al. Circulating immune complexes and immunoglobulin A rheumatoid factor in patients with mesangial immunoglobulin A nephropathies. *J. Clin. Invest.* 77: 1931, 1986.
46. D'Amico, G. Idiopathic Mesangial IgA Nephropathy. In T. Bertani and G. Remuzzi (eds.), *Glomerular Injury 300 Years after Morgagni*. Milan, Italy: 1983. Pp. 205–228.
47. D'Amico, G. The commonest glomerulonephritis in the world: IgA nephropathy. *Q. J. Med.* 64: 709, 1987.
48. Danielsen, H., Eriksen, E. F., Johansen, A., et al. Serum immunoglobulin sedimentation patterns and circulating immune complexes in IgA glomerulonephritis and Schönlein-Henoch nephritis. *Acta Med. Scand.* 215: 435, 1984.
49. Decoteau, W. E., Gerrard, J. W., and Cunningham, J. A. Glomerulitis in dermatitis herpetiformis. *Lancet* 2: 679, 1973.
50. Delacroix, D. L., Elkon, K. B., Geubel, A. P., et al. Changes in size, subclass, and metabolic properties of serum immunoglobulin A in liver diseases and other diseases with high serum immunoglobulin A. *J. Clin. Invest.* 71: 358, 1983.
51. Delacroix, D. L., Furtado-Barriera, G., Rahier, J., et al. Immunohistochemical localization of secretory component in the liver of guinea pigs and dogs versus rats, rabbits and mice. *Scand. J. Immunol.* 19: 425, 1984.
52. Demaine, A. G., Rambausek, M., Knight, J. F., et al. Relationship of mesangial IgA glomerulonephritis to polymorphism of immunoglobulin heavy chain switch region. *J. Clin. Invest.* 81: 611, 1988.
53. De Werra, P., Morel Maroger, L., Leroux-Robert, C., et al. Glomerulites à dépôts d'IgA diffus dans le mesangium Etude de 96 cas chez l'adulte. *Schweiz. Med. Wochenschr.* 103: 761, 1973.
54. Doi, T., Kanatsu, K., Magai, H., et al. Immuno-electron microscopic studies of IgA nephropathy. *Nephron* 36: 246, 1984.
55. Doi, T., Kanatsu, K., Sekita, K., et al. Circulating immune complexes of IgG, IgA and IgM classes in various glomerular diseases. *Nephron* 32: 335, 1982.
56. Doi, T., Kanatsu, K., Nagai, H., et al. An overlapping syndrome of IgA nephropathy and membranous nephropathy. *Nephron* 35: 24, 1983.
57. Doi, T., Kanatsu, K., Sekita, K., et al. Detection of IgA class circulating immune complexes bound to Anti-C_3d antibody in patients with IgA nephropathy. *J. Immunol. Methods* 69: 95, 1984.
58. Dosa, S., Cairns, S. A., Mallick, N. P., et al. Relapsing Henoch-Schönlein syndrome with renal involvement in a patient with an IgA monoclonal gammopathy. *Nephron* 26: 145, 1980.
59. Drew, P. A., Nieuwhof, W. N., Clarkson, A. R., et al. Raised IgA antibodies to pneumococcal polysaccharides in patients with IgA nephropathy. *Clin. Exp. Immunol.* 60: 124, 1987.
60. Droz, D. Natural history of primary glomerulonephritis with mesangial deposits of IgA. *Contrib. Nephrol.* 2: 150, 1976.
61. Druet, P., Bariety, J., and Lagrue, G. Les glomerulopathies primitives à dépôts mesangiaux d'IgA et IgG. *Presse Med.* 78: 583, 1970.
62. Dysart, N. K., Sisson, S., and Vernier, R. L. Immunoelectron microscopy of IgA nephropathy. *Clin. Immunol. Immunopathol.* 29: 254, 1983.
63. Egido, J., Blasco, R., Lozano, L., et al. Immunological abnormalities in the tonsils of patients with IgA nephropathy: Inversion in the ratio of IgA: IgG bearing lymphocytes and increased polymeric IgA synthesis. *Clin. Exp. Immunol.* 57: 101, 1984.
64. Egido, J., Blasco, R., Sancho, J., et al. T-cell dysfunctions in IgA nephropathy: Specific abnormalities in the regulation of IgA synthesis. *Clin. Immunol. Immunopathol.* 26: 201, 1983.
65. Egido, J., Sancho, J., Rivera, F., et al. The role of IgA and IgG immune complexes in IgA nephropathy. *Nephron* 36: 52, 1984.
66. Endoh, M., Suga, T., Miura, M., et al. In vivo alteration of antibody production in patients with IgA nephropathy. *Clin. Exp. Immunol.* 57: 564, 1984.
67. Evans, D. J., Williams, D. G., Peters, D. K., et al. Glomerular deposition of properdin in Henoch-Schönlein syndrome and idiopathic focal nephritis. *Br. Med. J.* 3: 326, 1973.
68. Fauchet, R., Lepogamp, P., Genetet, B., et al. HLA-DR4 antigen and IgA nephropathy. *Tissue Antigens* 16: 205, 1980.
69. Feehally, J., Beattie, T. J., Brenchley, P. E. C., et al. Sequential study of the IgA system in relapsing IgA nephropathy. *Kidney Int.* 30: 924, 1986.
70. Feiner, H. D., Cabili, S., Baldwin, D. S., et al. Intrarenal vascular sclerosis in IgA nephropathy. *Clin. Nephrol.* 18: 183, 1982.
71. Fellstrom, B., Dimeny, E., Bohman, S. O., et al. PDGF receptor expression in glomerular diseases. *Proceedings of the XIth International Congress of Nephrology*, Tokyo, 1990. P. 5A.
72. Frampton, G., Perry, G. J., and Cameron, J. S. Endothelial cell (EC) autoantigens and their partial characterization in IgA nephropathy (IgA-N). *Abstracts of the XIth International Congress of Nephrology*, Tokyo, 1990. P. 45A.
73. Frasca, G. M., Vangelista, A., Biagini, G., et al. Immunological tubulo-interstitial deposits in IgA nephropathy. *Kidney Int.* 22: 184, 1982.
74. Gairdner, D. The Schönlein-Henoch syndrome (anaphy-

lactoid purpura). *Q. J. Med.* 17: 95, 1948.

75. Galla, J. H., Kohaut, E. C., Alexander, R., et al. Racial difference in the prevalence of IgA associated nephropathies. *Lancet* 2: 522, 1984.
76. Garcia-Fuentes, M., Chantler, C., and Williams, D. G. Cryoglobulinemia in Henoch-Schönlein purpura. *Br. Med. J.* 2: 163, 1977.
77. Garcia-Fuentes, M., Martin, A., Chantler, C., et al. Serum complement components in Henoch-Schönlein purpura. *Arch. Dis. Child.* 53: 417, 1978.
78. Gartner, H. V., Hunlein, F., Traub, U., et al. IgA nephropathy (IgA-IgG Nephropathy, IgA nephritis) a disease entity? *Virchows Arch. A* [*Pathol. Anat.*] 385: 1, 1979.
79. Gluckman, J. C., Jacob, N., Beaufils, H., et al. Clinical significance of circulating immune complexes. Detection in chronic glomerulonephritis. *Nephron* 22: 138, 1978.
80. Guttierez Millet, V., Navas Palacios, J. J., Prieto, C., et al. Glomerulonephritis mesangial IgA idiopatica. Estudio clinico e immunopathologico de 40 casos y revision de la literatura. *Nefrologia* 2: 1, 1982.
81. Hale, G. M., Howarth, G. S., Aarons, I., et al. Quantitation of glomerular angiotensin II receptors in IgA nephropathy. *Clin. Nephrol.* 32: 5, 1989.
82. Hale, G. M., McIntosh, S. L., Hiki, Y., et al. Evidence for IgA-specific B cell hyperactivity in patients with IgA nephropathy. *Kidney Int.* 29: 718, 1986.
83. Hall, R. P., Stachura, I., Cason, J., et al. IgA containing circulating immune complexes in patients with IgA nephropathy. *Am. J. Med.* 74: 56, 1983.
84. Heaton, J. M., Turner, D. R., and Cameron, J. S. Localisation of glomerular "deposits" in Henoch-Schönlein nephritis. *Histopathology* 1: 93, 1977.
85. Heberden, W. Commentaries on the history and cure of diseases. London: 1806. P. 396.
86. Helin, H., Mustonen, J., Reunala, T., et al. IgA nephropathy associated with celiac disease and dermatitis herpetiformis. *Arch. Pathol. Lab. Med.* 107: 324, 1983.
87. Henoch, E. *Berl. Klin. Wochenschr.* 11: 641, 1874.
88. Heptinstall, R. H. Focal Glomerulonephritis and IgA Deposition. In R. H. Heptinstall (ed.), *Pathology of the Kidney*, Vol. II. 3rd ed. Boston: Little, Brown, 1983. Pp. 572 and 741.
89. Hiki, Y., Kobayashi, Y., Tateno, S., et al. Strong association of HLA-DR4 with benign IgA nephropathy. *Nephron* 32: 222, 1982.
90. Hood, S. S., Velosa, J. A., Holley, K. E., et al. IgA-IgG nephropathy: Predictive indices of progressive disease. *Clin. Nephrol.* 16: 554, 1981.
91. Hookerjee, B., Maddison, P. J., and Reichlin, M. Mesangial IgA-IgG deposition in mixed cryoglobulinemia. *Am. J. Med. Sci.* 276: 221, 1978.
92. Horii, Y., Iwano, M., Suematsu, S., et al. Interleukin 6 and Mesangial Proliferation: Generation and Characterization of IL-6 Transgenic Mice. In H. Sakai, O. Sakai, and Y. Nomoto (eds.), *Pathogenesis of IgA Nephropathy*. Tokyo: Harcourt Brace Jovanovich, 1990. P. 127.
93. Horii, Y., Muraguchi, A., Iwano, M., et al. Involvement of IL-6 in mesangial proliferative glomerulonephritis. *J. Immunol.* 143: 3949, 1989.
94. Iida, H., Izumino, K., Asaka, M., et al. IgA nephropathy and hepatitis B virus. *Nephron* 54: 18, 1990.
95. Iida, K., Koyama, A., Nakamura, H., et al. Abnormal expression of complement receptor (CRI) in IgA nephritis: Increase in erythrocytes and loss on glomeruli in patients with impaired renal function. *Clin. Immunol. Immunopathol.* 40: 393, 1986.
96. Jennette, J. C., Ferguson, A. L., Moore, M. A. IgA nephropathy associated with seronegative arthritis. *Arth. Rheum.* 25: 144, 1982.
97. Julian, B. A., Quiggins, P. A., Thompson, J. S., et al. Familial IgA nephropathy: Evidence for an inherited mechanism of disease. *N. Engl. J. Med.* 312: 202, 1985.
98. Julian, B. A., Wyatt, R. J., McMorrow, R. G., et al. Serum complement proteins in IgA nephropathy. *Clin. Nephrol.* 20: 251, 1983.
99. Kasahara, M., Hamada, K., Okuyama, T., et al. Role of HLA in IgA nephropathy. *Clin. Immunol. Immunopathol.* 25: 189, 1982.
100. Kashiwabara, H., Shishioo, H., Tomura, S., et al. Strong association between IgA nephropathy and HLA-DR4 antigen. *Kidney Int.* 22: 377, 1982.
101. Katz, A., Dyck, R. F., and Bear, R. A. Celiac disease associated with immune complex glomerulonephritis. *Clin. Nephrol.* 11: 39, 1979.
102. Katz, A., Walker, J. F., and Landy, P. J. IgA nephritis with nephrotic range proteinuria. *Clin. Nephrol.* 20: 67, 1983.
103. Kauffmann, R. H., Herrmann, W. A., Meyer, C. J. L. M., et al. Circulating IgA immune complexes in Henoch-Schönlein purpura. A longitudinal study of their relationship to disease activity and vascular deposition of IgA. *Am. J. Med.* 68: 859, 1980.
104. Kimura, M., Sato, I., Shiratori, Y., et al. Electron microscopic studies of IgA nephropathy. *Acta Pathol. Jpn.* 34: 289, 1984.
105. Kincaid-Smith, P., Bennett, W. M., Dowling, J. P., et al. Acute renal failure and tubular necrosis associated with haematuria due to glomerulonephritis. *Clin. Nephrol.* 19: 206, 1983.
106. Kincaid-Smith, P., and Nicholls, K. Mesangial IgA nephropathy. *Am. J. Kidney Dis.* 3: 90, 1983.
107. Kobayashi, Y., Fujii, K., Hiki, Y., et al. Steroid therapy in IgA nephropathy: A retrospective study in heavy proteinuric cases. *Nephron* 48: 12, 1988.
108. Komatsu, N., Nagura, H., Watanabe, K., et al. Mesangial deposition of J-chain linked polymeric IgA in IgA nephropathy. *Nephron* 33: 61, 1983.
109. Lagrue, G., Hirbec, G., Fournel, M., et al. Glomerulonéphrite mesangial à dépôts d'IgA: Étude des immunoglobulines seriques. *J. Urol. Nephrol.* (Paris) 80: 385, 1973.
110. Lagrue, G., Sadreux, T., Laurent, J., et al. Is there treatment of IgA glomerulonephritis? *Clin. Nephrol.* 14: 161, 1980.
111. Lai, K. N., Chan, K. W., Lai, F. M., Ho, C. W. R., et al. The immunochemical characterization of the light chains in the mesangial IgA deposits in IgA nephropathy. *Am. J. Clin. Pathol.* 85: 548, 1986.
112. Lai, K. N., Lai, F. M., Choi, S. H., et al. Studies of lymphocyte subpopulations and immunoglobulin production in IgA nephropathy. *Clin. Nephrol.* 28: 281, 1987.
113. Lai, K. N., Lai, F. M., Li, P. T. K., and Vallance-Owen, J. Cyclosporin treatment of IgA nephropathy, a short term controlled trial. *Br. Med. J.* 295: 1165, 1987.
114. Lai, K. N., Lai, F. M., and Tam, J. S. IgA nephropathy associated with chronic hepatitis B infection in adults: The pathogenetic role of Hbs Ag. *J. Pathol.* 157: 321, 1989.
115. Lai, K. N., Leung, J. C. K., Lai, F. M., and Tam, J. S. T-lymphocyte activation in IgA nephropathy: Serum soluble interleukin-2 receptor level, interleukin-2 production and interleukin-2 receptor expression by cultured lymphocytes. *J. Clin. Immunol.* 9: 485, 1989.
116. Lesavre, P. H., Digeon, M., and Bach, J. F. Analysis of circulating IgA and detection of immune complexes in

primary IgA nephropathy. *Clin. Exp. Immunol.* 48: 61, 1982.
117. Levinsky, R. J., and Barratt, T. M. IgA immune complexes in Henoch-Schönlein purpura. *Lancet* 2: 1100, 1979.
118. Levy, M., Broyer, M., Arsan, A., et al. Anaphylactoid purpura in childhood. *Adv. Nephrol.* 6: 183, 1976.
119. Levy, M., Bruyer, M., and Habib, R. Pathology and Immunopathology of Schönlein-Henoch Glomerulonephritis. In P. Kincaid-Smith, A. J. F. d'Apice, and R. C. Atkins (eds.), *Progress in Glomerulonephritis.* New York: Wiley, 1979. P. 261.
120. Levy, M., Moussa, R. A., Habib, R., Gagnadoux, M. F., et al. Anaphylactoid purpura nephritis and transplantation. *Kidney Int.* 22: 326, 1982.
121. Lomax-Smith, J. D., Zabrowarny, L., Howarth, G., et al. The immunochemical characterisation of mesangial IgA deposits. *Am. J. Pathol.* 113: 359, 1983.
122. Lopez-Trascasca, M., Egido, J., Sancho, J., et al. IgA glomerulonephritis (Berger's disease); evidence of high serum levels of polymeric IgA. *Clin. Exp. Immunol.* 42: 247, 1980.
123. Macdonald, I. M., Fairley, K. F., Hobbs, J. B., et al. Loin pain as a presenting symptom in idiopathic glomerulonephritis. *Clin. Nephrol.* 3: 129, 1975.
124. Magyarlarki, T., Davin, J. C., Szabados, E., et al. Peripheral B-lymphocyte markers and function in IgA nephropathy. *Clin. Nephrol.* 33: 123, 1990.
125. Mandreoli, M., Pasquali, S., Donini, U., et al. Correlazioni anatomo-cliniche in corso di malattia di Berger. *Nefrologia e Dialise* 1: 9, 1981.
126. Mathew, T. H., Mathews, D. C., Hobbs, J. B., et al. Glomerular lesions after renal transplantation. *Am. J. Med.* 59: 177, 1975.
127. Matsuda, S., Waldo, F. B., Czerkinsky, C., et al. Binding of IgA to erythrocytes from patients with IgA nephropathy. *Clin. Immunol. Immunopathol.* 48: 1, 1988.
128. McCombs, R. P., Patterson, J. F., and MacMahon, H. E. Syndromes associated with "allergic" vasculitis. *N. Engl. J. Med.* 255: 251, 1956.
129. McCoy, R. C., Abramowsky, C. R., and Tisher, C. C. IgA nephropathy. *Am. J. Pathol.* 76: 123, 1974.
130. McGhee, J. R., Mestecky, J., Elson, C. O., and Kiyono, H. Regulation of IgA synthesis and immune response by T cells and interleukins. *J. Clin. Immunol.* 9: 175, 1989.
131. McLean, R. H., Wyatt, R. J., and Julian, B. A. Complement phenotypes in glomerulonephritis, increased frequency of homozygous null C4 phenotypes in IgA nephropathy and Henoch-Schönlein purpura. *Kidney Int.* 26: 555, 1984.
132. Meadow, S. R. The prognosis of Henoch-Schönlein nephritis. *Clin. Nephrol.* 9: 87, 1978.
133. Meadow, S. R., Glasgow, E. F., White, R. H. R., et al. Schönlein-Henoch nephritis. *Q. J. Med.* 41: 241, 1972.
134. Mery, J. Ph., Dard, S., and Kenouch, S. (Letter) *Arthritis Rheum.* 26: 816, 1983.
135. Mihatsch, M. J., Imbasciati, E., Fogazzi, G., et al. Ultrastructural lesions of Henoch-Schönlein syndrome and of IgA nephropathy: Similarities and differences. *Contrib. Nephrol.* 40: 225, 1984.
136. Miyazaki, R., Kurdoa, M., Akiyama, T., et al. Glomerular deposition and serum levels of complement control proteins in patients with IgA nephropathy. *Clin. Nephrol.* 21: 335, 1984.
137. Montoliu, J., Darnell, A., Torras, A., et al. Familial IgA nephropathy. Report of two cases and brief review of the literature. *Arch. Intern. Med.* 140: 1374, 1980.
138. Moore, R. H., Hitman, G. A., Lucas, E. Y., et al. HLA DQ region gene polymorphism associated with primary IgA nephropathy. *Kidney Int.* 37: 991, 1990.
139. Moorthy, A. V., Zimmerman, S. W., and Maxim, P. E. Dermatitis herpetiformis and celiac disease: Association with glomerulonephritis, hypocomplementaemia and circulating immune complexes. *J.A.M.A.* 239: 2019, 1978.
140. Morita, M., and Sakaguchi, H. A quantitative study of glomerular basement membrane changes in IgA nephropathy. *J. Pathol.* 154: 7, 1988.
141. Morzycka, M., Croker, B. P., Seigler, H. F., et al. Evaluation of recurrent glomerulonephritis in kidney allografts. *Am. J. Med.* 72: 588, 1982.
142. Murakami, T., Furuse, A., Hattori, S., et al. Glomerular IgA_1 and IgA_2 deposits in IgA nephropathies. *Nephron* 35: 120, 1983.
143. Mustonen, J. IgA glomerulonephritis. (Academic Dissertation) *Acta Univ. Tamperensis* Vol. 170; 1984.
144. Mustonen, J., Helin, H., and Pasternack, A. IgA nephropathy associated with bronchial small cell carcinoma. *Am. J. Clin. Pathol.* 76: 652, 1981.
145. Mustonen, J., Pasternack, A., Helin, H., et al. Circulating immune complexes, the concentration of serum IgA and the distribution of HLA antigens in IgA nephropathy. *Nephron* 29: 170, 1981.
146. Mustonen, J., Pasternack, A., and Rantala, I. The nephrotic syndrome in IgA glomerulonephritis: Response to corticosteroid therapy. *Clin. Nephrol.* 20: 172, 1983.
147. Nagy, J., Fust, G., Ambrus, M., et al. Circulating immune complexes in patients with IgA glomerulonephritis. *Acta Med. Acad. Sci. Hung.* 39: 211, 1982.
148. Nagy, J., Uj, M., Szucs, G., et al. Herpes virus antigens and antibodies in kidney biopsies and sera of IgA glomerulonephritic patients. *Clin. Nephrol.* 21: 259, 1984.
149. Nakamoto, Y., Asano, Y., Dohi, K., et al. Primary IgA glomerulonephritis and Schönlein-Henoch purpura nephritis: Clinicopathological and immunohistological characteristics. *Q. J. Med.* 47: 495, 1978.
150. Nash, H., Binns, G. F., Clarkson, A. R., et al. Concomitant IgA nephropathy and cyclical neutropaenia. *Aust. N.Z. J. Med.* 8: 184, 1978.
151. Navas-Palacios, J. J., Gutierrez-Millet, V., Usera-Sarrago, G., et al. IgA nephropathy: An ultrastructural study. *Ultrastruct. Pathol.* 2: 152, 1981.
152. Ng, W.-L., Chan, K. W., and Ma, L. A scanning electron microscope study of isolated glomeruli in glomerulonephritis. *Pathology* 15: 139, 1983.
153. Nicholls, K., and Kincaid-Smith, P. Defective in vivo Fc and C3b receptor function in IgA nephropathy. *Am. J. Kidney Dis.* 4: 128, 1984.
154. Nochy, D., Callard, P., Bellon, B., et al. Association of overt glomerulonephritis and liver disease: A study of 34 patients. *Clin. Nephrol.* 6: 422, 1976.
155. Noel, L. H., Descamps, B., Jungers, P., et al. HLA antigens in three types of glomerulonephritis. *Clin. Immunol. Immunopathol.* 10: 19, 1978.
156. Nomoto, Y., Suga, T., Miura, M., et al. Characterization of an acidic nuclear protein recognized by autoantibodies in sera from patients with IgA nephropathy. *Clin. Exp. Immunol.* 65: 513, 1986.
157. Noriyuki, K., Yasuo, N., Hiroshi, N., et al. Application of immuno-electron microscopic technique for glomerular diseases: Particularly IgA nephropathy. *J. Clin. Electron Microscopy* 14: 5, 1981.
158. O'Donoghue, D. J., Darvill, A., Brenchley, P., and Ballardie, F. W. Localization and partial characterization of

the glomerular autoantigen(s) in IgA nephropathy. *Abstracts of XIth International Congress of Nephrology,* Tokyo, 1990. P. 44A.

159. Ooi, Y. M., Ooi, B. S., and Pollak, V. E. Relationship of levels of circulating immune complexes to histologic patterns of nephritis. *J. Lab. Clin. Med.* 90: 891, 1977.
160. Osborne, M. J., Droz, D., Meyer, P., and Morel, F. Angiotensin II: Renal localization in glomerular mesangial cells by autoradiography. *Kidney Int.* 8: 245, 1975.
161. Pape, J. F., Mellbye, O. J., and Oystese, B. Glomerulonephritis in dermatitis herpetiformis. *Acta Med. Scand.* 203: 445, 1978.
162. Pasternak, A., Mustonen, J., and Leinikki, P. Humoral immune responses in patients with IgA and IgM glomerulonephritis. *Clin. Exp. Immunol.* 63: 228, 1986.
163. Perl, I., Wilkinson, A., and Williams, D. G. IgA and IgG production by lymphocytes in IgA glomerulonephritis. *Kidney Int.* 28: 856, 1985.
164. Pettersson, E., Von Bonsdorff, M., Tornroth, T., et al. Nephritis among young Finnish men. *Clin. Nephrol.* 22: 217, 1984.
165. Power, D. A., Muirhead, N., Simpson, J. G., et al. Asymptomatic haematuria and IgA nephropathy: Results of a retrospective renal biopsy study (Abstract). *Kidney Int.* 22: 219, 1982.
166. Raij, L., and Keane, W. F. Glomerular mesangium: Its function and relationship to angiotensin II. *Am. J. Med.* 79: 24, 1985.
167. Rambausek, M., Rauterberg, E. W., Waldherr, R., et al. Evolution of IgA glomerulonephritis: Relation to morphology, immunogenetics and B.P. *Semin. Nephrol.* 7: 370, 1987.
168. Ramirez, G., Stinson, J. B., Zawada, E. T., et al. IgA nephritis associated with mycosis fungoides. *Arch. Intern. Med.* 141: 1287, 1981.
169. Richman, A. V., Mahoney, J. J., and Fuller, T. J. Higher prevalence of HLA-B12 in patients with IgA nephropathy. *Ann. Intern. Med.* 90: 201, 1979.
170. Rifai, A., and Millard, K. Glomerular deposition of immune complexes prepared with monomeric or polymeric IgA. *Clin. Exp. Immunol.* 60: 363, 1985.
171. Roccatello, D., Coppo, R., Piccoli, G., et al. Circulating Fc-receptor blocking factors in IgA nephropathies. *Clin. Nephrol.* 23: 159, 1985.
172. Roccatello, D., Coppo, R., Ropolo, R., et al. IgG co-presence in IgA containing immune complexes influences their removal from circulation. *Abstracts of XIth International Congress of Nephrology,* Tokyo, 1990. P. 4A.
173. Roccatello, D., Picciotto, G., Coppo, R., et al. Clearance of polymeric IgA aggregates in humans. *Am. J. Kidney Dis.* 14: 354, 1989.
174. Rothschild, E., and Chatenoud, L. T-cell subset modulation of immunoglobulin production in IgA nephropathy and membranous glomerulonephritis. *Kidney Int.* 25: 557, 1984.
175. Roy, L. P. Properdin and recurrent macroscopic haematuria. *Aust. N.Z. J. Med.* 5: 191, 1975.
176. Roy, L. P. Fish, A. J., and Vernier, R. L. Recurrent macroscopic hematuria, focal nephritis and mesangial deposition of immunoglobulin and complement. *J. Pediatr.* 82: 767, 1973.
177. Ruef, C., Budde, K., Lacy, J., et al. Interleukin 6 is an autocrine growth factor for mesangial cells. *Kidney Int.* 38: 249, 1990.
178. Sabatier, J. C., Genin, C., Assenat, H., et al. Mesangial IgA glomerulonephritis in HLA—Identical brothers. *Clin. Nephrol.* 11: 35, 1979.
179. Sakai, H., Miyazaki, M., Endoh, M., and Nomoto, Y. Increase in IgA-specific switch T cells in patients with IgA nephropathy. *Clin. Exp. Immunol.* 78: 378, 1989.
180. Sakai, H., Nomoto, Y., and Arimori, S. Decrease of IgA specific suppressor T cell activity in patients with IgA nephropathy. *Clin. Exp. Immunol.* 38: 245, 1979.
181. Sams, W. M., Thorne, E. G., Small, P., et al. Leukocytoclastic vasculitis. *Arch. Dermatol.* 112: 219, 1976.
182. Sancho, J., Egido, J., and Gonzalez, E. A simple method for determining polymeric IgA containing immune complexes. *J. Immunol. Methods* 60: 305, 1983.
183. Sancho, J., Egido, J., Revera, F., and Hernando, L. Immune complexes in IgA nephropathy: Presence of antibodies against diet antigens and delayed clearance of specific polymeric IgA immune complexes. *Clin. Exp. Immunol.* 54: 194, 1983.
184. Sanfilippo, F., Croker, B. P., and Bollinger, R. R. Fate of four cadaveric renal allografts with mesangial IgA deposits. *Transplantation* 33: 370, 1982.
185. Sato, M., Kojima, H., Takayama, K., and Koshikawa, S. Glomerular deposition of food antigens in IgA nephropathy. *Clin. Exp. Immunol.* 73: 295, 1988.
186. Sato, M., Takayama, K., Kojima, H., and Koshikawa, S. Sodium cromoglycate therapy in IgA nephropathy: A preliminary short-term trial. *Am. J. Kidney Dis.* 15: 141, 1990.
187. Scharschmidt, L. A., and Dunn, M. J. Prostaglandin synthesis by rat glomerular mesangial cells in culture: Effects of angiotensin II and arginine vasopressin. *J. Clin. Invest.* 71: 1756, 1983.
188. Schena, F. P., and Emancipator, S. N. Primary IgA associated nephropathy: A clue to pathogenesis. *J. Nephrol.* 2: 135, 1989.
189. Schena, F. P., Mastrolitti, G., Jirillo, E., et al. Increased production of interleukin 2 and expression of the IL-2 receptor by human peripheral blood mononuclear cells in primary IgA nephropathy. *Kidney Int.* 35: 875, 1989.
190. Schena, F. P., Pastore, A., Ludovico, N., et al. Increased serum levels of IgA1-IgG immune complexes and anti-$F(ab')_2$ antibodies in patients with primary IgA nephropathy. *Clin. Exp. Immunol.* 77: 15, 1989.
191. Schena, F. P., Pastore, A., Sinico, R. A., et al. Polymeric IgA and IgA rheumatoid factor decrease the capacity of serum to solubilize circulating immune complexes in patients with primary IgA nephropathy. *J. Immunol.* 141: 125, 1988.
192. Schonlein, J. L. *Allegemeine u. Specielle Pathologic u. Therapie.* 2: 48, 1837.
193. Shigematsu, H., Kobayashi, Y., Tateno, S., et al. Ultrastructure of acute glomerular injury in IgA nephritis. *Arch. Pathol. Lab. Med.* 104: 303, 1980.
194. Shigematsu, H., Kobayashi, Y., Tateno, S., et al. Ultrastructural glomerular loop abnormalities in IgA nephritis. *Nephron* 30: 1, 1982.
195. Siegler, H. F., Ward, F. E., Maccoy, R. E., et al. Long-term results with forty five living related renal allograft recipients genotypically identical for HLA. *Surgery* 81: 274, 1977.
196. Silva, F. G., Chanda, P., Pirani, C. L., et al. Disappearance of glomerular mesangial IgA deposits after renal allograft transplantation. *Transplantation* 33: 214, 1982.
197. Simon, P., Ang, K.-S., Bavay, P., et al. Glomerulonéphrite à immunoglobulines A. Epidemiologie dans une population de 250,000 habitants. *La Presse Med.* 13: 257, 1984.
198. Simon, P., Ramee, M.-P., Ang, K.-S., and Cam, G. Evolution de l'incidence annuelle des glomerulonéphritis

primitives dans un population de 400,000 au cours d'une periode de 10 ans (1976–1985). *Nephrologia* 5: 185, 1986.

199. Sinclair, R. A., Burns, J., and Dunnill, M. S. Immunoperoxidase staining of paraffin embedded renal biopsies. *Pathology* 14: 101, 1982.
200. Sinniah, R. Mucin secreting cancer with mesangial IgA deposits. *Pathology* 14: 303, 1982.
201. Sinniah, R. Occurrence of mesangial IgA and IgM deposits in a control necropsy population. *J. Clin. Pathol.* 36: 276, 1983.
202. Sinniah, R., Javier, A. R., and Ku, G. The pathology of IgA nephritis with clinical correlation. *Histopathology* 5: 469, 1981.
203. Sinico, R. A., Fornasieri, A., Oreni, N., et al. Polymeric IgA rheumatoid factor in idiopathic IgA mesangial nephropathy (Berger's disease). *J. Immunol.* 137: 536, 1986.
204. Sissons, J. G. P., Woodrow, D. F., Curtis, J. R., et al. Isolated glomerulonephritis with mesangial IgA deposits. *Br. Med. J.* 3: 611, 1975.
205. Sobel, A. T., Gabay, Y. E., and Lagrue, G. Analysis of glomerular complement receptors in various types of glomerulonephritis. *Clin. Immunol. Immunopathol.* 6: 94, 1976.
206. Southwest Pediatric Nephrology Study Group. A multicentric study of IgA nephropathy in children. *Kidney Int.* 22: 643, 1982.
207. Spargo, B. H., Seymour, A. E., and Ordonnez, N. G. *Renal Biopsy Pathology with Diagnostic and Therapeutic Implications.* New York: Wiley, 1980. Pp. 80–86.
208. Taguchi, T., Von Bassewitz, D. B., Grundmann, E., and Takebayashi, S. Ultrastructural changes in glomerular basement membrane in IgA nephritis: Relationship to haematuria. *Ultrastruct. Pathol.* 12: 17, 1988.
209. Thompson, A. J., Chan, Y.-L., Woodroffe, A. J., et al. Vascular IgA deposits in clinically normal skin of patients with renal disease. *Pathology* 12: 407, 1980.
210. Tolkoff-Rubin, N. E., Cosimi, A. B., Fuller, T., et al. IgA nephropathy in HLA—Identical siblings. *Transplantation* 26: 430, 1978.
211. Tomino, Y., Endoh, M., Suga, T., et al. Prevalence of IgA_1 deposits in Henoch-Schönlein purpura (HSP) nephritis. *Tokai J. Exp. Clin. Med.* 7: 527, 1982.
212. Tomino, Y., Miura, M., Suga, T., et al. Detection of IgA_1 dominant immune complexes in peripheral blood polymorphonuclear leukocytes by double immunofluorescence in patients with IgA nephropathy. *Nephron* 37: 137, 1984.
213. Tomino, Y., Sakai, H., Endoh, M., et al. Detection of immune complexes in polymorphonuclear leukocytes by double immunofluorescence in patients with IgA nephropathy. *Clin. Immunol. Immunopathol.* 24: 63, 1982.
214. Tomino, Y., Sakai, H., and Endoh, T. Cross reactivity of IgA antibodies between renal mesangial areas and nuclei of tonsillar cells in patients with IgA nephropathy. *Clin. Exp. Immunol.* 51: 605, 1983.
215. Tomino, Y., Sakai, H., Miura, H., et al. Detection of polymeric IgA in glomeruli from patients with IgA nephropathy. *Clin. Exp. Immunol.* 49: 419, 1982.
216. Tomino, Y., Sakai, H., Miura, M., et al. Effect of danazol on solubilization of immune deposits in patients with IgA nephropathy. *Am. J. Kidney Dis.* 4: 135, 1984.
217. Tomino, Y., Sakai, H., Miura, M., et al. Specific binding of circulating IgA antibodies in patients with IgA nephropathy. *Am. J. Kidney Dis.* 6: 149, 1985.
218. Tomino, Y., Sakai, H., Suga, T., et al. Impaired solubilisation of glomerular immune deposits by sera from patients with IgA nephropathy. *Am. J. Kidney Dis.* 3: 48, 1983.
219. Tomino, Y., Yagame, M., Omaja, F., et al. A case of IgA nephropathy associated with adeno- and herpes simplex viruses. *Nephron* 47: 258, 1987.
220. Turi, S., Belch, J. J. F., Beattie, T. J., and Forbes, C. D. Abnormalities of vascular prostaglandins in Henoch-Schönlein purpura. *Arch. Dis. Child.* 61: 173, 1986.
221. Ueda, Y., Sakai, O., Yamagata, M., et al. IgA glomerulonephritis in Japan. *Contrib. Nephrol.* 4: 32, 1977.
222. Uj, M., Szucs, G., Nagy, J., and Trinn, C. Antibodies to viruses of the herpes group in glomerulonephritis of membranous, membranoproliferative and IgA types. *Int. Urol. Nephrol.* 20: 201, 1988.
223. Vaerman, J. P., and Delacroix, D. L. Role of the liver in the immunobiology of IgA in animals and humans. *Contrib. Nephrol.* 40: 17, 1984.
224. Valentijn, R. M., Kauffmann, R. H., Riviere, G. B., et al. Presence of circulating macromolecular IgA in patients with haematuria due to primary IgA nephropathy. *Am. J. Med.* 74: 375, 1983.
225. Valentijn, R. M., Radi, J., Haaijman, J. J., et al. Circulating and mesangial secretory component binding IgA-1 in primary IgA nephropathy. *Kidney Int.* 26: 760, 1984.
226. Valles, M., Cantarell, C., Fort, J., et al. IgA nephropathy in leprosy. *Arch. Intern. Med.* 142: 1238, 1982.
227. Vanden Wall Bake, A. W. L., Daha, M. R., Valentijn, R., and Van, E. S. The bone marrow as a possible origin of the IgAI, deposited in the mesangium in IgA nephropathy. *Semin. Nephrol.* 7: 329, 1987.
228. Waldherr, R., Rambausek, M., Duncker, W. D., and Ritz, E. Frequency of mesangial IgA deposits in a nonselected autopsy series. *Nephrol. Dial. Transplant.* 4: 943, 1989.
229. Waldo, F. B., and Cochran, A. M. Systemic immune response to oral polio immunization in patients with IgA nephropathy. *J. Clin. Lab. Immunol.* 28: 109, 1989.
230. Walshe, J. J., Brentjens, J. R., Costa, G. G., et al. Abdominal pain associated with IgA nephropathy. *Am. J. Med.* 77: 765, 1984.
231. Wasserman, J., Santiago, R., Rifici, V., et al. Interactions of low density lipoprotein with rat mesangial cells. *Kidney Int.* 35: 1168, 1989.
232. Woodroffe, A. J. IgA, glomerulonephritis and liver disease. *Aust. J. Med.* 11: 109, 1981.
233. Woodroffe, A. J., Clarkson, A. R., Seymour, A. E., et al. Mesangial IgA nephritis. *Springer Semin. Immunopathol.* 5: 321, 1982.
234. Woodroffe, A. J., Gormly, A. A., McKenzie, P. E., et al. Immunologic studies in IgA nephropathy. *Kidney Int.* 18: 366, 1980.
235. Wyatt, R. J., Julian, B. A., Bhathena, D. B., et al. IgA nephropathy: Presentation, clinical course and prognosis in children and adults. *Am. J. Kidney Dis.* 4: 192, 1984.
236. Yasumoto, Y., Suga, T., Miura, M., et al. Subpopulations of $T\alpha$ cells in patients with IgA nephropathy: Correlation between $T\alpha$ 4 cells and in vitro IgA production. *Clin. Immunol. Immunopathol.* 51: 232, 1989.
237. Yum, M. N., Lamptom, L. M., Bloom, P. M., et al. Asymptomatic IgA nephropathy associated with pulmonary hemosiderosis. *Am. J. Med.* 64: 1056, 1978.

Antiglomerular Basement Membrane Antibody-Mediated Nephritis

Neil Turner
C. Martin Lockwood
Andrew J. Rees

The nephrotoxicity of antibodies to glomerular basement membrane (GBM) has been appreciated since the turn of the century [137], and the similarities between the injury they cause experimentally and human glomerulonephritis was remarked on more than 50 years ago [147]. However, the demonstration that similar autoantibodies could cause nephritis in humans had to await appropriate ways to detect them. Ortega and Mellors [169] described "linear staining of the GBM" in rats after injection of heterologous anti-GBM antibodies in 1956. Eight years later Scheer and Grossman [211] were able to describe similar appearances in immunofluorescence studies on autopsy material from patients who had died of crescentic glomerulonephritis in association with pulmonary hemorrhage. Finally, Lerner, Glassock, and Dixon [136] showed that immunoglobulin eluted from the kidneys of patients with linear staining could induce nephritis in primates.

This combination of fulminating lung and kidney disease, often occurring in young men, was labeled "Goodpasture's syndrome" by Stanton and Tange in 1958 [220]. Ernest Goodpasture [84] had described an 18-year-old man with this association of pathology in 1918, attributing it to the massive influenza epidemic of that year. Stanton and Tange [220] described 9 more patients and drew attention to 12 other cases in the literature. Since these original reports, it has become clear that the syndrome of lung hemorrhage and rapidly progressive glomerulonephritis (RPGN) has more than one cause. Anti-GBM, or Goodpasture's disease, accounts for perhaps one-third of cases of the syndrome in Europe and North America, although it is now clear that the disease may present with lung or renal disease alone. Most of the remaining two-thirds of those with the syndrome have systemic vasculitis of some type (Table 68-1), which may appear to be restricted to the lungs and kidneys or be obviously generalized. It is almost always possible to identify these cases by looking for the presence of antibodies to components of neutrophil cytoplasm (ANCA), described in detail in Chap. 71. Interestingly, Goodpasture's original report described arteritic lesions in the patient's spleen, so the original "Goodpasture's" patient may in fact have been suffering from systemic vasculitis. Nevertheless, the association of Ernest Goodpasture's name with autoantibodies to a specific component of GBM (often described as the Goodpasture antigen) is now firmly established, and here we use "Goodpasture's *disease*" to refer to the disorder associated with these antibodies, to distinguish it from the *syndrome* of lung hemorrhage and RPGN, which may have other causes (Table 68-1).

The term *anti-GBM disease* has been used to describe Goodpasture's disease but is misleading, as the antibodies are directed toward a basement membrane component that clearly has a much wider distribution [39, 127, 180], and furthermore, antibodies to other basement membrane components are found in various renal diseases [33, 68, 209, 253]. The distribution of the Goodpasture antigen includes the alveolar basement membrane; it is clear that the molecular target of the autoantibodies is the same in the lung as it is in the kidney and that the development of pulmonary hemorrhage depends on additional factors. Goodpasture's disease is therefore defined by the nature and specificity of the autoimmune response and has a clinical spectrum extending from mild pulmonary or renal disease in isolation to life-threatening combinations of both.

Epidemiology

INCIDENCE

In a large unselected series of renal biopsies reported from Europe and America, 1 to 2 percent of patients have anti-GBM (Goodpasture's) disease [10, 14, 36, 50], but it is not possible to estimate incidence accurately from these data. In the United Kingdom, the combined data from the Medical Research Council Glomerulonephritis Registry [50] and results from the main laboratories assaying sera for anti-GBM antibodies suggest an incidence of about 0.5 cases per million population per year. A recent estimate from Sweden gives an incidence of 0.9 cases per million [215]. There is an impression that the disease is less common in Asian and Afro-Caribbean races; Caucasoids accounted for more than 90 percent of cases surveyed by Wilson in the United States [260] and 97 percent of cases diagnosed in Britain over a 4-year period [205]. In New Zealand, it may be more common in Maoris [226].

Early reviews of Goodpasture's syndrome (many written before it was possible to make the distinction between those cases with anti-GBM antibodies and those associated with systemic vasculitis) described the disease as occurring predominantly in young men [12, 179]. As immunoassays for circulating autoantibodies in patients with RPGN and immunohistochemical analysis of renal biopsies have become standard, the true pattern of Goodpasture's disease has emerged. It can occur at extremes of age; the youngest and oldest cases known to us were 4 years [172] and 81 years old [239]. There is a bimodal incidence [205, 215] with peaks in the third and sixth decades (Fig. 68-1). Pulmonary hemorrhage is more common in younger patients, and the sex ratio is more uneven, giving rise to the earlier impression that it was a disease of young men. Overall the male-female ratio is less than 2:1 and approaches unity in some series [205, 215, 263]. Only about half of the patients diagnosed in more recent series have pulmonary hemorrhage, but it is much more common in men.

Table 68-1. Causes of acute renal and respiratory failure*

A: with alveolar hemorrhage
- Goodpasture's (anti-GBM) disease
- Primary systemic vasculitis
- Secondary systemic vasculitis
  - Systemic lupus erythematosus and related disorders
  - Churg-Strauss syndrome
  - Henoch-Schönlein purpura
  - Behçet's disease
  - Mixed essential cryoglobulinemia
  - Rheumatoid disease
  - Penicillamine therapy

B: without alveolar hemorrhage
- Hypervolemic pulmonary edema in acute renal failure of any cause
- Pulmonary edema in association with cardiac failure
- Severe pneumonia (e.g., caused by *Legionella*) with secondary renal failure
- Pneumonia in patients immunosuppressed for treatment of RPGN
- Pulmonary emboli with thrombosis of the inferior vena cava or renal veins
- Paraquat poisoning

*Causes of Goodpasture's syndrome (alveolar hemorrhage with RPGN) are listed under A. Group B, without alveolar hemorrhage, is more commonly encountered, but it is important to distinguish pulmonary hemorrhage promptly to instigate appropriate treatment. This distinction may not be straightforward. Alveolar hemorrhage is commonly exacerbated by hypervolemia or infection, so the clinical picture may be mixed.
Source: Data from [41, 61, 89, 99, 132, 133, 213].

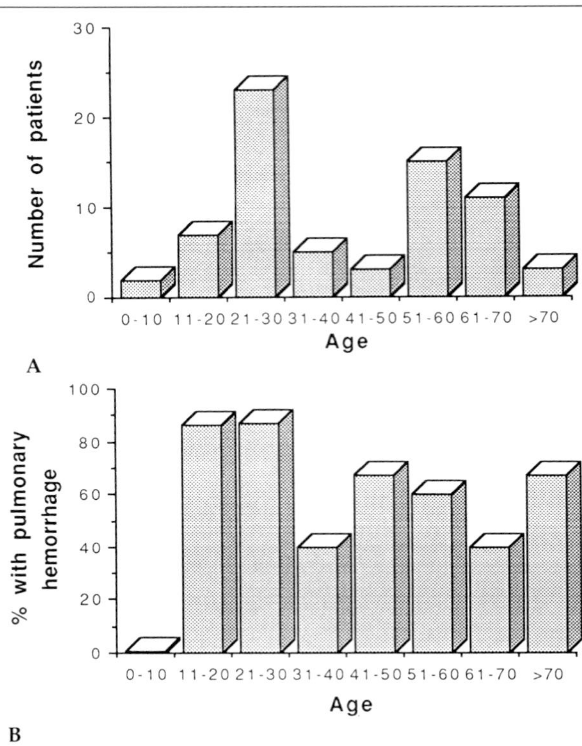

Fig. 68-1. A. Age distribution of 69 patients with Goodpasture's disease treated at Hammersmith hospital, 1974–1989. B. Proportion of patients with pulmonary hemorrhage in each age group.

Most centers would see cases of Goodpasture's disease relatively rarely if its incidence were evenly distributed. However, there have been repeated reports of temporal and geographic clustering of the disease, suggesting that a pathogen or environmental factor might be involved. In Britain, a seasonality was noted between 1980 and 1984, with peak incidence in spring and early summer [50, 205]. However, analysis of positive results from the same center in the 6 years since then no longer shows such a fluctuation. Geographic clusters have been noted in North America [170], New Zealand [218], and Britain [258].

GENETIC FACTORS

As in other autoimmune disease, there is evidence that genetic factors strongly influence susceptibility to Goodpasture's disease. It has been reported in identical twins [49, 217], in siblings [85, 220], and in first cousins [141]. The majority of patients' siblings are not affected, however, and discordance has also been reported in identical twins [5] (and in our series). Presumably some event or environmental influence must act in concert with an inherited trait to provoke the disease in susceptible individuals.

Inheritance of particular major histocompatibility complex molecules (MHC; HLA antigens in humans) has been associated with many human autoimmune diseases. These molecules facilitate the presentation of antigens to T cells, an interaction likely to be critical to the initiation and perpetuation of an autoimmune response. This is important not only for presentation of antigens in the periphery but also for elimination of potentially autoreactive T lymphocytes during ontogeny [13, 214]. However, the tight linkage disequilibrium between different genes in the HLA complex on chromosome 6 makes it difficult to establish with certainty whether one particular HLA gene product is critical to susceptibility. It may be possible to study such problems directly in in vitro experiments in the near future.

HLA-DR2 has been strongly associated with Goodpasture's disease in serologic studies [80, 171, 189, 190]. A recent molecular analysis of HLA class II genes has confirmed and extended this association [28]. HLA-DRw15(DR2)/DQw6 was carried by 75 percent of British patients (relative risk 6.8), and most of the remainder of the patients carried DR4/DQw7, so that 94 percent of patients carried one of these two haplotypes. A negative association with DR1 was also noted. In a serologic study, the inheritance of HLA-B7 with DR2 (which is common, as they are associated in a common haplotype) was associated with more severe nephritis [189]. Associations of autoimmune diseases with DR2 are uncommon, but multiple sclerosis [44] is another notable exception.

A second, but still immunologic genetic influence on susceptibility has been reported. Patients are more likely to have inherited specific variants of immunoglobulin heavy chains, encoded on chromosome 14, Gm allotypes [186]. These allotypes are determined by a series of very closely linked genes and are inherited as fixed haplotypes, of which three, designated by the alleles Gm 1,21, GM 1,2,21, and Gm 3,5,11, are common in Caucasoid populations [87, 144]. Inheritance of various combinations of these haplotypes has been associated with differences in immunologic functions, including the relative concentrations of IgG subclasses, the magnitude of antibody responses to exogenous antigens, and the susceptibility to various autoimmune diseases. The incidence of the haplotype Gm 1,2,21 was significantly increased in patients with Goodpasture's disease, especially when inherited as a heterozygote together with the haplotype Gm 3,5,11. However patients who were heterozygous at the Gm complex were found to have higher anti-GBM antibody titers than homozygotes, and this phenomenon of increased antibody concentrations in Gm heterozygotes has been reported previously in other situations [144, 186]. The association is weaker than that with MHC molecules, and the reasons why there should be differences between the different allotypes are not known.

DISEASE ASSOCIATIONS

Some diseases that have been associated with Goodpasture's disease are listed in Table 68-2. One interesting observation is that the disease is rarely associated with other autoimmune disorders or autoantibodies. The commonest association is with systemic vasculitis, a fascinating observation as the renal and pulmonary manifestations of the two can be so similar. The references in Table 68-2 are to cases in which there has been clinical evidence for two distinct disorders occurring in the same patient and antedate the ability to measure ANCA. A more common finding is the laboratory demonstration of autoantibodies characteristic of both Goodpasture's disease (anti-GBM) and systemic vasculitis (ANCA). The precise frequency with which this phenomenon has been reported varies. This could be due to different referral practices and/or to differing specificities of the assays used. In the Hammersmith laboratory, 8 percent of patients with specific antibodies to the Goodpasture antigen also have ANCA, and about 5 percent of those with ANCA have anti-Goodpasture antibodies. These observations were made on sera taken from patients at presentation, and cases have also been described of one disease leading to the other [167, 240], although these seem to be very rare. In the commonest situation, the anti-GBM antibodies may be detectable only fleetingly

Table 68-2. Diseases associated with Goodpasture's disease

Disease	Cases	Comments	References
AUTOIMMUNE DISORDERS			
Systemic vasculitis	5 (plus)	Plus many examples of immunologic, as opposed to clinical, association, described further in text	[191, 240, 263]
Hashimoto's thyroiditis	1		[113]
Myasthenia gravis	1	HLA-DR4,5	Hammersmith, unpublished
Partial lipodystrophy	1		[17]
Celiac disease	1		[205]
Penicillamine therapy	1	Many reports of vasculitis and anti-GBM negative RPGN with penicillamine, but no others of Goodpasture's disease	Lechler, unpublished
RENAL DISEASES			
Membranous nephropathy	6	Approximately an equal number have developed crescentic nephritis *without* anti-GBM antibodies	[10, 121, 157, 170, 194]
Cortical necrosis	1		[104]
Postlithotripsy	1	HLA-DR2	[90]
Postobstructive	1	HLA-DR2	[246]
MALIGNANT DISORDERS			
Lymphoma	6		[123, 140, 263]
Thymoma	1	Incidental autopsy finding	Hammersmith, unpublished
Carcinoma of bronchus	1	Antibody response predominantly IgA; HLA-DR3,4	Hammersmith, unpublished
INHERITED DISEASES			
Alport's syndrome	13	After renal transplantation (see text)	[75, 95, 149, 156, 185, 216] [83, 117, 227, 237]
Nail-patella syndrome	1		[46]

in a patient who seems clinically to fit the diagnosis of systemic vasculitis better; for example, there may be evidence of involvement of organs other than kidney and lung, and they may recover renal function despite being dialysis-dependent when treatment was started [107], a response that is distinctly unusual in typical Goodpasture's disease. Thus clinical evidence of overlap between the two disorders is even less common than evidence of overlap at the serologic level. It is possible that anti-GBM antibodies in this circumstance are a secondary phenomenon following damage to basement membranes in crescentic nephritis of different etiology and that they are not pathogenically important in these circumstances. The fact that both major ANCA subtypes (cytoplasmic and perinuclear, with specificities for proteinase 3 and myeloperoxidase respectively) may be associated with anti-GBM antibodies (G. Gaskin, unpublished observations) may support the hypothesis that the phenomenon is secondary to the pathology in the kidney and not related to the primary immune disturbance. It would be informative to study RPGN of other etiologies more closely and to investigate any relationship between MHC antigens and the development of such antibodies.

Membranous nephropathy occasionally undergoes a "crescentic transformation," usually leading rapidly to end-stage renal failure. A number of cases of this have now been described, and anti-GBM antibodies have been demonstrated in about half. It is tempting to suggest that here too, damage to the GBM leads to the development of an autoimmune response in genetically susceptible people. Little has been reported of MHC antigens in these patients, but it is interesting that in the two recent cases where Goodpasture's disease closely followed lithotripsy and an episode of urinary obstruction, either of which might have led to physical damage to the GBM, both patients carried HLA-DR2.

Six patients with Hodgkin's disease or other lymphoma are reported to have developed Goodpasture's disease, but only two have been described in any detail [123, 140]. Both developed the disease after successful treatment of their lymphoma, and neither had evidence of residual malignancy. One had been treated by upper mantle radiotherapy alone.

In Alport's syndrome, anti-GBM disease only occurs after renal transplantation, when it has been frequently described. The Goodpasture antigen is absent or diminished in the GBM of most patients with this disorder [149, 206], and it has previously been widely assumed that the Goodpasture antigen is the product of the gene that is mutated in Alport's syndrome (and therefore encoded on the X chromosome). It is now clear that this is not the case. Some features of the molecular basis of Alport's syndrome and the features of anti-GBM disease in patients with the syndrome are discussed later in this chapter.

One patient with the nail-patella syndrome is described as developing the disease. This is particularly interesting, as it has recently been suggested that some patients with this disorder may have abnormal expression of the Goodpasture antigen, similar to that described in Alport's [225]. However, the fact that the disease maps to chromosome 9q34 [67] precludes the primary involvement of the Goodpasture antigen or any of the currently known type IV collagen chains. In contrast, the Goodpasture antigen appears to be normal in another inherited nephropathy associated with GBM abnormalities, thin basement membrane nephropathy [55, 174], although linear binding of IgM in one case and IgA in another (associated with circulating IgA anti-GBM antibodies) has been reported in the absence of evidence of nephritis [51].

ENVIRONMENTAL FACTORS

Ever since Goodpasture's original report related the syndrome of lung hemorrhage and RPGN to influenza, there have been repeated suggestions that various infections or environmental exposures might cause or precipitate the disease. Such explanations could account for the disease clusters and seasonality just described. However, the search for specific pathogens or toxic agents has not been very fruitful.

Evidence implicating various environmental factors or pathogens comes from epidemiologic surveys and anecdotal accounts. The usual difficulties in assessing anecdotal accounts are compounded in this disease by the possibility that various nonspecific insults to the lung might precipitate pulmonary hemorrhage in people who already have circulating anti-GBM antibodies but have yet to develop symptoms. There is evidence from clinical examples and from animal experiments, described in more detail later, that this is an important mechanism of initiating pulmonary hemorrhage. A different problem affects the interpretation of the association of various infections with the onset of Goodpasture's disease. Infections may lead nonspecifically to amplification of the tissue damage caused by a given level of pathogenic antibodies. This is a well-described phenomenon in the clinical management of patients with Goodpasture's disease, but it may also lead to the acute presentation of a patient who previously had subclinical disease. A temporal association of the onset of symptoms of Goodpasture's disease with an apparent infection is therefore neither uncommon nor unexpected but does not mean that the infection was causative. Both these problems arise because the time of initiation of the autoimmune response cannot be determined, and the injury caused by (or associated with) low levels of autoantibodies can be very slight and may not be clinically detectable.

The strongest circumstantial evidence for environmental factors implicates exposure to organic solvents and hydrocarbon fumes. Heale et al. [93] described Goodpasture's disease after exposure to gasoline; Beirne and Brennan [9] later described heavy hydrocarbon exposure in seven of eight patients. Many case reports have followed, some describing patients with pulmonary hemorrhage [16, 37, 119, 122, 162, 258], others concerning nephritis alone [48, 123, 177]. A high level of awareness of the possible association makes it likely that a history of exposure will be keenly sought and that it is more likely to be reported. However, only a small proportion of patients in most series describe heavy exposures of this type. Exposure at lower levels must be almost universal in the Western world. Since the early reports, epidemiologic surveys have repeatedly suggested a more general risk of glomerulonephritis in those exposed to various solvents and hydrocarbons [48, 163]. As the disease is rare, firmer evidence that solvents can have this effect will probably only come from large, well-performed case-control studies.

Although evidence of specific infections, particularly influenza, has been repeatedly sought, there is not a strong case for suspecting any particular pathogen. Benoit et al. [12] and Proskey et al. [179] both remarked on the apparent increase in the disease during influenza epidemics and commented on the presence of an "influenza-like" illness in the histories of many patients. Specific cases definitely associated with influenza have been reported [265]. The problems in interpreting such accounts have been alluded to. Certainly, when systematic studies of the incidence of influenza [263] or other infections [10, 258, 264] have been performed, results have been negative.

A strong association of pulmonary hemorrhage with cigarette smoking has been described in Goodpasture's disease [56]. Its effect can be very rapid [56, 93], leading to a recurrence of bleeding within hours, as well as being a powerful influence on whether pulmonary hemorrhage occurs at all. Other anecdotal evidence indicates that various other inhaled toxins or irritants might precipitate lung hemorrhage [16, 258]. These effects seem certain to be mediated by direct effects on the pulmonary manifestations of the disease once the autoimmune process is established and not related to truly causative influences.

Clinical Features

Most patients present acutely with either lung hemorrhage or RPGN. Lung hemorrhage is an alarming symptom, so there is a tendency for patients with it to present earlier in the course of the disease. Renal disease may cause no or only nonspecifc symptoms until renal function is severely impaired. A minority of patients present subacutely, usually with manifestations related to chronic or recurrent pulmonary hemorrhage. The presenting complaint may then be episodes of hemoptysis, or it may just be breathlessness or the symptoms of iron deficiency anemia. The clinical and other manifestations are described in many series [15, 59, 93, 112, 152, 172, 188, 198, 211, 218, 241, 250, 263] (and large series listed in Table 68-3).

GENERAL

Some patients give a long history of nonspecific complaints, such as unexplained malaise, weight loss, and headaches of many months' duration. More specifically, a history of minor hemoptysis many weeks or months before presentation is not uncommon. Up to 50 percent describe symptoms suggestive of a recent upper respiratory tract or other infection. However, these symptoms are generally much less obvious than are found in

Table 68-3. Outcome of patients with Goodpasture's disease[a]

Series [reference]	Number of patients	Mortality, %	Patients with surviving renal function, %	Number with creatinine ≤ 600 μmol/L at presentation	Patients with surviving renal function at 1 year as % of previous column[b]
Benoit et al. (1964)[c,d,e] [12]	52	96	4	N/A	
Proskey et al. (1970)[c,d,e] [179]	56	77	≤23[f]	N/A	
Wilson and Dixon (1973)[d] [261]	53	25	11.5	N/A	
Beirne et al. (1977) [10]	26	54	15	15	27
Teague et al. (1978)[e] [226]	29	38	31	26[g]	35
Briggs et al. (1979) [25]	18	17	11	14	12
Johnson et al. (1985) [111]	17	6	55	13	69
Walker et al. (1985) [242]	22	41	45	11	91
Savage et al. (1986)[h] [205]	59	25	8.5	8	63
Savage et al. (1986)[i] [205]	49	16	35	19	89
Williams et al. (1988) [258]	10	10	20	1	100

N/A = not available.
[a]Series containing 10 or more cases are included. Differences in severity of renal disease at presentation and incidence of lung hemorrhage mean that figures are not strictly comparable.
[b]This column attempts to make a comparison between series by relating the proportion of patients alive and not requiring dialysis at 1 year to the proportion of patients with "potentially recoverable" renal function at presentation (creatinine ≤ 600 μmol/liter; see text).
[c]Patients in these series were not immunopathologically defined, but were diagnosed on the basis of the combination of focal necrotizing glomerulonephritis and pulmonary hemorrhage. A proportion will therefore have had systemic vasculitis.
[d]Included patients from multiple centers or from previous series.
[e]Excluded patients without lung hemorrhage.
[f]Maximum; figures not given.
[g]Figures refer to number of patients not requiring dialysis (creatinines not available).
[h]Patients from multiple British centers, 1980–1984.
[i]Patients treated at Hammersmith, 1974–1984.

patients with other causes of crescentic nephritis, and they are not generally accompanied by signs of systemic inflammation.

Anemia is common and frequently shows the features of iron deficiency. Biochemical and serologic tests are typically normal with the exception of abnormalities related to renal impairment. In particular, immunopathologic investigations including immunoglobulin concentrations, concentrations of complement components, tests for antinuclear factor, rheumatoid factor, and other autoantibodies are usually negative or normal.

Although features of the history and initial investigations often enable a probable diagnosis to be made, the clinical syndrome of fulminant lung and renal disease is indistinguishable from that caused by systemic vasculitis. Only the renal biopsy and tests for anti-Goodpasture antibodies and ANCA will distinguish the two groups of patients with certainty.

RENAL

Once significant nephritis develops in Goodpasture's disease, most patients experience a rapid progression to end-stage renal failure. In those with pulmonary hemorrhage, this phase of acceleration in the disease is usually associated with a simultaneous exacerbation of lung disease. The dismal prognosis of untreated patients was emphasized in Benoit's early clinical review [12], in which only 2 of 52 patients survived with useful renal function. This experience has been confirmed in other large series. In contrast, the stage of minimal renal disease, with episodes of pulmonary hemorrhage but normal renal function, can apparently exist for months or years before some event leads to a catastrophic deterioration. These patients often have microscopic hematuria, but renal biopsy shows no or only minimal abnormalities despite the presence of linear binding of immunoglobulin to the GBM [6, 37, 94, 148, 152, 202, 273]. Because of the very strong influence of early diagnosis on prognosis, it would be invaluable to diagnose more patients in this "prodromal" phase, which may seem to last for only days or occasionally for years. Rare patients fall between these two extremes, as described by McPhaul and Mullins [152]. As well as describing a number of patients with exceptionally mild disease, their report included six patients with a chronically progressive course, three of whom had the nephrotic syndrome.

With advanced renal disease, the manifestations are similar to those of RPGN of any etiology. Onset may be dramatic and associated with macroscopic hematuria and loin pain. The urinary findings reflect the severity of nephritis. Microscopic hematuria is the rule, and erythrocyte casts are common. Proteinuria is usually less than 5 gm/day but may be higher in rare patients with chronic disease. In our experience, hypertension is uncommon in the absence of fluid overload or chronic glomerular scarring.

Once renal disease is established, progression is usually relentless, but it may be extremely rapid, with complete loss of renal function occurring within hours [15, 25, 188]. Such rapid changes are clearly not caused by changes in antibody level and probably not by changes in levels of other effectors of the immune system, but are likely to be related to amplification of tissue damage by systemic influences, often originating in a remote infection (Fig. 68-2).

Renal size is normal. There are no specific changes in any tests of renal function or imaging to help with the diagnosis.

PULMONARY

Pulmonary hemorrhage almost always precedes or accompanies glomerulonephritis in those in whom it occurs. The incidence is highest in young adults and lower in older women. The relation of pulmonary hemorrhage to inhalation of toxins or irritants has been discussed; perhaps its incidence will fall if the proportion of the population smoking cigarettes continues to fall in the next decade.

Episodes of pulmonary hemorrhage may occur recurrently or chronically over months to years without the development of severe renal disease [48, 188, 211]. Such cases need to be distinguished from idiopathic pulmonary hemosiderosis and other causes of isolated lung hemorrhage [61, 131, 132, 158], by examination of the urine and estimation of circulating anti-GBM antibodies. Hemoptysis is usually present and may be profuse, but

Fig. 68-2. The clinical course of a patient with Goodpasture's disease. The renal function was relatively stable for the first 4 days after admission, and a renal biopsy showed only one of eight glomeruli surrounded by a crescent. Anuria occurred suddenly and immediately after bacteremia (*arrows*). The plasma creatinine rose exponentially, and renal function did not recover.

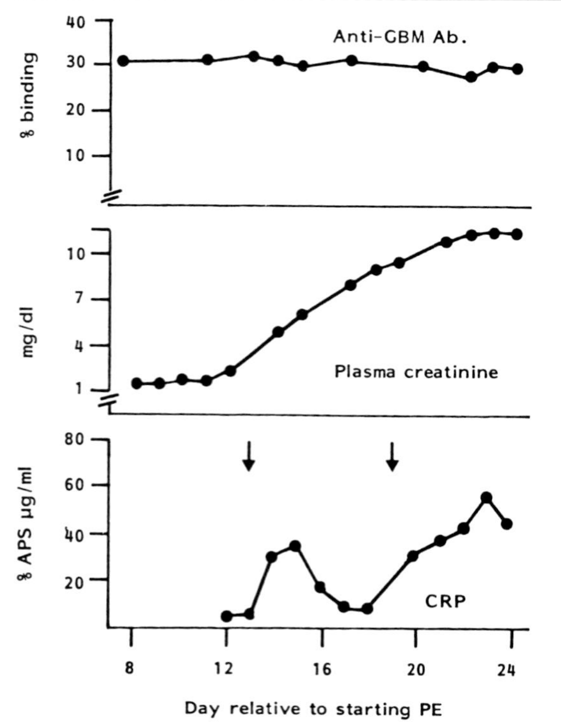

its volume is not closely related to the severity of the underlying hemorrhage—it may be absent in the most severe cases [72]. As the hemorrhage is alveolar, much of the blood never reaches the bronchi but instead is reabsorbed. When hemorrhage has been chronic, a large amount of iron may be sequestered in the lungs. Iron deficiency anemia at the time of diagnosis is common, even when the history is only short, suggesting that subclinical pulmonary hemorrhage may have been occurring for some time. At the opposite extreme, breathlessness rapidly progresses to respiratory failure, and ventilatory support is required. Clinical findings are of respiratory distress, usually with cough. The findings on auscultation are not specific, and there may be no audible abnormalities at all, but there are often dry-sounding inspiratory crackles and sometimes areas of bronchial breathing. It is often difficult to be clinically or radiologically certain how much of the clinical picture may be due to, or aggravated by, pulmonary edema associated with volume overload. Relapses of pulmonary hemorrhage can be precipitated by volume overload [6, 25, 188, 218, 258], by a resumption of smoking [56, 93] (Fig. 68-3) or reexposure to other pulmonary irritants [16, 258], or by local [25, 188, 218] or remote [112, 187] infection.

The radiologic features of pulmonary hemorrhage (Fig. 68-3) have been described by Bowley [21, 22] and Schwartz [213]. An important conclusion of both studies was that there were no unique features that distinguished pulmonary hemorrhage from other causes of alveolar shadowing, including pulmonary edema or infection. Typically, the lung apices and supradiaphragmatic regions are spared. The opacities are rarely bounded by fissures, and when they are it strongly suggests a concurrent infection; apical involvement is also suggestive of infection. Failure of the radiologic abnormalities to resolve within a few days strongly suggests continued bleeding. Although Schwartz described permanent abnormality of chest radiographs in patients with Goodpasture's disease, such hemosiderosis has not been seen in any of our patients.

A more sensitive way of detecting pulmonary hemorrhage than radiography, and of distinguishing other intrathoracic pathology, is by measuring the diffusing capacity for carbon monoxide. Corrected for lung volume and the patient's hemoglobin, this is expressed as the kCO. It can be measured serially (Fig. 68-4), and it has been shown that a rise of 30 percent above a stable baseline indicates fresh pulmonary hemorrhage [40, 65]. In renal failure, baseline values are somewhat depressed [134]. In episodes of lung hemorrhage detected by this technique, 5 of 23 were unsuspected clinically [65], and 5 of 27 were not accompanied by changes in the chest radiograph [21].

Patients presenting with predominantly pulmonary disease are often investigated by bronchoscopy. Usually appearances are either normal, or blood is seen to be coming from multiple bronchi. Hemosiderin-laden macrophages are a characteristic finding on bronchoalveolar lavage or transbronchial lung biopsy. However, despite some favorable reports [1, 8], transbronchial biopsies

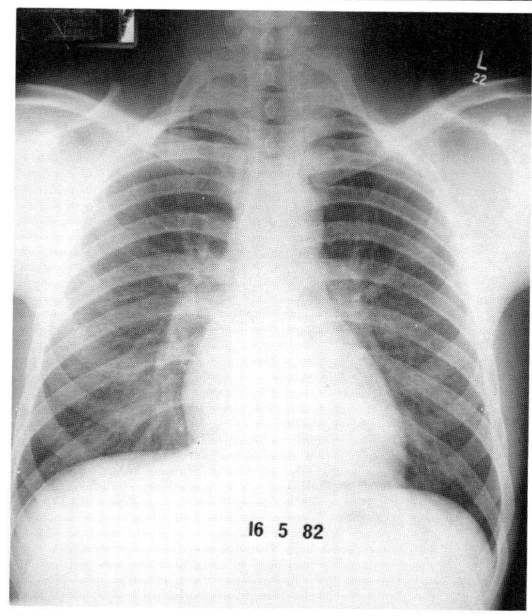

A

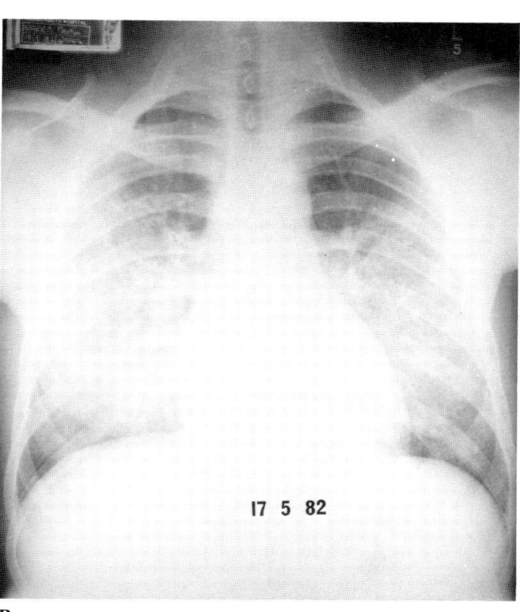

B

Fig. 68-3. Chest radiographs of a patient with Goodpasture's disease (A) before and (B) one day after he resumed smoking. Note diffuse shadowing, not bounded by fissures, spreading from the hilar region. The apical and supradiaphragmatic areas are clear.

have proved unreliable as a diagnostic tool [111]. Failure to demonstrate pathologic changes or linear binding of antibody to the alveolar basement membrane does *not* indicate that the diagnosis is incorrect.

OTHER ORGANS

The Goodpasture antigen is present in several other basement membranes throughout the body besides those of the glomerulus and the alveolus (Table 68-4). In

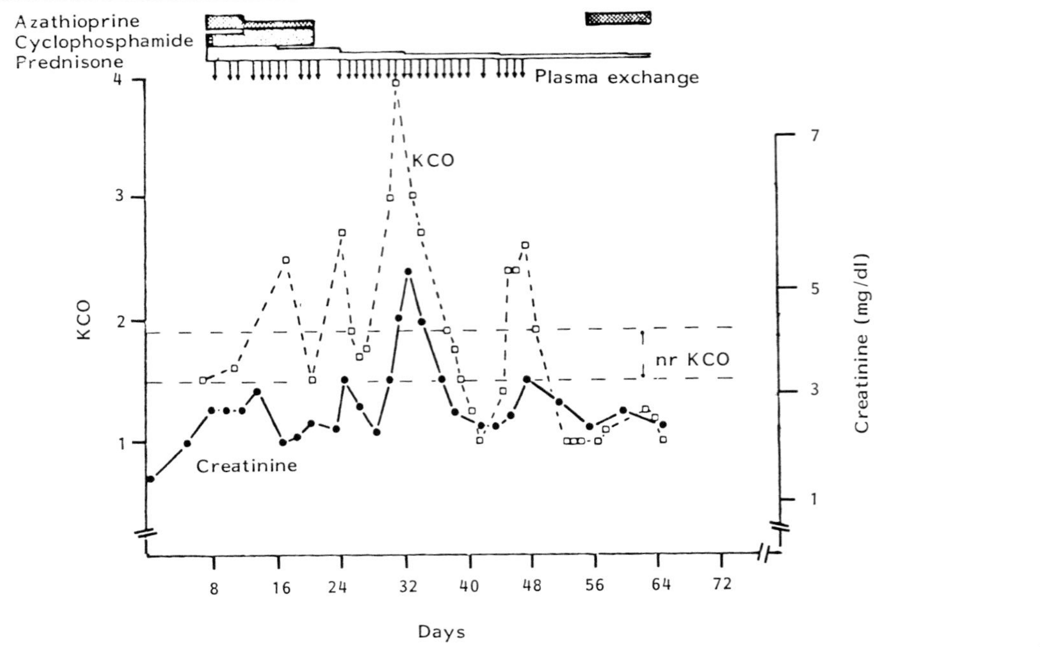

Fig. 68-4. Serial serum creatinine (*solid circles and lines*) and kCO (*dashed lines and open boxes*) measurements in a patient with Goodpasture's disease during treatment. The peaks of kCO coincided with clinical or radiologic evidence of renewed pulmonary hemorrhage. In this example, there is a close relationship between changes in renal function and kCO.

Table 68-4. Distribution of the Goodpasture antigen

Kidney	Glomerular basement membrane, distal tubular basement membrane, Bowman's capsule
Lung	Alveolar basement membrane
Eye	Choroid, ciliary body, Bruch's membrane, basement membranes of retinal capillaries, lens capsule, cornea
Ear	Cochlear basement membrane
Brain	Basement membrane of choroidal epithelium
Liver	Hepatic arteries in portal tract
Other	Adrenal, breast (ducts), pituitary, thyroid gland (follicular basement membrane)

Source: Data from [38, 39, 127, 180].

vivo binding of antibody to only some of these has been demonstrated in patients with Goodpasture's disease, probably because of differences in accessibility of the basement membrane to circulating antibodies. Binding to the choroid plexus [39, 150, 151] is probably common, and binding has been reported to various membranes in the eye [105]. In Jampol's report there was associated retinal detachment, and we have observed retinal changes in occasional patients that might be attributable to the disease [235], but these are rare. Although some patients have had convulsions during their acute illness, there does not appear to be a specific encephalopathy associated with Goodpasture's disease, and patients with acute renal failure tend already to have multiple risk factors for convulsions.

Pathology

RENAL

Morphologic appearances vary from almost no changes at all, progressing through a relatively mild focal proliferative glomerulonephritis, to a very severe nephritis in which all glomeruli are surrounded by cellular crescents [25, 94, 141, 152, 198, 226, 263] (Fig. 68-5). Severely affected glomeruli may contain multinucleated giant cells [114, 199]. Accompanying acute interstitial inflammation is usual. The crescents in Goodpasture's disease tend to have similar degrees of cellularity within one biopsy, suggesting that they were formed at about the same time. However, none of these findings are diagnostic unless combined with evidence of autoantibody formation to the GBM. Electron microscopy (Fig. 68-6) shows modest thickening of the GBM, often with a rarefied zone between the basement membrane and the endothelium. Fractures of the basement membrane may be seen, and epithelial and endothelial cells are often swollen [25, 94, 226].

The characteristic linear staining of the GBM on immunofluorescence (Fig. 68-7) or immunohistochemistry with anti-immunoglobulin reagents is very, but not absolutely, specific. IgG is almost invariably present and is accompanied by IgM and/or IgA in 10 to 20 percent of patients [152, 205, 226]. A number of patients have been reported to have linear staining with IgA predominantly or alone [20, 63, 205] (see Table 68-2) and one with IgM alone [205]. The GBM often shows linear binding of C3 as well. Linear staining may also be seen in the basement membrane of distal tubules in some patients. Bind-

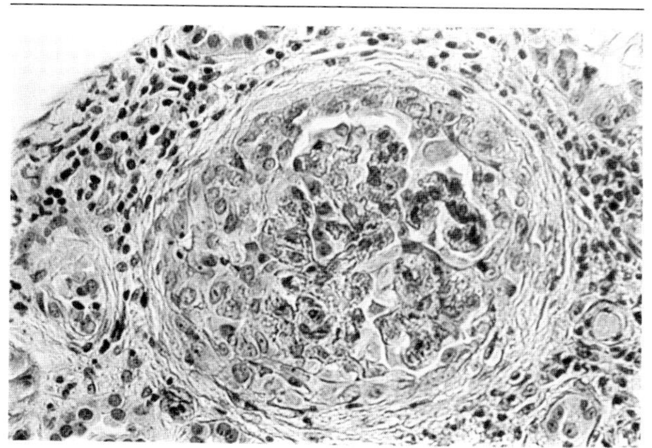

Fig. 68-5. Circumferential cellular crescent in a glomerulus from a patient with acute Goodpasture's disease.

ing fades slowly after disappearance of antibody from the circulation and is often detectable many months later [218, 226]; when this occurs, some patients develop a fine, superimposed granular staining [3]. In some patients, subepithelial, intramembranous, or subendothelial deposits of this type are present in the initial renal biopsy [108, 173, 184, 194, 207]. They may appear to increase in prominence as linear binding fades [3]; such appearances have been seen in four follow-up renal biopsies in our series. These cases are probably quite distinct from those in which anti-GBM disease complicates membranous nephropathy (see Table 68-2).

Vasculitic lesions have occasionally been described in the renal biopsies of patients with no other evidence of vasculitis (Wu et al. [268] and patients in our series). ANCA results on these patients are not generally known, but ANCA were not found in a patient we studied.

Linear binding of immunoglobulin to GBM is seen with low levels of antibody and can invariably be demonstrated, even in patients with apparently isolated lung disease. It can occasionally be seen in other diseases, in-

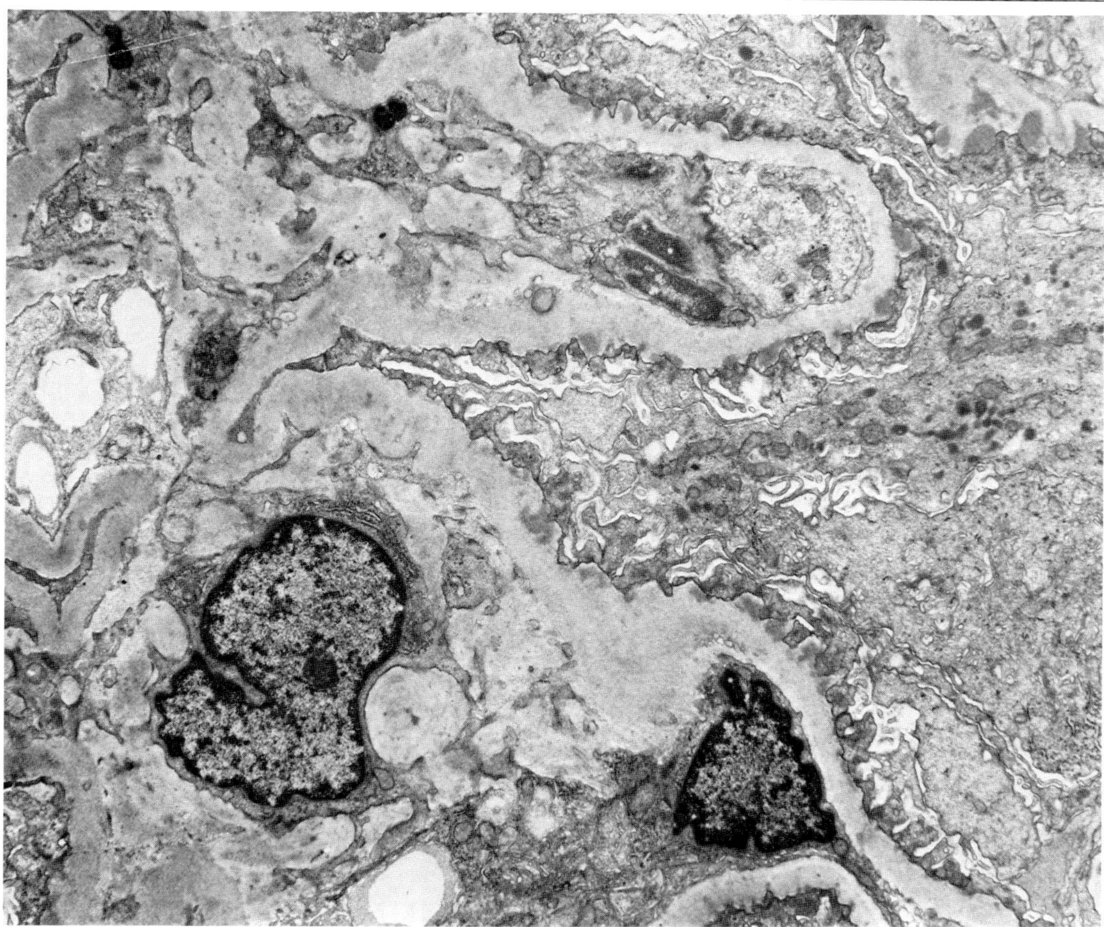

Fig. 68-6. Electron micrograph of GBM from a patient with Goodpasture's disease. This example shows electron-dense deposits within the GBM, mostly subepithelial. Immune deposits are seen by electron microscopy or immunohistology in a proportion of patients (see text) and may develop during resolution of the disease.

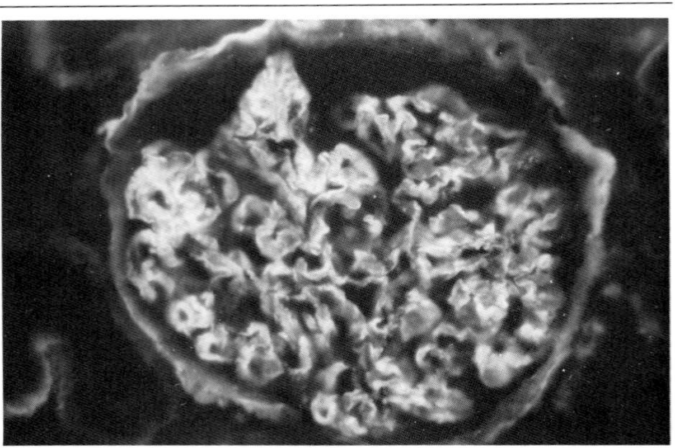

Fig. 68-7. Direct immunofluorescence study showing linear binding of IgG to the GBM in a renal biopsy taken from a patient with Goodpasture's disease. (Courtesy of S. J. Cashman.)

cluding systemic lupus erythematosus, diabetes mellitus, and in organs preserved for transplantation (see below). The specificity of the antibodies should always be confirmed by an assay for circulating anti-GBM antibodies or by the older method of elution studies [152, 208].

PULMONARY

At autopsy, the lungs of patients with severe disease are invariably firm and heavy. In badly affected areas, the alveoli are packed with erythrocytes, neutrophils, and macrophages, while in relatively unaffected parts, the alveoli may be normal except for a few hemosiderin-laden macrophages. Interstitial hemorrhage and edema are prominent, but the extent of inflammation in alveolar septa varies from one patient to another [8, 94]. On electron microscopy, the alveolar basement membrane is seen to be thickened, and it often contains breaks, but electron-dense deposits are not usual. There is evidence of proliferation of both types I and II pneumatocytes as well as injury to endothelial cells [57].

Antibodies eluted from affected lungs show the same binding properties as antibodies eluted from affected kidneys [129, 151, 261]. However, reports of direct immunofluorescence studies on affected lungs are conflicting. Some show diffuse linear staining of the alveolar basement membrane with IgG, but in many it is patchy or negative [39, 57, 98, 145, 224, 226]. In part this may be because autofluorescence makes such studies more difficult in the lung, but it is also likely to be explained by focal regional breakdowns in the normal barrier to IgG in the pulmonary capillaries. A variety of external stimuli, discussed later, are known to be capable of producing such an effect, but pathologic processes within the lungs (notably infection) may achieve the same.

IMMUNOLOGIC FEATURES AND DIAGNOSIS

The diagnosis of Goodpasture's disease is confirmed by demonstration of antibodies to Goodpasture antigen in the circulation or bound to basement membranes. The most straightforward way to do this is by direct immunohistochemical examination of kidney or lung. Linear fixation of immunoglobulin to the glomerular basement membrane is almost pathognomonic of the disease, especially in the setting of crescentic nephritis. Direct immunofluorescence is highly sensitive, and linear staining can be seen in patients with very low antibody titers. However, there are pitfalls and limitations to the technique. As mentioned, it is very slow to resolve and therefore cannot be used to monitor the disease. Difficulties in interpretation can arise in extensively damaged renal tissue, where the severity of inflammation can disrupt GBM to such an extent that only very short strips of linear staining can be recognized. Totally sclerosed glomeruli are also negative [152, 262]. False-positive results are occasionally obtained because of background immunofluorescence caused by a nonspecific increase in basement membrane immunoglobulin. This may occur in normal kidneys after interruption of blood flow and hence cause confusion in renal biopsies taken from cadaver kidneys before transplantation or in autopsy specimens [60, 262]. It may also be a problem in kidney specimens prepared in certain ways [262], in diabetic kidneys [79, 248], in lupus nephritis [128], and in renal allografts [183]. Nevertheless, in the setting of crescentic nephritis with or without lung hemorrhage, the demonstration of linear immunoglobulin on the GBM remains an almost certain indication that Goodpasture's disease is the diagnosis. Problems with interpretation are however greater in the lungs, as discussed earlier. Negative results on lung biopsy do not exclude the disorder.

Demonstration of circulating antibodies is an invaluable substitute for, and adjunct to, the demonstration of tissue-fixed antibodies in the diagnosis of Goodpasture's disease. The ability to measure the level of circulating antibodies has also been found to be valuable in monitoring the progress of the disease and the effects of treatment and in assessing the safety of renal transplantation. The earliest way of doing this, still used in many centers, is to overlay the patients' serum onto sections of normal kidney and look for the characteristic binding pattern by indirect immunofluorescence. The difficulties of interpreting binding of immunoglobulin to autopsy kidneys are relevant here, and many sera give high levels of background staining [263]. Appropriate positive and negative controls must be used. The method has limited sensitivity, is difficult to quantitate, and should by now have been largely replaced by solid-phase immunoassays. A number of such assays have been in use for over 10 years [24, 73, 143, 249, 254, 263]. Collagenase-solubilized human GBM is the usual substrate, but more recently, assays have been developed using highly purified Goodpasture antigen from bovine [210] or sheep kidney (Fig. 68-8). These assays appear to be more specific and more sensitive than their predecessors based on crude human antigen preparations. Our standard assay is now an ELISA based on highly purified antigen prepared from sheep kidney. Positive samples, or those giving equivocal results, can be verified by Western blotting using human GBM.

As described above, IgA and IgM antibodies are

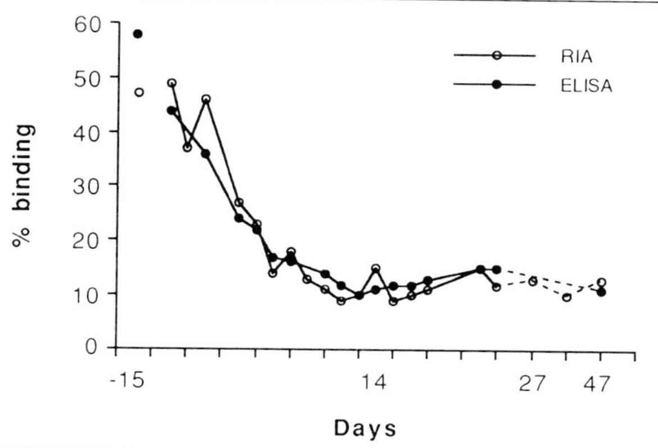

Fig. 68-8. Fall in titer of anti-GBM antibodies during treatment of a patient with lung hemorrhage and mild renal disease. The results obtained in a radioimmunoassay (RIA) using a crude collagenase digest of human GBM as the ligand are compared with the results in an enzyme-linked immunoassay (ELISA) using highly purified antigen from sheep kidney.

sometimes demonstrable in kidney sections, and IgA antibodies can make up a substantial proportion of circulating antibodies in some patients [20, 63, 205] (as in the case in Table 68-2 associated with carcinoma of the bronchus). Linear IgA deposition has also been reported in the absence of clinical Goodpasture's disease [74]—in one case in association with mild focal proliferative nephritis and the other in association with renal cell carcinoma but no evidence of nephritis. Neither had detectable circulating anti-GBM antibodies by indirect immunofluorescence. Binding of IgA (with circulating IgA antibodies) or IgM in the absence of nephritis has also been described in association with thin basement membrane nephropathy [51].

A number of studies have investigated the subclass of anti-GBM antibodies in Goodpasture's disease. All have shown a predominance of IgG1 [23, 164, 215, 244], and three of the four have found lesser amounts of IgG4. The IgG4 antibodies may be restricted to a subgroup of patients [215]. In one case report, a late rise in antibodies that was not associated with a clinical relapse was shown to consist mostly of IgG4 antibodies [96].

Treatment and Outcome

TREATMENT

In early series of cases of Goodpasture's disease, the prognosis was extremely poor. Benoit's 1964 series [12] (see Table 68-3) showed 96 percent mortality from lung hemorrhage and renal failure. In Wilson and Dixon's early, immunologically verified series [261], only 11 percent of patients who were not dialysis-dependent at presentation recovered or maintained renal function. With the increasing availability of dialysis treatment, pulmonary hemorrhage became the most immediate threat to life. In an attempt to staunch it, bilateral nephrectomy was frequently advocated and occasionally used, with variable effects [62, 141, 166, 261]. The rationale was to reduce the antigenic stimulus, but there is little evidence that it succeeded in reducing antibody titers. Corticosteroids and, later, immunosuppressive agents were introduced, sometimes with apparent effect but with many treatment failures as well [12, 25, 43, 261, 263, 267]. The poor outlook was especially disappointing because further work had shown that the anti-GBM response was transient and that it was possible to transplant patients safely. In the mid-1970s, combined treatment with immunosuppressive agents, corticosteroids, and intensive plasma exchange was introduced [138, 139]. The intention was to remove circulating antibodies as rapidly as possible by plasma exchange and to prevent their resynthesis with the chemotherapy. It was dramatically effective, arresting pulmonary hemorrhage within 24 to 48 hours and rescuing mild to moderate renal impairment. Others described similar results [25, 71, 112, 218, 242].

Our current regimen has changed little from the one described then, and similar regimens are widely used. It consists of daily 4-liter plasma exchanges for 14 days, or until the circulating antibody is suppressed, with replacement by 5% human albumin solution. In the presence of pulmonary hemorrhage, or within 48 hours of an invasive procedure, 300 to 400 ml of fresh frozen plasma is given at the end of each exchange. Oral cyclophosphamide, 3 mg/kg, is given daily, rounded down to the nearest 50 mg, along with prednisolone, 1 mg/kg/day up to a maximum of 60 mg daily. In the original study, patients under 55 years were also given azathioprine, 1 mg/kg/day, but this has not been found to be essential, and many centers use cyclophosphamide alone. Smaller doses of cyclophosphamide (2.0–2.5 mg/kg) are given to older patients. If antibody concentration has been suppressed and the patient is clinically stable, cytotoxic therapy is withdrawn completely at 8 weeks. Prednisolone is reduced in weekly steps to half the starting dose at 2 weeks and then tailed off over the ensuing 6 weeks. Close monitoring of hematologic indices and for any signs of recrudescence of disease activity or secondary infection is mandatory over this period. kCO measurements are useful for establishing a baseline above which pulmonary hemorrhage can be diagnosed (see Fig. 68-4). Serial monitoring of anti-GBM antibody titers is invaluable in monitoring the adequacy of treatment, but a falling antibody titer does not preclude a clinical relapse in the face of some disease-amplifying event, usually secondary infection. Most early deaths are related (in the era of dialysis) to fulminant pulmonary hemorrhage; most late deaths and morbidity are now related to secondary infections, either directly or in combination with the exacerbated disease that it causes. More specific immunotherapy would therefore be a major advance in the management of these patients, as the risk of such infections is increased by the intense immunosuppression required.

An important question is whether all patients need such intensive treatment. The majority of those who present to a nephrologist probably will. As has been mentioned, once significant renal disease has developed, its progression can be extremely rapid. Full treatment should therefore be given to anyone with severe lung hemorrhage or with deteriorating renal function and probably to anyone with significant renal disease. Older series and case reports dealing with isolated pulmonary hemorrhage have shown that very mild renal disease associated with mild to moderate pulmonary hemorrhage can relapse and remit spontaneously. These patients can probably be treated with cyclophosphamide and prednisolone alone. At the other extreme, there are patients with such severe renal damage (in the absence of pulmonary hemorrhage) that the risks of treatment seem to outweigh the unlikely chance of renal recovery. This is discussed again later.

While the treatment regimens were developed with the intention of removing the pathogenic autoantibodies, it is clear that cyclophosphamide and prednisolone have, in addition, much wider effects on cellular immunity and on mechanisms by which inflammation leads to tissue damage. Some of these pathways are discussed in more detail below. Because the disease is rare and there are other strong influences on outcome besides treatment, it is difficult to disentangle how much each component of this undoubtedly successful treatment is contributing. Johnson et al. [111] conducted the only controlled trial to look at a single aspect of the treatment, the role of plasma exchange. Their regimen involved less plasma exchange and lower doses of cyclophosphamide than those recommended above, and their overall results were rather disappointing (69% of those with creatinine < 600 recovered renal function, none with higher creatinines). The randomization process also led to the plasma exchange group having rather less severe disease at presentation, somewhat confounding interpretation of the results. However, they did clearly show that judged by the renal outcome, patients with mild renal disease (creatinine < 300, < 30% crescents) did well regardless of which treatment arm they were in, while patients with severe renal disease (creatinine > 600, > 70% crescents) did badly regardless of the treatment they received. Treatment with plasma exchange alone has only a very transient effect on autoantibody levels [179] and is ineffective.

A more specific alternative to plasma exchange is removal of circulating antibodies by immunoadsorption with protein A. This is certainly effective in removing autoantibodies [34], it prevents depletion of clotting factors, complement components, and other constituents of plasma, and it removes the requirement for reinfusion of large volumes of blood products. However, it still renders the patient hypogammaglobulinemic, requires anticoagulation, and is a complex and labor-intensive treatment. Specific immunoadsorption against the Goodpasture antigen is a hope for the future.

It has been suggested that large boluses of corticosteroids may be of value in the treatment of RPGN with pulmonary hemorrhage [19, 54]. Although 17 patients with Goodpasture's disease were included in Bolton and Sturgill's large study [19], most were treated late and fared uniformly badly regardless of treatment. Three potentially recoverable patients received bolus methylprednisolone treatment, and two retained renal function. de Torrente et al. originally advocated the treatment as an alternative to bilateral nephrectomy to control severe pulmonary hemorrhage [54], although their patient's renal disease also appeared to resolve. Johnson [111] felt that while such treatment appeared to arrest pulmonary hemorrhage, it had no impact on renal impairment. Williams et al. [258] found that neither pulmonary nor renal disease responded to such treatment. Such experiences do not suggest that bolus corticosteroid therapy is an adequate alternative to intensive plasma exchange in Goodpasture's disease, and the increased infection risk created by such treatment is particularly worrying in this group of patients.

PROGNOSIS

Although impressive reductions in mortality have been achieved by advances in ability to diagnose and treat Goodpasture's disease, it is disappointing that a majority of patients are still left with end-stage renal failure (Table 68-3). Analysis of the results shows that this is because aggressive treatment can only rescue renal function up to a certain degree of severity; indeed it is possible to say that patients with more than 80 percent of glomeruli showing crescent formation on a biopsy taken at the start of treatment or a serum creatinine of more than 600 μmol/liter have little chance of useful renal recovery. This is quite different from the picture in histologically or functionally similar cases of crescentic nephritis caused by systemic vasculitis [97]. It has been suggested that because of this, oliguric patients with Goodpasture's disease who do not have lung hemorrhage should not be exposed to the potential dangers of treatment with this type of regimen [77]. However, recovery can occur in dialysis-dependent patients [242] (and patients in our series). There are features that make it possible to predict those in whom renal function might be recoverable. First, some oliguric patients have superimposed acute tubular necrosis; the acutely ill patient with lung hemorrhage and hypoxia, and possibly inappropriate early treatment before the diagnosis was recognized, often has multiple reasons for developing acute tubular necrosis. Second, in some patients, the renal lesion looks surprisingly mild, or very recent, with cellular rather than fibrotic crescents and patent capillary loops (D. J. Evans, unpublished observations). An urgent renal biopsy is therefore essential before coming to the conclusion that the kidney is not salvageable—and treatment should not be delayed until the result is available.

Figure 68-9 shows the effects of creatinine and crescent score at presentation on the 1-year outcome in patients with Goodpasture's disease treated at Hammersmith since 1976. There is a clear relationship between severity of renal disease and outcome, confirming the effect on renal outcome mentioned above and showing that those who died from lung hemorrhage also had fulminant renal disease—usually patients in the "accelerated" phase of the disease in whom treatment was started late. In contrast, the different pattern of outcome associated with crescentic nephritis caused by systemic vasculitis (microscopic polyarteritis, Wegener's granulomatosis, and ANCA-positive idiopathic RPGN) is

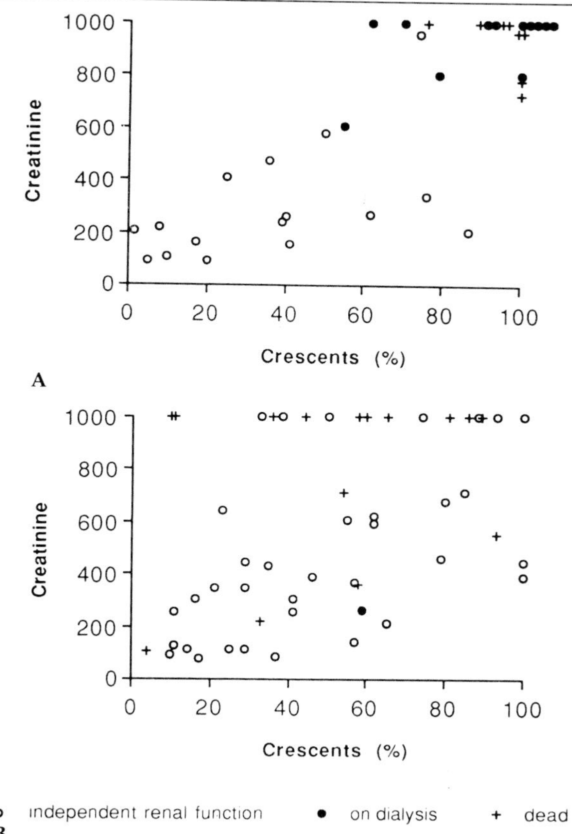

Fig. 68-9. Comparison of outcome at 1 year in patients treated at Hammersmith for RPGN due to (A) Goodpasture's disease and (B) systemic vasculitis (microscopic polyarteritis and Wegener's granulomatosis). Creatinine at presentation (*vertical axis*) is plotted against crescent score (*horizontal axis*) for all patients whose renal biopsy contained 10 or more glomeruli and who received intensive treatment with corticosteroids, cyclophosphamide, and (in Goodpasture's patients and some of those with vasculitis) plasma exchange. Different symbols indicate outcome at 1 year (see key). For Goodpasture's disease, there is a clear correlation between creatinine at presentation, or crescent score, and adverse outcomes. No such correlation is seen in the patients with systemic vasculitis.

shown. Renal function is often recoverable despite high creatinines and crescent scores at presentation. The reasons for these differences remain obscure.

There are few published large series reporting the effects of treatment in the last decade, and those that are available are not strictly comparable. Our results from the treatment of 57 patients with plasma exchange between 1976 and 1988 show a 1-year renal survival (i.e., alive and not requiring dialysis) of 90 percent for patients presenting with creatinine < 600 μmol/liter and 11 percent for those (the majority) presenting with creatinine > 600 μmol/liter. A similar regimen [242] achieved similar results, 82 and 18 percent respectively. It seems unlikely that much better results than these can be produced by minor changes in current therapy. More aggressive chemotherapy is likely to lead to higher risks of complications. Further improvements may depend on fundamental advances in ways of achieving more specific immunosuppression.

In marked contrast to the renal lesion, pulmonary damage in Goodpasture's disease appears to be capable of complete resolution without serious scarring. Survivors of fulminant disease usually have no detectable pulmonary deficit or radiologic abnormalities.

Renal transplantation is now known to be generally safe in those who are left with end-stage renal failure, as long as circulating antibodies have been undetectable for some months [15, 25, 152, 218, 261] and as long as immunosuppression is used after transplantation [5]. In some patients, treatment to accelerate the disappearance of antibodies may be justified, but this is only likely to be necessary if the patient was treated conservatively in their acute illness. Some cases of anti-GBM disease after renal transplantation are due to an immune response to new antigens present in kidneys transplanted into patients with Alport's syndrome (see reports listed in Table 68-2), as discussed later. The graft has inevitably been lost once crescentic nephritis has developed, but antibody formation without overt disease may be quite common [183]. Of five reported second grafts, two have been lost through recurrent anti-GBM disease [83, 116] and three have been successful [156, 185].

RELAPSE

A relapse is an exacerbation of tissue injury in patients who continue to have circulating anti-GBM antibodies and is distinct from a reactivation of the disease after the autoimmune response has subsided, defined here as a recurrence. Relapse may occur because therapy is inadequate to control the immune response (cessation of immunosuppression or plasma exchange) or because of some amplification of tissue injury initiated by a nonimmune process. This latter is more common; relapses have frequently been associated with intercurrent infections [112, 187]. Kidneys and lungs are equally affected, and the availability of simple tests (serum creatinine and kCO) to monitor both closely makes it easy to identify recrudescent disease in either organ promptly when it occurs (Fig. 68-4). Fluid overload and cigarette smoking can both precipitate fresh pulmonary hemorrhage without exacerbating renal injury. Both these phenomena are considered in more detail in the section on pathogenesis.

RESOLUTION AND RECURRENCE

Autoantibody synthesis usually declines after an acute episode of Goodpasture's disease, even when untreated. Once antibodies have become undetectable, recurrences are uncommon [111, 205, 263]. Treatment dramatically curtails the period of autoantibody synthesis [25, 205] (Figs. 68-10 and 68-11); how it might achieve this is fascinating but unclear. Some patients have episodes of pulmonary hemorrhage with intermittent evidence of

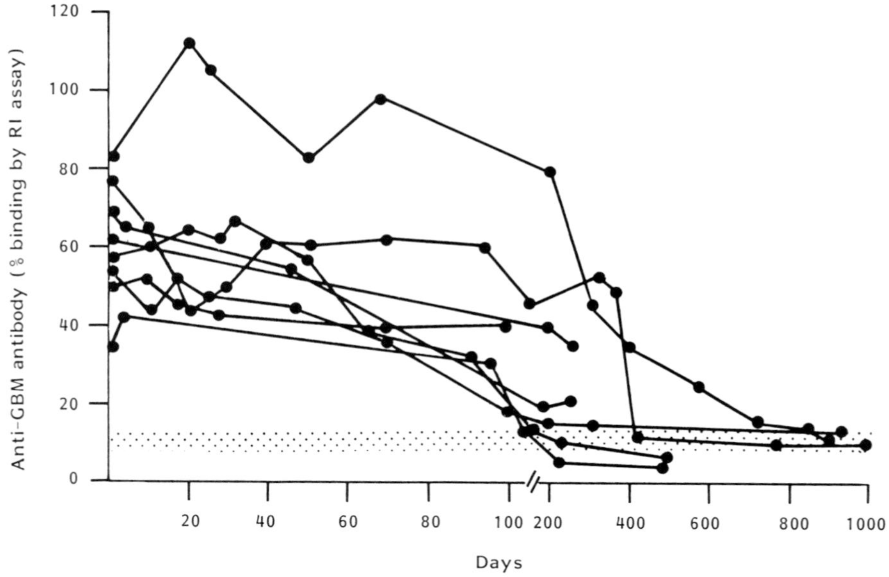

Fig. 68-10. Duration of circulating anti-GBM antibody synthesis in eight untreated patients. The antibody reaches undetectable levels only after more than a year. (Normal range in RIA is stippled.)

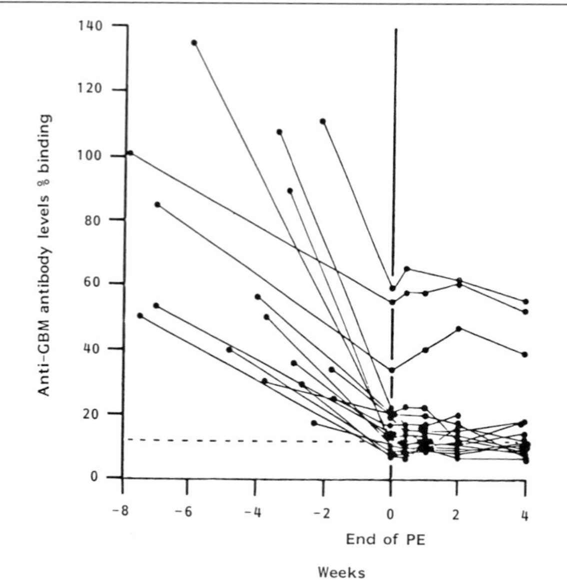

Fig. 68-11. Duration of circulating anti-GBM antibody synthesis in patients treated with corticosteroids, cytotoxic drugs, and plasma exchange. There was no rebound of antibody synthesis after levels had been reduced to normal and plasma exchange was discontinued.

mild nephritis over many years [27, 47, 153, 267], but recurrence after severe renal disease is extremely rare, except following renal transplantation. In this special case, it might be because of reimmunization of the patient with the Goodpasture antigen present in the donor kidney. The phenomenon is now very uncommon, as transplantation can be avoided until there is evidence that the autoimmune response has abated, although there are reports of recurrences despite this waiting period [11], including one in a graft from an identical twin in the absence of immunosuppressive agents [5]. There are instances of successful transplantation despite the presence of circulating antibodies [45, 261], but this is not to be recommended in view of previous experience. The incidence of recurrences of antibody synthesis without clinical manifestations [96] is unknown.

Pathogenesis

The pathogenicity of autoantibodies in Goodpasture's disease was shown by Lerner, Glassock, and Dixon [136] in primate transfer experiments. The antibody bound to the GBM, and the animals developed proteinuria and a severe proliferative (but not crescentic) nephritis with infiltration of neutrophils. The importance of antibody-mediated renal injury is also suggested by the correlation of antibody titers with the severity of renal disease at presentation [205, 218]. However, in the only account of the disease occurring in pregnancy, the fetus was apparently unaffected by the disease, although the mother later died [263]. The Goodpasture antigen is known to be present in fetal GBM from 10 weeks [38], and as typical anti-GBM antibodies are IgG1, they were almost certainly transported across the placenta. Possible explanations for the failure to produce fetal disease in this case include that the antigen is less accessible in the fetal GBM, or the inflammatory responses less activated, or that effector T cells are required for the induction of significant inflammation in Goodpasture's disease. The autoantibodies in Goodpasture's disease are a unique tool for the investigation of the pathogenetic mechanisms underlying the disorder. Here we review what is known of the interactions of various elements, including autoantibodies, that lead to the development of the disease.

A complete description of the pathogenesis of an autoimmune disorder would include accounts of (1) the initiation and the factors that determine individual susceptibility, (2) the components of the immune response that is generated and their targets and effector mechanisms, and (3) resolution of the disease process. This might make it possible to develop ways of specifically interfering with the processes involved, perhaps to induce early resolution, and ultimately to prevent the disease from developing.

In Goodpasture's disease, little is known of initiation, although some genetic susceptibility factors have been unusually well defined. Uniquely for a nephritis, a considerable amount is known about the target of immune injury, and there is increasing understanding of the immune effector mechanisms involved. Almost nothing definite is known about resolution.

Some of the clues to how the autoimmune response might be initiated in the disease have been discussed in the section on epidemiology. Thus, in patients with a genetic predisposition (those inheriting HLA-DR2, for example), an as yet undefined environmental influence could lead to exposure of the normally concealed antigen to the immune system (perhaps physical disruption in the case of membranous nephropathy or vasculitic disease) or, speculatively, to the development of cross-reacting immunity to a pathogen or to a disturbance of the immune system itself (lymphoma, or its treatment?).

The interaction between antigen and T helper lymphocyte is at the root of all immune responses. This interaction is fundamental to antibody synthesis by B cells as well as to cell-mediated immunity. At the molecular level, the antigen is taken up by antigen presenting cells and processed so that cleaved peptide fragments of the antigen combine with class II MHC molecules, which are then expressed on the cell surface. Here they react with the specific T-cell receptors of the lymphocyte. In the best understood animal model of autoimmune disease, experimental allergic encephalomyelitis, the autoantigen has been identified as myelin basic protein, and specific peptides within the sequence of the antigen have been shown to be critical to T-cell recognition. Immunization with these peptides alone can generate the disease. Specific interference with the autoimmune process has been effected by administration of antibodies to the T-cell receptor molecules predominantly involved in the interaction [266], by administration of peptides that can bind to the MHC molecule but not activate the T-cell receptor [106], and by giving antibodies that bind to the unique peptide/MHC complex involved in the disease [4]. It is the ultimate aim of research into human autoimmune diseases that it might be possible to reach this stage so that the knowledge can be exploited therapeutically. Knowledge of the autoantigen in Goodpasture's disease places it in a unique position for developing such knowledge in a human nephritis.

THE GOODPASTURE ANTIGEN

There is strong evidence that all patients with Goodpasture's disease form antibodies to the same component of GBM. Initially this came from studies using indirect immunofluorescence to show that circulating anti-GBM antibodies or those eluted from the kidneys of patients gave a characteristic binding pattern on tissue sections. Subsequently single monoclonal antibodies have been shown to replicate this pattern of binding both in tissue sections [39, 127, 180] (Fig. 68-12) and in binding to separated components of GBM, as described below.

Indirect immunohistochemical techniques show that the Goodpasture antigen is present in various basement membranes besides the GBM and alveolar basement membrane (Fig. 68-13 and Table 68-4). Many of these are basement membranes that are formed by the fusion of basement membranes of two cell types, endothelial cells and epithelial cells, lying on either side [2, 103]. In vivo binding of anti-GBM antibodies in patients with the disease is not as extensive as the distribution shown by these studies, probably because of differences in accessibility of basement membranes to circulating antibodies. It is probably quite common in the choroid plexus [39] and can occur in the eye, as mentioned above.

Basement membranes have many components. Major constituents are type IV collagen, heparan sulfate, proteoglycans, laminin, and entactin (nidogen), but there is a host of others, including some with restricted tissue distributions [146, 230]. The ultrastructural localization of the Goodpasture antigen has been studied by dual immunofluorescence and by immunoelectron microscopy [31, 54, 160]. Depending on the techniques used, the antigen is described as being distributed throughout the GBM, or limited to the lamina densa. A consistent finding has been that its distribution is different from that of the $\alpha 1$ and $\alpha 2$ chains of type IV collagen, found in all tissues, to which it is believed to be related. Antibodies to these components stain only the lamina rara interna in most studies, as well as the mesangial matrix, which contains no Goodpasture antigen at all.

Analysis of the components of basement membrane is hampered by their tightly cross-linked structure. Extraction of the antigen is usually achieved by collagenase digestion of lyophilized GBM prepared from glomeruli isolated by differential sieving. Treatment with most other proteolytic enzymes, or reduction of disulfide bonds, destroys the antigen or renders it nonantigenic, while other treatments fail to solubilize it from the membrane. A large body of evidence in the last decade has shown the antigen to be a part of the major C-terminal noncollagenous (NC1) domain of type IV collagen [29, 32, 103, 252, 256, 257], which makes up a large part of such collagenase digests. Solid-phase immunoassays using collagenase digests as the ligand are sensitive and specific (more so if combined with inhibition studies) for

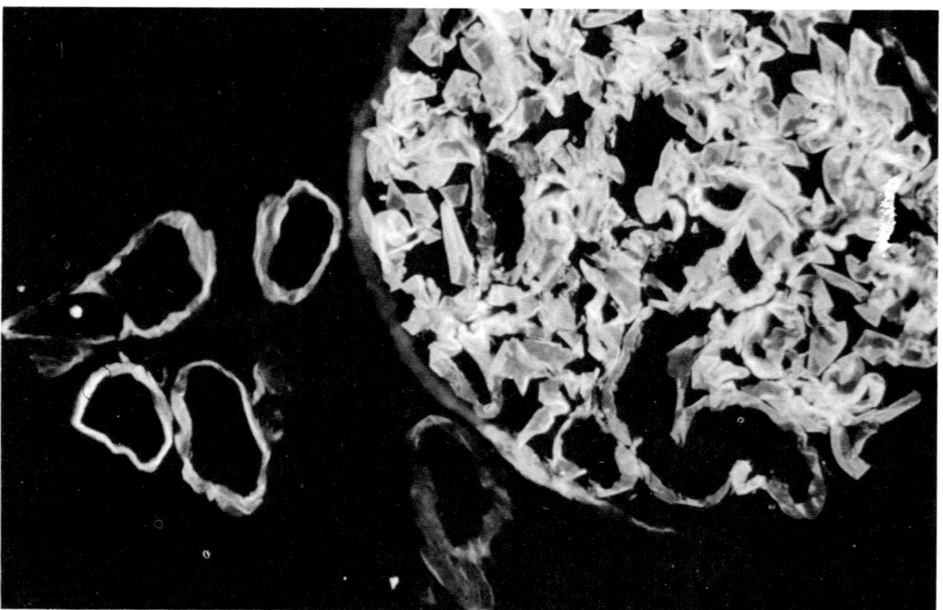

Fig. 68-12. Distribution of Goodpasture antigen in normal renal cortex demonstrated by indirect immunofluorescence. The GBM and basement membrane of the distal tubule are outlined, as is Bowman's capsule. Blood vessels do not bind the antibody, nor (in humans) does proximal tubular basement membrane. The section has been overlaid with a monoclonal antibody that precisely replicates the pattern of binding produced by patients' autoantibodies [180].

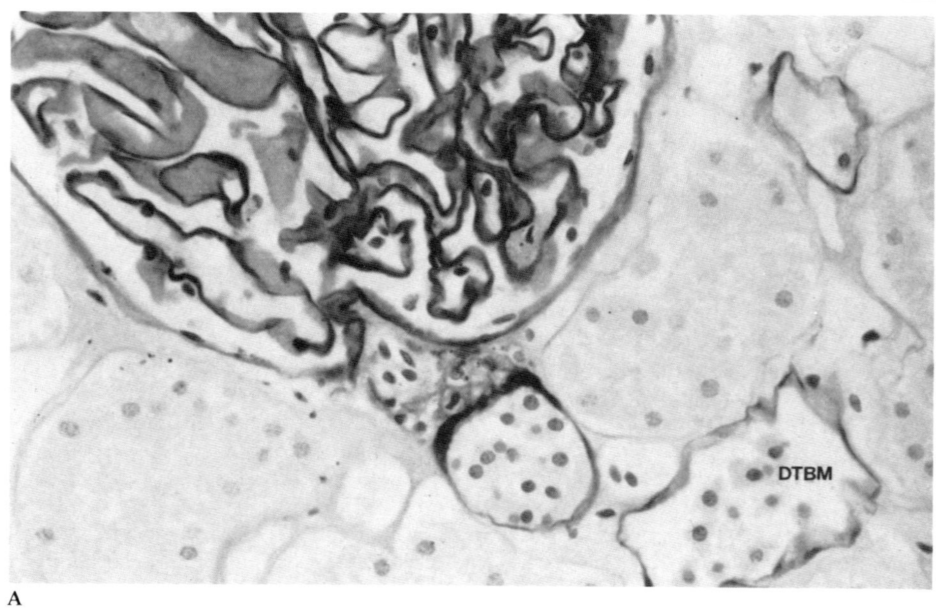

A

Fig. 68-13. Immunoperoxidase stain to show presence of the Goodpasture antigen in (A) glomerular and distal tubular basement membrane (DTBM) in the kidney, (B) alveolar basement membrane, (C) choroid plexus, and (D) basement membrane of the cochlea. (Courtesy of Professor L. Michael.)

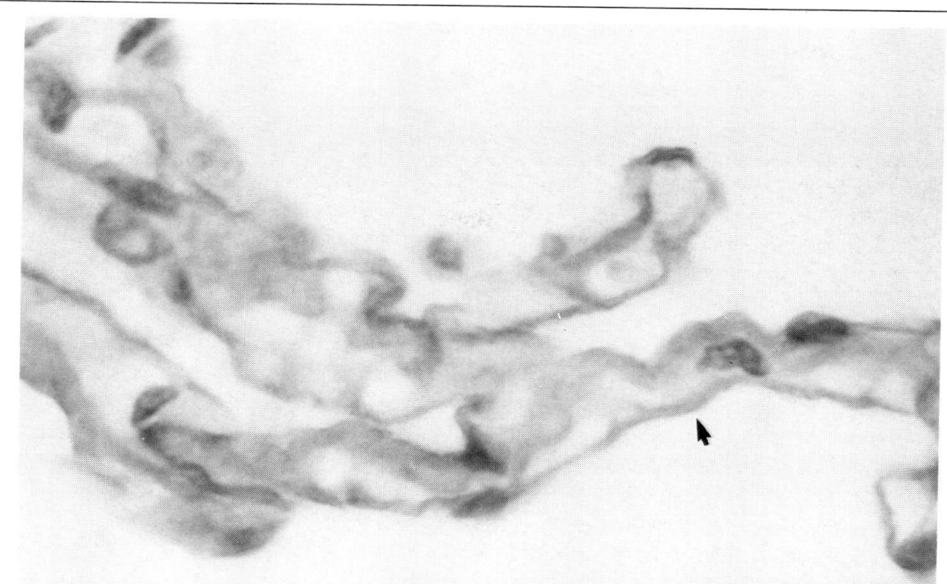
B

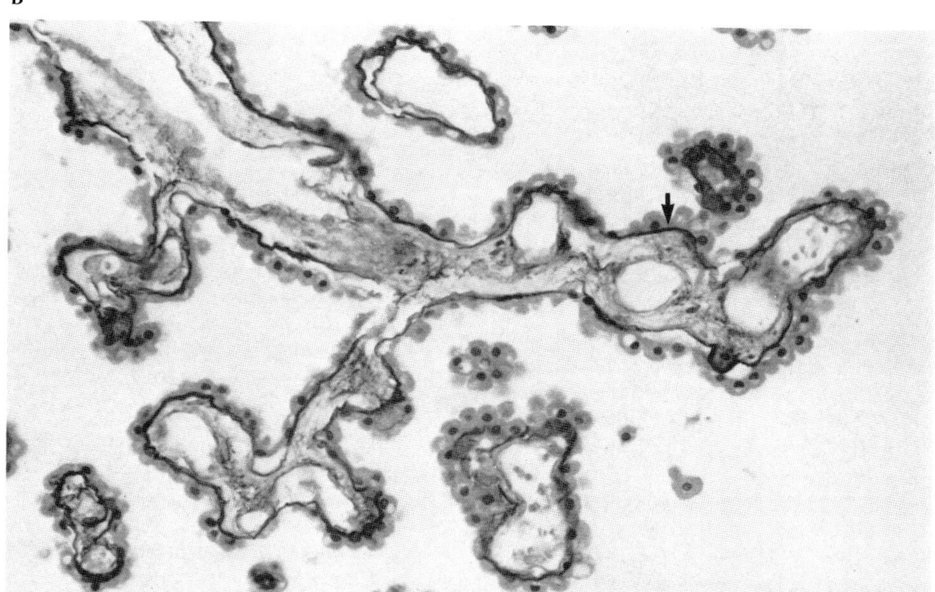
C

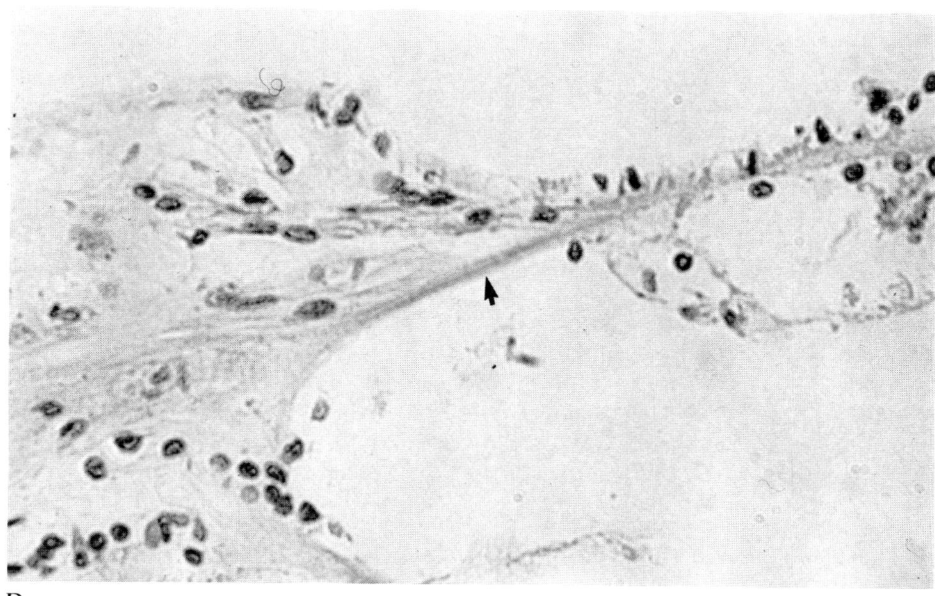
D

Goodpasture's disease. Now, assays that use a single highly purified component made from bovine or sheep GBM give even more sensitive and specific results than those using the crude human antigen preparation [210] (see Fig. 68-8). Some patients have additional antibodies to other basement membrane components, but these are inconsistent and usually of low titer [33, 78, 126, 215, 256].

The complexity of collagenase digests of basement membranes can be demonstrated by SDS-PAGE and immunoblotting. Autoantibodies bind to a "monomer" component of about 28 kd, and to a variety of "dimer" components of about 50 to 60 kd. This pattern can be replicated by single monoclonal antibodies [127, 180], showing that the multiple bands are due to the presence of a single epitope on various components of the antigen preparation, rather than to the existence of multiple antibody specificities. Two-dimensional electrophoresis (Fig. 68-14) shows that the antigenic component is a small proportion of the total protein and that it is strongly cationic (positively charged) in comparison with other constituents [52, 127]. It has been suggested that two-dimensional electrophoresis can show up different binding patterns with sera from different patients [271], but work in our laboratory has suggested that these differences are due to concentration effects, rather than differences in antibody specificity [52].

Type IV collagen makes up a chicken-wire-like network in basement membranes by cross-linking at the C-terminal and N-terminal ends of each molecule (Fig. 68-15). The majority of the molecule is triple helical, apparently made up in most tissues of two α1 and one α2 chains $(\alpha1)_2(\alpha2)_1$. The genes of these chains, and an unexpected α5 chain, have been cloned in humans [102, 161, 175]. Protein sequence obtained from components of bovine GBM implicated a novel and partially defined chain, α3, as the carrier of the Goodpasture antigen [30, 103, 203]. The existence of another novel chain, α4, was also demonstrated [91]. Interestingly, its distribution seems identical to that of the α3 chain [31, 127] and also in most tissues to that of a third new component, the "Alport antigen," identified by antibodies formed by a patient with Alport's syndrome after renal transplantation [120, 124]. By purifying antigenic material from sheep kidney and cleaving it with trypsin or cyanogen bromide, we have obtained protein sequence from within the antigenic domain. The sequences confirmed that the antigen resided in a novel type IV collagen chain and enabled oligonucleotides to be designed to amplify cDNA sequences encoding this molecule from sheep kidney mRNA, using the polymerase chain reaction. The sheep cDNA was then used to isolate human cDNA sequences encoding the entire NC1 domain of the same chain. Comparison of this sequence with that of the bovine α3(IV) cDNA [159] (isolated by similar methods but by using published bovine protein sequences) confirmed that this was the NC1 domain of the human α3 chain of type IV collagen. The derived amino acid sequence contained the peptides predicted by protein sequencing, and the high content of basic amino acids accounted for the strongly cationic nature of the antigen. The gene for the α3 chain maps to the tip of the long arm of chromosome 2. The Goodpasture antigen therefore resides in the NC1 domain of the α3 chain of type IV collagen, and its primary sequence is now known [159a, 233].

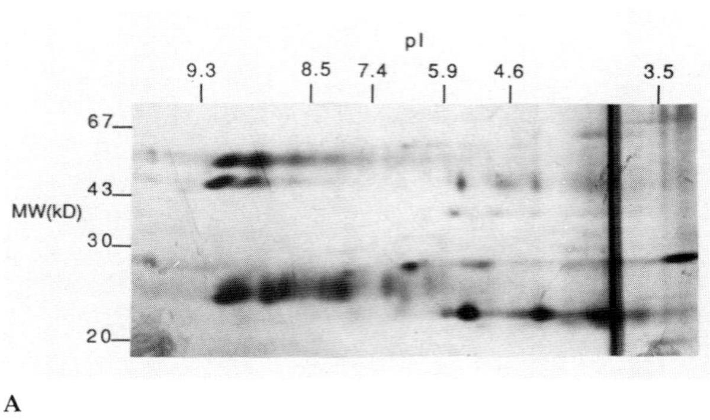

A

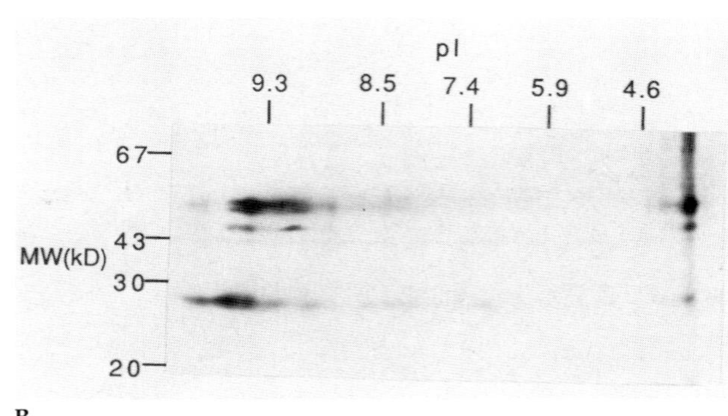

B

Fig. 68-14. Two-dimensional electrophoresis of collagenase-solubilized human GBM. Components are separated horizontally by isoelectric focusing and vertically by molecular weight (SDS-PAGE) and shown on a silver-stained gel (A) and by immunoblotting with a patient's serum (B). pI markers are shown along the upper border, and molecular weight markers down the left margin. The vertical line toward the right of the gel and the blot is an artefact from the loading point of the first (isoelectric focusing) stage. Components of interest fall into "monomer" (25–30 kd) and "dimer" (50–60 kd) groups, but each one shows "charge isoforms," with differing isoelectric points. The reason for this phenomenon is not known [130, 271]. The antigenic component is highly cationic (positively charged) and corresponds to a minority component of the digest; compare its position relative to the pI 9.3 marker on the Western blot (B) and gel (A). It is seen in both the monomer and dimer regions. The monomer component has a molecular weight of about 28 kd. (Courtesy of C. J. Derry. Reproduced from Turner and Pusey [234], with permission.)

EXPERIMENTAL MODELS OF ANTI-GBM DISEASE

A number of models have been described in which immunization or other manipulations lead to linear deposition of antibody along the GBM (Table 68-5), in association with nephritis of varying severity. They can be broadly divided into those associated with an autoimmune response specifically directed toward glomerular

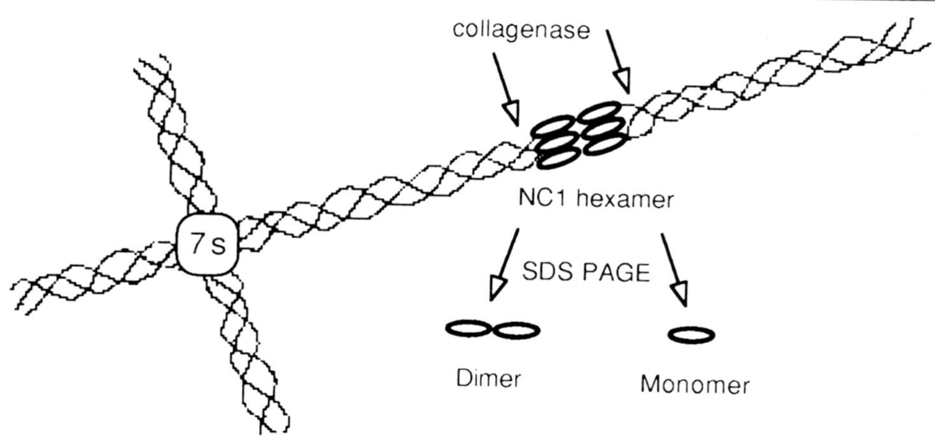

Fig. 68-15. Schematic representation of a type IV collagen molecule. A single, largely triple helical molecule is associated at N-terminal (7S) and C-terminal (NC1) ends with similar domains of adjacent molecules. The globular NC1 domain at the C-terminus contains the C-terminal ends of all three of the chains making up the molecule. Digestion with collagenase releases these domains from the collagenous region as "hexamers" composed of C-terminal domains of chains from adjacent molecules. SDS and other dissociating agents separate these hexamers into "monomers" (25–30 kd), each being the C-terminal end of a single type IV collagen chain, and dimers (50–60 kd), composed of covalently linked C-terminal domains from chains of two adjacent type IV collagen molecules [103, 247, 257]. These components can be best demonstrated by two-dimensional gel electrophoresis, as shown in Fig. 68-13.

Table 68-5. Active models of anti-GBM disease in animals compared with Goodpasture's disease in humans

Model species	Disease	Target	Genetic restriction	Comments
DISEASES ASSOCIATED WITH AUTOIMMUNITY TO GLOMERULUS-SPECIFIC ANTIGENS				
Human	Goodpasture's	α3(IV) NC1	DR2 (DR4)	Antibodies pathogenic in primates
Sheep	Steblay nephritis	α3(IV) NC1	Not known	Antibodies pathogenic in sheep
Rat (BN)	EAG	Not known	"Strain specific"	
Rat (WKY)	EAG	Not known	"Strain specific"	Antibodies pathogenic in rats
DISEASES ASSOCIATED WITH POLYCLONAL ACTIVATION [81, 82]				
Rat (BN)	$HgCl_2$	Various	MHC and other	Disease transferred by CD4+ T cells
Mouse	$HgCl_2$		MHC (H-2)	
Rat (BN)	Penicillamine, gold			Similar to $HgCl_2$ model
Mouse	LPS		LPS receptor	Granular glomerular deposits only
Mouse/rat	GVHD		Depends on MHC differences	Increased IgE and IgG as in $HgCl_2$ model
Mouse	Transplant tolerance			Increased IgE and IgG
Mouse	Trypanosomiasis		Not known	Malaria has similar effects, but granular deposits
Mouse	Schistosomiasis		Not known	

EAG = experimental allergic glomerulonephritis; $HgCl_2$ = mercuric chloride-induced disease; LPS = lipopolysaccharide; GVHD = graft-versus-host disease.

antigens and those in which nephritis occurs as part of a more generalized autoimmune disturbance, often associated with polyclonal activation.

Models produced by immunization with GBM (experimental allergic glomerulonephritis [EAG]) are the most clearly analogous to human disease and have been studied for the insights that they provide into the autoimmune response to GBM. A disadvantage of most is that the precise target of immunity is usually unknown. The prominent exception is Steblay nephritis, EAG produced in sheep by repeated immunization with human GBM in complete Freund's adjuvant. The animals develop a progressive glomerulonephritis with linear binding of complement-fixing immunoglobulin [221, 222]. As in

Goodpasture's disease, the antibodies react with alveolar basement membrane in vitro by indirect immunofluorescence, but they do not normally bind to it in vivo, and pulmonary hemorrhage is not seen. An identical disease can be induced by immunization with alveolar basement membrane, but not basement membranes of other tissues [223]. Passive transfer of antibodies eluted from affected kidneys to other sheep causes glomerular injury [135]. The major GBM target for these antibodies is probably the same molecule as the Goodpasture antigen [35, 39, 64, 110], although one study found it to be directed toward a less cationic species [126]. Two-dimensional electrophoretic studies in our laboratory implicate the α3 chain of type IV collagen, as in Goodpasture's disease (Derry and Pusey, unpublished observations). This is certainly the best animal model of Goodpasture's disease, but it is in an inconveniently large species, and one in which knowledge of MHC molecules and immunology is limited.

In some strains of rat, EAG can be induced by immunization with GBM prepared from different strains [181, 200]. Susceptibility is strain-dependent, and although linkage to MHC genes has not yet been demonstrated, such a genetic effect is strongly reminiscent of human disease. Cyclosporin inhibits the development of autoantibodies and proteinuria if administered before immunization [193]. The disease is more severe in Wistar-Kyoto WKY than in Brown Norway rats, and in this strain passive transfer of antibodies from affected animals can cause a similar renal disease in recipient animals [201]. The molecular targets of the antibodies in these models are not described.

Multiple glomerular antibody targets have been identified in those models associated with polyclonal activation, including antigens that may be trapped in the GBM and those normally located there [81, 82]. DNA, IgG, laminin, type IV collagen, and fibronectin antibodies are among those described. The most intensively studied model is that induced in Brown Norway rats by administration of mercuric chloride, but other agents (gold, penicillamine) can induce a similar disorder in this rat strain, and the mercuric chloride model has many features in common with others associated with polyclonal activation (Table 68-5). Several features are of particular interest because of parallels in human Goodpasture's disease. Susceptibility is at least partially MHC-dependent, but it appears to involve other genes as well. And although the disease proves fatal to about half of the diseased rats, in the survivors the autoimmune abnormalities all resolve after about 8 weeks [81].

Polyclonal activation in this model is evident from the development of a wide range of autoantibodies, including those to thyroglobulin, nuclear antigens, IgG, collagen II, and a variety of basement membrane antigens, as well as antibodies to extrinsic antigens such as sheep red blood cells and trinitrophenyl. Linear deposition of immunoglobulin along the GBM is seen in the second week; from the third week a membranous pattern develops. Nephritis is mild. Sjögren's syndrome and dermatitis may develop. There is an increase in total IgE and IgG and of B cells, but also of CD4+ T cells in spleen and lymph nodes. These T cells are required for polyclonal activation to occur. T cells from diseased animals can transfer disease to untreated syngeneic animals that have been depleted of CD8+ T cells. The mechanism of resolution is less clearly established. Transfer of spleen cells from convalescent to untreated animals attenuates the severity of subsequent mercuric chloride-induced disease. Induction is associated with a fall and recovery with a rise in circulating CD8+ T cells, but treatment with anti-CD8 monoclonal antibody fails to influence the course of the disease [81]. Observations on this model reinforce the importance of the abnormal T lymphocyte interactions that underly autoimmune disturbances.

Disentangling the respective roles of B and T cells in EAG by cell transfer experiments will clearly be important, and this has not yet been described in mammalian models. However, in a fascinating series of experiments in chickens, Bolton et al. [18] have shown that anti-GBM antibody binding can be completely dissociated from disease, which can be transferred by T-cell transfer without transfer of antibody formation. This may not say much about human disease, but it does warn against overinterpreting the visually striking signs of B-cell activity while ignoring the less obvious effects of T cells.

There is no direct evidence for the participation of cell-mediated immunity in Goodpasture's disease, but glomeruli of patients with crescentic nephritis contain increased numbers of T lymphocytes and macrophages [165]. In animal models, the influx of lymphocytes precedes that of macrophages in experimental models of anti-GBM disease [101, 231], and in other models, nephritis can be induced by cell-mediated immunity alone [168, 192]. Older experiments showed evidence of cellular sensitization to GBM antigens in anti-GBM and other nephritides [69, 70, 142, 197], and there is little doubt that such sensitization must exist for the disease to occur. The observation that cytokine-treated glomerular epithelial cells can process antigen and present it to specific T cells [155] provides a further pathway by which such processes can be initiated within the glomerulus. Now that the antigen (at least for B cells) is defined, it should be possible to begin to investigate these mechanisms in more detail.

MECHANISMS OF INJURY IN THE KIDNEY

Circulating antibodies must be able to reach their target to induce tissue damage. Differences in accessibility probably explain how disease can be restricted to a single organ while the antigen occurs in several basement membranes. Bound antibody must then engage humoral and cellular mediators, such as complement, neutrophils, and macrophages. And third, the capacity of these to release phlogistic molecules such as oxygen radicals and enzymes may need to be amplified for the development of inflammation, a coupling that is sensitive to various local and remote influences.

The major immunoglobulin subclass involved in Goodpasture's disease is IgG1, which is complement fixing, and the GBM is directly accessible to circulating antibodies. In the kidney, therefore, antibody-mediated damage may occur directly via complement activation [86], via recruitment of neutrophils with or without the assistance of complement [42, 176, 228], or via engaging macrophages [100, 212]. IgG4 makes up a significant proportion of anti-GBM antibodies in some patients. Although it is not complement fixing and has been considered a less tissue-damaging subclass, it has been shown to be the predominant pathogenic subclass in one human autoimmune disease, endemic pemphigus foliaceus [196]. Simple binding, without recruitment of other mediators, may be enough to achieve a pathogenic effect in this disease though [195].

In rabbits, the injury caused by injection of "nephrotoxic globulin" (heterologous antibodies to GBM) is dependent on the amount of antibody injected, but the relation between mass of antibody fixed and injury is not linear. Small amounts of antibody produce no detectable injury, but after a critical amount of antibody has been fixed, the severity of the lesion produced increases steeply as more antibody is administered [236]. Injury is also influenced by the rate of antibody deposition as well as the mass deposited [238], probably because the Fc piece of an antibody is only able to engage mediators for a short while after binding to its target. There is ample evidence from human disease that low levels of antibodies need not be associated with significant renal injury, as described earlier. However, the threshold at which injury occurs can be considerably reduced by, for example, the presence of systemic infection [238]. This effect can be replicated in rats by administering tiny quantities of lipopolysaccharide (endotoxin) or interleukin-1β or tumor necrosis factor [232] and is analogous to the ability of an infection to precipitate relapses in Goodpasture's disease. The phenomenon and these experiments draw attention to an important determinant of pathogenesis besides the existence of immunity to a particular antigen. It is possible that present treatments (corticosteroids in particular) may already exert some of their effects by modifying such effects.

INJURY IN THE LUNG

Although circulating antibodies have free access to the GBM, through the fenestrae in the glomerular capillary endothelial cells, they are excluded from the alveolar basement membrane by its more typical endothelium. Passive injection into animals of antibodies raised to the glomerular or alveolar basement membrane usually leads to binding to the GBM alone [136, 151, 223]. Certain interventions can alter this, leading to antibody binding to the alveolar basement membrane and pulmonary hemorrhage, as well as the renal lesion caused by the antibodies. The measures that have been shown to have this effect are likely to have directly toxic effects locally on the lungs: instillation of gasoline into the trachea [269], 2 weeks of exposure to cigarette smoke [Rees, unpublished results], and exposure to high concentrations of oxygen [58, 109]. It has recently been shown in mice that systemic administration of interferon-α and/or interleukin-2 achieves a similar effect [182].

Although differences in both pulmonary antigen and antibody have been postulated from elution and immunoblotting studies [151, 245, 255, 270], it is clear from immunohistochemical studies with monoclonal antibodies [39, 127] and from Western blotting studies [243, 255, 270, and Derry and Turner, unpublished observations] that the antigenic target is the same molecule in the lung as in the kidney. In Western blotting studies, relatively more of the antigen seems to be bound in "dimer" form than in the kidney.

Pulmonary hemorrhage is an inconstant or unusual [181, 201] feature of most models of anti-GBM disease, although it is a usual feature of some [251, 259]. Its presence in some of these models could be explained by coinjection of endotoxin or cytokines, of antibodies that damaged the alveolar capillary endothelium, or (in active models) of antigen that induced the development of such antibodies. It is possible that the variability observed in some models is related to coincident infections in recipient animals, acting to increase the permeability of the alveolar endothelium. These stimuli are presumed to increase the permeability of alveolar capillary endothelial cells to circulating antibodies or other mediators, and thus the normally concealed alveolar basement membrane becomes a target and site of injury. The mechanism of these effects explains why there is little relationship between antibody titers and severity of lung disease [218, 263] in contrast to the correlation observed for renal disease.

In clinical practice, these observations make it prudent to ensure avoidance of potential pulmonary toxins so far as is possible in patients with lung hemorrhage. This certainly involves not smoking; particular efforts to maintain reasonable concentrations of inspired oxygen in acutely ill patients are also justified. It is notable that such effects of inhaled toxins, including cigarette smoke, are not recognized for pulmonary hemorrhage caused by systemic vasculitis [92]. This presumably reflects basic differences in the pathogenesis of those disorders.

Anti-GBM Disease in Alport's Syndrome

The observation that patients with Alport's syndrome sometimes develop anti-GBM disease in their allografts led to the finding that the Goodpasture antigen was absent from the kidneys of many patients with the syndrome in indirect immunofluorescence studies [149]. Studies with monoclonal antibodies have confirmed this observation [124, 206], and it was widely supposed that patients with the disorder have mutations in the gene encoding the molecule bearing the Goodpasture antigen. As Alport's syndrome is usually X-linked [26, 76, 118], it was presumed to be encoded on the X chromosome. In 1990, a new type IV collagen chain, α5, was identified by cDNA cloning, and its gene mapped to the Alport region of the X chromosome [102, 175]. Mutations in this gene were subsequently described in 3 of 18 families studied by Barker et al. [7] and have since been identified in some families studied by other groups. However, the α5 chain did not seem to be the chain previously identified as the Goodpasture antigen, which had been labeled α3 from protein sequence data. An "Alport antigen," recognized by an antiserum from a patient with Alport's syndrome who developed anti-

GBM disease after renal transplantation, had, however, been previously postulated [115, 120, 124].

The specificities of antibodies formed by patients with Alport's syndrome who develop anti-GBM disease in their allograft after renal transplantation have not been studied as intensively as those of patients with Goodpasture's disease. Clinically the renal disease appears identical to the anti-α3 response seen in Goodpasture's disease, except that the patients never get pulmonary involvement. Fortunately, the development of nephritis is uncommon, but anti-GBM antibody formation may be much more common than clinical disease [183]. It is not known whether this or the expression of injury is influenced by immunosuppression or whether genetic (e.g., HLA) or other factors are important. The antibody response has seemed typical using standard techniques. When investigated by two-dimensional electrophoresis, however, the target of the autoantibodies in several patients has appeared to be a more neutral component of collagenase digests of human GBM than the α3 chain [95, 117, and Derry, unpublished observation]. This component could be the α4 or α5 chain, or possibly another as yet undefined component of collagenase digests of GBM. In the same reports though, two more patients are described as showing "anti-α3" two-dimensional immunoblotting patterns typical of Goodpasture's disease [95, 117]. By conventional immunoblotting, Savage et al. [204] also identified two distinct patterns of reactivity in three post-transplant Alport sera. Two patients gave a pattern typical of Goodpasture's disease, identifying a 28-kd band, while one identified a smaller (26-kd) component, probably the equivalent of the Alport antigen.

The distribution of the "Alport antigen" identified by one of these antisera has been closely studied by the Minnesota group [120, 124]. Like the Goodpasture antigen, it appears to be absent from the basement membranes of most patients with Alport's syndrome. In most tissues, it colocalizes with the α3 and α4 chains, as visualized by monoclonal antibodies or Goodpasture patients' (anti-α3) autoantibodies. This has been most strikingly shown in females with Alport's syndrome, where patchy absence of α3 [115, 229] and α4 chain antigens (a mosaicism presumably created by random inactivation of X chromosomes) is perfectly matched by absence of the Alport antigen at the same sites [124]. A plausible model to explain these observations hypothesizes that the α3, α4, and α5 chains must all unite to form a distinct network within certain basement membranes, separate from that involving the α1 and α2 chains of type IV collagen. In the glomerulus, the α3, α4, and α5 chains are probably synthesized by glomerular epithelial cells, while α1/α2 type IV collagen is produced by endothelial and mesangial cells [31, 160]. The α3/α4/Alport antigen network could be disrupted by a defect in the genes encoding any one of its constituents, and this might lead to the failure of antigenic expression of all its components. "Missing bands" in SDS-PAGE gels of collagenase digests of Alport's GBM provide evidence of this [125, 204]. Only in skin does the close relationship between the distribution of the three putative components of this complex appear to break down. The Alport antigen is easily demonstrable in epidermal basement membrane [115, 124], and while some find weak binding of certain Goodpasture sera in denatured tissue sections [272], this observation is not consistent [39, 115, 120, 124] and cannot be replicated by monoclonal antibodies to either the α3 or the α4 chain [38, 39, 124, 127]. Denaturing of sections may lead to Goodpasture autoantibodies binding to determinants other than those restricted to the α3 chain of type IV collagen [31].

If the α3 chain (gene on chromosome 2) is involved in a network with α5 and/or other type IV collagen chains, as suggested here, it is interesting that the vast majority of what we recognize as Alport's syndrome is X-linked. Very rare cases with a different pattern of inheritance have been described [66, 88], but none has yet been subjected to rigorous study. It is possible that other as yet unidentified components of GBM may also be involved in hereditary nephritis. The genes for the α1 and α2 chains of type IV collagen are located head-to-head in extremely close proximity on chromosome 13 [178, 219]. If the α5 chain shared a similar arrangement with another type IV collagen chain on the X chromosome, then mutations in this other gene could also lead to X-linked Alport's syndrome. Furthermore, it has been observed that amyloid P component is absent from the GBM in cases of Alport's syndrome [154]; is it also involved in the putative new network?

A little more needs to be uncovered about the genetics of type IV collagen, and a lot more about the expression of the type IV collagen gene products, before the molecular basis of Alport's syndrome is fully understood.

Conclusion

Goodpasture's disease remains rare, but continues to prove uniquely informative. Clinically, it is often a dramatic condition, affecting organs where tissue injury is particularly easy to monitor. The effects of treatment, infection, and other influences on the disease have been particularly easy to discern. Experimentally, investigation of the disease has taught us a great deal about mechanisms by which nephritis can be mediated and modulated. And at the molecular level, the pursuit of the molecular target of Goodpasture autoantibodies has led to the identification of several new molecules and significant advances in our understanding of basement membrane structure. It seems very likely that the disease will go on providing valuable information, the new knowledge leading toward a greater understanding of both the immunologic derangements underlying Goodpasture's disease and the structural derangements underlying Alport's syndrome.

References

1. Abboud, R. T., Chase, W. H., Ballon, H. S., et al. Goodpasture's syndrome: Diagnosis by transbronchial lung biopsy. *Ann. Intern. Med.* 89: 635, 1978.
2. Abrahamson, D. R. Structure and development of the glomerular capillary wall and basement membrane. *Am. J. Physiol.* 253: F783, 1987.
3. Agodoa, L. C. Y., George, C. R. P., Glassock, R., et al.

The appearance of nonlinear deposits of immunoglobulins in Goodpasture's syndrome. *Am. J. Med.* 61: 407, 1976.
4. Aharoni, R., Teitelbaum, D., Arnon, R., and Puri, J. Immunomodulation of experimental allergic encephalomyelitis by antibodies to the antigen-Ia complex. *Nature* 351: 147, 1991.
5. Almkuist, R. D., Buckalew, V. M., Jr., Hirszel, P., et al. Recurrence of anti-glomerular basement membrane antibody mediated glomerulonephritis in an isograft. *Clin. Immunol. Immunopathol.* 18: 54, 1981.
6. Bailey, R. R., Simpson, I. J., Lynn, K. L., et al. Goodpasture's syndrome with normal renal function. *Clin. Nephrol.* 15: 211, 1981.
7. Barker, D. F., Hostikka, S. L., Zhou, J., et al. Identification of mutations in the COL4A5 collagen gene in Alport syndrome. *Science* 248: 1224, 1990.
8. Beechler, C. R., Enquist, R. W., Hunt, K. K., et al. Immunofluorescence of transbronchial biopsies in Goodpasture's syndrome. *Am. Rev. Respir. Dis.* 121: 869, 1980.
9. Beirne, G. J., and Brennan, J. T. Glomerulonephritis associated with hydrocarbon solvents. *Arch. Environ. Health* 25: 365, 1972.
10. Beirne, G. J., Wagnild, J. P., Zimmerman, S. W., et al. Idiopathic crescentic glomerulonephritis. *Medicine* (Baltimore) 56: 349, 1977.
11. Beleil, O. M., Coburn, J. W., Shinaberger, J. H., et al. Recurrent glomerulonephritis due to anti-glomerular basement membrane antibodies in two successful allografts. *Clin. Nephrol.* 1: 377, 1973.
12. Benoit, F. L., Rulon, C. B., Theil, G. B., et al. Goodpasture's syndrome. A clinicopathologic entity. *Am. J. Med.* 37: 424, 1964.
13. Berg, L. J., Pullen, A. M., Fazekas de St Groth, M., et al. Antigen/MHC-specific T cells are preferentially exported from the thymus in the presence of their MHC ligand. *Cell* 58: 1035, 1989.
14. Berger, J., Yaneva, H., and Hinglais, N. Immunochemistry of glomerulonephritis. *Adv. Nephrol.* 1: 11, 1971.
15. Bergrem, H., Jervill, J., Brodwall, J., et al. Goodpasture's syndrome. A report of seven patients including long term follow-up of three who received a kidney transplant. *Am. J. Med.* 68: 54, 1980.
16. Bernis, P., Hamels, J., Quoidbach, A., et al. Remission of Goodpasture's syndrome after withdrawal of an unusual toxic. *Clin. Nephrol.* 23: 312, 1985.
17. Blake, D. R., Rashid, H., McHugh, M., and Morley, A. R. A possible association of partial lipodystrophy with anti-GBM nephritis (Goodpasture's syndrome). *Postgrad. Med. J.* 56: 137, 1980.
18. Bolton, W. K., Chandra, M., Tyson, T. M., et al. Transfer of experimental glomerulonephritis in chickens by mononuclear cells. *Kidney Int.* 34: 598, 1988.
19. Bolton, W. K., and Sturgill, B. C. Methylprednisolone therapy for acute crescentic rapidly progressive glomerulonephritis. *Am. J. Nephrol.* 9: 368, 1989.
20. Border, W. A., Baehler, R. W., Bhathema, D., et al. IgA antibasement membrane nephritis with pulmonary hemorrhage. *Ann. Intern. Med.* 91: 21, 1979.
21. Bowley, N. B., Hughes, J. M. B., and Steiner, R. E. The chest X-ray in pulmonary capillary haemorrhage: Correlation with carbon monoxide uptake. *Clin. Radiol.* 30: 413, 1979.
22. Bowley, N. B., Steiner, R. E., and Chin, W. S. The chest X-ray in antiglomerular basement membrane antibody disease (Goodpasture's syndrome). *Clin. Radiol.* 30: 419, 1979.
23. Bowman, C., Ambrus, K., and Lockwood, C. M. Restriction of human IgG subclass expression in the population of auto-antibodies to glomerular basement membrane. *Clin. Exp. Immunol.* 69: 341, 1987.
24. Bowman, C., and Lockwood, C. M. Clinical application of a radio-immunoassay for auto-antibodies to glomerular basement membrane. *J. Clin. Lab. Immunol.* 17: 197, 1985.
25. Briggs, W. A., Johnson, J. P., Teichman, S., et al. Antiglomerular basement membrane antibody-mediated glomerulonephritis and Goodpasture's syndrome. *Medicine* (Baltimore) 58: 348, 1979.
26. Brunner, H., Schroder, C., van Bennekom, C., et al. Localization of the gene for X-linked Alport's syndrome. *Kidney Int.* 34: 507, 1988.
27. Burke, B. R., and Bear, R. A. Recurrent Goodpasture's syndrome. *Can. Med. Assoc. J.* 129: 978, 1983.
28. Burns, A., Li, P., So, A., et al. HLA class II restrictions in Goodpasture's syndrome. *Nephrol. Dial. Transplant.* 5: 297, 1990.
29. Butkowski, R. J., Guo-Qui, S., Wieslander, J., et al. Characterization of type IV collagen NC1 monomers and Goodpasture antigen in human renal basement membranes. *J. Lab. Clin. Med.* 115: 365, 1990.
30. Butkowski, R. J., Langeveld, J. P. M., Wieslander, J., et al. Localization of the Goodpasture epitope to a novel chain of basement membrane collagen. *J. Biol. Chem.* 262: 7874, 1987.
31. Butkowski, R. J., Wieslander, J., Kleppel, M., et al. Basement membrane collagen in the kidney: Regional localization of novel chains related to collagen IV. *Kidney Int.* 35: 1195, 1989.
32. Butkowski, R. J., Wieslander, J., Wisdom, B. J., et al. Properties of the globular domain of Type IV collagen and its relationship to the Goodpasture antigen. *J. Biol. Chem.* 260: 3739, 1985.
33. Bygren, P., Cederholm, B., Heinegard, D., and Wieslander, J. Non-Goodpasture anti-GBM antibodies in patients with glomerulonephritis. *Nephrol. Dial. Transplant.* 4: 254, 1989.
34. Bygren, P., Freiburghaus, C., Lindholm, T., et al. Goodpasture's syndrome treated with staphylococcal protein A immunoadsorption (letter). *Lancet* 2: 1295, 1985.
35. Bygren, P., Wieslander, J., and Heinegard, D. Glomerulonephritis induced in sheep by immunization with human glomerular basement membrane. *Kidney Int.* 31: 25, 1987.
36. Cameron, J. S., and Williams, D. G. Glomerulonephritis. In E. J. Holborow and W. G. Reeves (eds.), *Immunology in Medicine,* 2nd ed. New York: Grune and Stratton, 1983.
37. Carre, P., Lloveras, J. J., Didier, A., et al. Goodpasture's syndrome with normal renal function. *Eur. Respir. J.* 2: 911, 1989.
38. Cashman, S. J., Pusey, C. D., and Evans, D. J. Immunohistochemical localization of Goodpasture antigen in human tissues. In M. C. Gubler and M. Sternberg (eds.), *Progress in Basement Membrane Research: Renal and Related Aspects in Health and Disease.* Paris: John Libbey Eurotext, 1988. Pp. 119–123.
39. Cashman, S. J., Pusey, C. D., and Evans, D. J. Extraglomerular distribution of immunoreactive Goodpasture antigen. *J. Pathol.* 155: 61, 1988.
40. Clark, E. H., Jones, H. A., and Hughes, J. M. B. Bedside rebreathing technique for measuring carbon-monoxide uptake by the lung. *Lancet* 1: 791, 1978.
41. Clutterbuck, E. J., and Pusey, C. D. Severe alveolar hae-

morrhage in Churg-Strauss syndrome. *Eur. J. Respir. Dis.* 71: 158, 1987.

42. Cochrane, C. G., Unanue, E. R., and Dixon, F. J. A role of polymorphonuclear leucocytes and complement in nephrotoxic nephritis. *J. Exp. Med.* 122: 99, 1965.
43. Cohen, L. H., Wilson, C. B., and Freeman, R. M. Goodpasture's syndrome: Recovery after severe renal insufficiency. *Arch. Intern. Med.* 136: 835, 1976.
44. Compston, A. *Multiple Sclerosis.* London: Butterworths, 1986. Pp. 56–73.
45. Couser, W. G., Wallace, A., Monaco, A. P., and Lewis, E. J. Successful renal transplantation in patients with circulating antibody to glomerular basement membrane: Report of two cases. *Clin. Nephrol.* 1: 381, 1973.
46. Curtis, J. J., Bhatena, D., Leach, R. P., et al. Goodpasture's syndrome in a patient with the nail-patella syndrome. *Am. J. Med.* 61: 401, 1976.
47. Dahlberg, P. J., Kurtz, S. B., Donadio, J. V., Jr., et al. Recurrent Goodpasture's syndrome. *Mayo Clin. Proc.* 53: 533, 1978.
48. Daniell, W. E., Couser, W. G., and Rosenstock, L. Occupational solvent exposure and glomerulonephritis: A case report and review of the literature. *J.A.M.A.* 259: 2280, 1988.
49. D'Apice, A. J. F., Kincaid-Smith, P., Becker, G. J., et al. Goodpasture's syndrome in identical twins. *Ann. Intern. Med.* 88: 61, 1978.
50. Davison, A. M. Seasonal incidence of glomerulonephritis: Findings of UK Medical Research Council's Glomerulonephritis Registry. *Abstracts of IX International Congress of Nephrology,* Los Angeles, 1984.
51. de Caestecker, M. P., Hall, C. L., and MacIver, A. G. Atypical antiglomerular basement membrane disease associated with thin membrane nephropathy. *Nephrol. Dial. Transplant.* 5: 909, 1990.
52. Derry, C. J., Dunn, M. J., Rees, A. J., and Pusey, C. D. Restricted specificity of the autoantibody response in Goodpasture's syndrome demonstrated by two-dimensional western blotting. *Clin. Exp. Immunol.* 86: 457, 1991.
53. Desjardins, M., Gros, F., Wieslander, J., et al. Heterogeneous distribution of monomeric elements from the globular domain (NC1) of type IV collagen in renal basement membranes as revealed by high resolution quantitative immunocytochemistry. *Lab. Invest.* 63: 637, 1990.
54. de Torrente, A., Popovtzer, M., Guggenheim, S. J., et al. Serious pulmonary hemorrhage, glomerulonephritis and massive steroid therapy. *Ann. Intern. Med.* 83: 218, 1975.
55. Dische, F. E., Brooke, I. P., Cashman, S. J., et al. Reactivity of monoclonal antibody P1 with glomerular basement membrane in thin-membrane nephropathy. *Nephrol. Dial. Transplant.* 4: 611, 1989.
56. Donaghy, M., and Rees, A. J. Cigarette smoking and lung haemorrhage in glomerulonephritis caused by autoantibodies to glomerular basement membrane. *Lancet* 2: 1390, 1983.
57. Donald, K. J., Edwards, R. L., and McEvoy, J. D. S. Alveolar capillary basement membrane lesions in Goodpasture's syndrome and idiopathic pulmonary hemosiderosis. *Am. J. Med.* 59: 642, 1975.
58. Downie, G. H., Roholt, O. A., Monte Blau, L. J., et al. Experimental anti-alveolar basement membrane antibody-mediated pneumonitis. II. Role of endothelial damage and repair, induction of autologous phase, and kinetics of antibody deposition in Lewis rats. *J. Immunol.* 129: 2647, 1982.
59. Duncan, D. A., Drummond, K. N., Michael, A. F., et al. Pulmonary hemorrhage and glomerulonephritis. Report of six cases and study of the renal lesion by the fluorescent antibody technique and electron microscopy. *Ann. Intern. Med.* 62: 920, 1965.
60. Dupont, E., Mendes da Costa, C. R., and Dupuis, F. Linear deposits of immunoglobulins on glomerular basement membrane of human stored kidneys. *Transplantation* 18: 458, 1974.
61. Editorial. Alveolar haemorrhage. *Lancet* 1: 853, 1985.
62. Eisinger, A. J. Goodpasture syndrome: Failure of nephrectomy to cure pulmonary hemorrhage. *Am. J. Med.* 55: 565, 1973.
63. Espinosa Melendez, E., Forbes, R. D., Hollomby, D. J., et al. Goodpasture's syndrome treated with plasmapheresis: Report of a case. *Arch. Intern. Med.* 140: 542, 1980.
64. Evans, D. J., Dash, A., and Lockwood, M. Role of Goodpasture antigen in Steblay nephritis. *J. Pathol.* 42: A17, 1984.
65. Ewan, P. R., Jones, H. A., Rhodes, C. G., et al. Detection of intrapulmonary hemorrhage with carbon monoxide uptake. Application in Goodpasture's syndrome. *N. Engl. J. Med.* 295: 1391, 1976.
66. Feingold, J., Bois, E., Chompret, A., et al. Genetic heterogeneity of Alport syndrome. *Kidney Int.* 27: 672, 1985.
67. Ferguson-Smith, M. A., Aitken, D. A., Turleau, C., and de Grouchy, J. Localisation of the human ABO:Np-1:AK-1 linkage group by regional assignment of AK-1 to 9q34. *Hum. Genet.* 34: 35, 1976.
68. Fillit, H., Damle, S. P., Gregory, J. D., et al. Sera from patients with poststreptococcal glomerulonephritis contain antibodies to glomerular heparan sulfate proteoglycan. *J. Exp. Med.* 161: 277, 1985.
69. Fillit, H. M., Read, S. E., Sherman, R. L., et al. Cellular reactivity to altered glomerular basement membrane in glomerulonephritis. *N. Engl. J. Med.* 298: 860, 1978.
70. Fillit, H. M., and Zabriskie, J. B. Cellular immunity in glomerulonephritis. *Am. J. Pathol.* 109: 227, 1982.
71. Finch, R. A., Rutsky, E. A., McGowan, E., et al. Treatment of Goodpasture's syndrome with immunosuppression and plasmapheresis. *South. Med. J.* 72: 1288, 1979.
72. Finley, T. N., Aronow, A., Cosentino, A. M., et al. Occult pulmonary hemorrhage in anticoagulated patients. *Am. Rev. Respir. Dis.* 112: 23, 1975.
73. Fish, A. J., Kleppel, M., Jeraj, K., and Michael, A. F. Enzyme immunoassay of anti-glomerular basement membrane antibodies. *J. Lab. Clin. Med.* 105: 700, 1985.
74. Fivush, B., Melvin, T., Solez, K., and McLean, R. H. Idiopathic linear glomerular IgA deposition. *Arch. Pathol. Lab. Med.* 110: 1189, 1986.
75. Fleming, S. J., Savage, C. O. S., McWilliam, L. J., et al. Anti-glomerular basement membrane antibody-mediated nephritis complicating transplantation in a patient with Alport's syndrome. *Transplantation* 46: 857, 1988.
76. Flinter, F. A., Cameron, J. S., Chantler, C., et al. Genetics of classic Alport's syndrome. *Lancet* 2: 1005, 1988.
77. Flores, J. C., Taube, D., Savage, C. O. S., et al. Clinical and immunological evolution of oligoanuric anti-GBM nephritis treated by haemodialysis. *Lancet* 1: 5, 1986.
78. Foidart, J. B., Pirard, Y., Foidart, J. M., et al. Anti-type IV procollagen and anti-laminin antibodies in Goodpasture syndrome. *Kidney Int.* 18: 126, 1980.
79. Gallo, G. R. Elution studies in kidneys with linear deposition of immunoglobulin in glomeruli. *Am. J. Pathol.* 61: 377, 1970.
80. Garovoy, M. R. Immunogenetic associations in nephrotic states. *Contemp. Issues Nephrol.* 9: 259, 1982.

81. Glotz, D., and Druet, P. Immune Mechanisms of Glomerular Damage. In J. S. Cameron, A. M. Davison, J. P. Grunfeld, et al. (eds.), *Oxford Textbook of Nephrology*. Oxford: Oxford University Press, 1991. Pp. 14–36.
82. Goldman, M., Baran, D., and Druet, P. Polyclonal activation and experimental nephropathies. *Kidney Int.* 34: 141, 1988.
83. Goldman, M., Depierreux, M., De Pauw, L., et al. Failure of two subsequent renal grafts by anti-GBM glomerulonephritis in Alport's syndrome: Case report and review of the literature. *Transplant. Int.* 3: 82, 1990.
84. Goodpasture, E. W. The significance of certain pulmonary lesions in relation to the etiology of influenza. *Am. J. Med. Sci.* 158: 863, 1919.
85. Gossain, V. V., Gerstein, A. R., and Janes, A. W. Goodpasture's syndrome: A familial occurrence. *Am. Rev. Respir. Dis.* 105: 621, 1972.
86. Groggel, G. C., Salant, D. J., Darby, C., et al. Role of terminal complement pathway in the heterologous phase of antiglomerular basement membrane nephritis. *Kidney Int.* 27: 643, 1985.
87. Grubb, R. The Genetic Markers on Human Immunoglobulins. Berlin: Springer Verlag, 1970.
88. Grunfeld, J. P. The clinical spectrum of hereditary nephritis. *Kidney Int.* 27: 83, 1985.
89. Grupe, W. E. Case record of the Massachusetts General Hospital: Case 12-1986. *N. Engl. J. Med.* 314: 834, 1986.
90. Guerin, V., Rabin, C., Noel, L. H., et al. Anti-glomerular basement membrane disease after lithotripsy. *Lancet* i: 856, 1990.
91. Gunwar, S., Saus, J., Noelken, M. E., and Hudson, B. G. Glomerular basement membrane: Identification of a fourth chain, α4, of type IV collagen. *J. Biol. Chem.* 265: 5466, 1990.
92. Haworth, S. J., Savage, C. O. S., and Carr, D., et al. Pulmonary haemorrhage complicating Wegener's granulomatosis and microscopic polyarteritis. *Br. Med. J.* 290: 1775, 1985.
93. Heale, W. F., Matthieson, A. M., and Niall, J. F. Lung haemorrhage and nephritis (Goodpasture's syndrome). *Med. J. Aust.* 2: 355, 1969.
94. Heptinstall, R. H. Schönlein-Henoch Syndrome: Lung Hemorrhage and Glomerulonephritis. In R. H. Heptinstall (ed.), *Pathology of the Kidney* (3rd ed.). Boston: Little, Brown, 1983. Pp. 761–791.
95. Heuvel, L. P. W. J., Schroder, C. H., Savage, C. S., et al. The development of antiglomerular basement membrane nephritis in two children with Alport's syndrome after renal transplantation: Characterisation of the antibody target. *Pediatr. Nephrol.* 3: 406, 1989.
96. Hind, C. R. K., Bowman, C., Winearls, C. D., et al. Recurrence of circulating anti-glomerular basement membrane antibody three years after immunosuppressive treatment and plasma exchange. *Clin. Nephrol.* 21: 244, 1984.
97. Hind, C. R. K., Paraskevakou, H., Lockwood, C. M., et al. Prognosis after immunosuppression of patients with crescentic nephritis requiring dialysis. *Lancet* 1: 263, 1983.
98. Hogan, P. G., Donald, K. J., and McEvoy, J. D. Immunofluorescence studies of lung biopsy tissue. *Am. Rev. Respir. Dis.* 118: 537, 1978.
99. Holdsworth, S., Boyce, N., Thomson, N. M., et al. The clinical spectrum of acute glomerulonephritis and lung haemorrhage (Goodpasture's syndrome). *Q. J. Med.* 55: 75, 1985.
100. Holdsworth, S. R., Neale, T. J., and Wilson, C. B. Abrogation of macrophage-dependent injury in experimental glomerulonephritis in the rabbit: Use of an antimacrophage serum. *J. Clin. Invest.* 68: 686, 1981.
101. Holdsworth, S. R., and Tipping, P. G. Cell Mediated Immunity in Glomerulonephritis. In C. D. Pusey (ed.), *Immunology of Renal Diseases*. Lancaster: Kluwer, 1991.
102. Hostikka, S. L., Eddy, R. L., Byers, M. G., et al. Identification of a distinct type IV collagen alpha chain with restricted kidney distribution and assignment of its gene to the locus of X chromosome-linked Alport syndrome. *Proc. Natl. Acad. Sci. U.S.A.* 87: 1606, 1990.
103. Hudson, B. G., Wieslander, J., Wisdom, B. J., and Noelken, M. E. Goodpasture syndrome: Molecular architecture and function of basement membrane antigen. *Lab. Invest.* 61: 256, 1989.
104. Hume, D. M., Sterling, W. A., Weymouth, R. J., et al. Glomerulonephritis in human renal homotransplants. *Transplant. Proc.* 2: 361, 1970.
105. Jampol, L. M., Lahar, M., Albert, D. M., et al. Ocular clinical findings and basement membrane changes in Goodpasture's syndrome. *Am. J. Ophthalmol.* 79: 452, 1975.
106. Janeway, C. A. Immunotherapy by peptides? *Nature* 341: 482, 1989.
107. Jayne, D. R. W., Marshall, P. D., Jones, S. J., and Lockwood, M. C. Autoantibodies to GBM and neutrophil cytoplasm in rapidly progressive glomerulonephritis. *Kidney Int.* 37: 965, 1990.
108. Jennette, J. C., Lamanna, R. W., Burnette, J. P., et al. Concurrent antiglomerular basement membrane antibody and immune complex mediated glomerulonephritis. *Am. J. Clin. Pathol.* 78: 381, 1982.
109. Jennings, L., Rohold, J. A., Pressman, D., et al. Experimental anti-alveolar basement membrane antibody-mediated pneumonitis. *J. Immunol.* 127: 129, 1981.
110. Jeraj, K., Michael, A. F., and Fish, A. J. Immunologic similarities between Goodpasture's and Steblay's antibodies. *Clin. Immunol. Immunopathol.* 23: 408, 1982.
111. Johnson, J. P., Moore, J., Austin, III, H. A., et al. Therapy of anti-glomerular basement membrane antibody disease: Analysis of prognostic significance of clinical, pathologic and treatment factors. *Medicine* 64: 219, 1985.
112. Johnson, J. P., Whitman, W., Briggs, W. A., and Wilson, C. B. Plasmapheresis and immunosuppressive agents in antibasement membrane antibody–induced Goodpasture's syndrome. *Am. J. Med.* 64: 354, 1978.
113. Kalderon, A. E., Bogaars, H. A., and Diamond, I. Ultrastructural alterations of the follicular basement membrane in Hashimoto's thyroiditis. *Am. J. Med.* 55: 485, 1973.
114. Kalowski, S., McKay, D. G., Howes, E. L., Jr., et al. Multinucleated giant cells in antiglomerular basement membrane antibody-induced glomerulonephritis. *Nephron* 16: 415, 1976.
115. Kashtan, C., Fish, A. J., Kleppel, M., et al. Nephritogenic antigen determinants in epidermal and renal basement membranes of kindreds with Alport-type familial nephritis. *J. Clin. Invest.* 78: 1035, 1986.
116. Kashtan, C. E., Atkin, C. L., Gregory, M. C., and Michael, A. F. Identification of variant Alport phenotypes using an Alport-specific antibody probe. *Kidney Int.* 36: 669, 1989.
117. Kashtan, C. E., Butkowski, R. J., Kleppel, M. M., et al. Posttransplant anti-glomerular basement membrane nephritis in related males with Alport syndrome. *J. Lab. Clin. Med.* 116: 508, 1990.
118. Kashtan, C. E., Rich, S. S., Michael, A. F., and de Mar-

tinville, B. Gene mapping in Alport families with different basement membrane antigenic phenotypes. *Kidney Int.* 38: 925, 1990.
119. Keogh, A. M., Ibels, L. S., Allen, D. H., et al. Exacerbation of Goodpasture's syndrome after inadvertent exposure to hydrocarbon fumes. *Br. Med. J.* 288: 188, 1984.
120. Kim, Y., Kleppel, M. M., Butkowski, R., et al. Differential expression of basement membrane collagen chains in diabetic nephropathy. *Am. J. Pathol.* 138: 413, 1991.
121. Klassen, J., Elwood, C., Grossberg, A. L., et al. Evolution of membranous nephropathy into anti-glomerular-basement-membrane glomerulonephritis. *N. Engl. J. Med.* 290: 1340, 1974.
122. Klavis, G., and Drommer, W. Goodpasture syndrome and the effects of petrol. *Arch. Toxicol.* 26: 40, 1970.
123. Kleinknecht, D., Morel-Maroger, L., Callard, P., et al. Anti-glomerular basement membrane nephritis after solvent exposure. *Arch. Intern. Med.* 140: 230, 1980.
124. Kleppel, M. M., Kashtan, C., Santi, P. A., et al. Distribution of familial nephritis antigen in normal tissue and renal basement membranes of patients with homozygous and heterozygous Alport familial nephritis. *Lab. Invest.* 61: 278, 1989.
125. Kleppel, M. M., Kashtan, C. E., Butkowski, R. J., et al. Alport familial nephritis: Absence of 28 kilodalton non-collagenous monomers of type IV collagen in glomerular basement membrane. *J. Clin. Invest.* 80: 263, 1987.
126. Kleppel, M. M., Michael, A. F., and Fish, A. J. Antibody specificity of human glomerular basement membrane type IV collagen NC1 subunits: Species variation in subunit composition. *J. Biol. Chem.* 261: 16547, 1986.
127. Kleppel, M. M., Santi, P. A., Cameron, J. D., et al. Human tissue distribution of novel basement membrane collagen. *Am. J. Pathol.* 134: 813, 1989.
128. Koffler, D., Agnello, V., Carr, R. I., et al. Variable patterns of immunoglobulin and complement deposition in the kidneys of patients with systemic lupus erythematosus. *Am. J. Pathol.* 56: 305, 1969.
129. Koffler, D., Sandson, J., Carr, R., et al. Immunologic studies concerning the pulmonary lesions in Goodpasture's syndrome. *Am. J. Pathol.* 54: 293, 1969.
130. Langeveld, J. P. M., Wieslander, J., Timoneda, J., et al. Structural heterogeneity of the noncollagenous domain of basement membrane collagen. *J. Biol. Chem.* 263: 10481, 1988.
131. Leatherman, J. W. Immune alveolar hemorrhage. *Chest* 91: 891, 1987.
132. Leatherman, J. W., Davies, S. F., and Hoidal, J. R. Alveolar hemorrhage syndromes: Diffuse microvascular lung hemorrhage in immune and idiopathic disorders. *Medicine* (Baltimore) 63: 343, 1984.
133. Leatherman, J. W., Sibley, R. K., and Davies, S. F. Diffuse intrapulmonary hemorrhage and glomerulonephritis unrelated to anti-glomerular basement membrane antibody. *Am. J. Med.* 72: 401, 1982.
134. Lee, H. Y., and Stretton, T. B. The lung in renal failure. *Thorax* 30: 46, 1975.
135. Lerner, R. A., and Dixon, F. J. Transfer of ovine experimental allergic glomerulonephritis (EAG) with serum. *J. Exp. Med.* 124: 431, 1966.
136. Lerner, R. A., Glassock, R. J., and Dixon, F. J. The role of anti-glomerular basement membrane antibody in the pathogenesis of human glomerulonephritis. *J. Exp. Med.* 126: 989, 1967.
137. Lindemann, W. Sur la mode d'action de certains poisons renaux. *Ann. Int. Pasteur* 14: 49, 1900.
138. Lockwood, C. M., Boulton Jones, J. M., Lowenthal, R. M., and Simpson, I. J. Recovery from Goodpasture's syndrome after immunosuppressive treatment and plasmapheresis. *South. Med. J.* 68: 635, 1975.
139. Lockwood, C. M., Rees, A. J., Pearson, T. A., et al. Immunosuppression and plasma-exchange in the treatment of Goodpasture's syndrome. *Lancet* i: 711, 1976.
140. Ma, K. W., Golbus, S. M., Kaufman, R., et al. Glomerulonephritis with Hodgkin's disease and herpes zoster. *Arch. Pathol. Lab. Med.* 102: 527, 1978.
141. Maddock, R. K., Jr., Stevens, L. E., Reemtsma, K., et al. Goodpasture's syndrome. Cessation of pulmonary hemorrhage after bilateral nephrectomy. *Ann. Intern. Med.* 67: 1258, 1967.
142. Mahieu, P., Dardenne, M., and Bach, J. F. Detection of humoral and cell-mediated immunity to kidney basement membranes in human renal diseases. *Am. J. Med.* 53: 185, 1972.
143. Mahieu, P., Lambert, P. H., and Miescher, P. A. Detection of anti-glomerular basement membrane antibodies by a radioimmunological technique. Clinical application in human nephropathies. *J. Clin. Invest.* 54: 128, 1974.
144. Male, D., Champion, B., and Cooke, A. *Advanced Immunology* (2nd ed.). Philadelphia: Lippincott/Gower, 1991.
145. Martinez, J. S., and Kohler, P. F. Variant "Goodpasture's syndrome?" The need for immunologic criteria in rapidly progressive glomerulonephritis and hemorrhagic pneumonitis. *Ann. Intern. Med.* 75: 67, 1971.
146. Martinez-Hernandez, A., and Amenta, P. S. The basement membrane in pathology. *Lab. Invest.* 48: 656, 1983.
147. Masugi, M. Uber die experimentelle glomerulonephritis durch das spezifische anti-nierenserum. Ein beitrag zur pathogenease der diffusen glomerulonephritis. *Beitr. Pathol.* 92: 429, 1934.
148. Matthew, T. H., Hobbs, J. B., Kaowshi, S., et al. Goodpasture's syndrome: Normal renal diagnostic findings. *Ann. Intern. Med.* 82: 215, 1975.
149. McCoy, R. C., Johnson, H. K., Stone, W. J., and Wilson, C. B. Absence of nephritogenic GBM antigen(s) in some patients with hereditary nephritis. *Kidney Int.* 21: 642, 1982.
150. McIntosh, R. M., Copack, P., Chernack, W. B., et al. The human choroid plexus and autoimmune nephritis. *Arch. Pathol.* 99: 48, 1975.
151. McPhaul, J. J., and Dixon, F. J. Characterization of human anti-glomerular basement membrane antibodies eluted from glomerulonephritic kidneys. *J. Clin. Invest.* 49: 308, 1970.
152. McPhaul, J. J., and Mullins, J. D. Glomerulonephritis mediated by antibody to glomerular basement membrane. *J. Clin. Invest.* 57: 351, 1976.
153. Mehler, P. S., Brunvand, M. W., Hutt, M. P., and Anderson, R. J. Chronic recurrent Goodpasture's syndrome. *Am. J. Med.* 82: 833, 1987.
154. Melvin, T., Kim, Y., and Michael, A. F. Amyloid P component is not present in the glomerular basement membrane in Alport-type hereditary nephritis. *Am. J. Pathol.* 125: 460, 1986.
155. Mendrick, D. L., Kelly, D. M., and Rennke, H. G. Antigen processing and presentation by glomerular visceral epithelium in vitro. *Kidney Int.* 39: 71, 1991.
156. Milliner, D. S., Pierides, A. M., and Holley, K. E. Renal transplantation in Alport's syndrome: Anti-glomerular basement membrane glomerulonephritis in the allograft. *Mayo Clin. Proc.* 57: 35, 1982.
157. Moorthy, A. V., Zimmerman, S. W., Burkholder, P. M.,

et al. Association of crescentic glomerulonephritis with membranous glomerulonephropathy: A report of three cases. *Clin. Nephrol.* 6: 319, 1976.

158. Morgan, P. G., and Turner-Warwick, M. Pulmonary haemosiderosis and pulmonary haemorrhage. *Br. J. Dis. Chest.* 75: 225, 1981.
159. Morrison, K. E., Germino, G. G., and Reeders, S. T. Use of the polymerase chain reaction to clone and sequence a cDNA encoding the bovine α3 chain of type IV collagen. *J. Biol. Chem.* 266: 34, 1991.

159a. Morrison, K. E., et al. Sequence and localization of a partial c DNA encoding the human α3 chain of type IV collagen. *Am. J. Hum. Genet.* 49: 545, 1991.

160. Mounier, F., Gros, F., Wieslander, J., et al. Glomerular Distribution of M1 and M2 Subunits of the Globular Domain of the Basement Membrane Collagen: An Immunohistochemical Study. In M. C. Gubler, and M. Sternberg (eds.), *Progress in Basement Membrane Research: Renal and Related Aspects in Health and Disease.* Paris: John Libbey Eurotext, 1988. Pp. 53–59.
161. Muthukumaran, G., Blumberg, B., and Kurkinen, M. The complete primary structure for the α1-chain of mouse collagen IV. *J. Biol. Chem.* 264: 6310, 1989.
162. Nathan, A. W., and Toseland, P. A. Goodpasture's syndrome and trichloroethane intoxication. *Br. J. Clin. Pharmacol.* 8: 284, 1979.
163. Nelson, N. A., Robins, T. G., and Port, F. K. Solvent nephrotoxicity in humans and experimental animals. *Am. J. Nephrol.* 10: 10, 1990.
164. Noel, L. H., Aucouturier, P., Monteiro, R. C., et al. Glomerular and serum immunoglobulin G subclasses in membranous nephropathy and anti-glomerular basement membrane nephritis. *Clin. Immunol. Immunopathol.* 46: 186, 1988.
165. Nolasco, F. E. B., Cameron, J. S., Hartley, B., et al. Intraglomerular T cells and monocytes in nephritis: Study with monoclonal antibodies. *Kidney Int.* 31: 1160, 1987.
166. Nowakowski, A., Grove, R. B., King, L. H., Jr., et al. Goodpasture's syndrome: Recovery from severe pulmonary hemorrhage after bilateral nephrectomy. *Ann. Intern. Med.* 75: 243, 1971.
167. O'Donoghue, D. J., Short, C. D., Brenchley, P. E. C., et al. Sequential development of systemic vasculitis with antineutrophil cytoplasmic antibodies complicating anti-glomerular basement membrane disease. *Clin. Nephrol.* 32: 251, 1989.
168. Oite, T., Shimizu, F., Kagami, S., and Morioka, T. Hapten-specific cellular immune response producing glomerular injury. *Clin. Exp. Immunol.* 76: 463, 1989.
169. Ortega, L. G., and Mellors, R. C. Analytical pathology. IV. The role of localized antibodies in the pathogenesis of nephrotic nephritis in the rat. *J. Exp. Med.* 104: 151, 1956.
170. Perez, G. O., Bjornsonn, S., Ross, A. L. I., et al. A mini epidemic of Goodpasture's syndrome. *Nephron* 13: 161, 1974.
171. Perl, S. I., Pussell, B. A., Charlesworth, J. A., et al. Goodpasture's (anti-GBM) disease and HLA-DRW2. (Letter) *N. Engl. J. Med.* 305: 463, 1981.
172. Peters, D. K., Rees, A. J., Lockwood, C. M., et al. Treatment and prognosis in anti-basement membrane antibody mediated nephritis. *Transplant. Proc.* 14: 513, 1982.
173. Pettersson, E., Tornroth, T., and Miettinent, A. Simultaneous anti-glomerular basement membrane and membranous glomerulonephritis: Case report and literature review. *Clin. Immunol. Immunopathol.* 31: 171, 1984.
174. Pettersson, E., Tornroth, T., and Wieslander, J. Abnormally thin glomerular basement membrane and the Goodpasture epitope. *Clin. Nephrol.* 33: 105, 1990.
175. Pihlajaniemi, T., Pohjolainen, E. R., and Myers, J. C. Complete primary structure of the triple-helical region and the carboxyl-terminal domain of a new type IV collagen chain, α5(IV). *J. Biol. Chem.* 265: 13758, 1990.
176. Pilia, P. A., Boackle, R. J., Swain, R. P., and Ainsworth, S. K. Complement-independent nephrotoxic serum nephritis in Munich Wistar rats: Immunologic and ultrastructural studies. *Lab. Invest.* 48: 585, 1983.
177. Polla, B., Pirson, Y., Cosyns, J. P., et al. Toxic anti-GBM glomerulonephritis. *Clin. Nephrol.* 19: 45, 1983.
178. Poschl, E., Pollner, R., and Kuhn, K. The genes for the α1(IV) and α2(IV) chains of human basement membrane collagen type IV are arranged head-to-head and separated by a bidirectional promoter of unique structure. *EMBO J.* 7: 2687, 1988.
179. Proskey, A. J., Weatherbee, L., Easterling, R. E., et al. Goodpasture's syndrome. A report of five cases and review of the literature. *Am. J. Med.* 48: 162, 1970.
180. Pusey, C. D., Dash, A., Kershaw, M. J., et al. A single autoantigen in Goodpasture's syndrome identified by a monoclonal antibody to human glomerular basement membrane. *Lab. Invest.* 56: 23, 1987.
181. Pusey, C. D., Holland, M. J., Cashman, S. J., et al. Experimental autoimmune glomerulonephritis induced by homologous and isologous glomerular basement membrane in Brown-Norway rats. *Nephrol. Dial. Transplant.* 6: 457, 1991.
182. Queluz, T. T., and Andres, G. Pathogenesis of an experimental model of Goodpasture's haemorrhagic pneumonitis. *Nephrol. Dial. Transplant.* [*Suppl.*] 1: 3, 1990.
183. Querin, S., Noel, L. H., Grunfeld, J. P., et al. Linear glomerular IgG fixation in renal allografts: Incidence and significance in Alport's syndrome. *Clin. Nephrol.* 25: 134, 1986.
184. Rajaraman, S., Pinto, J. A., and Cavallo, T. Glomerulonephritis with coexistent immune deposits and antibasement membrane activity. *J. Clin. Pathol.* 37: 176, 1984.
185. Rassoul, Z., Al-Khader, A. A., Al-Sulaiman, M., et al. Recurrent allograft antiglomerular basement membrane glomerulonephritis in a patient with Alport's syndrome. *Am. J. Nephrol.* 10: 73, 1990.
186. Rees, A. J., Demaine, A. G., and Welsh, K. I. Association of immunoglobulin Gm allotypes with antiglomerular basement membrane antibodies and their titre. *Hum. Immunol.* 10: 213, 1984.
187. Rees, A. J., Lockwood, C. M., and Peters, D. K. Enhanced allergic tissue injury in Goodpasture's syndrome by intercurrent bacterial infection. *Br. Med. J.* 2: 723, 1977.
188. Rees, A. J., Lockwood, C. M., and Peters, D. K. Nephritis Due to Antibodies to GBM. In P. Kincaid-Smith, A. J. F. d'Apice, and R. C. Atkins (eds.), *Progress in Glomerulonephritis.* New York: Wiley, 1979. P. 347.
189. Rees, A. J., Peters, D. K., Amos, N., et al. The influence of HLA-linked genes on the severity of anti-GBM antibody-mediated nephritis. *Kidney Int.* 26: 444, 1984.
190. Rees, A. J., Peters, D. K., Compston, D. A. S., et al. Strong association between HLA DRW2 and antibody mediated Goodpasture's syndrome. *Lancet* 1: 966, 1978.
191. Relman, A. S., Dvorak, H. F., and Colvin, R. B. Case records of the Massachusetts General Hospital: Weekly clinicopathological exercises. Case 46-1971. *N. Engl. J. Med.* 285: 1187, 1971.
192. Rennke, H. G., Klein, P. S., and Mendrick, D. L. Cell-mediated immunity in hapten-induced interstitial ne-

phritis and glomerular crescent formation in the rat (abstract). *Kidney Int.* 37: 428, 1990.

193. Reynolds, J., Cashman, S. J., Evans, D. J., and Pusey, C. D. Cyclosporin A in the prevention and treatment of experimental autoimmune glomerulonephritis in the brown Norway rat. *Clin. Exp. Immunol.* 85: 28, 1991.
194. Richman, A. I., Rifkin, S. I., and McAllister, C. J. Rapidly progressive glomerulonephritis. Combined antiglomerular basement membrane antibody and immune complex pathogenesis. *Hum. Pathol.* 12: 597, 1981.
195. Rock, B., Labib, R. S., and Diaz, L. A. Monovalent Fab' immunoglobulin fragments from endemic pemphigus foliaceus autoantibodies reproduce the human disease in neonatal Balb/c mice. *J. Clin. Invest.* 85: 296, 1990.
196. Rock, B., Martins, C. R., Theofilopoulos, A. N., et al. The pathogenic effect of IgG4 autoantibodies in endemic pemphigus foliaceus (fogo selvagem). *N. Engl. J. Med.* 320: 1463, 1989.
197. Rocklin, R. E., Lewis, E. J., and David, J. R. In vitro evidence for cellular hypersensitivity to glomerular basement-membrane antigens in human glomerulonephritis. *N. Engl. J. Med.* 283: 497, 1970.
198. Rusby, N. L., and Wilson, C. Lung purpura with nephritis. *Q. J. Med.* 29: 501, 1980.
199. Sabnis, S. G., Nandedkar, M. A., and Antonovych, T. T. Antiglomerular basement membrane antibody-induced glomerulonephritis with glomerular multinucleated giant cell reaction: A case study. *Am. J. Kidney Dis.* 12: 544, 1988.
200. Sado, Y., and Naito, I. Experimental autoimmune glomerulonephritis in rats by soluble isologous or homologous antigens from glomerular and tubular basement membranes. *Br. J. Exp. Pathol.* 68: 695, 1987.
201. Sado, Y., Naito, I., and Okigaki, T. Transfer of anti-glomerular basement membrane antibody-induced glomerulonephritis in inbred rats with isologous antibodies from the urine of nephritic rats. *J. Pathol.* 158: 325, 1989.
202. Saraf, P., Berger, H. W., and Thung, S. N. Goodpasture's syndrome with no overt renal disease. *Mt. Sinai J. Med.* 45: 451, 1978.
203. Saus, J., Wieslander, J., Langeveld, J. P. M., et al. Identification of the Goodpasture antigen as the α3(IV) chain of collagen IV. *J. Biol. Chem.* 263: 13374, 1988.
204. Savage, C. O. S., Noel, L. H., Crutcher, E., et al. Hereditary nephritis: Immunoblotting studies of the glomerular basement membrane. *Lab. Invest.* 60: 613, 1989.
205. Savage, C. O. S., Pusey, C. D., Bowman, C., et al. Antiglomerular basement membrane antibody mediated disease in the British Isles 1980–4. *Br. Med. J. (Clin. Res.)* 292: 301, 1986.
206. Savage, C. O. S., Pusey, C. D., Kershaw, M. J., et al. The Goodpasture antigen in Alport's syndrome: Studies with a monoclonal antibody. *Kidney Int.* 30: 107, 1986.
207. Savige, J. A., Dowling, J., and Kincaid-Smith, P. Superimposed glomerular immune complexes in anti-glomerular basement membrane disease. *Am. J. Kidney Dis.* 14: 145, 1989.
208. Saxena, R., Bygren, P., Butkowski, R., and Wieslander, J. Specificity of kidney-bound antibodies in Goodpasture's syndrome. *Clin. Exp. Immunol.* 78: 31, 1989.
209. Saxena, R., Bygren, P., Butkowski, R., and Wieslander, J. Entactin: A possible autoantigen in the pathogenesis of non-Goodpasture anti-GBM nephritis. *Kidney Int.* 38: 263, 1990.
210. Saxena, R., Isaksson, B., Bygren, P., and Wieslander, J. A rapid assay for circulating anti-glomerular basement membrane antibodies in Goodpasture syndrome. *J. Immunol. Methods* 118: 73, 1989.
211. Scheer, R. L., and Grossman, M. A. Immune aspects of the glomerulonephritis associated with pulmonary hemorrhage. *Ann. Intern. Med.* 60: 1009, 1964.
212. Schreiner, G. F., Cotran, R. S., Pando, V., and Unanue, E. R. A mononuclear cell component in experimental immunological glomerulonephritis. *J. Exp. Med.* 147: 369, 1978.
213. Schwartz, E. E., Teplick, J., Onesti, G., et al. Pulmonary hemorrhage in renal disease: Goodpasture's syndrome and other causes. *Radiology* 122: 39, 1977.
214. Scott, B., Bluthmann, H., Sia Teh, H., and Von Bohmer, H. The generation of mature T cells requires interaction of the aβ T-cell receptor with major histocompatibility antigens. *Nature* 338: 591, 1989.
215. Segelmark, M., Butkowski, R., and Wieslander, J. Antigen restriction and IgG subclasses among anti-GBM autoantibodies. *Nephrol. Dial. Transplant.* 5: 991, 1990.
216. Shah, B., First, M. R., Mendoza, N. C., et al. Alport's syndrome: Risk of glomerulonephritis induced by anti-glomerular-basement-membrane antibody after renal transplantation. *Nephron* 50: 34, 1988.
217. Simonsen, H., Brun, C., Frokjaer-Thomsen, O., et al. Goodpasture's syndrome in twins. *Acta Med. Scand.* 212: 425, 1982.
218. Simpson, I. J., Doak, P. B., Williams, L. C., et al. Plasma exchange in Goodpasture's syndrome. *Am. J. Nephrol.* 2: 301, 1982.
219. Soininen, R., Huotari, M., Hostikka, S. L., et al. The structural genes for α1 and α2 chains of human type IV collagen are divergently encoded on opposite DNA strands and have an overlapping promoter region. *J. Biol. Chem.* 263: 17217, 1988.
220. Stanton, M. C., and Tange, J. D. Goodpasture's syndrome: Pulmonary haemorrhage associated with glomerulonephritis. *Australas. Ann. Med.* 7: 132, 1958.
221. Steblay, R. W. Glomerulonephritis induced in sheep by injections of heterologous glomerular basement membrane and Freund's complete adjuvant. *J. Exp. Med.* 116: 253, 1962.
222. Steblay, R. W., and Rudofsky, U. H. Experimental autoimmune glomerulonephritis induced by anti-glomerular basement membrane antibody: II. Effects of injecting heterologous, homologous, or autologous glomerular basement membranes and complete Freund's adjuvant into sheep. *Am. J. Pathol.* 113: 125, 1983.
223. Steblay, R. W., and Rudofsky, U. H. Experimental autoimmune antiglomerular basement membrane antibody-induced glomerulonephritis. I. The effects of injecting sheep with human, homologous or autologous lung basement membranes and complete Freund's adjuvant. *Clin. Immunol. Immunopathol.* 27: 65, 1983.
224. Sturgill, B. C., and Westervelt, F. B. Immunofluorescence studies in a case of Goodpasture's syndrome. *J.A.M.A.* 194: 914, 1965.
225. Sutcliffe, N. P., Cashman, S. J., Savage, C. O. S., et al. Variability of the antigenicity of the glomerular basement membrane in nail-patella syndrome. *Nephrol. Dial. Transplant.* 4: 262, 1989.
226. Teague, C. A., Doak, P. B., Simpson, I. J., et al. Goodpasture's syndrome: An analysis of 29 cases. *Kidney Int.* 13: 492, 1978.
227. Teruel, J. L., Liano, F., Mampaso, F., et al. Allograft antiglomerular basement membrane glomerulonephritis in a patient with Alport's syndrome. *Nephron* 46: 43, 1987.
228. Thomson, N. M., Naish, P. F., Simpson, I. J., and Pe-

ters, D. K. The role of C3 in the autologous phase of nephrotoxic nephritis. *Clin. Exp. Immunol.* 24: 464, 1976.

229. Thorner, P. S., Baumal, R., Eddy, A., and Marrano, P. M. A study by immunofluorescence microscopy of the NC1 domain of collagen type IV in glomerular basement membranes of two patients with hereditary nephritis. *Virchows Arch.* [*A*] 416: 205, 1990.
230. Timpl, R., Paulsson, M., Dziadek, M., and Fujiwara, S. Basement membranes. *Methods Enzymol.* 145: 363, 1987.
231. Tipping, P. G., Neale, T. J., and Holdsworth, S. R. T lymphocyte participation in antibody-induced experimental glomerulonephritis. *Kidney Int.* 27: 530, 1985.
232. Tomosugi, N. I., Cashman, S. J., Hay, H., et al. Modulation of antibody-mediated glomerular injury in vivo by bacterial lipopolysaccharide, tumor necrosis factor, and IL-1. *J. Immunol.* 142: 3083, 1989.
233. Turner, N., Mason, P. J., Brown, R., et al. Molecular cloning of the Goodpasture antigen. *J. Clin. Invest.* 89: 592, 1992.
234. Turner, N., and Pusey, C. D. Anti-Glomerular Basement Membrane Disease. In C. D. Pusey (ed.), *The Immunology of Renal Disease*. Lancaster: Kluwer, 1991.
235. Turner, N., and Rees, A. J. Anti-Glomerular Basement Membrane Disease. In S. J. Cameron, A. M. Davison, J.-P. Grunfeld, et al. (eds.), *Oxford Textbook of Nephrology*. Oxford: Oxford University Press, 1991.
236. Unanue, E. R., and Dixon, F. J. Experimental glomerulonephritis: Immunological events and pathogenetic mechanisms. *Adv. Immunol.* 6: 1, 1967.
237. Vangelista, A., Frasca, G. M., Martella, D., and Bonomini, V. Glomerulonephritis in renal transplantation. *Nephrol. Dial. Transplant.* [*Suppl.*] 1: 42, 1990.
238. Van Zyl Smit, R., Rees, A. J., and Peters, D. K. Factors affecting the severity of injury during nephrotoxic nephritis in rabbits. *Clin. Exp. Immunol.* 54: 366, 1983.
239. Volpi, A., Battini, G., Conte, F., et al. Acute renal failure in elderly due to Goodpasture's syndrome. *Nephron* 57: 381, 1991.
240. Wahls, T. L., Bonsib, S. M., and Schuster, V. L. Coexistent Wegener's granulomatosis and anti-glomerular basement membrane disease. *Hum. Pathol.* 18: 202, 1987.
241. Walker, J. F., Watson, A. J., Garrett, P., et al. Goodpasture's syndrome—7 years' experience of two Dublin renal units. *Irish Med. J.* 75: 328, 1982.
242. Walker, R. G., Scheinkestel, C., Becker, G. J., et al. Clinical and morphological aspects of the management of crescentic anti-glomerular basement membrane antibody (anti-GBM) nephritis/Goodpasture's syndrome. *Q. J. Med.* 54: 75, 1985.
243. Weber, M., Kohler, H., Manns, M., et al. Identification of Goodpasture target antigens in basement membranes of human glomeruli, lung, and placenta. *Clin. Exp. Immunol.* 67: 262, 1987.
244. Weber, M., Lohse, A. W., Manns, M., et al. IgG subclass distribution of autoantibodies to glomerular basement membrane in Goodpasture's syndrome compared to other autoantibodies. *Nephron* 49: 54, 1988.
245. Weber, M., Meyer zum Buschenfelde, K. H., and Kohler, H. Immunological properties of the human Goodpasture target antigen. *Clin. Exp. Immunol.* 74: 289, 1988.
246. Weber, M., Pullig, O., and Boesken, W. H. Anti-glomerular basement membrane disease after renal obstruction. *Lancet* ii: 512, 1990.
247. Weber, S., Engel, J., Weidemann, H., et al. Subunit structure and assembly of the globular domain of basement membrane collagen type IV. *Eur. J. Biochem.* 139: 401, 1984.
248. Westberg, N. G., and Michael, A. F. Immunohistopathology of diabetic glomerulonephritis. *Diabetes* 21: 163, 1972.
249. Wheeler, J., Simpson, J., and Morley, A. R. Routine and rapid enzyme linked immunosorbent assays for circulating anti-glomerular basement membrane antibodies. *J. Clin. Pathol.* 41: 163, 1988.
250. Whitworth, J. A., Lawrence, J. R., and Meadows, R. Goodpasture's syndrome. A review of nine cases and an evaluation of therapy. *Aust. N.Z. J. Med.* 4: 167, 1974.
251. Wick, G., von der Mark, H., Dietrich, H., and Timpl, R. Globular domain of basement membrane collagen induces autoimmune pulmonary lesions in mice resembling human Goodpasture disease. *Lab. Invest.* 55: 308, 1986.
252. Wieslander, J., Barr, J. F., Butkowski, R. J., et al. Goodpasture antigen of the glomerular basement membrane: Localization to noncollagenous regions of type IV collagen. *Proc. Natl. Acad. Sci. U.S.A.* 81: 3838, 1984.
253. Wieslander, J., Bygren, P., and Heinegard, D. Antiglomerular basement membrane antibody: Antibody specificity in different forms of glomerulonephritis. *Kidney Int.* 23: 855, 1983.
254. Wieslander, J., Bygren, P. G., and Heinegard, D. Antibasement membrane antibody: Immunoenzymic assay and specificity of antibodies. *Scand. J. Clin. Invest.* 41: 763, 1981.
255. Wieslander, J., and Heinegard, D. The involvement of type IV collagen in Goodpasture's syndrome. *Ann. N.Y. Acad. Sci.* 460: 363, 1985.
256. Wieslander, J., Kataja, M., and Hudson, B. G. Characterization of the human Goodpasture antigen. *Clin. Exp. Immunol.* 69: 332, 1987.
257. Wieslander, J., Langeveld, J., Butkowski, R., et al. Physical and immunochemical studies of the globular domain of Type IV collagen: Cryptic properties of the Goodpasture antigen. *J. Biol. Chem.* 260: 8564, 1985.
258. Williams, P. S., Davenport, A., McDicken, I., et al. Increased incidence of anti-glomerular basement membrane antibody (anti-GBM) nephritis in the Mersey region, September 1984–October 1985. *Q. J. Med.* 68: 727, 1988.
259. Willoughby, W. F., and Dixon, F. J. Experimental hemorrhagic pneumonitis produced by heterologous antilung antibody. *J. Immunol.* 104: 28, 1970.
260. Wilson, C. B. Nephritogenic Immune Responses Involving Basement Membrane and Other Antigens in or of the Glomerulus. In N. B. Cummings, A. F. Michael, and C. B. Wilson (eds.), *Immune Mechanisms in Renal Disease*. New York: Plenum, 1983. P. 233.
261. Wilson, C. B., and Dixon, F. J. Anti-glomerular basement membrane antibody-induced glomerulonephritis. *Kidney Int.* 3: 74, 1973.
262. Wilson, C. B., and Dixon, F. J. Diagnosis of immunopathologic renal disease. (Editorial) *Kidney Int.* 5: 389, 1974.
263. Wilson, C. B., and Dixon, F. J. The Renal Response to Immunological Injury. In B. M. Brenner and F. C. Rector (eds.), *The Kidney*, 2nd ed. Philadelphia: Saunders, 1981.
264. Wilson, C. B., Dixon, F. J., Evans, A. S., and Glassock, R. J. Antiviral antibody responses in patients with renal diseases. *Clin. Immunol. Immunopathol.* 2: 121, 1973.
265. Wilson, C. B., and Smith, R. C. Goodpasture's syndrome associated with influenza A_2 virus infection. *Ann. Intern. Med.* 76: 91, 1972.
266. Wraith, D. C., McDevitt, H. O., Steinman, L., and Acha-Orbea, H: T cell recognition as the target for immune

intervention of autoimmune disease. *Cell* 57: 709, 1989.

267. Wu, M. J., Moorthy, A. V., and Beirne, G. J. Relapse in anti-glomerular basement membrane antibody mediated crescentic glomerulonephritis. *Clin. Nephrol.* 13: 97, 1980.
268. Wu, M.-J., Rajaram, R., Shelp, W. D., et al. Vasculitis in Goodpasture's syndrome. *Arch. Pathol. Lab. Med.* 104: 300, 1980.
269. Yamamoto, T., and Wilson, C. B. Binding of anti-basement membrane antibody to alveolar basement membrane after intratracheal gasoline instillation in rabbits. *Am. J. Pathol.* 126: 497, 1987.
270. Yoshioka, K., Iseki, T., Okada, M., et al. Identification of Goodpasture antigens in human alveolar basement membrane. *Clin. Exp. Immunol.* 74: 419, 1988.
271. Yoshioka, K., Kleppel, M., and Fish, A. J. Analysis of nephritogenic antigens in human glomerular basement membrane by two-dimensional gel electrophoresis. *J. Immunol.* 134: 3831, 1985.
272. Yoshioka, K., Michael, A. F., Velosa, J., and Fish, A. J. Detection of hidden nephritogenic antigen determinants in human renal and nonrenal basement membranes. *Am. J. Pathol.* 121: 156, 1985.
273. Zimmerman, S. W., Varanasi, M. R., and Hoff, B. Goodpasture's syndrome with normal renal function. *Am. J. Med.* 66: 163, 1979.

The Long-Term Outcome of Glomerular Diseases

J. Stewart Cameron

At first sight, the task of describing the outcome of a particular disease seems to be a simple one; but, in fact, nothing could be further from the truth.

First, we have the problem of definition, i.e., what the "disease" under consideration may be. Without getting into a deep philosophical discussion of what the word *disease* signifies, at a practical level, a number of difficulties arise. First, the very idea of a disease in its own right is an abstraction: as many clinicians emphasize, there are no diseases—only diseased patients—so that, in essence, we are describing the behavior and fate of groups of patients. But how are they to be defined for inclusion in a study?

Immediately, new problems arise, because there are no hard boundaries to the disease we are dealing with in the glomerulus. There are a variety of *clinical presentations* that can be defined but have, in real life, fluid boundaries; there are *histologic appearances,* both on optical and immunofluorescence microscopy, between which there is no one-to-one correspondence; and, finally, there are proved or (more usually) probable *precipitating events,* organisms, or multisystem diseases that affect other organs. I have discussed elsewhere [69], in more detail, the problems that arise from these different levels of description and the lack of one-to-one correspondence between them. To cite an example, when we come to consider the outcome of acute glomerulonephritis, we meet accounts in the literature of patients with the clinical presentation of acute glomerulonephritis, many or all of whom did not have a renal biopsy; we have other accounts of patients with a similar presentation, but in whom a streptococcal etiology was established by cultures or antibody titers, with or without biopsies; and we have accounts of patients with streptococcal glomerulonephritis, some of whom had mesangiocapillary glomerulonephritis on biopsy, or severe crescents. There will inevitably be discrepancies in the conclusions drawn as to outcome from these similar, but not identical, groups.

A further difficulty arises because, almost certainly, some of the histologic appearances seen in the diseased glomerulus—for example, membranous nephropathy—are no more single diseases than the broad clinical features they present to medical attention. We must think of these as appearances—*patterns of glomerular injury*—rather than diseases. There may be several different pathogenetic routes into a single histologic appearance, and each of these may have a different outcome. If we cannot distinguish, or are ignorant of, these subgroups, then a different mix of the subgroups inevitably will lead to different descriptions of outcome.

The second major problem is more obvious but equally neglected when looking at follow-up data from diverse sources: this is the question of *patient selection* (Fig. 69-1). The only unassailable data are those that derive from a population survey in which techniques that will select *all* the patients with a particular condition are applied, and those patients are followed up completely. Such studies do not exist in the study of glomerular diseases. Many of the conditions we discuss in this chapter exist undiagnosed in the population, such as IgA-associated glomerulopathy, minimal change disease, and membranous nephropathy, without ever being detected. The more diligently the population is examined, and the more frequently the urine is tested, the more such "patients" (who are, in fact, symptomless individuals) will be detected.

The second stage of selection is when these patients *are* discovered; just how far are they studied or referred for investigation? Many proteinurias and hematurias discovered on routine examination of healthy persons for insurance purposes may not be followed up.

Specialist centers also will attract, by their skills in management, patients who present considerable problems, and it is often from such centers that descriptions of outcome are published. It is usual for these first studies to present an over-pessimistic outlook for the disease, and subsequent recognition of milder, more indolent forms may restore the balance with, apparently, a decrease in the gravity of the condition. Thus the best outlook probably approximates more closely to the true description of outcome for the general population existing in the world as a whole.

Even if referred, a crucial question is whether or not a renal biopsy is performed. Since the criteria for many of the conditions discussed in this chapter depend on the availability of renal biopsy data, this point is crucial. It is often impossible to know exactly what the criteria for renal biopsy in a particular unit at a particular time may have been, because the authors do not tell us. Usually most adult patients with a nephrotic syndrome, or profuse proteinuria, are subjected to renal biopsy. The policy for biopsy in patients having isolated minor (0.5–1.5 gm per 24 hours) proteinuria, isolated hematuria, or hematuria with minor proteinuria is particularly variable, between units and in different countries, sometimes depending on nonmedical factors, such as the local availability of skills and funding structures for medical investigations. The presence or absence of routine screening of populations, e.g., military inductees, will depend on whether or not military service is obligatory.

Even when a population of patients, however gathered, is available for study, fall out begins as patients are lost to follow-up. Diligent work will often lead, even 10 to 40 years later, to more than 90 percent of "lost" patients being recovered, but very often the data available may be limited to those who are alive or dead or whether they are in good health or not. Built into any system of follow-up, however, is the inevitable fact that some patients enter the study early and some later, so that the length of follow-up may vary from 1 to 2 years or up to several decades. How can we best handle these incomplete data to extract the best information from them?

First, it is clear that, in the end, all diseases result in

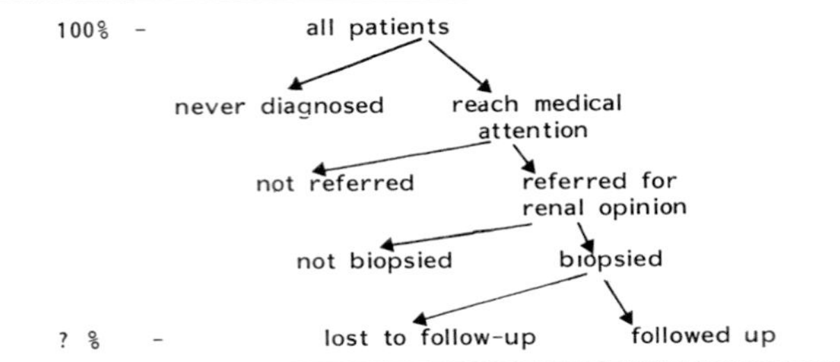

100% - all patients

never diagnosed — reach medical attention

not referred — referred for renal opinion

not biopsied — biopsied

? % - lost to follow-up — followed up

Fig. 69-1. The various levels of patient selection, which confuse descriptions of diseases and their outcome.

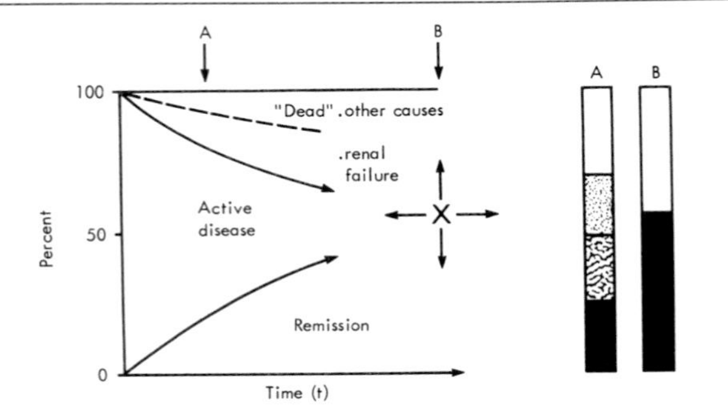

Fig. 69-2. A generalized diagram to describe the outcome of a glomerular disease. Vertically, the proportion of patients in a given state is shown: dead (either incidentally or as a result of the glomerular disease), with continued proteinuria, or in remission. The *time* (t) at which the final state of all patients being either in remission or dead will be reached will depend on the aggression of the disease; and the *proportion* dead or in remission, on its severity. If a cross section of patients is studied at times A or B, a proportion of patients will still have active disease, with or without impairment of renal function, as represented in the bar graphs at the right. Diagrams such as these can be used to summarize the outcome of glomerular diseases, the curves being calculated by the best estimate obtained from life table analysis of the necessarily incomplete data (see text).

one of two states: either the patient is dead (or on dialysis) or the disease is healed (Fig. 69-2). The proportion of patients that follow each of these two courses can vary from 1 : 99 to 99 : 1. Equally, the time that this evolution takes may vary: in practice, most glomerular diseases have run their course within 15 to 20 years at most of apparent onset, with the possible exception of IgA-associated nephropathies, which appear to have a slower evolution. This statement brings up yet another difficulty: When did the disease *really* start? What we actually have on record is the earliest point at which it reached clinical attention or, in retrospect, when the patient had symptoms, e.g., frothy urine or edema. In the case of symptomless hematuria and proteinuria, this point may be years or even decades from the true onset.

The next problem is to describe outcome. A technique that is much used in this area, and that will appear throughout this chapter, is that of the actuarial life table, usually presented in graphical form as a survival curve. It is worth discussing here the strengths and limitations of this technique, which is discussed in detail by Peto et al. [376], to which the reader is referred. It was first developed by actuaries to provide estimates of survival of populations—for example, at different ages—mainly for insurance purposes. It was first applied in medicine to studies of cancer data and was first used in renal disease in the middle 1960s to analyze transplant survival; finally in the early 1970s, it was introduced to the study of glomerular disease and has become popular as its advantages have been recognized.

Life tables were originally designed for large populations—thousands or tens of thousands—whereas in medical practice, it is rarely used for the analysis of more than a few hundred persons, especially for relatively rare diseases, such as those affecting the glomeruli; many series involve two figures only. The importance of this finding is that, like any statistical estimate, the potential error of the estimate achieved will increase sharply when small numbers are under consideration. In general terms, all the data on glomerular diseases deal only with small (or very small) numbers of patients.

The life table technique produces an *estimate* often referred to as Kaplan-Meier [266] estimate of what the behavior of the population at risk *might be* if all patients were followed for the full period under analysis. As already noted, this is almost never the case except for very short follow-up periods. The lines in a figure may be drawn in a bold fashion, but it is the possible error—usually expressed as the standard error for each point on the life table—that is crucial. For example, an estimated population survival at 10 years of 60 percent may have 95 percent confidence limits of from 20 to 90 percent, so that the estimate is almost useless for purposes of comparison; in fact, the only valid method of comparison between two life tables is to compare the whole curve with the contrasted one, that is, assuming that the two populations are comparable [376], which is almost never the case except in carefully randomized, prospective controlled studies.

With these reservations in mind, we can examine how a life table is constructed. There are several ways to do this in detail, and a number of computer programs are available. For any period under study, first the number of patients "at risk" of having the event in question is calculated. The event can be any event of interest—loss of proteinuria, entry into end-stage renal disease, or death, for example. The number of individuals at risk throughout the interval in question clearly is related to the number of patients being followed at the start of the interval. However, it will be less than this number, since some patients will be lost from follow-up during the interval.

The "risk" of experiencing the event is given by the number experiencing the event divided by the number at risk, which gives a figure somewhere between 0 and 1,000; subtracted from 1,000, this will give a survival rate for the period in question. A series of such ratios can be calculated for successive periods of any chosen length, the shortest being the best. A series of successive survival ratios will be generated, and when multiplied by each other sequentially, will give a cumulative survival ratio; this is the survival curve of the population under study. A life table looks like Table 69-1, which actually shows data for type I mesangiocapillary glomerulonephritis in our own unit, with the event being terminal renal failure.

The calculation of a standard error at any point on the curve is possible using the following formula:

$$\text{Cumulative survival rate}\sqrt{\frac{1 - \text{cumulative survival rate}}{\text{number at risk}}}$$

and two life-table curves can be compared for the statistical difference between them by statistics discussed by Kaplan and Meier [266] and, more recently, by Peto et al. [376] and Breslow [58]. In essence, this procedure is a X^2 test, weighted by the distribution of the data in the life table.

Obviously, it is possible, by drawing up a life table for terminal renal failure and another for loss of proteinuria, to generate a diagram of the type shown in Fig. 69-2 for any given glomerular condition or group of patients. Programs are available to construct life tables on microprocessors from raw data of dates of entry and the date of event or most recent follow-up. If doing it by hand, the first task is to arrange all the patients under study in order of decreasing follow-up, whatever the reason for exiting from the follow-up may be. If one wishes purely to examine the rate of entry into uremia, rather than true survival, then death from unrelated causes can be treated as "lost to follow-up" for the purposes of analysis. This may seem bizarre, but a similar problem arises in the analysis of transplantation data when immunologic graft loss is being examined and a patient dies of another cause with a functioning graft.

This, of course, raises the difficult problem of deaths from other causes in any study. Clearly, in the end all the patients in the study will be dead, including those who are in remission. Clearly also, the numbers of those dying within a decade or two of other causes than uremia will increase sharply if the mean age of the population under study is over 50 years. Ideally, any life-table analysis should include the expected life table for the population at risk, assuming no renal diseases were present. In Western countries, at 35 years of age, at least 95 percent of patients will survive 15 years and thus, in the case of most glomerular diseases that affect predominantly a young population, the effect of neglecting expected mortality is trivial. However, only 85 percent of 60-year-olds will survive a decade, the average survival being 20 years for females and 18 years for males; at 65 years, the corresponding figures are 16 and 12 years. Thus for some diseases, such as membranous nephropathy and vasculitis, some account of this issue may be considered.

It is not always clear what should be considered to be other causes of death and, especially, what role secondary hypertension may play, both as a direct cause of death and as a cause of accelerated decline in renal function. Vascular disease, similarly, would be considered by some as a possible complication of a persisting nephrotic syndrome. How should deaths from complications of

Table 69-1. Life table for 69 patients with type I mesangiocapillary glomerulonephritis*

Time interval (years)	Number entering interval	Number leaving interval	Number of events† during interval	Number "at risk" during interval‡	Interval event rate	Interval survival rate	Cumulative survival rate
0–1	69	66	2	68.5	0.029	0.971	0.971
1–2	66	63	1	65.5	0.015	0.985	0.956
2–3	63	55	4	62.0	0.065	0.935	0.894
3–4	55	98	4	53.5	0.075	0.925	0.827
4–5	48	43	5	48.0	0.104	0.896	0.741
5–6	43	38	1	41.0	0.024	0.976	0.723
6–7	38	34	2	36.5	0.054	0.946	0.684
7–8	34	31	2	33.5	0.060	0.940	0.643
8–9	31	26	1	29.0	0.034	0.966	0.621
9–10	26	23	0	24.5	0.000	1.000	0.621
10–11	23	19	4	23.0	0.174	0.826	0.512
11–12	19	15	0	16.5	0.000	1.000	0.512
12–13	15	13	0	14.0	0.000	1.000	0.512
13–14	13	11	0	12.5	0.000	1.000	0.512
14–15	11	11	0	11.0	0.000	1.000	0.512
15–16	11	7	0	9.0	0.000	1.000	0.512
16–17	7						

*Data of Cameron et al., 1983 [90].
†Death or terminal renal failure.
‡Enter + leave + events.

therapy be treated for statistical purposes? Clearly, they are the result of the disease, but the treatment may not be appropriate to some observers.

Thus the technique of life tables allows us to make a description of the general, average outcome of a glomerular disease or its appearances; but, of course, this is not what the patient wants to know. He or she wishes to know what their own *individual outcome* will be, and from the data on population, the doctor can make only the most general statements of risk. The possible evolution of the individual patients can be made more precise by attempting to assess the predictive value of various individual characteristics. At a clinical level, such observations as the presence or absence of hematuria in a proteinuric patient, the degree and persistence of proteinuria, and the presence or absence of hypertension or reduced renal function can be examined; and on histology, various glomerular and tubulointerstitial or vascular features can be assessed for their effect on prognosis. The crude way to do this is simply to examine the outcome of patients with and without a certain feature (*univariate* analysis), but this process ignores possible interactions, either purely statistical or causative, that may relate to certain features. This requires simultaneous *multivariate analysis,* for which a number of methods are available.

Perhaps the best technique for this analysis is Cox's method of proportional hazards [120]. This technique has been applied surprisingly little to the study of glomerular disease (but see [50, 130, 148, 316, 485]), perhaps because the number of patients under study are so small that the technique may not be appropriate, but perhaps also because of ignorance of the technique. Analysis by the Cox method can only be calculated by the use of a computer program, but it is included in the widely available SPSS and BDMP software packages. A discussion on the use of the Cox model and related statistics in renal data can be found in the paper of Beukhof and colleagues [50].

Obviously, the progress of proteinuria and indices of renal function, such as plasma creatinine and the glomerular filtration rate (GFR), followed sequentially, are some of the most powerful tools to allow individual prediction. For example, it has become apparent that functional progression rarely, if ever, occurs in proteinuric renal disease if the proteinuria falls to normal limits even for a short while [373], although hypertensive damage is possible subsequently. Also, the persistence of profuse proteinuria within or near the nephrotic range in patients with structurally disordered glomeruli (i.e., other than minimal change) is a clear indicator of a poorer prognosis in the majority of patients with this phenomenon (see Fig. 69-4).

The behavior of the plasma creatinine also has been the subject of much study. Mitch et al. observed [337] that GFR varies as $1/P_{creat}$ and several papers [403] have emphasized that the plot of $1/P_{creat}$ against time may be relatively linear, the slope being characteristic for each individual patient. In fact, the linearity of such plots has been greatly exaggerated, and the r value for plots, even with the best fit, rarely, if ever, exceeds 0.70 [201]. Study of glomerular diseases confirms this point, and while membranous nephropathy shows relatively linear plots [132], study of data from the Medical Research Council trial in the United Kingdom [86] showed that only 18 of 41 nephrotic membranous patients with a decline in renal function showed substantially linear falloff in reciprocal creatinine plots. Similarly, Fellin and colleagues [166] found few patients with IgA nephropathy whose decline in renal function could be described in a single slope of $1/P_{creat}$. Mesangiocapillary glomerulonephritis often shows a markedly nonlinear pattern [71] with sudden falloffs in renal function that are not associated with hypertension even after periods of relatively stable function. Also, the predictive value of the P_{creat} for the GFR has been overemphasized; changes occur with changes in diet and muscle mass, and conversely, a constant creatinine may conceal a falloff in GFR. The use and misuse of reciprocal and other functions of plasma creatinine have been reviewed by Walser [477], Hunsicker [245], and Levey [304].

One interesting observation [86, 132] is that for the main groups of progressive, proteinuric glomerular diseases (membranous nephropathy, focal segmental glomerulosclerosis, and mesangiocapillary glomerulonephritis), progressive disease usually reveals itself by a detectable falloff in GFR and a rise in plasma creatinine within 3 or so years of onset. Together with the observations on the presence and persistence of proteinuria mentioned previously, this information allows a better individual prognosis to be given quite early in the course of the disease.

In this chapter, for reasons of brevity, I have dealt mainly with recently published observations on the outcome of glomerular disease, published in 1979 or later. For a more detailed consideration of the literature up to 1978, the reader is referred to my previous chapter on the subject [71]. Given that an etiologic classification is still beyond our grasp, this chapter is organized in a conventional fashion around the usual histologic classification of glomerular disease [101], recognizing its limitations.

The Overall Prognosis of the Nephrotic Syndrome

Unlike symptomless patients with hematuria or proteinuria, patients who have the nephrotic syndrome are likely to be referred for medical attention and very likely to have a renal biopsy as part of their investigation. It is still usual to biopsy all adult patients with onset nephrotic syndrome, and older data exist for unselected series of biopsied children with nephrotic syndrome; however, it is now no longer usual to biopsy all cases, especially those between the ages of 1 and 5 years.

The outcome of a nephrotic syndrome depends on four sets of circumstances: complications of the nephrotic syndrome, the effects of proteinuria itself, the influence of underlying histopathology, and the response to treatment.

COMPLICATIONS OF THE NEPHROTIC STATE

Now only a minority of nephrotic children or adults die as a result of complications of the nephrotic state, because it is often forgotten how brief the nephrotic state may now be. In the study of Wass et al. [483], only one-third of adults with a nephrotic syndrome remained nephrotic 4 years later, the remainder having either progressed to renal failure with diminution of proteinuria and disappearance of edema or remitted spontaneously as a result of treatment. Today an even smaller proportion of children with nephrotic syndrome have a persistent course. The majority of children have minimal change lesions, and these will either remit within 3 years spontaneously (two-thirds) or have earlier remissions secondary to treatment with corticosteroids or cytotoxic agents (95%) (see below). In our own data, reviewed in Trompeter et al. [461], we found that after 15 to 20 years, only 3 percent of an unselected cohort of children with biopsy-proved minimal change nephrotic syndrome still had active disease.

Similarly, in a study of 89 adults with onset of minimal change nephrotic syndrome over the age of 15 years [361], after 2 to 24 years, follow-up of 80 percent of 74 surviving patients were in complete remission, and only 5 had a persisting nephrotic syndrome. Thus in contrast to the past experience, neither of these groups of patients is exposed to possible risks of complications for prolonged periods. However, the minority of adults and children who do suffer severe and prolonged proteinuria are very much at risk for complications. Many of these individuals, especially nephrotic patients in childhood and young adult life, have lesions of focal segmental glomerulosclerosis that is resistant to treatment with corticosteroids and cytotoxic drugs. In these unfortunates, a full nephrotic syndrome may progress to renal failure and even, on occasion, to dialysis, so that nephrectomy or renal infarction may be required [314]. This latter outcome is rarely seen with other forms of glomerular disease, but it may occur with primary amyloidosis, and we have seen it very rarely in mesangiocapillary glomerulonephritis.

Infections. Although their importance is still evident, in the past infections played an even more important role in determining the outcome for the nephrotic patient [89]. For example, the data of Arneil [21] from the Sick Children's Hospital in Glasgow, Scotland, suggest that during the preantibiotic era, more than half of nephrotic children were dead by 5 years from onset, the majority of infections within the first 2 years. There are no data from this period from a single source dealing with adult-onset nephrotic patients, but perusal of accounts in the literature of the 1920s and 1930s [100] suggests that the clinical picture was similar, although (as today) primary pneumococcal peritonitis seems to have been confined to children and adolescents. This is because they have yet to develop specific antibody against pneumococcal polysaccharides and thus are dependent on nonspecific immunity resting on the activity of the alternative pathway of complement, which is much reduced in nephrotics because of protein losses into the urine [89].

Hyperlipidemia. The most contentious area of risk is the possible danger of accelerated vascular disease from the hyperlipidemia of the nephrotic syndrome [89, 318, 482, 483]. In considering this problem, it may be forgotten that the majority of nephrotic patients with persistent nephrotic syndrome also have hypertension, and this is an even stronger risk factor for myocardial and other vascular disease than hyperlipidemia [425]. In almost all forms of progressive human glomerulonephritis with nephrotic syndrome, immune complexes will be present in the circulation to a greater or lesser extent. A further risk thus arises from possible interactions of immune complexes in the circulation, with dietary atherogenic stimuli, of themselves insufficient to induce disease. It has been shown in rabbits [329], baboons [240], monkeys [439], and mice [168] that such an interaction is present, and it is certain that long-term survivors of severe lupus nephritis suffer precocious and accelerated myocardial disease [57, 214, 332]. It is difficult in human nephrotic patients with lupus to dissect the various possible contributions of such interactions, such as hypertension, uremia, and corticosteroids, but the contribution of the hyperlipidemia—present in only a minority—does not seem to be a large one. In contrast to our carefully controlled population study in the United Kingdom [483], a similar-sized recent study in California did identify increased risk of myocardial infarction in a cohort of adult-onset nephrotic patients [368]; the many genetic and environmental differences between the two populations may, of course, be important.

On balance, it seems probable that the major hyperlipidemia of persisting severe nephrotic syndrome *does* lead to an increased risk of myocardial vascular disease, especially in the very small minority of nephrotic patients with low high-density lipoprotein (HDL) levels. Perhaps these unusual persons with prolonged nephrotic syndrome need to be identified and managed differently from those with relatively transient nephrotic syndromes lasting weeks, months, or a few years at most and with normal or even raised HDL concentrations in their serum, even though there may be considerable rises in both low-density lipoprotein (LDL) and very-low-density lipoprotein (VLDL) and, with them, total cholesterol and triglyceride fat [318, 482].

Thrombosis. The third major risk besides infection and vascular disease is thrombosis [76, 89]. This prothrombotic state arises mainly from platelet hyperaggregability, itself the result of platelet–von Willebrand factor interaction and possibly increased availability of arachidonic acid to form aggregant prostaglandins. Major alterations in fluid-phase coagulation proteins and their regulators (such as antithrombin III) seem to be almost confined to severe nephrotic syndromes, with a serum albumin concentration below 20 gm/dl. Unlike the risk of vascular disease, thrombosis may strike within only a few days or weeks of onset and, although rare, may attack most tragically those with the most reversible of nephrotic syndromes, because their proteinuria is great and their hypoalbuminemia and alterations in other proteins such as von Willebrand factor profound.

Prevention of Complications of the Nephrotic State. To what extent any of these risks can be minimized is controversial. Prophylactic treatment of children with a severe active nephrotic syndrome using penicillin seems sensible, and prompt treatment of cellulitis or septicemia is almost always successful. The role of hypolipidemic agents has until recently been doubtful because they were relatively ineffective, in turn because of unacceptable side effects. Now with the introduction of agents such as the statins, which are effective in reversing nephrotic hyperlipidemia in the short term [269, 391], the whole question of prophylaxis needs reexamination.

The question of prophylaxis against thrombosis of active severe nephrotic syndromes with anticoagulants remains contentious also [76, 89]. Warfarin seems to most observers too dangerous except in established thrombosis. Antiplatelet agents are attractive because of their low toxicity, but there are no long-term data to support their use. As a rule, 20 to 40 mg of acetylsalicylate per day would seem to be the most effective, since dipyridamole has not been proved to be effective alone in preventing thrombosis. What the risks of such treatment, together with high-dose or maintenance corticosteroids, may be has not been established, but they are probably low. Perhaps it is more important to remember that excessive use of diuretics may help to increase hematocrit and, with it, blood viscosity and thrombotic potential.

PROTEINURIA AS A FACTOR IN PROGRESSION

The second major area of risk in the nephrotic syndrome is the *proteinuria itself* [82]. It is well known that progression into renal failure in the absence of proteinuria almost never occurs in glomerular disease [373], although exceptions occur [324, 325, 458]. One exception is, of course, when secondary hypertension appears after apparent "healing" of the original disease. On the other hand, as shown in Figs. 69-3 and 69-4, progression is almost always accompanied by proteinuria in excess of 2 gm per 24 hours and usually within the nephrotic range. The prognosis of patients with the same glomerular histopathology is worse when a nephrotic syndrome is present, as demonstrated in Fig. 69-3 and confirmed by Williams et al. [492] and Hunt and colleagues [246]. In focal segmental glomerulosclerosis [42, 91], membranous nephropathy [74, 82, 156], and mesangiocapillary glomerulonephritis [96], the prognosis is markedly worse for nephrotic patients compared with patients who were never nephrotic. Further, if one plots proteinuria against rate of progression of renal disease [492], then the greater the proteinuria, the more rapid the falloff in renal function.

Two interpretations of these data are possible [82]. Either profuse continuing proteinuria is a marker for more severe and eventually more serious disease, or profuse persisting proteinuria is, of itself, damaging and leads to acceleration of the original disease process or to secondary glomerulosclerosis, for example by increased macromolecular traffic through the mesangial and/or epithelial cells, or to interstitial scarring by increased protein traffic through the tubular cells.

There is much current interest in these hypotheses, given that it has proved possible to reduce proteinuria in glomerular diseases using a variety of agents: nonsteroidal anti-inflammatory agents (NSAIDs), angiotensin converting enzyme (ACE) inhibitors, cyclosporin, dipyridamole, and low-protein diets (see [82] for review). One fact seems clear from all these studies: the reduction in proteinuria, when achieved, is always accompanied by a concomitant fall in glomerular filtration rate and filtration fraction, which, however, accounts for only about half the reduction of proteinuria with NSAIDs, less with ACE inhibitors and dipyridamole.

An interesting exception to these general rules may be lupus nephritis, however [92, 476], but the outcome of this disease is more affected by treatment than all the previously mentioned glomerular diseases, and, in most series, different treatments have been used for patients with severe nephritis and a nephrotic syndrome compared to those with neither. Thus today, survival of patients with severe diffuse proliferative lupus nephritis has improved to equal that of those beginning with focal or mesangial disease, some of whom may later develop more severe lesions (see the discussion later in this chapter).

Fig. 69-3. A. A plot of reciprocal creatinines from patients with three often progressive forms of glomerulopathy: focal segmental glomerulosclerosis, membranous nephropathy, and mesangiocapillary glomerulonephritis. The data are taken from a prospective study of glomerular disease undertaken in the South East Thames Region, 1972–1974 (Trounson et al., unpublished data). The proteinuria at the various follow-up points is indicated by the solid circle if over 2 gm per 24 hours. It can be seen that the majority of patients with a fall off in renal function during subsequent follow-up had persisting proteinuria above this level, whereas the majority of patients who did well (most of whom initially had proteinuria within this range) had proteinuria that diminished or disappeared. B. Life table survival of patients with the same three conditions as shown in *A* but drawn from patients seen at Guy's Hospital only. In each histological group (focal segmental glomerulosclerosis, membranous nephropathy, and mesangiocapillary glomerulonephritis), the prognosis of patients with a nephrotic syndrome at onset (NS+) is markedly poorer than those who were never nephrotic (NS−).

Sixty Adult Patients with MCGN, FSGS, or Membranous Nephropathy Followed Prospectively

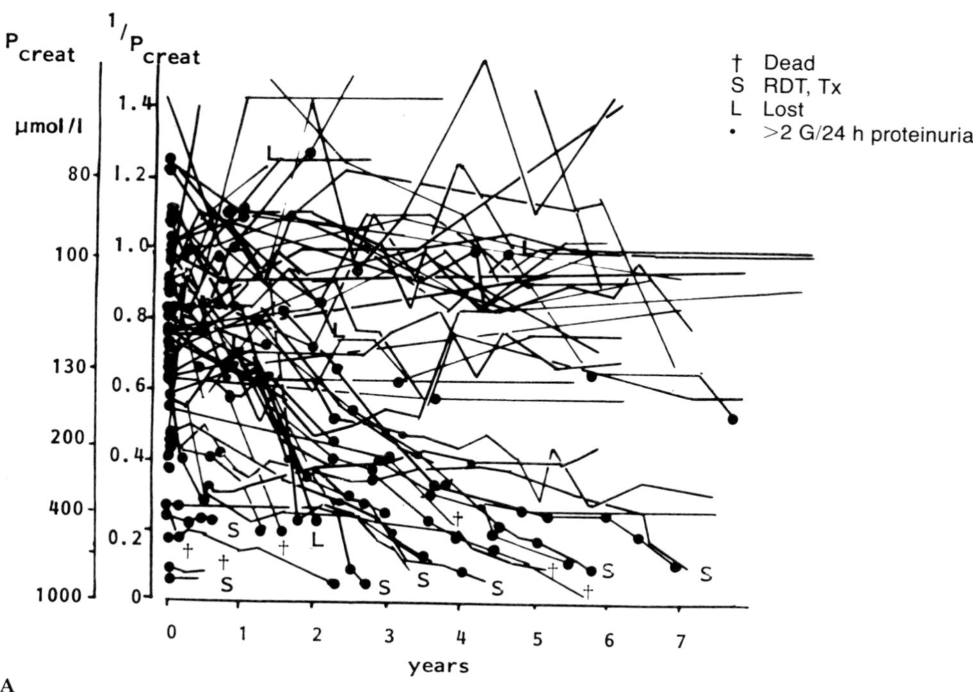

A

Survival in Patients with and without a Nephrotic Syndrome at Onset

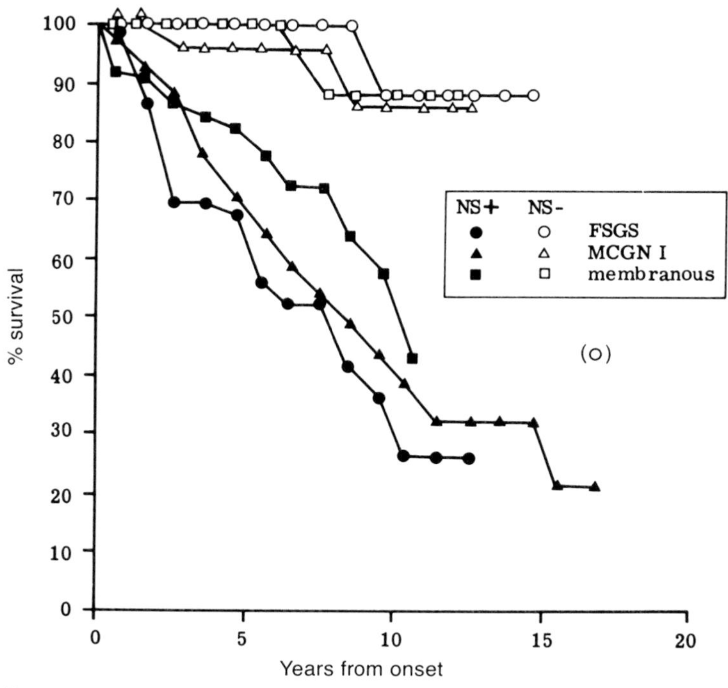

B

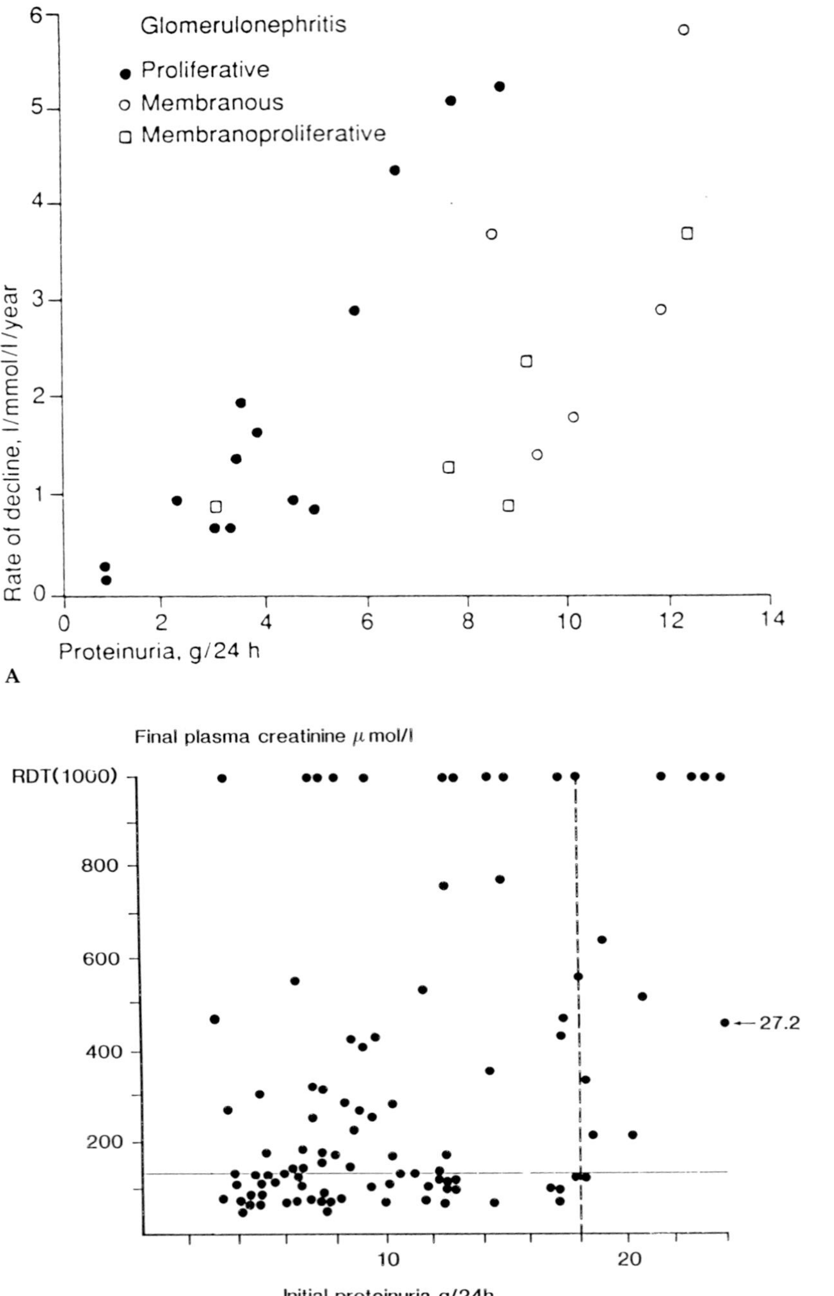

Fig. 69-4. The important relationship of outcome to quantity of proteinuria is further examined by correlating plasma creatinine concentration during follow-up and the quantity of proteinuria at presentation. A. Various forms of glomerular diseases. The relationship between initial proteinuria and rate of change in the $1/P_{creat}$ holds for all. (Data from Williams et al. [492].) B. Unpublished data from the trial of the British Medical Research Council trial [85] in membranous nephropathy. The plasma creatinine after a mean follow-up of 4 years is plotted against the mean of two consecutive 24-hour urine protein excretions taken before entry to the trial. Although the scatter is large, there is a highly significant correlation between the two sets of data ($r = 0.56$, $p < 0.01$). Note that all but 2 of patients excreting more than 18 gm/24 hour of protein developed renal insufficiency within 4 years. RDT = regular dialysis treatment.

RENAL HISTOPATHOLOGY

The third factor that determines prognosis for the nephrotic patient is, of course, the histologic appearances seen on renal biopsy, which, despite many reservations, remains overall the best guide to the nature and prognosis of the syndrome—although this has been challenged [245, 270, 304a]. I have reviewed the general prognosis of the various aspects of the histopathologic appearances in detail elsewhere [71] and in the following discussion. However, a number of general points may be made here.

The first point is to examine the *differing underlying histologic appearances*, especially because they are different at various ages and in different parts of the world. In Fig. 69-5 and Table 69-2 are shown data from the series of nearly 600 adult-onset nephrotic patients seen at Guy's Hospital in London between 1965 and 1990. The data for the childhood-onset cases in Figs. 69-5 and 69-6 are from the data of the International Study of Kidney Disease in Childhood (ISKDC) on 490 unselected nephrotic children and almost 200 childhood-onset patients seen at Guy's before 1970, during which time all children presenting with a nephrotic syndrome were biopsied. The main categories shown account for almost 99 percent of all nephrotic patients, and a few others are discussed later. The increase in the proportion of patients with membranous nephropathy with increasing age at onset is obvious. While amyloidosis is rare under the age of 40, primary amyloid is a relatively common cause of a nephrotic syndrome in the elderly. The younger patients (especially in countries with a significant incidence of familial Mediterranean fever) usually have secondary amyloidosis. Lupus has the usual distribution (from 15 to 50 years of age) in the nephrotic syndrome as in all lupus patients with or without a nephrotic syndrome. Focal segmental sclerosis is present at all ages, from neonates until old age, while the proportion of minimal change patients declines steadily from the age of 3 to the age of 20 years, but, thereafter, remains rather constant; about one-fifth of patients with the nephrotic syndrome at all ages in adult life show minimal change lesions in their renal biopsies.

In Fig. 69-5 is concealed, by its percentage format, the variation in the overall incidence of the nephrotic syndrome at various ages. In Fig. 69-6 is displayed the absolute numbers in the ISKDC study. The incidence of

Fig. 69-5. The underlying histopathologic appearances from a series of 607 nephrotic patients with onset over the age of 15 years, studied at Guy's from 1963 to 1984. The childhood data are derived from 521 patients studied by the ISKDC and 200 patients studied at Guy's before 1970, during which time all childhood nephrotic patients were biopsied. The curves have been smoothed to simplify the diagram, but the adult data are shown in Table 69-2, and the childhood data are shown in more detail in Fig. 69-5. (From [84] with permission of the publishers.)

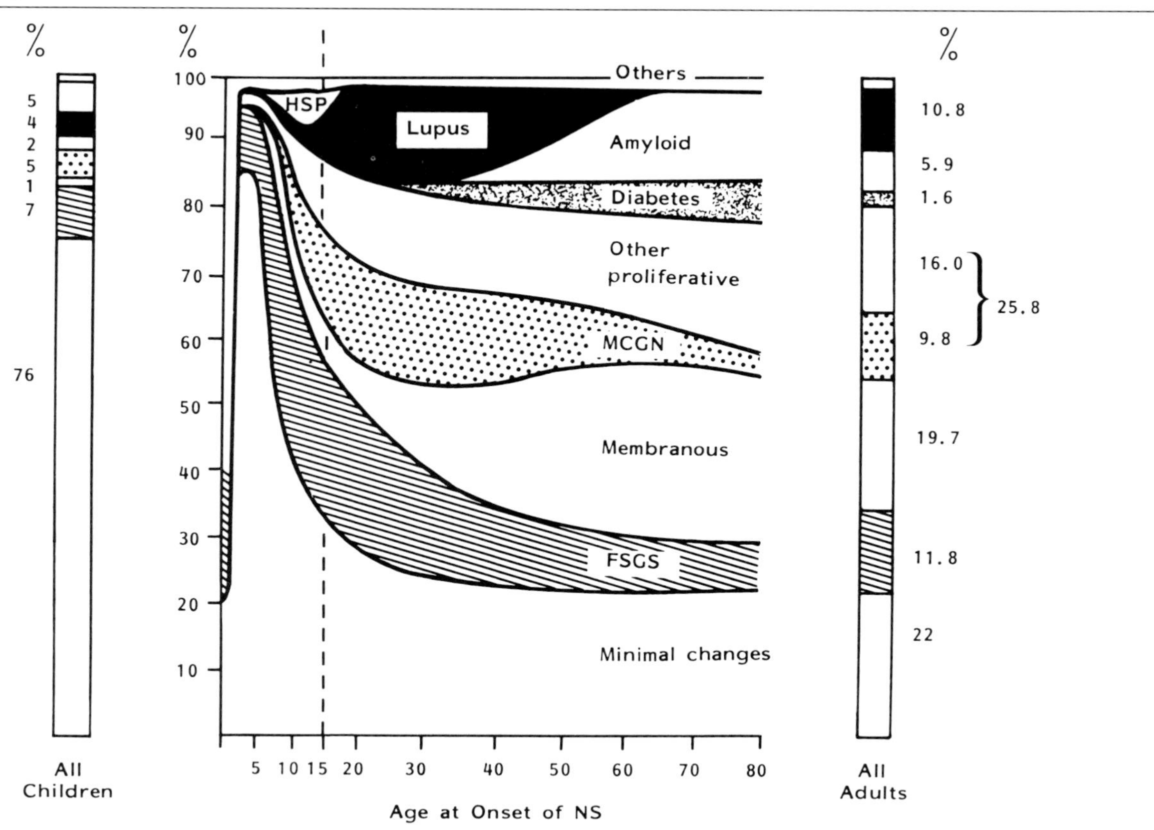

Table 69-2. Underlying histopathologic appearances in 607 adult-onset nephrotic syndromes seen at Guy's Hospital, 1964–1990

Age at onset	Minimal change	FSGS	Membrane	MCGN	Other proliferative GN[a]	Diabetes	Amyloid	Lupus	Other[b]	Total
15–19	24	14	3	10	15			9	0	75
20–29	31	18	5	19	17	1		21	0	112
30–39	21	9	22	4	15	2	2	13	2	90
40–49	24	4	25	6	14	2	4	12	4	95
50–59	15	16	31	8	15	2	15	5	4	111
60–69	16	3	30	4	14	3	11	1	3	85
70–79	9		13	1	5	1	5		2	36
>80	2		1							3
Total	142	64	130	52	95	11	37	61	15	607

FSGS = focal segmental glomerulosclerosis; MCGN = mesangiocapillary glomerulonephritis; GN = glomerulonephritis.
[a]IgA nephropathy, crescentic GN, mesangial proliferative, etc.
[b]Alport 3; light-chain nephropathy 4; vasculitis 5; Henoch-Schönlein purpura 3.

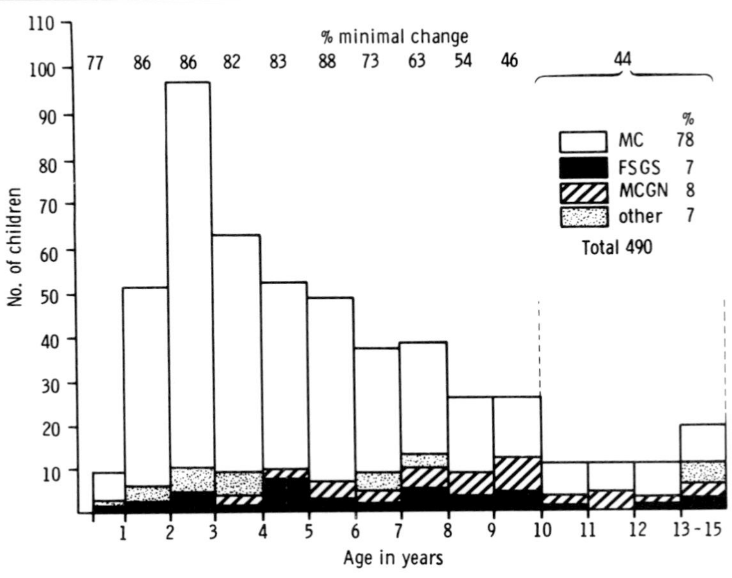

Fig. 69-6. The underlying histopathology in over 500 unselected nephrotic children studied by the International Study of Kidney Disease in Childhood, 1965–1980. Data from [24].

new cases in childhood has been estimated by several authors at between 1 and 2 cases per 100,000 children per year, and our own data from the southeast of England (W. W. Holland, R. H. R. White, and J. S. Cameron, unpublished data) suggest an incidence of about 2.1 per 100,000 children who were 1 to 14 years of age per annum. There are few published data on the incidence in adults of the nephrotic syndrome in the West, but our own recent unpublished data (W. Trounson et al.) suggest a minimum incidence of about 1.07 new cases per 100,000 adults who were 15 to 75 years of age among 2.45 million people living in southeast England. Of these, 0.87 cases were primary and 0.20 were secondary to systemic disorders, principally systemic lupus and amyloidosis. In this survey, the most prominent single underlying histopathology was membranous nephropathy (0.28 nephrotic cases per 100,000 per year) with minimal change a little behind (0.22 nephrotic cases per 100,000 per year), and mesangiocapillary glomerulonephritis, mesangial proliferative glomerulonephritis, and focal segmental glomerulosclerosis (FSGS) contributed about 0.1 cases per 100,000 per year each.

A number of factors will distort the incidence described. First, there is a tendency to under-refer older patients, at least for biopsy. Second, the proportion of diabetic patients seen with a nephrotic syndrome depends on the referral and biopsy policy in diabetic patients with proteinuria, with or without edema. Because there has been no effective treatment for diabetic nephropathy, and an 85 percent or better concordance between ocular and renal involvement in type I diabetes, it has been the policy in many units to avoid biopsy in diabetic nephrotic patients with retinopathy and to perform a biopsy only when there was some indication that the condition was unlikely to be diabetic nephropathy. For example, the presence of hematuria, or the absence or retinopathy, even by fluorescence angiography may be an indication for a biopsy. However, the proportion of all nephrotic patients with diabetic nephropathy, even where all nephrotic patients have been biopsied, does not exceed 10 percent in any published series. The coincidence or association of membranous nephropathy [268] and diabetes or with other forms of glomerular pathology needs emphasis, and many units are again performing biopsies more often in diabetic nephrotic patients.

These data apply, of course, only to developed Western communities, and there are many variations within the much higher incidence of nephrotic syndrome found in the tropics (see Seggie and Adu [420] for detailed discussion).

Although poorly documented for developing countries, the admission data analyzed by Kibukamusoke [273] suggest that while in the West the rate for the nephrotic syndrome is about 0.04 to 0.05 percent of all admissions (the former figure is our own from a population of 3.5 million in the southeast of England), in tropical countries it may range as high as 2, 3, or even 4 percent.

In the absence of firm data on incidence, it is difficult to judge whether minimal change disease is actually rare in the tropics or merely submerged in a much larger number of other forms of histopathology. It appears that, for example, in Malaysia [131], there may be a higher incidence of minimal change or very minor proliferative histology in adults. These patients are sensitive to corticosteroids so far as loss of proteinuria is concerned and constitute 40 to 50 percent of all nephrotic adults. Minor variations in incidence almost certainly occur throughout the Western world. For example, it is noticeable that higher proportions of nephrotic adult patients are reported from the United States to have membranous nephropathy (up to 50% or even 60%) than in comparable series from Europe. In the Interhospitals Study [111] of the nephrotic syndrome, 72 of 154 nephrotic patients had membranous nephropathy, while in our own series, the proportion of adult-onset cases with this appearance has been constant at about 20 to 22 percent over the past decade (Table 69-2).

Membranous nephropathy, unrelated to carriers of hepatitis B, also seems to be very common in Greece [473] and the Balkans. Incidences of mesangiocapillary glomerulonephritis also vary from one place to another; it is relatively rare in Japan, but in two series from Iran it was reported to account for 64 percent of the patients [59, 252]. We have also noted a high incidence of mesangiocapillary glomerulonephritis of both types I and II in nephrotic patients referred from Iran to the United Kingdom.

When one is considering the histopathology of diseases that underlie a nephrotic syndrome, the general prognosis of the group of patients with any given histopathologic pattern may have been estimated, but it remains the *individual prognosis* that is of primary concern to both the doctor and the patient. Within general statements, such as the 90 percent of adult type I mesangiocapillary glomerulonephritis patients with a nephrotic syndrome will be in renal failure before 10 years, or that 60 percent of adult-onset nephrotic patients with membranous nephropathy will have renal failure eventually, the prognosis and rate of progression of the individual are submerged.

EFFECTS OF TREATMENT

The fourth and final influence on prognosis is again an obvious one: the effect of specific treatment in removing the nephrotic syndrome or, at least, diminishing the proteinuria to the point at which edema no longer forms. The treatment of childhood and adult nephrotic patients has been discussed extensively elsewhere in this volume, but a few additional points are worth making here. Clearly, the response of the various histologic types of glomerulonephritis underlying the clinical presentations of glomerular disease differs. In broad terms, 90 percent of nephrotic patients with minimal changes, 25 percent of those with focal segmental glomerulosclerosis, and more doubtfully, 20 to 30 percent of those with membranous nephropathy will respond to treatment with corticosteroids, cytotoxic agents, or both, by complete or near-complete loss of proteinuria (see discussion in following sections). As noted previously, progression into renal insufficiency is almost unknown for any patient whose proteinuria remits completely, and thus these patients have almost universally a good prognosis in the long term, at least as far as renal function is concerned.

The prognosis for adult nephrotic patients with response to corticosteroids has been known for many years to be much superior to those who did not respond, irrespective of renal biopsy appearances, as demonstrated in Fig. 69-7 from Idelson et al. [247]. This distinction appeared by 1979 to be so clear to pediatric nephrologists that, since then, it has been almost universal practice to treat all but a minority of childhood-onset nephrotic patients with corticosteroids and only biopsy, at about 4 weeks, the remainder, who have failed to lose their proteinuria by this time. Recently, it has been argued [213, 270, 304a] that such a policy has merit also for nephrotic patients of adult onset, even though the proportion of adult nephrotic patients who will respond to the treatment is only some 30 to 35 percent at most, compared with 80 to 90 percent of younger and 50 to 60 percent of older children.

Such a suggestion involves balancing the relative risks of a continuing nephrotic syndrome against the risks of renal biopsy itself and of the corticosteroid treatment to be given. However, it is almost impossible to quantify such risks with accuracy, and any elaborate analysis [233, 270, 304a] erected on such dubious assumptions, however impeccable the mode of analysis, is bound to remain insecure.

To apply such a policy to adult patients, we also require firm data on the rate of response of loss of proteinuria in corticosteroid-responsive patients in order to time the biopsy optimally after a period of apparently ineffective treatment with corticosteroids. Hitherto,

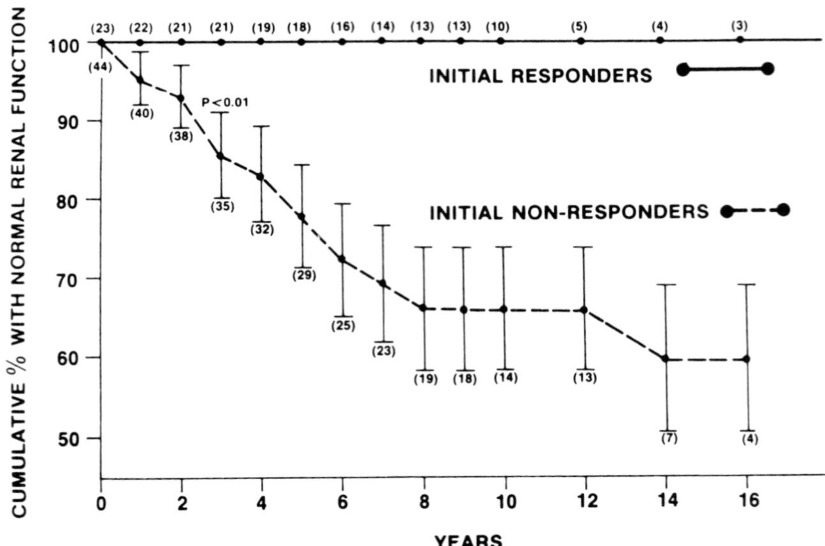

Fig. 69-7. The long-term outcome of unbiopsied adult patients with a nephrotic syndrome, all treated with prednisone. It is obvious that those who responded to this treatment with loss of proteinuria during the initial treatment fared much better than those who did not with respect to the outlook for renal function. (From Idelson et al. [247] with permission of the authors and publishers.)

such data, although present for children, have not been available for adult-onset patients. We [361] and Korbet et al. [288] have analyzed the rates of response to corticosteroids in adult-onset patients with a minimal change nephrotic syndrome treated with corticosteroids (see Fig. 69-10). As can be seen, the response rate for adults in our series is slower and less frequently complete than for children in the ISKDC study.

Thus if the "no biopsy first" policy is to be adopted in adult nephrotic patients [233, 270, 304a], the period of treatment would have to be longer than in children to identify with any comparable degree of security those resistant cases that are unlikely to have minimal changes on renal biopsy, with a corresponding increase in risk, which cannot at the moment be quantified exactly. Therefore, at the moment, a policy of performing a renal biopsy in all adult-onset nephrotic patients seems to remain preferable.

Prognosis of Individual Histologic Groups

MINIMAL CHANGE LESIONS

The majority of patients who are subjected to biopsy and show minimal change lesions have a full nephrotic syndrome, but it must not be forgotten that there are many symptomless patients with isolated proteinuria—especially adolescents and young adults [307] who may show minimal lesions in renal biopsies (see Chap. 64). By and large, these patients are *not* subjected to biopsies unless the proteinuria is over 2 gm per 24 hours or edema appears because of the excellent prognosis for these patients [15, 307] and the frequency of minimal changes in their renal biopsy specimens. We may, therefore, confine our discussion here to patients with a minimal change lesion and a nephrotic syndrome. The outcome of minimal change disease as observed today is very much modified from its "natural" history, both by control of infections (discussed above) and by the successful use of immunosuppressive agents to eliminate proteinuria.

Childhood-Onset Minimal Change Nephrotic Syndrome. As Figs. 69-4 and 69-6 demonstrate, minimal change is a lesion most commonly found in childhood nephrotic patients but accounts for 25 percent of adult nephrotic patients at all ages. As discussed previously [71], until the era of diuretics and antibiotics, death was common in nephrotic *children* from sepsis and occasionally from thrombosis. Now death from complications is rare, although we [461] and the International Study of Kidney Disease in Children (ISKDC) [251] have demonstrated that a small mortality from complications still exists. In our own study of 183 unselected children with a nephrotic syndrome and biopsy-proved minimal change lesions, there were 11 deaths during the subsequent 15 to 22 years, 7 of which were related to the nephrotic syndrome or its treatment, i.e., infections, septicemia, and hypovolemia. The only death in the past 8 years in this group has been one boy, who suffered brain infarction from sagittal sinus thrombosis during a relapse. Of 10 children who died from 389 studied by the ISKDC [251] for 7 to 15 years, 6 died from infection, 1 died of dural sinus thrombosis, 1 died from circulatory overload precipitated by intravenous albumin infusion, and 1 died in chronic renal failure; the cause of death in the final child was undetermined. Similar to our own series, all the deaths occurred in the early part of the study, i.e., before 1972. Krensky et al. [290] and Gorensek et al. [198]

confirm the continued importance of peritonitis as a complication of childhood nephrotic syndrome. In these two series, three children died of their sepsis.

Much attention has been directed to the relapsing pattern of patients with minimal change nephrotic syndrome. It has sometimes been said that this pattern is the result of "forcing" patients, whose disease would otherwise have continued, into remission with corticosteroids. This pattern of behavior was recorded, however, well before the introduction of corticosteroids; indeed, one of the first accounts of a childhood nephrotic patient, in Paris (1833–1834), describes two children whose urine became completely free of albumin between relapses [85]. The relapses themselves also may remit spontaneously [494]. There is little doubt from the data of Arneil [21] and others [418] that the natural evolution of childhood nephrotic syndrome progresses slowly toward remission; one can calculate a spontaneous remission rate of about 65 percent at 3 years from onset in Arneil's data. Today, this long-term natural evolution is obscured by early treatment with corticosteroids, almost always prednisone. From the data of the ISKDC [38], 93 percent of nephrotic children will go into remission within 6 to 8 weeks, taking 60 mg/m^2 per 24 hours of prednisone (see Fig. 69-10). Thirty-six percent will never experience a relapse, 18 percent will have infrequent relapses, but 39 percent will experience multiple relapses, either with a period off all treatment and free of proteinuria between relapses ("frequent relapser") or relapsing immediately when prednisone is withdrawn or even during modest doses of the drug (steroid-dependent).

What the exact influence of the initial treatment may be on subsequent outcome has been debated. Early claims were made that more prolonged initial treatment resulted in fewer relapses subsequently [294]. The German Arbeitsgeminschaft fur Padiatrische Nephrologie (APN) [19] examined the ISKDC regimen of 8 weeks' treatment contrasted with a shorter period of treatment, determined by how rapidly complete remission appeared. Sustained remission was significantly less frequent with the shorter course over the following 14 months of follow-up. In contrast, Choonara and colleagues [99] compared stability of remission in a group of relapsing children treated for similar lengths of time with lower doses (30 mg/24 hours) with those given the "standard" 60 mg/m^2 and found that duration of remission was similar in the two groups. Comparison of a longer treatment with the ISKDC 8-week regimen has not been made and would need careful evaluation of corticosteroid side effects if greater stability of remission were achieved. The French club for Pediatric Nephrology reexamined Lange et al.'s [294] suggestion but found that stability of remission was no greater after 1 year of alternate-day treatment compared with 16 weeks [283].

Much attention has been given to the optimum management of multiply relapsing or corticosteroid-dependent patients (see Chap. 64), and while there is no doubt that mustard and mustard-like agents, such as cyclophosphamide and chlorambucil, will induce a remission in such children (see [63a] and [460] for review), there is a greater tendency now to try carefully titrated alternate-day prednisone [380] or lower-dose prednisone [481] on an intermittent or continuous basis for longer periods, because of the undoubted side effects of these mustard-like drugs. This tendency has been strengthened by the observations of Garin et al. [186] and the German APN [18] that the patients who need the relief from steroid dosage the most, that is, the steroid-dependent patients, achieve the least benefit from cytotoxics in terms of duration of remission (Fig. 69-8). The optimum length of the course of cyclophosphamide has not been determined. Initial data suggested that a course of only 2 weeks was without effect and that 6 or 8 weeks of 3 mg/kg/24 hours would achieve as much as longer courses (see [460] for discussion). This view was challenged by the APN [19] who showed more stable remission when 12 weeks' treatment was used, but yet again no difference was found in a Japanese study [464]. Schulman et al. [416a] noted no difference in the proportion of prolonged remissions in those with or without IgM deposits or global sclerosis.

In recent years, cyclosporin A has been used in minimal change nephrotic children, on the reasonable assumption that the inhibition of activated T cells achieved by this drug could be useful. Accumulated data [63, 334, 356] show that the drug makes little difference to the longer-term evolution of the condition, since although remission may be induced in the majority of steroid-dependent or multiply relapsing patients, equal relapse occurs almost always on stopping or tapering the dosage of the drug. Cyclosporin A may of course be useful in permitting reduction in dosage or cessation of corticoste-

Fig. 69-8. The stability of response of nephrotic children who have become multiple-relapsing or steroid-dependent (see text for definitions) treated with mustard-like agents (cyclophosphamide or chlorambucil [18]). Those who are multiple-relapsing have a much superior response in the long term, compared with those who were steroid-dependent before treatment with cytotoxics. (From [18], with permission of the authors and publishers.)

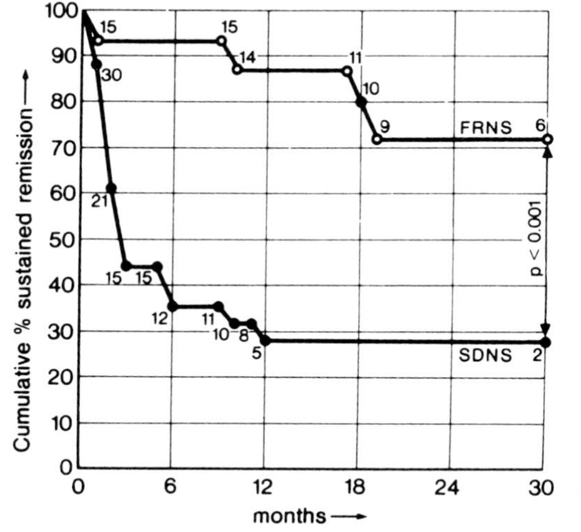

roids, but it substitutes the side effects of cyclosporin for those of corticosteroids. There is no evidence that it may induce prolonged remission, as nitrogen mustard–based drugs may achieve.

Although the tendency to relapse is prolonged, in most patients with minimal change nephrotic syndromes it is not indefinite. Siegel et al. [427] demonstrated a falloff in the frequency of relapses in an unbiopsied group of childhood nephrotic patients after 15 years, and it is striking how few childhood patients who are still relapsing are referred to adult clinics. These authors updated their experience more recently [49]. Sixty nephrotic children responsive to corticosteroids were studied for a mean of 14.5 years, with particular emphasis on the subset of 20 relapsers who received cyclophosphamide treatment. Those so treated had all gone into remission, while just over half (52%) of those treated with corticosteroids alone were still relapsing.

In our own long-term study [461], only 10 children, with a duration of disease from 15.0 to 20.5 years, were still relapsing out of 183 studied. By this time, they were aged from 17 to 27 years. A similar study was published by Lewis and colleagues from Manchester, England [310]. They studied 63 children with steroid-sensitive nephrotic syndromes for 10 to 21 years and again noted a tendency for relapses to become less frequent from 4 years following diagnosis, and the percentage of patients relapsing fell steadily with time. Two children only had died—one from sagittal sinus thrombosis and one from septicemia. The patient who has relapsed longest in our clinic (not in the series studies by Trompeter et al. [461]) has now been relapsing for 31 years, and another relapsed from the age of 3 years until his early thirties, when his proteinuria became persistent but mild, off all treatment; he finally became proteinuria-free at an age of 41 years. Niall [355] reported a patient who relapsed repeatedly between 4 and 53 years of age, at which point he died of tuberculosis.

Another observation of practical value is to determine after what period of remission a further relapse becomes unlikely. These data are influenced by the use of cytotoxic agents, but from our own and other published data [213], it appears that it is rare for a relapse to occur after more than 2 years in remission and almost unknown after 7 years of remission have passed. Nevertheless, reports have been published of relapses 10 to 25 years later [123, 213, 390, 424]. These late relapses are almost always responsive to treatment with corticosteroids, but an acquired resistance to treatment has been described [390].

It would, of course, be useful to be able to predict which children will be frequent relapsers at the outset, but no features of the initial nephrotic syndrome appear to distinguish frequent relapsers from those who will have no relapses or infrequent relapses. However, in the study of Trompeter et al. [461], we found a striking relation of persistent relapsing disease to the patient's age (Fig. 69-9). All the children with persisting disease had had an onset under the age of 6 years, and the younger the child at onset, the more likely they were to suffer a prolonged relapsing course. Data from the ISKDC have shown that the pattern of frequent relapses is usually established early following an attack, with two relapses within 6 months or three within 1 year in the majority

Fig. 69-9. The duration of relapsing course in relation to age at onset in minimal change nephrotic children initially treated with corticosteroids. (From Trompeter et al. [461], with permission of the publishers.)

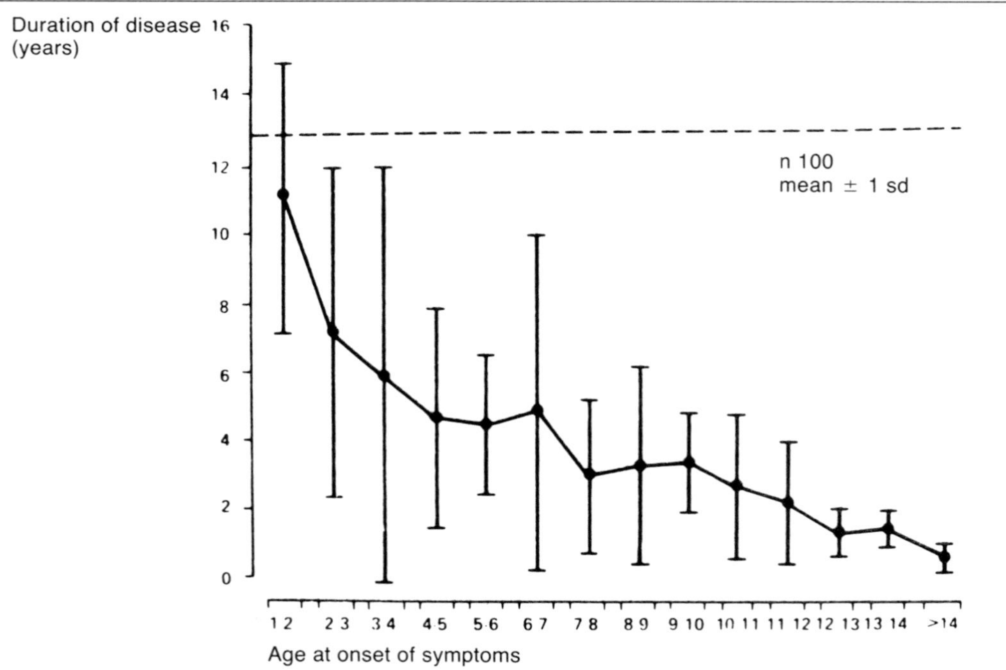

of cases; these data are useful in deciding what therapy to use before long-term corticosteroids have been used.

The terminal height attained by children with prolonged periods of relapse and consequent prolonged treatment with corticosteroids has been of interest. Our own data [461] showed that the height of 10 children relapsing for 20 to 25 years was within 2 standard deviations (SDs) of expected in all cases, although most were on the lower side of the mean. Similarly the Manchester data [175] showed a mean height of −0.22 SD in 80 patients, the majority relapsers, after 5 to 24 years; only 6 were more than 2 SDs below the mean. In both studies, hypertension was absent, and all patients had normal renal function. The results in Berns et al.'s study from Yale [49] were not so encouraging; the mean height of those treated with corticosteroids alone was −0.93 ± 0.3 SD, and those who had received cyclophosphamide −0.84 ± 0.4 SD, after a mean follow-up of 14.5 years.

Thus for most observers, the frequently relapsing corticosteroid-responsive nephrotic child, although unfortunate, rarely if ever goes into renal failure, even though later biopsies may show the appearance of focal segmental sclerosing lesions. Only a handful of cases have been published [222, 282, 351, 451, 454, 456], and we have experience of one patient only in our large series [420a]. However, Tejani's [451] experience of 48 children with minimal changes in their initial biopsy who relapsed repeatedly is at variance with this. Thirty-three of these patients, on second biopsies, showed segmental sclerosis [28], IgM [18], or both; of the remaining 9 children, second biopsies showed minimal changes, and third biopsies showed similar changes in 6. Twenty-five percent of the 30 children whose morphology had "converted" had already gone into renal failure, and actuarial calculations suggested that all might do so eventually. The reasons for this markedly poorer prognosis for multiply relapsing children, so much at variance with all other reports, is not clear, although the ethnic origins (predominantly American hispanic and black) of this group of patients are different from the majority of other published series, and black adults frequently show progressive focal segmental lesions [26] (see later discussion).

Minimal Change Nephrotic Syndrome in Adults. Far fewer data are available from adults than from children with minimal change disease [63, 105, 361]. The literature up to 1980 was reviewed by Coggins [105] and recently by Broyer et al. [63]. Recently, we have reviewed our own long-term follow-up in 89 adults with minimal change nephrotic syndrome [361]. It is often forgotten (Table 69-2) that at all ages, minimal changes account for one-quarter of adult nephrotic syndromes. Our first interesting observation was that adult-onset patients responded more slowly and more incompletely than children to corticosteroids (Fig. 69-10). This occurrence might reflect the lower dosage of prednisone normally in use on a body-weight or surface-area basis, when compared to pediatric use. However, the same effect was seen with cyclophosphamide, and here the dosage was identical (3 mg/kg per 24 hours for 8 weeks). In addition, a lower percentage of adult patients achieved complete response after corticosteroids. Fourteen (24%) or 58 patients who lost their proteinuria completely never relapsed, 56 percent relapsed on a single occasion or infrequently, and only 21 percent were frequent relapsers or steroid-dependent—a much lower proportion than in children. The same gradient of a less frequent relapsing course with age was seen in adult-onset minimal change patients, so that over the age of 60, relapses are rare—al-

Fig. 69-10. Rate of response (judged by loss of proteinuria) of adult-onset patients with minimal change nephrotic syndrome treated with corticosteroids, cyclophosphamide, or both, compared with data in children taken from the ISKDC. Data from 89 adults in the Guy's series are shown.

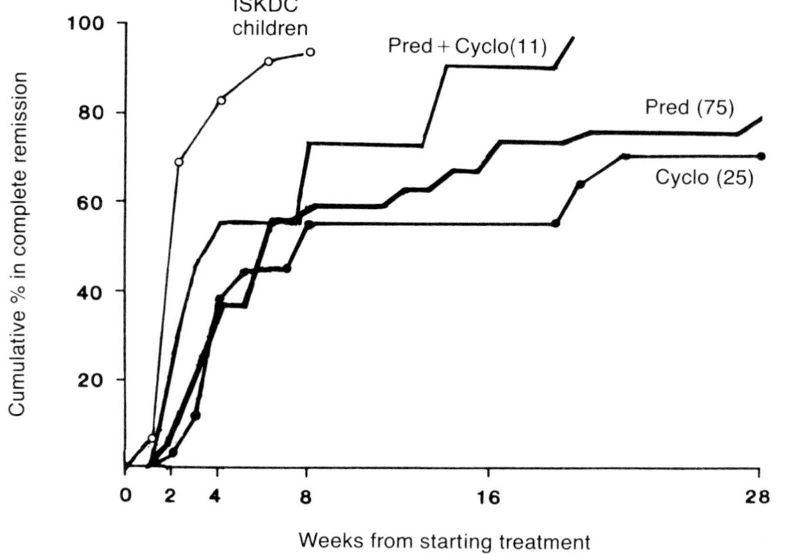

though we have seen this, in contrast to Zech et al. [503], who never observed any relapses in this age group. As in children, the first relapse was uncommon after 2 years of remission and never occurred more than 8 years later. Korbet et al. [288] described a similar study in 40 adult-onset patients. They confirmed the slower response of adults compared to children, and their data almost exactly parallel our own data.

Interestingly, in our study, stability of remission after treatment with cyclophosphamide (36 patients) was superior to that found in children, with 60 percent of patients still in remission at 10 to 15 years. Only patients over the age of 55 died, and only 5 of 15 deaths noted were related to the nephrotic syndrome, most in the period before 1975. At last follow-up, 1 to 24 years from onset, only 13 of 89 patients still had active disease, and only 6 were still manifesting nephrotic syndrome. As in children, cyclosporin has been used recently in multiply relapsing and steroid-dependent adults [334]. Seventy-seven percent of 31 steroid-sensitive adults reported in the literature responded with loss of proteinuria, but as in the children, relapses were observed on stopping the drug.

As with the childhood data, this information represents the modified history of the condition after treatment, including corticosteroids, cytotoxic agents, and cyclosporin. Data from untreated adult minimal change patients are available from two controlled trials, that of the Medical Research Council in Great Britain [53] and that of the Interhospitals study [111]. Both series suggest that after 3 years, about two-thirds of adult-onset patients will have gone into spontaneous remission, while one-third will still have proteinuria; there were no deaths among a total of 28 untreated patients in the two trials.

Evolution to Chronic Renal Failure in Corticosteroid-Sensitive Minimal Change Nephrotic Syndrome. It is clear that it is extremely rare—but not unprecedented—for a nephrotic patient with a minimal change biopsy and demonstrated responsiveness to prednisone, with complete loss of proteinuria to go into renal failure subsequently. In fact, only 11 such patients have been recorded in the literature [63, 222, 282, 420a, 451, 456], with the exception of Tejani's experience [351].

These exceptional patients are of great interest in thinking about the relationship between minimal change disease and focal segmental sclerosis (see the following discussion). Still rare, but slightly more frequent, is the patient who appears to have minimal changes on an initial biopsy but fails to respond either to corticosteroids or to cyclophosphamide [63]. Often, these patients have a rather prominent mesangium in their biopsies and, sometimes, mesangial deposits of IgM (see the following discussion). Subsequent biopsies may show obvious lesions of focal and segmental glomerulosclerosis, and the question arises as to whether these lesions may have already been present out of the plane of the biopsy section or out of the entire biopsy on the first occasion. Either way, the initial resistance to treatment with both agents is an important indicator of an adverse prognosis for renal function, and it exceeds in value the details of the histologic appearances on renal biopsy, which will be discussed next.

Primary Resistance to Treatment, Histologic Changes, and Acquired Resistance to Treatment. As just mentioned, resistance to treatment with both prednisone and cyclophosphamide is usually an ominous sign. Some patients, however, will fail to respond to steroids or have only a diminution, but not loss of, proteinuria with standard courses of prednisone; but they will then respond promptly to cyclophosphamide. They probably represent a rather resistant group who require more treatment but are at one end of the responsive spectrum and have a good prognosis in ISKDC data [249]; three-quarters of 31 initial nonresponders to prednisone (no loss of proteinuria by 8 weeks) lost their proteinuria. In data from the Hôpital des Enfants Malades [63, 182], 56 percent of 83 children with nonresponsive "nephrosis" eventually lost their proteinuria. It is often forgotten that the diagnosis of minimal changes is a diagnosis of *exclusion* made with varying certainty according to whether the juxtamedullary glomeruli (most frequently and earliest affected by focal segmental glomerulosclerosis) are included in the biopsy, and whether immunofluorescence or electron microscopy is available to distinguish a very early membranous pattern. Thus some patients in published series of "minimal changes" may have had focal segmental sclerosis from the start. However, within the ambit of what is usually regarded as minimal changes are patients with focal global sclerosis of glomeruli, sometimes accompanied by tubular atrophy, and varying mild degrees of mesangial matrix expansion and hypercellularity. The former appears to have no effect on prognosis when present in children with a nephrotic syndrome [249]. In adults, with increasing age, more and more global obsolescence of glomeruli is seen [264], together with tubulointerstitial damage and vessel changes that are probably the origin of these appearances. Thus interpretation of "minimal changes" in adults must take account of these changes, which occur with age.

The presence of mesangial expansion, proliferation, or both, is a more controversial topic. In childhood nephrotic syndrome, there seems to be little doubt that as the mesangial volume increases (as judged by its area in fixed material in histologic preparations), a higher proportion of patients with hematuria, hypertension, initial resistance to corticosteroid treatment, and ultimate entry into renal insufficiency is seen [224, 249, 282, 435, 474]. The presence or absence of IgM or minor mesangial deposits on electron microscopy does *not*, however, seem to alter the prognosis [244, 435]. Since fixation techniques affect the mesangial area, and there are no absolute criteria for normality, different observers may classify the same biopsy in different ways. However, a remarkable unanimity on the significance for prognosis has emerged, as just outlined. What is much less clear is what pathogenetic significance the mesangial expansion, proliferation, or deposits may have. Some patients with only mesangial expansion on initial biopsies, and no segmental lesions, will show segmental sclerosis on subsequent biopsies. This type of observation leads many [282, 474] to treat this group of patients as a variant of the minimal change–FSGS group and the whole as a spectrum of presentations of a single disease. The older German-American name, "lipoid nephrosis," is perhaps preferable for this group, since the name used by the Parisians [282, 474] (idiopathic nephrotic syndrome) could equally apply to other forms of primary glomerular disease.

Late nonresponsiveness to corticosteroid treatment in relapsing patients is an uncommon but well-recorded longer-term pattern of behavior in patients with minimal changes. In the ISKDC data [249], 43 of 311 initial responders acquired some degree of resistance to corticosteroid treatment during follow-up. Because only these troublesome patients usually have late biopsies and, in many, focal segmental sclerosing lesions were found [428], it was supposed at first that this evolution was confined to resistant patients. Since then, it has become apparent that the biopsy may remain normal in resistant patients [454] and show sclerosing lesions in responding relapsers (personal observations).

The value of the presence of IgM in predicting outcome is controversial, mainly because different authors have asked different questions. There seems little doubt that within the group of patients with minimal change biopsies, the presence of IgM makes no difference to short- or long-term outlook [63, 258, 471]. Mesangial proliferative glomerulonephritis with mesangial IgM deposition is dealt with in the following discussion.

FOCAL SEGMENTAL GLOMERULOSCLEROSIS (FSGS)

The relationship of this lesion to minimal changes has been much debated, and I have reviewed the controversy elsewhere in detail [71, 84] (see Chap. 64). In short, it is not likely that we will be able to decide whether these two appearances represent different aspects of what is pathogenetically the same lesion or two distinct diseases unless and until we understand the pathogenesis of either; at the moment, despite much speculation and experimentation, this remains unknown. New data from transplanted patients with recurrent disease, the occasional entry of patients with a completely responsive minimal change lesion into renal failure already mentioned, the more frequent appearance of focal segmental lesions in patients with mesangial expansion, and the occasional response of even the most severe form of focal segmental glomerulosclerosis to intense immunosuppression all support the thesis that the two represent two aspects of the same or a similar disease [63, 84, 282].

In adults, the prognosis is markedly better for patients with focal segmental glomerulosclerosis if proteinuria remains below the nephrotic range (Fig. 69-4). This is true also in the data of Beaufils et al. [42] and St. Hillier et al. [406]; few if any patients with subnephrotic proteinuria progress to renal failure within a decade. There are few data on children with FSGS [501] but without a nephrotic syndrome, perhaps because this is a rather rare finding (2 of 62 with FSGS in our own series). In Yoshikawa et al.'s series [501], there was no difference in outcome with degree of proteinuria, however.

In children, a proportion of patients with a full nephrotic syndrome respond to treatment with the conventional 6 to 8 weeks of prednisone, similar to those with minimal change (Table 69-3). In the published literature on 332 children, and including our own series of 62 nephrotic children with FSGS, 96 (29%) responded with complete loss of proteinuria [459]; many of these patients subsequently had a relapsing course, just as in the minimal change nephrotic syndrome, but some became corticosteroid-resistant later [20]. This pattern of behavior seems to be much less common in adult-onset nephrotic syndromes with FSGS; of 39 nephrotic patients reported by Beaufils et al. [42], 6 went into remission, but 2.5 to 10 years later, and only 3 of 26 treated with corticosteroids alone went into remission, plus 1 each treated with indomethacin and chlorambucil, respectively. In our own series [91], only two patients responded with loss of proteinuria out of 18 adults treated with corticosteroids.

Table 69-3. Initial responsiveness of nephrotic children with FSGS to corticosteroid treatment

Author	Year	Reference no.	Number treated	Number responded with loss of proteinuria	Percent
Siegel et al.	1974	428	22	16	73
Newman et al.	1976	354	15	9	60
Gubler et al.	1978	204	85	21	25
ISKDC	1980	250	16	5	31
Mongeau et al.	1981	339	31	6	19
Arbus et al.	1982	20	51	19	37
Schärer et al.	1982	412	51	10	20
SWPNG	1985	437	56	16	16
Trompeter (Guy's)	1987	459	62	10	16
Total			389	112	29%

Considering the long-term outcome of patients with FSGS and a nephrotic syndrome, one fact emerges with clarity from almost all studies: that is, the prognosis of those with complete loss of proteinuria in response to corticosteroids is much better than those who do not show this initial response (Table 69-4). In contrast, however, Tejani [453] and the South West Pediatric Nephrology Study Group [437] have reported recently that the outcome in terms of renal failure was no different in those who responded initially and those who did not, so the prognosis even for those who respond must remain guarded. Both these series contained, in contrast to the rest of the literature, a high proportion of black and hispanic children.

Thus the response to an initial treatment with corticosteroids may be an invaluable indicator of likely prognosis, at least in European caucasians. It also follows that the overall survival of a group of nephrotic patients with FSGS may depend on the proportion of steroid-responsive patients within the population under study. Finally, it supports the advisability of giving *all* nephrotic patients with FSGS a trial of 6 or 8 weeks of prednisone. It is less clear whether it is worth giving cyclophosphamide thereafter to those who do not respond; data scattered among the various papers in the literature [250] suggest that about another 10 percent of nephrotic children, over and above the 30 percent who respond to corticosteroids, will lose their proteinuria during or following cyclophosphamide treatment. There are no good data for adult-onset patients.

Table 69-4. Long-term outcome in nephrotic patients with FSGS in relation to initial responsiveness to corticosteroids[a]

	Responders[b]	Nonresponders	Total
All	49 (20%)	196 (80%)	245
In CRF	3 (10%)	49 (53%)	52 (45%)
"Death"[c]	2	55	57

[a]Summary of literature on adults and children 1969–1978 and personal cases; data from [72].
[b]Response = complete loss of proteinuria, usually within 8 weeks.
[c]Death = dead, dialyzed, or transplanted; mean follow-up, 6.4 years.

Cyclosporin has also been given to children [63, 356] and adults [344] with FSGS. A higher response rate than with either steroids or cyclophosphamide has been reported, although reduction in proteinuria (see above) has often been used as a criterion for "success." In corticoresistant cases, complete remission was obtained in 27 percent of 109 adults and 25 percent of 44 children [334]. Thus there may well be a role for this agent in the treatment of steroid-resistant FSGS (see Chap. 64).

The actuarially calculated (10-year) survivals for renal function in all patients with FSGS have been reported as 38 ± 12 percent (adults only) by Beaufils et al. [42]; and 45 ± 21 percent by Trompeter, unpublished (children only). In Fig. 69-11 are shown the survival curves for nephrotic adults and children in our unit, with either minimal change or FSGS. The two curves for 60 adults and 62 children with FSGS are not statistically different at a 1 : 20 level. Mongeau et al. [339] have emphasized the better prognosis of their children with FSGS, suggesting that the difference resides with the type of patient referred to some centers.

We [60] and St. Hillier et al. [406] have drawn attention to a group of patients that have come to be called "malignant" FSGS. These patients demonstrate complete resistance to corticosteroid and conventional cytotoxic therapy, usually have torrential proteinuria, with frequent hypovolemic episodes, are almost always under 20 years of age (the oldest we have seen were two girls, aged 22 and 24 years at onset). They run a relentless course to renal failure only 1 to 4 years from onset of the nephrotic syndrome, maintaining their proteinuria into terminal renal failure and even on to dialysis, so that bilateral nephrectomy or renal infarction may be needed [320]. Recurrence of equally torrential proteinuria in allografted kidneys may be immediate, with later

Fig. 69-11. Survival of nephrotic children or adults with either minimal changes (●) or focal segmental glomerulosclerosis (▲). From [85], with permission of the publishers. Unpublished data are from the Guy's series.

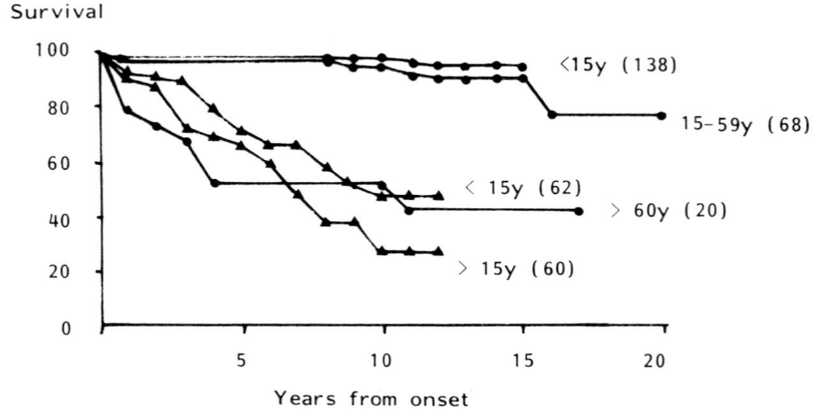

appearance of typical lesions of FSGS in the allograft and graft failure [420a].

Histologic Pattern. Almost all biopsies from patients with FSGS show some degree of tubular atrophy, so this is not of much use in determining prognosis within the group. However, if severe, this is usually not a good prognostic sign. The clinical correlate of this severe tubular disease is the finding of glycosuria, aminoaciduria [328], and excess losses of β_2-microglobulin in the urine [220], which may be a clinical indicator of the presence of FSGS. The lesions of FSGS have a characteristic distribution, often affecting either the perihilar area or the pole of the glomerulus opposite the hilus (*"glomerular tip" lesion*) [41, 271]. Ito et al. [253] have suggested that those children with perihilar lesions almost all progressed to renal failure, while those with "tip" lesions adjacent to the exit of the tubule from Bowman's capsule did well. These interesting observations have not been confirmed by others [342], although they agree with data on adults from Howie and Brewer [242]. However, our own data show no difference in the rather gloomy long-term outcome of both childhood and adult patients (Fig. 69-12).

It has also been suggested with more general agreement that *mesangial prominence* is an adverse finding [204, 416, 474], but our own data [60] again did not agree with this conclusion. Nor does the presence or absence of segmental IgM seem to make any difference in outlook, although being segmental this observation is peculiarly unreliable when absent from the sections examined (see discussion below).

Finally, we [60] noted precocious and prominent afferent arteriolar hyalinosis in our patients with a poor outcome for renal function, and this observation has been confirmed by Soon Lee and Spargo [433].

MESANGIAL GLOMERULONEPHRITIS

This is certainly *not* a histologic entity, since mesangial expansion is a feature without proliferation of mesangial cells and can be found in a number of circumstances, some of which may not be easy to distinguish from each other:

1. As part of the minimal change–FSGS complex [63, 474]
2. As an apparently idiopathic form of proliferative glomerulonephritis associated with mesangial aggregates of IgM, as first suggested by Cohen et al. [106] in 1978
3. As a sequel to poststreptococcal or other postinfective endocapillary glomerulonephritis [256]
4. In association with mesangial aggregates of IgA, or Berger's disease [125, 128, 129]
5. In association with isolated aggregates of C3 [369]

Fig. 69-12. Data on nephrotic children and adults showing focal segmental glomerulosclerosis in their renal biopsy seen at Guy's Hospital over a 20-year period. Survival curves (A) and status at most recent follow-up (B) are shown for 22 patients in whom the site of the lesion could be localized to the glomerular "tip," 63 patients in whom the lesion was perihilar, and 65 patients in whom on the sections available no statement as to localization could be made. Patients with both tip and perihilar lesions (12) were counted as perihilar. There is no difference in outcome between the groups. (From [69], with permission, and unpublished data of N. Chaudhury and J. S. Cameron.)

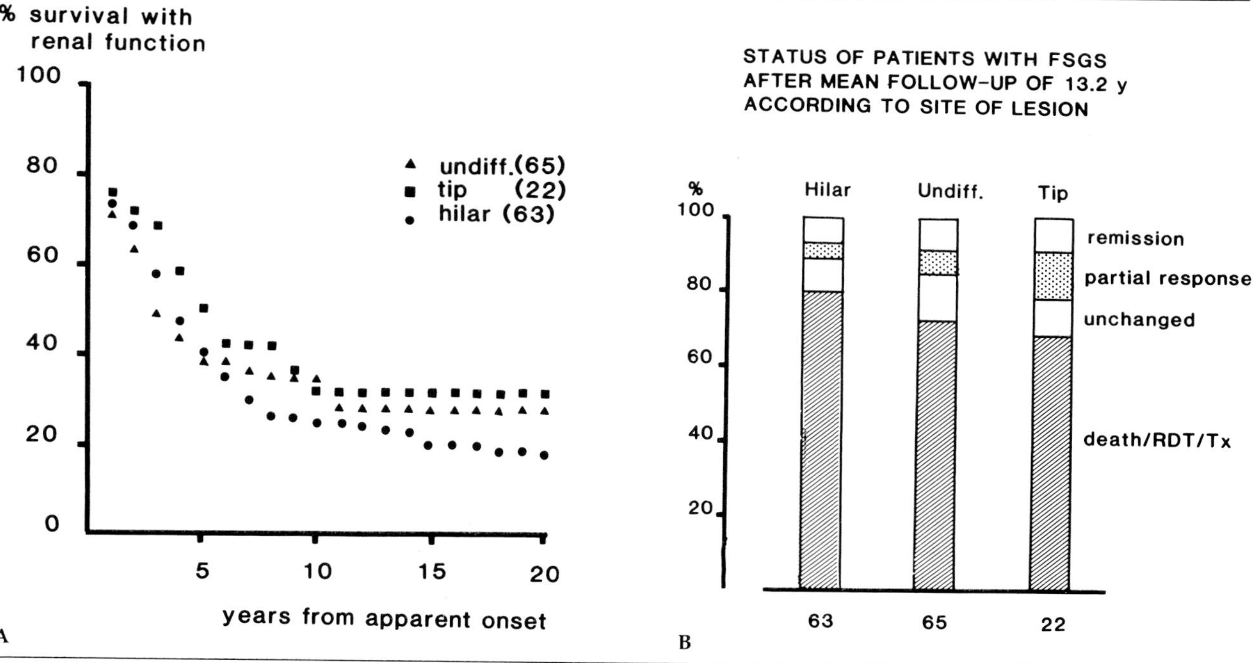

6. As an early manifestation of Alport's syndrome in children [180a]

The problem of mesangial expansion in nephrotic patients with minimal change, with or without aggregates of IgM, has already been discussed, as have those patients in whom subsequent biopsies reveal FSGS, either not present or missed in the first biopsy. Healing poststreptococcal glomerulonephritis will be discussed later. Thus, it is with those forms of mesangial glomerulonephritis presenting mainly with hematuria or hematuria plus proteinuria, usually without a nephrotic syndrome, that we are principally concerned with here. We can separate IgA-associated disease, but there remains an ill-defined and ill-assorted group of patients who do not fit clinically with any of the groups just listed.

Such patients not presenting with a nephrotic syndrome, but showing obvious mesangial expansion without obvious mesangial proliferation, have been discussed by Migone et al. [335]. Sixty-five of their 211 patients showed IgA and will be discussed in the next section, but 65 showed other immune aggregates, including IgM. Unfortunately, no long-term follow-up was available, but 9 percent of these patients already showed some degree of renal functional impairment.

The data of Brown et al. [62] do include long-term follow-up, but the value of their paper is greatly reduced by absence of any immunohistologic data, so that it is impossible to know how many of their patients had IgA-associated nephropathies or had IgM aggregates; all 8 of those presenting with symptomless proteinuria alone were well 10 to 119 months later, 3 without any proteinuria. Similarly, Uszyska-Karcz [467] noted no progression in 13 untreated children.

IgM-Associated Nephropathy. In 1974, Van de Putte et al. [469] drew attention for the first time to the fact that patients with hematuria as their first symptom might show, in the mesangium, diffuse aggregates of IgM, rather than the IgA described by Berger 6 years previously. This observation was confirmed by Pardo et al. [371]. Cohen et al. [106] extended these observations to patients presenting with a nephrotic syndrome and proteinuria in a paper published in 1978, which received wide attention. They suggested that the IgM had pathogenetic significance, and the term *IgM nephropathy* became current.

It is clear that at least some of the adult patients described by Cohen et al. [106] correspond to the nephrotic children described by Waldherr [474] and Gubler [204], and some of Cohen's original patients developed FSGS in subsequent biopsies (A. H. Cohen, personal communication). However, the position of those patients showing mesangial IgM and presenting with microscopic or macroscopic hematuria, or symptomless hematuria and proteinuria, is much less clear.

The presentation of these patients is similar to those with IgA-associated nephropathies [296] (see the following discussion) and, of course, if *all* patients with IgM are considered together, then patients with obvious FSGS on optical microscopy will be included, as well as some with apparently minimal change lesions. Thus the clinical and histologic boundaries of "IgM nephropathy" are ill-defined and include almost any presentation of which glomerular diseases are capable of showing.

If one goes a step further, one can then examine the effect of the presence or absence of IgM on a *given group defined by optical microscopy,* e.g., minimal changes, FSGS, or isolated mesangial expansion. If this is done, then the great mass of evidence suggests that the additional information on the presence or absence of IgM adds nothing to prognostic precision [51, 63, 225, 232, 243, 416a]. There is in addition no evidence that the circulating or glomerular IgM is pathogenetic, and it is well known that IgM may be seen as a nonspecific finding in tissue sections. Thus we should stop using the term "IgM nephropathy" unless it can be given precision or utility, both of which are lacking at present.

"Isolated C3 Disease." All that has just been said about IgM can be repeated for the proposed "entity" of C3-associated mesangial disease [200, 295, 369]. In some patients IgM was present also. At the moment, there seems to be no clinical or pathogenetic value in distinguishing these patients from others.

IgA-ASSOCIATED NEPHROPATHY (BERGER'S DISEASE)

It is with some relief that one turns now to a relatively well-defined form of glomerular disease—although it must be pointed out immediately that despite almost 25 years of research we still do not know whether the IgA present in the mesangium plays any role in glomerular injury, or what the significance of the raised serum IgA concentrations, the IgA-containing immune complexes, or the IgA autoantibodies in the serum may be [154, 165]. It must be admitted also that classifying patients with glomerular disease by the presence of predominant IgA on immunohistology cuts across both clinical presentation and conventional histologic classifications, as outlined above and elsewhere in this book.

Since IgA-associated nephropathy commonly presents without symptoms, through abnormal urine tests, there is considerable scope for variation in the population under study, depending on whether systematic urine testing of schoolchildren has been performed, as in some Japanese reports, or testing of the urine in all army recruits, as in Singapore. Second, the criteria for performing a renal biopsy become critical; if it is policy simply to watch patients with isolated hematuria, then a group with a generally favorable prognosis will be excluded. If, in contrast, all such patients are biopsied, then the group of patients with isolated hematuria and isolated mesangial IgA will be included and "improve" the prognosis of that particular series.

The prognosis of IgA nephropathy has been examined in more detail than for almost any other group of patients with glomerular disease, perhaps because of the large number of cases available worldwide [130]. Several conferences have been devoted to the subject of IgA nephropathy, that held in Milan in 1983 [129] containing the greatest quantity of clinical follow-up data, and other useful reviews have been published [125, 128, 130,

277, 413] to which the reader is referred, as well as Chap. 67 of this book.

All papers on IgA-associated disease in *adults* suggest a disease of indolent evolution toward healing or renal damage, although an aggressive course associated with extensive crescents may be seen in a few patients [127, 309]. In general, the entry into renal dysfunction and finally failure is slower in IgA nephropathy than in any of the other diseases discussed in this chapter [46, 414], occurring over a time scale of 30 years or more (Fig. 69-13), in contrast to the 5 to 15 years more usual in other glomerulopathies. In some part, this may reflect earlier diagnosis of macroscopic hematuria compared with symptomless proteinuria in the true course of indolent disease, but in fact many patients with the slowest evolution into renal failure present with symptomless urinary abnormalities on casual urine testing.

The long-term outcome of several large series of adult patients suffering from IgA nephropathy has been described [128, 143, 150, 348, 495] (see Schena [413] for a complete review of 68 series published between 1968 and 1988). Schena highlights the differing proportions of patients with hypertension, already raised plasma creatinine concentrations, macroscopic hematuria, and profuse proteinuria noted in differing parts of the world such as Europe, North America, East Asia, and Australia, which are bound to influence final data on follow-up (see discussion below). He also draws attention to the fact that in the papers from North America, follow-up has been notably shorter than in data from elsewhere in the world, which again will affect apparent outcome. Clearly at least 25 percent—and maybe as many as 50 percent—of adult patients with IgA nephropathy will end up in renal failure eventually (see Fig. 69-12); but what proportion of the remainder may develop renal insufficiency as well in their third, fourth, or fifth decades is quite unknown.

Fig. 69-13. Life table analysis of the survival of renal function in patients with IgA-associated nephropathy. Data from these series are shown: Droz, 1976 [143], D'Amico et al., 1984 [128], and Nicholls et al., 1984 [358]. It can be seen that, in general, the evolution of IgA-associated disease into renal failure in adults is slower than for other forms of idiopathic glomerulonephritis.

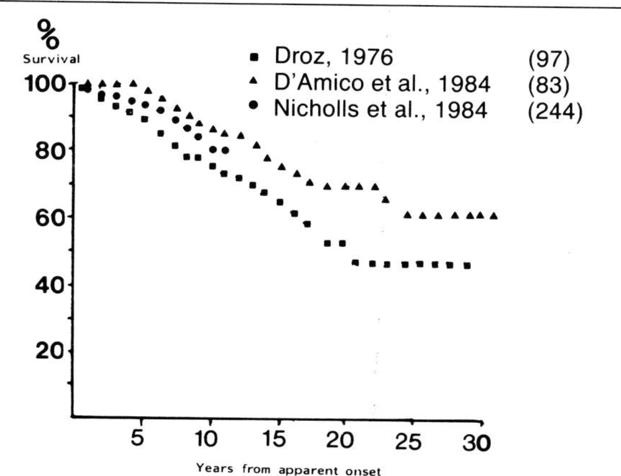

IgA nephropathy has been examined in more detail than any other form of glomerulopathy for factors that may predict prognosis, either for groups of patients [7, 130, 286, 353, 374, 495] or individuals [50] using both univariate and multivariate [30a, 86a] techniques. *Clinically,* male sex [358] proteinuria, especially if profuse, hypertension, and a raised plasma creatinine have appeared in all studies as determinants of a poorer prognosis. Macroscopic hematuria has given discordant results. On the one hand, Bennett and Kincaid-Smith [45] pointed to a *poorer* prognosis in those with macroscopic hematuria, a conclusion reinforced in their later paper [358]; however, all other studies, including those of D'Amico [130] and Beukhof [50], have shown that macroscopic hematuria is in contrast a *favorable* sign. In multivariate analyses [50, 130], proteinuria was the single most powerful clinical predictor of a poor outcome and the only independent clinical variable.

Pathologically, interstitial scarring is the most powerful predictor [50, 130], along with number of crescents [1], vascular hyaline lesions [239], the number of obsolescent glomeruli, and the degree of glomerular proliferation. Several groups [9, 403a] have counted and phenotyped the cells infiltrating the interstitium in IgA nephropathy and related these findings to prognosis. We [9], in a relatively short follow-up, found that only the rather small numbers of interstitial B cells correlated with rapid entry to renal failure, an interesting finding in view of the general B-cell overactivity in this condition. This area deserves further study.

There are surprisingly few data on entry into *complete remission* in IgA nephropathy. Nicholls et al. [358] noted that only 6 percent of their patients had entered remission after 5 years of follow-up, and Kitajima et al. [278], in a collaborative study of 1,394 adults, found only 6.5 percent after an average of 36 months; Schena [413] does not address the question in his otherwise admirable review, perhaps because so few authors comment on this aspect. Thus we simply do not know what proportion of adult patients will be in complete remission with normal urine after, say, 20 years. One is left with the impression that even in those with persisting normal renal function, at least for a decade or two, urinary abnormalities persist.

Although a common form of glomerulopathy in *children,* documentation of the longer-term outlook has not been extensive until recently. A relatively benign outlook for children presenting with hematuria, macroscopic or microscopic, had been noted in the past (see [19], [46], and [79] for summary of these earlier data) but did not include histologic data or information on the presence or absence of IgA. Levy et al. [309] described one of the larger follow-up studies on 91 children with IgA nephropathy, and their data are summarized in Table 69-5. Only 8 children developed renal failure (6 terminal, 2 more modest) within the follow-up period (mean 13.5 years); the 10-year survival was estimated to be 92 ± 2 percent. The majority of patients in this series had macroscopic hematuria at some point in their course, 66 at presentation, and only 7 had microscopic hematuria associated with proteinuria. Levy et al. [309]

Table 69-5. Prognosis of IgA-associated glomerulonephritis in children

Appearance on optical microscopy	*n*	Subsequent behavior 1–16 (mean 5.6) years: Number with recurrent macroscopic hematuria	Remission	NS	Renal failure
Minimal changes	26	25	16	0	0
Mesangial proliferation only	3	3	1	0	0
Focal segmental proliferative gn + mesangial proliferation	41	28	14	0	0
Proliferative gn plus crescents	21	13	2	0	8
	91	69	33	0	8

gn = glomerulonephritis.
Source: Data from [309].

noted that of 800 children previously described in the literature, only 8 patients entered renal failure 5 to 44 years from onset, and another 11 showed some degree of renal insufficiency 3 to 17 years from onset.

Data are also available from Japanese children, in which population IgA-associated nephropathy is particularly common. The study of Kitajima et al. [278], included in Levy's analysis of the literature, summarized data collected from 491 Japanese children; only 9 developed chronic renal failure or died. Kusumoto et al. [292] reported on 98 children with IgA nephropathy, with renal failure in only 9 and an estimated 10-year survival of 94 percent. Most of these children presented with both proteinuria and hematuria, and only 2 had isolated hematuria. Yoshikawa et al. [502] reported on follow-up of 200 Japanese children with IgA-associated nephropathy. Only 2 of 83 children less than 8 years of age at apparent onset had gone into renal failure, but follow-up was relatively short (5.5 ± 2.8 years). In 117 children aged 9 to 15 years at onset, 8 had gone into renal failure after a similar brief period. In Kusumoto's study [292], the outlook for renal function was significantly poorer in 86 adult-onset cases studied in parallel, so that a gradient of poorer prognosis with age at onset seems to be present.

Thus the overall prognosis in the medium term seems to be generally good for children with IgA-associated nephropathy. However, the very slow evolution of the disease must not be forgotten. After 10 years in Levy's study, only one-third of patients were in complete remission with normal urine, and the longer-term fate of such patients to 20 or 30 years has not been established. Other authors, however, have emphasized the poorer prognosis of children with IgA nephropathy seen in their units, probably because of referral and biopsy policies determining that only more severe cases reach tertiary referral centres. This has certainly been the case in our own unit (Afroze, Haycock et al. unpublished data): 16 percent of a small series of 32 children had progressive or continuing disease with hypertension, the outlook being poorer in those with an onset later than 10 years of age.

In children, the same prognostic indicators, although less extensively studied, have emerged as indicators of a poorer early prognosis as in adults. On histology, extensive crescent formation, interstitial fibrosis, and sclerosing glomerular lesions carry a poorer outlook. Clinically, proteinuria, hypertension, and greater age at onset seem the most important variables.

Unusual Patterns of Evolution in IgA Nephropathy. A particular feature of IgA-associated nephropathy is that while, in general, proteinuria has been an adverse factor in determining prognosis, a small but widespread number of patients have been described in whom a full nephrotic syndrome, normal renal function, and prompt response—and often a relapsing course—have followed corticosteroid therapy [103, 129, 196, 271, 309, 348]. These patients, more often children than adults, almost always show only minimal changes on optical microscopy, although some have shown mesangial expansion or even FSGS [196]. However, in the few patients examined by electron microscopy, characteristic IgA electron-dense aggregates have been absent.

Whether these patients represent a subset of IgA-associated nephropathy or the coincidence of minimal change nephropathy with symptomless IgA deposition within the mesangium, as may occur in the healthy population (e.g., organ donors), is not known. Many of the patients described in the literature, even from non-Oriental countries, are ethnic Chinese [e.g., 498]; in our own series in London, one case was Arab and one Chinese.

Another unusual pattern in IgA nephropathy is *recurrent attacks of acute renal failure* [364], first described by Talwalkar et al. [448] in 1978. It has been proposed that the acute hematuria is toxic to renal tubules [46, 358], and red cells ingested by the tubules have been demonstrated. These patients must be distinguished from those going into acute renal insufficiency because of crescentic glomerulonephritis, and thus a repeat renal biopsy is necessary.

MEMBRANOUS NEPHROPATHY

Membranous nephropathy is a well-documented histologic appearance, presenting in general with proteinuria and affecting principally middle-aged and elderly males (see Chap. 65). The short-term (<5 years) outcome of membranous nephropathy was extensively documented in adults during the late 1960s and 1970s; the data are reviewed in Cameron [71]. The appearance in its idiopathic form appeared to be a relatively indolent disease in the majority of patients, few patients either entering remission or progressing to renal failure within 5 years of apparent onset; although in contrast to this statement, several observers [153, 176, 177, 195, 215] reported 40 to 50 percent of patients dead or in renal failure within 5 to 6 years. In contrast, Pollak and colleagues [383] noted a relatively benign outcome within the first 5 years, other series (including our own [401]) falling somewhere between the two extremes.

All of these older data suffer from several handicaps. First, patients with idiopathic membranous nephropathy often were not separated from those with identifiable precipitating diseases, some of which (e.g., drugs) might improve the overall prognosis, some (e.g., malignancies) of which might make it worse. Second, a variable proportion had been treated for varying times with a number of agents believed to affect the outcome of the condition. Third, patients with only mild proteinuria were often mixed with those showing a full nephrotic syndrome.

Outlook in Untreated Patients. Over the past decade, data have become available on groups of patients that avoid some of these criticisms. First, the study of Noel et al. [360] described the outcome of a large group of patients, all with idiopathic membranous nephropathy, none of whom had received treatments believed to be specific. The outcome was notably better than that previously reported, actuarial survival at 10 years being estimated at 75 percent. The series included 48 percent of women (now known to do better, as discussed below), and only 78 percent had a nephrotic syndrome. Similarly, Nyberg et al. [365] reported a survival of 81 percent at 10 years in a small series of 22 untreated patients. The relatively good outlook reported in these papers contrasted with the control, untreated group in the Interhospitals study of the nephrotic syndrome reported from the United States in 1979 [111], in which 11 of 38 (29%) of untreated patients reached a renal failure end point (plasma creatinine > 4 mg/dl) within 48 months of entry.

These data stimulated us to perform a three-center retrospective analysis of untreated idiopathic nephrotic adult-onset patients from Guy's Hospital, Newcastle, and Leeds [132]. Sixty-four patients were identified, and an attempt was made not only to assess the survival of renal function but also the rate at which the plasma creatinine changed in those with progressive disease (Fig. 69-14). Fig. 69-14 shows the raw plasma creatinine data, plotted on reciprocal paper, so that no calculation is needed to assess the rate of change of $1/P_{creat}$. It can be seen that of 64 untreated idiopathic nephrotic patients followed for a mean of 4.5 years, only 32 (50%) showed a deterioration in renal function. The rate of change of plasma creatinine was only approximately linear for each patient, but the slopes of the data (Fig. 69-15) vary greatly from patient to patient. Three patients went into renal failure within 2 years of onset of a nephrotic syndrome, as previously described by Coggins and his colleagues [111] in untreated patients, and by the end of 5 years only 9 (14%) had started dialysis.

More recently data from untreated groups of nephrotic adults have become available from three further

Fig. 69-14. Plot of the serum creatinine (μmoles/L) on reciprocal paper, with time, for the 27 patients with membranous nephropathy who deteriorated (*solid line*) and for the five patients who had slow deterioration (*broken line*): (1) patients from Guy's Hospital, (2) patients from St. James's University Hospital, and (3) patients from the Royal Victoria Infirmary and Freeman Hospital. The remaining 30 patients, all with initial serum creatinines less than 120 μmoles/L, showed no significant changes throughout the study. (From Davison et al. [132], with permission of the editors and publishers.)

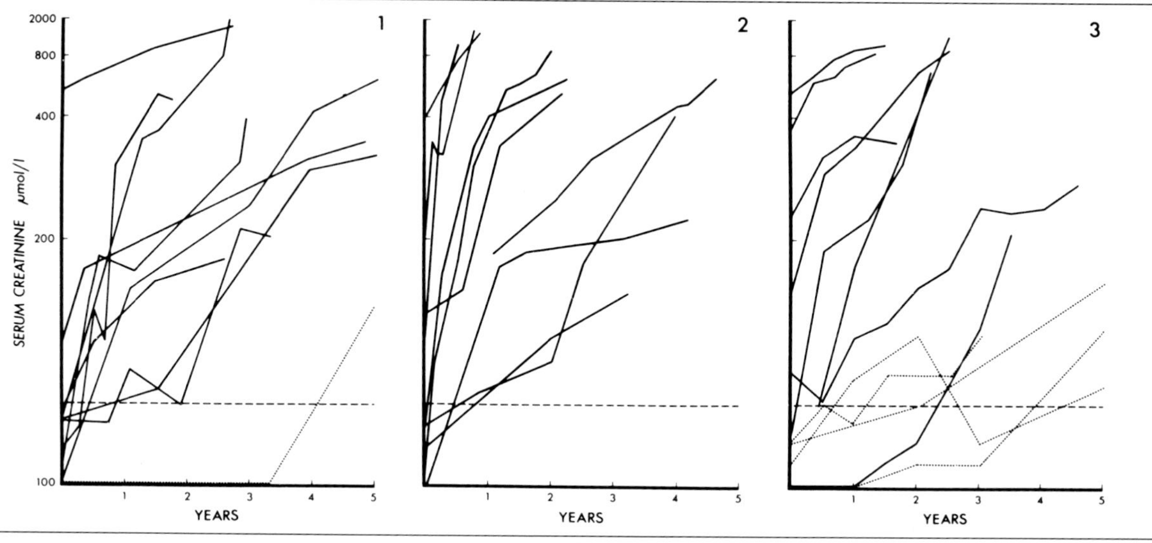

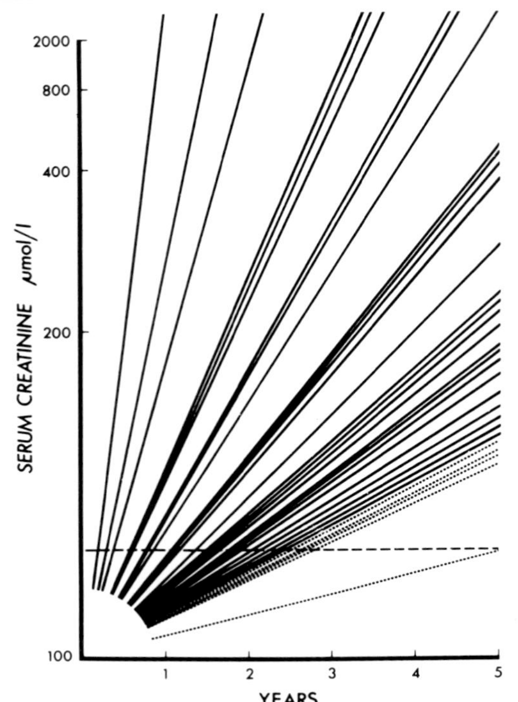

Fig. 69-15. Plot of the slope of the change in serum creatinine, with time, in 27 patients with membranous nephropathy and deterioration and 5 patients with slow deterioration, where the slope has been projected back to a uniform "starting point" of 100 μmoles/L. (From Davison et al. [132], with permission of the editors and publishers.)

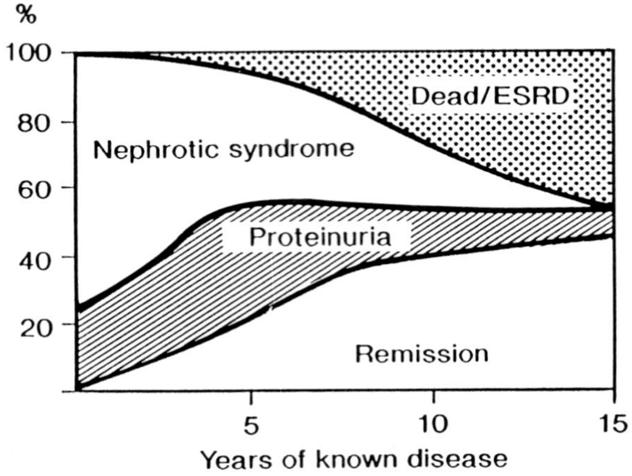

Fig. 69-16. The course of membranous nephropathy, summarized from personal data and the literature up to 1978. The evolution is relatively slow, and remissions and entry to uremia may occur more than 15 years from onset, although some patients evolve much more rapidly. (Modified from Cameron, 1979 [75], with permission of the editor and publishers.)

trials in membranous nephrotics in Italy [386], Canada [94], and the United Kingdom [85]. A total of 144 control patients were entered into these trials on roughly the same criteria (data from the Canadian trial are included here only for those patients with a nephrotic syndrome). After a follow-up averaging just under 5 years, a total of 16 patients (11%) had actually started dialysis, and a further 9 patients (6%) had plasma creatinines in excess of 400 μmol/liter.

Other series of untreated patients have also been published from individual units: Donadio et al. [141], 89 patients; Honkanen [236], 19 patients; Kida et al. [274], 45 patients; Murphy et al. [347], 79 patients; as well as a large collected series [484]. Although not all the patients in these studies had a nephrotic syndrome, these series in general confirm the apparently better prognosis—at least during the first decade—in recent studies of untreated membranous nephropathy. Estimated 10-year renal survivals were 77 percent [484], 81 percent [347], 64 percent [141], 82 percent [236], and 92 percent [274]. Figure 69-16 has thus been modified from that first published in Cameron [50] and reproduced in the previous edition of this book, in the light of these more recent data, to show that more than 40 percent of adult-onset patients will go into remission and only about 10 percent will go into renal failure or die within 10 years. Although some 10- to 15-year data are available from long-term studies of patients studied earlier [393, 507], which suggest a 50 percent renal failure/mortality rate at this time, the 20-year outcome is still not available. In the end, probably only at most 40 percent of all membranous patients go into renal failure, even if a nephrotic syndrome is present to begin with.

Another change in our evaluation of the outcome in membranous nephropathy has been the realization that relapses, and a relapsing course, are not that rare. For example, of a total of 104 patients who went into remission in the four controlled trials cited earlier [85, 94, 111, 386], either spontaneously or in apparent response to treatment, no less than 34 subsequently relapsed; of these 34, 8 were among 39 untreated patients, perhaps suggesting a higher relapse rate in patients with corticosteroid-induced remissions. Passerini and colleagues [373] have examined the prognostic implications of complete remission of proteinuria following treatment, even if it subsequently returns. In 33 patients followed for a median of 8 years, none had developed an abnormal plasma creatinine, although half (16) relapsed, 9 with a full nephrotic syndrome. Passerini and her colleagues estimate, using Kaplan-Meier statistics, that two-thirds of those who go into remission will have a further relapse of proteinuria before 10 years have gone by.

The realization that the prognosis for membranous nephropathy with regard to renal function is better than formerly supposed presents formidable problems in the design and conduct of therapeutic trials [86, 94, 111, 386]. First, the rather good survival and spontaneous tendency toward remission make it difficult to show improvement in terms of renal or patient survival, at least within the usual length of trials in practice. Trial end points must depend, therefore, on levels of renal function and proteinuria. Second, any trial that randomizes patients at apparent onset will result in the control limb including 3 or 4 in every 10 who will remit spontaneously and thus can only suffer side effects without benefit from the treatment.

Possible interventions and trials in membranous nephropathy are discussed in Chap. 65, but here we may consider which criteria might allow us to predict entry to renal failure at or near onset in idiopathic membranous nephropathy (see Zucchelli and Pasquali [505] for detailed discussion). *Clinically,* several features seem to carry a poorer prognosis in univariate analysis: male sex [132, 238], increasing age [132], proteinuria in excess of, rather than below, the nephrotic range [132, 360], reduced renal function [132, 360, 484], and raised blood pressure [141, 484]. Not all of these criteria, however, have emerged as significant in *all* the various studies that have examined them, with the exception of proteinuria. The prognosis of nonnephrotic patients with membranous nephropathy was considered in detail by Kobayashi and colleagues [287]. Of 123 patients with membranous nephropathy and subnephrotic proteinuria, including 18 of their own patients, only 13 (10%) had gone into renal failure over a mean follow-up of 4 years, even though 40 had later developed a full nephrotic syndrome. Twenty-five (22%) were in complete remission.

In white populations, a strong association between membranous nephropathy and the whole MHC haplotype HLA-A1-B8-DR3, and each of its component genes, has been described, while in Japanese populations the association is with HLA-DR2 (see Chap. 65 for discussion). Despite some earlier data that suggested correlations between outcome and MHC type among whites [370, 506], the largest study to date, that of the British MRC trial [85], failed to reveal any associations between either HLA or Bf allotypes and outcome in more than 100 patients with nephrotic syndrome and idiopathic membranous nephropathy.

On *histologic* examination, patients with milder (class I and II) glomerular disease [360, 484, 506] have been suggested to do better than those with class III and IV lesions, but several other groups have failed to find any correlation [132, 393, 462]. Bohle et al. [54] and our group [393] noted that interstitial lesions best predicted a poor outcome, and more recently Bohle's group [484] have performed a multivariate analysis that confirms that tubulointerstitial lesions predict a poor outcome better than any other criterion; Ponticelli and colleagues [386] came to the same conclusion. In addition, if the interstitial infiltrate is phenotyped, the numbers of both monocytes and T helper cells in the interstitium predict the GFR after 5 years follow-up [10] (Fig. 69-17).

Some patients show focal sclerosing lesions [181], and these may have some value in predicting outcome. Vascular lesions predicted outcome in our univariate analysis with long-term follow-up [462]. Finally, a few patients with membranous nephropathy develop crescentic nephritis [279, 340] with or without circulating antiglomerular basement membrane antibody. A poorer prognosis is experienced by these unfortunate patients, but luckily they are rare.

As in most glomerular diseases, in membranous nephropathy, once renal function has begun to fall, it usually continues to decline at a varying rate over the following years until end-stage renal disease is reached [132]. However, one or two circumstances may lead to acute *reversible* declines in renal function, such as renal venous thrombosis, the appearance of a spontaneous or drug-induced acute interstitial nephritis, or the formation of new crescents as just discussed. In the course of the tri-hospital study [132], it became apparent that some patients with membranous nephropathy might show a reversible decline in function without any of these circumstances being present. In the MRC trial [86], 6 patients showed remarkable slowing in renal function, and one reversal of decline, without any identifiable event or intervention such as control of hypertension, treatment with immunosuppressive agents, or use of low-protein diets. This obviously needs to be taken into account when evaluating data of serial renal function studies in relation to late treatment interventions.

In *children,* membranous nephropathy is rare in predominantly white populations, accounting for only 1 percent of nephrotic syndromes in childhood in the unselected data of the ISKDC. However, in some areas of the world, particularly the Far East and Poland, membranous nephropathy in association with hepatitis B carriage accounts for 5 to 15 percent of nephrotic syndromes in childhood [66, 447] (see Cameron [81] for detailed references). In children, up to 40 percent have some associated disease, principally infections [81], contrasting with only about 20 to 25 percent in adults [4, 68]. Because such forms of membranous nephropathy usually do well [283], it is not surprising that the overall prognosis for children with membranous nephropathy is good; however, even in the apparently idiopathic cases, the outlook is much better than in adults, with less than 10 percent going into renal failure. Such an evolution is almost unknown with onset under the age of 10 and rare with onset under the age of 20 [81, 211, 392, 455]. One interesting observation is that children with membranous nephropathy never, and adolescents very rarely, develop renal venous thrombosis.

MESANGIOCAPILLARY GLOMERULONEPHRITIS

Since the early 1970s, it has been usual to divide the optical microscopic appearances of mesangiocapillary (membranoproliferative) glomerulonephritis (see Chap. 66), often abbreviated MCGN or MPGN, into two categories: the commoner variety with *subendothelial* immune aggregates (type I); and a variety with extensive replacement of the lamina densa of the capillary basement membranes and those of the tubules and Bowman's capsule, with a birefringent, rather continuous material that takes stains avidly (type II). On optical microscopy, however, not all type I patients show a true mesangiocapillary pattern, that is, expansion of the mesangium with a complex thickening of the glomerular capillary walls by mesangial cell cytoplasm and new material. A "type III" MCGN has been distinguished by some authors [12, 13, 254, 441, 442] in which the immune aggregates are found not only at a subendothelial site, but also throughout the basement membrane itself on electron microscopy with subepithelial aggregates in

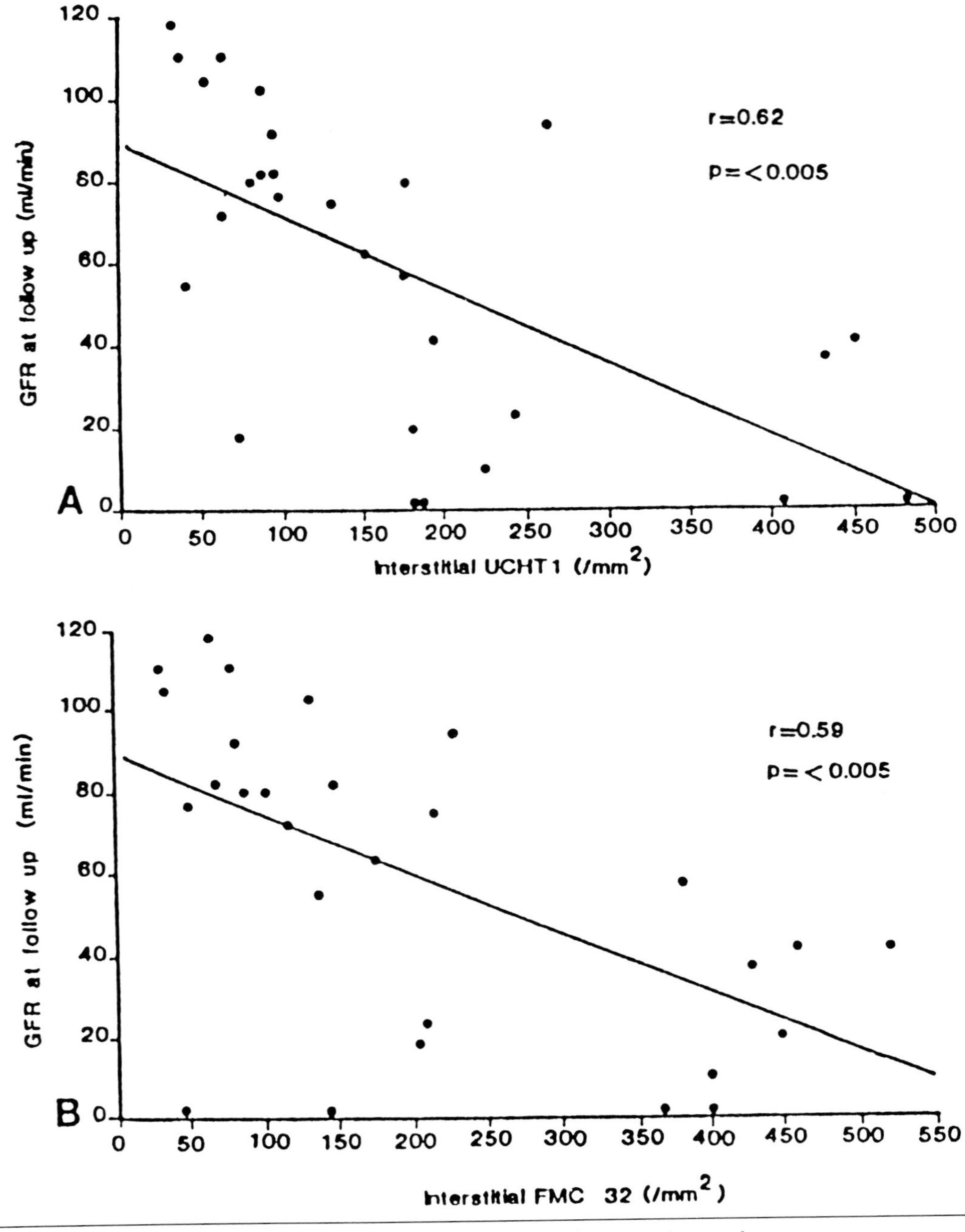

Fig. 69-17. In patients with membranous nephropathy, the relationship between the numbers of interstitial T lymphocytes (A) and monocytes (B) in the initial biopsy and the glomerular filtration rate (GFR) assessed by the single injection 51Cr− edetate method after an average of 5 years' follow-up is plotted. The numbers of cells predict the future course of the GFR with some accuracy. (Data from Alexopoulos et al. [9].) UCHT 1 = monoclonal antibody directed against CD14 (Dr. Hzola, Flinders Medical Center); FMC 32 = monoclonal antibody directed against CD3 (Dr. Beverly, University College Hospital).

addition, so that in isolation the appearances resemble those of an advanced membranous nephropathy. Some authors, including myself, regard this as a later stage of type I MCGN, and it will be so treated in this chapter.

One striking feature of data from Europe in recent years has been the decline in the numbers of new patients presenting with either type of MCGN [36, 429], suggesting that some precipitating environmental agent or agents, most probably infectious, has declined in frequency. The appearance has always been unusual in both adults and children in Japan, although it is very common in some other parts of the world; two series from Iran have shown MCGN to be the underlying histologic appearance of two-thirds of adult-onset nephrotic syndromes [59, 252].

The appearance may be seen complicating a variety of infections and as part of systemic disorders. The infection-related MCGN patients need to be separated from the apparently idiopathic disorder, since the outlook for infection-related MCGN, whether from endocarditis [275], infected juguloatrial shunts [22, 275], or deep sepsis [43], is in general good, providing that the infection can be controlled. The prognosis of MCGN in a setting of lupus or Henoch-Schönlein purpura is considered in later sections of this chapter.

The survival of patients with idiopathic types I and II MCGN was documented in a number of series during the 1970s, with a few more recent sets of data, summarized in Fig. 69-18. These show that, in general, MCGN of either type is usually a progressive disorder in both white and Chinese [96] populations, with estimated survival of renal function at 10 years being about 60 percent and 15-year survival no more than 50 percent. In agreement with this, a recent large collaborative study from Italy [169] on 246 patients gave an estimated 10-year survival of 57 percent. Since the patients are generally children or young adults [96], the effect of nonrenal deaths is lower than in membranous nephropathy, for example. The data from MCGN type I are rather concordant, while those for type II show much more varied outcomes, perhaps because of the small number of patients studied in individual series. In general, no form of treatment appears to affect the outcome in either form of MCGN, with the exception of a single series discussed below, and so untreated and treated patients are not separated in the data presented here.

In 1983, we [96] updated our follow-up on 104 patients (69 type I and 35 type II) who had an idiopathic disease. These data (Fig. 69-19) are in general agreement with the others published during the past two decades, with only 7 patients showing complete remission. The group of the Hôpital des Enfants Malades in Paris presented their data in the same year [206]. Complete remission was equally rare, only 1 type II and 4 type I patients achieving this out of 44 and 84 idiopathic cases respectively. In contrast, of the 44 type II patients, 18 were either dead or in end-stage renal disease, one was in uremia, 11 had a persisting nephrotic syndrome, and 11 had persisting proteinuria and normal renal function. Of the 84 type I patients, 21 were dead or in treatment for end-stage renal disease, 9 had chronic renal failure, 18 a persisting nephrotic syndrome, and 32 persisting proteinuria with normal renal function. Droz et al. [144] presented data in abstract from the adult series at the Hopital Necker, on 196 cases of type I followed 1 to 25 years; 13 went into complete remission, but 106 had gone into renal failure, while 54 remained unchanged with persisting proteinuria. In type II MCGN, only two groups have noted a better prognosis, in children: Klein et al. [280] found that 5 of 18 patients were in remission after 11 $\pm$ 1 years follow-up. Similarly Strife et al. [442] reported 17 children with type II MCGN, with only 4 showing progressive disease, 3 being nephrotic, while no child presenting with subnephrotic proteinuria showed progression.

Finally, the controlled trials in Canada [93] and the United States [136] gave some data on serial GFRs in adult patients with type I MCGN. In the former trial [93], over 18 months the control group lost 9 ml/minute, while the treatment group did marginally worse—14 ml/minute. In the Mayo Clinic trial [136], the control group lost a mean of 19 ml/minute over 1 year, while those treated with aspirin and dipyridamole lost only 5 ml/minute. However, long-term follow-up was identical in the two groups despite continued treatment [139]. The rate of falloff in renal function was, as in membranous nephropathy, very varied; Chan et al. [96] analyzed rates of change in $1/P_{creat}$ plasma, and noted similar wide variations in rates of decline in renal function. The frequency with which sudden changes in the GFR or its rate of decline may be seen in either type of MCGN has been noted earlier [71].

We [96] and Schmitt and colleagues [415], who studied only type I MCGN, were able to identify *clinical* indicators of poor prognosis using univariate analysis (Table 69-6). As in most forms of progressive glomerular disease, in our data and in most other series, a nephrotic syndrome, particularly if persistent, was a major clinical indicator of a poor outcome; but interestingly Schmitt et al. [415] did not confirm this conclusion. Hypertension was modestly predictive of poor outcome in both sets of data [96, 415], but there was (in sharp contrast to membranous nephropathy) no difference in outcome between adults and children. In our series, the presence, absence, or degree of hypocomplementemia had no relation to outcome in either type of MCGN, suggesting that the prominent in vivo complement breakdown is an epiphenomenon of the disease, although Swainson et al. [446] and Klein et al. [280] reported the opposite in smaller series. Magil et al. [316] found males did worse than females, as in other forms of glomerular disease, but this trend did not reach significance in our own or any other study.

Hardly surprising, both we and Schmitt found that reduced GFR [96] or raised plasma creatinine [415] at presentation had an adverse effect on outcome. Neither we nor the Parisians [206] found an onset with an acute nephritic syndrome and macroscopic hematuria (common in children) to be an adverse feature, but Donadio et al. [136] found the contrary, and Bennett et al. [46] noted a higher incidence of macroscopic hematuria in type II MCGN patients who did badly. The effect of hypertension is controversial; Schmitt et al. [415] found it to be a strong predictor of adverse outcome and a major direct cause of death, while we [96] and Valles Prats et al. [468] found no effect on outlook. Clearly the quality of blood pressure control will be a major factor here.

Histologically, Barbiano di Belgiojoso et al. [37] first suggested that the presence of crescents was an adverse feature, and we [96] and the Paris study [201] confirmed this. Schmitt et al. [415] performed a more elaborate analysis of the glomerular histology, with five grades, the last of which included crescent formation; these patients did worst of all. Although Barbiano di Belgiojoso et al. [37] noted a poorer prognosis for those patients with more lobular forms of glomerulonephritis, neither Schmitt's nor our data confirmed this suggestion. Schmitt et al. [415] also assessed interstitial changes

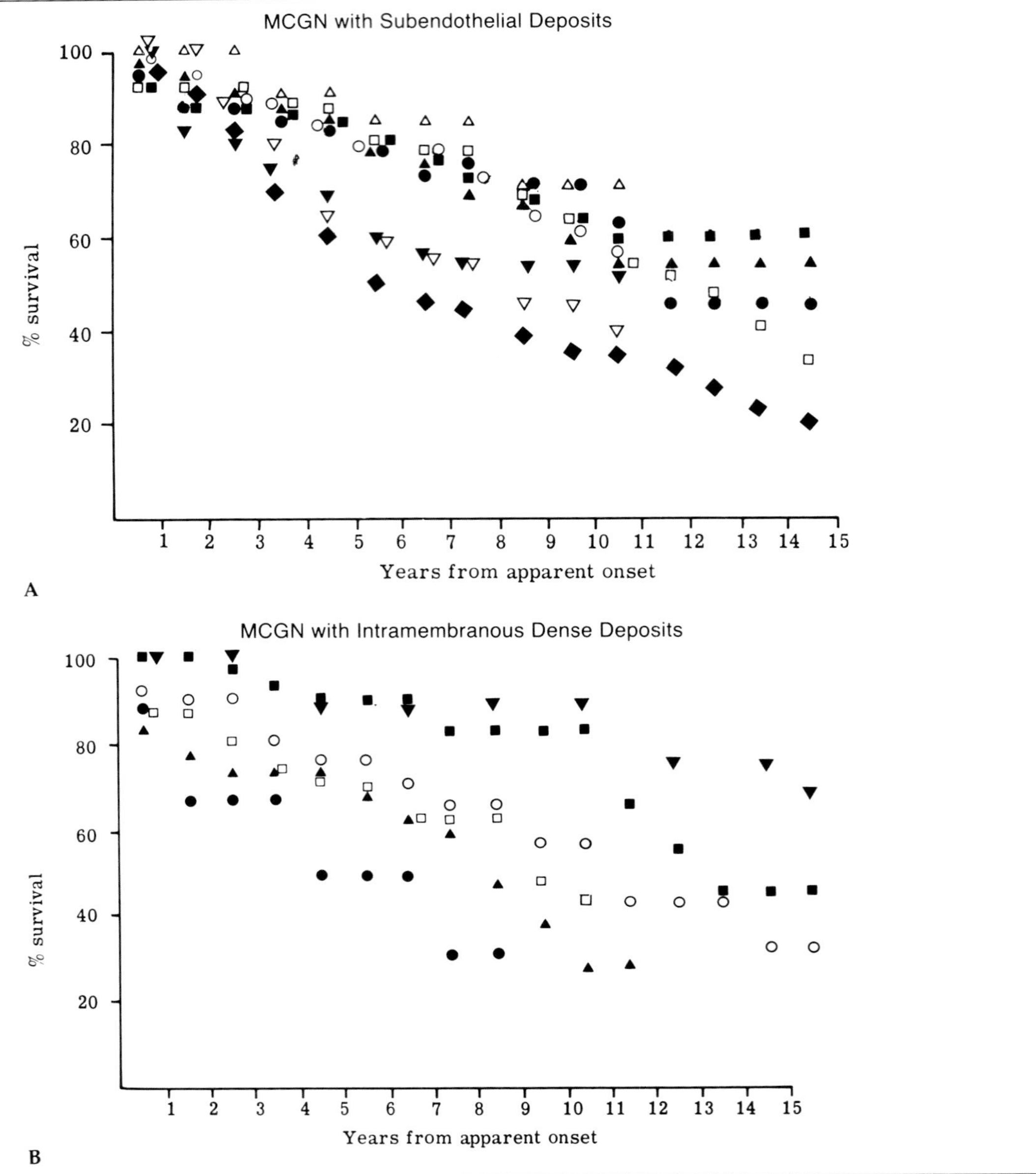

Fig. 69-18. Actuarially calculated probability of survival of renal function, or death from renal failure, in patients with mesangiocapillary glomerulonephritis types I (A) and II (B). In A, data are included from the following series: Herdman et al., 1970 [227], 22 children (△); Habib et al., 1975 [210], 84 children (▲); Cameron et al., 1983 [90], 75 adults and children (●); Nyberg et al., 1980 [365], 28 adults (■); Swainson et al., 1983 [446], 17 adults (○); Valles Prats et al., 1985 [468], 72 adults and children (□); Chan et al., 1989 [96], 46 adults (▽); Donadio and Offord, 1989 [139], 40 adults (▼); and Schmitt et al., 1990 [415], 220 adults (◆). In B, the following series of patients with type II MCGN are included: Antoine and Faye, 1972 [14], 34 adults (○); Galle and Mahieu, 1975 [183], 40 adults (■); Habib et al., 1975 [210], 44 children (▲); Cameron et al., 1983 [90], 25 children and adults (●); Swainson et al., 1983 [446], 23 adults (□); and Bennett et al., 1989 [46], 27 adults (▼).

carefully, which we did not, and found as in other glomerular diseases that the degree of tubulointerstitial changes was strongly predictive of outcome (Fig. 69-20).

One group has consistently claimed that their treatment results—using alternate-day, high-dose oral prednisolone—have been consistently better than in children with type I MCGN managed in other units [324, 325, 488], with a 10-year survival of renal function of almost 90 percent. However, the ISKDC [248] was unable to reproduce these challenging data in a prospective randomized controlled trial of this therapy, although a trend in favor of the treatment group was emerging

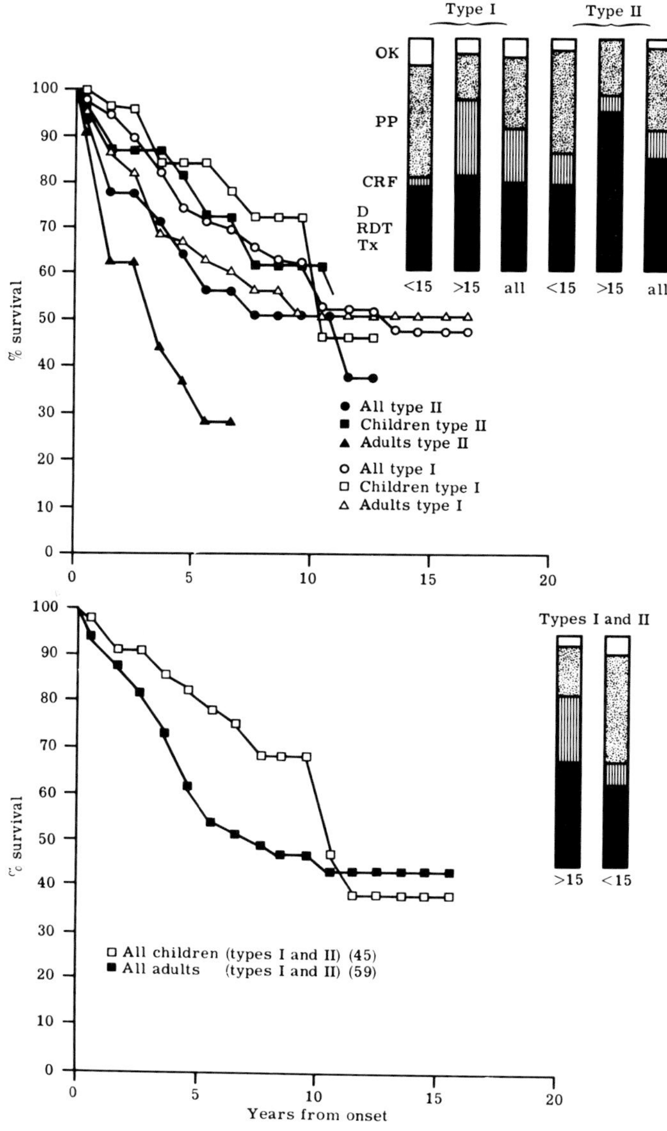

Fig. 69-19. (*Top*) Survival and status at last follow-up evaluation in patients with mesangiocapillary glomerulonephritis. The survival curves were calculated by the actuarial method and show data for patients of all ages with both types I and type II (*heavy lines*) and data for each of these two groups for children and for adults (*lighter lines*). None of the curves differ from each other when tested by the log-rank method (Peto et al. [376]), although the adult patients with type II mesangiocapillary glomerulonephritis approach significance when compared with similar children ($p = 0.08$). The most recent status is shown at top right: OK = well, normal urine, normal renal function; PP = persistent proteinuria with or without a nephrotic syndrome but with normal renal function; GFR = glomerular filtration rate of less than 80 ml/min/1.73 m^2 and persistent proteinuria with or without a nephrotic syndrome; D, RDT, Tx = dead, regular dialysis treatment, or transplantation. Data are presented for each of types I and II mesangiocapillary glomerulonephritis for patients above and below the age of 15 years at apparent onset. In type I mesangiocapillary glomerulonephritis, children have a significantly better prognosis than adults ($p < 0.01$) compared in this fashion. Similarly, data for types I and II together show a significant difference ($p = 0.003$). In the case of patients with type II alone, the differences between children ($n = 22$) and adults ($n = 13$) were not significant ($p = 0.12$) (see Table 69-8). (*Bottom*) Survival in children and adults with mesangiocapillary glomerulonephritis. For this analysis, types I and II have been considered together. There is no significant difference between the two curves, although there is an excess of early deaths among the adult patients. When the data for most recent status are examined, there is a significantly worse prognosis for adults than children ($\chi^2 = 7.74$, $p = 0.003$). (From Cameron et al. [90], with permission of the editors and publishers.)

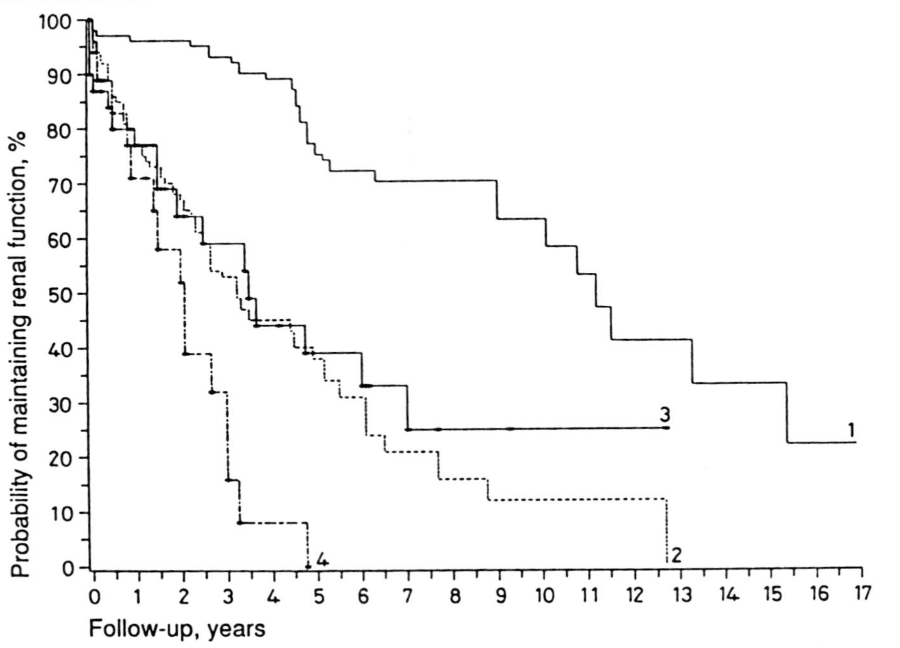

Fig. 69-20. Probability of entering renal failure in patients with mesangiocapillary glomerulonephritis type I, according to the degree of interstitial changes. Curve 1 is derived from 92 patients with a normal interstitium in the initial biopsy; curve 2 from 77 patients with interstitial fibrosis only; curve 3 from 32 patients with tubular damage only; and curve 4 from 19 patients with both tubular damage and interstitial fibrosis present. (From Schmitt et al. [415], with permission.)

when the trial was terminated, largely because of the high rate of withdrawal from the treatment group because of side effects, particularly severe hypertension. Lagrue [293] has also claimed that results in adults with type I MCGN using nonsteroidal anti-inflammatory drugs are much better than those from other units (10-year survival 78%). However, it is clear that many of the patients treated in this study were late survivors even before treatment was begun and thus intrinsically had a better outlook than the group as a whole. The general opinion is that no treatment reliably affects the long-term outlook of MCGN of either type.

ENDOCAPILLARY EXUDATIVE GLOMERULONEPHRITIS (POSTINFECTIOUS NEPHRITIS)

In this group of patients, we have particular problems with definition, as mentioned in the introduction to this chapter (see Chap. 63). Different observers may be talking about different types of patients, and it is essential to be absolutely clear about which are—and which are not—the subject of study. Three main sets of observation describe this group of patients, and these are best represented by the Venn diagram that forms Fig. 69-21. These sets are the *clinical presentation* (an acute nephritic syndrome), a *precipitating event* (e.g., documented antecedent streptococcal infection), and the *histopathology* of an exclusively, or at least predominant, endocapillary wall, and with infiltrates of leukocytes in the early stages (endocapillary glomerulonephritis, exudative glomerulonephritis).

Apart from core patients who satisfy all three criteria (A in diagram), there will be other patients who, variably, do not; in temperate climates, the majority of patients with an acute nephritic syndrome do not seem to have a renal disorder that has arisen from streptococcal infections, which are now rare with better hygiene and the absence of insect vectors (b, *bottom left,* and c, *top left*). Patients with an acute nephritic syndrome and streptococcal infection may present with mesangiocapillary patterns of nephritis or expansive crescent formation (d, *at top*). E and f on the right of the diagram represent rather rare occurrences, but set g spreads into the diverse group of mesangial and other proliferative glomerulonephritides discussed earlier in association with IgA-associated nephropathy and focal segmental sclerosis.

Obviously, different mixes of patients within these groups will lead to different impressions of outcomes. Since this chapter is predominantly organized according to appearances viewed by optical microscopy, we will discuss here only those patients with an exudative endocapillary pattern, since the prognosis of those streptococcal patients with acute nephritis who show either mesangiocapillary glomerulonephritis or extensive crescents on biopsy resembles closely that of nonstreptococcal cases with a similar histology. Even with the core

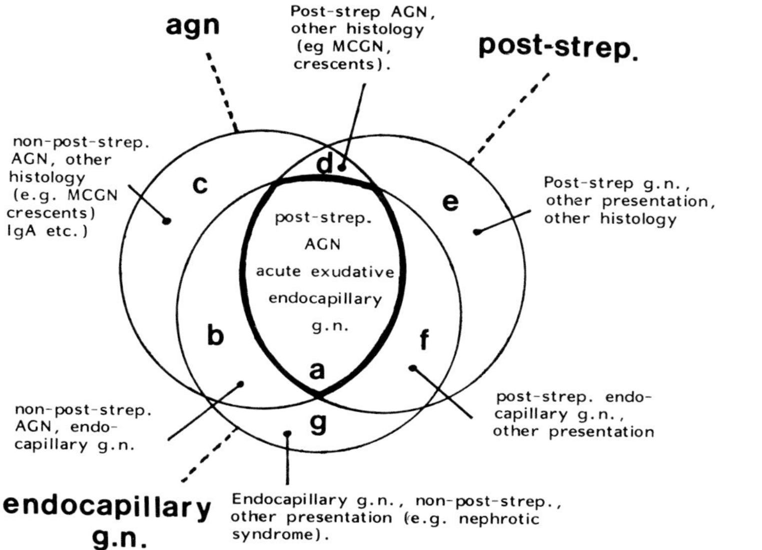

Fig. 69-21. A Venn diagram of the three sets of acute glomerulonephritis (clinical syndrome), streptococcal etiology, and endocapillary glomerulonephritis (histologic appearance), which together make seven subsets, as indicated by the letters a through g. The "core" subset of poststreptococcal acute glomerulonephritis (agn; AGN) with an acute exudative endocapillary glomerulonephritis is indicated in the center by a and the other groups, by b through g (see text).

group, we have two separate clusters to consider: those patients associated with epidemics of disease and those that appear to be sporadic. The prognosis of the latter may well be not so good as those observed in an epidemic setting.

Few subjects seem to have generated so much controversy as the frequency of occult or evident streptococcal glomerulonephritis as a cause of chronic renal failure [27] and on the other hand, the frequency with which persistent disease and an outcome in renal failure may be expected in patients with poststreptococcal or nonstreptococcal acute nephritis with diffuse exudative/proliferative changes [27, 149, 291]. Part of the problem arises from the fact that the mix of cases observed on the one hand in epidemics, mostly not in a Western urban environment, and the sporadic patients seen in city center referral specialist units is not the same.

As mentioned previously, most of the rather few cases of acute nephritis in the United Kingdom are now *not* the sequel of streptococcal infection [329]. As in Meadow's data [329], in less than one-third of patients with acute nephritis in our own series [88] was it possible to find any evidence of streptococcal infection. Conversely, an unknown number of patients may have subclinical attacks of poststreptococcal nephritis; these at least equal the obvious cases in the epidemic situation and may exceed them severalfold [135, 265, 397, 405]. The urine may show little or no abnormality [152, 262], and hypertension may be the principal feature. Unless these atypical cases are very thoroughly investigated with serology, serial complement estimations, and renal biopsy with electron microscopy, it may be difficult to exclude other forms of glomerulonephritis.

Occasional patients with a typical insidious nephrotic syndrome may show, on renal biopsy, typical active diffuse endothelial nephritis. Several patients with this appearance in our series of nephrotic proliferative glomerulonephritis patients had microscopic hematuria, all were 15 years old or older, and 2 had initially low plasma concentrations of the C3 component of complement. Some otherwise typical acute nephritic patients may have rather profuse proteinuria and show, rather briefly, a full nephrotic syndrome; this can certainly occur with the biopsy appearances discussed here, but it raises the suspicion of a mesangiocapillary glomerulonephritis. An occasional patient with only acute endothelial proliferative glomerulonephritis presents with anuria and acute renal failure [78].

My own reading of the data on long-term follow-up is that the majority of patients who suffer a typical acute nephritic syndrome, and have an active diffuse endocapillary glomerulonephritis on biopsy, heal clinically and histologically. Let us examine first the evidence for this statement in *childhood* cases. Many early statements of the prognosis of acute nephritis in children are difficult to evaluate, since in almost all cases, histology was not available, and the assumption was made (often without good evidence) that acute glomerulonephritis must necessarily be poststreptococcal. These early papers are summarized by Perlman et al. [375]. One paper is worthy of summary here, however, since it represents an early attempt to assess the very long-term prognosis of acute nephritic children [226]. Twenty-seven patients, who had acute nephritis in childhood severe enough to result in hospital admission, were studied 19 to 32 years later. These patients represented only 25 percent of the 130, which Herbert [226] set out to trace. None of the 27 showed evidence of disease, and all urine tests and blood pressure were normal; only 1 patient had died, from tuberculosis.

Epidemic Cases. The prognosis of epidemic, proved acute poststreptococcal glomerulonephritis appears to be equally benign. Perlman et al. [375] studied the children who had acute glomerulonephritis 10 years previously in the streptococcal epidemic in the Red Lake Indian reservation. All children had been studied initially and were shown to have streptococcal infection. After 10 years, renal function was normal in all, and the degree of proteinuria and hematuria did not differ from controls. Renal biopsies were performed in 12 of the 61 children; 12 were entirely normal and 4 showed minor mesangial changes.

Sanjad et al. [407] reported on 153 cases of acute glomerulonephritis from Florida. In this study, 103 patients were followed up, and none showed any clinical evidence of progressive disease up to 10 years later. However, 10 children showed minor urinary abnormalities, and all 6 who were biopsied had some glomerular abnormality.

Potter et al. [387], Nissenson et al. [359], and Potter et al. [388], in an important study, described the 2- to 6-, 7- to 12-, and 12- to 17-year follow-up of a group of mixed sporadic and epidemic cases of poststreptococcal nephritis, mostly children, collected in Trinidad in 1965 and the following years. This study involved over 700 persons, almost all of whom were still available in 1977 [359]. Only 2 patients had died in renal failure, 19 had proteinuria, 3 had hematuria, and 3 had both. The incidence of hypertension (16 cases) was no higher than expected from the Trinidadian population as a whole. The 1981 survey [388] was less complete, only 534 patients with urinary abnormalities were identified, all with normal plasma creatinine concentrations; it is worth noting that in the histories of the three patients who had died, it was not clear whether they died of renal failure or, if so, whether this was attributable to their nephritis. An interesting observation of Nissenson et al. [359] was of 13 persons who had abnormal urine, but no symptoms during the attack, i.e., subclinical nephritis; none showed abnormalities 7 to 12 years later. The other study of this type of patient is that of Smith et al. [430], who biopsied and followed up symptomless patients with acute poststreptococcal nephritis and minor urinary abnormalities. After 1 to 4 years, 8 of 28 patients showed persisting urinary abnormalities, and 2 had hypertension.

Rodriguez-Iturbe et al. [185, 396, 397] have summarized their experience of epidemic poststreptococcal glomerulonephritis in Maracaibo; only 1 patient of 71 followed for 11 to 12 years had gone into renal failure, but 21 percent still showed urinary abnormalities [185].

Sporadic Cases. Evidence is also available from patients with sporadic poststreptococcal glomerulonephritis in childhood. The most extensive study is that from Galveston [135, 457]. In this study, 60 patients were followed for at least 3 years, an important aspect in a condition with a relatively benign prognosis. Only 1 patient of 60 died after 2 years, and his initial biopsy showed an unstated number of epithelial crescents; another child died of causes unrelated to renal disease at 18 months. At 3 years, only 8 of 45 children had urinary abnormalities [135], and at 5 years, only 2 of 32 still under observation showed proteinuria. Similarly, in Lewy's study [311] of 46 children with sporadic poststreptococcal glomerulonephritis, only 4 patients died, all showing extensive crescent formation in their biopsies. Two children still showed proteinuria after 5 years' follow-up, one of whom had crescents in his initial biopsy; only 3 patients were lost to follow-up. Hinglais et al. [231] present evidence from 29 children with acute nephritic syndromes; 16 of their total of 65 had raised antistreptolysin levels, but it is impossible to deduce which of these were children. Of the 29 children, 25 had various forms of endocapillary glomerulonephritis, including exudative patterns with "humps" in 16. No patient with only endocapillary glomerulonephritis did poorly, and at the assessment point 2 years later, all those endocapillary cases with humps had normal urine. Evidence of persistent disease or progression was confined to those patients showing other than endocapillary lesions, as in the series of Mota-Hernandez et al. [344]. Baldwin et al. [30] included 37 children in their mainly adult study. One child required dialysis after 9 weeks, and her biopsy showed extensive epithelial crescents. In 6 children, glomerular filtration rates were measured 3 to 10 years from onset; all were more than 80 ml/min except one of 77 ml/min (uncorrected). Later, Schacht et al. [410] reviewed their experience of renal damage in childhood acute glomerulonephritis.

Finally, in our own series [102, 188], 38 children with acute poststreptococcal glomerulonephritis were first studied between 1962 and 1970. Two patients died during the acute illness with crescentic nephritis, and 33 of the remaining 36 were studied a mean of 9.4 years later (range 6–13 years) [188]. Two of the other 3 patients were known to be alive and in good health and only 1 was lost to follow-up entirely. One patient showed persistent hypocomplementemia, and a second biopsy in this child showed mesangiocapillary glomerulonephritis [193]. All others showed normal blood urea and plasma creatinine concentrations and, in 21, creatinine clearances were normal (mean 113 ml/min, range 80 to 170 ml/min/1.73 m^2). However, 9 patients showed persisting urinary abnormalities: hematuria plus proteinuria in 3, and isolated proteinuria in 6, ranging from 0.2 to 0.5 gm per day. Blood pressure was normal in all patients. All of these patients were recalled for restudy a mean of 19.4 (range 14.6–22.0) years later [102]. Only 1 was hypertensive, 3 patients had microscopic hematuria, and the patient with MCGN had proteinuria in addition. All showed normal plasma creatinine concentrations.

Thus the accumulated evidence suggests that in both epidemic and sporadic poststreptococcal glomerulonephritis and other acute nephritic syndromes in *childhood*, a similar pattern emerges. If the biopsy shows endocapillary changes only, whether or not "humps" are present, then healing within 5 years is the rule. The few patients who do badly almost always show some other histologic pattern and are usually associated with other adverse features, such as the appearance of a full nephrotic syndrome.

Turning to *adults*, the evidence is somewhat stronger that progression may occur in acute poststreptococcal glomerulonephritis, even in those with only an endocapillary glomerulonephritis on renal biopsy. In addition, other patterns of histology, such as the presence of extracapillary crescents, are more common. In Jennings and Earle's classic paper on poststreptococcal glomerulonephritis in 1961 [256], the only patient of the 36 who died, still anuric, had extensive crescent formation in his biopsy. Thirteen other patients had clinical evidence of continuing disease at follow-up 5 months to 4 years from onset. McCluskey and Baldwin [323] report on a mixed group of adults with an acute nephritic onset; 5 patients died and a further 14 showed evidence of progressive disease. Some of their patients showed evidence of diffuse crescentic glomerulonephritis or of mesangiocapillary glomerulonephritis. More recently, Baldwin and colleagues [27, 30, 32] have reported their findings in 89 adults with proved poststreptococcal glomerulonephritis, drawing the widely quoted conclusion that "up to one-half" of patients with this condition show evidence of progressive disease. This conclusion deserves careful examination.

Of the 10 patients over the age of 15 years at onset who died (or required dialysis), extensive crescent formation was present, and of these 10, 4 had a rapidly progressive course over 3 months into renal failure. The other patient with crescentic glomerulonephritis became uremic 6 months after a second attack of glomerulonephritis. Of the other 5 who died, only 2 died later, at 2 and 6 years of follow-up. Six of these 10 fatal patients showed a full nephrotic syndrome at presentation. These patients, therefore, although part of the spectrum of poststreptococcal nephritis, are not typical of this condition and were, of course, seen in a tertiary referral center.

In the remainder of the patients in this study, the evidence for persisting disease must be considered against the large fallout of patients that occurred during the study. Unlike the childhood series reported previously, only 56 of 126 patients completed even 1 year's follow-up, only 29 were still in contact after 5 years, and only 5 at 10 years or more. The fact that 50 percent of patients showed a raised blood pressure after 8 to 10 years is made less impressive when one remembers that the 10 patients studied at this time represented only *7 percent* of the whole group; the assumption cannot be made, as discussed in the introduction, that those patients lost to follow-up had the same characteristics as those retained. In most studies of relatively benign disease, as noted in the introduction, the more severe cases progressively concentrate in the follow-up group.

However, 8 of 16 adults whose glomerular filtration rate was measured 3 to 15 years after their attack of glomerulonephritis showed values of less than 80 ml/min. An inulin clearance of 100 ml/min was used as the lower limit of normality. These data are not corrected for sex, surface area, or age, and other published figures suggest that this would not represent the mean minus two standard deviations. Nor were the blood pressures compared with normal data for sex and age. Twenty patients still had proteinuria at 5 years, and 4 at 10 years, although the description of proteinuria as evidence of irreversible disease is not justified. Hypertension, judged as a diastolic blood pressure above 90 mm Hg was, however, equally common.

Baldwin and Schact [32] present further data on this group of patients: 125 of 176 patients in the study had a renal biopsy, and 105 had been followed for 2 years or more. By 1975, 9 patients had been observed to enter terminal renal failure within a maximum of 6 months from onset, while 6 others progressed to uremia from 1 to 12 years after onset; all this latter group showed typical acute endocapillary glomerulonephritis in their initial biopsy.

What have other authors reported? Hinglais et al. [231], in their study of 36 sporadic acute nephritic adults, found 25 with only endocapillary lesions on renal biopsy. Seven of these showed persisting proteinuria when restudied at 2 years. In contrast, the other 11 patients with changes other than endocapillary glomerulonephritis (mesangiocapillary, extracapillary) all had continuing disease except one. However, glomerular filtration rates were not measured in this study. In our own series, 17 adults showed acute exudative glomerulonephritis on biopsy; 14 presented with an acute nephritic syndrome, 8 being anuric or severely oliguric enough to require dialysis; and in 3 patients, the presentation was a nephrotic syndrome. Thus they represent the most severely affected end of the spectrum of acute exudative endocapillary glomerulonephritis. Two of the anuric patients died from infection before they obtained diuresis, a situation not different from other causes of acute reversible renal failure, especially in older patients. The remainder are well 1 to 10 years later, but only 4 have completely normal urine. Good evidence of streptococcal infection was present in 8 of the 17 patients.

Lien et al. [312] also studied 57 patients, 52 of them adults, suffering from sporadic poststreptococcal glomerulonephritis, for a mean range of 7 (±4) years. All had an initial biopsy, and 33 had repeat biopsies. Two patients died with abnormal renal function, while 11 showed evidence of some renal damage, and 4 additional patients had only hypertension. Vogel and colleagues [472] described 2 to 13 years' follow-up in 72 of 101 adult-onset sporadic cases of acute poststreptococcal nephritis in Germany, Luxemburg, and Austria. Only 3 patients entered terminal renal failure, one only 5 months after transformation into a diffuse crescentic ne-

Table 69-6. Effect of features at onset on prognosis for renal function in type I and type II mesangiocapillary glomerulonephritis

	Type I		Type II		All	
	"Dead"* versus alive	"Uremia"† versus persistent proteinuria and remission	"Dead" versus alive	"Uremia" versus persistent proteinuria and remission	"Dead" versus alive	"Uremia" versus persistent proteinuria and remission
Child or adult (< or >15 years)	NS‡	<0.001	(0.07)	NS	NS	0.003
Hematuria at onset	NS	NS	NS	NS	0.003	NS
Nephrotic syndrome at onset	0.01	NS	NS	NS	0.02	NS
Nephrotic syndrome at any time	0.001	0.06	0.04	NS	0.0001	0.003
Blood pressure elevated at onset	0.03	NS	NS	NS	NS	NS
Glomerular filtration rate decreased at onset	(0.07)	0.002	NS	NS	NS	NS

*"Dead" = dead, dialysis, or transplantation.
†"Uremia" = "dead" or persistent disease with glomerular filtration rate <80 ml/min/1.73 m^2.
‡NS = $p > 0.05$ (x^2 test).
Source: Cameron et al. [90].

phritis in a second biopsy, as others have described [338], including one case of our own [189]. Only 2 other patients had raised plasma creatinines and continued proteinuria. Four other patients died, however, 1 from accelerated hypertension after only 2 months, another of sepsis, and 2 others of unknown causes. They confirmed the suggestion of Hinglais et al. [231] and others that an onset with a nephrotic syndrome is an indication of a poorer prognosis.

Yet again the prognosis for renal function in this study does not accord with that reported by Baldwin's group. Baldwin and Schacht [32] discuss the problem of the interpretation of glomerulosclerosis found in subsequent biopsies. Previous authors, such as Lewy et al. [311] and Dodge et al. [135] had taken glomerulosclerosis as evidence of *healing;* Baldwin and his colleagues, in contrast, regard glomerulosclerosis as a sign of *progression*, and Baldwin and Schacht [32] report a frequency of just under 50 percent in those patients biopsied more than 2 years from onset. This important difference in interpretation can be resolved only by additional data on repeat biopsies.

Baldwin and colleagues [30, 411] indicate doubt also about the assumption that the disappearance of proteinuria suggests healing; 6 patients with normal urine in their series went into renal failure [410]. Although continuation of renal disease rarely occurs without urinary changes, this has been noted, for example, by Northway et al. [362] in mesangiocapillary glomerulonephritis and by Treser et al. [458] in acute nephritis itself. It may be that the "Dauerstadium," or chronic latent, phase of a progressive glomerulonephritis and that some of the undiagnosed patients entering dialysis and transplant programs, aged 30 to 50 years, represent the end result of acute poststreptococcal glomerulonephritis between the ages of 5 and 15 years. This once popular concept has, however, in general, fallen out of favor, but we must not forget that the evidence we have rarely extends beyond 10 years.

In addition to the prognostic value of the finding of mesangiocapillary or crescentic glomerulonephritis in renal biopsies, Sorger et al. [434] point out that what they term the "garland" type of immunofluorescence, contrasting with the more usual "starry sky" pattern and indicating densely packed subepithelial deposits along the basement membrane, carries a poorer prognosis in both children and adults and is correlated, in turn, with continuing profuse proteinuria, one of the clinical indicators of more severe disease. While emphasizing the evidence of glomerulosclerosis, Baldwin's group [184] also point to the fact that widespread vascular sclerosis of arterioles is also present and is a marker of progression. On the clinical side, apart from profuse proteinuria, anuria, or both, the persistence of a low complement level and hypertension beyond about 4 weeks from onset are valuable indicators of a poor outlook; many such patients show mesangiocapillary glomerulonephritis in their biopsies. Patients may begin with a biopsy that shows a pure endocapillary disease which then develops into mesangiocapillary nephritis [188, 193] or into severe crescentic nephritis [189, 338, 366]. However, it must be emphasized again that pure endocapillary glomerulonephritis may occur with anuria, and that anuria does not always indicate crescentic nephritis [78, 170].

One practical problem in uncomplicated childhood cases is to know just how long one has to wait before the urine can be expected to become free of hematuria, trace proteinuria, or both, and whether late renal biopsy should be performed. There are surprisingly few data on this important point, but it has been known for many years that it could take up to several years for complete clinical "healing" to take place. Joseph and Polani [260] provide evidence from a trial of bed rest (which showed no effect) that over 90 percent of children with sporadic poststreptococcal nephritis will be free of hematuria by 6 months.

In summary, the prognosis of acute glomerulonephritis, both epidemic and sporadic, postinfectious or poststreptococcal, probably becomes worse with ascending age. Recovery is almost invariable in the preschool child [135], there is some suggestion of chronicity in older children, and the disease becomes chronic in a significant minority of adults. Added to this, with increasing age, there is an increasing proportion of patients showing diffuse extracapillary proliferation of mesangiocapillary glomerulonephritis, which accounts for an increased incidence of precocious renal failure. It is difficult to generalize from these controversial figures, but of 100 acute nephritic children, 1 percent or less will show crescentic glomerulonephritis and go on to early uremia; 75 percent will be free of proteinuria in 2 to 3 years, and a further 20 percent by 5 years. Only 1 or 2 percent, usually older children, will develop uremia later. Some of these will have shown mesangiocapillary or crescent glomerulonephritis at onset. In adults, perhaps 5 percent will show persisting proteinuria, and some of these patients will have reduced renal function and hypertension. Their fate is not known, but some may progress to uremia within a decade or two.

Thus most of the difficulties and apparent inconsistencies in the various reports of the outcome of acute nephritic patients resolve themselves if the differences in age, etiology, epidemiology, and type of histology seen on renal biopsy are taken into account.

CRESCENTIC GLOMERULONEPHRITIS

It must be emphasized from the outset that this group of patients is neither pathologically nor clinically homogeneous (Table 69-7). Only the thesis that extensive crescent formation is a dominant determinant of prognosis, overriding that of the underlying glomerulopathy, justifies considering them together [394] (see Chap. 62). In practice, the outlook for patients with extensive crescent formation, whatever the underlying disease, is so much poorer than that noted for other forms of glomerulopathy [71] that this approach seems worthwhile, at least for the purposes of clinical management.

Some degree of extracapillary proliferation is relatively common in patients with primarily endocapillary proliferative glomerulonephritis. The changes are usually minor and often segmental. In some patients, however, a significant number of glomeruli show multilayered crescents affecting a large proportion of the glomerular circumference. In a minority of patients that are our concern in this section, most or all glomeruli show circumferential extracapillary proliferation.

It is impossible to draw a firm line at any point to distinguish what should be called *crescentic glomerulonephritis*. For purposes of discussion, 50, 60, 70, or 80 percent of glomeruli affected by crescents have been used by different authors as the definition of crescentic glomerulonephritis. Since the prognosis, at least of the untreated disease, may depend on the proportion of affected glomeruli, this is not an academic point. Expressing the percentage involvement from a total number of glomeruli less than, say, 10 may not seem to be a useful exercise, and reservations on the sampling error are certainly present. However, since the extent of the involvement in an individual glomerulus varies with the proportion affected [131, 491], the conclusions may be more secure than they at first appear.

The important point made earlier about crescentic nephritis is that while the presence of extensive crescent formation may dominate the histologic and clinical picture, justifying the separation of the group, the glomeruli themselves may show a variety of changes and the patient may show a variety of clinical pictures [144, 381, 438]. Apart from crescentic nephritis complicating vasculitis, the principal groups are anti-GBM disease, crescentic forms of glomerulonephritis with intraglomerular immune aggregates, and so-called idiopathic crescentic glomerulonephritis, usually associated with segmental necrotizing glomerulitis and collapsed, but otherwise normal, glomerular tufts [352, 440].

Interpretation of the distorted and compressed glomerulus is always difficult and may be impossible. Similarly, on immunohistologic examination, no glomerular aggregates may be visible or only fibrin may be visible within the crescents; this is particularly common in crescentic nephritis associated with vasculitis (see below). Linear deposits of IgG may be seen in anti-GBM disease along the capillary walls, or granular IgG and C3 in various distributions in other patients with endocapillary or mesangiocapillary nephritis, or IgA in crescentic IgA nephropathy [487].

The nature of so-called idiopathic crescentic glomerulonephritis [44, 440] was a subject of controversy, but now it is generally accepted by the majority of workers that these patients have in fact a single organ manifestation of some form of vasculitis. This may only be evident at detailed postmortem examination [353] but may

Table 69-7. Various glomerular conditions that may be associated with extensive crescent formation

- Primary crescentic glomerulonephritis
  - Common
    - Idiopathic* crescentic glomerulitis, usually necrotizing segmental
    - Endocapillary glomerulonephritis
    - Anti-GBM nephritis
    - Mesangiocapillary glomerulonephritis (I or II)
  - Uncommon
    - IgA nephropathy
    - Membranous nephropathy
- Secondary crescentic glomerulonephritis
  - Common
    - Henoch-Schönlein purpura
    - Microscopic polyarteritis
  - Uncommon
    - Systemic lupus erythematosus
    - Behçet's syndrome
    - Mixed cyroglobulinemia
    - Shunt nephritis
    - Subacute bacterial endocarditis
    - Neoplasia

*Considered by some always to represent microscopic polyarteritis (see text).

show itself later at a clinical level in patients with disease apparently confined to the kidney to begin with. Many of these patients have antineutrophil cytoplasmic antibody (ANCA) in their plasma, usually directed against myeloperoxidase (see below). However, a very few patients do not fit this description, do not have circulating ANCA, and if untreated do not go on to develop vasculitis. Some authors have never seen such cases [107], and certainly they are very uncommon.

Despite this heterogeneity, most patients with extensive crescent formation have a characteristic presentation and clinical course. The commonest presentation is with sudden onset of rapidly progressive renal failure, sometimes with anuria. Other patients present with a course over several months, but still quick enough to justify the description of rapidly progressive glomerulonephritis (RPGN). Of course, the apparent onset of the disease may not be anywhere near its true beginnings. RPGN may also supervene in a patient with an indolent course of nephritis, for example with membranous nephropathy, as discussed above.

Overall, the prognosis for patients with crescentic nephritis is poorer than for any other form of nephropathy and relates in broad fashion in the untreated patient to the extent and severity of the crescent formation (Table 69-8). Despite this generally poor outlook, there is no doubt that occasional patients make remarkable recoveries, sometimes without any specific intervention; however, today few patients with crescentic nephritis escape treatment! Even so, a search of the literature from 1964 to 1980 shows 115 patients with crescentic nephritis who received no specific treatment. Thirteen (11%) made a spontaneous recovery (Table 69-9), 5 of whom had streptococcal infection, while 4 had what was apparently idiopathic crescentic nephritis. These scanty historical data provide the basis against which the effects of treatments believed to modify the outcome may be judged.

Prognostic Features. Most authors [44, 107, 194, 343, 431, 438] reached the conclusion that within this severely affected group several features indicate a (relatively) favorable prognosis. These are (1) history of prior infection, (2) presence of a urine output, (3) lesser extent of crescent formation, (4) absent or mild tubular atrophy and interstitial fibrosis, (5) presence of glomerular immune aggregates on immunohistology or electron mi-

Table 69-8. Prognosis of crescentic glomerulonephritis in relation to proportion of glomeruli affected

			Number of glomeruli with crescents									
			100%		90–99%		80–89%		70–79%		60–69%	
	Number of patients	Reference	+	–	+	–	+	–	+	–	+	–
Berlyne (1964)	8	48	0	3	0	5						
Harrison (1964)	19	216	0	10	1	2	0	2	1	1	0	2
Leonard (1970)	20	303	1	14	1	1	0	1	0	0	0	2
Sonsino (1972)	31	431	0	8	3	4	4	1	4	4	2	1
Beirne (1977)	16	44	1	2	1	2	0	4	1	4	1	0
Morrin (1978)	25	343	1	9	4	0	3	3	3	0	2	0
Bolton (1979)	5	56	0	0	0	1	0	0	2	1	1	0
O'Neill (1979)	10	367	0	1	2	2	0	2	1	1	1	0
Nakamoto (1979)	22	349	1	2	1	6	1	1	3	1	3	3
Stilmant (1979)	5	440			0	1	1	0	1	1	0	1
Neild (1984)	39	353	6	7	1	5	9	4	4	2	1	0
Totals	200		10	56	14	29	18	18	20	15	11	9
Improvement in renal function			15%*		32%†		50%		56%		55%	

*100% vs. 60 to 89 percent crescents, $p < 0.001$ by χ^2 analysis.
†90 to 99 percent vs. 60 to 89 percent crescents $0.02 < p < 0.05$.
+ = improvement in renal function for >6 months.
– = no improvement.

Table 69-9. Prognosis of untreated and treated patients with crescentic glomerulonephritis

Total number of patients	Number not treated	Number judged to have "improved"	Total number treated	Number judged to have improved
328	115	13 (11.3%)	213	90 (42%)

Summary of treated and untreated patients with crescentic glomerulonephritis (>50 percent of glomeruli with crescents). (World literature 1964–1980), excluding patients with (1) anti-GBM disease, (2) known or suspected vasculitis, (3) SLE, and (4) Henoch-Schönlein purpura.

croscopy, (6) presence of endocapillary proliferation, and (7) intact Bowman's capsule.

Histology. The correlation with the proportion of glomeruli affected by extensive crescents has been mentioned already (Table 69-8). Note that, not surprisingly in view of the difficulty in defining crescents, the change in number and extent of crescents with time, and the small sample available, the correlation is only approximate; even when 100 percent of glomeruli are so affected, a proportion of patients may yet recover function. As usual, the extent and severity of tubulointerstitial disease correlates well with outcome, as reported in almost all other forms of glomerulonephritis. In our own series [353], using a scoring system for severity of tubular atrophy and interstitial fibrosis, of 26 patients with scores of less than 3 (out of 8), 14 of 26 patients showed improvement in renal function, which was sustained in 12. In contrast, of 13 patients with scores of greater than 3 of 8, only 5 of 13 patients showed improvement and this was sustained in only a single patient. Thus tubulointerstitial changes, together with the extent of crescent formation, can give a very good idea of which patients may respond to treatment and point to those whose disease has evolved to a point where recovery is likely.

The presence of subepithelial "humps" on electron microscopy, or obvious immune deposits on immunohistology, appears to carry a better prognosis also [231, 353, 431]. Paradoxically, as treatments have become more effective for glomerulonephritis with extensive crescents, these correlations have become less significant as the "natural" or untreated history of the condition is modified favorably.

Table 69-10. Frequency of an oligoanuric presentation in crescentic glomerulonephritis*

Percent crescents	Percent of patients with oligoanuria
60–70	0
70–80	40
80–90	44
90–100	72
100	92

*Excluding anti-GBM, polyarteritis, SLE, and Henoch-Schönlein purpura.

Clinical Course. Postinfectious nephritis, even when crescents are present, has a reputation of being more benign than comparable idiopathic disease; however, the apparently good prognosis in poststreptococcal nephritis, for example, is at least in part the result of the inclusion in published data of patients with relatively minor degrees of crescent formation. In Heaf et al.'s analysis [223], only 51 percent of patients in the infection-related group had >80 percent of glomeruli affected by crescents, compared with 69 percent in anti-GBM and 65 percent in the "idiopathic" group. It must be emphasized again that the prognosis for recovery only becomes less than even when the number of glomeruli affected by occluding crescents exceeds 60 percent; the literature on poststreptococcal crescentic nephritis is particularly poor in its definitions of "extensive crescent formation," as I have discussed elsewhere [71]. Thus the prognosis for postinfectious nephritis with really extensive crescent formation may not be as benign as supposed in the past.

Second, *oligoanuria* is a poor prognostic factor. In Table 69-10, the frequency of oligoanuria in relation to the extent of crescent formation is shown, in data taken from five papers in the literature and our own experience. Of 100 patients presenting with oligoanuria of less than 500 ml urine per 24 hours, GFR of less than 3 ml/min, only 20 showed any recovery of renal function, with or without treatment, which varied from series to series. Bolton and Couser [56] reach an even more pessimistic conclusion from their analysis of the literature: only 7 percent of oligoanuric patients recovered function. *Age,* surprisingly, does not appear to play a major part in determining recovery [223].

The prognosis of different groups of crescentic nephritis varies, as might be expected. In Glassock's analysis [194] (Table 69-11) dating from the early and mid 1970s, the prognosis for patients with vasculitis and "idiopathic" immune deposit negative crescentic glomerulonephritis, many of whom had vasculitis, was particularly poor. As will be shown in the next section, this "natural" history of vasculitic crescentic nephritis has now been much modified for the better.

Crescentic nephritis complicating proliferative glomerulonephritis, other than poststreptococcal nephritis, is rare, and few cases of crescentic MCGN [90] or IgA nephropathy [127, 357, 487] have been described. In general, the prognosis is worse than in those not affected by crescents (see discussions under IgA-Associated Nephropathy and Membranous Nephropathy), but the data are not extensive.

Table 69-11. Prognosis of crescentic glomerulonephritis in relation to associated glomerular disease

Histologic diagnosis	Number of patients	"Improved"	Death or dialysis
Postinfectious	47	23 (49%)	24 (51%)
No immune deposits/immune deposits	70	13 (19%)	57 (81%)
Anti-GBM disease	81	9 (11%)	72 (89%)
Vasculitis	69	4 (6%)	65 (94%)
All patients	521	124 (24%)	297 (76%)

Source: Data from Glassock, 1978 [194].

Crescentic nephritis is rather rare in *children* apart from Henoch-Schönlein purpura, and only two extensive series have been published [357, 436] on a total of 91 cases, which included 62 primary glomerulonephritides. Only 6 patients had anti-GBM nephritis (10%), emphasizing the rarity of this form of nephritis in childhood [305]. Ten children had crescentic nephritis without deposits and may have had occult vasculitis (17%); the remainder had various forms of glomerulonephritis including 7 cases of crescentic IgA nephropathy (11%), which thus appears relatively more common than in adults. Eleven children (18%) had postinfectious nephritis, and 11 MCGN (6 of these type II MCGN). One child had a juguloatrial shunt, and in 15 children the crescentic nephritis could not be further characterized.

Clinicopathologic correlations were similar to those found in adults. A total of 45 of 88 children with follow-up entered renal failure, more than half within 1 month of onset, the remainder from several months to 5 years later. No patient in the South West Pediatric Group series [436] appears to have gone into complete remission, but 7 of the series from Paris [357] did so. The remainder retained proteinuria and hematuria with varying degrees of renal dysfunction. Thus the outlook for children with crescentic nephritis does not differ greatly from that in adults, and even postinfectious cases may go into renal failure.

At several points in this section, the effects of treatment on the natural history of crescentic nephritis have been mentioned. Of course, dialysis alone without specific treatment may allow time for spontaneous healing, when otherwise an early death in uremia could be expected. Treatment of both vasculitic and anti-GBM nephritis (discussed later) have had dramatic effects. What evidence is there that treatment affects the outcome of other forms of crescentic nephritis? Heaf et al. [223] undertook an extensive analysis of the effects of treatment in all forms of crescentic nephritis, but their analysis includes cases with both anti-GBM and vasculitic nephritis (Table 69-12). The "best" results seem to be obtained with the use of intravenous methylprednisolone, which is relatively cheap, safe, and simple to administer, or with plasma exchange, which is none of these things. Bolton [55] and Couser [118] have reviewed the use and results of intravenous methylprednisolone and conclude that with its use about three-quarters of patients with idiopathic crescentic nephritis will maintain or recover renal function (44 of 59 in Couser's [118] analysis). Since these results are as good or better than from more complicated regimens including either prolonged anticoagulation or plasma exchange, this form of treatment seems preferable at the moment for all forms of crescentic nephritis, with the single exception of anti-GBM nephritis, in which it appears to have little or no effect [55] (see below).

The longer-term outcome of patients with crescentic nephritis has not been studied [65, 349], perhaps because until recently survival was unusual in severe cases. The series of Bruns et al. [65] included 8 cases of crescentic nephritis without immune deposits, i.e., probable vasculitis, and 2 cases of anti-GBM disease. However, the remaining 13 patients were immune complex related, and their evolution is of interest here. Seven patients entered chronic renal failure after temporary recovery, 2 within a few months, but 5 from 1 to 2 years later, and 4 remained in various degrees of renal failure (P_{creat} 2–4 mg/dl) for 2 to 11 years. In the study of Baldwin et al. [31a], 16 patients ran a protracted course of 2 to 10 years, sometimes with a prolonged period of nephritis before biopsy; 11 required dialysis eventually. However, 10 of their patients had only 17 to 44 percent of glomeruli affected by crescents and would not meet the criteria for extensive crescentic nephritis discussed above.

ANTI-GBM NEPHRITIS

The prognosis of anti-GBM nephritis, with or without pulmonary hemorrhage (Goodpasture's syndrome), is

Table 69-12. Apparent influence of treatment on prognosis in crescentic glomerulonephritis (all types)

Treatment	Number of patients	Results: Alive, normal renal function (%)	Alive, abnormal renal function (%)	In uremia (%)	In dialysis (%)	Death (%)		Uremia + dialysis + death
Symptomatic	82	3	7	3	42	45	=	90
Immunosuppression	144	11	15	4	22	47	=	71
Anticoagulation*	94	13	9	4	27	47	=	78
Plasma exchange	117	3	30	25	29	13	=	65
Methylprednisolone	39	20	36	7	24	12	=	43
Plasma exchange and methylprednisolone	7	0	42	0	42	14	=	56

*Often combined with immunosuppression.

Summary of the world literature, modified from Heaf et al., 1983 [223]. In regarding these data, it must be remembered that comparable patients were not allocated to all the treatment groups and that some data are predominantly recent (e.g., plasma exchange) and others less recent (e.g., immunosuppression alone).

now very different from that described two or three decades ago [463] (see Chap. 68). First, many of the older descriptions were unknowingly contaminated by patients who had pulmonary hemorrhage as part of vasculitic syndromes [235]. Second, as anti-GBM antibody assays have become widely available, a group of less severely affected patients with more indolent disease arising from anti-GBM antibody have been described [327] who do not have extensive crescent formation. Finally, treatment has modified the natural history of the condition in the past 15 years.

At first the prognosis for anti-GBM nephritis was worse than for almost any other form of nephritis, at least with regard to renal function (Table 69-11). Some additional patients with relatively good renal function died from pulmonary hemorrhage. Thus Benoit et al. [47] reported only 2 survivors out of 52 patients in 1964 (4%), and 6 years later Proskey et al. [389] reported 13 survivors out of 56 (23%); only 3 of 32 patients in Wilson and Dixon's series [493] survived off dialysis (9%). Even as recently as 1977, Beirne and colleagues [44] found only 3 patients of 17 who retained independent renal function and survived. Although occasional dramatic recoveries, even in those requiring dialysis, have been described [108], they usually related to patients without very extensive crescent formation (3 of 13 glomeruli in the case cited [108]).

Plasma exchange to remove the circulating antibody, together with cyclophosphamide to prevent its resynthesis, has changed the outlook for anti-GBM disease dramatically. Equally it has become evident that this is normally effective in protecting renal function only if the patient is treated early enough, before oligoanuria and a requirement for dialysis have become established (Table 69-13). Among patients already requiring dialysis [228, 305], very few recover renal function. Walker and colleagues [475], however, have reported more encouraging results; 5 of 11 oligoanuric patients in their series of 22 patients recovered renal function (45%). Savage and colleagues [408], as well as reviewing their extensive personal data from the Hammersmith Hospital (Table 69-13), reviewed collected data from other units (including our own) on 59 patients presenting between 1980 and 1984. Of a total of 58 patients out of 108 local and collected patients who were oligoanuric and who received treatment with plasma exchange and cyclophosphamide, 18 died and 51 continued on dialysis; thus only 7 patients (13%) requiring dialysis recovered function on aggressive treatment. More severe disease and a poorer outlook have been associated also with the HLA type, those with HLA-DR2 together with B7 doing badly [395].

We, together with the Hammersmith group, analyzed what happened to 9 patients who were not treated other than by dialysis for oligoanuria [173]; none recovered renal function, none died, and all lost their antibody eventually (although it took more than a year in some patients) and could then successfully undergo renal transplantation. Where the balance of benefit and risk lies between treating oligoanuric patients in the small hope of recovery, thus exposing them to the risks of intense immunosuppression while acutely uremic, is not clear. Of course, patients with lung hemorrhage require treatment even if anuric. The only group who appear not to have seen a clear benefit from plasma exchange are Johnson et al. [259], who saw little difference in outcome in 8 patients treated with immunosuppression and plasma exchange and 9 with immunosuppression alone.

There are few longer-term data on the survival of patients with anti-GBM disease; renal survival is obviously much poorer than patient survival, even although the latter is at risk from pulmonary hemorrhage and the effects of intensive immunosuppression. Turner and Rees [463] noted 8 deaths during the first year among 29 patients (28%) seen at the Hammersmith Hospital between 1976 and 1988. All were patients with extensive crescents, an initial plasma creatinine above 600 μmol/liter, and pulmonary hemorrhage. Eight of 22 patients in Walker's series [475] died within 12 months (36%). Savage et al. [408] noted 15 deaths within 8 weeks in their 59 collected British patients seen during 1980 to 1984 (25%), only half of which were the result of lung hem-

Table 69-13. Immediate outcome in patients with anti-GBM nephritis

Presentation P_{creat} (μmol/L)	n	Received full treatment*	Outcome after 8 weeks		
			Improved	Requiring dialysis	Dead
PATIENTS FROM BRITISH RENAL UNITS 1980–1984 (n = 59)					
Normal	3	2	3		
<600	5	5	2	2	1
>600	7	7		4	3
Dialysis dependent	44	33		33	11
PATIENTS SEEN AT THE ROYAL POSTGRADUATE MEDICAL SCHOOL 1974–1984 (n = 49)					
Normal	4	4	3		
<600	15	15	13	2	
>600	5	5	1	4	
Dialysis dependent	25	25		18	7

*Full treatment = at least 8 weeks of cyclophosphamide + plasma exchange for 2 weeks.
Data from Savage et al. [408].

orrhage, 14 in patients requiring dialysis. They also noted 8 deaths among 49 local patients seen from 1974–1984 (16%), all but one in patients requiring dialysis, the majority from lung hemorrhage. The later mortality is not given for either group, and so 1-year figures are not available.

Thus, mainly from the collected data of Savage et al. [408], one can predict that about one-quarter of patients with anti-GBM nephritis can be expected to retrieve or maintain renal function; in their series only 2 of 23 such patients died. However, about one-fifth of patients with anti-GBM nephritis requiring dialysis can be expected to die within 12 months, the majority within the first 3 months. Among those who recover or maintain renal function, a proportion subsequently develop uremia [259, 475] and require dialysis or transplantation later. This "late" deterioration presumably arises through whatever mechanisms operate in remnant kidneys, rather than through specific immunologic attack. Return of active disease during follow-up is exceptionally rare, although it has been described [124].

VASCULITIS: WEGENER'S GRANULOMA, MICROSCOPIC POLYARTERITIS, AND THE CHURG-STRAUSS SYNDROME

Until recently there were few data on the long-term survival of patients with vasculitis because untreated survival was so miserable [35, 145, 160, 161, 163, 422, 423, 478]. The 2-year survival of untreated vasculitis patients with severe nephritis was essentially zero, and there is overwhelming evidence—albeit uncontrolled—that aggressive treatment has modified the outlook dramatically over the past two decades (Table 69-14). Although Fauci and his colleagues [162, 163] reviewed the transformation from a 20 percent 2-year survival through to a *93 percent survival* at the same point, detailed scrutiny of this paper shows that most of these patients had no or only trivial renal disease.

This area in the study of nephritis has been particularly handicapped by difficulties in terminology and definition (see Chap. 76). Usually, a diagnosis of Wegener's granuloma has been based on clinical features of upper respiratory tract disease and not on biopsy, which is often equivocal because of extensive necrosis. Microscopic polyarteritis tends to be a diagnosis of exclusion made in vasculitic patients who do not have glomerular aggregates of IgA and who do not have clinical features of Wegener's. Recently, the suggestion that the form of crescentic nephritis showing necrotizing glomerular lesions without immune aggregates represents, in the majority of cases, a form of occult vasculitis [422, 423, 470, 486] has become widely accepted. The later appearance of overt vasculitis in untreated cases [496] and serum positivity for ANCA, usually of the P-ANCA type [255], strongly suggest that this is the case.

Modern aggressive treatment of vasculitic nephritis is

Table 69-14. Outcome in renal vasculitis, 1955–1990*

Treatment	5-year survival (%)		Author	Year	Ref.
Supportive only	13		Rose & Spencer	1957	398
	13		Frohnert & Sheps	1964	179
	12		Leib et al.	1979	301
Corticosteroids	62		MRC (U.K.)	1960	331
	48		Frohnert & Sheps	1967	179
	57		Sack et al.	1975	404
	61		Cohen et al.	1980	109
Corticosteroids plus cytotoxics	80		Leib et al.	1979	301
	55		Cohen et al.	1980	109
Corticosteroids plus cytotoxics methylprednisolone IV and plasma exchange in severe cases					
n					
53	38	Both	Serra et al.	1984	423
34	65	micro poly.	Savage et al.	1985	409
36	64	both	Coward et al.	1986	119
43	62	micro poly.	Adu et al.	1987	5
26	80	both	Fuiano et al.	1988	180
54	56	Wegener's	Gaskin & Rees	1991	187
49	64	micro poly.	Gaskin & Rees	1991	187
17	74	Wegener's	Cameron	1991	79
35	56	micro poly.	Cameron	1991	79

*In the earlier series (pre-1980, e.g., Leib et al. [301]), many patients had either no renal disease or only minor renal disease. In addition, most of these early series include some patients with large-vessel vasculitis (polyarteritis nodosa). Thus the data are not strictly comparable with more recent series consisting almost exclusively of patients with either Wegener's granuloma or microscopic polyarteritis, with severe (usually crescentic) glomerulonephritis.

centered on the use of cytotoxic agents (usually cyclophosphamide) as well as prednisolone [35, 82, 108, 229, 377, 409]. There is evidence that this more aggressive regimen improves results, decreasing the number of patients who die of the vasculitis in the acute phase [82, 180]. In patients in advancing or severe renal failure, most units employ intravenous methylprednisolone and/or plasma exchange as well [78, 82, 180, 218, 229, 323, 409], although there is only one controlled trial [390a] showing that these extra treatments confer benefit. Equally there is no evidence to suggest that giving the cyclophosphamide intravenously during the acute phase has any advantage [234], although intermittent intravenous cyclophosphamide *may* have benefits over long-term azathioprine in the longer term. No trial comparing the two has been performed, however.

Unlike anti-GBM nephritis, recovery of renal function in patients with vasculitis and crescentic nephritis but already dialysis-dependent and oligoanuric is common, almost the rule [82, 108, 119, 218, 219, 409]. Deaths still occur from other complications of the vasculitis, but the main cause of early death is sepsis from the intense immunosuppression in patients who are frequently elderly and often frail [5, 82, 229]. In earlier cases, reversal of mounting uremia is also usual. About three-quarters or more of patients can be expected to survive the early phases of the disease [5, 82, 119, 180, 409].

During the late 1980s, longer-term patient survival using these forms of treatment has been reported by several British groups [5, 82, 119, 180, 218, 377, 409] to be between 50 and 80 percent at 5 years (Fig. 69-22), with similar figures in the few patients studied for as long as 10 years. Unlike anti-GBM disease, rather few patients requiring dialysis survive following the acute attack. Thus of 60 patients with Wegener's granuloma, Gaskin and Rees [187] noted severe renal disease in 54. Eleven patients died during the first 2 weeks (20%), 7 among the 24 requiring dialysis, mostly the result of pulmonary complications (hemorrhage and infection); only 3 of the 24 continued on dialysis. There were three additional later deaths in those who recovered function, all the result of infection. Actuarial survival was estimated to be 70 percent at 1 year and 56 percent at 5 years. Similarly, in 49 patients with microscopic polyarteritis [187], 14 initially required dialysis, of whom 4 died without recovering function and 8 recovered function, 2 dying shortly thereafter, only 2 continuing on dialysis. Patient survival was 38 of 49 at 8 weeks, renal survival 36 of 49 (28% mortality). When Wegener's and microscopic polyarteritis are compared, even if the extent of renal damage is allowed for [82], then usually the Wegener's patients appear to do a little better, as in Gaskin and Rees's data [187], but the difference is not striking. The patients who die later [187, 423] are usually patients with their disease still active but suppressed—so-called smouldering disease [187]—but this mortality has been reduced in recent years.

Factors that predict outcome are now obscured by the relative success of treatment. Clinically, as already mentioned, oligoanuria does not predict failure of treatment, although as a group oligoanuric patients do rather worse. Histologically, the extent of crescent formation also has ceased to be a predictor of longer-term outcome in our own data, although it correlates with renal function at presentation [82] (Fig. 69-23). Falk [159] states that the presence and titer of ANCA makes no impact on long-term outcome as judged by life tables.

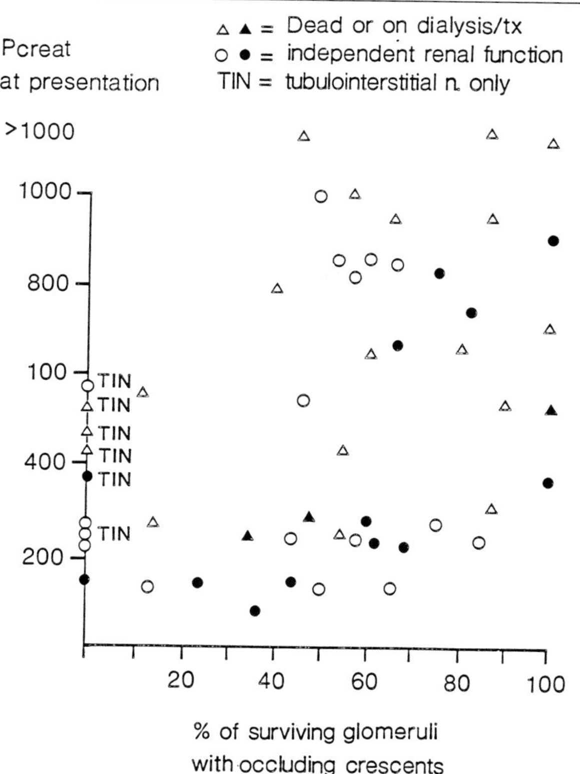

Fig. 69-22. Outcome in patients with renal vasculitis, showing the relation between the percentage of glomeruli affected by crescents and the plasma creatinine (P_{creat}) at presentation and outcome over an average of 5 years. Although there is a good correlation between the percentage of crescents and the plasma creatinine at presentation, with modern management of vasculitis there is no correlation between number of crescents and outcome. Note that six patients had normal glomeruli, vasculitis, and tubulointerstitial nephritis (TIN). (Data from [83].)

Patients with vasculitis who survive the initial illness may run a relapsing course, whose frequency depends very much on the intensity of the immunosuppression. Thus in our own series of 52 patients seen during the 1980s, almost all of whom were maintained on prednisolone and azathioprine for 5 years or more, relapses were rare [82]. ANCA titers may be of use in modulating immunosuppression, since relapse is unlikely when the ANCA titer is normal [110]. With recovery of glomerular function, a nephrotic syndrome (although almost unknown at presentation) may appear, as first reported by Akikusa and colleagues [6].

Vasculitis is rare in childhood [79], with the sole ex-

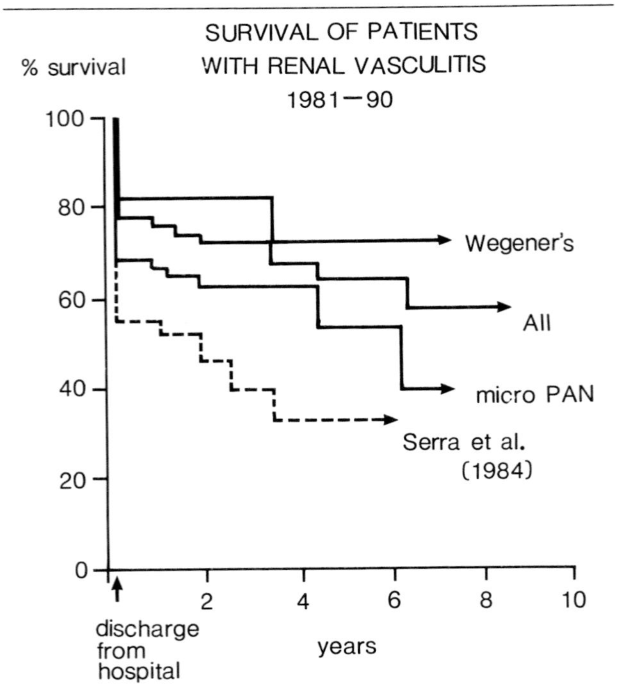

Fig. 69-23. Probability of survival of patients presenting with renal vasculitis, 1981–1990. Guy's Hospital data are from 1980–1989 [83]: Wegener's, 17 patients; microscopic polyarteritis (micro PAN), 34 patients; total, 51; mean age, 65 years; 19 requiring dialysis. Also shown are the data of Serra et al. [423] published in 1984 on the outcome of 53 patients presenting during the decade preceding the Guy's study. Overall survival has improved ($p < 0.05$) in association with more aggressive treatment (see text), and the major cause of death is no longer the vasculitis itself but side effects of the more intense immunosuppression. Early mortality during the acute illness, although reduced, remains the main problem.

ceptions of the infantile Kawasaki disease, which usually spares the kidney, and Henoch-Schönlein purpura, which is dealt with in the next section. Habib [207] reviews a relatively large experience of 16 children with Wegener's or polyarteritis, whose clinical picture did not differ from similar adults. We have seen only 5 patients with vasculitis in our busy pediatric nephrology service, three of whom had Wegener's.

There are few data on the outcome of renal disease in the *Churg-Strauss syndrome,* although it is now recognized that renal involvement is more common and more severe than thought in the past. Clutterbuck et al. [104] describe the outcome in 19 patients whose renal disease resembled histologically that of Wegener's or microscopic polyarteritis. The prognosis was better, however, only 1 patient requiring transplantation, while 5 had varying degrees of chronic renal failure and the remainder maintained renal function for up to a decade. Only 1 patient died, of a restrictive cardiomyopathy.

HENOCH-SCHÖNLEIN PURPURA NEPHRITIS

The prognosis of Henoch-Schönlein purpura (HSP) without clinical nephritis is excellent [219, 289], and nephritis forms the major cause of morbidity and mortality, apart from occasional problems with intussusception or other gastrointestinal complications (see Chap. 67). Nephritis may appear with the initial attack but is particularly associated with recurrent attacks of purpura [330], which may continue in exceptional cases for months or even years. Even so, compared with most other forms of glomerulonephritis in childhood or adults, the prognosis even with nephritis remains good [209]. Overall, after 2 years, half the children with HSP nephritis will be in complete remission, while a third show persisting urinary abnormalities with normal renal function (Fig. 69-24). A few children (perhaps 3%) progress to renal failure immediately, and their renal biopsies usually show extensive crescent formation. No more than 19 percent show continued urinary abnormalities with reduced renal function.

By the time 10 years have passed [116], most of the children who had urinary abnormalities but normal renal function at 2 years have gone into remission, but a proportion of those with decreased renal function have progressed to renal failure. It is difficult to judge how many will eventually do so, but Habib and Cameron [209] report that 32 of 188 patients (17%) had gone into renal failure, and the total would probably be about 20 percent eventually. It must not be forgotten that these data come from two highly specialized referral centers and that the proportion of children with more severe disease is inevitably exaggerated in these figures. The prognosis for unselected children with HSP nephritis is undoubtedly better than this, but by how much is impossible to say exactly. In Kobayashi's series [285], only 3 of 123 children (2.7%) with nephritis had died, while 86 percent were in complete remission, and in Koskimies' data [289], only one child of 39 still had signs of

Fig. 69-24. The state of 88 children with HSP at 6.5 to 15 (mean 9.9) years from onset (*left*). For 76 of these 88 children (*center* and *right*), follow-up data also were available at 2 years from the attack of nephritis: (□) = recovery; (⚄) = minimal renal signs; (▨) = persisting nephropathy; and (■) = terminal renal failure. At the time of follow-up, 17 percent of the children had reached terminal renal failure (data of Counahan et al. [117]). (Reproduced from Habib and Cameron, 1982 [209], with permission of the publishers.)

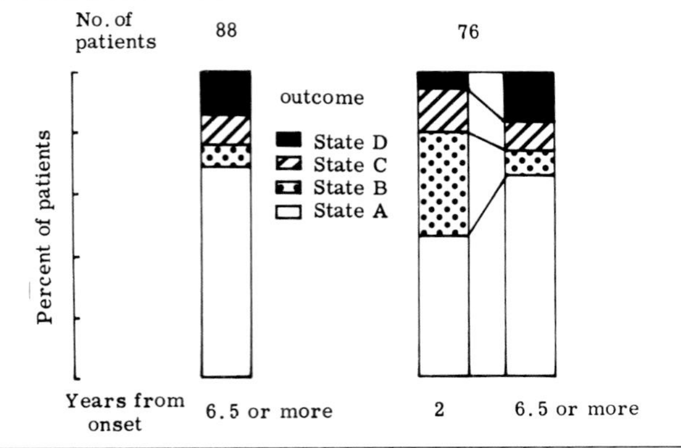

evident nephritis and another 2 had chronic disease. Kobayashi [285] calculated a final remission rate of 91 percent, with a 9 percent rate of renal failure/death. However, since (as here) the benign nature of the syndrome is usually emphasized, it is worth remembering that, on the other hand, HSP nephritis accounts for about 3 percent of children going into end-stage renal failure [205].

It would (as always) be useful to know at the outset which children would be most likely to have a severe course, so that treatment could be concentrated on the minority who might require it. There is some correlation between the clinical onset and outcome (Table 69-15 and Fig. 69-25). In general, patients with only symptomless urinary abnormalities do well, while those with a nephrotic syndrome, above all when combined with renal insufficiency, do poorly [116, 209, 308, 345]. However, there are exceptions in both directions. Another adverse feature is age at onset (Table 69-16); there was, however, no relation with serum IgA concentrations [208, 308].

The best guide to outcome is a combination of clinical data (see Table 69-15) and biopsy data (Table 69-17 and Figs. 69-25 and 69-26). Of those patients without diffuse glomerular proliferation, and less than 50 percent of glomeruli affected by segmental lesions or crescents, almost all did well. However, those with more extensive crescent formation tended to do poorly. In children *with* diffuse proliferative glomerulonephritis, only half of those who had less than 50 percent of glomeruli affected by segmental lesions healed clinically; the remainder showed persisting disease. In those with more than 50 percent of glomeruli affected by segmental lesions, the evolution was much less often favorable, and in those with more than 80 percent of glomeruli affected by crescents, evolution was usually into renal failure (12 of 19 patients). It is in this group that aggressive treatment with intravenous methylprednisolone and plasma exchange is usually concentrated [219]. Two children in this group, however, recovered completely without aggressive intervention. Overall, the greater the number of glomeruli affected by crescents, the poorer the prognosis.

Discussion of HSP nephritis in *adults* is made difficult by several circumstances. First, a number of older papers that purport to deal with the topic do not distinguish between HSP, other forms of vasculitis, or essential cryoglobulinemia, even with the technology available when the data were collected (e.g., Cream et al. [122]). Second, some papers deal with both adults and children, and it is impossible to separate the data. Third, in some papers, patients without renal involvement cannot be separated from those with nephritis. Finally, because of the relative rarity of HSP nephritis in adult life, no single series is large enough to form conclusions or do statistical analyses.

However, from the published literature and data from a national survey of 47 cases of HSP nephritis in the United Kingdom seen from 1976 to 1986 [284], the clinical manifestations do not differ much from those in children [76], although both a history of prior drug ingestion and severe arthralgia (80%) are more common, and abdominal signs and symptoms less common (35%). The purpura more frequently ulcerates in adults with HSP than in children, particularly in the elderly. The condition may be seen even in the ninth decade of life. There is some suggestion that in younger adults, the upper end of the childhood disease is present in decreasing numbers with increasing age; then there is a "bulge" of cases in the 50- to 70-year age group, corresponding to that for other forms of adult vasculitis. An association with malignancies has been reported [68], and in our own series, recurrent attacks have been associated with alcohol ingestion in two cases.

The renal histology in adults is again similar to the findings in children [63], and most interest has centered on whether the prognosis in the adult cases differs from that in childhood (Table 69-18). There is a suggestion that the adults do a little worse than the selected children seen in referral centers, but again the adults are even more highly selected. Overall 20 of 183 collected patients had gone into end-stage renal disease or died of renal failure (11%), although the duration of follow-up differs greatly in the various papers included in Table 69-17. Death, as might be expected in this older population, was sometimes from unrelated causes (14 of 183, 8%). In the U.K. study of 43 patients [284], after 1 to 7 years of follow-up, 15 were in complete remission, 17 had urinary abnormalities (12 with normal renal function), 4 were on end-stage renal disease treatment, and 7 had died, 2 with normal renal function.

Some patients with HSP nephritis may apparently

Table 69-15. Outcome in relation to clinical onset (10 years from onset) in Henoch-Schönlein nephritis

	Outcome (number of patients)				
	Recovery	Minor urinary abnormalities	Moderate nephropathy	Renal failure	Total
Hematuria only	4	0	1	0	5
Proteinuria + hematuria	31	3	3	3	40
Proteinuria + hypertension	7	0	0	1	8
NS + hematuria	8	0	0	1	9
"Nephritic-nephrotic" syndrome	11	3	5	7	26
Total	61	6	9	12	88

Source: Data from Counahan et al. [117].

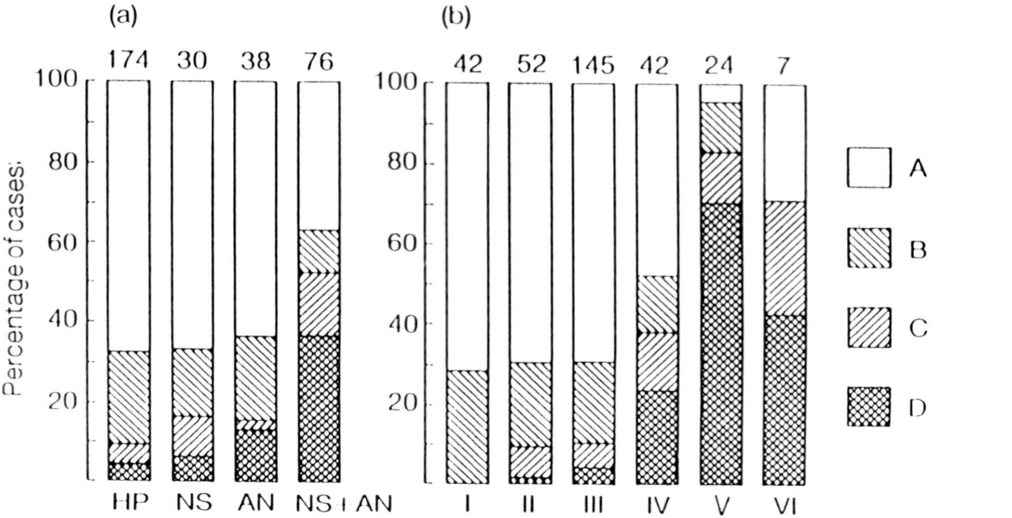

Fig. 69-25. Relationship between (a) the clinical presentation and (b) the histologic findings, and outcome in children with Henoch-Schönlein purpura. Outcome has been defined in terms of four states: A = complete recovery with normal renal function and urine; B = minor urinary abnormalities and normal renal function; C = active renal disease and proteinuria > 1 gm/24 hr; D = chronic renal insufficiency (GFR < 60 ml/min/1.73 m^2, renal death, or dialysis). Presentation is indicated by HP = hematuria and/or proteinuria; NS = nephrotic syndrome; AN = acute nephritic syndrome; and NS + AN = an acute nephritic-nephrotic syndrome. Histologic grades are those established by the International Study of Kidney Disease in Children, increasing in severity from I (minimal changes), II (mesangial disease only), III–V (increasing numbers of crescents), and VI (mesangiocapillary glomerulonephritis). Pooled data from several published series. (From G. Haycock, Henoch-Schönlein Purpura. In J. S. Cameron et al. [eds.], *The Oxford Textbook of Clinical Nephrology*. London: Oxford University Press, 1992.)

Table 69-16. Outcome in relation to age at onset in Henoch-Schönlein purpura nephritis

	Age at onset (years)		
	<6	6–11	<12
Recovery	19	38	3
Minor urinary abnormalities	2	4	0
Moderate nephropathy	2 (12.5%)	6 (26%)	1 (50%)
Renal failure	1	9	2
Total	24	57	6

Source: Data from Cameron [73].

heal but present again with severe hypertension 10 to 20 years later [116], so blood pressure should be checked at least once a year, indefinitely.

ESSENTIAL (MIXED) CRYOGLOBULINEMIA

Mixed cryoglobulinemia may arise from the formation of antiglobulins, either monoclonal as a result of proliferation of abnormal B-cell clones, or polyclonal as a result of antigen-driven B-cell proliferation [126] (see Chap. 78). In "essential" cryoglobulinemia, there is no associated plasma cell dyscrasia or lymphoproliferative disorder, rheumatologic or hepatic disease, or systemic lupus. The dominant finding in patients with renal involvement is a type II mixed cryoglobulinemia with a monoclonal IgM kappa antiglobulin. The most common type of glomerular involvement is an MCGN pattern with massive infiltration of monocytes, but crescentic nephritis may also supervene. The condition is particularly common in whites of Mediterranean origin [110a, 449].

Apart from the paper of Gorevic et al. [199], few accounts of the long-term outcome of patients with essential mixed cryoglobulinemia (see Chap. 78) had appeared until the comprehensive account of Tarantino and his colleagues, published in 1981 [449] and updated to 108 patients in 1986 [110a]. Between these two papers, a total of 84 patients were reviewed, the majority with renal disease either at the outset or appearing during the course of the condition. The clinical pattern was variable, but hypertension, often severe, was a prominent

Table 69-17. Outcome in relation to initial biopsy appearance in patients with Henoch-Schönlein nephritis followed for more than 1 year

	Recovery	Minimal urinary abnormalities	Persisting disease	Renal failure
Nonproliferative glomerulonephritis				
No crescents	1	0	0	0
Crescents < 50%	17	9	1	2
Crescents > 50%	0	0	1	3
Proliferative glomerulonephritis				
No crescents	1	1	1	0
Crescents < 50%	4	4	6	1
Crescents 50–80%	3	2	3	2
Crescents > 80%	2	4	1	12
Total	28	20	13	20

Source: Data from Levy et al. [308] and Habib et al. [208].

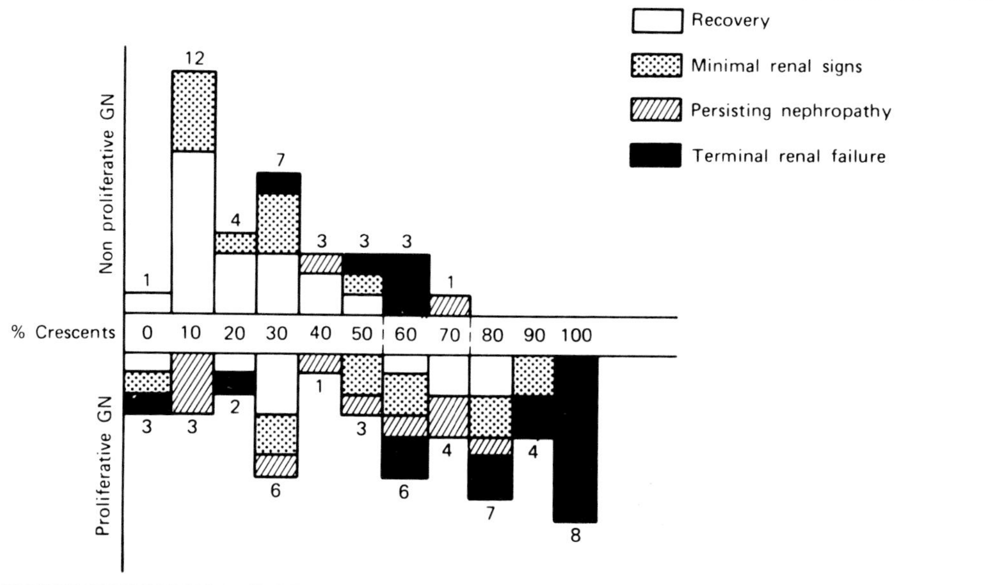

Fig. 69-26. The relationship between the extent of the glomerular segmental crescentic lesions and final status at follow-up in children with HSP. Above the line are children whose biopsies were otherwise apparently normal; below the line are those whose biopsies showed diffuse mesangial proliferation. GN = glomerulonephritis; (□) = recovery; (▩) = minimal renal signs; (▨) = persisting nephropathy; (■) = terminal renal failure. Terminal renal failure was commoner in those with more extensive crescent formation, especially against a background of diffuse mesangial proliferation. (From Levy et al. [308], courtesy of the authors.)

feature; 64% of Gorevic's patients were affected, and in Tarantino's study, hypertension was a major determinant of prognosis [110a, 449].

Chronic renal failure was surprisingly rare, although 13 of 59 patients with long-term follow-up experienced episodes of acute nephritis, amounting to acute renal failure, which was reversible in 9, a nephrotic syndrome, or both. Ten patients went into prolonged remission, while 19 had persisting urinary abnormalities. In the literature up to 1985, only 2 patients had been recorded as going into renal failure requiring dialysis [40, 121], and only 6 of Colasanti's [110a] 108 patients went into renal failure. The mortality displayed in Fig. 69-27 resulted almost entirely from vascular complications, associated in the majority of instances with severe uncontrolled hypertension. In the 1986 analysis [110a], 27 of 108 patients had died as a result of extrarenal complications, including vasculitis, infections, and cardiovascular and cerebrovascular events.

SYSTEMIC LUPUS ERYTHEMATOSUS

The outlook for patients with clinically evident nephritis in a setting of systemic lupus erythematosus (SLE) is difficult to summarize for several reasons (see Chap. 72).

Table 69-18. Follow-up in adult-onset patients with Henoch-Schönlein purpura nephritis

Ref.	Author	Country	Period	n	Age (years)	Male-female ratio	Outcome in those with f/u[a]: f/u (years)	Remitted	Persisting disease (reduced function)	ESRD/dead[b]
SERIES IN WHICH ALL PATIENTS HAD RENAL INVOLVEMENT										
33	Ballard	U.S.A.	1954–58	14	>20	14 : 0	?	8	1 (1)	5/0
172	Fillastre	France	1964–71	28	>20	22 : 6	?–13	8	7 (3)	2/1
261	Kalowski	Australia	1959–71	18	>16	13 : 5	mean 3.7	5	9 (2)	1/3
400	Roth	U.S.A.	1968–83	9	>16	9 : 0	?	7	2 (1)	0
298	Lee	Korea	1979–82	17	>16	9 : 8	mean 3.2	10	7 (0)	0
158	Esteve	Spain	?	11	>16	5 : 6	?	3	5 (0)	3
164	Faull	Australia	1975–85	27[c]	>12	16 : 11	0.16–9.0	6	16 (6)	2/3
284	Knight	U.K.	1976–86	47	>20	34 : 13	1–7	15	17 (5)	4/7
174	Fogazzi	Italy	1967–88	16	>15	11 : 5	1–20	2	11 (9)	3/0
				187		133 : 54		64	75 (27)	20/14
SERIES IN WHICH SOME PATIENTS HAD RENAL INVOLVEMENT										
133	Debray	France	?–1971	22 (10)	>15	12 : 10	4	5	2 (0)	0
39	Bar-On	Israel	1959–69	21 (12)	>15	12 : 9	0.5–6.0	4	2	2/0
Totals				209				73	79 (27)	22/14

f/u = follow-up; ESRD = end-stage renal disease.
[a]Normal urine plus hypertension counted as continuing disease in f/u.
[b]Dead = dead from causes other than renal failure.
[c]24 patients over 20 years old.

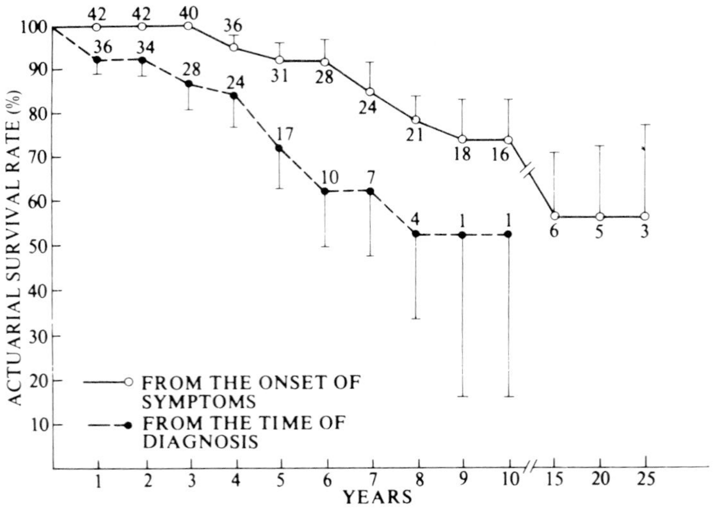

Fig. 69-27. Actuarial survival rate from the onset of symptoms and from the diagnosis of EMC. The bars indicate the standard error on the estimated survival. The number of patients still being followed at each point are indicated below and above the survival curves, respectively. (From Tarantino et al., 1981 [449], with permission of the authors and the publisher.)

First, being a multisystem disease, extrarenal organ involvement may have a major effect on mortality and morbidity in lupus, even in patients whose main involvement is in the kidney [73, 114, 146, 157, 267, 399]. Second, even in its "natural" untreated state, the disease may manifest itself over a very wide range of activity, from a limited indolent condition to a fulminant aggressive disorder affecting almost all major organ systems, including entry into acute renal failure. Third, if renal biopsies are performed, almost any pattern of glomerulopathy may be seen (see Chap. 72), and the terminology used to describe them differs from account to account. Within the past decade, the World Health Organization (WHO) classification of the pattern of injury [321, 322] has become almost universally used, but cutting across this is description according to the degree of histologic "activity" or sclerosis [24], which many now feel to be the more important determinant of prognosis. Fourth, even if an agreed description can be achieved, the appearances may transform in sequential biopsies, both spontaneously and in response to treatment [28, 191, 379, 432, 504]. Finally, most (although not all [8]) observers concur that treatment with corticosteroids and immunosuppressant drugs has had a major impact on the survival of patients with lupus during the past 20 to 30 years.

To illustrate this, Table 69-19 presents actuarially calculated estimates of survival at 5 years from onset, usually taken from the onset of the lupus nephritis but sometimes of the precedent lupus. The data are given where appropriate for all patients with lupus, for those with clinically evident nephritis irrespective of clinical severity or histologic appearances, and for those with the most severe form of lupus nephritis, WHO class IV or diffuse proliferative glomerulonephritis with or without crescent formation. In general, prognosis for lupus nephritis improved greatly during the 1960s and early 1970s and has remained rather static since. More recently, there has been a further improvement in survival of WHO class IV nephritis, to the point where even in this group renal failure is no longer the principal cause of mortality, at least during the first 5 years of evolution. Fig. 69-28 shows renal survival in patients seen at Guy's Hospital from 1980 to 1989. By this time survival was identical for those with WHO class IV to those with classes II, III, and V. During the last 20 to 30 years, the major differences in outlook for those with different WHO class nephritis, evident for example in the data of Pollak et al. [382, 384] and Baldwin et al. [29], have disappeared. In most series, however, including our own [92, 320], treatment has been more aggressive in those with clinically or histologically more severe forms of nephritis.

These data must of course be evaluated in the light of the fact that awareness of lupus as a diagnosis is much greater now than 25 years ago and that relatively specific tests for the condition are now widely available. Thus it is likely that some of the apparent "improvement" in the survival of all patients with lupus results from the inclusion of milder forms in more recent series. However, this is unlikely to apply to those with clinically evident nephritis to any extent and certainly not to those with severe proliferative lupus nephritis (WHO class IV), whose initial disease seems as savage as it was 25 years ago. What is different is the subsequent outcome. The small number of patients now dying or going into end-stage renal disease makes analysis of these events in detail difficult except in the largest data bases.

The *causes of death* in lupus of course are much more varied than in other forms of primary glomerulonephritis confined to the kidney in young adults, in whom renal failure is the dominant cause. Sepsis, not surprisingly, emerges as one of the major causes of death [114, 399, 402, 466], promoted or potentiated by immunosuppressive treatment. However other manifestations of extra renal lupus may prove fatal also [114, 399, 402, 466]. Rather surprisingly, however, recent survival curves for renal function and for the patient are almost identical in most series [203, 326]. A number of observers have commented that entry into chronic renal failure in lupus may be preceded by long periods of clinical quiescence [61, 98, 112, 319], suggesting that mechanisms other than continued activity of the nephritis determine the fate of the kidneys. A further cause of late death, even in young women with lupus, is severe atheromatous myocardial and other vascular disease; a number of our own patients have had coronary artery disease severe enough to require bypass surgery, and in two cases it was the major cause of death in women 28 and 35 years old. One boy died of a myocardial infarct of severe widespread atheroma at the age of only 19 while waiting to join our end-stage renal disease program. The pathogenesis of these late vascular lesions is not clear, but corticosteroid treatment, hyperlipidemia, and immune complexes may all play a part, since interactions between immune complexes and hyperlipidemia to accelerate atheroma formation are well described [168, 240, 336, 439] in experimental animals.

Nevertheless, as with other forms of nephritis, *clinical data* have been examined for clues to prognosis. An *age at onset* of greater than 55 years has been suggested by several series [24, 34] to be a determinant of prognosis, since in relatively older patients lupus is often a milder disease. This was not borne out, however, by the large series of Wallace et al. [476], who found the same survival in patients with onset before or after 50 years of age. Nor did age at onset affect the outcome in the very large collected series (>1,000 patients) of Ginzler et al. [190], or in Nossent's analysis [363].

The outcome of *lupus in childhood* has been the subject of some controversy, which I have reviewed in detail elsewhere [83]. In our own series of 80 patients with onset of lupus nephritis under the age of 20 years, 5- and 10-year estimates of renal survival were 88 and 85 percent, and in the data from Minneapolis [379] on 70 childhood-onset cases, the figures were 85 and 81 percent. Many other series, however, have reported poorer survival in children than in adults. Wallace et al. [476] describe outcome on 50 patients with onset before 16 years of age, being 73 percent at 5 years and 58 percent at 10 years; only one-third of these patients had nephritis, however, and the children were predominantly white, unlike in most North American series. Esdaile [148] performed a Cox analysis and noted no difference in renal failure or renal death in those above and below 24 years of age at onset (as Austin et al. [24] had done) in a series of 87 patients. In general, there seems to be little difference in the survival of adults and children or adolescents with lupus nephritis when other factors are taken into consideration [24, 146, 178, 196, 476], although some authors such as Ginzler and Schorn [192] have interpreted essentially the same data in the opposite fashion, sug-

Table 69-19. Calculated 5-year actuarial survival of patients with lupus, with clinical lupus nephritis of any type, and of severe diffuse proliferative lupus glomerulonephritis

			Five-year survival (%) life-table method		
Date of publication	Authors	Reference	All lupus	All lupus nephritis	Severe diffuse proliferative nephritis
1953	Jessar, Lamont-Havers, and Ragen	257	22		
1955	Merrill and Shulman	333	51		
1957	Muehrcke et al.	346			10
1964	Kellum and Haserick	272	69		
1964	Pollak, Pirani, and Schwartz	384	54	50	
1965	Dubois	146		41	
1969	Pollak and Pirani	382		42	25
1970	Drinkard et al.	142		46	
1970	Baldwin et al.	31	77	45	23
1971	Estes and Christian	157		53	25
1972	Hayslett et al.	221		60	
1973	Nanra and Kincaid-Smith	350		78	
1973	Striker et al.	443		82	76
1973	Mackay	314	68	74	
1973	Cheatum et al.	97		63	45
1974	Epstein and Grausz	155	95		74
1974	Fries, Weyl, and Holman	178		92	
1975	Decker et al.	134			65
1976	Morel-Maroger et al.	341	91	78	78
1977	Lee et al.	299			
1977	Baldwin et al.	29		54	30
1977	Urman and Rothfield	465	71		
1979	Albert, Hadler, and Ropes	8	91	65*	
1979	Cameron et al.	92		76	78
1981	Wallace et al.	476	86	78	
1982	Ginzler et al.	196	76		
1982	Donadio et al.	138			58
1985	Rubin et al.	402	88		
1986	Austin et al.	23		86–100*	
1987	Leaker et al.	297		83	74
1987	Hashimoto et al.	217	86		
1987	Appel et al.	16		88	
1987	Ponticelli et al.	385			97
1988	Magil et al.	315		69	
1989	Swaak et al.	445	94		
1989	Esdaile et al.	148		85	
1990	Worrall et al.	497	88		
1990	Nossent et al.	363		76	
1990	McLigeyo et al.	326		82	82
1992	Gruppo Italiano	203		87	82

*Depending on therapy used.

site fashion, suggesting that children still do worse than adults. Certainly the difference, if any, is not a major one.

Sex has been studied as a prognostic factor by several authors. Male patients, of course, form only a small minority of patients with lupus, which makes comparison difficult except in the largest series. In the series of Wallace et al. [476], only 39 percent of whose patients had evident nephritis, there was a significantly worse outcome for the 63 males they compared with 546 females, and the data of Austin et al. [24] were in agreement with this. In Swaak's study [445] 5 of 16 males but only 9 of 94 females died. Esdaile et al. [148] suggested in their Cox analysis a higher rate of renal failure in males, but

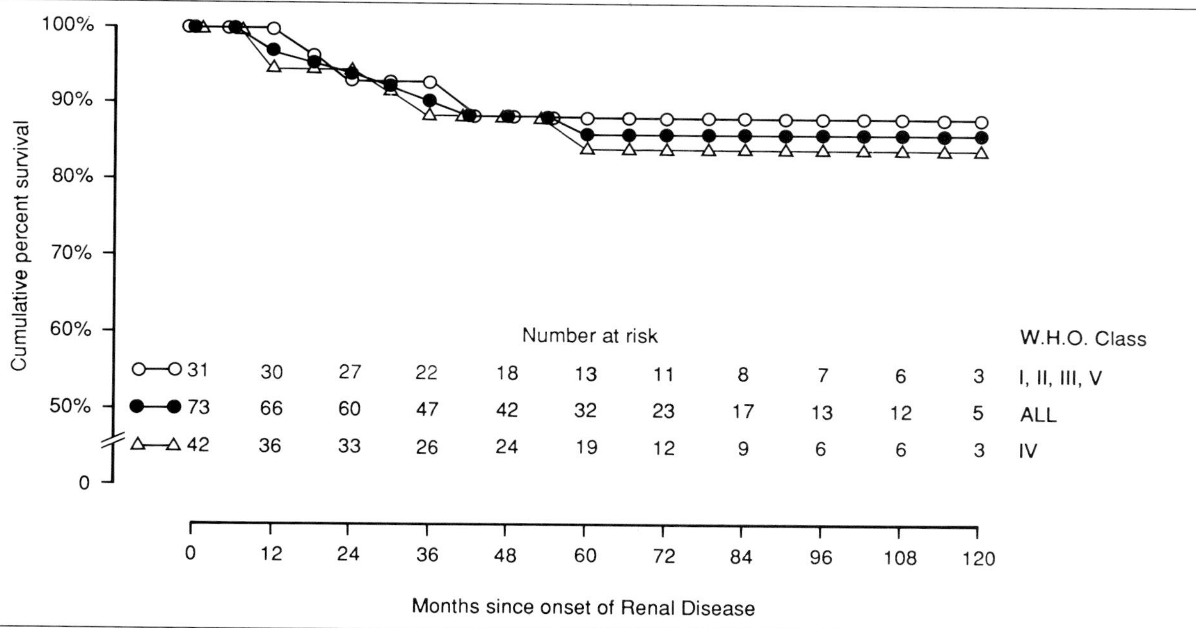

Fig. 69-28. Survival of renal function on patients with lupus nephritis seen at Guy's Hospital from 88 to 1989. The survival is shown for each of the WHO classes, arranged into two groups: milder disease (classes I, II, III, and V) and severe diffuse proliferative glomerulonephritis (class IV). Survival is identical irrespective of WHO class. Note that much more intensive immunosuppression was given in the early phases of disease to those with WHO class IV biopsies. (Data from S. McLigeyo et al., submitted for publication, 1992.)

no difference in nonrenal deaths. However, Ginzler et al. [190], using a stepwise linear regression model, found no difference in their large collected series. Tejani et al. [452] and other pediatricians [95] have suggested a poorer outcome for male children, especially those with a prepubertal onset, but the numbers are small, and other confusing factors such as race (see next section) are difficult to correct for.

Race is an obvious target for analysis, since the incidence and prevalence of lupus is so much higher in blacks and orientals compared with whites [171, 421, 426], although even within white groups the incidence seems to be highest in those with an origin in the Indian subcontinent. Many authors found no difference in outcome comparing black and white subjects [3, 148, 157, 178, 465]. The issue is complicated by the fact that black Americans differ in so many ways from whites, particularly in socioeconomic status [190]. Ginzler et al. [190] did, however, find a poorer outcome for blacks in their large study. Tejani et al. [452] suggested that black children with an onset before puberty form a particularly high-risk group. Gordon et al. [197], examining national mortality from lupus in the United States, also suggested a higher mortality among black females.

Ginzler et al. [190] also examined clinical criteria of *severity of nephritis* as predictors of outcome. Despite the undoubted fact that many patients with initially severe disease may have a favorable outcome, a raised plasma creatinine at onset in their and several other studies [148, 317, 363] was strongly associated with a poor outcome. Leaker et al. [297], however, saw no difference. The magnitude of proteinuria or the presence of a nephrotic syndrome is more controversial. We [3], Wallace et al. [476] and the Gruppo Italiano [203] noted no difference in outcome in those with nephrotic range or lesser degrees of proteinuria in univariate analyses. However, Esdaile et al. [148] and Appel et al. [16] found poorer survival in their nephrotic patients, in Appel's data particularly in those whose nephrotic syndrome persisted.

Hypertension, at least severe hypertension, is not as commonly present in lupus nephritis at apparent onset as in some other forms of glomerulopathy (e.g., 10 of 87 patients in Esdaile's [148] study; see also Budman and Steinberg [67]) and was neither examined as a prognostic factor in either of the two largest studies [196, 478] nor mentioned in the majority of follow-up studies. Esdaile et al. [148] did not find any association between outcome and high blood pressure itself, only with comorbid conditions, but the Gruppo Italiano [203] showed a markedly poorer survival in their hypertensive subgroup. Of course, in almost all patients, if hypertension is present at outset or appears later, it is usually treated vigorously. Nevertheless, it is interesting that, unlike IgA nephropathy for example, high blood pressure does not seem to be a powerful predictor of a poor outcome in lupus nephritis.

Esdaile et al. [148] found, as Ginzler et al. [190] had previously, that the total *number of American Rheumatological Association (ARA) criteria* for the diagnosis of lupus present at onset was a useful index of a poorer outcome. Swaak et al. [445] found a poorer prognosis in those with increasing *number of clinical relapses,* but this was in a population predominantly not under heavy immunosuppression. *Indices of activity* of the lupus itself have been examined in a number of studies (see [148] and [192] for discussion), many of which either do not deal with lupus nephritis or do not specify how many of the group studied had nephritis and are therefore of little use for our present purpose. Nevertheless, it is clear that at any time point, including presentation, there are correlations between immunologic tests, such as complement concentrations and levels of circulating anti-dsDNA antibody, and the severity of the clinical picture, judged in a variety of ways [2, 86, 115, 117, 224, 306, 313, 417, 444]. Their clinical utility in predicting outcome is small, however. When a group exclusively consisting of patients with nephritis was examined, *thrombocytopenia, hypocomplementemia,* and a *raised DNA binding* at onset predicted poor outcome also in Esdaile et al.'s [148] analysis.

At a *histologic* level, a considerable body of data is available. The WHO classification, which includes a category of sclerosing glomerulopathy [29, 341], has been the most studied. As indicated previously and in Table 69-19, although in the past considerable differences in outcome between milder and more severe forms were found [e.g., 38, 382], most recent reports find no or little difference in outcome between different WHO classes [148, 203, 297, 326]. However, Appel et al. [16] in a rather small study (56 patients studied 1976–1986) noted a better survival in those with class II (mesangial) nephritis compared to the other histologic classes, and the 1984 paper of Austin et al. [25] also reported a poorer survival in those with class IV nephritis, as did Nossent et al.'s recent analysis [363]. All authors [29, 31, 137, 302] are agreed that patients showing WHO class V pattern, i.e., membranous nephropathy, almost always run an indolent course, although renal failure occurs in a minority [479]. A particular problem exists with regard to patients classified as having WHO class III appearances—focal proliferative glomerulonephritis. A very diverse outcome has been reported for such individuals [17, 202, 315], which illustrates the great variation in severity within this group, to the point where division into IIIa (less severe focal nephritis) and IIIb (more severe) has been recommended. As noted, this lack of differentiation in outcome by WHO class has largely come about by an improvement in the survival of those with more severe disease, so that this now resembles the survival rate of milder forms of lupus nephritis, which remains essentially unchanged. In turn, this is presumably—although not certainly [23, 167]—the result of therapeutic decisions to treat those patients with more severe histologic appearances more aggressively.

Analyses have been performed also to assess the predictive value of individual elements of the histologic picture. Two observations appear to show some reliability in predicting a poor outcome. The first of these is *extensive subendothelial deposits,* especially if they persist in repeated biopsies [147, 450, 489, 490]. The value of this observation may have been vitiated by aggressive treatment of such patients. More consistent have been *tubulointerstitial changes,* which as noted by Muehrcke et al. [346] as long ago as 1957, point to a poor prognosis in a number of studies [25, 148, 372]. Magil et al. [317] found that the number of nonspecific esterase-positive cells (macrophages) correlated with outcome, and we [11] have shown, using monoclonal antibodies to phenotype the interstitial cells, correlations between both the numbers of infiltrating monocytes and T cells and subsequent glomerular filtration rates. *Crescents* have also been related to a poorer prognosis [500], as in other forms of nephritis, but very extensive crescentic disease is relatively uncommon in lupus. Renal vasculitis [52] and intraglomerular capillary thrombi [263] have been associated with unfavorable outcomes also, although the latter observation has been contested [297].

As a result of dissatisfaction with the data obtained by considering the morphologic aspects of the nephritis (which is in any case very variable between and within glomeruli in lupus nephritis and also varies in sequential biopsies [28, 191, 379, 432, 504]), an alternative approach has gained support: that of assessing the histologic *activity* of the nephritis on the one hand and its apparent *chronicity* on the other, as judged by the extent of sclerosis. This approach was pioneered by Pirani and Salinas-Madrigal [378], Morel-Maroger et al. [341], and others in the 1960s and 1970s but became popular after Austin et al. published a paper [25] describing the calculation of activity and chronicity indices using data from both glomeruli and interstitium in either case (Table 69-20). This approach allowed Austin et al. [25] to identify clear groups of high and low risk for a poor outcome and also permits therapeutic decisions, especially when and when not to use aggressive treatment. These data were supported by the analyses of Magil et al. [317], Esdaile et al. [148], and Nossent et al. [363], a high

Table 69-20. Renal pathology scoring system in lupus nephritis

Activity index	Chronicity index
Glomerular abnormalities	
1. Cellular proliferation	1. Glomerular sclerosis
2. Fibrinoid necrosis* karyorrhexis	2. Fibrous crescents
3. Cellular crescents*	
4. Hyaline thrombi wire loops	
5. Leukocyte infiltration	
Tubulointerstitial abnormalities	
1. Mononuclear cell infiltration	1. Interstitial fibrosis
	2. Tubular atrophy

*Fibrinoid necrosis and cellular crescents are weighted by a factor of 2. Maximum score of activity index is 24 and chronicity index is 12.
Source: Austin et al. [24], with permission.

chronicity index being in general the best predictor of subsequent renal failure; but several other authors have found poor or absent association of outcome with either index, or combinations of them [16, 297, 419], although the follow-up in Schwartz's study [419] was only 2 years.

Finally, the *additional value* for predicting outcome of the information in renal biopsies over that available from clinical studies has been examined by several authors [24, 148, 317, 489, 490] using different multivariate models and different sets of data to examine the question. Fries et al. [178] and others first suggested that there was only minimal extra value in the analysis of renal biopsy specimens in lupus nephritis, using then what approximates to the WHO classification now. Whiting-O'Keefe and colleagues [489, 490] came to less pessimistic conclusions, although only the degree of sclerosis and the presence/absence of subendothelial deposits seemed of any great value. Austin et al. [25] suggested more positively that not only did the WHO classification of biopsy data add useful information, but also the chronicity index was an even better predictor of outcome. Magil et al. [317] came to similar positive conclusions in their model, but later Esdaile et al. [148] found no biopsy information that added to the clinical predictions. The value of biopsy in directing more aggressive—and possibly more successful—therapeutic strategies is almost impossible to evaluate, but certainly this behavior interferes to a major extent with any or all of the analyses just discussed. Finally, it must not be forgotten that none of the outcome predictors discussed here and in relation to other forms of primary glomerulonephritis yet provides an accurate predictor for *individual* patients. Thus these comments do not address the question of whether a renal biopsy should be performed in patients with lupus, which has other goals besides predicting outcome.

A number of authors have noted that patients without clinical manifestations of nephritis have, on renal biopsy, changes in their glomeruli amounting to glomerular disease. There have been few follow-up studies on such patients, but the study of Leehey et al. [300] showed that the majority remain without clinical nephritis for some years, although even severe diffuse proliferative patterns may be observed in some patients. However, it is equally obvious that all patients with clinically evident nephritis must go through a period of absent or occult disease before this becomes evident; how many of these patients run a subclinical course for a prolonged period is not known.

Finally, the surprising frequency with which renal function may return in patients with lupus nephritis requiring dialysis [115, 276] has been commented on by many authors. Some of these respites are brief, but in others renal function capable of supporting life off dialysis persists for many years.

Conclusions

This chapter presents data suggesting that the great majority of patients with progressive forms of glomerulonephritis will have run their course to renal failure within 5 to 15 years from apparent clinical onset and that similarly those who will remit will usually have done so by the end of this time. A minority of patients show much more rapid evolution or remission, however.

A few patients show "grumbling" nephritis with proteinuria, hematuria, or both persisting at various levels of apparently stable renal function for 20 years or more. This is particularly common in membranous nephropathy and in IgA-associated disease. Now it may be seen also in treated patients with lupus nephritis.

One major task, along with introduction of effective treatments to slow or eliminate deterioration in renal function, is to identify patients who will run a progressive course as early as possible, so that treatments may be focused on this "high-risk" group. Several features emerge consistently [79] from multivariate analyses as predictors of a poor outcome in a broad range of glomerular diseases: (1) the magnitude and duration of proteinuria—although this must be interpreted in the light of renal biopsy findings, since of course minimal change nephrotic syndrome may show the highest figures; (2) a raised plasma creatinine that does not return to normal on control of the nephrotic syndrome, since reversible changes in K_f may depress the GFR temporarily; (3) tubulointerstitial damage in the renal biopsy—in general the severity of glomerular changes is a much poorer indicator of outlook with the sole exception of extensive crescent formation; and (4) a persistently raised blood pressure—again the transient hypertension of some patients with minimal change nephrotic syndrome or reversible acute nephritis makes a period of observation necessary and the first figures obtained on admission to the hospital relatively useless.

A number of other features are less consistently predictive of a poor outcome, male sex and increasing age among them. Some authors have suggested that the amount of hematuria in hematuric illnesses predicts poor outcome, but others have found just the opposite.

Thus the archetypal patient with glomerulopathy and a poor outlook is a middle-aged or elderly male with sustained hypertension, a raised plasma creatinine, persistent nephrotic range proteinuria, tubulointerstitial damage on renal biopsy, and crescents if a proliferative glomerulonephritis is present. On the contrary, a young normotensive female whose proteinuria remits or diminishes, who has normal renal function, and whose biopsy reveals only intraglomerular changes is likely to do well.

Glomerulonephritis remains the commonest single cause of end-stage renal failure in adults, and now we need 15-, 20-, and 30-year follow-up on patients with glomerular diseases to answer the many questions raised in this chapter about the fate of individual groups. Collecting such data is tedious, without glamor, and difficult to fund; changes in staff over the years result in many studies begun never being completed. Without such data, however, we will never be able to present even a 20-year picture of what happens to patients with glomerular disease.

References

1. Abe, T., Kida, H., Yishimura, H., et al. Participation of extracapillary lesions (ECL) in progression of IgA nephropathy. *Clin. Nephrol.* 25: 37, 1986.
2. Abrass, C. K., Nies, K. M., Louie, J. S., et al. Correlation and predictive accuracy of circulating immune complexes with disease activity in patients with systemic lupus erythematosus. *Arthritis Rheum.* 23: 273, 1980.
3. Adu, D., and Cameron, J. S. Lupus Nephritis. In G. R. V. Hughes (ed.), *Clinics in Rheumatic Diseases*, Vol. 8, No. 1. Philadelphia: Saunders, 1982. P. 153.
4. Adu, D., and Cameron, J. S. Aetiology of membranous nephropathy. *Nephrol. Dial. Transplant.* 4: 757, 1989.
5. Adu, D., Howie, A. J., Scott, D. G. I., et al. Polyarteritis and the kidney. *Q. J. Med.* 62: 221, 1987.
6. Akikusa, B., Suzuki, R., Irabu, N., and Yoshida, S. Nephrotic syndrome developed in the healing stage of necrotizing nephritis. *Am. J. Clin. Pathol.* 78: 873, 1982.
7. Alamartine, E., Sabatier, J. C., and Berthoux, F. C. Comparison of pathological lesions on repeated biopsies in 73 patients with primary IgA glomerulonephritis: Value of quantitative scoring and approach to prognosis. *Clin. Nephrol.* 34: 45, 1990.
8. Albert, D. A., Hadler, N. M., and Ropes, M. W. Does corticosteroid therapy affect the survival of patients with systemic lupus erythematosus? *Arthritis Rheum.* 22: 945, 1979.
9. Alexopoulos, E., Seron, D., Hartley, R. B., et al. The role of interstitial infiltrates in IgA nephropathy: A study with monoclonal antibodies. *Nephrol. Dial. Transplant.* 4: 187, 1989.
10. Alexopoulos, E., Seron, D., Hartley, R. B., et al. Immune mechanisms in idiopathic membranous nephropathy: The role of the interstitial infiltrates. *Am. J. Kidney Dis.* 13: 404, 1989.
11. Alexopoulos, E., Seron, D., Hartley, R. B., and Cameron, J. S. Lupus nephritis: Correlation of interstitial cells with glomerular function. *Kidney Int.* 37: 100, 1990.
12. Anders, D., Agricola, B., Sippel, M., et al. Basement membrane changes in membranoproliferative glomerulonephritis. II. Characterisation of a third type of silver impregnation of ultra-thin sections. *Virchow's Arch. A [Pathol. Anat.]* 376: 1, 1977.
13. Anders, D., and Thoenes, W. Basement membrane changes in membranoproliferative glomerulonephritis. A light and electron microscopic study. *Virchow's Arch. A [Pathol. Anat.]* 369: 87, 1975.
14. Antoine, B., and Faye, C. The clinical course associated with dense deposits in the kidney basement membranes. *Kidney Int.* 1: 420, 1972.
15. Antoine, B., Symvoulidis, A., and Dardenne, M. La stabilité evolutive des états de protéinurie. *Nephron* 6: 526, 1969.
16. Appel, G. B., Cohen, D. J., Pirani, C. L., et al. Long term follow up of patients with lupus nephritis: A study based on the classification of the World Health Organization. *Am. J. Med.* 83: 877, 1987.
17. Appel, G. B., Silva, F. G., Pirani, C. L., et al. Renal involvement in systemic lupus erythematosus (SLE). A study of 56 patients emphasising histologic classification. *Medicine* (Baltimore) 57: 371, 1978.
18. Arbeitsgemeinschaft für Pädiatrische Nephrologie. Effect of cytotoxic drugs in frequently relapsing nephrotic syndrome with and without steroid dependence. *N. Engl. J. Med.* 306: 451, 1982.
19. Arbeitsgemeinschaft für Pädiatrische Nephrologie. Short versus standard prednisone therapy for initial treatment of idiopathic nephrotic syndrome in children. *Lancet* 1: 380, 1988.
20. Arbus, G. S., Poucell, S., Bacheyie, G. S., et al. Focal segmental glomerulosclerosis with idiopathic nephrotic syndrome: Three types of clinical response. *J. Pediatr.* 101: 40, 1982.
21. Arneil, G. C. 164 children with nephrosis. *Lancet* 2: 1103, 1961.
22. Arze, R. S., Rashid, H., Morley, R., et al. Shunt nephritis: Report of two cases and review of the literature. *Clin. Nephrol.* 19: 48, 1983.
23. Austin, H. A., III, Klippel, J. H., Balow, J. E., et al. Therapy of lupus nephritis: Controlled trial of prednisone and cytotoxic drugs. *N. Engl. J. Med.* 314: 614, 1986.
24. Austin, K. A., III, Muenz, L. R., Joyce, K. M., et al. Prognostic factors in lupus nephritis. Contribution of renal histologic data. *Am. J. Med.* 75: 382, 1983.
25. Austin, K. A., III, Muenz, L. R., Joyce, K. M., et al. Diffuse proliferative lupus nephritis: Identification of specific pathologic features affecting outcome. *Kidney Int.* 25: 689, 1984.
26. Bakir, A. A., Bazilinski, N. G., Rhee, H. L., et al. Focal segmental glomerulosclerosis: A common entity in nephrotic Black adults. *Arch. Intern. Med.* 149: 1802, 1989.
27. Baldwin, D. S. Poststreptococcal glomerulonephritis. A progressive disease? *Am. J. Med.* 62: 1, 1979.
28. Baldwin, D. S. Clinical usefulness of the morphological classification of lupus nephritis. *Am. J. Kidney Dis.* (Suppl. I): 142, 1982.
29. Baldwin, D. S., Gluck, M. C., Lowenstein, J., et al. Lupus nephritis. Clinical course as related to morphologic forms and their transitions. *Am. J. Med.* 62: 12, 1977.
30. Baldwin, D. S., Gluck, M. C., Schacht, R. G., et al. The long-term course of post-streptococcal glomerulonephritis. *Ann. Intern. Med.* 80: 342, 1974.
31. Baldwin, D. S., Lowenstein, J., Rothfield, N. F., et al. The clinical course of the proliferative and membranous forms of lupus nephritis. *Ann. Intern. Med.* 73: 929, 1970.

31a. Baldwin, D. S., Neugarten, J., Feiner, H. D., et al. The existence of a protracted course in crescentic glomerulonephritis. *Kidney Int.* 31: 790, 1987.

32. Baldwin, D. S., and Schacht, R. G. Late sequelae of post-streptococcal glomerulonephritis. *Annu. Rev. Med.* 24: 49, 1976.
33. Ballard, H. S., Eisinger, R. P., and Gallo, P. Renal manifestations of Henoch-Schönlein syndrome in adults. *Am. J. Med.* 49: 328, 1970.
34. Ballou, S. P., Khan, M. A., and Kushner, I. Clinical features of systemic lupus erythematosus: Differences related to race and age of onset. *Arthritis Rheum.* 25: 55, 1982.
35. Balow, J. Nephrology forum: Renal vasculitis. *Kidney Int.* 27: 954, 1985.
36. Barbiano di Belgiojoso, G. B., Baroni, M., Pagliari, B., et al. Is membranoproliferative glomerulonephritis really decreasing? *Nephron* 40: 380, 1985.
37. Barbiano di Belgiojoso, G., Tarantino, A., Colasanti, G., et al. The prognostic value of some clinical and histological parameters in membranoproliferative glomerulonephritis (MPGN). *Nephron* 19: 250, 1977.
38. Barnett, H. L., Schoenmann, M., Bernstein, J., et al. Minimal Change Nephrotic Syndrome. In C. M. Edelmann (ed.), *Pediatric Kidney Disease*. Boston: Little, Brown, 1978. Pp. 195–211.
39. Bar-On, H., and Rosenmann, E. Schönlein-Henoch syn-

drome in adults. A clinical and histological study of renal involvement. *Isr. J. Med. Sci.* 8: 1702, 1972.

40. Bartlow, B. G., Oyama, J. H., Ing, T. S., et al. Glomerular abnormalities in patients with mixed IgG-IgM essential cryoglobulinemic nephritis. *Nephron* 14: 309, 1975.
41. Beaman, M., Howie, A. J., Hardwicke, J., et al. The glomerular tip lesion: A steroid responsive nephrotic syndrome. *Clin. Nephrol.* 27: 217, 1987.
42. Beaufils, H., Alphonse, J. C., Guedon, J., et al. Focal glomerulosclerosis: Natural history and treatment. A report of 70 cases. *Nephron* 21: 75, 1978.
43. Beaufils, M., Morel-Maroger, L., Sraer, J.-D., et al. Acute renal failure of glomerular origin during visceral abscesses. *N. Engl. J. Med.* 295: 185, 1976.
44. Beirne, G. J., Wagnild, J. P., Zimmerman, S. W., et al. Idiopathic crescentic glomerulonephritis. *Medicine* 56: 349, 1977.
45. Bennett, W. J., and Kincaid-Smith, P. S. Macroscopic hematuria in mesangial IgAN: Correlation with glomerular crescents and renal dysfunction. *Kidney Int.* 23: 393, 1983.
46. Bennett, W. M., Fassett, R. G., Walker, R. G., et al. Mesangiocapillary glomerulonephritis type II (dense deposit disease): Clinical features of a progressive disease. *Am. J. Kidney Dis.* 13: 469, 1989.
47. Benoit, F. L., Rulon, D. B., Theil, G. B., et al. Goodpasture's syndrome. A clinicopathologic entity. *Am. J. Med.* 34: 424, 1964.
48. Berlyne, G. M., and Baker, S. B. de C. Acute oliguric glomerulonephritis. *Q. J. Med.* 3: 105, 1964.
49. Berns, J. S., Gaudio, K. M., Krassner, L. S., et al. Steroid-responsive nephrotic syndrome of childhood: A long term study of clinical course histopathology, efficacy of cyclophosphamide therapy, and effects on growth. *Am. J. Kidney Dis.* 9: 108, 1987.
50. Beukhof, J. R., Kardaun, O., Schaafsma, W., et al. Toward individual prognosis of IgA nephropathy. *Kidney Int.* 29: 549, 1986.
51. Bhasin, H. K., Abuelo, J. G., Nayak, R., et al. Mesangial proliferative glomerulonephritis. *Lab. Invest.* 39: 21, 1978.
52. Bhuyan, U. N., Malaviya, A. N., Dash, S. C., et al. Prognostic significance of renal angiitis in systemic lupus erythematosus (SLE). *Clin. Nephrol.* 20: 109, 1983.
53. Black, D. A. K., Rose, G., and Brewer, D. B. Controlled trial of prednisone in adult patients with the nephrotic syndrome. *Br. Med. J.* 3: 421, 1970.
54. Bohle, A., Grund, K. E., Mackensen, S., et al. Correlations between renal interstitium and level of serum creatinine. Morphometric investigations of biopsies in per-membranous glomerulonephritis. *Virchow's Arch. A [Pathol. Anat.]* 373: 15, 1977.
55. Bolton, W. K. Use of Pulse Methylprednisone in Primary and Multisystem Glomerular Diseases. In R. R. Robinson (ed.), *Nephrology.* New York: Springer, 1984. Pp. 1454–1473.
56. Bolton, W. K., and Couser, W. G. Intravenous methylprednisolone therapy of acute crescentic rapidly progressive glomerulonephritis. *Am. J. Med.* 66: 495, 1979.
57. Bonfiglio, T. A., Botti, R. E., and Hagstrom, J. W. C. Coronary arteritis, occlusion and myocardial infarction due to lupus erythematosus. *Am. Heart J.* 83: 153, 1972.
58. Breslow, N. A. A generalized Kruskal-Wallis test for comparing K samples subject to unequal patterns of censorship. *Biometrika* 57: 579, 1970.
59. Broumand, B., and Antonovych, T. T. High incidence of membranoproliferative glomerulonephritis in Iran. *Abstracts, 9th Congress of the International Society of Nephrology,* Los Angeles, June, 1984. P. 273A.
60. Brown, C. B., Cameron, J. S., Turner, D. R., et al. Focal segmental glomerulonephritis with rapid decline in renal function ("Malignant" FSGS). *Clin. Nephrol.* 10: 51, 1978.
61. Brown, C. D., Rao, T. K. S., Maxey, R. I. N., et al. Regression of clinical and immunological expression of systemic lupus erythematosus consequent to development of uremia. *Kidney Int.* 16: 884, 1979.
62. Brown, E. A., Upadhyaya, K., Hayslett, J. P., et al. The clinical course of mesangial proliferative glomerulonephritis. *Medicine* 58: 295, 1979.
63. Broyer, M., Meyrier, A., Naiudet, P., and Habib, R. Minimal Changes and Focal Segmental Glomerular Sclerosis. In J. S. Cameron et al. (eds.), *The Oxford Textbook of Clinical Nephrology.* London: Oxford University Press, 1991.
64. Brun, C., Bryld, C., Fenger, L., et al. Glomerular lesions in adults with the Schönlein Henoch syndrome. *Acta Pathol. Microbiol. Scand. [A]* 79: 569, 1971.
65. Bruns, F. J., Adler, S., Fraley, D. S., and Segel, D. P. Long-term follow-up of aggressively treated idiopathic rapidly progressive glomerulonephritis. *Am. J. Med.* 86: 400, 1989.
66. Brzosko, W. J., Krauczynski, K., Nazarewicz, T., et al. Glomerulonephritis associated with hepatitis B surface antigen immune complexes in children. *Lancet* ii: 478, 1974.
67. Budman, D. R., and Steinberg, A. D. Hypertension and renal disease in systemic lupus erythematosus. *Arch. Intern. Med.* 136: 1003, 1976.
68. Cahen, R., Francois, B., Trolliet, P., et al. Aetiology of membranous glomerulonephritis: A prospective study of 82 adult patients. *Nephrol. Dial. Transplant.* 4: 172, 1989.
69. Cairns, S. A., Mallick, N. P., Lawler, W., et al. Squamous cell carcinoma of bronchus presenting with Henoch-Schönlein purpura. *Br. Med. J.* 3: 474, 1978.
70. Cameron, J. S. Clinicopathological correlations—Problems and limitations. *Clin. Nephrol.* 4: 1, 1977.
71. Cameron, J. S. The Natural History of Glomerulonephritis. In P. Kincaid-Smith, A. J. F. D'Apice, and R. C. Atkins (eds.), *Progress in Glomerulonephritis.* New York: Wiley, 1979. Pp. 1–25.
72. Cameron, J. S. The Problem of Focal Segmental Glomerulosclerosis. In P. Kincaid-Smith, A. J. F. D'Apice, and R. C. Atkins (eds.), *Progress in Glomerulonephritis.* New York: Wiley, 1979. Pp. 209–228.
73. Cameron, J. S. The Nephritis of Schönlein-Henoch Purpura: Current Problems. In P. Kincaid-Smith, A. J. F. D'Apice, and R. C. Atkins (eds.), *Progress in Glomerulonephritis.* New York: Wiley, 1979. Pp. 283–309.
74. Cameron, J. S. The Nephritis of Systemic Lupus Erythematosus. In P. Kincaid-Smith, A. J. F. D'Apice, and R. C. Atkins (eds.), *Progress in Glomerulonephritis.* New York: Wiley, 1979. Pp. 387–423.
75. Cameron, J. S. Pathogenesis and treatment of membranous nephropathy. *Kidney Int.* 15: 88, 1979.
76. Cameron, J. S. Coagulation and thrombotic complications in the nephrotic syndrome. *Adv. Nephrol.* 13: 137, 1983.
77. Cameron, J. S. Henoch-Schönlein purpura: Clinical presentation. *Contrib. Nephrol.* 40: 246, 1984.
78. Cameron, J. S. Acute Renal Failure in Glomerular Disease. In V. Andreucci (ed.), *Acute Renal Failure—Patho-*

physiology, Prevention, Treatment. The Hague: Martinus Nyhoff, 1984. Pp. 271–295.

79. Cameron, J. S. Renal disease and vasculitis. *Pediatr. Nephrol.* 2: 490, 1988.
80. Cameron, J. S. The natural history of glomerulonephritis. *Contrib. Nephrol.* 75: 68, 1989.
81. Cameron, J. S. Membranous nephropathy in childhood and its treatment. *Pediatr. Nephrol.* 4: 193, 1990.
82. Cameron, J. S. Proteinuria and progression in human glomerular diseases. *Am. J. Nephrol.* 10(Suppl. 1): 81, 1990.
83. Cameron, J. S. Renal vasculitis: Microscopic polyarteritis and Wegener's granuloma. *Contrib. Nephrol.* 94: 38, 1991.
84. Cameron, J. S. Nephritis of Systemic Lupus Erythematosis. In C. E. Edelmann, Jr., J. Bernstein, R. Meadow, A. Spitzer, and L. B. Travis (eds.), *Pediatric Kidney Disease*, 2nd ed. Boston: Little, Brown, 1992. Pp. 1407–1465.
85. Cameron, J. S., and Glassock, R. J. The Natural History and Outcome of the Nephrotic Syndrome. In J. S. Cameron and R. J. Glassock (eds.), *The Nephrotic Syndrome*. New York: Marcel Dekker, 1987.
86. Cameron, J. S., Healey, M. J. R., and Adu, D. The Medical Research Council trial of short-term high-dose alternate day prednisolone in idiopathic membranous nephropathy with nephrotic syndrome in adults. *Q. J. Med.* 74: 133, 1990.
87. Cameron, J. S., Lessof, M. H., Ogg, C. S., et al. Disease activity in the nephritis of systemic lupus erythematosus in relation to serum complement concentrations, DNA-binding capacity and precipitating anti-DNA antibody. *Clin. Exp. Immunol.* 25: 418, 1976.
88. Cameron, J. S., Ogg, C. S., Chantler, C., et al. Acute nephritic syndromes. *Bull. Acad. Med.* (Singapore) 4(Suppl.): 1, 1975.
89. Cameron, J. S., Ogg, C. S., and Wass, V. J. Complications of the Nephrotic Syndrome. In J. S. Cameron and R. J. Glassock (eds.), *The Nephrotic Syndrome*. New York: Marcel Dekker, 1988. Pp. 849–920.
90. Cameron, J. S., Turner, D. R., Heaton, J., et al. Idiopathic mesangiocapillary glomerulonephritis: Comparison of types I and II in children and adults and long-term prognosis. *Am. J. Med.* 74: 175, 1983.
91. Cameron, J. S., Turner, D. R., Ogg, C. S., et al. The long-term prognosis of patients with focal segmental glomerulosclerosis. *Clin. Nephrol.* 10: 213, 1978.
92. Cameron, J. S., Turner, D. R., Ogg, C. S., et al. Systemic lupus with nephritis. A long-term study. *Q. J. Med.* 48: 1, 1979.
93. Cattran, D. C., Cardella, C. J., Roscoe, J. M., et al. Results of a controlled drug trial in membranoproliferative glomerulonephritis. *Kidney Int.* 27: 436, 1985.
94. Cattran, D. C., Delmore, T., Roscoe, J., et al. A randomized controlled trial of prednisolone in patients with idiopathic membranous nephropathy. *N. Engl. J. Med.* 320: 210, 1989.
95. Celermajer, D. S., Thorner, P. S., Baumal, R., et al. Sex differences in childhood lupus nephritis. *Am. J. Dis. Child* 138: 586, 1984.
96. Chan, M. K., Chan, K. W., Chan, P. C. K., et al. Adult onset mesangiocapillary glomerulonephritis: A disease with a poor prognosis. *Q. J. Med.* 72: 599, 1989.
97. Cheatum, D. E., Hurd, E. R., Strunk, S. W., et al. Renal histology and clinical course of systemic lupus erythematosus: A prospective study. *Arthritis Rheum.* 16: 670, 1973.
98. Cheigh, J. S., Stenzel, K. H., Rubin, A. L., et al. Systemic lupus erythematosus in patients with chronic renal failure. *Am. J. Med.* 75: 602, 1983.
99. Choonara, I. A., Heney, D., and Meadow, S. R. Low dose prednisolone in nephrotic syndrome. *Arch. Dis. Child.* 64: 610, 1989.
100. Christian, H. A. Nephrosis—A critique. *J.A.M.A.* 93: 23, 1929.
101. Churg, J., and Sobin, L. H. Renal disease: Classification and atlas of glomerular disease. Tokyo: Igaku-Shoin, 1982.
102. Clark, G., White, R. H. R., Glasgow, E. F., et al. Poststreptococcal glomerulonephritis in children: Clinicopathological correlations and long term prognosis. *Pediatr. Nephrol.* 2: 381, 1988.
103. Clive, D. M., Galvanek, E. G., and Silva, F. G. Mesangial immunoglobulin A deposits in minimal change nephrotic syndrome: A report of a case and review of the literature. *Am. J. Nephrol.* 10: 31, 1990.
104. Clutterbuck, E. J., Evans, D. J., and Pusey, C. D. Renal involvement in Churg-Strauss syndrome. *Nephrol. Dial. Transplant.* 5: 161, 1990.
105. Coggins, C. H. Minimal Change Nephrosis in Adults. In W. Zurukzoglu et al. (eds.), *Proceedings of the 8th International Congress of Nephrology*. Basel: Karger, 1981. Pp. 336–344.
106. Cohen, A., Border, W., and Glassock, R. Nephrotic syndrome with glomerular mesangial IgM deposits. *Lab. Invest.* 38: 610, 1978.
107. Cohen, A. H., Border, W. A., Shankel, E., et al. Crescentic glomerulonephritis: Immune vs. nonimmune mechanisms. *Am. J. Nephrol.* 1: 78, 1981.
108. Cohen, L. H., Wilson, C. B., and Freeman, R. M. Goodpasture syndrome: Recovery after severe renal insufficiency. *Arch. Intern. Med.* 136: 835, 1976.
109. Cohen, R. D., Conn, D. L., and Ilstrup, D. M. Clinical features, prognosis and response to treatment in polyarteritis. *Mayo Clin. Proc.* 55: 146, 1980.
110. Cohen Tervaert, J. W., Huitema, M. G., Hene, R. J., et al. Prevention of relapses in Wegener's granulomatosis by treatment based on antineutrophil cytoplasmic antibody titre. *Lancet* 336: 709, 1990.

110a. Colasanti, G., Ferrario, F., Tarantino, A., et al. The Glomerulonephritis of Essential Mixed Cryoglobulinaemia. In L. Minetti, G. D'Amico, and C. Ponticelli (eds.), *The Kidney in Plasma Cell Dyscrasias*. Dordrecht: Kluwer, 1988. P. 183.

111. Collaborative study of the adult idiopathic nephrotic syndrome. A controlled study of short-term prednisone treatment in adults with membranous nephropathy. *N. Engl. J. Med.* 301: 1301, 1979.
112. Coplon, N. S., Diskin, C. J., Petersen, J., et al. The long-term clinical course of systemic lupus erythematosus in end-stage renal disease. *N. Engl. J. Med.* 308: 186, 1983.
113. Coppo, R., Bosticardo, G. M., Basolo, B., et al. Clinical significance of the detection of circulating immune complexes in lupus nephritis. *Nephron* 32: 320, 1982.
114. Correia, P., Cameron, J. S., Lian, J. D., et al. Why do patients with lupus nephritis die? *Br. Med. J.* 290: 126, 1985.
115. Correia, P., Cameron, J. S., Ogg, C. S., et al. End-stage renal failure in systemic lupus erythematosus with nephritis. *Clin. Nephrol.* 22: 293, 1984.
116. Counahan, R., and Cameron, J. S. Henoch-Schönlein nephritis. *Contrib. Nephrol.* 7: 143, 1977.
117. Counahan, R., Winterborn, M. H., White, R. H. R., et

al. Prognosis of Henoch-Schönlein nephritis in children. *Br. Med. J.* 2: 11, 1977.
118. Couser, W. G. Rapidly progressive glomerulonephritis: Classification, pathogenetic mechanisms, and therapy. *Am. J. Kidney Dis.* 11: 449, 1988.
119. Coward, R. A., Hamdy, N. A. T., Shortland, J. S., and Brown, C. B. Renal micropolyarteritis: A treatable condition. *Nephrol. Dial. Transplant.* 1: 31, 1986.
120. Cox, D. R. Regression models and life table (with discussion). *J. R. Stat. Soc.* 34: 187, 1972.
121. Cream, J. J. Cryoglobulins in vasculitis. *Q. J. Med.* 45: 255, 1976.
122. Cream, J. J., Gumpel, J. M., and Peachey, R. D. G. Henoch-Schönlein purpura in the adult: A study of 77 adults with anaphylactoid or Schönlein Henoch purpura. *Q. J. Med.* 39: 461, 1970.
123. Cuochi, D., Vangelista, A., Baraldi, A., et al. Relapsing nephrotic syndrome following remission for 20 years. *Int. J. Pediatr. Nephrol.* 4: 211, 1983.
124. Dahlberg, P. J., Kutz, S. B., Donadio, J. V., et al. Recurrent Goodpasture's syndrome. *Mayo Clin. Proc.* 53: 533, 1978.
125. D'Amico, G. Idiopathic IgA mesangial nephropathy. *Nephron* 41: 1, 1985.
126. D'Amico, G., Colasanti, G., Ferrario, F., and Sinico, R. A. Renal involvement in essential mixed cryoglobulinemia. *Kidney Int.* 35: 1004, 1989.
127. D'Amico, G., Ferrario, F., Colasanti, G., et al. IgA-mesangial nephropathy (Berger's disease) with rapid decline in renal function. *Clin. Nephrol.* 16: 251, 1981.
128. D'Amico, G., Imbasciati, E., Barbiano di Belgiojoso, G., et al. Idiopathic IgA mesangial nephropathy. Clinical and histological study of 374 patients. *Medicine* (Baltimore) 64: 49, 1985.
129. D'Amico, G., Minetti, L., and Ponticelli, C. (eds.). IgA Mesangial nephropathy. *Contrib. Nephrol.* 1984.
130. D'Amico, G., Minetti, L., Ponticelli, C., et al. Prognostic indicators in idiopathic IgA nephropathy. *Q. J. Med.* 59: 363, 1986.
131. Dash, S. C., Malhotra, K. K., Sharma, R. K., et al. Spectrum of rapidly progressive (crescentic) glomerulonephritis in Northern India. *Nephron* 30: 45, 1982.
132. Davison, A., Cameron, J. S., Kerr, D. N. S., et al. Natural history of renal function in untreated idiopathic membranous glomerulonephritis in adults. *Clin. Nephrol.* 22: 61, 1984.
133. Debray, J., Krulik, M., and Giorgi, H. Le purpura rhumatoïde (syndrome de Schönlein-Henoch) de l'adulte. *Sem. Hôp. Paris* 47: 1805, 1971.
134. Decker, J. L., Klippel, J. H., Plotz, P. K., et al. Cyclophosphamide and azathioprine in lupus glomerulonephritis. A controlled trial: Results at 28 months. *Ann. Intern. Med.* 832: 606, 1975.
135. Dodge, W. F., Spargo, B. K., Travis, L. B., et al. Poststreptococcal glomerulonephritis. A prospective study in children. *N. Engl. J. Med.* 286: 273, 1972.
136. Donadio, J. V., Anderson, C. F., Mitchell, J. C., III, et al. Membranoproliferative glomerulonephritis. A prospective trial of antiplatelet therapy. *N. Engl. J. Med.* 310: 1421, 1984.
137. Donadio, J. V., Burgess, J. H., and Holley, K. E. Membranous lupus nephropathy: A clinicopathologic study. *Medicine* 56: 527, 1977.
138. Donadio, J. V., Holley, K. E., and Ilstrup, D. M. Cytotoxic drug treatment of lupus nephritis. *Am. J. Kidney Dis.* 2(Suppl. 1): 178, 1982.
139. Donadio, J. V., and Offord, K. P. Reassessment of treatment results in membranoproliferative glomerulonephritis, with emphasis on life-table analysis. *Am. J. Kidney Dis.* 14: 445, 1989.
140. Donadio, J. V., Slack, T. K., Holley, K. E., et al. Idiopathic membranoproliferative (mesangiocapillary) glomerulonephritis. A clinicopathologic study. *Mayo Clin. Proc.* 54: 141, 1979.
141. Donadio, J. V., Torres, V. E., Velosa, J. A., et al. Idiopathic membranous nephropathy: The natural history of untreated patients. *Kidney Int.* 33: 708, 1988.
142. Drinkard, J. P., Stanley, T. M., Dornfield, L., et al. Azathioprine and prednisone in the treatment of adults with lupus nephritis. Clinical, histological and immunological changes with therapy. *Medicine* (Baltimore) 49: 411, 1970.
143. Droz, D. Natural history of primary glomerulonephritis with mesangial deposits of IgA. *(Proceedings of the 5th International Congress of Nephrology, Florence, 1975). Contrib. Nephrol.* 2: 150, 1976.
144. Droz, D., Noel, L. H., Barbanel, C., et al. Evolution of membranoproliferative glomerulonephritis with sub-endothelial deposits: Recovery in 13 cases (Abstract). *Kidney Int.* 29: 306, 1980.
145. Droz, D., Noel, L. H., Leibowitch, M., et al. Glomerulonephritis and necrotising angiitis. *Adv. Nephrol.* 9: 343, 1979.
146. Dubois, E. L. *Systemic Lupus Erythematosus,* 2nd ed. (revised). Los Angeles: University of California Press, 1976.
147. Dujovne, I., Pollak, V. E., Pirani, C. L., et al. The distribution and character of glomerular deposits in systemic lupus erythematosus. *Kidney Int.* 2: 33, 1972.
148. Esdaile, J. M., Levinton, C., Federgreen, W., et al. The clinical and renal biopsy predictors of long-term outcome in lupus nephritis: A study of 87 patients and review of the literature. *Q. J. Med.* 72: 779, 1989.
149. Editorial: Is post-streptococcal glomerulonephritis progressive? *Br. Med. J.* 3: 975, 1977.
150. Egido, J., Rivera Hernandez, F., Sandro, J., et al. Estudio del sistema HLA y factores de riesgo para la insuficencia renal en la glomerulonefritis mesangial IgA. *Nefrologia* 1: 21, 1981.
151. Egli, F., Zollinger, H. U., Geering, H. M., et al. Hypertensive Einzephalopathic bei akuter Glomerulonephritis mit minimalem Urinbefund. *Helv. Paediatr. Acta* 27: 381, 1972.
152. Egner, W., and Chapel, H. M. Titration of antibodies against neutrophil cytoplasmic antigens is useful in monitoring disease activity in systemic vasculitides. *Clin. Exp. Immunol.* 82: 244, 1990.
153. Ehrenreich, T., and Churg, J. Pathology of Membranous Nephropathy. In S. C. Sommers (ed.), *Pathology Annual,* Vol. 3. New York: Appleton-Century-Crofts, 1968. Pp. 145–186.
154. Emancipator, S. N. Immunoregulatory factors in the pathogenesis of IgA nephropathy. *Kidney Int.* 38: 1216, 1990.
155. Epstein, W. V., and Grausz, H. Favourable outcome in diffuse proliferative glomerulonephritis of systemic lupus erythematosus. *Arthritis Rheum.* 17: 129, 1974.
156. Erwin, D. T., Donadio, J. V., and Holley, K. E. The clinical course of idiopathic membranous nephropathy. *Mayo Clin. Proc.* 48: 697, 1973.
157. Estes, D., and Christian, C. The natural history of SLE by prospective analysis. *Medicine* (Baltimore) 50: 85, 1971.

158. Esteve, A. F., Garcia de Vinuesa, M., Alvarez de Lara, M. A., et al. Henoch Schönlein nephritis in adults. *Clin. Nephrol.* 26: 313, 1986.
159. Falk, R. J. ANCA-associated renal disease. *Kidney Int.* 38: 998, 1990.
160. Fauci, A. S. Vasculitis. *J. Allergy Clin. Immunol.* 72: 211, 1983.
161. Fauci, A. S., Haynes, B. F., and Katz, P. The spectrum of vasculitis: Clinical, pathologic and immunologic and therapeutic considerations. *Ann. Intern. Med.* 89: 660, 1978.
162. Fauci, A. S., Haynes, B. F., Katz, P., et al. Wegener's granulomatosis: Prospective clinical and therapeutic experience with 85 patients for 21 years. *Ann. Intern. Med.* 98: 76, 1983.
163. Fauci, A. S., Haynes, B. F., and Katz, P. Wegener's granulomatosis. Prospective clinical and therapeutic experience with 85 patients for 21 years. *Ann. Intern. Med.* 98: 76, 1983.
164. Faull, R. J., Woodroffe, A. J., Aarons, I., and Clarkson, A. R. Adult Henoch-Schönlein nephritis. *Aust. N.Z. J. Med.* 17: 396, 1987.
165. Feehally, J. Immune mechanisms of glomerular IgA deposition. *Nephrol. Dial. Transplant.* 3: 361, 1988.
166. Fellin, G., Gentile, M. G., Duca, G., and D'Amico, G. Renal function in IgA nephropathy with established renal failure. *Nephrol. Dial. Transplant.* 3: 17, 1988.
167. Felson, D. T., and Anderson, J. A. Evidence for the superiority of immunosuppressive drugs and prednisone over prednisone alone in lupus nephritis. *N. Engl. J. Med.* 311: 1528, 1984.
168. Fernandes, G., Alonso, D. R., Tanaka, J., et al. Influence of diet on vascular lesions in autoimmune-prone B/W mice. *Proc. Natl. Acad. Sci. U.S.A.* 80: 874, 1983.
169. Ferrario, F. Membranoproliferative glomerulonephritis (MPGN) type I: A correlation between treated (138) and untreated (108) patients. *Abstracts, XIth Congress of the International Society of Nephrology,* Tokyo, July 1990. P. 352A.
170. Ferrario, F., Kourilsky, O., and Morel-Maroger, L. Acute endocapillary glomerulonephritis in adults: A histologic and clinical comparison between patients with and without initial acute renal failure. *Clin. Nephrol.* 19: 17, 1983.
171. Fessel, J. Systemic lupus erythematosus in the community. *Arch. Intern. Med.* 143: 1027, 1974.
172. Fillastre, J.-P., Morel-Maroger, L., Ducroiset, B., et al. Atteinte renal du purpura rhumatoïde chez l'adulte. Étude de 20 biopsies renales. Interêt de l'examen glomerulaire en immunofluorescence. *Presse Méd.* 78: 2375, 1970.
173. Flores, J. C., Taube, D., Sarage, C. O. S., et al. Clinical and immunological evolution of oligoanuric anti-GBM nephritis treated by haemodialysis. *Lancet* 1: 5, 1986.
174. Fogazzi, G. B., Pasquali, S., Moroggi, M., et al. Long term outcome of Schönlein-Henoch nephritis in the adult. *Clin. Nephrol.* 31: 60, 1989.
175. Foote, K. D., Brocklebank, J. T., and Meadow, S. R. Height attainment in children with steroid-responsive nephrotic syndrome. *Lancet* 2: 917, 1985.
176. Forland, M., and Spargo, B. H. Clinicopathological correlations in idiopathic nephrotic syndrome with membranous nephropathy. *Nephron* 6: 498, 1969.
177. Franklin, W. A., Jennings, R. B., and Earle, D. P. Membranous glomerulonephritis. Long-term serial observations on clinical course and morphology. *Kidney Int.* 4: 36, 1973.
178. Fries, J. F., Weyl, S., and Holman, H. R. Estimating prognosis in systemic lupus erythematosus. *Am. J. Med.* 57: 561, 1974.
179. Frohnert, P. P., and Sheps, S. G. Long-term follow-up study of peri-arteritis nodosa. *Am. J. Med.* 43: 8, 1967.
180. Fuiano, G., Cameron, J. S., Raftery, M., et al. Improved prognosis of renal microscopic polyarteritis in recent years. *Nephrol. Dial. Transplant.* 3: 383, 1988.
180a. Gaboardi, F., Edelfonti, A., Imbasciati, E., et al. Alport's syndrome (progressive hereditary nephropathy). *Clin. Nephrol.* 2: 143, 1974.
181. Gaffney, E. F., and Panner, B. J. Membranous glomerulonephritis: Clinical significance of glomerular hypercellularity and parietal epithelial abnormalities. *Nephron* 29: 209, 1981.
182. Gagnadoux, M., Kleinknecht, C., Gubler, M. C., et al. Long-term prognosis of non-responsive nephrosis in children. *Abstracts, 9th International Congress of Nephrology,* Los Angeles, June, 1984. P. 88A.
183. Galle, P., and Mahieu, P. Electron-dense alteration of kidney basement membranes. A renal lesion specific of a systemic disease. *Am. J. Med.* 58: 749, 1975.
184. Gallo, G. R., Feiner, H. D., Steele, J. M., Jr., et al. Role of intrarenal vascular sclerosis in progression of post-streptococcal glomerulonephritis. *Clin. Nephrol.* 13: 49, 1980.
185. Garcia, R., Rubio, L., and Rodriguez-Iturbe, B. Long-term prognosis of epidemic post-streptococcal glomerulonephritis in Maracaibo: Follow-up studies 11–12 years after the acute attack. *Clin. Nephrol.* 15: 291, 1981.
186. Garin, E. H., Pryor, H. D., and Fennell, R. S. Pattern of response to prednisone in idiopathic minimal lesion nephrotic syndrome as a criterion for selecting patients for cyclophosphamide therapy. *J. Pediatr.* 92: 304, 1978.
187. Gaskin, G., and Rees, A. J. Systemic Vasculitis. In J. S. Cameron et al., *The Oxford Textbook of Clinical Nephrology.* London: Oxford University Press, 1991.
188. Gill, D., Richardson, H., Chantler, C., et al. The outcome of acute post-streptococcal nephritis ten years after the attack. *Arch. Dis. Child* 52: 423, 1977.
189. Gill, D. G., Turner, D. R., Chantler, C., et al. The progression of acute proliferative post-streptococcal glomerulonephritis to severe epithelial crescent formation. *Clin. Nephrol.* 8: 449, 1977.
190. Ginzler, E. M., Diamond, H. S., Weisner, M., et al. A multicentre study of outcome in systemic lupus erythematosus. I. Entry variables as predictors of prognosis. *Arthritis Rheum.* 25: 601, 1982.
191. Ginzler, E. M., Nicastri, A. D., Chen, C. K., et al. Progression of mesangial and focal to diffuse lupus nephritis. *N. Engl. J. Med.* 291: 693, 1974.
192. Ginzler, E. M., and Shorn, K. Outcome and prognosis in systemic lupus erythematosus. *Rheum. Dis. Clin. N. Am.* 14: 67, 1988.
193. Glasgow, E. F., and White, R. H. R. Acute Post-Streptococcal Glomerulonephritis with Failure to Resolve. In P. Kincaid-Smith, T. H. Mathew, and E. L. Becker (eds.), *Glomerulonephritis,* Vol. 1. New York: Wiley, 1973. Pp. 345–361.
194. Glassock, R. J. A clinical and immunopathologic dissection of rapidly progressive glomerulonephritis. *Nephron* 22: 253, 1978.
195. Gluck, M. C., Gallo, C., Lowenstein, T., et al. Membranous glomerulonephritis. Evolution of clinical and pathologic features. *Ann. Intern. Med.* 78: 1, 1973.
196. Gonzalo, A., Mampaso, F., Teruel, J. L., and Ortuno, J.

Steroid-responsive nephrotic syndrome with IgA deposits. *Nephron* 48: 84, 1988.
197. Gordon, M. F., Stolley, P. D., and Schinnar, K. Trends in recent systemic lupus erythematosus mortality rates. *Arthritis Rheum.* 24: 762, 1981.
198. Gorensek, M. J., Lebel, M. H., and Nelson, J. D. Peritonitis in children with nephrotic syndrome. *Pediatrics* 81: 849, 1988.
199. Gorevic, P. P., Kassab, H. J., Levo, Y., et al. Mixed cryoglobulinemia: Clinical aspects and long-term follow-up of 40 patients. *Am. J. Med.* 69: 287, 1980.
200. Grekas, D., Morley, A. R., Wilkinson, R., et al. Isolated C3 deposition in patients without systemic disease. *Clin. Nephrol.* 21: 270, 1984.
201. Gretz, N., Manz, F., and Strauch, M. Predictability of the progression of chronic renal failure. *Kidney Int.* 24(Suppl.): S2, 1983.
202. Grishman, E., and Churg, J. Focal segmental lupus nephritis. *Clin. Nephrol.* 17: 5, 1982.
203. Gruppo Italiano per lo Studio della Nefrite Lupica. The long term course of lupus nephritis. Unpublished data on 659 patients.
204. Gubler, M.-C., Broyer, M., and Habib, R. Signification des lesions de sclerose/hyalinose ségmentaire et focale (S?HSF) dans la néphrose. In *Proceedings of the 6th International Congress of Nephrology, Montreal.* Basel: Karger, 1978. Pp. 437–445.
205. Gurland, H. J., Brunner, F. P., Chantler, C., et al. Combined report on regular dialysis and transplantation in Europe VI, 1975. *Proc. Eur. Dial. Transplant Assoc.* 13: 3, 1978.
206. Habib, R. Glomerulonéphrite Membranoproliferative. In P. Royer, R. Habib, H. Matheiu, and M. Broyer (eds.), *Néphrologie Pediatrique*, 3rd ed. Paris: Flammarion, 1983. Pp. 316–328.
207. Habib, R. Periartérite noueuse et angéites necrosantes. In P. Royer, R. Habib, H. Mathieu, and M. Broyer (eds.), *Néphrologie Pediatrique*, 3rd ed. Paris: Flammarion, 1983. Pp. 368–374.
208. Habib, R., Broyer, M., and Levy, M. Schönlein-Henoch Purpura Glomerulonephritis in Children. In T. Strauss (ed.), *Pediatric Nephrology, 4*. New York: Garland Press, 1977. Pp. 155–195.
209. Habib, R., and Cameron, J. S. Schönlein-Henoch Purpura. In P. Bacon and N. Hadler (eds.), *The Kidney in Rheumatic Disease*. London: Butterworth, 1982. Pp. 178–201.
210. Habib, R., Gubler, M.-C., Loirat, C., et al. Dense deposit disease: A variant of membranoproliferative glomerulonephritis. *Kidney Int.* 7: 204, 1975.
211. Habib, R., Kleinknecht, C., and Gubler, M.-C. Extramembranous glomerulonephritis in children. Report of 50 cases. *J. Pediatr.* 82: 754, 1973.
212. Habib, R., Kleinknecht, C., Gubler, M.-C., et al. Idiopathic membranoproliferative glomerulonephritis in children. Report of 105 cases. *Clin. Nephrol.* 1: 193, 1978.
213. Habib, R., Kleinknecht, C., and Royer, P. The primary nephrotic syndrome of childhood: Classification and clinicopathologic study of 406 cases. *Pathol. Annu.* 417, 1971.
214. Haider, Y. S., and Roberts, W. V. Coronary arterial disease in systemic lupus erythematosus. *Am. J. Med.* 70: 775, 1981.
215. Hardwicke, J., Blainey, J. D., Brewer, D. B., et al. The Nephrotic Syndrome. *Proceedings of 3rd International Congress of Nephrology, Washington,* Vol. 3. Basel: Karger, 1966. Pp. 69–82.
216. Harrison, C. V., Loughridge, L. W., and Milne, M. D. Acute oliguric renal failure in acute glomerulonephritis and polyarteritis nodosa. *Q. J. Med.* 33: 39, 1964.
217. Hashimoto, H., Tsuda, H., Horano, T., et al. Differences in clinical and immunological findings of systemic lupus erythematosus related to age. *J. Rheumatol.* 14: 497, 1987.
218. Haworth, S. J. Renal Involvement in Wegener's Granulomatosis. The Hammersmith Experience. In G. D'Amico and G. Colosanti (eds.), *Nephrology '83*. Milan: Wichtig Editore, 1983. Pp. 33–43.
219. Haycock, G. B., and Cameron, J. S. Schönlein-Henoch Purpura. In R. J. Glassock (ed.), *Current Therapy in Nephrology and Hypertension*. Toronto: Decker, 1988. Pp. 129–131.
220. Haycock, G. B., Donaldson, M. D. C., Cobban, S., et al. β_2 microglobulin excretion in children with renal disease (Abstract). *Int. J. Pediatr. Nephrol.* 3: 132, 1984.
221. Hayslett, J. P., Kashgarian, M., Cook, C. D., et al. The effect of azathioprine in lupus nephropathy. *Medicine* (Baltimore) 51: 393, 1972.
222. Hayslett, J. P., Krassner, L. S., Bensch, K. G., et al. Progression of "lipoid nephrosis" to renal insufficiency. *N. Engl. J. Med.* 281: 181, 1969.
223. Heaf, J. G., Jorgensen, F., and Nielsen, N. P. Treatment and prognosis of extracapillary glomerulonephritis. *Nephron* 35: 217, 1983.
224. Hecht, B., Siegel, N., Adler, M., et al. Prognostic indices in lupus nephritis. *Medicine* 55: 163, 1976.
225. Helin, K., Mustonen, J., Pasternack, M., et al. IgM-associated glomerulonephritis. *Nephron* 31: 11, 1982.
226. Herbert, H. J. Acute glomerulonephritis in childhood, a study of the late prognosis in twenty-seven cases. *J. Paediatr.* 40: 549, 1952.
227. Herdman, R. C., Pickering, R. J., Michael, A. F., et al. Chronic glomerulonephritis associated with low serum complement activity (chronic hypocomplementemic glomerulonephritis). *Medicine* 49: 207, 1970.
228. Hind, C. R. K., Bowman, C., Winearls, C. G., et al. Recurrence of circulating antiglomerular basement membrane antibody three years after immunosuppressive treatment and plasma exchange. *Clin. Nephrol.* 21: 244, 1984.
229. Hind, C. R. K., Paraskevou, H., Lockwood, C. M., et al. Prognosis after immunosuppression of patients with crescentic nephritis requiring dialysis. *Lancet* 1: 263, 1983.
230. Hill, G. S., Hinglais, N., Tron, F., et al. Systemic lupus erythematosus: Morphologic correlations with immunologic and clinical data at the time of biopsy. *Am. J. Med.* 64: 61, 1979.
231. Hinglais, N., Garcia-Torres, R., and Kleinknecht, D. Long-term prognosis in acute glomerulonephritis. The predictive value of early clinical and pathologic features observed in 65 patients. *Am. J. Med.* 56: 52, 1974.
232. Hirszel, P., Yamase, H. T., Carney, W. R., et al. Mesangial proliferative glomerulonephritis with IgM deposits. *Nephron* 38: 100, 1984.
233. Hlatky, M. A. Is renal biopsy necessary in adults with nephrotic syndrome? *Lancet* 2: 1264, 1982.
234. Hoffman, G. S., Leavitt, R. Y., Fleisher, T. A., et al. Treatment of Wegener's granulomatosis with intermittent high-dose intravenous cyclophosphamide. *Am. J. Med.* 89: 403, 1990.
235. Holdsworth, S., Boyce, N., Thomson, N. M., et al. The

clinical spectrum of acute glomerulonephritis and lung haemorrhage (Goodpasture's syndrome). *Q. J. Med.* 55: 75, 1985.

236. Honkanen, E. Survival in idiopathic membranous nephropathy. *Clin. Nephrol.* 25: 122, 1986.
237. Hood, S. A., Velosa, J. A., Holley, K. E., et al. IgA-IgG nephropathy: Predictive indices of progressive disease. *Clin. Nephrol.* 16: 55, 1981.
238. Hopper, J., Jr., Trew, P. A., and Biava, C. G. Membranous nephropathy: Its relative benignity in women. *Nephron* 29: 18, 1981.
239. Hotta, O., Yoshizawa, N., Oshima, S., et al. Significance of renal hyaline arteriosclerosis and tubulo-interstitial change in IgA glomerulonephropathy and focal glomerular sclerosis. *Nephron* 47: 262, 1987.
240. Howard, A. N., Patelski, J., Bourger, D. E., et al. Atherosclerosis induced in hypercholesterolaemic baboons by immunological injury, and the effects of intravenous polyunsaturated phosphatidyl choline. *Atherosclerosis* 14: 17, 1971.
241. Howie, A. J., and Brewer, D. B. The glomerular tip lesion: A previously undescribed type of segmental glomerular abnormality. *J. Pathol.* 142: 205, 1984.
242. Howie, A. J., and Brewer, D. B. Further studies on the glomerular tip lesion: Early and late stages and life table analysis. *J. Pathol.* 147: 245, 1985.
243. Hsu, H.-C., Chen, W.-Y., Lin, G.-J., et al. Clinical and immunopathologic study of mesangial IgM nephropathy: Report of 41 cases. *Histopathology* 8: 435, 1984.
244. Hui, A., Poucell, S., Thorner, P., et al. Clinical features and glomerular immunofluorescence of renal biopsies from children with nephrotic syndrome due to minimal change disease and two variants of mesangial proliferative glomerulonephritis. *Int. J. Pediatr. Nephrol.* 5: 5, 1984.
245. Hunsicker, L. Studies of therapy of progressive renal failure in humans. *Semin. Nephrol.* 9: 380, 1989.
246. Hunt, L. P., Short, C. D., and Mallick, N. P. Prognostic indicators in patients presenting with the nephrotic syndrome. *Kidney Int.* 34: 382, 1988.
247. Idelson, B. A., Smithline, N., Smith, G. W., et al. Prognosis in steroid-treated idiopathic nephrotic syndrome in adults. *Arch. Intern. Med.* 137: 891, 1977.
248. International Study of Kidney Disease in Children. Membranoproliferative glomerulonephritis (MPGN). A double blind trial of alternate day prednisone (ADP). *Pediatr. Res.* 17: 1000 (abstract No. 140), 1980.
249. International Study of Kidneys in Children. Primary nephrotic syndrome in children: Clinical significance of histopathologic variants of minimal change and of diffuse mesangial hypercellularity. *Kidney Int.* 20: 765, 1981.
250. International Study of Kidney Disease in Children. Cyclophosphamide therapy in focal segmental glomerulosclerosis: A controlled clinical trial (Abstract). *Eur. J. Pediatr.* 140: 149, 1983.
251. International Study of Kidney Disease in Children. Minimal change nephrotic syndrome in children: Deaths occurring during the first five to fifteen years' observations. *Pediatrics* 173: 497, 1984.
252. Ipachki, E., Kashanian, B., Khanmohamadi, M., et al. Light microscopy in idiopathic proteinuria and nephrotic syndrome in Iran. Abstracts, *7th International Congress of Nephrology*, Montreal, June, 1978. Pp. 1–6.
253. Ito, H., Yoshikawa, N., Aozai, F., et al. Twenty-seven children with focal segmental glomerulosclerosis: Correlation between the segmental location of the glomerular lesion and prognosis. *Clin. Nephrol.* 22: 9, 1984.
254. Jackson, E. C., McAdams, A. J., Strife, F., et al. Differences between membranoproliferative glomerulonephritis type I and III in clinical presentation, glomerular morphology and complement perturbation. *Am. J. Kidney Dis.* 9: 115, 1987.
255. Jennette, J. C., Wilkman, A. S., and Falk, R. J. Anti-neutrophil cytoplasmic autoantibody associated glomerulonephritis and vasculitis. *Am. J. Pathol.* 135: 921, 1989.
256. Jennings, R. B., and Earle, D. P. Post-streptococcal glomerulonephritis, histopathologic and clinical studies of the acute, subsiding acute and early chronic latent phases. *J. Clin. Invest.* 40: 1525, 1961.
257. Jessar, R. A., Lamont-Havers, R. W., and Ragan, C. Natural history of lupus erythematosus disseminatus. *Ann. Intern. Med.* 138: 717, 1953.
258. Jiyun, Y., Melvin, T., Sibley, R., et al. No evidence for a specific role of IgM in mesangial proliferation of idiopathic nephritic syndrome. *Kidney Int.* 25: 100, 1984.
259. Johnson, J. P., Moore, J., Austin, H. A., III, et al. Therapy of anti-glomerular basement antibody disease: Analysis of prognostic significance of clinical pathologic and treatment factors. *Medicine* (Baltimore) 64: 219, 1985.
260. Joseph, M. C., and Polani, P. F. The effect of bed rest on acute haemorrhage nephritis in children. *Guy's Hosp. Rep.* 107: 500, 1958.
261. Kalowski, S., and Kincaid-Smith, P. Glomerulonephritis in Henoch-Schönlein Syndrome. In P. Kincaid-Smith, T. Mathew, and E. L. Becker (eds.), *Glomerulonephritis*. New York: Wiley, 1973. Pp. 1123–1132.
262. Kandall, S., Edelmann, C. M., Jr., and Bernstein, J. Acute post-streptococcal glomerulonephritis. A case with minimal urinary abnormalities. *Am. J. Dis. Child* 118: 426, 1969.
263. Kant, K. S., Pollak, V. E., Weiss, M. A., et al. Glomerular thrombosis in systemic lupus erythematosus: Prevalence and significance. *Medicine* 60: 71, 1981.
264. Kaplan, C., Pasternack, B., Shah, H., et al. Age-related incidence of sclerotic glomeruli in human kidneys. *Am. J. Pathol.* 80: 227, 1975.
265. Kaplan, E. L., Anthony, B. F., Chapman, S. S., et al. Epidemic glomerular nephritis associated with type 49 streptococcal pyoderma. I. Clinical and laboratory findings. *Am. J. Med.* 48: 9, 1970.
266. Kaplan, E. L., and Meier, P. Non-parametric estimation from incomplete observations. *J. Am. Stat. Assoc.* 53: 457, 1958.
267. Karsh, J., Klippel, J. H., Balow, J. E., et al. Mortality in lupus nephritis. *Arthritis Rheum.* 22: 764, 1979.
268. Kasinath, S. S., Mugais, S. K., Spargo, B. H., et al. Non-diabetic renal disease in patients with diabetes mellitus. *Am. J. Med.* 75: 613, 1983.
269. Kasiske, B. L., Velosa, J. A., Halstenson, C. E., et al. The effects of lovastatin in hyperlipidemic patients with the nephrotic syndrome. *Am. J. Kidney Dis.* 15: 8, 1990.
270. Kassirer, J. Nephrology forum: Is renal biopsy necessary for optimal management of the idiopathic nephrotic syndrome? *Kidney Int.* 24: 561, 1983.
271. Katz, A., Waller, J. F., and Landy, P. J. IgA nephritis with nephrotic range proteinuria. *Clin. Nephrol.* 20: 67, 1983.
272. Kellum, R. E., and Haserick, J. K. Systemic lupus erythematosus. A statistical evaluation of mortality based on a consecutive series of 299 patients. *Arch. Intern. Med.* 113: 200, 1964.

273. Kibukamusoke, J. W. Nephrotic syndrome of quartan malaria. Bristol: Edward Arnold, 1973.
274. Kida, H., Asamtoto, T., Yokoyama, H., et al. Long term prognosis of membranous nephropathy. *Clin. Nephrol.* 25: 64, 1986.
275. Kim, Y., and Michael, A. F. Chronic bacteremia and nephritis. *Annu. Rev. Med.* 29: 319, 1978.
276. Kimberly, R. P., Lockshin, M. D., Sherman, R. L., et al. Reversible "end-stage" lupus nephritis. Analysis of patients able to discontinue dialysis. *Am. J. Med.* 74: 361, 1983.
277. Kincaid-Smith, P. Mesangial IgA nephropathy. *Br. Med. J.* 290: 96, 1985.
278. Kitajima, T., Murakami, M., and Sakai, D. Clinicopathological features in the Japanese patients with IgA nephropathy. *Jpn. J. Med.* 22: 219, 1983.
279. Klassen, J., Elwood, C., Grossberg, A., et al. Evolution of membranous nephropathy into anti-glomerular basement membrane glomerulonephritis. *N. Engl. J. Med.* 290: 1340, 1974.
280. Klein, M., Poucell, S., Arbus, G. S., et al. Characteristics of a benign sub-type of dense deposit disease: Comparison with the progressive form of disease. *Clin. Nephrol.* 20: 163, 1983.
281. Kleinknecht, C. Glomerulonéphrite Extramembraneuse. In P. Royer, R. Habib, H. Mathieu, and M. Broyer (eds.), *Néphrologie Pédiatrique,* 3rd ed. Paris: Flammarion, 1983. Pp. 306–315.
282. Kleinknecht, C., and Gubler, M. C. La Néphrose. In P. Royer, R. Habib, H. Mathieu, and M. Broyer (eds.), *Néphrologie Pédiatrique,* 3rd ed. Paris: Flammarion, 1983. Pp. 274–293.
283. Kleinknecht, C., Levy, M., Gagnadoux, M.-F., et al. Membranous glomerulonephritis with extra-renal disorders in children. *Medicine* (Baltimore) 56: 219, 1979.
284. Knight, J. F., and Cameron, J. S. Unpublished data from the U.K. Medical Research Council glomerulonephritis registry, 1987.
285. Kobayashi, O., Wada, H., Okawa, K., et al. Schönlein-Henoch's syndrome in children. *Contrib. Nephrol.* 4: 48, 1977.
286. Kobayashi, Y., Tateno, S., Hiki, Y., et al. IgA nephropathy: Prognostic significance of proteinuria and histological alterations. *Nephron* 34: 146, 1983.
287. Kobayashi, Y., Tateno, S., Shigematsu, H., et al. Prednisone treatment in non-nephrotic patients with idiopathic membranous nephropathy. *Nephron* 30: 210, 1982.
288. Korbet, S. M., Schwartz, M. M., and Lewis, E. J. Minimal change glomerulopathy of adulthood. *Am. J. Nephrol.* 8: 291, 1988.
289. Koskimies, O., Mir, S., Rapola, J., et al. Henoch-Schönlein nephritis: Long-term prognosis of unselected patients. *Arch. Dis. Child.* 56: 482, 1981.
290. Krensky, A. M., Inglefinger, J. R., and Grupe, W. E. Peritonitis in childhood nephrotic syndrome. *Am. J. Dis. Child.* 136: 732, 1982.
291. Kurtzman, N. A. Does acute post-streptococcal glomerulonephritis lead to chronic renal disease? *N. Engl. J. Med.* 298: 795, 1978.
292. Kusumoto, Y., Takebayashi, S., Tagishi, T., et al. Long term prognosis and prognostic indices of IgA nephropathy in juvenile and in adult Japanese. *Clin. Nephrol.* 28: 118, 1987.
293. Lagrue, G. Les anti-inflammatoires et l'évolution des glomerulonéphrites primitives humaines. *Gaz. Méd. France* 86: 4371, 1979.
294. Lange, K., Wasserman, E., and Slobody, L. B. Prolonged intermittent steroid therapy for nephrosis in children and adults. *J.A.M.A.* 168: 377, 1958.
295. Larsen, S. Immunofluorescent microscopy findings in minimal or no-change disease and slight generalized mesangioproliferative glomerulonephritis. *Acta Pathol. Microbiol. Scand.* [A] 86: 531, 1978.
296. Lawler, W., Williams, G., Tarpey, P., et al. IgM-associated primary diffuse mesangial proliferative glomerulonephritis. *J. Clin. Pathol.* 37: 1029, 1980.
297. Leaker, B., Fairley, K. F., Dowling, J., and Kincaid-Smith, P. Lupus nephritis: Clinical and pathological correlation. *Q. J. Med.* 62: 163, 1987.
298. Lee, H. A., Koh, H. I., Kim, M. J., and Rha, H. Y. Henoch Schönlein nephritis in adults: A clinical and morphological study. *Clin. Nephrol.* 26: 125, 1986.
299. Lee, P., Urowitz, M. B., Bookman, A. M., et al. Systemic lupus erythematosus. A review of 110 cases with reference to nephritis, the nervous system, infections, aseptic necrosis and prognosis. *Q. J. Med.* 46: 1, 1977.
300. Leehey, D. J., Katz, A. I., Azaran, A. H., et al. Silent diffuse lupus nephritis: Long-term follow-up. *Am. J. Kidney Dis.* 2(Suppl. 1): 188, 1982.
301. Leib, E. S., Restivo, C., and Paulus, H. E. Immunosuppressive and corticosteroid therapy of polyarteritis nodosa. *Am. J. Med.* 67: 941, 1979.
302. Lentz, R. D., Michael, A. F., and Friend, P. F. Membranous transformation of lupus nephritis. *Clin. Immunol. Immunopathol.* 19: 131, 1981.
303. Leonard, C. D., Nagle, R. B., Striker, G. E., et al. Acute glomerulonephritis with prolonged oliguria. *Ann. Intern. Med.* 73: 703, 1970.
304. Levey, A. J. Use of measurement of GFR to assess the progression of renal disease. *Semin. Nephrol.* 9: 370, 1989.
304a. Levey, A. J., Lau, J., Panker, S. G., and Kassirer, J. P. Idiopathic nephrotic syndrome: Puncturing the biopsy myth. *Ann. Intern. Med.* 107: 697, 1987.
305. Levin, M., Rigden, S. P. A., Pincott, J. R., et al. Goodpasture's syndrome: Treatment with plasmapheresis, immunosuppression and anticoagulation. *Arch. Dis. Child.* 58: 697, 1983.
306. Levinsky, R. J., Cameron, J. S., and Soothill, J. F. Serum immune complexes and disease activity in lupus nephritis. *Lancet* 2: 564, 1977.
307. Levitt, J. I. The prognostic significance of proteinuria in young college students. *Ann. Intern. Med.* 66: 685, 1967.
308. Levy, M., Broyer, M., Arsan, A., et al. Anaphylactoid purpura nephritis in childhood: Natural history and immunopathology. *Adv. Nephrol.* 6: 182, 1976.
309. Levy, M., Gonzales Burchard, G., Broyer, M., et al. Berger's disease in children: Natural history and outcome. *Medicine* (Baltimore) 64: 151, 1985.
310. Lewis, M. A., Baildom, E. M., Davis, N., et al. Nephrotic syndrome: From toddlers to twenties. *Lancet* 1: 255, 1989.
311. Lewy, J. E., Salinas-Madrigal, L., Herdson, F. B., et al. Clinicopathological correlations in acute post-streptococcal glomerulonephritis. *Medicine* (Baltimore) 50: 453, 1971.
312. Lien, J. W. K., Mathew, T. H., and Meadows, R. Acute post-streptococcal glomerulonephritis in adults: A long-term study. *Q. J. Med.* 48: 99, 1979.
313. Lloyd, W., and Schur, P. H. Immune complexes, complement and anti-DNA in exacerbations of systemic lu-

pus erythematosus (SLE). *Medicine* (Baltimore) 60: 208, 1981.

314. Mackay, I. R. Chronic Lupus Erythematosus: Observations on Long-Term Survivors of "Suppressive" Therapy of Lupus Nephritis with Prednisone. In P. Kincaid-Smith, T. H. Mathew, and E. L. Becker (eds.), *Glomerulonephritis,* Vol. 11. New York: Wiley, 1973. Pp. 1211–1217.
315. Magil, A. B., Ballon, H. S., and Rae, A. Focal proliferative lupus nephritis. A clinicopathologic study using the W.H.O. classification. *Am. J. Med.* 72: 620, 1982.
316. Magil, A. B., Price, J. D. E., Bower, G., et al. Membranoproliferative glomerulonephritis type I: Comparison of natural history in children and adults. *Clin. Nephrol.* 11: 239, 1979.
317. Magil, A. B., Puterman, M. L., Ballon, H. S., et al. Prognostic factors in diffuse proliferative lupus glomerulonephritis. *Kidney Int.* 34: 511, 1988.
318. Mallick, N. P., and Short, C. D. The nephrotic syndrome and ischaemic heart disease. *Nephron* 27: 54, 1981.
319. Maxey, R. W., Rao, T. K. S., Butt, K. M. H., et al. Hemodialysis and transplantation in patients with uremia due to systemic lupus erythematosus. *Artif. Organs* 2(Suppl.): 470, 1978.
320. McCarron, D. A., Rubin, R. J., Barnes, B. A., et al. Therapeutic bilateral renal infarction in end-stage renal disease. *N. Engl. J. Med.* 294: 652, 1976.
321. McCluskey, R. T. Lupus Nephritis. In S. C. Sommers (ed.), *Kidney Pathology Decennial 1966–1975.* New York: Appleton-Century-Crofts, 1975. P. 435.
322. McCluskey, R. T. The value of the renal biopsy in lupus nephritis. *Arthritis Rheum.* 25: 867, 1982.
323. McCluskey, R. T., and Baldwin, D. S. The natural history of acute glomerulonephritis. *Am. J. Med.* 35: 213, 1965.
324. McEnery, P. T., McAdams, A. J., and West, C. D. Membranoproliferative glomerulonephritis: Improved survival with alternate day prednisone therapy. *Clin. Nephrol.* 13: 117, 1980.
325. McEnery, P. T., McAdams, A. I., and West, C. D. The effect of prednisone on the natural history of idiopathic membranoproliferative glomerulonephritis. *Medicine* (Baltimore) 64: 410, 1986.
326. McLigeyo, S., Cameron, J. S., Williams, D. G., et al. Improved survival in lupus nephritis 1979–89 using oral corticosteroids and azathioprine as maintenance therapy (submitted for publication), 1992.
327. McPhaul, J. J., and Mullins, J. D. Glomerulonephritis mediated by antibody to glomerular basement membrane. Immunological, clinical and histopathological characteristics. *J. Clin. Invest.* 57: 351, 1976.
328. McVicar, M., Exeni, R., and Susin, M. Nephrotic syndrome and multiple tubular defects in children; an early sign of focal segmental glomerulosclerosis. *J. Pediatr.* 97: 918, 1980.
329. Meadow, S. R. Poststreptococcal glomerulonephritis—A rare disease? *Arch. Dis. Child.* 50: 379, 1975.
330. Meadow, S. R., Glasgow, E. F., White, R. H. R., et al. Schönlein-Henoch nephritis. *Q. J. Med.* 41: 241, 1972.
331. Medical Research Council. Controlled trial of azathioprine and prednisone in chronic renal disease—Report of a Medical Research Council Working Party. *Br. Med. J.* 2: 239, 1971.
332. Meller, J., Conde, C. A., Deppesch, L. M., et al. Myocardial infarction due to coronary atherosclerosis in three young adults with systemic lupus erythematosus. *Am. J. Cardiol.* 35: 309, 1975.
333. Merrill, M., and Shulman, L. E. Determination of prognosis in chronic disease, illustrated by systemic lupus erythematosus. *J. Chronic Dis.* 1: 23, 1955.
334. Meyrier, A. Treatment of glomerular disease with cyclosporin A. *Nephrol. Dial. Transplant.* 4: 923, 1989.
335. Migone, L., Olivetti, G., Allegri, L., et al. Mesangioproliferative glomerulonephritis. *Clin. Nephrol.* 13: 219, 1980.
336. Minick, C. R., Murphy, G. E., and Campbell, W. G. Experimental induction of atherosclerosis by the synergy of allergic injury to arteries and lipid rich diet 1. Effect of repeated injections of horse serum in rabbits fed a dietary cholesterol supplement. *J. Exp. Med.* 124: 635, 1966.
337. Mitch, W. E., Walser, M., Buffington, A. A., et al. Simple method for estimating progression of chronic renal failure. *Lancet* 4: 1326, 1976.
338. Modai, D., Pik, A., Behar, M., et al. Biopsy proven evolution of post-streptococcal glomerulonephritis to rapidly progressive glomerulonephritis of a post-infectious type. *Clin. Nephrol.* 23: 198, 1985.
339. Mongeau, J.-G., Corneille, L., Robitaille, P., et al. Primary nephrosis in childhood associated with focal glomerular sclerosis: Is long-term prognosis that severe? *Kidney Int.* 20: 743, 1981.
340. Moorthy, A. V., Zimmerman, S. W., Burkholder, P. M., et al. Association of crescentic glomerulonephritis with membranous glomerulopathy: Report of three cases. *Clin. Nephrol.* 6: 319, 1976.
341. Morel-Maroger, L., Méry, J.-Ph., Droz, D., et al. The Course of Lupus Nephritis: Contribution of Serial Biopsies. In J. Hamburger, J. Crosner, and M. W. Maxwell (eds.), *Advances in Nephrology.* Chicago: Year Book, 1976. Pp. 79–118.
342. Morita, M., White, R. H. R., Coad, N. A. G., and Raafat, F. The clinical significance of the glomerular location of segmental lesions in focal segmental glomerulosclerosis. *Clin. Nephrol.* 33: 211, 1990.
343. Morrin, P. A. F., Hinglais, N., Nabarra, B., et al. Rapidly progressive glomerulonephritis. A clinical and pathological study. *Am. J. Med.* 65: 446, 1978.
344. Mota-Hernandez, F., Briseno-Mondragon, E., Gordillo-Paniagua, G. Glomerular lesions and final outcome in children with glomerulonephritis of acute onset. *Nephron* 16: 272, 1976.
345. Mota-Hernandez, F., Valbuena-Paz, R., and Gordillo-Paniagua, G. Long-term prognosis of anaphylactoid purpura nephropathy. *Paediatrician* 4: 52, 1975.
346. Muehrcke, R. C., Kark, R. M., Pirani, C. L., et al. Lupus nephritis: A clinical and pathologic study based on renal biopsies. *Medicine* (Baltimore) 36: 1, 1957.
347. Murphy, B. F., Fairley, K. F., and Kincaid-Smith, P. S. Idiopathic membranous glomerulonephritis: Long term followup in 139 cases. *Clin. Nephrol.* 30: 175, 1988.
348. Mustonen, J., Pasternack, A., and Rantala, I. The nephrotic syndrome in IgA nephropathy: Response to corticosteroid therapy. *Clin. Nephrol.* 20: 172, 1983.
349. Nakamoto, Y., Dohr, K., Fujioka, M., et al. Combined anticoagulant and immunosuppressive glomerulonephritis (RPGN). A long-term follow-up study. *Jpn. J. Med.* 18: 210, 1979.
350. Nanra, R. S., and Kincaid-Smith, P. Lupus Nephritis: Clinical Course in Relationship to Treatment. In P. Kincaid-Smith, T. H. Mathew, and E. L. Becker (eds.), *Glomerulonephritis,* Vol. 11. New York: Wiley, 1973. Pp. 1193–1210.
351. Nash, M. A., Bakara, M. A., D'Agate, V., et al. Late de-

velopment of chronic renal failure in steroid-responsive nephrotic syndrome. *J. Pediatr.* 101: 411, 1982.
352. Neelakantappa, K., Gallo, G., and Baldwin, D. S. Proteinuria in IgA nephropathy. *Kidney Int.* 33: 716, 1988.
353. Neild, G. H., Cameron, J. S., Ogg, C. S., et al. Rapidly progressive glomerulonephritis with extensive glomerular crescent formation. *Q. J. Med.* 52: 395, 1983.
354. Newman, W. J., Tisher, C. G., McCoy, R. C., et al. Focal glomerular sclerosis: Contrasting clinical patterns in children and adults. *Medicine* (Baltimore) 55: 67, 1976.
355. Niall, J. F. Prolonged survival in the nephrotic syndrome. *Med. J. Aust.* 2: 843, 1965.
356. Niaudet, P., Habib, R., Tete, M.-J., et al. Cyclosporin in the treatment of idiopathic nephrotic syndrome in children. *Pediatr. Nephrol.* 1: 566, 1987.
357. Niaudet, P., and Levy, M. Glomerulonephrite a Croissants Diffus. In P. Royer, R. Habib, H. Mathieu, and M. Broyer (eds.), *Néphrologie Pédiatrique,* 3rd ed. Paris: Flammarion, 1983. Pp. 381–394.
358. Nicholls, K. M., Fairley, K. F., Dowling, J. P., et al. The clinical course of mesangial IgA-associated nephropathy in adults. *Q. J. Med.* 210: 227, 1984.
359. Nissenson, A. R., Mayon-White, R., Potter, E. V., et al. Continued absence of clinical renal disease 7 to 12 years after post-streptococcal acute glomerulonephritis in Trinidad. *Am. J. Med.* 67: 255, 1979.
360. Noel, L. H., Zanetti, M., Droz, D., et al. Long-term prognosis of idiopathic membranous glomerulonephritis. Study of 116 untreated patients. *Am. J. Med.* 66: 32, 1979.
361. Nolasco, F., Cameron, J. S., Heywood, E. F., et al. Adult onset minimal change nephrotic syndrome: A long term follow-up. *Kidney Int.* 29: 1215, 1987.
362. Northway, J. D., McAdams, A. J., Forristal, J., et al. A 'silent' phase of hypocomplementaemic persistent nephritis detectable by reduced serum β1C-globulin levels. *J. Pediatr.* 74: 28, 1969.
363. Nossent, H. C., Henzen-Logmans, S. C., Vroom, T. M., et al. Contribution of renal biopsy data in predicting outcome in lupus nephritis. *Arthritis Rheum.* 33: 970, 1990.
364. Novoa, D., Romero, R., Arcocha, V., and Sanchez-Guisande, D. Relapsing acute renal failure in IgA nephropathy. *Nephron* 51: 438, 1990.
365. Nyberg, M., Pettersson, E., Tallqvist, G., et al. Survival in idiopathic glomerulonephritis. *Acta Pathol. Microbiol. Scand.* [*A*] 88: 319, 1980.
366. Old, C. W., Herrera, G. A., Reimann, B. E. F., et al. Acute poststreptococcal glomerulonephritis progressing to rapidly progressive glomerulonephritis. *South. Med. J.* 77: 1470, 1984.
367. O'Neill, W. M., Etheridge, W. M., and Bloomer, A. High-dose corticosteroids, their use in treating idiopathic rapidly progressive glomerulonephritis. *Arch. Intern. Med.* 139: 514, 1979.
368. Ordonez, J. D., Hiatt, R., Killebrew, E., and Fireman, B. The risk of coronary artery disease among patients with the nephrotic syndrome (Abstract). *Kidney Int.* 37: 243, 1990.
369. Orfila, C., Pieraggo, M.-T., and Suc, J.-M. Mesangial isolated C3 deposition in patients with recurrent or persistent hematuria. *Lab. Invest.* 43: 1, 1980.
370. Papiha, P. P., et al. HLA-A, B DR and Bf allotypes in patients with idiopathic membranous nephropathy. *Kidney Int.* 31: 130, 1987.
371. Pardo, V., Berian, M. G., Levi, D. F., et al. Benign primary hematuria. *Am. J. Med.* 67: 817, 1979.
372. Park, M. H., D'Agati, V., Appel, G. B., et al. Tubulointerstitial disease in lupus nephritis: Relation to immune deposits, interstitial inflammation, glomerular changes, renal function, and prognosis. *Nephron* 44: 309, 1986.
373. Passerini, P., Pasquali, S., Cesana, B., et al. Long term outcome of patients with membranous nephropathy after complete remission of proteinuria. *Nephrol. Dial. Transplant.* 4: 525, 1989.
374. Payton, C. D., McLay, A., and Boulton Jones, J. M. Progressive IgA nephropathy: The role of hypertension. *Nephrol. Dial. Transplant.* 2: 138, 1988.
375. Perlman, L. V., Herdman, R. C., Kleinman, H., et al. Poststreptococcal glomerulonephritis. A ten-year follow-up of an epidemic. *J.A.M.A.* 194: 63, 1965.
376. Peto, R., Pike, M. C., Armitage, P., et al. Design and analysis of randomised clinical trials requiring prolonged observation of each patient. II. Analysis and examples. *Br. J. Cancer* 35: 1, 1977.
377. Pinching, A. J., Lockwood, C. M., Pussell, B. A., et al. Wegener's granulomatosis: Observations on 18 patients with severe renal disease. *Q. J. Med.* 52: 435, 1983.
378. Pirani, C. L., and Salinas-Madrigal, L. Evaluation of percutaneous renal biopsy. *Pathol. Annu.* 3: 249, 1968.
379. Platt, J. L., Burke, B. A., Fish, A. J., et al. Systemic lupus erythematosus in the first two decades of life. *Am. J. Kidney Dis.* 2(Suppl. 1): 212, 1982.
380. Polito, C., et al. Normal growth of nephrotic children during long-term alternate day prednisone therapy. *Acta Paediatr. Scand.* 75: 245, 1986.
381. Pollak, V. E., and Mendoza, N. Rapidly progressive glomerulonephritis. *Med. Clin. North Am.* 55: 1397, 1971.
382. Pollak, V. E., and Pirani, C. L. Renal histologic findings in systemic lupus erythematosus. *Mayo Clin. Proc.* 44: 630, 1969.
383. Pollak, V. E., Pirani, C. L., and Clyne, D. H. The Natural History of Membranous Glomerulonephropathy. In P. Kincaid-Smith, T. H. Mathew, and E. L. Becker (eds.), *Glomerulonephritis.* New York: Wiley, 1973. Pp. 429–441.
384. Pollak, V. E., Pirani, C. L., and Schwartz, F. D. The natural history of the renal manifestation of systemic lupus erythematosus. *J. Lab. Clin. Med.* 63: 537, 1964.
385. Ponticelli, C., et al. Long-term prognosis of diffuse lupus nephritis. *Clin. Nephrol.* 28: 263, 1987.
386. Ponticelli, C., et al. A randomized trial of methylprednisolone and chlorambucil in membranous nephropathy. *N. Engl. J. Med.* 320: 8, 1989.
387. Potter, E. V., et al. Clinical healing two to six years after post-streptococcal glomerulonephritis in Trinidad. *N. Engl. J. Med.* 298: 767, 1978.
388. Potter, E. V., Lipschulz, S. A., Abidh, S., et al. Twelve to seventeen year follow-up of patients with post-streptococcal acute glomerulonephritis in Trinidad. *N. Engl. J. Med.* 307: 725, 1982.
389. Proskey, A. J., Weatherbee, L., Easterling, R. E., et al. Goodpasture's syndrome. A report of five cases and review of the literature. *Am. J. Med.* 48: 162, 1970.
390. Pru, C., Kjellstrand, C. M., Cohn, R. A., et al. Late recurrence of minimal change nephrotic syndrome. *Ann. Intern. Med.* 100: 69, 1984.
390a. Pusey, C. D., et al. Plasma exchange in focal necrotizing glomerular hepatitis without anti-GBM antibodies. *Kidney Int.* 40: 757, 1991.
391. Rabelink, A. J., Hene, R. J., Erkelens, D. W., et al. Effects of simvastatin and cholestyramine on lipoprotein profile in hyperlipidaemia of nephrotic syndrome. *Lancet* 2: 1335, 1988.
392. Ramirez, F., Brouhard, B. H., Travis, L. B., et al. Idio-

pathic membranous nephropathy in children. *J. Pediatr.* 101: 677, 1982.
393. Ramzy, M. K., Cameron, J. S., Turner, D. R., et al. The long-term outcome of idiopathic membranous nephropathy. *Clin. Nephrol.* 16: 13, 1981.
394. Rees, A. J., and Cameron, J. S. Crescentic Nephritis. In J. S. Cameron et al. (eds.), *The Oxford Textbook of Clinical Nephrology.* London: Oxford University Press, 1991.
395. Rees, A. J., Peters, D. K., Amos, N., et al. The influence of HL-A linked genes on the severity of anti-GBM and antibody-mediated nephritis. *Kidney Int.* 26: 444, 1984.
396. Rodriguez-Iturbe, B. Nephrology Forum: Epidemic post-streptococcal glomerulonephritis. *Kidney Int.* 25: 129, 1984.
397. Rodriguez-Iturbe, B., Rubio, L., and Garcia, R. Attack of post-streptococcal nephritis in families. A prospective study. *Lancet* 1: 401, 1981.
398. Rose, G. A., and Spencer, K. Polyarteritis nodosa. *Q. J. Med.* 26: 43, 1957.
399. Rosner, S., Ginzler, E. M., Diamond, H. S., et al. A multicenter study of outcome in systemic lupus erythematosus. II. Causes of death. *Arthritis Rheum.* 25: 612, 1982.
400. Roth, D. A., Wilz, D. R., and Theil, G. B. Schönlein-Henoch syndrome in adults. *Q. J. Med.* 55: 145, 1985.
401. Row, P. G., Cameron, J. S., Turner, D. R., et al. Membranous nephropathy. Long-term follow-up and association with neoplasia. *Q. J. Med.* 44: 207, 1975.
402. Rubin, L. A., Urowitz, M. B., and Gladman, D. D. Mortality in systemic lupus erythematosus: The bimodal pattern revisited. *Q. J. Med.* 55: 87, 1985.
403. Rutherford, W. E., Blondin, J., Miller, J. P., et al. Chronic progressive renal disease: Rate of change of serum creatinine. *Kidney Int.* 11: 62, 1977.
403a. Sabadini, E., Castiglione, A., Ferrario, F., et al. Characterization of interstitial infiltrates in IgA disease. *Am. J. Kidney Dis.* 12: 307, 1988.
404. Sack, M., Cassidy, J. T., and Bole, G. C. Prognostic factors in polyarteritis. *J. Rheumatol.* 2: 411, 1975.
405. Sagel, L., Triser, G., Ty, A., et al. Occurrence and nature of glomerular lesions after group A streptococci infections in children. *Ann. Intern. Med.* 79: 492, 1973.
406. St. Hillier, Y., Morel-Maroger, L., Woodrow, D., et al. Focal and segmental hyalinosis. *Adv. Nephrol.* 5: 67, 1975.
407. Sanjad, S., Tolaymat, A., Whitworth, J., et al. Acute glomerulonephritis in children: A review of 153 cases. *South. Med. J.* 70: 1202, 1977.
408. Savage, C. O. S., Pusey, C. D., Bowman, C., et al. Anti-glomerular basement membrane antibody mediated disease in the British Isles 1980–4. *Br. Med. J.* 292: 301, 1986.
409. Savage, C. O. S., Winearls, C. G., Evans, D. J., et al. Microscopic polyarteritis: Presentation, pathology and prognosis. *Q. J. Med.* 56: 467, 1985.
410. Schacht, R. G., Gallo, G. R., Gluck, M. C., et al. Irreversible disease following acute post-streptococcal glomerulonephritis in children. *J. Chronic Dis.* 32: 515, 1979.
411. Schacht, R. G., Gluck, M. C., Gallo, G. R., et al. Progression to uremia after remission of acute post-streptococcal glomerulonephritis. *N. Engl. J. Med.* 245: 977, 1976.
412. Schärer, K., Waldherr, R., Müller-Wiefel, D. E., et al. Idiopathic Nephrotic Syndrome Associated with Focal Segmental Glomerulosclerosis. In M. Bulla (ed.), *Renal Insufficiency in Children.* Berlin: Springer, 1982. Pp. 23–29.
413. Schena, F. P. A retrospective analysis of the natural history of primary IgA nephropathy worldwide. *Am. J. Med.* 89: 209, 1990.
414. Schena, F. P., and Cameron, J. S. Treatment of proteinuric glomerulonephritides in adults: A retrospective survey. *Am. J. Med.* 85: 315, 1988.
415. Schmitt, H., Bohle, A., Reineke, T., et al. Long term prognosis of membranoproliferative glomerulonephritis type I. Significance of clinical and morphological parameters: An investigation of 220 cases. *Nephron* 55: 242, 1990.
416. Schoenmann, M. J., Bennett, B., and Greifer, I. The natural history of focal segmental glomerulosclerosis with and without mesangial hyper-cellularity in children. *Clin. Nephrol.* 9: 45, 1978.
416a. Schulman, S. L., Kaiser, B. A., Polinsky, M. S., et al. Predicting the response to cytotoxic therapy for childhood nephrotic syndrome: Superiority of response to corticosteroid therapy over histopathologic patterns. *J. Pediatr.* 113: 996, 1988.
417. Schur, P. H., and Sandson, J. Immunologic factors and clinical activity in systemic lupus erythematosus. *N. Engl. J. Med.* 278: 533, 1968.
418. Schwartz, H., and Kohn, J. L. Lipoid nephrosis. A clinical and pathological study based on fifteen years' observation with special reference to prognosis. *Am. J. Dis. Child.* 49: 579, 1935.
419. Schwartz, M. M., Bernstein, J., Hill, G. S., et al. Predictive value of renal pathology in diffuse proliferative glomerulonephritis. *Kidney Int.* 36: 891, 1989.
420. Seggie, J., and Adu, D. Nephrotic Syndrome in the Tropics. In J. S. Cameron and R. J. Glassock, *The Nephrotic Syndrome.* New York: Marcel Dekker, 1988. Pp. 653–695.
420a. Senguttuvan, P., Cameron, J. S., Hartley, R. B., et al. Recurrence of focal glomerulosclerosis in transplanted kidney: Analysis of incidence and risk factors in 59 cases. *Pediatr. Nephrol.* 4: 21, 1990.
421. Serdula, M. K., and Rhoads, G. G. Frequency of systemic lupus erythematosus in different ethnic groups in Hawaii. *Arthritis Rheum.* 22: 328, 1979.
422. Serra, A., and Cameron, J. S. Clinical and pathologic aspects of renal vasculitis. *Semin. Nephrol.* 5: 15, 1985.
423. Serra, A., Cameron, J. S., Turner, D. R., et al. Vasculitis affecting the kidney. Presentation, histopathology, and long-term outcome. *Q. J. Med.* 53: 181, 1984.
424. Shearn, M. A., Tu, W. H., and Piel, C. F. Recurrent nephrotic syndrome. *Arch. Intern. Med.* 114: 525, 1964.
425. Shurtleff, D. Some Characteristics Related to the Incidence of Cardiovascular Disease and Death: Framingham Study, 18 Year Follow-Up. In *The Framingham Study: An Epidemiological Investigation of Cardiovascular Disease.* Washington: NIH publication 74-599. U.S. Dept. of Health, Education and Welfare, 1974, Sect. 10.
426. Siegel, M., and Lee, S. L. The epidemiology of systemic lupus erythematosus. *Semin. Arthritis Rheum.* 3: 1, 1973.
427. Siegel, N. J., Goldberg, B., Krassner, L. S., et al. Long-term follow-up of children with steroid-responsive nephrotic syndrome. *J. Pediatr.* 81: 251, 1972.
428. Siegel, N. J., Kashgarian, M., Spargo, B. H., et al. Minimal change and focal sclerotic lesions in lipoid nephrosis. *Nephron* 13: 125, 1974.
429. Simon, P., Ramee, M. P., Ang, K. S., and Cam, G. Variations of primary glomerulonephritis incidence in a rural area of 40,000 inhabitants in the last decade. *Nephron* 45: 171, 1987.
430. Smith, E. C., Co, Bun Shu, and Freedman, P. The evo-

lution of the focal post-streptococcal glomerular lesion. *J. Chronic Dis.* 27: 405, 1974.

431. Sonsino, E., Nabarra, B., Kazatchkine, M., et al. Extracapillary proliferative glomerulonephritis so-called malignant glomerulonephritis. *Adv. Nephrol.* 2: 121, 1972.
432. Soon Lee, H., Mujais, S. H., Kasinath, B. S., et al. Course of renal pathology in patients with systemic lupus erythematosus. *Am. J. Med.* 77: 612, 1984.
433. Soon Lee, H., and Spargo, B. H. Significance of renal hyaline arteriolosclerosis in focal segmental glomerulosclerosis. *Nephron* 41: 86, 1985.
434. Sorger, K., Balun, J., Hubner, F. K., et al. The 'garland' type of acute post-infectious glomerulonephritis: Morphological characteristics and follow-up studies. *Clin. Nephrol.* 20: 17, 1983.
435. South West Pediatric Nephrology Study Group. Childhood nephrotic syndrome associated with diffuse mesangial hypercellularity. *Kidney Int.* 23: 87, 1983.
436. South West Pediatric Nephrology Study Group. A clinicopathologic study of crescentic glomerulonephritis in 50 children. *Kidney Int.* 27: 450, 1985.
437. South West Pediatric Nephrology Study Group. Focal segmental glomerulosclerosis in children with idiopathic nephrotic syndrome. *Kidney Int.* 27: 442, 1985.
438. Spargo, B. H., Ordoñez, N. G., and Ringus, J. C. The differential diagnosis of crescentic glomerulonephritis. The pathology of specific lesions with prognostic implications. *Hum. Pathol.* 8: 187, 1977.
439. Stills, H. F., Bullock, B. C., and Clarkson, T. B. Increased atherosclerosis and glomerulonephritis in cynomolgus monkeys (*Macaca fascicularis*) given injections of BSA over an extended period of time. *Am. J. Pathol.* 113: 222, 1983.
440. Stilmant, M. M., Bolton, W. K., Sturgill, B. C., et al. Crescentic glomerulonephritis without immune deposits: Clinicopathologic features. *Kidney Int.* 15: 184, 1979.
441. Strife, C. F., Jackson, E. C., and McAdams, A. J. Type III membranoproliferative glomerulonephritis: Long-term clinical and morphologic evaluation. *Clin. Nephrol.* 21: 323, 1984.
442. Strife, C. F., McEnery, P. T., McAdams, A. J., et al. Membranoproliferative glomerulonephritis with disruption of the glomerular basement membrane. *Clin. Nephrol.* 7: 65, 1976.
443. Striker, G. E., Kelly, M. R., Quadracci, L. J., et al. The Course of Lupus Nephritis: A Clinical Pathological Correlation of Fifty Patients. In P. Kincaid-Smith, T. H. Mathew, and E. L. Becker (eds.), *Glomerulonephritis Morphology, Natural History and Treatment,* Vol. II. New York: Wiley, 1973. Pp. 1141–1166.
444. Swaak, A. J., Aarden, L. A., Statius van Eps, L. W., et al. Anti-dsDNA and complement profiles as prognostic guides in systemic lupus erythematosus. *Arthritis Rheum.* 22: 226, 1979.
445. Swaak, A. J. G., Nossent, J. C., Bronsfeld, W., et al. Systemic lupus erythematosus. I. Outcome and survival: Dutch experience with 110 patients studied prospectively. *Ann. Rheum. Dis.* 48: 447, 1989.
446. Swainson, C. P., Robson, J. S., Thomson, D., et al. Mesangiocapillary glomerulonephritis: A long-term study of 40 cases. *J. Pathol.* 141: 449, 1983.
447. Takekoshi, Y., Tanaka, M., Shida, N., et al. Strong association between membranous nephropathy and hepatitis B surface antigen anemia in Japanese children. *Lancet* ii: 1065, 1978.
448. Talwalkar, Y. B., Price, B. S., and Musgrave, J. E. Recurrent resolving acute renal failure in IgA nephropathy. *J. Pediatr.* 92: 596, 1978.
449. Tarantino, A., de Vecchi, A., Montagnino, G., et al. Renal disease in essential mixed cryoglobulinaemia. Long-term follow-up of 44 cases. *Q. J. Med.* 46: 1, 1981.
450. Tateno, S., Kobayashi, Y., Shigematsu, H., and Hiki, Y. Study of lupus nephritis: Its classification and the significance of subendothelial deposits. *Q. J. Med.* 52: 311, 1983.
451. Tejani, A. Morphological transition in minimal change nephrotic syndrome. *Nephron* 39: 157, 1985.
452. Tejani, A., Nicastri, A. D., Chen, C.-K., et al. Lupus nephritis in black and hispanic children. *Am. J. Dis. Child.* 137: 481, 1983.
453. Tejani, A., Nicastri, A. D., Sen, D., et al. Long-term evaluation of children with nephrotic syndrome and focal segmental glomerulosclerosis. *Nephron* 35: 225, 1983.
454. Trainin, E. B., Boichis, H., Spitzer, A., et al. Late nonresponsiveness to steroids in children with the nephrotic syndrome. *J. Pediatr.* 87: 519, 1975.
455. Trainin, E. B., Boichis, H., Spitzer, A., et al. Idiopathic membranous nephropathy. *N.Y. State J. Med.* 76: 357, 1976.
456. Trainin, E. B., and Gomez-Leon, G. Development of renal insufficiency after long standing steroid-responsive nephrotic syndrome. *Int. J. Pediatr. Nephrol.* 3: 55, 1982.
457. Travis, L. B., Dodge, W. F., Beathard, G. A., et al. Acute glomerulonephritis in children. A review of the natural history with emphasis on prognosis. *Clin. Nephrol.* 1: 169, 1973.
458. Treser, G., Ehrenreich, T., Ores, R. O., et al. Natural history of 'apparently healed' acute poststreptococcal glomerulonephritis. *Pediatrics* 43: 1005, 1969.
459. Trompeter, R. S. Steroid Resistant Nephrotic Syndrome: A Review of the Treatment of Focal Segmental Glomerulosclerosis (FSGS) in Children. In K. Murakami et al. (eds.), *Pediatric Nephrology.* Amsterdam: Elsevier, 1987. Pp. 363–371.
460. Trompeter, R. S. Immunosuppressive therapy in the nephrotic syndrome in children. *Pediatr. Nephrol.* 3: 194, 1989.
461. Trompeter, R. S., Lloyd, B. W., Hicks, J., et al. Long-term outcome for children with minimal change nephrotic syndrome. *Lancet* 1: 368, 1985.
462. Tu, W.-H., Pettit, D. B., Biara, C. G., et al. Membranous nephropathy: Predictors of terminal renal failure. *Nephron* 36: 118, 1984.
463. Turner, N., and Rees, A. J. Anti-glomerular Basement Membrane Disease. In J. S. Cameron et al. (eds.), *The Oxford Textbook of Clinical Nephrology.* London: Oxford University Press, 1991.
464. Ueda, N., Kuno, K., and Ito, S. Eight and twelve week courses of cyclophosphamide in nephrotic syndrome. *Arch. Dis. Child.* 65: 1147, 1990.
465. Urman, J. D., and Rothfield, N. F. Corticosteroid treatment in systemic lupus erythematosus. *J.A.M.A.* 238: 2272, 1977.
466. Urowitz, M. B., Bookman, H. A. M., Koehler, B. E., et al. The bimodal mortality pattern of systemic lupus erythematosus. *Am. J. Med.* 60: 221, 1976.
467. Uszycka-Karcz, M., Stolarczyk, J., Wrzolkowa, T., et al. Mesangial proliferative glomerulonephritis in children. *Int. J. Pediatr. Nephrol.* 3: 251, 1982.
468. Valles Prats, M., Espinel Garuz, E., Allcoza Gascon-Molins, J. L., et al. Glomerulonephritis mesangiocapilar idiopatica. Estudio de 72 casos. *Nefrologia* 5: 17, 1985.

469. Van de Putte, L. B. A., Britel de la Riviere, G., and van Breda Vriesman, P. J. C. Recurrent or persistent hematuria. Sign of mesangial immune complex deposition. *N. Engl. J. Med.* 290: 1165, 1974.
470. Velosa, J. A. Idiopathic crescentic glomerulonephritis or systemic vasculitis? *Mayo Clin. Proc.* 62: 145, 1987.
471. Vilches, A. R., Turner, D. R., Cameron, J. S., et al. Significance of mesangial IgM deposition in "minimal change" nephrotic syndrome. *Lab. Invest.* 46: 10, 1982.
472. Vogl, W., Renke, M., Mayer-Eichberger, D., et al. Long-term prognosis for endocapillary glomerulonephritis of post streptococcal type in children and adults. *Nephron* 44: 58, 1986.
473. Vosnides, G., Sotsiou, F., Papadakis, G., et al. Frequency of various forms of primary glomerulonephritis (GN) in Greek adults. *Abstracts IXth Congress of the International Society of Nephrology,* Los Angeles, June 1984. P. 129A.
474. Waldherr, R., Gubler, M.-C., Levy, M., et al. The significance of pure diffuse mesangial proliferation in idiopathic nephrotic syndrome. *Clin. Nephrol.* 10: 171, 1978.
475. Walker, R. G., Scheinkistel, C., Becker, G. J., et al. Clinical and morphological aspects of the management of crescentic anti-glomerular basement membrane antibody (anti-GBM) nephritis/Goodpasture's syndrome. *Q. J. Med.* 54: 75, 1985.
476. Wallace, D. J., Podell, T., Weiner, J., et al. Systemic lupus erythematosus—Survival patterns. Experience with 609 patients. *J.A.M.A.* 245: 934, 1981.
477. Walser, M. Progression of chronic renal failure in man. *Kidney Int.* 37: 1195, 1990.
478. Walton, E. W. Giant-cell granuloma of the respiratory tract (Wegener's granulomatosis). *Br. Med. J.* 2: 265, 1958.
479. Wang, F., and Looi, L. M. Systemic lupus erythematosus with membranous lupus nephropathy in Malaysian patients. *Q. J. Med.* 210: 209, 1989.
480. Wang, F., Looi, L. M., and Chua, F. T. Minimal change glomerular disease in Malaysian adults and use of alternate day steroid therapy. *Q. J. Med.* 203: 312, 1982.
481. Warshaw, B. L., and Hymes, L. C. Daily single-dose and daily reduced-dose prednisone therapy for children with the nephrotic syndrome. *Pediatrics* 83: 694, 1989.
482. Wass, V., and Cameron, J. S. Cardiovascular disease and the nephrotic syndrome: The other side of the coin. *Nephron* 27: 58, 1981.
483. Wass, V. J., Jarrett, R. J., Chilvers, C., et al. Does the nephrotic syndrome increase the risk of cardiovascular disease? *Lancet* 2: 664, 1979.
484. Wehrmann, M., Bohle, A., Bogenschutz, O., et al. Long term prognosis of chronic idiopathic membranous glomerulonephritis: An analysis of 334 cases with particular regard to tubulointerstitial changes. *Clin. Nephrol.* 31: 67, 1989.
485. Wehrmann, M., Bohle, A., Held, H., et al. Long term prognosis of focal sclerosing glomerulonephritis: An analysis of 250 cases with particular regard to tubulo-interstitial changes. *Clin. Nephrol.* 33: 115, 1990.
486. Weiss, M. A., and Crissman, J. D. Segmental necrotizing glomerulonephritis: Diagnostic, prognostic and therapeutic significance. *Am. J. Kidney Dis.* 6: 199, 1985.
487. Welch, T. R., McAdams, A. J., and Berry, A. Rapidly progressive IgA nephropathy. *Am. J. Dis. Child.* 142: 789, 1988.
488. West, C. D. Childhood membranoproliferative glomerulonephritis: An approach to management. *Kidney Int.* 29: 1077, 1986.
489. Whiting-O'Keefe, Q., Kenke, J. E., Shearn, M. A., et al. The information content from renal biopsy in systemic lupus erythematosus. *Ann. Intern. Med.* 96: 718, 1982.
490. Whiting-O'Keefe, Q., Riccardi, P. J., Henke, J. E., et al. Recognition of information in renal biopsies of patients with lupus nephritis. *Ann. Intern. Med.* 96: 723, 1982.
491. Whitworth, J. A., Morel-Maroger, L., Mignon, F., et al. The significance of extracapillary proliferation. Clinicopathological review of 60 patients. *Nephron* 16: 1, 1976.
492. Williams, P. S., Fass, G., and Bone, J. M. Renal pathology and proteinuria determine progression in untreated mild/moderate chronic renal failure. *Q. J. Med.* 67: 343, 1988.
493. Wilson, C. B., and Dixon, F. J. Antiglomerular basement membrane antibody-induced glomerulonephritis. *Kidney Int.* 3: 74, 1973.
494. Wingen, A.-M., Muller-Wiefel, D. E., and Scharer, K. Spontaneous remissions in frequently relapsing and steroid-dependent nephrotic syndrome. *Clin. Nephrol.* 23: 35, 1985.
495. Woo, K. T., Edmondson, R. P. S., Wu, A. Y. T., et al. The natural history of IgA nephritis in Singapore. *Clin. Nephrol.* 25: 15, 1986.
496. Woodworth, T. G., Abuelo, J. G., Austin, H. A., III, and Esparza, A. Severe glomerulonephritis with late emergence of classic Wegener's granulomatosis: Report of 4 cases and review of the literature. *Medicine* (Baltimore) 66: 181, 1987.
497. Worrall, J. G., Snaith, M. L., Batchelor, J. R., and Isenberg, D. A. SLE: A rheumatological view. Analysis of the clinical features, serology, and immunogenetics of 100 SLE patients during long term follow-up. *Q. J. Med.* 74: 319, 1990.
498. Wu, G., Katz, A., Cardella, and Oreopoulos, G. G. Spontaneous remission of nephrotic syndrome in IgA glomerular disease. *Am. J. Kidney Dis.* 6: 96, 1985.
499. Wu, M. J., Moorthy, A. V., and Beirne, G. J. Relapse in antiglomerular basement membrane antibody mediated crescentic glomerulonephritis. *Clin. Nephrol.* 13: 97, 1980.
500. Yeung, C. K., Wong, K. L., Wong, W. C., et al. Crescentic lupus glomerulonephritis. *Clin. Nephrol.* 21: 251, 1984.
501. Yoshikawa, N., Ito, H., Akamatsu, R., et al. Focal segmental glomerulosclerosis with and without nephrotic syndrome in children. *J. Pediatr.* 109: 65, 1986.
502. Yoshikawa, N., Ito, H., Yoshinara, S., et al. Clinical course of immunoglobulin A nephropathy in children. *J. Pediatr.* 110: 555, 1987.
503. Zech, P., Colon, S., Pointet, P. H., et al. The nephrotic syndrome in adults aged over 60—Etiology of 76 cases. *Clin. Nephrol.* 17: 232, 1982.
504. Zimmerman, S. W., Jenkins, P. G., Shelp, W. D., et al. Progression from minimal or focal to diffuse proliferative lupus nephritis. *Lab. Invest.* 32: 665, 1975.
505. Zucchelli, P., and Pasquali, S. Membranous Nephropathy. In J. S. Cameron et al. (eds.), *The Oxford Textbook of Clinical Nephrology.* London: Oxford University Press, 1991.
506. Zucchelli, P., Ponticelli, C., Cagnoli, L., and Passerini, P. Long term outcome of idiopathic membranous nephropathy with nephrotic syndrome. *Nephrol. Dial. Transplant.* 2: 73, 1987.
507. Zucchelli, P., Ponticelli, C., Cagnoli, L., et al. Prognostic value of T lymphocyte subset ratio in idiopathic membranous nephropathy. *Kidney Int.* 8: 15, 1988.

Chronic Tubulointerstitial Nephropathies

Garabed Eknoyan

Diseases of the kidney primarily affect the glomeruli, the vasculature, or the remainder of the renal parenchyma, i.e., the tubules and interstitium. It is the chronic forms of this latter category of diseases of the kidney that will be considered in this chapter. Initially referred to as *interstitial nephritis* [89, 182], the more descriptive term, *tubulointerstitial diseases* [421], or *nephropathies* [81], has been proposed as the preferred term to classify this heterogeneous group of disorders that affect primarily the renal interstitium and tubules and only secondarily involve the other structural components of the kidney. This term is preferred because inflammatory changes of the interstitium are not always clearly evident, and it is the tubules rather than the interstitium that comprise the bulk of the renal parenchyma that is affected [421]; more importantly, it is disorders of tubular function that constitute the most notable component of the disordered pathophysiology of these diseases and thereby differentiate them clinically from other forms of renal disease due to glomerular lesions [81]. This is not to imply that glomerular lesions do not occur or contribute to the loss of renal function in these diseases. For although the primary lesions originate in the tubules and interstitium, many of them eventually will develop structural and functional abnormalities of the glomeruli [421]. The structural alterations are characterized by glomerulosclerosis, whereas the functional changes are evidenced by progressive reduction in glomerular filtration rate, the development of glomerular proteinuria, and, ultimately, the onset of volume-dependent hypertension [47, 81, 82]. However, early in the course of chronic tubulointerstitial nephropathies, with their characteristic insidious onset and indolent course, tubular dysfunction is almost always out of proportion to glomerular dysfunction [81, 82]. It is in the later phases of tubulointerstitial nephropathies, when the glomerular lesions are quite advanced, that it may be difficult to differentiate them from the end-stage kidney disease of any etiology. Actually, although diseases of the glomeruli and vasculature are excluded by definition from this classification of tubulointerstitial diseases, interstitial injury can be an important component of primary diseases of the glomeruli and vasculature and, in fact, the extent and severity of concurrent tubulointerstitial changes contribute significantly to their clinical course to progressive renal failure [1, 48, 50, 441].

The frequency with which tubulointerstitial diseases affect the kidney is difficult to determine. Their importance, however, can be appreciated from the fact that some 20 to 40 percent of all patients undergoing treatment for end-stage renal disease have been estimated to have a primary tubulointerstitial disease as the cause of their renal failure [311, 364, 370]. Taken together with the demonstrated role of tubulointerstitial lesions in the deterioration of renal function and the progression of the renal disease in primary glomerular or vascular disease [370], it becomes evident why it is important to evaluate and appreciate lesions of the interstitium and tubules.

It must be noted that the preferential use of the term *tubulointerstitial* should in no way belittle the role of the interstitium, since it is at this site that the pathology is often initiated, and interstitial lesions may well account for many of the disorders of tubular function characteristic of these diseases. The renal interstitium as an important component of renal function has long been appreciated. The interstitial solute concentration in the cortex and in the medulla is an integral component of the regulatory mechanisms for proximal reabsorption and for concentration and dilution of urine, respectively [52, 339]. Furthermore, the endocrine functions of the interstitial cells, in the release of renin and possibly erythropoietin [227] in the cortex and of prostaglandins in the medulla, are essential modulators in the role of the kidney in maintaining homeostasis. Conceptually then, interstitial events could account for the pathogenesis of renal disease, in general, and of the tubulointerstitial nephropathies, in particular. Still, it is the tubular changes that bear the brunt of the insult and, being functionally more important, account for the clinical and functional manifestations of any interstitial nephritis.

Structural Features of the Interstitium

The interstitium of the kidney consists of peritubular and periarterial spaces. The relative contribution of each of these two spaces to interstitial volume varies, reflecting, in part, the arbitrary boundaries used in assessing them. In any case, the portion of the renal tissue occupied by interstitium increases from the cortex to the papilla. In the cortex, there is little interstitium, because the peritubular capillaries fill up the major part of the space between the tubules, and the cortical interstitial cells are scattered and relatively inconspicuous. In the medulla, however, there is a noticeable increase in interstitial space, and the interstitial cells have characteristic structural features and an organized arrangement. The ground substance of the renal interstitium contains different types of fibrils and a basement-like material embedded in a glycosaminoglycan-rich substance [58, 231, 251].

The relative volume of the interstitium of the cortex is approximately 7 percent, consisting of about 3 percent interstitial cells and 4 percent extracellular space [52, 338, 342]. The vasculature occupies another 6 percent; the remainder, i.e., some 85 percent or more, is occupied by the tubules. The cortical interstitial space is unevenly distributed and has been divided into "narrow" and "wide" structural components [338]. The tubules and peritubular capillaries are at several points closely apposed, sometimes to the point of sharing a common basement membrane or are separated by a very narrow space, the so-called narrow interstitium, that has been estimated to occupy 0.6 percent of cortical volume in the rat. The narrow interstitium occupies about one-half to two-thirds of the cortical peritubular capillary surface area and about one-fourth of the peritubular surface area. The remainder of the cortical interstitium consists of irregularly shaped clearly discernible larger areas, the so-called wide interstitium, which has been estimated to occupy 3.4 percent of cortical volume in the rat [338]. The capillary wall facing the narrow interstitium is significantly more fenestrated than that facing the wide interstitium [52, 338]. Evidence for a possible functional heterogeneity of these interstitial spaces has been advanced on the basis of studies of the interstitial albumin pool [344]. The actual significance of these findings, however, remains to be identified.

In the medulla, the relative size of the interstitium increases gradually from the outer medullary stripe to the tip of the papilla [52]. This occurrence is due to the increase in the relative volume contribution of both the interstitial cells and the extracellular space. Actually, in the outer stripe of the outer medulla, the relative volume of the interstitium is slightly less than that in the cortex and has been estimated to be approximately 5 percent in the rat. It is in the inner stripe of the outer medulla that the relative volume of the interstitium increases significantly in width, an increment that gradually becomes larger toward the papillary tip [52, 59]. The inner stripe of the outer medulla consists of the vascular bundles and the interbundle regions, which are occupied principally by tubules. Within the vascular bundles, the interstitial spaces are meager, whereas in the interbundle region, the interstitial spaces occupy some 10 to 20 percent of the volume. In the inner medulla, the differentiation into vascular bundles and interbundle region becomes gradually less obvious until the two regions merge. This is coupled by a gradual increase in the relative volume of the interstitial space from the base of the inner medulla to the tip of the papilla. In the rat, the increment in interstitial space is from 10 to 15 percent at the base to about 30 percent at the tip and in the rabbit, from 20 to 25 percent at the base to over 40 percent at the tip [223].

The cortex contains two types of interstitial cells. The more abundant variety of interstitial cells are the type I or fibroblastic cells. These have a prominent rough endoplasmic reticulum and elongated mitochondria. They probably produce the extracellular interstitial matrix and collagen fibrils and contribute to fibrosis in response to chronic irritation. The type II interstitial cells, mononuclear cells or macrophages, have an abundant chromatin, have no endoplasmic reticulum, and demonstrable phagocytic capacity; they are less common than the type I cells [52, 58]. An interstitial infiltrate of mononuclear cells is a prominent feature of interstitial nephritis, and some of the infiltrating cells are derived from these local precursors [52].

In the outer zone of the medulla, the interstitial cells are the same as in the cortex. In the inner zone of the medulla and the inner medulla, the cellular content is significantly altered. A unique type of cell that is present is the lipid-laden interstitial cell. The number of cytoplasmic lipid droplets in these cells varies from one cell to the other, and there are differences in the number of droplets among species as well as among individuals of the same species. A change in the number of droplets has been suggested, but not conclusively demonstrated, to occur in relation to the intake of salt and water and the level of blood pressure. Another characteristic feature of these medullary cells is their connection to each other. They also have a characteristic arrangement, similar to the rungs of a ladder, with a distinct close and regular transverse apposition to their surrounding structures, specifically the limbs of the loop of Henle and capillaries but not to the collecting duct cells [52, 58]. The other types of medullary cells are the mononuclear macrophages and the pericytes. The pericytes are prominent in the descending vasa recta in the outer medulla but become rare as the vascular bundles break up in the inner medulla. The number of macrophages increases beginning with the inner stripe of the outer medulla and is highest in the inner medulla [251].

The extracellular loose matrix is a hydrated gelatinous substance, which consists of glycoproteins and glycosaminoglycans (hyaluronic acid, heparin, dermatan sulfate, chondroitin sulfate) that are embedded within a fibrillar reticulum, which consists of collagen fibers (types I, III, and VI) and unbanded microfilaments. Collagen types IV and V are the principal components of the basement membrane lining the vessels and tubules. The relative increase in interstitial matrix of the medulla may be important for providing support to the delicate tubular and vascular structures in this region, and its alterations might well account for the susceptibility of the structures in this region to toxic reactive metabolites [18].

Functional Significance of the Interstitium

Exchange processes between the different segments of the renal tubular and vascular components are at the core of renal homeostatic functions. In most physiologic discussions, the transport of ions, water, and proteins is described as though it occurs directly from the tubule to the capillary, and the emphasis is on the permeability of the membranes concerned. In fact, a major part of the reabsorbed or secreted tubular fluid has to traverse a true interstitial space. The structure, composition, and permeability characteristic of the interstitial space must, of necessity, exert an effect on any such exchange. Several studies suggest that pressure and volume conditions of the interstitial space might modulate renal tubule function in response to fluid-balance disturbances. The normal interstitial hydrostatic pressure of about 3 mm Hg and protein concentration of about 2-gm percent changes with extracellular fluid volume expansion to 5 to 10 mm Hg and 0.5-gm percent protein, respectively [340]. Similarly, rapid transient changes in the hydrostatic pressure of the interstitial spaces occur following the intraaortic injection of albumin or saline solutions [340]. There also appears to be an increase in volume of the interstitial space during water diuresis and vasopressin-induced antidiuresis [433]. Although the normal structural and functional correlates of the interstitial space are poorly defined, changes in the interstitial composition and structure are bound to reflect themselves in changes of tubular function. Structural changes of the interstitium by delaying equilibration or exchange could well result in a significant alteration in the normal functions of the renal tubule. Correlation of the structural changes of the interstitium to those of renal function may be envisioned better when the rich but delicate capillary network of the renal microcirculation is taken into consideration. The periarterial loose connective tissue that envelops the intrarenal arteries is continuous with that of the sparse peritubular interstitium [52, 338]. It is possible that changes in the supporting interstitium could affect the blood flow to the adjacent tubule and thereby cause tubular dysfunction. In fact, angiographic studies of the renal microcirculation reveal that the number and volume of peritubular capillaries is markedly compromised in the areas of interstitial inflammation and fibrosis [258, 292]. Interstitial alterations also may be reflected in changes in glomerular capillary pressure and filtration rate through the tubuloglomerular feedback mechanism; specifically, as the function of the affected tubular segments becomes compromised secondary to interstitial disease, solute delivery to the macula densa may be altered [49, 339, 340, 376]. On the basis of studies correlating morphometric analysis of biopsy specimens to renal function, it has been suggested that obliteration of postglomerular capillaries secondary to interstitial injury and fibrosis may account for renal functional changes [51].

It is of special relevance, in this regard, that attempts to correlate renal function with histologic abnormalities of the glomeruli have been conflicting. Whereas some studies have found a relationship [56, 336], others were unable to document any correlation [376]. On the other hand, several studies of abnormalities of the interstitial tissue have shown a close correlation with abnormalities of renal function in an assortment of renal diseases [48, 133, 200, 308, 330, 359]. In a detailed study of 70 patients with a variety of renal diseases, the majority of which were glomerular in origin, the biopsy material was evaluated in regard to changes of glomerular, tubular, vascular, and interstitial components [384]. Studies of renal function, performed within 2 days of the biopsy, included measurements of glomerular filtration rate (GFR), effective renal plasma flow, acidifying ability, and maximal urinary concentrating ability. Glomerular filtration showed a higher correlation with both interstitial and tubular damage, regardless of the disease process (Fig. 70-1). Interstitial fibrosis and cellular infiltration were also well correlated with GFR, whereas interstitial edema was not. In contrast to these findings, there was only a modest correlation between GFR and the glomerular injury score. As might be expected, effective renal plasma flow showed a high correlation with the degree of vascular disease (Fig. 70-2); it was also highly correlated with tubular and interstitial damage but not to glomerular lesions. The urinary concentrating ability was

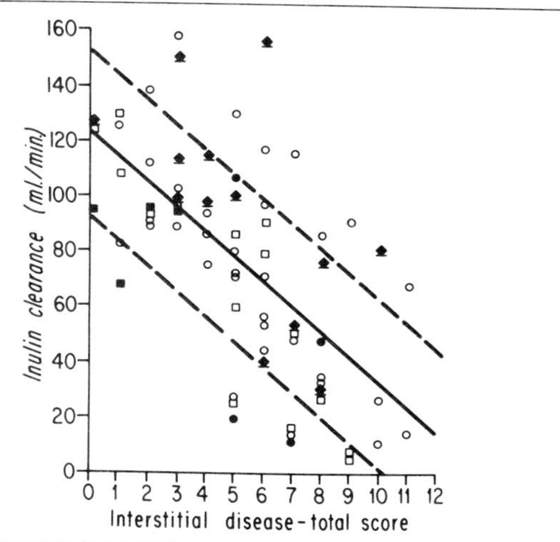

Fig. 70-1. Relationship of inulin clearance to the severity of tubulointerstitial lesions. The regression line is y = 122 − 8.8x. Symbols represent categories of kidney diseases studied: ◆ = acute glomerulonephritis; ○ = chronic glomerulonephritis; ● = tubulointerstitial nephropathy; ■ = nephrosclerosis; □ = miscellaneous. (Reproduced with permission from [384].)

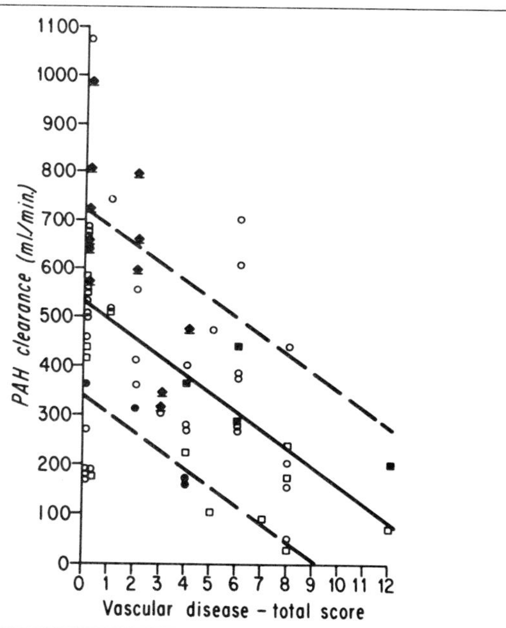

Fig. 70-2. Relationship of the effective renal plasma flow as measured by the clearance of paraaminohippurate (PAH) to the severity of vascular disease. The regression line is y = 553 − 38x. The symbols are the same as for Fig. 70-1. (Reproduced with permission from [384].)

found to be a very sensitive indicator of the presence or absence of tubular and interstitial abnormalities (Fig. 70-3). In fact, it was the severity of tubulointerstitial damage and not the basic disease process that seemed to be the determinant of impairment in urinary concentrating

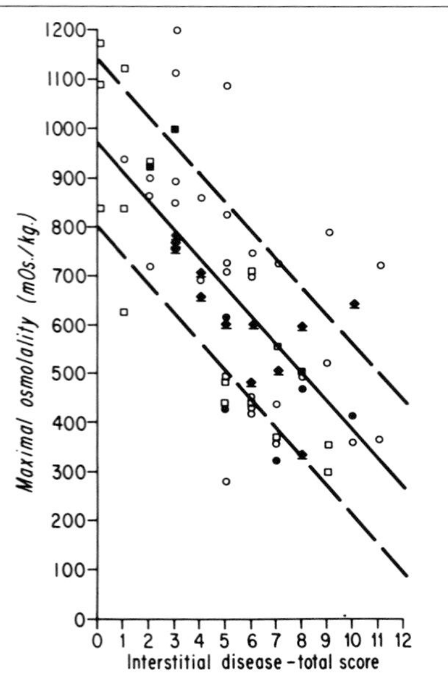

Fig. 70-3. Relationship of the maximum ability to concentrate the urine (maximal osmolality) to the severity of tubulointerstitial lesions. The regression line is y = 975 − 59x. The symbols are the same as for Fig. 70-1. (Reproduced with permission from [384].)

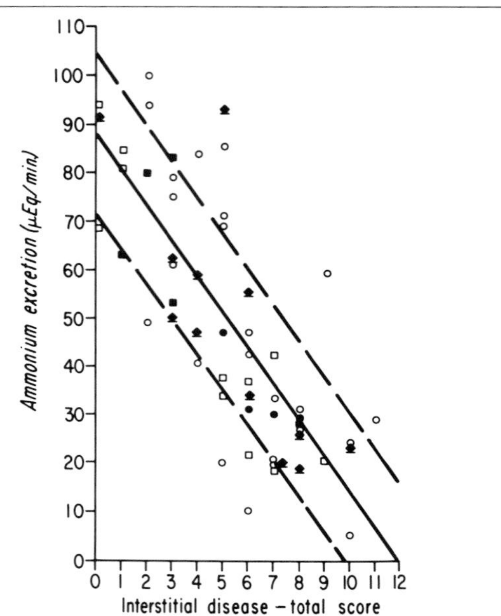

Fig. 70-4. Relationship between ammonium excretion in response to an acute acid load and the severity of tubulointerstitial lesions. The regression line is y = 90 − 7.6x. The symbols are the same as for Fig. 70-1. (Reproduced with permission from [384].)

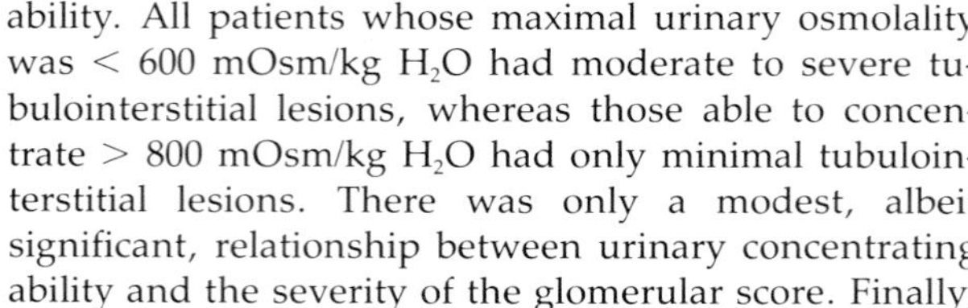

ability. All patients whose maximal urinary osmolality was < 600 mOsm/kg H_2O had moderate to severe tubulointerstitial lesions, whereas those able to concentrate > 800 mOsm/kg H_2O had only minimal tubulointerstitial lesions. There was only a modest, albeit significant, relationship between urinary concentrating ability and the severity of the glomerular score. Finally, the impairment in the ability to excrete titratable acid and ammonium in response to an acid load was highly correlated with the degree of interstitial and tubular lesions and, to a much lesser degree, with glomerular changes (Fig. 70-4). With increased awareness of the role of interstitial lesion, these studies have been expanded [1, 50, 194, 334, 456], and the presence of interstitial fi-

Fig. 70-5. Effect of the presence of cortical interstitial fibrosis noted at the time of the initial diagnostic kidney biopsy on the long-term prognosis of patients with mesangioproliferative glomerulonephritis (n = 455), membranous nephropathy (n = 334), and membranoproliferative glomerulonephritis (n = 220). (Data from [50].)

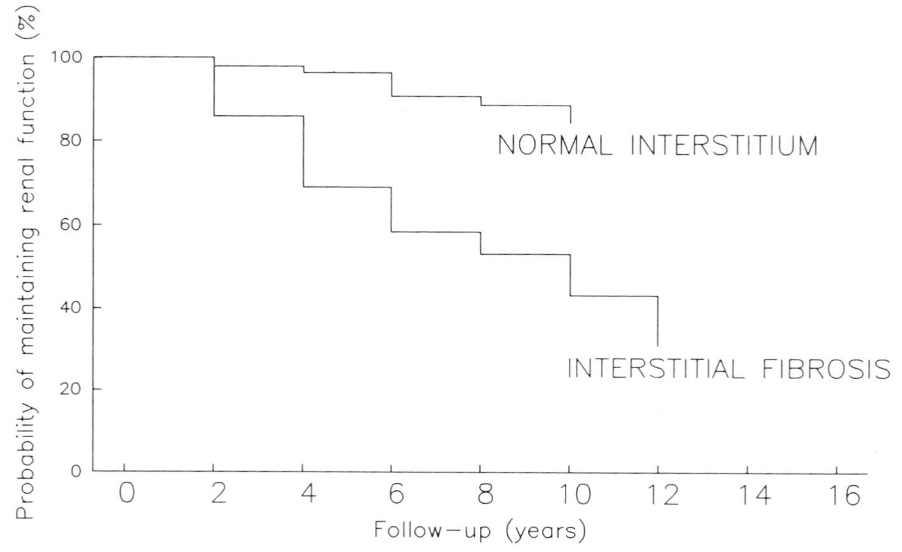

brosis has been shown to have a significant correlation with the progression of renal diseases of the glomeruli (Fig. 70-5). Thus, the presence of interstitial lesions in glomerular diseases not only shows a correlation with the altered renal function at the time of biopsy but also provides a prognostic index of the rate of progression to end-stage renal failure [50, 61, 92, 93, 441].

Proteinuria appears to be important in the development of tubulointerstitial lesions in primary glomerular diseases [92]. Interstitial nephritis has been induced by protein overload in uninephrectomized rats [108]. A significant cellular infiltration developed in the interstitium of experimental animals within 1 week of exposure to protein overload consisting of 1 gm of bovine serum albumin daily. The initial infiltrates consisting predominantly of macrophages were soon replaced by T lymphocytes, and by the fourth week, tubular atrophy and interstitial fibrosis were present. Iron loss in the tubular fluid also has been implicated in the pathogenesis of the tubulointerstitial injury associated with primary glomerular disease [4]. In a model of nephrotoxic serum nephritis in rats, the induction of iron deficiency prior to the development of proteinuria attenuated or prevented the development of tubulointerstitial lesions and attendant deterioration of renal function. Conceivably, iron, dissociated from filtered transferrin at the more acid pH of the tubule fluid or during its absorption in the proximal tubule, contributes to the formation of free hydroxyl radicals, which account for renal epithelial cell injury and consequent tubulointerstitial lesions. These experimental studies notwithstanding, a number of experimental and clinical forms of proteinuric glomerular diseases are not accompanied by severe tubulointerstitial lesions, and the search for additional factors contributory to the development of interstitial lesions must continue.

In summary, the available evidence would indicate that the normal interstitium plays an important role in maintenance of renal function and changes in the integrity of interstitial components show a significant correlation with abnormalities of renal function in a variety of diseases of the kidney. The further importance of the interstitium in the normal and diseased kidney remains to be explored.

Pathologic Features of Tubulointerstitial Nephropathies

Independent of its initiating process, the principal morphologic feature of chronic tubulointerstitial nephropathy is an increase in the interstitial volume, mainly because of interstitial fibrosis that is usually accompanied by varying degrees of infiltration with chronic inflammatory cells. Tubular atrophy and degeneration are also a common, if not invariable, finding. Depending on the duration, cause, and severity of the disease, the distribution of the lesions will vary from focal to diffuse but are generally patchy in distribution. This interstitial inflammatory reaction is a feature of several renal diseases, including some of glomerular origin [73, 92, 191, 272]. There are, however, several diseases of the kidney in which tubulointerstitial lesions are the principal, and early in the course of the disease usually the only, detectable lesion on morphologic examination of renal tissue [419]. Changes of glomerular sclerosis, periglomerular fibrosis, and glomerular atrophy, if not present at the onset, will ultimately occur in primary tubulointerstitial diseases of the kidney [343]. The final picture that emerges in the end-stage form of the disease may be undifferentiable from that of end-stage kidney disease of any etiology.

Immunohistologic examination utilizing monoclonal antibodies and immunoperoxidase analysis, coupled with conventional and electron microscopy, indicates that most of the mononuclear cells making up renal interstitial infiltrates are T cells [36, 270, 333]. Chronic inflammatory cell foci may be characterized by Ia antigen-positive T cells considered to be markers of activated lymphocytes [73, 199]. Interstitial infiltrates contain varying numbers of activated lymphocytes in the absence of tubulointerstitial immune deposits [92], even in classic examples of immune-complex mediated diseases such as systemic lupus erythematosus [334], and the extent of interstitial filtrates shows a direct correlation with the severity of tubular atrophy and interstitial fibrosis determined semiquantitatively [73]. The profile of immunocompetent cells suggests a major role for cell-mediated immunity in the tubulointerstitial lesions that are mediated by autoimmune mechanisms [262, 279]. Experimental studies show the sequential accumulation of T cells and monocytes after the initial immune insult, which would implicate an important role for T cells both as inflammatory cells and in the progression of subsequent injury [270]. The cells may be of the helper/inducer subset [333] or the cytotoxic/suppressor subset [36], although there generally seems to be a selective prevalence of the former variety [270]. Lymphocytes that are peritubular and are seen invading the tubular epithelial cells, so-called tubulitis, are generally of the cytotoxic (CD8+) variety [279]. Fine-needle aspiration of the kidney can be useful in the characterization of the cellular infiltrates [160] and their sequential evolution [64].

The fibroblastic (or type I) interstitial cells, which normally produce and maintain the extracellular matrix, proliferate and increase their well-developed rough endoplasmic reticulum in response to injury [317, 364]. The number of fibroblasts derived in cell culture from kidney biopsies obtained from patients with interstitial fibrosis is increased by a factor of 5 to 10 as compared to cultures derived from normal kidney biopsies [364]. Growth kinetic studies of these cells show a significant increase in proliferating capacity and generation time indicating hyperproliferative growth.

The type of infiltrate can be characteristic and, occasionally, diagnostic of the kidney disease. The presence of eosinophils can be diagnostic in cases of drug-induced acute allergic interstitial nephritis (see Chap. 50). Another cell type whose presence may be of diagnostic import is that of foam cells, with their characteristic vacuolated appearance. Studies utilizing monoclonal antibodies show them to be derived from macrophages

[326]. Isolated foam cells are frequently encountered in cases of heavy proteinuria of any etiology [368]. Their presence in large numbers in the glomeruli and interstitium has been considered to be indicative of Alport's nephritis [154]. Masses of interstitial foam cells, interspersed with inflammatory cells, occur in chronic forms of pyelonephritis and, when prominent, form the characteristic lesion of xanthogranulomatous interstitial nephritis [209]. A closely related condition is the appearance of large mononuclear cells with abundant cytoplasm, containing large and laminated phagolysosomes that show progressive mineralization and form the characteristic Michaelis-Gutmann (MG) bodies seen in cases of malacoplakia [209]. Although malacoplakia is commonly a lesion of the urinary bladder, it rarely involves the renal interstitium and usually occurs in the context of chronic urinary tract infection [120]. These peculiar cells have also been described in hemolytic-uremic syndrome [185] and transplanted kidneys [331].

The interstitial lesions of one group of tubulointerstitial diseases can be distinguished by the presence of a characteristic noncaseating granulomatous pattern, which, when present, is highly suggestive of sarcoidosis [260, 295]. Usually coexistent with extrarenal granulomata, there are rare reports of sarcoid granulomatous lesions localized to the kidney [216, 406]. Interstitial granulomatous reactions also occur in response to oxalate deposition [444] and to infection of the kidney by mycobacteria [242], fungus [167], or bacteria [138]. Renal granulomatous reactions to drugs, such as methicillin [295], sulfonamides [304], or narcotics [418] have been described in acute forms of tubulointerstitial disease. In experimental models of antibasement-membrane nephritis, granulomatous inflammation develops around immunologically altered tubular basement membrane. In the course of the granulomatous reaction, tissue monocytes evolve from blood monocytes and pursue one of two independent pathways of differentiation: (1) macrophages that evolve distant from the tubule or (2) epithelioid cells that are formed adjacent to tubules. The latter form through cell fusion and can develop into the multinucleated giant cells of Langhans [29, 240, 431]. Multinucleated giant cells also are a feature of renal involvement in multiple myeloma [252, 346].

Intracellular crystals can be diagnostic of some forms of tubulointerstitial diseases. Rhomboid-shaped crystals within the cell lysosomes are characteristic of cystinosis [389]. Tophaceous deposits and birefringent deposits of sodium biurate are seen in hyperuricemia and gout [221]. Birefringence on dark-field microscopy is observed in oxalosis [186, 444, 453]. Gold therapy for rheumatoid arthritis can result in characteristic lysosomal crystalloid aggregates that can be seen on electron microscopy [447].

The interstitial spaces may be invaded by proliferative malignant cells in leukemias and lymphomas [145]. Commonly found at postmortem in patients with clinically evident malignant disease, massive infiltration of the kidney with renal failure may rarely be an initial presenting feature of some cases [145, 204].

Functional Manifestations of Tubulointerstitial Nephropathies

The principal manifestations of interstitial lesions are those of tubular dysfunction, which is one reason that the term *tubulointerstitial disease* is preferred to that of interstitial nephritis. Because of the focal distribution of the lesions that occur and the segmental nature of normal tubular function, the pattern of tubular dysfunction that occurs will vary, depending on the major site of injury; whereas the extent of damage will determine the severity of tubular dysfunction. The hallmarks of glomerular disease, such as salt retention, edema, hypertension, proteinuria, and hematuria are characteristically absent in the early phases of the disease [47, 81, 82]. However, in keeping with the intact nephron hypothesis, glomerular damage ultimately will appear. As a rule, the magnitude of glomerular function reduction seems to correlate with the magnitude of interstitial fibrosis, whereas the enlargement of interstitium by cellular infiltrate has less of a bearing on the filtration rate [113, 263, 267, 384].

Basically, the tubulointerstitial lesions are localized either to the cortex or to the medulla. Cortical lesions will affect, in the main, either the proximal tubule or the distal tubule. Medullary lesions will affect the loop of Henle and the collecting duct. The change in the normal function of each of these affected segments will then determine the manifestations of tubular dysfunction (Table 70-1). Essentially, the proximal nephron segment reabsorbs the bulk of bicarbonate, glucose, amino acids, phosphate, and uric acid. Changes in the proximal tubular function, therefore, will result in bicarbonaturia (proximal RTA), β_2-microglobulinuria, glucosuria (renal glucosuria), aminoaciduria, phosphaturia, and uricosuria [335, 358]. The latter two can be valuable in suspecting tubulointerstitial disease when the serum phosphate and urate are noted to be lower than expected, particularly in individuals with renal insufficiency and azotemia [113]. Measurements of the fractional clearance of uric acid from a spot urine sample can also be helpful. The normal fractional clearance of urate is about 10 percent; values significantly higher than normal would suggest a defect in urate handling by the proximal tubule. The distal nephron segment secretes hydrogen and potassium and regulates the final amount of sodium chloride excreted. Lesions affecting primarily this segment, therefore, will result in the distal form of renal tubular acidosis, hyperkalemia, and salt wasting [25, 229, 278, 309]. Lesions that primarily involve the medulla and papilla will disproportionately affect the loops of Henle, collecting ducts, and the other medullary structures essential to attaining and maintaining medullary hypertonicity. Disruption of these structures, therefore, will result in different degrees of nephrogenic diabetes insipidus and clinically manifest themselves as polyuria and nocturia [114]. Although this general framework is useful in localizing the site of injury, considerable overlap in any one patient may be encountered clinically, with different degrees of proximal, distal, and medullary dysfunction present. Additionally, the ultimate develop-

Table 70-1. Principal sites of injury and patterns of tubular dysfunction in chronic tubulointerstitial nephropathies

Site of injury	Cause	Tubular dysfunction
I. *Cortex*		
A. Proximal tubule	1. Heavy metals 2. Multiple myeloma 3. Immunologic diseases 4. Cystinosis	↓ Reabsorption of: Bicarbonate Glucose Uric acid Phosphate Amino acids
B. Distal tubule	1. Immunologic diseases 2. Granulomatous diseases 3. Hereditary diseases 4. Hypercalcemia 5. Urinary tract obstruction 6. Sickle cell hemoglobinopathy 7. Amyloidosis	↓ Secretion of: Hydrogen ion Potassium ↓ Reabsorption of: Sodium
II. *Medulla*	1. Analgesic nephropathy 2. Sickle hemoglobinopathy 3. Uric acid disorders 4. Hypercalcemia 5. Infection 6. Hereditary disorders 7. Granulomatous diseases	Impaired ability to concentrate urine ↓ Reabsorption of: Sodium
III. *Papilla*	1. Analgesic nephropathy 2. Diabetes mellitus 3. Infection 4. Urinary tract obstruction 5. Sickle hemoglobinopathy 6. Transplanted kidney	Impaired ability to concentrate urine ↓ Reabsorption of: Sodium

ment of renal failure will complicate the issue further because of the added effect of urea-induced osmotic diuresis on tubular function in the remaining nephrons. In this later stage of tubulointerstitial diseases, the absence of glomerular proteinuria and the more common occurrence of hypertension in glomerular diseases can be helpful in the differential diagnosis [48, 81]. Under any circumstance though, the diagnosis of tubulointerstitial disease can only be established by morphologic examination of the renal tissue.

The type of insult will determine the segmental location of injury (Table 70-1). For example, agents secreted by the organic pathway in the pars recta (cephalosporins) or reabsorbed in the proximal tubule (aminoglycosides and light-chain proteins) will cause predominantly proximal tubular lesions. Conditions that cause hypersensitivity reactions (methicillin) or depositional disorders (amyloid and hypergammaglobulinemic states) will cause predominantly cortical distal tubular lesions. Finally, insulting agents that are affected by the urine concentrating mechanism (analgesics and uric acid) or medullary tonicity (sickle cell) will cause medullary injury [82].

The clinical course of tubulointerstitial diseases depends to a great extent on the primary cause and the magnitude of the insult. In general, acute exposure to a massive insult will result in the rapid deterioration of renal function [162], whereas sporadic exposure to small amounts of the same insult will result in a more indolent course, with a gradual but progressive loss of renal function [285]. In fact, tubulointerstitial diseases may be divided into acute or chronic forms on the basis of the clinical course and accompanying pathologic lesions (Table 70-2). The *acute* form is characterized by prominent interstitial edema and focal areas of varied cellular infiltrates. If the injury is severe, tubular damage and dilatation are also present, and azotemia and renal insufficiency are early presenting features (see Chap. 50). In the *chronic* form, interstitial fibrosis and tubular atrophy are present, and the cellular infiltrate is uniformly mononuclear. In this more indolent form, renal insufficiency is slow to develop and the early manifestations of the disease are those of tubular dysfunction that may go undetected unless specifically elicited in the history, noted in the laboratory results, or documented by specific testing. Ultimately, though, renal failure will occur. The onset of heavy proteinuria in tubulointerstitial disease is an ominous sign and indicative of the development of glomerulosclerosis [397, 419]. In contrast to glomerular disease, hypertension with tubulointerstitial disease is a late development and occurs after significant decrements in filtration rate have occurred [47]. In a study of 48 patients with biopsy-proven tubulointerstitial nephritis, hypertension was present in only half the cases [113]. In the other half, the blood pressure was normal even in the presence of severe renal failure. Of the 15 cases with a creatinine clearance of less than 15 ml/minute the blood pressure was normal in seven patients.

Table 70-2. Morphologic features of tubulointerstitial nephritis

Feature	Acute	Chronic
I. *Interstitium**		
Cellular infiltrate	+ → + + + +	+ → + +
Edema	+ → + + + +	± → + +
Fibrosis	±	+ + → + + + +
II. *Tubules*		
Epithelium	Injury → necrosis	Atrophy
Basement membrane	Injury → disruption	Thickened
Shape	Preserved	Atrophy Dilatation
III. *Glomerulus*		
Structure	None → MCD	Periglomerular fibrosis Sclerosis
IV. *Vascular*		
Structure	Minimal Reversible	Variable Sclerosis

MCD = minimal change disease.
*The severity of the changes is given as an estimate with + for minimal to + + + + as severe.

Etiologic Factors and Pathogenetic Mechanisms

Arbitrarily grouped together because the predominant morphologic involvement is in the tubules and interstitium, tubulointerstitial nephropathies are caused by a motley group of diseases of varied and diverse etiologies (Table 70-3). Nor is the mechanism of interstitial injury known and, hence, the many postulated and different pathogenetic mechanisms that have been proposed include immunologic mechanisms, infection, toxic and metabolic perturbations, mechanical obstruction to urine flow, neoplasia, and hereditary factors.

IMMUNOLOGIC DISEASES

Although the immune pathogenesis of tubulointerstitial nephritis remains uncertain, evidence exists for three different immunologic mechanisms of tubulointerstitial injury: immune-complex deposition, antibodies directed against the tubular basement membrane (TBM), and altered cell-mediated immunity [286, 288, 291]. The best studied experimental model is that of anti-TBM nephritis [22, 458]. However, anti-TBM antibodies are a rare cause of tubulointerstitial nephritis in humans, except in association with antiglomerular basement membrane (anti-GBM) disease [288]. Altered cell-mediated immunity seems to be the more likely central event in the majority of cases of tubulointerstitial nephritis in humans [322, 458].

Immune-Complex Deposition. The repeated injection of homologous renal tissue in Freund's adjuvant into rabbits [220] and rats [195] results in tubulointerstitial immune-complex disease characterized by tubule cell injury, interstitial fibrosis, and mononuclear cell infiltration, with only minimal changes noted in the glomeruli. Immunofluorescent staining reveals granular deposits of immunoglobulins and complement along the tubular basement membrane. Electron microscopy confirms the presence of focal electron-dense deposits along the tubule. The postulated mechanism for this model of tubulointerstitial disease is that the circulating antibodies, which are formed in response to the injection of homologous renal tissue, diffuse across the peritubular capillaries and combine in the interstitium with a tubular cell antigen that diffuses out of the epithelial cells, thereby forming the interstitial immune complexes seen on microscopy. A similar lesion can be produced in rats immunized with Tamm-Horsfall (TH) protein, a surface membrane glycoprotein of the epithelial cells of the ascending thick limb of the loop of Henle and distal tubules. These animals develop antibodies to Tamm-Horsfall protein and a tubulointerstitial nephritis that selectively involves the thick ascending limb [195, 281, 395]. In this model, the earliest electron-dense deposits are detected in the extracellular space between the basal infoldings of the cell membranes and the tubular basement membrane. Later, they are noted within the tubular basement membrane. Selective mononuclear cell infiltrates occur around the tubules at the site of the deposits. Tubulointerstitial immune-complex nephritis has been also produced by passive immunization of rats with antisera to rat TH protein [135]. In these studies, the antibodies were noted to combine with TH at the base of the cells lining the thick ascending limb of Henle's loop and to form granular immune-complexes in situ in the spaces between the basal cell surface membrane and the tubular basement membranes. The deposits were maximal in the juxtamedullary region and least prominent in the first portion of the ascending limb in the inner zone of the outer medulla. Immune complexes also were selectively formed, at the same sites, during perfusion of the isolated kidneys with antisera of TH. The deposits of immune complexes were maximal during the first week after injection, at a time that the levels of circulating antibody titers were highest. As the antibody titers subsequently fell to undetectable levels, tubular immune complexes cleared rapidly and were virtually absent by about 4 weeks after the injection of the

Table 70-3. Conditions associated with chronic tubulointerstitial nephropathy

I. Immunologic diseases
  A. Systemic lupus erythematosus
  B. Sjögren syndrome
  C. Transplanted kidney
  D. Cryoglobulinemia
  E. Goodpasture syndrome
  F. IgA nephropathy
  G. Amyloidosis
  H. Pyelonephritis ?
II. Infection
  A. Systemic
  B. Renal
    1. Bacterial
    2. Viral
    3. Fungal
    4. Mycobacterial
III. Urinary tract obstructions
  A. Vesicoureteral reflux
  B. Mechanical
IV. Drugs
  A. Analgesics
  B. Cyclosporin
  C. Nitrosourea
  D. *Cis*-platinum
  E. Lithium
  F. Miscellaneous
V. Hematopoietic diseases
  A. Sickle hemoglobinopathies
  B. Multiple myeloma
  C. Lymphoproliferative disorders
  D. Aplastic anemia
VI. Heavy metals
  A. Lead
  B. Cadmium
  C. Miscellaneous
VII. Vascular diseases
  A. Nephrosclerosis
  B. Atheroembolic disease
  C. Radiation nephritis
  D. Diabetes mellitus
  E. Sickle hemoglobinopathies
  F. Vasculitis
VIII. Metabolic disorders
  A. Hyperuricemia/hyperuricosuria
  B. Hypercalcemia/hypercalciuria
  C. Hyperoxaluria
  D. Potassium depletion
  E. Cystinosis
IX. Hereditary diseases
  A. Medullary cystic disease
  B. Hereditary nephritis
  C. Medullary sponge kidney
  D. Polycystic kidney disease
  E. Familial juvenile nephronophthisis
X. Granulomatous diseases
  A. Sarcoidosis
  B. Tuberculosis
  C. Wegener's granulomatosis
XI. Endemic diseases
  A. Balkan nephropathy
  B. Nephropathia epidemica
XII. Idiopathic diseases

anti-TH antibodies. This is in contrast to the prolonged persistence of glomerular immune complex deposits that occurs after the experimental injection of appropriate antiglomerular antisera and may account for the rapid reversibility of immune injury in tubulointerstitial nephritis when exposure to the antibody is limited [135]. Also, although immunoglobulin deposition in the glomeruli correlates with glomerular damage, a similar association is not found between the extent of tubulointerstitial deposits and interstitial inflammation and tubular injury [268, 286, 288]. It is also in contrast to the perpetuation of tubulointerstitial injury noted in guinea pigs injected with isologous antitubular basement-membrane sera [168].

A role for TH protein-mediated immune-complex disease has been implicated in certain forms of human renal diseases. Antibodies to TH are found in sera of patients with vesicoureteral reflux [190] and pyelonephritis [171] and are demonstrated in the interstitium of patients with medullary cystic disease [446], hydronephrosis [24], and hereditary nephritis [255, 472], and in the glomeruli of patients with obstructive uropathy [357]. However, immunoglobulins are not regularly associated with TH protein deposits noted in the interstitium of human kidneys [357]. Additionally, the frequent occurrence of round cell infiltrates surrounding the immune-complex deposits may reflect on a cell-mediated inflammatory or immune process to account for the progressive nature of the renal injury in some of these clinical conditions. Actually, in experimental tubulointerstitial nephritis induced in guinea pigs by immunization with homologous TH protein, the transfer of lymphocytes and spleen cells to nonimmunized animals induces tubulointerstitial nephritis in the recipients [380], indicating a causative role of cell-mediated immunity. Finally, it is not possible to attribute a primary role to antibodies to TH or to that of any other cellular antigenic component, since the immune deposits could have followed primary tubular injury by another mechanism, with the subsequent release of TH or other cellular antigenic components into the system and the secondary formation of autologous antibodies. In fact, evidence has been advanced that the rise of intrarenal ammonia concentration, engendered by the adaptation to chronic disease, could determine attendant immunologic effects [219]. Because ammonia attacks the reactive thioestel bond of C_3 [192], the direct reaction of ammonia with C_3 forms aminated C_3, which is sufficient to trigger the alternative complement pathway and thereby propagate the peritubular deposition of C_3 and C_{5b-9}, and the generation of other mediators of tubulointerstitial injury [152]. In a study of rats with surgically reduced renal mass, dietary supplementation with sodium bicarbonate resulted in lower tissue levels of ammonia, less deposition of complement components, and a diminution of tubulointerstitial damage [318]. It is possible, therefore, that local activation can contribute to the propagation of interstitial injury by an immune-mediated mechanism independent of the initial etiology of the renal disease [76].

Primary tubulointerstitial nephritis mediated by immune-complex deposition is rare in humans [288]. The condition in which tubulointerstitial deposits are most commonly found clinically is lupus nephritis in which interstitial infiltrates are detected by light microscopy in more than half of biopsied cases [55, 218, 249, 468]. The deposits may be focal or diffuse. They are located either along or within the tubular basement membrane, around the peritubular capillaries, or in the interstitium. They consist principally of IgG and C_3 and often of IgM or IgA. Evidence for immune-complex mediated injury is adduced from the demonstration of DNA in the deposits. In general, the tubular and interstitial changes correlate with the magnitude of the deposits, although interstitial mononuclear cell infiltrates can be present in the kidneys of patients who have few, if any, tubulointerstitial immune-complex deposits [218, 249, 468]. Moreover, even in the presence of tubulointerstitial deposits, there is no correlation between the prevalence of immune-complex deposits and the severity of interstitial reaction, indicating a role other than pathogenetic mechanisms [334]. Nevertheless, the severity of the interstitial changes, independent of their pathogenesis, correlates quite well with the degree of renal insufficiency in lupus nephritis [267, 330, 334], and appraisal of the disease activity may be possible by renal imaging with gallium-67_c [21]. Prominent tubulointerstitial nephritis also can occur in cases of systemic lupus erythematosus with only mild glomerular involvement and generally pursues a rapid fulminant course [68].

Tubulointerstitial immune-complex deposits have been also described in renal allografts [8], Sjögren's syndrome [279, 300, 369, 461], mixed cryoglobulinemia [218], crescentic glomerulonephritis [249], IgA nephropathy [133], and Wegener's granulomatosis [9]. In addition, sera of some patients with idiopathic tubular dysfunction have been reported to contain antibodies that react with distal tubular epithelium [72, 129, 337]. However, aside from systemic lupus erythematosus, where antigen (DNA) has been demonstrated in the deposits, and mixed cryglobulinemia, where anti-IgG antibodies and IgG have been identified, there is no evidence concerning the identity of the antigen responsible for the deposits. Thus direct proof of immune-complex mediated injury is lacking in most of the clinical instances where deposits are noted on examination of the renal tissue.

Antibodies Against TBM. Evidence for anti-TBM antibody disease was first obtained when guinea pigs were noted to develop a progressive, fatal tubulointerstitial kidney disease after they were injected with crude rabbit cortical tissue in Freund's adjuvant [412]. Morphologic examination of the kidneys from these animals revealed tubular cell injury, peritubular multinucleated giant cells, interstitial fibrosis, and mononuclear cell infiltration. The infiltrating cells consisted of monocytes, macrophages, and T-cell lymphocytes. Linear deposits of IgG were noted along the TBM on immunofluorescent study [412, 413]. Similar lesions were produced in guinea pigs immunized with bovine TBM [247] and in the Brown Norway strain of rats, but not Sprague-Dawley or Lewis rats, immunized with homologous or heterologous TBM [248, 417]. In both species, the lesion could be reproduced in normal recipients by injecting them with serum from the immunized animals [413, 417]. Independent of the initiating role of anti-TBM antibodies, cell infiltrates are a prominent feature in all models studied, implicating a role for cell-mediated immunity in the pathogenesis and modulation of the interstitial lesions [322, 458]. Although the disease cannot be transmitted by cells in all species, it can be transferred by the intravenous injection of lymph node and splenic cells from sensitized animals in other species [22, 458], suggesting a central role for cell-mediated immunity.

Evidence for anti-TBM antibodies causing tubulointerstitial disease in human diseases has been advanced from cases of Goodpasture's syndrome associated with anti-GBM antibodies [249] and cases of rapidly progressive glomerulonephritis that have associated anti-TBM antibodies [9, 268]. In both models, absorption of eluates with solubilized GBM has been shown to remove the anti-TBM activity [291]. The target antigen in human anti-TBM disease has been identified as a 48-kd glycoprotein [77, 127, 323], which in experimental models has been shown to be secreted by proximal tubular cells into the extracellular matrix, where it attaches to the tubular basement membrane [322]. Anti-TBM antibodies also have been reported in cases of glomerulonephritis without associated anti-GBM antibodies [40, 305, 411], in renal allografts [8, 219, 457], and in lupus nephritis [166, 265].

Cell-Mediated Immunity. While the presence of anti-TBM antibodies or immune-complex deposits is a variable feature of tubulointerstitial disease, interstitial cell infiltration is an almost invariable essential component of the lesion. Most of the mononuclear cells making up the renal interstitium are T cells and are generally characterized by markers of activated lymphocytes [73, 92, 199]. Hence the possibility that cell-mediated immunologic mechanisms are involved in tubulointerstitial diseases can be considered on a reasonably solid basis [287]. Since both immune-complex mediated and anti-TBM nephritis can both be transferred by lymph node and spleen cells, a cell-mediated response appears to be an essential component of the immunopathology of all tubulointerstitial nephropathies [322, 458]. It is evident that antibody-dependent cell-mediated toxicity plays a role in different forms of anti-TBM and immune-complex mediated interstitial lesions. In fact, some rats injected with homologous kidney tissue develop interstitial mononuclear cell infiltrates before there is evidence of autoantibody production [286, 288]. This was also noted in the early studies of nonimmunosuppressed dog experimental kidney transplants [420]. In a study of guinea pigs sensitized to bovine gamma globulin, the direct injection of the heterologous globulin into the renal cortex resulted in a mononuclear interstitial infiltrate with focal tubular destruction [443]. This reactivity could then be transferred to unsensitized animals with lymph node cells, but not with serum, providing direct evidence for cell-mediated tubulointerstitial injury in this experimental model.

Cellular reactivity to bacterial antigens has been implicated in the pathogenesis of interstitial lesions of pyelonephritis [390]. Utilizing an indirect fluorescent method for the detection of a common enterobacterial antigen in infected tissues, it was shown that bacterial antigen persisted in renal scars after the healing of experimental pyelonephritis [87, 378]. In one clinical study, bacterial antigen was found in 6 of 7 kidneys of patients with "abacterial" pyelonephritis who had not had clinical or bacteriologic evidence of infection for as long as 19 years preceding the study [11]. This finding, however, could not be substantiated in other studies where the antigen could be demonstrated in kidneys from acute pyelonephritis caused by enteric organisms, but not in those with chronic interstitial nephritis, nonspecific renal scars, or patients with pyelonephritis who were bacteriologically free of infecting organisms [390]. Experimental studies reveal that rats with acute enteric streptococcal pyelonephritis develop cellular reactivity to bacteria, as indicated by lymphocyte stimulation in vitro. In these animals, bacterial antigens can be shown by immunofluorescent studies within both the infiltrating leukocytes and the interstitium. However, after eradication of the infection, bacterial antigens are not demonstrable in the interstitium and, when present, are found only within macrophages [87, 390]. It would seem unlikely, therefore, that delayed reactivity against bacterial antigens could provide a mechanism for the perpetuation of pyelonephritis beyond the period when viable organisms are present in the kidney [87, 189, 378, 390].

INFECTION

Whereas the role of bacterial infection as the major determinant for the development of acute pyelonephritis is unequivocal, the role of recurrent infection as a cause of chronic renal damage remains doubtful. Progression from acute infection to chronic "atrophic" pyelonephritis does not appear to be a result of persistent or recurrent infection but, instead, may be due to immune mechanisms [10] or associated mechanical outflow obstruction [188–190]. Several studies of a large number of adult women and men with significant bacteriuria, who were followed over a decade, have shown that urinary tract infection does not lead to kidney damage, provided the condition is not associated with obstruction and there are no coexistent diseases, such as diabetes and hypertension [14, 134]. In children, however, bacteriuria does not necessarily pursue the relatively benign course it does in adults [147, 233, 362]. Chronic atrophic pyelonephritis, with classic tubulointerstitial lesions, is a disease of childhood that manifests itself clinically in adult life [362]. Children under the age of 5 to 6 years, in whom urinary tract infection coexists with vesicoureteral reflux and who develop pyelotubular back-flow appear to be the ones at risk of developing renal interstitial injury, scarring, and, ultimately, renal atrophy. In fact, reflux or obstruction without complicating infection can itself be detrimental to the tubules and interstitium [189, 190]. However, it is mainly children in whom coexistent infection and vesicoureteral reflux persist despite treatment who are the ones to develop renal scars and tubulointerstitial disease [405]. In one study [381], a 2-year follow-up revealed the formation of new scars in 3 out of 34 children whose infection was untreated as compared to only 1 out of 26 children whose bacteriuria was treated. Thus the role of infection is not to be discounted. Whether urinary tract infection uncomplicated by obstruction causes sufficient interstitial injury to result in irreversible changes and progressive renal disease is questionable [196, 362]. Nevertheless, obstruction or vesicoureteral reflux may produce renal injury either by causing recurrent infection or by back-pressure damage in the absence of infection [190].

Experimentally, the unmanipulated urinary tract is remarkably resistant to retrograde challenge with an infection inoculum, whereas direct intrarenal injection of organisms causes bacterial proliferation and elicits a local cellular reaction [298]. The initial inflammatory response to infection of the renal parenchyma is that of a classic tubulointerstitial nephritis characterized by edema, cellular infiltration, and tubular damage. To determine whether this initial response results in progressive injury after sterilization of the urinary tract, efforts have been made to characterize the local response and the immunologic activity to the lymphoid cells isolated from the experimentally infected kidney [250, 299, 300]. Within the first few days following infection, polymorphonuclear leukocytes predominate in the interstitium and tubular lumen, and the renal epithelial cells express class II major histocompatibility antigens [234] and the tumor necrosis alpha gene [466], indicating their ability to act as antigen presenting cells. Within the subsequent days, the neutrophilic infiltrate dissipates while a dense mononuclear lymphocytic infiltrate develops, indicating an active cellular response evident by presence of the B lymphocytes, a depression of the T lymphocytes' helper activity, while that of the T cell suppressor activity is increased [300]. There is also evidence for the local activation and deposition of the complement system [363] and for an increased local production of IgG, IgM, and IgA by the infected kidney [406]. During an acute infection, an increase in the level of circulating antibodies to TH have been reported [170, 171]. The level of antibodies decreases once the active infection is eradicated, and clearance studies have shown its rapid clearance from local deposits [135]. Whether these antibodies or the local cellular infiltrates play a role in the perpetuation of chronic renal injury and scarring is a possibility that has been proposed by some [11] but questioned by others [390]. The potential for ammonia production by urease-producing organisms has been implicated in the propensity of these organisms to produce renal injury [76, 192].

Preexisting renal disease or an immunocompromised host seems to predispose to the detrimental effect of infection [111, 403]. The latter is best exemplified by the unusual infections causing interstitial injury encountered in renal allografts [348, 403] and the kidney of patients with AIDS [53]. Actually, renal allografts and the kidney of patients with AIDS appear to be prone to tubulointerstitial nephritis even in the absence of superimposed infection [83, 396].

OBSTRUCTION AND REFLUX

Interstitial changes are a prominent feature of urinary tract obstruction of any etiology. The initial structural changes that follow are those of tubular dilatation and cortical infiltration with lymphocytes. Later, a network of fibrosis, extending from the capsule through the medulla of the affected pyramid, develops. Fibrosis gradually increases and causes contraction and scarring [189]. Proliferation of interstitial cells also occurs following ureteral obstruction [316, 317]. The whole process can occur in the absence of infection. If infection is deliberately induced, or occurs spontaneously, a polymorphonuclear reaction occurs and tubular casts are noted. More importantly, in the coexistence of infection, the fibrosis is more extensive.

Renal damage depends on the degree of incompetence of the ureterovesical valve, the magnitude of pressure that develops, and the length of time that the vesicoureteral reflux persists before correction. In persons with neurogenic bladder disorders, where a high-pressure condition develops, vesicoureteral reflux occurs as a secondary event. In one study, over 90 percent of children and 50 percent of adults with pyelonephritic scars had vesicoureteral reflux on voiding cystourethrogram. In 89 percent of adults with scars, cystoscopic examination revealed abnormal ureteral orifices, suggesting ureteral reflux [445].

The importance of reflux of infected urine in the causation of tubulointerstitial lesions and atrophic kidney is now well established [12, 189]. The role of sterile urine reflux, in doing so, although supported by experimental studies in pigs, remains to be documented in humans. A role for extravasation of TH protein in causing immune-mediated injury in the absence of infection has been postulated to occur in patients with vesicoureteral reflux, urine outflow obstruction, or inadequately draining transplanted kidneys [184, 266]. The tubular rupture responsible for extravasation is related to the increased pressure in the tubules when the intrapelvic pressure rises in the presence of urine flow obstruction [153]. Studies in 23 human neonatal kidneys obtained at autopsy have shown that the range of pressure needed to cause pyelotubular back-flow, with extravasation into the interstitial tissue, was 22 to 87 mm Hg, with a mean of 47 mm Hg [301]. Pyelovenous reflux occurs in about 50 percent of cases when intrapelvic pressures of 50 to 70 mm Hg are induced experimentally and in 100 percent of cases when pressures in excess of 70 mm Hg are attained [184, 302]. In humans, intrapelvic pressures of over 70 mm Hg are attained in patients with hydronephrosis and focal pyelotubular back-flow can be demonstrated radiologically [360]. Vesicoureteral reflux of a minor degree probably causes no renal damage. But vesicoureteral reflux in a high-pressure situation or in the presence of infection does appear to be associated with tubulointerstitial injury. Thus, whereas renal scarring as a result of intrarenal reflux, secondary to urinary outflow obstruction of any cause, does occur, no comprehensive uniform explanation has been advanced for the renal scarring and atrophy that develops.

Most of the experimental work attempting to explore the pathogenesis of scarring has been done on rats, where the unilobular pelvic anatomy is different from that of human kidney, which is multilobular and has 8 to 12 calyces [302]. The pig kidney used in some studies is multilobular and, therefore, considered more analogous to human anatomy [190]. About 75 percent of human kidneys have compound papillae, which fuse to drain several papillae and are generally in a polar location. The ducts of Bellini in some of the compound renal papillae have round or oval wide-open orifices, as opposed to the narrow slitlike orifices of the simple single papilla [427]. Thus, if the pressure of the refluxing urine is sufficient to overcome the pressure within the nephrons of the compound renal papillae, intrarenal reflux can occur [352, 356]. This accounts for the experimental and clinical observation that reflux can be demonstrated in only some segments of the kidney and that these are usually at a polar location. However, if the tubular flow is high and there is a large diuresis, intrarenal reflux may be prevented [122].

Of interest are the changes of the parenchymal cell content and function that accompany increased intrapelvic pressure. Mononuclear cell infiltration is one of the earliest responses of the kidney to ureteral obstruction. The infiltrating cells are macrophages and suppressor and cytotoxic lymphocytes [387]. Cultures of the fibroblastic type of cortical interstitial cells from explants of unilateral hydronephrotic rabbit kidneys, compared to those from the contralateral normal kidney, grow significantly faster and have increased prostaglandin E_2 production in response to bradykinin [96]. The release of various prostaglandins, by the infiltrating cells of the hydronephrotic kidney, appear to exert a significant modulating role in the transport processes and hemodynamic changes seen early in the course of obstruction [387, 388].

Also of note in reflux nephropathy are the glomerular changes that develop in the later phases of the disease in some cases. As a rule, the glomerular changes commonly encountered are ischemic in nature, consisting of sclerosis, periglomerular fibrosis, and obsolescence. In a few, focal and segmental glomerulosclerosis and hyalinosis will develop and are manifested clinically by massive proteinuria and rapidly progressive renal failure. The affected glomeruli commonly contain IgM and C_3 when examined by immunofluorescent microscopy, suggesting an immunologic mechanism [88, 214, 397, 436]. The nature of the immune reaction remains unclear. Autologous (TH protein, brush-border antigen) or bacterial antigen derivatives have been incriminated. The hemodynamic changes that develop in the glomeruli of remaining intact nephrons, adapting to reduction in renal mass by hyperfiltration, have also been implicated [88].

DRUGS

Drugs that are the major cause of acute tubulointerstitial disease also produce the chronic forms of tubulointerstitial nephropathy. Patients who develop the acute form of drug-induced tubulointerstitial nephritis generally recover fully. A few, however, do not recover and progress to chronic tubulointerstitial diseases, as best exemplified by cis-platinum [97, 266]. Most cases that develop drug-induced chronic tubulointerstitial nephritis do so insidiously, during or after the chronic use of one or more drugs. The latter is best exemplified by analgesic abuse nephropathy [110, 179], while the former includes cases due to prolonged exposure to cyclosporine [423], cis-platinum [46], nitrosurea [173], lithium [69, 169], methotrexate [347], and nonsteroidal anti-inflammatory agents [78, 178]. The risk of chronic tubulointerstitial nephropathy with these latter agents is quite small, often preventable, and their risk-benefit ratio is much too small to limit their clinical use beneficially.

The lesions of analgesic abuse deserve special consideration. In fact, it is, to a great extent, the appreciation of their role in the causation of chronic interstitial nephritis that had the greatest impact in questioning the wisdom of attributing all interstitial lesions to pyelonephritis. In the initial reports from Switzerland, the lesion was described as chronic interstitial nephritis (chronische interstielle nephritis), with a high incidence of papillary necrosis [410, 471]. Subsequent reports established papillary necrosis as a prominent lesion of analgesic-associated nephropathy (AAN) and documented the significance and occurrence of this problem worldwide [140, 141, 203, 241, 377, 386]. From the outset, it was evident that there was considerable variation in the incidence of AAN in different parts of the world (Australia > New Zealand > Scandinavia > England > Canada > U.S.A.), with wide regional differences within each country [110, 151, 159, 284, 311, 312, 349].

Because of the extremely common abuse of analgesic compounds, a common ingredient of which was phenacetin, the lesions of AAN were initially attributed to phenacetin [203, 351]. Subsequent clinical studies, however, questioned the role of any single agent as the cause of renal disease [213], and despite the withdrawal of phenacetin, AAN has remained one of the main causes of end-stage renal failure in Switzerland, Belgium, and Germany [159]. The preponderance of experimental studies indicate that phenacetin, paracetamol, or aspirin given alone are only moderately nephrotoxic, even in massive doses. Renal lesions can be much more readily induced when a mixture of aspirin and paracetamol or phenacetin is used, particularly when combined with water deprivation [19, 110]. In all experimental studies, the extent of renal injury was dose-dependent and, when examined, water diuresis was shown to protect from analgesic-induced renal injury [105, 110]. Actually, phenacetin itself is not toxic; it is rapidly metabolized by the liver to paracetamol (*N*-acetyl-*p*-aminophenol), which is then excreted by the kidneys either as the free compound or its conjugate. The bulk of the conjugate consists of the glucuronide and a smaller portion of the sulfate. Both paracetamol and its conjugate attain significant (four- to fivefold) concentrations in the medulla and papilla, depending on the state of hydration of the animal studied. Their toxic effect is apparently related to their intrarenal oxidation to reactive intermediates, which, in the absence of reducing substances, such as gluthathione, become cytotoxic by virtue of their capacity to induce oxidation [18, 105, 130]. Salicylates are also significantly (6- to 13-fold) concentrated in the medulla and papilla, where they attain a sufficient level to uncouple oxidative phosphorylation and reduce the ability of cells to generate reducing substances [105, 130]. Thus both agents attain sufficient renal medullary concentration to individually exert a detrimental and injurious effect on cell function. Their simultaneous presence results in an additive effect because of the salicylate-induced decrease in reducing capability at a time when the concentration of the reactive oxidative by-products of phenacetin are increased locally. Considered in this context, it is evident why water diuresis, by reducing the medullary tonicity and, therefore, that of the medullary concentration of drug attained, protects from analgesic-induced cell injury [95, 105, 110]. A direct role of analgesic-induced injury can be adduced from the arrest of the progress of renal dysfunction and, generally, improvement of renal function that are noted on cessation of analgesic abuse [32, 416].

The intrarenal distribution of analgesics provides an explanation for the medullary location of the pathologic lesions of analgesic abuse (Fig. 70-6). The initial lesions are patchy and consist of necrosis of the interstitial cells, thin loops of the loops of Henle, and vasa recta of the papilla. The collecting ducts are spared. The quantity of tubular and vascular basement membrane and ground substance are increased. At this stage, the kidneys are normal in size and there are no abnormalities in the renal cortex. With persistent drug exposure, the changes extend to the outer medulla. Again, the lesions are initially patchy, involving the interstitial cells, the loops of Henle, and vascular bundles. With continued drug abuse, the severity of the inner medullary lesions increases with sclerosis and obliteration of the capillaries, atrophy and degeneration of the loops of Henle and collecting ducts, and the beginning of calcification of the necrotic foci. Ultimately, the papillae become entirely necrotic, with sequestration and demarcation of the necrotic tissue. The necrotic papillae may then slough and are excreted into the urine or remain in situ, where they atrophy further and become calcified. Cortical scarring, characterized by interstitial fibrosis, tubular atrophy, and periglomerular fibrosis, develops over the necrotic medullary segments. The medullary rays traversing the cortex are usually spared and become hypertrophic, thereby imparting a characteristic cortical nodularity to the now shrunken kidneys. Examination of the renal tissue at this late stage of AAN reveals the classic features of cortical tubulointerstitial nephropathy [140, 149, 213, 215, 303].

As might be expected from the slow progressive nature of the lesion, the deterioration of renal function is insidious. In all cases, there is a relationship between renal function and the duration, intensity, and quantity

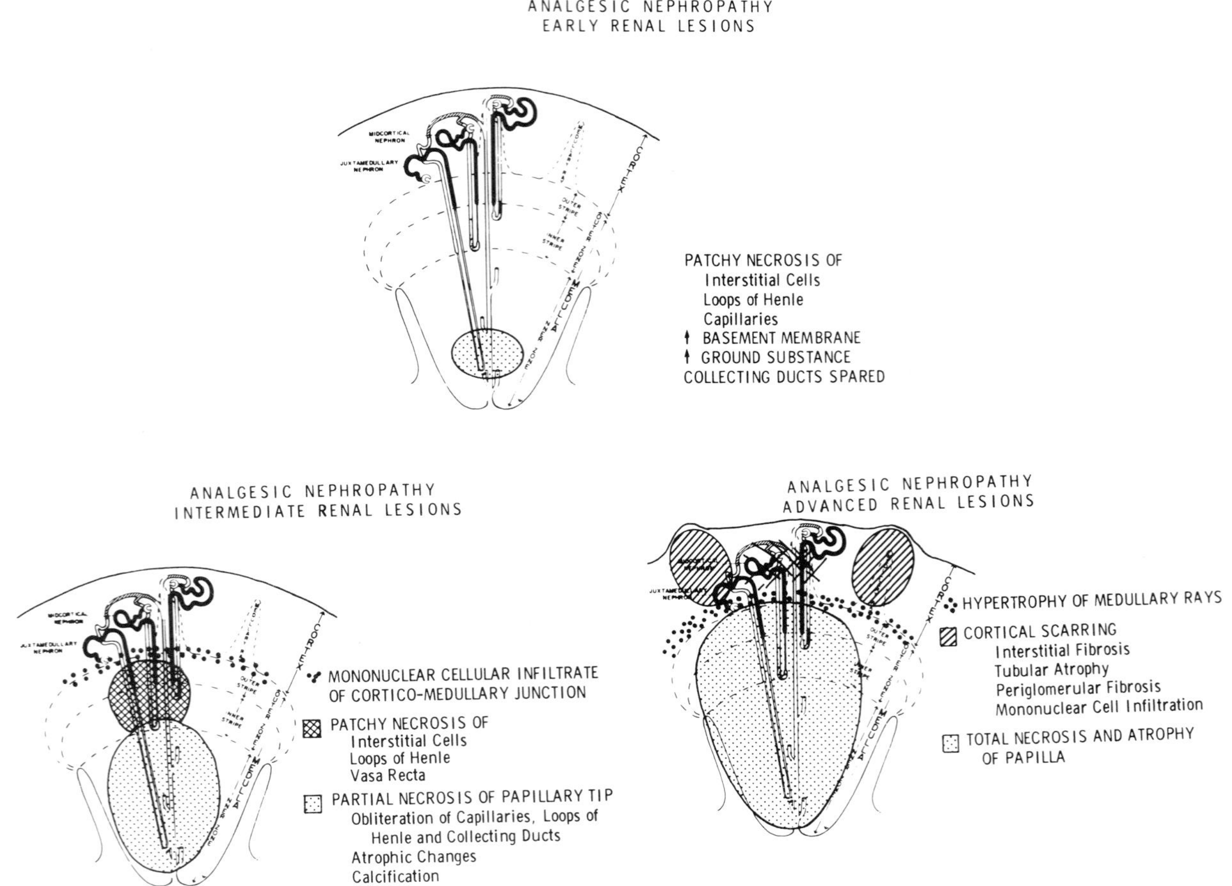

Fig. 70-6. The course and stages of analgesic nephropathy. (Reproduced with permission from [110].)

of analgesic consumed [102, 103]. The magnitude of injury is related to the quantity of analgesic ingested chronically over the years. In persons with significant renal impairment, the average dose ingested has been estimated at about 10 kg over a mean period of 13 years [60]. The minimum amount of drug consumption that results in significant renal damage is unknown. It has been estimated that a cumulative dose of 3 kg of the index compound, or a daily ingestion of 1 gm per day over 3 years or more, is a minimum that can result in detectable renal impairment [311]. Only a minority of persons who regularly take analgesic mixtures develop renal injury [103]. There is also considerable variation in the severity of the renal lesions in those who do develop renal injury. One reason for this variable response may be adduced from the experimental evidence for the medullary concentration of analgesics and the prevention of renal injury by hydration [105].

It is possible that those who develop renal lesions ingest lower quantities of fluid or are subjected to dehydration due to environmental conditions. This issue has not been investigated clinically, although a role for dehydration due to the climatic conditions has been proposed as one reason for the geographic variability in the incidence of analgesic nephropathy [110]. Other factors that might contribute to dehydration, such as laxative and diuretic use, have also been implicated [310, 447]. Differences in the content of the mixtures also could account for the geographic variation in the incidence of AAN [310, 328]. Finally, coexistent diseases, such as diabetes, sickle cell disease, and infection, which themselves cause tubulointerstitial nephritis, may predispose analgesic abusers to more severe renal injury [110].

Consumption of phenacetin-containing analgesics has been associated with a significant increase of urothelial tumors of the renal pelvis, ureters, and bladder [18]. The tumors occur after a latent period of decades, are typically multiple, are poorly differentiated, and spread rapidly. Epidemiologic and retrospective case control studies of the role of paracetamol association with urothelial tumors have yielded negative results [289, 345]. The presence of renal papillary necrosis in phenacetin abusers significantly increases the relative risk for urothelial cancer [290].

Tubulointerstitial nephritis has emerged as the most serious side effect of *cyclosporine* [296]. Cyclosporine-mediated vasoconstriction of the cortical microvasculature has been implicated in the development of an occlusive arteriolopathy and tubular epithelial cell injury [297, 321, 401, 462]. While these early lesions tend to be reversible upon cessation of therapy, an irreversible interstitial fibrosis and cellular infiltrate develop with prolonged use of the drug, especially in higher doses [148, 222, 373, 423]. The irreversible nature of this tubulointerstitial nephritis and its attendant reduction in renal function have raised serious concerns regarding the long-term use of this otherwise efficient immunosuppressive agent [315, 356], whose use has been proposed in the treatment of tubulointerstitial nephritis [322].

HEMATOPOIETIC DISORDERS

The renal lesion that develops in disorders of the hematopoietic system is generally that of a tubulointerstitial nephropathy. This is by far most common in persons with a sickle cell hemoglobinopathy. Although more frequent in those with sickle cell disease (SS), tubulointerstitial lesions also are common in those with sickle cell trait (SA), sickle cell hemoglobin C disease (SC), or sickle cell thalassemia (S thal) [398, 439]. The predisposing factors that lead to the propensity of renal involvement are the physicochemical properties of hemoglobin S that predispose its polymerization in an environment of low oxygen tension, hypertonicity, and low pH [398]. These are conditions that are characteristic to the renal medulla and, therefore, conducive to the intraerythrocyte polymerization of hemoglobin S and consequent erythrocyte sickling, which accounts for the development of typical vascular occlusive lesions [210, 411]. Although some of these lesions occur in the cortex, the lesions start and are predominantly located in the inner medulla and are at the core of the focal scarring and interstitial fibrosis [43, 57, 212, 439] and account for the common occurrence of papillary necrosis in these persons [110]. The incidence of radiographically demonstrable papillary necrosis has been reported to be as high as 33 to 65 percent [439]. Tubular function abnormalities such as impaired concentrating ability, depressed distal potassium and hydrogen secretion, tubular proteinuria, and decreased proximal reabsorption of phosphate and increased secretion of creatinine are common and detectable early in the course of the disease [6].

Disorders of plasma cell function also produce tubulointerstitial disease. Actually, the pathogenesis of renal involvement is of varied etiologies [278], and the renal complications of multiple myeloma are a major contributing factor in the morbidity and mortality of this neoplastic disorder [235]. However, it has become apparent that ultimate survival depends to a great extent on the hematologic response to chemotherapy and much less on the coexistent renal involvement that is amenable to dialytic therapy [201, 226]. The lesions that are directly the result of excessive production of light chains are those caused by the precipitation of the light-chain dimers in the distal tubules and result in what has been termed *myeloma cast nephropathy*. The affected tubules are surrounded by chronic inflammatory cells, interstitial fibrosis, and multinucleated giant cells [235, 252, 346]. Adjoining tubules show varying degrees of atrophy. The propensity of light chains to lead to myeloma cast nephropathy appears to be related to their concentration in the tubular fluid and the tubular fluid pH, rather than to their intrinsic physicochemical properties as was initially postulated [79, 236, 327]. This accounts for the observation that increasing the flow rate of urine or its alkalinization will prevent or reverse the casts in their early stages of formation. Direct tubular toxicity of light chains also may contribute to the tubular injury [346]. Lambda light chains appear to be more injurious than kappa light chains [79]. Binding of human kappa and lambda light chains to human and rat proximal tubule epithelial cell brush-border membrane has been demonstrated [26]. Analysis of the binding data reveals a single class of low-affinity, high-capacity binding sites that are specific to light chains. Another mechanism whereby plasma cell dyscrasias cause tubulointerstitial lesions is related to the interstitial and perivascular deposition of paraproteins, either as amyloid fibrils that are derived from lambda chains or as fragments of light chains that are derived from kappa chains and produce the so-called light-chain deposition disease [346]. Of these various lesions, myeloma cast nephropathy appears to be the most common, being observed in one-third of the autopsied cases, followed by amyloid deposition, present in 10 percent of cases, while intramembranous light-chain deposition is relatively rare, i.e., less than 5 percent of cases [202].

The kidney is one of the most common extranodal sites of metastatic lymphomas [275]. Infiltration of the kidney is frequent in patients with acute lymphoblastic leukemia and non-Hodgkin's lymphomas but less common in those with Hodgkin's disease [346]. Renal infiltrates are generally clinically silent and only result in renal failure either from vascular or ureteral compression or from extensive parenchyma infiltration [204].

HEAVY METALS

Environmental exposure to *cadmium* results in its accumulation in the body, where it is preferentially concentrated in the kidney, principally in the proximal tubule, in the form of a cadmium-metallothionein complex that has a biologic half-life of approximately 10 years [54]. Because of its chronic local toxic effect, an insidious form of chronic tubulointerstitial nephropathy results, the principal manifestations of which are proximal tubule dysfunction [2, 206, 255].

Exposure to *lead*, as an occupational hazard or its ingestion in moonshine whiskey, results in its insidious accumulation in the body [306, 452]. This subclinical accumulation of lead has been implicated in the causation of hyperuricemia, hypertension, and renal failure [27, 28]. Focal tubulointerstitial lesions are present in as many as half of such cases. The infusion of calcium disodium ethylene diaminetetraacetic acid (EDTA) to mobilize body stores of lead is a useful diagnostic tool for the detection and treatment of this disorder [28, 453]. Chelation therapy with EDTA is effective in reducing the total body load of lead but is not always effective in preventing progressive renal disease [143]. The lesions of gouty nephropathy have been attributed to lead overload [28]. Rare cases of tubulointerstitial nephropathy have been reported as being caused by exposure to *silicon, copper, bismuth, barium, uranium, arsenic* [350, 371], and possibly organic solvents [320].

VASCULAR DISEASES

Tubular degeneration, interstitial fibrosis, and mononuclear cell infiltration are part of the degenerative process that affects the kidneys in vascular diseases that involve the intrarenal vasculature with any degree of severity as to result in ischemia [437]. Rarely, if the insult is sudden and massive, the lesions are those of infarction and acute deterioration of renal function. More commonly, the vascular lesions develop gradually and will go undetected until renal insufficiency supervenes. It is this chronic form that accounts for the tubulointerstitial lesions of arteriolar nephrosclerosis and hypertension [47] and contributes to the renal interstitial lesions of patients with diabetes [142] and sickle cell hemoglobinopathy [439] and vasculitis [3, 325].

The renal injury caused by radiation, which is characteristically one of tubulointerstitial nephropathy, is also ischemic in origin because of the radiation-induced injury of the renal vasculature [207, 261]. The rash of cases that were reported in the 1940s and 1960s resulted from the failure to recognize the sensitivity of renal vessels to irradiation [15] and the then prevailing misconception that the kidney was resistant to radiation injury [13]. Recognition that the total dose and frequency of its administration are important determinants of nephrotoxicity has resulted in a dramatic decrease in the frequency with which radiation-induced tubulointerstitial lesions are currently encountered.

METABOLIC DISORDERS

Urate. The kidneys are the major organs for the excretion of uric acid and a primary target organ affected in disorders of urate metabolism. The renal lesions result from crystallization of uric acid either in the urine outflow tract or in the renal parenchyma [63, 128, 451]. The determinants of uric acid solubility are its concentration and the pH of the medium in which it is dissolved [217]. Consequently, the supersaturation of the tubular fluid, as the excreted uric acid becomes concentrated in the medulla, and the acidification of the urine in the distal tubule will, of necessity, be conducive to the precipitation of uric acid. Not unexpectedly then, the major sites of urate deposition are the renal medulla, the collecting tubules, and the urinary tract. The pK of uric acid is 5.4, and at the acid pH of the distal tubule fluid, the bulk of the filtered urate will be present in its nonionized form as uric acid, whereas at the more alkaline pH of the blood and interstitium, it is in its ionized form as urate salts. If deposition occurs in an acid medium, as in the tubular fluid, birefringent uric acid crystals are formed, whereas in an alkaline medium, as in the interstitium, amorphous urate salts are deposited [116, 118]. Depending on the load of uric acid presented to the kidneys, one of three disorders will result: acute uric acid nephropathy, uric acid nephrolithiasis, and chronic urate nephropathy. While either one of the former two forms can produce tubulointerstitial lesions, only the latter will be considered here, since uric acid nephropathy is an acute lesion and uric acid nephrolithiasis produces its effect by obstruction.

The principal lesion of chronic hyperuricemia is the deposition of microtophi of amorphous urate crystals in the interstitium, with a surrounding giant-cell reaction [23, 150, 221]. The earlier change, however, is probably due to the precipitation of birefringent uric acid crystals in the collecting tubules, with consequent tubular obstruction, dilatation, atrophy, and interstitial fibrosis [116, 393]. Experimental evidence in support for a role of tubular precipitation of uric acid has been advanced from studies on pigs fed an exogenous purine diet [124]. Additional support derives from the reported high incidence of uric acid crystals in the kidneys of patients with gout and those with Lesch-Nyhan syndrome [128, 426]. The proposal has, therefore, been made that the majority of patients whose hyperuricemia and gout are due to decreased uric acid excretion, rather than overproduction, should be spared from renal injury. However, this is not the case, since renal lesions are encountered in these "under excretors." The renal injury of these persons has been attributed to hyperacidity of the urine because of an inherent abnormality in their ability to produce ammonia [439]. The acidity of urine is important because uric acid is 17 times less soluble than urate and, therefore, it facilitates precipitation in the distal nephron of those who are not overproducers but have an acid urine.

The earlier notion that chronic renal disease was more common in patients with hyperuricemia [426] has been questioned in light of recent prolonged longitudinal studies of renal function in persons with hyperuricemia [430, 467, 468]. Renal dysfunction could be documented only when the serum urate was over 10 mg/dl in women and over 13 mg/dl in men for prolonged periods. The deterioration of renal function in those with hyperuricemia of a lower magnitude has been attributed to the higher-than-expected occurrence of concurrent hypertension, diabetes mellitus, abnormal lipid metabolism, and nephrosclerosis [104, 294]. Of particular interest in this regard has been the evidence presented for an association between renal disease and hyperuricemia in persons with a past history of exposure to lead and consequent subclinical lead toxicity [27, 28]. A series of studies from New Jersey have shown that patients with coexistent hyperuricemia and renal dysfunction have lead overload, whereas those with hyperuricemia and normal renal function had normal body lead stores. The mechanism whereby lead aggravates hyperuricemia is not clear [125].

Oxalate. The increased production or intestinal absorption of oxalate, with its consequent increased renal excretion, almost invariably results in its precipitation as calcium oxalate in the urine outflow tract [123, 186]. Microcrystallization first occurs in the proximal tubules where oxalate secretion occurs [123, 211, 432], but the lesions that develop are more severe in the renal medulla, where the increasing concentration of the tubular fluid and its acidification promote the precipitation of calcium oxalate [186, 187, 453]. This results in atrophy of the epithelial cells lining the affected tubules, interstitial edema, and inflammatory cell infiltration [186, 453].

Hyperoxaluria may be primary or acquired [186]. The primary form is a rare inherited disorder due to an enzymatic abnormality in the metabolism of glyoxylic acid. The acquired forms of hyperoxaluria are more common and result either from the ingestion of oxalate precursors, such as ethylene glycol [448], ascorbic acid [242], and exposure to methoxyflurane anesthesia [282]; or its increased absorption from the intestinal tract of persons with inflammatory bowel disease or who have undergone small bowel resection [71, 91]. When the hyperoxaluria is sudden and massive, such as after ethylene glycol ingestion, acute renal failure develops. Otherwise, as with most cases of hyperoxaluria, the overload is insidious and chronic; as a result, interstitial fibrosis, tubular atrophy, and dilatation result in a chronic tubulointerstitial nephritis, with progressive renal failure. The propensity to recurrent calcium oxalate nephrolithiasis and consequent obstructive uropathy contributes to the tubulointerstitial lesions.

Hypercalcemia. Given the many and vital roles of calcium in normal cell function, it is evident why changes in calcium concentration, either in the blood or urine, produce immediate reversible changes in renal function, which are followed by irreversible structural changes if calcium derangement goes undetected or remains unremedied [35]. In most instances, the severity and potential reversibility of the changes that occur are related to the degree and duration of the hypercalcemia [34, 117]. Acute changes in tubular function and renal hemodynamics have been noted to develop in several experimental studies [146, 253, 274, 420]. A defect in the urinary concentration is the most notable tubular dysfunction [34, 117, 420]. It is multifactorial in origin but results mainly from a direct inhibitory effect of calcium on the reabsorption of sodium in the tubule, in general, but the loop of Henle, in particular [34, 117, 420], and from an altered responsiveness of the collecting duct to antidiuretic hormone [30, 41, 101, 341]. The hemodynamic changes are due to an effect of calcium on the systemic as well as renal vasculature, either directly or indirectly through its effect on cardiac function [117, 274, 398].

Focal degeneration and necrosis of the tubular epithelium, primarily in the medulla where calcium is concentrated, occur shortly after persistent hypercalcemia and have been attributed to increased intracellular and mitochondrial calcium content [70, 139, 383]. The subsequent calcification and destruction of the tubular basement membrane results in proliferative and infiltrative changes of the adjacent interstitium, whereas the sloughing of necrotic cells results in tubular atrophy and obstruction with consequent dilatation and pressure injury to the proximal segments of the tubule [139, 316, 383]. Early changes in the proximal tubule also have been noted [70, 144]. Deposition of calcium in the necrotic and injured areas results in the characteristic nephrocalcinosis seen on radiography or noted at autopsy [34, 117, 144, 383]. The deposition of calcium in the glomerular capillaries and vasculature probably contributes to the further progression of the injury. The final lesion of focal scarified areas of tubular atrophy, increased interstitial fibrosis, and mononuclear cell infiltration is a classic example of chronic tubulointerstitial disease. The propensity to kidney stone formation and, therefore, to obstructive uropathy also can contribute to the tubulointerstitial lesions.

Potassium Depletion. A variety of well-documented abnormalities of renal function accompany the development of potassium depletion [355, 391], the hallmark of which is a vasopressin-resistant impairment of the ability to concentrate the urine [354, 355, 372], increased ammoniagenesis [428], and a modest reduction of the glomerular filtration rate [355, 372]. The characteristic structural change that accompanies potassium depletion in humans is that of vacuolation of the renal tubular epithelial due to the dilated cisternae of the endoplasmic reticulum and the basilar foldings of the cells [44]. The lesions are generally limited to the proximal tubule segments, with only focal changes in the distal segment. With potassium repletion, both the functional and structural changes appear to be reversible [355, 391]. Whether they can progress to a chronic tubulointerstitial nephropathy and result in persistent renal dysfunction is uncertain, but seems to depend on the duration and extent of potassium depletion [90, 355, 391]. A familial form of hypokalemic tubulointerstitial nephritis with progressive renal failure has been described [164, 450]. Experimental potassium depletion in rats has been reported to result in persistent interstitial fibrosis and scarring several months after potassium repletion [131]. Actually, in rats, the lesions of acute potassium depletion are more extensive than in humans, with vacuolation and tubular hyperplasia affecting both the proximal and distal tubule segments [434, 464]. These changes have been attributed to the susceptibility of potassium-depleted rats to chronic pyelonephritis [90, 464], although the evidence that potassium depletion predisposes to pyelonephritis is not well established and is controversial at best [66]. A principal cause of renal injury may well be the augmented ammoniagenesis associated with hypokalemia. Ammonia directly activates the alternate complement pathway and thereby sets off an immune-mediated process of progressive tubulointerstitial injury [76]. In hypokalemic rats, suppression of ammoniagenesis with bicarbonate supplementation has been shown to ameliorate the tubulointerstitial lesions [435].

Cystinosis. Cystinosis is a rare autosomal inherited disorder of amino acid metabolism that is characterized by the deposition of cystine crystals throughout the body [389]. The early lesions of the kidney in these persons is a "swan neck" deformity or atrophy of the proximal tubule segments that are adjacent to cystine-containing interstitial cells. The structural changes coincide with the development of proximal tubular dysfunction characteristic of the Fanconi syndrome [410], which is one of the eponyms used in describing this entity [389]. Progressive interstitial fibrosis, tubular atrophy, and interstitial inflammatory reaction result in progression to end-stage renal failure [429]. The characteristic rhomboid-shaped crystals of cystine that are generally seen in the interstitium also have been noted in the glomerular and tubular cells [176].

HEREDITARY DISEASES OF THE KIDNEY

Tubulointerstitial lesions are a prominent component of the renal pathology of a variety of hereditary diseases of the kidney, such as the medullary cystic disease, familial juvenile nephronephritis, medullary sponge kidney, polycystic kidney disease, and hereditary nephritis [42, 84]. The primary disorder of these conditions is a tubular defect that, in some cases, results in the cystic dilatation of the affected segment. Altered tubular basement membrane composition and associated epithelial cell proliferation account for cyst formation [65, 67, 157, 208]. It is the continuous growth of cysts and their progressive dilatation that cause pressure-induced ischemic injury of the adjacent renal parenchyma. A defect in urinary concentrating capacity is an early functional manifestation of experimental and clinical cystic diseases of the kidney [115, 137, 277]. Hypertension is common in these diseases, and the vascular lesions of nephrosclerosis contribute further to the course of the renal deterioration and development of tubulointerstitial lesions [33, 155, 156, 172, 394, 420].

GRANULOMATOUS DISEASES

Interstitial granulomatous reactions are a rare but characteristic hallmark of certain forms of tubulointerstitial disease [243, 295]. The two best known forms are sarcoidosis and tuberculosis. Granulomatous infiltration of the renal interstitium may be present in as many as 40 percent of the patients with sarcoidosis, but it is rarely extensive enough to cause renal dysfunction [80, 216, 260, 314]. They may develop after subsidence of the pulmonary lesions [440]. The lesions are usually responsive to steroid therapy [38, 163]. However, the regression of the active granulomatous reaction can result in interstitial fibrosis and progressive renal failure [313, 314]. Interstitial nephritis also has been noted in the absence of granulomatous lesions in some patients with sarcoidosis [314]; it may be due to the hypercalcemia, glomerular disease, and arteritis that occur in sarcoidosis [245, 259, 264].

A similar pathogenetic sequence of events occurs in tuberculosis of the kidney. The granulomatous reaction to the mycobacterial infection responds to antituberculous treatment, but the residual fibrosis can result in tubulointerstitial disease [75, 242]. A potential role for steroid treatment in conjunction with antituberculous therapy for the attenuation of the interstitial lesions has been suggested [269]. A contributory factor to the interstitial lesions of renal tuberculosis is the obstructive uropathy that follows ureteral and calyceal scarring caused by tuberculous involvement of the genitourinary tract [403].

Interstitial granulomatous reactions also have been noted in xanthogranulomatous pyelonephritis [138], Wegener's granulomatosis [452], renal candidiasis [167], heroin abuse [283], jejunoileal bypass surgery [425], and in association with anterior uveitis [99].

ENDEMIC DISEASES

The two endemic diseases in which tubulointerstitial lesions are a predominant component are Balkan nephropathy and nephropathia epidemica.

Endemic Balkan nephropathy is a progressive chronic tubulointerstitial nephritis, whose occurrence is limited to a geographic area bordering the Danube River as it traverses Bulgaria, Romania, and Yugoslavia [16, 463]. The etiology of the disease remains unknown but has been attributed to genetic factors, heavy metals, trace elements, and infectious agents [16, 417]. The regions where the disease occurs have a high ambient humidity and heavy rainfall and, hence, a propensity to fungal infection of food. A fungus-derived nephrotoxic component has been implicated on the basis of some preliminary epidemiologic and experimental animal studies [16, 232]. The disease evolves in emigrants from the endemic regions, suggesting a role for inheritance or the perpetuation of injury sustained prior to emigration. Actually, it has been hypothesized that the disease is clustered but may not be confined to the Balkans [417].

Nephropathia epidemica, initially thought to be restricted to the Scandinavian countries, and termed *Scandinavian acute hemorrhagic interstitial nephritis* [330], has been shown to have a more universal occurrence [98, 293] and has, therefore, been more appropriately termed by the World Health Organization as *hemorrhagic fever with renal syndrome* [86, 465]. As a rule the disease presents as a reversible acute interstitial nephritis but can progress to a chronic form [442]. It has been shown that it is caused by a rodent-transmitted virus of the genus of *Bunyaviride,* the hantavirus [246]. Humans are probably infected by respiratory aerosols contaminated by rodent excreta. Antibodies to the virus are detected in the serum [238], and virus-like structures have been demonstrated in the kidney of affected persons [85]. Tubulointerstitial nephropathy due to viral infection has also been reported with other agents including polyomavirus [367], cytomegalovirus [62, 451], herpes simplex [403], infectious mononucleosis [37], and human immunodeficiency virus [83, 396].

Papillary Necrosis

Renal papillary necrosis (RPN) develops in a variety of diseases that cause chronic tubulointerstitial nephropathy in which the lesion is more severe in the inner medulla [114]. The basic lesion is one of impairment of the vasculature and consequent focal or diffuse ischemic necrosis of the distal segments of one or more of the renal pyramids [215, 237, 318, 465]. In the affected papilla, the sharp demarcation of the lesion and the coagulative necrosis seen in the early stages of the disease closely resemble those of infarction [183]. The fact that the necrosis is anatomically limited to the papillary tips can be attributed to a variety of features, especially those of the vasculature, that are unique to this site. The renal papilla receives its blood supply from two sources: the vasa recta and branches of the arteries in the adventitia of the minor calyces. The importance of the latter is evidenced by the finding that the terminal portions of the papilla may be viable at a time that the remainder of it is necrotic, presumably because the blood supply from the minor calyceal arteries remains intact when the vascular involvement is limited to the vasa recta [20, 132] and the report of a case of RPN due to calyceal arteritis [177]. The vascular bundles formed by the vasa recta in the outer medulla and the interbundle region form distinct compartments; in the inner medulla, a subdivision into compartments is not obvious. Additionally, the vascular bundles, which are widest in the outer medulla, gradually decrease in size, and at the papillary tip only single or a few communicating vessels remain [31, 132]. The tapering away of the bundles is due to the gradual reduction of the vessels entering and leaving at different levels of the medullary capillary plexus. Measurements of medullary blood flow notwithstanding, it should be noted that much of the blood flow in the vasa rectae serves the countercurrent exchange mechanism. Nutrient blood supply is provided by small capillary vessels that originate in each given region. The net effect is that nutrient blood supply to the papillary tip is less than that to the rest of the medulla and, hence, its predisposition to ischemic necrosis [100].

Infection is usually, but not invariably, a concomitant finding of most cases of RPN [114, 198, 244, 385, 394, 404]. In fact, with few exceptions, most patients with RPN will ultimately develop a urinary tract infection. The infection has been considered by some to be the cause of the RPN and the suggestion has been made that RPN is a form of acute pyelonephritis that is more devastating than usual, because its natural course is altered by associated disease states, specifically diabetes mellitus and obstruction of the urinary tract [175, 244, 361]. However, angiographic studies reveal that vascular deficiency contributes even to the RPN associated with chronic pyelonephritis [237], and the necrosis of acute pyelonephritis has been attributed to compression of the thin-walled medullary vasculature by the inflammatory exudate of the interstitium [244]. Additionally, in considering infection as a cause of RPN, it should be taken into account that infection itself represents a complication of papillary necrosis [114], i.e., the infection develops after the primary underlying disease has initiated local injury to the renal medulla, with foci of impaired blood flow and poor tubular drainage. In any case, infection, if not the cause, is a frequent and important finding in most cases of RPN [114]. It contributes significantly to the symptomatology of cases of RPN, because fever and chills are the presenting symptoms of two-thirds of cases and a positive urine culture is obtained in 70 percent of the cases [114]. However, to consider RPN as an extension of severe pyelonephritis is inaccurate and simplistic. In the vast majority of cases of florid acute pyelonephritis, RPN does not occur. To classify RPN as a form of necrotizing pyelonephritis is archaic and has detracted from the recognition of RPN as a distinct clinicopathologic entity that can develop in the absence of pyelonephritis and urinary tract infection [114].

The necrotic lesion occurs in one of two forms. In the medullary form (Fig. 70-7), also termed *partial papillary necrosis,* the inner medulla is affected but the papillary tip and fornices remain intact; in the papillary form, also termed *total papillary necrosis,* the calyceal fornices and entire papillary tip are necrotic (Fig. 70-8) [165, 256, 257]. In the latter form, RPN is characterized by necrosis, demarcation, and sequestration of the papilla, which ultimately sloughs into the pelvis and may be recovered in the urine. In most of these cases, however, the necrotic papilla is not sloughed but is either resorbed or remains in situ, where it becomes calcified or forms the nidus of a calculus [198, 374]. In these, excretory radiologic examination is the only method by which diagnosis can be made during life. Unfortunately, these are not apparent

Fig. 70-7. Pathogenesis and radiologic changes in the medullary form of renal papillary necrosis. (Reproduced with permission from [114].)

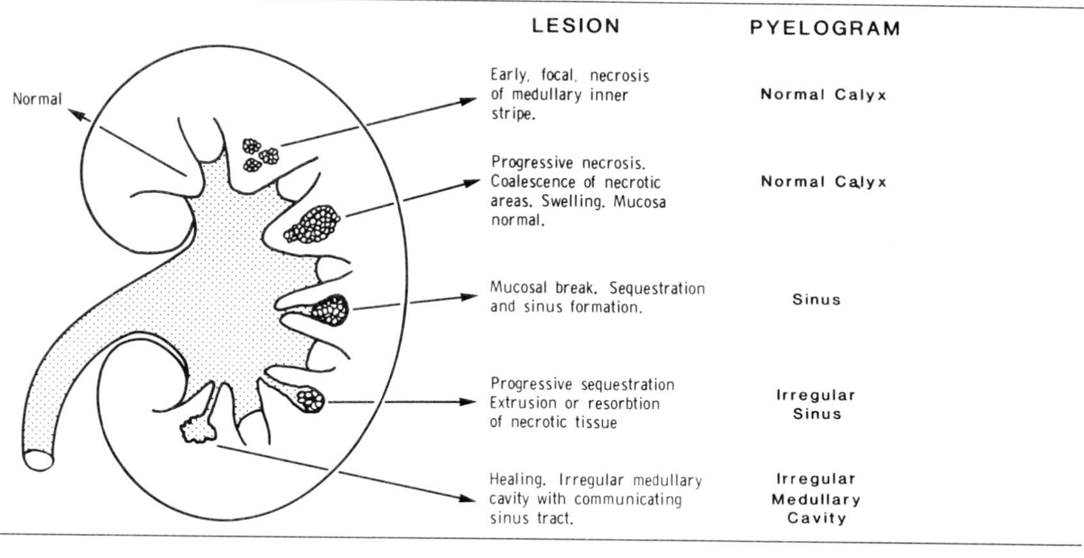

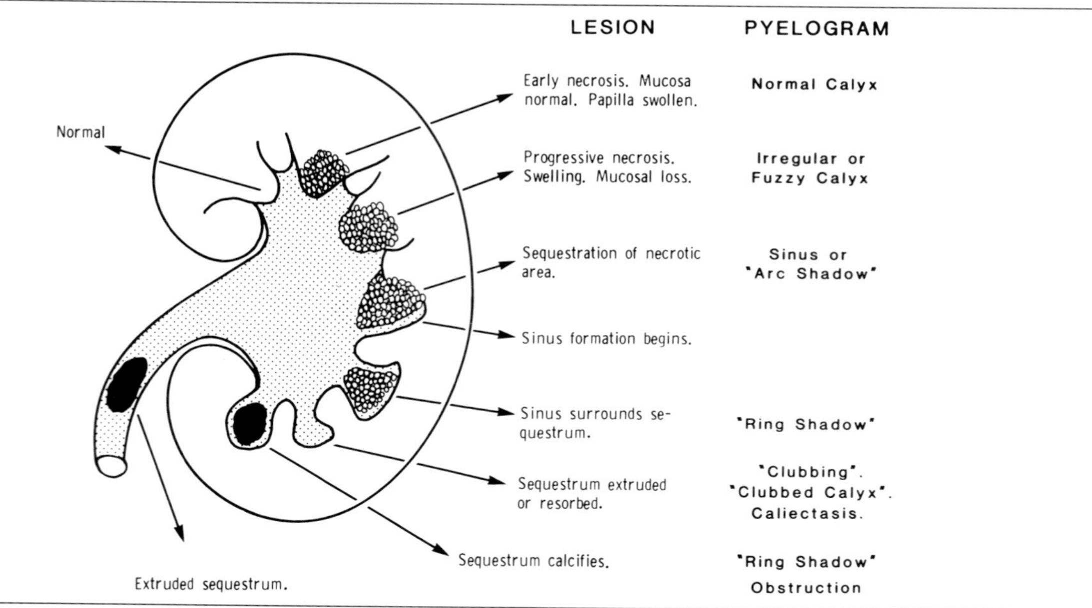

Fig. 70-8. Pathogenesis and radiologic changes in the papillary form of renal papillary necrosis. (Reproduced with permission from [114].)

until the late stages of RPN, when the papillae are shrunken and sequestered (Fig. 70-7). Actually, even when the papillae are sloughed out, excretory radiography can be negative [121, 239]. The passage of sloughed papillae is associated with lumbar pain, which is indistinguishable from ureteral colic of any cause and is present in about half of the cases [114]. Oliguria occurs in less than 10 percent of cases. Since a definitive diagnosis of RPN can be made on finding portions of necrotic papillae in the urine, a deliberate search should be made for papillary fragments in urine collected during or after attacks of colicky pain of all suspected cases, by straining the urine through filter paper or a piece of gauze [39, 254]. The separation and passage of papillary tissue may be associated with hematuria, which is microscopic in some 40 to 45 percent of the cases and gross in 20 percent of them [114]. The hematuria can be massive, and occasional instances of exsanguinating hemorrhage requiring nephrectomy have been reported [126, 158].

The necrotic lesions of RPN may be limited only to a few of the papillae or involve several of them in either one or both kidneys. In the majority of cases, the lesions are bilateral [114, 175, 198, 244, 374, 379, 402]. In cases where one kidney is involved at the time of initial presentation, RPN has been noted to develop in the other kidney within the ensuing 4 years [256]. This is not unexpected, considering the systemic nature of the diseases that are associated with RPN. RPN may be unilateral in cases where predisposing factors, such as infection and obstruction, are limited to one kidney [379]. Azotemia may be absent even in bilateral papillary necrosis, because it is the total number of papillae involved that ultimately determines the level of renal insufficiency that develops [114]. Each human kidney has an average of eight pyramids, such that even with bilateral RPN affecting one or two papillae in each kidney, sufficient unaffected renal lobules remain to maintain an adequate level of renal function. Moreover, in instances where several papillae in each kidney are necrotic, the localization of the lesion to the inner medulla results in the loss of the juxtamedullary nephrons only, whereas the cortical nephrons, which terminate in the outer medulla, are spared, such that even in the affected pyramids, there remain several intact nephrons that are capable of contributing to the maintenance of normal homeostasis [276, 374, 467]. Inability to concentrate the urine maximally is a more common development than is renal failure, as might be expected from the involvement of the inner medulla [276, 374]. Hence a long-standing history of polyuria and nocturia can be elicited from many of these patients. With the loss of several papillae and involvement of the cortex, however, renal failure will ultimately supervene.

The clinical course of renal papillary necrosis is variable. In its rare acute form, it may occur as a rapidly progressive devastating illness that results in the demise of the patient because of septicemia and renal failure [175, 361]. In its more common, chronic form, it will pursue a protracted course of months or years. These may remain totally asymptomatic, with the diagnosis made incidentally either at autopsy or excretory urography. Alternatively, it may be symptomatic, manifesting itself principally as epidoses of nephrolithiasis or pyelonephritis [45, 114, 198, 244, 256, 271]. In these conditions, fever and chills or renal colic are the presenting symptoms.

Diabetes mellitus is the most common condition associated with RPN, accounting for some 50 to 60 percent of the cases reported in the major series. The occurrence of RPN in diabetics may be more common than is generally appreciated. In an intravenous urographic study of 76 patients with long-standing insulin-dependent diabetes mellitus, RPN was observed in almost 25 percent of the cases [161]. *Obstructive uropathy* has been reported as the cause of RPN in 15 to 40 percent of the major reviews. *Pyelonephritis* can result in papillary necrosis, and infection is present in most cases of RPN, but its exact prevalence as the cause of RPN is difficult to determine, because infection may develop secondary to obstruction or diabetes, which remain the primary cause of RPN in the United States [114]. *Analgesic abuse* accounts for about 15 to 20 percent of the cases of RPN in the United States but for as many as 70 percent in countries where analgesic abuse is common [114, 159, 180], including children exposed to analgesics [5]. Radiologic evidence for RPN has been reported in over half of cases of *sickle cell hemoglobinopathy* [439]. The transplanted kidney appears to be vulnerable to developing RPN, either because of allograft rejection or secondary to the usual causes of RPN, which may have caused the end-stage kidney disease in the first place [205, 224, 438, 455]. The vasculitis of *allograft* rejection may lead to obliteration of the vessels supplying the papilla and result in ischemic necrosis of the papilla. Alternatively, RPN in renal allografts may be due to the primary disease that caused end-stage kidney disease, such as analgesic abuse, sickle cell disease, or diabetes mellitus.

As a rule, RPN is a disease of the older age group, the average age of patients being 53 years. Nearly half the cases occur in persons over 60 years of age, and more than 90 percent of cases in those over 40 years [114]. RPN is uncommon in persons below 40 years of age, except for those due to sickle cell hemoglobinopathy [439]. RPN is much less common in children, where the chronic conditions associated with RPN are rare, but it has been reported in association with hypoxia, dehydration, and septicemia [5, 74, 94, 136, 174, 230, 273, 280].

Other conditions in which RPN has been reported are renal vein thrombosis [45, 271], cryoglobulinemia [225], renal candidiasis [224], contrast media [7, 119], Wegener's granulomatosis [450], necrotizing angiitis [181], hypotensive shock [197, 228], pancreatitis [392], chronic alcoholism [102, 332], and aplastic anemia [460]. Most of these have been observed in individual cases and at least in some of them their association with RPN may have been coincidental. Actually, even in conditions commonly associated with RPN, more than one of the causative factors of RPN have been noted to be present in over half of the cases of RPN [114]. Thus in most cases of RPN, the lesion is multifactorial in origin and the pathogenesis of RPN may be considered the result of an overlap phenomenon, where a combination of detrimental factors are operating in concert to cause RPN (Fig. 70-9). As such, whereas each of the conditions alone can cause RPN, the coexistence of more than one predisposing factor in any one person significantly increases the risk for RPN. The contribution of any one of these factors to RPN would be expected to differ among individual cases and at various periods during the course of the disease. To the extent that the natural course of RPN itself predisposes to the development of infection of necrotic foci and obstruction by sloughed papillae, it may be difficult to assign a primary role for any of these processes in an individual case [19, 114]. Furthermore, the occurrence of any of these factors—necrosis, obstruction, or infection—may itself initiate a vicious cycle that can lead to the other and culminate in RPN. Evidence that this may well be the case can be adduced not only from clinical studies [114] but also from experimental models of RPN. For example, in the Gunn rat with congenital hyperbilirubinemia, RPN occurs spontaneously secondary to the deposition of unconjugated bilirubin in the renal papillae [17]. The administration of analgesics to these animals results in an acceleration of the papillary necrotic process and can be induced at doses of analgesics considerably less than those necessary to induce papillary lesions in other strains of rats [17].

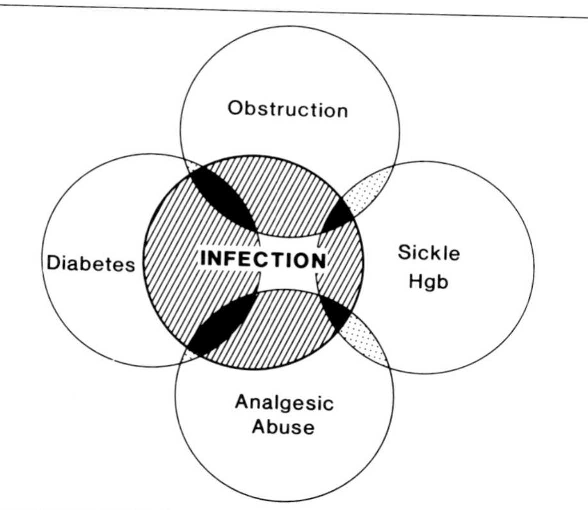

Fig. 70-9. Spectrum of diseases that are the major causes of renal papillary necrosis (RPN), illustrating the multifactorial pathogenesis of RPN. Whereas each of the conditions can, by itself, cause RPN, the coexistence of two (*striped areas*) or three (*black areas*) predisposing conditions increases the risk for RPN. (Reproduced with permission from [114].)

References

1. Abe, S., Amagasaki, Y., Iyori, S., et al. Significance of tubulointerstitial lesions in biopsy specimens of glomerulonephritic patients. *Am. J. Nephrol.* 9: 30, 1989.
2. Adams, R. G., Harrison, F., and Scott, P. The development of cadmium-induced proteinuria, impaired renal function, and osteomalacia in alkaline battery workers. *Q. J. Med.* 38: 425, 1969.
3. Akikusa, B., Irabu, N., Matsumura, R., et al. Tubulointerstitial changes in systemic vasculitic disorders: A quantitative study of 18 biopsy cases. *Am. J. Kidney Dis.* 16: 481, 1990.
4. Alfrey, A. C., Froment, D. H., and Stammond, W. S. Role of iron in the tubulo-interstitial injury in nephrotoxic serum nephritis. *Kidney Int.* 36: 753, 1989.
5. Allen, R. C., Petty, R. E., Lirenmann, D. S., et al. Renal papillary necrosis in children with chronic arthritis. *Am. J. Dis. Child.* 140: 20, 1986.
6. Allon, M. Renal abnormalities in sickle cell disease. *Arch. Intern. Med.* 150: 501, 1990.

7. Allwall, N., Erlanson, P., and Tornberg, A. The clinical course of renal failure occurring after intravenous urography and/or retrograde pyelography. *Acta Med. Scand.* 152: 163, 1955.
8. Andres, G. A., Accinni, L., Hus, K. C., et al. Human renal transplants. I. Immunopathologic studies. *Lab. Invest.* 22: 588, 1970.
9. Andres, G., Brentjens, J., Kohli, R., et al. Histology of human tubulo-interstitial nephritis associated with antibodies to renal basement membranes. *Kidney Int.* 13: 480, 1978.
10. Angell, M. E., Relman, A. S., and Robbins, S. L. Active chronic pyelonephritis without evidence of bacterial infection. *N. Engl. J. Med.* 278: 1303, 1968.
11. Aoki, S., Imamura, S., Aoki, M., et al. "Abacterial" and bacterial pyelonephritis: Immunofluorescent localization of bacterial antigen. *N. Engl. J. Med.* 281: 1375, 1969.
12. Arant, B. S. Vesicoureteric reflux and renal injury. *Am. J. Kidney Dis.* 17: 491, 1991.
13. Arruda, J. A. L. Radiation nephritis. *Contemp. Issues Nephrol.* 10: 275, 1983.
14. Asscher, A. W. Renal damage due to urinary tract infection. *Contrib. Nephrol.* 16: 5, 1979.
15. Asscher, A. W., Wilson, C., and Anson, S. G. Sensitization of blood-vessels to hypertensive damage by X-irradiation. *Lancet* 1: 580, 1961.
16. Austwick, P. K. C., Carter, R. L., Greig, J. B., et al. Balkan (endemic) nephropathy. *Contrib. Nephrol.* 16: 154, 1979.
17. Axelsen, R. A., and Burry, A. F. Papillary necrosis in the Gunn rat: Rapid induction by analgesics. *Pathology* 4: 225, 1972.
18. Bach, P. H., and Bridges, J. W. Chemically induced renal papillary necrosis and upper urothelial carcinoma: Parts 1 and 2. *Crit. Rev. Toxicol.* 15: 217, 1985.
19. Bach, P. H., and Hardy, T. L. Relevance of animal models to analgesic-associated renal papillary necrosis in humans. *Kidney Int.* 28: 605, 1985.
20. Baker, S. B. The blood supply of the renal papilla. *Br. J. Urol.* 31: 53, 1959.
21. Bakir, A. A., Lopez-Majano, V., Hryhorczuk, et al. Appraisal of lupus nephritis by renal imaging with gallium-67. *Am. J. Med.* 79: 175, 1985.
22. Bannister, K. M., Ulich, T. R., and Wilson, C. B. Induction, characterization and cell transfer of autoimmune tubulointerstitial nephritis. *Kidney Int.* 32: 642, 1987.
23. Barlow, K. A., and Beilin, K. J. Renal disease of primary gout. *Q. J. Med.* (New Series) 37: 79, 1968.
24. Barne, H. J. Herniations into the renal veins with special reference to hydronephrosis. *J. Pathol. Bacteriol.* 82: 177, 1961.
25. Battle, D. C., Arruda, J. A. L., and Kurtzman, N. A. Hyperkalemic distal renal tubular acidosis associated uropathy. *N. Engl. J. Med.* 304: 373, 1981.
26. Batuman, V., Dreishbach, A. W., and Cryan, J. Light-chain binding sites on renal brush-border membranes. *Am. J. Physiol.* 258: F1259, 1990.
27. Batuman, V., Landy, E., Maesaka, J. K., et al. Contribution of lead to hypertension with renal impairment. *N. Engl. J. Med.* 309: 17, 1983.
28. Batuman, V., Maesaka, J. K., Haddad, B., et al. The role of lead in gouty nephropathy. *N. Engl. J. Med.* 304: 520, 1981.
29. Baum, H. P., and Thoenes, W. Differentiation of granuloma cells (epithelioid cells and multinucleated giant cells): A morphometric analysis. Investigations using the model of experimental (anti-TBM) tubulo-interstitial nephritis. *Virchows Arch.* [*B*] 50: 181, 1985.
30. Beck, N., Singh, H., Reed, S. W., et al. Pathogenic role of cyclic AMP in the impairment of urinary concentrating ability in acute hypercalcemia. *J. Clin. Invest.* 54: 1049, 1974.
31. Beeuwkes, R., III, and Bonventre, J. V. Tubular organization and vascular-tubular relations in the dog kidney. *Am. J. Physiol.* 229: 695, 1975.
32. Bell, D., Kerr, D. N. S., Swinney, J., et al. Analgesic nephropathy. Clinical course after withdrawal of phenacetin. *Br. Med. J.* 3: 378, 1969.
33. Bell, P. E., Hossack, K. F., Gabow, P. A., et al. Hypertension in autosomal dominant polycystic kidney disease. *Kidney Int.* 34: 683, 1988.
34. Benabe, J., and Martinez-Maldonado, M. Hypercalcemic nephropathy. *Arch. Intern. Med.* 138: 777, 1978.
35. Benabe, J. E., and Martinez-Maldonado, M. Tubulointerstitial nephritis associated with systemic disease and electrolyte abnormalities. *Semin. Nephrol.* 8: 29, 1988.
36. Bender, W. L., Whelton, A., Beschorner, W. E., et al. Interstitial nephritis, proteinuria and renal failure caused by nonsteroidal anti-inflammatory drugs. Immunologic characterization of the inflammatory infiltrate. *Am. J. Med.* 76: 1006, 1984.
37. Bennett, W. M., Barry, J. M., and Joughton, D. C. Chronic tubulointerstitial nephritis from infectious mononucleosis. *West. J. Med.* 133: 248, 1980.
38. Berger, K. W., and Relman, A. S. Renal impairment due to sarcoid infiltration of the kidney. *N. Engl. J. Med.* 252: 44, 1955.
39. Bergnes, M. A. Recovery of papillae in renal papillary necrosis. Report of two cases. *Arch. Pathol.* 75: 501, 1963.
40. Bergstein, J. M., and Litman, N. Interstitial nephritis with antitubular basement membrane antibody. *N. Engl. J. Med.* 292: 875, 1975.
41. Berl, T. Cellular calcium uptake in the action of prostaglandins on renal water excretion. *Kidney Int.* 19: 15, 1981.
42. Bernstein, J., and Gardner, K. D. Hereditary tubulo-interstitial nephropathies. *Contemp. Issues Nephrol.* 9: 335, 1983.
43. Bernstein, J., and Whitten, C. F. A histologic appraisal of the kidney in sickle cell anemia. *Arch. Pathol.* 70: 409, 1960.
44. Biava, G. G., Dyrda, I., Genest, J., et al. Kaliopenic nephropathy: A correlated light and electron microscopy study. *Lab. Invest.* 12: 443, 1963.
45. Bittar, E. E., and Misanik, L. Renal necrotizing papillitis. *Am. J. Med.* 34: 82, 1963.
46. Blachley, J. D., and Hill, J. B. Renal and electrolyte disturbances associated with cisplatin. *Ann. Intern. Med.* 95: 628, 1981.
47. Blythe, W. B. Natural history of hypertension in renal parenchymal disease. *Am. J. Kidney Dis.* 5: A50, 1985.
48. Bohle, A., Christ, H., Grund, K. E., et al. The role of the interstitium of the renal cortex in renal disease. *Contrib. Nephrol.* 16: 109, 1979.
49. Bohle, A., Mackensen-Haen, S., and von Gise, H. Significance of tubulointerstitial changes in renal cortex for the excretory function and concentration ability of the kidney: A morphometric contribution. *Am. J. Nephrol.* 7: 421, 1987.
50. Bohle, A., Mackensen-Haen, S., von Gise, H., et al. The consequences of tubulo-interstitial changes for renal function in glomerulopathies: A morphometric and cytological analysis. *Pathol. Res. Pract.* 186: 135, 1990.
51. Bohle, A., von Gise, H., Mackensen-Haen, S., et al. The obliteration of the postglomerular capillaries and its in-

fluence upon the function of both glomeruli and tubuli: Functional interpretation of morphologic findings. *Klin. Wochenschr.* 59: 1043, 1981.
52. Bohman, S. The ultrastructure of the renal interstitium. *Contemp. Issues Nephrol.* 10: 1, 1983.
53. Bourgoignie, J. J. Renal complications of human immunodeficiency virus type I. *Kidney Int.* 37: 1571, 1990.
54. Bremmer, I. Mammalian absorption, transport and excretion of cadmium. *Top. Environ. Health* 2: 175, 1979.
55. Brentjes, J. R., Sepulveda, M., Baliah, T., et al. Interstitial immune complex nephritis in patients with systemic lupus erythematosus. *Kidney Int.* 7: 342, 1975.
56. Brod, J., and Benesova, D. A comparative study of functional and morphologic renal changes in glomerulonephritis. *Acta Med. Scand.* 157: 23, 1957.
57. Buckalew, V. M., Jr., and Someren, A. Renal manifestations of sickle cell disease. *Arch. Intern. Med.* 133: 660, 1974.
58. Bulger, R. E., and Nagle, R. B. Ultrastructure of the interstitium in the rabbit kidney. *Am. J. Anat.* 136: 183, 1973.
59. Bulger, R. E., Tisher, C. C., Myers, C. H., et al. Human renal ultrastructure. II. The thin limb of Henle's loop and the interstitium of healthy individuals. *Lab. Invest.* 16: 124, 1967.
60. Burry, A. F. The evolution of analgesic nephropathy. *Nephron* 5: 185, 1967.
61. Cameron, J. S. Immunologically mediated interstitial nephritis: Primary and secondary. *Adv. Nephrol.* 18: 207, 1989.
62. Cameron, J., Rigby, R. J., van Deth, A. G., et al. Severe tubulo-interstitial disease in a renal allograft due to cytomegalovirus infection. *Clin. Nephrol.* 18: 321, 1982.
63. Cameron, J. S., and Simmonds, H. A. Gout and crystal-related nephropathy. *Contrib. Nephrol.* 16: 147, 1979.
64. Capodicasa, G., De Santo, N. G., Nuzzi, F., et al. Sequential fine needle aspiration biopsy in glomerulonephritis. *Int. J. Pediatr. Nephrol.* 7: 3, 1986.
65. Carone, F. A. Functional changes in polycystic kidney disease are tubulo-interstitial in origin. *Semin. Nephrol.* 8: 89, 1988.
66. Carone, F. A., Kashgarian, M., and Epstein, F. H. Effect of acute potassium deficiency on susceptibility to infection with particular reference to the kidney. *Yale J. Biol. Med.* 32: 100, 1959.
67. Carone, F. A., Makino, H., and Kanwar, Y. S. Basement membrane antigens in renal polycystic kidney disease. *Am. J. Pathol.* 130: 466, 1988.
68. Case records of the Massachusetts General Hospital, Case 2-1976. *N. Engl. J. Med.* 294: 100, 1976.
69. Case records of the Massachusetts General Hospital, Case 17-1981. *N. Engl. J. Med.* 304: 1025, 1981.
70. Caulfield, J. B., and Shrag, P. E. Electron microscopic study of renal calcification. *Am. J. Pathol.* 44: 365, 1964.
71. Chadwick, V. S., Modha, K., and Dowling, R. H. Mechanisms for hyperoxaluria in patients with ileal dysfunction. *N. Engl. J. Med.* 289: 172, 1973.
72. Chanarin, I., Tavill, A. S., Loewi, G., et al. Defect of renal tubular acidification with antibody to loop of Henle. *Lancet* 2: 317, 1974.
73. Cheng, H. F., Nolasco, F., Cameron, J. S., et al. HLA-DR display by renal tubular epithelium and phenotype of infiltrate in interstitial nephritis. *Nephrol. Dial. Transplant.* 4: 205, 1989.
74. Chrispin, A. R., Hull, D., Lillie, J. G., et al. Renal tubular necrosis and papillary necrosis after gastroenteritis in infants. *Br. Med. J.* 1: 410, 1970.
75. Christensen, W. I. Genitourinary tuberculosis. Review of 102 cases. *Medicine* 53: 377, 1974.
76. Clark, E. C., Nath, K. A., Hostetter, M. K., et al. Role of ammonia in progressive interstitial nephritis. *Am. J. Kidney Dis.* 17(Suppl. 1): 15, 1991.
77. Clayman, M. D., Michaud, L., Brentjens, J., et al. Isolation of the target antigen of human anti-tubular basement membrane antibody-associated interstitial nephritis. *J. Clin. Invest.* 77: 1143, 1986.
78. Clive, D. M., and Stoff, J. S. Renal syndromes associated with nonsteroidal anti-inflammatory drugs. *N. Engl. J. Med.* 310: 563, 1984.
79. Clyne, D. H., Pesce, A. J., and Thompson, R. E. Nephrotoxicity of Bence-Jones protein in the rat. Importance of protein isoelectric point. *Kidney Int.* 16: 345, 1979.
80. Coburn, P. W., Hobbs, C., Johnston, G. S., et al. Granulomatous sarcoid nephritis. *Am. J. Med.* 42: 273, 1976.
81. Cogan, M. G. Tubulo-interstitial nephropathies: A pathophysiologic approach. *West. J. Med.* 132: 134, 1980.
82. Cogan, M. G. Classification and patterns of renal dysfunction. *Contemp. Issues Nephrol.* 10: 35, 1983.
83. Cohen, A. H., and Nast, C. C. HIV-associated nephropathy: A unique combined glomerular, tubular and interstitial lesion. *Mod. Pathol.* 1: 87, 1988.
84. Coles, G. A., Robinson, K., and Branch, R. A. Familial interstitial nephritis. *Clin. Nephrol.* 6: 513, 1976.
85. Collan, Y., and Lahdevirta, J. Electron microscopy of nephropathia epidemica. Cell nuclei in kidney biopsies. *Acta Pathol. Microbiol. Scand.* (Copenhagen) 87: 71, 1979.
86. Cosgriff, T. M. Hemorrhagic fever with renal syndrome: Four decades of research. *Ann. Intern. Med.* 110: 313, 1989.
87. Cotran, R. S. Retrograde proteus pyelonephritis in rats: Localization of antigen and antibody in treated sterile pyelonephrotic kidneys. *J. Exp. Med.* 117: 813, 1963.
88. Cotran, R. S. Glomerulosclerosis in reflux nephropathy. *Kidney Int.* 21: 528, 1982.
89. Councilman, W. T. Acute interstitial nephritis. *J. Exp. Med.* 3: 393, 1898.
90. Cremer, W., and Bock, K. D. Symptoms and causes of chronic hypokalemia nephropathy in man. *Clin. Nephrol.* 7: 112, 1977.
91. Cryer, P. E., Garber, A. J., Hoffsten, P., et al. Renal failure after small intestinal bypass for obesity. *Arch. Intern. Med.* 135: 1610, 1975.
92. D'Amico, G. Role of interstitial infiltration of leukocytes in glomerular diseases. *Nephrol. Dial. Transplant.* 3: 596, 1988.
93. D'Amico, G., Minetti, L., Ponticelli, C., et al. Prognostic indicators in idiopathic IgA mesangial nephropathy. *Q. J. Med.* 59: 363, 1986.
94. Davies, D. J., Kennedy, A., and Roberts, C. Renal medullary necrosis in infancy and childhood. *J. Pathol.* 99: 125, 1969.
95. Davis, B. B., Mattammal, M. B., and Zenser, T. V. Renal metabolism of drugs and xenobiotics. *Nephron* 27: 187, 1981.
96. Davis, B. B., Thomasson, D., and Zenser, T. V. Renal disease profoundly alters cortical interstitial cell function. *Kidney Int.* 23: 458, 1983.
97. Dentino, M., Luft, R. C., Yum, N. M., et al. Long-term effect of *cis*-diamminedichloride platinum (CDDP) on renal function and structure in man. *Cancer* 41: 1274, 1978.
98. Desmyter, J., Johnson, K. M., Deckers, C., et al. Laboratory rat associated with outbreak of hemorrhagic fever with renal syndrome due to Hantaan-like virus in Belgium. *Lancet* 2: 1445, 1983.

99. Dobrin, R. S., Vernier, R. L., and Fish, A. J. Acute eosinophilic interstitial nephritis and renal failure with bone marrow-lymph node granulomatous and anterior uveitis: A new syndrome. *Am. J. Med.* 59: 325, 1975.
100. Dobyan, D. C., and Jamison, R. L. Structure and function of the renal papilla. *Semin. Nephrol.* 4: 5, 1984.
101. Dousa, T. P., and Valtin, H. Cellular action of vasopressin in the mammalian kidney. *Kidney Int.* 10: 46, 1976.
102. Dubach, U. C., Rosner, B., Levy, P. S., et al. Epidemiological study in Switzerland. *Kidney Int.* 13: 41, 1978.
103. Dubach, U. C., Rosner, B., and Pfister, E. Epidemiologic study of analgesic containing phenacetin: Renal morbidity and mortality (1968–1979). *N. Engl. J. Med.* 308: 357, 1983.
104. Duffy, W. B., Senekjian, H. O., Knight, T. F., et al. Management of asymptomatic hyperuricemia. *J.A.M.A.* 246: 2215, 1981.
105. Duggin, G. G. Mechanisms in the development of analgesic nephropathy. *Kidney Int.* 18: 553, 1980.
106. Dunnil, M. S., and Millard, P. R. Segmental glomerulonephritis. *J. Clin. Pathol.* 28: 167, 1975.
107. Dykstra, M. J., and Hatchett, R. L. Ultrastructural events in early calcium oxalate crystal formation in rats. *Kidney Int.* 15: 640, 1979.
108. Eddy, A. E., McCulloch, L., Adams, J., et al. Interstitial nephritis induced by protein-overload proteinuria. *Am. J. Pathol.* 135: 719, 1989.
109. Edmondson, H. A., Reynolds, T. B., and Jacobson, A. Renal papillary necrosis with special reference to chronic alcoholism. A report of 20 cases. *Arch. Intern. Med.* 118: 255, 1966.
110. Eknoyan, G. Analgesic nephrotoxicity and renal papillary necrosis. *Semin. Nephrol.* 4: 65, 1984.
111. Eknoyan, G. The natural history of primary pyelonephritis. *Contrib. Nephrol.* 75: 82, 1989.
112. Eknoyan, G., Martinez-Maldonado, M., Suki, W. N., et al. Renal diluting capacity in the hypokalemic rat. *Am. J. Physiol.* 219: 933, 1970.
113. Eknoyan, G., McDonald, M., Appel, D., et al. Chronic tubulo-interstitial nephritis: Correlation between structural and functional findings. *Kidney Int.* 38: 736, 1990.
114. Eknoyan, G., Quinibi, W. Y., Grissom, R. T., et al. Renal papillary necrosis: An update. *Medicine* 61: 55, 1982.
115. Eknoyan, G., Weinman, E. J., Tsaparas, N., et al. Renal function in experimental cystic disease of the rat. *J. Lab. Clin. Med.* 88: 402, 1976.
116. Emmerson, B. T., and Row, P. G. An evaluation of the pathogenesis of the gouty kidney. *Kidney Int.* 8: 65, 1975.
117. Epstein, F. H. Calcium and the kidney. *Am. J. Med.* 45: 700, 1968.
118. Epstein, F. H., and Pigeon, G. Experimental urate nephropathy. Studies of the distribution of urate in renal disease. *Nephron* 1: 144, 1964.
119. Eskelund, V. Necrosis of renal papillae following retrograde pyelography. *Acta Radiol.* 26: 548, 1945.
120. Esparza, A. R., McKay, D. B., Cronan, J. J., et al. Renal parenchymal malakoplakia: Histologic spectrum and its relationship to megalocystic interstitial nephritis and xanthogranulomatous pyelonephritis. *Am. J. Surg. Pathol.* 13: 225, 1989.
121. Fairley, K. F., and Kincaid-Smith, P. Renal papillary necrosis with a normal pyelogram. *Br. Med. J.* 1: 156, 1968.
122. Fairley, K. F., and Roysmith, J. The forgotten factor in the evaluation of vesicoureteral reflux. *Med. J. Aust.* 2: 10, 1977.
123. Fanger, H., and Esparza, A. Crystals of calcium oxalate in the kidney in uremia. *Am. J. Clin. Pathol.* 41: 597, 1964.
124. Farebrother, D. A., Hatfield, P., Simmonds, H. A., et al. Experimental crystal nephropathy. One year study in the pig. *Clin. Nephrol.* 4: 243, 1975.
125. Farkas, W. R., Stanawitz, T., and Schneider, M. Saturnine gout: Lead-induced formation of guanine crystals. *Science* 199: 786, 1978.
126. Flasters, S., and Lowe, L. Urological complications of renal papillary necrosis. *J. Urol.* 5: 331, 1975.
127. Fliger, F. D., Wieslander, J., Brentjens, J. R., et al. Identification of a target antigens in human anti-tubular basement membrane nephritis. *Kidney Int.* 31: 800, 1987.
128. Foley, R. J., and Weinman, E. J. Urate nephropathy. *Am. J. Med. Sci.* 288: 208, 1984.
129. Ford, P. M. A naturally occurring human antibody to loops of Henle. *Clin. Exp. Immunol.* 14: 569, 1973.
130. Ford, S. M., and Hook, P. B. Biochemical mechanisms of toxic nephropathies. *Semin. Nephrol.* 4: 88, 1984.
131. Fourman, P., McCance, R. A., and Parker, R. A. Chronic renal disease in rats following a temporary deficiency of potassium. *Br. J. Exp. Pathol.* 37: 40, 1955.
132. Fourman, J., and Moffat, D. B. *The Blood Vessels of the Kidney.* Oxford, England: Blackwell Scientific Publications, 1971. Pp. 1–159.
133. Frasca, G. M., Vangelista, A., Biagini, G., et al. Immunological tubulo-interstitial deposits in IgA nephropathy. *Kidney Int.* 22: 184, 1982.
134. Freedman, L. R. Natural history of urinary infection in adults. *Kidney Int.* [*Suppl.*] 4: 96, 1975.
135. Friedman, J., Hoyer, J. R., and Seiler, M. W. Formation and clearance of tubulointerstitial immune complexes in kidneys of rats immunized with heterologous antisera to Tamm-Horsfall protein. *Kidney Int.* 21: 575, 1982.
136. Funston, M. R., Cremin, B. J., and Tidbury, I. J. K. Renal cortical necrosis and papillary necrosis in an infant. *Br. J. Radiol.* 49: 94, 1976.
137. Gabow, P. A., Kaehny, W. D., Johnson, A. M., et al. The clinical utility of renal concentrating capacity of polycystic kidney disease. *Kidney Int.* 35: 675, 1989.
138. Gammill, S., Rabinowitz, J. G., Peace, R., et al. New thoughts concerning xanthogranulomatous pyelonephritis (XP). *Am. J. Roentgenol. Rad. Ther. Nucl. Med.* 125: 154, 1975.
139. Ganote, C. E., Philipsborn, D. S., Chen, E., et al. Acute calcium nephrotoxicity: An electron microscopic and semiquantitative light microscopic study. *Arch. Pathol. Lab. Med.* 99: 650, 1975.
140. Gault, M. H., Blennerhasset, J., and Muehrcke, R. C. Analgesic nephropathy. A clinicopathologic study using electron microscopy. *Am. J. Med.* 51: 740, 1971.
141. Gault, M. H., Rudwal, T.-C., Engles, W. D., et al. Syndrome associated with the abuse of analgesics. *Ann. Intern. Med.* 68: 906, 1968.
142. Gellman, D. D., Pirani, C. L., Soothill, J. F., et al. Diabetic nephropathy. *Medicine* 38: 321, 1959.
143. Germain, M. J., Braden, G. L., and Fitzgibbons, J. P. Failure of chelation therapy in lead nephropathy. *Arch. Intern. Med.* 144: 2419, 1984.
144. Giacomelli, F., Spiro, D., and Wiener, J. A study of metastatic calcification at the cellular level. *J. Cell. Biol.* 22: 189, 1964.
145. Gilboa, N., Lum, G. N., and Urizar, R. E. Early renal involvement in acute lymphoblastic leukemia and non-Hodgkin's lymphoma in children. *J. Urol.* 129: 364, 1983.
146. Gill, J. R., and Bartter, F. C. On the impairment of renal concentrating ability in prolonged hypercalcemia and hypercalciuria in man. *J. Clin. Invest.* 40: 716, 1961.
147. Gillrnesyrt, J. Y., Harrison, R. B., and Kunnin, C. M.

Natural history of bacteriuria in school girls. *N. Engl. J. Med.* 301: 396, 1979.
148. Gillum, D. M., Truong, L., and Tasby, J. Characterization of the interstitial cellular infiltrate in experimental chronic cyclosporine nephropathy. *Transplantation* 49: 793, 1990.
149. Gloor, F. J. Changing concepts in the pathogenesis and morphology of analgesic nephropathy as seen in Europe. *Kidney Int.* 13: 27, 1978.
150. Gonick, H. C., Rubini, M. E., Glesson, I. U., et al. The renal lesion in gout. *Ann. Intern. Med.* 62: 667, 1965.
151. Gonwa, T. A., Hamilton, R. W., and Buckalew, V. A. Chronic renal failure and end-stage renal disease in northwest North Carolina. *Arch. Intern. Med.* 141: 462, 1981.
152. Gordon, D. L., Krueger, R. A., Quie, P. G., et al. Amidation of C_3 at the thiolester site: Stimulation of phagocytosis and chemiluminescence by a new inflammatory mediator. *J. Immunol.* 134: 3339, 1985.
153. Gottschalk, C. W., and Mylle, M. Micropuncture study of pressures in proximal tubules and peritubular capillaries of the rat kidney and their reaction to ureteral and renal venous pressures. *Am. J. Physiol.* 185: 430, 1956.
154. Grace, S. G., Suki, W. N., Spjut, H. J., et al. Hereditary nephritis in the Negro. Report of a kindred. *Arch. Intern. Med.* 125: 451, 1970.
155. Grantham, J. J. Polycystic kidney disease: A predominance of giant nephrons. *Am. J. Physiol.* 244: F3, 1983.
156. Grantham, J. J. Polycystic kidney disease—Hereditary and acquired. *The Kidney* 17: 19, 1984.
157. Grantham, J. J., Geiser, J. L., and Evan, A. P. Cyst formation and growth in autosomal dominant polycystic kidney disease. *Kidney Int.* 31: 1145, 1987.
158. Greenlaw, W. A. Renal papillary necrosis. *J. Maine Med. Assoc.* 70: 72, 1979.
159. Gregg, N. J., Elseviers, M. M., DeBroe, M. E., et al. Epidemiology and mechanistic basis of analgesic-associated nephropathy. *Toxicol. Lett.* 46: 141, 1989.
160. Grönhagen-Riska, C., von Willebrand, E., Honkanen, E., et al. Interstitial cellular infiltration detected by five-needle aspiration biopsy in nephritis. *Clin. Nephrol.* 34: 189, 1990.
161. Groop, L., Laasonen, L., and Egren, J. Renal papillary necrosis in patients with IDDM. *Diabetes Care* 12: 189, 1989.
162. Grunfeld, J. P., Ganeval, D., Chanard, J., et al. Acute renal failure in McArdle's disease. Report of two cases. *N. Engl. J. Med.* 286: 1237, 1972.
163. Guenel, J., and Chevet, D. Interstitial nephropathies in sarcoidosis: Effect of corticosteroid therapy and long-term evolution. Retrospective study of 22 cases. *Nephrologie* 9: 253, 1988.
164. Gullner, H. G., Bartter, F. G., Gill, J. R., et al. A sibship with hypokalemic alkalosis and renal proximal tubulopathy. *Arch. Intern. Med.* 143: 1534, 1983.
165. Gunther, G. W. Die papillennekrosen der niere bei diabetes. *Munchen Med. Wochnschr.* 84: 1695, 1937.
166. Gur, H., Kopolovic, Y., and Gross, D. J. Chronic predominant interstitial nephritis in a patient with systemic lupus erythematosus: A followup of three years and review of the literature. *Ann. Rheum. Dis.* 46: 617, 1987.
167. Guziel, L. P., Stone, W. J., Schaffner, W., et al. Primary renal candidiasis with renal granulomata and salt-losing nephropathy. *Am. J. Med. Sci.* 269: 123, 1975.
168. Hall, C. L., Calvin, R. T., Carey, K., et al. Passive transfer of autoimmune disease with isologous IgG, and IgG_2 and antibodies to the tubular basement membrane in strain XIII guinea pigs. Loss of self-tolerance induced by autoantibodies. *J. Exp. Med.* 146: 1246, 1977.
169. Hansen, H. E., Hestback, J., Sorenson, J. L., et al. Chronic interstitial nephropathy in patients on long-term lithium treatment. *Q. J. Med.* 48: 577, 1979.
170. Hanson, L. A., Ahlstedt, S., Fasth, A., et al. Antigens to *Escherichia coli,* human immune response and the pathogenesis of urinary tract infections. *J. Infect. Dis.* 136: S144, 1977.
171. Hanson, L. A., Fasth, A., and Jodal, U. Autoantibodies to Tamm-Horsfall protein, a tool of diagnosing the level of urinary tract infection. *Lancet* 1: 226, 1976.
172. Hansson, L., Karlander, L. E., Lundgren, W., et al. Hypertension in polycystic kidney disease. *Scand. J. Urol. Nephrol.* 8: 203, 1974.
173. Harmon, W., Cohen, H., Schneeberger, E., et al. Chronic renal failure in children treated with methyl CCNU. *N. Engl. J. Med.* 300: 1200, 1979.
174. Harris, V. J., Gooneratne, N. S., and White, H. Papillary necrosis in a child with homozygous sickle-cell anemia. *Radiology* 121: 156, 1976.
175. Harrison, J. H., and Bailey, O. T. The significance of necrotizing pyelonephritis in diabetes mellitus. *J.A.M.A.* 118: 15, 1942.
176. Haugulstaine, D., Corbeel, L., von Danne, B., et al. Glomerulonephritis in late-onset cystinosis. Report of two cases and review of the literature. *Clin. Nephrol.* 6: 529, 1976.
177. Heaton, J., and Bourke, E. Papillary necrosis associated with calyceal arteritis. *Nephron* 16: 57, 1976.
178. Henrich, W. L. Nephrotoxicity of nonsteroidal anti-inflammatory agents. *Am. J. Kidney Dis.* 2: 478, 1983.
179. Henrich, W. L. Analgesic nephropathy. *Am. J. Med. Sci.* 295: 561, 1988.
180. Henry, M. A., and Tange, J. D. Lesions of the renal papilla induced by paracetamol. *J. Pathol.* 151: 11, 1987.
181. Heppleston, A. G. Renal papillary necrosis associated with necrotizing angiitis and tubular necrosis. *J. Pathol. Bacteriol.* 70: 401, 1955.
182. Heptinstall, R. H. Interstitial nephritis. A brief review. *Am. J. Pathol.* 83: 214, 1976.
183. Heptinstall, R. H. *Pathology of the Kidney,* 3rd ed. Boston: Little, Brown, 1983. pp. 1149–1193.
184. Heptinstall, R. H., Bhagavan, B. S., and Solez, K. Urinary deposits in veins and interstitium of the kidney: Their possible role in causing renal damage. *Contrib. Nephrol.* 16: 70, 1979.
185. Hill, J. W., and Seedat, Y. K. The diagnosis of malakoplakia of the kidney by percutaneous renal biopsy. *S. Afr. Med. J.* 46: 953, 1972.
186. Hodgkinson, A. *Oxalic Acid in Biology and Medicine.* New York: Academic Press, 1977.
187. Hodgkinson, A., and Wilkinson, R. Plasma oxalate concentration and renal excretion of oxalate in man. *Clin. Sci. Mol. Med.* 46: 61, 1974.
188. Hodson, C. J. Vesico-ureteric reflux and renal scarring with and without infection. (Abstract) *Kidney Int.* 5: 308, 1974.
189. Hodson, C. J. Formation of renal scars with special reference to reflux nephropathy. *Contrib. Nephrol.* 16: 83, 1979.
190. Hodson, J., Maling, T. M. J., McManamon, P. J., et al. Reflux nephropathy. *Kidney Int.* 8: S50, 1975.
191. Hooke, D. H., Gee, D. C., and Atkins, R. C. Leukocyte analysis using monoclonal antibodies in human glomerulonephritis. *Kidney Int.* 31: 964, 1987.

192. Hostetter, M. K., Thoms, M. L., Rosen, F. S., et al. Binding of C_3b proceeds by a transesterification reaction at the thiolester site. *Nature* (London) 298: 72, 1982.

193. Hostetter, T. H., Nath, K. A., and Hostetter, M. K. Infection-related chronic interstitial nephropathy. *Semin. Nephrol.* 8: 11, 1988.

194. Hotta, O., Yoshizawa, N., Oshima, S., et al. Significance of renal hyaline arteriosclerosis and tubulo-interstitial change in IgA glomerulonephropathy and focal glomerular sclerosis. *Nephron* 47: 262, 1987.

195. Hoyer, J. R. Tubulo-interstitial immune complex nephritis in rats immunized with Tamm-Horsfall protein. *Kidney Int.* 17: 284, 1980.

196. Hucans, H., and Busch, R. Chronic pyelonephritis as a cause of end-stage disease. *J. Urol.* 127: 642, 1982.

197. Hullinghorst, R. L., and Steer, A. Pathology of epidemic hemorrhagic fever. *Ann. Intern. Med.* 38: 77, 1953.

198. Hultengren, N. Renal papillary necrosis. A clinical study of 103 cases. *Acta Chir. Scand.* (Suppl.) 277: 1, 1961.

199. Husby, G., Tung, K. S. K., and Williams, R. C. Characterization of renal tissue lymphocytes in patients with interstitial nephritis. *Am. J. Med.* 70: 31, 1981.

200. Hutt, M. S., Pinniger, J. L., and de Wardener, H. E. The relationship between the clinical and histological features of acute glomerular nephritis. *Q. J. Med.* 27: 265, 1958.

201. Iggo, N., Palmer, A. B., Severn, A., et al. Chronic dialysis in patients with multiple myeloma and renal failure: A worthwhile treatment. *Q. J. Med.* 73: 903, 1989.

202. Ivanyi, B. Frequency of light chain deposition nephropathy relative to renal amyloidosis and Bence Jones cast nephropathy in a necropsy study of patients with myeloma. *Arch. Pathol. Lab. Med.* 114: 986, 1990.

203. Jacobs, L. A., and Morris, J. G. Renal papillary necrosis and abuse of phenacetin. *Med. J. Aust.* 2: 531, 1962.

204. Kanfer, A., Vandewalle, A., Morel-Maroger, L., et al. Acute renal insufficiency due to lymphatomatous infiltration of the kidneys. *Cancer* 38: 2588, 1976.

205. Kaude, J. V., Stone, M., Fuller, T. J., et al. Papillary necrosis in kidney transplant patients. *Radiology* 120: 69, 1976.

206. Kazantzis, G. Cadmium nephropathy. *Contrib. Nephrol.* 16: 161, 1979.

207. Keane, W. F., Crosson, J. T., Staley, N. A., et al. Radiation-induced renal disease: A clinicopathologic study. *Am. J. Med.* 60: 127, 1976.

208. Kelly, C. J., and Neilson, E. G. Medullary cystic disease: An inherited form of autoimmune interstitial nephritis? *Am. J. Kidney Dis.* 10: 389, 1987.

209. Kelly, D. R., and Murad, T. M. Megalocytic interstitial nephritis, xanthogranulomatous pyelonephritis and malakoplakia. An ultrastructural comparison. *Am. J. Clin. Pathol.* 75: 333, 1981.

210. Khademi, M., and Marquis, J. R. Renal angiography in sickle cell disease: A preliminary report correlating the angiographic and urographic changes in sickle cell nephropathy. *Radiology* 107: 41, 1973.

211. Khan, S. R., Finlayson, B., and Hackett, R. L. Scanning electron microscopy of calcium oxalate crystal formation in experimental nephrolithiasis. *Lab. Invest.* 41: 504, 1979.

212. Kimmelstiel, P. Vascular occlusion and ischemic infarction in sickle cell disease. *Am. J. Med. Sci.* 216: 11, 1948.

213. Kincaid-Smith, P. Pathogenesis of the renal lesions associated with the abuse of analgesics. *Lancet* 1: 859, 1967.

214. Kincaid-Smith, P. Glomerular lesions in atrophic pyelonephritis and reflux nephropathy. *Kidney Int.* 8: S81, 1975.

215. Kincaid-Smith, P., Saker, B. M., and McKenzie, I. F. C. Lesions in the vasa recta in experimental analgesic nephropathy. *Lancet* 1: 24, 1968.

216. King, B. P., Esparza, A. R., Kahn, S. I., et al. Sarcoid granulomatous nephritis occurring as isolated renal failure. *Arch. Intern. Med.* 136: 241, 1976.

217. Kippen, I., Klinenberg, J. R., Weinberg, A., et al. Factors affecting urate solubility in vitro. *Ann. Rheum. Dis.* 33: 313, 1974.

218. Klassen, J., Andres, G. A., Brennan, J. C., et al. An immunologic renal tubular lesion in man. *Clin. Immunol. Immunopathol.* 1: 69, 1972.

219. Klassen, J., Kano, K., Milgrom, F., et al. Tubular lesions produced by autoantibodies to tubular basement membrane in human renal allografts. *Int. Arch. Allergy App. Immunol.* 45: 675, 1973.

220. Klassen, J., McCluskey, R. T., and Milgrom, F. Nonglomerular renal disease produced in rabbits by immunization with homologous kidney. *Am. J. Pathol.* 63: 333, 1971.

221. Klinenberg, J. R., Kippen, I., and Bluestone, R. Hyperuricemic nephropathy: Pathologic features and factors influencing urate deposition. *Nephron* 14: 88, 1975.

222. Klintmalm, G., Bohman, S. O., Sundelin, B., et al. Interstitial fibrosis in renal allografts after 12 to 46 months of cyclosporine treatment: Beneficial effects of low doses in early post-transplantation period. *Lancet* 2: 950, 1984.

223. Knepper, M. A., Danielson, R. A., Saidel, G. M., et al. Quantitative analysis of renal medullary anatomy in rats and rabbits. *Kidney Int.* 12: 313, 1977.

224. Knepshield, J. H., Feller, H. A., and Leb, D. E. Papillary necrosis due to *Candida albicans* in a renal allograft. *Arch. Intern. Med.* 122: 441, 1968.

225. Koelz, A. M., and Bourke, E. Cryoglobinaemic nephropathy with papillary necrosis. *Nephron* 19: 242, 1977.

226. Korzets, A., Tam, F., Russell, G., et al. The role of continuous ambulatory peritoneal dialysis in end-stage renal failure due to myeloma. *Am. J. Kidney Dis.* 16: 216, 1990.

227. Koury, S. T., Koury, M. J., Bondurant, M. C., et al. Quantitation of erythropoietin-producing cells in kidneys of mice by in situ hybridization: Correlation with hematocrit, renal erythropoietin mRNA, and serum erythropoietin concentration. *Blood* 74: 645, 1989.

228. Koutsaimanis, K. G., and De Wardener, H. E. Phenacetin nephropathy, with particular reference to the effect of surgery. *Br. Med. J.* 4: 131, 1970.

229. Kozeny, G. A., Barr, W., Bansal, V. K., et al. Occurrence of renal tubular dysfunction in lupus nephritis. *Arch. Intern. Med.* 147: 891, 1987.

230. Kozlowski, K., and Brown, R. W. Renal medullary necrosis in infants and children. *Pediatr. Radiol.* 7: 85, 1978.

231. Kriz, W., and Napiwotzky, P. Structural and functional aspects of the renal interstitium. *Contrib. Nephrol.* 16: 104, 1979.

232. Krogh, P., Hald, B., Plestina, R., et al. Balkan (endemic) nephropathy and foodborn ochratoxin. A. Preliminary results of a survey of foodstuffs. *Acta Pathol. Microbiol. Scand.* (Sect. B) 85: 238, 1977.

233. Kunin, C. M. Does kidney infection cause renal failure? *Annu. Rev. Med.* 36: 176, 1975.

234. Kurnick, J. T., McCluskey, R. T., Bhan, A. K., et al. *Escherichia coli* specific T lymphocytes in experimental pyelonephritis. *J. Immunol.* 141: 3220, 1988.

235. Kyle, R. A. Multiple myeloma. Review of 869 cases. *Mayo Clin. Proc.* 50: 29, 1975.
236. Kyle, R. A. Monoclonal gammopathies and the kidney. *Annu. Rev. Med.* 40: 53, 1989.
237. Lagergren, C., and Ljungqvist, A. The intrarenal arterial pattern in renal papillary necrosis. *Am. J. Pathol.* 41: 633, 1962.
238. Lahdevirta, J., Savala, J., Brummer, M., et al. Clinical and serological diagnosis of nephropathia epidemica, the mild type of haemorrhagic fever with renal syndrome. *J. Infect.* 9: 230, 1984.
239. Lalli, A. F. Renal papillary necrosis. *Am. J. Roentgenol. Rad. Ther. Nucl. Med.* 114: 741, 1972.
240. Langer, K. H., and Thoenes, W. Characterization of cells involved in the formation of granuloma. *Virchows Arch. [Cell Pathol.]* 36: 179, 1981.
241. Larsen, K., and Moller, C. E. Renal lesions caused by abuse of phenacetin. *Acta Med. Scand.* 165: 321, 1959.
242. Latimer, J. K. Renal tuberculosis. *N. Engl. J. Med.* 273: 208, 1975.
243. Laudet, J., Hiesse, C., Lucsko, M., et al. Nephropathie granulomateuse d'origine tuberculeuse revelle par une fievre au long cours. *Nouv. Presse Med.* 9: 3259, 1980.
244. Lauler, D. P., Schreiner, G. E., and David, A. Renal medullary necrosis. *Am. J. Med.* 29: 132, 1960.
245. Lebacq, E., Verhaegen, H., and Desmet, V. Renal involvement in sarcoidosis. *Postgrad. Med. J.* 46: 526, 1970.
246. Lee, H. W., Lee, P. W., Lahdevirta, J., et al. Aetiological relation between Korean hemorrhagic fever and nephropathia epidemica. *Lancet* 1: 186, 1979.
247. Lehman, D. H., Marquadt, H., Wilson, C. B., et al. Specificity of autoantibodies to tubular and glomerular basement membranes induced in guinea pigs. *J. Immunol.* 112: 241, 1974.
248. Lehman, D. H., Wilson, C. B., and Dixon, F. J. Interstitial nephritis in rats immunized with heterologous tubular basement membrane. *Kidney Int.* 5: 187, 1974.
249. Lehman, D. H., Wilson, C. B., and Dixon, F. J. Extraglomerular immunoglobulin deposits in human nephritis. *Am. J. Med.* 58: 765, 1975.
250. Lehman, J. D., Smith, J. W., Miller, T. E., et al. Local immune response in experimental pyelonephritis. *J. Clin. Invest.* 47: 2541, 1968.
251. Lemley, K. V., and Kriz, W. Anatomy of the renal interstitium. *Kidney Int.* 39: 370, 1991.
252. Levi, D. F., Williams, R. C., and Linstrom, F. D. Immunofluorescence studies of the myeloma kidney with special reference to light chain disease. *Am. J. Med.* 44: 922, 1968.
253. Levitt, M. F., Halpern, M. H., Polimeros, O. P., et al. The effect of abrupt changes in plasma calcium concentrations on renal function and electrolyte excretion in man and monkey. *J. Clin. Invest.* 37: 294, 1958.
254. Lindholm, T. On renal papillary necrosis with special reference to the diagnostic importance of papillary fragments in the urine, therapy and prognosis. *Acta Med. Scand.* 167: 319, 1960.
255. Lindquist, B., Nystrom, K., Stegmayr, B., et al. Cadmium concentration in human kidney biopsies. *Scand. J. Urol. Nephrol.* 23: 213, 1989.
256. Lindvall, N. Renal papillary necrosis. A roentgenographic study of 155 cases. *Acta Radiol.* 192(Suppl. 1): 1, 1960.
257. Lindvall, N. Radiological changes in renal papillary necrosis. *Kidney Int.* 13: 93, 1978.
258. Ljungqvist, A. The intrarenal arterial pattern in the normal and diseased human kidney. *Acta Med. Scand.* 174(Suppl. 401): 5, 1963.
259. Lofgren, S., Snellman, B., and Lindgren, A. G. H. Renal complications in sarcoidosis: Functional and biopsy studies. *Acta Med. Scand.* 159: 295, 1957.
260. Longcope, W. T., and Friedman, D. G. A study of sarcoidosis: Based on a combined investigation of 160 cases including 30 autopsies from the Johns Hopkins Hospital and Massachusetts General Hospital. *Medicine* 31: 1, 1952.
261. Luxton, R. W. Radiation nephritis. *Q. J. Med.* 22: 215, 1953.
262. Macdonegal, I. C., Isles, C. G., Whitworth, J. A., et al. Interstitial nephritis and primary biliary cirrhosis: A new association. *Clin. Nephrol.* 27: 36, 1987.
263. Mackensen, S., Grund, K. E., Sindjic, M., et al. Influence of the renal cortical interstitium on the serum creatinine concentration and creatinine clearance in different chronic sclerosing interstitial nephritis. *Nephron* 24: 30, 1979.
264. MacSearraigh, E. T., Twomey, M., Doyle, C. T., et al. Sarcoidosis with renal involvement. *Postgrad. Med. J.* 54: 528, 1978.
265. Makker, S. P. Tubular basement membrane antibody-induced interstitial nephritis in systemic lupus erythematosus. *Am. J. Med.* 69: 949, 1980.
266. Madias, N. E., and Harrington, J. T. Platinum nephrotoxicity. *Am. J. Med.* 65: 307, 1978.
267. Magil, A. B., and Tyler, M. Tubulo-interstitial disease in lupus nephritis. A morphometric study. *Histopathology* 8: 81, 1984.
268. Mahieu, P., Darderme, M., and Bach, J. F. Detection of humoral and cell-mediated immunity of kidney basement membranes in human renal diseases. *Am. J. Med.* 53: 185, 1972.
269. Mallinson, W. J. W., Fuller, R. W., Levisson, D. A., et al. Diffuse interstitial renal tuberculosis: An unusual cause of renal failure. *Q. J. Med.* 198: 137, 1981.
270. Mampaso, F. M., and Wilson, C. B. Characterization of inflammatory cells in autoimmune tubulointerstitial nephritis in rats. *Kidney Int.* 23: 448, 1983.
271. Mandel, E. E. Renal medullary necrosis. *Am. J. Med.* 13: 322, 1952.
272. Markovic-Lipkovski, J., Müller, C. A., Risler, T., et al. Association of glomerular and interstitial mononuclear leukocytes with different forms of glomerulonephritis. *Nephrol. Dial. Transplant.* 5: 10, 1990.
273. Marks, I. M. Renal medullary necrosis following exsanguination in infancy. *Lancet* 2: 680, 1960.
274. Marone, C., Beretta-Piccoli, C., and Weidman, P. Acute hypercalcemic hypertension in man: Role of hemodynamics, catecholamines and renin. *Kidney Int.* 20: 92, 1980.
275. Martinez-Maldonado, M., and Ramirez-Arillano, G. A. Renal involvement in malignant lymphoma. A survey of 49 cases. *J. Urol.* 95: 485, 1966.
276. Martinez-Maldonado, M., and Stitzer, O. Urine concentration and dilution in the rat. Contributions of papillary structures during high rates of urine flow. *Kidney Int.* 13: 194, 1978.
277. Martinez-Maldonado, M., Yium, J. J., Eknoyan, G., et al. Adult polycystic disease: Demonstration of a defect in urine concentration in patients without renal insufficiency and studies of its mechanism. *Kidney Int.* 2: 107, 1972.
278. Martinez-Maldonado, M., Yium, J., Suki, W. N., et al.

Renal complications in multiple myeloma. Pathophysiology and some aspects of clinical management. *J. Chronic Dis.* 24: 221, 1971.
279. Matsuma, R., Kondo, Y., Sugiyama, T., et al. Immunohistochemical identification of infiltrating mononuclear cells in tubulointerstitial nephritis associated with Sjögren's syndrome. *Clin. Nephrol.* 30: 335, 1988.
280. Mauer, S. M., and Nogredy, M. B. Renal papillary and cortical necrosis in a newborn infant. Report of a survivor with roentgenologic documentation. *J. Pediatr.* 74: 750, 1969.
281. Mayrer, A. R., Kashgarian, M., Ruddle, N. H., et al. Tubulo-interstitial nephritis and immunologic response to Tamm-Horsfall protein. *J. Immunol.* 128: 2634, 1982.
282. Mazzer, T., Shue, G. L., and Jackson, S. H. Renal dysfunction associated with methoxyflurane anesthesia. *J.A.M.A.* 216: 278, 1971.
283. McAllister, C. J., Horn, R., Havron, S., et al. Granulomatous interstitial nephritis: A complication of heroin abuse. *South. Med. J.* 72: 162, 1979.
284. McAnally, J. F., Winchester, J. F., and Schreiner, G. E. Analgesic nephropathy: An uncommon cause of end-stage renal disease. *Arch. Intern. Med.* 143: 1897, 1983.
285. McCarron, D. A., Royer, K. A., Houghton, D. C., et al. Chronic tubulo-interstitial nephritis caused by recurrent myoglobinuria. *Arch. Intern. Med.* 140: 1106, 1980.
286. McCluskey, R. T. Immunologically mediated tubulo-interstitial nephritis. *Contemp. Issues Nephrol.* 10: 121, 1983.
287. McCluskey, R. T., and Bhan, A. K. Cell mediated immunity in renal disease. *Hum. Pathol.* 17: 146, 1986.
288. McCluskey, R. T., and Colvin, R. B. Immunological aspects of renal tubular and interstitial diseases. *Annu. Rev. Med.* 29: 191, 1978.
289. McCredie, M., and Stewart, J. H. Does paracetamol cause urothelial cancer or renal papillary necrosis? *Nephron* 49: 296, 1988.
290. McCredie, M., Stewart, J. H., Carter, J. J., et al. Phenacetin and papillary necrosis: Independent risk factors for renal pelvic cancer. *Kidney Int.* 30: 81, 1986.
291. McPhaul, J. J., and Dixon, F. J. Characterization of human antiglomerular basement membrane antibodies eluted from glomerulonephritic kidneys. *J. Clin. Invest.* 49: 308, 1970.
292. Mellmann, J., Hess, K., Schnaidt, U., et al. Angiographic results in interstitial, vascular and glomerular kidney disease. *Contrib. Nephrol.* 16: 115, 1979.
293. Mery, J. P., Dard, S., Chamouard, J. M., et al. Mucoid virus nephropathies. *Lancet* 2: 845, 1983.
294. Messerli, F. H., Frohlich, E. D., Dreslinski, G. R., et al. Serum uric acid in essential hypertension. An indicator of renal vascular involvement. *Ann. Intern. Med.* 93: 817, 1980.
295. Mignon, F., Mery, J. P., Mougenot, B., et al. Granulomatous interstitial nephritis. *Adv. Nephrol.* 13: 219, 1984.
296. Mihatsch, M., Thiel, G., and Ryffel, B. Cyclosporin A: Action and side effects. *Toxicol. Lett.* 46: 125, 1989.
297. Mihatsch, M. J., Thiel, G., Spichtin, H. P., et al. Morphological finding in kidney transplants after treatment with cyclosporine. *Transplant. Proc.* 15: 2821, 1983.
298. Miller, T. E., and Robinson, K. B. Experimental pyelonephritis: A new method for inducing pyelonephritis in the rat. *J. Infect. Dis.* 127: 307, 1973.
299. Miller, T. E., Scott, L., Stewart, E., et al. Modification by suppressor cells and serum factors of cell-mediated immune response in experimental pyelonephritis. *J. Clin. Invest.* 61: 964, 1978.
300. Miller, T. E., Stewart, E., and North, J. D. K. Immunobacteriological aspects of pyelonephritis. *Contrib. Nephrol.* 16: 11, 1979.
301. Moffat, D. B., and Lawrence, K. M. The structure of the pelvis in the immature human kidney. *Nephron* 16: 205, 1976.
302. Moffat, D. B., and Lawrence, K. M. The pathomorphology of intrarenal reflux. *Contrib. Nephrol.* 16: 78, 1979.
303. Molland, E. A. Experimental renal papillary necrosis. *Kidney Int.* 13: 5, 1978.
304. More, R. H., McMillan, G. L., and Duff, G. L. The pathology of sulfonamide allergy in man. *Am. J. Pathol.* 22: 702, 1946.
305. Morel-Maroger, L., Kourilsky, O., Mignon, F., et al. Antitubular basement membrane antibodies in rapidly progressive post-streptococcal glomerulonephritis. Report of a case. *Clin. Immunol. Immunopathol.* 2: 185, 1974.
306. Morgan, J. M., and Hartley, M. N. Etiologic factors in lead nephropathy. *South. Med. J.* 69: 1445, 1976.
307. Mostoffi, F. K., Varder-Bruegge, C. F., and Diggs, L. W. Lesions in kidneys removed from unilateral hematuria in sickle cell disease. *Arch. Pathol. Lab. Med.* 63: 336, 1957.
308. Muehrcke, R. C., Kark, R. M., Pirani, C. L., et al. Lupus nephritis: A clinical and pathologic study based on renal biopsies. *Medicine* 36: 1, 1957.
309. Mujais, S., and Battle, D. C. Functional correlates of tubulointerstitial damage. *Semin. Nephrol.* 8: 94, 1988.
310. Murray, R. M. Patterns of analgesic use and abuse of medical patients. *Practitioner* 211: 639, 1973.
311. Murray, T., and Goldberg, M. Chronic interstitial nephritis. Etiologic factors. *Ann. Intern. Med.* 82: 453, 1975.
312. Murray, T. G., Stolley, P. D., Anthony, J. C., et al. Epidemiologic study of regular analgesic use and end-stage renal disease. *Arch. Intern. Med.* 143: 1687, 1983.
313. Muther, R. S., McCarron, D. A., and Bennett, W. M. Granulomatous sarcoid nephritis: A cause of multiple renal tubular abnormalities. *Clin. Nephrol.* 14: 190, 1980.
314. Muther, R. S., McCarron, D. A., and Bennet, W. B. Renal manifestations of sarcoidosis. *Arch. Intern. Med.* 141: 643, 1981.
315. Myers, B. D., Sibley, R., Newton, L., et al. The long-term course of cyclosporine-associated chronic nephropathy. *Kidney Int.* 33: 590, 1988.
316. Nagle, R. B., Bulger, R. E., Cutler, R. E., et al. Unilateral obstructive nephropathy in the rabbit. I. Early morphologic, physiologic, and histochemical changes. *Lab. Invest.* 28: 456, 1973.
317. Nagle, R. B., Johnson, M. E., and Jervis, H. R. Proliferation of renal interstitial cells following injury induced by ureteral obstruction. *Lab. Invest.* 35: 18, 1976.
318. Nanra, R. S., Chirawong, P., and Kincaid-Smith, P. Medullary ischemia in experimental analgesic nephropathy. The pathogenesis of renal papillary necrosis. *Aust. N.Z. J. Med.* 3: 580, 1973.
319. Nath, K. A., Hostetter, M. K., and Hostetter, T. H. Pathophysiology of chronic tubulo-interstitial disease in rats. Interaction of dietary acid load, ammonia and complement component C_3. *J. Clin. Invest.* 76: 667, 1985.
320. Navarte, J., Saba, S. R., and Ramirez, G. Occupational exposure to organic solvents causing chronic tubulointerstitial nephritis. *Arch. Intern. Med.* 149: 154, 1989.
321. Neild, G. H., Reuben, R., Hartley, R. B., et al. Glomerular thrombi in renal allografts associated with cyclosporine treatment. *J. Clin. Pathol.* 38: 253, 1985.
322. Neilson, E. G. Pathogenesis and therapy of interstitial nephritis. *Kidney Int.* 35: 1257, 1989.

323. Nielson, E. G., Sun, M. J., Kelly, C. J., et al. Molecular characterization of a major nephritogenic domain in the autoantigen of anti-tubular basement membrane disease. *Proc. Natl. Acad. Sci. U.S.A.* 88: 2006, 1991.
324. Nguyen, H. T., and Wodward, J. C. Intranephronic calculosis in rats. *Am. J. Pathol.* 100: 39, 1980.
325. Nojima, Y., Terai, C., Takano, K., et al. Tubulointerstitial immune complex nephritis in a patient with cutaneous vasculitis. *Clin. Nephrol.* 25: 48, 1986.
326. Nolasco, F., Cameron, J. S., Reuben, R., et al. Interstitial foam cells in the nephrotic syndrome belong to the monocyte/macrophage lineage. *Proc. Eur. Dial. Transplant. Assoc.* 21: 666, 1984.
327. Norden, A. G., Flynn, F. V., Fulcher, L. M., et al. Renal impairment of myeloma: Negative association with isoelectric point of excreted Bence Jones protein. *J. Clin. Pathol.* 42: 59, 1989.
328. Nordenfelt, O. Deaths from renal failure in abusers of phenacetin containing drugs. *Acta Med. Scand.* 191: 11, 1972.
329. Nystrom, K. Incidence and prevalence of endemic benign nephropathy in AC Country, Sweden, in relation to population density and prevalence of small rodents. *Acta Med. Scand.* [Suppl.] 609: 1, 1977.
330. O'Dell, J. R., Hays, R. C., Guggenheim, S. J., et al. Tubulointerstitial renal disease in systemic lupus erythematosus. *Arch. Intern. Med.* 145: 1996, 1985.
331. Osborn, D. E., Castro, J. E., and Ansell, I. D. Malakoplakia in a cadaver renal allograft: A case study. *Hum. Pathol.* 8: 341, 1977.
332. Pablo, N. C., Churg, J., Needle, M. A., et al. Renal papillary necrosis: Relapsing form associated with alcoholism. *Am. J. Kidney Dis.* 7: 88, 1986.
333. Pamukou, R., Moorthy, V., Singer, J. R., et al. Idiopathic acute interstitial nephritis: Characterization of the infiltrating cells in the renal interstitium as T helper lymphocytes. *Am. J. Kidney Dis.* 4: 24, 1984.
334. Park, M. H., D'Agati, V., Appel, G. B., et al. Tubulointerstitial disease in lupus nephritis: Relationship to immune deposits, interstitial inflammation, glomerular changes, renal function and progression. *Nephron* 44: 309, 1986.
335. Parrish, A. E., Kramer, N. C., Hatch, F. E., et al. Relationship between glomerular function and histology in acute glomerulonephritis. *J. Lab. Clin. Med.* 58: 197, 1961.
336. Partman, R. J., Kissane, J. M., and Robson, A. M. Use of B_2 microglobulin to diagnose tubulointerstitial lesions in children. *Kidney Int.* 30: 91, 1986.
337. Pasternack, A., and Linder, E. Renal tubular acidosis: An immunological study on four patients. *Clin. Exp. Immunol.* 7: 115, 1970.
338. Pedersen, J. C., Persson, A. E. G., and Maunsback, A. B. Ultrastructure and Quantitative Characterization of the Cortical Interstitium in the Rat Kidney. In A. B. Maunsback, T. S. Olsen, and A. I. Christensen (eds.), *Functional Ultrastructure of the Kidney.* London: Academic Press, 1980. Pp. 443–446.
339. Persson, A. E. G. Functional Aspects of the Renal Interstitium. In A. B. Maunsback, T. S. Olsen, and A. I. Christenson (eds.), *Functional Ultrastructure of the Kidney.* London: Academic Press, 1980. Pp. 399–410.
340. Persson, A. E. G., Muller-Swur, R., and Selen, G. Capillary oncotic pressure as a modifier for tubuloglomerular feedback. *Am. J. Physiol.* 236: F97, 1979.
341. Peterson, M. J., and Edelman, I. S. Calcium inhibition of the action of vasopressin on the urinary bladder of the toad. *J. Clin. Invest.* 43: 583, 1964.
342. Pfaller, W., and Rittinger, M. Quantitative morphology of the rat kidney. *Int. J. Biochem.* 12: 17, 1980.
343. Pfaltz, M., and Briner, J. Glomerular changes in interstitial kidney diseases. *Schweiz. Med. Wochenschr.* 114: 204, 1984.
344. Pinter, G. G., Wilson, P. D., Bell, D. R., et al. Interstitial Albumin Pool in the Renal Cortex: Its Turnover and Permeability of Peritubular Capillaries. In A. B. Maunsback, T. S. Olsen, and A. I. Christenson (eds.), *Functional Ultrastructure of the Kidney.* London: Academic Press, 1980. Pp. 411–422.
345. Piper, J., Tonascia, J., and Matanoshi, G. Heavy phenacetin use and bladder cancer in women aged 20 to 49 years. *N. Engl. J. Med.* 313: 292, 1985.
346. Pirani, C. L., Silva, F. G., and Appel, G. B. Tubulo-interstitial disease in multiple myeloma and other non-renal neoplasias. *Contemp. Issues Nephrol.* 10: 287, 1983.
347. Pitman, S. W., Parker, L. M., and Tattersall, M. H. N. Clinical trial of high dose methotrexate with citrovorum factor: Toxicologic and therapeutic observations. *Cancer Chemother. Rep.* 6: 43, 1975.
348. Platt, J. L., Sibley, R. K., and Michael, A. F. Interstitial nephritis associated with cytomegalovirus infection. *Kidney Int.* 28: 550, 1985.
349. Plotz, A. Analgesic nephropathy. For this time and this place. *Arch. Intern. Med.* 143: 1676, 1983.
350. Porter, G. A. (ed.). *Nephrotoxic Mechanisms of Drugs and Environmental Toxins.* New York: Plenum, 1982.
351. Ramsay, A. G., and Whick, D. F. Phenacetin nephropathy. *Can. Med. Assoc. J.* 92: 55, 1965.
352. Ransley, P. G., and Risdon, R. A. Renal papillary morphology and intrarenal reflux in the young pig. *Urol. Res. J.* 3: 105, 1975.
353. Ransley, P. G., and Risdon, R. A. Renal papillary morphology in infants and young children. *Urol. Res.* 3: 110, 1975.
354. Raymond, K. H., Davidson, K. K., and McKinney, T. D. In vivo and in vitro studies of urinary concentrating ability in potassium depleted rabbits. *J. Clin. Invest.* 76: 561, 1985.
355. Relman, A. S., and Schwartz, W. B. The kidney in potassium depletion. *Am. J. Med.* 24: 764, 1958.
356. Remuzzi, G., and Bertani, T. Renal vascular and thrombotic effects of cyclosporine. *Am. J. Kidney Dis.* 13: 261, 1989.
357. Resnick, J. S., Sisson, S., and Vernier, R. L. Tamm-Horsfall protein. Abnormal localization in renal disease. *Lab. Invest.* 38: 550, 1978.
358. Riley, A. L., Ryan, L. M., and Roth, D. A. Renal proximal tubular dysfunction and paroxysmal nocturnal hemoglobinuria. *Am. J. Med.* 62: 125, 1977.
359. Risdon, R. A., Slopper, J. C., and de Wardener, H. E. Relationship between renal function and histological changes found in renal biopsy specimens from patients with persistent glomerular nephritis. *Lancet* 2: 363, 1968.
360. Risholm, L. Studies in renal colic and its treatment by posterior splanchnic block. *Acta Chir. Scand.* [*Suppl.*] 184: 5, 1954.
361. Robbins, S. L., Mallory, G. K., and Kinney, D. T. Necrotizing renal papillitis. Form of acute pyelonephritis. *N. Engl. J. Med.* 235: 885, 1946.
362. Roberts, J. A. Etiology and pathophysiology of pyelonephritis. *Am. J. Kidney Dis.* 17: 1, 1991.
363. Roberts, J. A., Roth, J. K., Dominique, G., et al. Immu-

nology of pyelonephritis in primates: Model VI. Effect of complement depletion. *J. Urol.* 129: 193, 1983.
364. Rodeman, H. P., and Müller, G. H. Abnormal growth and clonal proliferation of fibroblasts derived from kidneys with interstitial fibrosis. *Proc. Soc. Exp. Biol. Med.* 195: 57, 1990.
365. Rosansky, S. J., and Eggers, P. W. Trends in the U.S. end-stage renal disease population 1973–1983. *Am. J. Kidney Dis.* 9: 91, 1987.
366. Rosebaum, J. L., Mikail, M., and Wiedmann, F. Further correlation of renal function with kidney biopsy in chronic renal disease. *Am. J. Med. Sci.* 254: 156, 1967.
367. Rosen, S., Harmon, W., Krensky, A. M., et al. Tubulointerstitial nephritis associated with polyoma-virus (BK type) infection. *N. Engl. J. Med.* 308: 1192, 1983.
368. Rosen, S., Pirani, C. L., and Muehrcke, R. C. Renal interstitial foam cells: A light and electron microscopic study. *Am. J. Clin. Pathol.* 45: 32, 1966.
369. Rosenberg, M. E., Schendel, P. B., McCurdy, F. A., et al. Characterization of immune cells in kidneys from patients with Sjögren's syndrome. *Am. J. Kidney Dis.* 11: 20, 1988.
370. Rostand, S., Kirk, K. A., Rutsky, E. A., et al. Racial differences in the incidence of treatment for end-stage renal disease. *N. Engl. J. Med.* 306: 1276, 1982.
371. Roxe, D. M., and Krumlovsky, F. A. Toxic interstitial nephropathy from metals metabolites and radiation. *Semin. Nephrol.* 8: 72, 1988.
372. Rubini, M. Water excretion in potassium deficient man. *J. Clin. Invest.* 40: 2215, 1961.
373. Ruiz, P., Kalbeck, P. C., Scroggs, M. W., et al. Associations between cyclosporine therapy and interstitial fibrosis in renal allograft biopsies. *Transplantation* 45: 91, 1988.
374. Rutner, A. B., and Smith, D. R. Renal papillary necrosis. *J. Urol.* 84: 462, 1961.
375. Sabatini, S. The pathophysiology of experimentally induced papillary necrosis. *Semin. Nephrol.* 4: 27, 1984.
376. Sahai, T., Harris, F. H., Marsh, D. J., et al. Extracellular fluid expansion and autoregulation in nephrotoxic nephritis in rats. *Kidney Int.* 25: 619, 1984.
377. Sanerkin, N. G. Chronic phenacetin nephropathy with particular reference to the relationship between renal papillary necrosis and "chronic interstitial nephritis." *Br. J. Urol.* 38: 361, 1966.
378. Sanford, J. P., Hunter, B. W., and Donaldson, P. Localization and fate of *Escherichia coli* in hematogenous pyelonephritis. *J. Exp. Med.* 116: 285, 1962.
379. Sargent, J. C., and Sargent, J. W. Unilateral renal papillary necrosis. *J. Urol.* 73: 757, 1955.
380. Sato, K., Oguchi, H., Yoshie, T., et al. Tubulointerstitial nephritis induced by Tamm-Horsfall protein sensitization in guinea pigs. *Virchows Arch.* [B] 58: 357, 1990.
381. Savage, D. C. L., Howie, G., Adler, K., et al. Controlled trial of therapy in covert bacteriuria in childhood. *Lancet* 1: 358, 1975.
382. Sawhney, A. S., Winer, R. L., Cohen, A. H., et al. Sjögren's syndrome with immune complex tubulointerstitial renal disease. (Abstract) *Kidney Int.* 6: 453, 1975.
383. Scarpelli, D. G. Experimental nephrocalcinosis. A biochemical and morphological study. *Lab. Invest.* 14: 123, 1965.
384. Schainuck, L. I., Striker, G. E., Cutler, R. E., et al. Structural-functional correlations in renal disease. Part II. The correlations. *Hum. Pathol.* 1: 631, 1970.
385. Schourup, K. Necrosis of the renal papillae: Post-mortem series. *Acta Pathol. Microbiol. Scand.* 41: 462, 1957.
386. Schreiner, G. E. The nephrotoxicity of analgesic abuse. *Ann. Intern. Med.* 57: 1047, 1962.
387. Schreiner, G. F., Jr., Harris, K. P. G., Purkerson, M. L., et al. Immunological aspects of acute ureteral obstruction: Immune cell infiltrate in the kidney. *Kidney Int.* 34: 487, 1988.
388. Schreiner, G. F., Jr., and Kohan, D. E. Regulation of renal transport processes and hemodynamics by macrophages and lymphocytes. *Am. J. Physiol.* 258: F761, 1990.
389. Schulman, J. D., and Schneider, J. A. Cystinosis and the Fanconi syndrome. *Pediatr. Clin. North Am.* 23: 779, 1976.
390. Schwartz, M. M., and Cotran, R. Z. Common enterobacterial antigen in human chronic pyelonephritis and interstitial nephritis. An immunofluorescent study. *N. Engl. J. Med.* 289: 830, 1973.
391. Schwartz, W. B., and Relman, A. S. Effect of electrolyte disorders on renal structure and function. *N. Engl. J. Med.* 276: 383, 1967.
392. Seedat, Y. K., and Schonland, M. Renal papillary necrosis associated with acute pancreatitis. *S. Afr. Med. J.* 49: 315, 1975.
393. Seegmiller, J. A., and Frazier, P. P. Biological considerations of the renal damage of gout. *Ann. Rheum. Dis.* 25(Suppl. 6): 668, 1966.
394. Seegal, A. J., Spataro, R. F., and Barbanic, Z. L. Adult polycystic disease. A review of 100 cases. *J. Urol.* 118: 711, 1977.
395. Seiler, M. W., and Hoyer, J. R. Ultrastructural studies of tubulointerstitial immune complex nephritis in rats immunized with Tamm-Horsfall protein. *Lab. Invest.* 45: 321, 1981.
396. Sency, F. D., Burns, D. K., and Silva, F. G. Acquired immunodeficiency syndrome and the kidney. *Am. J. Kidney Dis.* 16: 1, 1990.
397. Senekjian, H. O., Stinebaugh, B. J., Mattioli, C. A., et al. Irreversible renal failure following vesicoureteral reflux. *J.A.M.A.* 241: 160, 1979.
398. Sergeant, G. R. *The Clinical Features of Sickle Cell Disease.* New York: American Elsevier, 1974. Pp. 1–348.
399. Sheehan, H. L. Medullary necrosis of the kidneys. *Lancet* 2: 187, 1937.
400. Shiner, P. T., Harris, W. S., and Weissler, A. M. Effects of acute changes in serum calcium levels on the systolic time intervals in man. *Am. J. Cardiol.* 24: 42, 1969.
401. Shulman, H., Striker, G., Deeg, H. J., et al. Nephrotoxicity of cyclosporine A after allogenic marrow transplantation. *N. Engl. J. Med.* 305: 1392, 1981.
402. Sibley, R. K., and Kim, Y. Dense intramembranous deposit disease: New pathologic features. *Kidney Int.* 25: 660, 1984.
403. Silbert, P. L., Matz, L. R., Christiansen, K., et al. Herpes simplex virus interstitial nephritis in a renal allograft. *Clin. Nephrol.* 33: 264, 1990.
404. Simon, H. B., Bennett, W. A., and Emmett, J. L. Renal papillary necrosis. A clinicopathologic study of 42 cases. *J. Urol.* 77: 557, 1957.
405. Simon, H. B., Weinstein, A. J., Pasternak, M. S., et al. Genitourinary tuberculosis. Clinical features in a general hospital population. *Am. J. Med.* 63: 410, 1977.
406. Singere, D. R., and Evans, D. J. Renal impairment in sarcoidosis: Granulomatous nephritis as an isolated cause (two case reports and a review of the literature). *Clin. Nephrol.* 26: 250, 1986.
407. Smellie, J. M. Medical aspects of urinary infection in children. *J. R. Coll. Physicians Lond.* 1: 189, 1967.
408. Smith, J., Halmgren, J., Ahstedt, S., et al. Local antibody production in experimental pyelonephritis:

Amount, acidity and immunoglobulin class. *Infec. Immun.* 10: 411, 1974.
409. Solez, K., and Heptinstall, R. H. Intrarenal urinary extravasation in the formation of venous polyps containing Tamm-Horsfall protein. *J. Urol.* 119: 180, 1978.
410. Spear, G. S. Pathology of the kidney in cystinosis. *Pathol. Annu.* 9: 81, 1974.
411. Spital, A., Panner, B. J., and Sterns, R. H. Primary acute idiopathic tubulointerstitial nephritis: Report of two cases and review of the literature. *Am. J. Kidney Dis.* 9: 710, 1987.
412. Spuhler, O., and Zollinger, H. U. Die chronische interstitielle nephritis. *Z. Klin. Med.* 151: 1, 1953.
413. Statius van Eps, L. W., Pinedo-Veels, C., de Vries, G. H., et al. Nature of concentrating defect in sickle cell nephropathy: Microradioangiographic studies. *Lancet* 1: 450, 1970.
414. Steblay, R. W., and Rudofsky, U. Renal tubular disease and autoantibodies against tubular basement membrane induced in guinea pigs. *J. Immunol.* 107: 589, 1971.
415. Steblay, R. W., and Rudofsky, U. Transfer of experimental autoimmune renal cortical tubular and interstitial disease in guinea pigs by serum. *Science* 180: 966, 1973.
416. Steele, T. W., and Edwards, K. D. G. Analgesic nephropathy: Changes in various parameters of renal function following cessation of analgesic abuse. *Med. J. Aust.* 1: 181, 1971.
417. Stefanovic, V., and Polenakovic, M. H. Kidney disease beyond the Balkans. *Am. J. Nephrol.* 11: 1, 1991.
418. Steinmuller, D. R., Bolton, K., Stilmant, M. M., et al. Chronic interstitial nephritis and mixed cryoglobinemia associated with drug abuse. *Arch. Pathol. Lab. Med.* 103: 63, 1979.
419. Sugisaki, T., Klassen, J., Milgrom, F., et al. Immunopathologic study of an autoimmune tubular and interstitial renal disease in Brown Norway rats. *Lab. Invest.* 28: 658, 1973.
420. Suki, W. N. Polycystic kidney disease. *Kidney Int.* 22: 571, 1982.
421. Suki, W. N., and Eknoyan, G. Tubulo-Interstitial Disease. In B. Brenner and F. Rector (eds.), *The Kidney.* Philadelphia: Saunders, 1976. Pp. 1113–1137.
422. Suki, W. N., Eknoyan, G., Rector, F. C., et al. The renal diluting and concentrating mechanism in hypercalcemia. *Nephron* 6: 50, 1969.
423. Svenson, K., Bohman, S., and Hallgren, R. Renal interstitial fibrosis and vascular changes: Occurrence in patients with autoimmune diseases treated with cyclosporine. *Arch. Intern. Med.* 146: 2007, 1986.
424. Swartz, R. D., Wesley, J. R., Somermeyer, M. G., et al. Hyperoxaluria and renal insufficiency due to ascorbic acid administration during total parenteral nutrition. *Ann. Intern. Med.* 100: 530, 1984.
425. Sweet, R. M., Smith, C. L., Berkseth, R. O., et al. Jejunoileal bypass surgery and granulomatous disease of the kidney and liver. *Arch. Intern. Med.* 138: 626, 1978.
426. Talbott, J. H., and Terplan, K. L. The kidney in gout. *Medicine* 39: 405, 1960.
427. Tamminen, T. E., and Kapiro, E. A. The relationship of the shape of the renal papillae and of collecting duct openings to intrarenal reflux. *Br. J. Radiol.* 49: 345, 1977.
428. Tannen, R. L. The effect of uncomplicated potassium depletion on urine acidification. *J. Clin. Invest.* 49: 813, 1970.
429. Teree, T. M., Friedman, A. B., Kest, L. M., et al. Cystinosis and proximal tubular nephropathy in siblings. Progressive development of the physiological and anatomical lesions. *Am. J. Dis. Child.* 119: 481, 1970.
430. Tessel, W. J. Renal outcomes of gout and hyperuricemia. *Am. J. Med.* 67: 74, 1979.
431. Thoenes, W., Sonntag, W., Heine, W.-D., et al. Cell fusion as a mechanism for the formation of giant cells (Langhan's type): Autoradiographic findings in autoimmune tubulo-interstitial nephritis. *Virchows Arch [Cell. Pathol.]* 41: 45, 1982.
432. Thompson, C. S., and Weinman, E. J. The significance of oxalate in renal failure. *Am. J. Kidney Dis.* 4: 97, 1984.
433. Tisher, C. C., Bulger, R. E., and Valtin, H. Morphology of renal medulla in water diuresis and vasopressin-induced antidiuresis. *Am. J. Physiol.* 220: 87, 1971.
434. Toback, F. G., Ordonez, N. G., Bartz, S. C., et al. Zonal changes in renal structure and phospholipid metabolism in potassium deficient rats. *Lab. Invest.* 34: 115, 1976.
435. Tolins, J. P., Hostetter, M. K., and Hostetter, T. H. Hypokalemic nephropathy in the rat: Role of ammonia in chronic tubular injury. *J. Clin. Invest.* 79: 1447, 1987.
436. Torres, V. E., Velosa, J. A., Holley, K. E., et al. The progression of vesicoureteral reflux nephropathy. *Ann. Intern. Med.* 92: 776, 1980.
437. Truong, L. D., Farhood, A., Tasby, J., et al. Experimental chronic renal ischemia: Morphologic and immunologic studies. *Kidney Int.* 41: 1676, 1992.
438. Tuma, S., Chaimowitz, C., Erlik, D., et al. Fatal papillary necrosis in a kidney graft. *J.A.M.A.* 235: 754, 1976.
439. Vaamonde, C. A. Renal papillary necrosis in sickle cell hemoglobinopathies. *Semin. Nephrol.* 4: 48, 1984.
440. van Dorp, W. T., Jie, K., Lobatto, S., et al. Renal failure due to granulomatous interstitial nephritis after pulmonary sarcoidosis. *Nephrol. Dial. Transplant.* 2: 573, 1987.
441. Vangelista, A., Frasca, G. M., Severi, B., et al. Clinical factors in progressive renal damage: The role of interstitial fibrosis. *Am. J. Kidney Dis.* (Suppl. 1): 62, 1991.
442. van Ypersele de Strihou, C., and Mery, J. P. Hantavirus-related acute interstitial nephritis in Europe: Expansion of a world-wide zoonosis. *Q. J. Med.* 73: 941, 1989.
443. Van Zveiten, M. J., Lever, P. D., Bhan, A. K., et al. Experimental cell mediated interstitial nephritis induced with exogenous antigens. *J. Immunol.* 118: 589, 1977.
444. Verani, R., Nasir, M., and Foley, R. Granulomatous interstitial nephritis after a jejunoileal bypass: An ultrastructural and histochemical study. *Am. J. Nephrol.* 9: 51, 1989.
445. Vermillion, C. D., and Heale, W. F. Ureteral reflux in infancy. Relation to pyelonephritic scarring in adults. *Rocky Mt. Med. J.* 72: 200, 1975.
446. Vernier, R. L., and Resnick, J. Medullary cystic disease: The possible role of Tamm-Horsfall protein (Abstract). *Kidney Int.* 9: 450, 1976.
447. Viol, G. W., Minielly, J. A., and Bistricki, T. Gold nephropathy. *Arch. Pathol. Lab. Med.* 101: 635, 1977.
448. Wacker, W. E., Haynes, H., and Druyan, R. Treatment of ethylene glycol poisoning with ethyl alcohol. *J.A.M.A.* 194: 1231, 1965.
449. Wainscoat, J. S., and Finn, R. Possible role of laxatives in analgesic nephropathy. *Br. Med. J.* 4: 697, 1974.
450. Wallace, M. R., Bruton, D., North, A., et al. End-stage renal failure due to familial hypokalemic interstitial nephritis with identical HLA tissue types. *N.Z. Med. J.* 98: 5, 1985.
451. Warrell, M. J., Chinn, I., Morris, P. J., et al. The effects of viral infections on renal transplants and their recipients. *Q. J. Med.* 49: 219, 1980.
452. Watanabe, T., Nagafuchi, Y.. Yoshikawa, Y., et al. Renal

papillary necrosis associated with Wegener's granulomatosis. *Hum. Pathol.* 14: 551, 1983.

453. Wedeen, R. P., and Batuman, V. Tubulointerstitial nephritis induced by heavy metals and metabolic disturbances. *Contemp. Issues Nephrol.* 10: 211, 1983.
454. Wedeen, R. P., Maesaka, J. K., Weiner, B., et al. Occupational lead nephropathy. *Am. J. Med.* 59: 630, 1975.
455. Wedeen, R. P., Mallik, D. K., and Batuman, V. Detection and treatment of occupational lead nephropathy. *Arch. Intern. Med.* 139: 53, 1979.
456. Wehrmann, M., Bohle, A., Bogenschritz, O., et al. Long-term prognosis of chronic idiopathic membranous glomerulonephritis: An analysis of 334 cases with particular regard to tubulo-interstitial changes. *Clin. Nephrol.* 31: 67, 1989.
457. Whitworth, J. A., Leroux-Robert, C., Meyrier, A., et al. Papillary necrosis in renal allografts. Reports of two cases. *Aust. N.Z. J. Med.* 5: 69, 1975.
458. Wilson, C. B. Study of the immunopathogenesis of tubulointerstitial nephritis using model systems. *Kidney Int.* 35: 938, 1989.
459. Wilson, C. B., Lehman, D. H., McCoy, R. C., et al. Antitubular basement membranes after renal transplantation. *Transplantation* 18: 447, 1974.
460. Wind, E. S., and Platt, N. Renal papillary necrosis in aplastic anemia. *N.Y. State J. Med.* 70: 2117, 1970.
461. Winer, R. L., Cohen, A. H., Sawhney, A. S., et al. Sjögren's syndrome with immune complex tubulointerstitial renal disease. *Clin. Immunol. Immunopathol.* 8: 494, 1977.
462. Wolfe, J. A., McCann, R. L., and Sanfilipo, F. Cyclosporine-associated microangiopathy in renal transplantation: A severe but potentially reversible form of early graft injury. *Transplantation* 41: 541, 1986.
463. Wolstenholme, G. E. W., and Knight, J. (eds.). *The Balkan Nephropathy* (Ciba Foundation Study Group No. 33). Boston: Little, Brown, 1967.
464. Woods, J. W., Welt, L. G., Hollander, W., et al. Susceptibility of rats to experimental pyelonephritis following recovery from potassium depletion. *J. Clin. Invest.* 39: 28, 1960.
465. World Health Organization. Report of the working group on hemorrhagic fever with renal syndrome. Tokyo, Japan, February 22–24, 1982.
466. Wuthrich, R., Glincher, L., Yui, M., et al. MHC Class II, antigen presentation and tumor necrosis factor in renal tubular epithelial cells. *Kidney Int.* 37: 783, 1990.
467. Wylie, R. G., Hill, G. S., Murray, G., et al. Experimental papillary necrosis of the kidney. III. Effects of reserpine and other pharmacologic agents on the lesion. *Am. J. Pathol.* 68: 235, 1972.
468. Yeung, C. K., Wong, K. L., Ng, R. P., et al. Tubular dysfunction in systemic lupus erythematosus. *Nephron* 36: 84, 1984.
469. Yu, T. F., and Berger, L. Impaired renal function in gout. *Am. J. Med.* 72: 95, 1982.
470. Yu, T. F., Berger, L., Dorph, D. J., et al. Renal function in gout. *Am. J. Med.* 67: 766, 1979.
471. Yu, T. F., and Guttman, A. B. Uric acid nephrolithiasis in gout. Predisposing factors. *Ann. Intern. Med.* 67: 1133, 1967.
472. Zager, R. A., Cotran, R. S., and Hoyer, J. R. Pathologic localization of Tamm-Horsfall protein in interstitial deposits in renal disease. *Lab. Invest.* 38: 52, 1978.
473. Zollinger, H. U. Chronische interstitielle nephritis bei abusus von phenacetin hatingen analgetua. *Schweiz. Med. Woschenschr.* 85: 746, 1955.

XI

Collagen, Vascular, Hematologic, and Vasculitis-Related Renal Disease

sponses can be modulated by cyclooxygenase products such as prostaglandin I_2 (PGI_2, prostacyclin) and PGE_2, which have well-established roles in regulating platelet adhesion and in controlling blood flow and clot formation in the microvasculature [165].

PAF, a phosphoglyceride derived from choline-containing phospholipids, was first characterized by its ability to induce release of vasoactive amines from platelets [13, 65, 72]. However, it is also synthesized by inflammatory leukocytes such as neutrophils and monocyte/macrophages, by endothelial cells, and by interstitial cells, including those of smooth muscle and of the mesangium. Much of the PAF remains intracellular [117], but the significance of this is unknown. There is increasing evidence that, partly as a consequence of its rapid metabolic inactivation, PAF may have a "short-range" or "paracrine" role in neutrophil emigration from blood vessels, as will be discussed further. Administered PAF binds to cells via a specific receptor, which is a member of the rhodopsin receptor/G-protein–linked superfamily [76]. It can prime neutrophils in vitro, thus activating them; this leads to LTB_4 secretion as well as neutrophil aggregation and adhesion to surfaces. PAF also acts on both neutrophil and endothelial cells to promote adhesion. In vivo, PAF administration causes neutrophil accumulation, and the use of specific antagonists has indicated a role in a variety of models of inflammatory vascular injury, such as immune complex vasculitis and endotoxemia in the rat [219, 232].

Cytokines. Cytokines are a family of potent regulatory proteins synthesized and released by all the cell types involved in inflammatory vascular injury. They are active in the picomolar- to nanomolar-concentration range. Cytokines form another complex web of mediators that influence many stages of the inflammatory response. For example, they stimulate leukocyte production by the bone marrow, some are priming and chemotactic factors for leukocytes and modulate leukocyte-endothelial interaction, and they can govern processes of repair. They also have important effects on specific immune responses. Nathan and Sporn [145], recognizing the complexity of the cytokine network, suggested that these molecules should be regarded as elements of an intercellular language whose meaning is controlled by the "context" in which the cells are found, i.e., the surrounding extracellular matrix. In this view, cytokines are best regarded as acting on tissues rather than on individual cells. Their role is to coordinate the modeling and remodeling of tissues during development, during normal physiologic activity, and when driven by disease. A full review of cytokines is beyond the scope of this discussion, especially because most cytokines have a startling range of effects on isolated cells [6]. Nevertheless, the prospect of novel therapeutic agents that specifically interfere with cytokine action means that it is important to summarize the current state of knowledge by picking out individual molecules of particular importance in vascular injury.

IL-1 is not a chemoattractant for isolated neutrophils in vitro, but when injected intradermally, it induces neutrophil accumulation, albeit more slowly than C5a; presumably this is due to local release of chemotactic agents [164, 233]. IL-1 has a host of biologic actions, which suggest that it plays a central role in the initiation and regulation of inflammatory vascular injury. Furthermore, IL-1 is secreted by many of the cells involved in this process, be they leukocyte, vascular, or interstitial [41].

There are two distinct forms of IL-1, IL-1α, and IL-1β, which are homologous polypeptides that bind to the same receptors. The main difference between them is that IL-1α is predominantly membrane bound, whereas IL-1β is released. A wide range of stimuli, including important mediators such as lipopolysaccharide, complement fragments, and leukotrienes, induce synthesis of the 31-kd intracellular precursor peptides of IL-1α and IL-1β, which lack conventional N-terminal signal sequences and lack biologic activity. Subsequent cleavage by lysosomal enzymes releases "mature" 17.5-kd extracellular IL-1α and IL-1β. These may be further processed by inflammatory cell proteinases in the extracellular compartment to yield smaller, but still active, IL-1–derived peptides. However, depending on the cell and the stimulus, much IL-1 remains intracellular, where its function is poorly understood. Membrane-bound IL-1 also has potent effects on directly apposed cells. Indeed, the potential of IL-1 to have such highly localized effects of a "paracrine" or "autocrine" nature, in addition to its originally recognized systemic/"hormone" effects, is well demonstrated by its ability to stimulate its *own* production (and that of the related cytokines TNF and IL-6) in macrophages and endothelial cells [42, 231]. Finally, the potential complexity of IL-1 actions in vivo is exemplified by the observation that macrophages secrete a soluble IL-1 receptor antagonist as well as synthesizing IL-1 [48, 66].

The local and systemic activities of IL-1 have been extensively studied in vivo and modeled in vitro using pure recombinant IL-1. Table 71-3 shows some of the activities of particular relevance to the processes described in this chapter. An exhaustive dissection of the role of IL-1 in the inflammatory process would be inappropriate here; instead, in later sections we will concentrate specifically on mechanisms involving IL-1 that lead to leukocyte adhesion to endothelium and their emigration from blood vessels. Nevertheless, it should be clear that the properties of IL-1 imply a key role in the initiation and potentiation of vascular injury. Indeed, there is now direct evidence from animal models of disease that this is the case. For example, Tomosugi et al. [221] have shown that pretreatment with IL-1 exacerbates injury, as evidenced by albuminuria or capillary thrombus formation in rats with glomerular capillary injury induced by passive administration of heterologous antibody to glomerular basement membrane.

TNF-α, also known as cachectin, has many similarities to IL-1. It is a 17-kd polypeptide. Various proinflammatory stimuli elicit TNF-α synthesis from monocyte/macrophages, endothelial cells, and other cells implicated in vascular injury. Activated T cells secrete a distinct

Table 71-3. Activities of IL-1 relevant to vascular injury

Systemic	
Brain	Fever, anorexia
Liver	Increased synthesis of acute-phase proteins, C reactive protein, etc. Decreased synthesis of albumin
Muscle	Catabolism
Cardiovascular	Hypotension
Immune	Amplifies antigen-driven proliferation of B and T lymphocytes
Marrow	Increases neutrophil release
Local	
Leukocytes	Chemoattractant (in vivo) Stimulates synthesis of other mediators
Vessel wall	Increases expression of endothelial adhesion molecules for leukocytes Pro-coagulant effect on endothelium Promotes transendothelial passage of leukocytes Stimulates synthesis of other mediators
Interstitium	Stimulates proliferation of fibroblasts, mesangial cells, and keratinocytes Increases synthesis of collagen and collagenase Stimulates synthesis of other mediators

but structurally related polypeptide, lymphotoxin (also known as TNF-β), having similar biologic activities. In vivo, injection of TNF-α results in proinflammatory responses very similar to those observed with IL-1; it induces neutrophil accumulation and edema after intradermal administration, and the same systemic responses as IL-1 (see Table 71-3). However, TNF-α is more potent than IL-1 in inducing shock in rabbits [150] and appears to be one of the crucial mediators of this syndrome [19], as evidenced by the observation in baboons that passive immunization with antibodies to TNF-α prevents shock induced by intravenous infusion of live gram-negative bacteria [225]. Neutrophil adherence to vessel walls is prominent in this model, and it is tempting to relate the greater propensity of TNF-α to induce shock to its capacity to prime and activate neutrophils, an activity not shared with IL-1 [249]. TNF-α has also been shown to induce nitric oxide synthesis in mesangial cells and in vascular smooth muscle, resulting in decreased response of these cells to vasoconstrictor substances (see below).

TNF-induced neutrophil degranulation and activation of respiratory burst depend on concurrent signaling from a neutrophil receptor for matrix, the CR3 (CD11b/CD18) heterodimer, which mediates both adhesion and oscillations of cytosol free Ca^{2+} [173]; this is evocative of Nathan and Sporn's [145] concept that the information conveyed to a cell by cytokines depends on the "context" of the cell. Intracellular signal pathways activated by TNF-α and IL-1 have not been defined, so it is not known whether they use the same second messengers or why they are synergistic.

IL-1 and TNF induce cells to synthesize other cytokines, and many of their effects in vivo reflect this property. Some of the most important of these cytokines are of a family of cationic, chemotactic cytokines of molecular mass 8 to 10 kd that have been identified with startling rapidity and include polypeptides such as IL-8 and platelet factor 4 (PF 4). This family has been called the *intercrines* by Oppenheim [151] and subdivided into an α subfamily encoded on chromosome 4 and a β subfamily mapped to chromosome 17 (Table 71-4). The potential complexity of the interactions between intercrines is beyond the scope of this discussion, but the intercrines' power to initiate and amplify injury is clear, for example, by release of IL-8 from interstitial cells including resident macrophages, endothelial cells, and inflammatory leukocytes at the injured site [9].

As stated earlier, IL-1, TNF, and the intercrines are important mediators of the early stages of the classic acute inflammatory response. However, activated T cells can also initiate inflammation by secreting cytokines that are chemotactic for mononuclear cells rather than neutrophils. This may be important in the period after the first 8 hours of the acute inflammatory response or in the mediation of the predominantly mononuclear "inflammatory" response seen in delayed-type hypersensitivity.

Interferon-γ (IFN-γ) is a 40-kd, homodimeric glycoprotein released from antigen- or mitogen-stimulated T cells. It is probably the most important macrophage-activating factor [6] and was recently shown to stimulate adhesion of T cells (but not neutrophils) to cultured endothelial cells in vitro [216]. Unlike IL-1 and TNF-α, IFN-γ does not have a procoagulant effect on endothelium but instead induces major histocompatibility complex class II expression, as is seen in vivo in delayed hypersensitivity. Endothelial cells bearing class II molecules can present antigen to T cells in vitro and so may upregulate T-cell–driven responses in vivo [79].

IL-4 is another T-cell–derived cytokine with macrophage-activating properties. It enhances mononuclear cell adhesion to cultured endothelium selectively, albeit by a mechanism different than that of IFN-γ [217].

A number of other cytokines initiate an acute inflammatory response when they are injected in relatively large amounts in vivo; these include granulocyte-macrophage colony stimulatory factor (GM-CSF) and transforming growth factor-β (TGF-β). Both of these cytokines are more usually associated with other functions: GM-CSF is a growth factor for the bone marrow [135], and TGF-β is important for the repair of wounded tissue [51, 129, 204]. These observations emphasize the need for caution when interpreting the role of a cytokine in vascular injury. The demonstration of putatively proinflammatory effects on cells in vitro or following injection into an experimental animal is insufficient proof of a role in the inflammatory process in vivo. Proof demands that the mediator be shown to be present at the inflamed site, to have inflammatory effects when administered in

Table 71-4. Some members of the intercrine family

	Properties
α Subfamily	
Interleukin-8 (IL-8/NAP I)	Neutrophil chemoattractant Also acts on T cells, basophils, and monocytes
Platelet factor 4 (PF 4)	Chemoattractant (fibroblasts > neutrophils, monocytes) Immunostimulant
Platelet basic protein derivatives	
a. Higher molecular weight	
85 AA CTAP III 81 AA β thromboglobulin	Chemoattractants (fibroblast > neutrophil) "Connective tissue–activating peptide"
b. Lower molecular weight	
70 AA NAP II	Chemoattractant (neutrophil > fibroblast) "Neutrophil-activating peptide"
β Subfamily	
MCAP	"Monocyte chemotactic and activating factor"

doses providing local concentrations, and after inhibition by specific blockade, to result in abrogation of vascular injury.

CONTROL OF VASCULAR TONE

Vasodilatation is an early component of the inflammatory response and reflects a reduction in tone of resistant vessels. Vascular smooth muscle cells and glomerular mesangial cells contain contractile proteins. These elements are under the control of a number of the chemical messengers described in the previous section [134, 162]. Thus, PGI_2 and PGE_2 induce relaxation of vascular smooth muscle cells and mesangial cells, while PAF, thromboxane A_2 (TXA_2), and leukotriene C_4 (LTC_4) extend constrictor effects. An active role for the endothelium in control of vascular tone is suggested by its ability to synthesize PGI_2 from platelet-derived endoperoxides, LTC_4 from leukocyte-derived leukotriene A_4 (LTA_4), and PAF. It was also known that the endothelium can regulate the activity of other substances affecting vascular tone. For example, endothelium participates in the conversion of angiotensin I to angiotensin II, inactivates bradykinin, and is important in the uptake and metabolism of norepinephrine and serotonin [227]. The belief that the endothelium may be crucial in the regulation of local blood flow was strengthened by the identification of two powerful vasoactive substances synthesized by the endothelium, endothelin and endothelium-derived relaxing factor (EDRF). The endothelium synthesizes endothelin-1 (ET-1), one of the family of three vasoconstrictor peptides (ET-1, ET-2, and ET-3) [86, 246].

Endothelin. Preproendothelin-1 consists of 212 amino acids from which the 38–amino acid peptide "big ET-1" is cleaved. This is further converted to the biologically active 21–amino acid ET-1 by action of a peptidase named endothelin-converting enzyme. De novo synthesis of ET-1 is induced by several stimuli, including thrombin, hypoxia, and cytokines such as TGF-β and IL-1 [104, 246, 248]. Increased hemodynamic shear stress facilitates ET-1 release from the endothelium [247]. Activation of phospholipase C is part of the initial signaling events in the action of ET-1. In vascular smooth muscle cells and mesangial cells, ET-1 induces concentration-dependent mobilization of calcium, followed by contraction. ET-1 has also been shown to activate phospholipase A_2 [169]. In addition to vascular smooth muscle cell and mesangial cell contraction, ET-1 has been shown to exert a positive inotropic effect on cardiocytes [77, 96], to stimulate release of atrial natriuretic peptide (ANP) [54, 121], and to inhibit the release of renin [163, 210]. High-affinity specific binding sites for ET-1 have been found in vascular smooth muscle cells, mesangial cells, glomeruli in rats, renal papillae, heart, brain, and uterus [103, 118, 126, 209]. In the kidney, the highest concentration of immunoreactive ET-1 is in the papillae.

Intravenous infusion of ET-1 results in transient hypotension due to ET-1–induced release of EDRF and of vasodilatory prostaglandins [98, 137]. Increased release of ANP may also contribute to the initial hypotensive phase, which is followed by protracted hypertension due to severe peripheral vasoconstriction. There appears to be some heterogeneity in the vasoconstrictive response of different vascular beds to ET-1, with the coronary and renal territories being particularly sensitive [98, 115]. Moreover, ET-1 is mitogenic for vascular smooth muscle cells and mesangial cells, and this could be important in the vascular changes that occur in atherosclerosis and in those forms of glomerular injury accompanied by vascular smooth muscle cell and mesangial cell proliferation, respectively [8, 195].

ET-1 infused at low doses results in decreased renal blood flow without major changes in glomerular filtration rate, owing to a proportionately greater vasoconstrictive effect on the efferent than on the afferent glomerular arterioles [97]. A direct tubular effect of ET-1 is suggested by the natriuresis observed following doses of ET-1 that do not affect the glomerular filtration rate [97, 250]. Experimentally, ET-1 has been found to mediate, at least in part, the vasoconstriction that follows acute ischemic renal failure as well as that induced by cyclosporine [36, 156]. Clinically, increased plasma immunoreactive ET-1 is found in patients with acute and chronic renal failure [190, 220]. Elevated ET-1 has also been observed in septic shock [139], in patients with acute myocardial infarction, and in diabetics [211], but the clinical significance of these findings is at present unclear.

Endothelium-Derived Relaxing Factor. Nitrovasodilators such as nitroglycerin and sodium nitroprusside induce vascular smooth muscle relaxation in blood vessels in vitro, irrespective of whether they have been stripped of endothelium. This relaxation is mediated by modulation of the phosphorylation/dephosphorylation state of myosin light chains in response to increases in intracellular cyclic guanosine monophosphate (cGMP) and activation of cGMP-dependent protein kinases [85]. A substance similar to these vasodilators was found to be released by normal endothelium in response to a variety of agonists as well as to the mechanical stimulation of shear stress [227]. This diffusible, short-acting substance was termed EDRF [55]. Subsequent studies demonstrated that EDRF is nitric oxide released as such or in the form of a precursor that subsequently releases nitric oxide [143, 153].

Nitric oxide is formed from one of the two equivalent guanidine nitrogens of the amino acid L-arginine by an enzymatic oxidation process in which the primary products are nitric oxide and L-citrulline [153]. The nitric oxide synthase present in endothelial cells (nitric oxide–synthase II) is a dioxygenase [105], requires reduced NADP, and is dependent on calcium ions and calmodulin [125]. The nitric oxide–synthase II is inhibited by L-arginine analogues such as L-*N*-monomethylarginine and *N*-nitro-L-arginine. Nitric oxide is rapidly inactivated by superoxide anion but not by the other oxygen radical species. Hemoglobin also effectively inactivates nitric oxide, probably by binding the heme group [138].

Serotonin and adenosine diphosphate, released by platelets during aggregation, bind to specific receptors on endothelium to induce the release of EDRF/nitric oxide [227]. The same agonists induce vasoconstriction when released in the proximity of damaged endothelium. This may explain the abnormal vasospasm that may occur in different vascular territories such as the brain, heart, and kidney when intravascular coagulation is triggered in areas of damaged endothelial lining [116].

Recent studies give credence to the hypothesis that basal release of nitric oxide may help to maintain vascular tone [167]. A study by Tolins et al. [218] showed that intravenous administration of acetylcholine, an agonist of EDRF/nitric oxide, causes hypotension, renal vasodilation, and increased urinary levels of cGMP. These effects can be prevented by simultaneous administration of the inhibitor of EDRF/nitric oxide synthesis, L-*N*-monomethylarginine, whereas those of endothelium-independent vasodilators such as prostacyclin and sodium nitroprusside are unaffected. Moreover, systemic administration of L-*N*-monomethylarginine to normotensive animals results in protracted increases in blood pressure, suggesting that EDRF/nitric oxide contributes to the control of basal vascular tone [167, 218]. Although the existence of other EDRFs is suspected, their chemical nature has not been defined [227].

Recent studies have shown that in co-cultures of endothelial and mesangial cells, stimulation of the endothelium to release EDRF/nitric oxide results in increases in cGMP levels in mesangial cells [192]. In the same studies, nitric oxide was shown to attenuate angiotensin II–induced mesangial cell contraction. Since endothelial and mesangial cells are juxtaposed in the glomerulus, it is reasonable to assume that the release of vasoactive mediators by these cell types could act in an autocrine or paracrine fashion to influence the glomerular microcirculation. Nitric oxide also inhibits vascular smooth muscle cell and mesangial cell proliferation [58, 193]. Therefore, within the glomerular microenvironment, EDRF/nitric oxide, eicosanoids, and endothelin may act in concert, not only in the regulation of hemodynamic changes in response to other vasoactive substances but also in the modulation of thrombogenesis and growth-related events in response to glomerular injury.

Nitric oxide–synthase II has also been detected in neutrophils, platelets, and cerebellar cells, and nitric oxide affects several biologic functions in these cells. In macrophages and hepatocytes there is an isoform of the nitric oxide–synthase II termed *nitric oxide–synthase I.* This enzyme is not constitutive but is induced by lipopolysaccharide and by certain cytokines including TNF-α. Nitric oxide–synthase I is not dependent on calmodulin, but is dependent on tetrahydrobiopterin and on flavin-adenine dinucleotide [59, 128, 138]. Lipopolysaccharide and cytokines can also induce synthesis of nitric oxide in vascular smooth muscle and in mesangial cells, probably by induction of nitric oxide–synthase I [12, 194]. Nitric oxide synthesis by the inducible enzyme is more protracted (24–36 hours) and yields much larger amounts than those seen after receptor stimulation of endothelial cells by agonists such as acetylcholine.

Synthesis of nitric oxide by nitric oxide–synthase I is also inhibited by L-*N*-monomethylasparagine as well as by inhibitors of protein synthesis if given preceding induction of the enzyme. The biologic role of nitric oxide synthesis by nitric oxide–synthase I is at present unclear. However, it may be responsible for some of the changes in systemic and renal vascular tone that accompany gram-negative sepsis and those clinical situations in which circulating levels of cytokines are increased, such as in neoplastic disease [146, 194]. Protracted glomerular synthesis of nitric oxide by mesangial cells and/or by blood-borne macrophages could play an important role in glomerular injury due to either immune or nonimmune mechanisms. Potential renal pathophysiologic conditions in which nitric oxide and endothelin may play a role are summarized in Table 71-5.

LEUKOCYTE ADHESION TO THE VESSEL WALL

The cell-cell interaction between leukocytes and the endothelium is an important event in vascular injury. Advances in the understanding of the molecular mechanism of neutrophil-endothelial adhesion over the last 5 years have been remarkable. Among them are the finding that many of the mediators already discussed influ-

Table 71-5. Renal and extrarenal conditions in which nitric oxide and/or endothelin may be important

Nitric oxide
- Modulation of:
  - a. Systemic basal vascular tone
  - b. Glomerular microcirculation
  - c. Vascular smooth muscle proliferation
  - d. Mesangial cell proliferation
  - e. Platelet aggregation and adhesion
  - f. Natriuresis
- Acute renal failure
- Hypertension
- Septic shock
- Atherosclerosis

Endothelin
- Acute renal failure
- Malignant hypertension
- Septic shock
- Cyclosporine toxicity
- Modulation of vascular smooth muscle and mesangial cell proliferation
- Atherosclerosis

ence both leukocyte and endothelial cells to promote adhesion.

Site of Mediator Action. Over 100 years ago, Connheim [34] and Metchnikoff [136] provided seminal descriptions of the adherence of leukocytes to endothelium after injury and the subsequent leukocyte migration across vessel walls into the interstitium. However, they interpreted their results differently. Connheim believed that the primary event was increased adhesiveness of the endothelium, while Metchnikoff favored the hypothesis that the primary change was increased leukocyte stickiness. At about the same time, Thoma [215] suggested that neutrophil accumulation in the microvasculature reflected vasodilatation and reduced capillary blood flow. There is now evidence to suggest that all three mechanisms act in concert to promote leukocyte-endothelial adhesion, but this controversy seems set to continue on until there is a precise dynamic description of the molecular interactions responsible.

Important contributions to the understanding of these adhesion mechanisms have been made by vital microscopy of leukocyte-endothelial adhesion in living tissue subjected to trauma or injection of toxins/mediators. This type of observation was first made in rabbit ear chambers in the 1930s by the Clarks [27] and reinforced, using similar techniques, by Allison et al. [4] and Atherton and Born [7]. In these studies, neutrophils were seen to adhere to the walls of blood vessels and to migrate across them in minutes. Two types of neutrophil interaction with endothelium were distinguished. In the first, rounded "marginated" neutrophils rolled along the endothelium at about 10 μm/sec (one or two orders of magnitude slower than the blood flow), sometimes stopping transiently or dropping off into the faster flowing stream. In the second, tightly adherent, flattened neutrophils appeared destined to migrate across the vessel wall. Although slower blood flow did correlate with increased neutrophil margination [7], in keeping with Thoma's [215] concepts, local blood flow velocity alone did not predict which vessel leukocyte would adhere, indicating that other factors must be involved.

There is direct evidence to suggest that mediator-enhanced leukocyte adhesiveness is critical to the earliest stages of these phenomena. Nourshargh et al. [148] showed that treatment of purified, radiolabeled neutrophils with pertussis toxin (which inhibits receptor-mediated neutrophil responses in vitro by binding G-proteins) prevents neutrophil accumulation in rabbit skin injected with C5a, FMLP, or LTB_4. Furthermore, Nagai and Katori [144] provided confirmatory evidence in the hamster cheek pouch using leukocytes that had not been subjected to ex vivo manipulation. Injection of FMLP or LTB_4 by a very fine pipette into the interstitial space close to capillaries resulted in neutrophil adhesion to postcapillary venules *downstream.* However, direct administration of these mediators close to the venule did not induce leukocyte adhesion, suggesting that the effect of the mediators had been on the leukocyte, not the venular endothelium.

The rapidity of leukocyte adhesion to endothelium in vivo also suggests a primary change in the neutrophil, because neutrophil adhesiveness is upregulated by chemotactic peptides in less than a minute in vitro [223]. This is much faster than the increased expression of adhesion molecules on the surface of endothelial cells, which often takes an hour or more, as many are not constitutively expressed. A very rapid response does not preclude the endothelial cell from being responsible, because there are at least three situations in which adhesiveness of endothelial cells is rapidly upregulated: (1) Incubation of cultured endothelial cells with thrombin stimulates PAF production, which can induce neutrophil adhesion within a minute. This effect is maximal at 5 minutes, and rapidly wanes thereafter [252]; thrombin itself has no effect on neutrophil adhesion to inert surfaces. (2) Marks et al. [124] described another equally rapid but longer-lasting effect that depends on complement fixation to the endothelium. It peaks at 20 minutes and is maintained as long as a source of complement is available. However, it does not depend on complement-derived chemotactic factors, since components distal to C3 (i.e., C5 through C9) are not required. Instead, the evidence suggests that the complement activation product C3bi fixed to the endothelial cell acts as a bridge to neutrophil surface receptor CR3 (CD116/CD18). (3) Finally, the adhesion molecule, granule membrane protein 140 (GMP-140), is stored in Weibel-Palade bodies of endothelial cells and can be mobilized to the cell surface in seconds, promoting attachment of neutrophils [92, 106, 224].

To conclude, there are grounds for an eclectic view of the site of mediator action, since these agents can alter the adhesiveness of both leukocytes and endothelial cells almost simultaneously. It appears likely that coordinated changes in the surface properties of both cell types underlie leukocyte adherence to endothelial cells at inflamed sites in vivo.

Molecular Mechanisms of Leukocyte-Endothelial Adhesion. The molecular basis of leukocyte-endothelial adhesion is now well understood. The characterization, cloning, and sequencing of adhesion molecules that mediate biologic phenomena ranging from inflammation to differentiation have demonstrated that these structures can be grouped together in "supergene" families. Leukocyte-endothelial adhesion utilizes structures from three supergene families (Table 71-6), involved in a series of receptor/counterreceptor pairs (Table 71-7). Broadly speaking, integrins interact with members of the immunoglobulin family, and the selectins interact with a family of sugars [205].

The *leukocyte integrins* were the first family of proteins found to be important in leukocyte-endothelial interaction [84, 178], and the detailed molecular analysis of the rare heritable disorder leukocyte adhesion deficiency (LAD), was crucial to this discovery [5, 206]. Subjects affected with this disorder experience recurrent bacterial infections, impaired pus formation, and defective wound healing, features that reflect a severe impairment in the ability of leukocytes to migrate from blood vessels, even though histologic sections show abundant neutrophils and other leukocytes in the microvasculature [38].

In vitro, leukocytes from patients with LAD also have deficits in responses related to adherence, such as aggregation, chemotaxis, and adherence to inert substances or other cells. Leukocytes from these patients have a severe or total deficiency of a family of three leukocyte cell-surface glycoproteins known as the CD11/18 complex, or the β_2-integrins (see Tables 71-6 and 71-7). These are heterodimers containing different α chains combined with a common β chain. A variety of lesions are responsible for the defective β chain, which is required for surface expression of the otherwise normally synthesized α chains.

The critical role of these heterodimers in neutrophil adherence has been confirmed by studies showing the inhibitory effects of monoclonal antibodies to the CD11/18 complex. The studies indicated that the most important were lymphocyte function–associated antigen-1 (LFA-1) (originally identified by monoclonal antibodies inhibiting T-cell killing) and, for the neutrophil in particular, the integrin Mac-1 [57, 100, 160, 199, 206, 222]. In various systems it has been shown that CD11/18 adhesiveness is regulated by chemotactic factors in at least two ways: First, they mobilize Mac-1 to the cell surface by means of fusion of secondary granules containing preformed receptor within the plasma membrane. Second, they transiently increase the avidity of these structures for ligand. Clustering of receptors may also occur and further increase the affinity of binding.

Administration of anti-CD11/18 monoclonal antibodies to animals with experimentally induced inflammation inhibits leukocyte accumulation and attenuates leukocyte-related tissue injury in experimental models [175, 228] but does not inhibit neutrophil-endothelial adhesion universally. Thus, even when sufficient anti-CD18 monoclonal antibody was injected to inhibit neutrophil efflux into experimentally inflamed rabbit abdominal wall or peritoneum, it failed to inhibit neutrophil migration into the lungs after intratracheal installation of certain stimuli [43].

In vivo data therefore suggest that in addition to the CD11/18 complex, there must be other leukocyte surface molecules capable of mediating adhesion to endothelium at inflamed sites. A similar conclusion has been reached from in vitro studies of neutrophil interaction with endothelial cells under conditions of shear stress designed to mimic those calculated to be induced by blood flow in the postcapillary venule (thought to be about 2.0 dyne/cm^2) [109]. Under static conditions, or at very low shear stress (0.25 dyne/cm^2), monoclonal antibodies to CD11b and CD18 markedly inhibit neutrophil adhesion to endothelial cells, whether induced by exposure of neutrophils to chemotactic factors or by activation of endothelial cells by IL-1, TNF, or LPS. However, the same antibodies have virtually no effect on neutrophil adhesion to IL-1–stimulated endothelial cells at a wall shear stress of 2.0 dyne/cm^2, and cells from a CD18-deficient patient adhered to the same extent as did normal neutrophils [110, 189, 198].

Clues to the existence of a second class of leukocyte adhesion molecules, which appear to operate at high shear stress, came from studies of the mechanisms by which lymphocytes "home" to particular lymphoid organs, such as the peripheral node or gut and lung-associated lymphoid tissue [108, 213]. A monoclonal antibody MEL-14 was raised to a murine lymphocyte homing receptor for peripheral lymph nodes. It defined a 90-kd glycoprotein that bound certain sugars and was shown by cloning studies to be a founding member of what is now called the *selectin family* of adhesion molecules (see Tables 71-6 and 71-7). Murine neutrophils were found to bear a closely related, 100-kd molecule, designated gp100$^{MEL\text{-}14}$; the comparable molecule in humans has a variety of names (e.g., leukocyte adhesion molecule-1 [LAM-1], lectin adhesion molecule-1 [LECAM-1], DREG 56) [95, 101].

Monoclonal antibodies have been used to show that MEL-14/LAM-1 is involved in neutrophil interaction with endothelium in vitro, and systemic administration of MEL-14 to mice has been shown to inhibit (by over 60%) migration of ex vivo–labeled neutrophils into the experimentally inflamed peritoneal cavity [95]. Intriguingly, neutrophil surface MEL-14 appeared to be coordinately but inversely regulated with Mac-1 [61, 101]. Thus, in vitro exposure to chemotactic factors results in rapid (<10 minutes) shedding of MEL-14 into the medium, which is followed by progressively increasing Mac-1 expressions. In vivo, extravasated inflammatory neutrophils also have low levels of surface MEL-14 and high Mac-1 expression. Infused murine neutrophils (treated with chemotactic factors ex vivo to mimic this phenotype) circulate but do not accumulate at inflamed sites [95].

From these and other data, Kishimoto et al. [101] suggested that neutrophil adhesion to endothelial cells under inflammatory conditions involves two distinct adhesive mechanisms mediated by LAM-1/MEL-14 and the leukocyte integrins. They proposed that the LAM-1

Table 71-6. Supergene families in leukocyte-endothelial adhesion

Family	Structure and properties
Integrins	αβ Heterodimers; at least 11 α chains complexed in varying combinations with at least 5 β chains Many recognize Arg-Gly-Asp (RGD) tripeptide sequence in adhesive proteins; roles in cell-matrix and cell-cell interactions in inflammation, coagulation, metastasis, and differentiation; "activation" of avidity by mediators is important in function
Immunoglobulin	Generally single chain; variable numbers of immunoglobulin domains, each of 90–100 amino acids arranged in two β-pleated sheets; thus in leukocyte-endothelial adhesion, VCAM-1 has 6; ICAM-1 has 5; and ICAM-2 has 2 domains Also includes various T-cell molecules (CD3, CD4, CD8) and the MHC dimers indicating roles in immunoregulation, and the neural cell adhesion molecule N-CAM is a family member
Selectin	N-terminal domain homologous to Ca^{2+}-dependent lectins, next to which is epidermal growth factor motif, and then variable numbers of complement-regulatory protein repeats: LAM-1 has 2; ELAM-1 has 6; and GMP-140 has 9 Ligands are polylactosamine derivatives at termini of glycolipids and glycoproteins Roles in lymphocyte homing (MEL-14) and coagulation (GMP-140)

Table 71-7. Adhesion molecules in leukocyte-endothelial interaction

Name (alternatives)	Supergene family		Counterreceptor
Leukocytes			
LFA-1 (CD11a/CD18, α_L/β_2)	Integrin	LFA-1:	ICAM-1, ICAM-2
Mac-1 (CD11b/CD18, α_m/β_2; CR3)		Mac-1:	ICAM-1, iC3b, fibrinogen
p150, 95 (CD11c/CD18, α_x/β_2; CR4)		p150, 95:	iC3b
LAM-1 (LECAM-1, MEL-14, DREG)	Selectin		Unknown (?ELAM-1)
VLA-4 (α_4/β_1)	Integrin		VCAM-1
Endothelial cells			
ICAM-1 (CD54)	Immunoglobulin	ICAM-1:	LFA-1, Mac-1
ICAM-2		ICAM-2:	LFA-1
VCAM-1 (INCAM-110)	Immunoglobulin		VLA-4 on mononuclear cells
ELAM-1	Selectin		Sialylated Lewis x sugar on neutrophils and memory T cells
GMP-140 (PADGEM, CD62)	Selectin		Lewis x (CD15) on neutrophils/monocytes

mechanism is responsible for initial adhesion and that leukocyte integrins mediate continued adhesion and emigration. As the initial mechanism is "downregulated," the second mechanism is engaged, presumably by chemotactic factors.

Support for this hypothesis comes from elegant in vitro studies by Smith et al. [198–200], using a parallel-plate flow chamber to study human neutrophil adhesion to human endothelial cells under conditions of normal blood flow. Under the "CD18-independent" conditions of wall shear stresses on the order of 2 to 0 dyne/cm², there is strong evidence that LAM-1 mediates "tethering" of the neutrophils rolling along the IL-1–stimulated endothelial monolayer (in a manner reminiscent of "marginated" neutrophils seen in ear chamber vessels). This interaction is inhibited by antibody to LAM-1 and by prior shedding of the molecule in response to pretreatment with chemotactic factors. Furthermore, there is a close correlation between the degree of adhesion and the degree of LAM-1 expression. Tethered neutrophils spread and adhere tightly to the endothelium before migrating across the endothelial monolayer. The second process is not inhibited by antibodies to LAM-1 but is dependent on CD18, because neutrophils deficient in CD18 detach again, as do normal neutrophils in the presence of anti-CD18. It is intriguing that such neutrophils have been found to have shed LAM-1, while neutrophils in contact with unstimulated endothelium do not shed LAM-1. IL-8 and PAF induce LAM-1 shedding and could be the endothelial cell–derived factors responsible.

Thus, neutrophil adhesion and migration through endothelium appear to involve the following steps: (1) chemotactic factor–induced "activation" of LAM-1 by unknown mechanisms [202]; (2) LAM-1–mediated "tethering" of leukocytes to an unknown endothelial determinant (possibly endothelial-leukocyte adhesion molecule-1 [ELAM-1] [99]); (3) strengthening of adhesion by increased avidity and expression of leukocyte integrins, coincident with the shedding of LAM-1, mediated by endothelial-derived chemotactic factors; and (4) transendothelial migration, in which leukocyte integrins also play an important role (see below).

Rapid progress has also been made in the definition

of *endothelial cell adhesion molecules*, using human umbilical vein endothelial cells stimulated in culture by agents such as IL-1, TNF, or LPS. This leads to a time-related and protein synthesis–dependent increase in adhesiveness for neutrophils and other leukocytes [17, 46, 57, 160]. Newly synthesized adhesion molecules have been characterized using monoclonal antibodies to "activated" endothelial cells, and their functions have been defined by antibodies that inhibit leukocyte-endothelial interaction [100] or by using purified adhesion molecules incorporated into biplanar lipid membranes [127]. The molecules have also been studied using cells transfected with genes for particular adhesion molecules [152].

The first endothelial cell adhesion molecule to be identified in this manner was *intercellular cell adhesion molecule-1* (ICAM-1) [119, 127, 176]. This 90-kd monomeric member of the immunoglobulin supergene family was originally defined by a monoclonal antibody inhibiting phorbol ester–stimulated lymphocyte aggregation; later it was shown that ICAM-1 played a key role in T-cell killing of target cells [100, 206]. ICAM-1 has been shown to be the counterreceptor for LFA-1, both in this situation and in lymphocyte-endothelial interaction. LFA-1 also recognizes ICAM-2, a very similar molecule that is constitutively expressed by endothelial cells [207]. After some years of controversy, ICAM-1 (but not ICAM-2) was recently shown in vitro to be a counterreceptor for the neutrophil integrin Mac-1 (CD11b/CD18) [40]. This interaction is responsible for the adherence of chemotactically stimulated neutrophils to basal, unstimulated endothelial cells under static conditions which express small amounts of ICAM-1 constitutively [200]. However, in vivo immunohistochemical studies demonstrate ICAM-1 not only on endothelial cells in experimentally inflamed skin but also on fibroblasts, dendritic cells, and epithelial cells [142]. It is therefore likely that ICAM-1 has a more general role in inflammation and is particularly important in directing lymphocyte traffic. Nevertheless, a monoclonal antibody recognizing ICAM-1 inhibits neutrophil accumulation in rabbit lungs with PMA-induced inflammation [10].

The existence of a second class of endothelial cell adhesion molecules was suspected from the observation that increased endothelial cell adhesiveness for neutrophils was maximal at 4 to 6 hours after exposure to IL-1 or TNF (but not IFN-γ) [18], whereas the time course of ICAM-1 expression peaked at 24 hours and was sustained for as long as the cytokine remained in the culture medium. Subsequently, monoclonal antibodies raised to activated endothelial cells defined *ELAM-1*, an adhesion molecule not expressed by unstimulated endothelial cells in vitro [16]. The gene encoding ELAM-1 has been cloned, and the derived amino acid sequence shows it to be a member of the selectin family (see Table 71-6) [18]. The sugar sialylated Lewis x is a ligand for ELAM-1 and is found on the leukocyte surface [157, 230]. Consequently, the observed involvement of the ELAM-1 in endothelial adhesion to leukocytes other than the neutrophil (e.g., the memory T cell [158, 191]), is not unexpected. However, in vivo, ELAM-1 appears to be expressed in a manner compatible with a major role in cytokine-induced neutrophil accumulation. Unlike ICAM-1, it is found only on endothelial cells; in addition, immunohistochemical studies of baboon skin at various times after intradermal injection of TNF and IL-1 demonstrated ELAM-1 expression within 2 hours, which correlates with the earliest evidence of neutrophil accumulation [35].

Intriguingly, although of shorter duration than either ICAM-1 expression or mononuclear cell accumulation, both ELAM-1 expression and neutrophil accumulation persist longer in vivo than would be expected from in vitro studies; they were still prominent at 24 hours [113, 142, 159]. This finding underlines the difficulties of extrapolation from in vitro systems to living organisms, but it is reassuring that unpublished data (C. Smith. Personal communication, 1991) provide direct evidence for a role for ELAM-1 in neutrophil localization in vivo, since anti-ELAM antibodies attenuate neutrophil accumulation in injured canine lungs.

In vivo demonstration of a role for the third member of the selectin family, GMP-140, has yet to be provided. GMP-140 is stored in Weibel-Palade bodies and mobilized in less than 5 minutes to the surface of endothelial cells stimulated by thrombin or histamine. It adheres to neutrophils via Lewis x, and antibodies to GMP-140 inhibit attachment of neutrophils to endothelium stimulated by thrombin, suggesting a role in mediating neutrophil adhesion at the earliest stages of the inflammatory response [92, 106].

Vascular cell adhesion molecule-1 (VCAM-1) is a 110-kd cytokine-inducible molecule also known as inducible cell adhesion molecule-110 (INCAM-110) [152, 170]. It is a monomeric member of the immunoglobulin supergene family that is expressed by endothelial cells and other cells at inflamed sites in vivo in a manner analogous to ICAM-1. VCAM-1 is detectable on resting endothelial cells in vitro but can be induced by cytokines with maximal expression at about 12 hours. It is selectively upregulated by IL-1 and not induced by IFN-γ, unlike ICAM-1 [216]. VCAM-1 appears to mediate the binding of lymphocytes and monocytes by interacting with the integrin counterreceptor VLA-4 (α_4/β_1), a member of a subfamily of integrins different from the CD18/β_2 complex [49, 84, 179]. A direct demonstration of its role in vivo is pending, although VCAM-1 has been found to be expressed in human inflammatory disease [171].

The accumulated evidence shows that knowledge of factors in addition to the sequential expression of particular endothelial adhesion molecules is needed to explain why leukocyte infiltration of an inflamed site proceeds sequentially with neutrophils being followed by mononuclear cells. For example, although ELAM-1 expression correlates with neutrophil influx in vivo, in vitro data suggest that lymphocytes can also bind ELAM-1. Furthermore, lymphocytes and monocytes both express LAM-1, and yet this molecule appears to be involved in the earliest stages of neutrophil adhesion to the endothelium. It appears likely that sequential leukocyte influx is determined by cell lineage–specific chemotactic factors [202] that induce specific changes in individual leukocyte types and/or lead to expression of specific combinations of endothelial adhesion molecules, some of which have yet to be defined. It should also be emphasized that although most of the important *families* of adhesion molecules have been characterized, little is known of how their function is coordinated in vivo. In particular, improved understanding of the intracellular signaling mechanisms employed by adhesion receptors is needed and so attention is likely to turn to the intracellular portions of these molecules. For example, recent exciting data show that deletions of the cytoplasmic tail of the LFA-1β chain (i.e., CD18) prevent transient increases in activity induced by crosslinking other receptors [75]. Finally, the spatial distribution of various receptors in different vascular beds must be defined.

LEUKOCYTE PASSAGE THROUGH THE VESSEL WALL

Leukocyte attachment to the endothelium may lead to a number of events. In the 1930s, the Clarks [27] showed that adherent leukocytes can detach and return to the circulation. Alternatively, they may be incited to release histotoxic factors and injure the endothelium directly. However, in many instances leukocytes migrate across the vessel wall, and although the events involved in "leukodiapedesis" have been known for many years [2], the mechanisms responsible have been obscure.

Following attachment, most often to the wall of a postcapillary venule, leukocytes generally migrate on the surface of the endothelium to the region between endothelial cells. As shown in Fig. 71-2, pseudopodia from the leukocyte appear to pry apart the endothelial cells, allowing the migrating cell to squeeze into direct opposition with the basement membrane (Figs. 71-3 and 71-4). The basement membrane is then traversed and the cell enters the interstitium or migrates across the epithelium. This general scheme may be modified at particular sites, such as the glomerular capillary, where the basement membrane is more exposed by endothelial fenestrations. Passage through the substance of the endothelial cell does not generally occur but has been described across the specialized endothelial cells of lymph node venules [123] or during the passage of mature blood cells from bone marrow tissue into marrow sinuses [212].

Recent in vitro studies demonstrated shear stress–resistant "binding" of neutrophils to IL-1/TNF-treated endothelial cell monolayers [56, 141, 200]. Careful morphologic study revealed that the majority of such neutrophils had passed through the monolayer, presumably at intercellular junctions. Moser et al. [141] showed that this phenomenon is not an inevitable consequence of neutrophil attachment (e.g., via Fc receptor to antibody-coated endothelial cells). Furthermore, they found, using upside-down systems, that IL-1–stimulated traffic across the endothelial monolayer is polarized from "free" to attached surface and appears to depend on an endothelial cell-surface protein; no evidence of endothelial cell–derived chemotactic factors was found. Transendothelial migration is dependent on the CD11/18–ICAM-1 receptor pair [198–200]. This suggests that ICAM-1 induced on the endothelial cell as well as other adhesion molecules may form a "haptotactic" gradient

Fig. 71-2. A, B. Neutrophils lodged within glomerular capillaries. Neutrophils have put out small pseudopodia extending (apparently through fenestra) into the substance of the endothelial cell. (Courtesy of J. E. Henson, 1988.)

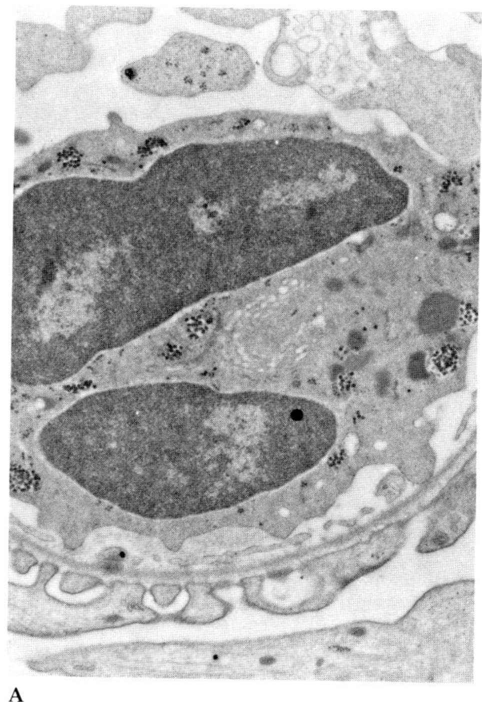

A

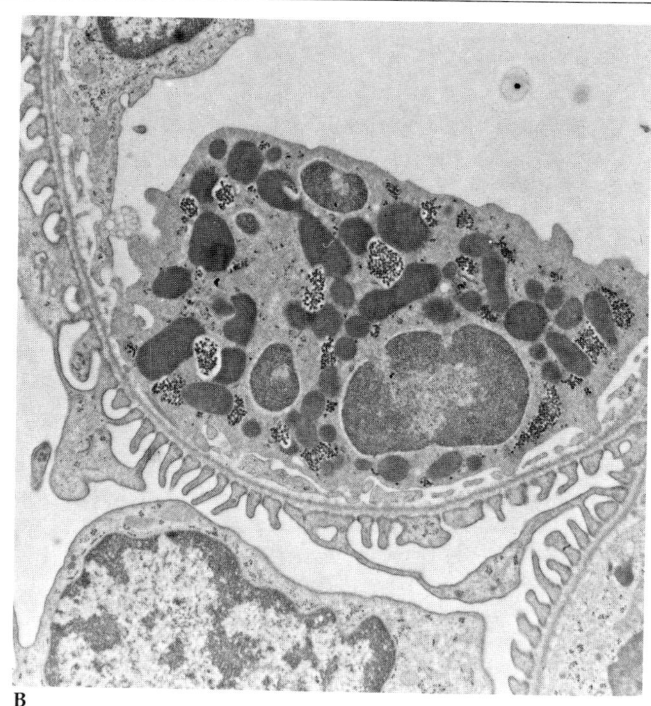

B

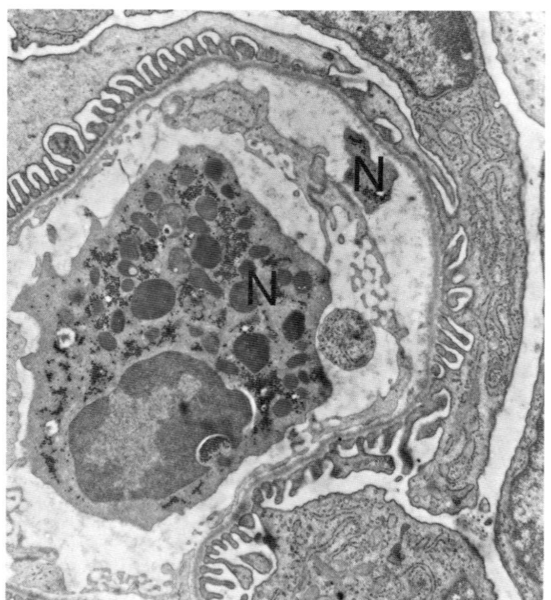

Fig. 71-3. Neutrophil and platelet within a glomerular capillary. Note that part of the neutrophil (labeled N) interposed between the capillary endothelium and the basement membrane. (Courtesy of J. E. Henson, 1988.)

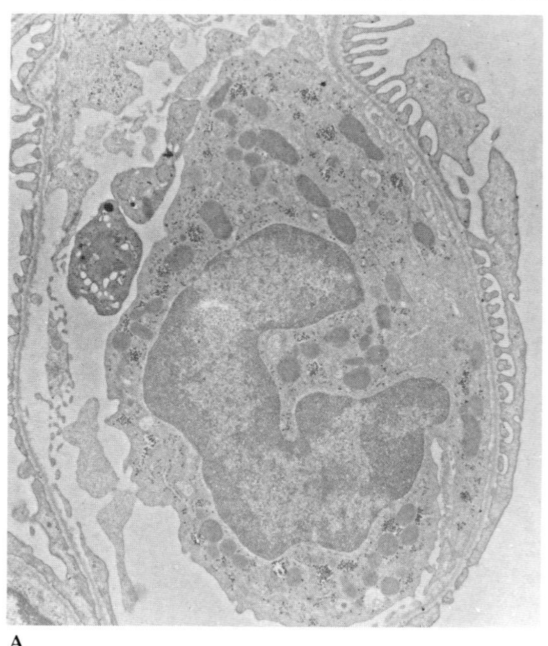
A

Fig. 71-4. A, B, C. Neutrophils in glomerular capillaries immediately adjacent to glomerular basement membrane (GBM). Note that the neutrophil is now interposed between endothelial cell and basement membrane. (Courtesy of J. E. Henson, 1988.)

guiding the leukocyte to the cell junction and beyond. Indeed, ICAM-1 expression is not restricted to the "luminal" surface of endothelial cells but also occurs on the underside, which contrasts with other adhesion molecules such as VCAM-1.

Morphologic studies by Hurley [82] and others showed that neutrophil passage across the endothelium is not associated with detectable damage to the monolayer or basement membrane. Similar observations were made in an in vitro model of the venular vessel wall devised by Huber and Weiss [78]. Culture of endothelial cells on a collagen matrix led to the formation of typical intercellular junctions and the secretion of a single-layer, continuous basement membrane. In plasma, complement-induced neutrophil migration across the monolayer led to leakiness of the basement membrane to colloidal pigment, even though there were no discernible changes morphologically. Migration was not abrogated by inhibitors of known neutrophil-degradative enzymes, which suggests involvement of a novel neutrophil enzyme. Interestingly, the impaired barrier function of the membrane was rapidly repaired by the overlying endothelial cells through a mechanism dependent on new RNA and protein synthesis. Many questions remain to be answered, but these data suggest that far from being a passive partner in neutrophil migration, the endothelial cell may play an important coordinating role in this event.

Leukocytes must employ a coordinated series of attachments and detachments with matrix molecules in order to breach the subendothelial barrier and migrate through the extracellular matrix of the interstitium. The CD11/18 integrins on leukocytes may interact with fibrinogen; in addition, leukocytes also express other receptors of the integrin superfamily with a specificity for matrix proteins such as laminins, collagens, fibronectins, vitronectin, and thrombospondin [84]. In the neutrophil, such receptors may be stored in a preformed state in "adhesomes" [197], ready to be mobilized to the cell surface. Adhesion receptors appear to be concentrated in "focal contacts," organized both by the actin cytoskeleton of the cell and by the matrix on which the cell is moving. Intermediate proteins (talin, vinculin, and α-actinin) probably link cytoskeleton to adhesion receptors, and it is likely that the ability to detach may reflect the transient nature of stimulated integrin adhesion first shown for LFA-1 by Dustin and Springer [47].

INJURY TO VASCULAR STRUCTURES

Thus far we have described mechanisms that bring leukocytes into close apposition to vascular structures, an event of central importance in vascular injury. The toxic potential of leukocytes, in particular the neutrophil, can induce damage in a number of different ways (see Table 71-1).

Reactive Oxygen Species. Oxygen radicals are generated by many cell types, but the most abundant sources are cells of myeloid lineage, particularly the neutrophil [73, 102, 240]. Neutrophils respond to phagocytosis of particles and to high concentrations of chemotactic factors with a large increase in oxygen consumption—the "extra respiration of phagocytosis" or "respiratory burst." This reaction utilizes a membrane-associated NADPH-oxi-

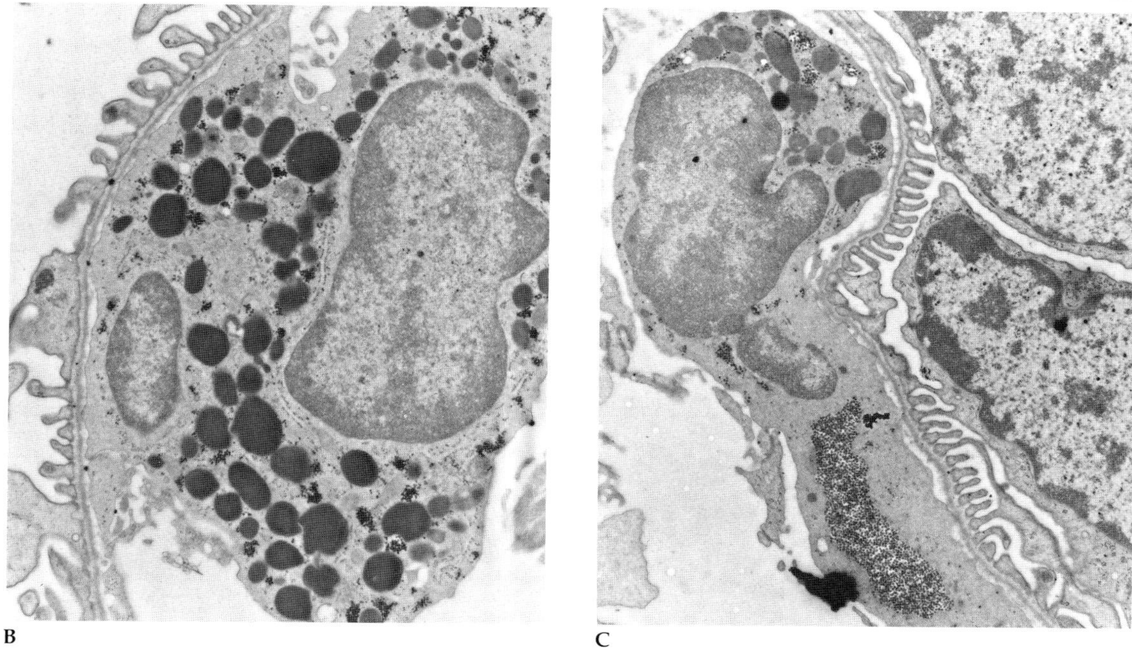

Fig. 71-4 (continued)

dase system to transfer electrons from cytosolic NADPH to oxygen, generating the highly reactive and unstable superoxide ion (O_2). The enzyme superoxide dismutase (SOD) converts two molecules of superoxide to one each of oxygen and hydrogen peroxide (H_2O_2), a stable and powerful oxidant. Further reactions generate other reactive species, such as the hydroxyl radical (OH), singlet oxygen, and most importantly, hypohalous acids. Klebanoff [102] showed that the neutrophil myeloperoxidase, in conjunction with H_2O_2, oxidizes halides (particularly chloride) to yield hypohalous acids such as HOCl. Finally, these acids can also generate toxic chloramines.

Reactive oxygen species (ROS) have enormous potential to disrupt tissue, since they can oxidize proteins, nucleic acids, and lipids, and alter their function. In vitro, they can injure a wide variety of cell types and have been implicated in injury in both isolated perfused organs and animal models of vascular injury. Thus, infusion of H_2O_2 and myeloperoxidase into rat renal arteries causes glomerular damage manifested by proteinuria and gross endothelial swelling [91]. Furthermore, vascular injury in skin and lung induced by injection of immune complexes can be abrogated by local administration of SOD, while catalase, which converts H_2O_2 to H_2O and O_2, inhibits lung injury induced by intratracheal installation of immune complexes [89, 131] and glomerular injury induced by cobra venom factor [168].

Recently, the primacy of ROS in mediating the ability of neutrophils to injure tissue was questioned [238], and in some experimental systems, neutrophil-derived proteinases appear more important. Furthermore, it may be difficult to demonstrate oxidant effects conclusively in vivo. Indeed, in an entertaining piece of scientific archeology, Weiss [238] revealed that direct perfusion of war wounds with high concentrations of hypohalous acid was found to be beneficial in the early twentieth century, even though the same preparation was known to reduce living tissue, such as tadpoles, "to a heap of sand" in vitro. Clearly, protective oxygen radical scavengers must be extremely powerful in vivo. These are compounds such as glutathione, methionine, ascorbic acid, and possibly uric acid [154] which can react with ROS without disrupting tissue function. The precise role of ROS in vascular injury remains uncertain.

Degradative Granule Enzymes. Neutrophil granules contain a number of degradative enzymes, the most important of which are listed in Table 71-1. Discharge of granules in a manner likely to cause vascular injury can be demonstrated in vivo (Fig. 71-5). Proteolytic enzymes may be classified according to the pH at which they are active. Thus, there are acid and neutral proteinases. Among the latter, the serine proteinases elastase and cathepsin G, and the metalloproteinases neutrophil collagenase and gelatinase (type IV collagenase), may be important in tissue injury [73, 74]; however, most attention has centered on the leukocyte *elastase,* a 35-kd cationic molecule that accounts for nearly all neutrophil-derived proteolytic activity in vitro [87]. It is located in azurophil granules and can cleave virtually all components of extracellular matrix, including elastin, fibronectin, collagen types III and IV, and proteoglycans. Furthermore, elastase can cleave complement components C3 and C5 to yield active fragments, thus increasing the phlogistic potential of the enzyme.

Plasma and interstitial fluids also contain a series of powerful antiproteinases that can regulate elastase and prevent this and other enzymes from attacking extracellular substrates. These inhibitors include α_2-macroglobulin, a large (~800-kd) broad-spectrum antiproteinase

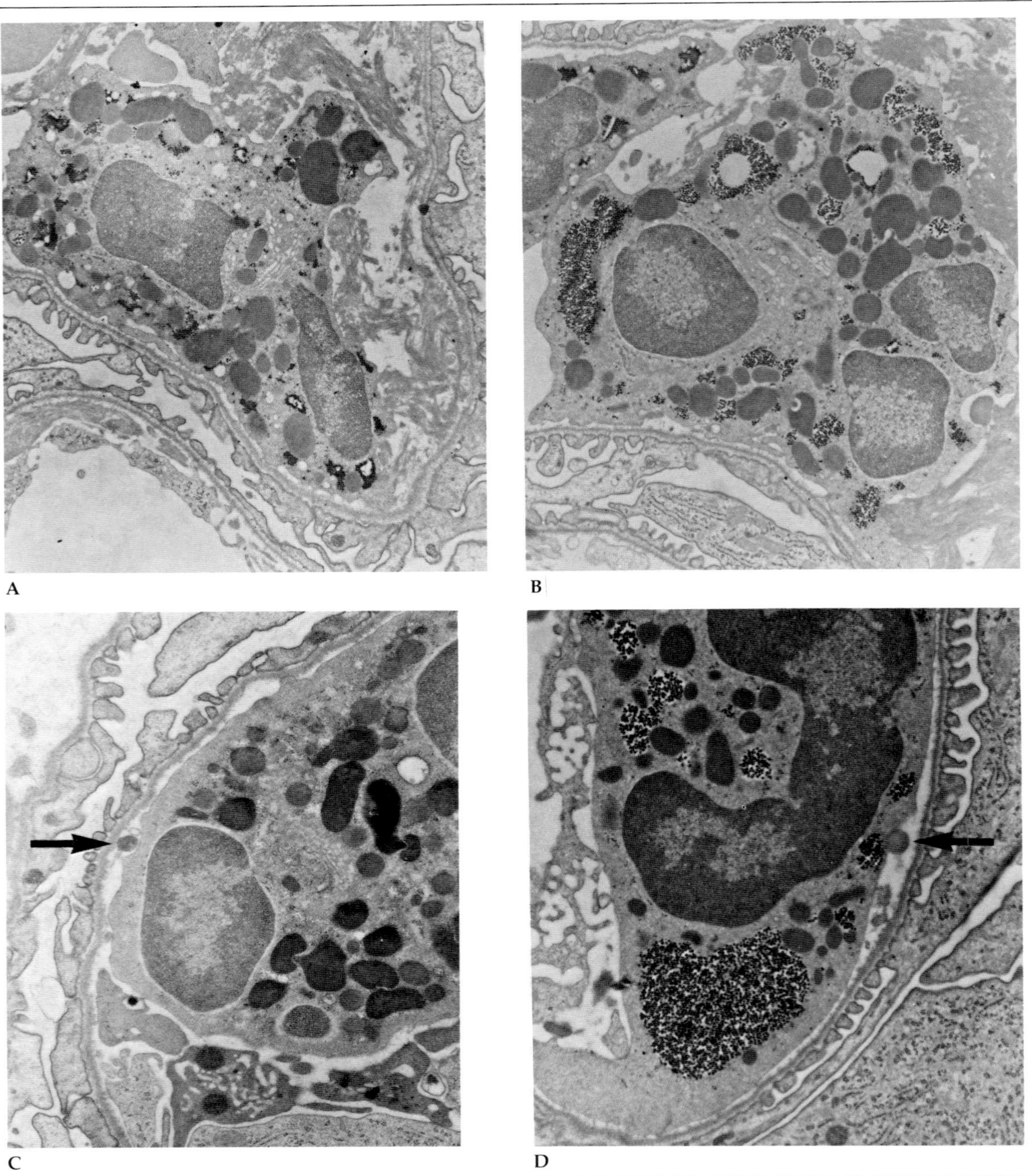

Fig. 71-5. A, B, C, D. Neutrophils are seen in glomerular capillaries immediately adjacent to glomerular basement membrane lodged within glomerular capillaries. It can be seen under the high magnification views in C and D that neutrophils appear to be releasing granules into the space immediately between the neutrophil and the basement membranes (arrows), evidence for neutrophil degranulation at the site of potential basement membrane injury. (Courtesy of J. E. Henson, 1988.)

that can inhibit nearly all mammalian proteinases, and the small (14-kd) secretory leukoproteinase inhibitor. The most powerful inhibitor of elastase is α_1-proteinase inhibitor (α_1-antitrypsin), a 52-kd glycoprotein that irreversibly inactivates the enzyme in milliseconds. Furthermore, various cells can synthesize tissue inhibitors of the metalloproteinases (TIMPs). Together these molecules constitute an "antiproteinase shield" capable of complete inhibition of isolated enzymes. Nevertheless, the ability of stimulated neutrophils to degrade protein substrates in the presence of proteinase inhibitors shows that this shield can be penetrated.

Weiss et al. [239] classified the mechanisms responsible as oxidative and nonoxidative. Adherent neutrophils can physically exclude the penetration of antiproteinase in highly circumscribed areas "sealed" by direct contact with the cell membrane [24], and local release of millimolar concentrations of enzyme that "swamp" local inhibitors may also be important [70, 71]. *Oxidative inhibition mechanisms* involve the direct inactivation of antiproteinases by ROS; for example, oxidation of a critical methionine in α_1-proteinase inhibitor reduces its affinity for elastase 2000-fold [87]. Indeed, ROS may enhance the tissue-destructive potential of leukocyte proteinases by other mechanisms, including activation of latent metalloproteinases, which include an enzyme-cleaving α_1-proteinase inhibitor.

These observations led Weiss [238] to propose an eclectic view of neutrophil-mediated tissue injury. He suggested that ROS and proteinases alone are only capable of mediating extremely localized injury, but when released in combination they inhibit the antiproteinase shield and lead to enhanced tissue injury. This hypothesis accords with various in vitro and in vivo models in which variably potent inhibitory effects of either proteinase inhibitors (e.g., Eglin C) or inhibitors of ROS generation (e.g., catalase) alone can be markedly increased by administration of the two classes of inhibitors together [114]. An important consequence of coordinate action of ROS and proteinases may be the generation of fibronectin fragments from degraded matrix that are chemotactic for monocytes [45] and may further amplify inflammatory injury by increasing leukocyte accumulation in inflamed sites.

Other Injurious Agents. Other leukocyte products have less well-defined roles in tissue injury. *Nonenzymatic cationic proteins* from neutrophil granules were implicated as a cause of vascular injury nearly 30 years ago [88, 166]. Intensive research, largely stimulated by their toxicity toward phagocytosed bacteria, has led to characterization of a number of such granule proteins. They include small (4-kd) cyclic polypeptides, which have been called defensins; bactericidal/permeability-increasing protein, also called cationic antimicrobial protein of 57-kd (CAP 57); and CAP 37/azurocidin, which also has monocyte-specific chemotactic properties [203]. At present, their role in vascular injury remains obscure, although they have potent effects on vascular elements in vitro and in vivo [29], presumably by binding and deranging polyanionic structures in the glycocalyx of cells and basement membrane/matrix. At high concentrations, TNF can lead to the death of endothelial cells [174] by inducing a "programmed" form of cell "suicide" called *apoptosis* (see below). Whether this mechanism is operative in vivo remains to be seen. *Complement proteins* generated by myeloid cells may also injure tissue.

Resolution and Repair

Inflammation evolved as a beneficial response to injury or perturbation of tissue. However, the mechanisms by which inflammation resolves and tissue damage is repaired are poorly understood. Improved knowledge of these mechanisms should provide new approaches toward limiting inflammatory tissue injury and preventing undesirable consequences such as scarring [68].

CESSATION OF LEUKOCYTE INFLUX

Given the complexity of the mechanisms involved in initiating leukocyte influx, there are likely to be equally complex mechanisms for "turning off" this response. The first step is removal of the initiating stimulus, for example, by phagocytosis of invading bacteria or deposited immune complexes. If this occurs, mediator generation may cease and the mediator may then be metabolized or dissipated. This mechanism appears to operate in C5a-induced acute experimental arthritis. Soon after intraarticular injection of C5a (detected by transfer into a fresh joint), there is a loss of chemoattractant activity that correlates with decreasing synovial fluid concentration of C5a [68]. Further administration of C5a leads to a fresh influx of leukocytes and provides evidence against the development of chemotactic factor–inhibiting systems [14, 93] or "desensitization" [33] to chemotactic factors described in other models of inflammation. Equally, these observations do not support other hypothetic mechanisms of cessation of leukocyte influx, such as (1) generation of a negative feedback signal or neutrophil immobilization factor dependent on accumulation of neutrophils at the inflamed site [234] or (2) development of some cellular "barrier" to leukocyte efflux. Whether similar mechanisms apply to other classes of mediator remains to be seen.

In addition to removal of stimulus and chemotactic factors, there must be mechanisms for downregulating the expression of adhesion molecules on the endothelium. Again, the transient nature of expression of such molecules following stimulation in vitro may imply that receptor downregulation could be an expected consequence of removal of mediators.

REMOVAL OF NEUTROPHILS

Neutrophils that fail to migrate across the vessel wall probably detach and are removed from the circulation by phagocytic cells in the liver, spleen, and bone marrow [183]. There is no evidence that extravasated neutrophils return to the circulation, and the polarized effect of IL-1 on transendothelial migration in vitro suggests that this is unlikely [141]. Nor is there evidence to suggest that sufficient neutrophils leave via the lymphatic system. The consensus was that the inevitable fate of the extravasated neutrophil is disintegration at the inflamed site, debris being cleared by macrophages [83], but this has not always been the case.

About 100 years ago, Metchnikoff [136] described an alternative neutrophil disposal mechanism. During the resolution of experimentally induced inflammation, he observed macrophage phagocytosis of apparently intact neutrophils, an observation since repeated by many other histopathologists. Henson's group [147] showed that freshly isolated neutrophils were not taken up by macrophages, but intact neutrophils "aging" in overnight culture became recognized and ingested. Haslett's group [186] observed that such aging neutrophils were spontaneously undergoing programmed cell death or "apoptosis," a process characterized by the cleavage of chromatin to internucleosomal fragments (presumptive evidence of endogenous endonuclease activation) and associated with nuclear chromatin condensation, cytoplasmic vacuolation, and other characteristic morphologic features [31, 243, 244]. Evidence exists of neutrophil apoptosis leading to uptake by macrophages at inflamed sites in vivo (e.g., human arthritis). It has been suggested that this may represent an injury-limiting neutrophil clearance mechanism; apoptotic neutrophils retain membrane integrity and phlogistic contents, and the uptake of such cells by macrophages does not induce secretion of proinflammatory mediators [133]. The changes in the apoptotic cell leading to recognition remain obscure, but the mechanism depends on negatively charged groups on the neutrophil surface and a macrophage integrin [184, 185]. The quantitative importance of this mechanism in neutrophil removal in various tissues is unknown, but in the inflamed peritoneum it appears to be the major route of neutrophil "disposal" [181].

MONOCYTE INFLUX AND MATURATION

Virtually all the mediators and adhesion molecules involved in neutrophil emigration from the blood also act on the monocyte. Even so, monocyte migration to inflamed sites in vivo generally occurs later than migration of the neutrophil and is dependent on it, as demonstrated by specific depletion and reconstitution experiments [44]. Possible explanations for this include a dependence on neutrophil-mediated generation of chemotactic fragments of fibronectin and other matrix proteins [45] or on release of monocyte chemotactic factors such as CAP 37 from neutrophil granules [203]. Furthermore, monocyte-specific members of the intercrine family could be implicated [151]. In common with lymphocytes, but unlike neutrophils, monocytes express the VLA-4 (α_4/β_1) integrin, which is the counterreceptor for endothelial VCAM-1. To some extent, therefore, monocyte recruitment may also be determined by "mononuclear cell"–specific endothelial adhesion molecules, which in turn can be regulated by T-cell–derived cytokines such as IL-4.

Monocytes undergo a remarkable change in phenotype on emigration from vessels. They undergo "maturation," over about 48 to 72 hours, to become inflammatory macrophages [172]. Such macrophages acquire a range of characteristics that appear adapted to the "scavenging" function of these cells first emphasized by Metchnikoff [136] and suited to a role in resolution, increased receptors for enzyme clearance, and development of the ability to take up apoptotic neutrophils. By acquiring the ability to clear the debris of the inflammatory response and to secrete reparative cytokines (such as TGF-β), macrophages occupy a central role in resolution and repair. However, the mechanisms controlling these functions need better definition, and the fate of the inflammatory macrophage is unknown.

REPAIR

The repair of inflammatory tissue injury was extensively reviewed by Clark and Hension [28] and only a few important principles will be discussed here. A central theme is that the extracellular matrix plays an active role in directing repair. However, other factors are involved and TGF-β is likely to be one of the most important *mediators* of repair. It originates mainly from platelets and monocytes/macrophages but is also secreted by resident cells [51, 129, 204]. It is a 25-kd dimeric cytokine secreted in a latent form that requires "activation" in vivo by enzymatic cleavage into a biologically active fragment, and another fragment "latency associated protein." The latter has the ability to bind and regulate activity of the active fragment, as do various proteoglycan molecules of extracellular matrix [177]. At low concentrations in vitro, TGF-β is chemotactic for fibroblasts and monocytes. At higher concentrations, it stimulates matrix protein synthesis and inhibits degradation of such proteins both by stimulating TIMP secretion metalloproteinase and by decreasing proteinase secretion. The matrix reciprocates by modulating the release of TGF-β as well as the activity of TGF-β and its effect on target tissue [145, 177]. In general, it can be seen that TGF-β augments healing, but sometimes this leads to "overexuberant" healing by granulation, to undesirable proliferation of local cells and matrix, and ultimately to scarring. For example, the mesangial proliferation following mesangiolysis in the rat induced by the administration of antiserum to Thy1.1 can be inhibited by antibody to TGF-β [20, 149]. However, it is obvious that TGF-β is but one part of the mechanism of repair. This point is well illustrated in the rat anti-Thy1.1 model where mesangial proliferation can also be inhibited by antibodies to platelet-derived growth factor [90], illustrating that other factors are involved.

A major *effector* cell in repair is the myofibroblast. Elegant morphologic studies of healing surgical wounds illustrate that from the fourth day after injury, fibroblasts begin to acquire characteristics of smooth muscle cells and to express α–smooth muscle actin and smooth muscle myosin [37]. Such "myofibroblasts" may also arise from vascular pericytes. They represent a mesenchymal cell phenotype that promotes wound healing and contraction, and that may play an important role, together with endothelial cells, in organizing angiogenesis with the affected area.

Finally, there is evidence that in some settings, epithelial cells *regulate* repair. In wounded skin, re-epithelialization heralds a wave of apoptosis in myofibroblasts and endothelial cells of the highly vascular granulation tissue [37].

Whether this results from impaired production of a growth factor or from the generation of a signal promoting cell death is unclear, but it leads to desirable remodeling of the wound. In other systems, epithelial cells promote healing and prevent excessive fibrosis. For example, Terzhagi et al. [214] showed that subcutaneous implantation of tracheal rings deprived of epithelium stimulated massive granulation tissue but that fibrosis could be prevented by co-implantation of isolated tracheal epithelial cells. Clearly, it would appear that exposed basement membrane can promote fibrosis unless some controlling influence from epithelial cells is present.

Conclusions and Prospects for Therapy

In this chapter we have described mechanisms involved in generating inflammatory vascular injury that promote resolution and repair. Particular attention has been paid to modern knowledge of the mediators involved, to the molecular mechanisms of neutrophil emigration from vessels, and to leukocyte factors that may injure cells. Improved understanding of these factors is already contributing to the development of a number of novel therapeutic agents. Before concluding with a brief description of these, we want to emphasize that existing treatments, such as steroids or nonsteroidal antiinflammatory drugs, have a wide range of effects on the processes under discussion. In some cases these are so effective that the goals of new therapies are improved specificity and reduced toxicity. However, in other situations (e.g., postinflammatory scarring) existing therapies are of no use, indicating a need for new approaches.

At the level of mediators, a number of interesting developments are taking place. An obvious approach is to use antibodies against mediators or against their receptors that inhibit their action, although problems of antigenicity mean that humanized antibody or single-chain antibodies may be needed. A prime example is the use of antibodies against LPS or TNF in patients at risk for septic shock from gram-negative bacteria [50, 251]. However, other innovative approaches include the use of recombinant DNA–derived proteins that inhibit mediator function. In this regard, the soluble IL-1 receptor antagonist has been found to inhibit neutrophil infiltration of the lungs or peritoneum of rats receiving local LPS or IL-1 [132, 226], while genetic engineering of the CR1 receptor for C3b has been found to yield a soluble complement receptor that can inhibit vascular injury following reperfusion of ischemic rat myocardium [237].

Agents inhibiting leukocyte adhesion are already undergoing clinical trials. Prominent among these is the monoclonal antibody to ICAM-1, reported to decrease eosinophil infiltration and bronchial hyperreactivity in a primate model of asthma [236] and to be protective in cardiac reperfusion injury and against rejection of renal transplants. Since ICAM-1–related functions of the leukocyte integrins are all that is blocked, it may be that the risk of inducing an undesirable state similar to leukocyte adhesion deficiency is less than the risk inherent in using antibodies to the CD18/β_2 integrin, which are also potent inhibitors of reperfusion injury in rabbit ear [228] and dog heart [196]. A further untested approach may be to administer soluble forms of ICAM-1. Nevertheless, it would appear that the potential side effects of interfering with the β_2-integrin–ICAM-1 counterreceptor pair on a long-term basis will limit the use of these agents to short-term inflammatory "crises."

The pharmaceutical industry has initiated a number of programs directed toward "oxygen radical scavengers" and specific inhibitors of proteinases such as elastase. The foregoing data suggest that combinations of these may be most effective. Actual manipulation of the resolution and repair of vascular injury seems a bit further away. However, the observation that the proteoglycan decorin can inhibit TGF-β function may lead to preliminary experiments to determine whether this molecule can inhibit TGF-β–related phenomena [245].

ACKNOWLEDGMENT. The authors would like to acknowledge the assistance of Morag Park and Marge Helgerson in preparing the manuscript.

References

1. Abbott, F., Jones, S. J., Lockwood, C. M., et al. Autoantibodies to glomerular antigens in patients with Wegener's granulomatosis. *Nephrol. Dial. Transplant.* 4: 1, 1989.
2. Addison, W. Experimental and practical researches on the structure and function of blood complexes on inflammation and the origin and nature of tuberdes in the lung. *Trans. Prov. Med. Surg. Assoc.* 11: 236, 1843.
3. Aida, Y., and Pabst, M. J. Priming of neutrophils by lipopolysaccharide for enhanced release of superoxide. Requirement for plasma but not for tumour necrosis factor-alpha. *J. Immunol.* 145: 3017, 1990.
4. Allison, F., Smith, M. W., and Wood, W. B. Studies of the pathogenesis of acute inflammation. I. The inflammatory reaction to thermal injury as observed in the rabbit ear chamber. *J. Exp. Med.* 102: 655, 1955.
5. Anderson, D. C., and Springer, T. A. Leukocyte adhesion deficiency: An inherited defect in the Mac1, LFA-1 and p150,95 glycoproteins. *Annu. Rev. Med.* 38: 175, 1987.
6. Arai, K-I., Lee, L., Miyajima, A., et al. Cytokines: Coordinators of immune and inflammatory conditions. *Annu. Rev. Biochem.* 59: 783, 1990.
7. Atherton, A., and Born, G. V. R. Quantitative investigations of the adhesiveness of circulating polymorphonuclear leucocytes to blood vessel walls. *J. Physiol.* 222: 447, 1971.
8. Badr, K. F., Murray, J. J., Breyer, M. D., et al. Mesangial cell, glomerular and renal vascular responses to endothelin in the rat kidney. *J. Clin. Invest.* 83: 336, 1989.
9. Baggiolini, M., Walz, A., and Kunkel, S. L. Neutrophil activating peptide 1/interleukin 8, a novel cytokine that activates neutrophils. *J. Clin. Invest.* 84: 1045, 1989.
10. Barton, R. W., Rothlein, R., Ksiazer, J., et al. The effect of anti-intercellular adhesion molecule-1 on phorbolester-induced rabbit lung inflammation. *J. Immunol.* 143: 1278, 1989.
11. Baytson, K. F., and Cohen, J. Bacterial endotoxin and current concepts in the diagnosis and treatment of endotoxinaemia. *J. Med. Microbiol.* 31: 73, 1990.
12. Beasley, D., Schwartz, J. H., and Brenner, B. M. Interleukin I induces prolonged L-arginine-dependent cyclic guanosine monophosphate and nitrite production in rat vascular smooth muscle cells. *J. Clin. Invest.* 87: 602, 1991.

13. Beneviste, J., Henson, P. M., and Cochrane, C. G. Leukocyte-dependent histamine release from rabbit platelets. The role of IgE, basophils and a platelet activating factor. *J. Exp. Med.* 136: 1356, 1972.
14. Berenberg, J. L., and Ward, P. A. Chemotactic factor inactivator in normal human serum. *J. Clin. Invest.* 52: 1200, 1973.
15. Berridge, M. J., and Irvine, R. F. Inositol phosphates and cell signalling. *Nature* 341: 197, 1989.
16. Bevilacqua, M. P., Pober, J. S., Mendrick, D. L., et al. Identification of an inducible endothelial leukocyte adhesion molecule. *Proc. Natl. Acad. Sci. U.S.A.* 84: 9238, 1987.
17. Bevilacqua, M. P., Pober, J. S., Wheeler, M. E., et al. Interleukin 1 acts on cultures of human vascular endothelium to increase the adhesion of polymorphonuclear leukocytes, monocytes and related cell lines. *J. Clin. Invest.* 76: 2003, 1985.
18. Bevilacqua, M. P., Stengelin, S., Gimbrone, M. A., Jr., et al. Endothelial leukocyte adhesion molecule 1: An inducible receptor for neutrophils related to complement regulatory proteins and lectins. *Science* 243: 1160, 1989.
19. Beutler, B., and Cerami, A. The biology of cachetin/TNF—A primary mediator of the host response. *Annu. Rev. Immunol.* 7: 625, 1989.
20. Border, W. A., Okuda, S., Languino, L. R., et al. Suppression of experimental glomerulonephritis by antiserum against transforming growth factor. *Nature* 346: 371, 1991.
21. Boulay, F., Tardif, M., Brouchon, L., et al. Synthesis and use of a novel N-formyl peptide derivative to isolate a human N-formyl peptide receptor cDNA. *Biochem. Biophys. Res. Commun.* 168: 1103, 1990.
22. Brain, S. D., and Williams, T. J. Prostaglandins, Leukotrienes, Related Compounds and Their Inhibitors. In S. Shuster and M. Greaves (eds.), *Handbook of Experimental Pharmacology,* Vol. 87. Berlin: Springer, 1989. P. 347.
23. Brasile, L., Kremer, J. M., Clarke, J. L., et al. Identification of an autoantibody to vascular endothelial cell-specific antigens in patients with systemic vasculitis. *Am. J. Med.* 87: 74, 1989.
24. Campbell, E. J., and Campbell, M. A. Cellular proteolysis by neutrophils in the presence of proteinase inhibitors: Effects of substrate opsonization. *J. Cell Biol.* 106: 667, 1988.
25. Chenoweth, D. E., and Hugli, T. E. Demonstration of specific C_{5a} receptor on intact human polymorphonuclear leukocytes. *Proc. Natl. Acad. Sci. U.S.A.* 75: 3943, 1978.
26. Clark, E., and Kaplan, B. J. Endocardial, arterial and other mesenchymal alterations associated with serum sickness disease in man. *Arch. Pathol.* 24: 458, 1937.
27. Clark, E. R., and Clark, E. L. Observations on changes in blood vascular endothelium in the living animal. *Am. J. Anat.* 57: 385, 1935.
28. Clark, R. A. F., and Hension, P. M. (eds.). *The Molecular and Cellular Biology of Wound Repair.* New York: Plenum, 1988.
29. Cochrane, C. G., and Aikin, B. S. Polymorphonuclear leukocytes in immunologic reactions. The destruction of vascular basement membrane in vivo and in vitro. *J. Exp. Med.* 124: 733, 1966.
30. Cochrane, C. G., and Koffler, D. Immune complex disease in experimental animals and man. *Adv. Immunol.* 16: 185, 1973.
31. Cohen, J. J., and Duke, R. C. Glucocorticoid activation of a calcium-dependent endonuclease in thymic nuclei leads to cell death. *J. Immunol.* 132: 38, 1984.
32. Colditz, I. G., and Movat, H. Z. Desensitization of acute inflammatory lesions to chemotazins and endotoxin. *J. Immunol.* 133: 2163, 1984.
33. Colditz, I. G., and Movat, H. Z. Kinetics of neutrophil accumulation in acute inflammatory lesions induced by chemotaxins and chemotaxinigens. *J. Immunol.* 133: 2169, 1984.
34. Connheim, J. *Lectures in General Pathology,* Vol. 1 (2nd ed., translated from 2nd German ed.). London: The New Sydenham Society, 1889.
35. Cotran, R. S., and Pober, J. S. Cytokine-endothelial interactions in inflammation, immunity and vascular injury. *J. Am. Soc. Nephrol.* 1: 225, 1990.
36. Cozza, E. N., Gomez-Sanchez, C. E., Foecking, M. F., et al. Endothelin binding to cultured calf adrenal zona glomerulosa cells and stimulation of aldosterone secretion. *J. Clin. Invest.* 84: 1032, 1989.
37. Darby, I., Skalli, O., and Gabbiani, G. α-Smooth muscle actin is transiently expressed by myofibroblasts during experimental wound healing. *Lab. Invest.* 63: 21, 1990.
38. Davies, K. A., Toothill, V. J., Savill, J., et al. A 19 year old man with leucocyte adhesion deficiency. In vitro and in vivo studies of leucocyte function. *Clin. Exp. Immunol.* 84: 223, 1991.
39. Devreotes, P. N., and Zigmond, S. H. Chemotaxis in eukaryotic cells: A focus on leukocytes and Dictyostelium. *Annu. Rev. Cell Biol.* 4: 649, 1988.
40. Diamond, N. S., Staunton, D. E., de Fougerolles, A. R., et al. ICAM-1 (CD54): A counter-receptor for Mac-1 (CD11b/CD18). *J. Cell Biol.* 111: 3129, 1990.
41. Dinarello, C. A. Interleukin-1 and its biologically related cytokines. *Adv. Immunol.* 44: 153, 1989.
42. Dinarello, C. A., Ikejima, T., Warner, S. J. C., et al. Interleukin-1 induces interleukin-1. 1) Induction of circulating interleukin-1 in rabbits in vivo and in human mononuclear cells in vitro. *J. Immunol.* 139: 1901, 1987.
43. Doerschuk, C. M., Winn, R. K., Coxon, H. O., et al. CD18-dependent and -independent mechanisms of neutrophil emigration in the pulmonary and systemic microcirculation of rabbits. *J. Immunol.* 144: 2327, 1990.
44. Doherty, D. E., Downey, G. P., Worthen, G. S., et al. Monocyte migration in pulmonary inflammation: Requirement for neutrophils. *Lab. Invest.* 59: 200, 1988.
45. Doherty, D. E., Henson, P. M., and Clark, R. A. F. Fibronectin fragments containing the RGDS cell binding domain mediate monocyte migration into the rabbit lung. A potential mechanism for C5 fragment-induced monocyte lung accumulation. *J. Clin. Invest.* 86: 1065, 1990.
46. Dunn, C. J., and Fleming, W. E. Increased adhesion of polymorphonuclear leukocytes to vascular endothelium by specific interaction of endogenous (interleukin-1) and exogenous (lipopolysaccharide) substances with endothelial cells "in vitro." *Eur. J. Rheumatol. Inflamm.* 7: 80, 1984.
47. Dustin, M. L., and Springer, T. A. T cell receptor cross-linking transiently stimulates adhesiveness through LFA-1. *Nature* 341: 619, 1989.
48. Eisenberg, S. P., Evans, R. J., Arend, W. P., et al. Primary structure and functional expression from complementary DNA of a human IL-1 receptor antagonist. *Nature* 343: 336, 1990.
49. Elices, M. J., Osborn, L., Takada, Y., et al. VCAM-1 on activated endothelium interacts with the leukocyte inte-

grin VLA-4 at a site distinct from the VLA-4/fibronectin binding site. *Cell* 60: 577, 1990.

50. Exley, A. R., Cohen, J., Burman, W., et al. Monoclonal antibody to TNF in severe septic shock. *Lancet* 335: 1275, 1990.
51. Fava, R. A., Olsen, N. J., Postlethwaite, A. E., et al. Transforming growth factor β1 (TGF-β1) induced neutrophil recruitment to synovial tissues: Implications for TGF-β-driven synovial inflammation and hyperplasia. *J. Exp. Med.* 173: 1121, 1991.
52. Forehand, J. R., Pabst, M. J., Phillips, W. A., et al. Lipopolysaccharide priming of human neutrophils for an enhanced respiratory burst—Role of intracellular free calcium. *J. Clin. Invest.* 83: 74, 1989.
53. Frampton, G., Jayne, D. R. W., Perry, G. J., et al. Autoantibodies to endothelial cells and neutrophil cytoplasm antigens in systemic vasculitis. *Clin. Exp. Immunol.* 82: 227, 1990.
54. Fukada, Y., Hirata, Y., Yoshimi, H., et al. Endothelin is a potent secretagogue for atrial natriuretic peptide in cultured rat atrial myocytes. *Biochem. Biophys. Res. Commun.* 155: 167, 1988.
55. Furchgott, R. F., and Zawadzki, J. V. The obligatory role of endothelial cells in the relaxation of arterial smooth muscle by acetylcholine. *Nature* 288: 373, 1980.
56. Furie, M. B., and McHugh, D. D. Migration of neutrophils across endothelial monolayers is stimulated by treatment of the monolayers with interleukin 1 or tumour necrosis factor-α. *J. Immunol.* 143: 3309, 1989.
57. Gamble, J. R., Harlan, J. M., Klebanoff, S. J., et al. Stimulation of adherence of neutrophils to umbilical vein endothelium by human recombinant tumour necrosis factor. *Proc. Natl. Acad. Sci. U.S.A.* 82: 8667, 1985.
58. Garg, U. C., and Hassid, A. Inhibition of rat mesangial cell mitogenesis by nitric oxide generating vasodilators. *Am. J. Physiol.* 257: F60, 1989.
59. Garg, U. C., and Hassid, A. Nitric oxide-generating vasodilators and 8-bromo-cyclic guanosine monophosphate inhibit mitogenesis and proliferation of cultured rat vascular smooth muscle cells. *J. Clin. Invest.* 83: 1774, 1989.
60. Gerard, N. P., and Gerard, C. The chemotactic receptor for human C5a anaphylatoxin. *Nature* 349: 614, 1991.
61. Griffin, J. D., Spertini, O., Ernst, T. J., et al. Granulocyte-macrophage colony stimulating factor and other cytokines regulate surface expression of the leukocyte adhesion molecule-1 on human neutrophils, monocytes and other precursors. *J. Immunol.* 145: 576, 1990.
62. Guthrie, L. A., McPhail, L. C., Henson, P. M., et al. Priming of neutrophils for enhanced release of oxygen metabolites by bacterial lipopolysaccharide. *J. Exp. Med.* 160: 1656, 1984.
63. Haeffner-Cavaillon, N., Cavallion, J., and Szabo, L. Cellular Receptors for Endotoxin. In L. J. Berry (ed.), *Handbook of Endotoxin: Cellular Biology of Endotoxin.* Amsterdam: Elsevier/North-Holland, 1985. P. 1.
64. Hampton, R. Y., Golenbock, D. T., Penman, M., et al. Macrophage binding and metabolism of endotoxin mediated by scavenger receptors. *Nature,* 352: 342, 1991.
65. Hanahar, D. J. Platelet activating factor: A biologically active phosphoglyceride. *Annu. Rev. Biochem.* 55: 483, 1986.
66. Hannum, C. H., Wilcox, C. J., Arend, W. P., et al. IL-1 receptor antagonist activity of a human IL-1 inhibitor. *Nature* 343: 336, 1990.
67. Hart, M. N., Tassell, S. K., Sadewasser, K. L., et al. Autoimmune vasculitis resulting from in vitro immunization of lymphocytes to smooth muscle cells. *Am. J. Pathol.* 119: 448, 1985.
68. Haslett, C., and Henson, P. M. Resolution of Inflammation. In R. A. F. Clark and P. M. Henson (eds.), *The Molecular and Cellular Biology of Wound Repair.* New York: Plenum, 1988. P. 185.
69. Henson, J. B., and Crawford, T. B. The pathogenesis of virus induced arterial disease—Aleutian disease and equine viral arteritis. *Adv. Cardiol.* 13: 183, 1974.
70. Henson, P. M. The immunologic release of constituents from neutrophil leukocytes. *J. Immunol.* 107: 1547, 1971.
71. Henson, P. M. Pathological mechanisms in neutrophil-mediated injury. *Am. J. Pathol.* 68: 593, 1972.
72. Henson, P. M. Release of vasoactive amines from rabbit platelets induced by sensitized mononuclear leukocytes and antigen. *J. Exp. Med.* 131: 287, 1970.
73. Henson, P. M., and Johnston, R. B., Jr. Tissue injury in inflammation: Oxidants, proteinases and cationic proteins. *J. Clin. Invest.* 79: 669, 1987.
74. Henson, P. M., Henson, J. E., Fitschen, C., et al. Phagocytic Cells: Degranulation and Secretion. In J. I. Gallin, I. M. Goldstein, and R. Synderman (eds.), *Inflammation: Basic Principles and Clinical Correlates.* New York: Raven, 1988. P. 363.
75. Hibbs, M. L., Hong, X., Stacker, S. A., et al. Regulation of adhesion to ICAM-1 by the cytoplasmic domain of LFA-1 integrin β subunit. *Science* 251: 1611, 1991.
76. Honda, Z-I., Nakamura, M., Miki, I., et al. Cloning by functional expression of platelet-activating factor receptor from guinea pig lung. *Nature* 349: 342, 1991.
77. Hu, J. R., Von Harsdorf, R., and Lang, R. E. Endothelin has potent inotropic effects in rat atrial. *Eur. J. Pharmacol.* 158: 275, 1988.
78. Huber, A. R., and Weiss, S. J. Disruption of the subendothelial basement membrane during neutrophil diapedesis in an in vitro construct of a blood vessel wall. *J. Clin. Invest.* 83: 1122, 1989.
79. Hughes, C. C. W., Savage, C. O. S., and Pober, J. S. Endothelial cells augment T cell interleukin-2 production by a contact-dependent mechanism involving CD2/LFA3 interaction. *J. Exp. Med.* 171: 1453, 1990.
80. Humphrey, J. H. The mechanisms of Arthus reactions. I. The role of polymorphonuclear leucocytes and other factors in reversed passive Arthus reactions in rabbits. *Br. J. Exp. Pathol.* 36: 268, 1955.
81. Hunter, J. (1794). Cited by Hurley, J. V. The Nature of Inflammation. In J. V. Hurley (ed.), *Acute Inflammation.* London: Churchill-Livingstone, 1983. P. 1.
82. Hurley, J. V. An electron microscopic study of leukocyte emigration and vascular permeability in rat strain. *Aust. J. Exp. Biol. Med. Sci.* 41: 171, 1963.
83. Hurley, J. V. Termination of Acute Inflammation 1. Resolution. In J. V. Hurley (ed.), *Acute Inflammation* (2nd ed.). London: Churchill-Livingstone, 1983. P. 109.
84. Hynes, R. O. Integrins: A family of cell surface receptors. *Cell* 48: 549, 1987.
85. Ignarro, L., Harbison, R., Wood, K., et al. Activation of purified soluble guanylate cyclase by endothelium-derived relaxing factor from intrapulmonary artery and vein. *J. Pharmacol. Exp. Ther.* 237: 893, 1986.
86. Inoue, A., Yanagisawa, M., Kimura, S., et al. The human endothelin family: Three structurally and pharmacologically distinct isopeptides predicted by three separate genes. *Proc. Natl. Acad. Sci. U.S.A.* 86: 2863, 1989.

87. Janoff, A. Elastase in tissue injury. *Annu. Rev. Med.* 36: 207, 1985.
88. Janoff, A., and Zweifach, B. W. Production of inflammatory changes in the microcirculation by cationic proteins extracted from lysosomes. *J. Exp. Med.* 120: 747, 1964.
89. Johnson, K. J., and Ward, P. A. Role of oxygen metabolites in immune complex injury of the lung. *J. Immunol.* 126: 2365, 1981.
90. Johnson, R., Iida, H., Yoshimura, A., et al. Platelet derived growth factor: A potentially important cytokine in glomerular disease. *Kidney Int.*, 41: 590, 1992.
91. Johnson, R. J., Couser, W. G., Chi, E. Y., et al. New mechanism for glomerular injury: Myeloperoxidase in hydrogen peroxide–halide system. *J. Clin. Invest.* 79: 1379, 1987.
92. Johnston, G. I., Cook, R. G., and McEver, R. P. Cloning of GMP 140, a granule membrane protein of platelets and endothelium: Sequence similarity to proteins involved in cell adhesion and inflammation. *Cell* 56: 1033, 1989.
93. Johnston, K. J., Anderson, T. P., and Ward, P. A. Suppression of immune complex-induced inflammation by the chemotactic factor inactivator. *J. Clin. Invest.* 59: 951, 1977.
94. Jose, P. J. Complement-derived peptide mediators of inflammation. *Br. Med. Bull.* 43: 336, 1990.
95. Jutila, M. A., Rott, L., Berg, E., et al. Function and regulation of the neutrophil MEL-14 antigen in vivo: Comparison with LFA-1 and Mac-1. *J. Immunol.* 143: 3318, 1989.
96. Karwatowska-Prokopczuk, E., and Wennmalm, A. Effects of endothelin on coronary flow, mechanical performance, oxygen uptake, and formation of purines and on outflow of prostacyclin in the isolated rabbit heart. *Circ. Res.* 66: 46, 1990.
97. King, A. J., Brenner, B. M., and Anderson, S. Endothelin: A potent renal and systemic vasoconstrictor peptide. *Am. J. Physiol.* 256: F1051, 1989.
98. King, A. J., Pfeffer, J. M., Pfeffer, M. A., et al. Systemic hemodynamic effects of endothelin in the rat. *Am. J. Physiol.* 258: H787, 1990.
99. Kishimoto, T. K., Anderson, D. C., Butcher, E., et al. The human neutrophil MEL-14 antigen and the endothelial antigen ELAM-1 are involved in the same CD18-independent adhesion pathway in vitro. Abstract. *J. Leukoc. Biol.* 48(Suppl. 1): 96, 1990.
100. Kishimoto, T. K., Jutila, M. A., Berg, E. L., et al. Neutrophil Mac-1 and MEL-14 adhesion proteins are inversely regulated by chemotactic factors. *Science* 245: 1238, 1989.
101. Kishimoto, T. K., Larson, R. S., Corbi, A. L., et al. The leukocyte integrins. *Adv. Immunol.* 46: 149, 1989.
102. Klebanoff, S. J. Phagocytic Cells: Products of Oxygen Metabolism. In J. I. Gallin, I. M. Goldstein, and R. Synderman (eds.), *Inflammation: Basic Principles and Clinical Correlates*. New York: Raven, 1988. P. 391.
103. Kohzuki, M., Johnston, C. I., Chai, S. Y., et al. Localization of endothelin receptors in rat kidney. *Eur. J. Pharmacol.* 160: 193, 1989.
104. Kurihara, H., Yoshizumi, M., Sugiyama, T., et al. Transforming growth factor-β stimulates the expression of endothelin mRNA by vascular endothelial cells. *Biochem. Biophys. Res. Commun.* 159: 1435, 1989.
105. Kwon, N. S., Nathan, C. F., Gilker, C., et al. L-Citrulline production from L-arginine by macrophage nitric oxide synthase. *J. Biol. Chem.* 265: 13442, 1990.
106. Larsen, E., Celi, A., Gilbert, G. E., et al. PADGEM protein: A receptor that mediates the interaction of activated platelets with neutrophils and monocytes. *Cell* 59: 305, 1989.
107. Larsen, G., and Henson, P. M. Mediators of inflammation. *Annu. Rev. Immunol.* 1: 335, 1983.
108. Lasky, L. A., Singer, M. S., Yednock, T. A., et al. Cloning of lymphocyte homing receptor reveals a lectin domain. *Cell* 56: 1045, 1989.
109. Lawrence, M. B., McIntire, L. V., and Eskin, S. G. Effect of flow on polymorphonuclear leukocyte endothelial cell adhesion. *Blood* 70: 1284, 1987.
110. Lawrence, M. B., Smith, C. W., Eskin, S. G., et al. Effect of venous shear stress on CD-18 mediated adhesion to cultured endothelium. *Blood* 75: 227, 1990.
111. Leung, D. Y. M., Collins, T., Lapierre, L. A., et al. Immunoglobulin M antibodies present in the acute phase of Kawasaki syndrome lyse cultured vascular endothelial cells stimulated by gamma interferon. *J. Clin. Invest.* 77: 1428, 1986.
112. Leung, D. Y. M., Geha, R. S., Newburger, J. W., et al. Two monokines, interleukin-1 and tumour necrosis factor, render vascular endothelial cells susceptible to lysis by antibodies circulating during acute Kawasaki syndrome. *J. Exp. Med.* 164: 1958, 1986.
113. Leung, D. Y. M., Pober, J. S., and Cotran, R. S. Expression of endothelial-leukocyte adhesion molecule-1 in elicited late phase allergic reactions. *J. Clin. Invest.* 87: 1805, 1991.
114. Linas, S. L., Whittenburg, D., and Repine, J. E. Role of neutrophil-derived oxidants and elastase in lipopolysaccharide-mediated renal injury. *Kidney Int.* 39: 618, 1991.
115. Lippton, H. L., Hauth, T. A., Summer, W. R., et al. Endothelin produces pulmonary vasoconstriction and systemic vasodilation. *J. Appl. Physiol.* 66: 1008, 1989.
116. Ludmer, P. L., Selwyn, A. P., Shook, T. L., et al. Paradoxical vasoconstriction induced by acetylcholine in atherosclerotic coronary arteries. *N. Engl. J. Med.* 315: 1046, 1986.
117. Lynch, J. M., and Henson, P. M. The intracellular retention of newly synthesized platelet activating factor. *J. Immunol.* 137: 2653, 1986.
118. MacCumber, M. W., Ross, C. A., and Snyder, S. H. Endothelin in brain: Receptors, mitogenesis, and biosynthesis in glial cells. *Proc. Natl. Acad. Sci. U.S.A.* 87: 2359, 1990.
119. Makgoba, M. W., Saunders, M. E., Luce, G. E. G., et al. ICAM-1: Definition by multiple antibodies of a ligand for LFA-1 dependent adhesion of B, T and myeloid cells. *Nature* 331: 86, 1988.
120. Malech, H. D., and Gallin, J. I. Neutrophils in human disease. *N. Engl. J. Med.* 37: 687, 1988.
121. Mantymaa, P., Leppaluoto, J., and Ruskoaho, H. Endothelin stimulates basal and stretch-induced atrial natriuretic peptide secretion from the perfused rat heart. *Endocrinology* 126: 587, 1990.
122. Marasco, W. A., Phan, S. H., Krutzsch, H., et al. Purification and identification of formyl-methionyl-leucyl-phenylalanine as the major peptide neutrophil chemotactic factor produced by *Escherichia coli*. *J. Biol. Chem.* 259: 5430, 1984.
123. Marchesi, V. T., and Gowans, J. L. The emigration of leucocytes through the endothelium of venules in lymph nodes. An electron microscopic study. *Proc. R. Soc. Biol.* 159: 283, 1964.
124. Marks, R. M., Todd, R. F., and Ward, P. A. Rapid induction of neutrophil-endothelial adhesion by endothelial

complement fixation. *Nature* 339: 314, 1989.

125. Marletta, M. A. Nitric oxide: Biosynthesis and biological significance. *Trends Biochem. Sci.* 14: 488, 1989.
126. Martin, E. R., Marsden, P. A., Brenner, B. M., et al. Identification and characterization of endothelin binding sites in rat renal papillary and glomerular membranes. *Biochem. Biophys. Res. Commun.* 162: 130, 1989.
127. Martin, S. D., and Springer, T. A. Purified intercellular adhesion molecule 1 (ICAM-1) is a ligand for lymphocyte function-associated antigen 1 (LFA-1). *Cell* 51: 813, 1987.
128. Martin, W., Vilani, G. M., Jothianandan, D., et al. Selective blockade of endothelium-dependent and glyceryl trinitrate-induced relaxation by hemoglobin and by methylene blue in the rabbit aorta. *J. Pharmacol. Exp. Ther.* 232: 708, 1985.
129. Massague, J. The transforming growth factor-β family. *Annu. Rev. Cell Biol.* 6: 597, 1990.
130. McArthy, J. B., Palm, S. L., and Furcht, L. T. Migration by haptotaxis of a Schwann cell tumour line to the basement membrane glycoprotein laminin. *J. Cell Biol.* 97: 772, 1983.
131. McCormack, R. J., Harkin, M. M., Johnson, K. J., et al. The effect of superoxide dismutase on pulmonary and dermal inflammation. *Am. J. Pathol.* 101: 55, 1980.
132. McIntyre, K. W., Stepan, G. J., Kolinsky, K. D., et al. Inhibition of interleukin-1 (IL-1) binding and bioactivity in vitro and modulation of acute inflammation in vivo by IL-1 receptor antagonists and anti-IL-1 receptor monoclonal antibody. *J. Exp. Med.* 173: 931, 1991.
133. Meagher, L. M., Savill, J. S., Baker, A., et al. Macrophage secretory responses to ingestion of aged neutrophils. *Biochem. Soc. Trans.* 17: 608, 1989.
134. Mene, P., Simonson, M. S., and Dunn, M. J. Physiology of the mesangial cell. *Am. Physiol. Soc.* 69: 1347, 1989.
135. Metcalf, D. The molecular biology and functions of the granulocyte-macrophage colony stimulating factors. *Blood* 67: 257, 1986.
136. Metchnikoff, E. *Lectures on the Comparative Pathology of Inflammation* (translated from the French by F. A. Starling and E. H. Starling). London: Kegan, Paul, Trench and Trubner, 1893.
137. Miller, W. L., Redfield, M. M., and Burnett, J. C. Integrated cardiac, renal and endocrine actions of endothelin. *J. Clin. Invest.* 83: 317, 1989.
138. Moncada, S., and Vane, J. R. Pharmacology and endogenous roles of prostaglandin endoperoxides, thromboxane A_2 and prostacyclin. *Pharmacol. Rev.* 30: 293, 1979.
139. Morel, D. R., Lacroix, J. S., Hemsen, A., et al. Increased plasma and pulmonary lymph levels of endothelin during endotoxin shock. *Eur. J. Pharmacol.* 167: 427, 1989.
140. Morrison, D. C., and Ryan, J. L. Endotoxins and disease mechanisms. *Annu. Rev. Med.* 38: 417, 1987.
141. Moser, R., Schleiffenbaum, B., Groscurth, P., et al. Interleukin 1 and tumour necrosis factor stimulate human vascular endothelial cells to promote transendothelial neutrophil passage. *J. Clin. Invest.* 83: 444, 1989.
142. Munro, J. M., Pober, J. S., and Cotran, R. S. Tumour necrosis factor and interferon-γ induce distinct patterns of endothelial activation and leukocyte accumulation in skin of *Papio anubis*. *Am. J. Pathol.* 133: 121, 1989.
143. Myers, P. R., Minor, R. L., Jr., Guerra, R., Jr., et al. Vasorelaxant properties of the endothelium-derived relaxing factor more closely resemble S-nitrosocysteine than nitric oxide. *Nature* 345: 161, 1990.
144. Nagai, K., and Katori, M. Possible changes in the leukocyte membrane as a mechanism of leucocyte adhesion to venular walls induced by leukotriene B4 and FMLP in the microvasculature of the hamster cheek pouch. *Int. J. Microcirc.* 7: 305, 1988.
145. Nathan, C., and Sporn, M. Cytokines in context. *J. Cell Biol.* 113: 981, 1991.
146. Nathan, C. F., and Stuehr, D. J. Does endothelium-derived nitric oxide have a role in cytokine-induced hypotension? *J. Natl. Cancer Inst.* 82: 762, 1990.
147. Newman, S. L., Henson, J. E., and Henson, P. M. Phagocytosis of senescent neutrophils by human monocyte-derived macrophages and rabbit inflammatory macrophages. *J. Exp. Med.* 156: 430, 1982.
148. Nourshargh, S., Edwards, A. J., and Williams, T. J. Effects of pertussis toxin on neutrophil accumulation in vivo. *Br. J. Pharmacol.* 96: 402, 1989.
149. Okuda, S., Languino, L. R., Ruoslahti, E., et al. Elevated expression of transforming growth factor-β and proteoglycan production in experimental glomerulonephritis. *J. Clin. Invest.* 86: 453, 1990.
150. Okusawa, S., Gelfand, J. A., Ikejima, T., et al. Interleukin-1 induces a shock-like state in rabbits. Synergism with tumour necrosis factor and the effect of cyclooxygenase inhibition. *J. Clin. Invest.* 81: 1162, 1988.
151. Oppenheim, J. J., Zacharie, C. O. C., Mukaida, N., et al. The intercrines. *Annu. Rev. Immunol.* 9: 617, 1991.
152. Osborn, L., Hession, C., Tizard, R., et al. Direct expression cloning of vascular cell adhesion molecule-1 (VCAM-1), a cytokine induced endothelial protein that binds to lymphocytes. *Cell* 59: 1203, 1989.
153. Palmer, R. M. J., Rees, D. D., Ashton, D. S., et al. L-Arginine is the physiological precursor for the formation of nitric oxide in endothelium-dependent relaxation. *Biochem. Biophys. Res. Commun.* 153: 1251, 1988.
154. Peden, D. B., Hohman, R., Brown, M. E., et al. Uric acid is a major antioxidant in human nasal airway secretions. *Proc. Natl. Acad. Sci. U.S.A.* 87: 7638, 1990.
155. Perez, H. D., Kelly, E., Chenoweth, D., et al. Identification of the C5a des Arg cochemotaxin. Homology with vitamin D-binding protein (group-specific component globulin). *J. Clin. Invest.* 82: 360, 1988.
156. Perico, N., Dadan, J., and Remuzzi, G. Endothelin mediates the renal vasoconstriction induced by cyclosporine in the rat. *J. Am. Soc. Nephrol.* 1: 76, 1990.
157. Phillips, M. L., Nudelman, E., Gaeta, F. C. A., et al. ELAM-1 mediates cell adhesion by recognition of carbohydrate ligand, Sialyl-Le^x. *Science* 250: 1130, 1990.
158. Picker, L. J., Kishimoto, T. K., Smith, C. W., et al. ELAM-1 is an adhesion molecule for skin-homing T cells. *Nature* 349: 796, 1991.
159. Pober, J. S., and Cotran, R. S. Cytokine-endothelial interactions in inflammation, immunity and vascular injury. *J. Am. Soc. Nephrol.* 1: 225, 1990.
160. Pohlman, T. H., Stanness, K. A., Beatty, P. G., et al. An endothelial cell surface factor(s) induced in vitro by lipopolysaccharide, interleukin 1 and tumour necrosis factor increases neutrophil adherence by a CD_w 18 (LFA)-dependent mechanism. *J. Immunol.* 136: 4548, 1986.
161. Pusey, C. D., and Lockwood, C. M. Autoimmunity in rapidly progressive glomerulonephritis. *Kidney Int.* 35: 929, 1989.
162. Raij, L., and Keane, W. F. Glomerular mesangium: Its function and relationship to angiotensin II. *Am. J. Med.* 79(3C): 24, 1985.
163. Rakugi, H., Nakamaaru, M., Saito, H., et al. Endothelin inhibits renin release from isolated rat glomeruli. *Biochem. Biophys. Res. Commun.* 155: 1244, 1988.
164. Rampart, M., and Williams, T. J. Evidence that neutro-

phil accumulation induced by interleukin-1 requires both local protein synthesis and neutrophil CD18 antigen expression in vivo. *Br. J. Pharmacol.* 94: 1143, 1988.

165. Rampart, M., and Williams, T. J. Polymorphonuclear leukocyte-dependent plasma leakage in the rabbit skin is enhanced or inhibited by prostacyclin depending on the route of administration. *Am. J. Pathol.* 124: 66, 1986.
166. Ranadive, N. S., and Cochrane, C. G. Basic proteins in rat neutrophils that increase vascular permeability. *Clin. Exp. Immunol.* 6: 905, 1970.
167. Rees, D. D., Palmer, R. M. J., and Moncada, S. Role of endothelium-derived nitric oxide in the regulation of blood pressure. *Proc. Natl. Acad. Sci. U.S.A.* 86: 3375, 1989.
168. Rehan, A., Wiggins, R. C., Kunkel, R. G., et al. Glomerular injury and proteinuria in rats after intrarenal injection of cobra venom factor. *Am. J. Pathol.* 123: 57, 1986.
169. Resink, T. J., Scott-Burden, T., and Buhler, F. R. Activation of phospholipase A_2 by endothelin in cultured vascular smooth muscle cells. *Biochem. Biophys. Res. Commun.* 158: 279, 1989.
170. Rice, G. E., Munro, J. M., and Bevilacqua, M. P. Inducible cell adhesion molecule 110 (INCAM 110) is an endothelial receptor for lymphocytes. *J. Exp. Med.* 171: 1369, 1990.
171. Rice, G. E., Munro, J. M., Corless, C., et al. Vascular and nonvascular expression of INCAM-110. A target for mononuclear leukocyte adhesion in normal and inflamed human tissue. *Am. J. Pathol.* 138: 385, 1991.
172. Riches, D. W. H. The Multiple Roles of Macrophages in Wound Healing. In R. A. F. Clark and P. M. Henson (eds.), *The Molecular and Cellular Biology of Wound Repair.* New York: Plenum, 1988. P. 213.
173. Richter, J., Ng-Sikorski, J., Olson, I., et al. Tumour necrosis factor-induced degranulation in adherent human neutrophils is dependent on $CD11_b$/CD18 integrin-triggered oscillations of cytosolic free Ca^{2+}. *Proc. Natl. Acad. Sci. U.S.A.* 87: 9472, 1990.
174. Robaye, B., Mosselmans, R., Fiers, W., et al. Tumour necrosis factor induced apoptosis (programmed cell death) in normal endothelial cells in vitro. *Am. J. Pathol.* 138: 447, 1991.
175. Rosen, H., and Gordon, S. Monoclonal antibody to the murine type 3 complement receptor inhibits adhesion of myelomonocytic cells in vitro and inflammatory cell recruitment in vivo. *J. Exp. Med.* 166: 1685, 1987.
176. Rothlein, R., Dustin, M. L., Marlin, S. D., et al. A human intercellular adhesion molecule (ICAM-1) distinct from LFA-1. *J. Immunol.* 137: 1270, 1986.
177. Ruoslahti, E. Integrins. *J. Clin. Invest.* 87: 1, 1991.
178. Ruoslahti, E., and Piersbacher, M. D. New perspectives in cell adhesion: RGD and integrins. *Science* 238: 491, 1987.
179. Ruoslahti, E., and Yamaguchi, Y. Proteoglycans as modulators of growth factor activities. *Cell* 64: 867, 1991.
180. Samuelson, B. Leukotrienes: Mediators of immediate hypersensitivity reactions and inflammation. *Science* 220: 568, 1983.
181. Sanui, H., Yoshida, S-I., Nomoto, K., et al. Peritoneal macrophages which phagocytose autologous polymorphonuclear leucocytes in guinea pigs. I. Induction by irritants and microorganisms and inhibition by colchucine. *Br. J. Exp. Pathol.* 63: 278, 1982.
182. Savage, C. O. S., Pottinger, B., Gaskin, G., et al. Vascular damage in Wegener's granulomatosis and microscopic polyarteritis: Presence of anti-endothelial cell antibodies and their relation to anti-neutrophil cytoplasm antibodies. *Clin. Exp. Immunol.*, 85: 14, 1991.
183. Saverymuttu, S. H., Peters, A. M., Danpure, H. T., et al. Lung transit of ^{111}In-labelled granulocytes: Relation to labelling cedmiques. *Scand. J. Haematol.* 30: 151, 1983.
184. Savill, J. S., Dransfield, I., Hogg, N., et al. Vironectin receptor-mediated phagocytosis of cells undergoing apoptosis. *Nature* 342: 170, 1990.
185. Savill, J. S., Henson, P. M., and Haslett, C. Phagocytosis of aged human neutrophils by macrophages is mediated by a novel "charge-sensitive" recognition mechanism. *J. Clin. Invest.* 84: 1518, 1989.
186. Savill, J. S., Wyllie, A. H., Henson, J. E., et al. Macrophage phacocytosis of aging neutrophils in inflammation. Programmed cell death in the neutrophil leads to its recognition by macrophages. *J. Clin. Invest.* 83: 865, 1989.
187. Schiffman, E., Corcoran, B. A., and Wahl, S. A. N-Formyl methionyl peptides as chemoattractants for leukocytes. *Proc. Natl. Acad. Sci. U.S.A.* 72: 1059, 1975.
188. Schumann, R. R., Leong, S. R., Flaggs, G. W., et al. Structure and function of lipopolysaccharide binding protein. *Science* 249: 1429, 1990.
189. Schwartz, B. R., Wayner, E. A., Carlos, T. M., et al. Identification of surface proteins mediating adherence of CD11/CD18 deficient lymphoblastoid cells to cultured human endothelium. *J. Clin. Invest.* 85: 2019, 1990.
190. Shichiri, M., Hirata, Y., Ando, K., et al. Plasma endothelin levels in hypertension and chronic renal failure. *Hypertension* 15: 493, 1990.
191. Shimizu, Y., Shaw, S., Graber, N., et al. Activation-independent binding of human memory T cells to adhesion molecule ELAM-1. *Nature* 349: 799, 1991.
192. Shultz, P., Ruble, D., and Raij, L. S-Nitroso-n-acetylpenicillamine (SNAP) inhibits mitogen-induced mesangial cell proliferation. Abstract. *Kidney Int.* 37: 203, 1990.
193. Shultz, P., Schorer, A. E., and Raij, L. Effects of endothelium-derived relaxing factor and nitric oxide on rat mesangial cells. *Am. J. Physiol.* 258: F162, 1990.
194. Shultz, P., Tayeh, M. A., Marletta, M. A., et al. Synthesis and action of nitric oxide in rat glomerular mesangial cells. *Am. J. Physiol.*, 261: F600, 1991.
195. Simonson, M. S., Wann, S., Mene, P., et al. Endothelin stimulates phospholipase C, NA^+/H^+ exchange, c-*fos* expression, and mitogenesis in rat mesangial cells. *J. Clin. Invest.* 83: 708, 1989.
196. Simpson, P. J., Todd, R. F., Fantone, J. C., et al. Reduction of experimental canine myocardial reperfusion injury by a monoclonal antibody (anti-Mo1, anti-CD11b) that inhibits leukocyte adhesion. *J. Clin. Invest.* 81: 624, 1988.
197. Singer, I. I., Scott, S., Kawka, D. W., et al. Human leukocyte specific granules contain receptors for laminin, fibronectin, vitronectin and C3bi/fibrinogen. *J. Leukoc. Biol.* 46: 331, 1989.
198. Smith, C. W., Kishimoto, T. K., Abbass, O., et al. Chemotactic factors regulate lectin adhesion molecule-1 (LECAM-1)-dependent neutrophil adhesion to cytokine-stimulated endothelial cells in vitro. *J. Clin. Invest.* 87: 609, 1991.
199. Smith, C. W., Marlin, S. D., Rothlein, R., et al. Co-operative interactions of LFA-1 and Mac-1 with intracellular adhesion molecule 1 in facilitating adherence and transendothelial migration of human neutrophils in vitro. *J. Clin. Invest.* 83: 2008, 1989.
200. Smith, C. W., Rothlein, R., Hughes, B. J., et al. Recog-

nition of an endothelial determinant for CD18-dependent human neutrophil adherence and transendothelial migration. *J. Clin. Invest.* 82: 1746, 1988.

201. Snyderman, R., and Pike, M. C. Chemoattractant receptors on phagocytic cells. *Annu. Rev. Immunol.* 2: 257, 1984.
202. Spertini, O., Kansas, G. S., Munro, J. M., et al. Regulation of leukocyte migration by activation of the leukocyte adhesion molecule-1 (LAM-1) selectin. *Nature* 349: 691, 1991.
203. Spitznagel, J. K. Antibiotic proteins of neutrophils. *J. Clin. Invest.* 86: 1581, 1990.
204. Sporn, M. B., Roberts, A. B., Wakefield, L. M., et al. Some recent advances in the chemistry and biology of transforming growth factor-β. *J. Cell Biol.* 105: 1039, 1987.
205. Springer, T. A. Adhesion receptors of the immune system. *Nature* 346: 425, 1990.
206. Springer, T. A., Thompson, W. S., Miller, L. J., et al. Inherited deficiency of the Mac-1, LFA-1, p150, 95 glycoprotein family and its molecular basis. *J. Exp. Med.* 160: 1901, 1984.
207. Staunton, D. E., Dustin, M. L., and Springer, T. A. Functional cloning of ICAM-2, a cell adhesion ligand for LFA-1 homologous to ICAM-1. *Nature* 339: 61, 1989.
208. Stephens, L. R., Hughes, K. T., and Irvine, R. F. Pathway of phosphatidylinositol (3,4,5)-tris phosphate synthesis in activated neutrophils. *Nature* 351: 33, 1991.
209. Sugiura, M., Snajdar, R. M., Schwartzberg, M., et al. Identification of two types of specific endothelin receptors in rat mesangial cells. *Biochem. Biophys. Res. Commun.* 162: 1396, 1989.
210. Takagi, M., Tsukada, H., Matsuoka, H., et al. Inhibitory effect of endothelin on renin release in vitro. *Am. J. Physiol.* 257: E833, 1989.
211. Takahashi, K., Ghatei, M. A., Lam, H. C., et al. Elevated plasma endothelin in patients with diabetes mellitus. *Diabetologia* 33: 306, 1990.
212. Tavassoli, M. The marrow-blood barrier. *Br. J. Haematol.* 41: 287, 1979.
213. Tedder, T. F., Isaacs, C. M., Ernst, T. J., et al. Isolation and chromosomal localization of cDNAs encoding a novel human lymphocyte cell surface molecule, LAM-1. Homology with the mouse lymphocyte cell surface molecule and other human adhesion proteins. *J. Exp. Med.* 170: 123, 1989.
214. Terzhagi, M., Nettesrheim, P., and Williams, M. L. Repopulation of denuded tracheal grafts with normal preneoplastic epithelial cell populations. *Cancer Res.* 38: 4551, 1978.
215. Thoma, R. Ueber entzundliche stonungen des capillarkreislaufes bei warmblutern. *Virchows Arch. B Pathol. Anat.* 74: 360, 1978.
216. Thornhill, M., Kyan-Aung, U., and Haskard, D. O. IL-4 increases human endothelial cell adhesion for T cells but not for neutrophils. *J. Immunol.* 144: 3060, 1990.
217. Thornhill, M., Williams, D., and Speight, P. Enhanced adhesion of autologous lymphocytes to gamma-interferon-treated human endothelial cells in vitro. *Br. J. Exp. Pathol.* 70: 59, 1989.
218. Tolins, J. P., Palmer, R. M. J., Moncada, S., et al. Role of endothelium-derived relaxing factor in regulation of renal hemodynamic responses. *Am. J. Physiol.* 258: H655, 1990.
219. Tolins, J. P., Vercellotti, G. M., Wilkowske, M., et al. Role of platelet activating factor in endotoxemic acute renal failure in the male rat. *J. Lab. Clin. Med.* 113: 316, 1989.
220. Tomita, K., Ujiie, K., Nakanishi, T., et al. Plasma endothelin levels in patients with acute renal failure. (Letter) *N. Engl. J. Med.* 321: 1127, 1990.
221. Tomosugi, N., Cashman, S. J., Hay, H., et al. Modulation of antibody-mediated glomerular injury in vivo by bacterial lipopolysaccharide, tumour necrosis factor and IL-1. *J. Immunol.* 142: 3083, 1989.
222. Tonnesen, M. G., Anderson, D. C., Springer, T. A., et al. Adherence of neutrophils to cultured human microvascular endothelial cells: Stimulation by chemotactic peptides and lipid mediators and dependence upon the Mac-1, LFA-1, p150,95. *J. Clin. Invest.* 83: 637, 1989.
223. Tonnesen, M. G., Smedly, L. A., and Henson, P. M. Neutrophil-endothelial cell interactions. Modulation of neutrophil adhesiveness induced by complement fragments C_{5a} and C_{5a} des arg and formyl-methionyl-leucyl-phenylalanine in vitro. *J. Clin. Invest.* 74: 1581, 1984.
224. Toothill, V. J., Van Mourik, J. A., Niewenhuis, H. K., et al. Characterization of the enhanced adhesion of neutrophil leukocytes to thrombin-stimulated endothelial cells. *J. Immunol.* 145: 243, 1990.
225. Tracey, K. J., Fong, Y., Hesse, D. G., et al. Anti-cachectin/TNF monoclonal antibodies prevent septic shock during lethal bacteraemia. *Nature* 330: 662, 1987.
226. Ulich, T. R., Yin, S., Guo, K., et al. Intratracheal administration of endotoxin and cytokines III. The interleukin-1 (IL-1) receptor antagonist inhibits endotoxin and IL-1-induced inflammation. *Am. J. Pathol.* 138: 521, 1991.
227. Vanhoutte, P. M., Rubany, G. M., Miller, V. M., et al. Modulation of vascular smooth muscle contraction by endothelium. *Annu. Rev. Physiol.* 48: 307, 1986.
228. Vedder, N. B., Winn, R. K., Rice, C. L., et al. Inhibition of leukocyte adherence by anti-CD18 monoclonal antibody attenuates reperfusion injury in the rabbit ear. *Proc. Natl. Acad. Sci. U.S.A.* 87: 2643, 1990.
229. Vosbeck, K., Tobias, P., Mueller, H., et al. Priming of polymorphonuclear granulocytes by lipopolysaccharide binding proteins and high density lipoprotein. *J. Leukoc. Biol.* 47: 97, 1990.
230. Walz, G., Aruffo, A., Kolanus, W., et al. Recognition by ELAM-1 of the Sialyl-Le^x determinant on myeloid and tumour cell lines. *Science* 250: 1132, 1990.
231. Warner, S. J. C., Auger, K. R., and Libby, P. Interleukin 1 induces interleukin 1. *J. Immunol.* 139: 1911, 1987.
232. Warren, J. S., Mandel, D. M., Johnson, K. J., et al. Evidence for the role of platelet-activating factor in immune complex vasculitis in the rat. *J. Clin. Invest.* 83: 669, 1989.
233. Watson, M. L., Lewis, G. P., and Westwick, J. Increased vascular permeability and polymorphonuclear leucocyte accumulation in vivo in response to recombinant cytokines and supernatants from IL-1 treated human synovial cell cultures. *Br. J. Exp. Pathol.* 70: 93, 1989.
234. Watt, K. W. K., Brightman, E. J., and Goetzl, E. J. Isolation of 2 polypeptides comprising the neutrophil immobilisation factor of human leucocytes. *Immunology* 48: 79, 1983.
235. Wedmore, C. V., and Williams, T. J. Control of vascular permeability by polymorphonuclear leukocytes in inflammation. *Nature* 289: 646, 1981.
236. Wegner, C. D., Gundel, R. H., Reilly, P., et al. Intercellular adhesion molecule-1 (ICAM-1) in the pathogenesis of asthma. *Science* 247: 456, 1990.
237. Weisman, H. F., Barlow, T., Leppo, M. K., et al. Soluble human complement receptor type 1: In vivo inhibitor of

complement suppressing post-ischaemic myocardial inflammation and necrosis. *Science* 249: 146, 1990.

238. Weiss, S. J. Tissue destruction by neutrophils. *N. Engl. J. Med.* 320: 365, 1989.
239. Weiss, S. J., Curnette, J. T., and Regani, S. Neutrophil-mediated solubilization of the subendothelial matrix: Oxidative and non-oxidative mechanisms of proteolysis used by normal and chronic granulomatous disease phagocytes. *J. Immunol.* 136: 636, 1986.
240. Wright, S. D., Levin, S. M., Jong, M. T. C., et al. CR3 (CD11b/CD18) expresses one binding site for Arg-Gly-Asp-containing peptides, and a second site for bacterial lipopolysaccharide. *J. Exp. Med.* 169: 175, 1989.
241. Wright, S. D., Ramos, R. A., Hermanowski-Vosatka, A., et al. Activation of the adhesive capacity of CR3 on neutrophils by endotoxin: Dependence on lipopolysaccharide binding protein and CD14. *J. Exp. Med.* 173: 1281, 1991.
242. Wright, S. D., Ramos, R. A., Tobias, P. S., et al. CD14, a receptor for complexes of lipopolysaccharide (LPS) and LPS binding protein. *Science* 249: 1431, 1990.
243. Wyllie, A., Kerr, J. F. R., and Currie, A. R. Cell death: The significance of apoptosis. *Int. Rev. Cytol.* 68: 251, 1980.
244. Wyllie, A. H. Glucocorticoid-induced thymocyte apoptosis is associated with endogenous endonuclease activation. *Nature* 284: 555, 1980.
245. Yamaguchi, Y., Mann, D. M., and Rucslahti, E. Negative regulation of transforming growth factor-β by the proteoglycan decorin. *Nature* 346: 281, 1990.
246. Yanagisawa, M., Kurihara, H., Kimura, S., et al. A novel potent vasoconstrictor peptide produced by vascular endothelial cells. *Nature* 332: 411, 1988.
247. Yoshizumi, M., Kurihara, H., Fumimaro, T., et al. Hemodynamic shear stress regulates endothelin gene expression in cultured endothelial cells. Abstract. *Circ. Res.* 78: 182, 1988.
248. Yoshizumi, M., Kurihara, H., Morita, T., et al. Interleukin I increases the production of endothelin-I by cultured endothelial cells. *Biochem. Biophys. Res. Commun.* 166: 324, 1990.
249. Yuo, A., Kitagawa, S., Suzuki, I., et al. Tumour necrosis factor as an activator of human granulocytes. Potentiation of the metabolisms triggered by the Ca^{2+}-mobilizing agonists. *J. Immunol.* 142: 1678, 1989.
250. Zeidel, M. L., Brady, H. R., Kone, B. C., et al. Endothelin, a peptide inhibitor of Na/K ATPase in intact renal tubular epithelial cells. *Am. J. Physiol.* 257: C1101, 1989.
251. Ziegler, E. J., Fisher, C. J., Sprung, C. L., et al. Treatment of gram-negative bacteraemia and septic shock with HA-IA human monoclonal antibody against endotoxin: A randomized, double-blind, placebo-controlled trial. *N. Engl. J. Med.* 324: 429, 1991.
252. Zimmerman, G. A., MacIntyre, T. M., and Prescott, S. M. Thrombin stimulates the adherence of neutrophils to endothelial cells in vitro. *J. Clin. Invest.* 76: 2235, 1985.

Nephropathy of Systemic Lupus Erythematosus

John P. Hayslett
Michael Kashgarian

Clinical Manifestations of Systemic Lupus Erythematosus (SLE)

DIAGNOSIS

Descriptions of lupus nephropathy were initially reported by Keith and Rowntree [62] in 1922, and the importance of renal involvement in SLE was detailed by Baehr in 1931. Prior to Hargrave's discovery of the lupus erythematosus (LE) cell in 1948 [48], the diagnosis of the disorder was confounded because of the nonspecificity of many of the clinical features of the disease and the difficulty of separating SLE from other rheumatic diseases. Discovery of the LE cell was a landmark event in the study of the disease because it rapidly led to the demonstration that SLE was an autoimmune disorder and provided a homogeneous population of patients for clinical study. In 1971 the American Rheumatism Association established criteria for the diagnosis of SLE based on 14 manifestations, which included 21 items [24]. The data base for this report was derived from rheumatology clinics and aimed to provide a useful means for distinguishing SLE from other rheumatic diseases in population studies and clinical trials. The criteria, which included both clinical and laboratory features of the disease, was updated in 1982 and showed 95 percent sensitivity and 96 percent specificity when tested with SLE and control data [103].

It should be emphasized that the diagnostic criteria established by the American College of Rheumatology apply to population studies when patients are observed over a long period and cannot always be relied on to establish the diagnosis at the onset of disease or even in all patients with SLE who have been followed for prolonged periods of time. Numerous reports have documented SLE in cases with isolated clinical features. Some patients, for example, initially present with apparent primary renal disease and exhibit systemic manifestations only after several years [75]. In these cases the serologic findings, renal biopsy changes, and exclusion of other disease entities serve to establish the probable diagnosis of SLE.

Antinuclear antibodies (ANAs) are found in nearly all patients with SLE, and a positive reaction is usually considered necessary for diagnosis. In addition, antibodies that recognize different cellular structures in the cytoplasm and on the cell surface are found. It is convenient to classify this broad array of antibodies according to whether they bind to a naked nucleic acid such as DNA, a chromatin component such as a histone, a ribonucleoprotein (RNP) particle, or some other cellular element. Despite the array of antibodies detectable in SLE, Hardin indicates that only a limited number of specificities, such as anti-DNA antibodies, antibodies to histones, and antibodies to small nuclear RNP (snRNP) and small cytoplasmic RNP (scRNP), are found in high titer with considerable frequency in individual patients [47]. Moreover, in regard to nucleoprotein structures, most prominently recognized autoantigens reside on only three types of nucleoprotein structures: the nucleosome, the U1 snRNP (uridylate-rich [U] RNAs), and the Ro scRNP, as shown in Fig. 72-1. Autoantibodies to each of these structures appear to occur in ordered sequences; anti-Sm antibodies, which recognize B, B', D, and D particles on U1 RNA, are accompanied by anti–U1 RNP antibodies, anti-La antibodies are accompanied by anti-Ro antibodies, and antibodies to histones H1 and H2B are almost always found together. In most cases, the epitopes are accessible on the surface of different particles, in contrast to internal components. A major unresolved question in SLE, as well as in other autoimmune disorders, is why these normally weak antigens escape tolerance mechanisms and induce antibody production. It is possible that an exogenous factor may play a role by altering the structure of macromolecules, as exemplified in drug-induced SLE.

Although a close correlation between antibodies to specific antigenic determinants and clinical features of SLE has not been established, certain antibodies are highly specific for different types of autoimmune disorders, as shown in Table 72-1 [84]. For example, anti-Sm and anti–native DNA are relatively specific for SLE, anti–transfer $tRNA^{His,Thr,Ala}$ synthetases for polymyositis, anti–Scl 70 for diffuse scleroderma, and anticentromere/kinetochore for CREST syndrome. It is of course possible that the names used clinically to label different diseases subserve a function to categorize different manifestations of the same disease.

CLINICAL FEATURES AND NATURAL COURSE

SLE occurs primarily in females (90 percent) who range in age at onset from 16 to 50 years. Several reports have summarized the clinical features in large numbers of patients [37, 49, 107]. The review of 150 patients by Estes and Christian in 1971 [37] provides typical data on a hospital-based population. Almost every patient (95 percent) had symptoms referable to the joints, usually the small joints, at some time during the course of the illness. Cutaneous manifestations were next in frequency (81 percent) and included a malar rash and/or dermal vasculitis most often. Hematologic findings were also frequent manifestations of disease in this series of patients, with an incidence of anemia in 73 percent, leukopenia (< 4500 per mm^{-3}) in 66 percent, and thrombocytopenia ($< 100{,}000$ per mm^{-3}) in 19 percent. Clinical manifestations reflecting involvement of the heart, kidneys, lung, and central nervous system occurred in 38 to 59 percent of patients during the course of their illness. Detailed descriptions of specific types of organ involvement are provided elsewhere [55, 110]. In the report by Estes and Christian [37] the 5-year survival rate was 76.9 percent, and for 10 years it was 59.1 percent. There was no difference in long-term outlook between

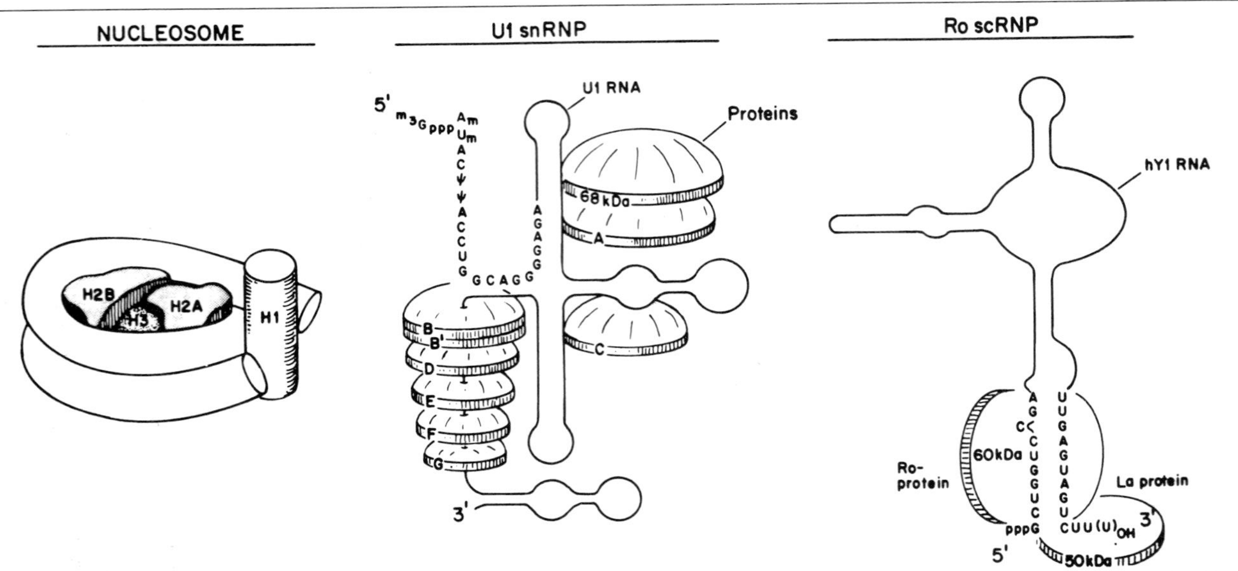

Fig. 72-1. The lupus autoantigens. In patients with systemic lupus erythematosus (SLE), immune responses to the nucleosome, the U1 small nuclear RNP (U1 snRNP), and Ro small cytoplasmic RNP (Ro scRNP) account for the majority of antinuclear antibodies that occur frequently and in high titers.

The nucleosome consists of 2 turns of DNA around a histone core comprised of an inner tetramer of 2 copies each of histones H3 and H4, and on each face, 1 copy each of histones H2B and H2A. Lupus antibodies recognize histone H1 (external) and the amino terminal (external), but not the carboxy terminal (internal) segments of H2B, and, to a lesser extent, the amino terminal segments of the other core histones (which are also exposed). The internal histone regions are rarely recognized by patient sera, although animal antisera to purified histones readily bind such sites. Thus, it appears that patients with SLE respond primarily to external features of relatively intact nucleosomal segments of chromatin as they produce antibodies to both histones and DNA.

The U1 snRNP consists of complex of 9 proteins and the U1 RNA. The extreme 5′ end of this RNA exhibits a base sequence that is complementary to splice junctions within newly transcribed messenger RNA (mRNA) molecules. Watson-Crick base pairing permits this structure to mediate the precise excision of introns during mRNA processing. The RNA secondary structure shown is that proposed by Mount and Steitz. The associated polypeptides are tentatively assigned to their present positions because the 3′ end of the RNA molecule appears to be protected from RNase digestion by the presence of the D, E, F, and G polypeptides; whereas, the ready removal of the 68 kDa, A, and C polypeptides suggest that their intervening RNA is accessible to this enzyme. In immunoblots, sera containing anti-U1 RNP antibodies usually recognize the 68 kDa, A, and C polypeptides; sera containing anti-Sm antibodies usually recognize the B, B′, and D polypeptides. Thus, it appears that the physical association of these antigens is responsible for the fact that anti-Sm antibodies are usually accompanied by anti-U1 RNP antibodies. However, anti-U1 RNP antibodies may be found alone. The order must be that anti-U1 RNP is primary, and in some patients, the response is propagated to include anti-Sm.

The Ro scRNP contains 1 of 5 small RNAs, known as human cytoplasmic 1-5 (hY1-5) RNA and, as shown, is complexed at the 3′ and 5′ ends with the Ro polypeptide. At some point, the Ro RNAs are also complexed with the La polypeptide, which recognizes a binding site constituted of oligo-U sequences with a terminal hydroxyl. Thus, the minute quantities of Ro particles can account for both anti-Ro and anti-La antibodies. As yet, there is no conclusive proof that the Ro and La proteins reside simultaneously on the Ro RNAs.

This figure is taken from reference [47], and is used with permission.

sexes or races. The lowest 5-year survival rates, however, involved patients with central nervous system disorders and clinical evidence of renal disease.

Since reports based on hospital patients or patients referred to specialty clinics are biased toward more severe complications, the spectrum of clinical manifestations of SLE is better defined by outpatient populations or demographic studies in geographic areas. Wallace summarized the long-term course of 609 private patients seen in private practice or in a lupus clinic [107]. In this series, the overall 10-year survival rate was 79 percent (87 percent without nephritis, 65 percent with nephritis). The most common causes of death were renal failure and sepsis. Female patients did better than males;

Table 72-1. Antinuclear antibody disease association

Antinuclear antibody type	Disease specificity
Anti-dsDNA	SLE
Anti-ssDNA	SLE, other rheumatic diseases
Both anti-ds and -ssDNA	SLE (60–70%)
Antihistones	SLE (30%), drug-induced SLE (95%), and rheumatoid arthritis (20%)
Anti-Sm	SLE (35%) and mixed connective tissue disease (95%)
Anti–U1 RNP	SLE
Anti–SS-A/Ro	SLE (35%) and systemic sclerosis
Anti–SS-B/La	SLE (15%) and systemic sclerosis
Anti-tRNA	Polymyositis
Anticentromere/ kinetochore	CREST
Anti-RNA	Rheumatoid arthritis
Anti–Scl 70	Systemic sclerosis

there were no racial differences. Interestingly, in this series 27 percent of all nephritic patients developed renal function impairment 5 years or longer after the onset of disease. In a recent report, Jonsson et al. described the course of all adult SLE patients (86 patients) in southern Sweden, during 1981 to 1986; the population was approximately 160,000 [60]. The mean incidence of new cases was 4 per 100,000 adults per year. Cumulative incidences of organ system involvement were 77 percent for mucocutaneous, 98 percent for musculoskeletal, 62 percent for serositis, and 49 percent for hematologic involvement. Major and minor clinical flares were common during the first year after the onset of disease and thereafter remained constant during the subsequent 5 years (minor flares, 20 percent; major flares, 10 percent). Of 26 patients with renal involvement, 16 had reduced renal function during active disease (glomerular filtration rate < 50 ml/min). Renal function returned to normal in 6, and 1 patient developed terminal renal failure. In this population, the 5-year patient survival rate was 95 percent, and full-time and part-time employment rates were similar to those for age-matched controls in Sweden.

Pathology of Lupus Nephritis

During the last 20 years, significant new knowledge has been acquired relative to the pathogenesis of lupus nephritis, and this has been extended to the diagnostic interpretation of renal biopsy specimens and to clinical pathologic correlations aimed at evaluating the natural history of this disease and its response to therapy. In the initial studies of renal biopsy specimens from patients with lupus nephritis, it was obvious that although the renal lesions were quite varied, the pattern of renal involvement correlated with clinical outcome [12, 13, 26, 86]. The use of light microscopy was extended by the addition of immunofluorescence microscopy and electron microscopy in the assessment of renal biopsy specimens, and various groups emphasized the utility of each or all of these morphologic methods in assessing the activity and severity of the renal lesions [12, 13, 26]. Although analysis of renal biopsy material has helped to define and classify subgroups of patients with differing therapeutic responses and natural histories, there are many controversies in the literature concerning the clinical pathologic correlations made with each of these modalities. In individual patients, however, the combination of clinical or laboratory tests is not an accurate predictor of the structural changes that are found in the kidney, and the findings by this morphologic modality (i.e., renal biopsy) alone did not always correlate with outcome. Despite these controversies and difficulties, it has become apparent that renal biopsy in lupus nephritis is an important part of the evaluation of patients with this disease and is of considerable value both in the choice of therapy and in predicting prognosis.

PATHOGENESIS

The pathogenesis of lupus nephritis is thought to be similar to that of experimental chronic immune complex glomerulonephritis. There are many theories about the immunologic mechanisms, and these have been the subject of extensive reviews [29, 51, 67, 69]. On the basis of earlier studies on the pathogenesis of SLE, it was proposed that there was faulty regulation of the immune response system, resulting in an autoimmune disease with antibodies directed toward a variety of cellular determinants, due to increased helper T-cell function, lack of T-cell suppression, and/or autonomous activity of B lymphocytes, all of which lead to excess antibody secretion by endogenously activated lymphoid cells [47]. Moreover, although many of the antigenic determinants subserve specific roles in cell function, such as RNA splicing (snRNPs), DNA replication (proliferating cell nuclear antigen), and transcription (ss-B/La), it seems unlikely that autoantibodies inhibit the function of their cognate antigens but rather induce altered tissue reactions, when immune complexes of antibody and antigens form in extracellular fluid [102].

The current paradigm for the pathogenesis of tissue injury in SLE, including lupus nephropathy, involves two linked components. The first component involves production of autoantibodies and the deposition of preformed antibody-antigen complexes on vascular or serosal surfaces, or formation of complexes in situ. These complexes, some of which activate the complement cascade, result in neutrophil and platelet infiltration and activation. The second component is characterized by cell proliferation, necrosis, and thrombus formation, secondary to factors released by infiltrating cells and platelets. For example, one of the major cytotoxic mechanisms of the neutrophil—the myeloperoxidase–hydrogen peroxide (H_2O_2)–halide system—has been shown to cause glomerular endothelial cell injury and proteinuria [59]. Platelets produce various chemotactic substances that increase neutrophil adherence and aggregation, phagocytosis, and release of reactive oxygen species and myeloperoxidase [80, 91]. In addition, platelets can release tissue factors, a major stimulus for fibrin deposition, and can activate the intrinsic pathway by both factor XII–dependent and factor XII–independent pathways [58]. The importance of the second component in the mechanism of tissue injury is highlighted by studies in experimental animals, in which immune glomerulonephritis, characterized by subendothelial immune complexes, was studied during platelet depletion [58]. Although immune complex deposition and neutrophil infiltration were similar in both platelet-depleted and nondepleted animals, platelet depletion was associated with a marked reduction in segmental glomerular necrosis and formation of intracapillary thrombi. Recognition and insights into the mechanism of the sequential roles of these components in the pathogenesis of immune complex nephritis provide the basis for treatment strategies in SLE.

In addition to autoantibodies that result in immune complex–induced tissue injury, recent studies have identified another type of autoimmune disorder, namely one that results in intravascular thrombosis. It is now established that the lupus anticoagulant, later shown to be associated with a tendency toward arterial and venous thrombosis, is an antiphospholipin [9]. The development of a radioimmunoassay and the subsequent enzyme-linked immunosorbent assay (ELISA) for the detection of antibodies against cardiolipin and other phospholipids has provided a means to assess their prevalence and the role of these autoantibodies in clinical disorders. In a recent report on 500 consecutive patients with SLE, antiphospholipid antibodies, isotypes IgG, IgM, and IgA, were found in 53 percent of patients and higher titers correlated with recurrent fetal loss, venous thrombosis, thrombocytopenia, hemolytic anemia, and livedo reticularis [8]. Not unexpectedly, there was also a strong correlation between the presence of lupus anticoagulant, and/or a false-positive result on the test for VDRL, and anticardiolipins. Other reports show an association with cerebrovascular occlusions and lupus anticoagulant in SLE, especially in patients with multiple infarctions and dementia [9]. These studies, together with reports that deep venous and arterial thrombosis and placental infarction correlate with high titers of anticardiolipin antibodies in other autoimmune diseases, as well as in patients with "lupuslike" disorders and in those with no evidence of immune complex disease, strongly suggest that anticardiolipin antibodies cause many of the vascular complications in SLE [56]. Furthermore, the demonstration of fibrin deposition in vascular structures and/or intraglomerular thrombi on renal biopsy specimens from patients with SLE and related disorders suggest that anticardiolipin antibody–induced thrombosis as well as immune complex deposition play an important role in the pathogenesis of lupus nephropathy [61]. Since anticardiolipin antibodies bind the phosphodiester group of negatively charged phospholipids, it has been proposed that thrombus formation is induced by antibody reaction with platelets directly or with vascular endothelial cell membranes, leading to decreased prostacyclin release.

A number of animal models that have some characteristics of human lupus have been studied, and information gained from these models has suggested that renal involvement is a prototype of experimental chronic immune complex nephritis [29, 44]. The variety of lesions seen in lupus nephritis have thus been attributed to individual differences in the immune response in different patients or in the same individual patient during the course of time. For example, mesangial deposition of immune complexes, resulting in a pure mesangial lupus glomerulonephritis, is probably the result of an immune response characterized by the presence of relatively small amounts of stable, intermediate-size complexes formed with high-affinity antibodies. These immune complexes are accumulated in the mesangium as part of filtration residues that may be adequately handled by the mesangial clearing system, resulting in a mild glomerular lesion. With larger numbers of intermediate-size complexes, or with large complexes formed by high-affinity antibodies, the capability of the mesangium to clear macromolecules is overloaded, resulting in accumulation of these complexes in a subendothelial location as well. This in turn may activate circulating inflammatory mediators, such as the complement system and the coagulation system. In such cases, a more severe diffuse histopathologic pattern can be seen, and may or may not be associated with areas of necrosis and deposition of fibrin. If the immune response is characterized by the presence of small, unstable circulating immune complexes formed by low-avidity or low-affinity antibodies in the presence of antigen excess, the complex may dissociate and reform in situ within the glomerular capillary wall. This mechanism may be particularly important in instances where antibodies to histones are present [42] since it has been demonstrated that histones are highly cationic and thus have a high affinity for the anionic sites of the glomerular basement membrane [92]. Once bound to the glomerular basement membrane, they can act as planted target antigens and a focus for in situ complex formation. This mechanism has been demonstrated to result in the development of a membranous glomerulonephropathy. While this hypothesis may be somewhat simplistic, experimental and clinical evidence suggests that it may have some validity [29, 51, 66, 69]. Additional factors that may relate to the severity and type of injury pattern include the nature of the antigen, the affinity and avidity of the antibodies formed, the class and subclass of the antibodies formed, and the valency and phlogogenic activity of the complexes.

CLASSIFICATIONS OF LUPUS NEPHROPATHY

The World Health Organization classification [79] of lupus nephritis (Table 72-2) has attempted to combine all morphologic modalities of biopsy interpretation and has added a semiquantitative assessment of severity as well. It is now in general use and has been widely accepted by clinical nephrologists and renal pathologists alike. This classification is a major improvement over previous classifications because it includes immunofluorescent and electron microscopic evaluations as well as light microscopic evaluation and therefore can differentiate patients with mild, purely mesangial patterns from those with peripheral capillary involvement and subendothelial deposits on electron microscopy, who generally have

Table 72-2. WHO classification of lupus nephritis

Patterns	Light microscopy		Immuno-fluorescence		Electron microscopy		
	Mes.	Perif.	Mes.	Perif.	Mes.	Endo.	Epi.
I Normal	0	0	0	0	0	0	0
IIA Mesangial deposits	0	0	+	0	+	0	0
IIB Mesangial hypercellularity	+	0	+	0	+	0	0
III Focal-segmental glomerulonephritis (< 50%)	+	+	+ +	+	+ +	+	±
IV Diffuse glomerulonephritis (> 50%)	+ +	+ +	+ +	+ +	+ +	+ +	±
V Membranous glomerulonephritis	+	+ +	+	+ +	+	±	+ +

Note: Mes., mesangial; Perif., peripheral capillary wall; Endo., subendothelial; Epi., subepithelial.

Table 72-3. International study of kidney disease in children: classification of lupus nephritis

I. Normal
  A. Nil
  B. Normal by light microscopy but deposits present
II. Pure mesangiopathy
  A. Mild (+)
  B. Moderate (+ +)
III. Segmental and focal proliferative glomerulonephritis
  A. Active necrotizing
  B. Active and sclerosing
  C. Sclerosing
IV. Diffuse proliferative glomerulonephritis
  A. Without segmental necrotizing lesions
  B. With segmental necrotizing lesions
  C. With segmental active and sclerotic lesions
  D. Inactive, sclerotic
V. Diffuse membranous GN
  A. Pure membranous
  B. Associated with lesions in group IIA or IIB
  C. Associated with lesions in group IIIA, IIIB, or IIIC
  D. Associated with lesions in group IVA, IVB, IVC, or IVD
VI. Advanced sclerosing GN

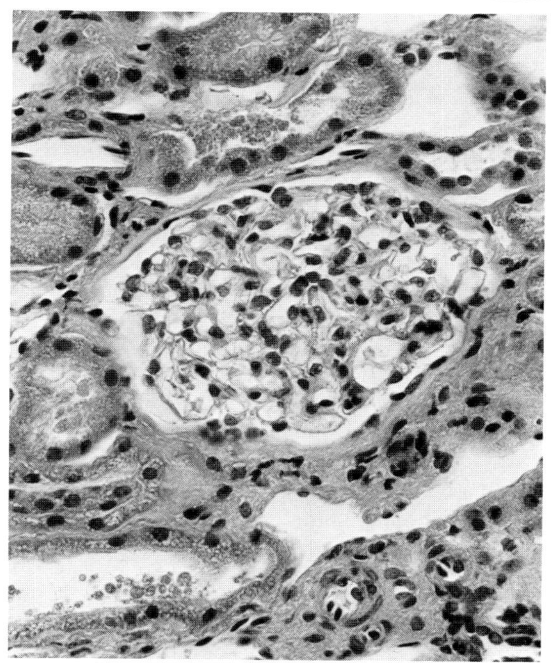

Fig. 72-2. Light photomicrograph of an essentially normal glomerulus in a patient with LE. This patient would be considered Class I. (×450.)

a more severe clinical course. A more detailed subclassification of the WHO system (Table 72-3) has been developed by the Pathology Advisory Group for the International Study of Kidney Diseases in Children (ISKDC) [23], but this appears to be of greater value for investigative purposes than for general clinical use. These classifications do have the limitation of emphasizing glomerular lesions and giving much less weight to tubular, interstitial, and vascular lesions. The relative importance of each of the classes and of tubular, vascular, and interstitial lesions will be discussed in greater detail later.

Class I. Class I (Fig. 72-2) is not a lesion that can be identified specifically. Renal biopsy reveals essentially a normal kidney by light, electron, and immunofluorescence microscopy, although minor nonspecific changes may be observed occasionally on electron microscopy. Since this class is really an absence of morphologic evidence of glomerular damage, it may not really represent a form of renal involvement.

Class II. This class (Fig. 72-3) is confined to purely mesangial lesions. It has been subdivided into class IIA, in which there are minimal or no significant changes by light microscopy, although there may be immunoflu-

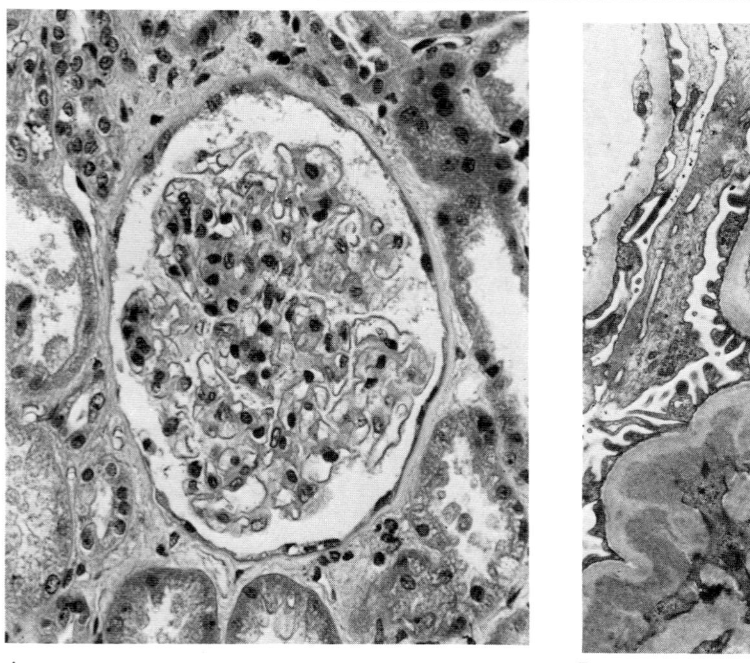

A

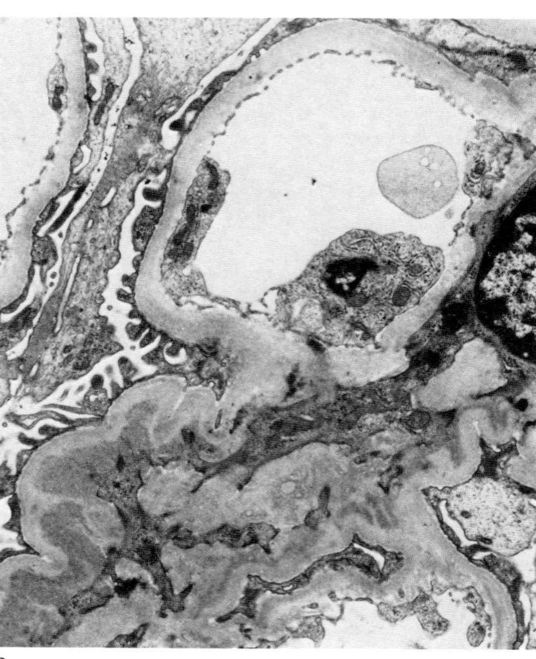

B

Fig. 72-3. Light micrograph (A) (×450) and electron micrograph (B) (×3,000) of a glomerulus with Class IIB lesion. There is mild mesangial hypercellularity and increase in matrix. The electron micrograph demonstrates mesangial dense deposits.

orescent evidence of immune deposits confined to the mesangium and/or dense deposits by electron microscopy. Class IIB shows definite glomerular mesangial hypercellularity by light microscopy, which is confined to the centrilobular regions away from the vascular pole. There are no significant changes in the peripheral glomerular capillary walls. Immune deposits are present by immunofluorescence and electron microscopy but are confined to the mesangial regions. Tubular, interstitial, or vascular changes are insignificant. Clinically, the majority of these patients have mild to moderate evidence of renal involvement and in general have a good prognosis.

Class III. Class III (Fig. 72-4) is represented by light microscopic findings of a focal and segmental glomerulonephritis. The changes may be proliferative, necrotizing, or sclerosing, or a combination of these. In addition to the mesangial prominence and deposits that are seen in class II lesions, segmental intracapillary and extracapillary cell proliferation with obliteration of the capillary lumina is found. The presence of necrosis and leukocytic infiltration suggests a higher degree of activity. Generally speaking, this category is assigned when less than 50 percent of the glomeruli are involved, and those that are involved show only focal damage occupying less than 50 percent of the glomerular surface. A major contrast to class II is the presence of subendothelial deposits in addition to mesangial deposits by electron microscopy. Interstitial and tubular changes are frequently encountered but are usually focal in distribution. The similarity of the immunofluorescence and electron mi-

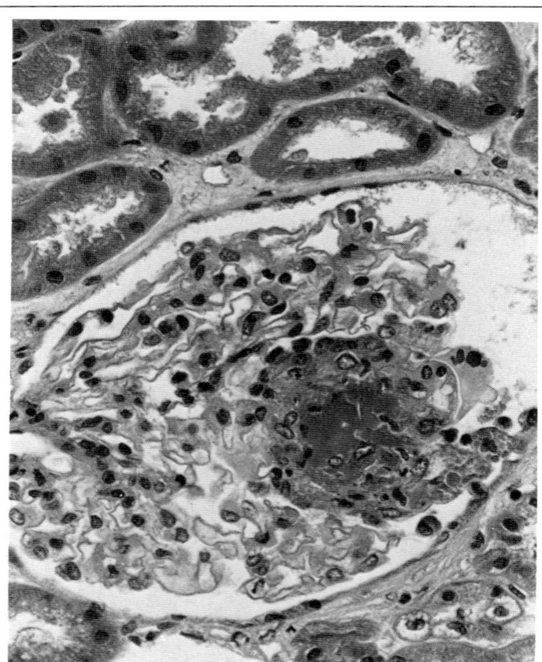

Fig. 72-4. Light photomicrograph of Class III glomerular lesion. There is segmental necrosis of the glomerular tuft. Less than 50 percent of glomeruli show this lesion. (×450.)

croscopic findings of class III with those of class IV suggests that the two may actually be part of a continuum of morphologic changes. The ISKDC classification subdivides this group into three subclasses, which include *active necrotizing* when necrotic lesions are present, *active* and *sclerosing* when sclerotic lesions are present in addition to necrosis, and *sclerosing* when necrotic lesions are not present. Clinically, these patients tend to have a more aggressive course and thus behave differently from patients in class II. The natural history of these patients is similar to that of patients in class IV. Thus on the basis of morphologic and clinical criteria, classes III and IV probably should not be considered separate forms of lupus nephritis but rather as continua of the same lesion [7].

Class IV. Class IV (Fig. 72-5) is characterized by a diffuse proliferative lupus glomerulonephritis. The majority or all of the glomeruli are involved, and each glomerulus shows diffuse hypercellularity. In addition, there may be focal areas of necrosis and crescent formation, and nuclear debris, which sometimes is represented by a "hematoxylin" body, may be present. Some areas of the peripheral capillary loops may be dramatically thickened to form what have been called "wire loop lesions." The range of glomerular lesions may extend from only diffuse mesangial hypercellularity without necrosis, sclerosis, or wire loops to a severe necrotizing and crescentic glomerulonephritis.

By immunofluorescence, immunoglobulins are present in a coarsely granular pattern, both in the mesangium and in the peripheral capillary wall. Immunoglobulins are generally accompanied by complement components, fibrinogen, and occasionally, properdin. Where sclerosis is prominent, immunofluorescence findings may be attenuated.

By electron microscopic examination the most prominent and distinguishing finding in this class is the presence of subendothelial deposits. The electron-dense deposits are larger and more abundant in class IV than in other classes and are always accompanied by mesangial deposits and, not infrequently, by subepithelial and intramembranous deposits. Mesangial hypercellularity with circumferential mesangial interposition in the basement membrane is frequently present, producing a pattern essentially identical to that seen in idiopathic mesangiocapillary glomerulonephritis. The electron-dense deposits may show a distinctive crystalline structure, which has been termed a *fingerprint* pattern. This organized crystalline structure is most frequently seen when there are abundant subendothelial and mesangial deposits but may also be present in all classes of lupus nephritis. The crystalline structure has been thought to suggest the presence of cryoglobulins because similar patterns are also seen in patients with idiopathic mixed cryoglobulinemia. It has also been thought that they may represent a pattern of crystalline DNA.

Endothelial cell swelling and proliferation are commonly seen, as are occasional mitotic figures. In addition, tubulovesicular structures, which resemble myxoviruslike particles, have been identified in a majority of patients with lupus nephropathy. The significance of these structures is unclear because similar structures can

Fig. 72-5. Class IV lupus nephritis (diffuse proliferative glomerulonephritis). The light micrograph (A) shows diffuse glomerular proliferation with lobular accentuation and thickening of the peripheral capillary walls. The electron micrograph (B) shows subendothelial electron-dense deposits in the peripheral capillary wall.

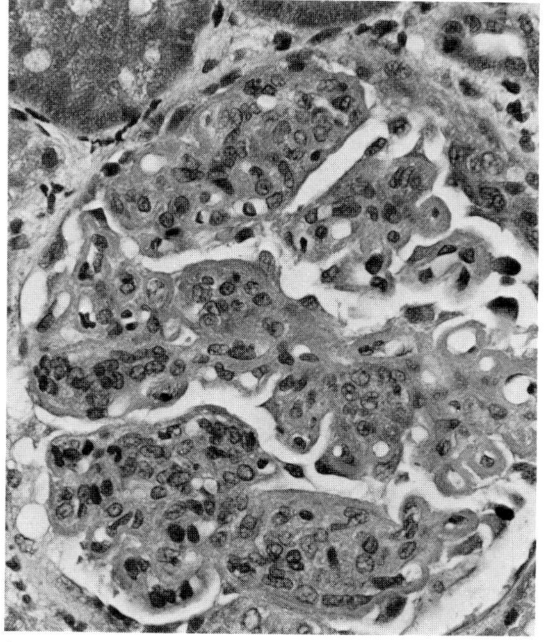

A

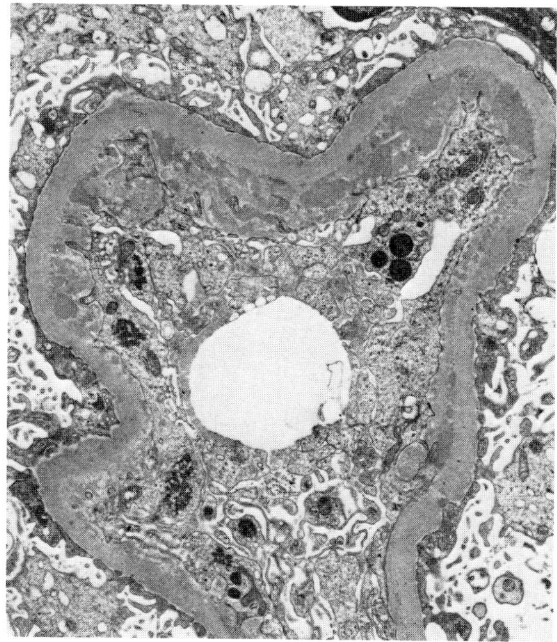

B

be seen in a small percentage of patients with other types of renal disease. Attempts at viral cultures have been unsuccessful.

Patients with class IV lesions generally have a relatively severe clinical picture with nephrotic-range proteinuria and an active sediment. Without therapy, these patients are considered to have the worst prognosis because a high percentage of them progress to renal failure.

Class V. This class (Fig. 72-6) is represented by a diffuse membranous glomerulonephropathy. By light microscopy there is generalized diffuse thickening of the peripheral capillary walls, which on silver methenamine Masson stain exhibits the so-called spike and dome pattern. The spikes are projections of basement membrane–like material, and the domes correspond to the subendothelial and intramembranous deposits. Immunofluorescence findings demonstrate a confluent, peripheral granular deposition of immunoglobulin, which is usually accompanied by mesangial granular deposits. Electron microscopy reveals numerous epimembranous and intramembranous deposits. The pattern is essentially identical to that of idiopathic membranous glomerulonephropathy and has the same stages of development that have been used to categorize that lesion. In lupus nephritis, however, mesangial deposits are usually prominent and may help to distinguish this lesion from idiopathic membranous glomerulonephropathy. In the ISKDC classification of lupus nephropathy, the membranous lesion is subclassified according to whether it is associated with lesions of class II, III, or IV. Such a subdivision seems, however, to be unnecessary, and the presence of subendothelial deposits or necrosis probably should take precedence over a superimposed membranous pattern. Clinically, these patients generally tend to have proteinuria, which may be in the nephrotic range, but this lesion tends to progress in a relatively indolent fashion similar to that of idiopathic disease.

Mixed Patterns and Transformation. It is likely that even these classes and subclasses may not be absolute and distinct clinical pathologic entities but may represent many differing points in a continuum of disease. This is particularly likely because transformation of the renal lesion from one class to another can occur both spontaneously and as a result of treatment. The exact incidence of spontaneous transformation is difficult to determine because relatively few serial biopsy studies have been carried out in untreated patients. A number of studies, however, suggest that transformation does occur and that it is not uncommon, particularly following treatment [12, 83, 52]. Transformation from class III to class IV has been commonly reported and supports the concept that these two classes are essentially the same. Transformation of diffuse proliferative glomerulonephritis to a predominantly membranous glomerulonephropathy or to a mesangial pattern has been observed in patients undergoing remission during therapy. The mechanism of the transformation is not known but may relate to the nature of the immune response or to the physical chemical characteristics of immune complexes.

Fig. 72-6. Membranous lupus glomerulonephropathy. There is diffuse thickening of the peripheral capillary walls, with a generalized increase in mesangial matrix by light microscopy (A). Electron microscopy (B) demonstrates characteristic epimembranous (subepithelial) and mesangial deposits.

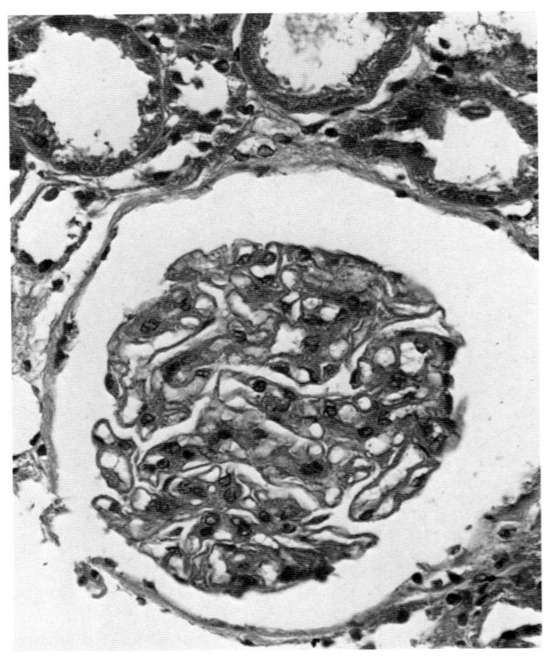

A

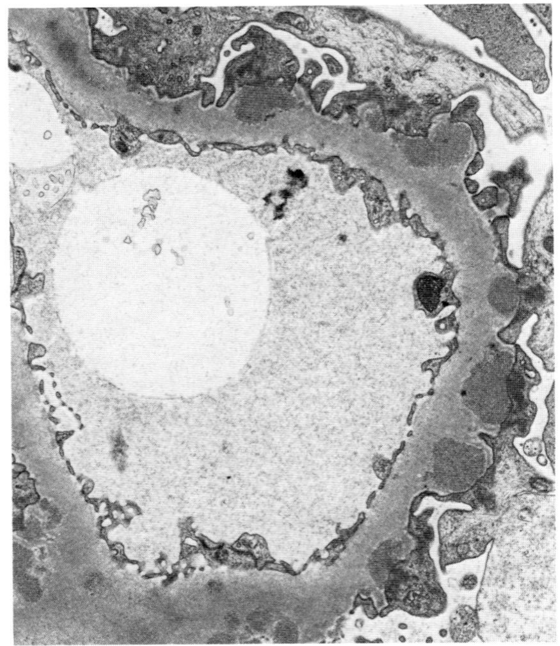

B

IMMUNOFLUORESCENCE FINDINGS

One factor that has not been given enough consideration in the histopathologic evaluation is the role of the immunoglobulin isotype and subclass [51]. Most studies of immunofluorescence findings in lupus nephropathy have emphasized the patterns of deposition rather than the classes of immunoglobulins found. IgG and IgM are the classes of immunoglobulin most commonly deposited; IgA, though frequently found, is not as common nor is its distribution as extensive or impressive as that of the other two immunoglobulins. In one study IgG2 was found more frequently than other subclasses. Since subclasses IgG2 and IgG4 do not readily activate complement, one might expect a milder lesion to occur with these classes than with IgG1 and IgG3. One analysis, however, showed a poor correlation between IgG subclass and the severity of the morphologic lesion. IgE is usually not commented on but when reported, it is found infrequently and is thought to reflect a part of the general autoimmune response that is associated with the clinical syndrome of lupus. Some recent reports have suggested that IgE deposits in lupus nephritis are associated with a poorer prognosis. The so-called full-house pattern or multiple immunoglobulin deposition is quite characteristic of lupus and does not predict any more severe disease than that characterized by IgG alone. Complement components including the membrane attack complex, fibrinogen, and properdin are usually associated with the presence of immunoglobulins, particularly in the more severe classes.

TUBULOINTERSTITIAL DISEASE

Severe tubulointerstitial nephritis is most commonly seen in patients with class III or class IV glomerular lesions. Although in most instances the interstitial inflammation is composed of lymphocytes and plasma cells, granulocytes and eosinophils are frequently found and probably reflect a more active lesion. Immunofluorescence occasionally reveals granular peritubular deposits and, very rarely, the presence of a linear deposit, suggesting an antitubular basement membrane antibody. Of interest is the observation that tubulointerstitial disease may progress independently from the glomerular disease in some patients.

VASCULAR LESIONS

Necrotizing vasculitis with vascular necrosis and leukocytic infiltration is a rare finding in the kidney. More commonly, evidence of venulitis is seen with a perivenular leukocytic infiltration, and this is generally found in association with tubulointerstitial nephritis. Nephrosclerotic lesions with intimal fibroplasia and medial sclerosis are also occasionally encountered, particularly in hypertensive patients. Immunofluorescence examination will occasionally demonstrate granular immune deposits in both arterioles and venules, and electron microscopy will reveal electron-dense deposits in the walls of both arteries and veins. Recently, attention has been drawn to a group of patients in whom there is prominent evidence of intravascular coagulation [61]. A pattern similar to that seen in adult hemolytic uremic syndrome, with multiple capillary thrombi containing fibrinogen, has been associated with a clinical picture of rapidly progressive renal failure. Recent studies have shown low levels of tissue-type plasminogen activator (t-PA) and elevated levels of plasmin inhibitor (α_2-antiplasmin) in patients with lupus nephropathy, associated with glomerular capillary deposition of fibrin or thrombus formation [45]. Since these alterations in plasma levels of t-PA and α_2-antiplasmin would be expected to retard fibrinolysis, and were corrected by administration of the fibrinolytic agent ancrod to patients with lupus glomerulonephritis, together with dissolution of the fibrin deposits by biopsy, it is proposed that a disorder in fibrinolysis predisposes some patients with SLE to renal microvascular thrombi.

ASSESSMENT OF SEVERITY AND CHRONICITY

Several studies (see next section, Clinical and Pathologic Correlations) have emphasized the importance of using semiquantitative analyses of biopsies to assess chronicity and severity. Activity has been related to the presence of necrosis, cellular proliferation, leukocytic infiltration, and hyaline thrombi in glomeruli. Chronicity has been graded according to the degree of glomerular sclerosis and fibrosis as well as the amount of interstitial scarring and tubular atrophy. Such an approach has been useful in studies of large groups of patients, and recent studies have suggested that quantitation may be of value in assessing the prognosis of individual patients [6, 36, 77, 95].

CLINICAL AND PATHOLOGIC CORRELATIONS

Clinical studies of relatively large numbers of patients with lupus nephritis first appeared in the late 1950s [review, 86]. Based on clinical signs of renal disease, the incidence of renal involvement in adult patients ranged from 50 to 80 percent. Clinicopathologic correlations demonstrated a significant relationship between the underlying histopathology and the subsequent clinical course. In patients with mild hypercellularity and membranous nephropathy renal function was preserved for long periods, although patients with membranous lesions commonly exhibited heavy proteinuria [86]. In contrast, the clinical course of patients with diffuse proliferative glomerulonephritis was usually hectic, and the 2-year patient survival rate was less than 30 percent despite the use of high-dose glucocorticoid treatment. In these reports there was little tendency for transformation of one category of histologic disease to other patterns of injury. The correlation between the renal histopathology and the clinical manifestations of renal disease was extended by Baldwin et al. [12] in an analysis of 52 patients in 1970, later expanded to 88 cases in 1977 [12]. In these studies three types of renal injury were recognized by light microscopy, including focal proliferative glomerulonephritis, membranous nephropathy, and diffuse proliferative glomerulonephritis. The focal lesion was characterized by sharply delineated segmental proliferation of some tufts, involving 12 to 55 percent of the glomeruli. In patients with this lesion there was a tendency toward preservation of renal function (92 percent), although the nephrotic syndrome was present in two-thirds, and all patients had proteinuria to some extent. The survival rate was 75 percent during the period of observation, and by life survival analysis the 5-year survival was estimated to be 70 percent. In the group with membranous nephropathy, proteinuria was present in nearly all patients and the nephrotic syndrome in 70 percent. In agreement with previous reports, renal function was preserved in the majority (70 percent). The 5-year survival was 79 percent. Patients with a diffuse proliferative glomerulonephritis had a poor outlook in regard to morbidity and progression to renal failure. The nephrotic syndrome was present in over 90 percent of these patients, and renal insufficiency existed in 82 percent. Life table analysis indicated a 5-year survival of 30 percent. Similar findings were obtained in subsequent studies [7, 26, 76].

Subsequent reports have emphasized the presence and location of electron-dense deposits as important indices of the clinical course in addition to the pattern of injury observed by light microscopy [34, 104]. Based on an analysis of clinical series, the presence of subendothelial electron-dense deposits, usually in association with changes of cellular proliferation, correlated with a higher incidence of heavy proteinuria and renal insufficiency regardless of whether the pattern of hypercellularity was focal or diffuse. In contrast, localization of deposits to the mesangial area or to subepithelial loci in peripheral capillary walls was associated with low rates of functional deterioration. Further evidence of the importance of the location of deposits was provided by Hecht et al. [54], who studied 31 patients with proliferative glomerulonephritis and subendothelial deposits on initial biopsy; they were treated with the same therapeutic regime, including low-dose prednisone and azathioprine. During follow-up, which averaged 40 months, a second renal biopsy demonstrated complete disappearance of subendothelial deposits in two-thirds of these patients; all these patients had normal renal function at the end of follow-up and either no proteinuria or low levels of proteinuria. It was of interest that on the second biopsy there was transformation of the histopathologic lesion to either normal histology (25 percent) or to a membranous lesion (75 percent). In patients with persistence of subendothelial deposits, the subsequent course was characterized by renal deterioration, defined by a urinary protein excretion of 3 gm per day and/or an increase in serum creatinine of more than 1.5 mg per dl^{-1}. The nature and composition of the interstitial infiltrate are also thought to be of predictive value in regard to the progression of lupus nephritis [4].

In addition to the histopathologic changes of acute nephritis, Austin et al. [11] have reported that glomerular sclerosis and interstitial fibrosis represent significant indicators for progression to renal failure. In their analysis of 102 adult patients entered in treatment trials at the National Institutes of Health, the presence of chronicity at the time of entry into the study correlated with a higher incidence of renal insufficiency than did the absence of those lesions. In a recent analysis of 87 consecutive patients with lupus nephritis, a tubulointerstitial index was devised to quantify mononuclear cell infiltrate in the interstitium and interstitial fibrosis or tubular atrophy, thus including both active and chronic types of tissue injury [36]. This analysis demonstrated that the tubulointerstitial index was superior to both the activity and chronicity indexes in predicting renal and patient death. As an extension of this study, Kant et al. [61] showed that thrombosis in the renal microvasculature of the kidney played an important role in the induction of chronic changes. The presence of glomerular thrombosis on the initial biopsy in patients with predominantly proliferative glomerulonephritis was found to correlate with glomerulosclerosis on a subsequent biopsy.

In summary, evidence obtained from analyses of clinical series suggests that the pattern of renal injury determines the long-term course of renal disease in lupus nephropathy. A proliferative glomerulonephritis accompanied by subendothelial electron deposits in the peripheral capillary loops reflects a more severe pattern of injury and one that is more likely to lead to irreversible tissue damage with subsequent glomerular sclerosis and interstitial fibrosis and eventually to renal failure. The lesion of diffuse proliferative glomerulonephritis, however, is potentially reversible, either because of therapy or because of variations in the severity of disease in individual patients and after transformation to a milder proliferative lesion or a membranous pattern, and it is often associated with improvement in the rate of protein excretion and preservation of renal function. Transformations between different patterns of renal injury are not uncommon. It is not known whether the type of renal lesion is determined by the rate of deposition of immune complexes on the glomerular capillary wall or by the physicochemical properties of the deposits. The aim of therapy, however, is directed toward prevention of necrosis because formation of fibrous tissue is an invariable consequence of tissue destruction.

SLE IN CHILDREN AND THE ELDERLY

Although the mean age at onset of SLE is approximately 28 years and the disease occurs primarily during the reproductive years, children and elderly individuals also are affected. In a report by Meislin and Rothfield, the onset of disease in 42 children occurred between 3 and 15 years of age, with a peak for girls during adolescence [81]. The systemic clinical features were similar in children and adults except for the involvement of the reticuloendothelial system in children, which was manifest as hepatosplenomegaly and lymphadenopathy and occurred in 69 percent of children and 35 percent of adults. The incidence of renal disease in children with SLE was approximately 70 percent and tended to be more severe than in adults. In the Meislin and Rothfield report, long-term survival was lower in children than in adults, both with and without nephritis. Fish et al. [40], however, reported on the long-term follow-up of 49 individuals with onset of disease during childhood who experienced an excellent outcome comparable to that seen in recent reports on adult patients. The average period of follow-up was 5.7 years, and patients were carefully monitored and treated with a similar therapeutic regimen throughout follow-up using prednisone and azathioprine. The initial clinical manifestations in these patients were severe, with prominent central nervous system involvement in 30 percent and renal insufficiency in 78 percent. The overall 10-year survival was 86 percent. A survival of 73 percent and 87 percent during this interval was achieved in patients with diffuse and focal proliferative glomerulonephritis, respectively.

In contrast to the often hectic clinical features of SLE in children in the early phase of disease, systemic manifestations are reported to be milder in elderly patients [41]. At onset, the most common symptoms are myalgia, loss of weight, and fatigue, suggesting a polymyalgia rheumatica-type syndrome or arthritis. Laboratory features of polymyalgia and rheumatic arthritis are absent. The incidence of clinical renal disease is reported to be lower than in children and young adults, and renal disease, when it occurs, is more indolent [107].

SILENT LUPUS NEPHRITIS

Although clinical signs of renal involvement develop in 50 to 80 percent of patients, as noted above, the disease involves the kidney in almost all cases in which adequate tissue analysis is available. Although the renal lesion is mild in the majority of patients with clinically silent lupus nephritis, several reports have described severe proliferative glomerulonephritis with subendothelial deposits in the absence of proteinuria or abnormalities of the urinary sediment [18, 35, 54, 111]. Mahajan et al. [77] performed renal biopsies on 27 patients with systemic lupus in which careful evaluation of urine specimens disclosed normal findings. The histopathologic changes in this series of patients included minimal glomerular damage in 11 percent, focal glomerulonephritis in 44 percent, and diffuse glomerulonephritis in 44 percent. In the series of patients without clinical renal involvement, electron-dense deposits were present in 16 of 19 patients examined by electron microscopy, including 3 with diffuse proliferative glomerulonephritis.

Although there is a consensus that more aggressive therapy is indicated in patients with diffuse proliferative and severe segmental lesions associated with overt signs of renal involvement, the clinical management of patients with similar histopathologic changes in the absence of clinical signs of renal involvement is less certain. Leehey et al. [70] followed 12 patients with clinically silent diffuse glomerulonephritis for intervals ranging from 5 to 11 years and reported a decrease in renal function in 3 cases and an increase in urinary protein excretion in 4. One patient died of renal failure. Although the group with silent lupus nephritis had a seemingly good prognosis compared with their own series of patients with overt renal disease, in which 8 of 37 patients progressed to end-stage renal disease, the authors caution that the number of patients analyzed was too small to state with certainty whether the prognosis was better in the subgroup without signs of renal disease. Moreover, it could not be determined whether treatment administered to the 12 patients (prednisone in 8 and combined prednisone-azathioprine in 4) may have mitigated the natural course of the renal injury.

CORRELATION OF DISEASE ACTIVITY WITH ANTINUCLEAR ANTIBODIES, COMPLEMENT, AND DETERMINANTS FOR CIRCULATING IMMUNE COMPLEXES

Since the pathogenesis of SLE involves the deposition of antigen-antibody complexes in affected tissues, there has been interest in determining whether specific serologic abnormalities correlate with certain types of tissue injury and whether fluctuating titers of antibodies to nuclear components, complement levels, or titers of circulating complexes correlate with disease activity. The general consensus is that patients with lupus nephritis have a higher incidence of positive reactions for anti-dsDNA, but tests for this antibody are relatively nonspecific as a marker for renal involvement in individual patients [67]. Although antibody to U1 snRNP was initially reported to have a high incidence in mixed connective tissue disease [100], this association has not been confirmed in subsequent analyses.

Regarding the use of serologic tests as markers of disease activity, several groups have reported that very low levels of hemolytic complement and high titers of DNA antibody were almost always associated with active disease, especially active renal disease, whereas the absence of these abnormalities usually indicated inactive renal disease [94]. Moreover, in serial studies, an increase in antibody titers to DNA and/or a fall in complement levels frequently heralded clinical relapses by several weeks. Similar studies also demonstrated a significant correlation between disease activity and the solid-phase C1q-binding assay used as a measure of circulating immune complex levels [1]. In addition, in the management of patients with lupus nephritis with aggressive drug therapy, normalization of serum hemolytic complement [5] or a fall in DNA-binding capacity [66] has been associated with a better clinical outcome than seen in patients without those serologic responses in some reports.

Subsets of the Lupus Syndrome

THE DRUG-INDUCED LUPUS SYNDROME

Since the discovery of the LE cell there have been reports that some drugs are capable of inducing a clinical syndrome similar to spontaneous SLE [3]. The more common drugs associated with this syndrome are hydralazine and procainamide and, to a lesser extent, other agents. The clinical features are similar to those seen in the spontaneous disease except for a lower incidence of renal involvement and more prominent pleuropulmonary manifestations in the drug-induced form of disease. Characteristically, clinical signs develop within a few months to about a year after initiating drug therapy and are usually found in subjects taking higher therapeutic doses. Serologic studies show that anti-DNA antibodies are usually absent. Craft et al. reported that sera from patients with procainamide-induced lupus exhibited antibodies to histone epitopes that were similar to those found in spontaneous SLE [27]. In contrast, a different set of antihistone antibodies was found in sera from patients with hydralazine-induced lupus.

Studies have demonstrated that as many as 65 percent of patients taking hydralazine and nearly 100 percent of patients taking procainamide develop antinuclear antibodies within 1 to several years. The incidence of the overt disease diathesis is lower, however, involving about 10 percent of patients on hydralazine and perhaps a somewhat higher incidence in the procainamide group. It has been shown that the likelihood of developing this syndrome is related to the acetylation pathway of drug metabolism. Evidence has been advanced to indicate that individuals with slow acetylation of the amine or hydrazine groups on many substances are at highest risk for developing the syndrome [90]. In addition, it seems likely that the amine or hydrazine groups may be the inciting agents that induce the drug-induced lupus syndrome. In subjects with procainamide-induced lupus, for example, the clinical and serologic manifestations of the syndrome receded when acetylprocainamide was substituted for procainamide.

The mechanism by which certain drugs cause a lupus-like syndrome has not been established. One proposal suggests that amines may covalently bind with or chemically react with endogenous macromolecules to form a foreign molecule that may stimulate antibody production. It is also possible that amines act pharmacologically on the immune system, making it more responsive to endogenous macromolecules. It is of interest that photo-oxidized DNA is more antigenic than native DNA and thus may offer an explanation of the occurrence of sun sensitivity in lupus patients as well as of the lupus-activating properties of ultraviolet light [19]. In individual patients it is apparent that several factors play a role in the pathogenesis. Most of the 65 percent of the population who develop antinuclear antibodies after exposure to agents possessing amine or hydrazine groups are slow acetylators, presumably because this allows longer or stronger action of the drugs. Since only a fraction of these individuals develop the clinical syndrome it is likely that a genetic predisposition also plays a role, as in spontaneous lupus.

MIXED CONNECTIVE TISSUE DISEASE

It has become increasingly evident that SLE is a mosaic with variations in the pattern of antibodies to specific nuclear components and in clinical manifestations. Sharp et al. [99] called attention to a group of patients with a syndrome composed of overlapping features of SLE, scleroderma, and polymyositis and characterized serologically by the presence of antibodies to a ribonuclease- and trypsin-sensitive antigen (RNP) present in a preparation of extractable nuclear antigens (ENA) and by an absence of Sm antibodies. Approximately 25 percent of these patients have hypocomplementemia. This syndrome has been termed *mixed connective tissue disease* (MCTD). Although there is some controversy about whether MCTD is a distinct entity, there is considerable agreement that high titers of RNP correlate with certain clinical manifestations. The most common features include positive fluorescent antinuclear antibodies, polyarthralgia, Raynaud's phenomenon, hyper-β gammaglobulinemia, polyarthritis, swollen hands, positive rheumatoid agglutinins, esophageal hypomotility, sclerodactyly, and inflammatory myositis. The polyarthritis is usually nondeforming but may resemble rheumatoid arthritis. These manifestations have a high sensitivity to treatment with glucocorticoids. In a series of patients with high titers of RNP antibodies described as SLE or MCTD, progressive renal disease was infrequent [100]. Follow-up studies of these patients have revealed that many develop the classic features of scleroderma.

CLINICAL COURSE OF SLE IN END-STAGE RENAL DISEASE AND AFTER TRANSPLANTATION

Although many patients have active systemic disease and serologic abnormalities at the time renal disease progresses to renal failure, several reports indicate that within a few months clinical activity of nonrenal systemic lupus markedly decreases. Caplan et al. [21] reported that only 3 of 28 patients on maintenance dialysis had evidence of continuing activity despite reduced dosages of immunosuppressive agents, and in those patients only mild arthralgia was present. Serologic parameters paralleled the nonrenal activity of disease. Patient survival was not different than that in patients on dialysis without systemic disease. In addition, in 8 patients a spontaneous remission occurred, permitting discontinuance of dialysis therapy. Similar results were observed in 30 patients from Dallas [112] and in 39 patients reported by Kimberly et al. [64]. In a report on 55 patients with end-stage renal failure from lupus nephropathy treated with hemodialysis or continuous ambulatory peritoneal dialysis (CAPD), maximal extrarenal disease activity and use of medication decreased markedly, but event rates for specific nonrenal manifestations of lupus did not decrease [85]. The overall survival rate with dialysis was 89 percent after 5 years, and no difference in survival rate or disease activity was found between patients treated with hemodialysis or CAPD.

With few exceptions, a reduction in systemic manifestations and lack of evidence of recurrent lupus nephritis have been characteristic features of lupus patients treated with renal transplantation. In the Caplan report [21] of 12 patients treated with transplantation, 3 lost their grafts owing to rejection, and in all cases with surviving grafts clinical activity of the underlying disorder was absent. In the report of the Advisory Committee to the Renal Transplant Registry, there were 37 of 56 transplant patients with long-term functioning grafts [2].

The mechanism responsible for the clinical and serologic improvement seen in this group of patients is unknown. Although it has been suggested that uremia may suppress the immune system, this mechanism would not be expected to explain the clinical findings in patients with successfully functioning renal grafts. These transplant patients are, however, receiving immunosuppressive agents.

EFFECT OF PREGNANCY IN WOMEN WITH SLE

Since SLE occurs primarily in women during the reproductive years the questions of whether the disease is affected by pregnancy and whether it alters the outlook for the products of conception are important concerns. There is strong evidence that estrogens have a potent influence on this disease process in both humans and animals. In humans, the ingestion of female hormones, normal menses, and pregnancy have been reported to exacerbate SLE [15]. In the B/W mouse model of SLE, sex hormones modulate the expression of autoimmunity and affect the concentration of antibodies to nucleic acid, the severity of glomerulonephritis, and, ultimately, mortality [82].

Two studies using patients as self-controls conclude that pregnancy increases exacerbations of SLE [43, 113]. In both reports the frequency of exacerbations was higher during pregnancy and postpartum than prior to conception. In a recent prospective study, however, in which 28 pregnant patients (33 pregnancies), matched for age, race, and severity of disease, were compared with nonpregnant patients with SLE, there was no evidence of an increased incidence of clinical flares [72]. In this series the activity of disease was reported to be mild.

Estes and Larsen [38] initially suggested that the effect of pregnancy on SLE correlated with the activity of disease at the time of conception. Recent studies have shown no relationship between exacerbation during pregnancy and activity of disease in the remote past [review, 50]. In women who have been in complete remission for several months prior to conception, clinical relapses occurred in 25 to 35 percent and activity subsided following delivery [53]. In contrast, in women with signs of active disease through the onset of pregnancy, exacerbations occurred in 50 to 60 percent of cases and tended to be more severe than in the former group. The effect of the maternal disease on the fetus paralleled the course of maternal disease activity. Fetal survival was more than 90 percent in women who were in clinical remission at conception but was reduced to 50 to 75 percent when conception was associated with active disease.

A high incidence of fetal intrauterine death and spontaneous abortions has been reported in women with a circulating lupus-anticoagulant (LE-anticoagulant). The LE-anticoagulant, an acquired immunoglobulin (IgG or IgM), is associated with reduction of prostacyclin release from vessel walls and interacts with the phospholipid fraction of platelets to predispose to thrombosis [105]. Fetal death is considered to be caused by thrombosis in the placenta. Recent studies showed that prednisone and aspirin therapy were successful in suppressing the anticoagulant in some patients and in those patients led to successful pregnancies despite a prior history of repeated spontaneous abortions [74]. Transmission of autoantibodies from the maternal circulation to the fetus is known to result in two types of phenomena that are either transient or result in permanent tissue injury. Some infants, for example, have exhibited discoid lupus or a syndrome of hemolytic anemia, neutropenia, and/or thrombocytopenia, which spontaneously disappeared in parallel with evidence of antinuclear antibodies [97]. A more important and often permanent complication of maternal SLE involves impairment of the fetal cardiac conduction system. The conduction defect arises from a diffuse and extensive endocardial fibrosis that may involve all four heart chambers and replace the septal musculature in the area of the atrial ventricular node [96]. It has been shown that mothers and affected offspring have circulating antibodies to a soluble tissue ribonucleoprotein antigen called R_o(SS-A). The fact that in children antibody is found after birth but not after 6 months of age suggests that anti-R_o(SS-A) reaches the body by placental transfer from the maternal circulation and induces a reaction in cardiac tissue during fetal life.

Treatment of Lupus Nephritis

TREATMENT WITH GLUCOCORTICOIDS

The introduction of glucocorticoids in the early 1950s had an important impact on the management of patients with SLE because many systemic manifestations such as fever, arthropathy, pleuropulmonary inflammation, and cutaneous lesions were very sensitive to those agents. The action of glucocorticoids on renal histopathologic lesions, however, remains uncertain even after 30 years of clinical experience. The early experience in patients with diffuse proliferative nephritis suggested that these agents were ineffective because 50 percent of patients died within 2½ years despite prolonged high-dose therapy [87]. In a subsequent study, however, Donadio et al. [31] demonstrated that high-dose prednisone administered at 60 mg per day^{-1} for 3 months followed by a taper to 20 mg at 6 months caused a significant increase in endogenous creatinine clearance and a reduction in urinary protein excretion and a decrease in glomerular proliferation. The toxic effects of long-term glucocorticoid therapy are well known and include the disfiguring effects of hypercortisonism, growth retardation in children, alopecia, and the probable increased risk to some infectious agents.

Because of reported success in treating renal transplant rejection and crescentic glomerulonephritis with large transient doses of glucocorticoids, pulse steroid therapy has been administered to patients with severe lupus nephropathy in uncontrolled trials. An improvement in renal function has been reported in 30 to 50 percent of patients after this form of therapy [22]. In the majority of responders, functional improvement was maintained for up to a year or more after low-dose oral therapy and/or immunosuppressive agents were resumed. The type of patient most likely to exhibit improvement with pulse steroid therapy was characterized by recent deterioration in function and acute diffuse glomerulonephritis and tended to have high titers of anti-DNA antibodies and low levels of total hemolytic complement [65]. In the only prospective trial that compared conventional oral steroid therapy with and without the addition of pulse steroids, the long-term effect of the two modes of therapy in children on renal function and morbidity was similar [16]. Toxic side effects have been reported to be low when methylprednisone (or an equivalent agent), 600 to 1000 mg per dose, was restricted to three to five doses. In summary, glucocorticoids remain the mainstay of treatment for the systemic features of SLE and have been demonstrated to suppress the renal inflammatory reaction, at least in part, in some patients. Aside from the well-established antiphlogistic action of these agents, their mechanism of action remains unknown.

TREATMENT WITH IMMUNOSUPPRESSIVE AGENTS

Cytotoxic drugs for the treatment of lupus nephritis were introduced on the premise that they might be useful in treating an autoimmune disorder such as the nephropathy of SLE. In the 1970s improvement was reported in patients with lupus nephritis taking various combinations of prednisone and immunosuppressive drugs [33, 52]. These cases, treated in uncontrolled and often retrospective studies, were usually selected because they had severe proliferative lupus nephritis or had been unresponsive to steroid therapy. In two recent studies, patients with diffuse proliferative and/or membranoproliferative lupus nephritis were randomized to groups taking prednisone alone or prednisone combined with azathioprine or cyclophosphamide. In the National Institutes of Health clinical trial, the combined mortality rate, death and development of renal failure, in 65 patients was 40 percent at 2.5 years and 57 percent at 5 years after diagnosis of nephritis [28]. In the study of 50 patients at the Mayo Clinic with diffuse proliferative glomerulonephritis, the combined mortality rate was 24 percent at 2.5 years and 40 percent at 5 years after diagnosis [30]. There was no significant difference, however, in either study between the groups taking prednisone alone or combined therapy. It was of interest, as recently reviewed by Donadio et al. [31], that these mortality rates were markedly better than the pre-1970 5-year survival rate of 25 percent. In an analysis of the role of immunosuppressive drugs in the management of lupus nephritis, the data of all eight published clinical trials in which patients were randomly assigned to specific treatment regimens were pooled [39]. This pool analysis showed that patients receiving immunosuppressive drugs had less renal deterioration, were less likely to have end-stage renal disease, and were less likely to die from kidney disease than patients receiving steroids alone. When cyclophosphamide and azathioprine were considered separately, both were associated with a 40 percent reduction in the rates of adverse renal outcomes, although the differences were not statistically significant owing to the smaller size of the treatment groups. An important observation of this report was that published trials may have reached false conclusions because of small sample size. In an analysis of a high-risk group with a 50 percent likelihood of renal insufficiency, the authors showed that at least 100 patients would be needed to show that immunosuppressive drugs were 50 percent superior to steroids alone in preventing renal deterioration. None of the published trials included a patient population of that size.

Using data derived from early randomized trials at the National Institutes of Health, Austin et al. [11] showed that patients with diffuse proliferative and membranoproliferative glomerulonephritis were at increased risk of end-stage renal disease compared to other histopathologic patterns of injury. Moreover, correlation of the specific histologic changes with the long-term clinical outcome (median follow-up of 53 months) demonstrated that the presence of chronic lesions on the initial biopsy, including tubular atrophy, glomerular sclerosis, and cellular crescents, identified a very high-risk group. Since chronicity appeared to herald functional deterioration, Balow et al. [14] evaluated 62 patients with a repeat renal biopsy after more than 18 months of observation to determine whether treatment affected the progression of chronic changes in the interval between biopsies. This analysis found that whereas the chronicity index for patients treated with conventional high-dose prednisone increased linearly with time, the index in the group receiving cytotoxic drug treatments did not increase over time. In 1986 Austin et al. [10] reported on an experience with cyclophosphamide administered intravenously in a dose of 0.5 to 1.0 gm per m^2 of body surface area, in the ongoing trials at the National Institutes of Health. The renal functional outcome in 20 patients was at least as good as in the groups treated with oral cyclophosphamide, azothiaprine, or both agents combined, but was not superior to that of the concurrent control group treated with prednisone alone. It should be noted that in addition to the small size of the treatment groups, all four groups treated with immunosuppressive agents were compared with a single group treated with prednisone alone. Further experience with this mode of therapy in a prospective randomized trial has not been reported.

Despite the lack of appropriately designed trials to evaluate the efficacy of glucocorticoids and immunosuppressive agents, it is useful to summarize a recent report on an uncontrolled trial with both classes of drugs, to illustrate recent experience with these categories of agents in the treatment of diffuse proliferative lupus nephritis. Ponticelli et al. [88] treated 43 patients with intravenous high-dose pulses of steroids, followed by low-dose prednisolone; 31 of these patients also were treated during relapse in the same manner as used in initial treatment. At 10 years the patient survival rate was 87 percent. The renal survival rate was 79 percent, but the actual 10-year kidney survival rate was 91 percent when extrarenal deaths were excluded. At the end of follow-up, serum creatinine was normal in 34 patients, elevated but stable in 3, and worsening in 2, and 1 patient was on dialysis.

Although cytotoxic drugs have been used in the treatment of lupus nephritis for nearly 20 years, there is still uncertainty about whether they are superior to glucocorticoid treatment. Attempts to pool data from several trials or to analyze material retrospectively from randomized trials, however, have in general supported the effectiveness of these agents in mitigating renal injury. Nevertheless, this group of drugs represents an important category in the current management of patients with lupus nephritis, especially those with severe proliferative lesions and subendothelial deposits. Like other categories of drugs used to treat the severe manifestations of lupus, important adverse complications attend their use. The acute complications of immunosuppressive agents include bone marrow depression, an increased susceptibility to infection, acute cystitis, and alopecia, whereas long-term treatment has been reported to cause infertility, pulmonary fibrosis, an increased incidence of malignancy, and chronic cystitis. These complications are apparently related to dose, since their frequency is reported to be low in studies in which lower oral doses were employed.

Other Treatment Regimens in the Treatment of Lupus Nephritis

PLASMAPHERESIS

Plasmapheresis has been used to treat patients with severe SLE on the premise that dilution of titers of circulating complexes increases the capacity of the reticuloendothelial system to clear complexes from plasma and decreases the absolute quantity of immunoglobulins in plasma. Several uncontrolled trials have reported clinical improvement in patients with severe SLE after pheresis treatment [73, 106]. In two prospective controlled trials, however, the frequency and degree of improvement were the same in both plasma exchange and control groups [71, 108]. In some patients treated with plasmapheresis alone, an increase in disease activity and clinical deterioration has actually been observed [106]. The lack of benefit may be attributable to a rebound phenomenon with an increased rate of synthesis of pathogenic antibodies following their removal by plasmapheresis. There has recently been a proposal to utilize this rebound effect positively in a therapeutic approach using sequential plasmapheresis followed by pulse cyclophosphamide to initially stimulate and then specifically delete the clones producing pathogenic antibodies [93]. Initial studies have reported positive results and a randomized prospective multicenter clinical trial is now under way.

EICOSAPENTAENOIC ACID

Eicosapentaenoic acid (EPA), a fatty acid analogue of arachidonic acid, is a constituent of lipids in marine animal tissue and has been shown to substitute for arachidonic acid in platelets of humans on a high marine diet [109]. Since administration of exogenous prostaglandins [114] and experimental production of essential fatty acid deficiency [57] were reported to improve or delay development of glomerulonephritis in NZB × NZW F_1 mice, a model for human SLE, experimental studies have been conducted to evaluate the effect of EPA in the same experimental model. Female animals were fed either a high EPA diet, such as menhadin oil, or a beef tallow diet [89]. This study demonstrated that the experimental diet prevented the development of glomerulonephritis and death from uremia. In addition, native DNA binding was also significantly reduced in animals fed EPA. Clinical trials based on these provocative observations have not been conducted.

ANCROD

As noted in the discussion on pathogenesis, there is substantial evidence that thrombus formation in intraglomerular capillaries plays an important role in the induction of tissue injury, due to both immune complex deposition and the action of antiphospholipins. Kant et al. [61] reported that the presence of anticardiolipins correlated with a high likelihood of fibrin deposition and thrombi in glomeruli of patients with lupus glomerulonephritis, and with a higher incidence of renal scarring during follow-up studies. In uncontrolled studies Glas-Greenwalt et al. [45] reported experience with the administration of ancrod to 18 patients with lupus glomerulonephritis and altered levels of plasminogen activator and/or an inhibitor of plasmin. Ancrod treatment was associated with prompt normalization of plasminogen activator in 13 patients, and in these responding patients, there was a striking decrease or disappearance of microvascular thrombosis. This series was subsequently expanded to 37 patients, with similar results [63]. The effect of ancrod was also studied in the male B × SB mouse with murine lupus glomerulonephritis and induced significantly reduced mortality and, at least in the early stages of nephritis, reduced severity of the renal lesion [25]. Ancrod is a purified fraction of Malayan pit viper venom, and is a thrombinlike enzyme that has a selective enzyme substrate specificity for fibrinogen; thus, it has a defibrinating action in the treatment of deep vein and retinal vein thrombosis in humans, and in experimental immune complex glomerulonephritis [17]. Clinical experience demonstrates that hemorrhagic side effects are rare, and therefore it is probably safer to use than aspirin [98]. This agent, therefore, has promising utility in lupus nephritis; randomized trials have not been conducted.

TOTAL LYMPHOID IRRADIATION

Total lymphoid irradiation has been shown to be a potent immunosuppressive regime that is accompanied by little increase in risk of bacterial infection or incidence of malignancy. Clinical improvement has followed this form of therapy in humans with rheumatoid arthritis [101] and in mice (NZB/NZW) with experimental lupus disease [68]. Improvement is associated with reduction in the absolute number of circulating helper T cells and in T-cell function. Strober et al. [101] recently reported the results of a feasibility trial in 10 patients with lupus nephritis and marked proteinuria who were unresponsive to conventional therapy. During follow-up, which ranged from 12 to 44 months in 8 patients, serum creatinine remained relatively stable in 70 percent and decreased in 25 percent. The fractional clearance of albumin, a measure of glomerular capillary wall permeability to albumin, declined to below irradiation values in 8 of 9 patients. In addition, levels of anti-DNA antibodies fell in all patients with elevated pretreatment values, and the concentration of serum C3 rose to normal levels in all cases. The authors suggest that total lymphoid irradiation may provide an alternative to cytotoxic agents in the treatment of lupus nephritis.

IMMUNOTHERAPY

Since SLE is an autoimmune disease that may stem from a failure of self-tolerance, experimental studies are underway to determine whether the induction of tolerance to autoantigens may lead to specific therapy of autoimmunity. Several approaches to this problem have been proposed, including (1) the use of tolerogens that specifically suppress humoral antibodies to nuclear components such as native DNA, (2) the generation of specific suppressor T cells that can abrogate cellular and humoral immunity, and (3) the use of antiidiotypic antibodies. Evidence that immunologic tolerance can be induced in adult animals is well established. As applied to the animal model of SLE, administration of nucleosides conjugated to isologous IgG to young female (NZB × NXW)F_1 mice prevented the development of nephritis [20]. This approach, however, has not been applied to patients with SLE.

Recent efforts in immunotherapy have used different experimental approaches. For example, two antibodies of rat origin, engineered to prevent an immune response in humans, were administered sequentially to a patient with chronic necrotizing vasculitis, and resulted in lasting remission [78]. One of these antibodies, Campath-1H, reacted with the Campath-1 antigen present on lymphocytes and monocytes, and acted to debulk lymphocytes, while the second antibody to CD4 on helper T cells was used to reduce cell-surface adhesion. In another approach, used in a murine model of SLE, treatment was aimed at the reduction of anti-DNA antibody production [46]. In this experiment, monoclonal anti-Id antibodies conjugated with the cytotoxic agent neocarzinostatin were directed to nephrogenic anti-DNA antibodies, and improved the survival rate, delayed the onset of nephritis, and reduced the number of anti-DNA–producing cells.

In contrast to all current modes of therapy for SLE that rely on nonspecific regimens that depress the immune system, it seems likely that SLE therapy in the future will incorporate the principles of immunotherapy that involve correcting specific defects in the immunoregulatory system. This approach will provide rational treatment for the underlying disorder and is likely to avoid severe complications of therapy that beset the currently available regimens.

References

1. Abrass, C. K., Nies, K. M., Louie, J. S., et al. Correlation and predictive accuracy of circulating immune complexes with disease activity in patients with systemic lupus erythematosus. *Arthritis Rheum.* 23: 273, 1980.
2. Advisory Committee to the Renal Transplant Registry. Renal transplantation in congenital and metabolic diseases: A report from the ASC/NIH Renal Transplant Registry. *J.A.M.A.* 232: 148, 1975.
3. Alarcon-Segovia, D. Drug-induced lupus syndromes. *Mayo Clin. Proc.* 44: 664, 1969.
4. Alarcon-Segovia, D., Deleze, M., Oria, C. V., et al. Anticardiolipid erythematosus. *Medicine* 68: 353, 1989.
5. Alexopoulos, E., Seron, D., Hartley, R. P., et al. Lupus nephritis correlation of interstitial cells with glomerular function. *Kidney Int.* 37: 100, 1990.
6. Appel, A. E., Sablay, L. B., Golden, R. A., et al. The affect of normalization on serum complement and anti-DNA antibody on the course of lupus nephritis. *Am. J. Med.* 64: 274, 1978.
7. Appel, G. B., Cohen, D. J., Pirani, C. L., et al. Long term follow-up of patients with lupus nephritis. A study based on classification of the World Health Organization. *Am. J. Med.* 83: 877, 1987.
8. Appel, G. B., Silva, F. G., Pirani, C. L., et al. Renal involvement in systemic lupus erythematosus. *Medicine* 57: 371, 1978.
9. Asherson, R. A., Mackworth-Young, C. G., Harris, E. N., et al. Multiple venous and arterial thrombosis associated with the lupus anticoagulant and antibodies to cardiolipin in the absence of SLE. *Rheumatol. Int.* 5: 91, 1985.
10. Austin, H. A., Klippel, J. H., Balow, J. E., et al. Therapy of lupus nephritis. Controlled trial of prednisone and cytotoxic drugs. *N. Engl. J. Med.* 314: 614, 1986.
11. Austin, H. A., Muenz, L. R., Joyce, K. M., et al. Diffuse proliferative lupus nephritis: Identification of specific pathologic features affecting renal outcome. *Kidney Int.* 25: 689, 1984.
12. Baldwin, D. S., Gluck, M. G., Lowenstein, J., et al. Lupus nephritis: Clinical causes as related to morphological forms and their transitions. *Am. J. Med.* 62: 12, 1977.
13. Baldwin, D. S., Lowenstein, J., Rothfield, N. F., et al. The clinical causes of the proliferative and membranous forms of lupus nephritis. *Ann. Intern. Med.* 73: 929, 1970.
14. Balow, J. E., Austin, H. A., Muenz, L. R., et al. Effect of treatment on the evaluation of renal abnormalities in lupus nephritis. *N. Engl. J. Med.* 311: 491, 1984.
15. Barmes, E. M., MacCuigh, A. C., Loudon, N. B., et al. Phytohemagglutinin-induced lymphocyte transformation and circulating autoantibodies in women taking oral contraceptives. *Lancet* 1: 898, 1974.
16. Barron, K. S., Person, D. A., Bremer, E. J., et al. Pulse methylprednisaline therapy in diffuse proliferative lupus nephritis. *J. Pediatr.* 101: 137, 1982.
17. Becker, G. J. Ancrod in glomerulonephritis. *Q. J. Med.* 69: 849, 1980.
18. Bennett, W. M., Bardana, E. J., Houghton, D. C., et al. Silent renal involvement in systemic lupus erythematosus. *Int. Arch. Allerg. Appl. Immunol.* 55: 420, 1977.
19. Blomgren, S. E., and Vaughn, J. N. The immunogenicity of photooxidized DNA and of the photoproduct of DNA and procainamide hydrochloride. *Arthritis Rheum.* 11: 470, 1968.
20. Borel, Y., Lewis, R. M., and Stollar, B. D. Prevention of murine lupus nephritis by carrier-dependent induction of immunologic tolerance to denatured DNA. *Science* 182: 76, 1973.
21. Caplon, N. S., Diskin, C. J., Petersen, J., et al. The long-term clinical course of systemic lupus erythematosus in end stage renal disease. *N. Engl. J. Med.* 308: 186, 1983.
22. Cathcart, E. S., Idelson, B. A., Scheinberg, M. A., et al. Beneficial effects of methylprednisone "pulse" therapy in diffuse proliferative lupus nephritis. *Lancet* 1: 163, 1976.
23. Churg, J., and Sobin, D. H. *Renal Disease. Classification and Atlas of Glomerular Diseases.* Tokyo: Igaku-Shoin, 1982. Pp. 127–149.
24. Cohen, A. S., Reynolds, W. E., Franklin, E. C., et al. Preliminary criteria for the classification of systemic lupus erythematosus. *Bull. Rheum. Dis.* 21: 643, 1971.
25. Cole, E. H., Glynn, M. F. X., Laskin, C. A., et al. Ancrod improves survival in murine systemic lupus erythematosus. *Kidney Int.* 37: 29, 1990.
26. Comerford, F. R., and Cohen, A. S. The nephropathy of systemic lupus erythematosus: An assessment of clinical, light and electron microscopic criteria. *Medicine* 46: 425, 1967.

27. Craft, J. E., Radding, J. A., Harding, M. W., et al. Autoantigenic histone epitopes: A comparison between procainamide and hydralazine-induced lupus. *Arthritis Rheum.* 30: 689, 1987.
28. Decker, J. L., Steinberg, A. D., and Reinertsen, J. L. Systemic lupus erythematosus: Evolving concepts. *Ann. Intern. Med.* 91: 587, 1979.
29. Dixon, F. J. The pathogenesis of murine systemic lupus erythematosus. *Am. J. Pathol.* 97: 10, 1979.
30. Donadio, J. V., Holley, K. E., Ferguson, M. D., et al. Treatment of diffuse proliferative lupus nephritis with prednisone and combined prednisone and cyclophosphamide. *N. Engl. J. Med.* 299: 1151, 1978.
31. Donadio, J. V., Holley, K. E., and Ilstrup, M. S. Cytotoxic drug treatment of lupus nephritis. *Am. J. Kidney Dis.* 2(Suppl. 1): 178, 1982.
32. Dosekun, A. K., Pollak, V. E., Glas-Greenwalt, P., et al. Ancrod in systemic lupus erythematosus with thrombosis. *Arch. Intern. Med.* 144: 37, 1984.
33. Drinkard, J. P., Stanley, T. M., Dornfield, L., et al. Azathioprine and prednisone in the treatment of adults with lupus nephritis. *Medicine* 49: 411, 1970.
34. Dujovne, I., Pollak, V. E., Pirani, C. L., et al. The distribution and character of glomerular deposits in systemic lupus erythematosus. *Kidney Int.* 2: 33, 1972.
35. Eiser, A. R., Katz, S. M., and Swartz, C. Clinically occult diffuse proliferative lupus nephritis: An age-related phenomena. *Arch. Intern. Med.* 139: 1023, 1979.
36. Esdaile, J. M., Levinton, C., Federgreen, W., et al. The clinical and renal biopsy predictors of long-term outcome in lupus nephritis: A study of 87 patients and review of the literature. *Q. J. Med.* 269: 779, 1989.
37. Estes, D., and Christian, C. L. The natural history of systemic lupus erythematosus by prospective analysis. *Medicine* 50: 85, 1971.
38. Estes, D., and Larsen, D. L. Systemic lupus erythematosus and pregnancy. *Clin. Obstet. Gynecol.* 8: 307, 1965.
39. Felson, D. T., and Anderson, J. Evidence for the superiority of immunosuppressive drugs and prednisone over prednisone alone in lupus nephritis. *N. Engl. J. Med.* 311: 1528, 1984.
40. Fish, A. J., Blau, E. B., Westberg, N. G., et al. Systemic lupus erythematosus within first two decades of life. *Am. J. Med.* 62: 99, 1977.
41. Foad, B. S. I., Shean, R. P., and Kirsner, A. B. Systemic lupus erythematosus in the elderly. *Arch. Intern. Med.* 130: 743, 1972.
42. Fournier, G. J. Circulation DNA and lupus nephritis. *Kidney Int.* 33: 487, 1988.
43. Garsenstein, M., Pollak, V. E., and Kark, R. M. Systemic lupus erythematosus and pregnancy. *N. Engl. J. Med.* 267: 165, 1962.
44. Germuth, F. G., and Rodriquez, E. *Immunopathology of the Renal Glomerulus.* Boston: Little, Brown, 1973. Pp. 15–44.
45. Glas-Greenwalt, P., Kant, K. S., Dosekum, A., et al. Ancrod: Normalization of fibrinolytic enzyme abnormalities in patients with systemic lupus erythematosus and lupus nephritis. *J. Lab. Clin. Med.* 105: 99, 1985.
46. Harata, N., Sasaki, T., Osaki, H., et al. Therapeutic treatment of New Zealand mouse disease by a limited number of anti-idiotypic antibodies conjugated to neocarzinostatin. *J. Clin. Invest.* 86: 769, 1990.
47. Hardin, J. A. The lupus autoantigen and the pathogenesis of systemic lupus erythematosus. *Arthritis Rheum.* 29: 457, 1986.
48. Hargraves, M. M., Richmond, H., and Morton, R. Presentation of two bone marrow elements: The "Tart" cell and the "L.E." cell. *Proc. Staff Meet. Mayo Clin.* 23: 25, 1948.
49. Harvey, A. M., Shulman, L. E., Tumulty, P. A., et al. Systemic lupus erythematosus: Review of the literature and clinical analysis of 138 cases. *Medicine* 33: 291, 1954.
50. Hayslett, J. P. Effect of pregnancy in patients with SLE. *Am. J. Kidney Dis.* 2(Suppl. 1): 223, 1982.
51. Hayslett, J. P., and Hardin, J. H. Advances in systemic lupus erythematosus. *Am. J. Kidney Dis.* 11: 97, 1982.
52. Hayslett, J. P., Kashgarian, M., Cook, C. D., et al. The effect of azathioprine on lupus glomerulonephritis. *Medicine* 49: 411, 1970.
53. Hayslett, J. P., and Lynn, R. I. Effect of pregnancy in patients with lupus nephropathy. *Kidney Int.* 18: 207, 1980.
54. Hecht, B., Siegel, N., Adler, M., et al. Prognostic indices in lupus nephritis. *Medicine* 55: 163, 1976.
55. Hejtmancik, M. R., Wright, J. C., Quint, R., et al. The cardiovascular manifestations of systemic lupus erythematosus. *Am. Heart J.* 68: 119, 1964.
56. Hughes, G. R. V., Harris, N. N., and Sharavi, A. E. The anticardiolipin syndrome. *J. Rheumatol.* 13: 486, 1986.
57. Hurd, E. R., Johnston, J. M., Okita, J. R., et al. Prevention of glomerulonephritis and prolonged survival in New Zealand Black/New Zealand White F_1 hybrid mice fed an essential fatty acid-deficient diet. *J. Clin. Invest.* 67: 476, 1981.
58. Johnson, R. J., Alpers, C. E., Pritzi, P., et al. Platelets mediate neutrophil-dependent immune complex nephritis in the rat. *J. Clin. Invest.* 82: 1225, 1988.
59. Johnson, R. L., Couser, W. G., Chi, E. Y., et al. New mechanisms for glomerular injury. Myeloperoxidase-hydrogen peroxide-halide system. *J. Clin. Invest.* 79: 1379, 1987.
60. Jonsson, H., Nived, O., and Sturfelt, G. Outcome in systemic lupus erythematosus: A prospective study of patients from a defined population. *Medicine* 68: 141, 1989.
61. Kant, K. S., Pollak, V. E., Weiss, M. A., et al. Glomerular thrombosis in systemic lupus erythematosus: Prevalence and significance. *Medicine* 60: 71, 1981.
62. Keith, N. M., and Rountree, L. G. A study of renal complications of disseminated lupus erythematosus. *Trans. Assoc. Am. Physicians* 37: 487, 1922.
63. Kim, S., Wadhwa, N. K., Kant, K. S., et al. Fibrinolysis in glomerulonephritis treated with ancrod: Renal functional, immunologic and histopathologic effects. *Q. J. Med.* 69: 879, 1988.
64. Kimberly, R. P., Lockshin, M. D., Sherman, R. L., et al. "End stage" lupus nephritis: Clinical course to and outcome on dialysis: Evidence with 39 patients. *Medicine* 60: 277, 1981.
65. Kimberly, R. P., Lockshin, M. D., Sherman, R. L., et al. High-dose intravenous methyl-prednisaline pulse therapy in systemic lupus erythematosus. *Am. J. Med.* 70: 817, 1981.
66. Koffler, D. Proceedings of the conference on current perspectives on the immunology of systemic lupus erythematosus. *Arthritis Rheum.* 25: 721, 1982.
67. Koffler, D., Shur, P. H., and Kunkel, H. G. Immunological studies concerning the nephritis of systemic lupus erythematosus. *J. Exp. Med.* 126: 607, 1967.
68. Kotzin, B. L., and Strober, S. Reversal of NZX4B/NZW disease with total lymphoid irradiation. *J. Exp. Med.* 150: 371, 1979.

69. Kunkel, A. G. The immunopathology of S.L.E. *Human Dev.* 15: 47, 1980.
70. Leehy, P. J., Katz, A. E., Azarum, A. H., et al. Silent diffuse lupus nephritis. Long-term followup. *Am. J. Kidney Dis.* 2(Suppl. 1): 188, 1982.
71. Lewis, E., and Tachin, J. Preliminary outcomes in the controlled trial of plasmapheresis therapy (PPT) in server lupus nephritis. *Kidney Int.* 31: 208, 1987.
72. Lockskin, N. D., Reinitz, E., Druzin, N. L., et al. Lupus pregnancy: Case control prospective study demonstrating absence of lupus exacerbation during and after pregnancy. *Am. J. Med.* 77: 893, 1984.
73. Lockwood, C. M., Rees, A. J., Russell, B., et al. Experience on the use of plasma exchange in the management of potentially fulminating glomerulonephritis and SLE. *Exp. Hematol.* 5: 117, 1977.
74. Lubbe, W. F., Palmer, S. J., Butter, W. S., et al. Fetal survival after prednisone suppression of maternal lupus anti-coagulant. *Lancet* 1: 1361, 1983.
75. Lynn, R. I., Siegel, N. J., and Hayslett, J. P. Lupus nephropathy as the initial manifestation of systemic lupus erythematosus. *Yale J. Biol. Med.* 53: 353, 1980.
76. Magil, A. B., Putterman, N. L., Ballon, H. S., et al. Prognostic factors in diffuse lupus glomerulonephritis. *Kidney Int.* 34: 511, 1988.
77. Mahajan, S. K., Ordonez, N. G., Feitelson, P. J., et al. Lupus nephropathy without clinical renal involvement. *Medicine* 56: 493, 1977.
78. Mathieson, P. W., Cobbold, S. P., Hale, G., et al. Monoclonal-antibody therapy in systemic vasculitis. *N. Engl. J. Med.* 323: 250, 1990.
79. McCluskey, R. T. Lupus Nephritis. In Summers, S. C. (ed.), *Kidney Pathology* (decennial). New York: Appleton Century Crofts, 1975. Pp. 456–459.
80. McCulloch, K. K., Powell, J., Johnson, K. J., et al. Enhancement by platelets of oxygen radical responses of human neutrophils. *Fed. Proc.* 45: 682, 1986.
81. Meislin, A. G., and Rothfield, N. Systemic lupus erythematosus in childhood: Analyses of 42 cases with comparative data on 200 adult cases followed concurrently. *Pediatrics* 42: 37, 1968.
82. Melez, K. A., Reeves, J. P., and Steinberg, A. D. Regulation of the expression of autoimmunity in NZB × N2W F_1 mice by sex hormones. *J. Immunopharmacol.* 1: 27, 1978–1979.
83. Morel-Maroger, L., Mery, J. P., Droz, D., et al. The course of Lupus nephritis: Contribution of serial renal biopsies. *Adv. Nephrol.* 6: 79, 1976.
84. Nakamura, R. M., Peebles, C. L., Rubin, R. L., et al. *Antibodies to Nuclear Antigens.* Chicago: American Society of Clinical Pathology Press, 1985. P. 4.
85. Nossent, H. C., Swaak, T. J. G., and Bergen, J. H. M. Systemic lupus erythematosus: Analysis of disease activity in 55 patients with end-stage renal failure treated with hemodialysis or continuous ambulatory peritoneal dialysis. *Am. J. Med.* 89: 169, 1990.
86. Pollak, V. E., and Pirani, C. L. Renal histologic findings in SLE. *Mayo Clin. Proc.* 44: 63, 1969.
87. Pollak, V. E., Pirani, C. L., and Kark, R. M. Effect of large doses of prednisone on the renal lesions and life span of patients with lupus glomerulonephritis. *J. Lab. Clin. Med.* 57: 495, 1961.
88. Ponticelli, C., Zucchelli, P., Morani, G., et al. Long term prognosis of diffuse lupus nephritis. *Clin. Nephrol.* 28: 263, 1987.
89. Prickett, J. D., Robinson, D. R., and Steinberg, A. D. Dietary enrichment with the polyunsaturated fatty acid eicosapentaenoic acid prevents proteinuria and prolongs survival in NZB × NZW F_1 mice. *J. Clin. Invest.* 68: 556, 1981.
90. Reidenberg, M. M. Aromatic amines and the pathogenesis of lupus erythematosus. *Am. J. Med.* 75: 1037, 1983.
91. Sakamoto, H., and Ooshima, A. Activation of neutrophil phagocytosis of complement coated and IgG coated sheep erythrocytes by platelet release products. *Br. J. Haematol.* 60: 173, 1985.
92. Schiedeke, T. M. J., Stockli, F. W., Weber, R., et al. Histones have high affinity for the glomerular basement membrane. *J. Exp. Med.* 169: 1879, 1989.
93. Schroeder, J. O., Euler, H. H., and Loffler, H. Synchronization of plasmapheresis and pulse cyclophosphamide in severe lupus erythematosus. *Ann. Intern. Med.* 107: 344, 1987.
94. Schur, P. N., and Sandson, J. Immunologic factors and clinical activity in systemic lupus erythematosus. *N. Engl. J. Med.* 278: 533, 1968.
95. Schwartz, M. M., Bernsten, J., Hill, G. S., et al. Predictive value of renal pathology in diffuse lupus glomerulonephritis. *Kidney Int.* 36: 891, 1989.
96. Scott, J. S., Maddison, P. J., Taylor, P. V., et al. Connective tissue disease, antibodies to ribonucleoprotein and congenital heart block. *N. Engl. J. Med.* 309: 209, 1983.
97. Seip, M. SLE in pregnancy with hemolytic anemia, leukopenia and thrombopenia in mother and her newborn infant. *Arch. Dis. Child.* 35: 364, 1960.
98. Sharp, A. A., Warren, B. A., and Paxton, A. M. Anticoagulation therapy with a purified fraction of Malayan pit viper venom. *Lancet* 1: 493, 1968.
99. Sharp, G. C., Irwin, W. S., LaRoque, R. L., et al. Association of autoantibodies to different nuclear antigens with clinical patterns of rheumatic disease and responsiveness to therapy. *J. Clin. Invest.* 50: 350, 1971.
100. Sharp, G. C., Irwin, W. S., Tan, E. M., et al. Mixed connective tissue disease—an apparent distinct rheumatic disease syndrome associated with a specific antibody to an extractable nuclear antigen (ENA). *Am. J. Med.* 52: 148, 1972.
101. Strober, S., Field, E., Hoppe, R. T., et al. Treatment of intractable lupus nephritis with total lymphoid irradiation. *Ann. Intern. Med.* 102: 450, 1985.
102. Tan, E. M. Interactions between autoimmunity and molecular and cell biology. Bridges between clinical and basic sciences. *J. Clin. Invest.* 84: 1, 1989.
103. Tan, E. M., Cohen, A. S., Fries, J. F., et al. The 1982 revised criteria for the classification of systemic lupus erythematosus. *Arthritis Rheum.* 25: 1271, 1982.
104. Tateno, S., Kobayaski, Y., Shigematsu, H., et al. Study of lupus nephritis: Its classification and the significance of subendothelial deposits. *Q. J. Med.* 52: 311, 1983.
105. Thiagarajan, P., Shapiro, S. S., and DeMarco, L. Monoclonal immunoglobulin M coagulation inhibitor with phospholipid specificity. *J. Clin. Invest.* 66: 397, 1980.
106. Verrier-Jones, J., Cummings, R. H., Bacon, P. A., et al. Evidence for a therapeutic effect of plasmapheresis in patients with systemic lupus erythematosus. *Q. J. Med.* 48: 555, 1979.
107. Wallace, D. J., Podell, T., Weiner, J., et al. Systemic lupus erythematosus—survival patterns: Experience with 609 patients. *J.A.M.A.* 245: 934, 1981.
108. Wei, N., Huston, D. P., Lawley, T. J., et al. Randomized trial of plasma exchange in mild systemic lupus erythematosus. *Lancet* I: 17, 1983.

109. Whitaker, M. O., Wyche, A., Fitzpatrick, F., et al. Triene prostaglandins: Prostaglandin D_3 and icosapentaenoic acid as potential antithrombotic substances. *Proc. Natl. Acad. Sci. U.S.A.* 76: 5919, 1979.
110. Wohlgelernter, D., Loke, J., Matthay, R. A., et al. Systemic and discoid lupus erythematosus: Analyses of pulmonary function. *Yale J. Biol. Med.* 51: 157, 1958.
111. Woolf, A., Croker, B., Osafsky, S. G., et al. Nephritis in children and young adults with systemic lupus erythematosus and normal urinary sediment. *Pediatrics* 64: 678, 1979.
112. Ziff, M., and Helderman, J. N. Dialysis and transplantation in end stage lupus nephritis. *N. Engl. J. Med.* 308: 218, 1983.
113. Zulman, J. I., Talal, N., Hoffman, G. S., et al. Problems associated with the management of pregnancies in patients with systemic lupus erythematosus. *J. Rheumatol.* 7: 37, 1980.
114. Zurier, R. B., Damjanov, D. M., Sayadoff, D. M., et al. Prostaglandin E_1 treatment of N2B/N2W F_1 hybrid mice II: Prevention of glomerulonephritis. *Arthritis Rheum.* 20: 1449, 1977.

Renal Involvement in Systemic Sclerosis

Alvin P. Shapiro
Thomas A. Medsger, Jr.
Virginia D. Steen

Systemic sclerosis is a generalized disorder classified as one of the connective tissue diseases. It is characterized by widespread fibrosis and degenerative changes and prominent proliferative and obliterative vascular lesions involving the skin (scleroderma), joints and tendon sheaths, muscles, and certain viscera, most notably the gastrointestinal tract, lungs, heart, and kidneys. Renal disease has been recognized as one of the most dramatic manifestations and, until recently, as the most common cause of death in virtually all case series reported.

Classification

Although systemic sclerosis represents a spectrum of cutaneous and visceral disease, certain common patterns of involvement have been recognized. The disorder is classified based on the degree and extent of cutaneous involvement and the presence of features frequently encountered in other connective tissue diseases (overlap syndromes) [27]. Individuals with symmetrical, widespread skin thickening that affects both the distal and proximal extremities and the trunk and face are considered to have *diffuse cutaneous* involvement or the classic form of this disease. In this variant, there tends to be rapid progression of the cutaneous induration with joint contractures and early appearance of visceral involvement, especially affecting the lungs, heart, and kidneys. In contrast, in the *limited cutaneous* involvement subtype, skin thickening remains relatively restricted, often confined to the fingers and face, and there is a prolonged delay before the appearance of visceral manifestations. In the past this variant was called the *CREST syndrome*, an acronym emphasizing its more distinctive features—i.e., *c*alcinosis, *R*aynaud's phenomenon, *e*sophageal hypomotility, *s*clerodactyly (thickening limited to the digits), and *t*elangiectasias. Of particular importance is the rarity of myocardial and renal involvement in individuals with limited cutaneous disease. Serum autoantibodies also aid in classification. Anti–topoisomerase I (anti–Scl 70) occurs in nearly 40 percent of patients with diffuse disease, while anticentromere antibody is present in 50 percent with limited disease and is relatively specific for this variant (Table 73-1).

Overlap syndrome refers to individuals who have either diffuse or limited skin thickening as well as features more consistent with another connective tissue disease, such as polymyositis-dermatomyositis or systemic lupus erythematosus.

Supported in part by National Heart, Lung, and Blood Institute grant 40962.

Epidemiology

Systemic sclerosis occurs in all races and is global in its distribution. In the United States, the most recent estimate of incidence approximates 20 new cases per million population annually [48]. Disease onset typically occurs between 30 and 50 years of age. Females are affected three times more frequently than males, especially during the childbearing and early menopausal years, and the disease is unusual in both children and young men [28]. However, systemic sclerosis occurs 10 times more frequently in young black as compared to young white females [49].

In most cases of limited cutaneous disease, the initial complaint is Raynaud's phenomenon. In contrast, patients with diffuse scleroderma most often have skin thickening or involvement of joints (arthritis) or tendons (tenosynovitis with palpable tendon friction rubs) as the first manifestation. In the few remaining patients, the earliest symptoms are gastrointestinal, or pulmonary. Dysphagia, gastroesophageal reflux, or other intestinal motility abnormalities may long precede the development of cutaneous changes. It is rare for renal involvement to antedate all other disease features. Thus the appearance of "scleroderma kidney" is virtually always accompanied by important clues by history or on physical examination of systemic sclerosis.

Renal Involvement

HISTORY

Auspitz [1] first reported involvement of the kidney by systemic sclerosis in 1863. He described a young locksmith with tightness and increased pigmentation of the skin who died of rapidly progressive uremia. However, Auspitz concluded that "there is no evidence to support a causal relationship between the kidney disease and the skin disease as such." Toward the end of the last century, Osler [37] observed that some patients with scleroderma may succumb to "nephritis." Masugi and Ya-Shu in 1938 [25] and Talbott et al. in 1939 [53] gave clear descriptions of intimal hyperplasia and fibrinoid degeneration in the interlobular renal arteries of two young women dying with diffuse scleroderma. In 1945, Goetz coined the term *progressive systemic sclerosis* and provided a classic description of the widespread pathologic changes seen in small blood vessels, including those of the kidney [15]. The causal relationship between systemic sclerosis and acute renal failure was generally accepted after Moore and Sheehan in 1952 described the clinical and renal histologic abnormalities in 3 patients with this connective tissue disease who died of uremia [32], and was considerably expanded by the research of Rodnan, Schreiner, and Black in 1957 [42].

CRITERIA AND FREQUENCY OF RENAL INVOLVEMENT

Widely varying frequencies of renal involvement in systemic sclerosis have been reported, depending on whether clinical and/or pathologic criteria were used and how these were defined. At one end of the spectrum is the distinct entity of acute *scleroderma renal crisis* (SRC), which is explosive and rapidly progressive, but a

Table 73-1. Comparison of clinical and laboratory features in systemic sclerosis subsets (University of Pittsburgh, 1972–1990)

	Diffuse cutaneous (N = 567)	Limited cutaneous (N = 551)
Demographic features		
Age (< 40 at onset)	36%	51%
Race (nonwhite)	10%	5%
Sex (female)	77%	84%
Duration of symptoms (years)	3.3	12.0
Organ system involvement		
Telangiectasias	67%	89%
Calcinosis	15%	38%
Raynaud's phenomenon	93%	97%
Arthralgias or arthritis	92%	70%
Tendon friction rubs	65%	7%
Joint contractures	90%	55%
Myopathy	23%	9%
Esophageal hypomotility	72%	75%
Pulmonary fibrosis	48%	42%
Pulmonary hypertension	1%	11%
Congestive heart failure	9%	2%
Renal "crisis"	19%	2%
Laboratory abnormalities		
Antinuclear antibody (1 : 16 or higher)	74%	69%
Anticentromere antibody (1 : 40 or higher)	2%	46%
Anti-Scl 70 antibody (any titer)	33%	14%
Cumulative survival		
(10 years from first physician diagnosis)	57%	75%

more slowly progressive form of chronic renal disease in which the relationship to systemic sclerosis is more tenuous may also occur. These two clinical situations are not always separated.

The more frequent clinical markers of renal disease in systemic sclerosis include proteinuria, hypertension, and azotemia. At least one of these three abnormalities was identified in 45 percent of 210 patients in the series of Cannon et al. [6]. These authors noted proteinuria (1 + or greater) in 36 percent, hypertension with blood pressure of more than 140/90 mm Hg in 24 percent, and azotemia with BUN higher than 25 mg per deciliter in 19 percent. Using these markers probably overestimates the frequency of renal involvement since essential hypertension and various causes of renal disease other than systemic sclerosis cannot be easily excluded. The frequency of these findings in our own series is shown in Table 73-2.

SRC is a distinctive clinical syndrome specific to systemic sclerosis. This complication is characterized by the explosive onset of malignant arterial hypertension, which is usually followed by rapidly progressive oliguric renal failure. Because of the precise definition of its criteria, its frequency is considerably more consistent than the chronic form of involvement, occurring in 5 to 15 percent of reported series [9, 29, 46]. However, in the opinion of many experts, SRC may have become a less frequent complication during the past decade, although no formal confirmation of this observation has been published.

CLINICAL FINDINGS IN SRC

Onset of SRC. Renal crisis may appear at any time in the course of the disease but most commonly (80%) occurs during the first 4 years after onset. It has a strong predilection for patients with diffuse scleroderma and rarely affects individuals with limited disease, as demonstrated in Tables 73-1 and 73-2. Several investigators have noted a tendency for this complication to appear during the winter months [6, 54] (vide infra).

Presenting Clinical Features. Striking clinical symptoms attend the onset of SRC. Severe headache, blurring of vision, encephalopathic symptoms, and convulsions may be presenting complaints, consequent to development of accelerated hypertension. Dyspnea, orthopnea, and other evidence of rapidly progressive left ventricular failure may ensue, and oliguria soon supervenes. Thus SRC is a true medical emergency requiring prompt therapeutic intervention.

Urinalysis. Proteinuria is almost a universal finding in SRC. As a clinical criterion of acute renal involvement by SRC, however, proteinuria is nonspecific because it may be present before SRC develops or be attributable to other causes such as diabetes mellitus, essential hypertension, and interstitial nephritis. Thus, proteinuria does not accurately predict the presence or subsequent development of SRC [50]. Proteinuria may increase in SRC, but usually not to the nephrotic range (i.e., not over 2 gm/24 hr). Microscopic hematuria and granular casts may be seen but red blood cell casts are uncommon.

Hypertension. Arterial hypertension is clearly a marker that suggests renal involvement and impending SRC in patients with systemic sclerosis. Cannon et al. [6] and Oliver and Cannon [35] reported hypertension in 24 percent and 52 percent of their patients, respectively. However, since the prevalence of hypertension in the general adult population between the ages of 18 and 74 years has been estimated to be 20 percent [33], one must assume that a similar prevalence of essential hypertension exists among patients with systemic sclerosis. Thus it is not surprising that some patients with systemic sclerosis and documented hypertension often do not develop SRC, whereas in a number of cases with SRC, antecedent high blood pressure (BP) had been present for

Table 73-2. Frequency of renal involvement in systemic sclerosis subsets (University of Pittsburgh, 1972–1990)

	Diffuse cutaneous (N = 567)	Limited cutaneous (N = 551)	Overlap syndrome (N = 100)
Proteinuria (2+ by dipstick or > 0.5 gm/24 hr)	20%	16%	12%
Hypertension (> 140/90 mm Hg)	25%	15%	25%
Azotemia (serum creatinine > 1.3 mg/dl)	28%	26%	10%
Scleroderma renal crisis	19%	2%	6%

several years, even preceding the first recognizable symptoms of scleroderma. Nevertheless, although hypertension lacks absolute specificity, it is a frequent and highly characteristic phenomenon in SRC, especially when the BP elevation is recent and its rate of rise is rapid. It should be used as part of the battery of inclusion criteria for SRC but not as an independent marker. The elevation of the BP as a manifestation of SRC is most often accompanied by both funduscopic changes indicating accelerated and malignant hypertension (i.e., hemorrhages, exudates, and papilledema) and by elevated peripheral renin activity (PRA).

In two of their three original cases, Moore and Sheehan had reported the BP as normal [32], and in a number of subsequent reports, cases of SRC without hypertension were noted, prompting the opinion that hypertension per se did not play a primary role in the genesis of the renal lesions [8]. Indeed, in a recent report by Helfrich et al. [17] of 131 patients with SRC, 11 percent had BPs recorded as normal during this complication. In comparison with SRC patients with hypertension, these normotensive individuals had a greater frequency of microangiopathic anemia, more exposure to corticosteroids, and a poorer 12-month survival rate.

In contrast, the "vascular disaster" observed in other types of malignant hypertension has been shown to correlate directly with acute increases in BP [4, 5, 30]. It should be pointed out, however, that extremely high BP is not present in occasional cases of malignant arterial hypertension including those developing from eclampsia and acute glomerulonephritis, even in the presence of clinical and pathologic changes compatible with malignant hypertension [11, 39, 57]. What seems to distinguish these cases from the usual instances of malignant hypertension is a low or normal BP prior to the vascular crisis, a sequence that also characterizes some patients with SRC [54]. In addition, it is possible that in certain patients with systemic sclerosis the arterial tree is particularly vulnerable and that a lesser degree of acute elevation of the BP may precipitate vascular damage. Indeed, an increased reactivity of blood vessels or BP to a number of mediators including cold exposure has been demonstrated in patients with systemic sclerosis [43, 59]. Thus, although it is likely that the initial pathologic lesions in the kidneys are the result of systemic sclerosis per se and are not a consequence of increased arterial pressure [7], rapid deterioration of renal function in SRC seems to be associated with a sudden, albeit occasionally modest, rise in BP.

We have noted a higher frequency of SRC and hypertension among black patients with systemic sclerosis (21 percent in comparison to 7 percent in whites), although its meaning is not clear [54]. It is perhaps in keeping with the twofold increase in prevalence of essential hypertension in the black population in this country and its usually more severe course, particularly in regard to the development of malignant hypertension and renal failure [33, 54].

The Renin-Angiotensin System. Marked elevation of the PRA level is clearly a clinical marker of the onset of renal deterioration in SRC. In our series, PRA was rarely less than twice the upper limit of normal, often increased tenfold, and occasionally was measured at up to 100 times normal, among the highest levels recorded in our laboratory [54].

These striking elevations of PRA, and consequently of angiotensin II, in SRC have led some investigators to consider them of prognostic importance in systemic sclerosis, portending the advent of the clinical stage of SRC [14, 22]. However, in our experience it is uncertain that a rise precedes and heralds this event [50, 54]. None of the 13 cases in which PRA was coincidentally measured from 1 week to 1 year prior to the development of SRC showed a significantly elevated PRA at that time, results that agree with those of other investigators [3, 10, 12]. It appears that although the basal PRA may not be elevated before SRC, it rises to extreme values very rapidly during the acute event itself. This sequence suggests that a functional, Raynaud-like renal vasoconstriction supervenes over and above the more chronic structural changes. The data of Kovalchik et al. [22] indicating a rise in PRA levels after cold pressor testing when renal microvascular changes are present are in keeping with this concept.

The idea of functional vascular narrowing in the kidneys of patients with systemic sclerosis has received support from the clearance studies done by Urai et al. [56] and by the investigations of Cannon et al. [6]. Using the xenon-133 washout technique, the latter authors demonstrated a decrease in renal cortical perfusion in patients with systemic sclerosis, a decrease that was much more severe in the subjects examined during SRC.

The immediate results of the decrease in cortical blood flow most likely are ischemia of the juxtaglomerular apparatus, enhanced renin secretion, and formation of large amounts of local and circulating angiotensin II. These high levels of angiotensin II further increase the renal and generalized vasoconstriction, with the disastrous consequences commonly encountered in malignant hypertension. Thus, while enhanced renin secretion seems to be a secondary factor, it participates in creating a "vicious cycle" of vascular constriction and damage in SRC.

Course of Renal Failure. As mentioned earlier, the only clinical manifestation of renal involvement in the more indolent form of renal disease may be proteinuria, which is nonspecific and often nonprogressive. When SRC develops, glomerular filtration rate (GFR) and renal blood flow rapidly fall, and oliguria and anuria supervene. The rise in serum creatinine is variable and sometimes volatile, climbing in the untreated case at a rate of 1 to 2 mg/dl/day. It is worth noting that since many patients with chronic systemic sclerosis have reduced muscle mass and thus "normal" serum creatinines in the range of 0.6 to 0.8 mg per deciliter, a rise to only 1.0 to 1.5 mg per deciliter may already represent a fall in GFR of up to 50 percent. Death from renal failure, usually punctuated by congestive heart failure due to volume overload, may occur within 7 to 10 days. With progressive renal failure, dialysis soon becomes necessary, but as we will discuss later, with continued treatment of the hyperreninemia and hypertension with angiotensin-converting enzyme (ACE) inhibition, it may not be required permanently.

Blood Abnormalities. Microangiopathic hemolytic anemia (MHA) may develop [44], contributing to the rapid progression of renal failure. The peripheral blood smear shows numerous red blood cell fragments, and a compensatory reticulocytosis is evident. Thrombocytopenia is part of this clinical picture. In this circumstance, there is no obvious immunologic mechanism; instead, accelerated arterial and arteriolar structural damage and platelet adhesion to damaged endothelial surfaces are responsible, leading to distortion and destruction of red blood cells. However, a similar phenomenon is often found in malignant hypertension of other types [21], rendering MHA nonspecific for SRC.

Combined Clinical Features. Rapidly progressive renal insufficiency in patients with systemic sclerosis is the hallmark of SRC; therefore, it can be considered sufficient even as a single criterion for diagnosis of this complication. However, in our series of patients with SRC, four of the characteristics we have mentioned (sudden renal failure, hypertension, grade III or IV retinopathy, and elevated PRA) were noted in 55 percent, and three or more of these signs were seen in 98 percent [54]. In fact, the appearance of any two of these criteria in a patient with systemic sclerosis should be considered as ominous.

HISTOPATHOLOGIC FINDINGS

The gross appearance of the kidneys at postmortem examination of subjects with systemic sclerosis is normal except in the circumstance of SRC. Then the capsule may show areas of hemorrhage and yellow-gray infarction, both on the surface and on cut section. In fulmi-

Fig. 73-1. Photomicrographs of the kidneys of two women who died of "renal crisis" associated with systemic sclerosis with diffuse scleroderma. A. Intimal hyperplasia with complete luminal occlusion of an interlobular artery. Note reduplication and fraying of the internal lamina (orcein stain). B. Fibrinoid necrosis of blood vessels in the glomerulus. (Reproduced with permission from [4].)

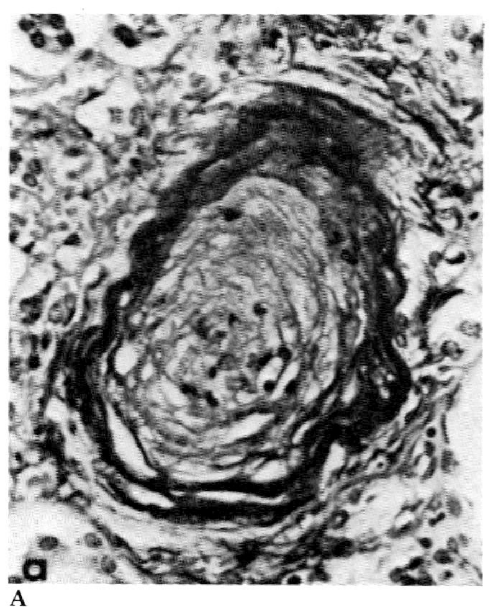

A

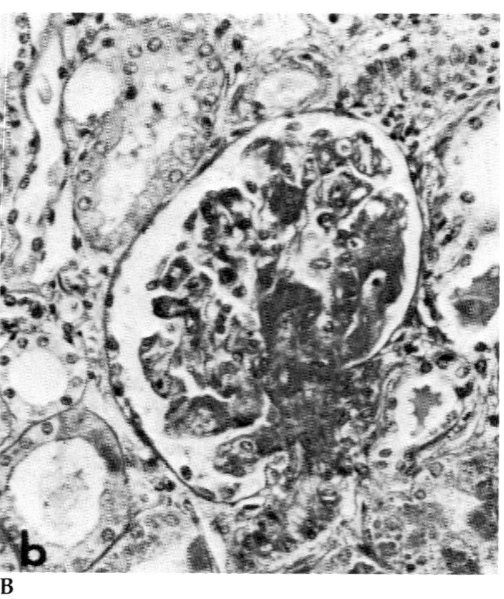

B

nant disease the picture of renal cortical necrosis may be seen. In individuals who have survived SRC, the kidneys become small and shrunken, as in other forms of chronic renal failure, and these changes are indistinguishable from those of malignant nephrosclerosis.

Acute Renal Disease. Microscopically, the characteristic lesions of systemic sclerosis are found in the cortical small interlobular and arcuate arteries (150 to 500 μ in outer diameter) [6]. Arteries larger than this are normal or show atherosclerotic changes consistent with the patient's age. The earliest change is intimal edema, followed by intense intimal cellular proliferation with mucoid ground substance composed of glycoproteins and both neutral and acid mucopolysaccharides [6]. In some instances these deposits separate the endothelium from the internal elastic lamina (Fig. 73-1A). One of the cells participating in intimal thickening has been identified by electron microscopy as having ultrastructural features of a smooth muscle (myointimal) cell, presumably having migrated from the media through gaps in the internal elastic lamina. These cells, not found in normal arteries, are capable of producing collagen fibrils and elastic tissue [16]. Of note is the absence of lymphocytes and other mononuclear cells in these arterial lesions.

Severe narrowing of vessels leads to ischemia and atrophy of tissue in the corresponding distribution, and thrombosis results in frank necrosis and hemorrhagic infarction of glomeruli and tubules. Although in some cases the media is thickened, more often it appears stretched and thinned around the expanded intima. Adventitial and periadventitial fibrosis, more distinguishing features of systemic sclerosis, are seldom present in nonsclerodermatous malignant hypertension; they are reminiscent of similar changes found in the digital arteries [41].

Small arteries and arterioles supplying glomeruli and glomerular capillaries are also involved. The typical lesion is fibrinoid necrosis, which may be located in the wall or subintimally (Fig. 73-1B), and in some cases intramural fibrin has been demonstrated. These changes are indistinguishable from those observed in malignant hypertension, but interestingly, they occur in some scleroderma patients who have never had elevated BP [7] or who have no clinical renal disease [22]. Such fibrinoid necrosis in systemic sclerosis is not associated with infiltration of either acute or chronic inflammatory cells, in contrast to the changes seen in polyarteritis nodosa and other forms of vasculitis. Swelling of endothelial cells is frequently noted on electron microscopy and contributes significantly to luminal narrowing in small arterioles. Eosinophilic and hyaline thrombi reminiscent of those found in the hemolytic-uremic syndrome are reported [18]. These arterial thrombi consist predominantly of fibrin-containing, fibrillar, electron-dense material, often with endothelial cell and red blood cell fragments, but rarely platelets.

Numerous glomerular changes have been reported. The capillary loops may be either thickened or obliterated, and focal or diffuse basement membrane thickening may occur, resulting in wire loop lesions. Hyperplasia of the juxtaglomerular apparatus is nonspecific to systemic sclerosis but is consistent with the marked hyperreninemia characteristic of SRC [52].

Tubules appear to be secondarily affected by the vascular insufficiency described above. Flattening and hyaline droplet degeneration of epithelial cells are the most prominent changes. The interlobular stroma may have increased fibrous tissue and variable small collections of lymphocytes and/or plasma cells.

Immunofluorescence microscopy has been reported to show deposits of immunoglobulins, most notably IgM, complement components (C1q, C3, and C4), and fibrinogen in small renal arteries [23]. Complement (C3) has also been seen in biopsies from patients without clinical renal disease [22]. Such changes are rarely seen in the kidneys of malignant hypertension patients without autoimmune disease. Immune reactants are less frequently found in glomeruli, but fibrinogen has been detected there and in arteries. Also, factor VIII–von Willebrand antigen has been identified in vessels, suggesting involvement of the coagulation cascade [19]. The nonspecificity of these findings may be attributable to gross disruption of vascular integrity with increased permeability. Elution of antinuclear antibodies from the kidney in a few cases has raised the possibility that immune complexes are involved in the pathogenesis [26], but electron microscopy has shown no electron-dense deposits or other evidence of immune complex deposition.

Chronic Renal Disease. With the prompt use of potent antihypertensive agents, patients with SRC can survive with reduction or normalization of serum creatinine. In this circumstance, similar but less cellular proliferative interlobular and arcuate artery changes are seen. However, histopathologic evidence of chronic renovascular disease is present in the majority of patients dying with scleroderma, even without SRC, compared with controls [55]. These changes include subintimal proliferation with luminal narrowing, most prominent in small and medium-size arteries [55]. Reduplication of elastic fibers is more frequent in long-standing scleroderma, especially in the limited cutaneous type, and is independent of hypertension. Tubular atrophy, glomerular obsolescence, and interstitial fibrosis are further evidence of chronicity, which is seen in patients with systemic sclerosis in whom SRC has not developed.

PATHOGENESIS OF RENAL INVOLVEMENT

The pathogenesis of the renal events in systemic sclerosis remains obscure, but seems to evolve from a series of insults to the kidney. The primary process may well be an immunologic injury with deposition of immune reactants in the intima of renal intralobular and arcuate arteries. Conspicuously absent are lymphocytes and other mononuclear cells. A relation to increased fibroblastic activity is suggested by rapid progression of skin thickening prior to the onset of SRC [50]. This "vasculopathy" proceeds at varying rates throughout most organs in systemic sclerosis, particularly of the diffuse type, and may account for the low-grade proteinuria and reduced renal blood flow noted in a high proportion of patients who do not develop the azotemia, significant hypertension, and high PRA levels associated with SRC.

The precipitation of SRC, with its acute and rapid progression of renal failure, indicates that some new and sudden event has supervened in the course of systemic sclerosis. A number of factors have been implicated, but their relative importance in producing the characteristic marked renal vasoconstriction is difficult to assess.

A role for hormonal factors is suggested by the predominance of systemic sclerosis among women. The description of SRC in pregnant women and during the early postpartum period [20, 38] supports this argument for hormonal or metabolic factors in its precipitation. However, the frequency of renal crisis was not noted to be increased during pregnancy in one large series [47] and several successful pregnancies have been reported in women who have recovered from SRC [2, 47]. A variety of other hormones with vasomotor properties including catecholamines, prostaglandins, the kallikrein-kinin system, and serotonin have been found in normal concentrations in the serum of patients suffering from systemic sclerosis [54]. On the other hand, onset of SRC following treatment of systemic sclerosis with corticosteroids has been noted, as emphasized by the patients with SRC without hypertension, mentioned earlier [17].

The deleterious effect of cold in systemic sclerosis was observed by Raynaud, who in 1865 described the phenomenon that bears his name in a patient with scleroderma [40]. Smooth muscle in arteries from sclerodermatous skin exhibits a normal response to catecholamines at 37°C, but its response is altered at lower temperatures [59], supporting the theory of abnormal vascular reaction to cold. Cannon et al. noted that 76 percent of deaths from renal failure among their patients with systemic sclerosis occurred in the fall and winter and that the induction of Raynaud's phenomenon by cooling was associated with a 32 percent reduction of renal cortical blood flow [6]. Our data confirm an association of cold weather with the occurrence of SRC, since 63 percent of our patients with SRC presented in the fall and winter months [54].

Other factors that may be involved in the precipitous onset of renal vasoconstriction include a sudden decrease in cardiac output, infection, reduced renal blood flow secondary to nonsteroidal antiinflammatory drugs, or other causes of hypotension. The imposition of a severe emotional crisis in the life situation of the patient was a possible triggering factor in some of our subjects.

To summarize, our present concept of the pathogenesis of renal involvement in systemic sclerosis is that immunologic and/or vascular mechanisms, as yet undefined, lead to enhanced deposition of connective tissue by fibroblasts and to intimal proliferation in the small arteries. These changes may be accompanied only by slight to modest proteinuria and a decrease in renal blood flow. The clinical course may be stable or only slowly progressive, thus accounting for patients with systemic sclerosis but no clinical renal impairment who have biopsy evidence of chronic renal disease. However, these changes may sensitize the small arteries to vasoconstriction, either directly or by serving as an antigenic stimulus in response to external factors (e.g., cold), circulating mediators (e.g., hormonal changes), or other types of stress. A "Raynaud-like phenomenon" in the kidneys may occur suddenly and then lead to cortical ischemia, which, if sustained, will drastically enhance the production of renin. The resulting high levels of angiotensin II can then perpetuate the generalized vasoconstriction with subsequent elevation of the BP, further renal ischemia, and azotemia.

SRC can be viewed as a form of malignant arteriolar nephrosclerosis, usually with hypertension, albeit a very special form, with a prognosis that is much worse than that of other etiologies. A markedly elevated BP per se is not always a prerequisite, since its ultimate level depends also on the efficiency of cardiac function and the size of circulating blood volume. The difference between SRC and other forms of malignant hypertension is essentially a quantitative one; thus vasoconstriction is more severe, the activation of the renin-angiotensin system is greater, the sequence of catastrophic events, especially deterioration of renal function, is more rapid, and control of BP without aggravating the renal failure is generally more difficult to accomplish. Renal failure is a function of the severity of both the renal vascular structural damage and vasoconstriction enhanced by elevated PRA. Thus unless the BP reduction is accompanied by effective renal vasodilatation and a reduction of circulating angiotensin II, a result not always possible with most antihypertensive agents, renal blood flow will fall further as BP is reduced.

Management of Renal Involvement in SRC

Prior to 1980, no treatment had been demonstrated to be effective in arresting or reversing renal involvement once significant azotemia had occurred. When azotemia was associated with severe hypertension, effective treatment of the hypertension had no beneficial effects on the rapidly progressive renal deterioration. In our series of 68 patients with SRC treated between 1955 and 1981, 84 percent were dead within 1 year, and in fact, prior to 1971, the average survival ranged from 1 to 3 months [29, 54]. However, with the knowledge concerning the central role of the renin-angiotensin system in the pathogenesis of renal failure in SRC, and the advent of the ACE inhibitors, this dire prognosis now has changed remarkably.

Prompt and aggressive treatment of the accelerated hypertension with potent vasodilators such as minoxidil and modest renin inhibitors such as the beta blockers do have some impact on survival. The vasodilators, however, cause avid sodium retention, while the beta blockers may have negative cardiac effects, so that heart failure, already a threat in these severely hypertensive patients, often supervenes. Calcium channel blockers, useful in peripheral Raynaud's phenomenon, are not particularly helpful in SRC; in some patients, they were being administered at the time SRC developed. Moreover, the renal failure makes the patient increasingly unresponsive to diuretics. Although associated congestive heart failure usually results from the hypertension and volume overload, systemic sclerosis also involves the myocardium [13], thus potentiating the likelihood of heart failure. If blood pressure control is poor, renal failure ensues and progresses, with dialysis soon becoming necessary. With antihypertensive agents ineffective against renin-angiotensin mechanisms, PRA levels may remain elevated and may even rise further during dialysis, with BP control continuing to be difficult. Under these circumstances, bilateral nephrectomy formerly was employed, resulting in an immediate decline in renin levels and allowing easier control of the hypertension and heart failure. Fortunately, this procedure is rarely, if ever, indicated today (vide infra). The restoration of normal BP by nephrectomy in SRC did, however, reinforce the concept that the elimination of the renin-angiotensin contribution to hypertension is a major goal of therapy.

Patients with SRC who require dialysis tolerate it equally well as those with other renal diseases. Both hemodialysis (80 percent) and peritoneal dialysis (20 percent) have been used without serious difficulty in access or clearance [34]. Kidney transplantation has led to disappearance of the clinical features of SRC in a number of instances, but recurrence of typical kidney lesions of systemic sclerosis in patients with renal allografts also has been noted [54]. Improvement in skin thickening and other nonrenal manifestations of systemic sclerosis may occur after control of SRC by drugs, dialysis, or transplantation [46, 54].

A new era in the management of SRC was opened with the advent of ACE inhibitors [36]. Since the original description of two patients with SRC in whom deterioration in renal function was prevented by the use of captopril [24], the first clinically available ACE inhibitor, treatment with these agents has become the standard of therapy. Prompt inhibition of angiotensin II production dramatically lowers BP, halts renal deterioration, and may indeed reverse it. If treatment is started before the serum creatinine has risen to a level of 4 mg per deciliter, renal function often returns to normal. When therapy is initiated at higher serum creatinine levels, renal function may still deteriorate and require dialysis [46, 58], but as noted below, a few such patients have resumed renal function after many months of dialysis, accompanied by continued BP control with ACE inhibition. Obviously, this potential has made bilateral nephrectomy an outmoded therapeutic modality, of historical interest only.

Recently, we reported on 20 patients who were on dialysis for at least 6 months but continued on ACE inhibitor therapy. In 11 of these patients, dialysis could be discontinued and 3 years after discontinuation, with maintenance of ACE inhibitor therapy, their mean creatinine level was 2.1 mg per deciliter. These 20 patients came from a series of 55 SRC patients treated with ACE inhibitors and 53 SRC patients not receiving this therapy (the latter mostly prior to 1980). There was a 76 percent cumulative survival rate at 1 year in the former group compared with only 20 percent in the latter group. Among the patients treated with ACE inhibitors, older age, male sex, congestive heart failure, and initiation of ACE inhibitor therapy when the serum creatinine was greater than 3.0 mg per deciliter were associated with poor survival [46].

Captopril, the prototype of the ACE inhibitors, does have a number of adverse effects, which are believed to be related to the sulfhydryl component of the molecule. These side effects include skin rashes, proteinuria, and occasionally leukopenia. In a situation as severe as SRC, these concerns do not mitigate against its use, but they do suggest some caution in administration of the drug in patients with only the lesser forms of chronic renal involvement in which azotemia is absent, PRA is not elevated, and the hypertension is not of the accelerated type. However, Beckett et al. [3] reported on seven patients with systemic sclerosis and hypertension, four of whom had no evidence of malignant hypertension (i.e., fundi less than grade III or IV), but all with creatinine levels of at least 1.5 mg per deciliter. Only four had elevated PRA, and renal biopsy specimens from six showed vascular changes but no fibrinoid necrosis. Treatment with captopril controlled BP in all seven patients and halted progression of renal deterioration in five over a 3-year period of observation [3]. These data are in keeping with our more recent experiences, and hence—and particularly since the transition from a "benign" hypertension and renal involvement to the explosive malignant hypertension of SRC is not always a clear-cut event—we are increasingly inclined to the early use of ACE compounds in scleroderma patients with hypertension.

Nevertheless, since the toxicity profile of captopril resembles that of D-penicillamine, which also has the sulfhydryl group, these two drugs should not be administered simultaneously. However, other compounds with ACE inhibition properties do not have the sulfhydryl radical, and their use in systemic sclerosis, even with only early renal involvement (e.g., proteinuria and nonaccelerated hypertension), may be in order. Our data and those of others [31, 45] using enalapril, an ACE inhibitor without the sulfhydryl group, indicate that it is as effective as captopril, and that it can be given to patients who have developed skin rashes with captopril without cross-sensitivity. However, angioneurotic edema, which has been noted with captopril, also occurs with enalapril, as does a troublesome cough, perhaps related to bradykinin, which may in fact be more common with enalapril. Enalapril is a longer-acting compound, with up to 24 hours of effect after single dosing—and longer if renal failure is present—but this presents disadvantages as well as advantages, particularly in titrating to an appropriate dose when initializing therapy.

The initial dose of captopril usually should be only 12.5 mg with careful observation of the BP effect over the next few hours. If patients are sodium depleted by previous diuretics or other causes of loss of extracellular volume, they may be quite sensitive to the drug because captopril has some diuretic effect of its own. Thereafter, the dose can be slowly increased by 12.5- to 25-mg increments and given every 6 to 8 hours with the goal of maintaining BP below 140/90 mm Hg. Usually 150 mg per day will suffice; occasionally as much as 300 mg per day has been given. Addition of a beta or calcium channel blocker and/or minoxidil may occasionally be needed, and in the latter instance a diuretic may be required. However, routine potassium supplementation is rarely necessary; in fact, captopril, by virtue of its blockade of the angiotensin II–aldosterone sequence, may result in rising concentrations of serum potassium. If the patient is unable to take oral medication, management of the hypertension may initially require intravenous titration with nitroprusside, as in other types of hypertensive crisis, but one should attempt to institute the ACE inhibitor as soon as possible. In fact, enalaprilat, a metabolized form of enalapril, is now available for parenteral use in doses of 1.5 mg every 6 hours and may be of value in such situations.

In occasional patients, serum creatinine may continue to rise despite adequate BP control with an ACE inhibitor and the question arises as to whether the drug is paradoxically contributing to such progression. Captopril has been reported rarely to produce an interstitial nephritis. Excessive lowering of BP, particularly in association with loss of renal glomerular efferent arterial constriction, may further depress GFR, especially if coincident renal artery stenosis is present. However, this sequence of events is most difficult to prove and we are quite hesitant to discontinue ACE inhibition, particularly since continued angiotensin suppression often results in significant return of renal function even after institution of dialysis, as described above. Furthermore, we have not observed improvement in the deterioration of renal function after discontinuation of these agents [54].

A number of older therapies advocated for treatment of SRC no longer have any place in its management. These include anticoagulants and antithrombotic drugs, therapies considered largely because of the presence of fibrin and microthrombi in the small vessels, which probably are secondary rather than primary events. Steroid therapy is ill-advised because of the aforementioned reports suggesting precipitation or even acceleration of SRC with such treatment. On the other hand, efforts to ameliorate fibroblastic proliferation by D-penicillamine, through immunosuppression, may help to prevent renal involvement [51].

Conclusions

Although some involvement of the renal vasculature may occur subclinically and may be relatively nonprogressive in patients with systemic sclerosis and diffuse scleroderma, the development of SRC should be viewed as a complication that is similar to malignant hypertension of other causes and has a rapid downhill course. A self-perpetuating cascade of events ensues in which the renin-angiotensin system has a paramount role. Renal deterioration is rapid and predictable, with heart failure a common concomitant. By blocking this cascade at one or more sites, reversal to a more "benign" stage of hypertensive disease can be achieved. Although minoxidil and other vasodilating antihypertensive agents and/or blockade of renin release by beta blockers may occasionally achieve this goal, ACE inhibition appears to be most promising because it specifically eliminates the synthesis of angiotensin II and its vasoconstrictive effects.

The urgency of treatment when the signs of SRC appear cannot be overemphasized since prompt and aggressive institution of therapy to block the renin-angiotensin sequence now offers hope to the patient with this formerly fatal condition. Use of ACE inhibition therapy in systemic sclerosis with any degree of hypertension, even without clinically evident renal involvement, may now be in order. Moreover, it appears likely that if the dramatic improvement of patients with potential and proven SRC continues to be evident, morbidity and mortality from this complication may be exceeded by those from other visceral involvement.

ACKNOWLEDGMENT. The authors dedicate this chapter to the late Gerald P. Rodnan, M.D., whose 30 years of detailed study of systemic sclerosis made possible many of the insights discussed herein.

References

1. Auspitz, H. Ein Beitrag zur Lehre vom Haut-Sklerem der Erwachsenen. *Wien Med. Wschr.* 13: 739, 1863. Quoted in Rodnan, G. P., and Benedek, T. G. An historical account of the study of progressive systemic sclerosis (diffuse scleroderma). *Ann. Intern. Med.* 57: 305, 1962.
2. Baethge, B. A., and Wolf, R. E. Successful pregnancy with scleroderma renal disease and pulmonary hypertension in a patient using angiotensin converting enzyme inhibitors. *Ann. Rheum. Dis.* 48: 776, 1989.
3. Beckett, V. L., Donadio, J. V., Brennan, L. A., et al. Use of captopril as early therapy for renal scleroderma: A prospective study. *Mayo Clin. Proc.* 60: 763, 1985.
4. Beilin, L. J., and Goldby, F. S. High arterial pressure versus humoral factors in the pathogenesis of the vascular lesions of malignant hypertension. *Clin. Sci.* 52: 111, 1977.
5. Byrom, F. B. *The Hypertensive Vascular Crisis. An Experimental Study.* London: Heinemann, 1969.
6. Cannon, P. J., Hassar, M., Case, D. B., et al. The relationship of hypertension and renal failure in scleroderma (progressive systemic sclerosis) to structural and functional abnormalities of the renal cortical circulation. *Medicine* 53: 1, 1974.
7. D'Angelo, W. A., Fries, J. F., Masi, A. T., et al. Pathologic observations in systemic sclerosis (scleroderma). A study of fifty-eight autopsy cases and fifty-eight matched controls. *Am. J. Med.* 46: 428, 1969.
8. Dichoso, C. C. The Kidney in Progressive Systemic Sclerosis (Scleroderma). In W. N. Suki and G. Eknoyan (eds.), *The Kidney in Systemic Disease.* Perspectives in Nephrology and Hypertension, Vol. 3. New York: Wiley, 1976.
9. Eason, R. J., Tan, P. L., and Gow, P. J. Progressive systemic sclerosis in Auckland: A ten-year review with emphasis on prognostic features. *Aust. N.Z. J. Med.* 11: 657, 1981.
10. Fiocco, U., Montanaro, D., Filippi, R., et al. Plasma renin activity in progressive systemic sclerosis. *Bull. Soc. Ital. Biol. Sper.* 54: 2507, 1978.
11. Fishberg, A. M. *Hypertension and Nephritis* (4th ed.). Philadelphia: Lea & Febiger, 1944. P. 463.

12. Fleischmajer, R., and Gould, A. P. Serum renin and renin substrate levels in scleroderma. *Proc. Soc. Exp. Biol. Med.* 150: 374, 1975.
13. Follansbee, W. P., Curtiss, E. I., Medsger, T. A., Jr., et al. Physiologic abnormalities of cardiac function in progressive systemic sclerosis with diffuse scleroderma. *N. Engl. J. Med.* 310: 142, 1984.
14. Gavras, H., Gavras, I., Cannon, P. J., et al. Is elevated plasma renin activity of prognostic importance in progressive systemic sclerosis? *Arch. Intern. Med.* 137: 1554, 1975.
15. Goetz, R. H. The pathology of progressive systemic sclerosis (generalized scleroderma) with special reference to changes in viscera. *Clin. Proc.* (Capetown) 4: 337, 1945.
16. Harker, L. A., Ross, R., and Glomset, J. A. The role of endothelial cell injury and platelet response in atherogenesis. *Thromb. Haemostas.* 39: 312, 1978.
17. Helfrich, D. J., Banner, B., Steen, V. D., et al. Normotensive renal failure in systemic sclerosis. *Arthritis Rheum.* 32: 1128, 1989.
18. Heptinstall, R. H. *Pathology of the Kidney* (2nd ed.). Boston: Little, Brown, 1974.
19. Kahaleh, M. B., Osborn, I., and LeRoy, E. C. Increased factor VIII/von Willebrand factor antigen and von Willebrand factor activity in scleroderma and in Raynaud's phenomenon. *Ann. Intern. Med.* 94: 482, 1981.
20. Karlen, J. R., and Cook, W. A. Renal scleroderma and pregnancy. *Obstet. Gynecol.* 44: 349, 1974.
21. Kincaid-Smith, P. Participation of intravascular coagulation in the pathogenesis of glomerular and vascular lesions. *Kidney Int.* 7: 242, 1975.
22. Kovalchik, M. T., Guggenheim, S. J., Silverman, M. H., et al. The kidney in progressive systemic sclerosis. A prospective study. *Ann. Intern. Med.* 89: 881, 1978.
23. Lapenas, D., Rodnan, G. P., and Cavallo, T. Immunopathology of the renal vascular lesion of progressive systemic sclerosis (scleroderma). *Am. J. Pathol.* 91: 243, 1978.
24. Lopez-Ovejero, J. A., Saal, S. D., D'Angelo, W. A., et al. Reversal of vascular and renal crises of scleroderma by oral angiotensin-converting enzyme blockade. *N. Engl. J. Med.* 300: 1417, 1979.
25. Masugi, M., and Ya-Shu. Die diffuse Sklerodermia und ihre Geffasveranderung. *Virchows Arch. (Pathol. Anat.)* 302: 39, 1938.
26. McGiven, A. R., de Boer, W. G. R. M., and Barness, A. J. Renal immune deposits in scleroderma. *Pathology* 3: 145, 1971.
27. Medsger, T. A., Jr. Systemic Sclerosis (Scleroderma), Localized Scleroderma, Eosinophilic Fasciitis and Calcinosis. In D. J. McCarty (ed.), *Arthritis and Allied Conditions* (11th ed.). Atlanta: Arthritis Foundation, 1988.
28. Medsger, T. A., Jr., and Masi, A. T. Epidemiology of progressive systemic sclerosis. *Clin. Rheum. Dis.* 5: 15, 1979.
29. Medsger, T. A., Jr., Masi, A. T., Rodnan, G. P., et al. Survival with systemic sclerosis (scleroderma). *Ann. Intern. Med.* 75: 396, 1971.
30. Menard, J., Louin, P. F., and Bariety, J. Accelerated (Malignant) Hypertension. In J. Hamburger, J. Crosnier, and J. P. Grunfeld (eds.), *Nephrology*. New York: Wiley, 1979. P. 225.
31. Milson, S. T., and Nicholls, M. G. Successful treatment of scleroderma renal crisis with enalapril. *Postgrad. Med. J.* 62: 1059, 1986.
32. Moore, H. C., and Sheehan, H. L. The kidney of scleroderma. *Lancet* 1: 68, 1952.
33. National Center for Health Statistics: *Blood Pressure Levels of Persons 6–74 Years, United States, 1971–1974.* By J. Roberts and K. Maurer. Vital and Health Statistics. Series 11, No. 203, DHEW Pub. No. (HRA) 78-1648. Health Resources Administration. Washington, D.C. U.S. Government Printing Office, 1977.
34. Nissenson, A. R., and Port, F. K. Outcome of end-stage renal disease in patients with rare causes in patients with renal failure III. Systemic/vascular disorders. *Q. J. Med.* 74: 63, 1990.
35. Oliver, J. A., and Cannon, P. J. The kidney in scleroderma. *Nephron* 18: 141, 1977.
36. Ondetti, M. A., Rubin, B., and Cushman, D. W. Design of specific inhibitors of angiotensin-converting enzyme: New class of orally active antihypertensive agents. *Science* 196: 441, 1977.
37. Osler, W. *The Principles and Practice of Medicine.* New York: Appleton Century Crofts, 1892. P. 993.
38. Palma, A., Sanchez-Palencia, A., Armas, J. R., et al. Progressive systemic sclerosis and nephrotic syndrome: An unusual association resulting in postpartum acute renal failure. *Arch. Intern. Med.* 141: 520, 1981.
39. Perera, G. A. Hypertensive Disease Without Hypertension. In G. E. W. Wolstenholme and M. P. Cameron (eds.), *Ciba Foundation Symposium on Hypertension; Humoral and Neurogenic Factors.* Boston: Little, Brown, 1954. P. 46.
40. Raynaud, M. Personal communication. In P. Horteloup (ed.), *De la Sclerodermie.* Paris: P. Asselin, 1865. P. 112.
41. Rodnan, G. P., Myerowitz, R. L., and Justh, G. P. Morphologic changes in the digital arteries of patients with progressive systemic sclerosis (scleroderma) and Raynaud's phenomenon. *Medicine* 59: 393, 1980.
42. Rodnan, G. P., Schreiner, G., and Black, R. Renal involvement in progressive systemic sclerosis (scleroderma). *Am. J. Med.* 23: 445, 1957.
43. Rodnan, G. P., Shapiro, A. P., and Krifcher, E. The occurrence of malignant hypertension and renal insufficiency in progressive systemic sclerosis (diffuse scleroderma). Abstract. *Ann. Intern. Med.* 60: 737, 1964.
44. Salyer, W. R., Salyer, D. C., and Heptinstall, R. H. Scleroderma and microangiopathic hemolytic anemia. *Ann. Intern. Med.* 78: 895, 1973.
45. Smith, C. D., Smith, R. D., and Korn, J. H. Hypertensive crisis in systemic sclerosis: Treatment with new oral angiotensin converting enzyme inhibitor MK 421 (enalapril) in captopril-intolerant patients. *Arthritis Rheum.* 27: 826, 1984.
46. Steen, V. D., Constantio, J. P., Shapiro, A. P., et al. Outcome of renal crisis in systemic sclerosis: Relation to availability of angiotensin converting enzyme (ACE) inhibitors. *Ann. Intern. Med.* 113: 352, 1990.
47. Steen, V. D., Conte, C., Day, N., et al. Pregnancy in systemic sclerosis. *Arthritis Rheum.* 32: 151, 1989.
48. Steen, V. D., Conte, C., Santora, D., et al. Twenty-year incidence survey of systemic sclerosis. Abstract. *Arthritis Rheum.* 31: S21, 1988.
49. Steen, V. D., and Medsger, T. A., Jr. Epidemiology and natural history of systemic sclerosis. *Rheum. Dis. Clin. North Am.* 16: 1, 1990.
50. Steen, V. D., Medsger, T. A., Jr., Osial, T. A., Jr., et al. Factors predicting the development of renal involvement in progressive systemic sclerosis. *Am. J. Med.* 76: 779, 1984.
51. Steen, V. D., Medsger, T. A., Jr., and Rodnan, G. P. D-penicillamine therapy in progressive systemic sclerosis (scleroderma). *Ann. Intern. Med.* 97: 652, 1982.
52. Stone, R. A., Tisher, C. C., Hawkins, H. K., et al. Juxtaglomerular hyperplasia and hyperreninemia in progres-

sive systemic sclerosis complicated by acute renal failure. *Am. J. Med.* 36: 119, 1974.

53. Talbott, J. H., Gall, E. A., Consolazio, W. V., et al. Dermatomyositis with scleroderma, calcinosis and renal endarteritis associated with focal cortical necrosis. *Arch. Intern. Med.* 63: 476, 1939.
54. Traub, Y. H., Shapiro, A. P., Rodnan, G. P., et al. Hypertension and renal failure (scleroderma renal crisis) in progressive systemic sclerosis. Review of a 25-year experience with 68 cases. *Medicine* 62: 335, 1983.
55. Trostle, D. C., Bedetti, C. D., Steen, V. D., et al. Renal vascular histology and morphometry in systemic sclerosis: A case control autopsy study. *Arthritis Rheum.* 31: 393, 1988.
56. Urai, L., Nagy, Z., Szinay, G., et al. Renal function in scleroderma: A clinical study of 727 cases. *Arch. Dermatol.* 84: 49, 1961.
57. Werko, L., and Brody, S. The blood pressure in toxemia of pregnancy. I. Spontaneous diurnal variability. *J. Obstet. Gynaecol. Br. Emp.* 60: 180, 1953.
58. Whitman, H. H., III, Case, D. B., Laragh, J. H., et al. Variable response to oral angiotensin-converting-enzyme blockade in hypertensive scleroderma patients. *Arthritis Rheum.* 25: 241, 1982.
59. Winkelmann, R. K., Goldyne, M. E., and Linscheid, R. L. Influence of cold on catecholamine response of vascular smooth muscle strips from resistance vessels of scleroderma skin. *Angiology* 28: 330, 1977.

Suggested Additional Readings

Claman, H. N. Mast cells, T cells, and abnormal fibrosis. *Immunology Today* 6: A2, 1985.

Kahaleh, M. B., and LeRoy, E. C. Progressive systemic sclerosis: kidney involvement. *Clin. Rheum. Dis.* 5: 167, 1979.

Medsger, T. A., Jr. Systemic Sclerosis (Scleroderma), Eosinophilic Fasciitis and Calcinosis. In D. J. McCarthy (ed.), *Arthritis and Allied Conditions.* Philadelphia: Lea & Febiger, 1984. P. 994.

Nussbaum, A. I., and LeRoy, E. C. Renal Involvement in Scleroderma (Systemic Sclerosis). In P. A. Bacon, and N. M. Hadler (eds.), *The Kidney and Rheumatic Disease,* London: Butterworth, 1982. P. 282.

Rheumatoid Arthritis, Sjögren's Syndrome, and Dermatomyositis-Polymyositis

Woodruff Emlen
James C. Steigerwald
William P. Arend

Rheumatoid Arthritis

Rheumatoid arthritis (RA) is a chronic inflammatory disease of unknown etiology, characterized primarily by symmetric polyarthritis. RA is, however, a systemic disease with extraarticular manifestations in up to 35 percent of patients, including constitutional symptoms, serositis, vasculitis, rheumatoid nodules, pulmonary lesions, and cardiac disease [50]. RA is the most common of the inflammatory rheumatic diseases, with a prevalence of 1 to 3 percent, reflecting over 4 million cases in the United States alone. The disease is more common in females by 2.5 : 1, and can occur at any age, although the peak onset is between 40 and 60 years old [50].

Although RA is often characterized by the presence of rheumatoid factors and circulating immune complexes, renal involvement is generally considered to be quite rare [50]. Clinically, renal disease in RA is usually mild and not a major problem in clinical management. However, recent studies showed that measurement of serum creatinine may underestimate renal impairment in patients with RA, possibly due to the decreased muscle mass of these patients [13, 80]. Furthermore, population-based studies have shown that patients with RA have an increased mortality over age-matched controls, and that a significant proportion of this increased mortality can be attributed to renal disease [11, 64]. These studies suggest that a combination of insults to the kidneys over time in patients with RA may contribute to renal compromise and make the kidneys more susceptible to subsequent diseases such as infection, hypertension, or atherosclerosis [11, 12, 14, 64].

Two broad categories of renal disorders can be distinguished in RA: lesions caused by the disease itself and side effects of therapeutic agents. Table 74-1 lists the types of renal lesions that have been found with RA. Because patients with RA are frequently treated with multiple drugs for many years, it is often difficult to distinguish between disease-associated and drug-associated renal lesions. Many studies in the literature suffer from a failure to make this distinction. In addition, many studies from the 1940s and 1950s included a significant number of patients with other connective tissue diseases such as systemic lupus erythematosus (SLE) in their series of patients with RA, thereby further confusing the definition of RA-associated renal disease. Nevertheless, a substantial literature exists describing renal lesions in RA and this literature will be reviewed in this chapter.

RENAL DISORDERS RELATED TO RHEUMATOID ARTHRITIS

Amyloidosis. Amyloidosis is a syndrome characterized by deposition of an insoluble proteinaceous material in the extracellular matrix of multiple organs. These deposits have a unique fibrillar ultrastructure characterized by a rigid, nonbranching filament of about 100 Å in diameter. Amyloidosis is generally classified according to the type of fibril deposited in tissue, being either secondary amyloidosis (AA amyloidosis) or primary amyloidosis associated with plasma cell dyscrasias (AL amyloidosis). RA is one of a number of chronic inflammatory or neoplastic diseases that may eventually lead to secondary amyloidosis (AA amyloidosis). The initial manifestation of renal involvement in amyloidosis is proteinuria; it progresses at a variable rate and most patients will eventually develop the nephrotic syndrome and/or uremia (see Chap. 80).

Amyloidosis as a complication of RA was apparently first described in 1856 by Wilks [139]. The frequency with which amyloidosis is found at postmortem examination ranges from 10 to 60 percent, although most authors report prevalence of 10 to 20 percent [3, 36, 37, 64, 125, 130]. Laakso et al. reported that amyloidosis was listed as the cause of death in 31 of 356 patients with RA who died during the period of 1958 to 1969 [64]. In living patients, the reported frequency of amyloidosis is variable. Using a Congo red stain on liver biopsies, Unger et al. found amyloidosis in 6 of 56 living patients with RA, all of whom had proteinuria [130]. Fearnley and Lackner surveyed 183 patients with RA, of whom 24 had persistent proteinuria [37]. Eight of these patients were found to have amyloidosis, giving an overall prevalence of 8 of 183, or 4 percent. Ennevaara and Oka studied 24 patients with RA and persistent proteinuria and found amyloidosis in 17 on renal, rectal, or lymph node biopsies [36]. Arapakis and Tribe performed rectal biopsies on 115 patients with RA in search of amyloidosis [3]. Six patients were positive, only three of whom had proteinuria. Thus, although more frequent at autopsy, clinically significant amyloid renal disease may occur in only 3 to 10 percent of living patients with RA.

Amyloidosis is seen with increasing frequency in patients with long-standing RA (> 10 years' duration) and is also more common in patients who are positive for rheumatoid factor (RF) and who have significant joint destruction [18]. This observation implies that if arthritis is kept under good control, the frequency of secondary amyloidosis can be reduced. Parkins and Bywaters described two patients in whom proteinuria and clinical renal disease improved when their arthritis went into remission, but renal disease recurred when the RA relapsed [82]. Wright and Calkins, in a more recent series of patients (1967 to 1979) where management of RA was presumably more aggressive and more successful, reported a lower frequency of amyloidosis at autopsy (3.6 percent) than in earlier studies [142]. These data are consistent with the hypothesis that aggressive management of active joint inflammation may be able to decrease the frequency of AA amyloidosis in RA patients.

The clinical course of amyloidosis in patients with RA is one of progressive renal failure. These patients gen-

Table 74-1. Renal involvement in rheumatoid arthritis

I. Renal disorders related to RA
   A. Amyloidosis
   B. Glomerular lesions
   C. Vascular lesions
   D. Tubulointerstitial lesions
II. Renal disorders related to drug therapy
   A. NSAIDs
   B. Analgesics
   C. Gold/penicillamine
   D. Cyclosporine

erally do poorly on dialysis, and recurrence of amyloid deposits has been reported in renal transplants [67]. However, because there are other causes of proteinuria in RA, the diagnosis of amyloidosis as a cause of clinical renal disease should be made only with biopsy confirmation and after other conditions have been excluded.

Glomerular Lesions. The existence of a glomerular lesion specific for RA has been debated for a number of years. One of the first articles describing renal involvement in RA was by Baggenstoss and Rosenberg in 1943 [5]. They reported autopsy findings in the kidneys of 30 RA patients, but a specific characteristic lesion was not identified. However, they observed that 19 of 30 rheumatoid patients demonstrated glomerular endothelial proliferation, a lesion that they designated a form of glomerulitis. In retrospect, a number of these patients may have had SLE, therefore casting doubt on some of the conclusions.

In the early 1960s, Sorensen studied renal function in patients with RA and reported reduced creatinine clearance in 33 percent as compared to 11 percent of controls [115–117]. The reduction in renal function in patients with RA seemed to be dependent on both the stage and the duration of disease and was thought to be independent of drug therapy. Patients who were RF positive had significantly poorer renal function compared to patients who were RF negative. No histologic or pathologic findings were described in this study.

In 1962 Pollak and co-workers described the results of renal biopsies and renal function tests in 41 patients with RA [86]. Histologically, vascular disease was found in 14, amyloidosis in 4, and lupus nephritis in 2. A specific rheumatoid glomerulitis was not found in any biopsies but was observed in 6 of 16 autopsy specimens. Clinical testing showed that 13 patients had persistent proteinuria, which was associated with renal amyloid in 4 patients, lupus nephritis in 2, and nephrosclerosis in 2 patients. Three patients had normal kidneys. Creatinine clearance, urine specific gravity, and serum creatinine were within normal limits in "almost all" of the patients. The authors concluded that renal involvement in RA, except for amyloidosis, was most probably not related to RA but was due to other conditions. Since a glomerulitis was found in 6 of 16 autopsy cases but not in renal biopsy material, they speculated glomerulitis may be a late or preterminal event of little clinical significance.

In 1974 Salomon et al. [97] performed renal biopsies on 18 patients with classic RA who demonstrated minimal to mild urine abnormalities. By light microscopy 11 biopsies were normal and 7 revealed an increase in mesangial cells and matrix. Electron microscopy of the 7 abnormal biopsies showed a slight increase in the mesangial matrix, with negative immunofluorescence findings for deposits of IgG and complement. Of these 18 patients, not one case of renal failure or elevated serum creatinine occurred. The authors concluded that renal function impairment in RA was uncommon.

In a review of the literature in 1977 Whaley and Webb concluded that few data existed to suggest a specific renal lesion in RA except for the rare occurrences of arteritis [137]. Most of the renal lesions associated with RA were thought to be either secondary to amyloidosis or due to the effects of medications.

In the late 1970s publications described membranoproliferative or membranous nephropathy in patients with RA who had not been treated with gold or penicillamine. Two patients with RA and membranous nephropathy who had never received gold or penicillamine were described [51, 126]. Renal biopsies demonstrated prominence of the mesangial matrix and thickening of the glomerular basement membrane on light microscopy, with dense subepithelial deposits and increased mesangial matrix on electron microscopy. Immunofluorescence showed deposits of complement and IgG in the basement membrane and mesangium. In a more recent study, Helin et al. examined renal biopsy specimens from 39 patients with RA and found signs of mild mesangial glomerulopathy in 11 patients; 2 of these patients had received neither gold nor penicillamine therapy [52]. Two additional publications described mesangial and membranous glomerulopathy in patients with RA not related to gold or penicillamine therapy [55, 103]. This lesion may be a cause of low-grade hematuria and proteinuria in rheumatoid patients.

Kelly et al. followed 21 patients who had isolated hematuria and mesangial nephropathy for a mean period of 7.7 years; 19 of these patients had no change in their renal function over the period of follow-up [61]. Two patients developed severe renal impairment, but both of these patients had significant additional renal disease at the time of initial biopsy. It thus appears that the natural history of isolated mesangial and/or membranous nephropathy associated with RA is benign. In a recent report by Pollet et al., mesangial nephropathy unrelated to drug therapy was described and the literature reviewed [87]. These authors speculated that mesangial nephropathy may be a common manifestation of RA and may arise as a result of clearance of RF–containing immune complexes by the renal mesangial matrix.

Proliferative glomerulonephritis is a rare cause of renal disease in RA. Davis and co-workers reviewed the records of 5,232 patients with the diagnosis of RA who were hospitalized over a 22-year period [27]. Proliferative glomerulonephritis was diagnosed in only 4 patients, all of whom met the criteria for SLE or mixed connective tissue disease. However, they did report a well-documented case of proliferative glomerulonephritis in RA in the absence of any other disorder [27]. Although this patient was on gold therapy at the time of the renal biopsy, proteinuria and hematuria both preceded initiation of gold therapy. The renal biopsy showed mesangial hypercellularity along with proliferative changes in the glomeruli, and electron microscopy revealed subendothelial deposits. The authors raised the question as to why a proliferative glomerulonephritis is not seen more often in RA since circulating immune complexes frequently are present in this disease. Weisman and Zvaifler speculated that reduced complement-fixing ability of the immune complexes in RA might explain the paucity of renal lesions [135]. However, the explanation as to why immune complex nephritis is not seen more often in RA remains unclear [73].

In summary, early studies describing a rheumatoid glomerulopathy are clouded by the inclusion of patients with diseases other than RA and by the inclusion of patients taking a variety of nephrotoxic drugs. Once these confounding variables are removed, it appears that proliferative glomerulonephritis is extremely rare in RA, occurring only in isolated cases. A mild form of mesangial and membranous glomerulopathy does appear to occur in RA independent of drug therapy. Functionally, this disease is usually mild, presents with microscopic hematuria and low-grade proteinuria, and follows a benign course. Thus, the decrease in renal function in RA described by Sorenson and others does not appear to be directly related to a specific lesion but is probably multifactorial.

Vascular Lesions. Systemic vasculitis is the most feared of all the complications of RA and is associated with an appreciable morbidity and mortality. Schmid and co-workers described 34 patients with RA in whom extraarticular disease was present [99]. The most common clinical symptoms were peripheral neuritis in 16 patients, episcleritis and pericarditis in 5, and hypertension in 4. Eight patients in their series were found to have proteinuria (24 percent), and this occurred in 43 percent of patients with extraarticular manifestations of RA summarized from the literature. No mention was made, however, of impaired renal function in any patient. Scott et al. reviewed 50 cases of systemic rheumatoid vasculitis; 12 (24 percent) of their cases had clinical features of renal disease [102]. Four patients had amyloidosis, 2 had chronic renal failure of undetermined cause, and 6 developed proteinuria or hematuria when typical lesions of cutaneous vasculitis appeared. Renal function was not impaired in these 6 patients. In a later study from the same group, 45 patients with systemic rheumatoid vasculitis were studied. No mention was made of any renal involvement in these patients.

There are, however, a few reports in which patients with RA developed a polyarteritislike clinical syndrome with renal vessel involvement. A case report described a patient with rheumatoid vasculitis who presented with abdominal pain and had intrarenal aneurysms on arteriography [74]. Ball reported 5 cases with rheumatoid arthritis and diffuse vasculitis [6]. Only 1 of the 5 patients had clinical renal involvement during life, but all had microscopic evidence of renal artery vasculitis. Two other cases, reported as clinicopathologic conferences in the *New England Journal of Medicine*, involved patients with RA, vasculitis, and rapidly progressive renal failure [65, 95]. Autopsy revealed acute and healing renal vasculitis and/or glomerulonephritis in both patients.

Tubulointerstitial Lesions. Tubulointerstitial disease of the kidneys is common in RA. However, the primary cause of these changes is Sjögren's syndrome, which is seen as a secondary manifestation in up to 50 percent of RA patients. The renal lesions of Sjögren's syndrome will be discussed later in this chapter. Another major cause of tubulointerstitial disease in RA is the use of nonsteroidal antiinflammatory drugs (NSAIDs). While interstitial nephritis may occur with any of these agents, it appears to be most frequently associated with fenoprofen. Investigators examining renal changes in biopsy or autopsy specimens described some degree of interstitial fibrosis in 20 to 46 percent of rheumatoid patients [20, 88]. However, none of these studies excluded patients taking NSAIDs or patients with Sjögren's syndrome. It is therefore unclear as to whether RA itself causes a tubulointerstitial lesion distinct from that associated with drugs or Sjögren's syndrome.

RENAL DISORDERS RELATED TO DRUG THERAPY

NSAIDs/Salicylates. NSAIDs are the mainstay of treatment of RA. The antiinflammatory properties of these drugs result, in part, from their ability to inhibit cyclooxygenase, one of the major enzymes involved in the synthesis of prostaglandins. Inhibition of renal prostaglandin synthesis by NSAIDs may result in reduced glomerular blood flow and elevation of serum creatinine levels [23] (discussed in more detail in Chap. 44). In addition to this reversible rise in serum creatinine, NSAIDs can also cause an interstitial nephritis. Interstitial nephritis has also been shown to be reversible when the drugs are discontinued (see Chap. 44). While all NSAIDs and salicylates [26] can induce a rise in serum creatinine and/or an interstitial nephritis, there is some evidence that sulindac may result in a less severe decrease in renal blood flow than found with other NSAIDs [21, 22, 138]. This point is controversial, however [89], and all NSAIDs should be regarded as potential inducers of renal dysfunction. As mentioned previously, the use of these drugs has made analysis of renal lesions in RA more difficult to interpret. Practically, when a patient with RA presents with evidence of decreased renal function or interstitial changes, discontinuation of NSAIDs should be one of the first steps before further diagnostic or therapeutic maneuvers are undertaken.

Analgesic Nephropathy. Analgesic nephropathy is characterized by a combination of papillary necrosis and interstitial nephritis (see Chap. 44). This type of injury is most widely attributed to phenacetin but may also be seen with NSAIDs [79, 98]. Papillary necrosis has been reported in association with ibuprofen, phenylbutazone, fenoprofen, and mefenamic acid as well as with several combinations of NSAIDs. The risk of rheumatoid patients developing analgesic nephropathy appears to be lower than would be expected on the basis of their regular consumption of NSAIDs [11]. This may be due to less frequent use of analgesic combinations or to more close physician monitoring. However, the frequency of subclinical renal disorders in patients with RA should raise the possibility that chronic NSAID therapy may cause some additional degree of renal damage.

Renal Lesions Associated with Gold Therapy. Gold salts have been advocated for the treatment of many diseases including pulmonary tuberculosis. In the belief that tuberculosis and RA had a common infectious etiology, Forestier used gold salts in the treatment of RA [38]. He noted improvement in 70 to 80 percent of over 500 cases, a finding that has been confirmed in multiple studies since that time. Gold injections are used primarily in patients with active synovitis after salicylates and/or NSAIDs have failed to control the disease. It is referred to as a "disease-modifying drug" since some studies have shown healing of bone erosions after its use [35]. The clinical effects of weekly gold injections do not develop until after 3 to 6 months of therapy, and the patient must be kept on maintenance monthly injections for years. Recent studies have shown that relatively few patients are able to remain on gold therapy for the long term, however, due to the cumulative incidence of side effects, including nephropathy, bone marrow suppression, rash, and stomatitis. The introduction of an oral form of gold (auranofin) in the early 1980s has decreased the frequency of side effects only minimally [53].

Clinically, the hallmark of renal toxicity from gold is proteinuria, occurring in 3 to 25 percent of RA patients receiving gold injections [25, 40, 41, 53, 104, 111]. While microscopic hematuria can accompany proteinuria, isolated hematuria or the appearance of cellular casts is rare and should prompt an investigation into other causes of renal disease. Nephrotic syndrome develops in up to one-third of patients with gold-induced proteinuria [11]. The onset of proteinuria is most common 4 to 6 months after the initiation of gold therapy (total dose 1,000–1,500 mg), although it may occur at any time during therapy. Furthermore, the severity of proteinuria is not proportional to the dose of gold received. The frequency of proteinuria in patients receiving oral gold (auranofin) appears to be very similar to the frequency in those patients receiving injectable gold [53].

The natural history of gold nephropathy has been studied extensively by Hall et al. [46–49]; the proteinuria resolves gradually with discontinuation of gold. Proteinuria resolved by 21 months in all 21 patients studied, with the mean time to resolution of proteinuria being 11 months [47]. In those patients who developed the nephrotic syndrome, treatment with a high-protein diet and diuretics was sufficient to control the symptoms; steroids were not required. No changes in creatinine clearance were observed in any patient during or after the resolution of proteinuria. Hall and Tighe examined the outcome of nephropathy when gold was continued after the onset of proteinuria [49]. Follow-up of these patients indicated an identical pattern of resolution of renal disease even when discontinuation of gold was delayed for up to 11 months after the onset of proteinuria. Indeed, a number of reports suggest that the continuation of gold after proteinuria develops does not necessarily lead to progressive proteinuria and renal deterioration. However, it is recommended that gold therapy be discontinued if proteinuria develops, since a number of alternative agents that are not nephrotoxic are now available for the treatment of RA.

The renal histology associated with gold-induced proteinuria and the nephrotic syndrome have been studied in detail over the past 30 years. In 1965 Lee and co-workers performed biopsies on three patients receiving gold who developed proteinuria [66]. They described changes consistent with membranous glomerulopathy in the basement membrane by light microscopy in one and by electron microscopy in all three. Vaamonde and Hunt reviewed the world's literature on patients with nephrotic syndrome secondary to gold therapy [131]. When available for study, renal tissue demonstrated membranous glomerulopathy as the predominant lesion in all patients. In a recent study, membranous glomerulopathy was demonstrated in 15 of 21 patients with gold-induced proteinuria, and increased mesangial matrix was present in 4 and minimal change nephropathy in 2 [47].

Silverberg and co-workers described subepithelial deposits on electron microscopy in patients receiving gold who developed the nephrotic syndrome [111], a finding also noted by Törnroth and Skrifvars [127]. When the disease was of short duration the only changes noted were subepithelial deposits on electron microscopy. With long-standing disease, however, basement membrane thickening could be detected on light microscopy. Of interest was the finding by Silverberg et al. that light and electron microscopy as well as histochemical studies revealed no difference in the site or degree of deposition of gold particles in the kidney, whether or not proteinuria was present. These observations suggest that gold nephropathy is an immune complex disease.

A potential explanation for the finding of proteinuria in only some patients with RA receiving gold has been offered by Wooley et al. [141]. They found that 14 of 15 episodes of gold-induced proteinuria occurred in patients who possessed the HLA antigens B8 and DR3. The relative risk of proteinuria during gold therapy was increased 32 times in patients with the DR3 antigen. Recent studies have confirmed the association of the HLA-B8/DR3 haplotype with gold-induced proteinuria, but have suggested a less strong correlation than was originally described [47]. Two possible explanations exist for the development of proteinuria. The first relates to the high nonspecific antibody responsiveness found in many patients with the B8/DR3 haplotype. For example, patients with RA bearing the B8/DR3 haplotype may have higher levels of circulating immune complexes. If gold inhibits removal of these complexes from the circulation, nephrotoxic levels of complexes could accumulate.

A second possible explanation is that gold may serve as a hapten leading to the formation of autoantibodies directed against proteins that have been altered by the drug. Patients with DR3 tend to form autoantibodies more readily and may therefore form immune complexes in the kidney, eventually resulting in membranous glomerulopathy.

Although these explanations are highly speculative, it appears that gold-induced glomerulopathy is mediated by immune complexes and is more prevalent in those patients with a genetic background that predisposes them to the development of autoantibodies and other autoimmune diseases. The association of gold-induced nephropathy with the B8/DR3 haplotype may also help to explain the predilection of patients with gold nephropathy to develop renal disease when treated subsequently with penicillamine, since penicillamine nephrotoxicity is associated with the same haplotype (see below). However, the relative risk of developing gold nephropathy in patients with the B8/DR3 haplotype does not merit HLA typing in rheumatoid patients before instituting gold therapy.

Renal Lesions Associated with Penicillamine Therapy. Penicillamine was introduced into clinical medicine in the 1950s for the treatment of Wilson's disease [134]. Within a few years it had been tried in RA and in the 1970s it became accepted as a disease-modifying drug. However, because of the recent addition of a number of other long-acting drugs to treat RA, the use of penicillamine has declined. Like gold therapy, penicillamine is also used after salicylates and/or NSAIDs have not controlled the disease; it is a slow-acting drug with responses generally not observed until after 3 to 6 months of therapy [43, 54, 119].

Clinically and histologically, penicillamine-induced nephropathy is similar to gold nephropathy. The initial clinical manifestation is hematuria or proteinuria, occurring in 5 to 30 percent of patients receiving penicillamine; nephrotic syndrome occurs in one-third to two-thirds of patients who develop proteinuria [4, 7, 43, 48, 54]. The onset of proteinuria is usually within the first 12 months of therapy (average, 8 months), but it may occur at any time. Initial studies using high doses of penicillamine (> 1,000 mg/day) indicated a rapid onset of proteinuria and higher frequency of this complication [4, 43, 54]. With newer treatment regimens starting therapy at lower doses, toxicity has decreased but proteinuria has been reported at doses as low as 125 mg/day. In a recent study the mean dose of penicillamine in those patients who developed proteinuria was 625 mg/day [48]. The natural history of penicillamine nephropathy was recently studied [46, 48]. In 33 patients with penicillamine-induced proteinuria, this abnormality resolved spontaneously after the discontinuation of penicillamine, with the mean time to resolution being 8 months (range, 1–21 months). No patients demonstrated changes in creatinine clearance due to penicillamine and no patients required steroid therapy. Continuation of penicillamine after the onset of proteinuria has been shown to have a benign outcome, similar to gold [49]. Several investigators have advocated that penicillamine can be continued in patients with proteinuria if renal function is closely monitored. However, as with gold therapy, this seems rarely justified in light of other agents presently available for the treatment of RA.

Histologically, penicillamine-induced renal lesions appear similar to those of gold-induced nephropathy. In the studies by Hall and co-workers, 29 of 33 patients with proteinuria secondary to penicillamine had membranous glomerulonephritis, 2 of 33 had minimal-change nephropathy, and 2 of 33 had only mesangial changes [46, 47]. Previous studies by Dische et al. showed glomerular wall thickening and increased mesangial matrix [30]. Electron microscopy revealed subepithelial deposits, similar to what was seen in gold-induced nephropathy or idiopathic membranous glomerulonephritis. The genetic predisposition to membranous glomerulopathy seen with gold therapy is also present with penicillamine. In one series, 9 of 13 patients with penicillamine-induced proteinuria were positive for the HLA-B8/DR3 haplotype [141].

In summary, although the pathogenesis of gold- or penicillamine-induced glomerulopathy is incompletely understood, the most likely hypothesis is that this is an immunologically mediated disease in which immune complexes form locally. These complexes may be a result of the induction of antibodies directed against renal constituents. The predisposition of patients with the B8/DR3 haplotype to develop nephropathy with gold or penicillamine therapy is thought to occur because of a predilection for these patients to develop autoantibodies when treated with these medications.

Cyclosporine. Cyclosporine is an immunosuppressive agent that primarily affects T cells, and has been used for a number of years in transplantation medicine to prevent allograft rejection [78]. Over the past 5 years it has been used with increased frequency in patients with autoimmune diseases including RA. A number of studies have shown that cyclosporine may be beneficial in refractory RA [1, 32, 33, 39, 70, 132, 143]. However, like gold and penicillamine, cyclosporine is a slow-acting drug and its use should be reserved for those patients who have not responded to more conventional therapy. The major factor preventing more widespread trials of cyclosporine in RA has been nephrotoxicity, which has been reported to occur in 30 to 70 percent of patients receiving this drug [8, 69, 78]. The mechanism of cyclosporine nephrotoxicity is not clear but appears to be primarily vascular, resulting in decreased glomerular filtration rate, decreased creatinine clearance, increased serum creatinine, hypertension, and hyperkalemia [58, 78]. The severity and frequency with which nephrotoxicity occurs are directly related to the dose of cyclosporine administered. Gordon et al. reported that nephrotoxicity correlated best with trough serum levels of cyclosporine [45]. Patients displaying cyclosporine nephrotoxicity showed trough levels greater than 200 ng/ml; 96 percent of patients who developed impaired renal function due to cyclosporine had trough levels greater than or equal to 250 ng/ml.

In RA, treatment regimens employing 2.5 to 10.0 mg/kg/day have been investigated. Berg et al. showed that patients receiving 5 mg/kg/day had a mean increase in serum creatinine of 19.7 percent and a decrease in creatinine clearance of 22 percent [8]. Patients receiving 10 mg/kg/day had a mean increase in serum creatinine of 59.5 percent. Renal dysfunction usually occurred within 2 to 3 weeks after the initiation of therapy and remained stable during the full course of treatment. After discontinuation of therapy, serum creatinine levels improved but remained slightly above baseline for up to 12 weeks. Of note is that in patients taking NSAIDs with cyclosporine, serum creatinine levels increased by 40 percent, whereas in patients taking no NSAIDs, serum creatinine levels increased by only 16.6 percent. Mean arterial blood pressure may also increase in patients taking cyclosporine, but blood pressure was elevated in only 5 of 24 patients. In addition, a clinically significant increase in serum potassium was observed. Dougados et al. recently studied 26 rheumatoid patients taking 5 mg/kg/day of cyclosporine and compared them with 26 patients receiving placebo over a 4-month time period [32, 33]. Serum creatinine levels increased by greater than 50 percent over baseline values in 13 of the 26 patients and there was a mean rise in plasma creatinine of 26 percent in the cyclosporine study group. Hypertension was not described in this group and only 1 of the 26 patients was forced to withdraw from the study because of nephrotoxicity. In a follow-up of RA patients treated with cyclosporine, Boers et al. demonstrated that renal function remained stable for up to 2 years after discontinuation of the drug [15]; no improvement was noted in those patients who had developed renal impairment, but no further deterioration occurred.

In summary, cyclosporine is still an experimental drug in RA. If prescribed, it should be used at a low initial dosage and plasma creatinine levels should be closely monitored during the course of therapy. Cyclosporine dosage should be decreased if serum creatinine levels increase by greater than 50 percent over baseline levels or above 150 μm/liter. Concurrent use of NSAIDs should be discouraged since this may exacerbate nephrotoxicity. Cyclosporine should be used with extreme caution in older patients with RA or in patients with preexisting hypertension or renal disease. Adjustment of cyclosporine dosage based on serum creatinine levels or (preferably) on trough plasma cyclosporine levels is mandatory to minimize renal toxicity.

Renal Disease in Juvenile Rheumatoid Arthritis

Juvenile rheumatoid arthritis (JRA) is defined as an inflammatory arthropathy occurring in individuals less than 16 years old. JRA can be divided into three subsets: (1) polyarticular arthritis, which resembles adult RA; (2) pauciarticular arthritis, which primarily affects young females and is associated with chronic iritis; and (3) systemic onset disease (Still's disease), characterized by fever, leukocytosis, splenomegaly, and serositis. Clinically significant renal disease in children with any of the forms of JRA is rare, although as in adults, proteinuria, hematuria, and amyloidosis have been reported. Studies in children suffer from the same problems as studies in adults with RA; frequently the effects of drug therapy are not separated from the effects of the disease itself.

In the largest study to date Anttila studied 165 children with JRA treated in Finland between 1967 and 1970 [2]. Proteinuria was observed in 42.5 percent of the children on at least one occasion during the 3-year period. Persistent proteinuria, however, occurred in only 4 patients or 2.4 percent of the total patient population. None of the children developed the nephrotic syndrome, although on biopsy 2 were found to have amyloidosis as a cause of proteinuria. Hematuria was found in 38 cases (23 percent). Seven of these children had two or more episodes of hematuria, while 31 had only one episode. Of the 7 cases with more than one episode of hematuria, amyloidosis was present in 2 cases, coagulopathy in 1, and 4 patients were receiving treatment with gold. Repeated episodes of pyuria occurred in 10 children, or 6 percent of the JRA patients. Creatinine clearance was diminished in 5.6 percent of the group who had only joint symptoms and in 18.5 percent of the group who had extraarticular manifestations of JRA. Creatinine clearance was more often depressed in patients receiving salicylate therapy.

Renal biopsies were performed on 57 of the 165 patients with JRA and autopsy specimens were obtained from 3 patients. Amyloidosis was observed in one biopsy and one autopsy specimen. Except for proteinuria, hematuria, and pyuria, amyloidosis had not caused major impairment of renal function. Glomerular changes were observed in 17 biopsies or 28 percent of the cases. In 13 cases it was described as a "local glomerulitis," which would now be described as mesangial changes. Twelve of these 13 patients had proteinuria or hematuria. Other changes included mild basement membrane thickening in 4 patients and interstitial changes in 8. No vascular abnormalities were noted in any biopsy. Overall, approximately 40 percent of JRA patients had an abnormal kidney biopsy, although renal function was not significantly compromised in any patient.

Amyloidosis in JRA is the subject of many reports [28, 100, 128]. Of 1,272 patients with JRA, Schnitzer and Ansell observed 51 who had developed amyloidosis, a cumulative incidence of 4 percent [100]. A large amount of geographic variation in the incidence of amyloidosis in JRA has been reported. In North America the frequency is estimated to be as low as 0.1 percent, compared to 0.25 percent in France, 3 percent in Germany, and up to 10 percent in Poland [28, 128]. Because of the poor prognosis of amyloidosis associated with JRA, Schnitzer and Ansell initiated therapy with chlorambucil in selected patients in 1967 [100]. Several studies since that time have indicated that chlorambucil can improve survival and decrease renal disease in a significant percentage of these patients. An 8-year survival rate of 80 percent was reported for those patients given chlorambucil, as compared to 55 to 60 percent for those receiving intermittent or no chlorambucil therapy. In a recent study by Deschênes et al., 8 patients with JRA and systemic amyloidosis were treated with chlorambucil [28]. After a mean 10-year follow-up period, 1 patient had died from renal disease, 2 had persistent nephrotic syndrome, and 5 were free of proteinuria or renal disease. It is of interest that the 3 patients who did poorly all had persistent activity of their arthritis, suggesting, as has been the experience in adult RA, that control of joint inflammation in JRA can improve renal amyloidosis.

In 1985 Stapleton et al. described 2 JRA patients who had hematuria, hypercalciuria, and urolithiasis [118]. They subsequently studied 38 children with JRA and found that 12 (32 percent) had increased urine calcium/creatinine ratios. Six of the 12 patients with hypercalciuria had hematuria, whereas only 3 of the 26 normocalciuric patients had hematuria. Detailed studies of calcium metabolism in 4 of the hypercalciuric patients showed normal serum calcium levels, normal parathyroid function, and no evidence of acidosis or vitamin D abnormalities. The authors speculated that the hypercalciuria in JRA may be due to immobilization and bone demineralization rather than to renal calcium wasting. In an earlier paper, Lorenz and Schnieder reported kidney stone formation in 6 of 89 German children with JRA [68]. Taken together, these reports suggest that hypercalciuria should be considered in the evaluation of children with JRA and that such children may be at risk for developing urolithiasis.

In conclusion, clinically significant renal disease in JRA is uncommon and reports of frequent proteinuria, hematuria, and mesangial nephropathy are clouded by the inclusion of patients taking a variety of nephrotoxic drugs. Renal amyloidosis can occur in JRA in frequencies ranging from as low as 0.1 percent in North America to 3 to 10 percent in Europe. There is some evidence that aggressive control of the inflammatory arthritis with chlorambucil in patients with amyloidosis can improve outcome. Finally, children with JRA may become hypercalciuric and be at risk for the development of renal stones.

Sjögren's Syndrome

Sjögren's syndrome is a chronic autoimmune disease characterized by the infiltration of lymphocytes into multiple organs, primarily the exocrine glands [60, 113, 121, 136]. The organs most frequently involved are the salivary and lacrimal glands, resulting in the clinical symptoms of dry eyes (keratoconjunctivitis sicca) and dry mouth (xerostomia). The presence of these two symptoms together is known as the sicca complex. While dry eyes and dry mouth are the major features of Sjögren's syndrome, in up to one-fourth of patients, other organs including the lung, gastrointestinal tract, pancreas, liver, central nervous system, and kidneys may also be infiltrated by lymphocytes. Infiltration of these organs results in varying degrees of organ dysfunction. Histologically, the infiltrating cells are CD4-positive T cells and B cells, leading to the hypothesis that Sjögren's syndrome may be triggered by an immune response to foreign antigens or altered self-antigens in the exocrine glands [77, 121]. Rarely, the lymphoid infiltrates may distort the normal architecture of the organ or of lymph nodes, resulting in a syndrome known as pseudolymphoma [122]. When this occurs, the distinction between benign and malignant tissue lesions can be difficult. Rarely, the lymphoid infiltrate may evolve into a malignant B-cell tumor.

In addition to the local cellular immune response, Sjögren's syndrome is characterized by the production of autoantibodies both to tissue-specific antigens (salivary duct antibody) and to non–tissue-specific antigens, such as antinuclear antibodies and RFs. Antibodies to two nuclear antigens, SS-A and SS-B, are particularly characteristic of this disease, although they may also be found in other autoimmune diseases including SLE. Patients with Sjögren's syndrome frequently have hypergammaglobulinemia and mild anemia indicative of a generalized inflammatory state [10, 60, 106].

The clinical and histologic complex known as Sjögren's syndrome can be broadly divided into two categories. Secondary Sjögren's syndrome occurs in conjunction with another autoimmune disease such as RA, SLE, or scleroderma. Primary Sjögren's syndrome is diagnosed when the symptom complex exists in isolation. Sjögren's syndrome has been reported to occur in up to 50 percent of patients with RA and is frequently seen in patients with SLE, mixed connective tissue disease, or progressive systemic sclerosis. In these diseases the presence of Sjögren's syndrome may be considered as an additional autoimmune feature of the underlying disease.

Primary Sjögren's syndrome, not associated with any other rheumatic disease, is characterized by the same histologic and clinical picture as is secondary Sjögren's syndrome. Like other autoimmune diseases, primary Sjögren's syndrome is more common in women, with the peak onset occurring in the 40- to 60-year age group.

RENAL ABNORMALITIES IN SJÖGREN'S SYNDROME

The renal abnormalities that have been described in Sjögren's syndrome arise as a result of either lymphocytic infiltration into the renal parenchyma or immune complex deposition in the glomeruli (Table 74-2). The renal abnormalities due to secondary Sjögren's syndrome are often minor in comparison to the renal abnormalities caused by primary rheumatic disease such as SLE or scleroderma [81]. For this reason the following discus-

Table 74-2. Renal abnormalities in Sjögren's syndrome

I. Tubulointerstitial disease
   A. Hyposthenuria
   B. Renal tubular acidosis
   C. Fanconi syndrome
   D. Interstitial nephritis
II. Glomerulonephritis

sion will focus on the renal abnormalities seen in primary Sjögren's syndrome. There is no evidence, however, that the renal abnormalities caused by primary Sjögren's syndrome differ in any way from those of secondary Sjögren's syndrome.

Tubular Dysfunction. Histologic studies of the kidneys in patients with Sjögren's syndrome have demonstrated mild to moderate interstitial infiltration of lymphocytes, with varying degrees of tubular atrophy and interstitial fibrosis [129]. Immunofluorescence studies of the infiltrating cells have indicated that they are CD4-positive T cells and B cells, a pattern identical to that seen in the exocrine glands [71, 93]. This pattern of cellular infiltration is different from that seen in many other forms of interstitial nephritis in which cytotoxic T cells are the predominant cell [71]. This finding has led several authors to postulate that the pathogenesis of renal disease in Sjögren's syndrome is similar to that seen in the salivary glands, and arises as a direct result of lymphocytic infiltration into the renal interstitium. The frequency with which lymphocytic infiltrates occur in the kidney in Sjögren's syndrome has not been extensively studied. Tu et al. studied 9 patients with Sjögren's syndrome and found interstitial changes in 6 [129]. There are numerous other small series of patients with Sjögren's syndrome and abnormal renal biopsy specimens, but while the presence of interstitial infiltrates appears to be common, the exact frequency cannot be determined from the present literature.

Clinically, renal dysfunction in Sjögren's syndrome is usually mild and subclinical. The most frequently reported functional abnormalities are hyposthenuria, renal tubular acidosis (RTA), Fanconi syndrome, and interstitial nephritis.

HYPOSTHENURIA. In 1962, a patient with Sjögren's syndrome who had nephrogenic diabetes insipidus was reported. Detailed studies on 8 additional patients demonstrated that 4 had a persistently impaired ability to concentrate urine with water deprivation [59]. This defect was not associated with proteinuria or other clinically apparent renal abnormalities. In 1965 Shearn and Tu reported a case of a young woman whose presenting manifestation of Sjögren's syndrome was vasopressin-resistant nephrogenic diabetes insipidus [107]. Her polydipsia and polyuria antedated the symptoms of dryness of the eyes and mouth by 10 years. Although hyposthenuria may exist as an isolated abnormality in Sjögren's syndrome, in many of the reported cases it has been associated with other tubular abnormalities including renal tubular acidosis and aminoaciduria.

RENAL TUBULAR ACIDOSIS. Distal RTA (type 1) has been reported to occur in up to 20 to 25 percent of patients with Sjögren's syndrome [120], and proximal RTA (type II) can also occur (although less frequently). Shearn and Tu used an acid-loading test to detect latent RTA in 10 patients with Sjögren's syndrome who lacked overt abnormalities of acid-base balance [108]. They found impairment of acid excretion in 3 of the 10 patients studied. Many of these patients also demonstrated a defect in renal concentrating ability. Urinary acidification was impaired in 6 of 12 patients with Sjögren's syndrome studied by Talal and co-workers [123]. The RTA was clinically evident in 3 patients, subclinical in 2, and associated with glomerulonephritis in 1 patient. Creatinine clearance was not altered in those patients with RTA.

In the largest study to date, 17 patients with primary Sjögren's syndrome who had no apparent clinical renal disease were examined for the presence of renal tubular acidification defects by ammonium chloride loading [109]. Seven (41 percent) of the 17 patients had an impaired ability to acidify the urine. In addition, 10 of 17 patients had an abnormal concentrating ability. The presence of RTA and abnormal concentrating ability did not necessarily correlate with one another, suggesting that Sjögren's syndrome may affect tubular function at multiple functional and anatomic sites. Siamopoulos et al. studied 15 patients with primary Sjögren's syndrome and demonstrated RTA in 5 (33 percent) with acid loading [110].

Hypergammaglobulinemia has also been associated with RTA [44, 72, 75, 83]. Morris and Fudenberg examined renal acidification in 22 patients with hypergammaglobulinemia and found impaired acidification in 12 of these patients [75]. Six were also noted to have impaired concentrating ability. Only 2 of the patients with hypergammaglobulinemia and abnormal tubular function had Sjögren's syndrome, suggesting that hypergammaglobulinemia may be an independent risk factor for tubular dysfunction. It is unlikely, however, that the development of RTA in Sjögren's syndrome is simply due to the associated hypergammaglobulinemia. Shioji and co-workers investigated 4 patients with Sjögren's syndrome complicated by RTA and 10 with Sjögren's syndrome without this complication [112]. Hypergammaglobulinemia was observed in 3 of 4 patients with RTA but was also found in the majority of patients without RTA. Thus, while hypergammaglobulinemia may contribute to tubular dysfunction in Sjögren's syndrome, it is probably not the only cause. Tubular dysfunction also can occur in the absence of hypergammaglobulinemia and tubular dysfunction is frequently not present despite significant degrees of hypergammaglobulinemia. Abnormal tubular function may, in large part, be due to lymphocytic infiltration into the renal interstitium.

OTHER TUBULAR DEFECTS. The Fanconi syndrome (aminoaciduria, glycosuria, and phosphaturia) has been reported in several patients with Sjögren's syndrome [133], although it appears to be uncommon. In Shiozawa's study, 6 of 17 patients with Sjögren's syndrome showed decreased tubular reabsorption of phosphate [109].

INTERSTITIAL NEPHRITIS. Although infiltration of the interstitium with lymphocytes is common in Sjögren's syndrome, severe interstitial nephritis resulting in impaired creatinine clearance is relatively rare. Gentric et al. recently reported on 5 patients with primary Sjögren's syndrome who developed severe interstitial nephritis with decreased creatinine clearance, proteinuria, and hematuria [42]. Two patients eventually required chronic hemodialysis, but 3 patients improved after taking corticosteroids. A recent case report by Rosenberg et al. described marked improvement in Sjögren's interstitial nephropathy with intravenous methylprednisolone [92]. Three other cases of severe interstitial nephritis have been reported in the literature [42, 129, 140]. However, this seems to be an unusual complication of Sjögren's syndrome.

Glomerulonephritis. Glomerulonephritis is rare in patients with primary Sjögren's syndrome, with only scattered cases reported in the literature [63, 76, 85, 96, 101]. Of these, approximately half have been membranous glomerulonephritis and half, membranoproliferative glomerulonephritis. These patients presented with either heavy proteinuria, active urinary sentiment, or renal insufficiency. Because of the rarity of glomerulonephritis in primary Sjögren's syndrome, the occurrence of nephritis should raise the question of an associated connective tissue disease such as SLE. Renal biopsy specimens in patients with Sjögren-associated glomerulonephritis have shown glomerular deposits of IgG and C3 on immunofluorescence studies [76]. Treatment with corticosteroids and cytotoxic drugs has been reported to be successful in some patients [63].

In summary, some form of renal involvement can occur in up to 50 percent of patients with Sjögren's syndrome. Inability to concentrate the urine, RTA, and other tubular dysfunctions can be demonstrated frequently with stress testing. However, clinically significant tubular dysfunction appears to be much less frequent. Severe interstitial nephritis resulting in renal insufficiency is rare. Glomerulonephritis is distinctly unusual and its presence should prompt consideration of an underlying connective tissue disorder in addition to the Sjögren's syndrome.

Polymyositis-Dermatomyositis

The inflammatory myopathies are a group of diseases in which the muscles are diffusely damaged by a perivascular and/or interstitial infiltration of inflammatory cells which are predominantly lymphocytes. The clinical syndrome associated with these pathologic changes is termed *polymyositis.* Although this syndrome is frequently pleomorphic in presentation, the cardinal feature in essentially all patients (98 percent) is muscle weakness. When the syndrome occurs in association with characteristic skin lesions it is termed *dermatomyositis.*

Five clinical or laboratory abnormalities are present in most patients with polymyositis and dermatomyositis and thus are used to define or diagnose the disease. The first criterion is symmetrical proximal muscle weakness, which is the initial manifestation in up to 69 percent of patients and is present overall in 98 percent at some time during the course of the disease. The second criterion is abnormal electromyographic (EMG) findings, present in 90 percent of patients. The third criterion is elevated serum muscle enzymes (creatine phosphokinase [CPK], aldolase), found in 95 percent of patients with myositis. The fourth criterion is the muscle biopsy, which should show evidence of necrosis of type 1 and type 2 muscle fibers, areas of degeneration and regeneration of fibers, phagocytosis, and an interstitial or perivascular inflammatory process. The fifth criterion consists of the characteristic skin changes seen in dermatomyositis. These include an erythematous, scaly involvement of the face, neck, and shawl area and the extensor surfaces of the knees, elbows, and medial malleoli; the heliotrope rash (a periorbital violaceous discoloration, often with associated edema), and Gottron's papules (scaly erythematous flat plaques over the dorsum of the metacarpophalangeal and proximal interphalangeal joints).

Although a number of different classification schemes of polymyositis-dermatomyositis have been suggested, that proposed by Bohan and Peter [16, 17] is the most widely used (Table 74-3).

Organ systems other than skin and muscle may be involved in patients with dermatomyositis or polymyositis. This is true even when those patients with overlap syndrome (group V) are excluded. The more common organ systems involved include the joints, with up to 35 percent of patients having some type of joint complaint. Gastrointestinal manifestations are also common, with involvement of both the proximal and distal esophagus in adults and abdominal crisis secondary to vasculitis sometimes seen in children [16, 17, 84]. Pulmonary involvement may be found in up to 50 percent of patients, with interstitial lung disease the most common abnormality [29]. Cardiac manifestations also occur, with reports of mild carditis occurring in up to 25 percent of patients in some series.

RENAL DISEASE

Involvement of the kidneys in polymyositis-dermatomyositis is distinctly uncommon and in fact is not mentioned in some references or chapters on polymyositis-dermatomyositis in standard textbooks [19, 90]. Some of the earlier references to renal disease with dermatomyositis have reported on patients who would now be rediagnosed as having mixed connective tissue disease. When examined carefully, all were found to have either scleroderma or SLE in association with myositis [81, 124]. Sheard reported proteinuria in up to 75 percent of patients with dermatomyositis but apparently found no evidence of impaired renal function [105]. More recently, Dyck et al. identified 5 patients with primary idiopathic polymyositis who had developed proteinuria associated with urine sediment abnormalities [34]. Renal biopsies

Table 74-3. Classification of polymyositis or dermatomyositis

Group I.	Primary idiopathic polymyositis
Group II.	Primary idiopathic dermatomyositis
Group III.	Dermatomyositis or polymyositis associated with malignancy
Group IV.	Childhood dermatomyositis or polymyositis often associated with vasculitis
Group V.	Dermatomyositis or polymyositis associated with another connective tissue disease

from these patients showed a focal mesangial proliferative glomerulonephritis with deposits of both immunoglobulin and complement. After treatment of the polymyositis with corticosteroids, the proteinuria and urine sediment changes disappeared as the muscle disease improved. These authors speculated that immune complexes may be implicated in the etiology of this renal disease, although serum complement studies and serum cryoglobulins were normal in all patients except one.

Membranous glomerulopathy is reported in up to 10 percent of all malignancies [94]. A case report by Rose describes a 58-year-old woman who presented with the nephrotic syndrome with renal biopsy features typical of membranous glomerulopathy [91]. Within the next year she developed dermatomyositis, and shortly thereafter an oat cell tumor was found in her lung. The relationship between these three conditions is unclear, although some interesting speculations are possible. Membranous nephropathy is thought to be an immune complex disease, which in this case may have resulted from the deposition of immune complexes induced by the tumor. Likewise, dermatomyositis is known to exhibit both humoral and cell-mediated abnormalities. In this patient soluble immune complexes could have formed between tumor antigens and antibodies that cross-reacted with muscle. Thus, membranous glomerulonephritis may be seen in conjunction with polymyositis-dermatomyositis because both may be associated with an underlying neoplasm (group III).

Myoglobinemia and myoglobinuria were first recognized in approximately 50 percent of a group of patients with dermatomyositis and polymyositis [57]. Their presence was associated with renal failure in 2 of the patients. In another study of patients with dermatomyositis and polymyositis, myoglobin was detected in 74 percent of sera taken from patients with active myositis prior to the initiation of treatment [56]. Most patients demonstrated rapid reduction in the level of sera myoglobin with prednisone therapy, usually before enzyme values had returned to normal. Kessler et al. reported a case of myoglobinuric acute renal failure in a 30-year-old woman with acute dermatomyositis [62]. Her kidney biopsy revealed degenerative and necrotic changes in the tubular epithelium with pigmented casts noted in the lumen of some tubules. The glomeruli were entirely normal. A similar case was described by Sloan and co-workers in which a 56-year-old man with polymyositis developed dark urine and acute renal failure [114]. Renal biopsy showed normal glomeruli but "myoglobin" casts in the tubules. With prednisone and dialysis both muscles and kidneys returned to normal.

Childhood dermatomyositis (group IV) is frequently associated with vasculitis involving the muscles and gastrointestinal tract. Bitnum et al. studied 13 children with dermatomyositis and performed percutaneous renal biopsy in 6 of these children because of proteinuria [9]. All six of the biopsies were abnormal, showing mild to moderate cellular proliferation of the glomerular tuft. In 2 patients the glomerular basement membrane was also thickened. The authors were unsure of the implications of their findings but did note that none of the patients developed signs of clinical renal failure. Others have also demonstrated diffuse glomerular changes in patients with juvenile dermatomyositis [31]. As in Bitnum's study [9], these authors also found that renal function was maintained, although proteinuria was present in the children.

In summary, renal involvement in dermatomyositis-polymyositis is distinctly uncommon. It may occur in the setting of another connective tissue disease (group V) in which the renal lesion is found to be that of either scleroderma or SLE, and membranous glomerulonephritis may occur in association with malignancy (group III). In acute fulminant myositis, tubular dysfunction or acute renal failure may be associated with myoglobinemia and myoglobinuria. This usually responds to treatment of the myositis, however, and progression to chronic renal disease is rare.

References

1. Amor, B., and Dougados, M. Cyclosporine: Therapeutic effects in rheumatic diseases. *Transplant. Proc.* 20(Suppl.): 218, 1988.
2. Anttila, R. Renal involvement in juvenile rheumatoid arthritis—a clinical and histopathological study. *Acta Paediatr. Scand. (Suppl.)* 227: 3, 1972.
3. Arapakis, G., and Tribe, C. R. Amyloidosis in rheumatoid arthritis investigated by means of rectal biopsy. *Ann. Rheum. Dis.* 22: 256, 1963.
4. Bacon, P. A., Tribe, C. R., Mackenzie, J. C., et al. Penicillamine nephropathy in rheumatoid arthritis. *Q. J. Med.* 45: 661, 1976.
5. Baggenstoss, A. H., and Rosenberg, E. F. Visceral lesions associated with chronic infectious (rheumatoid) arthritis. *Arch. Pathol.* 35: 503, 1948.
6. Ball, J. Rheumatoid arthritis and polyarteritis nodosa. *Ann. Rheum. Dis.* 13: 277, 1954.
7. Barraclough, D., Cunningham, T. J., and Muirden, K. D. Microscopic hematuria in patients with rheumatoid arthritis on D-penicillamine. *Aust. N.Z. J. Med.* 11: 706, 1981.
8. Berg, K. J., Forre, Ø., Djøseland, O., et al. Renal side effects of high and low cyclosporin A doses in patients with rheumatoid arthritis. *Clin. Nephrol.* 31: 232, 1989.
9. Bitnum, S., Daeschner, C. W., Jr., Travis, L. B., et al. Dermatomyositis. *J. Pediatr.* 64: 101, 1964.
10. Bloch, K. J., Wohl, M. J., Ship, I. I., et al. Sjögren's syndrome I. Serologic reactions in patients with Sjögren's syndrome with and without rheumatoid arthritis. *Arthritis Rheum.* 3: 287, 1960.
11. Boers, M. Renal disorders in rheumatoid arthritis. *Semin. Arthritis Rheum.* 20: 57, 1990.
12. Boers, M., Croonen, A. M., Dijkmans, B. A., et al. Renal findings in rheumatoid arthritis: Clinical aspects of 132 necropsies. *Ann. Rheum. Dis.* 46: 658, 1987.
13. Boers, M., Dijkmans, B. A. C., Breedveld, F. C., et al. Errors in the prediction of creatinine clearance in patients with rheumatoid arthritis. *Br. J. Rheumatol.* 27: 233, 1988.
14. Boers, M., Dijkmans, B. A. C., Breedveld, F. C., et al. Subclinical renal dysfunction in rheumatoid arthritis. *Arthritis Rheum.* 33: 95, 1990.
15. Boers, M., van Rijthoven, A. M., Goei Thè, H. S., et al. Serum creatinine levels two years later: Follow-up of a

placebo-controlled trial of cyclosporine in rheumatoid patients. *Transplant Proc.* 20(Suppl): 371, 1988.
16. Bohan, A., and Peter, J. B. Polymyositis and dermatomyositis. *N. Engl. J. Med.* 292: 344, 403, 1975.
17. Bohan, A., Peter, J. B., Bowman, R. L., et al. A computer-assisted analysis of 153 patients with polymyositis and dermatomyositis. *Medicine* 56: 255, 1977.
18. Bourke, B. E., Woodrow, D. F., and Scott, J. T. Proteinuria in rheumatoid arthritis—Drug-induced or amyloid? *Ann. Rheum. Dis.* 40: 240, 1981.
19. Bradley, W. G. Inflammatory Diseases of Muscle. In W. N. Kelley, E. D. Harris, Jr., S. Ruddy, et al. (eds.), *Textbook of Rheumatology* (3rd ed.). Philadelphia: Saunders, 1989.
20. Brun, C., Olsen, S., Raaschov, F., et al. Renal biopsy in rheumatoid arthritis. *Nephron* 2: 65, 1965.
21. Bunning, R. D., and Barth, W. F. Sulindac. *J.A.M.A.* 248: 2864, 1982.
22. Ciabattoni, G., Cinotti, G. A., Pierucci, A., et al. Effects of sulindac and ibuprofen in patients with chronic glomerular disease. *N. Engl. J. Med.* 310: 279, 1984.
23. Clive, D. M., and Stoff, J. S. Renal syndromes associated with nonsteroidal anti-inflammatory drugs. *N. Engl. J. Med.* 310: 563, 1984.
24. Cohen, A. H. Rheumatoid Arthritis and Acute Rheumatic Fever. In S. G. Massry and R. J. Glassock (eds.), *Textbook of Nephrology.* Baltimore: Williams & Wilkins, 1983.
25. The Cooperative Clinics Committee of the ARA. A controlled trial of gold salt therapy in rheumatoid arthritis. *Arthritis Rheum.* 16: 353, 1973.
26. Csuka, M. E., and McCarty, D. J. Aspirin and the treatment of rheumatoid arthritis. *Rheum. Dis. Clin. North Am.* 15: 439, 1989.
27. Davis, J. A., Cohen, A. H., Weisbart, R., et al. Glomerulonephritis in rheumatoid arthritis. *Arthritis Rheum.* 22: 1018, 1979.
28. Deschênes, G., Prieur, A. M., Hayem, F., et al. Renal amyloidosis in juvenile chronic arthritis: Evolution after chlorambucil treatment. *Pediatr. Nephrol.* 4: 463, 1990.
29. Dickey, B. F., and Meyers, A. R. Pulmonary disease in polymyositis/dermatomyositis. *Semin. Arthritis Rheum.* 14: 60, 1984.
30. Dische, F. E., Swinsox, D. R., Hamilton, E. B. D., et al. Immunopathology of penicillamine-induced glomerular disease. *J. Rheumatol.* 3: 145, 1976.
31. Dodge, W. F., Daeschner, C. W., Jr., Brennan, J. C., et al. Percutaneous renal biopsy in children—The collagen diseases, juvenile diabetes mellitus, and idiopathic hematuria and proteinuria. *Pediatrics* 30: 477, 1962.
32. Dougados, M., Awada, H., and Amor, B. Cyclosporin in rheumatoid arthritis: A double blind, placebo controlled study in 52 patients. *Ann. Rheum. Dis.* 47: 127, 1988.
33. Dougados, M., Duchesne, L., Awada, H., et al. Assessment of efficacy and acceptability of low dose cyclosporin in patients with rheumatoid arthritis. *Ann. Rheum. Dis.* 48: 550, 1989.
34. Dyck, R. F., Katz, A., Gordon, D. A., et al. Glomerulonephritis associated with polymyositis. *J. Rheumatol.* 6: 336, 1979.
35. Empire Rheumatism Council: Gold therapy in rheumatoid arthritis. *Ann. Rheum. Dis.* 19: 95, 1960.
36. Ennevarra, K., and Oka, M. Rheumatoid arthritis with amyloidosis. *Ann. Rheum. Dis.* 23: 131, 1964.
37. Fearnley, G. R., and Lackner, R. Amyloidosis in rheumatoid arthritis, and significance of "unexplained" albuminuria. *Br. Med. J.* I: 1129, 1955.
38. Forestier, J. Rheumatoid arthritis and its treatment by gold salts. *J. Lab. Clin. Med.* 20: 827, 1935.
39. Forre, Ø., Waalen, K., Rugstad, H. E., et al. Cyclosporine and rheumatoid arthritis. *Springer Semin. Immunopathol.* 10: 263, 1988.
40. Furst, D., Levine, S., Srenvasan, R., et al. A double-blind trial of high versus conventional dosages of gold salts for rheumatoid arthritis. *Arch. Rheum.* 20: 1473, 1977.
41. Ganley, C. J., Paget, S. A., and Reidenberg, M. M. Increased renal tubular cell excretion by patients receiving chronic therapy with gold and with nonsteroidal anti-inflammatory drugs. *Clin. Pharmacol. Ther.* 46: 51, 1989.
42. Gentric, A., Herve, J. P., Pennec, Y. L., et al. Severe renal involvement in primary Sjögren's syndrome. *Adv. Exp. Med. Biol.* 252: 73, 1989.
43. Golding, J. R., Wilson, J. V., and Day, A. T. Observations on the treatment of rheumatoid disease with penicillamine. *Postgrad. Med. J.* 46: 599, 1970.
44. Golding, P. L., and Mason, A. M. S. Hyperglobulinemic renal tubular acidosis: A report of nine cases. *Br. Med. J.* 3: 143, 1970.
45. Gordon, R. D., Iwatsuki, S., Shaw, B. W., Jr., et al. Cyclosporine-steroid combination therapy in 84 cadaveric renal transplants. *Am. J. Kidney Dis.* 5: 307, 1985.
46. Hall, C. L. The natural course of gold and penicillamine nephropathy: A long term study of 54 patients. *Adv. Exp. Med. Biol.* 252: 247, 1989.
47. Hall, C. L., Fothergill, N. J., Blackwell, M. M., et al. The natural course of gold nephropathy: Long term study of 21 patients. *Br. Med. J.* 295: 745, 1987.
48. Hall, C. L., Jawad, S., Harrison, P. R., et al. Natural course of penicillamine nephropathy: A long term study of 33 patients. *Br. Med. J.* 296: 1083, 1988.
49. Hall, C. L., and Tighe, R. The effect of continuing penicillamine and gold treatment on the course of penicillamine and gold nephropathy. *Br. J. Rheumatol.* 28: 53, 1989.
50. Harris, E. D., Jr. Rheumatoid Arthritis: The Clinical Spectrum. In W. N. Kelley, E. D. Harris, Jr., S. Ruddy, et al. (eds.), *Textbook of Rheumatology* (3rd ed.). Philadelphia: Saunders, 1989.
51. Heaney, D. J., Kupor, L. R., Gyorkey, F., et al. Membranous nephropathy associated with rheumatoid arthritis. *South. Med. J.* 71: 467, 1978.
52. Helin, H., Korpela, M., Mustonen, J., et al. Mild mesangial glomerulopathy—A frequent finding in rheumatoid arthritis patients with hematuria or proteinuria. *Nephron* 42: 224, 1986.
53. Heuer, M. A., Pietrusko, R. G., Morris, R. W., et al. An analysis of worldwide safety experience with auranofin. *J. Rheumatol.* 12: 695, 1985.
54. Hill, H. F. H. Treatment of rheumatoid arthritis with penicillamine. *Semin. Arthritis Rheum.* 6: 361, 1977.
55. Hordon, L. D., Sellars, L., Morley, A. R., et al. Haematuria in rheumatoid arthritis: An association with mesangial glomerulonephritis. *Ann. Rheum. Dis.* 43: 440, 1984.
56. Kagen, L. J. Myoglobinemia in inflammatory myopathies. *J.A.M.A.* 237: 1448, 1977.
57. Kagen, L. J. Myoglobinemia and myoglobulinemia in patients with myositis. *Arthritis Rheum.* 14: 457, 1971.
58. Kahan, B. D. Cyclosporine nephrotoxicity: Pathogenesis, prophylaxis, therapy, and prognosis. *Am. J. Kidney Dis.* 8: 323, 1986.

59. Kahn, M., Merritt, A. D., Wohl, M. J., et al. Renal concentrating defects in Sjögren's syndrome. *Ann. Intern. Med.* 56: 883, 1962.
60. Kassan, S. S., and Gardy, M. Sjögren's syndrome: An update and overview. *Am. J. Med.* 64: 1037, 1978.
61. Kelly, C. A., Mooney, P., Hordon, L. D., et al. Haematuria in rheumatoid arthritis: A follow up study. *Ann. Rheum. Dis.* 47: 993, 1988.
62. Kessler, E., Weinberger, I., and Rosenfeld, J. B. Myoglobinuric acute renal failure in a case of dermatomyositis. *Israel J. Med. Sci.* 8: 978, 1972.
63. Khan, M. A., Akhtar, M., and Taher, S. M. Membranoproliferative glomerulonephritis in a patient with primary Sjögren's syndrome. *Am. J. Nephrol.* 8: 235, 1988.
64. Laakso, M., Mutru, O., Isomäki, H., et al. Mortality from amyloidosis and renal diseases in patients with rheumatoid arthritis. *Ann. Rheum. Dis.* 45: 663, 1986.
65. Leaf, A. Case records of the Massachusetts General Hospital. *N. Engl. J. Med.* 272: 1069, 1965.
66. Lee, J. C., Dushken, M., Eyring, E. J., et al. Renal lesions associated with gold therapy—light and electron microscopic studies. *Arthritis Rheum.* 8: 1, 1965.
67. Light, P. D., and Hall-Craggs, M. Amyloid deposition in a renal allograft in a case of amyloidosis secondary to rheumatoid arthritis. *Am. J. Med.* 66: 532, 1979.
68. Lorenz, V. K., and Schneider, F. Nephrolithiasis bei juveniler rheumatoid-arthritis. *Kinderarztl. Prax.* 43: 450, 1975.
69. Ludwin, D., Bennett, K. J., Grace, E. M., et al. Nephrotoxicity in patients with rheumatoid arthritis treated with cyclosporine. *Transplant. Proc.* 20(Suppl.): 367, 1988.
70. Madhok, R., and Capell, H. A. Cyclosporine A in rheumatoid arthritis: Results in 30 months. *Transplant. Proc.* 20(Suppl.): 248, 1988.
71. Matsumura, R., Kondo, Y., Sugiyama, T., et al. Immunohistochemical identification of infiltrating mononuclear cells in tubulointerstitial nephritis associated with Sjögren's syndrome. *Clin. Nephrol.* 30: 335, 1988.
72. McCurdy, D. K., Cornwell, G. G., III, and DePratti, V. J. Hyperglobulinemic renal tubular acidosis. *Ann. Intern. Med.* 67: 110, 1967.
73. Miyazaki, M., Endoh, M., Suga, T., et al. Rheumatoid factors and glomerulonephritis. *Clin. Exp. Immunol.* 81: 250, 1990.
74. Moreland, L., DiBartolomeo, A., and Brick, J. Rheumatoid vasculitis with intrarenal aneurysm formation. *J. Rheumatol.* 15: 845, 1988.
75. Morris, R. C., Jr., and Fudenberg, H. H. Impaired renal acidification in patients with hypergammaglobulinemia. *Medicine* 46: 57, 1967.
76. Moutsopoulos, H. M., Balow, J. E., Lawley, T. J., et al. Immune complex glomerulonephritis in sicca syndrome. *Am. J. Med.* 64: 955, 1978.
77. Moutsopoulos, H. M., Chused, T. M., Mann, D. L., et al. Sjögren's syndrome (sicca syndrome): Current issues. *Ann. Intern. Med.* 92: 212, 1980.
78. Myers, B. D. Cyclosporine nephrotoxicity. *Kidney Int.* 30: 964, 1986.
79. Nanra, R. S. Pathology, aetiology and pathogenesis of analgesic nephropathy. *Aust. N.Z. Med.* 6(Suppl.): 33, 1976.
80. Nived, O., Sturfelt, G., Westling, H., et al. Is serum creatinine concentration a reliable index of renal function in rheumatic diseases? *Br. Med. J.* 286: 684, 1983.
81. O'Dell, J. R., Hays, R. C., Guggenheim, S. J., et al. Tubulo-interstitial disease in systemic lupus erythematosus. *Arch. Intern. Med.* 145: 1995, 1985.
82. Parkins, R. A., and Bywaters, E. G. L. Progression of amyloidosis secondary to rheumatoid arthritis. *Br. Med. J.* I: 536, 1959.
83. Pasternack, A., and Linder, E. Renal tubular acidosis: An immunopathological study on four patients. *Clin. Exp. Immunol.* 7: 115, 1970.
84. Pearson, C. M. Polymyositis and dermatomyositis. *Bull. Rheum. Dis.* 12: 269, 1962.
85. Perreau, P., Joubaud, F., Simard, C. L., et al. Syndrome de Gougerot-Sjögren et glomerulo-nephrite. *Semin. Hop. Paris* 48: 973, 1972.
86. Pollak, V. E., Pirani, C. L., Steck, I. E., et al. The kidney in rheumatoid arthritis: studies by renal biopsy. *Arthritis Rheum.* 5: 1, 1962.
87. Pollet, S., Depner, T., Moore, P., et al. Mesangial glomerulopathy and IgM rheumatoid factor in rheumatoid arthritis. *Nephron* 51: 107, 1989.
88. Raminez, G., Lambert, R., and Bloomer, H. A. Renal pathology in patients with rheumatoid arthritis. *Nephron* 29: 124, 1981.
89. Roberts, D. G., Gerber, J. G., Barnes, J. S., et al. Sulindac is not renal sparing in man. *Clin. Pharmacol. Ther.* 38: 258, 1985.
90. Rose, A. L., and Walton, J. N. Polymyositis: A survey of 89 cases with particular reference to treatment and prognosis. *Brain* 89: 747, 1966.
91. Rose, J. D. G. Membranous glomerulonephritis, dermatomyositis and bronchial carcinoma. *Br. Med. J.* 2: 641, 1979.
92. Rosenberg, A. M., Dyck, R. F., and George, D. H. Intravenous pulse methylprednisolone for the treatment of a child with Sjögren's nephropathy. *J. Rheumatol.* 17: 391, 1990.
93. Rosenberg, M. E., Schendel, P. B., McCurdy, F. A., et al. Characterization of immune cells in kidneys from patients with Sjögren's syndrome. *Am. J. Kidney Dis.* 11: 20, 1988.
94. Row, P. G., Cameron, J. S., Turner, D. R., et al. Membranous nephropathy. *Q. J. Med.* 44: 207, 1971.
95. Ruddy, S. Case records of the Massachusetts General Hospital. *N. Engl. J. Med.* 285: 1250, 1971.
96. Safar, M., Bariety, J., Lagrue, G., et al. Association D'Un syndrome nephrotique et D'un syndrome de Gougerot-Sjögren. *Semin. Hop. Paris* 24: 1425, 1964.
97. Salomon, M. I., Gallo, G., Poon, T. P., et al. The kidney in rheumatoid arthritis: A study based on renal biopsies. *Nephron* 12: 297, 1974.
98. Sandler, D. P., Smith, J. C., Weinberg, C. R., et al. Analgesic use and chronic renal disease. *N. Engl. J. Med.* 320: 1238, 1989.
99. Schmid, F. R., Cooper, N. S., Ziff, M., et al. Arthritis in rheumatoid arthritis. *Am. J. Med.* 30: 56, 1961.
100. Schnitzer, T. J., and Ansell, B. M. Amyloidosis in juvenile chronic polyarthritis. *Arthritis Rheum.* (Suppl.) 20: 245, 1977.
101. Schwartzberg, M., Burnstein, S. L., Calabro, J. J., et al. The development of membranous glomerulonephritis in a patient with rheumatoid arthritis and Sjögren's syndrome. *J. Rheumatol.* 6: 65, 1979.
102. Scott, D. G. I., Bacon, P. A., and Tribe, C. R. Systemic rheumatoid vasculitis: a clinical and laboratory study of 50 cases. *Medicine* 60: 288, 1981.
103. Sellars, L., Siamopoulos, K., Wilkinson, R., et al. Renal biopsy appearances in rheumatoid disease. *Clin. Nephrol.* 20: 114, 1983.
104. Sharp, J. T., Lidsky, M. D., Duggy, J., et al. Comparison

of two dosage schedules of gold salts in the treatment of rheumatoid arthritis. *Arthritis Rheum.* 20: 1179, 1977.
105. Sheard, C., Jr. Dermatomyositis. *Arch. Intern. Med.* 88: 640, 1951.
106. Shearn, M. A. Sjögren's syndrome. *Med. Clin. North Am.* 61: 271, 1977.
107. Shearn, M. A., and Tu, W. H. Nephrogenic diabetes insipidus and other defects of renal tubular function in Sjögren's syndrome. *Am. J. Med.* 39: 312, 1965.
108. Shearn, M. A., and Tu, W. H. Latent renal tubular acidosis in Sjögren's syndrome. *Ann. Rheum. Dis.* 27: 27, 1968.
109. Shiozawa, S., Shiozawa, K., Shimizu, S., et al. Clinical studies of renal disease in Sjögren's syndrome. *Ann. Rheum. Dis.* 46: 768, 1987.
110. Siamopoulos, K. C., Mavridis, A. K., Elisaf, M., et al. Kidney involvement in primary Sjögren's syndrome. *Scand. J. Rheumatol. Suppl.* 61: 156, 1986.
111. Silverberg, D. S., Kidd, E. G., Shnitka, T. K., et al. Gold nephropathy—a clinical and pathologic study. *Arthritis Rheum.* 13: 812, 1970.
112. Shioji, R., Furuyama, T., Onodera, S., et al. Sjögren's syndrome and renal tubular acidosis. *Am. J. Med.* 48: 456, 1970.
113. Sjögren, H. Zur Kenntis der Keraloconjunctivitis sicca. (Keratitio filemormis bei Hypunfunktion der Tranendrusen). *Acta Ophthalmol.* 11: 1, 1933.
114. Sloan, M. F., Franks, A. J., Exley, K. A., et al. Acute renal failure due to polymyositis. *Br. Med. J.* 1: 1457, 1978.
115. Sorensen, A. W. S. The Waaler-Rose test in patients suffering from rheumatoid arthritis in relationship to 24-hour endogenous creatinine clearance (III). *Acta Rheum. Scand.* 7: 304, 1961.
116. Sorensen, A. W. S. Investigation of the kidney function in rheumatoid arthritis (II). *Acta Rheum. Scand.* 7: 138, 1961.
117. Sorensen, A. W. S. Investigation of the kidney function in rheumatoid arthritis. *Acta Rheum. Scand.* 6: 115, 1960.
118. Stapleton, F. B., Hanissian, A. S., and Miller, L. A. Hypercalciuria in children with juvenile rheumatoid arthritis: Association with hematuria. *J. Pediatr.* 107: 235, 1985.
119. Stein, H. B., Patterson, A. C., Offer, R. C., et al. Adverse effects of D-penicillamine in rheumatoid arthritis. *Ann. Intern. Med.* 92: 24, 1980.
120. Talal, N. Sjögren's syndrome, lymphoproliferation, and renal tubular acidosis. *Ann. Intern. Med.* 74: 663, 1971.
121. Talal, N. Sjögren's syndrome. *Bull. Rheum. Dis.* 16: 404, 1966.
122. Talal, N., Sokoloff, L., and Barth, W. F. Extra-salivary lymphoid abnormalities in Sjögren's syndrome (reticulum cell sarcoma, "pseudolymphoma," macroglobulinemia). *Am. J. Med.* 43: 50, 1966.
123. Talal, N., Zisman, E., and Schur, P. H. Renal tubular acidosis, glomerulonephritis, and immunologic factors in Sjögren's syndrome. *Arthritis Rheum.* 11: 774, 1968.
124. Talbott, J. H., Gall, E. A., Consolazio, W. V., et al. Dermatomyositis with scleroderma, calcinosis and renal endarteritis associated with cortical necrosis. *Arch. Intern. Med.* 63: 476, 1939.
125. Teilum, G., and Lindahl, A. Frequency and significance of amyloid changes in rheumatoid arthritis. *Acta Med. Scand.* 149: 449, 1954.
126. Ting, H. C., and Wang, F. Mesangiocapillary (membranoproliferative) glomerulonephritis and rheumatoid arthritis. *Br. Med. J.* 1: 270, 1977.
127. Tornroth, T., and Skrifvars, B. Gold nephropathy prototype of membranous glomerulonephritis. *Am. J. Pathol.* 75: 573, 1974.
128. Trainin, E. B., Spitzer, A., and Greifer, I. Amyloidosis in juvenile rheumatoid arthritis. *N.Y. State J. Med.* 78: 72, 1978.
129. Tu, W. N., Shearn, M. A., Lee, J. C., et al. Interstitial nephritis in Sjögren's syndrome. *Ann. Intern. Med.* 69: 1163, 1968.
130. Unger, P. N., Zuckerbrod, M., Beck, G. J., et al. Amyloidosis in rheumatoid arthritis. *Am. J. Med. Sci.* 216: 51, 1948.
131. Vaamonde, C. A., and Hunt, F. R. The nephrotic syndrome as a complication of gold therapy. *Arthritis Rheum.* 13: 826, 1970.
132. van Rijthoven, A. W. A. M., Dijkmans, B. A. C., Goei Thè, H. S., et al. Cyclosporin treatment for rheumatoid arthritis: A placebo controlled, double blind, multicentre study. *Ann. Rheum. Dis.* 45: 726, 1986.
133. Walker, B. R., Alexander, F., and Tannebaum, P. J. Fanconi syndrome with renal tubular acidosis and light chain proteinuria. *Nephron* 8: 103, 1971.
134. Walshe, J. M. Wilson's disease—new oral therapy. *Lancet* i: 25, 1956.
135. Weisman, M., and Zvaifler, N. Cryoimmunoglobulins in rheumatoid arthritis. *J. Clin. Invest.* 56: 725, 1975.
136. Whaley, K., and Alspaugh, M. A. Sjögren's Syndrome. In W. N. Kelley, E. D. Harris, Jr., S. Ruddy, et al. (eds.), *Textbook of Rheumatology* (3rd ed.). Philadelphia: Saunders, 1989.
137. Whaley, K., and Webb, J. Liver and kidney disease in rheumatoid arthritis. *Clin. Rheum. Dis.* 3: 527, 1977.
138. Whelton, A., Stout, R. L., Spilman, P. S., et al. Renal effects of ibuprofen, piroxicam, and sulindac in patients with asymptomatic renal failure. *Ann. Intern. Med.* 112: 568, 1990.
139. Wilks, S. Cases of lardaceous disease and some allied affections: with remarks. *Guys Hosp. Rep.* (series 3) 2: 103, 1856.
140. Winer, R. L., Cohen, A. H., Sawhney, A. S., et al. Sjögren's syndrome with immune-complex tubulointerstitial renal disease. *Clin. Immun. Immunopathol.* 8: 494, 1977.
141. Wooley, P. N., Griffin, J., Panayi, G. S., et al. HLA-DR antigens and toxic reaction to sodium aurothiomalate and D-penicillamine in patients with rheumatoid arthritis. *N. Engl. J. Med.* 303: 300, 1980.
142. Wright, J. R., and Calkins, E. Clinical-pathologic differentiation of common amyloid syndrome. *Medicine* 60: 429, 1981.
143. Yocum, D. E., Klippel, J. H., Wilder, R. L., et al. Cyclosporin A in severe, treatment-refractory rheumatoid arthritis. *Ann. Intern. Med.* 109: 863, 1988.

Thrombotic Thrombocytopenic Purpura, Hemolytic-Uremic Syndrome, and Acute Cortical Necrosis

Giuseppe Remuzzi
Arrigo Schieppati
Piero Ruggenenti
Tullio Bertani

Definition of Thrombotic Thrombocytopenic Purpura and Hemolytic-Uremic Syndrome

Hemolytic-uremic syndrome (HUS) and thrombotic thrombocytopenic purpura (TTP) are syndromes of microangiopathic hemolytic anemia associated with variable signs of organ impairment [319].

In children the syndrome most commonly is dominated by renal failure and therefore is defined as HUS, whereas in older patients neurologic signs predominate and the disease is called TTP.

Microvascular thrombosis is the typical lesion [378] and endothelial injury is likely the inciting event [318]. Vascular endothelial injury may be triggered by viral [207] or bacterial agents [11, 183, 200] or drugs [32, 131, 359], or be the consequence of a genetic predisposition [247] or underlying disease [267]. Some authors believe that HUS and TTP are distinct entities [401]. However, the fact that there are no clear-cut clinical or laboratory features that differentiate HUS from TTP has led others to view the two syndromes as a clinical continuum [84, 177, 337].

Agents That Promote the Development of Thrombotic Microangiopathy and Their Effect on Cultured Endothelial Cells or Experimental Animal Models

INFECTIOUS AGENTS

In predisposed individuals, both HUS and TTP are sometimes triggered by bacteria [176, 182, 198, 200, 270, 271] or viruses [184, 207, 289, 317, 391, 402]. An association between *Shigella dysenteriae* type 1, severe colitis, and HUS in children was documented by Koster et al. [200] in 1978. This association is particularly frequent in the Indian subcontinent [315, 316] where HUS is epidemic. Recently Karmali et al. [182] detected a vero-cell cytotoxin (verotoxin) produced by *Escherichia coli* serotype 0157:H7 (VTEC) in the stools from 5 of 8 patients with sporadic HUS and demonstrated VTEC infection in 11 of the 15 cases they examined. The association between VTEC and HUS was then documented in 30 of 40 children, whereas no VTEC could be isolated from the stool cultures of healthy subjects [182]. At least two antigenically distinct verotoxins are described for *E. coli.* verotoxin 1 (VT 1), also designated Shiga-like toxin 1 (SLT-I), is neutralized by anti-Shiga toxin, whereas VT 2 (SLT-II) is not [374]. Endotoxins produced by *S. dysenteriae* 1 and *E. coli* 0157:H7 have similar biologic properties [198, 285] and, probably, share a common mechanism in the pathogenesis of the diarrheal prodrome and of the full clinical manifestation of HUS. Up to now, at least 60 serotypes of *E. coli* with verotoxin-producing ability have been identified [140]. Infection with the serotype 0157:H7 is also the cause of outbreaks of hemorrhagic colitis [329] complicated in some cases by full-blown HUS [283]. This and other reports support the evidence that VTEC infection may be a major cause of childhood HUS in North America and in Britain [145]. Neuraminidase-producing organisms including *Streptococcus pneumoniae,* influenza 2 virus, myxoviruses, streptococci, *Bacteroides, Pseudomonas, Klebsiella, Vibrio cholerae, Corynebacterium,* clostridia, and others have also been strongly related to the pathogenesis of childhood HUS [192, 312]. The underlying mechanism would be neuraminidase-induced exposure of the T antigen of erythrocytes, platelets, and renal endothelial cell surfaces that would result in interaction between the antigen and a complement-fixing IgM antibody and cause agglutination of cells [192, 312].

Enteric pathogens are being isolated with increasing frequency in postinfectious HUS. These include *Shigella, Salmonella, Yersinia, Campylobacter, E. coli, Streptococcus,* and a variety of enteroviruses [60, 135, 267, 283]. In a retrospective, population-based study of HUS in Minnesota residents less than 18 years old from 1979 through 1988, Martin et al. [241] identified 117 patients. The authors noted a mean annual incidence significantly increasing from 0.5 cases per 100,000 child-years among children less than 18 in 1979 (6 cases) to 2.0 cases per 100,000 in 1988 (26 cases). *E. coli* 0157:H7 was isolated from 13 of 28 patients who had stool specimens submitted for testing [198]. Hamburger was the major vehicle associated with food-borne outbreaks of *E. coli* 0157:H7 infection [16, 329, 344], and the increased incidence of HUS and *E. coli* 0157:H7 infection is consistent with an occurring epizootic infection. Adult HUS has been reported as a complication of hemorrhagic colitis associated with *E. coli* 0157:H7 characterized by severe renal failure and diffuse intestinal vasculopathy [283]. Of interest, *E. coli* 0157:H7 has been recognized as the inciting agent also of an adult case of TTP [270]. Associations between TTP and Coxsackie A [133], Coxsackie B [18], other unspecified viruses [402], Microtatobiotes [249], *Mycoplasma pneumoniae* [324], *Legionella pneumophila* [328], and with recent vaccinations [6, 34] have been described; and fatal simultaneous occurrences of TTP in a husband and wife [403] and in siblings [292] argue further for an infectious etiology in some cases. Neame hypothesized that viruses may cause the syndrome by producing platelet aggregation, endothelial cell damage, or the production of immune complexes [279]. Circulating immune complexes are probably involved in the pathogenesis of TTP associated with bacterial endocarditis [12]. HUS and TTP may complicate human immunodeficiency virus (HIV) type 1 infection as well as acquired immunodeficiency syndrome–related complex [23, 174, 212]. Elevated platelet-associated levels of IgG and IgM and of the third and fourth complement component suggest an immune-mediated pathogenesis of the syndrome [212].

Evidence is available that endotoxins and bacterial neuraminidase are toxic to endothelial cells in vitro. Yamada and co-workers [415] studied the effect of endotoxin on cultured endothelial cells in vitro and showed that endotoxin requires the presence of granulocytes to damage endothelial cells. Since the damage could be reduced by suppressing granulocyte adhesiveness or by oxygen free radical scavengers, the authors concluded that cytotoxic activity of endotoxin could be due in part to its capability of promoting granulocyte adhesion to endothelium and stimulating granulocyte production of toxic oxygen radicals. Recently Meyrick [251], using both in vitro and in vivo models, showed that endotoxin can cause a direct injury to pulmonary endothelium and that this damage is enhanced by activated complement and granulocytes by their interaction with the altered endothelium. Furthermore, lipopolysaccharides derived from *E. coli, Salmonella minnesota,* and *Salmonella typhosa* cause direct injury of bovine endothelial cells in culture, manifested initially by cell detachment from culture substrate with subsequent cell lysis [155]. In contrast to bovine endothelial cells, lipopolysaccharides did not induce direct lysis or detachment of cultured human endothelial cells exposed to endotoxin in vitro [156]. Inhibition of cell proliferation, a sensitive marker of sublethal injury, was observed after prolonged incubation with lipopolysaccharides, while cytotoxicity was induced by co-incubation with cycloheximide, a protein synthesis inhibitor. These findings suggest that protein synthesis may be required for detoxification of lipopolysaccharides, or that the latter may affect the catabolism of critical proteins [156].

Neuraminidase, produced by some bacteria and viruses, also can damage vascular endothelium. Klein et al. [192] found that neuraminidase exposes the Thomsen-Friedenreich receptor present on glomeruli, red blood cells, and platelets. The formation of an anti–Thomsen-Friedenreich IgM antibody would promote agglutination of red blood cells and platelets. Whether the antiendothelium antibodies occasionally found in some patients with HUS/TTP [396] also play a role in damaging endothelium in some forms of the disorder merits further investigation.

The few experimental models available further support the key role of endothelial damage in postinfectious HUS. The generalized Shwartzman reaction (GSR) is an experimental model of bilateral cortical necrosis of the kidneys induced in rabbits by two intravenous doses, spaced 18 to 24 hours apart, of endotoxin from gram-negative bacteria [383].

The earliest histologic lesion in the GSR is the deposition of a homogeneous, eosinophilic material with the staining properties of fibrinoid within the lumen of the glomerular capillaries of the kidneys [35]. Similar material is deposited in the vessels in other visceral organs in association with necrotizing and hemorrhagic lesions [35, 383].

There is experimental evidence that in pregnant animals (rabbits and rats) [118, 412] or in animals pretreated with corticosteroids [383], sympathomimetics (α-agonists) [407], or synthetic acid polymers [382], the GSR can be triggered by a single dose of endotoxin, whereas two spaced endotoxin injections are required in non-pregnant or untreated animals. Although recent studies have emphasized the role of endothelial injury that follows the exposure of endothelium to endotoxin, direct and definitive evidence of this mechanism is still lacking.

Raij et al. [317], in a model of unilateral cortical necrosis in rabbits, showed that after an in situ perfusion of one kidney with endotoxin followed by a systemic injection of endotoxin 24 hours later, the GSR was confined to that kidney. Thus it appears that endotoxin might have a specific local effect on the vascular endothelium that is sufficient as an initial event that predisposes to cortical necrosis. In agreement with this view is the finding of Arhelger [8] that in rats after an injection of nephrotoxic serum, which is known to induce immediate endothelial injury, a single dose of endotoxin was sufficient to elicit the GSR. Hoyer and co-workers [167] extended this experiment by infusing nephrotoxic serum into the left renal artery of pregnant rats and obtained a Shwartzman reaction restricted to the left kidney. More recently, Campos et al. [55] demonstrated that vascular prostacyclin (PGI_2) infusion prior to endotoxin significantly inhibited the GSR in pregnant rats. Although the lesions of the GSR were not completely abolished, the extent and severity of the histologic changes were significantly less than in PGI_2-untreated animals.

PGI_2 might exert its protective effect against the GSR by inhibiting platelet aggregation, regulating polymorphonuclear leukocyte adherence to endothelial cells, and influencing the participation of leukocytes in the GSR. The relevance of PGI_2 in antagonizing the occurrence of the GSR is strengthened by the observation that bradykinin, which increases the synthesis of renal prostaglandins [244], prevents the GSR elicited by a single injection of endotoxin in pregnant rats and cortisone-sensitized rabbits [209]. The protective effect of bradykinin on the GSR seems to be mediated by prostaglandins, since it is abolished after administration of aspirin.

IMMUNE REACTANTS

Antibodies [191, 228, 252, 280, 351] and immune complexes [194, 195, 281] can induce endothelial injury and trigger massive sequestration of platelets and polymorphonuclear leukocytes in the microvasculature [228] as in acute allograft rejection in humans [351]. It is likely that circulating antibodies or immune complexes or both play a pathogenetic role in the development of thrombotic microangiopathies in the course of connective tissue disorders, such as systemic lupus erythematosus (SLE) [83, 208], Sjögren's syndrome [370], rheumatoid arthritis [269], and polyarteritis [17], the most frequent association being with SLE, although the incidence varies in the different reports [219, 338].

Occasional patients with TTP have cytotoxic antibody to cultured endothelial cells in vitro [113, 396]. This cytotoxicity is complement dependent and related to the IgG fraction of immunoglobulins. That autoimmune-mediated endothelial damage may be the cause of microvascular injury is supported by the findings of Leung et al. [216], who recently described the consistent presence of cytotoxic anti–endothelial cell antibodies in the serum of patients in the acute phase of HUS/TTP. The same authors found that sera from 13 of 14 children with acute HUS contained complement-fixing IgG and IgM antibodies that specifically injured cultured human umbilical vein endothelial cells. The endothelial cell antigen was lost after treatment of the cells with interferon gamma. In contrast, only 3 of 5 adult patients with acute, nonrelapsing TTP had lytic antiendothelial antibodies and only 1 of these recognized an antigen lost on interferon gamma treatment. None of 32 control sera contained lytic anti–endothelial cell antibodies. These data suggest that at least in some children, HUS may involve a disorder of immunoregulation so that a unique class of anti–endothelial cell antibodies is detectable in such patients. The possibility of an antibody-mediated injury to endothelial cells is supported by the findings of Platt et al. [302], who recently showed that exposing cultured porcine endothelium to human serum as a source of natural antibodies and complement caused cleavage and release of endothelial cell proteoglycans that preceded irreversible cell injury. These in vitro findings might be interpreted as to indicate that the loss of endothelial cell proteoglycan is critical to the pathogenesis of vascular damage and that stimuli other than endotoxins can also induce endothelial injury.

Hyperacute renal allograft rejection and acute serum sickness are examples of immunologically mediated endothelial damage. Hyperacute rejection of the kidney is mediated by secondary injury following antigen-cytotoxic antibody reaction at the interface between the recipient's blood and the donor's endothelium [191, 252]. The earliest event after fixation of antibodies and complement to the endothelium is believed to be massive sequestration of platelets and, to a lesser extent, of polymorphonuclear leukocytes in the microvasculature of the graft [228, 351]. Widespread microthrombosis with concomitant vasoconstriction is a crucial event leading to vascular occlusion and ischemia [45]. The endothelial injury has been observed in several experimental models, such as hyperacute cardiac allograft rejection and skin allograft rejection; information obtained from rejection of these organs has greatly helped in our understanding of the mechanisms and targets of renal rejection. Dvorak et al. [92], in a model of skin allograft rejection, found diffuse microvascular damage preceding infarction of skin allograft. Vascular damage associated with hypertrophy, necrosis, and sloughing of endothelial cells was the major cause of skin graft rejection. Forbes and co-workers [112], studying cardiac allograft rejection in the rat, observed extensive endothelial injury that was complement dependent and associated with platelet aggregation.

Experimental endothelial damage can also be induced by immune complexes. A model of endothelial damage probably due to immune complex deposition has been described in rabbits treated with bovine serum albumin (BSA), which classically induces acute serum sickness [194, 281]. In this model endothelial damage is probably mediated by basophil and platelet activation. These cells release vasoactive amines responsible for increasing vascular permeability and facilitating the further localization of immune complexes at the level of endothelial injury. In these animals there is extensive endothelial destruction and exfoliation with fibrin deposits in the glomerular capillaries and mesangium [195].

DRUGS

HUS and TTP have been described in the course of neoplastic disease and are essentially the consequence of the use of some *anticancer drugs* [56, 153, 171, 313]. More than 100 cases of cancer-associated HUS/TTP have been described in the literature, and an analysis of a further 85 patients was recently published [215]. In this series of 75 (88 percent) of 85 patients had adenocarcinoma, including 26 percent with gastric cancer, and in all but one, mitomycin was part of the treatment regimen, at cumulative doses greater than 60 mg [215]. The risk to develop cancer-associated HUS/TTP after treatment with mitomycin was estimated to be between 4 and 15 percent. Interestingly, 35 percent of patients were without evidence of cancer at the time of syndrome development. These data are consistent with previous uncontrolled reports [199] and suggest a causal relationship between mitomycin and cancer-associated HUS/TTP [201]. The role of mitomycin in the pathogenesis of cancer-associated HUS/TTP was confirmed in two randomized trials comparing groups of patients receiving mitomycin with groups treated with other drugs. Proia et al. [311] reported findings of HUS in 4 of 26 patients with metastatic colorectal adenocarcinoma treated with 5-fluorouracil (5-FU), vincristine, and mitomycin, whereas none of the 27 control patients receiving lomustine instead of mitomycin developed HUS. An interim report by the British Stomach Cancer Group on 411 patients participating in a randomized study of adjuvant chemotherapy for operable cancer showed a case of HUS in 24 patients receiving mitomycin as part of the adjuvant chemotherapy and none in the control group receiving placebo [104]. Analysis of the data on cancer-associated HUS/TTP in a national registry [215] suggests an increased incidence of cancer-associated HUS at higher cumulative doses of mitomycin. Eighty-nine percent of the patients of the registry received a cumulative dose of mitomycin higher than 60 mg. The same incidence emerges from the review of the previously published reports. Although most of the available data support an etiologic role of mitomycin in cancer-associated HUS/TTP, it can not be ignored that in about 10 percent of the reported cases, the syndrome occurred in patients never exposed to mitomycin. Drugs other than mitomycin may trigger HUS and these include vinblastine, cisplatin, bleomycin, cytosine arabinoside, and daunorubicin [47, 157]. It also should be noted that most patients receive 5-FU in association with mitomycin and that a role of drug interaction in the pathogenesis of cancer-associated HUS can not be excluded.

Anticancer drugs inducing thrombotic microangiopathy in humans also alter endothelial cell function in vitro and in vivo. Mitomycin added to cultured human umbilical cord vein endothelial cells inhibits prostacyclin production and cell proliferation. This effect is dose dependent and is achieved at concentrations close to those found in sera of mitomycin-treated patients [91]. In vivo the perfusion of the renal artery with mitomycin induces ultrastructural changes similar to those found in patients with HUS [58]. The initial lesion is confined to vascular endothelium, but is followed in short order by deposition of platelets, obliteration of capillary lumens, and lucent subendothelial expansion. These observations are in keeping with the concept derived from morphologic data that endothelial damage represents a key lesion for the subsequent development of microangiopathic lesions [163].

Cyclosporine may also be involved in the pathogenesis of HUS and TTP [282]. Since 1981 an increasing number of case reports have documented that treatment with cyclosporine may be followed by severe renal failure, with pathologic changes characterized by glomerular thrombosis and severe arteriolar damage. These lesions resembling HUS have been mainly reported in patients receiving cyclosporine for bone marrow transplantation [308, 309]. Thus, thrombocytopenia, hemolytic anemia, and deterioration of renal function have been described in patients treated with cyclosporine for preventing graft-versus-host disease after allogeneic bone marrow transplantation [308]. Similar observations were made by Shulman et al. [359], who noted severe renal insufficiency and diffuse thrombi in the glomerular capillary tufts and arteries in 3 of 16 allogeneic bone marrow recipients treated with cyclosporine. De novo occurrence of HUS has been described also in recipients of solid-organ allografts treated with cyclosporine, including liver and heart [26, 93]. Thus, disseminated intravascular coagulation and renal function deterioration during cyclosporine treatment and recovery coincident with drug withdrawal have been reported in patients who underwent orthotopic liver transplantation for primary hepatocellular carcinoma [26]. By contrast, only anecdotal cases of well-identified de novo or recurrent cyclosporine-induced HUS in renal allograft recipients have been reported [132, 213, 390, 392, 410]. In these cases, HUS occurs in the first week after transplantation, and biopsy specimens show arteriolopathy and even thrombosis. Despite the striking nature of the histologic findings, a return of renal function has been noted with cessation of cyclosporine or the use of streptokinase and heparin.

Experimental evidence is also available in support of a direct toxic effect of cyclosporine on aortic cell cultures [419] and cultured endothelial cells of the microcirculation [210]. This is consistent with in vivo findings of vacuolization and scant endothelial cell necrosis in patients treated with cyclosporine. Endothelial damage may in turn promote platelet activation and microvascular thrombosis. Platelet activation at the site of endothelial damage may also be favored by cyclosporine-induced changes in the PGI_2–thromboxane A_2 (TXA_2) ratio. Studying the effect of cyclosporine on PGI_2 release by cultured human umbilical vein endothelial cells, Voss et al. [394] showed a cyclosporine-induced, time- and concentration-dependent reduction in unstimulated and Ca^{2+} ionophore–stimulated release of PGI_2. On the other hand, bovine endothelial cells in culture generate increased amounts of TXA_2 [419]. Moreover, the recent observation that human umbilical vein [42] and human glomerular [42] endothelial cells in culture, as well as bovine pulmonary artery endothelial cells in culture [197], release endothelin on stimulation with cyclosporine opens the possibility that this vasoactive peptide may also contribute to the process of thrombi formation by reducing locally the blood flow through its potent vasoconstrictor action. That this can indeed be the case is indicated by the fact that the main etiologic factor of HUS/TTP is bacterial endotoxin and that endotoxin-treated animals have much higher plasma endothelin than do controls [377]. In this context it is of interest that cultured endothelial cells exposed to endotoxin generate significantly higher amounts of endothelin than do cells challenged with the vehicle alone [377]. Recently, Perico et al. [296] demonstrated that the infusion of cyclosporine into an isolated perfused kidney preparation induces a dose-dependent decrease in renal perfusate flow associated with a concomitant increase in renal vascular resistance, and that these hemodynamic changes are prevented by the preexposition of the isolated kidneys to a specific antiendothelin antibody. The infusion of specific endothelin antiserum partially but significantly prevented the reduction of renal plasma flow and glomerular filtration rate induced by cyclosporine administration in a series of in vivo studies performed in normal rats, thus suggesting that endothelin is an important mediator of cyclosporine-induced renal vasoconstriction in the rat. The recent report of severe endothelial injury and acute renal failure associated with a dramatic increase in circulating endothelin levels in a renal transplant patient receiving high-dose cyclosporine [109] further supports that the endothelial cell can be a target for cyclosporine toxicity also in humans, and that cyclosporine-induced changes in the kidney may involve enhanced endothelin release from injured endothelial cells.

Oral contraceptives have also been suggested to cause HUS and TTP. HUS in women taking estrogen-containing oral contraceptives was first described by Brown et al. in 1973 [32] and confirmed in the following years [27, 267, 268, 304]. The reports of recurrent episodes in the same patient following the use of oral contraceptives [165] and in a post–renal transplantation patient inadvertently "challenged" with the birth control pill [67] suggest an association between the birth control pill and HUS. Other findings, however, argue against a clear cause-and-effect relationship. Some cases of "birth control pill–induced HUS" actually ensue shortly after pregnancy [27] or a flulike disease [32, 130] and could also be considered as pregnancy-associated or postinfectious HUS. Similarly, the episodes reported in women with a previous history of HUS [327] or with a positive familial history [57, 95, 100] could be diagnosed as cases of the chronic recurrent form of familial HUS. Moreover, hypertension is often reported in women on oral contraceptives developing HUS, and thus hypertension might actually be the real trigger of the syndrome [160, 346, 349]. Thus, one can speculate that oral contraceptives alone are unlikely to cause HUS, even if the possibility of a predisposing role can not be excluded [9].

Mechanisms Underlying the Development of a Microangiopathic Process

THE ROLE OF VASCULAR ENDOTHELIAL DAMAGE

The negative charge of platelets and endothelial cell membranes induces mutual repulsion, thus preventing platelets from reacting to vascular endothelium in physiologic conditions [78, 318]. Moreover, vascular endothelial cell membranes express thrombomodulin, a high-affinity thrombin receptor that acts as a physiologic anticoagulant, on their surface [98]. Vascular endothelium also synthesizes and releases a number of other factors including PGI_2, endothelial derived relaxing factors/nitric oxide (EDRF/NO), von Willebrand factor (vWf), and endothelin that modulate the interaction between circulating cells and the vessel wall and contribute to endothelial thromboresistance.

Following endothelial damage, a complex concert of abnormalities, including reduced PGI_2 bioavailability, defective EDRF/NO production, and altered endothelial synthesis and processing of vWf and endothelin, may contribute to the loss of thromboresistance and trigger a series of events at the endothelial cell surface that involve platelets, leukocytes, and plasma proteins and result in microvascular thrombosis.

Prostaglandin I_2. PGI_2, an inhibitor of platelet aggregation [258], is the major product of arachidonic acid formed by vascular endothelium. PGI_2 is devoid of systemic antithrombotic potential [369] since its circulating plasma levels are lower than required to inhibit platelet function [107]. However, at the site of endothelial injury, PGI_2 reaches the necessary concentrations to inhibit platelet-platelet interaction, thus limiting thrombus formation in cases of endothelial damage.

In 1978 it was reported that vascular tissues from adults with HUS/TTP failed to generate PGI_2 normally [320]. This observation has been confirmed by several investigators [81, 376]. A number of theories have been proposed to explain this finding and these include abnormally low plasma activity stimulating PGI_2 [81, 320, 387, 400, 409], the presence of an inhibitor of PGI_2 [217], or an excessively rapid PGI_2 degradation [61]. A defective plasma activity stimulating PGI_2 has been reconfirmed repeatedly in HUS [81, 175, 364, 376, 387, 400, 409] and this deficiency may possibly explain the beneficial effect of plasma infusions in some cases of HUS [253, 321]. The "factor" in plasma that normally stimulates endothelial PGI_2 synthesis [234, 293] has been purified and partially characterized [80]. This factor protects vascular PGI_2 from becoming exhausted during persistent endothelial injury [80]. Plasma from adult patients with HUS do not stimulate PGI_2 normally [320, 409]. The situation is more complex in children. Stuart et al. [376] described the occurrence of HUS in a 4-month-old infant who presented in an atypical manner with unexplained anemia that began in the neonatal period. The ability of this patient's plasma to regenerate PGI_2 activity was absent, and mixing experiments revealed the presence of an inhibitor in the plasma. Siegler et al. [364] studied 22 children with HUS and 22 healthy subjects matched for age and sex. They found that as a group, the sera from HUS patients were defective in their ability to support PGI_2 synthesis in vitro, as compared with control sera. However, a definite abnormality, defined as a value that was more than 2 standard deviations below the normal mean, was detected in only 6 of 22 patients. Unfortunately, no relationship can be deduced between defective PGI_2-stimulating activity (in 6 cases) and the type of HUS (typical or atypical) because of a lack of clinical information. This issue was addressed by Walters et al. [400] in an elegant study of a large number of children with HUS. They found normal PGI_2 synthesis by endothelial cells incubated with HUS plasma in 83 percent of typical cases. However, the plasma from most of the patients with atypical HUS failed to support PGI_2 synthesis. It would be important to know whether children with atypical HUS, who have low PGI_2-stimulating activity and a poor prognosis, represent a definite subset with a congenital defect that makes them more prone to develop HUS when exposed to a variety of environmental insults. These atypical cases more closely resemble adult HUS with respect to the clinical presentation (absence of a typical prodrome) and outcome (higher mortality and morbidity) than the typical HUS of childhood. Levin [217] also speculated that increased lipid peroxidation in the plasma of atypical cases might account for reduced vascular PGI_2 activity, and suggested that there is an inhibitor of PGI_2 production rather than a deficiency of a stimulating factor. Hope et al. [166] showed that endothelial cells have a receptor for β-thromboglobulin, and that the binding of β-thromboglobulin to its receptor results in decreased PGI_2 production. β-Thromboglobulin is released from platelets when they adhere to subendothelial collagen; this may be an additional mechanism contributing to the reduced availability of PGI_2 at sites of endothelial damage. PGI_2 deficiency might also result from an increased degradation rate as described in a case of TTP [61]. Treatment of that patient with plasma exchanges and plasma infusions slowed down the rate of PGI_2 degradation and this seemed to be associated with an increase in the platelet count, the disappearance of schistocytes, and an improvement in the neurologic status. It was speculated that this patient's plasma lacked a factor present in normal plasma that protects PGI_2 from too rapid degradation. Reduced availability of PGI_2 at the site of endothelial damage has been also explained as a defective binding of PGI_2 to serum proteins. In the normal state, such binding is rapid and readily reversible and is a function of proteins soluble in 60% saturated ammonium sulfate. Wu et al. [414] found defective PGI_2 binding, a markedly reduced PGI_2 half-life, and antiaggregatory activity in TTP sera. The decreased PGI_2 binding may contribute to the formation of microthrombi as a result of decreased PGI_2 at the site of injury. Thus, there is evidence that a primary or secondary defect in PGI_2

availability may have an important role in the pathogenesis of microthrombi in HUS (or HUS/TTP) and it is likely that a number of mechanisms act synergically to produce the defect. An altered PGI_2 bioavailability may also explain the high incidence of TTP and HUS in pregnancy. Patients with preeclampsia do not have the increase in PGI_2 that is observed in normal pregnancies [138]. This could account for the increased risk of thrombotic microangiopathy in this group of patients [325].

Endothelial Derived Relaxing Factors/Nitric Oxide. In addition to PGI_2, endothelial cells generate a labile activity generically termed *EDRF*, when stimulated with potent vasorelaxant substances such as acetylcholine, bradykinin, histamine, serotonin, and substance P [31, 169]. Bioassay studies convincingly documented that EDRF is distinct from PGI_2, and activates soluble guanylate cyclase in vascular smooth muscle cells with marked but transient cyclic guanosine monophosphate (cGMP) accumulation and concurrent relaxation of isolated strip of rabbit aorta [144, 170]. Chemically pure nitric oxide (NO) also activates soluble guanylate cyclase and induces accumulation of cGMP in vascular smooth muscle cells [142]. On the basis of pharmacologic and chemical similarities between NO and EDRF, recent evidence has been presented to indicate that NO is the major chemical form of EDRF. In response to agonists, NO is released not only from the endothelium of large and small arteries and veins [117] but also from microvessels. In this regard it has been documented that cultured endothelial cells from bovine renal glomeruli release NO after exposure to bradykinin, thrombin, platelet-activating factor, and ATP [240]. Once synthesized by vascular endothelial cells, NO rapidly diffuses into the immediately adjacent smooth muscle cells to cause relaxation and into nearly adhering platelets in the lumen of the blood vessels to inhibit platelet adhesion and aggregation [168, 290, 314, 323]. In this setting NO would function as an autoregulatory molecule that prevents thrombosis and maintains blood flow to critical organs such as the heart, brain, lungs, and kidneys. It has been suggested that loss of functional and/or morphologic integrity of endothelial cells, as it occurs in HUS and TTP, might result in a defect in NO production that would favor vasoconstriction, platelet aggregation and adhesiveness, and ultimately, vasoocclusion. This concept is supported by the recent demonstration in experimental animals that cyclosporine (CsA), which causes endothelial cell damage, diminished endothelium-dependent relaxation of renal resistance arteries [85], presumably reflecting impaired generation of NO. Of interest, an acute dramatic arteriolopathy resembling HUS has been reported in both experimental animals and humans given CsA [10, 282]. However, whether a defect in NO production also occurs in vivo in patients with thromboocclusive disorders, such as HUS, remains to be addressed.

Von Willebrand Factor. Endothelial cells form and release into the circulation vWf, a protein composed of protomeric subunits, arranged in a series of complex multimers with molecular masses ranging from 0.5 to 12.0 million daltons. vWf is required for platelets to adhere to subendothelial collagen [341]. Platelets possess receptors for vWf and glycoprotein II b-III 2 complex which are exposed on platelet activation. Following endothelial damage, vWf is released in the circulation and complex abnormalities in the multimeric structure of vWf have been reported in both HUS and TTP. Vascular damage can alter the mechanism modulating the synthesis and processing of vWf by endothelial cells and activated platelets [342, 420], and unusually large multimers of vWf (supranormal multimers) can be released in circulating plasma following endothelial injury. Supranormal multimers are potent inducers of platelet aggregation and predispose to microvascular thrombosis [187, 256, 339]. Moake et al. [256] found unusually large multimers of vWf in the plasma of 4 patients with relapsing TTP that were detected during clinical remission but not during relapses. They suggested that supranormal multimers in plasma of patients with the chronic relapsing form of TTP might be due to leakage from damaged endothelial cells. These large multimers would interact with activated platelets and would no longer be detected in the circulation [187, 255, 256, 334] during the acute phase of the disease while reappearing when remission ensues. Multimeric structure of vWf has been studied also in HUS [255, 334], and a variety of abnormalities have been reported. Moake et al. [255] found a relative decrease in the levels of the largest multimers in acute HUS, which then returned to normal when the platelet count normalized. To add to the confusion, increased concentrations of the high-molecular-weight multimers have been found in the plasma of children in the acute phase of HUS [334]. The abnormality disappeared in patients who improved clinically, but persisted in those who had relapses or had progressive renal failure. In 22 patients with acute HUS and TTP, plasma samples collected within the framework of an international registry showed a loss of larger multimers in 15 cases, normal multimers in 6, and supranormal multimers only in 1 (G. Remuzzi and P. M. Mannucci. Unpublished observations, 1989). This heterogeneous pattern of abnormalities in vWf multimeric structure in HUS and TTP is difficult to interpret. Proteolytic activity is increased in sera of patients with HUS/TTP [274], and enhanced in vivo activity of proteolytic enzymes such as plasmin, calcium-dependent cysteine protease, and elastase may account for the loss of larger multimers in acute HUS or TTP. However, vWf multimers are highly susceptible to proteolytic cleavage [101, 151, 203, 384], and the loss of the larger multimers might be an artifact related to in vitro proteolysis. To examine such a possibility, the multimeric structure of vWf was recently studied in 8 patients whose blood samples were collected into an anticoagulant containing a cocktail of protease inhibitors [236]. In all, enhanced proteolytic degradation was expressed as a relative decrease in the intact 225-kd subunit of vWf and a relative increase in the 176-kd fragment. However, instead of the loss of larger forms of normal multimers reported by Moake et al. [255, 256], the plasma of all but 1 of the patients contained a set of larger-than-normal (supranormal) multimers. Hence, although proteolytic fragmentation of vWf was enhanced during acute HUS/TTP, this was not associated with the loss of larger multimers. In the 5 patients who survived the acute phase of the disease, subunits and fragments returned to normal values and supranormal multimers were no longer detected in plasma. Thus, even though vWf proteolysis is enhanced in acute HUS/TTP, it does not lead to a loss of larger multimers. The following events can therefore be hypothesized to explain the presence of supranormal multimers during acute HUS/TTP and their disappearance after recovery. During the acute phase of the disease, supranormal multimers leak from endothelial cells, probably damaged by cytolytic antiendothelial antibodies [44, 216]. Effective therapy would stop the endothelial damage along with clinical remission. Supranormal multimers would reappear during remission only in patients with the chronic relapsing form of TTP, in which the process that maintains endothelial damage is still ongoing [256].

Evidence is also available that thrombin induces exposure of a specific receptor for vWf in human platelets, and PGI_2 can prevent this process [116]. Thus, an increase in large vWf might act synergistically with a concomitant reduction of vascular PGI_2, thus favoring microvascular thrombosis.

Endothelin. It was recently discovered that vascular endothelium synthesizes endothelin, a polypeptide that exhibits potent vasoconstrictor properties [416]. The fact that endothelin gene expression is augmented by shear stress [418] implies that local endothelial cell injury may be associated with enhanced endothelin release. The finding that endothelial cell injury may be associated with enhanced endothelin release [418] provides the rationale for looking to a possible role of endothelin in the pathogenesis of systemic disorders associated with endothelial damage, including HUS and TTP. That this can indeed be the case is indicated by the fact that the main etiologic factor of HUS and TTP is bacterial endotoxin and that endotoxin-treated animals have higher plasma endothelin levels than do controls [377]. In this context, it is of interest that cultured endothelial cells exposed to endotoxin generate significantly higher amounts of endothelin than do cells challenged with the vehicle alone [377]. The enhanced endothelin production during endothelial cell injury could participate in the process of thrombi formation by reducing locally the blood flow through its potent vasoconstrictor action.

THE ROLE OF PLATELET ACTIVATION

Although thrombocytopenia occurs in almost every patient with HUS, neither its cause nor the role of platelets in the pathogenesis of the syndrome is clear. The demonstration of normal megakaryocyte hyperplasia on bone marrow examination seems to exclude a thrombopoietic defect. It is likely that a number of processes including platelet destruction, increased consumption, and intrarenal aggregation contribute to the thrombocytopenia. The finding of a markedly shortened platelet survival, with normal fibrinogen survival [154], is consistent with the possibility that the reduced platelet half-life might be a consequence of platelet destruction during their passage through diseased renal microvessels. Indeed a prompt normalization of the platelet count follows bilateral nephrectomy, and increased uptake of infused labeled platelets by the spleen, liver, and to a lesser extent, the kidneys has been demonstrated [185, 250].

On the other hand, endothelial damage and initiation of coagulation could be responsible for platelet activation and release, followed by platelet aggregation at the site of injury. This is consistent with the description of "exhausted" circulating platelets during the acute phase of HUS. Intraplatelet β-thromboglobulin and serotonin were found to be significantly reduced and platelet-aggregating responses in vitro were markedly impaired [94, 111, 178]. Moreover, elevated plasma levels of platelet-derived proteins, β-thromboglobulin, and platelet factor 4, and low platelet-plasma serotonin ratios have been reported in children with HUS during the acute phase [14, 94], thereby indicating that intravascular platelet activation is a prominent pathophysiologic feature that may contribute considerably to the genesis of the thrombocytopenia.

A number of other mechanisms, in addition to the mechanical damage imparted during the passage of platelets through diseased vessels lined with fibrin, have been suggested as being responsible for intravascular platelet activation. Lian et al. [222] described the presence of a platelet-aggregating factor (PAF) in the plasma of patients with TTP and other authors confirmed this in HUS [263] and TTP [187]. This PAF induces aggregation of normal and TTP platelets. Of interest, the aggregating activity is inhibited by normal plasma or purified human adult IgG [223]. Moreover, Siddiqui and Lian purified a novel platelet agglutinating protein of 37,000 molecular weight from plasma of a patient with TTP [363]. This factor is not dialyzable, is absorbed by aluminum hydroxide, and is not inhibited by agents such as aspirin, prostacyclin, or heparin. At variance with acute TTP, this agglutinating protein was not detectable during recovery, or in patients with disseminated intravascular coagulation and idiopathic thrombocytopenic purpura. The finding that a preparation rich in large vWf multimers increased the capability of TTP serum to aggregate target platelets led to the suggestion that stimuli such as infections might induce the release of larger vWf multimers by endothelial cells [187]. These multimers might potentiate the activity of the PAF, thus causing microplatelet aggregation in TTP. This hypothesis is currently being debated. Lian and Siddiqui [224] stated that it is unlikely that vWf plays a major role in TTP plasma–induced platelet aggregation. They advanced several explanations for the decrease or disappearance of large vWf multimers from TTP plasma during acute episodes. These include the attachment of the multimers to exposed subendothelium in damaged vessels, decreased synthesis and release of vWf from endothelial cells, or accelerated proteolysis of large multimers by tissue plasminogen activator or other proteases. These authors' hesitation in accepting the speculation of Kelton et al. [187] was supported by the inability of anti–glycoprotein

IIb-IIIa complex and anti-vWf monoclonal antibodies to inhibit the platelet agglutination induced by TTP plasma in vitro [224]. Moake [254] holds the opposite point of view and favors the hypothesis that vWf is involved in the pathophysiology of TTP and closely related syndromes and raises doubt about the pathophysiologic relevance of the in vivo platelet clumping test of Lian and Siddiqui. A platelet-activating factor has also been demonstrated in HUS and, as in the case of TTP, it was suggested that the largest forms of vWf interact with platelets in the acute phase [263]. Although no correlation was found between the platelet-aggregating activity and the stage of the disease, this does not exclude the possibility that platelet-aggregating material is not of pathogenic significance. It may, however, merely reflect the widespread cell destruction and may be one of the many cellular constituents consequently released into the plasma.

THE ROLE OF OXIDANT INJURY TO ERYTHROCYTES

Thrombocytopenia and microangiopathic hemolytic anemia reflect the thrombotic process and appear when the number of lesions, regardless of distribution, reach the threshold required to produce changes in circulating blood. This traditional concept has been challenged by the recent finding of intrinsic changes in the erythrocyte membrane that would explain the hemolytic process [288]. Low levels of superoxide dismutase, together with peroxidative changes reflected by a lower red blood cell phosphatidylethanolamine content in HUS, increase the susceptibility of erythrocytes to oxidative hemolysis [368]. Of interest, metronidazole, which is known to sensitize tissues to oxidative changes, has been associated with the development of atypical HUS in 6 children given the drug either as prophylaxis after bowel surgery or as treatment for nonspecific diarrhea [305]. A link between HUS, membrane lipid peroxidation, and defective PGI_2 synthesis is suggested by the finding of reduced plasma levels of vitamin E in some HUS patients [288], who seem to benefit from management with this potent naturally occurring antioxidant [307].

Thrombotic Thrombocytopenic Purpura

The term *thrombotic thrombocytopenic purpura* was first introduced in 1925 by Moschcowitz [272], who described a 16-year-old female patient with a fulminant febrile attack, hemolytic anemia, bleeding, renal failure, and neurologic involvement. Pathologic changes were characterized by widespread hyaline thrombosis of small vessels. In Moschcowitz's view, thrombi were constituted by agglutinated hyalinized erythrocytes. The disease was believed to be due to a powerful "toxin that has both agglutinative and hemolytic properties" [272]. Since then and up to 1980 almost 500 cases of TTP have been reported in the literature, and several criteria have been proposed for the diagnosis [4, 77, 188]. The term *TTP* should be used when two of the three major criteria (thrombocytopenia, microangiopathic anemia, and neurologic involvement) are associated with two minor criteria (fever, renal changes, and presence of thrombi in the circulation) [37].

No objective clinical signs are available to differentiate TTP from HUS besides the age of onset [110, 319]. Generally, in young patients renal failure is frequent and the disease is typical of HUS, whereas in older patients the syndrome often has the clinical characteristics of TTP, particularly in regard to neurologic involvement [4, 365]. However, there are reports in which the same patient is classified as having HUS or TTP during two different episodes of disease exacerbation [235, 249, 360]. There are also cases with severe renal failure that have been classified as TTP, and cases of HUS often have neurologic symptoms [90, 357].

Idiopathic TTP has been separated from secondary TTP [37]. TTP may occur in pregnancy or may complicate the postpartum period [279, 348]. Cases of TTP have been discovered in association with neoplastic disorders such as lymphoma [72], Sjögren's syndrome [370], rheumatoid arthritis [269], polyarteritis [17], scleroderma [163], and systemic lupus erythematosus (SLE) [83, 208]. TTP has been recognized in patients with endocarditis [266] or after treatment with sulfonamide [43, 227], iodine [96], oral contraceptives [51], and some poisons [373].

The disease is more common in women, with a female-to-male ratio of 3:2 [4]. Although the peak incidence occurs in the third decade of life, cases of TTP have been described in patients ranging from 1 to 90 years [188, 264]. Recurrent episodes of TTP are not exceptions, but relapses cannot be predicted by any clinical or hematologic feature [61, 76, 246]. Based on cases of TTP occurring in siblings, a genetic predisposition has been suggested, and some reports indicate that there is a possibility that an autosomal recessive trait underlies TTP [115, 161, 397].

CLINICAL FEATURES

TTP is generally an acute illness; the symptoms appear 7 to 14 days before the diagnosis, and if therapy is not successful the patient dies within 3 months. In a minority of patients the disease follows a more chronic course and can progress with different signs or symptoms of disease activity from a few months [52] to several years [379].

The clinical presentation is dominated in most patients by hemorrhages and neurologic symptoms [4, 188]. In over 90 percent of cases purpura is the initial manifestation which may or may not be associated with retinal hemorrhage, epistaxis, gingival bleeding, hematuria, gastrointestinal hemorrhage, menorrhagia, and hemoptysis [4, 188, 204, 325]. More rare symptoms are malaise, fatigue, pallor, abdominal pain, arthralgia, myalgia, and jaundice [4, 188, 277]. Although fever is not frequently seen at onset, it is almost always present during the illness [4, 188, 204, 299, 325]. Anemia is severe, with average values between 7 and 9 gm per deciliter of hemoglobin [77, 188, 298]. Transient and fluctuating neurologic manifestations are present in almost all patients [365]. These include confusion, headache, paresis, aphasia, dysarthria, visual problems, and coma. Angiographic and electroencephalographic studies have not been extensively performed but do not appear to offer major diagnostic contributions. Ocular involvement is frequent, retinal and choroid hemorrhages being the most common manifestations [295].

Renal involvement is common, with proteinuria and microhematuria the most constant findings [188, 276, 298, 299]. Renal function is depressed in 40 to 80 percent of patients, although severe renal insufficiency is rare [77, 188, 299, 325]. Heart involvement is infrequent, although congestive heart failure and conduction disturbances have occasionally been reported [122, 326]. In rare instances lungs may contain some alveolar and interstitial infiltrates [25]. Abdominal pain has been reported in 10 to 30 percent of cases [4, 38, 188] and has been interpreted as secondary to the involvement of small vessels of the gastrointestinal tract [64, 408]. Pancreatitis has also been described [158].

Laboratory findings show microangiopathic hemolytic anemia in almost all patients (Table 75-1). A detailed analysis [37] of all the reported series of patients with TTP revealed that hemoglobin levels are less than 10 gm per deciliter in 99 percent of patients and less than 6.5 gm per deciliter in 38 percent. The peripheral smear shows fragmented red blood cells with the typical aspect of burr or helmet cells. Reticulocyte counts are elevated and in 35 percent of patients are greater than 20 percent of circulating red blood cells. Markers of the hemolytic process are elevated serum levels of lactate dehydrogenase (LDH), which are frequently correlated with the course of the disease [188, 380] and low or undetectable haptoglobin levels. Indirect bilirubin is usually higher than normal and the Coombs' test is usually negative. Leukocytosis is relatively frequent, but the white blood cell counts rarely exceed 20,000 per cubic millimeter [4]. The platelet count is generally low [77, 188, 204, 299, 325] and only rarely exceeds 60,000 per cubic millimeter. Platelet survival studies have shown reduced platelet survival suggesting peripheral destruction or consumption [18, 186, 278]. Coagulation studies have failed to detect disseminated intravascular coagulation (DIC). Prothrombin time, partial thromboplastin time (PTT), factor V, factor VIII, and fibrinogen are normal in the majority of patients although high levels of fibrin degradation products (FDP) and prolonged thrombin time are found in occasional cases [172, 188]. The complement system has not been extensively studied, but in most instances appears to be normal [5, 59, 279]. Positive LE cell preparations and antinuclear antibody (ANA) factors have been reported in a few cases [4, 38, 188].

PATHOLOGY

The typical pathologic changes of TTP are the thrombi that occlude capillaries and arterioles in many organs and tissues [139, 287]. These thrombi are constituted by fibrin and platelets and their distribution is widespread. They are most commonly detected in kidneys, pancreas, heart, adrenals, and brain [20, 139, 388]. Compared to HUS, pathologic changes of TTP are more extensively distributed, probably reflecting the more systemic nature of the disease.

Other types of lesions have been described in TTP; the subendothelial accumulation of hyaline material has led to the term *prethrombotic* lesions [139], and frequently microaneurysms [287] or glomeruloid structures [235] are found. Altogether thrombi, prethrombotic changes, aneurysmal dilatation of vessels, and glomeruloid structures have been considered typical of TTP, but recent studies cast doubt on the specificity of these lesions [137, 388]. Recently, it has been observed that gingival biopsies and bone marrow clot sections have the highest percentage of positivity for microthrombi [137, 299].

Fibrin has been detected in the thrombi by immunofluorescence [102, 237, 405]; although the presence of platelets in the thrombi has been shown by electron microscopy [102], staining with antiplatelet sera is often negative [71, 102, 237]. C3, C1q, and immunoglobulin deposits have been occasionally detected [204, 237]. In the kidney fibrin-platelet thrombi are more frequent in arterioles than in glomerular capillaries [1]. Reflecting the more chronic and relapsing character of the disease, proliferation of endothelial and myointimal cells (Fig. 75-1) is more pronounced in TTP than in HUS [301].

PROGNOSIS AND TREATMENT

The prognosis of the patients studied prior to 1965 was very poor. Of 271 cases reviewed by Amorosi and Ultmann [4] before 1965, survival was approximately 5 percent. During the last 20 years the clinical course of TTP has significantly improved. Ridolfi and Bell [325] reviewed 275 cases from 1965 and 1980 and found that survival was about 50 percent. However, the number of cases reported in each series is so limited that it is difficult to organize controlled studies to assess the best therapy for TTP. Therefore, it remains to be proved whether the better prognosis of patients treated after 1965 (46 percent versus 5 percent survival) is the consequence of a better diagnostic approach, including milder

Table 75-1. Clinical and laboratory findings from the major reported series of thrombotic thrombocytopenic purpura

Author	No. patients	Bleeding	Fever	Neurologic abnormalities	Anemia	Thrombocytopenia	Renal failure
Amorosi (1966)	246	44%	20%	60%	100%	nr	nr
Kwaan (1979)	12	100%	100%	100%	100%	100%	100%
Cuttner (1980)	20	nr	nr	100%	90%	90%	55%
Kennedy (1980)	48	45%	14%	45%	100%	100%	56%
Petitt (1980)	38	nr	86%	89%	100%	100%	39%
Ridolfi (1981)	25	100%	80%	100%	100%	96%	72%

nr = not reported.

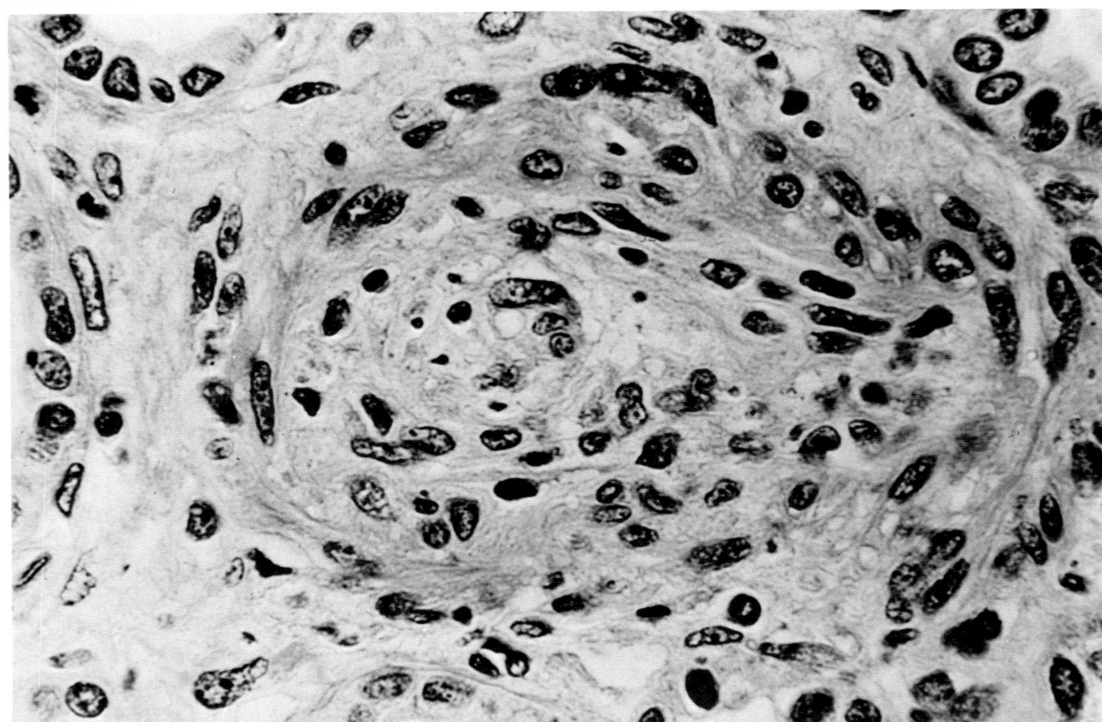

Fig. 75-1. Marked endothelial and myointimal cell proliferation with occlusion of the lumen of an interlobular artery in a case of thrombotic thrombocytopenic purpura. (Trichrome; ×375.)

forms, and better supportive care or an indication that new treatments employed have beneficial effects. Evaluation of new therapeutic approaches is even more complex because most patients have been treated with more than one agent. Recently, Bukowski et al. [39] reviewed the therapy of all the reported series and single cases with TTP. This analysis showed that plasma exchange was the treatment of choice, with 76 percent of patients responding. Almost all patients were simultaneously treated with other agents [275, 276]. The rationale for using plasma exchange is to remove injuring agents such as immune complexes or antiendothelial antibodies [37, 38] and possibly to add some lacking factor involved in the pathogenesis of the disease [48]. Plasma infusion for TTP patients has been extensively used since the report of Byrnes and Khurana in 1977 [48]. These authors described an 18-year-old patient with idiopathic relapsing TTP who had several relapses after plasma exchange but could be maintained with infusions of fresh frozen plasma. Others have confirmed the beneficial effect of plasma infusion alone in the therapy of TTP [46, 222]. There is experimental evidence that the efficacy of plasma infusion is probably related to the replacement of a deficient plasma factor, which either inhibits platelet aggregation [389] or is necessary for the generation of PGI_2 [322].

The side effects of plasma infusion have to be considered: Administration of plasma exposes patients to congestive heart failure and pulmonary edema consequent to oncotic volume overloading. An additional limitation is the large number of patients succumbing to non-A non-B post-transfusional hepatitis. The possible role of PGI_2 deficiency has provided a rationale for the use of PGI_2 infusion in the treatment of TTP [36, 67, 108, 162]. Few patients have been exposed to this treatment, and in all cases the use of antiplatelet agents, prednisone, and plasma exchange in association with PGI_2 makes it difficult to interpret the result. In a patient who did not respond to multiple other forms of therapy, the infusion of PGI_2 was followed by remission of the disease [108].

Antiplatelet agents such as aspirin (500 to 1,200 mg/day), dipyridamole (400 to 600 mg/day), sulfinpyrazone, and dextrans have been employed, often in combination with steroids, plasmapheresis, and splenectomy [21, 77, 99, 146, 239]. The pathologic finding of platelet thrombi in patients with TTP gave the rationale for the employment of antiplatelet agents. The overall response rate was approximately 50 percent [3, 39], with even better results if dextran was used. The finding of impaired fibrinolysis suggested the use of urokinase in TTP. This therapy was employed with apparent success in one patient but was accompanied by dramatic hemorrhages in others [205].

Steroids have been widely employed in TTP [4, 43, 218, 370], the rationale deriving from studies showing an improvement in platelet survival time in patients on steroids [154] and the response to steroids alone reported in occasional patients [299]. However, the effectiveness of steroids in the management of TTP has not been clearly documented [39].

As in other forms of thrombocytopenia, splenectomy has been tried in TTP as well, and several reports showed its efficacy [75, 77, 324, 343]. However, the majority of patients undergoing splenectomy received other concomitant forms of treatment [75]. No rationale is available for splenectomy in TTP, and Bukowski [37] has speculated that the results obtained with this procedure have been due to the intraoperative administration of a large amount of blood (Table 75-2).

As a means of neutralizing platelet-agglutinating activity present in TTP plasma, intravenous immunoglobulins (0.5 mg/kg/day for 5 consecutive days) have also been given in an uncontrolled way with a response rate similar to that reported following plasma exchange [62, 106, 127, 248, 411]. However, intravenous immunoglobulin infusions have been associated with anaphylaxis and infections secondary to inhibition of Fc receptor–mediated immune clearance [19, 74]. Fulminant *Candida* septicemia in a patient with acute myelocytic leukemia has been attributed to blockage of the reticuloendothelial system secondary to the use of intravenous immunoglobulins [73]. Recently, Sheth et al. [356] found in a double-blind, controlled study of 20 children with HUS, that intravenous infusion of gamma globulins (400 mg/kg/day for 5 days) had no benefits on platelet count and patient outcome. Persistence of severe central nervous system (CNS) symptoms and abnormal findings on computed tomography (CT) scans and radionuclide blood flow studies in 2 patients of the control group during the acute phase of the disease, compared to none in the treatment group, suggested a potential benefit of intravenous immunoglobulin infusion on CNS involvement of HUS. The limited number of cases, however, does not allow conclusions as to the effectiveness of this approach, whereas the severity of the reported side effects advise against the use of intravenous immunoglobulin as first-choice therapy for HUS and TTP.

Table 75-2. Therapeutic approaches in thrombotic thrombocytopenic purpura

	Author	Year	[Reference]
Steroids	Burke	1959	[43]
	Levin	1966	[218]
Splenectomy	Baehr	1936	[10a]
	Hill	1968	[163a]
	Bernard	1969	[20a]
	Scharoff	1969	[344a]
	Cuttner	1974	[75]
	Reynolds	1976	[324]
	Rutkow	1978	[343]
Heparin	Bernstock	1960	[20b]
	Richardson	1968	[324a]
Antiplatelet agents	Girouini	1972	[130a]
	Amir	1973	[2a]
	Rossi	1974	[337a]
	Amorosi	1977	[3]
	Eckel	1977	[93a]
	Gundlack	1977	[146]
	Birgens	1979	[21]
	Marmont	1980	[239]
Whole blood exchange transfusion	Rubinstein	1959	[339a]
	Gottschall	1981	[139a]
Plasma exchange	Bukowski	1976	[38]
	Taft	1979	[380]
	McLeod	1980	[245a]
	Petitt	1980	[299]
	Myers	1981	[275]
	Simon	1981	[365a]
Plasma infusion	Byrnes	1977	[48]
Prostacyclin infusion	Hensby	1979	[162]
	Budd	1980	[36]
	Fitzgerald	1981	[107]
	Cocchetto	1981	[67]
Immuno-Globulins	Messmore	1985	[248]
	Viero	1986	[392a]
	Wong	1986	[411]
	Gilcher	1987	[127]
	Chin	1987	[62]
	Finn	1987	[106]

Hemolytic-Uremic Syndrome

In 1955 Gasser [119] described a fatal syndrome of acute hemolytic anemia, thrombocytopenia, and renal failure that occurred in children. The following reports on this disorder, called *hemolytic-uremic syndrome* (HUS), focused on the gastrointestinal prodromes [2, 206, 360, 361]. The term *microangiopathic hemolytic anemia* [29] has also been used to indicate that the observed red cell fragmentation is the result of the passage of red cells through diseased blood vessels. Recent studies have led to a better knowledge of the epidemiology and clinical course of HUS, which represents the main cause of acute renal failure (ARF) in children [79a, 125, 226]; adults may also be affected [70, 114, 181, 350].

Whether TTP and HUS should be considered two distinct diseases or two different expressions of the same disease has not been established [337]. A recent comparison of TTP and HUS suggests that they are distinguishable by a different degree of renal involvement and a different localization of thrombotic changes [37, 110]. However, among the adult population it is very difficult to separate the two syndromes [337].

One of the best classifications of HUS has been proposed by Drummond [88], who considered the following categories of the disease: (1) Classic form, occurring in infants with diarrheal prodromes and good prognosis and not associated with abnormalities in PGI_2; (2) postinfectious form, associated with a well-recognized infection (*Shigella, Streptococcus, Salmonella*); (3) hereditary form, which may occur in children or adults, sometimes with recurrent episodes; vascular PGI_2 has been found to be abnormal in these cases; (4) immunologically mediated form, characterized by low plasma C3 levels; (5) secondary form, associated with SLE, scleroderma, and malignant hypertension or induced by radiation of the kidney, chemotherapy, and immunosuppressive drugs (mitomycin [202, 231] and cyclosporine [214, 360]; and finally (6) a form related to pregnancy or oral contraceptives.

CLINICAL FEATURES

Gastrointestinal prodromes often occur few days or weeks before the onset of HUS, especially in endemic or epidemic areas [88, 135, 189, 361]. Vomiting, diarrhea with soft mucus or blood in stools, and abdominal pain are common [119, 125]. Infections of the upper respiratory [86, 124] or urinary [225] tracts are found less frequently. It seems that the prognosis is worse in patients without the gastrointestinal prodrome [88, 334, 375].

Anemia and renal involvement are the keystone symptoms that are always present during the acute phase [110, 126]. Often anemia is severe and associated with signs of hemolysis—i.e., an increase in indirect bilirubin and LDH enzymes, a fall in haptoglobin, and reticulocytosis [1, 126]. Direct and indirect Coombs' tests are usually negative [110]. The peripheral smear shows the typical finding of fragmented red blood cells with helmet and burr cells [40, 41], whereas osmotic fragility and red blood cell enzymatic activities are normal [110, 173]. Bone marrow aspirate shows findings of marked erythroblastosis [126]. Occasionally in the vessels from tissue sections, fragmented red blood cells or cells at different degrees of hemolysis can be detected (Fig. 75-2A, B). Renal damage is a constant feature in all patients. ARF is reported in 92 percent of patients [126], and anuria is seen in one-third of cases [125]. Severe metabolic acidosis, hypercalcemia, and high blood levels of urea due to the high catabolic rate are present [125, 126]. Gross hematuria is infrequent, but microhematuria and proteinuria ranging from 1 to 2 gm per day are almost constant findings [126]. Hemoglobinuria is found during the severe hemolytic crisis [126]. Systemic arterial hypertension is found in about 60 percent of patients [152]. In a large percentage of patients, renal failure requires dialysis [22, 70, 97]. The mean duration of renal failure is about 14 days [126].

A bleeding tendency is described in the majority of patients. The gastrointestinal tract is the main source of bleeding, more frequently with melena and hematemesis [126]. Thrombocytopenia is the rule in all patients and is due to peripheral platelet destruction, platelets having a very short survival time [154, 250]. Prothrombin time may be prolonged, and fibrinogen degradation products are elevated in a significant number of patients [65, 68, 126, 372]. Plasma fibrinogen, however, is normal or even increased [28], whereas low levels of antithrombin III have been detected [30, 82a, 110]. Neurologic complications are detected in about 40 percent of patients and include generalized convulsions, obtundation, stupor, coma, and hemiparesis [126, 179, 242, 333].

Low levels of C3, C4 [53, 180, 259], and C3 activation with C3 breakdown products [190, 261] have been documented in patients with HUS. Both classic and alternate pathways of complement activation operate, but C5 levels are normal, implying that the phase fluid alone is activated and the membrane attack complex of complement is spared [135, 261].

PATHOLOGY

The kidneys are the main target organs involved in HUS. Pathologic changes originally described by Gasser [119] in children with HUS were consistent with a picture of cortical necrosis. Since then lesions of HUS have been described in more detail [123, 147, 149, 331, 393]. A term that successfully defines the characteristic pathologic changes of HUS is *thrombotic microangiopathy* [148]. The classic lesion is characterized by thickening of the capillary walls secondary to the presence of a fluffy material in the subendothelial space [135, 149, 393]. These changes, plus occasional thrombi, lead to occlusion of the glomerular capillary lumen. In the acute phase arteriolar and capillary thrombi are more common, whereas the subendothelial fluff is the dominant lesion seen days or weeks after the acute attack. A widening and fibrillar appearance of the mesangium coexists with the glomerular capillary wall alterations [148, 358]. The vascular lesions may be differently distributed [135, 221, 268], and the percentage of affected glomeruli may influence the prognosis [221].

The finding of pure thrombotic microangiopathic lesions derives mainly from studies in children, especially children under the age of 2 years. However, in older children and adults the histologic pattern is usually more complex and is characterized by a prevalence of arterial involvement with necrosis and thrombosis of interlobular arteries associated with ischemic changes in glomeruli.

According to a recent study [221], three patterns of renal lesions can be found in HUS—one with prevalent glomerular lesions of the microangiopathic type, one with predominant arterial involvement, and a third with simultaneous glomerular and arterial involvement. Other tentative classifications for HUS have been proposed. Recently, Thoenes and John [381] proposed the term *endotheliotropic haemolytic nephroangiopathy*. In the opinion of the authors, this term, in addition to including the main clinical features of the disease, also emphasizes the decisive pathogenetic role of endothelial damage. To emphasize the pathogenetic role of vascular changes in HUS Bohle et al. [24] used the definition *primary malignant nephrosclerosis*.

A detailed analysis of renal changes in younger children includes swelling of glomerular endothelial cells leading to narrowing or complete occlusion of glomerular capillary lumens (Fig. 75-3). Glomerular capillary walls are thickened, and often the endothelial cells are separated from the glomerular basement membrane (GBM). A fluffy material accumulates in the subendothelial space, giving a double-contoured appearance to the glomerular capillary walls (Fig. 75-4). Together with the swelling of the endothelial cells, the widening of the subendothelial space contributes to the occlusion of the glomerular lumen. Thrombi having the characteristic staining for fibrin are occasionally seen. Mesangial matrix has a fibrillar appearance without any sign of mes-

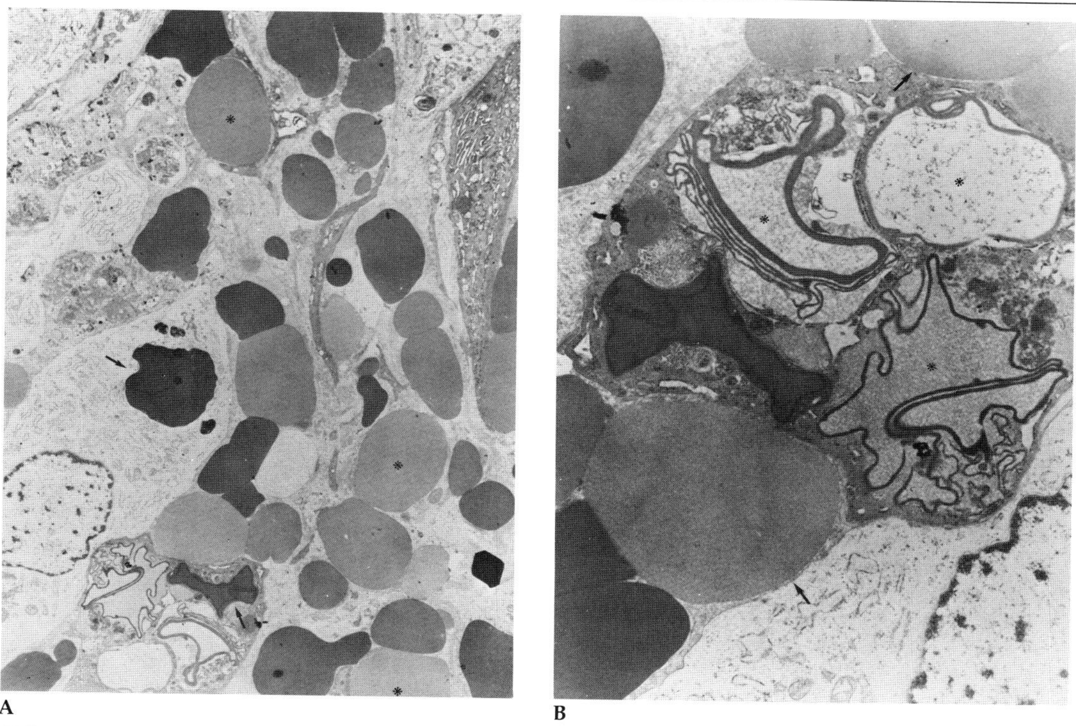

Fig. 75-2. A. Electron micrograph showing fragmented red blood cells (arrows) and red cells at different stages of hemolysis (asterisks) in a small renal vein from a patient with hemolytic uremic syndrome. (×5,000.) B. High magnification of inset of Fig. 75-2A showing red blood cells at different stages of hemolysis (arrow) and the presence of "ghosts" of red blood cells (asterisks) in a small renal vein from a patient with hemolytic-uremic syndrome. (×12,000.) (Both micrographs courtesy of Dr. C. L. Pirani and Dr. V. D'Agati.)

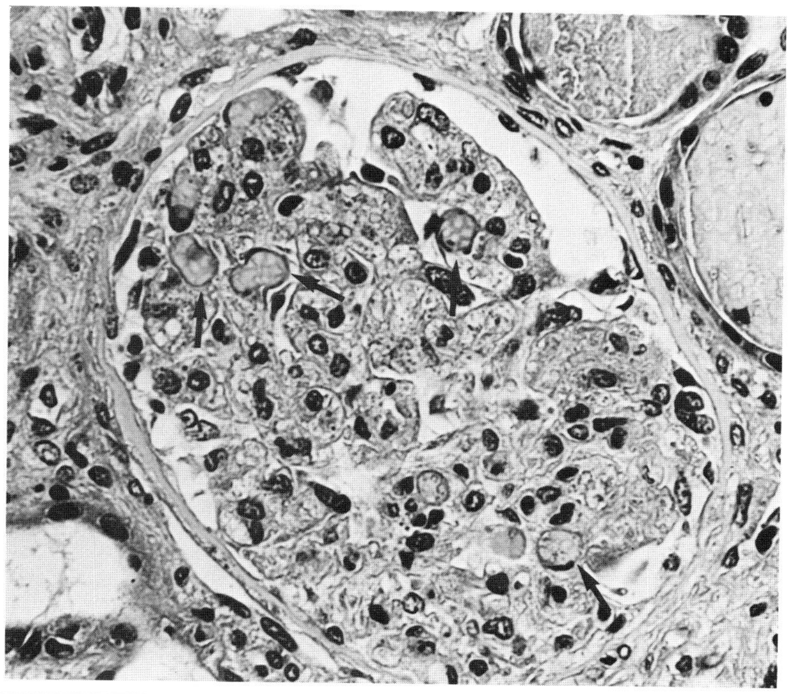

Fig. 75-3. Swelling of glomerular endothelial cells and occlusion of almost all capillary lumens packed with red blood cells (arrows) in a case of hemolytic-uremic syndrome. (Trichrome; ×250.)

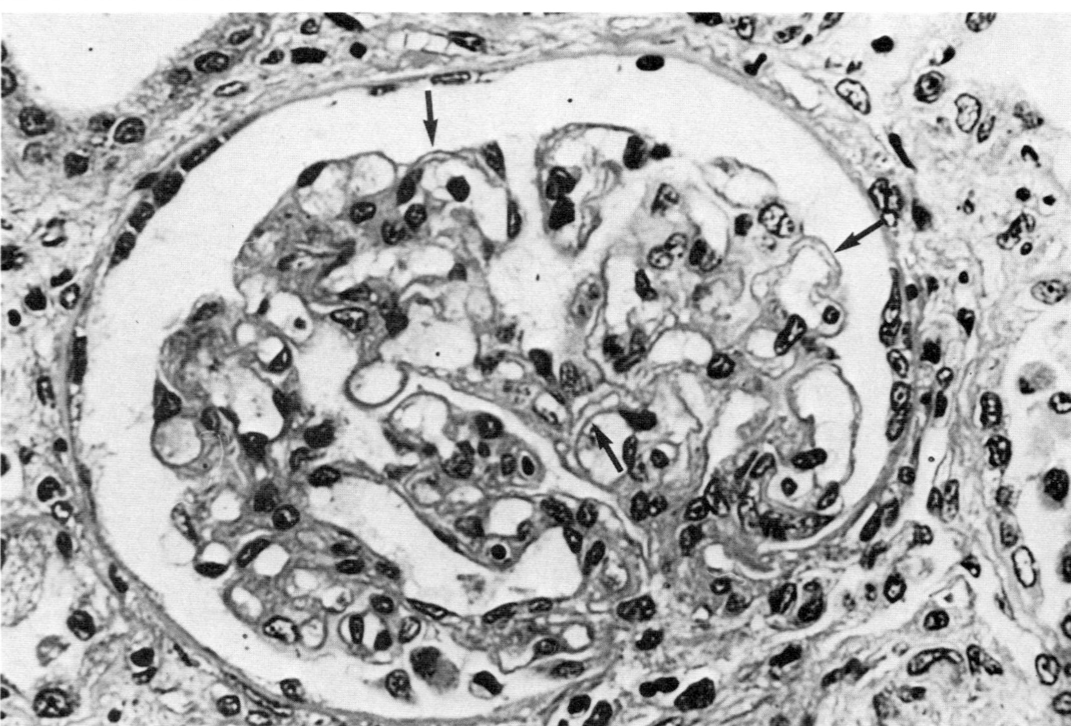

Fig. 75-4. Double tracks (arrows) in some areas of glomerular capillary walls of a patient with hemolytic-uremic syndrome. (Trichrome; ×375.)

angial hypercellularity. Occasionally red blood cells and platelets are seen in the glomerular capillary lumens. Not all glomeruli are equally affected. In some cases damage is more severe, whereas in others less pronounced changes (Fig. 75-4) are found. Arterial involvement is extremely variable, but some widening of the subendothelial space containing fluffy material is observed.

In older children and in adults the major changes are restricted to the arteries [176, 221]. Interlobular arteries are often occluded by thrombosis, necrosis, or intimal edema or proliferation [176] (Figs. 75-5 and 75-6). In the more chronic phases, fibroplasia of small arteries and arteriosclerotic changes are seen. In some cases glomeruloid structures of the small arteries are observed, probably as a result of endothelial and myointimal proliferation of small arteries adjacent to the glomeruli [301]. Glomerular lesions are ischemic, as shown by the thickening and wrinkling of the glomerular capillary walls, by atrophy of the glomerular tufts, and by thickening of Bowman's capsule (Fig. 75-7). In a small number of patients a histologic pattern of cortical or tubular necrosis is detected [221]. Not infrequently, however, the pattern of glomerular involvement coexists in the same patient with significant arterial damage [221, 268].

Immunofluorescence shows fibrinogen almost invariably present in the glomeruli, along the glomerular capillary walls and in the thrombi and vessel lumina [196]. Granular deposits of C3 and IgM are also found in glomeruli and vessels [136, 336]. Ultrastructural injury to glomerular endothelial cells is pronounced. Endothelial cells are swollen and are often detached from the underlying GBM (Fig. 75-8). Beneath, the endothelium is an electron-lucent fluffy material that may be associated with a thin, newly formed GBM (Fig. 75-9). The composition of this fluffy material is not known, but it has been suggested that it might consist of fibrinogen-fibrin breakdown products as well as fibronectin [301]. Glomerular capillary lumens are markedly narrowed by the combination of endothelial and subendothelial changes. Foam cells can be detected within the glomeruli, generally in the late stages of the disease, and contain lipid droplets and myelin figures. Glomerular mesangium may be the site of fibrin deposits, but the most common lesion is edema of the mesangial matrix leading to marked reticulation and even complete dissolution, called "mesangiolysis" [135]. Endothelial damage predominates in arteries and arterioles, which demonstrate detachment of endothelium, swelling of endothelial cells, and subendothelial fluffy deposits.

PROGNOSIS AND TREATMENT

The clinical course of HUS has significantly improved in recent years, probably because of a more efficient management of symptoms in the acute phase of the disease. This is particularly true in the pediatric population. In a classic study by Gianantonio and associates [126] the outcome of 678 patients with HUS was reported. The data clearly showed a trend toward a better prognosis from the late 1950s to 1972. Mortality rate was reported

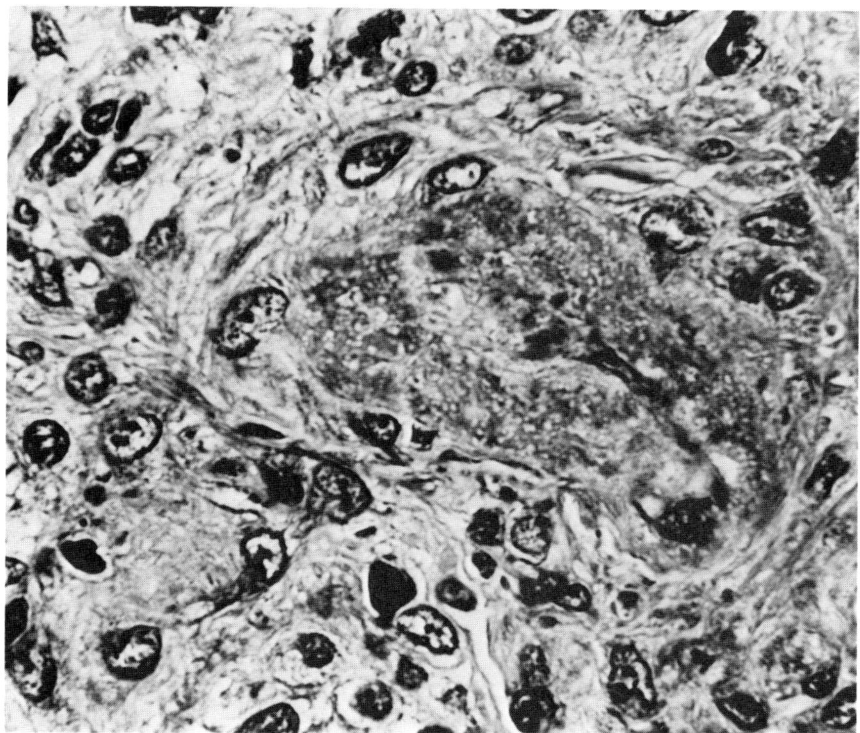

Fig. 75-5. Thrombotic and necrotic changes in a small artery from an adult patient with hemolytic-uremic syndrome. (Trichrome; ×375.)

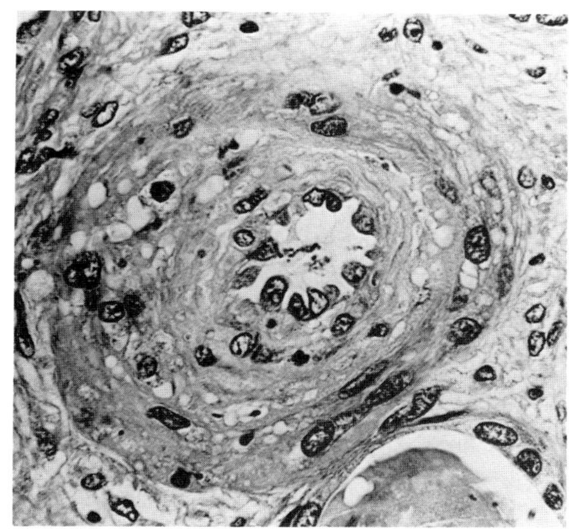

Fig. 75-6. Occlusion of an interlobular artery with intimal swelling and myointimal proliferation in a case of adult hemolytic-uremic syndrome. (Trichrome; ×375.)

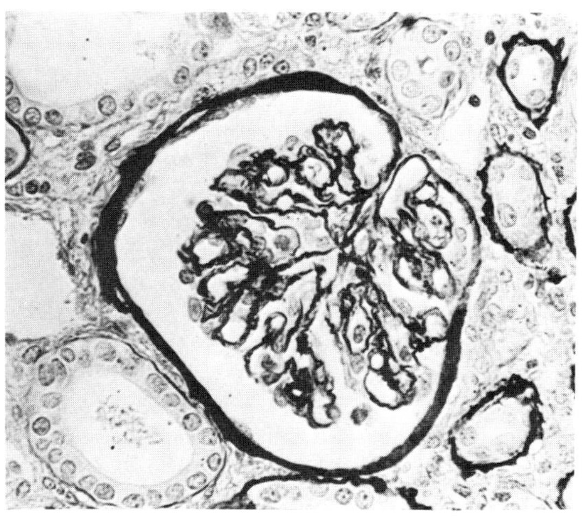

Fig. 75-7. Ischemic glomerular lesions characterized by thickening and wrinkling of glomerular capillary walls and atrophy of glomerular tuft in a case of adult hemolytic-uremic syndrome. (Silver; ×250.)

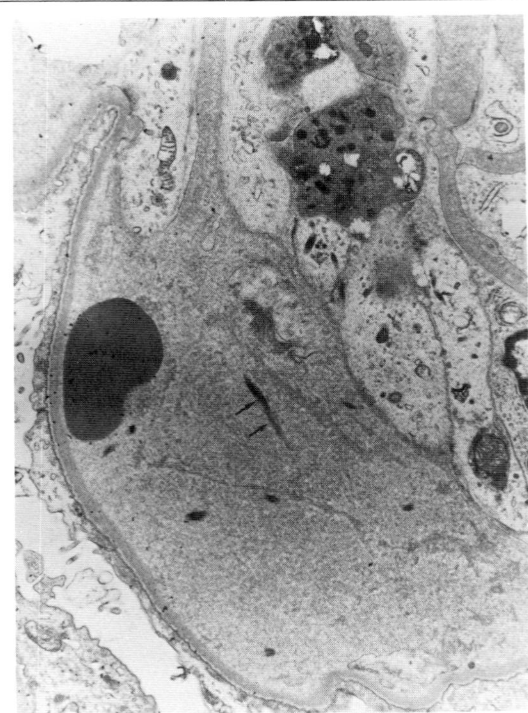

Fig. 75-8. Detachment of endothelial cell from the underlying glomerular basement membrane in a case of hemolytic-uremic syndrome. A red blood cell is in close contact with the glomerular basement membrane. Electron-lucent "fluffy" material and a few strands of fibrin (arrows) are present in subendothelial space. (×7,000.) (Courtesy of Dr. C. L. Pirani and Dr. V. D'Agati.)

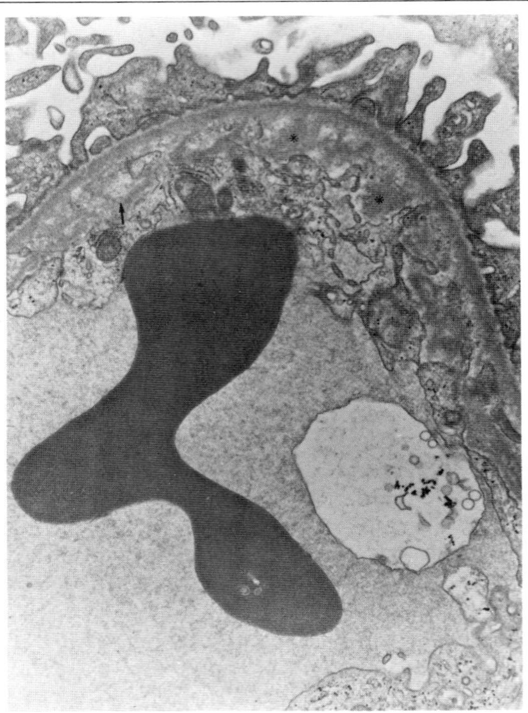

Fig. 75-9. Electron-lucent "fluffy" material (arrow) with some electron-dense deposits (asterisks) is located between the cytoplasm of an endothelial cell and the glomerular basement membrane in a segment of glomerular capillary from a patient with hemolytic-uremic syndrome. (×12,000.) (Courtesy of Dr. C. L. Pirani and Dr. V. D'Agati.)

as high as 47 percent in 32 children observed during the period from 1957 to 1961, but it dropped to only 6.25 percent in 1972.

Interest has recently focused on the evaluation of the role of specific prognostic factors on outcome patterns in HUS. Epidemiologic studies have shown that pediatric patients with HUS can be designated as affected by a typical or atypical form [399]. The typical form mostly affects younger children, who have a prodrome of bloody diarrhea, presents in warm seasons, and occurs in epidemic clusters. The atypical form of HUS affects older children in cold months and is not constantly announced by prodromal diarrhea. This classification, although not infallible, provides a relatively good index of outcome. In an elegant study in 1983 Trompeter and associates [386] examined retrospectively the clinical and laboratory data of 72 children with HUS seen between 1969 and 1980. They analyzed data with a stepwise logistic regression model, which allows an estimate of the prognostic value of each clinical or laboratory value. They found that the probability of complete recovery of renal function as predicted by this analysis was significantly higher in patients of younger age, presenting in summer, with diarrhea at onset, and with a short prodromal disease. In other words, patients classified as typical cases had a better prognosis than atypical ones. The overall recovery rate was, in any case, high; of 72 children, 50 (70 percent) completely recovered renal function, and 8 had residual hypertension or chronic renal failure.

In 1989 the same group of investigators [399] reviewed the clinical data of 79 patients with HUS and included polymorphonuclear leukocyte count among the potential prognostic factors. Patients with typical HUS had a significantly higher count as compared to atypical patients. When only typical cases were considered, logistic analysis showed that the higher the polymorphonuclear leukocyte count was, the higher the probability of an unfavorable outcome. Therefore the authors concluded that a high polymorphonuclear leukocyte count at onset in patients with typical HUS could be considered an indicator of poor prognosis. A recent study by Martin et al. [241] at Minnesota Department of Health confirmed the evidence that an elevated polymorphonuclear leukocyte count on hospital admission was associated with a more severe disease and could help in predicting outcome. This finding may reflect a more invasive disease or a higher infectious dose of verotoxin-producing *E. coli.* The authors concluded that the identification of these predictors may help clinicians to identify the treatment of choice. Few data are available on the long-term outcome of HUS in children. In a retrospective study by de Jong and Monnens [82] a 10-year follow-up of 73 patients who had HUS was presented. Patients were divided into three groups according to the increasing duration of oliguria and/or anuria. Only 10 percent of patients with the mild form of HUS had residual hypertension 10 years later. In group 2, 27.5 percent showed some degree of chronic renal damage (i.e., mild to moderate proteinuria and/or reduced renal function). All those who had severe renal impairment at onset had late renal sequelae. In adults HUS has a much worse prognosis than in children. In one of the largest published series [268], a mortality rate of 40 percent was reported. The authors could not find clinical features predictive of final outcome, whereas the severity of vascular lesions at the renal biopsy correlated well with the outcome [268]. We recently reviewed data on 43 adult patients with HUS who had been treated in several hospitals in Italy [345]. The overall mortality rate was 14 percent in this group; dialysis was required during the acute phase in 70 percent of the patients and as late as 1 year 25 patients were classified as having a "poor" outcome. More than half of the patients developed HUS in the setting of another disease (malignant hypertension, preeclampsia, scleroderma, or cancer). Our data confirm that HUS in adults is often a complication of some severe underlying disease, and this may explain its severity in terms of short- and long-term outcome [66, 105, 163, 229,268, 331].

Many therapeutic approaches have been proposed for HUS (Table 75-3). Steroids [125, 300], heparin [28, 128], dipyridamole and aspirin [7, 385], streptokinase [262], plasma exchange [13, 129], plasma infusion [253, 321], PGI_2 [14, 404], and vitamin E [307], have all been employed in various combinations. The overall results are difficult to interpret because almost all studies involve only small numbers of patients, and very few controlled prospective studies have been done. Reports of therapeutic success in isolated cases of HUS led during the 1960s and 1970s to extensive use of heparin, commonly associated with antiplatelet agents [28, 128, 164, 226]. However, the prospective study of Proesmans' group [310] did not confirm any useful effect of heparin alone or associated with antiplatelet agents in the short-term prognosis.

It is worth stressing the potentially serious risks of inducing anticoagulation in a disease that has serious hemorrhagic complications, often associated with severe hypertension [179]. Some beneficial effects of heparin therapy emerged from a retrospective analysis of uncontrolled studies in postpartum HUS [230, 331], which indicated a 53 percent survival in the treated group versus 17 percent in nontreated patients [303]. However, in postpartum HUS the lack of any controlled studies also makes it difficult to reach any definite conclusions.

Thrombolytic therapy has been employed, with conflicting results [15, 260, 262, 306, 375]. As in TTP, the use of exchange transfusion and plasmapheresis has been associated with remission of disease [13, 129]. However, reports are generally isolated, and once again no controlled studies have been done. Following the hypothesis that HUS patients might lack a plasma component that modulates vascular PGI_2 production [233, 320, 321], many patients have been treated by fresh plasma infusion with the aim of restoring normal plasma properties. Beneficial effects, especially in normalizing the hematologic abnormalities, have been reported by several authors [321, 376, 386]. Our group [253] recently considered the effect of plasma infusion associated with supportive measures alone in 10 children and 7 adults with HUS. All patients but 1 responded to the treatment with rapid disappearance of the hematologic abnormalities. Despite the anuria or oliguria present on admission in 15 of 17 patients, renal function recovered completely in 8 children and 2 adults. All the remaining 7 cases had chronic renal failure, but only 2 required chronic hemodialysis.

PGI_2 infusion has been used in occasional patients [14, 404], but to date the results are difficult to evaluate. Recently, vitamin E treatment has also been proposed [307] because of low plasma levels of vitamin E and the reported changes in membrane phospholipids suggestive of peroxidative damage in red blood cells and the reduced antioxidant power detected in HUS patients [288]. Powell and co-workers [307] reported a series of 16 children with HUS treated with vitamin E in whom, despite the presence of clinical features predictive of a poor prognosis, 100 percent survival and complete recovery of renal function were attained. These results are of sufficient interest to suggest a controlled trial.

Table 75-3. Therapeutic approaches in hemolytic-uremic syndrome

	Author	Year	Reference
Steroids	Gianantonio	1964	[125]
	Piel	1966	[300]
	Conte	1974	[68]
Heparin	Gilchrist	1969	[128]
	Luke	1970	[230]
	Vitacco	1973	[392b]
	Proesmans	1974	[309a]
	Khanh	1976	[189a]
	Ponticelli	1980	[303]
Antiplatelet agents	Arenson	1975	[7]
	Amorosi	1977	[3]
	Thorsen	1979	[385]
	O'Regan	1980	[289]
Fibrinolytic agents	Powell	1974	[306]
	Stuart	1974	[375]
	Monnens	1978	[262]
Plasma exchange	Beattie	1981	[13]
	Gillor	1983	[129]
Plasma infusion	Remuzzi	1979	[321]
	Misiani	1982	[253]
	Stuart	1983	[376]
	Trompeter	1983	[386]
Prostacyclin infusion	Webster	1980	[404]
	Beattie	1981	[14]
Vitamin E	Powell	1984	[307]
γ-Globulins	Sheth	1990	[356]

Treatment of Thrombotic Thrombocytopenic Purpura and Hemolytic-Uremic Syndrome: Conclusions

In summary all the proposed specific therapies for HUS and TTP need to be evaluated in controlled trials, taking into account the fact that the prognosis of the disease is extremely variable according to the age of onset and the different organs involved. It is likely that advances in the outcome of these patients are also due to the appropriate supportive treatments and to adequate management of life-threatening symptoms. Among nonspecific therapies, the crucial point appears to be the careful management of the acutely ill patient which includes intensive care for respiratory distress, dialysis, antihypertensive drugs, and blood transfusions when anemia is symptomatic. Among specific therapies, steroids, antiplatelet agents, human immunoglobulins, plasma infusion, and plasma exchange are the most commonly employed, in various combinations. However, none of these specific therapies has been formally tested in prospective controlled trials. Of interest in this context is the clinical history of a patient, now 22 years old, with repetitive occurrences of HUS and TTP [340]. During childhood, five episodes classified as HUS always recovered with blood transfusions. Since the age of 21 the patient has had eight episodes, classified as TTP, that always recovered following daily plasma exchange. In order to avoid exposure to large amounts of plasma, alternate forms of initial therapy, including aspirin (50 mg per day), prednisone (1 mg/kg/day), and human immunoglobulins (0.5 mg/kg/day) were employed during some of the relapses (Fig. 75-10). However, all these treatments were ineffective and plasma exchange was necessary on each occasion to achieve remission. On two more recent relapses, fresh frozen plasma was infused as initial therapy at a dose of 40 ml per kilogram the first day, followed by 20 mg per kilogram for 2 days, and produced complete clinical remission and normalized the platelet count within a few days, thus precluding the need for plasma exchange. Thus, in this individual patient, none of the suggested specific therapies except plasma infusion could be substituted for plasma exchange and achieve the desired response. The effectiveness of plasma infusion alone raises the question of whether plasma exchange is effective because it removes circulating toxins or because it gives to the patient putative "missing" factor(s) that may play a pathogenetic role. The invariable response to plasma manipulation stresses the concept that this is an essential part of the treatment of a potentially fatal disease; moreover, the virtually identical response to plasma exchange and infusion would indicate that infusing normal plasma is an important component of the procedure and that plasma exchange is probably not necessary in most patients with thrombotic microangiopathy. Since infusion imposes a limit on the amount of plasma a patient can receive, plasma exchange should be considered the treatment of choice unless there are clear indications that plasma infusion would be sufficient. The decision to treat a patient with large infusions of plasma has to be weighed against the potential side effects. Besides fluid overload, which can be easily controlled by hemodialysis, and hypersensitivity reactions, the possibility of transmitting hepatitis or other plasma-transmitted diseases (such as HIV infection) is of particular concern. In the management of adult TTP, plasma exchange remains the treatment of choice and, because of the high risk of sudden death in these patients, it should be instituted as soon as the diagnosis is made. Serum LDH concentration and platelet count are the most sensitive indicators of disease intensity and of therapy efficacy.

Fig. 75-10. Platelet count response to specific therapies in a patient with repetitive occurrences of hemolytic-uremic syndrome and thrombotic thrombocytopenic purpura.

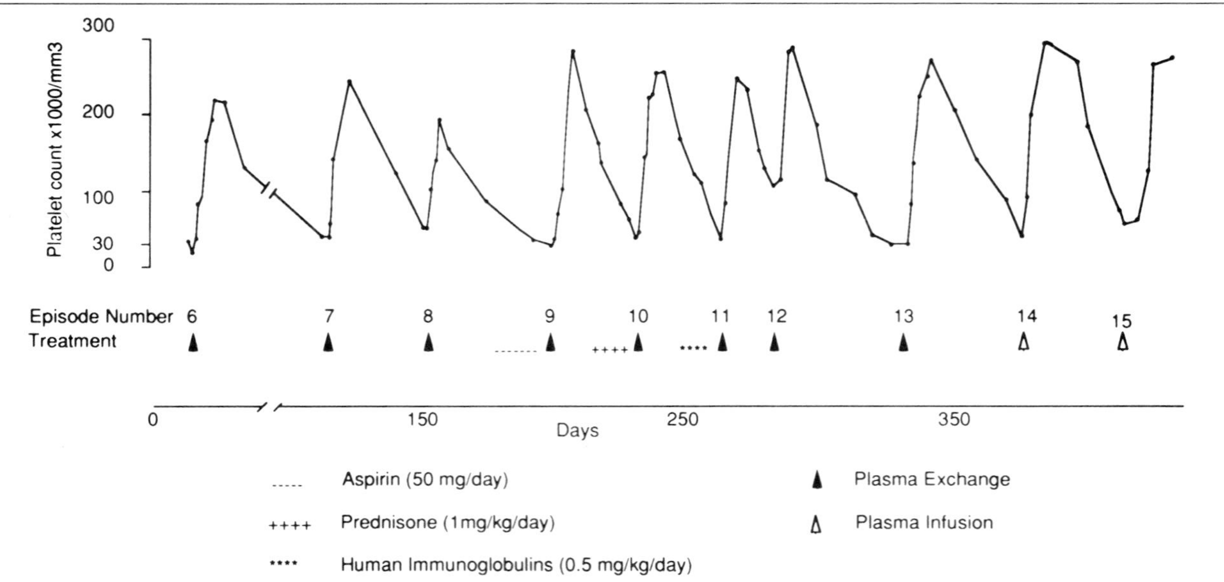

Acute Cortical Necrosis

Acute cortical necrosis represents a rare cause of ARF, occurring in about 2 percent of patients [193]. The term *acute cortical necrosis* defines a condition of destruction of the renal cortex except for a thin tissue rim under the capsule and usually a thicker layer under the corticomedullary junction. This phenomenon reflects a disturbed blood flow to interlobular and afferent arterioles, whereas the arcuate arteries, which supply blood to the juxtamedullary nephrons, are usually spared. The lack of necrosis in subcapsular nephrons is due to the presence of anastomoses with extrarenal vessels that allow minimal perfusion to superficial nephrons, just enough to prevent necrotic changes. In 50 to 70 percent of the series considered, acute cortical necrosis is a complication of pregnancy (especially in multiparous women over 30 years of age). Abruptio placentae is the most common prior complication of the illness [193, 354]. Preexisting toxemia seems to be an important predisposing factor [63, 103, 284], but there is no general agreement on this issue [193]. Intrauterine death, hemorrhage from placenta previa, septic abortion, postpartum hemorrhage, and occasionally hyperemesis are other conditions that may be complicated by acute cortical necrosis [193, 245, 265, 366, 417].

Recently, Donohoe [87] followed pregnant women throughout the two decades from 1961 to 1980. Comparing the incidence of acute cortical necrosis during these periods, he found that in the second group (1971 to 1980) abruptio placentae occurred almost three times less often than in the first group. Acute renal failure and acute cortical necrosis also decreased further in the following 10 years (1971 to 1980), proving that not only a better management of pregnancy but also a prompter and more appropriate approach may prevent the occurrence of necrotic changes in the cortex. In contrast, a recent experience [143] has indicated that cases of cortical necrosis associated with pregnancy are increasing despite an overall reduction in the number of patients suffering from ARF after pregnancy.

Bacterial and postoperative shock, pancreatitis, dissecting aneurysms, gastrointestinal hemorrhage, trauma, burns, phosphorous and diethylene glycol poisoning, snake venom bites, and sometimes HUS and TTP are other conditions that can be complicated by acute cortical necrosis [33, 79, 120, 134, 211, 243, 273, 286, 335, 354, 367, 398, 413]. In children, cases of cortical necrosis have been reported, most frequently after protracted vomiting and diarrhea with marked dehydration [54, 141, 421]. Moreover, as in adults, the disease has been seen concomitantly with infections such as peritonitis, septicemia, pharyngitis, transfusion reactions, and phosphorous poisoning [54, 141, 297, 395, 398, 421].

PATHOGENESIS

The pathogenesis of cortical necrosis still remains a mystery. The two major theories proposed so far only partially explain the disease. According to Sheehan and Moore [354], who studied specimens from patients who died after abruptio placentae, vasospasm is the primary event causing cortical necrosis. Alternatively, it has been suggested that acute vascular injury followed by activation of coagulation and thrombosis plays a key role in the development of cortical necrosis [332, 382]. Both these theories do not convincingly account for the fact that after the initial "trigger" a cascade of events takes place leading to a necrotic process localized at the renal cortex.

Sheehan and Davis [352] observed that prolonged experimental clamping of the renal pedicle can produce cortical necrosis. The same lesion was obtained in experimental animals by the infusion of a large amount of vasoactive substances such as epinephrine and oxytocin [49, 50, 294]. However, no convincing evidence is available so far to support the idea that vasospasm is the key event in acute cortical necrosis in man [87].

Experimental Shwartzman reaction produced in pregnant rabbits after a single injection of bacterial toxin supports the theory that vascular injury is the major etiologic event in cortical necrosis [362]. The Shwartzman reaction produces disseminated intravascular coagulation (DIC). The crucial role of the latter in the development of cortical necrosis is documented by the fact that heparin reduces the incidence of cortical necrosis in the model of GSR of nonpregnant rabbits [69]. However, the main difference between experimental Shwartzman reaction and cortical necrosis in humans is that in animals the necrotic process involves also the renal medulla and organs other than the kidney. Probably in humans selective damage of the cortical vasculature predisposes to the subsequent development of localized damage as soon as a "trigger event"—e.g., abruptio placentae—occurs. In this context recent experimental data are particularly relevant. Unilateral Shwartzman phenomenon confined to a single kidney has been produced by local perfusion of low-dose endotoxin before systemic injection of endotoxin [317]. Cortical necrosis in experimental animals has also been obtained using liquoid or diethylene glycol [120, 347]. The mechanisms by which these toxic agents lead to cortical necrosis are far from being understood, but these agents are known to cause endothelial damage.

Another intriguing issue is the significance of glomerular fibrin thrombi. Early reports have focused on the possible crucial role of glomerular thrombosis in the pathogenesis of the disease [238, 245]. However, a detailed analysis of the most representative series reported in the literature revealed that glomerular fibrin thrombi are relatively rare in cortical necrosis: Only occasionally have extensive intraglomerular thrombi been documented [193, 366]. Altogether, the available data do not support the idea that cortical necrosis is the consequence of a mechanical blockage of glomeruli by fibrin thrombi. Moreover, in the two largest series [330, 366] reported so far of patients affected by DIC with glomerular fibrin thrombi, the majority of which had bacterial sepsis, cortical necrosis was found in only 4 of the 63 cases studied.

Finally, it has been suggested that cortical necrosis might be a consequence of immunologic mechanisms. Most evidence in support of this hypothesis comes from the observation that pathologic findings similar to cortical necrosis have been found in hyperacute rejection of renal allografts [121]. Cortical necrosis in these cases presumably results from direct immunologic injury to transplanted cortical vessels by preformed antibodies. This event occurs in completely denervated allografts, and thus vascular endothelial damage rather than vasospasm may be the primary event in the overall pathogenesis of at least some forms of this dramatic disease.

CLINICAL FEATURES

The most typical clinical sign of acute cortical necrosis is sudden oligoanuria, the amount of urine ranging from 0 and 100 ml per day [220]. Sometimes this is preceded by gross hematuria. Lumbar pain, if present, constitutes a rather nonspecific symptom and may be associated with fever and leukocytosis. Urine contains proteins, red blood cells, white blood cells, epithelial cells, and various types of casts. Hypertension may occur, but generally the blood pressure is only slightly elevated. A picture of ARF with hyperazotemia, metabolic acidosis, and hyperkalemia emerges from laboratory data. LDH and glutamic oxaloacetic transaminases in serum are elevated during the first days of the disease [347]. DIC is frequent, especially in obstetric patients. Fibrinogen and platelet counts fall very low, prothrombin time is prolonged, and FDPs in serum are often elevated [87].

Acute cortical necrosis must be suspected when oliguria or anuria tends to persist for a long period. Renal biopsy provides the definitive diagnosis. However, the patient's clinical condition may not always permit the performance of a biopsy, and in some cases the diagnosis may be missed because, especially in the incomplete form of disease, the specimen does not detect the typical changes. Radiologic techniques are very useful in the evaluation of the diagnosis of acute cortical necrosis [193, 257, 406]. Renal echography may exclude obstruction. Selective arteriography may provide information about the extent of lesions, permitting a distinction between the complete and incomplete forms. The most typical radiologic sign of acute cortical necrosis is the renal cortical calcification, which, however, is uncommon and does not occur in the early phases of the disease [347].

Hemodynamic studies with krypton or xenon washout techniques indicate reduced renal blood flow; however, these techniques, except in cases of complete acute cortical necrosis, may not differentiate between patients with incomplete acute cortical necrosis and those with acute tubular necrosis [193].

PATHOLOGY

In 1953 Sheehan and Moore [354] described in detail the pathologic changes characteristic of cortical necrosis. In massive or complete cortical necrosis almost the whole cortex is affected by necrosis except the corticomedullary junction and a thin rim of cortical tissue under the capsule. On gross examination the kidneys are enlarged and weigh 200 to 300 gm. The cortex has a yellowish-white appearance, but congested areas are detected in the periphery. Moreover, the columns of Bertin are necrosed. The main renal arteries—the lobar and the arciform—are generally spared. Microscopic examination shows pathologic changes appearing 48 to 72 hours after the initial injury. Glomeruli and tubules show extensive necrotic changes, whereas the afferent arterioles are occluded by thrombi extending to the interlobular arteries. At the periphery of the necrosis, large-scale infiltration of polymorphonuclear leukocytes fully develops after 3 to 4 days.

In addition to the pattern of complete cortical necrosis, Sheehan and Moore [354] described other forms of acute cortical necrosis characterized by more limited necrotic changes, the so-called incomplete acute cortical necrosis. The latter includes the focal form, in which the necrotic lesion can reach a diameter ranging from 3.0 to 0.5 mm, and the patchy form, with much larger necrotic areas. The authors described an additional variant of acute cortical necrosis called confluent focal cortical necrosis, which differs from the forms previously described in the following aspects: (1) The focal lesions are so numerous that they merge with one another; (2) the typical changes are present in tubules and glomeruli but not in the arterioles and arteries and appear at different stages in the course of the disease; and (3) the pattern is not associated with abruptio placentae.

Histologically, the lesions of incomplete cortical necrosis are essentially the same as those in the complete form. The edge of the necrotic area forms a sharp border with normal renal tissue. In the late phases of the disease, kidneys are reduced in size; interstitial fibrosis occurs in the injured areas, and sclerotic substitutions occur in glomeruli and in vessels. Calcium deposits detected by Kossa stain can be found in glomeruli or in arteries.

Obviously the organ most often affected by acute cortical necrosis is the kidney; however, though to a lesser extent and more mildly, other organs are sometimes injured too, such as the adrenals, spleen, liver, large intestine, and particularly the pituitary gland sinusoids [89, 193, 232, 355].

PROGNOSIS AND TREATMENT

The course of acute cortical necrosis is characterized by death during the first days of the disease unless dialytic treatment is undertaken. Death was almost unavoidable in the past before dialysis and better management of ARF [193, 243]. In one of the largest series, reported by Kleinknecht et al. [193], 21 of 38 patients died. However, almost all these patients were seen before dialysis was available for the treatment of ARF. The most typical clinical course, especially in the obstetric forms, is characterized by prolonged oligoanuria requiring dialysis. After a period of 1 to 3 months, renal function may partially recover, so that patients become dialysis independent. Urine output progressively increases, and renal function may improve over a period of 1 to 2 years, to a final plateau of 20 to 25 ml per minute [87, 347]. Hypertrophy of the juxtamedullary nephrons has been suggested as a factor contributing to the partial restoration of renal function [87].

A large percentage of patients require chronic dialysis, and these patients are probably those with the most severe and diffuse form of acute cortical necrosis. In this context two opposite possibilities must be mentioned:

(1) the late return to dialysis a number of years after the occurrence of cortical necrosis; and (2) the late resumption of a degree of renal function sufficient to maintain patients off dialysis [87]. Many patients have received renal transplants, and the prognosis of such patients has greatly improved during the last few years [347].

No specific therapeutic approaches are available for acute cortical necrosis. All the supportive maneuvers commonly employed in ARF are performed. Substitutive treatment must be started as early as possible, and daily dialytic therapy may be necessary considering the high catabolic rate often present in these patients. In experimental models of cortical necrosis many measures favorably affect pathologic changes. These include employment of anticoagulants, general anesthesia, β-blocker agents, mannitol-induced diuresis, and the use of nitrogen mustards to induce leukopenia [69, 159, 291, 353, 371]. However, none of these measures has been employed with unequivocal beneficial effects in humans.

ACKNOWLEDGEMENTS. The authors thank Drs. Manuela Livio, Carla Zoja, Eliana Gotti, and Norberto Perico for fruitful cooperation. Judy Baggot, Paola Bossi, Cristina Signorelli, and Laura Piccoli helped prepare the manuscript.

References

1. Alfrey, A. C. The Renal Response to Vascular Injury. In B. M. Brenner, and F. C. Rector, Jr. (eds.), *The Kidney* (2nd ed.) Philadelphia: Saunders, 1981. P. 1668.
2. Allison, A. C. Acute haemolytic anaemia with distortion and fragmentation of erythrocytes in children. *Br. J. Haematol.* 3: 1, 1957.
2a. Amir J., Krauss, S. Treatment of thrombotic thrombocytopenic purpura with antiplatelet drugs. *Blood* 42: 27, 1973.
3. Amorosi, E. L., and Karpatkin, S. Antiplatelet treatment of thrombotic thrombocytopenic purpura. *Ann. Intern. Med.* 86: 102, 1977.
4. Amorosi, E. L., and Ultmann, J. E. Thrombotic thrombocytopenic purpura: Report of 16 cases and review of the literature. *Medicine* 45: 139, 1966.
5. Ansell, J., Beaser, R. S., and Pechet, L. Thrombotic thrombocytopenic purpura fails to respond to fresh frozen plasma infusion. *Ann. Intern. Med.* 89: 647, 1978.
6. Antes, E. H. Thrombotic thrombocytopenic purpura: A review of the literature with report of a case. *Ann. Intern. Med.* 48: 512, 1958.
7. Arenson, E. B., and August, C. S. Preliminary report. Treatment of the hemolytic-uremic syndrome with aspirin and dipyridamole. *J. Pediatr.* 86: 957, 1975.
8. Arhelger, R. B., Brunson, J. G., Good, R. A., et al. Influence of gram-negative endotoxin on pathogenesis of nephrotoxic serum nephritis in rats. *Lab. Invest.* 10: 669, 1961.
9. Ashouri, O. S., Marbury, T. C., Fullec, T. J., et al. Hemolytic uremic syndrome in two postmenopausal women taking a conjugated estrogen preparation. *Clin. Nephrol.* 17: 212, 1982.
10. Atkinson, K., Biggs, J. C., Hasyes, J., et al. Cyclosporin A associated nephrotoxicity in the first 100 days after allogeneic bone marrow transplantation: Three distinct syndromes. *Br. J. Haematol.* 54: 59, 1983.
10a. Baehr, G., Klemperer, P., Schifrin, A. An acute febrile anemia and thrombocytopenic purpura with diffuse platelet thromboses of capillaries and arterioles. *Trans. Assoc. Am. Phys.* 51: 43, 1936.
11. Baker, N. M., Mills, A. E., Rachman, I., et al. Haemolytic-uraemic syndrome in typhoid fever. *Br. Med. J.* 2: 84, 1974.
12. Bayer, A. S., Theofilopolous, A. N., and Eisenberg, R., et al. Thrombotic thrombocytopenic purpura-like syndrome associated with infective endocarditis: A possible immune complex disorder. *J.A.M.A.* 233: 408, 1977.
13. Beattie, T. J., Murphy, A. V., Willoughby, M. L. M., et al. Plasmapheresis in the haemolytic-uraemic syndrome in children. *Br. Med. J.* 282: 1667, 1981.
14. Beattie, T. J., Murphy, A. V., Willoughby, M. L. N., et al. Prostacyclin infusion in haemolytic-uraemic syndrome in children. *Br. Med. J.* 283: 470, 1981.
15. Beaufils, M., Beaufils, H., Lucsko, M., et al. Late streptokinase therapy in thrombotic microangiopathy. A case study. *Clin. Nephrol.* 4: 160, 1975.
16. Belongia, E. A., MacDonald, K. L., White, K. E., et al. Outbreak of *Escherichia coli* 0157:117 Colitis Associated with Precooked Hamburgers. *Program and Abstracts of the 29th Interscience Conference on Antimicrobial Agents and Chemotherapy.* Houston, September 17–20, American Society for Microbiology, 1989. P. 1.
17. Benitez, L., Mathews, M., and Mallory, G. K. Platelet thrombosis with polyarteritis nodosa: Report of a case. *Arch. Pathol.* 77: 116, 1964.
18. Berberich, F. R., Cuene, S. A., Chard, R. L., et al. Thrombotic thrombocytopenic purpura. Three cases with platelet and fibrinogen survival studies. *J. Pediatr.* 84: 503, 1974.
19. Berkman, S. A., Lee, M. E., and Gale, R. P. Clinical uses of intravenous immunoglobulins. *Ann. Intern. Med.* 112: 278, 1990.
20. Berkowitz, L. R., Dalldorf, F. G., and Blatt, P. M. Thrombotic thrombocytopenic purpura: A pathology review. *J.A.M.A.* 241: 1709, 1979.
20a. Bernard, R. P., Bauman, A. W., Schwartz, S. I. Splenectomy for thrombotic thrombocytopenic purpura. *Ann. Surg.* 169: 616, 1969.
20b. Bernstock, L., Hirson, C. Thrombotic thrombocytopenic purpura. Remission on treatment with heparin. *Lancet* I: 28, 1960.
21. Birgens, H., Ernst, P., and Hansen, M. S. Thrombotic thrombocytopenic purpura: Treatment with a combination of antiplatelet drugs. *Acta Med. Scand.* 205: 437, 1979.
22. Blaker, F., Altrogge, H., Hellwege, H. H., et al. Dialysebehandlung des schweren hamolytisch-uramischen Syndroms. *Dtsch. Med. Wochenschr.* 103: 1229, 1978.
23. Boccia, R. W., Gelmann, E. P., Baker, C. C., et al. A hemolytic uremic syndrome with the acquired immunodeficiency syndrome. *Ann. Intern. Med.* 101: 716, 1984.
24. Bohle, A., Helmchen, U., Grund, K. E., et al. Malignant nephrosclerosis in patients with hemolytic-uremic syndrome (primary malignant nephrosclerosis). *Curr. Top. Pathol.* 65: 81, 1977.
25. Bone, R. C., Henry, J. E., Petterson, J., et al. Respiratory dysfunction in thrombotic thrombocytopenic purpura. *Am. J. Med.* 65: 262, 1978.
26. Bonser, R. S., Adu, D., Franklin, I., et al. Cyclosporin-induced haemolytic uraemic syndrome in liver allograft recipient. *Lancet* 2: 1337, 1984.
27. Boyd, W. N., Burden, R. P., and Aber, G. M. Intrarenal vascular changes in patients receiving oestrogen-con-

taining compounds—A clinical, histological and angiographic study. *Q. J. Med.* 44: 415, 1975.
28. Brain, M. C., et al. Heparin therapy in the hemolytic-uremic syndrome. *Q. J. Med.* 36: 608, 1967.
29. Brain, M. C., Dacie, J. V., Hourihane, D. O. B. Microangiopathic haemolytic anaemia: The possible role of vascular lesions in pathogenesis. *Br. J. Haematol.* 8: 358, 1962.
30. Brandt, P., Jespersen, J., and Gregersen, G. Postpartum haemolytic-uraemic syndrome treated with antithrombin-III. *Nephron* 27: 15, 1981.
31. Brenner, B. M., Troy, J. L., and Ballermann, B. J. Endothelium-dependent vascular responses. *J. Clin. Invest.* 84: 1373, 1989.
32. Brown, C. B., Clarkson, A. R., Robson, J. S., et al. Haemolytic-uraemic syndrome in women taking oral contraceptives. *Lancet* 1: 1479, 1973.
33. Brown, C. E., and Crane, G. L. Bilateral cortical necrosis following severe burns. *J.A.M.A.* 122: 871, 1943.
34. Brown, R. C., Blecher, T. E., French, E. A., et al. Thrombotic thrombocytopenic purpura after influenza vaccination. *Br. Med. J.* 2: 303, 1973.
35. Brunson, J. G., Thomas, L., and Gamble, C. N. Morphological changes in rabbits following the intravenous administration of meningococcal toxin. II. Two appropriately spaced injections; the role of fibrinoid in the generalized Shwartzman reaction. *Am. J. Pathol.* 31: 655, 1955.
36. Budd, G. T., Bukowski, R. M., Lucas, F. V., et al. Prostacyclin therapy of thrombotic thrombocytopenic purpura. *Lancet* 2: 915, 1980.
37. Bukowski, R. M. Thrombotic Thrombocytopenic Purpura: A Review. In T. H. Spaet (ed.), *Progress in Hemostasis and Thrombosis.* New York: Grune & Stratton, 1982. P. 287.
38. Bukowski, R. M., Hewlett, J. S., Harris, J. W., et al. Exchange transfusions in the treatment of thrombotic thrombocytopenic purpura. *Semin. Hematol.* 13: 219, 1976.
39. Bukowski, R. M., Hewlett, J. S., Reimer, R. R., et al. Therapy of thrombotic thrombocytopenic purpura: An overview. *Semin. Thromb. Hemost.* 7: 1, 1981.
40. Bull, B. S., Rubenberg, M. L., Dacie, J. V., et al. Red-blood-cell fragmentation in microangiopathic haemolytic anaemia: In vitro studies. *Lancet* 2: 1123, 1967.
41. Bull, B. S., Rubenberg, M. L., Dacie, J. V., et al. Microangiopathic haemolytic anaemia: Mechanisms of red-cell fragmentation: in vitro studies. *Br. J. Haematol.* 14: 643, 1968.
42. Bunchman, T. E., and Brookshire, C. A. Cyclosporine stimulated synthesis of endothelin by human endothelial cells in tissue culture. *Kidney Int.* 37: 365, 1990.
43. Burke, H. A., and Hartmann, R. C. Thrombotic thrombocytopenic purpura. Two patients with remission associated with the use of large amounts of steroids. *Arch. Intern. Med.* 103: 105, 1959.
44. Burns, E. R., and Zucker-Franklin, D. Pathologic effects of plasma from patients with thrombotic thrombocytopenic purpura on platelets and cultured endothelial cells. *Blood* 60: 1030, 1982.
45. Busch, G. J., Martins, A. C. P., Hollenberg, N. K., et al. A primate model of hyperacute renal allograft rejection. *Am. J. Pathol.* 79: 31, 1975.
46. Byrnes, J. J. Plasma infusion in the treatment of thrombotic thrombocytopenic purpura. *Semin. Thromb. Hemost.* 7: 9, 1981.
47. Byrnes, J. J., Baquerizo, H., Gonzales, M., et al. Thrombotic thrombocytopenic purpura subsequent to acute myelogenous leukemia chemotherapy. *Am. J. Hematol.* 21: 299, 1986.
48. Byrnes, J. J., and Khurana, M. Treatment of thrombotic thrombocytopenic purpura with plasma. *N. Engl. J. Med.* 297: 1386, 1977.
49. Byrom, F. B. Morbid effects of vasopressin in the organs and vessels of rats. *J. Pathol. Bacteriol.* 45: 1, 1937.
50. Byrom, F. B., and Pratt, O. E. Oxytocin and renal cortical necrosis. *Lancet* 1: 753, 1959.
51. Caggiano, V., Chosney, B., and Way, L. W. Thrombotic thrombocytopenic purpura, cholangiocarcinoma, and oral contraceptives. *Lancet* 2: 365, 1980.
52. Cahalane, S. F., and Horn, R. C. Thrombotic thrombocytopenic purpura of long duration. *Am. J. Med.* 27: 333, 1959.
53. Cameron, J. S., and Vick, R. Plasma-C3 in haemolytic-uraemic syndrome and thrombotic thrombocytopenic purpura. *Lancet* 2: 975, 1973.
54. Campbell, A. C., and Henderson, J. L. Symmetrical cortical necrosis of the kidneys in infancy and childhood. *Arch. Dis. Child.* 24: 269, 1941.
55. Campos, A., Kim, Y., Azar, S. H., et al. Prevention of the generalized Shwartzman reaction in pregnant rats by prostacyclin infusion. *Lab. Invest.* 48: 705, 1983.
56. Cantrell, J. E., Phillips, T. M., and Schein, P. S. Carcinoma associated hemolytic-uremic syndrome: A complication of mitomycin-C chemotherapy. *J. Clin. Oncol.* 3: 723, 1985.
57. Carreras, L., Romero, R., Requesens, C., et al. Familial hypocomplementemic hemolytic uremic syndrome with HLA-A3, B7 haplotype. *J.A.M.A.* 245: 602, 1981.
58. Cattell, V. Mitomycin-induced hemolytic uremic kidney. An experimental model in the rat. *Am. J. Pathol.* 121: 88, 1985.
59. Celada, A., and Perrin, L. H. Circulating immune complexes in thrombotic thrombocytopenic purpura (TTP). *Blood* 52: 855, 1978.
60. Chamovitz, B. N., Hartstein, A. I., Alexander, S. R., et al. *Campylobacter jejuni*-associated hemolytic-uremic syndrome in a mother and daughter. *Pediatrics* 71: 253, 1983.
61. Chen, Y. C., McLeod, B., Hill, E. R., et al. Accelerated prostacyclin degradation in thrombotic thrombocytopenic purpura. *Lancet* 2: 267, 1981.
62. Chin, D., Chyczij, H., Etches, W., et al. Treatment of thrombotic thrombocytopenic purpura with intravenous gamma globulin. *Transfusion* 27: 115, 1987.
63. Churg, K. S., Singhal, P. C., Sharma, B. K., et al. Acute renal failure of obstetric origin. *Obstet. Gynecol.* 48: 642, 1976.
64. Civin, H., and Gotshalk, H. C. "Platelet thromboses" involving the gastrointestinal tract: Report of a case. *Hawaii Med. J.* 13: 119, 1953.
65. Clarkson, A. R., Lawrence, J. R., Meadows, R., et al. The haemolytic-uraemic syndrome in adults. *Q. J. Med.* 39: 227, 1970.
66. Clarkson, A. R., Meadows, R., and Lawrence, J. R. Post partum renal failure. The generalized Shwartzman reaction. *Austral. Ann. Med.* 18: 209, 1969.
67. Cocchetto, D. M., Cook, L., Cato, A. E., et al. Rationale and proposal for use of prostacyclin in thrombotic thrombocytopenic purpura therapy. *Semin. Thromb. Hemost.* 7: 43, 1981.
68. Conte, J., Deisol, J., Mignon-Conte, M., et al. Acute Renal Failure and Intravascular Coagulation. In J. Hamburger, J. Crosnier, and M. H. Maxwell (eds.), *Advances in Nephrology.* Chicago: Year Book, 1974. P. 197.

69. Corrigan, J. J., Jr. Effect of anticoagulating and non-anticoagulating concentrations of heparin on the generalized Shwartzman reaction. *Thromb. Diath. Haemorrh.* 24: 136, 1970.
70. Coulthard, M. G. An evaluation of treatment with heparin in the haemolytic-uraemic syndrome successfully treated by peritoneal dialysis. *Arch. Dis. Child.* 55: 393, 1980.
71. Craig, J. M., and Gitlin, D. The nature of the hyaline thrombi in thrombotic thrombocytopenic purpura. *Am. J. Pathol.* 33: 251, 1957.
72. Crain, S. M., and Choudhury, A. M. Thrombotic thrombocytopenic purpura in a splenectomized patient with Hodgkin's disease. *Am. J. Med. Sci.* 280: 35, 1980.
73. Cross, A. S., Alving, B. M., Sodoff, J. C., et al. Intravenous immune globulin: A cautionary note. *Lancet* 1: 912, 1984.
74. Cross, A. S., Siegel, G., Byrne, W. R., et al. Intravenous immune globulin impairs anti-bacterial defences of a cyclophosphamide-treated host. *Clin. Exp. Immunol.* 76: 159, 1989.
75. Cuttner, J. Splenectomy, steroids, and dextran 70 in thrombotic thrombocytopenic purpura. *J.A.M.A.* 227: 397, 1974.
76. Cuttner, J. Chronic thrombotic thrombocytopenic purpura: Report of a case with five relapses and review of the literature. *Mt. Sinai J. Med.* 45: 418, 1978.
77. Cuttner, J. Thrombotic thrombocytopenic purpura: A ten-year experience. *Blood* 56: 302, 1980.
78. Danon, D., and Skutelsky, E. Endothelial surface charge and its possible relationship to thrombogenesis. *Ann. N.Y. Acad. Sci.* 275: 47, 1976.
79. Da Silva, O. A., Lopez, M., and Godoy, P. Bilateral cortical necrosis and calcification of the kidney following snakebite: A case report. *Clin. Nephrol.* 11: 136, 1979.
79a. de Chadarevian, J. P., and Kaplan, B. S. The hemolytic uremic syndrome of childhood. *Perspect. Pediatr. Pathol.* 4: 465, 1978.
80. Deckmyn, H., Zoja, C., Arnout, J., et al. Partial isolation and function of the prostacyclin regulating plasma factor. *Clin. Sci.* 69: 383, 1985.
81. Defreyn, G., Proesmans, W., Machin, S. J., et al. Abnormal prostacyclin metabolism in the haemolytic uraemic syndrome: Equivocal effect of prostacyclin infusion. *Clin. Nephrol.* 18: 43, 1982.
82. De Jong, M., and Monnens, L. Haemolytic-uraemic syndrome: A 10-year follow-up study of 73 patients. *Nephrol. Dial. Transplant.* 3: 379, 1988.
82a. de Jong, M., Monnens, L., van Munster, P., et al. Antithrombin-III levels in children with the epidemic form of hemolytic-uremic syndrome. *Int. J. Pediatr. Nephrol.* 2: 150, 1981.
83. Dekker, A., O'Brien, M. E., and Cammarata, R. J. The association of thrombotic thrombocytopenic purpura with systemic lupus erythematosus. *Am. J. Med. Sci.* 267: 243, 1974.
84. De Sweet, M. Some rare medical complications of pregnancy. *Br. Med. J.* 290: 2, 1985.
85. Dieterich, D., Jameson, M., Dai Fu-Xiang, A., et al. Cyclosporine treatment impairs endothelial function in resistance arteries in rats. Abstract. *J. Am. Soc. Nephrol.* 1: 609, 1990.
86. Dolislager, D., and Tune, B. The hemolytic-uremic syndrome. Spectrum of severity and significance of prodrome. *Am. J. Dis. Child.* 132: 55, 1978.
87. Donohoe, J. F. Acute Bilateral Cortical Necrosis. In B. M. Brenner, and J. M. Lazarus (eds.), *Acute Renal Failure.* Philadelphia: Saunders, 1983. P. 252.
88. Drummond, K. N. Hemolytic uremic syndrome—then and now. *N. Engl. J. Med.* 312: 116, 1985.
89. Duff, G. L., and Murray, E. G. D. Bilateral cortical necrosis of the kidneys. *Am. J. Med. Sci.* 201: 428, 1941.
90. Dunea, G., Muerke, R. C., Nakamoto, S., et al. Thrombotic thrombocytopenic purpura with acute anuric renal failure. *Am. J. Med.* 41: 1000, 1966.
91. Duperray, A., Tranqui, L., Alix, J. L., et al. Effect of mitomycin C on the biosynthesis of prostacyclin by primary cultures of human umbilical cord vein endothelial cell. Abstract. *Kidney Int.* 25: 730, 1984.
92. Dvorak, H. F., Mihm, M. C., Dvorak, A. M., et al. Rejection of first-set skin allografts in man. The microvasculature is the critical target of the immune response. *J. Exp. Med.* 150: 322, 1979.
93. Dzik, W. H., Georgi, B. A., Khettry, U., et al. Cyclosporine-associated thrombotic thrombocytopenic purpura following liver transplantation—Successful treatment with plasma exchange. *Transplantation* 44: 570, 1987.
93a. Eckel, R. H., et al. Platelet-inhibiting drugs in thrombotic thrombocytopenic purpura. *Arch. Intern. Med.* 137: 735, 1977.
94. Edefonti, A., Tentori, F., Bettinelli, A., et al. Pattern of platelet serotonin (5TH), plasma beta-thromboglobulin (betaTG) and platelet factor (PG4) in hemolytic-uremic syndrome (HUS) in children. *Int. J. Pediatr. Nephrol.* 2: 149, 1981.
95. Edelsten, A. D., and Tuck, S. Familial haemolytic-uraemic syndrome. *Arch. Dis. Child.* 53: 255, 1978.
96. Ehrich, W. E., and Seifter, J. Thrombotic thrombocytopenic purpura caused by iodine. *Arch. Pathol.* 47: 446, 1949.
97. Ekberg, M., Holmberg, L., and Denneberg, T. Hemolytic uremic syndrome. Results of treatment with hemodialysis. *Acta Pediatr. Scand.* 66: 693, 1977.
98. Esmon, C. T. Protein-C: Biochemistry, physiology and clinical implications. *Blood* 62: 1155, 1983.
99. Faguet, G. B., and King, M. D. Thrombotic thrombocytopenic purpura: Treatment with antiplatelet agents. *Am. J. Med. Sci.* 268: 113, 1974.
100. Farr, M. J., Roberts, S., Morley, A. R., et al. The haemolytic-uraemic syndrome—A family study. *Q. J. Med.* 44: 161, 1975.
101. Federici, A. B., Elder, J. H., De Marco, L., et al. Carbohydrate moiety of von Willebrand factor is not necessary for maintaining multimeric structure and ristocetin cofactor activity but protects from proteolytic degradation. *J. Clin. Invest.* 76: 2049, 1984.
102. Feldman, J. D., Mardiney, M. R., Unanue, E. R., et al. The vascular pathology of thrombotic thrombocytopenic purpura: An immunohistochemical and ultrastructural study. *Lab. Invest.* 15: 927, 1966.
103. Ferris, T. F. The Kidney and Pregnancy. In L. E. Earley, and C. W. Gottschalk (eds.), *Strauss and Welt's Diseases of the Kidney.* Boston: Little, Brown, 1979. P. 1321.
104. Fielding, J. W., Fagg, S. L., Jones, B. G., et al. An interim report of a prospective, randomized, controlled study of adjuvant chemotherapy in operable gastric cancer: British Stomach Cancer Group. *World J. Surg.* 7: 390, 1983.
105. Finkelstein, F. O., Kashgarian, M., and Hayslett, J. P. Clinical spectrum of postpartum renal failure. *Am. J. Med.* 57: 649, 1974.
106. Finn, N. G., Wang, J. C., and Hong, K. J. High-dose in-

travenous γ-immunoglobulin infusion in the treatment of thrombotic thrombocytopenic purpura. *Arch. Intern. Med.* 147: 2165, 1987.
107. Fitzgerald, G. A., Brash, A. R., Falardeau, P., et al. Estimated rate of prostacyclin secretion into the circulation of normal man. *J. Clin. Invest.* 68: 1272, 1981.
108. Fitzgerald, G. A., Maas, R. L., Stein, R., et al. Intravenous prostacyclin in thrombotic thrombocytopenic purpura. *Ann. Intern. Med.* 95: 319, 1981.
109. Fogo, A., Hakim, R., Sugiura, M., et al. Severe endothelial injury in a renal transplant patient receiving cyclosporine. *Transplantation* 49: 1190, 1990.
110. Fong, J. S., De Chadarevian, J. P., and Kaplan, B. S. Hemolytic-uremic syndrome. Current concepts and management. *Pediatr. Clin. North Am.* 29: 835, 1982.
111. Fong, J. S. C., and Kaplan, B. S. Impairment of platelet aggregation in hemolytic uremic syndrome. Evidence for platelet 'exhaustion'. *Blood* 60: 564, 1982.
112. Forbes, R. D. C., Kuramochi, T., Guttmann, R. D., et al. A controlled sequential morphologic study of hyperacute cardiac allograft rejection in the rat. *Lab. Invest.* 33: 280, 1975.
113. Foster, P. A., and Anderson, J. C. Effects of plasma from patients with thrombotic thrombocytopenic purpura (TTP) on cultured human endothelial cells. *Blood* 54: 240a, 1979.
114. Franklin, W. A., Simon, N. M., Potter, E. W., et al. The hemolytic uremic syndrome. *Arch. Pathol.* 94: 230, 1972.
115. Fuchs, W. E., George, J. N., Dotin, L. N., et al. Thrombotic thrombocytopenic purpura—occurrence two years apart during late pregnancy in two sisters. *J.A.M.A.* 235: 2126, 1976.
116. Fujimoto, T., Ohara, S., and Hawiger, J. Thrombin induced exposure and prostacyclin inhibition of the receptor for factor VIII/von Willebrand factor in human platelets. *J. Clin. Invest.* 69: 1212, 1982.
117. Furchgott, R. F. The role of endothelium in the responses of vascular smooth muscle to drugs. *Annu. Rev. Pharmacol. Toxicol.* 24: 175, 1984.
118. Galton, M., Wong, T. C., and McKay, D. G. Vasomotor changes in the pregnant rabbit induced by bacterial endotoxin. *Fed. Proc.* 19: 246, 1960.
119. Gasser, C., Gautier, E., Steck, A., et al. Hamolytisch-uramische syndromes bilaterale nierenrindennekrosen bei akuten erworbenchenschr hamolytischen anamien. *Schweiz. Med. Wochenschr.* 85: 905, 1955.
120. Geiling, E. M. K., and Cannon, P. R. Pathologic effects of elixir of sulfanilamide (diethylene glycol) poisoning. A clinical and experimental correlation: Final report. *J.A.M.A.* 111: 919, 1938.
121. Gelfand, M. D., Friedman, E. A., Knapshield, J. H., et al. Detection of antiplatelet antibody activity in patients with renal cortical necrosis. *Kidney Int.* 6: 426, 1974.
122. Gendel, B. R., Young, J. M., and Kraus, A. P. Thrombotic thrombocytopenic purpura. *Am. J. Med.* 13: 3, 1952.
123. Gervais, M., Richardson, J. B., Chiu, J., et al. Immunofluorescent and histologic findings in the hemolytic uremic syndrome. *Pediatrics* 47: 352, 1971.
124. Gianantonio, C. A., Vitacco, M., Mendilaharzu, F., et al. Acute renal failure in infancy and childhood. Clinical course and treatment in 41 patients. *J. Pediatr.* 61: 660, 1962.
125. Gianantonio, C. A., Vitacco, M., Mendilaharzu, F., et al. The hemolytic-uremic syndrome. *J. Pediatr.* 64: 478, 1964.
126. Gianantonio, C. A., Vitacco, M., Mendilaharzu, F., et al. The hemolytic-uremic syndrome. *Nephron* 11: 174, 1973.
127. Gilcher, R. O., and Goldman, S. N. Refractory TTP responding to IV gamma globulin. *Blood* 64: 237a, 1987.
128. Gilchrist, G. S., Lieberman, E., Ekert, H., et al. Heparin therapy in the haemolytic-uraemic syndrome. *Lancet* 1: 1123, 1969.
129. Gillor, A., Bulla, M., Roth, B., et al. Plasmapheresis as a therapeutic measure in hemolytic-uremic syndrome in children. *Klin. Wochenschr.* 61: 363, 1983.
130. Giromini, M., and Hapenouza, C. Prolonged survival after bilateral nephrectomy in an adult with hemolytic-uremic syndrome. *Lancet* 2: 169, 1969.
130a. Girouini, M., et al. Effect of dipyridamole and aspirin in thrombotic microangiopathy. *Br. Med. J.* 1: 545, 1972.
131. Giroux, L., Bettez, P., and Giroux, L. L. Mitomycin-C nephrotoxicity: A clinico-pathologic study of 17 cases. *Am. J. Kidney Dis.* 6: 28, 1985.
132. Giroux, L., Smeesters, C., Corman, J., et al. Hemolytic uremic syndrome in renal allografted patients treated with cyclosporin. *Can. J. Physiol. Pharmacol.* 65: 1125, 1987.
133. Glasgow, L. A., and Balduzzi, P. Isolation of coxsackie virus group A, type 4 from a patient with hemolytic-uremic syndrome. *N. Engl. J. Med.* 273: 754, 1965.
134. Godwin, B., and McCall, A. J. Cortical necrosis complicating perforated gastric ulcer. *Lancet* 2: 512, 1941.
135. Goldstein, M. H., Churg, J., Strauss, L., et al. Hemolytic-uremic syndrome. *Nephron* 23: 263, 1979.
136. Gonzalo, A., Mampaso, F., Gallego, N., et al. Hemolytic uremic syndrome with hypocomplementemia and deposits of IgM and C3 in the involved renal tissue. *Clin. Nephrol.* 16: 193, 1981.
137. Goodman, A., Ramos, R., Petrelli, M., et al. Gingival biopsy in thrombotic thrombocytopenic purpura. *Ann. Intern. Med.* 89: 501, 1978.
138. Goodman, R. P., Killam, A. P., Brash, A. R., et al. Prostacyclin production during pregnancy. Comparison of production during normal pregnancy and pregnancy complicated by hypertension. *Am. J. Obstet. Gynecol.* 142: 817, 1982.
139. Gore, I. Disseminated arteriolar and capillary platelet thrombosis; a morphologic study of its histogenesis. *Am. J. Pathol.* 26: 155, 1950.
139a. Gottschall, J. L., et al. Thrombotic thrombocytopenic purpura: Experience with whole blood exchange transfusions. *Semin. Thromb. Hemost.* 7:25, 1981.
140. Gransden, W. R., Damm, M. A., Anderson, J. D., et al. Further evidence associating hemolytic uremic syndrome with infection by verotoxin-producing *Escherichia coli* 0157:H7. *J. Infect. Dis.* 154: 522, 1986.
141. Groshong, T. D., Taylor, A. A., Nolph, D. K., et al. Renal function following cortical necrosis in childhood. *J. Pediatr.* 79: 267, 1971.
142. Gruetter, C. A., Barry, B. K., McNamara, D. B., et al. Relaxation of bovine coronary artery and activation of coronary arterial guanylate cyclase by nitric oxide, nitroprusside and carcinogenic nitrosamine. *J. Cyclic Nucl. Res.* 5: 211, 1979.
143. Grunfeld, J. P., Ganeval, D., and Bournerias, F. Acute renal failure in pregnancy. *Kidney Int.* 18: 179, 1980.
144. Gryglewski, R. J., Moncada, S., and Palmer, R. M. J. Bioassay of prostacyclin and endothelium-derived relaxing factor (EDRF). *Br. J. Pharmacol.* 87: 685, 1986.
145. Gully, P. R. Haemolytic-uraemic syndrome: Epidemiology and report of an outbreak. *J. R. Soc. Health* 104: 214, 1984.
146. Gundlach, W. J., and Tarnasky, R. Thrombotic throm-

bocytopenic purpura—remission following treatment with aspirin and dipyridamole. *Minn. Med.* 60: 20, 1977.

147. Habib, R., Courtecuisse, V., Leclerc, F., et al. Etude anatomopathologique de 35 observations de syndrome hemolytique et uremique de l'enfant. *Arch. Franc. Pediatr.* 26: 391, 1969.
148. Habib, R., Mathieu, H., and Royer, P. Maladie thrombotique arteriolocapillaire due rein chez l'enfant. *Rev. Fr. Etud. Clin. Biol.* 3: 891, 1958.
149. Habib, R., Mathieu, H., and Royer, P. Le syndrome hemolytique et uremique de l'enfant: Aspects cliniques et anatomiques dans 27 observations. *Nephron* 4: 139, 1967.
150. Hadley, W. K., and Rosenan, W. Study of human renal disease by immunofluorescent methods. *Arch. Pathol.* 83: 342, 1967.
151. Hamilton, K. K., Fretto, L. S., Grierson, D. S., et al. Effects of plasmin on von Willebrand factor multimers. Degradation in vitro and stimulation of release in vivo. *J. Clin. Invest.* 76: 261, 1985.
152. Hammond, D., and Lieberman, E. The hemolytic-uremic syndrome. Renal cortical thrombotic microangiopathy. *Arch. Intern. Med.* 126: 816, 1970.
153. Hamner, R. W., Verani, R., and Weinman, E. J. Mitomycin-associated renal failure: Case report and review. *Arch. Intern. Med.* 143: 803, 1983.
154. Harker, L. A., and Slichter, S. J. Platelet and fibrinogen consumption in man. *N. Engl. J. Med.* 287: 999, 1972.
155. Harlan, J. M., Harker, L. A., Reidy, M. A., et al. Lipopolysaccharide-mediated bovine endothelial cell injury in vitro. *Lab. Invest.* 48: 269, 1983.
156. Harlan, J. M., Harker, L. A., Striker, G. E., et al. Effects of lipopolysaccharide on human endothelial cells in culture. *Thromb. Res.* 29: 15, 1983.
157. Harrel, M. N., Sibley, R., and Vogelzang, N. J. Renal vascular lesions after chemotherapy with vinblastine, bleomycin, and cisplatin. *Am. J. Med.* 73: 429, 1982.
158. Harrison, H. N. Thrombotic thrombocytopenic purpura occurring in the puerperium associated with pancreatic islet-cell necrosis. *Arch. Intern. Med.* 102: 124, 1958.
159. Hatcher, C. R., Jr., Gagnon, J. A., and Clarke, R. W. The effects of hydration in epinephrine-induced renal shutdown in dogs. *Surg. Forum* 9: 106, 1958.
160. Hauglustaine, D., Van Damme, B., Vanrenterghem, Y., et al. Recurrent hemolytic uremic syndrome during oral contraception. *Clin. Nephrol.* 15: 148, 1981.
161. Hellman, R. M., Jackson, D. V., and Buss, D. H. Thrombotic thrombocytopenic purpura and hemolytic uremic syndrome in HLA-identical siblings. *Ann. Intern. Med.* 93: 283, 1980.
162. Hensby, C. N., Lewis, P. J., Hilgard, P., et al. Prostacyclin deficiency in thrombotic thrombocytopenic purpura. *Lancet* 2: 748, 1979.
163. Heptinstall, R. H. Hemolytic Uremic Syndrome, Thrombotic Thrombocytopenic Purpura, and Systemic Scleroderma (Progressive Systemic Sclerosis). In R. H. Heptinstall (ed.), *Pathology of the Kidney.* Boston: Little, Brown, 1983. P. 907.

163a. Hill, J. B., and Cooper, W. M. Thrombotic thrombocytopenic purpura. Treatment with corticosteroids and splenectomy. *Arch. Intern. Med.* 122: 353, 1968.

164. Hitzig, W. H. Therapie mit Antikoagulantie in der Padiatrie. *Helv. Paediatr. Acta* 19: 213, 1964.
165. Hoorntje, S. J., Prins, E. J., Smit, A. J., et al. Reversal of long-lasting renal insufficiency by captopril in a patient with relapsing hemolytic uremic syndrome due to an oral contraceptive. *Ann. Intern. Med.* 94: 355, 1981.
166. Hope, W., Martin, T. J., Chesterman, C. N., et al. Human β-thromboglobulin inhibits PGI_2 production and binds to a specific site in bovine aortic endothelial cells. *Nature* 282: 210, 1979.
167. Hoyer, J. R., Bergstein, J. M., Michael, A. F., et al. Immunofluorescent localization of factor VIII-related antigen and fibrinogen in hyperacute xenograft rejection and in the Shwartzman reaction in the rat. *Clin. Immunol. Immunopathol.* 9: 454, 1978.
168. Ignarro, L. J. Biological actions and properties of endothelium-derived nitric oxide formed and released from artery and vein. *Circ. Res.* 65: 1, 1989.
169. Ignarro, L. J. Endothelium-derived nitric oxide: Actions and properties. *FASEB J.* 3: 31, 1989.
170. Ignarro, L. J., Harbison, R. G., Wood, K. S., et al. Activation of purified soluble guanylate cyclase by endothelium-derived relaxing factor from intrapulmonary artery and vein: Stimulation by acetylcholine, bradykinin and arachidonic acid. *J. Pharmacol. Exp. Ther.* 237: 893, 1986.
171. Jackson, A. M., Rose, B. D., Graff, L. G., et al. Thrombotic microangiopathy and renal failure associated with antineoplastic chemotherapy. *Ann. Intern. Med.* 101: 41, 1984.
172. Jaffe, E. A., Nachman, R. L., and Merskey, C. Thrombotic thrombocytopenic purpura: Coagulation parameters in twelve patients. *Blood* 42: 499, 1973.
173. Javett, S. N., and Senior, B. Syndrome of hemolysis, thrombocytopenia and nephropathy in infancy. *Pediatrics* 29: 209, 1962.
174. Jokela, J., Flynn, T., and Henry, K. Thrombotic thrombocytopenic purpura in a human immunodeficiency virus (HIV)-seropositive homosexual man. *Am. J. Hematol.* 25: 341, 1987.
175. Jorgensen, K. A., and Pedersen, R. S. Familial deficiency of prostacyclin production stimulating factor in the hemolytic uremic syndrome of childhood. *Thromb. Res.* 21: 311, 1981.
176. Kanfer, A., Morel-Maroger, L., Solez, K., et al. The Value of Renal Biopsy in Hemolytic-Uremic Syndrome in Adults. In G. Remuzzi, G. Mecca, and G. de Gaetano (eds.), *Hemostasis, Prostaglandins and Renal Disease.* New York: Raven Press, 1980. P. 399.
177. Kaplan, B. S., and Drummond, K. N. The hemolytic-uremic syndrome is a syndrome. *N. Engl. J. Med.* 298: 964, 1978.
178. Kaplan, B. S., and Fong, J. S. C. Reduced platelet aggregation in hemolytic uremic syndrome. *Thromb Haemost.* 43: 154, 1980.
179. Kaplan, B. S., Katz, J., Krawitz, S., et al. An analysis of the results of therapy in 67 cases of the hemolytic-uremic syndrome. *J. Pediatr.* 78: 420, 1971.
180. Kaplan, B. S., Thomson, P. D., and MacNab, G. M. Serum-complement levels in haemolytic-uraemic syndrome. *Lancet* 2: 1505, 1973.
181. Karlsberg, R. P., Lacher, J. W., and Bartecchi, C. Adult hemolytic-uremic syndrome: Familial variant. *Arch. Intern. Med.* 137: 1155, 1977.
182. Karmali, M. A., Petric, M., Lim, C., et al. The association between idiopathic hemolytic uremic syndrome and infection by verotoxin-producing *Escherichia coli. J. Infect. Dis.* 151: 775, 1985.
183. Karmali, M. A., Steele, B. T., Petric, M., et al. Sporadic cases of haemolytic-uraemic syndrome associated with faecal cytotoxin and cytotoxin-producing *Escherichia coli* in stools. *Lancet* 1: 619, 1983.
184. Karmali, M. A., Steele, B. T., Petric, M., et al. Enteroviruses associated with the hemolytic-uremic syndrome. *Pediatrics* 46: 378, 1970.

185. Katz, J., Krawitz, S., Sacks, P. V., et al. Platelet, erythrocyte, and fibrinogen kinetics in the hemolytic-uremic syndrome of infancy. *J. Pediatr.* 83: 739, 1973.
186. Keene, E., Willis, R., and Aster, R. H. Platelet kinetics (^{51}Cr) in thrombocytopenic purpura. *Lahey Clin. Found. Bull.* 17: 51, 1968.
187. Kelton, J. G., Moore, J., Santos, A., et al. Detection of a platelet-agglutinating factor in thrombotic thrombocytopenic purpura. *Ann. Intern. Med.* 101: 589, 1984.
188. Kennedy, S. S., Zacharski, L. R., and Beck, J. R. Thrombotic thrombocytopenic purpura: Analysis of 48 unselected cases. *Semin. Thromb. Hemost.* 6: 341, 1980.
189. Kibel, M., and Barnard, P. J. The haemolytic-uremic syndrome. A survey in South Africa. *S. Afr. Med. J.* 42: 692, 1966.
189a. Khanh, B. T., et al. Role of heparin therapy in the outcome of adult hemolytic uremic syndrome. *Nephron.* 16: 292, 1976.
190. Kim, Y., Miller, K., and Michael, A. F. Breakdown products of C3 and factor B in hemolytic-uremic syndrome. *J. Lab. Clin. Med.* 89: 845, 1977.
191. Kissmeyer-Nielsen, F., Olsen, S., Petersen, V. P., et al. Hyperacute rejection of kidney allografts, associated with pre-existing humoral antibodies against donor cells. *Lancet* 2: 662, 1966.
192. Klein, P. J., Bulla, M., Newman, R. A., et al. Thomsen-Friedenreich antigen in haemolytic uraemic syndrome. *Lancet* 2: 1024, 1977.
193. Kleinknecht, D., Grunfeld, J. P., Cia Gomez, P., et al. Diagnostic procedures and long-term prognosis in bilateral renal cortical necrosis. *Kidney Int.* 4: 390, 1973.
194. Kniker, W. T., and Cochrane, C. G. Pathogenetic factors in vascular lesions of experimental serum sickness. *J. Exp. Med.* 122: 83, 1965.
195. Kniker, W. T., and Cochrane, C. G. The localization of circulating immune complexes in experimental serum sickness. *J. Exp. Med.* 127: 119, 1968.
196. Koffler, D., and Paronetto, F. Fibrinogen deposition in acute renal failure. *Am. J. Pathol.* 49: 383, 1966.
197. Kon, V., Sugiura, M., Inagami, T., et al. Cyclosporine (CyA) causes endothelin-dependent acute renal failure. Abstract. *Kidney Int.* 37: 486, 1990.
198. Konowalchuk, J., Speirs, J. I., and Stavric, S. Vero response to a cytotoxin of *Escherichia coli*. *Infect. Immunol.* 18: 775, 1977.
199. Korec, S., Schein, P. S., and Smith, F. P. Treatment of cancer-associated hemolytic-uremic syndrome with staphylococcal protein A immunoperfusion. *J. Clin. Oncol.* 4: 210, 1986.
200. Koster, F., Levin, J., Walker, L., et al. Hemolytic-uremic syndrome after shigellosis: relation to endotoxemia and circulating immune complexes. *N. Engl. J. Med.* 298: 927, 1978.
201. Krauss, S., Sonoda, T., and Soloman, A. Treatment of advanced gastrointestinal cancer with 5-fluorouracil and mitomycin-C. *Cancer* 43: 1598, 1979.
202. Kressel, B. R., Ryan, K. P., Duong, A. T., et al. Microangiopathic hemolytic anemia, thrombocytopenia and renal failure in patients treated for adenocarcinoma. *Cancer* 48: 1738, 1981.
203. Kunicki, T. J., Montgomery, R. R., and Schullek, J. Cleavage of human von Willebrand factor by platelet calcium-activated protease. *Blood* 65: 352, 1985.
204. Kwaan, H. C. Role of fibrinolysis in thrombotic thrombocytopenic purpura. *Semin. Thromb. Hemostas.* 6: 395, 1979.
205. Kwaan, H. C., Gallo, G., Potter, E. V., et al. The nature of the vascular lesion in thrombotic thrombocytopenic purpura. *Ann. Intern. Med.* 68: 1169, 1968.
206. Lamvik, J. O. Acute glomerulonephritis with hemolytic anemia in infants. Report of three fatal cases. *Pediatrics* 29: 224, 1962.
207. Larke, R. P. B., Preiksaitis, J. K., and Devine, R. D. O. Hemolytic-uremic syndrome: Clustering of ten cases and association with multiple viral infections. *Lancet* 1: 479, 1973.
208. Laszlo, M. H., Alvarez, A., and Feldman, F. The association of thrombotic thrombocytopenic purpura and disseminated lupus erythematosus: Report of a case. *Ann. Intern. Med.* 42: 1308, 1955.
209. Latour, J. G., and Leger-Gauthier, C. Prostaglandins in the pathogenesis of the generalized Shwartzman reaction. *Am. J. Obstet. Gynecol.* 135: 577, 1979.
210. Lau, D. C. W., Wong, K. L., and Hwang, W. S. Cyclosporine toxicity on culture rat microvascular endothelial cells. *Kidney Int.* 35: 604, 1989.
211. Lauler, D. P., and Schreiner, G. E. Bilateral renal cortical necrosis. *Am. J. Med.* 24: 519, 1958.
212. Leaf, A. N., Laubenstain, L. J., Raphael, B., et al. Thrombotic thrombocytopenic purpura associated with human immunodeficiency virus type 1 (HIV-1) infection. *Ann. Intern. Med.* 109: 194, 1988.
213. Leithner, C., Sinzinger, H., Pohanka, E., et al. Recurrence of haemolytic uraemic syndrome triggered by cyclosporin A after renal transplantation. *Lancet* 2: 1470, 1982.
214. Leithner, C., Sinzinger, H., Schwartz, M., et al. Occurrence of Hemolytic Uremic Syndrome Under Cyclosporine Treatment: Accident or Possible Side Effect Mediated by Lack of Prostacyclin-Stimulating Plasma Factor? In B. D. Kahan (ed.), *Cyclosporine. Biological Activity and Clinical Applications.* New York: Grune & Stratton, 1984. P. 571.
215. Lesesne, J. B., Rothschild, N., Erickson, B., et al. Cancer-associated hemolytic-uremic syndrome: Analysis of 85 cases from a national registry. *J. Clin. Oncol.* 7: 781, 1989.
216. Leung, Y. D., Moake, J. L., Havens, P. L., et al. Lytic anti-endothelial cell antibodies in haemolytic-uraemic syndrome. *Lancet* 2: 183, 1988.
217. Levin, E. G. Latent tissue plasminogen activator produced by human endothelial cells in culture: Evidence for an enzyme-inhibitor complex. *Proc. Natl. Acad. Sci. USA* 80: 6804, 1983.
218. Levin, H., and Alfrey, C. P. Thrombotic thrombocytopenic purpura: Temporary remission induced by prednisone. *Texas Med.* 62: 72, 1966.
219. Levine, S., and Shearn, M. A. Thrombotic thrombocytopenic purpura and systemic lupus erythematosus. *Arch. Intern. Med.* 113: 826, 1964.
220. Levinsky, N. G., and Alexander, E. A. Acute Renal Failure. In B. M. Brenner, and F. C. Rector, Jr. (eds.), *The Kidney.* Philadelphia: Saunders, 1981. P. 1181.
221. Levy, M., Gagnadoux, M. F., and Habib, R. Pathology of Hemolytic-Uremic Syndrome in Children. In G. Remuzzi, G. Mecca, and G. de Gaetano (eds.), *Hemostasis, Prostaglandins and Renal Disease.* New York: Raven Press, 1980. P. 383.
222. Lian, E. C. Y., Harkness, D. R., Byrnes, J. J., et al. Presence of a platelet aggregating factor in the plasma of patients with thrombotic thrombocytopenic purpura (TTP) and its inhibition by normal plasma. *Blood* 53: 333, 1979.
223. Lian, E. C. Y., Mui, P. T. K., Siddiqui, F. A., et al. Inhibition of platelet-aggregating activity in thrombotic

thrombocytopenic purpura plasma by normal adult immunoglobulin G. *J. Clin. Invest.* 73: 548, 1984.
224. Lian, E. C. Y., and Siddiqui, F. A. Investigation of the role of von Willebrand factor in thrombotic thrombocytopenic purpura. *Blood* 66: 1219, 1985.
225. Lieberman, E. Hemolytic-uremic syndrome. *J. Pediatr.* 80: 1, 1972.
226. Lieberman, E., Heuser, E., Donnell, G. N., et al. Hemolytic-uremic syndrome. *N. Engl. J. Med.* 275: 227, 1966.
227. Lorber, J., and Emery, J. L. Thrombotic thrombocytopenic purpura. *Proc. R. Soc. Med.* 52: 301, 1959.
228. Lowenhaupt, R., and Nathan, P. The participation of platelets in the rejection of dog kidney allotransplants: Hematologic and electron microscopic studies. *Transplant. Proc.* 1: 305, 1969.
229. Luke, R. G. Treatment of adult hemolytic uremic syndrome. *N. Engl. J. Med.* 294: 396, 1976.
230. Luke, R. G., Siegel, R. R., Talbert, W., et al. Heparin treatment for post-partum renal failure with microangiopathic haemolytic anaemia. *Lancet* 2: 750, 1970.
231. Lyman, N. W., Michaelson, R., Viscuso, R. L., et al. Mitomycin-induced hemolytic uremic syndrome: Successful treatment with corticosteroids and intense plasma exchange. *Arch. Intern. Med.* 143: 1617, 1983.
232. MacGillivray, I. Combined renal and anterior pituitary necrosis. *J. Obstet. Gynaecol. Br. Commonw.* 57: 924, 1950.
233. Machin, S. J., Defreyn, G., Chamone, D. A. F., et al. Plasma 6-keto-$PGF_{1\alpha}$ levels after plasma exchange in thrombotic thrombocytopenic purpura. *Lancet* 1: 661, 1980.
234. MacIntyre, D. E., Pearson, J. D., and Gordon, J. L. Localisation and stimulation of prostacyclin production in vascular cells. *Nature* 271: 549, 1978.
235. MacWhinney, J. B., Packer, J. T., Miller, G., et al. Thrombotic thrombocytopenic purpura in childhood. *Blood* 19: 181, 1962.
236. Mannucci, P. M., Lombardi, R., Lattuada, A., et al. Enhanced proteolysis of plasma von Willebrand factor in thrombotic thrombocytopenic purpura and the hemolytic uremic syndrome. *Blood* 74: 978, 1989.
237. Mant, M. J., Couchi, M. N., and Medley, G. Thrombotic thrombocytopenic purpura; Report of a case with possible immune etiology. *Blood* 40: 416, 1972.
238. Marcussen, H., and Asnaes, S. Renal cortical necrosis: An evaluation of the possible relation to the Shwartzman reaction. *Acta Pathol. Microbiol. Scand.* (A) 80: 351, 1972.
239. Marmont, A. M., Damasio, E., Ross, E., et al. Thrombotic thrombocytopenic purpura successfully treated with a combination of dipyridamole and aspirin. *Haematologica* 65: 222, 1980.
240. Marsden, P. A., Brock, T. A., and Ballermann, B. J. Glomerular endothelial cells respond to calcium mobilizing agonists with release of endothelin derived relaxing factor. Abstract. *Clin. Res.* 37: 496a, 1989.
241. Martin, D. L., MacDonald, K. L., White, K. E., et al. The epidemiology and clinical aspects of the hemolytic uremic syndrome in Minnesota. *N. Engl. J. Med.* 323: 1161, 1990.
242. Mathieu, H., Leclerc, F., Habib, R., et al. Etude clinique et biologique de 37 observations de syndrome hemolytique et uremiques. *Arch. Franc. Pediatr.* 26: 369, 1969.
243. Matlin, R. A., and Gary, N. E. Acute cortical necrosis. Case report and review of the literature. *Am. J. Med.* 56: 110, 1974.
244. McGiff, J. C., Itskovitz, H. D., Terragno, A., et al. Modulation and mediation of the action of the renal kallikrein-kinin system by prostaglandins. *Fed. Proc.* 35: 175, 1976.
245. McKay, D. G. *Disseminated Intravascular Coagulation: An Intermediary Mechanism of Disease.* New York: Harper & Row, 1965. P. 431.
245a. McLeod, B. C., Wu, K. K., and Knospe, W. H. Plasmapheresis in thrombotic thrombocytopenic purpura. *Arch. Intern. Med.* 140: 1059, 1980.
246. Meacham, G. C., Orbison, J. L., Heinle, R. W., et al. Thrombotic thrombocytopenic purpura a disseminated disease of arterioles. *Blood* 6: 706, 1952.
247. Merrill, R. H., Knupp, C. L., and Jennette, J. C. Familial thrombotic microangiopathy. *Q. J. Med.* 57: 749, 1985.
248. Messmore, H. L., Yeshwant, C., Remlinger, K., et al. Intravenous gamma globulin in refractory thrombotic thrombocytopenic purpura (TTP). *Thromb. Haemost.* 54: 127, 1985.
249. Mettler, N. E. Isolation of a microtatobiote from patients with hemolytic-uremic syndrome and thrombotic thrombocytopenic purpura and from mites in the United States. *N. Engl. J. Med.* 281: 1023, 1969.
250. Metz, J. Observations on the mechanism of the haematological changes in the haemolytic-uraemic syndrome of infancy. *Br. J. Haematol.* 23(Suppl.): 53, 1972.
251. Meyrick, B. O. Endotoxin-mediated pulmonary endothelial cell injury. *Fed. Proc.* 45: 19, 1986.
252. Milgrom, F., Kano, K., and Klassen, J. Role of humoral antibodies in rejection of renal allografts. *Transplant. Proc.* 1: 1013, 1969.
253. Misiani, R., Appiani, A. C., Edefonti, A., et al. Haemolytic uraemic syndrome: Therapeutic effect of plasma infusion. *Br. Med. J.* 285: 1304, 1982.
254. Moake, J. L. Von Willebrand factor in thrombotic thrombocytopenic purpura. *Blood* 67: 1523, 1986.
255. Moake, J. L., Byrnes, J. J., Troll, J. H., et al. Abnormal VIII:von Willebrand factor patterns in the plasma of patients with the hemolytic-uremic syndrome. *Blood* 64: 592, 1984.
256. Moake, J. L., Rudy, C. K., Troll, J. H., et al. Unusually large plasma factor VIII:von Willebrand factor multimers in chronic relapsing thrombotic thrombocytopenic purpura. *Ann. Intern. Med.* 101: 589, 1985.
257. Moell, H. Gross bilateral renal cortical necrosis during long periods of oliguria-anuria. Roentgenologic observations in two cases. *Acta Radiol. (Stockholm)* 48: 355, 1957.
258. Moncada, S. Prostacyclin and Thromboxane A2 in the Regulation of Platelet-Vascular Interactions. In G. Remuzzi, G. Mecca, and G. de Gaetano (eds.), *Hemostasis, Prostaglandins and Renal Disease.* New York: Raven Press, 1980. P. 175.
259. Monnens, L., Hendrickx, G., van Wieringen, P., et al. Serum-complement levels in haemolytic-uraemic syndrome. *Lancet* 2: 294, 1974.
260. Monnens, L., Kleynen, F., van Munster, P., et al. Coagulation studies and streptokinase therapy in the haemolytic-uraemic syndrome. *Helv. Paediatr. Acta* 21: 45, 1972.
261. Monnens, L., Molenaar, J., Lambert, P. H., et al. The complement system in hemolytic-uremic syndrome in childhood. *Clin. Nephrol.* 13: 168, 1980.
262. Monnens, L., van Collenburg, J., de Jong, M., et al. Treatment of the hemolytic-uremic syndrome. *Helv. Paediatr. Acta* 33: 321, 1978.
263. Monnens, L., Van De Meer, W., Langenhuysen, C., et al. Platelet aggregating factor in the epidemic form of

hemolytic-uremic syndrome in childhood. *Clin. Nephrol.* 24: 135, 1985.

264. Monnens, L. A. H., and Retera, R. J. M. Thrombotic thrombocytopenic purpura in a neonatal infant. *J. Pediatr.* 71: 118, 1967.
265. Mookerjee, B. K., Bilefsky, R., Kendall, A. G., et al. Generalized Shwartzman reaction due to gram-negative septicemia after abortion: Recovery after bilateral cortical necrosis. *Can. Med. Assoc. J.* 98: 578, 1968.
266. Moore, M. R., and Poon, M. C. Syndrome resembling thrombotic thrombocytopenic purpura associated with bacterial endocarditis. *South. Med. J.* 73: 541, 1980.
267. Morel-Maroger, L. Adult hemolytic-uremic syndrome. *Kidney Int.* 18: 125, 1980.
268. Morel-Maroger, L., Kanfer, A., Solez, K., et al. Prognostic importance of vascular lesions in acute renal failure with microangiopathic hemolytic anemia (hemolytic uremic syndrome): Clinicopathologic study in 20 adults. *Kidney Int.* 15: 548, 1979.
269. Morey, D. A., White, J. B., and Daily, W. M. Thrombotic thrombocytopenic purpura diagnosed by random lymph node biopsy. *Arch. Intern. Med.* 98: 821, 1956.
270. Morrison, D. M., Tyrrel, D. L. J., and Jewell, L. D. Colonic biopsy in verotoxin-induced hemorrhagic colitis and thrombotic thrombocytopenic purpura (TTP). *Am. J. Clin. Pathol.* 86: 108, 1986.
271. Morton, A. R., Yu, R., Waldek, S., et al. Campylobacter induced thrombotic thrombocytopenic purpura. *Lancet* 2: 1133, 1985.
272. Moschcowitz, E. Acute febrile pleiochromic anemia with hyaline thrombosis of the terminal arterioles and capillaries: An undescribed disease. *Arch. Intern. Med.* 36: 89, 1925.
273. Moss, S. W., Gary, N. E., and Eisinger, R. P. Renal cortical necrosis following streptococcal infection. *Arch. Intern. Med.* 137: 1196, 1977.
274. Murphy, W. G., Moore, J. C., and Kelton, J. C. Calcium-dependent cysteine protease activity in the sera of patients with thrombotic thrombocytopenic purpura. *Blood* 70: 1683, 1987.
275. Myers, T. J. Treatment of thrombotic thrombocytopenic purpura with combined exchange plasmapheresis and anti-platelet agents. *Semin. Thromb. Hemost.* 7: 37, 1981.
276. Myers, T. J., Wakem, C. J., Ball, E. D., et al. Thrombotic thrombocytopenic purpura: Combined treatment with plasmapheresis and antiplatelet agents. *Ann. Intern. Med.* 92: 149, 1980.
277. Nalbandian, R. M., Henry, R. L., and Bick, R. L. Thrombotic thrombocytopenic purpura. An extended editorial. *Semin. Thromb. Hemost.* 5: 216, 1979.
278. Neame, P. B., Hirsh, J., Browman, G., et al. Thrombotic thrombocytopenic purpura: A syndrome of intravascular platelet consumption. *Can. Med. Assoc. J.* 114, 1108, 1976.
279. Neame, P. D. Immunologic and other factors in thrombotic thrombocytopenic purpura (TTP). *Semin. Thromb. Haemost.* 6: 416, 1980.
280. Neild, G. H. Mechanisms and Models of Endothelial Injury. In T. Bertani, and G. Remuzzi (eds.), *Glomerular Injury 300 Years After Morgagni.* Milano: Wichtig Editore, 1983. P. 139.
281. Neild, G. H., Ivory, K., Hiramatsu, M., et al. Cyclosporin A inhibits acute serum sickness nephritis in rabbits. *Clin. Exp. Immunol.* 52: 586, 1983.
282. Neild, G. H., Ivory, K., and Williams, D. G. Glomerular Thrombi and Infarction in Rabbits with Serum Sickness following Cyclosporine Therapy. In B. D. Kahan (ed.), *Cyclosporine, Biological Activity and Clinical Applications.* London: Grune & Stratton, 1984. P. 566.
283. Neill, M. A., Agosti, J., and Rosen, H. Hemorrhagic colitis with Escherichia coli 0157:H7 preceding adult hemolytic uremic syndrome. *Arch. Intern. Med.* 145: 2215, 1985.
284. Ober, W. E., Reid, D. E., Romney, S. L., et al. Renal lesions and acute renal failure in pregnancy. *Am. J. Med.* 21: 781, 1956.
285. O'Brien, A. D., and LaVeck, G. D. Purification and characterization of a Shigella dysenteriae 1-like toxin produced by Escherichia coli. *Infect. Immun.* 40: 675, 1983.
286. Oram, S., Ross, G., Pell, L., et al. Renal cortical calcification after snake bite. *Br. Med. J.* 1: 1647, 1963.
287. Orbison, J. L. Morphology of thrombotic thrombocytopenic purpura with demonstration of aneurysms. *Am. J. Pathol.* 28: 129, 1952.
288. O'Regan, S., Chesney, R. W., Kaplan, B. S., et al. Red cell membrane phospholipid abnormalities in the hemolytic-uremic syndrome. *Clin. Nephrol.* 15: 14, 1981.
289. O'Regan, S., Chesney, R. W., Mongeau, J. G., et al. Aspirin and dipyridamole therapy in the hemolytic-uremic syndrome. *J. Pediatr.* 97: 473, 1980.
290. Palmer, R. M. J., Ferrige, A. G., and Moncada, S. Nitric oxide release accounts for the biological activity of endothelium-derived relaxing factor. *Nature* 327: 524, 1987.
291. Palmerio, C., Ming, S. C., Frank, E., et al. The role of the sympathetic nervous system in the generalized Shwartzman reaction. *J. Exp. Med.* 115: 609, 1962.
292. Paz, R. A., Elijovic, F., Barcat, J. A., et al. Fatal simultaneous thrombocytopenic purpura in siblings. *Br. Med. J.* 4: 727, 1969.
293. Pearson, J. D. Plasma Factors Regulating Prostaglandin Biosynthesis and Catabolism. In A. G. Herman, P. M. Van Houtte, A. Goosens, et al. (eds.), *Prostaglandins and the Cardiovascular System.* New York: Raven Press, 1982. P. 23.
294. Penner, A., and Bernheim, A. I. Acute ischaemic necrosis of the kidney: A clinico-pathologic and experimental study. *Arch. Pathol.* 30: 465, 1940.
295. Percival, S. P. B. Ocular findings in thrombotic thrombocytopenic purpura (Moschowitz's disease). *Br. J. Ophthalmol.* 54: 73, 1970.
296. Perico, N., Dadan, J., and Remuzzi, G. Endothelin mediates the renal vasoconstriction induced by cyclosporine in the rat. *J. Am. Soc. Nephrol.* 1: 76, 1990.
297. Perry, J. W. Phosphorus poisoning with cortical necrosis of the kidney: A report of two fatal cases. *Aust. Ann. Med.* 2: 94, 1953.
298. Peterson, J., Amare, M., Henry, J., et al. Splenectomy and antiplatelet agents in thrombotic thrombocytopenic purpura. *Am. J. Med. Sci.* 277: 75, 1979.
299. Petitt, R. M. Thrombotic thrombocytopenic purpura: A thirty-year review. *Semin. Thromb. Hemostas.* 6: 350, 1980.
300. Piel, C. F., and Phibbs, R. H. The hemolytic-uremic syndrome. *Pediatr. Clin. North Am.* 13: 295, 1966.
301. Pirani, C. L. Coagulation and Renal Disease. In T. Bertani, and G. Remuzzi, (eds.), *Glomerular Injury 300 Years After Morgagni.* Milano: Wichtig Editore, 1983. P. 119.
302. Platt, J. L., Vercellotti, G. M., Lindman, B. J., et al. Release of heparan sulfate from endothelial cells. Implications for pathogenesis for hyperacute rejection. *J. Exp. Med.* 171: 1363, 1990.
303. Ponticelli, C., Imbasciati, E., Rivolta, E., et al. Long-term follow-up of postpartum hemolytic-uremic syndrome treated with heparin and antiplatelet agents. In

G. Remuzzi, G. Mecca, and G. de Gaetano (eds.), *Hemostasis, Prostaglandins and Renal Disease*. New York: Raven Press, 1980. P. 433.

304. Ponticelli, C., Rivolta, E., Imbasciati, E., et al. Hemolytic uremic syndrome in adults. *Arch. Intern. Med.* 140: 353, 1980.
305. Powell, H. R., Davidson, P. M., McCredie, D. A., et al. Haemolytic uraemic syndrome after treatment with metronidazole. *Med. J. Aust.* 149: 222, 1988.
306. Powell, H. R., and Ekert, H. Streptokinase and antithrombotic therapy in the hemolytic uremic syndrome. *J. Pediatr.* 84: 345, 1974.
307. Powell, H. R., McCredie, D. A., Taylor, C. M., et al. Vitamin E treatment of haemolytic uraemic syndrome. *Arch. Dis. Child.* 59: 401, 1984.
308. Powles, R. L., Clink, H. M., Spence, D., et al. Cyclosporin A to prevent graft-versus-host disease in man after allogeneic bone-marrow transplantation. *Lancet* 1: 327, 1980.
309. Powles, R. L., Kay, H. E. M., Clink, H. M., et al. Mismatched family donors for bone-marrow transplantation as treatment for acute leukaemia. *Lancet* 1: 612, 1983.

309a. Proesmans, W., Eeckels, R. Has Heparin changed the prognosis of the hemolytic-uremic syndrome. *Clin. Nephrol.* 2: 169, 1974.

310. Proesmans, W., ki Muaka, B., Van Damme, B., et al. The Use of Heparin in Childhood Hemolytic-Uremic Syndrome. In G. Remuzzi, G. Mecca, and G. de Gaetano (eds.), *Hemostasis, Prostaglandins and Renal Disease*. New York: Raven Press, 1980. P. 407.
311. Proia, A. D., Harden, E. A., and Silberman, H. R. Mitomycin-induced hemolytic-uremic syndrome. *Arch. Pathol. Lab. Med.* 108: 959, 1984.
312. Puspok, R., and Graninger, W. T. Antigen and Its Relation to Hemolytic Uremic Syndrome. *Contrib. Nephrol.* 35: 35, 1983.
313. Rabadi, S. J., Khandekar, J. D., and Miller, H. J. Mitomycin-induced hemolytic-uremic syndrome: Case presentation and review of literature. *Cancer Treat. Rep.* 66: 1244, 1982.
314. Radomski, M. W., Palmer, R. M. J., and Moncada, S. Comparative pharmacology of endothelium-derived relaxing factor, nitric oxide and prostacyclin in platelets. *Br. J. Pharmacol.* 92: 181, 1987.
315. Raghupathy, P., Date, A., Shastry, J. C. M., et al. Haemolytic-uraemic syndrome complicating shigella dysentery in south Indian children. *Br. Med. J.* 1: 1518, 1978.
316. Rahaman, M. M., Jamiulalam, A. K., Islam, M. R., et al. Shiga bacillus dysentery associated with marked leukocytosis and erythrocyte fragmentation. *Johns Hopkins Med. J.* 136: 65, 1975.
317. Raij, L., Keane, W. F., and Michael, A. F. Unilateral Shwartzman reaction: Cortical necrosis in one kidney following in vivo perfusion with endotoxin. *Kidney Int.* 12: 91, 1977.
318. Remuzzi, G. Thrombotic Thrombocytopenic Purpura and Allied Disorders. In M. Verstraete, J. Vermylen, H. R. Lijnen, et al. (eds.), *Thrombosis and Haemostasis*. Leuven: Leuven University Press, 1987. P. 673.
319. Remuzzi, G. HUS and TTP: Variable expression of a single entity. *Kidney Int.* 32: 292, 1987.
320. Remuzzi, G., Misiani, R., Marchesi, D., et al. Haemolytic-uraemic syndrome: deficiency of plasma factor(s) regulating prostacyclin activity? *Lancet* 2: 871, 1978.
321. Remuzzi, G., Misiani, R., Marchesi, D., et al. Treatment of the hemolytic-uremic syndrome with plasma infusion. *Clin. Nephrol.* 12: 279, 1979.
322. Remuzzi, G., Misiani, R., Mecca, G., et al. Thrombotic thrombocytopenic purpura. A deficiency of plasma factors regulating platelet-vessel-wall interaction? *N. Engl. J. Med.* 299: 311, 1978.
323. Remuzzi, G., Perico, N., Zoja, C., et al. Role of endothelium-derived nitric oxide in the bleeding tendency of uremia. *J. Clin. Invest.* 86: 1768, 1990.
324. Reynolds, P. M., Jackson, J. M., Brine, J. A. S., et al. Thrombotic thrombocytopenic purpura—remission following splenectomy. *Am. J. Med.* 61: 439, 1976.

324a. Richardson, J. H., and Smith, B. T. Thrombotic thrombocytopenic purpura. Survival in pregnancy with heparin sodium therapy. *J.A.M.A.* 203: 518, 1968.

325. Ridolfi, R. L., and Bell, W. R. Thrombotic thrombocytopenic purpura. Report of 25 cases and review of the literature. *Medicine* 60: 413, 1981.
326. Ridolfi, R. L., Hutchins, G. M., and Bell, W. R. The heart and cardiac conduction system in thrombotic thrombocytopenic purpura. *Ann. Intern. Med.* 91: 357, 1979.
327. Rifle, G., Chalopin, J. M., Genin, R., et al. Hemolytic uremic syndrome and recurrent uremia. Irreversible cortical necrosis due to estro-progestational hormones. Abstract. *J. Urol. Nephrol.* 85: 331, 1979.
328. Riggs, S. A., Wray, N. P., Waddell, C. C., et al. Thrombotic thrombocytopenic purpura complicating Legionnaires' disease. *Arch. Intern. Med.* 14: 2275, 1982.
329. Riley, L. W., Remis, R. S., Helgerson, S. D., et al. Hemorrhagic colitis associated with a rare *Escherichia coli* 0157:H7 serotype. *N. Engl. J. Med.* 308: 681, 1983.
330. Robboy, S. J., Major, M. C., Colman, R. W., et al. Pathology of disseminated intravascular coagulation (DIC): Analysis of 26 cases. *Human Pathol.* 3: 327, 1972.
331. Robson, J. S., Martin, A. M., Ruckley, V. A., et al. Irreversible post partum renal failure. *Q. J. Med.* 137: 423, 1968.
332. Rohrer, H. Kidney necrosis in acute hog cholera. *Virchows Arch. Pathol. Anat.* 284: 203, 1932.
333. Rooney, J. C., Anderson, R. M., and Hopkins, I. J. Clinical and pathological aspects of central nervous system involvement in the haemolytic uraemic syndrome. *Aust. Paediatr. J.* 7: 28, 1971.
334. Rose, P. E., Enayat, S. M., Sunderland, R., et al. Abnormalities of factor VIII related protein multimers in the haemolytic uraemic syndrome. *Arch. Dis. Child.* 59: 1135, 1984.
335. Rosello, S. G., Piulats, E. L., Gomez, I., et al. Renal cortical necrosis and right nephrectomy survival in a man. *Am. J. Med.* 45: 309, 1969.
336. Rosenmann, E., Kanter, A., Bacani, R. A., et al. Fatal late postpartum intravascular coagulation with acute renal failure. *Am. J. Med. Sci.* 257: 259, 1969.
337. Rossi, E. C., Carone, F. A., and del Greco, F. Hemolytic-Uremic Syndrome and Platelet-Endothelial Interactions. In G. Remuzzi, G. Mecca, and G. de Gaetano (eds.), *Hemostasis, Prostaglandins and Renal Disease*. New York: Raven Press, 1980. P. 321.

337a. Rossi, E. C., Redondo, D., and Borges, W. H. Thrombotic thrombocytopenic purpura. Survival following treatment with aspirin, dipyridamole and prednisone. *J.A.M.A.* 228: 1141, 1974.

338. Rothfield, N. F. Systemic lupus erythematosus. In D. J. McCarey (ed.), *Arthritis and Allied Conditions*. Philadelphia: Lea & Febiger, 1979. P. 706.
339. Rowa, J. M., Francis, C. W., Cyran, E. M., et al. Thrombotic thrombocytopenic purpura: Recovery after splenectomy associated with persistence of abnormally large

von Willebrand factor multimers. *Am. J. Hematol.* 20: 161, 1985.

339a. Rubinstein, M. A., et al. Unusual remission in a case of thrombotic thrombocytopenic purpura syndrome following fresh blood exchange transfusions. *Ann. Intern. Med.* 51: 1409, 1959.

340. Ruggenenti, P., Remuzzi, G., and Rossi, E. C. Epidemiology of hemolytic-uremic syndrome. *N. Engl. J. Med.*, 324: 1065, 1991.

341. Ruggeri, Z. M., De Marco, L., Gatti, L., et al. Platelets have more than one binding site for von Willebrand factor. *J. Clin. Invest.* 72: 1, 1983.

342. Ruggeri, Z. M., Mannucci, P. M., Lombardi, R., et al. Multimeric composition of factor VIII/von Willebrand factor following administration of DDAVP: Implications for pathophysiology and therapy of von Willebrand's disease subtypes. *Blood* 59: 1272, 1982.

343. Rutkow, I. M. Thrombotic thrombocytopenic purpura (TTP) and splenectomy. *Ann. Surg.* 188: 701, 1978.

344. Ryan, C. A., Tauxe, R. V., and Hosek, G. W. Escherichia coli 0157:H7 diarrhea in a nursing home: Clinical, epidemiological, and pathological findings. *J. Infect. Dis.* 154: 631, 1986.

344a. Scharoff, J. R., Serlin, N., and Atamer, M. A. Thrombotic thrombocytopenic purpura. Report of a case treated with splenectomy and steroids. *Acta. Hematol.* 41: 180, 1969.

345. Schieppati, A., Ruggenenti, P., Plata, R., et al. Renal function at hospital admission as a prognostic factor in adult haemolytic uraemic syndrome. *J. Am. Soc. Nephrol., in press.*

346. Schoolwerth, A. C., Sandler, R. S., Klahr, S., et al. Nephrosclerosis postpartum and in women taking oral contraceptives. *Arch. Intern. Med.* 136: 178, 1976.

347. Schreiner, G. E. La Necrose Corticale Bilaterale des Reins. In J. Hamburger, and J. Crosnier (eds.), *Nephrologie.* Paris: Editions Medicale Flammarion, 1979. P. 422.

348. Schwartz, M. L., and Brenner, W. E. The obfuscation of eclampsia by thrombotic thrombocytopenic purpura. *Obstetrics* 131: 18, 1978.

349. Sevitt, L. H., Evans, D. J., and Wrong, O. M. Acute oliguric renal failure due to accelerated (malignant) hypertension. *Q. J. Med.* 40: 127, 1971.

350. Shapiro, C. M., Kanter, A., Lopas, H., et al. Hemolytic-uremic syndrome in adults. *J.A.M.A.* 213: 567, 1970.

351. Sharma, H. M., Moore, S., Merrick, H. W., et al. Platelets in early hyperacute allograft rejection in kidneys and their modification by sulfinpyrazone (Anturan) therapy: An experimental study. *Am. J. Pathol.* 66: 445, 1972.

352. Sheehan, H. L., and Davis, J. C. Renal ischaemia with failed reflow. *J. Pathol. Bacteriol.* 78: 105, 1959.

353. Sheehan, H. L., and Davis, J. C. The protective effect of anesthesia in experimental renal ischaemia. *J. Pathol. Bacteriol.* 79: 337, 1960.

354. Sheehan, H. L., and Moore, H. C. *Renal Cortical Necrosis and the Kidney of Concealed Hemorrhage.* Springfield, Ill.: Charles C Thomas, 1953.

355. Sheldon, W. H., and Hertig, A. T. Bilateral cortical necrosis of the kidney: A report of 2 cases. *Arch. Pathol.* 34: 866, 1942.

356. Sheth, K. J., Gill, J. C., and Leichte, H. E. Randomized double blind controlled study of intravenous gamma globulin (IVGG) infusions in heolytic uremic syndrome (HUS). Abstract. *J. Am. Soc. Nephrol.* 1: 342, 1990.

357. Sheth, K. J., Swick, H. M., and Haworth, N. Neurological involvement in hemolytic-uremic syndrome. *Ann. Neurol.* 19: 90, 1986.

358. Shigematsu, H., Dikman, S. H., Churg, J., et al. Mesangial involvement in hemolytic-uremic syndrome. *Am. J. Pathol.* 85: 349, 1976.

359. Shulman, H., Striker, G., Deeg, H. J., et al. Nephrotoxicity of cyclosporin A after allogeneic marrow transplantation: Glomerular thrombosis and tubular injury. *N. Engl. J. Med.* 305: 1392, 1981.

360. Shumway, C. N., Jr., and Miller, G. An unusual syndrome of hemolytic anemia, thrombocytopenic purpura and renal disease. *Blood* 12: 1045, 1957.

361. Shumway, C. N., and Terplan, K. L. Hemolytic anemia, thrombocytopenia and renal disease in childhood: The hemolytic uremic syndrome. *Pediatr. Clin. North Am.* 11: 577, 1964.

362. Shwartzman, G. *Phenomenon of Local Tissue Reactivity.* New York: Hoebner, 1937. P. 193.

363. Siddiqui, F. A., and Lian, E. C. Y. Novel platelet-agglutinating protein from a thrombotic thrombocytopenic purpura plasma. *J. Clin. Invest.* 76: 1330, 1985.

364. Siegler, R. L., Smith, J. B., Lynch, M. B., et al. In vitro prostacyclin production in the hemolytic-uremic syndrome. *West. J. Med.* 144: 165, 1986.

365. Silverstein, A. Thrombotic thrombocytopenic purpura: The initial neurologic manifestations. *Arch. Neurol.* 18: 358, 1968.

365a. Simon, P., et al. Plasma exchange using filtration. Experience at the apropos of 21 patients. *Rev. Fr. Transfus. Immunohematol.* 24: 671, 1981.

366. Solez, K. Acute Renal Failure ("Acute Tubular Necrosis" Infarction, and Cortical Necrosis). In R. H. Heptinstall (ed.), *Pathology of the Kidney* (3rd ed.). Boston: Little, Brown, 1983. P. 1069.

367. Sporn, I. N. Renal cortical necrosis (letter). *Arch. Intern. Med.* 138: 1866, 1978.

368. Stamler, F. W. Fetal eclamptic disease of pregnant fed antivitamin E stress diet. *Am. J. Pathol.* 35: 1207, 1959.

369. Steer, M. L., MacIntyre, D. E., Levine, L., et al. Is prostacyclin a physiologically important circulating antiplatelet agent? *Nature* 283: 194, 1980.

370. Steinberg, A. D., Green, W. T., and Talal, N. Thrombotic thrombocytopenic purpura complicating Sjögren's syndrome. *J.A.M.A.* 215: 757, 1971.

371. Stetson, C. A., and Good, R. A. Studies on the mechanism of the Shwartzman phenomenon. *J. Exp. Med.* 93: 49, 1951.

372. Stiehm, E. R., and Trygstad, C. W. Split products of fibrin in human renal disease. *Am. J. Med.* 46: 774, 1969.

373. Stonesifer, L. D., Bone, R. C., and Hiller, F. C. Thrombotic thrombocytopenic purpura in carbon monoxide poisoning. *Arch. Intern. Med.* 140: 104, 1980.

374. Stockbine, N. A., Marques, L. R. M., Holmes, R. K., et al. Characterization of monoclonal antibodies against Shiga-like toxin from *Escherichia coli. Infect. Immun.* 50: 695, 1985.

375. Stuart, J., Winterborn, M. H., White, R. H. R., et al. Thrombolytic therapy in haemolytic uraemic syndrome. *Br. Med. J.* 3: 217, 1974.

376. Stuart, M. J., Spitzer, R. E., and Coppe, D. Abnormal platelet and vascular prostaglandin synthesis in an infant with hemolytic uremic syndrome. *Pediatrics* 71: 120, 1983.

377. Sugiura, M., Inagami, T., and Kon, V. Stimulatory effect of endotoxin on endothelin (ET) release in vivo and in vitro. *Biochem. Biophys. Res. Commun.* 161: 1220, 1989.

378. Symmers, W. S. C. Thrombotic microangiopathic haemolytic anemia (thrombotic microangiopathy). *Br. Med. J.* 2: 897, 1952.

379. Symmers, W. S. T. C., and Barrowcliff, D. F. Platelet thrombosis syndrome. *J. Pathol. Bacteriol.* 63: 552, 1951.
380. Taft, E. G. Thrombotic thrombocytopenic purpura and dose of plasma exchange. *Blood* 54: 842, 1979.
381. Thoenes, W., and John, H. D. Endotheliotropic (hemolytic) nephroangiopathy and its various manifestation forms (thrombotic microangiopathy, primary malignant nephrosclerosis, hemolytic-uremic syndrome). *Klin. Wochenschr.* 58: 173, 1980.
382. Thomas, L., Brunson, J., and Smith, R. T. Studies on the generalized Shwartzman reaction. VI. Production of the reaction by the synergistic action of endotoxin with three synthetic acid polymers (sodium polyanethol sulfonate, dextran sulfate, and sodium polyvinyl alcohol sulfonate). *J. Exp. Med.* 96: 249, 1952.
383. Thomas, L., and Good, R. A. Studies on the generalized Shwartzman reaction. I. General observations concerning the phenomenon. *J. Exp. Med.* 96: 605, 1952.
384. Thompson, E. A., and Howard, M. A. Proteolytic cleavage of human von Willebrand factor induced by enzyme(s) released from polymorphonuclear cells. *Blood* 67: 1281, 1986.
385. Thorsen, C. A., Rossi, E. C., Green, D., et al. The treatment of the hemolytic-uremic syndrome with inhibitor of platelet function. *Am. J. Med.* 66: 711, 1979.
386. Trompeter, R. S., Schwartz, R., Chantler, C., et al. Haemolytic-uraemic syndrome: An analysis of prognostic features. *Arch. Dis. Child.* 58: 101, 1983.
387. Turi, S., Beattie, T. J., Belch, J. J. F., et al. Disturbances of prostacyclin metabolism in children with hemolytic-uremic syndrome in first degree relatives. *Clin. Nephrol.* 25: 193, 1986.
388. Umlas, J., and Kaiser, J. Thrombohemolytic thrombocytopenic purpura (TTP): A disease or a syndrome? *Am. J. Med.* 49: 723, 1970.
389. Upshaw, J. D., Jr. Congenital deficiency of factor in normal plasma that reverses microangiopathic hemolysis and thrombocytopenia. *N. Engl. J. Med.* 298: 1350, 1978.
390. Van Buren, D., Van Buren, C. T., Flechner, S. M., et al. De novo hemolytic uremic syndrome in renal transplant recipients immunosuppressed with cyclosporin. *Surgery* 98: 54, 1985.
391. Van Wierengen, P. M. V., Monnens, L. A. H., and Schretlen, E. D. A. M. Haemolytic-uraemic syndrome. Epidemiological and clinical study. *Arch. Dis. Child.* 49: 432, 1974.
392. Verpooten, G. A., Paulus, G. J., Roels, F., et al. De novo occurrence of hemolytic-uremic syndrome in cyclosporine-treated renal allograft patient. *Transplant. Proc.* 19: 2943, 1987.
392a. Viero, P., et al. Thrombotic thrombocytopenic purpura and high-dose immunoglobulin therapy. *Ann. Intern. Med.* 104: 282, 1986.
392b. Vitacco, M., Sanchez-Avalos, J., and Gianantonio, C. A. Heparin therapy in the hemolytic-uremic syndrome. *J. Pediatr.* 83: 271, 1973.
393. Vitsky, B. H., Suzuki, Y., Strauss, L., et al. The hemolytic-uremic syndrome: A study of renal pathologic alterations. *Am. J. Pathol.* 57: 627, 1969.
394. Voss, B. L., Hamilton, K. K., Samara, E. N. S., et al. Cyclosporine suppression of endothelial prostacyclin generation. *Transplantation* 45: 793, 1988.
395. Wahle, G. H., Jr., and Muirhead, E. E. Bilateral renal cortical necrosis in a child associated with an incompatible blood transfusion. *Texas J. Med.* 49: 770, 1953.
396. Wall, R. T., and Harker, L. A. The endothelium and thrombosis. *Annu. Rev. Med.* 31: 361, 1980.
397. Wallace, D., Lovric, A., and Clubb, J., et al. Thrombotic thrombocytopenic purpura in four siblings. *Am. J. Med.* 58: 724, 1975.
398. Walls, J., Schorr, W. J., and Kerr, D. N. S. Prolonged oliguria with survival in acute bilateral cortical necrosis. *Br. Med. J.* 4: 220, 1968.
399. Walters, M. D. S., Matthei, I. U., Kay, R., et al. The polymorphonuclear leukocyte count in childhood haemolytic uraemic syndrome. *Pediatr. Nephrol.* 3: 130, 1989.
400. Walters, S., Levin, M., Smith, C., et al. Intravascular platelet activation in the hemolytic uremic syndrome. *Kidney Int.* 33: 107, 1988.
401. Wardle, E. N. Thrombotic micro-angiopathy. *Clin. Nephrol.* 20: 323, 1983.
402. Wasserstein, A., Hill, G., Goldfarb, S., et al. Recurrent thrombotic thrombocytopenic purpura after viral infection. Clinical and histological simulation of chronic glomerulonephritis. *Arch. Intern. Med.* 141: 685, 1981.
403. Watson, C. G., and Cooper, W. W. Thrombotic thrombocytopenic purpura: Concomitant occurrence in husband and wife. *J.A.M.A.* 215: 1821, 1971.
404. Webster, J., Rees, A. J., Lewis, P. J., et al. Prostacyclin deficiency in haemolytic-uraemic syndrome. *Br. Med. J.* 281: 271, 1980.
405. Weisenburger, D. D., O'Conner, M. L., and Hart, M. H. Thrombotic thrombocytopenic purpura with C3 vascular deposits: Report of an unusual case. *Am. J. Clin. Pathol.* 67: 61, 1977.
406. Whelan, J. G., Ling, J. T., and Davis, L. A. Antemortem roentgen manifestations of bilateral renal cortical necrosis. *Radiology* 89: 682, 1967.
407. Whitaker, A. N. Acute renal failure in disseminated intravascular coagulation. Experimental studies of the induction and prevention of renal fibrin deposition. *Progr. Biochem. Pharmacol.* 9: 45, 1974.
408. Whitington, P. F., Friedman, A. L., and Chesney, R. W. Gastrointestinal disease in the hemolytic uremic syndrome. *Gastroenterology* 76: 728, 1979.
409. Wiles, P. G., Solomon, L. R., Lawler, W., et al. Inherited plasma factor deficiency in haemolytic-uraemic syndrome. *Lancet* 1: 1105, 1981.
410. Wolfe, J. A., McCann, R. L., and San Filippo, F. Cyclosporin associated microangiopathy in renal transplantation: A severe but potentially reversible form of early graft injury. *Transplantation* 41: 541, 1986.
411. Wong, P., Itoh, K., and Yoshida, S. Treatment of thrombotic thrombocytopenic purpura with intravenous gamma globulin. *N. Engl. J. Med.* 314: 385, 1986.
412. Wong, T. C. A study on the generalized Shwartzman reaction in pregnant rats induced by bacterial endotoxin. *Am. J. Obstet. Gynecol.* 84: 786, 1962.
413. Woods, J. W., and Williams, T. F. Hypertension Due to Renal Vascular Disease, Renal Infarction, Renal Cortical Necrosis. In M. B. Strauss and L. G. Welt (eds.), *Diseases of the Kidney* (2nd ed.). Boston: Little, Brown, 1971. P. 769.
414. Wu, K. K., Hall, E. R., Rossi, E. C., et al. Serum prostacyclin binding defects in thrombotic thrombocytopenic purpura. *J. Clin. Invest.* 75: 168, 1985.
415. Yamada, O., Moldow, C. F., Sacks, T., et al. Deleterious effects of endotoxin on cultured endothelial cells: An in vitro model of vascular injury. *Inflammation* 5: 115, 1981.
416. Yanagisawa, M., Kurihara, H., Kimura, S., et al. A novel potent vasoconstrictor peptide produced by vascular endothelial cells. *Nature* 322: 411, 1988.
417. Yoshikawa, T., Tanaka, K. R., and Guze, L. B. Infection

and disseminated intravascular coagulation. *Medicine* 50: 237, 1971.

418. Yoshizumi, M., Kurihara, H., Sugiyama, F., et al. Hemodynamic shear stress stimulates endothelin production by cultured endothelial cells. *Biochem. Biophys. Res. Commun.* 161: 859, 1989.
419. Zoja, C., Furci, L., Ghilardi, F., et al. Cyclosporin-induced endothelial cell injury. *Lab. Invest.* 55: 455, 1986.
420. Zucker, M. B., Brockman, M. J., and Kaplan, K. Factor VIII-related antigen in human blood platelets. Localization and release by thrombin and collagen. *J. Lab. Clin. Med.* 94: 675, 1979.
421. Zuelzer, W. W., Charles, S., Kurnetz, R., et al. Circulatory diseases of the kidneys in infancy and childhood. *Am. J. Dis. Child.* 81: 1, 1951.

Vasculitic Diseases of the Kidney: Polyarteritis, Wegener's Granulomatosis, Necrotizing and Crescentic Granulomatosis, and Other Disorders

James E. Balow
Anthony S. Fauci

The kidney is affected by many types of systemic vasculitis. This chapter will focus on those forms of systemic vasculitis that are considered primary and usually involve the kidney: classic polyarteritis nodosa (PAN), microscopic polyarteritis, necrotizing and crescentic glomerulonephritis, and Wegener's granulomatosis. The types of primary vasculitis that less frequently affect the kidney will be only briefly discussed: allergic angiitis and granulomatosis (Churg-Strauss disease), polyangiitis overlap syndrome, lymphomatoid granulomatosis, temporal arteritis, Takayasu arteritis, Behçet's disease, relapsing polychondritis, and cutaneous vasculitis. Conditions that are considered to be secondary forms of renal vasculitis will be covered in other chapters: lupus nephritis, Henoch-Schönlein nephritis, and cryoglobulinemia.

The term *systemic vasculitis* has both clinical and pathologic implications. Pathologically, vasculitis denotes inflammation within the walls of blood vessels. Virtually any type or size of blood vessel may be involved. Fibrinoid necrosis is characteristic but not invariable. Clinically, systemic vasculitis designates a syndrome composed of generic features which different forms of vasculitis tend to express in common. When additional discrete and characteristic features are present, classification of systemic vasculitis is straightforward. Often, however, the patient presents with only the nonspecific features of the vasculitic syndrome, in which case classification may be difficult. Classification may be made additionally difficult by the simultaneous occurrence of specific elements of more than one type of systemic vasculitis (Table 76-1).

History and Approaches to Classification of Vasculitis

PAN was the first type of systemic vasculitis described in the German literature by Kussmaul and Maier in 1866. These authors observed gross aneurysms in several organ systems. Relatively few cases of PAN with such profound vascular disease have subsequently been reported. Whether the disease observed by Kussmaul and Maier should be considered pathogenetically distinctive because of the extreme nature of the vascular damage or whether comparable pathologic changes can evolve in any form of inadequately treated medium-sized vessel arteritis is uncertain.

The term *PAN* logically applies to patients with nodular irregularities of vessels. However, at the present time, the central element in the definition of classic PAN is necrotizing vasculitis of medium-sized arteries with or without gross aneurysm formation. Aneurysms are considered to be an index of the severity of the vasculitic process and their presence can be helpful in documenting arteritis; yet, aneurysms are not essential for the diagnosis of classic PAN. Because of the practical limitations in surveying the entire vascular tree for aneurysms, some clinicians prefer the unmodified term, polyarteritis, rather than PAN. However, for historical reasons, most investigators continue to use the terms *polyarteritis* and *polyarteritis nodosa* interchangeably.

Although Kussmaul and Maier considered that their patients with PAN succumbed to Bright's disease, they did not describe the exact nature of the renal disease. In subsequent literature, ischemia due to medium-sized vessel vasculitis, thrombosis, infarction, and aneurysms (rather than glomerulonephritis) were recognized to be the usual causes for renal dysfunction in patients with classic PAN.

The types of renal disease in polyarteritis were further elucidated by Davson et al. in 1948 [32]. They proposed that renal involvement in polyarteritis was of two distinct types: polyarteritis with predominantly extraglomerular vasculitis (classic PAN, Kussmaul-Maier disease, macroscopic PAN); and polyarteritis with glomerulonephritis, for which they proposed the term *microscopic polyarteritis.* They further noted that there were few clinical differences between classic PAN and microscopic polyarteritis in regard to extrarenal vasculitis. Both groups exhibited azotemia and moderate proteinuria. However, in classic PAN these renal features were due to severe hypertension, ischemia, and renal infarcts, while in microscopic polyarteritis the renal process was necrotizing and crescentic glomerulonephritis. It is important to emphasize that no sharp dichotomy existed: At autopsy, as many as one-third of the patients with microscopic polyarteritis had concomitant glomerulonephritis and medium-sized vessel vasculitis (including some aneurysms) in extraglomerular vessels.

This subclassification of polyarteritis has not been endorsed by all specialties since the distinction is based on the pathophysiology of the kidney. The separation of classic PAN and microscopic polyarteritis is used principally in nephrology and pathology [9, 122, 126, 129].

In the early 1950s Zeek suggested another approach to the classification of systemic vasculitis [144]. She observed that vasculitis induced by exogenous drugs, sera, or infections in humans tended to cause widespread cutaneous vasculitis, and less commonly, major organ vasculitis or glomerulonephritis. Similar changes in hyperimmunized animals led Zeek to propose the term *hypersensitivity angiitis* as a way to distinguish this condition from sporadic cases of polyarteritis. The terms *hypersensitivity angiitis* and *microscopic polyarteritis* have sometimes been used interchangeably, but at the present time the term *microscopic polyarteritis* is preferred in cases of polyarteritis with glomerulonephritis. The term

Table 76-1. Classification of systemic vasculitis

A. Polyarteritis group of systemic vasculitis
   1. Polyarteritis nodosa (classic PAN)
   2. Microscopic polyarteritis
   3. Necrotizing and crescentic glomerulonephritis

B. Polyangiitis overlap syndrome

C. Wegener's granulomatosis

D. Allergic angiitis and granulomatosis (Churg-Strauss disease)

E. Cutaneous vasculitis (hypersensitivity vasculitis)

F. Giant cell arteritis: temporal arteritis, Takayasu arteritis

G. Secondary and miscellaneous forms of vasculitis: systemic lupus erythematosus, Henoch-Schönlein purpura, cryoglobulinemia, rheumatoid vasculitis, vasculitis associated with malignancy, Behçet's syndrome, relapsing polychondritis, hypocomplementemic vasculitis

hypersensitivity angiitis is mostly used synonymously with cutaneous vasculitis [28, 47, 60].

A separate class of systemic vasculitis, designated *polyangiitis overlap syndrome,* has been proposed for patients with necrotizing vasculitis of multiple vessel sizes (e.g., classic PAN and cutaneous vasculitis) and for patients with mixed features of polyarteritis and other specific types of systemic vasculitis (e.g., classic PAN, Wegener's granulomatosis, Churg-Strauss disease) [88]. The reader should be aware that polyangiitis overlap syndrome has only recently been designated as a separate category of systemic vasculitis and that these patients have historically been included in reports on polyarteritis (nodosa).

There are numerous approaches to the classification of systemic vasculitis. The merits of lumping and splitting the categories of systemic vasculitis have been regularly debated. Given the diversity of clinical and pathologic features, it is difficult to envision a classification of systemic vasculitis that would serve all subspecialties equally well. The variations in terminology and classification have generated unfortunate levels of confusion in the literature.

Recent progress has been made through the efforts of the American College of Rheumatology and a panel of internationally recognized experts, who have developed a set of standard definitions for the classification of systemic vasculitis [74]. The formal criteria for diagnosis of the various forms of systemic vasculitis that are discussed in this chapter are summarized in Table 76-2.

The terminology used for the majority of systemic vasculitis syndromes enjoys a broad consensus because most entities are easily recognized and discrete (see Table 76-1). However, controversy has pervaded the terminology applied to the polyarteritis group of systemic vasculitis and, in particular, the merit of separating PAN and microscopic polyarteritis.

Additional controversy has been evoked recently by suggestions that many cases of what was traditionally called idiopathic necrotizing and crescentic glomerulonephritis should be considered a form of polyarteritis [9, 26, 41, 69, 103, 122, 126, 138]. These proposals are based on several observations. First, patients with idiopathic necrotizing and crescentic glomerulonephritis often have subtle clinical features that suggest an underlying systemic vasculitis, but they lack definitive evidence of extraglomerular vasculitis. Second, a substantial portion of patients presenting with necrotizing and crescentic glomerulonephritis develop full expressions of systemic vasculitis after prolonged follow-up [126, 142]. Third, the lesions of idiopathic necrotizing and crescentic glomerulonephritis are histologically indistinguishable from those of microscopic polyarteritis [27, 129]. Fourth, profiles of autoantibodies to neutrophil cytoplasmic antigens (ANCAs) are similar in patients with microscopic polyarteritis and in those with necrotizing and crescentic glomerulonephritis [5, 20, 39] (see below). Finally, if polyarteritis can affect any organ, then it follows logically that polyarteritis might affect only one organ, such as the kidney, skin, or central nervous system. In short, there is broad acceptance that necrotizing and crescentic glomerulonephritis is equivalent to renal-limited polyarteritis. The reader is reminded that many recent publications on diagnosis, treatment, and prognosis have lumped patients with microscopic polyarteritis and necrotizing and crescentic glomerulonephritis (and often Wegener's granulomatosis) together.

Table 76-2. The American College of Rheumatology criteria for classification of vasculitis [74]

Polyarteritis nodosa (3 or more)
1. Weight loss ≥ 4 kg
2. Livedo reticularis
3. Testicular pain or tenderness
4. Myalgias, weakness, or leg tenderness
5. Mononeuropathy or polyneuropathy
6. Diastolic blood pressure ≥ 90 mm Hg
7. Elevated BUN or creatinine
8. Hepatitis B virus
9. Arteriographic abnormality
10. Biopsy of small or medium-sized artery containing polymorphonuclear leukocytes

Wegener's granulomatosis (2 or more)
1. Nasal or oral inflammation
2. Abnormal chest radiograph
3. Urinary sediment: > 5 red blood cells or red blood cell casts
4. Granulomatous inflammation on biopsy

Churg-Strauss syndrome (4 or more)
1. Asthma
2. Eosinophilia > 10%
3. Mononeuropathy or polyneuropathy
4. Pulmonary infiltrates, nonfixed
5. Paranasal sinus abnormality
6. Extravascular eosinophils

Pathogenetic Considerations

The majority of clinical forms of systemic vasculitis are thought to be caused by immunologic processes, but information concerning the inciting stimuli in most human vasculitic diseases is less than compelling. A large number of anecdotal cases have been reported in which a causal link to some agent has been suspected. However, in most cases, definitive proof was lacking and it seems likely that the vasculitis and the putative inciting condition were coincidental. Some of the more recent studies on the possible causes, on abnormalities of the various mediators of inflammation, immune reactions, or clotting, and on the predisposing factors for vasculitis are summarized in Table 76-3.

The discovery in certain forms of systemic vasculitis of autoantibodies to enzymes in cytoplasmic granules of leukocytes has provided the first new clue to the immunopathogenesis of these diseases in some time (see below). Preliminary results raise the possibilities that other autoantibodies could be associated with vasculitic injury. Antibodies to normal human endothelial and epithelial [1, 51] cells have been detected in some cases of systemic vasculitis. Enthusiasm for accepting these antibody-dependent mechanisms must be tempered by the fact that immunoglobulins are rarely found in full-blown vasculitic lesions. Antiendothelial antibodies could theoretically function synergistically with autoantibodies to the leukocyte enzymes, to initiate and propagate vascular injury. Further studies are warranted before any of these preliminary observations can be accepted as relevant to the pathogenesis of systemic vasculitis.

The high frequency of exposure to potential etiologic agents in subjects who fail to develop vasculitis suggests, among other possibilities, that the development of systemic vasculitis requires one or more of the following conditions: an aberrant immunologic effector response (e.g., irregular antibody isotype), loss of immune regulatory controls (e.g., deficiency of antiidiotype or suppressor cell mechanisms), presence of a susceptibility factor (i.e., a two-step requirement for an immune reaction to occur), or the intersection of multiple inciting factors.

Spontaneous disease and induced disease in experimental models [25, 28, 67, 89, 115, 125] have provided some insights into the range of processes and mechanisms that may potentially cause vasculitic diseases. Few of the models are considered directly applicable to

Table 76-3. Possible causes, mediators, or predisposing factors in the pathogenesis of systemic vasculitis

1. Exogenous agents
   - Hepatitis B [35, 56, 65, 79, 100, 125]
   - Drugs/sera/vaccines [16, 28, 118]
   - Neoplasia [57, 63, 110]
2. Immune complexes and reticuloendothelial system dysfunction
   - Systemic lupus erythematosus, Wegener's granulomatosis, polyarteritis [82, 91, 96, 119]
3. Autoantibodies
   - Antibodies to neutrophil cytoplasmic antigens (ANCAs) [78, 121, 136], basement membrane [116], endothelial cells [51, 93], and epithelial cells [1]
4. Miscellaneous factors
   - Genetic predisposition [117]
   - Enhanced expression of tumor necrosis factor (TNF) genes in blood mononuclear cells [33]
   - Increased levels of circulating cytokines [25, 62, 93]
   - Deficient production of plasminogen activators [80]

the human vasculitic diseases; among the best models is that for Kawasaki disease [25, 90, 93], a form of vasculitis that does not affect the kidney.

The following is a hypothetical but working model for vasculitis which stems from clinical observations and from in vitro studies of leukocytes and endothelial cells. This model suggests that exogenous inciting factors (such as toxins, infectious agents, immune complexes, endothelial antibodies, or cytokines) could initiate a disturbance of the normal microenvironment of the vessel wall. A cascade of amplifying factors (including acute, chronic, and granulomatous inflammation, necrosis, clotting, and fibrosis) could increase the injury and compromise distal blood flow. Individual variations at any or all sites in this sequence could account for the diverse clinical and pathologic manifestations of systemic vasculitis. Unfortunately, experimental models have been mostly deficient for study of the pathogenesis of systemic vasculitis. Several excellent reviews of possible pathogenetic mechanisms in systemic vasculitis have appeared [24, 28, 47].

Antibodies to Neutrophil Cytoplasmic Antigens

The discovery of ANCAs has greatly facilitated the diagnosis and management of patients with certain forms of systemic vasculitis. Their role in pathogenesis is being intensively pursued but remains mostly speculative at the time of this writing.

ANCAs were described in 1982 [31]; serum samples from patients with necrotizing and crescentic glomerulonephritis were noted to stain the cytoplasm of normal human neutrophils. The diagnostic utility of these autoantibodies was espoused in 1985 [137]; sera from patients with generalized Wegener's granulomatosis were strikingly reactive with leukocyte cytoplasmic antigens [106, 131]. Subsequent studies have detected ANCAs in patients with polyarteritis and glomerulonephritis [19, 41, 123, 124], but rarely in those with secondary vasculitis. ANCAs occur in the highest titers in those forms of polyarteritis and Wegener's granulomatosis in which necrotizing and crescentic glomerulonephritis is a prominent feature. The frequency of ANCAs in classic PAN is low [19, 36, 106, 123, 137]. The relative frequencies and pattern of ANCA reactions in the more common forms of systemic vasculitis are shown in Table 76-4.

Two main types of indirect immunofluorescence staining patterns for ANCAs are recognized. The cytoplasmic pattern, or C-ANCA, (Fig. 76-1A) produces a diffuse staining of antigens throughout the cytoplasmic granules of neutrophils. The principal antigen in the C-ANCA reaction is a 29-kd serine protease called proteinase-3 [97]. A second pattern is seen in which the immunofluorescence appears in a perinuclear distribution, the so-called P-ANCA (Fig. 76-1B). The primary antigen in the P-ANCA reaction is myeloperoxidase. During the alcohol fixation of the neutrophils used for the indirect immunofluorescence assay, myeloperoxidase aggregates around the nuclear membrane [41]. In some instances, the pattern of P-ANCA may be mistaken for that of antinuclear antibodies (ANAs).

Table 76-4. Prevalence of autoantibodies to neutrophil cytoplasmic antigens (ANCAs) in systemic vasculitis

Entity	No.*	Frequency estimate		
		C-ANCA	P-ANCA	Negative
Polyarteritis nodosa (PAN)	144		< 10%	50–90%
Microscopic polyarteritis	202	< 10%	50–90%	< 10%
Necrotizing and crescentic granulomatosis	106	< 10%	50–90%	< 10%
Wegener's granulomatosis	346	> 90%	< 10%	

*Aggregate number of patients used for estimation of frequency of ANCA test results; compiled from [19, 20, 36, 39, 106, 123, 124, 131, 137].

Enzyme-linked immunosorbent assays (ELISAs) have been developed for testing antibodies to the purified antigens. Besides their reactivity to proteinase-3 and myeloperoxidase, ANCAs less frequently demonstrate specificity for other leukocyte enzymes, including elastase, lactoferrin, cathepsin, and others [21, 22, 86, 124]. ELISAs provide the means to quantitate the ANCA levels more precisely, which might be useful for monitoring disease activity as well as for studying the implications of autoantibodies to the various specific antigens.

ANCA levels tend to rise and fall with exacerbations and remissions of the vasculitic disease [36, 123, 131, 137]. Recent studies indicate that the rise of ANCA titer precedes the exacerbation of clinical activity [22], suggesting a cause rather than an effect relationship. The leading hypothesis is that ANCAs activate circulating leukocytes, which then respond in an excessively vigorous manner to perturbations of vascular integrity. The initial vascular disturbances may be caused by intercurrent infections [113] or other inciting factors [25, 33, 62], as might occur during the flulike prodromes that accompany many of the vasculitic diseases.

Some evidence obtained in vitro indicates that the ANCAs activate normal neutrophils, thereby augmenting the release of inflammatory mediators, such as lysosomal enzymes and reactive oxygen radicals [42]. Such mechanisms could fuel, if not initiate, the vasculitic process.

Fig. 76-1. ANCA test: characteristic patterns of indirect immunofluorescence of autoantibodies to neutrophil cytoplasmic antigens (ANCAs). A. Cytoplasmic, or C-ANCA, pattern. B. Perinuclear, or P-ANCA, pattern. (Courtesy of Dr. Thomas A. Fleisher, National Institutes of Health, Bethesda, Md.)

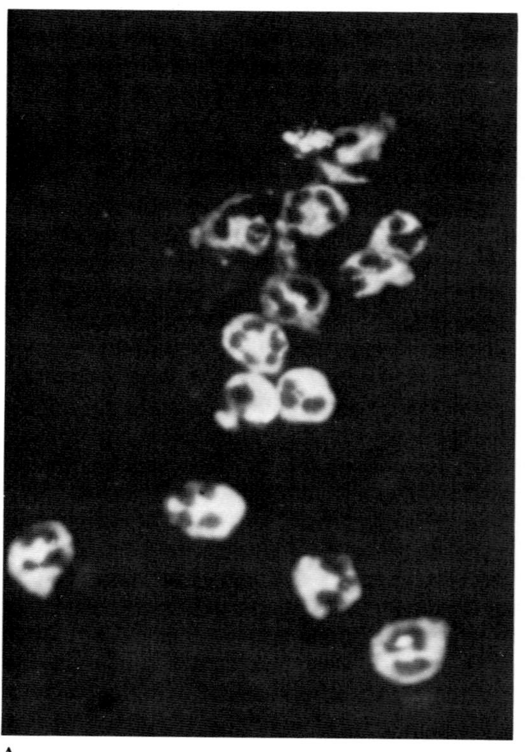

A

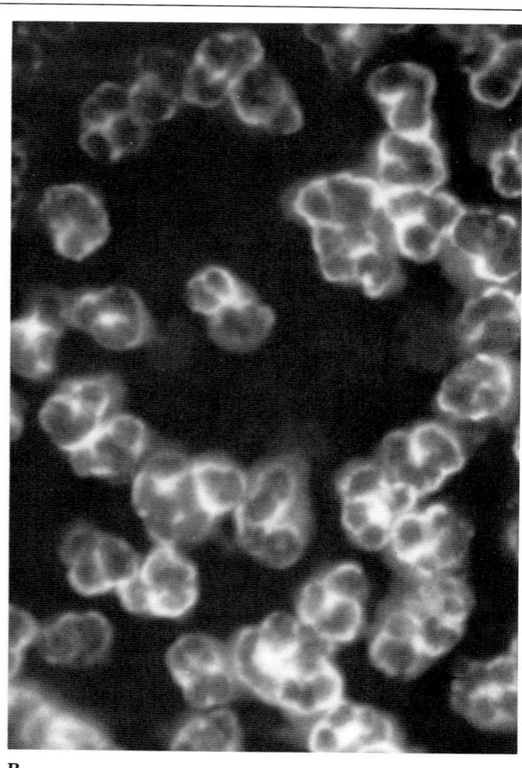

B

Polyarteritis

Polyarteritis encompasses a group of disorders that have in common a debilitating systemic illness in association with necrotizing arteritis. Polyarteritis is a great masquerader of infectious, neoplastic, toxic, allergic, and autoimmune diseases. It is rare, with an annual incidence between 4 and 10 per million and a prevalence estimated to be approximately 60 per million population [83, 101]. Polyarteritis exhibits a male predominance.

The nomenclature used to describe the polyarteritis group of diseases is not fully standardized. The following terminology will be used for the major forms of systemic vasculitis.

DEFINITIONS

Systemic Vasculitis Syndrome. This is a polymorphic clinical syndrome usually involving fever, weight loss, malaise, anorexia, myalgias, arthralgias, anemia, elevated erythrocyte sedimentation rate, leukocytosis, and thrombocytosis. It should be underscored that these features are nonspecific and constitute only a vasculitic syndrome. By. themselves, these clinical features have high sensitivity but low specificity for a correct diagnosis of one of the specific types of full-blown systemic vasculitis.

Classic Polyarteritis Nodosa. The concurrence of a clinical syndrome of systemic vasculitis, objective dysfunction of two or more major organ systems due to vascular insufficiency, and necrotizing arteritis (or the sequelae thereof) of small to medium-sized arteries constitutes a diagnosis of classic PAN.

Microscopic Polyarteritis. This form of polyarteritis is defined as a clinical syndrome of systemic vasculitis, usually including extrarenal features of PAN, but always including necrotizing and crescentic glomerulonephritis.

Necrotizing and Crescentic Glomerulonephritis. This form of glomerulonephritis is characterized by focal, segmental fibrinoid necrosis and crescents, but few or no immune complex deposits. The patients often present with a systemic vasculitic syndrome, but always exhibit nephritic urinary sediment and moderate proteinuria and either develop or carry a very high risk of developing rapidly progressive renal failure (defined as doubling or more of the serum creatinine within 3 months).

Polyangiitis Overlap Syndrome. This disorder is defined as a clinical syndrome of systemic vasculitis, with mixed features of polyarteritis and another discrete vasculitis (particularly cutaneous vasculitis, but also Wegener's granulomatosis, Churg-Strauss disease, or one of the secondary forms of vasculitis).

COMMON CLINICAL FEATURES OF POLYARTERITIS

The general clinical manifestations of classic PAN and microscopic polyarteritis, as well as most polyangiitis overlap syndromes, are comparable. The presenting vasculitic syndrome is typically vague and nonspecific, an aspect that is frequently responsible for serious delays in diagnosis. The majority of patients have fever, malaise, weakness, fatigue, anorexia, abdominal pain, weight loss, myalgias, and arthralgias. The emergence of certain clinical signs facilitates the diagnosis of polyarteritis: local neurologic deficits (especially mononeuritis multiplex), focal muscular tenderness, skin rashes, gastrointestinal bleeding, or other visceral ischemic episodes (see Table 76-2). Pulmonary involvement is uncommon but capillaritis can cause lung hemorrhage or interstitial infiltrates [68, 75, 98, 102]. Renal disease occurs in the great majority of patients but the clinical renal syndromes differ in classic PAN and microscopic polyarteritis [2].

CLASSIC POLYARTERITIS NODOSA

Renal Disease. In classic PAN renal disease is often indolent or eclipsed by manifestations of other visceral involvement. Renal ischemia due to medium-sized vessel arteritis is the major pathogenetic factor. Renin-mediated hypertension is nearly universal [61, 108]. Moderate proteinuria, rarely to the nephrotic range, without significant urinary sediment abnormalities is typical. Increased glomerular permeability to protein is due to ischemia and hypertension rather than to glomerulonephritis. Severe ischemic episodes produce renal infarction; the infarcts may be silent but may also produce flank pain and hematuria, which can be misinterpreted as glomerulonephritis. Rupture of aneurysms may produce parenchymal or perinephric hemorrhage, particularly in severely hypertensive patients [128]. Chronic ischemia can lead to focal irregularities of the renal cortex due to alternating atrophy and compensatory hypertrophy. Acute or rapidly progressive renal failure is very unusual in classic PAN. Slowly progressive renal insufficiency is common and is secondary to ischemic atrophy of nephrons due to combinations of active and sclerosing arteritis, as well as hypertensive nephrosclerosis.

Diagnosis. The most compelling reasons for considering the diagnosis of classic PAN come from a careful history and physical examination. Rarely, laboratory parameters or radiologic and pathologic examinations undertaken for routine or unrelated diagnostic purposes will result in an unexpected diagnosis of classic PAN. It is important that the clinician maintain a reasonable suspicion of systemic vasculitis when encountering patients with vague multisystem disorders. Subspecialty consultants are particularly vulnerable to error in diagnosis if they focus narrowly on isolated organ systems.

The diagnosis of classic PAN depends on recognition of the variegated clinical syndrome of systemic vasculitis outlined above. The objective clinical manifestations are occasionally so well delineated that the diagnosis is certain without supplemental studies. More commonly, however, additional evidence is needed to establish the diagnosis confidently. Standard clinical laboratory tests rarely provide results with adequate specificity for classic PAN. Elevated erythrocyte sedimentation rate, normochromic-normocytic anemia, leukocytosis, thrombocytosis, reversed albumin-globulin levels, and elevated acute phase reactants (e.g., fibrinogen, C-reactive protein, complement components) simply indicate a chronic inflammatory process. Hepatitis B antigenemia is associated with increased risk of polyarteritis [35, 79, 100], but the risk varies greatly in different populations.

The ANCA test can be helpful in the diagnosis of certain forms of polyarteritis. It is reasonable to obtain an ANCA test on all patients with a clinical syndrome of systemic vasculitis. However, the clinician should be aware that the ANCA test has relatively low sensitivity and that a negative ANCA test result does not rule out the diagnosis of classic PAN (see Table 76-4).

Routine kidney examinations are rarely indicative of classic PAN. Pyelography, ultrasonography, computed tomography, or magnetic resonance imaging of the kidneys may detect cortical scars from previous infarctions; however, these tests should not be considered routine components of the evaluation of systemic vasculitis because of their low yield, nonspecificity, and high expense. Vascular insufficiency due to active vasculitis is more effectively screened for by nuclear medicine scanning and, if suspected, verified by selective renal angiography (Fig. 76-2).

Angiographic studies, which are clearly the gold standard of radiologic diagnosis of classic PAN, should be considered regardless of the evidence of visceral functional abnormalities [4, 30, 38, 43, 134]. Arterial pruning and irregular tapering of vessels and particularly aneurysms in renal, hepatic, and mesenteric vascular beds can solidify the diagnosis of classic PAN. At the present time angiography of the abdominal viscera is favored over nondirected or blind tissue biopsies in patients who are suspected of having classic PAN but who lack clear-cut focal signs or symptoms of vasculitis. In most cases, the importance of a firm diagnosis of classic PAN should outweigh the modest risk of contrast medium nephrotoxicity following angiography.

Tissue biopsies provide the most direct evidence for diagnosis of classic PAN, but several practical considerations limit this objective. Blind biopsies of clinically silent sites are of low yield [4]. Yield from biopsies of some sites, such as the sural nerve, can be increased if there are abnormal findings on nerve conduction studies [70].

Needle biopsies are by nature small and contain few sizable vessels. This is of particular relevance when considering diagnostic renal biopsies. Occasionally the diagnosis of classic PAN can be made from percutaneous renal biopsies (Fig. 76-3). Although no comparative studies of the yield of open versus closed renal biopsies have appeared, the paucity and irregular distribution of necrotizing vasculitis seen at autopsy (even in cases of florid classic PAN) should prompt the nephrologist to be reserved about the role of renal biopsy in the diagnosis of classic PAN.

In short, a multidisciplinary perspective is warranted to consider thoughtfully the potential value, yield, safety, and expense of all diagnostic options related to classic PAN. The histologic features of classic PAN are quite similar in different organ systems and hence the

Fig. 76-2. Polyarteritis nodosa. A. Angiogram demonstrating extensive chains of aneurysms involving several hepatic arteries. B. Renal angiogram showing multiple aneurysms. Patient was a 23-year-old man with classic polyarteritis nodosa who exhibited severe hypertension and advanced renal insufficiency. (Courtesy of Drs. J. Moore and E. Marks, Nephrology Division, Walter Reed Army Medical Center, Washington, D.C.)

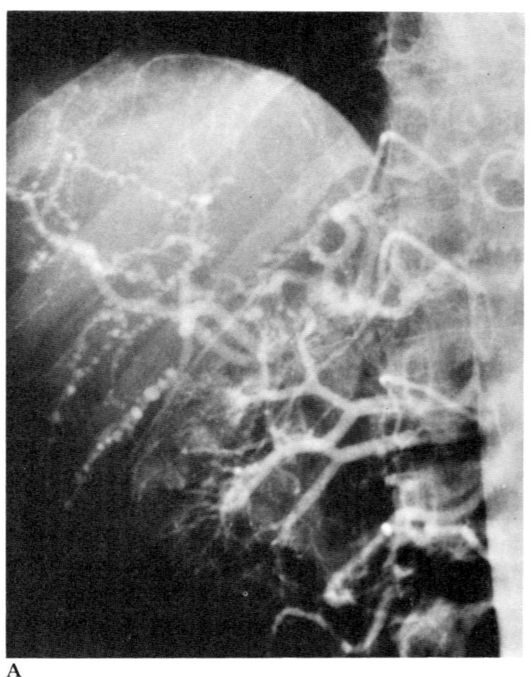
A

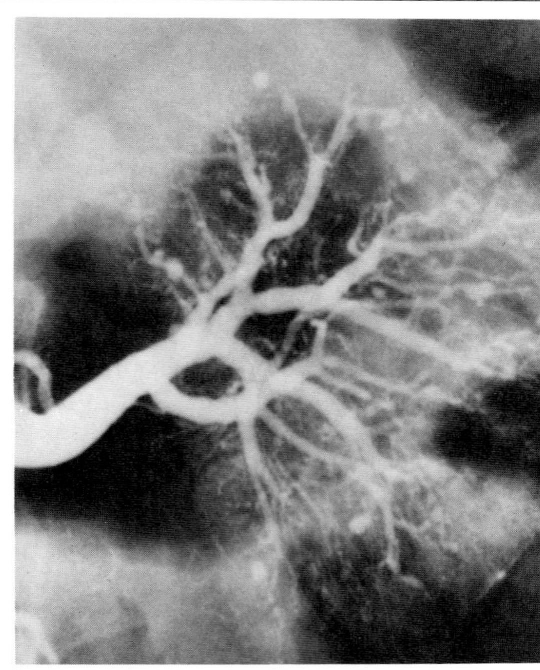
B

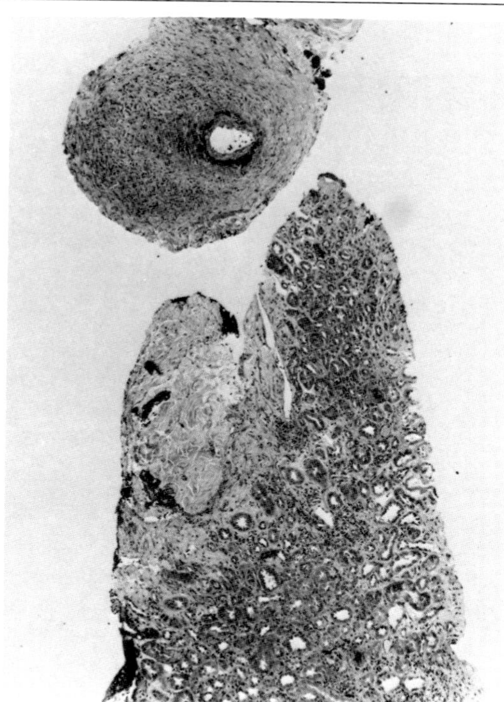

Fig. 76-3. Polyarteritis nodosa of the kidney evident in a needle biopsy specimen. The small artery showing fibrinoid necrosis is located in juxtamedullary tissue. (Hematoxylin and eosin [H&E]; ×60.) (Courtesy of Dr. T. Antonovych and Dr. S. Sabnis, Nephropathology Section, Armed Forces Institute of Pathology, Washington, D.C.)

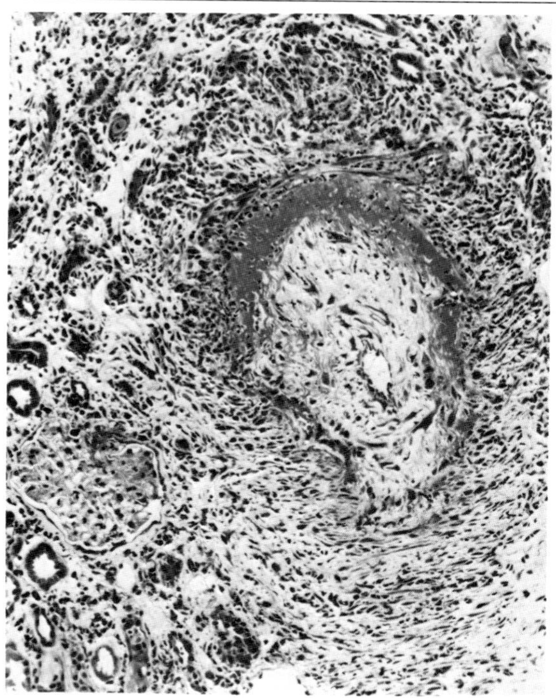

Fig. 76-4. Polyarteritis nodosa of a muscular renal artery. The biopsy specimen exhibits fibrinoid necrosis and marked reduction of the vessel lumen by inflammation, edema, and early fibrosis of the intima. (H&E; ×160.) (Courtesy of Dr. T. Antonovych and Dr. S. Sabnis, Nephropathology Section, Armed Forces Institute of Pathology, Washington, D.C.)

diagnosis can usually be made by examining the vascular pathology of any involved tissues.

Pathology of Classic Polyarteritis Nodosa. Characteristically, the arteritis of classic PAN is highly irregular in distribution and the lesions exhibit simultaneous stages of activity and healing. Any or all of the following vasculitic features may be seen, depending on the rate of disease progression, severity, and effects of therapy: leukocyte infiltration (polymorphonuclear and/or mononuclear cells), karyorrhexis, fibrinoid necrosis, disruption of the elastic lamina, aneurysm formation, rupture with hemorrhage, thrombosis, recanalization, and fibrosis [94, 129].

Renal vessels ranging in size from interlobar through arcuate to interlobular arteries are typically affected (Figs. 76-4 and 76-5). Afferent arterioles may be affected by hypertensive changes, and juxtaglomerular apparatus hyperplasia [61] may be evident. Glomeruli usually show no specific endocapillary or extracapillary changes except ischemic collapse of tufts. Interstitial lesions vary from mild to diffuse inflammatory cell infiltrates, including polymorphonuclear leukocytes, eosinophils, and mononuclear cells. Ischemia can lead to tubular atrophy. Areas of infarction and hemorrhage are common.

Immunofluorescence studies of necrotizing vasculitis demonstrate the escape of plasma constituents into vessel walls during the acute phase of disease. Albumin, immunoglobulins, complement components, and fibrin are readily demonstrated in active lesions, but these deposits are nonspecific. Some of these immunoreactants could represent immune complexes, though electron microscopy studies rarely show discrete deposits in the walls of certain affected vessels in classic PAN [6, 129].

Difficulty arises in the interpretation of vessels that show atypical features. Perivascular cuffing without fibrinoid necrosis suggests, but is not pathognomonic of, classic PAN. Extensive fibrosis of various layers of arterial walls in conjunction with disruption and/or duplication of elastic laminae may alternate with active arteritis. Thus, it is important to consider the innately uneven distribution of vascular pathology in classic PAN. It is imperative to examine serial sections of all pathology specimens for evidence of necrotizing arteritis when one is searching for definitive features of classic PAN. Certain special techniques, such as elastin and silver stains, are useful for detecting old or partially healed arteritis.

MICROSCOPIC POLYARTERITIS

Renal Disease. Microscopic polyarteritis is polyarteritis with glomerulonephritis. Asymptomatic hematuria or proteinuria may be present for long periods and may be associated with insidious loss of renal function. Nephritic urinary sediment denotes glomerular disease and is the

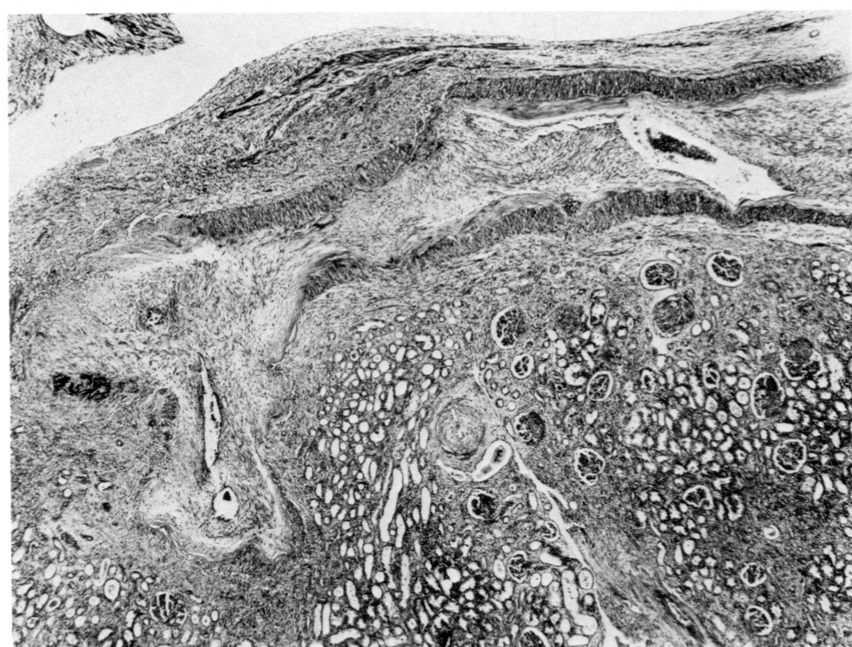

Fig. 76-5. Healing polyarteritis. The large muscular artery of the kidney shows partially recanalized lumens. Glomeruli show ischemia with collapse. (Masson trichrome; ×25.) (Courtesy of Dr. T. Antonovych and Dr. S. Sabnis, Nephropathology Section, Armed Forces Institute of Pathology, Washington, D.C.)

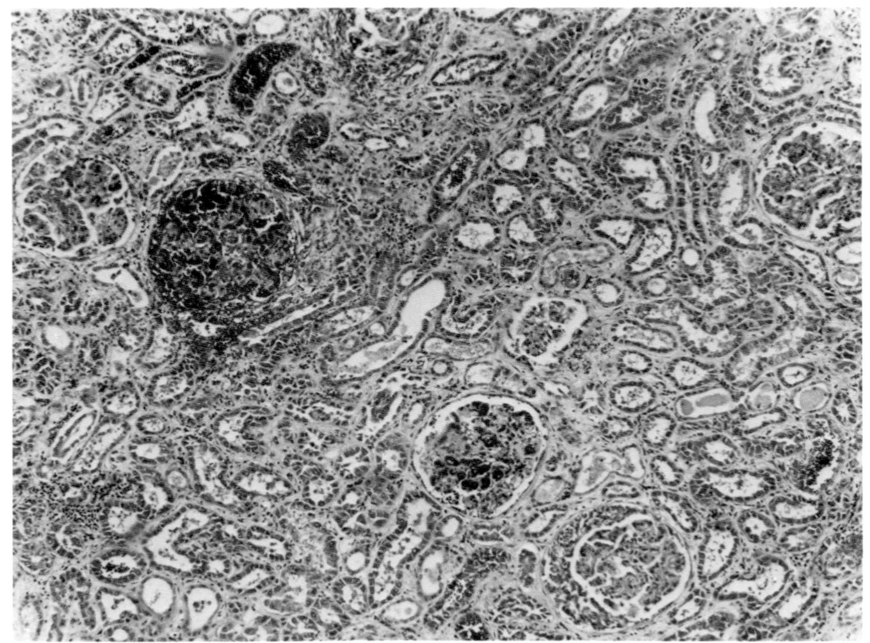

Fig. 76-6. Microscopic polyarteritis. Glomeruli show a range of changes: The lower central glomerulus shows segmental necrosis; the glomerulus at the lower right shows an eccentric cellular crescent; the glomerulus toward the left of center shows essentially global necrosis. Leukocytes are present in tubular lumina and in the interstitium. There is moderate tubular atrophy and interstitial fibrosis. (H&E; ×60.) (Courtesy of Dr. T. Antonovych and Dr. S. Sabnis, Nephropathology Section, Armed Forces Institute of Pathology, Washington, D.C.)

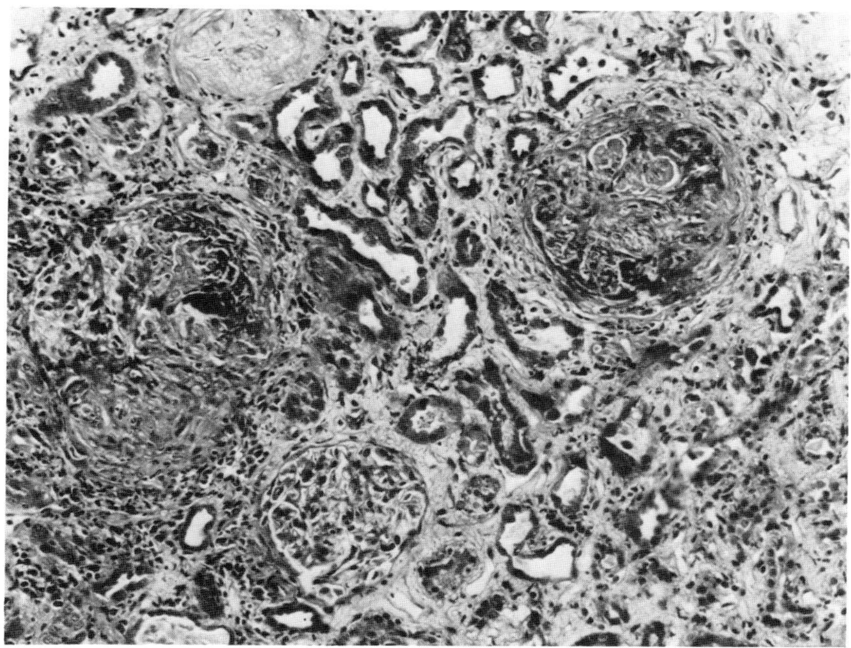

Fig. 76-7. Microscopic polyarteritis of the kidney, at a higher power. The glomerulus at the upper right shows severe segmental necrosis and a circumferential crescent. One normal glomerulus (bottom center) and one sclerotic glomerulus (top left) are present. (Masson trichrome; ×160.) (Courtesy of Dr. T. Antonovych and Dr. S. Sabnis, Nephropathology Section, Armed Forces Institute of Nephrology, Washington, D.C.)

usual indication for renal biopsy. Biopsy should be considered early for what some might consider trivial urinary findings (e.g., minimal hematuria, proteinuria) because microscopic polyarteritis carries a high risk of acceleration to rapidly progressive renal failure. Acute renal failure due to glomerulonephritis has been observed [14]. In contrast to classic PAN, hypertension is rarely a major clinical feature of microscopic polyarteritis.

Pathology of Microscopic Polyarteritis. The extraglomerular pathology of microscopic polyarteritis is similar to that of classic PAN, except for a predilection for smaller blood vessels [6, 27, 29, 129]. Aneurysms, if present, tend to be occult in microscopic polyarteritis [32, 119].

The glomerulonephritis of microscopic polyarteritis usually involves endocapillary and extracapillary changes (Figs. 76-6, 76-7, and 76-8). The glomerular lesions are typically focal and segmental in distribution. Hypercellularity of glomerular tufts tends to be modest, whereas fibrinoid necrosis and crescents are prominent and characteristic. Adhesions to Bowman's capsule commonly attend the segmental glomerular inflammation. Fibrin exudation, epithelial cell proliferation, and monocyte accumulation follow the rupture of glomerular capillaries and lead to the development of full-blown cellular crescents.

The typical glomerular lesions in microscopic polyarteritis have been described as uniform in age. The frequency of this finding has been overstated. The vast majority of cases with microscopic polyarteritis exhibit glomerular lesions of mixed types and stages. Notably, cellular and fibrous crescents as well as necrotizing and sclerosing endocapillary lesions are commonly seen in the same renal biopsy.

Interstitial inflammatory cells are seen in microscopic polyarteritis [3, 6]. The infiltrate is generally present in proportion to the severity and extent of glomerular reactions. The leukocytes are usually composed of lymphocytes, monocytes, and plasma cells; occasionally eosinophils are prominent, and rarely epithelioid and giant cells may produce a granulomatous reaction in an angiocentric pattern. Extraglomerular renal vasculitis of small arteries may be seen (Figs. 76-9 and 76-10), especially in open biopsy samples or at autopsy [126].

Immunofluorescent studies of glomeruli in microscopic polyarteritis generally show fibrin in association with cellular crescents. Other immunoreactants may be present in necrotizing lesions, but this is considered to result from a nonspecific increase in vascular permeability [119, 126, 129]. Immune complex deposits are usually absent by electron microscopy, a feature that supports the diagnosis of microscopic polyarteritis [6, 29, 129]. These observations have challenged the relevance of elevated circulating immune complexes in human disease, as well as the relevance of experimental models of vasculitis induced by immune complexes.

NECROTIZING AND CRESCENTIC GLOMERULONEPHRITIS

Necrotizing and crescentic glomerulonephritis can be primary or idiopathic, or it can be the renal lesion of

A

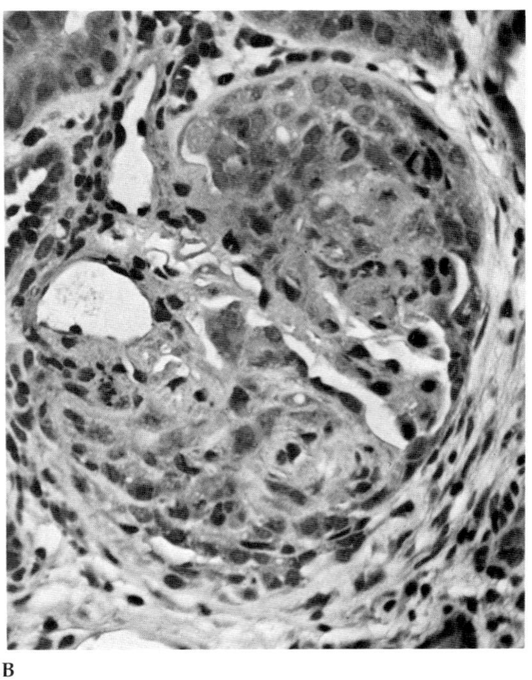

B

Fig. 76-8. Microscopic polyarteritis nodosa. A. Glomerulus showing mild segmental hypercellularity, with minimal karyorrhexis and a capsular adhesion. B. Glomerulus showing exuberant crescent formation. (H&E; ×400.)

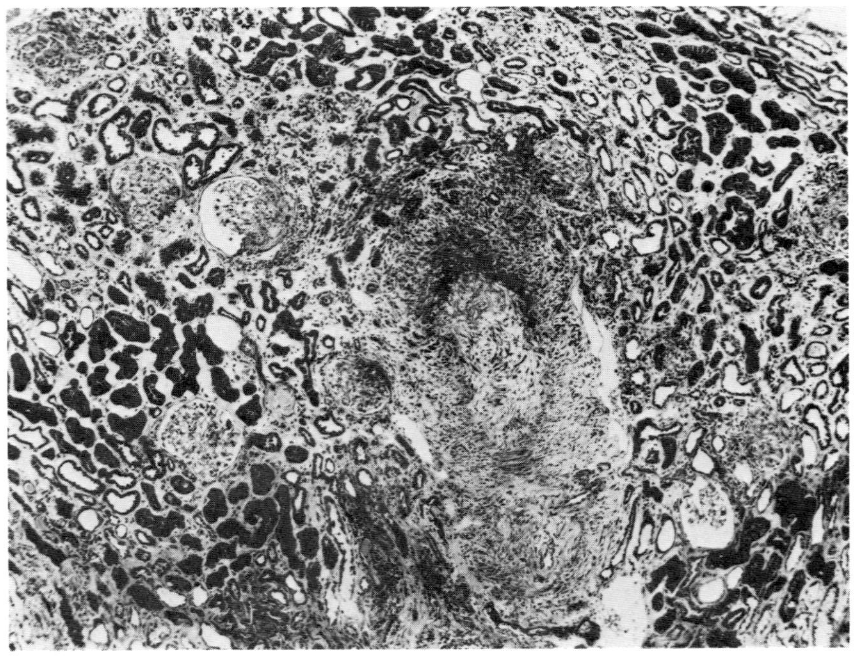

Fig. 76-9. Renal polyarteritis with features of extraglomerular vasculitis. The muscular artery in the center exhibits severe vasculitis, with fibrinoid necrosis, leukocyte infiltration, and luminal compromise due to intimal swelling and fibrosis. The glomeruli show a range of changes from normal to segmental necrosis to eccentric crescents. (Masson trichrome; ×60.) (Courtesy of Dr. T. Antonovych and Dr. S. Sabnis, Nephropathology Section, Armed Forces Institute of Pathology, Washington, D.C.)

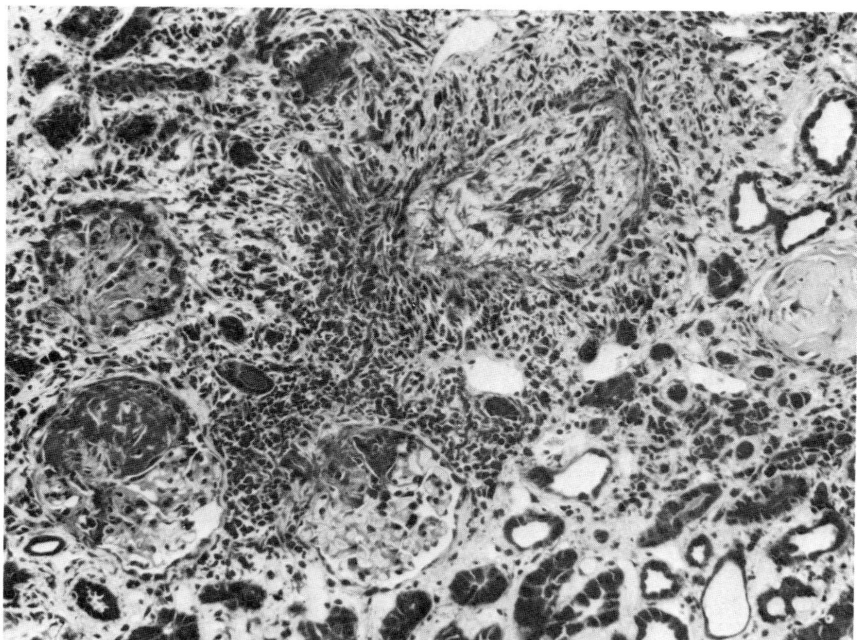

Fig. 76-10. Polyarteritis of the kidney showing both arteritis and glomerulonephritis. Large vessel toward the upper right shows healing arteritis with proliferation, edema, and fibrosis which compromises the lumen. Glomerular changes vary from a cellular crescent (upper left) to global sclerosis (center right). Two glomeruli at the bottom left and center show segmental fibrinoid necrosis. Leukocytes are present in the wall of the artery and are infiltrating the interstitium. Tubular atrophy and interstitial fibrosis are evident. (Masson trichrome; ×160.) (Courtesy of Dr. T. Antonovych and Dr. S. Sabnis, Nephropathology Section, Armed Forces Institute of Pathology, Washington, D.C.)

other conditions, in which case it is categorized as secondary [55, 111]. As previously discussed, there are numerous reasons for considering idiopathic necrotizing and crescentic glomerulonephritis to be a subset of polyarteritis. It is sometimes described as renal-limited polyarteritis.

Clinically, the development of necrotizing and crescentic glomerulonephritis is often accompanied by features of the vasculitic syndrome. As a rule, the systemic component mimics microscopic polyarteritis and tends to be milder and shorter-lived than in the other forms of polyarteritis. The vasculitic symptoms and signs are often mistaken for a simple intercurrent viral illness.

The ANCA test may be helpful in the evaluation of patients with suspected necrotizing and crescentic glomerulonephritis. As shown in Table 76-4, the ANCA profile of necrotizing and crescentic glomerulonephritis is basically the same as that of microscopic polyarteritis. The rate of positive test results is high. The P-ANCA pattern is more common that the C-ANCA pattern.

The pathology of necrotizing and crescentic glomerulonephritis is also indistinguishable from that of microscopic polyarteritis. The rarity of immune complex deposits by immunofluorescence or electron microscopy has led to suggestion of the term *pauci-immune glomerulonephritis* [41, 78], but this label has not been widely utilized. For further discussion of the pathology of necrotizing and crescentic glomerulonephritis, see Chap. 62.

COURSE AND TREATMENT OF POLYARTERITIS

As anticipated from the highly variable clinical presentation and organ involvement, it is difficult to describe a typical clinical course for patients with polyarteritis. In general, about one-fourth of patients with classic PAN manifest an early complicated and rapidly progressive course, with multisystem compromise and life-threatening complications. Often these patients are excluded from series that analyze treatment of classic PAN because death intervened before an adequate therapeutic regimen could be administered. A larger group, approximately one-half of patients with classic PAN, develop a more moderate disease with waxing and waning activity. Management of this latter group is constantly challenging because of the inherent difficulty of differentiating active vasculitis from the consequences of healing vascular scars. A minority of patients with polyarteritis develop a burst of active vasculitis, which spontaneously subsides or is well controlled on therapy without relapses. The course of the latter patients suggests the possibility that some vasculitic illnesses can be induced by transient exposure to an inciting agent; however, it is unusual to identify confidently any discrete etiologic agents in patients with polyarteritis.

There are notable differences between the courses and outcomes of patients with classic PAN and microscopic polyarteritis. Often it is difficult to extract data in this regard because these two forms of polyarteritis have rarely been clearly distinguished in many large clinical series. The reports from rheumatology centers include mainly patients with classic PAN, while those from nephrology units are dominated by patients with microscopic polyarteritis.

Renal involvement occurs in approximately three-fourths of patients with classic PAN, but only one-third develop progressive renal failure. The greater risk to patients with classic PAN stems from catastrophic complications of extrarenal disease due to the high prevalence of muscular artery disease with aneurysms and hypertension. All patients with microscopic polyarteritis have renal disease by definition. Approximately two-thirds of patients develop progressive renal insufficiency and one-half of these go on to end-stage renal failure.

The actuarial survival curves for patients with classic PAN are shown in Fig. 76-11. This graph was prepared from data on patients with classic PAN reported in the literature [18, 92, 120]. Patient death was the primary outcome. The shaded area represents the range of estimated survival of patients in these three series. The 1-year expected patient survival rate varies from 65 to 90 percent, while the 5-year survival rate is approximately 60 percent.

Survival estimates for patients with microscopic polyarteritis reported in the literature [40, 54, 122, 141] are shown in Fig. 76-12. Survival outcomes in these series include both patient death and end-stage renal failure. Overall, the 1-year expected survival rate without renal failure for patients with microscopic polyarteritis ranges between 65 and 80 percent, a figure that is slightly worse than that for classic PAN. At 5 years, the estimated survival rate is comparable for both groups.

Patients with all forms of polyarteritis have a high degree of debility and can be completely incapacitated by the general systemic features of vasculitis. Many of these constitutional symptoms improve promptly on initiation of corticosteroid therapy. It should be stressed that the improvement in symptoms can mask the more important management objectives. Control of the arteritis per se is the preeminent therapeutic issue. Smoldering activity of the vasculitis predisposes to continued high risks of mortality, major complications of vascular insufficiency, and renal failure.

There has been little controversy about the efficacy of corticosteroids in treatment of both classic PAN and microscopic polyarteritis [10, 18, 53, 92], even though there have been no concurrent comparisons of different treatments of this disease. In contrast, there has been controversy about the role of cytotoxic drugs [10], particularly azathioprine and cyclophosphamide [18, 24, 92]. As shown in Fig. 76-11, the experience of Leib and colleagues [92], shown by the separate curve above the shaded area, suggests the superior efficacy of cytotoxic drugs. However, Cohen and colleagues [18] found no difference in survival between patients treated with these agents and those treated with corticosteroids only. Neither is a controlled study.

Our own experience supports the benefits of cyclophosphamide over corticosteroids alone in certain circumstances [49]. The efficacy of cyclophosphamide has been particularly striking in patients responding poorly or incompletely to prednisone therapy. Complete remissions have been achieved, including reversion of severe aneurysm formation [45]. Cyclophosphamide has permitted reduction of corticosteroid doses and decreased the risk of complications of corticosteroids [49].

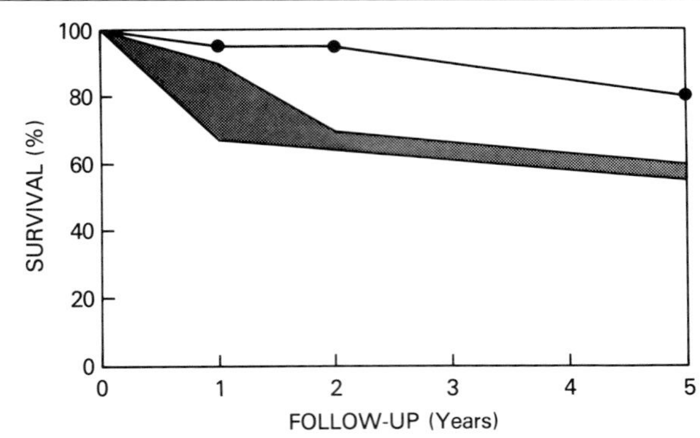

Fig. 76-11. Actuarial survival of patients with predominantly classic polyarteritis nodosa. The range of cumulative survival indicated by the hatched area is compiled from data in several series in which corticosteroids were the primary therapy [18, 92, 120]. The results with cytotoxic drug therapy of one of these groups [92] were substantially superior to the others and are depicted as a separate curve (solid line).

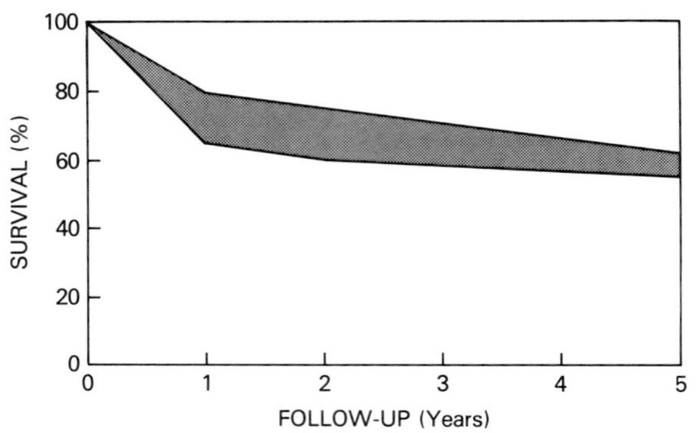

Fig. 76-12. Actuarial survival of patients with predominantly microscopic polyarteritis, but also including Wegener's granulomatosis, and necrotizing and crescentic glomerulonephritis. The range of cumulative survival indicated by the hatched area is compiled from data in several series [40, 54, 122, 141].

Treatment of Classic PAN. The major therapeutic options and protocols for their use in treatment of systemic vasculitis are summarized in Table 76-5. The initial therapy of active PAN always includes high-dose prednisone [10, 50]. We favor tapering to alternate-day therapy, although some authors contend that an extended course of daily prednisone is necessary [24]. Diligent observation is important during the prednisone tapering period. Cavalier dose reduction without careful monitoring may produce a major or even catastrophic flare. Equally problematic, however, can be the misinterpretation of

Table 76-5. Immunosuppressive drugs and treatment regimens used in polyarteritis

Prednisone: 1.0 mg/kg in single morning dose (or divided doses for 7–10 days for very aggressive disease). Taper to 1.0 mg/kg on alternate days by 2 mo. Continue tapering doses by 5 mg weekly as tolerated or to discontinuance over 3–6 mo.

Pulse methylprednisolone: 1.0 gm/m² infused over 15–30 min daily for 3 doses. May repeat in 1–2 wk for relapses or for unusually aggressive or persistent disease.

Cyclophosphamide: 2.0 mg/kg in single morning dose. Keep WBC > 3,000/μl. Reduce dose by increments of 50 mg as WBC falls below 4,000/μl, or hold temporarily for rapidly falling WBC or WBC < 2,000/μl. Encourage fluids to > 3 liters/day and frequent voiding.

Pulse cyclophosphamide: 1.0 gm/m² intravenously in 150 ml of saline over 60 min (0.5 gm/m² if GFR < one-third normal). Antiemetics as needed. Diurese with 3 liters of fluids (or irrigate bladder via three-way Foley catheter for 24 hr; or use mesna: Each dose of mesna is 60% of total cyclophosphamide dose intravenously or orally every 6 hr for 4 doses). Repeat cyclophosphamide monthly for 6 mo, then reduce stepwise to bi- and trimonthly doses. Adjust doses to achieve 10-day nadir WBC between 1,500 and 3,000/μl.

Azathioprine: Starting dose of 2 mg/kg/day. Avoid concurrent allopurinol. Monitor WBC frequently for first month; hold dose for declining WBC or platelets, as bone marrow depression may be precipitous and severe.

Plasma exchange: Daily 3–4-liter exchanges for severe or refractory disease; after first week, reduce exchanges to alternate days. Delay for several days after visceral (e.g., renal) biopsy. Concurrent use of cyclophosphamide recommended.

soft clinical findings that are due to minor fluctuations in activity or to corticosteroid withdrawal itself, rather than to relapse of vasculitis. The clinician should be circumspect about reinstitution of high doses of prednisone. At the same time, if intensification of prednisone therapy is clearly indicated, the clinician should not be reluctant to reinitiate tapering at the judicious time. In short, it is important that the dose and duration of corticosteroid therapy be as short and as low as necessary to control disease activity. Adjunctive treatments may help to minimize major short-term as well as insidious long-term corticosteroid side effects. It is not in the patient's best interest to consider alternative therapy only in desperation or only after serious corticosteroid toxicity has intervened.

Although no formal comparisons have been made among the various immunosuppressive agents, our experience with the treatment of systemic vasculitis has led us to favor cyclophosphamide over other cytotoxic agents. This preference is supported by considerable evidence from experimental and other clinical studies that cyclophosphamide is one of the most effective agents available for altering established, ongoing immunologic processes [28].

Cyclophosphamide in conventional oral doses is added to prednisone therapy in any of the following circumstances: (1) major vasculitis of organ systems that have a narrow window of tolerance to a vasculitic insult (e.g., cardiac, central nervous system, gastrointestinal tract, or kidneys); (2) unusually aggressive, progressive or persistently active vasculitis; (3) dependence on unacceptably high doses of prednisone; or (4) accelerated or debilitating corticosteroid complications.

The clinician should be mindful, on the one hand, that cautious dosing of cyclophosphamide is important since its therapeutic effects are delayed approximately 1 to 2 weeks from initiation and, on the other hand, that the side effects such as myelosuppression may continue to evolve for a comparable period after the drug is discontinued. It is imperative to monitor the white blood cell count in order to avoid an infectious diathesis [12]. Increased bone marrow sensitivity to cyclophosphamide may appear as prednisone is tapered. Conversely, increasing the dose of alternate-day prednisone can sometimes be used to improve neutrophil counts in patients who could benefit from increased doses of cyclophosphamide [28]. Experience with intermittent pulse cyclophosphamide in classic PAN has been limited [2].

Azathioprine has been extensively used for the treatment of aggressive cases of classic PAN or disease responding poorly to prednisone. We prefer to use azathioprine in patients who are intolerant of cyclophosphamide, or for maintenance therapy in patients who have been induced to remission with cyclophosphamide but who have cyclophosphamide intolerance or complications.

Ancillary medical therapy of classic PAN must include effective antihypertensives to minimize the risk of cardiovascular events and stroke. Antiplatelet drugs and vasodilators, particularly calcium channel blockers, might reduce some complications of vascular insufficiency [24].

Treatment of Microscopic Polyarteritis and Necrotizing and Crescentic Glomerulonephritis. The overall management of the vasculitic syndrome in patients with microscopic polyarteritis and in those with necrotizing and crescent glomerulonephritis is basically the same as for classic PAN, including the guidelines for the initiation, tapering, and discontinuance of prednisone therapy (see Table 76-5). Because of the threat of catastrophic, rapidly progressive renal failure in these conditions, we and others prefer to intensify the initial corticosteroid therapy by administering intravenous pulse methylprednisolone [9–11, 13, 126]. Some investigators use intensive plasma exchange and cyclophosphamide therapy in lieu of or in sequence with pulse methylprednisolone [13, 64, 95, 126]. Cyclophosphamide treatment seems to be important in reducing the risk of exacerbations after a course of plasma exchange [64]. After about 3 months of induction treatment with cyclophosphamide, some investigators switch routinely to azathioprine for maintenance therapy [122, 126].

At the present time, we believe that cyclophosphamide is among the key elements in the management of microscopic polyarteritis and necrotizing and crescentic glomerulonephritis. The largest experience is with the conventional regimen of daily oral cyclophosphamide that is basically the same as for classic PAN. Recently, Falk et al. [40] reported the use of monthly pulse cyclophosphamide for treatment of these diseases. They found this regimen to be comparable in efficacy to conventional oral cyclophosphamide; it was less certain that pulse therapy met the goal of reducing the toxicity of chronic, daily oral cyclophosphamide, as has been seen in patients with lupus nephritis [8]. Additional studies of the intermittent pulse method of administering cyclophosphamide to patients with these forms of renal vasculitis are clearly warranted.

Monitoring Therapy in Polyarteritis. Assessing disease activity is a major challenge in all forms of polyarteritis. Clinical features of vasculitis are often ambiguous and easily confused with superimposed infections. Certain laboratory features, such as anemia, leukocytosis, thrombocytosis, high sedimentation rate, and elevated C-reactive protein, are nonspecific but they can be helpful as indications of active vasculitis [72]. The urinary sediment provides the best information on activity of renal vasculitis and should be monitored personally by the attending physician. Renal biopsy can sometimes be useful if the activity of the urinary sediment is equivocal, but repeated renal biopsies are usually not warranted. The role of ANCA testing in monitoring disease activity is poorly defined; however, a rising titer calls for intensified follow-up, as it may herald an exacerbation of vasculitis.

In general, immunosuppressive therapies, described above and outlined in Table 76-5, should be continued for several months after the patient has demonstrated a sustained remission of polyarteritis, as defined by combinations of clinical evaluation and laboratory testing.

End-Stage Renal Failure. The development of renal failure in polyarteritis is often multifactorial. Glomerular obsolescence, due to underlying processes of either classic or microscopic polyarteritis, may be accelerated by aggressive hypertension. Hypertension can become even more difficult to control with severe uremia, but bilateral nephrectomy is rarely necessary with currently available antihypertensive agents. Maintenance dialysis is feasible for patients with polyarteritis. Recovery of renal function after several months of dialysis has been recorded [126]. Transplantation may be undertaken without untoward problems or risk of recurrence of polyarteritis in the renal allograft. Overall prognosis for patient survival during renal failure therapy appears to have improved in recent years [54, 105].

Wegener's Granulomatosis

Wegener's granulomatosis was originally described as a subset of PAN. Its clinical manifestations are variegated and reminiscent of both classic PAN and microscopic polyarteritis, but a certain constellation of clinical and pathologic features distinguishes this condition.

DEFINITION

Wegener's granulomatosis includes a clinical syndrome of systemic vasculitis with a specific triad of destructive chronic inflammation of the upper and lower respiratory tracts and glomerulonephritis (see Table 76-2). The diagnosis is verified by demonstration of necrotizing granulomas and arteritis in one or more of these sites. Necrotizing and crescentic glomerulonephritis is seen in the majority of cases, but a limited form of Wegener's granulomatosis occurs in which there is only airway disease.

CLINICAL FEATURES

Upper airway disease is typically the dominant clinical problem in Wegener's granulomatosis, with sinusitis, nasopharyngitis, epistaxis, or otitis media. Pulmonary disease tends to be asymptomatic in the majority, with migratory pulmonary infiltrates noted on chest radiographs. Computed tomography may detect lesions that are not seen or are indeterminate on conventional chest radiographs. Consolidation and cavitation of lung lesions associated with secondary infections and/or hemoptysis [68] may lead to serious pulmonary complications. Pulmonary function tests often show loss of flow, volume, and/or diffusion capacity. Biopsy of involved lung tissue usually provides the clearest evidence for diagnosis of Wegener's granulomatosis. Necrotizing granulomas and arteritis are typically seen concurrently, but either lesion may predominate. Open lung biopsy should be strongly considered in the presence of suspicious lesions on chest x-ray, especially in the absence of diagnostic pathology elsewhere. Upper airway biopsies tend to have lower diagnostic yield due to the paucity of vessels in superficial tissue samples and the high frequency of overriding chronic inflammation due to bacterial superinfections.

The extrarenal manifestations of Wegener's granulomatosis have been delineated in several reviews and monographs [7, 28, 48, 112]. Constitutional features such as fever, lassitude, anorexia, or weight loss are often present. The extrarenal symptoms and signs tend to dominate the clinical manifestations of Wegener's granulomatosis and easily overshadow the recognition of serious renal disease. Kidney involvement is an unusual first presentation of Wegener's granulomatosis, though its occurrence has been well documented [142]. As a working rule, all patients with Wegener's granulomatosis should be considered at risk for developing rapidly progressive glomerulonephritis until adequate therapy is administered.

LABORATORY PARAMETERS

As in most forms of systemic vasculitis, anemia of chronic disease, elevated erythrocyte sedimentation rate, increased platelets, and elevated acute phase reactants, especially C-reative protein [72], are common in Wegener's granulomatosis. Elevated immunoglobulins and rheumatoid factors may be present but are inconsistent [28, 48]. Circulating immune complexes are relatively common [48, 112, 119], especially in active disease.

The ANCA test has been a great boon for the diagnosis of Wegener's granulomatosis [22, 23, 137]. As noted previously, patients with active Wegener's granulomatosis demonstrate a very high rate of cytoplasmic staining, or the so-called C-ANCA pattern. Some investigators believe that the ANCA test may replace the need for tissue diagnosis in Wegener's granulomatosis. Thus, in the setting of a characteristic vasculitic syndrome, inflammatory disease of the upper and lower respiratory tracts, and glomerulonephritis and a strongly positive ANCA test result with the characteristic cytoplasmic or C-ANCA pattern and/or reaction to proteinase-3 by ELISA, one can be very confident of the diagnosis of Wegener's granulomatosis.

The most common manifestation of renal disease, seen in more than three-fourths of patients, is asymptomatic hematuria and proteinuria with a nephritic urinary sediment. As in other forms of polyarteritis with glomerulonephritis, hypertension is rarely a major clinical manifestation. Heavy proteinuria is unusual but, when present, it carries an ominous prognosis [7, 9].

RENAL PATHOLOGY

The glomerular pathology of Wegener's granulomatosis bears great similarity to that of microscopic polyarteritis [6, 129]. Necrotizing and crescentic glomerulonephritis is typical (Figs. 76-13 and 76-14). Fractures of Bowman's capsule and intense pericapsular inflammation dominated by T lymphocytes [6] are common. Immunofluorescent microscopy usually shows nonspecific immunoglobulin and complement deposits in necrotic areas. Fibrin is the dominant immunoreactant in the active glomerular lesions and especially in cellular crescents. Electron microscopy studies have not demonstrated significant local immune complex deposits in the kidney [6, 7, 59, 119, 129, 140]. Mononuclear cell infiltrates may become widespread throughout the renal interstitium. Necrotizing granulomas and/or small vessel vasculitis [112, 119] are rare in renal biopsies (Fig. 76-15), but their presence strongly supports the diagnosis of Wegener's granulomatosis.

COURSE AND TREATMENT

Early experience with Wegener's granulomatosis summarized by Walton in 1958 [139] emphasized the hopeless prognosis of this disease; only 20 percent of patients survived 1 year with available supportive treatment. The advent of corticosteroids produced only slight improvement. Survival increased in approximately 34 percent at 1 year [9, 28], and deaths due to progressive renal failure continued. Immunosuppressive drugs subsequently improved outcome dramatically [28].

Our own experience indicates that cyclophosphamide has improved the patient survival rate at 1 year to over 90 percent and at 5 years to approximately 80 percent [48]. Those with early-onset, necrotizing and crescentic glomerulonephritis have an estimated renal survival rate

Fig. 76-13. Wegener's granulomatosis. A. Glomerulus with segmental proliferation, fibrinoid necrosis, and adhesion to Bowman's capsule. B. Glomerulus with proliferation, fibrinoid necrosis, and a large cellular crescent. (Both: H&E; ×220.)

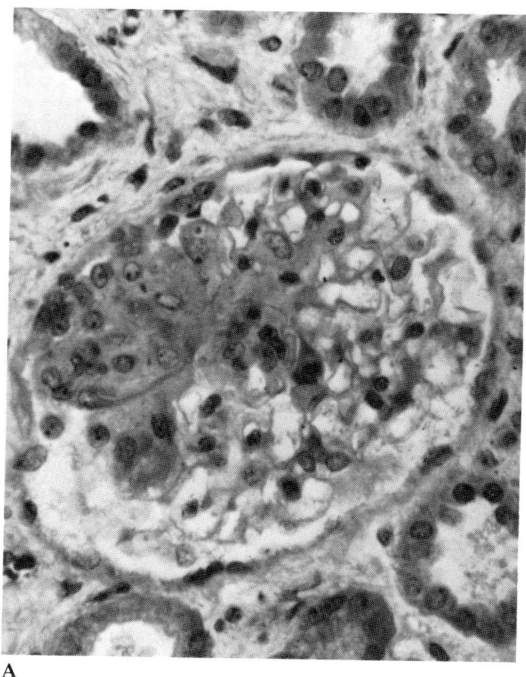

A

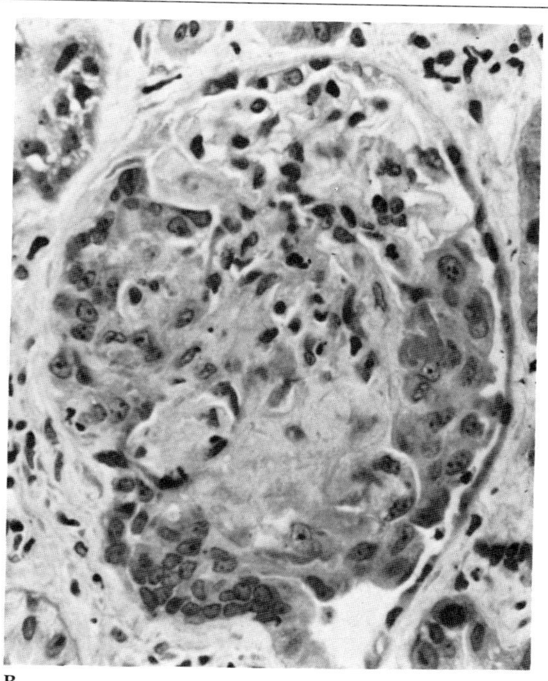

B

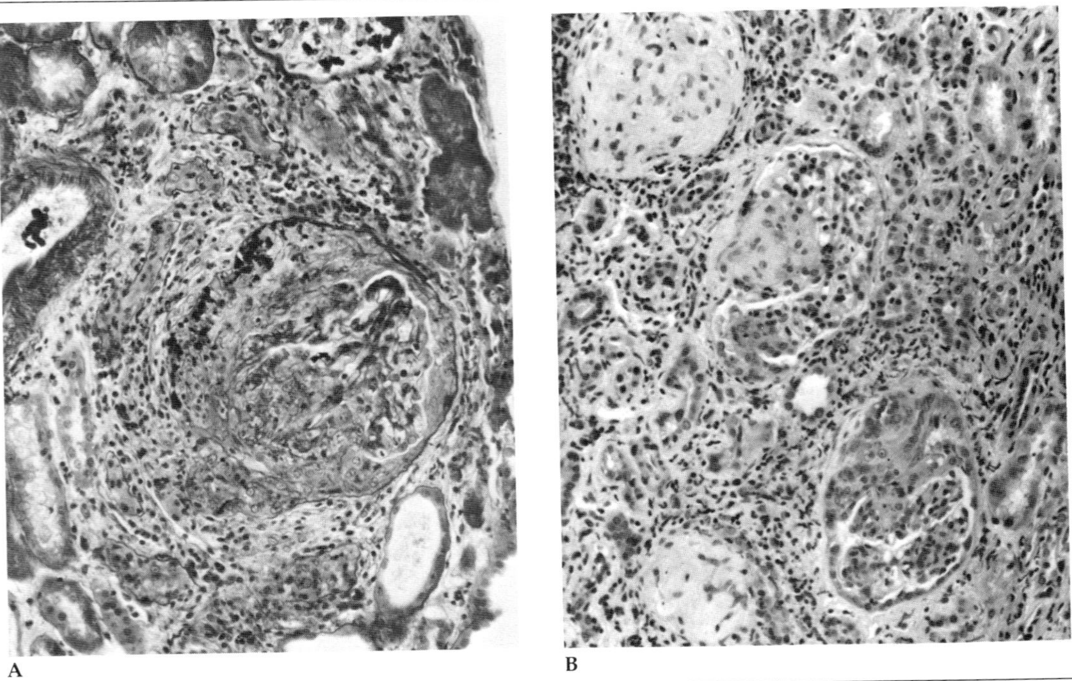

Fig. 76-14. Wegener's granulomatosis. A. Glomerulus, showing a circumferential fibroepithelial crescent associated with destruction of Bowman's capsule and periglomerular inflammatory cell infiltrate. (Masson trichrome; ×110.) B. Advanced renal disease with globally sclerotic glomeruli at the upper and lower left. The glomerulus just above center shows one segment with sclerosis. The glomerulus at the lower right shows proliferation as well as a cellular crescent. There is substantial tubular atrophy with extensive infiltration of the interstitium with mononuclear leukocytes. (H&E; ×100.)

of 50 to 60 percent at 5 years [9] (see Fig. 76-12). It is important to remember that prognosis is jeopardized by delays in the initiation of adequate treatment from onset of the earliest renal abnormality.

The most extensive experience with immunosuppressive drug treatment of Wegener's granulomatosis centers around cyclophosphamide. Cyclophosphamide is clearly efficacious in preventing progression of glomerulonephritis and in inducing general remission of Wegener's granulomatosis; as such, it has become the standard of treatment for this disease.

Treatment and drug monitoring (see Table 76-5) in patients with Wegener's granulomatosis are similar to those for polyarteritis and have been outlined in detail [10, 28, 50]. Cyclophosphamide is usually initiated in conventional daily doses for disease activity in essentially any organ system. Renal disease (other than fixed azotemia with inactive urinary findings) is an urgent indication for corticosteroid and cyclophosphamide therapy. High-dose prednisone is administered concurrently in the early phases of treatment, especially in patients with aggressive or destructive inflammatory lesions and in patients with necrotizing or crescentic glomerulonephritis. Some investigators use intravenous pulse methylprednisolone with favorable results [112]. Plasma exchange has been utilized as adjunctive therapy to prednisone and cyclophosphamide for early treatment of severe Wegener's granulomatosis [112] and in certain patients who are refractory to conventional drug therapy. The margin of additional efficacy provided by plasma exchange has not been clearly defined. At the present time, plasma exchange is not necessary or cost-effective for initial therapy of the typical patient with Wegener's granulomatosis.

Corticosteroids do not contribute substantially to the maintenance regimen of cyclophosphamide; prednisone is usually tapered to alternate day and discontinued as soon as tolerated. Cyclophosphamide is optimally continued for approximately 1 year after complete remission has been achieved. Certain long-term complications of cyclophosphamide [50] call for continued search for alternative maintenance therapies. In this regard, intermittent pulse cyclophosphamide is not completely satisfactory for long-term management of Wegener's granulomatosis [73]. Patients treated with intermittent pulse cyclophosphamide seemed to respond during the first few months of treatment but had higher rates of relapse than did patients treated with conventional, daily, oral cyclophosphamide.

Infections may precede exacerbations in certain patients [113], and a recent study suggested some control of flares of Wegener's granulomatosis with antibiotic treatment [34, 76]. However, we believe that antibiotic therapy should not be considered a sole therapy in Wegener's granulomatosis. Staphylococcal superinfections of the airways are easily mistaken for active vas-

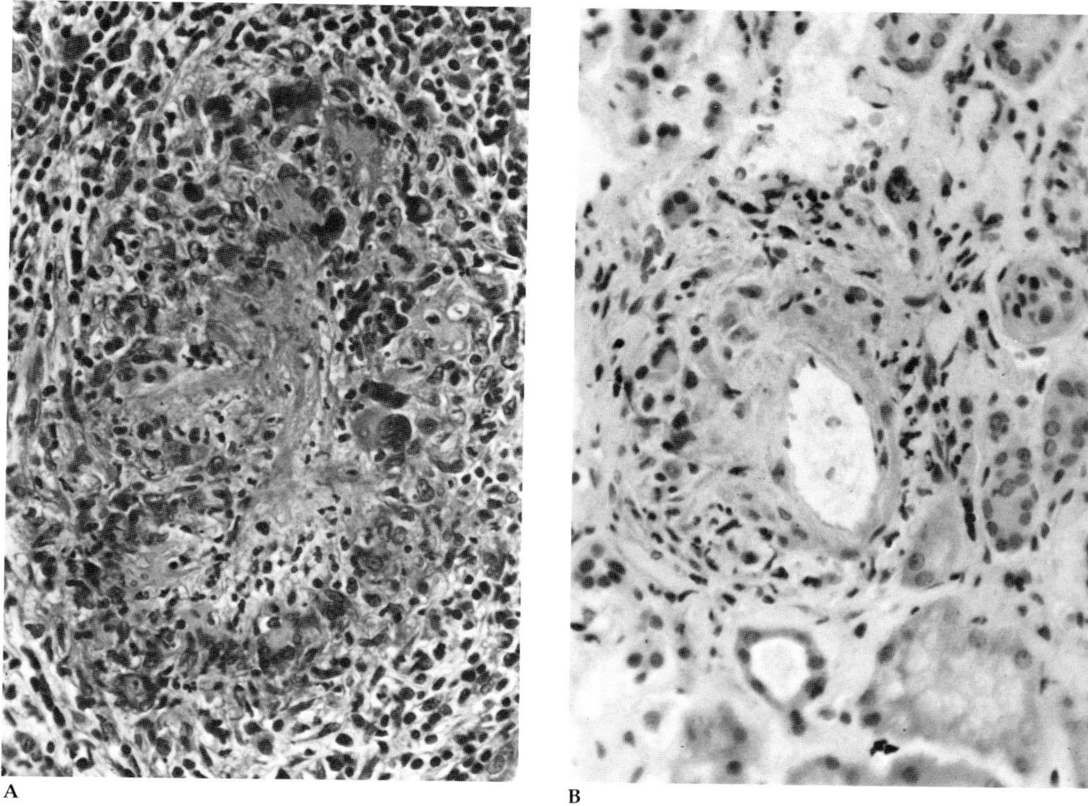

Fig. 76-15. Wegener's granulomatosis. A. Necrotizing granulomatous vasculitis of a renal artery with numerous giant cells. (Trichrome; ×220.) (Courtesy of Dr. Liliane Striker, National Institutes of Health, Bethesda, Md.) B. Necrotizing arteriolitis in a needle biopsy specimen of the kidney. (H&E; ×220.)

culitis and should be treated early with vigorous antibiotics.

RENAL FAILURE

Rapidly progressive renal failure may warrant temporary dialysis therapy in Wegener's granulomatosis. The prognosis is not generally favorable, but the reversibility of the renal disease depends on the severity of necrosis, the proportion of crescents, and the extent of irreversible sclerosing lesions. Gradual progression to end-stage renal disease may occur in spite of adequate control of the overall activity of Wegener's granulomatosis. During maintenance dialysis, retreatment of exacerbations of disease activity is sometimes required, but many patients enter a sustained remission on dialysis [84].

Patients with end-stage renal failure due to Wegener's granulomatosis are good candidates for renal transplantation after their disease becomes completely inactive [44, 84]. Recurrences of Wegener's granulomatosis in lung and in kidney have been documented following renal transplantation [132], but this appears to be rare [84].

Allergic Angiitis and Granulomatosis (Churg-Strauss Syndrome)

This condition was described by Churg and Strauss in 1951 [15] in an autopsy study of patients with a history of asthma and a clinical syndrome of systemic vasculitis. Certain features distinguished this entity from polyarteritis and Wegener's granulomatosis, to which it bears many resemblances [15, 17, 52, 87, 130].

DEFINITION

Allergic angiitis and granulomatosis is defined by the presence of the systemic vasculitic syndrome in patients with a history of asthma and atopic allergies and eosinophilia [74]. Paranasal sinus disease, mononeuropathy, and fleeting pulmonary infiltrates are seen in the majority and assist in diagnosis (see Table 76-2). Pathologic verification is based on extravascular granulomas associated with necrosis and prominent eosinophilic infiltration as well as necrotizing vasculitis of small arteries and veins (Fig. 76-16).

CLINICAL AND LABORATORY FEATURES

Asthma and atopic allergies usually present months to years before the emergence of the systemic vasculitic component of Churg-Strauss disease. Debilitating constitutional symptoms are prominent along with pneumonia and a high frequency of cutaneous granulomas and vasculitis [52]. The systemic vasculitis syndrome overlaps considerably with polyarteritis [28]. The distinguishing elements are asthma, eosinophilia, and gran-

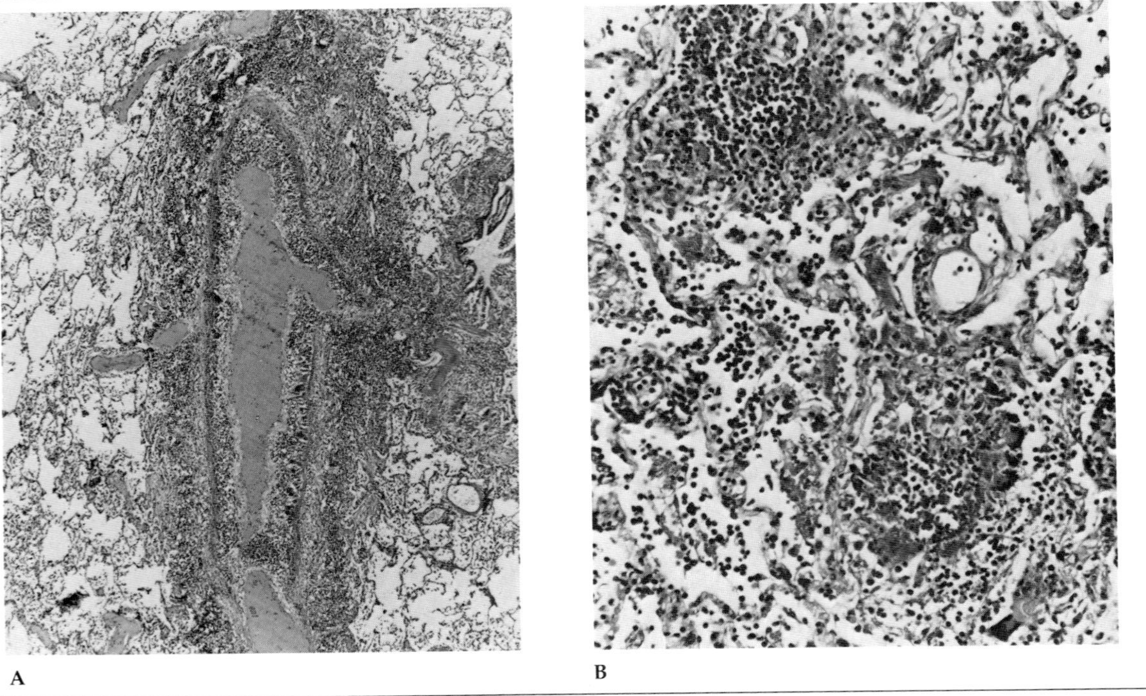

Fig. 76-16. Allergic angiitis and granulomatosis (Churg-Strauss disease). A. Lung vessel with severe necrotizing arteritis. The vasculitis is composed of neutrophils, mononuclear cells, and many eosinophils. (H&E; ×25.) B. Pulmonary granulomas near a vessel with severe arteritis. (H&E; ×160.) (Courtesy of Dr. T. Antonovych and Dr. S. Sabnis, Nephropathology Section, Armed Forces Institute of Pathology, Washington, D.C.)

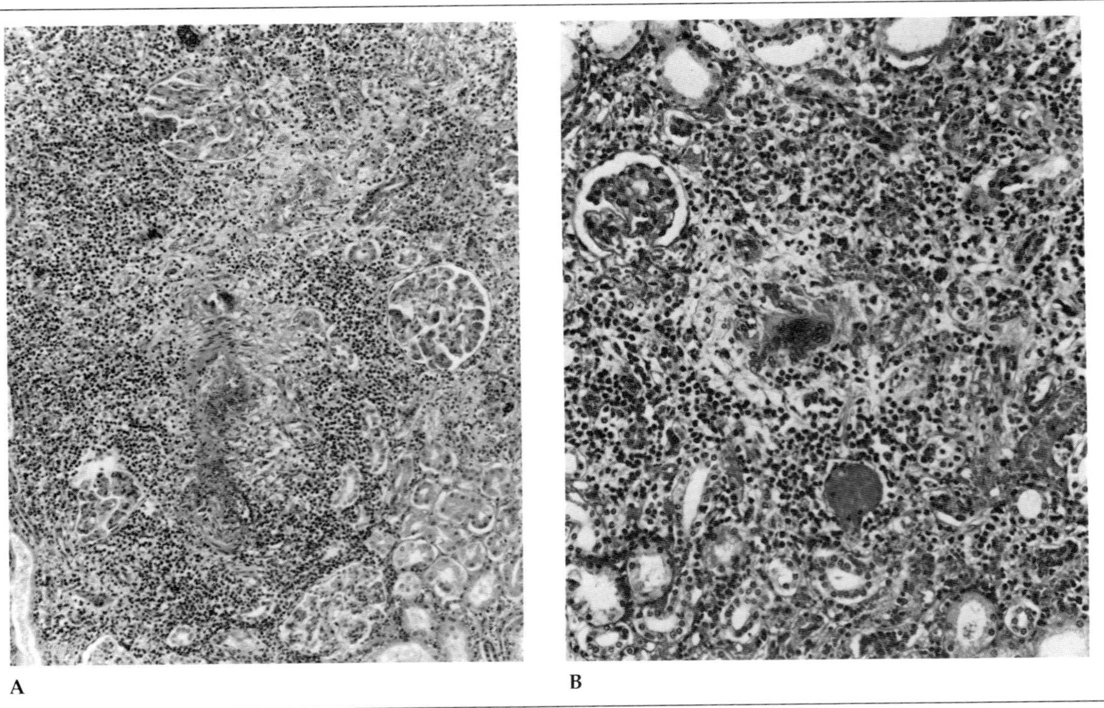

Fig. 76-17. Allergic angiitis and granulomatosis (Churg-Strauss disease). A. Renal tissue showing a longitudinally sectioned artery with fibrinoid necrosis in the center of the micrograph. The interstitium shows a dense infiltrate of eosinophils. The glomeruli show segmental proliferation. (H&E; ×100.) B. Renal tissue showing an early granuloma with a prominent giant cell. Eosinophils dominate the interstitial infiltrate. The glomerulus shows only ischemic collapse. (H&E; ×160.) (Courtesy of Dr. T. Antonovych and Dr. S. Sabnis, Nephropathology Section, Armed Forces Institute of Pathology, Washington, D.C.)

ulomas. Elevated IgE levels [87] and IgE-circulating immune complexes have been reported. About one-half of the patients have P-ANCAs [19].

RENAL DISEASE

The true frequency of renal involvement in Churg-Strauss syndrome is uncertain. Unselected series of patients seem to have a low prevalence of renal disease, but recent reports from a British renal unit indicated that over 80 percent of patients had glomerular disease [17, 87]. Hypertension, hematuria, and proteinuria have been most frequently observed, but the gamut of renal findings is quite similar to that of polyarteritis (classic and microscopic), including the risk of rapidly progressive renal failure.

The renal pathology of allergic angiitis and granulomatosis involves both the glomeruli and the extraglomerular vasculature and interstitium. Interstitial granulomas with eosinophilic infiltration are observed (Fig. 76-17), but effective immunosuppressive therapy seems to have reduced the prevalence of these lesions [17]. Necrotizing arteritis of the kidney and other viscera may be seen. Glomerular lesions are composed of focal and segmental endocapillary proliferation with necrosis and crescents. Ischemic changes may lead to cortical infarcts.

Management of Churg-Strauss syndrome is basically the same as that of polyarteritis. This includes high-dose corticosteroids and cyclophosphamide for major vasculitic disease. Cardiovascular complications are the most common cause of death. Rapidly progressive or necrotizing and crescentic glomerulonephritis is treated with pulse methylprednisolone and possibly with adjunctive plasma exchange [17]. Overall, the renal prognosis seems to be somewhat more favorable than in polyarteritis.

Miscellaneous Vasculitic Diseases

LYMPHOMATOID GRANULOMATOSIS

This rare and unusual condition encompasses a range of benign to malignant features [46, 81, 114]. Multiple organs, including the kidneys, are infiltrated by a polymorphic lymphoreticular collection of cells that have plasmacytoid and immunoblastoid features. The variegated morphology and extralymphatic predilection of this disease distinguish it from lymphoma, though malignant transformation is common [46, 81]. Granulomas are commonly seen without concomitant giant cells. In a strict sense, this disease is not a true vasculitis in that there is no inflammation and necrosis of vessel walls. However, the atypical cellular infiltrates are angiocentric and angiodestructive, giving rise to the vasculitic-like picture, which can involve necrosis, thrombosis, and recanalization.

Clinical renal disease is rare due to the sparing of glomeruli, but interstitial infiltrates and nodular masses of the atypical lymphoid cells are observed in one-third to one-half of patients at autopsy [133, 136]. Renal disease is rarely an important determinant of outcome and therefore it rarely dictates treatment for this disease [28, 46, 77, 114].

TEMPORAL ARTERITIS

This giant cell arteritis is a relatively common and debilitating illness that is frequently associated with polymyalgia rheumatica [28]. Diagnosis is established by the presence of three or more of the following criteria: age over 50 years, new headache, temporal artery abnormality, elevated erythrocyte sedimentation rate, or abnormal artery biopsy findings [74]. Vasculitis outside of the head and neck area is unusual. Renal vasculitis is extremely rare, but membranous glomerulonephritis has been described [135].

TAKAYASU ARTERITIS

Giant cell vasculitis of the aorta and major tributaries is a rare disease with a predilection for young females [28, 66, 127]. Decreased peripheral pulses, bruits, and abnormal angiograms are the main features of Takayasu arteritis.

Clinically, a systemic vasculitic syndrome is evident, and claudication and hypertension are major problems. Renovascular hypertension due to aortic involvement and/or renal artery stenosis is present in the majority of patients [66]. Renal insufficiency due to ischemia and infarction may develop. Glomerular disease is rare, but mild mesangial proliferative glomerulonephritis with sparse immune complex deposits has been reported [85, 133].

BEHÇET'S DISEASE

This condition is considered to be a systemic vasculitis with the following discrete features: recurrent aphthous stomatitis, genital ulcerations, and uveitis. Thrombophlebitis, arthritis, neuropsychiatric problems, and cutaneous vasculitic lesions are prominent features, but virtually any organ system seems to be susceptible to the underlying small vessel vasculitis [28]. The prevalence of kidney involvement appears to be high even in patients without clinical renal manifestations [71]. Immune complex deposits have been observed in the majority of renal biopsy samples, even those without significant alterations by light microscopy. More imposing, however, have been the reports of rapidly progressive and crescentic glomerulonephritis in Behçet's disease [58, 109]. The feature that distinguishes this glomerular disease from that of polyarteritis or Wegener's granulomatosis is the presence of mesangial and capillary loop (predominantly subendothelial) deposits of IgG and complement. Recent clinical trials suggest that azathioprine [143] and cyclosporine [107] are effective in the treatment of Behçet's disease.

RELAPSING POLYCHONDRITIS

This disorder is defined as a systemic vasculitis with three or more of the following discrete features: auricular chondritis, nonerosive polyarthritis, nasal chondritis, ocular inflammation, chondritis of the respiratory tract, and chondritis of the inner ear [99]. Relapsing polychondritis is likely to be related to polyarteritis nodosa and it has many features akin to Wegener's granulomatosis. Renal disease, expressed as rapidly progressive and crescentic glomerulonephritis with variable immune complex deposits, has been reported [37, 104].

CUTANEOUS VASCULITIDES

Many forms of cutaneous vasculitis have been described [28, 60]. The majority are associated with elevated circulating immune complexes, but renal disease is the exception, unless cutaneous vasculitis is simply one of the elements of a systemic vasculitis. A subset of disease called *hypocomplementemic urticarial vasculitis* has been described in which glomerulonephritis can occur, perhaps related to the complement abnormality. Type 1 membranoproliferative glomerulonephritis with subendothelial deposits has been reported [60].

ACKNOWLEDGEMENTS. The authors are deeply grateful to Dr. Tatiana Antonovych and Dr. Sharda Sabnis of the Armed Forces Institute of Pathology for their advice, contributions, and critical reviews of the portions of the manuscript pertaining to the renal pathology of the vasculitic diseases.

References

1. Abbott, F., Jones, S., Lockwood, C. M., et al. Autoantibodies to glomerular antigens in patients with Wegener's granulomatosis. *Nephrol. Dial. Transplant.* 4: 1, 1989.
2. Adu, D., Howie, A. J., Scott, D. G. I., et al. Polyarteritis and the kidney. *Q. J. Med.* 62: 221, 1987.
3. Akikusa, B., Irabu, N., Matsumura, R., et al. Tubulointerstitial changes in systemic vasculitic disorders: A quantitative study of 18 biopsy cases. *Am. J. Kidney Dis.* 16: 481, 1990.
4. Albert, D. A., Silverstein, M. D., Paunicka, K., et al. The diagnosis of polyarteritis nodosa. II. Empirical verification of a decision analysis model. *Arthritis Rheum.* 31: 1128, 1988.
5. Andrassy, K., Koderisch, J., Rufer, M., et al. Detection and clinical implication of anti-neutrophil cytoplasm antibodies in Wegener's granulomatosis and rapidly progressive glomerulonephritis. *Clin. Nephrol.* 32: 159, 1989.
6. Antonovych, T. T., Sabnis, S. G., Tuur, S. M., et al. Morphologic differences between polyarteritis and Wegener's granulomatosis using light, electron and immunohistochemical techniques. *Mod. Pathol.* 2: 349, 1989.
7. Appel, G. B., Kashigarian, M., and Hayslett, J. P. Wegener's granulomatosis-clinical-pathological correlations and long-term course. *Am. J. Kidney Dis.* 1: 27, 1981.
8. Balow, J. E. Lupus nephritis. *Ann. Intern. Med.* 106: 79, 1987.
9. Balow, J. E. Renal vasculitis. *Kidney Int.* 27: 954, 1985.
10. Balow, J. E., and Austin, H. A. III. Vasculitic Diseases of the Kidney. In W. N. Suki and S. G. Massry (eds.), *Therapy of Renal Diseases and Related Disorders.* Boston: Kluwer Academic, 1991, pp. 413–423.
11. Bolton, W. K., and Sturgill, B. C. Methylprednisolone therapy for acute crescentic rapidly progressive glomerulonephritis. *Am. J. Nephrol.* 9: 368, 1989.
12. Bradley, J. D., Brandt, K. D., and Katz, B. P. Infectious complications of cyclophosphamide treatment for vasculitis. *Arthritis Rheum.* 32: 45, 1989.
13. Bruns, F. J., Adler, S., Fraley, D. S., et al. Long-term follow-up of aggressively treated idiopathic rapidly progressive glomerulonephritis. *Am. J. Med.* 86: 400, 1989.
14. Cassidy, M. J., Gaskin, G., Savill, J., et al. Towards a more rapid diagnosis of rapidly progressive glomerulonephritis. *Br. Med. J.* 301: 329, 1990.
15. Churg, J., and Strauss, L. Allergic granulomatosis, allergic angiitis, and periarteritis nodosa. *Am. J. Pathol.* 27: 277, 1951.
16. Citron, B. P., Halpern, M., McCarron, M., et al. Necrotizing angiitis associated with drug abuse. *N. Engl. J. Med.* 283: 1003, 1970.
17. Clutterbuck, E. J., Evans, D. J., and Pusey, C. D. Renal involvement in Churg-Strauss syndrome. *Nephrol. Dial. Transplant.* 5: 161, 1990.
18. Cohen, R. D., Conn, D. L., and Ilstrup, D. M. Clinical features, prognosis and response to treatment in polyarteritis. *Mayo Clin. Proc.* 55: 146, 1980.
19. Cohen Tervaert, J. W., Goldschmeding, R., Elema, J. D., et al. Association of autoantibodies to myeloperoxidase with different forms of vasculitis. *Arthritis Rheum.* 33: 1264, 1990.
20. Cohen Tervaert, J. W., Goldschmeding, R., Elema, J. D., et al. Autoantibodies against myeloid lysosomal enzymes in crescentic glomerulonephritis. *Kidney Int.* 37: 799, 1990.
21. Lesavre, P. Antineutrophil cytoplasmic autoantibodies antigen specificity. *Am. J. Kidney Dis.* 10: 159, 1991.
22. Cohen Tervaert, J. W., Huitema, M. G., Hene, R. J., et al. Prevention of relapses in Wegener's granulomatosis by treatment based on antineutrophil cytoplasmic antibody titre. *Lancet* 336: 709, 1990.
23. Cohen Tervaert, J. W., van der Woude, F. J., Fauci, A. S., et al. Association between active Wegener's granulomatosis and anticytoplasmic antibodies. *Arch. Intern. Med.* 149: 2461, 1989.
24. Conn, D. L. Update on systemic necrotizing vasculitis. *Mayo Clin. Proc.* 64: 535, 1989.
25. Cotran, R. S., and Pober, J. S. Effects of cytokine on vascular endothelium: Their role in vascular and immune injury. *Kidney Int.* 35: 969, 1989.
26. Couser, W. G. Rapidly progressive glomerulonephritis: Classification, pathogenetic mechanisms, and therapy. *Am. J. Kidney Dis.* 11: 449, 1988.
27. Croker, B. P., Lee, T., and Gunnells, J. C. Clinical and pathologic features of polyarteritis nodosa and its renal-limited variant: Primary crescentic and necrotizing glomerulonephritis. *Human Pathol.* 18: 38, 1987.
28. Cupps, T. R., and Fauci, A. S. *The Vasculitides.* Philadelphia: Saunders, 1981.
29. D'Agati, V., Chandler, P., Nash, M., et al. Idiopathic microscopic polyarteritis nodosa: Ultrastructural observations on the renal vascular and glomerular lesions. *Am. J. Kidney Dis.* 7: 95, 1986.
30. Dahlberg, P. J., Lockhart, J. M., and Overholt, E. L. Diagnostic studies for systemic necrotizing vasculitis. *Arch. Intern. Med.* 149: 161, 1989.
31. Davies, D. J., Moran, J. E., Niall, J. F., et al. Segmental necrotizing glomerulonephritis with antineutrophil antibody: Possible arbovirus aetiology? *Br. Med. J.* 285: 606, 1982.
32. Davson, J., Ball, J., and Platt, R. The kidney in periarteritis nodosa. *Q. J. Med.* 17: 175, 1948.
33. Deguchi, Y., Shibata, N., and Kishimoto, S. Enhanced expression of the tumour necrosis factor/cachectin gene in peripheral blood mononuclear cells from patients with systemic vasculitis. *Clin. Exp. Immunol.* 81: 311, 1990.
34. DeRemee, R. A., McDonald, T. J., and Weiland, L. H. Wegener's granulomatosis: Observations on treatment

with antimicrobial agents. *Mayo Clin. Proc.* 60: 27, 1985.

35. Duffy, J., Kidsky, M. D., Sharp, J. T., et al. Polyarteritis, polyarthritis and hepatitis B. *Medicine* 55: 19, 1976.
36. Egner, W., and Chapel, H. M. Titration of antibodies against neutrophil cytoplasmic antigens is useful in monitoring disease activity in systemic vasculitides. *Clin. Exp. Immunol.* 82: 244, 1990.
37. Espinoza, L. R., Richman, A., Bocanegra, R., et al. Immune complex-mediated renal involvement in relapsing polychondritis. *Am. J. Med.* 71: 181, 1981.
38. Ewald, E. A., Griffin, D., and McCune, W. J. Correlation of angiographic abnormalities with disease manifestations and disease severity in polyarteritis nodosa. *J. Rheumatol.* 145: 952, 1987.
39. Falk, R. J. ANCA-associated renal disease. *Kidney Int.* 38: 998, 1990.
40. Falk, R. J., Hogan, S., Carey, T. S., et al. Clinical course of anti-neutrophil cytoplasmic autoantibody-associated glomerulonephritis and systemic vasculitis. *Ann. Intern. Med.* 113: 656, 1990.
41. Falk, R. J., and Jennette, J. C. Anti-neutrophil cytoplasmic autoantibodies with specificity for myeloperoxidase in patients with systemic vasculitis and idiopathic necrotizing and crescentic glomerulonephritis. *N. Engl. J. Med.* 318: 1651, 1988.
42. Falk, R. J., Terrell, R., Charles, L. A., et al. Antineutrophil cytoplasmic autoantibodies induce neutrophils to degranulate and produce oxygen radicals. *Proc. Natl. Acad. Sci. U.S.A.* 87: 4115, 1990.
43. Fan, P. T., Davis, J. A., Somer, T., et al. A clinical approach to systemic vasculitis. *Semin. Arth. Rheum.* 9: 248, 1980.
44. Fauci, A. S., Balow, J. E., Brown, R., et al. Successful renal transplantation in Wegener's granulomatosis. *Am. J. Med.* 60: 437, 1976.
45. Fauci, A. S., Doppman, J. L., and Wolff, S. M. Cyclophosphamide-induced remissions in advanced polyarteritis nodosa. *Am. J. Med.* 64: 890, 1978.
46. Fauci, A. S., Haynes, B. F., Costa, J., et al. Lymphomatoid granulomatosis: Prospective clinical and therapeutic experience over 10 years. *N. Engl. J. Med.* 306: 68, 1982.
47. Fauci, A. S., Haynes, B. F., and Katz, P. The spectrum of vasculitis. Clinical, pathologic, immunologic and therapeutic considerations. *Ann. Intern. Med.* 89: 660, 1978.
48. Fauci, A. S., Haynes, B. F., Katz, P., et al. Wegener's granulomatosis: Prospective and clinical therapeutic experience with 85 patients for 21 years. *Ann. Intern. Med.* 98: 76, 1983.
49. Fauci, A. S., Katz, P., Haynes, B. F., et al. Cyclophosphamide therapy of severe systemic necrotizing vasculitis. *N. Engl. J. Med.* 301: 235, 1979.
50. Fauci, A. S., and Leavitt, R. Y. Systemic Vasculitis. In L. M. Lichtenstein and A. S. Fauci (eds.), *Current Therapy in Allergy, Immunology, and Rheumatology*—3. Philadelphia: B. C. Decker, 1988.
51. Ferraro, G., Meroni, P. L., Tincani, A., et al. Anti-endothelial cell antibodies in patients with Wegener's granulomatosis and micropolyarteritis. *Clin. Exp. Immunol.* 79: 47, 1990.
52. Finan, M. C., and Winkelmann, R. K. The cutaneous extravascular necrotizing granuloma (Churg-Strauss granuloma) and systemic disease: A review of 27 cases. *Medicine* 62: 142, 1983.
53. Frohnert, P. P., and Sheps, S. G. Long-term follow-up study of periarteritis nodosa. *Am. J. Med.* 43: 8, 1967.
54. Fuiano, G., Cameron, J. S., Raftry, M., et al. Improved prognosis of renal polyarteritis in recent years. *Nephrol. Dial. Transplant.* 3: 383, 1988.
55. Furlong, T. J., Ibels, L. S., and Eckstein, R. P. The clinical spectrum of necrotizing glomerulonephritis. *Medicine* 66: 192, 1987.
56. Fye, K. H., Becker, M. J., Theofilopoulos, A. N., et al. Immune complexes in hepatitis B antigen-associated periarteritis nodosa. *Am. J. Med.* 62: 783, 1977.
57. Gabriel, S. E., Conn, D. L., Phyliky, R. L., et al. Vasculitis in hairy cell leukemia: Review of literature and consideration of possible pathogenic mechanisms. *J. Rheumatol.* 13: 1167, 1986.
58. Gamble, C. N., Wiesner, K. B., Shapiro, R. F., et al. The immune complex pathogenesis of glomerulonephritis and pulmonary vasculitis in Behçet's disease. *Am. J. Med.* 66: 1031, 1979.
59. Gephardt, G. N., Shah, L. F., Tubbs, R. R., et al. Wegener's granulomatosis. Immunomicroscopic and ultrastructural study of four cases. *Arch. Pathol. Lab. Med.* 114: 961, 1990.
60. Gibson, L. E. Cutaneous vasculitis: Approach to diagnosis and systemic associations. *Mayo Clin. Proc.* 65: 221, 1990.
61. Graham, P. C., and Lindop, G. B. The renin-secreting cell in polyarteritis—An immunocytochemical study. *Histopathology* 16: 339, 1990.
62. Grau, G. E., Roux-Lombard, P., Gysler, C., et al. Serum cytokine changes in systemic vasculitis. *Immunology* 68: 196, 1989.
63. Greer, J. M., Longley, S., Edwards, N. I., et al. Vasculitis associated with malignancy: Experience with 13 patients and literature review. *Medicine* 67: 220, 1988.
64. Guillevin, L. Treatment of polyarteritis nodosa and Churg-Strauss angiitis: Indications of plasma exchange. Results of three prospective trials in 162 patients. *Prog. Clin. Biol. Res.* 337: 309, 1990.
65. Gupta, R. C., and Kohler, P. F. Identification of HBsAg determinants in immune complexes from hepatitis B virus-associated vasculitis. *J. Immunol.* 132: 1223, 1984.
66. Hall, S., Barr, W., Lie, J. T., et al. Takayasu arteritis: A study of 32 North American patients. *Medicine* 64: 89, 1985.
67. Hart, M. N., Sadewasser, K. L., Cancilla, P. A., et al. Experimental autoimmune type of vasculitis resulting from activation of mouse lymphocytes to cultured endothelium. *Lab. Invest.* 48: 419, 1983.
68. Haworth, S. J., Savage, C. O., Carr, D., et al. Pulmonary hemorrhage complicating Wegener's granulomatosis and microscopic polyarteritis. *Br. Med. J.* 290: 1775, 1985.
69. Heilman, R. L., Offord, K. P., Holley, K. E., et al. Analysis of risk factors for patient and renal survival in crescentic glomerulonephritis. *Am. J. Kidney Dis.* 9: 98, 1987.
70. Hellman, D. B., Laing, T. J., Petri, M., et al. Mononeuritis multiplex: The yield of evaluations for occult rheumatic diseases. *Medicine* 67: 145, 1988.
71. Herreman, G., Beaufils, H., Godeau, P., et al. Bechçet's syndrome and renal involvement: A histological and immunofluorescent study of eleven renal biopsies. *Am. J. Med. Sci.* 284: 10, 1982.
72. Hind, C. R., Winearls, C. G., Lockwood, C. M., et al. Objective monitoring of activity in Wegener's granulomatosis by measurement of serum C-reactive protein concentration. *Clin. Nephrol.* 21: 341, 1984.
73. Hoffman, G. S., Leavitt, R. Y., Fleisher, T. A., et al. Treatment of Wegener's granulomatosis with intermittent high-dose intravenous cyclophosphamide. *Am. J. Med.* 89: 403, 1990.

74. Hunder, G. G., Arend, W. P., Bloch, D. A., et al. The American College of Rheumatology 1990 criteria for the classification of vasculitis. *Arthritis Rheum.* 33: 1065, 1990.
75. Imoto, E. M., Lombard, C. M., and Sachs, D. P. Pulmonary capillaritis and hemorrhage. A clue to the diagnosis of systemic necrotizing vasculitis. *Chest* 96: 927, 1989.
76. Israel, H. L. Sulfamethoxazole-trimethoprim therapy for Wegener's granulomatosis. *Arch. Intern. Med.* 148: 2293, 1988.
77. Jenkins, T. R., and Zaloznik, A. J. Lymphomatoid granulomatosis. A case for aggressive therapy. *Cancer* 64: 1362, 1989.
78. Jennette, J. C., and Falk, R. J. Antineutrophil cytoplasmic autoantibodies and associated diseases: A review. *Am. J. Kidney Dis.* 15: 517, 1990.
79. Johnson, R. J., and Couser, W. G. Hepatitis B infection and renal disease: Clinical, immunopathogenetic and therapeutic considerations. *Kidney Int.* 37: 663, 1990.
80. Jordan, J. M., Allen, N., and Pizzo, S. V. Defective release of tissue plasminogen activator in systemic and cutaneous vasculitis. *Am. J. Med.* 82: 397, 1987.
81. Katzenstein, A. A., Carrington, C. B., and Liebow, A. A. Lymphomatoid granulomatosis. A clinicopathologic study of 152 cases. *Cancer* 43: 360, 1979.
82. Kauffmann, R. H., Herrmann, W. A., Meijer, C. J., et al. Circulating and tissue-bound immune complexes in allergic vasculitis: Relationship between immunoglobulin class and clinical features. *Clin. Exp. Immunol.* 41: 459, 1980.
83. Kurland, L. T., Chuang, T. Y., and Hunder, G. G. The Epidemiology of Systemic Arteritis. In R. E. Laurence and L. E. Shulman (eds.), *Current Topics in Rheumatology: Epidemiology of the Rheumatic Diseases.* New York: Gower Medical, 1984.
84. Kuross, S., Davin, T., and Kjellstrand, C. M. Wegener's granulomatosis with severe renal failure: Clinical course and results of dialysis and transplantation. *Clin. Nephrol.* 16: 172, 1981.
85. Lai, K. N., Chan, K. W., and Ho, C. P. Glomerulonephritis associated with Takayasu's arteritis: Report of three cases and review of literature. *Am. J. Kidney Dis.* 7: 197, 1986.
86. Lai, K. N., Jayne, D. R. W., Brownlee, A., et al. The specificity of anti-neutrophil cytoplasm autoantibodies in systemic vasculitis. *Clin. Exp. Immunol.* 82: 233, 1990.
87. Lanham, J. G., Elkon, K. B., Pusey, C. D., et al. Systemic vasculitis with asthma and eosinophilia: A clinical approach to the Churg-Strauss syndrome. *Medicine* 63: 65, 1984.
88. Leavitt, R. Y., and Fauci, A. S. Polyangiitis overlap syndrome. *Am. J. Med.* 81: 79, 1986.
89. Lehman, T. J., and Mahnovski, V. Animal models of vasculitis. Lessons we can learn to improve understanding of Kawasaki disease. *Rheum. Dis. Clin. North Am.* 14: 479, 1988.
90. Lehman, T. J., Warren, R., Gietl, D., et al. Variable expression of Lactobacillus casei cell wall-induced coronary arteritis: An animal model of Kawasaki's disease in selected inbred mouse strains. *Clin. Immunol. Immunopathol.* 48: 108, 1988.
91. Leib, E. S., Hibrawi, H., Chia, D., et al. Correlation of disease activity in systemic necrotizing vasculitis with immune complexes. *J. Rheumatol.* 8: 258, 1981.
92. Leib, E. S., Restivo, C., and Paulus, H. E. Immunosuppressive and corticosteroid therapy of polyarteritis nodosa. *Am. J. Med.* 67: 941, 1979.
93. Leung, D. Y., Cotran, R. S., Kurt-Jones, E., et al. Endothelial cell activation and high interleukin-1 secretion in the pathogenesis of acute Kawasaki disease. *Lancet* 2: 1298, 1989.
94. Lie, J. T. Illustrated histopathologic classification criteria for selected vasculitis syndromes. *Arthritis Rheum.* 33: 1074, 1990.
95. Lockwood, C. M., Pinching, A. J., Sweny, P., et al. Plasma exchange and immunosuppression in the treatment of fulminating immune-complex crescentic glomerulonephritis. *Lancet* 1: 63, 1987.
96. Lockwood, C. M., Worlledge, S., Nicholas, A., et al. Reversal of impaired splenic function in patients with nephritis or vasculitis (or both) by plasma exchange. *N. Engl. J. Med.* 300: 524, 1979.
97. Ludemann, J., Utecht, B., and Gross, W. L. Anti-neutrophil cytoplasm antibodies in Wegener's granulomatosis recognize an elastinolytic enzyme. *J. Exp. Med.* 171: 357, 1990.
98. Mark, E. J., and Ramirez, J. F. Pulmonary capillaritis and hemorrhage in patients with systemic vasculitis. *Arch. Pathol. Lab. Med.* 109: 413, 1985.
99. McAdam, L. P., O'Hanlan, M. A., Bluestone, R., et al. Relapsing polychondritis: Prospective study of 23 patients and a review of the literature. *Medicine* 55: 193, 1976.
100. McMahon, B. J., Heyward, W. L., Templin, D. W., et al. Hepatitis B-associated polyarteritis nodosa in Alaskan Eskimos: Clinical and epidemiologic features and long-term follow-up. *Hepatology* 9: 97, 1989.
101. Michet, C. J. Epidemiology of vasculitis. *Rheum. Dis. Clin. North Am.* 16: 261, 1990.
102. Nada, A. K., Torres, V. E., Ryu, J. H., et al. Pulmonary fibrosis as an unusual clinical manifestation of pulmonary-renal vasculitis in elderly patients. *Mayo Clin. Proc.* 65: 847, 1990.
103. Neild, G. H., Cameron, J. S., Ogg, C. S., et al. Rapidly progressive glomerulonephritis with extensive glomerular crescent formation. *Q. J. Med.* 52: 392, 1983.
104. Neild, G. H., Cameron, J. S., Ogg, C. S., et al. Relapsing polychondritis with crescentic glomerulonephritis. *Br. Med. J.* 1: 743, 1978.
105. Nissenson, A. R., and Port, F. K. Outcome of end-stage renal disease in patients with rare causes of renal failure. III. Systemic/vascular disorders. *Q. J. Med.* 74: 63, 1990.
106. Nolle, B., Specks, U., Ludemann, J., et al. Anticytoplasmic autoantibodies: Their immunodiagnostic value in Wegener granulomatosis. *Ann. Intern. Med.* 111: 28, 1989.
107. Nussenblatt, R. B., Palestine, A. G., Chan, C. C., et al. Effectiveness of cyclosporin therapy for Behçet's disease. *Arthritis Rheum.* 6: 671, 1985.
108. O'Connell, M. T., Kubrusky, D. B., and Fournier, A. M. Systemic necrotizing vasculitis seen initially as hypertensive crisis. *Arch. Intern. Med.* 145: 265, 1985.
109. Olsson, P. J., Gaffney, E., Alexander, R. W., et al. Proliferative glomerulonephritis with crescent formation in Behçet's syndrome. *Arch. Intern. Med.* 140: 713, 1980.
110. O'Shea, J. J., Jaffe, E. S., Lane, H. C., et al. Peripheral T cell lymphoma presenting as hypereosinophilia with vasculitis. *Am. J. Med.* 82: 539, 1987.
111. Parfrey, P. S., Hutchinson, T. A., Jothy, S., et al. The spectrum of diseases associated with necrotizing glomerulonephritis and its prognosis. *Am. J. Kidney Dis.* 6: 387, 1985.
112. Pinching, A. J., Lockwood, C. M., Pussell, B. A., et al. Wegener's granulomatosis: Observations on 18 patients with severe renal disease. *Q. J. Med.* 52: 435, 1983.

113. Pinching, A. J., Rees, A. J., Pussell, B. A., et al. Relapses in Wegener's granulomatosis: The role of infection. *Br. Med. J.* 281: 836, 1980.
114. Pisani, R. J., and DeRemee, R. A. Clinical implications of the histopathologic diagnosis of pulmonary lymphomatoid granulomatosis. *Mayo Clin. Proc.* 65: 151, 1990.
115. Porter, D. D., and Larsen, A. E. Aleutian disease of mink. *Progr. Med. Virol.* 18: 32, 1974.
116. Pusey, C. D., and Lockwood, C. M. Autoimmunity in rapidly progressive glomerulonephritis. *Kidney Int.* 35: 929, 1989.
117. Reveille, J. D., Goodman, R. E., Barger, B. O., et al. Familial polyarteritis nodosa: A serologic and immunopathogenetic analysis. *J. Rheumatol.* 16: 181, 1989.
118. Rich, A. R., and Gregory, J. E. The experimental demonstration that periarteritis nodosa is a manifestation of hypersensitivity. *Bull. Johns Hopkins Hosp.* 72: 65, 1943.
119. Ronco, P., Verroust, P., Mignon, F., et al. Immunopathological studies of polyarteritis nodosa and Wegener's granulomatosis: A report of 43 patients with 51 renal biopsies. *Q. J. Med.* 52: 212, 1983.
120. Sack, M., Cassidy, J. T., and Bole, G. G. Prognostic factors in polyarteritis. *J. Rheumatol.* 2: 411, 1975.
121. Savage, C. O., and Lockwood, C. M. Antineutrophil antibodies in vasculitis. *Adv. Nephrol.* 19: 225, 1990.
122. Savage, C. O. S., Winearls, C. G., Evans, D. J., et al. Microscopic polyarteritis: Presentation, pathology and prognosis. *Q. J. Med.* 56: 467, 1985.
123. Savage, C. O. S., Winearls, C. G., Jones, S., et al. Prospective study of radioimmunoassay for antibodies against neutrophil cytoplasm in diagnosis of systemic vasculitis. *Lancet* 2: 1389, 1987.
124. Savige, J. A., Gallicchio, M., Georgiou, T., et al. Diverse target antigens recognized by circulating antibodies in anti-neutrophil cytoplasm antibody-associated renal vasculitides. *Clin. Exp. Immunol.* 82: 238, 1990.
125. Sergent, J. S. Vasculitides associated with viral infections. *Clin. Rheum. Dis.* 6: 339, 1980.
126. Serra, A., Cameron, J. S., Turner, D. R., et al. Vasculitis affecting the kidney: Presentation, histopathology and long-term outcome. *Q. J. Med.* 53: 181, 1984.
127. Shelhamer, J. H., Volkman, D. J., Parrillo, J. E., et al. Takayasu's arteritis and its therapy. *Ann. Intern. Med.* 103: 121, 1985.
128. Smith, D. L., and Wernick, R. Spontaneous rupture of a renal artery aneurysm in polyarteritis nodosa: Critical review of the literature and report of a case. *Am. J. Med.* 87: 464, 1989.
129. Spargo, B. H., Seymour, A. E., and Ordenez, N. G. Vasculitis. *Renal Biopsy Pathology with Diagnostic and Therapeutic Implications.* New York: Wiley, 1980.
130. Specks, U., and DeRemee, R. A. Granulomatous vasculitis, Wegener's granulomatosis and Churg-Strauss syndrome. *Rheum. Dis. Clin. North Am.* 16: 377, 1990.
131. Specks, U., Wheatley, C. L., McDonald, T. J., et al. Anticytoplasmic autoantibodies in the diagnosis and follow-up of Wegener's granulomatosis. *Mayo Clin. Proc.* 64: 28, 1989.
132. Steinman, T. I., Jaffe, B. F., Monaco, A. P., et al. Recurrence of Wegener's granulomatosis after kidney transplantation. Successful re-induction of remission with cyclophosphamide. *Am. J. Med.* 68: 458, 1980.
133. Takagi, M., Ikeda, T., Kimura, K., et al. Renal histological studies in patients with Takayasu's arteritis. *Nephron* 36: 68, 1984.
134. Travers, R. L., Allison, D. J., Brettle, R. P., et al. Polyarteritis nodosa: A clinical and angiographic analysis of 17 cases. *Semin. Arthritis Rheum.* 8: 184, 1979.
135. Truong, L., Kopelman, R. G., Williams, G. S., et al. Temporal arteritis and renal disease. *Am. J. Med.* 78: 171, 1985.
136. van der Woude, F. J., Daha, M. R., van den Wall Bake, W. A., et al. Antibodies directed against the cytoplasm of neutrophils and monocytes. *Adv. Nephrol.* 19: 211, 1990.
137. Van der Woude, F. J., Rasmussen, N., Lobatto, S., et al. Autoantibodies against neutrophils and monocytes: Tool for diagnosis and marker of disease activity in Wegener's granulomatosis. *Lancet* 1: 425, 1985.
138. Velosa, J. A. Idiopathic crescentic glomerulonephritis or systemic vasculitis? *Mayo Clin. Proc.* 62: 145, 1987.
139. Walton, E. W. Giant-cell granuloma of the respiratory tract (Wegener's granulomatosis). *Br. Med. J.* 2: 265, 1958.
140. Weiss, M. A., and Crissman, J. D. Renal biopsy findings in Wegener's granulomatosis: Segmental necrotizing glomerulonephritis with glomerular thrombosis. *Human Pathol.* 15: 943, 1984.
141. Wilkowski, M. J., Velosa, J. A., Holley, K. E., et al. Risk factors in idiopathic renal vasculitis and glomerulonephritis. *Kidney Int.* 36: 1133, 1989.
142. Woodworth, T. G., Abuelo, J. G., Austin, H. A., III, et al. Severe glomerulonephritis with late emergence of classic Wegener's granulomatosis. *Medicine* 66: 181, 1987.
143. Yazici, H., Pazarli, H., Barnes, C. G., et al. A controlled trial of azathioprine in Behçet's syndrome. *N. Engl. J. Med.* 322: 281, 1990.
144. Zeek, P. M. Periarteritis nodosa and other forms of necrotizing angiitis. *N. Engl. J. Med.* 248: 764, 1953.

Renal Thromboembolism, Atheroembolism, and Other Acute Diseases of the Renal Arteries

Jack W. Coburn
Keith L. Agre

The thromboembolic disorders and other conditions causing acute occlusion of the renal artery include several clinicopathologic entities: (1) acute thrombosis of the renal artery, most often arising from trauma; (2) thromboembolism, or the embolism of a thrombus to the renal artery from a distal site; (3) acute dissection of the renal artery; (4) atheroembolic disease of the kidneys; and (5) rupture of renal arterial aneurysms. Certain conditions, such as fibromuscular dysplasia and atherosclerotic disease of the renal vessels, which generally cause "renovascular" hypertension, are not considered in this chapter except as they relate to the differential diagnosis of the occlusive disorders noted above.

Acute Thrombosis of the Renal Artery

Acute thrombosis of the renal artery usually occurs as a result of blunt abdominal trauma, which most commonly results from vehicular accidents [165]; thrombosis can also develop following penetrating trauma. The thrombosis is most commonly unilateral with the left kidney more commonly involved [10]; bilateral thromboses also occur [108]. Thrombosis of the renal artery usually occurs in conjunction with injury to other intraabdominal organs, and this often obscures the diagnosis. Right-sided thrombosis occurs in association with injury to the duodenum and liver, while left-sided thrombosis is most often associated with damage to the spleen and pancreas [10]. The existence of a thrombosed renal artery is commonly missed at the time of the initial surgical exploration of the abdomen because the retroperitoneal areas are usually not visualized and because the finding of pulsations of the renal artery by palpation does not exclude the presence of such thrombosis [168]. The presence of oliguria suggests the presence of bilateral thrombosis, although acute tubular necrosis or a unilateral thrombosis combined with contralateral acute tubular necrosis secondary to shock and hemorrhage from the injury both cause acute renal failure with oliguria (Fig. 77-1). Abdominal tenderness and flank pain are usual [165], and vomiting is common [10]. Hematuria, either gross or microscopic, is common [167], but it may be absent in 25 percent of cases [165]; proteinuria is common.

A prompt diagnosis is important because of the need for early surgical intervention, particularly with bilateral thrombosis; thus, there is a certain window of opportunity for surgical revascularization to prevent total renal infarction [11]. The clinical and laboratory features of renal infarction, which are described below under thromboembolism, may be present; however, the clinical and laboratory findings are commonly modified by other sequelae of the original trauma.

An intravenous urogram remains the diagnostic radiologic procedure of choice, and it has been recommended that all patients with severe epigastric and/or flank pain after blunt trauma to the abdomen, flank, or back should have intravenous urography [10, 11, 164]. Negative urograms were reported in 12 percent of cases in an analysis of a large number of penetrating renal injuries [149], but it is not certain that all these cases really had renal artery thrombosis; perirenal hematomas and cortical contusions can impair the excretion of contrast media and lead to false-positive results [167]. Computed tomography that is accentuated by the injection of contrast material [88, 141, 150] and magnetic resonance scanning may provide better diagnostic accuracy than intravenous urography [135]. Computed tomography can help to delineate a renal infarction from subcapsular and perinephric hematomas, intrarenal hematomas, renal lacerations, or extravasation of contrast media [141]. However, if carrying out one of these specialized procedures creates any delay, it is advisable to proceed to early angiography, which can provide the definitive diagnosis [164], and will distinguish renal artery thrombosis from renal contusions [91].

Arteriography is useful for identifying the extent of the lesion and the presence or absence of collateral circulation [87]. Digital subtraction angiography, which can be done with smaller and safer quantities of radiographic contrast media than standard arteriography, may provide anatomic delineation in the safest manner [87].

The recent success in revascularization [8, 90, 91, 119, 163] and the spontaneous late recovery of renal function in nonoperated cases in rare instances [29, 61] indicate that early surgical revascularization should be undertaken unless there are major contraindications. This is particularly true since traumatic renal artery thrombosis occurs most commonly in young individuals with few underlying morbid conditions [11, 163, 165]. Most patients with successful restoration of renal function have undergone surgical repair within 20 hours [11, 29, 90] but cases have shown restoration of function with surgery after as long as 33 days of anuria [1]. The observations in the prior case and the spontaneous recovery of renal function after several weeks [29, 61] indicate that surgical repair may be indicated for an extended time after the injury. When successful restoration of renal function has followed surgical revascularization, autotransplantation [42] and resection of the damaged portion of the renal artery with a saphenous vein graft [92] have been the surgical procedures most commonly employed. In cases with renal infarction and with unsuccessful or no attempt at revascularization, nephrectomy has been recommended for symptoms of ileus, fever, pain, or hypertension [10]. On the other hand, others have recommended conservative nonintervention following renal trauma [115, 173]; few long-term conse-

Some of the work was supported by research funds from the Veterans Administration.

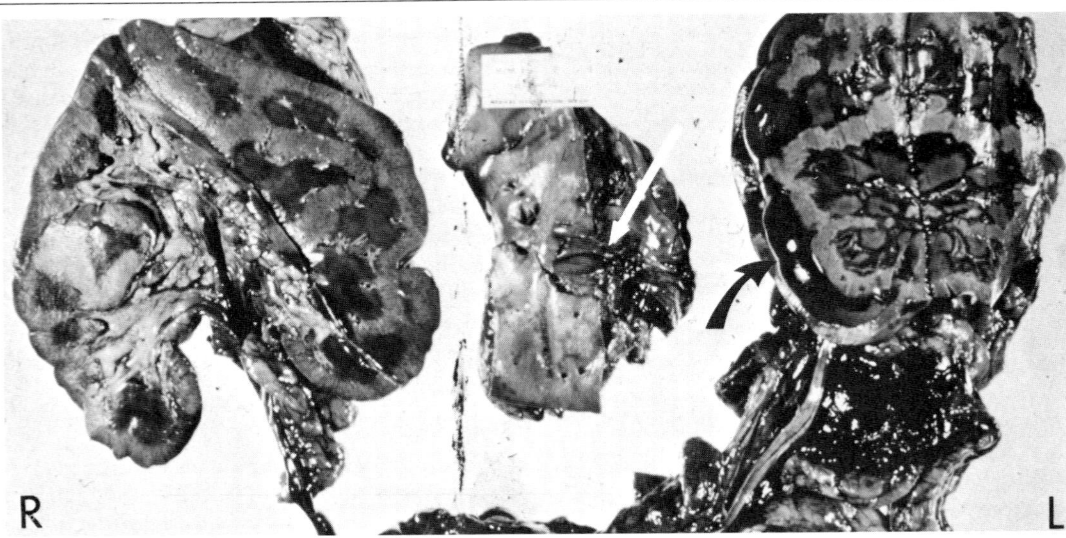

Fig. 77-1. Kidneys from a 41-year-old man with blunt trauma to the abdomen and fractures of the pelvis and femur due to an automobile accident. Laparotomy revealed intraabdominal bleeding and a ruptured spleen, and there was a typical course of oliguric acute renal failure. Nine days later, the patient died suddenly from fat emboli to the brain. Postmortem examination revealed thrombosis of the left renal artery (white arrow), a perirenal hematoma (curved black arrow), and infarction of the left kidney. The right kidney showed histologic features of acute tubular necrosis.

quences were noted after unilateral renal trauma [115], although diagnostic procedures to separate the specific types of renal damage were not carried out [115]; hence, many of these patients may have had milder types of renal injury. Intraarterial streptokinase has been utilized without success in one case report [171], although successful clot lysis and partial return of renal function were reported in one case of spontaneous unilateral renal artery thrombosis [122].

Thrombosis of the renal artery and renal infarction may also arise as a consequence of selective renal arteriography, although the patients reported had received large injections of highly concentrated contrast media [66]. With the concentrations and doses of contrast material employed more recently, there have been no reports of such cases. Renal arterial thrombosis with renal infarction and hemorrhage can occur spontaneously in patients with polyarteritis nodosa [73, 159]; under such conditions, the patient may have vascular collapse with marked flank pain and abdominal tenderness.

Renal infarction may arise from a thrombus dislodged from an aneurysm of the renal artery, leading to flank pain and hematuria [167]. Other rarer causes of renal artery occlusion and infarction include syphilis [74, 126] and other inflammatory diseases, such as phycomycosis [142], and cases have occurred following strenuous aerobic exercise [105]. Spontaneous renal artery thrombosis has been reported in association with intravenous injection of cocaine [67, 176], in a patient with neurofibromatosis [36], and as a result of an infiltrating urothelial carcinoma of the renal pelvis [70]. It has also occurred in association with the nephrotic syndrome [123], with the condition presumably arising as a consequence of the hypercoagulable state [123]; renal artery thrombosis has also occurred in newborn infants [178]. Acute renal failure has developed as a consequence of atherosclerotic occlusion of the renal artery in a patient with a solitary kidney; moreover, renal function rapidly improved after percutaneous transluminal recanalization [14]. Renal infarcts have been reported with sickle cell anemia [59, 68], in the loin-pain hematuria syndrome [132], and without any known cause [74, 132]; however, the methods of evaluation of some patients in the past were less discriminating than the procedures used more recently.

Patients with a functioning renal transplant may develop thrombosis of the renal artery [130]; this may develop because of the greater susceptibility of certain varieties of vascular anastomoses constructed between the iliac and renal arteries or because of unusual pressure on the graft. This type of thrombosis can occur owing to pressure from an automobile seat belt or following prolonged pressure to the graft site that may occur with positioning of the patient for certain surgical procedures, such as a total hip arthroplasty [181]. Cyclosporine therapy may predispose to renal artery thrombosis [139], and renal artery thrombosis has been reported to occur more commonly in renal allograft vessels when lupus anticoagulant is present [95].

Traumatic thrombosis of a segmental branch of the renal artery can also occur, and such a lesion can be identified more readily with radionuclide studies or accentuated computed tomography than with intravenous urography [87, 88]. Such a lesion may be detected quite commonly when angiography is done routinely after abdominal trauma [15]. If renal surgery is not required for a separate matter, the optimal treatment is conservative, nonoperative management [15, 23]. However, such a lesion must be distinguished from thrombosis of the main renal artery.

Thromboembolism of the Renal Arteries

The majority of emboli to the major renal arteries are associated with cardiac disease and arrhythmias, atrial fibrillation being the most common [74]. Emboli may occur following a myocardial infarction [74, 89] or from a mural thrombus or ventricular aneurysm [74]. Rheumatic valvular disease is a predisposing factor to thromboembolism of the kidney in a significant fraction of cases [89, 130]. Prosthetic heart valves can generate thrombi that can be the source of small emboli; in one case, renal failure arose from embolization of a disc from a prosthetic mitral valve [147]. Prior to the use of antibiotics, renal emboli often occurred as a consequence of subacute bacterial endocarditis; such cases were rarely diagnosed during life and were only noted at postmortem examination [74]. Under unusual circumstances, paradoxical renal emboli can pass from the venous system into the arterial tree through patent interatrial or interventricular septal defects [53]. Embolism to the renal artery has been reported to arise from tumors [120], and peripheral emboli to the kidney can arise from an aneurysm of the renal artery [97]. Embolism involving both the renal artery and the aorta has occurred as a complication of percutaneous intraarterial catheterization and aortography [107]. Iatrogenic embolism of the kidneys has been produced to control renal bleeding following a renal biopsy [155], and embolic renal infarcts have been induced in an effort to arrest the growth of renal malignancies [9, 128].

PATHOLOGY OF RENAL INFARCTION

When the main renal artery is occluded by an embolus, massive infarction of the entire kidney may result [68]; more commonly, renal function ceases but the kidney may remain viable because of the existence of collateral circulation [155]. Studies of experimental renal infarction in animals have shown that the kidney initially becomes darker in color with a grayish-red surface; this corresponds to increased numbers of red blood cells in glomerular and intertubular capillaries. There may be a rim of polymorphonuclear leukocytes surrounding the dead zone area, and the cellular cytoplasm then becomes abnormal. Subsequently, the polymorphonuclear leukocytes disappear, and the tubules become necrotic. At the margins of the infarction, the necrosis may be associated with proliferation of glomerular epithelial cells, and the necrosis may occupy only part of a glomerular tuft; moreover, the proliferation may be intense and produce an epithelial crescent [68]. Late changes involve partial or complete sclerosis of the glomeruli with atrophy and fibrosis of the tubules.

The ultimate course of experimental infarcts has been shown to depend on their initial size [94]. In rabbits with infarcts less than 5 mm in diameter initially, no infarct could be detected grossly after 2 weeks, and there was no fibrous scarring of the infarcted area; the histologic changes varied from slight atrophy to normal. Infarcts greater than 5 mm in diameter showed typical features of infarction after 2 weeks, and the degree of scarring depended on the initial size of the infarct. Whether a similar evolution occurs with renal infarcts of different sizes in man is uncertain; however, the absence of major clinical signs and symptoms following multiple small infarcts may be due to the complete healing noted above.

CLINICAL FEATURES OF RENAL ARTERIAL EMBOLIZATION

The clinical features of renal arterial embolization (Table 77-1) vary substantially, depending on (1) whether there is occlusion of both renal arteries or occlusion of the artery supplying a solitary kidney, (2) whether the embolism occurs in a single kidney with a contralateral functioning kidney, or (3) whether the embolus is peripheral and causes only a small segmental infarct. Acute anuria (urine volume < 50 ml/day) may be the presenting feature in patients following total occlusion of both vessels or occlusion of the main renal artery to a solitary kidney [120]. However, anuria or marked oliguria may occur and last for several days with unilateral embolization; presumably, this occurs because of arteriolar spasm of the unaffected kidney [89]. Patients commonly experience varying degrees of abdominal or flank pain, often with nausea and vomiting. The pain is often dull and unrelenting; it may be severe enough to lead a patient to seek medical attention. In as many as 25 percent of cases, flank pain is absent; hence, there may be no findings to direct the physician to consider the kidney as the source of the acute illness [89]. Gross hematuria can occur, but it is not usual. In some patients there is a history of prior embolic disease to other organs, and a small but significant fraction of these patients have had a previous embolism to the contralateral kidney [89].

Examination often discloses some degree of abdominal or flank tenderness. Abdominal tenderness and signs of peritoneal irritation may be present [89]. Fever of 101° to 103°F is common, and chills may occur; however, the fever may not develop until the second or third day after the onset of symptoms [167]. Hypertension, which may be severe and refractory to treatment, is prominent in a small fraction of cases [13, 94, 96]. Other organ systems, such as the brain or extremities, should be evaluated for signs of arterial embolization; however, these are usually absent. Cardiac arrhythmias, particularly atrial fibrillation, are common, and the presence of rheumatic valvular disease or a recent myocardial infarction should alert a clinician to the possibility of this disorder.

The diagnosis of thromboembolic disease to the kidney is not usually made at the onset of symptoms, and the disorder was correctly identified on the day of hospitalization in less than 30 percent of cases [89]; the initial diagnoses may include nephrolithiasis, pyelonephritis, acute myocardial infarction, acute cholecystitis, acute tubular necrosis, and congestive heart failure [89]. Thus, a patient with nausea, vomiting, abdominal tenderness, and signs of peritoneal irritation was mistakenly diagnosed as having acute cholecystitis and underwent cholecystectomy [89].

Laboratory findings include leukocytosis, varying from

Table 77-1. Clinical and laboratory features of thromboembolic disease of the kidney

Feature	Approximate incidence*
History and physical findings	
Pain and tenderness (flank, abdominal, chest, or back)	75%
Nausea and vomiting	50%
Gross hematuria	20%
Cardiac disease (myocardial infarction, atrial fibrillation, rheumatic valvular disease)	90%
Laboratory features	
Leukocytosis (11,000–32,000/mm^3)	95%
Microscopic hematuria (> 15 erythrocytes per high-power field)	90%
Pyuria (> 10 leukocytes per high-power field)	80%
Proteinuria (1+ to 4+)	95%
Increased enzymes (LDH, SGOT, SGPT, alkaline phosphatase)	95–100%
Special diagnostic procedures	**Finding**
Intravenous urogram	Decr. or absent function; delayed appearance
Renal ultrasound	No obstruction; rarely, wedge-shaped mass
Isotope renal flow scan	Decreased flow to all or part of kidney
Computed tomography (with contrast material)	Area of decreased accentuation; cortical rim of accentuation

*Refer to text. Abbreviations: LDH, lactic dehydrogenase; SGOT, glutamic oxaloacetic transaminase; SGPT, glutamic pyruvic transaminase; Decr., decreased.

15,000 to 30,000 per cubic millimeter; the urinalysis shows proteinuria, and most patients have microscopic hematuria [89]. The presence of acute anuria (urine volume < 50 ml/day) suggests but does not prove the presence of bilateral emboli or an embolus to a solitary kidney. There are few data reported on urinary indices, but a very low urinary sodium concentration has been observed (Fig. 77-2), a finding that may be consistent with the marked hypoperfusion of the partially functioning nephrons [102]. Increments in serum lactic dehydrogenase are almost universal, and elevated levels of serum glutamic-oxaloacetic transaminase (SGOT) and glutamic-pyruvic transaminase are common. Also, the degree of elevation of lactic dehydrogenase is greater than that of either transaminases [37, 89]. Moderate elevations of alkaline phosphatase occur in 30 to 50 percent of cases, and this abnormality may persist for up to 10 days [51, 89]. The course of changes of various serum enzymes in a patient with thromboembolic disease is shown in Fig. 77-3. Certain urinary enzymes are markedly increased following a renal artery embolism. Urinary lysozyme excretion is increased up to 5 to 6 times normal for several days [37], and other enzymes are increased to a greater extent. The urinary excretion of alanine aminopeptidase (AAP) and *N*-acetyl-β-D-glucosaminidase (NAG), expressed per creatinine excretion, is increased as much as 7 to 10 times above the normal range, and the augmented excretion persists for 2 to 3 weeks or longer [37].

Intravenous urography usually shows decreased or absent function of the affected kidney with a marked delay in the appearance of contrast material in the collecting system (Fig. 77-4). Ultrasound of the kidney is useful to exclude obstruction as a cause of decreased urinary output [167], making it unnecessary to carry out retrograde urographic evaluation. Occasionally, ultrasonography reveals a focal echogenic renal mass that has a triangular appearance suggesting an infarct [41, 118]. More commonly, renal ultrasonography reveals no mass and no changes in echogenicity [3, 140]. The intravenous administration of the sonographic contrast agent perfluorooctylbromide (PFOB), which remains within the vascular space for several hours and increases the echogenicity of the perfused tissues, was evaluated in rabbits 24 hours after partial renal infarcts [28]. In sonograms obtained without PFOB, the infarcts could not be identified; however, following PFOB administration all infarcts were readily and correctly identified by the sonographer. The application of this technique to clinical practice will be followed with interest.

Retrograde urography, often done to exclude nephrolithiasis or the possibility of ureteral obstruction, offers little for the diagnosis of embolism; however, if it is performed, it reveals a normal collecting system, but urine flow may be absent or decreased [167]. Rarely, gross hematuria will be found arising from one ureter [3]. Isotopic flow scans usually show absent or markedly reduced perfusion of the affected kidney or kidneys, as shown in Fig. 77-5 [49, 65]; however, such a decrease in perfusion may be nonspecific [51]. Isotopic flow scans, with the injection of a high-activity bolus of technetium 99m (^{99m}Tc)–labeled agent, such as dimethylenetriamine pentaacetic acid (DTPA), and a scintillation camera allow visualization of the abdominal aorta and kidneys during the first 30 seconds after injection. Such a flow scan usually shows absent or markedly reduced perfusion of the affected kidney(s), as shown in Fig. 77-5 [49, 65]; however, such an apparent decrease in "perfusion" can be nonspecific [51]. The infusion of ^{99m}Tc-labeled 2,3-dimer-

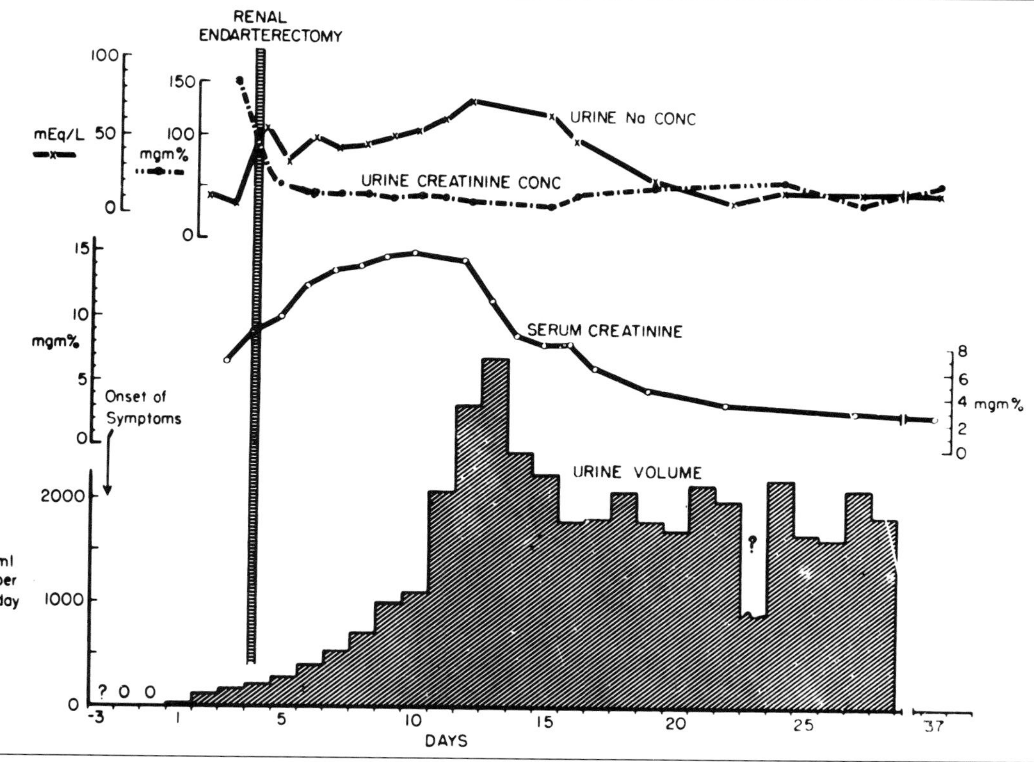

Fig. 77-2. Course of a 56-year-old woman with abrupt onset of anuria and right lower quadrant and low back pain; she had atrial fibrillation and mitral stenosis due to rheumatic heart disease. One year earlier she had undergone a left nephrectomy for malignant hypertension (earlier, she had suffered stroke and blindness of the left eye due to an embolism). A diagnosis of thromboembolism to the renal artery was confirmed by aortography (see Fig. 77-7), and surgery was performed with removal of the embolus and endarterectomy. The fractional excretion of sodium was 0.36% before surgery and increased to 7.3% after removal of the thrombus. There was ultimate recovery from acute tubular necrosis, as indicated. (Adapted from Lessman et al., case 7 [89].)

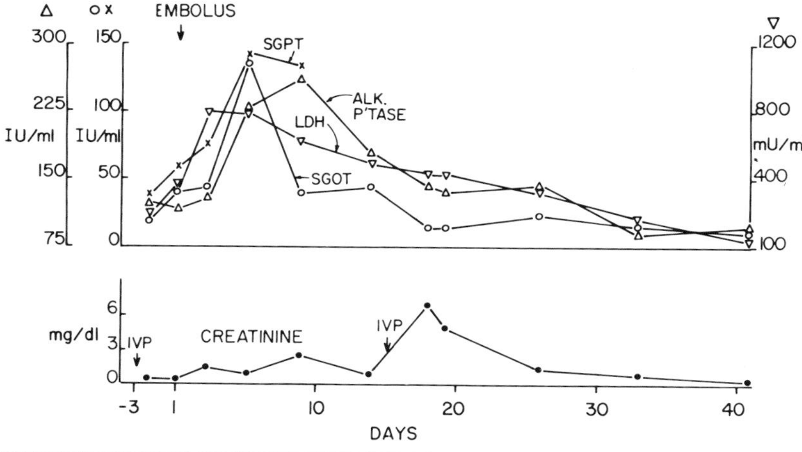

Fig. 77-3. Serial serum levels of glutamic-oxaloacetic transaminase (SGOT, ○), glutamic-pyruvic transaminase (SGPT, χ), lactic dehydrogenase (LDH, ▽), alkaline phosphatase (alk p'tase, △), and creatinine (●) in a 62-year-old man with thromboembolism to a single kidney 10 days after a myocardial infarction. Right flank and chest pain and lower abdominal tenderness appeared on day 1. The patient also exhibited an increase of serum creatinine following the second intravenous pyelogram (IVP). (Case 11 from Lessman et al. [89].)

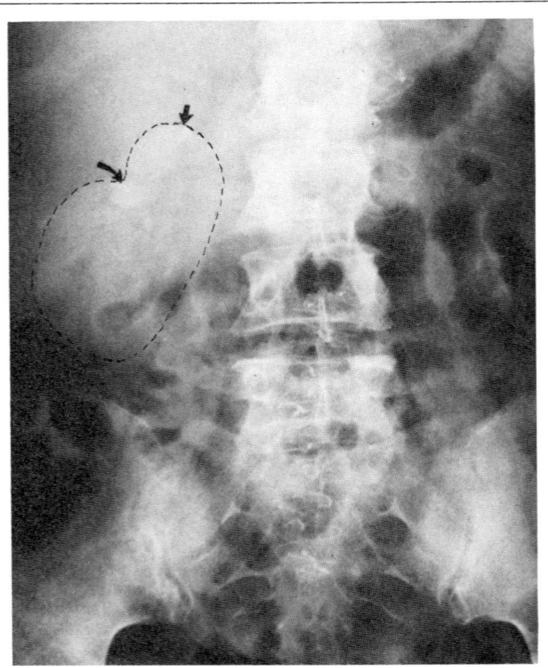

Fig. 77-4. Abdominal radiograph in a patient who had thromboembolism to a solitary kidney; taken 24 hours after an intravenous urogram showed no function in the remaining kidney. There was the delayed but faint appearance of contrast media in the renal pelvis (curved arrow). The renal outline is indicated by a dashed line. This patient's course is shown in Fig. 77-2.

captosuccinic acid (DMSA), which binds to the renal tubules, permits more precise definition of the functional morphology of the kidney and can identify infarcts that arise from embolism [48], as is shown in Fig. 77-6. Computed tomography, carried out with the injection of contrast material, may reveal areas of decreased enhancement and sometimes a thin rim of cortical accentuation of the contrast material [35, 131]. Computed tomographic scanning without injection of contrast material is less discriminating [64]. The view that persistent, wedge-shaped, low-density lesions on computed tomograms are specific for a renal infarct [55, 177] may be incorrect; thus, a patient with oliguric acute renal failure had multiple low-density lesions with a high-intensity rim on computed tomograms with contrast medium. When the patient died, postmortem examination revealed the recovery phase of acute tubular necrosis with no evidence of renal infarction. It was suggested that this lesion found by computed tomography can arise from patchy vasoconstriction and not require the presence of renal infarction [136]. Magnetic resonance imaging, particularly when done with an enhancing agent, may also be useful to identify renal infarcts [78]. Further studies may clarify the place for these various diagnostic procedures.

Renal arteriography and aortography are the definitive methods for the diagnosis of renal artery embolism, as shown in Fig. 77-7 [120, 167]. These procedures should be undertaken only if active therapeutic intervention is being considered (i.e., bilateral embolectomy or unilateral embolectomy in a solitary kidney with markedly impaired renal function). Because of the risk of acute renal damage from the injection of contrast ma-

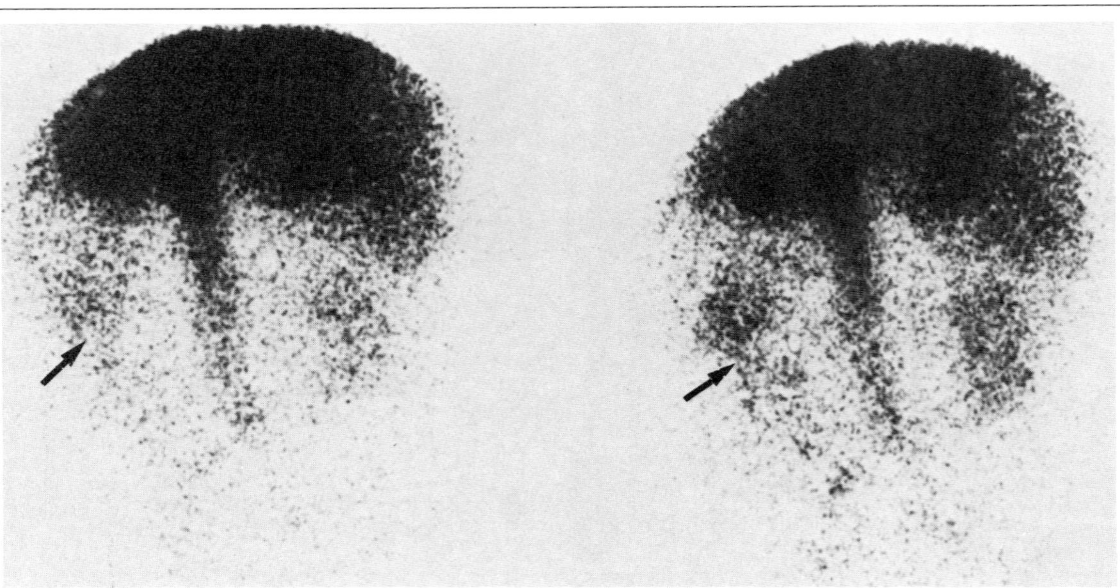

Fig. 77-5. A renal flow scan carried after the injection of technetium 99m DTPA. These scanning images were obtained 36 to 42 seconds after the injection. There is lack of perfusion of the lower part of the right kidney (arrow), and a segmental infarction of the right kidney was subsequently verified. (Courtesy of Drs. Coyle and William Blahd, Nuclear Medicine Service, Veterans Administration Center, West Los Angeles, Wadsworth Division.)

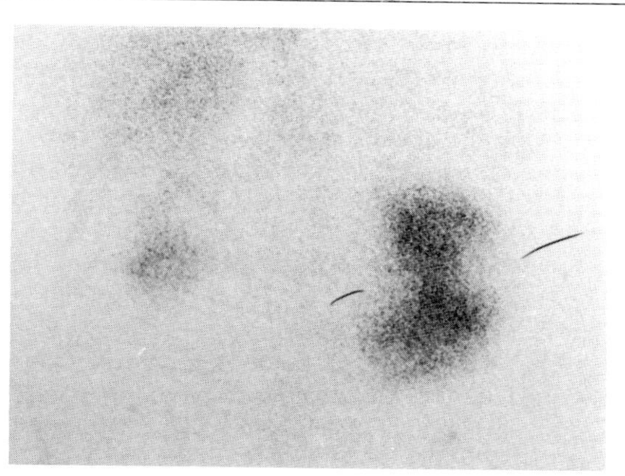

Fig. 77-6. Renal scan with technetium 99m–labeled DMSA showing evidence of segmental renal infarcts of the left kidney of a 74-year-old man who was hospitalized with abrupt appearance of a supraventricular tachycardia. There was a progressive rise in serum creatinine from a baseline value of 2.2 to 4.4 mg/dl over 5 successive days. He was never oliguric; urinalysis showed 2+ proteinuria with an occasional hyaline cast. His white blood cell count rose from $10,200/mm^3$ on admission to $15,400/mm^3$ after 4 days; there was no eosinophilia. His SGPT (ALT) rose from 33 to 42 U/L and his LDH from 49 to 173 U/L. A technetium-labeled EHDP "flow" scan disclosed markedly reduced flow bilaterally but more marked on the left than the right; however, there was no evidence of focal ischemia, and the DMSA scan was therefore done. There was a history of emboli to his feet, with the serum creatinine rising from 1.2 to 2.2 mg/dl in association with an acute myocardial infarction several years earlier. On the basis of the DMSA scan, a diagnosis of thromboembolism to the kidney was made; the patient received anticoagulants and his serum creatinine gradually fell to 2.4 mg/dl.

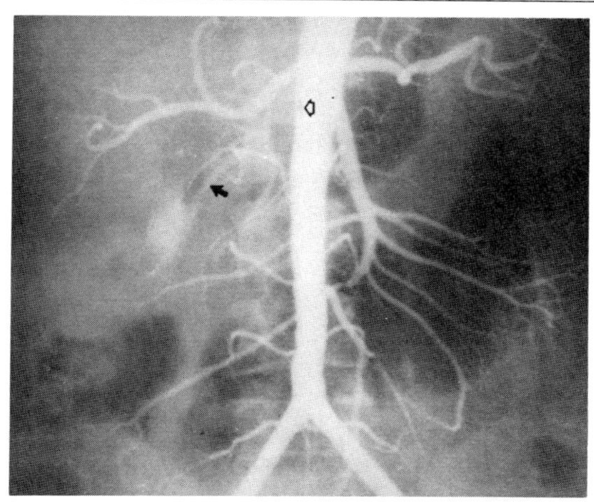

Fig. 77-7. Aortogram of a patient with an embolism to a solitary right kidney; her course is illustrated in Fig. 77-2. There is a faint lucency projecting into the lumen of the aorta (open arrow) at the site of an embolus to the right renal artery. The distal renal artery filled faintly (solid arrow), presumably via collaterals.

terial [2, 110], the dosage of such material should be kept to a minimum, and the noninvasive, safer procedures noted above should be done first. Thus ultrasonography, a renal flow scan, or a DMSA scan should be done initially; urography and computed tomography with the administration of contrast material may be done next; finally, arteriography or digital subtraction arteriography should be reserved for patients who are considered for thrombolytic therapy or surgical intervention or in cases that present special diagnostic problems [69, 97]. In some cases there may be difficulty in making the diagnosis of a segmental renal infarction; thus intravenous urography, ultrasonography, computed tomography, and radionuclide renography may all suggest a vascular mass, and the arteriogram may not reveal the thrombus in a segmental vessel. If a DMSA scan is nonrevealing, a renal biopsy, either percutaneous with guidance from computed tomography or an open biopsy at the time of surgery, may be the only means of making a specific diagnosis and excluding the presence of a malignancy [3]. Calcification has been reported in the site of a recent renal infarction, and the presence of such calcification may suggest a renal neoplasm [69].

THERAPY

The occurrence of segmental or unilateral renal embolization with little reduction in renal function can be managed effectively with anticoagulation with warfarin [89, 109]. Heparin should be administered intravenously, followed by oral anticoagulation. When oliguria exists due to bilateral embolization or embolization to a solitary kidney, there is disagreement about the optimal therapy [86, 167]; moreover, the availability of thrombolytic therapy, either with streptokinase or recombinant tissue-type plasminogen activator (rt-PA), has added to the therapeutic approaches available. The use of urokinase or streptokinase in 26 cases reported between 1979 and 1987 was reviewed by Mügge et al. [111], and other successful cases have been reported since that time [19]. In all but 2 of the cases receiving streptokinase, there was recanalization of the affected artery or branch, but renal function remained impaired in most of them. Also, in 4 of the 27 cases, percutaneous angioplasty was done in addition to the streptokinase infusion. In a review of patients treated between 1970 and 1982, Nicholas and DeMuth [112] considered both patient mortality and the salvage of the affected kidney. The salvage of renal function following oral anticoagulants or operative intervention varied from 67 to 97 percent, with no statistical difference between the two forms of therapy. With bilateral embolization or embolization to the main artery of a solitary kidney, renal salvage may be somewhat less following anticoagulation, although the number of patients managed in that manner was small. Earlier reports indicated an operative mortality as high as 25 percent following vascular reconstruction [109]; more recent reports have indicated an operative mortality of 11 percent [112]. Success with the intraarterial infusion of streptokinase has been reported [44, 143], and percutaneous transluminal angioplasty has been employed effectively, although the risk of peripheral embolization to the extremities following this procedure must be considered. Maxwell and Mispireta [99] combined the angiographic technique for the removal of the embolus from the renal artery with direct extraction of the embolus through a femoral arteriotomy.

On the basis of their review, Nicholas and DeMuth [112] developed an algorithm for the management of renal artery embolism: With unilateral embolism and a contralateral intact kidney, they recommend initial therapy with intraarterial streptokinase and/or transluminal angioplasty, followed by anticoagulation. They suggested that there is little or no benefit from surgery whether or not the medical therapy was successful. When there is an embolus to a solitary kidney or bilateral emboli, intraarterial streptokinase and/or transluminal angioplasty is recommended; if this results in effective restoration of renal blood flow, long-term anticoagulation is recommended. If there is failure of streptokinase or transluminal angioplasty, surgical reconstruction is considered to correct the arterial occlusion. Further experience with this approach is required.

Particular attention should be paid to the cause of embolization; long-term anticoagulant therapy may be required in some patients, since embolization to other vital organs, including the brain, has led to the sudden death of patients who had been successfully treated for renal arterial embolic disease [89, 112].

Renal Artery Aneurysms

Renal artery aneurysms are uncommon vascular abnormalities that are asymptomatic in most patients [169]. Clinical problems arise when they produce renovascular hypertension, when rupture occurs [124], when they lead to thrombosis and infarction [154], or when they cause renal embolism. The aneurysms are saccular in 80 percent and mostly occur in the main renal artery or at the bifurcation of the main artery [124, 169]; less than 10 percent are within the renal parenchyma [159]. Less commonly they are fusiform, have multiple stenoses and dilatations, or arise as dissecting aneurysms [124]; 61 percent involved the right kidney and 7 percent were bilateral in one survey of 83 patients found to have renal artery aneurysms among 8,525 Swedish patients having renal angiograms for all reasons [169]. The distribution between males and females was approximately equal; patients from age 4 to 86 years were affected. Renal artery aneurysms are associated with fibrous dysplasia for the most part, but they may be associated with arteriosclerosis or be posttraumatic [124]. Also, mycotic renal artery aneurysms can arise from bacterial endocarditis [38].

The most dangerous complication of a renal artery aneurysm is rupture. Estimates of this complication run as high as 14 to 30 percent [24a, 77]; the mortality may reach 80 percent [77]. There is a remarkable tendency for renal arterial aneurysms to rupture during pregnancy [93], with at least 19 cases reported [27, 146]; most of them occur during the last trimester [158]. Cases of rupture have also occurred during the postpartum period. Moreover, renal artery rupture has occurred during pregnancy in a renal transplant recipient [133a]. Love, Robinette, and Vernon [93] suggest that the pathogenic factors leading to rupture of a renal artery aneurysm during pregnancy include increased blood flow, particularly during the last trimester, the effect of steroid hormones on the vasculature, and increased intraabdominal pressure. Shoon et al. [146] stress the role of physical strain on the pelvic vasculature caused by the enlarged uterus, particularly in certain positions; this produces a "coarctation phenomenon" and leads to increased blood pressure above the uterus [103].

Patients with rupture of a renal artery aneurysm present with flank pain, vascular collapse, and shock; the abdominal size may increase or a flank mass may be detectable; the Grey Turner sign may appear. Hematuria may be a helpful finding in some cases, but its absence does not exclude this diagnosis.

Hypertension is often associated with renal artery aneurysms [179], but the high blood pressure can be the cause of the aneurysm or the aneurysm may be the renovascular mechanism of the hypertension [179]. It has been stated that this hypertension is often unresponsive to pharmacologic therapy [77]; however, many patients with renal artery aneurysms have no hypertension or few sequelae of hypertension [169]. A renovascular mechanism for hypertension has been documented with renal artery aneurysms [179], and appropriate surgical therapy often results in "cure" or marked improvement of the hypertension [116, 162, 179]. The topic of renovascular hypertension is reviewed in Chap. 55.

The only definitive method to diagnose a renal artery aneurysm is angiography, but for various reasons it may not be carried out. Computed tomography and radionuclide scanning may be useful when employed in the initial stages of the evaluation.

Despite the reported cases of renal artery rupture, the occurrence of this event in patients with known renal artery aneurysms is quite unusual. Tham et al. [169] point out that no deaths were attributed to ruptured renal arteries in 36,656 subjects autopsied in southern Sweden over a 10-year period, and no case of a ruptured renal artery aneurysm was found among 19,600 autopsied subjects in New York [100]. Also, a follow-up, which averaged 4 years, of 69 nonoperated patients with documented renal artery aneurysm revealed no deaths related to the aneurysm over this period of time [169]. Such observations indicate that the occurrence of rupture is quite rare.

A number of surgeons have attempted to provide a guide to the criteria for surgical intervention of renal artery aneurysm [12, 18, 100, 116]. The more commonly accepted criteria for surgical intervention include: (1) size greater than 1.5 to 2.0 cm; (2) the absence of calcifications, although rupture of a calcified saccular aneurysm can occur [151]; (3) occurrence in young females who may be pregnant or have a possibility of childbearing; (4) demonstration of serial expansion of an aneurysm by repeated angiography, computed tomography, or ultrasonography; (5) presentation of the aneurysm with symptoms of pain and an expanding mass, with or without hematuria—features that may suggest eminent rupture; (6) the presence of an aneurysm in a solitary kidney with the potential of embolization from a thrombus or a risk of dissection; and (7) hypertension with renal artery narrowing from an aneurysm, particularly with lateralization of renin levels.

The surgical approach varies with the type and location of the lesion. It would appear that nephrectomy should be reserved for patients with failure of an earlier revascularization, those with severe atrophy of one kidney, or as emergency surgery for spontaneous rupture and cardiovascular collapse [18]. With a variety of complex surgical repair methods employed for in situ vascular repair and with the use of aortofemoral bypass and inventive vascular reconstructive techniques, there is still a risk that nephrectomy will be required. Prior to the introduction of ex vivo vascular repair and autotransplantation, a nephrectomy was required in 7 to 30 percent of operated cases [34, 100, 162, 166]. Brugg-Asperheim et al. [18] pointed out that a complex situation with multiple arterial branches is better repaired with "bench" surgery. Novick et al. [113, 114] described autotransplantation and microsurgery in several surgical reports; avoiding "warm ischemia" by cold perfusion and microsurgery and use of in vitro techniques have reduced or eliminated the need for nephrectomy, with little risk of serious functional renal impairment [46]. However, Ortenberg et al. [116] recommend that extracorporeal microvascular branch arterial reconstruction be reserved for patients with complex intrarenal aneurysms.

Dissecting Lesions of the Renal Artery

Renal artery dissecting lesions are uncommon; such dissections can cause either acute or chronic occlusion of the renal artery and lead to malignant hypertension and/or loss of renal function [39]. Chronic renal artery dissection most commonly manifests itself as renovascular hypertension [157]; this problem is considered in Chap. 55. Acute renal artery dissection may be spontaneous, with atherosclerosis, fibromuscular dysplasia, or both processes being the predisposing factor, or the dissection can be iatrogenic and follow various angiographic procedures using guidewires, catheters, or angioplasty balloons [157]. Rarely, dissections can occur after blunt trauma to the kidney [52]. There are also a small number of acute dissections that are classified as agonal, in that they are detected at autopsy and showed no clinical features during life [157].

With an acute dissection, most patients have new or much worsened hypertension; flank pain is common and hematuria sometimes occurs. Headache may occur, perhaps as a result of the hypertension. In some cases, and more commonly in those who develop the lesion due to an angiographic procedure, there are no symptoms or signs other than the antecedent hypertension [134, 157].

The spontaneous dissecting lesions are about 3 times more common in males than females [39, 134, 157], and there is a predilection toward involvement of the right renal artery. Approximately 20 to 30 percent of cases are bilateral [39, 134]; renal artery dissection is most common in the 40- to 60-year age range, although patients as young as 20 to 30 years old can be affected.

Urinalysis shows proteinuria in some cases; only 20 to 35 percent of patients exhibit hematuria despite the importance of this finding in directing attention to this disorder [39, 157]. Impaired renal function, as indicated by serum creatinine levels above 1.5 mg per deciliter, was present in only 9 and 33 percent of two recent series [39, 156], although impaired renal function was more common in cases collected in earlier reports [157].

Intravenous urography may aid in the exclusion of ureteral obstruction; it may show decreased renal function, reduced renal size, delayed appearance or hyperconcentration of the contrast material, or even be normal. Selective arteriography, which is required for the diagnosis, reveals irregularity of the renal artery, and there may be aneurysmal dilatation associated with segmental stenosis. There is a predilection for the dissection to extend distally to the first bifurcation of the renal artery, and there may be cuffing at the branches. Follow-up arteriography often shows some degree of reversibility [167], and improved renal function and normal blood pressure have followed effective antihypertensive therapy only [106]. Renal function is generally relatively well maintained. In approximately 50 percent of cases, there was lateralization of renal vein renin levels, and the isotope renogram showed unilateral abnormalities in a similar fraction [39].

The appropriate therapy should depend on the severity of the hypertension and its ease of management. Edwards et al. [39] noted adequate response of the hypertension to medical therapy in the majority of patients; others [52] have emphasized the importance of vascular reconstruction when it can be carried out; indeed, "bench" surgery with autotransplantation is often the procedure that is done [156, 159]. However, a substantial fraction of the operated patients ultimately underwent uninephrectomy [52, 134].

Atheroembolic Disease of the Kidney

The clinical features of atheroembolic disease affecting the kidney differ significantly from those with renal infarction produced by thromboembolism of the major arteries. With atheroembolic disease, the injury to the kidney arises from occlusion of multiple small arteries; the latter leads to functional renal impairment that may be insidious and often lacks the clinical features of renal infarction. The vessels that are occluded are generally 150 to 200 microns in diameter, and the arcuate, interlobular, and terminal arteries are most commonly involved [40, 62, 82]. Pathologic examination of the occluded vessels reveals characteristic biconvex, needle-shaped clefts from cholesterol crystals present within the lumen of the affected artery (Fig. 77-8). In fresh samples, the crystals are birefringent, and they can be identified under polarized light. Specific histochemical methods that are specific for cholesterol can be employed for the identification of cholesterol [82].

During the early period after atheroembolization, cholesterol crystals may be surrounded by eosinophilic material with little inflammatory reaction in the sur-

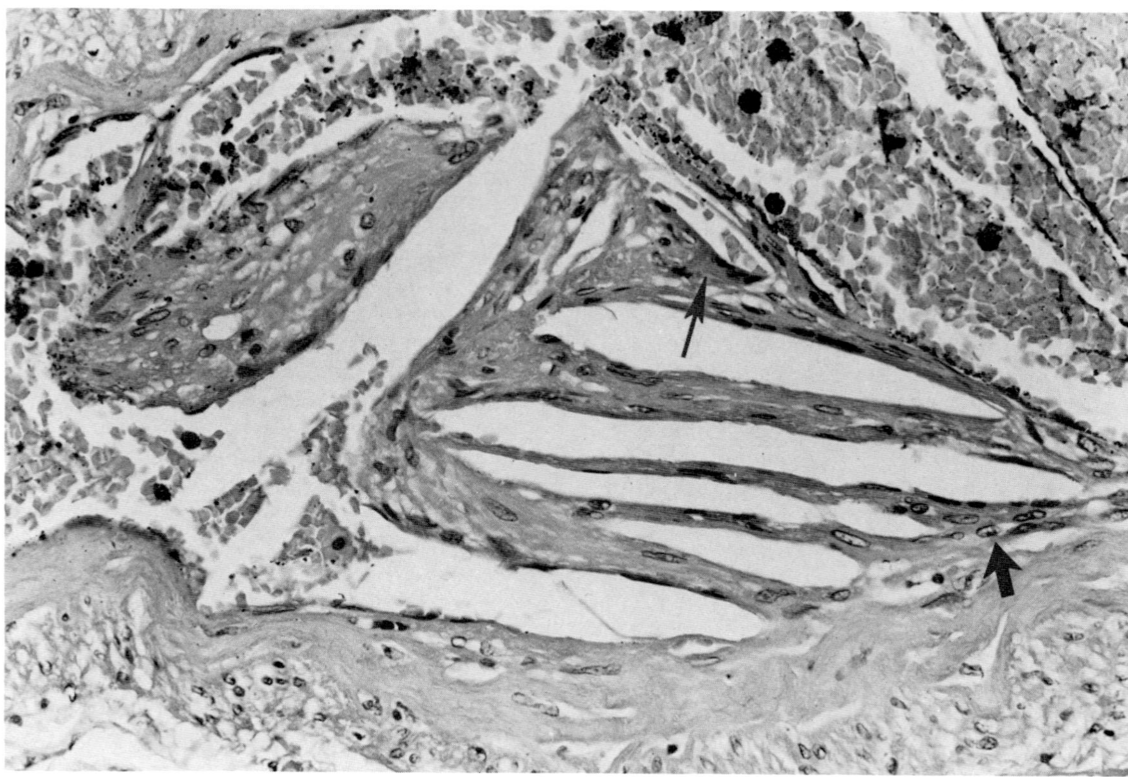

Fig. 77-8. Section of a renal artery containing the needle-shaped clefts of an atheroembolism to a renal arteriole. There are foreign-body giant cells (arrows) surrounding the cholesterol clefts. (Courtesy of Dr. Jerome Kassirer [83].)

rounding interstitium. Subsequently, there is intimal thickening, and the appearance of macrophages and multinucleated giant cells of the foreign-body type (Fig. 77-8). Later there may be marked intimal thickening with concentric fibrosis. There is no necrosis of the arterial wall despite the presence of a typical foreign-body reaction [82]. The occlusion of multiple small vessels from atheroemboli produces patchy areas of renal ischemia. Atrophy is usually predominant, and small areas of infarction can occur. The alterations produced by ischemia commonly evolve to produce a wedge-shaped lesion that involves all components of the renal cortex. With this atrophy, the glomeruli appear ischemic and may become hyalinized; occasionally, cholesterol crystals are found in glomerular capillaries. The tubules become atrophic, and the lesions may be distributed in a wedge-shaped pattern radiating toward the capsule. Grossly, the kidney may be reduced in size with a rough granular surface and wedge-shaped scars. The lesions produced by embolization with cholesterol crystals in experimental animals closely parallel the pathologic features observed in human tissue [57, 117, 161].

PATHOGENETIC FACTORS

When atheroembolic emboli occur, the resultant renal impairment arises from recurrent and multiple episodes of cholesterol microembolization. The features of the tissue reaction that surrounds the occluded vessels resemble the reaction to a foreign body, and the debris and cholesterol crystals found at the site of occlusion are identical to the material found in the severe atheromatous lesions observed in the aorta of these patients [40, 47, 133, 144]. Indeed, correlations have been shown between the incidence of atheroembolic renal disease and the severity of aortic atherosclerosis [133, 170]. Thus the internal surface of the aorta is commonly covered with atheromatous plaques that are shaggy and ulcerating and with fibrin and platelet thrombi [47, 58, 104, 144]. These thrombi are pliable and soft, and they can easily be dislodged. The intima may be completely eroded, revealing direct communications between an atheroma and the lumen of the aorta [62, 63, 80, 144].

Major predisposing factors are present in most cases of atheroembolic disease: Thus, manifestations or a history of significant atherosclerotic cardiovascular disease, aortic aneurysms, cerebrovascular disease, hypertension, renal failure, or diabetes were present in 86 percent of over 200 cases reviewed by Fine et al. [43]. Atheroemboli have also involved renal allografts [7, 79]. In fewer than 15 percent of reported cases, no preexisting disease was identified. Precipitating factors fall into three major categories: (1) various procedures involving vascular surgery, (2) numerous types of angiogram or arteriogram, and (3) therapy with anticoagulants. Thus, atheroembolic disease has occurred after aortic aneurysm resection, after coronary artery bypass graft [43], after carotid endarterectomy [31], and following renal artery angioplasty [43]. The interval between the onset of symptoms and such surgical procedures can vary from 1 to 14 days [31]. Various angiographic procedures can predispose to atheroemboli; the list includes aortogram, coronary angiography, and carotid and renal angiograms. The role of treatment with anticoagulant drugs or thrombolytic agents in predisposing to or actually precipitating thromboembolism is growing. Thus, 30 of the 68 patients who had at least one predisposing factor and were collected by Fine et al. [43] had been treated with anticoagulants; moreover, 4 of 14 patients reported by Dahlberg et al. [31] were receiving heparin or warfarin. The onset of symptoms was closely and temporally related to such treatment in a number of the cases [31, 76]. Atheroemboli have been reported in association with the intravenous administration of streptokinase [127, 148], including one patient who did not undergo angiography. It has been speculated that the inhibition of the further formation of thrombi or the dissolution of existing fibrin thrombi that overlie the ulcerated atheromas on the aorta or other vessels will predispose to the release of cholesterol crystals with subsequent embolization [104]. The appearance of this syndrome, with showers of cholesterol emboli being released into the lumen of the aorta or other vessels in association with anticoagulant therapy, may be coincidental, and the proof of a cause-and-effect relationship will be difficult. Occasionally, "spontaneous" atheroemboli may develop without any precipitating event [60, 80]. Emboli commonly occur in association with renal artery stenosis [172].

FEATURES OF THE CLINICAL SYNDROME

Atheroembolic diseases of the kidney (Table 77-2) are most common in patients over 60 years old, and the disease is rare in patients under 50 years of age. The disorder is more common in males than females [43], and for uncertain reasons, the syndrome is far more common in white than black patients [43, 137]. Evidence of aortic atherosclerosis is almost invariably present, and there is often evidence of symptomatic peripheral or cerebral vascular disease or a recent myocardial infarction. The peripheral pulses may be present and full, or they may be diminished or absent; vascular bruits are common. Proof of the diagnosis of atheroembolic disease is often made at postmortem examination, but the diagnosis can be made with the finding of cholesterol emboli

Table 77-2. Clinical and laboratory features in atheroembolic disease of the kidney

Feature	Approximate incidence*
History and physical findings	
Worsened and/or refractory hypertension	10–20%
Cholesterol plaques in renal arterioles	10–15%
Features of multisystem disease	Common
Strokes or transient ischemic episodes	
Gastrointestinal bleeding, abdominal pain	
Ischemia of digits (feet or hands)	
Livedo reticularis	
Progressive renal failure	
Weight loss	
Pancreatitis	
Predisposing factors	
Recent aortogram or angiogram	Common
Arteriosclerotic heart disease; generalized arteriosclerosis: cerebral artery or aorta; prior mild to moderate hypertension	
Recent anticoagulation or thrombolytic therapy	
Laboratory features	
Leukocytosis (10,000–20,000/mm^3)	25%
Eosinophilia (5–18%)	70–80%
Increased sedimentation rate	80–90%
Hypocomplementemia	50–70%
Proteinuria (1+ to 4+)	50–70%
Pyuria	> 50%
Hematuria	15%
Eosinophiluria	30%

Special diagnostic procedures	Finding
Biopsy of skin, muscle, or kidney	Emboli with cholesterol clefts and foreign-body-type giant cells

*Refer to text.

in histologic sections from skin, muscle, or renal biopsy [101]. Thus the specific diagnosis is often missed, although the clinical signs or features of multiorgan involvement often existed during life [20, 75, 82, 104, 133].

The organs that are frequently involved by atheroemboli include the kidneys, pancreas, gastrointestinal tract, spleen, and brain. The clinical features depend on which major organ is involved; thus permanent or transient focal neurologic defects occur in those with atheroembolic emboli to the brain; pancreatitis, either clinically overt or manifest only by an elevated plasma lipase or amylase, can occur when the pancreas is involved. Evidence of peripheral gangrene or hepatitis is common, and features of gastrointestinal ischemia with gastrointestinal bleeding may occur. An acute "surgical" abdomen may occur associated with a localized intestinal infarct with acute perforation. There may be involvement of the skeletal muscle or skin; thus ischemic necrosis of the toes may occur [75] with the "blue toe" syndrome [45, 180]; there may be marked livedo reticularis [26]. Renal involvement may be manifest by oliguric renal failure if there is extensive atheroembolism, or there may be an insidious and gradual decrease in renal function over a period of days to weeks [152]. The acute oliguric form may occur following aortic surgery or an angiographic study. Some patients with severe renal failure may require dialysis for some time, but renal function may be regained to a variable degree [22, 71, 152, 160]. The overall mortality from atheroembolism to the kidney has been high [82, 83], but the great majority of recognized cases were in autopsy series. The involvement of many organ systems and the likelihood of multiorgan failure combined with renal insufficiency undoubtedly contribute to the poor prognosis [160]. In some cases the blood pressure is markedly elevated and refractory to treatment [32]; more commonly, the hypertension is only moderate, and the finding of hypertension may antedate the atheroembolic episode.

The laboratory features are not particularly distinctive except to provide evidence to exclude the presence of other renal diseases. Occasionally, mild leukocytosis is present; moreover, significant eosinophilia may be common [21, 32, 75, 81, 121, 145]. The erythrocyte sedimentation rate is commonly quite elevated [26, 145], and hypocomplementemia has been observed [30]. Mild proteinuria is generally present and nephrotic-range proteinuria has been described [175]; microscopic hematuria occasionally occurs, and hyaline and granular casts may be found on urinalysis. Eosinophiluria has been described and may be common [138]. Few data are available on the biochemical characteristics of the urine in this syndrome. The lack of oliguria or a low urinary sodium concentration [22], which would be expected in conditions with substantial hypoperfusion of the kidney [102], is unexpected. An increase in the BUN-creatinine ratio in serum has been described [26]; this finding could be consistent with a decrease in the single nephron glomerular filtration rate, which would lead to enhanced urea reabsorption by the tubule [26]. Serum biochemical features similar to those described above under Renal Infarction, including elevated LDH, SGOT, SGPT, and alkaline phosphatase levels, are not common; however, such findings might be expected to occur in cases with marked atheromatous disease and rapidly progressive renal failure.

Occasional cases have shown increased renin generation from the more severely affected kidney [32], a finding indicating that the hypertension involves activation of the renin-angiotensin system. Some patients have shown transient improvement of severe hypertension after nephrectomy of the more severely involved kidney [21, 56].

DIAGNOSIS OF ATHEROEMBOLISM

The diagnosis of this condition can be made during life but only if it is considered in the original differential diagnosis. Particular suspicion of this disorder should exist in elderly patients, in those with evidence of arteriosclerotic heart disease, and when renal failure develops following arteriography or aortic or cardiac surgery, or when it appears soon after an anticoagulant or thrombolytic therapy is initiated [76, 127, 148]. The clinical course of renal failure due to atheroembolism arising after angiography or aortography may be characteristic: The decrease in renal function occurs over a longer time course than it does with either arterial embolic disease [89, 167] or exposure to radiocontrast material [160]. Thus renal insufficiency of varying degrees may develop over 1 to 4 weeks after angiography, and renal function may deteriorate even further during several more months [54, 63, 129]. Renal function partially recovers in some patients, although the mechanism for the recovery is uncertain [24, 25, 71, 101].

Occasionally the identification of cholesterol emboli on ophthalmoscopic examination has led to the diagnosis of this condition [21, 33, 72, 125]. They may be seen as bright copper yellow plaques (Fig. 77-9), which are usually lodged at the bifurcations of the retinal arterioles [33].

When "spontaneous" atheroembolic disease occurs with insidious renal insufficiency, the diagnosis will rarely be made unless the clinician considers atheroembolic disease in the initial differential diagnosis [6]. The other diagnoses that are frequently considered include renal failure due to bacterial endocarditis, vasculitis of various causes, including polyarteritis nodosa, renal artery thrombosis or thromboembolism, myoglobinuric acute renal failure, and nephrotoxicity secondary to the administration of radiographic contrast agents. Acute interstitial nephritis due to antibiotics [50] or reduced renal function from nonsteroidal antiinflammatory drugs must also be considered in the differential diagnosis. Thus impaired renal function due to these causes must be excluded. The diagnosis of atheroembolic disease represents a challenge for the clinician, particularly for the exclusion of other disorders with substantially different modes of therapy.

The definitive diagnosis of atheroembolic disease of the kidney requires the demonstration of characteristic cholesterol crystals within the lumen of arteries or arterioles within a histologic section (see Fig. 77-7). The biopsy of skeletal muscle or skin that is asymptomatic will

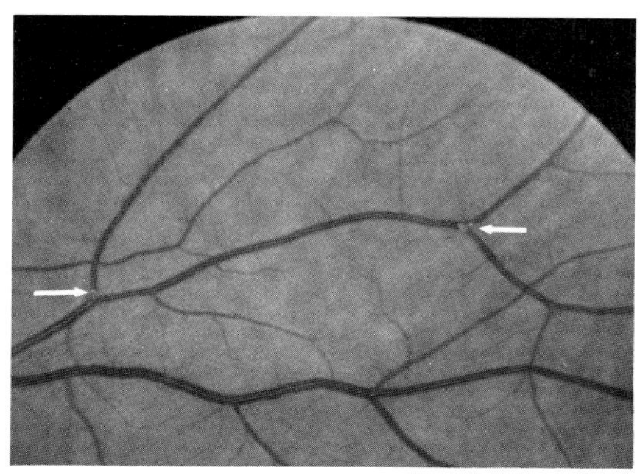

Fig. 77-9. Retinal photograph from a 68-year-old man with progressive renal insufficiency following cardiac catheterization and coronary angiography. The diagnosis of atheroembolic disease was confirmed by finding two bright yellow cholesterol plaques at two bifurcations (arrows) of the retinal arterioles. (Courtesy of Michael Goehagen, Ophthalmology Service, Veterans Administration Medical Center, West Los Angeles, Wadsworth Division.)

often provide the diagnosis [4, 5, 98, 101] and this seems the best approach for a definitive diagnosis. A bone marrow biopsy also has been positive [145]. A percutaneous renal biopsy can show the characteristic lesions [22], but the renal biopsy may be negative because of the patchy distribution of the atheroembolic disease within the kidney and the chance that the characteristic lesion will be missed in the small sample obtained [32]. Nonetheless, a renal biopsy may be positive more commonly than a muscle biopsy from an asymptomatic site [152]. A renal biopsy should be considered when renal insufficiency is marked and progressive and when there is a likelihood that a disorder such as vasculitis or periarteritis nodosa may be causing the impaired renal function. The antemortem diagnosis has also been made from other tissues, including a gastric biopsy [16] and from curettings from a transurethral resection of the prostate [85]. If histologic proof of this disorder is imperative, an open renal biopsy to obtain a wedge sample of adequate size may be considered but this is rarely needed. In the absence of any specific therapy for atheroembolic disease, the definitive diagnosis may not be absolutely imperative, except to exclude the other disorders noted above.

The management of this condition remains highly unsatisfactory. The adequate treatment of hypertension may slow progression of the renal insufficiency. The role of anticoagulation is particularly unsettled. Anticoagulation may predispose patients to the development of this condition [104, 174, 182], and anticoagulation certainly is not at all protective [43, 63, 82, 160]. It has been reported that the withdrawal of anticoagulants may be beneficial [17], but such observations are uncontrolled. When advanced renal failure develops secondary to atheromatous embolization, peritoneal dialysis rather than hemodialysis has been recommended in order to avoid the need for heparinization during the hemodialysis [84, 153]; in some cases, cholesterol-lowering agents are used as well [84]; anecdotal cases with a favorable outcome have been reported with the use of such techniques [84, 153]. However, further experience with the management of this difficult syndrome is needed.

References

1. Adovaso, R., and Pancrazio, F. Acute thrombosis of renal artery: Restoration of renal function after late revascularization. *Vasa* 18: 239, 1989.
2. Alexander, R. D., Berkes, S. L., and Abuelo, J. G. Contrast media-induced oliguric renal failure. *Arch. Intern. Med.* 138: 381, 1978.
3. Allibone, G. W. Renal infarction presenting as a mass: Diagnostic role of computerized tomography and ultrasound. *Urology* 19: 98, 1982.
4. Anderson, W. R. Necrotizing angiitis associated with embolization of cholesterol. Case report, with emphasis on the use of the muscle biopsy as a diagnostic aid. *Am. J. Clin. Pathol.* 43: 65, 1965.
5. Anderson, W. R., and Richards, A. M. Evaluation of lower extremity muscle biopsies in the diagnosis of atheroembolism. *Arch. Pathol.* 86: 535, 1968.
6. Arvold, D. S. Spontaneous atheromatous embolization—emphasis on the pitfalls of diagnosis. *Minn. Med.* 64: 141, 1981.
7. Aujla, N. D., Greenberg, A., Banner, B. F., et al. Atheroembolic involvement of renal allografts. *Am. J. Kidney Dis.* 13: 329, 1989.
8. Baichwal, K. S., and Waugh, D. Traumatic renal artery stenosis. *J. Urol.* 99: 14, 1968.
9. Bailey, G. A., Belis, J. A., Kandzari, S. J., et al. In vitro growth of renal cell carcinoma after preoperative renal infarction. *Urology* 24: 456, 1984.
10. Barlow, B., and Gandhi, R. Renal artery thrombosis following blunt trauma. *J. Trauma* 20: 614, 1980.
11. Bartsch, G., Flora, G., Buchsteiner, G., et al. Successful renal revascularization of unilateral renal artery thrombosis. *J. Urol.* 124: 115, 1980.
12. Bassi, P., Graziotti, P., Artibani, W., et al. Therapeutical aspects of intrarenal artery aneurysms. *Eur. Urol.* 14: 99, 1988.
13. Ben-Asher, S. Hypertension caused by renal infarction. *Ann. Intern. Med.* 23: 431, 1945.
14. Beraud, J. J., Calvet, B., Durand, A., et al. Reversal of acute renal failure following percutaneous transluminal recanalization of an atherosclerotic renal artery occlusion. *J. Hypertens.* 7: 909, 1989.
15. Bertini, J. E., Jr., Flechner, S. M., Miller, P., et al. The natural history of traumatic branch renal artery injury. *J. Urol.* 135: 228, 1986.
16. Bourdages, R., Prentice, R. S. A., Beck, I. T., et al. Atheromatous embolization to the stomach, an unusual cause of gastrointestinal bleeding. *Am. J. Dig. Dis.* 21: 889, 1978.
17. Bruns, F. J., Segel, D. P., and Adler, S. Control of cholesterol embolization by discontinuation of anticoagulant therapy. *Am. J. Med. Sci.* 275: 105, 1978.
18. Bugge-Asperheim, B., Sodal, G., and Flatmark, A. Renal artery aneurysm: Ex vivo repair and autotransplantation. *Scand. J. Urol. Nephrol.* 18: 63, 1984.
19. Campieri, C., Raimondi, C., Fatone, F., et al. Normalization of renal function and blood pressure after dissolution with intra-arterial fibrinolytics of a massive renal artery embolism in a solitary functioning kidney. *Nephron* 51: 399, 1989.
20. Carvajal, J. A., Anderson, W. R., Weiss, L., et al. Ath-

eroembolism: Etiologic factor in renal insufficiency, gastrointestinal hemorrhages and peripheral vascular diseases. *Arch. Intern. Med.* 119: 593, 1967.
21. Case Records of the Massachusetts General Hospital (Case 50-1977). *N. Engl. J. Med.* 297: 1337, 1977.
22. Case Records of the Massachusetts General Hospital (Case 4-1984). *N. Engl. J. Med.* 310: 244, 1984.
23. Cass, A. S., and Luxenberg, M. Traumatic thrombosis of a segmental branch of the renal artery. *J. Urol.* 137: 1115, 1987.
24. Chen, A., Ho, Y. S., Tu, Y., et al. Renal cholesterol embolization: Report of a case with emphasis on its improved prognosis. *Chin. Med. J.* 42: 329, 1988.
24a. Cerny, J. C., Chang, C. Y., and Fry, W. J. Renal artery aneurysms. *Arch. Surg.* 96: 653, 1968.
25. Clinicopathologic conference: Progressive renal failure with hematuria in a 62 year old man. *Am. J. Med.* 71: 468, 1981.
26. Clinicopathologic conference: Cyanotic feet and renal failure in a 67-year-old man. *Am. J. Med.* 75: 509, 1983.
27. Cohen, J. R., and Shamesh, F. S. Ruptured renal artery aneurysms during pregnancy. *J. Vasc. Surg.* 6: 51, 1987.
28. Coley, B. D., Mattrey, R. F., Roberts, A., et al. Potential role of PFOB enhanced sonography of the kidney. II. Detection of partial infarction. *Kidney Int.* 39: 140, 1991.
29. Cosby, R. L., Miller, P. D., and Schrier, R. W. Traumatic renal artery thrombosis. *Am. J. Med.* 81: 890, 1986.
30. Cosio, F., Zager, R., and Sharma, H. Atheroembolic renal disease causes hypocomplementemia. *Lancet* 2: 118, 1985.
31. Dahlberg, P. J., Frecentese, D. F., and Cogbill, T. H. Cholesterol embolization: Experience with 22 histologically proven cases. *Surgery* 105: 737, 1989.
32. Dalakos, T. G., Streeten, D. P. H., Jones, D., et al. "Malignant" hypertension resulting from atheromatous embolization predominantly of one kidney. *Am. J. Med.* 57: 135, 1974.
33. David, M. J., Klintworth, G. K., Friedberg, S. G., et al. Fatal atheromatous cerebral embolism associated with bright plaques in retinal arterioles: Report of a case. *Neurology* 13: 708, 1963.
34. DeBakey, M., Lafrak, E., Garcia-Rinaldi, R., et al. Aneurysm of the renal artery. A vascular reconstructive approach. *Arch. Surg.* 106: 438, 1973.
35. Dever, D. P., and Davis, R. S. Renal infarct. *N.Y. State J. Med.* 84: 258, 1984.
36. DiPrete, D. A., Abuelo, J. G., Abuelo, D. N., et al. Acute renal insufficiency due to renal infarctions in a patient with neurofibromatosis. *Am. J. Kidney Dis.* 15: 357, 1990.
37. Donadio, C., Auner, I., Giordani, R., et al. Serum and urinary enzyme activities in renal artery embolism. *Clin. Chim. Acta* 160: 145, 1986.
38. Dubrow, R. A., and Patel, S. K. Mycotic aneurysm of the renal artery. *Radiology* 138: 57, 1981.
39. Edwards, B. S., Stanson, A. W., Holley, K. E., et al. Isolated renal artery dissection: Presentation, evaluation, management, and pathology. *Mayo Clin. Proc.* 57: 564, 1982.
40. Eliot, R. S., Kanjuh, V. I., and Edwards, J. E. Atheromatous embolism. *Circulation* 30: 611, 1964.
41. Erwin, B. C., Carroll, B. A., Walter, J. F., et al. Renal infarction appearing as an echogenic mass. *Am. J. Roentgenol.* 138: 759, 1982.
42. Fay, R., Brosman, S. A., Lindstrom, R., et al. Renal artery thrombosis: A successful revascularization by autotransplantation. *J. Urol.* 111: 572, 1974.
43. Fine, M., Kapoor, W., and Falanga, V. Cholesterol crystal embolization: A review of 221 cases in the English literature. *Angiology* 38: 769, 1987.
44. Fischer, C. P., Konnak, J. W., Cho, K. J., et al. Renal artery embolism: Therapy with intra-arterial streptokinase infusion. *J. Urol.* 125: 402, 1981.
45. Fisher, D., Clagett, G. P., Brigham, R., et al. Dilemmas in dealing with the blue toe syndrome: Aortic versus peripheral source. *Am. J. Surg.* 148: 836, 1984.
46. Flatmark, A., Sodal, G., Jervell, J., et al. Preliminary experience with extracorporeal renal surgery and autotransplantation. *Eur. Surg. Res.* 9: 235, 1977.
47. Flory, C. M. Arterial occlusions produced by emboli from eroded aortic atheromatous plaques. *Am. J. Pathol.* 21: 549, 1945.
48. Freeman, L. M. The Radionuclide Renal Scan: Past, Present and Future. In M. D. Blaufox, N. K. Hollenberg, and C. Raynaud (eds.), *Radionuclides in Nephro-Urology.* Contributions to Nephrology. Basel: Karger, 1990. P. 87.
49. Freeman, L. M., Meng, C. H., Richter, M. W., et al. Patency of major renal vascular pathways demonstrated by rapid blood flow scintiphotography. *J. Urol.* 105: 473, 1971.
50. Galpin, J. E., Shinaberger, J. H., Stanley, T. M., et al. Acute interstitial nephritis due to methicillin. *Am. J. Med.* 65: 756, 1978.
51. Gault, M. H., and Steiner, G. Serum and urinary enzyme activity after renal infarction. *Can. Med. Assoc. J.* 93: 1101, 1965.
52. Gewertz, B. L., Stanley, J. C., and Fry, W. J. Renal artery dissection. *Arch. Surg.* 112: 409, 1977.
53. Gill, T. J., and Dammin, G. J. Paradoxical embolism with renal failure caused by occlusion of the renal arteries. *Am. J. Med.* 25: 780, 1958.
54. Gjesdal, K., Orning, O. M., and Smith, E. Fatal atheromatous emboli to the kidneys after left heart catheterization. *Lancet* 2: 405, 1977.
55. Glazer, G., Francis, I., Brady, T., et al. Computed tomography of renal infarction: Clinical and experimental observations. *A. J. R.* 140: 721, 1983.
56. Gore, I., and Collins, D. P. Spontaneous atheromatous embolization: Review of the literature and report of 16 additional cases. *Am. J. Clin. Pathol.* 33: 416, 1960.
57. Gore, I., McCombs, H. L., and Lindquist, R. I. Observations of the fate of cholesterol emboli. *J. Atherosclerosis Res.* 4: 427, 1964.
58. Goulet, Y., and MacKay, C. G. Atheromatous embolism: Entity with polymorphous symptomatology. *Can. Med. Assoc. J.* 88: 1067, 1963.
59. Granfortuna, J., Zamkoff, K., and Urrutia, E. Acute renal infarction in sickle cell disease. *Am. J. Hematol.* 23: 59, 1986.
60. Greendyke, R. M., and Akamatsu, Y. Atheromatous embolism as a cause of renal failure. *J. Urol.* 83: 231, 1960.
61. Greenholz, S. K., Moore, E. E., Peterson, N. E., et al. Traumatic bilateral renal artery occlusion: Successful outcome without surgical intervention. *J. Trauma* 26: 941, 1986.
62. Handler, F. P. Clinical and pathologic significance of atheromatous embolization, with emphasis on the aetiology of renal hypertension. *Am. J. Med.* 20: 366, 1956.
63. Harrington, J. T., Sommers, S. C., and Kassirer, J. P. Atheromatous emboli with progressive renal failure: Renal arteriography as the probable inciting factor. *Ann. Intern. Med.* 68: 152, 1968.

64. Harris, R. D., and Dorros, S. Computed tomographic diagnosis of renal infarction. *Urology* 17: 287, 1981.
65. Hartenbower, D. L., Winston, M. A., Weiss, E. R., et al. The scintillation camera in embolic acute renal failure. *J. Urol.* 104: 799, 1970.
66. Hartman, H. R., Newcomb, A. W., Barnes, A., et al. Renal infarction following selective renal arteriography. *Radiology* 86: 52, 1966.
67. Heng, M. C., and Haberfield, G. Thrombotic phenomena associated with intravenous cocaine. *J. Am. Acad. Dermatol.* 16: 462, 1987.
68. Heptinstall, R. H. *Pathology of the Kidney* (3rd ed.). Boston: Little, Brown, 1983. P. 1114.
69. Hicks, C. E., and Evans, C. Renal infarction as a cause of a calcified mass. *Br. J. Radiol.* 57: 840, 1984.
70. Hitti, I. F., Celmer, E. J., and Rapuano, J. Hemorrhagic infarction of the kidney. An uncommon presentation of infiltrating urothelial carcinoma of the renal pelvis. *Urol. Int.* 41: 212, 1986.
71. Ho, S. W., Thatcher, G. N., and Matz, L. R. Reversible renal failure due to renal cholesterol embolism. *Austr. N.Z. Med. J.* 12: 531, 1982.
72. Hollenhorst, R. W. Significance of bright plaques in the retinal arterioles. *Trans. Am. Ophthalmol. Soc.* 59: 252, 1961.
73. Hoover, L. A. Polyarteritis involving only the main renal arteries. *Am. J. Kidney Dis.* 11: 66, 1988.
74. Hoxie, H. J., and Coggin, C. B. Renal infarction. Statistical study of two hundred and five cases and detailed report of an unusual case. *Arch. Intern. Med.* 65: 587, 1940.
75. Hoye, S. J., Teitelbaum, S., Gore, I., et al. Atheromatous embolization. A factor in peripheral gangrene. *N. Engl. J. Med.* 261: 128, 1959.
76. Hyman, B., Landas, S., Ashman, R., et al. Warfarin-related purple toes syndrome and cholesterol microembolization. *Am. J. Med.* 82: 1233, 1987.
77. Ippolito, J. J., and Le Veen, H. H. Treatment of renal artery aneurysms. *J. Urol.* 83: 10, 1960.
78. Ishikawa, I., Masuzaki, S., Saito, T., et al. Magnetic resonance imaging in renal infarction and ischemia. *Nephron* 51: 99, 1989.
79. Jennings, W. C., Smith, J., and Corry, R. J. Atheromatous embolization as a cause of increasing creatinine levels in a renal transplant patient. *Transplant. Proc.* 22: 279, 1990.
80. Kaplan, K., Millar, J. D., and Cancilla, P. A. "Spontaneous" atheroembolic renal failure. *Arch. Intern. Med.* 110: 218, 1962.
81. Kasinath, B. S., and Lewis, E. J. Eosinophils as a clue to the diagnosis of atheroembolic renal disease. *Arch. Intern. Med.* 147: 1384, 1987.
82. Kassirer, J. P. Atheroembolic renal disease. *N. Engl. J. Med.* 280: 812, 1969.
83. Kassirer, J. P. Thrombosis and Embolism of the Renal Vessels. In L. E. Earley and C. W. Gottschalk (eds.), *Diseases of the Kidney* (3rd ed.). Boston: Little, Brown, 1979. P. 1385.
84. Kawakami, Y., Hirose, K., Watanabe, Y., et al. Management of multiple cholesterol embolization syndrome—A case report. *Angiology* 41: 248, 1990.
85. Knechtges, T. C., and Defever, B. A. Cholesterol emboli in transurethral curettings: Report of 4 cases. *J. Urol.* 114: 102, 1975.
86. Lacombe, M. Surgical versus medical treatment of renal artery embolism. *J. Cardiovasc. Surg.* 18: 281, 1977.
87. Lang, E. K. Arteriography in the assessment of renal trauma: The impact of arteriographic diagnosis on preservation of renal function and parenchyma. *Radiology* 15: 553, 1975.
88. Lang, E. K., Sullivan, J., and Frentz, G. Renal trauma: Radiological studies. Comparison of urographic, computed tomography, angiography, and radionuclide studies. *Radiology* 154: 1, 1985.
89. Lessman, R. K., Johnson, S. F., Coburn, J. W., et al. Renal artery embolism: Clinical features and long-term follow-up in 17 cases. *Ann. Intern. Med.* 89: 477, 1978.
90. Letsou, G. V., and Gusberg, R. Isolated bilateral renal artery thrombosis: An unusual consequence of blunt abdominal trauma—Case report. *J. Trauma* 30: 509, 1990.
91. Levine, E. F., and Hessl, J. M. Renal artery occlusion following blunt abdominal trauma. *J. Urol.* 112: 553, 1980.
92. Lohhse, J. R., Botham, R. J., and Waters, R. F. Traumatic bilateral renal artery thrombosis: Case report and review of literature. *J. Urol.* 127: 522, 1982.
93. Love, W. K., Robinette, M. A., and Vernon, C. P. Renal artery aneurysm rupture in pregnancy. *J. Urol.* 126: 809, 1981.
94. Magilligan, D. J., Jr., DeWeese, J. A., May, A. G., et al. The occluded renal artery. *Surgery* 78: 730, 1975.
95. Marcen, R., Pascual, J., Quereda, C., et al. Lupus anticoagulant and thrombosis of kidney allograft vessels. *Transplant. Proc.* 22: 1396, 1990.
96. Margolin, E. G., Merrill, J. P., and Harrison, J. H. Diagnosis of hypertension due to occlusions of the renal artery. *N. Engl. J. Med.* 256: 581, 1957.
97. Martin, D. C. Renal artery aneurysm with peripheral embolization of kidney. *Urology* 15: 590, 1980.
98. Maurizi, C. P., Barker, A. E., and Trueheart, R. E. Atheromatous emboli: A postmortem study with special reference to lower extremities. *Arch. Pathol.* 86: 528, 1968.
99. Maxwell, D. D., and Mispireta, L. A. Transfemoral renal artery embolectomy. *Radiology* 143: 653, 1982.
100. McCarron, J. P., Marshall, V. F., and Whitsell, J. C. Indications for surgery on renal artery aneurysms. *J. Urol.* 114: 177, 1975.
101. McGowan, J. A., and Greenberg, A. Cholesterol atheroembolic renal disease. Report of 3 cases with emphasis on diagnosis by skin biopsy and extended survival. *Am. J. Nephrol.* 6: 135, 1986.
102. Miller, T. R., Anderson, R. J., Linas, S. L., et al. Urinary diagnostic indices in acute renal failure. *Ann. Intern. Med.* 89: 47, 1978.
103. Milsom, I., and Forssman, L. Factors influencing aortocaval compression in late pregnancy. *Am. J. Obstet. Gynecol.* 148: 764, 1984.
104. Moldveen-Geronimus, M., and Merriam, J. C., Jr. Cholesterol embolization from pathological curiosity to clinical entity. *Circulation* 35: 946, 1967.
105. Montgomery, J. H., Moinuddin, M., Buchianan, J. S., et al. Renal infarction after aerobics. *Clin. Nucl. Med.* 9: 664, 1984.
106. Mori, H., Hayashi, K., Tasaki, T., et al. Spontaneous resolution of bilateral renal artery dissection: A case report. *J. Urol.* 135: 114, 1986.
107. Morrow, I., and Amplatz, K. Embolic occlusion of the renal artery during arteriography. *Radiology* 86: 57, 1966.
108. Morton, J. R., and Crawford, E. S. Bilateral traumatic renal artery thrombosis. *Ann. Surg.* 179: 62, 1972.
109. Moyer, J. D., Rao, C. N., Widrich, W. C., et al. Conser-

vative management of renal artery embolus. *J. Urol.* 109: 138, 1973.
110. Mudge, G. H. Nephrotoxicity of urographic radiocontrast drugs. *Kidney Int.* 18: 540, 1980.
111. Mügge, A., Gulba, D. C., Frei, U., et al. Renal artery embolism: Thrombolysis with recombinant tissue-type plasminogen activator. *J. Intern. Med.* 228: 279, 1990.
112. Nicholas, G. G., and DeMuth, W. E. Treatment of renal artery embolism. *Arch. Surg.* 119: 278, 1984.
113. Novick, A. Management of intrarenal branch arterial lesions with extracorporeal microvascular reconstruction and autotransplantation. *J. Urol.* 150: 54, 1981.
114. Novick, A., Straffon, R., and Stewart, B. Surgical management of branch renal artery disease: In situ versus extracorporeal methods of repair. *J. Urol.* 123: 311, 1981.
115. Opit, L. J., McKenna, K. P., and Nairn, D. E. Closed renal injury. *Br. J. Surg.* 48: 240, 1960.
116. Ortenberg, J., Novich, A. C., Straffon, R. A., et al. Surgical treatment of renal artery aneurysms. *Br. J. Urol.* 55: 341, 1983.
117. Otken, L. B., Jr. Experimental production of atheromatous embolization. *Arch. Pathol.* 68: 685, 1959.
118. Parker, M. D. Acute segmental renal infarction: Difficulty in diagnosis despite multimodality approach. *Urology* 18: 523, 1981.
119. Peterson, N. E. Traumatic bilateral renal infarction: Review article. *J. Trauma* 29: 158, 1989.
120. Peterson, N. E., and McDonald, D. F. Renal embolization. *J. Urol.* 100: 140, 1968.
121. Pierce, J. R., Jr., Wren, M. V., and Cousar, J. B., Jr. Cholesterol embolism: Diagnosis antemortem by bone marrow biopsy. *Ann. Intern. Med.* 89: 937, 1978.
122. Pineo, G. F., Thorndyke, W. C., and Steed, B. L. Spontaneous renal artery thrombosis: Successful lysis with streptokinase. *J. Urol.* 138: 1223, 1987.
123. Pochet, J. M., Bobrie, G., Basile, C., et al. Renal arterial thrombosis complicating nephrotic syndrome. *Presse Med.* 17: 2139, 1988.
124. Poutasse, E. F. Renal artery aneurysms: Their natural history and surgery. *J. Urol.* 95: 297, 1966.
125. Pribram, H. F. W., and Couves, C. M. Retinal embolism as a complication of angiography: The possible role of platelet and cholesterol emboli. *Neurology* 15: 188, 1965.
126. Price, R. K., and Skelton, R. Hypertension due to syphilitic occlusion of the main renal arteries. *Br. Heart J.* 10: 29, 1948.
127. Queen, M., Blem, H. J., Moe, G. W., et al. Development of cholesterol embolization after intravenous streptokinase for acute myocardial infarction. *Am. J. Cardiol.* 65: 1042, 1990.
128. Rabe, F. E., Yune, H. Y., Richmond, B. D., et al. Renal tumor infarction with absolute ethanol. *Am. J. Radiol.* 139: 1139, 1982.
129. Ramirez, G., O'Neill, W. M., Lambert, R., et al. Cholesterol embolization, a complication of angiography. *Arch. Intern. Med.* 138: 1430, 1978.
130. Rao, K. V., and Anderson, R. C. The incidence of thromboembolic disease in recipients of cadaver kidney transplants. *Am. J. Kidney Dis.* 6: A16, 1985 (Abstr.).
131. Reagan, K., Beckmann, C. F., Larsen, C. R., et al. Renal infarction: computerized tomographic appearance with angiographic correlation. *J. Urol.* 84: 258, 1984.
132. Regan, F. C., and Crabtree, E. G. Renal infarction: A clinical and possible surgical entity. *J. Urol.* 59: 981, 1948.
133. Richards, A. M., Eliot, R. S., Kanjuh, V. I., et al. Cholesterol embolism: A multiple system disease masquerading as polyarteritis nodosa. *Am. J. Cardiol.* 15: 696, 1965.
133a. Richardson, A. J., Liddington, M., Jaskowski, A., et al. Pregnancy in a renal transplant recipient complicated by rupture of a transplant renal artery aneurysm. *Br. J. Surg.* 77: 228, 1990.
134. Roa, C., and Blaivas, J. G. Primary renal artery dissecting aneurysm: A review. *J. Urol.* 118: 716, 1977.
135. Runge, M. M., Clanton, J. A., Harzer, W. A., et al. Intravascular contrast agents suitable for magnetic resonance imaging. *Radiology* 153: 171, 1984.
136. Sakemi, T., Kudo, S., Nagano, Y., et al. Persistent wedge-shaped low-density lesions on computed tomography of the kidneys without infarction. *Nephron* 51: 112, 1989.
137. Saklayen, M. G. Atheroembolic renal disease: Preferential occurrence in whites only. *Am. J. Nephrol.* 9: 87, 1989.
138. Salazer, T., Farkouh, M., and Wilson, D. Eosinophiluria in atheroembolic renal disease. *J. Am. Soc. Nephrol.* 1: 341, 1990.
139. Samara, E. N., Voss, B. L., and Pederson, J. A. Renal artery thrombosis associated with elevated cyclosporine levels: A case report and review of the literature. *Transplant. Proc.* 10: 119, 1990.
140. Sanders, R. C., Menon, S., and Sanders, A. D. The complementary uses of nuclear medicine and ultrasound in the kidney. *J. Urol.* 120: 521, 1978.
141. Sandler, C. M., and Toombs, B. D. Computed tomographic evaluation of blunt renal trauma. *Radiology* 141: 461, 1981.
142. Sane, S. Y., and Deshmukh, S. S. Total renal infarct and peri-renal abscess caused by phycomycosis (a case report). *J. Postgrad. Med.* 34: 448, 1988.
143. Sanfelippo, C. J., and Goldin, A. Intra-arterial streptokinase and renal artery embolization. *Urology* 11: 62, 1978.
144. Sayre, G. P., and Campbell, D. C. Multiple peripheral emboli in atherosclerosis of the aorta. *Arch. Intern. Med.* 103: 799, 1959.
145. Schipper, H., Gordon, M., and Beris, B. Atheromatous embolic disease. *Can. Med. Assoc. J.* 113: 640, 1975.
146. Schoon, I., Seeman, T., Niemand, D., et al. Rupture of renal arterial aneurysm in pregnancy: Case report. *Acta Chir. Scand.* 154: 593, 1988.
147. Schwarcz, T. H., Coffin, L. H., and Pilcher, D. G. Renal failure after embolization of a prosthetic mitral valve disc and review of systemic disc embolization. *J. Vasc. Surg.* 2: 697, 1985.
148. Schwartz, M. W., and McDonald, G. Cholesterol embolization syndrome. Occurrence after intravenous streptokinase therapy for myocardial infarction. *J.A.M.A.* 258: 1934, 1987.
149. Scott, R., Jr., Carloton, C. E., Jr., and Goldman, M. Penetrating injuries of the kidney: An analysis of 181 cases. *J. Urol.* 101: 247, 1969.
150. Seemann, W. R., Brambs, H. J., Mathias, K., et al. Value of angiography, sonography, and CT in renal infarction. *Eur. J. Radiol.* 4: 282, 1985.
151. Seppala, F. E., and Levey, J. Renal artery aneurysm: Case report of a ruptured calcified renal artery aneurysm. *Am. Surg.* 48: 42, 1982.
152. Sheehan, J., and Sweeney, E. Atheroembolic arteritis. *Irish J. Med. Sci.* 150: 319, 1981.
153. Siemons, L., van den Heuvel, P., Parizel, G., et al. Peritoneal dialysis in acute renal failure due to cholesterol embolization: Two cases of recovery of renal function and extended survival. *Clin. Nephrol.* 28: 205, 1987.

154. Sigelbaum, M. H., and Weiss, J. P. Renal infarction secondary to fibrous dysplasia and aneurysm formation of the renal artery. *Urology* 35: 73, 1990.
155. Silber, S. J., and Clark, R. E. Treatment of massive hemorrhage after renal biopsy with angiographic injection of clot. *N. Engl. J. Med.* 292: 1387, 1975.
156. Slavis, S., Hodge, E., Novick, A., et al. Surgical treatment for isolated dissection of the renal artery. *J. Urol.* 144: 233, 1990.
157. Smith, B., Holcomb, G. W., Richie, R., et al. Renal artery dissection. *Ann. Surg.* 200: 134, 1984.
158. Smith, J. A., and Macleish, D. G. Postpartum rupture of a renal artery aneurysm to a solitary kidney. *Aust. N.Z. J. Surg.* 55: 299, 1985.
159. Smith, J. N., and Hinman, F., Jr. Intrarenal arterial aneurysms. *J. Urol.* 97: 990, 1967.
160. Smith, M. C., Ghose, M. K., and Henry, A. R. The clinical spectrum of renal cholesterol embolization. *Am. J. Med.* 71: 174, 1981.
161. Snyder, H. E., and Shapiro, J. L. Correlative study of atheromatous embolism in human beings and experimental animals. *Surgery* 49: 195, 1961.
162. Soussou, I. D., Starr, D. S., Lawrie, G. M., et al. Renal artery aneurysm. Long term relief of renovascular hypertension by in situ operative correction. *Arch. Surg.* 114: 1410, 1979.
163. Spirnak, J. P., and Resnick, M. I. Revascularization of traumatic thrombosis of the renal artery. *Surg. Gynec. Obstet.* 164: 22, 1987.
164. Stables, D. P. Unilateral absence of excretion at urography after abdominal trauma. *Radiology* 121: 609, 1976.
165. Stables, D. P., Fouche, R. F., De Villers van Niekerk, J. P., et al. Traumatic renal artery occlusion: 21 cases. *J. Urol.* 115: 229, 1976.
166. Stanley, J. C., Rhodes, E. L., Bewertz, B. L., et al. Renal artery aneurysms: Significance of macroaneurysms exclusive of dissections and fibrodysplastic mural dilations. *Arch. Surg.* 110: 1327, 1975.
167. Stanley, J. C., and Whitehouse, W. M., Jr. Occlusive and aneurysmal disease of the renal arterial circulation. *Disease-a-Month* 30: 1, 1984.
168. Sullivan, M. F., Smalley, R., and Banowsky, L. H. Renal artery occlusion secondary to blunt abdominal trauma. *J. Trauma* 12: 509, 1972.
169. Tham, G., Ekelund, L., Herrlin, K., et al. Renal artery aneurysms: Natural history and prognosis. *Ann. Surg.* 197: 348, 1983.
170. Thurlbeck, W. M., and Castleman, B. Atheromatous emboli to the kidneys after aortic surgery. *N. Engl. J. Med.* 257: 442, 1957.
171. Toguri, A. B., Liu, T. T., Bayliss, C., et al. Traumatic bilateral renal artery thrombosis. *J. Urol.* 112: 430, 1974.
172. Vidt, D. G., Eisele, G., Gephardt, G. N., et al. Atheroembolic renal disease: Associated with renal artery stenosis. *Cleve. Clin. J. Med.* 56: 407, 1989.
173. Wein, A. J., Arger, P. H., and Murphy, J. J. Controversial aspects of blunt renal trauma. *J. Trauma* 17: 662, 1977.
174. Weissman, R. E., and Tobin, R. W. Arterial embolism occurring during systemic heparin therapy. *Arch. Surg.* 76: 219, 1958.
175. Williams, H. H., Wall, B. M., and Cooke, C. R. Reversible nephrotic range proteinuria and renal failure in atheroembolic renal disease. *Am. J. Med. Sci.* 299: 58, 1990.
176. Wohlman, R. A. Renal artery thrombosis and embolization associated with intravenous cocaine injection. *South. Med. J.* 80: 928, 1987.
177. Wong, W., Moss, A., Federle, M., et al. Renal infarction: CT diagnosis and correlation between CT findings and etiologies. *Radiology* 150: 201, 1984.
178. Woodard, J. R., Patterson, J. H., and Brinsfield, D. Renal artery thrombosis in newborn infants. *Am. J. Dis. Child.* 114: 191, 1967.
179. Youkey, J. R., Collins, G. J., Orecchia, P. M., et al. Saccular renal artery aneurysm as a cause of hypertension. *Surgery* 97: 498, 1985.
180. Zatuchni, J., Patel, H., and Chiemchanya, S. The "blue toe" syndrome with renal atheroembolism and failure. *Angiology* 36: 209, 1985.
181. Zimmerman, C. E., and Yett, H. S. Renal transplant infarction during total hip arthroplasty. *Clin. Orthopaed. Rel. Res.* 165: 195, 1982.
182. Zinn, W. J. Side reactions of heparin in clinical practice. *Am. J. Cardiol.* 14: 36, 1964.

Essential Mixed Cryoglobulinemia

Claudio Ponticelli
Giuseppe D'Amico

Cryoglobulins are immunoglobulins that reversibly precipitate in the cold, giving rise to high-molecular-weight aggregates [81, 128]. On the basis of immunochemical analysis, Brouet et al. [19] classified cryoglobulinemias into three types. Type I is composed of a single monoclonal immunoglobulin. Type II is composed of at least two immunoglobulins, of which one, usually of the IgM class, is a monoclonal antiglobulin that acts against polyclonal IgG. Type III is characterized by polyclonal immunoglobulins in both components of an immune complex. Single cryoproteins are usually found in association with multiple myeloma and Waldenström's macroglobulinemia [1, 56, 62, 98, 123, 146, 155], while type II and type III cryoglobulins may be associated with several disorders such as autoimmune diseases, infections, and liver diseases. However, in about one third of all mixed cryoglobulinemias, the etiology is unclear and the term *essential* is applied.

The clinical syndrome of essential mixed cryoglobulinemia (EMC) was first described by Meltzer et al. in 1966 [98]. It was characterized by purpura, weakness, arthralgias, and in several patients, proliferative glomerulonephritis (GN). Many subsequent reports further defined this syndrome, confirming that renal involvement is particularly frequent in EMC [13, 14, 22, 24, 25, 29, 30, 32, 33, 36, 41, 51, 54, 58, 60, 65, 69, 75, 77, 84, 92, 96, 103, 108, 111, 112, 117, 120, 122, 124, 125, 132, 133, 136, 139, 143, 147, 156]. Kidney involvement ranges from 8 to 58 percent in large series of patients [17, 70, 119] and is more frequent in women. The incidence of EMC nephritis varies in different geographic areas, suggesting an important role of genetic and environmental factors. The disease seems to be more frequent in some Mediterranean countries such as France, Spain, and particularly Italy, while it is very rare in northern Europe and in North America.

Renal Histology

LIGHT MICROSCOPY FINDINGS

Glomeruli. The GN frequently found in patients with type II EMC, termed *cryoglobulinemic glomerulonephritis* by Mazzucco et al. [94] is a membranoproliferative, exudative GN. It is different from the idiopathic type of membranoproliferative GN as well as from the diffuse proliferative GN of systemic lupus by having the following features:

1. Endocapillary hypercellularity mainly due to a frequently massive infiltration of monocytes and sometimes T lymphocytes [23, 42, 43, 88, 94, 103, 104] (Fig. 78-1). Some of the infiltrating monocytes express anti–tissue factor procoagulant activity and are therefore activated cells [23].
2. Large, amorphous, eosinophilic, periodic acid-Schiff (PAS)–positive, Congo red–negative deposits lying against the inner side of the glomerular capillary wall and filling the capillary lumen, the so-called *intraluminal thrombi,* seen in about one third of all patients and especially in those with more acute renal disease and more massive proliferation and exudation [25, 29, 43, 106, 107, 136] (Fig. 78-2).
3. Thickening of the glomerular basement membrane, with a "double contour" appearance, that is more diffuse and evident than in lupus nephritis and in idiopathic membranoproliferative GN (Fig. 78-3). As seen by electron microscopy, the double contour is mainly due to the peripheral interposition of monocytes, while mesangial matrix and cell interposition is less evident than in lupus nephritis and in idiopathic membranoproliferative GN [38, 43, 94, 157].

Not all patients with type II EMC have these characteristic glomerular lesions. In about 10 percent of patients only a mild segmental mesangial proliferation, without significant monocyte infiltration, is found. In another 10 percent of patients the glomerular pattern is that of a lobular GN, with mesangial expansion and centrolobular sclerosis. With the exception of this small group of patients, glomerular segmental and global sclerosis is rather mild and inconstant, even many years after the onset of the renal disease [43].

Interstitium and Vessels. Monocytes and T lymphocytes accumulate in the interstitium in the acute stages of EMC [23]. Interstitial fibrosis, however, is not a prominent finding, even in late biopsy specimens.

An acute vasculitis of small and medium-size arteries is present in at least one third of patients who are biopsied during the acute stage of the renal disease and in a larger percentage of postmortem specimens [29, 43, 60, 106]. It can be found even in the absence of obvious glomerular damage. The acute vasculitis is characterized by fibrinoid necrosis of the arteriolar wall, with infiltration of monocytes around the wall (Fig. 78-4).

ELECTRON MICROSCOPIC FINDINGS

Electron-dense deposits can be found in the capillary lumen, usually in a subendothelial position but sometimes also filling the capillary lumen. They are sometimes amorphous immune complex–like deposits, but often they have a peculiar fibrillar or crystalloid structure [13, 24, 29, 40, 94, 101, 136]. In IgG-IgM-κ EMC, the crystalloid structure, which is identical to that seen in the in vitro cryoprecipitate in the same patients [24, 40], consists of cylinders that are 100 or 1000 nm long and have a hollow axis (Fig. 78-5). In cross sections they look like annular bodies with a light center, a dense ring, and a lighter peripheral protein coat. The crystalloid deposits, when present, are often surrounded by areas of amorphous, weakly osmiophilic and translucent material, attributed to degradation of the deposits. Both types of deposits are infrequently seen in the mesangial area, and subepithelial deposits are quite unusual. Circulating aggregates or structured material can sometimes be

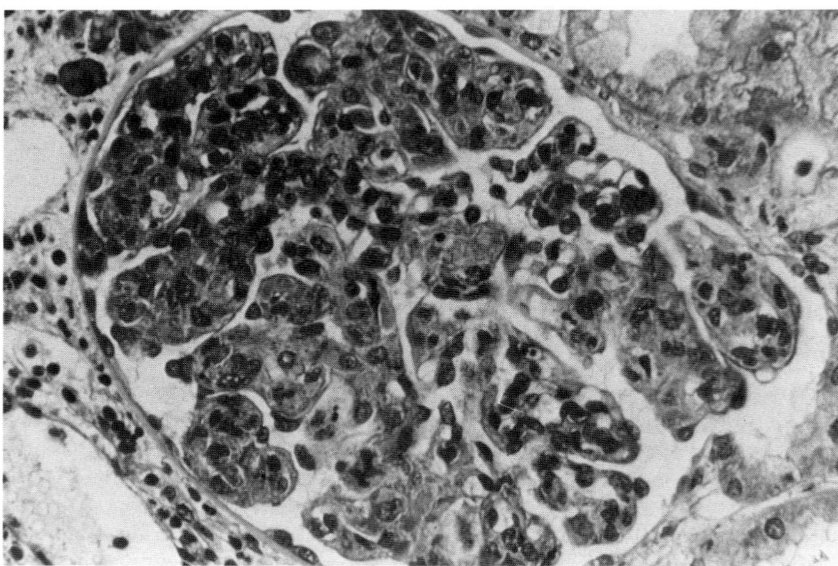

Fig. 78-1. Cryoglobulinemic glomerulonephritis. Marked infiltration of the glomerular tuft with mononuclear cells. Light microscopy. Masson trichrome, ×320.

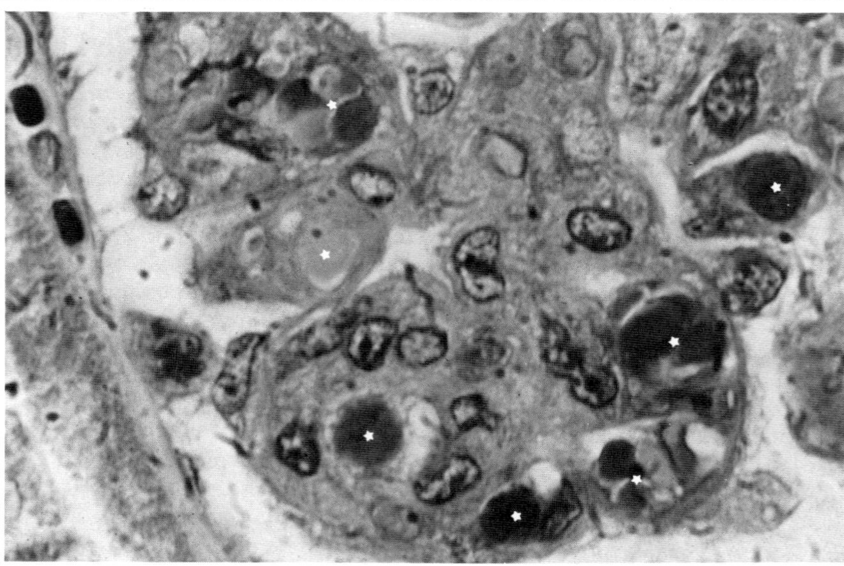

Fig. 78-2. Numerous hyaline thrombi (★) occluding many capillary lumina. Note their different tinctorial affinity. Light microscopy. Masson trichrome, ×750.

found in peritubular capillaries and arterioles. Ultrastructural examination confirms that monocytes in the capillary lumina are mainly responsible for the intracapillary proliferation, and mesangial matrix increases can also be found. Monocytes very often appear to be in close contact with subendothelial and intraluminal amorphous or crystalloid deposits. In fact, these cells appear to be filled with large amorphous protein droplets with different osmiophilia, which are probably products of phagocytosis (phagolysosomes) [101, 103, 104]. These intracellular protein droplets do not have a crystalloid structure, suggesting that the cryoglobulins lose their structure during phagocytosis. When a large number of these monocytes with giant protein droplets accumulate in the capillary lumen with the amorphous or crystalloid deposits, they contribute to the complete occlusion of the lumen. Monocytes can frequently be found interspersed with the subendothelial deposits, between the glomerular basement membrane and the endothelial cells or the newly formed basement mem-

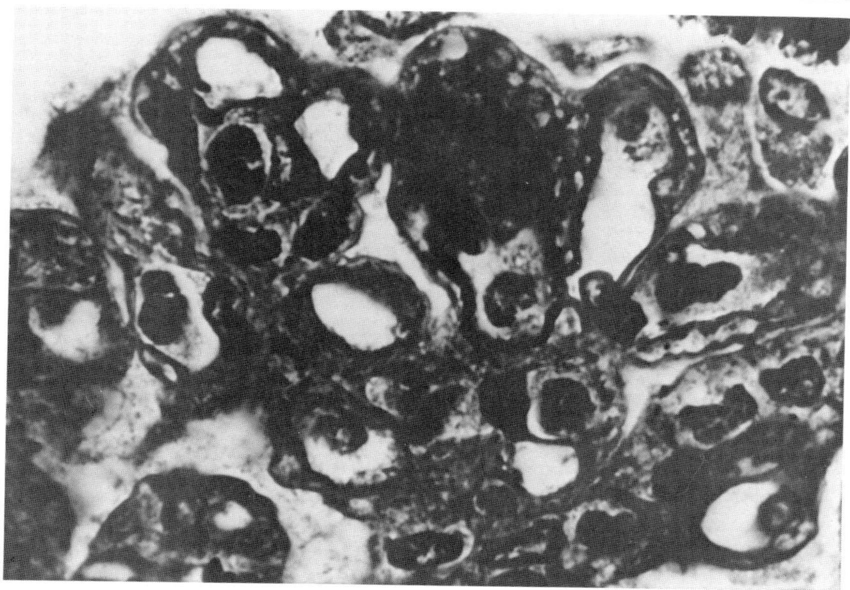

Fig. 78-3. Glomerular capillary walls with "double contour" appearance. Light microscopy. Jones silver methenamine, ×750.

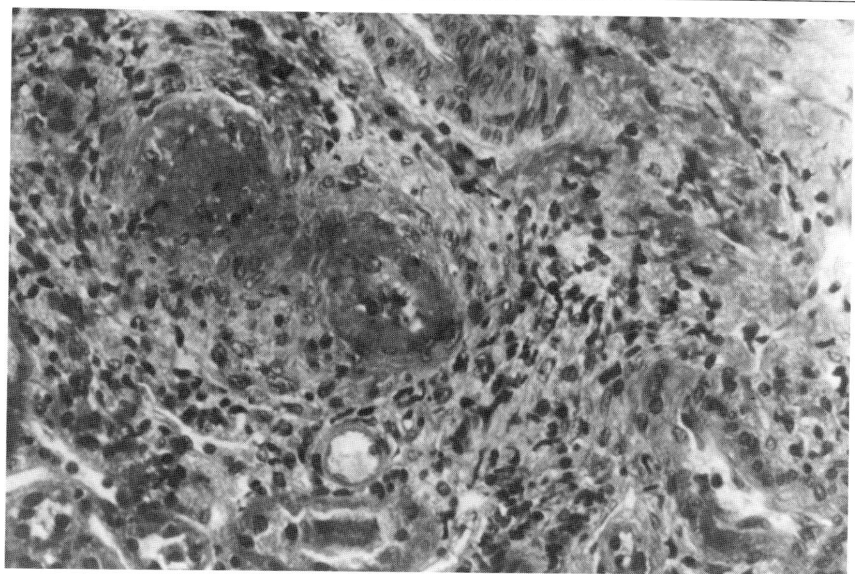

Fig. 78-4. Severe necrotizing arteritis involving an interlobular artery. Light microscopy. Masson trichrome, ×320.

brane–like material in those areas in which capillary walls are double-contoured.

IMMUNOHISTOLOGIC FEATURES

Three patterns of glomerular deposition can be seen by immunofluorescence [9, 10, 30, 106]:

1. Intensive, massive staining of huge deposits that fill the capillary lumen (intraluminal thrombi), usually associated with faint, irregular, segmental parietal staining of some peripheral loops, in a subendothelial position (Fig. 78-6).
2. The same pattern of faint, irregular, segmental parietal staining of some peripheral loops, in a subendothelial position, but without any intraluminal staining.
3. Intense granular diffuse staining of peripheral loops, with a subendothelial pattern (Fig. 78-7).

IgM and IgG are the prevailing immunoreactants in

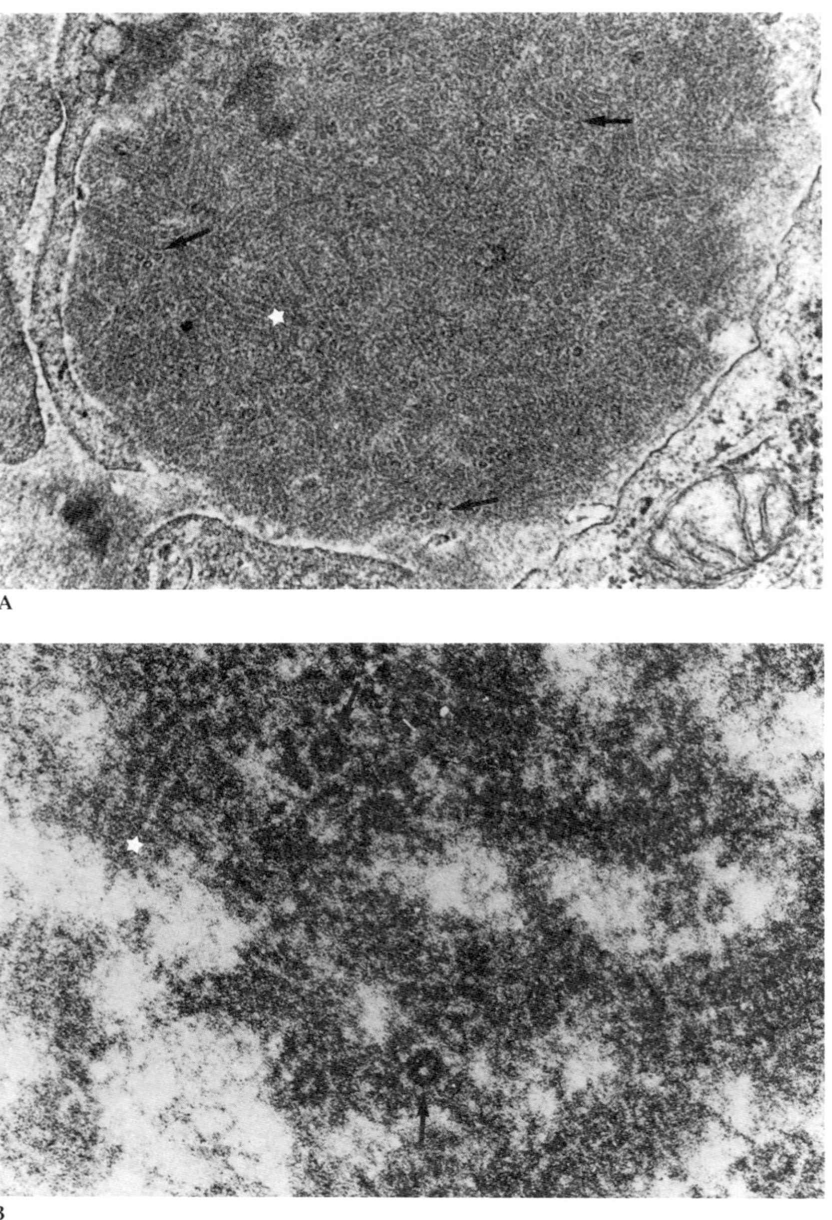

Fig. 78-5. A. Crystalloid structure of deposits in the glomerulus. B. Identical structure in the in vitro cryoprecipitate of the same patient. The deposits consist of straight or slightly curved paired cylinders (★) and annular structures (➞).

type II EMC, suggesting that they are locally trapped or precipitate cryoglobulins. This identity was confirmed by the demonstration [86] that the immune deposits have antiglobulin activity similar to that of the serum cryo-IgM. More recently, using monoclonal antibodies against cross-reactive idiotypes present on rheumatoid factors, we identified the same idiotype of the circulating monoclonal rheumatoid factors in renal biopsy specimens from patients with EMC-GN [131].

C3 is present very frequently in the parietal deposits, with a distribution similar to that of immunoglobulins, although with a lower intensity. Intraluminal thrombi only occasionally show positive fluorescence for complement components. Deposits of earlier complement components (C1q and C4) and fibrinogen are also found in the parietal deposits in about 30 percent of cases. Vascular deposits of IgM, IgG, C3, and fibrinogen are detected in about one third of cases.

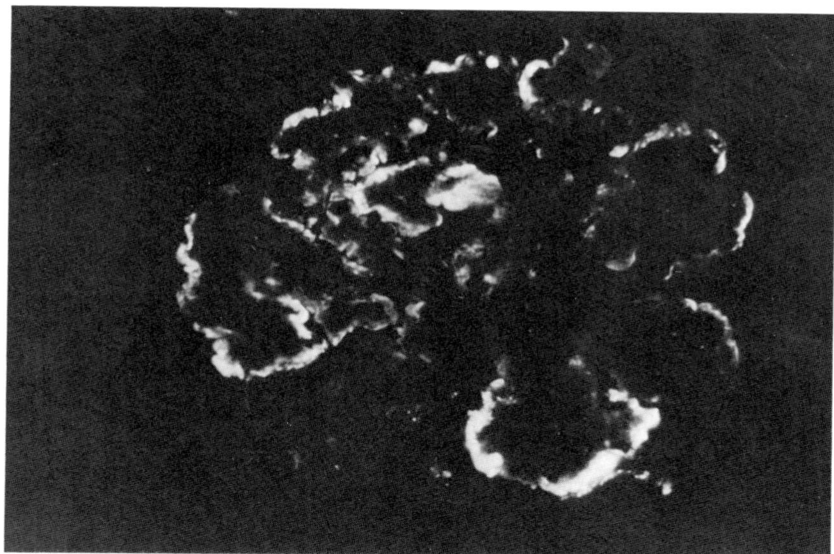

Fig. 78-6. Diffuse granular deposits irregularly distributed on peripheral capillary loops. Immunofluorescence study. Anti-IgM serum, ×320.

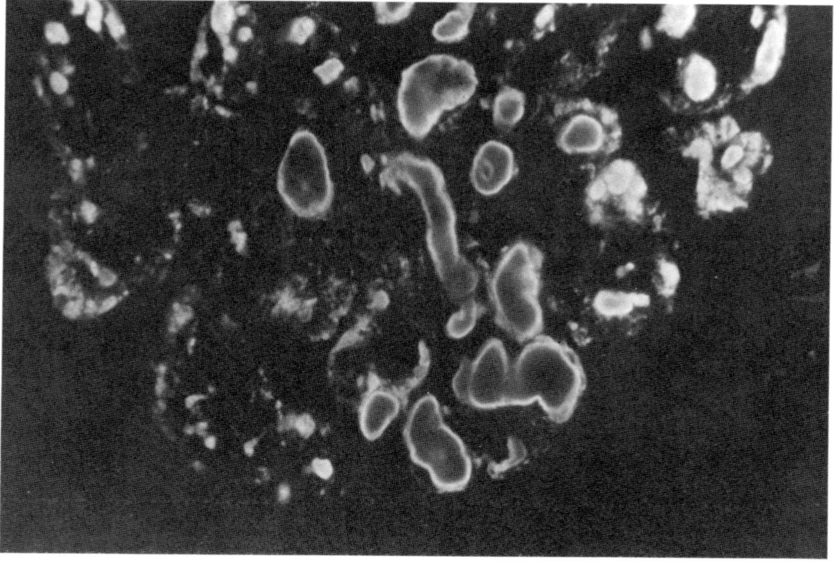

Fig. 78-7. Large thrombi in many capillary lumina and scanty deposits along glomerular basement membranes. The antiserum stains only the periphery of the thrombi. Immunofluorescence study. Anti-IgM serum, ×450.

Clinical Manifestations

CLINICAL FEATURES AT PRESENTATION

In most patients, type II EMC is diagnosed between the fourth and the fifth decade of life but in many patients some symptoms of the disease may first appear some 10 to 20 years before a correct diagnosis is made. Renal involvement usually manifests many years after the first symptoms appear. In some cases, however, renal and extrarenal manifestations appear concomitantly. More rarely, renal disease may be the first presenting manifestation.

The most frequent presenting renal syndrome is isolated proteinuria with microscopic hematuria, sometimes associated with signs of moderate chronic renal insufficiency. An acute nephritic syndrome characterized by severe proteinuria, microscopic or macroscopic hematuria, arterial hypertension, and a sudden rise in serum creatinine is the first renal manifestation in about 20 to 30 percent of patients and may be complicated by oligoanuria in some 5 percent of cases. In another 20 percent of patients, renal involvement presents with a nephrotic syndrome [25, 30, 136]. Arterial hypertension is observed in more than 80 percent of patients at the time of onset of renal disease [9]. Extrarenal symptoms and signs are usually observed at presentation (Table 78-1).

NATURAL HISTORY AND PROGNOSIS

Extrarenal symptoms may show a fluctuating course with alternations of quiescence and exacerbations. Most patients have recurrent, nonpruritic, palpable purpura or petechiae usually affecting the lower extremities [27]. Joints involved in EMC include the hands, knees, ankles, and elbows, often in a migratory fashion. Fever is a relatively frequent manifestation of EMC. About one fourth of patients in whom infection can be excluded may present with prolonged episodes of fever [31]. Liver involvement is frequent and can have serious consequences, but more characteristically, liver function abnormalities are mild and rarely symptomatic. Histology shows a chronic hepatitis with a striking mononuclear cell infiltrate [59]. The positive markers for hepatitis, especially hepatitis B surface antigen (HBsAg), have been found with increased incidence in some series [17, 52, 79, 89]. Anti–hepatitis B antibodies were also observed in both serum and cryoprecipitates of patients with EMC and hepatitis B particles were seen by electron microscopy in some cryoprecipitates [59, 79]. Immunofluorescent staining with anti-HBsAg antisera has been found in the glomeruli of some patients, but Maggiore et al. [84, 85] demonstrated that this staining is not specific. It is rather due to the interference of the antiglobulin IgM deposits present on the capillary walls. In fact, staining disappears after the inactivation of rheumatoid factor. Other series have not confirmed a high prevalence of markers for viral hepatitis [114, 136]. These differences are probably due to the criteria used for recruiting patients with EMC and to differences in the incidence of subclinical infection in different geographic areas. In rare cases patients with EMC may develop severe intestinal vasculitis with consequent ischemia, which can pose different problems of differential diagnosis. Lung involvement is frequent in EMC, probably as a consequence of immune complex deposition. Tests that are considered to be indicative of small airways disease frequently demonstrate abnormalities in EMC [17]. Several patients can show attacks of spasmodic asthma, pleurisy, and hemoptysis with roentgenographic or histologic abnormalities [17, 91]. An acute respiratory distress syndrome requiring mechanical ventilation may rarely occur [134].

In the past, kidney involvement in EMC was considered to have an ominous prognostic significance. However, it is clear today that renal disease may have a variable course. Some 30 percent of patients may attain complete or partial remission of renal symptoms even though some of them presented with an acute nephritic syndrome [136]. In another 30 percent of patients the renal disease follows an indolent course and does not progress to end-stage renal failure in spite of the persistence of urinary abnormalities and even of some degree of renal dysfunction. In about 20 percent of patients several episodes of an acute nephritic syndrome can occur, sometimes associated with flare-ups of the systemic signs of the disease. These episodes may be treated with high-dose corticosteroids and/or plasmapheresis but sometimes may spontaneously reverse and reappear. A moderate degree of renal insufficiency is rather frequent, usually long after the onset of the disease. However, the development of terminal renal failure is relatively rare. In the large series of patients with EMC nephritis studied in Milan, Tarantino et al. [138] reported that after a mean follow-up of 10 years, only 6 of 108 patients required regular dialysis and another 8 patients had chronic renal insufficiency. However, in the meantime, 27 patients died because of extrarenal complications. Cardiovascular complications, infections, liver failure, and neoplasia were the most important causes of death (Table 78-2). Cardiovascular and cerebrovascular accidents were particularly frequent in patients with arterial hypertension, which occurs early in EMC and is often severe and difficult to control. Patients with numerous systemic symptoms and those with severe renal disease were more likely to die, suggesting that a widespread vasculitis may have a major impact on the patients' prognosis. In the study with nephritic patients the mortality rate of 30 percent at 10 years was similar to that reported by others for EMC patients without kidney involvement [119]. Thus, one may conclude that the appearance of renal disease is not necessarily correlated with a poor prognosis. On the other hand, because of the late development of chronic renal failure, it is possible that longer follow-up periods might eventually reveal a higher incidence of end-stage renal disease. In summary, two groups of patients with EMC nephritis

Table 78-1. Extrarenal signs and symptoms in 116 patients with essential mixed cryoglobulinemia nephritis

Purpura	88%	Raynaud's phenomenon	35%
Hepatomegaly	88%	Nervous system involvement	31%
Arthralgias	78%	Abdominal pain	27%
Weakness	67%	Thrombocytopenia	26%
Fever	56%	Increase in liver enzymes	25%
Anemia	53%	Weight loss	23%
Splenomegaly	50%	Pleurisy	23%

Source: Tarantino, A., Montagnino, G., Baldassari, A., et al. Prognostic Factors in Essential Mixed Cryoglobulinemia Nephropathy. In C. Ponticelli, L. Minetti, and G. D'Amico (eds.), *Antiglobulins, Cryoglobulins and Glomerulonephritis*. Dordrecht: M. Nijhoff, 1986. Pp. 219–225.

Table 78-2. Causes of death in 30 patients with essential mixed cryoglobulinemia nephritis

Cardiovascular accidents	
Cerebral hemorrhage	4
Heart failure	3
Intestinal infarction	2
Myocardial infarction	2
Pulmonary embolism	1
Infections	
Sepsis	4
Tuberculosis	1
Meningitis	1
Pneumonia	1
Peritonitis	1
Liver failure	
HBsAg negative	4
Neoplasia	
Chronic lymphatic	
Leukemia	1
Non-Hodgkin's lymphoma	1
Laryngeal cancer	1
Acute respiratory distress	1
Unknown	2

Source: Tarantino, A., Montagnino, G., Baldassari, A., et al. Prognostic Factors in Essential Mixed Cryoglobulinemia Nephropathy. In C. Ponticelli, L. Minetti, and G. D'Amico (eds.), *Antiglobulins, Cryoglobulins and Glomerulonephritis.* Dordrecht: M. Nijhoff, 1986. Pp. 219–225.

can be identified: (1) those with multisystemic involvement including renal disease who may die before end-stage renal failure develops, and (2) those with fewer signs of systemic vasculitis who generally have a benign course without developing renal failure. Whether these differences are correlated to the nature of the immunoglobulins involved in the phenomenon of cryoprecipitation or to the physicochemical characteristics and other properties of cryoglobulins remains to be ascertained.

Laboratory Data

As already discussed, cryoglobulins in EMC are composed of two immunoglobulins, one of which is monoclonal and acts as an antiglobulin against polyclonal IgG. The monoclonal immunoglobulin is usually an IgM but can also be an IgG or an IgA [28, 50, 74, 142, 147]. Characterization of the cryoglobulins in patients with renal disease shows the exclusive monoclonal nature of the antiglobulin IgM, which is nearly always an IgM-κ [29, 136]. On the contrary, in rheumatologic surveys, patients with polyclonal IgM (type III cryoglobulinemia) outnumber those with monoclonal IgM. Serum titers of IgM rheumatoid factor activity are usually elevated [59, 132] and there are high serum levels of immune complex material as assessed by the C1q-binding assay [2, 78, 95]. The cryocrit value may vary considerably from 2 to 80 percent in different patients and can fluctuate over time in a single patient. Also characteristic, though not invariable, is the pattern of complement activation in serum with selective depletion of early components of the classic pathway and normal factor B levels [135]. The serum pattern of complement is rather specific for EMC. C1q, C4, and CH_{50} are usually low; C3 may be slightly low or normal; and the late components (C5-C9) C3PA and C1INH tend to be higher than in normal controls. The C3 breakdown product C3d is sometimes increased [55, 80, 135, 136, 138]. These complement component abnormalities have been attributed to complement hyposynthesis [127, 135], but it is also possible that the consumption of the early serum complement components with the characteristic sparing of C3 might be attributed to the C4-binding protein that controls the mechanism of the classic pathway C3 convertase [55, 66]. A retarded clearance of IgG-coated autologous erythrocytes, indicative of abnormal Fc receptor function, is specific for EMC patients with renal involvement or motor neuropathy [64]. A peculiar hematologic finding of all types of cryoglobulinemias is represented by pseudoleukocytosis and/or pseudothrombocytosis with an abnormal histogram as determined by a Coulter Counter [8, 105]. These abnormalities, which disappear if the blood sample is warmed at 37°C, can alert the clinician to the possible diagnosis of EMC. Thus, particular attention should be paid to the leukocytes and platelet counts in patients with EMC [153].

No correlation has been found between the degree of activity of EMC and the values for cryocrit, IgM rheumatoid factor, or early complement components [30, 80, 132, 135, 136]. However, patients who have died of EMC had significantly higher cryocrit values and lower levels of IgG than did those who have survived, thus suggesting a possible prognostic value of these parameters [138].

Pathogenesis

PATHOGENESIS OF TYPE II EMC

There is increasing evidence that the primary abnormality in type II EMC, the type of cryoglobulinemia associated with the renal lesions described above, is the production of a monoclonal IgM rheumatoid factor. Therefore this disease falls within the spectrum of lymphoproliferative disorders, even though, with rare exceptions of late progression to lymphoma, patients show very little evidence of lymphoid malignancy.

There is increasing evidence that the production of IgM-κ rheumatoid factor is due to a clonal B-cell expansion. An increased percentage of idiotype-positive ($\mu +$) B cells have been found in both peripheral blood and in morphologically normal bone marrow in most of the patients tested [151]. A specific expansion of μ heavy and κ light chain–bearing cells has been shown in some patients by flow cytometry [115]. The same investigators confirmed previous preliminary data [152] demonstrating immunoglobulin gene rearrangements in the DNA extracted from peripheral blood B cells. We have also found that peripheral blood B lymphocytes from EMC patients produce larger quantities of IgM rheumatoid factor than do normal mononuclear cells, both spontaneously and after in vitro stimulation with pokeweed mitogen [99]. Although it is likely that the polyclonal IgG to which monoclonal IgM binds is already bound to an antigen to form immune complexes (thus the IgM would act as an anti–immune complex antibody), no antigens have been identified in the majority of cases. HBsAg may, however, be such an antigen in a minority of patients. We recently demonstrated the presence of IgM anti–viral capsid antigen of Epstein-Barr virus in a great number of patients with type II EMC [47]. More recently, we detected by DNA studies that the Epstein-Barr virus genome was incorporated into the bone marrow cells of all tested individuals with type II, but not those with type III cryoglobulinemia, suggesting an association between type II EMC and persistent Epstein-Barr virus infection [48].

It is still debated whether monoclonal IgM rheumatoid factor of type II cryoglobulins is always bound to the Fc portion of polyclonal IgG or might react in some cases against the IgG's $F(ab')_2$ fragments, thus acting as antiidiotypic antibody [53]. The inverse possibility that IgG might react as an antiidiotype against the hypervariable portion of IgM light chains has also been proposed [76].

Whatever the mechanism of binding, the mechanism of cryoprecipitation of the immunoglobulins involved in type II cryoglobulinemia is still unclear [137]. Intrinsic physicochemical properties of the single components are not sufficient to explain the phenomenon [37, 100, 142, 148], since it has been demonstrated that both immunoglobulins must be present for cryoprecipitation to take place [26, 71, 83]. Factors such as antigen-antibody ratio [3, 63], Fc-Fc interactions [102], reduced solubility due to hypocomplementemia [61, 129, 140], binding with fibronectin [5, 11], and hydrophobic properties of proteins [149] have all been considered.

PATHOPHYSIOLOGY OF THE RENAL DAMAGE IN TYPE II EMC

EMC-GN is an immune complex GN. Electron microscopy provides evidence that lesions are produced by the same cryoprecipitating immunoglobulins that are present in the circulation. Moreover, the subendothelial deposition of immunoglobulins and complement seen by immunofluorescence, the frequent hypocomplementemia, and the association of this nephropathy with defective reticuloendothelial system Fc receptor function support the view that the kidney damage in EMC is caused by immune complex deposition [20]. However, when massive intraluminal accumulation of cryoglobulins is found histologically together with an immunofluorescence pattern of almost exclusively intraluminal staining of thrombi, it has been postulated [29, 30] that intraglomerular precipitation takes place because of high intracapillary cryoglobulin concentrations during glomerular filtration [83].

Whatever the prevailing mechanism for their deposition in the glomerulus may be, locally trapped cryoglobulins trigger intracapillary accumulation of monocytes from the bloodstream. The presence of a large number of monocytes in the capillary lumina and in the double-contoured capillary walls of the glomeruli is the hallmark of the disease. These cells accumulate not only during the more acute clinical-histologic syndrome (in these circumstances up to 80 cells/glomerulus may be counted), but also in the more chronic phases of the renal disease. Monocytes in the renal tissue act as scavenger cells, as suggested by the presence of large phagolysosomes in their cytoplasm [144] and by their close contact with the deposits of cryoglobulins. But it is highly likely that they also behave as mediators of the local damage, through liberation of lytic enzymes and other humoral factors able to induce proliferation of resident cells [35, 109, 110]. Since T lymphocytes, mainly cytotoxic-suppressor T lymphocytes, accumulate with monocytes both in the glomerulus and in the interstitium, the participation of cellular immunity in this type of renal damage must also be considered.

Treatment

There is no agreement at present about the optimal treatment of EMC, and some investigators even prefer to adopt only symptomatic measures for patients with this condition [59].

A dietary approach has been tried for controlling some immunologic abnormalities and some extrarenal symptoms and signs of EMC. It was recently shown that a low-antigen-content diet can decrease the circulating immune complex levels and reduce the cryocrit value in patients with EMC. Purpura, asthenia, and liver enzymes improved during the diet. These favorable effects have been suggested to be due to a decreased input of high-molecular-weight exogenous substances to the mononuclear phagocytic system, with consequent functional restoration of this system and better removal of circulating immune complexes. Unfortunately no changes in arterial hypertension or nephropathy occurred [46].

Since EMC nephritis is often characterized by alternating periods of quiescence with episodes of exacerbations, it is appropriate to consider the treatment of acute exacerbations separately from the maintenance treatment.

TREATMENT OF ACUTE EXACERBATIONS

The development of nephrotic syndrome and acute renal function impairment worsens the prognosis of EMC. From a retrospective analysis of the literature [11, 14, 25, 41, 49, 54, 57, 58, 73, 77, 82, 91, 92, 98, 111, 112, 117, 130, 132, 136, 145, 154], we have found that of 11 patients with nephritic syndrome who received supportive treatment alone, 4 (36%) died or showed progressive renal failure, renal insufficiency remained stable in 2 (18%), while spontaneous improvement occurred in the other 5 (45%). The outcome was very similar to that reported in 27 patients treated with oral corticosteroids and/or cytotoxic agents. In fact, of these 27 patients, (37%) died or had progressive impairment of renal function, 4 (15%) had persistent but unchanged renal failure, and improvement of renal function occurred in the other 13 patients (48%). Therefore, it appears from this analysis that spontaneous remission of the nephritic syndrome can occur, while the efficacy of corticosteroids and cytotoxic agents in influencing the natural course of this complication is unconvincing.

There is emerging evidence that two forms of treatment can favorably alter the course of rapidly progressive renal disease in EMC: intravenous high-dose methylprednisolone (MP) pulses and plasmapheresis. After promising preliminary results [34, 84, 117], we treated 27 episodes of acute renal function deterioration with MP pulses [118]. All patients had proteinuria and hypertension and many of them complained of extrarenal symptoms of different severity. Treatment consisted of three consecutive pulses of MP, 1 gm each, given every 24 hours. Subsequently, 0.5 mg/kg/day of oral prednisone was given and gradually tapered to 0.1 to 0.2 mg/kg/day within 3 to 6 months. In several cases prednisone was associated with a cytotoxic agent, usually cyclophosphamide, 1 to 2 mg/kg/day for at least 2 months. Dramatic improvement of extrarenal symptoms was the most immediate effect in all cases. Serum creatinine decreased within 7 days in 23 of 27 patients. One month after MP pulse therapy, serum creatinine levels were lower than the basal values in all patients but 3, in whom renal function remained almost unchanged. The mean plasma creatinine levels decreased from 3.3 ± 1.3 to 2.2 ± 0.7 mg/dl. Proteinuria and cryocrit were slightly reduced after 1 month. Although this was not a controlled study, and although acute renal failure can spontaneously improve in EMC patients, the observation that renal function improved within a week in most cases from MP pulse therapy favors this treatment approach. Theoretically, MP pulse therapy might influence the evolution of acute nephritic syndrome by one or more of the following mechanisms: reduced immune complex formation [113], decreased vasoactive inflammatory products [39], modification of renal plasma flow [12], vasodilatory effects [110], monocytopenia and reduced glomerular macrophage accumulation [68], inhibition of the amplification pathway of complement [150], an antioxidant effect [6], and inhibited production of the platelet-activating factor [21]. The greater effect on plasma creatinine than on proteinuria, together with the rapid and often long-lasting effect on extrarenal symptoms with little modification of cryocrit or complement levels, suggests that reduction of inflammation and enhancement of compensatory vasodilatory mechanisms played an important role in the beneficial response to MP pulse therapy.

Plasmapheresis has been extensively used for treating acute exacerbations of EMC. Significant amounts of cryoproteins can be removed with this technique, thus preventing local cryoprecipitation in small renal vessels and restoring reticuloendothelial system functions that have been saturated by the chronic overload of circulating cryoglobulins [30]. Many uncontrolled studies have reported good results with plasmapheresis, with improvements in serum creatinine, proteinuria, and cryocrit [15, 16, 22, 30, 33, 44, 69, 97, 121]. These results demonstrate that there is a role for plasmapheresis in acute exacerbations of EMC. However, in most trials, plasmapheresis was combined with corticosteroids (often given as MP pulses) and cyclophosphamide so that it is difficult to assess whether the beneficial effects were attributable to the plasmapheresis per se, to the concomitant immunosuppression, or to the combination of the two treatments. Another technique, called cryoapheresis, was suggested by Maggiore et al. [87] for the treatment of EMC. With this procedure, plasma removed by plasmapheresis is refrigerated at 4°C and then centrifuged. The cryoprecipitate is separated and the plasma is reinfused after warming to 37°C. Cooling of 5 to 6 liters of plasma should bring about a decrease in cryoglobulin levels, ranging from 50 to 60 percent of the pretreatment values. Maggiore et al. [86] treated 10 patients with cryoapheresis for periods ranging from 2 to 4 months. They also administered cyclophosphamide and prednisolone to restrain cryoglobulin rebound and to slow the frequency of cryoapheretic treatment. A wide spectrum of responses was observed, ranging from none to complete biologic and histologic remission. The mean creatinine clearance increased from an average pretreatment value of 45 ± 33 ml/min to 62 ± 36 ml/min. This improvement was related to the degree of reduction in cryocrit. Others, however, have found that cryoapheresis was of little help in removing cryoproteins [125].

It is thus difficult to draw a final conclusion about the treatment of choice for EMC exacerbations. However, MP pulse therapy can be administered even to outpatients, is economic, and is generally well tolerated. We believe, therefore, that whenever an acute nephritic episode occurs in a patient with EMC, a short course of intravenous MP pulses should be given as early as possible, while treatment with plasmapheresis should be reserved for the few nonresponders. Simultaneous use of intravenous MP pulses, cyclophosphamide, and plasma exchange can be considered in severe cases, especially when signs of systemic vasculitis are present.

MAINTENANCE THERAPY

Many patients with EMC nephritis have a long-lasting, symptomless clinical course even if they are not treated at all. Prolonged treatment with oral corticosteroids and/or cytotoxic agents has been tried in many uncontrolled studies but the results have been inconsistent. Moreover, long-term therapy with corticosteroids and immunosuppressive agents may worsen the spontaneous tendency of patients with EMC to develop cardiovascular diseases and infections and can expose them to an increased risk of neoplasia [138]. Therefore, because of the little efficacy and the potential toxicity, prolonged immunosuppression does not appear to be justified. Prolonged plasma exchange plus small amounts of prednisone was used in 9 patients by Ferri et al. [45]. Exchanges ranged in frequency from 15 to 113 over a period of 1.5 to 24.0 months. In 5 patients there was an improvement in renal function and/or proteinuria without clinical relapse following withdrawal of plasma exchange. Patients with histologically active disease and little or no evidence of irreversible lesions had better chances of responding. Nevertheless, plasma exchange alone must still be regarded as an unproven therapy in EMC [72]. Interferon alfa (an inhibitor of B-cell proliferation) reduced extrarenal symptoms and improved proteinuria and renal function in a pilot study [18]. This therapy, however, awaits further substantial study before recommending it in EMC patients.

Of great importance is the management of arterial hypertension, which is a frequent complication of EMC with its potential effect on cardiovascular diseases and renal function. Unfortunately, in EMC patients with renal diseases, arterial hypertension is often refractory to therapy. Moreover, some antihypertensive agents, such as β-blockers, can exacerbate the patients' Raynaud's phenomenon [126], and other agents, such as hydralazine, can be dangerous in patients with coronary artery disease. We obtained good results in treating the hypertension of EMC with calcium channels antagonists [4], often combined with a diuretic agent and a converting enzyme inhibitor. This latter group of agents also has the advantage of reducing proteinuria. In 7 EMC patients treated with captopril, at doses of 75 to 150 mg daily, we observed a decrease in proteinuria from 3.0 ± 1.9 gm/day to 0.7 ± 0.7 gm/day after 3 months of treatment [118]. This effect, which is dose and time dependent, is probably related to a modification of glomerular hemodynamics. However, it is also possible that captopril might exert an antiinflammatory effect either by removing hydroxyl radicals or by blocking the kinins, which allows increased production of prostaglandins [90]. For patients with refractory hypertension the combination of a converting enzyme inhibitor with the powerful vasodilator agent minoxidil should be considered [93, 141]. Because of platelet hyperaggregability in EMC [116], antiplatelet agents might be useful to prevent cardiovascular complications.

DIALYSIS AND TRANSPLANTATION

There is little information about the clinical outcome of patients with EMC nephritis when end-stage renal failure occurs. Some investigators reported that the clinical and serologic activity of EMC decreases when patients have started hemodialysis [67, 96]. In many cases no cryoprecipitate was detectable and serum C3 and C4 levels were normal after dialysis. This immunologic quiescence has been attributed to the impairment of immune responsiveness caused by uremia and hemodialysis. We observed a similar behavior in several patients submitted to regular hemodialysis or peritoneal dialysis. In a few patients, however, clinical flare-ups occurred even after starting dialysis, with cryocrit levels approaching 80 percent in some patients. Therefore, it is likely that as for other immune complex diseases, there are two subpopulations of EMC patients on dialysis. In most patients the disease is quiescent while a minority of patients can develop clinical symptoms and biologic signs of activity.

The outcome of 10 patients who underwent renal transplantation because of EMC nephritis has been reported [7, 67, 96]. In 5 patients cryoglobulinemia quickly recurred after transplantation, with clinical renal and extrarenal flares and reappearance of the biologic markers of the disease. Typical features of EMC-GN were seen at renal biopsy. The course was progressive in 4 of 5 patients. The activity of the disease tended to subside after patients returned to dialysis.

References

1. Abraham, G. N., Podell, D. N., Wistar, R., Jr., et al. Immunological structural properties of human monoclonal IgG cryoglobulins. *Clin. Exp. Immunol.* 36: 63, 1979.
2. Aho, K., and Simons, K. Studies of the nature of the rheumatoid factor. Reaction of the rheumatic factor with human specific precipitates and with native human gamma globulin. *Arthritis Rheum.* 6: 676, 1963.
3. Alkner, U., and Hansson, U. B. Effect of IgM fractions with or without rheumatoid factor activity on antigen-antibody reactions. *Scand. J. Immunol.* 10: 119, 1979.
4. Ambroso, G. C., Como, G., Scalamogna, A., et al. Treatment of arterial hypertension with nifedipine in patients with chronic renal insufficiency. *Clin. Nephrol.* 23: 41, 1985.
5. Anderson, B., Rucker, M., Entwistle, R., et al. Plasma fibronectin is a component of cryoglobulins from patients with connective tissue and other diseases. *Ann. Rheum. Dis.* 40: 50, 1981.
6. Anderson, D. K., and Means, E. D. Iron-induced lipid peroxidation in spinal cord: Protection with mannitol and methylprednisolone. *J. Free Radic. Biol. Med.* 1: 59, 1985.
7. Andrejak, M., Bariéty, J., Bedrassian, J., et al. Cryoglobulinemia in renal transplant recipients. *Transplantation* 24: 446, 1978.
8. Banfi, G., and Bonini, P. A. Detection of cryoglobulins by Coulter Counter model S.-Plus IV/D. *Clin. Lab. Haematol.* 10: 453, 1988.
9. Barbiano di Belgiojoso, G., Montoli, A., Tarantino, A., et al. Clinical and Histological Correlations in Essential Mixed Cryoglobulinemia (EMC) Glomerulonephritis. In C. Ponticelli, L. Minetti, and G. D'Amico (eds.), *Antiglobulins, Cryoglobulins and Glomerulonephritis.* Dordrecht: M. Nijhoff, 1986. Pp. 203–210.
10. Barbiano di Belgiojoso, G., Tarantino, A., Colasanti, G., et al. Immunohistological Patterns in Mixed IgG-IgM Essential Cryoglobulinemia Glomerulonephritis. In A. Leaf, G. Giebisch, L. Bolis, and S. Gorini (eds.), *Renal Pathophysiology.* New York: Raven Press, 1980. Pp. 245–252.
11. Bartlow, B. G., Oyama, J. H., Ing, T. S., et al. Glomerular ultrastructural abnormalities in a patient with mixed IgG-IgM essential cryoglobulinemic glomerulonephritis. *Nephron* 14: 309, 1975.
12. Bayliss, C., and Brenner, B. M. Mechanism of the glucocorticoid induced increase in glomerular filtration rate. *Am. J. Physiol.* 234: 166, 1978.
13. Ben Bassat, M., Boner, G., Rosenfeld, J., et al. The clinicopathologic features of cryoglobulinemic nephropathy. *Am. J. Clin. Pathol.* 79: 147, 1983.
14. Bengtsson, U., Larsson, O., Lindstedt, G., et al. Monoclonal IgG cryoglobulinemia with secondary development of glomerulonephritis and nephrotic syndrome. *Q. J. Med.* 175: 491, 1975.
15. Berkman, E. M., and Orlin, J. B. Use of plasmapheresis and partial plasma exchange in the management of patients with cryoglobulinaemia. *Transfusion* 20: 171, 1980.
16. Bombardieri, S., Ferri, C., Paleolongo, G., et al. Prolonged plasma exchange in the treatment of renal involvement in essential mixed cryoglobulinemia. *Int. J. Artif. Organs* 6: 47, 1983.
17. Bombardieri, S., Paoletti, P., Ferri, C., et al. Lung involvement in essential mixed cryoglobulinemia. *Am. J. Med.* 66: 748, 1979.
18. Bonomo, L., Casato, M., Alfetra, A., et al. Treatment of idiopathic mixed cryoglobulinemia with alpha interferon. *Am. J. Med.* 83: 726, 1987.
19. Brouet, J. C., Clauvel, J. P., Danon, F., et al. Biological and clinical significance of cryoglobulins. A report of 86 cases. *Am. J. Med.* 57: 775, 1974.

20. Cameron, J. S., and Clark, W. F. A role for insoluble antibody-antigen complexes in glomerulonephritis? *Clin. Nephrol.* 18: 55, 1982.
21. Camussi, G., Tetta, C., Bussolini, F., et al. Mediators of immune-complex induced aggregation of polymorphonuclear neutrophils. *Int. Arch. Allergy Appl. Immunol.* 64: 25, 1981.
22. Cassuto-Viguier, E., Quaranta, J. F., Ortonne, J. P., et al. Effect of Plasma Exchange on the Course of Cryoglobulinemia. In Y. Nosé, P. S. Malchesky, J. W. Smith, et al. (eds.), *Plasmapheresis. Therapeutic Applications and New Techniques.* New York: Raven Press, 1983. Pp. 299–308.
23. Castiglione, A., Bucci, A., Fellin, G., et al. The relationship of infiltrating renal leukocytes to disease activity in lupus and cryoglobulinemic glomerulonephritis. *Nephron* 50: 14, 1988.
24. Cordonnier, D., Martin, H., Groslambert, P., et al. Mixed IgG-IgM cryoglobulinemia with glomerulonephritis. Immunochemical fluorescent and ultrastructural study of kidney and in vitro cryoprecipitate. *Am. J. Med.* 59: 867, 1975.
25. Cordonnier, D., Vialtel, P., Renversez, J. Ch., et al. Lésions rénales chez 18 malades porteurs de cryoglobulines mixtes (IgM-IgG) de type II. In J. Hamburger, J. Crosnier, and J. L. Funck-Brentano (eds.), *Actualités Néphrologiques de Hôpital Necker.* Paris: Flammarion, 1982. Pp. 219–241.
26. Costanzi, J. J., Coltman, C. A., Jr., Clark, D. A., et al. Cryoglobulinemia associated with macroglobulin. Studies of a 17.5 S cryoprecipitating factor. *Am. J. Med.* 39: 163, 1965.
27. Cream, J. J. Clinical and immunological aspects of cutaneous vasculitis. *Q. J. Med.* 45: 255, 1976.
28. Cream, J. J., Howard, A., and Virella, G. IgG heavy chain subclasses in mixed cryoglobulins. *Immunology* 23: 405, 1972.
29. D'Amico, G., Colasanti, G., Ferrario, F., et al. Renal involvement in essential mixed cryoglobulinemia. *Kidney Int.* 35: 1004, 1989.
30. D'Amico, G., Ferrario, F., Colasanti, G., et al. Glomerulonephritis in Essential Mixed Cryoglobulinemia (EMC). In A. M. Davison and P. J. Guillon (eds.), *Proceedings of European Dialysis and Transplant Association.* European Renal Association. London: Pitman, 1984. Pp. 527–548.
31. Dammacco, F., Miglietta, A., Lobreglio, G., et al. Cryoglobulins and pyroglobulins: An overview. *Ricerca Clin. Lab.* 16: 247, 1986.
32. Dammacco, F., Scarpioni, L., Antonacci, S., et al. Cryoglobulinemia in four sisters. *Acta Haematol.* 59: 215, 1978.
33. Delaney, V. B., Fraley, D. S., Segal, D. P., et al. Plasmapheresis as sole therapy in a patient with essential mixed cryoglobulinemia. *Am. J. Kidney Dis.* 4: 75, 1984.
34. De Vecchi, A., Montagnino, G., Pozzi, C., et al. Intravenous methylprednisolone pulse therapy in essential mixed cryoglobulinemia nephropathy. *Clin. Nephrol.* 19: 221, 1983.
35. Dubois, C. H., Foidart, J. B., Hautier, M. B., et al. Proliferative glomerulonephritis in rats: Evidence that mononuclear phagocytes infiltrating the glomeruli stimulate the proliferation of endothelial and mesangial cells. *Eur. J. Clin. Invest.* 11: 91, 1981.
36. Edelman, G. M., Kunkel, H. G., and Franklin, E. C. Interaction of the rheumatoid factor with antigen-antibody complexes and aggregated gamma globulin. *J. Exp. Med.* 108: 105, 1958.
37. Erickson, B. W., Gerber-Jenson, B., Wang, A. C., et al. Molecular basis for the temperature-dependent insolubility of cryoglobulins-XI. Sequence comparison of the heavy-chain variable regions of the human cryoimmunoglobulins McE and Hil by metric analysis. *Mol. Immunol.* 19: 347, 1982.
38. Faraggiana, T., Parolini, C., Previato, G., et al. Light and electron microscopic findings in five cases of cryoglobulinemic glomerulonephritis. *Virchows Arch. Pathol. Anat.* 384: 29, 1979.
39. Fauci, A. S., Dale, D. C., and Balow, J. E. Corticosteroid therapy: Mechanism of action and clinical consideration. *Ann. Intern. Med.* 84: 304, 1976.
40. Feiner, H., and Gallo, G. Ultrastructure in glomerulonephritis associated with cryoglobulinemia. *Am. J. Pathol.* 88: 145, 1977.
41. Feizi, T., and Gitlin, N. Immune-complex disease of the kidney associated with chronic hepatitis and cryoglobulinaemia. *Lancet* 2: 873, 1969.
42. Ferrario, F., Castiglione, A., Colasanti, G., et al. The detection of monocytes in human glomerulonephritis. *Kidney Int.* 28: 513, 1985.
43. Ferrario, F., Colasanti, G., Barbiano di Belgiojoso, G., et al. Histological and Immunohistological Features in Essential Mixed Cryoglobulinemia Glomerulonephritis. In C. Ponticelli, L. Minetti, and G. D'Amico (eds.), *Antiglobulins, Cryoglobulins and Glomerulonephritis.* Dordrecht: M. Nijhoff, 1986. Pp. 193–202.
44. Ferri, C., Gremignai, G., Bombardieri, S., et al. Plasma exchange in mixed cryoglobulinemia: The effect on renal, liver and neurologic involvement. *Ricerca Clin. Lab.* 16: 403, 1986.
45. Ferri, C., Moriconi, L., Gremignai, G., et al. Treatment of the renal involvement in mixed cryoglobulinemia with prolonged plasma exchange. *Nephron* 43: 246, 1986.
46. Ferri, C., Pietrogrande, M., Cecchetti, R., et al. Low-antigen content diet in the treatment of patients with mixed cryoglobulinemia. *Am. J. Med.* 87: 519, 1989.
47. Fiorini, G., Bernasconi, P., Sinico, R. A., et al. Increased frequency of antibodies to ubiquitous viruses in essential mixed cryoglobulinemia. *Clin. Exp. Immunol.* 64: 65, 1986.
48. Fiorini, G., Sinico, R. A., Winearls, C., et al. Persistent Epstein-Barr virus in patients with type II essential mixed cryoglobulinemia. *Clin. Immunol. Immunopathol.* 47: 262, 1988.
49. Franklin, E. C. Cryoglobulinemia. *Am. J. Med. Sci.* 262: 50, 1971.
50. Franklin, E. C., and Frangione, B. Common structural and antigenic properties of human M anti-γ-globulins. *J. Immunol.* 107: 1527, 1971.
51. Gamble, C. N., and Ruggles, S. W. The immunopathogenesis of glomerulonephritis associated with mixed cryoglobulinemia. *N. Engl. J. Med.* 299: 81, 1978.
52. Garcia-Bragado, F., Vilardell, M., Fonollosa, V., et al. Cryoglobulinémie mixte essentielle: Relations avec le virus de l'hépatite B. *Nouv. Presse Med.* 10: 2955, 1981.
53. Geltner, D., Franklin, E. C., and Frangione, B. Antiidiotypic activity in the IgM fractions of mixed cryoglobulins. *J. Immunol.* 125: 1530, 1980.
54. Germain, M. J., Anderson, R. W., and Keane, W. F. Renal disease in cryoglobulinemia type II: Response to therapy. *Am. J. Nephrol.* 2: 221, 1982.
55. Gigli, I. Complement Activation in Patients with Mixed Cryoglobulinemia (Cryoglobulins and Complement). In C. Ponticelli, L. Minetti, and G. D'Amico (eds.), *Antiglobu-*

lins, Cryoglobulins and Glomerulonephritis. Dordrecht: M. Nijhoff, 1986. Pp. 135–146.
56. Gilboa, N., Durante, D., Guggenheim, S., et al. Immune deposits nephritis and single-component cryoglobulinemia associated with chronic lymphocytic leukemia. *Nephron* 24: 223, 1979.
57. Goldberg, L. S., and Barnett, E. V. Essential cryoglobulinemia. Immunologic studies before and after penicillamine therapy. *Arch. Intern. Med.* 125: 145, 1970.
58. Golde, D., and Epstein, W. Mixed cryoglobulins and glomerulonephritis. *Ann. Intern. Med.* 69: 1221, 1968.
59. Gorevic, P. D. Mixed Cryoglobulinemia: An Update of Recent Clinical Experience. In C. Ponticelli, L. Minetti, and G. D'Amico (eds.), *Antiglobulins, Cryoglobulins and Glomerulonephritis*. Dordrecht: M. Nijhoff, 1986. Pp. 179–192.
60. Gorevic, P. D., Kassab, H. J., Levo, Y., et al. Mixed cryoglobulinemia: Clinical aspects and long-term follow-up of 40 patients. *Am. J. Med.* 69: 287, 1980.
61. Gough, W. W., and Davis, J. S., IV. Effects of rheumatoid factor on complement levels in vivo. *Arthritis Rheum.* 9: 555, 1966.
62. Grey, H. H., and Kohler, P. F. Cryoimmunoglobulins. *Semin. Hematol.* 10: 87, 1973.
63. Griswold, W. R., and Brady, R. Cryoglobulins in acute experimental immune complex glomerulonephritis. *J. Lab. Clin. Med.* 92: 423, 1978.
64. Hamburger, M. J., Gorevic, P. D., Lawley, T. J., et al. Mixed cryoglobulinemia. Association of glomerulonephritis with defective reticuloendothelial system Fc-receptor function. *Trans. Assoc. Am. Physicians* 62: 104, 1979.
65. Hardin, J. A., and McCluskey, R. T. Case records of the Massachusetts General Hospital. *N. Engl. J. Med.* 292: 1285, 1975.
66. Haydey, R. P., Patarroyo de Royas, M., and Gigli, I. A newly described control mechanism of complement activation in patients with mixed cryoglobulinemia (cryoglobulins and complement). *J. Invest. Dermatol.* 74: 328, 1980.
67. Hiesse, C., Bastuji-Garin, S., Santelli, G., et al. Recurrent essential mixed cryoglobulinemia in renal allografts. Report of two cases and review of the literature. *Am. J. Nephrol.* 9: 150, 1989.
68. Holdsworth, S. R., and Bellomo, R. Differential effects of steroids on leukocyte-mediated glomerulonephritis in rabbit. *Kidney Int.* 26: 162, 1984.
69. Houwert, D. A., Hené, R. J., Struyvenberg, A., et al. Effect of Plasmapheresis (PP), Corticosteroids and Cyclophosphamide in Essential Mixed Polyclonal Cryoglobulinemia Associated with Glomerulonephritis. In B. H. B. Robinson, and J. B. Hawkins (eds.), *Proceedings of European Dialysis and Transplant Association*. London: Pitman, 1980. Pp. 650–654.
70. Invernizzi, F., Pioltelli, P., Cattaneo, R., et al. A long term follow-up study in essential mixed cryoglobulinemia. *Acta Haematol.* 61: 93, 1979.
71. Jacquot, C., Nochy, D., D'Auzac, C., et al. Glomerulonephritis, B monoclonal small lymphocytic lymphoma and mixed cryoglobulinemia. *Clin. Nephrol.* 27: 263, 1987.
72. Jordan, S. C., Jennette, J. C., Neale, T. J., et al. The Glomerular Diseases. In H. C. Gonick (ed.), *Current Nephrology*. Chicago: Year Book, 1990. Pp. 112–176.
73. Kaplan, N. G., and Kaplan, K. C. Monoclonal gammopathy glomerulonephritis and the nephritic syndrome. *Arch. Intern. Med.* 125: 696, 1970.
74. Klein, F., Van Rood, J. J., Van Furth, R., et al. IgM-IgG cryoglobulinemia with paraprotein component. *Clin. Exp. Immunol.* 3: 703, 1968.
75. Koelz, A. M., and Bourke, E. Cryoglobulinaemic nephropathy with papillary necrosis. *Nephron* 19: 242, 1977.
76. Lambert, P. H., Goldman, M., Renversez, J. C., et al. Pathological Consequences of Idiotype-Anti-Idiotype Interactions. In F. Milgrom (ed.), *Antibodies: Protective, Destructive and Regulatory Role*. Basel: Karger, 1985. Pp. 356–362.
77. Lapes, M. J., and Davis, J. S., IV. Arthralgia-purpura-weakness cryoglobulinemia. *Arch. Intern. Med.* 126: 461, 1980.
78. Lawley, T. J., Gorevic, L. D., Hamburger, M. I., et al. Multiple types of immune complexes in patients with mixed cryoglobulinemia. *J. Invest. Dermatol.* 75: 297, 1980.
79. Levo, Y., Gorevic, P. D., Kassab, H. J., et al. Association between hepatitis B virus and essential mixed cryoglobulinemia. *N. Engl. J. Med.* 296: 1501, 1977.
80. Linscott, W. D., and Kane, J. P. The complement system in cryoglobulinemia interaction with immunoglobulins and lipoproteins. *Clin. Exp. Immunol.* 21: 510, 1975.
81. Litman, G. W., Scheffel, C., Gerber-Jenson, B., et al. Molecular basis for the temperature-dependent insolubility of cryoglobulins. XII. *Immunol. Communications* 10: 707, 1981.
82. Lockwood, C. M. Lymphoma, cryoglobulinemia and renal disease. *Kidney Int.* 16: 522, 1979.
83. Lo Spalluto, J., Dorward, B., Miller, W., Jr., et al. Cryoglobulinemia based on interaction between a gamma macroglobulin and 7S gamma globulin. *Am. J. Med.* 32: 142, 1962.
84. Maggiore, Q., Bartolomeo, F., L'Abbate, A., et al. HBsAg glomerular deposits in glomerulonephritis: Fact or artifact? *Kidney Int.* 19: 579, 1981.
85. Maggiore, Q., Bartolomeo, F., L'Abbate, A., et al. Glomerular localization of circulating antiglobulin activity in essential mixed cryoglobulinemia. *Kidney Int.* 21: 387, 1982.
86. Maggiore, Q., L'Abbate, A., Bartolomeo, F., et al. Effects of Cryoapheresis on Plasma Cryoglobulins and Renal Function in Patients with EMC Glomerulonephritis. In C. Ponticelli, L. Minetti, and G. D'Amico (eds.), *Antiglobulins, Cryoglobulins and Glomerulonephritis*. Dordrecht: M. Nijhoff, 1986. Pp. 251–264.
87. Maggiore, Q., L'Abbate, A., Caccamo, A., et al. Cryopheresis in the treatment of essential mixed cryoglobulinemia (EMC) with glomerulonephritis. *Artif. Organs* (Suppl.)5: 47, 1981.
88. Magil, A. B. Monocytes and glomerulonephritis associated with remote visceral infection. *Clin. Nephrol.* 22: 169, 1984.
89. Markenson, J. H., Daniels, C. A., Notkins, A. L., et al. The interaction of rheumatoid factor with hepatitis B surface antigen-antibody complexes. *Clin. Exp. Immunol.* 19: 209, 1975.
90. Martin, M. F. R., Surrall, K. E., McKenna, F., et al. Captopril: A new treatment for rheumatoid arthritis? *Lancet* 1: 1325, 1984.
91. Martinez, J. S., and Kohler, P. F. Variant 'Goodpasture's syndrome'? The need for immunologic criteria in rapidly progressive glomerulonephritis and hemorrhagic pneumonitis. *Ann. Intern. Med.* 75: 67, 1971.
92. Mathison, D. A., Condemi, J. J., Leddy, J. P., et al. Purpura, arthralgia and IgM-IgG cryoglobulinemia with

rheumatoid factor activity. *Ann. Intern. Med.* 74: 383, 1971.

93. Matson, J. R., Norby, L. H., and Robillard, J. E. Interactions of minoxidil and captopril in the treatment of refractory hypertension. *Am. J. Dis. Child.* 135: 256, 1981.
94. Mazzucco, G., Monga, G., Casanova, S., et al. Cell interposition in glomerular capillary walls in cryoglobulinemic glomerulonephritis. Ultrastructural investigation of 23 cases. *Ultrastruct. Pathol.* 10: 355, 1986.
95. Mc Duffie, F. C., Hunder, G. G., and Clark, J. R. Complement-fixing material in the sera of patients with rheumatoid arthritis. *Clin. Exp. Immunol.* 32: 218, 1978.
96. Mc Intosh, R. M., Griswold, W. R., Chernack, W. B., et al. Cryoglobulins. III. Further studies in the nature, incidence, clinical, diagnostic and immunopathologic significance of cryoproteins in renal diseases. *Q. J. Med.* 44: 285, 1975.
97. McLeod, B. C., and Sassetti, R. J. Plasmapheresis with return of cryoglobulins-depleted autologous plasma (cryoglobulin-pheresis) in cryoglobulinaemia. *Blood* 55: 866, 1980.
98. Meltzer, M., Franklin, E. C., Elias, K., et al. Cryoglobulinemia—a clinical and laboratory study. II. Cryoglobulins with rheumatoid factor activity. *Am. J. Med.* 40: 837, 1966.
99. Meroni, P. L., Barcellini, W., Sinico, R. A., et al. In vitro synthesis of IgM rheumatoid factor by lymphocytes from patients with essential mixed cryoglobulinemia. *Clin. Exp. Immunol.* 65: 303, 1986.
100. Middaugh, C. R., Oshman, R. G., and Litman, G. W. Localization of anomaly to the Fabμ region of a monoclonal IgM cryoglobulin. *Clin. Exp. Immunol.* 31: 126, 1978.
101. Mihatsch, M. J., and Banfi, G. Ultrastructural Features in Glomerulonephritis in Essential Mixed Cryoglobulinemia. In C. Ponticelli, L. Minetti, and G. D'Amico (eds.), *Antiglobulins, Cryoglobulins and Glomerulonephritis.* Dordrecht: M. Nijhoff, 1986. Pp. 211–218.
102. Møller, N. P. H., and Steensgaard, J. Fc-mediated immune precipitation. II. Analysis of precipitating immune complexes by rate-zonal ultracentrifugation. *Immunology* 38: 641, 1979.
103. Monga, G., Mazzucco, G., Barbiano di Belgiojoso, G., et al. The presence and possible role of monocyte infiltration in human chronic proliferative glomerulonephritis. *Am. J. Pathol.* 94: 271, 1979.
104. Monga, G., Mazzucco, G., Coppo, R., et al. Glomerular findings in mixed IgG-IgM cryoglobulinemia. Light, electron microscopy, immunofluorescence and histochemical correlations. *Virchows Arch. Zell. Pathol.* 20: 185, 1976.
105. Montecucco, C., Cherie-Ligniere, E. L., and Ascari, E. Pseudo-leucocytosis in essential mixed cryoglobulinemia may simulate chronic lymphocytic leukemia. *Clin. Exp. Rheumatol.* 3: 278, 1985.
106. Morel-Maroger, L., and Méry, J. P. Renal lesions in mixed IgG-IgM essential cryoglobulinemia. In *Proceedings of the Fifth Congress of Nephrology,* Mexico, 1972. Basel: Karger, 1972. Pp. 249–252.
107. Morel-Maroger, L., and Verroust, P. Glomerular lesions in dysproteinemias. *Kidney Int.* 5: 249, 1974.
108. Moscicki, R. A., and Colvin, R. B. A 57 year old woman with recurrent skin lesions, arthritis and renal dysfunction. Case records of the Massachusetts General Hospital. *N. Engl. J. Med.* 320: 718, 1989.
109. Nathan, C. F., Murray, H. W., and Cohen, Z. A. Current concepts: The macrophage as an effector cell. *N. Engl. J. Med.* 303: 622, 1980.
110. Nayslett, A., McGiff, J. C., and Colina-Chourio, J. Interrelations of the renin-kallikrein-kinin system and renal prostaglandins in the conscious rat. *Circ. Res.* 43: 799, 1978.
111. Nightingale, S. D. Familial cryoglobulinemia. *Johns Hopkins Med. J.* 140: 267, 1977.
112. Ogihara, T., Saruta, T., Saito, I., et al. Finger print deposits of the kidney in pure monoclonal IgG kappa cryoglobulinemia. *Clin. Nephrol.* 12: 186, 1979.
113. Ooi, Y. M., Ooi, B. S., and Vallota, E. H. Circulating immunocomplexes after renal transplantation. Correlation of increased ^{125}I-C1q binding activity with acute rejection characterized by fibrin deposition in the kidney. *J. Clin. Invest.* 60: 611, 1977.
114. Perez, G. O., Pardo, V., and Fletcher, M. Renal involvement in essential mixed cryoglobulinemia. *Am. J. Kidney Dis.* 10: 276, 1987.
115. Perl, A., Gorevic, P. D., Ryan, D. H., et al. Clonal B cells expansion in patients with essential mixed cryoglobulinemia. *Clin. Exp. Immunol.* 76: 54, 1989.
116. Ponticelli, C., Canciani, M. T., Tarantino, A., et al. Acquired platelet dysfunction (Delta storage pool deficiency) in essential mixed cryoglobulinemia. *Thromb. Haemostas.* 50: 357, 1983.
117. Ponticelli, C., Imbasciati, E., Tarantino, A., et al. Acute anuric glomerulonephritis in monoclonal cryoglobulinaemia. *Br. Med. J.* 1: 948, 1977.
118. Ponticelli, C., Montagnino, G., Campise, R., et al. Treatment of Renal Disease in Essential Mixed Cryoglobulinemia. In C Ponticelli, L. Minetti, and G. D'Amico (eds.), *Antiglobulins, Cryoglobulins and Glomerulonephritis.* Dordrecht: M. Nijhoff, 1986. Pp. 265–272.
119. Pope, R. M., Fletcher, M. A., Mamby, A., et al. Essential mixed cryoglobulinemia without evidence for hepatitis B virus infection. *Ann. Intern. Med.* 92: 379, 1980.
120. Porush, J. G., Grishman, E., Alter, A. A., et al. Paraproteinemia and cryoglobulinemia associated with atypical glomerulonephritis and nephrotic syndrome. *Am. J. Med.* 47: 957, 1969.
121. Pusey, C. D., Schifferli, J. A., Lockwood, C. M., et al. Use of plasma exchange in the management of mixed essential cryoglobulinaemia. *Artif. Organs* (Suppl.) 5: 183, 1981.
122. Reza, M. J., Roth, B. E., Popps, M. A., et al. Intestinal vasculitis in essential mixed cryoglobulinemia. *Ann. Intern. Med.* 81: 632, 1974.
123. Rigo, P., De Leval-Rutten, F., and Salmon, J. Un cas de cryoglobulinémie mixte IgM-IgG chez une malade atteinte de macroglobulinémie de Waldenström. *Acta Clin. Belg.* 29: 20, 1974.
124. Robinson, D. R., and Kirkham, S. E. Case record of the Massachusetts General Hospital. *N. Engl. J. Med.* 311: 904, 1984.
125. Rock, G. A., Blanchette, V. A., McKendry, R. G., et al. Plasmapheresis and Cryoglobulinemia: An Evaluation of Cold Precipitation as a Method for Removing Abnormal Protein. In Y. Nosé, P. S. Malchesky, J. W. Smith, et al. (eds.), *Plasmapheresis: Therapeutic Applications and New Techniques.* New York: Raven Press, 1983. Pp. 217–218.
126. Rodeheffer, R. J., Rommer, J. A., Wigley, F., et al. Controlled double-blind trial of nifedipine in the treatment of Raynaud's phenomenon. *N. Engl. J. Med.* 308: 880, 1983.
127. Ruddy, S., Carpenter, G. B., Chin, K. W., et al. Human

complement metabolism: An analysis of 144 studies. *Medicine* 54: 165, 1975.

128. Saluk, P. A., and Clem, W. Studies on the cryoprecipitation of human IgG_3 cryoglobulin: The effects of temperature-induced conformational changes of the primary interaction. *Immunochemistry* 12: 29, 1975.
129. Schifferli, J. A., Amos, N., Pusey, C. D., et al. Metabolism of IgG in type II mixed essential cryoglobulinaemia-autologous cryoprecipitated and normal homologous IgG are incorporated into complexes and metabolized in vivo at similar rates. *Clin. Exp. Immunol.* 51: 305, 1983.
130. Scully, R. E., and Mc Nealy, B. U. Case records of the Massachusetts General Hospital. *N. Engl. J. Med.* 292: 1285, 1975.
131. Sinico, A. R., Winearls, C. G., Sabadini, E., et al. Identification of glomerular immune deposits in cryoglobulinemia glomerulonephritis. *Kidney Int.* 34: 109, 1988.
132. Skrifvars, B., Tallqvist, G., and Törnöth, T. Renal involvement in essential cryoglobulinemia. *Acta Med. Scand.* 194: 229, 1973.
133. Slatopolski, E. Mixed cryoimmunoglobulinemia. *Am. J. Med.* 61: 95, 1976.
134. Stagg, M. P., Lauber, J., and Michaliski, J. P. Mixed essential cryoglobulinemia and adult respiratory distress syndrome: A case report. *Am. J. Med.* 87: 445, 1988.
135. Tarantino, A., Anelli, A., Costantino, A., et al. Serum complement pattern in essential mixed cryoglobulinemia. *Clin. Exp. Immunol.* 32: 77, 1978.
136. Tarantino, A., De Vecchi, A., Montagnino, G., et al. Renal disease in essential mixed cryoglobulinemia. Long-term follow-up of 44 patients. *Q. J. Med.* 50: 1, 1981.
137. Tarantino, A., and Montagnino, G. The Pathogenesis of Essential Cryoglobulinemia. In T. Bertani, and G. Remuzzi (eds.), *Glomerular Injury 300 Years After Morgagni.* Milano: Wichtig, 1983. Pp. 245–254.
138. Tarantino, A., Montagnino, G., Baldassari, A., et al. Prognostic Factors in Essential Mixed Cryoglobulinemia Nephropathy. In C. Ponticelli, L. Minetti, and G. D'Amico (eds.), *Antiglobulins, Cryoglobulins and Glomerulonephritis.* Dordrecht: M. Nijhoff, 1986. Pp. 219–225.
139. Tarantino, A., and Ponticelli, C. Kidney Involvement in Essential Cryoglobulinemia. In P. A. Bacon, and N. M. Hadler (eds.), *The Kidney and Rheumatic Disease.* London: Butterworth Scientific, 1982. Pp. 128–149.
140. Tesar, J. T., and Schmid, F. R. Conversion of soluble immune complexes into complement-fixing aggregates by IgM-rheumatoid factor. *J. Immunol.* 105: 1206, 1970.
141. Traub, Y., and Levey, B. A. Combined treatment with minoxidil and captopril in refractory hypertension. *Arch. Intern. Med.* 143: 1142, 1983.
142. Trieshmann, H. W., Jr., Abraham, G. N., and Santucci, E. A. The characterization of human anti-IgG autoantibodies by liquid isoelectric focusing. *J. Immunol.* 114: 176, 1975.
143. Tubbs, R. R., Gephardt, G. N., Calabrese, L., et al. Primary ultrastructural diagnosis of cryoglobulinemic glomerulonephritis. *Arch. Pathol. Lab. Med.* 105: 474, 1981.
144. Unanue, E. R. Secretory function of mononuclear phagocytes: Review. *Am. J. Pathol.* 83: 396, 1976.
145. Verroust, P., Méry, J. P., Morel-Maroger, L., et al. Les Lésions Glomérulaires des Gammopathies Monoclonales et Des Cryoglobulinémies Idiopathiques IgG-IgM. In J. Hamburger, J. Crosnier, and J. L. Funck-Brentano (eds.), *Actualités Néphrologiques de l'Hôpital Necker.* Paris: Flammarion, 1971. Pp. 167–202.
146. Virella, G., and Hobbs, J. R. Heavy chain typing in IgG monoclonal gammopathies with special reference to cases of serum hyperviscosity and cryoglobulinaemia. *Clin. Exp. Immunol.* 9: 973, 1971.
147. Wager, O., Mustakallio, K. K., and Rasanen, J. A. Mixed IgA-IgG cryoglobulinemia. Immunological studies and case reports of three patients. *Am. J. Med.* 44: 179, 1968.
148. Wang, A. C., and Wang, I. Y. Intrinsic Properties Inducing Precipitation of Cryoglobulins. In C. Ponticelli, L. Minetti, and G. D'Amico (eds.), *Antiglobulins, Cryoglobulins and Glomerulonephritis.* Dordrecht: M. Nijhoff, 1986. Pp. 101–112.
149. Wang, A. C., Wells, J. V., and Fundemberg, H. H. Chemical analysis of cryoglobulins. *Immunochemistry* 11: 341, 1974.
150. Weiler, J. M., and Packard, B. D. Methylprednisolone inhibits the alternative and amplification pathways of complement. *Infect. Immunol.* 38: 122, 1982.
151. Winearls, C. G., Ono, M., Fiorini, G., et al. Identification of circulating MRF-producing cells in essential mixed cryoglobulinaemia. *Nephrol. Dial. Transplant.* 1: 78, 1986.
152. Winearls, C. G., and Sisson, J. P. Use of idiotype markers for cellular detection of monoclonal rheumatoid factor. *Springer Semin. Immunopathol.* 10: 67, 1988.
153. Zandeck, M., Dupriez, B., Demory, J. L., et al. Numération leucocytaire et plaquettaire artificiellement augmentées, révélatrices d'une cryoglobulinémie de type II. *Nouv. Presse Med.* 35: 1756, 1989.
154. Zimmerman, S. W., Dreher, W. H., Burkholder, P. M., et al. Nephropathy and mixed cryoglobulinaemia: Evidence for an immune complex pathogenesis. *Nephron* 16: 103, 1976.
155. Zinneman, H. H., Levi, D., and Seal, U. On the nature of cryoglobulins. *J. Immunol.* 100: 594, 1968.
156. Zlotnick, A., Slavin, S., and Eliamkin, M. Mixed cryoglobulinemia with monoclonal IgM component associated with chronic liver disease. *Israel J. Med. Sci.* 8: 1968, 1972.
157. Zollinger, H. U., and Miatsch, M. J. Immunohistopathologic Parameters. In H. U. Zollinger and M. J. Mihatsch (eds.), *Renal Pathology in Biopsy.* Berlin: Springer-Verlag, 1978. Pp. 152–172.

Index

Index

Abdomen, acute, in malignant hypertension, 1569
Abdominal tumor(s), acute renal vein thrombosis due to, in nephrotic syndrome, 1325
ABO incompatibility, renal transplantation and, 2920–2921
Abscess
 intrarenal, 959–966
 perinephric, 966–969
  angiography for, 968
  clinical features of, 967
  computed tomography for, 968, 969f
  diagnosis of, 967–968, 968f–969f
  emphysematous pyelonephritis in, 967–968
  etiology of, 966
  pathogenesis of, 966–967, 967f
  prognosis in, 969
  radionuclide imaging for, 968, 969f
  treatment of, 968–969
  ultrasonography in, 968, 968f
 renal, CT for, 451
 renal cortical, 959–963
  angiography for, 960, 962f
  clinical features of, 959–960
  computed tomography for, 961–962
  diagnosis of, 960–962, 961f–962f
  etiology of, 959
  laboratory findings in, 959–960
  pathogenesis of, 959, 960f
  physical examination in, 959
  radionuclide scan in, 960–961, 962f
  treatment of, 962–963
  ultrasonography for, 960, 961f
 renal corticomedullary, 963–966
  due to acute focal bacterial nephritis, 963
  due to acute multifocal bacterial nephritis, 963
  clinical features of, 963–964
  diagnosis of, 964–965
  etiology of, 963
  pathogenesis of, 963
  treatment of, 965–966
  due to xanthogranulomatous pyelonephritis, 963
 subcapsular, angiography for, 478
Acebutolol, pharmacology of, normal vs. in renal failure, 3236t–3237t
Acetaminophen
 as nephrotoxin, 1042
 pharmacology of, normal vs. in renal failure, 3236t–3237t
Acetoacetic acid, 2579
 decarboxylation of, 2570, 2571f
Acetone, metabolism of, 2579
Achilles reflex, loss of, in toxic neuropathies, 2805
Acid(s)
 amino. *See* Amino acid(s)
 endogenous production of, 2669
 inorganic, overproduction of, 2577
 net excretion of, determinants of, 211
 net transport of
  anatomic relationships among nephron segments and, 211f, 211–212
  in collecting ducts, 217–218
  in distal tubule, 216–217, 623f, 624
  in loop of Henle, 213f, 215–216
  in proximal tubule, 212–215, 623, 623f. *See also* Tubule(s), proximal
  renal handling of, 211–219
  in renal medulla, 218–219
 organic, overproduction of, 2577
Acid-base balance
 aging and, 2417–2418, 2418f
 altered, renal response to, 209–211, 210f
 bicarbonate concentration in, 208, 208f
 buffer base concentration in, 207, 208f
 disturbances of
  in cirrhosis, 2475
  complicating diabetes mellitus, 2563–2576
  in falciparum malaria, 2340
  metabolic, in diabetes mellitus, 2576–2592
 in extracellular fluid, 208–209
  bone buffering and, 209
  buffer systems for, 208
  carbon dioxide balance in, 208
  cellular buffering and, 209
  cellular metabolism and, 209
  diet and, 209
  nonrenal excretion and, 209
  total proton balance in, 208–209, 209f
  urinary net acid excretion in, 209
 hydrogen ion reactions in, 207
  buffer reactions in, 207
  metabolic reactions in, 207
 hypophosphatemia and, 2610
 mixed disorders of, 2583–2584, 2584t
 phosphorus absorption and, 2602
 potassium regulation and, 2648
 in pregnancy, 2288
 systemic, 207–211
Acid-base homeostasis, in chronic renal failure, 2728–2731
 pattern of, 2728–2729, 2729f
Acid-base transport, 207–228
 across apical membranes, 220–221
  acidification in, 220–221
   ammonium secretion for, 221
   proton transport for, 220–221
  alkalinization in, 221
  bicarbonate secretion in, 221
  NH_4^+ absorption in, 221
 across basolateral membranes, 221–222
  acidification and, 221–222
   ammonium transport for, 222
   bicarbonate for, 221
   bicarbonate-chloride exchange in, 222
   sodium-bicarbonate co-transport for, 221–222
  alkalinization and, 222
 cellular chemical reactions in, 222–223
  hydration of carbon dioxide as, 222–223
  metabolism of glutamine as, 222f, 223
 in cortical collecting duct, 226, 227f–228f
 in distal tubule, 623f, 624
 in inner and outer medullar collecting duct, 226–228, 228f
 luminal buffer reactions in, 223–225
  ammonium in, 223–224, 224f
  bicarbonate in, 223
  luminal carbonic anhydrase in, 224–225, 225f
  titratable acidity in, 224
 in proximal tubule, 225, 226f, 623, 623f
 summary and integration of, 225–228
 in thick ascending limb, 226, 227f
 transepithelial, 219–228
  principles of, 219–220
   net nonreactive ion flux in, 219–220
   net reactive ion concentration in, 219
   net reactive ion flux in, 219
Acidemia, treatment of, in hyperkalemia, 2659
Acidification
 renal, defect in, clinical implications of, 2421–2422
 of urine. *See* Urine acidification
Acidosis
 in experimental renal disease, 2719
 hyperchloremic, in diabetes mellitus, 2581–2582
 lactic
  anion gap in, 2577, 2577t
  diabetes mellitus and, 2580f, 2580–2581
 metabolic. *See* Metabolic acidosis
 respiratory. *See* Respiratory acidosis
 tubular. *See* Tubular acidosis
 uremic, 2671
  anion gap in, 2577, 2577t
  diabetes mellitus and, 2581
Acquired immunodeficiency syndrome (AIDS), 2361. *See also* Human immunodeficiency virus (HIV) infection
 acute renal failure in, 2362–2365
  drugs causing, 2363–2364
 adrenal abnormalities in, 2365–2366
 electrolyte abnormalities in, 2365
 failure to thrive syndrome in, 2370
 in heroin abusers, focal glomerulosclerosis and, 1219, 1225
 malignancy in, 2361
 membranoproliferative glomerulonephritis and, 1830–1831
 opportunistic infections in, 2361
 renal parenchymal abnormalities in, 2365
Acromegaly, hyperphosphatemia and, 2613
ACTH. *See* Adrenocorticotropic hormone (ACTH)
Acute renal failure, 1371–1394. *See also* Azotemia
 acute tubular necrosis in. *See* Tubular necrosis, acute
 age-related, 2424–2425, 2425f, 2426f
 in AIDS, 2362–2365
  acyclovir-induced, 2364
  aminoglycoside-induced, 2363
  amphotericin B-induced, 2363
  antineoplastic agents causing, 2364
  drugs causing, 2363–2364
  pentamidine-induced, 2363
  rifampin-induced, 2363–2364
  sulfadiazine-induced, 2364
  trimethoprim-sulfamethoxazole-induced, 2363
 amino acid intake predisposing to, 3196
 in analgesic-induced renal disease, 1112
 anemia in, 2743–2744
 in cancer, 1165–1168, 1166t. *See also* Cancer
 catabolism or malnourishment in, new techniques for, 3196
 causes of, 1371, 1372f
 causes of death in, 1373, 1373t
 clinical approach to, 1375, 1376f
 complications of, 1302t, 1302–1308
  cardiovascular, 1302
  endocrine, 1305–1306

Acute renal failure, complications of—Continued
gastrointestinal, 1303–1304
hematologic, 1308
infectious, 1305
neurologic, 1304–1305
pulmonary, 1303
contrast media-induced, 1187–1197. *See also* Contrast media-induced acute renal failure
copper sulfate poisoning and, 2332
definition of, 1287
diagnostic approach to, 1295–1302
anuria in, 1296
chart, review, and physical examination in, 1295–1296
nonoliguria in, 1296–1297
oliguria in, 1296–1297
renal biopsy in, 1301–1302
sequence for, 1295, 1295t
urinalysis in, 1296
urinary chemical indices in, 1298–1301, 1299t
urinary flow rate in, 1296–1298
urinary tract obstruction and, 1301
dietary therapy in, 3189–3196
amino acids in, 3193–3194
energy intake in, 3194t, 3194–3195
fluid and mineral intake in, 3193
general principles of, 3192–3193
glucose in, 3195
individualized by patient needs, 3192–3193
insulin in, 3193
lipids in, 3195
minerals in, 3195
nitrogen intake in, 3193–3194
recommended, 3192t, 3192–3196
recovery of renal function and, 3191
studies on, 3189–3190
unequal results of, 3191–3192
vitamins in, 3195–3196
differential diagnosis of, 1377–1380
duration of, metabolic acidosis and, 2670
in elderly, 1292
frequency of, 1287
geographic pattern of, 2331–2332, 2332t
hemolytic-uremic syndrome causing, 2388
high-risk settings for, 1287, 1288t
hypercalcemia in, 2774
idiopathic postpartum, 2301–2302
incidence of, 1371
malaria and, 2340
pathogenesis of, 2342–2345
medical, 2332, 2332t, 2333t
role of intravascular hemolysis in, 2332, 2333t
metabolic acidosis in
clinical features of, 2669–2670, 2671f
natural history of, 2671
pathophysiology of, 2669–2670
treatment of, 2670–2671
mortality in, 1287, 1288f, 1372
in multiple myeloma, 2204, 2204t
in neonates, 2385–2386
nonoliguric, 1296–1297
due to acute interstitial nephritis, 1297
due to burns, 1298
frequency of, 1297
due to glomerulonephritis, 1297–1298
due to heavy metals, 1298
due to ischemia, 1298
due to nephrotoxins, 1298
due to nontraumatic rhabdomyolysis, 1298
due to radiocontrast agent, 1298
due to nontraumatic rhabdomyolysis in drug abuse, 1230–1231
nutrient administration in, 3196–3198
enteral vs. parenteral, 3196–3198
obstetric, 2332, 2332t, 2334, 2335t
oliguric, in malignant hypertension, 1568
percutaneous renal biopsy for, 487
postrenal, 1290–1291
in cancer, 1168
due to extrarenal causes, 1288t, 1291
due to high filtered loads of insoluble crystalline substances, 1290–1291
due to intratubular obstruction, 1291
due to obstructive uropathy, 1290–1291
due to renal causes, 1288t
due to stone-induced obstruction, 1291
due to ureteric obstruction, 1291
due to uric acid nephropathy, 1291
in pregnancy, 2300t, 2300–2303
acute fatty liver and, 2301
bilateral cortical necrosis and, 2302
hyperemesis gravidarum and, 2301
intravascular coagulation and, 2302
prognosis of, 2302–2303
severe preeclampsia-eclampsia and, 2301
treatment of, 2303
tropical countries and, 2332, 2332t, 2334
uterine hemorrhage and, 2301
prerenal, 1287–1290
acute tubular necrosis vs., 1379, 1379t
due to burns or heat shock, 1290
in cancer, 1165, 1167
causes of, 1288t
due to congestive heart failure, 1289
due to decreased renal blood flow, 1289–1290
due to enhanced renal afferent arteriolar vasoconstriction, 1289–1290
due to extracellular fluid volume depletion, 1290
due to hemorrhagic shock, 1290
incidence of, 1287, 1289f
due to NSAIDs, 1288, 1338t
polyuric, 1297
renal autoregulation and, 1287–1288, 1289f
prognostic factors for survival in, 1373–1375
basic underlying disease as, 1373
demographic factors in, 1373
dialysis procedure as, 1374
multifactorial analysis of, 1374–1375, 1375t
organ system failure as, 1374
signs of infection as, 1374
type and degree of renal failure as, 1373–1374
prognostic factors in, 1308–1310, 1309t, 1310f
protein intake predisposing to, 3196
recovery of function in, 1392–1393, 1393f
renal, 1291–1295
due to abdominal aortic aneurysm surgery, 1293
due to acute tubular necrosis, 1292–1293
causes of, 1288t
due to nontraumatic rhabdomyolysis, 1294
due to open heart surgery, 1293–1294
due to renal artery thrombosis, 1295
due to renal artery thrombosis or embolism, 1295
due to traumatic rhabdomyolysis, 1294
respiratory failure and, 1865, 1865t
resuscitation in, 1375–1377
fluid overload and, 1376, 1377f
hyperkalemia and, 1376–1377, 1377f, 1378t
rhabdomyolysis and, 2332
in sickle cell disease, 2325
surgery and, 2332t, 2334
in transplanted kidney, 2930–2933
biopsy and, 2931–2933, 2932f–2935f
causes of, 2930t
differential diagnosis of, 2931, 2931t
fine-needle aspiration biopsy and, 2933, 2933f
radionuclide imaging and, 2931, 2931f
ultrasound and, 2931, 2932f
treatment of, 1380–1392
etiologic, 1380–1381
symptomatic dialysis, 1385–1392. *See also* Dialysis; Hemodialysis; Peritoneal dialysis
continuous peritoneal dialysis in, 1391–1392
hemodialysis in, 1386–1390, 1387f, 1389f
method of dialysis and, 1385t, 1385–1386
slow continuous hemofiltration/dialysis in, 1390–1391
when to start dialysis in, 1386
uremic encephalopathy and, 2790, 2791f
urinary concentrating defect in, 2512
wasting and malnutrition in, 3187–3189
net protein degradation in, 3187
other causes of, 3188–3189
due to uremia, 3187–3188
Acute tubular necrosis. *See* Tubular necrosis, acute
Acute tumor lysis syndrome, 1180
Acyclovir
acute interstitial nephritis due to, 1341
pharmacology of, normal vs. in renal failure, 3236t–3237t
in renal disease, 3228
renal failure due to, in AIDS patients, 2364
Addison's disease, sodium chloride for, 2548
Adenocarcinoma
renal. *See also* Renal cell carcinoma
angiography for, 475–476, 476f
urinary bladder, 815
Adenoma
adrenal
in Cushing's syndrome, 1541
management of, 1545
aldosterone-producing, malignant hypertension due to, 1561
parathyroid, 2273
renal
angiography for, 474–475
CT for, 454
villous, 2685

Adenosine, 314–315
cell membrane receptors and actions of, 314
cellular synthesis of, 314
glomerular receptors and actions of, 314
in renal hemodynamics, 97–98
renovascular receptors and actions of, 314
tubular receptors and actions of, 314
Adenosine diphosphate (ADP)
in experimental studies on ischemic renal injury, 1257–1260
in oxidative phosphorylation, 236, 236f–237f
Adenosine monophosphate, cyclic (cAMP)
age-related impairment in, 2417
as second messenger, in hormone activation, 284–286, 285f
Adenosine monophosphate (AMP), in experimental studies on ischemic renal injury, 1257–1260
Adenosine triphosphate (ATP)
decreased, in heart failure, 2829
degradation pathway to uric acid of, 1258, 1258f
in experimental studies on ischemic renal injury, 1257–1260, 1258f, 1260f
intracellular calcium and, 2619
in oxidative phosphorylation, 236, 236f–237f
renal synthesis of, 233, 234t
ADH. *See* Antidiuretic hormone (ADH)
Adipocyte(s), hormone-sensitive lipase in, 2570
Adolescent(s), peritoneal dialysis in, 3003–3004
Adrenal adenoma
in Cushing's syndrome, 1541
management of, 1545
Adrenal androgen blockade, for advanced prostatic carcinoma, 844t, 844–845
Adrenal carcinoma
in Cushing's syndrome, 1541
management of, 1545
Adrenal gland, abnormalities of, in AIDS patients, 2365–2366
Adrenal hormones, phosphorus absorption and, 2602–2603
Adrenal hyperplasia, congenital, malignant hypertension due to, 1561
Adrenal insufficiency, 2547–2552
antidiuretic hormone in, 2548, 2548f
glucocorticoid deficiency in, 2549–2551, 2550f–2551f, 2550t
vasopressin-independent effects of, 2551–2552
mineralocorticoid deficiency in, 2547–2548
vasopressin-independent effects of, 2548–2549, 2549f
Adrenalitis, due to cytomegalovirus, 2366
Adrenergic agent(s), in sodium absorption, in thick ascending limb of Henle, 159
Adrenocortical carcinoma, hyperaldosteronism due to, 1482
Adrenocorticotropic hormone (ACTH)
blood pressure effects of
experimental, 1546f–1548f, 1546–1547
physiologic mechanisms in, 1548–1550
deficiency of, in hyponatremic patient, 2554
excess. *See* Cushing's syndrome
polyuria after, 2523f, 2552
tumors producing, 2277
in uremia, 2857
Adrenocorticotropin-cortisol axis, dysfunction of, 2857
Afferent arteriole(s)
anatomic distribution of, 33, 34f
contractile processes in, structural-functional aspects of, 66–67, 67f
enhanced vasoconstriction of, prerenal acute renal failure due to, 1289–1290
hormonal effects on, 288f, 288–289
of juxtaglomerular apparatus, 30, 32f
light microscopy evaluation of, 496, 497f–498f
resistance model of, affecting GFR, 80–81, 81f
AFP, as tumor marker
in seminoma, 870
in testicular carcinoma, 860–861
A-G units, structure and classification of, 2406f
Age
renal transplantation and, 2913–2914
as survival factor, in diabetes mellitus, 2182
Aging. *See also* Elderly
kidneys and, 2405–2426
premature, due to analgesia abuse, 1111–1112
renal anatomy and, 2405, 2406f
renal disease and, clinical, 2422–2426
renal pathophysiology and, 2405, 2407–2420
clinical implications of, 2420–2422, 2421f–2422f
renal physiology and, 2405, 2407–2420
Aging kidney. *See also* Elderly
angiography for, 472
AIDS. *See also* Acquired immunodeficiency syndrome (AIDS)
AIDS-associated nephropathy (AAN), 2366
AIDS-related complex (ARC), 2361
Air embolism, in chronic hemodialysis, 3053–3054
Albumin
calcium binding and, 2616
glomerular filtration of, electrical charge in, 383
molecular weight and radius of, 381t, 382
for nephrotic syndrome, 2480
renal handling of, 384
urinary excretion of, in diabetes, variability of, 2158, 2159f, 2159t
Albumin-creatinine clearance ratio, 2380
Albuminuria
assessment of, in children, 2380
effect of lipid-lowering agents on, 2409, 2413f
exercise-induced, vs. resting baseline conditions, 2158
in renal metastasis, 2268
Alcohol-induced pseudo-Cushing's syndrome, 1542
Alcoholism
hypomagnesemia and, 2634
hypophosphatemia and, 2607
Aldosterone
in cirrhosis, 2468, 2470f, 2471
defective synthesis of, diabetes mellitus and, 2586–2587
deficiency of, diabetes mellitus and, 2585
effects on sodium excretion of, blood pressure and, 1412–1413
in idiopathic edema, 2495, 2497, 2498f
in renal function, 2714
in sodium transport, in collecting ducts, 163t, 163–164
spironolactone antagonism of, 2445–2446
Aldosterone-producing adenoma, malignant hypertension due to, 1561
Aldosterone-producing ovarian carcinoma, 1482
Aldosterone-renin ratio, plasma, in screening for primary aldosteronism, 1477
Aldosteronism, primary, 1475–1484
adenoma vs. hyperplasia in, biochemical distinction in, 1479f–1480f, 1479–1480
age/sex/race predilection in, 1475
clinical features of, 1475–1476
confirmation of inappropriate aldosterone production in, 1478, 1478f–1479f
definition of, 1475
diagnosis of, 1482–1483, 1483t
dietary sodium manipulation in, 1482, 1483t
recommended patient approach in, 1482–1483, 1484f
sensitivity and specificity of screening tests in, 1482, 1483t
endocrine disorders associated with, 1482
glucocorticoid-remediable, 1482
hypertension and, 1425, 1475, 1476f
management of, 1484
mineralocorticoid excess syndromes mimicking, 1481–1482
screening for, 1476–1477
captopril test for, 1477
plasma aldosterone-renin ratio in, 1477
plasma renin activity in, 1477, 1477f–1478f
serum potassium concentration in, 1476f, 1476–1477
signs and symptoms of, 1475–1476
tumor localization in, 1480–1481
adrenal CT scan in, 1480, 1480f–1481f
adrenal vein sampling for plasma aldosterone in, 1481
scintigraphy with radiolabeled iodocholesterol in, 1480–1481
Alkali therapy
for classic distal tubular acidosis, 2682
metabolic alkalosis secondary to, 2684–2685
Alkaline phosphatase, in bone studies, 2765
Alkalinizing agent(s), in dietary therapy in chronic hemodialysis, 3184–3185
Alkalosis
contraction, 2685
gastric, 2582–2583
metabolic. *See* Metabolic alkalosis.
respiratory. *See* Respiratory alkalosis.
Alkylating agent(s). *See specific types*
Allergic angiitis and granulomatosis, 2111–2113, 2112f

Allergy, minimal change nephrotic syndrome and, 1733–1734
Alloantibody, role of, 2887
Allograft(s), 2881. *See also* Graft(s); Transplantation
 clinical histocompatibility testing of, 2881–2882
 glomerulonephritis in, 2934–2935, 2937, 2937t
 HIV transmission through, 2372
 HLA typing of, 2881–2882, 2882f
 immunodeficient host and, reconstitution of, 2888–2890
 infiltrate
  experimental models of, 2883t, 2883–2886, 2884f–2885f, 2884t
  in renal transplantation, 2886–2887
 presensitivity testing of, 2881
 rejection of
  accelerated, 2930
  acute, 2930–2931
  cellular, 2883
   acute, 2888t, 2889
  cytotoxic T lymphocytes in, 2884f–2885f, 2884–2885
  humoral immunity response in, 2887
  hyperacute, 2930
  immune elements in, 2888–2889
  model of events in, 2891
 response of, 2882–2891
  immunologic specificity of, 2883
 suppressor cells in, 2887
Allopurinol
 acute interstitial nephritis due to, 1340
 for gout, 2252–2253, 2259
 pharmacology of, normal vs. in renal failure, 3236t–3237t
Alpha-blocker(s)
 for heart failure, 2834
 for severe hypertension in pregnancy, 1526
Alpha-fetoprotein (AFP), as tumor marker
 in seminoma, 870
 in testicular carcinoma, 860–861
Alpha-receptor(s), 299
 of kidney, 299–300
Alport antigen, 1886, 2170
Alport syndrome, 571–584
 antiglomerular basement membrane antibody–mediated nephritis and, 1868, 1885–1886
 canine model of, hereditary nephritis as, 576–577
 chronic renal failure in, incidence of, 574
 clinical classification of, 573–574
  diseases relevant to, 572t
  indeterminant type, 574
  juvenile vs. adult type in, 573
  type I, 573
  type II, 573
  type III, 573
  type IV, 573
  type V, 573–574
  type VI, 574
 clinical findings in, 579–582
  esophageal and genital leiomyomatosis in, 581
  hematuria in, 579
  ocular features of, 580f, 580–581
  platelets in, 581
  proteinuria in, 579
  rare or chance associations in, 581, 582t
  renal function in, 579
  sensorineural hearing loss in, 579f, 579–580
 diagnosis of, 583–584
 disease definitions in, 571–574
  affected individuals and, 572
  affected kindreds and, 572–573
  complications of, 571–572
 end-stage renal disease in, 571, 573f
 familial thin basement membrane disease vs., 583
 gene frequency in, 574
 gene mutations in, 575
 genetic counseling in, 575
 modes of inheritance of, 574–575
  autosomal dominant inheritance in, 575
  penetrance and dominance in, 574
  X-linked dominant inheritance in, 574–575
 pathogenesis of, 578–579
 pathologic findings in, 575–578
  in cochlea, 577
  in eye, 577–578
  glomerular ultrastructural, 576, 577f
  gross renal, 575
  immunopathology in, 576
  light microscopic renal, 575–576
  in nonrenal tissues, 577–578
  in platelets and granulocytes, 578
  in skin, 578, 578f
 renal transplantation and, 2916
 reproductive fitness in, 575
 treatment of, 584
Aluminum, 3156–3161
 in acute tubular necrosis, 1308
 biliary excretion of, 3156
 in bone disease, 2760–2761, 2770f–2772f, 2770–2772
 elevated levels of
  causing hypercalcemia, 2774
  in dialysis dementia, 2800, 2801f
  in uremia, 3157, 3157f
 food sources of, 3156
 gastrointestinal tract absorption of, 3156
 inhalation of, 3156
 renal excretion of, 3156
 skin absorption of, 3156
Aluminum assays, 2766, 2766t
Aluminum phosphate antacids, for hypophosphatemia, 2610
Aluminum salts, for hyperphosphatemia, 2615
Aluminum toxicity, 2615
 Alzheimer's disease and, 2801
 in children, 2773
 in chronic hemodialysis, 3075–3079
  contamination of dialysate in, 3156
  management of hyperphosphatemia and, 3160–3161
  treatment of, 3161
 diagnosis of, 2767t
 erythropoiesis and, 2746–2747
 hematologic, 3160
  in chronic hemodialysis, microcytic anemia due to, 3078
 vs. hyperparathyroidism, 2766t
 neurotoxic, 3158–3159
  acute form, in uremic patients, 3158–3159
  Alzheimer's disease and, 3158
  diagnosis of, 3159
  dialysis encephalopathy and, 3078–3079, 3158–3159
 skeletal, 3159f, 3159–3160
  in chronic hemodialysis, 3074f–3077f, 3075
  diagnosis of, 3160
  mechanism of, 3160
  parathyroid hormone and, 3159
  pathologic features of, 3159, 3159f
  in uremia, 3159–3160
 speciation and, 3160
Aluminum-associated osteodystrophy, 2777–2778, 2778t, 2779f, 2779t
Alzheimer's disease, aluminum toxicity and, 2801
Amantadine, pharmacology of, normal vs. in renal failure, 3236t–3237t
Amdinocillin, pharmacology of, normal vs. in renal failure, 3236t–3237t
Amikacin
 chemical structure of, 1135f
 pharmacology of, normal vs. in renal failure, 3236t–3237t
Amiloride
 mechanism of action of, 2444–2445, 2445f
 pharmacology of, normal vs. in renal failure, 3236t–3237t
Amine precursor uptake and decarboxylation (APUD) cell tumors, 2277
Amino acid(s)
 essential. *See also* Protein
  analogues of, in chronic renal failure, 3145–3147
  in chronic renal failure, 3144–3145
  in dietary therapy in acute renal failure, 3193–3194
  predisposing to acute renal failure, 3196
 supplements of, for anemia, 2752
 in uremia, 2852–2853, 2853t
Amino acid transport, renal, 611
 measurement of, 613
Aminoaciduria, 611–617
 dibasic, in cystinuria, 614
 dicarboxylic, 616–617
  hereditary, characteristics of, 612t
 hereditary, 623t
 mechanisms of, 611, 613
α-Aminoaciduria, 617
ε-Aminocaproic acid, in sickle cell disease, 2324
Aminoglutethimide, pharmacology of, normal vs. in renal failure, 3236t–3237t
Aminoglycoside(s)
 causing renal failure, in AIDS patients, 2363
 chemical structure of, 1134, 1135f
 net charge of, 1134, 1135t
 renal pharmacology of, 1134–1139
  apical membrane binding in, 1137
  apical membrane transport mechanisms in, 1137–1138
  basolateral membrane transport mechanisms in, 1138, 1138f
  determinants of renal cortical concentration in, 1138–1139
  intrarenal distribution in, 1138
  kinetics of renal cortical accumulation in, 1136–1137

renal tubular transport in, 1135–1136
transtubular flux in, 1136
ultrafilterability in, 1134–1135
Aminoglycoside nephrotoxicity, 1131–1155. *See also specific drugs*
clinical aspects of, 1131–1132
enzymuria as, 1131
GFR in, 1131–1132
nonoliguric renal failure in, 1131
proteinuria as, 1131
clinical risk factors for, 1153–1155, 1154t
drugs causing, 1131
experimental modifications of, 1151–1153
calcium and parathyroid hormone in, 1151
polyamino acids in, 1152f–1153f, 1152–1153
pyridoxal 5′-phosphate in, 1153
incidence of, 1131
morphologic alterations in, 1132–1134, 1133f
lysosomal, 1132, 1133f
proximal tubular, 1134
scarring and regeneration in, 1134
tubular epithelial, 1132, 1133f, 1134
pathogenesis of, 1134–1153
aminoglycoside-basolateral membrane interactions in, 1140t, 1142–1143
aminoglycoside-brush border membrane interactions in, 1140–1142, 1141t
aminoglycoside-lysosome-phospholipid interactions in, 1143–1147, 1144f–1147f
aminoglycoside-microsomal interactions in, 1150–1151
aminoglycoside-mitochondrial interactions in, 1149–1150
aminoglycoside-model membrane interactions in, 1139–1140
aminoglycoside-phosphoinositide interactions in, 1147–1149, 1148f–1149f
aminoglycoside-plasma membrane interactions in, 1140t, 1140–1143
free radicals in, 1151
membrane interactions in, 1139–1151
treatment and prevention of, 1153–1155
p-Aminohippurate (PAH) transport, 262–268
across apical cell membranes, 267–268
across basolateral cell membranes, 265–266, 266f
renal localization of, 263, 264f
Amiodarone, pharmacology of, normal vs. in renal failure, 3236t–3237t
Ammoniagenesis, 243–249
in acute metabolic acidosis, 246f–248f, 246–248, 247t
calcium transport and, 249
in chronic metabolic acidosis, 248–249
in chronic renal failure, 249, 2673
compensatory role of, 249
glutamine in, 244–245, 245f
pH effects on, 243–244
potassium level effects on, 244
in renal hypertrophy, 2710
succinate dehydrogenase in, 247–248, 248f
in tubular acidosis, 249
Ammonium
apical membrane transport of, 221
basolateral membrane transport of, 222, 222f
collecting duct transport of, 217, 217f
countercurrent multiplication of, by loop of Henle, 223, 224f
excretion of
alterations in, 2729–2731, 2730f
in elderly, 2418–2419, 2419f
loop of Henle transport of, 216
proximal tubule transport of, 214–215
renal medulla transport of, 218
as tubular fluid buffer, 223–224, 224f
Ammonium chloride, for renal tubular acidosis, in children, 2381
Amoxicillin
clavulanate-potentiated, for cystitis and urethritis, 1015
for cystitis and urethritis, 1015
pharmacology of, normal vs. in renal failure, 3236t–3237t
Amphetamine abuse, parenteral, systemic necrotizing vasculitis due to, 1231–1232
Amphotericin B
for candidiasis, 941–942
causing renal failure, in AIDS patients, 2363
pharmacology of, normal vs. in renal failure, 3236t–3237t
Ampicillin
cystic fluid concentration of, in autosomal dominant polycystic kidney disease, 551t
for cystitis and urethritis, 1015
pharmacology of, normal vs. in renal failure, 3236t–3237t
Amputation, in diabetes mellitus, 2181
Amrinone, pharmacology of, normal vs. in renal failure, 3236t–3237t
Amylase, molecular weight, radius, and renal handling of, 381t
Amyloid(s), 2209
AA, 2210t, 2211
AF, 2210t, 2211
AL, 2210t, 2210–2211
AP, 2211–2212
AS, 2210t, 2211
β-microglobulin, 2210t, 2212
immunohistochemistry of, 2219–2220
morphologic characteristics of, 2217
β-2-Amyloid, in bone disease, 2773
Amyloidosis, 2209–2226
biochemistry of, 2210–2212
in chronic hemodialysis, 3079
classification of, 2209–2210, 2210t
clinical features of, 2212t, 2212–2213
Congo red-negative glomerular fibrils in, 2218t, 2219
cystic fibrosis and, 2220
definition of, 2209
diagnosis of, 2213, 2214t, 2215
histologic, 2217, 2218f, 2218t, 2219
diseases associated with, 2220, 2221t
in drug abusers, 2220
electron microscopy of, 2216f, 2217
familial, 2210, 2210t, 2222
classification of, 2223t
clinical and diagnostic features of, 2214t
with renal lesions, classification of, 2222, 2223t
gout in, 2256–2257
histopathology of, 2215, 2216f, 2217
Hodgkin's disease and, 2221
hypertension in, 2220
immunochemistry of, 2219–2220
immunofluorescence microscopy of, 2217
in juvenile rheumatoid arthritis, 2054–2055
light microscopy of, 2215, 2216f, 2217
multiple myeloma and, 2200
nephrotic syndrome and, 2220
paraplegia and, 2220
pathogenesis of, 2210–2212
prognosis of, 2222, 2224, 2224f
proteinuria in, 2220
in renal cell carcinoma, 787, 2221
renal failure in, 2222
renal involvement in, 2215, 2216f
renal syndromes and, 2220
renal transplantation and, 2916
in rheumatoid arthritis, 2049–2050, 2220
schistosomal infection and, 2348
skin poppers'. *See* Heroin abuse, subcutaneous
due to subcutaneous heroin abuse, 1226–1229. *See also* Heroin abuse, subcutaneous.
systemic, 2220–2221
treatment of, 2224–2225
tubular dysfunction in, 2221
of urinary tract, 2221–2222
Analgesic(s)
in renal disease, 3229
for rheumatoid arthritis, renal damage due to, 2051–2052
in severe preeclampsia, 1529
Analgesic nephropathy. *See* Analgesic-induced renal disease
Analgesic syndrome, 1105–1106, 1106t
with active abuse, 1109, 1110t, 1111
with cessation of abuse, 1110t, 1113
natural history of, 1113
with NSAID-associated abuse, 1110t, 1113
Analgesic-induced renal disease, 1104–1118. *See also* NSAID nephrotoxicity
acute interstitial nephritis in, 1339
chronic tubulointerstitial, 1971–1972, 1972f
clinical features of, 1109–1113
in active abuse, 1109, 1110t, 1111
cardiovascular, 1111
in cessation of abuse, 1110t, 1113
gastrointestinal, 1111
gonadal, 1111
hematologic, 1111
nonrenal, 1111–1112
in NSAID-associated abuse, 1110t, 1113
pigmentation, 1111
pregnancy-associated, 1111
premature aging, 1111–1112
psychologic and psychiatric, 1111
renal manifestations in, 1112–1113
definition of, 1105–1106
diagnosis of, 1115–1117, 1116f, 1116t–1117t
end-stage renal failure in, 1118
etiology of, 1106–1107
animal studies of, 1107, 1108t
aspirin in, 1107
caffeine in, 1107
NSAIDs in, 1107, 1109t

Analgesic-induced renal disease, etiology of—Continued
phenacetin in, 1107
studies on, 1106
gout in, 2258
historical, 1104–1105
malignant hypertension due to, 1560
management of, 1117–1118
natural history of, 1113
papillary necrosis in, 1113–1115, 1979
animal studies on, 1113–1115
aspirin and, 1113–1114
medullary ischemia in, 1114
NSAIDs and, 1114
paracetamol and, 1114
phenacetin and, 1114
radiographic findings in, 1116f, 1116t–1117t, 1116–1117
renal concentrating mechanism and, 1114
stages in pathogenesis of, 1114–1115
pathologic findings in, 1107–1109
macroscopic, 1107, 1109f
microscopic, 1107–1109
due to phenacetin, 1104, 1105t
prognosis in, 1118
reflux nephropathy vs., 1117, 1117t
renal transplantation and, 2918
uroepithelial tumors and, 1115
Androgen(s), anemia and, 2752
Anemia
in acute renal failure, 2743–2744
in acute tubular necrosis, 1308
aluminum-associated, 3160
amino acid supplements for, 2752
due to analgesia abuse, 1111
androgens for, 2752
blood loss in, 2746
in chronic renal failure, 2744–2746, 2745f
in children, 2397
correction of, hemodynamic effects of, 2817–2818, 2819f
in dialysis patients, 2746–2748
epoetin therapy for, 2748–2752
administration of, 2749, 2750
diastolic blood pressure and, 2752
inflammation and, 2751f, 2751–2752
iron availablility and, 2750f–2751f, 2750–2751
pharmacokinetics of, 2749–2750, 2750f
response to, 2748f–2749f, 2748–2749
erythropoietin deficiency in, 2743
exercise and, 2752
folic acid for, 2752
in heart failure, 2829
hematologic findings in, 2744
hemolysis in, 2746, 2746f
hemolytic, microangiopathic
in hemolytic-uremic syndrome, 2073
in malignant hypertension, 1569
improved dialysis clearance for, 2752
iron overload in, 2753
microcytic, due to aluminum toxicity, in chronic hemodialysis, 3078
in myeloma kidney, 2744
pathogenesis of, 2744, 2745f
red cell survival in, 2752
red cell transfusions for, 2752
in renal disease, 2743–2753
management of, 2748–2752
pathophysiology of, 2743–2748
sickle cell, 2311. *See also* Sickle cell disease
vitamins for, 2752
Anesthesia
in cancer, acute renal failure due to, 1168
in severe preeclampsia, 1529
stocking-glove, in toxic neuropathies, 2805
Aneurysm
cerebral, in autosomal dominant polycystic kidney disease, 553f, 553–554
renal artery, 2126–2127
angiography for, 472–473, 473f
rupture of, 2126
surgical intervention in, 2126–2127
Angiitis
allergic, granulomatosis and, 2111–2113, 2112f
hypersensitivity, 2095–2096
Angiography, 465–478
for adult malignant renal tumors, 475–477, 476f–477f
for aging kidney, 472
for chronic glomerulonephritis, 478
for chronic pyelonephritis, 478
complications of, 467
diagnostic, 472–478
digital subtraction, 465–467
advantages of, 465
indications for, 465
for percutaneous transluminal angioplasty, 467
for renal cell carcinoma, 790
for renal transplantation, 467
for renovascular hypertension, 465, 467
in screening for renovascular hypertension, 1461
technique in, 465, 467f
indications for, 465, 466f
for juxtaglomerular tumors, 475
for mesoblastic nephroma, 477
for multilocular cystic nephroma, 477
for nephroblastomatosis, 477
for pediatric renal tumors, 477
for perinephric abscess, 968
for polycystic kidney disease, 478
radionuclide, in heart failure, 2833
for renal adenocarcinoma, 475–476, 476f
for renal adenoma, 474–475
for renal angiomyolipoma, 475, 475f
for renal arteriovenous malformation, 473
for renal artery aneurysm, 472–473, 473f
for renal artery atherosclerosis, 472
for renal artery fibromuscular dysplasia, 472, 472f
for renal artery stenosis, in children, 472, 473f
for renal cell carcinoma, 475–476, 476f
for renal cortical abscess, 960, 962f
for renal hemangioma, 474
for renal lymphoma, 476–477
for renal metastasis, 477
for renal necrotizing angiitis, 474, 474f
for renal oncocytoma, 475
for renal polyarteritis nodosa, 474, 474f
for renal venous thrombosis, 478
for simple renal cyst, 478
for subcapsular abscess, 478
for subcapsular hematoma, 477–478, 478f
for Takayasu's disease, 472
technique for, 465, 466f
for uroepithelial carcinoma, 477
for Wilms' tumor, 477
Angiokeratoma, in Fabry's disease, 594
Angiomyolipoma, renal
angiography for, 475, 475f
computed tomography for, 453–454, 454f
ultrasonography for, 429f, 430
Angioplasty
percutaneous transluminal
for atherosclerosis, 468–469
complications of, 470–471
digital subtraction angiography for, 467
for fibromuscular dysplasia, 469
for neurofibromatosis, 469–470
for renal insufficiency, 470
for renal transplantation, 470
for Takayasu's disease, 469
technique for, 468, 469f
renal, 1464–1467
complications of, 1466–1467
hemodynamic and hormonal factors in, 1465
mechanisms of, 1465
for preservation of renal function, 1466
results with, 1465t, 1465–1466, 1466f
surgery vs., 1467
technique in, 1464–1465
Angiotensin converting enzyme (ACE), localized sites of, 87
Angiotensin converting enzyme (ACE) inhibitor
in diabetic nephropathy, 2179
in end-stage renal disease, 2824
in heart failure, 2834
in renovascular hypertension, 1468
in severe hypertension in pregnancy, 1526
Angiotensin II. *See also* Renin-angiotensin system.
in acute tubular necrosis, 1306
in ADH secretion, 122
adrenal actions of, 305
CNS and pituitary actions of, 305
effects of, 88
effects on blood pressure of, 1417
effects on sodium excretion of, blood pressure and, 1412–1413, 1413f
GFR effects of, 88, 89f
GFR reduction and, in urinary tract obstruction, 665–666, 666f
major actions of, 304–305
in medullary blood flow regulation, 100
in proximal tubule sodium reabsorption, 151
renal actions of, 304–305
renal blood flow effects of, 88, 89f
in renin secretion, 303
synthesis of, 87
vascular actions of, 304
vasoconstriction due to, cellular mechanisms in, 90
Anion gap
in distal nephron acidification defects, 2679
elevated, metabolic acidosis with, 2577t, 2577–2581
normal, metabolic acidosis with, 2577t, 2581–2582
plasma, 2381
urinary, 2381, 2581

Anion transport, 261–275
 across apical cell membranes, 267–268, 268f
 across basolateral cell membranes, 265–267, 266f, 268f
 compound types in, 262, 262t, 263f
 compounds transported by, 273–274
 inhibition of, 275
 passive, 263–264
 in renal failure, 274
 renal tubular localization of, 262–264, 264f
 study techniques for, 261–262, 262t
AAN (AIDS-associated nephropathy), 2366
Anodic antigen(s), circulating, 2347, 2349
Anorexia, in chronic renal failure, 2395
Antacid(s)
 drug interactions of, in renal disease, 3230
 for hypophosphatemia, 2610
Antibody(ies)
 anti-GBM. *See* Antiglomerular basement membrane antibody–mediated nephritis
 anti-IL-2 receptor, in immunosuppression, 2903–2904
 monoclonal
  in immunosuppression, 2902–2903, 2903t
  MRC OX8, 2890
Antibody-coated bacteria test, for upper urinary tract infection, 985
Anticoagulant(s), lupus, 2022
Anticonvulsant(s), in renal disease, 3230
Antidepressant(s), tricyclic, pharmacology of, normal vs. in renal failure, 3260t–3261t
Antidiuretic hormone (ADH)
 in adrenal insufficiency, 2548, 2548f
 for assessment of renal concentrating capacity, 379
 cellular actions of, 123f–124f, 124–125
 chemical structure of, 120–121
 in diabetes insipidus, 2503, 2508t
 extrarenal effects of, 291
 in fluid balance, 121–125
 in fluid transport, 48–51
  apical membranes and cytosolic vesicles and, 49–50
  collecting ducts and, 48–49
  morphologic effects on nephron and, 50–51
 function of, 121
 glomerular and renovascular receptors and actions of, 291–292
 in glucocorticoid deficiency, 2549–2551, 2550f–2551f, 2551t
  independent effects of, 2551–2552
 in idiopathic edema, 2495
 inappropriate secretion of. *See* Syndrome of inappropriate antidiuretic hormone (SIADH) secretion.
 major actions of, 291–292, 292f
 in malignant hypertension, 1580–1581
 in medullary blood flow regulation, 100
 in mineralocorticoid deficiency, 2548, 2548f
  independent effects of, 2548–2549, 2549f
 in myxedema, 2543–2545, 2544f–2546f
 permeability increase due to, mechanism of, 123f, 124–125
 receptor mechanisms of, 123f, 124, 291, 375
 release of, in hypernatremic patients, 2513, 2513f
 in renal hemodynamics, 99
 secretion of
  angiotensin effects on, 122
  effect of blood osmolality vs. blood volume on, 122, 123f
  extracellular fluid osmolality and, 373, 374f
  nausea effects on, 122–123
  neural impulse effects on, 123–124
  nonosmotic factors in, 122–124
  osmotic control of, 121f–122f, 121–122
  pharmacologic effects on, 123–124
 SIADH secretion and. *See* Syndrome of inappropriate antidiuretic hormone (SIADH) secretion
 in sodium absorption, in thick ascending limb of Henle, 158t, 158–159
 in sodium transport, in collecting ducts, 164
 synthesis of, 121
 tubular receptors and actions of, 292f, 292–293
 in uremia, 2857
 in urine concentration, 374–375
  effect of ADH absence in, 375
 in urine dilution, 374–375
  effect of ADH excess in, 376
 in vascular reactivity in preeclampsia, 1512
Antiglomerular basement membrane antibody–mediated nephritis, 1865–1886
 Alport's syndrome and, 1868, 1885–1886
 clinical features of, 1869–1872
  general, 1869–1870
  other organs in, 1871–1872, 1872t
  pulmonary hemorrhage in, 1870–1871, 1871f
  renal, 1870, 1870f
 disease associations with, 1867t, 1867–1868
 environmental factors in, 1868–1869
  cigarette smoking as, 1869
  infections as, 1869
  organic solvents and hydrocarbon fumes as, 1868–1869
 epidemiology of, 1865–1869
 genetic factors in, 1866–1867
 Goodpasture's disease and, 1865
 historical, 1865
 Hodgkin's disease and, 1868
 immunopathology of, 1654–1657, 1655t
 incidence of, 1865–1866, 1866f
 membranous nephropathy and, 1868
 nail-patella syndrome and, 1868
 outcome in, 1869t
 pathogenesis of, 1878–1885
  experimental models of, 1882–1884, 1883t
  Goodpasture antigen in, 1879, 1880f–1883f, 1882
  immune response in, 1879
  mechanisms of kidney injury and, 1884–1885
  mechanisms of lung injury and, 1885
 pathologic findings in, 1872–1875
  immunologic, 1874–1875, 1875f
  pulmonary, 1874
  renal, 1872–1874, 1873f
 prognosis in, 1876–1877, 1877f, 1932–1934, 1933t
 relapse in, 1877
 renal transplantation and, 2917
 resolution and recurrence in, 1877–1878, 1878f
 treatment in, 1875–1876
Antihypertensive agent(s)
 in diabetic nephropathy, 2178f, 2178–2179
 in end-stage renal disease, 2823–2824
 in pregnancy. *See* Pregnancy, antihypertensive therapy in
 withdrawal of, hypertensive crisis in, 1615
Anti-IL-2 receptor antibody(ies), in immunosuppression, 2903–2904
Antilymphocyte globulin, 2929
Antimetabolite(s). *See also specific types*
 nephrotoxicity due to, 1176–1178
Antimicrobial(s), in cancer, acute renal failure due to, 1168
Antineoplastic agent(s)
 acute uric acid nephropathy due to, 1180
 hyperphosphatemic nephropathy due to, 1181
 hyponatremia associated with, 2520
 nephrotoxicity due to, 1170–1180, 1171t. *See also specific drugs*
 renal failure due to, in AIDS patients, 2364
 xanthine nephropathy due to, 1180–1181
Antineutrophil cytoplasmic antigen(s), in systemic vasculitis, 2097–2098, 2098f, 2098t
Antipsychotic agent(s), hyponatremia associated with, 2519t, 2520
Antireflux surgery, controlled trials for, 718–719. *See also* Reflux nephropathy; Vesicoureteral reflux
Antisera, polyclonal, 2929
Antithrombin-III, in acute renal vein thrombosis, in nephrotic syndrome, 1321–1322
Antithymocyte globulin, 2929
Antitubercular drug(s), acute interstitial nephritis due to, 1337
Antitubular basement membrane disease, acute interstitial nephritis and, 1345–1346
Antitubular basement membrane tubulointerstitial nephropathy, 1968
Antitumor antibiotic(s). *See also specific types*
 nephrotoxicity of, 1178–1179
Antiviral agent(s), acute interstitial nephritis due to, 1341
Anuria, in diagnosis of acute renal failure, 1296
Aortic aneurysm surgery, acute tubular necrosis and, 1293
Aortic coarctation, repair of, hypertension after, 1613
Aortic dissection
 classification of, 1608, 1608f
 clinical features of, 1609
 diagnosis of, 1609
 hypertension and, 1607–1610
 long-term medical management of, 1610
 pathogenesis of, 1608–1609
 treatment of, 1609–1610
Apolipoprotein, in uremia, 2850

Arachidonate metabolism, in nephrotoxicity, 1037
Arachidonic acid metabolism
 pathway of, 90, 90f
 in renal vasculature, 90–91
Arachidonic acid pathway, in hormonal activation, 286–287
Arachnoid cyst, in autosomal dominant polycystic kidney disease, 553
ARC (AIDS-related complex), 2361
Arginine vasopressin. *See* Antidiuretic hormone (ADH)
Armani-Ebstein lesion, 2574
Arrhythmia(s), in dialysis patients, 2830
Arsenic poisoning, renal manifestations of, 1248f, 1248–1249
Arterial vasodilation, peripheral
 in hepatorenal disease, 1360–1364, 1361f–1364f
 renal sodium and water retention in, 1361f
Arteriography, renal
 in acute renal vein thrombosis in nephrotic syndrome, 1325–1326
 in renal cell carcinoma, 789, 789f
 in screening for renovascular hypertension, 1462
Arteriolosclerosis, hyaline
 in nephrosclerosis, 1433, 1434f
 in primary nephrosclerosis, 1433–1434
Arteriosclerosis
 in diabetic nephropathy, 2573
 renal, clinicopathologic correlations of, 505
 retinal, in malignant hypertension, 1564f, 1564t, 1564–1565
Arteriovenous graft(s), in chronic hemodialysis, 3033
Arteriovenous malformation, renal, angiography for, 473
Arteritis. *See also* Polyarteritis; Vasculitis
 Takayasu, 2113
  angiography for, 472
  renal artery, in renovascular hypertension, 1456
  renal percutaneous transluminal angioplasty for, 469
 temporal, 2113
Arthritis
 gouty, lead nephropathy and, 2254–2255, 2256f
 in long-term hemodialysis patients, 2226
 rheumatoid. *See* Rheumatoid arthritis
Arthropathy
 in chronic hemodialysis, 3079–3080
 crystal-induced, 2763
Ascites
 in chronic hemodialysis, 3087t, 3087–3088
 diuretics for, 2473–2474
 neonatal, urinary tract obstruction and, 660
 overfill theory of, 2467f, 2467–2468
 paracentesis for, 2473
 peritoneal shunting for, 2473–2474
 sodium restriction for, 2474
 underfill theory of, 2466f, 2466–2467
Ask-Upmark kidney, malignant hypertension due to, 1560
L-Asparaginase, pharmacology of, normal vs. in renal failure, 3248t–3249t
Aspergillosis
 as complication of transplantation, 2946, 2946f, 2947
 opportunistic, 946t–947t, 946–947
Aspirin
 analgesic-induced renal disease due to, 1107. *See also* Analgesic-induced renal disease
 effect of
  in preeclampsia, 2292
  in pregnancy-induced hypertension, 2292
 for hypercalcemia, 2629, 2630t
 low-dose, for preeclampsia prevention, 1530
 pharmacology of, normal vs. in renal failure, 3258t–3259t
 urate excretion and, 2240
Atenolol, pharmacology of, normal vs. in renal failure, 3236t–3237t
Atheroembolic disease of kidney, 2127–2131
 clinical findings in, 2129t, 2129–2130
 diagnosis of, 2130–2131, 2131f
 laboratory findings in, 2129t, 2130
 management of, 2131
 pathogenesis of, 2128–2129
 pathologic findings in, 2127–2128, 2128f
 predisposing factors in, 2128–2129
Atherogenesis, in uremia, 2851
Atheromatous plaque(s), in renal arteries, in renovascular hypertension, 1455f, 1456
Atherosclerosis
 accelerated, in chronic hemodialysis, 3082–3083
 due to analgesia abuse, 1111
 lipids in, 2851
 renal artery
  angiography for, 472
  percutaneous transluminal angioplasty for, 468–469
 systemic, age and, 2409, 2411f
Atopy, minimal change nephrotic syndrome and, 1733–1734
Atrial natriuretic factor. *See* Atrial natriuretic peptide
Atrial natriuretic peptide, 294–296
 actions of, 295
 age-related increase in, 2414, 2415f–2416f, 2416
 in cirrhosis, 2471
 in congestive heart failure, 2460
 in edema formation, in nephrotic syndrome, 1756
 endocrine effects of, 296
 GFR reduction and, in urinary tract obstruction, 667, 668f
 glomerular filtration rate effects of, 295–296
 in medullary blood flow regulation, 100
 peripheral vascular effects of, 296
 regulation and sites of action of, 294, 295f
 renal blood flow effects of, 295–296
 in renal function, 2713–2714
 in renal hemodynamics, 97
 secretion of, 294–295
 in sodium transport, in collecting ducts, 164
 synthesis and structure of, 294
 in uremia, 2861–2862
 volume expansion due to, in hypertension, 1409
 in water and solute secretion, 295
Autonomic hyperreflexia, hypertensive crisis in, 1616–1617
Autonomic nerves, dysfunction of, uremic nephropathy and, 2809
Avascular necrosis, posttransplant, 2951, 2952f
5-Azacytidine nephrotoxicity, 1178
Azathioprine
 in immunosuppression, 2897, 2897f, 2898t, 2926
 pharmacology of, normal vs. in renal failure, 3238t–3239t
 side effects of, 2926t
Azlocillin, pharmacology of, normal vs. in renal failure, 3238t–3239t
Azotemia. *See also* Acute renal failure
 postrenal, 1290–1291
 prerenal, 1287–1290
  nonoliguric, 1297
 renal, 1291–1295
AZT (zidovudine)
 for HIV-associated nephropathy, 2370
 in renal disease, 3228
Aztreonam, pharmacology of, normal vs. in renal failure, 3238t–3239t

Bacampicillin, pharmacology of, normal vs. in renal failure, 3238t–3239t
Bacteremia, in upper urinary tract infection, 983
Bacteria, urinalysis for, 336
Bacterial cast(s), 351
Bacterial endotoxin, in vascular inflammatory injury, 1996
Bacterial infection. *See also specific infections*
 in acute renal failure, etiologic role of, 2332, 2333t
 in tropical countries, renal disease and, 2338–2339
Bacteriuria. *See also* Cystitis; Urethritis; Urinary tract infection
 asymptomatic
  definition of, 973
  in diabetes mellitus, 978
  management of, 1013, 1016, 1017f
  in pregnancy, 1019, 1020f
  prevalence and incidence of, 976–978
  in reflux nephropathy, 709–710
  urine culture in, 981
  in vesicoureteral reflux, 709–710
 automated methods for, 1012–1013
  bioluminescence, 1013
  filtration, 1013
  photometric, 1012–1013
 catalase test for, 1012
 definition of, 973, 1007
 in elderly, 978
 glucose oxidase test for, 1012
 Griess test for, 1012
 leukocyte esterase test for, 1012
 in pregnancy, 978, 2299
 in sickle cell disease, 2324
 significant, definition of, 973, 1007
 symptomatic, management of, 1013–1014
 urine culture for, 1013
Balkan nephropathy, 1976
Baroreceptor(s)
 hepatic, 2456–2457

high-pressure, 2454–2456
intrarenal, 2457
low-pressure, 2456
renal vascular, in renin release, 88
Bartter's syndrome, 627–628
characteristics of, 612t
classification of, 627–628
definition of, 627
differential diagnosis of, 628
gout in, 2258
metabolic alkalosis in, 2684, 2686
pathophysiology of, 627
treatment of, 628
Basement membrane. *See* Glomerular basement membrane
BCG, intravesical, for urinary bladder carcinoma, 822
Bed rest
for preeclampsia, 2295
for renal osteodystrophy, 2774
Behçet's disease, 2113
Bence Jones protein
in dysproteinemias, 2190
in proteinuria, 355
Bence Jones proteinuria, 2189. *See also* Proteinuria, light chain
Bence Jones test, for light chain proteinuria, 389
Benzbromarone, urate excretion and, 2240
Berger's disease. *See* IgA nephropathy
Beta-blocker(s)
for end-stage renal disease, 2824
for hypertension, 2296
for moderate hypertension in pregnancy, 1523t, 1523–1524
Beta-receptor(s), 299
of kidney, 299–300
Bezoar(s)
due to *Candida* cystitis, 934–935
in "primary" renal candidiasis, 936
Bicarbonate
concentration of, in acid-base balance, 208, 208f
reabsorption of, 2435–2437, 2436f
alterations in, 2731
as tubular fluid buffer, 223
Bicarbonate transport
across apical membranes, 221
across basolateral membranes, 221
collecting duct, 217, 217f
distal tubule, 623f, 624
loop of Henle, 215–216
proximal tubule, 212–214, 213f–214f, 623, 623f
renal medulla, 218–219
Biliary tract, cancer of, nephrotic syndrome in, 2265
Bingeing, idiopathic edema and, 2500, 2501
Biomembrane(s), properties of, 139, 140f
Biopsy
bone, 2766–2767
brush
for renal pelvic carcinoma, 804
for ureteral carcinoma, 803
fine-needle aspiration renal, 487
for renal transplantation monitoring, 487, 489–490
technique in, 487
in multiple myeloma, indications for, 2200
percutaneous renal, 485–507
for acute interstitial nephritis, 1332, 1334, 1334f–1335f, 1335t
for acute renal failure, 487, 1301–1302
for acute tubular necrosis, 487
clinicopathologic correlations in, 503–507
capillary wall thickening in, 504, 505f–506f
crescents in, 503–504
glomerulosclerosis in, 504
interstitial inflammation in, 504–505
mesangial expansion in, 503
neutrophilic exudates in, 503, 504f–505f
renal allografts in, 505–507
vascular lesions in, 505
complications of, 485
contraindications in, 490
for diabetic nephropathy, 489
electron microscopy evaluation of, 499–500, 500f–502f
gross examination in, 491
for hematuria, 488
historical, 485
immunohistochemical evaluation of, 500–503
glomerular immunoglobulin staining patterns in, 500–502
immunoperoxidase staining in, 502–503
indications for, 487–490
kidney localization for, 486, 486f
light microscopy evaluation of, 493–499, 494f–499f
Bowman's capsule in, 496
estimation of chronic nephron loss in, 494
glomerular capillary evaluation in, 495, 496f
glomerular cellular composition in, 495, 495f
juxtaglomerular arterioles in, 496, 497f–498f
mesangial evaluation in, 495–496, 497f
relative degrees of pathologic involvement in, 498–499
renal arteries in, 498
renal veins in, 498
sample adequacy in, 494
terminology for, 493–494
tubules in, 496–498, 498f–499f
for lupus nephritis, 489
molecular biology and, 493
for nephrotic syndrome, 487–488
in nephrotic syndrome, 1736–1737, 1737t
postoperative care in, 486–487
processing for histologic examination in, 491–493
dividing tissue core in, 491, 491f
for electron microscopy, 491
fixatives for electron microscopy in, 492
fixatives for light microscopy in, 492
frozen section procedures in, 493
immunofluorescence staining in, 493
for immunohistochemistry, 491
immunoperoxidase staining in, 493
for light microscopy, 491
tissue preservation for immunohistochemistry in, 492–493
in transplant biopsy, 492
wax embedding and staining in, 492
for proteinuria, 488
for renal transplantation, 489–490
for secondary malignant hypertension, 1592–1593
technique for, 485–487
Travenol Tru-cut needle for, 486
for vasculitis, 489
Vim-Silverman needle for, 486
of transplanted kidney, 2931–2933, 2932f–2935f
Bismuth poisoning, renal manifestations of, 1248
Blackwater fever, 2342
Bladder. *See* Urinary bladder
Blastomycosis, 944, 945t–946t
Bleeding. *See* Hemorrhage
Bleomycin
intravesical, for urinary bladder carcinoma, 822
pharmacology of, normal vs. in renal failure, 3238t–3239t
phase specificity and mechanism of action of, 821t
Blindness, in diabetes mellitus, 2180–2181
Block Design Learning Test, 2791, 2792
Blood flow, renal. *See* Renal blood flow
Blood pressure, 1407–1428. *See also* Hypertension; Hypotension
ACTH effects on
experimental, 1546f–1548f, 1546–1547
physiologic mechanisms in, 1548–1550
in diabetic nephropathy, 2166, 2167t, 2168f
diastolic, epoetin therapy and, 2752
effect of increasing sodium intake on, 1410
effect of reducing sodium intake on, 1410–1411
measurement of, in children, 2379, 2380t
neural control of, 1485–1486, 1486f
in normal pregnancy, 2289f, 2289–2290
in pheochromocytoma, 1485f, 1485–1486
in pregnancy, 1505–1508. *See* Pregnancy, blood pressure in
renal mechanisms of, 1412–1420
hypotensive hormones from renal papilla as, 1417–1420, 1418f
renal control of interstitial space compliance as, 1420
renin-angiotensin system as, 1416f, 1416t, 1416–1417
sodium excretion as, 1412–1416
acquired or imposed restraints on, 1412–1414
aldosterone and, 1412–1413
angiotensin and, 1412–1414, 1413f
inherited restraint on, 1414–1415
renal mass and, 1412
renal perfusion pressure and, 1412
sodium intake and, 1409–1412
Blood transfusion. *See* Transfusion
Blood urea nitrogen (BUN), 369–371
in acute tubular necrosis, 1306, 1306t
in chronic renal failure, 3132
clinical utility of, 371
creatinine clearance vs., 371
diuretic state effects on, 370
GFR and, 370
nitrogen load effects on, 370–371, 371f

Blood urea nitrogen (BUN)—Continued
"normal," 370
serum creatinine vs., 371
urea metabolism and, 370
uremic inhibitors and, 2747
Bochdalek ectopic kidney, 654
Bone
calcium in, 2616, 2617–2618
calcium mobilization from, hypercalcemia secondary to, 2625–2626
cancellous (trabecular), 2617
compact, 2617
decreased calcium mobilization from, hypocalcemia secondary to, 2623
hypermineralization of, 2617
lamellar, 2617
measurement of, 2764–2765
woven, 2617
Bone disease. *See also* Osteodystrophy, renal
aluminum-associated, 2769–2772, 2777–2778, 2778t
aplastic, 2769
high turnover
histology of, 2767–2768, 2768f–2769f
pathogenesis of, 2760, 2762f, 2762–2763
low turnover
histology of, 2768–2772, 2770f–2772f
pathogenesis of, 2760, 2763
mixed-transitional, pathogenesis of, 2763
posttransplant, 2951
Bone lesion(s)
amyloidosis and, 2226
cystic, 2764, 2764f–2765f
Bone pain, and fracture, 2774
Bowman's capsule
anatomy of, 6, 8f
light microscopy evaluation of, 496
visceral epithelium (podocytes) of, 7–8, 11f–12f, 381. *See also* Epithelial foot process(es)
Bowman's space, anatomy of, 6, 8f
Bradykinin
in renal hemodynamics, 92–93, 93f
in sodium transport, in collecting ducts, 164
Brain
biochemical changes in, 2792f–2793f, 2792–2794
calcium in, acute renal failure and, 2798, 2798f
mitochondria in, 2797–2798
Breast cancer
nephrotic syndrome in, 2265
renal metastasis from, 2268
Brescia-Cimino fistula, native, 3032f, 3032–3033
Bronchogenic carcinoma
diffuse membranous glomerulopathy in, 2266
nephrotic syndrome in, 2265
SIADH associated with, 2522–2524
Brown tumor, of hyperparathyroidism, 2773
Brucella species, upper urinary tract infection due to, 974
Buffer base concentration, 207, 208f
Bumetanide
mechanism of action of, 2443
pharmacology of, normal vs. in renal failure, 3238t–3239t
BUN. *See* Blood urea nitrogen (BUN)
Burkitt's lymphoma
hyperphosphatemia and, 2274, 2613
tumor lysis syndrome and, 2274, 2274t
Burn(s), prerenal acute renal failure due to, 1290
Burning foot syndrome, 2805
Burr cell(s), 2744

C3
in focal glomerulosclerosis due to heroin abuse, 1222, 1223t
in vascular inflammatory injury, 1996
C5, in vascular inflammatory injury, 1996
Cacitriol (1,25-dihydroxyvitamin D), in renal osteodystrophy, 2775–2776
Cadaver kidney
for transplantation
evaluation of, 2922, 2922t
graft survival and, 2921f
vs. living donor kidney, 2921–2922, 2922t
removal of, 2922
results of, 2939, 2939f
unsuspected nephritis in, 2935
Cadmium, metabolism of, 1242
Cadmium nephropathy, 1242–1245
calcium wasting in, 1243
chronic interstitial nephritis in, 1243–1245, 1244f
chronic tubulointerstitial, 1973
clinical findings in, 1242–1243
diagnosis of, 1245
historical, 1242
itai-itai disease and, 1243
β_2-microglobulin excretion in, 1242–1243
treatment of, 1245
Caffeine, analgesic-induced renal disease due to, 1107
Calbindin, 2619
Calcifediol, in renal osteodystrophy, 2775
Calciferol (vitamin D_3)
in hypercalcemia of malignancy, 2273
in renal osteodystrophy, 2775
Calcific periarthritis, in chronic renal failure, 3154
Calcification
conjunctival, in chronic renal failure, 3154
metastatic, 2625
in chronic renal failure, due to hyperphosphatemia, 3154f–3155f, 3154t, 3154–3155
myocardial, in heart failure, 2830
soft tissue, periarticular, 2762, 2762f
vascular, 2762, 2762f
in chronic renal failure, 3155
visceral, in chronic renal failure, 3154–3155
Calcinosis, tumoral, hyperphosphatemia and, 2613
Calcitonin, for hypercalcemia, 2629, 2630t
Calcitriol
for hypercalcemia of malignancy, 2273
for osteitis fibrosa, 2777
for renal osteodystrophy, 2395, 2775–2776
renal synthesis of, after transplantation, 2778
Calcium, 2615–2630. *See also* Hypercalcemia; Hypocalcemia
albumin binding to, 2616
ATPase activity of, 2619
in bone, 2616, 2617–2618
in brain, acute renal failure and, 2798, 2798f
in collecting duct, 2620–2621
in collecting tubule, 2621
cytosolic
in hormonal activation, 286
in renal vascular contraction and relaxation, 70–71, 71f
in dietary therapy in chronic hemodialysis, 3182–3183
in distal convoluted tubule, 2620–2621
distribution of, 2615–2616
elemental, for hypocalcemia, 2628
endogenous fecal, 2618
extracellular, 2616, 2616f
in glomerular filtrate, 2620–2621
intake of, in vascular reactivity in preeclampsia, 1513
intestinal absorption of, 2618–2619
increased, hypercalcemia secondary to, 2627–2628
intracellular, 2616–2617
potassium regulation and, 2648
in loop of Henle, 2620
metabolism of
in cirrhosis, 2475
treatment of disorders of, 2628–2630, 2630t
miscible pool of, 2616
mitochondrial accumulation of, 2617
mitochondrial metabolism of, nephrotoxicity and, 1048
mobilization of, from bone, hypercalcemia secondary to, 2625–2626
for modification of aminoglycoside nephrotoxicity, 1151
parathyroid hormone and, 2621
in pars recta, 2620
plasma, in children, 2382
in proximal convoluted tubule, 2620
in proximal straight tubule, 2620
renal handling of, 2617f, 2619–2620
reservoir of, skeleton as, 2617–2618
serum, 2616, 2616f
supplement of, 2775
for preeclampsia prevention, 1530
transfer of, across intestinal brush border, 2618–2619
transport of
ammoniagenesis and, 249
factors regulating, 2621–2622
parathyroid hormone in, 293–294
in synaptosomes, 2797
ultrafilterable, 2616
uptake of, in synaptosomes, 2795, 2796f–2797f
urinary excretion of, 2619, 2619f
in children, 2382
decreased, hypercalcemia secondary to, 2628
hypocalcemia secondary to, 2624
in urinary tract obstruction, 673
in vascular reactivity in preeclampsia, 1513
Calcium antagonist(s), in treatment of renovascular hypertension, 1468
Calcium balance, 2618f, 2618–2619
aging and, 2419
in continuous ambulatory peritoneal dialysis, 3176–3177, 3177t

Calcium carbonate, hypercalcemia and, 2628
Calcium channel blocker, in end-stage renal disease, 2824
Calcium gluconate, for hypocalcemia, 2628
Calcium homeostasis
in acute tubular necrosis, 1305
cellular, nephrotoxicity and, 1050–1055. *See also* Nephrotoxicity
Calcium ion(s), in experimental studies of ischemic renal injury, 1263f, 1263–1265
Calcium oxalate crystal(s), urinalysis for, 356, 357f
"Calcium pump," 2616, 2618
Calcium wasting, in cadmium nephropathy, 1243
Calculus(i)
cystine, after renal transplantation, 2915
prostatic, in chronic prostatitis, 751
renal. *See also* Nephrolithiasis
in autosomal dominant polycystic kidney disease, 551
chemical analysis of, 729–730, 730t
chemical composition of, 729, 730t
CT for, 451, 451f
formation of, 729
determinants of crystallization in, 729
process of crystallization in, 729, 730f
in gout, 2252
imaging studies of, 426
in medullary sponge kidney, 527
MRI for, 458
obstructive atrophy due to, imaging studies in, 426, 427f
plain film of, 407
in pregnancy, 2300
in reflux nephropathy, 714–715
management of, 720
ultrasonography for, 422, 422f
ureteral obstruction due to, treatment of, 681
ureteropelvic obstruction due to, treatment of, 681
urinary tract infection due to, 900
urinary tract obstruction due to, 660
in vesicoureteral reflux, 714–715
ureteral, plain film of, 407
Calicectasis, in sickle cell disease, 2324–2325
Calyceal diverticulum(a)
congenital, 650–651
cystic appearance of, 521, 522f
medullary sponge kidney vs., 531
Calyceal/papillary abnormality, imaging studies of, 422–427
with diffuse parenchymal loss, 426–427, 427f
with focal parenchymal loss, 425–426, 426f
without parenchymal loss, 422–425, 423f–426f
Calyx(ces)
intravenous urography for, 409–410
minor renal, anatomy of, 3, 4f
cAMP
age-related impairment in, 2417
as second messenger, in hormone activation, 284–286, 285f
Cancer. *See also* Malignancy; Tumor; *and specific types*
acute interstitial nephritis in, 1344
acute renal failure in, 1165–1168
due to anesthetic agents, 1168
due to antimicrobials, 1168
etiology of, 1166t
glomerular abnormalities in, 1167
due to hemoglobinuria, 1168
due to hypercalcemia, 1168
due to immunoglobulins, 1168
interstitial abnormalities in, 1168
intrarenal blood vessels in, 1168
due to intravascular contrast agents, 1167–1168
intrinsic, 1167–1168
postrenal, 1168
prerenal, 1165, 1167
due to rhabdomyolysis, 1168
tubular abnormalities in, 1167–1168
in chronic hemodialysis, 3088–3089
chronic renal failure in, 1166t–1167t, 1168–1169
etiology of, 1166t–1167t
glomerular abnormalities in, 1168–1169
interstitial abnormalities in, 1169
obstruction in, 1169
renovascular disease in, 1169
as complication of transplantation, 2947t, 2947–2948
glomerulopathy in, 2265–2267
hematologic, renal involvement in, 2269f, 2269–2271
hypercalcemia in, 2271t, 2271–2273
hyperkalemia in, 2276–2277
hyperphosphatemia in, 2274, 2274t, 2275t
hypocalcemia in, 2273–2274
hypokalemia in, 2277–2278
hypophosphatemia in, 2275–2276, 2276f
immune complexes in, 2265–2266
lymphatic, renal involvement in, 2270–2271
membranoproliferative glomerulonephritis and, 1829–1830
membranous nephropathy and, 1793–1794
metastatic, to kidney, 2268
molecular mechanisms of, 777–782. *See also* Oncogene(s)
nephrotic syndrome and, 1733, 1733t, 2265, 2267–2268
proteinuria in, 2265
renal abnormalities in, 2265–2278, 2266t
specific tubular dysfunction in, 1169–1170
antineoplastic agents and, 1170
intrinsic disorders and, 1170
tumor products and metabolites as, 1170
tumor-induced inappropriate hormone concentration as, 1169–1170
tubular abnormalities in, 2266t
unusual, in AIDS patients, 2361
Candida, characteristics of, 929–930
Candidemia, in "primary" renal candidiasis, 935
Candidiasis, 929–944
Candida in, 929–930
clinical manifestations of, 933–937
asymptomatic candiduria as, 933–934, 934t
candiduria as, 933
cystitis as, 934–935
genitourinary, 934, 934t
hematogenous renal candidiasis as, 937
primary renal candidiasis as, 935–937, 936f
cutaneous, 929
cystitis due to
clinical manifestations of, 934–935
diagnosis of, 939
definition of, 929
diagnosis of, 937–941
antibody coating of fungi in, 938
bladder irrigation in, 938–939
Candida casts in, 938
fungal morphology in urine in, 937–938
papillary necrosis and, 938
quantification of candiduria in, 937
relative value of techniques for, 937, 938t
serology in, 939
epidemiology of, 930
in cystitis, 930
in lower urinary tract, 930
in upper urinary tract, 930
esophageal, posttransplant, 2948
etiology of, 929–930
genitourinary, clinical manifestations of, 934
immunology in, 930–931
pathogenesis of, 931–933, 932f
adherence factors in, 931
experimental studies on, 931–933
hematogenous spread in, 931
in lower urinary tract, 931–932
species differences in, 931
in upper urinary tract, 931
renal
disseminated, 937
hematogenous, 937
blood cultures in, 940
diagnosis of, 940–941
endophthalmitis in, 940
macronodular skin lesions in, 940
in neonates, 937
"primary"
ascending route for, 936
bezoars in, 936–937
candidemia and, 935
clinical manifestations of, 936–937
controversy over, 935–936
criteria for, 935
diagnosis of, 939–940
fungal masses in, 936
intravenous pyelography for, 939–940
percutaneous antegrade pyelography for, 940
renal papillary necrosis in, 936
retrograde ureteral catheterization for, 940
sonography for, 940
treatment of, 941–944
amphotericin B in, 941–942
fluconazole in, 942–943
flucytosine in, 942
imidazole in, 942
itraconazole in, 943
ketoconazole in, 942
miconazole in, 942
in specific urinary tract syndromes, 943t, 943–944
triazole in, 942
urine alkalization in, 943
urethral, clinical manifestations of, 934
Candiduria, 933–934
asymptomatic, 933–934
catheterized urine sample for, 933

Candiduria—Continued
clean-catch midstream urine sample for, 933
pyuria in, 933
quantification of, 933, 937–938
suprapubic aspiration sample for, 933
CAPD. *See* Peritoneal dialysis, continuous ambulatory, (CAPD)
Capillary(ies)
abnormal permeability of, in idiopathic edema, 2496
in edema formation, 2453–2454, 2454t
glomerular. *See* Glomerular capillary(ies)
Capreomycin, for urinary tract tuberculosis, 923t
Captopril
acute interstitial nephritis due to, 1341
for hypertension, 1626–1627, 2390t
membranous nephropathy and, 1796
pharmacology of, normal vs. in renal failure, 3238t–3239t
for scleroderma renal crisis, 2045–2046
for sodium and water retention, in congestive heart failure, 2463–2464
Captopril test
in screening for primary aldosteronism, 1477
in screening for renovascular hypertension, 1459t, 1459–1460, 1461, 1461f
Carbamazepine
acute interstitial nephritis due to, 1340
for diabetes insipidus, 2508t
hyponatremia associated with, 2519t, 2519–2520
pharmacology of, normal vs. in renal failure, 3238t–3239t
Carbenicillin, pharmacology of, normal vs. in renal failure, 3238t–3239t
Carbohydrate(s)
in dietary therapy in chronic hemodialysis, 3180
idiopathic edema and, 2499, 2499f
intravenous administration of, hypophosphatemia and, 2607
Carbohydrate metabolism
continuous ambulatory peritoneal dialysis and, 2848–2849
glucose intolerance in, 2845–2848, 2846f, 2848f
hormones in, 2845
in hypophosphatemia, 2609
in nephrotic syndrome, 1762
renal, 240f, 240–243, 242f. *See also* Gluconeogenesis
in uremia, 2845–2849
abnormal, 2849
Carbon dioxide, hydration of, in acid-base balance, 222–223
Carbon tetrachloride, as nephrotoxin, 1042–1043
Carbonic anhydrase
apical membrane area and, in hydrogen transport in distal nephron, 47–48
localization of, in nephron, 46, 47t
as luminal buffer, 224–225, 225f
in proximal tubule bicarbonate reabsorption, 622–623
role of, in proximal nephron and loop, 46–47
Carbonic anhydrase inhibitor(s)
mechanism of action of, 2435–2437, 2436f
in proximal tubular acidosis, 624
Carboplatin
pharmacology of, normal vs. in renal failure, 3238t–3239t
toxicity of, 1172–1173
Carbuncle, renal, 959–963. *See also* Abscess, renal cortical
Carcinoembryonic antigen, in cancers, 2266
Carcinoma. *See* Cancer; Malignancy; Tumor(s).
renal cell. *See* Renal cell carcinoma
Carcinomatosis, disseminated, renal metastasis in, 2268
Cardiac disease, in Fabry's disease, 595
Cardiac failure. *See* Heart failure
Cardiac output
low, in sodium retention, 1361f, 2455
in preeclampsia, 1518
role of anemia in, correction of, 2817–2818
Cardiac tamponade, in pericarditis, 2826–2827
Cardiac valve abnormality(ies), in autosomal dominant polycystic kidney disease, 554
Cardiomyopathy
causes of, 2830t
in end-stage renal disease, 2829–2834
Cardiovascular drug therapy, in renal disease, 3229
Cardiovascular system
complications of
in end-stage renal disease, 2817–2834
posttransplant, 2949–2951
evaluation of, prior to renal transplantation, 2919
in hypercalcemia, 2625
in hypophosphatemia, 2608–2609
Carmustine nephrotoxicity, 1174
Carnitine
deficiency, in uremic dyslipoproteinemia, 2851
in dietary therapy in chronic hemodialysis, 3179–3180
Carpal tunnel syndrome, 2226
amyloidosis and, 2213, 2213t
in chronic hemodialysis, 3080
Cast(s)
bacterial, 351
Candida, in diagnosis of candidiasis, 938
erythrocyte, 349, 351f–352f
granular, 347, 351, 351f
leukocyte, 348
in upper urinary tract infection, 982
light chain. *See also* Light chain cast nephropathy
in multiple myeloma, 2195f, 2195–2196
in proteinuria, 2193f, 2194
protein composition of, 346, 347t
in glomerulonephritis, 347t
size and shape of, 348
tubular epithelial cell, 348f, 349, 351
urine microscopy for, 346f–352f, 346–351
waxy, 351, 352f
Catabolism
in acute renal failure, 1383
increased, hyperphosphatemia and, 2614
uremic, clinical management of, 2855
Catalase test, for bacteriuria, 1012
Cataract(s)
in Alport syndrome, 580–581
posttransplant, 2953
Catecholamine(s), 299–300. *See also* *specific types*
biochemistry of, 1488f, 1488–1489
in cirrhosis, 2469–2471
diabetes mellitus and, 2585
excess, hypertensive crisis in, 1555
major renal actions of, 299
malaria and, 2343
mode of action of, 284
organic anion and cation transport pathways for, 273–274
plasma, for pheochromocytoma, 1490–1491, 1491f
platelet, for pheochromocytoma, 1493
potassium regulation and, 2646–2647, 2647t
renal effects of, 2575
renal function and, 2715–2716
in renal hemodynamics, 96–97
in renal neurologic control, 299
in renovascular hypertension, 1454
in uremia, 2861
urinary, for pheochromocytoma, 1491–1492, 1492f, 1492t
in vascular reactivity in preeclampsia, 1513
Catheter(s), indwelling urinary, prostatitis due to, 744
Catheter-associated urinary tract infection
lower, 1020–1021
pathogenesis of, 1020
prevention of, 1021, 1021t
treatment of, 1021
upper, treatment and prevention of, 994, 996
Catheterization
femoral vein, in chronic hemodialysis, 3033
in heart failure, 2833
ureteral
retrograde, for renal candidiasis, 940
for for urinary tract infection, 983
urinary, for treatment of renal failure, 1382
Cathodic antigen(s), circulating, 2347, 2349
Cation transport, 268–275
across apical cell membranes, 272–273, 274f
across basolateral cell membranes, 270–272, 272f
compounds transported by, 273–274
inhibition of, 275
renal tubular localization of, 269–270, 270f–271f
study techniques for, 261–262, 262t
types of, 268–269, 269f, 269t
Cecal urinary reservoir, continent, 829, 829f
Cecoureterocele, 647
Cefaclor, pharmacology of, normal vs. in renal failure, 3238t–3239t
Cefamandole, pharmacology of, normal vs. in renal failure, 3238t–3239t
Cefazolin, pharmacology of, normal vs. in renal failure, 3238t–3239t
Cefixime, pharmacology of, normal vs. in renal failure, 3238t–3239t
Cefonicid, pharmacology of, normal vs. in renal failure, 3238t–3239t
Cefoperazone, pharmacology of, normal vs. in renal failure, 3238t–3239t

Ceforanide, pharmacology of, normal vs. in renal failure, 3238t–3239t
Cefotaxime, pharmacology of, normal vs. in renal failure, 3240t–3241t
Cefotetan, pharmacology of, normal vs. in renal failure, 3240t–3241t
Cefoxitin, pharmacology of, normal vs. in renal failure, 3240t–3241t
Ceftazidime, pharmacology of, normal vs. in renal failure, 3240t–3241t
Ceftizoxime, pharmacology of, normal vs. in renal failure, 3240t–3241t
Ceftriaxone, pharmacology of, normal vs. in renal failure, 3240t–3241t
Cell membrane, hypopolarization of, in diabetes mellitus, 2572
Central core model of Stephenson, 131–132, 132f
Central nervous system (CNS)
gap junctions in, 2794
infections of, as complication of transplantation, 2946–2947
in SIADH secretion, 2524t, 2524–2525
Central pontine myelinolysis, 2525
Cephadroxil, pharmacology of, normal vs. in renal failure, 3240t–3241t
Cephalexin, pharmacology of, normal vs. in renal failure, 3240t–3241t
Cephaloridine, as nephrotoxin, 1042
Cephalosporin(s)
mitochondrial effects of, 1047
nephrotoxicity of, 1042
acute interstitial nephritis and, 1336–1337
tubular cell uptake in, 1035–1036
Cephalothin, pharmacology of, normal vs. in renal failure, 3240t–3241t
Cephapirin
cystic fluid concentration of, in autosomal dominant polycystic kidney disease, 551t
pharmacology of, normal vs. in renal failure, 3240t–3241t
Cephradine, pharmacology of, normal vs. in renal failure, 3240t–3241t
Cerebral aneurysm, in autosomal dominant polycystic kidney disease, 553f, 553–554
Cerebral hemorrhage
hypertension and, 1604–1605
in preeclampsia and eclampsia, 1517, 1518t
Cerebral infarction, hypertension and, 1603–1604
Cerebral perfusion, reduced, metabolic alkalosis and, 2583
Cerebrospinal fluid, altered, dialysis dementia and, 2803
Cerebrovascular accident(s)
as complication of dialysis, 2803–2804
hypertension and, 1603–1606
cGMP, as second messenger, in hormonal activation, 286–287
Charcot-Marie-Tooth disease, nephritis in, 581
Chemical(s), in acute renal failure, etiologic role of, 2332, 2333t
Chemotherapy. *See also specific drugs*
for amyloidosis, 2224
hyperphosphatemia and, 2613
for multiple myeloma, 2205
Chest pain, in pericarditis, 2826
Children. *See also* Infant(s); Neonate(s).
acute nephrotic syndrome in, 2391–2392, 2392t
aluminum toxicity in, 2773
autosomal dominant polycystic kidney disease in, 555t, 555–556
blood pressure in, measurement of, 2379, 2380t
bone disease in, 2773–2774
calcium excretion in, 2382
chronic lead nephropathy in, 1239
chronic renal failure in, 2394–2398
dialysis for, 2397
epidemiology of, 2394, 2394t
growth hormone therapy for, 2396
growth retardation and, 2394–2395
nutritional therapy for, 2395–2396
organization of services and, 2394
psychosocial problems and, 2396–2397
transplantation for, 2397
treatment of, selection of children for, 2398
cystitis and urethritis in, management of, 1019–1020
electrolytes in, plasma and urine, 2382
endocapillary exudative glomerulonephritis in, 1925–1926, 1927, 1928t
fluid and electrolyte status in, 2384, 2384t
clinical management of, 2384–2385
focal segmental glomerulosclerosis in, 1911
fractional excretion of phosphate in, 2380
glomerular filtration rate in, 2379–2380, 2384t
glomerulonephritis in, 2391–2393, 2392t
growth and nutrition in, 2383–2384
hematuria in, 2392
causes of, 2392t
hemolytic-uremic syndrome in, 2074–2075, 2075f–2076f, 2388–2389
Henoch-Schönlein nephritis in, 2393
hypernatremia in, 2382
hypertension in, 2389–2390
causes and investigation of, 2389, 2389t
essential, 2390
treatment of, 2389–2390, 2390t
hyponatremia in, 2382
IgA nephropathy in, 1915–1916
membranous nephropathy in, 1793–1794, 1919
minimal change nephrotic syndrome in, 1906–1909, 1907f–1908f
nephritis in Henoch-Schönlein purpura and, 1936f–1939f, 1936–1937, 1937t–1939t
nephrotic syndrome in, 2392–2393
obstructive uropathy in, 2387–2388
peritoneal dialysis in, 3003–3004
plasma phosphate concentration in, 2382
polycystic kidney disease in, 2387
posttransplant growth retardation in, 2953
proteinuria in, 2380
symptomless, 2393
prune-belly syndrome in, 2387
rapidly-progressive glomerulonephritis in, 1932
renal agenesis in, 2383, 2383f, 2387
renal artery stenosis in, angiography for, 472, 473f
renal disease in, 2379–2399
identification and investigation of, 2379–2382
polymyositis-dermatomyositis in, 2058
renal function testing in, 2379
renal physiology in, 2382–2385, 2384t
renal tubular acidosis in, 2381
renal tubular function in
distal, 2381–2382
proximal, 2380–2381
renovascular hypertension in, 1458
systemic lupus erythematosus in, 1941–1942, 2028–2029
upper urinary tract infection in
clinical presentation in, 989
natural history of, 978–979
urinary oxalate-creatinine ratio in, 2382
urinary tract infection in, 2379, 2390t, 2390–2391
diagnosis and investigation of, 2391, 2391t
management of, 2391
urine acidification in, 2381
urine albumin-creatinine concentration in, 2380
urine collection in, 2379
urine concentrating capacity in, 2381–2382
Chlamydia trachomatis infection
cystitis and urethritis vs., 1011
prostatitis due to, 752
Chloral hydrate, pharmacology of, normal vs. in renal failure, 3240t–3241t
Chloramphenicol
cystic fluid concentration of, in autosomal dominant polycystic kidney disease, 551t
pharmacology of, normal vs. in renal failure, 3240t–3241t
Chlordiazepoxide, pharmacology of, normal vs. in renal failure, 3240t–3241t
Chloride, in metabolic alkalosis, 2685–2686
Chloridorrhea, congenital, 2685
Chloroform, as nephrotoxin, 1041–1042
Chloroquine, pharmacology of, normal vs. in renal failure, 3240t–3241t
Chlorothiazide acute interstitial nephritis due to, 1340
for hypertension, 2390t
Chlorpromade, for essential hypernatremia, 2514
Chlorpromazine, pharmacology of, normal vs. in renal failure, 3240t–3241t
Chlorpropamide
for diabetes insipidus, 2508t
for diabetes mellitus, 2576
hyponatremia associated with, 2519, 2519t
Chlorthalidone, pharmacology of, normal vs. in renal failure, 3242t–3243t
Cholemia, in hepatorenal disease, 1359
Cholesterol, high-density lipoprotein, in CAPD, 2851
Cholesterol embolism
in elderly, 2422
renal
in malignant hypertension, 1560

Cholesterol embolism, renal—Continued
in renovascular hypertension, 1456–1457
Choriocarcinoma, testicular
classification and pathogenesis of, 853–855, 854f, 854t
natural history of, 855
Choroidopathy, hypertensive, 1566, 1566f
Chromogranin A, plasma, for pheochromocytoma, 1492
Chromomycosis, 946
Chronic renal failure
acid-base homeostasis in, 2728–2731, 2729f
age-related, 2425–2426
in Alport syndrome, 574
ammoniagenesis in, 249
in analgesic-induced renal disease, 1112
anemia in, 2744–2746, 2745f
assessment of progression in, 3132–3135
creatinine clearance for, 3133–3134
diet manipulation and, 3134
frequency of GFR measurement for, 3134–3135
serum creatinine for, 3132–3134
blood loss in, 2746
blood urea nitrogen in, 3132
in cancer, 1166t–1167t, 1168–1169. *See also* Cancer
in children, 2394–2398. *See also* Children, chronic renal failure in
creatinine clearance in, 3131
in diabetes mellitus, 2585–2586, 2586f
dietary therapy in, 3139–3147, 3170–3187. *See also* Protein restriction
assessment of compliance and, 3139–3141, 3140f
essential amino acid analogues and, 3145–3147
essential amino acids and, 3144–3145
general approach to, 3170–3172
goals of, 3170
nitrogen balance in uremia and, 3141
nutritional adequacy and, 3140–3141
phosphate restriction for, 3155–3156
progression of diabetic renal disease and, 3143–3144
progression of disease and, 3142–3143
protein, amino acids, and ketoacids in, 3173–3178
background information in, 3173–3175, 3175t
for GFR 25–70 ml/min/1.72m^2, 3176
for GFR less than 25 ml/min/1.72m^2 without dialysis, 3176
types of diets with, 3174, 3175t
protein catabolic rate in, 3140–3141
protein turnover in uremia and, 3141–3142
recommended dietary nutrient intake in, 3170, 3170t–3171t
serum urea nitrogen-serum creatinine ratio in, 3172–3173
urea generation in, 3140–3141
urea nitrogen appearance in, 3172–3173
glomerular filtration rate in, 2707–2708
assessment of, 3131
homeostasis in, 2705–2706, 2706f
hypercalcemia and, 2627
hypergastrinemia in, 2862
hyperphosphatemia in, 3153–3156
management of, aluminum intoxication and, 3160–3161
metastatic calcification due to, 3154f–3155f, 3154t, 3154–3155
progressive renal damage due to, 3155–3156
secondary hyperparathyroidism due to, 3153–3154
hyperprolactinemia in, 2857–2858
hypertrophic response modification in, 2708
hypertrophy in
ammoniagenesis and, 2710
cellular mechanisms in, 2708–2709
cyclic nucleotide metabolism and, 2710
DNA metabolism and, 2710
early cellular changes in, 2709–2712
gene expression patterns and, 2712
GFR changes and, 2709
growth factors and, 2711–2712
morphologic changes and, 2709
neural stimuli and, 2711
phospholipid metabolism and, 2710
protein metabolism and, 2711
renal plasma flow and, 2709
RNA metabolism and, 2710–2711
transport systems and, 2709–2710
without increase in filtration rate, 2708
loss of mass vs. loss of function in, 2708
metabolic acidosis in
clinical features of, 2671–2673, 2672f
pathophysiology of, 2673–2674
treatment of, 2674
β_2-microglobulin in, 3132
in multiple myeloma, 2203–2204
natural history of, 3131–3135
time to end-stage renal disease in, 3131, 3132f
nephron adaptation in, 2703–2704
general principles of, 2704
patterns of, 2704f, 2704–2705
structural, 2706–2713
nutrient administration in, 3196–3198
enteral vs. parenteral, 3196–3198
nutritional disorders in, 3167
osteodystrophy of, 2759–2779. *See also* Osteodystrophy, renal
potassium homeostasis in, 2651, 2725–2726, 2726f
protein losses in, 3167–3169, 3169t
protein-calorie malnutrition in, 3167, 3168t
psychological testing and, 2791–2792
due to radiation nephropathy, 1169
red cell survival in, 2746, 2746f
renotropin in, 2707
salt-losing tendency of, 2722, 2722f, 2723t
serum creatinine in, 3131–3132
sodium homeostasis in, 2720–2725
sodium-hydrogen exchange in, 2707–2708
solute homeostasis in, 2720–2731
thyroid hormone metabolism in, 2858t
treatment challenges in, 3059
uremic encephalopathy and, 2790–2791
urinary concentrating defect in, 2512
wasting and malnutrition in, 3167–3169, 3169t
water homeostasis in, 2727–2728
Churg-Strauss syndrome, 1936, 2111–2113, 2112f
Chvostek's sign, 2635
Cigarette smoking
malignant hypertension and, 1562
renovascular hypertension and, 1458
urinary bladder carcinoma and, 811–812
Cilastatin, pharmacology of, normal vs. in renal failure, 3242t–3243t
Cimetidine
acute interstitial nephritis due to, 1340
for hypophosphatemia, 2610
organic anion and cation transport pathways for, 273–274
pharmacology of, normal vs. in renal failure, 3242t–3243t
Ciprofloxacin
cystic fluid concentration of, in autosomal dominant polycystic kidney disease, 551t
pharmacology of, normal vs. in renal failure, 3242t–3243t
Circulating anodic antigen, 2347, 2349
Circulating cathodic antigen, 2347, 2349
Circulating schistosomal antigen, 2348, 2349
Cirrhosis. *See also* Hepatorenal disease
aldosterone and, 2471
ascites in
overfill theory of, 2467f, 2467–2468
underfill theory of, 2466f, 2466–2467
biochemical features of, 2467t, 2475t
catecholamines in, 2469–2471
edema formation in, 2465, 2466f
enhanced tubular sodium reabsorption in, 2469
glomerular filtration rate in, 2469
kallikrein in, 2471
maladaptive responses in, 1360, 1362f
membranoproliferative glomerulonephritis and, 1831
natriuretic factors in, 2471
prostaglandins in, 2471
renal blood flow in, 2469
sodium retention in
nephron sites of, 2468–2469
sympathetic nervous system in, 2469–2471
stages of progression in, 1360, 1362f
CIsplatin, pharmacology of, normal vs. in renal failure, 3242t–3243t
Cisplatin nephrotoxicity, 1043–1044, 1170–1173
clinical manifestations of, 1171
histopathology and pathogenesis of, 1170–1171
mitochondrial effects of, 1047
prophylactic measures in, 1171–1173
saline infusion as, 1171–1172
thiosulfate as, 1172
tubular cell uptake in, 1036
Cisplatinum, phase specificity and mechanism of action of, 821t
Citrate, renal handling of, 238, 239f
Citric acid cycle, in renal metabolism, 238, 239f
Clavulanic acid, pharmacology of, normal vs. in renal failure, 3242t–3243t
Clearance, formula for, 364
Clindamycin
cystic fluid concentration of, in autosomal dominant polycystic kidney disease, 551t

pharmacology of, normal vs. in renal failure, 3242t–3243t
Clinidine, pharmacology of, normal vs. in renal failure, 3242t–3243t
Cloaca
congenital malformations of, 637
faulty partition of, 654
normal embryologic development of, 637
Clofibrate
for diabetes insipidus, 2508t
pharmacology of, normal vs. in renal failure, 3242t–3243t
Clofibric acid, effect of, on proteinuria and focal glomerulosclerosis, 2409, 2413f
Clonidine
for hypertension, 1627
in treatment of renovascular hypertension, 1468
Clonidine suppression test, for pheochromocytoma, 1494f, 1494–1495
Cloxacillin, pharmacology of, normal vs. in renal failure, 3242t–3243t
CNS. *See* Central nervous system (CNS)
Coagulation. *See also* Platelet(s)
disturbances of, in preeclampsia, 2291–2292
intravascular
in acute renal failure, 2302
in malaria, 2344
in sickle cell disease, 2323
Coagulation abnormality(ies)
in acute tubular necrosis, 1308
in preeclampsia, 1514
Coagulation inhibitor(s), in acute renal vein thrombosis, in nephrotic syndrome, 1321
Cocaine abuse, nontraumatic rhabdomyolysis in, acute renal failure due to, 1230–1231
Coccidioides, as complication of transplantation, 2947
Coccidioidomycosis, 944, 945t–946t
Cochlea, in Alport syndrome, 577
Codeine
pharmacology of, normal vs. in renal failure, 3242t–3243t
in renal disease, complications of, 3231
Colchicine
for amyloidosis, 2224
pharmacology of, normal vs. in renal failure, 3242t–3243t
Colitis, pseudomembranous, posttransplant, 2949
Collagen, 2759
Collagen disease(s), in pregnancy, 2304
Collecting duct(s)
ADH effects on, in fluid transport, 48–49
ADH receptors in, 292
calcium absorption in, 2621
cellular structure of, 27f–31f, 27–29, 160f, 161
collecting duct (principal) cells in, 27f–28f, 27–28, 160f, 161
intercalated cells in, 27f, 28–29, 30f, 160f, 161
congenital malformations of, 650–651
cortical
acid-base transport in, summary and integration of, 226, 227f–228f
potassium transport in
aldosterone in, 194
basolateral membrane amplification in, 194
cellular mechanisms of, 192–195, 193f
mineralocorticoids in, 194
principal cells in, 193–194
inner medullary, sodium transport in, 164–165, 165f
medullary, acid-base transport in, summary and integration of, 226–228, 228f
net acid transport in, 217–218
ammonium and, 217, 217f
bicarbonate and, 217, 217f
limiting luminal pH and, 218
titratable acid and, 217, 218f
outer medullary
potassium transport in, cellular mechanisms of, 195
sodium transport in, 164
potassium in, 2649
sodium transport in, 162–165
ADH in, 164
aldosterone in, 163t, 163–164
atrial natriuretic peptide, 164
bradykinin in, 164
control of, 163t, 163–164
electrophysiologic aspects of, 162
general considerations in, 162
mechanisms of, 162f, 162–163
prostaglandin in, 164
Collecting duct system
morphology of, 26
regions of, 4, 5f
Colloid osmotic pressure, total plasma protein concentration for prediction of, 75, 75f
Colon
cancer of, nephrotic syndrome in, 2265
diverticula of, in autosomal dominant polycystic kidney disease, 554
Coma, with hyperglycemia, as complication of dialysis, 2803
Complement deficiency, in membranoproliferative glomerulonephritis, 1821–1822, 1828–1829
Complement fragments, in vascular inflammatory injury, 1996
Complement system, in membranoproliferative glomerulonephritis, 1820–1821
Computed tomography (CT), 449–456
for acquired cystic disease, 453
for acute pyelonephritis, 451
for acute renal vein thrombosis in nephrotic syndrome, 1326
adrenal, for tumor localization in primary aldosteronism, 1480, 1480f–1481f
for adult polycystic kidney disease, 452–453, 453f
of bone mass, 2764–2765
for congenital anatomic variants, 450, 450f
contrast media in, 449–450
for focal bacterial nephritis, 451
MRI vs., 461
for nephrolithiasis, 451, 451f
for normal anatomy, 450
for obstructive disease, 450–541, 451f
for parapelvic cyst, 452
for pheochromocytoma, 1495f, 1495–1496
for renal adenoma, 454
for renal angiomyolipoma and hamartoma, 453–454, 454f
for renal artery thromboembolism, 2124
for renal cell carcinoma, 454, 454f, 789–790, 790f
for renal cortical abscess, 961–962
for renal fungal infection, 451–452
for renal lymphoma/leukemia, 455
for renal metastatic tumors, 455, 455f
for renal oncocytoma, 454
for renal pelvic transitional cell carcinoma, 455
for renal sarcoma, 455, 455f
for renal transplantation, 453, 453f
for renal trauma, 455–456, 456f
for renal tumors, 453–455, 454f–455f
for renal vascular disease, 453, 453f
for simple renal cyst, 452, 452f
technical considerations in, 449
for urinary tract obstruction, 679, 679f
for urinary tract tuberculosis, 920, 921f
for xanthogranulomatous pyelonephritis, 452, 452f
Concentration, urine. *See* Glomerular filtrate; Renal concentrating capacity; Urine, concentration of
Congenital disorder(s), renal transplantation and, 2915
Congenital nephrotic syndrome, 2386
Congestive heart failure, 2454–2465
amyloidosis and, 2213, 2213t
diabetes mellitus and, 2576
in malignant hypertension, 1569
neuroendocrine activation in, 2464
sodium retention in, 2461f
afferent mechanisms for, 2454t, 2454–2457
hepatic receptors in, 2456–2457
high-pressure receptors in, 2454–2456
intrarenal receptors in, 2457
low-pressure receptors in, 2456
backward theory of, 2454
efferent mechanisms for
atrial natriuretic factor in, 2460
filtration fraction in, 2458
glomerular filtration rate in, 2457
prostaglandins in, 2459–2460
proximal tubular sodium reabsorption in, 2458
renal blood flow in, 2457–2458
renal nerves in, 2458–2459
renin-angiotensin-aldosterone system in, 2459
forward theory of, 2454
treatment of, 2463–2465
water retention in, 2461f
afferent and efferent pathways for, 2463, 2464f
mechanisms for, 2461–2463
treatment of, 2463–2465
Conjunctiva
calcification of, in chronic renal failure, 3154
irritation of, hypercalcemia and, 2625
Continuous Performance Test, 2791
Contraceptive(s), oral
acute renal vein thrombosis due to, in nephrotic syndrome, 1324
malignant hypertension due to, 1560
microvascular thrombosis due to, 2066

Contrast media
  for computed tomography, 449–450
  dimeric, 1192f
  hazards of, 408
  for intravenous urography, 407
  ionic, 1192f
  management of reactions to, 408
  for MRI, 457–458
  nonionic
    advantages of, 1196–1197
    chemical structure of, 1192f
    indications for, 408
  precautions for, 408
  renal complications of, 408
  steroid prophylaxis prior to, 408
Contrast media-induced acute renal failure, 1187–1197
  in cancer, 1167–1168
  clinical features of, 1190
  diagnosis of, 1190–1191, 1191f
  incidence of, 1187–1188
  nonoliguric, 1298
  pathogenesis of, 1191–1196
    allergic and immunologic reactions and, 1194
    altered glomerular permeability in, 1196
    direct toxicity in, 1194–1196, 1195f
    enzymuria in, 1194
    hemodynamic factors in, 1192–1193, 1193f
    proteinuria in, 1193–1194
    tubular obstruction in, 1194
  pathologic findings in, 1191
  prevention of, 1197
  risk factors for, 1188t, 1188–1190, 1189f
    diabetes mellitus as, 1189f, 1189–1190
    multiple myeloma as, 1190
Converting enzyme inhibitor(s), 2588
  for hypertension, 1626–1627
Copper sulfate poisoning
  acute renal failure and, 2332
  renal manifestations of, 1248
Corneal calcification, hypercalcemia and, 2625
Corneal opacity, in Fabry's disease, 595
Coronary artery disease
  in heart failure, 2829
  treatment of, 2833
Corpuscle, renal. *See* Glomerulus
Cortex, renal
  anatomy of, 3, 4f
  interstitium of, 35, 35f, 1959–1960
  ischemia of, malaria and, 2342–2343
  necrosis of
    bilateral, 2302
    in pregnancy, incidence of, 2334, 2335t
  oxygen gradient between medulla and, 233, 234f, 235
Cortical abscess, renal, 959–963. *See also* Abscess, renal cortical
Cortical labyrinth, renal, 3
Cortical necrosis
  acute, 2081–2083
    clinical features of, 2082
    conditions associated with, 2081
    definition of, 2081
    pathogenesis of, 2081–2082
    pathologic findings in, 2082
    prognosis and treatment in, 2082–2083
  bilateral, 2302
  in pregnancy, 2334, 2335t
Corticomedullary abscess, 963–966. *See also* Abscess, renal corticomedullary.
Corticosteroid(s). *See also* Glucocorticoid(s); Mineralocorticoid(s).
  in distal nephron sodium transport, 43–44
  in immunosuppression, 2895–2897, 2896, 2896t, 2926
  major renal effects of, 296–299
  in pericarditis, 2827
  in proximal tubule sodium reabsorption, 151
Cortisol, in uremia, 2857
Corynebacterium parvum nephrotoxicity, 1180
Co-transporter blockers, 2441f–2442f, 2441–2443
Countercurrent mechanism. *See* Loop of Henle; Urine, concentration of
Cowper syringocele, 639
Cowper's gland, ducts of, cyst of, 639
Coxsackie virus infection, renal manifestations of, 998
Cranial nerves, dysfunction of, uremic nephropathy and, 2809
Craniotabes, hypophosphatemia and, 2605
Creatinine
  plasma, age and, 2380
  serum, 367–369, 368f–369f
    accuracy of, 369
    in acute tubular necrosis, 1306t, 1306–1307
    age effects on, 367, 368
    BUN vs., 371
    in chronic renal failure, 3131–3132
    diet effects on, 367
    GFR and, 367–368, 368f–369f
    methods for measurement of, 367
    muscular size effects on, 367
    normal concentration of, 367
    reciprocal, 369
Creatinine clearance, 365–367
  advantages of, 365–366
  age-related decline in, 2408f, 2408t
  BUN vs., 371
  in chronic renal failure, 3131
  combined
    in continuous ambulatory peritoneal dialysis, calculation of, 2981–2982, 2982t–2983t
    in intermittent peritoneal dialysis, calculation of, 2981–2982, 2982t–2983t
  in continuous ambulatory peritoneal dialysis, 2977–2978, 2978f
  dietary effects on, 366
  in elderly, 2407–2408, 2408t, 2409f
  erroneous measurement of, 366–367
  GFR and, 366
  inulin clearance vs., 366
  organic anion and cation pathways in, 273
  in renal failure, for drug dosage regimen alterations, 3221–3222
  total chromogen method for, 366
  urine collection for, 366–367
^{51}Cr-EDTA clearance, for GFR, 372
Crescent(s), clinicopathologic correlations of, 503–504
CREST syndrome, 2039
Cryoglobulinemia
  classification of, 1829t, 2137
  essential mixed, 2137–2146
    clinical manifestations of, 2141–2142, 2142t
    laboratory data in, 2143
    natural history and prognosis in, 2142–2143, 2143t
    pathogenesis of, 2143–2144
      IgM rheumatoid factor in, 2143–2144
      renal damage and, 2144
    prognosis in, 1938–1940, 1940t
    renal histology in, 2137–2140
      electron microscopy in, 2137–2138, 2140f
      immunohistology in, 2139–2140, 2141f
      light microscopy in, 2137, 2138f–2139f
    treatment of, 2144–2146
      in acute exacerbations, 2144–2145
      dialysis and transplantation in, 2146
      maintenance, 2145–2146
  membranoproliferative glomerulonephritis and, 1828, 1829t
  nephritis in, immunopathology of, 1662–1663
Cryptococcosis
  as complication of transplantation, 2947
  opportunistic, 946t–947t, 946–947
Cryptorchidism, testicular carcinoma and, 851–853
CT. *See* Computed tomography (CT)
Cushing's disease
  classification of, 1541
  management of, 1545
Cushing's syndrome, 1541–1550
  ACTH-dependent, 1541
    ectopic, 1541
    exogenous, 1541
    pituitary, 1541
  ACTH-independent, 1541–1542
    adrenal adenoma in, 1541
    adrenal carcinoma in, 1541–1542
    exogenous glucocorticoids in, 1542
  ACTH-producing tumors causing, 2277
  classification of, 1541–1542, 1542t
  clinical features of, 1542
  diagnosis of, 1542–1544, 1543f
  historical, 1541
  hypertension in, 1545
  imaging studies in, 1544f, 1544–1545
    for adrenal gland, 1544, 1544f
    for pituitary macroadenoma, 1544, 1544f
  malignant hypertension due to, 1561
  management of, 1545
  in pregnancy, 1542
  steroid excesses in, 1542
Cutaneous entries. *See* Skin
Cyclacillin, pharmacology of, normal vs. in renal failure, 3242t–3243t
Cyclic nucleotide metabolism, in renal hypertrophy, 2710
Cyclooxygenase metabolic pathway, 90, 90f
Cyclophilin, in immunosuppression, 2899
Cyclophosphamide
  hyponatremia associated with, 2520
  nephrotoxicity of, 1173
  pharmacology of, normal vs. in renal failure, 3242t–3243t
Cycloserine, for urinary tract tuberculosis, 923t
Cyclosporin A
  in gout, 2253
  in renal transplantation, 2397
  side effects of, 2926t

Cyclosporine
analgesic-induced renal disease due to, 1972–1973
drug interactions with, 2927, 2927t
in renal disease, 3230–3231
in hypoaldosteronism, 2588
in immunosuppression, 2897–2899, 2898f, 2899t
levels of, monitoring, 2927–2928
microvascular thrombosis due to, 2066
nephrotoxicity of, 1044
acute, 2928
chronic, 2928–2929
differential diagnosis of, 2929
pharmacodynamics of, 2900
pharmacokinetics of, 2927
pharmacology of, normal vs. in renal failure, 3242t–3243t
for rheumatoid arthritis, renal damage due to, 2053–2054
side effects of, 2927
Cyst. *See also* Polycystic kidney disease
arachnoid, in autosomal dominant polycystic kidney disease, 553
of ducts of Cowper's gland, 639
hepatic, in autosomal dominant polycystic kidney disease, 552f–553f, 552–553
intrarenal, congenital, 650
medullary, simple, 521, 522f
parapelvic, CT for, 452
peripelvic, congenital, 650
pyelogenic, 521, 522f
renal
complicated
MRI for, 458
ultrasonography for, 428f, 429
diagnostic puncture of, in renal cell carcinoma, 789
infected, 966
simple
angiography for, 478
characteristics of, 547t
CT for, 452, 452f
MRI for, 458
ultrasonography for, 428f, 429
urographic diagnosis of, 428, 428f
Cysteine conjugate(s), as nephrotoxin, 1044–1045
Cysteine metabolism, in nephrotoxicity, 1038
Cystic bone lesions, 2764, 2764f–2765f
Cystic fibrosis
amyloidosis and, 2220
growth retardation in, 2395
Cystic kidney disease, acquired, 521, 559–561. *See also* Polycystic kidney disease
autosomal dominant polycystic kidney disease vs., 547
characteristics of, 547t
in chronic hemodialysis, 3088
clinical and radiologic diagnosis of, 560
description of, 559–560
diagnosis and treatment of, 521
due to hemodialysis, 521
management of, 560
pathologic findings in, 560, 560f
renal tumors in, 560
Cystic nephroma, multilocular, angiography for, 477
Cystine crystal(s), urinalysis for, 356, 357f
Cystine nephrolithiasis, 737, 738
Cystinosis
in chronic tubulointerstitial nephropathy, 1975–1976
renal transplantation and, 2915
Cystinuria, 613–616
clinical findings in, 614
definition of, 613–614
dibasic aminoaciduria in, 614
genetic patterns of, clinical manifestations of, 614
hereditary, characteristics of, 612t
incidence of, 614
nephrolithiasis due to, 731, 731t
therapy in, 614–616, 615t
dietary, 614
medical, 614–616
Cystitis, 1007–1021. *See also* Urinary tract infection
due to candidiasis
bezoar formation in, 934–935
clinical manifestations of, 934–935
diagnosis of, 930
epidemiology of, 930
clinical manifestations of, 1011–1012
definition of, 1007
diagnosis of, 1012–1013
automated tests for, 1012–1013
bioluminescence methods for, 1013
filtration methods for, 1013
photometric methods for, 1012–1013
rapid diagnostic tests for, 1012
catalase test for, 1012
glucose oxidase test for, 1012
Griess test for, 1012
leukocyte esterase test for, 1012
urine culture for, 1013
epidemiology of, 1010–1011
management of, 1013–1020
in acute dysuria, 1016–1017, 1018f
amoxicillin for, 1015
ampicillin for, 1015
in asymptomatic bacteriuria, 1013, 1016, 1017f
in children, 1019–1020
clavulanate-potentiated amoxicillin for, 1015
duration of therapy in, 1016
fluoroquinolones for, 1015–1016
general principles of, 1013–1014
nitrofurantoin for, 1015
in pregnancy, 1019, 1020f
in recurrent infection, 1017–1019, 1018t
in relapsing infection, 1017
specific antimicrobial therapy in, 1014t, 1014–1016
sulfonamides for, 1014–1015
in symptomatic bacteriuria, 1013–1014
trimethoprim for, 1015
trimethoprim-sulfamethoxazole for, 1015
in uncomplicated presentation, 1014t, 1014–1016
pathogenesis of, 1008–1010
host factors in, 1009–1010
pathogens in, 1008f, 1008–1009
route of infection in, 1008
virulence factors in, 1009
sexually transmitted disease vs., 1011
urine culture in, 1011
vaginitis vs., 1011
Cystography, radionuclide micturition, for vesicoureteral reflux, 701–702, 702f
Cystometrogram
filling, in lower urinary tract dysfunction, 767–768
voiding, in lower urinary tract dysfunction, 768
Cystoprostatectomy, radical, complications of, 823–824, 824t–825t
Cystoscopy, with ureteral catheterization, for upper urinary tract infection, 983
Cystourethrography, voiding, for vesicoureteral reflux, 700f–701f, 700–701
Cytarabine, pharmacology of, normal vs. in renal failure, 3242t–3243t
Cytochrome P450 monooxygenase metabolic pathway, 90, 90f
products of, 309–310
Cytokine(s)
malaria and, 2343
in vascular inflammatory injury, 1996
Cytomegalovirus (CMV) infection
adrenalitis due to, 2366
gancyclovir for, 2364, 2944t
of lungs, as complication of transplantation, 2945, 2946f
in renal transplantation, 2943–2944, 2944t
of allograft, 2937
percutaneous renal biopsy for, 506
Cytosine arabinoside nephrotoxicity, 1177
Cytoskeleton, in experimental studies on ischemic renal injury, 1274–1275
Cytosolic calcium, in renal vascular contraction and relaxation, 70–71, 71f
Cytosolic vesicle(s), in apical membrane, ADH effects on fluid transport and, 49–50
Cytotoxicity, lymphocyte-mediated, 2884, 2884f

Dactinomycin, pharmacology of, normal vs. in renal failure, 3242t–3243t
Daunorubicin, pharmacology of, normal vs. in renal failure, 3244t–3245t
DDAVP test, for assessment of renal concentrating capacity, 379, 380f
Decubitus ulcer(s), amyloidosis and, 2220
Deferoxamine, aluminum chelation with, 2777–2778, 2779f
Deferoxamine challenge, in renal osteodystrophy, 2766, 2767t
Dehydration. *See also* Fluids
acute renal vein thrombosis due to, in nephrotic syndrome, 1324
associated with acute renal failure, 2204
renal hemodynamic effects of, 101
Demeclocycline
diabetes insipidus associated with, 2511–2512
for hyponatremia, 2474
polyuria and polydipsia caused by, 2527
vasopressin secretion and, 2545
Dementia, dialysis. *See* Dialysis dementia.
Dense deposit disease, 1817–1820. *See also* Glomerulonephritis, membranoproliferative
Densitometry, single-photon, of bone mass, 2764

Deoxycorticosterone excess syndrome(s), 1481–1482
15-Deoxyspergualin, in immunosuppression, 2901
Desoxycorticosterone acetate
in glucocorticoid deficiency, 2549–2550, 2550t
in mineralocorticoid deficiency, 2548
Detrusor hyperreflexia, 763
treatment of, 768–769
Detrusor instability, 763
treatment of, 768–769
vesicoureteral reflux and, 702–704, 703t
Detrusor-sphincter dyssynergia
treatment of, 770
vesicoureteral reflux and, 702–704, 703t
Dextran, glomerular filtration of
electrical charge in, 382, 382f
molecular size in, 381, 382f
Diabetes insipidus
anterior pituitary insufficiency and, 1523f, 2552
central
assessment of, 379
clinical features of, 2503–2505
diagnosis of, 2505–2508, 2506t, 2507f, 2508t
etiology of, 2505, 2506t
pathophysiology of, 2503
treatment of, 2508t, 2508–2509
dipsogenic, 2505
nephrogenic
ADH absence in, 375
assessment of, 379
characteristics of, 612t
neurogenic, 2509–2513
acquired causes of, 2509t, 2510–2516
ADH absence in, 375
congenital, 2509–251o
pregnancy-associated, 375
Diabetes mellitus
acid-base complications in, 2563–2576
pathogenetic mechanisms and related principles in, 2563–2564, 2564f, 2564t
acid-base syndromes in, 2576–2592
acidemia in, 2585
advanced renal failure in, 2572–2573
aldosterone deficiency in, 2585
aldosterone synthesis defect and, 2586–2587
asymptomatic bacteriuria in, 978
casts in, protein composition of, 347t
catecholamines in, 2585
chronic renal failure in, 2585–2586, 2586f
compartmental fluid and electrolyte shift in, 2564–2567, 2566f
congestive heart failure in, 2576
continuous ambulatory peritoneal dialysis in, 3001–3003. *See also* Peritoneal dialysis, continuous ambulatory (CAPD)
contrast media-induced acute renal failure and, 1189–1190
control of, 2177
flow sheet outlining, 2176t–2177t
diarrhea in, 2575
diuretics in, 2588
drug therapy and, 2585
fluid-electrolyte complications in, 2563–2576
pathogenetic mechanisms and related principles in, 2563–2564, 2564f, 2564t
fluid-electrolyte syndromes in, 2576–2592
gastrointestinal disorders in, 2574
gastrointestinal losses in, 2588–2589
gastroparesis diabeticorum in, 2574–2575
hepatic glucogenesis in, 2563
hepatic ketogenesis in, 2570, 2571f
hyperglycemia in, 2563–2564, 2564f, 2585
hyperkalemia in, 2584
due to impaired potassium excretion, 2585
due to maldistribution, 2585
hyperlipidemia in, 2568
hypernatremic disorders in, 2590–2591, 2591f
hypoaldosteronism in, 2586, 2587f
clinical features and management of, 2587–2588
hypokalemia in, 2588
from diminished intake, 2588
due to redistributuion, 2588
hyponatremic disorders in, 2589–2590, 2590f, 2591t
hypophosphatemia in, 2592
hyporeninemia in, 2586
idiopathic edema and, 2496
insulin deficiency in, 2563, 2564t, 2565f, 2585
insulin-dependent
examination of, during high-risk period, 2160, 2161f–2163f, 2161t
renal changes in, 2153, 2155
reversal of, 2159–2160
ketogenesis in
hepatic, 2570
overview of, 2568, 2569t
ketone consumption in, 2570, 2571f
ketone metabolism in, 2568
lactic acidosis and, 2580–2581
long-term, renal changes in, 2161
membrane hypopolarization in, 2572
membranous nephropathy and, 1796
metabolic acidosis and
with elevated anion gap, 2577–2581, 2578f, 2580f
general features of, 2576–2577, 2577f, 2577t
with normal anion gap, 2581–2582
metabolic alkalosis and, 2582–2583
nephrogenic, in cancer, 1170
nephropathy of. *See* Diabetic nephropathy
nephrosclerosis in, pathologic findings in, 1433–1434
nephrotic syndrome in, 2574
non–insulin-dependent, renal changes in, 2153, 2155
obstructive nephropathy in, 2573–2574
osmotic diuresis in, 2567–2568
papillary necrosis and, 1978–1979
potassium disorders in, 2584
primary nephrosclerosis in, 1433
pseudohyperkalemia in, 2584
pseudohyponatremia in, 2568, 2568f
renal disease in, 2153
progression of, 3143–3144
hypertension and, 3143
protein restriction and, 3143–3144
stages of, 2155t
renal function in, measurement of, 2155–2158
renal ketone handling in, 2571–2572
renal transplantation and, 2914f, 2914–2915
renal tubular secretory defect and, 2587
renin-angiotensin-aldosterone system in, deranged, 2573
respiratory acid-base disorders in, 2583–2584, 2584t
respiratory acidosis in, 2583
respiratory alkalosis in, 2583
sodium disorders in, 2589–2591
substrate delivery in, 2568, 2570
tubulointerstitial disease in, 2574
uremic acidosis and, 2581
urinary tract infection in, 900–901, 2572
Diabetic ketoacidosis, 2588
anion gap in, 2577–2578, 2578f
euglycemic, 2579
hyperglucagonemia complicating, 2570
hypophosphatemia in, 2591
treatment of, hypophosphatemia and, 2607
Diabetic ketogenesis, pathogenetic forces in, 2569t
Diabetic nephropathy, 2153–2183
blood pressure in, 2166, 2167t, 2168f
classification of, 2173, 2174t–2175t
diagnosis of, 2153
end-stage renal failure in, 2153, 2154f
treatment of
complications in, 2180–2181, 2181t
results and problems of, 2179
hyperfiltration in, 2165–2166, 2166f
incidence of, 2153
management of
antihypertensive treatment in, 2178f, 2178–2179
continuous subcutaneous insulin infusion in, 2179
establishment of diabetes control and complication follow-up system in, 2176t–2177t, 2178
general comments in, 2173
results of, 2179
mechanisms responsible for, 2163–2166
general concepts in, 2163–2164
mesangial expansion in, 2170–2171, 2171f, 2171t
microalbuminuria in, 2164–2166, 2165t
pancreas transplantation for, role of, 2182
pathogenesis related to, 2165t
pathology of, 2166, 2168t, 2169f–2170f, 2169–2170
patient survival and, 2179–2180, 2180f, 2180t
prognostic factors for, 2181–2182
percutaneous renal biopsy for, 489
in pregnancy, 2304–2305
prognosis of, 2173
proteinuria in, 2153
renal function in, 2154–2158
examination of, 2160, 2161f–2163f
in long-term diabetes, 2160
newly diagnosed patients and, 2158–2159, 2159t
problems regarding patient condition and, 2158, 2159f, 2159t
reversal of renal changes and, 2159–2160, 2160f
stages of, 2173, 2174t–2175t
structural-functional relationships in, 2170–2172, 2171f–2172f, 2171t, 2172t

systemic hypertension in, 2166, 2167t, 2168f
Dialysate(s)
aluminum contamination of, 3157
for chronic hemodialysis, 3037–3038
acetate vs. bicarbonate in, 3038, 3038f
composition of, 3037–3038
calcium in, 3037
glucose in, 3037–3038
magnesium in, 3037
potassium in, 3037
sodium in, 3037
in chronic hemodialysis, overheated, 3053
for hemodialysis, 1387–1388
bicarbonate in, 1388
calcium concentration in, 1388
chloride in, 1388
dextrose in, 1388
magnesium concentration in, 1388
phosphorus concentration in, 1388
potassium concentration in, 1387–1388
sodium concentration in, 1387
improper proportioning of, complications of, 2804
for peritoneal dialysis, 1391–1392, 2992–2993
additives to, 2993
composition of, 2992–2993
acetate in, 2993
calcium in, 2992
dialysate buffers in, 2992–2993
divalent cations in, 2992
glucose in, 2992
lactate in, 2992–2993
magnesium in, 2992
monovalent cations in, 2992
osmolality in, 2993
osmotic agents in, 2992
pH in, 2993
sodium in, 2992
conditioning of, 2993
contaminants of, 2993
toxicity of, peritoneal cavity defense mechanisms and, 2985–2986
Dialysis. *See also* Hemodiafiltration; Hemodialysis; Hemofiltration; Peritoneal dialysis
anemia and, 2746–2748
chronic, hypercalcemia in, 2774
continuous ambulatory peritoneal. *See* Peritoneal dialysis, continuous ambulatory (CAPD)
effect of, on uremic nephropathy, 2808
in end-stage renal disease, 2823
gastrointestinal bleeding due to, 1384
hypersplenism and, 2748
hypertension in, 1425–1427, 1426f
improved clearance in, anemia and, 2752
methods of, 1385t, 1385–1386
pericarditis and, 2825, 2826t
peritoneal. *See* Peritoneal dialysis
relative indications for, 1385–1386
uremic inhibitors and, 2747
Dialysis dementia, 2789, 2799–2803, 3078–3079 *See also* Encephalopathy, uremic
altered cerebrospinal fluid and, 2803
due to aluminum neurotoxicity, 3158–3159
differential diagnosis of, 2802t
elevated aluminum levels in, 2800, 2801f
etiology of, 2799–2800
initial reports of, 2800
neurofibrillary tangles in, 2800
prevention of, 2802
senile plaques in, 2800
slow virus infection and, 2803
subgroups of, 2799t
trace element contamination and, 2803
treatment of, 2802
Dialysis disequilibrium syndrome, 2789, 2798–2799
differential diagnosis of, 2799t
treatment of, 2799
Dialysis encephalopathy-dementia, 3078–3079
due to aluminum neurotoxicity, 3158–3159
Dialysis index model, 3071
Dialysis-related amyloidosis, 2210, 2210t, 2212, 2225–2226. *See also* Amyloidosis
clinical and diagnostic features of, 2214t
clinical manifestations of, 2226
pathogenesis of, 2225
treatment of, 2226
Diarrhea, in diabetes mellitus, 2575
Diazepam
for convulsion in eclampsia, 1527
pharmacology of, normal vs. in renal failure, 3244t–3245t
Diazoxide
for hypertension, 1621–1622, 2296–2297, 2390t
in neonates, 2386
in pregnancy, 1526
pharmacology of, normal vs. in renal failure, 3244t–3245t
Dicarboxylic aminoaciduria, hereditary, characteristics of, 612t
Dicloxacillin, pharmacology of, normal vs. in renal failure, 3244t–3245t
Diet
creatinine clearance effects of, 366
in end-stage renal disease, 2823
in hyperkalemia, 2659
phosphorus absorption and, 2603–2604
serum creatinine effects of, 367
Dietary therapy. *See also specific disorders*
in acute renal failure, 3189–3196
in chronic renal disease, 3139–3147
in chronic renal failure, in children, 2395–2396
in lipid disorders, 2852
in nephrotic syndrome, 3186–3187
in renal transplantation, 3198–3199
DiGeorge syndrome, 2623
Digitalis
action of, magnesium deficiency and, 2634
for heart failure, 2834
intoxication, metabolic alkalosis and, 2583
Digitalis-like factors, endogenous, 2862
Digitoxin, pharmacology of, normal vs. in renal failure, 3244t–3245t
Dihydrocodeine, in renal disease, complications of, 3231–3232
Dihydrotachysterol, for osteitis fibrosa, 2776
1,25-Dihydroxycholecalciferol, for renal osteodystrophy, 2395
1,25-Dihydroxyvitamin D. *See* Calcitriol
1,25-Dihydroxyvitamin D_3
metabolism of, age-related impairment in, clinical implications of, 2422
in phosphorus absorption, 2599
24,25-Dihydroxyvitamin D, for osteomalacia, 2776
25-Dihydroxyvitamin D_3, in phosphorus absorption, 2599
Diltiazem, in end-stage renal disease, 2824
Dilution, urine. *See* Glomerular filtrate; Urine
Dimethyl sulfoxide (DMSO), for amyloidosis, 2224
Diphenhydramine, pharmacology of, normal vs. in renal failure, 3244t–3245t
Diphenylhydantoin
acute interstitial nephritis due to, 1340–1341
vasopressin secretion and, 2545
Diphosphonate(s)
hyperphosphatemia and, 2613
in osteoporosis, 2779
Disequilibrium pH, 2435
Disequilibrium syndrome, dialysis. *See* Dialysis disequilibrium syndrome
Disodium dichloromethylene diphosphonate, for hypercalcemia, 2629, 2630t
Disodium ethrythronate, hyperphosphatemia and, 2613
Disopyramide, pharmacology of, normal vs. in renal failure, 3244t–3245t
Disseminated intravascular coagulation, in malaria, 2344
Diuresis
osmotic, in diabetes mellitus, 2567–2568
postobstructive, 667–670. *See also* Urinary tract obstruction, postobstructive diuresis after
Diuretic(s)
acute interstitial nephritis due to, 1340
acute renal vein thrombosis in nephrotic syndrome due to, 1323
for ascites, 2473–2474
in distal tubule
amiloride and, 2444–2445, 2445f
mechanism of action of, 2444–2446, 2446f
spironolactones and, 2445–2446, 2446f
thiazides and, 2447
triamterene and, 2445
for edematous state, in nephrotic syndrome, 2480
in elderly, 2420–2421
hypercalcemia and, 2627
hyperkalemia and, 2659
for hypertension, in diabetic patient, 2588
idiopathic edema and, 2496–2497, 2497f–2499f, 2499–2500
loop
co-transporter blockers and, 2441f–2442f, 2441–2443
ethacrynic acid and, 2443–2444
mechanism of action of, 2439–2444
in nephrotic patients, 2480
in thick ascending limb, 244of, 2439–2441
mechanism of action of, 2435–2447

Diuretic(s)—Continued
metabolic alkalosis as complication of, 2582
potassium-sparing, 2444
in preeclampsia, 2296
for preeclampsia prevention, 1529
in proximal tubule
carbonic anhydrase inhibitors and, 2435–2437, 2436f
ethacrynic acid and, 2438–2439
mechanism of action of, 2435–2439
sulfamoyl benzoates and, 2437–2438
thiazides and, 2437
in renal disease, 3229
Diverticulitis, posttransplant, 2949
Diverticulum(a)
calyceal
congenital, 650–651
cystic appearance of, 521, 522f
medullary sponge kidney vs., 531
colonic, in autosomal dominant polycystic kidney disease, 554
paraureteral, 642
saccular, of male urethra, 639, 640f
urachal, 641
urinary bladder, 641
Dobutamine, pharmacology of, normal vs. in renal failure, 3244t–3245t
Donor
cadaver
vs. living donor, 2921–2922, 2922t
transplant results of, 2939, 2939f
living-related, transplant results of, 2938–2939
living-unrelated, transplant results of, 2939
Dopamine
pharmacology of, normal vs. in renal failure, 3244t–3245t
receptor types for, 299
in renal hemodynamics, 96–97
renal receptors for, 300
in thirst, 120
Doppler ultrasonography, 413
Down's syndrome, 2801
Doxorubicin
nephrotoxicity of, 1179
pharmacology of, normal vs. in renal failure, 3244t–3245t
phase specificity and mechanism of action of, 821t
Doxycycline, pharmacology of, normal vs. in renal failure, 3244t–3245t
Drug(s). *See also specific drugs*
associated with water retention, 2519t, 2519–2521
causing hyperkalemia, discontinuation of, 2659
causing sodium and water retention, 2494
effect of, on urinary urate excretion, 2240
immunosuppressive. *See* Immunosuppression
to lower lipid levels, 2852
nephrotoxicity of, in AIDS patients, 2363–2364
prolonged use of, diabetes insipidus and, 2511–2512
Drug abuse, 1219–1233. *See also* Heroin abuse
amyloidosis and, 2220
end-stage renal disease and, 3121–3133
intravenous, HIV-associated nephropathy and, 2366–2367
nontraumatic rhabdomyolysis in, acute renal failure due to, 1230–1231
renal disease associated with, 1219, 1220t
Drug therapy, 3211–3232
in continuous ambulatory peritoneal dialysis, 3228
with decreased renal function, 3216–3221
pharmacodynamics in, 3221, 3222f
pharmacokinetics in, 3216–3221
absorption and bioavailability in, 3216–3217
biotransformation and metabolism in, 3218–3220, 3220t–3221t
elimination in, 3218–3221
protein binding in, 3217t, 3217–3218
renal excretion in, 3220–3221
volume of distribution in, 3218, 3219t
in dialysis
pharmacokinetic factors in, 3227–3228
quantitation of drug removal in, 3226–3228
in high-flux hemodialysis, 3228
with normal renal function, 3211–3216
pharmacodynamics in, 3216, 3217f
pharmacokinetics in, 3211–3216
absorption and bioavailability in, 3212
biotransformation and metabolism in, 3213–3214
distribution in, 3212–3213
drug disposition in, 3211, 3212f
elimination in, 3213–3216
parameters of elimination in, 3215–3216
plasma and tissue protein binding in, 3213
renal excretion in, 3214f, 3214–3215, 3215t
in renal failure
analgesic drugs as, 3229
anticonvulsant agents as, 3230
cardiovascular agents as, 3229
diuretic drugs as, 3229
dosage regimen alterations in, 3221–3228
altering dose and interval as, 3225, 3225f
creatinine clearance and, 3221–3222
decreasing dose as, 3223–3225, 3224f–3225f
general approach to, 3223–3226, 3224f–3225f
general equation method for dose adjustment in, 3226
pharmacokinetics and pharmacodynamics in, 3222
plasma concentrations and, 3222–3223, 3223f
varying dosage interval as, 3223, 3224f
drug–disease complication interactions in, 3231–3232
CNS, 3231–3232
uremic bleeding as, 3232
drug-drug interactions in, 3230–3231
antacids and, 3230
cyclosporine and, 3230–3231
phenobarbitol-vitamin D, 3230
prednisolone, 3231
immunosuppressive drugs as, 3230
psychotherapeutic drugs as, 3230
sedative-hypnotic drugs as, 3230
for urinary tract infection, 3228
for vascular access infection, 3228
for viral infection, 3228–3229
Dry weight, definition of, 2823
DTPA scan, of transplanted kidney, 2931, 2931f
Dysgenesis, renal, classification of, 652–653
Dyslipoproteinemia, in uremia
atherogenic, 2851
clinical management of, 2851–2852
pathogenesis of, factors in, 2850–2851
pathomechanisms of, 2850–2851
treatment modality in, influence of, 2851
Dysplasia, renal
in children, 2387
classification of, 652–653
definition of, 652
pathogenesis of, 652
ureteral orifice position and, 651f, 651–652
Dyspnea, in heart failure, 2832
Dysproteinemia(s), 2189–2226. *See also specific types*
clinical manifestations of, 2189
human, 2190t
Dysuria, acute. *See also* Cystitis; Urethritis; Urinary tract infection
management of, 1016–1017, 1018f

EABV. *See* Effective arterial blood volume (EABV)
Echocardiography
in heart failure, 2833
in pericardial effusion, 2825
Eclampsia, 1509. *See also* Preeclampsia; Pregnancy, hypertension in
cerebral hemorrhage in, 1517, 1518t
clinical findings in, 1517–1518
coagulation, fibrinolysis, and platelet disorders in, 2291–2292
convulsion in, 1517–1518
prevention and treatment of, 1526–1527
diazepam for, 1527
magnesium sulfate for, 1526–1527
phenytoin for, 1527
definition of, 2293
postpartum, late, 1511, 1517
remote prognosis in, 1530–1531
severe, acute renal failure in, 2301
survival following, 2297, 2297f
Edema
formation of, capillary mechanisms in, 2453–2454, 2454t
idiopathic, 2493–2501
clinical features of, 2493
diagnosis of, 2493–2494
etiology of, 2494–2500
management of, 2500t, 2500–2501
of legs, vs. idiopathic, 2494
in liver disease, 2465–2472
nephritic (overflow), 2453
nephrotic (underflow), 2453
in nephrotic syndrome, 1754f, 1754–1756
pitting, 2493
pulmonary
in malignant hypertension, 1600–1603, 1601f–1602f

in renovascular hypertension, 1458
in severe benign hypertension, 1600–1603, 1601f–1602f
EDRF-nitric oxide system, interactions of, with intrarenal neurohumoral systems, 93, 93f
EDTA (ethylenediaminetetraacetate), for hypercalcemia, 2629, 2630t
Effective arterial blood volume (EABV), 2454
diminished, in nephrotic syndrome, 2476
influence of, in renal sodium excretion, 2455
Effective filtration pressure, calculation of, 74, 76
Effective renal plasma flow (ERPF), radionuclide studies for, 419–420
Efferent arteriole(s)
anatomic distribution of, 33, 34f
contractile processes in, structural-functional aspects of, 67f, 67–68
hormonal effects on, 288f, 288–289
resistance model of
affecting GFR, 80–81, 81f
affecting peritubular capillary hydrostatic pressure, 82
Effusion, pericardial, 2825, 2826
Eicosanoid(s), 305–306
renal actions of, 307t
in renal function, 2715
renal synthesis of, 305f, 305–306
synthetic pathways of, 90, 90f
Elderly. *See also* Aging
acid-base balance in, 2417–2418, 2418f
acute pyelonephritis in, 988
acute renal failure in, 1292
ammonium excretion in, 2418–2419, 2419f
autosomal dominant polycystic kidney disease in, 556
bacteriuria in, 978
calcium balance in, 2418
creatinine clearance in, 2407–2408, 2408t, 2409f
cystitis in, 1011
1,25-dihydroxyvitamin D_3 metabolism in, 2422
electrolyte balance in, 2412
fluid balance in, 2412
glomerular filtration rate in, 2407–2409, 2408f–2413f, 2409t
clinical implications of, 2420, 2421f
glomerulonephritis in, 2423, 2423t
glomerulosclerosis in, 2423, 2423t
hyperkalemia in, 2422
hypertension in, 2422–2423
hyporeninemic hypoaldosteronism in, 2421
minimal change disease in, 2423, 2423t
nephrotic syndrome in, 2423t, 2423–2424
potassium balance in, 2418–2420
primary nephrosclerosis in, 1435
renal acidification in, 2421–2422
renal blood flow in, 2405, 2407f, 2420, 2421f
renal concentrating ability in, 2416, 2417, 2420
renal diluting ability in, 2417, 2420–2421
renal failure in
acute, 2424–2425, 2426f
chronic, 2425–2426
renal phosphate transport in, 2422
renin-angiotensin-aldosterone activity in, 2422
renovascular hypertension in, treatment in, 1463
sodium conserving ability in, 2412, 2414f–2425f, 2420
sodium excreting ability in, 2412, 2414, 2415f–2416f
systemic lupus erythematosus in, 2028–2029
urethritis in, 1011
urinary tract infections in, 901, 2426
vascular disorders in, 2422–2423
Electroencephalogram, in acute renal failure, 2790, 2791f
Electrolyte(s)
depletion of, in acute renal failure, 2332, 2333t
disorders of
in AIDS patients, 2365
in diabetes insipidus, 2510–2511
in diabetes mellitus, 2563–2592
in falciparum malaria, 2339
in malignant hypertension, 1570
in multiple myeloma, 2201
in nephrotic syndrome, 1756–1757
posttransplant, 2951–2952
excretion of, prolactin and, 2556–2557
plasma and urine, in children, 2382
Electrolyte balance
aging and, 2412
compartmental fluid shifts in, 2564–2567, 2566f
Electron microscopy evaluation, 499–500, 500f–502f
ELISA (enzyme-linked immunosorbent assay), HIV testing with, 2361
Elschnig's spots, in hypertensive choroidopathy, 1566, 1566f
Embolism
air, in chronic hemodialysis, 3053–3054
cholesterol, in elderly, 2422
renal artery
in acute renal failure, 1295
cholesterol
in malignant hypertension, 1560
in renovascular hypertension, 1456–1457
Embolization, percutaneous transcatheter renal, technique and indications for, 470f–471f, 471–472
Embryonal carcinoma, testicular
classification and pathogenesis of, 853–855, 854f, 854t
natural history of, 855
Emphysematous pyelonephritis, in perinephric abscess, 967–968
Enalapril, pharmacology of, normal vs. in renal failure, 3244t–3245t
Encainide, pharmacology of, normal vs. in renal failure, 3244t–3245t
Encephalopathy
dialysis. *See* Dialysis dementia
hypertensive, 1555, 1594–1600
clinical presentation in, 1595
etiologies of, 1595t, 1595–1596
hypertensive neuroretinopathy in, 1595
pathogenesis of, 1597–1599, 1598f–1599f
breakthrough theory in, 1597–1598, 1598f
overregulation theory in, 1597, 1598f
structural theory in, 1599, 1599f
pathologic findings in, 1596f–1597f, 1596–1597
treatment of, 1599–1600
uremic, 2789–2804. *See also* Dialysis dementia
acute renal failure and, 2790, 2791f
biochemical brain changes in, 2792f–2793f, 2792–2794
chronic renal failure and, 2790–2791
diagnosis of, 2789
differential diagnosis of, 2789–2790
drug interactions in, 3231
parathyroid hormone in, 2798, 2798f
pathology of, 2798
pathophysiology of, 2798
physiology of neurotransmission in, 2794–2798, 2796f–2797f
psychologic testing in, 2791–2792
synaptosomes in, 2794
treatment of
acute hypernatremia and, 2804
acute hyponatremia and, 2804
cerebrovascular accidents and, 2803–2804
coma with hyperglycemia and, 2803
dialysis dementia and, 2799t, 2799–2803, 2801f, 2802t
dialysis disequilibrium syndrome and, 2798–2799, 2799t
neurologic complications in, 2798–2804
subdural hematoma and, 2803
Encephalopathy-dementia, dialysis. *See* Dialysis dementia
Endocarditis, bacterial, 2831
glomerulonephritis with, 1681–1685
antibiotic therapy in, 1682
focal and diffuse, 1681–1682
due to heroin abuse, 1229–1230
incidence of, 1681
laboratory findings in, 1682
pathologic changes in, 1682–1685, 1683f–1684f
renal findings in, 1681, 1682t
treatment of, 2833
Endocrine disorder(s), in uremia, 2855–2863
Endophthalmitis, candidiasis, 940
Endothelial cell adhesion molecule, 2004
Endothelial-leukocyte adhesion molecule, 2004
Endothelin, 312–313
in chronic renal failure, 2715
in fluid balance, 313
in malignant hypertension, 1583
in microvascular thrombosis, 2069
receptors for, 312
in renal hemodynamics, 94, 312–313
subtypes of, 312
in uremia, 2863
in vascular inflammatory injury, 1999–2000
Endothelin proteinuria, 389
Endotheliotropic hemolytic nephroangiopathy, 2074. *See also* Hemolytic-uremic syndrome
Endothelium
in experimental studies on ischemic renal injury, 1270–1273
vascular, in end-stage renal disease, 2823

Endothelium-derived contracting factor, 72
Endothelium-derived relaxing factor, 72, 313, 2823
in chronic renal failure, 2715
major renal actions of, 313
in malignant hypertension, 1583
in microvascular thrombosis, 2068
in vascular inflammatory injury, 2000
Endothelium-derived vasoactive factor, in renal hemodynamics, 93–94
Endotoxemia
in chronic hemodialysis, 3053
hepatorenal disease due to, 1359–1360
malaria and, 2343
Endotoxin, bacterial, in vascular inflammatory injury, 1996
End-stage renal disease
in Alport syndrome, 571, 573f
in analgesic-induced renal disease, 1118
in autosomal dominant polycystic kidney disease, 556t, 556–557
in benign hypertension, 1593–1594
cardiovascular complications of, 2817–2833
causes of
in adults, 2390t
in children, 2390t
in diabetic nephropathy, 2153
dialysis in, neurologic disorders and, 2789
epidemiology of, 2394, 2394t
ethical considerations in, 3097–3124
allocation of resources as, 3098–3101
demographics in, 3102–3108
patient selection and, 3103, 3106–3108, 3107f
statistics on, 3102–3103, 3103t–3106t
genetics and, 3122–3123
health care costs and, 3097
HIV infection as. *See also* Human immunodeficiency virus (HIV) infection
initiation and withdrawal of dialysis and, 3109–3111
issues in, 3097–3098
kidney transplantation and, 3111–3115, 3112f
age criteria and, 3112
case study on, 3113–3115
foreign nationals and, 3112
living unrelated donors and, 3112–3115
religious views and, 3115
shortage of donor kidneys and, 3111–3112
legal issues in, 3115–3119
advance health care directives as, 3118–3119
background in, 3115–3116
dialysis for noncompliant patients as, 3117–3118
HIV infection as, 3119–3121
termination of dialysis as, 3116–3117
principles and models for, 3108–3109, 3109t
starting and stopping treatment as, 3101–3102
substance abuse as, 3121–3122
world heath resources and, 3099f, 3099–3101, 3100t–3101t
heart failure and cardiomyopathy in, 2829–2834
causes of, 2830t
clinical features and laboratory findings and, 2832–2833
management of, 2833–2834
morphologic and functional abnormalities and, 2831–2832
HIV infection and, 2371–2373
hypertension in, 2817–2824. *See also* Hypertension, in end-stage renal disease
in hypertensive nephrosclerosis, 1441, 1441t, 1593–1594
kidney transplantation for, 2179
patient survival following, 2179–2180, 2180f, 2180t
prognostic factors in, 2181–2182
success and complications of, 2180–2181, 2181t
in lupus nephritis, 2030
in malignant hypertension, 1568
pancreas transplantation for, 2182
pericarditis in, 2824–2829
clinical features and laboratory findings in, 2825–2827, 2826t
incidence of, 2824–2825
management of, 2827–2829, 2828f
pathogenesis of, 2825
in polyarteritis, 2108
prevalence and treatment modalities in, 2911, 2912t
renal transplantation for. *See* Transplantation, renal
Energy expenditure, during illness, 3194, 3194t
Energy intake
in dietary therapy in acute renal failure, 3194t, 3194–3195
in dietary therapy in chronic hemodialysis, 3178–3179
in dietary therapy in continuous ambulatory peritoneal dialysis, 3178–3179
in dietary therapy in renal transplantation, 3199
Enteral alimentation, for acute or chronic renal failure, 3196–3198
Enteral hyperalimentation, for urinary bladder carcinoma, 825–826
Enterococcus fecalis, in upper urinary tract infection, 974
Enuresis, nocturnal, in vesicoureteral reflux, 717
Enzyme-linked immunosorbent assay (ELISA), HIV testing with, 2361
Enzymuria
in aminoglycoside nephrotoxicity, 1131
in contrast media-induced acute renal failure, 1194
Eosinophilia, peritoneal, 3004–3005
Epidermal growth factor, major renal actions of, 301–302
Epididymitis, 755–756
acute
nonsexually transmitted, 755
sexually transmitted, 756
chronic, 756
clinical manifestations of, 755
pathogenesis of, 755
Epinephrine
biosynthesis of, 1488, 1488f
metabolism of, 1488–1489, 1489f
receptor types for, 299
Epithelial foot process(es), 7–8, 11f–12f, 381
cell contents in, 7
cell membrane of, 7
filtration-slit membrane of, 7, 11f–12f, 381
functions of, 8
fusion effacement of, proteinuria and, 386
pedicels of, 7, 11f
podocalyxin in, 7–8, 382
in protein handling, 384
Epodyl, phase specificity and mechanism of action of, 821t
Epoetin therapy
administration of, 2749
diastolic blood pressure and, 2752
inflammation and, 2751f, 2751–2752
iron availability and, 2750f, 2750–2751
pharmacokinetics of, 2750f, 27492750
response to, 2748f–2749f, 2748–2749
Epstein-Barr virus (EBV), as complication of transplantation, 2944
Erythrocyte(s)
casts of, 349, 351f–352f
parasitized, in malaria, 2344, 2344f
sickling of, 2311, 2312f, 2317
survival of
in anemia, 2752
factors decreasing, 2747–2748
urinalysis for, 335–336, 336t
urine microscopy for, 341–343, 342f–346f
in acid urine, 341, 345f
due to exercise, 343
due to glomerular bleeding, 341, 342f–344f
due to nonglomerular bleeding, 341, 344f–345f
Erythrocytosis
definition of, 2753
vs. polycythemia vera, 2753
in renal cell carcinoma, 786
Erythromycin
acute interstitial nephritis due to, 1337
pharmacology of, normal vs. in renal failure, 3244t–3245t
Erythrophagocytosis, urine microscopy for, 343, 346f
Erythropoiesis, 2743
factors decreasing, 2746–2747
Erythropoietic stimulating factor, 2743
Erythropoietin, 316–317, 2743
deficiency of, 2746
prostaglandins and, 309
recombinant human
for anemia, in children, 2397
in multiple myeloma, 2206
renal production of, 316–317
serum, in autosomal dominant polycystic kidney disease, 549
in sickle cell disease, 2321
in uremia, 2860
Escherichia coli. *See also* Urinary tract infection
adherence properties of, 886t, 886–887
in cystitis, 1008f, 1008–1009
epithelial cell receptors of, 888–889
fimbriae of, 886t, 886–887
mannose-resistant, 888, 888t
mannose-sensitive, 888, 888t
Tamm-Horsfall protein and, 890, 891f
X-type, 888
in upper urinary tract infection, 974
in urethritis, 1008f, 1008–1009
in urinary tract infection, 886t, 886–887

uropathogenic, virulence factors of, 1009
Escherichia coli 0157:H7, microvascular thrombosis due to, 2063
Esophageal leiomyomatosis, in Alport syndrome, 581
Esophagitis, posttransplant, 2948
Estrogen(s)
for advanced prostatic carcinoma, 844, 844t
idiopathic edema and, 2495–2496
Ethacrynic acid, mechanism of action of, 2438–2439, 2443–2444
Ethambutol
acute interstitial nephritis due to, 1337
pharmacology of, normal vs. in renal failure, 3244t–3245t
for urinary tract tuberculosis, 923t
Ethchlorvynol, pharmacology of, normal vs. in renal failure, 3244t–3245t
Ethionamide, for urinary tract tuberculosis, 923t
Ethosuximide, pharmacology of, normal vs. in renal failure, 3246t–3247t
Ethylenediaminetetraacetate (EDTA), for hypercalcemia, 2629, 2630t
Etoposide, pharmacology of, normal vs. in renal failure, 3246t–3247t
Euglycemia, diabetic ketoacidosis and, 2579
Excretory duct, common, embryonic development of, 642
Exercise
anemia and, 2752
hematuria due to, urine microscopy for, 343
to lower lipid levels, 2852
Exercise renography, in screening for renovascular hypertension, 1461–1462
Extracellular fluid
acid-base balance in, 208–209
osmolality of, 373, 374f
reduced, thirst and, 120
Extraglomerular mesangium, 29–30
Eye(s)
in Alport syndrome, 577–578, 580f, 580–581
in Fabry's disease, 595
in nail-patella syndrome, 603

Fabry's disease, 593–603
carrier identification in, 602
clinical manifestations and course in, 594–595
biochemical findings in, 595
cardiac findings in, 595
crisis in, 594
gastrointestinal findings in, 595
ocular findings in, 595
pain, 594
renal concentration defect in, 596
renal findings in, 595–596
renal size in, 596
skin eruptions in, 594
urinalysis in, 595, 596f
definition of, 593
diagnosis of, 602
frequency of, 593
in heterozygotes, 598–602
metabolic defect in, 593
molecular genetics of, 593–594
pathologic findings in, 596–597, 597f–601f
pathophysiology of, 597–598
renal transplantation and, 2916
renal transplantation in, 602–603
treatment of, 602–603
Failure to thrive syndrome, in AIDS patients, 2370
Fairley washout test, for upper urinary tract infection, 984
Falciparum malaria, 2339–2345. *See also* Malaria, falciparum
Famotidine, pharmacology of, normal vs. in renal failure, 3246t–3247t
Fanconi syndrome, 621–622
acute lead nephropathy and, 1239
amyloidosis and, 2221
characteristics of, 612t
clinical findings in, 622
etiology of, 621, 621t
multiple myeloma and, 2200
pathogenesis of, 621–622
protein aggregates causing, 2194
in Sjögren's syndrome, 2056
therapy in, 622
Waldenström's macroglobulinemia and, 2207
Fasting, idiopathic edema and, 2500, 2501
Fatty acid metabolism, 251f–252f, 251–253
compartmentation in, 251f–252f, 251–252
distribution in, 252
sodium transport in, 252–253
Fatty liver, acute, in pregnancy, 2301
Fechtner syndrome, 581
Femoral vein catheterization, in chronic hemodialysis, 3033
Fenoprofen, acute interstitial nephritis due to, 1338
Ferritin, and renal handling of, 381t
Fetal lobation, intravenous urography for, 409
Fetus
effect of antihypertensive therapy on, 1522
obstructive uropathy in, in utero diagnosis of, 2388
in preeclampsia, 1520
renal ultrasonography of, for vesicoureteral reflux, 717
Fever, in acute renal failure, 1381, 1382f
Fiber, in dietary therapy in chronic hemodialysis, 3186
Fibrinogen, plasma, in acute renal vein thrombosis, in nephrotic syndrome, 1321
Fibrinolysis, in preeclampsia, 2291–2292
Fibrinolytic system, in acute renal vein thrombosis, in nephrotic syndrome, 1321
Fibroblast(s), interstitial, cellular structure of, 35–36, 36f
Fibromuscular dysplasia, renal artery
angiography for, 472, 472f
percutaneous transluminal angioplasty for, 469
in renovascular hypertension, 1456, 1456f
Fibrosarcoma, renal, 798
Filtration-slit membrane
of Bowman's capsule, 7, 11f–12f, 381
in protein handling, 384
Fine-needle aspiration biopsy
of kidney, technique in, 487
of transplanted kidney, 2933, 2933f
Fingernail(s), in nail-patella syndrome, 603, 604f
Fistula, congenital, 637
FK-506, in immunosuppression, 2899
Flecainide, pharmacology of, normal vs. in renal failure, 3246t–3247t
Fluconazole
for candidiasis, 942–943
pharmacology of, normal vs. in renal failure, 3246t–3247t
Flucytosine
for candidiasis, 942
pharmacology of, normal vs. in renal failure, 3246t–3247t
Fludrocortisone acetate, for hypoaldosteronism, 2588
Fluid(s)
aging and, 2412
conservation of, renal mechanisms of, 373–375
depletion of, in acute renal failure, 2332, 2333t
disturbances of, in falciparum malaria, 2339
excretion of
in edema-forming disorders, 2453
in myxedema, 2540f–2541f, 2540t, 2541–2543, 2543f
prolactin and, 2556–2557
prostaglandin effects on, 1207
renal, 2727–2728
renal mechanisms of, 373–375
extracellular
acid-base balance in, 208–209
hyperconcentrated, 2564
osmolality of, 373, 374f
volume expansion of, hypophosphatemia and, 2605
homeostasis of, in chronic renal failure, 2727–2728
retention of
in congestive heart failure, 2461f
afferent and efferent pathways and, 2463, 2464f
mechanisms for, 2461–2463
treatment of, 2463–2465
drugs associated with, 2519t, 2519–2521
drugs causing, 2494
idiopathic edema and, 2494
in liver disease, 2465–2468, 2466f–2467f
in nephrotic syndrome, 2479
treatment of, 2479–2481
orthostatic, 2495
Fluid and electrolyte(s)
disorders of, complicating diabetes mellitus, 2563–2592
in nephrotic syndrome, 1756–1757
Fluid balance
compartmental shift in, 2564–2567, 2566f
endothelin in, 313
kallikrein-kinin system in, 311
NSAID nephrotoxicity and, 1213
prostaglandins in, 308–309
Fluid deprivation test, for assessment of renal concentrating capacity, 379
Fluid intake
in dietary therapy in acute renal failure, 3193
in dietary therapy in chronic hemodialysis, 3180–3181
Fluid loading, renal hemodynamics in, 102

Fluid overload, in acute renal failure, treatment of, 1376
Fluid space, intracellular, in sodium homeostasis, 2721–2723, 2722f
Fluid transport
  angiotensin II effects on, 305
  antidiuretic hormone effects on, 48–51
   apical membranes and cytosolic vesicles and, 49–50
   collecting ducts and, 48–49
   morphologic effects on nephron and, 50–51
  structure-function relationships in, 48–51
Fluid volume
  extracellular
   reduced, thirst and, 120
   in sodium homeostasis, 2720–2721, 2721f
  homeostasis of, in preeclampsia, 1514
  during pregnancy, alteration of, 2287, 2288f
Fluoroquinolone, for cystitis and urethritis, 1015–1016
5-Fluorouracil
  nephrotoxicity of, 1177
  pharmacology of, normal vs. in renal failure, 3246t–3247t
  phase specificity and mechanism of action of, 821t
Flurazepam, pharmacology of, normal vs. in renal failure, 3246t–3247t
Flushing solutions, in renal preservation, composition of, 2923t
Focal and segmental glomerulosclerosis (FSGF). *See* Glomerulosclerosis, focal segmental
Folate, deficiency of, erythropoiesis and, 2747
Folic acid, for anemia, 2752
Follicle-stimulating hormone, in idiopathic edema, 2495
Foot process(es), epithelial. *See* Epithelial foot process(es)
Foscarnet, nephrotoxicity of, 2364
Fractional excretion of phosphate ($FEPO_4$), in children, 2380
Fracture(s), bone pain and, 2774
Free radical(s)
  aminoglycoside nephrotoxicity due to, 1151
  definition of, 1036
  nephrotoxicity due to, 1036–1041. *See also* Nephrotoxicity
  oxygen, in experimental studies on ischemic renal injury, 1267–1270, 1269f, 1271f
Friction rub, in pericarditis, 2826
Fungal infection
  as complication of transplantation, 2946, 2946f
  renal, 929–947. *See also* Candidiasis
   CT for, 451–452
  urinary tract, 929–947
Fungal peritonitis, due to continuous peritoneal dialysis, 3009, 3011
Furosemide
  acute interstitial nephritis due to, 1340
  for cirrhotic ascites, 2474
  for distal nephron acidification defects, 2679
  for hypercalcemia, 2629, 2630t
  for hypertension, 2390t
  for hyponatremia, 2527
  for idiopathic edema, 2497
  mechanism of action of, 2441–2443, 2442f
  for nephrotic syndrome, 2480
  pharmacology of, normal vs. in renal failure, 3246t–3247t
  in protection against nephrotoxicity, 1067

G protein(s), in hormonal action, 284
G protein-coupled receptor(s), 70
Gamma globulin, 381t
  renal handling of, 384
Ganciclovir
  for cytomegalovirus, 2364, 2944t
  pharmacology of, normal vs. in renal failure, 3246t–3247t
  in renal disease, 3228
Gap junctions, in central nervous system, 2794
Gastric cancer, nephrotic syndrome in, 2265
Gastrin, in uremia, 2862
Gastrointestinal hormone(s), in uremia, 2862
Gastrointestinal tract
  calcium absorption from, 2618–2619
  cancer of, nephrotic syndrome in, 2265
  complications of, posttransplant, 2948–2949
  decreased magnesium absorption by, hypomagnesemia secondary to, 2634
  disorders of, in diabetes mellitus, 2574–2575
  evaluation of, pretransplant, 2919
  in hypercalcemia, 2625
  hypophosphatemia and, 2609–2610
  increased calcium absorption from, hypercalcemia and, 2627–2628
  phosphorus absorption by, 2599, 2600f
  potassium losses from, 2588–2589
  reduced calcium absorption by, hypocalcemia secondary to, 2623–2624
Gastroparesis diabeticorum, 2574–2575
Genital herpes simplex infection, cystitis and urethritis vs., 1011
Genital leiomyomatosis, in Alport syndrome, 581
Genitourinary candidiasis, clinical manifestations of, 934
Gentamicin
  acute interstitial nephritis due to, 1337
  chemical structure of, 1135f
  cystic fluid concentration of, in autosomal dominant polycystic kidney disease, 551t
  mitochondrial effects of, 1046
  nephrotoxicity of, 1043. *See also* Aminoglycoside nephrotoxicity
   calcium homeostasis and, 1055
   lysosomal damage and, 1062, 1063f
   membrane phospholipid effects of, 1056–1057
  pharmacology of, normal vs. in renal failure, 3246t–3247t
Gentofte-Montecatini Convention definition, of microalbuminuria, 2164, 2165t
GFR. *See* Glomerular filtration rate (GFR)
Glafenin, acute interstitial nephritis due to, 1339
Glomerular barrier permselectivity
  in animal models, 2716–2717, 2717f
  in human disease, 2718
Glomerular basement membrane. *See also* Antiglomerular basement membrane antibody–mediated nephritis
  anatomy of, 6, 8f, 10f–11f, 381
  biochemical constituents of, 12
  cellular structure of, 10f, 10–12
  collagen types in, 12
  in diabetic nephropathy, 2163
  as filtration barrier, 14–15, 381
  in focal glomerulosclerosis due to heroin abuse, 1221
  lamina of, 12, 381
  leaky, proteinuria due to, 387
Glomerular capillary(ies)
  anatomic distribution of, 32–33
  contractile processes in, structural-functional aspects of, 67t, 68
  electron microscopy evaluation of, 499, 500f–501f
  endotheliosis of, in preeclampsia, 1516
  leaky, proteinuria due to, 386
  light microscopy evaluation of, 495, 496f
  ultrafiltration in, 74–77, 75f–76f, 381–384
   Bowman's space pressure and, 75–76
   colloid osmotic pressure and, 74–75, 75f
   filtration disequilibrium in, 76, 76f
   filtration equilibrium in, 76, 76f
   hemodynamic effects on, 383
   macromolecular permeability in, 77f, 77–78, 381–383
    electrical charge and, 77, 382–383
    molecular configuration and, 77–78, 381t, 381–382, 382f
    quantitation of, 77–78
    sieving coefficient in, 77, 77f
   physical forces affecting, 74–77, 75f–76f
   Starling filtration-reabsorption principle in, 74
Glomerular capillary wall
  components of, 361
  thickening of, clinicopathologic correlations of, 504
Glomerular cystic disease, 558–559
Glomerular disease. *See also specific disorders*
  geographic distribution of, 2334–2335, 2335t, 2336f, 2337t, 2337–2338
  long-term outcome in, 1895–1945
   statistical complications of, 1895–1898
    actuarial life tables and, 1896–1898, 1897t
    Cox's method of proportional hazards and, 1898
    defining disease and, 1895
    patient follow-up and outcome in, 1895–1896, 1896f
    patient selection and, 1895, 1896f
    plasma creatinine levels and, 1898
    renal biopsy and, 1895
  minimal change. *See* Nephrotic syndrome, minimal change
  due to NSAID nephrotoxicity, 1211–1212, 1212t
Glomerular fibrils
  Congo red-negative, in amyloidosis, 2219
  morphologic characteristics of, 2218t

Glomerular filtrate. *See also* Urine
calcium in, 2620–2621
dilution or concentration of, 374–375
ADH in, 374–375
in ascending limb of loop of Henle, 374
in descending limb of loop of Henle, 374
in distal tubule, 374
in proximal tubule, 374
osmolality of, 126f–127f, 126–127
Glomerular filtration
normal, 361
of peptide hormones, 318f, 318–319
Glomerular filtration barrier, 14–15
basement membrane in, 14–15, 381
blood flow and, 15
heteroporous membrane theory of, 382
in molecular transport, 380–381
morphology of, 15
size- and charge-dependency of, 361
structure of, 380–381
Glomerular filtration coefficient (K_f)
angiotensin antagonist effects on, 90
formula for, 74
hemodynamic effects on, 81
vasoconstrictor and vasodilator effects on, 81–82
Glomerular filtration rate (GFR)
age-related decline in, 2407–2409, 2408f–2413f, 2409t, 2412
clinical implications of, 2420, 2421f
in aminoglycoside nephrotoxicity, 1131–1132
in analgesic-induced renal disease, 1112
angiotensin II effects on, 88, 89f
assessment of, 3131
atrial natriuretic peptide effects on, 295–296
autoregulation of, 361–363
Bowman's space pressure in, 363
intrinsic glomerular myogenic system in, 362
prerenal acute renal failure and, 1287–1288, 1289f
renal artery pressure and, 361–362, 362f
renin-angiotensin system in, 363
tubuloglomerular feedback mechanism in, 362–363
blood urea nitrogen for, 369–371. *See also* Blood urea nitrogen (BUN)
changes in, during pregnancy, 2288, 2288f
in children, 2379–2380, 2384t
in chronic renal failure, 2707–2708, 2709
reduction of, 2704
solute elimination and, 2704f, 2704–2705
in cirrhosis, 2469
creatinine clearance for, 365–367. *See also* Creatinine clearance
in diabetes mellitus, 2154f, 2155, 2158–2160, 2162f
in edema formation, in nephrotic syndrome, 1756
estimation of, formulas for, 2407, 2409t
fall in, gout and, 2252
formula for, 74
in hepatorenal disease, 1356
in hypercalcemia, 2624–2625
in hypertrophy, 2708
in infants, 2384t
in lithium-induced renal disease, 1101
measurement of, 364–365
clearance in, 364
inulin clearance in, 364
in neonates, 2383, 2384t
newer techniques for, 371–372
^{51}Cr-EDTA as, 372
external counting over kidneys and bladder as, 372
^{125}I-iothalamate as, 372
modified infusion technique as, 372
radiolabeled isotopes as, 372
single (bolus) IV technique as, 372
Tc-DTPA as, 372
normal values for, 364–365, 365f
in obstructive nephropathy, 675
oral protein feeding effects on, 365, 365f
physiologic alterations in, 364–365
prostaglandins and, 308
quantitative analysis of, 79–82, 80f–81f
afferent and efferent arteriolar resistance model in, 80–81, 81f
single capillary model for, 70f, 79–80
filtration coefficient in, 79, 80f
glomerular plasma flow in, 80, 80f
plasma protein concentration in, 79, 80f
transcapillary hydrostatic pressure in, 79, 80f
radionuclide studies for, 372, 419
regulation of, 361–364
glomerular membrane properties in, 363–364
hydrostatic and oncotic pressures in, 361, 362f
major factors in, 361
oncotic pressure in, 363
renal plasma flow in, 363
renal blood flow and, 65, 66t
in renal disease, models of, 2717–2718
serum creatinine for, 367–369, 368f–369f. *See also* Creatinine, serum
single nephron, 2716–2718
sodium retention and, 2457
in urinary tract obstruction, 661, 662–667. *See also* Urinary tract obstruction
Glomerular lesions
malaria and, pathogenesis of, 2342
schistosomal antigens in, 2348
Glomerular macrophage, propagation of, schema for, 2409, 2411f
Glomerular membrane, in regulation of GFR, 363–364
Glomerular myogenic system, intrinsic, in autoregulation of GFR, 362
Glomerular proteinuria, 335, 385
protein selectivity in, 392
Glomerular stalk, anatomy of, 6
Glomerular tuft. *See under* Glomerulus
Glomerulonephritis. *See also* Nephritis
acute
age-related, 2423
MRI for, 459, 459f
in pregnancy, 2303
acute poststreptococcal, 1715–1726
acute nephritic syndrome in, 1720–1722
differential diagnosis of, 1722, 1722t
pathophysiology of, 1720–1722, 1721f
clinical manifestations of, 1718–1720, 1719t
nephritis in, 1718f, 1718–1719, 1719t
serologic findings in, 1719–1720, 1720t
streptococcal infection in, 1718
epidemiology of, 1715
etiopathogenesis of, 1715–1718
autoimmune reactivity in, 1716–1717
genetic aspects of, 1718
humoral and cellular immune mechanisms in, 1717–1718
streptococcal antigens in, 1716
historical, 1715
pathologic findings in, 1722, 1723f, 1724, 1724t
prognosis in, 1724–1725, 1725t
terminology in, 1715
treatment of, 1725–1726
for acute nephritic syndrome, 1725–1726
for streptococcal infection, 1725
in allografts, 2934–2935, 2937, 2937t
animal models of, chemically induced, 1652
in cancer, 1167
casts in, protein composition of, 347t
in children, 2391–2393, 2392t
chronic
angiography for, 478
malignant hypertension in, 1560
pathologic findings in, 1576
in pregnancy, 2303
crescentic
age-related, 2423
definition of, 2099
Hodgkin's disease and, 2267
idiopathic, 1689
urinary findings in, 354, 355f
endocapillary exudative, prognosis in, 1924–1929
adult disease and, 1927–1928, 1928t
childhood disease and, 1925–1926, 1927, 1928t
epidemic cases and, 1926
problems with definition in, 1924–1925, 1925f
sporadic cases and, 1926–1929
endocarditis-associated, 1681–1685. *See also* Endocarditis, bacterial
focal necrotizing, immunopathology of, 1664f, 1664–1665
focal segmental, membranous, 1789
glomeruli in, 2716–2727f
Henoch-Schönlein, 2744
hepatitis B-related, due to heroin abuse, 1233
hereditary, non-Alport, 582
IgA-associated, immunopathology of, 1659–1660, 1660f
lipiduria in, quantitation of, 353, 354f
malaria and, 2340
membranoproliferative, 1815–1832
carcinoma and, 1830
chronic liver disease and, 1831
chronic lymphocytic leukemia and, 1830
classification of, 1815, 1816t
clinical manifestations of, 1823–1825, 1824t
in type I disease, 1823
in type II disease, 1823–1824
in type III disease, 1824–1825
disorders associated with, 1827–1828
hereditary deficiency of complement components and, 1828–1829
Hodgkin's disease and, 1830
immunopathology of, 1658–1659
infectious disease and, 1830–1831

Glomerulonephritis—Continued
light-chain nephropathy and, 1829–1830
mixed cryoimmunoglobulinemia and, 1828, 1829t
monoclonal cryoimmunoglobulinemia and, 1830
neoplastic diseases and, 1829–1830
non-Hodgkin's lymphoma and, 1830
pathogenesis of, 1820–1823
cellular immune function in, 1822
complement system in, 1820–1821
dense deposits in, 1822
hereditary complement deficiency in, 1821–1822
nephritic factor in, 1821
platelets in, 1822–1823
pathologic findings in, 1815–1820
in dense-deposit or type II disease, 1817–1820, 1819f–1820f
in diffuse or type I disease, 1815–1817, 1816f–1817f
endocapillary cellular proliferation in, 1815, 1816f–1817f
membranous thickening in, 1815–1816, 1816f–1817f
mesangial expansion in, 1815, 1816f–1817f
in type III disease, 1820, 1820f
prognosis in, 1919–1924
actuarial survival probability and, 1921, 1922f–1923f
histologic findings and, 1921–1922
subtyping in, 1919–1920
treatment effects on, 1922, 1924
renal transplantation and, 1831–1832, 2917, 2918f
in schistosomiasis, 2347–2349, 2348f
systemic lupus erythematosus and, 1828
treatment of, 1825t–1826t, 1825–1827, 1827f
clinical studies of, 1826t, 1826–1827, 1827f
cyclophosphamide, dipyridamole, and warfarin in, 1825, 1825t
platelet inhibitors in, 1825–1826
prednisone in, 1826
in tropical countries, 2336f, 2337, 2337t
type I, renal transplantation and, 2917
type II, renal transplantation and, 2917
urinary findings in, 354, 355f
membranous
renal transplantation and, 2917, 2918f
in tropical countries, 2336f, 2337, 2337t
urinary findings in, 354, 355f
mesangial
prognosis in, 1913–1914
urinary findings in, 353–354, 354f
mesangiocapillary. *See* Glomerulonephritis, membranoproliferative
in nail-patella syndrome, 605–606
necrotizing, definition of, 2099
necrotizing and crescentic
polyarteritis and, 2103, 2105
treatment of, 2107–2108
nonoliguric, 1297
pauci-immune, 2105
proliferative
in rheumatoid arthritis, 2050–2051
in tropical countries, 2335
rapidly progressive, 1689–1706
clinical features of, 1701t, 1701–1702
factors determining outcome in, 1704t
laboratory findings in, 1702, 1702t
mechanism of crescent formation in, 1697–1699
fibrin in, 1699
leukocyte infiltration in, 1699
macrophages in, 1697
studies of, 1697, 1699
underlying common pathway in, 1699
natural history of, 1702–1704
extent of crescent formation and, 1703, 1703t
glomerular tuft and, 1703–1704
immunopathogenesis in, 1704
interstitial fibrosis and, 1704
tubular atrophy and, 1704
urine output at presentation and, 1703, 1703t
pathogenesis of, 1696–1697
absent glomerular immune deposits in, 1696–1697
anti-GBM antibody deposit in, 1696
glomerular immune complex deposit in, 1696
pathologic findings in, 1689–1696
animal studies of, 1690–1692
crescents in, 1689, 1691f–1692f
glomerular tuft hypercellularity in, 1693
immune deposits in, 1694f–1695f, 1695–1696
inflammatory cell infiltrate in, 1693f–1694f, 1693–1695
macrophage in, 1689, 1692f
T cells in, 1690
prognosis in, 1929–1932
associated conditions and, 1929, 1929t
associated glomerular disease and, 1931, 1931t
childhood disease and, 1932
clinical course in, 1931t–1932t, 1931–1932
definition of disease in, 1929
histologic features and, 1930t, 1930–1931
oligoanuria and, 1931
prognostic features and, 1930
proportion of glomeruli affected and, 1930, 1930t
treatment and, 1932, 1932t
in untreated vs. treated patients, 1930, 1931t
synonyms for, 1689
treatment in, 1704–1706, 1705t
anticoagulants for, 1705–1706
antiplatelet agents for, 1706
corticosteroids for, 1704–1705
cytotoxic agents for, 1705
factors in, 1706
plasma exchange for, 1706
renal transplantation for, 1706
renal transplantation and, 2616f–2617f, 2616–2618
in Sjögren's syndrome, 2057
with ventriculovascular shunts, 1685
with visceral infection, 1685–1686
clinical findings in, 1685–1686
pathologic findings in, 1686
Glomerulopathy
in cancer, 2265–2267
de novo, 2937
immunotactoid, 2219
light chain. *See* Light chain deposition disease
membranous
acute renal vein thrombosis in, 1319, 1320t
in cancer, 1169
in polymyositis-dermatomyositis, 2058
in rheumatoid arthritis, 2050–2051
mesangial, in rheumatoid arthritis, 2050–2051
transplant, 2937
Glomerulosclerosis
clinicopathologic correlations of, 504
diabetes mellitus and, 2572
diffuse diabetic, 2169
effect of lipid-lowering agents on, 2409, 2413f
in elderly, 2423, 2423t
focal
effect of lipid-lowering agents on, 2409, 2413f
due to heroin abuse, 1219–1226. *See also* Heroin abuse.
due to HIV infection, FGS due to heroin abuse vs., 1225
immunopathology of, 1663
focal segmental, 1739–1740. *See also* Nephrotic syndrome.
after renal transplantation, 1750–1751
diseases associated with, 1740, 1740t
in HIV-associated nephropathy, 2367–2369
mechanism of progression to, 1742–1743
hemodynamic changes in, 1742
high-protein diet and, 1742
hypercoagulable state in, 1742
immune complexes in, 1742
intrinsic glomerular factors in, 1742
lipid nephrotoxicity in, 1743
minimal change nephrotic syndrome vs., 1740–1741, 1741f
pathologic findings in, 1739–1740
prognosis in, 1750, 1911–1913
adult disease and, 1911
childhood disease and, 1911
corticosteroid responsiveness and, 1912, 1912t
histologic pattern in, 1913, 1913f
survival curves for, 1912, 1912f
due to reflux nephropathy, 697f, 697–698
renal transplantation and, 2916f, 2916–2917
synonyms for, 1739
treatment of, 1748
in tropical countries, 2335, 2336f, 2337t
nodular (Kimmelstiel-Wilson lesions), 2168t, 2169f, 2169–2170
in sickle cell disease, 2315
Glomerulotubular balance, 150
Glomerulus
adenosine receptors of, 314
ADH receptors in, 291–292
cellular structure of, 494f, 495
changes of, malaria and, 2341, 2341f
components of, 6–21. *See also specific parts*
endothelium of, 8–10, 13f
function of, in renal disease, 2716–2718, 2717f
growth of, in experimental renal disease, 2719
hemodynamic adaptations of, in experimental renal disease, 2718–2719

hormonal effects on, 288f, 288–289
involvement of, in typhoid fever, 2338
parathyroid hormone receptors in, 293
potassium filtrate in, 2648–2649
potassium transport in, 184
structural-functional relationships in, 5–6, 8f–10f
vascular anatomy of, 67, 68f
Glucagon
major renal actions of, 300
role of, in uremia, 2848
in sodium absorption, in thick ascending limb of Henle, 159
in uremia, 2845
Glucagon stimulation test, for pheochromocytoma, 1493–1494, 1494f
Glucocorticoid(s), 296–297
deficiency of
in adrenal insufficiency, 2549–2552, 2550f–2551f, 2550t
in anterior pituitary insufficiency, 2555–2556
role of vasopressin in, 2549–2551, 2550f–2551f, 2550t
vasopressin-independent effects of, 2551–2552
in immunosuppression, 2897
major renal actions of, 296–297
physiologic effects of, 1548–1550
adrenergic activity and, 1549
body fluid distribution and, 1548
membrane ion transport and, 1549
preoptic hypothalamic area and AVP and, 1549
renin-angiotensin system and, 1549
sodium and potassium status and, 1549–1550
vascular response to epinephrine and, 1548–1549
receptors for, 296, 297f
in renal transplantation, 2778
in uremic hypercatabolism, 2854
Glucocorticoid-remediable aldosteronism, 1482
Gluconeogenesis
hepatic, 2563
ion transport and, 243
metabolic pathway of, 240, 240f
renal regulation of, 241–242, 242f
in vitro, 241
in vivo, 241
Glucose
in dietary therapy in acute renal failure, 3195
tubular reabsorption of, maximum, 621
urinalysis for, 336
Glucose intolerance, uremia and, 2845–2848
Glucose oxidase test, for bacteriuria, 1012
Glucose threshold, renal, 2563
Glucose-6-phosphate deficiency, malaria and, 2340
Glue "sniffers", nephropathy in, 1232–1233
Glutamate transport, 245–246
Glutamine, in ammoniagenesis, 244–245, 245f
Glutamine metabolism, 244–245
in acid-base balance, 222f, 223
pathways of, 244, 244f
regulation of, 244–245
Glutamine transport, 246
Glutathione
as antioxidant, 1039
metabolism of, in nephrotoxicity, 1038
Glutethimide, pharmacology of, normal vs. in renal failure, 3246t–3247t
Glycine, in modulation of toxic injury, 1040
Glycogenolysis, insulin and, 2563
Glycolysis
aerobic vs. anaerobic, 241
metabolic pathway of, 240, 240f
red cell, 2748
renal sites of, 240–241
Glycoprotein hormone(s), renal metabolism of, 319
Glycosuria, hereditary, 620–621
characteristics of, 612t
GnRH analogue(s), for advanced prostatic carcinoma, 842, 843f, 844, 844t
Goiter, in uremia, 2859
Gold therapy
membranous nephropathy and, 1795
for rheumatoid arthritis, renal damage due to, 2052–2053
Gonorrhea, cystitis and urethritis vs., 1011
Goodpasture antigen, 1879, 1880f–1883f, 1882, 2170
Goodpasture's disease. *See also* Antiglomerular basement membrane antibody-mediated nephritis
antiglomerular basement membrane antibody-mediated nephritis and, 1865
Goodpasture's syndrome, iron deficiency in, 2744
Gout
in amyloidosis, 2256–2257
analgesic nephropathy and, 2258
in analgesic-induced renal disease, 1112
in Bartter syndrome, 2258
in bilateral hydronephrosis, 2258
familial, hyperuricemia, interstitial nephritis, and, 582
in familial nephropathy, 2257
glomerular filtration rate in, fall of, 2252
hypertension in, 2252
hyperuricemia and, 2239–2240
renal interaction with, 2242
lead and, vs. primary gout, 2255–2256
in medullary cystic disease, 2257
medullary microtophi in, 2258–2259
obesity in, 2252
in polycystic kidney disease, 2256
primary, 2248–2253
clinical features of, 2251–2252
vs. lead gout, 2255–2256
management of, 2252–2253
pathogenesis of, 2250–2251
pathology of, 2249–2250, 2250f–2251f
renal involvement in, 2248–2249
proteinuria in, 2252
secondary, 2253–2259
management of, 2259
tophaceous deposits in, 2252
urate underexcretion in, 2239, 2240t
urolithiasis in, 2252
vascular nephrosclerosis in, 2252
Gout nephropathy
chronic lead nephropathy and, 1241
hypertensive nephrosclerosis vs., 1442
Gouty arthritis, lead nephropathy and, 2254–2255, 2256f
Gouty nephrolithiasis, 737
Graft(s). *See also* Allograft(s); Transplantation
rejection of
immunosuppression in, 2895–2905. *See also* Immunosuppression
anti-IL-2 receptor antibodies in, 2903–2904
azathioprine and, 2897, 2897f, 2898t
corticosteroids and, 2895–2897, 2896f, 2896t
cyclophilin and, 2899
cyclosporine/FK-506 and, 2897–2901, 2898f, 2899t
15-deoxyspergualin and, 2901
experimental solutions in, 2904–2905
FK-506 and, 2899–2900
future prospects and, 2905
monoclonal antibodies and, 2902–2903, 2903t
multiple drug protocols and, 2901
polyclonal immune globulins and, 2902, 2902t
rapamycin and, 2900
RS-61443 and, 2900–2901
selective, 2902–2905
papillary necrosis and, 1979
in renal transplantation, 2892–2905
T cell activation in, 2891f, 2892–2895, 2893f–2895f
survival of, 2938, 2938f
Granulocyte(s), in Alport syndrome, 578
Granulocyte-macrophage colony-stimulating factor, in vascular inflammatory injury, 1998
Granuloma(s)
in acute interstitial nephritis, 1332, 1335f, 1335t
in chronic tubulointerstitial nephropathy, 1976
Wegener's, prognosis in, 1934
Granulomatosis
allergic angiitis and, 2111–2113, 2112f
lymphomatoid, 2113
Wegener's, 2108–2111
renal transplantation and, 2917–2918
Griess test, for bacteriuria, 1012
Griseofulvin, pharmacology of, normal vs. in renal failure, 3246t–3247t
Growth factor(s)
kidney-specific, 2707
in renal hypertrophy, 2711–2712
transforming, in hypercalcemia of malignancy, 2272
Growth hormone
for chronic renal failure, in children, 2396
hyporesponsiveness of, in uremia, 2855
phosphorus absorption and, 2603
recombinant human, in uremia, 2855
in uremia, 2856–2857
Growth retardation
in chronic renal failure, 2394–2395
posttransplant, in children, 2953
Guanabenz, pharmacology of, normal vs. in renal failure, 3246t–3247t
Guanethidine, pharmacology of, normal vs. in renal failure, 3246t–3247t
Guanosine monophosphate, cyclic (cGMP), as second messenger, in hormonal activation, 286–287
Gut antigen, 2348
Gynecomastia, uremia and, 2855

Hairy cell leukemia, 2269f
Hamartoma, renal, CT for, 453–454, 454f
Hantavirus nephropathy, acute interstitial nephritis due to, 1343
Harris-Benedict equations, 3194
Hartnup disease, 612t, 616
β-HCG, as tumor marker
in seminoma, 870
in testicular carcinoma, 860–861
HDL (high-density lipoprotein), 2849, 2849t
Head, cancer of, nephrotic syndrome in, 2265
Head trauma, hypertension and, 1605–1606
Hearing loss
renal disease and, miscellaneous causes of, 581–582
sensorineural, in Alport syndrome, 579f, 579–580
Heart failure
biochemical features of, 2475t
causes of, 2830t
congestive. *See* Congestive heart failure
in end-stage renal disease, 2829–2834
morphologic and functional abnormalities and, 2831–2832
Heart murmur, diastolic, in heart failure, 2832
Heat shock, prerenal acute renal failure due to, 1290
Heat shock protein(s), in protection against nephrotoxicity, 1069
Heavy chain(s), in overproduction proteinuria, 388–389
Heavy chain disease, 2208
Heavy metal(s), 1237–1249. *See also specific types*
in chronic tubulointerstitial nephropathy, 1973–1974
nephrotoxic, 1237
nonoliguric acute renal failure due to, 1298
HELLP syndrome, 1517
Helmet cells, 2744
Helper T lymphocyte(s), 2891f, 2892
Hemangioma, renal, angiography for, 474
Hematoma
subcapsular, angiography for, 477–478, 478f
subdural, as complication of dialysis, 2803
Hematopoietic system
cancer of, renal involvement in, 2269f, 2269–2271
hypophosphatemia and, 2609
Hematuria
in acute interstitial nephritis, 1331–1332
in Alport syndrome, 579
in analgesic-induced renal disease, 1112
in autosomal dominant polycystic kidney disease, 548
in children, 2392, 2392t
due to exercise, urine microscopy for, 343
in familial thin basement membrane disease, 583
in IgA nephropathy, 1858
in malignant hypertension, 1568
in medullary sponge kidney, 527
percutaneous renal biopsy for, 488
in renal metastasis, 2268
in sickle cell disease, 2323–2324
in upper urinary tract infection, 983
Hemihypertrophy, congenital, medullary sponge kidney and, 525
Hemi-Kock pouch, as urinary reservoir, 830, 831f
Hemodiafiltration, 3042
advantages of, 1385
disadvantages of, 1385
Hemodialysis, 1386–1390
acquired polycystic kidney disease due to, 521
CT for, 453
in acute renal failure
elderly and, 2425
neonates and, 2385–2386
advantages of, 1385
in AIDS patients, 2372
in amyloidosis, with renal failure, 2225
anticoagulation in, 1388–1389
in autosomal dominant polycystic kidney disease, 557
chronic, 3031–3059
accelerated atherosclerosis in, 3082–3083
acquired cystic disease of kidney in, 3088
acute complications of, 3049–3056
adequacy of, 3044–3049
adequate dialysis dose and, 3048–3049
adequate treatment vs., 3048
blood concentration concept and, 3046–3047
clearance concept and, 3045–3046, 3046t
clinical condition concept and, 3047
correct dialysis dose and, 3047f, 3047–3048
cramps due to, 3055
Kt/V and, 3045–3046
measurement of, 3044–3047
nutrition and, 3048
urea kinetic modeling and, 3045–3046
urea reduction and, 3046
adverse effects of improvements in, 3069, 3070t
air embolism in, 3054–3055
aluminum toxicity and, 3075–3079
bone disease due to, 3074f–3077f, 3075
dialysis encephalopathy-dementia due to, 3078–3079
microcytic anemia due to, 3078
amyloidosis in, 3079
anticoagulation for, 3040–3041
alternative agents in, 3040
heparin in, 3040
arthropathy in, 3079–3080
biochemical complications in, 3052–3053
biocompatibility in, 3079
particulate accumulation and, 3079
plasticizers and, 3079
saline and, 3079
silicone spallation and, 3079
blood circuit for, 3034
bowel infarction in, 3052
carpal tunnel syndrome in, 3080
causes of death on, 3081t, 3082
causes of failure of, 3069, 3070t
causes of underdialysis in, 3069–3070, 3071t
circulatory access for, 3031–3034
arteriovenous grafts as, 3033
diagnostic procedures for, 3033–3034
extrarenal shunts as, 3033
femoral vein catheterization as, 3033
native Brescia-Cimino fistula as, 3032f, 3032–3033
subclavian vein cannulation as, 3033
temporary, 3033
dialysate circuit for, 3034
dialysate for, 3037–3038
acetate vs. bicarbonate for, 3038, 3038f
composition of, 3037–3038
dialysate-related problems in, 3053
dialysis ascites in, 3087t, 3087–3088
dialysis disequilibrium in, 3055–3056
dialysis prescription in, 3071t, 3071–3072
kinetic modeling for, 3072–3073
dietary therapy in
alkalinizing agents and, 3185–3186
calcium in, 3182–3183
carbohydrates in, 3180
energy in, 3178–3179
fiber in, 3186
iron in, 3183
lipids and cartinine in, 3179–3180
magnesium in, 3181
phosphate binders in, 3181–3182
phosphorus in, 3181–3182
potassium in, 3181
prioritizing goals for, 3186
protein, amino acids, and ketoacids in, 3176, 3178, 3178f
recommended dietary nutrient intake in, 3170, 3170t–3171t
selenium in, 3184
sodium and water in, 3180–3181
trace elements in, 3183–3184
vitamins in, 3184–3195
zinc in, 3183–3184
equipment for, 3034–3040
evolutionary improvements in, 3069, 3070t
fever and endotoxemia in, 3053
hemodialyzer for, 3034–3037, 3035f
biocompatibility issues in, 3036, 3036t
clearance of, 3034
dialyzer reuse and, 3036–3037
first use syndrome and, 3036
interleukin-1 effects and, 3036, 3036t
membrane material in, 3035, 3035f
performance of, 3034–3035
physical aspects of, 3035, 3035f
ultrafiltration characteristics of, 3035
home, 3056–3058
patient selection for, 3057
patient survival for, 3058
psychologic impact of, 3090
quality of life with, 3058
reimbursement for, 3056
special issues with, 3058
support services for, 3058
training for, 3058
hypercalcemia in, 3053
hyperkalemia in, 3053
hypermagnesemia in, 3053, 3161–3162
hypernatremia in, 3052
hypertension in, 3084–3085
hypokalemia in, 3053
hyponatremia in, 3052

hypotension in, 3049–3051
antihypertensive medications and, 3051
autonomic neuropathy and, 3051
bicarbonate dialysis and, 3051
cardiac factors and, 3051
extracorporeal blood volume and, 3050
due to hemorrhage, 3050
hypoxemia and, 3051
plasma osmolality and, 3050
prevention of, 3051
time of onset of, 3051
treatment of, 3051
ultrafiltration and, 3050
due to volume depletion, 3050
intravenous nutrition in, 3197
life expectancy with, 3031
liver disease in, 3086–3087
long-term survival on, 3082
muscle cramps in, 3054–3055
nausea and vomiting in, 3056
neoplasia in, 3088–3089
neuropathy in, 3085–3086, 3086f
nutritional, 3197–3198
outcome and complications of, 3069–3090
recirculation and, 3073
underdialysis in, 3069–3071
overheated dialysate in, 3054
protein losses in, 3168
psychological failure and, 3089–3090
recovery of renal function and, 3089
rehabilitation in, degree of, 3083–3084
safety of, 3073–3074, 3074t
sexual function in, 3085–3086
sudden death in, 3056
survival statistics on, 3080–3082, 3081t–3082t
techniques for, 3041–3044
hemodiafiltration as, 3043
hemofiltration as, 3042
high-flux dialysis as, 3043–3044, 3043f–3044f, 3044t
isolated ultrafiltration as, 3041–3042
traditional, 3041
urea appearance rate in, 3168
water purity and, 3074–3075
water quality in, 3038–3040, 3039t
in chronic renal failure, children and, 2397
complications of, 1389f, 1389t–1390t, 1389–1390
incidence of, 1389, 1389t
pathogenesis of, 1389, 1389f
in diabetes mellitus, 2179
success and complications of, 2180–2181, 2181t
survival effects of, 2179–2180, 2180f, 2180t
dialysate in, 1387–1388
dialysis dementia in, 2799t, 2799–2803, 2801f, 2802t
dialysis disequilibrium syndrome in, 2799, 2799t
dialyzer in, 1387
disadvantages of, 1385
high-efficiency, 3072
high-flux, 3072
drug therapy in, 3228
in HIV-associated nephropathy, 2370, 2371
in hypercalcemia, 2630t
hypertension in, 1425–1427, 1426f
hypotension in, 1389–1390
pathogenesis of, 1389–1390
treatment of, 1390, 1390t
method of dialysis in, 1388
in multiple myeloma, 2206
nutritional, 2855
in pregnancy, 2305
vascular access in, 1386–1387
Hemodynamics
of hypertension, in end-stage renal disease, 2817–2818, 2818f–2820f
renal. *See* Renal hemodynamics.
Hemofiltration, 3042
slow continuous, 1390–1391
access in, 1391
advantages of, 1385
anticoagulation in, 1391
complications of, 1391
disadvantages of, 1385
filter for, 1391
when to start, 1386
theoretic considerations in, 3042
ultrafiltration vs., 3042
Hemoglobin, urinalysis for, 335–336, 336t
Hemoglobin C disease, 2311
Hemoglobin SD disease, 2311
Hemoglobinuria, in cancer, acute renal failure due to, 1168
Hemolysis
acute, 2748
in acute renal failure, role of, 2332, 2333t
chronic, 2747–2748
in chronic renal failure, 2746, 2746f
intravascular, malaria and, 2340, 2344–2345
Hemolytic anemia, microangiopathic
in hemolytic-uremic syndrome, 2073
in malignant hypertension, 1569
Hemolytic nephroangiopathy, endotheliotropic, 2074. *See also* Hemolytic-uremic syndrome
Hemolytic-uremic syndrome, 2073–2080, 2744
in children, 2388–2389
classification of, 2073–2074
clinical features of, 2074, 2075f
definition of, 2063
diarrheal form of, 2388
historical, 2073
HIV-associated, 2365
nondiarrheal form of, 2389
pathologic features of, 2074–2076, 2075f–2078f
in older children and adults, 2076, 2077f–2078f
thrombotic microangiopathy in, 2074
in younger children, 2074–2075, 2075f–2076f
prognosis and treatment in, 2076–2079
evaluation of, 2080, 2080f
long-term outcome in, 2078–2079
prognostic factors in, 2078
therapeutic approaches in, 2079, 2079t
renal transplantation and, 2917
thrombotic thrombocytopenic purpura vs., 2070, 2073
Hemopoietine, 2743
Hemorrhage
cerebral
hypertension and, 1604–1605
in preeclampsia and eclampsia, 1517, 1518t
in chronic renal failure, 2746
as complication of transplantation, 2940
gastrointestinal, in acute tubular necrosis, 1303–1304
nonhypotensive, renal hemodynamics in, 101–102
pulmonary, in antiglomerular basement membrane antibody-mediated nephritis, 1870–1871, 1871f
striate, in hypertensive neuroretinopathy, 1565, 1656f
subarachnoid
as complication of dialysis, 2803–2804
hypertension and, 1605
uterine, 2301
Hemorrhagic fever
renal manifestations of, 998–999
with renal syndrome
acute interstitial nephritis due to, 1343
chronic tubulointerstitial nephritis due to, 1976
Hemorrhagic shock, prerenal acute renal failure due to, 1290
Henle's loop. *See* Loop of Henle; Tubule(s)
Henoch-Schönlein purpura, 1839–1858. *See also* IgA nephropathy
clinical course of, 1842
clinical findings in, 1842, 1842f
glomerulonephritis and, 2744
historical, 1839
laboratory features of, 1843
nephritis and, 2393
nephritis in, prognosis in, 1936f–1939f, 1936–1938, 1937t–1940t
adult disease and, 1937, 1939f
childhood disease and, 1936f–1939f, 1936–1937, 1937t–1939t
nomenclature in, 1839
renal transplantation and, 2917
Heparin
for chronic hemodialysis, 3040
inhibitors of, 2588
pericarditis and, 2825
pharmacology of, normal vs. in renal failure, 3246t–3247t
Hepatitis
CMV-associated, as complication of transplantation, 2945
as complication of transplantation, 2944–2945
Hepatitis B
as complication of transplantation, 2945
membranous nephropathy and, 1795
Hepatitis B surface antigen (HBsAG), screening for, prior to renal transplantation, 2919–2920
Hepatitis B-related glomerulonephritis, due to heroin abuse, 1233
Hepatitis C, as complication of transplantation, 2945
Hepatorenal disease, 1355–1365
clinical course in, 1355–1356
definition of, 1355
historical, 1355
pathogenesis of, 1357–1364
arterial hypotension in, 1357
cholemia in, 1359
endotoxinemia in, 1359–1360
false neurotransmitters in, 1360
kallikrein-kinin system in, 1358–1359

Hepatorenal disease, pathogenesis of—Continued
liver transplantation in, 1359
peripheral arterial vasodilation hypothesis in, 1360–1364, 1361f–1364f
renal prostaglandin production in, 1357–1358
renin-angiotensin-aldosterone axis in, 1358
vasoactive intestinal peptides in, 1359
pathologic findings in, 1356–1357
renal function in, 1356
therapy in, 1364–1365
dialysis in, 1364
LeVeen peritoneojugular shunt in, 1365
pharmacologic intervention in, 1364–1365
portacaval shunt in, 1365
Hernia
hiatal, 642, 642f
perihiatal, 642, 642f
Heroin abuse
endocarditis-associated glomerulonephritis due to, 1229–1230
clinical features of, 1229–1230
outcome in, 1230
pathologic findings in, 1229
focal glomerulosclerosis due to, 1219–1226
clinical findings in, 1224, 1224t
electron microscopic findings in, 1223
epidemiology of, 1225–1226
etiology and pathogenesis of, 1223–1224
historical, 1219–1220
HIV infection and, 1219
HIV related FGS vs., 1225
idiopathic form vs., 1225
immunofluorescence findings in, 1222, 1223t, 1228f
morphology and natural history of, 1223
outcome in, 1224–1225
pathogenesis of, 1226
pathologic findings in, 1220f–1222f, 1220–1224, 1223t
global sclerosis in, 1220, 1221f
glomerular basement membrane in, 1220–1221, 1221f
hyalinosis in, 1220f, 1221
hypercellularity in, 1221, 1221f
idiopathic form vs., 1223
segmental sclerosis in, 1220, 1220f
talc deposits in, 1224
tubulointerstitial lesions in, 1222, 1222f
treatment in, 1225
hepatitis B-related glomerulonephritis due to, 1233
nontraumatic rhabdomyolysis in, acute renal failure due to, 1230–1231
subcutaneous, amyloidosis due to, 1226–1229
clinical features of, 1227–1229, 1228t
frequency of, 1226
pathogenesis of, 1227
pathologic findings in, 1227, 1228f
tubular disorders and, 1229
Heroin-associated nephropathy (HAN), 2368
vs. HIV-associated nephropathy, 2369
Herpes simplex infection
as complication of transplantation, 2944
genital, cystitis and urethritis vs., 1011
Hexobarbital, pharmacology of, normal vs. in renal failure, 3246t–3247t
Heyman nephritis, 2717
Heymann nephritis, 1652–1653, 1653f, 1790
HGPRT (hypoxanthine-guanine phosphoribosyltransferase)
deficiency of, 2242
acute renal failure with, 2244
mutations of, urate overproduction and, 2239, 2242
Hiatal hernia, 642, 642f
High-density lipoprotein (HDL), 2849, 2849t
High-pressure baroreceptor(s), in sodium retention, 2454–2456
Hilus, renal, anatomy of, 3
Histamine, in renal hemodynamics, 98
Histidinuria, 617
Histocompatibility, 2879–2882
clinical testing of, 2881–2882, 2882f
molecular organization in, 2879–2881, 2880f
structural relationship in, 2880f, 2881
Histoplasmosis, 944, 945t–946t
as complication of transplantation, 2946
HIV infection. *See* Human immunodeficiency virus (HIV) infection.
HIV-associated nephropathy (HIVAN), 2366–2370. *See also* Human immunodeficiency virus (HIV) infection
AZT therapy for, 2370
clinical features of, 2369
focal segmental glomerulosclerosis in, 2367–2369
vs. heroin-associated nephropathy, 2369
intravenous drug addiction and, 2366–2367
maintenance dialysis therapy for, 2370
malignant nature of, 2368
Mycoplasma fermentans antigen in, 2369–2370
pathogenesis of, 2369
pathologic features of, 2369
proteinuria in, 2367
treatment options for, 2370
tubuloreticular inclusions in, 2368
ultrasound examination in, 2367
HLA antigen, 2879
class-I, 2879
class-II, 2880
determination of, prior to renal transplantation, 2920
molecular organization of, 2879–2881, 2880f
presensitivity testing for, 2881
in reflux nephropathy, 716–717
structural relationship of, 2880f, 2881
typing, 2881–2882, 2882f
HLA antigen A, 2879, 2880f
HLA antigen B, 2879, 2880f
HLA antigen C, 2879, 2880f
HLA antigen D, 2879–2880, 2880f
HLA antigen DP, 2880
HLA antigen DQ, 2880
HLA antigen DR, 2880
HLA type
in antiglomerular basement membrane antibody-mediated nephritis, 1866–1867
in membranous nephropathy, 1919
in nephrotic syndrome, 1734, 1735t
HLA-identical siblings, renal transplant results in, 2938
HLA-nonidentical parents or siblings, renal transplant results in, 2939
HMG CoA reductase inhibitors, in lipid reduction, 2852
Hodgkin's disease
amyloidosis and, 2221
antiglomerular basement membrane antibody-mediated nephritis and, 1868
nephrotic syndrome in, 2267
Hodson scar, definition of, 652
Hormone(s), 283–319. *See also specific types.*
general mechanisms of, 283–288
glomerular function and, 288f, 288–289
lipid-soluble, 287–288
mode of action of, 288
receptor recognition of, 287–288, 288f
tubular function and, 289–291, 290f, 291t
water-soluble, 283–287
arachidonic acid pathway for, 286–287
cAMP as second messenger for, 284–286, 285f
cGMP as second messenger for, 287
cytosolic calcium concentration and, 286
guanine nucleotide-binding regulatory proteins and, 284
mode of action of, 284
phosphoinositide pathway for, 286, 287f
phospholipid-derived pathway for, 286
receptor concentration and affinity and, 284
receptor interactions of, 283–284
Horseshoe kidney, 653–654
asymmetric renal fusion in, 653
CT for, 450, 450f
definition of, 653
embryogenesis of, 653
lateral renal fusion in, 653
midline renal fusion in, 653
Hospital-acquired upper urinary tract infection, pathogens in, 974
Howship's lacunae, 2617
HTLV-associated nephropathy, 2366
Human immunodeficiency virus (HIV) infection, 2361–2373. *See also* Acquired immunodeficiency syndrome (AIDS)
acute renal failure in, 2362–2365
drugs causing, 2363–2364
hemolytic uremic syndrome and, 2365
thrombotic thrombocytopenia purpura and, 2365
adrenal abnormalities in, 2365–2366
as complication of transplantation, 2944
electrolyte abnormalities in, 2365
end-stage renal disease and, 2371–2373
epidemiology of, 2361–2362
ethical issues in, 3119–3121
HIV testing as, 3120
initiation and termination of dialysis as, 3120–3121

limitation of dialysis services as, 3120
renal transplantation as, 3121
resistance of medical workers as, 3119–3120
in heroin abusers, focal glomerulosclerosis and, 1219, 1225
membranoproliferative glomerulonephritis and, 1830–1831
renal disease in
classification of, 2361–2362, 2362t
unrelated, 2370–2371
renal parenchymal abnormalities in, 2365
screening for, prior to renal transplantation, 2920
transmission of, modes of, 2371, 2372–2373
Human leukocyte antigen. *See* HLA *entries.*
Humoral immunity, graft rejection and, 2887
Hungry bone syndrome, 2624
Hyaline arteriolosclerosis
in nephrosclerosis, 1433, 1434f
in primary nephrosclerosis, 1433–1434
Hydralazine
for hypertension, 1624–1625, 2296, 2390t
lupus-like syndrome due to, 2029–2030
for moderate hypertension in pregnancy, 1524
pharmacology of, normal vs. in renal failure, 3246t–3247t
for severe hypertension in pregnancy, 1524–1525
Hydrochlorothiazide
acute interstitial nephritis due to, 1340
pharmacology of, normal vs. in renal failure, 3248t–3249t
Hydrogen ion reaction(s), 207. *See also* Acid-base balance
buffer, 207
metabolic, 207
Hydrogen transport
in distal nephron, carbonic anhydrase and apical membrane in, 47–48
in nephron, structural-functional relationships in, 45–46
Hydronephrosis. *See also* Obstructive nephropathy; Obstructive uropathy; Urinary tract obstruction
bilateral, gout in, 2258
causes of, 659
definition of, 657
incidence of, 657
renal parenchymal atrophy in, 659
Hydrops, nonimmune, in neonates, 2386
β-Hydroxybutyric acid, 2579
1α-Hydroxyvitamin D, in renal failure, 2776
Hyperaldosteronemia, in cardiac failure, 2459
Hyperaldosteronism. *See also* Aldosteronism
in adrenocortical carcinoma, 1482
in malignant hypertension, 1592
in renovascular hypertension, 1454–1455
Hyperalimentation, in acute renal failure, 1383
Hyperammonemia, in multiple myeloma, 2201
Hyperamylasemia, in acute tubular necrosis, 1304
Hyper-apolipoprotein B, in uremia, 2850
Hyperbilirubinemia, in malaria, 2345
Hypercalcemia, 2624–2630
in acute renal failure, 2774
in acute tubular necrosis, 1308
in AIDS patients, 2365
associated with acute renal failure, 2204
in cancer, 2271t, 2271–2273
acute renal failure due to, 1168
renal complications of, 1170
cardiovascular effects of, 2625
causes of, 2626t
in chronic hemodialysis, 3052–3053
in chronic tubulointerstitial nephropathy, 1975
clinical symptoms of, 2624t, 2624–2625
diabetes insipidus and, 2510–2511
gastrointestinal manifestations of, 2625
humoral, of malignancy, 2625–2626
hydration therapy for, 2205
hyperthyroidism and, 2627
immobilization and, 2627
metastatic calcification and, 2625
milk-alkali syndrome and, 2628
multiple myeloma and, 2199, 2201
neurologic effects of, 2625
posttransplant, 2952
primary hyperparathyroidism and, 2626–2627
psychiatric effects of, 2625
in renal cell carcinoma, 786–787
renal disease and, 2627
renal effects of, 2624–2625
renal transplantation and, 2627
sarcoidosis and, 2627–2628
secondary to decreased urinary calcium excretion, 2628
secondary to increased bone calcium mobilization, 2625–2626
secondary to increased calcium absorption from gastrointestinal tract, 2627–2628
secondary to malignancies, 2625–2626
thiazide diuretics and, 2627
treatment of, 2628–2630, 2630t
vitamin A intoxication and, 2627
vitamin D intoxication and, 2627, 2628
Hypercalciuria
absorptive, 733, 734f
treatment of, 736
due to hyperparathyroidism, 733–734, 734f
treatment of, 734, 736
in medullary sponge kidney, 528–529
nephrolithiasis due to, 730, 731t, 733–736
pathogenesis of, 733–734, 734f
renal, 733, 734f
treatment of, 736
renal phosphate leak, treatment of, 736
resorptive, 733–734, 734f
treatment of, 734, 736
treatment of, 734–736, 735t
Hyperchloremic acidosis
in diabetes mellitus, 2581–2582
renal tubular potassium and, 2657–2658
Hyperemesis gravidarum, 2301
Hyperfiltration, in diabetic nephropathy, 2165–2166, 2166f
Hypergastrinemia, in chronic renal failure, 2862
Hyperglucagonemia, complicating diabetic ketoacidosis, 2570
Hyperglycemia
coma with, as complication of dialysis, 2803
in diabetes mellitus, 2585
insulin and, 2563–2564, 2565f
posttransplant, 2952–2953
symptoms of, 2567
Hyperkalemia
acidemia therapy in, 2659
in acute renal failure, treatment of, 1376–1377, 1377f–1378f, 1378t
in acute tubular necrosis, 1307
in AIDS patients, 2365
ammoniagenesis and, 244
in cancer, 2276–2277
chronic
pathophysiologic approach to, 2658f
treatment of, 2658f, 2658–2659
in chronic hemodialysis, 3052
in diabetes mellitus, 2584
due to impaired potassium excretion, 2585
due to maldistribution, 2585
dietary intervention in, 2659
distal tubular acidosis in, 2682–2684, 2683t
diuretic therapy in, 2659
drugs causing, dicontinuation of, 2659
in elderly, 2422
in end-stage renal disease, 2830
in falciparum malaria, 2339–2340
mineralocorticoids in, 2659
in multiple myeloma, 2200
NSAID nephrotoxicity and, 1213
in renal insufficiency, 2650t
renin-angiotensin-aldosterone system defect and, 2653f, 2653–2657, 2654t
sodium-potassium exchange resins in, 2659
tubular secretory defect and, 2653f, 2654t, 2656–2657
volume expansion in, 2659
Hyperlipidemia
in diabetes mellitus, 2568
in nephrotic syndrome, 1757–1759, 1758f
posttransplant, 2949–2950
Hypermagnesemia, 2532–2633
in acute tubular necrosis, 1308
in chronic hemodialysis, 3052–3053, 3161–3162
in end-stage renal disease, 2831
signs and symptoms of, 2633
treatment of, 2635
Hypermetabolism, 2709
Hypernatremia, 2503, 2504f, 2504t
acute, as complication of dialysate abnormality, 2804
adipsic, causes of, 2513t
in children, 2382
in chronic hemodialysis, 3052
consequences of, 2515
diabetes mellitus and, 2590–2591
diagnostic approach to, 2591f
essential, 2503, 2513f, 2513t, 2513–2514
treatment of, 2514
in falciparum malaria, 2339
hypervolemic, 2591
hypovolemic, 2590–2591
isovolemic, 2591
in mineralocorticoid excess, 2514–2515
morbidity and mortality in, 2515
neurologic sequelae of, 2515
treatment of, 2515–2516

Hypernephroma, acute renal vein thrombosis due to, in nephrotic syndrome, 1325
Hyperosmolar thirst, 119–120
Hyperoxaluria
in chronic tubulointerstitial nephropathy, 1974–1975
nephrolithiasis due to, 731, 731t, 736
Hyperparathyroid bone disease, treatment of, 2776–2777, 2777f
Hyperparathyroidism
vs. aluminum toxicity, 2766t
brown tumor of, 2773
ennervation in, 2762
erythropoiesis and, 2747
hypercalciuria due to, pathogenesis of, 733–734, 734f
malignancy associated with, 2273
medullary sponge kidney and, 528–529
posttransplant, 2951
primary
hypercalcemia and, 2626–2627
hypophosphatemia and, 2604
secondary
growth retardation in, 2395
due to hyperphosphatemia, in chronic renal failure, 3153–3154
hypophosphatemia and, 2604
pathogenesis of, 2761f
sequential treatment of, 2775t
Hyperphosphatemia, 2611–2615
acromegaly and, 2613
in acute tubular necrosis, 1307
in cancer, 2274, 2274t, 2275t
causes of, 2611t, 2611–2614
in chronic renal failure, 3153–3156
management of, aluminum intoxication and, 3160–3161
metastatic calcification due to, 3154f–3155f, 3154t, 3154–3155
progressive renal damage due to, 3155–3156
secondary hyperparathyroidism due to, 3153–3154
clinical manifestations of, 2614f, 2614–2615
diphosphonate administration and, 2613
in end-stage renal disease, 2831
increased catabolism and, 2614
ingestion of phosphate salts and, 2614
parathyroid hormone and
abnormal circulating, 2613
decreased or absent levels of, 2611–2612
pathophysiologic changes in, 2614f
phosphate and, 2614
preventive therapy for, 2774–2775, 2775t
pseudohypoparathyroidism and, 2612–2613
respiratory acidosis and, 2614
treatment of, 2615
tumor lysis syndrome and, 2613–2614
tumoral calcinosis and, 2613
vitamin D and, 2614
Hyperphosphatemic nephropathy, due to antineoplastic agents, 1181
Hyperprolactinemia, in chronic renal failure, 2857–2858
Hyperreflexia, autonomic, hypertensive crisis in, 1616–1617
Hyperreninemia, in cardiac failure, 2459
Hypersensitivity angiitis, 2095–2096
Hypersplenism, dialysis and, 2748
Hypertension. *See also* Blood pressure
accelerated. *See also* Malignant hypertension
malignant hypertension vs., 1566–1567, 1567f
acquired, 1424–1427
causes of, 1424
mechanism of, 1424–1425
in primary aldosteronism, 1425
in unilateral renal artery stenosis, 1425
ACTH effects on, 1546f–1548f, 1546–1547
after aortic coarctation repair, 1613
in amyloidosis, 2220
in analgesic-induced renal disease, 1112–1113
aortic dissection and, 1607–1610
in autosomal dominant polycystic kidney disease, 548–549
benign
with acute complications, 1555
acute pulmonary edema in, 1600–1603, 1601f–1602f
with chronic stable complications, 1557
end-stage renal disease and, 1593–1594
malignant hypertension vs., 1593–1594
in cancer, renovascular disease due to, 1169
cerebral infarction and, 1603–1604
cerebrovascular accident and, 1603–1606
in children, 2389–2390
causes of, 2389, 2389t
treatment of, 2389–2390, 2390t
in chronic hemodialysis, 3084–3085
chronic lead nephropathy and, 1241
complicating postoperative bleeding, 1613
in Cushing's syndrome, 1545
dialysis and, 1425–1427, 1426f
in elderly, 2422–2423
in end-stage renal disease, 2817–2824
hemodynamics of, 2817–2818, 2818f–2820f
management of, 2823–2824
pathophysiology of, 2818–2819, 2820f, 2821
renin-angiotensin system in, 2821–2822
sympathetic nervous system in, 2823
vascular endothelium in, 2823
vasodepressors in, 2822–2823
volume factors and, 2818–2819, 2820f, 2821
essential, 1420–1421, 1436–1440
in blacks vs. whites, 1436
casts in, protein composition of, 347t
in children, 2390
definition of, 1436
effect of treatment of, 1437, 1437t
Guyton's hypothesis for renal mechanisms of, 1437f–1438f, 1437–1438
historical, 1407–1408
incidence of, 1436
natural history of, 1437
plasma renin levels in, 1437
pregnancy in, 1519
proposed pathogenesis of, 1438–1440
barriers to, 1438
genetic defects in, 1438–1439
rat model of, 1439
renal transplantation and, 1439–1440
sodium loading and, 1440
renal function abnormality in, 1420–1421
in early disease, 1421
in late disease, 1421
primary, 1420
secondary, 1420–1421
sodium excretion in, 1415–1416
studies of renal function in, 1436
glucocorticoid-suppressible, familial, 1542
in gout, 2252
head trauma and, 1605–1606
inherited, 1420–1424
rat strains of, 1421–1424
hypothesis on mechanism of, 1421–1422
Na-K-ATPase inhibitor in, 1423–1424, 1424f
natriuretic hormone and, 1422–1423, 1423f
sodium excretion in, 1414–1416
intracerebral hemorrhage and, 1604–1605
malignant. *See* Malignant hypertension
mineralocorticoid-induced, 1475, 1476f
moderate, treatment of, 2296
myocardial infarction and, 1606–1607
in neonates, 2386
nephrosclerosis in, pathologic findings in, 1433–1434
paradoxical, 1613
poorly controlled, emergency surgery and, 1556
postcarotid endarterectomy, 1613
postcoronary bypass, 1612–1613
postpartum, 1511
posttransplant, 2950
in pregnancy, 1505–1531, 2290–2298. *See also* Preeclampsia; Pregnancy, hypertension in
prevalence of, sodium intake vs., 1411f, 1411–1412
primary aldosteronism and, 1475, 1476f
primary nephrosclerosis and, 1433–1434
in reflux nephropathy, 711
management of, 720
peripheral plasma renin activity and, 712
renal vein renin activity in, 712–713
renin-dependent, 2822
renovascular. *See* Renovascular hypertension
salt-and-water-dependent, 2822
in scleroderma renal crisis, 2040–2041
secondary, historical, 1407–1408
severe
clinical spectrum of, 1555–1557, 1556t
definition of, 2389
postoperative, 1556
treatment of, 2296–2297
uncomplicated, 1557, 1627–1629
oral antihypertensive loading regimen in, 1628
urgency of treatment in, 1627–1628
sickle cell disease and, 2323
subarachnoid hemorrhage and, 1605
in surgical patient, 1610–1612
anesthesia in, 1611–1612
endotracheal intubation in, 1612
intraoperative and postoperative control of, 1612
preoperative control of, 1610–1611
systemic, in diabetic nephropathy, 2166, 2167t, 2168f
treatment of
clonidine in, 1627

converting enzyme inhibitors, 1626–1627
diazoxide in, 1621–1622
gradual vs. rapid reduction in, 1617–1619
hydralazine in, 1624–1625
intravenous nitroglycerine in, 1623
labetolol in, 1623–1624
methyldopa in, 1627
minoxidil in, 1625–1626
nifedipine in, 1625
phentolamine in, 1624
reserpine in, 1627
sodium nitroprusside in, 1619–1621
trimethaphan in, 1622–1623
in unilateral reflux nephropathy, 711–712
nephrectomy for, 711–712
peripheral plasma renin activity and, 712
renal vein renin activity in, 712–713
in upper urinary tract infection, 980
in urinary tract obstruction, 660, 682
in urinary tract tuberculosis, 916
in vesicoureteral reflux, 711
volume expansion in, 1409
atrial natriuretic peptide and, 1409
sodium excretion and, 1409
Hypertensive choroidopathy, 1566, 1566f
Hypertensive crisis, 1555. *See also* Malignant hypertension
in antihypertensive therapy withdrawal, 1615
in autonomic hyperreflexia, 1616–1617
catecholamine-related, 1613–1616
in miscellaneous conditions, 1616
in monoamine oxidase inhibitor interactions, 1615–1616
in nonprescription sympathomimetic amine reactions, 1616
in pheochromocytoma, 1613–1615
in renal allograft recipients, 1617
Hypertensive encephalopathy. *See* Encephalopathy, hypertensive
Hypertensive nephrosclerosis. *See* Nephrosclerosis, hypertensive
Hypertensive neuroretinopathy. *See* Neuroretinopathy, hypertensive
Hypertensive syndrome, hyponatremic, in malignant hypertension, 1570
Hyperthyroidism, hypercalcemia and, 2627
Hypertransfusion, erythropoiesis and, 2747
Hypertrophy
definition of, 2706
renal
ammoniagenesis in, 2710
cellular, 2709–2710
cellular mechanisms in, 2708–2709
compensatory, 2706–2713
DNA metabolism in, 2710
gene expression patterns in, 2712
growth factors and, 2711–2712
neural stimuli and, 2711
phospholipid metabolism in, 2710
protein metabolism in, 2711
RNA metabolism in, 2710–2711
without increase in filtration rate, 2708
"work," 2706
Hyperuricemia
in acute tubular necrosis, 1307
in chronic tubulointerstitial nephropathy, 1974
disproportionate, 2258
familial, gout, interstitial nephritis, and, 582
familial nephropathy and, 2257
gout and, 2239–2240
renal interaction with, 2242
intense physical training and, 2245
medullary cystic disease and, 2257
multiple myeloma and, 2201
complications from, 2199
pathogenesis of, 2240t
posttransplant, 2952
sickle cell anemia and, 2244–2245, 2320
tumor lysis syndrome and, 2274
urate in, 2239, 2240t
Hyperuricosuria, 2245
nephrolithiasis due to, 730–731, 731t
Hyperuricosuric calcium nephrolithiasis, 737
Hyperviscosity syndrome
diagnosis of, 2208
in Waldenstrom's macroglobulinemia, 2207–2208
Hypervolemia, in malaria, 2343
Hypoaldosteronism
clinical features and management of, 2587–2588
diabetes mellitus and, 2586, 2587f
hyporeninemia, 2654–2655
hyporeninemia in, 2656
elderly and, 2421
metabolic acidosis and, 2657
potassium in, 2655–2656
Hypobicarbonatemia, 2577, 2669–2670
Hypocalcemia, 2622–2624
acute pancreatitis and, 2624
in acute tubular necrosis, 1307–1308
in AIDS patients, 2365
in cancer, 2273–2274
causes of, 2622t
clinical symptoms of, 2622
in end-stage renal disease, 2831
hungry bone syndrome and, 2624
secondary to decreased calcium mobilization from bone, 2623
secondary to increased urinary excretion of calcium, 2624
secondary to low or absent levels of PTH, 2623
secondary to reduced intestinal calcium absorption, 2623–2624
secondary to translocation of calcium into different compartments, 2624
treatment of, 2628
Hypocitraturia, nephrolithiasis due to, 731, 731t, 736
Hypocomplementemic urticarial vasculitis, 2114
Hypodipsia, 2514
Hypodysplasia, renal
classification of, 652–653
definition of, 652
etiology of, 652
ureteric orifice ectopy and, 652
Hypoglycemia
postdialysis, 2848
spontaneous, 2848
Hypokalemia
ammoniagenesis and, 244
cancer and, 2277–2278
in chronic hemodialysis, 3052
diabetes insipidus and, 2510
diabetes mellitus and, 2588–2589
from diminished potassium intake, 2588
in end-stage renal disease, 2830–2831
due to increased potassium excretion, 2588
due to intracellular potassium redistribution, 2588
liver disease and, 2474–2475
Hypomagnesemia, 2623, 2633–2635
in AIDS patients, 2365
causes of, 2633t
clinical manifestations of, 2634
development of, mechanisms responsible for, 2634–2635
in end-stage renal disease, 2831
ketoacidosis and, 2634
secondary to decreased intestinal magnesium absorption, 2634
secondary to decreased magnesium intake, 2634
secondary to increased urinary losses of magnesium, 2634–2635
treatment of, 2635
Hyponatremia, 2516–2521
acute
as complication of dialysate abnormality, 2804
treatment of, 2525–2526, 2526f
in acute tubular necrosis, 1307
anterior pituitary insufficiency and, 2554, 2554f–2555f
approach to, 2517, 2518f
in children, 2382
chronic, treatment of, 2526–2527
in chronic hemodialysis, 3052
clinical disorders resulting in, 2517–2518
diabetes mellitus and, 2589–2590
diagnostic approach to, 2590f
drugs associated with, 2519t, 2519–2521
factitious, 2516
in falciparum malaria, 2339
in HIV infection, 2365
hypertonic, 2589
hypotonic, 2589–2590
increasing solute excretion in, 2527
in liver disease, 2472–2473
treatment of, 2474
in malignant hypertension, 1570
in myxedema, 2539–2541
plasma osmolality and, 2516–2517, 2517t
postoperative, 2521
psychiatric disorders and, 2521
SIADH secretion and, 2521–2527
treatment of, 2525–2527
vasopressin antagonists in, 2527
Hyponatremic hypertensive syndrome, in malignant hypertension, 1570
Hypophosphatemia, 2604–2611
acid-base disturbances in, 2610
acute alcoholism and, 2607
acute tubular necrosis and, diuretic phase of, 2605
after renal transplantation, 2605
associated with tumors, 2607
biochemical manifestations of, 2608, 2609t
cancer and, 2275–2276, 2276f
carbohydrate administration and, 2607
carbohydrate metabolism and, 2609
cardiovascular manifestations of, 2608–2609
causes of, 2604t, 2604–2608
clinical manifestations of, 2608, 2609t
craniotabes and, 2605
decreased gastrointestinal phosphate absorption and, 2607

Hypophosphatemia—Continued
diabetes mellitus and, 2591
diabetic ketoacidosis therapy and, 2607
differential diagnosis of, 2610
in end-stage renal disease, 2831
extracellular fluid volume expansion and, 2605
falciparum malaria and, 2340
gastrointestinal disturbances in, 2609–2610
hematologic manifestations of, 2609
hyperparathyroidism and
primary, 2604
secondary, 2604
hypothermia and, 2608
leukemia and, 2608
malabsorption and, 2607
malnutrition and, 2607
neurologic manifestations of, 2609
osteomalacia and, 2605
phosphate binders and, 2607
postobstructive diuresis and, 2605
posttransplant, 2952
renal manifestations of, 2610
renal tubular defects and, 2605
respiratory alkalosis and, 2607–2608
skeletal abnormalities in, 2609
skeletal muscle manifestations of, 2608–2609
sodium bica rbonate administration and, 2608
toxic shock syndrome and, 2608
treatment of, 2610–2611
vitamin D metabolism and, 2605
in vitamin D-deficient rickets, 2605–2606
in vitamin D-dependent rickets, 2606–2607
in X-linked rickets, 2606
Hypophosphatemic nonrachitic bone disease, 618t, 619–620. *See also* Rickets
Hypoplasia, renal
classification of, 652
definition of, 652
Hyporeninemia
in diabetes mellitus, 2586
in hypoaldosteronism, 2656
Hyporeninism, 2654–2655
Hyposthenuria
obligatory, in children, 2387
in Sjögren's syndrome, 2056
Hypotension. *See also* Blood pressure
in chronic hemodialysis, 3049–3051. *See also* Hemodialysis, chronic
due to hemodialysis, 1389–1390, 1390t
orthostatic, in amyloidosis, 2213, 2213t
in pericarditis, 2826
renal, 1427f, 1427–1428
Hypotensive crisis, in pheochromocytoma, 1615
Hypothalamic disorders, idiopathic edema and, 2495
Hypothermia, hypophosphatemia and, 2608
Hypothyroidism
idiopathic edema and, 2496
in uremia, 2859
Hypouricemia, 2245
Hypovolemia, in malaria, 2343
Hypoxanthine-guanine phosphoribosyltransferase (HGPRT)
deficiency of, 2242
acute renal failure with, 2244
mutations of, urate overproduction and, 2239, 2242

Ibuprofen, pharmacology of, normal vs. in renal failure, 3248t–3249t
Ifosfamide, pharmacology of, normal vs. in renal failure, 3248t–3249t
IgA
in focal glomerulosclerosis due to heroin abuse, 1223t
immunobiology of, 1855–1856
IgA nephropathy, 1839–1858
after renal transplantation, 1843
classification of and disease associations in, 1842–1843, 1843t
clinical course of, 1842
clinical findings in, 1840–1842, 1841f, 1841t
clinicopathologic correlation in, 1855, 1855t
diagnosis of, 1840
geographic distribution of, 1840
historical, 1839
incidence of, 1840, 1840f–1841f
laboratory features of, 1843
nomenclature in, 1839
pathogenesis of, 1855–1858
defective immune clearance in, 1856–1857
environmental agents in, 1856
genetic factors in, 1856
humoral immune abnormalities in, 1856
immunobiology of IgA in, 1855–1856
increased IgA production in, 1856
mediation of glomerular injury in, 1857, 1857t
summary of, 1857–1858, 1858f
pathologic findings in, 1844–1850
electron microscopy in, 1849–1850, 1850f–1854f
immunologic studies in, 1848f–1849f, 1849
light microscopy in, 1844, 1844f–1848f, 1848
prognosis in, 1914–1916
in adults, 1915, 1915f
in children, 1915–1916
complete remission and, 1915
life table analysis in, 1915, 1915t
pathologic findings and, 1915
in unusual patterns, 1916
renal transplantation and, 2917
treatment of, 1858–1859
diet in, 1858
hypertension and, 1858
macroscopic hematuria in, 1858
pathogenetic factors and, 1858t, 1858–1859
primary vs. secondary disease and, 1858
systemic symptoms in, 1858
vasculitis in, 1854f–1855f, 1854–1855
IgG, in focal glomerulosclerosis due to heroin abuse, 1222, 1223t
IgG myeloma, malignant hypertension due to, 1561
IgM, in focal glomerulosclerosis due to heroin abuse, 1222, 1223t
IgM nephropathy
mesangial, 1737
prognosis in, 1914
^{125}I-Iothalamate clearance, for GFR, 372
Ileocecal urinary reservoir, 829, 830f
Imidazole, for candidiasis, 942
Iminoglycinuria, 616
hereditary, characteristics of, 612t
Imipenem, pharmacology of, normal vs. in renal failure, 3248t–3249t
Immune complex(es)
in cancer, 2265–2266
in chronic tubulointerstitial nephropathy, 1966–1968
in preeclampsia, 1515–1516
in tubulointerstitial nephritis, acute interstitial nephritis and, 1346, 1347
Immune mechanism(s), of urinary tract, 897–899. *See also* Urinary tract, immune mechanisms of
Immunity
elements of
in acute cellular rejection, 2888t, 2889
in allograft rejection, 2888–2889
humoral, graft rejection and, 2887
Immunodeficient host, reconstitution of, 2888–2890
Immunofluorescence microscopy, of amyloidosis, 2217
Immunoglobulin(s)
in cancer
acute renal failure due to, 1168
chronic renal failure due to, 1169
in pyelonephritis, 897–898
urinary, in urinary tract infection prevention, 898
Immunoglobulin A. *See* IgA
Immunoglobulin A nephropathy. *See* IgA nephropathy
Immunoglobulin G. *See* IgG
Immunoglobulin M. *See* IgM
Immunohistochemical evaluation, 500–503
glomerular immunoglobulin staining patterns in, 500–502
immunoperoxidase staining in, 502–503
Immunoperoxidase labeling with monoclonal antibodies, for urinalysis, 354–356, 355f
Immunosuppression, 2925–2930
anti-IL-2 receptor antibodies in, 2903–2904
antilymphocyte globulin in, 2929
antithymocyte globulin in, 2929
azathioprine in, 2897, 2897f, 2898t, 2926
corticosteroids in, 2895–2897, 2896f, 2896t, 2926
cyclophilin in, 2899
cyclosporine in, 2897–2899, 2898f, 2899t, 2926–2929, 2927t, 2928t
cyclosporine/FK-505 in, 2897–2900, 2898f, 2899t
15-deoxyspergualin in, 2901
experimental solutions in, 2904–2905
FK-506 in, 2899
future prospects for, 2905
in graft rejection, 2895–2901
induction and maintenance of, 2925
monoclonal antibodies in, 2902–2903, 2903t, 2929t, 2929–2930
multiple drug protocols in, 2901
new agents in, 2930
OKT3 therapy in, 2903, 2903t, 2929t, 2929–2930
plasma exchange in, 2930
polyclonal antisera in, 2929
polyclonal immune globulins in, 2902, 2902t
rapamycin in, 2900

in renal disease, 3230
RS-61443 in, 2900–2901
selective, 2902–2905
T lymphocyte activation and impact in, 2890–2891, 2891f
total lymphoid irradiation in, 2930
Immunotactoid glomerulopathy, 2219
Impotence
due to radical prostatectomy, 841–842
uremia and, 2855
Incontinence, 763
functional, 763
overflow, 763
stress, 763
urge, 763
Indomethacin
acute interstitial nephritis due to, 1338
for hypercalcemia, 2629, 2630t
for pericarditis, 2827
pharmacology of, normal vs. in renal failure, 3248t–3249t
in sickle cell disease, 2318, 2318f, 2322
Infant(s). *See also under* Children; Neonate(s)
cystitis and urethritis in, 1019–1020
fluid and electrolytes in, 2383–2384, 2384t
glomerular filtration rate in, 2384t
growth and nutrition in, 2383
peritoneal dialysis in, 3003–3004
upper urinary tract infection in
clinical presentation in, 989
natural history of, 978–979
Infarction
cerebral, hypertension and, 1603–1604
lobar, imaging studies in, 427, 427f
myocardial, hypertension and, 1606–1607
renal, CT for, 453
renal segmental, in renovascular hypertension, 1458
Infection
associated with acute renal failure, 2204
bacterial. *See* Bacterial infection
as complication of transplantation, 2942–2947, 2943t
HIV. *See* Human immunodeficiency virus (HIV) infection
opportunistic, in AIDS patients, 2361
parasitic. *See* Parasitic infection
susceptibility to, multiple myeloma and, 2199–2200
viral. *See* Viral infections
Infectious mononucleosis, renal manifestations of, 998
Infective endocarditis. *See* Endocarditis, bacterial
Inflammation, historical concepts of, 1993
Inorganic acid, overproduction of, 2577
Insulin
in carbohydrate metabolism, 2845
continuous subcutaneous infusion of, in diabetes mellitus, 2179
in diabetes mellitus, deficiency of, 2585
in dietary therapy in acute renal failure, 3193
diminished effect of, hyperglycemia and, 2563–2564, 2565f
effect of, on protein synthesis, 2855
effect of hyperkalemia on, 2645–2646
intraperitoneal, 3002
major renal actions of, 300–301
metabolic actions of, 2564t
molecular weight, radius, and renal handling of, 381t
in potassium regulation, 2645–2646
resistance to, 2845
in acute tubular necrosis, 1305–1306
cellular mechanism of, 2845–2847
clamp studies in, 2845, 2846f
site of, 2845
uremic milieu and, 2847
secretion of, 2847–2848, 2848f
in uremic dyslipoproteinemia, 2850
Insulin infusion system, continuous subcutaneous, in diabetes mellitus, 2179
Insulin-dependent diabetes mellitus. *See* Diabetes mellitus, insulin-dependent
Insulin-like growth factor, 2856
major renal actions of, 301
receptors for, 301
in renal hypertrophy, 2712
Integrin, in leukocyte-endothelial adhesion, 2002, 2003t
Intercalated cell(s)
cellular structure of, 27f, 28–29, 30f, 160f, 161
potassium depletion effects on, 44–45
in potassium transport, 194–195
Intercellular cell adhesion molecule, 2004
Interferon
acute interstitial nephritis due to, 1341
for HIV infection, 2364
nephrotoxicity of, 1179–1180
pharmacology of, normal vs. in renal failure, 3248t–3249t
in vascular inflammatory injury, 1998
Interleukin(s), for HIV infection, 2364
Interleukin-1 (IL-1), 2272
activation of, corticosteroids and, 2897, 2897f
in uremia, 2862
in vascular inflammatory injury, 1997, 1998t
Interleukin-2 (IL-2)
activation of, cyclosporine in, 2898, 2898f
interaction of, with antigen-activated T lymphocytes, 2895, 2896f
Interleukin-4 (IL-4), in vascular inflammatory injury, 1998
Interleukin-2 (IL-2) receptor positive T cells, 2890–2891, 2891f
Interleukin-2 rich conditioned media (IL-2CM), 2888
Interstitial inflammatory infiltrate(s), clinicopathologic correlations of, 504–505
Interstitial nephritis. *See also* Tubulointerstitial nephropathy
acute, 1331–1347
acute tubular necrosis and, 1345
acute tubulointerstitial nephropathy vs., 1331
due to acyclovir, 1341
due to allopurinol, 1340
due to analgesics, 1339
analysis of cellular infiltrate in, 1331
due to antiviral agents, 1341
due to captopril, 1341
due to carbamazepine, 1340
causes of, 1331, 1332t
due to cephalosporin, 1336–1337
due to cimetidine, 1340
clinical renal features of, 1331
definition of, 1331
differential diagnosis of, 1331
due to diphenylhydantoin, 1340–1341
due to diuretics, 1340
due to drug therapy, 1332–1342
clinical and pathologic findings in, 1332–1336
clinical course in, 1334–1336
diagnosis of, 1341–1342
drugs associated with, 1332, 1333t
granulomas in, 1332, 1335f, 1335t
incidence of, 1332, 1333t
laboratory findings in, 1334
renal biopsy findings in, 1332, 1334, 1334f–1335f, 1335t
steroid therapy for, 1335–1336
due to erythromycin, 1337
due to ethambutol, 1337
due to fenoprofen, 1338
due to gentamicin, 1337
due to glafenin, 1339
due to Hantavirus nephropathy, 1343
hematuria in, 1331–1332
due to hemorrhagic fever with renal syndrome, 1343
idiopathic, 1344–1345
immunopathology of, 1665
incidence of, 1331
due to indomethacin, 1338
due to interferon, 1341
due to isoniazid, 1337
laboratory findings in, 1331
due to β-lactam antibiotics, 1332, 1334t, 1336, 1336t
due to leptospirosis, 1342–1343
in lymphoma, 1344
in malignancy, 1344
due to methicillin, 1336
due to netilmicin, 1337
nonoliguric acute renal failure in, 1297
due to NSAIDs, 1211–1212, 1212t, 1332, 1334t, 1337–1339
pathophysiology of, 1345–1347
antitubular basement membrane disease and, 1345–1346
cell-mediated tubulointerstitial disease and, 1346, 1347
experimental models of, 1345–1346
immune complex-mediated tubulointerstitial nephritis and, 1346, 1347
due to penicillin, 1336
due to penicillin derivatives, 1336
due to phenindione, 1341
due to polymyxin B, 1337
due to polymyxin E, 1337
due to propionic acid derivatives, 1338
proteinuria in, 1331–1332
due to rifampin, 1337
in sarcoid granulomatous nephritis, 1344
due to scarlet fever, 1343
due to septicemia, 1342
in Sjögren's syndrome, 1344, 2056–2057
due to spiramycin, 1337
due to sulfinpyrazone, 1339
due to sulfonamides, 1337
due to systemic infection, 1342–1344
in systemic lupus erythematosus, 1344
with uveitis, 1344f, 1344–1345
due to vancomycin, 1337
chronic, cadmium nephropathy in, 1243–1245, 1244f
megalocytic, 1345

Interstitium, renal
in cancer, 1168, 1169
cell types in, 35–37, 36f–37f
cortical, 35, 35f
volume of, 1959–1960
in diabetes mellitus, 2572
extracellular components of, 37
functional significance of, 1960–1963, 1961f–1962f
ammonium excretion and, 1962, 1962f
fibrosis and, 1962f, 1962–1963
inulin clearance and, 1961, 1961f
proteinuria and, 1963
renal plasma flow and, 1961, 1961f
urinary concentrating ability and, 1961–1962, 1962f
in malaria, 2341–2342, 2342f
medullary, 35
volume of, 1960
morphology of, 34–37
peritubular, 35
structural features of, 1959–1960
volume of, 35
Intracranial aneurysm, in autosomal dominant polycystic kidney disease, 553f, 553–554
Intrarenal baroreceptor(s), in sodium retention, 2457
Intrarenal reflux
historical, 692
in hydronephrosis, 659
in reflux nephropathy, 691–693, 692f
renal papillae and, 693
Intravenous urography. *See* Urography, intravenous
Intravesical chemotherapy, for urinary bladder carcinoma, 820–822, 821t
Inulin, molecular weight, radius, and renal handling of, 381t
Inulin clearance, 2410f
creatinine clearance vs., 366
for measurement of GFR, 364
Iron
in bone disease, 2760
complex deposits of, in sickle cell disease, 2325
deficiency of
erythropoiesis and, 2746
in Goodpasture's syndrome, 2744
in dietary therapy in chronic hemodialysis, 3183
overload of, in anemia, 2753
stores of, epoetin therapy and, 2750f, 2750–2751
Irradiation, total lymphoid, 2930
Ischemic renal injury, 1257–1277
biochemical and ionic disturbances in, 1258t
experimental studies on, 1257–1277
acidosis in, 1265–1266
activated platelets in, 1274
ADP in, 1257–1260
AMP in, 1257–1260
ATP in, 1257–1260, 1258f, 1260f
cell repair in, 1275–1276
cytoskeletal changes in, 1274–1275
endothelium in, 1270–1273
ion gradients in, 1260–1265
calcium ions and, 1263f, 1263–1265
magnesium ions and, 1265
potassium ions and, 1262f–1263f, 1262–1263
sodium ions and, 1261–1262
lactate dehydrogenase release in, 1265
mesangial cells in, 1274
model differences in, 1257
oxygen free radicals in, 1267–1270, 1269f, 1271f
phospholipases in, 1266–1267, 1268f
time-dependent changes in cellular Ca^{2+} in, 1276, 1276f
vascular smooth muscle in, 1273–1274
malaria and, 2342–2343
Isolated C3 disease, 1914
Isoniazid
acute interstitial nephritis due to, 1337
pharmacology of, normal vs. in renal failure, 3248t–3249t
for urinary tract tuberculosis, 923t
Isosorbide dinitrate, pharmacology of, normal vs. in renal failure, 3248t–3249t
Itai-itai disease, cadmium nephropathy and, 1243
Itraconazole, for candidiasis, 943

Jaundice
in acute tubular necrosis, 1304
in malarial renal failure, 2345
in renal failure, 2345
Jejunal urinary conduit, 828
Jugular vein, distention of, in heart failure, 2832
Juvenile rheumatoid arthritis
amyloidosis in, 2054–2055
renal disease in, 2054–2055
subsets of, 2054
Juxtaglomerular apparatus
afferent arteriole and granular cells in, 30, 32f
arterioles of, light microscopy examination of, 496, 497f–498f
extraglomerular mesangium in, 31, 32f
macula densa of, 30, 32f
morphology of, 29–32
peripolar cells in, 31
receptor mechanisms of, in renin release, 87
renin release by, 31–32, 303
structures of, 30, 32f
vascular anatomy of, 67, 68f
Juxtaglomerular tumor(s), angiography for, 475

Kallidin, in renal hemodynamics, 92
Kallikrein
in cirrhosis, 2471
metabolism of, 310–311
Kallikrein-kinin system, 310–312
actions of, 311
components of, 310, 310f
in end-stage renal disease, 2822–2823
in hepatorenal disease, 1358–1359
interactions of, with intrarenal neurohumoral systems, 93, 93f
interrelationships with other hormones and, 311–312
in malignant hypertension, 1583
in renal hemodynamics, 92–93, 93f, 311
salt and water excretion and, 311
in uremia, 2861
Kanamycin
chemical structure of, 1135f
pharmacology of, normal vs. in renal failure, 3248t–3249t
for urinary tract tuberculosis, 923t
Kaposi's sarcoma
in AIDS patients, 2361, 2366
as complication of transplantation, 2947t, 2948
Keratopathy, band, in hypercalcemia, 2625
Ketoacid, anions of, tubular reabsorption of, 2572
Ketoacidosis
anion gap in, 2577–2578, 2578f
diabetic. *See* Diabetic ketoacidosis
hypomagnesemia and, 2634
Ketoconazole
for candidiasis, 942
pharmacology of, normal vs. in renal failure, 3248t–3249t
Ketogenesis
diabetic, pathogenetic forces in, 2569t
hepatic, 2570
overview of, 2568
substrate delivery in, 2569, 2570
Ketone
consumption of, in diabetes mellitus, 2570, 2571f
renal handling of, 2571–2572
Ketone acid metabolism, pseudohyponatremia and, 2568
Ketone body(ies), 253, 253f
interplay of, 2570, 2571f
renal absorption and excretion of, 253
renal metabolism of, 253, 253f
Ketone precursors, 2570
Kidney(s)
ablation of, partial, 2716
abnormal, nonrenal neoplasms and, 266t, 2265–2278
aging and, 2405–2426. *See also* Elderly
anatomy of, 3, 4f. *See also specific anatomic parts*
antimicrobial defense mechanisms of, 896–897
cancer of. *See* Renal cell caricinoma
developmental physiology of, 2382–2383, 2383f, 2384t
diseased, hormonal modulation of, 2713–2716
ectopic
Bochdalek, 654
crossed fused, 653–654
superior (thoracic), 654
embryonic development of, 3–4, 648–650, 649f
handling of light chain proteins by, 2190–2191
horseshoe. *See* Horseshoe kidney
length of, ultrasonography for, 412
metastasis to, 2268
myeloma, 1169, 2195
anemia in, 2744
Page, 477
position of, intravenous urography for, 409
size of, 3
intravenous urography for, 409
supernumerary, 654
for transplantation. *See also* Allograft(s); Graft(s); Transplantation
cadaver, 2921–2922, 2922t
living donor, 2921–2922, 2922t
preservation of, 2923t, 2923–2924
ultrasonography of, technique for, 411f, 411–412
in urate overproduction, 2242–2248
Kidney stone. *See* Calculus(i), renal; Nephrolithiasis

Kidney transplantation. *See* Transplantation, renal
Kimmelstiel-Wilson lesions (nodular glomerulosclerosis), 2168t, 2169f, 2169–2170
Kinin, metabolism of, kininogen and, 311
Kininogen, kinin metabolism and, 311
Kock pouch, as urinary reservoir, 830, 830f

Labetalol
 for hypertension, 1623–1624, 2390t
  in neonates, 2386
 for moderate hypertension in pregnancy, 1524
 pharmacology of, normal vs. in renal failure, 3248t–3249t
 for severe hypertension in pregnancy, 1525–1526
Laboratory examination, of renal function, 361–392. *See also* Glomerular filtration rate (GFR)
β-Lactam antibiotics, acute interstitial nephritis due to, 1332, 1334t, 1336, 1336t
Lactate, renal metabolism of, 239, 239f
Lactate dehydrogenase, in experimental studies on ischemic renal injury, 1265
Lactic acidosis
 anion gap in, 2577, 2577t
 diabetes mellitus and, 2580f, 2580–2581
Lacuna magna, 639–640
Lamina densa, of glomerular basement membrane, 381
Lamina rara externa, of glomerular basement membrane, 381
Lamina rara interna, of glomerular basement membrane, 381
Landis-Pappenheimer relationship, 75
Laxative(s), idiopathic edema and, 2500
LDH, as tumor marker
 in seminoma, 870
 in testicular carcinoma, 861–862
LDL (low-density lipoprotein), 2849t, 2849–2850
Lead
 gout and, 2255–2256
 moonshine and, 2254–2255
Lead nephropathy, 1237–1242
 acute, 1239
  Fanconi syndrome and, 1239
 chronic, 1239–1241, 1240f
  childhood, 1239
  gout nephropathy and, 1241
  hypertension and, 1241
  due to "moonshine" consumption, 1239
  pathogenesis of, 1240
  renal biopsy findings in, 1240, 1240f
  renal function in, 1240–1241
  tubulointerstitial, 1973–1974
  types of lead exposure in, 1239
 diagnosis of, 1237–1239, 1238f
  blood lead concentration for, 1237–1238
  bone lead for, 1238, 1238f
  EDTA test for, 1238, 1238f
  in vivo tibial K x-ray fluorescence for, 1238f, 1238–1239
 gouty arthritis and, 2254–2255, 2256f
 historical, 1237
 hypertensive nephrosclerosis vs., 1442
 treatment of, 1241–1242
Lead poisoning
 chronic, malignant hypertension due to, 1561
 gouty arthritis and, 2254–2255
Legionella pneumonia, as complication of transplantation, 2946
Leiomyomatosis
 esophageal, in Alport syndrome, 581
 genital, in Alport syndrome, 581
Leiomyosarcoma, renal, 798–799
Leishmaniasis
 clinical course of, 2351
 pathogenesis of, 2350–2351
 pathology of, 2350, 2350f
 prognosis of, 2351
 renal involvement in, 2349–2351
Lenticonus, anterior, in Alport syndrome, 580, 580f
Leptospirosis, 2332, 2338–2339
 acute interstitial nephritis due to, 1342–1343
 upper urinary tract infection due to, 974
Leukemia
 acquired overproduction of urate associated with, 2244, 2245f–2246f
 acute myelomonocystic, hypophosphatemia in, 2275
 chronic lymphocytic, membranoproliferative glomerulonephritis and, 1830
 hairy cell, 2269f
 hyperphosphatemia in, 2274
 hypokalemia in, 2277–2278
 hypophosphatemia in, 2275, 2608
 lysozymuria in, 389
 nephrotic syndrome in, in pregnancy, 2268
 renal infiltration in, CT for, 455
 renal involvement in, 2270–2271
Leukocyte(s), urinalysis for, 336
Leukocyte adhesion molecule, 2002–2003, 2003t
Leukocyte cast(s), 348
 in upper urinary tract infection, 982
Leukocyte count, urine microscopy for, 339t, 339–340, 340f
Leukocyte esterase test, for bacteriuria, 1012
Leukocyte-endothelial adhesion, in vascular injury. *See also* Vascular injury
Leukoplakia, of urinary bladder, 815
Leukotriene(s)
 actions of, 309
 renal vasoconstrictor effects of, 92
 synthesis of, 90f, 92
LeVeen shunt, 2474
 in hepatorenal syndrome, 1365
Levodopa, pharmacology of, normal vs. in renal failure, 3248t–3249t
Liddle's syndrome, metabolic alkalosis in, 2686
Lidocaine, pharmacology of, normal vs. in renal failure, 3248t–3249t
Light chain(s)
 Bence Jones test for, 389
 excretion of, in tubular proteinuria, 388
 molecular weight and radius of, 381t
 in overproduction proteinuria, 388–389
 renal handling of, 384
Light chain cast nephropathy
 chronic tubulointerstitial, 1973
 factors influencing formation of, 2202t
 isoelectric point of, 2202–2203
 vs. light chain deposition disease, 2199
 membranoproliferative glomerulonephritis and, 1829–1830
 in multiple myeloma, 2195f, 2195–2196
 in proteinuria, 2193f, 2194
Light chain deposition disease
 clinical and laboratory features of, 2198–2199, 2199t
 vs. light chain cast nephropathy, 2199
 in multiple myeloma, 2196f–2198f, 2196–2199
 pathogenesis of, 2198
Light chain nephropathy. *See* Light chain cast nephropathy
Light chain proteinuria. *See* Proteinuria, light chain
Lincomycin, pharmacology of, normal vs. in renal failure, 3248t–3249t
Lipase, hormone-sensitive, in adipocytes, 2570
Lipid(s)
 in dietary therapy in acute renal failure, 3195
 in dietary therapy in chronic hemodialysis, 3179–3180
 status of, 2849–2850
 synthesis of, 2850
 in uremia, abnormalities of, 2849t
Lipid metabolism
 disorders of, in uremia, 2849t, 2849–2852
 in nephrotic syndrome, 1758f, 1758–1759
 in obstructive nephropathy, 675
Lipid-laden interstitial cell(s), cellular structure of, 36–37, 37f
Lipiduria
 in glomerulonephritis, quantitation of, 353, 354f
 urine microscopy in, 353, 353f–354f
Lipoid nephrosis, 1737
Lipomatosis, renal sinus, 410
Lipoprotein
 degradation of, 2850
 high-density, 2849, 2849t
 low-density, 2849t, 2849–2850
 very-low-density, 2849t, 2849–2850
Lipoprotein injury cycle, 2412f
Lipotropin, in uremia, 2863
Lipoxygenase pathway, 90, 90f
 products of, 309
Listeria monocytogenes, as complication of transplantation, 2947
Lithium
 for diabetes insipidus, 2511
 pharmacology of, normal vs. in renal failure, 3248t–3249t
 for SIADH secretion, 2527
Lithium-induced renal disease, 1099–1104
 acute changes in, 1099–1100
  renal functional abnormalities as, 1100
   renal water handling and, 1100
   urine acidification and, 1100
  reversible tubular effects as, 1099, 1100f
 chronic damage in, 1102–1104, 1103f
 clinical features of, 1102
 historical, 1099
 management of, 1104
 prevention or detection of, 1102
  renal function tests in, 1102
  serum lithium levels in, 1102

Lithium-induced renal disease—Continued
progressive damage in, 1101–1102
concentrating capacity and, 1101
GFR and, 1101
histologic studies of, 1101f, 1102
Littre's gland(s), ectatic ducts of, 639
Liver. *See also* Hepatitis
acute fatty, in pregnancy, 2301
baroreceptors of, in sodium retention, 2456–2457
cirrhosis of. *See* Cirrhosis
cysts of, in autosomal dominant polycystic kidney disease, 552f–553f, 552–553
fibrosis of, nephronophthisis-medullary cystic disease and, 517
gluconeogenesis in, 2563
impression of, intravenous urography for, 409
ketogenesis in, 2570
transplantation of, hepatorenal disease due to, 1359
Liver disease, 2465–2475. *See also* Hepatitis
acid-base balance in, 2475
calcium metabolism in, 2475
chronic, membranoproliferative glomerulonephritis and, 1831
in chronic hemodialysis, 3086–3087
edema formation in, 2465–2472
hypokalemia in, 2474–2475
hyponatremia in, 2472–2473, 2474
magnesium metabolism in, 2475
phosphorus metabolism in, 2475
potassium metabolism in, 2474–2475
in preeclampsia, 1516
sodium and water retention in
ascites formation in
overfill theory of, 2467f, 2467–2468
underfill theory of, 2466f, 2466–2467
effector mechanisms for, 2468–2471
aldosterone and, 2471
blood flow and, 2469
catecholamines and, 2469–2471
enhanced tubular reabsorption and, 2469
filtration fraction and, 2469
glomerular filtration rate and, 2469
kallikrein and, 2471
natriuretic factors and, 2471
nephron sites and, 2468–2469
norepinephrine and, 2469–2471
peritubular physical factors and, 2469
prostaglandins and, 2471
renal nervous system and, 2469–2471
peripheral arterial vasodilation with, 2468, 2469f
stimulus for, 2465–2468
treatment of, 2473–2474
Liver function
in autosomal dominant polycystic kidney disease, 550
in renal cell carcinoma, 786
Living donor kidney, for transplantation
evaluation of, 2921–2922, 2922t
removal of, 2922
Lobar infarct, imaging studies in, 427, 427f
Lobe(s), renal, embryonic development of, 650
Lobule(s), renal
anatomy of, 6
embryonic development of, 650
Lomustine nephrotoxicity, 1174, 1176
Loop diuretic(s). *See* Diuretic(s), loop
Loop of Henle
ascending limb of
decreased NaCl reabsorption in, urine dilution and, 377
fluid conservation and excretion in, 374
urea in, 135
calcium absorption in, 2620
countercurrent multiplication theory and, 128f–129f, 128–130
descending limb of, fluid conservation and excretion in, 374
impaired solute transport in, elderly and, 2416
morphology of, 21–23
net acid transport in, 213f, 215–216
ammonium and, 216
bicarbonate and, 215–216
titratable acidity and, 216
potassium transport in, 185, 2649
regions of, 4, 5f
sodium transport in, as function of perfusion rate, 152f, 152–153
straight part of proximal tubule, cellular structure of, 18f, 21–22
thick ascending limb of
acid-base transport in, summary and integration of, 226, 227f
cortical, transport properties of, 154t
electrophysiologic parameters of, 154t
function of, 130
medullary, transport properties of, 154t
potassium transport in, cellular mechanisms of, 190–191, 191f
sodium absorption in, 154–160
ADH and, 158t, 158–159
adrenergic agents and, 159
apical K^+ conductance in, 156–157, 157f
apical Na^+-K^+-$2Cl^-$ co-transport in, 156
basolateral membrane Cl^- transport in, 156–157, 157f
general features of, 154t–155t, 154–156, 155f
glucagon and, 159
mineralocorticoids and, 159–160
origin of transepithelial voltage in, 158
osmolality and, 159
peptide hormones and, 159
prostaglandins and, 159
regulation of, 158–160
synchronous Na^+-H^+-Cl^-/HCO_3^- exchange in, 157–158
structure of, 152
thin ascending limb of, 22
countercurrent multiplication in, 130–131, 131f
sodium transport in, 153t, 153–154
structure of, 152
thin descending limb of
in long-looped nephrons, 22
in short-looped nephrons, 22
sodium transport in, 153t, 153–154
structure of, 152
thin limb of
sodium-potassium-ATPase and basolateral membrane in, 45
types of, 22
Lorazepam, pharmacology of, normal vs. in renal failure, 3250t–3251t
Low-density lipoprotein (LDL), 2849t, 2849–2850
Low-pressure baroreceptor(s), in sodium retention, 2456
Lung cancer
diffuse membranous glomerulopathy in, 2266
nephrotic syndrome in, 2265
SIADH secretion associated with, 2522–2524
Lupus anticoagulant, 2022
Lupus erythematosus, systemic, 2019–2034
autoantibody mechanisms in, 2019, 2020f
in children, 2028–2029
clinical features of, 2019–2021
diagnosis of, 2019
in elderly, 2028–2029
membranoproliferative glomerulonephritis and, 1828
membranous nephropathy and, 1796
natural course of, 2019–2021
nephritis in. *See* Lupus nephritis
pregnancy and, 2030–2031, 2304
prognosis in, 1940–1945
actuarial survival tables in, 1941, 1942t
age at onset and, 1941
causes of death vs., 1941
childhood disease and, 1941–1942
extensive subendothelial deposits and, 1944
histologic activity and chronicity and, 1944t, 1944–1945
histologic findings and, 1944
hypertension and, 1943
indices of lupus activity and, 1944
race and, 1943
renal biopsies and, 1944
renal pathology scoring system in, 1944t, 1944–1945
severity of nephritis and, 1943
sex and, 1942–1943
tubulointerstitial changes in, 1944
renal transplantation and, 2917
renal tubular potassium and, 2657
Lupus nephritis, 2021–2034
acute interstitial, 1344
after renal transplantation, 2030
assessment of severity and chronicity in, 2027
classifications of, 2022–2026, 2023t
class I, 2023, 2023f
class II, 2023–2024, 2024f
class III, 2024f, 2024–2025
class IV, 2025f, 2025–2026
class V, 2026, 2026f
mixed patterns and transformation in, 2026
clinical and pathologic correlations in, 2027–2028
glomerular sclerosis and interstitial fibrosis in, 2028
location of electron-dense deposits in, 2028
disease activity in, antinuclear antibodies, complement, and immune complexes in, 2029
end-stage renal disease in, clinical SLE and, 2030
immunofluorescence findings in, 2026
immunopathology of, 1661–1662

membranous, 1789
murine, 1654
pathogenesis of, 2021–2022
anticardiolipin antibodies in, 2022
autoantibodies in, 2021
immune complex accumulation in, 2022
lupus anticoagulant in, 2022
platelet factors in, 2021–2022
percutaneous renal biopsy for, 489
silent, 2029
treatment of, 2031–2034
ancrod in, 2033
eicosapentaenoic acid in, 2033
glucocorticoids in, 2031
immunosuppressive agents in, 2032–2033
immunotherapy in, 2033–2034
plasmapheresis in, 2033
total lymphoid irradiation in, 2033
tubulointerstitial, 2026
vascular lesions in, 2027
Lupus-like syndrome, drug-induced, 2029–2030
Luteinizing hormone, in idiopathic edema, 2495
Lymph, hepatic, formation vs. removal of, 2465–2466
Lymphatic capillary(ies)
macromolecular and fluid reabsorption by, 79
morphology of, 35
Lymphatic system
anatomy of, 35
cancer of, renal involvement in, 2270–2271
Lymphocele, as complication of transplantation, 2942
Lymphocyte(s), T. *See* T lymphocyte(s).
Lymphocyte-mediated cytotoxicity, allograft response and, 2884, 2884f
Lymphocytosis, peritoneal, 3005
Lymphoid irradiation, total, 2930
Lymphoma
acute interstitial nephritis in, 1344
Burkitt's
hyperphosphatemia and, 2274, 2613
tumor lysis syndrome and, 2274, 2274t
as complication of transplantation, 2947t, 2948
Hodgkin's, antiglomerular basement membrane antibody-mediated nephritis and, 1868
hyperphosphatemia and, 2613
metastatic, in chronic tubulointerstitial nephropathy, 1973
nephrotic syndrome in, 2267–2268
non-Hodgkin's, membranoproliferative glomerulonephritis and, 1830
renal, 2270
angiography for, 476–477
CT for, 455
management of, 2270–2271
ultrasonography for, 429, 429f
Lymphomatoid granulomatosis, 2113
Lymphotoxin, in hypercalcemia of malignancy, 2272
Lypressin, for diabetes insipidus, 2508t
Lysinuria, 617
Lysosome(s)
in aminoglycoside nephrotoxicity, 1132, 1133f, 1143–1147, 1144f–1147f
in nephrotoxicity, 1061–1066. *See also* Nephrotoxicity
Lysozyme, molecular weight, radius, and renal handling of, 381t
Lysozymuria
in cancer, renal complications of, 1170
hypokalemia and, 2277
in leukemia, 389
in tubular proteinuria, 388

Macroglobulinemia, Waldenström's
clinical features of, 2206–2208, 2207, 2207f
hyperviscosity syndrome in, 2207–2208
Macrophage(s), interstitial, 36f, 37
Macula densa
anatomy of, 4–5
cellular structure of, 30, 32f
receptor mechanisms of, in renin release, 87–88
sodium chloride delivery to, renin release and, 1416
Macular lesion(s), in Alport syndrome, 580
Magnesium, 2630–2635. *See also* Hypermagnesemia; Hypomagnesemia
balance of, 2631, 2631f
in continuous ambulatory peritoneal dialysis, 3176–3177, 3177t
body stores of, 2630–2631
decreased intake of, hypomagnesemia secondary to, 2634
deficiency of, digitalis action and, 2634
in dietary therapy in chronic hemodialysis, 3181
excretion of, in urinary tract obstruction, 673
metabolism of
alterations in, treatment for, 2635
in cirrhosis, 2475
in regulation of PTH secretion, 2630
renal handling of, 2631–2632, 2632f
in vascular reactivity in preeclampsia, 1513
Magnesium chloride, for hypomagnesemia, 2635
Magnesium ion(s)
in experimental studies on ischemic renal injury, 1265
mitochondrial effects of, 1046–1047
Magnesium oxide, for hypomagnesemia, 2635
Magnesium sulfate
for convulsion in eclampsia, 1526–1527
for eclampsia, 2297
for hypomagnesemia, 2635
Magnetic resonance imaging (MRI), 456–461
for acute glomerulonephritis, 459, 459f
for acute renal vein thrombosis in nephrotic syndrome, 1326
for congenital anatomic variants, 458
contrast media for, 457–458
CT vs., 461
for nephrolithiasis, 458
for normal anatomy, 457, 457f
for obstructive disease, 458, 458f
for pheochromocytoma, 1496, 1496f
for renal cell carcinoma, 459–460, 460f–461f
for renal cystic disease, 458, 459f
for renal failure, 459
for renal inflammatory disease, 458
for renal neoplasms, 459–460, 460f–461f
for renal transplantation, 459, 460f
for renal vascular disease, 458–459
technical considerations in, 456–457
of transplanted kidney, 2933, 2936f
for urinary tract obstruction, 679
Major histocompatibility complex (MHC), 2879–2881
Malabsorption, hypophosphatemia and, 2607
Malakoplakia, renal, 998
Malaria
falciparum, 2339–2345
acid-base disturbances in, 2340
acute intravascular hemolysis in, 2340
acute renal failure in, 2340
catecholamine activity in, 2343
cytokines in, 2343
disseminated intravascular coagulation in, 2344
endotoxemia in, 2343
fluid and electrolyte disturbances in, 2339–2340
glomerular lesions in, 2341, 2341f
pathogenesis of, 2342
glomerulonephritis in, 2340
hemorrheologic changes in, 2344
hyperbilirubinemia in, 2345
hyperkalemia in, 2339–2340
hypernatremia in, 2339
hypervolemia in, 2343
hyponatremia in, 2339
hypophosphatemia in, 2340
hypovolemia in, 2343
inflammatory effects in, 2343
intravascular hemolysis and, 2344–2345
kidney disease in, 2339–2345
parasitemia and, 2340–2341
parasitized erythrocytes in, 2344, 2344f
pathogenesis of, 2342–2345
pathology of, 2341–2342
tubulointerstitial changes in, 2341–2342, 2342f
vascular changes in, 2342
kidney disease in, 2339–2346
Plasmodium causing, 2339
quartan, 2345–2346
kidney disease in, 2345–2346
clinical manifestations of, 2345–2346
pathogenesis of, 2346
pathology of, 2346
Malignancy. *See also* Cancer; Tumor(s); *specific neoplasms*
acquired overproduction of urate associated with, 2244, 2245f–2246f
diabetes insipidus and, 2505
humoral hypercalcemia of, 2625–2626
hypercalcemia secondary to, 2625–2626
SIADH secretion associated with, 2522–2524
Malignant hypertension, 1555–1629
accelerated vs., 1562
acute pulmonary edema in, 1600–1603, 1601f–1602f
pathophysiology of, 1600–1602, 1601f–1602f
treatment of, 1602–1603
due to aldosterone-producing adenoma, 1561
due to analgesic nephropathy, 1560
due to Ask-Upmark kidney, 1560
asymptomatic presentation in, 1562
benign vs., 1593–1594
cardiac manifestations of, 1569
due to chronic glomerulonephritis, 1560, 1576

Malignant hypertension—Continued
due to chronic lead poisoning, 1561
due to chronic pyelonephritis, 1560, 1576
clinical features of, 1562–1570
due to congenital adrenal hyperplasia, 1561
due to congenital unilateral renal hypoplasia, 1560
due to Cushing's syndrome, 1561
de novo, 1559
definition of, 1555
electrolyte abnormalities in, 1570
epidemiology of, 1561–1562
age in, 1561
gender in, 1561
preceding duration of benign hypertension in, 1562
race in, 1561–1562
smoking as risk factor in, 1562
etiologies of, 1559t, 1559–1561
fundoscopic manifestations of, 1563–1567
accelerated hypertension and, 1566–1567
cotton-wool spots in, 1565f, 1566
diagnostic guidelines in, 1567
Elschnig's spots in, 1566, 1566f
hypertensive choroidopathy in, 1566, 1566f
hypertensive neuroretinopathy in, 1565f, 1565–1566
Keith and Wagener classification in, 1563–1564
macular star figure in, 1565f, 1566
papilledema in, 1566–1567, 1567f
retinal arteriosclerosis in, 1564f, 1564t, 1564–1565
striate hemorrhages in, 1565, 1565f
gastrointestinal manifestations of, 1569
acute abdomen in, 1569
acute pancreatitis in, 1569
hematologic manifestations of, 1569
historical, 1407–1408, 1557–1558
due to IgG myeloma, 1561
incidence of, 1561
level of blood pressure in, 1563, 1563f
natural history of, 1558–1559
neurologic manifestations of, 1568–1569
due to oral contraceptives, 1560
pathologic findings in, 1570–1577
adrenal, 1577
cardiac, 1577
distribution of vascular lesions in, 1577
gastrointestinal, 1577
ophthalmic, 1577
pulmonary, 1577
renal, 1570–1577
accelerated glomerular obsolescence in, 1573, 1574f–1575f, 1575
antihypertensive therapy and, 1575–1576
fibrinoid necrosis of afferent arteriole in, 1570f, 1570–1571
focal and segmental fibrinoid glomerular necrosis in, 1573
interlobular arteries in, 1571, 1571f–1572f
juxtaglomerular hypertension in, 1575
musculomucoid intimal hyperplasia in, 1571, 1573f
myointimal cell in, 1571, 1573
pathophysiology of, 1577–1585, 1584f
dietary potassium in, 1582
endothelin in, 1583
endothelium-derived relaxing factor in, 1583
fibrinoid necrosis in, 1583
glucocorticoids in, 1582–1583
immunologic mechanisms in, 1583
intracellular calcium in, 1582
kallikrein-kinin system in, 1583
localized intravascular coagulation in, 1581–1582
proliferative endarteritis in, 1583
prostacyclin in, 1582
renin-angiotensin axis in, 1579–1580
role of increased blood pressure per se in, 1577–1578
vasculotoxic theory in, 1578–1579
vasopressin in, 1580–1581
volume depletion in, 1581
due to polyarteritis nodosa, 1560, 1576–1577
presenting symptoms in, 1562–1563
headache as, 1562
visual symptoms as, 1562–1563
weight loss as, 1563
primary (essential), 1559
due to radiation nephritis, 1560
due to renal cholesterol embolization syndrome, 1560
renal manifestations of, 1567–1568
hematuria in, 1568
protein excretion in, 1568
pyuria in, 1568
renal size in, 1568
spectrum of, 1568
renin-angiotensin-aldosterone axis in, 1569–1570
due to renovascular hypertension, 1560
due to scleroderma renal crisis, 1560–1561, 1577
secondary, 1559–1561
evaluation of, 1592–1593
renal biopsy in, 1592–1593
renal pathology in, 1576–1577
therapeutic response in, 1588–1592
mechanism of recovery of renal function and, 1592
prognostic significance of renal function and, 1589–1592, 1590f
reversal of hypertensive neuroretinopathy and, 1592
treated vs. untreated patients and, 1588–1589, 1589f
treatment of, 1585–1588
indications for, 1585, 1586t
long-term management in, 1588
nephrectomy in, 1587–1588
oral therapy in, 1586, 1588
parenteral therapy in, 1586
in renal insufficiency, 1587
volume status and diuretics in, 1586–1587
untreated prognosis in, 1558–1559
Malnutrition
in acute renal failure, 1383
in chronic renal failure, causes of, 3167–3169, 3169t
hypophosphatemia and, 2607
protein, in chronic renal failure, 2395
protein-calorie, in chronic renal failure, 3167, 3168t
in uremia, 2853–2855
Mannitol, in protection against nephrotoxicity, 1066–1067
Meatal stenosis, penile, 640
Mebendazole, pharmacology of, normal vs. in renal failure, 3250t–3251t
Mediterranean fever, familial, 2222
classification of, 2223t
renal transplantation and, 2916
Medulla, renal
anatomy of, 3, 4f
inner, countercurrent multiplication in, 130–135, 131f–134f
interstitium of, 35, 1960
net acid transport in, 218–219
ammonium and, 218
bicarbonate and, 218–219
oxygen gradient between cortex and, 233, 234f, 235
subdivisions of, 3, 5f
tonicity of, effect on urine concentration of, 375–376
Medullary blood flow, regulation of, 100
angiotensin II in, 100
atrial natriuretic peptide in, 100
kinins in, 100
prostaglandins in, 100
vasopressin in, 100
Medullary cyst, simple, 521, 522f
Medullary cystic disease, 513, 514t. *See also* Nephronophthisis–medullary cystic disease
autosomal dominant polycystic kidney disease vs., 547
gout in, 2257
hyperuricemia and, 2257
Medullary microtophus(i), in gout, 2258–2259
Medullary ray(s), renal, anatomy of, 3
Medullary sponge kidney, 525–532
autosomal dominant polycystic kidney disease vs., 547
autosomal recessive polycystic kidney disease vs., 531
calyceal diverticula vs., 531
clinical features in, 526–527
hematuria as, 527
hypertension as, 527
nephrolithiasis as, 527
urinary tract infection as, 527
congenital abnormalities associated with, 525
congenital hemihypertrophy and, 525
course prognosis, treatment in, 531–532
differential diagnosis of, 531
hereditary basis of, 525
historical, 525
hypercalciuria in, 528–529
causes of, 528–529
parathyroid hormone and, 528–529
prevalence of, 528
imaging studies of, 424–425, 425f
papillary necrosis vs., 531
pathogenesis of, 525–526
congenital anomalies as, 525
defective acidification as, 525–526
hereditary factors as, 525
stone formation in, 526
urine apatite excretion in, 526
urine oxalate excretion in, 526
pathologic findings in, 525, 526f
prevalence of, 526–527
pyelotubular stasis vs., 531
pyelovenous backflow vs., 531

radiographic diagnosis of, 529f–530f, 529–531
characteristic findings in, 529, 529f
difficulties of, 529–531, 530f
lesions simulating, 530
papillary blush in, 530f, 530–531
preliminary x-ray film in, 529, 530f
renal function in, 527–528
potassium balance in, 528
sodium excretion in, 527–528
urinary acidification and, 527
urine concentrating capacity and, 527
renal tuberculosis vs., 531
Megacalyx(ces), imaging studies of, 425
Megalocytic interstitial nephritis, 1345
Megalourethra, diffuse nonobstructive, 639, 640f
Megaureter, 645–646
classification of, 645
nonreflux, nonobstructed, 645–646
primary obstructed, 645, 646
reflux, 645
Melphalan, for amyloidosis, 2224
Membrane amplification principle, in transcellular transport, 40–41
Membrane phospholipid metabolism, in nephrotoxicity, 1056–1057
Membrane transport, 139–142
active transport processes in, 141f, 141–142
convective processes in, 141
diffusion processes in, 139–140, 140f
facilitated diffusion in, 141
membrane properties and, 139, 140f
Membranoproliferative glomerulonephritis. *See* Glomerulonephritis, membranoproliferative
Membranous glomerulopathy
acute renal vein thrombosis in, 1319, 1320t
in cancer, 1169
in polymyositis-dermatomyositis, 2058
in rheumatoid arthritis, 2050–2051
Membranous nephropathy, 1785–1801
after renal transplantation, 1797–1798
age and sex in, 1793
antiglomerular basement membrane antibody-mediated nephritis and, 1868
captopril and, 1796
in childhood, 1793–1794
course of, 1798–1799
diabetes mellitus and, 1796
drugs and, 1795–1796
geographic locations of, 1793
gold therapy and, 1795
hepatitis B and, 1795
hereditary, 1794
historical, 1785
immunopathology of, 1657f, 1657–1658
incidence of, 1793
infection and, 1795
lupus erythematosus and, 1796
malignancy and, 1794–1795
mercury exposure and, 1796
nonsteroidal prostaglandin antagonists and, 1796
pathogenesis of, 1789–1793
brush-border antigens in, 1792
causative antigens in, 1792–1793
circulating immune complex hypothesis in, 1789–1790
complement in, 1791
DNA antigens in, 1792
hepatitis antigens in, 1792
Heymann model in, 1790
host susceptibility in, 1791
in situ immune complex formation in, 1790
immunogenetics in, 1791–1792
physical properties of deposited antigens in, 1790–1791
thyroid antigens in, 1792
tumor antigens in, 1792–1793
pathologic findings in, 1785–1789, 1798–1799
atypical, 1789
electron microscopy in, 1785, 1786f–1788f, 1789
immunofluorescence microscopy in, 1789, 1789f
light microscopy in, 1785, 1786f
penicillamine and, 1795–1796
prognosis in, 1916–1919
in children, 1919
histologic findings and, 1919, 1920f
HLA type and, 1919
relapse rate and, 1918
reversible decline in function and, 1919
therapeutic trials and, 1918–1919
in untreated patients, 1917f–1918f, 1917–1918
prognostic factors in, 1799
proteinuria in
asymptomatic, 1794
selective, 1794
remissions in, 1798
renal failure in, 1798
renal transplantation and, 2917, 2918f
renal vein thrombosis and, 1796–1797
rheumatoid arthritis and, 1795
secondary, 1789
sickle cell disease and, 1796
thyroid disease and, 1796
transformation of, 1797
treatment of, 1799–1801
corticosteroid, 1799–1800
cytotoxic, 1800–1801
general, 1799
Meningoencephalitis, as complication of transplantation, 2946–2947
Meningomyelocele, vesicoureteral reflux due to, 694
Meperidine, pharmacology of, normal vs. in renal failure, 3250t–3251t
Meprobamate, pharmacology of, normal vs. in renal failure, 3250t–3251t
Mercaptopurine, pharmacology of, normal vs. in renal failure, 3250t–3251t
Mercuric chloride, as nephrotoxin, 1043
Mercury poisoning, 1245–1248
acute tubular necrosis due to, 1246–1247
diagnosis of, 1245
membranous nephropathy and, 1796
Minimata disease due to, 1247
nephrotic syndrome due to, 1247, 1247f
renal manifestations of, 1245, 1246f
treatment of, 1247–1248
Mesangial cell(s)
contents of, 12
contraction or relaxation of, mechanisms of, 71f, 71–72
in experimental studies on ischemic renal injury, 1274
in phagocytosis, 14
processes of, GBM and, 10f, 12
Mesangial expansion, clinicopathologic correlations in, 503
Mesangial glomerulonephritis
prognosis in, 1913–1914
urinary findings in, 353–354, 354f
Mesangial glomerulopathy, in rheumatoid arthritis, 2050–2051
Mesangial IgM nephropathy, 1737
Mesangial interposition, clinicopathologic correlations of, 504, 506f
Mesangial lysis, light microscopy evaluation of, 496, 497f
Mesangiocapillary glomerulonephritis. *See* Glomerulonephritis, membranoproliferative
Mesangium
anatomy of, 6, 9f–10f
capillary tuft and, 13–14
cellular structure of, 12–14
contractility of, 13–14
expansion of, in diabetic nephropathy, 2170–2171, 2171f, 2171t
extraglomerular, 29–30
light microscopy evaluation of, 495–496, 497f
matrix of, 13
in schistosomal nephropathy, 2347, 2348f
Mesoblastic nephroma, angiography for, 477
Mesonephric duct, normal embryologic development of, 637
Mesonephros, embryonic development of, 4, 642–643, 643f
Metabolic acidosis
acute, ammoniagenesis in, 246f–248f, 246–248, 247t
in acute tubular necrosis, 1307
ammoniagenesis in, 243
chronic, ammoniagenesis in, 248–249
diabetes mellitus and
with elevated anion gap, 2577t, 2577–2581
general features of, 2576–2577, 2577f
with normal anion gap, 2577t, 2581–2582
hyperchloremic, renal tubular potassium and, 2657–2658
in loss of nephron function, 2669–2685
in multiple myeloma, 2201
uremic, 2728–2729
pathogenesis of, 2729–2731
Metabolic alkalosis
in Bartter's syndrome, 2684, 2686
chloride-resistant, 2686
chloride-responsive, 2685–2686
classification of, 2582t
diabetes mellitus and, 2582–2583
hypokalemic, in malignant hypertension, 1570
in Liddle's syndrome, 2686
miscellaneous causes of, 2686
in renal disease, 2684–2686
secondary to alkali administration, 2684–2685
Metabolism
acetone, 2579
arachidonate, in nephrotoxicity, 1037
arachidonic acid, in renal vasculature, 90–91

Metabolism—Continued
cadmium, 1242
carbohydrate. *See* Carbohydrate metabolism
cellular, in extracellular fluid acid-base balance, 209
cyclic nucleotide, in renal hypertrophy, 2710
cysteine, in nephrotoxicity, 1038
disorders of, renal transplantation and, 2915
DNA, in renal hypertrophy, 2710
epinephrine, 1488–1489, 1489f
fatty acid, compartmentation in, 251f–252f, 251–252
glutamine. *See* Glutamine metabolism
glutathione, in nephrotoxicity, 1038
ketone acid, pseudohyponatremia and, 2568
lipid, 2849–2852
in nephrotic syndrome, 1758f, 1758–1759
in obstructive nephropathy, 675
magnesium, in cirrhosis, 2475
membrane phospholipid, in nephrotoxicity, 1056–1057
mineral, in protein restriction in experimental renal failure, 3138
norepinephrine, 1488–1489, 1489f
phosphate, in experimental renal disease, 2719
phospholipid, in renal hypertrophy, 2710
potassium. *See* Potassium metabolism
protein. *See* Protein metabolism
renal, 233–253. *See also* Renal metabolism
RNA, in renal hypertrophy, 2710–2711
trace metal, in nephrotic syndrome, 1762
tubular cell energy, in nephrotoxicity, 1045–1050
urea, 370
uric acid, in acute tubular necrosis, 1307
vitamin D, in primary hypophosphatemic rickets, 619
xanthine oxidase, in nephrotoxicity, 1037–1038
Metallothionein(s), in protection against nephrotoxicity, 1069
Metanephros, embryonic development of, 4, 642–643, 643f
Methadone, pharmacology of, normal vs. in renal failure, 3250t–3251t
Methaqualone, pharmacology of, normal vs. in renal failure, 3250t–3251t
Methenamine, pharmacology of, normal vs. in renal failure, 3250t–3251t
Methicillin
acute interstitial nephritis due to, 1336
pharmacology of, normal vs. in renal failure, 3250t–3251t
Methotrexate
nephrotoxicity of, 1176–1177
clinical course in, 1177
pathogenesis of, 1176f, 1176–1177
pharmacology of, normal vs. in renal failure, 3250t–3251t
phase specificity and mechanism of action of, 821t
Methyldopa
for hypertension, 1627, 2296
for moderate hypertension in pregnancy, 1523, 1523t
pharmacology of, normal vs. in renal failure, 3250t–3251t
Methylprednisolone, in immunosuppression, 2896
Methylprylon, pharmacology of, normal vs. in renal failure, 3250t–3251t
Metolazone, pharmacology of, normal vs. in renal failure, 3250t–3251t
Metoprolol, pharmacology of, normal vs. in renal failure, 3250t–3251t
Metronidazole, pharmacology of, normal vs. in renal failure, 3250t–3251t
Mevinolin, effect of, on proteinuria and focal glomerulosclerosis, 2409, 2413f
Mexiletine, pharmacology of, normal vs. in renal failure, 3250t–3251t
Mezlocillin, pharmacology of, normal vs. in renal failure, 3252t–3253t
MHC (major histocompatibility complex), 2879–2881
Miconazole
for candidiasis, 942
pharmacology of, normal vs. in renal failure, 3252t–3253t
Microalbuminuria
acute reversible, 2165
Gentofte-Montecatini Convention definition of, 2164, 2165t
measurement of, 390, 2155
pathogenesis of, 2164, 2165t
persistent, 2166
Microangiopathy, thrombotic, renal, clinicopathologic correlations of, 505
β-2-Microglobulin
in chronic renal failure, 3132
deposition of, in bone disease, 2763
excretion of, in cadmium nephropathy, 1242–1243
metabolism of, 2225
in sickle cell disease, 2320
in uremia, 2766
β-Microglobulin amyloidosis. *See* Dialysis-related amyloidosis
Microtophus(i), medullary, in gout, 2258–2259
Microvascular thrombosis, 2063–2070. *See also* Hemolytic-uremic syndrome; Thrombosis, microvascular; Thrombotic thrombocytopenic purpura
Micturition, disorders of, 759–771. *See also* Urinary tract dysfunction, lower
Milk-alkali syndrome, hypercalcemia and, 2628
Mineral(s)
in dietary therapy in acute renal failure, 3195
in dietary therapy in renal transplantation, 3199
metabolism of, in protein restriction in experimental renal failure, 3138
Mineralization front, 2605, 2617
Mineralocorticoid(s), 297–299
deficiency of
in adrenal insufficiency, 2547–2548
in anterior pituitary insufficiency, 2554–2555, 2556f
role of vasopressin in, 2548, 2548f
vasopressin-independent effects of, 2548–2549, 2549f
diminished activity of, syndromes of, 2587f
in hydrogen ion transport, 298–299
in hyperkalemia, 2659
major renal actions of, 297
potassium regulation and, 2647–2648
in potassium transport, 297–298, 298f
receptors for, 297
in sodium absorption, in thick ascending limb of Henle, 159–160
in sodium transport, 297
Mineralocorticoid excess syndrome(s), mimicking primary aldosteronism, 1481–1482
Mineralocorticoid-induced hypertension, 1475, 1476f
Minimal change glomerular disease. *See* Nephrotic syndrome, minimal change.
Minimal change nephrotic syndrome. *See* Nephrotic syndrome, minimal change.
Minimata disease, due to mercury poisoning, 1247
Minocycline
acute interstitial nephritis due to, 1337
pharmacology of, normal vs. in renal failure, 3252t–3253t
Minoxidil
in end-stage renal disease, 2824
for hypertension, 1625–1626, 2390t
pharmacology of, normal vs. in renal failure, 3252t–3253t
Mithramycin
for hypercalcemia, 2629, 2630t
nephrotoxicity of, 1178–1179
Mitochondria
in aminoglycoside nephrotoxicity, 1149–1150
in brain, 2797–2798
in nephrotoxicity, 1045–1050. *See also* Nephrotoxicity
oxidative phosphorylation in, 236, 236f–237f
of proximal convoluted tubule, 16–17, 17f–21f
substrates and carriers of, 234, 234t
Mitomycin C
causing renal failure, in AIDS patients, 2364
intravesical, for urinary bladder carcinoma, 822
microvascular thrombosis due to, 2066
nephrotoxicity of, 1178
pharmacology of, normal vs. in renal failure, 3252t–3253t
phase specificity and mechanism of action of, 821t
Mitoxantrone, pharmacology of, normal vs. in renal failure, 3252t–3253t
Mixed connective tissue disease, 2030
Monoamine oxidase inhibitor interactions, hypertensive crisis in, 1615–1616
Monoclonal antibody(ies)
in immunosuppression, 2902–2903, 2903t, 2929t, 2929–2930
MRC OX-8, 2890
Monoclonal gammopathy(ies), diagnosis of, 2209t
Monoclonal gammopathy of undetermined significance (MGUS), 2208–2209
vs. smoldering myeloma, 2208
Mononucleosis, infectious, renal manifestations of, 998
Monosodium urate monohydrate (MSUM). *See* Urate

Monozygotic twins, renal transplant results in, 2938
Moonshine, lead nephropathy due to, 2254–2255
Moricizine, pharmacology of, normal vs. in renal failure, 3252t–3253t
Morphine
 pharmacology of, normal vs. in renal failure, 3252t–3253t
 in renal disease, complications of, 3231
Motor nerve conduction, slowing of, in toxic neuropathies, 2805
Motor nerve conduction velocity (MNCV) test, 2804
Moxalactam, pharmacology of, normal vs. in renal failure, 3252t–3253t
mRHA, erythropoietin-specific, 2743
MRI. *See* Magnetic resonance imaging (MRI)
MSUM (monosodium urate monohydrate). *See* Urate
Mucoprotein, Tamm-Horsfall, 2190. *See also* Tamm-Horsfall protein
Mucormycosis, opportunistic, 946t–947t, 946–947
Multiple myeloma, 2194–2206
 amyloidosis and, 2200
 clinical features of, 2194
 as contraindication to urography, 408
 contrast media-induced acute renal failure and, 1190
 diagnosis of, 2194
 electrolyte abnormalities in, 2201
 Fanconi syndrome and, 2200
 hyperammonemia in, 2201
 hypercalcemia in, 2199, 2201
 hyperkalemia in, 2200
 hyperuricemia in, 2201
  complications from, 2199
 immunochemical classes of, 2190t
 incidence of, 2194
 infection and, susceptibility to, 2199–2200
 light chain deposition disease in, 2196f–2198f, 2196–2199, 2199t
 light chain nephropathy in, 2195f, 2195–2196
 light chain proteinuria in, 2194–2195
 metabolic acidosis in, 2201
 nephrotic syndrome and, 2200
 pseudohyperphosphatemia in, 2201
 pseudohyponatremia in, 2201
 renal, fluid, and electrolyte disturbances associated with, 2190t
 renal biopsy in, indications for, 2200
 renal concentrating defects in, 2200
 renal failure in, 2202–2204
  acute, 2204
  chronic, 2203–2204
  pathogenesis of, 2202–2203
  prevention of, 2205
  reversibility of, 2204t
 renal function in, 2200
 renal morphology in, 2195–2220
 treatment of, 2205–2206
 tubular disorders in, 2200
 urologic manifestations in, 2205
Mumps, renal manifestations of, 998
Muscle, skeletal, in hypophosphatemia, 2608–2609
Muzolimine, mechanism of action of, 2442–2443
Mycetoma, 946
Mycobacterial infection, as complication of transplantation, 2946
Mycobacterium tuberculosis, 909–910
Mycoplasma fermentans antigen, in HIV-associated nephropathy, 2369–2370
Mycoplasma hominis, in upper urinary tract infection, 974
Mycoses, 944–947. *See also* Candidiasis
 cutaneous, 944, 946
 endemic, renal manifestations of, 944, 945t–946t
 opportunistic, 946t–947t, 946–947
 primary (systemic), 944
 subcutaneous, 946
Myelinolysis, central pontine, 2525
Myelodysplasia, vesicoureteral reflux due to, 694
Myeloma
 chronic renal failure in, 1169
 IgG, malignant hypertension due to, 1561
 multiple. *See* Multiple myeloma
 smoldering, 2208
Myeloma cast nephropathy, 2195
 chronic tubulointerstitial, 1973
 Tamm-Horsfall protein in, 2203
Myeloma kidney, 1169, 2195
 anemia in, 2744
Myocardial calcification, 2762
Myocardial ectopy, alkalemia and, 2583
Myocardial infarction, hypertension and, 1606–1607
Myocarditis, 2826
Myoglobulin, molecular weight, radius, and renal handling of, 381t
Myointimal hypertrophy, in nephrosclerosis, 1433, 1434f
Myxedema, 2539–2547
 antidiuretic hormone in, 2543–2545, 2544f–2546f
 hyponatremia in, 2539–2541
 natriuresis in, 2545–2546
 SIADH secretion and, 2539–2541
 urine osmolality in, 2541–2543
 water excretion in, 2540f–2541f, 2540t, 2541–2543, 2543f

Nadolol, pharmacology of, normal vs. in renal failure, 3252t–3253t
Nafcillin, pharmacology of, normal vs. in renal failure, 3252t–3253t
Nail-patella syndrome, 603–606
 antiglomerular basement membrane antibody-mediated nephritis and, 1868
 clinical findings in, 603, 604f
  eyes in, 603
  nails in, 603, 604f
  patella in, 603, 604f
 genetics and pathogenesis of, 606
 incidence of, 603
 renal manifestations of, 604–606
  clinical presentation in, 605
  glomerulonephritis in, 605–606
  incidence of, 604–605
  nephropathy as, 606
  pathologic findings in, 605, 605f
 renal transplantation for, 606
 synonyms for, 603
Nalidixic acid
 pharmacology of, normal vs. in renal failure, 3252t–3253t
 for urinary tract infection, 2391
Naloxone, pharmacology of, normal vs. in renal failure, 3252t–3253t
Naproxen, pharmacology of, normal vs. in renal failure, 3252t–3253t
Narcotics. *See also* Drug abuse; Heroid abuse
 hyponatremia associated with, 2520
Nash antigen, 2348
Natriuresis, in myxedema, 2545–2546
Natriuretic factor, 2725
 atrial. *See* Atrial natriuretic peptide
Natriuretic hormone, idiopathic edema and, 2496
Nausea, in ADH secretion, 122–123
Neck, cancer of, nephrotic syndrome in, 2265
Necrotizing angiitis, renal, angiography for, 474, 474f
Neomycin
 chemical structure of, 1135f
 pharmacology of, normal vs. in renal failure, 3252t–3253t
Neonate(s). *See also* Children; Infant(s)
 acute renal failure in, 2385–2386
 ascites in, urinary tract obstruction and, 660
 congenital nephrotic syndrome in, 2386
 fluid and electrolytes in, 2383–2384, 2384t
 glomerular filtration rate in, 2383, 2384t
 growth and nutrition in, 2383
 hematogenous renal candidiasis in, 937
 hypertension in, 2386
 nonimmune hydrops in, 2386
 renal problems in, 2385–2386
 renal venous thrombosis in, 2386
 restricted renal cortical blood flow in, 2383
Neoplasm(s). *See specific types*; Cancer; Malignancy; Tumor
Nephrectomy
 bilateral, erythropoiesis and, 2746
 of cadaver donor kidney, 2922
 of living donor kidney, 2922
 for malignant hypertension, 1587–1588
 prior to renal transplantation, 2920
 unilateral, kidney weight after, 2706
 for unilateral reflux nephropathy, with hypertension, 711–712
 for urinary tract obstruction, 681
 for urinary tract tuberculosis, 924
Nephritic (overflow) edema, 2453
Nephritic factor, in membranoproliferative glomerulonephritis, 1821
Nephritic syndrome, acute
 in acute poststreptococcal glomerulonephritis, 1720–1722, 1721f, 1722t, 1725–1726
 in children, 2391–2392, 2392t
Nephritis. *See also* Glomerulonephritis
 acute focal bacterial
  diagnosis of, 964
  pathogenesis of, 963
  treatment of, 965
 acute multifocal bacterial
  diagnosis of, 964
  pathogenesis of, 963
  treatment of, 965
 animal models of, 1650–1654
  chemically induced, 1652
  induction of autoimmunity in, 1650–1654
  interstitial, 1653–1654

Nephritis, animal models of—Continued
spontaneous, 1654
spontaneous nephritis in, 1654
antiglomerular basement membrane antibody–mediated, 1865–1886. *See also* Antiglomerular basement membrane antibody–mediated nephritis
of donor origin, 2935
experimental, 1647–1654
autoimmune, immunopathologic features of, 1651t
due to exogenous antibody or antigen, 1647–1650
glomerular cell antibodies in, 1650
IgA-dependent, 1649–1650
immune complex, 1648f, 1648–1649
nephrotoxic, 1647–1648, 1648f
planted antigens in, 1649, 1649f
focal bacterial, CT for, 451
hereditary. *See also* Alport syndrome
immune, 582
interstitial
with hearing loss, 581
hyperuricemia, gout, and, 582
with hypokalemia, 582
without hearing loss, 582
Heymann, 1652–1653, 1653f, 1790
immune deposit, immunopathology of, 1654–1663, 1655t
immunopathology of, 1654–1665, 1655t
interstitial. *See* Interstitial nephritis
chronic, in pregnancy, 2300
lupus. *See* Lupus nephritis
postinfective. *See also* Glomerulonephritis, endocapillary exudative
immunopathology of, 1661
prognosis in, 1924–1929
radiation, malignant hypertension due to, 1560
salt-losing, 1427, 2722
sarcoid granulomatous, acute interstitial nephritis in, 1344
Steblay, 1650, 1651
trench, 1685
tubulointerstitial
acute, in cancer, 1168
animal model of, 1653–1654
immune complex–mediated, acute interstitial nephritis and, 1346, 1347
murine progressive, 1654
without immune deposits, immunopathology of, 1663–1665
Nephroangiopathy, endotheliotropic hemolytic, 2074. *See also* Hemolytic-uremic syndrome
Nephroblastoma. *See* Wilms tumor
Nephroblastomatosis, angiography for, 477
Nephrogenic diabetes insipidus
ADH absence in, 375
assessment of, 379
Nephrogenic rest(s), Wilms tumor and, 782
Nephrogram, definition of, 407
Nephrolithiasis, 729–738. *See also* Calculus(i), renal
classification of, 731t, 731–732
conservative management of, 733, 733t
cystine, 737, 738
diagnostic protocol for, 732, 732t
extensive vs. simple evaluation in, 732
gouty diathesis in, 737
due to hypercalciuria, 733–736. *See also* Hypercalciuria
hyperoxaluria, 736
hyperuricosuric calcium, 737
hypocitraturia, 736
infection stones in, 737–738
noncalcareous stones in, 737–738
pathogenesis of, 737–738
treatment of, 738
nonhypercalciuric calcium, 736–737
pathogenesis of, 736–737
treatment of, 735t, 737
pathogenesis of, 730–731, 731t
stone-provoking medications in, 732
upper urinary tract infection and, 980
uric acid, 737, 738
tubulointerstitial, 1974
in urinary tract tuberculosis, 916
Nephroma
mesoblastic, angiography for, 477
multilocular cystic, angiography for, 477
Nephron(s)
adaptation of, 2703
general principles in, 2704
patterns of, 2704f, 2704–2705
structural, 2706–2713
anatomy of, 4, 5f
calcium reabsorption by, 2619, 2619f
congenital malformations of, 650–651
distal. *See also specific parts*
acidification defects in, 2677–2679
furosemide administration and, 2679
infusion of neutral phosphate and, 2678–2679
infusion of sodium sulfate and, 2678–2679
urinary anion gap and, 2679
urine-blood PCO_2 in, 2678
anatomic segments of, 160f, 160–161
embryonic development of, 650
heterogeneity of, ADH effects on, 50
intact, 2703
juxtamedullary, 5, 5f
long-looped, 5
loss of function of, metabolic acidosis in, 2669–2685
midcortical, 5, 5f
morphology of, 4–5, 5f
in potassium transport, 181–183, 182f
regions of, 4
short-looped, 5
sodium retention sites in, 2468–2469, 2477
superficial, 5, 5f
transcellular transport processes in, 40–48
carbonic anhydrase activity in
apical membrane area and H^+ transport and, 47–48
localization of, 46, 47t
in proximal nephron and loop, 46–47
cytoplasm and, 40
H^+ transport and, 45–46
membrane amplification principle and, 40–41
Na^+-K^+-ATPase and, 41–43, 42f–43f
basolateral membrane and corticosteroids and, 43–44
potassium restriction and, intercalated cells and apical membrane changes in, 44–45
transepithelial acid-base transport in, 219–228. *See also* Acid-base transport
transit times in, 415f
Nephronia, lobar, acute, pathogenesis of, 963
Nephronophthisis, juvenile, 513, 514t
Nephronophthisis–medullary cystic disease, 513–523
acystic, 519
aortography in, 515
clinical features of, 513–515
conditions associated with, 516–517
diagnosis of, 519–520, 520t
diagnostic studies in, 514f–515f, 515
differential diagnosis of, 520
general signs and symptoms of, 513–515
genetic factors in, 513
hair color and, 516
hepatic fibrosis and, 517
intravenous pyelography in, 514f, 515
negative findings in, 517
pathologic anatomy in, 517f–519f, 518–519
gross examination in, 517f–518f, 518
microscopic examination in, 518f–519f, 518–519
pathophysiology and pathogenesis of, 521
physical and laboratory findings in, 514f, 515
prognosis and treatment in, 520–521
renal arteriography in, 515, 515f
renal sodium wasting in, 516, 516f
renal-retinal dysplasia and, 517
synonyms for, 513
urinary concentrating ability in, 515–516
variants of, 513, 514t
Nephropathia epidemica, 1976
Nephropathy
AIDS-associated, 2366
analgesic. *See* Analgesic-induced renal disease
Balkan, 1976
cadmium, 1242–1245. *See also* Cadmium nephropathy
diabetic. *See* Diabetic nephropathy
familial
gout in, 2257
hyperuricemia in, 2257
in glue "sniffers," 1232–1233
gouty, 2248–2253
chronic lead nephropathy and, 1241
hypertensive nephrosclerosis vs., 1442
Hantavirus, acute interstitial nephritis due to, 1343
heroin-associated, 2368
vs. HIV-associated nephropathy, 2369
HIV-associated, 2366–2370. *See also* HIV-associated nephropathy (HIVAN)
HTLV-associated, 2366
hypercalcemic, in multiple myeloma, 2199
hyperphosphatemic, due to antineoplastic agents, 1181
hyperuricemic, 2248
hypokalemic, impaired renal concentrating ability in, 376
IgA. *See* IgA nephropathy
IgM
mesangial, 1737
prognosis in, 1914
lead, 1237–1242. *See also* Lead nephropathy
light chain cast. *See* Light chain cast nephropathy
membranous. *See* Membranous nephropathy

minimal change. *See also* Nephrotic syndrome, minimal change
immunopathology of, 1663
myeloma cast, 2195
chronic tubulointerstitial, 1973
Tamm-Horsfall protein in, 2203
obstructive. *See* Obstructive nephropathy
radiation
chronic renal failure due to, 1169
chronic tubulointerstitial, 1974
reflux. *See* Reflux nephropathy
in solvent "sniffers," 1232–1233
tropical, 2331–2351
bacterial infection and, 2338–2339
geographic patterns in, 2331–2338
parasitic infection and, 2339–2351
snakebite-associated disease and, 2351
tubulointerstitial. *See* Tubulointerstitial nephropathy
uric acid, 2244
acute, due to antineoplastic agents, 1180
acute postrenal failure due to, 1291
chronic tubulointerstitial, 1974
syndrome of, 2247
vasomotor, in AIDS, 2362
xanthine, due to antineoplastic agents, 1180
Nephroptosis, in renovascular hypertension, 1454
Nephrosclerosis, 1433–1445
diseases associated with, 1434
hypertensive, 1440–1445
antihypertensive drug therapy in, 1443–1445
principles of, 1444
renal effects of, 1444–1445
in blacks vs. whites, 1443–1444, 1444t
definition of, 1433
diagnosis of, 1441, 1441t
differential diagnosis of, 1442
end-stage renal disease due to, 1441, 1441t, 1593–1594
gouty nephropathy vs., 1442
high-protein diet and, 1443
hypertension secondary to renal disease and, 1443
incidence of, 1441, 1441t
lead nephropathy vs., 1442
progressive nephron loss in, 1442–1443
urinalysis in, 1441–1442
malignant, pathologic findings in, 1575
pathogenesis of, 1435
pathologic findings in, 1433–1435, 1434f
in diabetes mellitus, 1433–1434
gross, 1433
hyaline arteriolosclerosis as, 1433, 1434f
in hypertension, 1433–1434
myointimal hypertrophy as, 1433, 1434f
postpartum, 2301
primary, 1435–1436
aging and, 1433
definition of, 1433
diabetes mellitus and, 1433
hyaline arteriolosclerosis in, 1433–1434
hypertensive, 1433–1434
malignant, 2074
mechanisms of, 1433, 1433t
primary malignant. *See also* Hemolytic-uremic syndrome
vascular, in gout, 2252
Nephrosis, lipoid, 1737
Nephrotic (underflow) edema, 2453
Nephrotic syndrome, 1731–1766, 2475–2481. *See also* Glomerulosclerosis, focal segmental
acute renal vein thrombosis in, 1319–1327, 1320t. *See also* Thrombosis, renal vein
admission for, in different world regions, 2334, 2335t
age-related, 2423t, 2423–2424
amyloidosis and, 2213, 2213t, 2220
treatment of, 2224
biochemical features of, 2475t
cancer and, 2265, 2267–2268
caused by disease other than MCNS, 1737t
in children, 2392t, 2392–2393
classification of, 1731, 1732t
clinical findings in, 1731–1734
edema in, 1732–1733
history in, 1731–1732
physical findings in, 1732–1733
complications of, 1749
congenital, 1743, 2386
diabetes mellitus and, 2574
dietary therapy for, 3186–3187
etiology of, 1320t
factors precipitating, 1732, 1732t
in first year of life, 1743, 1744t
geographic distribution of, 2334–2335, 2337, 2337t
histopathology of, 1737–1743
variants of, 1737–1740, 1738f–1739f
HLA type and, 1734, 1735t
inheritance patterns in, 1734, 1735t
laboratory findings in, 1734–1737
blood studies in, 1736
hyperlipidemia in, 1736
hypoalbuminemia in, 1736
renal biopsy in, 1736–1737, 1737t
serum electrolyte concentrations in, 1736
urinalysis in, 1734–1736
malignancy and, 1733, 1733t
due to mercury poisoning, 1247, 1247f
mesangial changes in, mechanism of, 1741–1742
minimal change
after renal transplantation, 1750–1751
atopy and, 1733–1734
in cancer, 1169
complications of, 1749
definitions in, 1744t
drugs causing, 1732, 1732t
in elderly, 2423, 2423t
epidemiology of, 1732
focal segmental glomerulosclerosis vs., 1740–1741, 1741f
frequent relapsing, 1744t
histopathology of, 1737, 1738f
immune complex deposits in, 1738–1739
incidence of, 1732–1733
inheritance patterns in, 1734
malignancy and, 1733, 1733t
mesangial IgM deposits in, 1737–1738
mesangial proliferation in, 1739
outcome in, 1749–1751, 1750f
percutaneous renal biopsy for, 487
prognosis in, 1906–1911
in adults, 1909f, 1909–1910
childhood-onset disease and, 1906–1909, 1907f–1908f
frequency of relapse and, 1908
initial treatment in, 1907
optimal management of, 1907f, 1907–1908
relapsing pattern in, 1907
chronic renal failure and, 1910
resistance to treatment and, 1910–1911
steroid dependent, 1744t
steroid resistant, 1748
steroid responsive, 1744t
treatment of, 1743–1748
adjunct, 1748–1749
chlorambucil in, 1746–1747
cyclophosphamide in, 1746
cyclosporine in, 1747
immunization in, 1747–1748
levamisole in, 1747
methylprednisolone in, 1746
NSAIDs in, 1747
prednisone in, 1744–1746, 1745f
in steroid-resistant disease, 1748
symptomatic, 1747
in tropical countries, 2334–2335, 2336f, 2337t
urinalysis in, 1734–1736
multiple myeloma and, 2200
NSAID nephrotoxicity and, 1211–1212, 1212t, 1338–1339
nutritional disorders in, 3186–3187
pathophysiology of, 1751–1766
carbohydrate metabolism in, 1762
drug toxicity in, 1762
edema formation in, 1754f, 1754–1756
atrial natriuretic factor in, 1756
blood volume and, 1755
GFR in, 1756
mechanism of, 1754–1755, 1755f
renin-angiotensin system and, 1755–1756
fluid and electrolyte metabolism in, 1756–1757
hemostatic disorders in, 1759–1761, 1760f
blood viscosity in, 1761
deep vein thrombosis in, 1759–1760
hypercoagulable state in, 1760f, 1760–1761
platelet abnormalities in, 1761
renal vein thrombosis in, 1760
hyperlipidemia in, 1757–1759
clinical significance of, 1759
lipid classifications in, 1757
lipid metabolism in, 1758f, 1758–1759
lipid transport in, 1757–1758
lipoprotein synthesis in, 1757
immunologic abnormalities in, 1762–1765, 1763t
abnormal lymphokine activity in, 1764–1765
cellular immunity in, 1764
immune complexes in, 1765
immunoglobulin synthesis and, 1763
lymphocyte surface marker expression in, 1763–1764
minimal change nephrotic syndrome and, 1765
infections in, 1761–1762
loss of other proteins in, 1762
proteinuria in, 1751–1756
consequences of, 1753–1756
glomerular electrostatic charge and, 1753
hypoalbuminemia in, 1753–1754

Nephrotic syndrome, pathophysiology of, proteinuria in—Continued
renal handling of macromolecules and, 1751f–1752f, 1751–1753
reduced serum calcium in, 1762
thyroid hormone losses in, 1762
trace metal metabolism in, 1762
percutaneous renal biopsy for, 487–488
in pregnancy, 2303–2304
primary
definition of, 1731
renal histologic findings in, 1731
prognosis in, 1898–1906
complications and, 1899–1900
hyperlipidemia as, 1899
infection as, 1899
prevention of, 1900
thrombosis as, 1899–1900
effect of treatment on, 1905–1906, 1906f
proteinuria and, 1900, 1901f–1902f
renal histopathology and, 1903f–1904f, 1903–1905, 1904t
sickle cell disease and, 2325
pathologic changes in, 2315
sodium retention in, 2476–2479
clearance studies and, 2477–2478
edema formation and, 2476–2478
effector mechanisms for, 2477–2478
enhanced tubular reabsorption and, 2478–2479
stimulus for, 2476–2477
treatment of, 2479–2481
terminology in, 1731
treatment of, 1743–1749. *See also* Nephrotic syndrome, minimal change, treatment of
vitamin D deficiency in, 3186–3187
water retention in, 2479
treatment of, 2479–2481
Nephrotomography
indications for, 409
in renal cell carcinoma, 787–788
Nephrotoxicity, 1031–1069
alkylating agent, 1170–1176
altered membrane phospholipid metabolism and, 1056–1057
decreased degradation as, 1056–1057
increased degradation as, 1056
aminoglycoside, 1131–1155. *See also* Aminoglycoside nephrotoxicity
antibiotic-induced, 2204
antimetabolite, 1176–1178
antineoplastic agent, 1170–1180, 1171t
antitumor antibiotic, 1178–1179
5-azacytidine, 1178
carmustine, 1174
cell pH alterations in, 1058–1059
cell protease abnormalities in, 1059
cell volume regulation in, 1058
cisplatin, 1170–1173
Corynebacterium parvum, 1180
cyclophosphamide, 1173
cyclosporine
acute, 2928
chronic, 2928–2929
differential diagnosis of, 2929
cytosine arabinoside, 1177
cytoskeletal disruption in, 1059–1061
disrupted cell calcium homeostasis in, 1050–1055
calcium overload and, 1051, 1051f
cytosolic free calcium ions and, 1053f–1054f, 1053–1054
gentamicin nephrotoxicity and, 1055
high-calcium diet and, 1055
impaired cellular mechanisms for sequestering and extruding calcium and, 1054
prelethal, 1051–1053, 1052f
cisplatin model of, 1052
gentamicin model of, 1051–1052, 1052f
mercuric chloride model of, 1051–1052, 1052f
disruption of cell monovalent cations in, 1057–1058
doxorubicin, 1179
endogenous protective measures against, 1069
acquired insensitivity as, 1069
heat shock proteins as, 1069
metallothioneins as, 1069
extent of tubular cell injury in, renal clearance function and, 1032–1033
5-fluorouracil, 1177
functional manifestations of, 1032
heavy metal, 1237–1249. *See also specific types*
interferon, 1179–1180
intrinsic protective measures against, 1066–1069
amino acid infusions as, 1068
calcium channel blockers as, 1068
chelators as, 1068
chronic saline loading and, 1067
furosemide and, 1067
mannitol and, 1066–1067
pyridoxal-5-phosphate as, 1068
selenium as, 1068–1069
streptozotocin-induced diabetes as, 1067–1068
thyroxine as, 1068
of light chain proteins, 2191–2194, 2192f–2193f
lomustine, 1174, 1176
lysosomes and, 1061–1066
compromised integrity of, 1065–1066
effects of various drugs on, 1062–1063
functional effects of, 1063–1065
gentamicin effects on, 1062, 1063f
methods for assessment of, 1062
myeloid body formation and, 1062–1063
phospholipid accumulation and, 1064
toxin accumulation in, 1062–1063, 1063f
mechanisms of, 1031, 1036–1045
biochemical pathways in, 1036, 1037f
direct toxicity as, 1031
dose in, 1031–1032
free radical production as, 1036–1041
abnormal calcium production and, 1040
acetaminophen and, 1042
agents altering, 1040
arachidonate metabolism and, 1037
carbon tetrachloride and, 1042–1043
cephalosporin and, 1042
chloroform and, 1041–1042
cisplatin and, 1043–1044
cyclosporine and, 1044
cysteine conjugates and, 1044–1045
cysteine metabolism and, 1038
distribution of metabolites and, 1041
Fenton reaction and, 1036–1037
gentamicin and, 1043
glutathione as antioxidant and, 1039
glutathione depletion and, 1039–1040
glutathione metabolism and, 1038
glycine modulation and, 1040
hydroxyl radical and, 1037
intrinsic mechanisms in modulation of, 1039
leukocytes and, 1037
lipid peroxidation and, 1038–1039
measurement techniques for, 1039
mercuric chloride and, 1043
nucleic acid oxidant damage and, 1039
pathways for, 1036, 1037f
phenobarbitol response and, 1040
phospholipase activation and, 1040–1041
protein oxidant damage and, 1039
specific nephrotoxins and, 1041–1045
superoxide ions and, 1036
ultimate cell death and, 1040
vitamin E as antioxidant and, 1039
xanthine oxidase metabolism and, 1037–1038
metabolic activation as, 1031
time frame in, 1031–1032
due to metabolic tumor lysis products, 1180–1181
methotrexate, 1176–1177
mithramycin, 1178–1179
mitomycin-C, 1178
nonoliguric acute renal failure due to, 1298
NSAID, 1207–1213. *See also* NSAID nephrotoxicity
protein and nucleic acid synthesis abnormalities in, 1061
radiocontrast. *See* Contrast media-induced acute renal failure
renal factors in, 1031
semustine, 1174, 1175f
silicon, 1237
streptomycin, 1131
streptozotocin, 1173–1174
sublethal, pathologic findings in, 1032
6-thioguanine, 1177
tubular cell energy metabolism in, 1045–1050
mitochondria and, 1045–1050
altered enzyme function in, 1048
ATP levels and, 1045
cephalosporin effects on, 1047, 1048
cisplatin effects on, 1047
criteria for, 1050
disrupted calcium ion metabolism in, 1048–1049
gentamicin toxicity and, 1046
ischemia and, 1049–1050
magnesium ion effects on, 1046–1047
metal toxin effects on, 1047
organic toxin effects on, 1047
tert-butyl hydroperoxide effects on, 1048
tissue slice studies of, 1046
in vitro vs. in vivo studies of, 1045–1046
tubular cell uptake in, 1033–1036
of aminoglycosides, brush-border membrane in, 1033–1035, 1034f–1035f
cephalosporins and, 1035–1036
cisplatin and, 1036
competitive, amelioration of toxicity and, 1035

complexed toxins and, 1035
membrane mechanisms in, 1033
tubular factors in, 1031, 1032f
Nervous system
central. *See* Central nervous system (CNS)
in hypercalcermia, 2625
in hypophosphatemia, 2609
in renal failure, 2789–2809
sympathetic. *See* Sympathetic nervous system (SNS)
Netilmicin
acute interstitial nephritis due to, 1337
chemical structure of, 1135f
Neurofibrillary tangles, in dialysis dementia, 2800
Neurofibromatosis, renal percutaneous transluminal angioplasty for, 469–470
Neurogenic bladder
management of, in vesicoureteral reflux, 719
upper urinary tract infection in, 981
prevention of, 996–997
vesicoureteral reflux due to, 694
Neurogenic diabetes insipidus, ADH absence in, 375
Neuron, structure of, 2794
Neuropathy
in chronic hemodialysis, 3085–3086, 3086f
diabetes mellitus and, 2575–2576
peripheral, in amyloidosis, 2213, 2213t
uremic, 2804–2809
autonomic and cranial nerve dysfunction in, 2809
clinical manifestations of, 2804–2805
effects of dialysis on, 2808
effects of renal transplantation on, 2808–2809
etiology of, 2805–2806
insidious onset of, 2805
manifestations of, 2804–2805
metabolic, 2805
nerve conduction in, 2806, 2807t
parathyroid hormone and, 2806–2808, 2808f
peripheral, 2805
toxins in, 2806, 2807t
Neuropeptide Y, in renal hemodynamics, 97
Neuroretinopathy, hypertensive, 1555, 1565f, 1565–1566
cotton-wool spots in, 1565f, 1566
in hypertensive encephalopathy, 1595
macular star figure in, 1565f, 1566
papilledema in, 1566–1567, 1567f
pathophysiology of, 1584
reversal of, prognostic value of, 1592
striate hemorrhage in, 1565, 1565f
Neurotoxicity, of aluminum, 3158–3159. *See also under* Aluminum
Neurotransmitter(s)
false, hepatorenal disease due to, 1360
physiology of, 2794–2798, 2796f–2797f
Neutrophil(s)
in acute renal failure, 1381
in vascular inflammatory injury, 1994, 1994t, 1995f
Neutrophilic exudate(s), clinicopathologic correlations in, 503
Nicardipine, in end-stage renal disease, 2824
Nifedipine
in end-stage renal disease, 2824
for hypertension, 1625, 2390t
pharmacology of, normal vs. in renal failure, 3252t–3253t
for severe hypertension in pregnancy, 1526
Nissl granules, 2505
Nitric oxide, vasodilator, in renal hemodynamics, 93–94
Nitrofurantoin
for cystitis and urethritis, 1015
pharmacology of, normal vs. in renal failure, 3254t–3255t
for urinary tract infection, 2391
Nitrogen balance
for assessment of protein intake, 3139–3140
in continuous ambulatory peritoneal dialysis, 3176–3177, 3177t
in renal transplantation, 3198
in uremia, 3141
Nitrogen intake, in dietary therapy in acute renal failure, 3193–3194
Nitrogen load, BUN and, 370–371, 371f
Nitroglycerin
intravenous, for hypertension, 1623
pharmacology of, normal vs. in renal failure, 3254t–3255t
Nitroprusside, pharmacology of, normal vs. in renal failure, 3254t–3255t
Nocardia, as complication of transplantation, 2947
Nocturnal enuresis, in vesicoureteral reflux, 717
Non-A, non-B hepatitis (hepatitis C), as complication of transplantation, 2945
Nonglomerular disease, sodium homeostasis in, 2723–2724, 2724f
Non-Hodgkin's lymphoma
membranoproliferative glomerulonephritis and, 1830
nephrotic syndrome in, 2267
Nonimmune hydrops, in neonates, 2386
Non–insulin-dependent diabetes mellitus. *See* Diabetes mellitus, non–insulin-dependent.
Nonsteroidal antiinflammatory drug(s) (NSAIDs). *See* NSAID(s)
Norepinephrine
biosynthesis of, 1488, 1488f
in chronic renal failure, 2716
in cirrhosis, 2469
increased arteriolar resistance and, in congestive heart failure, 2458
metabolism of, 1488–1489, 1489f
receptor types for, 299
Norepinephrine/DHPG ratios, for pheochromocytoma, 1493
Norfloxacin
cystic fluid concentration of, in autosomal dominant polycystic kidney disease, 551t
pharmacology of, normal vs. in renal failure, 3254t–3255t
Normonatremia, 2504f, 2518f
Nortriptyline, pharmacology of, normal vs. in renal failure, 3254t–3255t
NSAID(s)
chemical classification of, 1208t
hyponatremia associated with, 2520
for pericarditis, 2827
in renal disorders, effects on vasodilator prostaglandins and, 91–92
renal failure due to, 2204
in elderly, 2424
types of, 1207–1208
NSAID nephrotoxicity, 1207–1213
acute interstitial nephritis due to, 1337–1339
clinical and pathologic features of, 1338, 1338t
diagnosis of, 1338t, 1338–1339
incidence of, 1337
acute tubular necrosis due to, 1338t
analgesic-induced renal disease due to, 1107, 1109t, 1110t, 1113
clinical consequences of, 1208, 1209t
fluid balance and, 1213
frequency of, 1208
due to glomerular and interstitial disease, 1211–1212, 1212t
hyperkalemia and, 1213
nephrotic syndrome and, 1338–1339
prerenal acute renal failure due to, 1288
prerenal failure due to, 1338t
due to renal vasoconstriction, 1209t, 1209–1211, 1210f, 1212t
in rheumatoid arthritis therapy, 2051
sodium balance and, 1212–1213
Nuclear medicine, 413–421. *See also* Radionuclide study(ies)
Nutraphos, for hypophosphatemia, 2610
Nutrient administration. *See also* Dietary therapy
in acute or chronic renal failure, 3196–3198
enteral vs. parenteral, 3196–3198
intravenous, in hemodialysis, 3197
Nutrition, preoperative, for urinary bladder cancer surgery, 824–826. *See also* Urinary bladder carcinoma
Nutritional disorder(s)
in chronic renal failure, 3167. *See also* Chronic renal failure, dietary therapy in
in nephrotic syndrome, 3186–3187
in renal transplantation, 3198–3199

Obesity, in gout, 2252
Obstructive nephropathy. *See also* Hydronephrosis; Obstructive uropathy; Urinary tract obstruction
clinical syndromes in, 657–658, 658t
definition of, 657
diabetes mellitus and, 2573–2574
GFR decrease in, 675
imaging studies of, 430
lipid metabolism in, 675
parathyroid hormone responsiveness in, 675
renal hormonal abnormalities in, 675
renal metabolism in, 675–676
renin-angiotensin system in, 675
Obstructive uropathy. *See also* Hydronephrosis; Obstructive nephropathy; Urinary tract obstruction
acute postrenal failure due to, 1290–1291
causes of, 657, 658t
in children, 2387–2388
clinical syndromes in, 657–658, 658t
definition of, 657
effect of age on, 674–675
imaging studies of, 430
incidence of, 657
in multiple myeloma, 2205

Obstructive uropathy—Continued
papillary necrosis and, 1979
renal tubular potassium and, 2657
stone-induced, 1291
in utero diagnosis of, 2387–2388
OKT3 therapy
in immunosuppression, 2903, 2903t, 2929–2930
recommended protocol for, 2929t
side effects of, 2926t
Oligohydramniosis, in renal agenesis, 2383
Oligonephronia
classification of, 652
definition of, 652
Oliguria
in acute renal failure, in malignant hypertension, 1568
in diagnosis of acute renal failure, 1296–1297
Oncocytoma, renal, 799
angiography for, 475
CT for, 454
Oncogene(s), 777–782
cellular, 777
class I: protein kinases, 778t, 778–779
class II: receptors lacking tyrosine activity, 778t, 779
class III: growth factors, 778t, 779
class IV: ras oncogenes, 778t, 779
class V: nuclear oncogenes, 778t, 779
classification of, 778t, 778–779
dominantly acting, 777–778
historical, 777
unclassified, 779
urologic neoplasia and, 779–780
viral, 777
Oncotic pressure, in regulation of GFR, 361, 362f, 363
Opioid agonists, for hyponatremia, with congestive heart failure, 2465
Opioid peptides, in uremia, 2863
Opportunistic infection(s), as complication of transplantation, 2945–2946
Opportunistic mycoses, 946t–947t, 946–947
Oral contraceptive(s)
acute renal vein thrombosis due to, in nephrotic syndrome, 1324
malignant hypertension due to, 1560
microvascular thrombosis due to, 2066
Orchiopexy, for cryptorchidism, testicular carcinoma and, 852
Orchitis, 754–755
granulomatous, 755
ischemic, 755
pyogenic, 754–755
traumatic, 755
viral, 754
Organic acid, overproduction of, 2577
Orthopnea, in heart failure, 2832
Os-Cal, for hypocalcemia, 2628
Osmolality
of body fluids, control of, 373, 374f
of glomerular ultrafiltrate, 126f–127f, 126–127
of plasma, hyponatremia and, 2516–2517, 2517t
potassium regulation and, 2648
of urine
measurement of, 377
in myxedema, 2541–2543
volume vs., 377
Osmole(s), idiogenic, 2567
Osmotic diuresis, in diabetes mellitus, 2567–2568
Osteitis fibrosa
bone reabsortpion in, 2768
dihydrotachysterol for, 2776
treatment of, 2776–2777, 2777f
vitamin D metabolites for, 2776
Osteoblast(s), 2759
Osteoclast(s)
bone reabsorption by, 2759
calcium in, 2617
Osteoclast-activating factor, 2273
Osteocyte(s), 2617
Osteodystrophy, renal, 2759–2779
aluminum assay in, 2766, 2766t
aluminum-associated, treatment of, 2777–2778, 2778t, 2779f
bed rest for, 2774
beta-2-amyloid in, 2773
beta-2-microglobulin assay in, 2766
beta-2-microglobulin deposition in, 2763
biochemical studies of, 2765–2767
biopsy in, 2766–2767
bone mass measurements in, 2764–2765
bone pain and, 2774, 2775t
calcifediol in, 2775
calciferol in, 2775
calcitriol in, 2775–2776
calcium supplementation in, 2775
in children, 2773–2774
clinical features of, 2761
deferoxamine challenge in, 2766, 2767t
diagnostic problems in, 2774
dihydrotachysterol in, 2776
24,25-dihydroxyvitamin D in, 2776
early manifestations of, 2761–2762
fracture and, 2774, 2775t
growth retardation in, 2395
high turnover, 2760, 2762f, 2762–2763
histology of, 2767–2768, 2768f–2769f
histology of, 2767–2774
1-alpha-hydroxyvitamin D in, 2776
hypercalcemia and, 2774
hyperphosphatemia in, treatment of, 2774–2775, 2775t
low turnover, 2760–2761, 2763
histology of, 2768–2772, 2770f–2772f
mixed, uremic, 2761
mixed-transitional, 2763
histology of, 2773
nutritional therapy for, 2395
pathogenesis of, 2760–2765
posttransplant, 2951
preventive therapy for, 2774–2776
PTH measurements in, 2765t, 2765–2766
PTH stimulation in, 2766
radiographs of, 2763f–2765f, 2763–2764
serum chemistry of, 2765
transplantation in, 2778–2779
treatment of, 2776–2779
types of, 2760t
Osteogenesis imperfecta, abnormal collagen synthesis in, 2759
Osteoid, woven, 2759, 2767–2768
Osteomalacia. *See also* Rickets
bone disease and, 2763
24,25-dihydroxyvitamin D for, 2776
growth retardation in, 2395
hypophosphatemia in, 2605
hypophosphatemic, adult sporadic, 618t, 620
in low turnover bone disease, 2768–2770
oncogenic, 2607
hypophosphatemic, 2275–2276, 2276f
Osteomalacia-rickets, pseudofracture in, 2763, 2764f
Osteomyelitis, amyloidosis and, 2220
Osteonecrosis, posttransplant, 2951
Osteoporosis, posttransplant, 2951
Ovarian carcinoma
aldosterone-producing, 1482
nephrotic syndrome in, 2265
Overflow incontinence, 763
Overlap syndrome, 2039
Oxacillin, pharmacology of, normal vs. in renal failure, 3254t–3255t
Oxalate disorder(s), in chronic tubulointerstitial nephropathy, 1974–1975
Oxalosis, renal transplantation and, 2915, 2915f
Oxazepam, pharmacology of, normal vs. in renal failure, 3254t–3255t
Oxidative phosphorylation, in renal metabolism, 236, 236f–237f
Oxygen consumption
renal, 235t, 235–238
basal vs. suprabasal, 235–236
oxidative phosphorylation in, 236, 236f–237f
rates of, 235, 235t
sodium transport and, 237f–238f, 237–238
renal blood flow and, 65, 66f
Oxygen delivery, reduced, metabolic alkalosis and, 2583
Oxygen free radical(s), in experimental studies of ischemic renal injury, 1267–1270, 1269f, 1271f
Oxygen gradient, between renal cortex and medulla, 233, 234f, 235
Oxytocin, hyponatremia associated with, 2520–2521
Ozolinone, mechanism of action of, 2441, 2441f

Page kidney, 477
Paget's disease, hypercalcemia and, 2627
Pain, chest, in pericarditis, 2826
Pancreas
cancer of, nephrotic syndrome in, 2265
transplantation of, in diabetic nephropathy, 2182
Pancreatitis
acute
hypocalcemia and, 2624
in malignant hypertension, 1569
in acute tubular necrosis, 1304
posttransplant, 2949
Papilla, renal
anatomy of, 3, 4f
intrarenal reflux and, 693
Papillary blush, in medullary sponge kidney, 530f, 530–531
Papillary necrosis, 1976–1979
age of onset, 1979
in analgesic-induced renal disease, 1113–1115. *See also* Analgesic-induced renal disease
blood supply in, 1976–1977
clinical course in, 1978
conditions associated with, 1978–1979, 1979f
cyst-like defect in, 521, 522f
diabetes mellitus and, 1978–1979
in diagnosis of candidiasis, 938

distribution of necrotic lesions in, 1978
imaging studies of, 422–423, 423f–424f
infection in, 1977
medullary sponge kidney vs., 531
partial (medullary), 1977, 1977f
in "primary" renal candidiasis, 936
in sickle cell disease, 2324–2325
total (papillary), 1977, 1978f
Papovavirus infection, renal manifestations of, 998
Para-aminosalicylic acid, for urinary tract tuberculosis, 923t
Paracellular transport route, 38
Paracentesis, for ascites, 2473
Parapelvic cyst, CT for, 452
Paraplegia, amyloidosis and, 2220
Parasitemia, 2340–2341
Parasitic infection. *See also specific infections*
in acute renal failure, etiologic role of, 2332, 2333t
in tropical countries, renal disease and, 2339–2351
Parasitized erythrocyte(s), in malaria, 2344, 2344f
Parathyroid adenoma, 2273
Parathyroid gland
aluminum deposits in, 2761
dysfunction of, 2858
Parathyroid hormone, 293–294
abnormal circulating, 2613
aluminum skeletal toxicity and, 3159
assays for, 2765t, 2765–2766
in calcium transport, 2621
glomerular receptors and actions of, 293
hypercalcemia and, cancer-related, 2271–2272
hyperphosphatemia and, 2611–2612
low or absent levels of, hypocalcemia secondary to, 2623
major renal effects of, 293
for modification of aminoglycoside nephrotoxicity, 1151
in obstructive nephropathy, 675
potassium regulation and, 2648
in proximal tubule sodium reabsorption, 151
in pseudohypoparathyroidism, 2622
in renal calcium excretion, 293–294
renal phosphorus absorption and, 2601–2602, 2602t
role of
in CNS function, 2798, 2798f
in uremia, 2847–2848
stimulation of, in renal bone disease, 2766
tubule receptors and actions of, 293
in uremia, 2858
in uremic dyslipoproteinemia, 2850
uremic neuropathy and, 2806–2808, 2807t, 2808f
Parathyroidectomy, for osteitis fibrosa, 2777
Paraureteral diverticula, 642
Parenchymal atrophy, in hydronephrosis, 659
due to intrarenal reflux, 659
due to ischemia, 659
due to pressure atrophy, 659
due to urinary tract infection, 659
Parenchymal disease. *See also specific disorders*
in AIDS patients, 2365
imaging studies for, 423f–427f, 423t, 423–427
malaria and, 2340
urographic diagnosis of, 423t
Parenchymal thickness, intravenous urography for, 409
Parenteral alimentation
for acute or chronic renal failure, 3196–3198
for urinary bladder carcinoma, 826
Parenthood, posttransplant, 2953, 2953t
Pars recta, calcium absorption in, 2620
Patella, in nail-patella syndrome, 603, 604f
PCBC, mitochondrial effects of, 1048
PCO_2, urine-blood, in distal nephron acidification defects, 2678
Pelvicalyceal cyst, imaging studies of, 425, 426f
Pelvicalyceal system, intravenous urography for, 409–410, 410f
Pelvis, renal, carcinoma of, 801–805
brush biopsy in, 804
causes of, 801
chemotherapy in, 805
diagnostic evaluation of, 802f–803f, 802–804
features at presentation in, 801
five-year survival rate in, 804t
grading and staging of, 801–802, 802f
intravenous pyelography for, 802, 802f
radiation therapy in, 805
retrograde pyelography for, 802–803, 803f
treatment of, 804–805
radical operative therapy in, 804–805
urine cytology in, 803
Pelviureteric junction obstruction, imaging studies in, 432, 433f
Penicillamine
membranous nephropathy and, 1795–1796
for rheumatoid arthritis, renal damage due to, 2053
Penicillin, acute interstitial nephritis due to, 1336
Penicillin derivatives, acute interstitial nephritis due to, 1336
Penicillin G, pharmacology of, normal vs. in renal failure, 3254t–3255t
Penis
meatal stenosis of, 640
tuberculosis of, 916
Pentamidine
causing renal failure, in AIDS patients, 2363
pharmacology of, normal vs. in renal failure, 3254t–3255t
in renal disease, 3228
Pentazocine, pharmacology of, normal vs. in renal failure, 3254t–3255t
Pentobarbital, pharmacology of, normal vs. in renal failure, 3254t–3255t
Peptic ulcer disease, due to analgesia abuse, 1111
Peptide hormone(s)
glomerular filtration of, 318f, 318–319
metabolism of, 317–319
mode of action of, 284
peritubular removal of, 319
renal regulatory mechanisms of, 317, 317f
Periarterial connective tissue, morphology of, 35, 35f–36f
Periarthritis, calcific, in chronic renal failure, 3154
Pericardial effusion, 2826
echocardiography in, 2825
Pericardiectomy, for pericarditis, 2829
Pericardiocentesis, 2828, 2829
Pericardiotomy, subxiphoid, for pericarditis, 2828–2829
Pericarditis
dialysis-associated, 2825, 2826t
in end-stage renal disease, 2824–2829
clinical features and laboratory findings in, 2825–2827, 2826t
incidence of, 2824–2825
management of, 2827–2829, 2828f
pathogenesis of, 2825
mortality from, 2826
subacute constrictive, 2826
Perihiatal hernia, 642, 642f
Perimacular lesion(s), in Alport syndrome, 580
Perinephric abscess, 966–969. *See also* Abscess, perinephric
Perineum, antimicrobial defense mechanisms of, 894–895
Peripelvic cyst, congenital, 650
Peripheral arterial vasodilation
in hepatorenal disease, 1360–1364, 1361f–1364f
renal sodium and water retention in, 1361f
Peripheral nerves, dysfunction of, 2805
Peripheral vasculature, atrial natriuretic peptide effects on, 296
Peritoneal cavity, host defense mechanisms in, 2984–2986
effect of CAPD on, 2985
toxicity of dialysis fluid and, 2985–2986
Peritoneal dialysis, 2969–3019
in acute renal failure, in neonates, 2385
advantages of, 1385
alternate regimens for, 2994f, 2995
assessment of dialysis efficiency in, 2981–2984
clearance measurements for, 2981–2982, 2982t–2983t
Kt/V in, 2982–2984, 2984t
mass transfer area coefficient in, 2984
protein catabolic rate in, 2983–2984, 2984t
solute transport curves in, 2982, 2983f
urea kinetic parameters in, 2982–2984, 2984t
catheter break-in in, 2989–2990
catheter care in, 2990
exit-site care in, 2990
catheter placement in, 2988
bedside access for acute peritoneal dialysis and, 2988
creation of subcutaneous tunnel in, 2988–2989
long-term peritoneal access and, 2988
postoperative care in, 2989
preinsertion patient preparation in, 2988
surgical technique for, 2988
catheter removal in, 2992
catheter revision in, 2992
catheter survival in, 2992
complications after CAPD discontinuation in, 2992
complications of long-term catheter use in, 2991
catheter malfunction as, 2991

Peritoneal dialysis, complications of long-term catheter use in—Continued
  cuff extrusion as, 2991
  pericatheter hernia as, 2991
  skin-exit infection as, 2991
  tunnel infection as, 2991
 complications related to peritoneal access in, 2990t, 2990–2992
  bleeding as, 2990–2991
  bowel perforation as, 2991
  catheter placement and, 2990–2991
  exit-site infection as, 2991
  leakage of dialysis fluid as, 2990
  pain in perineal area as, 2990
  reflex ileus as, 2990
 continuous, 1391–1392
  complications of, 1392, 1392t
  peritoneal access in, 1391
  peritoneal dialysis solution in, 1391–1392
 continuous ambulatory (CAPD)
  for AIDS patients, 2372
  calcium balance in, 3176–3177, 3177t
  carbohydrate metabolism in, 2848–2849
  for chronic renal failure, in children, 2397
  combined creatinine clearance in, 2981–2982, 2982t–2983t
  complications of, 3004t, 3004–3018
   abdominal hernia as, 3017
   back pain as, 3017
   cardiovascular, 3018
   chronic hypotension as, 3018
   dialysate leak as, 3017
   increased abdominal pressure as, 3017–3018
   lipid metabolic abnormalities as, 3016
   loss of ultrafiltration as, 3015
   massive hydrothorax as, 3017–3018
   metabolic, 3016–3017
   nutritional problems as, 3016–3017
   peripheral vascular disease as, 3018
   peritoneal adhesions and loss of surface area as, 3015–3016
   peritonitis as, 3004–3015. *See also* Peritonitis
  connecting devices for, 2995–2996
  continuous cyclic vs., 2995, 2996t
  contraindications for, 3000
  creatinine clearance in, 2977–2978, 2978f
  development of, in North America and Europe, 3018
  in diabetes mellitus, 3001–3003
   blood sugar control in, 3002, 3002t
   dialysis regimens for, 3001–3002
   glucose as osmotic agent in, 3001
   indications for, 3001
   intraperitoneal insulin in, 3002
   peritoneal access for, 3001
   short-term and long-term outcomes in, 3002–3003
  dietary therapy in
   energy in, 3178–3179
   recommended dietary nutrient intake in, 3170, 3170t–3171t
  drug therapy in, 3228
  future of, 3018
  high-dose
   high-volume, 2995
   standard-volume, 2995
  historical development of, 2969
  home cycler technique vs., 2995, 2996t
  host defense mechanisms in, 2985
  indications for, 2999
  in infants, children, and adolescents, 3003–3004
  integration with other treatment modalities of, 3018
  kinetics of peritoneal transport in, 2978–2979
  Kt/V in, 2982–2984, 2984t
  long-term results of, 3000
  magnesium balance in, 3176–3177, 3177t
  nitrogen balance in, 3176–3177, 3177t
  nutritional, 3197–3198
  pediatric, technical aspects of, 2997
  peritoneal equilibration test in, 2980t–2981t, 2980–2981
  peritoneal irrigation technique in, 2996
  peritoneal membrane transport characteristics in, 2979f, 2980
  peritoneal ultrastructure in, 2972f–2973f, 2972–2973
  phosphorus balance in, 3176–3177, 3177t
  potassium balance in, 3176–3177, 3177t
  prescription for, 2995
  program organization for, 2997
  protein catabolic rate in, 2983–2984, 2984t
  protein intake in, 3167
  protein losses in, 3168, 3169t
  red cell survival and, 2747
  removal of small solutes with, 2977–2978, 2978f
  side effects of, 2997–2999
   amino acid losses as, 2998
   hypercholesterolemia as, 2998
   hyperglycemia as, 2998
   hyperlipidemia as, 2998
   increased intraabdominal pressure as, 2998–2999, 2999f
   metabolic disturbances as, 2997–2998
   protein losses as, 2997–2998
   vitamin losses as, 2998
  solute equilibrium in, 2979f, 2980
  standard-dose, high-volume, 2995
  ultrafiltration volumes in, 2979f, 2980
  urea clearance in, 2977–2978, 2978f
  uremic inhibitors and, 2747
 continuous cyclic
  complications of, 3004t, 3004–3018
   abdominal hernia as, 3017
   back pain as, 3017
   cardiovascular, 3018
   chronic hypotension as, 3018
   dialysate leak as, 3017
   increased abdominal pressure as, 3017–3018
   lipid metabolic abnormalities as, 3016
   loss of ultrafiltration as, 3015
   massive hydrothorax as, 3017–3018
   metabolic, 3016–3017
   nutritional problems as, 3016–3017
   peripheral vascular disease as, 3018
   peritoneal adhesions and loss of surface area as, 3015–3016
   peritonitis as, 3004–3015. *See also* Peritonitis
  continuous ambulatory vs., 2995, 2996t
  contraindications for, 3000
  creatinine clearance in, 2977–2978, 2978f
  cyclers for, 2997
  development and future of, 3018–3019
  in diabetes mellitus, 3001–3002
  future of, 3018
  high-dose, 2995
  indications for, 3000
  in infants, children, and adolescents, 3003–3004
  kinetics of peritoneal transport in, 2978–2979
  pediatric, technical aspects of, 2997
  prescription for, 2995
  program organization for, 2997
  removal of small solutes with, 2977–2978, 2978f
  side effects of, 2997–2999
   amino acid losses as, 2998
   hypercholesterolemia as, 2998
   hyperglycemia as, 2998
   hyperlipidemia as, 2998
   increased intraabdominal pressure as, 2998–2999, 2999f
   metabolic disturbances as, 2997–2998
   protein losses as, 2997–2998
   vitamin losses as, 2998
  techniques for, 2996–2997
  urea clearance in, 2977–2978, 2978f
 continuous regimens for, 2994f, 2995
 daytime ambulatory, 2993
 disadvantages of, 1385
 flow techniques for, 2993, 2994f
 intermittent, 2994
  combined creatinine clearance in, steps for calculation of, 2981–2982, 2982t–2983t
  in diabetes mellitus, 3001
  high-dose nightly, 2995
  nightly, 2994–2995
  regimens for, 2993–2995, 2994f
 nightly tidal, 2995
 optimum catheter function in, 2986–2988
  catheter material in, 2986
  catheter tip migration in, 2987
  direction of catheter tunnel and skin exit in, 2986–2987
  foreign body tissue reaction in, 2987–2988
  material for cuff in, 2986
  role of catheter cuff in tunnel in, 2986
  sinus tract length in, 2987
  uninterrupted dialysis solution flow in, 2987
 peritoneal access for, 2986–2992
 solutions for, 2992–2993. *See also* Dialysate(s)
 ultrafiltration in, physiologic mechanism of, 2977, 2977f
Peritoneal eosinophilia, 3004–3005
Peritoneal equilibration test, 2980t–2981t, 2980–2981
Peritoneal lymphocytosis, 3005
Peritoneal shunting, for ascites, 2473–2474
Peritoneum, 2969–2977
 capillary blood flow in, 2969–2971
 gross anatomy of, 2969
 lymphatic drainage of, 2975–2976
 physiology of, 2976–2984
  in dialysis. *See* Peritoneal dialysis
  normal, 2985
  solute and water transport in, 2976–2977
   bulk or convective flow in, 2976

diffusion in, 2976
osmotic pressure in, 2976
pinocytotic or vesicular transport in, 2976–2977
ultrastructure of, 2971–2975
after recovery from peritonitis, 2974f, 2974–2975
basement membrane changes as, 2974
stromal cellular desert as, 2974f, 2974–2975
in CAPD patients, 2972f–2973f, 2972–2973
nonenzymatic glycosylation of structural protein in, 2975
parietal, 2970f–2971f, 2971–2972
in peritonitis, 2973–2974
uremic, 2972, 2972f
Peritonitis
due to continuous peritoneal dialysis, 3004–3015
antibiotics and dosing guidelines for, 3012t–3014t
causes of, 3005
clinical diagnosis of, 3004
"cloudy bag" and cell counts in, 3004
consequences of, 3004
differential diagnosis of "cloudy bag" in, 3004–3005
fecal peritonitis and, 3011, 3014
fungal peritonitis and, 3009, 3011
incidence of, 3008, 3014
management of, 3007–3008
microbiologic aspects of, 3005, 3006t
microbiologic methods for, 3005–3007
direct examination of dialysis effluent in, 3006
effluent fluid culture in, 3006–3007
mortality in, 3008
nontuberculous peritonitis and, 3014
outcome in, 3008
peritoneal eosinophilia vs., 3004–3005
peritoneal lymphocytosis vs., 3005
prevention of, 3014–3015
sclerosing (chronic inflammatory), 3014–3015, 3015f
sterile peritonitis and, 3007
treatment decision tree in, 3009f–3012f
tuberculous peritonitis and, 3014
peritoneal ultrastructure in, 2973–2974
recovery from, peritoneal ultrastructure in, 2974f, 2974–2975
basement membrane changes as, 2974
stromal cellular desert as, 2974f, 2974–2975
Peritubular capillary(ies)
anatomy of, 6
fluid reabsorption in, hemodynamics of, 78–79
hydrostatic pressure in, efferent arteriolar resistance and, 82
macromolecular permeability of, 78–79
in peptide hormone removal, 319
Peritubular reabsorptive coefficient (K_r), formula for, 78
Periurethral region, antimicrobial defense mechanisms of, 894–895
pH
ammoniagenesis and, 243–244
disequilibrium, 2435
of urine. *See also* Urine acidification
antimicrobial therapy and, 1014
nephrolithiasis due to, 731, 731t
urinalysis for, 336
Phagocytosis, mesangial cells in, 14
Phenacetin, analgesic-induced renal disease due to, 1104, 1105t, 1107, 1971–1972
Phenindione, acute interstitial nephritis due to, 1341
Phenobarbital, pharmacology of, normal vs. in renal failure, 3254t–3255t
Phenobarbital–vitamin D drug interaction, in renal disease, 3230
Phentolamine, for hypertension, 1624
Phenytoin
for convulsion in eclampsia, 1527
pharmacology of, normal vs. in renal failure, 3254t–3255t
Pheochromocytoma, 1484–1499
associated clinical syndromes in, 1487
biochemical diagnostic tests in, 1490–1493
norepinephrine/DHPG ratios in, 1493
plasma catecholamines and, 1490–1491, 1491f
plasma chromogranin A in, 1492
platelet catecholamine levels in, 1493
sensitivity and specificity of, 1493, 1493t
urinary catecholamines and metabolites in, 1491–1492, 1492f, 1492t
biochemistry of, 1489–1490, 1490f
clinical recognition of, 1486–1487
clinical setting leading to confusion in, 1487, 1487t
definition of, 1484
diagnostic considerations in, 1488–1490
hypertensive crises in, 1613–1615
hypotensive crises in, 1615
malignant, 1499
malignant hypertension due to, 1561
management of, 1498–1499
follow-up, 1499
medical, 1498
surgical, 1498–1499
pathophysiology of, 1485–1486, 1490
neural regulation of blood pressure and, 1485–1486
regulation of blood pressure and, 1485, 1485f
patient evaluation in, 1498, 1498f
pharmacologic diagnostic tests in, 1493–1495
clonidine suppression test in, 1494f, 1494–1495
glucagon stimulation test in, 1493–1494, 1494f
in pregnancy, 1509–1510, 1510f
preoperative localization of, 1495–1498
arteriography in, 1497f, 1498
comparison of imaging techniques in, 1496–1498, 1497t
CT scanning for, 1495f, 1495–1496
MRI for, 1496, 1496f
possible sites of, 1495, 1495f
renal scintigraphy for, 1496, 1497f
prevalence of, 1484
signs and symptoms of, 1486–1487
undiagnosed, prevalence of, 1487–1488
Phimosis, 640
Phosphate
excretion of
alterations in, 2731
in urinary tract obstruction, 673
for hypercalcemia, 2629, 2630t
infusion of, in distal nephron acidification defects, 2678–2679
metabolism of, in experimental renal disease, 2719
plasma concentration of, in children, 2382
restriction of, for chronic renal failure, 3155–3156
transport of
age-related impairment in, clinical implications of, 2422
disorders of, 617–620. *See also* Rickets
in proximal tubule, 617
Phosphate binders, 2607
in dietary therapy in chronic hemodialysis, 3181–3182
Phosphate salt, in hyperphosphatemia, 2614
Phosphoinositide pathway, in hormonal activation, 286, 287f
Phospholipase(s), in experimental studies on ischemic renal injury, 1266–1267, 1268f
Phospholipid(s)
membrane, nephrotoxicity and, 1056–1057
metabolism of, in renal hypertrophy, 2710
Phosphoribosyl pyrophosphate synthetase (PRPPS), mutations of, urate overproduction and, 2239
Phosphorus, 2599–2615. *See also* Hyperphosphatemia; Hypophosphatemia
balance of
aging and, 2419–2420
in continuous ambulatory peritoneal dialysis, 3176–3177, 3177t
in dietary therapy in chronic hemodialysis, 3181–3182
extracellular, 2613
gastrointestinal absorption of, 2599, 2600f
intracellular, 2613
metabolism of, 2599, 2600f
in cirrhosis, 2475
normal renal handling of, 3153
physiologic concentration of, 2599
renal absorption of, growth hormone and, 2603
renal reabsorption of, 2599–2604
acid-base balance in, 2602
adrenal hormones and, 2602–2603
cellular mechanisms in, 2601, 2601f
dietary intake in, 2603–2604
effects of PTH om, 2601–2602, 2602t
vitamin C and, 2603
tubular fluid, ultrafilterable, 2600
urinary excretion of
decreased, 2611
factors affecting, 2601–2604
increased, 2604
Physical training, intense, hyperuricemia and, 2245
PIAP, as tumor marker
in seminoma, 870
in testicular carcinoma, 862
Pindolol, pharmacology of, normal vs. in renal failure, 3254t–3255t
Piperacillin, pharmacology of, normal vs. in renal failure, 3254t–3255t
Piretanide, mechanism of action of, 2443

Pituitary ACTH excess, 1541. *See also* Cushing's syndrome
Pituitary gland, anterior, insufficiency of, 2552–2556
glucocorticoid deficiency in, 2555–2556
hyponatremia in, 2554, 2554f–2555f
mineralocorticoid deficiency in, 2554–2555, 2556f
Pituitary-gonadal axis, dysfunction of
in females, 2856
in males, 2855–2856
Placenta, in preeclampsia
blood flow in, 1517
perfusion of, 2296
role of, 2291
Plaques, senile, in dialysis dementia, 2800
Plasma protein
molecular weight, radius, and renal handling of, 381t
for prediction of colloid osmotic pressure, 75, 75f
in quantitative analysis of GFR, 79, 80f
renal handling of, 384
Plasma volume
in acute renal vein thrombosis, in nephrotic syndrome, 1323
effective, definition of, 2468
Plasmacytoma, in multiple myeloma, 2205
Plasmapheresis
in immunosuppression, 2930
in multiple myeloma, 2206
Platelet(s)
activated
in experimental studies on ischemic renal injury, 1274
in microvascular thrombosis, 2069–2070
in acute renal failure, 1384
in acute renal vein thrombosis, in nephrotic syndrome, 1322
in Alport syndrome, 578, 581
in membranoproliferative glomerulonephritis, 1822–1823
in preeclampsia, 1514, 2291–2292
in urine, immunoperoxidase labeling with monoclonal antibodies for, 355f–356f, 356
Pneumocystis carinii pneumonia
in AIDS patients, 2361
as complication of transplantation, 2945–2946
Pneumonia
CMV, as complication of transplantation, 2945, 2946f
Legionella, as complication of transplantation, 2946
Pneumocystis carinii
in AIDS patients, 2361
as complication of transplantation, 2945–2946
Podocalyxin, 7–8
electrical charge of, 382
Poisoning, lead. *See also* Lead nephropathy
chronic, malignant hypertension due to, 1561
gouty arthritis and, 2254–2255
Polyamino acids, for modification of aminoglycoside nephrotoxicity, 1152f–1153f, 1152–1153
Polyangiitis overlap syndrome, 2096, 2099
Polyarteritis, 2099–2108. *See also* Vasculitis
common clinical features of, 2099
course and treatment of, 2105–2108, 2106f, 2107t
crescentic and necrotizing glomerulonephritis and, 2103, 2105
definition of, 2099
end-stage renal failure in, 2108
incidence of, 2099
microscopic, 2101–2103
classification of, 2095
clinical course of, 2105–2106, 2106f
definition of, 2099
pathologic findings in, 2102f–2104f, 2103
renal disease in, 2101, 2103
treatment of, 2107–2108
monitoring therapy in, 2108
Polyarteritis nodosa
classic, 2099–2101
clinical course of, 2105–2106, 2106f
definition of, 2099
diagnosis of, 2099–2101, 2100f–2101f
ANCA test in, 2100
angiography in, 2100, 2100f
biopsy in, 2100
pathologic findings in, 2101, 2101f–2102f
renal disease in, 2099
treatment of, 2106–2107, 2107t
azathioprine in, 2107
cyclophosphamide in, 2107
classification of, 2095
malignant hypertension in, 1560
pathologic findings in, 1576–1577
renal, angiography for, 474, 474f
Polyarteritis-like syndrome, in rheumatoid arthritis, 2051
Polychondritis, relapsing, 2113–2114
Polyclonal antisera, 2929
Polyclonal immune globulins, in immunosuppression, 2902, 2902t
Polycystic kidney disease, 535–561
acquired. *See* Cystic kidney disease, acquired
autosomal dominant, 535–558
acquired cystic kidney disease vs., 547
angiography for, 478
antibiotic concentrations in cysts in, 550–551, 551t
characteristics of, 547t
in childhood, 555t, 555–556
autosomal recessive vs., 555, 555t
extrarenal manifestations of, 555–556
renal manifestations of, 556
clinical features of, 547–549
CT for, 452–453, 453f
definition of, 535
diagnosis of, 543–547
computed axial tomography in, 546, 546t
family history in, 544
gene linkage techniques for, 546–547
magnetic resonance imaging in, 546
physical examination in, 544
radioisotope scanning in, 546
renal biopsy in, 546
studies in, 544t
ultrasonography in, 544–546, 545f
differential diagnosis of, 547, 547t
in elderly, 556
epidemiology of, 535
flank and back pain in, 548
genetic counseling and screening in, 557
hematuria in, 548
hemodialysis in, 557
hypertension in, 548–549
inheritance of, 535–536, 536f
kidney enlargement in, 549
liver enlargement in, 549
liver function in, 550
medullary cystic disease vs., 547
medullary sponge kidney vs., 547
nonrenal complications of, 551t, 551–555
arachnoid cysts as, 553
cardiac valve abnormalities in, 554
colon diverticula as, 554
intracranial aneurysm as, 553–554, 554f
liver cysts as, 552f–553f, 552–553
other organ cysts as, 553
sundry other types of, 554–555
pathogenesis of, 538–539
abnormal cell proliferation in, 538
abnormal extracellular matrix metabolism in, 538–539
abnormal fluid accumulation in, 538
pathologic findings in, 536–538, 537f–542f
electron microscopy in, 537–538, 538f–543f
gross inspection in, 536–537, 537f
microdissection studies in, 537
pathophysiology of, 539–543
cyst fluid composition in, 540, 544t
cyst sodium concentrations in, 539, 544f
cyst wall characteristics in, 540–541
cystic solute transport in, 541–543
percutaneous cyst puncture for, 548
renal complications of, 550t, 550–551
calculi as, 551
cyst infection as, 550–551
pyelonephritis as, 550
renal cell carcinoma as, 551
urinary tract infection as, 550
renal concentrating defect in, 549–550
renal disease in, natural history of, 556t, 556–557
renal dysplasia vs., 547
renal transplantation in, 557–558
Rovsing's procedure for, 548
serum erythropoietin levels in, 549
symptoms of, 547–548, 548t
systolic murmurs in, 549
uric acid homeostasis in, 550
urinalysis in, 550
urine acidification in, 549
autosomal recessive, 558–559
in childhood, autosomal dominant vs., 555, 555t
complications of, 559
description of, 558
diagnosis of, 558f, 558–559
disorders associated with, 559
genetic counseling in, 559
medullary sponge kidney vs., 531
treatment of, 559
urinary tract infection in, 559
in children, 2387
gout in, 2256
due to hemodialysis, CT for, 453
MRI for, 458, 459f
in pregnancy, 2300
renal transplantation and, 2916

Polycythemia
posttransplant, 2951
urinary tract obstruction and, 660
Polycythemia vera, vs. erythrocytosis, 2753
Polydipsia
demeclocycline causing, 2527
diabetes insipidus and, 2512
due to lithium-induced renal disease, 1100
Polymyositis-dermatomyositis, 2057–2058
classification of, 2057, 2057t
clinical and laboratory abnormalities in, 2057
renal disease in, 2057–2058
in childhood disease, 2058
membranous glomerulopathy as, 2058
myoglobinemia and myoglobinuria in, 2058
Polymyxin B
acute interstitial nephritis due to, 1337
pharmacology of, normal vs. in renal failure, 3254t–3255t
Polymyxin E, acute interstitial nephritis due to, 1337
Polyneuropathy
dying-back, 2805
uremic, in chronic hemodialysis, 3085–3086, 3086f
Polyp, of verumontanum, 638–639
Polysaccharide antigen, 2348
Polyuria, 2503
after adrenocorticotropic hormone, 2523f, 2552
demeclocycline causing, 2527
diabetes insipidus and, 2512
due to lithium-induced renal disease, 1100
during pregnancy, 2512
Pontine myelinolysis, central, 2525
Portacaval shunt, in hepatorenal syndrome, 1365
Postcarotid endarterectomy hypertension, 1613
Postcoronary bypass hypertension, 1612–1613
Postinfective nephritis, immunopathology of, 1661
Postoperative bleeding, hypertension complicating, 1613
Postpartum eclampsia, late, 1511, 1517
Postpartum hemolytic-uremic syndrome, 2301
Postpartum hypertension, 1511
Postpartum nephrosclerosis, 2301
Postrenal failure. *See* Acute renal failure, postrenal
Poststreptococcal glomerulonephritis, acute, 1715–1726. *See also* Glomerulonephritis, acute poststreptococcal
Posture, upright, idiopathic edema and, 2494–2495
Potassium. *See also* Hyperkalemia; Hypokalemia
in dietary therapy in chronic hemodialysis, 3181
diminished intake of, hypokalemia due to, 2588
intracellular redistribution of, hypokalemia due to, 2588
plasma, reduced, distal tubular acidosis in, 2679f, 2679–2682, 2680t
in renal failure
external, 2651–2652
internal, 2651
intestinal excretion of, 2652–2653
total body and cellular, 2650–2651
serum, in screening for primary aldosteronism, 1476f, 1476–1477
Potassium balance
aging and, 2418–2419
in continuous ambulatory peritoneal dialysis, 3176–3177, 3177t
in idiopathic edema, 2497, 2497f
internal and external, 2645, 2646f
in medullary sponge kidney, 528
Potassium depletion
in chronic tubulointerstitial nephropathy, 1975
effects on intercalated cells and apical membrane, 44–45
Potassium excretion
factors affecting, 183t, 183–184
acid-base balance as, 184
adrenal cortex as, 183–184
diuretic drugs as, 183
extracellular fluid volume as, 183
non-chloride anions as, 184
plasma potassium concentration as, 183
potassium intake as, 183
sodium intake as, 183
hypokalemia due to, 2588
prostaglandin effects on, 1207
renal, 2648–2650, 2649f
in urinary tract obstruction, 673
Potassium homeostasis, 2645–2653
acid-base balance in, 2648
catecholamines in, 2646–2647, 2647t
in chronic renal failure, 2725–2726, 2726f
diabetes mellitus and, 2584
insulin in, 2645–2646
internal, 2645–2648
intracellular calcium in, 2648
Ki:Ko ratio in, 2645
mineralocorticoids in, 2647–2648
osmolality in, 2648
parathyroid hormone in, 2648
renal excretion of potassium in, 2648–2650, 2649f
in severe renal failure, 2650t, 2650–2653
external, 2651–2652
internal, 2651
intestinal potassium excretion and, 2652–2653
total body and potassium content and, 2650–2651
Potassium ion(s), in experimental studies on ischemic renal injury, 1262f–1263f, 1262–1263
Potassium metabolism
in cirrhosis, 2474–2475
disorders of, 2645–2659
in sickle cell disease, 2320
Potassium phosphate, for hypophosphatemia, 2610
Potassium transport, 181–196
cellular mechanisms of, 188–195
active transport in, 189
basolateral membrane voltage in, 189–190
conductive pathways of, 189
leakage mechanisms in, 189
sodium-potassium exchange in, 189
in distal tubule, 186–188. *See also* Tubule(s), distal
general mechanisms of, 181
in glomerulus, 184
in loop of Henle, 185
mineralocorticoids in, 297–298, 298f
nephron segments in, 181–183, 182f
in proximal convoluted tubule, 184–185
regulatory factors in, interactions among, 195–196
sodium-potassium-ATPase in, basolateral membrane area and, 41–43, 42f–43f
Potassium-sparing diuretics, 2444
Potter's syndrome (renal agenesis), 2383, 2383f, 2387
Prazosin, pharmacology of, normal vs. in renal failure, 3254t–3255t
Prazosin, for sodium and water retention, in congestive heart failure, 2463–2464
Prealbumin, in familial amyloidosis, 2212
Prednisolone
drug interactions with, in renal disease, 3230–3231
pharmacology of, normal vs. in renal failure, 3256t–3257t
Prednisone
for hypercalcemia, 2629, 2630t
in maintenance immunosuppression, 2925, 2925t
Preeclampsia, 2290–2298. *See also* Eclampsia; Pregnancy, hypertension in
causes of, 2290–2292
clinical and biochemical findings in, 2292–2293, 2293f
clinical manifestations of, 1509
clinical sequelae of, 1516–1519
cardiovascular hemodynamics and, 1518–1519
central nervous system and, 1517–1518
glomerular capillary endotheliosis and, 1516
kidneys and, 1516–1517
liver and, 1517
placenta and, 1517
proteinuria and, 1516
renal hemodynamics and, 1516
uric acid clearance and, 1516
coagulation disorders in, 2291–2292
differential diagnosis of, 1519t
vs. essential hypertension, 2294
etiology of, 1514–1516
decreased uteroplacental perfusion in, 1515
endothelial cell damage in, 1515
genetic factors in, 1516
immunologic mechanisms of, 1515–1516
familial influences in, 2291
fibrinolysis in, 2291
hereditary influences in, 2291
immunohistology of, 2294, 2296f
immunologic factors in, 2291
incidence of, 2290, 2290f
management of, 2295–2298
pathology of, 2293–2294, 2294f–2296f
pathophysiology of, 1511–1514
vascular reactivity in, 1511–1514
calcium in, 1513
catecholamines in, 1513
hormones in, 1512
infection theory in, 1513

Potassium transport, pathophysiology of—Continued
magnesium in, 1513
progesterone in, 1512
prolactin in, 1512
prostaglandins in, 1512
renin-angiotensin system in, 1511–1512
serotonin in, 1513
"unknown humoral substances" in, 1513
vasopressin in, 1512
VIP in, 1512–1513
placenta in, role of, 2291
platelet and coagulation abnormalities in, 1514, 2291–2292
prevention of, 1529–1530
antihypertensive therapy for, 1522
calcium in, 1530
diuretics in, 1529
low-dose aspirin in, 1530
treatment of hypertension in, 1529
proteinuria in, 1509
remote prognosis in, 1530–1531
renal pathologic findings in, 1516–1517
renin-angiotensin-aldosterone system and, 2291
severe
acute renal failure in, 2301
anesthesia and analgesia in, 1529
blood transfusion in, 1529
signs and symptoms of, 1519, 1520t
sodium retention in, 2291
superimposed on chronic hypertension, 1510
synonyms for, 1508
treatment of
anticoagulant therapy in, 1527–1528
antihypertensive therapy in. *See also* Pregnancy, antihypertensive therapy in
prostaglandin therapy in, 1528–1529
volume expansion in, 1528
uterus in, role of, 2291
volume homeostasis and sodium retention in, 1514
Pregnancy
acid-base balance during, 2289
acute fatty liver of, 2301
acute glomerulonephritis in, 2303
acute pyelonephritis in, 981, 988, 2299
acute renal failure in, 2300t, 2300–2301. *See also* Acute renal failure, in pregnancy
acute tubular necrosis in, incidence of, 2334, 2335t
antihypertensive therapy in, 1521–1526
approved agents in, 1520, 1521t, 1523t
indications for, 1521
in mild or moderate presentation, 1522–1524
beta-adrenergic blocking agents for, 1523–1524
drugs for, 1523t, 1523–1524
fetal benefits of, 1522
hydralazine for, 1524
labetalol for, 1524
maternal benefits of, 1522
methyldopa for, 1523
preeclampsia prevention and, 1522
uteroplacental blood flow in, 1522
risk assessment classification in, 1521t, 1521–1522
in severe presentation, 1524–1526
alpha blockers for, 1526
angiotensin converting enzyme inhibitors for, 1526
diazoxide for, 1526
hydralazine for, 1524–1525
labetalol for, 1525–1526
near term or during labor, 1524, 1525t
nifedipine for, 1526
serotonin blockers for, 1526
sodium nitroprusside for, 1526
bacteriuria in, 978, 2299
asymptomatic, 1019, 1020f
bilateral cortical necrosis in, incidence of, 2334, 2335t
blood pressure in, 2289f, 2289–2290
control of, 1505–1508
measurement of, 1505
chronic glomerulonephritis in, 2303
chronic interstitial nephritis in, 2300
collagen diseases in, 2304
Cushing's syndrome in, 1542
cystitis and urethritis in, management of, 1019, 1020f
diabetes insipidus and, 2512–2513
diabetic nephropathy in, 2304–2305
fluid volume during, alterations in, 2287
glomerular filtration rate during, 2288, 2288f
hemodialysis during, 2305
hyperemesis gravidarum in, 2301
hypertension in, 1505–1531, 2290–2298. *See also* Eclampsia; Preeclampsia
assessment and management of, 1519–1521
aims of antenatal care in, 1519–1520, 1520t–1521t
fetal surveillance and delivery in, 1520
special considerations in, 1521
chronic, 1509–1510, 1510f
differential diagnosis of, 1519t
essential, 1519
initial evaluation in, 1519–1520, 1520t
with superimposed preeclampsia, 1510
classification of, 1508, 2290
clinical sequelae of, 1516–1519
cardiovascular hemodynamics and, 1518–1519
central nervous system and, 1517–1518
kidneys and, 1516–1517
liver and, 1517
placenta and, 1517
clinical vs. pathologic diagnosis in, 1508, 1509t
diagnostic criteria for, 1505
essential, 2294
incidence and prevalence of, 1511, 1511t
management of, 2295–2297
remote prognosis of, 2297f–2298f, 2297–2298
significance of, 2294–2295
transient or late, 1510–1511
nephrotic syndrome in, 2303–2304
pheochromocytoma and, 1509–1510, 1510f
polycystic kidney disease in, 2300
preeclampsia in. *See* Preeclampsia
proteinuria in, 2289
reflux nephropathy in, 713
renal calculi in, 2300
renal cortical necrosis in, bilateral, 2302
renal disease in, 2287–2306
renal plasma flow during, 2287–2288, 2288f
renal sodium handling in, factors affecting, 2287, 2288t
renal transplantation and, 2305–2306
renal tuberculosis in, 2299–2300
renal tubular function during, 2288–2289
sickle cell disease in, 2305
sickle cell trait in, 2305
sodium excretion in, 1508t
systemic lupus erythematosus in, 2030–2031, 2304
toxemia of, 2290
upper urinary tract infection in, 981
prevention of, 996
urinary tract in, 2287–2290
anatomic changes of, 2287
infections of, 2299
malformations of, 2300
obstruction of, 2300
physiologic changes of, 2289
uterine hemorrhage during, 2301
vascular reactivity in, 1505–1507
baroreceptor function in, 1507
blood vessel wall factors in, 1507
hormones in, 1506–1507
neurogenic factors in, 1507
prostaglandins in, 1506
renin-angiotensin system and, 1505–1506
uterine renin and, 1506
venous factors in, 1507
volume homeostasis in, 1507–1508
Pregnancy-associated diabetes insipidus, 375
Pregnancy-induced hypertension. *See* Preeclampsia
Prerenal failure. *See* Acute renal failure, prerenal
Primidone, pharmacology of, normal vs. in renal failure, 3256t–3257t
Probenecid
pharmacology of, normal vs. in renal failure, 3256t–3257t
urate excretion and, 2240
Procainamide
lupus-like syndrome due to, 2029–2030
pharmacology of, normal vs. in renal failure, 3256t–3257t
Progesterone
idiopathic edema and, 2495–2496
in vascular reactivity in preeclampsia, 1512
Prolactin
electrolyte excretion and, 2556–2557
in uremia, 2857–2858
in vascular reactivity in preeclampsia, 1512
water excretion and, 2556–2557
Pronephros, embryonic development of, 3–4, 642–643, 643f
Propafenone, pharmacology of, normal vs. in renal failure, 3256t–3257t
Propantheline, pharmacology of, normal vs. in renal failure, 3256t–3257t
Propionic acid derivative(s), acute interstitial nephritis due to, 1338

Propoxyphene, pharmacology of, normal vs. in renal failure, 3256t–3257t
Propranolol
for hypertension, 2390t
in neonates, 2386
pharmacology of, normal vs. in renal failure, 3256t–3257t
Propylthiouracil, pharmacology of, normal vs. in renal failure, 3256t–3257t
Prostacyclin, in sickle cell disease, 2323
Prostaglandin(s), 306–309
in cirrhosis, 2471
compartmentalization of, 1203
in congestive heart failure, 2459–2460
in disease states, 309
NSAID effects on, 91–92
effects on renal fluid excretion of, 1207
effects on renal potassium excretion, 1207
effects on renal sodium excretion of, 1206–1207
effects on renal vascular tone of, 1204–1206, 1205f–1206f
effects on renin release of, 1207
endothelial, in microvascular thrombosis, 2067–2068
in end-stage renal disease, 2822
in erythropoietin production, 309
in fluid balance, 308–309
glomerular filtration rate and, 308
in hepatorenal disease, 1357–1358
hypercalcemia and, cancer-related, 2272–2273
interactions of, with intrarenal neuro-humoral systems, 93, 93f
localization of synthesis and destruction of, 307
major renal actions of, 307–308
in medullary blood flow regulation, 100
metabolism of, 307
in preeclampsia, 1528–1529
renal blood flow and, 308
renal effects of, 1203–1207
in renal function, 2715
in renal physiologic processes, 1203–1204
renal synthesis of
location and effects of, 1203, 1204t
pathways of, 1203, 1204f
renin release and, 91
in renin secretion, 303–304, 309, 1416–1417
in renovascular hypertension, 1454
in sickle cell disease, 2321–2322
in sodium absorption, in thick ascending limb of Henle, 159
in sodium transport, 308
in collecting ducts, 164
stimuli for synthesis of, 91
synthesis of, 306t, 306–307
inhibitors of, 2588
in uremia, 2860
in vascular reactivity
in preeclampsia, 1512
in pregnancy, 1506
vasoconstrictor, GFR reduction and, in urinary tract obstruction, 665–666, 666f–667f
vasodilator
effects of, 91f, 91–92
GFR reduction and, in urinary tract obstruction, 665
Prostaglandin antagonists, nonsteroidal, membranous nephropathy and, 1796
Prostate, ultrasonography of, technique for, 412, 412f–413f
Prostatic antibacterial factor, 749
Prostatic carcinoma, 835–847
advanced
chemotherapy for, 845–847, 846t
hormonal manipulations for, 842–845, 843t–845t, 844f
adrenal androgen blockade as, 844t, 844–845
costs of, 845, 845t
estrogens for, 844, 844t
GnRH analogues for, 842, 843f, 844, 844t
historical, 842
treatment of, 842–847
diagnosis of, 837–838, 838f
epidemiology of, 835
etiology of, 835
localized
radiation therapy in, 840, 841f, 841t
radical prostatectomy in, 840–842
advantage of, 842, 842t
complications of, 841–842
impotence due to, 841–842
staging for treatment in, 838t, 840
treatment of, 840–842
screening for, 835–837
controversy over, 836–837
digital rectal exam in, 835–836, 836f
serum PSA values in, 836, 837f, 837t
transrectal ultrasound in, 836, 837f
staging of, 838t–840t, 838–840, 839f
ultrasonography for, 412, 413f
Prostatic hypertrophy, benign, ultrasonography for, 412, 412f
Prostatic secretory dysfunction, 749, 749t
Prostatitis, 743–754
acute, 750–751
clinical manifestations of, 750
pathologic features of, 750–751
treatment of, 751
bacteriologic localization cultures in, 746f, 746–747
culture interpretation in, 747, 748t
quantitative culture method for, 747
specimen collection for, 746f, 746–747
chronic, 751–752
clinical manifestations of, 751
infected prostatic calculi in, 751
medical treatment of, 751–752
pathologic findings in, 751
surgical treatment of, 752
chronic vs. acute, 745
clinical features of, 744t, 744–745
diagnostic methods in, 744–749
eosinophilic granulomatous, 754
etiology and pathogenesis of, 743–744
due to ascending urethral infection, 743
due to indwelling catheters, 744
pathogens in, 743
routes of infection in, 743–744
due to urine reflux, 743–744
histologic findings in, 745
immune markers in, 747–749
miscellaneous types of, 753–754
nonbacterial, 752–753
due to *Chlamydia trachomatis*, 752
clinical manifestations of, 752
due to *Mycoplasma*, 752
putative causative agents in, 752–753
treatment of, 752
due to *Ureaplasma*, 752
noneosinophilic granulomatous, 754
pharmacokinetics in, 749–750, 750t
physicochemical markers in, 747
prostate expressate microscopy and culture in, 745–746
prostatic antibacterial factor and, 749
prostatic secretory dysfunction and, 749, 749t
semen microscopy and culture in, 746
tuberculous, 916, 917f
types of, 743, 744t
urine microscopy and culture in, 745
x-ray and endoscopic findings in, 745
Prostatodynia, 753
Protein
Bence Jones
in dysproteinemias, 2190
in proteinuria, 355
calcium-binding, 2619
dietary
BUN effects of, 371, 371f
GFR effects of, 365, 365f
renal hemodynamic effects of, 102
light chain
nephrotoxicity of, 2191–2194, 2192f–2193f
renal handling of, 2190–2191
plasma
molecular weight and radius of, 381t
for prediction of colloid osmotic pressure, 75, 75f
in quantitative analysis of GFR, 79, 80f
renal handling of, 384
predisposing to acute renal failure, 3196
proximal tubular reabsorption of, 383
Tamm-Horsfall. *See* Tamm-Horsfall protein
turnover of, 2853
Protein C, in acute renal vein thrombosis, in nephrotic syndrome, 1322
Protein catabolic rate
calculation of, 3140
in peritoneal dialysis, 2983–2984, 2984t
Protein intake
in continuous ambulatory peritoneal dialysis, 3167
in dietary therapy in renal transplantation, 3199
Protein loss(es)
in chronic hemodialysis, 3168
in chronic renal failure, 3167–3169, 3169t
in continuous ambulatory peritoneal dialysis, 3168, 3169t
Protein malnutrition, in chronic renal failure, 2395
Protein metabolism
in renal hypertrophy, 2711
in uremia, 2852–2855
amino acid levels and, 2852–2853, 2853t
clinical observations and, 2852
disturbed
clinical management of, 2855
mechanisms of, 2853–2855
protein turnover and, 2853
Protein restriction. *See also* Chronic renal failure, dietary therapy in
in experimental renal failure, 3135–3139

Protein restriction, in experimental renal failure—Continued
compensatory renal growth and, 3135–3136
hypertension and, 3135
immune mechanisms and, 3137
intrarenal hemodynamics and, 3135–3137
lipids and coagulation and, 3137–3138
metabolic effects of, 3138–3139
mineral metabolism and, 3138
neurohumoral hemodynamic control and, 3136
nutritional adequacy of, 3140–3141
progression of diabetic renal disease and, 3143–3144
progression of renal insufficiency and, 3142–3143
Protein S, in acute renal vein thrombosis, in nephrotic syndrome, 1322
Proteinase activity, increased, 2854
Protein-calorie malnutrition, in chronic renal failure, 3167, 3168t
Proteinuria, 380–392
in acute interstitial nephritis, 1331–1332
in Alport syndrome, 579
in aminoglycoside nephrotoxicity, 1131
in amyloidosis, 2220
in analgesic-induced renal disease, 1112
asymptomatic, 391
Bence Jones, 2189
in cancer, 2265
categories of, 385
in children, 2380, 2392t, 2393
clinical implications of, 335
in contrast media-induced acute renal failure, 1193–1194
in diabetic nephropathy, 2153
effect of lipid-lowering agents on, 2409, 2413f
endothelin, 389
in experimental renal disease, 2719
functional, 385, 391
hemodynamic alterations and, 385
prostaglandin synthetase activity and, 385
in various disorders, 385
glomerular, 335, 385
protein selectivity in, 392
in gout, 2252
in HIV-associated nephropathy, 2367
in hypertensive nephrosclerosis, 1441–1442
as index of clinical course, 392
intermittent, 391
light chain, 388–389, 2189–2194
causes of, 2190, 2191t
clinical consequences of, 388–389
identification and quantification of, 2189
in multiple myeloma, 2194–2195
nephrotoxicity of, 2191–2194, 2192f–2193f
renal handling of, 2190–2191
in malignant hypertension, 1568
measurement techniques in, 389–390
dipstick test as, 390
excretion in 24-hour collection as, 390
excretion in single voided specimen as, 390
quantitative tests for, 390
semiquantitative, 389–390
in nephrotic syndrome, 1751–1756. *See also* Nephrotic syndrome, pathophysiology of
in nonglomerular renal disease, 387–388
of nonplasma origin, 389
overproduction, 385
clinical consequences of, 389
light chains and heavy chains in, 388–389
pathophysiology of, 388–389
pathophysiology of, 385–387
percutaneous renal biopsy for, 488
persistent, 391–392
postural, 391
prognosis in, 391
tests for, 391
in preeclampsia, 1509, 1516
in pregnancy, 2289
in reflux nephropathy, 713
in renal disease, 385–387
basement membrane and, 387
charge disruption and, 387
endothelial cells and, 387
epithelial foot process fusion effacement and, 386
focal epithelial denudation and, 386–387
increased protein filtration and, 385–386, 386f
leaky glomerular capillary wall and, 386
morphologic abnormalities and, 386
in renovascular hypertension, 1458
selective, 335
in sickle cell disease, 2325
significance of, 391–392
Tamm-Horsfall, 389
tubular, 385
diseases associated with, 335
light chain excretion in, 388
lysozyme excretion in, 388
measurement of, in children, 2381
pathophysiology of, 388
in upper urinary tract infection, 983
urinalysis for, 335
in vesicoureteral reflux, 713
Proteus mirabilis, in upper urinary tract infection, 974
Proton transport, across apical membranes, 220
Proto-oncogene(s), 777
Protoplast(s), upper urinary tract infection due to, 974
PRPPS (phosphoribosyl pyrophosphate synthetase), mutations of, urate overproduction and, 2239
Prune-belly syndrome, 654, 2387
Pseudoaneurysm, renal artery, percutaneous transcatheter embolization for, 470f, 471
Pseudo-Cushing's syndrome, alcohol-induced, 1542
Pseudohyperkalemia, in diabetes mellitus, 2584
Pseudohyperphosphatemia, in multiple myeloma, 2201
Pseudohypertension, 1629
Pseudohyponatremia, 2516
ketone metabolism and, 2568
multiple myeloma and, 2201
pathogenesis of, 2568f
Pseudohypoparathyroidism, parathyroid hormone in, 2622
Pseudoparathyroidism, hyperphosphatemia and, 2612–2613
Psychological disorders
analgesia abuse and, 1111
hyponatremia and, 2521
Psychological testing, chronic renal failure and, 2791–2792
Psychosocial problems
in children, with chronic renal insufficiency, 2396–2397
in diabetes mellitus, 2181
Psychotherapeutic drugs, in renal disease, 3230
PTH. *See* Parathyroid hormone
Pulmonary capillary wedge pressure, in preeclampsia, 1518
Pulmonary edema
in malignant hypertension, 1600–1603, 1601f–1602f
in renovascular hypertension, 1458
in severe benign hypertension, 1600–1603, 1601f–1602f
Pulmonary hemorrhage, in antiglomerular basement membrane antibody–mediated nephritis, 1870–1871, 1871f
Pulmonary infection, as complication of transplantation, 2945–2946, 2946f
Pulsus alternans, in heart failure, 2832
Purpura
Henoch-Schönlein. *See* Henoch-Schönlein purpura.
thrombotic thrombocytopenic, HIV-associated, 2365
Putnam test, in light chain proteinuria, 2189
Pyelogenic cyst, 521, 522f
Pyelography
definition of, 407–408
intravenous
in acute renal vein thrombosis in nephrotic syndrome, 1324f, 1325
in renal pelvic carcinoma, 802, 802f
in screening for renovascular hypertension, 1460–1461
in ureteral carcinoma, 802, 802f
in urinary tract obstruction, 677, 677f–678f
retrograde
in renal cell carcinoma, 788
in renal pelvic carcinoma, 802–803, 803f
in ureteral carcinoma, 802–803, 803f
Pyelonephritis. *See also* Urinary tract infection, upper
acute
adult, clinical presentation in, 987–988
CT for, 451
definition of, 973
in elderly, clinical presentation in, 988
imaging techniques in, 986
management of, 990–992, 991f
pathologic findings in, 975
in pregnancy, 981, 988, 2299
urine culture in, 981–982
atrophic, chronic, imaging studies of, 425–426, 426f
in autosomal dominant polycystic kidney disease, 550
chronic. *See also* Reflux nephropathy
angiography for, 478
clinical presentation in, 988
definition of, 973

imaging techniques in, 986–987
malignant hypertension due to, 1560, 1576
management of, 991f
pathologic findings in, 975
renal transplantation and, 2918
emphysematous, in perinephric abscess, 967–968
glomeruli in, 2716–2727
immunoglobulins in, 897–898
papillary necrosis and, 1979
in sickle cell disease, 2324
symptomatic, prevalence and incidence of, 976, 977f
xanthogranulomatous, 997–998
clinical findings and diagnosis in, 997
CT for, 452, 452f
diagnosis of, 964–965
incidence of, 997
pathogenesis of, 963, 997
treatment of, 966
Pyelotubular stasis, medullary sponge kidney vs., 531
Pyelovenous backflow, medullary sponge kidney vs., 531
Pyrazinamide
urate excretion and, 2240
for urinary tract tuberculosis, 923t
Pyridoxal-5-phosphate, in protection against nephrotoxicity, 1068
Pyruvate, renal metabolism of, 239–240
Pyrvinium pamoate, pharmacology of, normal vs. in renal failure, 3256t–3257t
Pyuria
definition of, 973
laboratory assessment of, 982
in malignant hypertension, 1568
screening method for, 1012
in upper urinary tract infection, 982
urine microscopy for, 340

Quartan malaria, 2345–2346. *See also* Malaria
Quinacrine, pharmacology of, normal vs. in renal failure, 3256t–3257t
Quinidine, pharmacology of, normal vs. in renal failure, 3256t–3257t

Radiation nephritis, malignant hypertension due to, 1560
Radiation nephropathy
chronic renal failure due to, 1169
chronic tubulointerstitial, 1974
Radiation therapy, for leukemia and lymphoma, with renal involvement, 2270
Radiocontrast media. *See* Contrast media
Radiography, plain film
in renal cell carcinoma, 787, 788f
in urinary tract obstruction, 677
in urinary tract tuberculosis, 918, 918f
Radionuclide micturition cystography, for vesicoureteral reflux, 701–702, 702f
Radionuclide study(ies), 413–421
compartmental model for, 413–414
for effective renal plasma flow, 419–420
for GFR, 372, 419
hazards of, 416
indications for, 421
isomorphic model for, 413
normal and abnormal images in, 416, 417f
normal and abnormal measurements in, 416–417, 419
patient preparation for, 415
for perinephric abscess, 968, 969f
for pheochromocytoma, 1496, 1497f
principles of, 413–414
radionuclide injection and data collection in, 415–416
radiopharmaceuticals for, 413, 414, 415t, 416t
for reflux nephropathy, 705f–706f, 705–706
for relative renal function, 420–421
for renal artery thromboembolism, 2122–2124, 2124f–2125f
for renal cortical abscess, 960–961, 962f
renal transit times in, 414, 415f, 415t
for renal transplantation, 441
for renovascular hypertension, 439–441
for screening in renovascular hypertension, 1461
for static renal imaging, 421
techniques for, 414–416
of transplanted kidney, 2931, 2931f
for tumor localization, in primary aldosteronism, 1480–1481
for upper urinary tract obstruction, 435f–437f, 436–437
for urinary tract obstruction, 678–679
Rantidine, pharmacology of, normal vs. in renal failure, 3256t–3257t
Rapamycin, in immunosuppression, 2900
Raynaud's phenomenon, in Waldenstrom's macroglobulemia, 2207
Receptor(s), 69–70
affinity constant of, 69
agonists of, 70
antagonists of, 70
down regulation of, 70
G protein-coupled, 70
ligands and, 69
subtypes of, 70
up regulation of, 69–70
Recombinant human erythropoietin
for anemia, in children, 2397
in multiple myeloma, 2206
Recombinant human growth hormone, in uremia, 2855
Rectobulbar fistula, congenital, 637
Rectocloacal fistula, congenital, 637
Rectoprostatic urethral fistula, congenital, 637
Rectourinary fistula, congenital, 637
Rectovaginal fistula, congenital, 637
Rectovesical fistula, congenital, 637
Rectovestibular fistula, congenital, 637
Rectum
blind, congenital, 637
cancer of, nephrotic syndrome in, 2265
Red blood cell(s). *See* Erythrocyte(s)
Reflux, vesicoureteral. *See* Vesicoureteral reflux
Reflux megaureter, 645
Reflux nephropathy, 689–721
analgesic nephropathy vs., 1117, 1117t
in chronic tubulointerstitial nephropathy, 1970
clinical presentation in, 709t, 709–717
coincidental findings in, 717
definition of, 652
diffuse or generalized, imaging studies in, 426–427
end-stage, 713–714, 714f, 715t
experimental, 699–700
familial associations in, 715–717, 716f
focal, imaging studies of, 425–426
glomerular lesions due to, 697f, 697–698
historical, 689–690, 691f
HLA antigens in, 716–717
hypertension in, 711
management of, 720
peripheral plasma renin activity and, 712
renal vein renin activity in, 712–713
imaging techniques for, 704–707
intravenous urography in, 704f–705f, 704–705
radionuclide techniques in, 705f–706f, 705–706
ultrasonography in, 706–707
intrarenal reflux in, 691–693, 692f
mechanisms of damage in, 698–699
Tamm-Horsfall glycoprotein in, 698–699
urodynamic factors in, 698–699
pathologic findings in, 696f, 696–697
in pregnancy, 713
proteinuria in, 713
unilateral, hypertension in, 711–712
nephrectomy for, 711–712
peripheral plasma renin activity and, 712
renal vein renin activity in, 712–713
urinary calculi in, 714–715
management of, 720
urinary tract infection in, 709–711, 710f
asymptomatic bacteriuria vs., 709–710
imaging techniques for, 710–711
incidence of, 709, 710f
vesicoureteral reflux in, anatomic considerations in, 690–691, 691f–692f
Refractive index, of urine, 378
Rehabilitation, following renal transplantation, 2181
Rejection
allograft. *See* Allograft(s), rejection of
graft. *See* Graft(s), rejection of
Relaxing factor, endothelium-derived. *See* Endothelium-derived relaxing factor
Renal acidification. *See also* Urine acidification
defect in, clinical implications of, 2421–2424
Renal agenesis (Potter's syndrome), 2383, 2383f, 2387
Renal angioplasty. *See* Angioplasty, renal
Renal arteriography
in acute renal vein thrombosis in nephrotic syndrome, 1325–1326
in renal cell carcinoma, 789, 789f
in screening for renovascular hypertension, 1462
Renal arteriosclerosis, clinicopathologic correlations of, 505
Renal arteriovenous malformation, angiography for, 473
Renal artery(ies)
adenosine receptors of, 314
dissecting lesions of, 2127
chronic vs. acute, 2127
diagnosis of, 2127
therapy in, 2127

Renal artery(ies)—Continued
divisions of, 32–33, 34f
fibromuscular dysplasia of
angiography for, 472, 472f
percutaneous transluminal angioplasty for, 469
light microscopy evaluation of, 498
percutaneous transcatheter embolization of, 470f–471f, 471–472
for renal cell carcinoma, 471f, 471–472
techniques and agents for, 471
for traumatic renal artery pseudoaneurysm, 470f, 471
in renovascular hypertension, 1455f–1456f, 1455t, 1455–1457
anatomic configuration of, 1455t, 1455–1456
arteritis in, 1456
atheromatous lesions in, 1455f, 1456
cholesterol emboli in, 1456–1457
fibromuscular dysplasia in, 1456, 1456f
Renal artery aneurysm, 2126–2127
angiography for, 472–473, 473f
rupture of, 2126
surgical intervention in, 2126–2127
Renal artery atherosclerosis
angiography for, 472
percutaneous transluminal angioplasty for, 468–469
Renal artery embolism, acute renal failure due to, 1295
Renal artery pressure, GFR and, 361–362, 362f
Renal artery pseudoaneurysm, traumatic, percutaneous transcatheter embolization for, 470f, 471
Renal artery stenosis
in children, angiography for, 472, 473f
in elderly, 2422
posttransplant, 2950–2951
unilateral, hypertension and, 1425
Renal artery thromboembolism, 2121–2126. *See also* Thromboembolism, renal artery
Renal artery thrombosis, 2119–2121. *See also* Thrombosis, renal artery
Renal blood flow. *See also* renal hemodynamics
aging and, 2405, 2407f
clinical implications of, 2420, 2421f
angiotensin II effects on, 88, 89f
atrial natriuretic peptide effects on, 295–296
in cirrhosis, 2469
in congestive heart failure, 2457–2458
contrast media-induced acute renal failure and, 1192–1193
decreased
in hydronephrosis, 659
prerenal acute renal failure due to, 1289–1290
glomerular filtration rate and, 65, 66t
in hepatorenal disease, 1356
oxygen consumption and, 65
prostaglandins and, 308
regional differences in, 69
Renal calculus(i). *See* Calculus(i), renal
Renal capsular sarcoma, angiography for, 477
Renal cell carcinoma, 785–798
adult, molecular mechanisms of, 781–782
amyloidosis and, 2221
angiography for, 475–476, 476f
in autosomal dominant polycystic kidney disease, 551
clinical staging of, 790–791, 791f
CT for, 454, 454f
diagnosis of, 787–790
CT scan in, 789–790, 790f
cyst puncture in, 789
digital subtraction angiography in, 790
flow sheet for, 787, 788f
intravenous urography with nephrotomography in, 787–788
plain abdominal film in, 787, 788f
renal arteriography in, 789, 789f
retrograde pyelography in, 788
ultrasonography in, 788–789
features at presentation in, 785t, 785–786
immunotherapy in, 798
incidence of, 785
metastatic
chemotherapy for, 795, 796t–797t
cytokinetics of, 794f, 794–795, 795t
hormonal therapy for, 795, 795t
interferon for, 795–796
interleukin-2 for, 796
radiotherapy for, 794
surgical therapy in, 796–798
in multiple metastasis, 797–798, 798f
in solitary metastasis, 796–797, 797t
MRI for, 459–460, 460f–461f
nephrotic syndrome in, 2265
paraneoplastic syndromes in, 786–787
amyloidosis as, 787
anemia as, 786
erythrocytosis as, 786
fever as, 786
frequency of, 786, 786t
hepatic dysfunction as, 786
hypercalcemia as, 786–787
other effects as, 787
pathologic grading of, 791
pathologic staging of, 791–792, 792f, 793t
radiotherapy in, 794
adjuvant, 794
for metastatic disease, 794
renal percutaneous transcatheter embolization for, 471f, 471–472
surgical management of, 792–794
in bilateral simultaneous tumor, 793
preoperative arterial embolization and, 794
prognosis with, 793
regional lymphadenectomy in, 793
renal vein and/or inferior vena cava involvement and, 793
in tumor in solitary kidney, 793
terminology in, 785
ultrasonography for, 428f, 429, 429f, 430
Renal cholesterol embolization syndrome, malignant hypertension due to, 1560
Renal circulation. *See specific vascular structures;* Renal vasculature
Renal concentrating capacity. *See also* Urine, concentration of
age-related decline in, 2416–2417, 2420
in analgesic-induced renal disease, 1112
assessment of, 379
ADH administration for, 379
DDAVP test for, 379, 380f
water deprivation test for, 379
in autosomal dominant polycystic kidney disease, 549–550
in Fabry's disease, 596
in lithium-induced renal disease, 1101
in medullary sponge kidney, 527
in nephronophthisis-medullary cystic disease, 515–516
in upper urinary tract infection, 985
in urinary tract obstruction, 670–672, 672f
Renal cortex. *See* Cortex, renal
Renal diluting capacity, assessment of, 379–380. *See also* Urine, dilution of
Renal disease
acid-base disorders in, 2669–2686
anemia in, 2743–2753
management of, 2748–2752
pathophysiology of, 2743–2748
bacterial infection and, 2338–2339
in children, 2379–2399. *See also* Children
experimental, 2718–2719
geographic patterns of, 2331–2338
glomerular function in, 2716–2718, 2717f
hypercalcemia and, 2627
impaired concentrating and diluting function in, 2728
metabolic acidosis association in, 2669–2684
metabolic alkalosis association in, 2684–2686
nephron adaptation to, 2718–2720
acidosis in, 2719
glomerular growth in, 2719
glomerular hemodynamic adaptations in, 2718–2719
phosphate matabolism in, 2719
proteinuria in, 2719
parasitic infection and, 2339–2351
potassium metabolism disorders associated with, 2645–2659
in pregnancy, 2287–2306. *See also* Pregnancy
primary, recurrence of, transplantation and, 2935, 2937t
snakebite and, 2351
tubulointerstitial, diabetes mellitus and, 2574
underlying, renal transplantation and, 2914–2918
urinary concentrating defect in, 2512
Renal dysplasia, autosomal dominant polycystic kidney disease vs., 547
Renal failure
acute. *See* Acute renal failure
advanced, diabetes mellitus and, 2572–2573
amyloidosis and, 2222, 2224–2225
anion transport in, 274
chronic. *See* Chronic renal failure
contrast-induced, 2204
drug elimination by nonrenal pathways and, 3219, 3221t, 3222f
drug therapy. *See* Drug therapy; *specific drugs*
end-stage. *See* End-stage renal disease
experimental, dietary protein restriction in, 3135–3139
compensatory renal growth and, 3135–3136
hypertension and, 3135
immune mechanisms and, 3137
intrarenal hemodynamics and, 3135–3137
lipids and coagulation and, 3137–3138
metabolic effects of, 3138–3139
mineral metabolism and, 3138

neurohumoral hemodynamic control and, 3136
high-dose urography for, 438–439, 439f
imaging studies in, 437–439, 438f–439f
in leptospirosis, 2338–2339
malarial
jaundice in, 2345
pathogenesis of, 2342–2345
pathology of, 2341–2342
MRI in, 459
multiple myeloma and, 2202–2204
pathogenesis of, 2202–2203
prevention of, 2205
reversibility of, 2204t
treatment of, 2206
nervous system manifestations of, 2789–2809
nonoliguric, in aminoglycoside nephrotoxicity, 1131
potassium in, 2650–2653
external homeostasis, 2651–2652, 2652t
internal homeostasis, 2651
intestinal excretion of, 2652–2653
total body and cellular, 2650–2651
in scleroderma renal crisis, 2042
due to snake poisoning
pathogenesis of, 2351
treatment and prognosis of, 2351
treatment of, conservative symptomatic, 1381–1384
bleeding abnormalities and, 1383t, 1383–1384
catabolism, nutrition, and immunologic problems and, 1383
drug usage and, 1384
fever and, 1381, 1382f
infections and, 1381–1382, 1382f
metabolic abnormalities and, 1384
neutrophil count and, 1381
surgical complications and, 1382
urinary catheterization and, 1382
ultrasonography in, 438, 438f
in urinary tract obstruction, 682
volume of distribution of drugs in, 3218, 3219t
Renal function
in Alport syndrome, 579
alterations of, hormonal modulation in, 2713–2716
effect of urate concentration on, 2247–2248
in Fabry's disease, 595–596
hyperphosphatemia and, 2611, 2612f
laboratory examination of, 361–392. *See also* Glomerular filtration rate (GFR)
in medullary sponge kidney, 527–528
in multiple myeloma, 2200
reduced, urate excretion and, 2241, 2241f
regulation of, intrinsic vs. extrinsic, 2705
relative, radionuclide studies for, 420–421
in sickle cell disease, 2315–2321
hemodynamics of, 2314f, 2315–2317
testing of, in children, 2379
Renal glucose threshold, 2563
Renal hemodynamics, 66f, 66t, 82–102. *See also* Renal blood flow
adenosine in, 97–98
in altered physiologic states, 100–102
atrial natriuretic peptide in, 97
autoregulation in, 82–86, 83f
cellular mechanisms in, 86
myogenic theory of, 83, 84f
tubuloglomerular feedback mechanism of, 83–86, 84f–86f
in dehydration, 101
dietary protein effects on, 102
dopamine in, 96–97
endothelin in, 94, 312–313
endothelium-derived vasoactive factors in, 93–94
in fluid loading, 102
histamine in, 98
intrinsic control mechanisms in, 82–86
kallikrein-kinin system in, 92–93, 93f, 311
medullary blood flow in, 100
neuropeptide Y in, 97
in nonhypotensive hemorrhage, 101–102
in preeclampsia, 1516
renal eicosanoids in, 90f, 90–92
renin-angiotensin system in, 86–90
serotonin in, 99–100
in sodium depletion, 100–101, 101f
sympathetic nervous system and catecholamines in, 94–97
vasodilator nitric oxide in, 93–94
vasodilator prostaglandins in, 91f, 91–92
vasopressin in, 99
Renal hypoplasia, congenital unilateral, malignant hypertension due to, 1560
Renal insufficiency
chronic
clinical features of, 2671–2673
pathophysiology of, 2673–2674
treatment of, 2674
hyperkalemia in, 2650t
metabolic alkalosis in, 2685
percutaneous transluminal angioplasty for, 470
Renal mass lesion(s)
imaging studies in, 427–430
ultrasonography for, 428f–429f, 429–430
urography in, 428, 428f
Renal medulla. *See* Medulla, renal
Renal metabolism, 233–253
acid-base balance and, 249–251, 250f
ammoniagenesis in, 243–249. *See also* Ammoniagenesis
ATP synthesis in, 233, 234t
carbohydrates in, 240f, 240–243, 242f. *See also* Gluconeogenesis
citric acid cycle in, 238, 239f
fatty acid, 251f–252f, 251–253
compartmentation in, 251f–252f, 251–252
distribution in, 252
sodium transport in, 252–253
fuels for, 233
glutamate transport in, 245–246
glutamine transport in, 246
ketone body turnover and, 253, 253f
lactate in, 239, 239f
metabolite transport and specific carriers in, 234t, 234–235
in organic ion production, 274
oxygen consumption in, 235t, 235–238
basal vs. suprabasal, 235–236
oxidative phosphorylation in, 236, 236f–237f
rates of, 235, 235t
sodium transport and, 237f–238f, 237–238
pyruvate in, 239–240
substrate compartmentation and, 233, 234f
substrate utilization in, 233–234
Renal microcirculation. *See specific vascular structures;* Renal vasculature
Renal microvasculature, basic pattern of, 32–35, 34f
Renal nerve(s), role of, in sodium retention, 2458–2459
Renal nervous system, hormonal mediation of, 299
Renal parenchyma. *See* Parenchymal
Renal perfusion rate, age-related decline in, 2407f
Renal plasma flow
changes in, during pregnancy, 2287–2288, 2288f
effective (ERPF), radionuclide studies for, 419–420
in regulation of GFR, 363
Renal sinus lipomatosis, 410
Renal thrombotic microangiopathy, clinicopathologic correlations of, 505
Renal tubular acidosis. *See* Tubular acidosis
Renal tubule(s). *See* Tubular; Tubule
Renal vasculature. *See also* Renal artery(ies); Renovascular
abnormalities of, in cancer, 1168, 1169
anatomy of, 66, 66f
contractile processes of, 66–74
endothelial cells and smooth muscles in, 72–74, 73f
receptors and receptor activation in, 69f, 69–70
regulation of, 70f, 70–72
cytosolic calcium in, 70–71, 71f
mesangial cells and, 71f, 71–72
smooth muscle cells and, 70–71, 71f
structural-functional aspects of, 66f–69f, 66–69
prostaglandin effects on, 1204–1206, 1205f–1206f
sites of arachidonic acid metabolism in, 90–91
transcapillary exchange in, 74–82
capillary uptake by vasa recta in, 79
macromolecular permeability and, 77f, 77–78
peritubular capillaries and fluid reabsorption in, 78–79
quantitative analysis of, 79–82, 80f–81f
ultrafiltration at glomerulus and, 74–77, 75f–76f
Renal vasculitis, 1934t, 1934–1936, 1935f–1936f
Renal vasoconstriction, due to NSAID nephrotoxicity, 1209t, 1209–1211, 1210f, 1212t
Renal vein(s)
anatomic distribution of, 34–35
light microscopy evaluation of, 498
thrombosis of. *See* Thrombosis, renal vein
Renal vein renin
measurement technique for, 468
in reflux nephropathy, with hypertension, 712–713
in screening for renovascular hypertension, 1460, 1460f
Renal venography, 467–468
in acute renal vein thrombosis in nephrotic syndrome, 1325

Renal-retinal dysplasia, 513, 514t
  nephronophthisis-medullary cystic disease and, 517
Renin
  idiopathic edema and, 2497, 2498f
  juxtaglomerular apparatus in release of, 31–32, 303
  peripheral plasma, in reflux nephropathy, with hypertension, 712
  plasma
    in screening for primary aldosteronism, 1477, 1477f–1478f
    in screening for renovascular hypertension, 1459, 1459f
    in sickle cell disease, 2321
  prostaglandin effects on, 1207
  release of
    mechanisms for, 87f, 87–88
    prostaglandin effects on, 91
  renal vein
    in reflux nephropathy, with hypertension, 712–713
    sampling for, 468
    in screening for renovascular hypertension, 1460, 1460f
  secretion of, 303–304
    angiotensin II and, 303
    factors influencing, 1416–1417
    intracellular calcium concentration and, 1416, 1416t
    prostaglandins and, 303–304, 309, 1416–1417
    renal perfusion pressure and, 303
    sodium chloride delivery to macula densa and, 1416
    sodium chloride load and, 303
    sympathetic nerve effects on, 303, 1416
  synthesis of, 87, 302–303
  uterine, in vascular reactivity in pregnancy, 1506
Renin-angiotensin system, 302–305. *See also* Angiotensin II
  angiotensin antagonist effects on, 88, 90
  in autoregulation of GFR, 363
  blood pressure effects of, 1416f, 1416t, 1416–1417
  components of, 302, 302f
  in edema formation, in nephrotic syndrome, 1755–1756
  end-stage renal disease and, 2821–2822
  GFR reduction and, in urinary tract obstruction, 666–667
  glucocorticoid effects on, 1549
  interactions of, with intrarenal neurohumoral systems, 93, 93f
  in malignant hypertension, 1579–1580
  in obstructive nephropathy, 675
  renal hemodynamic effects of, 86–90
  renin release mechanisms of, 87f, 87–88
  in renovascular hypertension, 1453–1454, 1454f
  in scleroderma renal crisis, 2041–2042
  in thirst response, 120
  in treatment of renovascular hypertension, 1468
  tubuloglomerular feedback mechanism and, 88, 89f
  in vascular reactivity in preeclampsia, 1511–1512
  vascular reactivity in pregnancy and, 1505–1506
Renin-angiotensin-aldosterone system
  age-related alterations in, 2412, 2415f
  in congestive heart failure, 2459
  deranged, diabetes mellitus and, 2573
  in hepatorenal disease, 1358
  hyperkalemia and, 2653f, 2653–2657, 2654t
  idiopathic edema and, 2497, 2499
  in malignant hypertension, 1569–1570
  in pathogenesis of nephrotic sodium retention, 2478
  in preeclampsia, 2291
  in renal function, 2714
  in sickle cell disease, 2321
  in uremia, 2860–2861
Renin-dependent hypertension, 2822
Renography, isotopic, for urinary tract obstruction, 678–679
Renotropin, in chronic renal failure, 2707
Renovascular disease
  in chronic tubulointerstitial nephropathy, 1974
  due to hypertension, in cancer, 1169
Renovascular hypertension, 1451–1468
  animal model of, 1451–1453
    acute phase of, 1451
    chronic phase of, 1451, 1452t
    Goldblatt hypertension in, 1451–1453, 1452f, 1452t
    one-kidney, one-clip hypertension in, 1451, 1453
    two-kidney, one-clip hypertension in, 1451–1452, 1452f, 1453
    unclipping of ischemic kidney in, 1452–1453
  in children, 1458
  cigarette smoking and, 1458
  clinical signs and symptoms of, 1457t, 1457–1458
  diagnosis of, 1458–1462
  digital subtraction angiography for, 465, 467
  imaging studies in, 439–441
  laboratory investigations of, 1458
  malignant hypertension due to, 1560
  pathophysiology of, 1453–1457
    catecholamines in, 1455
    hemodynamics in, 1454
    hormonal factors in, 1454–1455
    hyperaldosteronism in, 1454–1455
    nephroptosis in, 1454
    posture in, 1454
    prostaglandins in, 1455
    renal artery pathology in, 1455f–1456f, 1455t, 1455–1457. *See also* Renal artery(ies)
    renin-angiotensin system in, 1453–1454, 1454f
  physical examination in, 1457–1458
  prevalence of, 1457
  proteinuria in, 1458
  pulmonary edema in, 1458
  radionuclide studies in, 439–441
  renal biopsy complications in, 490
  renal segmental infarction in, 1458
  screening for, 1458–1462, 1459t
    arteriography in, 1462
    captopril renography in, 1461, 1461f
    captopril test in, 1459t, 1459–1460
    differential renal vein determinations in, 1460, 1460f
    digital subtraction angiography in, 1461
    duplex Doppler imaging in, 1462
    exercise renography in, 1461–1462
    intravenous pyelography in, 1460–1461
    peripheral plasma renin activity in, 1459, 1459f
    renal scan in, 1461
    sequence of testing for, 1462
    split renal function studies in, 1462
  treatment of, 1462–1468
    in elderly, 1463
    medical, 1467–1468
      angiotensin-converting enzyme inhibitors in, 1468
      beta-blockers in, 1467–1468
      calcium antagonists in, 1468
      clonidine in, 1468
      renin-angiotensin system and, 1468
    options in, 1462–1463
    renal angioplasty in, 1464–1467, 1465t, 1466f. *See also* Renal angioplasty
    revascularization in, 1464
    surgical, 1463–1464
      results of, 1463–1464, 1464t
      techniques for, 1463
  ultrasonography in, 441
  urography in, 440f, 441
Reserpine, for hypertension, 1627
Respiratory acidosis
  ammoniagenesis in, 243–244
  diabetes mellitus and, 2583
  hyperphosphatemia and, 2614
Respiratory alkalosis
  diabetes mellitus and, 2583
  hypophosphatemia and, 2607
Respiratory failure
  acute renal failure and, 1865, 1865t
  acute tubular necrosis and, 1292
Restless leg syndrome, 2805
Retinal arteriosclerosis, in malignant hypertension, 1564f, 1564t, 1564–1565
Rhabdomyolysis
  acute renal failure and, 23332
  in cancer, acute renal failure due to, 1168
  nontraumatic
    acute renal failure and, 1294
    in drug abuse, acute renal failure due to, 1230–1231
    nonoliguric acute renal failure due to, 1298
  traumatic, acute renal failure and, 1294
Rheumatoid arthritis, 2049–2054
  amyloidosis and, 2220
  juvenile
    amyloidosis in, 2054–2055
    renal disease in, 2054–2055
    subsets of, 2054
  membranous nephropathy and, 1795
  renal disorders in, 2049–2054, 2050t
    amyloidosis as, 2049–2050
    due to analgesics, 2051–2052
    due to cyclosporine, 2053–2054
    due to drug therapy, 2051–2054
    glomerular lesions as, 2050–2051
    due to gold therapy, 2052–2053
    membranous glomerulopathy as, 2050–2051
    mesangial glomerulopathy as, 2050–2051
    due to NSAIDs/salicylates, 2051
    due to penicillamine therapy, 2053
    polyarteritis-like syndrome in, 2051
    proliferative glomerulonephritis as, 2050–2051
    systemic vasculitis in, 2051

tubulointerstitial disease in, 2051
vascular disorders as, 2051
Ribavirin, pharmacology of, normal vs. in renal failure, 3256t–3257t
Rickets
autosomal recessive, vitamin-D dependent
type I, 620
type II, 620
hypophosphatemic
hereditary, with hypercalciuria, 618t, 620
primary, 617–619
animal model of, 619
biochemical findings in, 617, 619
classification of, 618t
clinical findings in, 617
defective vitamin D metabolism in, 619
pathogenesis of, 619
therapy in, 619
oncogenous, with phosphaturia, 618t, 620
pseudofracture in, 2763, 2764f
vitamin D-deficient, 2605–2606
vitamin D-dependent, 2606–2607
X-linked hypophosphatemic, 2606
Rifampin
acute interstitial nephritis due to, 1337
causing renal failure, in AIDS patients, 2363–2364
pharmacology of, normal vs. in renal failure, 3256t–3257t
for urinary tract tuberculosis, 923t
Rocaltrol, for hypocalcemia, 2628
RS-61443, in immunosuppression, 2900–2901
Russell's viper venom, 2351

Salicylate(s). *See also* Aspirin
pharmacology of, normal vs. in renal failure, 3258t–3259t
for rheumatoid arthritis, renal damage due to, 2051
Saline, for hypercalcemia, 2629, 2630t
Salmonella infection, in tropical countries, 2338
Salt. *See also* Sodium
human appetite for, 1409–1410
restriction of, in end-stage renal disease, 2823
and water-dependent hypertension, 2822
Salt-losing nephritis, 1427
Sarcoid granulomatous nephritis, acute interstitial nephritis in, 1344
Sarcoidosis
in chronic tubulointerstitial nephropathy, 1976
hypercalcemia and, 2627–2628
Sarcoma
Kaposi's
in AIDS patients, 2361, 2366
as complication of transplantation, 2947t, 2948
renal, 798–799
CT for, 455, 455f
renal capsular, angiography for, 477
Scandinavian acute hemorrhagic interstitial nephritis, 1976
Scarlet fever, acute interstitial nephritis due to, 1343
Schistosoma mansoni, 2347
Schistosoma mansoni infection, membranoproliferative glomerulonephritis and, 1830
Schistosomal antigen(s), circulating, 2348, 2349
Schistosomiasis
clinical presentation of, 2347
histologic findings in, 2347–2348, 2348f
membranoproliferative glomerulonephritis in, 2347–2349, 2348f
natural history of, 2349
prevalence of, 2347
renal involvement in, 2346–2349
Scleroderma, renal transplantation and, 2918
Scleroderma renal crisis, 1556, 2039–2046. *See also* Sclerosis, systemic
clinical findings in, 2040t, 2040–2042
blood abnormalities in, 2042
combined, 2042
hypertension in, 2040–2041
presenting symptoms in, 2040
renal failure in, 2042
renin-angiotensin system in, 2041–2042
urinalysis in, 2040
criteria and frequency of, 2039–2040, 2041t
histopathologic findings in, 2042–2043
in acute renal disease, 2042f, 2043
in chronic renal disease, 2043
malignant hypertension in, 1560–1561
pathologic findings in, 1577
management of, 2044–2046
ACE inhibitors in, 2045
captopril in, 2045–2046
dialysis and transplantation in, 2045
hypertension and, 2044–2045
onset of, 2040
pathogenesis of, 2043–2044
cold in, 2044
hormonal factors in, 2044
immune factors in, 2043–2044
Sclerosis, systemic, 2039–2046
classification of, 2039
diffuse cutaneous, 2039
epidemiology of, 2039
limited cutaneous, 2039
progressive (scleroderma), renal transplantation and, 2918
renal involvement in, 2039–2046. *See also* Scleroderma renal crisis
clinical findings in, 2040t, 2040–2042, 2042f
criteria and frequency of, 2039–2040, 2041t
histopathologic findings in, 2042–2043
historical, 2039
management of, 2044–2046
pathogenesis of, 2043–2044
Sebastian syndrome, 581
Sedative-hypnotic drugs, in renal disease, 3230
Seizure(s)
in eclampsia, 1517–1518
prevention and treatment of, 1526–1527
metabolic alkalosis and, 2583
Selectin, in leukocyte-endothelial adhesion, 2002, 2003t
Selenium
in dietary therapy in chronic hemodialysis, 3184
in protection against nephrotoxicity, 1068–1069
Seminoma, 869–874
chemotherapy in, 872t, 872–873
classification and pathogenesis of, 853–855, 854f, 854t
cryptorchidism and, 852
incidence of, 869
natural history of, 855
postchemotherapy residual mass in, 873–874
radiotherapy in, 870–872
for bulky disease, 871–872
for retroperitoneal metastasis, 872
for stage A disease, 871
for stage B disease, 871
for stage C disease, 873
treatment fields in, 870–871, 871f
staging of, 869–870
tumor markers in, 861, 870
AFP as, 870
HCG as, 870
LDH as, 870
PIAP as, 870
Semustine nephrotoxicity, 1174, 1175f
Senile amyloidosis, 2210, 2210t. *See also* Amyloidosis
Senile plaques, in dialysis dementia, 2800
Sensory conduction velocity (SCV) test, 2804
Septicemia, acute interstitial nephritis due to, 1342
Septum of Bertin, intravenous urography for, 409, 410f
Serotonin, in renal hemodynamics, 99–100
Serotonin blocker(s), for severe hypertension in pregnancy, 1526
Sexual dysfunction, in uremia, 2855–2856
Sexual function, in chronic hemodialysis, 3085–3086
Sexually transmitted disease
cystitis vs., 1011
urethritis vs., 1011
Sheehan's syndrome, 2505, 2513
Shigella dysenteriae, microvascular thrombosis due to, 2063
Shohl's solution, 2677
Sia test, for macroglobulins, 2207
Sickle cell anemia, 2311
Sickle cell disease, 2311–2325
acute renal failure in, 2325
bacteriuria in, 2324
blood coagulation in, 2323
calicectasis in, 2324–2325
chronic tubulointerstitial nephropathy and, 1973
clinical manifestations of, 2323–2325
erythropoietin levels in, 2321
generation of negative free water in, 2319
glomerulosclerosis in, 2315
gross anatomy of, 2313, 2314f
hematuria in, 2323–2324
heterozygous form of, 2311
homozygous form of, 2311
hypertension and, 2323
hyperuricemia in, 2244–2245, 2320
incidence of, 2312–2313
kidneys in, 2313
membranous nephropathy and, 1796
nephrotic syndrome and, 2325
pathologic changes in, 2315

Sickle cell disease—Continued
papillary necrosis and, 1979, 2324–2325
pathologic features of, 2313, 2314f, 2315
microscopic, 2313, 2315
ultrastructural, 2315
potassium metabolism in, 2320
in pregnancy, 2305
prostaglandins and, 2321–2322
proteinuria in, 2325
proximal tubular reabsorption in, 2320–2321, 2321f
proximal tubular secretion in, 2320
pyelonephritis in, 2324
renal function in, 2315–2321
hemodynamics of, 2314f, 2315–2317
renal hormones in, 2321–2323
renal transplantation and, 2916
renal tubular potassium and, 2657
renin-angiotensin-aldosterone system in, 2321
sickled red blood cells in, 2311, 2312f
urinary acidification in, 2319–2320
urinary tract infections and, 2324
urine concentrating capacity in, 2316f–2318f, 2317–2319
effect of indomethacin in, 2318, 2318f
loss of zonation in, 2318
urine diluting capacity in, 2319
urosepsis in, 2324
variants of, 2311–2312
vasa recta occlusion in, 2323
Sickle cell syndrome, benign, 2311–2312
Sickle cell trait, 2311
in pregnancy, 2305
Sickle cell-beta thalassemia disease, 2311
Sickle cell-hemoglobin C disease (Hb-SC), 2311
Sigmoid urinary conduit, 828
Silicon nephrotoxicity, 1237
Sinus, renal
anatomy of, 3
intravenous urography for, 410
lipomatosis of, 410
Sjögren's syndrome, 2055–2057
acute interstitial nephritis in, 1344
clinical findings in, 2055
primary vs. secondary, 2055
renal abnormalities in, 2055t, 2055–2057
Fanconi syndrome and, 2056
glomerulonephritis in, 2056–2057
hyposthenuria in, 2056
interstitial nephritis in, 2056–2057
renal tubular acidosis in, 2056
tubular dysfunction in, 2056–2057
Skeletal muscle, in hypophosphatemia, 2608–2609
Skeletal toxicity, of aluminum, 3159f, 3159–3160
Skeleton. *See also* Bone
as calcium reservoir, 2617–2618
in hypophosphatemia, 2609
Skene's duct, blocked, 640
Skene's gland(s), 640
Skin
in Alport syndrome, 578, 578f
in Fabry's disease, 594
mycoses of, 944, 946
pigmentation of, due to analgesia abuse, 1111
vasculitides of, 2114
Skin cancer
as complication of transplantation, 2947t, 2947–2948
nephrotic syndrome in, 2265
Skin poppers' amyloidosis. *See* Heroin abuse, subcutaneous
Small intestine, perforation of, posttransplant, 2949
Smooth muscle cell(s)
contraction or relaxation of, mechanisms of, 70–71, 71f
interactions between vascular endothelial cells and, 72–74, 73f
Snake venom, 2351
Snakebite, renal disease associated with, 2351
SNS. *See* Sympathetic nervous system (SNS)
Sodium. *See also* Hypernatremia; Hyponatremia; Salt
concentration of
aging and, 2412, 2414f–2415f, 2420
disorders of, 2589–2591
renal handling of, deranged, 2453
uptake of, in synaptosomes, 2795, 2796f
Sodium adaptation, mechanisms of, 2723
Sodium balance
in dietary therapy in chronic hemodialysis, 3180–3181
in idiopathic edema, 2497, 2497f
NSAID nephrotoxicity and, 1212–1213
Sodium bicarbonate
hypophosphatemia and, 2608
for renal tubular acidosis, in children, 2381
Sodium chloride
for Addison's disease, 2548
decreased reabsorption by ascending limb of, urine dilution and, 377
in renin secretion, 303
Sodium depletion, renal hemodynamic effects of, 100–101, 101f
Sodium excretion
aging and, 2412, 2414, 2415f–2416f
aspects of, at different levels of GFR, 2723t
blood pressure effects of, 1412–1416. *See also* Blood pressure, renal mechanisms of
fractional, in children, 2382
in medullary sponge kidney, 527–528
in pregnancy, 1508t, 2287, 2288f
prostaglandin effects on, 1206–1207
in uremia, regulation of, 2724–2725
volume expansion and, in hypertension, 1409
Sodium homeostasis, 2720–2725
in chronic renal failure, 2720–2725
excretion regulation and, 2724–2725
extracellular fluid volume and, 2720–2721, 2721f
in glomerular disease, 2724
intracellular fluid space and, 2721–2723, 2722f, 2723t
mechanisms of, 2723
in nonglomerular disease, 2723–2724, 2724f
Sodium intake
decreased, blood pressure and, 1410–1411
increased, blood pressure and, 1410
prevalence of hypertension vs., 1411f, 1411–1412
Sodium ion(s), in experimental studies on ischemic renal injury, 1261–1262
Sodium nitroprusside, 1619–1621
adverse effects of, 1620–1621
dosage and administration of, 1620
for hypertension, 2390t
in neonates, 2386
mechanism of action in, 1619–1620
pharmacokinetics of, 1620
for severe hypertension in pregnancy, 1526
Sodium reabsorption, in proximal tubule, 146–151. *See also* Tubule(s), proximal, sodium reabsorption in
Sodium restriction, for ascites, 2474
Sodium retention
in congestive heart failure
afferent mechanisms of, 2454–2457
efferent mechanisms of, 2457–2461
treatment of, 2463–2465
drugs causing, 2494
idiopathic edema and, 2494
in liver disease, 2465–2472. *See also* Liver disease
effector mechanisms for, 2468–2471
stimulus for, 2465–2468, 2466f–2467f, 2469f
nephron sites of, 2468–2469, 2477
in nephrotic syndrome, 2476–2479
treatment of, 2479–2481
orthostatic, 2495
in preeclampsia, 1514, 2291
Sodium sulfate infusion, in distal nephron acidification defects, 2678–2679
Sodium transport
active transport processes in, 141f, 141–142
in collecting ducts, 162–165. *See also* Collecting duct(s)
in connecting tubule, 161–162. *See also* Tubule, connecting
in distal convoluted tubule, 161–162. *See also* Tubule, distal convoluted
kallikrein-kinin system in, 311
in loop of Henle, 153–160. *See also* Loop of Henle
mineralocorticoids in, 297
prostaglandins in, 308
in proximal tubule, 142–151. *See also* Tubule, proximal, sodium transport in
renal oxygen consumption and, 237f–238f, 237–238
sodium-potassium-ATPase in, basolateral membrane area and, 41–43, 42f–43f
corticosteroid effects on, 43–44
Sodium wasting, in nephronophthisis–medullary cystic disease, 516, 516f
Sodium-bicarbonate co-transport, across basolateral membranes, 221–222
Sodium-hydrogen exchange, in chronic renal failure, 2707
Sodium-potassium exchange resins, in hyperkalemia, 2659
Sodium-potassium-ATPase
active transport processes and, 141f, 141–142
basolateral membrane area and
in sodium and potassium transport, 41–43, 42f–43f
in sodium transport, corticosteroid effects on, 43–44
in thin limbs of loop of Henle, heterogeneity of, 45
Soft tissue calcification, periarticular, 2762, 2762f

Solute elimination
by filtration, 2704
by filtration and tubular absorption, 2704f, 2704–2705
increasing, in hyponatremia, 2527
by tubular secretion, 2705
Solute free water clearance (CH_2O), age-related impairment in, 2418
Solute homeostasis, in chronic renal failure, 2720–2731
Solvent "sniffers," nephropathy in, 1232–1233
Somatotropin-somatomedin axis, dysfunction of, 2856–2857
Spinal cord injury, vesicoureteral reflux due to, 694–695, 695f
Spine, "rugger jersey," 2763f
Spiramycin, acute interstitial nephritis due to, 1337
Spironolactone
for cirrhotic ascites, 2474
for hypertension, 2390t
mechanism of action of, 2445–2446, 2446f
pharmacology of, normal vs. in renal failure, 3258t–3259t
Splenic impression, intravenous urography for, 409, 409f
Sporotrichosis, 946
Squamous metaplasia, of urinary bladder, 815
Staphylococcus epidermidis infection, membranoproliferative glomerulonephritis and, 1830
Staphylococcus saprophyticus
in cystitis, 1009
in upper urinary tract infection, 974
in urethritis, 1009
uropathogenic, virulence factors of, 1009
Starling filtration-reabsorption principle, in glomerular capillary ultrafiltration, 74
Steblay nephritis, 1650, 1651
Stenosis, renal artery. *See* Renal artery stenosis
Steroid(s). *See also* Corticosteroid(s).
acute renal vein thrombosis due to, in nephrotic syndrome, 1324–1325
in immunosuppression, 2896t
renal metabolism of, 319
side effects of, 2926t
Steroid-sensitive nephrotic syndrome, in children, 2392t, 2393
Stocking-glove sensory loss, in toxic neuropathies, 2805
Stone, renal. *See* Calculus(i), renal; Nephrolithiasis
Streptomycin
chemical structure of, 1135f
nephrotoxicity of, 1131
pharmacology of, normal vs. in renal failure, 3258t–3259t
for urinary tract tuberculosis, 923t
Streptozocin
nephrotoxicity of, 1173–1174
pharmacology of, normal vs. in renal failure, 3258t–3259t
Stress incontinence, 763
Subarachnoid hemorrhage
as complication of dialysis, 2803–2804
hypertension and, 1605
Subcapsular abscess, angiography for, 478
Subcapsular hematoma, angiography for, 477–478, 478f
Subclavian vein cannulation, in chronic hemodialysis, 3033
Subdural hematoma, as complication of dialysis, 2803
Substance abuse. *See* Drug abuse
Succinate dehydrogenase, in ammoniagenesis, 247–248, 248f
Sulbactam, pharmacology of, normal vs. in renal failure, 3258t–3259t
Sulfadiazine, causing renal failure, in AIDS patients, 2364
Sulfamethoxazole
cystic fluid concentration of, in autosomal dominant polycystic kidney disease, 551t
pharmacology of, normal vs. in renal failure, 3258t–3259t
Sulfamoyl benzoates, mechanism of action of, 2437–2438
Sulfasalazine, pharmacology of, normal vs. in renal failure, 3258t–3259t
Sulfinpyrazone
acute interstitial nephritis due to, 1339
pharmacology of, normal vs. in renal failure, 3258t–3259t
urate excretion and, 2240
Sulfisoxazole, pharmacology of, normal vs. in renal failure, 3258t–3259t
Sulfonamide(s)
acute interstitial nephritis due to, 1337
for uncomplicated cystitis, 1014–1015
for urinary tract infection, 2391
Sulindac, pharmacology of, normal vs. in renal failure, 3258t–3259t
Superalimentation, in acute renal failure, 1383
Suppressor cells, in engraftment, 2887
Sympathetic nervous system (SNS)
in cirrhosis, 2469–2471, 2470f
in end-stage renal disease, 2823
of kidney, 299
in renal hemodynamics, 95f, 95–96
in renin secretion, 303
Sympathomimetic amine reaction(s), nonprescription, hypertensive crisis in, 1616
Synapse(s), 2795
Synaptosome(s), 2794, 2795
calcium transport in, 2797
calcium uptake in, 2795, 2796f–2797f
sodium uptake in, 2795, 2796f
Syndrome of inappropriate antidiuretic hormone (SIADH) secretion, 2521–2527
clinical characteristics of, 2521
clinical setting for, 2522–2524, 2524f
CNS symptoms of, 2524t, 2524–2525
disorders associated with, 376, 2523t
hyponatremia and, 2521–2527
increasing solute excretion in, 2527
malignancy-associated, 2522–2524
mortality and morbidity in, 2524–2525
myxedema and, 2539–2541
pathophysiology of, 2521–2522, 2522f
potential etiologies of, 2590, 2591t
treatment of, 2525–2527
vasopressin antagonists and, 2527
Syringocele, Cowper, 639
Systemic lupus erythematosus. *See* Lupus erythematosus, systemic
Systemic sclerosis. *See* Sclerosis, systemic
Systolic murmur(s), in autosomal dominant polycystic kidney disease, 549

T cell(s). *See* T lymphocyte(s)
T lymphocyte(s)
activated, in graft rejection, 2892–2895, 2893f–2895f
alloantigen-specific, immune activation of, 2893, 2894f
antigen-activated, interaction of IL-2 with, 2895, 2896f
cytotoxic, in allograft rejection, 2884f–2885f, 2884–2885
helper, 2891f, 2892
IL-2 receptor positive, 2890–2891, 2891f
proliferation of, 2893, 2894f
suppressor, in engraftment, 2887
in urinary tract infection prevention, 898
Takayasu arteritis, 2113
angiography for, 472
renal artery, in renovascular hypertension, 1456
renal percutaneous transluminal angioplasty for, 469
Talc deposit(s), in focal glomerulosclerosis due to heroin abuse, 1224
Tamm-Horsfall protein, 889–891, 890f–891f, 2190
autoantibodies to, 891
biochemical structure of, 889
in casts, 346
cellular secretion of, 335
in chronic tubulointerstitial nephropathy, 1967
in dysproteinemias, 2190
exfoliated uroepithelial cells and, 890
furosemide binding and, 2442
immunomodulatory effects of, 891
in light chain casts, 2195, 2196
MS-fimbriated *E. coli* and, 890, 891f
in myeloma casts, 2203
in persistent immune response, 898–899
in reflux nephropathy, 699
secretion of, 889–890
Tamm-Horsfall proteinuria, 389
Tamoxifen, pharmacology of, normal vs. in renal failure, 3258t–3259t
Taurine, intracellular levels of, 2853
Tc-DTPA clearance, for GFR, 372
$^{99}Tc^{m}$DMSA, static renal imaging with, 421
Temazepam, pharmacology of, normal vs. in renal failure, 3258t–3259t
Temporal arteritis, 2113
Teratoma, testicular
classification and pathogenesis of, 853–855, 854f, 854t
natural history of, 855
Testicular carcinoma, 851–874
advanced
central nervous system metastasis in, 869
chemotherapy for, 864–867
CBDCA for, 867
clinical remission and, 865
historical, 864
maintenance, 865
new studies on, 866–867
PVB vs. BEP for, 864–865
relapse after remission and, 866
salvage, 865

Testicular carcinoma, advanced, chemotherapy for—Continued
VAB-6 program for, 864, 864t
various regimens for, 865
VIP for, 865–866, 866t
management of, 864–869
surgery for, 867–869
in advanced disease, 869
complete surgical resection in, 868–869
mature teratoma and, 869
preoperative chemotherapy in, 867–868
technique for, 868
classification of, 853, 854t
clinical features of, 856
cryptorchidism and, 851–853
orchidectomy for, 852
orchiopexy and, 852
as risk factor, 851–852
second testicular carcinoma and, 852
diagnosis of, 856–857
epidemiology of, 851
extranodal metastasis in, 856
familial factors in, 851
fertility issues in, 863
chemotherapy and, 863
preexisting infertility and, 863
incidence of, 851
low-stage
management of, 862–864
retroperitoneal lymph node dissection for, 862–864
controversy over, 863
infertility due to, 862–863
modified surgical boundaries in, 862f, 863
preservation of ejaculate in, 862–863
results of, 863
surgical boundaries for, 862, 862f
low-volume, retroperitoneal lymph node dissection for, 863
lymphatic metastasis in, 855
mixed cell types in, classification and pathogenesis of, 853–855, 854f, 854t
natural history of, 855–856
pathologic findings in, 853–855
retroperitoneal nodal metastasis in, 855
risk factors for, 851
staging of, 857t–859t, 857–860
chest CT for, 859–860
chest x-ray for, 859
laboratory studies in, 859
lymphangiography for, 859–860
physical examination in, 859
staging procedures for, 858–859
tomography for, 859
subdiaphragmatic metastasis in, 855–856
tumor markers for, 860–862
AFP as, 860–861
β-HCG as, 860–861
LDH as, 861–862
PIAP as, 862
Testicular carcinoma in situ
classification and pathogenesis of, 855
cryptorchidism and, 852
Testicular choriocarcinoma
classification and pathogenesis of, 853–855, 854f, 854t
natural history of, 855
Testicular embryonal carcinoma
classification and pathogenesis of, 853–855, 854f, 854t
natural history of, 855
Testicular seminoma. *See* Seminoma
Testicular teratoma
classification and pathogenesis of, 853–855, 854f, 854t
natural history of, 855
Tetany, treatment of, 2628
Tetracycline
acute interstitial nephritis due to, 1337
pharmacology of, normal vs. in renal failure, 3258t–3259t
Theophylline, pharmacology of, normal vs. in renal failure, 3258t–3259t
Thiabendazole, pharmacology of, normal vs. in renal failure, 3260t–3261t
Thiazide
in diabetes insipidus, 2509
hypercalcemia and, 2627
mechanism of action of
in distal tubules, 2447
in proximal tubules, 2437
nondiuretic, 2447
Thin basement membrane disease
familial, 583
Alport syndrome vs., 583
hematuria in, 583
pathologic findings in, 583
urinary findings in, 353–354, 354f
6-Thioguanine nephrotoxicity, 1177
Thiopental, pharmacology of, normal vs. in renal failure, 3260t–3261t
Thiotepa
intravesical, for urinary bladder carcinoma, 821–822
pharmacology of, normal vs. in renal failure, 3260t–3261t
phase specificity and mechanism of action of, 821t
Thirst
dopamine in, 120
hyperosmolar, 119–120
reduced extracellular fluid volume and, 120
renin-angiotensin system in, 120
water intake and, 119
Thoracic kidney, 654
Thrombocytopenia, macrothrombocytopathic, in Alport syndrome, 581
Thromboembolism, renal artery, 2121–2126
causes of, 2121
clinical findings in, 2121–2125, 2122t
CT and MRI in, 2124
intravenous urography in, 2122, 2124f
laboratory findings in, 2121–2122, 2123f
pathologic findings in, 2121
radioisotopic scan in, 2122–2124, 2124f–2125f
renal arteriography and aortography in, 2124–2125
serum enzymes in, 2122, 2123f
therapy in, 2125–2126
urinary indices in, 2122, 2123f
Thrombosis
deep venous, in nephrotic syndrome, 1759–1760
microvascular, 2063–2070. *See also* Hemolytic-uremic syndrome; Thrombotic thrombocytopenic purpura
drugs causing, 2065–2067
anticancer drugs as, 2065–2066
cyclosporine as, 2066
mitomycin as, 2066
oral contraceptives as, 2066–2067
due to erythrocyte oxidant injury, 2070
immune reactants causing, 2064–2065
autoimmune mechanisms in, 2064–2065
immune complexes in, 2064–2065
renal allograft rejection and, 2065
infectious agents causing, 2063–2064
bacterial endotoxin as, 2064
bacterial neuraminidase as, 2064
Escherichia coli 0157:HT as, 2063
Shigella dysenteriae as, 2063
due to platelet activation, 2069–2070
due to vascular endothelial damage, 2067–2069
endothelial derived relaxing factors/nitric oxide and, 2068
endothelin and, 2069
prostaglandin I_2 and, 2067–2068
von Willebrand factor and, 2068–2069
renal artery
acute, 2119–2121
causes of, 2120
clinical manifestations of, 2119
diagnosis of, 2119
in renal transplant, 2120
revascularization in, 2119–2120
traumatic, 2120
acute renal failure due to, 1295
as complication of transplantation, 2940
renal vein
acute, 1319–1327
etiology of, 1319
historical, 1319
incidence of, 1319, 1320t
in membranous glomerulopathy, 1319, 1320t
in nephrotic syndrome, 1319, 1320t
due to abdominal tumors, 1325
anticoagulant therapy for, 1327
AT-III levels in, 1321–1322
clinical course and treatment in, 1326–1327, 1327t
clinical manifestations of, 1323–1326
coagulation inhibitors in, 1321
co-factor levels in, 1320–1321
computed tomography in, 1326
due to dehydration, 1324
diuretics causing, 1323
fibrinolytic system in, 1321
hypercoagulability and, 1319–1323
intravenous pyelography in, 1324f, 1325
magnetic resonance imaging in, 1326
due to oral contraceptives, 1324
pathogenesis of, 1323f
pathophysiology in, 1319–1323
plasma fibrinogen levels in, 1321
plasma volume in, 1323
platelet abnormalities in, 1322
protein C in, 1322
protein S in, 1322
radiologic manifestations of, 1325
renal arteriography in, 1325–1326
renal ultrasonography in, 1326
renal venography in, 1325
due to steroid therapy, 1323, 1324–1325
surgical treatment in, 1327
due to trauma, 1324
zymogen abnormalities in, 1320
angiography for, 478

as complication of transplantation, 2940–2941
CT for, 453
in membranous nephropathy, 1789, 1796–1797
in neonates, 2386
in nephrotic syndrome, 1760
in sickle cell disease, 2325
Thrombotic microangiopathy
in hemolytic-uremic syndrome, 2074
renal, clinicopathologic correlations of, 505
Thrombotic thrombocytopenic purpura, 2070–2073
clinical features of, 2070–2071, 2071t
definition of, 2063
hemolytic-uremic syndrome vs., 2070, 2073
historical, 2070
HIV-associated, 2365
laboratory findings in, 2071, 2071t
pathologic findings in, 2071, 2072f
prognosis and treatment in, 2071–2073, 2073t
antiplatelet agents in, 2072
evaluation of, 2080, 2080f
intravenous immunoglobulins in, 2073
plasma exchange in, 2072
splenectomy in, 2073
steroids in, 2072–2073
Thromboxane, 2860
enhanced production of, in renal disease, 92
GFR reduction and, in urinary tract obstruction, 665–666, 666f
Thymus, congenital absence of, 2623
Thyroid disease, membranous nephropathy and, 1796
Thyroid function, in acute tubular necrosis, 1305
Thyroid gland, in uremia, 2858–2859
Thyroid hormone
in proximal tubule sodium reabsorption, 151
in uremia, 2858t, 2858–2859, 2859t
in uremic dyslipoproteinemia, 2851
Thyrotropin-releasing hormone, in idiopathic edema, 2495
Thyroxine, in protection against nephrotoxicity, 1068
Ticarcillin
cystic fluid concentration of, in autosomal dominant polycystic kidney disease, 551t
pharmacology of, normal vs. in renal failure, 3260t–3261t
Tienilic acid, acute interstitial nephritis due to, 1340
Tight junction(s)
functions of, 38
leak pathway of, 38
lipid and protein compositions of, 38
morphologic classification of, 38
functional significance of, 38–39
permeability characteristics of
control of, 39
cyclic AMP and, 39–40
cytoskeletal proteins and, 40
extracellular calcium and, 40
in transepithelial solute and water transport, 39
Timolol, pharmacology of, normal vs. in renal failure, 3260t–3261t
Tinsel's sign, 2226
Tissue renin-angiotensin system, hypertension and, 2822
Titralac, for hypocalcemia, 2628
Tobramycin
chemical structure of, 1135f
cystic fluid concentration of, in autosomal dominant polycystic kidney disease, 551t
pharmacology of, normal vs. in renal failure, 3260t–3261t
Tocainide, pharmacology of, normal vs. in renal failure, 3260t–3261t
Tophaceous deposits, in gout, 2252
Torulopsis glabrata, 930
renal infection due to, 937
Toxemia, 1509. *See also* Preeclampsia
of pregnancy, 2290
Toxic shock syndrome, hypophosphatemia and, 2608
Toxicity, aluminium. *See* Aluminum toxicity.
Toxin(s)
in acute renal failure, etiologic role of, 2332, 2333t
uremic, and nerve conduction, 2806
Trace element(s)
dialysis dementia and, 2803
in dietary therapy in chronic hemodialysis, 3183–3184
Trace metal metabolism, in nephrotic syndrome, 1762
Trailmaking Test, 2791
Transcellular transport processes, in nephron, 40–48. *See also* Nephron(s), transcellular transport processes in
Transcellular transport route, 38
Transforming growth factor
in hypercalcemia of malignancy, 2272
in vascular inflammatory injury, 1998
Transfusion
for chronic renal failure, in children, 2397
donor-specific, 2920
HIV transmission by, 2371
prior to renal transplantation, 2920
red cell, for anemia, 2752
in severe preeclampsia, 1529
in sickle cell disease, 2316, 2317
Transplantation
pancreas, in diabetic nephropathy, 2182
renal, 2911–2954. *See also* Allograft(s); Graft(s)
acute tubular necrosis in, prevention of, 2923–2924, 2924f
age of recipient and donor in, 2913–2914
alloantibody in, 2887
allograft infiltrate in, 2886–2887
allograft rejection in. *See* Allograft(s), rejection of.
allograft response to, 2882–2891
experimental models of, 2882–2886, 2883t, 2884f–2885f, 2884t
Alport syndrome and, 2916
amyloidosis and, 2916
with renal failure, 2225
analgesic nephropathy and, 2918
antiglomerular basement membrane disease and, 2917
in autosomal dominant polycystic kidney disease, 557–558
cadaver vs. living donor kidney in, 2921–2922, 2922t
cardiovascular evaluation in, 2919
chronic pyelonephritis and, 2918
for chronic renal failure, in children, 2397
complication(s) of, 2939–2953
cancer as, 2947t, 2947–2948
cardiovascular, 2949–2951
cataracts as, 2953
electrolyte and tubular, 2951–2953
gastrointestinal, 2948–2949
hemorrhage as, 2940
infection as, 2942–2947, 2943t, 2944t, 2946f
lymphocele as, 2942
osseous, 2951
polycythemia as, 2951
retarded growth as, in children, 2953
surgical, 2939–2940
urologic, 2941–2942, 2942f
vascular, 2940–2941
wound, 2940
contraindications to, 2914t
CT for, 453, 453f
cystinosis and, 2915
diabetes mellitus and, 2914f, 2914–2915
in diabetic nephropathy, 2179
patient survival following, 2179–2180
prognostic factors for, 2181–2182
success and complications of, 2180–2181, 2181t
dietary therapy in, 3198–3199
energy intake in, 3199
mineral intake in, 3199
protein intake in, 3199
recommended nutrient intake in, 3199
vitamin intake in, 3199
digital subtraction angiography for, 467
engraftment in, suppressor cells in, 2887
in essential mixed cryoglobulinemia, 2146
ethical issues in
age criteria and, 3112
case study on, 3113–3115
end-stage renal disease and, 3111–3115, 3112f
foreign nationals and, 3112
living unrelated donors and, 3112–3115
religious views and, 3115
shortage of donor kidneys and, 3111–3112
in Fabry's disease, 602–603, 2916
familial Mediterranean fever and, 2916
fine-needle aspiration biopsy for, 487, 489–490
focal segmental glomerulosclerosis after, 1750–1751
gastrointestinal evaluation in, 2919
genitourinary evaluation in, 2919
glomerulonephritis and, 2916f, 2916–2917
graft rejection in. *See* Graft(s), rejection of
graft survival and, 2938, 2938f
HBsAg screening in, 2919–2920
hemolytic uremic syndrome and, 2917
Henoch-Schönlein purpura and, 2917
histocompatibility and, 2879–2882
clinical testing of, 2881–2882
HIV infection and, 3121
HIV screening in, 2920
HIV transmission by, 2371, 2372–2373
HLA typing for, 2881–2882

Transplantation, pancreas—Continued
hypercalcemia and, 2627
hypertensive crisis in, 1617
hypophosphatemia and, 2605
IgA nephropathy and, 1843
imaging studies in, 441–442
in immunodeficient host, 2888–2890
immunologic evaluation in, 2920–2921
immunosuppression in, 2895–2905, 2925–2930. *See also* Immunosuppression
experimental solutions in, 2904–2905
future prospects of, 2905
induction and maintenance of, 2925
multiple drug protocols and, 2901
new agents and, 2930
plasma exchange and, 2930
recommended regimens in, 2925t, 2925–2926
selective, 2902–2905
side effects of, 2926t
kidney preservation in, 2923t, 2923–2924, 2924f
life expectancy with, 3031
lupus nephritis after, 2030
membranoproliferative glomerulonephritis and, 1831–1832, 2917
membranous nephropathy and, 1797–1798, 2917, 2918f
metabolic and congenital disorders and, 2915–2916
minimal change nephrotic syndrome after, 1750–1751
MRI for, 459, 460f
in multiple myeloma, 2206
in nail-patella syndrome, 606
nephrectomy in, 2920
cadaver donor, 2922
living donor, 2922
nutritional disorders in, 3198–3199
due to glucocorticoids, 3198
nitrogen balance in, 3198
serum folate levels in, 3198–3199
serum triglycerides and cholesterol in, 3198
zinc levels in, 3198
for osteodystrophy, 2778–2779
oxalosis and, 2915, 2915f
patient selection for, 2911–2913
patient survival and, 2937
percutaneous renal biopsy for, 489–490
cellular infiltrates in, 506
cellular rejection and, 506
chronic rejection and, 506–507
clinicopathologic correlations in, 505–507
hyperacute rejection and, 506
systemic CMV infection and, 506
vascular rejection and, 506
percutaneous transluminal angioplasty for, 470
plasma protein binding of drugs in, 3218
polycystic kidney disease and, 2916
postoperative management of, 2924–2925
pregnancy and, 2305–2306, 2953, 2953t
preparation for, 2920–2921
pretransplant evaluation and, 2911–2920
problem(s) related to, 2930–2937
acute renal failure as, 2930–2933
differential diagnosis of, 2931f–2936f, 2931t, 2931–2933
acute tubular necrosis as, 2930
allograft rejection as, 2930–2931
chronic rejection as, 2933–2934, 2937f
glomerulonephritis in allograft as, 2934–2935, 2937, 2937t
progressive systemic sclerosis and, 2918
radionuclide studies in, 441
recipient for, evaluation of, 2918–2920, 2919t
rejection of. *See* Allograft(s), rejection of; Graft(s), rejection of
renal tubular potassium and, 2657
results of, 2937–3939, 2938f–2939f
from cadaver donor, 2939, 2939f
from living-related donor, 2938–2939
from living-unrelated donor, 2939
risk factors in, 2918–2919
sickle cell disease and, 2916
surgical technique of, 2924
systemic lupus erythematosus and, 2917
transfusions in, 2920
ultrasonography for, 441f–442f, 441–442
underlying renal disease and, 2914–2918
uremic nephropathy and, 2808–2809
U.S. Healthcare Finance Administration Annual Facility Survey of, 2912t
vesicoureteral reflux in, 695
Wegener's granulomatosis and, 2917–2918
Trauma
acute renal vein thrombosis due to, in nephrotic syndrome, 1324
renal, CT for, 455–456, 456f
Trench nephritis, 1685
Triad syndrome, 654–655
Triamterene
acute interstitial nephritis due to, 1340
mechanism of action of, 2445
pharmacology of, normal vs. in renal failure, 3260t–3261t
Triazolam, pharmacology of, normal vs. in renal failure, 3260t–3261t
Triazole, for candidiasis, 942
Trichosporon 3, 944, 946
Triglyceride, serum, in CAPD, 2851
Trigone, embryonic development of, 640
Trimethaphan, for hypertension, 1622–1623
Trimethoprim
cystic fluid concentration of, in autosomal dominant polycystic kidney disease, 551t
for cystitis and urethritis, 1015
pharmacology of, normal vs. in renal failure, 3260t–3261t
for urinary tract infection, 2391
Trimethoprim-sulfamethoxazole
causing renal failure, in AIDS patients, 2363
for cystitis and urethritis, 1015
Tropical nephropathy
bacterial infection and, 2338–2339
geographic patterns in, 2331–2338
parasitic infection and, 2339–2351
snakebite-associated disease and, 2351
Trousseau's sign, 2634
Trypanosoma cruzi infection, 2346
Tuberculosis
amyloidosis and, 2220
granuloma formation in, 913
hematogenous dissemination in, 913
immune response to, 912
pathogenesis of, 912–913
renal
chronic tubulointerstitial nephropathy in, 1976
imaging studies of, 423–424, 424f
medullary sponge kidney vs., 531
in pregnancy, 2299–2300
urinary tract, 909–924. *See also* Urinary tract tuberculosis
Tubular abnormality(ies), in cancer, 2266t
Tubular absorption, solute elimination by, 2704f, 2704–2705
Tubular acidosis, 622–627, 2674–2677
ammoniagenesis in, 249
in children, 2381
classic, 2679–2682
distal, 624–625
causes of, 626, 626t
characteristics of, 625t
classic, 2679–2682
clinical features of, 2680–2681
diagnosis of, 2681f, 2681–2682
differential diagnosis of, 2681f
disorders associated with, 2680t
etiology of, 2681
general characteristics of, 2679–2681
pathophysiology of, 2679f, 2679–2681
treatment of, 2682
clinical approach to, 626–627
defects associated with, 625t, 626
diagnosis of, 625–626
hyperkalemic, 2682–2684
amyloidosis and, 2221
clinical features of, 2683–2684
diagnosis of, 2684
disorders associated with, 2683t
etiology of, 1683t, 2683–2684
general characteristics of, 2682–2683
pathophysiology of, 2682–2683
treatment of, 2684
pathogenesis of, 624–625
animal model for, 625
sodium sulfate infusion for, 625
urine minus blood PCO_2 for, 625
treatment of, 627
hereditary, type 1, characteristics of, 612t
phosphate wasting in, 2762
proximal, 623–624
carbonic anhydrase inhibition in, 624
characteristics of, 625t
clinical findings in, 623, 2676, 2676f
diagnosis of, 625–626, 2676–2677
disorders associated with, 2677t
etiology of, 2676, 2677t
general characteristics of, 2674–2676
pathogenesis of, 623
pathophysiology of, 2674–2676, 2675f–2676f
primary, 623
treatment of, 627, 2677
in Sjögren's syndrome, 2056
Tubular cell energy metabolism, in nephrotoxicity, 1045–1050
Tubular disorder(s)
in amyloidosis, 2221
due to subcutaneous heroin abuse, 1229

isolated, 611–629, 612t. *See also specific disorders*
multiple myeloma and, 2200
Tubular epithelial cell(s), urine microscopy for, 340, 340f–341f
Tubular epithelial cell cast(s), 348f, 349, 351
Tubular necrosis, acute, 1287–1310. *See also* Acute renal failure; Azotemia
acute interstitial nephritis and, 1345
acute prerenal failure vs., 1379, 1379t
acute renal failure due to, 1292–1293
in AIDS, 2362
biochemical abnormalities in, 1306t, 1306–1307
BUN in, 1306, 1306t
creatinine in, 1306t, 1306–1307
in cancer, 1167
causes of, 1292
causes of death in, 1373, 1373t
complications of, 1302–1306
angiotensin II levels as, 1306
calcium homeostasis and, 1305
cardiovascular, 1302
endocrine, 1305–1306
frequency of, 1302t
gastrointestinal hemorrhage as, 1303–1304
gonadal function as, 1305
hyperamylasemia as, 1304
infectious, 1305
insulin resistance as, 1305–1306
jaundice as, 1304
neurologic, 1304–1305
pancreatitis as, 1304
PTH levels as, 1305
pulmonary, 1303
thyroid function as, 1305
electrolyte abnormalities in, 1307–1308
etiologic treatment of, 1380–1381
atrial natriuretic peptide in, 1380
clinical management in, 1381
dopamine in, 1380
intracellular damage and, 1381
loop diuretics in, 1380–1381
hematologic status in, 1308
hypophosphatemia and, 2605
light microscopy evaluation of, 496, 498f
due to mercury poisoning, 1246–1247
metabolic acidosis in, 1307
due to NSAIDs, 1338t
pathophysiology of, 1371–1372
percutaneous renal biopsy for, 487
postoperative, 1292–1293
posttransplant, prevention of, 2923–2924, 2924f
in pregnancy, incidence of, 2334, 2335t
prognostic factors in, 1308–1310, 1309t, 1310f
respiratory failure and, 1292
risk factors for, 1292
in transplanted kidney, 2930
uric acid metabolism in, 1307
Tubular obstruction, in contrast media-induced acute renal failure, 1194
Tubular proteinuria, 385
diseases associated with, 335
light chain excretion in, 388
lysozyme excretion in, 388
pathophysiology of, 388
Tubular reabsorption, in urinary tract obstruction, 661–662
Tubular secretion, solute elimination by, 2705
Tubular transport, hormonal modulation of, 289–291, 290f, 291t
Tubular vacuolization, light microscopy evaluation of, 497, 499f
Tubule(s)
adenosine receptors of, 314
ADH receptors in, 292f, 292–293
anatomy of, 3–6, 6f–11f
collecting
ADH receptors in, 292f, 292–293
calcium absorption in, 2620–2621
connecting
anatomy of, 4, 5f
cellular structure of, 26–27, 27f, 160f, 160–161
potassium transport in, cellular mechanisms of, 194
sodium transport in, 161–162
apical conductive sodium channels in, 162
apical NaCl co-transport in, 162
basolateral electrogenic sodium pump in, 161–162
electrophysiologic considerations in, 161
general characteristics of, 161
mechanism of, 161–162
convoluted, in neonate, 2383
defects of, hypophosphatemia and, 2605
disorders of, posttransplant, 2951–2952
distal
acid-base transport in, 623f, 624
cortical thick ascending limb of, cellular structure of, 24, 26
diuretics in, 2444–2447
fluid conservation and excretion in, 374–375
function of, in children, 2381–2382
functional and anatomic subdivisions of, 186
medullary thick ascending limb of, cellular structure of, 23–24, 25f
morphology of, 23–26, 24f–25f
net acid transport in, 216–217, 623f, 624
potassium transport in, 186–188
ADH and, 188
barium inhibition to, 188
calcium ions and, 188
factors affecting, 186–188, 187t
apical, 187t, 187–188
peritubular, 187t, 188
functional and anatomic considerations in, 186–187
inhibition of, 188
luminal chloride concentration and, 187
luminal fluid acidity and, 187–188
luminal potassium concentration and, 187
luminal sodium concentration and, 187
plasma acidity and, 188
plasma potassium concentration and, 188
potassium-sparing diuretics and, 188
tubule fluid flow rate and, 187
regions of, 4, 5f
segments of, 23
distal convoluted
calcium absorption in, 2620–2621
cellular structure of, 25f, 26, 160, 160f
potassium transport in, cellular mechanisms of, 191–192
sodium transport in, 161–162
apical conductive sodium channels in, 162
apical NaCl co-transport in, 162
basolateral electrogenic sodium pump in, 161–162
electrophysiologic considerations in, 161
general characteristics of, 161
mechanism of, 161–162
parathyroid hormone receptors in, 293–294
potassium in, 2649, 2649f
hyperchloremic metabolic acidosis and, 2657–2658
proximal
acid-base transport in, 623, 623f
summary and integration of, 225, 226f
cellular morphology of, 143, 144f
cellular structure of, 15–16, 17f–19f
diuretics in, 2435–2439
electrophysiology of, 145t, 145–146
electrical resistance and, 145t, 145–146
ion selectivity and, 146, 146t
transepithelial potential difference and, 145, 145f
fluid conservation and excretion in, 374
function of, in children, 2380–2381
isotonic fluid absorption in, 151–152
light microscopy evaluation of, 496–498, 498f–499f
morphology of, 15f–21f, 15–16
net acid transport in, 212–215, 623, 623f
ammonium and, 214–215
bicarbonate and, 212–214, 213f–214f
sites of, 212, 212f
titratable acid and, 215
permeability characteristics of, 146t
phosphate transport in, 617
potassium transport in, cellular mechanisms of, 190, 190f
protein reabsorption in, 383–384
reabsorption of, in sickle cell disease, 2320–2321, 2321f
regions of, 4, 5f
secretion of, in sickle cell disease, 2320
sodium reabsorption in, 146–151, 2458
angiotensin II in, 151
apical membrane sodium entry in, 146
basolateral membrane sodium entry in, 149–150
control of, 150–151
corticosteroids in, 151
glomerulotubular balance in, 150–151
mechanisms of, 146–150
NaCl transport in, 147–148, 148f, 148t
Na^+-H^+ exchange in, 146–147
parathyroid hormone in, 151
passive sodium absorption in, 149
renal innervation in, 151
simple electrogenic sodium entry in, 149
sodium-amino acid co-transport in, 147
sodium-glucose co-transport in, 147
thyroid hormone in, 151
sodium transport in, 142–152
active transport processes for, 142–143

Tubule(s), proximal, sodium transport in—Continued
axial changes in fluid composition in, 143, 145f
general features of, 142–143
nephron heterogeneity and, 143, 144f, 144t
passive transport processes for, 143
subdivisions of, 15, 17f–19f
proximal convoluted
calcium absorption in, 2620
cell junctions of, 18, 21f
cells and mitochondria of, 16–17, 17f–21f
cellular cytoplasm of, 21
cellular structure of, 15f–20f, 16
cross section of, 2707f
intracellular digestive tract of, 15f, 18f, 18–19
lateral intracellular space of, 17f–18f, 17–18, 21f
microbodies of, 18f, 19, 21
microvilli of, 18
potassium transport in, 184–185
proximal straight, calcium absorption in, 2620
reabsortive maximum of, 2563
secretory defect of
diabetes mellitus and, 2587
hyperkalemia and, 2653f, 2654t, 2656–2657
segmentation of, 4
sodium reabsorption by
in cirrhosis, 2469
in nephrotic syndrome, 2478–2479
Tubuloglomerular feedback mechanism
in autoregulation of GFR, 362
GFR reduction and, in urinary tract obstruction, 667
in renal hemodynamic autoregulation, 83–86, 84f–86f
renin-angiotensin system and, 88, 89f
Tubulointerstitial disease
cell-mediated, acute interstitial nephritis and, 1346, 1347
diabetes mellitus and, 2574
in rheumatoid arthritis, 2051
Tubulointerstitial nephritis
acute, in cancer, 1168
animal model of, 1653–1654
immune complex-mediated, acute interstitial nephritis and, 1346, 1347
lupus, 2026
murine progressive, 1654
Tubulointerstitial nephropathy. *See also* Interstitial nephritis
acute, acute interstitial nephritis vs., 1331
chronic, 1959–1979
etiologic and pathogenetic mechanisms in, 1966–1976, 1967t
analgesics in, 1971–1972, 1972f
anti-TBM antibody in, 1968
Balkan nephropathy in, 1976
cadmium in, 1973
cell-mediated immunity in, 1968–1969
cyclosporine in, 1972–1973
cystinosis in, 1975–1976
drugs in, 1971–1973
endemic diseases in, 1976
granulomatous diseases in, 1976
heavy metals in, 1973–1974
hematopoietic disorders in, 1973
hereditary kidney diseases in, 1976
hypercalcemia in, 1975
immune-complex deposition in, 1966–1968
immunologic diseases in, 1966–1969
infection in, 1969–1970
lead in, 1973–1974
light-chain deposition disease in, 1973
metabolic disorders in, 1974–1976
metastatic lymphoma in, 1973
myeloma cast nephropathy in, 1973
nephropathia epidemica in, 1976
obstruction and reflux in, 1970
oxalate disorders in, 1974–1975
phenacetin in, 1971–1972
potassium depletion in, 1975
radiation-induced injury in, 1974
sarcoidosis in, 1976
sickle cell hemoglobinopathy in, 1973
Tamm-Horsfall protein in, 1967
tuberculosis in, 1976
urate disorders in, 1974
vascular diseases in, 1974
frequency of, 1959
functional manifestations of, 1964–1965, 1965t
cortical lesions in, 1964, 1965t
medullary lesions in, 1964–1965, 1965t
morphologic features of, 1965, 1966t
papillary lesions in, 1964–1965, 1965t
primary cause and magnitude of insult and, 1965
type of insult and, 1965, 1965t
functional significance of interstitium in, 1960–1963, 1961f–1962f
ammonium excretion and, 1962, 1962f
fibrosis and, 1962f, 1962–1963
inulin clearance and, 1961, 1961f
proteinuria and, 1963
renal plasma flow and, 1961, 1961f
urinary concentrating ability and, 1961–1962, 1962f
pathologic features of, 1963–1964
fibroblastic interstitial cells in, 1963
granulomatous lesions in, 1964
immunohistologic findings in, 1963
increase in interstitial volume in, 1963
infiltrate in, 1963–1964
intracellular crystals in, 1964
structural features of interstitium in, 1959–1960
terminology in, 1959
Tubulointerstitium, changes of, malaria and, 2341–2342, 2342f
Tubuloreticular inclusions, in HIV-associated nephropathy, 2368
Tumor(s). *See also individual types*
brown, of hyperparathyroidism, 2773
hypophosphatemia associated with, 2607
nonrenal, and kidney, 2265–2278
renal
angiography for, 474–477
CT for, 453–455, 454f–455f
metastatic
angiography for, 477
CT for, 455, 455f
MRI for, 459–460, 460f–461f
pediatric, angiography for, 477
urographic diagnosis of, 428
Tumor lysis syndrome, 2274
acute, 1180
hyperphosphatemia and, 2613
management of, 2275t
risk for, 2274t
Tumor necrosis factor
in hypercalcemia of malignancy, 2272
in uremia, 2863
in vascular inflammatory injury, 1997–1998
Tumor suppressor gene(s)
loss of heterozygosity and, 780–781
recessive, 780t, 780–781
Wilms tumor and, 781
Tumor-induced inappropriate hormone concentration, 1169–1170
Turner's syndrome, 2505
Twins, monozygotic, renal transplant results in, 2938
Typhoid fever, 2338

Ulcer(s), decubitus, amyloidosis and, 2220
Ultrafiltration
hemofiltration vs., 3042
isolated, 3041–3042
complications of, 3041–3043
technique for, 3041
underdialysis with, 3041–3042
pure, 2799
Ultrasonography, 410–413
in acute renal vein thrombosis in nephrotic syndrome, 1326
of bladder, 412, 412f
Doppler, 413
in HIV-associated nephropathy, 2367
indications for, 421–422
of kidney, 411f, 411–412
for perinephric abscess, 968, 968f
of prostate, 412, 412f–413f
for reflux nephropathy, 706–707
for renal calculi, 422, 422f
for renal cell carcinoma, 788–789
for renal cortical abscess, 960, 961f
for renal failure, 438, 438f
for renal mass lesions, 428f–429f, 429–430
for renal transplantation, 441f–442f, 441–442
for renovascular hypertension, 441
technique in, 410–411
of transplanted kidney, 2931, 2932f
for upper urinary tract obstruction, 432–436, 434f
of ureter, 412
for urinary tract obstruction, 677–678, 678f
for vesicoureteral reflux, 702
Urachal ligament, 641
Urachus, diverticula of, 641
Uranium poisoning, renal manifestations of, 1248
Urate. *See also* Uric acid
effect of, on renal function, 2247–2248
overproduction of
acquired, malignancy associated with, 2244, 2245f–2246f
animal studies in, 2245, 2247
genetic, 2239, 2242–2244, 2243f
hyperuricemia and, 2239, 2240t
kidney in, 2242–2248
uric acid nephropathy and, 2244
renal deposition of, gout and, 2250, 2251f
renal excretion of, 2240, 2241
renal homeostasis of, 2240–2241, 2241f
underexcretion of, in gout, 2239, 2240t
Urate nephropathy, chronic, tubulointerstitial, 1974

Urate transport
across apical cell membranes, 267–268
across basolateral cell membranes, 266–267
mechanisms of, 264–265
Urea
in ascending limb of loop of Henle, 135
metabolism of, 370
renal excretion of, 370
Urea appearance rate, 3139
in chronic hemodialysis, 3168
Urea clearance
in chronic renal failure, measurement of, 3139
in continuous ambulatory peritoneal dialysis, 2977–2978, 2978f
Urea generation, calculation of, 3140
Urea kinetic parameter(s), in peritoneal dialysis, 2982–2984, 2984t
Urea nitrogen appearance, in dietary therapy in chronic renal failure, 3172–3173
Urea nitrogen-creatinine ratio, serum, in dietary therapy in chronic renal failure, 3172–3173
Uremia. *See also* Acute renal failure; Chronic renal failure
aluminum absorption in, 3157, 3157f
aluminum neurotoxicity in, 3158–3159
aluminum skeletal toxicity in, 3159–3160
amino acid metabolism in, 2852–2853, 2853t
bleeding complications in, 1383t, 1383–1384
carbohydrate metabolism in, disorders of, 2845–2849
dyslipoproteinemia in
atherogenic, 2851
clinical management of, 2851–2852
pathogenesis of, factors in, 2850–2851
pathomechanisms of, 2850–2851
treatment modality of, influence of, 2851
endocrine disorders in, 2855–2863
glucagon in, role of, 2848
glucose intolerance and, 2845–2848
goiter in, 2859
hypothyroidism in, 2859
insulin metabolism in, 2845–2847, 2846f
insulin secretion in, 2848
lipid metabolism in, disorders of, 2849t, 2849–2852
nitrogen balance in, 3141
nutritional status and nutritional requirements in, 3167–3170
parathyroid hormone in, role of, 2847–2848
peritoneal ultrastructure in, 2972, 2972f
pituitary-gonadal axis in, 2855–2856
plasma protein binding of drugs in, 3217, 3217t
protein metabolism in, disorders of, 2852–2855
protein turnover in, 3141–3142
in renal metastasis, 2268
sodium excretion in, regulation of, 2724–2725
sodium in, renal handling of, 2721–2723, 2722f
spontaneous hypoglycemia in, 2849
treatment of
alternative etiologies and, 2803
cerebrovascular accidents and, 2803–2804
coma with hyperglycemia and, 2803
dialysis dementia and, 2799t, 2799–2803, 2801f, 2802t
dialysis disequilibrium syndrome and, 2789–2799, 2799t
neurologic complications in, 2789–2804
subdural hematoma and, 2803
wasting and malnutrition due to, in acute renal failure, 3187–3188
zinc deficiency in, 3162
Uremic acidosis, 2671, 2728–2729
anion gap in, 2577, 2577t
diabetes mellitus and, 2581
pathogenesis of, 2729–2731
Uremic bleeding, drug therapy complicating, 3232
Uremic catabolism, clinical management of, 2855
Uremic encephalopathy. *See* Encephalopathy, uremic
Uremic inhibitors, erythropoiesis and, 2747
Uremic neuropathy. *See* Neuropathy, uremic
Uremic osteodystrophy, mixed, 2761
Uremic pericarditis. *See* Pericarditis.
Uremic polyneuropathy, in chronic hemodialysis, 3085–3086, 3086f
Ureter(s)
agenesis of, 643
atresia of, 643
blind, 643
calculi of, plain film of, 407
dilatation of, due to urinary tract obstruction, 661
duplex, 646–647
complications of, 646
embryogenesis of, 647
dysfunction of, diabetes mellitus and, 2572
ectopic, 643–645, 644f
caudal, 644
intravesical caudal, 644
lateral, 643–644
urethral, 644
vaginal, 645
vestibular, 644–645
embryonic development of, 642–643, 643f
musculature and competence of, 641–642
retrocaval, 654
superficial sheath of, 641
ultrasonography of, technique for, 412
Ureteral carcinoma, 801–805, 812–815
brush biopsy in, 803
causes of, 801
classification and staging of, 813, 814t
clinical presentation in, 812–813
diagnosis of, 802f–803f, 802–804, 813
features at presentation in, 801
five-year survival rate in, 804t
grading and staging of, 801–802, 802f
intravenous pyelography for, 802, 802f, 812f–813f, 812–813
results of treatment of, 815, 815t
retrograde pyelography for, 802–803, 803f
treatment of, 804–805, 813–815
chemotherapy in, 805
radiation therapy in, 805
radical operative therapy in, 804–805
urine cytology in, 803
Ureteral catheterization
retrograde, for renal candidiasis, 940
for urinary tract infection, 983
Ureteral obstruction
acute postrenal failure due to, 1291
as complication of transplantation, 2941–2942, 2942f
CT for, 450–451, 451f
MRI for, 458, 458f
due to renal calculi, treatment of, 681
Ureteral orifice
renal dysplasia correlations with, 651f, 651–652
vesicoureteral reflux and, 690–691, 691f–692f
Ureteral peristalsis, 661
Ureterocele, 647–648
ectopic, 647, 648f
etiology of, 648
intravesical, 647
Ureteroileal urinary conduit, 828, 828f
Ureteropelvic obstruction
congenital, 654
treatment of, 680–681
due to renal calculi, treatment of, 681
Ureteropyelography, for urinary tract obstruction, 679–680
Ureterosigmoidostomy, 828–829
Ureterovesical valve, competence of, 642
Urethra
antimicrobial defense mechanisms of, 894–895
dysfunction of, diabetes mellitus and, 2572
female
anatomy of, 759, 760f
embryonic development of, 640–641
neurophysiology of, 759–761, 760f–762f
male
anatomy of, 759, 760f
neurophysiology of, 759–761, 760f–762f
posterior valves of, 638
saccular diverticula of, 639, 640f
tuberculosis of, 916
Urethral syndrome, 1007. *See also* Cystitis; Urethritis
Urethritis, 1007–1021. *See also* Urinary tract infection
due to candidiasis, 934
clinical manifestations of, 1011–1012
definition of, 1007
diagnosis of, 1012–1013
automated tests for, 1012–1013
bioluminescence methods for, 1013
filtration methods for, 1013
photometric methods for, 1012–1013
urine culture for, 1013
rapid diagnostic tests for, 1012
catalase test for, 1012
glucose oxidase test for, 1012
Griess test for, 1012
leukocyte esterase test for, 1012
epidemiology of, 1010–1011
management of, 1013–1020
in acute dysuria, 1016–1017, 1018f
amoxicillin for, 1015
ampicillin for, 1015
in asymptomatic bacteriuria, 1013, 1016, 1017f
in children, 1019–1020
clavulanate-potentiated amoxicillin for, 1015
duration of therapy in, 1016
fluoroquinolones for, 1015–1016

Urethritis, management of—Continued
general principles of, 1013–1014
nitrofurantoin for, 1015
in pregnancy, 1019, 1020f
in recurrent infection, 1017–1019, 1018t
in relapsing infection, 1017
specific antimicrobial therapy in, 1014t, 1014–1016
sulfonamides for, 1014–1015
in symptomatic bacteriuria, 1013–1014
trimethoprim for, 1015
trimethoprim-sulfamethoxazole for, 1015
in uncomplicated presentation, 1014t, 1014–1016
pathogenesis of, 1008–1010
host factors in, 1009–1010
pathogens in, 1008f, 1008–1009
route of infection in, 1008
virulence factors in, 1009
sexually transmitted disease vs., 1011
urine culture in, 1011
vaginitis vs., 1011
Urge incontinence, 763
Urgency, urinary, definition of, 763
Uric acid. *See also* Hyperuricemia; Hypouricemia; Urate
clearance of, in preeclampsia, 1516
homeostasis of, in autosomal dominant polycystic kidney disease, 550
levels of, in normal pregnancy, preeclampsia, and hypertension, 2293, 2293f
metabolism of, in acute tubular necrosis, 1307
renal deposition of, gout and, 2250, 2251f
Uric acid crystal(s), urinalysis for, 356, 356f
Uric acid nephrolithiasis, 737, 738
tubulointerstitial, 1974
Uric acid nephropathy, 2244
acute, due to antineoplastic agents, 1180
acute postrenal failure due to, 1291
chronic tubulointerstitial, 1974
syndrome of, 2247
Urinalysis, 335–357
in acute renal failure, 1296
in autosomal dominant polycystic kidney disease, 550
for bacteria, 336
in crescentic glomerulonephritis, 354, 355f
in Fabry's disease, 595, 596f
for formed elements, 356, 356f–358f
calcium oxalate crystals as, 356, 357f
cystine crystals as, 356, 357f
uric acid crystals as, 356, 356f
for glucose, 336
for hemoglobin, 335–336, 336t
in hypertensive nephrosclerosis, 1441–1442
immunoperoxidase labeling with monoclonal antibodies in, 354–356
nucleated cells and, 354, 356
platelets and, 355f–356f, 356
for leukocytes, 336
in lower urinary tract dysfunction, 766
in membranous glomerulonephritis, 354, 355f
in mesangial proliferative glomerulonephritis, 353–354, 354f
in mesangiocapillary glomerulonephritis, 354, 355f
microscopic examination in. *See* Urine microscopy
in nephrotic syndrome, 1734–1736
for proteinuria, 335
in scleroderma renal crisis, 2040
specimen collection for, 337
in thin basement membrane disease, 353–354, 354f
in urinary tract obstruction, 676
in urinary tract tuberculosis, 917
for urine pH, 336
Urinary albumin excretion, variability of, in diabetes, 2158, 2159f, 2159t
Urinary bladder
anatomy of, 759, 760f
antimicrobial defense mechanisms of, 895t, 895–896
diverticula of, 641
dysfunction of, diabetes mellitus and, 2572
embryonic development of, 640–641
emptying capacity of, 761–762
filling/storage capacity of, 761–762
incomplete emptying of, urinary tract infection due to, 900
irrigation of, in diagnosis of candidiasis, 938–939
leukoplakia of, 815
neurogenic
management of, in vesicoureteral reflux, 719
upper urinary tract infection in, 981
prevention of, 996–997
vesicoureteral reflux due to, 694
neurophysiology of, 759–761, 760f–762f
squamous cell carcinoma of, 815
squamous metaplasia of, 815
ultrasonography of, technique for, 412, 412f
Urinary bladder adenocarcinoma, 815
Urinary bladder carcinoma, 811–832, 815–832
biochemical studies predicting progression in, 818–819
blood group antigens for, 818–819
tumor karyotyping for, 819
cigarette smoking and, 811–812
clinical presentation and diagnosis in, 816
epidemiology of, 811–812
invasive
noninvasive vs., treatment results in, 817
treatment recommendations in, 823
nodal disease in, staging of, 827t–828t
noninvasive
external beam radiation therapy for, 820
immunotherapy for, 822
intravesical agents for, 820–822, 821t
comparison between, 822, 822t
intravesical BCG for, 822
intravesical bleomycin for, 822
intravesical mitomycin C for, 822
intravesical thiotepa for, 821–822
invasive vs., treatment results in, 817
radical surgery for, 820
transurethral resection for, 819–820
treatment of, 819–823
treatment recommendations in, 822–823
preoperative nutritional status in, 824–825
determination of, 825
enteral hyperalimentation for, 825–826
hypermetabolism and, 824
hyperosmotic intravenous nutrition for, 826
isosmotic intravenous nutrition for, 826
nutritional requirements and, 825
preoperative patient management in, 824
radiation as single or adjunctive treatment in, 827
radical cystoprostatectomy for, complications of, 823–824, 824t–825t
recurrence vs. progression in, 817–818, 818f
staging classifications in, 816, 817t
surgical therapy in, 827–831
continent cecal reservoir in, 829, 829f
hemi-Kock pouch in, 830, 831f
ileocecal urinary reservoir in, 829, 830f
jejunal urinary conduit in, 828
Kock pouch in, 830, 830f
lymphadenectomy in, 827, 827t–828t
sigmoid urinary conduit in, 828
ureteroileal urinary conduit in, 828, 828f
ureterosigmoidostomy in, 828–829
urethrectomy in, 827–828
urinary diversions in, 828f–831f, 828–831
systemic chemotherapy in, 831–832
combination therapy in, 832, 832t
single agent, 831t, 831–832
treatment of, 819
Urinary bladder carcinoma in situ, 815–816, 816f
intravesical agents for, 822
studies for predicting progression in, 819
treatment recommendations in, 823
Urinary bladder contraction, uninhibited, 763
treatment of, 768–769
Urinary bladder neck
anatomy of, 759, 760f
hypermobility of, treatment of, 769–770
neurophysiology of, 759–761, 760f–762f
Urinary bladder outlet obstruction, 763
Urinary diversions, for urinary bladder carcinoma surgery, 828f–831f, 828–831
Urinary frequency, definition of, 762–763
Urinary incontinence, 763
functional, 763
overflow, 763
stress, 763
urge, 763
Urinary oxalate-creatinine ratio, in children, 2382
Urinary tract
amyloidosis of, 2221–2222
changes in, during pregnancy, 2287–2290
anatomic, 2287
physiologic, 2289
immune mechanisms of, 897–899
immunoglobulin response to infection as, 897–898
T lymphocytes in, 899

lower. *See also specific parts*
anatomy of, 759, 760f
emptying capacity of, 761–762
filling/storage capacity of, 761–762
neurophysiology of, 759–761, 760f–762f
normal function of, 761–762, 762f
malformations of, in pregnancy, 2300
structural abnormalities of, in children, 2386–2388
Urinary tract dysfunction, lower
emptying disorders in, 763
evaluation in, 764–768
family history in, 765
filling/storage disorders in, 762–763, 763t
genital/pelvic examination in, 765–766
history in, 764–765
neurologic examination in, 766
neurologic history in, 764
physical examination in, 765–766
therapy in, 768–771
for filling disorders, 768–770
for voiding disorders, 770
urinalysis in, 766
urodynamic evaluation in, 767–768
filling cystometrogram in, 767–768
uroflowmetry for, 767, 768f
voiding cystometrogram in, 768
in vesicoureteral reflux, 702–704, 703f
visual analogue pain scale in, 764, 765f
voiding diary in, 766–767
Urinary tract infection. *See also* Cystitis; Urethritis
in analgesic-induced renal disease, 1112
antiadherence mechanisms in, 889t, 889–892
bacterial interference as, 889
bladder mucopolysaccharide layer as, 891
Tamm-Horsfall protein as, 889–891, 890f–891f. *See also* Tamm-Horsfall protein
urinary oligosaccharides in, 891–892
in autosomal dominant polycystic kidney disease, 550
in autosomal recessive polycystic kidney disease, 559
catheter-associated, 1020–1021
pathogenesis of, 1020
prevention of, 1021, 1021t
treatment of, 1021
in children, 2379, 2390t, 2390–2391
diagnosis and investigation of, 2391, 2391t
management of, 2391
as complication of transplantation, 2947
diabetes mellitus and, 2572
E. coli in, 886–887
virulence factors of, 886, 886t
in elderly, 2426
host defense mechanisms in, 885–901. *See also specific types*
abnormalities interfering with, 899–901
calculi as, 900
diabetes mellitus as, 900–901
elderly patients and, 901
incomplete bladder emptying as, 900
obstruction as, 899–900
vesicoureteral reflux as, 900
antiadherence mechanisms as, 889t, 889–892
bladder in, 895t, 895–896
immune mechanisms in, 897–899
kidney in, 896–897
natural, 893–897
perineum in, 894–895
periurethral region in, 894–895
urethra in, 894
urine in, 893–894
in hydronephrosis, 659
in medullary sponge kidney, 527
pathogenesis of, 885–886
ascending route in, 885–886
bacterial adherence in, 887–893
animal studies of, 892–893
blood group and, 892
epithelial cell receptors in, 888–889
fimbria in, 887–888, 888t
immunoglobulin deficiencies and, 892
importance of, 887
increased susceptibility to, 892
properties of, 887–888, 888t
receptor density and, 892
selection of uropathogens and, 887
therapeutic implications of, 893
hematogenous route in, 885
lymphatic route in, 885
pathogens in, 886–887
in pregnancy, 2299
recurrent, definition of, 1007–1008
in renal disease, drug therapy for, 3228
in sickle cell disease, 2324
upper, 973–999. *See also* Pyelonephritis
bacteremia in, 983
clinical presentation in, 987–989
in adults, 987–989
in infants and children, 989
metastatic infection in, 988–989
definitions in, 973
etiology of, 974–975
anaerobes in, 974
Brucella species in, 974
Enterococcus fecalis in, 974
Escherichia coli in, 974
hospital-acquired, 974
leptospirosis in, 974
Mycoplasma hominis in, 974
Proteus mirabilis in, 974
protoplasts in, 975
various bacterial pathogens in, 974
hematuria in, 983
historical, 973–974
hypertension and, 980
imaging techniques in, 986–987
in acute pyelonephritis, 986
in chronic pyelonephritis, 986–987
indications for, 987
infection localization in, 983t–984t, 983–986
ACB test for, 985
antibody response for, 984
biopsy or necropsy for, 984
cystoscopy with ureteral catheterization for, 983
Fairley washout test for, 984
intravenous pyelography for, 984
radionuclide imaging for, 984
renal concentrating capacity and, 985
urinary enzymes in, 984
laboratory diagnosis of, 981–983
leukocyte casts in, 982
mortality in, 981
natural history of, 978–981
in adult onset, 979–980
in infancy and childhood, 978–979
nephrolithiasis and, 980
neurogenic bladder and, 981
pathologic findings in, 975
acute presentation and, 975
chronic presentation and, 975
pregnancy and, 981
prevalence and incidence of, 976–978, 977f
asymptomatic pyelonephritis and, 976–978
symptomatic pyelonephritis and, 976, 977f
prevention of, 995–997
in catheter-associated infection, 996
continuous suppression in, 995–996
in neurogenic bladder, 996–997
in pregnancy, 996
prophylaxis in, 995
proteinuria in, 983
pyuria in, 982
recurrent, 993–994
bacterial resistance in, 994
ileal conduits and, 994
long-term indwelling catheters and, 994
in males, 993–994
unilateral renal impairment and, 994
urine culture in, 993
urologic abnormalities in, 993
virulent invasive organisms and, 994
treatment of, 989–995
in acute invasive infection, 990–992
drug therapy for, 990t
follow-up for, 992
with impaired renal function, 994–995
inpatient therapy in, 990–992
outpatient therapy in, 992
in recurrent infection, 993–994
therapeutic principles of, 989–990
urine culture in, 981–982
viral, 998–999
in urinary tract obstruction, 659–660, 682
in vesicoureteral reflux
management of, 719–720
in reflux nephropathy, management of, 719–720
Urinary tract obstruction, 657–682. *See also* Hydronephrosis; Obstructive nephropathy; Obstructive uropathy
in analgesic-induced renal disease, 1113
calcium excretion in, 673
in cancer, 1169
causes of, 657, 658t
in chronic tubulointerstitial nephropathy, 1970
clinical syndromes in, 657–658, 658t
defects in urinary acidification in, 672–673
diagnosis of, 676–680
diagnostic approach to, in acute renal failure, 1301
diagnostic imaging in, 676–680
computed tomography in, 679
intravenous urography in, 677, 677f–678f
isotopic renography in, 678–679
magnetic resonance imaging in, 679
plain films in, 677
tomography in, 677
ultrasonography in, 677–678, 678f
ureteropyelography in, 679–680
effect of age on, 674–675

Urinary tract obstruction—Continued
GFR reduction in, 662–667
after relief of obstruction, 664–665
atrial natriuretic factor and, 667, 668f
factors affecting, 662
mechanisms of, 665–667
during obstruction, 662–664, 663f, 663t
renal nerve activity and, 667
renin-angiotensin system and, 666–667
tubuloglomerular feedback mechanism and, 667
urine hemodynamics and, 661
vasoconstrictor prostaglandins and, 665–666, 666f–667f
vasodilator prostaglandins and, 665
hypertension in, 660, 682
incidence of, 657
laboratory findings in, 676
lower, treatment of, 681
magnesium excretion in, 673
pathophysiology of, 660–676
urine hemodynamics in, 661–662
phosphate excretion in, 673
physical examination in, 676
polycythemia and, 660
postobstructive diuresis after, 667–670
after relief of complete obstruction, 669t, 669–670
during and after relief of partial obstruction, 667–670
due to defect in tubular reabsorption of sodium, 670, 671f
glomerular filtration recovery and, 670
hypophosphatemia and, 2605
due to impaired water reabsorption, 670
osmotic
due to excessive IV solutions, 669–670
due to urea retention, 669
saline, due to extracellular fluid volume expansion, 669
potassium excretion in, 673
in pregnancy, 2300
recovery of tubular function after, 673–674, 674f
renal calculi and, 660
renal failure in, 682
symptoms and signs of, 676
treatment of, 680–682
medical, 681–682
natural history of disorder and, 680
nephrectomy for, 681
principles of, 680
surgical, 680–681
tubular reabsorption in, 661–662
upper
imaging studies of, 430–437
radionuclide studies for, 435f–437f, 436–437
ultrasonography for, 432–436, 434f
urography for, 430f–433f, 431–432
ureteral dilatation due to, 661
urinalysis in, 676
urinary concentration impairment in, 670–672, 672f
due to increased osmotic load, 672
due to insensitivity of tubule to vasopressin, 671–672
due to lack of hypertonicity in medullary interstitium, 671
mechanisms of, 671, 672f
urinary tract infection in, 659–660, 682, 899–900
Urinary tract tuberculosis, 909–924
atypical mycobacterial infection in, 917
clinical features of, 915–917
bladder in, 916
genital infection in, 916–917
female, 916–917
male, 916
hypertension in, 916
nephrolithiasis in, 916
penile involvement in, 916
prostatitis in, 916, 917f
renal dysfunction in, 916
urethral involvement in, 916
urinary tract inflammation in, 915–916
clinical management of, 922–924
chemotherapy in, 922–924, 923t
drug resistance and, 922
nephrectomy in, 924
recommendations for, 924
short-course drug regimens in, 922–923
surgical, 924
ureteral strictures and, 924
diagnosis of, 917–918
epidemiology of, 910–912
in HIV-infected individuals, 911–912
in non–HIV-infected individuals, 910–911
etiology of, 909–910
Mycobacterium tuberculosis in, 909–910
pathogenesis of, 913f, 913–914
pathologic findings in, 914, 914f–915f
radiologic findings in, 918f–921f, 918–922
computed tomography in, 920, 921f
excretory urography in, 918–920, 919f–921f
plain film in, 918, 918f
urinalysis in, 917
Urinary urgency, definition of, 763
Urine. *See also* Glomerular filtrate
alkalization of, for candidiasis, 943
antimicrobial defense mechanisms of, 893–894
bacteria in. *See* Bacteriuria; Urinary tract infection
collection of, 2155, 2157–2158
in children, 2379
overnight, 2157–2158
random sampling in, 2155, 2157
short-term, 2157
twenty-four hour sampling in, 2157
concentrating capacity of
in children, 2381–2382
impaired, mechanisms of, 2727–2728
in sickle cell disease, 2316f–2318f, 2317–2319
concentration of
ADH in, 374–375
defects in, disorders causing, 376
effect of ADH absence on, 375
effect of diabetes insipidus on, 375
effect of medullary tonicity on, 375–376
mechanisms for, 125–126
renal mechanisms in, 373–375
urine volume vs., 377
diluting capacity of
age-related decline in, 2417
clinical implications of, 2420–2421
impaired, mechanisms of, 2727–2728
in sickle cell disease, 2319
diluting mechanism of, components of, 2517, 2518f
dilution of
ADH in, 374–375
effect of ADH excess in, 376
effect of decreased fluid delivery to loop of Henle and distal nephron on, 376–377
effect of decreased NaCl reabsorption by ascending limb on, 377
mechanisms for, 125
renal mechanisms in, 373–375
hypertonic, definition of, 373
hypotonic, definition of, 373
leakage of, as complication of transplantation, 2941
normal values of, 2158
osmolality of
measurement of, 377
in myxedema, 2541–2543
volume vs., 377
pH of. *See also* Urine acidification
antimicrobial therapy and, 1014
nephrolithiasis due to, 731, 731t
urinalysis for, 336
protein in, normal, 380. *See also* Proteinuria
refractive index of, 378
specific gravity of, measurement of, 377–378, 378f
tonicity of, measurement of, 377–378
volume vs. osmolality of, 377
Urine acidification
antimicrobial therapy and, 1014
in autosomal dominant polycystic kidney disease, 549
in children, 2381
distal nephron dysfunction in, 2677–2679
in lithium-induced renal disease, 1100
in medullary sponge kidney, 527
in sickle cell disease, 2319–2320
in urinary tract obstruction, 672–673
Urine albumin–creatinine concentration ratio, 2380
Urine collection, 24-hour, 366–367
Urine culture
in acute pyelonephritis, 981–982
in asymptomatic bacteriuria, 981
for bacteriuria, 1013
in cystitis, 1011
in recurrent upper urinary tract infection, 993
in upper urinary tract infection, 981–982
in urethritis, 1011
Urine cytology
in renal pelvic carcinoma, 803
in ureteral carcinoma, 803
Urine excretion
of calcium, 2619
hypercalcemia secondary to, 2628
hypocalcemia secondary to, 2624
of magnesium, hypomagnesemia secondary to, 2634–2635
of phosphorus, factors affecting, 2601–2604
Urine flow
in acute renal failure, 1296–1298
hemodynamics of, 661
Urine microscopy, 336–356
for cast(s), 346f–352f, 346–351
bacterial, 351
erythrocyte, 349, 351f–352f
granular, 347, 351, 351f
leukocyte, 348
protein contents of, 347t

size and shape in, 348
tubular epithelial cell, 348f, 349, 351
waxy, 351, 352f
cells per milliliter vs. cells per hour in, 338, 338f
counting chamber for, 337, 337f
for erythrocyte(s), 341–343, 342f–346f
in acid urine, 341, 345f
dysmorphic cells in, 341, 342f, 343
erythrophagocytosis in, 343, 346f
due to exercise, 343
due to glomerular bleeding, 341, 342f–344f
due to nonglomerular bleeding, 341, 344f–345f
for leukocyte count, 339t, 339–340, 340f
for lipiduria, 353, 353f–354f
specific gravity and, 338t, 339
specimen collection for, 337
technical aspects of, 337f–338f, 337–339, 338t
for tubular epithelial cells, 340, 340f–341f
urine pH and specific gravity in, 336
Urine specimen
collection technique for, 337
for diagnosis of candidiuria, 933
midstream, 337
Uriniferous tubule. *See* Tubule(s)
Urodilatin, 313–314
Uroepithelial carcinoma, 811–832
due to analgesic-induced renal disease, 1115
angiography for, 477
epidemiology of, 811–812
upper urinary tract, 812–815
classification and staging of, 813, 814t
clinical presentation in, 812–813
diagnosis of, 813
intravenous pyelography in, 812f–813f, 812–813
results of treatment of, 815, 815t
treatment of, 813–815
urinary bladder, 815–832. *See also* Urinary bladder carcinoma
Uroflowmetry, in lower urinary tract dysfunction, 767, 768f
Urography, intravenous, 407–410
contrast media for, 407
excretory phase of, 407–408
for fetal lobation, 409
hazards of, 408
indications for, 421
management of reactions in, 408
normal findings and common variants in, 409, 409f
for parenchymal disease, 423t
for pelvicalyceal system and papillae, 409–410, 410f
plain film prior to, 407
renal calcifications and, 407
ureter calcifications and, 407
postcontrast films in, 409
precautions in, 408
for reflux nephropathy, 704f–705f, 704–705
for renal cell carcinoma, 787–788
renal complications of, 408
for renal failure, 438–439, 439f
for renal mass lesions, 428, 428f
for renal parenchyma/outline, 409
for renal position, 409
for renal sinus, 410
for renal size, 409
for renovascular hypertension, 440f, 441
for septum of Bertin, 409, 410f
for splenic hump, 409, 409f
technique in, 408–409
for upper urinary tract obstruction, 430f–433f, 431–432
for urinary tract obstruction, 677, 677f–678f
for urinary tract tuberculosis, 918–920, 919f–921f
Urolithiasis. *See* Calculus(i), renal; Nephrolithiasis
Urologic anomalies, congenital, 637–655, 638t. *See also specific types;* Kidney; Ureter; Urethra; Urinary bladder
Uropathy, obstructive. *See* Obstructive uropathy
Urosepsis, in sickle cell disease, 2324
U.S. Healthcare Finance Administration Annual Facility Survey, of renal transplantation, 2912t
Uterine renin, in vascular reactivity in pregnancy, 1506
Uteroplacental perfusion
effect of antihypertensive therapy on, 1522
in preeclampsia, 1515
Uterus
hemorrhage of, 2301
preeclampsia and, 2291
Uveitis, acute interstitial nephritis with, 1344f, 1344–1345

Vacuolization, tubular, light microscopy evaluation of, 497, 499f
Vaginitis, cystitis and urethritis vs., 1011
Valine, intracellular levels of, in uremia, 2853
Valproic acid, pharmacology of, normal vs. in renal failure, 3260t–3261t
"Valve" of Guérin, 639–640
Vancomycin
acute interstitial nephritis due to, 1337
cystic fluid concentration of, in autosomal dominant polycystic kidney disease, 551t
pharmacology of, normal vs. in renal failure, 3260t–3261t
Varicella zoster, as complication of transplantation, 2944
Vasa recta
anatomic distribution of, 33–34, 34f
ascending
macromolecular and fluid reabsorption by, 79
morphology of, 34, 34f, 68
as countercurrent diffusion exchangers, 127f, 127–128
descending
macromolecular and fluid reabsorption by, 79
morphology of, 34, 34f, 68
occlusion of, in sickle cell disease, 2323
Vascular access infection, in renal disease, drug therapy for, 3228
Vascular calcification, in chronic renal failure, 3155
Vascular cell adhesion molecule-1, 2004
Vascular disease
malaria and, 2342
renal
age-related, 2422–2423
CT for, 453, 453f
MRI for, 458–459
in renal transplantation, 2182, 2182t
Vascular endothelial cell(s), interactions between smooth muscle cells and, 72–74, 73f
Vascular injury, 1993–2011
acute inflammation in
chemical mediators of, 1994–1999
bacterial, 1995–1996
complement fragments as, 1996
cytokines as, 1997–1999
endotoxin as, 1996
GM-CSF as, 1998
IL-1 as, 1997, 1998t
IL-4 in, 1998
interferon-γ as, 1998
lipid mediators in, 1996–1997
lipopolysaccharide as, 1996
N-formyl-methionyl-leucyl-phenylalamine as, 1995
PAF as, 1997
TGF-β as, 1998
TNF-α as, 1997–1998
initiation and potentiation of, 1993–2009
leukocyte adhesion to vessel walls in, 2000–2005
endothelial cell adhesion molecule in, 2004
endothelial-leukocyte adhesion molecule in, 2004
integrin family in, 2002, 2003t
intercellular cell adhesion molecule in, 2004
leukocyte adhesion molecule in, 2002–2003, 2003t
molecular mechanisms of, 2002–2005, 2003t
selectin family in, 2002, 2003t
site of mediator action in, 2001–2002
vascular cell adhesion molecule-1 in, 2004
leukocyte injury to vascular structures in, 2006–2009
degradative granule enzymes in, 208f, 2007, 2009
nonenzymatic cationic proteins in, 2009
reactive oxygen species in, 2006–2007
leukocyte passage through vessel wall in, 2005f–2006f, 2005–2006
neutrophils in, 1994, 1994t, 1995f
stimuli initiating, 1994
circulating antibodies as, 1994
immune complexes as, 1994
vascular tone in, 1999–2000
chemical mediators of, 1999
endothelin in, 1999–2000
endothelium-derived relaxing factor in, 2000
endothelial, microvascular thrombosis due to, 2067–2069. *See also* Thrombosis, microvascular
historical concepts of inflammation and, 1993
in lupus nephritis, 2027
resolution and repair in, 2009–2011
cessation of leukocyte influx in, 2009
monocyte influx and maturation in, 2010
removal of neutrophils in, 2009–2010
repair of inflammatory tissue in, 2010–2011
therapeutic prospects in, 2011

Vascular smooth muscle, in experimental studies on ischemic renal injury, 1273–1274
Vasculature
 endothelial, in end-stage renal disease, 2823
 peripheral, atrial natriuretic peptide effects on, 296
 renal. *See* Renal vasculature
Vasculitides, cutaneous, 2114
Vasculitis, 2095–2114. *See also* Polyarteritis
 cutaneous, 2114
 hypocomplementemic urticarial, 2114
 percutaneous renal biopsy for, 489
 renal, prognosis in, 1934t, 1934–1936, 1935f–1936f
 systemic
  antibodies to neutrophil cytoplasmic antigens in, 2097–2098, 2098f, 2098t
  classification of, 2095–2096, 2096t
  definition of, 2095
  in IgA nephropathy, 1854f–1855f, 1854–1855
  immunopathology of, 1664f, 1664–1665
  necrotizing, due to parenteral amphetamine abuse, 1231–1232
  pathogenesis of, 2096–2097, 2097t
  in rheumatoid arthritis, 2051
Vasculitis syndrome, systemic, definition of, 2099
Vasoactive intestinal peptide (VIP)
 in hepatorenal disease, 1359
 in vascular reactivity in preeclampsia, 1512–1513
Vasodepressor(s), in hypertension, with end-stage renal disease, 2822–2823
Vasodilation, peripheral, of edematous states, 2468, 2469f
Vasodilator(s)
 for heart failure, 2834
 for hypertension, in neonates, 2386
Vasomotor nephropathy, in AIDS, 2362
Vasopressin. *See* Antidiuretic hormone (ADH)
Vasopressin analogues, hyponatremia associated with, 2520–2521
Vasopressin antagonists, in hyponatremia, 2527
Vasopressin escape, 2522
Vena cava
 constriction of, thoracic, 2455
 inferior, constriction of, 2455
Venom
 Russell's viper, 2351
 snake, 2351
Ventriculovascular shunts, glomerulonephritis with, 1685
Verapamil, pharmacology of, normal vs. in renal failure, 3260t–3261t
Verumontanum, polyp of, 638–639
Very-low-density lipoprotein (VLDL), 2849t, 2849–2850
Vesicoureteral hiatus, normal and abnormal, 641
Vesicoureteral reflux, 689–721
 anatomic considerations in, 690–691, 691f–692f
 bladder pressure and, 702
 clinical presentation in, 709t, 709–717
 coincidental findings in, 717
 as complication of transplantation, 2942
 familial associations in, 715–717, 716f
 fetal ultrasonography for, 717
 in healthy children and infants, prevalence of, 693–694
 hypertension in, 711
 imaging techniques in, 700–702
  indirect, 701
  radionuclide micturition cystography for, 701–702, 702f
  ultrasonography for, 702
  voiding cystourethrography in, 700f–701f, 700–701
 loin pain in, 717
 lower urinary tract dysfunction in, 702–704, 703f
  assessment of, 702–703, 703f
  reflux and, 703–704
 management of, 717–720
  controlled antireflux surgery trials in, 718–719
  hypertension and, 720
  indications for surgery in, 717–718
  investigation of family members in, 720
  neurogenic bladder and, 719
  surgical technique in, 719
  in urinary calculi, 720
  urinary tract infection and, 719–720
 natural history of, 707–708, 708f
 due to neurogenic bladder, 694
 nocturnal enuresis in, 717
 proteinuria in, 713
 in renal transplantation, 695
 secondary, 694
 due to spinal cord injury, 694–695, 695f
 urinary calculi in, 714–715
 urinary tract infection in, 709–711, 710f, 900
  asymptomatic bacteriuria vs., 709–710
  imaging techniques for, 710–711
  incidence of, 709, 710f
Vidarabine, pharmacology of, normal vs. in renal failure, 3260t–3261t
Villous adenoma, 2685
Vinblastine, pharmacology of, normal vs. in renal failure, 3262t–3263t
Vincristine, pharmacology of, normal vs. in renal failure, 3262t–3263t
Viral infection(s)
 as complication of transplantation, 2943–2946
 in renal disease, drug therapy for, 3228–3229
 slow, dialysis dementia and, 2803
Viruria, in upper urinary tract infection, 998
Visceral calcification, in chronic renal failure, 3154–3155
Vitamin(s)
 for anemia, 2752
 in dietary therapy in acute renal failure, 3195–3196
 in dietary therapy in chronic hemodialysis, 3184–3185
 in dietary therapy in renal transplantation, 3199
Vitamin A
 in dietary therapy in acute renal failure, 3195–3196
 intoxication, hypercalcemia and, 2627
Vitamin B_6 deficiency, in chronic uremia, 3184–3185
Vitamin B_{12} deficiency, in chronic uremia, 3184
Vitamin C, in dietary therapy in chronic hemodialysis, 3184
Vitamin D, 315–316
 deficiency of
  hypocalcemia secondary to, 2623
  in nephrotic syndrome, 3186–3187
 in dietary therapy in acute renal failure, 3196
 hyperphosphatemia and, 2614
 for hypocalcemia, 2628
 intoxication, hypercalcemia and, 2627, 2628
 metabolic pathways of, 315, 315f
 metabolism of
  hypophosphatemia and, 2605
  in primary hypophosphatemic rickets, 619
 metabolites of, in uremia, 2859–2860
 for osteitis fibrosa, 2776
 phosphorus absorption and, 2603
 renal actions of, 316
 for renal osteodystrophy, 2395
 synthesis, activation, and metabolism of, 315–316
Vitamin D_3
 in hypercalcemia of malignancy, 2273
 in renal osteodystrophy, 2775
Vitamin D-deficient rickets, 2605–2606
Vitamin D-dependent rickets, 2606–2607
Vitamin D-phenobarbitol drug interaction, in renal disease, 3230
Vitamin E, as antioxidant, 1039
Vitamin K, in dietary therapy in acute renal failure, 3196
VLDL (very-low-density lipoprotein), 2849t, 2849–2850
VM-26, phase specificity and mechanism of action of, 821t
Voiding diary, in lower urinary tract dysfunction, 766
Vomiting, surreptitious, idiopathic edema and, 2500
von Hippel-Lindau disease, 782
von Willebrand factor, in microvascular thrombosis, 2068–2069

Waldenstrom's macroglobulinemia, 2206–2208, 2207f
 clinical features of, 2207
 hyperviscosity syndrome in, 2207–2208
Waldeyer's fascia, 641
Walton-Black Modified Word Learning Test, 2791
Warfarin, pharmacology of, normal vs. in renal failure, 3262t–3263t
Water. *See also* Fluid(s)
 deionization of, in prevention of dialysis dementia, 2802
 negative free, in sickle cell disease, 2319
 restriction of, in end-stage renal disease, 2823
Water deprivation test, 2508t
Water excretion
 in edema-forming disorders, 2453
 in myxedema, 2540f–2541f, 2540t, 2541–2543, 2543f
 prolactin and, 2556–2557
 renal, 2727–2728
Water homeostasis, in chronic renal failure, 2727–2728
Water intake
 thirst and, 119
 and vasopressin release, 2726

Water retention
in congestive heart failure, 2461–2465, 2461f, 2464f
drugs causing, 2494, 2519t, 2519–2521
idiopathic edema and, 2494
in liver disease, 2465–2468, 2466f–2467f
in nephrotic syndrome, 2479–2481
orthostatic, 2495
Waxy cast(s), 351, 352f
Wegener's granuloma, 1934
Wegener's granulomatosis, 2108–2111, 2505
clinical features of, 2108
course and treatment in, 2109–2111, 2109f–2111f
definition of, 2108
laboratory parameters in, 2108–2109
renal pathology in, 2109, 2109f–2110f
renal transplantation and, 2917–2918
Weight, dry, definition of, 2823
Weight gain, in idiopathic edema, 2497, 2497f, 2499, 2499f
Weil's syndrome, 2338
Weschler Adult Intelligence Scale, 2791, 2792
Western blot method, of HIV testing, 2361
Wilms gene, isolation of, 781
Wilms tumor, 799–801
angiography for, 477
clinical findings in, 799
evaluation and staging in, 799–800, 800t
hypokalemia in, 2277
nephrogenic rests and, 782
treatment of, 800–801
chemotherapy, 800–801
radiation, 800
surgical, 800
tumor suppressor genes and, 781
Wolffian body, embryonic development of, 642–643, 643f
Wolffian duct, embryonic development of, 641, 641f
Wolfram syndrome, 2505
Wound(s), complication of, in renal transplantation, 2940

Xanthine nephropathy, due to antineoplastic agents, 1180–1181
Xanthine oxidase metabolism, in nephrotoxicity, 1037–1038
Xanthogranulomatous pyelonephritis, 997–998
clinical findings and diagnosis in, 997
diagnosis of, 964–965
incidence of, 997
pathogenesis of, 963, 997
treatment of, 966
Xenograft(s), 2881. *See also* Allograft(s); Graft(s)
clinical histocompatibility testing of, 2881–2882
HLA typing of, 2881–2882, 2882f
presensitivity testing of, 2881
X-linked hypophosphatemic rickets, 2606

Zidovudine (AZT)
for HIV-associated nephropathy, 2370
pharmacology of, normal vs. in renal failure, 3262t–3263t
in renal disease, 3228
Zinc
abnormal excretion of, in sickle cell disease, 2320–2321
in dietary therapy in chronic hemodialysis, 3183–3184
Zinc deficiency
in renal transplantation, 3198
in uremia, 3162
Zygomycosis, opportunistic, 946t–947t, 946–947
Zymogen(s), in acute renal vein thrombosis, in nephrotic syndrome, 1320